The 5-Minute Clinical Consult Premium 2015

23RD EDITION

The 5-Minute Clinical Consult Premium 2015

23RD EDITION

1-Year Enhanced Online Access + Print

Editor-in-Chief

Frank J. Domino, MD
Professor
Director of Predoctoral Education
Department of Family Medicine and Community Health
University of Massachusetts Medical School
Worcester, Massachusetts

Associate Editors

Robert A. Baldor, MD, FAAFP
Professor and Vice-Chairman, Educational Affairs
Department of Family Medicine and Community Health
University of Massachusetts Medical School
Worcester, Massachusetts

Jeremy Golding, MD, FAAFP
Professor of Family Medicine and Obstetrics &
  Gynecology
University of Massachusetts Medical School
Quality Officer
Department of Family Medicine and Community Health
University of Massachusetts Memorial Health Care
Hahnemann Family Health Center
Worcester, Massachusetts

Jill A. Grimes, MD, FAAFP
Clinical Instructor
Department of Family Medicine
University of Massachusetts Medical School
Worcester, Massachusetts
Attending Physician
University of Texas Health Services
Austin, Texas

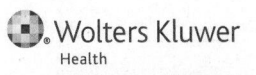
Health
Philadelphia · Baltimore · New York · London
Buenos Aires · Hong Kong · Sydney · Tokyo

Acquisitions Editor: Rebecca Gaertner
Product Development Editor: Leanne Vandetty
Production Project Manager: Priscilla Crater
Senior Manufacturing Coordinator: Beth Welsh
Strategic Marketing Manager: Stephanie Manzo
Design Coordinator: Teresa Mallon
Production Service: Aptara, Inc.

© 2014 Wolters Kluwer Health
Two Commerce Square
2001 Market Street
Philadelphia, PA 19103 USA
LWW.com

Printed in China

Library of Congress Cataloging-in-Publication Data

ISBN-13: 978-1-4511-9215-5
ISBN-10: 1-4511-9215-0

Care has been taken to confirm the accuracy of the information presented and to describe generally accepted practices. However, the authors, editors, and publisher are not responsible for errors or omissions or for any consequences from application of the information in this book and make no warranty, expressed or implied, with respect to the currency, completeness, or accuracy of the contents of the publication. Application of the information in a particular situation remains the professional responsibility of the practitioner.

The authors, editors, and publisher have exerted every effort to ensure that drug selection and dosage set forth in this text are in accordance with current recommendations and practice at the time of publication. However, in view of ongoing research, changes in government regulations, and the constant flow of information relating to drug therapy and drug reactions, the reader is urged to check the package insert for each drug for any change in indications and dosage and for added warnings and precautions. This is particularly important when the recommended agent is a new or infrequently employed drug.

Some drugs and medical devices presented in the publication have Food and Drug Administration (FDA) clearance for limited use in restricted research settings. It is the responsibility of the health care provider to ascertain the FDA status of each drug or device planned for use in their clinical practice.

To purchase additional copies of this book, call our customer service department at (800) 638-3030 or fax orders to (301) 223-2320. International customers should call (301) 223-2300.

Visit Lippincott Williams & Wilkins on the Internet: at LWW.com. Lippincott Williams & Wilkins customer service representatives are available from 8:30 am to 6 pm, EST.

10 9 8 7 6 5 4 3 2 1

As I sat down to write this, the radio announced the passing of Nelson Mandela. Imagine being imprisoned for your beliefs for 27 years! Nelson Mandela stood quietly and soundly on his beliefs, knowing the world would be a better place for his personal turmoil. History's high points occur when someone comes forward to take an unpopular stand, believing the world will be a better place for their suffering. *Is the world of medicine ready to step up?*

Choosing Wisely (http://www.choosingwisely.org/). These two words made a huge impact this past year, as most every medical specialty and health care–related group (over 60!) found consensus on what tests and treatments were of use and beneficial to society…. and which were wasteful and harmful. Despite each group's involvement, many called this heresy. It is not. This effort is the beginning of applying evidence-based medicine and a cost effective approach to care of our patients.

Like it or not, the Affordable Care Act, complete with flaws and technological blunders, was brought forward in an effort to bring health insurance to 47 million US citizens who were previously uninsured; that is 1 in 6 people. President Obama voluntarily addressed something most Americans believe to be necessary—health insurance coverage for all. The Congressional Budget Office, a nonpartisan group that provides the US Congress with real numbers, continues to report lower than expected costs, with significant patient benefits (https://www.cbo.gov/topics/health-care/affordable-care-act).

Other changes are rapidly occurring in health care. In some, solid, evidence-based medical research has yielded results that shake up the status quo, directing us toward changes that will prevent long term morbidity and mortality:

—Head trauma from sports-related activities during adolescence and early adulthood causes permanent damage. Concussion prevention is the priority. *Will football soon be a sport played only in college and after?*

—Prescription narcotics had a rough year: First, a call for training in appropriate use of long-term agents for nonmalignant pain and a systematic review of data showing no benefit of opioids for chronic low back pain. Accidental prescription opioid death is the most common cause of death in those under the age of 50 in the US and *is our responsibility. Pulling back on prescribing these agents will be a challenge we must accept with the grace and strength of Mandela.*

—Curing hepatitis C can be at hand, and doing so will move cirrhosis and hepatoma from their leading role as causes of cancer death worldwide. Screen those born between 1945 and 1965 once and all who practice high-risk behaviors (blood transfusion before 1992, long-term hemodialysis, born to an HCV-infected mother, incarceration, intranasal drug use, getting an unregulated tattoo, and other percutaneous exposures).

—HIV has become a chronic disease and like hepatitis C *should now be part of our universal routine adult health screening;* **the new guidelines recommend screening all** adolescents and adults ages 15 to 65 years, all pregnant women, and those younger adolescents and older adults who are at increased risk.

—Bacteria in our gut may play a huge role in our degree of health, influencing illness from viral URIs to coronary artery disease… and even maybe obesity! In our efforts to overcome obesity, we will need to advocate a more vegetarian-based diet as an intervention to alter the gut microbiome and prevent illness.

—Prevention of cardiovascular morbidity and mortality is clearly benefited by use of statins where cardiovascular risk is high *but is not achieved by reaching a simple LDL goal. Again, we will need to prioritize helping patients to stop smoking and to start exercising. The benefit of medications to prevent heart disease hinges on these interventions, not just a pill.*

Mandela said "resentment is like drinking poison and then hoping it will kill your enemies." Clinicians in all disciplines should remember that our differences in opinion are so much smaller than our common goal of helping others.

This year's **5-Minute Clinical Consult** is dedicated to those who have suffered long and risked much to m~ our patients better. Let's make certain their efforts were just the beginning of a better future.

PREFACE

> **Any man may easily do harm but not every man can do good to another.**
>
> —PLATO

Born in the 3rd century BC, Plato understood the essential role of providing care to those in need. And when you hold this book, you too have enormous potential to serve humanity, one person at a time.

Welcome to *The 5-Minute Clinical Consult 2015.* Our editorial team has collaborated with hundreds of authors so that you may deliver your patients the best care. Each topic provides you with quick answers you can trust, where and when you need them most, either in print or online at www.5minuteconsult.com.

This highly organized content provides you with:

- Differential diagnosis support from an accessible, targeted search, delivering the answers you need quickly
- Current evidence-based designations highlighted in each topic
- A revised and updated Health Maintenance section
- 880+ commonly encountered diseases and disorders in print, and more than 1,200 additional topics online, including 500 topics from *The 5-Minute Pediatric Consult* and over 620 topics from *The 5-Minute Emergency Medicine Consult*
- FREE Point of Care CME and CE: 1/2 hour credit for every digital search
- 200+ diagnostic and treatment algorithms
- Color images and videos for procedures, treatment, and physical therapy
- A to Z Drug Database from Facts & Comparisons®
- More than 1,250 patient handouts in English and Spanish from the AAFP
- ICD-10 Codes and DSM-V criteria; in addition, ICD-9 and SNOMED codes are available online.

5minuteconsult.com delivers quick access to continually updated online content—an ideal resource when you're treating patients. Integrate 5-Minute content into your workflow, with online access, so you never have to skip a beat. If you purchased the Premium Edition your access includes 1 year FREE; the Standard Edition includes a free 30-day trial! The site promises an easy-to-use interface, allowing smooth maneuverability between topics, algorithms, images, videos, and patient education materials, as well as over 1,200 online-only topics.

Evidence-based health care is the integration of the best medical information *with* the values of the patient and your skill as a clinician. We have updated our EBM content and its visibility, so you can focus on how to best apply it in your practice.

The Health Maintenance 1-page summaries have been updated through December 2013 and are based on the US Preventive Services Task Force recommendations.

The Algorithm section includes both diagnostic and treatment algorithms. This easy-to-use graphic method helps you evaluate an abnormal finding and prioritize treatment. They are also excellent *teaching tools*, so share them with the learners in your office.

In our role as clinicians, caring for those who are ill or helping to prevent illness, we use tests and prescribe treatments, hoping they improve outcomes. As importantly, our words and actions, even a shared smile, can make a huge difference. We can "do good" for our patients, especially when we meet them at their most vulnerable. Thank you for making a difference.

The 5-Minute Clinical Consult editorial team values your observations, so please share your thoughts, suggestions, and constructive criticism through our Web site, www.5mintueconsult.com.

FRANK J. DOMINO, MD
January 1, 2014

EVIDENCE-BASED MEDICINE

WHAT IS EVIDENCE-BASED MEDICINE?

Remember when we used to treat every otitis media with antibiotics? These recommendations came about because we applied logical reasoning to observational studies. If bacteria cause an acute otitis media, then antibiotics should help it resolve sooner, with less morbidity. Yet, when rigorously studied (via a systematic review), we found little benefit to this intervention.

The underlying premise of evidence-based medicine (EBM) is the evaluation of medical interventions, and the literature that supports those interventions, in a systematic fashion. EBM hopes to encourage treatments proven to be effective and safe. And when insufficient data exists, it hopes to inform you on how to safely proceed.

EBM uses as endpoints of real patient outcomes; morbidity, mortality and risk. It focuses less on intermediate outcomes (bone density) and more on patient conditions (hip fractures).

Implementing EBM *requires* 3 components: The best medical evidence, the skill and experience of the provider, and the values of the patients. Should this patient be screened for prostate cancer? It depends on what is known about the test, on what you know of its benefits and harms, your ability to communicate that information, and that patient's informed choice.

This book hopes to address the first EBM component, providing you access to the best information in a quick format. While not every test or treatment has this level of detail, many of the included interventions here use systematic review literature support.

The language of medical statistics is useful to interpreting the concepts of EBM. Below is a list of these terms, with examples to help take the confusion and mystery out of their use.

Prevalence: *Proportion of people* in a population who have a disease (in the US, 0.3% [3 in 1,000] people over the age 50 have colon cancer).

Incidence: How many *new cases of a disease* occur in a population during an interval of time; for example, "the estimated incidence of colon cancer in the US is 104,000 in 2005."

Sensitivity (Sn): Percent of people with disease who test positive; for mammography, the sensitivity is 71–96%.

Specificity (Sp): Percent of people without disease who test negative; for mammography, the specificity is 94–97%.

Now suppose you saw ML, a 53-year-old woman, for a Health Maintenance visit, ordered a *screening* mammogram, and the report demonstrates an irregular area of microcalcifications. She is waiting in your office to receive her test results; what can you tell her?

Sensitivity and specificity refer to characteristics of people who are *known to have disease* (sensitivity) or those that are *known not to have disease* (specificity). But, what you have is an abnormal test result. To better explain this result to ML, you need to know the positive predictive value.

Positive predictive value (PPV): Percent of *positive* test results that are truly positive; the PPV for a woman aged 50–59 is approximately 22%. That is to say that only 22% of abnormal screening mammograms in this group truly identified cancer. The other 78% are false positives.

You can tell ML only 1 out of 5 abnormal mammograms correctly identify cancer; the 4 are false positives, but the only way to know which mammogram is correct is to do further testing.

The corollary of the PPV is the Negative predictive value (NPV), which is the percent of negative test results that are truly negative.

The PPV and NPV tests are population dependent, while the Sensitivity and Specificity are characteristics of the test, and have little to do with the patient in front of you. So when you receive an abnormal lab result, especially a screening test like mammography, understand their limits based on their PPV and NPV.

Treatment Information is a little different. In discerning the statistics of randomized, controlled trials of interventions, first consider an example. The Scandinavian Simvastatin Survival Study (4S) (*Lancet.* 1994;344[8934]:1383–1389) found using simvastatin in patients at high risk for heart disease for 5 years resulted in deaths in 8% of patients vs. 12% of those on placebo; this results in a relative risk of 0.70, a relative risk reduction (RRR) of 33%, and a number needed to treat of 25.

There are two ways of considering the benefits of an intervention with respect to a given outcome. The absolute risk reduction (ARR) is the difference in the percent of people with the condition before and after the intervention. Thus, if the incidence of MI was 12% for the placebo group and 8% for the simvastatin group, the ARR is 4% (12% − 8% = 4%).

The RRR reflects the improvement in the outcome as a percentage of the original rate and is commonly used to exaggerate the benefit of an intervention. Thus, if the risk of MI were reduced by simvastatin from 12% to 8%, then the RRR would be 33% (4%/12% = 33%); 33% may appear better than 4%, the 4% that reflects the true outcome.

ARR is usually a better measure of *clinical* significance of an intervention. For instance, in one study, the treatment of mild hypertension was been shown to have a RRR of 40% over 5 years (40% fewer strokes in the treated group). However, the ARR was only 1.3%. Because mild hypertension is not strongly associated with strokes, aggressive treatment of mild hypertension yields only a small clinical benefit. Don't confuse Relative Risk Reduction with Relative Risk.

Absolute (or attributable) risk (AR): The percent of people in the placebo or intervention group who reach an end point; in the simvastatin study, the absolute risk of death was 8%.

Relative risk (RR): The risk of disease of those treated or exposed to some intervention (i.e., simvastatin) divided by those in the placebo group or who were untreated.

—If RR < 1.0, it reduces risk—the smaller the number, the greater the risk reduction.

—If RR > 1.0, it increases the risk—the greater the number, the greater the risk increase.

Relative risk reduction (RRR): The relative decrease in risk of an end point compared to the percent of that end point in the placebo group.

If you are still confused, just remember the RRR is an overestimation of the actual effect.

Number needed to treat (NNT): This is the number of people who need to be treated by an intervention to prevent one adverse outcome. A "good" NNT can be a large number (>100) if risk of serious outcome is great. If the risk of an outcome is not that dangerous, then lower (<25) NNTs are preferred.

The NNT should be compared to a similar statistic, the Number Needed to Harm (NNH). This is the number of people who have to be given treatment before one excess side effect or harm occurs. When the NNT is compared to the NNH, you and the patient can judge whether the benefit of the intervention is great enough to outweigh the risk of harm.

EVIDENCED-BASED GRADING:

To help you interpret diagnostic and treatment recommendations within *The 5-Minute Clinical Consult*, we have graded the best information within the text, and highlighted this content.

An "A" grade means the reference is from the highest-quality resource, like a systematic review. A *systematic review* is a summary of the medical literature on a given topic that uses strict, explicit methods to perform a thorough search of the literature and then provides a critical appraisal of individual studies, concluding in a recommendation. The most prestigious collection of systematic reviews is from the Cochrane Collaboration (www.cochrane.org).

A "B" grade means the data referenced comes from high-quality randomized controlled trials performed to minimize bias in their outcome. Bias is anything that interferes with the truth; in the medical literature, it is often unintentional, but it is much more common than we appreciate. In short, always assume some degree of bias exists in any research endeavor.

A "C" grade implies the reference used does not meet the A or B requirements; they are often treatments recommended by consensus groups (like the American Cancer Society). In some cases, they may be the standards of care. But implicit in a group's recommendation is the bias of the author or the group that supports the reference. For example, the American Urological Society's recommendation around screening for prostate cancer may be motivated by their narrow scope and financial benefit. Compare this to the recommendations of the US Preventive Services Task Force (www.ahrq.gov), who recommends against screening for prostate cancer.

BIAS:

Bias is anything that interferes with the truth. There are many types of bias that should be considered by the publishers of medical information. Below describes a number of bias types that often affect our care without us knowing it is present:

Publication bias occurs when research is not published; this is often when a study finds data that does *not* support an intervention. The motivation to publish information that "didn't work" is low. It is estimated that up to 40% of all medical research never gets published. So when you read of an intervention that "works," wonder if other studies were done that did not show benefit and went unpublished.

Comparator bias occurs when research compares an intervention to placebo, when placebo is not the standard of care. Knowing a new antibiotic is more effective than placebo for treating acute otitis media is not helpful if you typically use amoxicillin.

Why not release research comparing the new drug to the standard of care? Often, the research has been done, and the new drug proved no better. If this study does not get published, you have an example of publication bias.

Selection bias involves either using a tool that does not discriminate between populations selected or just reporting a just subset of study participants from a study. Either will result in the data being skewed because it can only be applied to small subset of people.

Attrition bias and the concept of intention to treat. Attrition bias is when researchers do not fully acknowledge and address how a study deals with participants who do not adhere to the research protocol or drop out completely. Intention to treat analysis hopes to diminish attrition bias by statistically considering the nonadhering or dropped out patients as unsuccessfully benefiting from the intervention.

Commercial (funder) bias involves who paid for the research being done, and do they have a vested interest in the outcome. Despite its size and scope, the recent *Jupiter* trial on treating low-risk adults with a statin has been called into question, as the company who funded the study makes the brand name drug used in the study and the lead author is part owner of the unique test employed in the trial. The data may be accurate, but until this is studied by less vested interests, some feel its outcome cannot be clinically applied.

Have you been annoyed how one week you learn of a randomized controlled trial that supports a treatment, to be followed the next week with a contradictory article? Statisticians have figured out how to resolve this using something called a systematic review.

Systematic reviews take all the literature on a topic, say using antibiotics to treat otitis media, and combines the data to determine if the sum of all the trials tells a different story than any single trial. The large number of participants in this type of research results in a much more statistically (and clinically) significant conclusion than any single paper. Want more? Check this out: http://musculoskeletal.cochrane.org/what-systematic-review.

A **meta-analysis** is a quantitative systematic review, and demonstrates it outcomes in the form of a forest plot. The bottom line with interpretation of a forest plot is look for the diamond on the bottom. If it is to LEFT of the vertical line, it means risk of an outcome was reduced by the intervention. If it is fully to the RIGHT, then risk of that outcome was increased. And if the diamond touches the vertical line, it means there was no statistical influence of the intervention on the outcome. To understand these concepts better, here is a great resource: http://www.cochrane-net.org/openlearning/html/mod3-2.htm.

I hope this brief introduction to EBM has been informative, clear, and helpful. If any of the information above seems unclear, or if you have a question, please contact us via www.5minuteconsult.com.

ACKNOWLEDGMENTS

This is the 23rd edition of *The 5-Minute Clinical Consult*, a comprehensive point-of-care tool to assist in the care of patients. From beginning to end, one cannot find a more current and easy-to-use collection of clinically useful content.

Developing and maintaining a book and Web site of this magnitude requires an equally broad effort from its supporting team. I wish to thank the dedication and tireless efforts of many: Product Development Editor, Leanne Vandetty; Executive Editor, Rebecca Gaertner; Program Manager, Katy McSurdy; and Publisher, Lisa McAllister.

This 2015 edition is the direct result of the dedication and insights of our associate editors. I wish to thank Drs. Robert Baldor, Jeremy Golding, and Jill Grimes for their hard work, and overwhelming commitment to *The 5-Minute Clinical Consult*.

I wish to especially thank my wife, Sylvia, and my daughter, Molly, who have given greatly for this book.

The challenge of completing a book covering this broad a spectrum of medicine requires insights and skills far beyond my own.

Many thanks to my mentors Bob Baldor and Mark Quirk who are an enormous support—always there to encourage, reassure, and impart wisdom.

Many in the academic and health care worlds are due thanks for support, insight, and friendship: Daniel Lasser, Alan Chuman, Michele Pugnaire, Karen Rayla, Phil Fournier, Erik Garcia, Jeff Stovall, Jim Comes, Len Levin, Judy Norberg, J. Herb Stevenson, Bob Jenal, Mick Godkin, Susanna Guzman, Michael Kidd, Zainab Nawab, Sanjiv and Amita Chopra, Vasilios (Bill) Chrisostomidis, James (Jay) Broadhurst, Danuta Antkowiak, Atreyi Chakrabarti, Kerry Morse, Mark Powicki, Steve Messineo, and the faculty and students of the University of Massachusetts Medical School.

Medicine is a challenge I have fortunately not had to meet alone. Thanks to my parents, Frank and Angela (Jean); my brother John and his family, Marylou, Cate, and Jane; Frank, Mary Anne, Diane, and David Christian; the Diana and Hymie Lipschitz family; and the Bob and Ruth Pabreza family; they are responsible for who I am and my success in life.

I am blessed with the best of friends; without them, I would not be a physician. Thanks to Bob Bacic, Ron Jautz, Richard Onorato, John Horcher, Auguste Turnier, Bob Smith, Paul Saivetz, Bob and Nancy Gallinaro, Drew and Jill Grimes, Louay Toma, Laurie, Alan, Daniel, Jenny and Matt Bugos, Alan Ehrlich, Teri and Andy Jennings, Bill Demianiuk, Mark Steenbergen, John and Kathleen Polanowicz, Phil and Carol Pettine, Mark Shelton, Steve Bennett, Vicki Triolo, Michael Bernatchez, and a happier Milo.

—FRANK J. DOMINO, MD

CONTRIBUTING AUTHORS

Thomas L. Abell, MD
Arthur M. Schoen, MD Chair in
    Gastroenterology
University of Louisville
Louisville, Kentucky

Humaira Abid, MD
Associate Professor
University of Texas Health Science Center
Houston, Texas

George M. Abraham, MD, MPH
Associate Chief of Medicine
Saint Vincent Hospital
Professor of Medicine
University of Massachusetts Medical
    School
Worcester, Massachusetts

Luis K. Abrishamian, MD
Attending Physician
Little Company of Mary
Torrance Department of Emergency
    Medicine
Torrance, California

Gabriela F. Abrishamian-Garcia
Clinical Research Assistant
Endocrine Unit
Massachusetts General Hospital
Boston, Massachusetts

Reem Abu-Sbaih, DO
Assistant Professor
Department of Osteopathic Manipulative
    Medicine
New York College of Osteopathic Medicine
Old Westbury, New York

**Abdulrazak Abyad, MPH, MBA, AGSF,
AFCHSE**
Chairman
Medical Education and Training
Prince Mohammed Bin Abdulaziz Hospital
Middle-East Academy for Medicine of
    Aging
Riyadh, Saudi Arabia

William B. Adams, MD
Division of Dermatology
University of Louisville
Louisville, Kentucky

Ehiozogie Adu
Brooklyn, New York

Maria I. Aguilar, MD
Associate Professor of Neurology
Program Director, Vascular Neurology
    Fellowship
Mayo Clinic Arizona
Phoenix, Arizona

Sumera R. Ahmad, MD
Department of Pulmonary and Critical
    Care
UMass Memorial Medical Center
Worcester, Massachusetts

Yasir Ahmed, MD
Penn State Hershey Eye Center
Penn State College of Medicine
Hershey, Pennsylvania

Jamil A. Alarafi, DO
Attending Staff
Case Western Reserve Richmond Medical
    Campus
Emergency Medicine Residency Program
Cleveland, Ohio

Christina N. Alavian, MD
Assistant Professor
Department of Medicine, Division of
    Dermatology
University of Massachusetts Medical
    School
Worcester, Massachusetts

Kelly Alberda, MD
Faculty
Family and Community Medicine
University of Texas Southwestern, Austin
    Programs
Blackstock Family Health Center
Austin, Texas

Fozia Akhtar Ali, MD
Assistant Professor
Family & Community Medicine
University of Texas Health Science
    Center San Antonio
San Antonio, Texas

Andrew Allegretti, MD
Fellow in Nephrology
Massachusetts General Hospital/Brigham
    and Women's Hospital Division of
    Nephrology
Boston, Massachusetts

Richard W. Allinson, MD
Associate Professor
Department of Ophthalmology
The Texas A&M University System, Health
    Sciences Center
College Station, Texas
Senior Staff Physician
Department of Ophthalmology
Baylor Scott & White Clinic
Waco, Texas

Ziad Alnabki, MD
University of Louisville
Louisville, Kentucky

Jowhara Hamad Al-Qahtani, MD
General Surgery Resident
New York Presbyterian Hospital
New York, New York

Bree Alyeska, MD
Resident, Emergency Medicine
University of Massachusetts
Worcester, Massachusetts

Bradley T. Anderson, MD
Department of Gastroenterology
The George Washington University
School of Medicine and Health Sciences
Washington, DC

Mark Andrews, MD
Rhode Island Hospital
Warwick, Rhode Island

Tanya E. Anim, MD
Fellow in Women's Health with Obstetrics
    Focus
Florida Hospital Family Medicine
    Residency Program
Winter Park, Florida

David Anthony, MD, MSc
Assistant Professor of Family Medicine
Warren Alpert Medical School of Brown
    University
Pawtucket, Rhode Island

Kashif Syed Anwar, MD, MMS
Resident Physician
Department of Family Medicine
Summa Barberton Hospital
Barberton, Ohio

Vlad Apostol, DO
University Hospitals Richmond Medical
    Center
Cleveland, Ohio

Paul M. Arguin, MD
Chief, Domestic Malaria Unit
Centers for Disease Control and
    Prevention
Atlanta, Georgia

James J. Arnold, DO
Family Medicine Faculty Physician
Family Medicine Residency
Fort Belvoir, Virginia

Michael Arnold, MD, CDR, MC
United States Navy
United States Naval Hospital
Naples, Italy

Rajiv Arya, MD, FACEP
Assistant Professor
Vice Chair, Department of Emergency
    Medicine
Rutgers-Robert Wood Johnson Medical
    School
Medical Director, Division of Emergency
    Care
Robert Wood Johnson University Hospital
New Brunswick, New Jersey

Armand Asarian, MD

Asma Ashraf, MD
Department of Family Medicine
University of Texas Southwestern
Dallas, Texas

Aneel A. Ashrani, MD, MS
Assistant Professor
Division of Hematology
Department of Internal Medicine
Mayo Clinic
Rochester, Minnesota

Atena Asiaii, MD, MPH
Resident in Obstetrics & Gynecology
Thomas Jefferson University Hospital
Philadelphia, Pennsylvania

Shumaila Athar, MD
Department of Family Medicine
University of Texas Southwestern Medical
    Center
Dallas, Texas

Nicholas Atudonyang, MD
Senior Resident
University of Texas Southwestern
Dallas, Texas

Gerard P. Aurigemma, MD
Professor of Medicine and Radiology
University of Massachusetts Medical School
Director, Noninvasive Cardiology
University of Massachusetts Memorial
    Medical Center
Worcester, Massachusetts

Philip H. Aurigemma, MD
Orthopedic Surgery
University of Massachusetts Medical School
Worcester, Massachusetts

Swati B. Avashia, MD, FAAP
Assistant Professor, Internal Medicine and
    Pediatrics
Family Medicine Residency Program
University of Texas Southwestern Austin
Austin, Texas

Thomas R. Avonda, MD
Assistant Professor
Department of Family Medicine
East Tennessee State University
Johnson City, Tennessee

Patrick Axtmayer, MD
Emergency Medicine Resident
Brown/Rhode Island Hospital
Providence, Rhode Island

Jennifer L. Ayres, PhD
Director of Behavioral Health Services
University of Texas Southwestern Medical
    Center Austin
Family Medicine Residency Program
Austin, Texas

Holly L. Baab, MD
Assistant Director
Bayfront Family Medicine Residency
St. Petersburg, Florida

Sultan M. Babar, MD
Resident Physician
Department of Family Medicine
East Carolina University Brody School of
    Medicine
Greenville, North Carolina

Kavita Babu, MD
Associate Professor
Department of Emergency Medicine
Division of Medical Toxicology
University of Massachusetts Memorial
    Medical Center
Worcester, Massachusetts

Elisabeth L. Backer, MD
Clinical Associate Professor
Department of Family Medicine
University of Nebraska Medical Center
Omaha, Nebraska

Melissa Badowski, PharmD
Section of Infectious Diseases,
    Pharmacotherapy
University of Illinois at Chicago
College of Pharmacy
Chicago, Illinois

Sangeetha Balasubramanian, MD
Consultant Rheumatologist
South Bay Joint Care, Inc.
San Jose, California

Robert A. Baldor, MD, FAAFP
Professor and Vice-Chairman, Educational
    Affairs
Department of Family Medicine and
    Community Health
University of Massachusetts Medical
    School
Worcester, Massachusetts

Katherine L. Ball, MD
Department of Family Medicine
University of Washington
Seattle, Washington

Rahul Banerjee, MD
Warren Alpert Medical School of Brown
    University
Providence, Rhode Island

Brent J. Barber, MD
Associate Professor, Pediatric Cardiology
University of Arizona College of Medicine
Tucson, Arizona

Wendy Brooks Barr, MD, MPH, MSCE
Associate Residency Director
Lawrence Family Medicine Residency
Assistant Professor of Family Medicine
Tufts University School of Medicine
Lawrence, Massachusetts

**Michael C. Barros, PharmD, BCPS,
BCACP**
Clinical Assistant Professor of Pharmacy
    Practice
Temple University School of Pharmacy
Clinical Pharmacy Specialist, Ambulatory
    Care
Temple University Hospital
Division of Cardiology and Internal
    Medicine
Philadelphia, Pennsylvania

Adam Barta, MD
Assistant Professor
Department of Family Medicine
University of Texas Southwestern, Austin
Austin, Texas

Saurabh Basundhra, MD
Family Medicine Residency Program
University of Cincinnati Family Medicine
    Program
Clinton Memorial Hospital
Wilmington, Ohio

Kay A. Bauman, MD, MPH
Medical Director
New Mexico Department of Corrections
Professor
Department of Family and Community
    Medicine
University of New Mexico School of
    Medicine
Albuquerque, New Mexico

Dennis J. Baumgardner, MD
Clinical Adjunct Professor of Family
    Medicine
University of Wisconsin School of
    Medicine and Public Health
Aurora University of Wisconsin Medical
    Group
Milwaukee, Wisconsin

Jeffrey Baxter, MD
Assistant Professor
Department of Family Medicine and
    Community Health
University of Massachusetts Medical
    School
Worcester, Massachusetts

Cheryl B. Bayart, MD, MPH
Dermatology Resident
Cleveland Clinic Foundation
Cleveland, Ohio

Francesca L. Beaudoin, MD, MS
Assistant Professor of Emergency
    Medicine
The Alpert Medical School of Brown
    University
Rhode Island Hospital and The Miriam
    Hospital
Providence, Rhode Island

Angela Leigh Beeler, MD
Clinical Associate Professor
Department of Pediatrics
University of Massachusetts Medical
    School
Worcester, Massachusetts

Kelly H. Beers, DO
New York Institute of Technology College
    of Osteopathic Medicine
Old Westbury, New York

Hershey S. Bell, MD, MS, FAAFP
Vice President of Academic Affairs and
    Dean
Lake Erie College of Osteopathic
    Medicine School of Pharmacy
Erie, Pennsylvania and Bradenton, Florida

Paul P. Belliveau, PharmD, RPh
Professor of Pharmacy Practice
Department of Pharmacy Practice
Massachusetts College of Pharmacy and
    Health Sciences University
Worcester, Massachusetts

Kara Keating Bench, MD, MPH
University of Massachusetts Medical School
Worcester, Massachusetts

Crystal Benjamin, MD, MPH
Resident Physician, Family Medicine
University of Massachusetts Medical School
Fitchburg, Massachusetts

Sheldon Benjamin, MD
Professor of Psychiatry and Neurology
Department of Psychiatry
University of Massachusetts Medical
    School
Worcester, Massachusetts

Terrell B. Benold, MD
Clinical Assistant Professor
Department of Family and Community
    Medicine
University of Texas Southwestern Medical
    School
Austin Programs
Austin, Texas

Andrew Bentley
Herbalist
Director, Natural Health Clinic
Lexington, Kentucky

Lionel Bercovitch, MD
Department of Dermatology
Warren Alpert Medical School
Brown University
Providence, Rhode Island

Jasmine S. Beria, DO, MPH, MS
College of Osteopathic Medicine
Old Westbury, New York

Louis J. Berk, MD
Assistant Clinical Instructor
Department of Family Medicine
State University of New York-Downstate
    Medical Center
Brooklyn, New York

Jamie Lee Berkes, MD
Assistant Professor of Medicine
Medical Director of Liver Transplant
Loyola University
Maywood, Illinois

Bettina Bernstein, DO
Clinical Assistant Professor
Department of Psychiatry and
    Neurosciences
Philadelphia College of Osteopathic
    Medicine
Philadelphia, Pennsylvania

Sandra New Berryman, DNP
Clinical Assistant Professor
University of Arkansas Medical Science
    College of Nursing
Little Rock, Arkansas

John F. Bertagnolli, Jr., DO
Associate Professor, Family Medicine
Rowan University School of Osteopathic
    Medicine
Glassboro, New Jersey

Sandra Katlyn Beverly, MD
Resident
Department of Emergency Medicine
Carolinas Medical Center
Charlotte, North Carolina

Neela Bhajandas, PharmD
Clinical Assistant Professor of Pharmacy
Critical Care and Pulmonary Clinical
    Specialist
Temple University School of Pharmacy
Philadelphia, Pennsylvania

Varun Kumar Bhalla, MD
Georgia Regents University
Department of Surgery
Augusta, Georgia

Rekha Bhandari, MD
Chief of Geriatrics
Kingsbrook Jewish Medical Center
Brooklyn, New York

Nirmanmoh Bhatia, MD
Resident, Internal Medicine
University of Louisville
Louisville, Kentucky

Kenneth M. Bielak, MD, FACSM, MBA
Associate Director of Sports Medicine
Health Science Center
University of Tennessee Medical Center
Knoxville, Tennessee

Ghazaleh Bigdeli, MD, FCCP
Pulmonary Rehab Associates
Youngstown, Ohio

Melissa Phillips Black, MD
Assistant Professor
Department of Internal and Geriatric
    Medicine
Emory University
Atlanta, Georgia

Jocelyn F. Blackwell, MD, MAJ, MC
Kempner, Texas

Lewis S. Blevins, Jr., MD
Professor of Neurological Surgery and
    Medicine
Director
California Center for Pituitary Disorders at
    University of California, San Francisco
San Francisco, California

Sandeep Bodige, DO
Resident Physician, Family Medicine
University of Texas Southwestern Medical
    Center
Dallas, Texas

Elise Bognanno, MD

Aaron Robert Bolduc, MD
Surgery Department
Georgia Regents University
Augusta, Georgia

Caitlin Bonney, MD
General Surgery Resident
University of Massachusetts Medical
    School
Worcester, Massachusetts

Nancy A. Bono, DO, FACOFP
Associate Professor/Chair of Family
    Medicine
New York Institute of Technology College
    of Osteopathic Medicine
Old Westbury, New York

Bryan C. Bordeaux, DO, MPH
Instructor
Harvard Medical School
Department of Population Medicine
Harvard Vanguard Medical Associates
Boston, Massachusetts

Susan Borisuk-Ratay, DO
Family Practice Resident
University Hospitals Regional Hospitals
Richmond Heights, Ohio

Jessica L. Borowicz, DO, FAOCD
Dermatologist and Dermatologic Surgeon
The Derm
Glenview & Park Ridge, Illinois

Marie L. Borum, MD, MPH, EdD
Professor of Medicine
Division of Gastroenterology and Liver
    Diseases
George Washington University
Washington, DC

Christopher M. Bositis, MD, AAHIVS
Clinical Program Director, HIV Program
Greater Lawrence Family Health Center
Lawrence, Massachusetts

Naomi F. Botkin, MD
Associate Professor of Medicine
University of Massachusetts Medical
    School
Worcester, Massachusetts

Thaddeus S. Boucree II, MD, DDS
Chairman, Department of Oral and
    Maxillofacial Surgery
Larkin Community Hospital
South Miami, Florida

Andre Joseph Boustani, MD
Resident Physician
Department of Emergency Medicine
Rhode Island Hospital/Brown University
Providence, Rhode Island

Crystal C. Bowe, MD, MPH
Family Medicine Physician
Caromont Medical Group
Gastonia, North Carolina

Rachel Bramson, MD
Department of Family Medicine
Texas A&M Health Science Center
    College of Medicine
Bryan, Texas

Doreen B. Brettler, MD
Professor of Medicine
Director, New England Hemophilia Center
Department of Medicine
University of Massachusetts Medical
    Center
Worcester, Massachusetts

Renata T. Brindise, DO
Dermatology Resident
Oakwood Southshore Medical Center
Trenton, Michigan

Ekaterina Brodski-Quigley, MD, EdM

Amy L. Brodsky, MD

Goran Broketa, MD
Staff Oncologist
VA Medical Center Manchester
Manchester, New Hampshire

Emma Brooks, MD
Assistant Professor
Department of Family Medicine
Oregon Health Sciences University
Portland, Oregon

Benjamin P. Brown, MD
Resident
Department of Obstetrics and Gynecology
University of Chicago Medical Center
Chicago, Illinois

Jimmy J. Brown, DDS, MD, FACS
Chief, Head & Neck Surgery
Georgia Regents University
Augusta, Georgia

Joyce Brown, DO, CHSE
Assistant Professor of Emergency
    Medicine
Department of Primary Care
Touro College of Osteopathic Medicine
New York, New York

Michael L. Brown, MD
Director, Psychiatry and Psychology
Scott & White Healthcare - College
    Station
College Station, Texas

Samuel Luke Brown, DO
Emergency Medicine Resident
Dartmouth Hitchcock Medical Center
Lebanon, New Hampshire

Theodore R. Brown, DO, MPH, FAAFP
Division Surgeon
25th Infantry Division
Schofield Barracks, Hawaii

Timothy S. Brown, MD
Director, Dermatologic Surgery
Division of Dermatology
University of Louisville School of Medicine
Louisville, Kentucky

Karen Browning, MD
Obstetrics & Gynecology
Women & Infants Hospital
Brown University
Providence, Rhode Island

Nitin Budhwar, MD, FAAFP
Department of Family & Community
    Medicine
University of Texas Southwestern Health
    Center
Dallas, Texas

Han Q. Bui, MD, CDR, MC, USN
Uniformed Service University
Bethesda, Maryland

Tiffany Burca, DO
University of Nebraska Medical Center
    Family Medicine Residency
Omaha, Nebraska

K. John Burhan, MD
Faculty
Department of Family Medicine
Creighton University School of Medicine
Omaha, Nebraska

John R. Burk, MD
Texas Pulmonary and Critical Care
    Consultants, PA
Fort Worth, Texas

Kristin Burke, MD
Resident, Internal Medicine
Beth Israel Deaconess Medical Center
Boston, Massachusetts

Harold J. Bursztajn, MD
Associate Clinical Professor of Psychiatry
Co-founder, Program in Psychiatry and
    the Law
Beth Israel Deaconess Medical Center
    Psychiatry of Harvard Medical School
President of the American Unit of the
    UNESCO Bioethics Chair
Boston, Massachusetts

Nancy Byatt, DO, MBA, FAPM
University of Massachusetts Medical
    School
UMass Memorial Medical Center
Worcester, Massachusetts

Mitchell A. Cahan, MD, FACS
Associate Professor of Surgery
Department of Surgery
University of Massachusetts Medical
    School
Worcester, Massachusetts

Elizabeth M. Cain, MD, FAAFP
Assistant Professor of Family Medicine
Assistant Program Director
Louisiana State University Rural Family
    Medicine Residency Program at
    Bogalusa
Bogalusa, Louisiana

Katherine M. Callaghan, MD
Resident
Department of Obstetrics and Gynecology
University of Massachusetts Memorial
Worcester, Massachusetts

Maya Campara, PharmD, BCPS
Clinical Assistant Professor
Department of Pharmacy Practice
University of Illinois Medical Center at
    Chicago
Clinical Pharmacist
Division of Solid Organ Transplant
University of Illinois at Chicago Medical
    Center
Chicago, Illinois

Tyler V. Campbell, DO
Radiology Resident
Larkin Community Hospital
South Miami, Florida

Jennifer Caragol, MD
University of Colorado Family Medicine
    Residency
Denver, Colorado

Jennifer L. Carey, MD
Assistant Professor of Emergency Medicine
University of Massachusetts Medical School
Worcester, Massachusetts

Samuel B. Carli, MD
Department of Internal Medicine
University of Arizona
Tucson, Arizona

Laurie Carrier, MD
Assistant Professor
Department of Community and Family
    Medicine
Northwestern University, Feinberg School
    of Medicine
Director of Behavioral Health Integrated
    Care
Heartland Health Center
Chicago, Illinois

Stephanie J. Carroll, MD
Resident
Department of Family Medicine
David Grant Medical Center
Travis Air Force Base, California

Ana I. Casanegra, MD, ABVM, RPVI
Assistant Professor
Vascular Medicine Program
Cardiovascular Section
Department of Medicine
Vascular Medicine Program
University of Oklahoma Health Sciences
    Center
Oklahoma City, Oklahoma

Casandra Cashman, MD
Assistant Director
Community Health Network
Family Medicine Residency
Indianapolis, Indiana

Mary Cataletto, MD, MMM
Pediatric Pulmonology
Winthrop University Hospital
Mineola, New York

Jeanne M. Cawse-Lucas, MD
Acting Assistant Professor
Department of Family Medicine
University of Washington
Seattle, Washington

Lorena Ceci
University of Massachusetts Medical
    School
Worceser, Massachusetts

Jan Cerny, MD, PhD, FACP
Assistant Professor of Medicine
Division of Hematology/Oncology
Department of Medicine
Director, Leukemia Program
University of Massachusetts Medical
    School
Associate Medical Director, Cancer
    Research Office
University of Massachusetts Memorial
    Cancer Center
Worcester, Massachusetts

Olga M. Ceron, MD
Staff Physician
Retina Specialist
Massachusetts Eye Research & Surgery
    Institution (MERSI)
Cambridge, Massachusetts

Catherine Chamberlain, MD
Brown Medical School
Providence, Rhode Island

Jacquelyn Chambers, MD

Aditya Chandrasekhar, MD, MPH
Internal Medicine Resident
Department of Medicine
University of Massachusetts Medical
    School
Worcester, Massachusetts

Christopher Chang, MD
Chief Resident
University of Massachusetts Worcester
    Family Medicine Residency Program
Worcester, Massachusetts

Felix B. Chang, MD, DABMA
Director, Inpatient Service
UMass Fitchburg Family Medicine
    Residency Program
UMass Memorial Health Alliance Hospital
Assistant Professor
Department of Family Medicine and
    Community Health
Attending Physician
UMass Memorial Medical Group
Leominster Community Health
    Connections
Leominster, Massachusetts

Joanne Chan, MD

Joann Yuen Chang, MD
Family Medicine Resident
Long Beach Memorial Family Medicine
Long Beach, California

Jason Chao, MD, MS
Professor
Department of Family Medicine and
    Community Health
Case Western Reserve University
University Hospitals Case Medical Center
Cleveland, Ohio

Arka Chatterjee, MD
Department of Cardiovascular Medicine
University of Alabama at Birmingham
Birmingham, Alabama

Nida Chaudhary, MD
Rheumatology Fellow
UMass Memorial Hospital
Worcester, Massachusetts

Sarah H. Cheeseman, MD
Division of Infectious Diseases and
    Immunology
UMass Memorial Healthcare
Clinical Professor of Medicine, Pediatrics,
    Microbiology, and Applied Physiologic
    Systems
University of Massachusetts Medical
    School
Worcester, Massachusetts

Amy Chen, MD, PhD
Assistant Professor
Department of Neurology
University of Rochester
Rochester, New York

Andy H. Chen, MD
Resident Physician
Department of Emergency Medicine
Brown University/Rhode Island Hospital
Providence, Rhode Island

Suma Chennubhotla, MD
Combined Internal Medicine and
    Pediatrics Residency Training Program
University of Louisville
Louisville, Kentucky

Karen Cherian, MD
Department of Family Medicine
Bayfront Health
Saint Petersburg, Florida

Manjula Cherukuri, MD, FAAFP
Medical Director
Community Medicine
University of North Texas Health Science
    Center
Dallas - Fort Worth, Texas

Edward Cheung, MD
Orthopaedic Surgery Resident
University of California, Los Angeles
Los Angeles, California

Sonia Nagy Chimienti, MD
Clinical Associate Professor of Medicine
Medical Director, Solid Organ Transplant
    Program
Co-Director, Organ System Diseases
University of Massachusetts School of
    Medicine
UMass Memorial Medical Center
Worcester, Massachusetts

Vasilios Chrisostomidis, DO
Assistant Professor
University of Massachusetts Medical
    School
Department of Family Medicine and
    Community Health
Worcester, Massachusetts

Felicia Chu, MD
Assistant Professor
Department of Neurology
University of Massachusetts Memorial
    Medical Center
Worcester, Massachusetts

Connie Yooran Chung, MD, Capt.
Family Medicine Resident
David Grant Medical Center
Travis Air Force Base, California

Lee T. Church, MD
David Grant Medical Center
Family Medicine Residency Program
Travis Air Force Base, California

Tara Chute, MD
Obstetrics and Gynecology
University of Massachusetts Medical
    Center
Worcester, Massachusetts

S. Lindsey Clarke, MD, FAAFP
MUSC AHEC Professor
Department of Family Medicine
Self Regional Healthcare Family Medicine
    Residency Program
Greenwood, South Carolina

Lisa Clemons, MD
Faculty
Family and Community Medicine
University of Texas Southwestern—Austin
Blackstock Family Health Center
Austin, Texas

David M. Clive, MD
Professor of Medicine
Department of Renal Medicine
University of Massachusetts Medical
    School
Worcester, Massachusetts

Kara M. Coassolo, MD
Attending Perinatologist
Lehigh Valley Health Network
Allentown, Pennsylvania

Jason Cohn
New York Institute of Technology College
    of Osteopathic Medicine
Old Westbury, New York

Timothy J. Coker, MD
Assistant Program Director
Ehrling Bergquist Family Medicine
    Residency
Offutt Air Force Base, Nebraska

Irene C. Coletsos, MS, MD
Associate Professor in Psychiatry
University of Massachusetts Medical
    School
Community Healthlink
Worcester, Massachusetts

Dana Collaguazo, MD
Clinical Assistant Professor
Department of Emergency Medicine
University of Iowa Hospitals & Clinics
Iowa City, Iowa

Jamie N. Colombo, DO
Pediatric Resident
Department of Pediatrics
University of Arizona
Tucson, Arizona

Jennifer C. Colvin, MD
Hematology/Oncology Fellow
University of Minnesota
Minneapolis, Minnesota

Brittany Conahan, PharmD

Jiadi Cook, MD
Christiana Care Family Medicine
    Department
Wilmington, Delaware

Maryann R. Cooper, PharmD, BCOP
Assistant Professor of Pharmacy Practice
Massachusetts College of Pharmacy and
    Health Sciences
University School of
    Pharmacy-Worcester/Manchester
Manchester, New Hampshire

Marco Cornelio, MD
Resident
Department of Family Medicine and
    Community Health
University of Massachusetts
Worcester, Massachusetts

Macario C. Corpuz, Jr., MD, FAAFP
Assistant Professor
Department of Family Medicine and
Community Health
University of Massachusetts Medical
School
Medical Staff
Department of Family Medicine
University of Massachusetts Memorial
Hospital
Worcester, Massachusetts

Danton Spohr Correa, MD, PhD
Attending Surgeon, Department of
Surgery
Federal University of Santa Catarina
Medical School
Florianopolis, Santa Catarina, Brazil

Jack Cossman, MD
Providence, Rhode Island

Ryan F. Coughlin, MD
Department of Emergency Medicine
Yale New Haven Hospital
New Haven, Connecticut

Alissa Craft, DO, MBA
Associate Professor and Vice Chair,
Pediatrics
Western University of Health Sciences
College of Osteopathic Medicine of the
Pacific-Northwest
Lebanon, Oregon

Neil E. Crittenden, MD
Instructor of Medicine
Department of Internal Medicine
University of Louisville
Louisville, Kentucky

Justin J. Crivelli, DO
University Hospitals Richmond Medical
Center
Richmond Heights, Ohio

Alan Cropp MD, FCCP
Department of Pulmonary Medicine
St. Elizabeth Hospital Health Center
Youngstown, Ohio

Katie M. Crowder, MD
Faculty Family Medicine Physician
Travis Family Medicine Residency
Travis Air Force Base, California

Eric J. Csernyik, DO
Director of Emergency Medicine
University Hospitals Richmond Medical
Center
Cleveland, Ohio

Sandra Cuellar, PharmD, BCOP
Clinical Assistant Professor
Clinical Oncology Pharmacist
Department of Pharmacy Practice
University of Illinois Hospital & Health
Sciences System
Chicago, Illinois

Hongyi Cui, MD, PhD, FACS, FICS
Assistant Professor of Surgery
Department of General and Laparoscopic
Surgery
University of Massachusetts Medical
School
Associate Director, Acute Care Surgery
University of Massachusetts Memorial
Medical Center
Worcester, Massachusetts

John Curington, MD
Assistant Clinical Professor in Family
Medicine
University of California San Diego School
of Medicine
San Diego, California

Michael P. Curry, MD
Medical Director, Liver Transplantation
Beth Israel Deaconess Medical Center
Assistant Professor of Medicine
Harvard Medical School
Boston, Massachusetts

Kevin M. Curtis, MD, MS
Program Director, Emergency Medicine
Residency
Dartmouth-Hitchcock Medical Center
Associate Professor of Medicine
The Geisel School of Medicine at
Dartmouth
Lebanon, New Hampshire

Megan H. Curtis, MD
Resident
Swedish Family Medicine Residency First
Hill
Seattle, Washington

Tyler Cymet, DO, FACP, FACOP
Associate Vice President for Medical
Education
Chief of Clinical Medical Education
American Association of Colleges of
Osteopathic Medicine
Chevy Chase, Maryland

Jessica Dalby, MD
Assistant Professor
Department of Family Medicine
University of Wisconsin
Madison, Wisconsin

Jennifer S. Daly, MD
Clinical Chief, Infectious Diseases and
Immunology
Professor of Medicine, Microbiology and
Physiological Systems
University of Massachusetts Medical
School
Worcester, Massachusetts

Anthony Dambro, MD
Camp Lejeune Family Medicine Residency
Camp Lejeune, North Carolina

Jayaprakash R. Dasari, MD
Nephrology Fellow
University of Massachusetts
Worcester, Massachusetts

Akhil Das, MD, FACS
Assistant Professor
Department of Urology
Thomas Jefferson University
Philadelphia, Pennsylvania

**Janice E. Daugherty, MD, FAAFP,
DABIHM**
Diplomate of American Board of Family
Medicine
Certificate of Added Qualifications in
Geriatric Medicine
Diplomate of American Board of
Integrative Holistic Medicine
Medical Acupuncture
Associate Professor
Department of Family Medicine
The Brody School of Medicine at East
Carolina University
Greenville, North Carolina

Joel David, DO
Resident, Medicine
University Hospitals Regional Hospitals
Cleveland, Ohio

Robert C. Day
Milford, Massachusetts

Sondra M. De Antonio, MD
Neurology
Adjunct Assistant Professor
Internal Medicine Department
Rowan University School of Osteopathic
Medicine
Glassboro, New Jersey

Lauren de Leon, MD
Providence, Rhode Island

Garreth C. Debiegun, MD
Assistant Clinical Professor
Department of Emergency Medicine
Maine Medical Center
Tufts University School of Medicine
Portland, Maine

Alexei DeCastro, MD
Assistant Professor
Program Director
MUSC/Trident Family Medicine
  Residency
Medical University of South Carolina
Charleston, South Carolina

Sophia L. Delano, MD, MPP
Dermatology Resident
Division of Dermatology
UMass Memorial Health Care
Worcester, Massachusetts

Konstantinos E. Deligiannidis, MD, MPH
Assistant Professor of Family Medicine
  and Community Health
University of Massachusetts Medical
  School
UMass Memorial Health Care
Worcester, Massachusetts

Marie DeLuca, ScB
Alpert Medical School
Providence, Rhode Island

Deborah M. DeMarco, MD
Senior Associate Dean for Clinical Affairs
Professor of Medicine
Division of Rheumatology
University of Massachusetts Medical
  School
Worcester, Massachusetts

Gautam J. Desai, DO, FACOFP, CPI
Professor, Department of Family &
  Community Medicine
Kansas City University of Medicine and
  Biosciences
Kansas City, Missouri

Tarina Desai, MD
Family Medicine
University of Texas Health Science
  Center at San Antonio
San Antonio, Texas

Mathew J. Devine, DO
Assistant Professor
Associate Medical Director
Department of Family Medicine
University of Rochester
Highland Family Medicine
Rochester, New York

Howard Dickey-White, MD, FACEP
Hudson, Ohio

Ashley Dickinson, MD
University of Louisville School of Medicine
ouisville, Kentucky

Gretchen M. Dickson, MD, MBA
Assistant Professor
Department of Family and Community
  Medicine
University of Kansas—School of Medicine,
  Wichita
Wichita, Kansas

Robert J. Dimeff, MD
Professor Orthopedic Surgery, Pediatrics,
  and Family & Community Medicine
Medical Director of Sports Medicine
University of Texas Southwestern Medical
  Center
Dallas, Texas

Michael K. Ditkoff, MD, FACS
Progressive Ear, Nose & Throat
  Associates
Manhasset, New York

Frank J. Domino, MD
Professor
Director of Predoctoral Education
Department of Family Medicine and
  Community Health
University of Massachusetts Medical
  School
Worcester, Massachusetts

John N. Dorsch, MD
Associate Professor
Department of Family & Community
  Medicine
University of Kansas School of
  Medicine-Wichita
Wichita, Kansas

Kristin D'Orsi, DO
Resident
Department of Obstetrics and Gynecology
University of Massachusetts
Worcester, Massachusetts

Cassandra Dorvil, DO, MBA
Family Medicine Resident
University of Massachusetts Family
  Medicine Residency
Fitchburg, Massachusetts

Hobie Dotson, PsyD
Licensed Clinical Psychologist
Assistant Professor
University of Kentucky
Hazard, Kentucky

Elizabeth Dougherty, MD
Internal Medicine/Pediatrics Resident
Maine Medical Center
Portland, Maine

Kathleen A. Downey, MD
Associate Professor of Family and
  Community Medicine
Department of Family and Community
  Medicine
University of Cincinnati
Cincinnati, Ohio

Emily Drummond, DO
Emergency Medicine Physician
Emergency Department
University Hospital
Richmond Heights Medical Center
Richmond Heights, Ohio

Kristina M. Duarte, MD, ScM
Clinical Assistant Professor of Family
  Medicine
Alpert School of Medicine
Brown University
Memorial Hospital of Rhode Island
Pawtucket, Rhode Island

Maurice Duggins, MD
Clinical Associate Professor
Department of Family and Community
  Medicine
Kansas University School of
  Medicine-Wichita
Associate Director, Via Christi Family
  Medicine Residency Program
Wichita, Kansas

Kaelen C. Dunican, PharmD
Associate Professor
Department of Pharmacy Practice
Massachusetts College of Pharmacy and
  Health Sciences University
Worcester, Massachusetts

Cheryl Durand, PharmD
Assistant Professor of Pharmacy Practice
Massachusetts College of Pharmacy and
  Health Sciences University
Manchester, New Hampshire

Omar Durani, MD
Family & Community Medicine
University of Texas Southwestern
Dallas, Texas

William Jerry Durbin, MD
Professor of Pediatrics and Internal
  Medicine
University of Massachusetts Medical
  School
Worcester, Massachusetts

Nathalie Duroseau
New York Institute of Technology College
  of Osteopathic Medicine
Old Westbury, New York

Muhammad Durrani
New York Institute of Technology College
  of Osteopathic Medicine
Old Westbury, NY

Kylee Eagles, DO
Instructor
Department of Family Medicine and
  Community Health
University of Massachusetts Medical
  School
Fellow, Sports Medicine
Department of Family Medicine
University of Massachusetts
Fitchburg, Massachusetts

Phillip Marks Ecker, MD
Dermatologist
Minnesota Dermatology, PA
Plymouth, Minnesota

Samuel Ecker, DO
Traditional Rotating Intern
Larkin Community Hospital
Miami, Florida

Alan M. Ehrlich, MD
Assistant Professor of Family Medicine
University of Massachusetts Medical
  School
Worcester, Massachusetts

Jordan Eisenstock, MD
Departments of Neurology & Psychiatry
University of Massachusetts Memorial
  Healthcare
Assistant Professor
University of Massachusetts Medical
  School
Director of Neurorehabilitation
Fairlawn Rehabilitation Hospital
Worcester, Massachusetts

William G. Elder, Jr., PhD
Professor of Family and Community
  Medicine
University of Kentucky College of
  Medicine
Chandler Medical Center
Lexington, Kentucky

Darryl Elefan, MD
Nephrology Fellow
University of Massachusetts Medical
  School
Worcester, Massachusetts

Nancy Elliott, MD, FACS
Montclair Breast Center
Montclair, New Jersey

Carrie Lynn Ellis, DVM, MS
Associate Veterinarian
Animal Hospital on Mt. Lookout Square
Cincinnati, Ohio

Robert Ellis, MD
Associate Professor
Department of Family and Community
  Medicine
University of Cincinnati
Cincinnati, Ohio

Pamela Ellsworth, MD
Professor of Urology
UMass Memorial Medical Center
University of Massachusetts Medical
  School
Worcester, Massachusetts

Lacey Beth Elwyn, DO
Traditional Rotating Intern with
  Dermatology Emphasis
University Hospitals
Regional Hospitals
Richmond Medical Center
Richmond Heights, Ohio

Julia M. Emanuel, MD, MSc
The George Washington University School
  of Medicine and Health Sciences
Washington, DC

Dawnielle C. Endly, DO

Fallon Enfinger, PharmD, CDE
Assistant Professor of Pharmacy Practice
Lake Erie College of Osteopathic
  Medicine School of Pharmacy
Bradenton, Florida

Kevin Engelhardt, MD
Resident
Department of Pediatrics
University of Arizona
Tucson, Arizona

Mark W. English, MD
Associate Professor
Texas A&M Health Science Center
Department of Family and Community
  Medicine
Bryan, Texas

Elizabeth A. Erban, MD
Assistant Professor, Family Medicine and
  Community Health
University of Massachusetts Memorial
  Health Care
Worcester, Massachusetts

Rasai L. Ernst, MD
Assistant Professor
Department of Family Medicine and
  Community Health
University Hospitals Case Medical Center
Case Western University School of
  Medicine
Cleveland, Ohio

Justin Ertle
School of Medicine and Health Sciences
George Washington University
Washington, DC

Landrey Fagan, MD, MS
Family Medicine with Obstetrics
  Fellowship
Associate Clinical Professor
Tufts Medical School
Physician
Lynn Community Health Center
Lynn, Massachusetts

Kristyn T. Fagerberg, MD
Private Practice
Austin, Texas

Margaret Fairhurst, DO
Resident
University Hospitals Richmond Medical
  Center
Richmond Heights, Ohio

Nathan P. Falk, MD, CAQSM
Director, Primary Care Sports Medicine
Offutt Air Force Base/University of
  Nebraska Medical Center Family
  Medicine Residency
Omaha, Nebraska

Pang-Yen Fan, MD
Associate Professor of Medicine
Division of Renal Medicine
University of Massachusetts School of
  Medicine
Worcester, Massachusetts

Rami Farhat, DO
Graduate Medical Education
Meadowlands Hospital Medical Center
Secaucus, New Jersey

Olusola Fasusi, MD

Rhonda A. Faulkner, PhD
Director of Behavioral Medicine
Department of Family Medicine
Saint Joseph Hospital/University of Illinois
Chicago, Illinois

Jeffrey P. Feden, MD
Assistant Professor
Department of Emergency Medicine
Alpert Medical School of Brown University
Providence, Rhode Island

Ryan B. Feeney, PharmD
Community Staff Pharmacist
Philadelphia, Pennsylvania

Patricia Feito, MD
Family Medicine
Bayfront Health St. Petersburg
St. Petersburg, Florida

Neil J. Feldman, DPM
Private Practice
Central Massachusetts Podiatry, PC
Worcester, Massachusetts

Edward Feller, MD, FACP, FACG
Clinical Professor of Medicine and Health
    Services, Policy and Practice
Brown University
Providence, Rhode Island

Warren J. Ferguson, MD
Associate Professor
Department of Family Medicine and
    Community Health
University of Massachusetts Medical
    School
Vice Chair
Department of Family Medicine and
    Community Health
UMass Memorial Medical Center
Worcester, Massachusetts

Laura Ferraro, MD
University of Massachusetts Medical
    School
Worcester, Massachusetts

Kathleen Ferrer, MD, FAAP, AAHIVS
Children's National Medical Center
Department of Pediatrics
George Washington University School of
    Medicine
Washington, DC

Scott A. Fields, MD, MHA
Professor and Vice Chair
Department of Family Medicine
Oregon Health and Science University
Portland, Oregon

Sara J. Fine, MD
University of Massachusetts Medical
    School
Worcester, Massachusetts

Stanley Fineman, MD
Adjunct Associate Professor
Department of Pediatrics
Emory University School of Medicine
Atlanta Allergy & Asthma Clinic
Atlanta, Georgia

Judy Fingergut, MD
Clinical Assistant Professor
Department of Family Medicine
Stony Brook University Medical Center
Stony Brook, New York

Jonathon M. Firnhaber, MD
Assistant Professor
Residency Program Director
Department of Family Medicine
Brody School of Medicine
East Carolina University
Greenville, North Carolina

Marc Fisher, MD
Department of Neurology
University of Massachusetts Medical School
Worcester, Massachusetts

Timothy P. Fitzgibbons, MD, PhD
Assistant Professor of Medicine
Division of Cardiovascular Medicine
University of Massachusetts Medical School
Worcester, Massachusetts

Jonathan M. Flacker, MD, AGSF
Chief, Section of Geriatrics and
    Gerontology
Emory University School of Medicine
Atlanta, Georgia

John P. Flaherty, DO
New York Institute of Technology College
    of Osteopathic Medicine
Old Westbury, New York

Theodore B. Flaum, DO, FACOFP
Assistant Professor
Department of Osteopathic Manipulative
    Medicine
New York Institute of Technology College
    of Osteopathic Medicine
Old Westbury, New York

Joseph A. Florence, MD
Director of Rural Programs
Department of Family Medicine
James H. Quillen College of Medicine
East Tennessee State University
Johnson City, Tennessee

Emily K. Flores, PharmD, BCPS
Bill Gatton College of Pharmacy
East Tennessee State University
Johnson City, Tennessee

Mary K. Flynn, MD
Assistant Professor
Department of Family Medicine and
    Community Health
University of Massachusetts Medical School
Plumley Village Health Services
Worcester, Massachusetts

Harry W. Flynn, Jr., MD
Ophthalmology Department
Bascom Palmer Eye Institute
University of Miami Miller School of
    Medicine
Miami, Florida

Jay Fong, MD
Assistant Professor
Department of Pediatrics
University of Massachusetts Medical
    Center
Worcester, Massachusetts

Joao C.S. Fontoura, Jr., MD
Florida International University
Miami, Florida

James J. Foody, MD, FACP
Vice Chairman and Professor of Medicine
Northwestern University Feinberg School
    of Medicine
Chicago, Illinois

Emily Forbes, DO
New York Institute of Technology
College of Osteopathic Medicine
Old Westbury, New York

Lorna Fountain, MD
Associate Director
Bayfront Family Medicine Residency
    Program
St. Petersburg, Florida

Phillip Fournier, MD
Associate Professor of Family Medicine
    and Community Medicine
University of Massachusetts Medical
    School
UMass Memorial Healthcare
Worcester, Massachusetts

Robert Lee Frachtman, MD
Austin Gastroenterology, PA
Austin, Texas

Mony Fraer, MD, FACP, FASN
Assistant Professor, Internal Medicine and
    Nephrology
University of Iowa Hospital and Clinics
Iowa City, Iowa

Brian E. Frank, MD
Assistant Professor
Department of Family Medicine
Oregon Health and Science University
Portland, Oregon

Jennifer Frank, MD
ThedaCare Physicians
Neenah, Wisconsin

Robert S. Freelove, MD
Clinical Associate Professor
Department of Family and Community
 Medicine
University of Kansas School of Medicine,
 Wichita
Wichita, Kansas

Tara Futrell, MD
Sports Medicine Fellow
University of Massachusetts
Worcester, Massachusetts

Heidi L. Gaddey, MD
Family Medicine Residency
University of Nebraska
Omaha, Nebraska

Steven Gale, MD
Family Medicine Resident
Department of Family Medicine
University of Nebraska Medical Center/
 Ehrling Bergquist Family Medicine
 Residency
Omaha, Nebraska

Christina Gallagher, PharmD
Post-Doctoral Fellow
Global Medical Affairs
Sanofi Oncology
Massachusetts College of Pharmacy and
 Health Sciences University
Boston, Massachusetts

Sumanth Gandra, MD, MPH
Post-doctoral Fellow
Center for Disease Dynamics, Economics
 & Policy
Washington, DC

Jennifer Gao, MD
Department of Medicine
Massachusetts General Hospital
Boston, Massachusetts

Andrew Gara, MD
University of Massachusetts Medical
 School
Worcester, Massachusetts

William T. Garrison, PhD
Professor of Pediatrics
University of Massachusetts Medical
 School
Worcester, Massachusetts

Jewell Victoria Gaulding, MD
University of Louisville School of Medicine
Louisville, Kentucky

Gerald Gehr, MD
Assistant Professor of Medicine
Dartmouth Medical School
Hanover, New Hampshire

B. Chance Gentry, MD, CDR, MC, USN
Staff Family Physician
Family Medicine Residency Program
Naval Hospital Camp Lejeune
Camp Lejeune, North Carolina

Shari L. Gentry, MD
Faculty, Naval Hospital Camp Lejeune
Family Medicine Residency
Camp Lejeune, North Carolina.

Bethany Gentilesco, MD
Assistant Professor of Medicine (Clinical)
Warren Alpert Medical School of Brown
 University
Providence, Rhode Island

Paul George, MD, MHPE
Assistant Professor of Family Medicine
The Warren Alpert Medical School of
 Brown University
Providence, Rhode Island

Fereshteh Gerayli, MD, FAAFP
Professor, Family Medicine
Johnson City Family Medicine Residency
 Program
East Tennessee State University
Quillen College of Medicine
Johnson City, Tennessee

Amaninderapal Ghotra, MD, MS
Department of Internal Medicine
Division of Cardiovascular Disease
University of Louisville
Louisville, Kentucky

Juliana E. Gilbert, MD
University of Louisville School of Medicine
Louisville, Kentucky

David B. Gilchrist, MD, FAAFP
Assistant Professor in Family Medicine
 and Community Health
University of Massachusetts Memorial
 Health Care
Worcester, Massachusetts

Neil A. Gilchrist, PharmD, BCPS
Manager, Pharmacy Operations
Department of Pharmacy
UMass Memorial Medical Center
Worcester, Massachusetts

Megan Dianne Gillem, DO
Family Medicine Residency
University of Texas Southwestern
Dallas, Texas

Wolfgang G. Gilliar, DO, FAAPMR
Dean and Professor
New York Institute of Technology College
 of Osteopathic Medicine
Old Westbury, New York

Margaret Gilmore, MD
Resident Physician, Family Medicine
University of Texas Southwestern
Austin, Texas

Nora E. Gimpel, MD
Assistant Professor
Chief, Division of Community Medicine
University of Texas Medical Center at
 Dallas
Department of Family and Community
 Medicine
Parkland Family Medicine Clinic
Dallas, Texas

Jonathan Giordano, DO, MS
New York Institute of Technology College
 of Osteopathic Medicine
Old Westbury, New York

Dori Goldberg, MD
Assistant Professor of Medicine
Division of Dermatology
University of Massachusetts Medical
 School
Worcester, Massachusetts

Elizabeth M. Goldberg, MD
Assistant Professor of Emergency
 Medicine
The Alpert Medical School of Brown
 University
Providence, Rhode Island

Ankur Goel, MD
Department of General Surgery
Georgia Regents Univeristy
Augusta, Georgia

Jeremy Golding, MD, FAAFP
Professor of Family Medicine and
 Obstetrics & Gynecology
University of Massachusetts Medical
 School
Quality Officer
Department of Family Medicine and
 Community Health
University of Massachusetts Memorial
 Health Care
Hahnemann Family Health Center
Worcester, Massachusetts

Michael Golding, MD
Headquarters Senior Psychiatrist
California Department of Corrections
Elk Grove, California

Matthew J. Goldman, MD
Family Medicine Resident Physician
University Hospital Case Medical Center
Cleveland, Ohio

Rayna Goldstein, MD
Mount Sinai Hospital
New York, New York

Walter K. Goljan, MD
Webster Square Medical
Worcester, Massachusetts

Mercedes E. Gonzalez, MD
Clinical Assistant Professor
Department of Dermatology
University of Miami School of Medicine
Florida International University School of
 Medicine
Miami, Florida

Herbert P. Goodheart, MD
Associate Clinical Professor
Department of Dermatology
Mount Sinai College of Medicine
New York, New York

Geetha Gopalakrishnan, MD
Associate Professor of Medicine
Alpert Medical School of Brown University
Providence, Rhode Island

Farzan Gorgani, MS
Department of Biomedical Sciences
New York Institute of Technology College
 of Osteopathic Medicine
Old Westbury, New York

Edward A. Gotfried, DO, FACOS
Associate Professor
New York Institute of Technology College
 of Osteopathic Medicine
Old Westbury, New York

Archana Govindan, MD, MS
University of Texas Southwestern
Family Medicine Residency
Dallas, Texas

Parag Goyal, MD
New York Presbyterian Hospital
Weill Cornell Medical Center
New York, New York

Shami Goyal, MD, MS
Assistant Professor
Department of Family Medicine
University of Pittsburgh Physicians
Piitsburgh, Pennsylvania

Scott F. Graham, MD
Assistant Director
Bayfront Family Medicine Residency
St. Petersburg, Florida

Jane M. Grant-Kels, MD
Professor of Dermatology, Pathology, and
 Pediatrics
Chair, Department of Dermatology
Director of Dermatopathology
Director of the Cutaneous Oncology
 Program and Melanoma Center
Dermatology Residency Director
Assistant Dean of Clinical Affairs
University of Connecticut Health
 Center
Farmington, Connecticut

Michael Gray, MD, MS, MA
Attending Physician
Emergency Department
Harrington Hospital
Southbridge, Massachusetts

Ellen Greenblatt, MD, FRCSC

David A. Greenwald, MD
Gastroenterology Fellowship Program
 Director
Associate Division Director,
 Gastroenterology
Montefiore Medical Center
Professor of Clinical Medicine
Albert Einstein College of Medicine
Bronx, New York

Andrew Grimes, MD
Medical Director
Capitol Anesthesiology Association
Austin, Texas

Jill A. Grimes, MD, FAAFP
Clinical Instructor
Department of Family Medicine
University of Massachusetts Medical
 School
Worcester, Massachusetts
Attending Physician
University of Texas Health Services
Austin, Texas

Michael W. Groves, MD, FACS
Assistant Professor
Department of Otolaryngology - Head and
 Neck Surgery
Georgia Regents University
Augusta, Georgia

John A. Guisto, MD, FACEP
Professor, Clinical Emergency Medicine
Department of Emergency Medicine
University of Arizona College of Medicine
University of Arizona Health Network
Tucson, Arizona

Adarsh K. Gupta, DO, MS, FACOFP
Director, Center for Medical Weight Loss
 & Metabolic Control
Director, Center for Information Mastery
Associate Professor
Department of Family Medicine
Stratford, New Jersey

Neena R. Gupta, MD
Assistant Professor of Pediatrics
Medical Director, Pediatric Kidney
 Transplant Program
Division of Pediatric Nephrology
University of Massachusetts Memorial
 Children's Medical Center
Worcester, Massachusetts

Neha Gupta, MD
Department of Family Medicine
Western Michigan University School of
 Medicine
Kalamazoo, Michigan

Sergey G. Gurevich, MD
Department of Medicine
New York Presbyterian Hospital
New York, New York

M. Tye Haeberle, MD
Resident
Department of Medicine
Division of Dermatology
University of Louisville
Louisville, Kentucky

Laura Hagopian, MD, FAWM
Resident Physician
Department of Emergency Medicine
Boston Medical Center
Boston, Massachusetts

Zahraa Fayez Hajjiri, MD
Nephrology Fellow
Department of Nephrology
University of Massachusetts
Worcester, Massachusetts

Ihab Hamzeh, MD, FACC
Section of Cardiology
Department of Medicine
Baylor College of Medicine
Houston, Texas

Edward Han, PharmD
Adjunct Assistant Professor
Department of Pharmacy Practice
Massachusetts College of Pharmacy and
 Health Sciences University
Worcester, Massachusetts

Vanessa Hand, MD

Thomas J. Hansen, MD
Chief Academic Officer
Advocate Health Care
Downers Grove, Illinois

David M. Hardy, MD
Vascular Surgery Fellow
Department of Vascular Surgery
Cleveland Clinic
Cleveland, Ohio

Allison Hargreaves, MD

Sarah L. Harkness, MD
Department of Emergency Medicine
Alpert Medical School of Brown University
Providence, Rhode Island

Angela D. Hart, DO
Department of Osteopathic Manipulative
   Medicine
New York Institute of Technology
College of Osteopathic Medicine
Old Westbury, New York

Amena Hashmi, DO
Family Practice Physician
Denton, Texas

Fern R. Hauck, MD, MS

Spencer P. Bass, MD
Twenty-First Century Professor of Family
   Medicine
Department of Family Medicine
University of Virginia School of Medicine
Charlottesville, Virginia

James C. Haug, DO
Resident Physician
Diagnostic Radiology
San Antonio Military Medical Center
San Antonio, Texas

Aaron Hauptman, MD
Resident
University of Texas Southwestern
Austin, Texas

Peter J. Hayes, MD
Division of Dermatology
University of Louisville
Louisville, Kentucky

Kevin Heaton, DO, CAQSM
Primary Care Sports Medicine
Access Sports Medicine and Orthopaedics
Exeter, New Hampshire

Janet Odry Helminski, PT, PhD
Professor, Physical Therapy Program
Midwestern University
Downers Grove, Illinois

Scott T. Henderson, MD
Director, Medical Services
Student Health Center
University of Missouri
Columbia, Missouri

Jaroslaw T. Hepel, MD
Department of Radiation Oncology
Rhode Island Hospital
Brown University
Providence, Rhode Island

Jennifer P. Herbert, MD
Assistant Professor
Associate Director for Medical Student
   Education
Department of Family Medicine
Georgia Health Sciences University
Augusta, Georgia

Nicolas Hernandez, MD
Family Medicine Senior Resident
   Physician
UMass Family Residency Program
Fitchburg, Massachussetts

David N. Herrmann, MBBCh
Professor of Neurology, Pathology, and
   Laboratory Medicine
University of Rochester
Rochester, New York

Brian D. Hertz, MD

Luisa Amanda Hiendlmayr, MD
Chief Resident
University of Massachusetts
Fitchburg Family Medicine Residency

Benjamin J. Hilliker, MD
Department of Obstetrics &
   Gynecology
Aultman Hospital
Canton, Ohio

Michael P. Hirsh, MD, FACS, FAAP
Professor
Department of Surgery
Chief, Division of Pediatric Surgery
University of Massachusetts Medical
   School
Worcester, Massachusetts

**Crystal L. Hnatko, DO, LtCol, MC,
USAFR**
Family and Sports Medicine
Kaiser Permanente
Vacaville, California
Adjunct Faculty
David Grant Medical Center Family
   Medicine Residency
Travis Air Force Base, California

Brian Ho, MD

Brandi Hoag, DO
Director
St. Vincent Ambulatory Care Center
Worcester, Massachusetts

Abigail Weil Hoffman, MD
General Surgery Resident
Georgia Regents University
Augusta, Georgia

Holly Milne Hofkamp, MD
Assistant Professor
Department of Family Medicine
Oregon Health & Science University
Portland, Oregon

Christopher Hogan, MD
Director of Trauma
Co-Director of Intensive Care Unit
Doctors Hospital
Augusta, Georgia

N. Wilson Holland, MD, FACP, AGSF
Associate Professor of Medicine
Division of General Medicine and
   Geriatrics
Department of Medicine
Emory University School of Medicine
Atlanta Veterans Affairs Medical Center
Decatur, Georgia

Michael B. Holliday, MD
Assistant Professor
Department of Family and Community
   Medicine
University of Cincinnati
Cincinnati, Ohio

David Holmes, MD
Clinical Associate Professor
Director of Global Health Education
Department of Family Medicine
State University of New York at Buffalo
Buffalo, New York

Steven B Holsten, Jr., MD
Associate Professor of Surgery
Georgia Regents University
Augusta, Georgia

Amer Homsi, MD
General Surgery Resident
Department of Surgery
The Brooklyn Hospital Center
Brooklyn, New York

Serena Hon, MD
University of Massachusetts Family
   Medicine Residency/Hahnemann
   Family Health Center
Worcester, Massachusetts

Vincent F. Honrubia, MD, FACS
South Texas Sinus Institute
Doctor's Hospital at Renaissance
Edinburgh, Texas

Michael P. Hopkins, MD, MEd
Professor and Chairman
Department of Obstetrics and Gynecology
Northeast Ohio Medical University
Rootstown, Ohio
Director
Aultman Health Foundation
Canton, Ohio

Jennifer L. Hopp, MD
Resident Physician
Department of Family Medicine and
    Community Health
University of Pennsylvania
Philadelphia, Pennsylvania

James M. Horowitz, MD, FACC
Associate Director, Critical Care Unit
Assistant Professor of Medicine
Division of Cardiology
Weill Cornell Medical College
New York, New York

Evan R. Horton, PharmD
Assistant Professor
Department of Pharmacy Practice
School of Pharmacy
Massachusetts College of Pharmacy and
    Health Sciences University
Worcester, Massachusetts

Robert Hostoffer, DO, FACOP, FAAP
Clinical Associate Professor
Case Western Reserve University
Program Director, Allergy/Immunology
    Fellowship
University Hospital Regional Medical
    Centers
Richmond Heights, Ohio

Adam B. Howes, MD
Resident Physician
Family Medicine Residency Clinic
David Grant Medical Center
Travis AFB, California

Heather J. Hue, MD, MPH
Department of Hematology and Medical
    Oncology
Denver, Colorado

Dennis E. Hughes, DO
Medical Director
Emergency Medical Services
Fayetteville, Arkansas

Karen Hulbert, MD
Associate Professor
Department of Family and Community
    Medicine
The Medical College of Wisconsin
Milwaukee, Wisconsin

John C. Huscher, MD
Assistant Professor
Department of Family Medicine
University of Nebraska Medical Center
Omaha, Nebraska

Christopher J. Husko
New York Institute of Technology College
    of Osteopathic Medicine
Old Westbury, New York

Carol Hustedde, PhD
Assistant Professor
Department of Family and Community
    Medicine
University of Kentucky
Lexington, Kentucky

Eric J. Hwang, DO
Emergency Department
St. Joseph's Regional Medical Center
Paterson, New Jersey

Benjamin Hyatt, MD
Assistant Professor of Medicine
Division of Gastroenterology
UMass Memorial Medical Center
Worcester, Massachusetts

Sara Hyatt
New York Institute of Technology College
    of Osteopathic Medicine
Old Westbury, New York

Robert J. Hyde, MD, MA
Assistant Professor of Medicine
Section of Emergency Medicine
Dartmouth-Hitchcock Medical Center
Lebanon, New Hampshire

Marsela Hyska, MD
Homestead, Florida

P. Charles Inboriboon, MD, MPH
Assistant Professor of Emergency
    Medicine
University of Missouri Kansas City
Kansas City, Missouri

Adam Anthony Ingraffea, MD
Assistant Professor
Department of Dermatology
University of Cincinnati
Cincinnati, Ohio

Pablo Hernandez Itriago, MD, MHCM,
FAAFP
Assistant Clinical Professor
Department of Family Medicine
Boston University Medical Center
Boston, Massachusetts

J. Mark Jackson, MD
Clinical Professor of Medicine and
    Dermatology
Division of Dermatology
University of Louisville
Louisville, Kentucky

Christine K. Jacobs, MD, FAAFP
Associate Professor, Family and
    Community Medicine
Saint Louis University School of Medicine
St. Louis, Missouri

Rebecca Khezri Jacobson, MD
Resident, Internal Medicine
University of Chicago Medical Center
Chicago, Illinois

Neha Jakhete, MD
Department of Medicine
Johns Hopkins Hospital
Baltimore, Maryland

Omer M. Jamal, DO
Resident at Parkland Memorial
    Hospital/University of Texas
    Southwestern Medical Center
Department of Family and Community
    Medicine
University of Texas Southwestern Medical
    Center
Dallas, Texas

Catherine James, MD
Assistant Professor of Pediatrics
University of Massachusetts Medical
    School
Attending Physician
Pediatric Emergency Medicine
University of Massachusetts Memorial
    Medical Center
Worcester, Massachusetts

Daniel Sabido Jamorabo, MD
The Warren Alpert Medical School of
    Brown University
Providence, Rhode Island

Kyu K. Jana, MD
Assistant Professor
University of Texas Medical Branch
Galveston, Texas

Maissaa Janbain, MD
Tulane School of Medicine
New Orleans, Louisiana

Carrie R. Janiski, DO, MS, ATC
Resident Physician
Osteopathic Manipulative Medicine
University of New England College of
Osteopathic Medicine
Biddeford, Maine

Danielle Janosevic, DO, MS
New York Institute of Technology College
of Osteopathic Medicine
Old Westbury, New York

Courtney I. Jarvis, PharmD
Associate Professor
Department of Pharmacy Practice
Massachusetts College of Pharmacy and
Health Sciences University–Worcester/
Manchester
Worcester, Massachusetts

Sakshi Jasra, MD
Resident Physician
Department of Internal Medicine
University at Buffalo
Buffalo, New York

Salmaan A. Jawaid, MD
Resident Physician
Department of Internal Medicine -
Pediatrics
University of Massachusetts Medical Center
Worcester, Massachusetts

Sarah I. Jawed, MD
School of Medicine & Health Sciences
The George Washington University
Washington, DC

Pim Jetanalin, MD
Assistant Professor
Department of Internal Medicine, Division
of Rheumatology
University of Missouri Kansas City
Kansas City, Missouri

Cynthia Jeremiah, MD
Assistant Professor
Department of Family Medicine
University of Massachusetts Memorial
Medical Center
Worcester, Massachusetts

Zaiba Iqbal Jetpuri, DO, MBA
Assistant Professor, Family Medicine –
Primary Care
University of Texas Southwestern
Dallas, Texas

Kevin C. Jillson, MD
Resident
Internal Medicine-Pediatrics
University of Massachusetts Medical School
Worcester, Massachusetts

Samuel W. Joffe, MD
Cardiology Fellow
University of Massachusetts Medical
School
Worcester, Massachusetts

Julia V. Johnson, MD
Professor and Chair
Department of Obstetrics & Gynecology
University of Massachusetts Medical
School
Worcester, Massachusetts

Chiedza Jokonya, MD, MRCPCH
Wentworth Health Partners
South Berwick, Maine

Marci D. Jones, MD
Associate Professor
Department of Orthopedics and Physical
Rehabilitation
University of Massachusetts
Worcester, Massachusetts

Stacy Jones, MD
Capitol Anesthesiology Association
Austin, Texas

Maurice F. Joyce, MD, EdM
Resident
Department of Anesthesiology
Tufts Medical Center
Boston, Massachusetts

LCDR Patrick Wakefield Joyner, MD,
MS
Bone & Joint/Sports Medicine Institute
Naval Medical Center Portsmouth
Portsmouth, Virginia

Monica Juarez-Gonzalez, DO
University of Texas Southwestern
Dallas, Texas

Tya-Mae Y. Julien, MD
Gastroenterology and Hepatology
Baylor Regional Medical Center at Plano
Plano, Texas

Manjula Julka, MD, FAAFP
Associate Professor & Medical Director
Dr. John L. & Louise Roan Professorship
in Family Medicine
Family Medicine-Primary Care
University of Texas Southwestern Medical
Center
Dallas, Texas

Tipsuda Junsanto-Bahri, MD, FCAP
Chair, Basic Biomedical Sciences
Course Director, Pathology
Touro College of Osteopathic Medicine
New York, New York

Jigar Kadakia, MD
Summa Barberton Family Practice
Barberton, Ohio

Jenna M. Kahn, MD
Warren Alpert Medical School at Brown
University
Providence, Rhode Island

Monica Kaitz, MD, MPH
Resident, Internal Medicine & Preventive
Medicine
Kaiser Permanente San Francisco
University of California San Francisco
University of California Berkeley
San Francisco, California

Daniel Kapner, DO, MS
New York College of Osteopathic
Medicine
Old Westbury, New York

Rahul Kapur, MD, CAQSM
Associate Professor, Family Medicine and
Sports Medicine
Chief Medical Physician, Penn Athletics
Department of Family Medicine and
Community Health
Penn Sports Medicine Center
University of Pennsylvania
Philadelphia, Pennsylvania

Atil Y. Kargi, MD
Assistant Professor of Medicine
Department of Medicine
Division of Endocrinology, Diabetes and
Metabolism
University of Miami Miller School of
Medicine
Miami, Florida

Niraj Karki, MD
Fellow, Infectious Disease
Baystate Medical Center
Springfield, Massachusetts

Deirdre L. Kathman, DO
Fellow
Division of Pulmonary, Allergy, and Critical
Care Medicine
University of Massachusetts Medical
School
Worcester Massachusetts

Anubhav Kaul, MD, MPH
Internal Medicine
Lajey Medical Center
Burlington, Massachusetts

Jennifer Tickal Keehbauch, MD
Associate Professor, Family Medicine
Loma Linda University
Loma Linda, California

Clara Keegan, MD, FAAFP
Assistant Professor of Family Medicine
University of Vermont/Fletcher Allen
   Health Care
Burlington, Vermont

Eve Kellner, DO
Resident Psychiatrist
Westchester Medical Center
Valhalla, New York

Brendan Kelly, MD

Paul Kenyan, MD
University of Massachusetts Medical
   School
Worcester, Massachusetts

Glenn R. Kershaw, MD
Professor of Clinical Medicine
Department of Renal Medicine
University of Massachusetts Medical
   School
Worcester, Massachusetts

Robert M. Kershner, MD, MS, FACS
Eye Physician and Surgeon, Refractive
   and Cataract Surgery
Professor and Chairman
Department of Ophthalmic Medical
   Technology
Palm Beach State College
Consultant Specialist, Biomedical,
   Pharmaceutical, and Ophthalmic
   Medical Devices
Eye Laser Consulting
Palm Beach Gardens, Florida

Sujin Key, PharmD
Adjunct Assistant Professor
Department of Pharmacy Practice
Massachusetts College of Pharmacy and
   Health Sciences University
Worcester, Massachusetts

Anila Khaliq, MD
Faculty
Family Medicine Residency Program
St. Elizabeth Medical Center
Utica, New York

Mahpara B. Khaliq, MD
Resident Physician
Department of Internal Medicine and
   Pediatrics
Stony Brook University Medical Center
Stony Brook, New York.

Muhammad Imran Khan, MD
Karachi, Pakistan

Omar A. Khan, MD, MHS, FAAFP
Associate Vice-Chair
Department of Family & Community
   Medicine
Medical Director
Community Health & Eugene DuPont
   Preventive Medicine & Rehabilitation
   Institute
Christiana Care Health System
Clinical Assistant Professor
Departments of Family & Community
   Medicine
University of Pennsylvania & Jefferson
   Medical College.
Wilmington, Delaware

Rabeea Khan, MD
University of Texas Medical Branch
Galveston, Texas

Salwa Khan, MD, MHS, FAAP
Associate Director, Pediatric Hospitalist
   Program
Johns Hopkins Bayview Medical Center
Johns Hopkins University School of
   Medicine
Baltimore, Maryland

Andrew Kim, MD
Department of Medicine
Lenox Hill Hospital
New York, New York

Daniel Y. Kim, MD, FACS
Chair
Department of Otolaryngology–Head and
   Neck Surgery
University of Massachusetts Medical
   School
Worcester, Massachusetts

Jessica J. Kim, MD
Department of Family Medicine
University of Vermont
Burlington, Vermont

Walter M. Kim, MD, PhD
Internal Medicine Resident
Department of Medicine
University of Massachusetts Medical
   School
Worcester, Massachusetts

Brian James Kimbrell, MD, FACS
Trauma/Surgical Critical Care Medical
   Director
Blake Medical Center
Bradenton, Florida
Assistant Professor of Surgery
University of South Florida
Tampa, Florida

Franklin King, IV, MD
Resident
Massachusetts General Hospital/McLean
   Adult Psychiatry Program
Boston, Massachusetts

Ray King, MD

Rebecca G. Kinney, MD
Partnership Health Center
Missoula, Montana
Clinical Instructor
Family Medicine Residency of Western
   Montana
University of Washington School of
   Medicine
Missoula, Montana

Jeffery T. Kirchner, DO, FAAFP, AAHIVS
Associate Director, Family Medicine
   Residency Program
Department of Family and Community
   Medicine
Lancaster General Hospital
Lancaster, Pennsylvania

Brandon Kirsch, MD
Mayo Clinic
Jacksonville, Florida

Gloria J. Klapstein, PhD
Associate Professor
Department of Basic Sciences
College of Osteopathic Medicine
Touro University California
Vallejo, California

Jason D. Klein, DO
Director of Emergency Medicine
University Hospitals at Richmond Medical
   Center
Richmond Heights, Ohio

Jacob W. Kleinman, MD
Resident Physician
Department of Emergency Medicine
University of Pittsburgh Medical Center
Pittsburgh, Pennsylvania

Dagmar Klinger, MD
Department of Medicine, Renal Medicine
   Division
University of Massachusetts Memorial
   Health Care
Worcester, Massachusetts

Laura Klug, PharmD
Assistant Professor
Departments of Pharmacy Practice and
   Family Medicine
Creighton University
Omaha, Nebraska

Christopher J. Klunk, MD
Resident, Department of Pediatrics
Hasbro Children's Hospital
Providence, Rhode Island

Ryan R. Knapp, MD, MS
Lebanon, New Hampshire

Kevin Ko, MD
Family Medicine Resident
University of Texas Southwestern
Dallas, Texas

Sharon L. Koehler, DO., FACS
Assistant Professor
Breast Surgical Oncology
Department of Medicine, Division of
    Surgery
New York Institute of Technology College
    of Osteopathic Medicine
Old Westbury, New York

Aaron Kofman, MD
The Warren Alpert Medical School
Brown University
Providence, Rhode Island

Oleg Kotelskiy, DO

Nathalee Kong, MD
Massachusetts General Hospital
Department of Medicine
Boston, Massachusetts

Patricia S. Kooyman, DO
Assistant Professor
Department of Osteopathic Manipulative
    Medicine
New York Institute of Technology College
    of Osteopathic Medicine
Old Westbury, New York

Scott E. Kopec, MD
Associate Professor of Medicine
Division of Pulmonary, Allergy, and Critical
    Care
University of Massachusetts Medical School
Worcester, Massachusetts

Sathya S. Krishnasamy, MD
Associate Professor
Department of Medicine
Division of Endocrinology, Diabetes, and
    Metabolism
University of Louisville
Louisville, Kentucky

Allana M. Krolikowski, MD
Resident Physician
Greater Lawrence Family Health Center
Lawrence, Massachusetts

David C. Krulak, MD, MPH, MBA, FAAFP
Pensacola, Florida

David William Kruse, BS, MD
Primary Care Sports Medicine
Orthopaedic Specialty Institute
Orange, California

E. James Kruse, DO, FACS
Associate Professor
Surgical Oncology Section, Department of
    Surgery
Georgia Regents University
Augusta, Georgia

Rebecca Kruse-Jarres, MD, MPH
Associate Professor of Medicine
Section of Hematology/Oncology
Tulane University
New Orleans, Louisiana

Archana Kudrimoti, MD (MBBS), MPH
Assistant Professor
Department of Family and Community
    Medicine
University of Kentucky
Lexington, Kentucky

Vishnu Kulasekaran, MD
General Internal Medicine
Denver Health
Denver, Colorado

Ajoy Kumar, MD, FAAFP
Chair
Department of Family Medicine
Bayfront Health
Assistant Director
Bayfront Family Medicine Residency
St. Petersburg, Florida

Barrett J. Kumar, DO, MSBA

Jason M. Kurland, MD
Assistant Professor of Medicine
Division of Renal Medicine
University of Massachusetts Memorial
    Medical Group
Worcester, Massachusetts

Daniel Barr Kurtz, PhD
Associate Professor of Biology
Biology Department
Utica College
Utica, New York

Kyle Kutsche, MD
Family Medicine Resident
David Grant Medical Center
Travis Air Force Base, California

SreyRam Kuy, MD, MHS
Department of Surgery
Medical College of Wisconsin
Milwaukee, Wisconsin

Dylan C. Kwait, MD
Department of Radiology
Brigham and Women's Hospital
Harvard Medical School
Boston, Massachusetts

Howsen Kwan, MD, MRCS
Family & Community Medicine
University of Texas Southwestern Medical
    Center
Dallas, Texas

Melinda Y. Kwan, DO, MPH
Family Medicine Resident
Department of Family Medicine
University Hospitals Regional Medical
    Center
Richmond Heights, Ohio
Family Medicine/Urgent Care Physician
Urgent Care Department
Southwest Medical Associates
Las Vegas, Nevada

Patricia May Lacsina, MD
Department of Family and Community
    Medicine
University of Texas Health Science
    Center
San Antonio, Texas

Alisha Lakhani, MPH
Alpert Medical School
Brown University
Providence, Rhode Island

Aaron Lambert, MD
Assistant Clinical Professor
Assistant Residency Director
Department of Family Medicine
East Carolina University
Greenville, North Carolina

Rahele Lameh, MD
Family Medicine
Dallas, Texas

Amy BW LaMothe, PharmD, BCPS
Assistant Professor of Pharmacy
    Practice
Massachusetts College of Pharmacy and
    Health Sciences University
Worcester, Massachusetts

Stephen K. Lane, MD, FAAFP
Scituate, Massachusetts

Christine J. Langenberg, MD
University of Massachusetts Primary Care
    Sports Medicine Fellowship
Worcester, Massachusetts

Eduardo Lara-Torre, MD
Vice Chair for Academic Affairs
Residency Program Director
Department of Obstetrics and Gynecology
Associate Professor of Obstetrics and
  Gynecology and Pediatrics
Virginia Tech-Carilion School of Medicine
Roanoke, Virginia

Deborah Lardner, DO, DTM&H
Assistant Professor
Department of Family Medicine
New York Institute of Technology
College of Osteopathic Medicine
Old Westbury, New York

Austin Larson, MD
Fellow
Medical Genetics
Children's Hospital Colorado
Aurora, Colorado

Richard A. Larson, MD
Professor
Department of Medicine
The University of Chicago
Chicago, Illinois

Shane L. Larson, MD
Staff Family Physician
United States Army
Fort Carson, Colorado

Lakshmi Devi Nelson Lattimer, MD
Department of Medicine
George Washington University
Washington, DC

Emily S. Lau, MD
Internal Medicine Resident
Department of Medicine
Brigham & Women's Hospital
Boston, Massachusetts

Justin P. Lavin, Jr., MD, FACOG
Chairman, Department of Obstetrics and
  Gynecology
Akron General Medical Center
Professor Emeritus of Obstetrics and
  Gynecology
Northeastern Ohio Medical University
Akron, Ohio

Alexis Lawrence, MD
University of Massachusetts Medical
  School
Worcester, Massachusetts

Ashik Lawrence, MD

Jeffrey J. Lawrence, MD
Chief Resident
University of Massachusetts Combined
  Internal Medicine and Pediatrics
  Residency
Worcester, Massachusetts

Naomi Lawrence-Reid, MD
Children's Hospital at Montefiore
Bronx, New York

Mary Le, MD

Tinh Le, DO, MBA
Arlington, Texas

Erika L. LeBaron, DO, MSN
Family Medicine Resident Physician
University Hospitals–Richmond Medical
  Center
Richmond Heights, Ohio

James J. Ledwith Jr., MD, FAAFP
Residency Director
University of Massachusetts Fitchburg
  Family Medicine Residency Program
University of Massachusetts Medical
  School
Fitchburg, Massachusetts

Stephanie LeBourdais, MD

Andrew G. Lee, MD
Chair of Ophthalmology
Houston Methodist Hospital
Professor of Ophthalmology, Neurology
  and Neurosurgery
Weill Cornell Medical College
Adjunct Professor
Baylor College of Medicine and the
  University of Iowa
Clinical Professor
University of Texas Medical Branch at
  Galveston
University of Texas MD Anderson Cancer
  Center
Houston, Texas

Bianca Lee
New York Institute of Technology
College of Osteopathic Medicine,
Old Westbury, New York

Damon F. Lee, MD
Assistant Director, Office of Student
  Affairs
Assistant Clinical Professor
Department of Family Medicine and
  Community Health
University of Hawaii, John A. Burns
  School of Medicine
Honolulu, Hawaii

Daniel T. Lee, MD, MA
Clinical Professor of Family Medicine
David Geffen School of Medicine at
  University of California Los Angeles
Clinical Faculty
UCLA-Santa Monica Family Medicine
  Residency Program
Santa Monica, California

Ginny H. Lee, MD
Department of Emergency Medicine
Summa Health System
Akron, Ohio

Justin Lee, MD, CAQSM
Clinical Assistant Professor
Family and Sports Medicine
Family Medicine Department
East Carolina University
Brody School of Medicine
Greenville, North Carolina

Woo Jung Lee, MD, MS
Clinical GI Fellow
Department of Medicine
Division of Gastroenterology
The George Washington University
Washington, DC

Frederic Stuart Leeds, MD
Assistant Professor of Family Medicine
Wright State University
Boonshoft School of Medicine
Dayton, Ohio

Jaclyn E.A. Legg, DO, MA
Psychiatry Resident
University of Kansas Medical Center
Kansas City, Kansas

Carrie Geisberg Lenneman, MD, MSCI
Assistant Professor, Cardiovascular
  Medicine
University of Louisville
Louisville, Kentucky

Alexa Leone
Ohio University Heritage College of
  Osteopathic Medicine
Athens, Ohio

Louis D. Leone, DO, FAOASM
University Hospitals Richmond Medical
  Center
Richmond Heights, Ohio

Ariel Marissa LeRoy, MD
Geisel School of Medicine at Dartmouth
Hanover, New Hampshire

Maya Leventer-Roberts, MD, MPH
Pediatric Environmental Health Fellow
Department of Preventive Medicine
Icahn School of Medicine at Mount Sinai
New York, New York

Jay H. Levin, MD
Department of Neurology
Rhode Island Hospital
Brown University
Providence, Rhode Island

Nikki A. Levin, MD, PhD
Associate Professor of Medicine
Division of Dermatology
University of Massachusetts Medical
    School
Worcester, Massachusetts

David C. Levine, MD, FACS
Assistant Dean, Clinical Education
Assistant Professor of Surgery
New York Institute of Technology College
    of Osteopathic Medicine
Old Westbury, New York

Gary I. Levine, MD
Associate Professor
Department of Family Medicine
The Brody School of Medicine at East
    Carolina University
Greenville, North Carolina

Brent J. Levy, MD
Resident in Emergency Medicine
Dartmouth Hitchcock Medical Center
Lebanon, New Hampshire

Erik E. Lewis, MD
University of Massachusetts Medical
    School
Resident, Department of Surgery
St. Luke's-Roosevelt Hospital Center
New York, New York

James H. Lewis, MD, FACP, FACG,
AGAF
Professor of Medicine
Division of Gastroenterology
Georgetown University Hospital
Washington, DC

To Shan Li, DO
Assistant Professor
Department of Osteopathic Manipulative
    Medicine
New York Institute of Technology College
    of Osteopathic Medicine
Old Westbury, New York

Charmiane Lieu, MD
Resident
Department of Emergency Medicine
Alpert Medical School of Brown University
Providence, Rhode Island

Jennifer Lin, DO
Family Medicine Resident
University of Massachusetts
Fitchburg, Massachusetts

Jonathan T. Lin, MD
Housestaff, Internal Medicine
Department of Medicine
Mount Sinai Hospital
New York, New York

Adriana C. Linares, MD, MPH, DrPH
Physician
Family Medicine Southwest
Peacehealth Southwest Medical Center
Vancouver, Washington

Mary Segraves Lindholm, MD
Clinical Associate Professor
Department of Family Medicine and
    Community Health
University of Massachusetts Medical
    School
Worcester, Massachusetts

Kimberly Ellen Liu, MD, FRCSC, MSL
Assistant Professor
University of Toronto
Department of Obstetrics & Gynecology
Centre for Fertility & Reproductive Health
Mount Sinai Hospital
Toronto, Ontario, Canada

Nancy Y.N. Liu, MD
Associate Clinical Professor of Medicine
Division of Rheumatology
University of Massachusetts Medical
    School
Worcester, Massachusetts

Jenifer R. Lloyd, DO
Program Director
Dermatology Residency
Department of Dermatology
University Hospitals Regional Hospitals
    Richmond Campus
Richmond Heights, Ohio

Meredith Loh
New York Institute of Technology
College of Osteopathic Medicine
Old Westbury, New York

M. Chantel Long, MD
Clinical Assistant Professor
Department of Family and Community
    Medicine
University of Kansas School of
    Medicine-Wichita
Wichita, Kansas
Associate Director
Smoky Hill Family Medicine Residency
Salina, Kansas

David Longstroth, MD
Family Medicine-Surgery Registrar
Contra Costa Regional Medical Center
Martinez, California

Mary L. Lopresti, DO
Department of Hematology and Oncology
University of Massachusetts Medical
    Center
Worcester, Massachusetts

Bency Louidor-Paulynice, MD
Family Medicine
UMASS Medical School
Worcester, Massachusetts

Zhen Lu, MD
Pacific Urgent Care & Family Medicine
Orange, California

John R. Luksch, DO

Marie Luksch, DO
Resident
Department of Family Medicine
Rowan University - School of Osteopathic
    Medicine
Stratford, New Jersey

Ann M. Lynch, PharmD, RPh, AE-C
Associate Professor of Pharmacy Practice
Massachusetts College of Pharmacy and
    Health Sciences University
Worcester, Massachusetts

Jonathan MacClements, MD, FAAFP
Professor and Chairman, Family Medicine
    Department
University of Texas Health Center at Tyler
Tyler, Texas

Marina MacNamara, MD, MPH
Resident Physician
Mountain Area Health Education Center
    Family Residency Program
Asheville, North Carolina

Douglas W. MacPherson, MD,
MSc(CTM), FRCPC
Migration Health Consultants Inc.
Qualicum Beach, British Columbia,
    Canada
Department of Pathology and Molecular
    Medicine
Michael G. DeGroote School of Medicine
McMaster University
Hamilton, Ontario, Canada
International Centre for Migrant Health
    and Development
Geneva, Switzerland

Michelle Magid, MD
Clinical Associate Professor
University of Texas Southwestern in
    Austin
Clinical Assistant Professor
University of Texas Medical Branch
Texas A&M Health Science Center
Austin, Texas

Maricarmen Malagon-Rogers, MD
Associate Professor of Family Medicine
Pediatric Nephrology
University of Tennessee Graduate School
    of Medicine
Knoxville, Tennessee

Melanie J.S. Malec, MD
Family Physician
Lake Health Chardon Family Practice
Chardon, Ohio

Uzma Malik, MD
Glen Cove, New York

Samir Malkani, MD, MRCP (UK)
Associate Clinical Professor of Medicine
University of Massachusetts Medical
    School
Worcester, Massachusetts

Michael Malone, MD
Assistant Professor and Co-Medical
    Director
Penn State Hershey Department of
    Family and Community Medicine
Pennsylvania State Hershey College of
    Medicine Medical Center
Hershey, Pennsylvania

Alison Mancuso, DO
Assistant Professor
Department of Family Medicine
Rowan University School of Osteopathic
    Medicine
Stratford, New Jersey

Mark J. Manning, DO, MsMEL
Assistant Professor
Department of Obstetrics and Gynecology
University of Massachusetts Medical
    School
Worcester, Massachusetts

Mariann Manno, MD
Division Director, Pediatric Emergency
    Medicine
UMass Memorial Children's Medical
    Center
Professor of Pediatrics and Emergency
    Medicine
University of Massachusetts Medical
    School
Worcester, Massachusetts

Kenia Mansilla-Rivera, MD
Assistant Professor,
Department of Family Medicine
University of Connecticut
School of Medicine
Farmington, Connecticut

Eric J. Mao, MD
Internal Medicine Resident
Department of Medicine
Rhode Island Hospital/Brown
    University
Providence, Rhode Island

Murat Mardirossian, MD
Department of Family Medicine
University of California, Irvine
University of California Irvine Douglas
    Hospital
Orange, California

Katherine L. Margo, MD
Associate Professor of Family Medicine
    and Community Health
University of Pennsylvania School of
    Medicine
Philadelphia, Pennsylvania

Rachel A. Marinch, MD
Resident
Department of Family Medicine
Exempla Saint Joseph Hospital
Denver, Colorado

Robert A. Marlow, MD, MA
Professor of Clinical Family Medicine
Department of Family and Community
    Medicine
University of Arizona College of
    Medicine
Phoenix, Arizona
Associate Director
Family Medicine Residency Program
Scottsdale Healthcare
Scottsdale, Arizona

Wendy K. Marsh, MD, MSc
Associate Professor
Department of Psychiatry
University of Massachusetts
Worcester, Massachusetts

Cara Marshall, MD
Faculty, Lawrence Family Medicine
    Residency
Lawrence, Massachusetts

Lawrence Martin, MD
Department Chairman, Internal
    Medicine
Co-Chief, Division Critical Care &
    Pulmonology
University Hospitals Regional Hospitals -
    Richmond Campus
Richmond, Ohio

**Michelle T. Martin, PharmD, BCPS,
BCACP**
Clinical Pharmacist
University of Illinois Hospital and Health
    Sciences System
Clinical Assistant Professor
Department of Pharmacy Practice
University of Illinois at Chicago College of
    Pharmacy
Chicago, Illinois

Stephen A. Martin, MD, EdM
Assistant Professor
Department of Family Medicine and
    Community Health
University of Massachusetts Medical
    School
Barre Family Health Center
Barre, Massachusetts

Neil B. Marya, MD
Department of Internal Medicine
University of Massachusetts Medical
    School
Worcester, Massachusetts

Mohamad Masoumy, MD, MS
General Surgery Resident
Department of General Surgery
Medical College of Georgia at Georgia
    Regents University
Augusta, Georgia

Jerin Mathew, MD

Sally Mathew, DO
Holbrook, New York

Donnah Mathews, MD, FACP
Attending Physician
Department of Medicine
Rhode Island Hospital
Assistant Professor, Clinician Educator
Alpert School of Medicine at Brown
    University
Providence, Rhode Island

Brandon C. Maughan, MD, MHS
Department of Emergency Medicine
Veterans Affairs Medical Center
Robert Wood Johnson Clinical Scholars
    Program
Perelman School of Medicine
Fellow
Leonard Davis Institute of Economics
University of Pennsylvania
Philadelphia, Pennsylvania

George H. Maxted, MD
Associate Program Director
Tufts University Family Medicine
    Residency at Cambridge Health Alliance
Malden, Massachusetts

Beth Mazyck, MD
Chief Medical Officer
South End Community Health Center
Boston, Massachusetts

Kelly McCants, MD

Margaret J. McCormick, MS, RN
Clinical Associate Professor, Nursing
Towson University
Towson, Maryland

Michelle McCreary, MD

Melissa McEnery-Stonelake, MD
School of Medicine
University of Massachusetts Medical
    School
Worcester, Massachusetts

Tamara McGregor, MD
Assistant Professor
University of Texas Southwestern Family
    Medicine
Dallas, Texas

Bridget E. McIlwee, DO
Dermatology-Focused Osteopathic
    Traditional Intern
University Hospitals Regional Medical
    Centers
Cleveland, Ohio

Juliet M. McKee, MD
Assistant Professor
Department of Family Medicine
University of Texas Medical Branch
Galveston, Texas

Elizabeth C. McKeen, MD
Clinical Instructor in Pediatrics
Harvard Medical School
Boston, Massachusetts

Riley E. McLean, MD
University of Massachusetts Medical
    School
Worcester, Massachusetts

Geoffrey A. McLeod

Donna-Marie McMahon, DO, FAAP
Assistant Professor, Medicine
Division of Pediatrics
Director of the Doctor Patient Continuum
New York Institute of Technology College
    of Osteopathic Medicine
Old Westbury, New York

Erin M. McMaster, MD
Assistant Professor of Pediatrics
University of Massachusetts Medical
    School
Worcester, Massachusetts

Roger L. McRoberts, III, MD
Assistant Professor of Psychiatry
University of Texas Southwestern
Austin, Texas

Melissa K. Meghpara
Rutgers University
New York Institute of Technology College
    of Osteopathic Medicine
Old Westbury, New York

Michelle L. Mellion, MD
Assistant Professor of Neurology
Director, Clinical Neurophysiology
    Fellowship
Warren Alpert Medical School of Brown
    University
Rhode Island Hospital
Providence, Rhode Island

Daniel Elias Melville, MD
Destination Health
Southlake, Texas

Caleb J. Mentzer, DO
Resident
Department of General Surgery
Medical College of Georgia
Georgia Reagents University
Augusta, Georgia

Miesha Merati, DO
Traditional Internship
University Hospitals Regional Hospitals
Cleveland, Ohio

Theo E. Meyer, MD, DPhil
Professor
Department of Cardiovascular Medicine
University of Massachusetts Medical
    School
Director
Cardiac Cath Lab
Department of Cardiology
University of Massachusetts Medical
    School
Worcester, Massachusetts

Christina Mezzone
New York Institute of Technology College
    of Osteopathic Medicine
Old Westbury, New York

Alyssa Miceli, DO
Glen Cove, New York

Athanasios Michos, MD, PhD
Assistant Professor of Pediatrics and
    Infectious Diseases
1st Department of Pediatrics
University of Athens
Athens, Greece

Tracy O. Middleton, DO
Chair and Associate Professor, Family
    Medicine
Midwestern University
Arizona College of Osteopathic Medicine
Glendale, Arizona

Mariya Milko, DO, MS
New York Institute of Technology College
    of Osteopathic Medicine
Old Westbury, New York

James P. Miller, MD
Medical Director, Pediatric Surgery
Cook Children's Medical Center
Fort Worth, Texas

Luke R. Miller, MD
University of Colorado Family Medicine
Denver, Colorado

Nathan Miller, MD, CAPT, MC
Department of Family Medicine
David Grant (USAF) Medical Center
Travis Air Force Base, California

Sandra Miller, MD
Clinical Faculty
Banner Good Samaritan Family Medicine
    Residency
Phoenix, Arizona

Suzanne Minor, MD, FAAFP
Assistant Professor
Department of Humanities, Health, &
    Society
Florida International University Herbert
    Wertheim College of Medicine
Miami, Florida

Jeffrey F. Minteer, MD
Program Director
Washington Health System Family
    Medicine Residency
Washington, Pennsylvania

Mona Mislankar, MD
Resident
University Hospitals Case Medical Center
Cleveland, Ohio

Jesse Wm. Mix, DO

Payal Modi, MD, MSc
Department of Emergency Medicine
Brown University Medical School
Providence, Rhode Island

Justin B. Moore, MD
Department of Internal Medicine
University of Kansas
School of Medicine-Wichita
Wichita, Kansas

Tiffany A. Moore Simas, MD, MPH, MEd, FACOG
Associate Professor of Obstetrics & Gynecology and Pediatrics
Department of Obstetrics & Gynecology
University of Massachusetts Medical School
UMass Memorial Health Care
Worcester, Massachusetts

Wynne Morgan, MD
Child Psychiatry Fellow
Department of Psychiatry
University of Massachusetts Medical School
Worcester, Massachusetts

Kelvin A. Moses, MD, PhD
Assistant Professor of Urology
Department of Urologic Surgery
Vanderbilt University
Nashville, Tennessee

Sarah E. Mowry, MD
Assistant Professor
Georgia Regents University
Department of Otolaryngology
Augusta, Georgia

Mohammad Ansar Mughal, MD
Assistant Professor
University Health System
San Antonio, Texas

Shani Muhammad, MD
Family Medicine Physician
Fresno, California

Joshua Mularella, DO
Wilderness and Expedition Medicine Fellow
Department of Emergency Medicine
Upstate Medical Center
Syracuse, New York

Herbert L. Muncie, Jr., MD
Professor of Family Medicine
Department of Family Medicine
Louisiana State University School of Medicine
New Orleans, Louisiana

Amanda Murchison, MD
Assistant Professor
Virginia Tech–Carilion School of Medicine
Roanoke, Virginia

Gregory Murphy, MD
Sports Medicine Fellow
Department of Sports Medicine
University of Massachusetts Department of Family and Community Medicine
Worcester, Massachusetts

Eleftherios Mylonakis, MD, PhD, FIDSA
Dean's Professor of Medical Science (Medicine, and Molecular Microbiology and Immunology)
Chief, Infectious Diseases Division
Alpert Medical School/Brown University
Rhode Island Hospital
Providence, Rhode Island

Jonathan Nadler, MD
Brookline, Massachusetts

Urooj Najm, MBBS
Pueblo, Colorado

Nisha Nathan, MD
Frederick, Maryland

Tabasum Nazir, MD
Family Medicine
University of Texas Southwestern
Dallas, Texas

Mark John Neavyn, MD
Clinical Instructor
Department of Emergency Medicine
University of Massachusetts Medical School
Worcester, Massachusetts

Tara J. Neil, MD
Associate Director
Via Christi Family Medicine Residency Program
Clinical Assistant Professor
Department of Family and Community Medicine
University of Kansas School of Medicine-Wichita
Wichita, Kansas

Donald Nelson, MD, FAAFP, MS
Professor Emeritus
Director of Informatics
Cedar Rapids Medical Education Foundation
Cedar Rapids, Iowa

Elizabeth A. Nelson, MD
Associate Professor
Department of Medicine
Baylor College of Medicine
Houston, Texas

Carla M. Nester, MD
Director, Pediatric Glomerular Disease Clinic
University of Iowa
Iowa City, Iowa

Anne Newbold, DO
Department of Emergency Medicine
Midwestern University
Swedish Covenant Hospital
Chicago, Illinois

Sabrina Newman, MD
Department of Dermatology
George Washington University School of Medicine
Washington, DC

Maria De La Luz Nieto, MD
Fellow
Urogynecology and Reconstructive Pelvic Surgery
University of North Carolina
Chapel Hill, North Carolina

Neil Nixdorff, MD, MA, MS, MPH
Resident
Department of Family and Community Health
The University of Pennsylvania
Philadelphia, Pennsylvania

Thomas Noh, MD
Department of Neurological Surgery
Henry Ford Hospital
Detroit, Michigan

Rocio I. Nordfeldt, MD
Assistant Professor
Family Medicine Department
University of Massachusetts Medical School
Leominster, Massachusetts

David R. Norris, MD
Assistant Professor
Department of Family Medicine
University of Mississippi Medical Center
Jackson, Mississippi

Bakr Nour, MD, FACS

Laura Novak, MD
Associate Director
Summa Barberton Residency
Barberton, Ohio

J. Michael O'Connell, Jr., MD
Primary Care Physician
Department of Veterans Affairs
Sacramento, California

Michael Ryan Odom, MD
Family Medicine
David Grant Medical Center
Travis Air Force Base, California

John B. O'Donnell, MD, MS
Associate Professor
Department of Medicine
College of Human Medicine
Michigan State University
Grand Rapids, Michigan

Annie Lee Oh, MD
Department of Medicine
Division of Hematology/Oncology
University of Illinois at Chicago
Chicago, Illinois

Arthur Ohannessian, MD
Assistant Clinical Professor
David Geffen School of Medicine at UCLA
Los Angeles, California

Smriti Ohri, MD
Assistant Professor
Department of Family Medicine
Oregon Health and Science University
Portland, Oregon

Jacqueline L. Olin, MS, PharmD, BCPS,
CPP, CDE
Associate Professor of Pharmacy
Wingate University School of Pharmacy
Wingate, North Carolina

Jill SM Omori, MD
Associate Professor of Family Medicine
    and Community Health
Office of Medical Education
University of Hawaii John A. Burn School
    of Medicine
Honolulu, Hawaii

David Y. Ong, MD
Andover, Massachusetts

Edward Onusko, MD
Associate Professor
Department of Family and Community
    Medicine
University of Cincinnati
Cincinnati, Ohio

Amimi S. Osayande, MD, FAAFP
Department of Family and Community
    Medicine
University of Texas
Dallas, Texas

Cindy England Owen, MD
Assistant Professor Dermatology
University of Louisville
Louisville, Kentucky

Kelly Pagidas, MD
Women and Infants Hospital
Providence, Rhode Island

Balakumar Pandian, MD
Assistant Professor
Departments of Internal Medicine and
    Pediatrics
University of Texas Southwestern-Austin
    Residency Program
Austin, Texas

Linda Paniagua, MD
Warren Alpert Medical School of Brown
    University
Providence, Rhode Island

Jon S. Parham, DO, MPH
Associate Professor
Department of Family Medicine
Graduate School of Medicine
University of Tennessee
Knoxville, Tennessee

Mamta H. Parikh, MD, MPH
Internal Medicine
St. Charles Hospital
New York, New York

Douglas S. Parks, MD
Associate Professor
Family Medicine Residency
University of Wyoming
Cheyenne, Wyoming

David Parrish, MS, MD, FAAFP
Director
Bayfront Family Medicine Residency
Affiliate Associate Professor
University of South Florida College of
    Medicine
Bayfront Health St. Petersburg
St. Petersburg, Florida

Julia Parzych, MD

Michael D. Passafaro, DO, DTM&H,
FACEP, FACOEP
Assistant Professor
Division of Emergency Medicine
New York Institute of Technology
College of Osteopathic Medicine
Old Westbury, New York

Paul Pastor, MD
Guayaquil, Ecuador

Birju B. Patel, MD, FACP, AGSF
Assistant Professor of Medicine
Director of the Bronze Geriatric Clinic and
    the Mild Cognitive Impairment Clinic
Atlanta Veterans Affairs Medical Center
Emory University School of Medicine
Department of Medicine
Division of General Medicine and
    Gerontology
Atlanta, Georgia

Deepak Patel, MD
Assistant Professor
Department of Family Medicine
Rush Medical College
Chicago, Illinois
Director of Sports Medicine
Rush-Copley Family Medicine Residency
Aurora, Illinois

Dilip Patel, MD

Kiki Chandni Patel, PharmD
Adjunct Assistant Professor of Pharmacy
    Practice
Massachusetts College of Pharmacy and
    Health Sciences University
Boston, Massachusetts

Krunal Patel, MD
Resident, Internal Medicine
University of Massachusetts Medical
    School
Worcester, Massachusetts

Mahesh C. Patel, MD
Assistant Professor
Department of Internal Medicine
Division of Infectious Diseases
University of Illinois College of Medicine
Chicago, Illinois

Mayha Patel, DO
Intern
Department of Medicine
College Medical Center
Long Beach, California

Mohita A. Patel, MD
Family Medicine
University of Texas Southwestern Medical
    Center
Dallas, Texas

Neepa Patel, MD
Assistant Professor
Department of Neurology and
    Neurotherapeutics
Clinical Center for Movement Disorders
University of Texas Southwestern
Dallas, Texas

Neil Patel, DO
Internal Medicine
University Hospitals
Cleveland, Ohio

Nihal Patel, MD
Department of Medicine
Montefiore Medical Center
Albert Einstein College of Medicine
Bronx, New York

Pramesh Patel, MD
Villa Park, Illinois

Seema Patel, PharmD
Oncology Specialty Resident
Department of Pharmacy Practice
University of Illinois at Chicago College of
    Pharmacy
Chicago, Illinois

Yogi Patel, MD

Abhijeet Patil, MD, MS
Assistant Professor
Department of Family Medicine and
    Geriatric Medicine
Umass Memorial and Fitchburg Family
    Medicine Residency Program
Fitchburg, Massachusetts

Vinit Patil, MD
Department of Medicine
University of Arizona
Tucson, Arizona

Rosanne M. Paul, DO
Department of Medical Education
University Hospitals
Richmond Heights, Ohio

Gisela Lopez Payares, MD
Department of Family and Community
    Medicine
University of Texas - Health Science
    Center
San Antonio, Texas

Amrutha Pavle, MD
Family Medicine
University of Texas Southwestern Medical
    Center
Dallas, Texas

**Erica F. Pearce, PharmD, BCPS,
BCACP**
Assistant Professor of Pharmacy Practice
St. Louis College of Pharmacy
Clinical Pharmacist and Assistant Clinical
    Professor
Department of Family and Community
    Medicine
Saint Louis University School of Medicine
Saint Louis, Missouri

Ryan D. Pearson, MD, FAAFP
Family Medicine Faculty Physician
David Grant Medical Center Family
    Medicine Residency
Travis Air Force Base, California

Helio F. Pedro, MD
Section Chief, Genetics
Hackensack University Medical Center
Hackensack, New Jersey

Rade N. Pejic, MD, MMM
Assistant Professor of Family Medicine
Tulane University
New Orleans, Louisiana

Timothy D. Pelkowski, MD, MS, FAAFP
Assistant Director
Family Medicine Residency Program
Saint Vincent Hospital
Erie, Pennsylvania

Rod Pellenberg, MD

Randall Pellish, MD
Assistant Professor of Medicine
Program Director, Gastroenterology
    Fellowship
Division of Gastroenterology
University of Massachusetts Medical
    School
Worcester, Massachusetts

Cinthya Pena-Orbea, MD
Staten Island, New York

**E. E. Anderson Penno, MD, MS, FRCSC,
Diplomate ABO**
Western Laser Eye Associates
Calgary, Alberta, Canada

Brian Patrick Peppers, DO, PhD
Pediatric Resident
Department of Pediatrics
University Hospitals Regional Hospitals
Richmond Heights, Ohio

Ruben Peralta, MD, FACS
Director of Trauma and Critical Care
    Fellowship Program
Senior Consultant in Surgery, Trauma, and
    Critical Care Medicine
Department of Surgery
Hamad General Hospital
Department of Medical Education
Hamad Medical Corporation
Doha, Qatar

Eric Perez, MD
St. Luke's Roosevelt Hospital
New York, New York
Hunterdon Medical Center
Flemington, New Jersey

Christine S. Persaud, MD
Primary Care Sports Medicine Fellow
University of Rochester Medical Center
Rochester, New York

Bobby Peters, MD, FAAEM
Assistant Professor
Emergency Department
University of Iowa Hospitals
Iowa City, Iowa

Hugh Peterson, MD, FACP
Associate Professor of Medicine
Department of Medicine
School of Medicine
University of Louisville
Louisville, Kentucky

Teny Anna Philip, MD
Department of Community and Family
    Medicine
University of Texas Health Science
    Center San Antonio
San Antonio, Texas

Jeffrey W. Phillips, MD
Faculty
University of Massachusetts Medical
    School
Tufts University School of Medicine
Family Doctors Clinician
Swampscott, Massachusetts

Kantima Phisitkul, MD
Clinical Assistant Professor
Division of Nephrology
Department of Internal Medicine
University of Iowa Hospital and Clinics
Iowa City, Iowa

Warren W. Piette, MD
Chair, Division of Dermatology
John H. Stroger, Jr. Hospital of Cook
    County
Professor, Department of Dermatology
Rush Medical School
Chicago, Illinois

Maria A. Pino, PhD, MS, RpH
Assistant Professor of Pharmacology
Department of Basic Biomedical Science
Touro College of Osteopathic Medicine
New York, New York

Maria M. Plummer, MD
Assistant Professor
Medical Education
New York Institute of Technology College
    of Osteopathic Medicine
Old Westbury, New York

Phyllis Pollack, MD
Associate Clinical Professor of Pediatrics
University of Massachusetts Medical
    School
Worcester, Massachusetts

Diana Ponsky, MD
Assistant Professor
Department of Otolaryngology
Case Western University School of
    Medicine
University Hospitals
Cleveland, Ohio

Anna C. Porter, MD
Assistant Professor of Medicine
Department of Medicine
Section of Nephrology
University of Illinois at Chicago
Chicago, Illinois

Stacy Potts, MD, MEd
Associate Professor
Department of Family Medicine and
    Community Health
University of Massachusetts
Worcester, Massachusetts

Anne Powell, MD

Jennifer Luo Powell, DO
Resident Physician
Department of Family Medicine
University of Massachusetts
Worcester, Massachusetts

James E. Powers, DO, FACEP
Associate Dean for Clinical Affairs
Associate Professor of Emergency
    Medicine
Edward Via College of Osteopathic
    Medicine, Virginia Campus
Blacksburg, Virginia

Pia Prakash, MD
Department of Gastroenterology and Liver
    Diseases
The George Washington University
Washington, DC

Tharani Vadivelu Prasad, MD
Resident
Department of Family and Community
    Medicine
University of Texas Health Science
    Center San Antonio
San Antonio, Texas

Bethany Prater, DO
Brooklyn, New York

Colleen M. Prinzivalli, PharmD, BCPS,
CGP
Pharmacist Care Manager
Dovetail Health
Needham, Massachusetts

Barbara J. Provo, MSN, RN, FNP-BC,
CWON
Nurse Practitioner
Coordinator
Wound & Ostomy Program
Froedtert and Medical College of
    Wisconsin
Milwaukee, Wisconsin

George Gunter A. Pujalte, MD, FACSM
Assistant Professor
Division of Sports Medicine
Departments of Family and Community
    Medicine, and Orthopaedics and
    Rehabilitation
Penn State Milton S. Hershey Medical
    Center
Hershey, Pennsylvania

Juan Qiu, MD, PhD
Associate Professor
Department of Family and Community
    Medicine
Pennsylvania State University College of
    Medicine
Penn State Hershey Medical Group -
    Colonnade
State College, Pennsylvania

Katherine Quayle, MD
Pediatrics Resident
Primary Children's Medical Center
University of Utah
Salt Lake City, Utah

Diane M. Radford, MD, FACS, FRCSEd
Breast Surgical Oncologist
Mercy Clinic
St. Louis Cancer and Breast Institute
St. Louis, Missouri

Naureen Rafiq, MD
Assistant Professor
Department of Family Medicine
Creighton University School of Medicine
Omaha, Nebraska

Jyoti Ramakrishna, MBBS, MD
Chief
Pediatric Gastroenterology and Nutrition
Floating Hospital for Children/Tufts
    Medical Center
Boston, Massachusetts

Muthalagu Ramanathan, MD
Division of Hematology/Oncology
University of Massachusetts Medical
    Center
Worcester, Massachusetts

Alex Ramirez, MD
University of Massachusetts Medical
    School
Worcester, Massachusetts

Laura K. Randolph, DO, MS
Resident Physician
Department of Obstetrics and Gynecology
Aultman Hospital
Northeast Ohio Medical University
Canton, Ohio

Swathi A.N. Rao, MD
Internal Medicine
University of Louisville
Louisville, Kentucky

Brandon L. Raudenbush, DO
University Hospitals Richmond Medical
    Center
University Hospitals Regional Hospitals
Richmond Heights, Ohio

Elenee M.P. Raudenbush, DO
University Hospitals Regional Hospitals
    Richmond Medical Center
Richmond, Ohio

Edwin Q. Ravano, MD, MPH
Hospitalist
University of Pittsburgh Medical Center
Pittsburgh, Pennsylvania

Wasiq Faraz Rawasia, MD
Resident
Department of Medicine
University of Louisville
Louisville, Kentucky

Tejesh Srinivasa Reddy, MD
Program Director and Hospitalist
St. Alphonsus Medical Center
Ontario, Oregon

Jennifer Reidy, MD, FAAHPM
Co-Chief
Division of Palliative Care
University of Massachusetts Memorial
    Medical Center
Worcester, Massachusetts

Emmanuel Reyes-Ramos, MD

Harlan G. Rich, MD
Associate Professor of Medicine
The Warren Alpert Medical School of
    Brown University
Gastroenterology Division
University Medicine Foundation, Inc.
Director of Endoscopy
Rhode Island Hospital
Providence, Rhode Island

Alexander Mark Richardson, MD
Wake Forest School of Medicine
Winston-Salem, North Carolina

Tara Richardson, MD
Pediatric Resident
University of Massachusetts
Worcester, Massachusetts

Elizabeth C. Riley, MD, FACP
Assistant Professor of Medicine
Division of Hematology/Oncology
University of Louisville
Louisville, Kentucky

Sonia Rivera-Martinez, DO, FACOFP
Assistant Professor
Department of Family Medicine
New York Institute of Technology College
    of Osteopathic Medicine
Old Westbury, New York

Michele Roberts, MD, PhD
Paxton, Massachusetts

Caroline Nyenke Robinson, MD
Resident, Division of Dermatology
Southern Illinois University School of
  Medicine
Springfield, Illinois

Scott W. Rodi, MD, MPH
Associate Professor of Medicine,
  Emergency Medicine
Geisel School of Medicine at Dartmouth
Section Chief and Medical Director
Section of Emergency Medicine
Dartmouth Hitchcock Medical Center
Lebanon, New Hampshire

Robert Eugene Rogers
Texas A&M Health Science Center
  College of Medicine
Bryan, Texas

**Mark S. Rosenberg, DO, MBA, FACEP,
FACOEP-D**
Chairman Emergency Medicine
Chief Geriatric Emergency Medicine and
  Palliative Medicine
St. Joseph's Healthcare System
Paterson, New Jersey

Noah M. Rosenberg, MD
Resident
Family Medicine Residency
University of Massachusetts
Worcester, Massachusetts

Montiel Teresa Rosenthal, MD
Associate Clinical Professor and Director
  of Maternity Services
Department of Family and Community
  Medicine
University of Cincinnati College of
  Medicine
Cincinnati, Ohio

Steven E. Roskos, MD
Associate Professor
Department of Family Medicine
Michigan State University
College of Human Medicine
East Lansing, Michigan

Patricio Rossi, MD

**Michael P. Rowane, DO, MS, FAAFP,
FAAO**
Associate Clinical Professor of Family
  Medicine and Psychiatry
Director of Medical Education
Case Western Reserve University
University Hospitals Regional Hospitals
Director of Osteopathic Medical Education
University Hospitals Case Medical Center
Richmond Heights, Ohio

Sani Ann Mathew Roy, MD
Pediatric Endocrinology Fellow
Division of Pediatric Endocrinology and
  Diabetes
The Children's Hospital of Philadelphia
Philadelphia, Pennsylvania

Vibin Roy, MD
Faculty Instructor
Family and Community Medicine
Thomas Jefferson University
Philadelphia, Pennsylvania

Anna G. Rudnicki, MD
Assistant Professor of Medicine
Division of Pulmonary, Allergy, and Critical
  Care
University of Massachusetts Medical
  School
Worcester, Massachusetts

Stephanie M. Ruest, MD
Pediatric Resident
Boston, Massachusetts

Jennifer Ruskis, MD
Department of Emergency Medicine
Alpert Medical School of Brown University
Providence, Rhode Island

Emilio A Russo, MD
Assistant Professor and Program Director
Department of Medicine
Section Rural Family Medicine
  Residency—Bogalusa
Louisiana State University
Bogalusa, Louisiana

Anup Sabharwal, MD, MBA, FACE, CCD
Endocrinology, Diabetes, and Metabolism
Herbert Wertheim College of Medicine
Florida International University
Miami, Florida

Komel Safdar, MBBS
Dubai, United Arab Emirates

Paul F. Sahd, DO

Afshin Sam, MD
Department of Medicine
University of Arizona
Tucson, Arizona

Kathryn Samai, PharmD, BCPS
Assistant Professor
Lake Erie College of Osteopathic
  Medicine
School of Pharmacy
Bradenton, Florida

Juan Sanabria, MD, MSc, FRCSC, FACS
Assistant Professor of Surgery & Nutrition
Case Western Reserve University
Cleveland, Ohio

Arthur B. Sanders, MD, MHA
Professor
Department of Emergency Medicine
University of Arizona College of Medicine
Tucson, Arizona

**Mark Allen Sanders, DO, JD, MPH, LLM,
FACOFP**
President and Chief Executive Officer
The Physician's Group
Fort Worth, Texas

Scott M. Sandilands, DO
Resident, Department of Surgery
Larkin Community Hospital
South Miami, Florida

Shailendra K. Saxena, MD, PhD
Assistant Professor
Department of Family Medicine
Creighton University School of Medicine
Omaha, Nebraska

**L. Michelle W. Seawright, DO, LT, MC,
USN**
Family Medicine Intern
Naval Hospital Camp Lejeune
Camp Lejeune, North Carolina

Durr-e-Shahwaar Sayed, DO
Faculty Physician
Inspira Health Network
Glassboro, New Jersey

Henry A. Schaeffer, MD
Clinical Professor of Pediatrics
State University of New York-Downstate
  Medical Center
Brooklyn, New York
New York Institute of Technology College
  of Osteopathic Medicine
Old Westbury, New York

Courtney R. Schadt, MD, FAAD
Associate Professor
Division of Dermatology
University of Louisville
Louisville, Kentucky

Matthew Schear, DO, MS
Department of Osteopathic Manipulative
  Medicine
New York Institute of Technology College
  of Osteopathic Medicine
Old Westbury, New York

Fred J. Schiffman, MD
Sigal Family Professor of Humanistic
  Medicine
Warren Alpert Medical School of Brown
  University
Providence, Rhode Island

Benjamin N. Schneider, MD
Assistant Professor
Department of Family Medicine
Oregon Health & Science University
Portland, Oregon

Lisa M. Schroeder, MD
Assistant Director
Summa Barberton Family Practice
    Residency Program
Barberton, Ohio

Jennifer Schwartz, MD
Steward Medical Group
Boston, Massachusetts

Christopher J. Scola, MD
Assistant Clinical Professor of Medicine
University of Connecticut School of
    Medicine
Chief, Rheumatology Division
Hartford Hospital
Hartford, Connecticut

Ingrid U. Scott, MD, MPH
Professor of Ophthalmology and Public
    Health Sciences
Penn State Hershey Eye Center
Penn State College of Medicine
Hershey, Pennsylvania

Stephen M. Scott, MD, MPH
Associate Professor of Family Medicine
Weill Cornell Medical College in Qatar
Doha, Qatar

Gail Scully, MD, MPH
University of Massachusetts Memorial
    Medical Center
University of Massachusetts Medical School
Worcester, Massachusetts

David P. Sealy, MD
AHEC Professor
Greenwood Medical University South
    Carolina
Director, Primary Care Sports Medicine
    Fellowship
Associate Director
Self Regional Healthcare Family Medicine
    Residency
Greenwood, South Carolina

Margaret R. Seaver, MD, MPH
Palliative Medicine Service
Lahey Hospital and Medical Center
Burlington, Massachusetts

Sheila M. Seed, PharmD, MPH, RPh
Associate Professor
Department of Pharmacy Practice
Massachusetts College of Pharmacy and
    Health Sciences University
Worcester, Massachusetts

Amy Seery, MD
Assistant Professor
Department of Family and Community
    Medicine
University of Kansas School of
    Medicine-Wichita
Pediatrics Faculty
Via Christi Family Medicine Residency
Wichita, Kansas

Dan Sepdham, MD, FAAFP
Assistant Professor
Department of Family & Community
    Medicine
University of Texas Southwestern Medical
    Center at Dallas
Dallas, Texas

Anna Serur, MD, FACS, FASCRS
Chief
Colon and Rectal Surgery
Maimonides Medical Center
Brooklyn, New York

Tarsheen Kaur Sethi, MBBS
Post-doctoral Fellow
Department of Radiology
Stanford University School of Medicine
Palo Alto, California

Patricia L. Seymour, MS, MD
University of Massachusetts Medical
    School
Memorial Hospital
Worcester, Massachusetts

Samir A. Shah, MD, FACG, FASGE,
AGAF
Clinical Professor of Medicine
The Warren Alpert Medical School of
    Brown University
Providence, Rhode Island

Kevin C. Shannon, MD, MPH, FAAFP
Associate Professor
Department of Family Medicine
Loma Linda University School of Medicine
Loma Linda, California

Sanjeev Sharma, MBBS
Associate Professor
Creighton University School of Medicine
Omaha, Nebraska

Shannon Sharpe, DO
Dermatology Focused Traditional Intern
University Hospitals Richmond Medical
    Center
Cleveland, Ohio

Karen Sheflin, DO
Assistant Professor
Department of Family Medicine
New York Institute of Technology
College of Osteopathic Medicine

Douglas Shermin, MD
Associate Professor of Medicine
Alpert Medical School of Brown University
Providence, Rhode Island

Tisamarie B. Sherry, PhD
Harvard Medical School
Boston, Massachusetts

Nicole Shields, MD
Harrogate, Tennessee

Ryan Yoshimura Shields
Johns Hopkins University School of
    Medicine
Baltimore, Maryland

Jeffrey A. Shih, MD
Assistant Professor of Medicine
Advanced Heart Failure and Cardiac
    Transplantation
Cardiovascular Medicine
University of Massachusetts
Worcester, Massachusetts

Natasha Shur, MD
Assistant Professor
Warren Alpert Medical School at Brown
    University
Clinical Genetics Attending
Rhode Island Hospital
Providence, Rhode Island

Aamir Siddiqi, MD
Director of Clinical Services
Norris Health Center
University of Wisconsin-Milwaukee
Milwaukee, Wisconsin

Najm Hasan Siddiqui, MD
Hospitalist Physician
Parkview Medical Center
Pueblo, Colorado

Sarah Siddiqi, MD
Resident, Family Medicine
University of Texas Southwestern
Dallas, Texas

Hugh J. Silk, MD, MPH
Clinical Associate Professor
Department of Family Medicine and
    Community Health
University of Massachusetts Medical
    School
Worcester, Massachusetts

Matthew Silva, PharmD, RPh, BCPS
Professor of Pharmacy Practice
Massachusetts College of Pharmacy and
    Health Sciences University
Worcester, Massachusetts

Phillip Silva, MD, MPH
Department of Family Medicine
University of Texas Southwestern Medical
    Center
Dallas, Texas

Ashley Simela, DO
Orthopaedic Spine Surgeon
Cedars Sinai Medical Center
West Hollywood, California

Tracey G. Simon, MD
Warren Alpert Medical School of Brown
    University
Providence, Rhode Island

Parminder Singh, MD
Assistant Professor, Department of
    Medicine
Division Hematology and Oncology
University of Arizona Cancer Center
Tucson, Ariona

Avani Sinha, MD
The Warren Alpert Medical School of
    Brown University
Providence, Rhode Island

Nga Yan Siu
New York Institute of Technology College
    of Osteopathic Medicine
Old Westbury, New York

Brian G. Skotko, MD, MPP
Co-Director
Down Syndrome Program
Division of Medical Genetics
Massachusetts General Hospital
Boston, Massachusetts

Glenn Skow, MD, MPH
Chief of Staff
Medical Director, Emergency Department
Fayette County Hospital
Vandalia, Illinois

Adam J.T. Smith, MD, PhD
Resident Physician
Department of Radiation Medicine
University of Kentucky
Lexington, Kentucky

Jennifer N. Smith, MD
Family Medicine
University of Massachusetts
Fitchburg, Massachusetts

John C. Smulian, MD, MPH
Vice-Chair, Department of Obstetrics and
    Gynecology
Chief, Division of Maternal Fetal Medicine
Lehigh Valley Health Network
Allentown, Pennsylvania
Professor
University of South Florida-Morsani
    College of Medicine
Tampa, Florida

Rachel Sneed, MD
Associate Professor of Family Medicine
University of Cincinnati College of Medicine
Cincinnati, Ohio

L. Michael Snyder, MD
Professor of Medicine and Pathology
University of Massachusetts Medical School
Worcester, Massachusetts

Kristeina Sole, MD

David B. Sommer, MD, MPH

Adam J. Sorscher, MD
Department of Psychiatry
Sleep Medicine Division
Department of Community and Family
    Medicine
The Geisel School of Medicine at
    Dartmouth
Lebanon, New Hampshire

Andres F. Sosa, MD
University of Massachusetts Medical School
Division of Pulmonary, Allergy and Critical
    Care Medicine
UMass Memorial Medical Center
Worcester, Massachusetts

Marie Anne Sosa, MD
Worcester, Massachusetts

Alison Southern MD, MS, FACEP
Associate Program Director
Department of Emergency Medicine
Summa Akron City Hospital
Akron, Ohio

Sara Hope Soshnick
New York Institute of Technology College
    of Osteopathic Medicine
Old Westbury, New York

Mikayla Spangler, PharmD, BCPS
Assistant Professor
Department of Family Medicine
Department of Pharmacy Practice and
    School of Medicine
School of Pharmacy and Health
    Professions
Creighton University
Omaha, Nebraska

Jack Spittler, MD
Sports Medicine Fellow
Department of Sports Medicine
University of Colorado
Aurora, Colorado

Jacoby D. Spittler, DO
Resident Physician
Department of Obstetrics and Gynecology
Akron General Medical Center
Akron, Ohio

Kellie A. Sprague, MD
Assistant Professor of Medicine
Tufts University School of Medicine
Director
Bone Marrow Transplant Program
Tufts Medical Center
Boston, Massachusetts

Dana Sprute, MD, MPH, FAAFP
Associate Professor
University of Texas Southwestern Austin
    Family Medicine Residency
Austin, Texas

Daniel Stein, MD, MPH
Resident Physician
University of Virginia Health System
Charlottesville, Virginia

Gillian S. Stephens, MD, MSc
Assistant Professor
Department of Family and Community
    Medicine
St. Louis University
St. Louis, Missouri

Nate Stepp, DO
Lieutenant Commander
United States Navy
Family Medicine Physician
Naval Hospital Camp Lejeune
Family Medicine Residency Staff
Camp Lejeune, North Carolina

Kevan M. Sternberg, MD
Assistant Professor
Department of Surgery
Division of Urology
University of Vermont
Burlington, Vermont

J. Herbert Stevenson, MD
Director of Sports Medicine
Director of the Sports Medicine
    Fellowship Program
Associate Professor
Department of Family Health
Joint Appointment Department of
    Orthopedics
University of Massachusetts
Worcester, Massachusetts

Lara E. Stewart, DO, MPH
Pleasanton, California

Sheila O. Stille, DMD, MAGD
Associate Professor
Department of Surgical Dentistry
University of Colorado School of Dental
    Medicine
Aurora, Colorado

James A. Stober, MD
Senior Resident
David Grant Medical Center Family
    Medicine Residency Program
Travis Air Force Base, California

Marcus F. Stoddard, MD
Director, Non-invasive Cardiology
Professor of Medicine
Division of Cardiovascular Medicine
Department of Medicine
University of Louisville
Louisville, Kentucky

Jeffrey G. Stovall, MD
Associate Professor
Department of Psychiatry
Vanderbilt University School of Medicine
Nashville, Tennessee

Karyn M. Sullivan, PharmD, MPH
Associate Professor of Pharmacy Practice
Massachusetts College of Pharmacy and
    Health Sciences University
Worcester, Massachusetts

Heather Summe, MD
Division of Dermatology
University of Massachusetts Memorial
    Health Center
Worcester, Massachusetts

Kevin Svancara, DO
Glendale, Arizona

Alexander E. Swift, MD
Assistant Professor of Medicine
Department of Pulmonary and Critical
    Care
Temple University Hospital/School of
    Medicine
Philadelphia, Pennsylvania

Vassiliki P. Syriopoulou, MD
Emeritus Professor of Pediatrics
University of Athens
Aghia Sophia Children's Hospital
Athens, Greece

Julie M. Tabroff, MD
Sharon, Massachusetts

Alfonso J. Tafur, MD
Oklahoma University Health and Science
    Center
Oklahoma City, Oklahoma

Denisse V. Tafur, MD
Guayaquil, Ecuador

Komal Talati, MD
Radiology Resident
Department Radiology
Beth Israel Deaconess Medical Center
Boston, Massachusetts

Irene J. Tan, MD, FACR
Associate Professor of Clinical Medicine
Department of Medicine, Section of
    Rheumatology
Temple University School of Medicine
Philadelphia, Pennsylvania

Weizhen Tan, MD
Resident, Pediatrics
Yale-New Haven Hospital
New Haven, Connecticut

Horace Tang, MD
Assistant Professor of Medicine
University of Massachusetts Medical
    School
Worcester, Massachusetts

Annette Taranowicz, MS, DO
Department of Neuromusculoskeletal
    Medicine
New York Institute of Technology
College of Osteopathic Medicine
Old Westbury, New York

Dawn S. Tasillo, MD
Assistant Professor and Clerkship
    Director
Department of Obstetrics and Gynecology
University of Massachusetts School of
    Medicine
University of Massachusetts Memorial
    Medical Center
Worcester, Massachusetts

Eugene M. Tay, MD, MS
Clinical Assistant Professor
Department of Family Medicine
College of Human Medicine
Michigan State University
Grand Rapids, Michigan

Randolph Taylor, II, MD, CAQSM
Memorial Family Medicine Residency
    Program
Physicians at Sugar Creek
Sugar Land, Texas

David H. Tegay, DO, FACMG, FACOI
Associate Professor and Chair
Department of Medicine
New York Institute of Technology College
    of Osteopathic Medicine
Old Westbury, New York

Meaghan Tenney, MD
Assistant Professor
Department of Obstetrics and
    Gynecology
Section of Gynecologic Oncology
University of Chicago Medicine
Chicago, Illinois

Diana Teplitsky, DO
New York Institute of Technology College
    of Osteopathic Medicine
Westbury, New York

Michael J. Terzella, DO
Assistant Professor
Department of Osteopathic Manipulative
    Medicine
New York Institute of Technology College
    of Osteopathic Medicine
Old Westbury, New York

Pardeep Thandi, MD
Emergency Medicine
The Brooklyn Hospital Center
Brooklyn, New York

Richard J. Thomas, MD, MPH, FACOEM
Associate Professor, Occupational
    Medicine
Uniformed Services University of the
    Health Sciences
Bethesda, Maryland

Robin A. Thomas, DO
Department of Internal Medicine
University Hospitals Richmond Medical
    Center
Richmond Heights, Ohio

Margaret E. Thompson, MD
Associate Professor of Family
    Medicine
Michigan State University College of
    Human Medicine
Grand Rapids, Michigan

Richard Tibbetts, MD
Intern, Internal Medicine
University of Massachusetts Medical
    School
Worcester, Massachusetts

Michelle Tinitigan, MD
Assistant Clinical Professor
Department of Family and Community
  Medicine
University of California, San Francisco
Associate Physician
Adult and Family Medicine
Kaiser Permanente
San Francisco, California

Adam Z. Tobias, MD, MPH
Assistant Professor of Emergency
  Medicine
University of Pittsburgh School of
  Medicine
Pittsburgh, Pennsylvania

Elizabeth M. Tocci
University of Massachusetts Medical
  School
Worcester, Massachusetts

Louay Toma, MD
Walnut Creek, California

Sebastian Tong, MD, MPH
Family Medicine Resident
Greater Lawrence Family Health Center
Lawrence, Massachusetts

Moshe S. Torem, MD
Professor of Psychiatry
Northeast Ohio Medical University
Chief of Integrative Medicine
Akron General Medical Center
Medical Director
Center for Mind-Body Medicine
Akron, Ohio

Khasha Touloei, DO
Broward Health
Dermatology
Largo, Florida

Carmen Tran, MD
Resident, Internal Medicine
University of Texas at Tyler
Good Shepherd Medical
Longview, Texas

Hayden Tran, DO, MS
Resident, Internal Medicine
University Hospitals Regional Hospitals
Richmond Medical Center
Richmond Heights, Ohio

Kashyap Trivedi, MD
Los Alamitos, California

Zoltan Trizna, MD, PhD
Austin, Texas

Katherine M. Tromp, PharmD
Assistant Professor
Lake Erie College of Osteopathic
  Medicine
School of Pharmacy
Bradenton, Florida

Caroline Y. Tschibelu, MD
Emergency Medicine Resident
Robert Wood Johnson Medical School
New Brunswick, New Jersey

Tomoki Tsukahara, MD

Clint M. Tucker, MD
Division of Dermatology
University of Louisville
Louisville, Kentucky

Deepali Nivas Tukaye, MD, PhD
Fellow, Cardiovascular Medicine
Department of Medicine/Division of
  Cardiology
The Ohio State University – Wexner
  Medical Center
Columbus, Ohio

Auguste Turnier, MD
Internist/Gastroenterologist, Private
  Practice
Haddonfield, New Jersey

Lawrence E. Udom, MD, MPH
Dayton, Ohio

John K. Uffman, MD, MPH
Pediatric Surgery
Cook Childrens Medical Center
Fort Worth, Texas

Katherine S. Upchurch, MD
Clinical Professor of Medicine
University of Massachusetts Medical
  Group
Clinical Chief
Division of Rheumatology
University of Massachusetts Memorial
  Medical Group
Worcester, Massachusetts

Diana P. Vaca, MD
Newark, New Jersey

Santiago O. Valdes, MD, FAAP
Assistant Professor of Pediatrics
Section of Pediatric Cardiology,
  Electrophysiology, and Pacing
Baylor College of Medicine
Houston, Texas

**Anthony F. Valdini, MD, MS, FACP,
FAAFP**
Director of Research and Faculty
  Development
Lawrence Family Medicine Residency
Greater Lawrence Family Health Center
Lawrence, Massachusetts

Olga Valdman, MD
Assistant Professor
Department of Family Medicine
University of Massachusetts Medical
  School
Worcester, Massachusetts

William E. Valencia, MD
Family Medicine
Travis Air Force Base, California

Sara Valente, MD
University of Massachusetts
Worcester, Massachusetts

Virginia J. Van Duyne, MD
Department of Family Medicine and
  Community Health
University of Massachusetts
Worcester, Massachusetts

Chad Van Ginkel, MD, MPH
Resident Physician
Department of Emergency Medicine
Alpert Medical School of Brown University
Providence, Rhode Island

Elizabeth Varadian, DO, MS
Family Practice Residency
Natividad Medical Center
Salinas, California

Jose F. Vargas, MD
Newark, New Jersey

Kathleen M. Vazzana
Academic Medicine Scholar
New York Institute of Technology
College of Osteopathic Medicine
Old Westbury, New York

W. Brooke Veith, MD, MS
Preliminary Intern, Internal Medicine
University of Kentucky College of
  Medicine
Lexington, Kentucky

Maria Montanez Villacampa, MD
Family and Community Medicine
The University of Texas Health Science
  Center at San Antonio
San Antonio, TX

Jeffery Villanueva, MD
Urology Resident
Georgetown University Medstar
    Washington Hospital Center
Washington, DC

Siva Vithananthan, MD, FACS
Associate Professor of Surgery (Clinical)
Site-Director, Surgical Residency and
    Medical Student Program at Miriam
    Hospital
Alpert Medical School of Brown University
Providence, Rhode Island

Stacey Vitiello, MD
Breast Imaging Specialist
Montclair Breast Center
Montclair, New Jersey

Katherine Vlasica, DO
Emergency Department
Saint Joseph's Regional Medical Center
Patterson, New Jersey

Yongkasem Vorasettakarnkij, MD, MSc
Faculty of Medicine
Department of Medicine
Chulalongkorn University Cardiac Center
King Chulalongkorn Memorial Hospital
Thai Red Cross Society
Bangkok, Thailand

Athena Vuong, DO
University Hospitals
Cleveland, Ohio

Cynthia M. Waickus, MD, PhD
Associate Professor
Associate Chair for Predoctoral Education
Department of Family Medicine
Rush Medical College
Chicago, Illinois

John B. Waits, MD, FAAFP
Program Director, Cahaba Family
    Medicine Residency
CEO, Cahaba Medical Care Foundation
Centreville, Alabama

Annie R. Wang, MD
Warren Alpert Medical School of Brown
    University
Providence, Rhode Island

Jeff Wang, MD, MPH
University of Massachusetts Family
    Medicine Fitchburg
Fitchburg, Massachusetts

HY Janey Wang, MD
Resident, Family Medicine
University of Texas Health Science
    Center at San Antonio
San Antonio, Texas

Ryan Wargo, PharmD, BCACP
Assistant Professor/Clinical Pharmacist
Lake Erie College of Osteopathic
    Medicine School of Pharmacy
Bradenton, Florida

Terri Warren, BSN, MSN, MEd
Owner and Nurse Practitioner
Westover Heights Clinic
Portland, Oregon

Donald E. Watenpaugh, PhD
Adjunct Professor
Department of Integrative Physiology
University of North Texas Health Science
    Center
Fort Worth, Texas

Andrea N. Watson, DO, MS
Assistant Professor
Department of Family Medicine
New York Institute of Technology
College of Osteopathic Medicine,
Old Westbury, New York

Brandon Weeks, DO, MPH
University of Texas Southwestern
Austin Family Medicine Residency
Austin, Texas

Eilene Weibley, MD
Bayfront Family Medicine Residency
St. Petersburg, Florida

Jodi J. Weinstein, MD
Psychiatrist
Department of Psychiatry
Vanderbilt University Medical Center
Nashville, Tennessee

Daniel Weiss, MD, CDE, FACP, PNS, CPI
Director
Your Diabetes Endocrine Nutrition Group,
    Inc.
Mentor, Ohio

Patrice M. Weiss, MD, FACOG
Chair and Professor
Carilion Clinic/Virginia Tech Carilion
    School of Medicine
Roanoke, Virginia

Fred Weitendorf, RPH, RN
ICCU Clinical Pharmacist
Department of Pharmacy
Robley Rex VA Medical Center
Louisville, Kentucky

Jennifer Greene Welch, MD
Assistant Professor of Pediatrics
The Warren Alpert Medical School of
    Brown University
Providence, Rhode Island

Nathan Weldon, MD
Department of Family Medicine
Southern California Permanente Medical
    Group
Moreno Valley, California

Jeremy Blake Wells, MD
Chief Resident
Department of Family Medicine
University of Mississippi Medical Center
Jackson, Mississippi

Andrew J. Westwood, MD, MRCP(UK)
Assistant Professor of Clinical Neurology
Neurological Institute of New York
Division of Epilepsy and Sleep
New York, New York

Tyler H. Wheeler, MD
Primary Care Sports Medicine Fellow
Family Medicine Residency of Idaho
Boise, Idaho

Chris Wheelock, MD
PeaceHealth Southwest Washington
    Family Medicine
Clinical Assistant Professor
University of Washington
Vancouver, Washington

Brett White, MD
Associate Clinical Professor
Medical Director, Lewis Family Medicine
    Clinic
Associate Program Director, Family
    Medicine Residency
Associate Director, Combined Family
    Medicine/Psychiatry Residency
Department of Family & Preventive
    Medicine
University of California, San Diego
San Diego, California

Christopher C. White, MD, JD
Adjunct Assistant Professor
Departments of Family Medicine &
    Psychiatry
University of Cincinnati College of
    Medicine
Cincinnati, Ohio

Rebecca M. Wight, MD
Department of Surgery
University of Massachusetts Medical
    School
Worcester, Massachusetts

Judith Wilber, MD
University of Massachusetts Medical
    School
Worcester, Massachusetts

Elaina C. Wild, MD
United States Air Force
Fairfield, California

Susanne Wild, MD
Clinician Educator
Banner Good Samaritan Family Medicine
    Center
Clinical Assistant Professor
Department of Family and Community
    Medicine
University of Arizona College of Medicine
Phoenix, Arizona

Anna T. Wiley
University of Cincinnati College of
    Medicine
Cincinnati, Ohio

Eric C. Wilkerson, MD
Resident
Department of Internal Medicine
University of Louisville
Louisville, Kentucky

Faren H. Williams, MD, MS
Chief, Physical Medicine & Rehabilitation
Clinical Professor
Department of Orthopedics and Physical
    Rehabilitation
University of Massachusetts Medical
    School
Worcester, Massachusetts

Tasscia Williams MD, MPH
Obstetrics & Gynecology
Nassau University Medical Center
East Meadow, New York

Tracy L. Williams, MD
Assistant Professor
Family & Community Medicine
University of Kansas School of
    Medicine–Wichita
Associate Director
Via Christi Family Medicine Residency
Wichita, Kansas

Alan J. Williamson, MD
Medical Director
Family Health Clinic
Ehrling Bergquist Clinic
Offutt Air Force Base, Nebraska

Leah C. Wilson, MD
Obstetrics & Gynecology Resident
Department of Obstetrics and Gynecology
University of Massachusetts Medical
    School
Worcester, Massachusetts

Shenelle Wilson, MD
Section of Urology
Department of Surgery
Georgia Regents University
Augusta, Georgia

Norton Winer, MD
Department of Neurology
University Hospitals Case Medical Center
Cleveland, Ohio

Robyn D. Wing, MD
Pediatric Chief Resident
Department of Pediatrics
University of Massachusetts Medical School
Worcester, Massachusetts

James Winger, MD, CAQ
Primary Care Sports Medicine
Department of Family Medicine
Loyola Stritch School of Medicine
Maywood, Illinois

Fawn Winkelman, DO
Coral Springs, Florida

Aaron M. Winnick, MD
Department of Surgery
Maimonides Medical Center
Brooklyn, New York

Christopher M. Wise, MD
W. Robert Irby Professor of Medicine
Division of Rheumatology, Allergy, and
    Immunology
Department of Medicine
Virginia Commonwealth University Health
    System
Richmond, Virginia

Jeffrey D. Wolfrey, MD
Chair, Department of Family Medicine
Banner Good Samaritan Medical Center
Clinical Professor
Department of Family and Community
    Medicine
University of Arizona College of Medicine
Phoenix, Arizona

Christi Woods, DO

J. Andrew Woods, PharmD, BCPS
Assistant Professor of Pharmacy
Wingate University School of Pharmacy
Wingate, North Carolina

Dawna H. Woodyear, MD
Assistant Professor
University of Pittsburgh School of Medicine
Department of Family and Community
    Medicine
Medical Director
University of Pittsburgh Medical Center
    Matilda Theiss Health Center
Pittsburgh, Pennsylvania

Adrian Scott Worthen
Universidad Central Del Este
Escuela de Medicina
Dominican Republic

David Ryan Worthen
American University of the Caribbean
    School of Medicine
St. Maarten, Netherlands, Antilles

Mary Lauren Worthen, MD
Department of Otolaryngology
University of Louisville School of Medicine
Louisville, Kentucky

Frances Y. Wu, MD
Assistant Director
Somerset Family Medicine Residency
    Program
Robert Wood Johnson Medical Center at
    Somerset
Somerville, New Jersey

Kaiming Wu, MD
Florida International University Herbert
    Wertheim College of Medicine
Miami, Florida

Roger Y. Wu, MD, MBA
Resident
Department of Emergency Medicine
Brown University
Providence, Rhode Island

Ewa M. Wysokinska, MD
Willmar Cancer Center
Willmar, Minnesota

Sheldon C. Yao, DO
Acting Chair, Assistant Professor
Department of Osteopathic Manipulative
    Medicine
New York Institute of Technology–College
    of Osteopathic of Medicine
Old Westbury, New York

Brian Yokers, DO
Emergency Medicine Resident
St. Joseph's Regional Medical Center
Paterson, New Jersey

James R. Yon, MD
General Surgery Resident
Georgia Regents University
Augusta, Georgia

Robert A. Yood, MD
Chief of Rheumatology
Reliant Medical Group
Clinical Professor of Medicine
University of Massachusetts Medical
    School
Worcester, Massachusetts

Jocelyn C. Young
New York Institute of Technology -
   College of Osteopathic Medicine
Old Westbury, New York.

Edward L. Yourtee, MD, FACP
Chief Medical Officer
Parkland Medical Center
Derry, New Hampshire

Edlira Yzeiraj, DO, MS
New York Institute of Technology College
   of Osteopathic Medicine
Old Westbury, New York

Isabel Zacharias, MD
Staff Physician
Department of Gastroenterology
UMass Memorial Medical Center
Worcester, Massachusetts

Amy M. Zack, MD, FAAFP
Department of Family Medicine
MetroHealth Medical Center
Cleveland, Ohio

Bita Haji Zadeh, MD

Leanne Zakrzewski, MD
Clinical Instructor
Department of Family Medicine
David Geffen School of Medicine at
   University of California, Los Angeles
Los Angeles, California

Isheeta Zalpuri, MD
Resident, Psychiatry Department
University of Massachusetts Medical
   School
Worcester, Massachusetts

Matthew Zanghi, MD

Katrina Darlene Zedan, MSPAS, PA-C
Masters of Science in Physician Assistant
   Studies
South Texas Sinus Institute
San Antonio, Texas

Steven Zeddun, MD
Assistant Professor of Medicine
Department of Medicine, Division of
   Gastroenterology
The George Washington University
Washington, DC

Anne Marie C. Zeller, DO
University Hospitals Richmond
   Heights-Regional Hospitals
Richmond Heights, Ohio

Youhua Zhang, MD, PhD
Assistant Professor
Department of Biomedical Sciences
New York Institute of Technology College
   of Osteopathic Medicine
Old Westbury, New York

Derek Zickgraf, DO
Family Medicine Physician
United States Army
Schofield Barracks, Hawaii

D. Matthew Ziegler, MD
Sports Medicine Fellow
Department of Family Medicine
University of Utah
Salt Lake City, Utah

Peter J. Ziemkowski, MD
Associate Dean for Student Affairs
Associate Professor
Department of Family and Community
   Medicine
Western Michigan University School of
   Medicine
Kalamazoo, Michigan

Gennine M. Zinner, RNCS, ANP
Boston Health Care for the Homeless
   Program
Instructor, Massachusetts General
   Hospital of Health Professions
Boston, Massachusetts

Susan L. Zweizig, MD
Associate Professor and Director
Division of Gynecologic Oncology
University of Massachusetts
Worcester, Massachusetts

CONTENTS

Contents

US Preventive Services Task Force Recommendations

This section is designed to be a quick reference to the best screening and prevention recommendations from the least biased sources. They are the US Preventive Services Task Force (USPSTF), the US Centers for Disease Control (CDC), the American Academy of Pediatrics, and the American Academy of Family Physicians.

The recommendations below should be tailored to patients' preferences. For example, **"The USPSTF recommends biennial screening mammography for women aged 50 to 74 years"** recommendation is just that, a recommendation; screening every year or starting earlier is a decision to be made between you and the patient. *An Informed Consent* discussion for screening empowers the patient and the clinician to use these recommendations in a patient-centered manner.

Absent in these recommendations are "vested interests." Many disease-specific groups (the American Cancer Society, the American Heart Association, the National Osteoporosis Foundation, etc.) suggest interventions that serve *their* goals but do not always have a strong evidence base. The USPSTF provides the most unbiased, evidence-based recommendations.

—Frank J. Domino, MD
Editor-in-Chief

Each intervention receives an evidence-based grading set by the USPSTF. They are:

2005 TASK FORCE RATINGS
Strength of Recommendations

The USPSTF grades its recommendations according to 1 of 5 classifications (A, B, C, D, I) reflecting the strength of evidence and magnitude of *net benefit* (benefits minus harms).

- **A.** The USPSTF strongly recommends clinicians provide [the service] to eligible patients. The USPSTF found good evidence that [the service] improves important health outcomes and concludes that benefits substantially outweigh harms.

- **B.** The USPSTF recommends clinicians provide [this service] to eligible patients. The USPSTF found at least fair evidence that [the service] improves important health outcomes and concludes that benefits outweigh harms.

- **C.** The USPSTF makes no recommendation for or against routine provision of [the service]. The USPSTF found at least fair evidence [the service] can improve health outcomes but concludes the balance of benefits and harms is too close to justify a general recommendation.

- **D.** The USPSTF recommends against routinely providing [the service] to asymptomatic patients. The USPSTF found at least fair evidence that [the service] is ineffective or that harms outweigh benefits.

- **I.** The USPSTF concludes the evidence is insufficient to recommend for or against routinely providing [the service]. Evidence the [service] is effective is lacking, of poor quality, or conflicting and the net benefit cannot be determined.

In 2008, the USPSTF updated their rating system for *all new recommendations*; they are:

GRADE DEFINITIONS AFTER MAY 2007
What the Grades Mean and Suggestions for Practice

The USPSTF has updated its definitions of the grades it assigns to recommendations and now includes "suggestions for practice" associated with each grade. The USPSTF has also defined levels of certainty regarding net benefit. These definitions apply to USPSTF recommendations voted on after May 2007.

Grade	Definition	Suggestions for Practice
A	The USPSTF recommends the service. There is high certainty that the net benefit is substantial.	Offer or provide this service.
B	The USPSTF recommends the service. There is high certainty that the net benefit is moderate or there is moderate certainty that the net benefit is moderate to substantial.	Offer or provide this service.
C	The USPSTF recommends against routinely providing the service. There may be considerations that support providing the service in an individual patient. There is at least moderate certainty that the net benefit is small.	Offer or provide this service only if other considerations support the offering or providing the service in an individual patient.
D	The USPSTF recommends against the service. There is moderate or high certainty that the service has no net benefit or that the harms outweigh the benefits.	Discourage the use of this service.
I Statement	The USPSTF concludes that the current evidence is insufficient to assess the balance of benefits and harms of the service. Evidence is lacking, of poor quality, or conflicting, and the balance of benefits and harms cannot be determined.	Read the clinical considerations section of the USPSTF Recommendation Statement. If the service is offered, patients should understand the uncertainty about the balance of benefits and harms.

Levels of Certainty Regarding Net Benefit

Level of Certainty*	Description
High	The available evidence usually includes consistent results from well-designed, well-conducted studies in representative primary care populations. These studies assess the effects of the preventive service on health outcomes. This conclusion is, therefore, unlikely to be strongly affected by the results of future studies.
Moderate	The available evidence is sufficient to determine the effects of the preventive service on health outcomes, but confidence in the estimate is constrained by such factors as: • The number, size, or quality of individual studies. • Inconsistency of findings across individual studies. • Limited generalizability of findings to routine primary care practice. • Lack of coherence in the chain of evidence. As more information becomes available, the magnitude or direction of the observed effect could change, and this change may be large enough to alter the conclusion.
Low	The available evidence is insufficient to assess effects on health outcomes. Evidence is insufficient because of: • The limited number or size of studies. • Important flaws in study design or methods. • Inconsistency of findings across individual studies. • Gaps in the chain of evidence. • Findings not generalizable to routine primary care practice. • Lack of information on important health outcomes. More information may allow estimation of effects on health outcomes.

*The USPSTF defines certainty as "likelihood that the USPSTF assessment of the net benefit of a preventive service is correct." The net benefit is defined as benefit minus harm of the preventive service as implemented in a general, primary care population. The USPSTF assigns a certainty level based on the nature of the overall evidence available to assess the net benefit of a preventive service. *Current as of May 2008.*

HEALTH MAINTENANCE: BIRTH TO 10 YEARS
(www.uspreventiveservicestaskforce.org/uspstopics.htm)

Leading causes of death:
- Perinatal infections
- Congenital anomalies
- Sudden infant death syndrome (SIDS)
- Accidents (drowning, abuse)
- Motor vehicle accidents

Recommended counseling, testing, or interventions

Height, weight, growth chart	
Immunizations (*http://www.cdc.gov/vaccines/schedules/hcp/child-adolescent.html* or *www.immunizationed.org*)	(DPaT, IPV, Hib, hepatitis A, hepatitis B, MMR, pneumococcal, rotavirus, varicella, influenza 6 months–18 years)
Counseling:	Injury prevention: –Car seats –Seat belts –Bicycle helmets –Smoke and carbon monoxide detector –Window/stair guards –Firearm storage
Breast-fed infants	400 IU vitamin D started within a few days of birth
Congenital hypothyroidism	At birth
Dental caries in preschool children	Oral fluoride supplementation for children older than 6 months whose primary water source is deficient in fluoride: –6 months–3 years 0.25 mg, –3–6 years 0.5 mg, –6–16 years 1 mg/d
Diet	Low-saturated-fat diet and physical exercise
Hearing screening	At birth
Lead screening	High risk: Minority, urban residency, low SES, house built before 1950, recent immigration
Obesity	Screen children ≥6 years for obesity and offer/refer to comprehensive, intensive behavioral interventions to promote improvement in weight status
Substance abuse prevention	Tobacco, alcohol counseling
Tuberculosis screening	High risk: Urban residency, low SES, recent immigration or exposure to recent immigrant
Vision screening: Strabismus, amblyopia, visual acuity	To be completed between ages 3 and 5 years
Gonococcal ophthalmia neonatorum	Prophylactic ocular topical medication for all newborns

Insufficient to recommend for or against

Dysplasia of the hip	By physical examination

HEALTH MAINTENANCE: 11–24 YEARS

(www.uspreventiveservicestaskforce.org/uspstopics.htm)

Leading causes of death:

- Motor vehicle accidents
- Unintentional injuries (over 15 homicide)
- Suicide
- Malignant neoplasms

Immunizations *(http://www.cdc.gov/vaccines/schedules/hcp/child-adolescent.html, www.cdc.gov/vaccines/schedules/hcp/adult.html or www.immunizationed.org)*

Tetanus-diphtheria-pertussis (Tdap), meningococcal (MCV4), human papilloma virus (females), varicella (2 total for those without immunity), influenza

Disease	Recommended intervention (A or B grade)
General	Height, weight, BMI, BP, injury prevention (seat belts, firearms), low-saturated-fat diet, physical exercise
Alcohol and substance abuse screening	Screen those 18 and older for alcohol and substance misuse and provide those at risk with brief counseling to reduce misuse (see below for screening tools)
Breast and ovarian cancer by BRCA mutation	If high risk: Ashkenazi, or 2 first-degree relatives with breast or ovarian cancer at <50 years of age
Cervical cancer screening	Age 21 by cytology (no HPV)
Chlamydia, gonorrhea, syphilis screening	If sexually active, pregnancy, IV drug use
Depression	In clinical practices that have systems in place to assure accurate diagnosis, effective treatment, and follow-up
Diabetes mellitus (non–fasting glucose)	If BP >135/80
Domestic/family violence	Screen all women of childbearing age
HIV screening	Screen all aged 15–65 years, including all pregnant women, and those younger and older who are at increased risk
Hepatitis B	If high risk: Sexually active, pregnancy, IV drug use
Lipid disorders	One fasting lipid panel to identify familial hypercholesterolemia during adolescence
Tuberculosis screening	If high risk: Travel, immigrant, alcohol abuse, IV drug use
Obesity (counseling for obese patients)	Screen children ≥6 years for obesity and offer/refer to comprehensive, intensive behavioral interventions to promote improvement in weight status.
Folic acid for women	All women planning or capable of pregnancy take a daily supplement of 0.4–0.8 mg (400–800 µg) of folic acid
Tobacco cessation	Screen all school-aged children and adults about tobacco use and provide tobacco cessation interventions for those who use tobacco
Suicide screening	Depression*

*Additional screening

Alcohol abuse	"Risky"/"hazardous" alcohol use: >7 drinks per week or >3 drinks on any one occasion for women, and >14 drinks per week or >4 drinks on any one occasion for men. OR Screen: "On any occasion during the last 3 months, have had >5 alcohol drinks" or CAGE: Tried to CUT down, been ANGERED by questions about your drinking, felt GUILTY about your drinking, had an EYE OPENER (drink in the morning)
Domestic violence	Screen all women of childbearing age, and provide intervention or refer those who screen positive "Do you feel safe in your present relationship?" "Have you been hit, kicked, punched, or otherwise hurt in the last year?"
Substance abuse	Question about drug use and related problems should be considered in all adolescents and adults.
Suicide	Risk factors include history of mood or other mental disorder, substance abuse, and history of "deliberate self-harm."

Against (D grade)

Coronary heart disease via ECG, ETT, etc.	D: Do Not Screen
Hemochromatosis	D: Do Not Screen
Scoliosis screening	D: Do Not Screen
Testicular cancer	D: Do Not Screen

HEALTH MAINTENANCE: 25–45 YEARS

(www.uspreventiveservicestaskforce.org/uspstopics.htm)

Leading causes of death:

- Unintentional injury (especially accidental overdose [narcotics])
- Suicide
- Cardiovascular disease
- Malignant neoplasm

Immunizations *(www.cdc.gov/vaccines/schedules/hcp/adult.html* or *www.immunizationed.org)*

Tetanus	Tdap every 10 years or just at age 50 (if completed primary series)
Influenza	All adults

Disease	Recommended intervention (A or B grade)
General	Height, weight, BMI, BP, injury prevention (seat belts, firearms), low-saturated-fat diet, physical exercise
Alcohol and substance abuse	Screen all for alcohol and substance misuse and provide those at risk with brief counseling to reduce misuse (see below for tools)
Breast and ovarian cancer by genetic testing	Refer for genetic counseling if: Ashkenazi heritage, or 2 first-degree relatives with breast or ovarian cancer at <50 years of age
Breast cancer screening by mammography	For those who are at increased risk, have an informed consent discussion about medications (i.e., tamoxifen or raloxifene) to lower their risk
Cervical cancer screening	Age 21–65: every 3 years with cytology OR Age 30–65: every 5 with cytology and HPV
Coronary heart disease	—Screen all men starting at 35 years and all women at 45 years (or 10 years younger if at high risk) —Evidence is insufficient to recommend using nontraditional risk factors (high-sensitivity C-reactive protein [hs-CRP], ankle-brachial index [ABI], leukocyte count, fasting blood glucose level, periodontal disease, carotid intima-media thickness [carotid IMT], coronary artery calcification [CAC] score on electron-beam computed tomography [EBCT], homocysteine level, and lipoprotein[a] level) to screen asymptomatic men and women with no history of CHD to prevent CHD events
Depression	In clinical practices that have systems in place to assure accurate diagnosis, effective treatment, and follow-up
Diabetes mellitus, type II (if BP >135/80)	Random serum glucose if sustained BP (either treated or untreated) >135/80 mm Hg
Domestic/family violence	Screen all women of childbearing age
Diet/obesity	Intensive behavioral dietary counseling for patients with known risk factors for cardiovascular and diet-related chronic disease
Chlamydia, gonorrhea, syphilis testing	All adults who are at increased risk (multiple partners, IV drug use, etc. and all pregnant women)
HIV screening	Screen all aged 15–65 years, including all pregnant woman, and those younger and older who are at increased risk
Hepatitis B	All pregnant women and those with multiple sexual partners, IV drug use, etc.
Lipid disorders	Men: 35 and older for lipid disorders Women: 45 and older for lipid disorders
Suicide screening	If depressed*
Tobacco abuse	Ask all adults about tobacco use and provide tobacco cessation interventions for those who use tobacco
Tuberculosis screening	If high risk: Travel, immigrant, alcohol abuse, IV drug use

*Additional screening

Alcohol abuse	"Risky"/"hazardous" alcohol use: >7 drinks per week or >3 drinks on any one occasion for women, and >14 drinks per week or more than 4 drinks on any one occasion for men. OR Screen: "On any occasion during the last 3 months, have had more than 5 alcohol drinks" or CAGE: Tried to CUT down, been ANGERED by questions about your drinking, felt GUILTY about your drinking, had an EYE OPENER (drink in the morning)
Domestic violence	Screen all at-risk patients (all women, especially when pregnant) "Do you feel safe in your present relationship?" "Have you been hit, kicked, punched, or otherwise hurt in the last year?"
Substance abuse	Questioning about drug use and related problems should be considered in all adolescents and adults.
Suicide	Risk factors include history of mood or other mental disorder, substance abuse, and history of "deliberate self-harm."

Recommends against

Aspirin	The USPSTF recommends against the use of aspirin for stroke prevention in women younger than 55 years and for myocardial infarction prevention in men younger than 45 years.
Testicular cancer	The USPSTF recommends against testicular exam to screen for testicular cancer.

HEALTH MAINTENANCE: 45–65 YEARS

(www.uspreventiveservicestaskforce.org/uspstopics.htm)

Leading causes of death:

- Cardiovascular disease
- Malignant neoplasm
- Accidents
- Cirrhosis

Immunizations *(www.cdc.gov/vaccines/schedules/hcp/adult.html or www.immunizationed.org)*

Tetanus	Tdap every 10 years or just at age 50 (if completed primary series)
Influenza	All adults

Disease	Recommended intervention (A or B grade)
General	Height, weight, BMI, BP, injury prevention (seat belts, firearms), low-saturated-fat diet, physical exercise
Alcohol and substance abuse	Screen all for alcohol and substance misuse and provide those at risk with brief counseling to reduce misuse (see below for tools)
Aspirin	Recommends use of aspirin for men age 45–79 and women age 55–79 years when potential benefit due to a reduction in myocardial infarctions outweighs the potential harm due to an increase in GI hemorrhage
Breast and ovarian cancer by genetic testing	Refer for genetic counseling if: Ashkenazi heritage, or 2 first-degree relatives with breast or ovarian cancer at <50 years of age
Breast cancer screening by mammography	—For those who are at increased risk, have an informed consent discussion about medications (i.e., tamoxifen or raloxifene) to lower their risk —Mammography starting at age≥50; repeat every 2 years
Cervical cancer screening	Age 21–65: every 3 years with cytology *OR* Age 30–65: every 5 years with cytology and HPV
Chlamydia, gonorrhea, syphilis testing	All adults who are at increased risk (multiple partners, IV drug use, etc.) and all pregnant women)
Colon cancer	Start at age 50–75 by fecal occult blood testing, sigmoidoscopy, or colonoscopy
Coronary heart disease	Evidence is insufficient to recommend using nontraditional risk factors (high-sensitivity C-reactive protein [hs-CRP], ankle-brachial index [ABI], leukocyte count, fasting blood glucose level, periodontal disease, carotid intima-media thickness [carotid IMT], coronary artery calcification [CAC] score on electron-beam computed tomography [EBCT], homocysteine level, and lipoprotein[a] level) to screen asymptomatic men and women with no history of CHD to prevent CHD events
Depression	In clinical practices that have systems in place to assure accurate diagnosis, effective treatment, and follow-up
Diabetes mellitus, type II if BP >135/80	Random serum glucose if sustained BP (either treated or untreated) >135/80 mm Hg
Domestic/family violence	Screen all women of childbearing age
Diet/obesity	Intensive behavioral dietary counseling for patients with known risk factors for cardiovascular and diet-related chronic disease
HIV screening	Screen all aged 15–65 years, including all pregnant women, and those younger and older who are at increased risk
Hepatitis B	All pregnant women and those with multiple sexual partners, IV drug use, etc.
Hepatitis C	Screen all adults born between 1945 and 1965 once for hepatitis C
Lipid disorders	All adults over 45 should be screened
Suicide screening	If depressed*
Osteoporosis	Only screen in women younger than 65 years if their fracture risk is equivalent to that of a 65-year-old
Tobacco abuse	Ask all adults about tobacco use and provide tobacco cessation interventions for those who use tobacco
Tuberculosis screening	If high risk: Travel, immigrant, alcohol abuse, IV drug use

*Additional screening

Alcohol abuse	"Risky"/"hazardous" alcohol use: >7 drinks per week or >3 drinks on any one occasion for women, and >14 drinks per week or >4 drinks on any one occasion for men. OR Screen: "On any occasion during the last 3 months, have had more than 5 alcohol drinks" or CAGE: Tried to CUT down, been ANGERED by questions about your drinking, felt GUILTY about your drinking, had an EYE OPENER (drink in the morning)
Domestic violence	Screen all at-risk patients (all women, especially when pregnant) "Do you feel safe in your present relationship?" "Have you been hit, kicked, punched, or otherwise hurt in the last year?"
Substance abuse	Questioning about drug use and related problems should be considered in all adolescent and adult.
Suicide	Risk factors include history of mood or other mental disorder, substance abuse, and history of "deliberate self-harm."

Recommends against

Prostate cancer	The USPSTF recommends against PSA-based screening for prostate cancer.
Ovarian cancer	The USPSTF recommends against screening for ovarian cancer in women.

HEALTH MAINTENANCE: 65 YEARS AND ABOVE

(www.uspreventiveservicestaskforce.org/uspstopics.htm)

Leading causes of death:

- Cardiovascular disease
- Malignant neoplasm
- COPD
- Stroke
- Dementia

Immunizations *(www.cdc.gov/vaccines/schedules/hcp/adult.html or www.immunizationed.org)*

Tetanus	Tdap every 10 years (if completed primary series)
Influenza	All adults

Disease	Recommended Intervention (A or B Grade)
General	Height, weight, BMI, BP, injury prevention (seat belts, firearms), low-saturated-fat diet, physical exercise
Alcohol and substance abuse	Screen all for alcohol and substance misuse and provide those at risk with brief counseling to reduce misuse (see below for tools)
Aspirin	Recommends use of aspirin for men age 45–79 and women age 55–79 years when potential benefit due to a reduction in myocardial infarctions outweighs the potential harm due to an increase in GI hemorrhage
Breast and ovarian cancer by genetic testing	Refer for genetic counseling if: Ashkenazi heritage, or 2 first-degree relatives with breast or ovarian cancer at <50 years of age
Breast cancer screening by mammography	Mammography through age 75; repeat every 1–2 years; after age 75, at discretion
Cervical cancer screening	May cease to screen if had adequate recent screening and are not at high risk
Chlamydia, gonorrhea, syphilis testing	All adults who are at increased risk (multiple partners, IV drug use, etc.)
Colon cancer	Start at age 50–75 by fecal occult blood testing, sigmoidoscopy, or colonoscopy
Coronary Heart Disease	Evidence is insufficient to recommend using nontraditional risk factors (high-sensitivity C-reactive protein [hs-CRP], ankle-brachial index [ABI], leukocyte count, fasting blood glucose level, periodontal disease, carotid intima-media thickness [carotid IMT], coronary artery calcification [CAC] score on electron-beam computed tomography [EBCT], homocysteine level, and lipoprotein[a] level) to screen asymptomatic men and women with no history of CHD to prevent CHD events
Depression	In clinical practices that have systems in place to assure accurate diagnosis, effective treatment, and follow-up
Diabetes mellitus, type II if BP >135/80	Random serum glucose if sustained BP (either treated or untreated) >135/80 mm Hg
Domestic/family violence	*If sexually active
Diet/obesity	Intensive behavioral dietary counseling for patients with known risk factors for cardiovascular and diet-related chronic disease
Fall prevention	The USPSTF recommends exercise or physical therapy and vitamin D supplementation (>800 IU/d)
HIV screening	Screen all until age 65 years, and those older who are at increased risk
Hepatitis B	All pregnant women and those with multiple sexual partners, IV drug use, etc.
Hepatitis C	Screen all adults born between 1945 and 1965 once for hepatitis C
Lipid disorders	All adults over 45 should be screened
Osteoporosis	All women at 65; insufficient evidence to support screening men
Suicide screening	If depressed*
Tobacco abuse	Ask all adults about tobacco use and provide tobacco cessation interventions for those who use tobacco
Tuberculosis screening	If high risk: Travel, immigrant, alcohol abuse, IV drug use

*Additional screening

Alcohol abuse	"Risky"/"hazardous" alcohol use: >7 drinks per week or >3 drinks on any one occasion for women, and >14 drinks per week or >4 drinks on any one occasion for men. OR Screen: "On any occasion during the last 3 months, have had more than 5 alcohol drinks" or CAGE: Tried to CUT down, been ANGERED by questions about your drinking, felt GUILTY about your drinking, had an EYE OPENER (drink in the morning)
Domestic violence	Screen all at-risk patients (all women, especially when pregnant) "Do you feel safe in your present relationship?" "Have you been hit, kicked, punched, or otherwise hurt in the last year?"
Substance abuse	Questioning about drug use and related problems should be considered in all adolescent and adult.
Suicide	Risk factors include history of mood or other mental disorder, substance abuse, and history of "deliberate self-harm."

Recommends against

Prostate cancer	The USPSTF recommends against PSA-based screening for prostate cancer.
Ovarian cancer	The USPSTF recommends against screening for ovarian cancer in women.

Diagnosis and Treatment: An Algorithmic Approach

This section contains flowcharts (or algorithms) to help the reader in the diagnosis of clinical signs and symptoms, and treatment of a variety of clinical problems. They are organized by the presenting sign, symptom, or diagnosis.

These algorithms were designed to be used as a quick reference and adjunct to the reader's clinical knowledge and impression. They are not an exhaustive review of the management of a problem, nor are they meant to be a complete list of diseases.

ABDOMINAL PAIN, CHRONIC

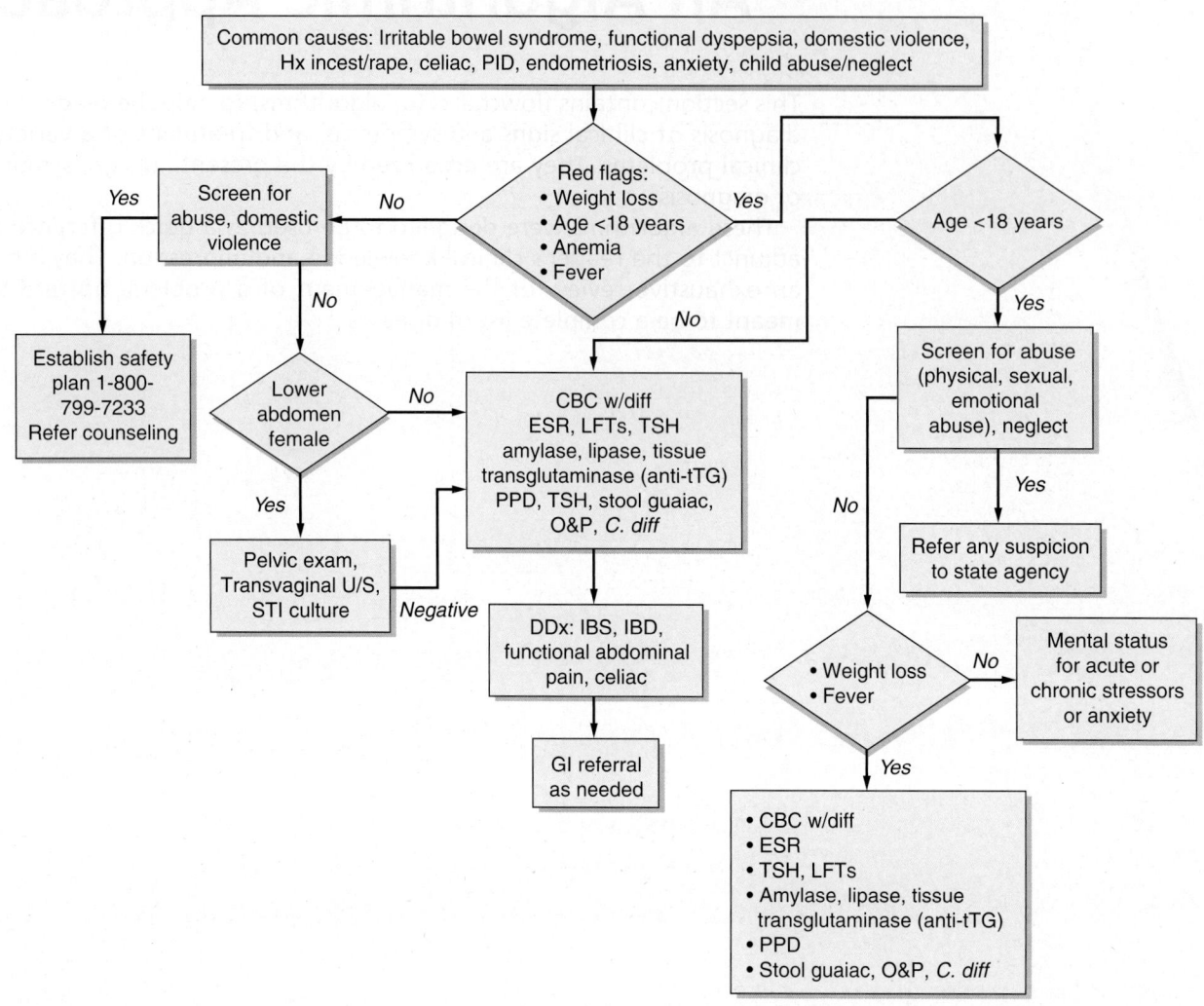

Frank J. Domino, MD and Bree Alyeska Huning

Camilleri M. Management of patients with chronic abdominal pain in clinical practice. *Neurogastroenterol Motil.* 2006;18(7):499–506.

ABDOMINAL PAIN, LOWER

Common causes: Appendicitis, ovarian cyst, diverticulitis, UTI, cholecystitis, IBS, IBD, constipation, pregnancy, PID, ruptured AAA pancreatitis

Check labs/imaging: CBC, amylase, lipase, UA, abdominal XR [pelvic U/S, colonoscopy, abdominal CT]

Right lower

Hypogastric

Left lower

Gradual onset

Sudden onset

Sigmoid diverticulitis
IBD
Constipation
Pyelonephritis
Crohn disease

Mesenteric adenitis
Appendicitis
Pyelonephritis
Crohn disease

Ovarian torsion/ ruptured cyst
Cecal diverticulitis
Meckel's diverticulitis

Genitourinary

Gastrointestinal

Ruptured AAA
Abdominal wall hematoma
Psoas or Abdominal abscess
Incarcerated or strangulated hernia

Cystitis
Pyelonephritis
Nephrolithiasis
PID
Endometriosis
Mittelschmerz
Ovarian torsion
Ectopic pregnancy

Constipation
IBD
Ischemic colitis

Nihal Patel, MD and Siva Vithananthan, MD

Heading RC. Prevalence of upper gastrointestinal symptoms in the general population: A systematic review. *Scand J Gastroenterol Suppl.* 1999;231:3–8.

ABDOMINAL PAIN, UPPER

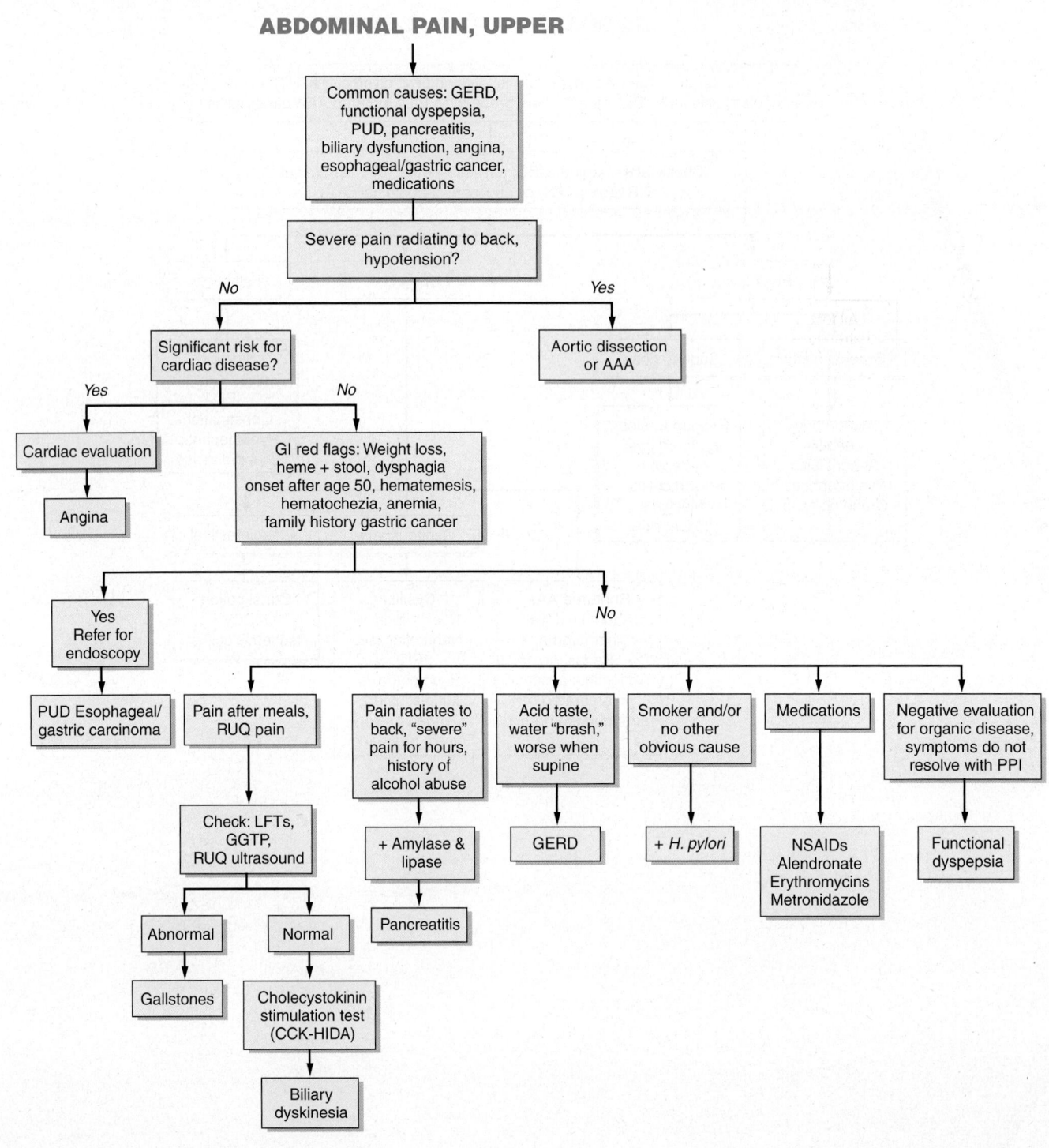

Matthew Zanghi, MD and Frank J. Domino, MD

Ford AC, Moayyedi P. Managing dypepsia. *Curr Gastroenterol Rep.* 2009;11(4):288–294.

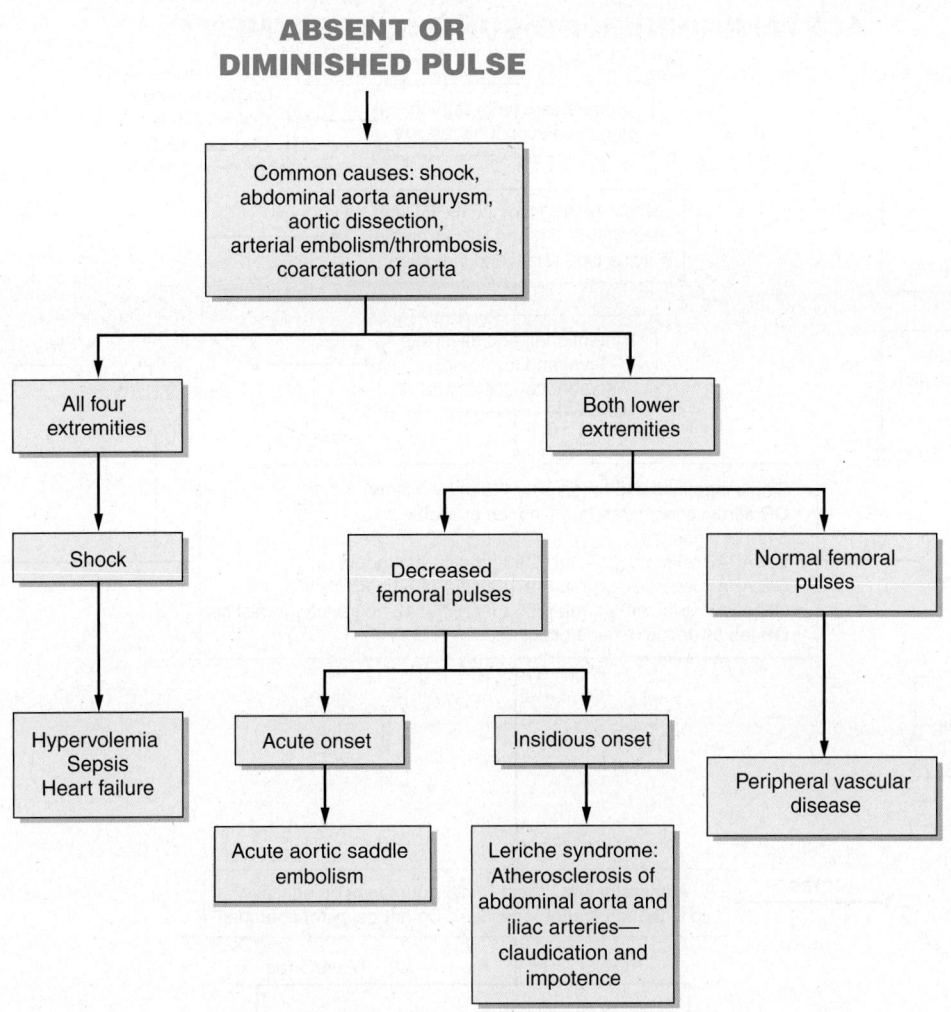

ABSENT OR DIMINISHED PULSE

Common causes: shock, abdominal aorta aneurysm, aortic dissection, arterial embolism/thrombosis, coarctation of aorta

All four extremities → Shock → Hypervolemia, Sepsis, Heart failure

Both lower extremities →
- Decreased femoral pulses
  - Acute onset → Acute aortic saddle embolism
  - Insidious onset → Leriche syndrome: Atherosclerosis of abdominal aorta and iliac arteries—claudication and impotence
- Normal femoral pulses → Peripheral vascular disease

Robert A. Baldor, MD and Alan M. Ehrlich, MD

O'Connell JB, Quiñones-Baldrich WJ. Proper evaluation and management of acute embolic versus thrombotic limb ischemia. *Semin Vasc Surg.* 2009;22(1):10–16.

ACETAMINOPHEN POISONING, TREATMENT

Secure airway, breathing, and circulation if necessary → Contact Poison Control Center 800-222-1222

Obtain APAP level, LFTs, PT/INR, electrolytes, Cr, and HCG (female). Note time relative to ingestion.

If intentional, add salicylate level and toxicology screen, consult psych.

<2 hours since ingestion — **Yes** → Give 50 g activated charcoal (PO, NG)

No

Single ingestion? — **No** →
- Single ingestion >150 mg/kg (or 7.5 g) by history
- **OR** serum concentration will not be available by 8 hrs of ingestion
- **OR** APAP level >150 μg/mL (993 μmol/L) at 4 hours
- **OR** APAP level >75 μg/mL (497 μmol/L) at 8 hours
- **OR** APAP level >40 μg/mL (265 μmol/L) at 12 hours after ingestion
- **OR** lab evidence of hepatotoxicity

Yes ↓

If extended-release product suspected, repeat at least one additional level 4 hours after first. Administer NAC in interim if significant overdose suspected.

If no extended-release APAP ingested, ingestion likely not significant. Observe.

Yes ↑ (Single ingestion?)

No ↓

Repeated supratherapeutic ingestion (RSTI)

APAP >10 μg/ml OR elevated AST or ALT — **Yes** → Administer NAC (best w/in 8 hours may be effective up to 36 hours after ingestion). Do not delay for charcoal!

No ↓

Aggressive patient education

Administer NAC →
- *PO/NG* → **72-hour PO regimen:** 140 mg/kg loading dose THEN 70 mg/kg q4h × 17 total doses for 17 total doses
- *IV preferred* → **IV regimen:** 150 mg/kg in 200 mL D5W over 60 minutes THEN 50 mg/kg in 500 mL D5W over 4 hours THEN 100 mg/kg in 1 L D5W over 16 hours

Check APAP, ALT, AST, PT/INR every 4 hours

APAP ≤10 μg/ml, ALT/AST have peaked are improving, INR ≤1.3
- **Yes** → Discontinue NAC
- **No** → **Extended IV regimen:** 150 mg/kg in 200 mL D5W over 60 minutes THEN 50 mg/kg in 500 mL D5W over 4 hours THEN 100 mg/kg in 1 L D5W over 16 hours, then 6.25 mg/kg/hr until INR <2.0 or death. Monitor for hypoglycemia* Vitamin K for coagulopathy* (FFP only if active bleeding)
  *Consider transport to transplant center.
  Fulminant hepatic failure is rare. King's College Hospital

  Transplant criteria: Lactate >3.0 OR pH <7.3 OR creatinine >3.2 and INR >6.5 and encephalopathy

*APAP = Acetaminophen NAC = N-acetylcysteine

Christine Jacobs, MD, FAAFP

Hodgman MJ, Garrard AR. A review of acetaminophen poisoning. *Crit Care Clin.* 2012;28(4):499–516.

ACID PHOSPHATASE ELEVATION

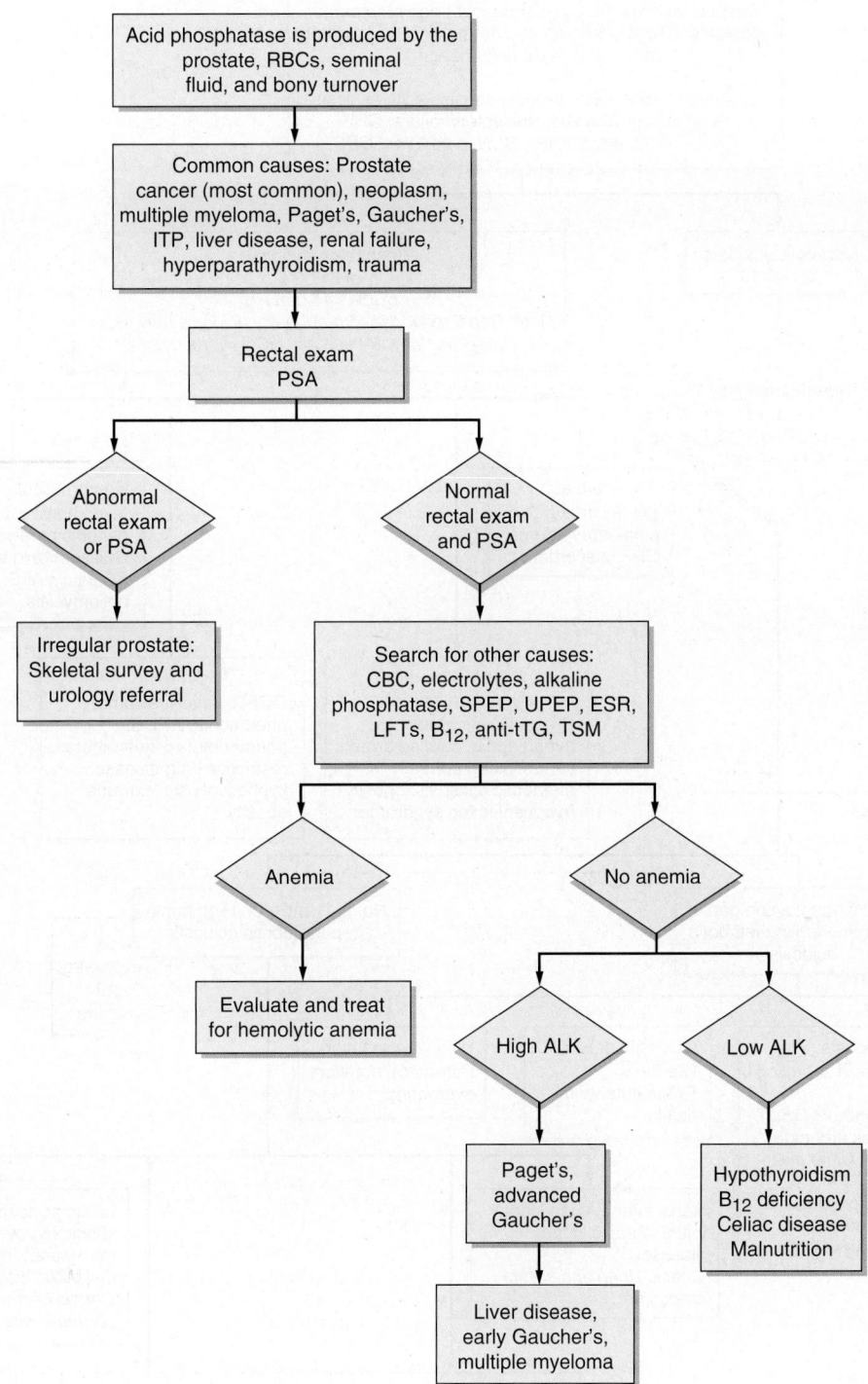

Laura Hagopian, MD and Michael Snyder, MD

Scarnecchia L, Minisola S, Pacitti MT, et al. Clinical usefulness of serum tartrate-resistant acid phosphatase activity determination to evaluate bone turnover. *Scand J Clin Lab Invest.* 1991;51(6):517–524.

ACIDOSIS

Suspect with low HCO_3 (<24 mmol/L) and respiratory disorders. If high suspicion and normal HCO_3, consider mixed acid-base disturbance.

Common causes: DKA, uremia, sepsis, lactic acidosis, renal tubular acidosis, respiratory failure, CHF
Check: ABG, electrolytes, BUN, creatinine, CBC

Metabolic acidosis: pH <7.33

Respiratory acidosis:
pH <7.33
pCO_2 >44 mm Hg
Note: Renal response to respiratory acidosis may occur over days. May not see low HCO_3 immediately.

Serum anion gap normal?
$[Na] - ([Cl] + [HCO_3]) = 3-11$ mEq/L

Cardiac:
Acute cardiogenic pulmonary edema, CHF exacerbation

Neuromuscular disorders: Myasthenia gravis, periodic paralysis, Guillain-Barré syndrome, SC injury, ALS, MS, poliomyelitis

Inhibition of medullary respiratory center:
Drugs, O_2 in chronic hypercapnia, cardiac arrest, central sleep apnea, metabolic alkalosis, obesity-hypoventilation syndrome

Pulmonary:
COPD, severe asthma, pneumonia, ARDS, pneumothorax–hemothorax, restrictive lung disease, kyphoscoliosis, extreme obesity

Yes: Normal anion gap (hyperchloremic) metabolic acidosis

No: (>11 mEq/L): High anion gap metabolic acidosis

Renal tubular acidosis:
• RTA type 1: Failure of acid secretion distally. *Hypokalemia, inappropriately high urine pH (>5.3).*
• RTA type 2: Failure of bicarbonate reabsorption proximally. *Urine can acidify to pH <5.3.*
• RTA type 4: Decreased proximal ammonia production secondary to hypoaldosteronism. *Hyperkalemia*

GI losses of HCO_3:
Diarrhea, Enterocutaneous fistula

Hyperalimentation:
Parenteral nutrition, overeating

Renal injury: Acute kidney injury, chronic kidney disease
Check: Urine and serum creatinine

Lactic acidosis: Sepsis, cardiogenic shock, hypovolemic shock, malignancy, medications, hereditary metabolic disorders
Check: Lactate levels (may not correlate with severity)

Toxin: Methanol, ethylene glycol, acetaminophen overdose, salicylate overdose
Check: Urine toxicology screen

Ketoacidosis: DKA, alcoholic ketoacidosis.
Check: Urine and plasma ketones

Judith Wilber, MD and Stacy E. Potts, MD, MEd

Reddy P, Mooradian AD. Clinical utility of anion gap in deciphering acid-base disorders. *Int J Clin Pract.* 2009;63:1516–1525.

ACNE

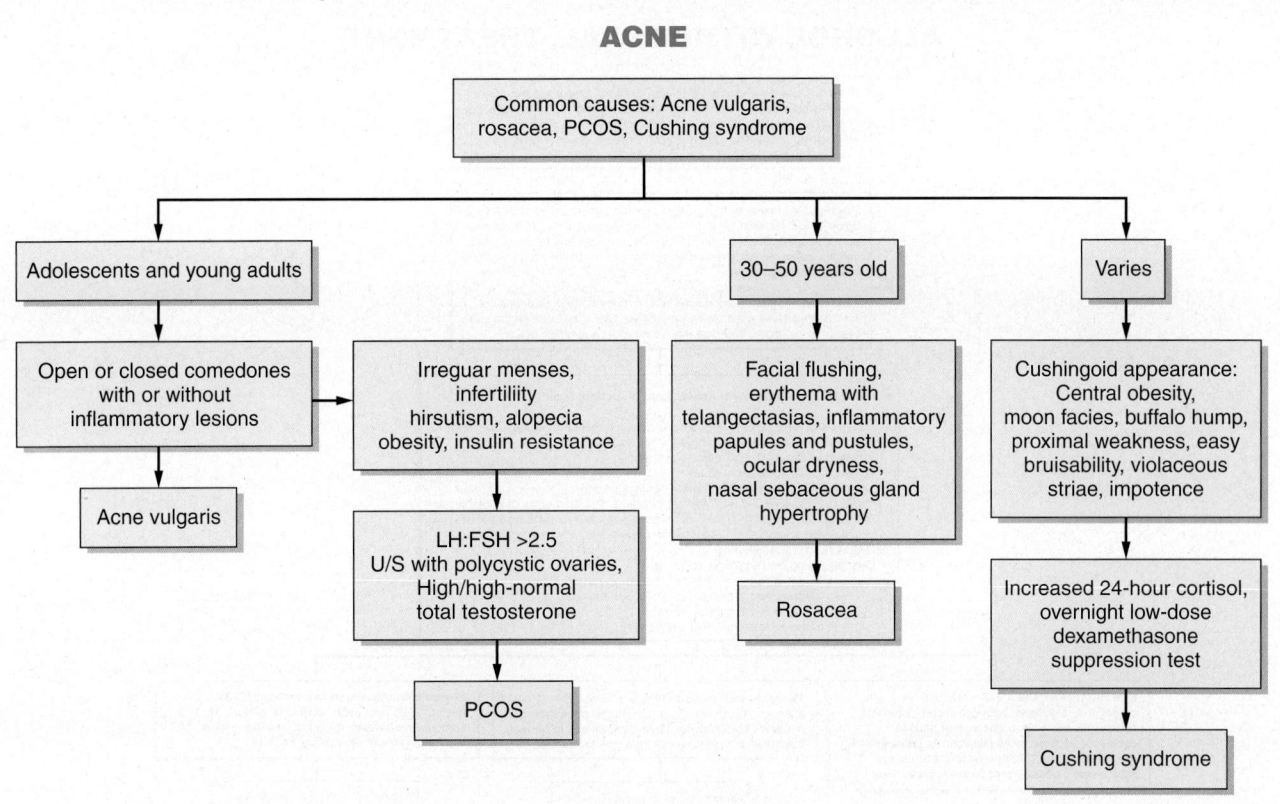

Elise Bognanno, MD and Frank J. Domino, MD

Titus S, Hodge J. Diagnosis and treatment of acne. *Am Fam Physician*. 2012;86:734–740.

ALCOHOL WITHDRAWAL, TREATMENT

History: Duration and quantity of alcohol intake, time since last drink, previous episodes of alcohol withdrawal, concurrent substance use, pre-existing medical and psychiatric conditions, prior detoxification admissions, prior seizure activity, living situation, social supports, stressors, triggers, etc.

Physical: VS (fever, tachycardia, tachypnea, hypertension), **CIWA** (see below), MSE (arousal, orientation, hallucinations), HEENT (diaphoresis, scleral icterus), CV (arrhythmias, M/R/G), eval s/sx liver failure (ascites, varices, caput medusae, asterixis, palmar erythema), neuro (nystagmus, tremor, seizure activity)

Include assessment of conditions likely to *complicate, exacerbate* or *precipitate* alcohol withdrawal: Arrhythmias, CHF, CAD, dehydration, GI bleeding, infections, liver disease, pancreatitis, neurologic deficits

Clinical Institute Withdrawal Assessment of Alcohol Scale (CIWA)

– Nausea and vomiting 0–7; (7-constant nausea, frequent dry heaves/vomiting)
– Tremor 0–7; (7-severe, even with arms not extended)
– Paroxysmal sweats 0–7; (7-drenching sweats)
– Anxiety 0–7; (7-acute panic state)
– Agitation 0–7; (7-constantly thrashing about or pacing)
– Tactile disturbances 0–7; (4–7 for hallucinations, 1–3 for pruritus or paresthesias)
– Auditory disturbances 0–7; (4–7 for hallucinations, 1–3 for increased sensitivity)
– Visual disturbances 0–7; (4–7 for hallucinations, 1–3 for increased sensitivity)
– Headache, fullness in head 0–7
– Orientation and clouding of sensorium 0–4:
 o Cannot do serial additions or is uncertain about date
 o Disoriented to date but within 2 calendar days
 o Disoriented to date by >2 days
 o Disoriented to place or person

Mild withdrawal; CIWA 0–7 (onset 5–8 hours after cessation or significant decrease in consumption): Anxiety, restlessness, agitation, mild nausea, decreased appetite, sleep disturbance, facial sweating, mild tremulousness, fluctuating tachycardia and hypertension, possible mild cognitive impairment

May be monitored as outpatient, *unless* pregnant, history of seizures or withdrawal seizures, chronic or acute comorbid illness requiring inpatient observation, lack of ability to follow-up

– Admit to inpatient detox program for monitoring
– Vital signs q4h; CIWA q1–3h

Moderate withdrawal; CIWA 8–14 (onset 24–72 hours after cessation): Marked restlessness and agitation, moderate tremulousness with constant eye movement, diaphoresis, nausea, vomiting, anorexia, diarrhea

– Admit to inpatient detox program
– Private room if possible
– Vital signs q4h
– CIWA q1–3h
– Institute seizure precautions
– IVF

Diazepam 20 mg PO q1–2h until CIWA<8, **OR**
Diazepam 2–5 mg IV/min–maximum 10–20 mg q1h
If severe liver disease, severe asthma or respiratory failure, elderly, debilitated, or low serum albumin:
Lorazepam SL, PO 1–2 mg q2–4h PRN

Long-acting benzodiazepines (diazepam) have rapid onset of action, and provide smooth treatment course with fewer breakthrough symptoms.
Short-acting (lorazepam) may have lower risk when there is concern about prolonged sedation, e.g., elderly patients or those with severe hepatic insufficiency.

Severe withdrawal/delirium tremens; CIWA >15 (onset 72–96 hours after alcohol cessation): Marked tremulousness, fever, drenching sweats, severe hypertension and tachycardia, delirium

– Admit to ICU for inpatient detox
– VS q30h
– CIWA q1h
– NPO, IVF
– Lateral decubitus position, restrain if necessary
– Glucose, Na, K, PO4, Mg replacement as needed

Diazepam 5–20 mg IV q10min until calm, then q1h to maintain light somnolence for duration of delirium
If severe liver disease, severe asthma or respiratory failure, elderly, debilitated, or low serum albumin:
Lorazepam 1–4 mg IV q10min until calm, then q1h to maintain light somnolence for duration of delirium

Labs: Tox screen/BAL to assess need for and timing of withdrawal regimen; electrolytes, phos, Mg with severe withdrawal [B12 and folate repleted regardless of levels], amylase/lipase if sx pancreatitis, PT, PTT if suspect liver failure; CBC if suspect infection
Imaging: Head CT if history of trauma or mental status changes out of range expected for degree of withdrawal. Seizure workup if no history of withdrawal seizures. Head CT and EEG if focal neurologic signs or prolonged post-ictal state

– **Thiamine** 100 mg IM/IV/PO q24h × 5 days; up to 1,000 mg/d if oculogyric crisis

– Sympatholytic adjunctive therapy: Atenolol 50–100 mg q24
Beta blockers and clonidine may be used only in conjunction with benzodiazepines because they *may mask symptoms of alcohol withdrawal and artificially lower CIWA score*, reduce peripheral signs and symptoms of alcohol withdrawal but have not been shown to prevent or treat delirium or seizures

– Phenothiazines for hallucinosis: Haloperidol 2–5 mg IM/PO q1–4h max 5 mg/d
used only in conjunction with benzodiazepines. May lower seizure threshold, use with extreme caution.

Discharge Planning:
– CIWA scores <8–10 for 24 hours
– Begin 1:1 or group therapy
– Discharge to treatment center, day program, home
– Facilitate entry into Alcoholics Anonymous
– Do not discharge with benzodiazepine rx
– Nutrition consult
– Social work consult

Alexis Lawrence, MD and Warren J. Ferguson, MD

Kosten TR, O'Connor PG. Management of drug and alcohol withdrawal. *N Engl J Med.* 2003;348:1786.

ALKALINE PHOSPHATASE ELEVATION

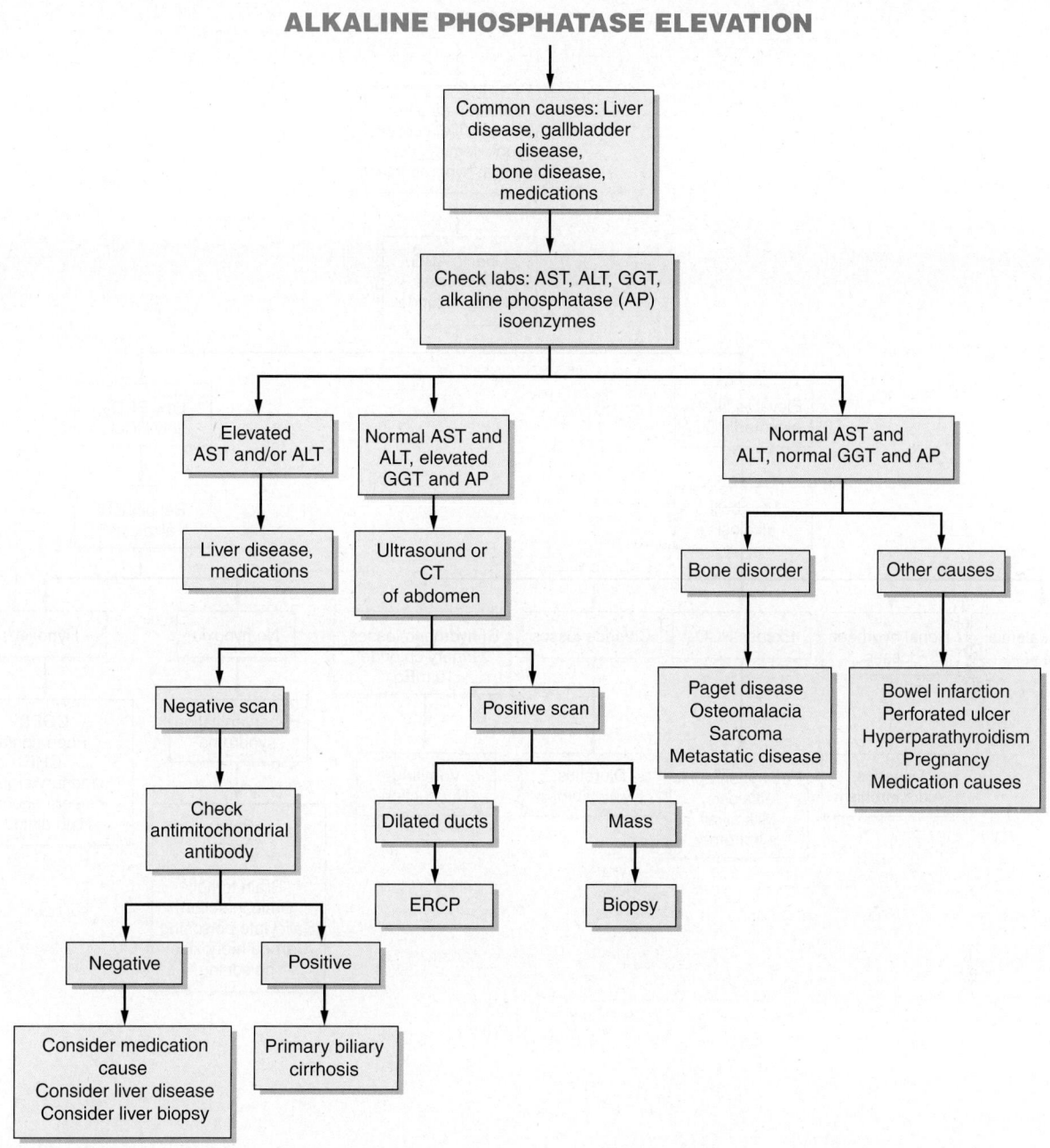

Common causes: Liver disease, gallbladder disease, bone disease, medications

↓

Check labs: AST, ALT, GGT, alkaline phosphatase (AP) isoenzymes

- Elevated AST and/or ALT → Liver disease, medications
- Normal AST and ALT, elevated GGT and AP → Ultrasound or CT of abdomen
  - Negative scan → Check antimitochondrial antibody
    - Negative → Consider medication cause / Consider liver disease / Consider liver biopsy
    - Positive → Primary biliary cirrhosis
  - Positive scan
    - Dilated ducts → ERCP
    - Mass → Biopsy
- Normal AST and ALT, normal GGT and AP
  - Bone disorder → Paget disease / Osteomalacia / Sarcoma / Metastatic disease
  - Other causes → Bowel infarction / Perforated ulcer / Hyperparathyroidism / Pregnancy / Medication causes

Tya-Mae Y. Julien, MD

Reust CE, Hall L. Clinical inquiries. What is the differential diagnosis of an elevated alkaline phosphatase (AP) level in an otherwise asymptomatic patient? *J Fam Pract.* 2001;50:496–497.

ALKALOSIS

Robert A. Baldor, MD and Alan M. Ehrlich, MD

Ayers P, Warrington L. Diagnosis and treatment of simple acid-base disorders. *Nutr Clin Pract.* 2008;23(2):122–127.

AMENORRHEA, SECONDARY

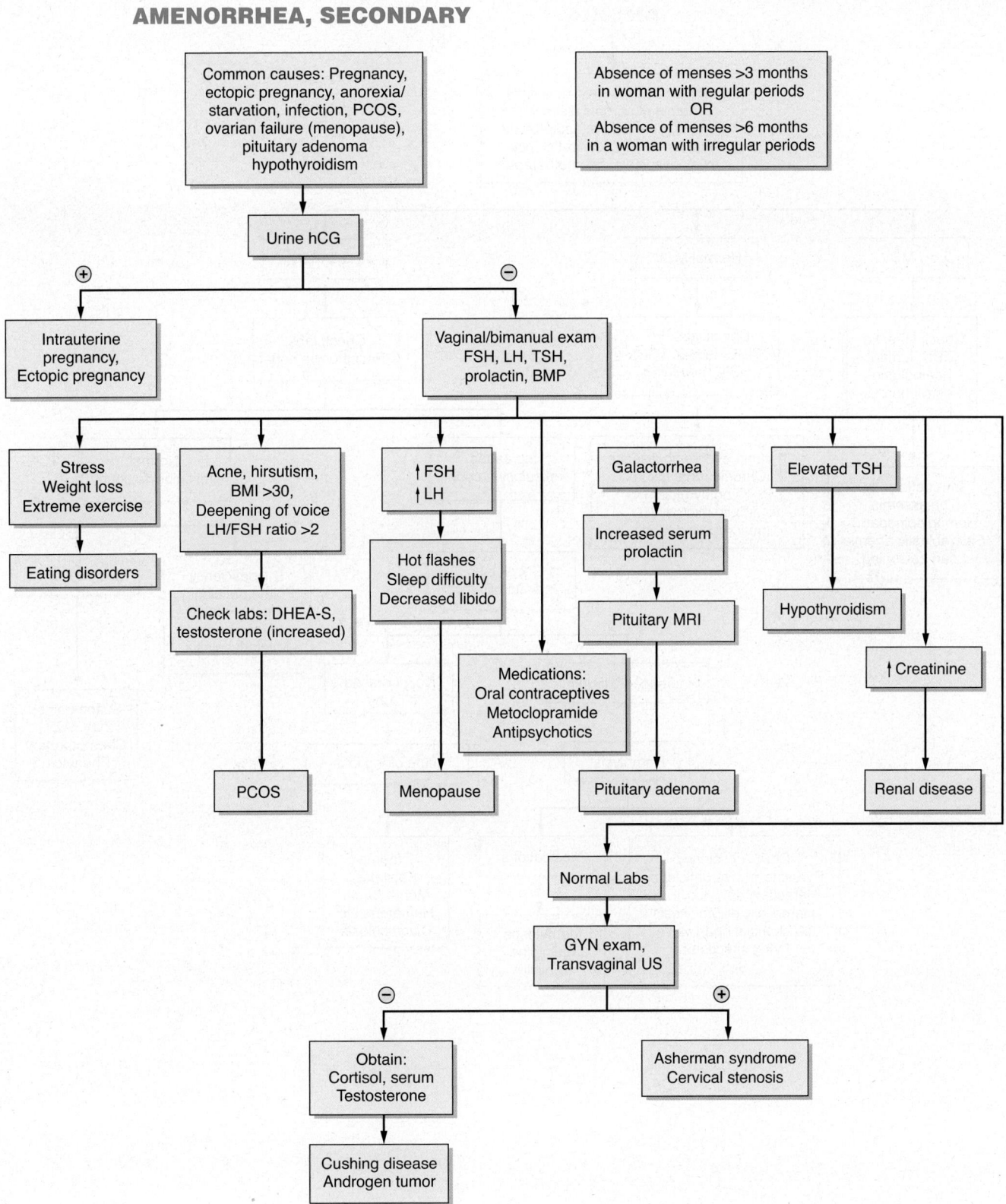

Maria Montanez, MD and Fozia Akhtar Ali, MD

Master-Hunter T, Heiman DL. Amenorrhea: Evaluation and treatment. *Am Fam Physician.* 2006;73:1374–1382.

ANEMIA

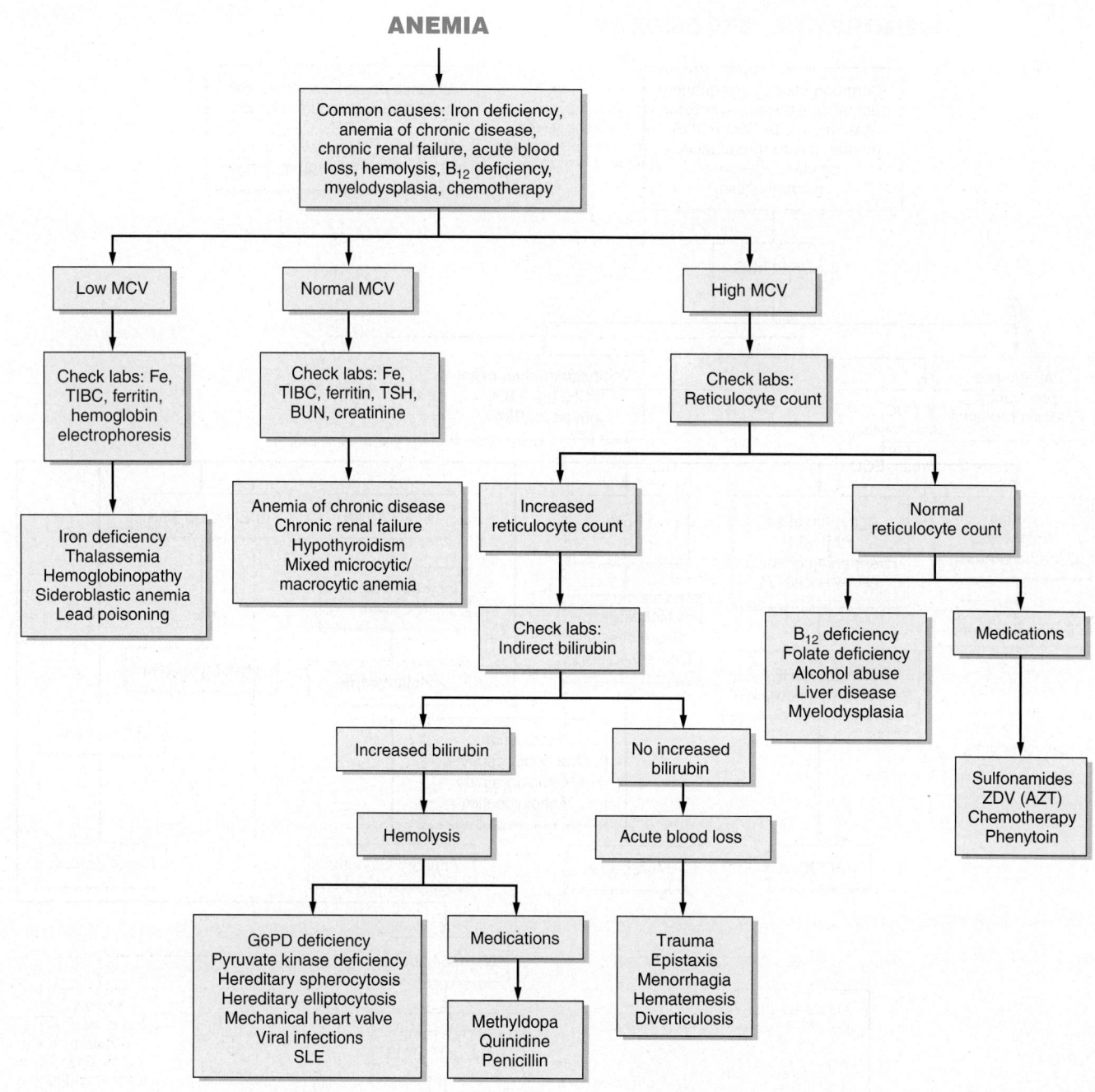

Common causes: Iron deficiency, anemia of chronic disease, chronic renal failure, acute blood loss, hemolysis, B_{12} deficiency, myelodysplasia, chemotherapy

Low MCV

Check labs: Fe, TIBC, ferritin, hemoglobin electrophoresis

Iron deficiency
Thalassemia
Hemoglobinopathy
Sideroblastic anemia
Lead poisoning

Normal MCV

Check labs: Fe, TIBC, ferritin, TSH, BUN, creatinine

Anemia of chronic disease
Chronic renal failure
Hypothyroidism
Mixed microcytic/macrocytic anemia

High MCV

Check labs: Reticulocyte count

Increased reticulocyte count

Check labs: Indirect bilirubin

Increased bilirubin

Hemolysis

G6PD deficiency
Pyruvate kinase deficiency
Hereditary spherocytosis
Hereditary elliptocytosis
Mechanical heart valve
Viral infections
SLE

Medications

Methyldopa
Quinidine
Penicillin

No increased bilirubin

Acute blood loss

Trauma
Epistaxis
Menorrhagia
Hematemesis
Diverticulosis

Normal reticulocyte count

B_{12} deficiency
Folate deficiency
Alcohol abuse
Liver disease
Myelodysplasia

Medications

Sulfonamides
ZDV (AZT)
Chemotherapy
Phenytoin

Robert A. Baldor, MD and Alan M. Ehrlich, MD

Smith DL. Anemia in the elderly. *Am Fam Physician*. 2000;62:1565–1572.

ANXIETY

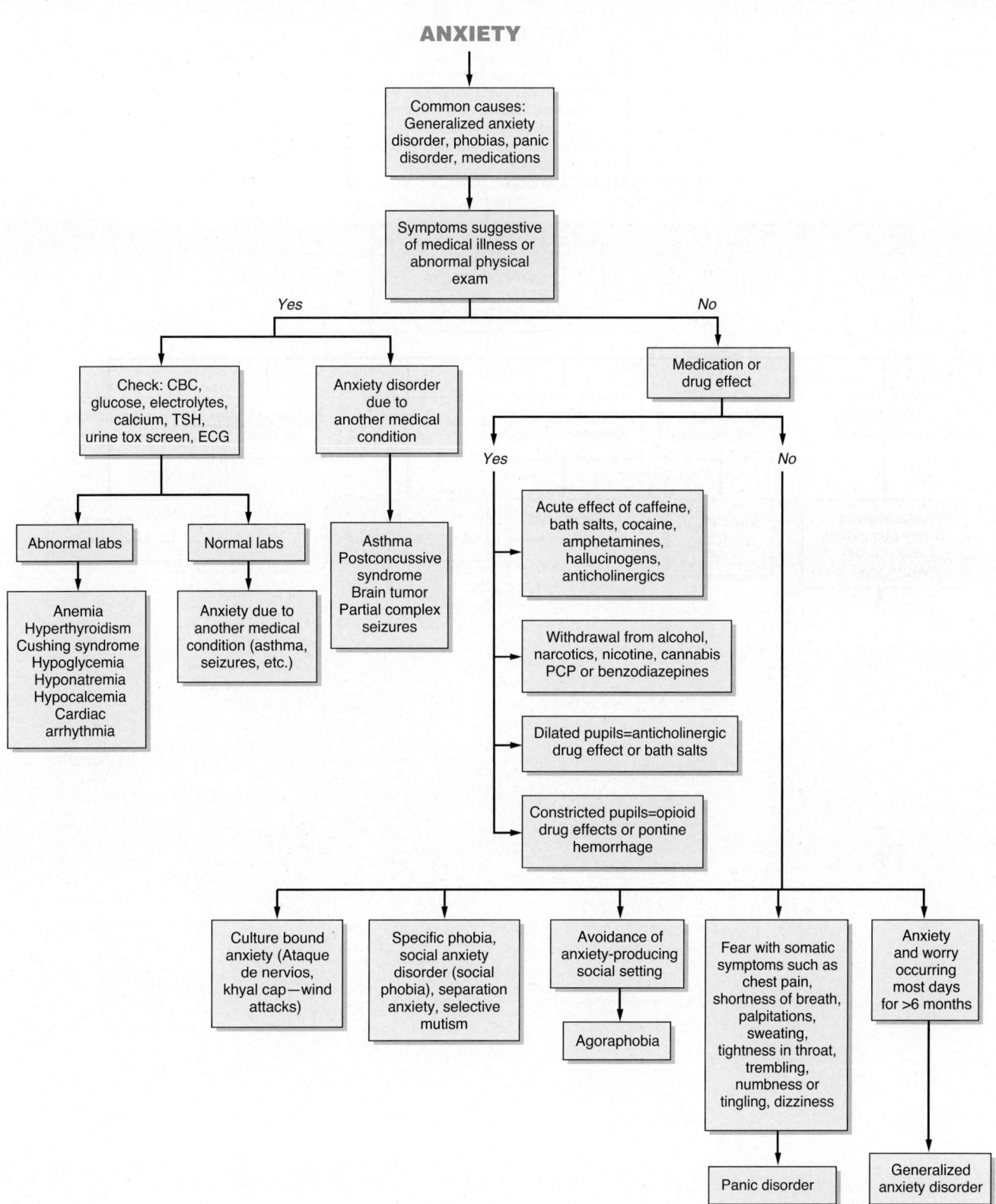

Bettina Bernstein, DO

Kavan MG, Elsasser G, Barone EJ. Generalized anxiety disorder: Practical assessment and management. *Am Fam Physician*. 2009;79(9):785–791.

AST ELEVATION

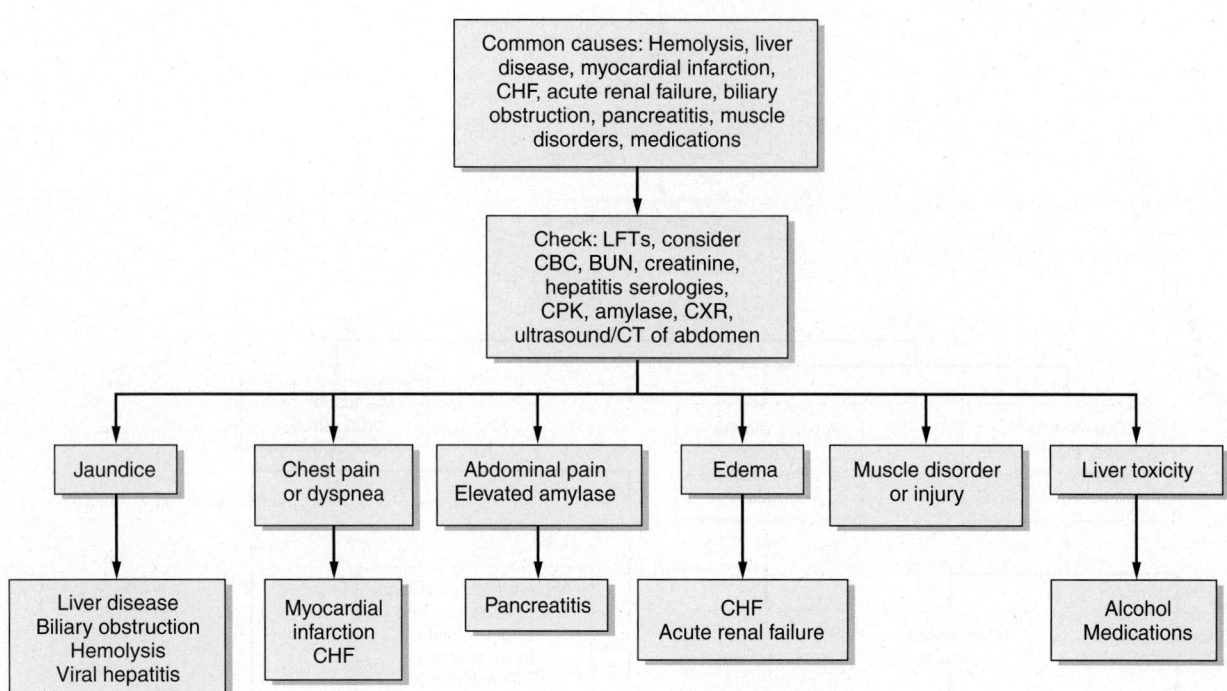

Common causes: Hemolysis, liver disease, myocardial infarction, CHF, acute renal failure, biliary obstruction, pancreatitis, muscle disorders, medications

Check: LFTs, consider CBC, BUN, creatinine, hepatitis serologies, CPK, amylase, CXR, ultrasound/CT of abdomen

Jaundice → Liver disease / Biliary obstruction / Hemolysis / Viral hepatitis

Chest pain or dyspnea → Myocardial infarction / CHF

Abdominal pain / Elevated amylase → Pancreatitis

Edema → CHF / Acute renal failure

Muscle disorder or injury

Liver toxicity → Alcohol / Medications

Robert A. Baldor, MD and Alan M. Ehrlich, MD

Giboney PT. Mildly elevated liver transaminase levels in the asymptomatic patient. *Am Fam Physician.* 2005;71:1105–1110.

ASTHMA EXACERBATION, PEDIATRIC ACUTE

Initial evaluation: Brief history, physical exam
History: Emergency department visits, hospital and ICU admissions, repeated courses of oral steroids, history of intubation, rapidly progressive episodes, or food allergy
Physical exam: Auscultation, use of accessory muscles, ability to speak, heart rate, respiratory rate

Severity	Respiratory rate (<6 yr)	(>6 yr)	Wheezing	Inspiratory expiratory ratio	Accessory muscle use	Oxygen saturation (room air)
Normal	30	20	None	2:1	None	99–100%
Mild	31–45	21–35	End expiration	1:1	+	96–98%
Moderate	46–60	36–50	Entire expiration	1:2	++	93–95%
Severe	>60	>50	Inspiration and expiration	1:3	+++	<93%

Mild exacerbation:
Inhaled β-agonist (nebulized or MDI with spacer) ×1
Consider systemic corticosteroid PO/IM if no immediate response or history of recent course of corticosteroids.
Check initial oxygen saturation level; no need for continuous pulse-ox monitoring.

Moderate exacerbation:
Inhaled β-agonist (nebulized or MDI with spacer) q20min, up to 3 doses in 1 hour
Inhaled ipratropium ×3 doses
Systemic corticosteroids PO/IM
Supplemental O_2 to achieve SaO_2 >90%

Severe exacerbation:
Inhaled β-agonist (nebulized or MDI with spacer) q20min ×3 doses or continuous ×1 hr.
Inhaled ipratropium ×3 doses
Systemic corticosteroids (PO/IM/IV)
Supplemental O_2 to achieve SaO_2 >90%
Consider IM epinephrine if imminent respiratory failure

Discharge criteria met?
In first 2 hours:
– Decreased/absent wheezing and retractions;
– Sustained SaO_2 >90% at least 60 minutes after last albuterol dose

Yes   *No*

Moderate exacerbation:
Inhaled β-agonist q20min
Continue treatment 1–3 hours, provided there is improvement.
Make admit decision in <4 hours; reassess after each treatment.

Severe exacerbation:
Severe symptoms at rest, accessory muscle use, no improvement after initial treatment
Nebulized β-agonist hourly or continuous
Consider magnesium sulfate IV.
Consider terbutaline infusion.
Consider heliox.
Consider endotracheal intubation for presumed or actual respiratory failure.
Make admit decision in <4 hours.

Discharge home
Patient education: Asthma action plan + inhaler technique.
Instructions for close follow-up.
Continue treatment with inhaled β-agonist and PO corticosteroid.
Continue or consider initiation of inhaled corticosteroid.

Discharge criteria met?
– Decreased/absent wheezing and retractions
– Sustained SaO_2 >90% on room air at least 60 minutes after last albuterol dose

No

Admission: ICU or closely monitored on floor

Yes

Catherine A. James, MD

National Asthma Education and Prevention Program. Expert Panel Report 3 (EPR-3): Guidelines for the Diagnosis and Management of Asthma-Summary Report. *J Allergy Clin Immunol.* 2007;120(5 Suppl):S94–S138.

ASTHMA, INITIAL TREATMENT

Management of Chronic Asthma
Classification of Asthma Severity in Youths ≥12 Years of Age and Adults

Components of Severety	Intermittent	Mild Persistent	Moderate Persistent	Severe Persistent
Symptoms	≤2 days/week	>2 days/week but not every day	Daily	Throughout the day
Nighttime awakenings	≤2 times/month	3 or 4 times/month	>1 time weekly, but not nightly	Often 7 times weekly
Short-acting β_2-agonist use for symptom control	≤2 days/week	>2 days/week, but not daily, and not more than 1 time on any day	Daily	Several times daily
Interference with normal activity	None	Minor limitation	Some limitation	Extremely limited
Lung function	• Normal FEV_1 between exacerbations • FEV_1 >80% predicted • FEV_1/FVC normal	• FEV_1 >80% predicted • FEV_1/FVC normal	• FEV_1 >60% but <80% predicted • FEV_1/FVC reduced 5%	• FEV_1 predicted • FEV_1/FVC reduced >5%
Astma exacerbations requiring oral steroids	0–1 year	≥2/year	≥2/year	≥2/year

Recommended step for initiating treatment	Step 1	Step 2	Step 3	Step 4 or 5
Preferred and alternative pharmacotherapy based on step	**Preferred:** Short-acting β_2-agonist as needed	**Preferred:** Low-dose ICS **Alternative:** Leukotriene modifier or theophylline	**Preferred:** Low-dose ICS + LABA or medium-dose ICS **Alternative:** Low-dose ICS + leukotriene modifier, theophylline or zileuton	**Step 4** **Preferred:** Medium-dose ICS + LABA **Alternative:** Medium-dose ICS + leukotriene modifier, theophylline or zileuton **Step 5** **Preferred:** High-dose ICS + LABA and consider omalizumab for patients with allergies **Step 6** **Preferred:** High-dose ICS + LABA + oral corticosteroid and consider omalizumab for patients with allergies

Michael C. Barros, PharmD, BCPS, BCACP, Colleen M. Prinzivalli, PharmD, BCPS, and J. Michael O'Connell, Jr., MD

Elward KS, Pollart SM. Medical Therapy for Asthma: Updates from the NAEPP Guidelines. *Am Fam Physician*. 2010;82:1242–1251.

ASTHMA, MAINTENANCE

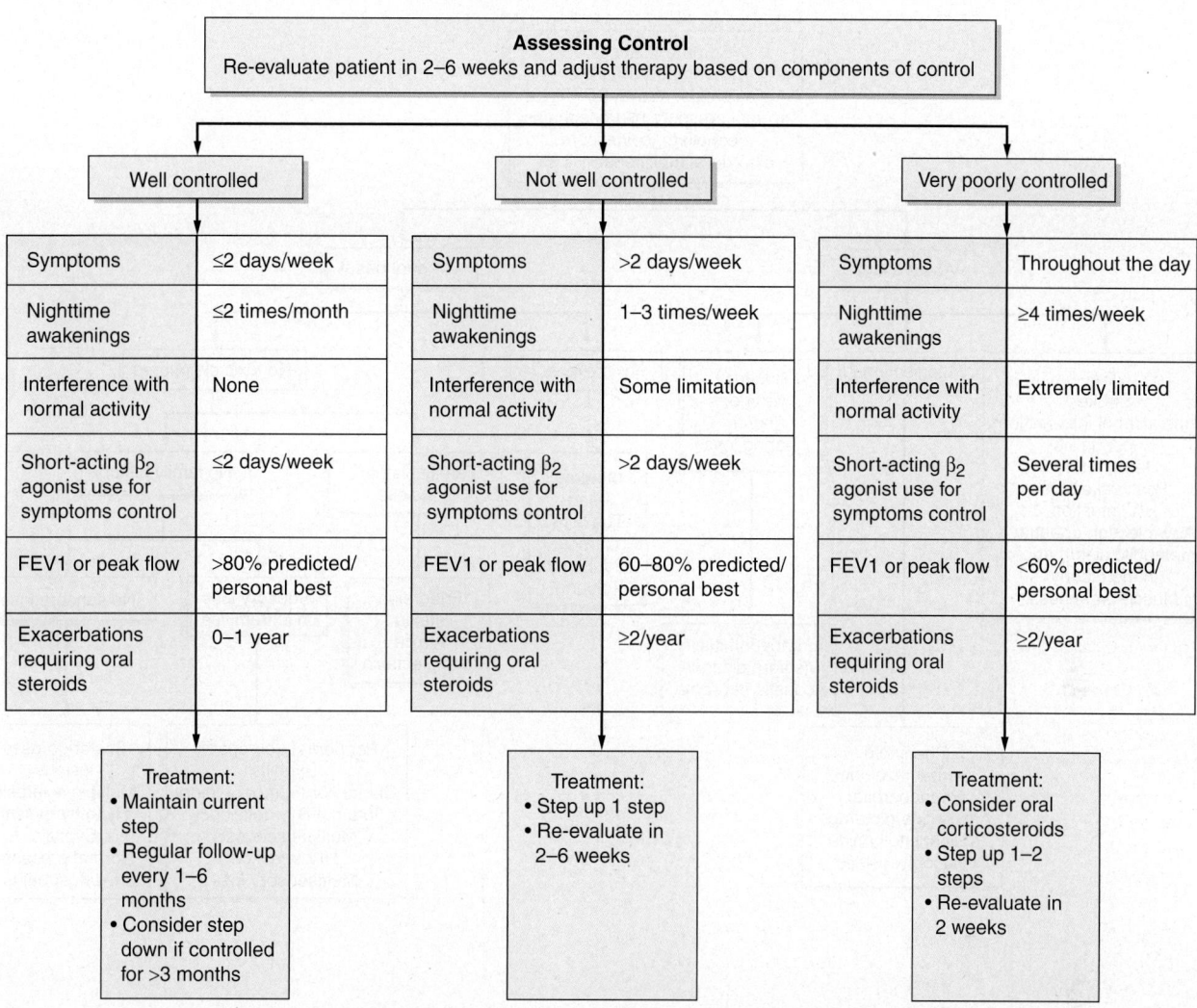

Assessing Control
Re-evaluate patient in 2–6 weeks and adjust therapy based on components of control

Well controlled

Symptoms	≤2 days/week
Nighttime awakenings	≤2 times/month
Interference with normal activity	None
Short-acting β₂ agonist use for symptoms control	≤2 days/week
FEV1 or peak flow	>80% predicted/ personal best
Exacerbations requiring oral steroids	0–1 year

Treatment:
• Maintain current step
• Regular follow-up every 1–6 months
• Consider step down if controlled for >3 months

Not well controlled

Symptoms	>2 days/week
Nighttime awakenings	1–3 times/week
Interference with normal activity	Some limitation
Short-acting β₂ agonist use for symptoms control	>2 days/week
FEV1 or peak flow	60–80% predicted/ personal best
Exacerbations requiring oral steroids	≥2/year

Treatment:
• Step up 1 step
• Re-evaluate in 2–6 weeks

Very poorly controlled

Symptoms	Throughout the day
Nighttime awakenings	≥4 times/week
Interference with normal activity	Extremely limited
Short-acting β₂ agonist use for symptoms control	Several times per day
FEV1 or peak flow	<60% predicted/ personal best
Exacerbations requiring oral steroids	≥2/year

Treatment:
• Consider oral corticosteroids
• Step up 1–2 steps
• Re-evaluate in 2 weeks

FVC = forced vital capacity; FEV_1 = forced expiratory volume in 1 second; ICS = inhaled corticosteroid; LABA = long acting

Michael C. Barros, PharmD, BCPS, BCACP, Colleen M. Prinzivalli, PharmD, BCPS, and J. Michael O'Connell, Jr., MD

Elward KS, Pollart SM. Medical Therapy for Asthma: Updates from the NAEPP Guidelines. *Am Fam Physician.* 2010;82:1242–1251.

ATAXIA

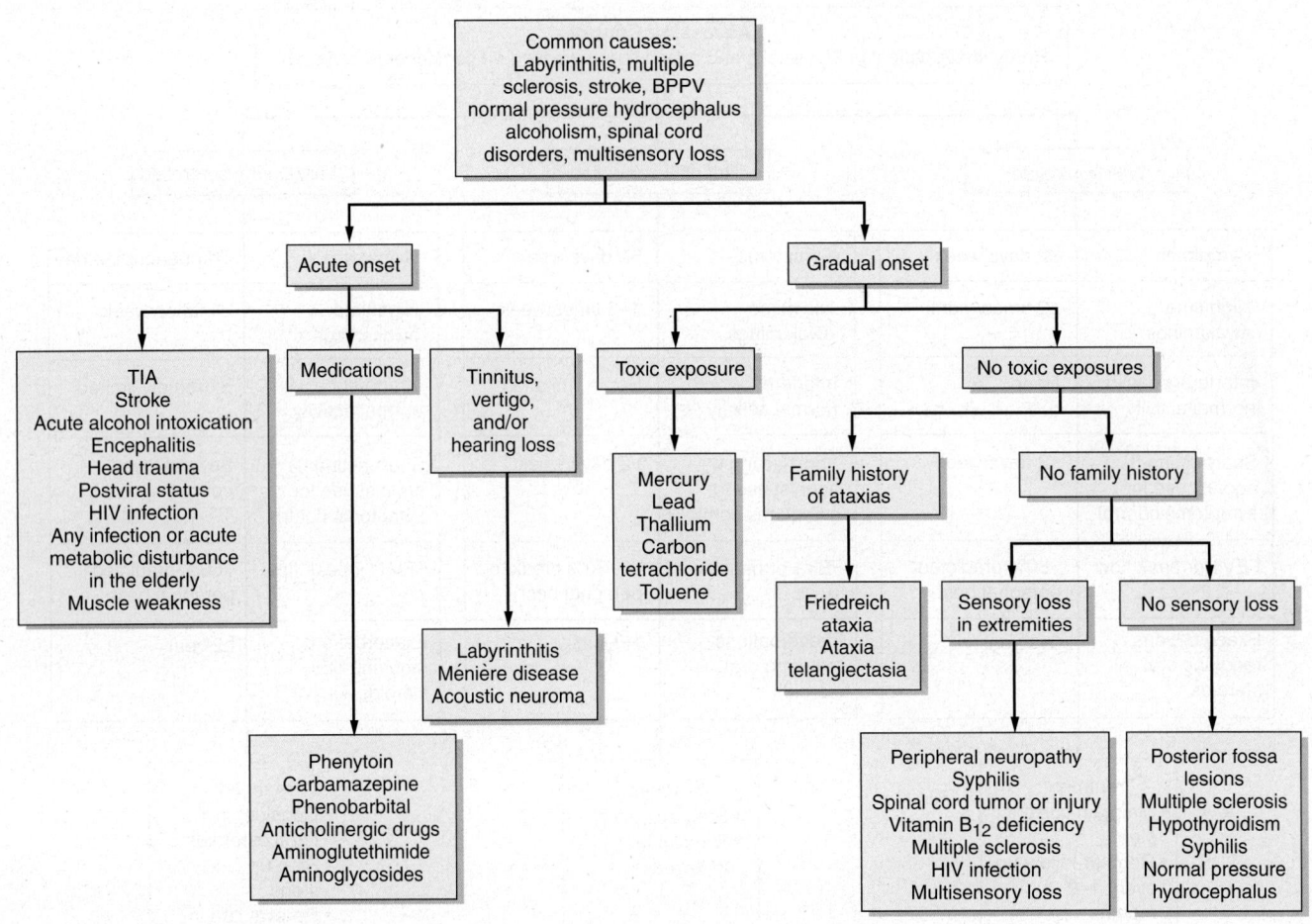

Robert A. Baldor, MD and Alan M. Ehrlich, MD

Pandolfo M. Friedreich ataxia. *Arch Neurol.* 2008;65(10):1296–1303.

BREAST DISCHARGE

Abigail Hoffman, MD, Ankur Goel, MD, and Edward Kruse, DO

Sabel MS, Helvie MA, Breslin T, et al. Is duct excision still necessary for all cases of suspicious nipple discharge? *Breast J.* 2012;18:157–162.

BREAST PAIN

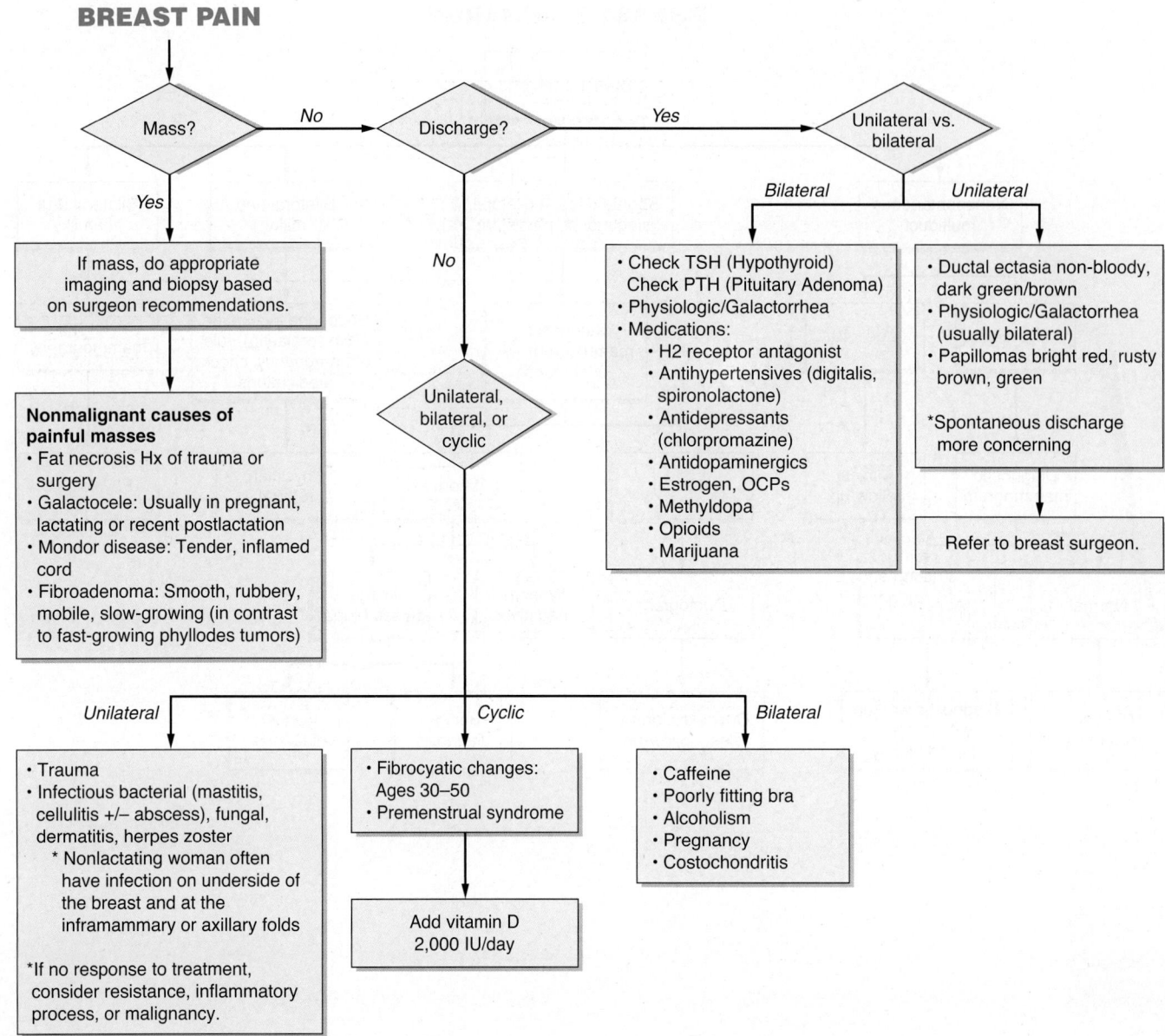

Nonmalignant causes of painful masses
- Fat necrosis Hx of trauma or surgery
- Galactocele: Usually in pregnant, lactating or recent postlactation
- Mondor disease: Tender, inflamed cord
- Fibroadenoma: Smooth, rubbery, mobile, slow-growing (in contrast to fast-growing phyllodes tumors)

If mass, do appropriate imaging and biopsy based on surgeon recommendations.

Mass? — No → **Discharge?** — Yes → **Unilateral vs. bilateral**

Yes

No

Bilateral / *Unilateral*

Unilateral, bilateral, or cyclic

Bilateral
- Check TSH (Hypothyroid) Check PTH (Pituitary Adenoma)
- Physiologic/Galactorrhea
- Medications:
  - H2 receptor antagonist
  - Antihypertensives (digitalis, spironolactone)
  - Antidepressants (chlorpromazine)
  - Antidopaminergics
  - Estrogen, OCPs
  - Methyldopa
  - Opioids
  - Marijuana

Unilateral
- Ductal ectasia non-bloody, dark green/brown
- Physiologic/Galactorrhea (usually bilateral)
- Papillomas bright red, rusty brown, green

*Spontaneous discharge more concerning

Refer to breast surgeon.

Unilateral
- Trauma
- Infectious bacterial (mastitis, cellulitis +/– abscess), fungal, dermatitis, herpes zoster
  * Nonlactating woman often have infection on underside of the breast and at the inframammary or axillary folds

*If no response to treatment, consider resistance, inflammatory process, or malignancy.

Cyclic
- Fibrocyatic changes: Ages 30–50
- Premenstrual syndrome

Add vitamin D 2,000 IU/day

Bilateral
- Caffeine
- Poorly fitting bra
- Alcoholism
- Pregnancy
- Costochondritis

Mohamad Masoumy, MD, Varun K. Bhalla, MD, and E. James Kruse, DO

Salzman B, Fleegle S, Tully AS. Common breast problems. *Am Fam Physician.* 2012;86(4):343–349.

CARDIAC ARRHYTHMIAS

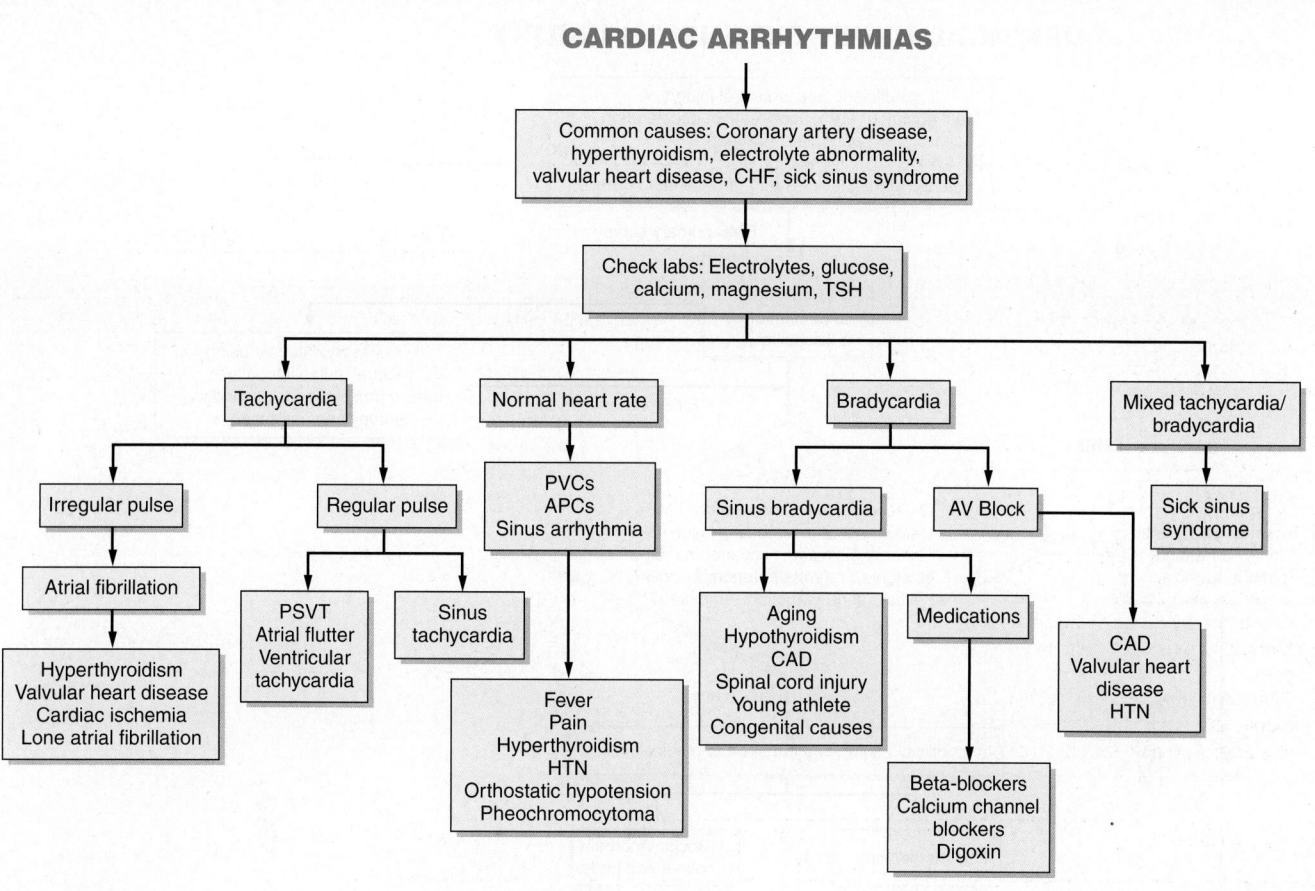

Amaninderapal Ghotra, MD, Suma Chennubhotla, MD, and Kelly McCants, MD

Link M. Evaluation and Initial Treatment of superventricular tachycardia. *N Engl J Med.* 2012;367:1438–1448.

CERVICAL HYPEREXTENSION INJURY

Sufficient mechanism of injury:
Most common: MVA, acceleration–deceleration,
sports, falls (>3 feet)
and/or
Trauma above the clavicles (e.g., frontal head or face)

EMS primary survey

Airway
Breathing
Circulation
Disability

If necessary, intubate using
manual in-line intubation
before proceeding to secondary
survey/immobilization.

EMS primary survey

On-Scene (EMS)

On-scene/side-line evaluation (EMS):
Assessment of mechanism—high risk?
Neurologic exam—impaired motor,
sensory or reflexes? Nonambulatory?
Neck range of motion—impaired?

No to all → Restrict activity until follow up without patient physician.

Yes to any

Immobilize C-spine and transport to medical facility.

No helmet/pads

Hockey/football helmet and pads

*Leave helmet/pads in place.
Remove facemask.*

Rigid collar, spine board

Physician primary survey

ABCDs → Hemodynamically unstable → IV crystalloid, blood transfusion, pressors search for hemorrhagic source Intubate with MLI if necessary

Hemodynamically stable

Goal MAP 90 mmHg?
Yes
No

Physician secondary survey

Imaging for clinically significant spinal injury?

Neurogenic shock
Administer IV steroids
Emergent surgical decompression
with postop imaging

NEXUS low-risk criteria:
No posterior cervical midline tenderness
No abnormal level of alertness
No evidence of intoxication
No painful/distracting injuries
No abnormal neurologic symptoms
(unconscious, numbness, weakness,
paralysis, or neck pain/cervical
tenderness)

Meets all 5 criteria

OR

Fails any 1 of the criteria

Yes to ≥1

No

Neurologic symptoms indicative of cord compression or central cord syndrome?

Yes

No

Conservative Management: NSAIDs, analgesics, muscle relaxants Rest with possible soft collar Follow up in 3 weeks.

Canadian cervical spine rules: High Risk?: Dangerous/high-speed mechanism Age: >65 or <9 Extremity parasthesias or focal neurologic symptoms

Yes to ≥1

IV methylprednisolone bolus 30 mg/kg over 15 minutes

Time from injury?

Persistent symptoms?

No to all

<3 hours

3–8 hours

Low risk?: Simple rear-end MVA Able to sit up in ED Able to ambulate any point after injury Delayed onset of neck pain

No to all

5.4 mg/kg/hr IV for 24 hours

5.4 mg/kg/hr IV for 48 hours

Yes to ≥1

Yes

Neck active ROM 45° to left and right?

No

C-spine plain films—3 views: AP, lateral, and odontoid (flexion–extension only if asymptomatic, without neurologic deficits or mental impairment)

Fracture or stenosis

Cervical CT, spinal MRI, or CT myelogram

Persistent clinical suspicion

No

Yes

Central cord syndrome, hangman fracture, Odontoid fracture, C3–C7 hyperextension fracture

Rest and immobilization

No

Unstable?

Yes

Surgical decompression, fixation, and immobilization. IV methylprednisolone if not already given

Kevin Jillson, MD and Kylee Eagles, DO

Pimentel L, Diegelmann L. Evaluation and management of acute cervical spine trauma. *Emerg Med Clin North Am.* 2010;28(4):719–738.

CHEST PAIN/ACUTE CORONARY SYNDROME

Sandra Beverly, MD and Naomi F. Botkin, MD

2005 International Consensus on Cardiopulmonary Resuscitation and Emergency Cardiovascular Care Science with Treatment Recommendations. Part 5: Acute Coronary Syndromes. *Circulation.* 2005;112:III-55–III-72.

CHILD ABUSE

BE SUSPICIOUS FOR INTENTIONAL TRAUMA IF:
• A vague explanation for an injury
• An important detail of caregiver's explanation changes significantly
• Caregiver's or patient's story is inconsistent with pattern, age, or severity of injury
• Explanation is inconsistent with child's physical and/or developmental capabilities
• Different witnesses provide different explanations for the injury
• Caregiver(s) refuse to permit child to be interviewed alone

MEDICAL HISTORY
(When interviewing children, it is important to ask open ended questions that do not introduce concepts of abusive acts/abuser. Document direct quotes of child and caretaker as part of the history.)
1. Routine past medical history (trauma, hospitalizations, congenital/chronic illnesses)
2. Family history (bleeding, bone, metabolic, genetic)
3. Developmental history
4. Previous hospitalizations/ED visits for injury
*Note: The history-taking is the most important part of the child abuse exam—documenting who, what, when, where (and how the stories differ between caregivers and patient).

PHYSICAL EXAM
1. General assessment—child's alertness, demeanor, degree of pain, growth chart parameters, evidence of neglect (severe dental caries, diaper dermatitis, neglected wound care, cachexia)
2. Complete head-to-toe exam (skin: bruises, lacerations, burns, bites)
3. Consider photographs and/or sketches of physical signs.
4. Complete a neurological exam.

DIAGNOSTIC TESTS
(As indicated based on exam)
1. "Skeletal survey" (mandatory for suspected abuse in children <2 years old)
2. Hematologic tests (CBC, platelets, PT/PTT/INR, bleeding time)
3. Retinal exam
4. Liver enzymes
5. Pancreatic enzymes
6. Urinalysis
7. MRI (head/neck)
8. CT (head/abdomen)
9. Cardiac enzymes
10. Radionuclide bone scan
11. Skin biopsy for fibroblast culture or DNA analysis of blood (osteogenesis imperfecta)
12. Calcium, ALP, phosphorus, vitamin D, PTH (bone-mineralization disorders)
*Note: Obtain neuroimaging in children if nonaccidental head injury suspected, and consider in all children <6 months in whom any inflicted injury suspected.

MANAGEMENT
1. Referral to investigative agencies/child-protection agencies according to state-specific mandated reporting laws (800-442-4453). In most states, health care providers are mandated to report suspected abuse/neglect. State reporting statutes and other resources are available from the Child Welfare Information Gateway (www.childwelfare.gov).
2. Referral to appropriate medical providers (such as pediatric trauma center)
3. Medicolegal documentation

Jaclyn EA Legg, DO and Gautam J. Desai, DO, FACOFP

Lamb ME, Orbach Y, Hershkowitz I, et al. A structured forensic interview protocol improves the quality and informativeness of investigative interviews with children: A review of research using the NICHD Investigative Interview Protocol. *Child Abuse Negl.* 2007;31:1201.

CHRONIC OBSTRUCTIVE PULMONARY DISEASE (COPD), DIAGNOSIS AND TREATMENT

Suspect COPD if:
- Chronic cough and/or sputum production
- History of smoking or chemical exposure
- Dyspnea at rest and exertion

Spirometry with pre- and postbronchodilator

Severity of change 1

	FEV1/FVC	FEV1
Mild	<0.7	>00
Moderate	<0.7	50–80
Severe	<0.7	30–50
Very severe	<0.7	<50

Functional Dyspnea Scale

0 Not troubled with breathlessness except with strenuous exercise.
1 Troubled by shortness of breath when hurrying or walking up a slight hill.
2 Walks slower than people of same age due to breathlessness or has to stop for breath when walking at own pace on the level.
3 Stops for breath after walking ~100 m or after a few minutes on the level.
4 Too breathless to leave the house or breathless when dressing or undressing.

Diagnosis confirmed, initiate preventative measures:
Influenza vaccine (yearly), pneumococcal vaccine one dose before age 65, one after age 65, at least 5 years after previous dose

Aggressive smoking cessation counseling if actively smoking

Mild COPD

– FEV1 >50%
– FDS = 0 or 1

Treatment:
– Short-acting beta-agonist or anti-cholinergic PRN

Moderate COPD

– FEV1 >50%
– FDS ≥2

Treatment:
– Long-acting beta-agonist or anti-cholinergic

Severe COPD

– FEV1 ≤50%
– FDS = 0 or 1

Treatment:
– Inhaled corticosteroid plus
– Long-acting anticholinergic
– Pulmonary rehabilitation
– Assess for supplemental Oxygen*
– Short-acting beta-agonist

Very severe COPD

– FEV1 ≤50%
– FDS ≥2

Treatment:
– Inhaled corticosteroids plus
– Long-acting anticholinergic plus
– Long-acting beta-agonist
– Pulmonary rehabilitation
– Assess for supplemental oxygen*
– Consider surgical options and/or adding a phosphodiesterase inhibitor

*Supplemental Oxygen Determination:

– $PaO_2 \leq 55$ mm Hg OR $SaO_2 \leq 88\%$
    OR
– $PaO_2 \leq 59$ mm Hg OR $SaO_2 \leq 89\%$ AND Symptoms of Cor Pulmonale, Right Heart Failure or HCT >55%

No

Yes

Continue current treatment

Consider long-term supplemental oxygen therapy

Scott Kopec, MD

Global Strategy for the Diagnosis, Management and Prevention of COPD, Global Initiative for Chronic Obstructive Lung Disease (GOLD) 2013. Available at: http://www.goldcopd.org/

CONCUSSION, PEDIATRIC

Concussion: Traumatic event AND change in neurologic function OR one of the following signs/ symptoms: **Somatic** (HA, N/V, dizziness, vertigo, visual problems, sensitivity to light or sound, numbness/ tingling), **cognitive** (LOC, memory problems, feeling "foggy," slower reaction times, confusion), **emotional/behavioral** (i.e., irritability, sadness), **sleep** (i.e., drowsiness, difficulty falling asleep)

Evaluate ABCs, check for C-spine injury. Remove from play.

Stable | *Unstable*

Assess with standardized tool (SCAT2, SAC, Maddock's Questions, BESS, etc.): Vital signs, GCS, orientation, past and immediate memory, concentration, balance, coordination, delayed recall
-SCAT2 available at www.cces.ca/en/files-116

Transfer to ED. Activate trauma team if needed. C-spine precautions if indicated. Continue to assess ABCs. Continue First Aid.

Full history and PE (head and neck evaluation, complete neurological exam).

Vital Signs q5min: Do not leave patient alone.

GCS ≤14, signs of altered mental status,* or signs of skull fracture

Condition back to baseline | Condition not back to baseline

No | *Yes*

Continued monitoring at home and evaluation by medical professional within 24 hours.

Occipital or parietal or temporal scalp hematoma, or LOC ≥5 sec, or severe mechanism of injury,‡ or not acting normally per parent

Noncontrast head CT (or less commonly, MRI)

Abnormal | *Normal*

No | *Yes*

No imaging.

Appropriate treatment (neurosurgical consult for bleeding or edema)

A. Follow up with medical professional in next 24 hours
  • History and PE (including complete neurological exam)
  • Consider neuropsych testing.
  • If at neurologic baseline, review Return to Play protocol.
  • If not at neurologic baseline, consider ED evaluation, close follow-up, and symptomatic treatment.
B. Consider neuropsych testing (paper-and-pencil, ImPACT, CogState, HeadMinder, etc.).
  • The ideal timing, frequency, and type of neuropsych testing have not been determined
  • Most concussions can be managed appropriately without the use of neuropsych testing
  • Neuropsych testing may be most helpful for high-risk athletes, those with prior concussions, and those who may downplay symptoms in an effort to return to play sooner
C. Return to Play protocol:
  • No athlete may return to play the same day.
  • Once asymptomatic at a stage for 24 hours, may move on to next stage; if symptoms arise, must take a 24-hour period of complete rest before dropping back one stage and starting from there.
  • Most athletes should return no sooner than 6 days after concussion.
      o Stage 1: No activity (complete physical AND cognitive rest)
      o Stage 2: Light aerobic exercise (walking, swimming, or stationary cycling at <70% max HR)
      o Stage 3: Sport-specific exercise (sport-specific drills such as skating or running, no head impact activities)
      o Stage 4: Noncontact training drills (progression to more complex training drills such as passing, may start progressive resistance training)
      o Stage 5: Full contact practice
      o Stage 6: Return to game play (should also be free of any medicines that could mask symptoms of concussion)
  • Please note initial cognitive rest and a graded resumption of typical cognitive activity is also important. Patients may require accommodations such as a shortened school day, reduced academic workload, extended time for tests, etc. when recovering from a concussion.
D. Symptom management: If concussive symptoms (typically HA, sleep, cognitive, and mood disturbances) are persistent and interfering with function, consider symptomatic treatment.
  • In the acute setting, ASA and NSAIDs should be used with caution due to increased risk of intracranial bleeding. Acetaminophen and physical modalities are OK.
  • If HA persists for a few days, consider typical abortive treatment. There is no established role for pharmacotherapy in the acute treatment of concussion-induced sleep, cognitive, or mood disturbances.
  • If symptoms persist beyond a few weeks, consider referral to specialist (neurology, sports medicine, etc.). Multidisciplinary approach is often needed.
  • If symptoms do not resolve despite appropriate evaluation and treatment, consider terminating athletic season or athletic career (no clear guidelines have been established; this decision should be made on a case-by-case basis).

*Signs of altered mental status: Agitation, somnolence, repetitive questioning, or slow response to verbal communication
‡Severe mechanism of injury: Motor vehicle crash with patient ejection, death of another passenger, or rollover; pedestrian or bicyclist without helmet struck by motorized vehicle; falls of >3 ft for patients <2 years old or >5 ft for patients ≥2 years old; or head struck by high-impact object

Michelle McCreary, MD and Frank J. Domino, MD

Kuppermann N, Holmes JF, Dayan PS, et al. Identification of children at very low risk of clinically-important brain injuries after head trauma: A prospective cohort study. *Lancet.* 2009;374:1160–1170.

CONGESTIVE HEART FAILURE: DIFFERENTIAL DIAGNOSIS

Common causes: CAD, HTN, MI, cardiomyopathy, AFib, aortic valve dysfunction

History: Orthopnea, paroxysmal nocturnal dyspnea, nocturia, dyspnea on exertion or rest, nocturnal cough.

Physical exam: Elevated jugular venous pressure, hepatojugular reflex, S3 gallop, rales, pedal edema.

Check: Chest x-ray, ECG, echocardiogram, BNP, troponin (if suspicion of acute coronary syndrome)

Diagnosis of CHF requires presence of 2 major criteria or 1 major + 2 minor criteria.

Major criteria:
• Paroxysmal nocturnal dyspnea
• Neck vein distention
• Rales
• Radiographic cardiomegaly (increasing heart size on chest radiography)
• Acute pulmonary edema
• S3 gallop
• Increased central venous pressure (>16 cm H_2O at right atrium)
• Hepatojugular reflux
• Weight loss >4.5 kg in 5 days in response to treatment

Minor criteria:
• Bilateral ankle edema
• Nocturnal cough
• Dyspnea on ordinary exertion
• Hepatomegaly
• Pleural effusion
• Decrease in vital capacity by 1/3 from maximum recorded
• Tachycardia (heart rate >120 beats/min)

Minor criteria are acceptable only if they can not be attributed to another medical condition.

Not CHF

Look for alternative diagnosis:
• Asthma
• COPD
• Pulmonary embolus
• Interstitial lung disease

CHF

Evaluate for causes of CHF:
• Ischernic: CAD/MI
• Nonischemic: HTN, valvular disease, thyrotoxicosis, HIV/infections, tachycardia-mediated, medications, drugs, chemotherapeutic agents, stress induced cardiomyopathy, vitamin deficiencies (thiamine, selenium), alcohol.

• History of angina/CAD
• Positive troponins
• Positive stress test
• Obstructive CAD on coronary angiogram

Nonischemic cardiomyopathy

Ischemic cardiomyopathy

Mitral regurgitation, aortic stenosis or aortic regurgitation on echo

Atrial fibrillation/flutter, SVT, very frequent PVC's on ECG or telemetry

HTN, thyrotoxicosis, alcoholism, medications (chemotherapy), drugs (cocaine), autoimmune and collagen vascular disorders, infiltrative disorders (amyloidosis, hemochromatosis), disordered sleep

Nonspecific viral-mediated or idiopathic cardiomyopathy

Cardiomyopathy secondary to valvular heart disease

Tachycardia-mediated cardiomyopathy

Nirmanmoh Bhatia, MD and Carrie G. Lenneman, MD, MSCI

King M, Kingery J, Casey B. Diagnosis and Evaluation of Heart Failure. *Am Fam Physician.* 2012;85(12):1161–1168.

CONSTIPATION, DIAGNOSIS AND TREATMENT (ADULT)

Rome III Criteria:
- 2 of the following for 12 weeks in past 6 months
  - <3 stools/week
  - For 25% of time, any of the following:
    - Hard stools
    - Straining
    - Manual assist
    - Sense of incomplete evacuation
    - Sense of anorectal blockade
- Rare loose stools without laxative use

Common causes: Primary—functional, slow transit, pelvic floor dysfunction; Secondary—IBS, diabetes mellitus, hypothyroidism, hypercalcemia, pregnancy, obstruction, medication side effect

History & Physical:
Diet, fluid intake, exercise, Rome III criteria, digital rectal exam, abdominal exam, neurological exam

Red flags:
Unintentional weight loss, Hematochezia, Family Hx IBD or colon cancer, positive fecal occult, anemia, new onset in age >50, Change in stool size, neurological findings

Yes → Colonoscopy

No

Consider medication effect: Adjust and/or begin with empiric treatment

Yes

Medication Hx: Anticholinergics, opiates, calcium channel blockers, antidepressants, antacids

No

Diagnostic testing: CBC, glucose, creatinine, calcium, TSH

Negative

Positive

Anemia

Hypothyroidism

Hypercalcemia

Diabetes mellitus

Empiric treatment: Increase exercise and water intake. Trial of fiber of bulk-forming laxatives

Symptoms improved

No → Add polyethylene glycol and/or stimulant laxative.

Yes

Functional constipation

Yes ← Symptoms improved

No

Treatment failure

Diagnostic testing: Colonic transit time study (CTT) Balloon expulsion test (BET) Anorectal manometry (AM)

Abnormal CTT

Normal CTT, abnormal BET, AM

Slow transit constipation

Pelvic floor dysfunction

Treatments above, enemas biofeedback

Treatments above, biofeedbacks, also Botox, surgery

Jacquelyn Cambers, MD and Robert A. Baldor, MD

Longstreth GF, Thompson WG, Chey WD, et al. Functional bowel disorders. *Gastroenterology.* 2006;130:1480–1491.

CONSTIPATION, TREATMENT (PEDIATRIC)

Child with hard stools, ≤2 bowel movements per week, or incontinence after toilet trained

Do careful H&P including Digital Rectal Exam-assess rectal tone and determine the presence of rectal distention or impaction

Any of the following present on history?
- Passage of meconium >48 hours after birth
- Onset after introduction to cow's milk
- Weight loss/poor weight gain
- Delayed growth/failure to thrive
- Fever, vomiting, diarrhea, alternating with constipation
- Urinary incontinence (bladder disease)
- Bloody stools

Physical exam findings?
- Decreased muscular tone
- Presence of pilonidal dimple or hair tuft (Spinal abnormalities)
- Abnormal anatomical appearance of anus

Yes (<5%)   *No*

Organic causes:
- Hirschsprung's
- Cystic fibrosis
- Gluten enteropathy or lactose intolerance
- Congenital anorectal malformations
- Heavy metal poisoning
- Developmental delay
- Spinal cord abnormalities (myelomeningocele)

Metabolic causes:
- Hypothyroidism
- Diabetes insipidus
- Hypokalemia
- Hypercalcemia

Other causes:
- Pseudo-obstruction
- Medication side effect

Functional constipation

Dietary changes and family education
- High-fiber diet (1–5 years: 14 g/d; 5–13 years: 17–25 g/d; 13 years: 25–31 g/d). Fiber increased gradually to minimize flatulence.
- Limit caffeine and milk products (>16 oz/d of milk)

Persists?

Yes   *No*

1. Disimpaction with enemas, rectal suppositories, or oral agents (polyethylene glycol: Maximum dose of MiraLAX or Go-Lytely 1.5 g/kg in 4–6 oz of water).

2. Maintenance: ≤6 months sorbitol-containing juices, lactulose; >6 months lactulose (0.7–2 g/kg/d [1–3 mL/kg/d], max 40 g/d [60 mL/d]) or MiraLAX (0.5–1 g/kg max 17 g/d).

Follow up on compliance to dietary changes

Persists?

Yes   *No*

Adjust meds for ≥3 BMs per week. Start maintenance program—Goal is to maintain soft bowel movements once or twice a day.

Continue treatment.

Tarina Desai, MD and Fozia Akhtar Ali, MD

Constipation Guideline Committee of the North American Society for Pediatric Gastroenterology, Hepatology and Nutrition. Evaluation and treatment of constipation in infants and children: Recommendations of the North American Society for Pediatric Gastroenterology, Hepatology and Nutrition. *J Pediatr Gastroenterol Nutr.* 2006;43(3):e1–e13.

CONTRACEPTION

Does she want short- or long-term contraception?

→ Short-term
→ Long-term

Short-term branch

Any contraindications against using estrogen?

Yes:

Condoms:
Male Condom: 82% effective
Female Condom: 79% effective
– Both provide STD protection

Other Barrier Methods:
– Diaphragm
– Sponge
– Cervical Cap
– +/– Spermicide
– Efficacy 72.88%
– Less widely used
– Efficacy ↑ with dual contraceptive use for all barrier methods

Fertility Awareness Methods:
– Less effective (76%)
– Nonhormonal, nonsurgical, natural methods
– Based on avoiding prime ovulation days during cycle
– Ovulation
– Standard Day
– Two Day
– Symptothermal

Progestin Only Pills/Mini Pill:
– Good efficacy (91%)
– Must be taken at same time everyday
– Likely to cause breakthrough bleeding

No:

Can she reliably take medication daily?

Yes →

Breastfeeding <1 month

Yes → Progestin Only Pills/Mini Pill

No →

Combined Oral Contraceptive Methods:
– Good efficacy (91%)
– Many non conctraceptive benefits, ↓ dysmenorrhea, cycle control
– Continuous cycling/extended formulations available
– Daily dosing
– Estrogen-related AE, ↑ risk of VTE

No (can't take daily):

Transdermal Method:
– Ortho-Evra
– Good efficacy (91%)
– Nonconctraceptive benefits, ↓ dysmenorrhea, cycle control
– Once-weekly dosing
– 48-hour "window of forgiveness"
– Contraindicated in women >90 kg
– **Black Box Warning:** Increased estrogen-related AE, especially VTE

Intravaginal Method:
– Nuva-Ring
– Good efficacy (91%)
– Lower hormone doses
– Simple to use
– Once a month dosing
– Many nonconctraceptive benefits, ↓ dysmenorrhea, cycle control

Long-term branch

Does she want to have children in the future?

No:

Permanent Methods

Sterilization Methods:
– Very effective (>99%)
– **Tubal ligation**—can be done laparoscopically or after a C-section
– **Vasectomy**—outpatient procedure

Yes:

Long-Acting Reversible Methods

Injectable Method: Depo-Provera
– Good efficacy (94%), good for 3 months
– High likelihood of unscheduled bleeding

Implantable Methods:
– Implanon, Nexplanon
– Sino-Implant
– Very effective (>99%), good for 3–5 years
– Simple office procedure with no ongoing effort required
– High likelihood of unscheduled bleeding and/or prolonged amenorrhea

Intrauterine Methods:
– Mirena IUD
– Copper T 380A IUD—nonhormonal
– Very effective (>99%) good for 5–10 years
– Outpatient office procedure with no ongoing effort required
– Prompt return to fertility
– Good when breastfeeding
– May cause irregular bleeding and cramping for first 3–6 months
– Option for adolescents and nulliparous women

Combined oral contraceptive methods

Acne/Hirsutism/PCOS → 3rd-generation combined oral contraceptive
Progestin: Norgestimate
• Ortho-tricyclen,
• Ortho-cyclen
• Srintec
• Tri-sprintec
• Othens
Progestin: Desogestrel
• Apri
• Desogen
• Ortho-cept
• Othens
(slight ↑ VTE rish)

Abnormal uterine bleeding → Age ≤35 years
— No → Evaluate for endometrial CA:
• TVUS Endometrial biopsy
— Yes → • Take OCP same time each day
• Rule out STI
• Stop smoking

Bleeding day 5–14 → Proliferative (follicular) phase → Use OCP containing >20 mcg estrogen or vaginal ring

Midcycle → Ovulation

Bleeding day 14–28 → Luteal phase defect (progestin insufficiency) → Use OCP with progestin norgestrel or levonorgestrel

Initiation and no special concerns → Combined OCP (use pill with ≤35 mcg EE)

• Severe dysmenorrhea
• Leiomyomata
• Adenomyosis
• Endometriosis
• PMD/PMDD
• Menstrual migraine
→ Offer continuous pill formulations
• Seasonale
• Seasonique

Mary Le, MD and Anne Powell, MD

Blenning CE, Paladine H. An approach to the postpartum office visit. *Am Fam Physician.* 2005;72(12):2491–2496.

COUGH, CHRONIC

Common causes: GERD, medications, postviral status, allergic rhinitis, mediastinal mass, TB, sarcoid, anxiety

↓

ACE inhibitor use

- *No* →
- *Yes* → ACE inhibitor–induced chronic cough

No → Dyspnea at rest

- *No* → Weight loss
- *Yes* → Trauma

Weight loss
- *Yes* → Mediastinal mass | Tuberculosis
- *No* → GERD | Sarcoid | Postviral status | Postnasal drip: Sinusitis, allergic rhinitis

Postnasal drip → Bronchiectasis

Trauma
- *Yes* → Pneumothorax
- *No* → History of cardiac disease
  - *Yes* → CHF
  - *No* → History of tobacco abuse → COPD

Robert A. Baldor, MD and Alan M. Ehrlich, MD

Pratter MR. Unexplained (idiopathic) cough: ACCP evidence-based clinical practice guidelines. *Chest.* 2006;129(1 Suppl):220S–221S.

DEEP VENOUS THROMBOSIS, DIAGNOSIS AND TREATMENT

Diagnosis

Determine Wells Score

• Active cancer	+1
• Calf swelling >3 cm	+1
• Collateral superficial veins	+1
• Pitting edema	+1
• Previous DVT	+1
• Swelling of entire leg	+1
• Pain along venous system	+1
• Paralysis or recent immobilization (cast)	+1
• Recently bedridden or general anesthesia	+1
• Alternate diagnosis	−2

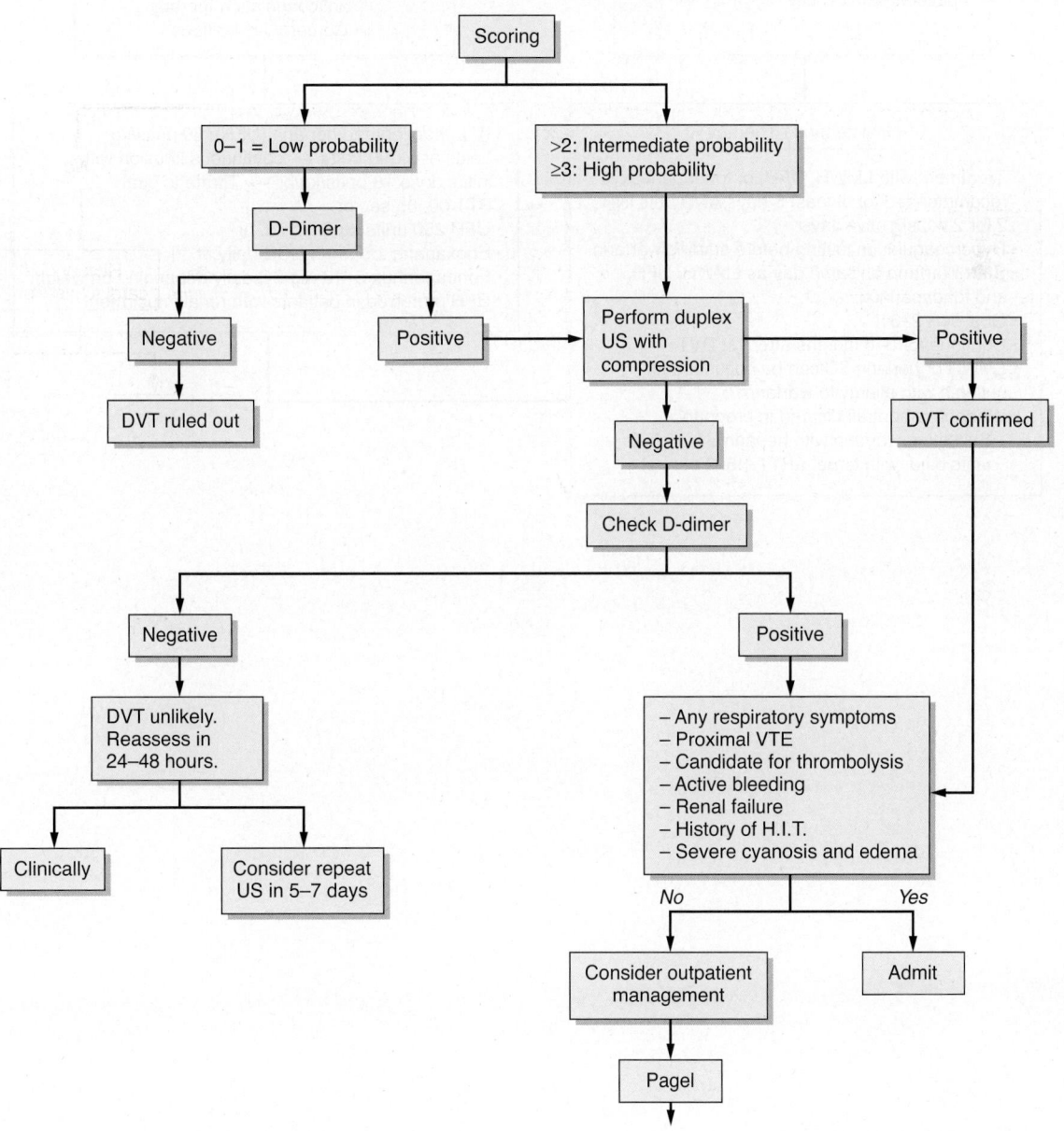

DEEP VENOUS THROMBOSIS, DIAGNOSIS AND TREATMENT
Treatment

Outpatient management

Low-molecular-weight heparin (LMWH)
• Enoxaparin 1 mg/kg SC BID or
• Dalteparin 200 units/kg SC daily for patients with cancer

Maintenance Therapy

• Treatment with LMWH, UFH, or fondaparinux is recommended for at least 5 days **AND** until INR 2 for 2 consecutive days.
• Hypercoagulation testing before starting warfarin
• Start Warfarin on same day as LMWH, UFH, and fondaparinux.
• Goal INR 2–3
• Continue for 3–6 months after 1st DVT
• LMWH or heparin SC can be continued for patients with allergy to warfarin
• Warfarin is contraindicated in pregnancy
  – Substitute warfarin with heparin SC 15,000 units b.i.d. with target aPTT 1.5–2 control

Inpatient management indications

• Massive DVT
• Symptomatic PE
• High-risk bleeding with anticoagulation therapy
• Comorbid conditions

• IV unfractionated heparin (UFH): 80 units/kg bolus or 5,000 units → continuous infusion with initial dose 18 units/kg/hr → Titrate to goal PTT 60–85 sec or
• UFH 250 units/kg SC b.i.d. or
• Enoxaparin 1.5 mg/kg SC daily or
• Fondaparinux 5–10 mg SC daily depending on weight
• UFH preferred in patients with renal impairment

Bency K. Louidor-Paulynice, MD and Elizabeth A. Erban, MD

Wilbur J, Shian B. Diagnosis of deep venous thrombosis and pulmonary embolism. *Am Fam Physician*. 2012;86:913–919.

DEHYDRATION, PEDIATRIC

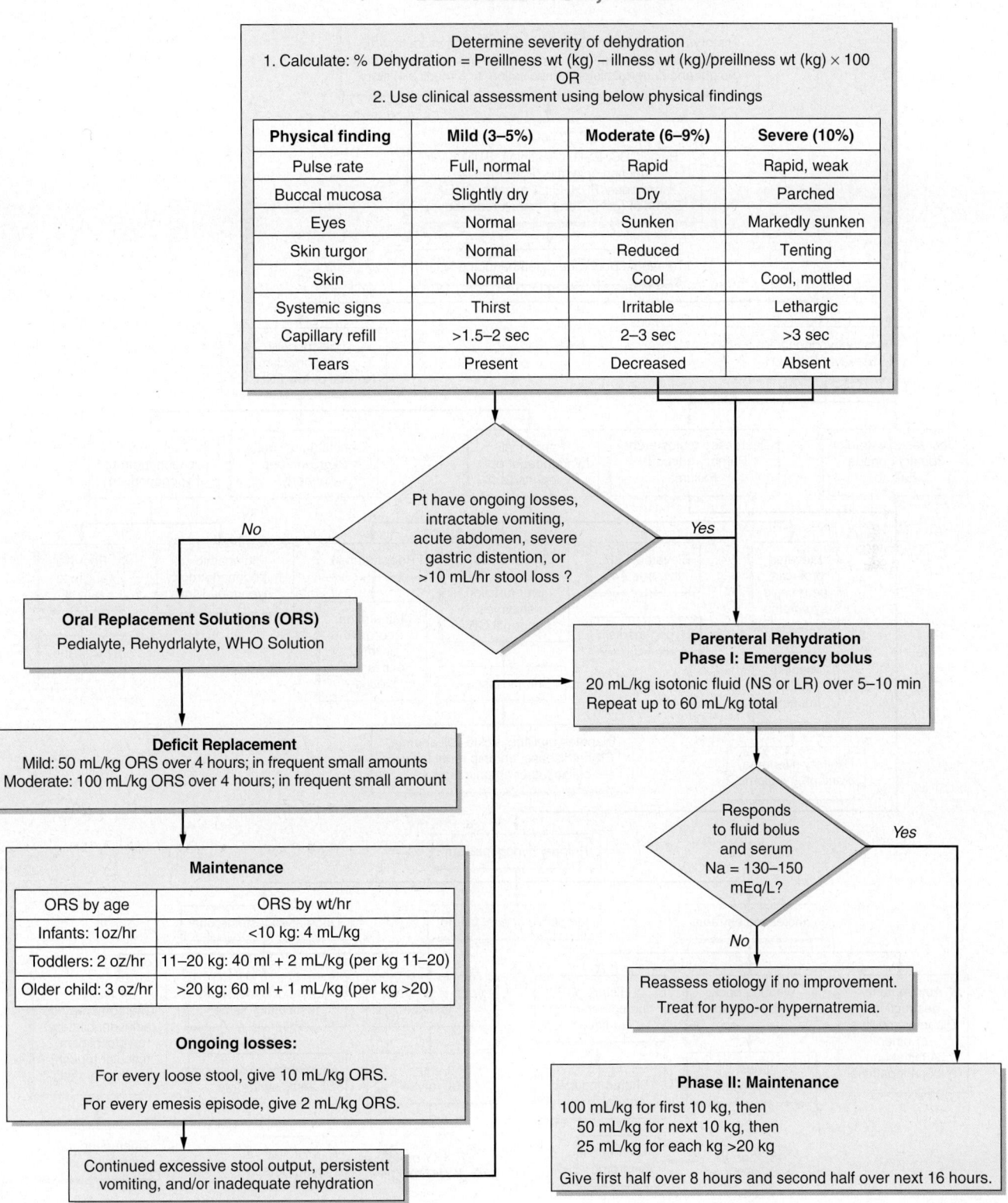

Determine severity of dehydration

1. Calculate: % Dehydration = Preillness wt (kg) − illness wt (kg)/preillness wt (kg) × 100

OR

2. Use clinical assessment using below physical findings

Physical finding	Mild (3–5%)	Moderate (6–9%)	Severe (10%)
Pulse rate	Full, normal	Rapid	Rapid, weak
Buccal mucosa	Slightly dry	Dry	Parched
Eyes	Normal	Sunken	Markedly sunken
Skin turgor	Normal	Reduced	Tenting
Skin	Normal	Cool	Cool, mottled
Systemic signs	Thirst	Irritable	Lethargic
Capillary refill	>1.5–2 sec	2–3 sec	>3 sec
Tears	Present	Decreased	Absent

Pt have ongoing losses, intractable vomiting, acute abdomen, severe gastric distention, or >10 mL/hr stool loss ?

No

Yes

Oral Replacement Solutions (ORS)
Pedialyte, Rehydrlalyte, WHO Solution

**Parenteral Rehydration
Phase I: Emergency bolus**
20 mL/kg isotonic fluid (NS or LR) over 5–10 min
Repeat up to 60 mL/kg total

Deficit Replacement
Mild: 50 mL/kg ORS over 4 hours; in frequent small amounts
Moderate: 100 mL/kg ORS over 4 hours; in frequent small amount

Responds to fluid bolus and serum Na = 130–150 mEq/L?

Yes

No

Maintenance

ORS by age	ORS by wt/hr
Infants: 1oz/hr	<10 kg: 4 mL/kg
Toddlers: 2 oz/hr	11–20 kg: 40 ml + 2 mL/kg (per kg 11–20)
Older child: 3 oz/hr	>20 kg: 60 ml + 1 mL/kg (per kg >20)

Ongoing losses:

For every loose stool, give 10 mL/kg ORS.

For every emesis episode, give 2 mL/kg ORS.

Reassess etiology if no improvement.

Treat for hypo-or hypernatremia.

Continued excessive stool output, persistent vomiting, and/or inadequate rehydration

Phase II: Maintenance
100 mL/kg for first 10 kg, then
50 mL/kg for next 10 kg, then
25 mL/kg for each kg >20 kg

Give first half over 8 hours and second half over next 16 hours.

L. Michelle W. Seawright, DO and Nathaniel Stepp, DO

Tschudt M, Arcara K. *Harriet Lane Handbook*, 19 ed. Philadelphia: Elsevier; 2012:271–291.

DELAYED PUBERTY

History/Physical Exam: Growth pattern (stalled vs. delayed), sexual development, nutrition and exercise habits, family history (height and pubertal history), medication, and medical history

Labs:
*Basic CBC, ESR, Creatinine, BUN, Liver function enzymes, TSH/FreeT4
*Hormones: FSH, LH, Prolactin, DHEA, Estrodiol (girls), Total Testosterone (boys)

Images: Bone age of left hand and wrist

Primary hypogonadism: Elevated FSH, LH

Secondary hypogonadism: Normal or low FSH, LH

Decreased estradiol Primary gonadal Failure:

Decreased testosterone Primary gonadal Failure:

Functional hypogonadotropic hypogonadism

Constitutional delay of growth and puberty

Permanent hypogonadotropic hypogonadism

Elevated prolactin, neurologic symptoms

Elevated TSH, low free T4

Elevated ESR, creatinine, BUN, liver function enzymes, abnormal CBC

Poor nutrition

Idiopathic hypogonadotropic hypogonadism

Poor/No ability to smell

Imaging: CNS Imaging

Hypogonadism

Malnutrition, anorexia, bulimia, excessive exercise

Kallmann syndrome

Chronic disease

Pituitary adenoma, craniopharyngioma

Diabetes mellitus, sickle cell anemia, Crohn disease, chronic renal failure, celiac, other chronic disease

Primary hypogonadism

Decreased estradiol

Idiopathic gondal failure

Decreased testosterone

Autoimmune destruction: Diabetes mellitus or other autoimmune endocrinopathies

Webbed neck, short stature

History of chemotherapy or radiation

Long legs, small testes

Absent or diminishing testicular volume

History: Chemotherapy or radiation, bilateral cryptochidism, teticular torison, mumps orchitis

Labs: Karyotype

Chemo-induced gondal toxicity

Labs: Karyotype

Anorchism or vanishing testis syndrome

45, X or 45, X/46,XX

Turner syndrome

47, XXY or 46, XY/47XXY

Klinfelter syndrome

Chemo-induced gondal toxicity

Vanessa Hand, MD and Frank J. Domino, MD

Master-Hunter T, Heiman DL. Amenorrhea: evaluation and treatment. *Am Fam Physician.* 2006;73(8):1374–1382.

DELIRIUM

Common causes: Medications, infection, electrolyte abnormality, toxic ingestion, hypoxia, neurologic disorder, psychiatric illness, hepatic encephalopathy, uremia, sundowning

Check all medications

Yes — *No*

Benzodiazepines
Anticholinergic drugs
Narcotics
Digoxin
Anticonvulsants
Diabetes drugs
Cimetidine
Numerous others

No medication used

Check: CBC, electrolytes, renal function, urinalysis, TSH, pulse ox, ABG (arterial blood gas), CXR, LFTs, toxic substance screen

Abnormal — Normal

Infection
Thyroid dysfunction
Hyponatremia
Hypernatremia
Hypoglycemia
Hepatic encephalopathy
Hypoxia
Uremia
Toxic ingestion

Check brain CT or MRI

Normal (consider LP or EEG) — Abnormal

Psychiatric illness
Hypertensive
Concussion
Alcohol withdrawal
Seizure disorder
Cerebral infection

Subdural hematoma
Brain tumor
Stroke

Jaclyn EA Legg, DO and Gautam J. Desai, DO, FACOFP

Gleason OC. Delirium. *Am Fam Physician.* 2003;67:1027–1034.

DEMENTIA

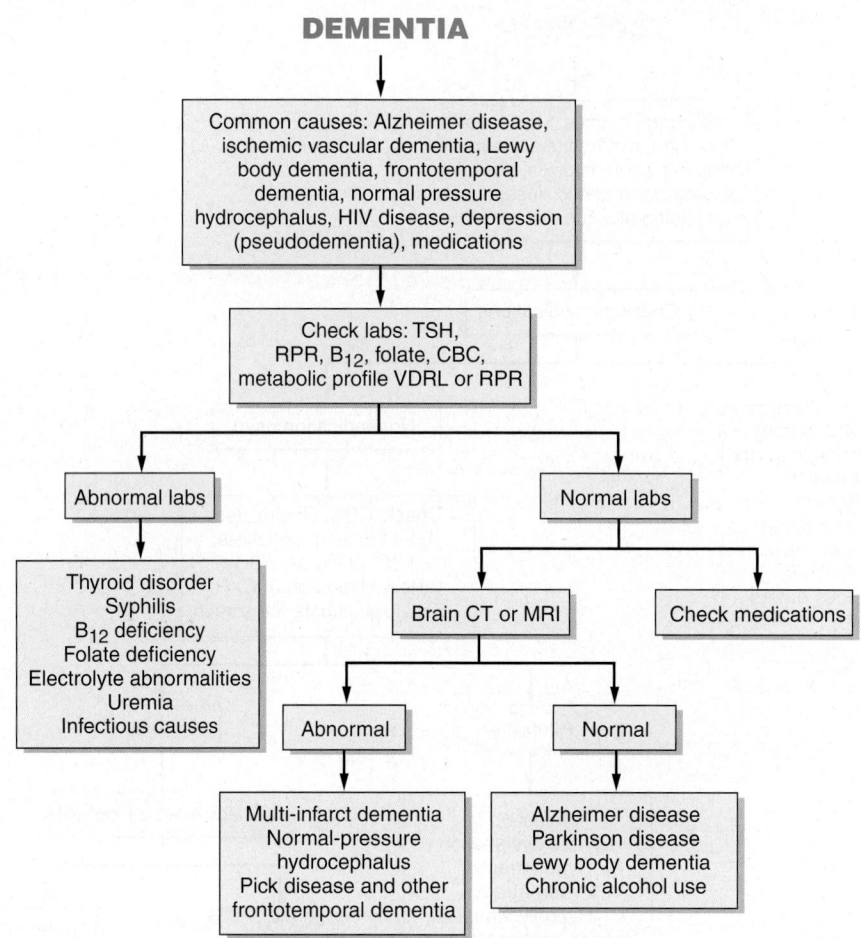

Common causes: Alzheimer disease, ischemic vascular dementia, Lewy body dementia, frontotemporal dementia, normal pressure hydrocephalus, HIV disease, depression (pseudodementia), medications

Check labs: TSH, RPR, B_{12}, folate, CBC, metabolic profile VDRL or RPR

Abnormal labs

Thyroid disorder
Syphilis
B_{12} deficiency
Folate deficiency
Electrolyte abnormalities
Uremia
Infectious causes

Normal labs

Brain CT or MRI

Check medications

Abnormal

Multi-infarct dementia
Normal-pressure hydrocephalus
Pick disease and other frontotemporal dementia

Normal

Alzheimer disease
Parkinson disease
Lewy body dementia
Chronic alcohol use

Robert A. Baldor, MD and Alan M. Ehrlich, MD

Knopman DS, DeKosky ST, Cummings JL, et al. Practice parameter: Diagnosis of dementia (an evidence-based review). Report of the Quality Standards Subcommittee of the American Academy of Neurology. *Neurology.* 2001;56(9):1143–1153.

DEPRESSIVE EPISODE, MAJOR

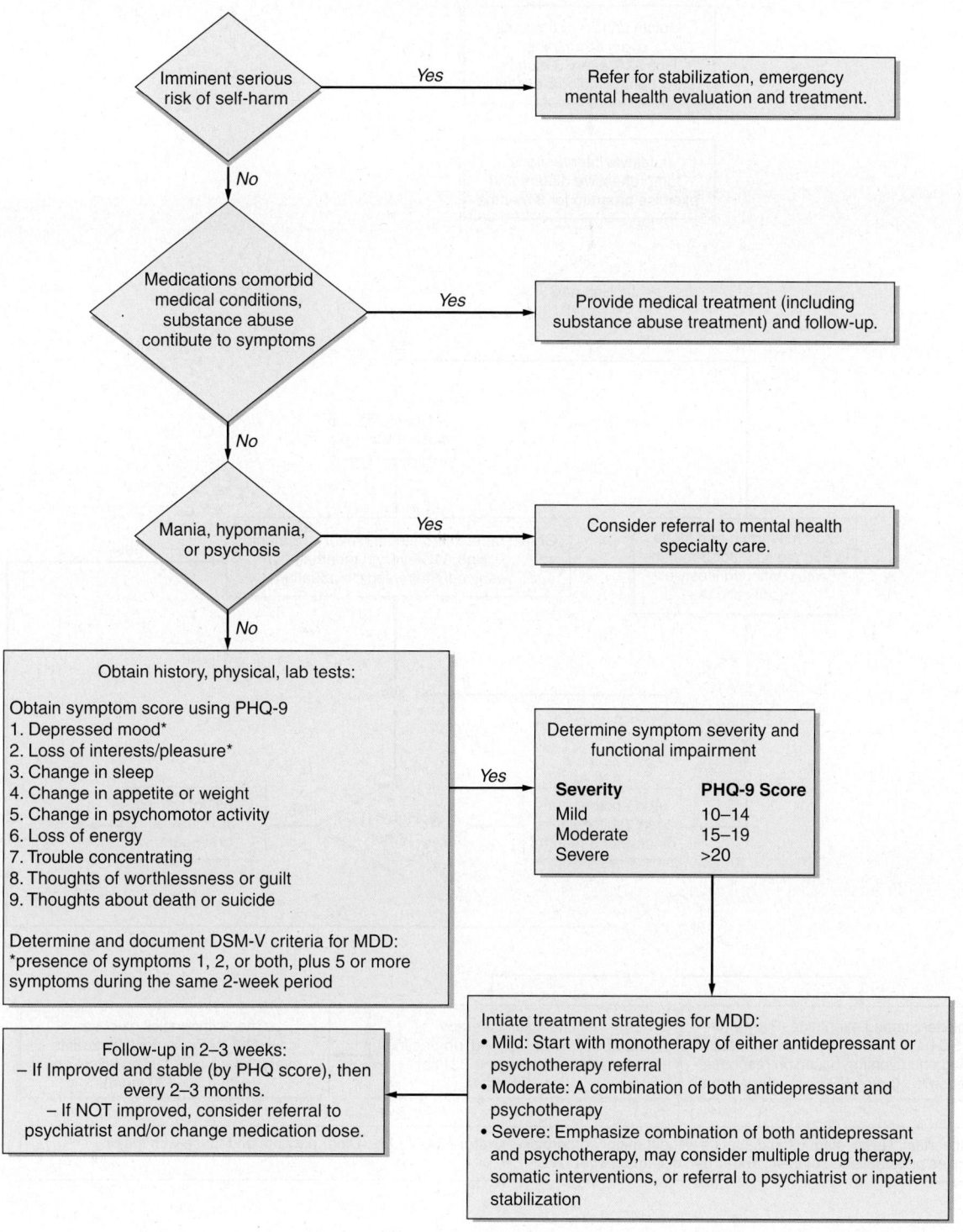

Imminent serious risk of self-harm — Yes → Refer for stabilization, emergency mental health evaluation and treatment.

No ↓

Medications comorbid medical conditions, substance abuse contribute to symptoms — Yes → Provide medical treatment (including substance abuse treatment) and follow-up.

No ↓

Mania, hypomania, or psychosis — Yes → Consider referral to mental health specialty care.

No ↓

Obtain history, physical, lab tests:

Obtain symptom score using PHQ-9
1. Depressed mood*
2. Loss of interests/pleasure*
3. Change in sleep
4. Change in appetite or weight
5. Change in psychomotor activity
6. Loss of energy
7. Trouble concentrating
8. Thoughts of worthlessness or guilt
9. Thoughts about death or suicide

Determine and document DSM-V criteria for MDD:
*presence of symptoms 1, 2, or both, plus 5 or more symptoms during the same 2-week period

Yes →

Determine symptom severity and functional impairment

Severity	PHQ-9 Score
Mild	10–14
Moderate	15–19
Severe	>20

Intiate treatment strategies for MDD:
- Mild: Start with monotherapy of either antidepressant or psychotherapy referral
- Moderate: A combination of both antidepressant and psychotherapy
- Severe: Emphasize combination of both antidepressant and psychotherapy, may consider multiple drug therapy, somatic interventions, or referral to psychiatrist or inpatient stabilization

Follow-up in 2–3 weeks:
– If Improved and stable (by PHQ score), then every 2–3 months.
– If NOT improved, consider referral to psychiatrist and/or change medication dose.

Wendy K. Marsh, MD, MSc

US Department of Verterans Affairs. *VA/DoD Clinical Practice Guideline for Management of Major Depressive Disorder.* Washington, DC: Department of Veteran Affairs; 2010.

DIABETES MELLITUS, TYPE 2

Obtain urine microalbumin
every 12 months
Hgb A1C every 6 months
Yearly ophthalmologic evaluation

Lifestyle interventions
Comprehensive dietary and
exercise program for 3 months

Is Hgb A1C ≤ target*

No

Yes

Continued close follow-up

Start metformin and titrate to 850 mg b.i.d. for 3 months with continued lifestyle modifications

Obtain urine micro albumin every 12 months
Hgb A1C every 6 months
Yearly ophthalmologic evaluation

Yes

Is Hgb A1C ≤ target*

Yes

No

Add another oral agent (sulfonylurea, others) for 3 months

Is Hgb A1C ≤ target*

No

Consider adding 3rd class of oral agent

A1C ≤ target*

No

BMI >30

Consider starting exenatide (Byetta) 5 mcg SC b.i.d. within 1 hour before meals in morning and evening, based on response, may increase to 10 mcg SC b.i.d. after 1 month

Initiate insulin therapy Start bedtime or morning long-acting insulin (10 units or 0.2 U/kg) for 3 months

Check fingerstick glucose daily and increase dose by 2 units every 3 days until fasting levels are within 70–130 mg/dL

*Target uncertain. Newly diagnosed diabetics without major comorbidities, target likely <7%. Older patients and those with major comorbidities or established diabetic end-organ disease, target <8%

Frank J. Domino, MD

Ripsin CM, Kang H, Urban RJ. Management of blood glucose in type 2 diabetes mellitus. *Am Fam Physician*. 2009;79(1):29–36.

DIABETIC KETOACIDOSIS (DKA), TREATMENT

DKA diagnostic criteria: serum glucose >250 mg/dL, arterial pH <7.3, serum bicarbonate <18 mEq/L, and moderate ketonuria or ketonemia.
Complete initial evaluation. Check capillary glucose and serum/urine ketones to confirm hyperglycemia and ketonemia/ketonuria.

IV Fluids

Start 1.0 L of 0.9% NaCl/hr

Severe/Shock

Administer 0.9 percent NaCl (at least 10–20 mL/kg over first hour)

Hemodynamic monitoring/pressors

Mild dehydration

Evaluate corrected serum Na*

Serum Na* normal or high → 0.45% NaCl (250–500 mL/hr)

Serum Na* low → 0.9% Na/Cl (250–500 mL/hr)

Serum glucose <200 mg/dL

5% dextrose with 0.45% NaCl at 150–250 mL/hr

Decrease insulin to 0.05–0.1 U/kg/hr IV

Keep serum glucose between 150 and 200 mg/dL until resolution of DKA

Insulin

Regular insulin 0.1 U/kg IV bolus

...then 0.1 U/kg/hr IV

If serum glucose does not fall by 50–70 mg/dL in first hour, double IV dose.

Potassium

Urine output >50 mL/hr

K^* <3.3 mEq/L

K^+ ≥3.3 & <5.3 mEq/L

K^* ≥5.3 mEq/L

NO K^+ Recheck every 2 hours.

Add 20–30 mEq K^* to each liter of IV fluid. Goal is K^* between 4 and 5 mEq/L

Assess need for bicarbonate

pH <7.0

$NaHCO_3$ (50 mmol) in 200 mL H_2O with 10 mEq KCL. Give over 1 hour

Repeat IV $NaHCO_3$ dose q2h until pH >7.0 and check serum K^*

Laboratory Evaluation

Initial: CBC, CMP, ABG, serum ketones, phos, UA, EKG, CXR, BCx.

Serial: in addition to clinical, glucose, electrolytes, venous blood gas, urine output

Calculated: effective osmolality, anion gap, corrected Na^+, urine output

Frequency: q1h initially, then q2–4h once stable until DKA resolution

Resolution of DKA:

Glucose <200 mg/dL, serum bicarbonate ≥18 mEq/L and venous pH >7.3

Feed and initiate subcutaneous insulin regimen (0.5–0.8 U/kg/d), keeping IV insulin going 1–2 hours after SC doses. Look for precipitating cause(s).

John B. Waits, MD

Trachetenbarg DE. Diabetic ketoacidosis. *Am Fam Physician.* 2005;71(9):1705–1714.

DIARRHEA, CHRONIC

Common causes: Infectious (bacterial, viral, parasitic), inflammatory bowel disease, malignancy, irritable bowel syndrome, medications, thyroid dysfunction, food additives, malabsorption syndromes (celiac disease, pancreatic insufficiency)

History: Bloody stools, medications, recent antibiotics, recent travel, family history, floating stools, relationship to food intake, surgical history (cholecystectomy, bowel resections) sexual history, recent hospitalizations

Medications

Yes

Acid-reducing agents (PPIs, H2-blockers), antacids (containing magnesium), antibiotics, NSAIDs, colchicine, herbal medications, vitamin and mineral supplements, antineoplastic agents, antiretroviral agents, sorbitol, fructose abuse, chronic laxative abuse

No

Labs: Stool studies (culture, C. diff ova + parasites), TSH, glucose, fecal fat, celiac serologies (TTG IgA), HIV

Abnormal

Stool positive for ova and parasites-Parasitic infections (e.g., *Cryptosporidium, Giardia, Microsporidium*)

Positive C. diff Antigen/Toxin or PCR- Clostridium difficile infection

Positive fecal fat: See "Malabsorption" algorithm

Hyperthyroidism Diabetes

Positive stool cultures-bacterial infection (*Escherichia coli, Salmonella, Shigella, Campylobacter*)

Positive celiac serologies (tissue transglutaminase IgA, anti-endomysial antibiodies)

Upper endoscopy to confirm diagnosis of celiac disease

Normal

Colonoscopy, sigmoidoscopy + biopsy

Abnormal exam and/or abnormal biopsies

Normal exam and biopsies

Inflammatory bowel diseases, malignancy, ischemic colitis, infectious colitis, microscopic colitis

Irritable bowel syndrome

Lakshmi D.N. Lattimer, MD and Marie L. Borum, MD, MPH, EdD

Schiller L, Sellin J. Diarrhea. In Feldman M, Friedman L, Brandt, L, eds. *Sleisenger and Fordtran's Gastrointestinal and Liver Disease*, 9th ed. Philadelphia: Elsevier; 2010:2257–2274.

DISCHARGE, VAGINAL

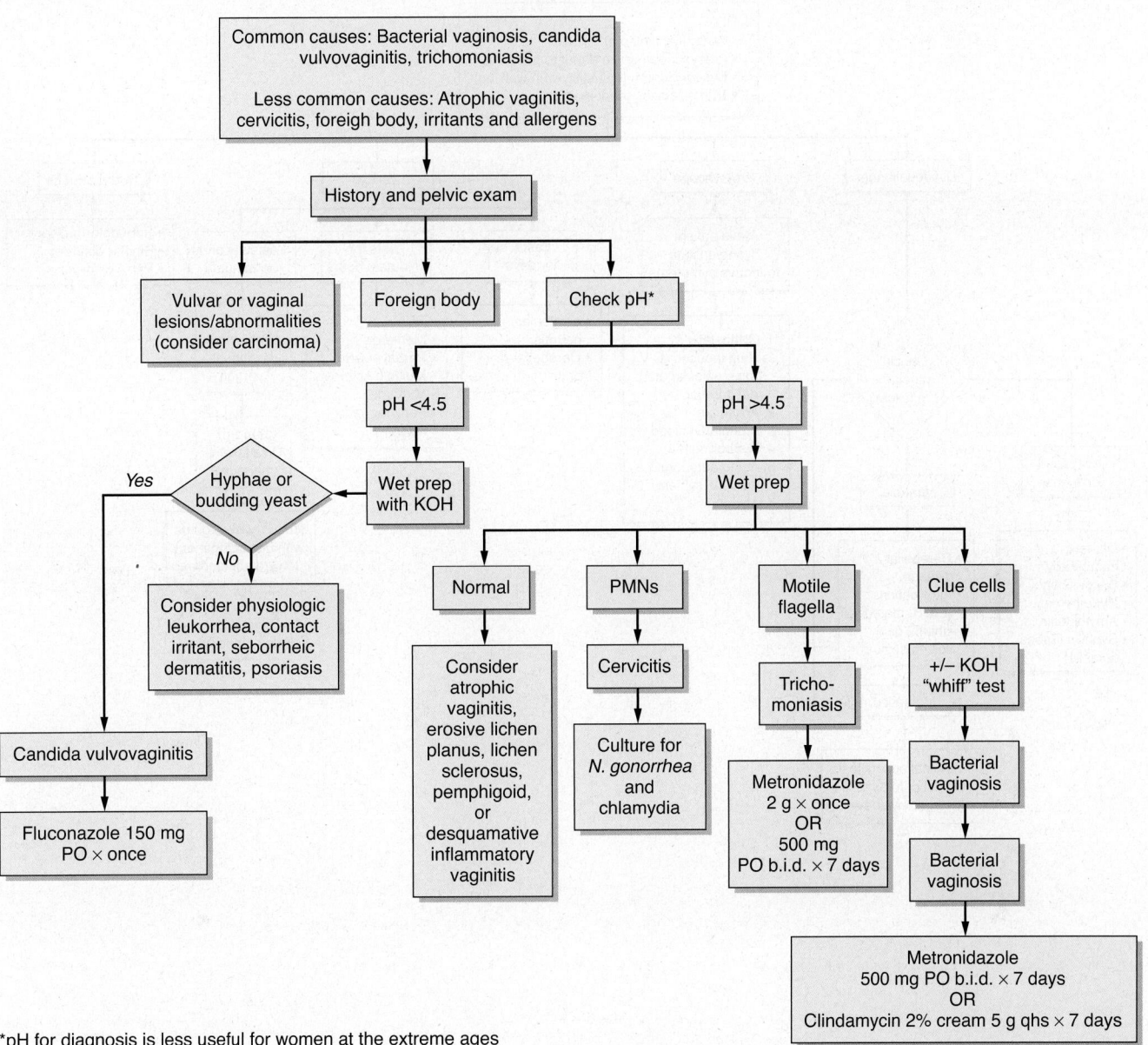

*pH for diagnosis is less useful for women at the extreme ages

Nicole Shields, MD

Hainer BL, Gibson MV. Vaginitis. *Am Fam Physician.* 2011;83:807–815.

DIZZINESS

DDX:
- Vertigo (room spin)
- Presyncope (sense about to pass out)
- Dysequilibrium (instability with walking)
- True dizziness (nonorganic)

Dysequalibrium

Pre-syncope

Vertigo

True dizziness
- Somatoform disorder
- Bipolar disorder
- Panic disorder

Have patient hyperventilate to induce symptoms

Check patellar reflexes

Lasts for days
- Vestibular neuritis
- Cerebellar or brain stem stroke

Lasts for minutes–hours
- T.I.A.
- Meniere's
- Partial seizure
- Multiple sclerosis
- Migraine
- Perilymphatic fistula

Lasts seconds to minutes

1. Orthostatic
   - drug induced (C.V. drugs, opioids, etc.)
   - dehydration
2. Arrythmia
3. Anemia/GI bleed
4. Hypoglycemia
5. Aging autonomic nervous system
6. Anxiety

Decreased reflexes

Variable

Benign paroxysmal positional vertigo

Perform Dix-Hallpike maneuver

- Diabetic neuropathy
- B₁₂ deficiency
- Hypothyroid
- Amyloidosis
- Syphilis (Tabes dorsalis)

- Cerebellar disease
- Intoxication (EtOH, mercury, lithium, gas, solvents, glue)

Rotatory nystagmus with last component toward affected ear

Treat with Epley maneuver

Increased

- Cervical spondylosis
- Spinal cord tumor
- Multiple myeloma

James J. Foody, MD, FACP

Post RE, Dickerson LM. Dizziness: A diagnostic approach. *Am Fam Physician.* 2010;82(4):361–368.

DYSPEPSIA

Robert A. Baldor, MD and Alan M. Ehrlich, MD

Fennerty MB, Finke KB, Kushner PR, et al. Short- and long-term management of heartburn and other acid-related disorders: Development of an algorithm for primary care providers. *J Fam Pract.* 2009;58(7 Suppl Short):S1–S12.

DYSPHAGIA

Parag Goyal, MD

Lind CD. Dysphagia: Evaluation and treatment. *Gastroenterol Clin North Am.* 2003;32(2):553–575.

DYSPNEA

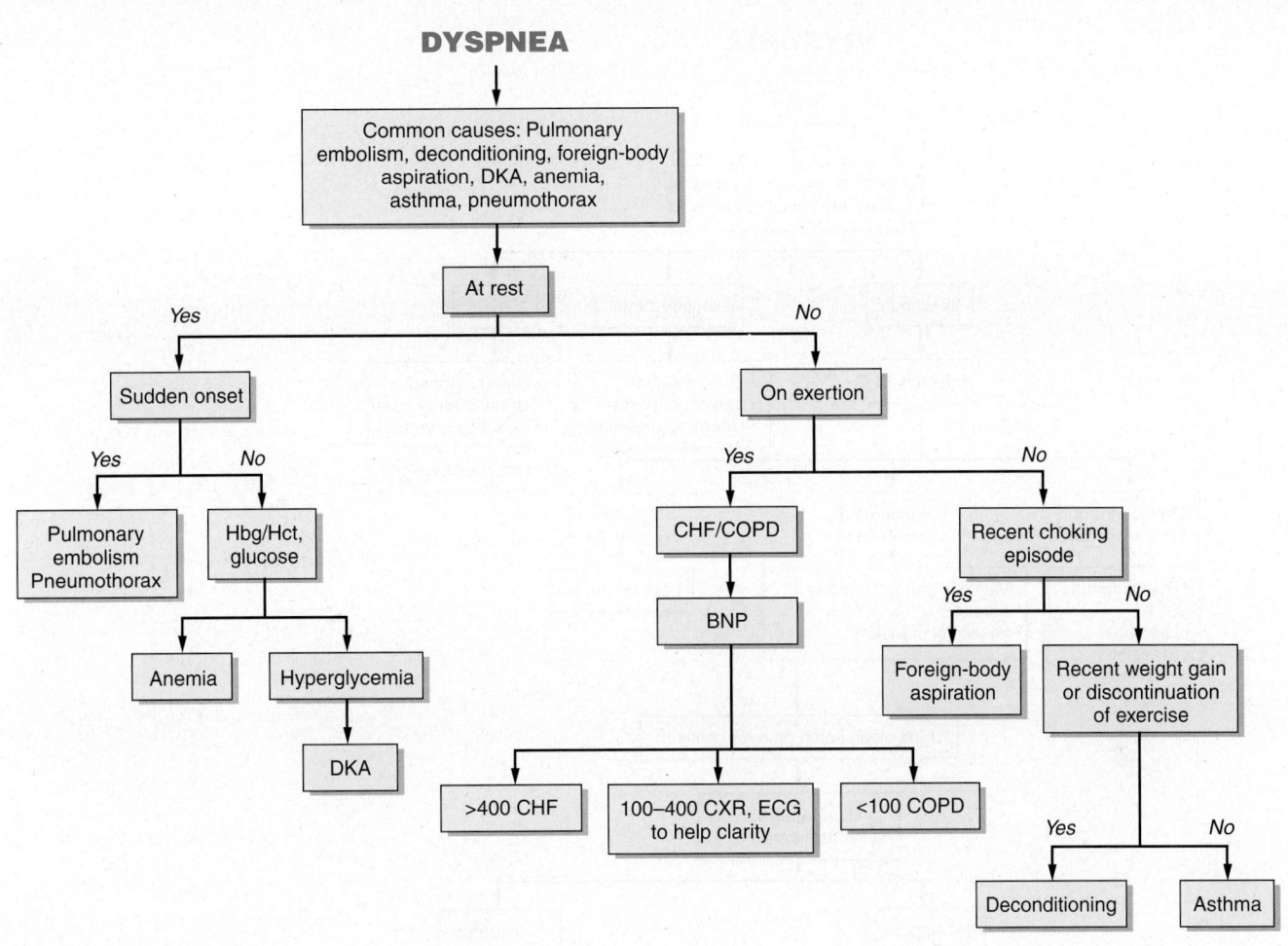

Common causes: Pulmonary embolism, deconditioning, foreign-body aspiration, DKA, anemia, asthma, pneumothorax

At rest

Yes — *No*

Sudden onset

Yes — *No*

Pulmonary embolism Pneumothorax

Hbg/Hct, glucose

Anemia

Hyperglycemia

DKA

On exertion

Yes — *No*

CHF/COPD

BNP

>400 CHF

100–400 CXR, ECG to help clarity

<100 COPD

Recent choking episode

Yes — *No*

Foreign-body aspiration

Recent weight gain or discontinuation of exercise

Yes — *No*

Deconditioning

Asthma

Vinit Patil, MD and Afshin Sam, MD

Wahls SA. Causes and evaluation of chronic dyspnea. *Am Fam Physician.* 2012;86(2):173–180.

DYSURIA

Causes

Common causes: Cystitis, STIs, vaginitis, prostatitis

- Infectious
  - Infection of
    - Genitourinary
      - Pyelonephritis
      - UTI
      - Urethritis
      - Prostatitis
    - Perineum
      - Vaginitis (fungal, bacterial)
      - Balanitis
      - Pelvic inflammatory
    - Systemic
      - Less common
- Noninfectious
  - Local trauma
  - Labial adhesions
  - Chemical urethritis
- Others
  - Urinary stones
  - Urethral strictures
  - Reactive arthritis
  - Behçet disease
  - Lichen sclerosus

Urine clean catch on every patient.

Urine analysis
Urine pregnancy test

(+) Nitrates
(+) Pyuria
- Acute bacterial cystitis

(–) Nitrates
(–) Pyuria
- Vaginal discharge
- Urethral discharge
- Cervical discharge

Yes
- Nucleic acid amplification test for STI.
- Cultures for gonorrhea/chlamydia.
- PCR/viral culture for genital herpes simplex.

Positive

Male
- Urethritis
- Acute bacterial prostatitis
- Chronic bacterial prostatitis
- Epididymitis

Female
- Pelvic inflammatory disease
- Atrophic vaginitis
- Vulvar disease
- Vaginal warts

No

Female
Cystoscopy for interstitial cystitis.

Male
ESR for Reiter syndrome.

Shami Goyal, MD and Dawna Woodyear, MD

Mehnert-Kay SA. Diagnosis and management of urinary tract infections. *Am Fam Physician.* 2005;72(3):451–456.

EAR PAIN

Common causes: Acute otitis media, serous otitis media, otitis externa, perforated tympanic membrane, eustachian tube dysfunction, cerumen impaction, foreign body, cholesteatoma. Secondary causes: TMJ syndrome, mastoiditis, pharyngitis, referred pain

↓

Periauricular pain?

Yes →

Discharge from EAC?

Yes → Otitis externa → If immuno-compromised, (diabetes, HIV) consider malignant otitis externa; order ESR and CT or MRI

No → TMJ syndrome

No →

Recent URI

Yes → Physical exam

Red TM w/effusion and fever → Acute otitis media

Postauricular erythemia, tenderness or swelling? Consider mastoiditis & obtain CT

Age <2 years or immuno-compromised or w/otorrhea

Yes → Treat:
- Amoxicillin 50 mg/kg divided bid × 7–10 d
- If PCN allergic, cefdinir 14 mg/kg divided bid
- If severe PCN allergy, azithromycin

No → Watchful waiting

Air–fluid levels → Serous otitis media → At risk for language delay?

Yes → Refer to ENT

No → Watchful waiting for 3 months

No → Recent air travel or SCUBA diving?

Severe pain or bloody discharge → Perforate TM, barotrauma

Intact TM, hearing loss? → Eustacian tube dysfunction, foreign body, cerumen impaction, cholesteotoma

Stephanie LeBourdais, MD and Frank J. Domino, MD

Lieberthal AS, Carroll AE, Chonmaitree T, et al. The diagnosis and management of acute otitis media. *Pediatrics.* 2013;131:e964–e999.

ENURESIS

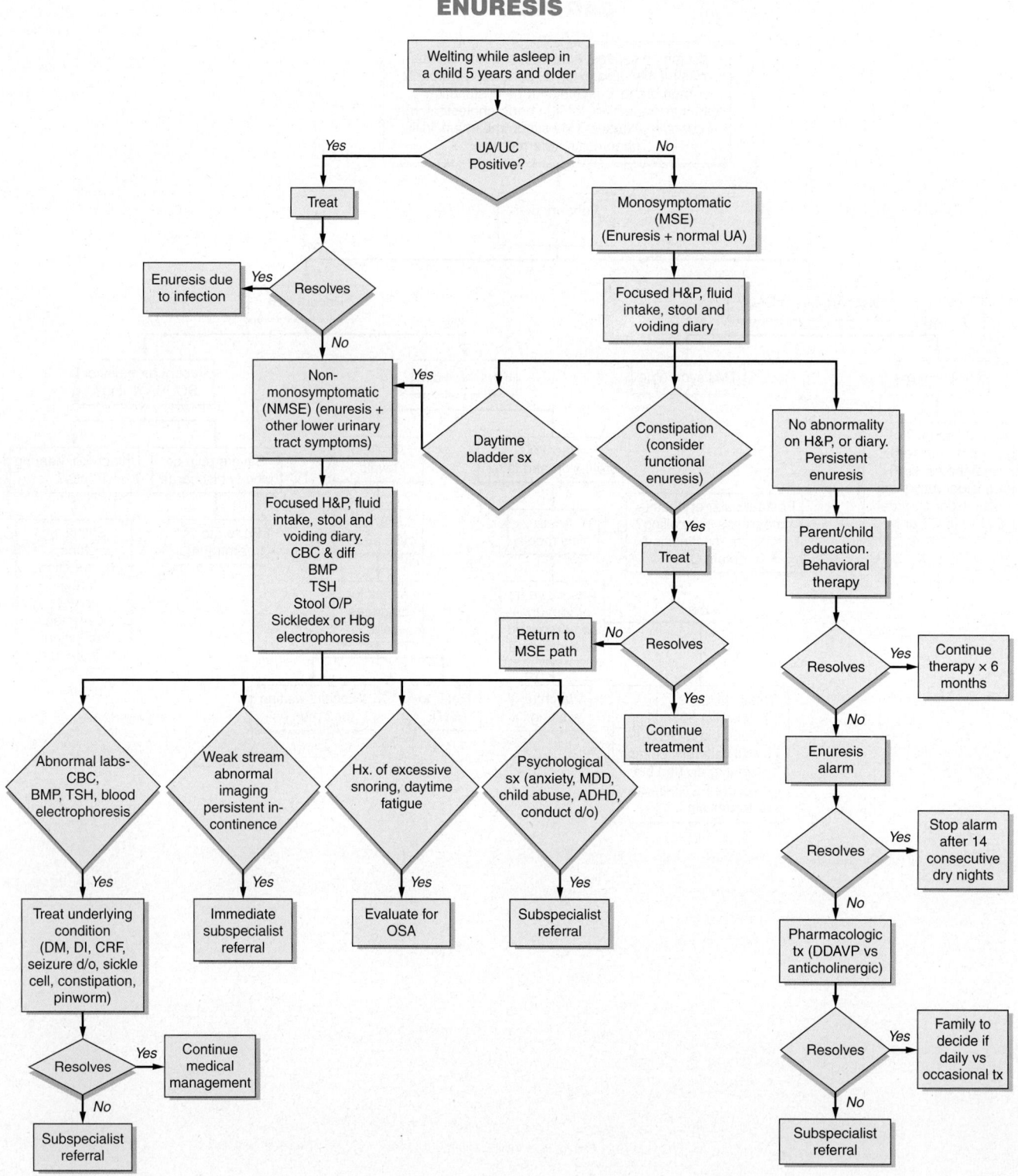

Monica Juarez-Gonzalez, DO and Amimi Osayande, MD

Franco I, von Gontard A, De Gennaro M, et al. Evaluation and treatment of non monosymptomatic nocturnal enuresis: A standardization document from the International Children's Continence Society. *J Pediatr Urol.* 2013;9:234–243.

Neveus T, Eggert P, Evans J, et al. Evaluation and treatment for monosymptomatic enuresis: A standardization document from the International Children's Continence Society. *J Urol.* 2010;183:441–447.

ERYTHROCYTOSIS

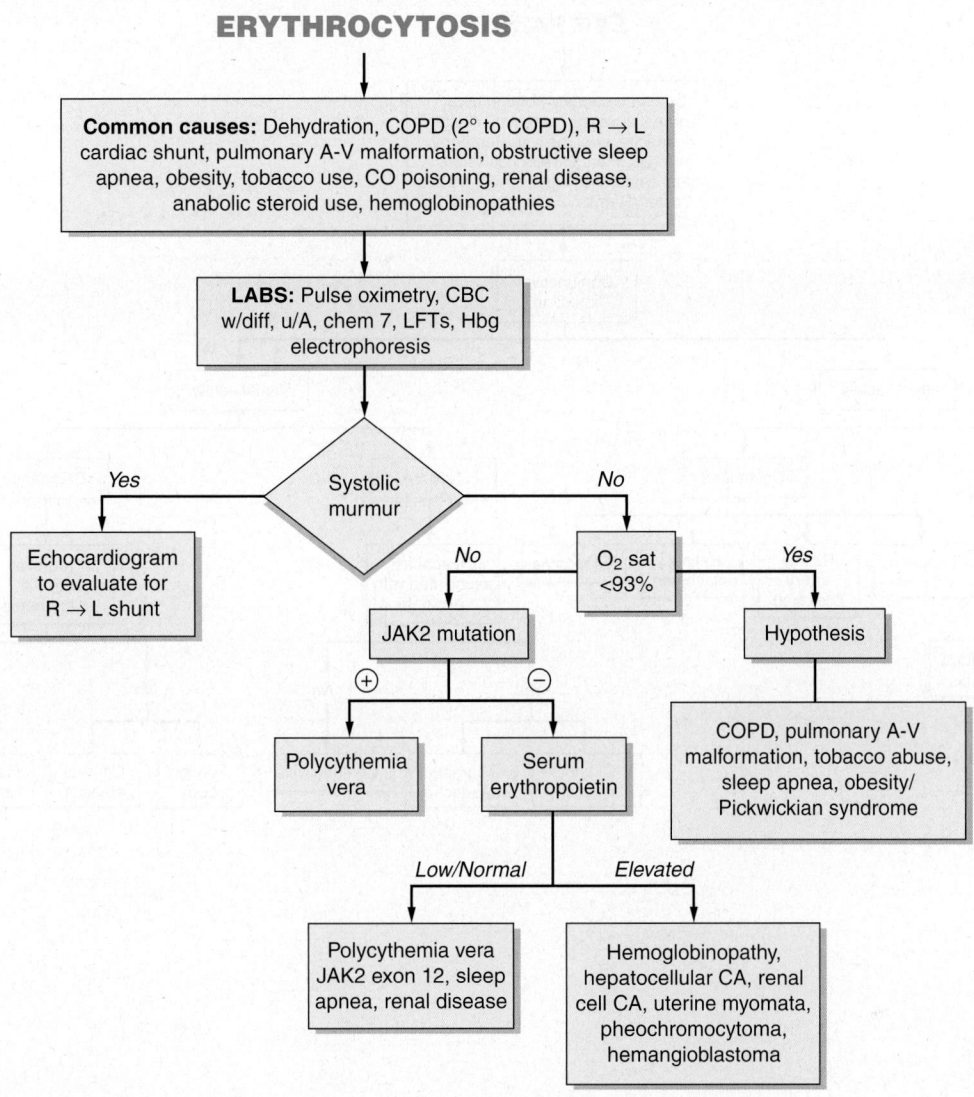

Common causes: Dehydration, COPD (2° to COPD), R → L cardiac shunt, pulmonary A-V malformation, obstructive sleep apnea, obesity, tobacco use, CO poisoning, renal disease, anabolic steroid use, hemoglobinopathies

LABS: Pulse oximetry, CBC w/diff, u/A, chem 7, LFTs, Hbg electrophoresis

Systolic murmur

Yes — Echocardiogram to evaluate for R → L shunt

No — O₂ sat <93%

No — JAK2 mutation

Yes — Hypothesis — COPD, pulmonary A-V malformation, tobacco abuse, sleep apnea, obesity/Pickwickian syndrome

JAK2 mutation:
(+) Polycythemia vera
(−) Serum erythropoietin

Serum erythropoietin:
Low/Normal — Polycythemia vera JAK2 exon 12, sleep apnea, renal disease
Elevated — Hemoglobinopathy, hepatocellular CA, renal cell CA, uterine myomata, pheochromocytoma, hemangioblastoma

Alexis Ramirez, MD and Michael Snyder, MD

Tefferi A. JAK2 mutations in polycythemia vera–molecular mechanisms and clinical applications. *N Engl J Med.* 2007;356:444.

EYE PAIN

Common causes: Foreign body, corneal abrasion, migraine, cluster headache, conjunctivitis, temporal arteritis, retinal artery occlusion, retinal detachment, glaucoma, herpes zoster (Ramsay Hunt syndrome)

Conjunctival injection

No — *Yes*

Visual acuity | Visual acuity

Normal — Decreased | Normal — Decreased

Migraine | Temporal arteritis

Temporal arteritis | Retinal artery occlusion | Retinal detachment | Glaucoma

Headache associated with eye pain

Yes — *No*

Cluster headache | Migraine headache | Conjunctivitis

Preorbital edema or erythema

No — *Yes*

Foreign body | Corneal abrasion | Herpes zoster | Periorbital cellulitis

Robert A. Baldor, MD and Alan M. Ehrlich, MD

Friedman DI. Headache and the eye. *Curr Pain Headache Rep.* 2008;12(4):296–304.

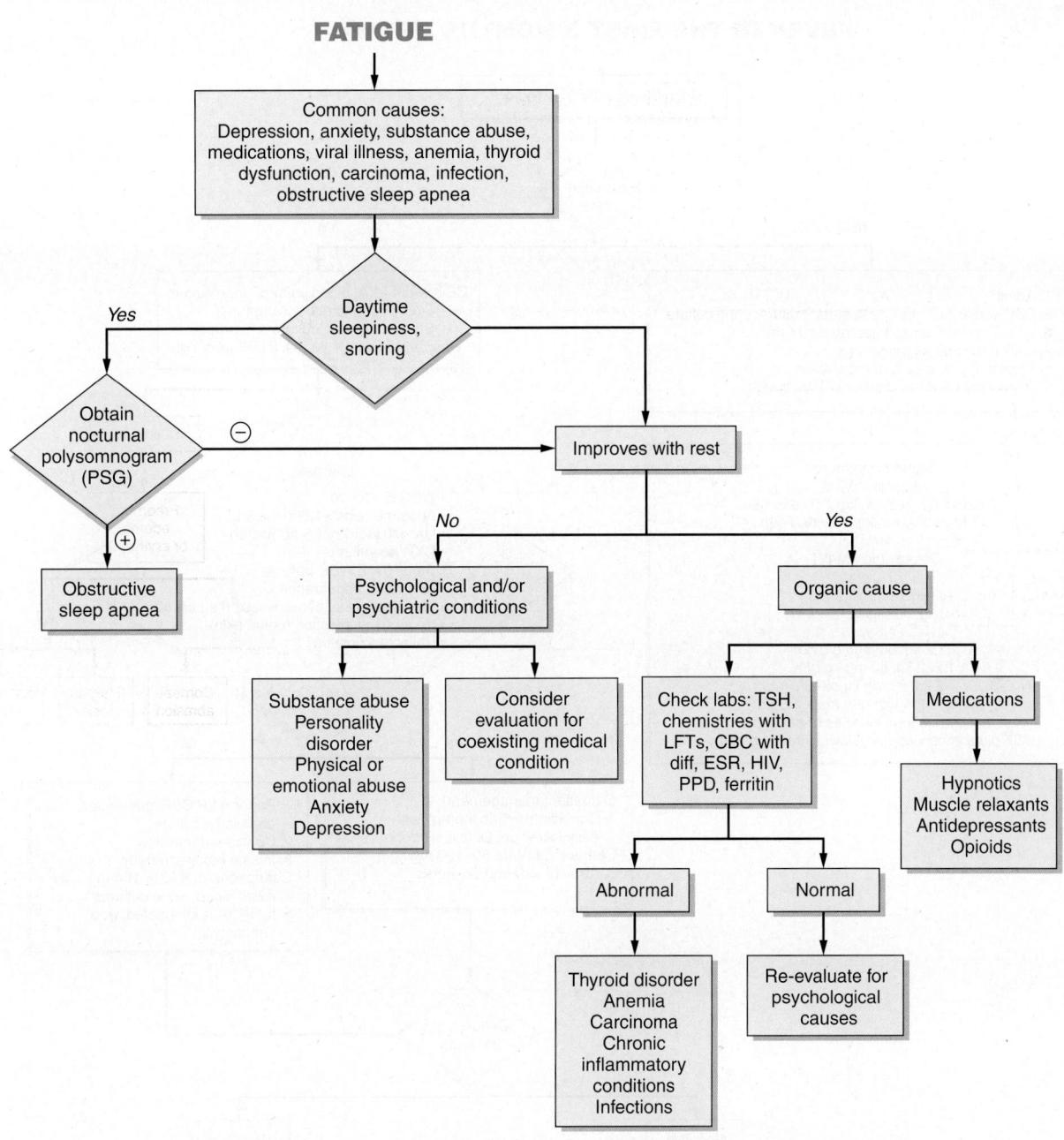

Robert A. Baldor, MD and Alan M. Ehrlich, MD

Nijrolder I, van der Windt D, de Vries H, et al. Diagnoses during follow-up of patients presenting with fatigue in primary care. *CMAJ.* 2009;181:683–687.

FEVER IN THE FIRST 3 MONTHS OF LIFE

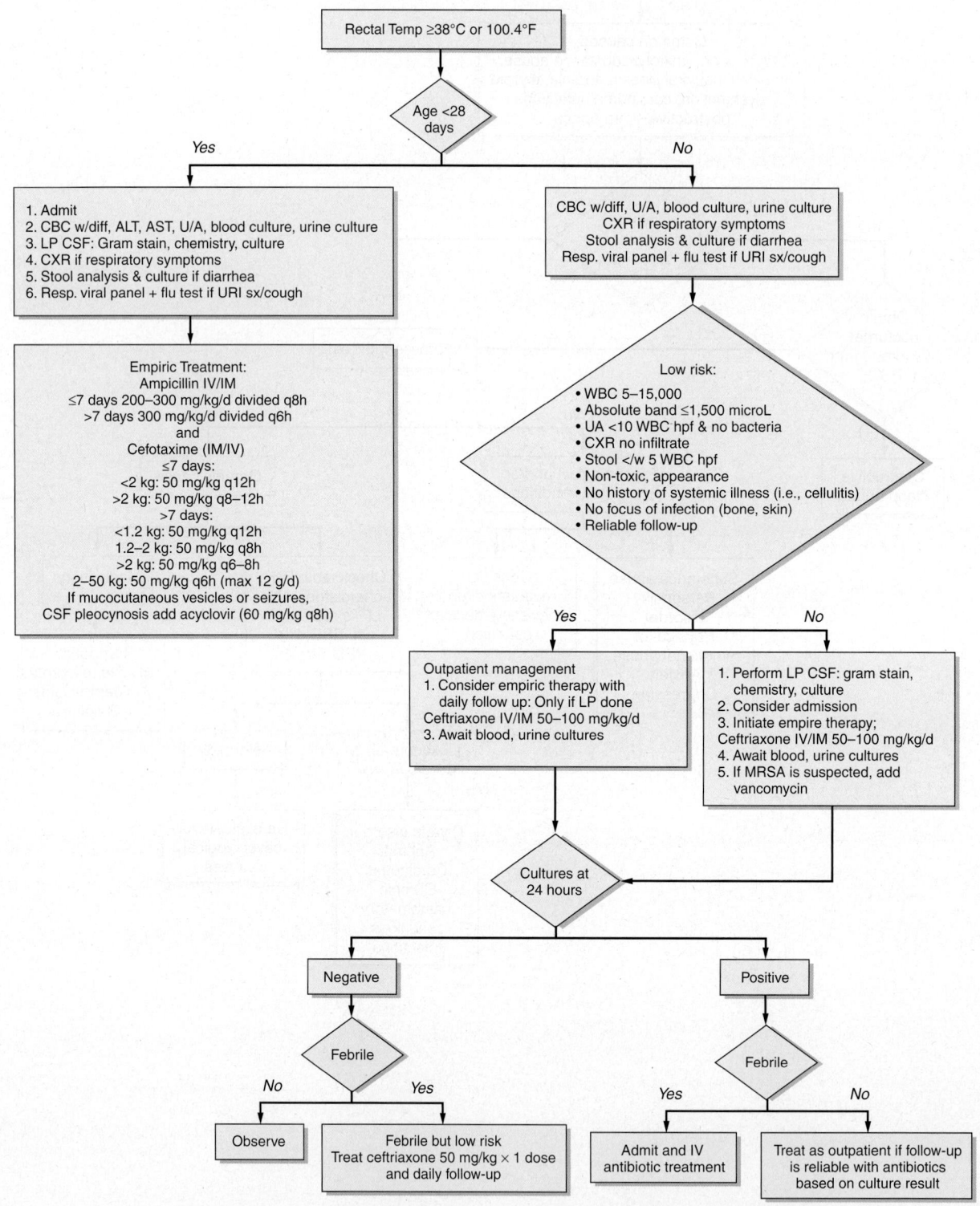

Rectal Temp ≥38°C or 100.4°F

Age <28 days

Yes

1. Admit
2. CBC w/diff, ALT, AST, U/A, blood culture, urine culture
3. LP CSF: Gram stain, chemistry, culture
4. CXR if respiratory symptoms
5. Stool analysis & culture if diarrhea
6. Resp. viral panel + flu test if URI sx/cough

Empiric Treatment:
Ampicillin IV/IM
≤7 days 200–300 mg/kg/d divided q8h
>7 days 300 mg/kg/d divided q6h
and
Cefotaxime (IM/IV)
≤7 days:
<2 kg: 50 mg/kg q12h
>2 kg: 50 mg/kg q8–12h
>7 days:
<1.2 kg: 50 mg/kg q12h
1.2–2 kg: 50 mg/kg q8h
>2 kg: 50 mg/kg q6–8h
2–50 kg: 50 mg/kg q6h (max 12 g/d)
If mucocutaneous vesicles or seizures,
CSF pleocynosis add acyclovir (60 mg/kg q8h)

No

CBC w/diff, U/A, blood culture, urine culture
CXR if respiratory symptoms
Stool analysis & culture if diarrhea
Resp. viral panel + flu test if URI sx/cough

Low risk:
• WBC 5–15,000
• Absolute band ≤1,500 microL
• UA <10 WBC hpf & no bacteria
• CXR no infiltrate
• Stool </w 5 WBC hpf
• Non-toxic, appearance
• No history of systemic illness (i.e., cellulitis)
• No focus of infection (bone, skin)
• Reliable follow-up

Yes

Outpatient management
1. Consider empiric therapy with
   daily follow up: Only if LP done
   Ceftriaxone IV/IM 50–100 mg/kg/d
3. Await blood, urine cultures

No

1. Perform LP CSF: gram stain, chemistry, culture
2. Consider admission
3. Initiate empire therapy; Ceftriaxone IV/IM 50–100 mg/kg/d
4. Await blood, urine cultures
5. If MRSA is suspected, add vancomycin

Cultures at 24 hours

Negative

Febrile

No

Observe

Yes

Febrile but low risk
Treat ceftriaxone 50 mg/kg × 1 dose
and daily follow-up

Positive

Febrile

Yes

Admit and IV
antibiotic treatment

No

Treat as outpatient if follow-up
is reliable with antibiotics
based on culture result

Robyn Wing, MD, William Jerry Durbin, MD, and Mariann Manno, MD

American College of Emergency Physicians Clinical Policies Committee; American College of Emergency Physicians Clinical Policies Subcommittee on Pediatric Fever. Clinical policy for children younger than three years presenting to the emergency department with fever. *Ann Emerg Med.* 2003;42(4):530–545.

FEVER OF UNKNOWN ORIGIN (FUO)

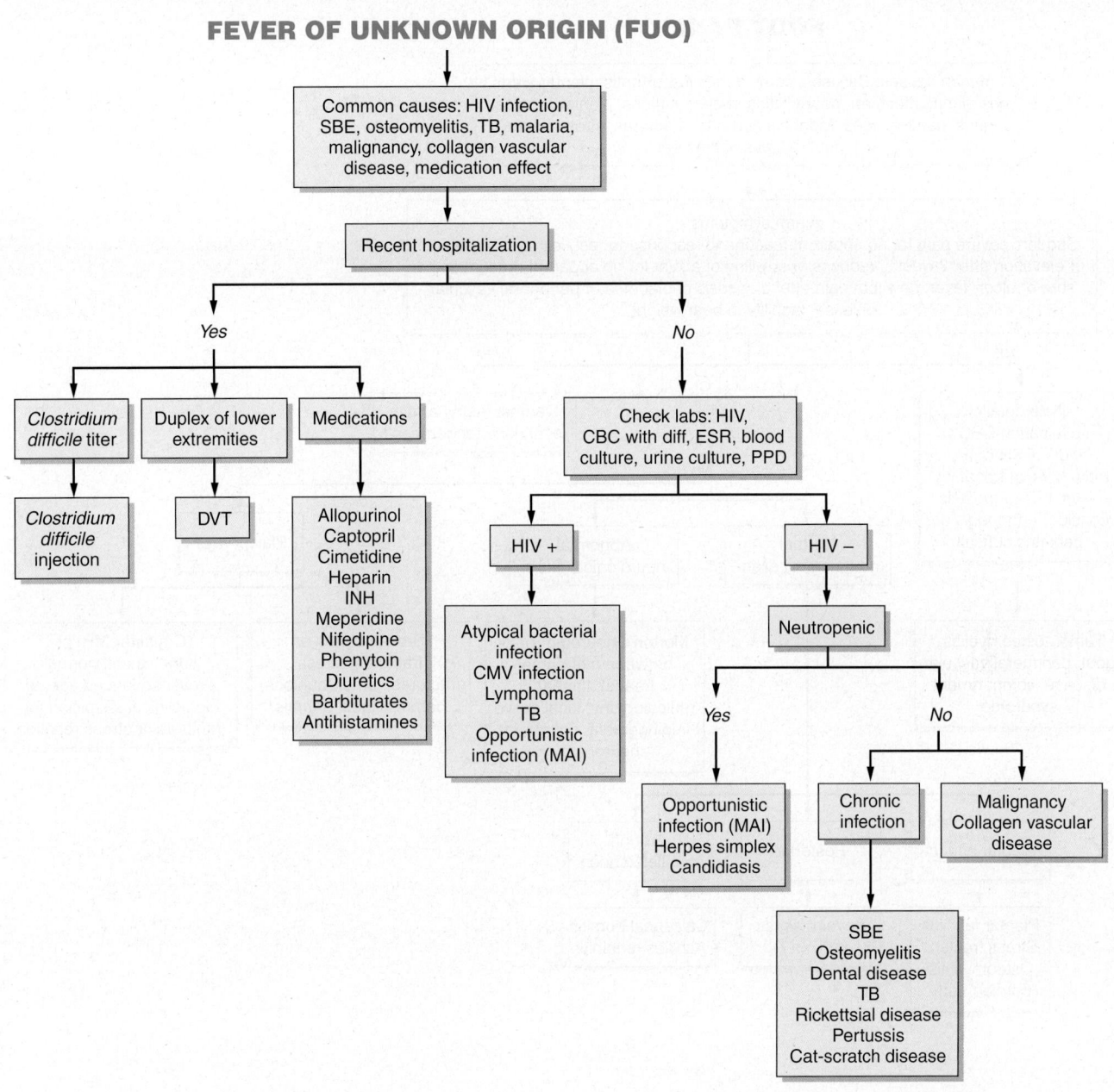

Robert A. Baldor, MD and Alan M. Ehrlich, MD

Mintegi S, Garcia-Garcia JJ, Benito J, et al. Rapid influenza test in young febrile infants for the identification of low-risk patients. *Pediatr Infect Dis J.* 2009;28(11):1026–1028.

FOOT PAIN

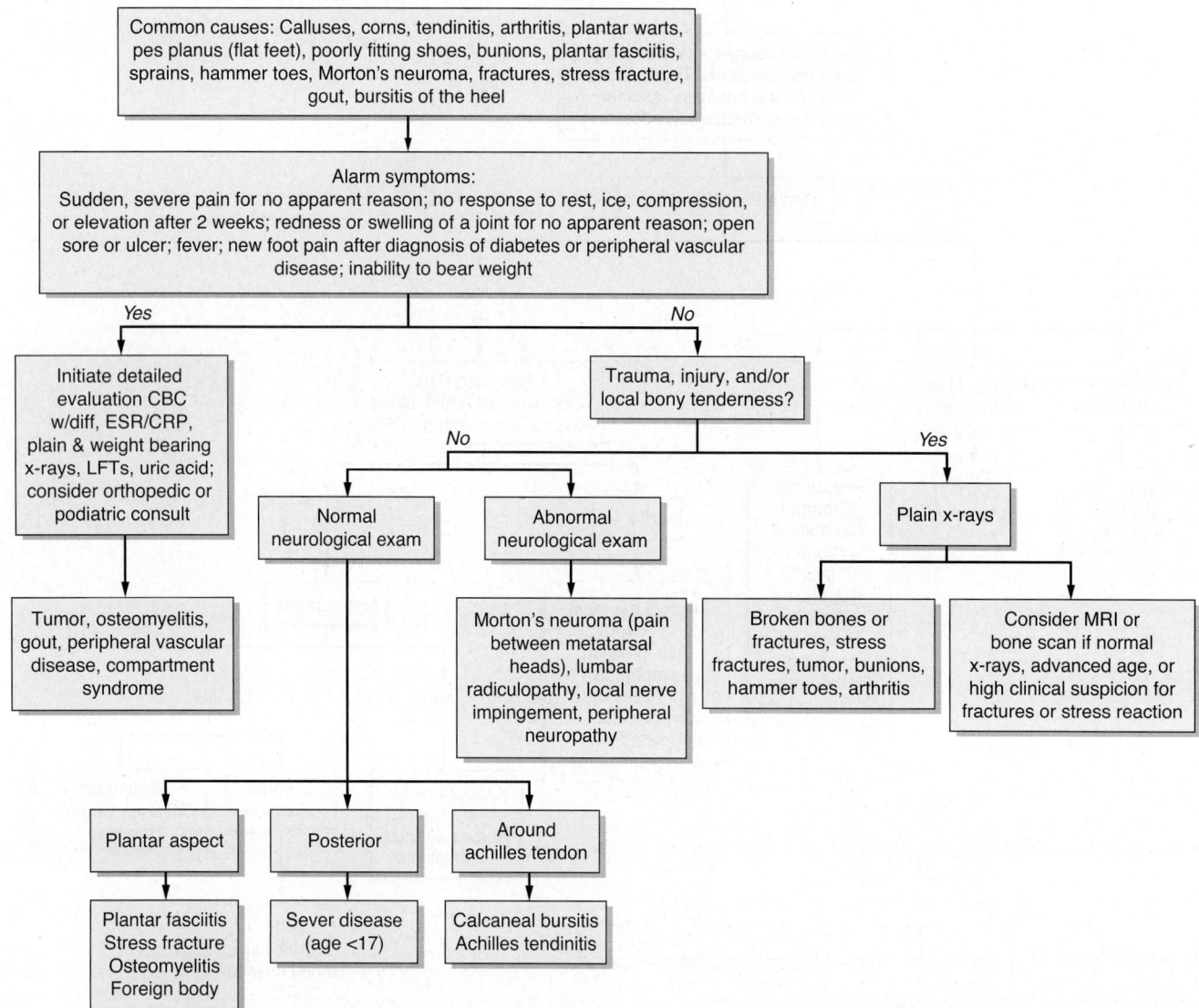

George Gunter A. Pujalte, MD

Bachmann LM, Kolb E, Koller MT, et al. Accuracy of Ottawa ankle rules to exclude fractures of the ankle and mid-foot: Systematic review. *Br Med J.* 2003;326:417.

GAIT DISTURBANCE

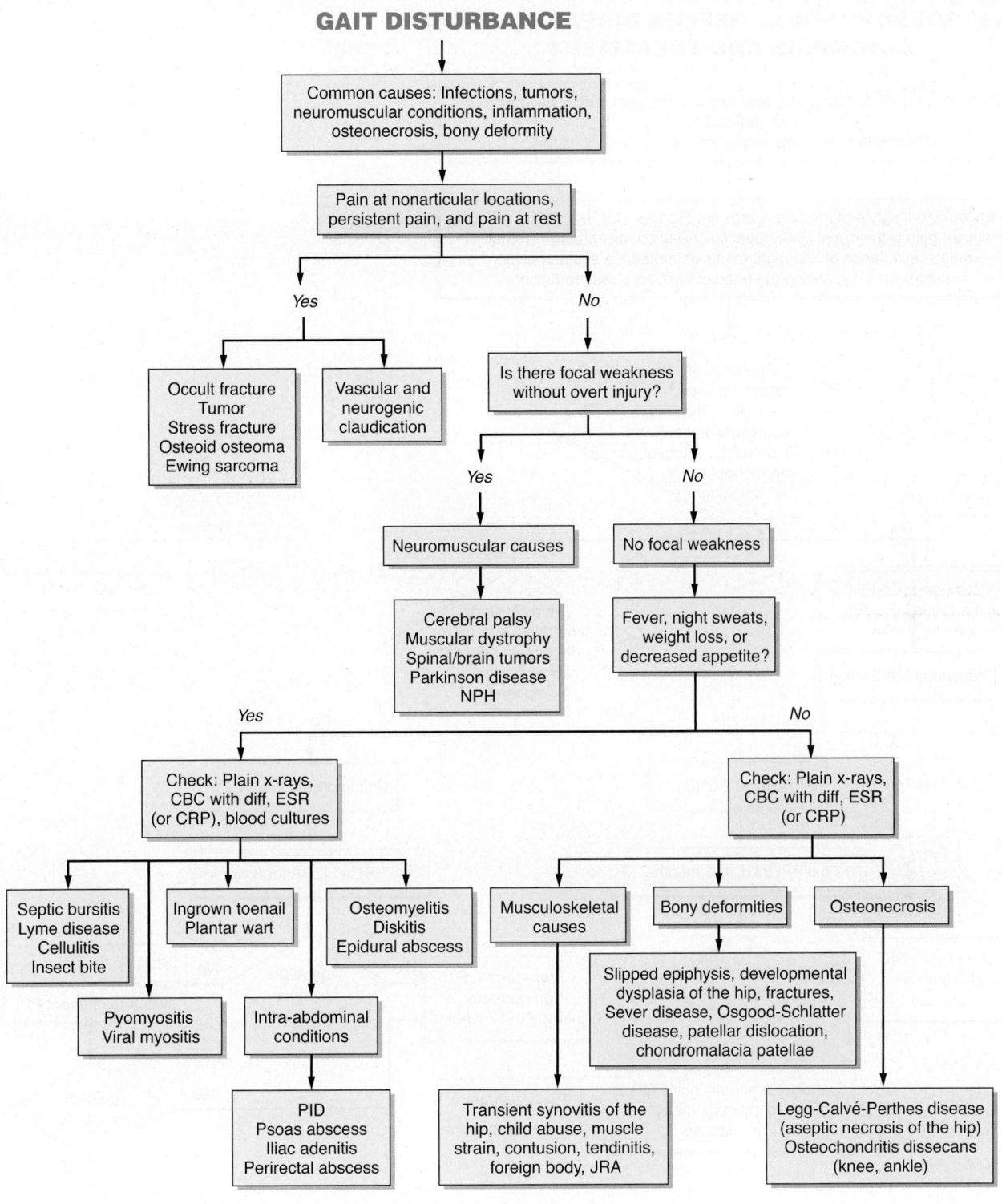

Robert A. Baldor, MD and Alan M. Ehrlich, MD

Bhadelia RA, Price LL, Tedesco KL, et al. Diffusion tensor imaging, white matter lesions, the corpus callosum, and gait in the elderly. *Stroke*. 2009;40(12):3816–3820.

GASTROESOPHAGEAL REFLUX DISEASE (GERD), DIAGNOSIS AND TREATMENT

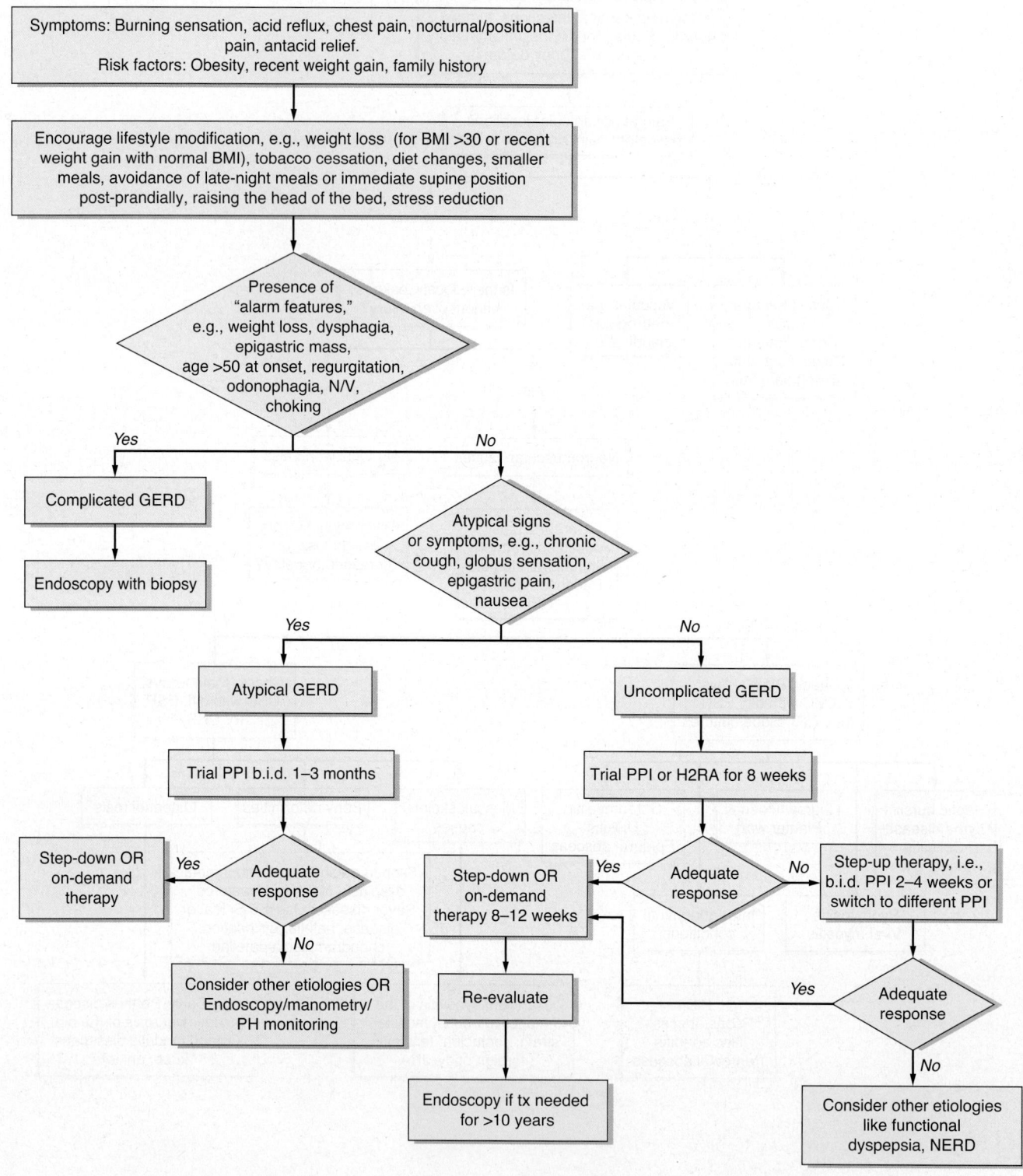

Suma Chennubhotla, MD, Amaninderapal Singh Ghotra, MD, and Thomas L. Abell, MD

Katz PO, Gerson LB, Vela MF. Guidelines for the diagnosis and management of gastroesophageal reflux disease. *Am J Gastroenterol.* 2013;108:308–328.

GENITAL ULCERS

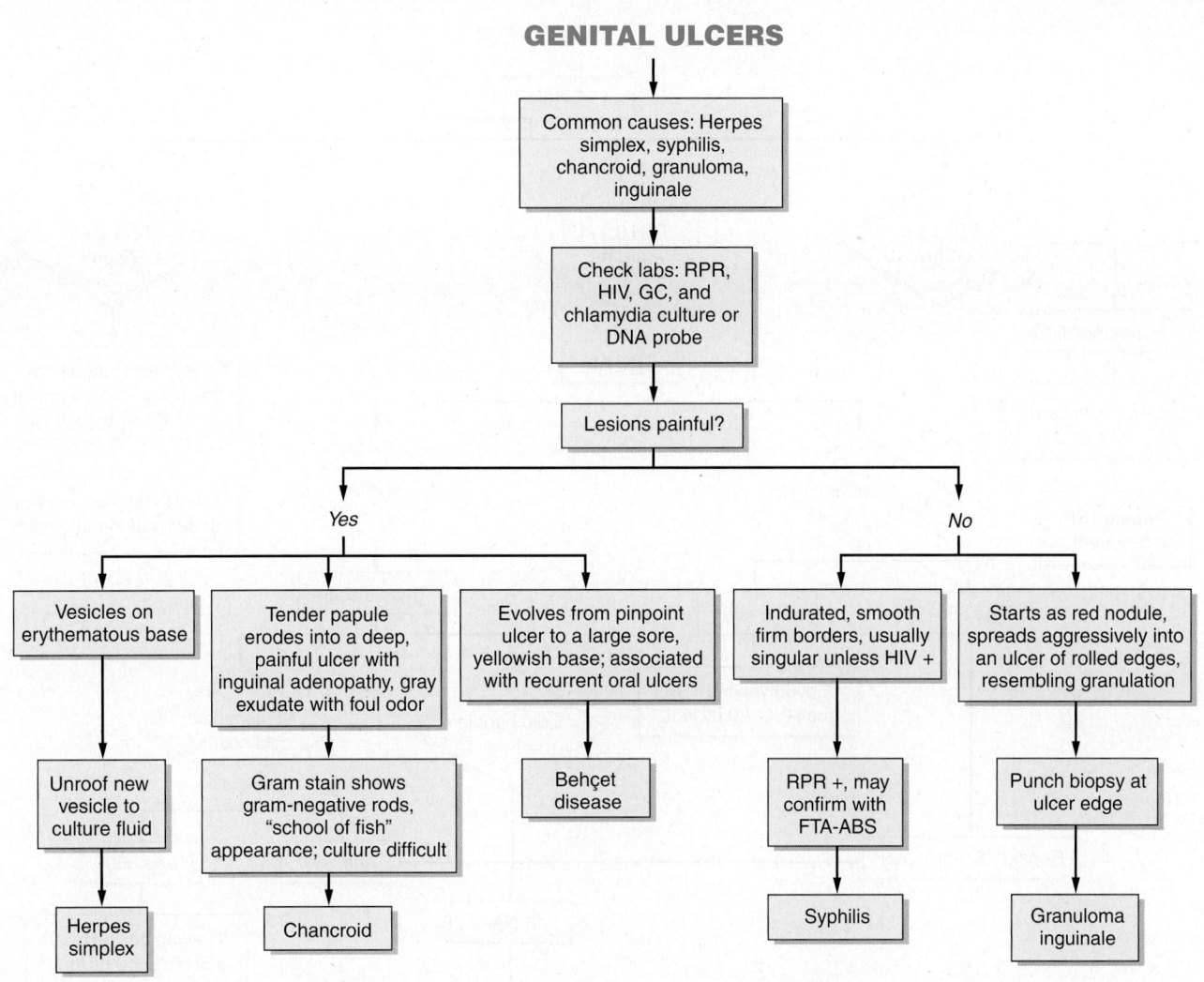

Common causes: Herpes simplex, syphilis, chancroid, granuloma, inguinale

Check labs: RPR, HIV, GC, and chlamydia culture or DNA probe

Lesions painful?

Yes

Vesicles on erythematous base

Tender papule erodes into a deep, painful ulcer with inguinal adenopathy, gray exudate with foul odor

Evolves from pinpoint ulcer to a large sore, yellowish base; associated with recurrent oral ulcers

Unroof new vesicle to culture fluid

Gram stain shows gram-negative rods, "school of fish" appearance; culture difficult

Behçet disease

Herpes simplex

Chancroid

No

Indurated, smooth firm borders, usually singular unless HIV +

Starts as red nodule, spreads aggressively into an ulcer of rolled edges, resembling granulation

RPR +, may confirm with FTA-ABS

Punch biopsy at ulcer edge

Syphilis

Granuloma inguinale

Robert A. Baldor, MD and Alan M. Ehrlich, MD

O'Farrell N, Morison L, Moodley P, et al. Genital ulcers and concomitant complaints in men attending a sexually transmitted infections clinic: Implications for sexually transmitted infections management. *Sex Transm Dis.* 2008;35(6):545–549.

GOITER

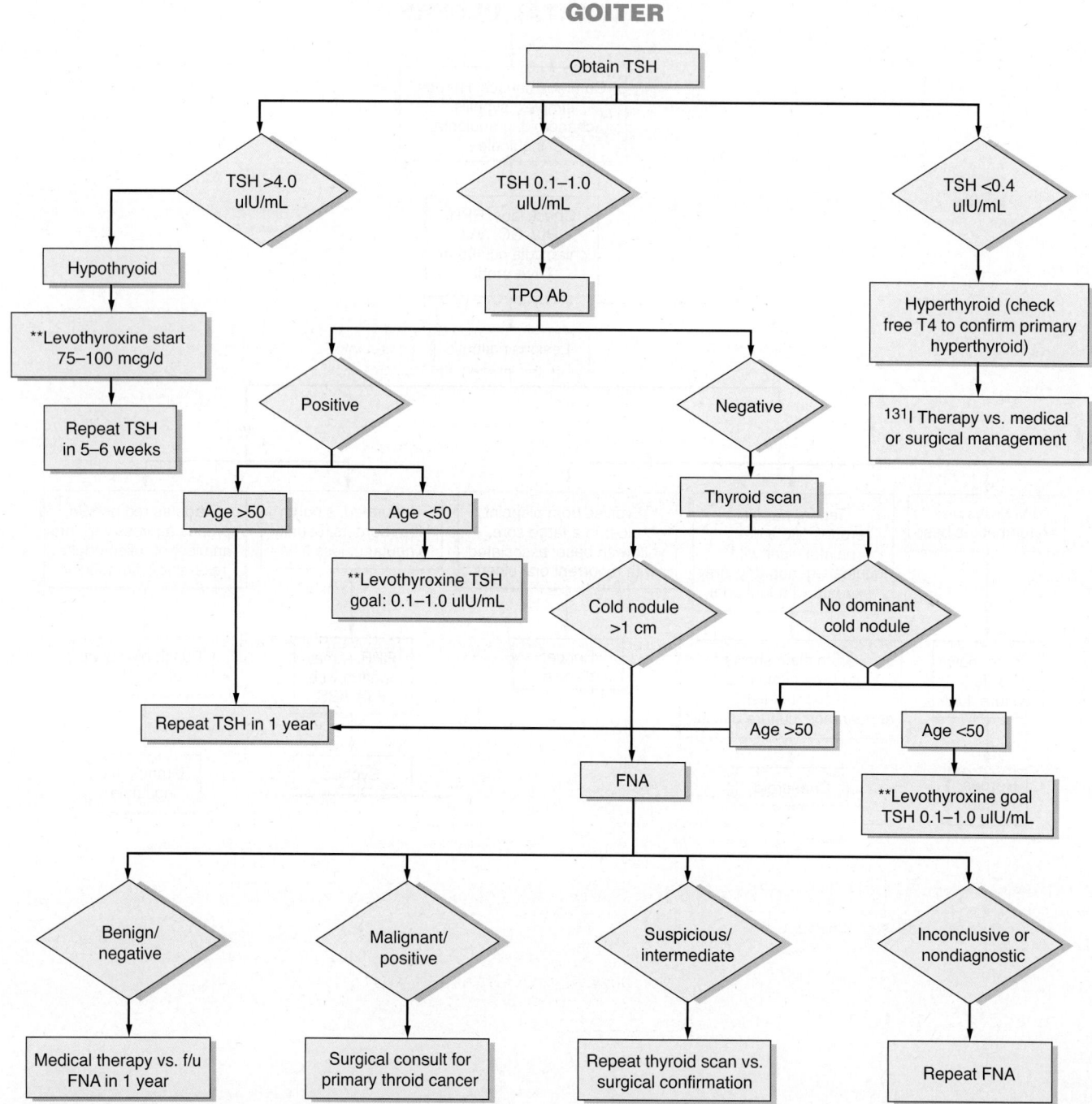

Obtain TSH

TSH >4.0 uIU/mL
- Hypothryoid
- **Levothyroxine start 75–100 mcg/d
- Repeat TSH in 5–6 weeks

TSH 0.1–1.0 uIU/mL
- TPO Ab
  - Positive
    - Age >50 → Repeat TSH in 1 year
    - Age <50 → **Levothyroxine TSH goal: 0.1–1.0 uIU/mL
  - Negative
    - Thyroid scan
      - Cold nodule >1 cm → FNA
      - No dominant cold nodule
        - Age >50 → Repeat TSH in 1 year
        - Age <50 → **Levothyroxine goal TSH 0.1–1.0 uIU/mL

TSH <0.4 uIU/mL
- Hyperthyroid (check free T4 to confirm primary hyperthyroid)
- 131I Therapy vs. medical or surgical management

FNA:
- Benign/negative → Medical therapy vs. f/u FNA in 1 year
- Malignant/positive → Surgical consult for primary throid cancer
- Suspicious/intermediate → Repeat thyroid scan vs. surgical confirmation
- Inconclusive or nondiagnostic → Repeat FNA

** Caution with cardiovascular disease or osteoperosis.

Katie Crowder, MD and Elaina C. Wild, MD

Hoffman MR, Meadows SE, Langlois JP. Clinical inquiries. What is the best approach to goiter for euthyroid patients? *J Fam Pract*. 2007;56(6):479–480.

HALLUCINATIONS

Definition: A false perception that occurs in the waking state in the absence of a sensory stimulus

Common causes: Delirium, hypnogogic state (transition from sleep to awake)

Visual

DDx: Migraine, seizure, stroke, glaucoma, cataract, toxic/metabolic disorders, major affective disorders, conversion disorders, sleep deprivation, acute situational stress, EtOH/drug intoxication/withdrawal, Lewy body dementia, Parkinson disease

Mental status exam abnormal or clouding of consciousness

Does the patient have clouding of consciousness?

No — Are the hallucinations complex?

Yes — Delirium

No — Salicylate use or other (tinnitus, whistling, clicking)?

Yes (e.g., voices, music) — Do the hallucinations occur within 48 hours of cessation of alcohol use?

No — Workup for lesions of superior temporal gyrus, middle ear, auditory nerve

Yes — Salicylate toxicity

No — Recent hallucinogen use?

Yes — Workup for alcohol withdrawal

No — Are the hallucinations brief, stereotyped, acute onset?

Yes — Hallucinogen abuse

No — Consider psychotic disorder

Yes — See "Seizure, New Onset" algorithm

Jaclyn EA Legg, DO and Gautam J. Desai, DO, FACOFP

Gleason OC. Delirium. *Am Fam Physician.* 2003;67(5):1027–1034.

HEAD INJURY, DIAGNOSIS AND MANAGEMENT

Risk Factors:
- Anticoagulation therapy or hemophilia
- Known or suspected skull fracture
- Posttraumatic seizures
- Hx of shunt-treated hydrocephalus
- Multiple injuries (especially above clavicles)
- Age >60
- Drug or alcohol intoxication
- Amnesia, headache, or vomiting

ICU care:
- Seizure prophylaxis
- Sedation
- SBP >90
- Ventilator management (PCO_2 35–40; pulse ox >90%)
- Frequent neurological assessment
- INR <1.4
- Cerebral perfusion pressure >60
- Maintain normothermia
- Platelets $>75 \times 10^3/mm^3$
- Hgb >8 g/dL

Michael J. Gray, MD

Swadron SP, LeRoux P, Smith WS, et al. Emergency neurological life support: Traumatic brain injury. *Neurocit Care.* 2012;17:S112–S121.

HEADACHE, CHRONIC

*Red flags include onset of headache after age 50, altered mental status (including confusion, personality changes), papilledema, report of "worst headache of my life," and focal neurologic deficits such as weakness or ataxia.

Naomi Lawrence-Reid, MD and David B. Sommer, MD, MPH

National Guidelines Clearinghouse. *Diagnosis and Treatment of Headache.* http://www.guideline.gov/content.aspx?id=14440&search=chronic+headache
Sobri M, et al. Red flags in patients presenting with headache: Clinical indications for neuroimaging. *Br J Radiol.* 2003;76:532–535.

Nirmanmoh Bhatia, MD, Amaninderapal S. Ghotra, MD and Marcus F. Stoddard, MD

Biancaniello T. Innocent murmurs. *Circulation.* 2005;111:e20–e22.

HEMATEMESIS (BLEEDING, UPPER GI)

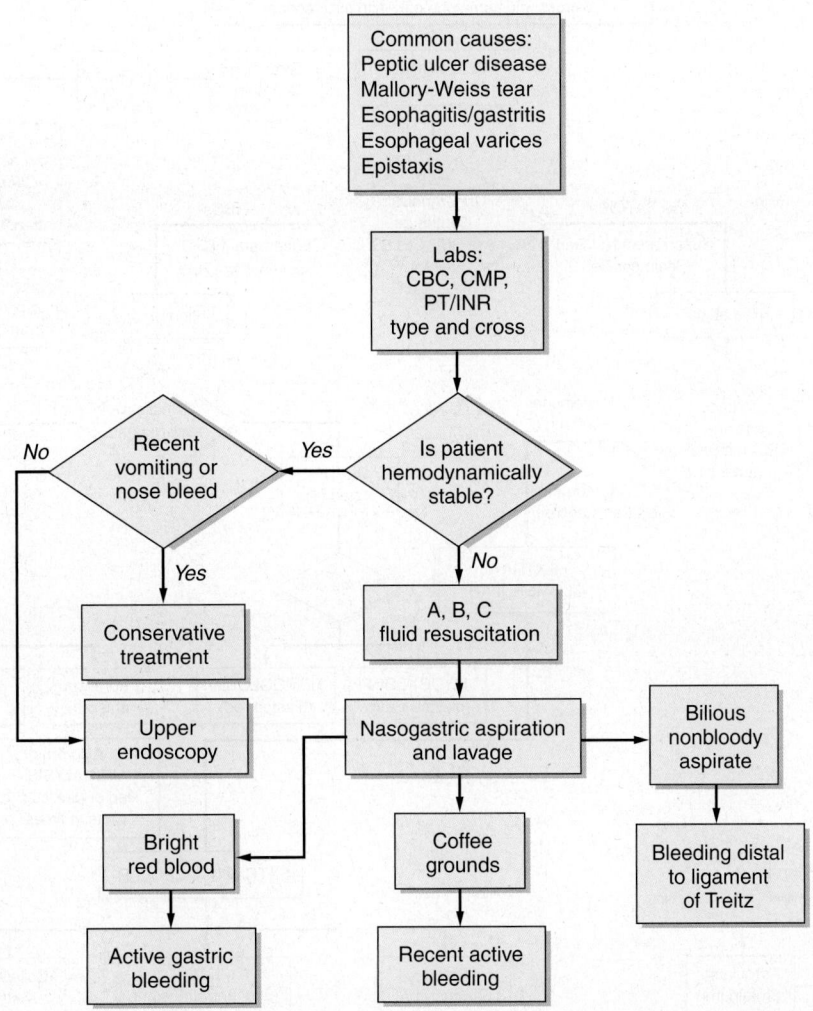

Sanjeev Sharma, MD

Barkun A, Fallone CA, Chiba N, et al. A Canadian clinical practice algorithm for the management of patients with nonvariceal upper gastrointestinal bleeding. *Can J Gastroenterol.* 2004;18(10):605–609.

HEMATURIA

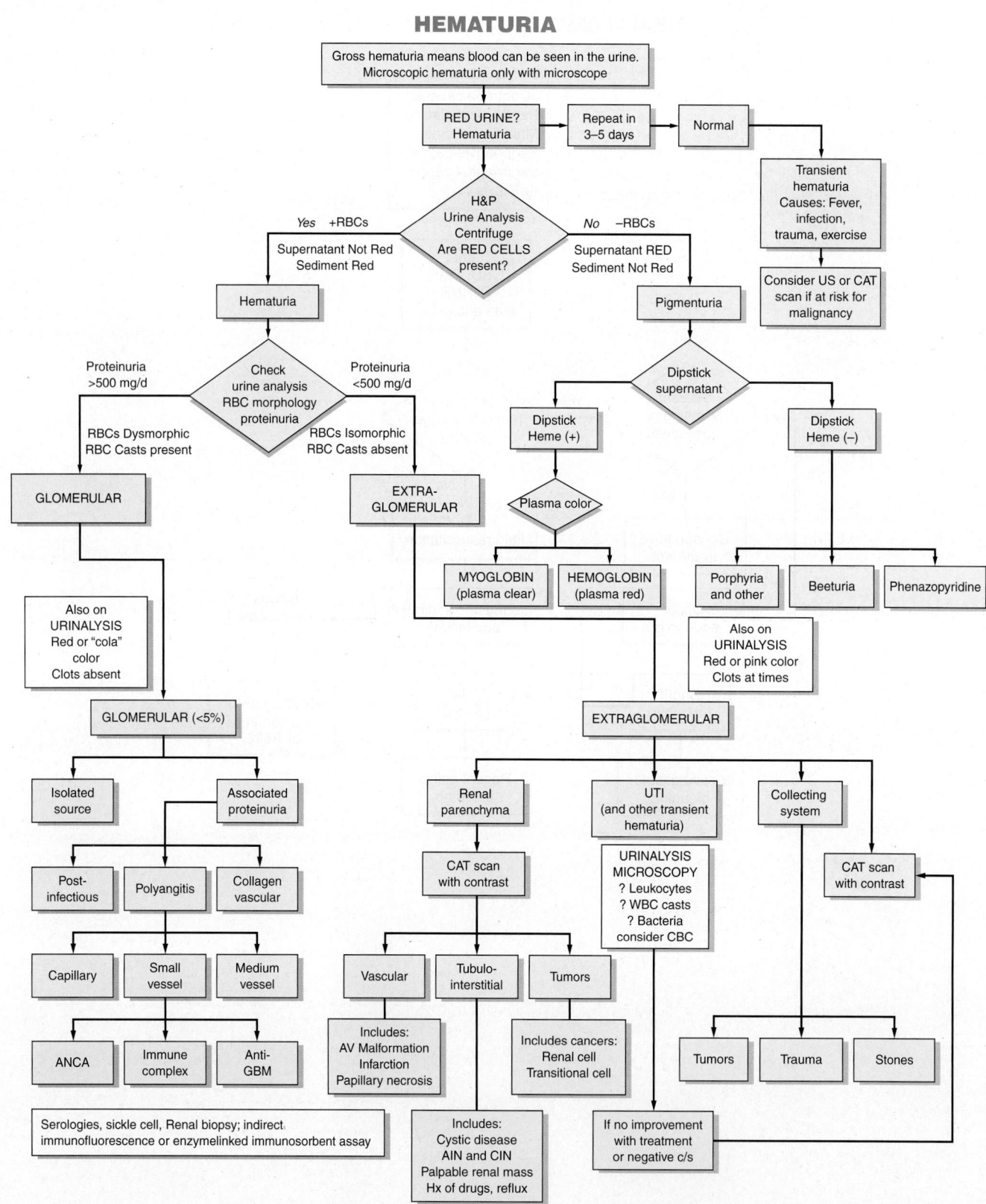

Nathalee Kong, MD and Marie Anne Sosa, MD

McDonald MM, Swagerty D, Wetzel L. Assessment of microscopic hematuria in adults. *Am Fam Physician.* 2006;73(10):1748–1754.

HEMOCHROMATOSIS

Hemochromatosis Evaluations

- Family history of liver disease or diabetes mellitus
- Early signs: Arthralgias, fatigue, decreased libido, persistently elevated AST and ALT, elevated serum Fe
- Late signs: Cirrhosis, diabetes mellitus, cardiomyopathy, pseudogout

Obtain
Fasting serum Fe*, TIBC

*Off multivitamin
or iron supplement

$$\text{Transferrin Saturation} = \frac{\text{Serum Fe}}{\text{TIBC}} \times 100$$

<55%

>55%

Consider other etiology of symptoms

Possible hemochromatosis

Obtain C282Y
(HFE gene)
H63D mutation

Negative

Positive

Consider other diagnosis

Hemochromatosis confirmed

Does patient have ANY of the following?
- Age >40 years
- Hepatomegaly
- ↑AST or ACT
- Ferritin >1,000

No

Yes

Cirrhosis unlikely biopsy not indicated

Liver biopsy to determine if cirrhosis is present

- Screen family members for genetic mutation
- Phlebotomy

Kristin Burke, MD

Brandhagen DJ, Fairbanks VF, Baldus W. Recognition and management of hereditary hemochromatosis. *Am Fam Physician.* 2002;65(5):853–860.

HEPATOMEGALY

Neha Jekhete, MD and Marie L. Borum, MD, EdD, MPH

Starr SP, Raines D. Cirrhosis: Diagnosis, management, and prevention. *Am Fam Physician.* 2011;84:1353–1359.

HIP/GROIN PAIN

Common causes: OA, osteonecrosis, sciatica, stress fracture

↓

Traumatic — Yes → Fracture dislocation labral tear loose body

No ↓

History of childhood pathology (such as developmental dysplasia, slipped capital femoral epiphysis, Legg-Calve-Perthes) — Yes → Labral tear osteoarthritis/ chondral damage

No ↓

Groin pain Can be elicited by ranging hip in flexion, internal rotation or flexion external rotation, or a resisted straight leg raise — Yes → Intra-articular → **History of trauma** — Yes → Osteoarthritis / Labral tear / Femoroacetabular impingement / Capsular laxity / Ligamentum teres tears / Osteomyelitis / Osteonecrosis / Occult fracture

No ↓ (from History of trauma)

Synovitis / Hernia / Osteonecrosis / Occult fracture / Inflammatory arthritis / Neoplasm

No ↓ (from Groin pain)

Extra-articular

↓

Numbness, paresthesias or shooting pain — Yes → Sciatica / Piriformis syndrome / Sacroiliac joint pathology / Meralgia peresthetica (lateral femoral cutaneous nerve entrapment)

No ↓

Location

- Other: Inability to reproduce pain at site with physical exam, but examination at another site reproduces pain
- Anterior: Iliopsoas tendinitis
- Medial: Athletic pubalgia (sports hernia) / Adductor strain / Muscle contracture / Osteitis pubis
- Lateral: Trochanteric Bursitis / Iliotibial band tendonitis / Iliotibial band contracture / Gluteal tears / Hip osteonecrosis

(from Other) ↓

Exercise induced?

No → Abdominal pathology must be ruled out (such as PID, nephrolithiasis, appendicitis, ovarian cysts, aneurysms, etc.)

Yes → Stress fracture / Aorto-occlusive disease

Edward Cheung, MD and Paul George, MD

Kuhlman GS, Domb BG. Hip impingement: Identifying and treating a common cause of hip pain. *Am Fam Physician.* 2009;80:1429–1434.

HYPERBILIRUBINEMIA AND CIRRHOSIS

Robert A. Baldor, MD and Alan M. Ehrlich, MD

Porter ML, Dennis BL. Hyperbilirubinemia in the term newborn. *Am Fam Physician.* 2002;65(4):599–606.

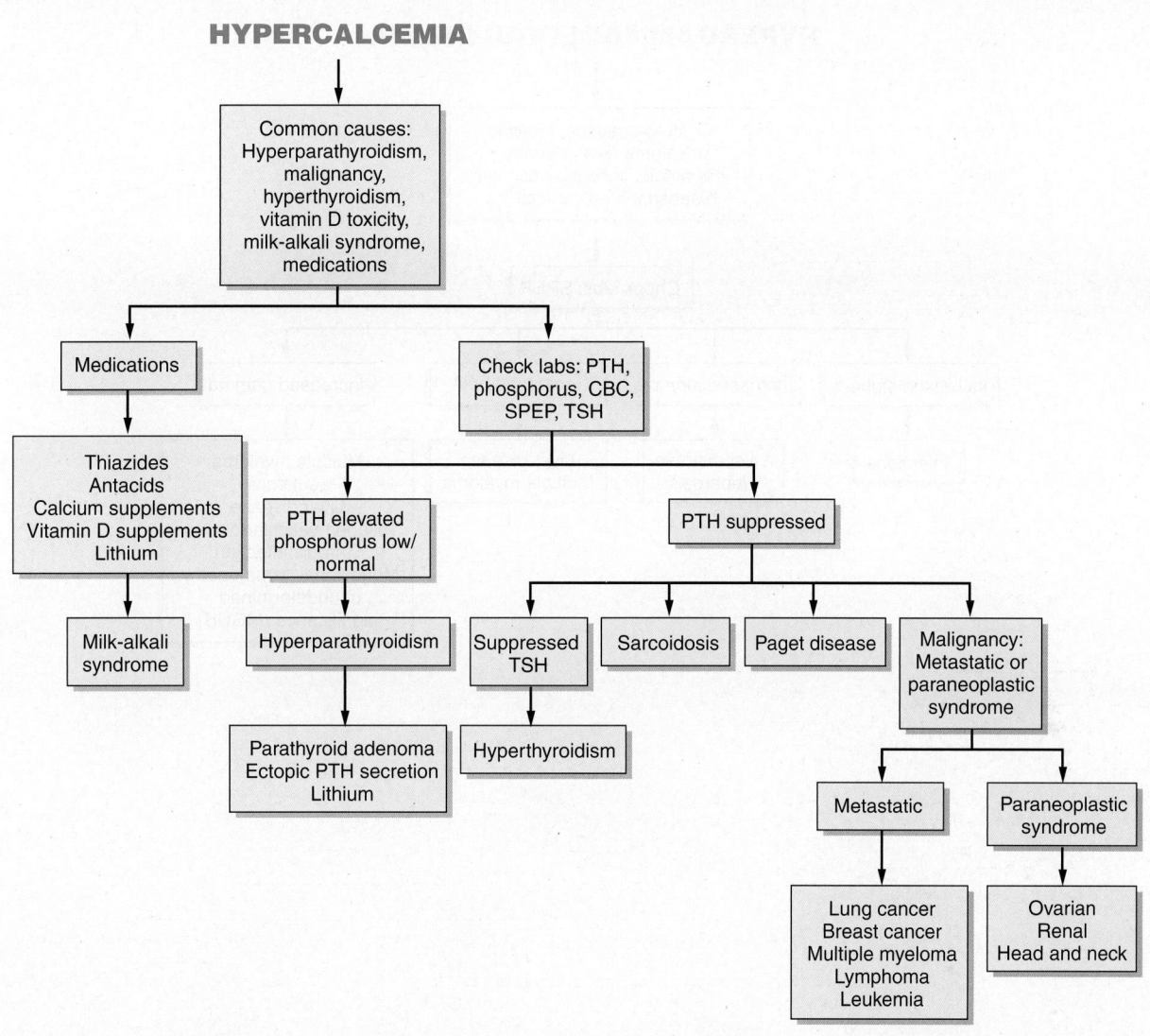

HYPERCALCEMIA

Common causes: Hyperparathyroidism, malignancy, hyperthyroidism, vitamin D toxicity, milk-alkali syndrome, medications

Medications → Check labs: PTH, phosphorus, CBC, SPEP, TSH

Medications:
Thiazides
Antacids
Calcium supplements
Vitamin D supplements
Lithium

Milk-alkali syndrome

PTH elevated phosphorus low/normal → Hyperparathyroidism → Parathyroid adenoma / Ectopic PTH secretion / Lithium

PTH suppressed → Suppressed TSH → Hyperthyroidism
Sarcoidosis
Paget disease
Malignancy: Metastatic or paraneoplastic syndrome

Metastatic → Lung cancer / Breast cancer / Multiple myeloma / Lymphoma / Leukemia

Paraneoplastic syndrome → Ovarian / Renal / Head and neck

Robert A. Baldor, MD and Alan M. Ehrlich, MD

Carroll MF, Schade DS. A practical approach to hypercalcemia. *Am Fam Physician.* 2003;67(9):1959–1966.

HYPERGAMMAGLOBULINEMIA

Robert A. Baldor, MD and Alan M. Ehrlich, MD

Baimpa E, Dahabreh IJ, Voulgarelis M, et al. Hematologic manifestations and predictors of lymphoma development in primary Sjögren syndrome: Clinical and pathophysiologic aspects. *Medicine (Baltimore)*. 2009;88(5):284–293.

HYPERKALEMIA

Rocio Nordfeldt, MD and Felix B. Chang, MD

Palmer BF. A physiologic-based approach to the evaluation of a patient with hyperkalemia. *Am J Kidney Dis.* 2010;56(2):387–393.

HYPERKINESIS

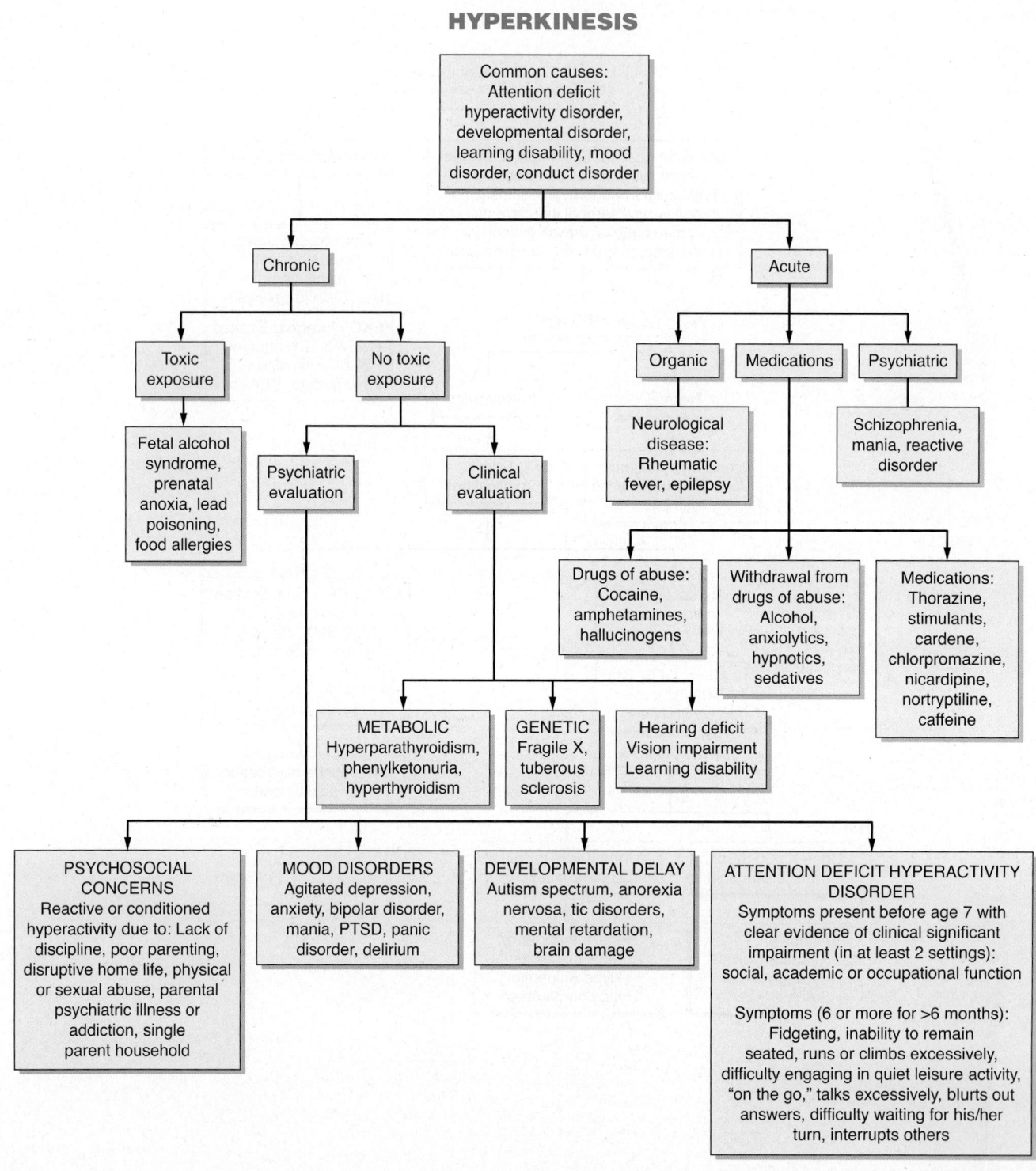

Carrie Janiski, DO, MS, ATC and Peter Ziemkowski, MD

Modesto-Lowe V, Meyer A, Soovajian V. A clinican's guide to adult attention-deficit hperactivity disorder. *Conn Med.* 2012;76(9):517–523.

HYPERLIPIDEMIA

Rade N. Pejic, MD and Frank J. Domino, MD

Stone NJ, Robinson J, Lichtenstein C, et al. 2013 ACC/AHA Guideline on the Treatment of Blood Cholesterol to Reduce Atherosclerotic Cardiovascular Risk in Adults: A Report of the American College of Cardiology/American Heart Association Task Force on Practice Guidelines. *Circulation.* 2013 Nov 12. [Epub ahead of print]

HYPERNATREMIA

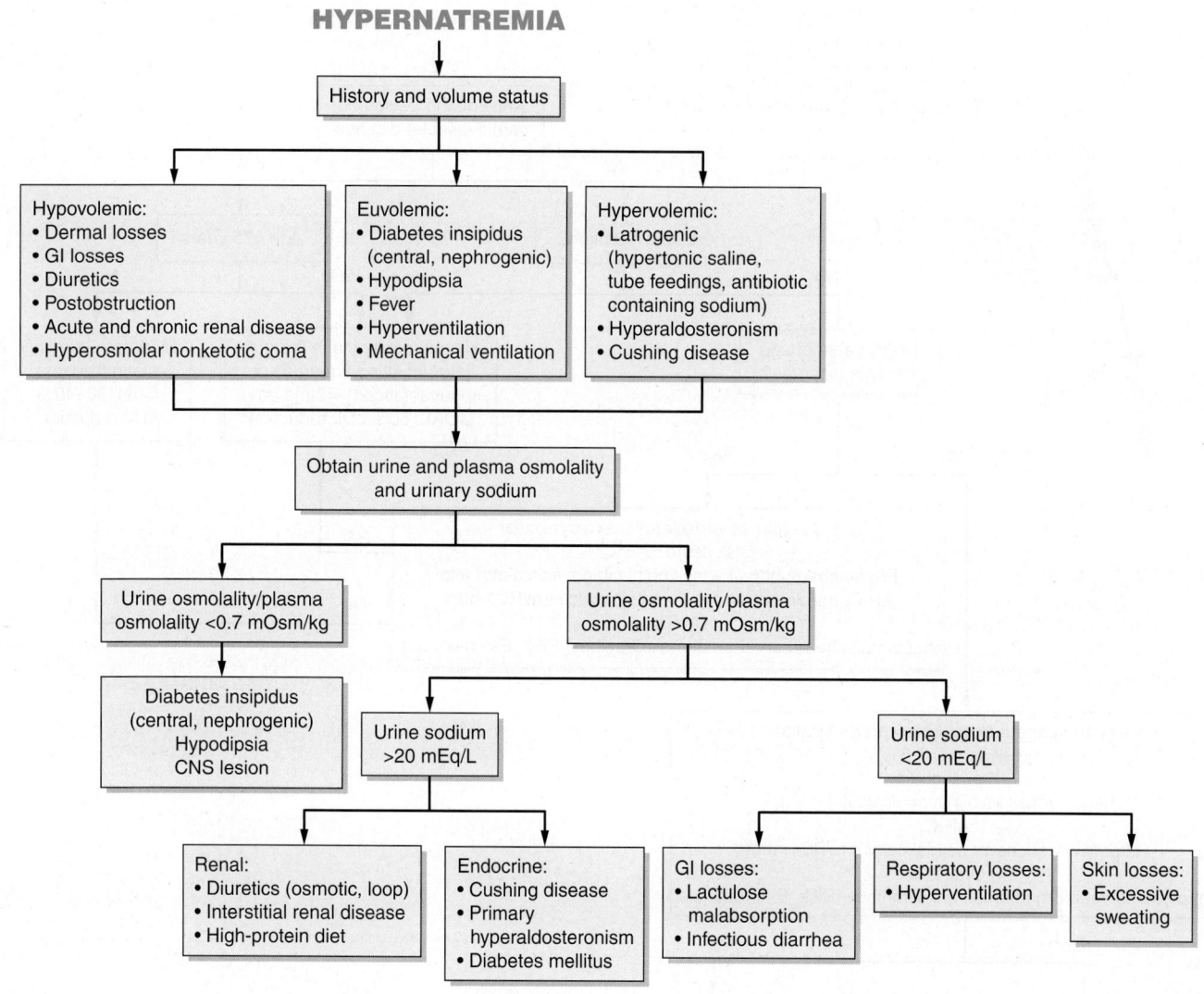

Timothy J. Coker, MD

Reynolds RM, Padfield PL, Seckl JR. Disorders of sodium balance. *Br Med J.* 2006;332:702–705.

HYPERTENSION AND ELEVATED BLOOD PRESSURE, TREATMENT

Nicolas Hernandez, MD and Felix B. Chang, MD

National Heart, Lung, and Blood Institute. *The Seventh Report of the Joint National Committee on Prevention, Detection, Evaluation, and Treatment of High Blood Pressure (JNC 7).* Bethesda, MD: National Heart, Lung, and Blood Institute. 2004.

HYPOACTIVE REFLEXES

Common causes: Hyperthyroidism, hypoglycemia, peripheral nerve injury, peripheral neuropathy, Guillain-Barré syndrome, herniated disk, Lyme disease, normal aging

Check labs: TSH, calcium, B_{12}, Lyme titer, consider monospot, RPR

Abnormal labs

- Infections
  - Lyme disease
    Infectious mononucleosis
    Syphilis
    West Nile virus infection
    Postpolio syndrome
- Elevated TSH → Hyperthyroidism
- Low calcium → Hypocalcemia
- Low vitamin B_{12} → Pernicious anemia Strict vegan diet

Normal labs

- Focal hyporeflexia → Herniated disk Peripheral neuropathy Peripheral nerve injury
- Diffuse hyporeflexia → Peripheral neuropathy Guillain-Barré syndrome Myasthenia gravis Muscle diseases Normal aging
- Upper extremity hyporeflexia with lower extremity hyperreflexia → Syringomyelia and other cervical spine disorders

Robert A. Baldor, MD and Alan M. Ehrlich, MD

Pascuzzi RM. Peripheral neuropathy. *Med Clin North Am.* 2009;93(2):317–342, vii–viii.

HYPOALBUMINEMIA

Albumin <3.5 g/dL

History: Edema, jaundice, alcoholism, hepatitis, foamy urine, muscle atrophy, ascitis, weight gain, loss of appetite, malnutrition, decreased PO intake, hyperlipidemia, diarrhea, vomiting, burns, inflamation

DECREASE PROTEIN SYNTHESIS

ABNORMAL PROTEIN DISTRIBUTION

PROTEIN LOSS

Cirrhosis stigmass ascites, spider angiomas

Physiological stress (infection, surgery, trauma)

Hemodilutional States

URINE DIPSTICK ANALYSIS
≥3-4+protein

↑CRP ESR

Peripheral edema, dyspnea, fatigue, ↑BNP crackles

Flank dullness, abdominal distension, fluid wave

SPOT URINE Random urine protein/Cr ratio ≥3–3.5

24-HOUR URINE If ≥3.5 g/24 hr

Plt <160,000/mm³

Elevated LFTs (esp. AST)

Positive Hepatitis

INR ≥1.5

Elevated GGT

Alkaline phosphatase

Nodular liver on abdominal U/S

ACUTE & CHRONIC INFLAMMATION

CHF

ASCITES

NEPHROTIC SYNDROME

Diminished height
Poor weight gain
Deficit in lean body mass
Wasted
Stunted linear growth
Alopecia
Frequent infection
Vitamin deficiencies

Enteral Protein Loss Alpha-1-antitrypsin in Stool

Skin burns and tissue damage

LIVER CIRRHOSIS

Upper GI endoscopy

EXTENSIVE SKIN BURNS

Decreased lymphocyte count, BUN, transferrin, Prealbumin

PROTEIN-LOSING GASTROENTEROPATHY WORKUP

MALNUTRITION & STARVATION

Crystal Benjamin, MD and Felix B. Chang, MD, DABMA

Kodner C. Nephrotic syndrome in adults: diagnosis and management. *Am Fam Physician.* 2009;80(10):1129–1134.

Tiffany Burca, DO and Timothy Coker, MD

Michels TC, Kelly KM. Parathyroid disorders. *Am Fam Physician.* 2013;88:249–257.

HYPOGLYCEMIA

Robert A. Baldor, MD and Alan M. Ehrlich, MD

Murad MH, Coto-Yglesias F, Wang AT, et al. Clinical review: Drug-induced hypoglycemia: A systematic review. *J Clin Endocrinol Metab.* 2009;94(3):741–745.

HYPOKALEMIA

HISTORY TAKING

INADEQUATE INTAKE
Potassium deficient diet:
Tea and toast diet
Eating disorders:
Anorexia, bulimia, starvation, pica
Inability to eat
Potassium-poor TPN

MEDICATIONS
Diuretics
Laxatives
Bicarbonate
Methylxanthines OD
Amphotericin B
Cisplatin
Chloroquine intoxication
Verapamil OD
Beta agonist intoxication
Ephedrine

SPURIOUS
leukocytosis
>100K
AML
Severe lipemia

TRANSCELLULAR SHIFT
DRUG INDUCED:
β2-adrenergic agonists:
Epinephrine
Decongestants:
Pseudoephedrine,
phenylpropanolamine
Bronchodilators: Albuterol,
terbutaline, isoprotenerol,
ephedrine, metaproterenol
Tocolytic: ritrodrine, nylidin
Theophylline
Chloroquine
Caffeine
Verapamil
Insulin
Alkalosis
**Increased anabolic state-
increased in RBC production:**
Pernicious anemia (Vit B_{12})
Neutropenia (G-CSF)
Thyrotoxic periodic paralysis
Barium intoxication
Pheochromocytoma
**Hypokalemic periodic
paralysis**
Refeeding syndrome
Hypothermia
Delirium Tremens

**No transcellular shift, Adequate K intake.
Obtain serum electrolytes, BUN, Cr, Urine
Na, K, and osmolality**

GI LOSS

Vomiting
Diarrhea
GI suction
Draining GI fistula
laxatives
**Secretory
tumors:**
Villous adenoma,
VIPoma,
Zolinger-Ellison

RENAL LOSS

**UK <25 mEq/d
TTKG <3**

**UK >30 mEq/d
TTKG** ** >7**

INSENSIBLE LOSS
Profuse sweating

**Hyponormotensive
Acid-base status**

Hypertensive
Primary hyperaldonerism: Conn
syndrome
Secondary hyperaldosteronism:
renovascular disease, renin-secreting
tumor
Nonaldosterone mineralocorticoid:
Cushing's, Liddle's, exogenous
mineralocorticoid, licorice

ACIDEMIC

DKA
RTA type II
Some distal
RTA type I

VARIABLE

Mg deficiency:
Amphotericin B
Cisplatinum
Aminoglycosides
Foscarnet
Poor Mg intake

ALKALEMIC

UCl

<20
Vomiting
NGT

>20
Diuretics
Barter's
Gitelmans's

TTKG ** →? (urine K+ x p osm) x (serum K+ x Uosm)
<3 kidney is not wasting excessive potassium >7 significant renal loss

AML: Acute myelogenous leukemia, **OD:** Overdose
GI: Gastrointestinal, **UK:** Urine potassium; **TTKG:** transtubular potassium gradient, **UCl:** urine chloride

Nicolas Hernandez, MD and Felix B. Chang, MD

Unwin RJ, Luft FC, Shirley DG. Pathophysiology and management of hypokalemia: A clinical perspective. *Nat Rev Nephrol.* 2011;7(2):75–84.

HYPOMAGNESEMIA

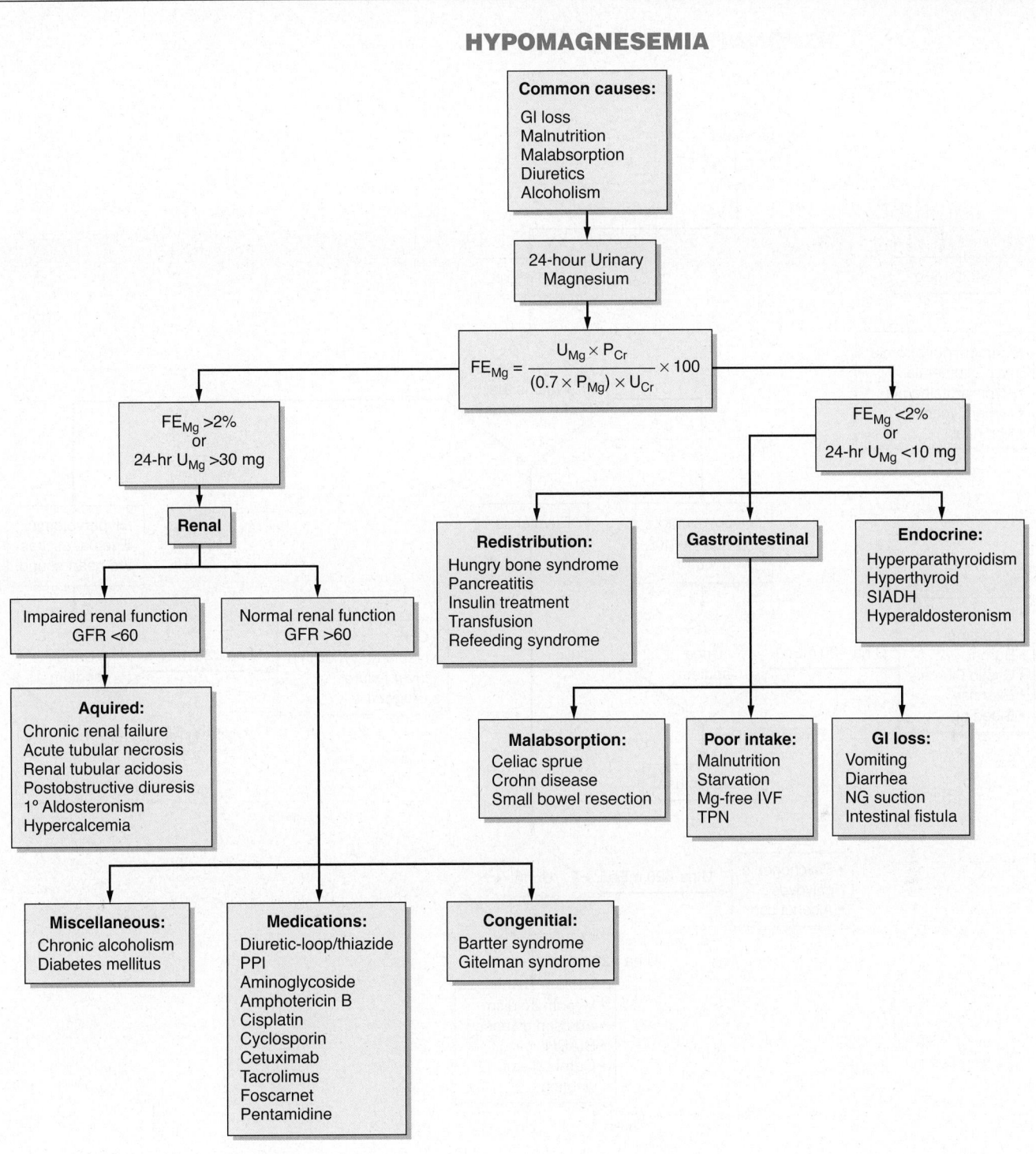

Common causes:

GI loss
Malnutrition
Malabsorption
Diuretics
Alcoholism

24-hour Urinary Magnesium

$$FE_{Mg} = \frac{U_{Mg} \times P_{Cr}}{(0.7 \times P_{Mg}) \times U_{Cr}} \times 100$$

$FE_{Mg} > 2\%$
or
24-hr $U_{Mg} > 30$ mg

$FE_{Mg} < 2\%$
or
24-hr $U_{Mg} < 10$ mg

Renal

Impaired renal function GFR <60

Normal renal function GFR >60

Redistribution:

Hungry bone syndrome
Pancreatitis
Insulin treatment
Transfusion
Refeeding syndrome

Gastrointestinal

Endocrine:

Hyperparathyroidism
Hyperthyroid
SIADH
Hyperaldosteronism

Aquired:

Chronic renal failure
Acute tubular necrosis
Renal tubular acidosis
Postobstructive diuresis
1° Aldosteronism
Hypercalcemia

Malabsorption:

Celiac sprue
Crohn disease
Small bowel resection

Poor intake:

Malnutrition
Starvation
Mg-free IVF
TPN

GI loss:

Vomiting
Diarrhea
NG suction
Intestinal fistula

Miscellaneous:

Chronic alcoholism
Diabetes mellitus

Medications:

Diuretic-loop/thiazide
PPI
Aminoglycoside
Amphotericin B
Cisplatin
Cyclosporin
Cetuximab
Tacrolimus
Foscarnet
Pentamidine

Congenitial:

Bartter syndrome
Gitelman syndrome

Jesse Wm. Mix, DO and Katie Crowder, MD

Martin KJ, Gonzalez EA, Slatopolsky E. Clinical consequences and management of hypomagnesemia. *J Am Soc Nephrol.* 2009;20:2291–2295.

HYPONATREMIA

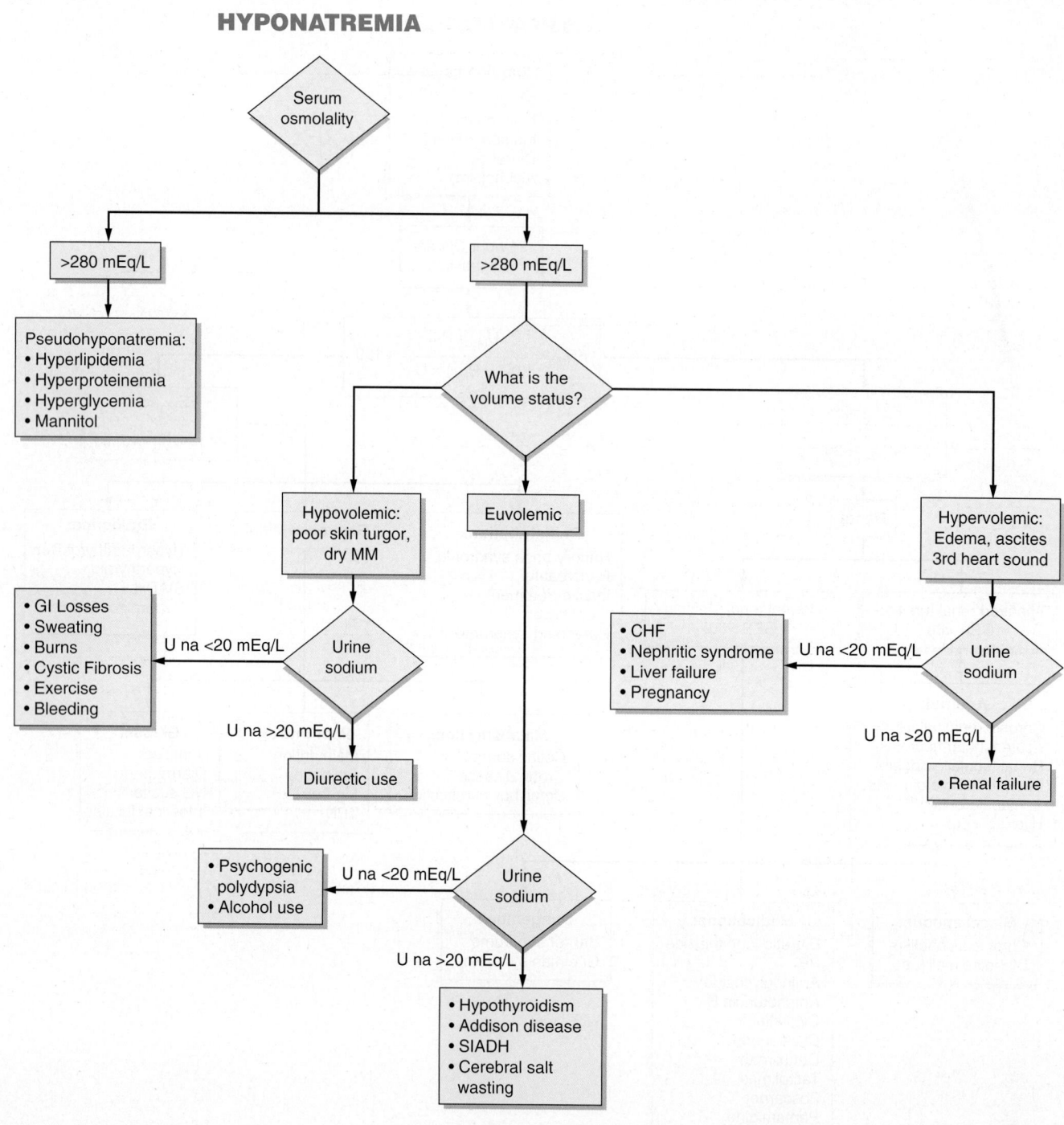

Sultan M. Babar, MD and R. Aaron Lambert, MD

Lien YH, Shapiro JI. Hyponatremia: Clinical diagnosis and management. *Am J Med.* 2007;120(8):653–658.

HYPOTENSION

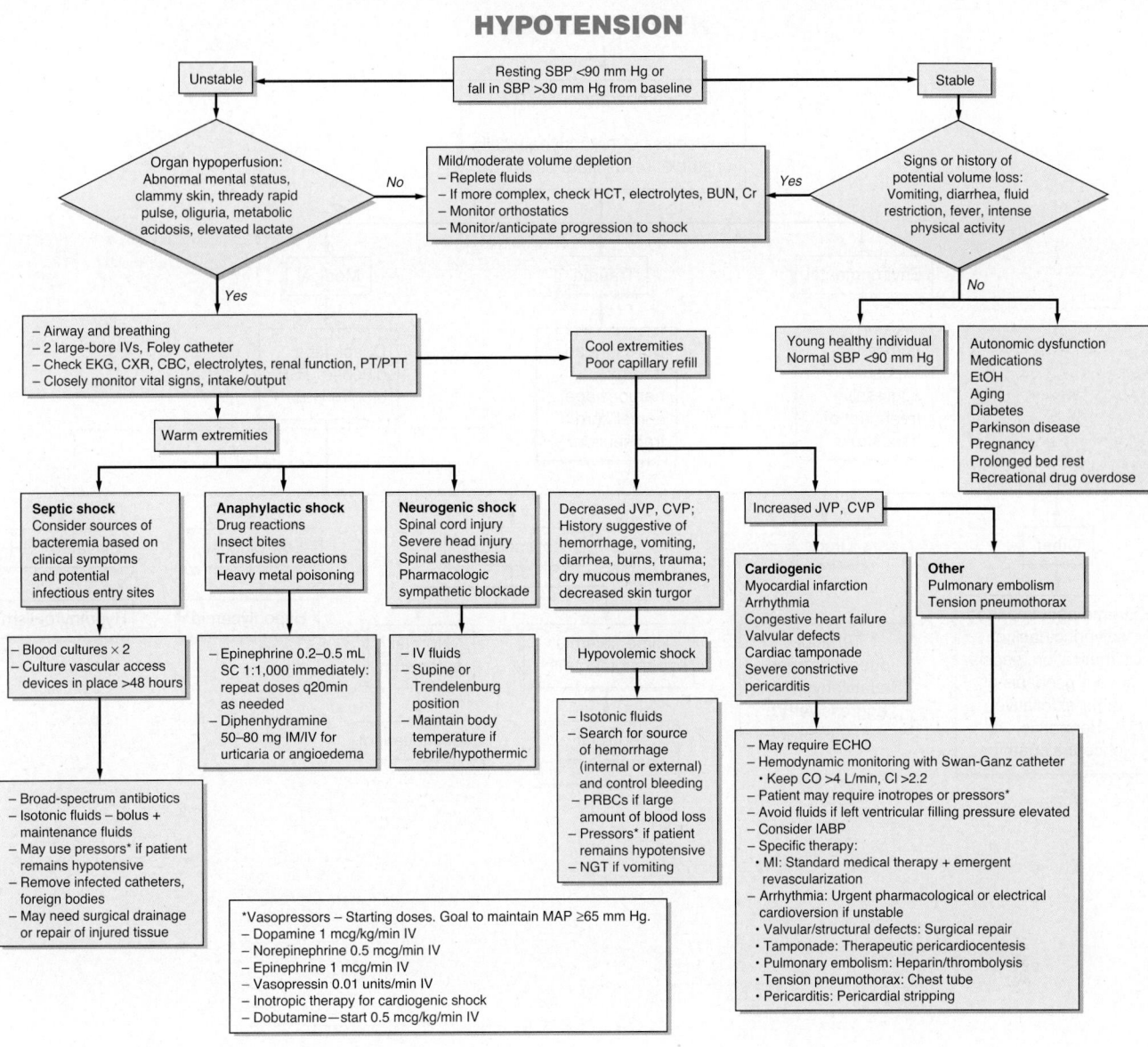

Septic shock
Consider sources of bacteremia based on clinical symptoms and potential infectious entry sites

– Blood cultures × 2
– Culture vascular access devices in place >48 hours

– Broad-spectrum antibiotics
– Isotonic fluids – bolus + maintenance fluids
– May use pressors* if patient remains hypotensive
– Remove infected catheters, foreign bodies
– May need surgical drainage or repair of injured tissue

Anaphylactic shock
Drug reactions
Insect bites
Transfusion reactions
Heavy metal poisoning

– Epinephrine 0.2–0.5 mL SC 1:1,000 immediately: repeat doses q20min as needed
– Diphenhydramine 50–80 mg IM/IV for urticaria or angioedema

Neurogenic shock
Spinal cord injury
Severe head injury
Spinal anesthesia
Pharmacologic sympathetic blockade

– IV fluids
– Supine or Trendelenburg position
– Maintain body temperature if febrile/hypothermic

Cool extremities
Poor capillary refill

Decreased JVP, CVP;
History suggestive of hemorrhage, vomiting, diarrhea, burns, trauma; dry mucous membranes, decreased skin turgor

Hypovolemic shock

– Isotonic fluids
– Search for source of hemorrhage (internal or external) and control bleeding
– PRBCs if large amount of blood loss
– Pressors* if patient remains hypotensive
– NGT if vomiting

Increased JVP, CVP

Cardiogenic
Myocardial infarction
Arrhythmia
Congestive heart failure
Valvular defects
Cardiac tamponade
Severe constrictive pericarditis

Other
Pulmonary embolism
Tension pneumothorax

– May require ECHO
– Hemodynamic monitoring with Swan-Ganz catheter
  • Keep CO >4 L/min, CI >2.2
– Patient may require inotropes or pressors*
– Avoid fluids if left ventricular filling pressure elevated
– Consider IABP
– Specific therapy:
  • MI: Standard medical therapy + emergent revascularization
– Arrhythmia: Urgent pharmacological or electrical cardioversion if unstable
  • Valvular/structural defects: Surgical repair
  • Tamponade: Therapeutic pericardiocentesis
  • Pulmonary embolism: Heparin/thrombolysis
  • Tension pneumothorax: Chest tube
  • Pericarditis: Pericardial stripping

*Vasopressors – Starting doses. Goal to maintain MAP ≥65 mm Hg.
– Dopamine 1 mcg/kg/min IV
– Norepinephrine 0.5 mcg/min IV
– Epinephrine 1 mcg/min IV
– Vasopressin 0.01 units/min IV
– Inotropic therapy for cardiogenic shock
– Dobutamine—start 0.5 mcg/kg/min IV

Kristin Burke, MD and Frank J. Domino, MD

Krassioukov A, Eng JJ, Warburton DE, et al. A systematic review of the management of orthostatic hypotension after spinal cord injury. *Arch Phys Med Rehabil.* 2009;90(5):876–885.

HYPOTHERMIA

Joshua Mularella, DO

Smith DL. Anemia in the elderly. *Am Fam Physician*. 2000;62:1565–1572.

INFERTILITY

Common causes: Endocrine disorders (PCOS, thyroid disease, hyperprolactinemia), pelvic structural abnormalities, azosperima/oligospermia, unexplained infertiity, poor coital timing/frequency

↓

Evaluate coital timing and frequency

Female factor

Patient history, physical, pelvic exam

- Uterine/tubal evaluation hysterosalpingogram
- Assess ovulation using basal body temperature chart, urine LH ovulation predictor kit, and mid-luteal serum progesterone
- Positive for gonorrhea/chlamydia → Evaluate and treat for PID

Uterine/tubal: Normal → In the presence of pelvic pain, consider laparoscopy; Tubal abnormality → Consider laparoscopy/in vitro fertilization; Uterine abnormality → Consider surgery

Ovulatory → If >30 y/o evaluate ovarian resistance with menses day-3 serum FSH or clomiphene citrate challenge test

Oligoovulation → Measure serum FSH, LH, TSH, and PRL levels → Progestin challenge test
- Positive → If hirsutism present determine serum 17-hydroxyprogesterone and testosterone levels to evaluate for PCOS and CAH
- Negative → If low/normal FSH/LH or high PRL, perform CT scan or MRI to evaluate for hypothalamic/pituitary disorder

Male factor

Semen analysis
- Normal semen
- Abnormal semen

Consider genetic evaluation; Consider testicular biopsy; History and physical exam → Structural abnormalities → Evaluate for varicocele, undescended testes, retrograde ejaculation, congenital absence of vas deferens; Endocrine evaluation → Measure serum FSH, LH, testosterone, PRL

Sara J. Fine, MD and Julia V. Johnson, MD

Jose-Miller AB, Boyden JW, Frey KA. Infertility. *Am Fam Physician.* 2007;75(6):849–856.

A-91

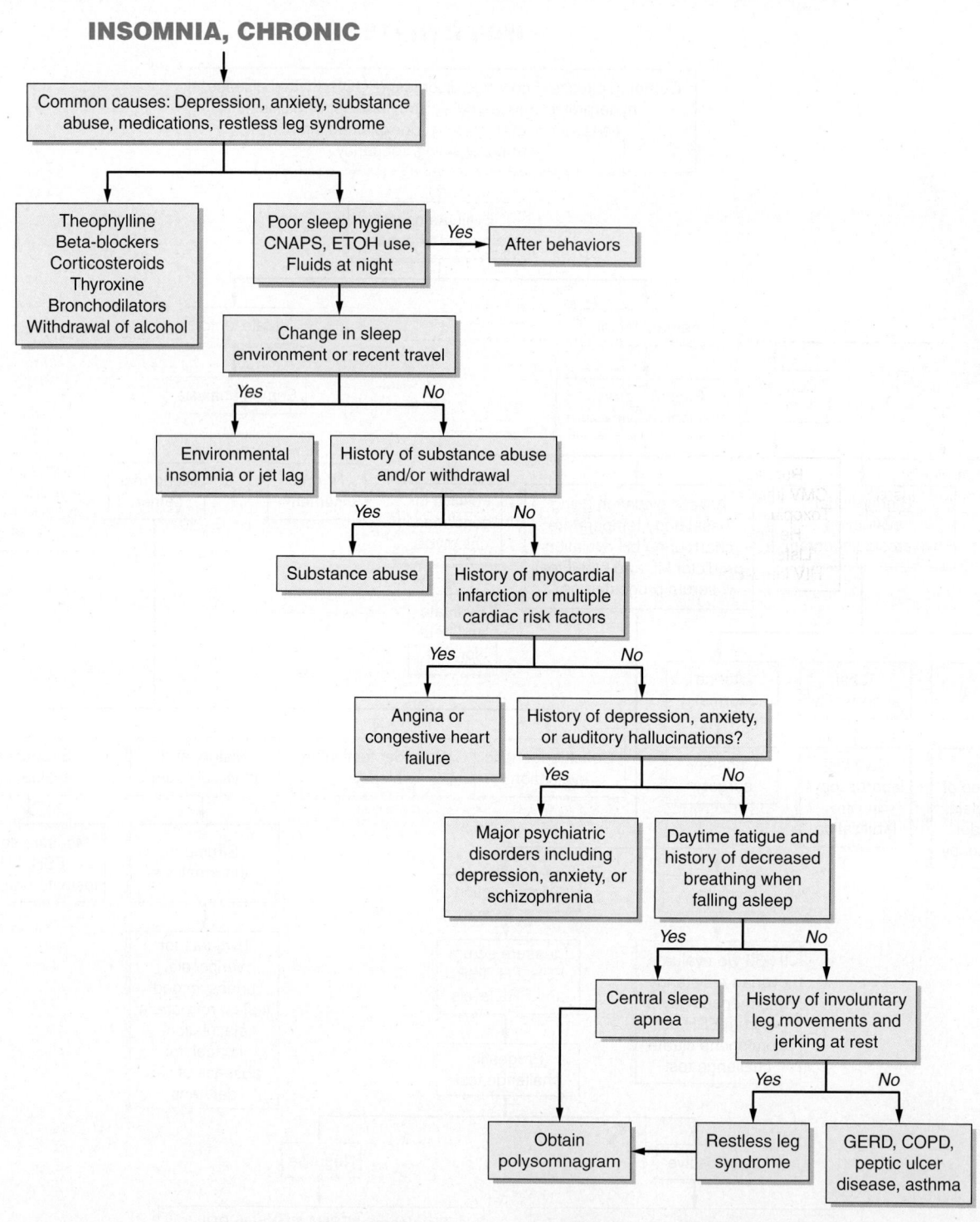

INSOMNIA, CHRONIC

Common causes: Depression, anxiety, substance abuse, medications, restless leg syndrome

**Theophylline
Beta-blockers
Corticosteroids
Thyroxine
Bronchodilators
Withdrawal of alcohol**

Poor sleep hygiene CNAPS, ETOH use, Fluids at night — *Yes* → After behaviors

Change in sleep environment or recent travel

Yes → Environmental insomnia or jet lag

No → History of substance abuse and/or withdrawal

Yes → Substance abuse

No → History of myocardial infarction or multiple cardiac risk factors

Yes → Angina or congestive heart failure

No → History of depression, anxiety, or auditory hallucinations?

Yes → Major psychiatric disorders including depression, anxiety, or schizophrenia

No → Daytime fatigue and history of decreased breathing when falling asleep

Yes → Central sleep apnea

No → History of involuntary leg movements and jerking at rest

Yes → Restless leg syndrome

No → GERD, COPD, peptic ulcer disease, asthma

Obtain polysomnagram

Franklin King, MD and Frank J. Domino, MD

Ramakrishnan K, Scheid DC. Treatment options for insomnia. *Am Fam Physician.* 2007;76(4):517–526.

INTELLECTUAL DISABILITY

Common causes: Trauma, infections, genetic abnormalities, toxic exposures, metabolic abnormalities, environmental factors

Check labs: TORCH studies, chromosomal analysis, genetic testing

Trauma	Congenital infections	Metabolic disorders	Genetic abnormalities	Environmental factors	Toxins
Head injury Anoxic brain insult	Rubella CMV infection Toxoplasmosis Herpes Listeriosis HIV infection	Kernicterus Congenital hypothyroidism Hypoglycemia	Down syndrome Fragile X syndrome Velocardiofacial syndrome Rett syndrome Tuberous sclerosis Angelman syndrome >500 genetic disorders identified	Malnutrition Deprivation syndrome	Fetal alcohol syndrome Lead poisoning Mercury poisoning

Crystal C. Bowe, MD, MPH

Carbone PS, Farley M, Davis T. Primary care for children with autism. *Am Fam Physician*. 2010;81:453–460.

JAUNDICE

Jaundice: A yellow discoloration of skin, sclera and mucous membranes by bilirubin, a bile pigment formed by the breakdown of heme rings; detected when the serum bilirubin level >3 mg/dL. Bilirubin is a product of hemoglobin breakdown in the spleen. Heme is converted to unconjugated bilirubin, bound to albumin and then sent to the liver where it is then conjugated.

Common causes: Gilbert syndrome, hemolysis, hepatitis and choledocholithiasis

CBC with diff, LFTs: ALT, AST, serum alkaline phosphatase (AP), total bilirubin (TB) and direct bilirubin (DB), haptoglobin, hepatitis serologies, amylase, lipase, hCG, urinalysis with urine bilirubin. Ultrasound or CT

Unconjugated hyperbilirubinemia — No — Direct bilirubin >0.3 mg/dL — Yes — Conjugated hyperbilirubinemia

Elevated AP — Yes — Intrahepatic — No — Obstruction on imaging — Yes — Extrahepatic

Elevated AP — No — Prehepatic

Prehepatic

• **Hemolytic anemia**
• **Reabsorption of large hematoma**

Labs: Anemia, possible reticulocytosis, mild TB elevation (5 mg/dL), increased indirect bilirubin, normal DB levels and negative urine bilirubin. All other LFTs are normal.

Unconjugated hyperbilirubinemia

° **Gilbert syndrome:** Mild defect in UDP glucuronosyltransferase (UGT, responsible for conjugation of bilirubin)
° **Crigler-Najjar syndromes:** More severe defect in UGT, usually presents during infancy

Conjugated hyperbilirubinemia
° **Dublin-Johnson syndrome:** Defective secretion of conjugated bilirubin
° **Rotor syndrome**

Both conjugated & unconjugated hepatocellular injury:

° **Hepatitis:** Viral, alcohol, or autoimmune insult leading to inflammation that impedes or prevents transport/secretion of conjugated bilirubin
° **Medication/drug:** Acetaminophen
° **Cirrhosis**
° **Congestive heart failure:** Hypoxia/anoxia of hepatocytes leads to cellular injury.

Intrahepatic cholestasis (No elevated LFTs, (primarily AP), US shows normal sized bile ducts)

Other:
° **Medication/drug induced**
° **Total parenteral nutrition (TPN)**
° **Sepsis**
° **Sarcoidosis**
° **Pregnancy**

Extrahepatic cholestasis (Labs: Elevated TB and DB, elevated AP and positive urine bilirubin. US shows dilated bile duct(s).

• **Choledocholithiasis**
• **Chronic pancreatitis:** Alcohol
• **Cholangitis:** Fever, pain and jaundice, altered mental status, sepsis
• **Biliary structure:** History of surgical/invasive procedure
• **Primary biliary cirrhosis**
• **Primary sclerosing cholangitis**
• **Biliary tract tumor/cholangiocarcinoma:** Hepatomegaly, weight loss, abdominal pain
• **Pancreatic tumor:** Painless jaundice, palpable gallbladder (rare)

Krunal Patel, MD and Isabel Zacharias, MD

Roche SP, Kobos R. Jaundice in the adult patient. *Am Fam Physician.* 2004;69(2):299–304.

KNEE PAIN

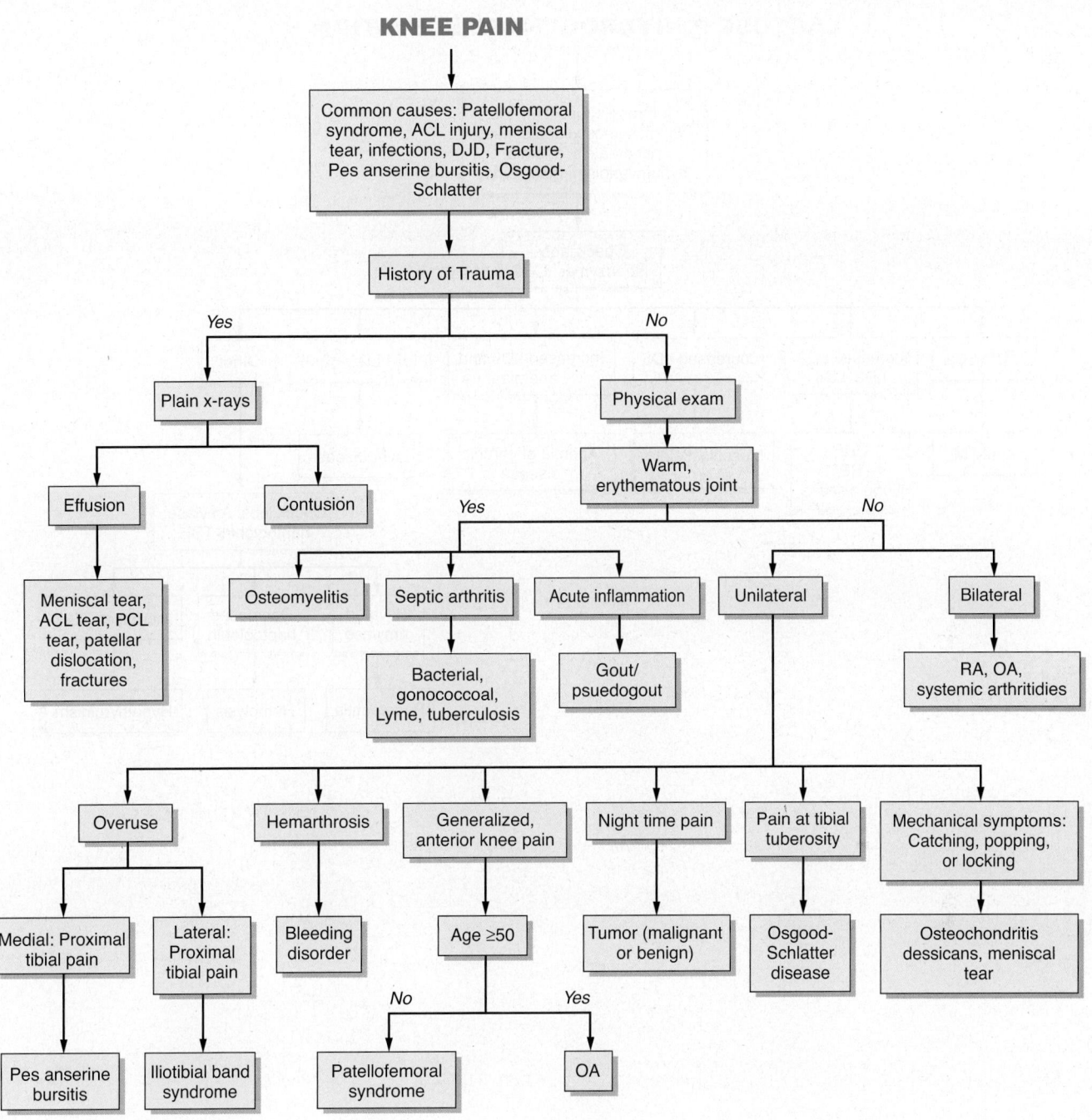

Common causes: Patellofemoral syndrome, ACL injury, meniscal tear, infections, DJD, Fracture, Pes anserine bursitis, Osgood-Schlatter

History of Trauma

Yes → Plain x-rays
- Effusion → Meniscal tear, ACL tear, PCL tear, patellar dislocation, fractures
- Contusion

No → Physical exam → Warm, erythematous joint

Yes
- Osteomyelitis
- Septic arthritis → Bacterial, gonococcoal, Lyme, tuberculosis
- Acute inflammation → Gout/psuedogout

No
- Unilateral
- Bilateral → RA, OA, systemic arthritidies

Unilateral:
- Overuse
  - Medial: Proximal tibial pain → Pes anserine bursitis
  - Lateral: Proximal tibial pain → Iliotibial band syndrome
- Hemarthrosis → Bleeding disorder
- Generalized, anterior knee pain → Age ≥50
  - **No** → Patellofemoral syndrome
  - **Yes** → OA
- Night time pain → Tumor (malignant or benign)
- Pain at tibial tuberosity → Osgood-Schlatter disease
- Mechanical symptoms: Catching, popping, or locking → Osteochondritis dessicans, meniscal tear

Alec DeCastro, MD

Calmbach WL, Hutchens M. Evaluation of patients presenting with knee pain: Part I. History, physical examination, radiographs, and laboratory tests. *Am Fam Physician.* 2003;68(5):907–912.

LACTOSE DEHYDROGENASE ELEVATION

Common causes: MI, PE, hepatitis, muscular diseases, pancreatitis, anemia, hypothyroidism, malignancy

Check labs: Isoenzymes, CBC

LDI >LD2	Increased LD2, LD3, LD4	Increased LD5	Increased LD5 and anemia	LD4/LD5 <1.05	Other

Acute MI

CHF PE Lung disease

Musculoskeletal disorder

Anemia of chronic disease

Liver disease

Check labs: Amylase, haptoglobin, TSH

Elevated amylase — Decreased haptoglobin — Increased TSH

Pancreatitis — Hemolysis — Hypothyroidism

Robert A. Baldor, MD and Alan M. Ehrlich, MD

Dimopoulos MA, Barlogie B, Smith TL, et al. High serum lactate dehydrogenase level as a marker for drug resistance and short survival in multiple myeloma. *Ann Int Med.* 1991;115(12):931–935.

LEAD TOXICITY, DIAGNOSIS AND TREATMENT (ADULT)

* If pregnant, reduce lead exposure for BLL 5–9 mcg/dL and remove lead exposure for BLL >10 mcg/dL

Pardeep Thandi, MD and Jennifer Carey, MD

Kosnett MJ, Wedeen RP, Rothenberg SJ, et al. Recommendations for medical management of adult lead exposure. *Environ Health Perspect.* 2007;115(3):463–471.

LEG ULCER

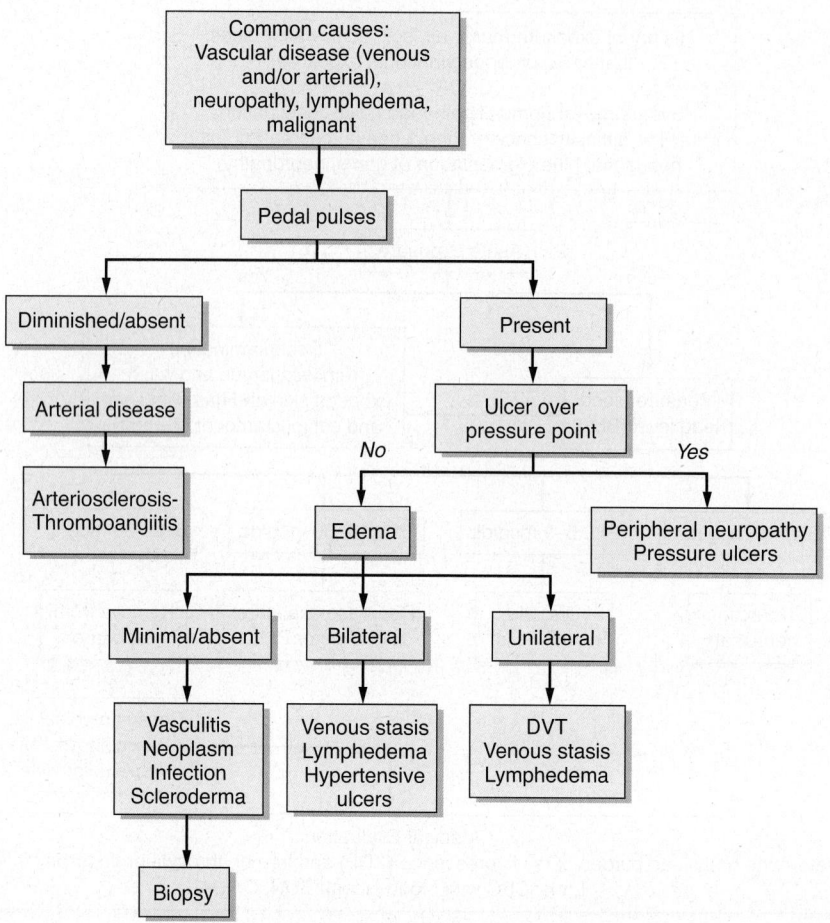

Olusola O. Fasusi, MD and Ankur Goel, MD

Senet P, Combemale P, Debure C, et al. Malignancy and chronic leg ulcers: The value of systematic wound biopsies: A prosepective, multicenter, cross-sectional study. *Arch Dermatol.* 2012;148:704.

LEUKOPENIA

Robert A. Baldor, MD and Alan M. Ehrlich, MD

Tefferi A, Hanson CA, Inwards DJ. How to interpret and pursue an abnormal complete blood cell count in adults. *Mayo Clin Proc.* 2005;80(7):923–936.

LOW BACK PAIN, CHRONIC

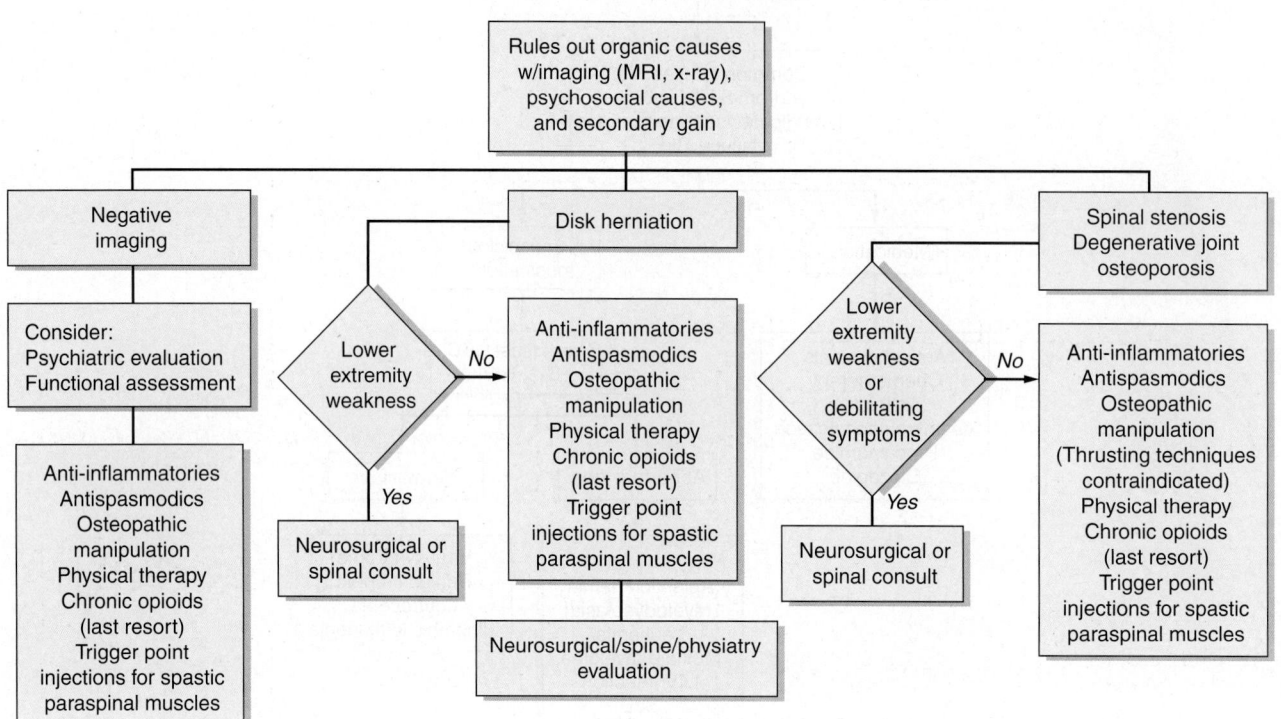

Ashley Simela, DO

Carey TS, Freburger JK, Holmes GM, et al. A long way to go: Practice patterns and evidence in chronic low back pain care. *Spine*. 2009;34(7):718–724.

LYMPHADENOPATHY

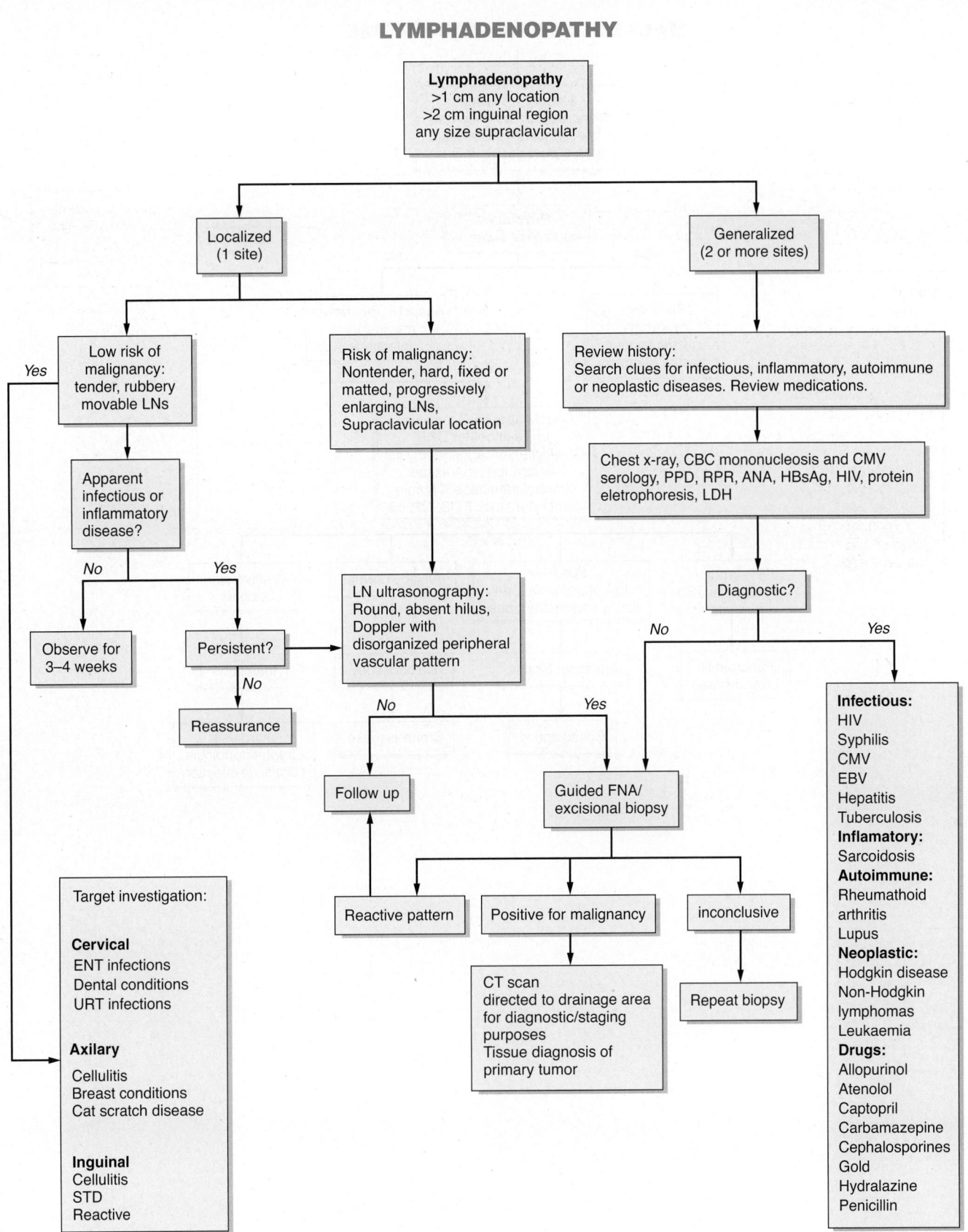

Danton S. Correa, MD and Felix B. Chang, MD, DABMA

Motyckova G. Steensma DP. Why does my patient have lymphadenopathy or splenomegaly? *Hematol Oncol Clin North Am.* 2012;26(2):395–408.

MALABSORPTION SYNDROME

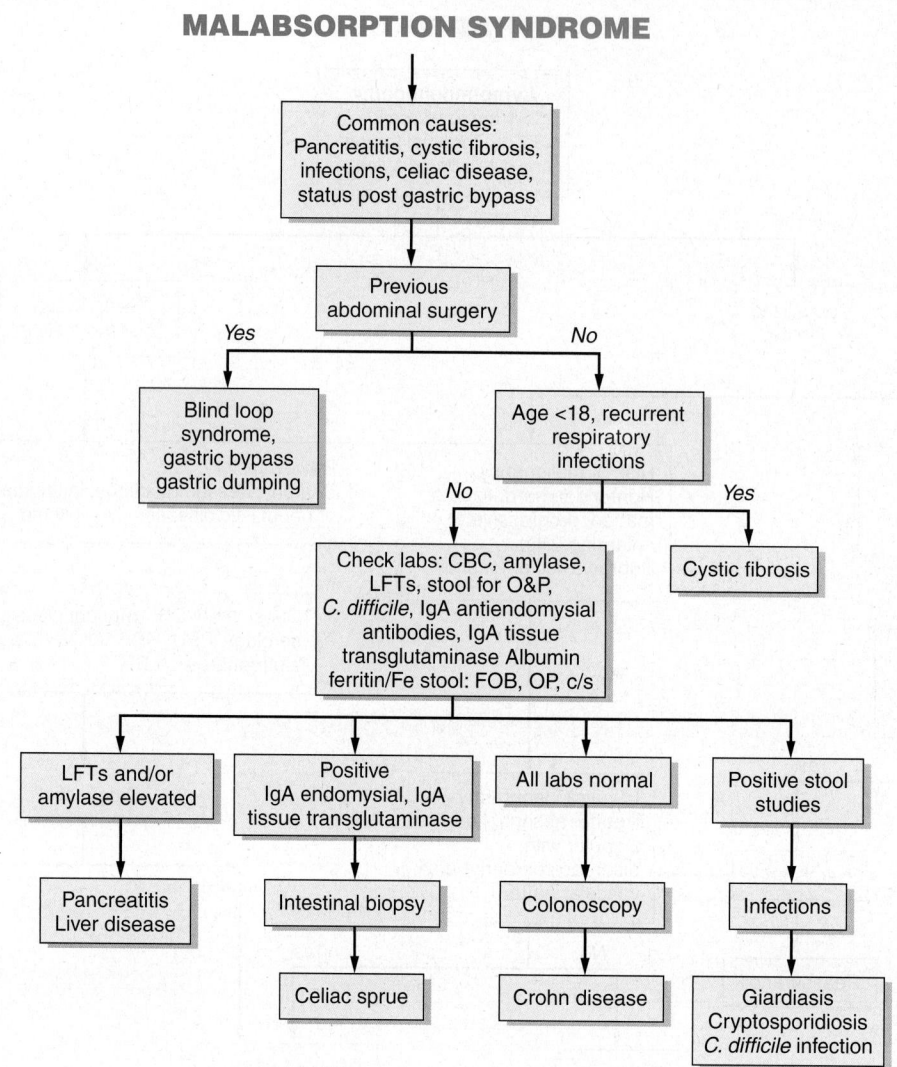

Tya-Mae Y. Julien, MD

Xanthakkos SA. Nutritional deficiencies in obesity and after bariatric surgery. *Pediatr Clin North Am.* 2009;56(5):1105–1121.

MENOPAUSE, EVALUATION AND MANAGEMENT

Menopause:
The permanent end of menstruation and fertility, defined as occurring 12 months after last period.
Average age = 51.3 years

Symptomatic? — *No* → **Age ≥65 years** — *No*

Yes

Hot flashes and/or night sweats

Vaginal dryness and/or vaginal atrophy

Known osteopenia or osteoporosis

Yes → **Age ≥65 years** — *Yes*

Assess bone health
DEXA scan at age 65 if no risk factors[2]; age 60 if risk factors

Hormone Replacement Therapy (HRT) desired and no contraindications[1] present?

See guidelines for bone health at right

Yes

HRT
(see Hormone Replacement Therapy information in the following section)

No

Nonhormonal therapy

* **Hot flashes:**
  * Avoid triggers: Stress, caffeine, alcohol, spicy foods, cigarette smoke, and heat.
  * Dress in layers
  * Medications: Off-label medications can be considered on an individual basis.
  *Herbs: Soy-based products

* **Vaginal symptoms:**
  *Vaginal moisturizers & lubricants: As needed and before intercourse
  * Topical estrogen: See next page

Osteoporosis
(T-score < –2.5)

Exclude other causes: CBC, K, Ca, 25(OH)-vitamin D, 24h urine Ca & Cr.
-AND-
Weight-bearing exercise, vit. D & Ca2+
-AND-
First-line agents are Bisphosphonates:
Alendronate (10 mg/d or 70 mg/wk), **Risedronate** (5 mg/d, 35 mg/wk or 150 mg/mo), **Zoledronic acid** (5 mg/yr IV), Ibandronate (150 mg/mo or 3 mg IV q3mo)
-OR-
If high risk of breast cancer use SERM:
Raloxifene (60 mg po qday)
-OR-
If very severe or continued bone loss on bisphosphonates use synthetic
PTH: **Teriparatide** (20 or 40 mcg/d SQ)
-OR-
HRT: not first line.
-AND-
DEXA monitoring of hip and spine q2yr.

Osteopenia
(T-score –1.0 to –2.5)

Further assess fracture risk with FRAX tool:
http://www.shef.ac.uk/FRAX/

Weight-bearing exercise, Ca2+ & vit D.

DEXA monitoring q2yr.

If FRAX shows 10-yr fracture risk ≥3% at the hip or ≥20% for major osteoporosis related fracture recommend pharmacologic treatment.

Medications: See osteoporosis.

Normal
(T-score > –1)

Prevent bone loss with weight-bearing exercise. Vitamin D: supplementation with 800 IU/d with consideration for higher doses (1,000–4,000 IU).

Hormone Replacement Therapy (HRT):
(use lowest effective dose for shortest duration possible.
Short-term use = 2–3 years; generally do not exceed 5 years.)

Intact uterus?

Yes

No

Transdermal, oral, spray, gel, vaginal or injectable estrogen + progesterone:

Transdermal estrogen: Start 0.05 mg/d; max 0.10 mg/d.

-OR-

Oral estrogen: 0.3, 0.45 mg, max 0.625 mg/d conjugated estrogens; 0.5–1 mg/d micronized estradiol

-OR-

Spray or gel: estradiol spray 0.021 mg delivered per spray; max 3 spray/d; 0.75 mg/d estradiol gel applied to large skin area.

-OR-

Vaginal estrogen: 1 ring PV q3mos releases 50 or 100 mcg/d estradiol

-OR-

Injectable estrogen: 10–20 mg estradiol valerate IM q4wks.

PLUS

Concomitant administration of one of the following:
1. **Medroxyprogesterone acetate (MPA)** 2.5 mg/d PO.

-OR-

2. **Natural progesterone** 100–200 mg/d PO.

Combined estrogen progesterone HRT:

Combined estrogen and progesterone transdermal patches:

Estradiol/levonorgestrel (delivers 0.045 mg/0.015 mg/d)

Estradiol/norethindrone acetate (delivers 0.05 mg/0.14 mg/d or = 0.05 mg/0.25 mg/d)

-OR-

Combined estrogen and progesterone pills:

Estradiol 1 mg and drospirenone 0.5 mg

Ethinyl estradiol 2.5 or 5 mcg & norethindrone acetate 0.5 or 1 mg

Conjugated estrogen 0.3, 0.45, or 0.625 mg and MPA 1.5, 2.5, or 5 mg

Estradiol 1 mg/norgestimate 0.9 mg

Topical estrogen therapy:

Little or no estrogen is absorbed in bloodstream → lower risk of side effects, but no effect on vasomotor symptoms. For use in patients with vaginal symptoms only.

Vaginal creams:
0.01% estradiol cream PV daily equiv. to 0.1 mg

0.625 mg conjugated estrogen/gm: 0.5 g PV daily x21 d then off for 7 d.

Vaginal tablet:
Vaginal estradiol 10 mcg tablet PV qday x 2 weeks, then 10 mcg tablet PV twice weekly.

Vaginal ring:
Vaginal estradiol that delivers 7.5 mcg/d estradiol. Insert 1 ring PV q3mos.

Estrogen-only therapy:
Transdermal
Oral
Spray/gel
Vaginal
Injectable

Do not use progesterone in women without a uterus.

Karen Browning, MD and Kelly Pagidas, MD

Hutzinger A. Practice Guidelines. AHRQ Releases Evidence Report on Managing Menopause-Related Symptoms. *Am Fam Physician.* 2005;72(4):709–710.

METABOLIC SYNDROME, TREATMENT

Identify Risk Factors
Abdominal obesity, insulin resistance, physical inactivity, high BMI, high-carb diet, cigarette smoking, Western diet, 1–2 sugar sweetened beverages/day, patients with known cardiovascular disease.

Is waist circumference ≥40″ (102 cm) - men or ≥35″ (88 cm) - women?

Yes → Assess

No → **Consider and Treat Alternative Individual Conditions**
Hypertension, hyperlipidemia, diabetes, obesity

Assess
1. Serum triglycerides ≥1.7 mmol/L (150 mg/dL) or on lipid lowering therapy.
2. Serum HDL <1.03 mmol/L (40 mg/dL) in men or <1.3 mmol/L (50 mg/dL) in women.
3. SBP ≥130 mm Hg or DBP ≥85 mm Hg or treatment of previously diagnosed HTN.
4. Fasting plasma glucose ≥5.6 mmol/L (100 mg/dL) or previously diagnosed DM2.

Does patient meet 2 of 4 criteria above?

No →

Yes →

Treat Physical Inactivity
Recommend:
Regular moderate-intensity physical activity; 30–60 min of continuous or intermittent exercise 5 days/week.
(Level 3)

Treat Abdominal Obesity
Recommend:
7% to 10% body weight reduction in 1st year of therapy. Weight maintenance/reduction through balanced physical activity, reduced caloric intake, and lifestyle changes.
(Level 3)

Intensive Lipid Therapy/ Reduce Insulin Resistance
Recommend:
Total fat 25% to 35% of total calories-saturated fat <7% of total calories; reduce *trans* fat; dietary cholesterol <200 mg/dL. Limit simple sugars. Lipid lowering medications if necessary. (Level 3)

Treat Elevated BP
Recommend:
Physical activity (see above)
Weight reduction
Pharmacotherapy if indicated for BP >140/90.
(Level 3)

Treat Elevated Glucose
Recommend:
Physical activity (see above)
Weight reduction
Pharmacotherapy if necessary to delay progression to DM.
(Level 3)

Amimi S. Osayande, MD

Grundy SM, Cleeman JI, Daniels SR, et al. Diagnosis and management of the metabolic syndrome: An American Heart Association/National Heart, Lung, and Blood Institute Scientific Statement. *Circulation.* 2005;112:2735–2752.

MIGRAINE, TREATMENT

```
Suspected migraine headache
            │
            ▼
Sudden onset
Age >55
Abnormal neurological exam
Increasing frequency or intensity
Awakens from sleep
Altered mental status
Localized neurological findings
Fever, weight loss, etc.
```

Yes →

Consider alternate diagnosis and workup.

(temporal arteritis, tumor, infection, cluster headache, etc.)

No →

POUND:

Pulsatile quality
One-day duration (4–24 hours)
Unilateral location
Nausea or vomiting
Disabling intensity

No →

Consider other headache syndrome.

Yes →

Nausea and vomiting?

No →

Avoid triggers
Sleep hygiene (critical for prevention)
Acetaminophen/aspirin/caffeine combination
Acetaminophen/isometheptene/ dichloralphenazone combination
NSAID
Triptans: Sumatriptan, zolmitriptan, rizatriptan, naratriptan, frovatriptan, eletriptan, almotriptan
(SQ, intranasal and ODT available)
NSAID/triptan combination
Intranasal lidocaine
Intranasal dihydroergotamine

Yes →

Consider IM/IV therapy:
Metoclopramide
Ketorolac
Dihydroergotamine
Dexamethasone

Chance Gentry, MD and Shari Gentry, MD

Gilmore B, Michael M. Treatment of acute migraine headache. *Am Fam Physician.* 2011;83(3):271–280.

NAIL ABNORMALITIES

Miesha Merati, DO and Jenifer Lloyd, DO

Tully AS, Trayes KP, Studdiford JS. Evaluation of nail abnormalities. *Am Fam Physician.* 2012;85:779–787.

NEPHROTIC SYNDROME

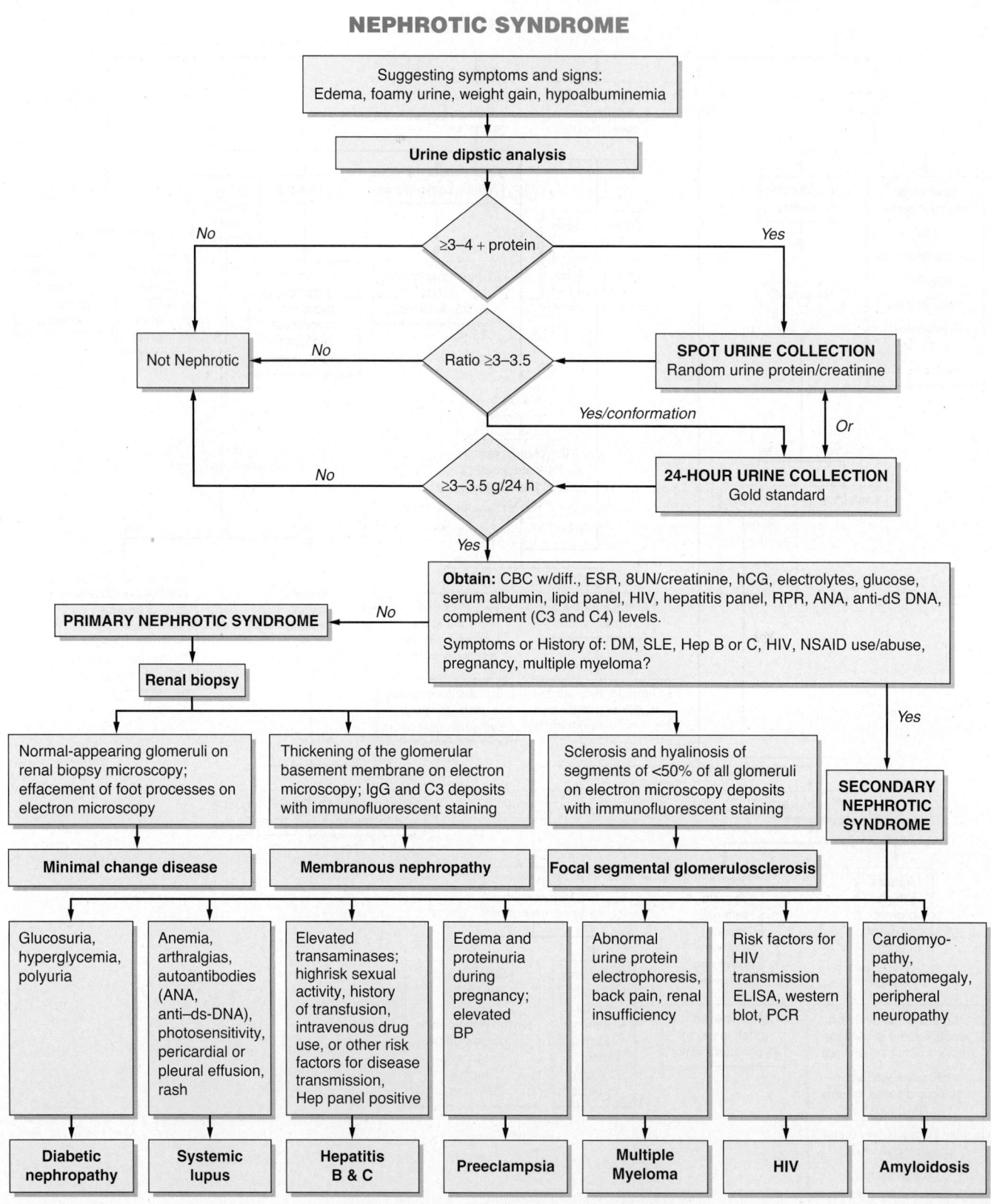

Jeff Wang, MD and Felix B. Chang, MD

Kodner C. Nephrotic Syndrome in adults: Diagnosis and management. *Am Fam Physician.* 2009;80(10):1129–1134.

NEVUS, ABNORMAL

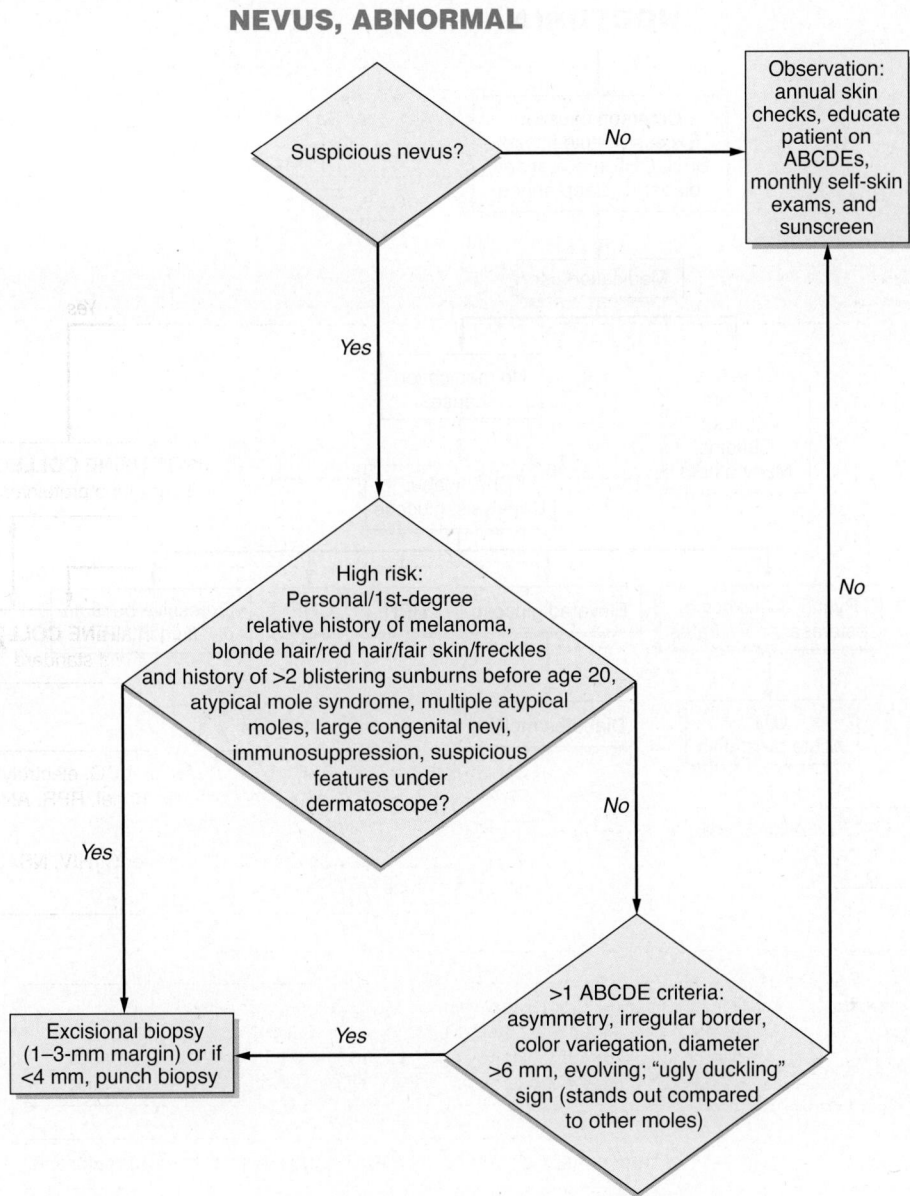

Miesha Merati, DO and Jenifer Lloyd, DO

Shenenberger DW. Cutaneous malignant melanoma: A primary care perspective. *Am Fam Physician.* 2012;85:161–168.

NOCTURIA

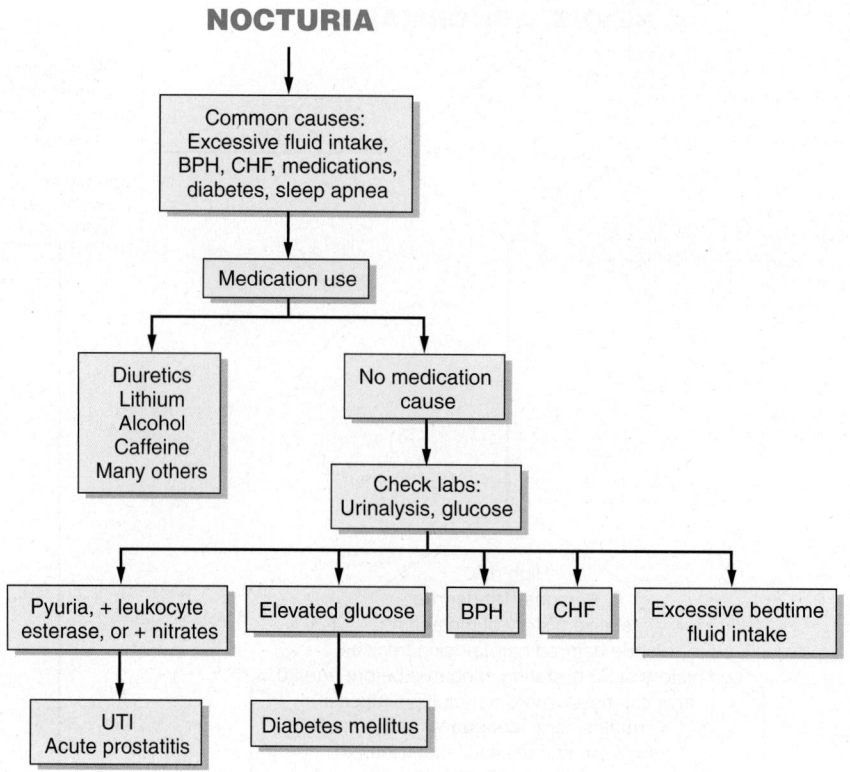

Robert A. Baldor, MD and Alan M. Ehrlich, MD

Marinkovic SP, Gillen LM, Stanton SL. Managing nocturia. *BMJ*. 2004;328(7447):1063–1066.

NYSTAGMUS

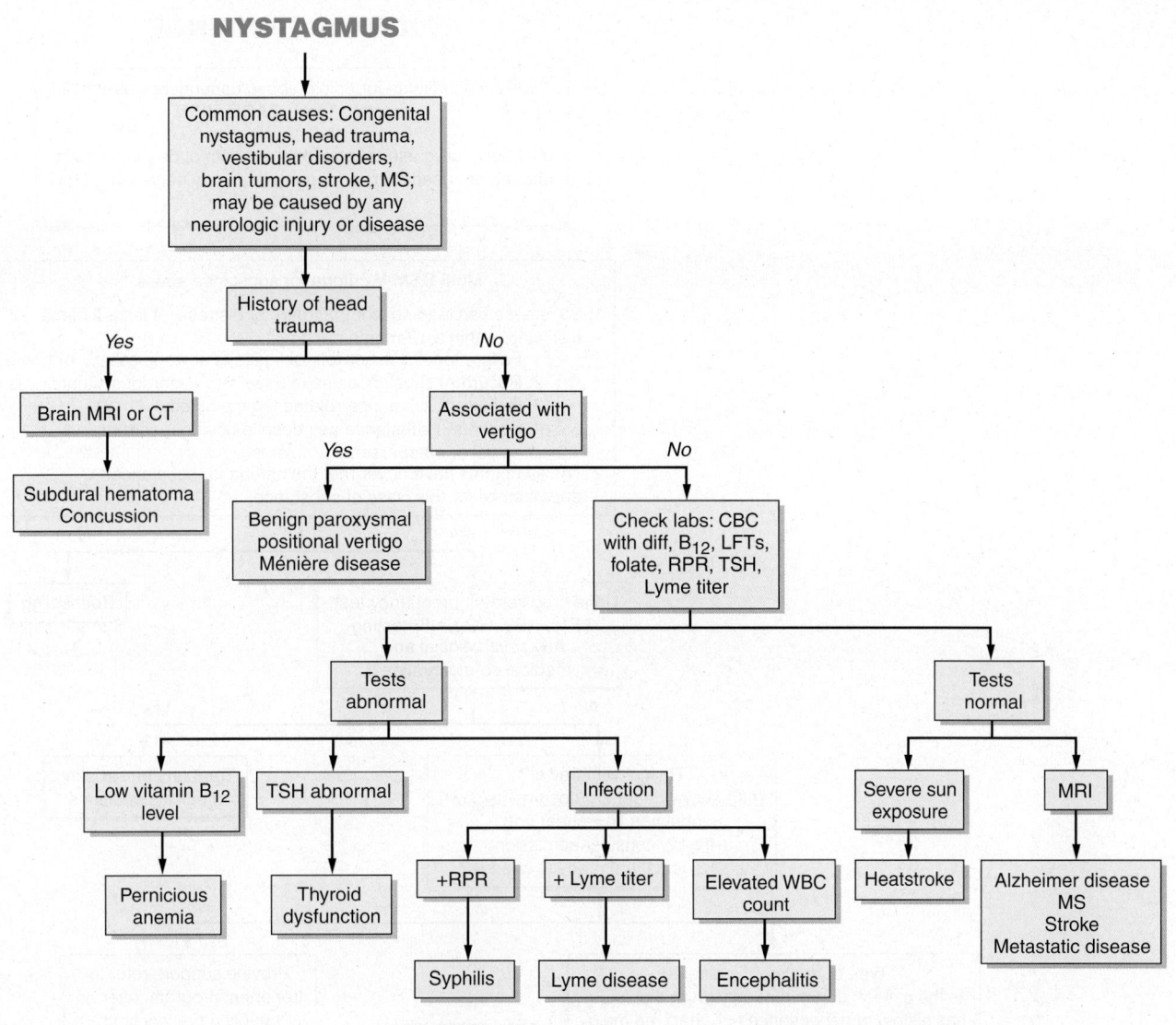

Common causes: Congenital nystagmus, head trauma, vestibular disorders, brain tumors, stroke, MS; may be caused by any neurologic injury or disease

History of head trauma

Yes → Brain MRI or CT → Subdural hematoma / Concussion

No → Associated with vertigo

- **Yes** → Benign paroxysmal positional vertigo / Ménière disease
- **No** → Check labs: CBC with diff, B_{12}, LFTs, folate, RPR, TSH, Lyme titer

Tests abnormal
- Low vitamin B_{12} level → Pernicious anemia
- TSH abnormal → Thyroid dysfunction
- Infection
  - +RPR → Syphilis
  - + Lyme titer → Lyme disease
  - Elevated WBC count → Encephalitis

Tests normal
- Severe sun exposure → Heatstroke
- MRI → Alzheimer disease / MS / Stroke / Metastatic disease

Robert A. Baldor, MD and Alan M. Ehrlich, MD

Tusa RJ. Dizziness. *Med Clin North Am.* 2009;93(2):263–271, vii.

OPIOID DEPENDENCE

Screen all patients for opioid abuse/dependence every 12 months. Tools: CAGE AID

(Cut down drug use, annoyed by criticism of drug use, guilty about drug, used drug in morning to steady nerves or get rid of hangover?)

Meet DSM-V criteria for substance abuse?

1. Substance use leading to impairment or distress, at least 2 of the following, within a 12-month period:
   1. Failure to fulfill major role obligations at work, school, or home
   2. Recurrent substance use in physically hazardous situations is
   3. Recurrent substance-related legal problems
   4. Continued substance use despite having recurrent social or interpersonal problems
2. The symptoms have never met the criteria for substance dependence for this class of substance.

Yes → Urine drug screen, pregnancy test, LFTs, HBV, HCV, HIV testing. Any psychosocial and medical co-morbidities?

No → Counseling

Urine drug screen... :

No → Risk of withdrawal? (http://www.naabt.org/documents/cows induction flow sheet.pdf); If >12, consider admission. If ≤12, is patient ready to change?

Yes → Treat any pre-existing medical conditions

Risk of withdrawal?:

Yes → Type of treatment indicated: Is the patient: dependent only on oral opioids, has history of dependence (<1 year), no major psychiatric co-morbidity, and is socially stable with a supportive network?

No → Provide support, refer to treatment program, offer no enabling prescriptions

Type of treatment indicated → If pregnant, use methadone

Yes →
Office based:
1. Buprenorphine/Naloxone
2. Rapid naloxone with clonidine and/ or buprenorphine/naloxone
3. Clonidine

Hospital based:
1. Methadone
2. Buprenorphine/naloxone
3. Rapid naloxone with clonidine and/or buprenorphine

Failure? →

No → Consider maintence therapy in patients with long history of abuse or repeated failed attempts

Opioid treatment program:
1. Methadone
2. Naltrexone
3. Buprenorphine/Naloxone

Office based: Buprenorphine/naloxone

Failure? →

Andrea Watson, DO and Nathalie Duroseau

Krantz MJ, Mehler PS. Treating opioid dependence. Growing implications for primary care. *Arch Intern Med.* 2004;164:277–288.

Pain, Chronic

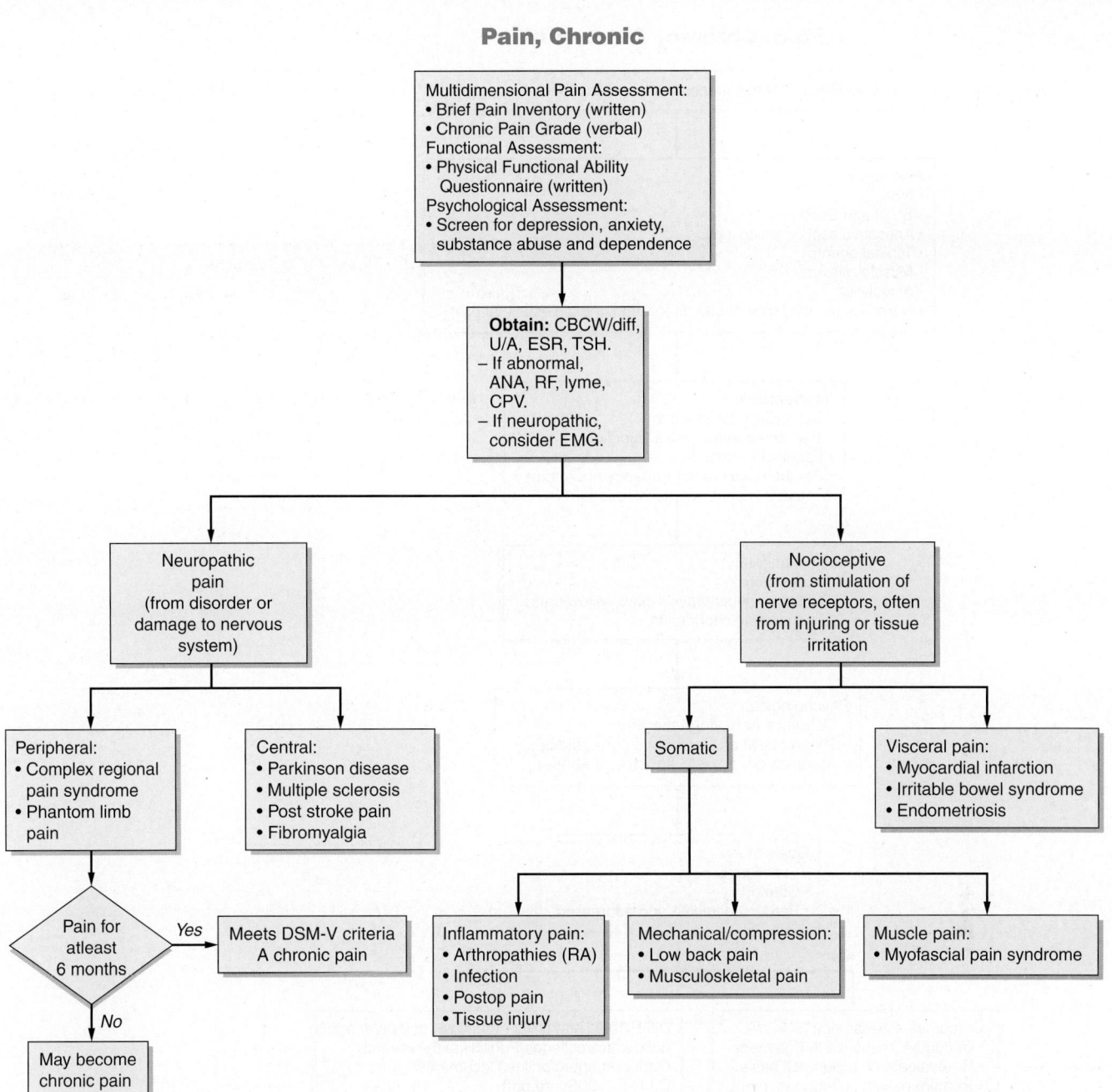

Multidimensional Pain Assessment:
• Brief Pain Inventory (written)
• Chronic Pain Grade (verbal)
Functional Assessment:
• Physical Functional Ability Questionnaire (written)
Psychological Assessment:
• Screen for depression, anxiety, substance abuse and dependence

Obtain: CBCW/diff, U/A, ESR, TSH.
– If abnormal, ANA, RF, lyme, CPV.
– If neuropathic, consider EMG.

Neuropathic pain (from disorder or damage to nervous system)

Nocioceptive (from stimulation of nerve receptors, often from injuring or tissue irritation

Peripheral:
• Complex regional pain syndrome
• Phantom limb pain

Central:
• Parkinson disease
• Multiple sclerosis
• Post stroke pain
• Fibromyalgia

Somatic

Visceral pain:
• Myocardial infarction
• Irritable bowel syndrome
• Endometriosis

Pain for atleast 6 months

Yes → Meets DSM-V criteria A chronic pain

No → May become chronic pain

Inflammatory pain:
• Arthropathies (RA)
• Infection
• Postop pain
• Tissue injury

Mechanical/compression:
• Low back pain
• Musculoskeletal pain

Muscle pain:
• Myofascial pain syndrome

Ashik Lawrence, MD, Anubhav Kaul, MD and Margaret Seaver, MD

Institute for Clinical Systems Improvement. *Health Care Guideline: Assessment and Management of Chronic Pain,* 5th ed. Bloomington, MN: Institute of Clinical System Improvement; 2011.

Pain, Chronic, Treatment

Level I Management (Conservative and Standard Approach)

Pharmacology:
• NSAIDs
• SSRI and SNRI
• Anticonvulsant or antiepileptic
• Topical agents
• Muscle relaxers
• Anxiolytics
• Narcotics (no evidence of benefit for most musculoskeletal pain)

Interventional:
• Sacroiliac joint injection
• Transforaminal epidural injection
• Facet joint injection
• Percutaneous radiofrequency neurotomy

Complementary:
• Acupuncture
• Herbal products (devil's claw, willow bark)
• Glucosamine/chondroitin

Psychological:
– Cognitive behavioral therapy
– Dx and treat all psychiatric comorbidities
  (depression, anxiety, substance abuse)

Goals met?
• Functional
• Comfort
• Barriers identified and addressed

Yes — No

Outcomes assessment:
• Document response to treatment
• Re-evaluate on scheduled basis
• Require patient self-management
  (exercise, counseling, etc.)

DIRE Tool (Add URL: http://www.ucdenver.edu/
academics/colleges/PublicHealth/research/
centers/maperc/online/Documents/
D.I.R.E.%20Score.pdf)

May be chronic opioid candidate

Yes — Score ≥14 — No

Level II Management
• Biopsychosocial assessment
• Refer to multidisciplinary team
• Consider surgery
  (spinal cord stimulator,
  intrathecal pump)

Ashik Lawrence, MD, Anubhav Kaul, MD and Margaret Seaver, MD

Institute for Clinical Systems Improvement. *Health Care Guideline: Assessment and Management of Chronic Pain,* 5th ed. Bloomington, MN: Institute of Clinical System Improvement; 2011.

PALPABLE BREAST MASS (AGE <30 OR PREGNANT OR LACTATING)

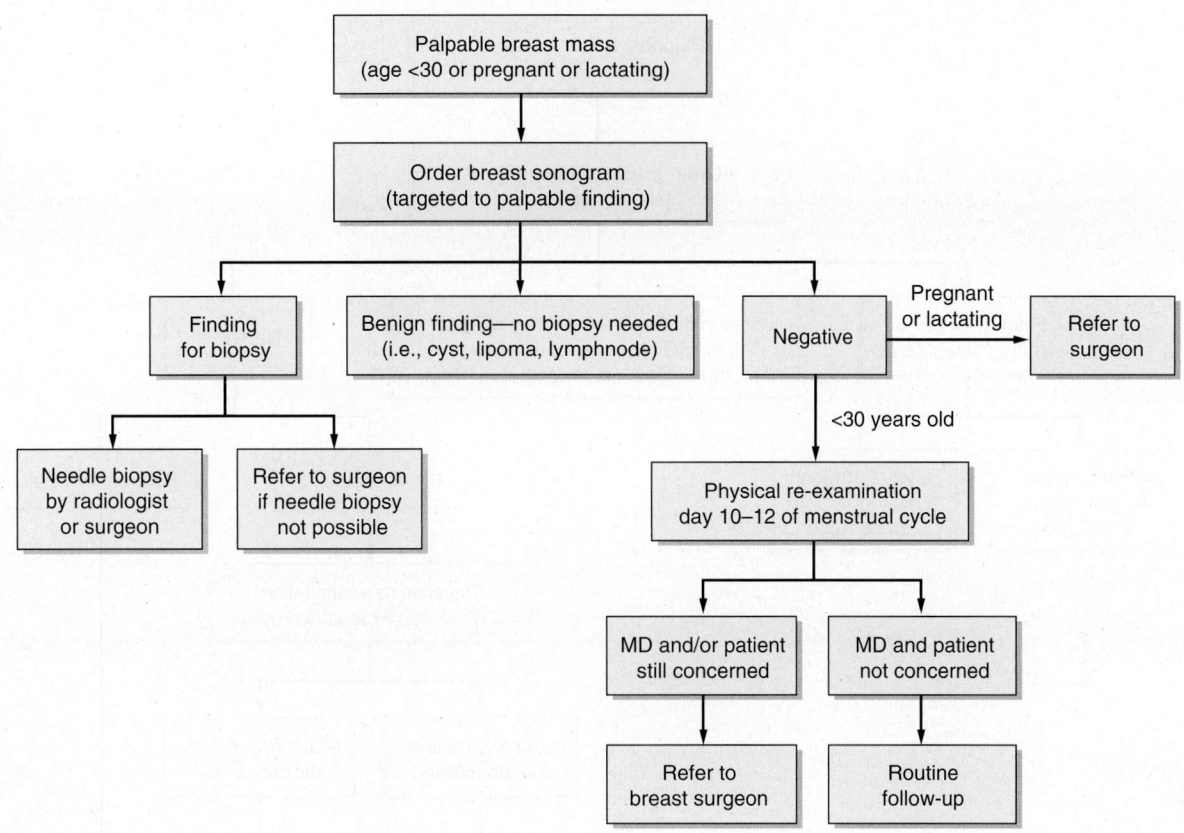

Stacey Vitiello, MD and Nancy Elliot, MD, FACS

Salzman B, Fleegle S, Tully AS. Common breast problems. *Am Fam Physician*. 2012;8(4):343–349.

PALPABLE BREAST MASS (AGE ≥30)

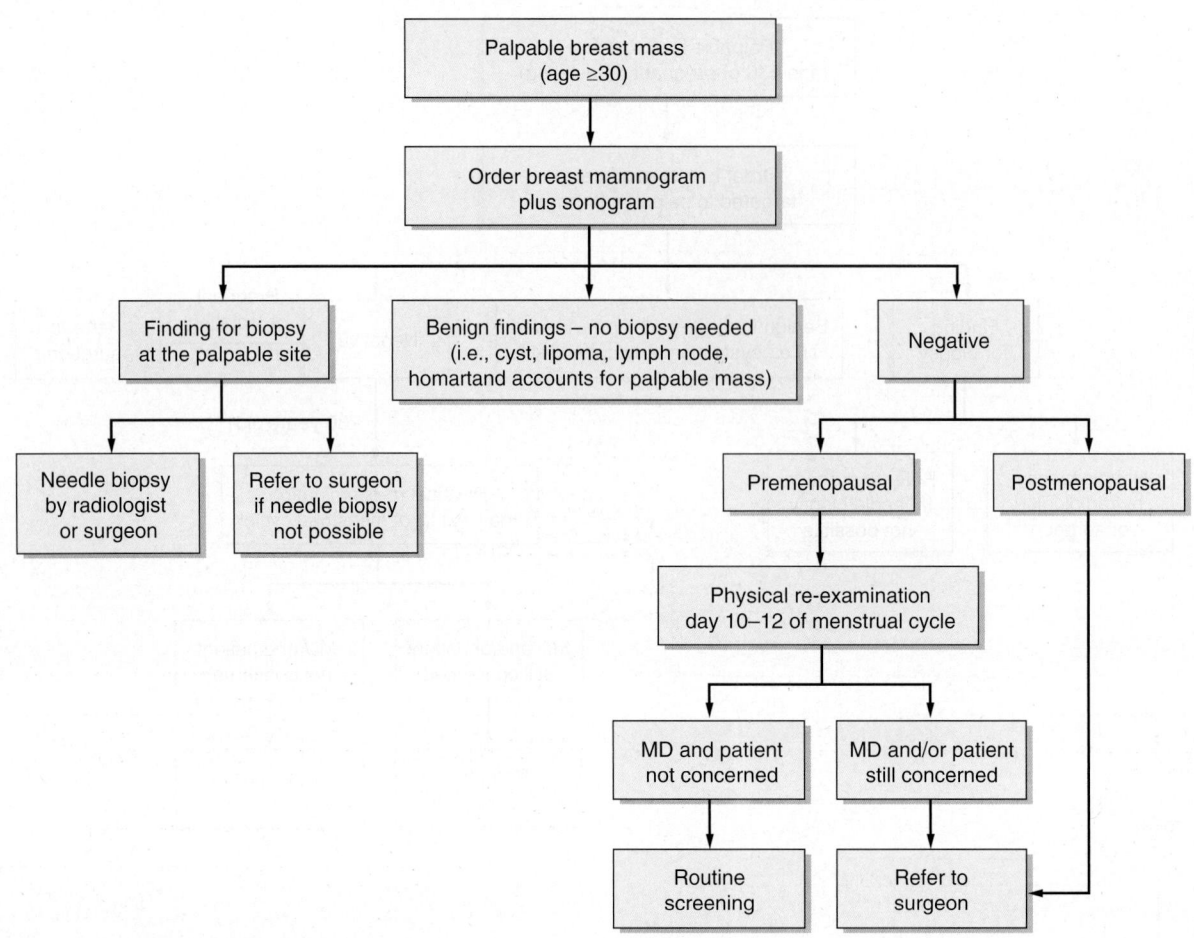

Stacey Vitiello, MD and Nancy Elliot, MD

Salzman B, Fleegle S, Tully AS. Common breast problems. *Am Fam Physician*. 2012;86(4):343–349.

PALPITATIONS

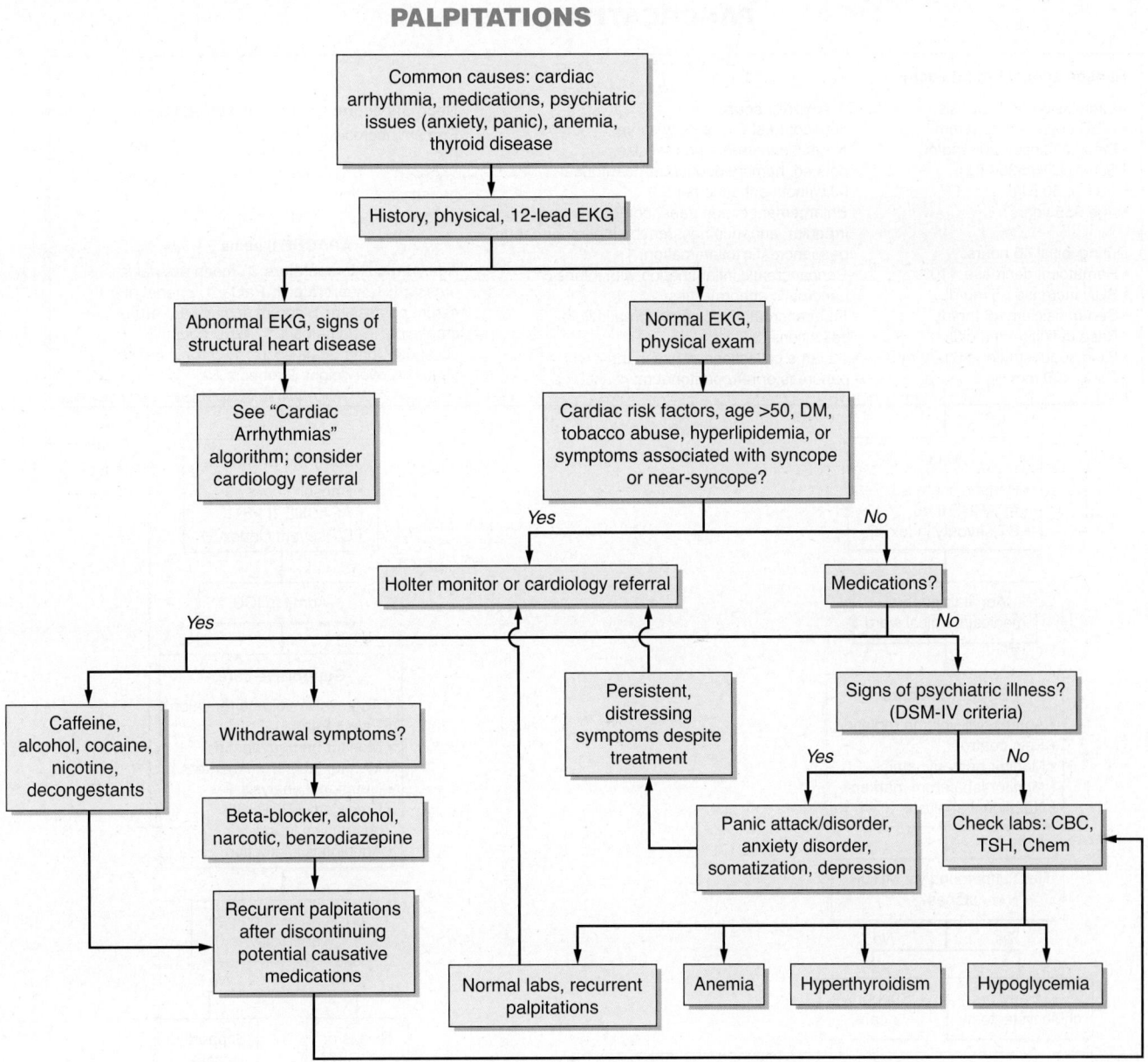

Elizabeth Dougherty, MD and Frank J. Domino, MD

Wexler RK, Pleister A, Raman, S. Outpatient approach to palpitations. *Am Fam Physician.* 2011;84(1):63–69.

PANCREATITIS, ACUTE

Ranson score (1 point each)

At admission or diagnosis:
- WBC count >16,000/mm^3
- Blood glucose >200 mg/dL
- Scrum LDH >350 IU/L
- AST >250 IU/L
- Age >55 years

During initial 48 hours:
- Hematocrit decrease >10%
- BUN increase >5 mg/dL
- Serum calcium <8 mg/dL
- Base deficit >4 mmol/L
- Fluid sequestration >6,000 mL
- PaO$_2$ <60 mm Hg

CT severity score*
*Non–contrast CT severity score
- Normal pancreas—normal size, defined, homogeneous, retroperitoneal fat without enhancement: 0
- Enlargement of pancreas, contour maybe irregular, enhancement maybe inhomogeneous, peripancreatic inflammation: 1
- Peripancreatic inflammation with intrinsic pancreatic abnormalities: 2
- Intrapancreatic or extrapancreatic fluid collections: 3
- ≥2 large collections of gas in the pancreas or retroperitoneum: 4

Necrosis score: Contrast-enhanced CT

Percent necrosis	Points
0%	0
<33%	2
33–55%	4
50%	6

APACHE II scale
Age: 1, rectal temperature: 1, mean arterial pressure: 1, heart rate: 1, PaO$_2$: 1, arterial pH: 1, serum potassium: 1, serum sodium: 1, serum creatinine: 1, hematocrit: 1, WBC count: 1, Glasgow Coma Scale score: 1, chronic health status: 1, overweight: 2, obese: 2

http://www.sfar.org/scores2/apache22.html#calcul

Mild
- Ranson score ≤3
- APACHE II <8
- CT severity index <7

↓

Admit to general medical/surgical ward

↓

Supportive care
- Aggressive volume repletion
- Pain control
- Monitor hemodynamics
- Monitor lab/serum markers
- Nutritional analysis

↓

RUQ ultrasound vs. MRCP: stones?

Yes / *No*

Early cholecystectomy / Supportive care

Moderate or severe
- Ranson score >3
- APACHE II ≥8
- CT severity index ≥7

↓

Admit to ICU

↓

Supportive care
- Aggressive volume repletion
- Pain control
- Monitor hemodynamics
- Monitor lab/serum markers
- Nutritional analysis
- Emergent ERCP with obstructive jaundice
- Antibiotics if infection

↓

CT scan of abdomen: necrosis?

Yes / *No*

Sepsis or MOSF? / Supportive care

No / *Yes*

Expectant management with frequent reassessment /
- CT-guided aspiration and culture
- Surgical consultation for possible surgical debridement (if infected)

APACHE II = Acute Physiology and Chronic Health Evaluation
CT = Computed Tomography
ERCP = Endoscopic Retrograde Cholangiopancreatography
RUQ = Right Upper Quadrant
MOSF = Multiorgan System Failure
WBC = White Blood Cell
BUN = Blood Urea Nitrogen
LDH = Lactate Dehydrogenase
AST = Aspartate Transaminases
PaO$_2$ = Partial Arterial Oxygen Tension

Maurice F. Joyce, MD, EdM and Mitchell A. Cahan, MD, FACS

Wu BU, Banks PA. Clinical management of patients with acute pancreatitis. *Gastroenterology.* 2013;144:1272–1281.

PAP, NORMAL AND ABNORMAL IN NONPREGNANT WOMEN AGES 25 AND OLDER

Pap, normal and abnormal in nonpregnant women ages 25 and older (excludes women with HIV, DES exposure immunosuppression, history of high-grade dysplasia [CIN 2,3, or higher])

Pap cytology shows

Normal: If age is <30: No HPV, repap **3** years. If age is ≥30 and HR-HPV is…

AGC, HSIL, LSIL cro HSIL, ASC-HG

LSIL, HR-HPV is…

Positive → Colposcopy

Or unknown

Negative

Positive / Negative

ASC-US. Reflex HR-HPV is…

Co-test 1 year

2 acceptable strategies / Re-Pap no sooner than 5 years

Positive / Negative

HR-HPV AND Cyto Negative / ≥ ASC OR HR-HPV Positive

COLPOSCOPY (with endometrial and endocervical sampling for AGC)

Co-test in 3 years

COLPOSCOPY

Abbreviations:
Co-test: Pap cytology AND HR-HPV testing
HR-HPV: High-risk HPV DNA probe testing
ASC: Atypical squamous cells (-US of uncertain significance; -HG cannot exclude high grade)
HSIL: High-grade squamous intraepithelial lesion
LSIL: Low-grade squamous intraepithelial lesion
AGC: Atypical glandular cells
cro: Cannot rule out
Cyto: Pap cytology

OR

HPV 16/18 probe → Negative → Co-test at 12 months

Positive

COLPOSCOPY

Positive

HR-HPV DNA ← Negative ← Pap result is…

Negative / Positive

Re-Pap in 3 years

Pap ≥ ASC to COLPOSCOPY

Pap Smear Frequency:
Age <21 Screening not recommended
Age 21–24 3 years. See separate Algorithm
Age 25–29 Every 3 years
Age 30–65 Every 5 years if cyto and HR-HPV is negative, or every 3 years if cyto is normal, HR-HPV not done, and pt prefers more frequent screening

Jeremy Golding, MD

Adapted from ASCCP 2013 Guidelines.

PAP, NORMAL AND ABNORMAL
IN WOMEN AGE 21–24

Pap cytology shows

ASC-US or LSIL

HSIL
LSIL cro HSIL
ASC-HG

Normal
Do not order
HPV

Reflex HPV Testing
*Acceptable for
ASC-US only*

Colposcopy

Re-Pap 3 years

HPV Positive   *HPV Negative*

Repeat Cytology
at 12 months
Preferred

**Routine
Screening**

Negative, ASC-US,   *ASC-H, AGC, HSIL*
or LSIL

Repeat cytology
at 12 months

Negative × 2   *≥ASC*

Routine Screening   Colposcopy

Abbreviations:

ASC: Atypical squamous Cells (-US of uncertain)
significance; -HG cannot exclude high grade)
HSIL: High-grade squamous intraepithelial lesion
LSIL: Low-grade squamous intraepithelial lesion
AGC: Atypical glandular cells
cro: Cannot rule out

Jeremy Golding, MD

Adapted from ASCCP 2013 Guideline.

A-120

PARATHYROID HORMONE, ELEVATED SERUM

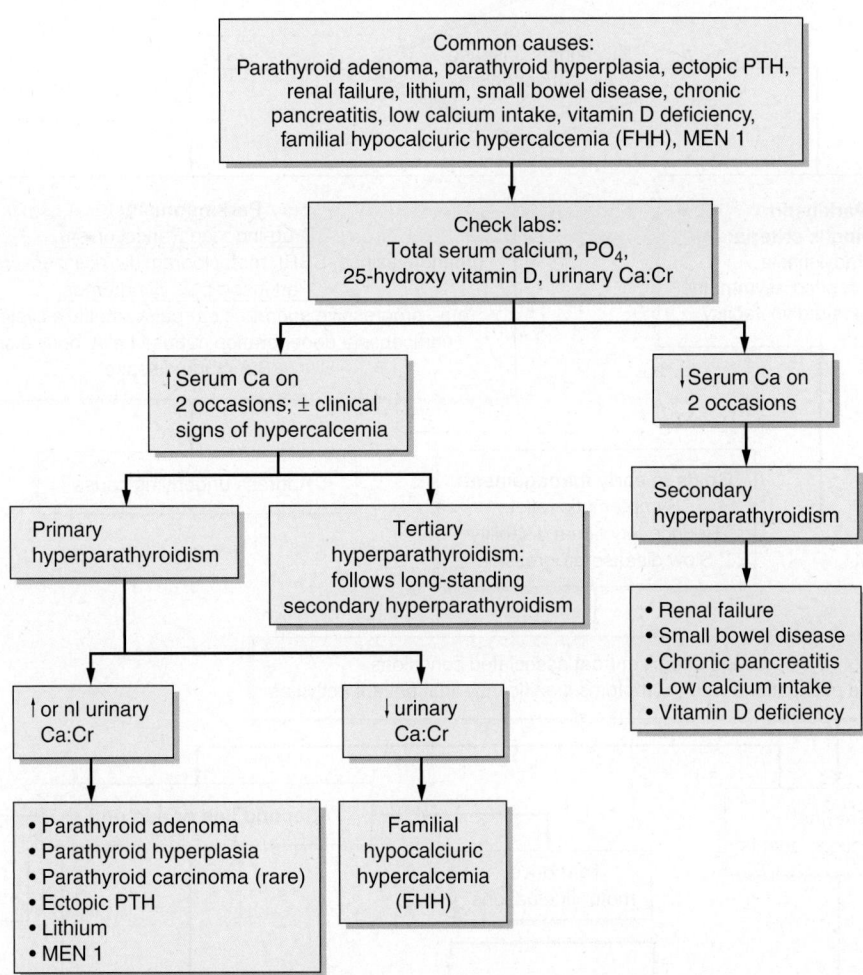

Common causes:
Parathyroid adenoma, parathyroid hyperplasia, ectopic PTH, renal failure, lithium, small bowel disease, chronic pancreatitis, low calcium intake, vitamin D deficiency, familial hypocalciuric hypercalcemia (FHH), MEN 1

Check labs:
Total serum calcium, PO_4, 25-hydroxy vitamin D, urinary Ca:Cr

↑Serum Ca on 2 occasions; ± clinical signs of hypercalcemia

↓Serum Ca on 2 occasions

Secondary hyperparathyroidism

Primary hyperparathyroidism

Tertiary hyperparathyroidism: follows long-standing secondary hyperparathyroidism

• Renal failure
• Small bowel disease
• Chronic pancreatitis
• Low calcium intake
• Vitamin D deficiency

↑ or nl urinary Ca:Cr

↓ urinary Ca:Cr

• Parathyroid adenoma
• Parathyroid hyperplasia
• Parathyroid carcinoma (rare)
• Ectopic PTH
• Lithium
• MEN 1

Familial hypocalciuric hypercalcemia (FHH)

Andrew Gara, MD and Auguste Turnier, MD

Mikhail N, Cope D. Evaluation and treatment of primary hyperparathyroidism. *JAMA*. 2005;294(21):2700.

PARKINSON DISEASE, TREATMENT

Parkinson disease vs. parkinsonism?

Parkinson diagnostic criteria:
Bradykinesia
Rest tremor, often asymmetric
rigidity, postural instability

Parkinsonism:
Drug-induced Parkinsonism
(phenothiazines, SSRI, metoclopramide, diltiazem, valproic acid)
Parkinson-plus Syndromes
(e.g., progressive supranuclear palsy, multiple system atrophy,
corticobasal degeneration, diffuse Lewy body disease)
Structural disease

Address underlying cause

Goals in early management:
Symptomatic relief
Reduce functional disability
Slow disease progression

Encourage exercise; treat associated conditions
Initiate medications when symptoms significantly limit patient activities

First line:
Dopaminergic agents

Second line or add on:

To reduce
motor fluctuations

To reduce
tremor/drooling

MAO-B Inhibitors:
Rasagiline
Selegiline

COMT inhibitors:
Entacapone

Antipsychotics:
Trihexyphenidyl
Benztropine

Acute hypomobility
episodes

To treat
psychosis

Young
or old?

Apomorphine

Antipsychotics:
Quetiapine
Clozapine

Younger patient
(Age <65)
Dopamine agonist
monotherapy:
Pramipexole
Ropinirole
Bromocriptine

Older patient
(Age >65)
Carbidopa/levodopa
most effective; dopamine
agonist can also be added

Surgery?
Severe, unresponsive to medications—consider
deep-brain stimulation with the use of implanted electrodes

James J. Arnold, DO and Nathan Miller, MD, CAPT, MC

Diaz NL, Waters CH. Current strategies in the treatment of Parkinson's disease and a personalized approach to management.
Expert Rev Neurother. 2009;9(12):1781–1789.

PEDIATRIC EXANTHEMS, DIAGNOSTIC

URI symptoms present?

No →

Roseola (Sixth Disease, Exanthem Subitim)
- Rash: Erythematous maculopapular rash develops as fever resolves; starts on trunk and progresses to neck, extremities, (rarely) face
- Prodrome: Fever
- Enanthem: Erythematous macules on soft palate
- Peak prevalence 7–13 months

Yes →

Enanthem (involvement of mucous membranes)?

No → **Vesicular?**

Yes → **Vesicular?**

Vesicular? (No branch)

No →

Erythema Infectiosum (Fifth Disease)
- Rash: Intensely red malar rash followed in 1–2 days by reticular erythematous maculopapular rash on trunk, extremities, and buttocks); recrudescence can last up to months
- Prodrome: Generally mild, may have 1–4 days of headache, chills, URI symptoms
- Enanthem: None

Yes →

Varicella (Chicken Pox)
- Rash: Macules form on trunk and spread to face and extremities; progress quickly in clusters to papules then tear-dropped shaped vesicles ("dew drops on a rose petal") that crust over or umbilicate
- Prodrome: 1–2 days of fever, malaise, anorexia
- Enanthem: Rarely, vesicles can lead to erosions of hard palate

Vesicular? (Yes branch)

No →

Yes →

Coxsackie (Hand, Foot, Mouth Disease)
- Rash: Erythematous macules and papules ~2–3 mm found on palmar surface of hand, plantar surface of feet, and oral mucosa; progresses quickly through vesicular phase to form central gray ulcer
- Prodrome: 12–36 hours of cough, fever, malaise, anorexia, abdominal pain
- Enanthem: Occurs with exanthema as painful ulcerative lesions commonly found on tongue, hard palate, and buccal mucosa

Koplik spots (white papules on buccal muscos)?

No → **Fast-spreading rash?**

Yes →

Measles (First Disease, Rubeola)
- Rash: Erythematous maculopapular rash with downward progression from face and brownish hue during resolution.
- Prodrome: 3–4 days of conjunctivitis, coryza, fever, cough
- Enanthem: Koplik spots

Fast-spreading rash?

No →

Rubella (Third Disease, German Measles)
- Rash: Erythematous maculopapular rash with downward progression from face
- Prodrome: 1–7 days of malaise, painful lymphadenopathy
- Enanthem: Forchheimer spots

Yes →

Scarlet Fever (Second Disease)
- Rash: Rapidly progressing erythematous macules and pinpoint, blanchable papules ("goose pimples") with sandpaper texture, greatest intensity at skin folds
- Prodrome: 1–2 days of fever, sore throat, vomiting, abdominal pain
- Enanthem: Progression from white to red strawberry tongue

Phillip Fournier, MD

Sands R, Shanmugavadivel D, Stephenson T, et al. Medical problems presenting to paediatric emergency departments: 10 years on. *Emerg Med J.* 2012;29(5):379–382.

PELVIC PAIN

Common causes: Menstrual cramps, PID, ectopic pregnancy, fibroid uterus, endometriosis, ovarian cyst

+ Pregnancy test

Ectopic pregnancy
Normal gestation

− Pregnancy test

Cyclic pain

Menstrual cramps
Endometriosis
Adenomyosis

Acute pain

PID
Ovarian torsion
UTI
Appendicitis
Diverticulitis

Gradual onset

Uterine fibroids
Ovarian tumor
Functional disorder

Robert A. Baldor, MD and Alan M. Ehrlich, MD

Ortiz DD. Chronic pelvic pain in women. *Am Fam Physician.* 2008;77(11):1535–1542.

PHARYNGITIS

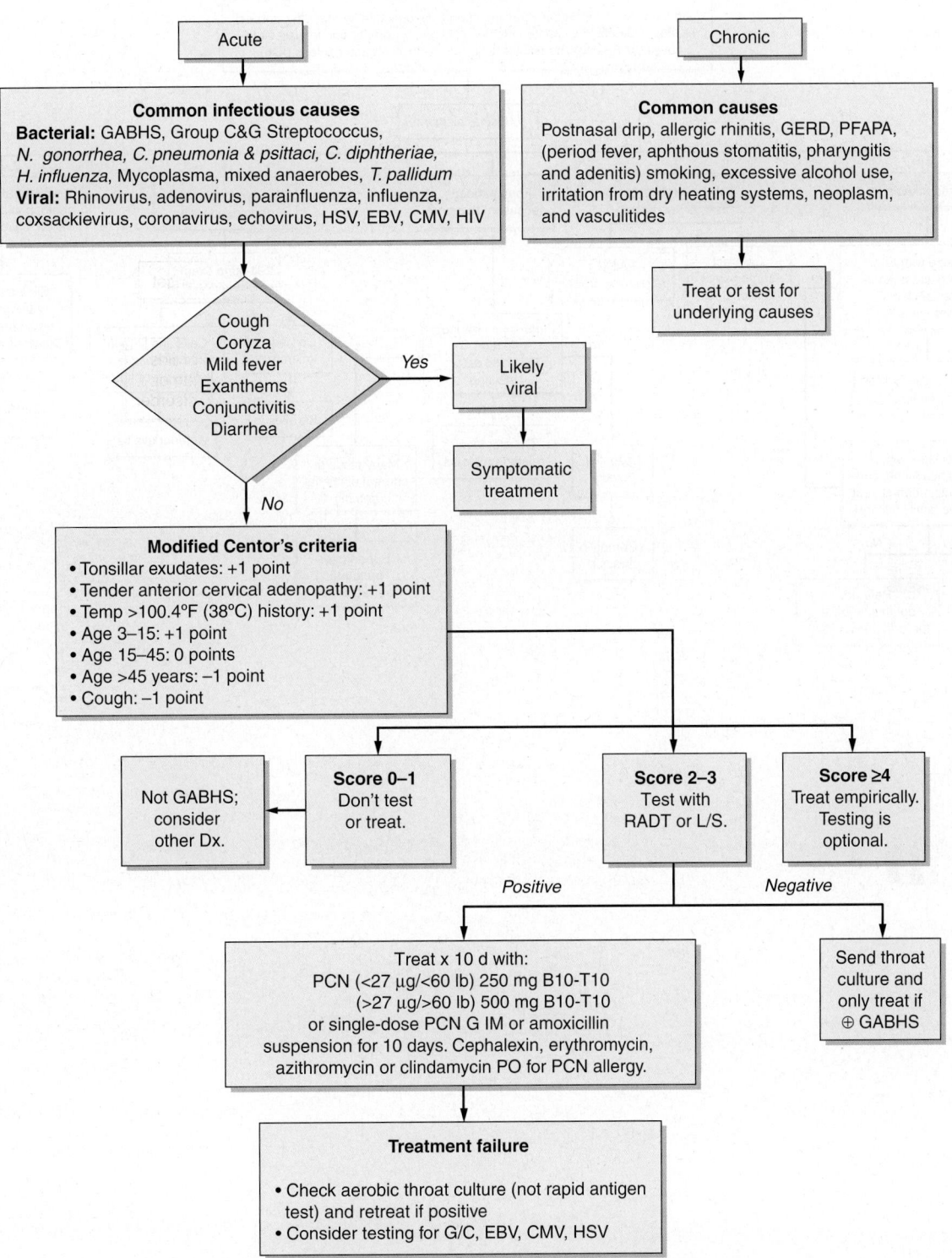

Acute

Common infectious causes
Bacterial: GABHS, Group C&G Streptococcus, *N. gonorrhea, C. pneumonia & psittaci, C. diphtheriae,* *H. influenza,* Mycoplasma, mixed anaerobes, *T. pallidum*
Viral: Rhinovirus, adenovirus, parainfluenza, influenza, coxsackievirus, coronavirus, echovirus, HSV, EBV, CMV, HIV

Chronic

Common causes
Postnasal drip, allergic rhinitis, GERD, PFAPA, (period fever, aphthous stomatitis, pharyngitis and adenitis) smoking, excessive alcohol use, irritation from dry heating systems, neoplasm, and vasculitides

Treat or test for underlying causes

Cough
Coryza
Mild fever
Exanthems
Conjunctivitis
Diarrhea

Yes → Likely viral → Symptomatic treatment

No

Modified Centor's criteria
• Tonsillar exudates: +1 point
• Tender anterior cervical adenopathy: +1 point
• Temp >100.4°F (38°C) history: +1 point
• Age 3–15: +1 point
• Age 15–45: 0 points
• Age >45 years: –1 point
• Cough: –1 point

Score 0–1
Don't test or treat.

Not GABHS; consider other Dx.

Score 2–3
Test with RADT or L/S.

Score ≥4
Treat empirically. Testing is optional.

Positive

Negative

Treat x 10 d with:
PCN (<27 µg/<60 lb) 250 mg B10-T10
(>27 µg/>60 lb) 500 mg B10-T10
or single-dose PCN G IM or amoxicillin suspension for 10 days. Cephalexin, erythromycin, azithromycin or clindamycin PO for PCN allergy.

Send throat culture and only treat if ⊕ GABHS

Treatment failure

• Check aerobic throat culture (not rapid antigen test) and retreat if positive
• Consider testing for G/C, EBV, CMV, HSV

Bency Louidor-Paulynice, MD and Hugh J. Silk, MD, MPH

Gerber MA, Baltimore RS, Eaton CB, et al. Prevention of rheumatic fever and diagnosis and treatment of acute Streptococcal pharyngitis: A scientific statement from the American Heart Association Rheumatic Fever, Endocarditis, and Kawasaki Disease Committee of the Council on Cardiovascular Disease in the Young, the Interdisciplinary Council on Functional Genomics and Translational Biology, and the Interdisciplinary Council on Quality of Care and Outcomes Research: Endorsed by the American Academy of Pediatrics. *Circulation.* 2009;119(11):1541–1551.

PHOTOPHOBIA

Yasir Ahmed, MD, Ingrid U. Scott, MD, MPH, and Harry W. Flynn, Jr., MD

Digre KB, Brennan KC. Shedding light on photophobia. *J Neuroophthalmol.* 2012;32(1):68–81.

POISON EXPOSURE AND TREATMENT
POISON EXPOSURE

Personal protective equipment; secure airway, breathing, circulation
*Consider prolonged resuscitation effort (60 minutes) as intact neurologic survival is possible

Check blood sugar (treat with 1 amp D50); administer thiamine (100 mg IV/IM)
and naloxone (0.4–2 mg q2–3min) if unresponsive

Seizure Control
1st-line benzodiazepines (BZD), 2nd-line barbiturates, avoid phenytoin
consider lorazepam 4 mg or Diazepam 8 mg IV then phenobarbital 10–20 mg/kg IV or
Propofol 1 mg/kg IV
*Pyridoxine 5 g IV if suspect isoniazid or mushroom poisoning

Correct hyperthermia (antipyretics ineffective)
evaporative cooling, ice water immersion, ice packing, gastric lavage, peritoneal lavage

Collateral history from patient, family, or EMS; thorough physical exam

Contact Poison Control Center at 800-222-1222

Initial workup: Electrocardiogram, Tylenol level, ASA level, urinalysis with pH, hepatic function panel,
comprehensive metabolic panel, pregnancy test (female), lactate, coagulation blood tests,
salicylates, serum osmolality, serum ethanol level, blood gas (arterial or venous),
chest x-ray, creatine kinase, carboxyhemoglobin, expanded urine drug screen

Consider drug immunoassay and drug levels for the following if indicated: Digoxin, valproic
acid, methotrexate, theophylline, carbamazepine, iron, lithium, phenobarbital, phenytoin,
carbon monoxide, methemoglobin

Bicarbonate for severe
metabolic acidosis or widened
QRS interval
*Instructions for drip below—
titrate infusion to a target serum
pH of 7.45–7.50

GI decontamination only if
supportive care not satisfactory and airway
is secure. Consider activated charcoal
1 g/kg PO × 1 within an hour of ingestion or
whole-bowel irrigation with polyethylene
glycol at 1–2 L/hr via NGT

Enhanced clearance with dialysis
(aspirin, methanol, ethylene glycol,
lithium, theophylline, isoniazid) or with
urine alkalinization (urine pH >7.5)
*Instructions for drip below—titrate
infusion to a target urine pH of >7.50

Go to "Poison Treatment" algorithm.

POISON TREATMENT

Opioid: • Sedation • Miosis • Decreased respirations	Anticholinergic: • Hallucinations • Mydriasis • Dry skin • Urinary retention	Sedative/ Hypnotic: • Normal pupils • Decreased respirations	Sympathomimetic: • Mydriasis • Tachycardia • Hypertension • Hyperthermia • Diaphoresis	Cholinergic: • Seizures • Miosis • Lacrimation • Vomiting/Diarrhea • Bradycardia	Serotonin: • Tachycardia • Hypertension • Clonus • Hyperthermia
Naloxone: 0.4–2 mg q2–3min	• BZD (midazolam 5–10 mg IV, lorazepam 2 mg IV) • Physostigmine (2 mg IV over 4 min)	Consider flumazenil 0.2 mg IV q1min (max 5 mg) *Caution in BZD patients may cause seizure	BZD (midazolam 5–10 mg IV, lorazepam 2 mg IV)	• Atropine 1–2 mg IV bolus, glycopyrrolate 1–2 mg/kg PRN • Pralidoxime 1–2 g in 100 mL 0.9% NaCl/D5W over 15–30 min IV • BZD (midazolam 5–10 mg IV, lorazepam 2 mg IV)	• BZD (midazolam 5–10 mg IV, lorazepam 2 mg IV) • Consider cyproheptadine 4–8 mg PO t.i.d. • Aggressive cooling measures

Observe for 12–24 hours until stable with continuous cardiac monitoring.

Psychiatry consult for intentional overdose

*How to mix a bicarbonate drip: 150 mEq (3 amps) NaHCO3 in 1 L of D5W, then start at a rate of 150–200 mL/hr.

PEDIATRIC DOSING (adult doses in algorithm):
- Activated charcoal (0.5–1 g/kg PO)
- Atropine (0.02 mg/kg IV)
- Bicarbonate (1–2 mEq/kg IV*)
- Chlorpromazine (not recommended)
- Cyproheptadine (0.25 mg/kg/d divided b.i.d. or t.i.d.)
- Dextrose (2.5 mL/kg of 10% or 1 mL/kg of 25% IV)
- Flumazenil (5 mcg/kg IV)
- Glycopyrrolate (0.025 mg/kg IV)
- Lorazepam (0.05–0.1 mg/kg IV)
- Midazolam (0.1 mg/kg IV)
- Phenobarbital (10–20 mg/kg IV)
- Physostigmine (10–30 mcg/kg IV)
- Polyethylene glycol (250–500 mL/h PO/NG)
- Pralidoxime (20–40 mg/kg IV)
- Pyridoxine (same as adults)
- Naloxone (0.1 mg/kg IV q2–3min)
- Thiamine (not routinely given)

Mark Neavyn, MD and Jonathan Nadler, MD

Frithsen IL, Simpson WM Jr. Recognition and management of acute medication poisoning. *Am Fam Physician.* 2010;81(3):316–323.

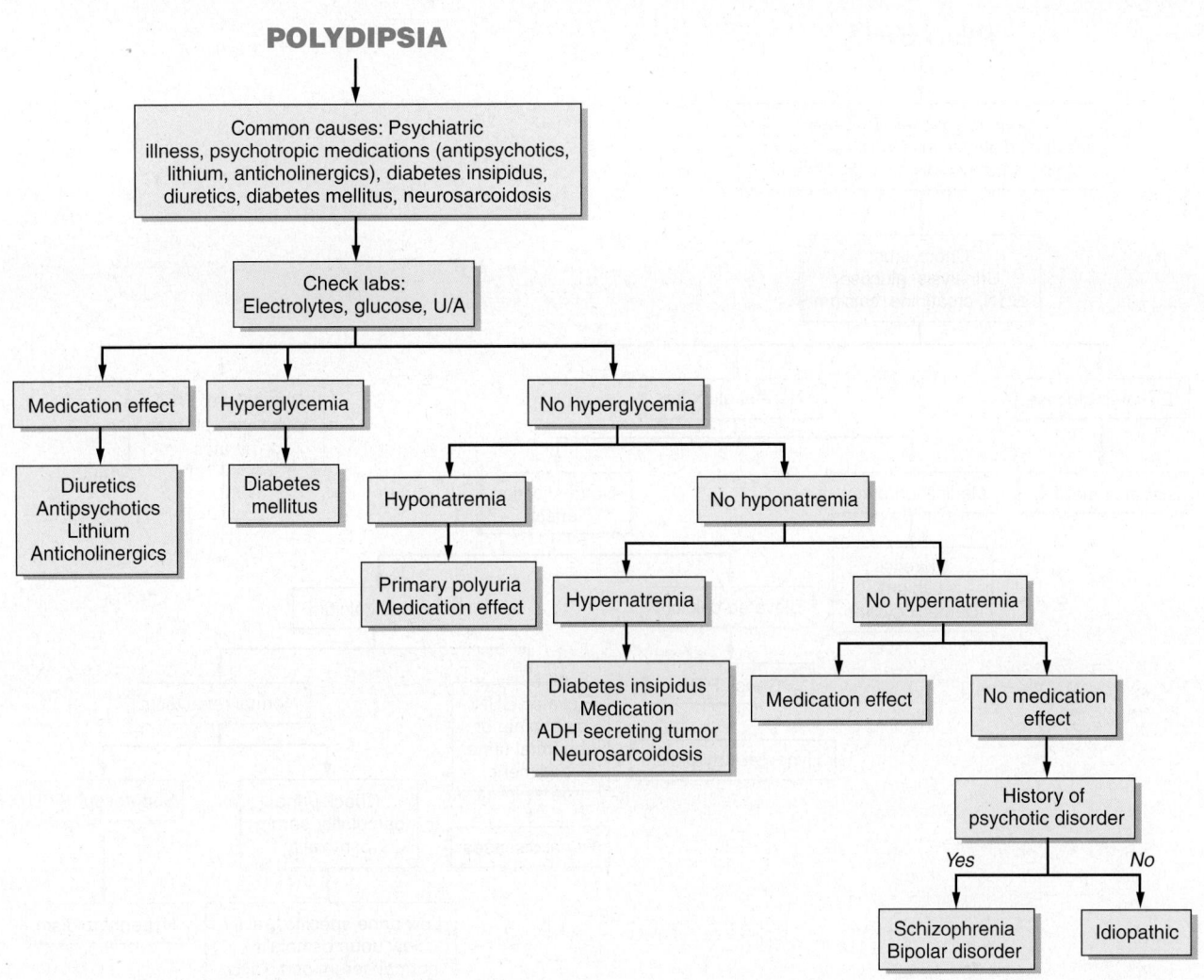

POLYDIPSIA

Common causes: Psychiatric illness, psychotropic medications (antipsychotics, lithium, anticholinergics), diabetes insipidus, diuretics, diabetes mellitus, neurosarcoidosis

Check labs: Electrolytes, glucose, U/A

- Medication effect
  - Diuretics
    Antipsychotics
    Lithium
    Anticholinergics
- Hyperglycemia
  - Diabetes mellitus
- No hyperglycemia
  - Hyponatremia
    - Primary polyuria
      Medication effect
  - No hyponatremia
    - Hypernatremia
      - Diabetes insipidus
        Medication
        ADH secreting tumor
        Neurosarcoidosis
    - No hypernatremia
      - Medication effect
      - No medication effect
        - History of psychotic disorder
          - *Yes* — Schizophrenia
            Bipolar disorder
          - *No* — Idiopathic

Robert A. Baldor, MD and Alan M. Ehrlich, MD

Moritz ML, Ayus JC. Hospital-acquired hyponatremia—why are hypotonic parenteral fluids still being used? *Nat Clin Pract Nephrol.* 2007;3:374–382.

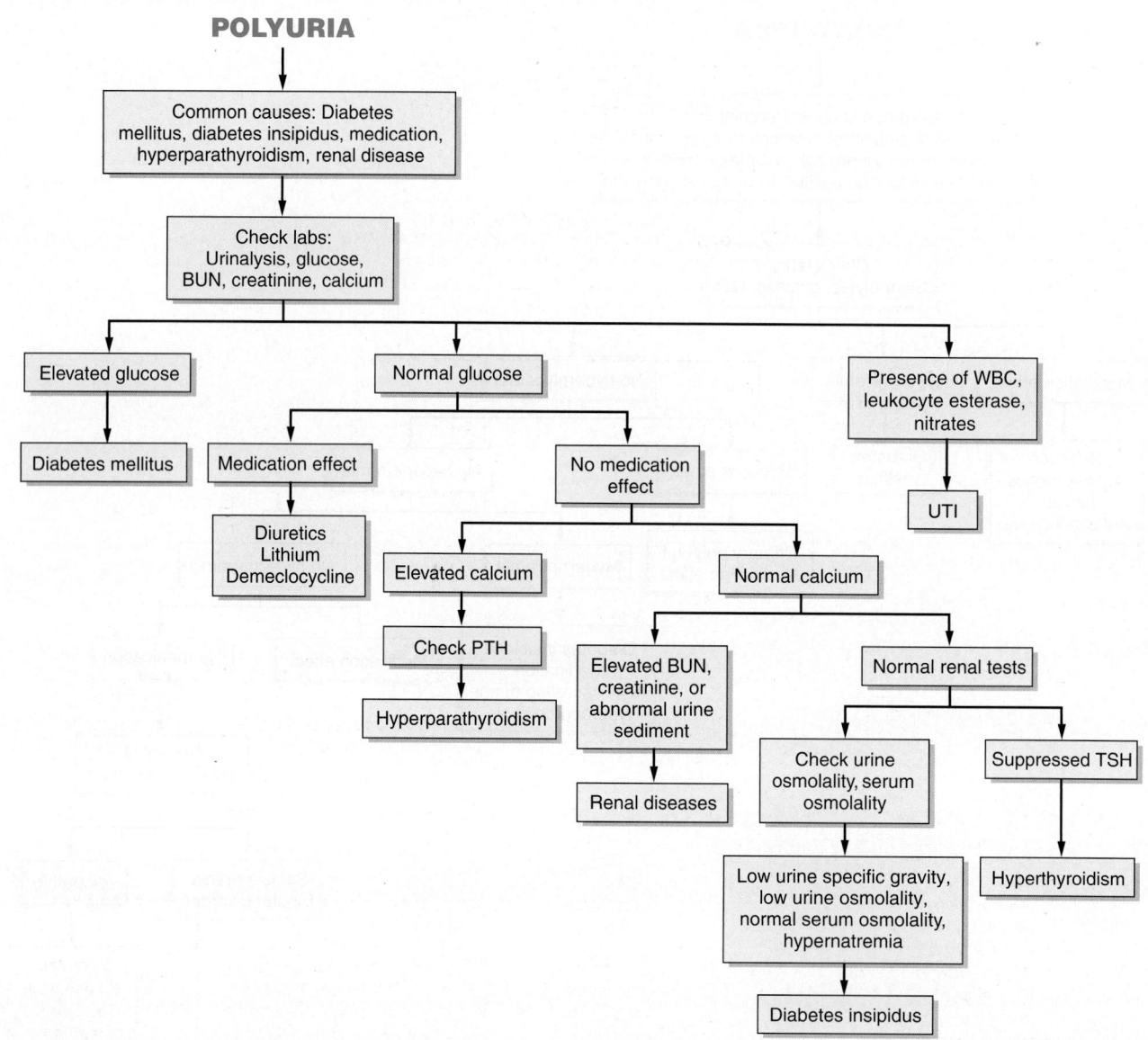

POLYURIA

Common causes: Diabetes mellitus, diabetes insipidus, medication, hyperparathyroidism, renal disease

Check labs: Urinalysis, glucose, BUN, creatinine, calcium

- Elevated glucose → Diabetes mellitus
- Normal glucose
  - Medication effect → Diuretics, Lithium, Demeclocycline
  - No medication effect
    - Elevated calcium → Check PTH → Hyperparathyroidism
    - Normal calcium
      - Elevated BUN, creatinine, or abnormal urine sediment → Renal diseases
      - Normal renal tests
        - Check urine osmolality, serum osmolality → Low urine specific gravity, low urine osmolality, normal serum osmolality, hypernatremia → Diabetes insipidus
        - Suppressed TSH → Hyperthyroidism
- Presence of WBC, leukocyte esterase, nitrates → UTI

Robert A. Baldor, MD and Alan M. Ehrlich, MD

Kujubu DA, Aboseif SR. An overview of nocturia and the syndrome of nocturnal polyuria in the elderly. *Nat Clin Pract Nephrol.* 2008;4(8):426–435.

PRECOCIOUS PUBERTY

Nicole Shields, MD

Nwosu BU, Lee MM. Evaluation of short and tall stature in children. *Am Fam Physician.* 2008;78(5):597–604.

PREOPERATIVE EVALUATION OF NONCARDIAC SURGICAL PATIENT

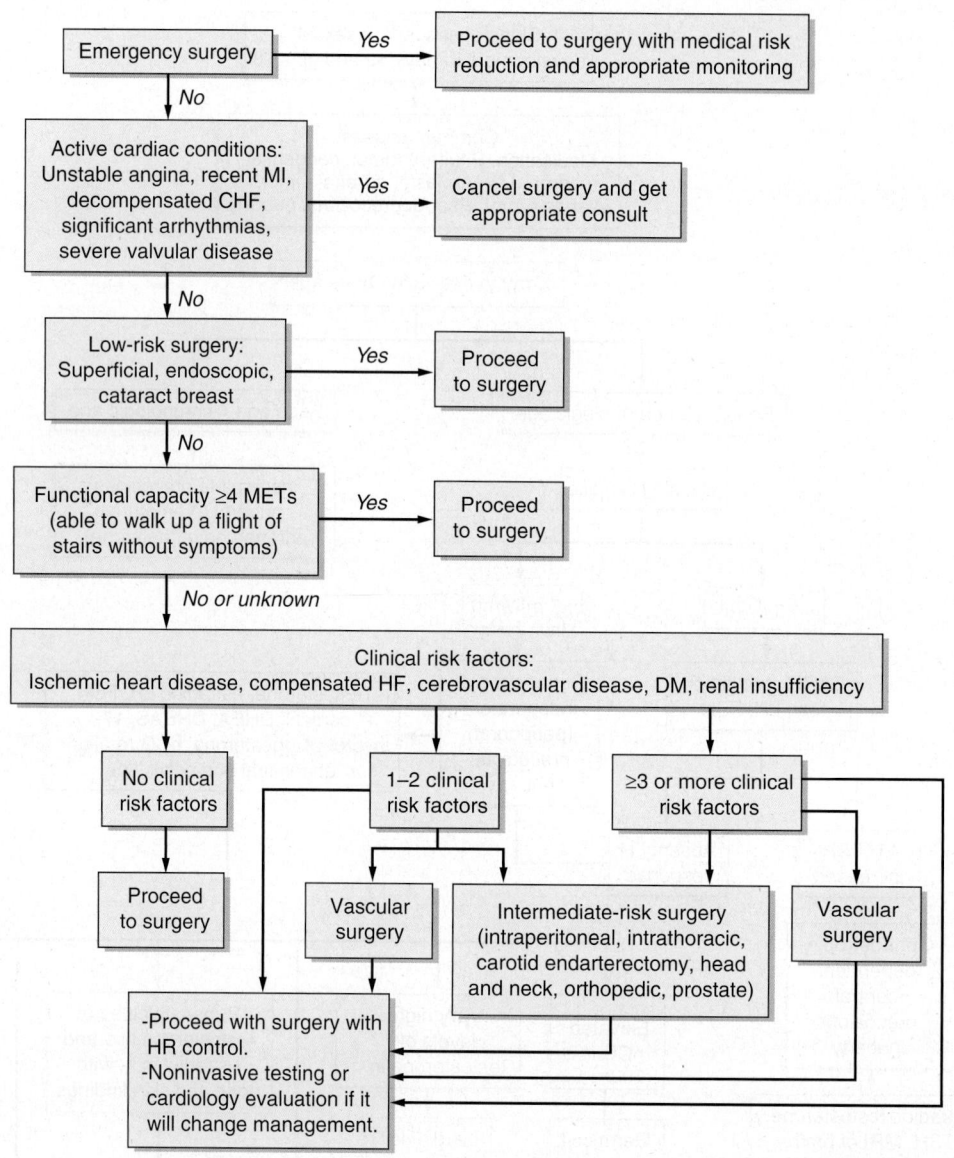

Drew Grimes, MD and Stacy Jones, MD

Fleisher LA, Beckman JA, Brown KA, et al. ACC/AHA 2007 guidelines on perioperative cardiovascular evaluation and care for noncardiac surgery: A report of the American College of Cardiology/American Heart Association Task Force on Practice Guidelines (Writing Committee to Revise the 2002 Guidelines on Perioperative Cardiovascular Evaluation for Noncardiac Surgery): Developed in collaboration with the American Society of Echocardiography, American Society of Nuclear Cardiology, Heart Rhythm Society, Society of Cardiovascular Anesthesiologists, Society for Cardiovascular Angiography and Interventions, Society for Vascular Medicine and Biology, and Society for Vascular Surgery. *Circulation.* 2007;116(17):e418-e499.

PROTEINURIA

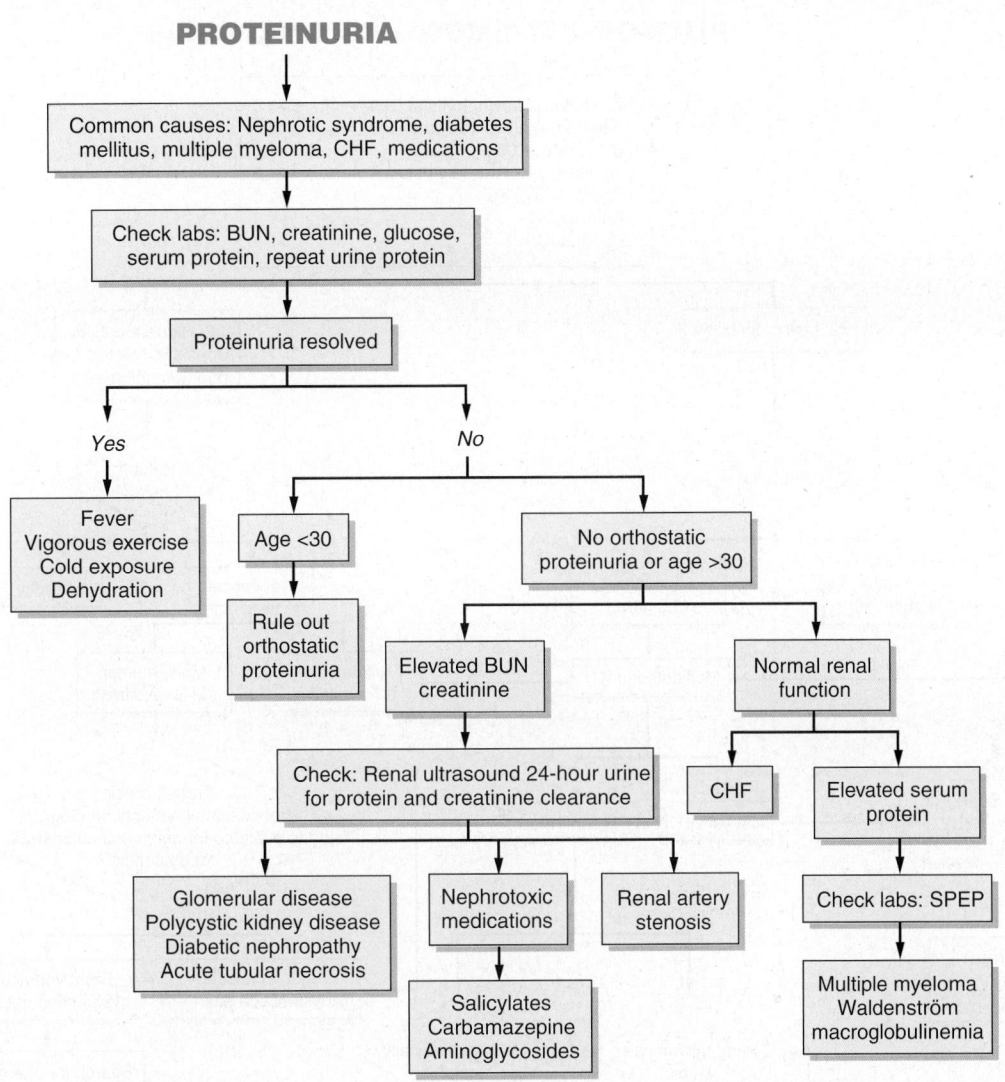

Common causes: Nephrotic syndrome, diabetes mellitus, multiple myeloma, CHF, medications

Check labs: BUN, creatinine, glucose, serum protein, repeat urine protein

Proteinuria resolved

Yes

Fever
Vigorous exercise
Cold exposure
Dehydration

No

Age <30

Rule out orthostatic proteinuria

No orthostatic proteinuria or age >30

Elevated BUN creatinine

Check: Renal ultrasound 24-hour urine for protein and creatinine clearance

Glomerular disease
Polycystic kidney disease
Diabetic nephropathy
Acute tubular necrosis

Nephrotoxic medications

Salicylates
Carbamazepine
Aminoglycosides

Renal artery stenosis

Normal renal function

CHF

Elevated serum protein

Check labs: SPEP

Multiple myeloma
Waldenström macroglobulinemia

Robert A. Baldor, MD and Alan M. Ehrlich, MD

Carroll MF, Temte JL. Proteinuria in adults: A diagnostic approach. *Am Fam Physician.* 2000;62:1333–1340.

PULMONARY EMBOLISM, DIAGNOSIS

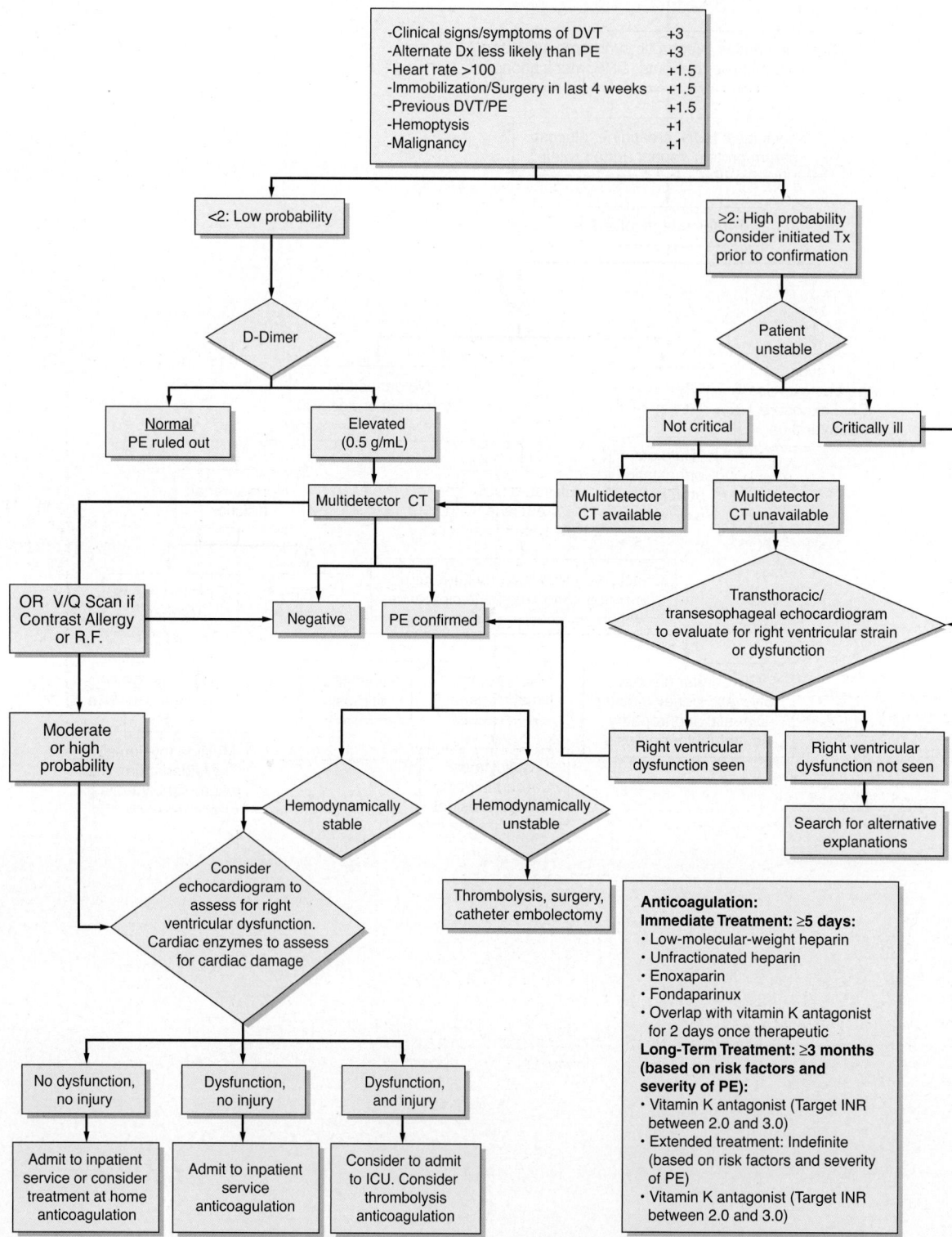

-Clinical signs/symptoms of DVT	+3
-Alternate Dx less likely than PE	+3
-Heart rate >100	+1.5
-Immobilization/Surgery in last 4 weeks	+1.5
-Previous DVT/PE	+1.5
-Hemoptysis	+1
-Malignancy	+1

<2: Low probability

≥2: High probability Consider initiated Tx prior to confirmation

D-Dimer

Patient unstable

Normal PE ruled out

Elevated (0.5 g/mL)

Not critical

Critically ill

Multidetector CT

Multidetector CT available

Multidetector CT unavailable

OR V/Q Scan if Contrast Allergy or R.F.

Negative

PE confirmed

Transthoracic/ transesophageal echocardiogram to evaluate for right ventricular strain or dysfunction

Moderate or high probability

Right ventricular dysfunction seen

Right ventricular dysfunction not seen

Hemodynamically stable

Hemodynamically unstable

Search for alternative explanations

Consider echocardiogram to assess for right ventricular dysfunction. Cardiac enzymes to assess for cardiac damage

Thrombolysis, surgery, catheter embolectomy

Anticoagulation:
Immediate Treatment: ≥5 days:
· Low-molecular-weight heparin
· Unfractionated heparin
· Enoxaparin
· Fondaparinux
· Overlap with vitamin K antagonist for 2 days once therapeutic
Long-Term Treatment: ≥3 months (based on risk factors and severity of PE):
· Vitamin K antagonist (Target INR between 2.0 and 3.0)
· Extended treatment: Indefinite (based on risk factors and severity of PE)
· Vitamin K antagonist (Target INR between 2.0 and 3.0)

No dysfunction, no injury

Dysfunction, no injury

Dysfunction, and injury

Admit to inpatient service or consider treatment at home anticoagulation

Admit to inpatient service anticoagulation

Consider to admit to ICU. Consider thrombolysis anticoagulation

After PE is diagnosed, follow up and monitor for 2 years in office, as there is a high rate of recurrence.

Patricia Seymour, MS, MD and Jeremy Golding, MD

Kearon C, Kahn SR, Agnelli G, et al. Antithrombotic therapy for venous thromboembolic disease: American College of Chest Physicians Evidence-Based Clinical Practice Guidelines (8th edition). *Chest.* 2008;133(6 Suppl):454S–545S.

PULMONARY EMBOLISM, TREATMENT

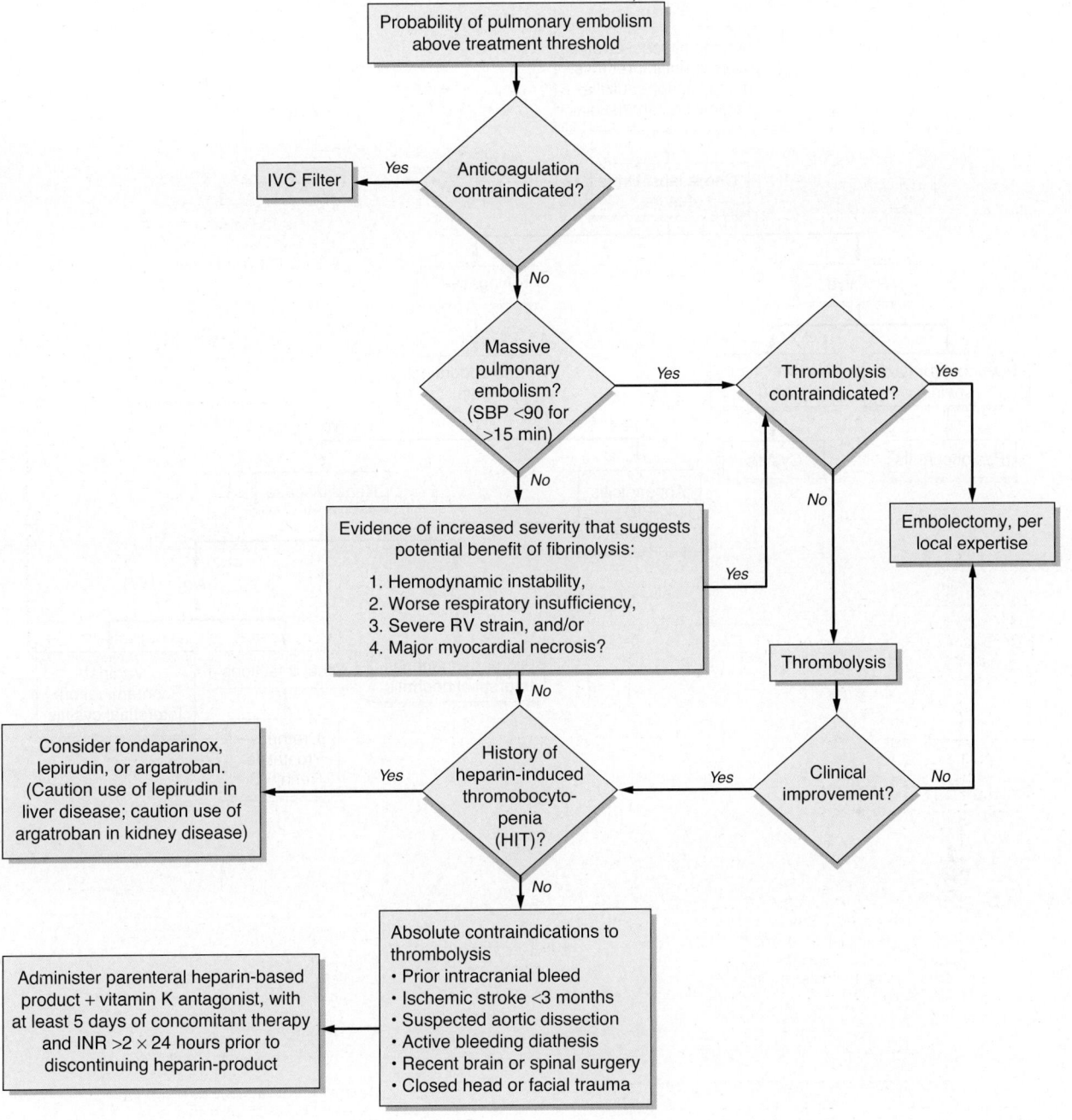

Parag Goyal, MD

Jaff MR, McMurtry MS, Archer SL, et al. Management of massive and submassive pulmonary embolism, iliofemoral deep vein thrombosis, and chronic thromboembolic pulmonary hypertension: A scientific statement from the American Heart Association. *Circulation.* 2011;123:1788–1830.

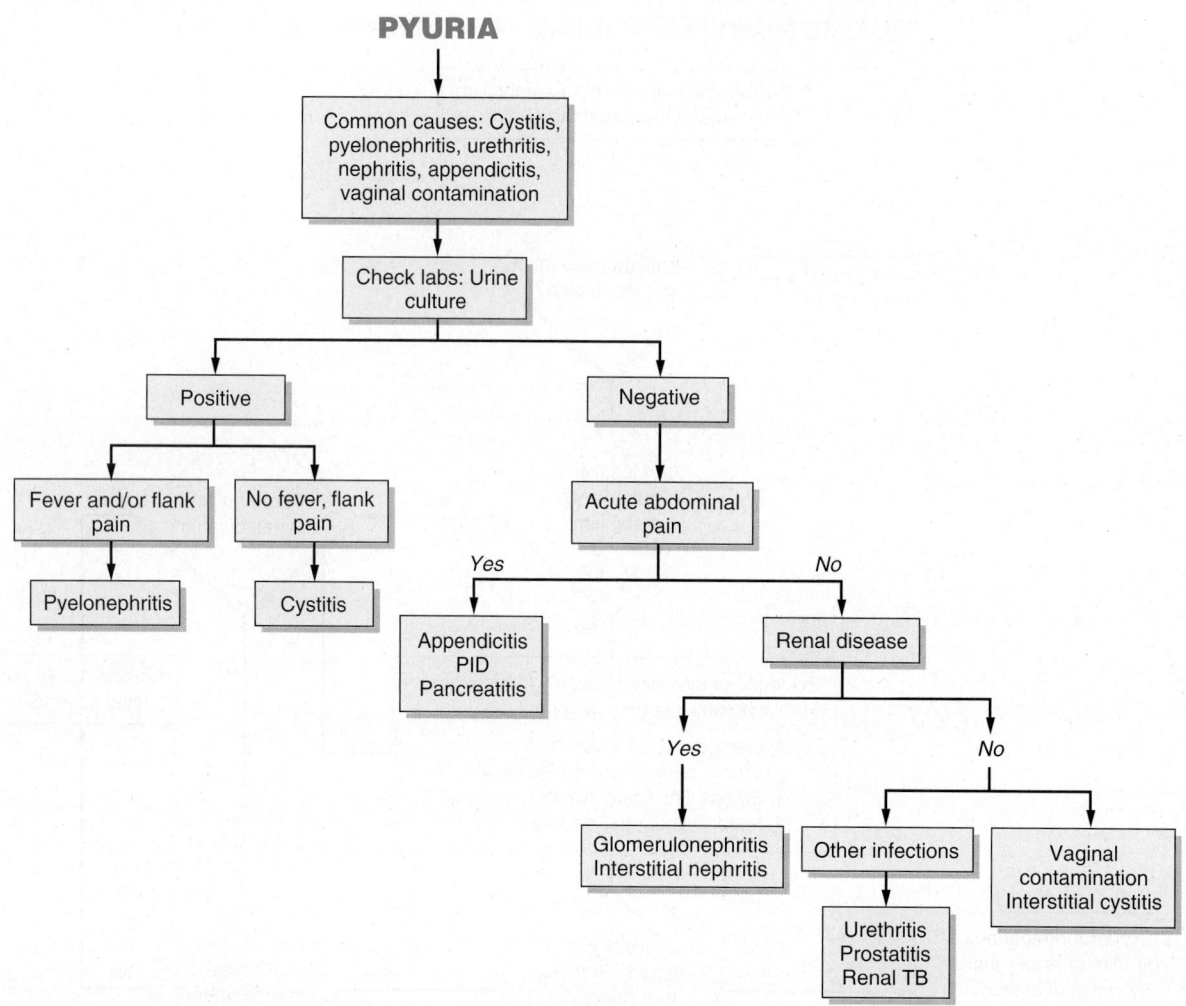

PYURIA

Common causes: Cystitis, pyelonephritis, urethritis, nephritis, appendicitis, vaginal contamination

Check labs: Urine culture

Positive

Negative

Fever and/or flank pain

No fever, flank pain

Acute abdominal pain

Pyelonephritis

Cystitis

Yes

Appendicitis PID Pancreatitis

No

Renal disease

Yes

Glomerulonephritis Interstitial nephritis

No

Other infections

Vaginal contamination Interstitial cystitis

Urethritis Prostatitis Renal TB

Robert A. Baldor, MD and Alan M. Ehrlich, MD

Simerville JA, Maxted WC, Pahira JJ. Urinalysis: A comprehensive review. *Am Fam Physician.* 2005;71:1153–1162.

RASH, FOCAL

Robert A. Baldor, MD and Alan M. Ehrlich, MD

Federman DG, Reid M, Feldman SR, et al. The primary care provider and the care of skin disease: The patient's perspective.
Arch Dermatol. 2001;137:25–29.

RECTAL BLEEDING AND HEMATOCHEZIA

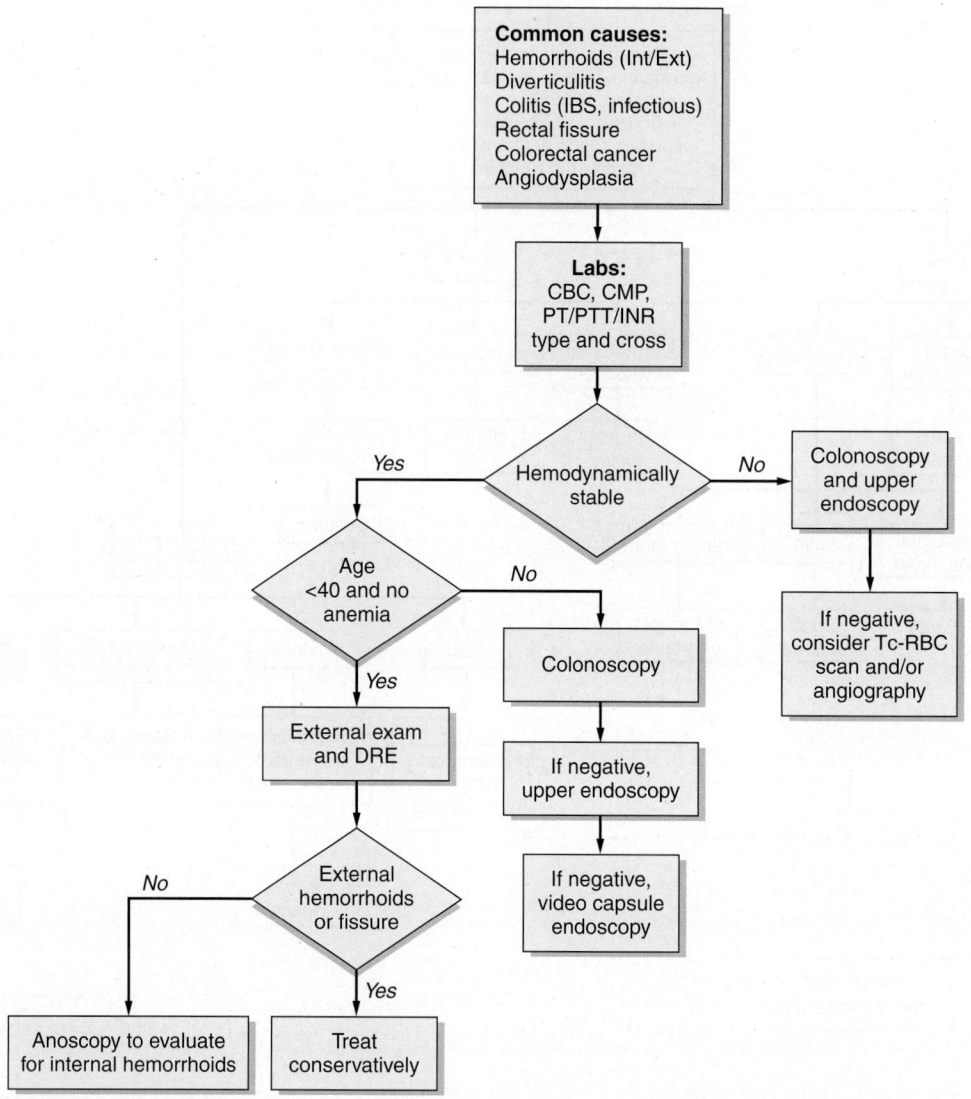

Common causes:
Hemorrhoids (Int/Ext)
Diverticulitis
Colitis (IBS, infectious)
Rectal fissure
Colorectal cancer
Angiodysplasia

Labs:
CBC, CMP,
PT/PTT/INR
type and cross

Hemodynamically stable

Yes — Age <40 and no anemia

No — Colonoscopy and upper endoscopy

If negative, consider Tc-RBC scan and/or angiography

No — Colonoscopy

If negative, upper endoscopy

If negative, video capsule endoscopy

Yes — External exam and DRE

External hemorrhoids or fissure

No — Anoscopy to evaluate for internal hemorrhoids

Yes — Treat conservatively

Mohammad Ansar Mughal, MD

Hoedema RE, Luchtefeld MA. The management of lower gastrointestinal hemorrhage. *Dis Colon Rectum.* 2005;48(11):2010–2024.

RECTAL PAIN

Common causes: Hemorrhoids, anal fissure, fistula, infections (HSV, syphilis, GC, chlamydia, HPV), perianal abscess, inflammation, malignancy, trauma, rectal prolapse

History: Bleeding, masses, discharge, change in bowel habits (diarrhea, constipation, tenesmus), pruritis, rectal fullness, sexual history, trauma

Physical Exam: Lesions, discharge, inflammation, tenderness, masses, blood, digital rectal examination, Valsava maneuver

Abnormal Hx and exam findings

Normal Hx and exam findings

Hemorrhoids, anal fissure, fistula, abscess, mass, foreign body, pilonidal cyst, hidradenitis supurrativa, rectal prolapse, anal skin tag, trauma, perianal abscess

Labs: CBC, ESR, CRP, GC/Chl, HSV, VRDL, HPV, UA, urine cx, stool cx, FOBT

Treat accordingly ← Abnormal

Normal

Hemorrhoids, fissure, proctitis, rectal cancer, ulcer(s), abscess ← Abnormal exam — Proctoscopy, anoscopy, sigmoidoscopy ± biopsy

Normal exam

Abnormal imaging — Ultrasound, CT scan pelvis, MRI pelvis, LS spinal x-ray, defocography

Normal imaging

Malignancy, fistula, abscess, pelvic abscess, coccydynia (fracture, dislocation), foreign body

Proctalgia fugax, levator ani syndrome, IBS, anismus, pruritis ani, coccydynia (nonfracture), endometriosis

Lakshmi D.N. Lattimer, MD and Marie L. Borum, MD, MPH, EdD

Fargo MV, Latimer KM. Evaluation and management of common anorectal conditions. *Am Fam Physician.* 2012;85:624–630.

RECURRENT PREGNANCY LOSS

Defused: 2 or more failed clinical pregnancies

Common causes: Thyroid dysfunction, diabetes, pituitary disorders, genetic issues, uterine dysfunction, thrombophilic disorders, substance abuse, obesity

Labs: TSH, glucose/Hbg A1C, prolactin, transvaginal ultrasound

Labs normal?

No → Thyroid disease, diabetes mellitus, pituitary disorder

Yes

Labs:
Anticardiolipin antibodies, lupus, Anticoagulant, Factor V (Ceirten) mutation, protein C, protein S antigen, prothrombin G20210A, karyotype of parents

Julia Parzych, MD and Frank J. Domino, MD

Practice Committee of the American Society for Reproductive Medicine. Evaluation and treatment of recurrent pregnancy loss: A committee opinion. *Fertil Steril.* 2012;98(5):1103–1111.

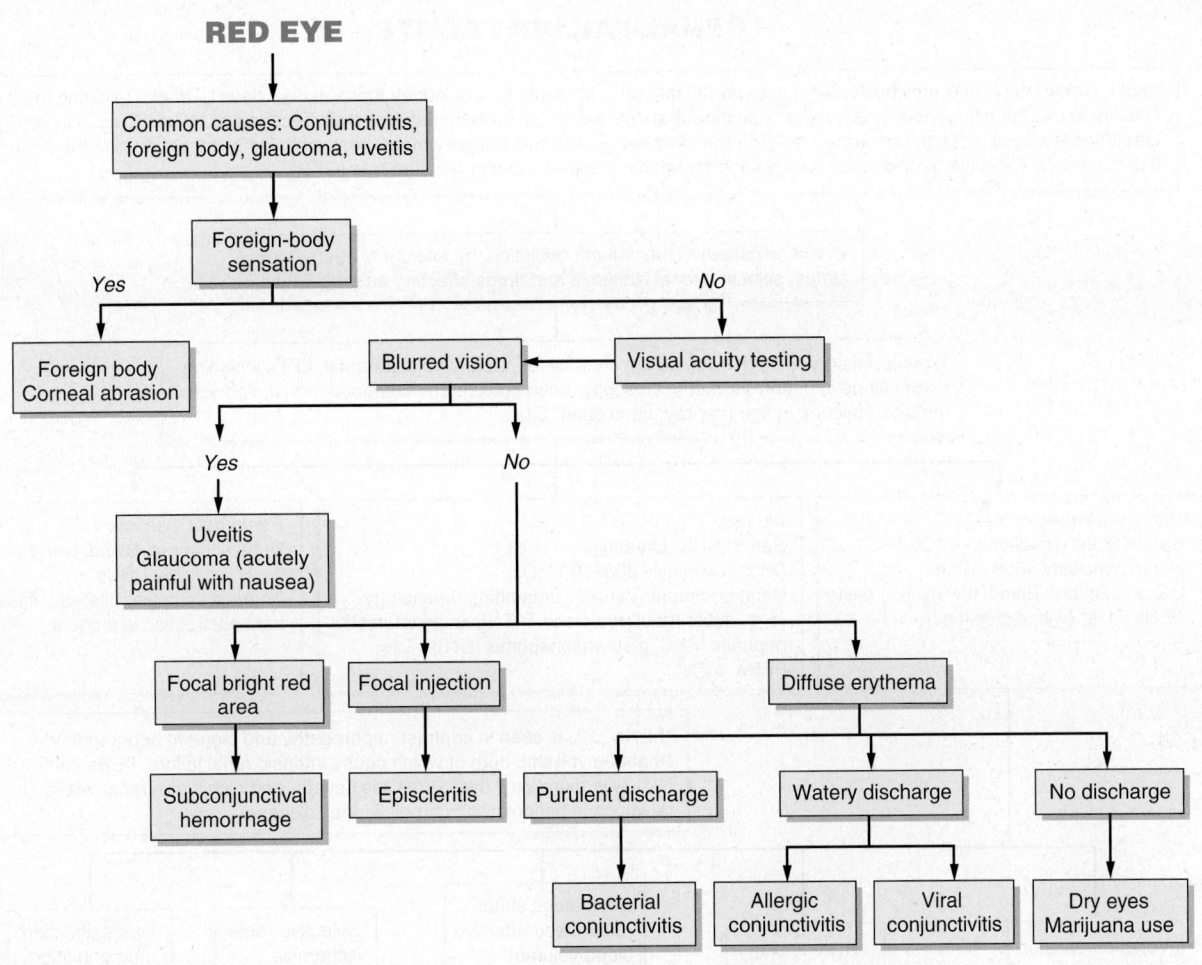

RED EYE

Common causes: Conjunctivitis, foreign body, glaucoma, uveitis

Foreign-body sensation

Yes → Foreign body / Corneal abrasion

No → Visual acuity testing → Blurred vision

Blurred vision — Yes → Uveitis / Glaucoma (acutely painful with nausea)

Blurred vision — No:
- Focal bright red area → Subconjunctival hemorrhage
- Focal injection → Episcleritis
- Diffuse erythema:
  - Purulent discharge → Bacterial conjunctivitis
  - Watery discharge → Allergic conjunctivitis / Viral conjunctivitis
  - No discharge → Dry eyes / Marijuana use

Robert A. Baldor, MD and Alan M. Ehrlich, MD

Leibowitz HM. The red eye. *NEJM.* 2000;343(5):345–351.

RENAL FAILURE, ACUTE

Acute kidney injury (AKI, previously called acute renal failure) is an acute loss of kidney function over days to weeks resulting in an inability to excrete nitrogenous wastes and creatinine. Patients are often asymptomatic, and are recognized by an increase in serum creatinine level (>0.5 mg/dL from baseline). Prerenal disease (PD) is one category of AKI where the injury occurs outside the nephron; it is marked by diminished renal blood flow leading to a decrease in glomerular filtration rate (GFR).

Common causes: True volume depletion, hypotension, edematous states, selective renal ischemia and drugs affecting autoregulation

Workup: History and physical, serum chemistries, CBC with differential, LFTs including serum albumin urinalysis with microscopy, urine sodium and creatinine and if diagnosis remains obscure, imaging (x-ray, ultrasound, CT)

Prerenal disease
Serum BUN: Creatinine → ≥20:1
Urine osmolality >500 mOsm
Urine sediment: Bland, few hyaline casts
FENa <1%* (with exceptions)

Intrinsic
Serum BUN: Creatinine → <20:1
Urine osmolality 200–300 mOsm
Urine sediment: Variable depending on etiology (e.g., acute tubular necrosis [ATN], acute interstitial nephritis [AIN], glomerulonephritis [GN])
FENa: >2%*

Postrenal/Obstructive
Urine sediment: Bland, few hyaline casts, possible RBCs
Anuria if complete bilateral urinary tract obstruction is present

*FENa <1% is seen in contrast nephropathy and pigment nephropathy (rhabdomyolysis), both of which cause intrinsic renal failure. FENa can be >1% with diuretics if overdiuresis is severe, and also if pre–renal failure develops in patients with chronic kidney disease

Volume depletion

Hypotension

Edematous states (decreased effective blood volume)

Selective renal ischemia

Drugs affecting autoregulation

Dehydration/Poor PO intake: Dry mucous membranes, pallor, orthostatic hypotension, weight loss, perspiration, decreased skin turgor
GI losses: Emesis, diarrhea
Renal losses: Overdiuresis with Diuretics, osmotic diuresis with hyperglycemia
Infectious: Fever, chills, leukocytosis (with left shift)
Hemorrhage
Insensible losses: Perspiration, burns
Large vessel diseases: Arterial thrombus (hypercoagulable syndromes), emboli (atherosclerotic disease), aortic dissection (connective tissue disease, trauma)

Shock
Sepsis: Evidence of infection, hypotension, acidosis, constitutional symptoms, leukopenia or leukocytosis, bandemia, tachycardia, tachypnea

CHF: JVD, pulmonary rales, pitting edema, hepatomegaly, dyspnea
Cirrhosis: Ascites, varices, pruritus, jaundice, asterixis, bruising, edema, elevated LFTs, hypoalbuminemia
Nephrotic syndrome: Hypoalbuminemia, proteinuria, foamy urine, hypertension, facial and peripheral edema

Hepatorenal syndrome: Portal hypertension, oliguria, hyponatremia, constitutional symptoms
Bilateral renal artery stenosis: Possible history of hypertension, atherosclerosis, fibromuscular dysplasia/worsened by ACE inhibitors or ARBs

ACE inhibitors: Vasodilation of efferent arterioles
NSAIDs: Vasoconstriction of afferent arterioles
Calcineurin inhibitors: Vasoconstriction of afferent arterioles

Krunal Patel, MD and Dagmar Klinger, MD

Needham E. Management of acute renal failure. *Am Fam Physician.* 2005;72:1739–1746.

SALICYLATE POISONING, ACUTE, TREATMENT

Assess Airway, Breathing, Circulation
Provide appropriate ABC management. Avoid intubation unless patient is unable to protect airway because intubation may increase salicylate Neurotoxicity associated may result in cardiovascular collapse.

Early Toxicity: Tachypnea, hyperpnea, nausea, vomiting, Unnitus.
Late Toxicity: Fever, hypotension, altered mental status.

H+P
Obtain careful history of ingestion (time, reported ingestion, coingestants, etc.) and perform thorough physical exam for hemodynamic instability, alterations in respiratory pattern, and changes in mental status.

Does the patient exhibit evidence of severe toxicity?* — No → (H+P) / Yes →

Initiate Emergent Hemodialysis
Begin volume resuscitation and alkalinization unless prohibited by cerebral/pulmonary edema. Administer 25 g (1 amp) D50 for altered mental status. Do not delay treatment for diagnostic studies.

***Note:** Clinical manifestations of severe toxicity at presentation include altered mental status/coma, seizures, pulmonary edema, need for endotracheal intubation and mechanical ventilation.

Is the patient asymptomatic, stable, and known to liave ingested <150 mg/kg? — Yes → / No →

Evaluation/Observation
Obtain first salicylate level nothing time since ingestion occured.

Initial Treatment
1. Early volume resuscitation with normal saline.
2. Urinary alkalinization using 150 mEq (3 amps) NaHCO3 mixed in 1 L D5W and add 40 mEq KCl per L infused at 2–3 mL/kg/hr.
3. Administer first dose activated charcoal at 1 g/kg (max 50 g) ONLY IF patient is alert, cooperative, and can tolerate. Consider additional doses of 25 g q4h If patient can tolerate and has bowel sounds on exam.

ASA Detectable
Recheck levels q2h until persistently within therapeutic range, trending down, or nondetectable. Routinely reassess for changes in clinical status and initiate treatment if indicated.

ASA Non-detectable
Recheck if within 2 hours of presentation. Discharge after 6 hours observation if patient remains asymptomatic and levels are nondetectable.

Note: Volume resuscitation and alkalinization are the mainstays of therapy and should be given to all symptomatic patients unless pulmonary or cerebral edema is present. Respiratory alkalosis (pH >7.5) is NOT a contraindication to therapy. Do not delay for charcoal or diagnostic studies.

Obtain Diagnostic Studies
Lab: Salicylate level (note time since ingestion), ABG/VBG, basic electrolytes, BUN, Creatinine, LFTs, coags, UA. Obtain APAP level. Obatain tox screen if polysubstance overdose suspected.
Imaging: Chest radiograph (evaluate for pulmonary edema). Consider head CT if Altered Mental Status to evaluate for cerebral edema.

Maintenance Therapy and Evaluation
1. Continue bicarbonate infusion at ~2–3 mL/kg/hr to maintain urine output of 1–2 mL/kg/hr.
2. Measure urine pH hourly and titrate infusion to goal pH of 7.5–8.
3. Measure ABG or VBG hourly and decrease rate of bicarbonate drip if serum pH exceeds 7.6.
4. Measure serum salicylate level every 2 hours until salicylate level begins to decline and acid-base status is normal.
5. Measure serum K hourly and replete if <4.5 mEq/L.

Presence of slicylate level >100 mg/dL, arterial pH <7.3 renal insufficiency, pulmonary or cerebral edema, or has patient deteriorated? — No → / Yes → **Initiate Hemodialysis**

Disposition
Treatment should be continued with frequent clinical assessment for improvement. Treatment and testing may be stopped ONLY when patient is asymptomatic acid-base status is stable, AND salicylate level has fallen into therapeutic range (10–30 mg/dL).

Mark Andrews, MD and Kavita Babu, MD

O'Malley GF. Emergency department management of the salicylate-poisoned patient. *Emerg Med Clin North Am.* 2007;25:333–346.

SEIZURE, NEW ONSET

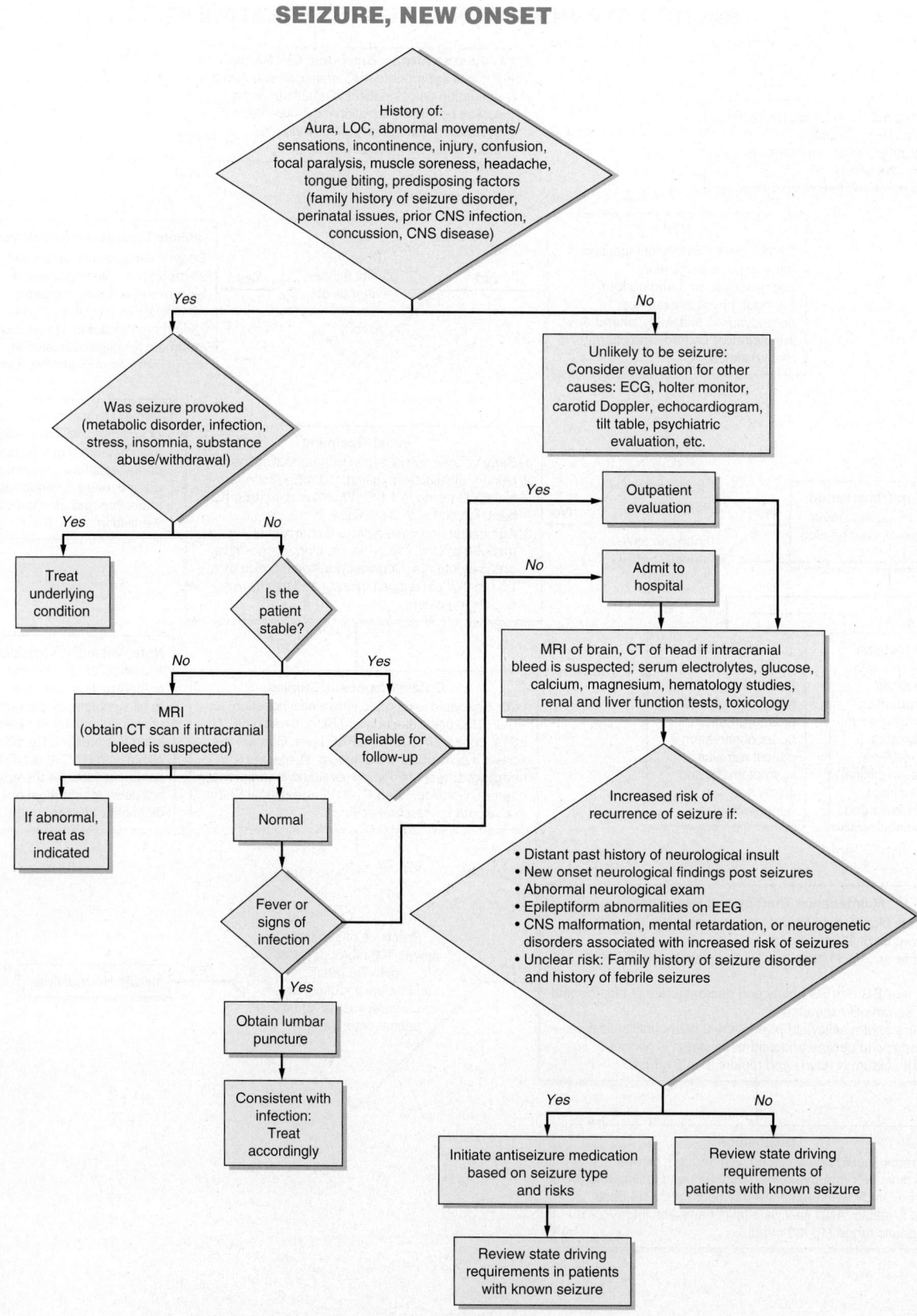

History of:
Aura, LOC, abnormal movements/sensations, incontinence, injury, confusion, focal paralysis, muscle soreness, headache, tongue biting, predisposing factors (family history of seizure disorder, perinatal issues, prior CNS infection, concussion, CNS disease)

Yes → Was seizure provoked (metabolic disorder, infection, stress, insomnia, substance abuse/withdrawal)

No → Unlikely to be seizure: Consider evaluation for other causes: ECG, holter monitor, carotid Doppler, echocardiogram, tilt table, psychiatric evaluation, etc.

Was seizure provoked:
- Yes → Treat underlying condition
- No → Is the patient stable?

Is the patient stable?
- No → MRI (obtain CT scan if intracranial bleed is suspected) → If abnormal, treat as indicated / Normal
- Yes → Reliable for follow-up?

Reliable for follow-up?
- Yes → Outpatient evaluation
- No → Admit to hospital

Outpatient evaluation / Admit to hospital → MRI of brain, CT of head if intracranial bleed is suspected; serum electrolytes, glucose, calcium, magnesium, hematology studies, renal and liver function tests, toxicology

Normal → Fever or signs of infection
- Yes → Obtain lumbar puncture → Consistent with infection: Treat accordingly

Increased risk of recurrence of seizure if:
- Distant past history of neurological insult
- New onset neurological findings post seizures
- Abnormal neurological exam
- Epileptiform abnormalities on EEG
- CNS malformation, mental retardation, or neurogenetic disorders associated with increased risk of seizures
- Unclear risk: Family history of seizure disorder and history of febrile seizures

Increased risk:
- Yes → Initiate antiseizure medication based on seizure type and risks → Review state driving requirements in patients with known seizure
- No → Review state driving requirements of patients with known seizure

Neepa Patel, MD

Chang BS, Lowenstein DH. Epilepsy. *N Engl J Med.* 2003;349:1257–1266.

SHOULDER PAIN, DIAGNOSIS

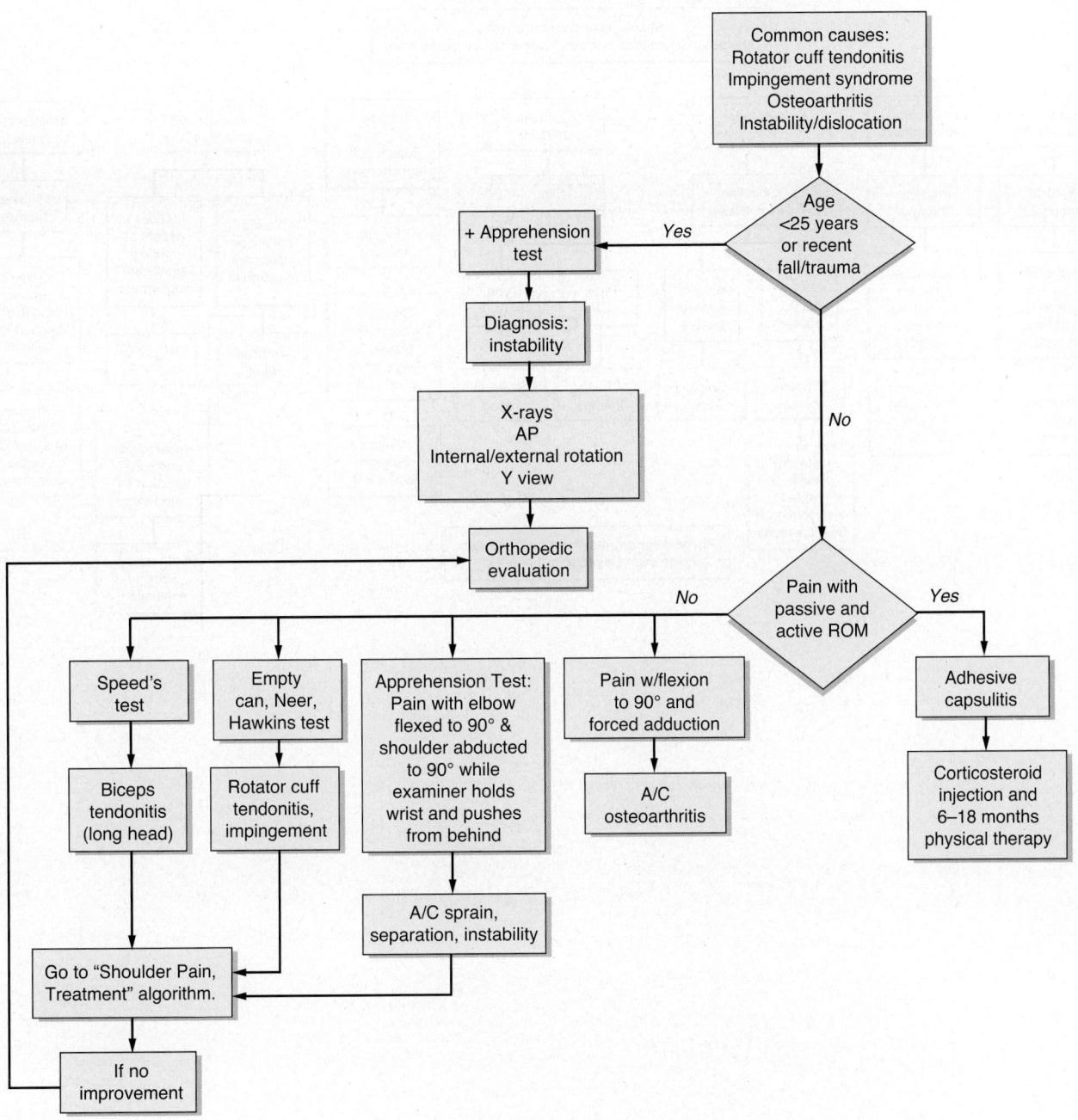

David W. Kruse, MD and Murat Mardirossian, MD

Woodward TW, Best TM. The painful shoulder: Part I. Clinical evaluation. *Am Fam Physician*. 2000;61:3079–3088.

SHOULDER PAIN, TREATMENT

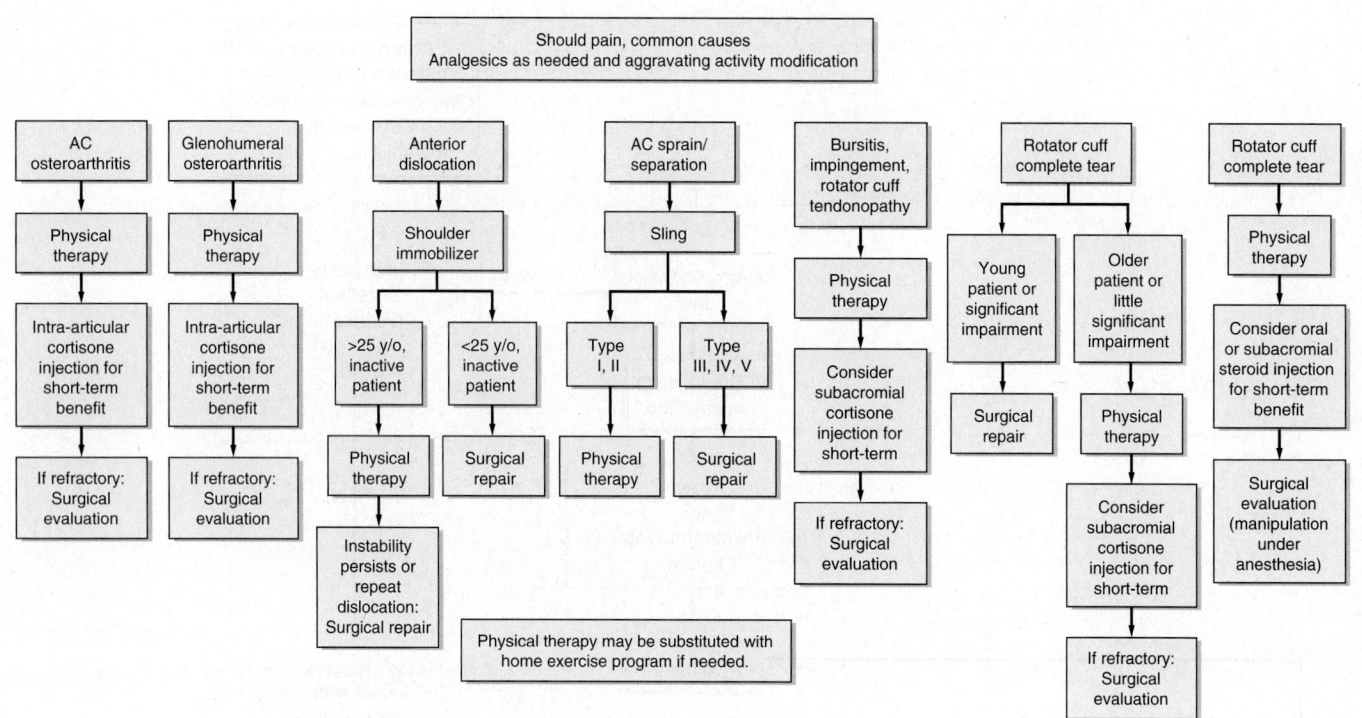

Should pain, common causes
Analgesics as needed and aggravating activity modification

AC osteroarthritis → Physical therapy → Intra-articular cortisone injection for short-term benefit → If refractory: Surgical evaluation

Glenohumeral osteroarthritis → Physical therapy → Intra-articular cortisone injection for short-term benefit → If refractory: Surgical evaluation

Anterior dislocation → Shoulder immobilizer → >25 y/o, inactive patient → Physical therapy → Instability persists or repeat dislocation: Surgical repair; <25 y/o, inactive patient → Surgical repair

AC sprain/separation → Sling → Type I, II → Physical therapy; Type III, IV, V → Surgical repair

Physical therapy may be substituted with home exercise program if needed.

Bursitis, impingement, rotator cuff tendonopathy → Physical therapy → Consider subacromial cortisone injection for short-term → If refractory: Surgical evaluation

Rotator cuff complete tear → Young patient or significant impairment → Surgical repair; Older patient or little significant impairment → Physical therapy → Consider subacromial cortisone injection for short-term → If refractory: Surgical evaluation

Rotator cuff complete tear → Physical therapy → Consider oral or subacromial steroid injection for short-term benefit → Surgical evaluation (manipulation under anesthesia)

Deepak Patel, MD

Favejee MM, Huisstede BM, Koes BW. Frozen shoulder: The effectiveness of conservative and surgical interventions–systematic review. *Br J Sports Med.* 2011;45(1):49–56.

SICKLE CELL ANEMIA, ACUTE, EVALUATION AND MANAGEMENT

This algorithm is meant to assist clinicians in the workup and management of common complications of sickle cell disease. It should not replace a physician's clinical judgment or be considered a standardized protocol for all patients.

Known Sickle Cell Patient (Part I of II)

Chief Complaint: Joint/Musculoskeletal Pain

Possible Causes: Vaso-occlusive crisis (VOC) Infection

No specific physical findings:
• Likely VOC

Warmth, swelling/effusion over joint/skin:
• In addition to VOC, consider infection (cellulitis, osteomyelitis, septic joint) or dactylitis if over hands/feet
• Erythema may be seen with infection but is less likely with VOC

Localized hip pain or difficulty with ambulation:
• Possible aseptic necrosis of femoral head

Tests:
• CBC w/diff & retic[a]
• Type & Crossmatch
• Blood cultures if febrile or concern for osteomyelitis
• If bone infarct or aseptic necrosis suspected, consider MRI
• Aspiration/analysis of joint fluid if effusion present
• If osteomyelitis suspected, consult radiology for MRI &/or bone marrow scan

Treatment*:
• Pain control **within 30 min of presentation**; start with PO meds, then IV
• Supplemental O2 (adults); for peds, only if hypoxia is present
• IV hydration[b]
• Abx if possible infectious cause (cover *Salmonella*, *E. coli*, staph/strep)
• May need simple/exchange transfusion
• Ortho consult for aseptic necrosis or osteomyelitis

Mild/Moderate Pain:
• Manage as outpatient or admit if other concerns
• Acetaminophen, ibuprofen, or PO narcotics
• Bowel regimen while on narcotics

Severe Pain:
• Admit for IV pain control–NSAIDs (ketorolac), narcotics, consider patient-controlled analgesia (PCA)
• Bowel regimen while on narcotics

Chief Complaint: Acute Neurologic Change or Deficit

Possible Causes: TIA Stroke Subarachnoid hemorrhage

Tests:
• Full neuro exam
• CBC w/diff & retic
• Chem10
• Type & Crossmatch
• Noncontrast head CT to rule out bleed ASAP
• MRI/MRA w/ diffusion-weighted images of brain to look for ischemia (may be deferred until after exchange transfusion)
• Consider LP after imaging if signs of infection

Treatment*:
• Neurology &/or neurosurgery consults as indicated
• Hematology & transfusion medicine consults
• IV hydration[b] (maintenance or less if concern for increased ICP)
• Supplemental O2 (adults); for peds, only if hypoxia is present
• Simple/exchange transfusion ASAP (do not wait for MRI or LP to be completed if stroke suspected)
• Abx if infectious cause suspected
• ADMIT (likely ICU)

• ADMIT for treatment of any serious bacterial infection, if IV pain meds are needed to control pain, or if patient not tolerating oral hydration

---

Chief Complaint: Fever >101°F (38.3°C)

Possible Causes: Viral illness (respiratory, GI, or systemic viral infection, including parvovirus B19)
Pneumonia (esp. *S. pneumo* & atypicals)
Osteomyelitis (esp. *Salmonella, E. coli, S. aureus*)
Meningitis
UTI/pyelonephritis
Acute chest syndrome
Port/line infection
Other bacterial infections/sepsis (especially encapsulated bacterial organisms)

Initial Assessment:
MUST HAVE RAPID TRIAGE, exam, labs, and empiric antibiotics – goal within 1 hour of presentation

Tests:
• CBC w/ diff & retic (if H&H down & retic <0.5% consider aplastic crisis)
• Blood cultures (draw off port or central line if present)
• UA C&S if GU sx & all males <6 mo/females <2 years
• Type & Crossmatch
• CXR even if no respiratory sx (acute chest may first present w/ fever)
• Throat cultures, viral panel, LP, stool studies if clinically indicated
• Imaging if osteomyelitis suspected

Treatment*:
• Supplemental O2 (adults); for peds, only if hypoxia is present
• IV hydration[b]
• Immediate empiric treatment w/ broad-spectrum abx; consider additional coverage if port or line is present
• May require simple/exchange transfusion for aplastic crisis
• ADMIT for severe bacterial infection, new chest infiltrate, or high-risk patient–hematology to determine risk based on age, appearance, exam, labs, & past medical history
• Low-risk patient may be discharged home with follow-up per hematology's recommendations

Known Sickle Cell Patient (Part II of II)

Chief Complaint:
Abdominal pain

Possible Causes:
Visceral pain from vaso-occlusive crisis Cholelithiasis/cholestasis Constipation 2°/2 narcotic use Visceral infarct appendicitis Splenic sequestration UTI/pyelonephritis/renal infarct Pancreatitis

Physical Exam:
• If LUQ pain &/or splenomegaly, think splenic sequestration (may also have tachycardia, pallor, hypoTN, lethargy)
• If focal pain, work up focal causes (appendicitis, cholecystitis, etc)
• Acute jaundice + abd pain, think hepatic infarct, vs. hepatitis, vs. cholecystitis, vs. intrahepatic cholestasis vs. liver sequestration

Tests:
• CBC w/ diff & retic
• Type & Crossmatch
• Consider blood culture
• AST, ALT, Alk Phos, LDH, Tbili/Dbili[c]
• Amylase, Lipase
• UA C&S if GU sx or flank pain
• Abdominal imaging if needed (KUB, U/S, or CT)

Treatment*:
• Supplemental O2 (adults); for peds, only if hypoxia is present
• IV hydration[b]
• Pain control
• Treat appropriately once cause is determined
• Likely ADMIT
• If splenic sequestration is suspected, call hematology immediately for directions regarding transfusion

Chief Complaint:
Respiratory symptoms (chest pain, tachypnea, SOB, non-productive/productive cough, wheezing, +/− fever)

Possible Causes:
Acute chest syndrome (ACS) Pneumonia Pulmonary embolus or infarctReactive airways/asthma exacerbation +/− above

Tests:
• Pulse oximetry
• CXR
• CBC w/ diff & retic
• Blood culture
• Type & Crossmatch
• ABG as needed
• CT PE protocol if PE suspected

Treatment*:
• ADMIT anyone with infiltrate on CXR
• IV hydration[b] – avoid over hydration
• Supplemental O2 (adults); for peds, only if hypoxia is present
• Incentive spirometry
• Pain control (avoid respiratory depression)
• Broad spectrum IV abx (ex: Ceftriaxone, Cefuroxime) + PO macrolide
• Severe cases of acute chest may need transfusion
• Brochodilators for active wheezing or hx of reactive airways disease (RAD)/asthma
• Consider steroids for symptomatic RAD
• Closely monitor respiratory status–watch for impending respiratory failure

Chief Complaint:
Genitourinary symptoms

Possible Causes:
Priapism
UTI
Pyelonephritis
Renal infarct

Tests if Priapism:
• CBC w/ diff & retic
• Type & Crossmatch
• UA +/− C&S

Tests if other GU Sxs:
• CBC w/ diff & retic
• Type & Crossmatch
• UA C&S
• Blood cx if fever or signs of urosepsis or UTI

Treatment:
• Supplemental O2 (adults); for peds, only if hypoxia is present
• IV hydration[b]
• Pain control
• Abx to cover common urinary tract pathogens

Treatment*:
prolonged priapism is a urologic emergency
• Supplemental O2 (adults); for peds, only if hypoxia is present
• IV hydration[b]
• Pain control (opioids may cause urinary retention; NEVER use ice packs)
• Pseudoephedrine
• Consult urology for possible drainage if no improvement after 3 hours
• May require simple or exchange transfusion
• Consider catheterization if difficulty voiding

[a]Typical Hgb 6–9%, Hct 20–30%, retic 5–25%, slight leukocytosis 12,000–15,000, mild thrombocytosis; consider infection of there is a left shift and/or WBC >20,000

[b]Preferred fluid is 1/2 NS at 1–1.5× maintenance in pediatrics and NS in adults (consider bolus first if dehydrated)

[c]Bilirubin and LDH are often slightly to moderately elevated due to chronic and acute hemolysis

*Always call heme/onc for further recommendations

Stephanie Ruest, MD and Doreen Brettler, MD

New England Pediatric Sickle Cell Consortium Practice Guidelines. Available at: http://www.nepscc.org/nepscc.html

STROKE

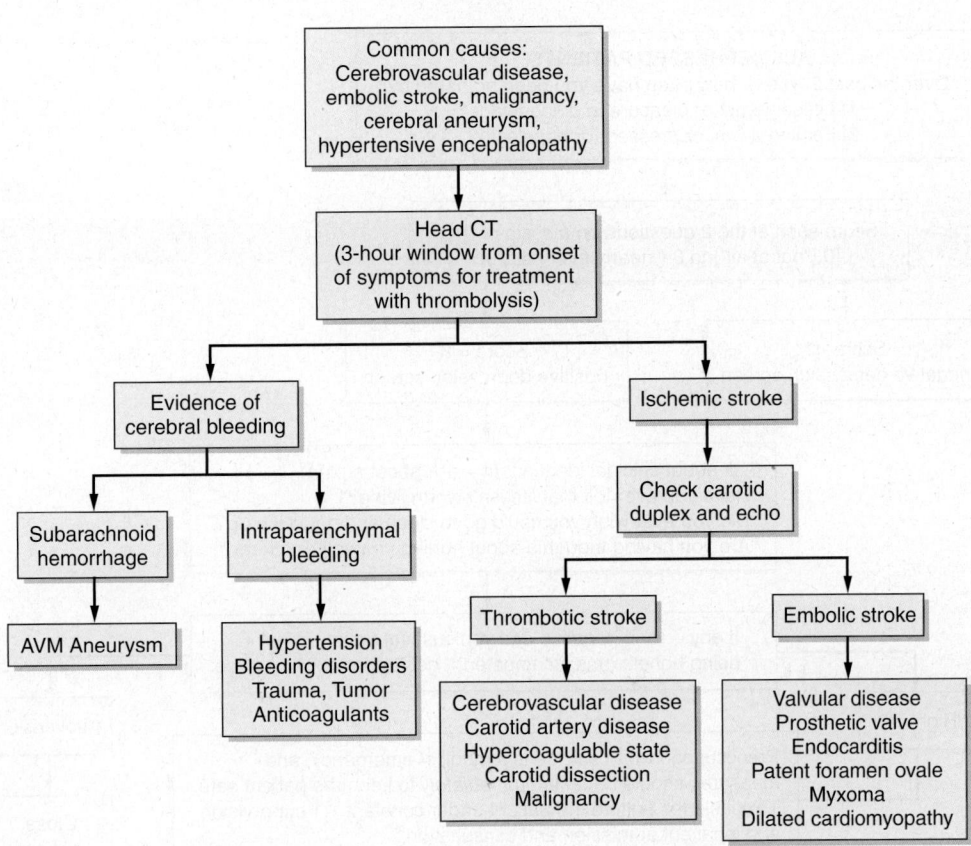

Common causes:
Cerebrovascular disease, embolic stroke, malignancy, cerebral aneurysm, hypertensive encephalopathy

Head CT
(3-hour window from onset of symptoms for treatment with thrombolysis)

Evidence of cerebral bleeding

Ischemic stroke

Subarachnoid hemorrhage

Intraparenchymal bleeding

Check carotid duplex and echo

AVM Aneurysm

Hypertension
Bleeding disorders
Trauma, Tumor
Anticoagulants

Thrombotic stroke

Embolic stroke

Cerebrovascular disease
Carotid artery disease
Hypercoagulable state
Carotid dissection
Malignancy

Valvular disease
Prosthetic valve
Endocarditis
Patent foramen ovale
Myxoma
Dilated cardiomyopathy

Robert A. Baldor, MD and Alan M. Ehrlich, MD

Adams HP Jr, del Zoppo G, Alberts MJ, et al. Guidelines for the early management of adults with ischemic stroke: A guideline from the American Heart Association/American Stroke Association Stroke Council, Clinical Cardiology Council, Cardiovascular Radiology and Intervention Council, and the Atherosclerotic Peripheral Vascular Disease and Quality of Care Outcomes in Research Interdisciplinary Working Groups: The American Academy of Neurology affirms the value of this guideline as an educational tool for neurologists. *Stroke.* 2007;38:1655–1711.

SUICIDE, EVALUATING RISK FOR

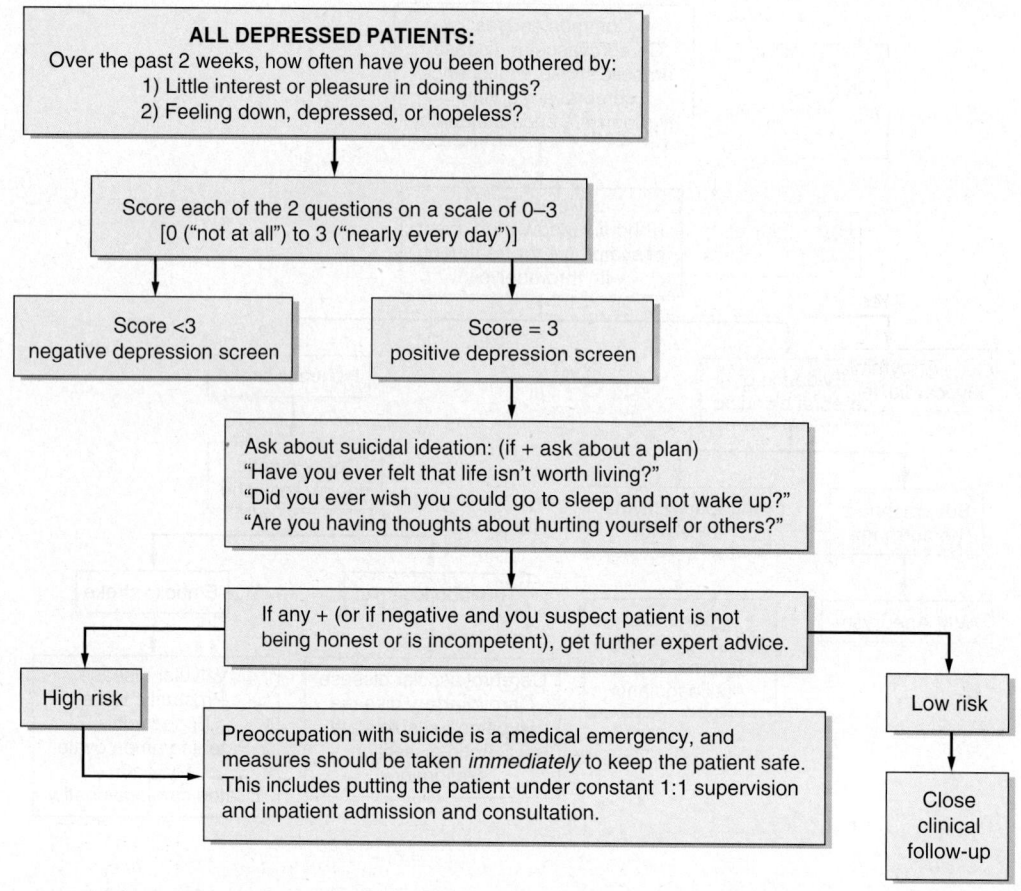

ALL DEPRESSED PATIENTS:
Over the past 2 weeks, how often have you been bothered by:
1) Little interest or pleasure in doing things?
2) Feeling down, depressed, or hopeless?

Score each of the 2 questions on a scale of 0–3
[0 ("not at all") to 3 ("nearly every day")]

Score <3
negative depression screen

Score = 3
positive depression screen

Ask about suicidal ideation: (if + ask about a plan)
"Have you ever felt that life isn't worth living?"
"Did you ever wish you could go to sleep and not wake up?"
"Are you having thoughts about hurting yourself or others?"

If any + (or if negative and you suspect patient is not being honest or is incompetent), get further expert advice.

High risk

Low risk

Preoccupation with suicide is a medical emergency, and measures should be taken *immediately* to keep the patient safe. This includes putting the patient under constant 1:1 supervision and inpatient admission and consultation.

Close clinical follow-up

Irene C. Coletsos, MD and Harold J. Bursztajn, MD

Posner K, Oquendo MA, Gould M, et al. Columbia Classification Algorithm of Suicide Assessment (C-CASA): Classification of suicidal events in the FDA's pediatric suicidal risk analysis of antidepressants. *Am J Psych.* 2007;164:1035–1043.

SYNCOPE

Common causes:
Vasovagal syncope (faint), seizure, arrhythmia, orthostatic (drop attack), psychiatric illness, narcolepsy

History of palpitations or onset without preceding symptoms

Yes — Arrhythmia / Myocardial infarction

No — Abnormal neurologic examination

Yes — Stroke / Brain tumor / Seizure

No — Precipitating event: Excessive heat, change in posture, acute stressful event, prolonged standing

Yes — Vasovagal syncope / Orthostatic hypotension / Anxiety

No — Obesity

Yes — Obstructive sleep apnea / Pickwickian syndrome

No — Seizure / Drop attack / Narcolepsy / Psychiatric disorder

Amaninderapal Ghotra, MD, Nirmanmoh Bhatia, MD, and Kelly McCants, MD

Strickberger SA, Benson DW, Biaggioni I, et al. AHA/ACCF Scientific Statement on the evaluation of syncope: From the American Heart Association Councils on Clinical Cardiology, Cardiovascular Nursing, Cardiovascular Disease in the Young, and Stroke, and the Quality of Care and Outcomes Research Interdisciplinary Working Group; and the American College of Cardiology Foundation: In collaboration with the Heart Rhythm Society: Endorsed by the American Autonomic Society. *Circulation.* 2006;113:316.

THROMBOCYTOPENIA

Common causes:
Idiopathic thrombocytopenic purpura (ITP), medications, DIC, pernicious anemia, collagen-vascular disease, hypersplenism, thrombotic thrombocytopenic purpura (TTP), ICU patient/sepsis hemolytic-uremic syndrome

Platelet clumping? → Consider artifact thrombocytopenia

Check peripheral smear

Giant platelets? → Consider hereditary thrombocyopenia

Lymphocytes, atypical cells or toxic granulation? → Consider infection and check ESR, CRP, CXR, virology as deemed necessary

Blasts, nucleated RBCs or Pelger-Heut? → Check bone marrow aspirate or Bx → Consider primary BM disorder

Are there schistocytes? → Check LDH, bilirubin, haptoglobin, coags, D-dimer, fibrinogen → TTP/HUS or DIC

Spherocytes? → Confirm hemolysis: Positive DAT, retic count, LDH, nili → Evan syndrome

Isolated? → Consider ITP, HIV, HCV, DIC, GT and continue workup based on history → Consider drug-induced thrombocytopenia

Common offending agents: Chemotherapy, anticonvulsants, heparin, PCN, sulfonamides, NSAIDs, diuretics and GP IIb/IIIa inhibitors

Samuel B. Carli, MD and Parminder Singh, MD

Reese JA, Li X, Hauben M, et al. Identifying drugs that cause acute thrombocytopenia: An analysis using 3 distinct methods. *Blood.* 2010;116:2127–2133.

THYROID NODULE

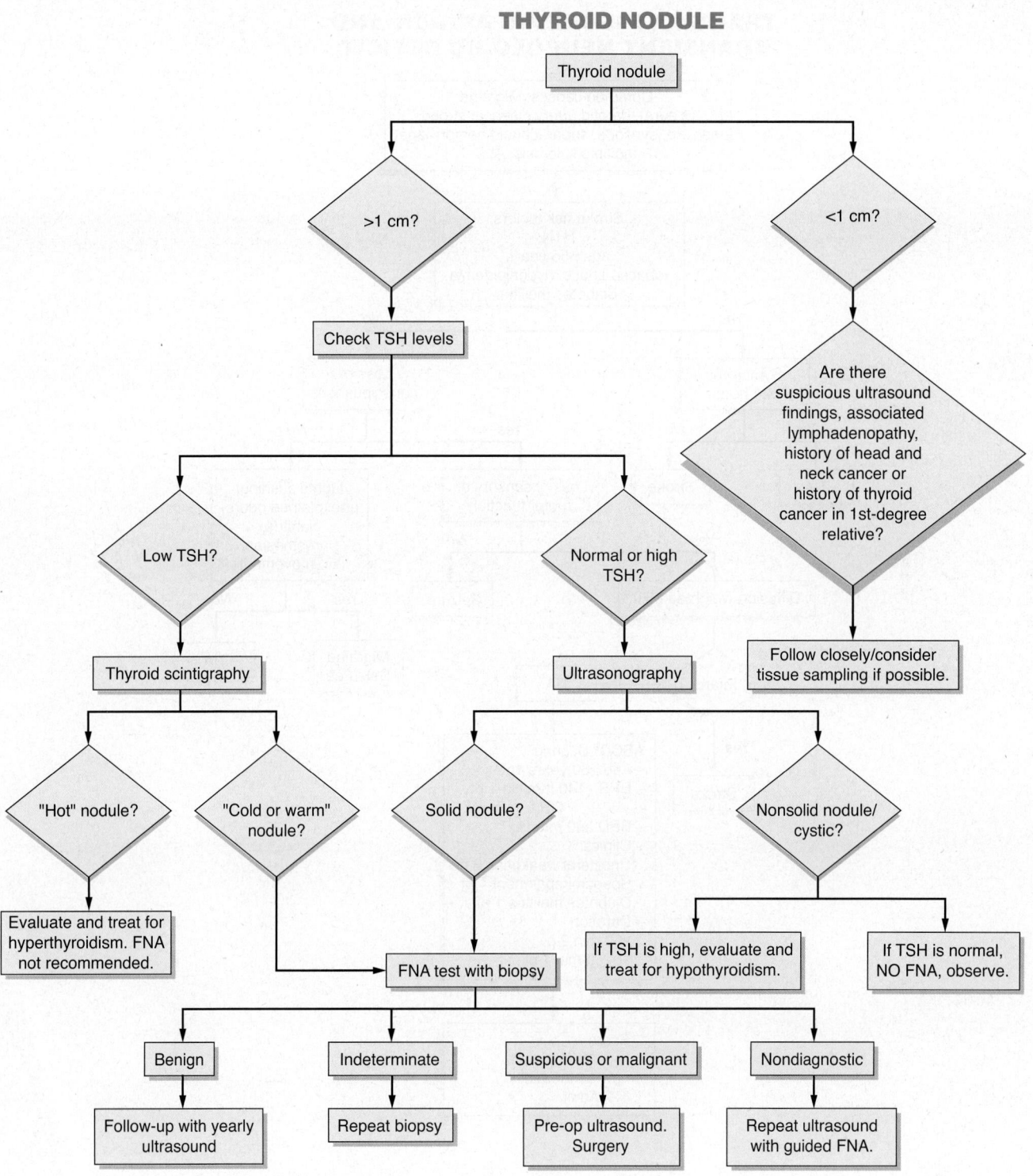

Maria Plummer, MD and Ehiozogie Adu

American Thyroid Association (ATA) Guidelines Taskforce on Thyroid Nodules and Differentiated Thyroid Cancer, Cooper DS, Doherty GM, et al. Revised American Thyroid Association management guidelines for patients with thyroid nodules and differentiated thyroid cancer. *Thyroid.* 2009;19:1167–1214.

TRANSIENT ISCHEMIC ATTACK AND TRANSIENT NEUROLOGIC DEFICIT

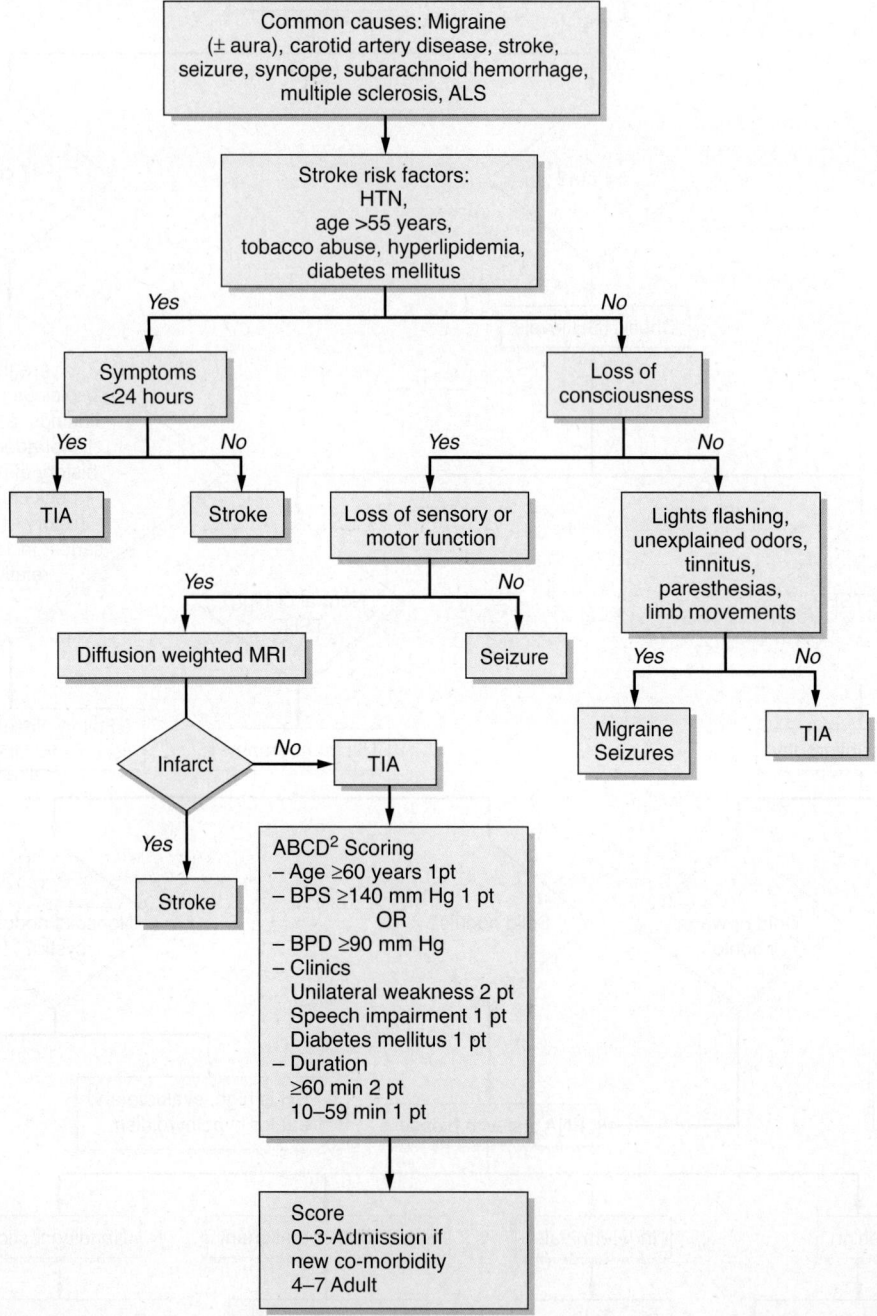

Robert A. Baldor, MD and Alan M. Ehrlich, MD

Solenski NJ. Transient ischemic attacks: Part I. Diagnosis and evaluation. *Am Fom Physician*. 2004;69:1665–1674.

TREMOR

Andrew J. Westwood, MD, MRCP(UK)

Smaga S. Tremor. *Am Fam Physician.* 2003;68(8):1545–1552.

TUBERCULOSIS, TREATMENT

Suspicion of latent infection with *Mycobacterium tuberculosis*:
– Known close contact with TB+ individual.
This may include working in high-risk area such as health care facility.
– Originating from TB endemic area.

- Unlikely to follow up for TST read
- History of BCG

Child <5 years

For everyone else targeted for testing

Tuberculin skin test (TST)

Interferon-γ release assay (IGRA)

TST or IGRA

Positive — Yes → CXR / No → TB unlikely

CXR → Abnormal / Normal

Abnormal:
Contact Department of Health.

Conduct sputum smear × 3/Nucleic acid amplification test (NAAT) on 1st smear sample/culture (at least 8 hours apart).

Presenting with respiratory symptoms

Normal → No respiratory symptoms

- Consider INH daily × 9 months
- If concerned about adherence, consider INH-RIF × 4 months
- If concerned about drug resistance/adherence, consider RIF × 4 months

Baseline LFTs should be measured in patients who are pregnant or with any history of liver disease, alcohol abuse, or HIV.

Negative:
Consider bronchoscopy, if amenable, for lavage/biopsy

Positive:
Start treatment: INH/RIF/PZA/EMB. Also, test drug susceptibility; if full susceptibility, can discontinue EMB.

Baseline LFTs should be measured in patients who are pregnant or with any history of liver disease, alcohol abuse, or HIV.

Negative histology / Positive histology

Consider alternative diagnosis or extrapulmonary TB.

Treat

Monthly follow-up visits for physical assessment of hepatitis, adherence, side effects. Periodically repeat LFTs for those with history of liver disease. Patients should be aware of signs of hepatitis and advised to stop treatment immediately and see a physician should they occur.

Repeat smears every 2 weeks until 2 consecutive negative results.

Continue INH/RIF only for another 4 months (total treatment time: 6 months).

Negative culture by 2 months / Positive culture by 2 months

(Consider second-line therapy if continues to be positive by 3 months).

Continue INH/RIF only for another 4 months (total treatment time: 6 months).

Negative cavitation on original CXR.

Positive cavitation on original CXR.

Continue INH/RIF only for another 7 months (total treatment time: 9 months).

Marina MacNamara, MPH, MD and Paul George, MD, MHPE

Vernon A. Treatment of latent tuberculosis infection. *Semin Respir Crit Care Med.* 2013;34(1):67–86.

UREMIA

Common causes: Chronic renal failure, obstructive uropathy, prerenal azotemia, medications

Acute renal failure

Chronic renal failure

Renal ultrasound

Diabetes mellitus
HTN
Glomerulonephritis
Amyloidosis
SLE

Obstructive uropathy

No obstruction

BPH
Neoplasm

Prerenal azotemia

Renal azotemia

Sepsis
CHF
Shock
Cirrhosis

Drug-induced renal failure

Acute tubular necrosis
Renal artery stenosis
Collagen-vascular disease
Rhabdomyolysis

Aminoglycosides
Sulfonamides
Lithium
ACE inhibitors
NSAIDs
Contrast media

Robert A. Baldor, MD and Alan M. Ehrlich, MD

Diagnosis and management of adults with chronic kidney disease. Michigan Quality Improvement Consortium - Professional Association. 2006 Nov (revised 2008 Nov). 1 page. NGC:007054.

URETHRAL DISCHARGE

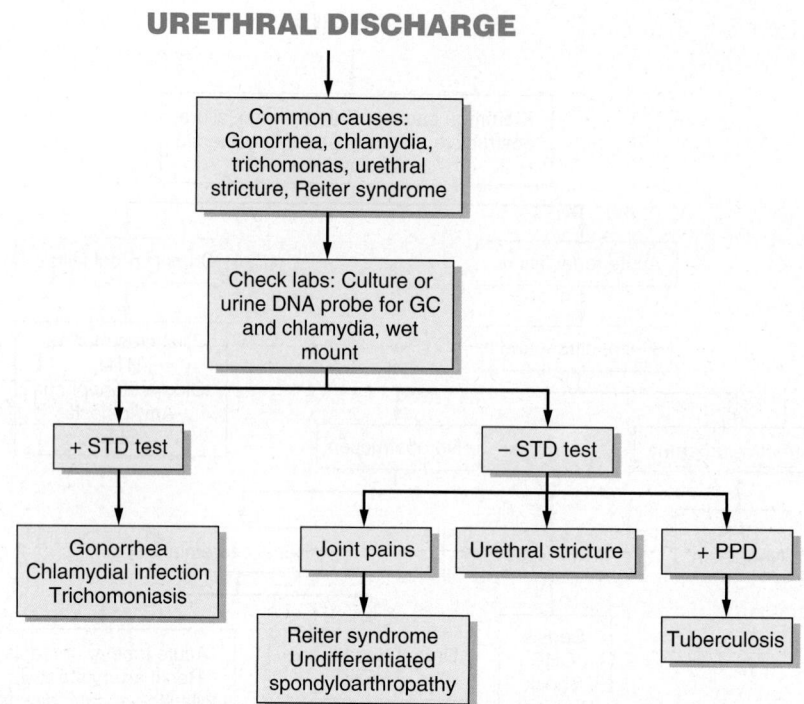

Robert A. Baldor, MD and Alan M. Ehrlich, MD

Djajakusumah T, Sudigdoadi S, Keersmaekers K, et al. Evaluation of syndromic patient management algorithm for urethral discharge. *Sex Transm Infect.* 1998;74(Suppl 1):S29–33.

VAGINAL BLEEDING DURING PREGNANCY

Robert A. Baldor, MD and Alan M. Ehrlich, MD

Deutchman M, Tubay AT, Turok D. First trimester bleeding. *Am Fam Physician.* 2009;79:985–994.

VAGINAL BLEEDING, ABNORMAL

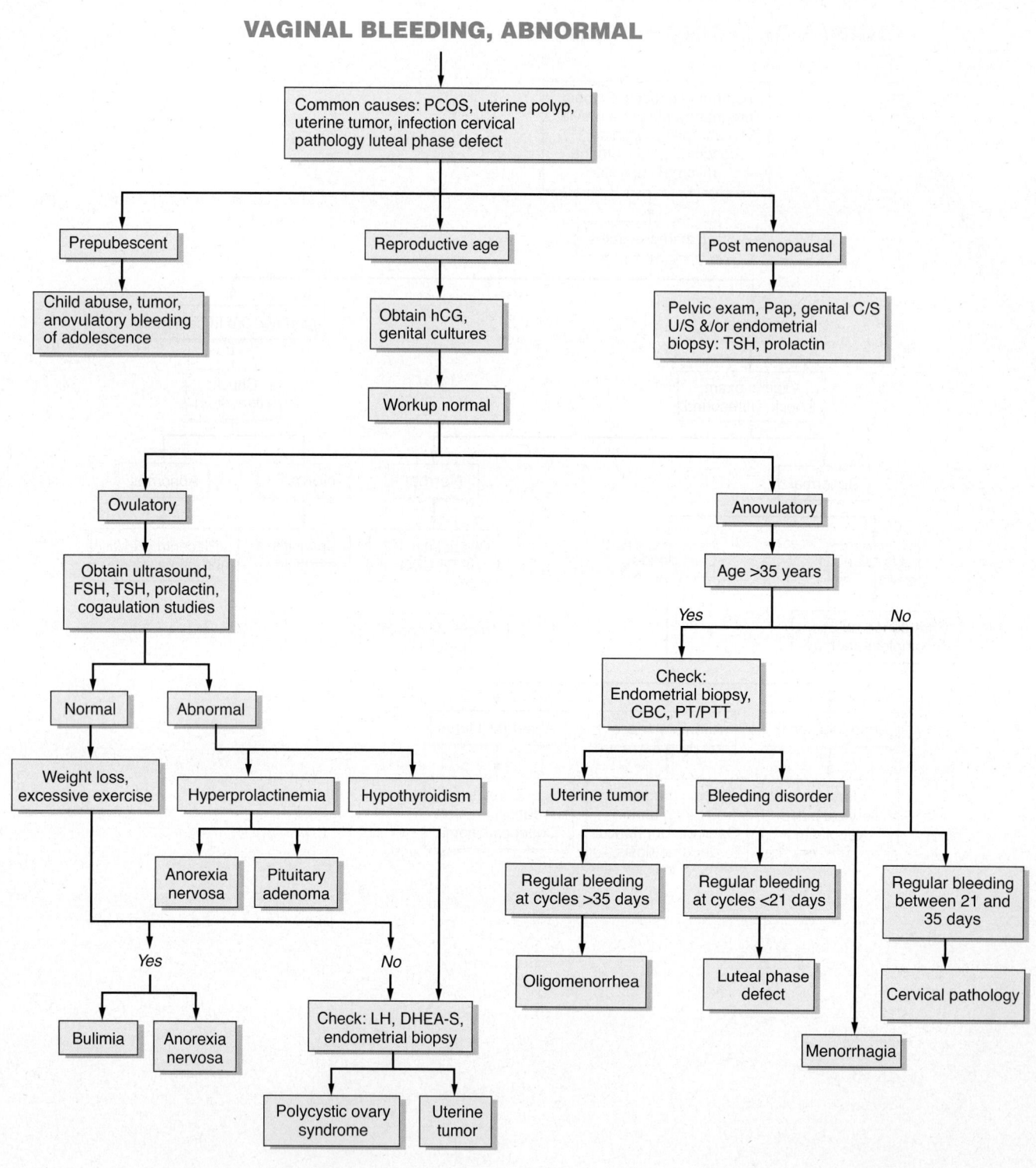

Tanya E. Anim, MD and Jennifer Keehbauch, MD

Keehbauch J, Nystrom J. Diagnosis and management of abnormal uterine bleeding. *Female Patient.* 2007;32(7):38–40.

VITAMIN D DEFICIENCY

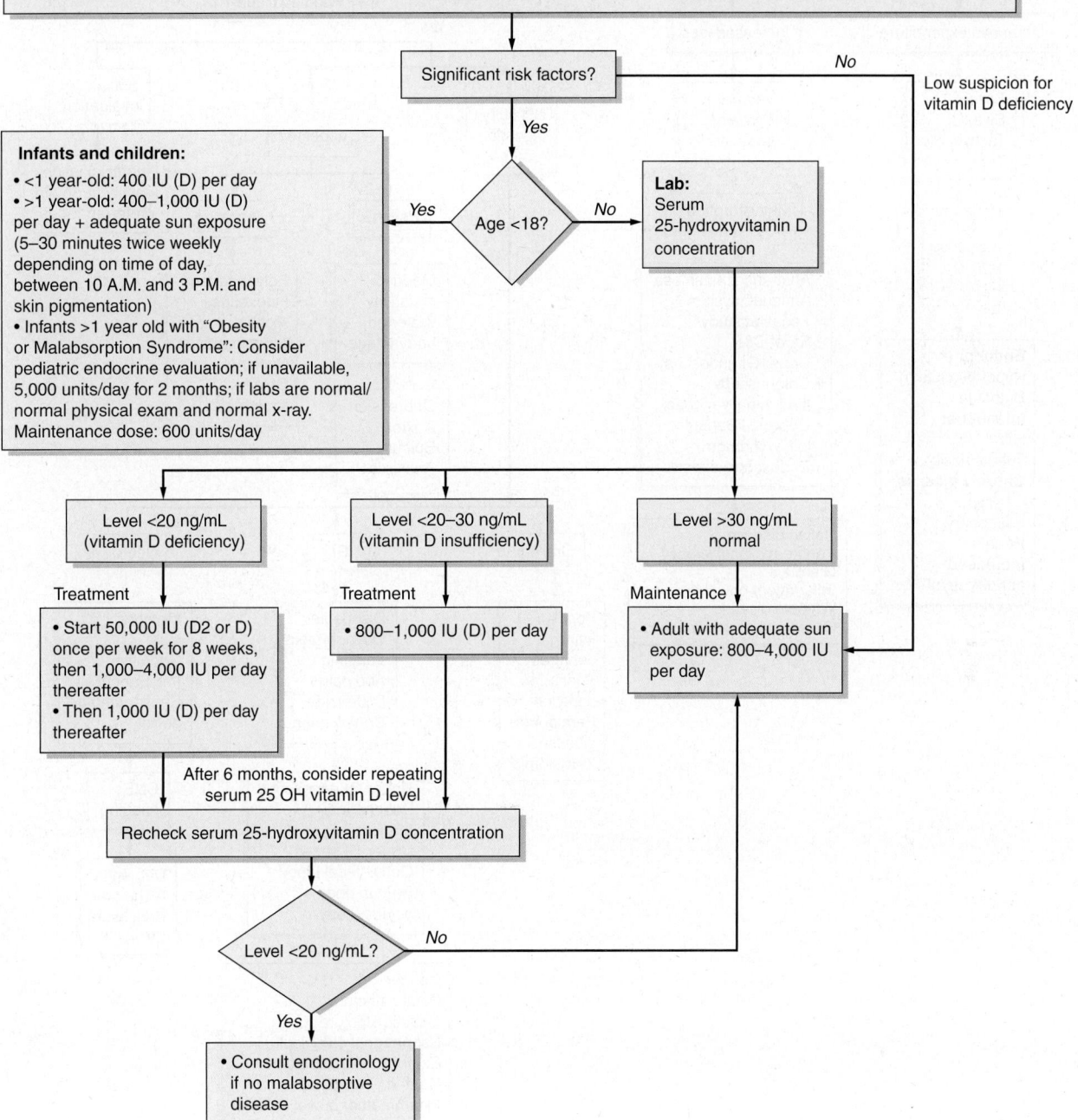

Risk Factors/Common Causes:

- Age >65
- Insufficient sunlight exposure (homebound, veiled)
- Renal disease
- Liver disease
- Depression
- Chronic use of anticonvulsants

- Dark skin
- Insufficient dietary intake
- GI malabsorption
- Obesity (BMI >30)
- Immigrants to colder climates
- Chronic use of glucocorticoids
- Periosteal bone pain (e.g., sternum, tibia)

- GI malabsorption: (Celiac, cystic fibrosis, inflammatory bowel disease)
- Pregnancy
- Medications: Anticonvulsants, antiretroviral and glucocorticoids
- Gastrectomy or extensive bowel surgery

Significant risk factors? — No → Low suspicion for vitamin D deficiency

Yes ↓

Age <18?
- Yes → Infants and children:
- No → **Lab:** Serum 25-hydroxyvitamin D concentration

Infants and children:
- <1 year-old: 400 IU (D) per day
- >1 year-old: 400–1,000 IU (D) per day + adequate sun exposure (5–30 minutes twice weekly depending on time of day, between 10 A.M. and 3 P.M. and skin pigmentation)
- Infants >1 year old with "Obesity or Malabsorption Syndrome": Consider pediatric endocrine evaluation; if unavailable, 5,000 units/day for 2 months; if labs are normal/normal physical exam and normal x-ray. Maintenance dose: 600 units/day

Level <20 ng/mL (vitamin D deficiency)

Treatment
- Start 50,000 IU (D2 or D) once per week for 8 weeks, then 1,000–4,000 IU per day thereafter
- Then 1,000 IU (D) per day thereafter

Level <20–30 ng/mL (vitamin D insufficiency)

Treatment
- 800–1,000 IU (D) per day

Level >30 ng/mL normal

Maintenance
- Adult with adequate sun exposure: 800–4,000 IU per day

After 6 months, consider repeating serum 25 OH vitamin D level

Recheck serum 25-hydroxyvitamin D concentration

Level <20 ng/mL? — No

Yes ↓

- Consult endocrinology if no malabsorptive disease

Gisela M. Lopez Payares, MD and Fozia Akhtar Ali, MD

Bordelon P, Ghetu MV, Langan RC. Recognition and management of vitamin D deficiency. *Am Fam Physician.* 2009;80(8):841–846.

WEIGHT LOSS, UNINTENTIONAL

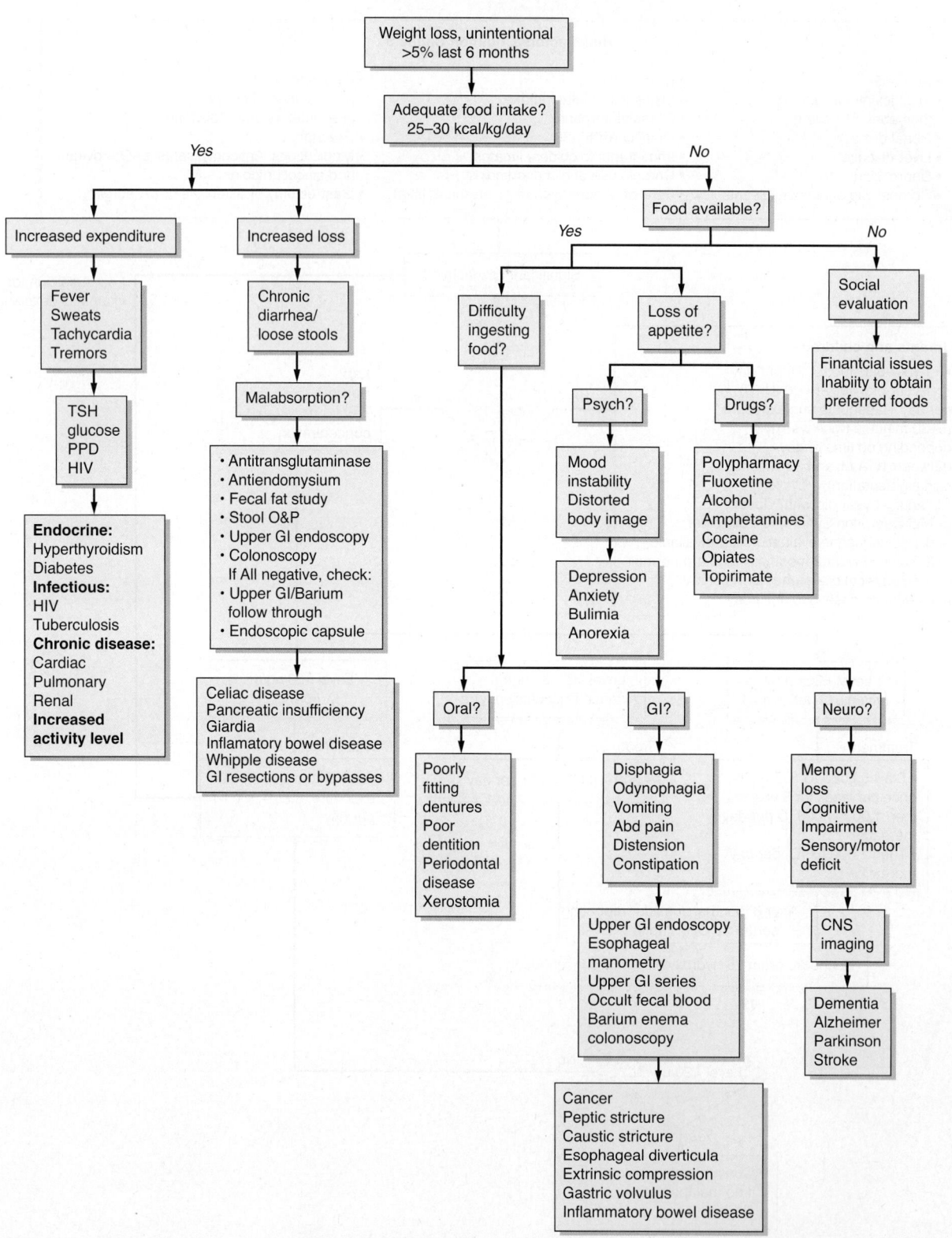

Danton S. Correa, MD and Felix B. Chang, MD, DABMA

Scolapio JS. Rational approach to patients with unintentional weight loss. *Mayo Clin Proc.* 2001;76(9):923–929.

The 5-Minute Clinical Consult Premium
2015
23RD EDITION

ABNORMAL PAP AND CERVICAL DYSPLASIA

Fozia Ali, MD • Tharani Vadivelu Prasad, MD

BASICS

DESCRIPTION
- Cervical dysplasia: Premalignant cervical disease that is also called cervical intraepithelial neoplasia (CIN). Precancerous epithelial changes in the transformation zone of the uterine cervix almost always associated with human papilloma virus (HPV) infections.
- Cervical intraepithelial neoplasia (CIN) encompasses a range of histologic diagnoses:
  - CIN I: Mild dysplasia. Low-grade lesion. Cellular changes are limited to the lower 1/3 of the squamous epithelium.
  - CIN II: Moderate dysplasia. High-grade lesion. Cellular changes are limited to the lower 2/3 of the squamous epithelium.
  - CIN III or carcinoma in situ: Severe dysplasia. High-grade lesion. Cellular changes involve the full thickness of the squamous epithelium.
- System(s) affected: Reproductive

ALERT
Incidence of cervical cancer has decreased by >50% in the last 30 years due to cervical cytology screening.

Pediatric Considerations
Cervical cancer is rare before age 21 years. Screening women younger than age 21 years (regardless of sexual history) does not reduce cervical cancer incidence and mortality compared with beginning screening at age 21 years. Screenings of adolescents lead to unnecessary evaluation and overtreatment of cervical lesions, which are highly likely to regress spontaneously (1).

Geriatric Considerations
- Women age >65 years who have had adequate prior screening and no history of CIN II+ in the last 20 years should not be screened for cervical cancer. Adequate prior screening is defined as 3 consecutive negative cytology results or 2 consecutive negative HPV results within 10 years before cessation of screening (with the most recent test within the last 5 years).
- Routine screening should continue for at least 20 years after spontaneous regression or appropriate management of a high-grade precancerous lesion, even if this extends screening past age 65 years.

Pregnancy Considerations
- Squamous intraepithelial lesions can progress during pregnancy, but often regress postpartum.
- Colposcopy only to exclude the presence of invasive cancer in high-risk women.
- Endocervical curettage is contraindicated during pregnancy.
- Unless cancer is identified or suspected, treatment of cervical intraepithelial neoplasia is contraindicated during pregnancy

EPIDEMIOLOGY
- Cervical cancer is the 3rd most common cancer among women worldwide, and ranks 14th for cancer deaths in women (2).

- Predominant age: Can occur at any age, but incidence of CIN III peaks between ages 25 and 29; invasive disease peaks 15 years later. Cervical cancer most commonly occurs in women age 35–55 years.

Incidence
The American Cancer Society estimates that 12,340 women will be diagnosed with invasive cervical cancer in 2013 (2). Since 2004, cervical cancer incidence rates have decreased by 2.1% per year in women younger than 50 years, and by 3.1% per year in women age 50 years and older.

Prevalence
- ~80% of sexually active women will have acquired a genital HPV infection by age 50 years.
- Overall, 26.8% of women are HPV positive. Point prevalence of HPV positivity is highest in those age 18–22 years (as high as 70%), falling off rapidly as women enter their 30s.

PATHOPHYSIOLOGY
HPV DNA is found in virtually all cervical carcinomas and precursor lesions worldwide.
- High-risk HPV types: 16, 18, 31, 33, 35, 45, 52, and 58 are common oncogenic virus types for cervical cancer.
- HPV16 is the most carcinogenic HPV genotype, accounting for 55–60% of all cervical cancers
- HPV18 is the next most carcinogenic HPV genotype. HPV18 causes a greater proportion of glandular cancers, adenocarcinoma and adenosquamous carcinoma, than squamous cell carcinoma.
- Most HPV infections are transient, becoming undetectable within 1–2 years. Persistent infections are what place women at significant risk for developing precancerous lesions.
- Low-risk types: HPV viral types 6, 11, 42, 43, and 44 are considered common low-risk types and may cause genital warts. HPV 6 and 11 (cause 90% of benign anogenital warts) can lead to low-grade squamous intraepithelial lesion (LSIL) and CIN I.

RISK FACTORS
- Previous or current HPV infection
- HIV infection and other immunosuppressive conditions
- In utero exposure to diethylstilbestrol
- Previous treatment of a high-grade precancerous lesion or cervical cancer
- Cigarette smoking
- Early age at first coitus (<20 years), and multiple sexual partners
- Some correlation with low socioeconomic status, high parity, oral contraceptive use, and poor nutrition

GENERAL PREVENTION
- Immunization: Immunization decreases high-risk HPV infections and cervical pathology.
  - Ideally, HPV immunization of girls, boys, and women should be initiated prior to first intercourse:
    - Gardasil (quadrivalent: HPV4):
      - Reduces dysplasia due to HPV types 16 and 18 (70% of cervical cancer) and types 6 and 11 (anogenital warts).
      - 3 doses at 0, 2, 6 months, approved for use in women age 9–26. Only the quadrivalent vaccine is approved for males (ages 9–26) for prevention of anogenital warts.

- Cervarix (bivalent: HPV2): Reduces dysplasia due to HPV 16 and 18 infection and CIN. 3 doses at 0, 1, 6 months, approved for use in females age 10–25.
- Safe sex practices: Condom use
- Screening:
  - Pap smear is the main screening test for cervical cellular pathology.
  - Screening recommendations by age and source:
    - <21 years: Do not screen. (Grade D) (USPSTF/ASCCP/ACS/ASCP/ACOG)
  - Frequency of screening recommendation: USPSTF/ASCCP/ACS/ASCP generally agree by age and screen:
    - 21–29 years: Screen with cytology (Pap smear) every 3 years (Grade A). Do not screen with HPV testing alone or combined with cytology (Grade D).
    - 30–65 years: Screen with cytology every 3 years (acceptable) or co-testing (cytology/HPV testing) every 5 years (preferred).
    - >65 years (who have had adequate prior screening and are not high risk): Do not screen (Grade D).
- Special circumstances: Women after hysterectomy with removal of the cervix and with no history of CIN II+: Do not screen.

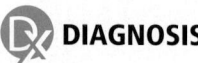

DIAGNOSIS

HISTORY
Usually asymptomatic until there is invasive disease. Patients may present with vaginal discharge, abnormal vaginal bleeding, postcoital bleeding, pelvic pain, cervical mass, or bladder obstruction.

PHYSICAL EXAM
Pelvic exam occasionally reveals external HPV lesions. Examine for exophytic or ulcerative cervical lesions, with or without bleeding.

DIFFERENTIAL DIAGNOSIS
Acute or chronic cervicitis; cervical glandular hyperplasia; cervical polyp; cervical fibroid; HPV infection; invasive cervical malignancy; uterine malignancy.

DIAGNOSTIC TESTS & INTERPRETATION
- Current evidence indicates no clinically important differences between conventional cytology and liquid-based cytology in detecting cervical cancer precursors: Conventional Pap smear involves a cervical sample plated on a microscope slide with fixative. ThinPrep is a liquid-based collection and thin-layer preparation.
- Sensitivity of a single Pap smear for HSIL ~60–70%; specificity of ~90%. Pap smears done routinely at recommended intervals further increases the sensitivity.
- HPV viral typing: High-risk HPV subtype testing is more sensitive, but less specific for identifying women with prevalent CIN III+.
- Co-testing: HPV typing in combination with Pap smear for women age ≥30 years
- Cytology report component: Specimen type (conventional Pap smear or liquid based), adequacy (presence of endocervical cells), and categorization (negative for intraepithelial lesion or malignancy or epithelial cell abnormality; i.e., squamous/glandular)

- Bethesda system (cytologic grading) epithelial cell abnormalities:
  - Squamous cell:
    - ASC (atypical squamous cells) [ASC-US (of undetermined significance), ASC-H (cannot exclude high-grade squamous intraepithelial lesion)]
    - HPV, mild dysplasia, CIN I
    - Moderate/severe dysplasia CIS, CIN II, and CIN III
  - Glandular cell:
    - AGC (atypical glandular cells):
      - AGCs: Not otherwise specified
      - AGCs: Favor neoplasia
    - AIS (adenocarcinoma in situ)
    - Adenocarcinoma

Diagnostic Procedures/Other
Algorithms differ for women age 21–24 years; see ASCCP Guideline (3). Below recommendations for ages as noted.
HPV positive, cytology negative (30 years of age and older):

- Option 1: HPV DNA typing: If HPV 16 or 18+, proceed to colposcopy; if negative, repeat co-testing at 1 year
- Option 2: Repeat co-testing at 1 year: If ≥ASC or HPV positive, proceed to colposcopy; if negative, repeat co-testing at 3 years

ASC-US (>24 years of age)

- Option 1: HPV testing (preferred)
  - If HPV positive, proceed to colposcopy
  - If HPV negative, repeat co-testing at 3 years
- Option 2: Repeat cytology at 1 year (acceptable)
  - If repeat cytology ASC or greater, proceed to colposcopy
  - If repeat cytology is negative, proceed to routine screening in 3 years

ASC-H: Colposcopy required
LSIL (>24 years of age)

- LSIL with negative HPV test: Repeat co-testing at 1 year (preferred)
  - If repeat co-testing is negative, repeat co-testing in 3 years
  - If co-testing is positive, proceed to colposcopy
- LSIL with no HPV test or positive HPV test: Proceed to colposcopy

HSIL: LEEP or colposcopy
Atypical glandular cells: Colposcopy with endocervical sampling and endometrial sampling
(if age 35 years or older or at risk for endometrial neoplasia)
Atypical endometrial cells: Endometrial and endocervical sampling.

- If negative, perform colposcopy

Women with no lesion on colposcopy or CIN I (preceded by "lesser abnormalities," such as ASC-US, LSIL, HPV 16+, 18+, and persistent HPV):

- Follow-up without treatment: Co-testing at 12 months
- If both HPV and cytology negative, age-appropriate retesting 3 years later
- If either positive, proceed to colposcopy. If persistent CIN I for at least 2 years, proceed to treatment with ablative or excisional methods

Test Interpretation
Histopathology: Atypical squamous or columnar cells; coarse nuclear material; increased nuclear diameter; koilocytosis (HPV hallmark)

 TREATMENT

ASCCP guidelines: Evidence-based management algorithms guide Pap smear and post colposcopic diagnostics and therapeutics and are available online (3).

GENERAL MEASURES
Office evaluation and observation; promote smoking cessation, protected intercourse, and immunization

MEDICATION

- Infective/reactive Pap smear: Treat trichomoniasis, symptomatic candida, or shift in flora suggestive of bacterial vaginosis found on Pap smear results.
- *Condyloma acuminatum*: May be treated with cryotherapy, or: Podophyllin topically q1–2wk or podofilox 0.5% applied b.i.d. ×3 days then off 4 days, repeated for 1–4 weeks OR trichloroacetic acid, applied topically by a physician and covered for 5–6 days OR imiquimod cream 3×/wk at bedtime up to 16 weeks

SURGERY/OTHER PROCEDURES

- Persistent CIN I, CIN II or III: Ablative or excisional methods. If inadequate colposcopy for CIN II or III or recurrent CIN II or III, diagnostic excisional procedure is done. For adenocarcinoma in situ, hysterectomy is preferred.
- Cryotherapy, laser ablation, LEEP/large loop excision of transition zone, or cold-knife conization all effective, but require different training and with different side effects for patient. If cervical malignancy, see "Cervical Malignancy."

 ONGOING CARE

FOLLOW-UP RECOMMENDATIONS
After treatment (excision or ablation) of CIN II or III, women may re-enter routine screening only after negative co-testing at 12 and 24 months. Screening should be continued for 20 years (4).

DIET
Promote increased intake of antioxidant-rich foods.

PATIENT EDUCATION
HPV vaccination, smoking cessation, protected intercourse, regular screening with Pap smear per guidelines.

PROGNOSIS

- Progression of CIN to invasive cervical cancer is slow, and the likelihood of regression is high: Up to 43% of CIN II and 32% of CIN III lesions may regress. CIN III has a 30% probability of becoming invasive cancer over a 30-year period, although only about 1% of treated
- CIN III will become invasive (4). Lesions discovered early are amenable to treatment with excellent results and few recurrences.
- One- and 5-year relative survival rates for cervical cancer patients are 87% and 68%, respectively. The 5-year survival rate for patients diagnosed with localized disease is 91% (2).

COMPLICATIONS
Aggressive cervical surgery may be associated with cervical stenosis, cervical incompetence, and scarring affecting cervical dilatation in labor.

REFERENCES

1. Yang KY. Abnormal pap smear and cervical cancer in pregnancy. *Clin Obstet Gynecol*. 2012;55(3): 838–848.
2. Cancer Facts and Figures 2013: American Cancer Society 2013. Accessed May 16, 2013 at http://www.cancer.org/acs/groups/content/@epidemiologysurveilance/documents/document/acspc-036845.pdf.
3. Massad S, Eienstein MH, Warner KH. 2012 Updated Consensus Guidelines for the Management of Abnormal Cervical Cancer Screening Tests and Cancer Precursors. *J Lower Genital Tract Dis*. 2013;17(5):S1–S27.
4. McCredie MR, Sharples KJ, Paul C, et al. Natural history of cervical neoplasia and risk of invasive cancer in women with cervical intraepithelial neoplasia 3: A retrospective cohort study. *Lancet Oncol*. 2008;9(5):425–434.

ADDITIONAL READING
Screening for Cervical Cancer: U.S. Preventive Services Task Force Recommendation Statement. Accessed May 16, 2013 at http://www.uspreventiveservicestaskforce.org/uspstf11/cervcancer/cervcancerrs.pdf.

 SEE ALSO

- Cervical Malignancy; Condyloma Acuminata; Trichomoniasis; Vulvovaginitis, Prepubescent
- Algorithm: Pap (Abnormal), >21 Years of Age; Pap (Abnormal), Pap, Use of HPV DNA Co-Testing in Women Over 30

 CODES

ICD10

- N87.1 Moderate cervical dysplasia
- N87.9 Dysplasia of cervix uteri, unspecified
- R87.619 Unspecified abnormal cytological findings in specimens from cervix uteri

CLINICAL PEARLS

- HPV is present in virtually all cervical cancers (99.7%), but most HPV infections are transient.
- Vaccine should be offered prior to onset of any sexual activity for maximum effectiveness.
- Know and adhere to recognized screening guidelines to avoid the harms of over screening.

ABORTION, SPONTANEOUS (MISCARRIAGE)

Clara Keegan, MD

 BASICS

DESCRIPTION
- Spontaneous abortion (SAb) (miscarriage) is the separation of products of conception from the uterus prior to the potential for fetal survival outside the uterus, generally defined as expulsion from the uterus of an embryo or fetus weighing ≤500 g. A number of other related terms:
  - Threatened abortion: Vaginal bleeding in the first trimester of pregnancy
  - Inevitable abortion: Cervical dilatation, rupture of membranes, or expulsion of products of conception in the presence of vaginal bleeding
  - Complete abortion: Entire contents of uterus expelled
  - Incomplete abortion: Abortion with retained products of conception, generally placental tissue; more common after 12 weeks' gestation
  - Early pregnancy failure: Nonviable pregnancy identified by ultrasound (anembryonic or without embryonic cardiac activity)
  - Induced abortion: Evacuation of uterine contents or products of conception medically or surgically
  - Septic abortion: A spontaneous or therapeutic abortion complicated by pelvic infection; common complication of illegally performed induced abortions
  - Recurrent abortion: ≥2 consecutive pregnancy losses at <15 weeks' gestation
- Synonym(s): Miscarriage; Habitual abortion; Involuntary pregnancy loss:
  - Missed abortion and blighted ovum are older terms that do not represent the pathophysiology of the process.

EPIDEMIOLOGY
Predominant age: Increases with advancing age, especially >35 years; at age 40, the loss rate is twice that of age 20

Incidence
- Threatened abortion (1st-trimester bleeding) occurs in 20–25% of clinical pregnancies.
- Between 10% and 15% of all clinically recognized pregnancies end in SAb, with 80% of these occurring within 12 weeks after last menstrual period (LMP).
- When both clinical and biochemical (β-hCG detected) pregnancies are considered, up to 50% of pregnancies end in spontaneous abortion.

ETIOLOGY AND PATHOPHYSIOLOGY
- Chromosomal anomalies (50–65% of cases)
- Congenital anomalies
- Trauma
- Maternal factors: Uterine abnormalities, infection (toxoplasma, other viruses, rubella, cytomegalovirus, herpesvirus), maternal endocrine disorders, hypercoagulable state

Genetics
~50–65% of 1st-trimester spontaneous abortions have significant chromosomal anomalies, with 50% of these being autosomal trisomies and the remainder being triploidy, tetraploidy, or 45X monosomies.

RISK FACTORS
Most cases of spontaneous abortion occur in patients without identifiable risk factors; however, risk factors listed in order of importance include:
- Chromosomal abnormalities
- Advancing maternal age

- Uterine abnormalities
- Maternal chronic disease (diabetes mellitus, polycystic ovarian syndrome, obesity, systemic lupus erythematosus, hypertension, antiphospholipid antibodies, thyroid disease, renal disease)
- Other possible contributing factors include smoking, alcohol, infection, and luteal phase defect, although conclusive data are currently lacking.

GENERAL PREVENTION
- Insufficient evidence supports the use of aspirin and/or other anticoagulants, bed rest, hCG, immunotherapy, progestogens, uterine muscle relaxants, or vitamins for general prevention of SAb, before or after threatened abortion is diagnosed.
- By the time hemorrhage begins, 1/2 of pregnancies complicated by threatened abortion already have no fetal cardiac activity.
- Recurrent abortion: Women with a history of ≥3 prior SAbs may benefit from progestogens (OR 0.38, 95% CI 0.20–0.70) (1)[A].
- Antiphospholipid syndrome: The combination of unfractionated heparin and aspirin reduces risk of SAb in women with antiphospholipid antibodies and a history of recurrent abortion (RR 46%, 95% CI 0.29–0.71) (2)[A].

 DIAGNOSIS

HISTORY
- Consider any reproductive-age woman with vaginal bleeding to be pregnant until such is proven otherwise.
- Vaginal bleeding:
  - Characteristics (amount, color, consistency, associated symptoms), onset (abrupt or gradual), duration, intensity/quantity, and exacerbating/precipitating factors
  - Document LMP if known: Allows calculation of estimated gestational age if no ultrasound (US) documentation of intrauterine pregnancy (IUP)
- Abdominal pain/uterine cramping, as well as associated nausea/vomiting/syncope
- Rupture of membranes
- Passage of products of conception
- Prenatal course: Toxic or infectious exposures, family or personal history of genetic abnormalities, past history of ectopic pregnancy or spontaneous abortion, endocrine disease, autoimmune disorder, bleeding/clotting disorder

PHYSICAL EXAM
- Orthostatic vital signs to estimate hemodynamic stability
- Abdominal exam for tenderness, guarding, rebound, bowel sounds (peritoneal signs more likely with ectopic pregnancy)
- Speculum exam for visual assessment of cervical dilation, blood, and products of conception; bimanual exam for uterine size/tenderness and presence of adnexal mass

DIFFERENTIAL DIAGNOSIS
- Ectopic pregnancy: Potentially life-threatening; must be considered in any woman of childbearing age with abdominal pain and vaginal bleeding
- Physiologic bleeding in normal pregnancy (implantation bleeding)

- Cervical polyps, neoplasia, and/or inflammatory conditions
- Hydatidiform mole pregnancy
- hCG-secreting ovarian tumor

DIAGNOSTIC TESTS & INTERPRETATION
Initial Tests (lab, imaging)
- Quantitative human chorionic gonadotropin (hCG)
  - Particularly useful if IUP has not been documented by US
  - Serial quantitative serum hCG measurements can assess viability of the pregnancy. Serum hCG should rise at least 67% every 48 hours through 7 weeks after LMP. An inappropriate rise/plateau of hCG suggests abnormal IUP or possible ectopic pregnancy.
- CBC with differential
- Rh type
- Cultures: Gonorrhea/Chlamydia
- US exam to evaluate fetal viability and to rule out ectopic pregnancy:
  - hCG >2,000 mIU/mL necessary to detect IUP via transvaginal US (TVUS), >6,500 mIU/mL for abdominal ultrasound
- TVUS criteria for nonviable intrauterine gestation: 5-mm fetal pole without cardiac activity or 16-mm gestational sac without a fetal pole
- Structures and timing: With TVUS, gestational sac of 2–3 mm generally seen by 4 weeks +1–3 days; yolk sac by 5 weeks; fetal pole with cardiac activity by 5.5–6 weeks

Follow-Up Tests & Special Considerations
- In the case of vaginal bleeding with no documented IUP, follow serum hCG levels weekly to zero.
- If levels plateau, consider ectopic pregnancy, retained products of conception, or gestational trophoblastic disease.
- If initial hCG level does not permit documentation of IUP by TVUS, follow serum hCG in 48 hours to document appropriate rise.
- Repeat US once hCG is at a level commensurate with visualization on US (see above).
- Provide patient with ectopic precautions in interim: Worsening abdominal pain, dizziness/syncope, nausea/vomiting.

Diagnostic Procedures/Other
- Fetal heart tones can be auscultated with Doppler starting between 10 and 12 weeks' gestation in a viable pregnancy.
- In threatened abortion, fetal cardiac activity at 7–11 weeks' gestation is 90–96% predictive of continued pregnancy.

Test Interpretation
Products of conception, placental villi

TREATMENT

GENERAL MEASURES
Discuss contraception plan at the time of diagnosis of SAb, as ovulation can occur prior to resumption of normal menses.

MEDICATION
- Long-term conception rate and pregnancy outcomes are similar for women who undergo medical or surgical evacuation.
- Postinfection rates are lower with medical vs. surgical management.

First Line

- Misoprostol: Most common agent for inducing passage of tissue in missed or incomplete abortion:
  - Not approved by the FDA for treatment of early pregnancy failure
  - Efficacy: Complete expulsion of products of conception in 71% by day 3, 84% by day 8
  - Efficacy depends on route of administration, gestational age of pregnancy, and dose.
  - Recommended dose is 800 μg vaginally (3)[A]; alternate regimens include the World Health Organization (WHO) regimen of 600 μg sublingually q3h for up to 3 doses; multidose regimens and oral dosing (including buccal and sublingual) may result in increased side effects. Concerns related to possible increased risk for *C. sordelii* infection with vaginal route are unproven but many protocols have switched to the buccal route as a result.
- Common adverse effects include abdominal pain/cramping, nausea, and diarrhea. Pain increases at higher doses, but is manageable with oral analgesia. There is no increase in nausea/diarrhea with a higher dose.
- Recommended for stable patients who decline surgery, but do not want to wait for spontaneous passage of products of conception

Second Line

Rh-negative patients should be given Rh immunoglobulin (RhoGAM) following a spontaneous abortion.

ISSUES FOR REFERRAL

Patients should be monitored for up to 1 year for the development of pathologic grief. Insufficient evidence indicates that counseling prevents development of anxiety or depression related to grief following SAb.

SURGERY/OTHER PROCEDURES

- Uterine aspiration (suction dilation and curettage (D&C) or manual vacuum aspiration) is the conventional treatment.
- Indications: Septic abortion, heavy bleeding, hypotension, patient choice
- Risks: Anesthesia (usually local), uterine perforation, intrauterine adhesions, cervical trauma, infection that may lead to infertility or increased risk of ectopic pregnancy
- When compared with expectant management, surgical intervention leads to fewer days of vaginal bleeding, with a lower risk of incomplete abortion and heavy bleeding, but a higher risk of infection (4)[A].
- Vacuum aspiration (manual or electric) is considered preferable to sharp curettage as aspiration is less painful, takes less time, involves less blood loss, and does not require general anesthesia (5)[A]. The WHO supports use of suction curettage over rigid metal curettage (4)[A].
- Data from induced abortions suggest that antibiotic prophylaxis with doxycycline 100 mg b.i.d. substantially reduces postprocedure infection risk; however, data for incomplete abortions treated surgically is inconclusive (6)[A].
- For patients who desire contraception after completion of a spontaneous abortion, immediate insertion of an intrauterine device is both acceptable and safe.

COMPLEMENTARY AND ALTERNATIVE MEDICINE

A systematic review of Chinese herbal medicine alone and in conjunction with Western medicine showed benefit over Western medicine alone in achieving continued viability at 28 weeks (NNT = 4.8 pregnancies with combined therapy) (7)[A]. However, the available studies did not meet international standards for reporting quality.

IN-PATIENT CONSIDERATIONS

Admission Criteria/Initial Stabilization

If the patient has orthostatic vital signs, initiate resuscitation with IV fluids and/or blood products, if needed.

IV Fluids

Hemodynamically unstable patients may require IV fluids and/or blood products to maintain BP.

 ONGOING CARE

FOLLOW-UP RECOMMENDATIONS

All patients should be seen in 2–6 weeks to monitor for resolution of bleeding, return of menses, and symptoms related to grief, as well as to review the contraception plan.

Patient Monitoring

- Identification of products of conception within material expelled from the uterus or D&C specimen
- If abortion is complete, observe the patient for further bleeding
- Pelvic rest until 2 weeks after evacuation
- If spontaneous abortion occurs in setting of previously documented IUP and abortion is completed with resumption of normal menses, it is not necessary to check or follow serum hCG to 0.

DIET

NPO if patient is to undergo D&C

PATIENT EDUCATION

Patient pamphlet (no. AP090) available from the American College of Obstetricians and Gynecologists, 409 12th St., SW, Washington, DC 20090-6290; (800) 762-2264 or online at http://www.acog.org

PROGNOSIS

- Prognosis is excellent once bleeding is controlled.
- Recurrent abortion: Prognosis depends on etiology. Up to 70% rate of success with subsequent pregnancy.

COMPLICATIONS

- D&C: Uterine perforation, bleeding, adhesions, cervical trauma, and infection that may lead to infertility or increased risk of ectopic pregnancy
- Retained products of conception

REFERENCES

1. Haas DM, Ramsey PS. Progestogen for preventing miscarriage. *Cochrane Database Syst Rev.* 2008;(2): CD003511.
2. Empson M, Lassere M, Craig J, et al. Prevention of recurrent miscarriage for women with antiphospholipid antibody or lupus anticoagulant. *Cochrane Database Syst Rev.* 2005;(2):CD002859.
3. Neilson JP, Gyte GM, Hickey M, et al. Medical treatments for incomplete miscarriage (less than 24 weeks). *Cochrane Database Syst Rev.* 2010;(1): CD007223.
4. Nanda K, Lopez LM, Grimes DA, et al. Expectant care versus surgical treatment for miscarriage. *Cochrane Database Syst Rev.* 2012;3:CD003518.
5. Tunçalp O, Gülmezoglu AM, Souza JP. Surgical procedures for evacuating incomplete miscarriage. *Cochrane Database Syst Rev.* 2010;(9):CD001993.
6. May W, Gülmezoglu AM, Ba-Thike K. Antibiotics for incomplete abortion. *Cochrane Database Syst Rev.* 2007;(4):CD001779.
7. Li L, Dou L, Leung PC, et al. Chinese herbal medicines for threatened miscarriage. *Cochrane Database Syst Rev.* 2012;5:CD008510.

ADDITIONAL READING

- Grimes DA, Lopez LM, Schulz KF, et al. Immediate postabortal insertion of intrauterine devices. *Cochrane Database Syst Rev.* 2010;(6):CD001777.
- Murphy FA, Lipp A, Powles DL. Follow-up for improving psychological well being for women after a miscarriage. *Cochrane Database Syst Rev.* 2012; 3:CD008679.
- Prevention of Rho(D) alloimmunization. American College of Obstetricians and Gynecologists Practice Bulletin No. 4. American College of Obstetricians and Gynecologists, Washington, DC; 1999.

 SEE ALSO

- Ectopic Pregnancy
- Algorithm: Abortion, Recurrent

 CODES

ICD10

- O02.1 Missed abortion
- O03.4 Incomplete spontaneous abortion without complication
- O03.9 Complete or unspecified spontaneous abortion without complication

CLINICAL PEARLS

- Any reproductive-age woman or pregnant woman with abdominal pain and vaginal bleeding must be evaluated to rule out ectopic pregnancy, which is potentially life threatening.
- As all options have similar long-term outcomes, patient preference should determine whether management is expectant, medical, or surgical.

ABSCESS, PSOAS
Megan Curtis, MD • Louay Toma, MD

BASICS

Psoas abscess is a rare and potentially life-threatening suppurative myositis of the iliopsoas compartment.

DESCRIPTION
- The iliopsoas compartment is an anatomic space composed of the psoas major, psoas minor, and iliacus muscles, which mediate hip flexion and are innervated by L2–4.
- The muscle group originates from the lateral borders of the 12th thoracic to 5th lumbar vertebrae, passes posterior to the inguinal ligament and anterior to the hip joint, and inserts on the lesser trochanter of the femur.
- Abscesses of the iliopsoas compartment are considered primary (hematogenous/lymphatic spread, idiopathic) or secondary (extension of nearby infection).
- Synonym(s): Iliopsoas abscess; Ilio-psoas abscess

EPIDEMIOLOGY
- In developed countries, >75% of psoas abscesses are secondary, usually originating from bone or inflammatory bowel disease (1–3).
- Primary psoas abscess is most common in developing and tropical countries.
- *Mycobacterium tuberculosis* (TB) with secondary vertebral osteomyelitis is a common cause of psoas abscess in countries where TB is prevalent, with about 5% of patients with vertebral TB developing psoas abscess.
- About 83% of primary psoas abscesses occur in patients <30 years of age.
- In neonates and pediatric patients, psoas abscess is more likely to be primary, predominantly due to *Staphylococcus aureus*.
- Older patients are more predisposed to secondary psoas abscess due to increased incidence of age-related diseases, such as diverticulitis.
- 3–12% occur unilaterally.
- A male preponderance for psoas abscess has been reported.

Incidence
- 0.5 cases per 10,000 hospital admissions 1993–2004 to 6.5 cases per 10,000 hospital admissions 2005–2007 (urban, tertiary care center) (4)
- Rising incidence from increased prevalence of risk factors (e.g., immunosuppressant therapy, diabetes)
- Increased detection from improvement in quality and interpretation of cross-sectional imaging

ETIOLOGY AND PATHOPHYSIOLOGY
- Primary psoas abscess results from hematogenous or lymphatic spread of infection from a distant source:
  - Primary abscesses are often monomicrobial, with 80% of infections due to *S. aureus* bacteremia or sepsis.
  - The rich blood supply of the iliopsoas muscles are thought to predispose these muscles to infection by hematogenous spread.
  - *Mycobacterium tuberculosis* and *S. aureus* are the most common organisms causing iliopsoas abscess in patients with HIV/AIDS, with primary abscesses more common than secondary.
  - *Pseudomonas aeruginosa, Haemophilus aphrophilus,* and *Proteus mirabilis* infections have also been reported.

- Secondary psoas abscess results from contiguous spread of infection from nearby structures of the musculoskeletal system, GI tract, genitourinary tract, and vasculature:
  - Secondary psoas abscesses are often polymicrobial, most commonly involving *S. aureus* from skeletal origins and *Escherichia coli* and other enteric organisms, such as *Bacteroides* spp. and *Enterococcus faecalis,* from GI and urinary sources (1).
  - Secondary psoas abscesses have also been reported with *Salmonella* from aortic aneurysm infection as well as fungal infections in immunocompromised patients.
- In recent years, MRSA has become the predominant pathogen in psoas abscesses with definitive microbiologic diagnosis, accounting for up to 25% of cases (4).
- Most psoas abscesses are unilateral and single, although multiple abscesses may be found in up to 25% of cases (2).

RISK FACTORS
- Primary psoas abscess:
  - IV drug use
  - Diabetes
  - HIV/AIDS
  - Active malignancy
  - Other immunodeficiency states
- Other factors include trauma to the lumbar spinous processes incurring psoas muscle damage, and hematoma formation, as in the setting of hematologic disorders.
- Secondary psoas abscess: Skeletal infections (vertebral and pelvic osteomyelitis, spondylodiscitis), GI infections (Crohn disease, ulcerative colitis, appendicitis, diverticulitis), genitourinary and gynecologic infections, and infections of aortic aneurysms (2,4):
  - Complications of hip arthroplasty, spinal surgery, aortic surgery, and kidney transplantation (2)
  - Paraspinal abscess, anastomotic leak, and hematoma set the stage for postoperative infection and abscess formation.
  - Cases have been reported of psoas abscess following acupuncture, secondary to spinal infection or bowel perforation.

COMMONLY ASSOCIATED CONDITIONS
- Primary psoas abscess: IV drug use, diabetes, HIV/AIDS and other immunocompromised states, renal failure
- Secondary psoas abscess: Common: Inflammatory bowel disease, appendicitis, diverticulitis, and osteomyelitis. Infrequently: septic arthritis, colorectal carcinoma, trauma, endocarditis, hepatocellular carcinoma, pancreatitis, traumatic hematoma, bowel perforation by foreign body, and Henoch-Schönlein purpura.

DIAGNOSIS

Diagnosis of psoas abscess can be difficult; it involves a thorough history, physical examination, and appropriate imaging studies.
- CT scan is the preferred imaging modality for identification of psoas abscess; definitive diagnosis is made by image-guided drainage and microbial culture.
- A definitive microbiological diagnosis occurs in ~75% of cases (1).

HISTORY
- Reported symptoms are often nonspecific indicators of generalized infection: Fever, flank or abdominal pain, with or without radiation to the anterior hip and thigh
- Additional symptoms: Limp, nausea, anorexia, malaise, and weight loss
- The classic symptom triad described by Myntner in 1881 of fever, abdominal or flank pain, and limp is present in <8% of cases.
- Most patients will present with pain (~50%), whereas persistent low-grade fever is found in 25–75% of cases (1,2,5).

PHYSICAL EXAM
- Maneuvers that stretch or contract the inflamed psoas compartment result in considerable pain on the affected side.
- Pain with extension and internal rotation of the hip (the "psoas sign") is the most common physical exam finding:
  - A positive psoas sign may be elicited by the examiner by placing a hand proximal to the patient's knee on the affected side and asking the patient to raise the ipsilateral thigh against resistance.
  - A second psoas test is performed by asking the patient to lay on the unaffected side and hyperextend the contralateral hip, eliciting pain with stretching of affected psoas muscle.
- These maneuvers may also be positive in the setting of other conditions causing iliopsoas inflammation, including retrocecal appendicitis. Sensitivity and specificity of the psoas sign have been reported at 16% and 95%, respectively (6).
- Rectal examination may aid in differentiating psoas abscess from retrocecal appendicitis, with pain on palpation of the retrovesical pouch more consistent with appendicitis.
- Whereas patients with psoas abscess may find relief from pain with full hip flexion, patients with hip pathology experience persistent or heightened pain.
- Distal extension of a psoas abscess may yield a painful or painless mass palpable below the inguinal ligament.
- ~50% of patients report abdominal tenderness; guarding and rebound are uncommon.
- Most common findings in neonates include leg or groin swelling, limitation of leg motion, and pain, with fever occurring in a few cases.

DIFFERENTIAL DIAGNOSIS
Retrocecal appendicitis, diverticulitis, bacterial infection or avascular necrosis of the hip, renal colic, pyelonephritis, arthritis, S1 disc herniation, inflammatory bowel disease, epidural abscess, vertebral osteomyelitis, endometriosis, pelvic inflammatory disease, hematoma, tumor, and noninfectious inflammation of the iliopsoas compartment.

DIAGNOSTIC TESTS & INTERPRETATION
Initial Tests (lab, imaging)
- WBC >10,000/mL
- Anemia (hemoglobin <11 g/L)
- Thrombocytosis is less common.
- Elevations in BUN, sedimentation rate, and C-reactive protein (CRP) have been reported (2). CRP level has been shown to correspond with the severity of infection.

- CT is the gold standard imaging modality:
  - Sensitivity rate between 88% and 100%
  - Typically reveals a focal, hypodense lesion consistent with an abscess
  - May demonstrate:
    - Enlargement of the iliopsoas muscle
    - Gas or air fluid levels within the muscle and fat stranding
  - Contrast CT may show rim enhancement of the abscess wall.
- Although not integral to the diagnosis of psoas abscess, MRI and technetium 99m scintigraphy may elucidate local infectious sources, such as vertebral osteomyelitis.
- Plain abdominal radiographs occasionally reveal the outline of an inflammatory mass.
- Chest plain films may identify scant pleural effusions or raised hemidiaphragm.
- US may disclose evidence of an inflammatory mass and is often diagnostic in cases of pediatric psoas abscess.
- US should be used as the initial imaging modality in neonates, followed by CT or MRI to further classify the abscess (7).
- An IV pyelogram may show deviation of the kidney and ureter, and barium studies may reveal bowel loop displacement and associated GI disease.

Diagnostic Procedures/Other
- Gram stain and culture of blood and aspirated abscess fluid confirm the diagnosis and guide antimicrobial treatment.
- AFB stain and mycobacterial culture if TB infection suspected

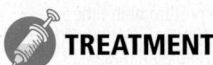 TREATMENT

- Most cases of psoas abscess will require percutaneous or surgical drainage, as well as parenteral antibiotic treatment (20% success rate with antibiotics alone) (8)[B].
- CT-guided percutaneous drainage is the initial procedure of choice, leading to successful decompression in at least 50% of cases, with up to 100% success after a second drainage (8,9)[B].
- Open drainage may be indicated:
  - For large, complex, and multiloculated abscesses
  - If imaging shows gross involvement of adjacent structures
  - When percutaneous drainage fails
- Psoas abscess associated with conditions such as inflammatory bowel disease or diverticulitis may be effectively managed with open drainage and surgical treatment of the underlying disease process.
- For complicated tuberculous psoas abscess, may consider retroperitoneoscopic drainage (in addition to antituberculous medical therapy) to minimize radiation exposure and shorten recovery (10)[B].
- For neonatal and pediatric psoas abscess, may consider US-guided percutaneous drainage as an alternative to surgical drainage (7)[B].

MEDICATION
- Broad-spectrum empiric antibiotics targeting staphylococcal (primary and secondary due to skeletal infections) and enteric organisms (secondary to intra-abdominal infection) are indicated in most cases.

- IV monotherapy with Unasyn, Zosyn, or a carbapenem is effective as initial treatment.
- Dual therapy with a 3rd-generation cephalosporin, such as ceftriaxone with metronidazole, is also adequate.
- Suspected MRSA infection is best treated with vancomycin, and, alternatively, linezolid or daptomycin.
- Coverage should be determined by culture sensitivity results from aspirated fluid.
- Although most psoas abscesses require drainage, abscesses ≤3 cm have been successfully managed by antibiotics alone.

 ONGOING CARE

Following drainage, pigtail catheter placement permits continued decompression of the abscess cavity and monitoring of purulent output for improvement.

FOLLOW-UP RECOMMENDATIONS
Duration of antibiotic treatment should be tailored to the patient and may be continued for 2–6 weeks.

Patient Monitoring
Follow-up imaging may be warranted to verify adequate resolution of the fluid collection.

DIET
Patients should be kept NPO for percutaneous and surgical drainage procedures.

PROGNOSIS
- A high index of suspicion for abscess in the iliopsoas compartment is crucial, as early intervention is associated with favorable outcomes.
- Delays in diagnosis can lead to serious complications, including septic shock, reported in up to 20% of cases.
- Mortality is reported at 2.4–19% for treated patients with primary and secondary abscesses, respectively. Untreated cases face a near 100% mortality rate (2).
- Mortality is significantly increased with age >65, bacteremia, and growth of E. coli in cultures (1).

COMPLICATIONS
- Risk factors for unfavorable outcomes include delays in treatment, bacteremia, and inadequate treatment (percutaneous drainage or antibiotics only) in patients with advanced age. About 40% of patients require >1 drainage procedure for full recovery.
- Incomplete drainage or suboptimal antibiotic treatment may lead to relapses of psoas abscess up to a year after initial presentation in 15–36% of cases.
- Spinal cord compression has been reported via direct extension of psoas abscess.
- Most cases of relapse occur within 6 months of follow-up, but may occur after 1 year (1).

REFERENCES
1. Navarro López V, Ramos JM, Meseguer V, et al. Microbiology and outcome of iliopsoas abscess in 124 patients. Medicine (Baltimore). 2009;84(2):120–130.
2. Tabrizian P, Nguyen SQ, Greenstein A, et al. Management and treatment of iliopsoas abscess. Arch Surg. 2009;144:946–949.
3. Yacoub WN, Sohn HJ, Chan S, et al. Psoas abscess rarely requires surgical intervention. Am J Surg. 2008;196:223–227.
4. Alonso CD, Barclay S, Tao X, et al. Increasing incidence of iliopsoas abscesses with MRSA as a predominant pathogen. J Infect. 2011;84(1):1–7.
5. Wong OF, Ho PL, Lam SK. Retrospective review of clinical presentations, microbiology, and outcomes of patients with psoas abscess. Hong Kong Med J. 2013;19(5):416–423.
6. Navarro Fernández JA, Tárraga López PJ, Rodríguez Montes JA, et al. Validity of tests performed to diagnose acute abdominal pain in patients admitted at an emergency department. Rev Esp Enferm Dig. 2009;101:610–618.
7. Yano T, Takamatsu H, Noguchi H, et al. Iliopsoas abscess in the neonate. J Pediatr Surg. 2004;84(7):e13–e15.
8. Dietrich A, Vaccarezza H, Vaccaro CA. Iliopsoas abscess: Presentation, management, and outcomes. Surg Laparosc Endosc Percutan Tech. 2013;23(1):45–48.
9. Gupta S, Suri S, Gulati M, et al. Ilio-psoas abscesses: Percutaneous drainage under image guidance. Clin Radiol. 1997;52:704–707.
10. Büyükbebeci O, Seçkiner I, Karsl B, et al. Retroperitoneoscopic drainage of complicated psoas abscesses in patients with tuberculous lumbar spondylitis. Eur Spine J. 2012;84(3):470–473.

 CODES

ICD10
K68.12 Psoas muscle abscess

CLINICAL PEARLS
- Psoas abscess is a rare, retroperitoneal collection of pus resulting from hematogenous, lymphatic, or contiguous spread of infection. Primary and secondary psoas abscesses have different underlying causes that may affect treatment strategy.
- The classic presentation of fever, limp, and pain is found in <8% of patients with psoas abscess. A high level of clinical suspicion and CT imaging can effectively diagnose psoas abscess and delineate gross involvement of adjacent anatomic structures. Gram stain and culture of aspirated abscess fluid provide definitive diagnosis of causative organisms.
- Favorable treatment outcomes are associated with appropriate antibiotic selection and prompt abscess drainage. Percutaneous drainage is the preferred approach. This method is much less invasive than surgical drainage and is often effective at draining uniloculated and multiloculated abscesses.
- Diagnosis of psoas abscess should prompt consideration of associated conditions such as Crohn disease, skeletal infection, HIV, or other immunocompromised states.

ACETAMINOPHEN POISONING

Lars C. Larsen, MD

 BASICS

DESCRIPTION

- A disorder characterized by hepatic necrosis following large ingestions of acetaminophen. Symptoms may vary from initial nausea, vomiting, diaphoresis, and malaise to jaundice, confusion, somnolence, coma, and death. The clinical hallmark is the onset of symptoms within 24 hours of ingestion of acetaminophen-only or combination products.
- Acetaminophen poisoning is most often encountered following large, single ingestions of acetaminophen-containing medications. Usual toxic doses are >10 g in adults and >150 mg/kg in children. However, poisoning also occurs after acute and chronic ingestions of lesser amounts in susceptible individuals, including those who regularly abuse alcohol, are chronically malnourished, or take medications that affect hepatic metabolism of acetaminophen.
- Therapeutic adult doses are 0.5–1 g q4–6h, up to a maximum of 4 g/d. Therapeutic pediatric doses are 10–15 mg/kg q4–6h, not to exceed 5 doses in 24 hours.
- System(s) affected: Gastrointestinal; Cardiovascular; Renal/Urologic:
  - Multisystem organ failure can occur.
- Synonym(s): Paracetamol poisoning

Geriatric Considerations
Hepatic damage may be increased if chronically taking hepatotoxic medications.

Pediatric Considerations
Hepatic damage at toxic acetaminophen levels is decreased in children <6 years.

Pregnancy Considerations
- Increased incidence of spontaneous abortion, especially with overdose at early gestational age
- Incidence of spontaneous abortion or fetal death appears to be increased when N-acetylcysteine (NAC) treatment is delayed.
- IV NAC is generally preferred in pregnancy since it may offer greater bioavailability.

EPIDEMIOLOGY
- Predominant age: Children and adults
- Predominant sex: No reported association

Incidence
- >88,000 single-substance ingestions of acetaminophen or acetaminophen combination products reported by poison control centers in 2011
- 139 deaths in 2011; none in children <6 years of age

Prevalence
>48% of single-substance exposures in 2011 were in children <6 years.

ETIOLOGY AND PATHOPHYSIOLOGY
- Accidental or intentional ingestion of acetaminophen or combination medications containing acetaminophen

- 96% of ingested acetaminophen is metabolized in the liver, with only 2–4% excreted unchanged in the urine. When taken in therapeutic doses, 90–95% of hepatic metabolism occurs via glucuronidation and sulfation and results in the formation of benign metabolites. 5–10% of hepatic metabolism is by oxidation through the cytochrome P_{450} enzyme system (CYP 3A4 and CYP 2E1), which results in the formation of the toxic metabolite N-acetyl-p-benzoquinoneimine (NAPQI). NAPQI is rapidly conjugated with glutathione to form a nontoxic metabolite. The metabolites are excreted in the urine along with a small amount of unchanged drug. Hepatocellular damage typically occurs when toxic doses of acetaminophen result in saturation of the glucuronidation and sulfation pathways with subsequent production of excessive amounts of NAPQI. Available glutathione stores become depleted, NAPQI accumulates, and hepatocellular damage occurs.

RISK FACTORS
- Age >6 years
- Concurrent poisoning with other substances
- Psychiatric illness
- Previous toxic ingestions or suicide attempts
- Regular ingestion of large amounts of alcohol

GENERAL PREVENTION
Parent/caregiver education essential:
- Education during well-child exams regarding poisoning prevention
- Emergency telephone numbers

 DIAGNOSIS

- Signs and symptoms develop over the first 24 hours following large ingestions; may last as long as 8 days.
- Symptoms may develop gradually following long-term ingestion of near maximal-therapeutic amounts of acetaminophen. Such patients may present in stages 1–3, without a history of ingestion of the usual toxic doses.
- Severe symptoms indicate large ingestions or coingestants:
  - Stage 1: First 24 hours after time of ingestion:
    ○ Nausea
    ○ Vomiting
    ○ Diaphoresis
  - Stage 2: 24–48 hours:
    ○ Right upper quadrant pain
    ○ Typically less nausea, vomiting, diaphoresis, and malaise than in stage 1
  - Stage 3: 72–96 hours:
    ○ Nausea, vomiting, and malaise reappear.
    ○ Severe poisonings may result in jaundice, confusion, somnolence, and coma.
  - Stage 4: 7–8 days:
    ○ Resolution of clinical signs in survivors
- Fulminant hepatic failure occurs in <1% of adults and is very rare in children <6 years of age.
- Patients with an unexplained rise in liver function tests (LFTs) with negative acetaminophen levels may be overdose patients presenting in stage 3.

HISTORY
Ingestion or suspected ingestion of acetaminophen-containing product

DIFFERENTIAL DIAGNOSIS
- Consider presence of coingestants, especially alcohol and aspirin.
- Other ingested toxins that produce severe acute hepatic injury, including the mushroom *Amanita phalloides* and products containing yellow phosphorus or carbon tetrachloride

DIAGNOSTIC TESTS & INTERPRETATION
Initial Tests (lab, imaging)
- Plasma acetaminophen levels should be drawn on all patients ≥4 hours after ingestion (levels prior to 4 hours not helpful).
- AST, ALT, PT/NR, bilirubin, lactate dehydrogenase (LDH)
- Electrolytes, glucose, BUN, creatinine
- Pregnancy screen in females (urine or serum)
- Urinalysis
- Consider arterial blood gas (ABG) if pH disturbance suspected on clinical or lab grounds.
- Screens for suspected coingestants (aspirin, iron, and others) may be positive (especially when suicide attempt is a possibility).
- With toxic ingestions, aspartate transaminase (AST; serum glutamic-oxaloacetic transaminase), alanine transaminase (ALT; serum glutamic-pyruvic transaminase), and bilirubin levels begin to rise in stage 2 and peak in stage 3.
- In severe poisonings, the prothrombin time (PT)/international normalized ratio (INR) will parallel these changes and should be monitored.
- AST levels >1,000 IU/L are consistent with the diagnosis, and levels of 20,000 IU/L are not uncommon.
- Laboratory abnormalities usually resolve by stage 4.
- Renal function abnormalities are common in patients with hepatotoxicity.
- Evidence of damage to pancreas and heart may present following severe poisonings.
- Anion-gap metabolic acidosis due to accumulation of 5-oxoprolene may rarely be seen.
- Drugs that may alter lab results: None with clinically significant cross-reactivity with plasma acetaminophen assay
- Disorders that may alter lab results: Diseases or toxic substances that damage the liver, particularly alcohol
- No specific imaging required

Follow-Up Tests & Special Considerations
ABG after hydration if pH is acidotic

Test Interpretation
Centrilobular hepatic necrosis

TREATMENT

- Contact a regional/local poison control center for management recommendations. In the US: (800) 222-1222.
- NAC should be given when plasma acetaminophen concentrations measured ≥4 hours after ingestion are in the "possible risk" or higher levels on the Rumack-Matthew nomogram. This corresponds to acetaminophen levels >150 μg/mL (993 μmol/L), >75 μg/mL (497 μmol/L), and >37 μg/mL (244 μmol/L) at 4, 8, and 12 hours after ingestion, respectively. See http://www.ars-informatica.ca/toxicity_nomogram.php?calc=acetamin or http://www.merckmanuals.com/professional/resources/clinical_calculators/name/calculator.html?WT.z_resource=Clinical Calculators.
- NAC should be started within 8 hours of ingestion for best chance of hepatic protection. Patients presenting near 8 hours should empirically receive NAC while waiting for labs.
- All patients with acetaminophen liver injury (even after 8 hours) should receive NAC.
- NAC therapy may be effective up to ≥36 hours after ingestion.
- Single-dose activated charcoal may be used if given within 1 hour of ingestion (especially in cases of coingestants) (1,2)[C],(3)[A], but not within 1 hour of administration of the antidote NAC. Never delay NAC for activated charcoal.
- NAC should be initiated within 8 hours of ingestion whenever possible.
- Ipecac and gastric lavage are no longer recommended for routine use at home or in health care facilities (4)[C].

MEDICATION
First Line
- Acetylcysteine (NAC, Mucomyst) should be initiated within 8 hours of ingestion whenever possible; single-dose activated charcoal (1 g/kg PO) may be effective if given within 1 hour of ingestion. *Never delay oral NAC for activated charcoal.*
- Acetylcysteine may be given PO or IV, depending on situation and availability:
  – Currently, IV administration is often preferred:
    ○ IV loading dose of Acetadote 150 mg/kg over 60 minutes followed by an infusion of 50 mg/kg over 4 hours (12.5 mg/kg/hr); this is followed by an infusion of 100 mg/kg over the next 16 hours (6.25 mg/kg/hr). Oral loading dose of 140 mg/kg, followed by 70 mg/kg q4h for 17 additional doses.
- Contraindications: Medication allergies
- Precautions:
  – Oral NAC may cause significant nausea and vomiting due to its sulfur content; consider IV administration or by nasogastric tube.
  – Nausea can be treated with metoclopramide (Reglan), 1–2 mg/kg IV, or ondansetron (Zofran), 0.15 mg/kg IV (for age >4 years, usually 4 mg/dose).
  – IV NAC (Acetadote) may cause anaphylactoid reactions, including rash, bronchospasm, pruritus, angioedema, tachycardia, or hypotension (higher rates seen in asthmatics and those with atopic history) (5,6)[C].

- Reactions usually occur with loading dose. Slow or temporarily stop the infusion; may concurrently treat with antihistamines.
- Significant possible interactions: Activated charcoal given within 1 hour of oral NAC may adsorb NAC, limiting its effectiveness.

Second Line
Oral racemethionine (methionine)

ISSUES FOR REFERRAL
- Psychiatric and psychological evaluation in emergency room and close follow-up after intentional ingestions
- Consider child abuse reporting if neglect led to overdose.

IN-PATIENT CONSIDERATIONS
Admission Criteria/Initial Stabilization
- Toxic and intentional ingestions
- Any reported ingestion with increased LFTs, acidosis on ABG, elevated creatinine, etc.

Aggressive age- and weight-appropriate IV hydration

 ONGOING CARE

FOLLOW-UP RECOMMENDATIONS
- All patients should be evaluated at a health care facility.
- Patients with evidence of organ failure, increased LFTs, or coagulopathy should be evaluated for transfer to a site capable of liver transplant.
- Outpatient for nontoxic accidental ingestions
- Activity may be restricted if significant hepatic damage is present.

Patient Monitoring
Ask about possible ingestion by others (i.e., suicide pacts).

DIET
No special diet, except with severe hepatic damage

PATIENT EDUCATION
- Patients should be counseled to avoid Tylenol if already using combination product(s) containing acetaminophen.
- Education of parents/caregivers during well-child visits
- Anticipatory guidance for caregivers, family, and cohabitants of potentially suicidal patients
- http://familydoctor.org/familydoctor/en/kids/home-safety/child-safety-keeping-medicines-out-of-reach.html
- Education of patients taking long-term acetaminophen therapy

PROGNOSIS
- Complete recovery with early therapy
- <1% of adult patients develop hepatic failure. King criteria (pH <7.3, PT >100 s [INR >65], creatinine >3.4 mg/dL [>300 μmol/L]) is associated with a poor prognosis and possible need for liver transplant (7)[C]. Early referral increases the chance for transplant success (8)[A].
- Hepatic failure is very rare in children <6 years of age.

COMPLICATIONS
Rare following recovery from acute poisoning

REFERENCES
1. Gaudreault P. Activated charcoal revisited. *Clin Ped Emerg Med*. 2005;6:76–80.
2. Heard K. Gastrointestinal decontamination. *Med Clin North Am*. 2005;89:1067–1078.
3. Brok J, Buckley N, Gluud C. Interventions for paracetamol (acetaminophen) overdose. *Cochrane Database Syst Rev*. 2009;1.
4. American Academy of Pediatrics Committee on Injury, Violence, and Poison Prevention. Poison treatment in the home. American Academy of Pediatrics Committee on Injury, Violence, and Poison Prevention. *Pediatrics*. 2003;112: 1182–1185.
5. Acetylcysteine (Acetadote) for acetaminophen overdosage. *Med Lett*. 2005;47:70–71.
6. Culley CM, Krenzelok EP. A clinical and pharmacoeconomic justification for intravenous acetylcysteine: A US perspective. *Toxicol Rev*. 2005;24:131–143.
7. O'Grady JG, Alexander GJ, Hayllar KM, et al. Early indicators of prognosis in fulminant hepatic failure. *Gastroenterology*. 1989;97:439–445.
8. Ferner RE, Dear JW, Bateman DN. Management of paracetamol poisoning. *BMJ*. 2011;342.

 SEE ALSO

Acetaminophen Poisoning, Treatment

 CODES

ICD10
- T39.1X4A Poisoning by 4-Aminophenol derivatives, undetermined, init
- T39.1X4D Poisoning by 4-Aminophenol derivatives, undetermined, subs
- T39.1X4S Poisoning by 4-Aminophenol derivatives, undet, sequela

CLINICAL PEARLS
- Contact a regional poison control center for management recommendations. In the US: (800) 222-1222.
- NAC should be given when plasma acetaminophen concentrations measured ≥4 hours after ingestion are in the "possible risk" or higher levels on the Rumack-Matthew nomogram. This corresponds to acetaminophen levels >150 μg/mL (993 μmol/L), >75 μg/mL (497 μmol/L), and >40 μg/mL (265 μmol/L) at 4, 8, and 12 hours after ingestion, respectively.
- NAC should be started within 8 hours of ingestion for best chance of hepatic protection. Patients presenting near 8 hours should empirically receive NAC while waiting for labs.
- All patients with acetaminophen liver injury (even after 8 hours) should receive NAC.

ACL INJURY
Kylee Eagles, DO • J. Herbert Stevenson, MD

 BASICS

DESCRIPTION
- The anterior cruciate ligament (ACL) is a major stabilizer of the knee:
  - It prevents excessive anterior translation and internal rotation of the tibia in relation to the femur.
  - During dynamic movement, the ACL and posterior cruciate ligament (PCL) work together to stabilize the knee.
- ACL injuries are common and can occur through noncontact or contact mechanisms. >70% of ACL injuries are caused by noncontact forces (1).
- Partial tears of the ACL can occur, but complete tears are far more common.
- Female athletes are at 2–5 times higher risk of ACL tear, particularly in soccer, basketball, and skiing.
- ACL injury is associated with early onset of knee osteoarthritis, regardless of surgical or nonsurgical treatment (2)[B].

EPIDEMIOLOGY
Incidence
- 250,000 ACL injuries annually in the US (1)
- Female athletes incidence 2–5-fold > male athletes
- Greater incidence of noncontact ACL injuries in sports requiring cutting, pivoting, and rapid deceleration, such as basketball and soccer

Prevalence
- Young athletes aged 15–25 years sustain >50% of all ACL injuries.
- >2/3 of patients with complete ACL tear have associated menisci and/or articular cartilage injury (1).

Pediatric Considerations
- Rule out physeal injuries in the skeletally immature.
- The incidence of ACL tears in patients with open physes has increased in recent years.
- ACL injury rates increase for both boys and girls beginning at age 11 years.

ETIOLOGY AND PATHOPHYSIOLOGY
- Noncontact mechanisms (torsional or hyperextension forces)
- Direct trauma (player, object on playing field), most often a valgus blow to the knee

Genetics
Familial tendency has been identified.

RISK FACTORS
- Female athletes have increased risk likely due to multiple variables.
  - Sex hormones:
    - Increased rate may be due to monthly hormonal fluctuations.
    - No conclusive evidence links a menstrual cycle phase to ACL injury risk.
  - Anatomic gender differences:
    - Increased Q angle, increased genu valgum, narrower femoral notch size, smaller ACL
    - Neuromuscular imbalances (increased quadriceps activation, decreased hamstring activity during landings)
  - Movement patterns (sudden deceleration, change-of-direction cutting movements, landing from a jump in hyperextension)

GENERAL PREVENTION
- Neuromuscular training with proprioceptive, plyometric, and strength exercises may reduce noncontact ACL injuries by 72% in female athletes if performed more than once per week for >6 weeks (1,3)[B].
- No evidence shows that prophylactic knee bracing prevents ACL injuries.
- Educate the patient about possible risk factors for ACL injury and provide instruction on neuromuscular training exercises.

COMMONLY ASSOCIATED CONDITIONS
- Meniscal tear
- Collateral ligament tear
- PCL tear
- Tibia or femur fractures
- Osteochondral injury
- Loose bodies
- Early-onset degenerative joint disease

 DIAGNOSIS

HISTORY
May recall mechanism:
- Noncontact:
  - Sudden deceleration
  - Cutting, sudden change in direction
  - Landing from a jump in extension
- Contact with player, object
- May recall sudden pop or snap
- Sudden pain and giving way
- Marked effusion/hemarthrosis within 4–12 hours

PHYSICAL EXAM
- Inspect for malalignment (fracture, dislocation)
- Pain
- Palpate for effusion
- Decreased range of motion (ROM)
  - Deficits may be secondary to pain, effusion, mechanical blocks (meniscal tear, loose body, torn ACL stump).
- Joint instability
- Difficulty bearing weight
- Evaluate extensor mechanism integrity

DIFFERENTIAL DIAGNOSIS
- Fracture
- Meniscal injury
- Patellar dislocation/subluxation
- Tendon disruption
- PCL injury
- Collateral ligament injury

DIAGNOSTIC TESTS & INTERPRETATION
Initial Tests (lab, imaging)
- Lachman test: Most sensitive and highly specific diagnostic test for ACL injury, especially in acute setting (4)[A]:
  - Knee placed in 20–30 degrees of flexion. Tibia is translated anteriorly while the femur is stabilized with the opposite hand. Increased anterior translation compared with uninjured knee indicates injury. Lack of a solid endpoint indicates rupture.
- Pivot shift test: Lower sensitivity, but more specific for ACL tear than Lachman test (4)[B]:
  - Knee placed in extension. Knee is flexed while applying a valgus and internal rotation stress. A positive test is subluxation at 20–40 degrees of flexion.
- Anterior drawer test:
  - Low sensitivity for ACL integrity, especially in acute setting (4)[A]
- Posterior drawer test assesses PCL integrity.
- McMurray test assesses for meniscal tears.
- Valgus/Varus stress test for medial collateral ligament/lateral collateral (MCL/LCL) integrity
- Radiographs to rule out associated bony injury
- Anterior-posterior (AP), lateral, and tunnel views:
  - Segond fracture: Avulsion fracture of the lateral capsular margin of the tibia
  - Tibial eminence avulsion fracture
  - Fracture of proximal tibia or distal femur
  - Osteochondral injuries

Follow-Up Tests & Special Considerations
- MRI is the gold standard for imaging ligamentous and intra-articular structures; MRI may show secondary signs of ACL injury. The sensitivity of MRI is 87–94%, specificity 88–93% (5).
- Secondary signs include: Bone contusion of the anterior femoral condyle and/or posterior tibial plateau, anterior translation of the tibia, an uncovered or displaced posterior horn of the lateral meniscus, PCL buckling, or a Segond fracture (an avulsion fracture of the lateral tibial condyle).

Diagnostic Procedures/Other
Surgical management should be considered in the active population, young or old.

 TREATMENT

GENERAL MEASURES
- Acute injury: PRICEMM therapy: Protection, Relative rest, Ice, Compression, Elevation, Medications, Modalities
- Crutches may be indicated until patient is able to ambulate without pain.
- Locked knee brace may be used initially for comfort. Use with caution and transition to a hinged knee brace as soon as possible. Quadriceps atrophy and stiffness develop quickly.
- Aspiration of large effusion may be indicated to alleviate pain and increase ROM.

MEDICATION
First Line
- NSAIDs:
  - Acute ligament sprains:
    - Ibuprofen: 200–800 mg t.i.d.
    - Naproxen: 375–500 mg b.i.d.
    - Indomethacin: 25–50 mg t.i.d.
- Acetaminophen: 3–4 g/d
- Narcotics for severe pain (e.g., acetaminophen-hydrocodone)
- Contraindications/Precautions/Interactions: Refer to the manufacturer's profile of each drug.

ISSUES FOR REFERRAL
Surgical management should be considered in the active population.
- Physical therapy is recommended whether an athlete chooses nonsurgical or surgical treatment. Nonsurgical physical therapy is focused on restoring ROM, strength, and proprioception.
- Preoperative phase:
  - Increase ROM and quad strength, minimize inflammation
- Early postoperative phase: Weeks 2–4:
  - ROM: Full extension is the most important goal. Rehabilitation begins immediately.
  - Progress to full weight bearing.
- Intermediate postoperative phase: Weeks 4–12:
  - ROM: Full flexion, hyperextension
  - Quadriceps and hamstring strengthening proprioceptive training, normalize gait
- Late postop phase: >3 months postop:
  - Straight-line running
  - Increase speed, duration over 6–8 weeks.
  - Progress to cutting and sport-specific drills.
  - Strength and proprioceptive training (6,7).

Geriatric Considerations
Management is based on anticipated activity level, associated injuries, coexisting medical conditions, and acute vs. long-standing ACL deficiency.

SURGERY/OTHER PROCEDURES
- Surgical vs. conservative management depends on patient's activity level, age, associated injuries, and presence of osteoarthritis.
- Insufficient evidence for ACL reconstructive surgery vs. conservative management in the skeletally immature patient
- Insufficient evidence from randomized trials comparing surgical vs. nonoperative management of ACL injuries in adults based on studies in the 1980s (8)[A]
- In young, active adults with acute ACL tears, rehabilitation plus early ACL repair was not superior to a strategy of initial rehabilitation with delayed repair if rehab alone failed. In fact, the latter strategy led to an overall reduction of ACL reconstructions (9)[A].

- Reconstruction techniques:
  - Bone-patella tendon-bone autograft
  - Hamstring autograft
  - Allograft tendon (from cadaver)
- No consistent significant differences in outcome between patellar tendon and hamstring tendon autografts (10)[A]
- Concomitant meniscal tears are repaired at the time of ACL reconstruction.

IN-PATIENT CONSIDERATIONS
Admission Criteria/Initial Stabilization
Outpatient

 ## ONGOING CARE

FOLLOW-UP RECOMMENDATIONS
- ROM exercises to regain full flexion and extension
- Advance activity as tolerated.

Patient Monitoring
Assess functional status, rehabilitative exercise compliance, and pain control at follow-up visit.

PROGNOSIS
- Athletes typically are out of competitive play for 6–9 months after injury to undergo ACL reconstructive surgery and rehabilitation.
- High prevalence of OA, even in those with early ACL reconstruction (2)[B]
- Delay of surgical reconstruction of torn ACL raises risk of secondary meniscal injury

COMPLICATIONS
- Instability
- Secondary meniscal and articular cartilage injury
- Early-onset degenerative arthritis
- Surgical risks:
  - Infection, pulmonary embolism (PE), subsequent ACL graft rupture, laxity due to failure of graft remodeling

REFERENCES

1. Silvers HJ, Mandelbaum BR. Prevention of anterior cruciate ligament injury in the female athlete. *Br J Sports Med.* 2007;41(Suppl 1):i52–i59.
2. Christiansen BA, Anderson MJ, Lee CA, et al. Musculoskeletal changes following non-invasive knee injury using a novel mouse model of post-traumatic osteoarthritis. *Osteoarthr Cartil.* 2012;20(7):773–782. Epub 2012 Apr 21.
3. Hewett TE, Ford KR, Myer GD. Anterior cruciate ligament injuries in female athletes: Part 2, a meta-analysis of neuromuscular interventions aimed at injury prevention. *Am J Sports Med.* 2006;34:490–498.
4. Jain DK, Amaravati R, Sharma G. Evaluation of the clinical signs of anterior cruciate ligament and meniscal injuries. *Indian J Orthop.* 2009;43(4):375–378.
5. Vincken PW, ter Braak BP, van Erkell AR, et al. Effectiveness of MR imaging in selection of patients for arthroscopy of the knee. *Radiology.* 2002;223(3):739–746.
6. White K, Di Stasi SL, Smith AH, et al. Anterior cruciate ligament- specialized post-operative return-to-sports (ACL-SPORTS) training: A randomized control trial. *BMC Musculoskelet Disord.* 2013;14:108.
7. Hewett TE, Di Stasi SL, Myer GD. Current concepts for injury prevention in athletes after anterior cruciate ligament reconstruction. *Am J Sports Med.* 2013;41(1):216–224.
8. Linko E, Harilainen A, Malmivaara A, et al. Surgical versus conservative interventions for anterior cruciate ligament rupture in adults. *Cochrane Database Syst Rev.* 2005;Issue 4.
9. Frobell RB, Roos EM, Roos HP, et al. A randomized trial of treatment for acute anterior cruciate ligament tears. *N Engl J Med.* 2010; 363(4):331–342.
10. Mohtadi NG, Chan DS, Dainty KN, et al. Patellar tendon versus hamstring tendon autograft for anterior cruciate ligament rupture in adults. *Cochrane Database Syst Rev.* 2011;(9): CD005960. Epub 2011 Sep 7.

ADDITIONAL READING
- Cascio BM, Culp L, Cosgarea AJ. Return to play after anterior cruciate ligament reconstruction. *Clin Sports Med.* 2004;23(3):395–408, ix.
- Spindler KP, Kuhn JE, Freedman KB, et al. Anterior cruciate ligament reconstruction autograft choice: Bone-tendon-bone versus hamstring: does it really matter? A systematic review. *Am J Sports Med.* 2004;32(8):1986–1995.

 ## SEE ALSO

Algorithm: Knee pain

 ## CODES

ICD10
- S83.519A Sprain of anterior cruciate ligament of unsp knee, init
- S83.519D Sprain of anterior cruciate ligament of unsp knee, subs
- S83.519S Sprain of anterior cruciate ligament of unsp knee, sequela

CLINICAL PEARLS
- Lachman test is the most sensitive and highly specific diagnostic test for ACL injury, especially in acute setting (4)[A].
- Pivot shift test is less sensitive but more specific for ACL tear than the Lachman test (4)[B].
- Anterior drawer test has low sensitivity for ACL integrity, especially in acute setting (4)[A].
- Bone contusion of the anterior femoral condyle and/or posterior tibial plateau on MRI is highly suggestive of ACL tear even if it appears intact on imaging.
- 2/3 of complete ACL tears have associated meniscal or articular injuries.

ACNE ROSACEA

Adarsh K. Gupta, DO, MS, FACOFP

 ## BASICS

DESCRIPTION
- Rosacea is a chronic condition characterized by recurrent episodes of facial flushing, erythema (due to dilatation of small blood vessels in the face), papules, pustules, and telangiectasia (due to increased reactivity of capillaries) in a symmetrical, facial distribution. Sometimes associated with ocular symptoms (ocular rosacea).
- System(s) affected: Skin/Exocrine
- Synonym(s): Rosacea

Geriatric Considerations
- Uncommon >60 years of age
- Effects of aging might increase the side effects associated with oral isotretinoin (at present, data are insufficient due to lack of clinical studies in elderly patients ≥65)

EPIDEMIOLOGY
Prevalence
- Predominant age: 30–50 years
- Predominant sex: Female > Male. However, males are at greater risk for progression to later stages.

ETIOLOGY AND PATHOPHYSIOLOGY
- No proven cause
- Possibilities include:
  – Thyroid and sex hormone disturbance
  – Alcohol, coffee, tea, spiced food overindulgence (unproven)
  – Demodex follicular parasite (suspected)
  – Exposure to cold, heat, hot drinks
  – Emotional stress
  – Dysfunction of the GI tract

Genetics
People of Northern European and Celtic background commonly afflicted

RISK FACTORS
- Exposure to cold, heat, hot drinks
- Environmental trigger factors: Sun, wind, cold

GENERAL PREVENTION
No preventive measures known

COMMONLY ASSOCIATED CONDITIONS
- Seborrheic dermatitis of scalp and eyelids
- Keratitis with photophobia, lacrimation, visual disturbance
- Corneal lesions
- Blepharitis
- Uveitis

 ## DIAGNOSIS

HISTORY
- Usually have a history of episodic flushing with increases in skin temperature in response to heat stimulus in mouth (hot liquids), spicy foods, alcohol, sun (solar elastosis).
- Acne may have preceded onset of rosacea by years; nevertheless, rosacea usually arises de novo without preceding history of acne or seborrhea.
- Excessive facial warmth and redness are the predominant presenting complaints. Itching is generally absent.

PHYSICAL EXAM
- Rosacea has typical stages of evolution:
  – The rosacea diathesis: Episodic erythema, "flushing and blushing"
  – Stage I: Persistent erythema with telangiectases
  – Stage II: Persistent erythema, telangiectases, papules, tiny pustules
  – Stage III: Persistent deep erythema, dense telangiectases, papules, pustules, nodules; rarely persistent "solid" edema of the central part of the face (phymatous)
- Facial erythema, particularly on cheeks, nose, and chin. At times, entire face may be involved.

- Inflammatory papules are prominent; pustules and telangiectasia may be present.
- Comedones are absent (unlike acne).
- Women usually have lesions on the chin and cheeks, whereas nose is commonly involved in men.
- Ocular findings (mild dryness and irritation with blepharitis, conjunctival injection, burning, stinging, tearing, eyelid inflammation, swelling, and redness) are present in 50% of patients.

DIFFERENTIAL DIAGNOSIS
- Drug eruptions (iodides and bromides)
- Granulomas of the skin
- Cutaneous lupus erythematosus
- Carcinoid syndrome
- Deep fungal infection
- Acne vulgaris
- Seborrheic dermatitis
- Steroid rosacea (abuse)
- Systemic lupus erythematosus

DIAGNOSTIC TESTS & INTERPRETATION
Diagnosis is based on physical exam findings.

Test Interpretation
- Inflammation around hypertrophied sebaceous glands, producing papules, pustules, and cysts
- Absence of comedones and blocked ducts
- Vascular dilation and dermal lymphocytic infiltrate

 ## TREATMENT

GENERAL MEASURES
- Use of mild, nondrying soap is recommended; local skin irritants should be avoided.
- Reassurance that rosacea is completely unrelated to poor hygiene
- Treat psychological stress if present.
- Avoid oil-based cosmetics:
  – Others are acceptable and may help women tolerate symptoms.
- Electrodesiccation or chemical sclerosis of permanently dilated blood vessels
- Cyclosporine 0.05% ophthalmic emulsion may be more effective than artificial tears for rosacea of the eyes (1).
- Possible evolving laser therapy
- Support physical fitness

MEDICATION

First Line

- Topical metronidazole preparations once or twice daily for 7–12 weeks was significantly more effective than placebo in patients with moderate to severe rosacea (1)[A]. A rosacea treatment system (cleanser, metronidazole 0.75% gel, hydrating complexion corrector, and sunscreen SPF30) may offer superior efficacy and tolerability to metronidazole (2).
- Azelaic acid (Finacea) with oral doxycycline is very effective as initial therapy; azelaic acid topical alone is effective for maintenance (3)[A].
- Doxycycline 40-mg dose is at least as effective as 100-mg dose and has a correspondingly lower risk of adverse effects (1), but is much more expensive.
- Precautions: Tetracycline may cause photosensitivity; sunscreen is recommended.
- Significant possible interactions:
  - Tetracycline: Avoid concurrent administration with antacids, dairy products, or iron.
  - Broad-spectrum antibiotics: May reduce the effectiveness of oral contraceptives; barrier method is recommended.

Pediatric Considerations

Tetracycline: Not for use in children <8 years

Pregnancy Considerations

- Tetracycline: Not for use during pregnancy
- Isotretinoin: Teratogenic; not for use during pregnancy or in women of reproductive age who are not using reliable contraception

Second Line

- Topical erythromycin
- Topical clindamycin lotion preferred
- Possible utility of calcineurin inhibitors (tacrolimus 0.1%; pimecrolimus 0.1%). Pimecrolimus 1% is effective to treat mild to moderate inflammatory rosacea (4).
- Permethrin 5% cream (5)[A]; similar efficacy compared to metronidazole
- Topical steroids should not be used, as they may aggravate rosacea.
- For severe cases, isotretinoin PO for 4 months

ADDITIONAL THERAPIES

Surgery/Other Procedures

Laser treatment is an option for progressive telangiectasias or rhinophyma.

 ONGOING CARE

FOLLOW-UP RECOMMENDATIONS

Outpatient treatment

Patient Monitoring

- Occasional and as needed
- Close follow-up for women using isotretinoin

DIET

Avoid alcohol, excessive sun exposure, and hot drinks of any type.

PROGNOSIS

- Slowly progressive
- Subsides spontaneously (sometimes)

COMPLICATIONS

- Rhinophyma (dilated follicles and thickened bulbous skin on nose), especially in men
- Conjunctivitis
- Blepharitis
- Keratitis
- Visual deterioration

REFERENCES

1. van Zuuren EJ, Kramer SF, Carter BR, et al. Effective and evidence-based management strategies for rosacea: Summary of a Cochrane systematic review. *Br J Dermatol*. 2011;165(4):760–781. Epub 2011 Sep 15.
2. Leyden JJ. Efficacy of a novel rosacea treatment system: An investigator-blind, randomized, parallel-group study. *J Drugs Dermatol*. 2011; 10(10):1179–1185.
3. Thiboutot DM, Fleischer AB, Del Rosso JQ, et al. A multicenter study of topical azelaic acid 15% gel in combination with oral doxycycline as initial therapy and azelaic acid 15% gel as maintenance monotherapy. *J Drugs Dermatol*. 2009;8:639–648.
4. Kim MB, Kim GW, Park HJ, et al. Pimecrolimus 1% cream for the treatment of rosacea. *J Dermatol*. 2011;38(12):1135–1139. Epub 2011 Sep 28.
5. Koçak M, Yali S, Vahapoolu G, et al. Permethrin 5% cream versus metronidazole 0.75% gel for the treatment of papulopustular rosacea. A randomized double-blind placebo-controlled study. *Dermatology*. 2002;205:265–270.

ADDITIONAL READING

- Del Rosso JQ, Webster GF, Jackson M, et al. Two randomized phase III clinical trials evaluating anti-inflammatory dose doxycycline (40-mg doxycycline, USP capsules) administered once daily for treatment of rosacea. *J Am Acad Dermatol*. 2007;56:791–802.
- Liu RH, Smith MK, Basta SA, et al. Azelaic acid in the treatment of papulopustular rosacea: A systematic review of randomized controlled trials. *Arch Dermatol*. 2006;142:1047–1052.

 SEE ALSO

- Acne Vulgaris; Blepharitis; Dermatitis, Seborrheic; Lupus Erythematosus, Discoid; Uveitis
- Algorithm: Acne

 CODES

ICD10

L71.9 Rosacea, unspecified

CLINICAL PEARLS

- Rosacea usually arises de novo without any preceding history of acne or seborrhea.
- Rosacea may cause chronic eye symptoms, including blepharitis.
- Avoid alcohol, sun exposure, and hot drinks.
- Medication treatment resembles that of acne vulgaris, with oral and topical antibiotics.

ACNE VULGARIS

Gary I. Levine, MD

BASICS

DESCRIPTION
- Acne vulgaris is a disorder of the pilosebaceous units. It is a chronic inflammatory dermatosis notable for open/closed comedones, papules, pustules, or nodules.
- System(s) affected: Skin/Exocrine

Geriatric Considerations
Favre-Racouchot syndrome: Comedones on face and head due to sun exposure

Pregnancy Considerations
- May result in a flare or remission of acne
- Erythromycin can be used in pregnancy; use topical agents when possible.
- Isotretinoin is teratogenic; Class X
- Avoid topical tretinoin, although no good evidence exists that its use is teratogenic; Class C
- Contraindicated: Isotretinoin, tazarotene, tetracycline, doxycycline, minocycline

Pediatric Considerations
- Neonatal acne (neonatal cephalic pustulosis) (1):
  – Newborn to 8 weeks, lesions limited to face
- Infantile acne:
  – Newborn to 1 year, lesions on face, neck, back, and chest
- Early childhood acne:
  – 1–7 years; rare, consider underlying hormonal pathology
- Preadolescent acne:
  – 7–11 years; common, 47% of children, usually due to adrenal awakening
- Do not use tetracyclines <8 years of age

EPIDEMIOLOGY
- Predominant age: Early to late puberty, may persist into 4th decade
- Predominant sex:
  – Male > Female (adolescence)
  – Female > Male (adult)

Prevalence
- 80–95% of adolescents affected. A smaller percentage will seek medical advice.
- 8% of adults aged 25–34; 3% at 35–44 years

ETIOLOGY AND PATHOPHYSIOLOGY
- Androgens (testosterone and dehydroepiandrosterone sulfate [DHEA]) stimulate sebum production and proliferation of keratinocytes in hair follicles.
- Keratin plug obstructs follicle os, causing sebum accumulation and follicular distention.
- *Propionibacterium acnes*, an anaerobe, colonizes and proliferates in the plugged follicle.
- *P. acnes* promote chemotactic factors and proinflammatory mediators, causing inflammation of follicle and dermis.

Genetics
- Familial association in 50%
- If a family history exists, the acne may be more severe and occur earlier.

RISK FACTORS
- Increased endogenous androgenic effect
- Oily cosmetics
- Rubbing or occluding skin surface (e.g., sports equipment such as helmets and shoulder pads), telephone, or hands against the skin

- Polyvinyl chloride, chlorinated hydrocarbons, cutting oil, tars
- Numerous drugs, including androgenic steroids (e.g., steroid abuse, some birth control pills)
- Endocrine disorders: Polycystic ovarian syndrome, Cushing syndrome, congenital adrenal hyperplasia, androgen-secreting tumors, acromegaly
- Stress
- High glycemic load diets and milk may exacerbate acne.
- Severe acne may worsen with smoking

COMMONLY ASSOCIATED CONDITIONS
- Acne Fulminans, Pyoderma faciale
- Acne Conglobata, Hidradenitis suppurativa
- Pomade acne
- SAPHO syndrome: synovitis, acne pustulosis
- PAPA syndrome: Pyogenic sterile arthritis, pyoderma gangrenosum, cystic acne
- Behçet syndrome, Apert syndrome
- Dark-skinned patients: 50% keloidal scarring and 50% acne hyperpigmented macules

DIAGNOSIS

HISTORY
- Ask about duration, medications, cleansing products, stress, smoking, exposures, diet, family history.
- Females may worsen prior to menses.

PHYSICAL EXAM
- Closed comedones (whiteheads)
- Open comedones (blackheads)
- Nodules or papules
- Pustules ("cysts")
- Scars: Ice pick, rolling, boxcar, atrophic macules, hypertrophic, depressed, sinus tracts
- Grading system (American Academy of Dermatology, 1990):
  – Mild: Few papules/pustules; no nodules
  – Moderate: Some papules/pustules; few nodules
  – Severe: Numerous papules/pustules; many nodules
  – Very severe: Acne conglobata, acne fulminans, acne inversa.
- Most common areas affected are face, chest, back, and upper arms (areas of greatest concentration of sebaceous glands).

DIFFERENTIAL DIAGNOSIS
- Folliculitis: Gram negative and gram positive
- Acne (rosacea, cosmetica, steroid-induced)
- Perioral dermatitis
- Chloracne
- Pseudofolliculitis barbae
- Drug eruption
- Verruca vulgaris and plana
- Keratosis pilaris
- Molluscum contagiosum
- Sarcoidosis
- Seborrheic dermatitis
- Miliaria

DIAGNOSTIC TESTS & INTERPRETATION
Initial Tests (lab, imaging)
Only indicated if additional signs of androgen excess; if so: Free testosterone, DHEA-sulfate (DHEA-S), LH and FSH (2)[A]

TREATMENT

- Comedonal (grade 1): Keratolytic agent (3)[A]
- Moderate inflammatory acne (grade 3): Add systemic antibiotic to grade 2 regimen.
- Mild inflammatory acne (grade 2): Benzoyl peroxide ± topical antibiotic. Keratolytic if needed.
- Topical retinoid plus a topical antimicrobial agent is first-line treatment (4) for more than mild disease.
- Topical retinoid + antibiotic (topical or PO) is better than either alone for mild/moderate acne (3)[A].
- Topical retinoids are first-line agents for maintenance. Avoid long-term antibiotics for maintenance.
- Severe inflammatory acne (grade 4): As in grade 3, or isotretinoin (3)[A]
- Recommended vehicle type:
  – Dry or sensitive skin: Cream or ointment
  – Oily skin, humid weather: Gel, solution, pledget, or wash
  – Hair-bearing areas: Lotion, hydrogel, or foam
- Apply topical agents to entire affected area, not just visible lesions.
- Mild soap daily to control oiliness; avoid abrasives
- Avoid drying agents with keratolytic agents.
- Gentle cleanser and noncomedogenic moisturizer helps decrease irritation.
- Oil-free, noncomedogenic sunscreens
- Stress management if acne flares with stress

MEDICATION

ALERT
Most prescription topical medications are expensive. Review cost.
- Keratolytic agents (alpha-hydroxy acids, salicylic acid, azelaic acid)(side effects include dryness, erythema, scaling, and photosensitivity; start with lower strength; increase as tolerated) (2,3)[A].
- Tretinoin (Retin-A, Retin A Micro, Avita): Apply at bedtime; wash skin and let skin dry 30 minutes before topical application:
  – Retin-A Micro and Avita are less irritating; produce less phototoxicity.
  – May cause an initial flare of lesions; may be eased by 14-day course of oral antibiotics.
- Adapalene (Differin): 0.1%, apply topically at night:
  – Effective; less irritation than tretinoin or tazarotene (3)[A]
  – May be combined with benzoyl peroxide.
- Tazarotene (Tazorac): Apply at bedtime:
  – Most effective and most irritating; teratogenic
- Azelaic acid (Azelex, Finevin): 20% topically, b.i.d.:
  – Keratolytic, antibacterial, anti-inflammatory
  – Reduces postinflammatory hyperpigmentation in dark-skinned individuals
  – Side effects: Erythema, dryness, scaling, hypopigmentation
  – Less effective in clinical use than in studies
- Salicylic acid: 2%, less effective and less irritating than tretinoin
- Alpha-hydroxy acids: Available over-the-counter

- Topical antibiotics and anti-inflammatorie:
  – Topical benzoyl peroxide:
    ○ 2.5% as effective as stronger preparations
    ○ Gel penetrates better into follicles
    ○ When used with tretinoin, apply benzoyl peroxide in morning and tretinoin at night
    ○ Side effects: Irritation; may bleach clothes
- Topical antibiotics (2,3)[A]:
  – Erythromycin 2%
  – Clindamycin 1%
  – Metronidazole gel or cream: Apply once daily.
  – Azelaic acid (Azelex, Finevin): 20% cream: Enhanced effect and decreased risk of resistance when used with zinc and benzoyl peroxide
  – Benzoyl peroxide-erythromycin (Benzamycin): Especially effective with azelaic acid
  – Benzoyl peroxide-clindamycin (BenzaClin, DUAC, Clindoxyl)
  – Benzoyl peroxide-salicylic acid (Cleanse & Treat, Inova): Similar in effectiveness to benzoyl peroxide-clindamycin
  – Sodium sulfacetamide (Sulfacet-R, Novacet, Klaron): Useful in acne with seborrheic dermatitis or rosacea
  – Dapsone (Aczone) 5% gel: May cause yellow/orange skin discoloration when mixed with benzoyl peroxide
- Oral antibiotics (2,3)[A]: Use for at least 6–8 weeks after initiation, discontinue after 12–18 weeks duration; indicated when acne is more severe, trunk involvement, unresponsive to topical agents, or at greater risk for scarring
  – Tetracycline: 500–2,000 mg/d divided b.i.d.–q.i.d.; high dose initially, taper in 6 months, as tolerated (3). Side effects: Photosensitivity, esophagitis
  – Minocycline: 50–200 mg/d, divided daily–b.i.d.; side effects include photosensitivity, urticaria, gray-blue skin, vertigo, autoimmune hepatitis (2)[A],(5).
  – Doxycycline: 50–200 mg/d, divided daily– b.i.d.; side effects include photosensitivity.
  – Erythromycin: 500–1,000 mg/d; divided b.i.d.–q.i.d.; decreasing effectiveness as a result of increasing *P. acnes* resistance
  – Trimethoprim-sulfamethoxazole (Bactrim DS, Septra DS): 1 daily or b.i.d.
  – Azithromycin (Zithromax): 500 mg 3 days/week × 1 month, then 250 mg every other day × 2 months
- Oral retinoids:
  – Isotretinoin (2,3)[A]: 0.5–1.0 mg/kg/d divided b.i.d to max 2.0 mg/kg/d divided b.i.d for very severe disease; 60–90% cure rate; usually given for 12–20 weeks; maximum cumulative dose = 120–150 mg/kg; 20% of patients relapse and require retreatment:
    ○ Side effects: Highly teratogenic, pancreatitis, hypertriglyceridemia, hepatitis, blood dyscrasias, hyperostosis, premature epiphyseal closure, night blindness, erythema multiforme, Stevens-Johnson syndrome, suicidal ideation, psychosis
    ○ Avoid tetracyclines or vitamin A preparations during Isotretinoin therapy.
    ○ Monitor for pregnancy, CBC, lipids, and liver function tests at baseline and every month.
    ○ Should be registered member of manufacturer's iPLEDGE program; (www.ipledgeprogram.com)

- Isotretinoin is teratogenic; Class X.
- Medications for women only:
  – Oral contraceptives (2,3)[A]:
    ○ Norgestimate/Ethinyl estradiol (OrthoTricyclen), norethindrone acetate/ethinyl estradiol (Estrostep), drospirenone/ethinyl estradiol (Yaz, Yasmin) are approved by US FDA for this indication.
    ○ Levonorgestrel/Ethinyl estradiol (Alesse) and most combined contraceptives effective.
  – Spironolactone (Aldactone); 25–200 mg/d; antiandrogen; reduces sebum production
  – Flutamide (Eulexin) 250–500 mg/d; hepatotoxic

ISSUES FOR REFERRAL
Consider referral/consultation to dermatologist:
- Refractory lesions despite appropriate therapy
- Consideration of isotretinoin therapy
- Management of acne scars

ADDITIONAL THERAPIES
- Acne hyperpigmented macules:
  – Topical hydroquinones (1.5–10%)
  – Azelaic acid (20%) topically
  – Topical retinoids as, above
  – Corticosteroids: Low dose, suppresses adrenal androgens (2)[B]
  – Dapsone 5% gel (Aczone): Topical, anti-inflammatory use in patients >12 years
- Light-based treatments:
  – Ultraviolet A/Ultraviolet B (UVA/UVB), blue or blue/red light, pulse dye laser, KTP laser, infrared laser
  – Photodynamic therapy for 30–60 minutes with 5-aminolevulinic acid × 3 sessions is effective for inflammatory lesions:
    ○ Greatest utility when used as adjunct to medications or if can't tolerate medications

SURGERY/OTHER PROCEDURES
- Comedo extraction after incising the layer of epithelium over closed comedo (2)[C]
- Inject large cystic lesions with 0.05–0.3 mL triamcinolone (Kenalog 2–5 mg/mL); use 30-g needle to inject and slightly distend cyst (2)[C].
- Acne scar treatment: Retinoids, steroid injections, cryosurgery, electrodessication, micro/dermabrasion, chemical peels, laser resurfacing

COMPLEMENTARY AND ALTERNATIVE MEDICINE
- Topical tea tree oil is effective, slow onset (2)[B].
- Nicotinamide 4% gel (Nicam): As effective as clindamycin in moderate inflammatory acne

 ## ONGOING CARE

FOLLOW-UP RECOMMENDATIONS
Use oral or topical antibiotics for 3 months; taper as inflammatory lesions resolve Do not use topical and oral antibiotic together.

Patient Monitoring
- Pretreatment and monthly lipids, liver function tests, and pregnancy tests when on isotretinoin
- Consider antibiotic resistance (60% overall) or gram-negative folliculitis if treatment fails.

DIET
Special diets do not diminish acne (2)[B].

PATIENT EDUCATION
- There may be a worsening of acne during first 2 weeks of treatment.
- Results are typically seen after a minimum of 4 weeks of treatment

PROGNOSIS
Gradual improvement over time (usually within 8–12 weeks after beginning therapy)

COMPLICATIONS
- Acne conglobata: Severe confluent inflammatory acne with systemic symptoms
- Facial scarring and psychological distress
- Gram-negative folliculitis: Superinfection due to long-term oral antibiotic use; treatment with ampicillin, trimethoprim-sulfa, or isotretinoin

REFERENCES
1. Williams HC, Dellavalle RP, Garner S. Acne vulgaris. *Lancet* 2012;379(9813):361–372.
2. Strauss JS, Krowchuk DP, Leyden JJ, et al. Guidelines of care for acne vulgaris management. *J Am Acad Dermatol*. 2007;56:651–663.
3. Titus S, Hodge J. Diagnosis and treatment of acne. *Am Fam Physician*. 2012;86(8):734–740.
4. Thiboutot D, Gollnick H, Bettoli V, et al. New insights into the management of acne: An update from the Global Alliance to Improve Outcomes in Acne Group. *J Am Acad Dermatol*. 2009; 60(5 Suppl):S1–S50.
5. Leyden JJ, Del Rosso JQ, Webster GF, et al. Clinical considerations in the treatment of acne vulgaris and other inflammatory skin disorders: A status report. *Dermatol Clin*. 2009;27:1–15.

ADDITIONAL READING
- Del Rosso JQ, Kim G. Optimizing use of oral antibiotics in acne vulgaris. *Dermatol Clin*. 2009;27:33–42.
- Heymann WR. Oral contraceptives for the treatment of acne vulgaris. *J Am Acad Dermatol*. 2007;56: 1056–1057.

 ## SEE ALSO

- Acne Rosacea
- Algorithm: Acne

CODES

ICD10
L70.0 Acne vulgaris

CLINICAL PEARLS

- Expect worsening for the first 2 weeks of treatment. Full results take 8–12 weeks.
- Decrease topical frequency from b.i.d. to every day or to every other day for irritation.

ACOUSTIC NEUROMA

Mary Lauren Worthen, MD • David Worthen • Adrian Worthen

BASICS

DESCRIPTION
- Acoustic neuromas (vestibular schwannomas) are slow-growing, benign intracranial, extra-axial tumors originating from the vestibulocochlear nerve:
  - Originate from Schwann cells of the nerve sheath
  - Usually arise in the internal auditory canal near the cerebellopontine angle
  - Most are unilateral; bilateral seen in neurofibromatosis type II
- Patients commonly present with hearing loss, tinnitus, and balance dysfunction. Rarely associated facial paralysis, brain stem compression, and even death.

EPIDEMIOLOGY
- 6–10% of all intracranial tumors
- 80–90% of cerebellopontine angle tumors
- 95% of cases are unilateral
- Present most commonly in the 5th–6th decade
- Female predominance
- Bilateral acoustic neuroma occurring in neurofibromatosis II present before age 30

Incidence
- 1/100,000 per year
- Asymptomatic lesions may be more common

Prevalence
3,000 diagnosed annually in the US

ETIOLOGY AND PATHOPHYSIOLOGY
- Compresses local structures rather than invading
- Exerts pressure on the surrounding structures
- Compression of acoustic and facial nerve when located within internal acoustic canal
- Compression of brain stem, 4th ventricle, and trigeminal nerve when tumor at the cerebellar pontine angle
- Vestibular schwannomas are related to the NF2 gene and its product merlin. Merlin acts as a tumor suppressor and as a mediator of contact inhibition. Thus, deficiencies in both NF2 genes lead to vestibular schwannoma development (1).

Genetics
- Unknown for unilateral acoustic neuroma
- Neurofibromatosis type II: Bilateral acoustic neuromas:
  - Autosomal dominant
  - Gene located on chromosome 22q1

RISK FACTORS
- High-dose ionizing radiation.
- Pregnancy and epilepsy may increase risk (2)[C].
- Smoking may decrease the risk (2)[C].
- No proven increase in risk of acoustic neuroma with regular use of a mobile phone (3)[C],(4)[A].

COMMONLY ASSOCIATED CONDITIONS
- Neurofibromatosis type II
- Pregnancy may accelerate the growth of the tumor

DIAGNOSIS

HISTORY
- Common:
  - Sensorineural hearing loss (unilateral), often progressive
  - Loss of speech discrimination
  - Tinnitus
  - Balance problems are common, but vertigo is less common
- Less common:
  - Weakness/loss of facial muscle functions
  - Headache with hydrocephalus and increased intracranial pressure
  - Trigeminal nerve involvement when tumor is large and compressing on cranial nerve V
  - Ataxia due to cerebellar or brain stem compression from large tumor

PHYSICAL EXAM
- Exclude other causes of hearing loss (e.g., middle-ear effusion, infection, wax, cholesteatoma, or tympanic membrane rupture) with otoscopic exam
- Neurologic exam of cranial nerves
- Weber and Rinne tests to confirm sensorineural hearing loss versus conductive hearing loss
- Contralateral ear exam in patients <30 years; suspect neurofibromatosis type II

DIFFERENTIAL DIAGNOSIS
- Cerebellopontine lesions:
  - Meningioma
  - Glioma
  - Facial nerve schwannoma
  - Epidermoid
  - Hemangioma
  - Arachnoid cyst
- Sensorineural hearing loss:
  - Ménière disease
  - Ototoxicity
  - Presbycusis
  - Cerebellar pathology

DIAGNOSTIC TESTS & INTERPRETATION
Initial Tests (lab, imaging)
- MRI with gadolinium (gold standard):
  - 100% specificity
  - Detects tumors starting at 2 mm
  - Tumor has marked enhancement with gadolinium
- Noncontrast T2-weighted fast spin-echo MRI:
  - 98% specificity
  - Less expensive than MRI with gadolinium
- CT:
  - Detect tumors as small as 1 cm
  - Up to 37% false-negative findings
  - Provides good information about surrounding bony structures of the tumor

Diagnostic Procedures/Other
- Pure-tone and speech audiometry (asymmetrical, high-frequency sensorineural hearing loss)
- Speech discrimination
- Stacked auditory brain stem response (ABR): 95% sensitivity and 88% specificity. Can detect tumors <1 cm.
- Standard ABR: Can only detect tumors >1 cm

Test Interpretation
- Well-demarcated and encapsulated mass attached to neural structures without direct invasion
- The mass may be dense or cystic
- Diagnostic microscopy: Densely packed spindle cells (Schwann cells) mixed in with myxoid and collagenous matrix:
  - Zones of alternatively dense and sparse areas of Antoni type A and B patterns of tissue
  - Palisading nuclei (Verocay bodies)
  - S-100 antibody immunoreactivity

TREATMENT

GENERAL MEASURES
- Treatment options include observation, stereotactic radiosurgery, fractionated radiotherapy, and microsurgery (5)[B].
- Without intervention, 16–26% of patients require additional treatment, with 54–63% preserving functional hearing.
- With radiosurgery, only 2–4% of patients require additional treatment and hearing preservation is accomplished in 44–66%.
- With fractionated radiotherapy 3–7% of patients will require additional treatment; hearing preservation is reported at 59–94% of patients, although long-term outcomes are not known.
- Up to 57% of acoustic neuromas may not grow or shrink without treatment (6)[B].
- Up to 70% of extracanalicular tumors may never have a growth rate exceeding 2 mm per year (7)[B].

MEDICATION
A greater understanding of the molecular mechanisms behind vestibular schwannoma tumorigenesis has begun to yield novel therapies. These advances may reduce morbidity and mortality by decreasing tumor burden, tumor volume, hearing loss, and cranial nerve deficits seen in vestibular schwannomas. The following have been suggested therapies (1)[C]:
- Avastin induces regression of progressive schwannomas by >40% and improves hearing.
- An inhibitor of VEGF synthesis, PTC299, is currently in phase II trials as a potential agent to treat vestibular schwannoma.
- In vitro studies have shown that trastuzumab (an ERBB2 inhibitor) reduces vestibular schwannoma cell proliferation.

ISSUES FOR REFERRAL
If an asymptomatic tumor becomes symptomatic, intervention is indicated.

ADDITIONAL THERAPIES
Geriatric Considerations
Conservative management is suitable for elderly patients with contraindications to surgery and radiotherapy:

- Conservative therapy is more likely to preserve hearing than radiotherapy or surgery (8)[C].
- Of patients, 69% with 100% speech discrimination at diagnosis have maintained good hearing, even after 10 years of observation (9)[B].
- Stereotactic radiosurgery:
  - Gamma knife single-dose stereotactic radiosurgery:
    - Performed on an outpatient basis
    - Alternative for those with smaller tumor (<3 cm) or contraindications to microsurgery
    - Shown to have better tumor control rates than conservative management (10)[A]
    - Lower-dose radiation has fewer complications, but unclear whether this is as effective as high-dose radiation in tumor control (11)[A].
    - Higher-dose radiation significantly influences hearing preservation rates (12)[C].
    - Complications (radiation damage): trigeminal, and/or facial nerve neuropathy, hydrocephalus
  - Fractionated stereotactic radiosurgery:
    - Conformal radiation delivers a higher dose of radiation within the tumor and less damage to surrounding healthy tissue.
    - Requires multiple treatments and total radiation dose is higher than single-dose radiation
    - Suitable for all sizes of tumor

SURGERY/OTHER PROCEDURES
- Surgery is recommended definitive treatment (13)[A].
- Lowest rate of recurrence, with up to 97.5% complete tumor removal (13)[A]
- 3 standard operating microscope approaches:
  - Retromastoid/retrosigmoid: Can be used for all acoustic tumors, especially tumors located mostly outside the internal auditory canal and adjacent to the brain stem. May require retraction of cerebellum.
  - Middle cranial fossa: For small tumors with aim of preserving hearing. Involves retraction of temporal lobe and has higher risk of facial nerve injury.
  - Translabyrinthine: For larger tumors. Hearing not preserved. Completely exposes the distal internal auditory canal and has more favorable facial nerve results. A fat graft must be used, with chance of complications, such as infections and bleeding.
  - Transpetrous approaches are safe for acoustic neuroma removal and the postoperative complication rate is low (14)[B].
  - The retrolabyrinthine approach seems to be a good hearing preservative approach, regardless of tumor volume (14).
- Endoscopic approach may be used in some centers
- Surgical complications:
  - Hearing loss
  - CSF leakage
  - Facial nerve injury
  - Headache
  - Meningitis

 ONGOING CARE

FOLLOW-UP RECOMMENDATIONS
- Yearly MRI follow-up for slow-growing tumors is advised.
- MRI and audiometric follow-up for those treated by surgical excision, radiotherapy and conservative management.

Patient Monitoring
- Preoperative practice of physical activity promotes the neuroplasticity of neural networks involved in motor learning, which allows benefit of physical therapy more rapidly and efficiently (15).
- Physical activity allows the implementation of new sensorimotor and behavioral strategies leading to an improvement of balance control.

COMPLICATIONS
Predominantly local pathology due to pressure effects:
- Cranial nerve compression
- Hydrocephalus
- Brain stem compression
- Cerebellar tonsil herniation

REFERENCES

1. Fong B, Barkhoudarian G, Pezeshkian P, et al. The molecular biology and novel treatments of vestibular schwannomas. *J Neurosurg.* 2011; 115(5):906–914. Epub 2011 Jul 29.
2. Schoemaker MJ, Swerdlow AJ, Auvinen A, et al. Medical history, cigarette smoking and risk of acoustic neuroma: An international case-control study. *Int J Cancer.* 2007;120:103–110.
3. INTERPHONE Study Group. Acoustic neuroma risk in relation to mobile telephone use: Results of the INTERPHONE international case-control study. *Cancer Epidemiol.* 2011;35(5):453–464. Epub 2011 Aug 23.
4. Repacholi MH, Lerchl A, Röösli M, et al. Systematic review of wireless phone use and brain cancer and other head tumors. *Bioelectromagnetics.* 2012;33(3):187–206. Epub 2011 Oct 21.
5. Arthurs BJ, Fairbanks RK, Demakas JJ, et al. A review of treatment modalities for vestibular schwannoma. *Neurosurg Rev.* 2011;34(3): 265–277; discussion 277–279. Epub 2011 Feb 9.
6. Smouha EE, Yoo M, Mohr K, et al. Conservative management of acoustic neuroma: A meta-analysis and proposed treatment algorithm. *Laryngoscope.* 2005;115:450–454.
7. Stangerup SE, Caye-Thomasen P, Tos M, et al. The natural history of vestibular schwannoma. *Otol Neurotol.* 2006;27:547–552.
8. Lin VY, Stewart C, Grebenyuk J, et al. Unilateral acoustic neuromas: Long-term hearing results in patients managed with fractionated stereotactic radiotherapy, hearing preservation surgery, and expectantly. *Laryngoscope.* 2005;115:292–296.
9. Stangerup SE, Thomsen J, Tos M, et al. Long-term hearing preservation in vestibular schwannoma. *Otol Neurotol.* 2010;31:271–275.
10. Maniakas A, Saliba I. Conservative management versus stereotactic radiation for vestibular schwannomas: A meta-analysis of patients with more than 5 years' follow-up. *Otol Neurotol.* 2012;33(2):230–238.
11. Battaglia A, Mastrodimos B, Cueva R. Comparison of growth patterns of acoustic neuromas with and without radiosurgery. *Otol Neurotol.* 2006;27:705–712.
12. Combs SE, Welzel T, Schulz-Ertner D, et al. Differences in clinical results after LINAC-based single-dose radiosurgery versus fractionated stereotactic radiotherapy for patients with vestibular schwannomas. *Int Radiat Oncol Biol Phys.* 2010;76:193–200.
13. Weil RS, Cohen JM, Portarena I, et al. Optimal dose of stereotactic radiosurgery for acoustic neuromas: A systematic review. *Br J Neurosurg.* 2006:195–202.
14. Enée V, Guérin J, Bébéar JP, et al. [Acoustic neuroma surgery. Results and complications in 348 cases]. *Rev Laryngol Otol Rhinol (Bord).* 2003;124(1):45–52.
15. Gauchard GC, Parietti-Winkler C, Lion A, et al. Impact of pre-operative regular physical activity on balance control compensation after vestibular schwannoma surgery. *Gait & Posture.* 2013; 37(1):82–87.

 CODES

ICD10
D33.3 Benign neoplasm of cranial nerves

CLINICAL PEARLS
- A bone-anchored hearing aid can improve hearing for those patients with sensorineural hearing loss, which may be present before or after the surgery.
- Conservative management is suitable for elderly patients with contraindications to surgery and radiotherapy.

BASICS

DESCRIPTION

Acute myocardial infarction (AMI) is the rapid development of myocardial necrosis resulting from a sustained and complete absence of blood flow to a portion of the myocardium. ST-segment elevation myocardial infarction (STEMI) occurs when coronary blood flow ceases following thrombotic occlusion of a large coronary artery (usually) affected by atherosclerosis, causing transmural ischemia. This is accompanied by release of serum cardiac biomarkers and ST elevation (and likely a Q wave when infarction occurs) on an ECG.

EPIDEMIOLOGY

Incidence

In the US, estimated annual incidence of MI is 600,000 new and 320,000 recurrent attacks. In 2009, ~683,000 patients were discharged from US hospitals diagnosed with ACS.

Prevalence

- Leading cause of morbidity and mortality in the US
- ~7.5 million people in the US are affected by MI.
- Prevalence increases with age and is higher in men (5.5%) than in women (2.9%).

ETIOLOGY AND PATHOPHYSIOLOGY

- Atherosclerotic coronary artery disease (CAD)
- Nonatherosclerotic:
  - Emboli: For example, thrombi from left ventricle or atrium
  - Mechanical obstruction: Chest trauma, dissection of aorta or coronary arteries
  - Increased vasomotor tone, variant angina
  - Arteritis, others: Hematologic (disseminated intravascular coagulation [DIC]), aortic stenosis, cocaine, IV drug use, severe burns, prolonged hypotension
- Atherosclerotic lesions may be smooth and concentric or rough, eccentric, and fissured. Plaques that are rough and eccentric are more unstable, thrombogenic, and prone to rupture.

RISK FACTORS

Advancing age, hypertension, tobacco use, diabetes mellitus, dyslipidemia, family history of premature onset of CAD, sedentary lifestyle

GENERAL PREVENTION

Smoking cessation, healthy diet, weight control, regular physical activity, maintain goal BP

COMMONLY ASSOCIATED CONDITIONS

Abdominal aortic aneurysm, extracranial cerebrovascular disease, atherosclerotic peripheral vascular disease

DIAGNOSIS

HISTORY

- Classically, sudden-onset of chest heaviness/tightness, with or without exertion, lasting at least minutes
- Pain/discomfort radiating to neck, jaw, interscapular area, upper extremities, and epigastrium
- Previous history of myocardial ischemia (stable or unstable angina, MI, coronary bypass surgery, or percutaneous coronary intervention [PCI])
- Assess risk factors for CAD, history of bleeding, noncardiac surgery, family history of premature CAD.

- Medications: Phosphodiesterase-5 inhibitors (if recent use, avoid concomitant nitrates)
- Alcohol and drug abuse (especially cocaine)

PHYSICAL EXAM

- General: Restless, agitated, hypothermia, fever
- Neurologic: Dizziness, syncope, fatigue, asthenia, disorientation (especially in the elderly)
- Cerebrovascular (CV): Dysrhythmia, hypotension, widened pulse pressure, S_3 and S_4, jugular venous distention (JVD)
- Respiratory: Dyspnea, tachypnea, crackles
- GI: Abdominal pain, nausea, vomiting
- Musculoskeletal: Pain in neck, back, shoulder, or upper limbs
- Skin: Cool skin, pallor, diaphoresis

Geriatric Considerations

Elderly patients may have an atypical presentation, including silent or unrecognized MI, often with complaints of syncope, weakness, shortness of breath, unexplained nausea, epigastric pain, altered mental status, or dementia. Patients with diabetes mellitus may have fewer and less dramatic chest symptoms.

DIFFERENTIAL DIAGNOSIS

Unstable angina, aortic dissection, pulmonary embolism (PE), perforating ulcer, pericarditis, dysrhythmias, gastroesophageal reflux disease (GERD) and spasm, biliary/pancreatic pain, hyperventilation syndrome

DIAGNOSTIC TESTS & INTERPRETATION

ALERT

The third universal definition for MI issued in 2012 by the American College of Cardiology, American Heart Association, European Society of Cardiology, and World Heart Federation revises older definitions of MI. It establishes the level of troponin necessary to diagnose MI in various clinical situations (e.g., after cardiac and noncardiac procedures). According to the definition, an MI diagnosis requires a cardiac troponin (I or T) level above the 99th percentile of a normal reference population, plus one or more of the following:
- Symptoms of ischemia
- New significant ST/T wave changes or left bundle branch block
- Pathologic Q waves on ECG
- New loss of viable myocardium or regional wall motion abnormality, as observed on imaging
- Intracoronary thrombus diagnosed by angiography or autopsy

Initial Tests (lab, imaging)

- Coronary angiography
- 12-lead ECG: ST-segment elevation in a regional pattern ≥1 mm ST elevation, with or without abnormal Q waves. ST depression ± tall R wave in V_1/V_2 may be STEMI of posterior wall. Absence of Q waves represents partial or transient occlusion or early infarction. New ST- or T-wave changes indicative of myocardial ischemia or injury. Consider right-sided and posterior chest leads if inferior MI pattern (examine V_3R, V_4R, V_7-V_9).
- ECG with continuous monitoring:
  - 2-D and M-mode echocardiography is useful in evaluating regional wall motion in MI and left ventricular function.

- Portable echo can clarify diagnosis of STEMI if concomitant left bundle branch block (LBBB).
- Useful in assessing mechanical complications and mural thrombus

Follow-Up Tests & Special Considerations

- Serum biomarkers:
  - Troponin I and T (cTnI, cTnT) rise 3–6 hours after onset of ischemic symptoms. Elevations in cTnI persist for 7–10 days, while those in cTnT persist for 10–14 days after MI.
  - Myoglobin fraction of creatine kinase (CK-MB): Rises 3–4 hours after onset of myocardial injury; peaks at 12–24 hours and remains elevated for 2–3 days. CK-MB adds little diagnostic value in assessment of possible acute coronary syndromes (ACS) to troponin testing.
  - Myoglobin: Early marker for myocardial necrosis. Rises 2 hours after onset of myocardial necrosis, reaches peak at 1–4 hours, and remains elevated for 24 hours. Myoglobin adds little diagnostic value in assessment of possible ACS to troponin testing.
- Fasting lipid profile, CBC with platelets, electrolytes, magnesium, BUN, serum creatinine, and glucose. International normalized ratio (INR) if anticoagulation contemplated. Brain natriuretic peptide (BNP) is elevated in acute MI; may or may not indicate heart failure.

Pregnancy Considerations

Findings mimicking acute MI in pregnancy: ST-segment depression after anesthesia, increase in CK-MB after delivery, and mild increase in troponin I levels in preeclampsia and gestational hypertension

Diagnostic Procedures/Other

High-quality portable chest x-ray. Transthoracic and/or transesophageal echocardiography, contrast chest CT scan, or MRI may occasionally be of value acutely. Coronary angiography is definitive test.

ALERT

Isosmolar contrast medium or low-molecular-weight contrast medium other than ioxaglate or iohexol is indicated in patients with chronic kidney disease undergoing angiography who are not having chronic dialysis.

Test Interpretation

Myocardial necrosis and atherosclerosis, if etiologic

TREATMENT

GENERAL MEASURES

- Admit to telemetry/coronary care unit (CCU) with continuous ECG monitoring and bed rest. Anxiolytics, if needed. Stool softeners.
- Antiarrhythmics, as needed, for unstable dysrhythmia. Deep vein thrombosis (DVT) prophylaxis
- Continuation of aspirin and clopidogrel or prasugrel or ticagrelor, BB, ACE inhibitors (or ARB if ACE-intolerant), lipid-lowering therapy, tight BP control, progressively increased physical activity, smoking cessation, annual influenza vaccine
- Elicit symptoms or signs of depression and treat with an SSRI or psychotherapy if present.

MEDICATION

Medication recommendations based on 2009 ACC/AHA focused guideline updates (1) and 2012 ESC STEMI guidelines (2)

First Line

- Supplemental oxygen 2–4 L/min for patients with arterial oxygen saturation <90% or respiratory distress
- Nitroglycerin (NTG) sublingual 0.4 mg q5min for total of 3 doses, followed by nitroglycerin IV if ongoing pain and/or hypertension and/or management of pulmonary congestion if no contraindications exist (systolic BP <90 mm Hg or 30 mm Hg below baseline, right ventricle (RV) infarct, use of sildenafil within 24 hours or within 48 hours of tadalafil)
- Morphine sulfate 2–4 mg IV (with increments of 2–8 mg IV repeated at 5–15-minute intervals to relieve pain or pulmonary congestion
- Antiplatelet agents:
  – Aspirin (ASA), nonenteric-coated, initial dose 162–325 mg chewed
  – A loading dose of a thienopyridine is recommended for patients with STEMI for whom PCI is planned:
    ○ 600 mg of clopidogrel should be given as early as possible before or at the time of primary or nonprimary PCI or
    ○ Prasugrel 60 mg should be given as soon as possible for primary PCI. Do not use in patients likely to undergo coronary artery bypass graft (CABG) or with active bleeding, history of transient ischemic attack (TIA) or stroke, or additional risk factors for bleeding (body weight <60 kg or concomitant use of medications that increase risk of bleeding). (Generally, not recommended for patients age ≥75 years.) or
    ○ Ticagrelor 180 mg loading dose
    ○ Duration of therapy with a thienopyridine varies. At least 12 months for patients receiving drug-eluting stent (DES) during PCI for ACS and up to 12 months for patients receiving bare-metal stent (BMS). Consider earlier discontinuation if risk of morbidity due to bleeding outweighs the benefits of therapy. May continue clopidogrel or prasugrel or ticagrelor for longer than 15 months in patients undergoing DES placement. Discontinue clopidogrel for at least 5 days or prasugrel at least 7 days prior to planned CABG.
  – For patients with STEMI undergoing nonprimary PCI:
    ○ Continue clopidogrel in a patient who has received fibrinolytic therapy and has been given clopidogrel.
    ○ Administer loading dose of clopidogrel 600 mg if patient received a fibrinolytic without a thienopyridine, or, ticagrelor 180 mg or once the coronary anatomy is known and PCI is planned, administer a loading dose of prasugrel as soon as possible, but no later than 1 hour after PCI. Administer loading dose of clopidogrel 300 mg in patients <75 years of age who received fibrinolytic therapy or who do not receive reperfusion therapy.
    ○ Clopidogrel 75 mg should be given with aspirin in patients with STEMI regardless of reperfusion therapy.
- β-blocker (BB) within 24 hours, if no contraindications exist (signs of congestive heart failure [CHF], low output state)
- Glycoprotein IIb/IIIa receptor antagonists at time of primary PCI in selected patients: Abciximab, eptifibatide, or tirofiban

- ACE inhibitors should be initiated orally within 24 hours of STEMI in patients with anterior infarction, HF or ejection fraction (EF ≤0.40 unless contraindicated
- Coronary reperfusion therapy:
  – Primary PCI:
    ○ Symptom onset of ≤12hours
    ○ Symptom onset of ≤12hours and contraindication to fibrinolytic therapy irrespective of time delay
    ○ Cardiogenic shock or acute severe HF irrespective of time delay from onset of MI
    ○ Evidence of ongoing ischemia 12–24 hours after symptom onset
    ○ If substantial risk for intracranial hemorrhage (ICH)
    ○ Age <75 with STEMI or LBBB who develop shock within 36 hours of acute MI (AMI)
- Fibrinolysis:
  – If presenting at a hospital without PCI capability and cannot be transferred to a PCI-capable facility to undergo PCI within 90 minutes of first medical contact
  – If no contraindications, administer within 12 hours, but not beyond 24 hours, of onset of symptoms to patients with STEMI in ≥2 contiguous leads and new or presumably new LBBB:
    ○ Alteplase (rt-PA): 15-mg IV bolus, followed by 0.75 mg/kg (up to 50 mg) IV over 30 minutes, then 0.5 mg/kg (up to 35 mg) over 60 minutes; maximum 100 mg over 90 minutes
    ○ Reteplase (r-PA): 10 units IV bolus over 2 minutes, give 2nd bolus 30 minutes later.
    ○ Tenecteplase (TNK-tPA): 30–50 mg (based on weight) IV bolus over 5–10 seconds
  – Combination reperfusion with abciximab and half-dose r-PA or TNK-tPA
  – Use anticoagulants (unfractionated heparin [UFH], enoxaparin, or fondaparinux) as ancillary therapy to reperfusion therapy for minimum 48 hours and duration of admission (up to 8 days). Avoid UFH if >48 hours of anticoagulant required: Recommend supportive anticoagulant regimens in patients proceeding to primary PCI who have been treated with ASA and thienopyridine. Administer additional boluses of UFH as needed to maintain therapeutic clotting time levels in patients who received prior treatment with UFH. Bivalirudin recommended as a supportive measure for primary PCI in patients with or without prior treatment with UFH.

Second Line

- Long-acting nondihydropyridine calcium channel blocker (CCB) when BB is ineffective or contra-indicated if eEF is normal. Use of immediate release nifedipine is contraindicated in patients with STEMI.
- Initiate aldosterone blockers if already on an ACE inhibitor and BB in patients with STEMI with EF ≤0.40 and either symptomatic HF or diabetes
- Lipid-lowering therapy: Statin (preferred because of additional nonlipid effects on vascular function), niacin, or fibrate

SURGERY/OTHER PROCEDURES

Intra-aortic balloon pump for cardiogenic shock. PCI of the left main coronary artery with stents as an alternative to CABG in patients with favorable anatomy and comorbid conditions that may increase risk of adverse surgical outcomes if CABG chosen.

IN-PATIENT CONSIDERATIONS

Admission Criteria/Initial Stabilization

- Definitive/suspected acute MI, ongoing pain, positive cardiac markers, ST deviations, hemodynamic abnormalities
- All patients with STEMI should be admitted to a CCU for evaluation and treatment. Transfer high-risk patients who receive fibrinolytic therapy as primary reperfusion therapy at a non–PCI-capable facility to a PCI-capable facility as soon as possible.

IV Fluids

Right ventricular infarction may need fluid resuscitation for hypotension.

 ### ONGOING CARE

FOLLOW-UP RECOMMENDATIONS

Follow up in 3–6 weeks of discharge. Identify high-risk patients for implantable cardioverter defibrillator (ICD) placement (especially those with EF <30%).

DIET

NPO for first 4–12 hours due to risk of emesis or aspiration; request dietary consult if lipid, weight, or glucose issues

PATIENT EDUCATION

May resume sexual activity within 10 days, consistent with current exercise capacity. Driving can resume 1 week after discharge. Low-fat diet.

COMPLICATIONS

Heart failure, myocardial rupture/left ventricular aneurysm, pericarditis, dysrhythmias, acute mitral regurgitation, severe depression (common)

REFERENCES

1. O'Gara PT. 2013 ACC/AHA guideline for the management of ST-elevation myocardial infarction and ACC/AHA/SCAI guidelines on percutaneous coronary intervention. *J Am Coll Cardiol*. 2013; 127:529–555.
2. Task Force on the management of ST-segment elevation acute myocardial infarction of the European Society of Cardiology (ESC), Steg PG, James SK, et al. ESC Guidelines for the management of acute myocardial infarction in patients presenting with ST-segment elevation. *Eur Heart J*. 2012;33(20):2569–2619. Epub 2012 Aug 24.

 ## CODES

ICD10

- I21.3 ST elevation (STEMI) myocardial infarction of unspecified site
- I21.09 STEMI involving oth coronary artery of anterior wall
- I21.19 STEMI involving oth coronary artery of inferior wall

CLINICAL PEARLS

Discontinue clopidogrel at least 5–7 days before elective CABG. Do not administer nitrates to patients who have recently used PDE-5 inhibitors.

ACUTE CORONARY SYNDROMES: UNSTABLE ANGINA AND NSTEMI

Samuel W. Joffe, MD • Louis Berk, MD

BASICS

DESCRIPTION
- Unstable angina (UA) and non–ST-segment elevation myocardial infarction (NSTEMI) are acute coronary syndromes (ACS) without ST-segment elevation.
- NSTEMI typically presents with anginal symptoms, may demonstrate ST-segment depressions and/or T-wave inversions on ECG, and is defined by the presence of elevated cardiac biomarkers, typically troponin (I or T) above the 99th percentile of normal or elevated MB fraction of creatinine kinase (CKMB). Elevated cardiac biomarkers may not be detectable for several hours following the onset of symptoms (1).
- UA, although clinically indistinguishable from NSTEMI (in an appropriate clinical setting, chest discomfort or anginal equivalent), can be differentiated from NSTEMI by a persistent lack of elevation in cardiac biomarkers. Just as with NSTEMI, nonspecific ECG changes, such as ST-segment depressions or T-wave inversions, may be present (1).

EPIDEMIOLOGY
- Incidence of UA/NSTEMI increases with age (2).
- Presentation of coronary events in women is, on average, 10 years later than in men, with comparable rates of occurrence (2).

Incidence
Age-adjusted CHD incidence rates (per 1,000 person-years): White men, 12.5; black men, 10.6; white women, 4.0; and black women, 5.1 (2)

Prevalence
For adults ≥20 years of age: 8.3% for men and 6.1% for women (2)

ETIOLOGY AND PATHOPHYSIOLOGY
- Platelet-rich thrombus forming on a disrupted plaque
- Coronary vasospasm, often caused by cocaine or methamphetamine abuse
- Dynamic obstruction (coronary spasm, vasoconstriction, muscle bridge)
- Progressive mechanical limitation of coronary flow
- Coronary arterial inflammation
- Coronary dissection/rupture and thrombogenesis
- Myocardial oxygen demand exceeds supply

UA/NSTEMI is usually caused by acute rupture of an atherosclerotic plaque, causing thrombosis and partial or total occlusion of a coronary artery.

RISK FACTORS
- Age
- Hypertension
- Tobacco use
- Diabetes mellitus
- Dyslipidemia
- Family history of early coronary artery disease (CAD)
- Sedentary lifestyle
- Overweight/Obesity

GENERAL PREVENTION
- Smoking cessation, healthy diet, weight control, physical activity
- If risk factors are present: BP control, lipid-lowering therapy, daily aspirin (in select patients)

COMMONLY ASSOCIATED CONDITIONS
- Cardiovascular disease (atherosclerotic, aneurysmal, autoimmune, peripheral)
- Other forms of heart disease (myocardial, valvular, high-output states)

DIAGNOSIS

HISTORY
- Chest heaviness/tightness, with or without exertion, and increasing in frequency
- Pain or discomfort radiating to the neck, jaw, interscapular area, upper extremities, or epigastrium
- Associated symptoms of dyspnea, nausea, diaphoresis, light-headedness, dysphoria
- History of myocardial ischemia (stable or unstable angina, MI, coronary bypass surgery, or percutaneous coronary intervention [PCI])
- Family history of CAD or MI
- Risk factors for CAD and bleeding
- Use of phosphodiesterase-5 inhibitors (e.g., Viagra) and concomitant nitrates
- Use of cocaine or amphetamines
- Medications and recent medication changes

PHYSICAL EXAM
- General: Abnormal vital signs including tachycardia or bradycardia, hypertension or hypotension, widened pulse pressure, tachypnea, fever
- Neuro: Dizziness, syncope, fatigue, weakness, altered mental status
- Cardiovascular: Dysrhythmia, jugular venous distention (JVD), new murmur, rub or gallop, diminished peripheral pulses, carotid bruits
- Respiratory: Tachypnea, increased work of breathing, crackles
- Musculoskeletal: Sharp pain reproducible with movement or palpation is unlikely to be cardiac.
- Skin: Cool skin, pallor, diaphoresis, signs of dyslipidemia (xanthomas, xanthelasma)

DIFFERENTIAL DIAGNOSIS
- Aortic dissection
- Pulmonary embolism
- Pleuropericarditis
- Perforating ulcer
- Gastroesophageal reflux disease (GERD) and spasm
- Esophageal perforation
- Biliary or pancreatic pain
- Dysrhythmia

Geriatric Considerations
Elderly patients, as well as women and those with diabetes, may have an atypical presentation without classic anginal symptoms.

DIAGNOSTIC TESTS & INTERPRETATION
Initial Tests (lab, imaging)
- 12-lead ECG (1): Applies to both UA and NSTEMI:
  - ST-segment depression and/or T-wave inversion:
    - ≥1-mm ST depression in ≥2 contiguous leads
    - T-wave inversions, other changes
    - ST depression and/or tall R-wave in V1/V2 with upright T waves may indicate transmural STEMI of posterior wall.
    - If initial ECG is nondiagnostic but symptoms persist with suspicion for ACS, perform serial ECGs at 15–30-minute intervals (1).
- Serum biomarkers (negative in UA):
  - NSTEMI is strictly defined as elevated serum biomarkers (usually troponin I or T, as they are more sensitive for detecting NSTEMI) exceeding the 99th percentile of a normal reference population in the absence of evidence of STEMI.
  - Troponin concentration rises 3–6 hours after onset of ischemic symptoms, but can be delayed to 8–12 hours (troponin T is not specific in patients with renal dysfunction).
  - CK-MB increases 3–4 hours after onset of myocardial injury.
  - Myoglobin: Early marker for myocardial necrosis; increases 2 hours after onset of myocardial necrosis.
  - Patients with negative biomarkers within 6 hours of the onset of symptoms should have biomarkers remeasured 8–12 hours from onset of symptoms (1)[B]
- Chest x-ray
- Consider transthoracic echocardiography if not recently performed (1)[B].

Follow-Up Tests & Special Considerations
- Fasting lipid profile
- CBC, basic metabolic panel, activated partial thromboplastin time (aPTT)
- Other laboratory tests:
  - Lactate dehydrogenase: Increases within 24 hours, peaks 3–6 days, baseline 8–12 days (not routinely ordered)
  - Leukocytes: Increase within several hours after MI, peak in 2–4 days
  - Brain natriuretic peptide (BNP): Increases with MI, may not indicate heart failure

Pregnancy Considerations
Findings mimicking NSTEMI in pregnancy: ST depression after anesthesia, increase in CK-MB after delivery, and mild increase in troponin in preeclampsia and gestational hypertension. Spontaneous coronary dissection is a rare cause of ST elevation in pregnancy.

Diagnostic Procedures/Other
- Coronary angiography (discussed below under "Treatment")
- If serial cardiac enzymes are negative and symptoms have resolved, consider stress testing, including either standard exercise treadmill test (ETT), stress echocardiography, or stress nuclear study (1)[B].
- Transesophageal echocardiography, contrast chest CT scan, or MRI generally are reserved for differentiating STEMI and other causes of chest pain from aortic dissection.

Test Interpretation
- Subendocardial myocardial necrosis may be present.
- Atherosclerosis

TREATMENT

GENERAL MEASURES

- Bed/Chair rest with continuous ECG monitoring
- Antiarrhythmics as needed
- Anxiolytics as needed
- Deep vein thrombosis prophylaxis
- Continuation of aspirin, clopidogrel or prasugrel or ticagrelor, beta-blockers, ACE inhibitors (or ARBs if ACE-intolerant), lipid-lowering therapy
- Tight BP control
- Treatment for depression PRN (common post-MI)
- Cardiac rehabilitation and increased physical activity
- Smoking cessation
- Annual influenza vaccine

MEDICATION
First Line

- Aspirin, nonenteric-coated, initial dose of 162–325 mg PO or chewed (1)[A]:
  – For ASA-intolerant patients, as well as for patients planned for PCI who are not at high risk for complex disease requiring coronary artery bypass graft (CABG) surgery, administer clopidogrel loading dose 300–600 mg followed by 75 mg/d (1)[A], or prasugrel, loading dose 60 mg followed by 10 mg/d (1)[B], or ticagrelor, loading dose 180 mg followed by 90 mg bid (1)[B]. (Ticagrelor increases the risk of fatal ICH compared with clopidogrel and should be avoided in those with a prior history of ICH (1)).
- Nitroglycerin sublingual 0.4 mg q5min for total of 3 doses, then assess need for IV NTG (1)[C]
- Supplemental oxygen 2–4 L/min, maintaining arterial oxygen saturation >90% (1)[B]
- Morphine sulfate 2–4 mg IV (with increments of 2–8 mg IV repeated at 5–15-minute intervals (1)[A]
- Oral beta-blocker (cardioselective agent such as metoprolol or atenolol preferred) if no contraindication (1)[B]
- Risk stratify using the TIMI or GRACE score to select use of early invasive approach (within 12–24 hours of admission) vs. medical therapy.
- Risks and benefits of the early invasive approach:
  – 33% relative risk reduction for both the endpoints of refractory angina and rehospitalization at 6–12 months (2)[A]
  – 27% and 22% relative risk reduction in rates of MI at 6–12 months and 3–5 years, respectively (2)[A]
  – Doubled risk of procedure-related MI and increased risk of minor periprocedural bleeding (1)[A]
- Invasive management:
  – Benefits are more pronounced in higher risk patients, such as those with ECG changes or diabetes (2).
- Subsequent recommendations all (1)[A]: For patients with elevated risk for clinical events or refractory angina or hemodynamic or electrical instability, initiate anticoagulant: Enoxaparin or unfractionated heparin (UFH) or bivalirudin. Prior to angiography, add GP IIb/IIIa inhibitor (eptifibatide or tirofiban) or thienopyridine (clopidogrel or prasugrel) or ticagrelor.

- Medical management:
  – For low-risk or selected intermediate-risk patients; based on patient or physician preference; or in chronic renal insufficiency stage IV: Initiate anticoagulant therapy: Enoxaparin or UFH or fondaparinux; enoxaparin or fondaparinux preferable. Initiate clopidogrel or prasugrel or ticagrelor.
- Contraindications: Prasugrel and ticagrelor is contraindicated in patients >75 or those with history of CVA/TIA or increased bleeding risk. Enoxaparin is contraindicated in patients with renal insufficiency.

Second Line

- ACE inhibitor in patients with pulmonary congestion or left ventricular ejection fraction (EF) ≤40%. (1)[A].Substitute angiotensin receptor blocker (ARB) for ACE-intolerant patients
- Nondihydropyridine calcium channel blocker (CCB) (verapamil or diltiazem) to reduce myocardial oxygen demand when beta-blockers are contraindicated if normal EF (1)[B]. Use oral long-acting CCB only after beta-blockers and nitrates have been fully used (1)[C].
- Long-term nitrate therapy for recurrent angina/ ischemia or heart failure (1)[C]
- Sublingual NTG at discharge (1)[C]
- Lipid-lowering therapy: High-dose statin (preferred due to nonlipid benefit on vascular function) (1)[A], niacin, or fibrate (1)[C]

ISSUES FOR REFERRAL
Cardiology consultation is appropriate for likely UA/NSTEMI, particularly regarding the complexities of anticoagulation/antiplatelet therapy.

SURGERY/OTHER PROCEDURES
- Coronary reperfusion:
  – PCI with stent placement
  – CABG surgery
- Intra-aortic balloon pump for severe ischemia, hypotension, refractory pain

IN-PATIENT CONSIDERATIONS
Admission Criteria/Initial Stabilization
- All patients with definite or suspected acute MI, ongoing pain, positive cardiac markers, ST deviations, hemodynamic abnormalities, probable or definite acute coronary syndrome (ACS)
- Bed rest with continuous ECG monitoring, assess for reperfusion therapy, relieve ischemic pain, treat life-threatening complications, admit to coronary care unit.

ONGOING CARE

FOLLOW-UP RECOMMENDATIONS
- Follow-up within 2–6 weeks (low risk) and 14 days (high risk).
- Refer to cardiac rehabilitation.

DIET
- Diet low in saturated fat, cholesterol, and sodium
- Request dietary consult

PATIENT EDUCATION
- Education on new medications, diet, exercise, smoking cessation, lifestyle modification
- Resume exercise, sexual activity after outpatient re-evaluation

PROGNOSIS
UA/NSTEMI patients have a lower in-hospital mortality than those with STEMI, but a similar or worse long-term outcome.

COMPLICATIONS
- Cardiogenic shock
- Heart failure
- Myocardial rupture
- Ventricular aneurysm
- Dysrhythmia
- Acute pulmonary embolism
- Acute thromboembolic stroke
- Pericarditis/Dressler syndrome
- Depression (increases mortality risk)
- Hyperglycemia

REFERENCES

1. Jneid H, Anderson JL, Wright RS, et al. 2012 ACCF/AHA focused update of the guideline for the management of patients with unstable angina/ non–ST-elevation myocardial infarction (updating the 2007 guideline and replacing the 2011 focused update): A report of the American College of Cardiology Foundation/American Heart Association Task Force on Practice Guidelines. *Circulation*. 2012;126:875–910.
2. Roger VL, Go AS, Lloyd-Jones DM, et al. Heart disease and stroke statistics–2012 update: A report from the American Heart Association. *Circulation*. 2012;125(1):e2–e220

ADDITIONAL READING

- Anderson JL, Adams CD, Antman EM, et al. 2011 ACCF/AHA Focused Update Incorporated Into the ACC/AHA 2007 Guidelines for the Management of Patients With Unstable Angina/Non-ST-Elevation Myocardial Infarction: A report of the American College of Cardiology Foundation/American Heart Association Task Force on Practice Guidelines. *Circulation*. 2011;123:e426–e579.
- Hoenig MR, Aroney CN, Scott IA. Early invasive versus conservative strategies for unstable angina and non-ST elevation myocardial infarction in the stent era (review). *Cochrane Database Syst Rev*. 2010;3.

CODES

ICD10
- I20.0 Unstable angina
- I21.4 Non-ST elevation (NSTEMI) myocardial infarction
- I24.9 Acute ischemic heart disease, unspecified

CLINICAL PEARLS

- Discontinue NSAIDs, nonselective or selective cyclooxygenase (COX)-2 agents, except for ASA, due to increased risks of mortality, reinfarction, hypertension, heart failure, and myocardial rupture.
- Discontinue clopidogrel or prasugrel or ticagrelor 5–7 days before elective CABG.
- Do not use nitrate products in patients who recently used a phosphodiesterase-5 inhibitor (24 hours of sildenafil or 48 hours of tadalafil).
- Duration of antithrombotic therapy after NSTEMI depends on type of stent received and medications administered.
- Avoid beta-blockers in cocaine users

ACUTE KIDNEY INJURY

Darryl Elefan, MD • Jason M. Kurland, MD

BASICS

DESCRIPTION
Abrupt loss of kidney function, defined as a rise in serum creatinine of ≥ 0.3 mg/dL or a 50% increase within 48 hours, resulting in retention of nitrogenous waste as well as electrolyte, acid–base, and volume homeostasis abnormalities, with or without oliguria (urine output <500 mL/d).

EPIDEMIOLOGY
Incidence
5% of hospital and 30% of ICU admissions have a diagnosis of acute kidney injury (AKI). 25% of patients develop AKI while in the hospital, and 50% of those cases are iatrogenic. Development of AKI in the inpatient setting is associated with a >4-fold increased risk of death (1).

ETIOLOGY AND PATHOPHYSIOLOGY
- Prerenal (~55%): Hypotension; volume depletion (GI losses, excessive sweating, dehydration, hemorrhage); renal artery stenosis/embolism; burns; heart failure; liver failure
- Intrarenal (~40%): Acute tubular necrosis (ATN) (from prolonged prerenal insufficiency, radiographic contrast material, aminoglycosides, NSAIDs, or other nephrotoxic substances); glomerulonephritis; acute interstitial nephritis (drug-induced); arteriolar insults; vasculitis; accelerated hypertension; cholesterol embolization (common after arterial procedures); intrarenal deposition/sludging (uric acid nephropathy and multiple myeloma [Bence-Jones proteins])
- Postrenal (~5%): Extrinsic compression (e.g., benign prostatic hypertrophy [BPH], carcinoma, pregnancy); intrinsic obstruction (e.g., calculus, tumor, clot, stricture, sloughed papillae); decreased function (e.g., neurogenic bladder)

Can be divided into 3 categories: Prerenal, intrarenal, and postrenal:

- Prerenal: Secondary to decreased renal perfusion (often due to hypovolemia) leading to a decrease in glomerular filtration rate (GFR); reversible if factors decreasing perfusion are corrected; otherwise, it can progress to an intrarenal pathology known as *ischemic acute tubular necrosis*.
- Intrarenal: Secondary to intrinsic damage within the kidney; ATN is the most common cause via ischemic/nephrotoxic kidney injury; 75% of ATN is a complication of a prerenal etiology (2). Intrarenal causes divided into glomerular, vascular, and tubular/interstitial.
- Postrenal: Secondary to extrinsic (e.g., BPH) or intrinsic (e.g., stones) obstruction of the urinary collection system

Genetics
No known genetic pattern

RISK FACTORS
- Chronic kidney disease (CKD)
- Comorbid conditions (e.g., diabetes, hypertension, heart failure, liver failure)
- Advanced age
- Radiographic contrast material exposure
- Nephrotoxic medications (e.g., aminoglycoside antibiotics, NSAIDs, ACE inhibitors)
- Volume depletion (e.g., sepsis, hemorrhage, dehydration)
- Surgery

- Rhabdomyolysis
- Solitary kidney (risk in nephrolithiasis)
- BPH
- Malignancy (e.g., multiple myeloma)

GENERAL PREVENTION
See "Treatment; General Measures."

COMMONLY ASSOCIATED CONDITIONS
Hyperkalemia, hyperphosphatemia, hypercalcemia, hyperuricemia, hydronephrosis, BPH, nephrolithiasis, congestive heart failure (CHF), uremic pericarditis, cirrhosis, chronic renal insufficiency, malignant hypertension, vasculitis, drug reactions, sepsis, severe trauma, burns, transfusion reactions, recent chemotherapy, rhabdomyolysis, internal bleeding, dehydration

DIAGNOSIS

HISTORY
- General: PO intake, urine output, body weight, and baseline creatinine (to assess how far from baseline the current creatinine is), medication use
- Prerenal: Thirst, orthostatic dizziness
- Intrarenal: Nephrotoxic medications, radiocontrast material, other toxins:
  - Fever, arthralgias, and pruritic rash suggest *allergic interstitial nephritis (AIN)*, although systemic effects are not always seen in this pathology (only ~10% present with this triad).
  - Edema, hypertension, and oliguria with nephritic urine sediment (RBCs and RBC casts) point to *glomerulonephritis* or *vasculitis*.
  - Livedo reticularis, SC nodules, and ischemic digits despite good pulses suggest *atheroembolization*.
  - Flank pain suggests *occlusion of the renal artery or vein*.
- Postrenal: Colicky flank pain that radiates to the groin suggests a *ureteric obstruction* such as a stone; nocturia, frequency, and hesitancy suggest *prostatic disease*; suprapubic and flank pain are usually secondary to *distension* of the bladder and collecting system; ask about anticholinergic drugs that could lead to *neurogenic bladder*.
- Symptoms of uremia: Lethargy, nausea/vomiting, anorexia, pruritus, restless legs, sleep disturbance, hiccups

PHYSICAL EXAM
- Signs of uremia: Mental status changes, seizures, asterixis, myoclonus, pericardial friction rub, peripheral neuropathies
- Prerenal signs: Tachycardia, decreased jugular venous pressure (JVP), orthostatic hypotension, dry mucous membranes, decreased skin turgor; look for stigmata of associated comorbid conditions such as liver and heart failure, as well as sepsis.
- Intrinsic renal signs: Pruritic rash, livedo reticularis, SC nodules, ischemic digits despite good pulses
- Postrenal signs: Suprapubic distension, flank pain, enlarged prostate

DIFFERENTIAL DIAGNOSIS
See "Etiology."

DIAGNOSTIC TESTS & INTERPRETATION
Initial Tests (lab, imaging)
- Urinalysis: Dipstick for blood and protein; microscopy for cells, casts, and crystals

- Casts: Transparent hyaline casts—prerenal etiology; pigmented granular/muddy brown casts—ATN; WBC casts—acute interstitial nephritis; RBC casts—glomerulonephritis
- Urine eosinophils: $\geq 1\%$ eosinophils by Hansel's stain suggestive of acute interstitial nephritis (sensitivity, 67%; specificity, 83%)
- Urine electrolytes in an oliguric state:
  - $FE_{Na} = [(U_{Na} \times P_{Cr})/(P_{Na} \times U_{Cr})] \times 100$, where U = urine, P = plasma, Na = sodium, Cr = creatinine; $Fe_{Na} <1\%$, likely prerenal etiology; >2%, likely intrarenal.
  - If patient is on diuretics, use FE_{urea} instead of FE_{Na}: $FE_{urea} = [(U_{urea} \times P_{Cr})/(P_{BUN} \times U_{Cr})] \times 100$; $FE_{urea} <35\%$ suggests prerenal etiology (3).
- CBC, BUN, creatinine, electrolytes (including Ca/Mg/Phos), consider arterial blood gases (ABGs)
- Common lab abnormalities in AKI:
  - Increased: K^+, phosphate, Mg, uric acid
  - Decreased: Hematocrit (Hct), Na, Ca
- Calculate creatinine clearance (CrCl) to ensure that medications are dosed appropriately:
  - Cockcroft-Gault equation for CrCl (mL/min) = $(140-age) \times$ (weight in kilograms) $\times$ (0.85 if female)/($72 \times$ serum creatinine)
  - Note that estimating equations of CrCl/GFR are only valid when renal function (serum Cr) is at steady-state; anuria implies CrCl of 0.
  - Renal ultrasound (US): First line; excludes postrenal causes if negative; identifies kidney size, hydronephrosis, and nephrolithiasis
  - Doppler-flow renal US: Rules out renal artery stenosis/thrombosis
  - Abdominal x-ray (kidney, ureter, bladder [KUB]): Identifies calcification, renal calculi, and kidney size
- Several novel biomarkers, such as urinary IL-18, NGAL (neutrophil gelatinase associated lipocalin), KIM-1 (kidney injury molecule) and plasma cystatin C, are currently being validated for their role in the initial evaluation and management of AKI (4).

Follow-Up Tests & Special Considerations
- Consider CK (if suspect rhabdomyolysis) and immunology antibodies (if suspect vasculitis).
- More advanced imaging techniques should be considered if initial tests do not reveal etiology:
  - Radionucleotide renal scan: Evaluates renal perfusion, function (GFR), and presence of obstructive uropathy and extravasation
  - CT scan: Limited use due to need for radiographic contrast material, which can worsen AKI, although noncontrast helical scan is test of choice for suspected lithiasis
  - MRI: Acute tubulointerstitial nephritis can show an increased T2-weighted signal.

Diagnostic Procedures/Other
Cystoscopy with retrograde pyelogram evaluates for bladder tumor, hydronephrosis, obstruction, and upper tract abnormalities, and poses no threat of radiocontrast toxicity.

Test Interpretation
Kidney biopsy: Last resort if patient does not respond to therapy or other tests do not reveal a diagnosis; most useful for evaluation of intrinsic AKI of unclear cause, such as AIN, glomerulonephritis, vasculitis, or renal transplant rejection.

TREATMENT

GENERAL MEASURES

Identify and correct all prerenal and postrenal causes:

- Stop nephrotoxic drugs and renally dose others.
- Strictly record intake/output and daily weights.
- Optimize cardiac output to maintain renal perfusion.
- Follow nutrition suggestions and be aware of infections; treat aggressively if they occur.
- Avoid aspirin to reduce bleeding tendency (5)[A].
- Indications for initiation of hemodialysis in patients with AKI: Fluid overload refractory to conservative management; severe hyperkalemia (serum K^+ >6.5 mmol/L), or rapidly increasing serum K^+; metabolic acidosis (serum pH <7.1); advanced uremic complications (pericarditis, encephalopathy)

MEDICATION

First Line

- Focus on treating the underlying cause and associated complications.
- Monitor and adjust fluids and electrolytes to prevent fluid overload, hyperkalemia, hyperphosphatemia, hypermagnesemia:
  – If patient is oliguric and not volume overloaded, a *fluid challenge* may be appropriate with diligent monitoring for volume overload (5)[C].
- Furosemide is ineffective in preventing and treating AKI (5–7)[A].
- Dopamine, natriuretic peptides, insulin-like growth factor, and thyroxine also have no benefit in the treatment of AKI (3,5)[A].
- Fenoldopam, a dopamine agonist, may decrease dialysis need and mortality in setting of AKI.
- Hyperkalemia with ECG changes: Give IV calcium, sodium bicarbonate (if acidemic), and glucose with insulin (to drive K^+ into cells); can be supplemented with Kayexalate, which removes K^+ from the body; hemodialysis if severe/refractory (8)[A]
- Oliguric patients should have a fluid restriction of 400 mL + yesterday's urine output (if they are euvolemic) (8)[A].
- Acidosis (serum bicarbonate <15–18 mmol/L): Small amounts of sodium bicarbonate can be given; be aware of volume overload (8)[A].
- Effective strategies for AKI prevention: IV isotonic hydration, once-daily dosing of aminoglycosides, use of lipid formulations of amphotericin B, use of iso-osmolar nonionic contrast media (9)[A]
- Risk of contrast-induced AKI may be reduced by N-acetylcysteine 600 mg PO b.i.d. on day prior to and day of contrast (10)[A] and isotonic NaHCO₃ 3 mL/kg/hr × 1 hour before and 1 mL/kg/hr × 6 hours after contrast administration (11)[B].

Second Line

- Flomax or other selective α-blockers for bladder outlet obstruction secondary to BPH
- Calcium channel blockers may have a protective effect in posttransplant ATN.

ISSUES FOR REFERRAL

- Nephrology should be consulted for all cases as soon as patient is found with AKI.
- Urology consult for obstructive nephropathies

SURGERY/OTHER PROCEDURES

- Relief of obstruction with retrograde ureteral catheters/percutaneous nephrostomy
- Hemodialysis catheter placement

COMPLEMENTARY AND ALTERNATIVE MEDICINE

Many supplements not approved by the FDA can be nephrotoxic.

IN-PATIENT CONSIDERATIONS

Admission Criteria/Initial Stabilization

All patients with AKI should be admitted.

- ABCs of resuscitation
- Treat hyperkalemia emergently, especially if ECG changes present.
- If volume depleted, give isotonic IV fluids.
- Place a Foley catheter.

IV Fluids

Isotonic fluids should be used in patients with volume depletion.

Nursing

Place a Foley catheter; strict recording of intakes and outputs and daily weights.

Discharge Criteria

Stabilization of renal function and a concrete plan for continued treatment, if necessary
Some patients may require dialysis until renal recovery.

 ONGOING CARE

FOLLOW-UP RECOMMENDATIONS

Patient Monitoring

As needed

DIET

- Total caloric intake should be 35–50 kcal/kg/d to avoid catabolism.
- Restrict sodium to 2 g/d (8)[A].
- Consider potassium restriction if hyperkalemic.
- If hyperphosphatemic, consider dietary phosphorus restriction and/or use of phosphate binders.
- Avoid magnesium compounds.

PATIENT EDUCATION

Keep well-hydrated. Avoid nephrotoxic drugs, such as NSAIDs, ACE inhibitors, and aminoglycosides.

PROGNOSIS

- Depending on the cause, comorbid conditions, and age of patient, mortality ranges from 5–80%.
- In cases of prerenal and postrenal failure, very good rates of recovery are positively correlated with shorter duration of AKI. Intrarenal etiologies usually take more time to recover. Overall, average recovery takes from days to months.

COMPLICATIONS

Death, sepsis, infection, seizures, paralysis, peripheral edema, CHF, arrhythmias, uremic pericarditis, bleeding, hypotension, anemia, hyperkalemia, uremia

REFERENCES

1. Wang HE, Muntner P, Chertow GM, et al. Acute kidney injury and mortality in hospitalized patients. *Am J Nephrol*. 2012;84(4):349–355. Epub 2012 Apr 2.
2. Lameire N. The pathophysiology of acute renal failure. *Crit Care Clin*. 2005;21:197–210.
3. Schrier R. Acute renal failure: Definitions, diagnosis, pathogenesis, and therapy. *J Clin Invest*. 2004;114:5–14.
4. McCullough PA, Kellum JA, Mehta RL, et al. ADQI consensus on AKI biomarkers and cardiorenal syndromes. Karger, 2013;182:45–64.
5. Hilton R. Acute renal failure. *BMJ*. 2006;333: 786–790.
6. Ho KM, Sheridan DJ. Meta-analysis of furosemide to prevent or treat acute renal failure. *BMJ*. 2006;84(7565):420. Epub 2006 Jul 21.
7. Cantarovich F, Rangoonwala B, Lorenz H, et al. High-dose furosemide for established ARF: A prospective, randomized, double-blind, placebo-controlled, multicenter trial. *Am J Kidney Dis*. 2004;84(3):402–409.
8. Lameire N, Van Biesen W, Vanholder R. Acute renal failure. *Lancet*. 2005;365:417–430.
9. Venkataraman R. Prevention of acute renal failure. *Chest*. 2007;131:300–308.
10. Birck R, Krzossok S, Markowetz F. Acetylcysteine for prevention of contrast nephropathy: Meta-analysis. *Lancet*. 2003;362:598–603.
11. Merten GJ, Burgess WP, Gray LV. Prevention of contrast-induced nephropathy with sodium bicarbonate: A randomized controlled trial. *JAMA*. 2004;291:2328–2334.

 SEE ALSO

- Glomerulonephritis, Acute; Hepatorenal Syndrome; Hyperkalemia; Prostatic Hyperplasia, Benign (BPH); Renal Failure, Chronic; Reye Syndrome; Rhabdomyolysis; Sepsis
- Algorithm: Anuria or Oliguria

CODES

ICD10

- N17.0 Acute kidney failure with tubular necrosis
- N17.9 Acute kidney failure, unspecified

CLINICAL PEARLS

- Can be divided into 3 categories: Prerenal, intrarenal, and postrenal:
  – Prerenal: Decreased renal perfusion (often from hypovolemia) leading to a decrease in GFR; reversible if factors decreasing perfusion are corrected.
  – Intrarenal: Intrinsic kidney damage; ATN is the most common cause via ischemic/nephrotoxic injury to the kidney.
  – Postrenal: Secondary to extrinsic/intrinsic obstruction of the urinary collection system.
- Recognize the need for emergent hemodialysis: Severe hyperkalemia, metabolic acidosis, or volume overload refractory to conservative therapy; uremic pericarditis, encephalopathy, or neuropathy; and alcohol and drug intoxications.

ADDISON DISEASE

Robert A. Baldor, MD

 BASICS

DESCRIPTION
- Adrenal gland insufficiency from partial or complete destruction of the adrenal cells with inadequate secretion of glucocorticoids and mineralocorticoids
- 80% of cases are caused by an autoimmune process, followed by tuberculosis (TB), AIDS, systemic fungal infections, and adrenoleukodystrophy
- Addison disease (primary adrenocortical insufficiency) can be differentiated from secondary (pituitary failure) and tertiary (hypothalamic failure) causes because mineralocorticoid function usually remains intact in secondary and tertiary causes.
- Addisonian (adrenal) crisis: Acute complication of adrenal insufficiency (circulatory collapse, dehydration, hypotension, nausea, vomiting, hypoglycemia); usually precipitated by an acute physiologic stressor(s) such as surgery, illness, exacerbation of comorbid process, and/or acute withdrawal of long-term corticosteroid therapy
- System(s) affected: Endocrine/Metabolic
- Synonym(s): Adrenocortical insufficiency; Corticoadrenal insufficiency; Primary adrenocortical insufficiency

EPIDEMIOLOGY
- Predominant age: All ages; mean age at diagnosis in adults is 40 years
- Predominant sex: Females > Males (slight)

Incidence
0.6:100,000

Prevalence
4:100,000

ETIOLOGY AND PATHOPHYSIOLOGY
- Autoimmune adrenal insufficiency (80% of cases in the US)
- Infectious causes: TB (most common infectious cause worldwide), HIV (most common infectious cause in the US), Waterhouse-Fredrickson syndrome, fungal disease
- Bilateral adrenal hemorrhage and infarction (for patients on anticoagulants, 50% are in the therapeutic range)
- Antiphospholipid syndrome
- Lymphoma, Kaposi sarcoma, metastasis (lung, breast, kidney, colon, melanoma); tumor must destroy 90% of gland to produce hypofunction
- Drugs (ketoconazole, etomidate)
- Surgical adrenalectomy, radiation therapy
- Sarcoidosis, hemochromatosis, amyloidosis
- Congenital enzyme defects (deficiency of 21-hydroxylase enzyme is most common), neonatal adrenal hypoplasia, congenital adrenal hyperplasia, familial glucocorticoid insufficiency, autoimmune polyglandular syndromes 1 and 2, adrenoleukodystrophy
- Idiopathic

Destruction of the adrenal cortex resulting in deficiencies in cortisol, aldosterone, and androgens

Genetics
- Autoimmune polyglandular syndrome (APS) type 2 genetics are complex. It is associated with adrenal insufficiency, type 1 diabetes, and Hashimoto disease. It is more common than APS type 1.
- APS type 1 is caused by mutations of the autoimmune regulator gene. Nearly all have the following triad: Adrenal insufficiency, hypoparathyroidism, and mucocutaneous candidiasis before adulthood.
- Adrenoleukodystrophy is an X-linked recessive disorder resulting in toxic accumulation of unoxidized long-chain fatty acids.
- Increased risk with cytotoxic T-lymphocyte antigen 4 (CTLA-4)

RISK FACTORS
- 40% of patients have a 1st- or 2nd-degree relative with associated disorders.
- Chronic steroid use, then experiencing severe infection, trauma, or surgical procedures

GENERAL PREVENTION
- No preventive measures known for Addison disease; focus on prevention of complications:
  - Anticipate adrenal crisis and treat before symptoms begin.
- Elective surgical procedures require upward adjustment in steroid dose.

COMMONLY ASSOCIATED CONDITIONS
- Diabetes mellitus
- Graves disease
- Hashimoto's thyroiditis
- Hypoparathyroidism
- Hypercalcemia
- Ovarian failure
- Pernicious anemia
- Myasthenia gravis
- Vitiligo
- Chronic moniliasis
- Sarcoidosis
- Sjögren syndrome
- Chronic active hepatitis
- Schmidt syndrome

DIAGNOSIS

HISTORY
- Weakness, fatigue
- Dizziness
- Anorexia, nausea, vomiting
- Abdominal pain
- Chronic diarrhea
- Depression (60–80% of patients)
- Decreased cold tolerance
- Salt craving

PHYSICAL EXAM
- Weight loss
- Low BP, orthostatic hypotension
- Increased pigmentation (extensor surfaces, hand creases, dental-gingival margins, buccal and vaginal mucosa, lips, areola, pressure points, scars, "tanning," freckles)
- Vitiligo
- Hair loss in females

DIFFERENTIAL DIAGNOSIS
- Secondary adrenocortical insufficiency (pituitary failure):
  - Withdrawal of long-term corticosteroid use
  - Sheehan syndrome (postpartum necrosis of pituitary)
  - Empty sella syndrome
  - Radiation to pituitary
  - Pituitary adenomas, craniopharyngiomas
  - Infiltrative disorders of pituitary (sarcoidosis, hemochromatosis, amyloidosis, histiocytosis X)
- Tertiary adrenocortical insufficiency (hypothalamic failure):
  - Pituitary stalk transection
  - Trauma
  - Disruption of production of corticotropic-releasing factor
  - Hypothalamic tumors
- Other:
  - Myopathies
  - Syndrome of inappropriate antidiuretic hormone
  - Heavy-metal ingestion
  - Severe nutritional deficiencies
  - Sprue syndrome
  - Hyperparathyroidism
  - Neurofibromatosis
  - Peutz-Jegher syndrome
  - Porphyria cutanea tarda
  - Salt-losing nephritis
  - Bronchogenic carcinoma
  - Anorexia nervosa

DIAGNOSTIC TESTS & INTERPRETATION
Initial Tests (lab, imaging)
- Basal plasma cortisol and adrenocorticotropic hormone (ACTH) (low cortisol and high ACTH indicative of Addison disease)
- Standard ACTH stimulation test: Cosyntropin 0.25 mg IV, measure preinjection baseline and 60-minute postinjection cortisol levels (patients with Addison disease have low to normal values that do not rise)
- Insulin-induced hypoglycemia test
- Metapyrone test
- Autoantibody tests: 21-hydroxylase (most common and specific), 17-hydroxylase, 17-alpha-hydroxylase (may not be associated), and adrenomedullin
- Circulating very-long-chain fatty acid levels if boy or young man
- Low serum sodium
- Elevated serum potassium
- Elevated BUN, creatinine, calcium, thyroid-stimulating hormone (TSH)
- Low serum aldosterone
- Hypoglycemia when fasting
- Metabolic acidosis
- Moderate neutropenia
- Eosinophilia
- Relative lymphocytosis
- Anemia, normochromic, normocytic

Follow-Up Tests & Special Considerations
- Plasma ACTH levels do not correlate with treatment and should not be used for routine monitoring of replacement therapy (1)[C].
- TSH: Repeat when condition has stabilized:
  – Thyroid hormone levels may normalize with the treatment of Addison disease.
- Drugs that may alter lab results: Digitalis
- Disorders that may alter lab results: Diabetes

Diagnostic Procedures/Other
- Abdominal CT scan: Small adrenal glands in autoimmune adrenalitis; enlarged adrenal glands in infiltrative and hemorrhagic disorders
- Abdominal radiograph may show adrenal calcifications.
- Chest x-ray may show small heart size and/or calcification of cartilage.
- MRI of pituitary and hypothalamus if secondary or tertiary cause of adrenocortical insufficiency is suspected
- CT-guided fine-needle biopsy of adrenal masses may identify diagnoses (2)[C].

Test Interpretation
- Atrophic adrenals in autoimmune adrenalitis
- Infiltrative and hemorrhagic disorders produce enlargement with destruction of the entire gland.

 TREATMENT

GENERAL MEASURES
Consider the 5 Ss for the management of adrenal crisis:
- Salt, sugar, steroids, support, and search for a precipitating illness (usually infection, trauma, recent surgery, or not taking prescribed replacement therapy)

MEDICATION
First Line
- Chronic adrenal insufficiency:
  – Glucocorticoid supplementation:
    ○ Dosing: Hydrocortisone 15–20 mg (or therapeutic equivalent) PO each morning upon rising and 10 mg at 4–5 PM each afternoon (3)[C]; dosage may vary and is usually lower in children and the elderly
    ○ Precautions: Hepatic disease, fluid disturbances, immunosuppression, peptic ulcer disease, pregnancy, osteoporosis
    ○ Adverse reactions: Immunosuppression, osteoporosis, gastric ulcers, depression, hyperglycemia, weight gain, glaucoma
    ○ Drug interactions: Concomitant use of rifampin, phenytoin, or barbiturates
  – Mineralocorticoid supplementation:
    ○ Dosing: Fludrocortisone 0.05–0.2 mg/d PO
  – May require salt supplementation
- Addisonian crisis:
  – Hydrocortisone 100 mg IV followed by 10 mg/hr infusion, or hydrocortisone 100 mg IV bolus q6–8h
  – IV glucose, saline, and plasma expanders
  – Fludrocortisone 0.05 mg/d PO (may not be required; high-dose hydrocortisone is an effective mineralocorticoid)

- Acute illnesses (fever, stress, minor trauma):
  – Double the patient's usual steroid dose, taper the dose gradually over a week or more, and monitor vital signs and serum sodium.
- Supplementation for surgical procedures:
  – Administer hydrocortisone 25–150 mg or methylprednisolone 5–30 mg IV on the day of the procedure in addition to maintenance therapy; taper gradually to the usual dose over 1–2 days.

Second Line
Addition of androgen therapy:
- Dehydroepiandrosterone (DHEA) 25–50 mg PO once daily may be considered in women to improve well-being and sexuality (4)[B].

Admission Criteria/Initial Stabilization
Addisonian crisis:
- Airway, breathing, and circulation management
- Establish IV access; 5% dextrose and normal saline.
- Administer hydrocortisone 100 mg IV bolus q6–8h; replacement with fludrocortisone is not necessary (high-dose hydrocortisone is an effective mineralocorticoid).
- Correct electrolyte abnormalities.
- BP support for hypotension
- Antibiotics if infection suspected

IN-PATIENT CONSIDERATIONS
Admission Criteria/Initial Stabilization
- Presence of circulatory collapse, dehydration, hypotension, nausea, vomiting, hypoglycemia
- ICU admission for unstable cases

IV Fluids
IV saline containing 5% dextrose and plasma expanders

 ONGOING CARE

FOLLOW-UP RECOMMENDATIONS
Patient Monitoring
- Verify adequacy of therapy: Normal BP, serum electrolytes, plasma renin, and fasting blood glucose level
- Periodically assess for the development of long-term complications of corticosteroid use, including screening for osteoporosis, gastric ulcers, depression, and glaucoma
- Lifelong medical supervision for signs of adequate therapy and avoidance of overdose

DIET
Maintain water, sodium, and potassium balance.

PATIENT EDUCATION
- National Adrenal Disease Foundation, Great Neck, NY 11021, (516) 487-4992 (http://www.medhelp.org/nadf)
- Patient should wear or carry medical identification about the disease and the need for hydrocortisone or other replacement therapy.
- Instruct patient in self-administration of parenteral hydrocortisone for emergency situations.

PROGNOSIS
Requires lifetime treatment: Life expectancy approximates normal with adequate replacement therapy; without treatment, the disease is 100% lethal.

COMPLICATIONS
- Hyperpyrexia
- Psychotic reactions
- Complications from underlying disease
- Over- or underuse of steroid treatment
- Hyperkalemic paralysis (rare)
- Addisonian crisis

REFERENCES
1. Nieman LK, Chanco Turner ML. Addison's disease. *Clin Dermatol.* 2006;24:276–280.
2. Oelkers W. Adrenal insufficiency. *N Engl J Med.* 1996;335:1206–1212.
3. Coursin DB, Wood KE. Corticosteroid supplementation for adrenal insufficiency. *JAMA.* 2002;287:236–240.
4. Arlt W, Callies F, van Vlijmen JC, et al. Dehydroepiandrosterone replacement in women with adrenal insufficiency. *N Engl J Med.* 1999;341:1013–1020.

 SEE ALSO

Algorithm: Adrenocortical Insufficiency

CODES

ICD10
- A18.7 Tuberculosis of adrenal glands
- E27.1 Primary adrenocortical insufficiency

CLINICAL PEARLS
- 80% of cases are caused by an autoimmune process; the average age of diagnosis in adults is 40 years.
- Consider the 5 Ss for the management of Addison disease: Salt, sugar, steroids, support, and search for an underlying cause.
- The goal of steroid replacement therapy should be the lowest dose that alleviates patient symptoms while preventing adverse drug events.
- Plasma ACTH levels do not correlate with treatment and should not be used for routine monitoring for efficacy of replacement therapy.
- Long-term use of steroids predisposes patients to the development of osteoporosis; screen accordingly and encourage calcium and vitamin D supplementation.

ADENOVIRUS INFECTIONS

Scott Graham, MD

BASICS

DESCRIPTION
- Usually self-limited, febrile illnesses characterized by inflammation of various mucous membranes including the conjunctivae, and the respiratory and GI tracts.
- Adenovirus infections occur in epidemic and endemic situations:
  - Common types:
    - Acute febrile respiratory illness, affecting primarily children
    - Acute respiratory disease, affecting adults
    - Viral pneumonia, affecting children and adults
    - Acute pharyngo-conjunctival fever, affecting children, particularly after summer swimming
    - Acute follicular conjunctivitis, affecting all ages
    - Epidemic kerato-conjunctivitis, affecting adults
    - Intestinal infections leading to enteritis, mesenteric adenitis, and intussusception
  - Conjunctivitis, sometimes called "pink eye"
- System(s) affected: Cardiovascular; Gastrointestinal; Hematologic/Lymphatic/Immunologic; Musculoskeletal; Nervous; Pulmonary; Renal/Urologic; Ophthalmologic

Geriatric Considerations
Complications more likely

Pediatric Considerations
Viral pneumonia in infants and neonates may be fatal.

EPIDEMIOLOGY
- Predominant age: <10, but epidemics in all ages
- Predominant sex: Male = Female
- Occurs worldwide and throughout the year

Incidence
- Very common infection, estimated at 2–5% of all upper respiratory infections (URIs) and >10% of URIs in children
- Most individuals show evidence of prior adenovirus infection by age 10.
- As many as half the infections with adenovirus are subclinical or asymptomatic.
- 15–70% of conjunctivitis worldwide (1)

ETIOLOGY AND PATHOPHYSIOLOGY
- Adenovirus (DNA viruses 60–90 nm in size, six species (A-F) with 53 known serotypes)
- Transmission:
  - Aerosol droplets, fecal–oral, contact with contaminated fomites
  - Virus can survive long periods on skin and environmental surfaces
  - Median incubation period is 5.6 days (2)[A]
- Most common known pathogens:
  - Types 1, 2, 3, 4, 5, 7, 14, and 21 cause upper respiratory illness and pneumonia.
  - Types 3, 7, and 21 cause pharyngo-conjunctival fever.
  - Types 31, 40, and 41 cause gastroenteritis.
  - Types 8, 19, and 37 cause epidemic kerato-conjunctivitis.
  - Types 5, 7, 14, and 21 cause the most severe illnesses.

RISK FACTORS
- Large number of people gathered in a small area (e.g., military recruits, college students, daycare centers, summer camps, community swimming pools)
- Immunocompromised persons are at risk for severe disease.

GENERAL PREVENTION
- Live, enteric-coated oral type 4 and type 7 adenovirus vaccine is available for military personnel ages 17–50; reduces incidence of acute respiratory disease (3)
- Frequent handwashing among office personnel and family members
- Decontamination of environmental surfaces using chlorine, bleach, formaldehyde, or heat
- Vigorous handwashing and use of gloves when examining patients with epidemic kerato-conjunctivitis; add droplet precautions if suspected adenoviral respiratory infection
- Health care providers with suspected adenoviral conjunctivitis should avoid direct patient contact for 14 days after onset (in 2nd eye).

COMMONLY ASSOCIATED CONDITIONS
- Otitis media
- Conjunctivitis
- Bronchiolitis
- Viral enteritis
- Less frequent syndromes seen primarily in immunocompromised individuals include meningo-encephalitis, hepatitis, myocarditis, pancreatitis, genital infections, Intussusception and mesenteric adenitis hemorrhagic cystitis, and interstitial nephritis (4)

DIAGNOSIS

HISTORY
Depends on type (see "Differential Diagnosis").
Common symptoms with most respiratory forms (5):
- Headache
- Malaise
- Sore throat
- Cough
- Coryza
- Fever (moderate to high)
- Vomiting
- Diarrhea
- Abdominal pain
- Ear pain
- Urinary symptoms/hematuria
- Eye redness and pain

PHYSICAL EXAM
- Mucosa exhibiting patches of white exudates
- Cervical adenitis
- Otitis media
- Conjunctivitis

DIFFERENTIAL DIAGNOSIS
- Depends on clinical presentation
- The following are the primary characteristics of the major adenovirus infections:
  - Acute respiratory illness:
    - Mostly in children
    - Incubation period: 2–5 days
    - Malaise, fever, chills, headache, pharyngitis, hoarseness, dry cough
    - Fever lasting 2–4 days
    - Illness subsiding in 10–14 days
    - DDx: Rhinovirus, influenza, parainfluenza, RSV
  - Viral pneumonia:
    - Sudden onset of high fever, rapid infection of upper and lower respiratory tracts, skin rash, diarrhea
    - Occurs mostly in children aged a few days up to 3 years
    - DDx: Bacterial pneumonia, RSV, influenza, parainfluenza
  - Acute pharyngo-conjunctival fever:
    - Spiking fever lasting several days, headache, pharyngitis, conjunctivitis, rhinitis, cervical adenitis
    - Conjunctivitis, usually unilateral
    - Subsides in 1 week
    - DDx: Bacterial conjunctivitis, enterovirus, herpes simplex virus (HSV)
  - Epidemic kerato-conjunctivitis:
    - Usually unilateral onset of ocular redness and edema, periorbital edema, periorbital swelling, local discomfort suggestive of foreign body
    - Lasts 3–4 weeks
    - DDx: Bacterial conjunctivitis, enterovirus, HSV
  - Viral enteritis:
    - Nausea/vomiting, diarrhea, abdominal pain
    - DDx: Bacterial enteritis, bowel obstruction

DIAGNOSTIC TESTS & INTERPRETATION
Initial Tests (lab, imaging)
- Diagnosis only needs to be confirmed in severe cases and epidemics
- Viral cultures from respiratory, ocular, or fecal sources can establish diagnosis:
  - Pharyngeal isolate suggests recent infection.
- Adenovirus-specific ELISA; more rapid, but less sensitive than culture (6)
- Adenovirus DNA detection through polymerase chain reaction (PCR)
- Rapid pathogen screening, adeno-detector, is available for detecting adenoviral conjunctivitis (sensitivity, 89%; specificity, 94%); results in 10 minutes (7)
- Antigen detection in stool for enteric serotypes is available.
- Serologic procedures, such as complement fixation, with a 4-fold rise in serum antibody titer, identify recent adenoviral infection.
- Radiographs: Bronchopneumonia in severe respiratory infections

Diagnostic Procedures/Other
Biopsy (lung or other) may be needed in severe or unusual cases; usually only in immunocompromised patients

Test Interpretation
- Varies with each virus:
  - Severe pneumonia may be reflected by extensive intranuclear inclusions.
- *Bronchiolitis obliterans* may occur.

TREATMENT

GENERAL MEASURES
- Treatment is supportive and symptomatic.
- Infections are usually benign and of short duration.

MEDICATION
First Line
- Acetaminophen 10–15 mg/kg PO for analgesia (avoid aspirin)
- Cough suppressants and/or expectorants
- Antihistamine/Decongestant combos may reduce symptoms.
- Antivirals and immunotherapy are reserved for immunocompromised individuals and patients with severe disease:
  - No controlled trials showing benefit of any antiviral agents against human adenovirus infection; however, cidofovir (1 mg/kg every other day) is most commonly used.
  - For adenoviral conjunctivitis, topical ganciclovir 0.15% ophthalmic gel has been suggested for "off-label" use (1).

COMPLEMENTARY AND ALTERNATIVE MEDICINE
Echinacea has not been shown to be better than placebo for treatment of viral upper respiratory infections.

IN-PATIENT CONSIDERATIONS
Admission Criteria/Initial Stabilization
Severely ill infants or immunocompromised patients with severe illness

Nursing
Hospitalized patients with adenoviral infections should be placed on contact precautions; add droplet precautions for those with respiratory illness.

ONGOING CARE

FOLLOW-UP RECOMMENDATIONS
Rest during febrile phases

Patient Monitoring
For severe infantile pneumonia and conjunctivitis, daily physical exam until well

DIET
No special diet

PATIENT EDUCATION
- Avoid aspirin in children
- Give instructions for saline nasal spray, cough preparations, frequent handwashing, and surface cleaning.

PROGNOSIS
- Self-limited, usually without sequelae
- Severe illness and death in neonates and in immunocompromised hosts can occur; severe pneumonia in children under 2 can have a mortality rate as high as 16% (8).

COMPLICATIONS
Few, if any, recognizable long-term problems

REFERENCES

1. AM Pihos. Epidemic keratoconjunctivitis: A review of current concepts in management. *J Optom*. 2013;06:69–74.
2. Lessler J, Reich NG, Brookmeyer R, et al. Incubation periods of acute respiratory viral infections: A systematic review. *Lancet Infect Dis*. 2009;9(5): 291–300.
3. Lyons A, Longfield J, Kuschner R, et al. A double-blind, placebo-controlled study of the safety and immunogenicity of live, oral type 4 and type 7 adenovirus vaccines in adults. *Vaccine*. 2008; 26:2890.
4. Houlihan C, Valappil M, Waugh S, et al. Severe adenovirus infection: An under-recognized disease with limited treatment options. *JICS*. 2012;13 (4), October.
5. Dominguez O, Rojo P, de Las Heras S, et al. Clinical presentation and characteristics of pharyngeal adenovirus infections. *Pediatr Infect Dis J*. 2005; 24:733.
6. Goto E. Meta-analysis of evaluating diagnostic accuracy of adenoclone (ELISA) for adenoviral infection among Japanese people. *Rinsho Byori*. 2010;58(2):148–155.
7. Kaufman HE. Adenovirus advances: New diagnostic and therapeutic options. *Curr Opin Ophthalmol*. 2011;22:290–293.
8. Majeed A, Naeem Z, Khan DA, et al. Epidemic adenoviral conjunctivitis report of an outbreak in a military garrison and recommendations for its management and prevention. *J Pak Med Assoc*. 2005;55:273–275.

ADDITIONAL READING
- Barrett BP, Brown RL, Locken K, et al. Treatment of the common cold with unrefined Echinacea. A randomized, double-blind, placebo-controlled trial. *Ann Intern Med*. 2002;137:939–946.
- Pratter MR. Cough and the common cold: ACCP evidence-based clinical practice guidelines. *Chest*. 2006;129:72S–74S.
- Spurling GKP, Del Mar CB, Dooley L, et al. Delayed antibiotics for symptoms and complications of respiratory infections. *Cochrane Database Syst Rev*. 2004;(4):CD004417.

 SEE ALSO

Conjunctivitis, Acute; Intussusception; Pneumonia, Viral

 CODES

ICD10
- B30.1 Conjunctivitis due to adenovirus
- B34.0 Adenovirus infection, unspecified
- J12.0 Adenoviral pneumonia

CLINICAL PEARLS
- Can present like streptococcus pharyngitis with white exudates and cervical adenitis, but negative strep test
- Most common cause of strep-negative tonsillitis in young children
- Diagnosis only needs to be confirmed in severe cases and epidemics.
- Average incubation time is 5.6 days (2)[A].
- Adenovirus conjunctivitis is highly contagious; cold compresses may help relieve symptoms (8)[A].

ADOPTION, INTERNATIONAL

Kara Keating Bench, MD, MPH • Christopher M. Bositis, MD, AAHIVS

BASICS

DESCRIPTION
Adoption of children from foreign countries into the US has tripled in the past 15 years, and the demographics of those children and their homelands have also shifted significantly during that time. The diverse birth countries, disease exposures, and unknown health histories of these children make them a population that requires special attention.

EPIDEMIOLOGY

Incidence
- 9.504 children were adopted internationally in 2011
- In 2011, the most common countries of origin for internationally adopted children were, in descending order, China, Ethiopia, Russia, South Korea, Ukraine, India, Philippines, Colombia, Taiwan, Uganda, Haiti, and Nigeria.
- In 2011, 15% of internationally adopted children were aged <1 year, 55% were ages 1–4 years, and 30% were ages ≥ 5 years. 56% were girls. (1)

RISK FACTORS
- Unknown birth history, medical history, and vaccination status
- Possible exposure to toxins and/or inadequate nutrition in utero
- Exposures to infectious diseases not commonly seen in the US
- Previous living conditions:
  - Overcrowding
  - Institutionalization (orphanages)
  - Environmental toxins
- History of neglect, deprivation, or abuse

GENERAL PREVENTION
- Required to be examined by a US State Department physician in their native country before immigration to the US (2). This is a limited examination targeted at identifying diseases that would exclude qualifying for a visa.
- Should be examined by a US physician within 2 weeks of arrival or sooner if indicated.
- A follow-up visit 4–6 weeks after their postadoption appointment is recommended.
- All internationally adopted children should be screened for hearing, vision, growth, and developmental delays.

COMMONLY ASSOCIATED CONDITIONS
- Infectious diseases, including (2,3):
  - Hepatitis B
  - Intestinal parasites
  - Tuberculosis (TB)
  - Syphilis
  - HIV
  - *Helicobacter pylori*
- Emotional or behavioral problems
- Developmental delay
- Fetal alcohol syndrome
- Feeding difficulties
- Anemia
- Congenital conditions, including:
  - Cleft lip/palate
  - Orthopedic deformities
- Prematurity or low birth weight
- Malnutrition, rickets
- Inadequate immunizations
- Lead poisoning

- Sensorineural and conductive hearing loss
- Strabismus, blindness

DIAGNOSIS

HISTORY
- Immunization records and titers (most helpful when dates of administration are included)
- Birth/Prenatal history
- Known family history of birth parents
- Prenatal and perinatal disease or toxin exposures
- Documented history of emotional or nutritional deprivation, or physical or sexual abuse
- Duration of time, if any, spent in orphanage. (Studies have suggested every 3–5 months spent in orphanage is associated with 1 month delay in developmental milestones, although quality of care can vary widely (4).)
- Growth charts when available: Failure to gain weight appropriately (or weight loss) is the earliest sign of malnutrition, followed by slowed linear growth, and finally lagging head circumference (brain growth).
- Development, behavior, attachment, parent stress, and parent–child interactions should also be routinely monitored.

PHYSICAL EXAM
- Age-appropriate complete physical exam, with particular attention to growth, evaluation for microcephaly, facial features (red flag for fetal alcohol syndrome, genetic disorders, or perinatal brain injury), vision, and hearing
- Evaluate for signs of dental decay and refer for prompt treatment.
- Developmental assessment, especially for those with unknown date of birth
- Skin exam for signs of scabies, pediculosis, and tinea

DIAGNOSTIC TESTS & INTERPRETATION
- Developmental screening: Denver II Test and/or PEDS parent questionnaire or other validated developmental screening tools at each visit to screen for potential developmental delay and to assess improvement, decline, and need for additional services
- Age-appropriate hearing screening
- Age-appropriate vision screening

Initial Tests (lab, imaging)
- Obtain (2,3):
  - Hepatitis A (Hep A IgM, Hep A IgG)
  - Hepatitis B (HBsAg, HBsAb, HBcAb)
  - Hepatitis C (enzyme immunoassay [EIA])
  - HIV 1,2 antibody testing/ELISA; consider DNA polymerase chain reaction (PCR) for those <6 months
  - Syphilis: Nontreponemal (RPR, VDRL, or ART) and treponemal (MHA-TP, FTA-ABS, or TPPA)
  - Tuberculin skin test in all ages or interferon-gamma release assay ages ≥5 years
  - 3 stool specimens for ova and parasites, and single specimen for *Giardia intestinalis* and *Cryptosporidium parvum* antigens
  - CBC with indices and differential
  - Lead
  - Thyroid-stimulating hormone (TSH)
  - Urinalysis
  - G6PD deficiency screen
  - Hemoglobin Electrophoresis
- Consider based on clinical presentation (2,3)

- Stool cultures for bacterial pathogens (for children with diarrhea)
- *H. pylori* testing (for children with dyspepsia, abdominal pain, or anemia)
- Ca^{++}, PO_4, alkaline phosphate, and 25 vitamin D level (if signs of rickets)
- >12 months of age: For Chagas disease via *Trypanosoma cruzi* serologic testing in adoptees from endemic countries (Mexico, Central and South America)
- >24months of age: serologic testing for lymphatic filariasis with circulating filarial antigen if from endemic countries
- Provide age-appropriate immunization if unreliable record of DTaP, polio, measles-mumps-rubella (MMR), or pneumococcal.
- Conduct serologic testing and immunize for Hep A, varicella. If no record of MMR, can immunize with MMR or check measles, mumps antibodies and if positive give one dose MMR for rubella coverage.

Follow-Up Tests & Special Considerations
Follow-up testing (3,5):
- Hep B: Repeat at 6 months.
- HIV: Transplacentally acquired maternal antibody may be present in uninfected infants up to 18 months: If antibody positive, confirm with DNA PCR for children <18 months.
- Hep C: Positive tests should be confirmed with recombinant immunoblot assay (RIBA) testing and/or HCV RNA PCR. Transplacentally acquired maternal antibody may be present in uninfected infants up to 18 months, so if positive <18 months, repeat after this age.
- TB: Positive tuberculin skin test should NOT be attributed to bacille Calmette-Guérin (BCG) vaccine, and must be investigated. Give preventive therapy if known exposures. Repeat testing at 6 months, as poor nutrition may result in false-negative (anergic) skin test. No CXR indicated.
- GI tract signs or symptoms occurring years after immigration: Test for intestinal parasites.
- Eosinophilia: Eosinophilia >450 cells/mm³ with negative stool ova and parasites, serologic testing for *Schistosoma*; and add *Strongyloides* for adoptees from sub-Saharan African, Latin American, and Southeast Asian countries
- Developmental screening: Repeat at each visit and follow progress. 50–90% of all internationally adopted children are delayed upon adoption; however, most of them have normal cognition at long-term follow-up.
- Social history screening: Behavioral concerns may first present during adolescence, even for children adopted in infancy (6).

TREATMENT

GENERAL MEASURES
- Regular diet for children who arrive malnourished
- Monitor linear growth.
- If developmental delay is diagnosed, consider early services (e.g., Early Intervention) or referral to developmental specialist.
- Recommend local support groups for parents.
- Attention to parental interactions: Postadoption depression may occur.

MEDICATION
- Immunizations per CDC schedule with catch-up as needed: http://www.cdc.gov/vaccines/recs/schedules/
- If no records or records do not comply with the US or WHO guidelines, treat as unimmunized.
- Checking antibody titers is acceptable in children >12 months if doubt regarding immunization status
- Adoptive parents, caretakers, and household members should be up to date on TdaP, Hep A, Hep B

ISSUES FOR REFERRAL
- Individual or family counseling considered for all adoptive families for adjustment support.
- Many internationally adopted children show sensory-seeking behaviors early on thought to be related to the sensory-depriving orphanage experience. These behaviors typically improve without treatment. Child may appear similar to autistic-like features (e.g., hand-flapping, rocking), but if child is otherwise developing normally (socially, emotionally), no action needed (2).
- If a child continues to have disruptive behaviors, or would rather self-soothe than seek nurturing human interaction, consider a thorough developmental evaluation.
- Persistent behavioral issues in the parent–child interactions should be evaluated by a pediatric psychologist or psychiatrist.
- Vision (higher rates of strabismus): Refer to pediatric ophthalmology (2).
- Hearing (higher rates of conductive and sensorineural hearing loss): Refer to audiology and/or ENT (2).
- Pediatric dental evaluation by 12 months of age, sooner if signs of dental pathology.

ONGOING CARE

FOLLOW-UP RECOMMENDATIONS
Patient Monitoring
- Regular well-child visits, particularly within first months of entry into the US
- Close monitoring of developmental milestones, behavior, and individual attachment

DIET
- Regular diet
- Weight catch-up will occur with a normal diet, barring other medical conditions, and eating habits should normalize using parenting methods discussed below (7).

PATIENT EDUCATION
- Eating: The recommended approach is to allow access to as much healthy food as the child wants, as often as he or she wants it, so that the child can learn the important self-regulatory behaviors of eating that may not have been learned in an institution (hunger, satiety) and can build trust with the parent(s) who feed him or her.
- Toileting: While some children may simply not be trained yet, others may have accidents in their new home because of regression. Time and positive reinforcement and avoiding punishment will resolve this issue as the child becomes comfortable with his or her new surroundings.
- Sleeping: Children must learn to trust their new home and parents, and thus this is not a time for aggressive sleep rules (i.e., ferberization). Parents should be present, physically and emotionally, just enough to let the child know he or she is safe,

establish a bedtime ritual upon arrival, and then gently reinforce this ritual.
- Language: As the child experiences a myriad of changes, it may be helpful for the adoptive family to have learned some key phrases in the child's native language for the first few weeks after adoption. Depending on the child's age and language proficiency, an interpreter may also be useful in the home and at medical appointments until English becomes more comfortably understood and familiar (2).
- Adopted children may experience grieving of lost family, relationships, and culture, which is common and expected behavior; encourage parents to acknowledge and work through this loss with their children, and consider formal counseling, if needed.
- At 3–4 years of age, adopted children will begin to recognize physical differences between themselves and adoptive family if they are of different racial origin.
- Children and families should be encouraged to learn about the culture of the birth country and the ethnic group of origin.
- Relationships with others of the same racial or ethnic group may be very helpful to the adopted child.

PROGNOSIS
Long-term issues include (4,7):
- Children who experienced early neglect, deprivation, or loss prior to adoption are more likely to have developmental delay or behavioral or attachment problems.
- These issues decrease with time the child has spent within the adoptive family, although those with significant histories of deprivation are at risk for difficulties that may persist for life.
- Although most adopted children are healthy, as a group, they have been found to have higher rates of moderate to severe physical and mental health problems, hearing and visual impairment, learning disability, developmental delay, and special health care needs when compared with biologic children of the same parents.
- Developmental delay, in particular, is found to be more likely in an internationally adopted child than in his or her nonadopted peers. However, recent studies show marked catch-up development reported after living in adoptive homes, with many children achieving normal-range development later in life (depending on length of time spent in an institution prior to adoption).
- Fortunately, international adoption pairs some of the most vulnerable, potentially high-risk children with the lowest-risk parents (usually financially stable, well educated, with relatively extremely low divorce rates).
- Most families have found the process of international adoption deeply rewarding, while acknowledging the potential challenges.

REFERENCES

1. Centers for Disease Control and Prevention. *CDC Health Information for International Travel 2014*. New York: Oxford University Press; 2014.
2. Schulte EE, Springer SH. Health care in the first year after international adoption. *Pediatr Clin North Am*. 2005;52:1331–1349, vii.
3. Miller LC. International adoption: Infectious diseases issues. *Clin Infect Dis*. 2005;40(2): 286–293. Epub 2004 Dec 17.
4. Weitzman C, Albers L. Long-term developmental, behavioral, and attachment outcomes after international adoption. *Pediatr Clin North Am*. 2005;52:1395–1419, viii.
5. American Academy of Pediatrics. Medical evaluation of internationally adopted children for infectious diseases. In: Pickering LK, ed. *Red Book: 2012 Report of the Committee on Infectious Diseases*, 29th ed. Elk Grove Village, IL.
6. Hawk B, McCall RB. CBCL behavior problems of post-institutionalized international adoptees. *Clin Child Fam Psychol Rev*. 2010;13(2):199–211.
7. Van Ijzendoorn MH, Bakermans-Kranenburg MJ, Juffer F. Plasticity of growth in height, weight, and head circumference: Meta-analytic evidence of massive catch-up after international adoption. *J Dev Behav Pediatr*. 2007;28:334–343.

ADDITIONAL READING

- Juffer F, van Ijzendoorn MH. Behavior problems and mental health referrals of international adoptees: A meta-analysis. *JAMA*. 2005;293(20):2501–2515.
- US Department of State, Bureau of Consular Affairs. The Hague Convention on Intercountry Adoption: A Guide for Prospective Adoptive Parents. Available at: http://www.travel.state.gov/pdf/Prospective_Adoptive_Parents_Guide.pdf.

 CODES

ICD10
Z02.82 Encounter for adoption services

CLINICAL PEARLS
- Initial labs: Hepatitis B (HBsAg, HBsAb, HBcAb), hepatitis A (HepA IgM, Hep A IgG), hepatitis C (EIA), HIV 1,2 Ab (ELISA), syphilis (RPR, VDRL, or ART AND MHA-TP, FTA-ABS or TPPA) CBC, TSH, lead, G6PD deficiency, hemoglobin electrophoresis; tuberculin skin test for ages ≥5 interferon-gamma release assay; 3 stool specimens for ova and parasites, and single specimen for *Giardia intestinalis* and *Cryptosporidium parvum* antigens; urinalysis
- Immunizations per CDC schedule with catch-up, as needed: Ensure adoptive family, caretakers current on Tdap, Hep A, Hep B (http://www.cdc.gov/vaccines/recs/schedules/)
- Immunization versus serologic testing: Age-appropriate immunization if unclear on record of DTaP, polio, MMR, or pneumococcal. Conduct serologic testing and immunize appropriately for Hep A, varicella. If no record of MMR, can immunize with MMR or check measles, mumps antibodies and, if positive, give 1 dose MMR for rubella coverage. Reimmunization for unknown is appropriate.
- >12 months of age: *Trypanosoma cruzi* serologic testing for adoptees from endemic countries.
- >24 monts of age, serologic testing for lymphatic filariasis with circulating filarial antigen if from endemic countries.
- Many internationally adopted children show sensory-seeking that typically improve without treatment but may benefit from work with occupational therapy if significant. They may appear quite similar to autistic-like features on exam (e.g., hand-flapping, rocking), but as long as the child is otherwise developing normally (socially, emotionally), they should not raise significant levels of concern.

ALCOHOL ABUSE AND DEPENDENCE

Gennine M. Zinner, RNCS, ANP

BASICS

DESCRIPTION
- Any pattern of alcohol use causing significant physical, mental, or social dysfunction; key features are tolerance, withdrawal, and persistent use despite problems
- Alcohol abuse: Maladaptive pattern of alcohol use manifested by ≥1 of:
  - Failure to fulfill obligations at work, school, or home
  - Recurrent use in hazardous situations
  - Recurrent alcohol-related legal problems
  - Continued use despite related social or interpersonal problems
- Alcohol dependence: Maladaptive pattern of use manifested by ≥3 of the following:
  - Tolerance
  - Withdrawal
  - Using more than intended
  - Persistent desire or attempts to cut down/stop
  - Significant amount of time obtaining, using, or recovering from alcohol
  - Social, occupational, or recreational activities sacrificed for alcohol use
  - Continued use despite physical or psychological problems
- National Institute on Alcohol Abuse and Alcoholism criteria for "at-risk" drinking: Men >14 drinks a week or >4 per occasion. Women: >7 drinks a week or >3 per occasion.
- System(s) affected: Nervous; Gastrointestinal (GI)
- Synonym(s): Alcoholism; Alcohol abuse; Alcohol dependence

Geriatric Considerations
- Common and underdiagnosed in elderly; less likely to report problem; may exacerbate normal age-related cognitive deficits and disabilities
- Multiple drug interactions
- Signs and symptoms may be different or attributed to chronic medical problem or dementia.
- Common assessment tools may be inappropriate.

Pediatric Considerations
- Children of alcoholics are at increased risk.
- In 2004, 28% of persons 12–20 years reported use in past month, 1 in 5 binge drink; binge drinkers are 7 times more likely to report illicit drug use.
- Negative effect on maturation and development
- Early drinkers are 4 times more likely to develop a problem than those who begin >21.
- Depression, suicidal or disorderly behavior; family disruption; violence or destruction of property; poor school or work performance; sexual promiscuity; social immaturity; lack of interests; isolation; moodiness

Pregnancy Considerations
- Alcohol is teratogenic, especially during the 1st trimester; women should abstain during conception and throughout pregnancy.
- 10–50% of children born to women who are heavy drinkers will have fetal alcohol syndrome.
- Women experience harmful effects at lower levels and are less likely to report problems.

EPIDEMIOLOGY
- Predominant age: 18–25, but all ages affected
- Predominant sex: Male > Female (3:1)

Prevalence
- Lifetime prevalence: 13.6%
- 20% in primary care setting
- 48.2% of 21-year-olds in the US reported binge drinking in 2004.

ETIOLOGY AND PATHOPHYSIOLOGY
Multifactorial: Genetic, environment, psychosocial
Alcohol is a CNS depressant, facilitating γ-aminobutyric acid (GABA) inhibition and blocking N-methyl-d-aspartate receptors.

Genetics
50–60% of risk is genetic.

RISK FACTORS
- Family history
- Depression (40% with comorbid alcohol abuse)
- Anxiety
- Other substance abuse
- Tobacco
- Male gender
- Low socioeconomic status
- Unemployment
- Peer/social approval
- Family dysfunction or childhood trauma
- Posttraumatic stress disorder
- Antisocial personality disorder
- Bipolar disorder
- Eating disorders
- Criminal involvement

GENERAL PREVENTION
Counsel with family history and risk factors

COMMONLY ASSOCIATED CONDITIONS
- Cardiomyopathy, atrial fibrillation
- Hypertension
- Peptic ulcer disease/gastritis
- Cirrhosis, fatty liver, cholelithiasis
- Hepatitis
- Diabetes mellitus
- Pancreatitis
- Malnutrition
- Upper GI malignancies
- Peripheral neuropathy, seizures
- Abuse and violence
- Trauma (falls, motor vehicle accidents [MVAs])
- Severe psychiatric disorders (depression, bipolar, schizophrenia): >50% of patients with these disorders have a comorbid substance abuse problem.

DIAGNOSIS

HISTORY
- Behavioral issues:
  - Anxiety, depression, insomnia
  - Psychological and social dysfunction, marital problems
  - Social isolation/withdrawal
  - Domestic violence
  - Alcohol-related legal problems
  - Repeated attempts to stop/reduce
  - Loss of interest in nondrinking activities
  - Employment problems (tardiness, absenteeism, decreased productivity, interpersonal problems, frequent job loss)
  - Blackouts
  - Complaints about alcohol-related behavior
  - Frequent trauma, MVAs, emergency department visits

- Physical symptoms:
  - Anorexia
  - Nausea, vomiting, abdominal pain
  - Palpitations
  - Headache
  - Impotence
  - Menstrual irregularities
  - Infertility

PHYSICAL EXAM
- Physical exam may be completely normal.
- General: Fever, agitation, diaphoresis
- Head/Eyes/Ears/Nose/Throat: Plethoric face, rhinophyma, poor oral hygiene, oropharyngeal malignancies
- Cardiovascular: Hypertension, dilated cardiomyopathy, tachycardia, arrhythmias
- Respiratory: Aspiration pneumonia
- GI: Stigmata of chronic liver disease, peptic ulcer disease, pancreatitis, esophageal malignancies, esophageal varices
- Genitourinary: Testicular atrophy
- Musculoskeletal: Poorly healed fractures, myopathy, osteopenia, osteoporosis, bone marrow suppression
- Neurologic: Tremors, cognitive deficits (e.g., memory impairment), peripheral neuropathy, Wernicke-Korsakoff syndrome
- Endocrine/Metabolic: Hyperlipidemias, cushingoid appearance, gynecomastia
- Dermatologic: Burns (e.g., cigarettes), bruises, poor hygiene, palmar erythema, spider telangiectasias, caput medusa, jaundice

DIFFERENTIAL DIAGNOSIS
- Other substance use disorders
- Depression
- Dementia
- Cerebellar ataxia
- Cerebrovascular accident (CVA)
- Benign essential tremor
- Seizure disorder
- Hypoglycemia
- Diabetic ketoacidosis
- Viral hepatitis

DIAGNOSTIC TESTS & INTERPRETATION
- CAGE Questionnaire: (Cut down, Annoyed, Guilty, and Eye opener): >2 "yes" answers is 74–89% sensitive, 79–95% specific for alcohol use disorder; less sensitive for white women, college students, elderly. Not an appropriate tool for less severe forms of alcohol abuse (1)[A].
- AUDIT: Alcohol Use Disorders Identification Test: 10 items, if >4: 70–92% sensitive, better in populations with low incidence of alcoholism (2)[A]: http://www.nams.sg/addictions/Alcohol/Pages/Self-Assessment-Tool.aspx
- Single question for unhealthy use screening: "How many times in the last year have you had X or more drinks in one day" (X = 5 for men, 4 for women); 81.8% sensitive, 79% specific for alcohol use disorders (3)[C]

Initial Tests (lab, imaging)
- CBC, liver function tests (LFTs), electrolytes, BUN/creatinine, lipid panel, thiamine, folate, hepatitis A, B, C serology
- Serum levels increased in chronic abuse:
  - AST/ALT ratio >2.0
  - γ-glutamyl transferase (GGT)

- Carbohydrate-deficient transferrin
- Elevated mean corpuscular volume (MCV)
- Prothrombin time
- Uric acid
- Triglycerides and cholesterol (total)
- Often decreased:
  - Calcium, magnesium, potassium, phosphorus
  - BUN
  - Hemoglobin, hematocrit
  - Platelet count
  - Serum protein, albumin
  - Thiamine, folate
- Blood alcohol concentration:
  - >100 mg/dL in outpatient setting
  - >150 mg/dL without obvious signs of intoxication
  - >300 mg/dL at any time
- CAT scan or MRI of brain: Cortical atrophy, lesions in thalamic nucleus and basal forebrain
- Abdominal US: Ascites, periportal fibrosis, fatty infiltration, inflammation

Test Interpretation
- Liver: Inflammation or fatty infiltration (alcoholic hepatitis), periportal fibrosis (alcoholic cirrhosis occurs in only 10–20% of alcoholics)
- Gastric mucosa: Inflammation, ulceration
- Pancreas: Inflammation, liquefaction necrosis
- Heart: Dilated cardiomyopathy
- Immune system: Decreased granulocytes
- Endocrine organs: Elevated cortisol levels, testicular atrophy, decreased female hormones
- Brain: Cortical atrophy, enlarged ventricles

TREATMENT

For management of acute withdrawal, please see "Alcohol Withdrawal."

GENERAL MEASURES
- Brief interventions and counseling by clinicians have proven efficacy for problem drinking (4)[B].
- Treat comorbid problems (sleep, anxiety, etc.); use caution if prescribing medications with cross-tolerance to alcohol (benzodiazepine).
- Group programs and/or 12-step programs may have benefit in helping patients accept treatment.
- Research shows the benefit of referring patients with alcohol dependence to an addiction specialist or treatment program (2)[A].

MEDICATION
First Line
- Adjuncts to withdrawal regimens:
  - Naltrexone: 50–100 mg/d PO or 380 mg IM once every 4 weeks; opiate antagonist reduces craving and likelihood of relapse (IM route may enhance compliance and thus efficacy) (2,5)[A].
  - Acamprosate (Campral): 666 mg PO t.i.d. beginning after completion of withdrawal; reduces relapse risk. If helpful, recommended to use for 1 year (6)[A].
  - Topiramate (Topamax): 25–300 mg/d PO or divided b.i.d.; enhances abstinence (2)[B] (not approved by FDA for use in alcohol dependence; off-label use)
- Supplements to all:
  - Thiamine: 100 mg/d (1st dose IV prior to glucose to avoid Wernicke encephalopathy)
  - Folic acid: 1 mg/d
  - Multivitamin daily

- Contraindications:
  - Naltrexone: Pregnancy, acute hepatitis, hepatic failure
  - Monitor liver function tests.
- Precautions: Organic pain, organic brain syndromes
- Significant possible interactions: Alcohol, sedatives, hypnotics, naltrexone, and narcotics

ALERT
Treat acute symptoms if in alcohol withdrawal; give thiamine 100 mg/d with 1st dose prior to glucose.

Second Line
- Disulfiram: 250–500 mg/d PO; unproven efficacy; may provide psychologic deterrent
- Selective serotonin reuptake inhibitors may be beneficial if comorbid depression exists.

ISSUES FOR REFERRAL
Addiction specialist, 12-step or long-term program, psychiatrist

IN-PATIENT CONSIDERATIONS
Assess medical and psychiatric condition.

Admission Criteria/Initial Stabilization
- Correct electrolyte imbalances, acidosis, hypovolemia (treat if in alcohol withdrawal).
- Thiamine: 100 mg IM, followed by 100 mg PO, and folic acid: 1 mg/d
- Benzodiazepines used to lower risk of alcohol withdrawal, seizures

ONGOING CARE

FOLLOW-UP RECOMMENDATIONS
Patient Monitoring
- Outpatient detoxification: Daily visits (not recommended for heavy alcohol abuse)
- Early outpatient rehabilitation: Weekly visits
- Detoxification alone is not sufficient.

PATIENT EDUCATION
- American Council on Alcoholism: (800) 527-5344 or http://www.aca-usa.com (treatment facility locator, educational information)
- National Clearinghouse for Alcohol and Drug Information: (800) 729-6686 or http://www.health.org
- Center for Substance Abuse Treatment: (800) 662-HELP or http://www.csat.samhsa.gov
- Alcoholics Anonymous: http://www.aa.org
- Rational Recovery: http://www.rational.org
- Secular Organizations for Sobriety: www.cfiwest.org/sos/index.htm
- http://www.alcoholanswers.org/list: An evidence-based Web site for those seeking credible information on alcohol dependence and online support forums
- National Institute on Alcohol Abuse and Alcoholism (NIAAA) Guide for clinicians: "Helping Patients Who Drink Too Much." http://www.niaaa.nih.gov/guide

PROGNOSIS
- Chronic relapsing disease; mortality rate more than twice general population, death 10–15 years earlier
- Abstinence benefits survival, mental health, family, employment
- 12-step programs, cognitive behavior, and motivational therapies are often effective during 1st year following treatment.

COMPLICATIONS
- Cirrhosis (women sooner than men)
- GI malignancies
- Neuropathy, dementia, Wernicke-Korsakoff syndrome
- CVA
- Ketoacidosis
- Infection
- Adult respiratory distress syndrome
- Depression
- Suicide
- Trauma

REFERENCES
1. Dhalla S, Kopec JA. The CAGE questionnaire for alcohol misuse: A review of reliability and validity studies. *Clin Invest Med.* 2007;30:33–41.
2. Willenbring M, Massey S, Gardner M. Helping patients who drink too much: An evidence-based guide for primary care physicians. *Am Fam Physician.* 2009;80(1):44–50.
3. Smith PC, Schmidt SM, Allensworth-Davies D, et al. Primary care validation of a single-question alcohol screening test. *J Gen Intern Med.* 2009;24(7): 783–788.
4. McQueen J, Howe TE, Allan L, et al. Brief interventions for heavy alcohol users admitted to general hospital wards. *Cochrane Database Syst Rev.* 2011;10(8):CD005191.
5. Pettinati HM, Gastfriend DR, Dong Q, et al. Effect of extended-release naltrexone (XR-NTX) on quality of life in alcohol-dependent patients. *Alcohol Clin Exp Res.* 2009;33(2):350–356.
6. Rosner S, Hackl-Herrwerth A, Leucht S, et al. Acamprosate for alcohol dependence. *Cochrane Database Syst Rev.* 2010;9: CD004332.

SEE ALSO

Substance Use Disorders; Alcohol Withdrawal

CODES

ICD10
- F10.10 Alcohol abuse, uncomplicated
- F10.20 Alcohol dependence, uncomplicated
- F10.99 Alcohol use, unsp with unspecified alcohol-induced disorder

CLINICAL PEARLS
- CAGE Questionnaire: (Cut down, Annoyed, Guilty, and Eye opener): >2 "yes" answers is 74–89% sensitive, 79–95% specific for alcohol use disorder; less sensitive for white women, college students, elderly. Not an appropriate tool for less severe forms of alcohol abuse
- Single question for unhealthy use screening: "How many times in the last year have you had X or more drinks in one day" (X = 5 for men, 4 for women); 81.8% sensitive, 79% specific for alcohol use disorders
- National Institute on Alcohol Abuse and Alcoholism criteria for "at-risk" drinking: Men >14 drinks a week or >4 per occasion. Women: >7 drinks a week or >3 per occasion.

ALCOHOL WITHDRAWAL

Brittany Conahan, PharmD • Neela Bhajandas, PharmD • Alexander Swift, MD

BASICS

DESCRIPTION
Alcohol withdrawal syndrome (AWS) is a spectrum of symptoms that results from abrupt cessation of alcohol in a dependent patient. Symptoms can begin within 5 hours of the last drink and persist for 5–10 days, ranging in severity.

EPIDEMIOLOGY
Each year, 8.2 million Americans meet diagnostic criteria for alcohol dependence. It is more prevalent among men, whites, Native Americans, younger and unmarried adults, and those with lower socioeconomic status; only 24% of those with dependence are ever treated. <5% of US adults will experience withdrawal.

ETIOLOGY AND PATHOPHYSIOLOGY
- Consumption of alcohol potentiates the effect of the inhibitory neurotransmitter gamma-aminobutyric acid (GABA). With chronic alcohol ingestion, this repeated stimulation down-regulates the inhibitory effects of GABA.
- Concurrently, alcohol ingestion inhibits the stimulatory effect of glutamate on the CNS, with chronic alcohol use up-regulating excitatory NMDA glutamate receptors.
- When alcohol is abruptly stopped, the combined effect of a down-regulated inhibitory neurotransmitter system (GABA-modulated) and up-regulated excitatory neurotransmitter system (glutamate-modulated) results in brain hyperexcitability when no longer suppressed by alcohol; clinically seen as AWS.

Genetics
There is some evidence for a genetic basis of alcohol dependence.

RISK FACTORS
- High tolerance, prolonged use, high quantities
- Previous alcohol withdrawal episodes, detoxifications, alcohol withdrawal seizures, and delirium tremens (DTs)
- Serious medical problems
- Concomitant benzodiazepine dependence

Geriatric Considerations
Elderly dependent on alcohol are more susceptible to withdrawal, and chronic comorbid conditions place them at higher risk of complications from withdrawal.

Pregnancy Considerations
Hospitalization or inpatient detoxification is usually required for treatment of acute alcohol withdrawal.

GENERAL PREVENTION
- Routinely screen all adults for alcohol misuse (1)[B].
- Screen with the **CAGE** or similar questionnaire:
  - Feeling the need to **C**ut down
  - **A**nnoyed by criticism about alcohol use
  - **G**uilt about drinking/behaviors while intoxicated
  - "**E**ye opener" to quell withdrawal symptoms
  - Useful to detect problematic alcohol use, positive screen is ≥2 "yes" responses
- 10-question AUDIT screening test is also useful to identify problem drinking.
- The "5 A's" is a screening tool used in primary care settings (Assess, Advise, Agree, Assist, Arrange).

COMMONLY ASSOCIATED CONDITIONS
- General: Poor nutrition, electrolyte abnormalities (hyponatremia, hypomagnesemia, hypophosphatemia), thiamine deficiency, and dehydration
- GI: Hepatitis, cirrhosis, varices, GI bleed
- Heme: Splenomegaly, thrombocytopenia, macrocytic anemia
- Cardiovascular: Cardiomyopathy, hypertension, atrial fibrillation, other arrhythmias
- CNS: Trauma, seizure disorder, generalized atrophy, Wernicke-Korsakoff syndrome
- Peripheral nervous system: Neuropathy, myopathy
- Pulmonary: Aspiration pneumonitis or pneumonia; increased risk of anaerobic infections
- Psychiatric: Depression, posttraumatic stress disorder, bipolar disease, polysubstance abuse

DIAGNOSIS

- *Diagnostic and Statistical Manual of Mental Disorders* AWS criteria are diagnosed when ≥2 of the following present within a few hours to several days after the cessation or reduction of heavy and prolonged alcohol ingestion:
  - Autonomic hyperactivity (sweating, tachycardia)
  - Increased hand tremor
  - Insomnia
  - Psychomotor agitation
  - Anxiety
  - Nausea
  - Vomiting
  - Grand mal seizures
  - Transient (visual, auditory, or tactile) hallucinations or illusions
- These should cause clinically significant distress or impair functioning and not be secondary to an underlying medical condition or mental disorder.
- There are 3 stages to AWS:
  - Stage 1 (minor withdrawal; onset 5–8 hours after cessation):
    - Mild anxiety, restlessness, and agitation
    - Mild nausea/GI upset and decreased appetite
    - Sleep disturbance
    - Sweating
    - Mild tremulousness
    - Fluctuating tachycardia and hypertension
  - Stage 2 (major withdrawal; onset 24–72 hours after cessation):
    - Marked restlessness and agitation
    - Moderate tremulousness with constant eye movements
    - Diaphoresis
    - Nausea, vomiting, diarrhea, anorexia
    - Marked tachycardia and hypertension
    - Alcoholic hallucinosis (auditory, tactile, or visual); may have mild confusion but can be reoriented
  - Stage 3 (DTs; onset 72–96 hours after cessation):
    - Fever
    - Severe hypertension, tachycardia
    - Delirium
    - Drenching sweats
    - Marked tremors
    - Persistent hallucinations
- Alcohol withdrawal–associated seizures are often brief, generalized tonic-clonic seizures and can occur 6–48 hours after last drink.

HISTORY
Essential historical information should be:
- Duration and quantity of alcohol intake, time since last drink
- Previous episodes/symptoms of alcohol withdrawal, prior detox admissions
- Concurrent substance use
- Pre-existing medical and psychiatric conditions, prior seizure activity
- Social history: Living situation, social support, stressors, triggers, etc.

PHYSICAL EXAM
Should include assessment of conditions likely to complicate or that are exacerbated by AWS:
- Cardiovascular: Arrhythmias, heart failure, coronary artery disease
- GI: GI bleed, liver disease, pancreatitis
- Neuro: Oculomotor dysfunction, gait ataxia, neuropathy
- Psych: Orientation, memory
- General: Hand tremor, infections

DIFFERENTIAL DIAGNOSIS
- Cocaine intoxication
- Opioid, marijuana, and methamphetamine withdrawal
- Anticholinergic drug toxicity
- Neuroleptic malignant syndrome
- Liver failure
- Sepsis, CNS infection or hemorrhage
- Mania, psychosis
- Thyroid crisis (2)[C]

DIAGNOSTIC TESTS & INTERPRETATION
Initial Tests (lab, imaging)
- Blood alcohol level, urine drug screen
- CBC; comprehensive metabolic panel
- CNS imaging if acute mental status changes

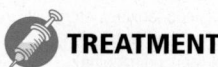

TREATMENT

- The goal is to prevent and treat withdrawal symptoms (e.g., seizures, DTs, cardiovascular events). This is done primarily with benzodiazepines (BZDs), which reduce the duration of symptoms and raise the seizure threshold:
  - Exclude other medical and psychiatric causes.
  - Provide a quiet, protective environment.
  - The Clinical Institute Withdrawal Assessment for Alcohol Scale revised (CIWA-Ar) is useful for determining medication dosing and frequency of evaluation for AWS. Severity of symptoms are rated on a scale from 0–7, with 0 being without symptoms and 7 being the max score (except orientation and clouding of sensorium, scale 0–4):
    - Nausea and vomiting
    - Tremor
    - Paroxysmal sweats
    - Anxiety
    - Agitation
    - Tactile disturbances
    - Auditory disturbances
    - Visual disturbances
    - Headache or fullness in head
    - Orientation and clouding of sensorium
- Frequent re-evaluation with CIWA-Ar score is crucial.

MEDICATION
First Line
- BZD monotherapy remains the treatment of choice (3)[A]; it is associated with fewer complications compared with neuroleptics (4)[A].
- BZD should be chosen by the following considerations:
  – Agents with rapid onset control agitation more quickly (e.g., IV diazepam [Valium]).
  – Long-acting BZDs (diazepam, chlordiazepoxide [Librium]) are more effective at preventing breakthrough seizures and delirium management.
  – Short-acting BZDs (lorazepam [Ativan], oxazepam [Serax]) are preferable when prolonged sedation is a concern (e.g., elderly patients or other serious concomitant medical illness) and preferable when severe hepatic insufficiency may impair metabolism (4)[A].
- BZD dosages will vary by patients. Given as symptom-triggered or fixed-schedule regimens. Symptom-triggered regimens have been found to require less BZD amounts and reduce hospitalization time (2)[A].
- Symptom-triggered regimen: Start with chlordiazepoxide 50–100 mg PO, repeat CIWA-Ar hourly and if score is ≥8, give additional dose of chlordiazepoxide 50 mg PO. Continue to re-evaluate with CIWA-Ar hourly until adequate sedation achieved (score <8). May substitute chlordiazepoxide with respective doses of diazepam, lorazepam, or oxazepam (2)[C].

Second Line
- Thiamine: 100 mg daily IV or IM for at least 3 days (4)[C]:
  – Note that IV glucose administered before treatment with thiamine may precipitate Wernicke encephalopathy and Korsakoff psychosis.
- β-blockers (e.g., atenolol [Tenormin]) and α2 agonists (e.g., clonidine [Catapres]) help to control hypertension and tachycardia and can be used with BZDs (2)[C]. Not used as monotherapy, due to their inability to prevent DTs and seizures.
- Carbamazepine: Not recommended as first-line therapy; associated with reduced incidence of seizures but more studies are needed (3,5)[C].
- If the patient exhibits significant agitation and alcoholic hallucinosis, an antipsychotic (haloperidol [Haldol]) can be used, but this requires close observation, as it lowers the seizure threshold (2)[C].

ADDITIONAL THERAPIES
Peripheral neuropathy and cerebellar dysfunction merit physical therapy evaluation.

IN-PATIENT CONSIDERATIONS
Patients in withdrawal stages 1 and 2 can be treated as outpatients unless medical comorbidities require inpatient care. A reliable and supportive social environment should be in place with frequent follow-up.

Admission Criteria/Initial Stabilization
- CIWA score >15, or severe withdrawal
- Concurrent acute illness requiring in patient care
- Poor ability to follow-up or no reliable social support
- Pregnancy
- Seizure disorder or history of severe alcohol-related seizures

- Suicide risk
- Concurrent BZD dependence
- Age >40 years old
- Prolonged heavy drinking >8 years
- Consumes >1 pint of alcohol or 12 beers per day
- Random blood alcohol level >200 mg/dL
- Elevated MCV, BUN
- Cirrhosis, liver failure

Discharge Criteria
CIWA scores of <10 on 3 consecutive determinations

 ## ONGOING CARE

FOLLOW-UP RECOMMENDATIONS
- Discharge arrangements include transfer to a treatment facility (e.g., sober house or residential program), outpatient substance abuse counseling, peer support groups (Alcoholics Anonymous), and the use of adjuvant treatment such as disulfiram (Antabuse), acamprosate (Campral), or naltrexone (ReVia, Vivitrol).
- Disulfiram: Irreversibly inhibits aldehyde dehydrogenase, blocking alcohol metabolism, leading to an accumulation of acetaldehyde; therefore, it reinforces the individual's desires to stop drinking by providing a disincentive associated with increase acetaldehyde:
  – 250–500 mg/day PO × 1–2 weeks; maintenance 250 mg/day PO
  – Contraindications: Concomitant use of metronidazole and ethanol-containing products, psychosis, severe myocardial disease, and coronary occlusion
- Acamprosate (666 mg PO t.i.d.): Glutamate and GABA modulator indicated to reduce cravings:
  – Contraindications: Renal impairment (CrCl <30 mL/min)
- Naltrexone (50 mg/day PO; 380 mg IM every 4 weeks): Opiate receptor antagonist, theorized to attenuate pleasurable effects of alcohol and reduce craving. Initiate therapy after patient is opioid-free for at least 7 days:
  – Contraindications: Acute hepatitis/liver failure, concomitant opioid therapy

Patient Monitoring
Frequent follow-up to monitor for relapse

PATIENT EDUCATION
- Alcoholics Anonymous at www.aa.org
- SMART Recovery (Self-Management and Recovery Training) at www.smartrecovery.org (not spiritually based)
- National Institute on Alcohol Abuse and Alcoholism at www.niaaa.nih.gov
- FamilyDoctor.Org: Alcoholism (Spanish resources available)

PROGNOSIS
Mortality from severe withdrawal (DTs) is 1–5%.

COMPLICATIONS
Occurs more frequently in individuals who have prior episodes of withdrawal or concomitant illnesses.

REFERENCES
1. Rockville MD. Screening and Behavioral Counseling Interventions in Primary Care to Reduce Alcohol Misuse: Recommendation Statement. *USPSTF*. May 2013.
2. Mayo-Smith MF. Pharmacological management of alcohol withdrawal: a meta-analysis and evidence-based practice guideline. *JAMA*. 1997; 278:144–1451.
3. Amato L, Minozzi S, Vecchi S, et al. Benzodiazepines for alcohol withdrawal. *Cochrane Database Syst Rev*. 2010;(3):CD005063. Epub 2010 Mar 17.
4. Amato L, Minozzi S, Davoli M, et al. Efficacy and safety of pharmacological interventions for the treatment of the alcohol withdrawal syndrome. *Cochrane Database Syst Rev*. 2011;(6):CD008537.
5. Minozzi S, Amato L, Vecchi S, et al. Anticonvulsants for alcohol withdrawal. *Cochrane Database Syst Rev*. 2010;(3):CD005064. Epub 2010 Mar 17.

ADDITIONAL READING
Sarff M, Gold JA. Alcohol withdrawal syndromes in the intensive care unit. *Crit Care Med*. 2010;38(9 Suppl):S494–S501.

 ## SEE ALSO

Substance Use Disorders

CODES

ICD10
- F10.230 Alcohol dependence with withdrawal, uncomplicated
- F10.231 Alcohol dependence with withdrawal delirium
- F10.239 Alcohol dependence with withdrawal, unspecified

CLINICAL PEARLS
- The *kindling phenomenon* has postulated that long-term exposure to alcohol affects neurons, resulting in increased alcohol craving and progressively worse withdrawal episodes.
- The CIWA-Ar is a useful tool for managing the symptoms and treatment of alcohol withdrawal.
- Any BZD dose should be patient-specific, sufficient to achieve and maintain a "light somnolence" (e.g., sleeping but easily arousable), and should be tapered off carefully even after AWS resolves.
- Administer thiamine before patient receives glucose, so as not to precipitate Wernicke encephalopathy.
- There should be frequent outpatient follow-up to monitor for relapse.
- Counsel patients taking disulfiram to avoid over-the-counter products that contain alcohol (i.e., mouthwashes).
- Avoid IM administration (i.e. IM diazepam and IM lorazepam) because of erratic absorption.

ALOPECIA
Amy M. Zack, MD, FAAFP

 BASICS

DESCRIPTION
- Alopecia: Absence of hair from areas where it normally grows:
  - Anagen phase: Growing hairs, 90% scalp hair follicles at any time, lasts 2–6 years
  - Catagen phase: Regression of follicle, <1% follicles, lasts 3 weeks
  - Telogen phase: Resting phase, lasts 2–3 months, 50–150 telogen hairs shed per day
- Classified as scarring (cicatricial), nonscarring, or structural
- Scarring (cicatricial) alopecia:
  - Inflammatory disorders leading to *permanent* hair loss and follicle destruction
  - Includes lymphocytic, neutrophilic, and mixed subtypes
- Nonscarring alopecia:
  - Lack of inflammation, no destruction of follicle
  - Includes focal, patterned and diffuse hair loss such as androgenic alopecia, alopecia areata, telogen effluvium, anagen effluvium, syphilitic hair loss
- Structural hair disorders:
  - Brittle or fragile hair from abnormal hair formation or external insult

EPIDEMIOLOGY
- Androgenic alopecia: Onset in males between 20 and 25 years. Onset in females prior to 40 years, affecting as many as 70% of women over 65 years (1)
- Alopecia areata: Onset usually prior to 30 years; men and women are equally effected. Well-documented genetic predisposition.

Incidence
Incidence greatest in Caucasians, followed by Asians, African Americans, and Native Americans. In females, 13% premenopausal, with as many as 70% females over 65 years of age (1)

Prevalence
- Androgenic alopecia: In males, 30% Caucasian by 30 years, 50% by 50 years and 80% by 70 years.
- Alopecia areata: 1/1000 with lifetime risk of 1–2%
- Scarring alopecia: rare, 3–7% of all hair disorder patients

ETIOLOGY AND PATHOPHYSIOLOGY
- Scarring (Cicatricial) alopecia:
  - Slick smooth scalp without follicles evident
  - Inflammatory disorders leading to permanent destruction of the follicle; it is not known what causes inflammation to develop.
  - Three major subtypes based on type of inflammation: Lymphocytic, neutrophilic and mixed
  - Primary scarring includes discoid lupus, lichen planopilaris, dissecting cellulitis of scalp, among others.
  - Secondary scarring from infection, neoplasm, radiation, surgery, and other physical trauma, including tinea capitis
- Nonscarring alopecia:
  - Focal alopecia
  - Alopecia areata:
    - Patchy hair loss, usually autoimmune in etiology, T-cell-mediated inflammation resulting in premature transition to catagen then telogen phases

- May occur with hair loss in other areas of the body (alopecia totalis [entire scalp]), alopecia universalis (rapid loss of all body hair).
    - Nail disease frequently seen
    - High psychiatric comorbidity (2)
  - Alopecia syphilitica: "Moth-eaten" appearance, secondary syphilis
  - Postoperative, pressure-induced alopecia: From long periods of pressure on one area of scalp
  - Temporal triangular alopecia: Congenital patch of hair loss in temporal area, unilateral or bilateral
  - Traction alopecia: Patchy, due to physical stressor of braids, ponytails, hair weaves
- Pattern hair loss:
  - Androgenic alopecia: Hair transitions from terminal to vellus hairs
  - Male pattern hair loss: Androgen-mediated hair loss in specific distribution; bitemporal, vertex occurs where androgen sensitive hairs are located on scalp (3).
    - Increased androgen receptors, increased 5-alpha reductase leads to increased testosterone conversion in follicle to DHT. This leads to decreased follicle size and vellus hair (3).
    - Norwood Hamilton Classification type I–VII
    - Female pattern hair loss: Thinning on frontal and vertex areas. (Ludwig Classification, grade I–III). Females with low levels of aromatase have more testosterone available for conversion to DHT (4).
    - Polycystic ovarian syndrome, adrenal hyperplasia, pituitary hyperplasia all lead to androgen changes and can result in alopecia.
  - Drugs (testosterone, progesterone, danazol, adrenocorticosteroids, anabolic steroids)
- Trichotillomania: Intentional pulling of hair from scalp. May present in variety of patterns.
- Diffuse alopecia:
  - Telogen effluvium: Sudden shift of many follicles from anagen to telogen phase resulting in decreased hair density but not bald areas
    - May follow major stressors, including childbirth, injury, illness. Occurs 2–3 months after event.
    - Can be chronic with ongoing illness, including SLE, renal failure, IBS, HIV, thyroid disease, pituitary dysfunction.
    - Adding or changing medications (oral contraceptives, anticoagulants, anticonvulsants, SSRIs, retinoids, β-blockers, ACE inhibitors, colchicine, cholesterol-lowering medications, etc.)
    - Malnutrition from malabsorption, eating disorders; poor diet can contribute
  - Anagen effluvium:
    - Interruption of the anagen phase without transition to telogen phase. Days to weeks after inciting event.
    - Chemotherapy is most common trigger.
    - Radiation, poisoning, and medications can also trigger.
- Structural hair disorders:
  - Multiple inherited hair disorders including Menkes disease, monilethrix, etc. These result in the formation of abnormal hairs that are weakened.
  - May also result from chemical or heat damaging from hair processing treatments

Genetics
- Family history of early patterned hair loss is common in androgenic alopecia, also in alopecia areata.
- Rare structural hair disorders may be inherited.

RISK FACTORS
- Genetic predisposition
- Chronic illness including autoimmune disease, infections, cancer
- Physiologic stress including pregnancy
- Poor nutrition
- Medication, chemotherapy, radiation
- Hair treatments, braids, weaves

GENERAL PREVENTION
Minimize risk factors where possible.

COMMONLY ASSOCIATED CONDITIONS
See "Etiology and Pathophysiology"

 DIAGNOSIS

HISTORY
- Description of hair loss problem: Rate of loss, duration, location, degree of hair loss, other symptoms including pruritus, infection, hair care, and treatments
- Medications
- Medical illness including chronic disease, recent illness, surgeries, pregnancy, thyroid disorder, iron deficiency, poisonings, exposures
- Psychological stress
- Dietary history and weight changes
- Family history of hair loss or autoimmune disorders

PHYSICAL EXAM
- Pattern of hair loss:
  - Generalized, patterned, focal
  - Assess hair density, vellus vs. terminal hairs, broken hair
- Scalp scaling, inflammation, papules, pustules
- Presence of follicular ostia to determine class of alopecia
- Hair pull test:
  - Pinch 25–50 hairs between thumb and forefinger and exert slow, gentle traction while sliding fingers up:
    - Normal: 1–2 dislodge
    - Abnormal: ≥6 hairs dislodged
    - Broken hairs (structural disorder)
    - Broken-off hair at the borders patch that are easily removable (in alopecia areata)
- Hair loss at other sites, nail disorders, skin changes
- Clinical signs of thyroid disease, lupus, or other diseases
- Clinical signs of virilization: Acne, hirsutism, acanthosis nigrans, truncal obesity

DIFFERENTIAL DIAGNOSIS
Search for type of alopecia and then for reversible causes.

DIAGNOSTIC TESTS & INTERPRETATION
Initial Tests (lab, imaging)
- No testing may be indicated depending on clinical appearance.
- Nonandrogenic alopecia:
  - TSH, CBC, ferritin
  - Consider: LFT, BMP, zinc, VDRL, ANA, prolactin all depending on clinical history and exam
- Androgenic alopecia: Especially in females:
  - Consider free testosterone and dehydroepiandrosterone sulfate

Diagnostic Procedures/Other

- Light hair-pull test: Pull on 25–50 hairs; ≥6 hairs dislodged is consistent with shedding (effluvium, alopecia areata).
- Direct microscopic exam of the hair shaft:
  - Anagen hairs: Elongated, distorted bulb with root sheath attached
  - Telogen hairs: Rounded bulb, no root sheath
  - Exclamation point hairs: Club-shaped root with thinner proximal shaft (alopecia areata)
  - Broken and distorted hairs may be associated with multiple hair dystrophies
- Biopsy: Most important in scarring alopecia
- Ultraviolet light fluorescence and potassium hydroxide prep (to rule out tinea capitis)

 TREATMENT

GENERAL MEASURES

- Stop any possible medication causes if possible; this will often resolve telogen effluvium (5)[C].
- Treat underlying medical causes (e.g., thyroid disorder, syphilis).
- Traction alopecia: Change hair care practices; education.
- Trichotillomania: Often requires psychological intervention to induce behavior change

MEDICATION

Non-scarring:

- Androgenic alopecia: Treatment must be continued indefinitely. Can use in combination.
- Minoxidil (Rogaine): 2% topical solution (1 mL b.i.d.) for women, 5% topical solution (1 mL b.i.d.) or foam (daily) for men. Works in 60% of cases (3,4)[A]
  - Unclear mechanism of action; appears to prolong anagen phase (2)[A]
  - Adverse effects: Skin irritation, hypertrichosis of face/hands, tachycardia. Category C in pregnancy (3,4)[A]
- Finasteride (Propecia): 1 mg/d for men and women (1)[A],(4)[A]
  - 5-alpha reductase inhibitor, reduces DHT in system, increases total and anagen hairs, slows transition of terminal to vellus hairs
  - Works best on vertex, least in anterior, temporal areas (3)[A]
  - Adverse effects: Loss of libido, gynecomastia, depression. Caution in liver disease. Absolutely no use or contact during pregnancy, category X, reliable contraception required in female use (6)[A]
- Spironolactone (Aldactone): 100–200 mg/d (off-label) (4)[C]:
  - Aldosterone antagonist, antiandrogen; blocks the effect of androgens, decreasing testosterone production
  - Adverse effects: Dose-dependent, hyperkalemia, menstrual irregularity, fatigue; Category D in pregnancy.
- Ketoconazole: Decreases DHT levels at follicle, works best with minoxidil in female androgenic alopecia (6)[A]

- Alopecia areata: No FDA-approved treatment; high rate of spontaneous remission in patchy AA.

Intralesional steroids:

- Triamcinolone: 2.5–5 mg/mL (4,6)[C]:
  - First line if <50% scalp involved
  - Inject 0.1 mL into deep dermal layer at 0.5–1 cm intervals with 1/2 in 30-gauge needle, every 4–6 weeks. Max. 20 mg/session (2)[C]
  - Adverse effects: Local burning, pruritus, skin atrophy
- Topical steroids: Very limited evidence for efficacy
- Betamethasone: 0.1% foam shows limited hair regrowth (2)[C]:
  - Adverse effects: Folliculitis, high relapse rate after discontinuation

- Systemic glucocorticoids: Use in extensive AA. May induce regrowth, but requires long-term monthly treatment to maintain growth (2)[B]:
  - Adverse effects: Hyperglycemia, adrenal insufficiency, osteoporosis, cataracts, obesity
  - Psychiatric: SSRIs, psychiatric care, support groups
- Tinea capitis: See "Tinea (Capitis, Corporis, Cruris)"

SURGERY/OTHER PROCEDURES

- Hair transplantation
- Wigs, hairpieces, extensions
- Surgical: Graft transplantation, flap transplantation, or excision of the scarred area; used primarily in scarring alopecia

- Laser therapies to promote growth: Lacks evidence (3)[A]

COMPLEMENTARY AND ALTERNATIVE MEDICINE

- Many herbal medications are available; no clear evidence at this time.
- Volumizing shampoos can help remaining hair look fuller.

 ONGOING CARE

DIET

If nutritional deficit noted, supplementation may be necessary.

PATIENT EDUCATION

National Alopecia Areata Foundation: www.naaf.org

PROGNOSIS

- *Androgenic alopecia*: Prognosis depends on response to treatment
- *Alopecia areata*: Often regrows within 1 year even without treatment. Recurrence common. 10% have severe, chronic form. Poor prognosis more likely with long duration, extensive hair loss, autoimmune disease, nail involvement, and young age (2)[A].
- *Telogen effluvium*: Maximum shedding 3 months after the inciting event and recovery following correction of the cause. Usually subsides in 3–6 months but takes 12–18 months for cosmetically significant regrowth. Rarely, permanent hair loss, usually with long-term illness.
- *Anagen effluvium*: Shedding begins days to a few weeks after the inciting event, with recovery following correction of the cause. Rarely, permanent hair loss.

- *Traction alopecia*: Excellent prognosis with behavior modification
- *Cicatricial alopecia*: Hair follicles permanently damaged; prognosis depends on type of alopecia and available treatments (7).
- *Tinea capitis*: Excellent prognosis with treatment

REFERENCES

1. BMJ Best Practice. Accessed 5/30/2013. http://bestpractice.bmj.com/best-practice/monograph/223/basics/epidemiology.html
2. Alkhalifah A. Alopecia areata update. *Dermatol Clin*. 2013;31:93–108.
3. Banka N, Bunagan K, Shapiro, J. Pattern hair loss in men: Diagnosis and medical treatment. *Dermatol Clin*. 2013;31:129–140.
4. Rathnayake D, Sinclair R. Innovative use of spironolactone as an antiandrogen in the treatment of female pattern hair loss. *Dermatol Clin*. 2010;20:611–618.
5. Harrison S, Bergfeld W. Diffuse hair loss: Its triggers and management. *Cleve Clin J Med*. 2009;76:361–367.
6. Mesinkovska N, Bergfled W. Hair: What's new in diagnosis and management? Female pattern hair loss update: Diagnosis and treatment. *Dermatol Clin*. 2013;31:119–127.
7. Otberg N. Primary cicatricial alopecias. *Dermatol Clin*. 2013;31:155–166.

 SEE ALSO

- Tinea (Capitis, Corporis, Cruris); Syphilis; Systemic Lupus Erythematosus; Polycystic Ovarian Syndrome; Lichen Planus; Hyperthyroidism
- Algorithm: Alopecia

 CODES

ICD10
- L63.9 Alopecia areata, unspecified
- L64.9 Androgenic alopecia, unspecified
- L65.9 Nonscarring hair loss, unspecified

CLINICAL PEARLS

- History and physical are necessary in determining type of alopecia for appropriate treatment.
- Treatment of underlying medical condition or removal of triggering medication will often resolve hair loss.
- Educating the patient about the nature of the condition and expectations is key to care.
- Alopecia can affect the psychological condition of the patient, and it may be necessary to address this in any type of hair loss.

ALTITUDE ILLNESS
Robert J. Hyde, MD, MA

BASICS

DESCRIPTION
- Altitude illness is a spectrum of medical problems ranging from mild discomfort to fatal illness that may occur on ascent to higher altitudes (elevations >1,500 m [4,921 feet]). It is divided into three categories: high, 1,500–3,500 m; very high, 3,500–5,500 m; and extreme, 5,500–8,850 m (1). Altitude illness can affect anyone, including the most experienced and fit individual (2). For most, it is an unpleasant, but self-limiting syndrome that will not require physician intervention.
- Acute mountain sickness (AMS): Symptoms associated with a physiologic response to a hypobaric, hypoxic environment. Onset occurs within 24 hours of arrival at altitude, often within 1–4 hours. Neurologic symptoms are predominant and range from a mild to moderate headache and malaise to severe impairment.
- High-altitude pulmonary edema (HAPE): Noncardiogenic pulmonary edema. Onset 1–4 days at altitude. Rare <8,000 feet (2,438 m).
- High-altitude cerebral edema (HACE): A potentially fatal neurologic syndrome; considered the end stage of AMS. Onset within 3–5 days at elevations as low as 9,022 feet (2,750 m), but may be more abrupt at higher altitudes. Death results from brain herniation.
- System(s) affected: Nervous/Pulmonary
- Synonym(s): Mountain sickness

Geriatric Considerations
- Risk does not increase with age.
- Age alone should not preclude travel to high altitude; allow extra time to acclimate.
- Pre-existing medical problems are made worse; referred to as altitude-exacerbated conditions.

Pediatric Considerations
- Altitude illness seems to have the same incidence in children as in adults, but diagnosis may be delayed in younger children.
- Any child who experiences behavioral symptoms after recent ascent should be presumed to be suffering from altitude illness.

Pregnancy Considerations
- The risk during pregnancy is unknown.
- No evidence suggests that exposure to high altitudes (1,500–3,500 m) poses a risk to a pregnancy.
- It may be prudent to advise a low-altitude dwelling for any pregnant woman experiencing complications.

EPIDEMIOLOGY
Most epidemiologic studies are limited to relatively homogeneous populations of men.

Incidence
- AMS: 10–90% of travelers ascending to higher altitudes may experience symptoms.
- HAPE/HACE: These conditions occur in 0.01–1% of sojourner ascents at typical mountain resorts, although incidence increases with rapid and higher ascents (3).

ETIOLOGY AND PATHOPHYSIOLOGY
Individuals with a prior episode of HAPE have an increased risk of recurrence (4):
- Not completely understood
- Hypobaric hypoxia and hypoxemia are the pathophysiologic precursors to altitude illness.
- Symptoms of AMS may be the result of cerebral swelling, either through vasodilatation induced by hypoxia or through cerebral edema.
- Other mechanisms include impaired cerebral autoregulation, release of vasogenic mediators, and alteration of the blood–brain barrier.
- HAPE is a noncardiogenic pulmonary edema characterized by exaggerated pulmonary hypertension leading to vascular leakage through overperfusion, stress failure, or both.

RISK FACTORS
- Rapid rate of ascent
- Maximum altitude attained
- Increased duration at high altitude
- Failure to acclimatize at lower altitude
- Higher altitude during sleep cycle
- Prior history of altitude illness
- Cardiac congenital abnormalities

GENERAL PREVENTION
- General guidelines:
  - Preacclimatization affords some protection against altitude illness.
  - A staged or graded ascent (rest every 600–1,200 m) and a slow ascent rate (maximum 600 m/d) should allow adequate time for acclimatization.
  - Sleeping elevation: "Climb high and sleep low" is a prudent practice for anyone going above 3,500 m.
  - Avoid heavy exertion for the first 1–3 days.
  - Avoid respiratory depressants such as alcohol and soporifics.
  - Preascent physical conditioning is not preventive.
- Drug prophylaxis:
  - Acetazolamide, dexamethasone, and ibuprofen (see below)
  - For HAPE only:
    - Consider nifedipine and beta agonists (see "Treatment" section).

DIAGNOSIS

HISTORY
- AMS, mild to moderate symptoms:
  - Headache, plus at least 1 of the following:
    - Anorexia
    - Nausea or vomiting
    - Dizziness or lightheadedness
    - Insomnia

- AMS, severe symptoms:
  - Increased headache
  - Irritability
  - Marked fatigue
  - Dyspnea with exertion
  - Nausea and vomiting
  - HAPE (Lake Louise diagnostic criteria):
    - At least 2 of the following symptoms: Dyspnea at rest, cough, weakness, decreased exercise performance, chest tightness, congestion
    - AND at least 2 of the following signs: Crackles or wheezing in at least 1 lung field, central cyanosis, tachycardia, tachypnea. (Note: Fatigue may be pulmonary edema.)
  - HACE symptoms: Mental status changes (irrational behavior, lethargy, obtundation, coma)

PHYSICAL EXAM
- HAPE:
  - Lung crackles or wheezing
  - Central cyanosis
  - Tachycardia
  - Tachypnea
- HACE:
  - Abnormal mental status exam (behavioral change, lethargy, obtundation, coma)
  - Truncal ataxia
  - Papilledema, retinal hemorrhage, cranial nerve palsies
  - Focal neurologic deficits (rare)

DIFFERENTIAL DIAGNOSIS
- Onset of symptoms >3 days at a given altitude, the absence of headache, or the lack of rapid response to oxygen or descent suggest other diagnoses.
- AMS/HACE:
  - Subarachnoid hemorrhage, CNS mass, cerebrovascular accident
  - Migraine headache
  - Dehydration
  - Ingestion of toxins, drugs, or alcohol
  - Carbon monoxide exposure
  - CNS infection
  - Acute psychosis
- HAPE:
  - Pneumonia
  - Cardiogenic pulmonary edema
  - Spontaneous pneumothorax
  - Pulmonary embolism
  - Asthma
  - Bronchitis
  - Myocardial infarction
  - Hyperventilation syndrome

DIAGNOSTIC TESTS & INTERPRETATION
An ECG may show sinus tachycardia or right-sided heart strain.

Initial Tests (lab, imaging)
- AMS: Laboratory studies are nonspecific and rarely required for diagnosis.
- HAPE: Severe hypoxemia demonstrated with oximetry or blood gas analysis.
- No radiographic feature is specific to HAPE.

TREATMENT

GENERAL MEASURES

- Therapy must be tailored to fit disease severity.
- Early recognition is critical.
- Stop ascent, acclimatize at the same altitude, and/or descend if symptoms do not abate over 24 hours. Definitive treatment is to descend to a lower altitude. Dramatic improvement accompanies even modest reductions in altitude.
- Oxygen helps relieve symptoms. Give continuously by cannula or mask initially, and then titrate to SaO_2 >90%.
- AMS:
  - Acetazolamide is effective in reducing mild to moderate symptoms of AMS, but the optimum dosage is unknown. Consider 125–500 mg PO b.i.d. until symptoms resolve.
  - Dexamethasone may also be effective in treating moderate AMS. Consider 4 mg PO/IM/IV q6h.
  - Analgesics and antiemetics as needed for symptomatic relief
- HAPE:
  - Oxygen therapy
  - Minimize exertion and keep patient warm.
  - Immediate descent or evacuation to a lower altitude
  - Portable hyperbaric therapy (2–15 psi), such as the Gamow bag or Chamberlite, is an effective and practical alternative when descent is not possible.
  - Consider nifedipine 10 mg PO, then 20–30 mg extended-release PO b.i.d.
- HACE:
  - Immediate descent
  - Supplemental oxygen (highest flow available; maintain SaO_2 >90%)
  - Dexamethasone: 8 mg IV/IM/PO initially, then 4 mg q6h
  - Hyperbaric therapy if unable to descend

MEDICATION

First Line

- Oxygen: 2–15 L/min to maintain SaO_2 >90% until symptoms improve
- Acetazolamide: If patient has a history of problems at altitude and/or plans to ascend >500 m/d. Dosage is usually 125–500 mg PO b.i.d. starting 2 days before ascent and continued for 3 days at maximum altitude. Patients with a drug allergy to sulfonamides should avoid acetazolamide (5)[C]:
  - Primary prevention of AMS: 125–500 mg PO b.i.d. starting 1 day before ascent and continued for 2 days at maximum altitude
  - Treatment of AMS: 125–500 mg PO b.i.d. until symptoms resolve

- Dexamethasone: May significantly reduce the incidence and severity of AMS. Dosage is 2–4 mg PO q6h, begun the day of ascent, continued for 3 days at the higher altitude, then tapered over 5 days. Adverse side effects are rare:
  - Prevention of AMS: 2 mg PO q6h or 4 mg PO q12h, starting 1 day before ascent and discontinued cautiously after 2 days at maximum altitude
  - Treatment of AMS: 4 mg PO/IV/IM q6h
  - Treatment of HACE: 8 mg PO/IV/IM initially, then 4 mg q6h
- Nifedipine (reduces pulmonary arterial pressure):
  - Prevention of HAPE: 20–30 mg extended-release PO b.i.d. starting 1 day prior to ascent and continued for 2 days at maximum altitude
  - Treatment of HAPE: 10 mg, then 20–30 mg extended-release PO b.i.d.
- Salmeterol:
  - Prevention and possible treatment of HAPE: 125 μg inhaled b.i.d. starting 1 day before ascent and continued for 2 days at maximum altitude
- NSAIDs:
  - Prevention and treatment of headache
  - Aspirin: 325 mg PO q4h for total 3 doses
  - Ibuprofen: 400–600 mg PO (6)
  - Prevention of AMS: Dose unknown. Begin 1–5 days before ascent.
- Antiemetics:
  - Prochlorperazine: 10 mg PO/IM q6–8h
  - Promethazine: 25–50 mg PO/IM/PR q6h

Second Line

Furosemide: Consider for treatment of AMS or HACE, 20–80 mg PO/IV q12h for a total of 2 doses. Currently out of favor; not recommended for prophylaxis; not established for use in HAPE.

IN-PATIENT CONSIDERATIONS

Admission Criteria/Initial Stabilization

Outpatient treatment for mild cases

 ONGOING CARE

FOLLOW-UP RECOMMENDATIONS

Patient Monitoring

- For mild cases, no follow-up is needed.
- For more severe cases, follow until symptoms subside.

PATIENT EDUCATION

Patients should be counseled about the risks of high-altitude travel and how to recognize high-altitude illnesses.

PROGNOSIS

Most cases of mild to moderate AMS are self-limiting and do not require physician intervention. Patients may resume ascent once the symptoms subside. HAPE and HACE respond well to descent, evacuation, and/or pharmacologic treatment if identified early.

COMPLICATIONS

A patient may experience a high-altitude retinal hemorrhage, which can cause visual changes, but this is usually asymptomatic.

REFERENCES

1. Gallagher SA, Hackett PH. High-altitude illness. *Emerg Med Clin North Am*. 2004;22:329–355, viii.
2. Schoene RB. Illnesses at high altitude. *Chest*. 2008;134:402–416.
3. Maloney JP, Broeckel U. Epidemiology, risk factors, and genetics of high-altitude-related pulmonary disease. *Clin Chest Med*. 2005;26:395–404, v.
4. Basnyat B, Murdoch DR. High-altitude illness. *Lancet*. 2003;361:1967–1974.
5. Luks AM, Swenson ER. Medication and dosage considerations in the prophylaxis and treatment of high-altitude illness. *Chest*. 2008;133:744–755.
6. Lipman GS, Kanaan NC, Holck PS, et al. Ibuprofen prevents altitude illness: A randomized controlled trial for prevention of altitude illness with nonsteroidal anti-inflammatories. *Ann Emerg Med*. 2012;59(6):484–490. Epub 2012 Mar 21.

ADDITIONAL READING

Imray C, Booth A, Wright A, et al. Acute altitude illnesses. *BMJ*. 2011;343:d4943.

CODES

ICD10

- T70.20XA Unspecified effects of high altitude, initial encounter
- T70.20XD Unspecified effects of high altitude, subsequent encounter
- T70.20XS Unspecified effects of high altitude, sequela

CLINICAL PEARLS

- Slow ascent and timely descent are important tenets in the prevention and treatment of high-altitude illnesses, respectively.
- High-flow oxygen, followed by oxygen titrated to maintain SaO_2 >90%, is the first-line treatment for all patients with more than a mild illness.

ALZHEIMER DISEASE

Jill A. Grimes, MD, FAAFP

 BASICS

DESCRIPTION
- Alzheimer disease (AD) is the most common cause of dementia in the elderly.
- Degenerative neurologic disease with progressive impairment in ≥2:
  - Memory, executive function, attention, language, or visuospatial skills
  - With significant interference in ability to function in work, home, or social interactions
- *New diagnostic criteria* released in 2011 emphasize full spectrum of disease (1)[A]:
  - Preclinical AD (*research purposes only:* Biomarkers present; subtle decline evident to patient, but cognitive tests in "normal" range)
  - Mild cognitive impairment (MCI): Social, occupational, and functional skills preserved despite significant decline in cognition
  - Alzheimer dementia
- System(s) affected: Nervous
- Synonym(s): Presenile dementia; Senile dementia of the Alzheimer type

Geriatric Considerations
Asymptomatic screening is not recommended.

EPIDEMIOLOGY
- Predominant age: >65 years
- 2/3 Female, 1/3 Male in US

Incidence
1 in 8 Americans age >65 years (13%); nearly 50% once >85

Prevalence
>5.4 million in US:
- 200,000 younger onset (<65 years)

ETIOLOGY AND PATHOPHYSIOLOGY
- Unknown, but involves amyloid beta accumulation initially, then synaptic dysfunction, neurodegeneration, and eventual neuronal loss
- Age, genetics, systemic disease, behaviors (smoking), and other host factors may influence the response to amyloid beta and/or the pace of progression toward the clinical manifestations of AD.

Genetics
- Positive family history in 50%, but 90% of AD is sporadic:
  - APOE4 increases risk, but full role unclear
- Familial/autosomal-dominant AD accounts for <5% AD:
  - Amyloid precursor protein (APP), presenilin-1 (PS-1), and presenilin-2 (PS-2)

RISK FACTORS
- Aging, family history, APOE4, Down syndrome
- Cardiovascular and carotid artery disease
- Smoking (2–4-fold increase) (1)
- Head trauma

GENERAL PREVENTION
- NSAIDs, estrogen, and vitamin E do NOT delay AD (2)[A]; insufficient evidence for statins (3)[A].
- Intellectual challenge (puzzles) and regular physical exercise may offer preventive benefit.
- Control vascular risk factors (e.g., hypertension); lowering cholesterol may retard pathogenesis of AD.
- Ginkgo biloba may be beneficial for cognition, but not activities of daily living (4).

- Physical activities and omega-3 fatty acids may help to prevent or delay cognitive decline (5).
- US may help to identify asymptomatic patients at increased risk with chronic brain hypoperfusion secondary to cardiovascular or carotid artery pathology (6).

COMMONLY ASSOCIATED CONDITIONS
- Down syndrome
- Depression

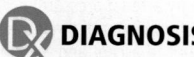 **DIAGNOSIS**

Degenerative neurologic disease with progressive impairment in ≥2 areas:
- Memory, executive function, attention, language, or visuospatial skills AND
- Significant interference in ability to function in work, home, or social interactions

HISTORY
- Include family members in interview (for accuracy and for behavioral assessment).
- Progressive and disruptive memory loss
- Depression, anhedonia, or apathy
- Intellectual decline, difficulty with calculations, multiple missed appointments
- Loss of interest, social withdrawal
- Date or time confusion
- Occupational dysfunction or personality change
- Restlessness and sleep disturbances

PHYSICAL EXAM
- Neurologic exam to rule out other causes
- Folstein Mini Mental Status Exam (MMSE): Copyrighted, but available (http://www.aafp.org/afp/20010215/703.html)
- Counting coins test: "If I gave you a nickel, quarter, dime, and penny, how much is that?"
- No focal neurologic signs
- Short-term memory loss
- Acalculia (e.g., cannot balance checkbook)
- Agnosia: Inability to recognize objects
- Apraxia: Inability to carry out movements
- Confabulation
- Delusions
- Impaired abstraction
- Decreased attention to hygiene
- Visuospatial distortion
- Late signs: Psychotic features, mutism

DIFFERENTIAL DIAGNOSIS
- Depression
- Vascular dementia, multi-infarct dementia
- Lewy body disease
- Dementia associated with Parkinson disease
- Normal-pressure hydrocephalus
- Creutzfeldt-Jakob disease
- End-stage multiple sclerosis
- Brain tumor: Primary or metastatic
- Subdural hematoma
- Progressive multifocal leukoencephalopathy
- Metabolic dementia (hypothyroidism)
- Drug reactions, alcoholism, other addictions
- Dementia pugilistica
- Toxicity from liver and kidney failure
- Vitamin and other nutritional deficiencies
- Vasculitis
- Neurosyphilis

DIAGNOSTIC TESTS & INTERPRETATION
Neuropsychologic testing: If clinical picture is confusing, or to help determine level of independence for skills such as balancing checkbooks, driving, or managing medicines

Initial Tests (lab, imaging)
To help rule out other causes of dementia:
- CBC, ESR
- Chemistry panel
- Thyroid-stimulating hormone
- Folate and B_{12} levels
- Venereal disease reaction level (VDRL) or rapid plasma reagin (RPR)
- HIV antibody (selected cases)
- APOE4 or biomarker testing is not routine.
- Controversy exists; consider MRI or CT scan if:
  - Cognitive decline is recent and rapid; age <60; history of stroke; gait disturbance or focal neurologic signs
  - Cancer, urinary incontinence, bleeding disorder, or current use of anticoagulants
- Single-photon emission computed tomography (SPECT) and photon emission tomography (PET): Only if diagnostic uncertainty after CT or MRI; insufficient evidence to use alone

Follow-Up Tests & Special Considerations
- Genetic testing for APOE4 or for familial AD types; discuss with genetic counselor (2)[A]
- CT scan/MRI: Moderate cortical atrophy, ventricular enlargement
- MRI: Hippocampal volumetry; PET and SPECT not indicated
- Medicare pays for PET to distinguish AD from frontotemporal dementia.

Test Interpretation
- Gross: Diffuse cerebral atrophy in hippocampus, amygdala, and some subcortical nuclei
- Micro:
  - Neuritic senile plaques
  - Neurofibrillary tangles
  - Pyramidal cell loss
  - Decreased cholinergic innervation (other neurotransmitters variably decreased)
  - Degeneration of locus ceruleus and basal forebrain nuclei of Meynert; amyloid angiopathy

 TREATMENT

GENERAL MEASURES
- Optimize treatment of associated comorbid conditions (including hearing and vision loss).
- Analyze environment for safety and security, and avoid sudden changes in environment.
- Assess spouse/caregiver burnout.
- Advance directives planning, living will, power of attorney

MEDICATION
First Line

- May reduce symptoms, but do not prevent disease progression (7)[A]:
  - Cholinesterase inhibitors (8)[A]:
    ○ Equally effective; all have significant GI side effects

○ When used for at least 6 months, provide mild benefit in cognition, daily function, and behavior. Also shown to reduce nursing home placement by 20% after 25 months of treatment. No deterioration over 6–12 months is evidence of efficacy.

○ Best in mild-to-moderate disease (Folstein MMSE scores 10–24); drugs *may* be effective in Lewy body dementia.

○ Donepezil (Aricept): Start at 5 mg/d PO; may increase to 10 mg/d after 1 month:

○ Tablets or orally disintegrating tablets; generic available

○ Caution with digoxin or beta-blockers (can cause 3rd-degree heart block)

○ Aricept 23-mg tablet approved in 2010

○ Rivastigmine (Exelon): Start 1.5 mg PO b.i.d., increase by 1.5 mg b.i.d. every 2 weeks; maintenance 6–12 mg/d total:

○ Capsule, solution, or patch (patch greatly reduces side effects)

○ Indicated for both AD and Parkinson dementia

○ Galantamine (Razadyne): Start 4 mg b.i.d. for 4 weeks, then increase by 4 mg b.i.d. every month with goal 16–24 mg/d dose:

○ Tablets, solution, and extended-release (ER) capsule (ER has daily dosing)

– *N*-methyl-D-aspartate (NMDA) receptor antagonists (for moderate-to-severe AD; MMSE 5–14):

○ Monotherapy or in combination with acetylcholinesterase inhibitors

○ Memantine (Namenda): Start at 5 mg/d, with starter pack titrating to target dose of 10 mg b.i.d. after 4 weeks

○ Often improves behavioral issues

○ Beneficial for cognition and physician's global impression; increases risk of somnolence, weight gain, confusion, hypertension, nervous system disorders, and falling (9)[A]

- For depression (occurs in 1/3 of patients), use SSRIs.
- Insomnia:
  – Trazodone 25–100 mg at bedtime, zolpidem (Ambien) 5 mg at bedtime, zaleplon (Sonata) 5–10 mg at bedtime, ramelteon (Rozerem) 8 mg at bedtime
  – Avoid diphenhydramine in elderly, due to negative cognitive effects and risk of urinary retention (males).
- Moderate anxiety/restlessness: Consider low-dose, short-acting benzodiazepines, buspirone, or SSRIs (efficacy unproven).
- Severe aggressive agitation:
  – Behavioral techniques and environmental modification help more than medications for wandering, restlessness, uncooperativeness, hoarding, and irritability:
    ○ Consider changing environment, rewards, behavioral redirection, hearing aids, and bright light therapy.
  – Memantine (Namenda) (8)[A]: Start at 5 mg/d, with starter pack titrating to target dose of 10 mg b.i.d. after 4 weeks.
  – Antipsychotics (both conventional and atypical) are associated with increased mortality and acute care hospital admissions in elderly patients with dementia.
- Precautions:
  – Avoid anticholinergic drugs, such as tricyclic antidepressants and antihistamines.
  – Ginkgo biloba: Avoid anticoagulants and aspirin.

– Benzodiazepines may produce paradoxical excitation or daytime drowsiness.
– Triazolam (Halcion) can produce confusion, memory loss, and psychotic behavior.
– Benzodiazepines may increase serum phenytoin concentration.
– Cimetidine may increase benzodiazepine concentration.
– Donepezil (Aricept): Use with caution with anticholinergic medication, in sick sinus syndrome or history of peptic ulcers.
– Paroxetine increase donepezil levels.

Second Line
Vitamin E, statins, estrogen, and NSAIDs should not be routinely recommended due to lack of evidence and safety concerns (10)[A].

ISSUES FOR REFERRAL
- Assess driving safety (vision, spatial relations, hearing, judgment):
  – http://www.nhtsa.gov/people/injury/olddrive/ Driving%20Safely%20Aging%20Web/
- Support groups for patient and family: Alzheimer Association: http://www.alz.org

ADDITIONAL THERAPIES
- Exercise to reduce restlessness
- Cognitive challenge; traditional and computerized training both effective (11)[A]
- Occupational therapy, music therapy, aroma therapy, pet therapy

COMPLEMENTARY AND ALTERNATIVE MEDICINE
- Huperzine A 400 mg (herbal cholinesterase inhibitors) may improve cognition with minimal side effects.
- Ginkgo biloba extracts (120 mg/d) show conflicting efficacy in treatment of AD, but may be beneficial (4).
- Coenzyme Q10 is not effective.

 ## ONGOING CARE

FOLLOW-UP RECOMMENDATIONS
Patient Monitoring
- Schedule regular follow-up (3 months) to assess medical complications, provide support for family, and assess need for placement.
- Serial mental status testing is potentially helpful, but bedside tests (Folstein MMSE) offer wide variability and lack of sensitivity.

PATIENT EDUCATION
- Alzheimer Association: http://www.alz.org/
- Explain progressive nature of the disease and start advance directives planning as early as possible.

PROGNOSIS
Poor: Average survival from diagnosis is 4–8 years (diagnosis is often delayed).

COMPLICATIONS
- Behavioral: Hostility, agitation, wandering, falls
- Metabolic: Infection, dehydration, drug toxicity
- "Sundowning" (increase full-spectrum lights) Depression (1/3 of patients); suicide

REFERENCES
1. McKhann GM, Knopman DS, Chertkow H, et al. The diagnosis of dementia due to Alzheimer's disease: Recommendations from the National Institute on Aging-Alzheimer's Association workgroups on diagnostic guidelines for Alzheimer's disease. *Alzheimers Dement.* 2011;7(3):263–269.
2. Cataldo JK, Prochaska JJ, Glantz SA. Cigarette smoking is a risk factor for Alzheimer's disease: An analysis controlling for tobacco industry affiliation. *J Alzheimers Dis.* 2010;19:465–480.
3. McGuinness B, O'Hare J, Craig D, et al. Cochrane review on 'Statins for the treatment of dementia.' *Int J Geriatr Psychiatry.* 2013;28(2):119–126. Epub 2012 Apr 2.
4. Weinmann S, Roll S, Schwarzbach C, et al. Effects of Ginkgo biloba in dementia: Systematic review and meta-analysis. *BMC Geriatr.* 2010;10:14.
5. Daviglus ML, Bell CC, Berrittini W, et al. NIH State-of-the-Science Conference: Preventing Alzheimer's Disease and Cognitive Decline. 2010.
6. de la Torre JC. Vascular risk factor detection and control may prevent Alzheimer's disease. *Ageing Res Rev.* 2010;10.
7. Herrmann N, Chau SA, Kircanski I, et al. Current and emerging drug treatment options for Alzheimer's disease: A systematic review. *Drugs.* 2011;71(15):2031–2065.
8. Segal-Gidan F, Cherry D, Jones R, et al. Alzheimer's disease management guideline: Update 2008. *Alzheimers Dement.* 2011;7(3):e51–e59.
9. Yang Z, Zhou X, Zhang Q. Effectiveness and safety of memantine treatment for Alzheimer's disease. *J Alzheimers Dis.* 2013 May 1
10. Work group on Alzheimer's Disease and Other Dementias. Treatment of patients with Alzheimer's disease and other dementias, 2nd ed. *Am J Psychiatry.* 2007;164(12 Suppl):5–56.
11. Kueider AM, Parisi JM, Gross AL, et al. Computerized cognitive training with older adults: A systematic review. *PLoS ONE.* 2012;7(7): e40588. Epub 2012 Jul 11.

 ## SEE ALSO

Substance Use Disorders; Hypothyroidism, Adult; Depression

CODES

ICD10
- F02.80 Dementia in other diseases classified elsewhere without behavioral disturbance
- F02.81 Dementia in oth diseases classd elswhr w behavioral disturb
- G30.9 Alzheimer's disease, unspecified

CLINICAL PEARLS
- Daily intellectual stimulation, such as puzzles, and moderate physical exercise may help prevent AD.
- Imaging studies have low yield in patients with a history typical of AD.
- Encourage families to join a chapter of the Alzheimer Association and to pursue advanced directive planning early in the course of the disease.
- Atypical antipsychotic medications increase mortality.

AMBLYOPIA
Robert M. Kershner, MD, MS, FACS

 BASICS

DESCRIPTION
- Amblyopia is a reduction in visual acuity as a result of abnormal visual development in the absence of a structural or pathologic abnormality of the eye; it cannot be corrected by eyeglasses or contact lenses.
- The abnormality is in the brain's visual pathways and interpretative areas, not in the eye itself, although it is the eye that triggers the perceptual change.
- Functional amblyopia is potentially reversible with occlusion therapy.
- Organic amblyopia is irreversible.
- The visual acuity deficit is typically unilateral; rarely, it may be bilateral.
- The reduction in vision is usually apparent in the eye with the greater refractive error or with abnormal position of gaze (strabismus).
- Identification of abnormal visual pathway development became the basis of the 1981 Nobel Prize in Physiology or Medicine awarded to David H. Hubel and Torsten Wiesel.
- System(s) affected: Nervous
- Synonym(s): Lazy eye, Squint

Pediatric Considerations
More commonly seen in the pediatric age group. The mean age at presentation is 3–6 years.

EPIDEMIOLOGY
- Predominant age: Onset may be present from birth or can appear in early childhood. If diagnosed in adulthood, it is most likely permanent and uncorrectable. The condition often goes undiagnosed but can be detected at any age.
- Predominant gender: Male > Female

Incidence
Amblyopia carries a projected lifetime risk of visual loss of 1.2%.

Prevalence
~2–3% of children

ETIOLOGY AND PATHOPHYSIOLOGY
- Strabismus causes disparate retinal images whereby 1 eye sees the object of regard in the fovea and the other in a different part of the retina.
- Inability to fuse the 2 images from each eye results in the brain ignoring the less preferred image (this does not necessarily need to be the less clear image).
- Refractive errors such as anisometropia (a difference in refractive error between the 2 eyes) can cause the 2 retinal images to be of unequal clarity.
- An obstruction to the visual axis, such as cataracts, causes unequal clarity of the retinal image. Cataract in an infant or child, therefore, is a medical emergency warranting surgical intervention and prompt removal.
- The result of 1 eye seeing better than the other interrupts the development of fine visual perception, which can contribute to the development of amblyopia.
- Individuals with amblyopia do not have normal degrees of stereo vision and often complain of not appreciating 3D images.
- Strabismic amblyopia is a loss of visual acuity due to suppression of the images from an eye that turns in or out in an individual with misalignment of the visual axis.

- Anisometropic amblyopia is present when 1 eye has a significantly different refractive error than the other, especially if that error is hyperopia; it leads to visual blurring and therefore suppression of the image from that eye.
- Refractive amblyopia is due to uncorrected high refractive error, resulting in visual blurring in either or both eyes.
- Deprivation amblyopia (amblyopia ex anopsia) is due to relatively complete visual deprivation in 1 eye, which may be caused by a congenital abnormality such as a corneal scar or cataract.
- Deficiency amblyopia is also known as nutritional optic neuropathy or tobacco–alcohol amblyopia. Deficiencies of vitamin B_1, B_{12}, or riboflavin may be responsible.
- Amblyopia can only occur early in life:
  – When the brain detects unequal images, for any reason, it is forced to ignore one.
  – The ability of the brain to suppress the unwanted image can only occur when the development of neuroadaptive responses is in a critical "plastic" period, usually the 1st several years of life.
  – If amblyopia has not developed after that period, the individual will be unable to "suppress" the unwanted image, and diplopia or double vision will result.

Genetics
Increased incidence in children with a parent or sibling with a history of amblyopia

RISK FACTORS
- Pre-existing refractive error, such as myopia, hyperopia, or astigmatism
- More common with a pre-existing occlusion of the visual pathway, such as abnormal eyelid position, hemangioma, or malposition of the eye
- Conditions that cause anisometropia (unequal refractive difference between the eyes) or obstruction to clear vision (i.e., cataract, corneal abnormalities) can lead to permanent amblyopia.

GENERAL PREVENTION
- All infants and children should be screened from birth for normal visual acuity and development. Refractive errors or abnormal position of the eyes should be promptly evaluated by an ophthalmologist and treated if permanent visual loss is to be avoided.
- Children do not grow out of refractive errors or strabismus and should always be evaluated and treated by a specialist in pediatric ophthalmology.

COMMONLY ASSOCIATED CONDITIONS
Neurological abnormalities, Down syndrome, cerebral palsy

 DIAGNOSIS

HISTORY
- Squinting of 1 eye in bright light is the most common symptom, hence the alternative term for strabismus, "squint."
- Rubbing the eyes
- Sitting close to television or computer screen
- Problems in sports
- Preference for front-row seating
- Covering or closing an eye
- Eye turns in or out, wandering eye
- Poor vision in an eye without apparent explanation or a diagnosable organic cause

- Poor vision that does not correct with glasses
- Often, because 1 eye is seeing properly, parents, schools, and physicians are not aware of a potentially amlyopic eye.
- Absence of "red reflex," such as that seen with flash photography in both eyes

PHYSICAL EXAM
- All children should have complete visual exams prior to starting school, with each eye tested individually (this is critical, children peak under cover) (1)[B].
- Children from families with a known history of amblyopia or strabismus should have dilated exams performed by an ophthalmologist.
- The corneal light reflex test (shining a light into the child's eyes and noting the location of the light in relation to the pupil) may be used to assess ocular alignment in young children. Observing a photograph of the child looking into the camera can often reveal the abnormality as well (2)[C].

DIFFERENTIAL DIAGNOSIS
- The diagnosis of amblyopia can be confused with an organic lesion, causing decreased visual acuity, and must always be excluded before amblyopia is considered.
- Intraocular tumors, glaucoma, congenital abnormalities, and trauma can result in and be mistaken for amblyopia.

DIAGNOSTIC TESTS & INTERPRETATION
Specialized tests such as Worth Four Dot, steroscopic testing, and monocular vs. binocular acuity testing can reveal abnormalities in acuity between the 2 eyes.

Initial Tests (lab, imaging)
- There is no lab test for amblyopia.
- External photographs can reveal an obstruction to the visual pathway or a malalignment in the positions of the eyes.
- At the first examination, the face and position of the eyes should be documented with flash photography.

Follow-Up Tests & Special Considerations
- Any of the above conditions indicate prompt evaluation and ophthalmologic referral. In a young child, the earlier the diagnosis, the better the therapeutic outcome.
- Children with cataract may require cataract surgery.
- Unequal refractive errors need to be promptly treated with glasses or contact lenses to improve sight before amblyopia sets in.
- Any concern regarding the positions of the eyes or visual acuity requires a prompt referral to an ophthalmologist.

Diagnostic Procedures/Other
- Measurement of visual acuity (this can be accomplished even in infants and nonverbal children)
- Measurement of the alignment and position of the eyes (Krimsky, prism testing, cover-uncover tests)

Test Interpretation
The presence of a pathologic abnormality of the eye, cataract, or retinal lesion precludes the diagnosis of amblyopia but necessitates prompt evaluation and intervention.

TREATMENT

GENERAL MEASURES
- Correction of the underlying disorder should be instituted promptly, as the condition may become irreversible if the child is >4–6 years of age.
- Patching of the stronger eye to encourage visual development of the amblyopic eye is warranted. There may be resistance from the child to wearing a patch, which may lessen benefit. Various patching regimens have been studied (from 2 to 23 hours of patching per day for 4–6 months, and alternate patching). Close follow up is necessary. Should the "good" eye be patched excessively, the risk of development of amblyopia in that eye increases.
- An alternative therapy to patching is pharmacologic blurring, usually achieved with atropine eye drops. Similar efficacy is achieved compared to patching, with improved compliance. The risk associated with systemic effects from the antimuscarinic effects of the drug cannot be ignored (3,4)[A].
- Corrective lenses should be prescribed for refractive errors.
- Correction of anatomic obstructions, including cataracts or ptosis, may improve vision and minimize recurrence.
- Amblyopia never corrects itself spontaneously and will always require treatment. Children do not outgrow amblyopia.
- Deficiency amblyopia: Balanced diet, vitamins, and avoidance of alcohol and tobacco
- All treatments for amblyopia, regardless of cause, need to be instituted promptly and early if success is to be achieved. Studies have shown that intervention after the age of 8 greatly lessens the outcome, although treatment of amblyopia has met with limited success in adults.

MEDICATION
Cycloplegia is often utilized to pharmacologically paralyze the ability of the eye to accommodate, necessitating the use of the "weaker" or nondominant amblyopic eye.

ISSUES FOR REFERRAL
Obstruction of vision in the infant or toddler is a medical emergency. Failure to refer can result in irreversible loss of vision in an otherwise healthy eye.

SURGERY/OTHER PROCEDURES
Surgical correction of an abnormal eye position or intraocular obstruction may be required.

COMPLEMENTARY AND ALTERNATIVE MEDICINE
- There are no effective homeopathic remedies for amblyopia.
- Vision training can be an effective adjunct only if the underlying organic causes are addressed and patching therapy instituted.

ONGOING CARE

FOLLOW-UP RECOMMENDATIONS
- All children diagnosed with amblyopia need to be followed for years to prevent recurrence.
- Amblyopia treatment is not a 1-time therapy; lapses and recurrences are common, and therefore continued monitoring and intervention are required for years.

Patient Monitoring
Once the diagnosis of amblyopia has been made, the patient must be seen frequently until complete resolution of the problem occurs.

DIET
There are no known dietary effects on amblyopia.

PATIENT EDUCATION
Advise all parents to have children's eyes examined as infants and again prior to starting school if no abnormalities are noted.

PROGNOSIS
- A treatable condition in most cases if the diagnosis is made early:
  - Patching therapy, pharmacologic blurring, eyeglasses, and surgical correction of abnormal eye positions can result in near-normal vision when instituted early.
  - Visual development occurs during the first several years of life, and amblyopia therapy can be effective until 12 years.
- The risk of recurrence is 24% after 1 year; reinstitution of treatment is warranted.
- The recovery of vision depends on how mature the visual connections are, the length of deprivation, and at what age the therapy is begun. It is important to rule out any organic cause of decreased vision because many diseases may not be detectable on routine exam.
- The best outcome is achieved if treatment is started before age 8. Research has shown that children >12 and some adults can also show improvement with treatment (5)[B].
- Children from 9–11 who wore an eye patch and performed near-point activities (vision therapy) were 4 times as likely to show a 2-line improvement on a standard 11-line eye chart than amblyopic children who did not receive treatment.
- Adolescents aged 13–17 showed limited improvement, not as great as when treatment was instituted at a younger age.
- A 2004 study showed that perceptual learning can improve vision in amblyopic adults (6)[B].
- Virtual reality computer games, especially when each eye receives different images, has shown limited success in improving monocularity in the affected eye.

COMPLICATIONS
- Failure to institute therapy early in life can lead to permanent, irreversible, unilateral visual loss:
  - Unilateral amblyopia causes an increased risk of severe visual impairment due to loss of vision in the nonamblyopic eye.

- Psychosocial complications include difficulty in schooling, work, or physical activity and an increased risk of depression and anxiety.

REFERENCES
1. Schmucker C, Grosselfinger R, Riemsma R, et al. Diagnostic accuracy of vision screening tests for the detection of amblyopia and its risk factors: A systematic review. *Graefes Arch Clin Exp Ophthalmol*. 2009;247:1441–1454.
2. Teed RG, Bui CM, Morrison DG, et al. Amblyopia therapy in children identified by photoscreening. *Ophthalmology*. 2010;117:159–162.
3. Kushner BJ. Atropine vs patching for treatment of amblyopia in children. *JAMA*. 2002;287: 2145–2146.
4. Li T, Shotton K. Conventional occlusion versus pharmacologic penalization for amblyopia. *Cochrane Database Syst Rev*. 2009;4:CD006460.
5. Schmucker C, Kleijnen J, Grosselfinger R, et al. Effectiveness of early in comparison to late(r) treatment in children with amblyopia or its risk factors: A systematic review. *Ophthalmic Epidemiol*. 2010;17:7–17.
6. Levi DM, Li RW. Perceptual Learning as a potential treatment for amblyopia: A mini-review. *Vision Res*. 2009;49:2535–2549.

ADDITIONAL READING
National Eye Institute. Amblyopia. Available at: www.nei.nih.gov/health/amblyopia/index.asp

SEE ALSO
Refractive Errors; Strabismus

CODES

ICD10
- H53.009 Unspecified amblyopia, unspecified eye
- H53.029 Refractive amblyopia, unspecified eye
- H53.039 Strabismic amblyopia, unspecified eye

CLINICAL PEARLS
- Amblyopia typically presents between 3 and 6 years, but it needs to be diagnosed as soon as possible if treatment is to be effective.
- Referral should always be considered if an inequality in the appearance of the alignment of the eyes or visual function is suspected.
- Due to increased incidence in families where there is a history of amblyopia, all related children should be screened.
- In some children with prominent nasal folds, pseudostrabismus can be mistaken for strabismus: If in doubt, referral is always recommended.

AMENORRHEA

Heidi L. Gaddey, MD

 BASICS

DESCRIPTION
- Primary amenorrhea:
  - No menses by age 13–14 with absence of secondary sexual characteristics OR
  - No menses by age 15–16 with normal secondary characteristics
- Secondary amenorrhea: Absence of menses for 3 months in a woman with previously normal menstruation or 6 months in a woman with a history of irregular cycles
- System(s) affected: Endocrine/Metabolic; Reproductive

Pregnancy Considerations
Pregnancy is by far the most common cause of secondary amenorrhea.

EPIDEMIOLOGY
Prevalence
- Primary amenorrhea: <1% of female population
- Secondary amenorrhea: 3–5% of female population
- No evidence for race and ethnicity affecting prevalence

ETIOLOGY AND PATHOPHYSIOLOGY
- Primary amenorrhea:
  - Hypothalamic–pituitary abnormalities:
    - Constitutional delay of puberty
    - Functional hypothalamic amenorrhea
    - Eating disorder
    - Stress/Exercise
    - Central lesions (tumors, hypophysitis, granulomas)
    - Pituitary dysfunction (hyperprolactinemia, abnormal secretion of follicle-stimulating hormone [FSH], luteinizing hormone [LH], or GnRH)
    - Thyroid dysfunction
  - Gonadal abnormalities:
    - Chromosomal abnormalities (androgen insensitivity syndrome)
    - Euchromosomal gonadal agenesis or dysgenesis (Turner syndrome, Swyer syndrome, and pure gonadal dysgenesis)
    - Polycystic ovarian syndrome (PCOS)
    - Abnormal gonadotropin function
    - Autoimmune gonadal failure
    - Idiopathic gonadal failure
  - Anatomic abnormalities:
    - Imperforate hymen
    - Transverse vaginal septum
    - Congenital absence of the cervix
    - Müllerian agenesis
- Secondary amenorrhea:
  - Pregnancy
  - Thyroid disease
  - Hyperprolactinemia (altered metabolism, ectopic production, breastfeeding/stimulation, hypothyroidism, medications, empty sella syndrome, pituitary adenoma)
  - If pregnancy, thyroid disease, and hyperprolactinemia are ruled out, consider:
    - Normogonadotropic amenorrhea: Hyperandrogenic anovulation (acromegaly, androgen-secreting tumors, Cushing disease, exogenous androgens, nonclassical congenital adrenal hyperplasia, PCOS); outflow tract obstruction (Asherman syndrome, cervical stenosis, fibroids or polyps)

- Hypergonadotropic hypogonadism: Normal menopause; premature ovarian failure (autoimmune, chemotherapy, galactosemia, fragile X premutation and other genetic causes, 17-hydroxylase deficiency, idiopathic, mumps oophoritis, pelvic radiation)
- Hypogonadotropic hypogonadism: Eating disorders, CNS tumors, chronic illness, cranial radiation, excessive weight loss/exercise/malnutrition, hypothalamic or pituitary destruction, Sheehan syndrome
- Pathophysiology varies, depending on etiology.
- Primary amenorrhea should be evaluated in the context of presence or absence of secondary sexual characteristics.
- Can result from dysfunction in hypothalamic-pituitary-gonadal axis, anatomic abnormalities, or another endocrine gland disorder

Genetics
May occur with Turner syndrome or testicular feminization

RISK FACTORS
- Obesity
- Overtraining (prolonged, excessive exercise)
- Eating disorders
- Malnutrition
- Anovulatory disorders
- Psychosocial crisis
- Treatment with antipsychotic medications

GENERAL PREVENTION
Maintenance of proper body mass index (BMI) and healthy lifestyle with respect to food and exercise

COMMONLY ASSOCIATED CONDITIONS
- Premature ovarian failure may be associated with autoimmune abnormalities (autoimmune thyroiditis, type 1 diabetes).
- Polycystic ovarian syndrome is associated with insulin resistance and obesity.
- Decreased exposure to estrogen may increase risk for osteopenia or osteoporosis.

DIAGNOSIS

HISTORY
- Review of systems, including recent weight changes, symptoms of early pregnancy or menopause, virilizing changes, cyclic pelvic pain, galactorrhea, headaches, vision changes, fatigue, palpitations
- Growth and pubertal development history, including age of breast development, pubertal growth spurt, and adrenarche
- History of chronic illness, trauma, surgery, medications, prior chemotherapy or radiation
- Psychiatric history
- Social history, including diet and exercise history, drug abuse, and sexual history

PHYSICAL EXAM
- General appearance
- Vital signs, height, weight, growth percentile and BMI, hypotension, bradycardia, hypothermia (anorexia nervosa)
- HEENT exam: Evidence of dental erosions, trauma to palate (bulimia), visual field defect, funduscopic changes, cranial nerve findings (prolactinoma), webbed neck (Turner syndrome), thyromegaly

- Skin exam: Evidence of androgen excess (acne, hirsutism), acanthosis nigricans (PCOS), fine downy hair on body (anorexia nervosa)
- Breast: State of development, evidence of galactorrhea (prolactinoma)
- Pelvic exam: Presence or absence of pubic hair (if sparse: Androgen insensitivity or deficiency); clitoromegaly (androgen excess); distention or bulging of external vagina (imperforate hymen); thin, pale vaginal mucosa without rugae (estrogen deficiency and ovarian failure); presence of cervical mucus (evidence for estrogen production); blind vaginal pouch (müllerian agenesis, androgen insensitivity syndrome); ovarian enlargement (tumors, PCOS, autoimmune oophoritis)

DIAGNOSTIC TESTS & INTERPRETATION
Initial Tests (lab, imaging)
- Primary amenorrhea:
  - Serum prolactin (PRL) and thyroid-stimulating hormone (TSH)
  - If no secondary sexual characteristics, measure serum FSH and (LH):
    - FSH/LH <5 IU/L suggests primary hypothalamic or pituitary etiology
    - FSH >20 and LH >40 IU/L suggests gonadal failure, and karyotype analysis should be performed
  - If secondary sexual characteristics present, evaluate for anatomic abnormalities. If uterus is absent or abnormal, perform karyotype analysis, testosterone level and DHEA-S.
- Secondary amenorrhea:
  - Exclude pregnancy with HCG.
  - Serum TSH: Elevated in hypothyroidism, decreased in hyperthyroidism
  - Consider (low yield): Serum chemistry, CBC, urinalysis to rule out underlying disease
  - PRL:
    - >100 ng/mL suggests empty sella syndrome or pituitary adenoma; perform MRI for evaluation.
    - <100 ng/mL: Evaluate for other etiologies, of which medications are most common.
- If PRL and TSH are normal, perform progestin challenge (see "Treatment"):
  - If withdrawal bleed: Normogonadotropic amenorrhea related to hyperandrogenic chronic anovulation, most commonly PCOS
  - If no withdrawal bleed: Follow-up with estradiol priming (see "Diagnostic Procedures/Other" and "Treatment") and repeat progestin challenge:
    - If no bleed: Consider outflow tract obstruction.
    - If bleed occurs: Check FSH/LH: Elevated in hypergonadotropic hypogonadism, decreased in pituitary tumors or hypogonadotropic hypogonadism
- If virilizing signs and significant acne present, measure free testosterone, DHEA-S, and 17-OH progesterone levels. Initiate evaluation for androgen secreting tumor if testosterone >200 ng/dL.
- Imaging is not generally indicated as a first-line approach.
- US may show ovarian cysts (PCOS), presence or absence of uterus, and endometrial thickness.
- An MRI of the pelvis can clarify any uterine or vaginal anomalies suggested by US, or if pediatric patient is unable to tolerate transvaginal US probe.
- An MRI of the sella turcica if prolactinoma suspected (elevated PRL >100), and consider with functional hypothalamic amenorrhea (other adenomas)

Follow-Up Tests & Special Considerations
- Women <30 with ovarian failure (see below) should have karyotype analysis and be investigated for premutations of FMR1 gene (fragile X syndrome) and for adrenal antibodies.
- If absence of uterus or foreshortened vagina, karyotype analysis should also be performed.
- Laparoscopy: Diagnosis of streak ovaries (Turner syndrome) or polycystic ovaries
- Hysterosalpingogram: Rule out Asherman syndrome and other etiologies of outflow obstruction.

Diagnostic Procedures/Other
- If constitutional delay suspected, obtain bone age.
- If hypothalamic amenorrhea from functional suppression suspected, consider dual-energy x-ray absorptiometry (DEXA) scan to assess for bone loss.

 TREATMENT

GENERAL MEASURES
Treatment depends on the underlying cause.

MEDICATION
- Progesterone challenge and replacement: Medroxyprogesterone (Provera): 10 mg/d for 10 days will result in withdrawal bleed if hypothalamic–pituitary–gonadal axis is intact.
- Estrogen replacement: Cycling with a combination oral contraceptive (containing 35 or 50 mcg of estrogen) or conjugated estrogen (Premarin) 0.625 mg for 25 days with progesterone added as above for the last 10 days will result in a withdrawal bleed if the uterus and lower genital tract are normal.
- Use of hormonal therapies will not correct the underlying problem. Other drugs might be required to treat specific conditions (e.g., bromocriptine for hyperprolactinemia).
- Use of hormonal replacement therapy is *not* recommended for long-term management of amenorrhea in older women (1)[A]:
  – It may be safe for symptom management in young women (1)[C].
  – Give to maintain secondary sex characteristics and to prevent osteoporosis in adolescents and young women.
- Combination estrogen/progesterone contraceptives (oral contraceptive pills [OCPs], patch, ring) replace estrogen and prevent pregnancy:
  – Have a positive effect on bone mineral density in oligo-/amenorrheic women (2)[B].
  – Can decrease hirsutism in PCOS
- Calcium supplementation: 1,500 mg/d if cause is hypoestrogenism
- Because PCOS is related to insulin resistance, metformin (Glucophage) has been used (start at 500 mg b.i.d.) to correct metabolic abnormalities, improve ovulation, and restore normal menstrual patterns. Of note, treatment with metformin has shown an increase in clinical pregnancy rates but not in live birth rates (3).
- Functional hypothalamic amenorrhea appears to improve with administration of exogenous leptin (still under investigation) (4).
- Contraindications to estrogen administration:
  – Pregnancy, thromboembolic disease, previous myocardial infarct or cerebrovascular accident, estrogen-dependent malignancy, severe hepatic impairment or disease

- Precautions:
  – Patients with amenorrhea who desire pregnancy should not be given hormone replacement therapy but should receive treatment for infertility based on the specific cause.

ISSUES FOR REFERRAL
Many causes of amenorrhea require referral to specialists in ob/gyn, endocrine, surgery, and/or psychiatry.

SURGERY/OTHER PROCEDURES
- Hymenectomy for primary amenorrhea if due to imperforate hymen
- Lysis of adhesions in Asherman syndrome is often effective in restoring regular menses and fertility.
- If karyotype is XY, gonads must be removed due to increased risk of tumors.
- Patients with congenital short vagina can undergo surgery to create a functioning vagina.

 ONGOING CARE

FOLLOW-UP RECOMMENDATIONS
If overtraining is suspected, activity level should be reduced by 25–50%.

Patient Monitoring
- Depends on the cause and treatment chosen
- If hormonal replacement is used, discontinue after 6 months to assess spontaneous resumption of menses.

DIET
- Correct overweight or underweight by dietary management and behavior modification.
- If PCOS is the etiology, a weight-loss diet will help restore ovulation.

PATIENT EDUCATION
- Educate the patient on the circumstances and complications of her condition and its underlying etiology.
- Specific educational resources are helpful (e.g., prenatal classes and menopause support groups).
- Discuss the expected duration of amenorrhea (temporary or permanent), effect on fertility, and the long-term sequelae of untreated amenorrhea (e.g., osteoporosis, vaginal dryness).
- Appropriate contraceptive advice should be given because fertility returns before menses.
- Additional support may be needed if the amenorrhea is associated with a reduction in, or loss of, fertility.

PROGNOSIS
Reflects the underlying cause. In functional hypothalamic amenorrhea, 1 study demonstrated 83% reversal rate in presence of obvious contributing factor.

COMPLICATIONS
- Estrogen-deficiency symptoms (e.g., hot flashes, vaginal dryness) and osteoporosis in prolonged hypoestrogenic amenorrhea
- Increased risk of endometrial cancer in patients whose amenorrhea is secondary to anovulation with estrogen excess (obesity, PCOS)
- Premature ovarian failure may increase cardiovascular risk.

REFERENCES

1. Farquhar CM, Marjoribanks J, Lethaby A. Long term hormone therapy for perimenopausal and postmenopausal women. *Cochrane Database Syst Rev*. 2005:CD004143.
2. Liu SL, Lebrun CM. Effect of oral contraceptives and hormone replacement therapy on bone mineral density in premenopausal and perimenopausal women: A systematic review. *Br J Sports Med*. 2006;40:11–24.
3. Tang T, Lord JM, Norman RJ, et al. Insulin-sensitising drugs (metformin, rosiglitazone, pioglitazone, D-chiro-inositol) for women with polycystic ovary syndrome, oligo amenorrhoea and subfertility. *Cochrane Database Syst Rev*. 2012;5:CD003053. Epub 2012 May 16.
4. Chou SH, Chamberland JP, Liu X, et al. Leptin is an effective treatment for hypothalamic amenorrhea. *Proc Natl Acad Sci USA*. 2011;108(16): 6585–6590. Epub 2011 Apr 4.

ADDITIONAL READING
- Gordon CM. Clinical practice. Functional hypothalamic amenorrhea. *N Engl J Med*. 2010;363:365–371.
- Practice Committee of American Society for Reproductive Medicine. Current evaluation of amenorrhea. *Fertil Steril*. 2008;90(5 Suppl): S219–S225.
- Santoro N. Update in hyper- and hypogonadotropic amenorrhea. *J Clin Endocrinol Metab*. 2011;96(11): 3281–3288.

 SEE ALSO

Algorithms: Amenorrhea, Primary; Amenorrhea, Secondary; Delayed Puberty; Thyroid Disorders; Osteoporosis

 CODES

ICD10
- N91.0 Primary amenorrhea
- N91.1 Secondary amenorrhea
- N91.2 Amenorrhea, unspecified

CLINICAL PEARLS
- First evaluate whether amenorrhea is primary or secondary and exclude pregnancy. TSH and PRL are usual first blood tests.
- Progestin challenge will cause withdrawal bleeding in women with an intact hypothalamic-pituitary-gonadal axis.

AMNESTIC DISORDER

Umer Farooq, MD, MBBS • Najm Hasan Siddiqui, MD

BASICS

- Memory is an arbitrary term that encompasses:
  - Knowledge of facts (*semantic* memory)
  - Knowledge of previous self-experiences (*episodic* memory)
  - Exercise of a learned skill (*procedural* memory)
  - Temporary knowledge for immediate use (*working* memory)
- Coded for by various regions of the brain, with significant involvement of the following:
  - Medial temporal lobe, including:
    ○ Amygdaloid nucleus
    ○ Hippocampus
    ○ Parahippocampal region
  - Thalamus, especially the dorsomedial nuclei
  - Hypothalamus
  - Basal forebrain
- Amnestic disorder is marked by memory impairment and forgetfulness

DESCRIPTION
- Amnestic disorder, amnestic syndrome, or simply amnesia comes from the Greek for forgetfulness.
- Essential feature of amnestic disorder is the acquired impaired ability to learn and recall new information or the inability to recall previously learned knowledge or past events
- *DSM-IV* TR recognizes amnestic disorders as:
  - Amnestic disorder due to general medical condition
  - Substance induced persisting amnestic disorder
  - Amnestic disorder for amnestic disorder not otherwise specified

EPIDEMIOLOGY
- No adequate studies have reported on the incidence or prevalence of amnestic disorder
- Memory impairment due to head trauma is probably most common cause
- Transient global amnesia (TGA) is one type of amnestic disorder found in 1 study to occur at of rate of 6.8/100,000 people per year (1).

ETIOLOGY AND PATHOPHYSIOLOGY
- In general, metabolic or structural changes that cause an imbalance in the memory-related regions of the brain can cause an amnestic disorder
- Amnestic disorders have many potential causes
  - Thiamine deficiency(Korsakoff syndrome)
  - Hypoglycemia
- Primary brain conditions
  - Seizures
  - Cerebral tumors
  - Head trauma
  - Chronic alcoholism
  - Nutritional disorders
  - Cebrovascular disease
  - TGA
  - Electroconvulsive therapy, hypoxia
  - Multiple sclerosis
- Substance-related causes
  - Alcohol use disorders
  - Benzodiazepines

- The exact cause of TGA is not well understood, but it has been associated with:
  - Physical exertion, emotional stress, pain, exposure to cold water, sexual intercourse, Valsalva maneuver
  - Malingering and factitious disorder should also be considered.
- Amnestic disorder is a syndrome that can be caused by many distinct disease processes, including head trauma, global hypoxia, cardiovascular accident (CVA), alcohol consumption/abuse, seizure, dissociative amnesia, TGA, encephalitis, tumor, and paraneoplastic limbic encephalitis.
- In most causes of amnesia, some damage or disruption (either temporary or permanent) occurred to the limbic structures in the brain responsible for memory.
- TGA is well studied, but is not fully understood, and may be related to venous congestion of the brain.

Genetics
Recent evidence supports the possibility of a genetic predisposition to developing TGA (2).

COMMONLY ASSOCIATED CONDITIONS
- No data available of TGA association with focal neurological features or any psychiatric disorder
- History of headaches may constitute important risk factors (3)[B]

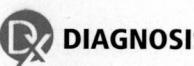

DIAGNOSIS

HISTORY
- A thorough history can help elucidate the underlying cause of the amnestic disorder.
- Onset may be sudden or gradual depending on the etiology. Confabulation is often associated with amnestic disorder.
- Most patients with amnestic disorder lack insight into their deficits and deny the presence of memory impairment, obtaining corroborative history from an acquaintance may be helpful.
- Amnestic disorders, by definition, are significant enough to impair social/occupational functioning
- A history of heavy alcohol consumption associated with poor nutrition can present acutely as Wernicke encephalopathy marked by confusion, memory deficits, ataxia and ophthalmoplegia, or with chronic short-term memory loss, often associated with compensatory confabulation: Korsakoff dementia.
- Heavy alcohol or substance abuse also raises the risk for traumatic brain injury and hypoxia-associated cortical damage.
- Use of short-acting benzodiazepines is commonly associated with amnesia. Most common offender triazolam (4)[B]
- A history of head trauma and a period of loss of consciousness would suggest that this was the cause of amnesia.

- Cerebral hypoxia often presents with a period of lost consciousness followed by a period of anterograde amnesia that usually resolves within several days. Remote memory and registration are generally preserved.
- CVA following posterior cerebral artery occlusion could present with sudden onset memory disruption and would likely involve additional neurologic deficits.
- In TGA, patients present with sudden onset anterograde amnesia and may also complain of a period of retrograde amnesia. Amnesia lasts for minutes to hours, ending with spontaneous restoration of intact cognitive function. Deficits usually fully resolve within 24 hours. TGA more common in men, common after age 50.

PHYSICAL EXAM
- Memory testing is important to determine whether the patient has deficits in recent or remote memory.
- A detailed neurologic exam will help identify whether additional deficits present might indicate a specific organic cause. Patients presenting with TGA often have no focal abnormalities on exam.
- If the neurologic exam demonstrates more than memory dysfunction, other differential diagnoses should be further explored.
- In dissociative forms of amnesia, the memory loss usually does not involve deficits in learning and recalling new information.

DIFFERENTIAL DIAGNOSIS
- Head trauma
- CVA (vertebrobasilar system, posterior cerebral artery)
- Global hypoxia (carbon monoxide poisoning)
- Seizure or status epilepticus
- Alcohol-related (alcoholic blackout, Wernicke encephalopathy)
- Encephalitis
- Tumor
- Paraneoplastic limbic encephalitis
- TGA
- Dissociative amnesia, presents as loss of select memories following a traumatic or stressful event. In contrast to many organic causes of amnesia, dissociative amnesia tends to cause loss of remote memories with relatively preserved recent memory

DIAGNOSTIC TESTS & INTERPRETATION
Initial Tests (lab, imaging)
- CBC with differential
- Basic metabolic profile, including serum glucose
- Toxicology screen
- Oxygenation level

- PT/PTT to rule out hypercoagulable state
- Diffusion-weighted MRI can be useful in distinguishing between various causes of the amnestic syndrome (5,6)[C]
- In TGA, MRI may reveal small 1–2-mm dot-like hyperintensities in the lateral aspect of the hippocampus.
- In ischemic stroke, hippocampal hyperintensity would be seen within a specific vascular territory.
- In prolonged seizures or status epilepticus, there may be hyperintensity of the unilateral or bilateral hippocampus, thalamus, and/or cortex, not restricted to a particular vascular territory.
- In global hypoxia and encephalitis, MRI would likely reveal extensive abnormalities in both hemispheres, not restricted to a particular vascular territory.

Diagnostic Procedures/Other
EEG if seizure is suspected

TREATMENT

- Treatment is to identify and treat the underlying cause.
- No definitively effective treatment for amnestic disorder aimed at reversing memory deficits
- Supportive care and reassurance for TGA, as symptoms usually resolve within 24 hours (7)[B].

MEDICATION
If Wernicke encephalopathy is suspected, thiamine should be promptly administered. Insufficient evidence exists to guide dosing, frequency, route, and duration of treatment, but 1 study recommends 500 mg IV thiamine hydrochloride given t.i.d. daily for 2–3 days (8,9)[A].

ONGOING CARE

FOLLOW-UP RECOMMENDATIONS
Follow up with a primary care provider and/or specialist may be indicated, depending on the identified cause of the amnestic disorder.

DIET
No restrictions on diet

PROGNOSIS
The amnestic syndrome has a variable prognosis depending on the underlying cause. In many cases (TGA, head trauma), memory deficits will fully resolve. In other cases (CVA, hypoxia), neurologic symptoms may persist long term. TGA has good prognosis with only 8% experiencing a 2nd episode.

REFERENCES

1. Berli R, Hutter A, Waespe W, et al. Transient global amnesia—not so rare after all. *Swiss Med Wkly*. 2009;139:288–292.
2. Segers-van Rijn J, de Brujin SF. Transient global amnesia: A genetic disorder? *Eur Neurol*. 2010;63: 186–187.
3. Quinette P, Guillery-Girard B, Dayan J, et al: What does transient global amnesia really mean? Review of the literature and thorough study of 142 cases. *Brain*. 2006;129:1640–1658.
4. Lida R, Kajiwara K, Kashiwai A, et al. [Comprehensive evaluation of the effect of triazolam on amnesia during the preoperative period]. *Masui*. 2011;60:67–74.
5. Förster A, Griebe M, Gass A, et al. Diffusion weighted imaging for the differential diagnosis of disorders affecting the hippocampus. *Cerebrovasc Dis*. 2012;33:104–115.
6. Greer DM, Schaefer PW, Schwamm LH. Unilateral temporal lobe stroke causing ischemic transient global amnesia: Role for diffusion-weighted imaging in the initial evaluation. *J Neuroimaging*. 2001;11:317–319.
7. Jäger T, Bäzner H, Kliegel M, et al. The transience and nature of cognitive impairments in transient global amnesia: A meta-analysis. *J Clin Exp Neuropsychol*. 2009;31:8–19.
8. Sechi G, Serra A. Wernicke's encephalopathy: New clinical settings and recent advances in diagnosis and management. *Lancet Neurol*. 2007;6: 442–455.
9. Day E, Bentham P, Callaghan R, et al. Thiamine for Wernicke-Korsakoff syndrome in people at risk from alcohol abuse. *Cochrane Database Syst Rev*. 2004;1:CD004033.

 SEE ALSO

Algorithm: Amnesia

 CODES

ICD10
- R41.1 Anterograde amnesia
- R41.2 Retrograde amnesia
- R41.3 Other amnesia

CLINICAL PEARLS

- Amnestic disorder is a clinical syndrome that can have a variety of causes.
- A detailed history, neurologic exam, and imaging can help rule out some causes of the amnestic syndrome.
- Management will depend on the underlying cause of amnesia.
- TGA is a diagnosis of exclusion, and supportive care and reassurance are appropriate management.
- Amnestic sleep-related eating disorders may also be seen, with transient amnesia for nocturnal eating.
- Diagnosis is made by *Diagnostic and Statistical Manual of Mental Disorders* criteria.

AMYOTROPHIC LATERAL SCLEROSIS

Ajoy Kumar, MD • Ryan Wargo, PharmD

 BASICS

Amyotrophic lateral sclerosis (ALS) is a progressive neurodegenerative disease of the brain and spinal cord. It is relentless in progression and is currently incurable.

DESCRIPTION
- Average survival ranges from 2–5 years from the time of diagnosis.
- 50% live >3 years, 25% live >5 years, 10% live >10 years, 5% live up to 20 years.
- Sporadic ALS is the most common form of the disease. It includes a number of overlapping syndromes, such as pseudobulbar palsy, progressive bulbar palsy, progressive muscular atrophy, and primary lateral sclerosis.
- Familial ALS is an autosomal-dominant or autosomal-recessive disease, which is clinically similar to sporadic ALS but probably represents a distinct entity pathologically and biochemically.
- Guam ALS and Parkinson-dementia complex are ALS-like syndromes often, but not always, associated with Parkinson syndrome and dementia. Guam ALS is prevalent among the Chamorro Indians of Guam and rare in the US.
- System(s) affected: Nervous
- Synonym(s): Motor neuron disease, MND, Lou Gehrig disease, ALS

ALERT
- Infantile and juvenile spinal muscular atrophies are conditions distinct from ALS, both clinically and pathologically.
- Symptoms of ALS may inappropriately be attributed to age.

Pregnancy Considerations
- Uncommon among affected individuals
- If pregnancy did occur, the only foreseeable difficulties would be related to weakness.

EPIDEMIOLOGY
Incidence
- In US, 5,600 newly diagnosed per year
- Rate = 2/100,000 per year

Prevalence
- Estimated 30,00 Americans may have the disease at any given time
- No racial, ethnic, or socioeconomic boundaries
- Predominant age: Uncommon before age 40
- Predominant sex: Male > Female in sporadic ALS:
  – After 70: Male = Female

ETIOLOGY AND PATHOPHYSIOLOGY
- Sporadic ALS: Unknown cause, but elevated levels of glutamate have been found in serum and CSF.
- Familial ALS: Neurodegenerative disease passed on directly or indirectly by skipping generation
- Guam ALS and Parkinson-dementia complex: Possible relationship to ingestion of the cycad nut or to some other environmental toxin
- Degeneration of the UMN and LMN with gliosis replacing lost neurons. Leads to spinal cord atrophy, thin ventral roots, and loss of large myelinated fibers in motor nerves.
- Progressive weakness of both skeletal and smooth muscles that leads to progressive loss of function

related to movement, speech, swallowing, and breathing.

Genetics
- Currently 18 types of genetic mutations
- Familial ALS, most common (5% of cases); can be autosomal-dominant or autosomal-recessive; X-linked cases have been reported.
- Gene locus has been localized to the long arm of chromosome 21 and encodes the superoxide dismutase (SOD1) enzyme in 20% of familial ALS cases.
- Mutation in the gene encoding fused in sarcoma (FUS) was identified in familial ALS type 6.
- Mutations in the angiogenin gene (ANG) have been recently discovered to be associated with sporadic ALS.
- Mutations in TARDP region encoding TAR DNA-binding protein TDP-43 have also been identified in familial and sporadic ALS.
- C9ORF72 repeat expansions found in 2011 is a major cause of ALS.

RISK FACTORS
- Family history
- Age >40
- Smoking (1)[B]

GENERAL PREVENTION
Genetic counseling is advised if there is a family history of ALS.

Dx DIAGNOSIS

- Diagnosis can be established according to Revised El Escorial World Federation of Neurology criteria.
- The presence of:
  – Evidence of LMN degeneration by clinical, electrophysiological, or neuropathological examination
  – Evidence of UMN degeneration by clinical examination
  – Progressive spread of symptoms or signs within a region or to other regions, as determined by history or examination
- The absence of:
  – Electrophysiological and pathological evidence of other disease processes that might explain the signs of LMN and/or UMN degeneration
  – Neuroimaging evidence of other disease processes that might explain the observed clinical and electrophysiological sign
- The newer Awaji criteria may offer higher sensitivity and earlier diagnosis of ALS (2)[B].

HISTORY
ALS is suggested when symptoms are consistent with UMN and LMN dysfunction that worsens over time. Symptoms include:
- Loss of muscle strength and coordination
- Difficulty opening and closing the jaw, drooling
- Voice change, hoarseness
- Muscle cramps, difficulty breathing, difficulty swallowing, paralysis

PHYSICAL EXAM
Variable combinations of:
- Unexplained weight loss
- Limb weakness with variable symmetry and distribution

- Gait disorder (steppage-waddling)
- Slurring of speech
- Inability to control affect (inappropriate laughing, crying, yawning)
- Focal atrophy of muscle groups (initially in a myotomal distribution)
- Fasciculations (other than calves)
- Hyperreflexia (including jaw jerk—Hoffmann sign)
- Babinski sign, present in 50% of patients
- Spasticity
- Sialorrhea
- Spares cognitive, oculomotor, sensory, and autonomic functions

DIFFERENTIAL DIAGNOSIS
- Multifocal motor neuropathy
- Cervical radiculomyelopathy
- Cervical spondylosis
- Lead intoxication
- Spinal muscular atrophy (adult form)
- Primary lateral sclerosis
- Familial spastic paraparesis
- Benign fasciculations
- Lyme disease
- Spinal multiple sclerosis
- Tropical spastic paraparesis
- Myasthenia gravis

DIAGNOSTIC TESTS & INTERPRETATION
Initial Tests (lab, imaging)
- No simple reliable laboratory test is available that confirms the diagnosis. Creatinine kinase levels may be elevated.
- Rule out other conditions (i.e., check SPEP/UPEP, TSH, PTH, 24-hour urine for heavy metals, HIV, HTLV, Lyme, syphilis, tick-borne encephalitis):
  – Elevated levels of glutamate in CSF and serum
  – Anti-monosialoganglioside autoantibodies in low titer commonly found (of unclear significance)
  – Possibly reduced levels of nerve growth factor
- MRI is used to exclude other possible diagnoses in the evaluation of suspected ALS:
  – MRI is usually normal in ALS, although increased signal in the corticospinal tracts on T2-weighted and FLAIR images and hypointensity of the motor cortex on T2-weighted images have been reported.

Diagnostic Procedures/Other
- Electromyography: EMG findings include evidence of ongoing denervation, fibrillation or positive sharp waves, and chronic partial reinnervation implying frequently unstable, increased duration motor unit action potentials with a reduced interference pattern (2).
- Nerve conduction studies: Usually elicit normal values in recordings from relatively unaffected muscles. However, during disease progression, compound motor action potential (CMAP) amplitude elicited by distal stimulation may induce greater physiological phase cancellation, such as a pathological conduction block (2).
- Motor unit number estimation: Attractive end-point measure in clinical drug trials in ALS, because it directly assesses loss of lower motor neurons and is sensitive to disease progression (2).
- Muscle biopsy: Not a routine part of the diagnostic evaluation of ALS but may be performed if myopathy is suspected on clinical, electrodiagnostic, or serological grounds:

− Muscle biopsy will show groups of shrunken angulated muscle fibers (grouped atrophy) amid other groups of fibers with a uniform fiber type (fiber type grouping).

Test Interpretation
- Loss of Betz cells in the motor cortex
- Atrophic or absent anterior horn cells of spinal cord
- Atrophic or absent neurons within the motor nuclei of the medulla and pons
- Degeneration of the lateral columns of the spinal cord
- Atrophy of the ventral roots
- Grouped atrophy of muscle (motor units)

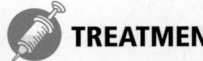 # TREATMENT

GENERAL MEASURES
- Multidisciplinary care should be available as this may extend survival, decrease medical complications, and improve quality of life (3)[C].
- Outpatient may ultimately need nursing home placement or hospice.
- Supportive care is necessary for complicating emergencies (aspiration, respiratory failure). Use of a respirator is a major ethical dilemma. Consideration should be given to those with selective respiratory dysfunction.
- Discussion of advance directives, focusing on patient's specific values about which interventions are to be used, is critical to meeting the patient's needs.
- Prosthetic devices

MEDICATION
Riluzole: 50 mg PO b.i.d.: The only FDA-approved drug for ALS. It produces a slight prolongation in life expectancy by decreasing the release of glutamate (4)[A],(5)[C], and it slows the disease progression.

ALERT
Riluzole withhold should be considered for patients developing fatigue. Monitor LFTs for hepatic dysfunction and CBC for neutropenia (5)[C].

ISSUES FOR REFERRAL
- Early exam by a neurologist can confirm diagnosis of ALS.
- Tracheostomy or G-tube placement may be performed by surgeon or gastroenterologist.
- Pulmonologist and respiratory therapist for ventilator assistance and management of concurrent infections and tracheostomy
- Referral to ongoing clinical trials may be beneficial (ClinicalTrials.gov)
- Palliative care management is beneficial to both patient and patient's family at end stage.

ADDITIONAL THERAPIES
- These drugs may be used to relieve severe spasticity:
  − Baclofen: 5 mg PO t.i.d. initially, followed by gradual increase of 5 mg/d every 4–7 days; not to exceed 80 mg/d divided q.i.d.
  − Tizanidine: 4–8 mg PO q8h PRN; not to exceed 36 mg/d
- Treatment for refractory sialorrhea:
  − Botulinum toxin B
  − Low-dose radiation therapy to the salivary glands

SURGERY/OTHER PROCEDURES
- Percutaneous endoscopic gastrostomy (PEG) tube should be considered with early signs of malnutrition to stabilize weight and prolong survival.
- Noninvasive ventilation (NIV) can lengthen survival and improve quality of life.
- Elective tracheostomy should be considered in patients with early signs of respiratory difficulty.

COMPLEMENTARY AND ALTERNATIVE MEDICINE
- Currently, insufficient evidence to recommend disease-modifying treatment other than Riluzole.
- Research offering therapy with stem cells is evolving, providing a new approach in cellular replacement and support for patients (6)[B].
- Several therapy options are under current investigation, including ceftriaxone, dexpramipexole, memantine, tamoxifen, and insulin-like growth factor.
- Therapeutic trials of the efficacy of antioxidants (vitamin E and vitamin C and β-carotene), nerve growth factor, gabapentin, Myotrophin, thyrotropin-releasing hormone, and creatine have been undertaken. Reports are not encouraging (7)[A].

 # ONGOING CARE

FOLLOW-UP RECOMMENDATIONS
Patients should be involved in regular exercise and a physical therapy program.

Patient Monitoring
- Initially every 3 months; frequency to be increased as needed for symptomatic therapy
- Patients with a presumed diagnosis of ALS should have neuroimaging and electrodiagnostic studies.

DIET
- Evaluate swallowing to quantify any dysphagia.
- Modify the patient's diet to prevent aspiration.
- Consider a gastrostomy tube when patient cannot swallow fluids or soft foods (8)[B].

PATIENT EDUCATION
Printed material for patients (and reference lists for physicians) available from:
- The Muscular Dystrophy Association: (520) 529-2000; (800) 572-1717; http://www.mdausa.org
- The ALS Association: (800) 782-4747; http://www.alsa.org
- Families of Spinal Muscular Atrophy: http://www.fsma.org

PROGNOSIS
- ALS usually results in death within 5 years.
- Patients who predominantly manifest progressive muscular atrophy have a better prognosis.
- There have been reports of spontaneous arrest of the disease.

COMPLICATIONS
- Aspiration pneumonia
- Pulmonary embolism
- Nutritional deficiency
- Complications from wheelchair-bound or bedridden states, including decubitus ulcers and skin infections

REFERENCES

1. Wang H, O'Reilly ÉJ, Weisskopf MG, et al. Smoking and risk of amyotrophic lateral sclerosis: A pooled analysis of 5 prospective cohorts. *Arch Neurol.* 2011;68(2):207–213.
2. Inghilleri M, Iacovelli E. Clinical neurophysiology in ALS. *Arch Ital Biol.* 2011;149(1):57–63.
3. Anderson PM, Abraham S, Borasio GD, et al. EFNS guidelines on the clinical management of amyotrophic lateral sclerosis (MALS)—revised report of an EFNS task force. *Eur J Neurol.* 2012;19:360-375. Epub 2011 Sep 14.
4. Bensimon G, Lacomblez L, Meininger V. A controlled trial of riluzole in amyotrophic lateral sclerosis. ALS/Riluzole Study Group. *N Engl J Med.* 1994;330:585–591.
5. Morren JA, Galvez-Jimenez N. Current and prospective disease-modifying therapies for amyotrophic lateral sclerosis. *Expert Opin Investig Drugs.* 2012;21(3):297–320. Epub 2012 Feb 6.
6. Kim SU, de Vellis J. Stem cell-based cell therapy in neurological diseases: A review. *J Neurosci Res.* 2009;87(10):2183–2200.
7. Pastula DM, Moore DH, Bedlack RS, et al. Creatine for amyotrophic lateral sclerosis/motor neuron disease. *Cochrane Database Syst Rev.* 2010;6:CD005225.
8. Andersen PM, Borasio GD, Dengler R, et al. Good practice in the management of amyotrophic lateral sclerosis: Clinical guidelines. An evidence-based review with good practice points. EALSC Working Group. *Amyotroph Lateral Scler.* 2007;8:195–213.

ADDITIONAL READING
- Kiernan MC, Vucic S, Cheah BC, et al. Amyotrophic lateral sclerosis. *Lancet.* 2011;377(9769):942–955. Epub 2011 Feb 4.
- Miller RG, Jackson CE, Kasarskis EJ, et al. Practice parameter update: The care of the patient with amyotrophic lateral sclerosis: Drug, nutritional, and respiratory therapies (an evidence-based review): Report of the Quality Standards Subcommittee of the American Academy of Neurology. *Neurology.* 2009;73(15):1218–1226.
- Miller RG, Jackson CE, Kasarskis EJ, et al. Practice parameter update: The care of the patient with amyotrophic lateral sclerosis: Multidisciplinary care, symptom management, and cognitive/behavioral impairment (an evidence-based review): Report of the Quality Standards Subcommittee of the American Academy of Neurology. *Neurology.* 2009;73(15):1227–1233.

 # CODES

ICD10
G12.21 Amyotrophic lateral sclerosis

CLINICAL PEARLS
- ALS is a progressive upper and lower motor neuron degenerative disease.
- Diagnosis is made by history, physical exam, EMG, and NCS.
- Riluzole is the only available treatment that might increase survival.

ANABOLIC STEROID ABUSE

Adam Howes, MD • Ryan Pearson, MD

 BASICS

Anabolic steroid abuse is the misuse of testosterone and closely related compounds, which are commonly used together in supratherapeutic dosages to increase lean muscle mass and improve athletic performance.

DESCRIPTION
- Anabolic steroids are compounds that increase muscle mass; primarily anabolic-androgenic steroids (AAS). They include exogenous testosterone, synthetic androgens, synthetic androgen receptor modulators, androgen precursors, and multiple other androgen stimulators.
- On the street they may be referred to as "roids" or "juice," and are administered primarily via oral, transdermal, or intravenous routes.
- When used in supraphysiologic doses, they result in varying degrees of muscle building and masculinization.
- Patients often "stack" steroids, in that they will use a cocktail of multiple steroids at high doses, then cycle off for a period of weeks to prevent significant side effects as well as to avoid detection.
- The effects of the steroids are typically dose dependent, and most reverse after weeks of discontinuation.
- Although there is not the immediate "high" as experienced in illicit drug usage, dependence has been increasingly recognized.
- Growth hormone is another commonly abused substance; however, its effects on increasing lean muscle mass are minimal, and it has not been shown to improve athletic performance (1).

EPIDEMIOLOGY
Incidence
- Most studies have indicated at least 3–11% of young men in the US and other Western countries have used AAS at some time in their lives. The number is much higher in sports such as weight lifting.
- Incidence is ~1% of young men in Asian countries, thought to be due to less emphasis on muscle mass by media and society.
- Usage is much less common in women (2).

Prevalence
- Prevalence varies on age; however, estimate for high school males is ~2.7%.
- In power sports or weight lifting, the prevalence has ranged from 20–50% (3).

ETIOLOGY AND PATHOPHYSIOLOGY
- Natural testosterone is produced in small amounts in the adrenal gland and ovaries, and in large amounts by the testes.
- AAS increase protein production, particularly in muscle cells.
- Additionally, they decrease catabolism by blocking the effects of cortisol.
- Administration of exogenous testosterone suppresses the hypothalamic-pituitary-gonadal (HPG) axis, thereby causing testicular hypotrophy and suppressed spermatogenesis.
  - Patients will oftentimes use human chorionic gonadotropin (HCG) as well, to prevent this side effect.

- Additionally, aromatase inhibitors may be used to counteract gynecomastia which occurs due to peripheral conversion of testosterone to estradiol.
- This peripheral conversion to estradiol also may lead to accelerated cartilage formation and premature closure of the epiphyses when used in adolescents.
- Muscle mass decreases after cessation of use within weeks.

Genetics
No identified association

RISK FACTORS
- Male gender
- Age: Mean age of onset mid 20s
- Participation in power sports, weight lifting
- Residing in Western country
- Consumption of legal performance enhancing substances
- Use of alcohol, illicit drugs

GENERAL PREVENTION
- The US Preventative Task Force concluded that insufficient evidence exists to recommend screening for anabolic steroid abuse (4).
- Education of young adults and athletes, focusing on the negative side effects of anabolic steroid abuse, is imperative.

COMMONLY ASSOCIATED CONDITIONS
Major depressive disorder, body dysmorphic syndrome, substance abuse

 DIAGNOSIS

- History and physical exam
- Laboratory studies to detect use are limited by timing of consumption and advanced administration techniques to avoid detection and, thus, are not routinely performed.

HISTORY
- Duration, dosage, frequency, route of usage
- Ask about side effects, including impotence, mood disturbance, and amenorrhea in females.
- Concurrent substances, including OTC supplements, illegal drugs, alcohol, and prescription drug use
- Social situation, including stressors, support
- Preexisting medical and psychiatric conditions
- Body image: Screen for features of muscle dysmorphia and body-checking behavior.
- Assess for suicidality.

PHYSICAL EXAM
- General:
  - Increased muscle mass
  - Decreased body fat
  - Deepening of voice and hirsutism in women
  - Height velocity change in adolescents
- Cardiovascular: Hypertension
- Breast: Gynecomastia
- Gastrointestinal: Hepatomegaly
- Dermatology: Acne, male pattern baldness
- Genitourinary: Testicular atrophy, clitoromegaly
- Psychiatric: Anxiety, depression, mania, psychosis

DIFFERENTIAL DIAGNOSIS
- Cushing syndrome
- Congenital adrenal hyperplasia
- Adrenal neoplasm
- Polycystic ovarian syndrome
- Precocious puberty
- Drug-induced hirsutism

DIAGNOSTIC TESTS & INTERPRETATION
- Initial evaluation should focus on side effects of anabolic steroid usage and any comorbid medical conditions:
  - Initial Tests (lab, imaging)
  - Urine testosterone:Epitestosterone ratio >3:1
  - Elevated ratio of 13C to 12C
  - HDL decreased, LDL increased (5)
  - Hemoglobin, hematocrit increased (5)
  - AST, ALT elevated
  - Use of GH: Elevated HgbA1c, fasting glucose
- Obtain fasting lipid profile. Consider CBC, CMP, UA:
  - No imaging studies are required unless symptomatic, or evidence of liver dysfunction.
  - Studies have been unable to demonstrate any difference in echocardiogram results, thus this imaging modality is not necessary unless clinically indicated (5).

Diagnostic Procedures/Other
- Renal function is difficult to assess given increased muscle mass and frequent ingestion of creatine supplements, which is readily converted to creatinine.
- Evaluation for proteinuria may also assist in diagnosis of renal disease.

 TREATMENT

- Limited by few abusers who seek assistance.
- Dependence is complicated by the following:
  - Hypogonadism, which typically resolves in weeks to months after withdrawal of the AAS. This makes reinitiating the steroid more desirable in order to reverse the effects of HPG dysfunction.
  - High frequency of comorbid body image disorders including "muscle dysmorphia," which requires recognition and treatment.
  - Small proportion of patients develops marked depressive symptoms upon withdrawal of AAS.
  - Neurologic basis for dependence, possibly related to opioid receptors, which also needs to be overcome to produce sustained abstinence.

GENERAL MEASURES
Goals of therapy are to have patients acknowledge that anabolic steroid usage is detrimental to their health, and discontinue and remain abstinent from the substances:
- The physician should attempt to minimize withdrawal side effects, and treat any comorbid psychiatric or substance abuse conditions.
- Assure adequate social support and coping mechanisms.

MEDICATION

- Medications are limited to treating any underlying psychiatric illness and the clinical manifestations of hypogonadism.
- Naltrexone, which blocks opioid-mediated positive reinforcement, has been shown successful in reducing testosterone usage in animal studies only (6).
- Many of the studies on medications are small in size.

First Line

Depressive symptoms and body dysmorphism may be treated as typically performed for depression, particularly with SSRIs (6)[B]:
- Fluoxetine 20 mg PO daily

Second Line

- An endocrinologist may prescribe HCG to help accelerate testicular testosterone production.
- Clomiphene supplementation may be used to stimulate pituitary function.
- Less frequently, Tamoxifen, HCG, and phosphodiesterase inhibitors, such as Sildenafil are used to symptomatically improve hypogonadism (6).
- Severe medication refractory depression associated with anabolic steroid discontinuation has been treated successfully with electroconvulsive therapy.

ISSUES FOR REFERRAL

- Endocrinology: Prolonged HPG suppression, management of hypogonadal symptoms
- Psychiatry: Psychosis, grandiosity, suicidal ideation
- Additional side effects should be managed by their corresponding system.

ADDITIONAL THERAPIES

- Cognitive-behavioral therapy
- Couples therapy, family therapy

IN-PATIENT CONSIDERATIONS

- In-patient psychiatric hospitalization for those with significant mood alterations.
- In-patient stay may be required for other complications of AAS.

 ONGOING CARE

Patients who abuse AAS should have close follow-up with their primary care physician, and other specialists, including a psychiatrist or addiction specialist based on their clinical picture.

FOLLOW-UP RECOMMENDATIONS

Determined by side effects, comorbid psychiatric illness

PATIENT EDUCATION

- National Institute on Drug Abuse: The Science of Drug Abuse & Addiction: findtreatment.samhsa.gov or 1-800-662-HELP
- National Center for Drug Free Sport, Inc: www.drugfreesport.com or 816-474-8655
- Substance Abuse and Mental Health Services Administration: www.samhsa.org

PROGNOSIS

Most side effects resolve with discontinuation of the AAS, and prognosis is generally good. Given the recent widespread usage, long-term side effects have not been completely characterized. ~30% of patients who abuse anabolic steroids become chronic users; however, AAS use is more often problematic and chronic when polypharmacy is present (7)

COMPLICATIONS

- Testicular atrophy
- Decreased sperm count
- Decreased fertility index
- Impotence
- Premature epiphyseal closure in adolescents
- Hypertension
- Myocardial infarction
- Cardiomyopathy (unclear causation)
- Sudden cardiac death
- Thrombosis
- Dyslipidemia
- Depression
- Substance abuse
- Suicide
- Violent behavior
- Anxiety
- Paranoia
- Hepatotoxicity
- Cholestasis
- Hepatocarcinoma
- Tendon rupture
- Hepatitis C, HIV, blood-borne illnesses
- Local site infections
- GH specific: Carpal tunnel syndrome, acromegaly, diabetes mellitus

REFERENCES

1. Liu H, Bravata DM, Olkin I, et al. Systematic review: The effects of growth hormone on athletic performance. *Ann Intern Med*. 2008;148(10): 747–758. Epub 2008 Mar 17.
2. Kanayama G, Hudson JI, Pope HG. Illicit anabolic-androgenic steroid use. *Horm Behav*. 2010;58(1):111–121. Epub 2009.
3. Dodge T, Hoagland MF. The use of anabolic androgenic steroids and polypharmacy: A review of the literature. *Drug Alcohol Depend*. 2011; 114(2–3):100–109. Epub 2011.
4. Polen MR, Whitlock EP, Wisdom JP, et al. *Screening in primary care settings for illicit drug use: Staged systematic review for the United States Preventive Services Task Force [Internet]*. Rockville, MD: Agency for Healthcare Research and Quality (US); 2008 Jan. Report No.: 08–05108-EF-1.
5. Bonetti A, Tirelli F, Catapano A, et al. Side effects of anabolic androgenic steroids abuse. *Int J Sports Med*. 2008;29(8):679–687. Epub 2007.
6. Kanayama G, Brower KJ, Wood RI, et al. Treatment of anabolic-androgenic steroid dependence: Emerging evidence and its implications. *Drug Alcohol Depend*. 2010;109(1–3):6–13. Epub 2010.
7. Hildebrandt T, Lai J, et al. The diagnostic dilemma of pathological appearance and performance enhancing drug use. *Drug Alcohol Depend*. 2011;114(1):1–11.

ADDITIONAL READING

- Angoorani H, Narenjiha H, Tayyebi B, et al. Amphetamine use and its associated factors in body builders: A study from Tehran, Iran. *Arch Med Sci*. 2012;8(2):362–367.
- Eaton DK, Kann L, Kinchen S, et al. Youth risk behavior surveillance—United States, 2009. *MMWR Surveill Summ*. 2010;59(5):1–142.
- Herlitz LC, Markowitz GS, Farris AB, et al. Development of focal segmental glomerulosclerosis after anabolic steroid abuse. *J Am Soc Nephrol*. 2010;21(1):163–172. Epub 2009.
- Kersey RD, Elliot DL, Goldberg L, et al; National Athletic Trainers' Association. National Athletic Trainers' Association position statement: anabolic-androgenic steroids. *Journal of Athletic Training*. 2012 Sep-Oct;47(5):567–588. doi: 10.4085/1062-6050-47.5.08
- Lundmark J, Gårevik N, Thörngren JO, et al. Non-steroidal anti-inflammatory drugs do not influence the urinary testosterone/epitestosterone glucuronide ratio. *Front Endocrinol (Lausanne)*. 2013 May 16;4:51. doi: 10.3389/fendo. 2013.00051. Print 2013.

 SEE ALSO

Substance Use Disorders

 CODES

ICD10

F55.3 Abuse of steroids or hormones

CLINICAL PEARLS

- Anabolic steroid abuse is common, and not limited to elite athletes.
- Suspect anabolic steroid abuse in patients with clinical features consistent with side effects, and ask in a judgment-free manner.
- Treating symptoms of withdrawal will greatly improve the patient's ability to remain abstinent.
- Monitor closely for concerning psychiatric signs suggestive of psychosis, mania, violence, or severe depression, as well as for cardiac risk factors.

ANAL FISSURE

Anne Walsh, PA-C, MMSc • Kashyap Trivedi, MD

 BASICS

DESCRIPTION
Anal fissure/Fissure in ano: Longitudinal tear in the lining of the anal canal distal to the dentate line, most commonly at the posterior midline. Characterized by a knifelike tearing sensation upon defecation, often associated with bright red blood per rectum. This very common benign anorectal condition is often confused with hemorrhoids. May be acute (<6 weeks) or chronic (>6 weeks) in duration.

EPIDEMIOLOGY
- Affects all ages. Common in infants 6–24 months; not common in older children, suspect abuse or trauma. Elderly less common due to lower resting pressure in the anal canal.
- Sex: Male = Female; but women are more likely to get anterior midline tears (25% vs. 8%).

Incidence
Exact incidence is unknown. Patients often treat with home remedies and do not seek medical care.

Prevalence
- 80% of infants, usually self-limited
- 20% of adults, most of whom do not seek medical advice

ALERT
- Lateral fissure: Rule out infectious disease
- Atypical fissure: Rule out Crohn disease

ETIOLOGY AND PATHOPHYSIOLOGY
High resting pressure within the anal canal (usually as a result of constipation/straining) leads to ischemia of the anoderm, resulting in splitting of the anal mucosa during defecation and spasm of the exposed internal sphincter.

Genetics
None known

RISK FACTORS
- Constipation (25% of patients)
- Diarrhea (6% of patients)
- Passage of hard or large-caliber stool
- High resting tone of internal anal sphincter (prolonged sitting, obesity)
- Trauma (sexual abuse, childbirth, mountain biking)
- Inflammatory bowel disease (Crohn disease)
- Infection (chlamydia, syphilis, herpes, tuberculosis)

GENERAL PREVENTION
All measures to prevent constipation and prolonged sitting on toilet

COMMONLY ASSOCIATED CONDITIONS
Constipation, Irritable bowel syndrome, Crohn disease, tuberculosis, leukemia, and HIV

 DIAGNOSIS

HISTORY
- Severe, sharp rectal pain, often with and following defecation, but can be continuous; some patients will see bright red blood on the stool or when wiping.
- Occasionally, anal pruritus or peri-anal irritation

PHYSICAL EXAM
- Gentle spreading of the buttocks with close inspection of the anal verge will reveal a tear in the anodermal tissue, typically posterior midline, occasionally anterior midline, rarely eccentric to midline.
- Minimal edema, erythema, or bleeding may be seen.
- In chronic fissure, hypertrophic papillae may be seen at proximal end, and a sentinel pile (tag) may be seen at distal end.

DIFFERENTIAL DIAGNOSIS
- Thrombosed external hemorrhoid: Swollen, painful mass at anal verge
- Perirectal abscess: Tender, warm erythematous induration or fluctuance
- Perianal fistula: Abnormal communication between rectum and perianal epithelium with purulent drainage
- Pruritus ani: Shallow excoriations rather than true fissure

DIAGNOSTIC TESTS & INTERPRETATION
Diagnostic Procedures/Other
- Avoid anoscopy or endoscopy initially unless necessary for other diagnoses.
- Rarely, some patients may require exam under anesthesia due to pain in order to confirm the diagnosis.

 TREATMENT

The goal of treatment is to avoid repeated tearing of the anal mucosa with resultant spasm of the internal anal sphincter by decreasing the patient's high sphincter tone and addressing its underlying cause.

GENERAL MEASURES
- Wash area with warm water; consume a high-fiber diet; avoid constipation, maintain healthy weight.
- Medical therapy is usually initiated in a stepwise manner: Nitrates, calcium channel blockers, botulinum toxin (1)[B].

MEDICATION
First Line
Acute fissures:
- Stool softeners (docusate) daily
- Osmotic laxatives if needed (polyethylene glycol)
- Fiber supplements (psyllium, methylcellulose, inulin e.g.) and increased fluid intake
- Topical analgesics (2% lidocaine gel)
- Topical lubricants/emollients (Balneol cream)
- Sitz baths (sit in hot water bath for 20 minutes 2–3 times daily)

Second Line
Chronic fissures:
- Chemical sphincterotomy:
  - Topical nitroglycerin ointment 2% diluted to 0.2% applied q.i.d.: Marginally but significantly better than placebo in healing (48.6% vs. 37%); late recurrence was common (50%) (2)[A]; effect is to reduce resting anal pressure through the release of nitric oxide (2)[B].
  - Calcium channel blockers (e.g., nifedipine, diltiazem), oral or topical: No better than nitrates but with fewer side effects (2)[A]; effect is to relax the internal sphincter muscle, thereby reducing the resting anal pressure (3)[A].
  - Botulinum toxin 4 mL injected into the internal sphincter muscle: No better than topical nitrates but with fewer side effects (2)[A]; effect is to inhibit the release of acetylcholine from nerve endings to inhibit muscle spasm (4)[B].

ISSUES FOR REFERRAL
- Late recurrence is common (50%) particularly if the underlying issue remains untreated (constipation, irritable bowel, etc.).
- Medical therapy usually is tried for 90–120 days prior to colorectal surgery referral.

ADDITIONAL THERAPIES
Anococcygeal support (modified toilet seat) may offer some advantage in chronic fissures to avoid surgery.

SURGERY/OTHER PROCEDURES
- Reserved for failure of medical therapy; involves division of the internal sphincter muscle
- Lateral internal sphincterectomy is the surgical procedure of choice (5)[B].
- Risk for fecal incontinence: 45% short term, 6–8% long term
- Anal stretching/dilation: Unlikely to benefit (2)[C]

 ## ONGOING CARE

DIET
High fiber (>25 g/d; augment with daily fiber supplements); increase fluid intake.

PATIENT EDUCATION
- Avoid prolonged sitting or straining during bowel movements; drink plenty of fluids; avoid constipation, weight loss if obese.
- Avoid use of triple antibiotic ointment to anal area.

PROGNOSIS
Most acute fissures heal within 6 weeks with conservative therapy. Medical therapy is less likely to be successful for chronic anal fissures; 40% failure rate (6)[A].

COMPLICATIONS
Fecal incontinence and incontinence to flatus; primarily associated with surgery (30% post op, which may become permanent).

REFERENCES
1. Altomare DF, Binda GA, Canuti S, et al. The management of patients with primary chronic anal fissure: A position paper. *Tech Coloproctol.* 2011;15:135–141.
2. Madoff RD, Fleshman JW. AGA technical review on the diagnosis and care of patients with anal fissure. *Gastroenterology.* 2003;124:235–245.
3. Samim M, Twigt B, Stoker L, et al. Topical diltiazem cream versus botulinum toxin A for the treatment of chronic anal fissure: A double-blind randomized clinical trial. *Ann Surg.* 2012;255(1):18–22.
4. Madalinski MH. Identifying the best therapy for chronic anal fissure. *World J Gastro Pharm Ther.* 2011;2:9–16.
5. Mousavi SR, Sharifi M, Mehdikhah Z. A comparison between the results of fissurectomy and lateral internal sphincterotomy in the surgical management of chronic anal fissure. *J Gastrointest Surg.* 2009;13:1279–1282.
6. Shao WJ, Li GC, Zhang ZK. Systematic review and meta-analysis of randomized controlled trials comparing botulinum toxin injection with lateral internal sphincterotomy for chronic anal fissure. *Int J Colorectal Dis.* 2009;24:995–1000.

ADDITIONAL READING
- Gee T, Hisham RB, Jabar MF et al. Ano-coccygeal support in the treatment of idiopathic chronic posterior anal fissure: A prospective randomized controlled pilot trial. *Tech Coloproctol* 2013;17: 181–186.
- Sinha R, Kaiser AM. Efficacy of management algorithm for reducing need for sphincterotomy in chronic anal fissures. *Colorectal Dis.* 2012;14(6): 760–764.
- Yiannakopoulou E. Botulinum toxin and anal fissure: Efficacy and safety systematic review. *Int J Colorectal Dis.* 2012;27(1):1–9.

 ## CODES

ICD10
- K60.0 Acute anal fissure
- K60.1 Chronic anal fissure
- K60.2 Anal fissure, unspecified

CLINICAL PEARLS
- Avoid anoscopy or endoscopy initially unless necessary for other diagnoses.
- Best chance to prevent recurrence is to treat the underlying cause.
- No medical therapy approaches the cure rate of surgery for chronic fissure.

ANAPHYLAXIS

Bobby Peters, MD, FAAEM

 BASICS

DESCRIPTION
- An IgE-mediated, acute systemic reaction following antigen exposure in a sensitized person
- A non–IgE-mediated idiopathic anaphylactoid reaction also may occur. Anaphylactoid reactions are clinically indistinguishable from anaphylaxis and are treated in the same manner.
  - System(s) affected: Cardiovascular; Endocrine/Metabolic; Gastrointestinal; Hematologic/Lymphatic/Immunologic; Pulmonary; and Skin/Exocrine
- Synonym(s): Anaphylactoid reactions

EPIDEMIOLOGY
- Predominant age: All ages
- Predominant sex: Male = Female

Incidence
- Up to 40,000 cases of idiopathic anaphylaxis with no identifiable cause occur each year.
- Drug-induced anaphylaxis occurs in 1/2,700 hospitalized patients.
- Anaphylaxis deaths: 0.3–0.7/100,000 per year
- Food allergic reactions constitute 1/3–1/2 of all anaphylactic reactions worldwide.
- Anaphylaxis may occur secondary to allergy skin testing.
- Asthmatics are more prone to anaphylaxis than nonasthmatics. Female asthmatics are at greater risk of anaphylaxis than their male counterparts.

ETIOLOGY AND PATHOPHYSIOLOGY
- IgE-mediated mast cell degranulation
- Complement activation (C3a, C4a, C5a) by antigen–antibody complexes that contain complement-fixing antibodies
- Other non–IgE-dependent anaphylaxislike syndromes may be caused by modulators of arachidonic acid metabolism, sulfiting agents, exercise-induced anaphylaxis, and idiopathic recurrent anaphylaxis.
- Some important causes of anaphylaxis are:
  - Antimicrobials (e.g., penicillin)
  - Blood products (especially in IgA deficiency)
  - Iodinated contrast media
  - Ethylene oxide gas (dialysis tubing, other sterilized products)
  - Exercise
  - Foods (commonly peanuts, nuts, fish, crustaceans, mollusks, cow's milk, eggs, and soy)
  - Immunotherapy
  - Insect stings (e.g., honeybees, wasps, kissing bugs, and deer flies)
  - Latex rubber (gloves, catheters)
  - Macromolecules (e.g., chymopapain, insulin, dextran, glucocorticoid, and protamine)
  - Vaccines

Genetics
Genetic predisposition for sensitization to antigens

RISK FACTORS
- Previous anaphylaxis
- History of atopy or asthma

GENERAL PREVENTION
- Avoid inducing drugs and foods.
- For those with history of anaphylaxis, carry a prefilled epinephrine syringe. Keep a syringe at home, work/school, and in vehicle, although syringe should be protected from temperature extremes.
- Avoid areas where insect exposure is likely. Avoid wearing insect attractants (e.g., perfumes, colored clothing); avoid bare feet outdoors.
- Carry or wear a medical alert ID about the anaphylaxis-causing substance or event.
- When radiologic contrast is unavoidable, use of low-osmolar contrast agents (e.g., iothalamate) reduces the risk of contrast reactions to 3.1%:
  - Only 0.22% were considered severe.
  - Stop beta-blockers before administering contrast materials.
  - Pretreat with diphenhydramine (50 mg IV) and a steroid (e.g., methylprednisolone 60 mg IV q6h) until procedure. Start methylprednisolone the day before the procedure is scheduled.
  - Those with frequent (>6 per year) episodes of idiopathic anaphylaxis should be treated prophylactically with prednisone (40–60 mg/d in a single morning dose), hydroxyzine (25 mg t.i.d.), and albuterol (2 mg PO t.i.d.). The prednisone should be rapidly tapered to an every-other-day regimen.

ALERT
- Have a latex-free kit (gloves, etc.) available for the treatment of latex-allergic patients. Some latex-allergic patients will react to tropical fruits, such as kiwi, bananas, avocados, and chestnuts.
- Avoid beta-blockers.

COMMONLY ASSOCIATED CONDITIONS
- Asthma
- Atopy

 DIAGNOSIS

HISTORY
Rapid progression within minutes to hours of the signs and symptoms of anaphylaxis, with or without an obvious trigger, including but not limited to cutaneous symptoms (90% of cases), respiratory symptoms (70%), GI symptoms (40%), and cardiovascular symptoms (35%)

PHYSICAL EXAM
- Pruritus, flushing, urticaria, angioedema
- Dyspnea, cough, rhonchi
- Rhinorrhea, bronchorrhea, wheezing, stridor
- Difficulty swallowing
- Nausea, vomiting, diarrhea, cramps, bloating
- Tachycardia, hypotension, shock, syncope
- Malaise, shivering
- Mydriasis

DIFFERENTIAL DIAGNOSIS
- Anaphylactoid reactions:
  - May occur after the first contact with a substance such as polymyxin, pentamidine, radiographic contrast media, and aspirin
- Carcinoid syndrome
- Globus hystericus:
  - May mimic pharyngeal edema
- Hereditary angioedema:
  - C1q esterase deficiency with painless, pruritus-free angioedema without urticaria, flushing, or wheezing
- Pheochromocytoma:
  - Paradoxically, because of β_2 stimulation, some patients have hypotensive attacks accompanied by tachycardia.
  - Urticaria, angioedema, and wheezing are absent.
- Pseudoanaphylactic reaction:
  - After injection of procaine penicillin:
    - Is a drug effect of procaine and not a penicillin allergy
- Scombroid poisoning:
  - From ingestion of dark meat fish (e.g., tuna, mackerel, and mahi-mahi)
  - Histaminelike mediator: Symptoms include flushing, sweating, nausea, vomiting, diarrhea, headache, palpitations, dizziness, rash, swelling of face and tongue, respiratory distress, and vasodilatory shock.
- Serum sickness:
  - Occurs several days after exposure
- Systemic mastocytosis:
  - Benign or malignant overgrowth of mast cells
  - Urticaria pigmentosa seen in the benign form and the presence of reddish-brown macular–papular cutaneous lesions, which urticate after trauma (Darier sign)
- Vasovagal reactions:
  - Bradycardia and hypotension without tachycardia, flushing, urticaria, angioedema, pruritus, and wheezing
- Pulmonary embolism, foreign body aspiration, and arrhythmia

DIAGNOSTIC TESTS & INTERPRETATION
Initial Tests (lab, imaging)
- Little data to support extensive testing; targeted IgE antibodies of little value due to low sensitivity and specificity
- Often found when severe: Hypoxemia, hypercarbia, acidosis
- Acidosis may cause apparent hyperkalemia by moving potassium extracellularly
- Elevated serum tryptase, a mast cell enzyme for allergic and anaphylactic reactions (1)[B]
- Drugs that may alter lab results: Epinephrine and albuterol may cause apparent hypokalemia by shifting K^+ intracellularly.

 TREATMENT

GENERAL MEASURES
- Treatment depends on severity.
- Maintain a patent airway:
  - Endotracheal intubation and assisted ventilation may be necessary.
  - Possibly tracheostomy or needle cricothyrotomy in children <12 years
- Oxygen
- IV fluids (normal saline/lactated Ringer's)

MEDICATION
First Line
- Epinephrine:
  - Less severe reaction: 0.3–0.5 mg (0.01 mg/kg in children) = (0.3–0.5 mL of a 1:1,000 solution, 0.01 mL/kg in children), SQ q20–30min PRN, up to 3 doses
  - Life-threatening reactions: 0.5 mg (5 mL of a 1:10,000 solution) (for children: 0.05–0.1 mL/kg per dose) IV, slowly: q5–10min as needed. If IV access is not possible, endotracheal or intraosseous may be effective.
- Diphenhydramine: An H1 blocker: 25–50 mg IV (IM or PO) q6h for 72 hours (children 1.25 mg/kg to 25 mg)
- Cimetidine: An H2 blocker: 300 mg IV over 3–5 minutes (children 5–10 mg/kg per dose) and then 400 mg PO b.i.d. is helpful and may be more effective than diphenhydramine.
- Corticosteroids: Although routinely used, no immediate effect and no evidence for their use in the emergency department (2)[B]:
  - Hydrocortisone sodium succinate: 250–500 mg IV q4–6h (4–8 mg/kg for children)
  - Prednisone: 1 mg/kg in children, up to 60 mg
  - Methylprednisolone: 60–125 mg IV in adults (1–2 mg/kg in children)
- Bronchodilator, if persistent bronchospasm:
  - Inhaled β_2 agonists. Continuous nebulized albuterol of 10 mg/hr or 2.5 mg q15–20min is safe, effective, and preferable to aminophylline as a first line.
- Laryngeal edema:
  - Epinephrine: 5 mL 1:1,000 by nebulizer is more effective than racemic epinephrine and is usually available.
- Persistent hypotension:
  - Dopamine: 200 mg in 500 mL of dextrose in water given by infusion pump; titrate to BP (3–20 mcg/kg/min)
  - Glucagon: May be beneficial for resistant hypotension caused by concurrent beta-blockade therapy; 50 mcg/kg IV bolus over 1 minute, or alternatively, give as continuous infusion at 5–15 mcg/min
- Normal saline or Ringer's lactate: As necessary to maintain tissue perfusion
- Oral antihistamines for 72 hours

Geriatric Considerations
Epinephrine may induce myocardial ischemia in those with cardiac disease, but is the drug of choice. Be alert for anticholinergic and CNS side effects after giving diphenhydramine or cimetidine.

Pediatric Considerations
Epinephrine could reduce the placental blood flow, but may save the life of the mother and fetus. It also increases the risk of congenital malformation.

Second Line
- Several reports of tranexamic acid: 1,000 mg IV or sigma-aminocaproic acid for refractory anaphylaxis
- These drugs are not standard care; use only in patients who do not respond to other therapy.
- Aminophylline: 5–6 mg/kg IV in 100 mL D₅W over 20 minutes, then maintenance at 1 mg/kg/hr drip

- Anti-IgE monoclonal antibody may have a role in long-term management of food-induced anaphylaxis.
- Venom immunotherapy has been effective in the prevention of sting anaphylaxis, but with a high side-effect risk (3)[A].

ISSUES FOR REFERRAL
- Allergist referral if anaphylaxis cause unclear
- Patients with anaphylaxis from insect stings benefit from desensitization immunotherapy.

IN-PATIENT CONSIDERATIONS
Admission Criteria/Initial Stabilization
Moderate–severe anaphylaxis, admit for observation.

Discharge Criteria
Outpatient: Patients with cutaneous angioedema, urticaria, and minimal bronchospasm may be released when symptoms and signs have cleared.

 ONGOING CARE

FOLLOW-UP RECOMMENDATIONS
Bed rest until anaphylaxis clears and patient is hemodynamically stable

DIET
NPO until acute symptoms are controlled

PATIENT EDUCATION
- Asthma and Allergy Foundation of America, 1717 Massachusetts Avenue, Suite 305, Washington, DC 20036; (800)-7-ASTHMA or American Allergy Association, P.O. Box 7273, Menlo Park, CA 94026, (415) 322-1663
- Medic-Alert–type tags (Medic-Alert Foundation, Turlock, CA 95381-1009)
- Avoid beta-blockers, if possible.
- Instruct patient in the use of the bee sting kit.

PROGNOSIS
- Good prognosis if treated immediately; worse outcome with a delay of >30 minutes in administration of epinephrine.
- Of those with idiopathic anaphylaxis, 60% are free of anaphylactic episodes at 2.5 years; most others are steroid-free.

COMPLICATIONS
- Hypoxemia
- Cardiac arrest
- Death

REFERENCES
1. Brown SG, Blackman KE, Heddle RJ. Can serum mast cell tryptase help diagnose anaphylaxis? *Emerg Med Australas*. 2004;2:120–124.
2. Choo KJ, Simons E, Sheikh A. Glucocorticoids for the treatment of anaphylaxis. *Allergy*. 2010;65(10):1205–1211. Epub 2010.
3. Brown SG, Wiese MD, Blackman KE, et al. Ant venom immunotherapy: A double-blind, placebo-controlled, crossover trial. *Lancet*. 2003;(361)9362:1001–1006.

ADDITIONAL READING
- Arias K, Waserman S, Jordana M. Management of food-induced anaphylaxis: Unsolved challenges. *Curr Clin Pharmacol*. 2009;4(2):113–125.
- González-Pérez A, Aponte Z, Vidaurre CF, et al. Anaphylaxis epidemiology in patients with and patients without asthma: A United Kingdom database review. *J Allergy Clin Immunol*. 2010;125(5):1098–1104.e1. Epub 2010 Apr 14.
- Pitsios C, Dimitriou A, Stefanaki EC, et al. Anaphylaxis during skin testing with food allergens in children. *Eur J Pediatr*. 2010;169(5):613–615. Epub 2009 Sep 23.
- Sheikh A, Shehata YA, Brown SG, et al. Adrenaline (epinephrine) for the treatment of anaphylaxis with and without shock. *Cochrane Database Syst Rev*. 2008;(4):CD006312. Epub 2008 Oct 8.
- Sheikh A, ten Broek V, Brown SG, et al. H1-antihistamines for the treatment of anaphylaxis with and without shock. *Cochrane Database Syst Rev*. 2007;(1):CD006160. Epub 2007 Jan 24.
- Tanus T, Mines D, Atkins PC, et al. Serum tryptase in idiopathic anaphylaxis: A case report and review of the literature. *Ann Emerg Med*. 1994;24(1):104–107.
- Wittbrodt ET, Spinler SA. Prevention of anaphylactoid reactions in high-risk patients receiving radiographic contrast media. *Ann Pharmacother*. 1994;28(2):236–241.

 SEE ALSO

Arthropod Bites and Stings; Food Allergy

 CODES

ICD10
- T78.00XA Anaphylactic reaction due to unspecified food, init encntr
- T78.2XXA Anaphylactic shock, unspecified, initial encounter
- T88.6XXA Anaphylactic reaction due to adverse effect of correct drug or medicament properly administered, initial encounter

CLINICAL PEARLS
- Allergy to one species of legume (e.g., peanuts) or one type of seafood (e.g., shrimp) does not mean allergy to all products in that category. Skin testing is prudent.
- Measles, mumps, rubella (MMR) vaccine can be safely administered to those with a history of egg allergy; most egg allergies are related to the albumin.
- Penicillin-allergic patients can generally tolerate 2nd- and 3rd-generation cephalosporins as well as monobactams (e.g., aztreonam). Generally, they will be allergic to carbapenems (e.g., imipenem) and 1st-generation cephalosporins.
- IgA-deficient patients should have washed RBCs for transfusion.
- Those allergic to seafood are not allergic to iodine-based radiocontrast. Shellfish allergy is protein-related.

ANEMIA, APLASTIC
Muthalagu Ramanathan, MD • Jan Cerny, MD, PhD

BASICS

DESCRIPTION
- Pancytopenia with hypocellular bone marrow without infiltrates or fibrosis. Classified as acquired (much more common) and congenital
- Acquired aplastic anemia: Insidious onset; due to exogenous insult triggering an autoimmune reaction; often responsive to immunosuppression.
- Congenital forms: Rare, mostly in childhood (exception is atypical presentation of Fanconi syndrome in adults; 30s for males and 40s for females).
- The occurrence of specific mutations in genes of the telomere complex in acquired aplastic anemia has blurred the distinction between the congenital and acquired forms.
- System(s) affected: Heme/Lymphatic/Immunologic
- Synonym(s): Hypoplastic anemia; Panmyelophthisis; Refractory anemia; Aleukia hemorrhagica; Toxic paralytic anemia

ALERT
- Early intervention for aplastic anemia greatly improves the chances of treatment success.
- Hematopoietic growth factors require close monitoring in newly diagnosed patients.

Geriatric Considerations
The elderly are often exposed to large numbers of drugs and therefore may be more susceptible to acquired aplastic anemia.

Pediatric Considerations
- Congenital forms of aplastic anemia require different treatment regimens than acquired forms.
- Acquired aplastic anemia is seen in children exposed to ionizing radiation or treated with cytotoxic chemotherapeutic agents.

Pregnancy Considerations
- Pregnancy is a real but rare cause of aplastic anemia. Symptoms may resolve after delivery and with termination.
- Complications in pregnancy likely from low platelet counts and paroxysmal nocturnal hemoglobinuria-associated aplastic anemia.

EPIDEMIOLOGY
- Predominant age: Biphasic 15–25 (more common) and >60
- Predominant sex: Male = Female

Incidence
- 2–3 new cases per million per year in Europe and North America
- The incidence is 3-fold higher in Thailand and China vs. the Western world.

ETIOLOGY AND PATHOPHYSIOLOGY
- Idiopathic (~70% of the cases)
- Drugs: Phenylbutazone, chloramphenicol, sulfonamides, gold, cytotoxic drugs, antiepileptics (felbamate, carbamazepine, valproic acid, phenytoin)
- Viral: HIV, Epstein-Barr virus (EBV), nontypeable postinfectious hepatitis (not A, B, or C), parvovirus B19 (mostly in the immunocompromised), atypical mycobacterium
- Toxic exposure (benzene, pesticides, arsenic)

- Radiation exposure
- Immune disorders (systemic lupus erythematosus, eosinophilic fascitis, graft vs. host disease)
- Pregnancy (rare)
- Congenital (Fanconi anemia, dyskeratosis congenita, Shwachman-Diamond syndrome, amegakaryocytic thrombocytopenia)
- The immune hypothesis: Bone marrow suppression through activation of T cells with associated cytokine production leading to destruction or injury of hematopoietic stem cells. This leads to a hypocellular bone marrow without marrow fibrosis.
- The activation of T cells likely occurs because of both genetic and environmental factors. Exposure to specific environmental precipitants, diverse host genetic risk factors, and individual differences in characteristics of immune response likely account for variations in its clinical manifestations and patterns of responsiveness to treatment.
- Telomerase deficiency leads to short telomeres. This leads to impaired regenerative capacity and hence a reduction in marrow progenitors and likely a qualitative deficiency in the repair capacity of hematopoietic tissue.
- Reduction of natural killer cells in the bone marrow

Genetics
- Telomerase mutations found in a small number of patients with acquired and congenital forms. These mutations render carriers more susceptible to environmental insults.
- Mutations in genes called TERC and TERT were found in pedigrees of adults with acquired aplastic anemia who lacked the physical abnormalities or a family history typical of inherited forms of bone marrow failure. These genes encode for the RNA component of telomerase.
- HLA-DR2 incidence in aplastic anemia is twice that in the normal population.

RISK FACTORS
- Treatment with high-dose radiation or chemotherapy
- Exposure to toxic chemicals
- Use of certain medications
- Certain blood diseases, autoimmune disorders, and serious infections
- Tumors of thymus (red cell aplasia)
- Pregnancy, rarely

GENERAL PREVENTION
- Avoid possible toxic industrial agents.
- Use safety measures when working with radiation.

DIAGNOSIS

HISTORY
- Solvent and radiation history, family, environmental, travel, and infectious disease history
- Patients often asymptomatic, but may have frequent infections, fatigue, shortness of breath, headache, or bleeding/bruising.

PHYSICAL EXAM
- Mucosal hemorrhage, petechiae
- Pallor
- Fever
- Hemorrhage, menorrhagia, occult stool blood, melena, epistaxis
- Dyspnea

- Palpitations
- Progressive weakness
- Retinal flame hemorrhages
- Systolic ejection murmur
- Weight loss
- Signs of congenital aplastic anemia:
  - Short stature
  - Microcephaly
  - Nail dystrophy
  - Abnormal thumbs
  - Oral leukoplakia
  - Hyperpigmentation (café au lait spots) or hypopigmentation

DIFFERENTIAL DIAGNOSIS
Includes other causes of bone marrow failure and pancytopenia:
- Marrow replacement:
  - Acute lymphoblastic leukemia
  - Lymphoma
  - Hairy cell leukemia (increased reticulin and infiltration of hairy cells)
  - Large granular lymphocyte leukemia
  - Fibrosis
- Megaloblastic hematopoiesis:
  - Folate deficiency
  - Vitamin B$_{12}$ deficiency
- Paroxysmal nocturnal hemoglobinuria, hemolytic anemia (dark urine), pancytopenia and venous thrombosis (classically hepatic veins)
- Systemic lupus erythematosus
- Prolonged starvation or anorexia nervosa (bone marrow is gelatinous with loss of fat cells and increased ground substance)
- Transient erythroblastopenia of childhood
- Drug-induced agranulocytosis that may be reversible on withdrawal of drug
- Overwhelming infection:
  - HIV with myelodysplasia
  - Viral hemophagocytic syndrome

DIAGNOSTIC TESTS & INTERPRETATION
Screening tests to exclude other etiologies:
- CBC and absolute reticulocyte count
- Blood smear exam
- Cytogenetic studies of peripheral lymphocytes if <35 years of age to exclude Fanconi anemia
- Liver function test
- Viral serology: Hepatitis A, B, C; EBV; cytomegalovirus (CMV); HIV
- Vitamin B$_{12}$ and folate levels
- Autoantibody screening antinuclear antibody (ANA) and anti-DNA
- Flow cytometry looking for GPI, negative neutrophils and RBCs for paroxysmal nocturnal hemoglobinuria
- Fetal hemoglobin in children
- Red cell adenosine deaminase (pure red cell aplasia)
- Cytogenetic analysis of bone marrow

Initial Tests (lab, imaging)
- CBC: Pancytopenia, anemia (usually normocytic), leucopenia, neutropenia, thrombocytopenia
- Decreased absolute number of reticulocytes
- Increased serum iron secondary to transfusion
- Normal total iron-binding capacity (TIBC)
- High mean corpuscular volume (MCV) >104
- CD 34+ cells decreased in blood and marrow
- Urinalysis: Hematuria

- Abnormal liver function tests (hepatitis)
- Increased fetal hemoglobin (Fanconi)
- Increased chromosomal breaks under specialized conditions (Fanconi)
- Molecular determination of abnormal gene (Fanconi)
- CT of thymus region if thymoma-associated RBC aplasia suspected
- Radiographs of radius and thumbs (if congenital anemia suspected)
- Renal ultrasound (to rule out congenital anemia or malignant hematologic disorder)
- Chest x-ray to exclude infections such as mycobacterial infection

Diagnostic Procedures/Other
Bone marrow aspiration and biopsy

Test Interpretation
- Normochromic RBC
- Bone marrow:
  - Decreased cellularity (<10%): No fibrosis, no malignant cells seen
  - Decreased megakaryocytes
  - Decreased myeloid precursors
  - Decreased erythroid precursors
  - Prominent fat spaces and marrow stroma, polyclonal plasma cells

 # TREATMENT

Early treatment increases the chance of success. 2 major options: Immunosuppressive therapy and hematopoietic stem cell transplantation. Treatment decisions are based on age of the patient, severity of disease, and availability of a human leukocyte antigen (HLA)-matched sibling donor for transplantation (1).

GENERAL MEASURES
- Supportive measures: RBC and platelet transfusions. Use only irradiated leukoreduced or CMV-negative blood initially if patient is a candidate for hematopoietic stem cell transplantation.
- Antibiotics, antifungals, antivirals when appropriate, especially if ANC <200 cells/μL
- Oxygen therapy for severe anemia
- Good oral hygiene
- Control menorrhagia with norethisterone or oral contraceptive pills.
- Avoid causative agents/isolation if necessary.
- HLA testing on all patients and their immediate families
- Transfusion support (judiciously prescribed RBCs for severe anemia; platelets for severe thrombocytopenia):
  - Transfuse when platelet count is <10 × 10^9 or if <20 × 10^9 with fever

MEDICATION
First Line
- Immunosuppressive therapy:
  - A combination of antithymocyte globulin (ATG) plus cyclosporine. ATG eliminates lymphocytes, and cyclosporin blocks T-cell function (2).
- Antithymocyte globulin (ATG):
  - A horse serum containing polyclonal antibodies against human T cells
  - 1st-choice treatment for patients >40 years of age and for younger patients without a compatible donor. Consider in patients 30–40 years of age.
  - May be used as a single agent but has better response in combination with cyclosporine

- Cyclosporine following initial ATG therapy for minimum of 6 months:
  - Monitor through blood levels. Normal values for assays vary.
  - Granulocyte colony-stimulating factor (G-CSF):
    ○ May be used in conjunction with ATG and cyclosporine
    ○ Shows faster neutrophil recovery, but survival is not improved
    ○ Treatment is costly and is disputed in 2 randomized trials.
  - Note: Relapses may occur after the initial response to the immunosuppressive therapy if cyclosporine is discontinued too early. Restarting cyclosporine can lead to a response in up to 25% of patients.
- Stem cell transplant: Matched sibling allogeneic stem cell transplant for age <20 and absolute neutrophil count (ANC) <500 or age 20–40 and ANC <200

Second Line
- Rabbit ATG + cyclosporine
- Campath
- Androgen in a subset of patients who have anemia as a predominant feature
- Matched unrelated donor stem cell transplant
- Clinical trials: TPO receptor agonists (3) http://patientrecruitment.nhlbi.nih.gov/AplasticAnemia.aspx

SURGERY/OTHER PROCEDURES
- First-line hematopoietic stem cell transplantation is recommended for patients with an HLA-identical donor and severe aplastic anemia when age <20 and ANC <500 or age 20–40 and ANC <200. Consider in patients 40–50 years in good general medical condition.
- Patients >40 have higher rates of graft vs. host disease and graft rejection (4).
- Unrelated donor transplants should be considered for patients age <40 without HLA-matched sibling donor who failed 2nd-line immunosuppressive therapy
- Thymectomy for thymoma

IN-PATIENT CONSIDERATIONS
Nursing
If neutropenic, use antiseptic mouthwash such as chlorhexidine.

 # ONGOING CARE

DIET
If neutropenic, avoid foods that can expose patient to bacteria, such as uncooked foods.

PATIENT EDUCATION
- Stay away from people who are sick; avoid large crowds.
- Wash your hands often.
- Brush and floss your teeth; get regular dental care to reduce risk of infections.
- Yearly flu shot and pneumonia vaccine.
- Printed patient information available from Aplastic Anemia & MDS International Foundation, Inc., 800-747-2828. Web site: www.aamds.org/aplastic

PROGNOSIS
- Hematopoietic stem cell transplantation with HLA-matched sibling:
  - Age <16, 91%
  - Age >16, 70–80%
- Immunosuppressive therapy using ATG and cyclosporine: Overall survival of 75%; 90% among responders at 5 years

COMPLICATIONS
- Infection (fungal, sepsis)
- Graft vs. host disease in bone marrow transplant recipients (acute 18%; chronic 26%)
- Side effects of immunosuppressant medications
- Hemorrhage
- Transfusion hemosiderosis
- Transfusion hepatitis
- Heart failure
- Development of secondary cancer: Leukemia or myelodysplasia (15–19% risk at 6–10 years)
- Refractory pancytopenia

REFERENCES
1. Scheinberg P, Young NS. How I treat acquired aplastic anemia. *Blood*. 2012;120(6):1185–1196. Epub 2012 Apr 19.
2. Bacigalupo A, Passweg J. Diagnosis and treatment of acquired aplastic anemia. *Hematol Oncol Clin N Am*. 2009;23:159–170.
3. Townsley DM, Desmond R, Dunbar CE, Young NS. Pathophysiology and management of thrombocytopenia in bone marrow failure: Possible clinical applications of TPO receptor agonists in aplastic anemia and myelodysplastic syndromes. *Int J Hematol*. Epub 2013 May 21.
4. Brodsky RA, Jones RJ. Aplastic anaemia. *Lancet*. 2005;365:1647–1656.

SEE ALSO
- Myelodysplastic Syndromes; Systemic Lupus Erythematosus (SLE)
- Algorithm: Anemia

CODES
ICD10
- D61.01 Constitutional (pure) red blood cell aplasia
- D61.89 Oth aplastic anemias and other bone marrow failure syndromes
- D61.9 Aplastic anemia, unspecified

CLINICAL PEARLS
- Acquired aplastic anemia has an insidious onset and is caused by an exogenous insult triggering an autoimmune reaction. This form is usually responsive to immunosuppressive therapy.
- Immunosuppressive therapy using ATG and cyclosporine: Overall survival of 75%; 90% among responders at 5 years

ANEMIA, AUTOIMMUNE HEMOLYTIC

Heather J. Hue, MD, MPH • Emily Lau, MD • Rahul Banerjee

BASICS

DESCRIPTION
- Autoimmune Hemolytic Anemia (AIHA): Accelerated destruction of RBCs in the presence of anti-RBC autoantibodies (1)
- Classified into 3 main groups (1,2,3):
  - Warm AIHA (antibodies optimally bind at 37°C): Mainly IgG-mediated; triggers are either idiopathic or secondary to an underlying process
  - Cold AIHA (antibodies optimally bind at 4–18°C): Mainly IgM-mediated (although IgG or IgA possible); includes cold agglutinin syndrome or paroxysmal cold hemoglobinuria
  - Mixed AIHA (antibodies bind from 4–37°C): Primarily IgM-mediated, linked to lymphomas; has features of both warm and cold AIHA
- Drug-induced autoimmune hemolytic anemia: Related to drug exposure, behaves similarly to warm AIHA (mainly IgG-mediated)

EPIDEMIOLOGY
Incidence
- Adults: 10–30 cases per million, Female > Male (1,3)
  - Warm AIHA: 70–80% cases, age of onset: 40–60
  - Cold AIHA: 20–30% cases, age of onset: >65
- Pediatric: 0.2–1 cases per million, Male > Female (3,4)
  - Warm AIHA: Average age of onset: 4; 40% of cases associated with Evans syndrome
- Cold AIHA: Typically after Mycoplasma or Epstein-Barr virus (EBV) infection
- Mixed AIHA: 10% of cases, mainly in adults (3)

Prevalence
Total AIHA prevalence approaches 170 cases per million (5)

ETIOLOGY AND PATHOPHYSIOLOGY
- General concepts (1,2,3):
  - IgG, IgA, and IgM target RBC antigens, resulting in direct opsonization and/or the triggering of complement fixation
  - Antibody-triggered complement fixation can lead to cell opsonization (via C3b) or cell lysis (via the C5–C9 membrane attack complex)
  - Result: intravascular or extravascular hemolysis
  - Extravascular hemolysis: Phagocytosis of RBCs by tissue macrophages within liver or spleen
    - Mediator: Opsonization of RBCs by autoantibody binding and/or antibody-induced complement fixation (e.g., C3b)
    - IgG-opsonized cells (e.g., in warm AIHA) primarily phagocytosed within the spleen
    - IgM-opsonized cells (e.g., in cold AIHA) primarily phagocytosed within the liver
  - Intravascular hemolysis: Direct destruction of circulating RBCs within bloodstream
    - Mediator: Membrane attack complex insertion triggered by complement fixation (as a result of autoantibody-RBC binding)
    - Not as common as extravascular hemolysis because of protective RBC surface proteins (specifically, CD55 and CD59)
  - Pathogenicity of autoantibodies depends on circulating antibody titer, antibody class, avidity for RBC antigens, and ability to fix complement
  - Clinical symptoms depend on rate of hemolysis, ability of body to process breakdown products, and bone marrow capacity to regenerate RBCs

- Warm AIHA (1,3):
  - Pathophysiology: Autoantibody formation (typically IgG targeting Rh peptide on RBCs) leading to extravascular hemolysis
  - Causes:
    - Idiopathic: 50% of cases
    - Acquired lymphoproliferative disorders: CLL, lymphomas, Castleman disease
    - Autoimmune disorders: systemic lupus erythematosus (SLE), rheumatoid arthritis (RA), ulcerative colitis (UC)
    - Autoimmune lymphoproliferative syndrome
    - Infections: EBV, brucella
  - Predisposing risk factors for anti-RBC autoantibody formation:
    - Common variable immunodeficiency
    - Allogeneic stem cell transplant
- Cold AIHA (2,3):
  - Pathophysiology: Autoantibody formation (typically IgM targeting I-i peptide on RBCs) leading primarily to extravascular hemolysis
    - IgM binds RBCs at low temperatures (e.g., acral areas) and can trigger permanent complement fixation even if IgM later detaches at warmer temperatures
  - Intravascular hemolysis possible in states of CD55/CD59 deficiency; also common in Paroxysmal Cold Hemoglobinuria
  - Causes:
    - Idiopathic cold agglutinin syndrome
    - Infections: Mycoplasma, EBV (rarer: CMV, Legionella, Chlamydia)
    - Lymphoproliferative disorders/dyscrasias: Waldenström's macroglobulinemia, non-Hodgkin's lymphoma
  - Paroxysmal cold hemoglobinuria (PCH) (6,7):
    - Rare type of cold AIHA historically linked to syphilis in adults; in children, linked to varicella or other viral infections
    - Mediator: Donath-Landsteiner antibodies (IgG, not IgM) against P antigen on RBCs
    - Primarily intravascular hemolysis
- Mixed AIHA (3):
  - Linked to the lymphomas, involves autoantibodies with wide range of RBC-binding temperatures
- Drug-Induced AIHA (5,8):
  - Pathophysiology: RBC opsonization by antidrug antibodies or immune complexes; rarely, de novo anti-RBC antibody production
  - Causes:
    - Antimicrobials: Cefotetan, ceftriaxone, penicillin, piperacillin, quinine
    - Antineoplastics: Fludarabine, cladribine, oxaliplatin, alkylating agents
    - Others: Methyldopa, interferon, ibuprofen, sulfa drugs, procainamide

Genetics
- No genetic component in majority of cases (7)
- Inherited: Autoimmune Lymphoproliferative Syndrome (rare disorder of lymphocyte apoptosis involving *Fas* or *FasL* genes) (9)

RISK FACTORS
- Malignancy, lymphoproliferative disorders, infection, autoimmune disorders, CVID, medications

GENERAL PREVENTION

COMMONLY ASSOCIATED CONDITIONS
- Warm AIHA (5):
  - CLL, SLE, RA, UC, ITP (Evans syndrome)

- Cold AIHA (5):
  - Mycoplasma or EBV infection
- Dyscrasias (e.g., monoclonal gammopathies)

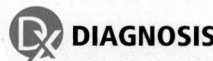

DIAGNOSIS

HISTORY
- Symptoms of anemia: Fatigue/weakness, palpitations, dyspnea, dizziness
- Symptoms of hemolysis: Jaundice (+/– dark urine in intravascular hemolysis, e.g. PCH)
- Temperature-related symptoms: Discoloration, rash, or pain in acral surfaces (cold AIHA)
- Predisposing factor assessment:
  - Recent infections or medication use
  - History or risk factors for underlying causes
  - Concurrent lymphoproliferative disorder or blood dyscrasia

PHYSICAL EXAM
- Signs of anemia: Tachycardia, conjunctival pallor, flow murmur
- Signs of hemolysis: Scleral icterus, splenomegaly and/or hepatomegaly from extravascular hemolysis
- Temperature-related signs: Blue-gray discoloration or livedo reticularis on acral surfaces (cold AIHA)
- Predisposing factor assessment:
  - Fevers (infection, autoimmune, malignancy)
  - Lymphadenopathy, splenomegaly, or hepatomegaly (infection, malignancy)

DIFFERENTIAL DIAGNOSIS
- Allo-antibody syndromes (pregnancy, post-RBC transfusion, post–stem cell transplant)
- Microangiopathic hemolytic disorders (e.g., TTP)
- Other hemolytic anemias (e.g., G6PD deficiency or paroxysmal nocturnal hemoglobinuria)
- Other anemias (e.g., aplastic, megaloblastic)
- Other hemoglobin disorders (e.g., thalassemia)
- Evans Syndrome (if ITP also present)

DIAGNOSTIC TESTS & INTERPRETATION
Initial Tests (lab, imaging)
- CBC and blood smear (1,3):
  - Anemia, +/– mild leukocytosis
  - Reticulocytosis
  - Blood smear examination: anisocytosis, polychromasia, macrocytosis
  - Warm AIHA-specific: Spherocytes
  - Cold AIHA-specific: Agglutinated RBCs
- Hemolytic workup (1,3):
  - Elevated lactate dehydrogenase (LDH), indirect bilirubinemia, decreased haptoglobin
  - Hemoglobinuria in cases of intravascular hemolysis (e.g., PCH)
- Gold Standard: Direct antiglobulin test (DAT), also known as the Coombs reaction (1,2,3)
  - Warm AIHA: DAT+ for IgG +/– C3d
  - Cold AIHA: DAT+ for C3d alone, although weak IgG signal in 20% of patients
    - Confirmatory test: Cold agglutinin titers (with incubation at 4°C) at least 1:64
  - Mixed AIHA: DAT+ for IgG and C3d
  - PCH: Test for Donath-Landsteiner antibody

Follow-up tests and special considerations
Targeted workup based on clinical suspicion for underlying associated conditions (SLE, CLL, EBV, Mycoplasma) (1,3)

Diagnostic Procedures/Other
Bone marrow biopsy not routinely required (2)

TREATMENT

GENERAL MEASURES
- Treatment of underlying condition if identified (2)[C]
- Avoidance or discontinuation of triggering agents (cold weather or fluids for cold AIHA, offending medication for drug-induced AIHA) (2)[C]
- Warm AIHA: Vitamin supplementation (folate; calcium/vitamin D if on long-term steroids) (1)[C]

MEDICATION
First Line
- Warm/mixed AIHA:
  – Glucocorticoids (1,3)[B]:
    ○ Effective, but 3–12 months required for complete response
    ○ Side effects include weight gain, hyperglycemia, depression, osteoporosis
    ○ Dosing: Oral prednisone 1 mg/kg for 3–4 weeks, or IV methylprednisolone 250–1,000 mg/day for 1–3 days if continued hemolysis
  – Danazol (1,3)[C]:
    ○ Synergistic with prednisone
    ○ Black-box warning in pregnancy, androgenic side effects in females
    ○ Long-term hepatotoxicity risk
    ○ Dosing: 400–800 mg PO daily
  – Alemtuzumab: Highly effective for patients with underlying CLL (1,3)[C]
- Cold AIHA:
  – Rituximab (2,3)[B]:
    ○ Partial response in 54–58% of patients
    ○ Side effects uncommon but include hypotension, fevers, infection
    ○ Dosing: 375 mg/m^2 IV infusion repeated periodically
  – Fludarabine: Synergistic with rituximab, but higher immunosuppression risk when used together (2,3)[B]
  – Glucocorticoids have low efficacy (14%) and high side effect profile (2)[B]

Second Line
- Warm/mixed AIHA:
  – Rituximab (1)[C]:
    ○ 25–100% response rates in both primary and secondary warm AIHA
    ○ Delayed efficacy, with weeks to months required before maximum response
    ○ Dosing: 375 mg/m^2 IV infusion weekly
  – IVIG (1,3)[C]:
    ○ Indication: Glucocorticoid-refractory or transfusion-dependent patients; presplenectomy temporizing measure
    ○ Potentially synergistic with glucocorticoids
    ○ Dosing: 400–1,000 mg/kg IV daily × 5 days
  – Other agents in refractory illness (1)[C]:
    ○ Cyclophosphamide, azathioprine, cyclosporin A, mycophenolate mofetil
- Cold AIHA:
  – Chlorambucil or cyclophosphamide (2)[C]
  – No benefit from immunosuppressive drugs (3)[C]
  – Investigational agents (2,3)[C]:
    ○ Darbepoetin as transfusion-sparing strategy
    ○ Eculizumab (no benefit to PCH) (6)[C]

SURGERY/OTHER PROCEDURES
- RBC transfusions:
  – Warm AIHA (1,3)[C]:
    ○ Urgent setting: Transfuse with typed and crossed blood; however, 33% risk of exacerbating hemolysis due to alloantibodies to minor RBC antigens
    ○ Nonurgent setting: Extended RBC pretransfusion workup, including RBC phenotyping and antibody detection
  – Cold AIHA (2)[C]:
    ○ Typed and crossed blood transfusions; extended testing generally not required
    ○ All RBC compatibility tests should be performed at 37°C
    ○ Use prewarmed blood products (or in-line blood warmer) to avoid hemolytic crises
- Splenectomy (1,3)[C]:
  – 38–70% success rate in warm/mixed AIHA
  – Not effective in cold AIHA
  – Pediatric considerations: Splenectomy not recommended given typically self-limited course
  – Laparoscopic approach preferred due to significant difference in mortality (1.6% vs. 6%)

ALERT
Vaccinate against encapsulated bacteria (*S. pneumoniae, N. meningitidis, H. influenzae*) before splenectomy (at least 2 weeks) (1,3)[A]:
- Allogenic Stem Cell Transplant: investigational in warm AIHA (1)[C]
- Plasmapheresis: Investigational; use before transfusions (warm AIHA) or surgeries that require cold exposure (cold AIHA) (1,3)[C]
- Vincristine-loaded platelet transfusions: Consider in refractory AIHA or Evans syndrome (1)[C]

IN-PATIENT CONSIDERATIONS
Admission Criteria
- Symptomatic patients (tachycardia, dyspnea)
- Unstable patients (significant anemia or hemolysis with end-organ damage)
- Patients requiring surgery or patients requiring stabilization with transfusions/plasmapheresis

ALERT
Use prewarmed IV fluids in cold AIHA to avoid major hemolytic crises.

Discharge Criteria
- Cessation or reduction in hemolysis
- Uneventful posttransfusion or operative course

ONGOING CARE

FOLLOW-UP RECOMMENDATIONS
Patient Monitoring
- Serial hemoglobin measurements to evaluate degree of anemia and/or ongoing hemolysis
- Avoidance of hypothermic fluids, blood products, or surgeries for cold AIHA

PATIENT EDUCATION
- Behavior modification in cold AIHA

PROGNOSIS
- Primary AIHA: Good with appropriate lifestyle changes and pharmacologic treatment (1,3)
- Secondary AIHA: Dependent on prognosis of underlying disorder

COMPLICATIONS
- End-organ damage related to severe anemia
- Hepatic or splenic dysfunction
- Morbidity from underlying diseases
- Treatment side-effects (see above)

REFERENCES

1. Barros M, Blajchman M, Bordin J. Warm autoimmune hemolytic anemia: Recent progress in understanding the immunobiology and treatment. *Transfusion Med Rev*. 2010;24(3):195–210.
2. Berenstein S, Tjønnfjord GE. Diagnosis and treatment of cold agglutinin mediated autoimmune hemolytic anemia. *Blood Rev*. 2012;26:107–115.
3. Michel M. Classification and therapeutic approaches in autoimmune hemolytic anemia: an update. *Expert Rev Hematol*. 2011;4:607–618.
4. Aladjidi N, Leverger G, Leblanc T, et al. New insights into childhood autoimmune hemolytic anemia: A French national observational study of 265 children. *Haemotologica*. 2011;96(5):655–663.
5. Lechner K, Jäger U. How I treat autoimmune hemolytic anemias in adults. *Blood*. 2010;116(11):1831–1838.
6. Gregory GP, Opat S, Quang H, et al. Failure of eculizumab to correct paroxysmal cold hemoglobinuria. *Ann Hematol*. 2011;90:989–990.
7. Lambert F, Nydegger U. Geoepidemiology of autoimmune hemolytic anemia. *Autoimmun Rev*. 2010;9:A350–354.
8. Garratty G. Immune hemolytic anemia caused by drugs. *Expert Opin Drug Saf*. 2012;11(4):635–642. Epub 2012 Apr 16.
9. Seif AE, Manno CS, Sheen C, et al. Identifying autoimmune lymphoproliferative syndrome in children with Evans Syndrome: A multi-institutional study. *Blood*. 2010;115:2142–2145.

SEE ALSO
- Lymphoma, Non-Hodgkin's; Leukemia; Systemic Lupus Erythematosus (SLE)
- Algorithm: Anemia

CODES

ICD10
- D59.0 Drug-induced autoimmune hemolytic anemia
- D59.1 Other autoimmune hemolytic anemias

CLINICAL PEARLS
- AIHA is a rare cause of anemia; diagnosis requires evidence of hemolytic anemia and a positive direct antiglobulin test (Coombs)
- In AIHA secondary to an underlying process (e.g., CLL, SLE, EBV, Mycoplasma), treatment of the underlying process determines prognosis
- For primary warm AIHA, corticosteroids are first-line; alternatives include rituximab, IVIG, and splenectomy
- For primary cold AIHA, avoidance of hypothermic conditions (weather, fluids, surgery) is preventative

ANEMIA, CHRONIC DISEASE
Carmen Tran, MD • Matthew Goldman, MD

 BASICS

DESCRIPTION
- During chronic systemic infection, inflammation, or malignancy, the production of proinflammatory mediators causes the inhibition of erythropoiesis as well as the imbalance in iron homeostasis (1).
- Anemia of chronic disease (ACD) is characterized as a normocytic, normochromic, hypoproliferative anemia, and classically has low serum iron (SI) levels, elevated ferritin levels, and an elevated total iron-binding capacity (TIBC) (1).

EPIDEMIOLOGY
Incidence
ACD is the 2nd most common anemia, after iron-deficiency anemia (IDA), due to the high rate of infectious diseases in developing countries as well as the high rate of inflammatory and malignant disorders in developed countries (1).

Prevalence
For isolated causes of anemia, ACD was found in ~20% of adults, especially those >65 years of age and with cancer (1,2).

ETIOLOGY AND PATHOPHYSIOLOGY
- In general, the severity of the anemia will correspond with the severity of the underlying disease (1).
- Proinflammatory cytokines such as interleukins, tumor necrosis factor (TNF), and interferons create changes in iron homeostasis in several ways (1,3):
  - Dysregulating iron homeostasis
  - Diminishes proliferation as well as differentiation of red blood cell progenitor cells
  - Diminished erythropoietin response
  - Increased erythrocyte phagocytosis and apoptosis
- The production of interleukin-6 (IL-6), a proinflammatory cytokine, acts to increase the production of an iron-regulating hormone called hepcidin from the hepatocytes (3,4,5,6).
  - Hepcidin acts to decrease both iron-absorption within the GI tract as well as the release of iron from macrophages. Increased retention of iron within the reticuloendothelial cells also occurs (5,6).
  - Hepcidin accomplishes these by specifically negatively regulating ferroportin (5,6).
  - This downregulation results in low serum iron levels and inhibited erythropoiesis, known as iron-restricted erythropoiesis.
  - As a result, iron delivery to erythroid progenitor cells within bone marrow is reduced and erythropoiesis is diminished, causing anemia.
- Erythropoietin (EPO) production and the response to EPO by erythroid bone marrow is suppressed by proinflammatory cytokines such as IL-1, TNF, and interferon-γ (IFN-γ) (1)
- Increased production of hemolysins causes increased erythrocyte apoptosis

COMMONLY ASSOCIATED CONDITIONS
- Chronic systemic diseases
  - Rheumatoid arthritis (RA), systemic lupus erythematosus (SLE), sarcoidosis, temporal arteritis, inflammatory bowel disease (IBD), systemic inflammatory response syndrome (SIRS)
- Hepatic disease or failure
- Congestive heart failure or coronary artery disease
- Chronic kidney disease (CKD)

- Acute or chronic infections
  - Viral
    ○ HIV
  - Bacterial
    ○ Abscess, subacute bacterial endocarditis, tuberculosis, osteomyelitis
  - Fungal
  - Parasitic
- Malignancies
  - Lymphomas, myelomas, carcinomas
- Cytokine dysregulation
  - Anemia of aging
- Hypometabolic states
  - Protein malnutrition, thyroid disease, Panhypopituitarism, diabetes mellitus, Addison disease

 DIAGNOSIS

HISTORY
- The spectrum of causes for ACD is so broad that there is no classical presentation.
- ACD symptoms resemble those of the causative infectious, inflammatory, or malignant process without any source of occult bleeding; often mild and general for anemic symptoms, such as fatigue, dizziness and palpitations (1).
- ACD is often discovered incidentally on a routine CBC with differential.
- Those with a cardiovascular condition may experience symptoms of angina, shortness of breath, and reduced exercise capacity with a moderate hemoglobin level (10–11 g/dL).

PHYSICAL EXAM
Physical exam findings are associated with the causative underlying condition.

DIFFERENTIAL DIAGNOSIS
- Iron deficiency anemia
- Anemia of CKD
- Drug-induced marrow suppression or hemolysis
- Endocrine disorders
- Thalassemia
- Sideroblastic anemia
- Dilutional anemia

DIAGNOSTIC TESTS & INTERPRETATION
Initial Tests (lab, imaging)
- Hemoglobin (Hb) (1):
  - Typically 8.5–9.5 g/dL; may be 10–12 g/dL within 2 days of an acute bacterial infection
  - May produce a drop in Hb levels of 2–3 g/dL within 2 days due to hemolysis
  - A Hb of <8 g/dL typically suggests a 2nd underlying cause for the anemia
- Hematocrit (Hct) (1):
  - Rarely <60% of baseline (unless in the presence of kidney failure)
- Mean corpuscular volume (MCV):
  - Usually normal 80–100 fL
  - Microcytosis (<80 fL) may occur
- RBC morphology:
  - Normocytic and normochromic
  - Increased protoporphyrin levels
- Serum ferritin levels (1):
  - Elevated, 30–200 μg/L
  - Levels <30 μg/L is suggestive of coexisting iron deficiency

- Serum iron (SI) levels:
  - Low due to increased retention and decreased release from the reticuloendothelial system <50
- Total iron binding capacity (TIBC):
  - Extremely low, < 300
- Serum transferrin levels (1):
  - Low
- Transferrin saturation levels:
  - Extremely low, 10–20%
- Absolute reticulocyte count:
  - Inappropriately low (reticulocyte index <20,000–25,000/μL) due to reduced erythropoiesis
    ○ Serum B12 and folate
      ■ Diminished due decreased absorption or lacking in diet

Diagnostic Procedures/Other
- Distinguishing anemia of chronic disease (ACD) from absolute iron-deficiency anemia (IDA) (1,6):
  - Determining type of anemia is necessary when ACD is associated with a cause of iron deficiency (e.g., hemodialysis, chronic blood loss):
    ○ Administration of iron will typically correct IDA but will leave ACD unresolved
  - Bone marrow biopsy with iron stain:
    ○ Gold standard for diagnosis; necessary if pancytopenia is present, as serum tests do not provide a diagnosis, there is progression of the anemia, or there is no response to empirical treatment
    ○ Localized iron within macrophages of the bone marrow is indicative of ACD
    ○ Absent iron staining is indicative of IDA
  - Reticulocyte hemoglobin concentration of <28 pg (3)
  - Soluble serum transferrin (sTfR):log ferritin (1):
    ○ Ratio used reflects erythropoiesis within bone marrow and to differentiate ACD from IDA
    ○ ACD without IDA, ACD with IDA, or IDA without ACD can be determined from ratio
  - Functional test:
    ○ The response of Hb to oral or parenteral iron
- Iron, B12, and folate deficiencies should still be ruled out.

 TREATMENT

GENERAL MEASURES
- Primary management should address the disorder causing the ACD (1):
  - Treatment of the underlying disorder will generally restore basal Hb levels as well as the normal production of erythrocytes.
- In some cases, where treatment of the underlying disease (e.g., cancer, end-stage kidney disease) is not possible, symptomatic anemia will require treatment:
  - Two dominant forms of treatment are transfusions and EPO (1)
  - Studies have shown that ACD is frequently responsive to EPO in pharmacologic doses (1):
    ○ Epoetin-α
    ○ Darbepoetin
  - Evaluation of iron status and repletion of iron must be performed for maximal effects from EPO.
  - Indications for recombinant EPO are a Hb of <10 g/dL

- Coexisting iron deficiency or folic acid (FA) deficiency should be considered in severe cases of anemia:
  - A reduced dietary intake of iron or FA is common among patients who are chronically ill.
  - Patients who regularly undergo hemodialysis will often lose both iron and FA during treatment.

MEDICATION

- Epoietin-α (1,4,7):
  - Indications:
    - Hemoglobin (Hb) is <10g/dL
    - Fatigue or exertional intolerance
    - Anemia due to IBD, RA, hepatitis C
    - Administration of zidovudine or dapsone in HIV-positive patients may result in an increase of Hb levels
    - Chemotherapy in patients with a solid malignancy (palliative therapy)
    - CKD (eGFR <60 mL/min)
  - Dosing and schedule:
    - Individualized to maintain an Hb level between 10–12 g/dL; usually reached within 4–6 weeks when iron levels are adequate; ~90% of patients respond.
    - When target Hb level is obtained, EPO dose can be decreased; if Hb level decreases with EPO therapy, consider iron deficiency or infection
    - Dialysis patients, CKD-associated; start 50–100 U/kg SC/IV 3 × week; Use lowest dose to maintain Hb level sufficient to reduce RBC transfusion need
    - Nondialysis patients: Start 50–100 U/kg SC/IV 3 × week for patients with Hb <10 g/dL and when rate of decline indicates RBC transfusion needed; use lowest dose to maintain Hb level sufficient to reduce RBC transfusion need
    - Patients with cancer who are undergoing chemotherapy; 150 U/kg 3 × week or 450–600 U/kg 1 × week. Use in cancer patients restricted to certified prescribers and facilities (contact via www.esa-apprise.com or call 1-866-284-8089); due to evidence of tumor progression in patients with cancer who are undergoing chemotherapy, EPO administration must be approached with caution.
  - Adverse effects:
    - Increased risk of cardiovascular complications and mortality in CKD patients
    - Increased risk of thromboembolism
    - Rare red cell aplasia
    - Elevated risk of mortality with possible tumor progression in cancer patients
  - Specific benefits:
    - Usually well tolerated
    - Relatively safe
- Darbepoetin-α (7,8):
  - Longer-acting, molecularly modified EPO preparation with a half-life 3–4 times longer than recombinant human EPO, reduces the frequency of injections to weekly or biweekly.
  - Dosing and schedule:
    - CKD associated; conversion from epoetin, >1 year old; Start: See package insert based on current epoetin therapy; administer SC/IV q1–2 wk; for patients with Hb <10 g/dL; IV route preferred in hemodialysis patients; use the lowest dose to maintain Hb level sufficient to reduce RBC transfusion need
  - Adverse effects:
    - Increased risk of thromboembolism

- Epoetin-α or darbepoetin-α dose adjustments:
  - Follow FDA-approved labeling
  - Treatment beyond 6–8 weeks without appropriate rise of Hb (>1–2 g/dL) is not recommended

ADDITIONAL THERAPIES

- Iron (1,4):
  - Indications:
    - Coexisting iron deficiency
    - Resistance to EPO
  - Adverse effects:
    - Gastrointestinal side effects (oral)
    - Systemic and/or local reactions (parenteral)
  - Benefits:
    - Relatively safe
    - Inexpensive
- Transfusions (1,4):
  - Indications
    - Cardiac ischemia with a Hb <10 g/dL
    - Chest pain, shortness of breath, reduced exercise capacity and/or ECG changes
    - Lack of response to medical therapy
  - Possible adverse effects:
    - Infection
    - Volume overload
    - Transfusion reaction
  - Specific benefits:
    - Rapid correction of anemia
  - In general, patients without serious pulmonary or cardiovascular disease can tolerate Hb levels >8 g/dL and would only require intervention when the level falls below.
  - Transfusion is typically justifiable when the Hb level is <7 g/dL.
  - Patients with underlying physiologic compromise, such as cardiac or pulmonary disease, elderly patients, or patients who have symptoms interfering with daily functioning, may require a Hb level maintained >10 g/dL.
  - When an infection occurs during EPO therapy, it is best to cease EPO therapy and rely on transfusion therapy instead until infection is properly treated.

 ## ONGOING CARE

FOLLOW-UP RECOMMENDATIONS
Referral to a hematologist is not always warranted.

Patient Monitoring
- Hb should be raised to near 12 g/dL at which dosages should be managed to maintain that level of Hb (1).
- Baseline and periodic monitoring of iron, TIBC, transferring saturation, and/or ferritin levels may be of value:
  - Iron repletion may be indicated for patients requiring EPO therapy (1)

PATIENT EDUCATION
- Patients receiving medical therapy should be advised about the following possible risks:
  - Mortality, cardiovascular complications, blood clots, progression of tumor
  - Patients can access more information at www.esa-apprise.com or by calling 866-284-8089.

PROGNOSIS
Anemia of chronic disease does not typically progress.

COMPLICATIONS
Adverse effects of EPO (7)
- Heightened risk of mortality and/or cardiovascular complications in CKD patients
- Heightened risk of mortality and/or tumor progression in cancer patients
- Elevated risk of thromboembolism
- Arterial thrombotic episodes

REFERENCES

1. Weiss G, Goodnough LT. Anemia of chronic disease. *N Engl J Med*. 2005;352:1011.
2. Knight K, Wade S, Balducci L. Prevalence and outcomes of anemia in cancer: A systematic review of the literature. *Am J Med*. 2004;116(Suppl 7A): 11S–26S.
3. Roy CN. Anemia of inflammation. *Hematol Am Soc Hematol Educ Prog*. 2010;2010:276–280.
4. Goodnough LT, Nemeth E, Ganz T, et al. Detection, evaluation, and management of iron-restricted erythropoiesis. *Blood*. 2010;116:4754–4761.
5. Ganz T. Hepcidin and iron regulation, 10 years later. *Blood*. 2011;117:4425.
6. Cheng PP, Jiao XY, Wang XH, et al. Hepcidin expression in anemia of chronic disease and concomitant iron-deficiency anemia. *Clin Exp Med*. 2011;11:33–42.
7. Rizzo JD, Somerfield MR, Hagerty KL, et al: Use of epoetin and darbepoetin with cancer: 2007 American Society of Hematology/American Society of Clinical Oncology clinical practice guideline update. *Blood*. 2008;111:25.
8. Bloomfield M, Jaresko G, Zarek J, et al. Guidelines for using darbepoetin alfa in patients with chemotherapy-induced anemia. *Pharmacotherapy*. 2003;23(Pt 2):110S–118S.

 ### SEE ALSO

Iron-Deficiency Anemia; Normocytic Anemia; Microcytic Anemia; Iron, Studies

CODES

ICD10
- D63.0 Anemia in neoplastic disease
- D63.1 Anemia in chronic kidney disease
- D63.8 Anemia in other chronic diseases classified elsewhere

CLINICAL PEARLS

- ACD is one of the most common anemias clinically seen.
- One of the most common diagnostic problems encountered within the clinical setting is making the distinction between anemia of chronic disease and iron-deficiency anemia. Iron values will usually make a clear distinction.
- Although there are no clinical tests yet, classic ACD has elevated hepcidin levels.
- Iron should be given to all patients treated with EPO.

ANEMIA, IRON DEFICIENCY
Frank J. Domino, MD

 BASICS

DESCRIPTION
- Deficiency in red blood cells, hemoglobin, or blood volume due to decreased iron stores
- Onset may be acute, with rapid blood loss, or chronic, with nutrition derangement or slow blood loss.
- System(s) affected: Heme; Lymphatic; Immunologic
- Synonym(s): Anemia of chronic blood loss; Hypochromic; Microcytic anemia; Chlorosis

Geriatric Considerations
60% of anemias occur in people >65 years of age.

Pediatric Considerations
Problematic in infants whose major source of nutrition is unfortified cow's milk and/or juices

Pregnancy Considerations
Iron supplements (15–30 mg/d) are recommended during pregnancy.

EPIDEMIOLOGY
- Iron deficiency anemia (IDA) is the most common cause of anemia in the US.
- Predominant age: All ages, but especially toddlers and menstruating women
- Predominant sex: Female > Male
- More likely in the poor and in underimmunized children

Incidence
- Adults: Men 2%, women 15–20% annually
- Infants and toddlers: 3–5% annually
- Pregnant patients: Unclear; maybe as high 20% (pseudoanemia common during pregnancy as plasma volume expands faster than red cell mass)

Prevalence
- Infants and children age <12 years: 4–7%
- Men: 2–5%
- Women: 9–16% (18–50% in menstruant blood donors) (1)

ETIOLOGY AND PATHOPHYSIOLOGY
Depletion of iron stores leads to decrease in both reticulocyte count and production of hemoglobin:
- Blood loss (e.g., menses, GI bleeding, trauma)
- Poor iron intake
- Poor iron absorption (e.g., atrophic gastritis, postgastrectomy, celiac disease)
- Increased demand for iron (e.g., infancy, adolescence, pregnancy, and breastfeeding)

RISK FACTORS
- Premenopausal woman
- Frequent blood donor
- Pregnancy and breastfeeding
- Strict vegan diet
- Use of NSAIDs

GENERAL PREVENTION
- Screen asymptomatic pregnant women (2)[B].
- Supplementation in asymptomatic children aged 6–12 months if at risk for IDA (e.g., malnutrition, abuse, cow's milk <12 months) (2)[B]

COMMONLY ASSOCIATED CONDITIONS
- GI tract malignancy, peptic ulcer disease (PUD), *Helicobacter pylori* infection, irritable bowel disease
- Hookworm or other parasitic infestations
- Hypermetrorrhagia
- Pregnancy
- Obesity treated with Gastric Bypass Surgery

 DIAGNOSIS

HISTORY
- Asymptomatic in most cases
- Weakness, fatigue, and/or malaise
- Exertional dyspnea
- Palpitations
- Angina in patients with coronary artery disease
- Headaches or inability to concentrate
- Melena
- Pica

PHYSICAL EXAM
- Pallor
- Cheilosis
- Tachycardia
- Tachypnea
- Koilonychia (spoon-shaped, brittle nails)

DIFFERENTIAL DIAGNOSIS
- GI bleeding (e.g., gastritis, PUD, carcinoma, varices)
- Chronic intravascular hemolysis (e.g., paroxysmal nocturnal hemoglobinuria, malfunctioning prosthetic valve)
- Defective iron utilization (e.g., thalassemia trait, sideroblastosis, G6PD deficiency)
- Defective iron reutilization (e.g., infection, inflammation, cancer, other chronic diseases)
- Hypoproliferation (e.g., decreased erythropoietin from hypothyroidism, renal failure)

DIAGNOSTIC TESTS & INTERPRETATION
Initial Tests (lab, imaging)
- Hemoglobin: <13 g in men and <12 g in women (3). Patients with higher premorbid hemoglobin (e.g., those with chronic hypoxia, smokers, those who live at high altitudes) may be anemic at higher hemoglobin levels.
- Mean corpuscular volume (MCV): <80 fL
- Ferritin: <41 ng/mL (98% sensitivity and specificity); gold standard, noninvasive test for diagnosis in adults, but may miss some deficient patients (e.g., cirrhosis) because ferritin is an acute-phase reactant.
- Total iron-binding capacity (TIBC): Increased
- Transferrin saturation: <9%
- CBC with differential, peripheral smear, reticulocyte count, and index. A peripheral smear usually shows hypochromia and microcytosis, but may be normal, and reticulocyte production index is low.
- Iron-to-TIBC (transferrin ratio) is usually not recommended because it is less sensitive and less specific than ferritin.
- Consider testing for G6PD deficiency: Assay at least 6 weeks after the last drop in hemoglobin.

- Rule out thalassemia:
  - Review prior CBCs for persisting mild anemia and marked micro-ovalocytosis, elevated hemoglobin A2 or hemoglobin F, family history, and especially high or high normal RBC count.
  - A low RBC count in patients with chronic bleeding helps to distinguish it from the thalassemia trait, where the count is high or high-normal.
  - Microcytosis with ovalocytosis and anemia unresponsive to iron suggests the thalassemia trait.
- MCV may be normal in mild anemia or hidden by the population of larger cells (e.g., reticulocytes or macrocytes). Red cell distribution width will be increased if a mixed population of cells is present (e.g., mixed iron deficiency anemia and B_{12} deficiency).
- An empiric trial of iron at 3 mg/kg/d may be the best way to diagnose decreased iron stores in infants and children; reticulocytes become elevated in 7–10 days or hemoglobin increases >1 g/dL weekly, indicating iron deficiency.
- Drugs that may alter lab results: Iron supplements or multivitamin–mineral preparations that contain iron
- Disorders that may alter lab results:
  - Elevated ferritin: Acute or chronic liver disease, Hodgkin disease, acute leukemia, solid tumors, fever, acute inflammation, renal dialysis
  - Elevated hemoglobin: Smoking, chronic hypoxemia, long-term residency at high altitude
  - Stool guaiac (1)[C]; if high index of suspicion of GI bleed, perform GI endoscopy. Under appropriate circumstances, check stool for ova and parasites.
  - Rule out poor reutilization: Trial of iron, bone marrow aspiration, and iron stain
  - Rule out colorectal cancer and gastric carcinoma, especially in the elderly

Diagnostic Procedures/Other
- GI endoscopy to evaluate for bleeding sites
- Bone marrow aspiration confirms diagnosis, but is rarely performed

Test Interpretation
- Absent or decreased marrow iron stores
- Marrow: Hyperplastic, micronormoblastic

 TREATMENT

GENERAL MEASURES
- Search for the cause and correct it.
- Occult GI malignancy should be suspected in all men and postmenopausal women with iron deficiency.
- Avoid transfusions, except in rare cases.

MEDICATION

- Ferrous sulfate 325 mg t.i.d. on an empty stomach 1 hour before meals provides 180 mg of elemental iron per day:
  - Reduce dose as needed for GI symptoms, which affect 25% of patients receiving standard iron therapy; or, the dose can be taken with meals, which may reduce the delivery of iron by 50%. Constipation will occur in ~1/4 patients using various iron formulations (4).
  - Drugs that increase gastric pH (e.g., proton pump inhibitors, H_2 antagonists) also reduce iron absorption (5).
  - Individuals with moderate anemia need only a total of 1,500–2,000 mg of elemental iron replacement; reducing the iron per dose as much as necessary to abate adverse effects will make parenteral iron therapy unnecessary in almost all cases.
  - Special oral iron formulations (including enteric-coated iron) and compounds are expensive and reduce symptoms only to the degree that they reduce the delivery of iron.
- Liquid iron preparations are useful for children, with a recommended dose of 3 mg/kg/d; can also be used in adults when tablets are not absorbed or low tolerance requires a dose reduction.
- Foods and beverages containing ascorbic acid (vitamin C) enhance iron absorption when taken simultaneously with the iron.
- Continued bleeding and untreated hypothyroidism are causes for "failure to respond" to iron.
- Consider parenteral iron for patients with a hemoglobin level <6 g/dL, malabsorption, or if higher oral doses and use of vitamin C fail:
  - Anaphylaxis to parenteral iron therapy has occurred; ferric gluconate or iron sucrose may be safer alternatives to iron dextran (6,7)[B]. Dimercaprol increases risk of nephrotoxicity.
  - Iron sucrose 200 mg IV, 5 doses over 2 weeks, or 500 mg IV, 2 doses every 2 weeks (less experience with this regimen); total dose is 1,000 mg, then re-evaluate. 1 mL = 20 mg elemental iron. Hemodialysis-dependent patients should receive 100 mg 1–3×/week for total of 10 doses.
- Reserve blood transfusion for severe acute blood loss or severely symptomatic patients (e.g., demand ischemia due to anemia). Hemoglobin threshold varies by risk factors and clinical scenario.
- Contraindications (oral iron):
  - Antacids concomitantly
  - Dairy products concomitantly
  - Tetracycline concomitantly
- Significant possible interactions (oral iron):
  - Allopurinol
  - Antacids
  - Penicillamine
  - Quinolones
  - Tetracyclines
  - Vitamin E
- Precautions:
  - Iron preparations may cause black bowel movements and constipation.
  - Iron overdose is highly toxic; patients should be instructed to keep tablets and liquids out of the reach of small children.

ISSUES FOR REFERRAL

- Pregnant women with a hemoglobin (Hgb) level <9 g/dL
- Failure to respond to a 4–6-week trial of oral iron therapy
- Nonpregnant women or other patients with an Hgb level <6 g/dL

IN-PATIENT CONSIDERATIONS
Admission Criteria/Initial Stabilization
Outpatient

 ## ONGOING CARE

FOLLOW-UP RECOMMENDATIONS
Patient Monitoring
- Regularly after Hgb returns to normal (to detect recurrences).
- Hgb increases 1 g/dL every 2–3 weeks.
- Iron stores may take up to 4 weeks to correct after Hgb returns to normal.

DIET
- Do not consume milk or other dairy products, antacids, quinolones, or tetracycline within 2 hours of iron supplement ingestion.
- Limit tea, coffee, and caffeinated beverages.
- Limit milk to 16 oz/d (adults).
- Emphasize protein and iron-containing foods (meat, beans, and leafy green vegetables).
- Taking iron with orange juice or ascorbic acid increases absorption, but decreases GI tolerability.
- Increase fluid and dietary fiber to decrease likelihood of constipation during iron replacement therapy.

PATIENT EDUCATION
National Heart, Lung & Blood Institute, Communications & Public Information Branch, National Institutes of Health, Building 31, Room 41–21, 9000 Rockville Pike, Bethesda, MD 20892; (301) 251–1222.

PROGNOSIS
- Can be resolved with iron therapy if the underlying cause can be discovered and appropriately treated.
- Treat subclinical hypothyroidism and IDA together when these conditions coexist. Failure to treat hypothyroidism results in poor response to iron therapy (8)[B].

COMPLICATIONS
- Neglecting to identify hidden bleeding points, particularly a bleeding malignancy
- Maternal iron deficiency negatively affects mother–child interactions. Iron supplementation protects against these negative effects (9).

REFERENCES

1. Dubois RW, Goodnough LT, Ershler WB, et al. Identification, diagnosis, and management of anemia in adult ambulatory patients treated by primary care physicians: Evidence-based and consensus recommendations. *Curr Med Res Opin*. 2006;22:385–395.
2. Mabry-Hernandez IR. Screening for iron deficiency anemia–including iron supplementation for children and pregnant women. *Am Fam Physician*. 2009;79(10):897–898.
3. de Benoist B, McLean E, Egli I, et al., eds. Worldwide prevalence of anaemia 1993–1995. *WHO Global Database on Anaemia*. Geneva: World Health Organization; 2008. http://whqlibdoc.who.int/publications/2008/9789241596657_eng.pdf. Accessed October 19, 2011.
4. Melamed N, Ben-Haroush A, Kaplan B, et al. Iron supplementation in pregnancy—does the preparation matter? *Arch Gynecol Obstet*. 2007;276:601–604.
5. Killip S, Bennett JM, Chambers MD. Iron deficiency anemia. *Am Fam Physician*. 2007;75:671–678.
6. Chertow GM, Mason PD, Vaage-Nilsen O, et al. On the relative safety of parenteral iron formulations. *Nephrol Dial Transplant*. 2004;19:1571–1575.
7. Chertow GM, Mason PD, Vaage-Nilsen O, et al. Update on adverse drug events associated with parenteral iron. *Nephrol Dial Transplant*. 2006;21: 378–382.
8. Cinemre H, Bilir C, Gokosmanoglu F, et al. Hematologic effects of levothyroxine in iron-deficient subclinical hypothyroid patients: A randomized, double-blind, controlled study. *J Clin Endocrinol Metab*. 2009;94(1):151–156. Epub 2008 Nov 4.
9. Murray-Kolb LE, Beard JL. Iron deficiency and child and maternal health. *Am J Clin Nutr*. 2009;89: 946S–950S.

ADDITIONAL READING

- Short MW, Domagalski JE. Iron deficiency anemia: evaluation and management. *Am Fam Physician*. 2013 Jan 15;87(2):98–104.
- Tefferi A, Hanson CA, Inwards DJ. How to interpret and pursue an abnormal complete blood cell count in adults. *Mayo Clin Proc*. 2005;80:923–936.
- Zhu A, Kaneshiro M, Kaunitz JD. Evaluation and treatment of iron deficiency anemia: A gastroenterological perspective. *Dig Dis Sci*. 2010;55(3):548–559.

 ## SEE ALSO

Algorithm: Anemia

 ## CODES

ICD10
- D50.0 Iron deficiency anemia secondary to blood loss (chronic)
- D50.8 Other iron deficiency anemias
- D50.9 Iron deficiency anemia, unspecified

CLINICAL PEARLS

- IDA due to poor dietary intake is the most common type of anemia in the US and in the world.
- Blood loss and reduced iron stores due to malabsorption or poor utilization are major risk factors for IDA.
- Premenopausal women and children are at the greatest risk for IDA.
- Recommend no cow's milk to any child age <12 months.
- Oral iron supplementation is the standard treatment option for patients with IDA.

ANEMIA, SICKLE CELL
Rami Farhat, DO • Tipsuda Junsanto-Bahri, MD, FCAP

BASICS

DESCRIPTION
- Hereditary chronic hemoglobinopathy marked by chronic hemolytic anemia, periodic acute episodes of painful "crises," and increased susceptibility to intercurrent infections; generally manifesting in first 6–12 months of life
- The heterozygous condition (Hb A/S), sickle cell trait, is usually asymptomatic without anemia.
- Among the compound heterozygotes, sickle-hemoglobin C disease (HbSC) and Sβ+ thalassemia are clinically similar to the heterozygous condition, whereas Sβ° thalassemia is clinically similar to the homozygous condition.
- Synonym(s): Sickle cell disease (SCD); Hb SS disease

Pediatric Considerations
- Sequestration crises and hand–foot syndrome seen typically in infants/young children
- Adolescence/Young adulthood:
  - Frequency of complications and organ/tissue damage increases with age (except for strokes, which occur mostly in childhood).
  - Psychological complications: Body image, interrupted schooling, restriction of activities; stigma of disease; low self-esteem

Pregnancy Considerations
- Usually complicated and hazardous, especially 3rd trimester and delivery:
  - Fetal survival is >90% if the fetus reaches the 3rd trimester.
- Increased risk of pain, toxemia, infection, pulmonary infarction, phlebitis
- Fetal mortality 35–40%
- Partial exchange transfusion in 3rd trimester may reduce maternal morbidity and fetal mortality, but this is controversial.
- Chronic transfusions have been effective in diminishing pain episodes in pregnant women. However, this method should be used with caution due to risk of alloimmunization.

EPIDEMIOLOGY
Prevalence
- ~90,000 Americans have sickle cell anemia (SCA) and 10% of African Americans carry the trait. ~1/500 African Americans and 1/1,000 Hispanics have homozygous SCA. Each year in the US, about 1/400 African American infants are born with SCD.
- Lesser risk: Middle East, Mediterranean area, and populations in India may be affected.

ETIOLOGY AND PATHOPHYSIOLOGY
- Substitution of valine for glutamic acid in 6th amino acid of hemoglobin β-chain. Mutation → RBCs change from biconcave to sickle shape when deoxygenated due to poor solubility of mutated hemoglobin chain.
- Sickle RBCs are inflexible, causing increased blood viscosity, stasis, obstruction of small arterioles and capillaries, and ischemia. Sickle RBCs are fragile, leading to hemolysis.
- Chronic anemia; crises:
  - Vaso-occlusive crisis ("painful crisis"): Tissue ischemia and necrosis; progressive organ failure/tissue damage from repeated episodes
  - Hand–foot syndrome: Vessel occlusion/ischemia affects small blood vessels in hands or feet.

- Aplastic crisis: Suppression of RBC production by severe infection (e.g., parvoviral and other viral infections)
  - Suppression of RBC production
  - Hyperhemolytic crisis: Accelerated hemolysis with reticulocytosis; increased RBC fragility/shortened lifespan
  - Sequestration crisis: Splenic sequestration of blood (only in young children as spleen is later lost to autoinfarction)
- Susceptibility to infection: Impaired/absent splenic function leading to decreased ability to clear infection; defect in alternate pathway of complement activation
- Sickle cells are abnormally shaped, fragile RBCs. Increased red cell destruction causes an inability to maintain adequate hemoglobin levels and results in anemia and fatigue.
- Sickle cells exhibit increased adhesion and decreased ability to maneuver small vessels, leading to vaso-occlusion.

Genetics
Autosomal recessive. Homozygous presence of Hb S, or sickle hemoglobin (genotype SS). Heterozygous condition Hb AS. The heterozygote condition can also be combined with other hemoglobinopathies, the most common of which are HbC and β thalassemia.

RISK FACTORS
- For vaso-occlusive crisis ("painful crisis"): Pain results from tissue ischemia and necrosis: Hypoxia, dehydration, fever, infection, acidosis, cold, anesthesia, strenuous physical exercise, smoking
- For aplastic crisis (suppression of RBC production): Severe infections, human parvovirus B19 infection, folic acid deficiency
- Hyperhemolytic crisis (accelerated hemolysis with reticulocytosis) (existence is controversial): Acute bacterial infections, exposure to oxidant drugs

GENERAL PREVENTION
- Prevention of crises:
  - Avoid hypoxia, dehydration, cold, infection, fever, acidosis, and anesthesia.
  - Prompt management of fever, infections, pain
  - Hydration
  - Avoid alcohol and smoking.
  - Avoid high-altitude areas.
- Minimizing trauma: Aseptic technique is imperative.

DIAGNOSIS

A chronic hemolytic anemia. Increased infection risk (e.g., pneumococcal sepsis, *Salmonella* osteomyelitis), with functional asplenia by ~5–6 years of age, and delayed physical/sexual maturation. Diagnosis now often made by newborn screening programs.

HISTORY
- Often asymptomatic in early months of life due to presence of fetal hemoglobin
- >6 months of age, earliest symptoms are irritability and painful swelling of the hands and feet (hand–foot syndrome). May also see pneumococcal sepsis or meningitis, severe anemia and acute splenic enlargement (splenic sequestration), acute chest syndrome, pallor, jaundice, or splenomegaly.
- Major manifestations in older children include anemia, severe or recurrent musculoskeletal or abdominal pain, aplastic crisis, acute chest

syndrome, splenomegaly or splenic sequestration, and cholelithiasis.
- Painful crises in bones, joints, abdomen, back, and viscera account for 90% of all hospital admissions.
- Acute chest syndrome: Tachycardia, fever, bilateral infiltrates caused by pulmonary infarctions

PHYSICAL EXAM
Fever, pale skin and nail beds, mild jaundice

DIFFERENTIAL DIAGNOSIS
Anemia: Other hemoglobinopathies

DIAGNOSTIC TESTS & INTERPRETATION
Initial Tests (lab, imaging)
- Screening test: Sickledex test:
  - Hb electrophoresis (diagnostic test of choice). Sickle cell anemia (FS pattern):
    - 80–100% Hb S, variable amounts of Hb F and no Hb A1
    - Sickle cell trait (FS pattern): 30–45% Hb S, 50–70% Hb A1, minimal Hb F
- Hemoglobin ~5–10 g/dL; RBC indices: MCV normal to increased; MCHC increased; HgSS, reticulocytes 3–15%
- Leukocytosis; bands in absence of infection, platelets elevated; peripheral smear: sickled RBCs, nucleated RBCs, Howell-Jolly bodies
- Serum bilirubin mildly elevated (2–4 mg/dL); ferritin very elevated in multiply transfused patients; serum lactate dehydrogenase (LDH) elevated
- Fecal/urinary urobilinogen high
- Haptoglobin absent or very low
- Need for imaging depends on clinical circumstances:
  - Bone scan to rule out osteomyelitis
  - CT/MRI to rule out CVA; high index of suspicion required for any acute neurologic symptoms other than mild headache
  - Chest x-ray: May show enlarged heart; diffuse alveolar infiltrates in acute chest syndrome
  - Transcranial Doppler: Start at age 2; repeat yearly (1,2)[B]. Transcranial Doppler ultrasound identifies children age 2–16 at higher risk of stroke.
  - ECG to detect pulmonary hypertension (2)[C] and echocardiogram every other year from age 15 on.

Test Interpretation
Hyposplenism due to autosplenectomy is common; hypoxia/infarction in multiple organs

TREATMENT

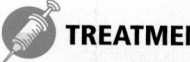

GENERAL MEASURES
- Painful crises: Hydration, analgesics; oxygen regardless of whether the patient is hypoxic
- Retinal evaluation starting at school age to detect proliferative sickle retinopathy
- Occupational therapy, cognitive and behavioral therapies, support groups
- Special immunizations (1,2)[B]:
  - Influenza vaccine yearly starting at age 2
  - Heptavalent conjugated pneumococcal vaccine at 2, 4, 6 months; booster at 15 months, 2 years, 5 years
  - 23-valent pneumococcal vaccine at 2 years; booster at age 5; always separate this by 8 weeks from heptavalent vaccine

- Meningococcal vaccine >2 years of age
- H1N1 vaccination
- G-CSF use is contraindicated as it may lead to vaso-occlusive episodes and multiorgan failure (3)[B]

MEDICATION
First Line
- Supplemental oxygen
- Painful crises (mild, outpatient):
  – Nonnarcotic analgesics (ibuprofen, tramadol) (1,2)[C]
- Painful crises (severe, hospitalized) (1,2)[B]:
  – Parenteral narcotics (e.g., morphine on fixed schedule); patient-controlled analgesia (PCA) pump may be useful.
- Hydroxyurea is indicated for prevention of painful acute chest syndrome, vaso-occlusive episodes, and very severe anemia. Start with 15 mg/kg/d single daily dose; titrate upward every 12 weeks if blood counts satisfactory (avoid severe neutropenia)
- Acute chest syndrome
  – May deteriorate quickly; aggressive management with oxygen, analgesics, antibiotics, simple or exchange transfusion (1)
- Empiric antibiotics (2) to cover *S. pneumoniae*, *H. influenzae*, *Mycoplasma pneumoniae*, and *Chlamydia pneumoniae* (cephalosporins or azithromycin). If osteomyelitis, cover for *Staphylococcus aureus* and *Salmonella* (e.g., ciprofloxacin). If apparent pneumonia not promptly responding to antibiotics, consider diagnosis of acute chest syndrome and initiate simple or exchange transfusion.
- Prophylactic penicillin is indicated in all infants and children starting at 2 months (1,4)[A]: For children younger than 5 years of age, a dose of 125 mg b.i.d. is recommended. Unless the patient has a history of severe pneumococcal sepsis, administration may be stopped at 5 years as there is no longer any significant benefit for continued treatment. If a history of pneumococcal sepsis is present, a dose of 250 mg b.i.d. is suggested (5)[A]; if high risk remains, continue until puberty. Rising pneumococcal resistance to penicillin may change future recommendations.
- Precautions: Avoid high-dose estrogen oral contraceptives; consider Depo-Provera.

Second Line
Folic acid (1,2)[C]: 0–6 months: 0.1 mg/d; 6–12 months: 0.25 mg/d; 1–2 years: 0.5 mg/d; >2 years of age 1 mg/d

ADDITIONAL THERAPIES
Transfusions and additional therapies:
- Transfusion for aplastic crises, severe complications (i.e., CVA), prophylactically before surgery, and treatment for acute chest syndrome
- Transfusions carry risk of iron overload, resulting in damage to heart, liver, and other organs. Avoid blood hyperviscosity.
- Prophylactic transfusions for primary or secondary stroke prevention in children
- Preoperative transfusions have been shown to reduce the risk of perioperative complications (6)[C].
- Consider chelation with Deferasirox, an oral agent, if the patient is multiply transfused (after age 2).

SURGERY/OTHER PROCEDURES
- Experimental gene therapy: Replace normal gene and inactivate Hgb S while reactivating Hgb F (fetal hemoglobin).
- Hematopoietic stem cell transplant (HSCT): Curative, but with significant morbidity and mortality

IN-PATIENT CONSIDERATIONS
Admission Criteria/Initial Stabilization
Severe pain, suspected infection or sepsis, evidence of acute chest syndrome

IV Fluids
The preferred maintenance IV fluid is 1/2 NS, as NS may theoretically increase the risk of sickling.

 ## ONGOING CARE

FOLLOW-UP RECOMMENDATIONS
Patient Monitoring
- Treat infections early. Parents/patients: Any temperature of ≥101°F (38.3°C) requires immediate medical attention.
- For patients who receive chronic transfusions, monitor for hepatitis and hemosiderosis.
- Periodic eye evaluations: Starting age 5 to detect proliferative sickle retinopathy (1,2)[C].
- Biannual examination for hepatic, renal, and pulmonary dysfunction
- Baseline pulmonary evaluation at each visit to assess for wheezing, shortness of breath, or cough as these may be indicators of disease severity and prognosis (7)[B]

DIET
- Folic acid supplementation; avoid alcohol (leads to dehydration); maintain hydration
- Multivitamin without iron is recommended as there is high incidence of vitamin D deficiency and decreased bone marrow density in patients with SCD (8)[B].

PATIENT EDUCATION
- Sicklecellkids.org—Education Web site for children with sickle cell anemia: http://www.sicklecelldisease.org
- American Sickle Cell Anemia Association: http://www.ascaa.org

PROGNOSIS
- In 2nd decade of life, fewer crises, but more complications. Median age of death is 42 for men and 48 for women. Causes: Infections, thrombosis, pulmonary emboli, pulmonary hypertension, and renal failure
- Children become anemic in infancy and begin to have sickle cell crises at 1–2 years of age; some children die in their 1st year.

COMPLICATIONS
- Alloimmunization, bone infarct and osteomyelitis, aseptic necrosis of femoral head
- CVA (peak age 6–7), impaired mental development, even without history of stroke
- Cholelithiasis/abnormal liver function
- Chronic leg ulcers, poor wound healing
- Impotence, priapism, hematuria/hyposthenuria, renal concentrating, and acidifying defects
- Retinopathy, splenic infarction (by age 10 years)
- Acute chest syndrome (infection/infarction) leading to chronic pulmonary disease

- Infections (pneumonia, osteomyelitis, meningitis, pyelonephritis); sepsis (leading cause of morbidity and mortality)
- Hemosiderosis (secondary to multiple transfusions). Substance abuse related to chronic pain

REFERENCES
1. Section on Hematology/Oncology Committee on Genetics, American Academy of Pediatrics. Health supervision for children with sickle cell disease. *Pediatrics*. 2002;109:526–535.
2. National Institutes of Health. *The Management of Sickle Cell Disease*, 4th ed. 2002. NH Publ No. 02–2117.
3. Fitzhugh CD, Hsieh MM, Bolan CD, et al. Granulocyte colony-stimulating factor (G-CSF) administration in individuals with sickle cell disease: Time for a moratorium? *Cytotherapy*. 2009;11(4):464–471.
4. Bonds DR. Three decades of innovation in the management of sickle cell disease: The road to understanding the sickle cell disease clinical phenotype. *Blood Rev*. 2005;19:99–110.
5. Cober MP, Phelps SJ. Penicillin prophylaxis in children with sickle cell disease. *J Pediatr Pharmacol Ther*. 2010;15(3):152–159.
6. Howard J, Malfroy M, Llewelyn C, et al. The transfusion alternatives preoperatively in sickle cell disease (TAPS) study: A randomised, controlled, multicentre clinical trial. *The Lancet*, 2013;381 (9870), 930–938.
7. Cohen RT, Madadi A, Blinder MA, et al. Recurrent, severe wheezing is associated with morbidity and mortality in adults with sickle cell disease. *Am J Hematol*. 2011;86(9):756–761. Epub 2011 Aug 2.
8. Lal A, Fung EB, Pakbaz Z, et al. Bone mineral density in children with sickle cell anemia. *Pediatr Blood Cancer*. 2006;47(7):901–906.

 ## SEE ALSO
Algorithm: Anemia

CODES
ICD10
- D57.00 Hb-SS disease with crisis, unspecified
- D57.1 Sickle-cell disease without crisis
- D57.3 Sickle-cell trait

CLINICAL PEARLS
- Almost 90,000 Americans have SCA, ~1/500 African Americans and 1/1,000 Hispanics have SCA; 10% carry the trait
- The preferred maintenance IV fluid is 1/2 NS, as NS may theoretically increase the risk of sickling.
- Painful crises in bones, joints, abdomen, back, and viscera account for 90% of all hospital admissions.
- Acute chest syndrome: Tachycardia, fever, bilateral infiltrates caused by pulmonary infarctions

ANEMIA, SIDEROBLASTIC

Pia Prakash, MD • Marie L. Borum, MD, EdD, MPH

BASICS

DESCRIPTION
- Sideroblastic anemia is a defect in heme synthesis affecting red blood cell production, resulting in anemia. It is characterized by the presence of ringed sideroblasts in the bone marrow. This disease process can be congenital or acquired.
- Although the body has available iron stores, iron cannot be incorporated into the hemoglobin, resulting in granules of iron that accumulate in the mitochondria where heme is produced.

EPIDEMIOLOGY
- Sideroblastic anemias (SAs) are uncommon. Incidence and prevalence are not well studied.
- Acquired forms are more common than hereditary forms (1) and usually occur in older adults; present in 25–30% of alcoholics with anemia, most commonly with folate and B_6 deficiency.
- Hereditary forms vary in severity, usually manifesting in childhood.

ETIOLOGY AND PATHOPHYSIOLOGY
- Inability to utilize iron for the production of hemoglobin due to inherited or acquired impairment
- Ineffective erythropoiesis despite abundance of iron in the body
- Increased GI absorption of iron leading to iron overload
- Inability to utilize iron for heme synthesis results in sideroblasts, which are abnormal erythroblasts with granules of iron accumulated in the mitochondria, forming a ring around the nucleus.
- Congenital SAs are inherited forms of SA resulting from genetic defects:
  – X-linked sideroblastic anemia is caused by mutation in 5-aminolevulinate synthase, which is the first enzyme in the heme biosynthesis pathway. This is the most common congenital form. More prevalent in males.
  – X-linked sideroblastic anemia with spinocerebellar ataxia results from defect in *ABCB7* gene.
  – Mitochondrial defects:
    ○ Defect of mitochondrial transporter *SLC25A38*; usually autosomal recessive
    ○ Deficiency in mitochondrial *GXRL5*, which effects iron-sulfur cluster synthesis
  – Deficiency of ferrochelatase, a necessary enzyme in the heme biosynthesis pathway
  – Roger syndrome results from defect in thiamine transporter protein, usually improved with administration of thiamine
  – Pearson syndrome results from defect in mitochondria of erythroblasts.
- Acquired SA is usually reversible when the inciting factor is removed. Acquired SA is more common than congenital SA. Acquired SA can be caused by:
  – Alcohol
  – Isoniazid
  – Pyrazinamide
  – Pyridoxine deficiency
  – Chloramphenicol
  – Cycloserine
  – Azathioprine
  – D-penicillamine
  – Copper deficiency
  – Zinc toxicity leading to copper deficiency
  – Lead poisoning
  – Hypothermia affecting mitochondrial functions

- Refractory anemia with ring sideroblasts (RARS) and pure SA (PSA) are subtypes of the myelodysplastic syndromes related to clonal overproliferation of hematopoietic cell lines:
  – RARS is more commonly associated with acute leukemia than is PSA.

Genetics
- Congenital form can arise from multiple gene defects:
  – Defect in aminolevulinic acid synthase (ALAS-2 mutation): The first and rate-limiting enzyme in heme biosynthesis
  – Defect in mitochondrial amino acid transporter (*SLC25A38*)
  – Defect in ferrochelatase
  – Defect in glutaredoxin 5
  – Defect in thiamine transporter 1
  – Defect in mitochondrial proteins and exporters
- Can be X-linked or autosomal recessive

RISK FACTORS
- Male gender (X-linked SA)
- Family history of hereditary SA
- Chronic alcohol abuse

GENERAL PREVENTION
Pyridoxine should be given to all patients on isoniazid to avoid anemia.

COMMONLY ASSOCIATED CONDITIONS
- Iron overload or secondary hemochromatosis from transfused blood products
- Transformation into acute leukemia is rare.
- Alcohol abuse

DIAGNOSIS

Moderate to severe anemia with symptoms of fatigue, dizziness, and dyspnea should prompt an evaluation for sideroblastic anemia (2)[B].

HISTORY
- Symptoms of anemia, including fatigue, dizziness, and dyspnea
- Alcohol or drug exposures as listed above
- Toxin exposures
- Developmental delays in children
- Symptoms of iron overload
- Cardiac arrhythmias or heart failure related to iron overload
- Family history of anemia or myopathy, especially in men
- Patients can present with peripheral neuropathy or dermatitis if SA related to pyridoxine deficiency.

PHYSICAL EXAM
- No pathognomonic physical findings
- Signs of anemia, including tachycardia, conjunctival pallor, etc.
- Mild to moderate hepatosplenomegaly may be present.

DIFFERENTIAL DIAGNOSIS
- Thalassemias
- Iron deficiency anemia
- Folate or B_{12} deficiency
- Anemia of chronic disease
- Myelodysplastic syndromes
- Lead toxicity with anemia

DIAGNOSTIC TESTS & INTERPRETATION
Initial Tests (lab, imaging)
- CBC:
  – Microcytosis with low mean corpuscular volume (MCV) in most cases
  – Hypochromia with low mean corpuscular hemoglobin (MCH)
  – Increased red cell distribution width (RDW)
  – Normal leukocytes and platelets
  – It is important to note that in SA related to myelodysplastic syndromes, normocytosis or macrocytosis may be seen.
- Peripheral smear showing siderocytes. Anisocytosis and poikilocytosis may be present (3)[B]:
  – Basophilic stippling may be seen in lead poisoning.
- Iron studies are consistent with iron overload:
  – Ferritin increased
  – Serum iron levels increased
  – Transferrin saturation increased
  – Serum transferrin decreased
  – Total iron-binding capacity (TIBC) normal

Follow-Up Tests & Special Considerations
- Serum copper, ceruloplasmin, serum zinc if suspected as cause
- Bone marrow evaluation reveals ringed sideroblasts, which is diagnostic for SA. Prussian blue staining also reveals ringed sideroblasts. Electron micrograph shows iron-filled mitochondria clustered around the nucleus.
- Abnormal liver function tests may be seen if cause is related to alcohol, cirrhosis, or iron overload.
- Molecular studies may be done to identify specific mutations causing hereditary SA syndromes.
- Serum erythrocyte protoporphyrin is low in X-linked SA. This level is increased in X-linked SA with ataxia.
- Liver biopsy is helpful to assess degree of iron overload.

Diagnostic Procedures/Other
Bone marrow biopsy confirms the diagnosis of sideroblastic anemia.

Test Interpretation
- Bone marrow exam is the key diagnostic modality (1)[C]:
  – Normoblastic erythroid hyperplasia
  – Prussian blue iron stain showing ringed sideroblasts, >10% of erythroblasts with increased number of abnormally large granules ringing the nucleus
  – Electron microscopy reveals iron-overloaded mitochondria within erythroblasts.
  – Iron-laden macrophages
- Liver biopsy:
  – Iron deposition indistinguishable from hereditary hemochromatosis

TREATMENT

MEDICATION

First Line
- Treatment is largely supportive.

- Pyridoxine (1)[B]:
  – Will improve anemia only in X-linked SA and alcohol-related SA
  – Initial dose should be 50–100 mg PO daily.
  – Supplement folate to compensate for increased erythropoiesis if pyridoxine is effective.
  – Positive clinical response if reticulocytosis is seen within 2 weeks followed by increase in hemoglobin level over several months
- Combination therapy with erythropoietin and G-CSF can be helpful in acquired SA (1)[B].

- Blood transfusion based on symptoms of anemia. May worsen iron overload and create need for iron chelation therapy (1)[C]
- Treatment for iron overload:
  – Therapeutic phlebotomy can be considered.
  – Iron chelation therapy (4)[A]:
    ○ Deferoxamine 50 mg/kg/d in continuous 8–24-hour daily infusions (4)[B]:
    ○ Iron removal improved with addition of ascorbate. Due to cardiac, visual, auditory toxicity, limit ascorbate intake to ≤200 mg/d.
    ○ Deferasirox is an oral once-daily iron chelator (5)[B]:
    ○ Recommended dose 20–40 mg/kg/d
    ○ Long-term safety profile not well studied
    ○ Side effects include skin rash, GI symptoms, and acute kidney injury.
    ○ Goal of chelation therapy is to maintain serum ferritin <500 μg/L (4)[A,B].

- Removal of causative factors, such as alcohol, drugs, or toxins, should fully reverse SA.
- Repletion of copper in patients with copper deficiency

Second Line
Chemotherapeutic agents may have a role.

ISSUES FOR REFERRAL
- Hematology consultation
- Genetic counseling is important for patients with heritable cause of SA.

ADDITIONAL THERAPIES
Allogeneic stem cell transplantation has been successful in a few cases in younger patients with myelodysplastic syndromes.

SURGERY/OTHER PROCEDURES
Splenectomy is contraindicated due to frequent postoperative thromboembolic complications.

IN-PATIENT CONSIDERATIONS
Admission Criteria/Initial Stabilization
Most patients without cardiac complications can be treated in the outpatient setting.

 ONGOING CARE

FOLLOW-UP RECOMMENDATIONS
Patient Monitoring
- Annual ferritin and transferrin saturation to monitor for Fe overload.
- Patients given pyridoxine should be followed for response to treatment. As above, lab results should show reticulocytosis within 2 weeks and improved hemoglobin within 1–2 months.
- Correction of nutritional deficiency
- Ensure withdrawal of reversible cause.

DIET
- Patients may need to avoid excessive alcohol intake.
- Patients with copper deficiency may need oral copper repletion.

PROGNOSIS
- 75% of X-linked SA with *ALAS-2* mutations are pyridoxine-responsive.
- Prognosis is better if iron overload is prevented.
- RARS: Median survival 3–6 years, <10% progression to leukemia
- When only the erythroid line is affected (PSA), progression to acute leukemia is not usually seen.
- If SA follows treatment for malignancy, leukemic transformation is common.

COMPLICATIONS
- Iron overload may cause organ damage:
  – Cardiac arrhythmia or CHF
  – Hepatic dysfunction
- Complication may arise from blood transfusions.

REFERENCES

1. Alcindor T, Bridges KR. Sideroblastic anaemias. *Br J Haematol*. 2002;116:733–743.
2. Cuijpers ML, van Spronsen DJ, Muus P, et al. Need for early recognition and therapeutic guidelines of congenital sideroblastic anaemia. *Int J Hematol*. 2011;94:97–100.
3. Rovó A, Stüssi G, Meyer-Monard S, et al. Sideroblastic changes of the bone marrow can be predicted by the erythrogram of peripheral blood. *Int J Lab Hematol*. 2010;32(3):329–335.
4. Olivieri NF, Brittenham GM. Iron-chelating therapy and the treatment of thalassemia. *Blood*. 1997;89: 739–761.
5. Porter J, Galanello R, Saglio G, et al. Relative response of patients with myelodysplastic syndromes and other transfusion-dependent anaemias to deferasirox (ICL670): A 1-yr prospective study. *Eur J Haematol*. 2008;80: 168–176.

ADDITIONAL READING

- Camaschella C. Hereditary sideroblastic anemias: Pathophysiology, diagnosis, and treatment. *Semin Hematol*. 2009;46(4):371–377.
- Müller-Berndorff H, Haas PS, Kunzmann R, et al. Comparison of five prognostic scoring systems, the French-American-British (FAB) and World Health Organization (WHO) classifications in patients with myelodysplastic syndromes: Results of a single-center analysis. *Ann Hematol*. 2006;85(8): 502–513. Epub 2006 May 20.

 SEE ALSO

Algorithms: Anemia, Sideroblastic; Anemia

CODES

ICD10
- D64.0 Hereditary sideroblastic anemia
- D64.2 Secondary sideroblastic anemia due to drugs and toxins
- D64.3 Other sideroblastic anemias

CLINICAL PEARLS

- Sideroblastic anemia results from inability to incorporate iron during heme synthesis in the mitochondria, leading to microcytic anemia and sideroblasts in the bone marrow.
- Multiple inherited forms are linked to genetic mutations, as well as acquired forms of SA.
- Patients may present with symptomatic anemia, with blood tests revealing iron overload.
- Bone marrow biopsy is required for diagnosis. Prussian blue staining reveals ringed sideroblasts.
- Treatment includes blood transfusions for symptomatic anemia, chelation therapy for iron overload, pyridoxine in X-linked SA and alcohol-related SA, and removal of causative factors if present.

ANEURYSM OF THE ABDOMINAL AORTA

Michael Gray, MD

BASICS

DESCRIPTION
- An infrarenal aorta ≥3 cm in diameter is considered aneurysmal.
- Types:
  - Fusiform aneurysm: Involves the whole circumference or wall of the artery
  - Saccular aneurysm: Does not involve the full circumference; often appears as an asymmetrical bleb or blister on side of aorta. Clinical presentation relates to aneurysm location, size, type, and comorbid factors affecting patient. The majority are asymptomatic. May present with rupture, embolism, or thrombosis. Treatment and indications for surgical repair are dictated by risk of rupture, risk of surgical repair, and estimated patient life expectancy.
- System(s) affected: Cardiovascular; Neurologic; Heme/Lymphatic/Immunologic
- Synonym(s): Aortic aneurysms; AAA

Geriatric Considerations
Incidence of AAA, risk of rupture, and operative morbidity and mortality all rise with age.

Pediatric Considerations
Rare in children; may be associated with umbilical artery catheters, connective tissue diseases, arteritides, or congenital abnormalities.

EPIDEMIOLOGY
- Frequency increases >50 years of age
- Predominant sex: Male > Female (5:1) (1)

Incidence
- >15,000 deaths per year in US
- 10th leading cause of death in men 65–75
- 8% of men age >65

Prevalence
- Depends on risk factors associated with AAA
- Prevalence of AAAs 2.9–4.9 cm in diameter ranges from 1.3% for men aged 45–54 to 12.5% for men 75–84. Data for women are 0% and 5.2%, respectively (2); however, when detected, women presented at an older age and were more likely to present with a ruptured AAA. Female sex is an independent risk factor for *death* from AAA (3).

ETIOLOGY AND PATHOPHYSIOLOGY
- Vascular inflammatory degenerative disease, with major role of matrix metalloproteinases and inflammatory markers that result in aortic medial degeneration (2)
- Gradual and/or sporadic expansion of aneurysm and accumulation of mural thrombus
- Mural thrombus can contribute to an area of localized hypoxia, thus further weakening the aneurysm.
- Aneurysms tend to expand over time. (Laplace law: T (wall tension) = pressure × radius. Wall tension directly related to BP and radius of artery.) When wall tension exceeds wall tensile strength, rupture occurs (3).
- Average small AAA (<5.5 cm) grows at rate of 2.6–3.2 mm/yr. Larger aneurysms grow faster rate, as do aneurysms in current smokers; otherwise no identifiable risk factors to assess which small AAAs will advance to require further intervention.
- Annual growth rate of 2.2 mm/yr average for small aneurysms but increased in smokers; decreased in diabetics (4)

- 60–80% of AAAs between 40 and 49 mm will enlarge and require surgery in 5 years.
- Degenerative: Atherosclerotic (80%); other causes: Inflammatory diseases (5%), trauma, connective tissue disorders, infection (*Brucella, Salmonella*, staph, tuberculosis)

Genetics
- Familial aggregations exist: Aneurysms may develop at an earlier age.
- 2× risk of AAA if 1st-degree relative with AAA (1)
- Marfan syndrome
- Ehlers-Danlos syndrome
- Polycystic kidney disease
- Tuberous sclerosis

RISK FACTORS
Older age, male, Northern European ethnicity, family history, smoking, hypertension (HTN), hyperlipidemia, peripheral vascular disease, peripheral aneurysms, chronic obstructive peripheral disease (COPD), obesity (3)

GENERAL PREVENTION
- Address cardiovascular disease risk factors.
- Follow screening guidelines: US screening for detection of AAA in male patients, 65–75, who have ever smoked and men >60 who are siblings or offspring of patients with AAA (USPSTF Guideline).

COMMONLY ASSOCIATED CONDITIONS
- HTN, myocardial infarction (MI), heart failure, carotid artery, and/or lower extremity peripheral arterial disease
- Screening for thoracic aneurysm should also be considered.

DIAGNOSIS

- Screening: Recommended 1-time US for AAA in men 65–75 who have ever smoked. Men >60 years old who are siblings or offspring of AAA patients should undergo physical exam and US screening (2)[B]. US Preventive Services Task Force recommends against routine screening for women.
- Most often asymptomatic: Discovered during exams for other complaints
- Symptomatic: Embolization, thrombosis, vague abdominal or back pain, syncope, lower extremity paralysis
- Rupture

ALERT
- The triad of shock, pulsatile mass, and abdominal pain always suggests rupture of AAA:
  - Shock may be absent if rupture is contained.
  - Palpable pulsatile mass may be absent in up to 50% of patients with rupture.
  - Pain may radiate to the back, groin, flank (mimics urolithiasis), buttocks, or legs.
- Unusual presentations:
  - Primary aortoenteric fistula: Erosion/rupture of AAA into duodenum
  - Aortocaval fistula: Erosion/Rupture of AAA into vena cava or left renal vein: 3–6%
  - Inflammatory aneurysm: Encasement by thick inflammatory rind; can cause chronic abdominal pain, weight loss, and elevated ESR. Surrounding viscera densely adherent.

HISTORY
Abdominal or back pain; AAA risk factors

PHYSICAL EXAM
- Pulsatile supraumbilical mass
- Only 30–40% of AAA detected by physical exam
- 14% of AAA associated with femoral or popliteal aneurysms (1)
- Vague abdominal tenderness: May radiate to the back or flank
- Encroachment by aneurysm:
  - Vertebral body erosion, gastric outlet obstruction, ureteral obstruction
  - Lower extremity ischemia secondary to embolization of mural thrombus
- Rupture leads to tachycardia, hypotension, evidence of shock and anemia, possible flank contusion (Grey-Turner sign).

DIAGNOSTIC TESTS & INTERPRETATION
Initial Tests (lab, imaging)
- If rupturing AAA is considered: Complete blood chemistry, chemistries, coags, type and cross, ECG
- US: Simplest and least expensive diagnostic procedure
- Multiple studies have demonstrated high sensitivity (94–100%) and specificity (98–100%) of US diagnosis of AAA by emergency physicians.
- Additional studies confirm family physicians trained in US also with high sensitivity and specificity for AAA detection.
- Although effective in detecting AAA, US is a poor test to show leakage or rupture if bleeding is into the retroperitoneal space.
- Surveillance of asymptomatic aneurysm (1)[C]:
  - 2.6–2.9 cm: Screen at 5-year intervals.
  - 3.0–3.4 cm: Screen at 3-year intervals.
  - 3.5–4.4 cm: Screen every 12 months.
  - 4.4–5.4 cm: Screen every 6 months.
- CT scans are preferred preoperative study (caution with IV contrast in renal failure).
- MRI/MRA can visualize AAA, but is often not possible in emergent situations.
- Aortography: Does not define outer dimensions of aneurysm
- Abdominal x-rays can be diagnostic if calcifications exist; not a diagnostic tool of choice
- Ongoing research is exploring alternative diagnostic measurements, including measurement of total aortic volume vs. single axial diameter measurement and measurement of total thrombus burden associated with AAA since this appears to have a greater risk association (3).

Follow-Up Tests & Special Considerations
Evaluation for coronary artery disease is appropriate prior to elective AAA repair (i.e., cardiac clearance), including stress test, echocardiography, and ECG if appropriate (1).

Diagnostic Procedures/Other

ALERT
Use clinical judgment: Patients with known AAA having abdominal or back pain symptoms may be rupturing despite a negative CT scan.

DIFFERENTIAL DIAGNOSIS
- Other abdominal masses
- Other causes of abdominal or back pain (e.g., peptic ulcer disease, renal colic, diverticulitis, appendicitis, incarcerated hernia, GI hemorrhage, arthritis, metastatic disease)

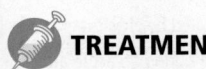

TREATMENT

GENERAL MEASURES
- Treat atherosclerotic risk factors (2,5)[C].
- Medical optimization of cardiac, renal, and pulmonary conditions
- Smoking cessation (increased rate of expansion of 20–25% with continued smoking) and exercise (5)
- Emergent treatment in unstable or symptomatic patients is immediate vascular surgery consultation, adequate IV access and resuscitation, type and cross for multiple units, and rapid bedside US.
- Less acute treatment of AAA/prevention of rupture is elective repair and risk factor modification.

MEDICATION
- Beta-blockers may be initiated to reduce the rate of aneurysm expansion (2)[C].
- Beta-blockers should be used perioperatively in absence of contraindications (2)[A]; bronchodilators should be used for 2 weeks prior to repair for patients with COPD (1)[C].
- Statin therapy may be effective in decreasing the growth rate of small AAA according to a meta-analytic study. More data and trials are still needed.
- Aspirin may inhibit expansion by inhibiting thrombus growth.
- Doxycycline may also inhibit expansion; further studies are needed. Early animal studies indicate possible role for ACE-I/ARBs, mast cell stabilizers, prostaglandin inhibitors, and novel gene therapy (2).

SURGERY/OTHER PROCEDURES
Current recommendations (5)[C]:
- Elective:
  – 5.5-cm diameter is threshold for repair in "average" patient.
  – Younger, low-risk patients with long life expectancy may prefer early repair.
  – Women or AAA with high risk of rupture: Consider elective repair at 4.5–5 cm
  – Consider delayed repair in high-risk patients.
  – 5% perioperative mortality for open elective repair (3)
- High risk of rupture:
  – Expansion >0.6 cm/yr
  – Smoking/COPD severe/steroids
  – Family history; multiple relatives
  – Hypertension poorly controlled
  – Shape nonfusiform
- High-risk patients for elective repair:
  – Risk factors for open repair include age >70 years, COPD, chronic renal insufficiency (CRI), suprarenal clamp site, with 1-year mortality if 0 risk factors present of 1.2% and 67% for all 4 risk factors present.
  – Other poor prognostic factors include inactive/poor stamina, congestive heart failure, significant coronary artery disease, liver disease, family history of AAA.
  – Consider coronary revascularization prior to aneurysm repair if coronary artery disease (CAD) (1)[B]

- Discontinue thienopyridine (clopidogrel and others) use 10 days prior to AAA repair and restart immediately postoperatively (1)[C].
  – Transfusion to hematocrit >28.0 if elective open repair planned (1)[C]
- Emergent/Symptomatic repair: Traditionally, open repair; however, candidates with appropriate anatomy can have endovascular repair, with an estimated mortality of 32% for endovascular vs. 44% open.
- Open repair vs. endovascular repair (EVAR):
  – Open repair or EVAR in patients who are good or average surgical candidates (6)[A]
  – Open repair for patients who are unable to comply with the recommended periodic long-term surveillance (6)[B]
  – EVAR for patients at high surgical risk due to significant cardiac, pulmonary, or renal disease [C] but no significant mortality improvement compared with no therapy (6)
  – EVAR tends to have improved procedural mortality (1.8% vs. 4.3%), but long-term mortality over 6 years is similar (7.5 deaths/patient–years for EVAR vs. 7.7 deaths/patient-years for open repair) (6).

IN-PATIENT CONSIDERATIONS
Risk of abdominal compartment syndrome after repair, 4–12%; usually associated with large fluid resuscitation

ONGOING CARE

FOLLOW-UP RECOMMENDATIONS
- CT or MRI evaluation of the graft for EVAR surveillance at 1 month, 6 months, then annually (6)

Patient Monitoring
BP and fasting lipid values: Control as for atherosclerotic disease (2)[C]

DIET
Low-fat, low-salt, and low-caffeine diet; nutrition optimized prior to elective repair; parenteral nutrition started within 7 days postoperatively if unable to have enteral feeds (1)[B]

PATIENT EDUCATION
Smoking cessation (2)[B], aerobic exercise

PROGNOSIS
- Annual risk of rupture (5):
  – <4 cm diameter: ~0%. 4–4.9 cm: ~0.5–5%
  – 5–5.9 cm: ~3–15% 6–6.9 cm: ~10–20%
  – 7–7.9 cm: ~20–40% >8 cm: 30–50%
- Patients with AAAs measuring ≥5.5 cm should undergo repair (2)[B], as should all patients with symptomatic AAA (2)[C]. Recommended routine surveillance at 1 year and every 5 years following repair (3)
- Only ~18% of patients with ruptured AAA survive.
- Despite a 5:1 ratio of AAA between males and females, women have higher AAA-associated mortality and morbidity, regardless of open or endovascular repair (3).

COMPLICATIONS
- Nonoperative: Rupture, dissection, thromboembolization. Elective operative (conventional): Death 2–8%, all cardiac 10–12% (MI 2–8%)
- 5.1% of patients with EVAR repair required reintervention compared with 1.7 for open repair group (6).

- Pulmonary 5–10%; renal 5–7%; wound infection >5%; colon ischemia 1%; spinal cord ischemia <1%

REFERENCES

1. Chaikof EL, Brewster DC, Dalman RL, et al. The care of patients with an abdominal aortic aneurysm: The Society for Vascular Surgery practice guidelines. *J Vasc Surg.* 2009;50:S2–S49.
2. Hirsch AT, Haskal ZJ, Hertzer NR, et al. ACC/AHA 2005 Practice Guidelines for the management of patients with peripheral arterial disease: A collaborative report. *Circulation.* 2006;113: e563–e601.
3. Moxon JV, Parr A, Emeto TI, et al. Diagnosis and monitoring of abdominal aortic aneurysm: Current status and future prospects. *Curr Probl Cardiol.* 2010;35:512–548.
4. Sweeting MJ, Thompson SG, Brown LC, et al. Meta-analysis of individual patient data to examine factors affecting growth and rupture of small abdominal aortic aneurysms. *Br J Surg.* 2012;99:655–665. Epub 2012 Mar 5.
5. Aggarwal S, Qamar A, Sharma V, et al. Abdominal aortic aneurysm: A comprehensive review. *Exp Clin Cardiol.* 2011;16:11–15.
6. Rooke TW, Hirsch AT, Misra S, et al. 2011 ACCF/AHA Focused Update of the Guideline for the Management of Patients with Peripheral Artery Disease (Updating the 2005 Guideline). *J Am Coll Cardiol.* 2011;58:2020–2045.

SEE ALSO

Aortic Dissection; Ehlers-Danlos; Giant Cell Arteritis; Marfan Syndrome; Polyarteritis Nodosa; Turner Syndrome

CODES

ICD10
- I71.3 Abdominal aortic aneurysm, ruptured
- I71.4 Abdominal aortic aneurysm, without rupture

CLINICAL PEARLS

- US is procedure of choice for screening for AAA in any male >65 with any history of tobacco use.
- Suspect AAA for any elderly patient with back, abdominal, or groin pain. Triad of hypotension/shock, pulsatile abdominal mass, and abdominal/back pain always suggests rupture, which requires emergent evaluation for surgery.
- 5.5 cm is threshold diameter for elective surgical treatment (with some exceptions).

ANGIOEDEMA

Michelle T. Martin, PharmD, BCPS, BCACP • Jamie Berkes, MD

BASICS

DESCRIPTION
- Angioedema (AE) is an acute, localized swelling of skin, mucosa, and submucosa caused by extravasation of fluid into the affected tissues. It often resolves in hours to days, but it can be life threatening if the upper airway is involved.
- Hereditary AE (HAE) and acquired AE (AAE) are diseases of the complement cascade that result in recurrent episodes of AE of the skin, upper airway, and GI tract.
- Synonym(s): Angioneurotic edema; Quincke edema

EPIDEMIOLOGY
- Predominant age:
  - Allergen, medication, or other triggers can affect all ages.
  - HAE: Infancy to 2nd decade of life
  - AAE: Typically patients in 4th decade of life
- Predominant gender: Male = Female (except type III HAE, which affects more women than men)

Prevalence
- AE occurs in ~15% of the population over a lifetime.
- AE: 0.1–2.2% of patients receiving ACE inhibitors: African Americans have a 4–5 times greater risk of ACE inhibitor–induced AE than Caucasians.
- HAE: 1:10,000–50,000 population in the US

ETIOLOGY AND PATHOPHYSIOLOGY
- Idiopathic
- Medication-induced:
  - ACE inhibitors cause 10–25% of AE cases, mostly occurring within the 1st month of use. However, onset may be delayed by years.
  - Angiotensin-receptor blockers (ARBs) also can cause AE, but more rarely than ACE inhibitors.
- Allergic triggers:
  - Food allergens such as shellfish, nuts, eggs, milk, wheat, soy
  - Medications such as aspirin, NSAIDs, antibiotics, narcotics, and oral contraceptives
  - Latex, venom
- Physically induced: Cold, heat, pressure, vibration, trauma, emotional stress, ultraviolet light
- Hereditary or acquired C1 INH deficiency
- Thyroid autoimmune disease–associated AE
- Type I hypersensitivity reaction
- Increase in vascular permeability secondary to IgE-mediated mast cell–stimulated histamine release or from activation of the complement system and an elevation in bradykinin (HAE)
- Attacks of HAE are triggered by prolonged mechanical pressure, cold, heat, trauma, emotional stress, menses, illness, and inflammation:
  - Type I HAE, the most common form, caused by decreased production of C1 esterase inhibitor (C1 INH), has autosomal-dominant inheritance.
  - Type II HAE has functionally impaired C1 INH and autosomal-dominant inheritance.
  - Type III (HAE-FXII) involves mutations in coagulation factor XII gene (occurs more frequently in women, often estrogen-dependent, associated with estrogen administration); also type III HAE-unknown exists.

- AAE is a rare condition:
  - Type I is associated with lymphoproliferative diseases or paraneoplastic diseases.
  - Type II is due to autoimmune disorders (anti-C1 INH antibody).
  - Affected patients have circulating antibodies directed either against specific immunoglobulins expressed on B cells (type I) or against C1 INH (type II).
  - AAE typically presents later in life (>40), and patients lack family history of AE.

Genetics
- HAE types I and II are autosomal dominant, whereas type III is dominant X-linked.
- HAE occurs in 25% of patients as a result of spontaneous genetic mutations.

RISK FACTORS
- Consuming medications and foods that can cause allergic reactions
- Pre-existing diagnosis of HAE or AAE

GENERAL PREVENTION
- Avoid known triggers.
- Do not use ACE inhibitors in patients with C1 esterase inhibitor (C1 INH) deficiency.

COMMONLY ASSOCIATED CONDITIONS
- Quincke disease (AE of the uvula)
- Urticaria

DIAGNOSIS

HISTORY
- Identify potential triggers, including medication history, recent exposure to allergens, physical elements, or trauma (1)[C].
- In comparison with urticaria, AE typically is nonpruritic, but it can cause a burning sensation.
- Family history

PHYSICAL EXAM
- Acute onset of asymmetric localized swelling, usually of the face (eyelids, lips, ears, nose), tongue, larynx, and, less often, of the extremities or genitalia.
- GI tract involvement may manifest as intermittent unexplained abdominal pain.

ALERT
10–35% of patients present with severe respiratory compromise requiring endotracheal intubation.

DIFFERENTIAL DIAGNOSIS
Urticaria (with AE in 40–50% of patients); allergic contact dermatitis; connective-tissue disease: Lupus, dermatomyositis; anaphylaxis; cellulitis; erysipelas; lymphedema; diffuse SC infiltrative process

DIAGNOSTIC TESTS & INTERPRETATION
Initial Tests (lab, imaging)
- If AE with urticaria and/or anaphylaxis, check for allergen-specific IgE to verify suspected trigger. Serum tryptase is elevated during acute AE (1)[C].
- Without a clear etiology and recurrence in AE and urticaria, check CBC and ESR:
  - Macrocytosis implies a pernicious anemia.
  - Eosinophilia may imply atopy or, rarely, a parasitic infection.
  - Elevated ESR may imply systemic disorders (1)[C].

- In recurrent AE without a clear etiology and without urticaria, consider ordering serum C4 level:
  - Low serum C4 is a sensitive, but nonspecific screening test for hereditary and acquired C1 INH deficiency.
  - If C4 is normal, determine C1 INH level and function, and recheck C4 during an acute attack.
  - If C4 level and C1 INH level and function are still normal, consider other causes (i.e., medications or HAE type III) for AE (2)[C].
  - If C4 level, C1 INH level, and C1 INH function are low, this indicates HAE type I.
  - HAE type II is characterized by low C4 and low C1 INH function, but C1 INH level can be normal or elevated (2)[C].
- C1q is decreased in ~75% of AAE, but is usually normal in all types of HAE (2)[C].

Follow-Up Tests & Special Considerations
- If C4 and C1q are low (as in AAE), neoplastic and autoimmune workup is warranted. CBC, a peripheral smear, protein electrophoresis, immunophenotyping of lymphocytes, and imaging studies are often undertaken to rule out hematologic malignancies or cancer (1)[C].
- Abdominal radiographs and CT scan can demonstrate GI AE or ileus.
- C1 INH deficiency may occur in association with internal malignancy, so AE rarely can be a paraneoplastic disease. Imaging (CT scan, radiography, etc.) then would be done as part of a neoplastic workup for patients with AAE.

Diagnostic Procedures/Other
Skin biopsy (may be nonspecific)

Test Interpretation
- Edema of deep dermis and SC tissue
- Variable perivascular and interstitial infiltrate

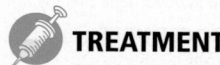

TREATMENT

GENERAL MEASURES
Intubation if airway is threatened

MEDICATION
First Line
- Acute allergic AE (with airway compromise):
  - Epinephrine 1:1,000, 0.3 mL IV or SC (1)[C]
  - Glucocorticoids (hydrocortisone 200 mg IV or Solu-Medrol 40 mg IV) (1)[C]
  - Diphenhydramine 50 mg IV
  - If medication-induced, stop the causative agent.
- Idiopathic recurrent AE:
  - 1st-generation antihistamines for acute AE (cause drowsiness)
  - Older children and adults: Hydroxyzine (Vistaril) 5 mg/5 mL, 25-mg tablets 10–25 mg t.i.d., or diphenhydramine (Benadryl) 25–50 mg q6h (3)[C]
  - Children <6 years of age: Diphenhydramine 12.5 mg (elixir) q6–8h (5 mg/kg/d) (2)[C]
  - 2nd-generation H_1 blockers: Fexofenadine (Allegra) 180 mg/d b.i.d., loratadine (Claritin) 10 mg/d, cetirizine (Zyrtec) 10 mg/d, desloratadine (Clarinex) 5 mg/d (3)[C]; use with caution in pregnancy and in the elderly.

- HAE chronic prophylaxis:
  - A nanofiltered plasma-derived C1 INH (pdC1 INH) concentrate (Cinryze) dosed at 1,000 units/10 mL IV, rate of 1 mL/min (for 10 min) q3–4d. Administration setting options include clinic, home health care, and after proper training, home self-administration (4,5)[B].
  - Attenuated androgens increase hepatic production of C1 INH: Oral Danazol 50–200 mg/d or oral stanozolol 2 mg/d; use lowest effective dose. Side effects include, but are not limited to, headache, weight gain, liver dysfunction, hirsutism, and menstrual disturbances. Monitor CBC, liver function tests, creatinine kinase, lactic dehydrogenase, fasting lipid profile, and urinalysis at baseline and q6mo. Abdominal US to be performed annually or q6mo. if dose of danazol >200 mg/d. Danazol is not to be used in children, during first 2 trimesters of pregnancy, during lactation, and in patients with hepatitis or cancer (2)[C].
- HAE short-term prophylaxis:
  - Minor procedures (dental work): If C1 INH is available, no prophylaxis; otherwise: Danazol 2.5–10 mg/kg/d (maximum 600 mg/d), stanozolol 4–6 mg/d, for 5 days prior to and 2–5 days after event (2)[C].
  - Major procedures (including intubation): C1 INH 1 (max. 6) hour prior with additional dose on hand during procedure. If unavailable, danazol 2.5–10 mg/kg/d (max. 600 mg/d) and solvent/detergent treated plasma (SDP). If SDP unavailable, use fresh-frozen plasma (FFP) 10 mL/kg; 2–4 units (400–800 mL) for an adult 1–6 hours prior.
- Acute HAE treatment:
  - C1 INH concentrate IV, dosed at 1,000 units if <50 kg; 1,500 units if 50–100 kg; 2,000 units if >100 kg (2)[C].
  - Pasteurized human pdC1 INH (Berinert), dosed at 20 units/kg (available in 500 units/10 mL, max. infusion rate of 4 mL/min IV via peripheral vein. DO NOT SHAKE (will denature the protein). Worsening of HAE pain was reported as the most severe adverse event (4,6)[B].
  - Ecallantide (Kalbitor), a kallikrein inhibitor, is dosed in patients age ≥16 years at 30 mg SC with 3 separate 10 mg/mL injections in the abdomen, thigh, or upper arm, and a second 30 mg dose may be repeated within 24 hours if needed. Injection-site rotation not necessary, but must be 2 inches away from attack site. A black box warning of anaphylaxis (potential adverse event) mandates administration in health care setting (4,7)[B].
  - Icatibant (Firazyr), a bradykinin receptor-2 antagonist, is dosed at 30 mg SC over at least 30 seconds in the abdomen in patients age ≥18 years and supplied in a prefilled 10 mg/mL (3 mL) syringe for home administration. Subsequent doses of 30 mg may be repeated in 6-hour intervals (max. 90 mg/24 hours) (4,8)[B].
  - Antihistamines and glucocorticoids typically do not benefit patients with HAE. Epinephrine can offer transient stabilization/improvement in laryngeal AE, but is not sufficient for full treatment, and does not alter the course of attack.

- New therapies are under investigation for acute HAE treatment:
  - Other C1 INH replacement therapy: A recombinant human C1 INH isolated from the milk of transgenic rabbits (Rhucin), dosed IV, studied at 50 or 100 units/kg. Treatment is approved in Europe: Ruconest (8)[C].
  - Cinryze is awaiting FDA approval for use during acute attacks (4)[C].
- Acute AAE treatment:
  - C1 INH concentrate and FFP
  - Treatment of underlying lymphoproliferative disease is often curative in AAE type I.
  - Immunosuppressive therapy to suppress antibody production
  - Clinical trials under way with recombinant human C1 INH (Rhucin) (4)[C]

Second Line
- HAE chronic prophylaxis: If pdC1 INH is unavailable and if patient cannot tolerate attenuated androgens, antifibrinolytic agents (plasmin inhibitors), such as tranexamic acid (not approved by the FDA in US) 25–50 mg/kg/d divided b.i.d. or t.i.d. (3–6 g/d max.) or ε-aminocaproic acid could be used. They are less effective than attenuated androgens and have many side effects. On rare occasions, they have been linked to (but not proven to cause) thrombophlebitis, embolism, or myositis (2)[C],(8).
- Acute HAE: FFP if C1 INH concentrate is not available, but it can potentially worsen attack (8)
- Idiopathic AE: Oral Doxepin (Sinequan) may be effective for AE (10–25 mg at bedtime).
- H2RA: Oral Ranitidine (Zantac) 150 mg/d b.i.d.

SURGERY/OTHER PROCEDURES
Tracheostomy if progressive laryngeal edema prevents endotracheal intubation

IN-PATIENT CONSIDERATIONS
Admission Criteria/Initial Stabilization
Ensure patent airway. If anaphylaxis, epinephrine (1:1,000) SC 0.3–0.5 mg q10–15min

IV Fluids
Given if needed to stabilize patient

 ## ONGOING CARE

FOLLOW-UP RECOMMENDATIONS
Patient Monitoring
- Diagnostic workup if symptoms are severe, persistent, or recurrent
- Protect airway if mouth, tongue, or throat is involved

DIET
Avoid known dietary allergens.

PATIENT EDUCATION
Educate on avoidance of triggers (i.e., food, medication, other physical stimuli), types of treatment, when to seek emergency care, and wearing Medic Alert bracelet.

PROGNOSIS
- AE symptoms often resolve in hours to 2–4 days. If airway is compromised, AE can be life threatening.
- Patients with HAE have an average of 20 attacks/yr; each may last 3–5 days. Prophylaxis can decrease the frequency of events and number of missed days of school or work.

COMPLICATIONS
Anaphylaxis

REFERENCES
1. Temiño VM, Peebles RS. The spectrum and treatment of angioedema. *Am J Med*. 2008;121:282–286.
2. Bowen T, Cicardi M, Farkas H, et al. 2010 International consensus algorithm for the diagnosis, therapy and management of hereditary angioedema. *Allergy Asthma Clin Immunol*. 2010;6(1):24. Epub 2010 Jul 28.
3. Frigas E, Park M. Idiopathic recurrent angioedema. *Immunol Allergy Clin North Am*. 2006;26:739–751.
4. Levy JH, Freiberger DJ, Roback J. Hereditary angioedema: Current and emerging treatment options. *Anesth Analg*. 2010;110(5):1271–1280.
5. Zuraw BL, Busse PJ, White M, et al. Nanofiltered C1 inhibitor concentrate for treatment of hereditary angioedema. *N Engl J Med*. 2010;363(6):513–522.
6. Craig TJ, Levy RJ, Wasserman RL, et al. Efficacy of human C1 esterase inhibitor concentrate compared with placebo in acute hereditary angioedema attacks. *J Allergy Clin Immunol*. 2009;124:801–808.
7. Cicardi M, Levy RJ, McNeil DL, et al. Ecallantide for the treatment of acute attacks in hereditary angioedema. *N Engl J Med*. 2010;363(6):523–531.
8. Lumry WR, Li HH, Levy RJ, et al. Randomized placebo-controlled trial of the bradykinin-receptor antagonist icatibant for the treatment of acute attacks of hereditary angioedema: The FAST-3 trial. *Ann Allergy Asthma Immunol*. 2011;107(6):529–537. Epub 2011 Oct 5.

ADDITIONAL READING
Craig T, Riedl M, Dykewicz MS, et al. When is prophylaxis for hereditary angioedema necessary? *Ann Allergy Asthma Immunol*. 2009;102:366–372.

 ## SEE ALSO

Urticaria; Anaphylaxis

 ## CODES

ICD10
- T78.3XXA Angioneurotic edema, initial encounter
- T78.3XXD Angioneurotic edema, subsequent encounter
- T78.3XXS Angioneurotic edema, sequela

CLINICAL PEARLS
- Angioedema (AE) is an acute, localized swelling of skin, mucosa, and submucosa caused by extravasation of fluid into the affected tissues. It often resolves in hours to days, but it can be life threatening if the upper airway is involved
- Hereditary AE (HAE) and acquired AE (AAE) are diseases of the complement cascade that result in recurrent episodes of AE of the skin, upper airway, and GI tract.
- Trigger identification and avoidance are key in the prevention of AE.
- Patients with a history of allergies and AE should be prescribed an epinephrine autoinjector

ANKLE FRACTURES

Elizabeth M. Goldberg, MD

BASICS

- Bones: Tibia, fibula, talus
- Mortise: Tibial plafond (horizontal surface of the tibia), medial malleolus, and lateral malleolus
- Ligaments: Syndesmotic, lateral collateral, and medial collateral ligaments

DESCRIPTION

- Fractures involve the distal fibula (lateral malleolus) and/or distal tibia (medial malleolus and plafond).
- Lateral malleolus fractures are the most common.
- Common fractures with ligamentous injury:
  - Maisonneuve fracture: Proximal fibular fracture with distal ligamentous rupture and avulsion of medial malleolus
  - Osteochondral fracture of the talar dome
  - Avulsion fracture of the 5th metatarsal
- 2 common classification systems are useful for describing fractures; however, Lauge Hansen has recently been shown to be superior for detecting syndesmotic injury after comparison with MRI as a gold standard (1)[B]:
  - Danis-Weber system: Type A, B, C based on the location of the fibular fracture in relationship to the syndesmosis:
    - Type A: Below the level of syndesmosis (of tibiofibular joint)
    - Type B: At the level of the syndesmosis; both usually stable
    - Type C: Above syndesmosis; usually unstable;
    - Lauge Hansen: Fracture type based on foot position and applied force, with the most basic nomenclature referring to the number of fractures:
      - Unimalleolar:
        - Lateral malleolus if type C, unstable
        - Medial malleolus fracture usually occurs in conjunction with ligamentous or lateral/posterior malleolus injury.
      - Bimalleolar: Both the medial and lateral malleolus; usually unstable
      - Trimalleolar: Lateral, medial, and posterior malleoli; unstable
- Pilon fracture: Intra-articular fracture of the tibial plafond; usually axial loading mechanism; unstable

Pediatric Considerations

- The distal tibial and fibular physis is the third most common fracture in children.
- Distal tibia is most common site of pathologic fracture.
- Injuries are more likely to affect the growth plate.
- Juvenile Tillaux: Isolated Salter-Harris (SH) III fracture of anterolateral portion of the distal tibia epiphysis
- Triplane fracture: SH IV; occurs in adolescence; 2-, 3-, and 4-part fractures:
  - Most commonly epiphyseal fragment anteriorly and metaphyseal fragment posteriorly

EPIDEMIOLOGY

- Predominant ages: Even age distribution
- Predominant sex:
  - Age <50: Male > Female
  - Age >50: Female > Male
- Unimalleolar (fibular fractures) = 60–70%; bimalleolar = 15–20%; trimalleolar = 7–12%

Incidence

- 1–2 cases per 1,000 people per year
- Rising incidence and severity in the elderly; seen in as many as 8.3 Medicare patients per 1,000 (2)[B]

RISK FACTORS

- Obesity
- History of smoking or osteoporosis

ETIOLOGY AND PATHOPHYSIOLOGY

- Fall or twisting injury to the ankle
- Alcohol or slippery surfaces (1/3 of injuries, each)
- Sports: The ankle is the most commonly injured joint among athletes.
- Location and pattern of injury depend on foot position and the direction of force applied.
- Most commonly, the foot is plantar flexed and inverted, and the force is external rotation.
- Axial loading can cause a tibial plafond or pilon fracture.

GENERAL PREVENTION

- Proper shoe wear (i.e., flat, supportive shoes)
- Fall precautions in the elderly

COMMONLY ASSOCIATED CONDITIONS

- Ligamentous injury (sprains):
  - Lateral collateral sprains are the most common (85–90%); medial collateral sprains and distal syndesmotic are uncommon.
- Syndesmosis injury
- Ankle or subtalar dislocation
- Fractures of metatarsals, talus, or calcaneus
- Osteochondral fractures
- Posterior ankle impingement (os trigonum)
- Peroneal tendon dislocation
- Compartment syndrome (rare)
- Neurovascular injury (rare)
- Other axial loading or shearing injuries (i.e., vertebral compression fractures or contralateral pelvic fractures)

DIAGNOSIS

HISTORY

- Location of pain
- Timing/mechanism of injury
- Weight-bearing status after injury
- History of ankle injury or surgery

Geriatric Considerations

- Assess for safety and fall risk.
- More likely to have increased BMI, polypharmacy, and deconditioning

PHYSICAL EXAM

- Examine for swelling, ecchymosis, possible deformity, point of maximal tenderness.
- Assess ability to bear weight.
- Skin integrity: Tenting, lacerations, or blistering
- Check neurovascular status: Motor/Sensory exam of foot/ankle, check capillary refill, and assess dorsalis pedis and posterior tibial pulses. If equivocal vascular exam, use Doppler.
- Evaluate for compartment syndrome: Swelling, pain out of proportion, pain with passive extension. Pallor, coolness to the touch, pulselessness, paralysis, and parathesias are late signs.

- Palpate ankle, foot, leg, and knee. Examine for other associated injuries (i.e., Pilon fractures: Vertebral injuries, contralateral tibial plateau).
- Assess ankle stability with the anterior drawer test for the ATFL, the talar tilt test for lateral and medial ligaments, and the squeeze test for the tibiofibular syndesmosis.

DIFFERENTIAL DIAGNOSIS

- Ankle sprain
- Other fractures: Talus, 5th metatarsal, calcaneus

DIAGNOSTIC TESTS & INTERPRETATION

- Plain radiographs are the standard.
- Ottawa Ankle Rules (OAR) has an overall sensitivity of 98% and, when applied within 48 hours after trauma, it rises to 99.6% in adults (3)[A].
- X-rays indicated in patients aged 18–55 only when malleolar pain AND:
  - Bone tenderness at the posterior edge or tip of the medial malleolus, OR
  - Bone tenderness at the posterior edge or tip of the lateral malleolus, OR
  - Inability to bear weight both immediately and in the emergency department, OR
  - Pain at navicular or along 5th metatarsal
- If OAR criteria not met for immediate x-ray, but symptoms persist beyond 48–72 hours, obtain films.
- For pediatric patients: A head-to-head comparison of the OAR vs. the Malleolar Zone Algorithm vs. the Low-Risk Exam found the OAR to be most sensitive and the Low Risk Exam most specific. Of note, the OAR did not miss any clinically important fractures, whereas the Low Risk Exam missed 13% (4)[B].
- OAR is not valid in intoxicated patients, patients with multiple injuries, or sensory deficits (diabetics with neuropathy).
- 3 standard views:
  - Anteroposterior (AP)
  - Lateral: Instability depicted by talar dome and distal tibia incongruity
  - Mortise (15–25-degree internal rotation view): Look for parallel lines between joint spaces; space between the medial malleolus and talus should not exceed 4 mm.

Follow-Up Tests & Special Considerations

- CT is useful for Tillaux, triplane, and pilon fractures or fractures with intra-articular involvement.
- CT imaging changed operative strategy in 24% of cases and was most useful in (5)[B]:
  - Fracture dislocations
  - Cases where radiographs were obscured due to plaster, trimalleolar fractures, and suprasyndesmotic fractures
- MRI should be limited to chronic instability, suspicion for osteochondral lesions, occult fractures, or injuries to the tibiofibular syndesmosis (3)[A].
- US not included in standard protocol as its sensitivity is highly operator-dependent (3)[A].

Diagnostic Procedures/Other

Arthroscopy is an option in cases of persistent pain or suspicion of any cartilaginous lesions.

TREATMENT

GENERAL MEASURES
- If there is a suspected open fracture, remove any debris from the wound and place a moist dressing over the wound. Will require immediate orthopedic consultation.
- Immobilization:
  – Noncircular cast; short leg posterior splint, stirrup or sugar tong
  – Jones compression bandage
  – Crutches
- Ice and elevate the extremity.
- Do not reduce the fracture or dislocation unless neurovascular compromise is apparent.

Medication, joint support, consultation, surgical repair, physical therapy

MEDICATION
In general, ankle fractures are painful, particularly in the first 5–7 days following an injury.

First Line
- Acetaminophen 1,000 mg q.i.d.
- NSAIDs
- Opioid analgesics
- For suspected open fractures, tetanus booster, broad-spectrum cephalosporin and aminoglycoside; penicillin G for farm injuries at risk for *Clostridium perfringens*

Second Line
Nonopioid analgesics (i.e., tramadol)

ISSUES FOR REFERRAL
- Send to emergency department for surgical evaluation if:
  – Neurovascular compromise
  – Tenting of skin/open fracture
  – Displaced fracture of malleoli
  – Intra-articular fracture
  – Bi- or trimalleolar, Pilon fractures
  – Unstable fracture or unstable ligament exam
  – Signs of compartment syndrome
  – Pediatric Salter types III, IV, V
  – Maisonneuve or Jones fractures
- All other fractures, orthopedic follow-up within 1 week and be non–weight-bearing EXCEPT:
  – Isolated avulsion fractures of the tip of the lateral malleolus may be weight-bearing as tolerated.
  – Pediatric Salter-Harris I, II of the distal fibula

SURGERY/OTHER PROCEDURES
- Surgical options:
  – Open reduction internal fixation
  – External fixation for comminuted distal tibia fractures
  – Isolated unstable nondisplaced fractures of the lateral malleolus recently shown to have equivalent functional outcomes after operative and nonoperative treatment (6)[A].
- Timing of surgery:
  – Within 6–8 hours for emergent cases (i.e., open fractures)
  – After swelling decreased in all other cases (preferably not >1 week)
- Circular cast or protective boot:
  – Isolated nondisplaced medial malleolar: Non–weight-bearing 3 weeks + 6–8 weeks in a cast
  – Posterior malleolar with no instability: 6-week cast
  – Bimalleolar: Surgery vs. cast; orthopedic follow-up

- Length of recovery:
  – In general, 6–8 weeks for healing
  – 6–8 weeks in a cast or splint (longer if fracture involves both medial and lateral malleoli)
  – 2–4 months for syndesmotic injury
  – Orthopedist may allow range of motion after 4 weeks and place in removable cast boot (fracture pattern and surgeon dependent)

IN-PATIENT CONSIDERATIONS
Admission Criteria/Initial Stabilization
Admit to the hospital if:
- Patient will require emergency surgery (e.g., open fracture, neurovascular injury, compartment syndrome)
- Cannot maintain non–weight-bearing status and requires physical therapy consultation
- Concern because of mechanism of injury (i.e., syncope, myocardial infarction [MI], head injury)

Nursing
Non–weight-bearing, maintain splint/cast, apply ice, and instruct patient to keep leg elevated

Discharge Criteria
When patient has completed the following:
- Able to ambulate with walker/crutches
- Medical workup (if needed) is completed
- Appropriate orthopedic follow-up is arranged
- Elderly patients may require a short stay in a rehabilitation facility.

ONGOING CARE

FOLLOW-UP RECOMMENDATIONS
If the fracture does not require emergent orthopedic consultation; most ankle fractures require an orthopedic consultation within <1 week and close follow-up.

Patient Monitoring
- Orthopedic follow-up:
  – Serial x-rays should be performed weekly for 4 weeks if there is any question about stability.
  – Otherwise, x-rays should be performed at 2, 4, and 8 weeks or until the fracture is healed.
- Physical therapy: Once healing begins, at orthopedic surgeon's discretion:
  – Encourage toe and knee motion as soon as possible and start ankle range of motion (ROM).
  – Recovery of strength and proprioception is critical for return to prior functional status.

DIET
NPO if surgery is being considered

PATIENT EDUCATION
- Ice and elevate the affected leg for 2–3 weeks following the injury to decrease swelling.
- Prevent splint/cast from getting wet.
- Use crutches/cane as instructed.
- Call physician if:
  – Swelling increases
  – Toes become numb, painful, or change color
  – Pain increases despite elevation/pain medication

PROGNOSIS
- Good results can be achieved in many ankle fractures without surgery provided there is no disruption of the ankle mortise or the fibulotalar, interosseous, or deltoid ligaments; disruption to any of these structures can limit the function and stability of the ankle (7)[B]:
  – Back to activities, except sports, in 3–4 months

- Long term, 30% of patients may develop ankle arthritis; timing is unpredictable.
- Effusion or pain can persist for up to 1 year.

COMPLICATIONS
- Displace fracture or instability
- Malunion or nonunion
- Skin breakdown or necrosis (early)
- Deep venous thrombosis (DVT)
- Complex regional pain syndrome
- Infection (osteomyelitis)
- Loss of fixation (postop)
- Osteoarthritis (late)

REFERENCES
1. Hermans JJ, Wentink N, Beumer A, et al. Correlation between radiological assessment of acute ankle fractures and syndesmotic injury on MRI. *Skeletal Radiol*. 2012;41(7):787–801. Epub 2011 Oct 20.
2. Strauss EJ, Egol KA. The management of ankle fractures in the elderly. *Injury*. 2007;38(Suppl 3):S2–S9.
3. Polzer H, Kanz KG, Prall WC, et al. Diagnosis and treatment of acute ankle injuries: Development of an evidence-based algorithm. *Orthop Rev (Pavia)*. 2012;4(1):e5. Epub 2011 Dec 14.
4. Gravel J, Hedrei P, Grimard G, et al. Prospective validation and head-to-head comparison of 3 ankle rules in a pediatric population. *Ann Emerg Med*. 2009;54(4):534–540.e1. Epub 2009 Aug 3.
5. Black EM, Antoci V, Lee JT, et al. Role of preoperative computed tomography scans in operative planning for malleolar ankle fractures. *Foot Ankle Int*. 2013;34(5):697–704. Epub 2013 Feb 4.
6. Sanders DW, Tieszer C, Corbett B, et al. Operative versus nonoperative treatment of unstable lateral malleolar fractures: A randomized multicenter trial. *J Orthop Trauma*. 2012;26(3):129–134.
7. Mayer D. The injured ankle and foot. *BMJ*. 2009;339:b2901. Epub 2009 Aug 7.

ADDITIONAL READING
Lin CW, Hiller CE, de Bie RA. Evidence-based treatment for ankle injuries: A clinical perspective. *J Man Manip Ther*. 2010;18(1):22–28.

CODES

ICD10
- S82.891A Oth fracture of right lower leg, init for clos fx
- S82.892A Oth fracture of left lower leg, init for clos fx
- S82.899A Oth fracture of unsp lower leg, init for clos fx

CLINICAL PEARLS
- OAR has nearly 100% sensitivity in determining which adult patients require ankle x-rays.
- Check neurovascular status: Motor/Sensory exam of foot/ankle, check capillary refill, and assess dorsalis pedis and posterior tibial pulses. *If equivocal vascular exam, use Doppler.*
- Distal tibia is most common site of pathologic fracture.

ANKYLOSING SPONDYLITIS

Sangeetha Balasubramanian, MD • Nancy Y. N. Liu, MD

 BASICS

DESCRIPTION

- Ankylosing spondylitis (AS) is a chronic inflammatory seronegative arthritis affecting mainly the axial skeleton and sacroiliac (SI) joints, but hips and shoulders may also be involved.
- System(s) affected: Musculoskeletal; Eyes; Cardiac; Neurologic; Pulmonary
- Synonym(s): Marie-Strümpell disease

EPIDEMIOLOGY

- Predominant age: Onset usually in early 20s; rarely occurs after age 40
- Predominant sex: Male > Female (2–3:1)

Incidence
Age- and gender-adjusted rate of 6.3–7.3/100,000 person-years

Prevalence
~0.1–1% in the US

ETIOLOGY AND PATHOPHYSIOLOGY

- Interaction between genetic factors and unknown trigger(s) – evidence for role of enteric bacteria in trigger (1)
- Inflammation at the insertion of tendons (enthesitis), ligaments, and fasciae to bone, causing inflammation, erosion, and new bone formation

Genetics
About 90–95% of Caucasian patients with AS are HLA-B27–positive.

RISK FACTORS

- HLA-B27:
  - However, only 1–8% of HLA-B27–positive adults have AS
- Positive family history:
  - A HLA-B27–positive child of a parent with AS has a 10–30% risk of developing the disease.

COMMONLY ASSOCIATED CONDITIONS

- Uveitis/Iritis (up to 40%)
- Aortitis
- Cardiac conduction defects
- Spondylitis and sacroiliitis also seen in psoriatic arthritis, reactive arthritis, and arthropathy associated with inflammatory bowel disease

 DIAGNOSIS

HISTORY

- Insidious onset of back pain
- Duration >3 months
- Morning stiffness in spine lasting >1 hour
- Frequent awakenings at night secondary to back pain
- Increased pain and stiffness with rest and improvement with activity
- Alternating buttock pain is a common symptom.
- Constitutional symptoms (fatigue, weight loss, low-grade fever)

PHYSICAL EXAM

- Sacroiliac joint tenderness, loss of lumbar lordosis, and cervical spine rotation
- Diminished range of motion in the lumbar spine in all 3 planes of motion
- Modified Wright-Schober test for lumbar spine flexion is abnormal or <5 cm:

- Mark the patient's back over the L5 spinous process (or at dimples of Venus) and measure 10 cm above and 5 cm below this point. Have the patient bend
- forward. The normal exam is at least 5 cm of expansion between these 2 marks.
- Thoracocervical kyphosis (rarely occurs before 10 years of symptoms)
- Chest pain with inspiration due to enthesitis at costochondral junction and chest wall expansion
- Measurement of respiratory excursion of chest wall:
  - Normal is >5 cm of maximal respiratory excursion of chest wall measured at fourth intercostal space
  - <2.5 cm is virtually diagnostic of ankylosing spondylitis.
- Aortic regurgitation murmur (1%)
- Acute anterior uveitis (usually unilateral on initial presentation, but can recur on contralateral side)
- Achilles tendonitis
- Plantar fasciitis
- Peripheral oligoarthritis, rare; seen mostly with psoriatic arthropathy, reactive arthritis, and arthropathy associated with inflammatory bowel disease
- Cauda equina syndrome is rare, but well recognized late in the disease.

DIFFERENTIAL DIAGNOSIS

- Osteoarthritis of the axial spine
- Diffuse idiopathic skeletal hypertrophy (DISH)
- Psoriatic arthritis
- Reactive arthritis
- Spondylitis associated with inflammatory bowel disease
- Osteitis condensans illi: Benign sclerotic changes in the iliac portion of the SI joint found in women after pregnancies
- Infectious arthritis or discitis, especially unilateral sacroiliitis: Tuberculosis, brucellosis, bacterial (in IV drug users)

DIAGNOSTIC TESTS & INTERPRETATION
Initial Tests (lab, imaging)

- Since up to 10% of Caucasian population and 4% of African American population are HLA-B27–positive, gene testing is not recommended as part of initial evaluation.
- ESR and C-reactive protein (CRP) may be mildly elevated or normal; if high, correlates poorly with disease activity and prognosis
- Absent rheumatoid factor
- Mild normochromic anemia (15%)
- Synovial fluid: Mild leukocytosis
- SI joints: Preferred position for imaging the SI joints with plain films is oblique projection:
  - X-ray changes may not be apparent for up to 10 years after disease onset. MRI is more sensitive in documenting changes; increased signal from the bone and bone marrow suggests osteitis and edema.
  - Sequential plain radiographic changes with time: Widening, erosions, sclerosis on both sides of joint not extending >1 cm from articular surface and finally ankylosis of sacroiliac joint
- Spine:
  - Early plain radiograph changes include "shiny corners" due to osteitis and sclerosis at site of annulus fibrosus attachments to the corners of vertebral bodies and "squaring" due to erosion and remodeling of vertebral body;

contrast-enhanced MRI imaging is more sensitive in revealing these early changes.
  - Late changes include ossification of annulus fibrosis resulting in bony bridging between vertebral bodies (syndesmophytes) to give the classic "bamboo spine" appearance; ankylosis of apophyseal joints, ossification of spinal ligaments, and/or spondylodiscitis also occurs.
- Peripheral joints:
  - Rare; asymmetric involvement of joints of lower extremities
  - Pericapsular ossification, sclerosis, loss of joint space, and erosions may occur.

Diagnostic Procedures/Other
- ECG: Conduction defects; echocardiogram: Aortic valvular abnormalities
- Dual-energy x-ray absorptiometry scan may reveal osteopenia/osteoporosis.

Test Interpretation
- Erosive changes coupled with new bone formation at the attachment of the tendons and ligaments to the bone, resulting in ossification of periarticular soft tissues
- Synovial hypertrophy and pannus formation, mononuclear cell infiltrate into subsynovium and subchondral bone marrow inflammation in the SI joint with erosions is followed by granulation tissue formation and, finally, obliteration of joint space by fusion of joint and sclerosis of para-articular bone.

 TREATMENT

Aggressive physical therapy, with referral to a physical therapist for daily home exercises, as well as group programs, is the most important nonpharmacologic management.

MEDICATION

- Posture training and range-of-motion exercises for the spine are essential.
- Firm bed; sleep in supine position without a pillow
- Breathing exercises 2–3×/d
- Smoking cessation

First Line
Anti-inflammatory drugs:
- NSAIDs provide rapid and dramatic symptomatic relief, which can be virtually diagnostic of AS. NSAIDs chosen empirically, but most importantly, in high doses. May be disease modifying (2)
- Injection of intra-articular corticosteroids into SI joints and prostheses can provide relief, but systemic corticosteroids are usually ineffective.

Pregnancy Considerations

- Infants exposed to NSAIDs in 1st trimester may have higher incidence of cardiac malformations (3)[A].
- Precautions:
  - All patients on long-term NSAIDs should have their hepatic and renal function monitored.
  - NSAIDs may aggravate peptic ulcer disease or cause gastritis; such patients and all patients >60 years of age should receive prophylactic proton pump inhibitors (PPIs) or misoprostol while on NSAIDs.
  - NSAIDs should be used with caution in patients with a bleeding diathesis or patients receiving anticoagulants.

Second Line
- Disease-modifying agents:
  - Used in those patients who have persistently high disease activity (BASADAI score >4), fail, or become intolerant of NSAIDs
  - Biologic disease-modifying agents: Anti-tumor necrosis factor (TNF)-α-blocking agents that are approved by FDA for AS include etanercept (recombinant TNF receptor fusion protein) (4)[A], infliximab (chimeric monoclonal IgG1 antibody to TNF-α) (5)[A], adalimumab (fully humanized IgG1 monoclonal antibody to TNF-α) (6), and golimumab (human IgG1 kappa monoclonal antibody to TNF-α) (7).
  - The TNF blockers listed above have been shown to effectively reduce the signs and symptoms of the axial component of AS (8)[A]
  - Pamidronate may also help function and decrease disease activity.
  - Nonbiologic disease-modifying antirheumatic drugs, such as methotrexate and sulfasalazine, are ineffective for axial disease; sulfasalazine may be effective for peripheral arthritis (9).
- Precautions:
  - Anti-TNFs increase the risk for serious and even fatal, bacterial, mycobacterial, fungal, opportunistic, and viral infections.
  - It is imperative to screen and treat latent tuberculosis before initiation of treatment.
  - Screening for hepatitis B is also required.
  - Monitoring for reactivation of tuberculosis in all patients and invasive fungal infections, such as histoplasmosis, especially with travel to, or residence in, endemic areas
  - Lymphomas, nonmelanoma skin cancers, and other malignancies have been reported in patients receiving anti-TNFs.
  - Immunizations (especially live vaccines) should be updated before initiation of anti-TNFs since live vaccines are contraindicated once patients receive anti-TNFs.

ISSUES FOR REFERRAL
Management of aortic regurgitation, uveitis, spinal fractures, pulmonary fibrosis, hip joint involvement, renal amyloidosis, and, cauda equina syndrome may require referral to appropriate specialty.

ADDITIONAL THERAPIES
- May need treatment with antiresorptive medications if osteopenia or osteoporosis is present
- Monitoring and management of cardiovascular risk factors and comorbidities

SURGERY/OTHER PROCEDURES
- Crucial to evaluate for C-spine ankylosis/instability before intubation
- Total hip replacement should be considered to restore mobility and to control pain.
- Vertebral osteotomy can improve posture for those patients with severe cervical or thoracolumbar flexion.

 ONGOING CARE

FOLLOW-UP RECOMMENDATIONS
- Maintaining physical activity and posture is critical in preventing disability.
- Swimming, tai chi, walking, and maintenance of active lifestyle are recommended.
- Avoid trauma/contact sports.
- Appropriate work ergonomics

Patient Monitoring
- Visits every 6–12 months to monitor posture and range of motion
- Counsel about risk of spinal fracture.

PATIENT EDUCATION
- Arthritis Foundation: http://www.arthritis.org
- Spondylitis Association of America: http://www.spondylitis.org

PROGNOSIS
- Extent and rapidity of progression of ankylosis are highly variable.
- Progressive limitation of spinal mobility necessitates lifestyle modification.

COMPLICATIONS
- Spine:
  - Spinal fusion causing kyphosis
  - Cervical spine fracture carries high mortality rate; fracture can occur at any level of ankylosed spine.
  - C1–C2 subluxation
  - Cauda equina syndrome (rare)
- Pulmonary:
  - Restrictive lung disease
  - Upper lobe fibrosis (rare)
- Cardiac:
  - Conduction defects at atrioventricular (AV) node
  - Aortic insufficiency
  - Aortitis
  - Pericarditis (extremely rare)
- Uveitis and cataracts
- Renal:
  - IgA nephropathy
  - Amyloidosis (<1%)
- GI: Microscopic, subclinical ileal, and colonic mucosal ulcerations in up to 50% of patients, mostly asymptomatic

REFERENCES
1. Syrbe U, Scheer R, Wu P, et al. Differential synovial Th1 cell reactivity towards *Escherichia coli* antigens in patients with ankylosing spondylitis and rheumatoid arthritis. *Ann Rheum Dis*. 2012;71:1573–1576.
2. Kroon F, Landewé R, Dougados M, et al. Continuous NSAID use reverts the effects of inflammation on radiographic progression in patients with ankylosing spondylitis. *Ann Rheum Dis*. 2012;71:1623–1629.
3. Adams K, Bombardier C, van der Heijde DM. Safety of pain therapy during pregnancy and lactation in patients with inflammatory arthritis: A systematic literature review. *J Rheumatol Suppl*. 2012;90:59–61.
4. Davis JC, van der Heijde DM, Braun J. Sustained durability and tolerability of etanercept in ankylosing spondylitis for 96 weeks. *Ann Rheum Dis*. 2005;64:1557–1562.
5. Baraliakos X, Braun J, et al. Continuous long-term anti-TNF therapy does not lead to an increase in the rate of new bone formation over 8 years in patients with ankylosing spondylitis. *Ann Rheum Dis*. 2012;71:1623–1629.
6. Haibel H, Rudwaleit M, Brandt HC. Adalimumab reduces spinal symptoms in active ankylosing spondylitis: Clinical and magnetic resonance imaging results of a fifty-two-week open-label trial. *Arthritis Rheum*. 2006;54:678–681.
7. Inman RD, Davis JC, Heijde DV. Efficacy and safety of golimumab in patients with ankylosing spondylitis: Results of a randomized, double-blind, placebo-controlled, phase III trial. *Arthritis Rheum*. 2008;58:3402–3412.
8. Machado MA, Barbosa MM, Almeida AM, et al. Treatment of ankylosing spondylitis with TNF blockers: a meta-analysis. *Rheumatol Int*. 2013 May 18. Epub ahead of print.
9. Braun J, Zochling J, Baraliakos X, et al. Efficacy of sulfasalazine in patients with inflammatory back pain due to undifferentiated spondyloarthritis and early ankylosing spondylitis: A multicentre randomised controlled trial. *Ann Rheum Dis*. 2006;65:1147–1153.
10. Sieper J, Rudwaleit M. Early referral recommendations for ankylosing spondylitis (including pre-radiographic and radiographic forms) in primary care. *Ann Rheum Dis*. 2005;64:659–663.

ADDITIONAL READING
- Gaujoux-Viala C, Fautrel B. Cost effectiveness of therapeutic interventions in ankylosing spondylitis: A critical and systematic review. *Pharmacoeconomics*. 2012;30(12):1145–1156.
- Ozgocmen S, Akgul O, Altay Z, et al. Expert opinion and key recommendations for the physical therapy and rehabilitation of patients with ankylosing spondylitis. *Int J Rheum Dis*. 2012;15(3):229–238. Epub 2011 Dec 12.

 SEE ALSO

Arthritis, Psoriatic; Arthritis, Rheumatoid (RA); Crohn Disease; Reiter Syndrome; Ulcerative Colitis

 CODES

ICD10
- M45.0 Ankylosing spondylitis of multiple sites in spine
- M45.8 Ankylosing spondylitis sacral and sacrococcygeal region
- M45.9 Ankylosing spondylitis of unspecified sites in spine

CLINICAL PEARLS
- HLA-B27 antigen exists in 8–10% of Caucasians and 4% of African Americans in the general US population.
- Diagnosis is based on history of inflammatory back pain and morning stiffness for >1 hour, alternating buttock pain, and evidence of limitation of chest wall expansion and spinal movements in all planes; evidence of sacroiliitis and response to NSAIDs (10).
- HLA-B27 testing is an expensive and unnecessary test when clinical diagnosis is clear, but it may help support the diagnosis when clinical features are less definitive.
- Plain radiography may fail to reveal changes of sacroiliitis or axial changes for up to 10 years.
- MRI is sensitive for detecting early changes of sacroiliitis or enthesitis in the axial spine.
- Physical therapy to maintain posture and mobility remains the most important nonpharmacologic intervention.
- NSAIDs and TNF-α blockers are the mainstay of treatment and improve symptoms and function, but unfortunately, no current evidence indicates that the latter treatment prevents progressive bony ankylosis.

ANORECTAL FISTULA

Nihal Patel, MD • David Greenwald, MD

 BASICS

DESCRIPTION
- An anorectal fistula is a connection between an anal abscess and the perirectal skin.
- Most commonly, anorectal fistulas form due to rupture or drainage of an anorectal abscess at the level of the anal crypt glands.
- The classification of fistulas is crucial in devising a treatment plan and understanding the severity.
- Five categories exist:
  – Submucosal or superficial: The fistula tracks beneath the submucosa and does not involve the sphincter mechanism (not classified under original Parks' classification)
  – Intersphincteric: The fistula travels along the intersphincteric plane (Parks' type 1)
  – Transsphincteric: The fistula transverses through both the internal and external sphincter muscles (type 2).
  – Suprasphincteric: The fistula originates at the dentate line but loops over the external sphincter, terminating in the ischiorectal fossa (type 3)
  – Extrasphincteric (rare): The fistula is very high in the anal canal, proximal to dentate line, does not involve sphincter complex (type 4)
- Fistulas can be further classified as low or high:
  – Low fistulas involve only the outer or distal 1/3 of the external sphincter muscle.
  – High fistulas have greater involvement of the external sphincter muscle.
- Fistulas may be simple or complex:
  – Simple fistulas are low and include superficial, intersphincteric, or low transsphincteric fistulas. They also involve only 1 communicating tract and are not associated with inflammatory bowel disease (IBD) or with any other organs such as the bladder.
  – Complex fistulas are high fistulas, may have multiple tracts, involve other organs, be recurrent, or be associated with IBD or radiation
  – System(s) affected: Gastrointestinal; Skin/Exocrine
  – Synonym(s): Fistula-in-ano; Anal fistula

EPIDEMIOLOGY
- True prevalence is unknown because anorectal pain is commonly attributed to symptomatic hemorrhoids
- Mean age of presentation for anal abscess and fistula is 40 years (range 20–60)
- Predominant sex: Males twice as likely to develop an abscess and/or fistula compared with females
- Lifetime risk of developing fistula in Crohn disease patients is 20–40%

ETIOLOGY AND PATHOPHYSIOLOGY
- An infection in the anal crypt glands occurs due to an obstruction with inspissated debris and results in suppuration and abscess formation along the path of least resistance in the perianal and perirectal spaces (cryptoglandular theory)
- Rupture or drainage of this anorectal abscess leads to an epithelialized track or fistula formation in ∼1/3 of patients
- Other causes for fistulas include IBD such as Crohn disease
- Radiation proctitis in patients undergoing pelvic radiation can also predispose patients to fistula formation.

- Immunocompromised patients can rarely develop primary perianal actinomycosis, which can cause fistula-in-ano.
- Anorectal mucosal laceration due to rectal foreign bodies can result in abscess and fistula formation. Rarely, retained rectal foreign bodies can cause anorectal fistulas.

RISK FACTORS
- Inflammatory bowel disease (Crohn disease)
- Pelvic radiation
- Trauma via rectal foreign bodies
- Previous anorectal abscess
- Pelvic carcinoma or lymphoma
- Ruptured anal hematoma
- Abscess formation due to acute appendicitis, salpingitis or diverticulitis
- Tuberculosis (rare)
- Syphilis
- Lymphogranuloma venereum (chronic infection with chlamydia trachomatis causing inflammatory perirectal masses with possible fistula formation)
- Immunocompromised state (actinomycosis)

GENERAL PREVENTION
Prevention or prompt treatment of anorectal abscess. Management of commonly associated conditions or risk factors.

COMMONLY ASSOCIATED CONDITIONS
- Anorectal abscess
- IBD (Crohn)

 DIAGNOSIS

HISTORY
- Diagnosis based on perianal pain, perianal purulent drainage, and perirectal skin lesions
- Intermittent rectal pain, worse with defecation or sitting may also be described
- Perianal drainage may be malodorous and may be accompanied by pruritus

PHYSICAL EXAM
- Excoriations or inflammation around perianal skin
- Perineal or perianal external orifice may be palpated or visualized or may exist as an induration if opening is incomplete or blind.
- Anoscopy may reveal an internal opening in anus
- Anorectal abscess may be felt as an indurated or fluctuant tender perianal mass or small tender palpable lesion felt on rectal exam at level of anal crypt
- Fever most common with abscesses, generally not common with fistulas:
  – Goodsall rule is commonly cited to assist in determining course of the fistula tract (not always accurate but more predictive with posterior external anal openings):
    ○ If external opening is *anterior* to an imaginary line drawn transversely through anal canal, fistula usually runs directly (radially) into anal canal.
    ○ If external opening is within 3 cm of anal verge and *posterior* to line, fistula leads to a curved tract, with an internal opening in posterior commissure (except for a long anterior fistula)
    ○ In children, tract is usually straight.

DIFFERENTIAL DIAGNOSIS
- Pilonidal sinus
- Hidradenitis suppurativa
- Anal fissure, ulcer, or sores
- Infected inclusion cyst
- Urethroperineal fistulas
- Ischiorectal or high muscular abscess
- Rule out: Crohn disease, carcinoma, lymphoma, tuberculosis, chronic chlamydia trachomatis infection, actinomycosis in immunocompromised, acute untreated pelvic inflammatory condition

DIAGNOSTIC TESTS & INTERPRETATION
Initial Tests (lab, imaging)
- Imaging studies are crucial in accurate assessment of perianal anatomy
- MRI and endoscopic ultrasound are preferred imaging tests in the evaluation of perianal fistulas
- MRI has ∼80–90% overall concordance with surgical examination under anesthesia, accuracy improves with dedicated pelvic MRI coils to allow better spatial resolution in the pelvis.
- Angulation of fistula from internal opening on MRI correlates with the type of fistula (acute angle likely high transsphincteric; obtuse angle likely lower fistula) (1)
- Fistulography (insertion of catheter into external opening of fistula and injection of radiographic contrast material) is *not* preferred and generally not accurate when evaluating perianal disease.
- Fistulography is reserved for patients who may have a fistula between the rectum and another organ (such as bladder).
- CT is limited in evaluating perianal fistula tracts; more helpful when looking for large perianal abscesses and inflammation

Follow-Up Tests & Special Considerations
- Can consider testing to rule out inflammatory bowel disease (Crohn disease) if suspected
- Consider testing for syphilis for recurrent fistulas in sexually active patients.

Diagnostic Procedures/Other
- Anoscopy or sigmoidoscopy
- Colonoscopy and esophagogastroduodenoscopy if Crohn disease suspected
- Probing into the tract may be done under anesthesia prior to surgery to determine course of fistula
- Injection of dilute methylene blue or hydrogen peroxide intraoperatively may be helpful in identifying internal opening

TREATMENT

GENERAL MEASURES
- Surgical treatment is the mainstay of therapy
- Optimal surgical treatment based on correctly classifying the fistula
- Goals of treatment include resolving the inflammatory process, maintaining continence and preventing future recurrence
- Sitz baths 3–4 times per day until definitive surgery

MEDICATION
- Medical management with antibiotics and immunosuppressive agents plays a role in the treatment of fistulas due to Crohn disease, particularly if patients are minimally symptomatic.
- Studies have shown improvement (reduced pain, discharge, and induration) and healing in up to 80% of patients with 8 weeks of treatment using oral metronidazole (1)
- Use of infliximab has also been shown to be effective in healing perianal Crohn's fistulas but has been associated with a high rate of recurrence (1)
- Antibiotics may be indicated if patients have signs of sepsis or an active infection with a concurrent anorectal abscess
- Surgery may be reserved for Crohn's patients who fail long-term medical therapy

SURGERY/OTHER PROCEDURES
- Choice of surgical procedure is a balance between achieving cure without recurrence or persistence of the fistula, but at the cost of fecal incontinence with use of more aggressive interventions
- Low transsphincteric and intersphincteric simple fistulas can be treated with simple fistulotomy or fibrin sealant (fistula plug)
- Fistula plugs can be used as initial treatment for high transsphincteric fistulas. If the fistula recurs, then an advancement flap may be performed.
- Complex fistulas should be treated with an endorectal advancement flap, which involves closing off the internal opening of the fistula with a mobilized flap of healthy mucosal and submucosal tissue.
- Fistulotomy involves laying open the entire fistula tract in its entirety (unroofing) (2)
  - Fistula tract is cauterized or curetted and tract is marsupialized with absorbable stitch to promote healing
  - Lower rate of recurrence compared to incision and drainage alone
  - Fistulotomy for treatment of simple fistulas results in incontinence in about 12% of patients, compared with almost 50% of patients with complex fistulas (2)
- Setons may be placed for complex fistulas treated with fistulotomy, including those that involve >30% of the external sphincter, are proximal to the dentate line, or are categorized as high transsphincteric fistulas

- A seton is a reactive suture or elastic that is used for drainage (noncutting seton) or to allow scarring of the tract (cutting seton). Cutting setons are tightened at regular intervals to allow slow cutting through the tract and causing scarring.
- Postoperative: Patients discharged on day of procedure. Sitz baths several times per day (sit in warm bath 20 minutes 3–4 times per day and after bowel movements)
- Aggressive bowel regimen to prevent constipation
- Patients undergoing anal fistulotomy may benefit postoperatively from the use of topical application of sucralfate (3)[A].

ONGOING CARE

FOLLOW-UP RECOMMENDATIONS
Resumption of activity as tolerated after surgery

Patient Monitoring
Anoscopy at 3–6 months following procedure. Frequent follow up to ensure complete healing and assess continence.

DIET
High fiber diet

PROGNOSIS
- Postoperative healing:
  - 4–5 weeks for perianal fistulas
  - 12–16 weeks for deeper fistulas
  - Postoperative healing may occur within 2–3 weeks in children.
  - Healing may be significantly delayed in patients with Crohn disease

COMPLICATIONS
- Fecal incontinence
- Constipation
- Rectovaginal fistula
- Delayed wound healing
- Low-grade carcinoma may develop in long-standing fistulas
- Recurrent anorectal fistula if fistula is incompletely treated

REFERENCES

1. Rizzo JA, Naig LA, Johnson EK. Anorectal abscess and fistula-in-ano: Evidence-based management. *Surg Clin North Am*. 2010;90:45–68.
2. Whiteford MH, Kilkenny J, Hyman N, et al. Practice parameters for the treatment of perianal abscess and fistula-in-ano (revised). *Dis Colon Rectum*. 2005;48:1337–1342.
3. Gupta PJ, Heda PS, Shrirao SA, et al. Topical sucralfate treatment of anal fistulotomy wounds: a randomized placebo-controlled trial. *Dis Colon Rectum*. 2011;54:699–704.

ADDITIONAL READING

- A ba-bai-ke-re MM, Wen H, Huang HG, et al. Randomized controlled trial of minimally invasive surgery using acellular dermal matrix for complex anorectal fistula. *World J Gastroenterol*. 2010;16: 3279–3286.
- Cirocchi R, Farinella E, La Mura F, et al. Fibrin glue in the treatment of anal fistula: A systematic review. *Ann Surg Innov Res*. 2009;3:12.
- Jacob TJ, Perakath B, Keighley MR. Surgical intervention for anorectal fistula. *Sao Paulo Med J*. 2011;129:120–121.
- Lewis RT, Maron DJ. Anorectal Crohn's disease. *Surg Clin North Am*. 2010;90:83–97.
- Malik AI, Nelson RL. Surgical management of anal fistulae: A systematic review. *Colorectal Dis*. 2008; 10:420–430.
- Mishra A, Shah S, Nar AS, et al. The role of fibrin glue in the treatment of high and low fistulas in ano. *J Clin Diagn Res*. 2013;7:876–879.
- Niyogi A, Agarwal T, Broadhurst J, et al. Management of perianal abscess and fistula-in-ano in children. *Eur J Pediatr Surg*. 2010;20:35–39.

SEE ALSO

Anorectal Abscess; Crohn's Disease

CODES

ICD10
- K60.3 Anal fistula
- K60.4 Rectal fistula
- K60.5 Anorectal fistula

CLINICAL PEARLS

- Suspect anorectal fistula when a patient complains of perianal pain, perianal purulent drainage, and perirectal skin lesions.
- Surgery is the mainstay of treatment unless patients have fistulas related to Crohn's disease.
- MRI or endoscopic ultrasound are the imaging modalities of choice for evaluating anorectal fistulas.

ANOREXIA NERVOSA
Umer Farooq, MD, MBBS • Najm Hasan Siddiqui, MD

BASICS

DESCRIPTION
- Refusal to maintain normal body weight (less than 85% of expected), with associated fear of weight gain, body-image disturbance, and amenorrhea (At least 3 consecutive cycles)
- *Diagnostic and Statistical Manual of Mental Disorders, Fourth Edition,divides anorexia in to 2 types*
  - Restricting type: Not engaged in binge eating or purging behaviors
  - Binge eating/purging type: Regularly engages in binge eating or purging behaviors (see bulimia information related to these behaviors)
- System(s) affected: Cardiovascular; Endocrine; Metabolic; Gastrointestinal; Nervous; Reproductive

EPIDEMIOLOGY
- Predominant age: 13–20 years
- Predominant sex: Female > Male (10–20 times more common in females)
- Global distribution

Incidence
8–19 women/2 men per 100,000 per year

Prevalence
- 0.9% in women
- 0.3% in men (higher in gay and bisexual men)

ETIOLOGY AND PATHOPHYSIOLOGY
- Complex relationship among genetic, biological, environmental, psychological, and social factors that results in an unrealistic perception of fatness
- Subsequent malnutrition leads to disorder of multiple organs
- Serotonin, norepnephrine and dopamine neuronal systems are implicated.

Genetics
- Underlying genetic vulnerability likely but not well understood, some evidence of higher concordance rates in monozygotic twins than in dizygotic
- 1st-degree female relative with eating disorder increases risk 6–10-fold.

RISK FACTORS
- Female gender
- Adolescence
- Body dissatisfaction
- Perfectionism
- Negative self-evaluation
- Academic and other achievement pressure
- Severe life stressors
- Participation in sports or artistic activities that emphasize leanness or involve subjective scoring: Ballet, running, wrestling, figure skating, gymnastics, cheerleading, weight lifting
- Type I diabetes mellitus
- Family history of substance abuse, affective disorders, or eating disorder

GENERAL PREVENTION
Prevention programs can reduce risk factors and future onset of eating disorders (1)[C]:
- Target adolescents and young women 15 years of age or older.
- Encourage realistic and healthy weight-management strategies and attitudes.
- Decrease body dissatisfaction.

- Promote self-esteem.
- Reduce focus on thin as ideal.
- Moderate overly high self-expectations.
- Decrease anxiety/depressive symptoms and improve stress management.

COMMONLY ASSOCIATED CONDITIONS
- Mood disorder (Major depression)
- Social phobia, obsessive–compulsive disorder
- Substance abuse disorder
- High rates of cluster C personality disorders

DIAGNOSIS

HISTORY
- Patient unlikely to self-identify problem (lack of insight in to the illness), corroborate with family
- Fear of weight gain and/or distorted body image
- Report feeling fat even when emaciated
- Preoccupation with body size, weight control
- Onset may be insidious or stress-related.
- Elaborate food preparation and eating rituals
- Extensive exercise
- Amenorrhea (primary or secondary)
- Weakness, fatigue, cognitive impairment
- Cold intolerance
- Constipation, bloating, early satiety
- Growth arrest, delayed puberty
- History of fractures (decreased bone density)

PHYSICAL EXAM
- May be normal
- Vital signs: Hypothermia, bradycardia, orthostatic hypotension, body weight <85% of expected
- Cardiac: Dysrhythmias, midsystolic click of mitral valve prolapse
- Skin/Extremities: Dry skin; lanugo hair on extremities, face, and trunk; hair loss; edema
- Neurologic and abdominal exams: To rule out other causes of weight loss and vomiting

DIFFERENTIAL DIAGNOSIS
- Hyperthyroidism, adrenal insufficiency
- Inflammatory bowel disease, malabsorption
- Immunodeficiency, chronic infections
- Diabetes
- CNS lesion
- Bulimia; body dysmorphic disorder
- Depressive disorders with loss of appetite
- Anxiety disorder, food phobia
- Conversion disorder

DIAGNOSTIC TESTS & INTERPRETATION
- No specific test for anorexia nervosa (AN)
- Diagnosis based upon "Diagnostic and Statistical Manual of Mental Disorder" criteria (see description for Summary of criteria)
- Most findings are related directly to starvation and/or dehydration.
- All findings may be within normal limits.
- Psychological self-report screening tools:
  - Eating Attitudes Test
  - Eating Disorder Inventory
  - Eating Disorder Screen for Primary Care
  - SCOFF (Sick, Control, One, Fat, Food) Questionnaire

Initial Tests (lab, imaging)
- CBC: Anemia, leukopenia, thrombocytopenia
- Low serum luteinizing hormone, follicle-stimulating hormone; low serum testosterone in men
- Thyroid function tests: Low thyroid-stimulating hormone with normal T_3/T_4
- Liver function tests: Abnormal liver enzymes
- Chem 7: Altered BUN, creatinine clearance; electrolyte disturbances
- Hypoglycemia, hypercholesterolemia, hypercortisolemia, hypophosphatemia
- Low sedimentation rate
- 12-lead electrocardiogram to assess for prolonged QT interval
- Dual-energy x-ray absorptiometry of bone to assess for diminished bone density, only if underweight for >6 months

Test Interpretation
- Osteoporosis/Osteopenia, pathologic fractures
- Sick euthyroid syndrome
- Cardiac impairment

ALERT
AN may exist concurrently with chronic medical disorders such as diabetes and cystic fibrosis.

TREATMENT

GENERAL MEASURES
- Initial treatment goal geared to weight restoration; most managed as outpatients
- Outpatient treatment:
  - Interdisciplinary team (primary care physician, mental health provider, nutritionist) (2,3)[C]
  - Average weekly weight gain goal: 0.5–1.0 kg (2,3)[C], with stepwise increase in calories
  - Cognitive-behavioral therapy, interpersonal psychotherapy, family-based therapy (2,4,5,6)[B]
  - Focus on health, not weight gain alone.
  - Build trust and a treatment alliance.
  - Involve the patient in establishing diet and exercise goals.
  - Challenge fear of uncontrolled weight gain; help the patient to recognize feelings that lead to disordered eating.
  - In chronic cases, goal may be to achieve a safe weight rather than a healthy weight.
- Inpatient treatment:
  - If possible, admit to a specialized eating disorders unit (3)[C].
  - Assess risk for refeeding syndrome (weight loss >10% in 2–3 months; current weight <70% ideal body weight).
  - Monitor vital signs, electrolytes, cardiac function, edema, and weight gain.
  - Initial supervised meals may be necessary.
  - Stepwise increase in activity
  - Tube feeding or total parenteral nutrition is used only as a last resort.
  - Supportive symptomatic care as needed
- Most patients should be treated as outpatients using an interdisciplinary team (2,3)[C].
- Behavioral therapies (e.g., cognitive-behavioral, interpersonal, or family therapy) should be offered (2,4,5,6)[B].
- Pharmacotherapy should not be used as the sole treatment modality (2,3,7)[C].

MEDICATION

First Line

- No medications are available that effectively treat patients with AN, but pharmacotherapy may be used as an adjuvant to cognitive-behavioral therapies (2,3,6,7)[C].
- SSRIs may:
  - Help to prevent relapse after weight gain
  - Treat co morbid depression or obsessive–compulsive disorder (2,3,6,7)[C]
  - Use of atypical antipsychotics is being studied with mixed findings to date. Olanzapine potentially beneficial as an adjuvant treatment of underweight individuals in the inpatient settings.
- Attend to black-box warnings concerning antidepressants

Second Line

- Management of osteopenia:
  - Primary treatment is weight gain (3)[C].
  - Elemental calcium 1,200–1,500 mg/d plus multiple vitamin injection containing 800 IU of vitamin D (3)[C]
  - No indication for bisphosphonates in AN (3)[C]
  - Weak evidence for use of hormone-replacement therapy (3)[C]
- Psyllium (Metamucil) preparations (1 T) to prevent constipation

ISSUES FOR REFERRAL

Patients with AN require an interdisciplinary team (primary care physician, mental health provider, nutritionist). An important step in management is to arrange OP mental health therapist.

IN-PATIENT CONSIDERATIONS

Admission Criteria/Initial Stabilization

- Suggested physiologic values: Heart rate, <40 beats/min; BP, <90/60 mm Hg; symptomatic hypoglycemia; potassium, <3 mmol/L; temperature, <97.0°F (36.1°C); dehydration; other cardiovascular abnormalities; weight, <75% of expected; rapid weight loss; lack of improvement while in outpatient therapy
- Suggested psychological indications: Poor motivation/insight, lack of cooperation with outpatient treatment, inability to eat, need for nasogastric feeding, suicidal intent or plan, severe coexisting psychiatric disease, problematic family environment

Pediatric Considerations

- Children often present with nausea, abdominal pain, fullness, and inability to swallow.
- Additional indications for hospitalization: Heart rate, <50 beats/min; orthostatic BP; hypokalemia or hypophosphatemia; rapid weight loss even if weight not <75% below normal
- Children and adolescents should be offered family-based treatment (5)[C].

Geriatric Considerations

Late-onset AN (>50 years of age) may be long-term disease or triggered by death of loved one, marital discord, or divorce.

Discharge Criteria

Discharge when medically stable. Arrange OP appointment with mental health provider and primary care provider

 ONGOING CARE

FOLLOW-UP RECOMMENDATIONS

- Close follow-up until patient demonstrates forward progress in care plan
- Family and individual therapy extremely important for the long-term benefits/outcomes.
- CBT is very helpful for the treatment of AN, and may be helpful for the prevention of relapse (8)[C]
- Emphasize importance of moderate activity for health, not thinness.

Patient Monitoring

- Level of exercise activity
- Weigh weekly until stable, then monthly.
- Depression, self-esteem, suicidal ideation

DIET

- Importance of adherence to prescribed diet
- Goal is stabilization at a healthy weight on a balanced diet with a normal eating pattern.

PATIENT EDUCATION

- Provide patients and families with information about the diagnosis and its natural history, health risks, and treatment strategies.
- The National Alliance on Mental Illness: www.nami.org/helpline/anorexia.htm

PROGNOSIS

- Prognosis: ~50% recover, 30% improve, 20% are chronically ill
- Outcomes in men likely better than for women.
- Mortality: 3%
- Suicide is the cause of death in 1 in 5 individuals who die with AN

COMPLICATIONS

- Refeeding syndrome
- Cardiac arrhythmia, cardiac arrest
- Cardiomyopathy, congestive heart failure
- Delayed gastric emptying, necrotizing colitis
- Seizures, Wernicke encephalopathy, peripheral neuropathy, cognitive deficits
- Osteopenia, osteoporosis

Pregnancy Considerations

- Fertility may be affected.
- Behaviors may persist, decrease, or recur during pregnancy and the postpartum interval.
- Increased risk for preterm labor, operative delivery, and infants with low birth weight, anemia; genitourinary infections; and labor induction; should be managed as high risk

REFERENCES

1. Stice E, Shaw H, Marti CN. A meta-analytic review of eating disorder prevention programs: Encouraging findings. *Ann Rev Clin Psychol*. 2007;3:207–231.
2. NICE. *Eating disorders—core interventions in the treatment and management of anorexia nervosa, bulimia nervosa and related eating disorders. NICE Clinical Guideline no 9*. London: NICE, 200.
3. American Psychiatric Association. *Practice Guideline for the Treatment of Patients with Eating Disorders*, 3rd ed. Arlington, VA: American Psychiatric Publishing; 2006.
4. Hay P, Bacaltchuk J, Claudino A, et al. Individual psychotherapy in the outpatient treatment of adults with anorexia. *Cochrane Database Syst Rev*. 2003;(4):CD003909.
5. Fisher CA, Hetrick SE, Rushford N. Family therapy for anorexia nervosa. *Cochrane Database Syst Rev*. 2010;(4):CD004780. Epub 2010 Apr 14.
6. Bulik CM, Berkman ND, Brownley KA, et al. Anorexia nervosa treatment: A systematic review of randomized controlled trials. *Int J Eat Disord*. 2007;40:310–320.
7. Claudino AM, Hay P, Lima MS, et al. Antidepressants for anorexia nervosa. *Cochrane Database Syst Rev*. 2006;(1):CD004365. Epub 2006 Jan 25.
8. Kleifield EI, Wagner S, Halmi KA. Cognitive-behavioral treatment of anorexia nervosa. *Psychiatr Clin North Am*. 1996;19(4):715–737.

ADDITIONAL READING

Dalle Grave R. Eating disorders: progress and challenges. *Eur J Intern Med*. 2011;22:153–160.

 SEE ALSO

- Amenorrhea; Osteoporosis; Bulimia Nervosa
- Algorithm: Weight Loss

 CODES

ICD10

- F50.00 Anorexia nervosa, unspecified
- F50.01 Anorexia nervosa, restricting type
- F50.02 Anorexia nervosa, binge eating/purging type

CLINICAL PEARLS

- "Are you satisfied with your eating patterns?" and/or "Do you worry that you have lost control over how you eat?" may help to screen those with an eating problem.
- Studies have shown patients with AN will not accept medications unless combined with psychotherapy.
- To care for a patient with AN, an interdisciplinary team that includes a medical provider, a dietician, and a behavioral health professional is the most accepted approach.
- Family analysis is necessary for the Pts with AN, to determine what kind of therapy would be most helpful.
- Diagnosis is made by "Diagnostic and Statistical Manual of Mental Disorders" criteria

ANTHRAX

Richard J. Thomas, MD, MPH • Han Q. Bui MD

 BASICS

DESCRIPTION
- Anthrax is a highly infectious disease of animals, especially ruminants (hooved animals such as cows, goats, and sheep) that is caused by the bacteria *Bacillus anthracis*. Cutaneous (95% of US cases), inhalational, and GI forms can be transmitted to humans by contact with the animals or their products (typically hair or hides).
- Synonym(s) for cutaneous anthrax: Charbon; Malignant pustule; Siberian ulcer; Malignant edema; Splenic fever; Milzbrand
- Synonym(s) for inhalational anthrax: Ragpicker disease; Woolsorter disease

EPIDEMIOLOGY
- Total of 235 anthrax cases (224 cutaneous and 11 inhalational) occurred in the US between 1955 and 1994, resulting in 20 fatalities.
- Cutaneous: 95% of cases in the US; cases of cutaneous anthrax without occupational risk should raise concern for bioterrorism:
  - ~5–20% of untreated cases result in death; case fatality rate is <1% with antibiotic therapy.
- GI: Very rare in the US (a few documented cases in the last 50 years):
  - Mortality rate is estimated to be 25–60%.
- Inhalational anthrax is rare in the US; if no occupational exposures to animal hides or products, it should be considered a bioterrorist event in the US until proven otherwise:
  - Death results in 99% of untreated cases and in 45–80% of patients with severe symptoms who are treated in a state-of-the-art medical facility.
  - From October to November 2001, the first 11 cases of intentional inhalational anthrax along with 11 cutaneous cases were caused by bioterrorist releases of *B. anthracis* in the US.
- A new route of anthrax exposure termed "Injectional Anthrax" has occurred over the past several years where *B. anthracis* was a contaminant in the drug injected; >50 recognized cases occurred in the United Kingdom between December 2009 and December 2010, with a 33% case fatality rate.
- Anthrax is most common in agricultural regions, where it occurs in animals. These regions include the Middle East, Asia, Southern and Eastern Europe, Africa, South and Central America, and the Caribbean.

ETIOLOGY AND PATHOPHYSIOLOGY
- *B. anthracis* is a spore-forming, gram-positive bacterium found in the soil worldwide. The word *anthracis* is derived from a Greek word meaning "coal," which is used to describe the cutaneous form of the disease that leads to a characteristic black lesion.
- *B. anthracis* has 3 known virulence factors: An antiphagocytic capsule and 2 protein toxins (known as edema factor and lethal factor):
  - The capsule provides resistance to phagocytosis.
  - Lethal factor and edema factor are named for the effects they induce when injected into experimental animals.
  - A protein called *protective antigen* binds to the host cell's surface; when cleaved by a protease on the cell surface, it creates a site to which the lethal factor and edema factor can bind; protective antigen is required for the action of the 2 protein toxins.

- *B. anthracis* spores introduced into the host are ingested at the exposed site by macrophages and then germinate into vegetative forms that produce the virulence factors.
- Cutaneous: Occurs when *B. anthracis* enters the skin through a cut or abrasion during the handling of animal products (e.g., meat, wool, or hides infected with *B. anthracis*)
- GI: Ingestion of bacillus-contaminated meat
- Inhalational: Inhalation of aerosolized *B. anthracis* spores

RISK FACTORS
- Contact with infected animals or their products
- Drug users
- Bioterrorist event

GENERAL PREVENTION
- Anthrax vaccine protects against all forms of anthrax and is as safe as other vaccines, according to the FDA, CDC, and the National Academy of Sciences.
- A 2009 review by the Cochrane Infectious Disease Group concluded that the anthrax vaccine is effective in reducing the risk of contracting anthrax and has a low rate of adverse effects (1)[A].
- A longitudinal study published in 2012 of United Kingdom military personnel who were offered anthrax vaccination showed no overall adverse health effect from the vaccination in follow-up data ranging from 3–6 years (2)[B].
- Anthrax vaccine should be effective against all known strains of *B. anthracis* as well as against any strains that might be bioengineered by terrorists or others.
- Vaccine schedule and route: Vaccine is given IM in 5 doses at 0, 4 weeks, and 6, 12, and 18 months plus annual boosters. IM vs. SC injection greatly reduces the incidence of injection-site adverse events (3)[A]:
  - Anthrax vaccine adsorbed (trade name BioThrax) is FDA approved for ages 18–65 and is pregnancy Category D.
  - If behind schedule, do not start the series over; begin where left off (delays do not reduce the resulting protection).
  - Individuals are not considered protected until they have completed the full vaccination series.
  - The most common (>10%) local (injection-site) adverse reactions observed in clinical studies were tenderness, pain, erythema, and arm motion limitation. The most common (>5%) systemic adverse reactions were muscle aches, fatigue, and headache.
  - The Advisory Committee on Immunization Practices recommends vaccination for the following groups:
    - Persons who work directly with the organism in the laboratory
    - Persons who work with imported animal hides or furs in areas where standards are insufficient to prevent exposure to anthrax spores
    - Persons who handle potentially infected animal products in high-incidence areas
    - Military personnel deployed to areas with high risk for exposure to organisms (when used as a biologic warfare weapon)
    - Pregnant women should be vaccinated for anthrax only if absolutely necessary.

- Patients with a likely inhalational exposure history, but no symptoms, are candidates for postexposure prophylaxis with either ciprofloxacin 500 mg PO b.i.d. or doxycycline 100 mg PO b.i.d. for 60 days. Levofloxacin is also FDA approved for patients age ≥18. CDC guidelines state patients should also receive 3 doses of anthrax vaccine (0, 2 weeks, 4 weeks), but since BioThrax is not licensed for postexposure prophylaxis or for a 3-dose series, this would need to be conducted under an Investigational New Drug application. Prophylactic medications are not indicated for prevention of cutaneous anthrax.

 DIAGNOSIS

- Cutaneous: Incubation period is usually immediate up to 1 day. Begins as a pruritic spot, followed by a red–brown papule that enlarges with peripheral erythema, vesiculation, and induration, followed by black eschar formation within 7–10 days of the initial lesion:
  - The papule, blister, and eschar are painless, and cutaneous symptoms may be accompanied by fever, malaise, and headache.
  - A black eschar with massive edema is nearly pathognomonic for cutaneous anthrax.
- GI: Incubation period is usually 1–7 days. Presents as 1 of 2 distinct syndromes—oropharyngeal and abdominal:
  - Oropharyngeal syndrome presentation can include fever, edema, ulcer, severe sore throat, and lymphadenopathy, resulting in marked unilateral or bilateral neck swelling.
  - Abdominal syndrome may present with fever, malaise, hematemesis, anorexia, severe abdominal pain, and hematochezia or melena; 2–4 days after onset of symptoms, pain begins to subside and ascites develops, with shock and death within just a few days.
- Inhalational: Incubation period is usually <1 week, but may be up to 60 days. Biphasic presentation, with initial phase featuring nonspecific influenzalike symptoms (e.g., low-grade fever, chills, headache, nonproductive cough, diaphoresis, malaise, chest discomfort, nausea, vomiting, diarrhea, abdominal pain):
  - This initial phase is followed by a 2nd fulminant phase that begins 1–5 days after onset of the initial phase symptoms. Signs and symptoms of the fulminant phase include abrupt onset of high fever, severe dyspnea, hypoxia, hypotension, and death within 24–36 hours.

HISTORY
- Cutaneous: Crucial clinical clues are rapid evolution of symptoms, lack of pain, occasional massive edema, and the near pathognomonic black eschar. Incubation period is usually immediate, but may last up to 1 day.
- GI: Incubation period usually 1–7 days; 2–4 days after onset of symptoms, ascites develops as abdominal pain decreases. Shock and death occur within 2–5 days after onset of symptoms.
- Inhalational: Incubation period is usually <1 week, but may be as long as 2 months. 2nd portion of the biphasic presentation begins 1–5 days after onset of initial symptoms. There may be a 1–3-day period of improvement after the 1st phase and before the 2nd phase begins. Shock and death occur within 24–36 hours after onset of the 2nd phase.

PHYSICAL EXAM
- Cutaneous: Red–brown papule, vesicles, or black eschar
- GI: Acute abdomen with rebound tenderness may occur. Ascites presents later in course.
- Inhalational: Rhonchi may be present.

DIFFERENTIAL DIAGNOSIS
- Skin cellulitis
- Brown recluse spider bite
- Cat-scratch disease
- Rat bite fever
- Rickettsial spotted fever
- Carbuncle
- Cowpox
- Bullous erysipelas
- Tularemia vasculitides
- Ecthyma gangrenosum
- Orf (a transmissible viral disease of goats and sheep)

DIAGNOSTIC TESTS & INTERPRETATION
Initial Tests (lab, imaging)
Gram stain and culture. Obtain specimens for culture before initiating antimicrobial therapy. *B. anthracis* is easily isolated from blood cultures in <24 hours. A presumptive diagnosis can be made if gram-positive rods are present that are nonmotile, nonhemolytic, and encapsulated (usually seen with India ink). If antibiotics have been given for >24 hours, perform immunohistochemical staining and/or polymerase chain reaction (PCR).
- Inhalational: Widened mediastinum on chest x-ray (CXR) may be present; pleural effusions frequently present; infiltrates are rare.
- CXR is indicated for suspected inhalational anthrax (4)[A].
- CT chest for patients with suspected anthrax, but normal CXR (4)[A]
- GI: Mesenteric adenopathy on CT scan is likely.

TREATMENT
GENERAL MEASURES
- Inhalational and GI anthrax are not known to spread from person to person, so communicability concerns are not an issue during treatment of the patient.
- Although cutaneous anthrax is also considered noncontagious, avoidance of contact with the wound or wound drainage seems prudent.

MEDICATION
First Line
- Cutaneous: Ciprofloxacin 500 mg PO b.i.d. or doxycycline 100 mg PO b.i.d. for 7–10 days for localized or uncomplicated cases of naturally acquired cutaneous anthrax. Treat for 7–10 days with IV instead for severe cases of naturally acquired cutaneous anthrax with signs of systemic involvement, extensive edema, or lesions of the head and neck:
  - If cutaneous case is localized or uncomplicated but is bioterrorism-related, patients must be treated for 60 days with PO ciprofloxacin or doxycycline because they are at risk for inhalational anthrax.
  - Patients with bioterrorism-related cutaneous anthrax who show signs of systemic involvement, massive edema, or lesions on the head or neck should be treated per inhalational anthrax recommendation (below) (5,6)[C].

- A shorter course of antibiotics lasting just 3–5 days may be as effective as the standard 7–10-day course in uncomplicated cutaneous anthrax (7)[B].
- Inhalational and GI: IV ciprofloxacin 400 mg q12h (first line) or doxycycline 100 mg q12h (second line) and 1 or 2 additional antimicrobials, such as rifampin, vancomycin, penicillin, ampicillin, chloramphenicol, imipenem, clindamycin, and clarithromycin:
  - May switch to PO when clinically appropriate
  - Must complete 60-day course (combined PO and IV) (5)[C]
  - Early and aggressive pleural fluid drainage is recommended for all cases of inhalational anthrax (6)[C].

Second Line
- Patients being treated for anthrax may also benefit from vaccination as part of their regimen.
- Cethromycin (a new ketolide antibiotic) has an orphan drug designation for anthrax prophylaxis (Mansour)

ONGOING CARE
FOLLOW-UP RECOMMENDATIONS
Patient Monitoring
Patient must be monitored for 60 days to ensure completion of the treatment course.

PROGNOSIS
- Cutaneous: Death in 5–20% of untreated cases, but the case fatality rate is <1% with antibiotic therapy
- GI: Mortality rates as high as 50% reported
- Inhalational: Death in 45–80% of patients with severe symptoms who are treated in a state-of-the-art facility; case fatality rate approaches 99% in untreated cases.

REFERENCES
1. Donegan S, Bellamy R, Gamble CL. Vaccines for preventing anthrax. *Cochrane Database Syst Rev*. 2009;2:CD006403.
2. Murphy D, Marteau TM, Wessely S. A longitudinal study of UK military personnel offered anthrax vaccination: Informed choice, symptom reporting, uptake and pre-vaccination health. *Vaccine*. 2012;30(6):1094–1100. Epub 2011 Dec 16.
3. Wright JG, Quinn CP, Shadomy S, et al. Use of anthrax vaccine in the United States: Recommendations of the Advisory Committee on Immunization Practices (ACIP), 2009. *MMWR Recomm Rep*. 2010;59:1–30.
4. Kirsch J, Ramirez J, Mohammed TL, et al. ACR Appropriateness Criteria® acute respiratory illness in immunocompetent patients. *J Thorac Imaging*. 2011;26:W42–W44.
5. Centers for Disease Control and Prevention. Update: Investigation of bioterrorism-related anthrax and interim guidelines for exposure management and antimicrobial therapy, October 2001. *MMWR Morb Mortal Wkly Rep*. 2001;50:909–919.
6. Stern EJ, Uhde KB, Shadomy SV, et al. Conference report on public health and clinical guidelines for anthrax. *Emerg Infect Dis*. 2008;14.
7. Kayabas U, Karahocagil MK, Ozkurt Z, et al. Naturally occurring cutaneous anthrax: Antibiotic treatment and outcome. *Chemotherapy*. 2012;58(1):34–43. Epub 2012 Feb 10.

ADDITIONAL READING
- Centers for Disease Control and Prevention, Emergency Preparedness and Response. http://www.bt.cdc.gov/agent/anthrax/
- Durning SJ, Roy MJ. Anthrax. In: Roy MJ, ed. *Physician's Guide to Terrorist Attack*. Totowa, NJ: Humana, 2003.
- Jernigan DB, Raghunathan PL, et al. Investigation of Bioterrorism-Related Anthrax, United States 2001; *Epidemiological Findings Emerg Inf Dis*. 2002;8(10): 1019–1028.
- Marano N, Plikaytis BD, Martin SW, et al. Effects of a reduced dose schedule and intramuscular administration of anthrax vaccine adsorbed on immunogenicity and safety at 7 months: A randomized trial. *JAMA*. 2008;300:1532–1543.
- Sweeney DA, Hicks CW, Cui X, et al. Anthrax infection. *Am J Respir Crit Care Med*. 2011;184(12):1333–1341. Epub 2011 Aug 18.
- The anthrax vaccination immunization program. http://www.anthrax.mil
- Mansour H, Chahine EB, Karaoui LR, et al. Cethromycin: A new ketolide antibiotic. *Ann Pharmacother*. 2013;47(3):368–379.

CODES
ICD10
- A22.0 Cutaneous anthrax
- A22.1 Pulmonary anthrax
- A22.9 Anthrax, unspecified

CLINICAL PEARLS
- Anthrax vaccine (only recommended for high-risk groups) protects against all forms of anthrax and is as safe as other vaccines, according to the FDA, CDC, and the National Academy of Sciences.
- Inhalational anthrax is rare in the US; if no occupational exposures to animal hides or products, it should be considered a bioterrorist event even in the US until proven otherwise:
  - Death results in 99% of untreated cases and in 45–80% of patients with severe symptoms who are treated in a state-of-the-art facility.
- Widened mediastinum on CXR may be present; pleural effusions frequently present; infiltrates are rare.
- Early detection and reporting of the potential use of pathogens as bioterrorism agents may be identified by astute clinicians, public health syndromic surveillance, laboratory surveillance reporting, outbreak investigations, and air monitoring pathogen detectors such the US DHS, EPA, & CDC BioWatch program.

ANTIPHOSPHOLIPID ANTIBODY SYNDROME

Tarsheen Kaur Sethi, MD • Elizabeth C. Riley, MD, FACP

 BASICS

DESCRIPTION

Antiphospholipid antibody syndrome (APS) is an autoantibody-mediated thrombophilic disorder characterized by recurrent arterial or venous thrombosis and/or recurrent fetal loss in the presence of antiphospholipid antibodies (APAs) (1). The APAs enhance clot formation by interacting with phospholipid-binding plasma proteins. The resulting APS can cause significant morbidity and mortality in both pregnant and nonpregnant individuals:

- Types of APS (based on clinical presentation):
  - Primary: Occurs without an associated underlying disease
  - Secondary: Associated with autoimmune diseases (systemic lupus erythematosus [SLE] is most common). Transient APAs may be associated with certain infections, drugs, and malignancy.
  - Catastrophic APS (CAPS) a.k.a Asherson syndrome (<1%):
    ○ Most severe form of disease; characterized by thrombotic microangiopathy. It is associated with multiorgan involvement and a high mortality rate if treatment is delayed.
    ○ Severe thrombocytopenia, hemolytic anemia, and DIC may be additional features.
  - Associated clinical features: Livedo reticularis, cardiac valve disease, thrombocytopenia, nephropathy
  - Of note, the 2006 updated criteria recommend that additional risk factors, such as age, atherosclerosis, and inherited thrombophilia, should be used to risk-stratify patients for APS.

Pregnancy Considerations

- Complications include maternal thrombosis (stroke, venous thromboembolism [VTE]) fetal death, pre-eclampsia and placental insufficiency, fetal growth retardation, and preterm birth.
- Low-dose aspirin and low-molecular-weight heparin (LMWH) or unfractionated heparin are the drugs of choice in pregnancy.
- Prophylactic-dose heparin is recommended in the postpartum period (unless patient is on therapeutic anticoagulation) given high risk of thrombosis during this time.

EPIDEMIOLOGY

- The prevalence of APAs increases with age, but is not necessarily associated with a higher risk of thrombosis.
- For APS, Female > Male

Incidence

- In patients with positive APAs without prior risk of thrombosis, the annual incident risk of thrombosis is 0–3.8%. This risk is up to 5.3% in those with triple positivity (anticardiolipin antibodies, lupus anticoagulant, and anti-β2-glycoprotein I antibodies positive).
- 10–15% of recurrent abortions are attributable to APS.

Prevalence

APAs are present in 1–5% of the general population and in ~40% of those with SLE. A higher prevalence is also seen in those with venous thromboembolism and those with stroke.

ETIOLOGY AND PATHOPHYSIOLOGY

- It is now known that the anti-β2-glycoprotein-1 antibodies play a central role in the pathogenesis of APS. The procoagulant effect is mediated by various possible mechanisms:
  - Endothelial effects: Inhibition of prostacyclin production and loss of the annexin V cellular shield.
  - Platelet activation resulting in adhesion and aggregation
  - Interference of innate anticoagulant pathways, such as inhibition of protein C
  - Complement activation
- Pregnancy-related complications are also a result of autoantibody-mediated effects:
  - Interference with expression of trophoblastic adhesion molecules resulting in abnormal placentation
  - Placental thrombosis
- Proposed mechanisms: Excess production of natural antibodies, molecular mimicry due to infections, exposure of phospholipid antigens during platelet activation, cardiolipin peroxidation, and genetic predisposition (2)
- A "second hit" by environmental factors may be required to produce thrombosis.

Genetics

Most cases of APS are acquired. There are a few studies of familial occurrence of anticardiolipin (aCL) antibodies and lupus anticoagulant (LAC). A valine 247/leucine polymorphism in β2-glycoprotein I could be a genetic risk for the presence of anti-β2GPI antibodies and APS.

RISK FACTORS

The following may contribute to a higher risk of thrombosis in these patients:

- Age >55 in males, >65 in females
- Cardiovascular risk factors (hypertension, diabetes, obesity, smoking, combined oral contraceptive use)
- Inherited thrombophilia
- Surgery, immobilization, pregnancy.

GENERAL PREVENTION

Risk factor modification: Control HTN and diabetes; smoking cessation; avoidance of oral contraceptives. Thromboprophylaxis in established cases.

COMMONLY ASSOCIATED CONDITIONS

- Autoimmune diseases: SLE (most common), scleroderma, Sjögren syndrome, dermatomyositis, and rheumatoid arthritis
- Malignancy
- Various infections, including viral, bacterial, parasitic, and rickettsial
- Certain drugs may be associated with APA production without increased risk of thrombosis; these include phenothiazines, hydralazine, procainamide, and phenytoin
- HELLP syndrome (hemolysis, elevated liver enzymes, and low platelet count in association with pregnancy)
- Sneddon syndrome (APS variant syndrome with livedo reticularis, HTN, and stroke)

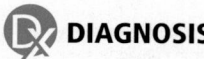 **DIAGNOSIS**

Sapporo criteria, revised 2006 (1)[A]:

- The presence of at least one of the following clinical criteria:
  - Vascular thrombosis:
    ○ ≥1 clinical episodes of arterial, venous, or small vessel thrombosis, occurring within any tissue or organ. Thrombosis should be confirmed by unequivocal imaging studies or histopathology.
  - Complications of pregnancy (any one of the following):
    ○ ≥3 consecutive spontaneous abortions before the 10th week of pregnancy, unexplained by maternal/paternal chromosomal abnormalities or maternal anatomic/hormonal causes
    ○ ≥1 unexplained deaths of morphologically normal fetuses at or after the 10th week of gestation
    ○ ≥1 premature births of morphologically normal newborn babies at or before the 34th week of pregnancy due to severe pre-eclampsia, eclampsia, or placental insufficiency
- *AND* the presence of at least one of the three laboratory findings (confirmed on ≥2 occasions at least 12 weeks apart):
  - Lupus anticoagulant (LAC) detected in blood
  - Anticardiolipin (aCL) IgG and/or IgM antibodies present at moderate or high levels in the blood (>40 GPL or MPL or 99th percentile) via a standardized ELISA.
  - Anti-β2 GP1 IgG and/or IgM antibodies in blood at a titer >99th percentile via a standardized ELISA

HISTORY

- History of VTE or arterial thrombosis (stroke, MI)
- History of fetal loss or other obstetric complications
- Bleeding from thrombocytopenia if severe, or acquired factor II deficiency
- Personal or family history of autoimmune disease

PHYSICAL EXAM

- Signs of venous thrombosis in extremities
- Skin manifestations, including a vasculitic rash in the form of palpable purpura or livedo reticularis or lower-extremity ulcers
- Cardiac murmurs
- Focal neurologic or cognitive deficits

DIFFERENTIAL DIAGNOSIS

- Thrombophilic conditions, such as:
  - Inherited: Deficiency of protein C, protein S, antithrombin III; mutation of factor V Leiden, prothrombin gene mutation
  - Acquired: Neoplastic and myeloproliferative disorders, hyperviscosity syndromes, nephrotic syndrome
- Embolic disease secondary to atrial fibrillation, marked LV dysfunction, endocarditis, cholesterol emboli
- Heparin-induced thrombocytopenia
- Atherosclerosis
- For CAPS: Conditions that cause thrombotic microangiopathy, such as hemolytic-uremic syndrome, TTP, or malignant hypertension

DIAGNOSTIC TESTS & INTERPRETATION

- The recommended tests for diagnosis are the LAC assay, and ELISA for aCL antibodies and anti-β2-GP1 antibodies.
- The LAC assay combines at least 2 out of 3 screening tests (prolongation of aPTT, dilute Russel's viper venom time [dRVVT], and kaolin clotting) followed by 2 confirmatory tests. The latter includes the mixing study (clotting time is not corrected by addition of healthy plasma and thus is due to an inhibitor). The final step demonstrates that the prolongation is phospholipid-dependent (3).
- The anti-β2-GP1 antibodies are important in the pathogenesis of thrombosis. Of note, the positive LAC assay is thought to recognize antibodies against β2-glycoprotein 1 (GP1) and prothrombin.
- The clinical significance of other autoantibodies, including those directed against annexin V, phosphatidylserine, and phosphatidylinositol, remains unclear.

Initial Tests (lab, imaging)

- CBC, PT/INR, aPTT, LAC, anticardiolipin antibodies, anti-β2-GP1 antibodies
- Further testing for secondary causes such as SLE when clinically suspected
- Imaging is based on clinical picture, suspected sites of thrombosis, and organ involvement.

Follow-Up Tests & Special Considerations

- The results of LAC are difficult to interpret in patients treated with warfarin. Unfractionated heparin or LMWH and fondaparinux do not affect the LAC assay.
- Repeat testing at 12 weeks for persistence of antiphospholipid antibodies as noted above.

Diagnostic Procedures/Other

Biopsy of the affected organ system may be necessary to distinguish from vasculitis.

Test Interpretation

Usual finding is thrombosis and minimal vascular or perivascular inflammation:

- Acute changes: Capillary congestion and noninflammatory fibrin thrombi
- Chronic changes: Ischemic hypoperfusion, atrophy, and fibrosis

 ## TREATMENT

Treatment of APS encompasses primary thromboprophylaxis, secondary prevention of clots (secondary thromboprophylaxis), treatment of acute thrombotic microangiopathy and pregnancy-related APS.

MEDICATION

First Line

- Primary thromboprophylaxis: Low-dose aspirin is indicated in asymptomatic carriers of APAs with SLE and in pregnancy. It may be considered in other asymptomatic carriers. Control of vascular factors is an important intervention in all these patients (2)[A].
- Secondary thromboprophylaxis: All symptomatic, nonpregnant patients with definite APS will need indefinite anticoagulation. The goal INR will depend on the severity and type of thrombosis (2)[A]:
  – Venous thrombosis (1st episode): Warfarin for goal INR of 2.0–3.0.
  – Arterial thrombosis or recurrent venous thrombosis despite anticoagulation: Warfarin for goal INR 3.0–4.0.
  – LMWH and fondaparinux are alternatives.

– Prospective treatment considerations: These include new oral anticoagulants such as rivaroxaban and dabigatran; rivaroxaban has recently been approved for treatment of DVT/PE; studies in APS are lacking, a prospective randomized controlled trial of warfarin versus rivaroxaban in patients with thrombotic APS and with a target INR or 2.5 is underway (4). Rituximab may be an option in severe cases (2)[B].

- Newer oral anticoagulants such as dabigatran and rivaroxaban have the potential of being a reliable alternative to warfarin with few drug interactions and obviating the new for frequent monitoring. The presence of APA is known to interfere with hemostatic mechanisms and can modulate the effects of anticoagulants. Ongoing Phase III trials in patients with APS will yield valuable information to help define the role of new oral anticoagulants.
- CAPS: Anticoagulants and high-dose steroids may suffice in less severe cases. However, timely and aggressive treatment with either IVIG or plasmapheresis is often required in this life-threatening condition. These measures have improved survival to 66%.
- Treatment in pregnancy (2)[A]:
  – For women with no prior history of thrombosis and ≥2 early miscarriages, either 81 mg ASA alone or in combination with unfractionated heparin (5,000–10,000 units SC q12h) or LMWH (prophylactic dose). In those with a previous late pregnancy loss (>10 weeks' gestation) or preterm (<34 weeks) delivery due to severe pre-eclampsia, a combination of ASA and heparin is recommended.
  – In those with a history of thrombosis, low-dose ASA plus either therapeutic low-dose heparin (dosed 8–12 hours to maintain mid-interval aPTT or factor Xa levels) or LMWH (therapeutic dose)
  – Refractory cases: Up to 30% of patients have recurrent pregnancy loss despite the use of ASA and heparin. There is no role for warfarin due to risk of teratogenicity (early pregnancy) and fetal bleeding (late pregnancy). Prednisolone has been discarded as a treatment option in the past due to higher risk of complications and uncertain benefit, but a recent study showed benefit with low-dose (10 mg) prednisolone when given in the 1st trimester. Further studies are required to validate this intervention (5)[B]. IV immunoglobulin was found to provide no benefit.

SURGERY/OTHER PROCEDURES

Patients with thrombosis may require thrombectomy or an IVC filter (depending on site) when anticoagulation is contraindicated.

 ## ONGOING CARE

FOLLOW-UP RECOMMENDATIONS

Patient Monitoring

- Standard guidelines for monitoring to maintain INR at goal with warfarin therapy
- Close monitoring is required during pregnancy.

DIET

Atherosclerotic risk factor control with a low-fat and low-sodium diet. Avoid large consumption of vitamin K intake while on warfarin.

PATIENT EDUCATION

- Compliance with warfarin therapy to keep INR at goal.
- Awareness of drug and diet interactions with warfarin.
- Avoid oral hormonal contraceptives.

PROGNOSIS

- Pulmonary HTN, neurologic involvement, myocardial ischemia, nephropathy, gangrene of extremities, and catastrophic APS are associated with a worse prognosis.
- 30% risk of recurrent thrombosis in the absence of adequate anticoagulation

COMPLICATIONS

- In addition to the above-mentioned pregnancy complications, pulmonary HTN is associated with high maternal mortality.
- Thrombotic complications are the most common cause of death.

REFERENCES

1. Miyakis S, Lockshin MD, Atsumi T, et al. International consensus statement on an update of the classification criteria for definite antiphospholipid syndrome (APS). *J Thromb Haemost*. 2006;4:295–306.
2. Ruiz-Irastorza G, Crowther M, Branch W, et al. Antiphospholipid syndrome. *Lancet*. 2010;376: 1498–1509.
3. Giannakopoulos B, Passam F, Ioannou Y, et al. How we diagnose the antiphospholipid syndrome. *Blood*. 2009;113(5):985–994. Epub 2008 Aug 28.
4. Arachchillage DJ, Cohen H. Use of new oral anticoagulants in antiphospholipid syndrome. *Curr Rheumatol Rep*. 2013;15(6):331.
5. Branham K, Thomas M, Nelson-Piery C, et al. First-trimester low-dose prednisolone in refractory antiphospholipid antibody-related pregnancy loss. *Blood*. 2011;117:6948–6951.

ADDITIONAL READING

Baker WF, Bick RL, Fareed J. Controversies and unresolved issues in antiphospholipid syndrome pathogenesis and management. *Hematol Oncol Clin North Am*. 2008;22(1):155–174, viii.

CODES

ICD10

- D68.61 Antiphospholipid syndrome
- D68.62 Lupus anticoagulant syndrome
- D68.69 Other thrombophilia

CLINICAL PEARLS

- APS can be either primary, secondary, or present as a severe microvascular disease known as CAPS.
- Both clinical and laboratory criteria are required for diagnosis. The latter must be confirmed on 2 separate occasions at least 12 weeks apart.
- Thrombotic manifestations of APS can be either venous or arterial and need lifelong anticoagulation.

ANTITHROMBIN DEFICIENCY

Ryan Wargo, PharmD • Patricia Feito, MD • Holly Baab, MD

 BASICS

DESCRIPTION

- Antithrombin is a protease that inhibits thrombin by forming an irreversible thrombin–antithrombin complex.
- There are 2 active sites: One that binds to heparin and one that binds to thrombin/target enzyme. Antithrombin can also inhibit factors Xa, IXa, and XIa. This process is catalyzed by the presence of heparin.
- Patients deficient in antithrombin have an increased incidence of venous thrombosis, including deep vein thrombosis (DVT) of the lower extremity. Arterial thrombosis is much less common in patients deficient in antithrombin.
- System(s) affected: Cardiovascular; Nervous; Pulmonary; Reproductive; Hematologic; Lymphatic/Immunologic Hemic/Lymphatic/ Immunologic
- Synonym(s): Antithrombin III deficiency

EPIDEMIOLOGY

- Predominant age: Mean age of 1st thrombosis is in 2nd decade, usually after puberty
- Predominant sex: Male = Female
- No racial or ethnic predisposition

Incidence

4% of patients with thrombophilia

Prevalence

0.16% of normal individuals

ETIOLOGY AND PATHOPHYSIOLOGY

- Hereditary deficiency:
  – Type I deficiency is characterized by low levels of antigen (decreased synthesis). Plasma levels of antithrombin are often <50%.
  – Type II deficiency is found when the antithrombin molecule is dysfunctional (decreased function).
  – Type II deficiencies are due to mutations in either the active center of antithrombin that binds the target enzyme or the heparin-binding site.
  – No patients homozygous for defects in the active center have been described, suggesting that this is a lethal condition. Patients heterozygous for mutations in the heparin-binding site rarely have thrombotic episodes.
- Acquired deficiency:
  – Many clinical conditions are associated with antithrombin deficiency, such as those listed under special considerations, but limited evidence suggests these deficiencies contribute to increased thrombosis.

Genetics

Autosomal dominant

RISK FACTORS

- Oral contraceptives, pregnancy, and the use of hormone replacement therapy (HRT) increase the risk of venous thrombosis in patients with antithrombin deficiency.
- Patients with antithrombin deficiency and another prothrombotic state, such as factor V Leiden or the prothrombin G20210A mutation, have increased rates of thrombosis.
- Heterozygotes have an odds ratio of venous thrombosis of 10–20.

Pregnancy Considerations

Increases thrombotic risk in patients with antithrombin deficiency and specific complications may include: Pre-eclampsia, eclampsia, placental abruption, HELLP, premature birth and recurrent pregnancy loss.

GENERAL PREVENTION

Patients with antithrombin deficiency without a history of thrombosis do not require prophylactic treatment.

COMMONLY ASSOCIATED CONDITIONS

Venous thromboembolism

 DIAGNOSIS

HISTORY

- Previous thrombosis
- Family history of thrombosis
- Family history of antithrombin deficiency

PHYSICAL EXAM

Signs consistent with a deep or superficial venous thrombosis or pulmonary embolism

DIFFERENTIAL DIAGNOSIS

- Factor V Leiden
- Protein C deficiency
- Protein S deficiency
- Dysfibrinogenemia
- Dysplasminogenemia
- Homocystinemia
- Prothrombin G20210A mutation
- Elevated factor VIII levels

DIAGNOSTIC TESTS & INTERPRETATION
Initial Tests (lab, imaging)

- For evaluation of a new clot in a patient at risk: CBC with peripheral smear, PT/INR, aPTT, thrombin time, lupus anticoagulant, antiphospholipid antibodies, factor VIII, anticardiolipin antibody, anti-B2 glycoprotein I antibody, activated protein C resistance, protein S antigen and resistance, antithrombin III assay, fibrinogen, factor V Leiden, prothrombin G20210A, homocysteine
- Testing should be done off heparin and at least 2 weeks after the 3–6 months course of oral anticoagulation.

- Another test to consider in the workup of antithrombin deficiency:
  – Antithrombin-heparin cofactor assay measures the ability of heparin to bind to antithrombin, which neutralizes the action of thrombin and factor Xa. This is an indirect measure of factor Xa and thrombin inhibition, the factor Xa inhibition activity being more specific. This assay will detect all currently recognized subtypes of hereditary antithrombin deficiency.
- Drugs that may alter lab results: Heparin (increased clearance), estrogen, and L-asparaginase (decreased synthesis) can lower antithrombin levels.

Follow-Up Tests & Special Considerations

- The role of family screening for antithrombin deficiency is unclear because most patients with this mutation do not have thrombosis. Screening may be offered to pregnant women with a family history of factor protein S deficiency considering using oral contraceptives or pregnancy(1)[C].
- Antithrombin levels are low in:
  – DIC
  – Sepsis
  – Burns
  – Severe trauma
  – Acute thrombosis
  – Pregnancy or postpartum
  – Liver disease
  – Nephrotic syndrome
  – Malignancy
  – Myeloproliferative disorders
- Antithrombin levels could be elevated by oral contraceptive pills.
- US to diagnose DVT if clinically indicated
- If DVT diagnosis in question, a negative D-dimer will help to rule out DVT.
- Spiral CT or V/Q scan to diagnose pulmonary embolism (PE) if clinically indicated
- V/Q scan may be difficult to interpret in patients with other lung disease.

Test Interpretation

Venous thrombosis

 TREATMENT

GENERAL MEASURES

Routine anticoagulation for asymptomatic patients with antithrombin deficiency is not recommended (1)[A].

MEDICATION
First Line

- Patients with antithrombin deficiency and a first thrombosis should be anticoagulated initially with unfractionated heparin followed by oral anticoagulation with warfarin (1)[A].
- Heparin can be stopped after 5 total days of therapy provided the INR is 2–3 (1)[A].
- Oral anticoagulant should be started with the initial administration of heparin. Warfarin (Coumadin) 10 mg/d PO for the first 2 days, then adjusted to INR of 2–3. Patients should be maintained on warfarin for at least 6 months (2)[A].
- Recurrent thrombosis requires indefinite anticoagulation (1)[A].

- Contraindications:
  - Active bleeding precludes anticoagulation; risk of bleeding is a relative contraindication to long-term anticoagulation.
- Precautions:
  - Observe patient for signs of embolization, further thrombosis, or bleeding.
  - Avoid IM injections.
  - Periodically check stool and urine for occult blood and monitor CBCs, including platelets.
  - Heparin-thrombocytopenia and/or paradoxical thrombosis with thrombocytopenia
- Significant possible interactions:
  - Agents that intensify the response to oral anticoagulants: Common antiinfective agents that potentially increase the effect of warfarin include: ciprofloxacin, clarithromycin, erythromycin, metronidazole, trimethoprim-sulfamethoxazole, and azole antifungals. Additional interacting agents include: Alcohol, allopurinol, amiodarone, anabolic steroids, androgens, cimetidine, chloral hydrate, disulfiram, all NSAIDs, sulfinpyrazone, tamoxifen, thyroid hormone, vitamin E, ranitidine, salicylates, acetaminophen.
  - Agents that diminish the response to oral anticoagulants: Aminoglutethimide, antacids, barbiturates, carbamazepine, cholestyramine, diuretics, griseofulvin, rifampin, oral contraceptives
  - See DIET

Second Line
- Argatroban: 0.4–0.5 μg/kg/min. Case reports describing the use of this direct thrombin inhibitor in patients with antithrombin deficiency have been published (3)[C].
- Antithrombin III (ATnativ, Thrombate III): 50–100 IU/min IV titrated to antithrombin level desired. Precise role in therapy remains unclear (1)[C].
- LMWH is difficult to manage in this population (1)[C].

ISSUES FOR REFERRAL
- Recurrent thrombosis on anticoagulation
- Difficulty anticoagulating
- Genetic counseling

ADDITIONAL THERAPIES
- Patients with severe antithrombin deficiency may require plasma replacement of thrombin in order for heparin to be effective (4)[C].
- Compression stockings for prevention

SURGERY/OTHER PROCEDURES
Thrombectomy may be indicated in complicated cases.

IN-PATIENT CONSIDERATIONS
Admission Criteria/Initial Stabilization
Complicated thrombosis, such as pulmonary embolism. Heparin initial bolus of 80 U/kg followed by infusion of 18 U/kg/hr. Frequent monitoring of the partial thromboplastin time (PTT) is important, as ~50% of patients deficient in antithrombin require >40,000 U of heparin daily to adequately prolong PTT (1)[C].

Discharge Criteria
Stable on anticoagulation

 ## ONGOING CARE

FOLLOW-UP RECOMMENDATIONS
Patient Monitoring
Warfarin use requires periodic INR measurements (monthly after initial stabilization) with a goal of 2–3 (1)[A].

DIET
Foods high in vitamin K may interfere with anticoagulation on warfarin. Consider nutrition consultation.

PATIENT EDUCATION
- Patients should be educated about:
  - Use of oral anticoagulant therapy
  - Avoidance of NSAIDs while on warfarin
- The role of family screening is unclear, as most patients with this mutation do not have thrombosis. In a patient with a family history of factor V Leiden, consider screening during pregnancy or if considering oral contraceptive use.

PROGNOSIS
- The odds ratio of thrombosis in a patient with antithrombin deficiency is much higher than in patients with other thrombophilic conditions. The recurrence rate is similarly high.
- There is no difference in clinical severity between patients with type I defects and type II mutations.
- Overall, prognosis is good, if appropriately anticoagulated.

COMPLICATIONS
Recurrent thrombosis (requires indefinite anticoagulation)

REFERENCES
1. Vinazzer H. Hereditary and acquired antithrombin deficiency. *Semin Thromb Hemost.* 1999;25: 257–263.
2. Guyatt GH, Akl EA, Crowther M, et al. Executive summary: Antithrombotic Therapy and Prevention of Thrombosis, 9th ed.: American College of Chest Physicians Evidence-Based Clinical Practice Guidelines. *Chest.* 2012;141(2 Suppl):7S–47S.
3. Dager WE, Gosselin RC, Owings JT. Argatroban therapy for antithrombin deficiency and mesenteric thrombosis: Case report and review of the literature. *Pharmacotherapy.* 2004;24:659–663.
4. Maclean PS, Tait RC. Hereditary and acquired antithrombin deficiency: Epidemiology, pathogenesis and treatment options. *Drugs.* 2007;67:1429–1440.

ADDITIONAL READING
- Kottke-Marchant K, Duncan A. Antithrombin deficiency: Issues in laboratory diagnosis. *Arch Pathol Lab Med.* 2002;126:1326–1336.
- Vossen CY, Conard J, Fontcuberta J, et al. Risk of a first venous thrombotic event in carriers of a familial thrombotic defect. The European Prospective Cohort on Thrombophilia (EPCOT). *J Thromb Heamost.* 2005;3:459–464.

 ### SEE ALSO

Deep Vein Thrombophlebitis (DVT)

 ### CODES

ICD10
D68.59 Other primary thrombophilia

CLINICAL PEARLS
- Antithrombin levels will be low on heparin and during acute thrombosis.
- Diagnosis can be difficult. Conditions causing low levels of antithrombin III, such as pregnancy, liver disease, sepsis, and DIC, must be ruled out.
- Testing should be done off heparin and at least 2 weeks after the 3–6 month course of oral anticoagulation.
- For pregnant women with antithrombin deficiency but no prior history of VTE, antepartum and postpartum vigilance are recommended. Postpartum prophylaxis with prophylactic or intermediate-dose LMWH or vitamin K antagonists with target INR 2–3 for 6 weeks is only recommended if there is positive family history of VTE (2)[C].

ANXIETY

Mary K. Flynn, MD

 BASICS

DESCRIPTION
- Persistent, excessive, and difficult-to-control worry associated with significant symptoms of motor tension, autonomic hyperactivity, and/or disturbances of sleep or concentration
- System(s) affected: Nervous (resulting in increased sympathetic tone and increased catecholamine release)

EPIDEMIOLOGY
Prevalence
- 12-month prevalence rate: 3.1%
- Lifetime prevalence rate: 5.7%
- Onset can occur any time in life, from adolescence to adulthood; median age of onset in the US is 31 years.
- Predominant sex: Female > Male (2:1)
- Anxiety accounts for 5–8% of primary care office visits.

ETIOLOGY AND PATHOPHYSIOLOGY
fMRI studies display decreased amygdala connectivity bilaterally.
Mediated by abnormalities of neurotransmitter systems (i.e., serotonin, norepinephrine, and γ-aminobutyric acid [GABA])
Genetics
- Strongly linked to depression in heritability studies
- A variant of the serotonin transporter gene (*5HT1A*) may contribute to both conditions; other genes (such as that for glutamic acid decarboxylase) also may play a role.

RISK FACTORS
- Caucasian race
- Adverse life events: Stress, medical illness, disability, unemployment, childhood physical and mental abuse
- Family history
- Lack of social support
- Depression
- Lesbian/Bisexual women at increased risk

GENERAL PREVENTION
Regular exercise is associated with decreased anxiety and depression.

COMMONLY ASSOCIATED CONDITIONS
- Major depressive disorder (>60%), dysthymia, bipolar disorder
- Alcohol/Drug abuse (37.6%/27.6%)
- Cigarette smoking in adolescence
- Panic disorder, agoraphobia, simple phobia, social anxiety disorder, anorexia nervosa

 DIAGNOSIS

HISTORY
- History and evaluation should carefully identify generalized anxiety disorder (GAD) from other anxiety disorders (1)[C]
- Symptoms of excessive anxiety and worry must occur more often than not for at least 6 months.

- At least 3 additional criteria are required for diagnosis of GAD in adults; only 1 is required in children:
  – Restlessness or feeling keyed up or on edge
  – Easily fatigued
  – Difficulty concentrating or mind going blank
  – Irritability
  – Muscle tension
  – Sleep disturbances (difficulty falling or staying asleep)
  – Difficulty controlling worry
- Persistent worry must cause significant distress or impairment in social, occupational, or other areas of functioning.
- Focus of anxiety and worry is not consistent with or limited to the occurrence of other types of psychiatric disorders and is not directly related to posttraumatic stress disorder (PTSD).
- All other causes of anxiety and worry have been eliminated (see "Differential Diagnosis").
- Patient may report symptoms of dyspnea, palpitations, diaphoresis, nausea, or diarrhea, or may experience tremor.

PHYSICAL EXAM
No specific physical findings, but patient may be noted to be irritable or easily startled and observable findings of bitten nails, a tremor, or clammy hands may also be present.

DIFFERENTIAL DIAGNOSIS
- Cardiovascular: Ischemic heart disease, valvular heart disease (mitral valve prolapse), cardiomyopathies, arrhythmias, congestive heart failure
- Respiratory: Asthma, chronic obstructive pulmonary disease, pulmonary embolism
- CNS: Stroke, seizures, dementia, migraine, vestibular dysfunction, neoplasms
- Metabolic and hormonal: Hyper- or hypothyroidism, pheochromocytoma, adrenal insufficiency, Cushing syndrome, hypokalemia, hypoglycemia, hyperparathyroidism
- Nutritional: Thiamine, pyridoxine, or folate deficiency; iron-deficiency anemia
- Drug-induced anxiety: Alcohol, sympathomimetics (cocaine, amphetamine, caffeine), corticosteroids, herbals (ginseng)
- Withdrawal: Alcohol, sedative-hypnotics
- Psychiatric: Other disorders (e.g., panic disorder, obsessive–compulsive disorder, PTSD, social phobia, adjustment disorder, and somatization disorder)

DIAGNOSTIC TESTS & INTERPRETATION
Initial Tests (lab, imaging)
- Laboratory tests are normal. Initial tests should include thyroid-stimulating hormone, CBC, basic metabolic panel, and ECG
- See "Differential Diagnosis" for other conditions to consider, especially in patients with many physical symptoms.
- GAD-2: 2-question self-reporting scale (22% positive predictive value [PPV]/78% negative predictive value [NPV]) (2)[B]

Diagnostic Procedures/Other
Psychological testing:
- GAD-7: 5 additional questions; provides more detailed information for treatment (29% PPV/71% NPV); also may be indicative of panic disorder (GAD-7: 29% PPV/71% NPV).

- Hamilton Anxiety Scale (HAM-A), Anxiety Disorders Interview Schedule (ADIS-IV)
- In pediatric populations: ADIS-IV Parent and Child Version, Multidimensional Anxiety Scale for Children (MASC), Screen for Child Anxiety Related Emotional Disorders (SCARED)

 TREATMENT

GENERAL MEASURES
- Assess for suicidality given increased risk.
- Identify and treat coexisting substance abuse and other psychiatric conditions.

MEDICATION
First Line
- Antidepressants take longer to have effect (2–4 weeks) but outperform benzodiazepines in the long term.
- SSRIs (2,3)[A]:
  – Escitalopram (Lexapro): Initially 10 mg/d; may titrate to a maximum of 20 mg/d
  – Paroxetine (Paxil): Initially 10–20 mg/d; may titrate to a maximum of 50 mg/d (no added benefit above 20 mg/d)
  – Sertraline (Zoloft): Initially 25 mg/d; may titrate to a maximum of 200 mg/d
- Selective-norepinephrine reuptake inhibitors (SNRIs) (2,3)[A]:
  – Duloxetine (Cymbalta): Initially 30 mg/d; may titrate to a maximum of 120 mg/d
  – Venlafaxine XR (Effexor XR): Initially 37.5–75 mg; may titrate up by 75 mg every 4 days to a maximum of 225 mg/d
- Tricyclic antidepressants (TCAs): Imipramine (Tofranil): Initially 25–50 mg/d; maximum of 300 mg/d, 100 mg/d in the elderly (2,3)[A]
- Azapirones: Buspirone (BuSpar): 15 mg/d divided b.i.d.–t.i.d. initially; maximum of 60 mg/d divided b.i.d.–t.i.d. (2,3)[A]

Second Line
- Benzodiazepines (best for short-term use) (2,3)[A]:
  – Clonazepam (Klonopin): 0.25 mg b.i.d.; may increase to 4 mg/d divided b.i.d.
  – Diazepam (Valium): 2–5 mg b.i.d.–q.i.d.; may increase to a maximum of 40 mg/d
  – Lorazepam (Ativan): 0.5 mg b.i.d.–t.i.d.; may increase to 6 mg/d divided t.i.d.
- Hydroxyzine (Vistaril, Atarax): CNS depressant, antihistamine, anticholinergic; decreased risk of dependence compared with benzodiazepines: Usual dose: 50–100 mg PO q.i.d.
- Pregabalin (Lyrica): Has shown promise in decreasing anxiety scores and preventing relapse at 75–300 mg b.i.d.

Geriatric Considerations
- Avoid TCAs and long-acting benzodiazepines. Benzodiazepines may cause delirium.
- Pregabalin may cause dizziness and somnolence.

Pediatric Considerations
- Black box warning (SSRIs): Antidepressants increase the risk of suicidal thinking and behavior in children, adolescents, and young adults.
- Medications other than SSRIs have not been well-tested in pediatric populations.
- Anxiety often exists comorbid with ADHD.

Pregnancy Considerations
- Buspirone: Category B: Secreted in breast milk; inadequate studies to assess risk
- Benzodiazepines: Category D: May cause lethargy and weight loss in nursing infants; avoid breastfeeding if the mother is taking chronically or in high doses.
- SSRIs: If possible, taper and discontinue. After 20 weeks' gestation, there is increased risk of pulmonary hypertension; mild transient neonatal syndrome of CNS; and motor, respiratory, and GI signs. One small study has raised concern about increased autism risk (4). Most are Category C:
  – Paroxetine: Category D: Conflicting evidence regarding the risk of congenital cardiac defects and other congenital anomalies.
- Hydroxyzine: Category C: Case reports of neonatal withdrawal exist.

ALERT
Precautions:
- Benzodiazepines: Age >65 years, hepatic insufficiency, respiratory disease/sleep apnea, renal insufficiency, suicidal tendency, contraindicated with narrow-angle glaucoma, precaution with open-angle glaucoma. Sudden discontinuation, especially of alprazolam, increases seizure risk. Long-term use has potential for tolerance and dependence; use with caution in patients with history of substance abuse.
- Buspirone: Hepatic and/or renal dysfunction; monoamine oxidase inhibitor (MAOI) treatment
- TCAs: Advanced age, glaucoma, benign prostate hypertrophy, hyperthyroidism, cardiovascular disease, liver disease, urinary retention, MAOI treatment
- SSRIs: Use caution in those with comorbid bipolar disorder; may trigger mania. Avoid with medications that may increase risk of serotonin syndrome.

ISSUES FOR REFERRAL
Concomitant depression may warrant a psychiatric evaluation in light of increased suicide risk.

ADDITIONAL THERAPIES
- Psychological:
  – Cognitive-behavioral therapy (CBT): Has shown comparable benefit to medical management; may improve comorbid conditions such as depression.
- Mindfulness-based cognitive therapy and stress-reduction studies have been limited. A 2010 meta-analysis showed promise in reducing acute symptoms of anxiety in individuals diagnosed with anxiety disorders and in other populations with high anxiety (i.e., the chronically ill) (5)[B].

- Relaxation training (various subtypes exist): Historical treatment of choice; has been shown to reduce anxiety symptoms.
- Psychodynamic psychotherapy: Treatment is focused on patient discovering and verbalizing unconscious content of the psyche.

COMPLEMENTARY AND ALTERNATIVE MEDICINE
- Patients frequently engage in CAM; providers should be familiar with common therapies.
- Yoga and meditation may help; additional studies are needed, but few adverse effects are known.
- Kava: Some evidence for benefit over placebo in mild to moderate anxiety, but concern regarding potential hepatotoxicity:
  – May consider for short-term use (up to 24 weeks) at doses 70–240 mg/d (6,7,8)[C].
  – Must avoid concomitant use of alcohol or other medications metabolized via the liver (CYP 450 inhibitor); other adverse effects include dermatopathy (usually reversible), ataxia, hearing loss, and loss of appetite.
- St. John's wort, passionflower, valerian, inositol: little evidence to support use.
  – In combination with SSRI or buspirone, St. John's wort may lead to serotonin syndrome. Rarely, photosensitivity or triggering of mania.
  – Others have benign side-effect profile.

IN-PATIENT CONSIDERATIONS
Patients at risk of suicide should be treated as inpatients; consider as well for patients with comorbid substance use.

 ## ONGOING CARE

FOLLOW-UP RECOMMENDATIONS
Patient Monitoring
- Follow up within 2–4 weeks from starting new medications.
- Monitor mental status on benzodiazepines, and avoid drug dependence.
- Monitor BP, heart rate, and anticholinergic side effects of TCAs.
- Monitor all patients for suicidal ideation, but especially those on SSRIs, SNRIs, and imipramine.

DIET
- Limit caffeine intake.
- Avoid alcohol (drug interactions, high rate of abuse, potential for increased anxiety).

PATIENT EDUCATION
- Regular exercise, especially yoga, may be beneficial for both anxiety and comorbid conditions.
- Continue with meditation, CBT, and other therapies that provide relief.
- www.familydoctor.org
- National Institute of Mental Health (NIMH): www.nimh.nih.gov/health/publications/index.shtml

PROGNOSIS
- A chronic disease, with many patients experiencing continued symptoms or relapse
- Successful treatment is possible but must be carried out over the long term.
- Relapse is more likely with the discontinuation of medications, particularly in the first year of treatment and during periods of increased stress.

REFERENCES
1. American Psychiatric Association. *Diagnostic and Statistical Manual of Mental Disorders*, 5th ed. Arlington, VA: American Psychiatric Association; 2013.
2. Kavan MG, Elsasser GN, Barone EJ. Generalized anxiety disorder: Practical assessment and management. *Am Fam Physician*. 2009;79: 785–791.
3. Davidson JR. First-line pharmacotherapy approaches for generalized anxiety disorder. *J Clin Psychiatry*. 2009;70(Suppl 2):25–31.
4. Croen LA, Grether JK, Yoshida CK, et al. Antidepressant use during pregnancy and childhood autism spectrum disorders. *Arch Gen Psychiatry*. 2011;68(11):1104–1112.
5. Hofmann SG, Sawyer AT, Witt AA, et al. The effect of mindfulness-based therapy on anxiety and depression: A meta-analytic review. *J Consult Clin Psychol*. 2010;78:169–183.
6. Saeed SA, Bloch RM, Antonacci DJ. Herbal and dietary supplements for treatment of anxiety disorders. *Am Fam Physician*. 2007;76:549–556.
7. Pittler MH, Ernst E. Kava extract for treating anxiety. *Cochrane Database Syst Rev*. 2003;(1):CD003383.
8. Ernst E. The risk-benefit profile of commonly used herbal therapies: Ginkgo, St. John's Wort, Ginseng, Echinacea, Saw Palmetto, and Kava. *Ann Intern Med*. 2002;136:42–53.

 ## SEE ALSO

Algorithms: Depression, Adult; Anxiety

 ## CODES

ICD10
- F41.1 Generalized anxiety disorder
- F41.8 Other specified anxiety disorders
- F41.9 Anxiety disorder, unspecified

CLINICAL PEARLS
- Psychiatric comorbidities, especially depression, are extremely common with GAD; patients are at increased risk for suicidality.
- SSRIs are the treatment of choice, although they require up to 4 weeks for full effect.
- Benzodiazepines may be used initially but should be tapered and withdrawn if possible.
- Psychological therapy should be used in conjunction with medications if patients are agreeable.
- CAM use is common, and certain therapies may be effective.

AORTIC VALVULAR STENOSIS

Nirmanmoh Bhatia, MD • Amaninderapal S. Ghotra, MD • Marcus F. Stoddard, MD

BASICS

DESCRIPTION
Aortic stenosis (AS) is a narrowing of the aortic valve area causing obstruction to left ventricular (LV) outflow. The disease has a long asymptomatic latency period, but development of severe obstruction or onset of symptoms such as syncope, angina, and CHF are associated with a high mortality rate without surgical intervention.

EPIDEMIOLOGY
- Most common valvular disease in developed countries
- Predominant age:
  - <30 years: Congenital
  - 30–65 years: Congenital or rheumatic fever
  - >65 years: Degenerative calcification of aortic valve

Prevalence
- Affects 1.3% of population 65–74 years old, 2.4% 75–84 years old, 4% >84 years old (1)
- Bicuspid aortic valve: 1–2% of population. Bicuspid aortic valve predisposes to development of aortic stenosis at an earlier age (1)

ETIOLOGY AND PATHOPHYSIOLOGY
- Progressive stiffening of aortic valve results in LV outflow obstruction. Obstruction causes increased afterload and decreased cardiac output.
- Increase in left ventricular pressure is required to preserve cardiac output; this leads to development of concentric left ventricular hypertrophy (LVH). LVH preserves ejection fraction but adversely affects heart functioning:
  - LVH impairs coronary blood flow during diastole by compression of coronary arteries and reduced capillary ingrowth into hypertrophied muscle.
  - LVH results in diastolic dysfunction by reducing ventricular compliance.
- Diastolic dysfunction necessitates stronger left atrial (LA) contraction to augment preload and maintain stroke volume. Loss of LA contraction by atrial fibrillation can induce acute deterioration.
- Angina: Myocardial demand is elevated due to increased LV pressure. Myocardial supply is compromised due to LVH.
- Syncope (exertional): Can be multifactorial from inability to augment cardiac output due to the fixed obstruction to LV outflow, ventricular arrhythmias, or, most commonly, abnormal vasodepressor reflexes.
- Heart failure: Eventually LVH cannot compensate for increasing afterload, resulting in high LV pressure and volume, which are accompanied by an increase in LA and pulmonary pressures.
- Degenerative calcific changes to aortic valve (2):
  - Mechanism involves mechanical stress to valve leaflets as well as atherosclerotic changes to the valve tissue. Bicuspid valves are at higher risk for mechanical stress.
  - Early lesions: Subendothelial accumulation of oxidized LDL and macrophages and T-lymphocytes (inflammatory response)
  - Disease progression: Fibroblasts undergo transformation into osteoblasts. Protein production of osteopontin, osteocalcitonin, and BMP-2, which modulate calcification of leaflets

- Congenital: Unicuspid valve, bicuspid valve, tricuspid valve with fusion of commissures, hypoplastic annulus
- Rheumatic fever: Chronic scarring with fusion of commissures

RISK FACTORS
- Congenital unicommissural valve or bicuspid valve (1):
  - Unicommissural valve: Most cases detected during childhood
  - Bicuspid valve: Predisposes to development of aortic stenosis earlier in adulthood (4th–5th decade) compared to tricuspid valve (6th–8th decade)
- Rheumatic fever (1):
  - Prevalence of chronic rheumatic valvular disease has declined significantly in the US.
  - Most cases are associated with mitral valve disease
- Degenerative calcific changes:
  - Most common cause of acquired aortic stenosis in the US
  - Shares same risk factors as coronary artery disease due to similar pathophysiology: Hypercholesterolemia, hypertension, smoking, male gender, age, diabetes mellitus
- Rare causes:
  - Metabolic diseases (e.g., Fabry's disease), systemic lupus erythematosus, Paget's disease, and alkaptonuria. Calcific AS has also been associated with chronic kidney disease.

COMMONLY ASSOCIATED CONDITIONS
- Coronary artery disease (50% of patients)
- Hypertension (40% of patients): Results in "double-loaded" LV (dual source of obstruction from AS and hypertension)
- Aortic regurgitation (common in calcified bicuspid valves and rheumatic disease)
- Mitral valve disease: 95% of patients with AS from RF also have mitral valve disease.
- LV dysfunction and congestive heart failure (CHF)
- Acquired von Willebrand disease: Impaired platelet function and decreased vWF results in bleeding (ecchymosis and epistaxis) in 20% of AS patients. Severity of coagulopathy is directly related to severity of AS.
- Gastrointestinal arteriovenous malformations (AVM)

DIAGNOSIS

HISTORY
- Primary symptoms: Angina, syncope, and heart failure (3). Angina is most frequent symptom. Syncope is often exertional. Heart failure symptoms include fatigue, exertional dyspnea, orthopnea, paroxysmal nocturnal dyspnea, shortness of breath.
- Palpitations
- Neurological events (transient ischemic attack or cerebrovascular accident) secondary to embolization
- Geriatric patients may have subtle symptoms such as fatigue and exertional dyspnea.
- Note: Symptoms do not always correlate with valve area (severity of AS) but most commonly occur when AV area is <1 cm^2.

PHYSICAL EXAM
- Auscultation (3):
  - Harsh, systolic crescendo-decrescendo murmur best heard at 2nd intercostal space on the right sternal border, radiates into carotid arteries. Peak of murmur correlates with severity of stenosis: Later peaking murmur suggests greater severity
  - High-pitched diastolic blow, suggests associated aortic regurgitation
  - Paradoxically split S2 or absent A2. Note: Normally split S2 reliably excludes severe AS.
  - S4 due to stiffening of left ventricle
- Other associated signs (3): include *Pulsus parvus et tardus:* Decreased and delayed carotid upstroke. LV heave. Findings of CHF: Crackles at lung bases, lower extremity edema
- Three findings most useful for ruling in AS:
  - A slow rate of rise in the carotid pulse
  - Mid to late peak intensity of the murmur
  - Reduced intensity of the second heart sound

DIFFERENTIAL DIAGNOSIS
- Mitral regurgitation: Either primary (such as mitral valve prolapse or a flail mitral valve) or secondary to underlying coronary artery disease or dilated cardiomyopathy. Usually an apical, high-frequency, pansystolic murmur, often radiating to axilla.
- Hypertrophic obstructive cardiomyopathy: Also systolic crescendo-decrescendo murmur, but best heard at left sternal border and may radiate into axilla. Murmur intensity increases by changing from squatting to standing and/or by Valsalva maneuver.
- Discrete fixed subaortic stenosis: 50–65% have associated cardiac deformity (PDA, VSD, coarctation of aorta).
- Aortic supravalvular stenosis: Williams syndrome, homozygous familial hypercholesterolemia

DIAGNOSTIC TESTS & INTERPRETATION
Initial Tests (lab, imaging)
- Chest x-ray (1):
  - May be normal in compensated, isolated valvular aortic stenosis.
  - Boot-shaped heart reflective of concentric hypertrophy
  - Poststenotic dilatation of ascending aorta, and calcification of aortic valve (seen on lateral PA CXR)
- ECG: Often normal ECG (ECG is nondiagnostic), or may show LVH, left atrial enlargement, and nonspecific ST and T-wave abnormalities
- Echo indications:
  - Initial workup:
    - Doppler echocardiogram is mainstay of diagnosis
    - Assesses the severity of AS
    - Assesses left ventricular wall thickness, size, function
  - In known AS and changing signs/symptoms
  - In known AS and pregnancy due to hemodynamic changes of pregnancy
- Echo findings:
  - Aortic valve morphology, thickening, calcifications
  - Decreased aortic valve excursion
  - Aortic valve area
  - Transvalvular gradient across aortic valve
  - LV hypertrophy and diastolic dysfunction
  - LV ejection fraction
  - Wall-motion abnormalities suggesting CAD

- Evaluate for concomitant aortic valve insufficiency or mitral valve disease
- Aortic stenosis severity based on echo values (assumes normal cardiac output):
  - Normal: Area: 3–4 cm^2; Mean pressure gradient: 0 mm Hg; Jet vel. <2.5 m/s
  - Mild: Area: 1.5–2 cm^2; Mean pressure gradient: <25 mm Hg; Jet vel. 2.5–2.9 m/s
  - Mod: Area: 1–1.5 cm^2; Mean pressure gradient: 25–40 mm Hg; Jet vel. 3–4 m/s
  - Severe: Area: <1 cm^2; Mean pressure gradient: >40 mm Hg; Jet vel. >4 m/s
  - Extremely severe: Area <0.6 cm^2; Mean pressure gradient >60 mm Hg; Jet vel. >5 m/s
- Patients with severe AS and low cardiac output may have a relatively low transvalvular pressure gradient (i.e., mean pressure gradient <30 mm Hg).

Diagnostic Procedures/Other
- Exercise stress testing:
  - Asymptomatic patients (4)[B]: Helpful to uncover subtle symptoms or changes, abnormal BP (increase <20 mm Hg), and ECG changes (ST depressions). 1/3 of patients develop symptoms with exercise testing; STOP testing at this point.
  - Symptomatic patients (4)[B]: DO NOT perform exercise stress testing as may induce hypotension or ventricular tachycardia.
  - CHF patients (4)[B]: Dobutamine stress echocardiography is reasonable to evaluate patients with low-flow/low-gradient AS and LV dysfunction.
- Cardiac catheterization:
  - Perform prior to aortic valve replacement in patients with suspected CAD (4)[B]. Determines need for coronary artery bypass graft (CABG). If unambiguous diagnosis of AS, perform only coronary angiography.
  - Use if noninvasive testing is inconclusive or if there is discrepancy between severity of symptoms and findings on ECG
  - Measures transvalvular flow, transvalvular pressure gradient, and effective valve area
  - Hemodynamic measurements with infusion of dobutamine can be useful for evaluation of patients with low-flow/low-gradient AS and LV dysfunction.

Test Interpretation
- Aortic valve: Nodular calcification on valve cusps (initially at bases), cusp rigidity, cusp thickening, and fibrosis.
- LV hypertrophy, myocardial interstitial fibrosis
- 50% incidence of concomitant CAD

 # TREATMENT

MEDICATION
- NO medical therapy for severe or symptomatic aortic stenosis
- Prevention: Currently no recommended medical therapy. Statins have been thought to slow progression if initiated during mild disease. However, this has not been supported by large, randomized controlled trials.
- Antibiotic prophylaxis against recurrent RF is indicated for patients with rheumatic AS (Penicillin G 1,200,000 U IM q4wk, duration varies with age and history of carditis).

- Antibiotic prophylaxis is no longer indicated for prevention of infective endocarditis (4).
- Comorbidities: Hypertension: ACE inhibitors, start with low dose and increase cautiously. Be cautious of vasodilators, which may cause hypotension.

SURGERY/OTHER PROCEDURES
- The only proven treatment for aortic stenosis is valve replacement.
- Indications for aortic valve replacement (AVR) surgery:
  - Symptomatic and severe AS (4)[B]
  - Asymptomatic, severe AS and:
    ○ Requires aortic root surgery or other valve surgery (4)[C]
    ○ Requires CABG (4)[C]
    ○ EF Positive stress test (4)[C]
    ○ Risk of rapid progression (moderate to severe calcification, age, CAD) (4)
  - In addition, it is reasonable to perform AVR in patients with moderate stenosis and undergoing CABG or other valve surgery (4)[B].
  - AVR may be considered for patient with asymptomatic, extremely severe AS (4)[C] or mild AS and CABG and high risk of rapid progression (4)[C], however this is controversial.

ALERT
Note: If the AV area is >1.5 cm^2 and the gradient is <15 mm Hg, there is no benefit from AVR.
- Transcatheter aortic valve replacement (TAVR) may be indicated in patients with symptomatic, severe AS who are high surgical risk (5).
- Percutaneous balloon valvuloplasty may have role as bridge to valve replacement in hemodynamically unstable or high-risk patients (4)[C], but is not recommended as an alternative to valve replacement.
  - May be used as palliative therapy for patients who are not surgical candidates (4)[C].
  - Indicated in young adults and others without calcified valves and no AR if:
    ○ Symptoms of angina, syncope, CHF and peak gradients >50 mm Hg on catheterization (4)[C]
    ○ ST or T-wave changes in the left precordial leads and catheter peak gradient >60 mm Hg (4)[C]
    ○ Patient plays competitive sports or may become pregnant and has catheter peak gradient >50 mm Hg (4)[C].

 # ONGOING CARE

FOLLOW-UP RECOMMENDATIONS
- Advise patient to immediately report symptoms referable to AS.
- Asymptomatic patients: Yearly history and physical (4)[C]
- Serial echo: Yearly for severe AS, every 1–2 years for moderate AS, every 3–5 years for mild AS (4)[B]

PATIENT EDUCATION
Physical activity limitations:
- Asymptomatic mild AS: No restrictions.
- Asymptomatic moderate-to-severe AS: Avoid strenuous exercise. Consider exercise stress test prior to starting exercise program.

PROGNOSIS
- 25% mortality/yr in symptomatic patients who do not undergo valve replacement; average survival is 2–3 years without AVR surgery.
- Median survival in symptomatic AS (3): Heart failure: 2 years; syncope: 3 years; angina: 5 years
- Perisurgical mortality: AVR surgery has 4% mortality rate; AVR + CABG has 6.8% mortality rate.
- Adverse postoperative prognostic factors: Age, HF NYHA III/IV, cerebrovascular disease, renal dysfunction, CAD

REFERENCES
1. Carabello BA, Paulus WJ. Aortic stenosis. *Lancet.* 2009;373:956–966.
2. Otto CM. Calcific aortic stenosis—time to look more closely at the valve. *N Engl J Med.* 2008;359: 1395–1398.
3. Grimard BH, Larson JM. Aortic stenosis: Diagnosis and treatment. *Am Fam Physician.* 2008;78: 717–724.
4. Bonow RO, Carbello BA, Chatterjee K, et al. ACC/AHA 2006 guidelines for the management of patients with valvular heart disease: A report of the American College of Cardiology/American Heart Association Task Force on Practice. Guidelines. *Circulation.* 2006;114:e84–e231.
5. Smith CR, Leon MB, Mack MJ, et al. Transcatheter versus surgical aortic-valve replacement in high-risk patients. *N Engl J Med.* 2011;364(23):2187–2198. Epub 2011 Jun 5.

 ## CODES

ICD10
- I06.0 Rheumatic aortic stenosis
- I35.0 Nonrheumatic aortic (valve) stenosis
- Q23.0 Congenital stenosis of aortic valve

CLINICAL PEARLS
- Aortic stenosis is diagnosed on physical exam by a systolic crescendo-decrescendo murmur and delayed and diminished pulses.
- Symptomatic AS most commonly presents as angina, syncope, and heart failure.
- Symptomatic AS has a very poor prognosis unless treated with surgical intervention.

APPENDICITIS, ACUTE
Francesca L. Beaudoin, MD, MS • Andy H. Chen, MD

 BASICS

DESCRIPTION
- Acute inflammation of the vermiform appendix, first described by Reginald Fitz in 1886
- Arising from the base of the cecum in right lower quadrant (RLQ); can be localized anterior, posterior, medial, lateral to the cecum, as well as in the pelvis. Vascular supply by appendicular artery, a branch of the ileocolic artery. Nerve supply derived from the superior mesenteric plexus.
- Most common cause of the acute surgical abdomen

EPIDEMIOLOGY
- Predominant age: 10–30 years: Rare in infancy
- Predominant sex: Slight male predominance:
  – Ages 10–30: Male > Female (3:2)
  – Age >30: Male = Female

Incidence
- 1 case per 1,000 people per year
- Lifetime incidence 1 in every 15 persons (7%)

Pregnancy Considerations
- Most common extrauterine surgical emergency
- No more common in pregnant vs. nonpregnant women
- Higher rate of perforation; more likely to present with peritonitis

ETIOLOGY AND PATHOPHYSIOLOGY
The cause is thought to be obstruction of the appendiceal lumen. This leads to distention, ischemia, and bacterial overgrowth. Without intervention, most cases of appendicitis will lead to perforation and subsequently abscess formation or generalized peritonitis. Causes of obstruction:
- Fecaliths (most common)
- Lymphoid tissue hyperplasia (in children)
- Vegetable, fruit seeds, and other foreign bodies
- Intestinal worms (ascarids)
- Strictures, fibrosis, neoplasms

Genetics
1st-degree relative with history of appendicitis increases risk, although no direct genetic link has been found.

RISK FACTORS
Adolescent males, familial tendency, intra-abdominal tumors

 DIAGNOSIS

Diagnosis of acute appendicitis relies on the history and physical examination with supporting laboratory studies and imaging. Scoring systems, including the Alvarado Score and the Pediatric Appendicitis Score, have been developed to help predict the likelihood of acute appendicitis, although diagnosis is still considered a clinical decision.

HISTORY
- Classic history is vague periumbilical pain, followed by anorexia/nausea/vomiting. Over the next 4–48 hours, pain migrates to the RLQ.
- Only 50% of patients present with this classic history.
- Pain before vomiting (~100% sensitive), abdominal pain (~100%), pain migration (50%)
- Anorexia (~100%), nausea (90%), vomiting (75%), obstipation
- Atypical symptoms and pain associated with a retrocecal or pelvic appendix

PHYSICAL EXAM
- Fever; temp >100.4°F (may be absent). Tachycardia.
- RLQ tenderness. Maximal tenderness at McBurney point (1/3 the distance from the anterior superior iliac spine to the umbilicus)
- Voluntary and involuntary guarding
- Rovsing sign: RLQ pain with palpation of left lower quadrant
- Psoas sign: Pain with right thigh extension (retrocecal appendix)
- Obturator sign: Pain with internal rotation of flexed right thigh (pelvic appendix). Local and suprapubic pain on rectal exam (pelvic appendix)
- Pelvic and rectal exams are necessary to rule out other causes of lower abdominal pain (e.g., pelvic inflammatory disease, prostatitis).
- Serial exams can be useful in indeterminate cases.

DIFFERENTIAL DIAGNOSIS
- GI:
  – Gastroenteritis, inflammatory bowel disease
  – Diverticulitis, ileitis
  – Cholecystitis, pancreatitis
  – Intussusception, volvulus
- Gynecologic:
  – Pelvic inflammatory disease, ectopic pregnancy
  – Ovarian cyst, ovarian torsion, tubo-ovarian abscess
  – Endometriosis
  – Ruptured graafian follicle
- Urologic:
  – Testicular torsion, epididymitis
  – Kidney stones, prostatitis, cystitis, pyelonephritis
- Systemic:
  – Diabetic ketoacidosis
  – Henoch Schönlein purpura
  – Sickle cell crisis
  – Porphyria
- Other:
  – Acute mesenteric lymphadenitis
  – No organic pathologic condition
  – Hernias
  – Psoas abscess
  – Rectus sheath hematoma
  – Epiploic appendagitis
  – Pneumonia (basilar)

Pediatric Considerations
- Decreased diagnostic accuracy of history and physical exam
- Higher fever, more vomiting and diarrhea

Pregnancy Considerations
- Difficult diagnosis
- Normal response to infection/inflammation is suppressed.
- Appendix displaced out of pelvis by gravid uterus

Geriatric Considerations
Decreased diagnostic accuracy, more likely to be atypical presentation

DIAGNOSTIC TESTS & INTERPRETATION
Initial Tests (lab, imaging)
- Leukocytosis: WBC >10,000/mm^3 (70%)
- Polymorphonuclear predominance or "left shift" (>90%)
- Human chorionic gonadotropin (hCG) (if negative, rules out ectopic pregnancy)
- Urinalysis: Hematuria, pyuria (~30%)
- C-reactive protein: Nonspecific inflammatory marker. When paired with an elevated WBC can increase the likelihood of appendicitis.
- Drugs may alter lab results: Antibiotics, steroids
- Imaging used in cases of suspected appendicitis when the diagnosis is not clear; is helpful to detect complications (abscess, perforation)
- Plain films: Little utility, nonspecific findings, may visualize fecalith
- CT scan with contrast: Sensitivity ~91–98%; specificity 95–99%; imaging modality of choice However, growing concern regarding radiation dose, particularly in young patients (1)[A].
- Ultrasound: Alternative in pregnant patients, children, and in women with suspected gynecologic pathology. Sensitivity and specificity vary by report and accuracy depends on the skill of the ultrasonographer. Can rule in appendicitis, but cannot reliably exclude the diagnosis. Starting with an ultrasound and, if negative, obtaining a CT scan has been proposed as an effective workup strategy (2)[B].
- MRI: Growing in popularity for diagnosing pregnant patients, but also may be useful for patients with contrast allergies and/or patients with renal failure. Limitations include cost, availability, and time required to complete study.
- Radioisotope-labeled WBC scans: May be used in patients with indeterminate CT scans and suspected appendicitis as an alternative to observation or surgery. Limitations include availability and time required to complete study.

Diagnostic Procedures/Other
- Exploratory laparotomy/laparoscopy: Acceptable nontherapeutic appendectomy rates vary based on age and gender and may be higher for females of child-bearing age than males.

Test Interpretation
- Acute appendiceal inflammation, local vascular congestion, obstruction
- Gangrene, perforation with abscess (15–30%)
- Fecalith

TREATMENT

GENERAL MEASURES
- Surgery (appendectomy) is the standard of care for acute, uncomplicated appendicitis.
- Nonoperative management with antibiotics has been studied as an alternative (3)[A]. However, this approach carries recurrent appendicitis rates of 14–20% in the 1st year.
- In the case of acute appendicitis complicated by abscess formation or phlegmon in pediatric patients, some studies show initial conservative management with antibiotics alone to carry fewer risks and complications than emergent appendectomy (4)[A].

MEDICATION
First Line
- Uncomplicated acute appendicitis: Perioperative dose of antibiotic (5)[A]: Single dose of cefoxitin or ampicillin/sulbactam (Unasyn) or cefazolin plus metronidazole
- Gangrenous or perforating appendicitis:
  - Broadened antibiotic coverage for aerobic and anaerobic enteric pathogens
  - Piperacillin and tazobactam (Zosyn) or ticarcillin and clavulanate (Timentin) or a third-generation cephalosporin plus metronidazole are initial options
  - Adjust dosage and choice of antibiotic based on intraoperative cultures.
  - Continue antibiotics for at least 7 days postoperatively or until patient becomes afebrile with normal WBC count.

Second Line
- Uncomplicated acute appendicitis: clindamycin plus one of the following: ciprofloxacin, levofloxacin, gentamicin, or aztreonam
- Gangrenous or perforated appendicitis: ciprofloxacin or levofloxacin plus metronidazole or monotherapy with a carbapenem (imipenem and cilastatin, meropenem, ertapenem)

ISSUES FOR REFERRAL
All cases of appendicitis require emergent surgical consultation.

SURGERY/OTHER PROCEDURES
- Inpatient surgery is indicated
- Patients presenting within 72 hours of onset:
  - Immediate appendectomy; laparoscopic favored unless perforation (6)[A]
  - Drainage of abscess, if present
- Patients who present late (>4–5 days after symptom onset) may be treated initially with antibiotics, bowel rest, and drainage of any abscess. Later (4–10 weeks) appendectomy can then be performed in this subgroup only.

IN-PATIENT CONSIDERATIONS
Admission Criteria/Initial Stabilization
All patients with appendicitis should be admitted.

IV Fluids
Fluid resuscitation with normal saline (NS) or lactated Ringer's (LR) solution. Correct fluid and electrolyte deficits.

Nursing
Preoperative preparation

Discharge Criteria
Tolerating PO; return of bowel function; afebrile; normal WBC

 ONGOING CARE

FOLLOW-UP RECOMMENDATIONS
- Return to work is usually possible 1–2 weeks following most uncomplicated appendicitis.
- Restrict activity for 4–6 weeks after surgery: No heavy lifting (>10 lbs) or strenuous physical activity.

PATIENT EDUCATION
Contact physician for postoperative development of:

- Anorexia, nausea, vomiting
- Abdominal pain, fever, chills
- Signs/symptoms of wound infection

PROGNOSIS
- Generally uncomplicated course in young adults with unruptured appendicitis
- Factors increasing morbidity and mortality: Extremes of age, presence of appendiceal rupture
- Morbidity rates:
  - Nonperforated appendicitis: 3%
  - Perforated appendicitis: 47%
- Mortality rates:
  - Unruptured appendicitis: 0.1%
  - Ruptured appendicitis: 3%
  - Patients >60 years of age make up 50% of total deaths from appendicitis.
  - Older patients with ruptured appendix: 15%

Pediatric Considerations
- Rupture earlier
- Rupture rate: 15–60%

Pregnancy Considerations
- Rupture rate: 40%
- Fetal mortality rate: 2–8.5%

Geriatric Considerations
Rupture rate: 67–90%

COMPLICATIONS
- Wound infection, intra-abdominal abscess; lower rate with antibiotic prophylaxis (3)[A], intestinal fistulas
- Intestinal obstruction, paralytic ileus, incisional hernia
- Liver abscess (rare), pyelophlebitis

REFERENCES

1. Hlibczuk V, Dattaro JA, Jin Z, et al. Diagnostic accuracy of noncontrast computed tomography for appendicitis in adults: A systematic review. *Ann Emerg Med.* 2010;55:51–59.e1.
2. Poortman P, Oostvogel HJ, Bosma E, et al. Improving diagnosis of acute appendicitis: Results of a diagnostic pathway with standard use of ultrasonography followed by selective use of CT. *J Am Coll Surg.* 2009;208:434–441.
3. Wilms IM, de Hoog DE, de Visser DC, et al. Appendectomy versus antibiotic treatment for acute appendicitis. *Cochrane Database Syst Rev.* 2011;(11):CD008359. Epub 2011 Nov 9.
4. Simillis C, Symeonides P, Shorthouse AJ, et al. A meta-analysis comparing conservative treatment versus acute appendectomy for complicated appendicitis (abscess or phlegmon). *Surgery.* 2010;147:818–829.
5. Andersen BR, Kallehaue FL, Andersen HK. Antibiotics versus placebo for prevention of postoperative infection after appendectomy. *Cochrane Database Syst Rev.* 2005;(3):CD001439.
6. Sauerland S, Lefering R, Neugebauer EA. Laparoscopic versus open surgery for suspected appendicitis. *Cochrane Database Syst Rev.* 2004;(4):CD001546. Epub 2004 Oct 18.

 SEE ALSO

Algorithm: Abdominal Rigidity

CODES

ICD10
- K35.2 Acute appendicitis with generalized peritonitis
- K35.3 Acute appendicitis with localized peritonitis
- K35.80 Unspecified acute appendicitis

CLINICAL PEARLS
- Classic history of anorexia with periumbilical pain localizing to RLQ is the cornerstone of diagnosis for acute appendicitis.
- Diagnosis is much more challenging in children, pregnant patients, and the elderly due to varying symptoms and signs.
- In equivocal cases, CT of abdomen and pelvis is the diagnostic test of choice, although ultrasound and MRI are useful alternatives.
- Acute appendicitis is the most common surgical emergency during pregnancy.

ARTERITIS, TEMPORAL
Cynthia M. Waickus, MD, PhD

BASICS

DESCRIPTION
- Technically termed giant cell arteritis (GCA)
- A chronic, generalized, cellular and humoral immune-mediated vasculitis of large and medium-sized vessels, predominantly affecting the cranial arteries originating from the aortic arch, although vascular involvement may be wide spread. Inflammation of the aorta is observed in 50% of cases (1).
- Frequent features include fatigue, headaches, jaw claudication, loss of vision, scalp tenderness, polymyalgia rheumatica (PMR), and aortic arch syndrome (decreased or absent peripheral pulses, discrepancies of blood pressure, arterial bruits) (2).

EPIDEMIOLOGY
- The mean age of onset is approximately 70 years.
- Women are affected about 3 times as often as men.
- Most common vasculitis in individuals of Northern European descent.
- Rare in Asians and African Americans

Incidence
- Prevalence in individuals >50: 1 in 500 (1)
- Cyclic incidence: Peaking every 5–7 years

ETIOLOGY AND PATHOPHYSIOLOGY
- The exact etiology of GCA remains unknown, although current theory suggests that advanced age, ethnicity, and specific genetic predisposition lead to a maladaptive response to endothelial injury, intimal hyperplasia, and ultimately vascular stenosis.
- Temporal arteritis (TA) is a chronic, systemic vasculitis primarily affecting the elastic lamina of medium- and large-sized arteries. Histopathology of affected arteries is marked by transmural inflammation of the intima, media, and adventitia, as well as patchy infiltration by lymphocytes, macrophages, and multinucleated giant cells. Mural hyperplasia can result in arterial luminal narrowing, resulting in subsequent distal ischemia.
- Current theory regarding the etiology of TA: A maladaptive response to endothelial injury leads to an inappropriate activation of cell-mediated immunity via immature antigen-presenting cells. The subsequent release of cytokines within the arterial vessel wall can attract macrophages and multinucleated giant cells, which gives diseased vessels their characteristic histology. This also leads to an oligoclonal expansion of T-cells directed against antigens in or near the elastic lamina. Ultimately, this cascade results in vessel wall damage, intimal hyperplasia, and eventual stenotic occlusion.
- In recent years, GCA and polymyalgia rheumatica (PMR) have increasingly been considered to be closely related conditions (2,3).

Genetics
The gene for HLA-DRB1–04 has been identified as a risk factor for TA, and polymorphisms of ICAM-1 have also been implicated (4).

RISK FACTORS
- Increasing age >70 is the greatest risk factor
- Genetic predisposition

- Possible infective pathogens function as initial inciting agents
- Heavy smoking and atherosclerotic disease are risk factors for females, but not for males.

COMMONLY ASSOCIATED CONDITIONS
PMR may develop either before or after the arteritis (3,5).

DIAGNOSIS

HISTORY
- Most common presenting symptom is headache (2/3 of patients) (1,2,5)[A].
- Scalp tenderness or sensitivity
- Jaw claudication (presence of symptom significantly increases likelihood of a positive biopsy)
- Claudication of upper extremities
- Constitutional symptoms (fever, fatigue, weight loss)
- Symptoms of polymyalgia rheumatica (shoulder and hip girdle pain and stiffness)
- Any visual disturbances (amaurosis fugax, diplopia)
- Vision loss (20% of patients)
- Distal extremity swelling/edema
- Upper respiratory symptoms

PHYSICAL EXAM
- Temporal artery abnormalities (beading, prominence, tenderness)
- Typically appear "ill"
- Decreased peripheral pulses in the presence of large vessel diseases
- Funduscopic exam shows pale and edema of the optic disk, scattered cotton-wool patches, and small hemorrhages.
- Unlike other forms of vasculitis, GCA rarely involves the skin, kidneys, and lungs.

DIFFERENTIAL DIAGNOSIS
- Classification Criteria:
  - Age >70 years
  - New localized headache
  - Temporal artery abnormality (tenderness to palpation, decreased or absent pulses)
  - ESR >50 mm/hr
  - Abnormal temporal artery biopsy showing vasculitis with predominance of mononuclear cell infiltration or granulomatous inflammation
- ≥3 of the above symptoms: 95% sensitivity/91% specificity for GCA diagnosis (The American College of Rheumatology criteria for the classification of GCA)

DIAGNOSTIC TESTS & INTERPRETATION
Initial Tests (lab, imaging)
- ESR >50 (86% sensitivity), although nonspecific (27%); infrequently, may be normal (1,5)[A].
- C-reactive protein (CRP) >2.45 mg/dL is a more sensitive marker of inflammation (97% sensitivity); it is associated with increased odds of a positive biopsy result.
- Platelet count >400 × 10^3
- A normal ESR and/or CRP renders the diagnosis of GCA unlikely.

- Elevated acute-phase reactants (fibrinogen, interleukin-6) are frequently elevated, but very nonspecific, and reserved for diagnostically difficult cases.
- Mild anemia: Very nonspecific, but may be associated with a lower rate of ischemic complications.
- Color Doppler US of the temporal artery may identify vascular occlusion, stenosis, or edema ("halo-sign"); it is low cost and noninvasive, but also very operator dependent and does not significantly improve on the clinical exam. It may aid in the diagnosis of larger vessel involvement (6).
- MRI and MRA allow for noninvasive evaluation of both the vessel lumen and the vessel wall and assess mural thickness (edema) and lumen diameter (occlusion). The information may aid in diagnosis, but results are affected by prior glucocorticoid treatment, perhaps indicating more value in assessing the disease course or relapse. Cost, logistics, and lack of validity data preclude its routine usefulness.
- Positron emission tomography (PET), like MRI/MRA and color Doppler, may be useful in diagnostically difficult cases, and early in the course of disease as the metabolic changes occur prior to structural vascular damage, but it also lacks studies to support its use (7).

Follow-Up Tests & Special Considerations
- Development of aortic aneurysms (late and potentially serious complication of GCA) can lead to aortic dissection.
- Due to the risk of irreversible vision loss, treatment with high-dose steroids should be started on strong clinical suspicion of TA, prior to the temporal biopsy being done.

Diagnostic Procedures/Other
- Gold standard diagnostic study: Histopathologic examination of the temporal artery biopsy specimen
- Overall sensitivity is 87%.
- The temporal artery is chosen because of its accessibility in the systemic disease, but any accessible cranial artery may be chosen.
- Length of biopsy specimen should be at least 2 cm to avoid false–negative results, as skip lesions may occur.
- Diagnostic yield of biopsy may be increased if procedure is coupled with imaging (high-resolution MRI or color Doppler US).
- Bilateral temporal artery biopsy should not be performed unless the initial histopathology is negative and the suspicion for GCA remains high.
- May be negative in up to 42% of patients, especially in large vessel disease.
- Biopsy results are not affected by prior glucocorticoids, so treatment should not be delayed.

Test Interpretation
- Inflammation of the arterial wall, with fragmentation and disruption of the internal elastic lamina
- Multinucleated giant cells are found in <50% of cases and are not specific for the disease.
- TA occurs in 3 histologic patterns: Classic, atypical, and healed.

TREATMENT

MEDICATION

First Line

Glucocorticoids:

- Prolonged treatment with glucocorticoids has been the mainstay of treatment, and should be initiated immediately when the diagnostic suspicion for GCA is high (1)[A](8)[B].

ALERT

- Because of the risk of irreversible vision loss, treatment with high-dose steroids should be started on strong clinical suspicion of temporal arteritis, prior to the temporal biopsy being done.
- The typical dose of prednisone is 60 mg/d (or 1 mg/kg/d). Steroids should not be in the form of alternate day therapy, as this is more likely to lead to a relapse of vasculitis.
- The initial dose of steroids is continued for 2–4 weeks and slowly tapered over 9–12 months. Tapering may require ≥2 years.
- Oral steroids are at least as effective as IV steroids, except in the treatment of acute visual loss where IV steroids appear to offer significant benefit over oral steroids.
- It has been suggested that low-dose aspirin might be effective for patients with GCA (9)[B].
- Patients on corticosteroids should be placed on therapy to minimize osteoporosis unless there are contraindications.

Second Line

Methotrexate has a modest effect in TA (10)[B],(11)[A].

ONGOING CARE

FOLLOW-UP RECOMMENDATIONS

Sun avoidance and protection of the head and the face from photodamage may eventually prove to be important preventive measures for TA.

Patient Monitoring

- TA is typically self-limited and lasts several months or years.
- Overall, TA does not seem to decrease longevity. Nevertheless, it may lead to serious complications, such as visual loss, which occurs in about 15–20% of patients.
- Another complication of GCA is the development of aortic aneurysms, usually affecting the ascending aorta. Yearly chest x-rays may be useful to identify this problem.
- About 50% of the patients with GCA will eventually develop polymyalgia rheumatica (stiffness of shoulder and hip girdle).

DIET

Calcium and vitamin D supplementation

PATIENT EDUCATION

- Consequences of discontinuing steroids abruptly: adrenal insufficiency, disease relapse
- Risks of long-term steroid use: infection, hyperglycemia, weight gain, impaired wound healing, osteoporosis, hypertension
- Possibility of relapse and importance of reporting new headaches and vision changes to provider immediately

PROGNOSIS

- Once vision loss has occurred, it is unlikely to be recovered, but treatment resolves the other symptoms and prevents future vision loss and stroke.
- In most patients, glucocorticoid therapy can eventually be discontinued without complications. In a few patients, however, the disease is chronic and prednisone must be continued for years.
- Disease relapse is a distinct possibility.

COMPLICATIONS

- Vision loss with delayed diagnosis
- Glucocorticoid-related toxicity

REFERENCES

1. Salvarani C, Cantini F, Hunder GG. Polymyalgia rheumatica and giant-cell arteritis. *Lancet*. 2008; 372(9634):234–245.
2. Waldman CW, Waldman SD, Waldman RA. Giant cell arteritis. *Med Clin North Am*. 2013;97(2): 329–335.
3. Cantini F, Niccoli L, Storri L, et al: Are polymyalgia rheumatica and giant cell arteritis the same disease? *Semin Arthritis Rheum*. 2004;33: 294–301.
4. González-Gay MA, Amoli MM, Garcia-Porrua C, et al. Genetic markers of disease susceptibility and severity in giant cell arteritis and polymyalgia rheumatica. *Semin Arthritis Rheum*. 2003;33(1): 38–48.
5. Kermani TA, Warrington KJ. Recent advances in diagnostic strategies for giant cell arteritis. *Curr Neurol Neurosci Rep*. 2012;12(2):138–144.
6. Arida A, Kyprianou M, Kanakis M, et al. The diagnostic value of ultrasonography-derived edema of the temporal artery wall in giant cell arteritis: A second meta-analysis. *BMC Musculoskelet Disord*. 2010;11:44.
7. Blockmans D, de Ceuninck L, Vanderschueren S, et al. Repetitive 18F-fluorodeoxyglucose positron emission tomography in giant cell arteritis: A prospective study of 35 patients. *Arthritis Rheum* 2006;55:131–137.
8. Villa-Forte A. Giant cell arteritis: Suspect it, treat it promptly. *Cleve Clin J Med*. 2011;78(4):265–270.
9. Lee MS, Smith SD, Galor A, et al. Antiplatelet and anticoagulant therapy in patients with giant cell arteritis. *Arthritis Rheum*. 2006;54:3306–3309.
10. Mahr AD, Jover JA, Spiera RF, et al. Adjunctive methotrexate for treatment of giant cell arteritis: An individual patient data meta-analysis. *Arthritis Rheum*. 2007;56:2789–2797.
11. Borchers AT, Gershwin ME. Giant cell arteritis: A review of classification, pathophysiology, geoepidemiology and treatment. *Autoimmun Rev*. 2012;11(6–7):A544–A554. Epub 2012 Jan 21.

ADDITIONAL READING

- Gonzalez-Gay MA, Vazquez-Rodriguez TR, Lopez-Diaz MJ, et al. Epidemiology of giant cell arteritis and polymyalgia rheumatica. *Arthritis Rheum*. 2009;61:1454–1461.
- Mukhtyar C, Guillevin L, Cid MC, et al. EULAR recommendations for the management of large vessel vasculitis. *Ann Rheum Dis*. 2009;68:318–323.

SEE ALSO

Depression; Fibromyalgia; Headache, Cluster; Headache, Tension; Polymyalgia Rheumatica; Polymyositis/Dermatomyositis

CODES

ICD10

- M31.5 Giant cell arteritis with polymyalgia rheumatica
- M31.6 Other giant cell arteritis

CLINICAL PEARLS

- Due to the risk of irreversible vision loss, treatment with high-dose steroids (prednisone 60 mg/d) should be started immediately in patients suspected of temporal arteritis.
- Temporal artery biopsy is the gold standard for diagnosis. Temporal artery biopsy is not likely to be affected by a few weeks of treatment.
- Treatment consists of a very slow steroid taper. Bone protection therapy and low-dose aspirin should be considered.
- Normal ESR level = value of age/2 for men and (age + 10)/2 for women

ARTHRITIS, INFECTIOUS, BACTERIAL

Jennifer Ruskis, MD • Jeffrey Feden, MD

BASICS

DESCRIPTION
- Invasion of joints by bacteria
- Associated morbidity and mortality necessitates early diagnosis and treatment
- System(s) affected: Musculoskeletal
- Synonym(s): Suppurative arthritis; Septic arthritis; Pyarthrosis; Pyogenic arthritis; Bacterial arthritis

EPIDEMIOLOGY
- Occurs at any age, but higher incidences found at the extremes of age.
- Incidence:
  - 2–10 cases/100,000 persons annually
  - Higher in those with lower socioeconomic status, rheumatoid arthritis, HIV
  - 1/3 of cases occur in children under age 2 (1,2).
- Prevalence: In patients presenting with monoarticular arthritis, 27% have nongonococcal septic arthritis (2).
- Gender differences:
  - Gonococcal: Female > Male
  - Nongonococcal: Male > Female

ETIOLOGY AND PATHOPHYSIOLOGY
- Almost any organism can be pathogenic but main causative organisms are:
- Nongonococcal:
  - *S. aureus* (37–56% of cases for age >2 yrs) (1)
    - MRSA risk: Elderly, intravenous drug users (IVDU), postsurgical (3)
  - *Streptococcus* spp.
  - Gram-negative bacilli
- Gonococcal
- Other: Lyme, fungal, mycobacterium
- Risk by age (1):
  - <2 months: *S. aureus* and *S. agalactiae*
  - 2 months–5 years: *S. aureus, S.pyogenes, Kingella kingae*
- Specific high risk groups:
  - Rheumatoid Arthritis: *S. aureus*
  - IVDU: *S. aureus,* gram-negative bacilli, opportunistic pathogens
  - Elderly: group B streptococci
  - Chronic disease: group B streptococci
  - Immunocompromised: gram-negative bacilli
- Pathogenesis:
  - Hematogenous invasion (most common)
  - Contiguous spread
  - Direct penetration by micro-organisms secondary to trauma or iatrogenic cause(i.e., joint surgery)
- Pathophysiology:
  - High vascularity of synovium allows easy access. Low fluid shear forces and production of matrix proteins promote adherence and rapid replication.
  - Intense inflammatory response results in severe joint destruction (1).

RISK FACTORS
- Extremes of age (especially age >80) (4)
- Prosthetic joint and overlying cellulitis are most highly associated with septic arthritis (2)[A]
- Prior violation of joint capsule:
  - Prior surgery
  - Steroid injection
  - Trauma

- History of joint disease:
  - Inflammatory arthritis (rheumatoid arthritis [RA]: 10-fold increased risk)
  - Noninflammatory arthritis (osteoarthritis)
  - Crystal arthritis
- Systemic Illness:
  - Diabetes mellitus, liver disease, HIV, malignancy, ESRD/hemodialysis, immunosuppressive therapy, sickle cell anemia, immunodeficiency
- Risks for hematogenous spread:
  - Dental procedures, poor dental hygiene, systemic infection elsewhere, intravenous drug use
- Risks for contiguous spread:
  - Adjacent skin or soft tissue infection, trauma

GENERAL PREVENTION
- Prompt treatment of skin and soft tissue infections
- Control of risk factors
- Immunization

DIAGNOSIS

HISTORY
- General: Painful swelling of joint with decreased range of motion
  - Predominantly monoarticular (90%)
  - Recent joint surgery or cellulitis overlying a prosthetic hip or knee increases risk (2)[A].
  - Typically large joints, 60% knee or hip
  - Fever present in >50% of patients (5), low-grade fever seen in 90% (4)
  - Symptoms generally present for <2 weeks
- Pediatric consideration:
  - Infants may present with refusal to walk or bear weight
- Gonococcal:
  - Bacteremic phase: Migratory polyarthritis, tenosynovitis, high fever, chills, pustules
  - Localized phase: Monoarticular, low-grade fever

PHYSICAL EXAM
- Limited or loss of joint use/motion
- Joint effusion and tenderness
- Joint warmth and redness
- Hip and shoulder involvement may reveal severe pain on range of motion with less obvious joint swelling on exam.
- Pediatric consideration: Infants with septic hip will typically sit with hip flexed and externally rotated

DIFFERENTIAL DIAGNOSIS
- Crystal arthritis: Gout, pseudogout, calcium oxalate, cholesterol
- Infectious arthritis: Fungi, spirochetes, rheumatic fever, HIV, bacterial endocarditis
- Inflammatory arthritis: RA, spondyloarthropathy, systemic lupus erythematosus
- Osteoarthritis
- Cellulitis
- Other: Foreign body, fracture, hemarthrosis, traumatic effusion, avascular necrosis

DIAGNOSTIC TESTS & INTERPRETATION
Initial Tests (lab, imaging)
- Imaging: Helpful to identify effusions and inflammation; not helpful in differentiating septic from other forms of arthritis (3).

- X-ray:
  - Nondiagnostic for septic arthritis but indicated as basic screening for underlying osteomyelitis or other pathology (4,6).
  - Identify trauma, soft tissue swelling, osteoarthritis or osteopenia
  - Nonspecific changes of inflammatory arthritis may be appreciated: Erosions, joint destruction, joint-space loss (4).
- Ultrasound:
  - Can identify effusions especially in joints difficult to examine, such as the hip (4).
  - Pediatric consideration: Ultrasound is the most sensitive imaging modality for hip effusions in children (7).
- MRI:
  - Highly sensitive for effusions and superior to CT for soft tissue inflammation and pathology (4,8).
- Other imaging techniques (nuclear scans):
  - Technetium joint scans: Reveal distribution of inflammation; sensitive, not specific (1,6)
- Laboratory tests:
  - Serum tests:
    - WBC counts do not have sufficient sensitivity or specificity to use elevated WBC count alone for diagnostic purposes (2)[A].
    - ESR with cutoff of >30 mm/h has sensitivity up to 96% but poor specificity (9)[C]; however, may be useful in monitoring course of disease
    - CRP also may be useful but no studies have found adequate sensitivity or specificity. May be used with ESR to follow course (2)[A].
    - Procalcitonin may have diagnostic utility, however, insufficient evidence to support routine use (10)[A]
    - Blood cultures have sensitivities ranging from 23–36% (2)[A].
  - Other tests:
    - Disseminated gonococcus: Send urethral or cervical GC swabs
    - Suspected Lyme arthritis: Send serum Lyme titers
  - Synovial fluid analysis:
    - Must be done prior to antibiotic therapy
    - Fluid typically cloudy
    - Gram stain with reported sensitivities ranging from 29–63% (2)[A].
    - >50,000 WBCs/HPF is accepted cutoff, however, *synovial WBC (sWBC) count alone is insufficient to rule in or rule out septic arthritis* (11)[A]. With a +LR of 4.7, it can significantly augment clinical suspicion but should not be used in isolation (2)[A].
    - Polymorphonuclear leukocytes usually predominate in synovial fluid (>90%) though this is not diagnostic (2)[A].
    - Crystals (e.g., urate or calcium pyrophosphate) do not exclude infectious arthritis.
    - Joint fluid: For Gram stain (positive in 50%); culture (positive in 50–70%) should be sent with understanding of limitations (2)[A].
    - Prosthetic joint: sWBC count extremely unreliable for indicating septic arthritis. A much lower number of sWBCs may indicat infection and should be taken very seriously.

- Pediatric consideration: There is no single lab test that can distinguish septic arthritis from transient synovitis (12)[A].
  - The combination of fever, non–weight-bearing, CRP >20, or ESR >40 and a WBC >12 is suspicious for septic arthritis (12)[B].

Diagnostic Procedures/Other
- Arthrocentesis with Gram stain and culture is standard of practice.
- Shoulder or hip joints may require image-guided aspiration
- Arthrocentesis should be performed prior to initiation of antibiotics whenever possible.
- Arthrocentesis approach must avoid contaminated tissue (e.g., overlying cellulitis) when possible

Test Interpretation
- Synovial biopsy will reveal polymorphonuclear leukocytes and possibly the causative organism, if synovial fluid and blood cultures are negative.

TREATMENT

GENERAL MEASURES
- All patients should be hospitalized for parenteral antibiotics and monitoring. Antibiotics should begin immediately after appropriate cultures sent (4).
- Removal of purulent material is *required* and needle aspiration may be preferred over surgical management in certain cases (1,6)[A].
  - Pediatric consideration: Arthrotomy is recommended for septic hip due to high morbidity (7)[A].
- If prosthetic joint is involved, removal of the prosthesis by an orthopedic surgeon must be considered.
- Continue treatment for 1–2 weeks after total resolution of all signs of inflammation, for a total of 4–6 weeks for most organisms
  - Exception: Gonococcal (2–3 weeks)
- Intra-articular antibiotics are not necessary.

MEDICATION
First Line
- Empiric therapy guided by Gram stain when possible (4)
- Nongonococcal:
  - Gram-positive cocci in clusters:
    - Vancomycin IV
  - Gram-positive cocci in chains:
    - Ceftriaxone
  - Gram-negative bacilli:
    - Cefepime or piperacillin-tazobactam IV.
    - Penicillin allergic: Aztreonam or ciprofloxacin IV.
  - Negative Gram stain:
    - Vancomycin or linezolid plus 3rd-generation cephalosporin
  - Therapy duration typically 3–4 weeks with transition to PO after resolution of symptoms.
- Gonococcal (3):
  - Ceftriaxone 1 g IM or IV every day for 14 days (and at least 24–48 hours after symptoms resolve).
  - Fluoroquinolone or oral 3rd-generation cephalosporin for 14 days depending on local resistance.
  - Concomitant treatment for chlamydia
- Other considerations:
  - Narrow antibiotic therapy based on culture results when possible
  - Short course of dexamethasone IV at onset of treatment may decrease length of hospital stay and symptoms (13)[A]

- If Lyme arthritis considered: Doxycycline PO is first-line treatment.
- Significant possible interactions:
  - Broad-spectrum antibiotics: May reduce effectiveness of oral contraceptives and barrier method is recommended

ISSUES FOR REFERRAL
- Infectious disease and orthopedic consultations are strongly encouraged.
- Involvement of prosthetic joint mandates orthopedic consultation.
- IVDU, immunosuppression warrants infectious disease consultation to guide therapy.

SURGERY/OTHER PROCEDURES
- Arthroscopy indicated if fluid accumulated is loculated and/or not amenable to needle drainage.
- Surgical drainage typically is required for shoulder or hip involvement.

ONGOING CARE

FOLLOW-UP RECOMMENDATIONS
Patient Monitoring
- Repeat arthrocentesis (once) if fluid reaccumulates to verify sterilization of joint and reversion of inflammatory signs to normal.
- If no improvement within 24 hours, re-evaluate and consider arthroscopy.
- Follow up 1 week and 1 month after stopping antibiotics to detect any relapse.

PROGNOSIS
- Early treatment should allow cure
- Delayed recognition/treatment is complicated by morbidity and mortality.

COMPLICATIONS
- High morbidity (9–33% in elderly)
- Case fatality rate estimated at 11% (1)
- Limited joint range of motion
- Secondary osteoarthritis
- Flail or fused or dislocated joint
- Septic necrosis
- Sinus formation
- Ankylosis
- Osteomyelitis
- Postinfectious synovitis
- Shortening of limb (in children)

REFERENCES

1. García-Arias M, Balsa A, Mola EM. Septic arthritis. *Best Pract Res Clin Rheumatol*. 2011;25: 407–421.
2. Carpenter CR, Schuur JD, Everett WW, et al. Evidence-based diagnostics: Adult septic arthritis. *Acad Emerg Med*. 2011;18:781–796.
3. Mathews CJ, Weston VC, Jones A, et al. Bacterial septic arthritis in adults. *Lancet*. 2010;375: 846–855.
4. García-De La Torre I, Nava-Zavala A. Gonococcal and nongonococcal arthritis. *Rheum Dis Clin North Am*. 2009;35:63–73.
5. Margaretten ME, Kohlwes J, Moore D, et al. Does this adult patient have septic arthritis? *JAMA*. 2007;297:1478–1488.
6. Matthews CJ, Kingsley G, Field M, et al. Management of Septic Arthritis: a systematic review. *Ann Rheum Dis*. 2007;66:440–445.
7. Kang SN, Sanghera T, Magwani J et al. The management of septic arthritis in children: A systematic review of the English language literature. *J Bone Joint Surg*. 2009;91:1127–1133.
8. Paakkonen M, Pelota H. Bone and joint infections. *Pediatr Clin North Am*. 2013;60: 425–436.
9. Li SF, Cassidy C, Chang C et al. Diagnostic utility of laboratory tests in septic arthritis. *Emerg Med J*. 2007;24:75–77.
10. Wang CH, Yen ZS. Best evidence topic report. BET 3. Is there a role for serum procalcitonin in the differentiation between septic and non-septic arthritis. *Emerg Med J*. 2010;27:144–145.
11. O'Malley A, Svinos H. Towards evidence based emergency medicine: Best BETs from the Manchester Royal Infirmary. BET 3: Is the white cell count of the joint aspirate sufficiently sensitive/specific to rule in/out septic arthritis? *Emerg Med J*. 2009;26:435–437.
12. Taekema HC, Landham PR, Maconochie I. Towards evidence based medicine for paediatricians. Distinguishing between transient synovitis and septic arthritis in the limping child: How useful are clinical prediction tools? *Arch Dis Child*. 2009;94:167–168.
13. Harel L, Prais D, Bar-on E, et al. Dexamethasone therapy for septic arthritis in children: Results of a randomized double-blind placebo-controlled study. *J Pediatr Orthop*. 2011;31:211–215.

ADDITIONAL READING

- Clerc O, Prod'hom G, Greub G, et al. Adult native septic arthritis: A review of 10 years of experience and lessons for empirical antibiotic therapy. *J Antimicrob Chemother*. 2011;66:1168–1173.
- Fangtham M, Baer AN. Methicillin-resistant Staphylococcus aureus arthritis in adults: Case report and review of the literature. *Semin Arthritis Rheum*. 2012;41:604–610.
- Mathews CJ, Coakley G. Septic arthritis: Current diagnostic and therapeutic algorithm. *Curr Opin Rheumatol*. 2008;20:457–462.

 CODES

ICD10
- M00.9 Pyogenic arthritis, unspecified
- M00.80 Arthritis due to other bacteria, unspecified joint
- M00.89 Polyarthritis due to other bacteria

CLINICAL PEARLS
- The ability to definitively diagnose septic arthritis based on history, physical exam, and laboratory analysis is limited.
- If the diagnosis is considered, arthrocentesis and synovial fluid analysis are mandatory to help guide treatment.
- Early IV antibiotics and washout of purulent material are the cornerstones of treatment.
- Crystalline process can mimic or coexist with septic arthritis.
- Prosthetic joint infection can be very difficult to identify and warrants early orthopedic consultation when considered.

ARTHRITIS, JUVENILE IDIOPATHIC

Donna-Marie McMahon, DO, FAAP • Kathleen M. Vazzana

 BASICS

DESCRIPTION
- Juvenile idiopathic arthritis (JIA): Most common chronic pediatric rheumatologic disease
- A cause of significant short- and long-term disability
- General characteristics:
  - Age of onset: <16 years
  - Signs of arthritis: Joint swelling, restricted range of motion, warmth, redness, or pain
  - At least 6 weeks of symptoms
- Division of 7 subtypes exist, according to the International League of Associations for Rheumatology, determined by clinical characteristics in the first 6 months of illness (1):
  - Systemic (Still disease): 10%; preceded by febrile onset of at least 2 weeks with one of the following: rash, serositis, hepatosplenomegaly, lymphadenopathy (1)
  - Polyarticular rheumatoid factor (RF) (+): 5–10%; ≥5 joints involvement (1). Large and small joints. RF positive on 2 tests at least 3 months apart (2)
  - Polyarticular RF(–): 10–30%; ≥5 joint involvement (1); large and small joints affected; RF negative (2)
  - Oligoarticular: 30–60%; involvement of 1–4 joints; Risk for chronic uveitis in ANA(+) females (1) and axial skeletal involvement in older boys (2). Types: (a) Monoarthritis (50%) knee, ankle, elbow; (b) extended type = >4 joints after first 6 months
  - Psoriatic arthritis: 5%; arthritis with psoriasis or arthritis with >2 of following: Dactylitis, nail changes, psoriasis in a 1st-degree relative (1)
  - Enthesitis arthritis: 1–7%; oligo- or polyarthritis in small or large joints and enthesis plus 2 of the following: Sacroiliac or lumbosacral pain, Reiter syndrome, family history or presence of acute anterior uveitis, HLA-B27(+), ankylosing spondylitis, inflammatory bowel disease
  - Undifferentiated arthritis: Arthritis that does not fulfill above categories or in ≥2 categories (2).
- System(s) affected: Musculoskeletal, Hematologic, Lymphatic, Immunologic
- Synonym(s): Juvenile chronic arthritis; Juvenile arthritis; Juvenile rheumatoid arthritis (JRA); Still disease (2)

EPIDEMIOLOGY
- Systemic: Incidence = 0.4–0.9 per 100,000. Prevalence 3.5 per 100,000; Male = Female (1); onset throughout childhood; 54% = 0–5 yrs (3)
- Polyarticular RF(+): Female > Male (3:1) (2); onset late childhood or adolescence (1)
- Polyarticular RF(–): Female > Male (3:1); onset early peak = 2–4 yrs, late peak = 6–12 yrs (2)
- Oligoarticular: Female > Male (5:1); onset 2–4 yrs (2)
- Psoriatic: Female > Male (1:0.95) (2); onset early peak = 2–3 yrs; late peak = 10–12 yrs (1)
- Enthesitis: Female > Male (1:7); onset early peak = 2–4 yrs; late peak: 6–12 yrs (2)
- Affected patients have an increased risk of developing cancer compared to healthy children, although short-term risk is found to be low (4)

Incidence
2–20/100,000 children <16 yrs/year in developed nations

Prevalence
16–150/100,000 children <16 yrs in developed nations (1)

ETIOLOGY AND PATHOPHYSIOLOGY
Multifactorial, including:
- Immunodysregulation
- Genetic predisposition
- Environmental triggers, possibly infectious:
  - Rubella or parvovirus B19 (5)
  - Heat shock proteins (5)
- Immunoglobulin or complement deficiency

Genetics
- Human leukocyte antigen (HLA) class I and II alleles
- HLA-A2: Early-onset oligoarthritis in females
- HLA-DRB1*11: Increased risk of systemic and oligo-JIA.
- HLA-B27: Risk of enthesitis-related arthritis
- HLA-DR4: Associated with polyarthritis RF(+) (5)

RISK FACTORS
Female gender

GENERAL PREVENTION
No known preventive measures

COMMONLY ASSOCIATED CONDITIONS
Other autoimmune disorders, chronic anterior uveitis (iridocyclitis), nutritional impairment, growth issues (5)

 DIAGNOSIS

Clinical diagnostic criteria: Age of onset <16 years and >6 weeks duration of objective arthritis in ≥1 joints, defined as swelling or restricted range of motion of a joint accompanied by heat, pain, or tenderness with no other form of childhood arthritis

HISTORY
- Arthralgias, fever, fatigue, malaise, myalgias, weight loss, morning stiffness, rash
- Limp if lower extremity involvement
- Arthritis for ≥6 weeks
- Behavioral and compliance problems frequent in toddlers and teenagers

PHYSICAL EXAM
- Joints: Swelling, effusion, limited range of motion, tenderness, pain with motion, warmth
- Rash, rheumatoid nodules, lymphadenopathy, hepato- or splenomegaly, enthesitis, dactylitis

DIFFERENTIAL DIAGNOSIS
- Musculoskeletal: Legg-Calve-Perthes, toxic synovitis, growing pains, Perthes disease
- Infectious: Septic arthritis, osteomyelitis, viral infection, mycoplasma infection, Lyme disease
- Reactive arthritis: Postinfectious, rheumatic fever, Reiter syndrome
- Inflammatory bowel disease: Crohn disease or ulcerative colitis
- Hemoglobinopathies; rickets
- Malignancy: Leukemia, bone tumors (osteoid osteoma), neuroblastoma
- Vasculitis, Henoch-Schönlein Purpura, Kawasaki disease
- Systemic lupus erythematosus, dermatomyositis, mixed connective tissue disease, sarcoidosis, systemic sclerosis, collagen disorders
- Trauma: Accidental or nonaccidental; abuse

DIAGNOSTIC TESTS & INTERPRETATION
Initial Tests (lab, imaging)
- CBC: Leukocyte count normal or markedly elevated (systemic), lymphopenia, reactive thrombocytosis, anemia
- Joint-fluid aspiration/analysis: Exclude infection
- Inflammatory markers: ESR and C-reactive protein may be elevated
- Antinuclear antibodies (ANA) positive (>1:80): 40% (polyarticular, oligoarticular, psoriatic early onset); increased risk of uveitis
- RF (+): 2–10% (usually polyarticular); poor prognosis
- HLA-B27 positive: Enthesitis-related arthritis
- Diagnostic radiography, MRI, US, and CT, play a role in diagnosing and monitoring, but no one modality has been found to have superior diagnostic value (6)[A]
- Radiograph of affected joint(s): Early radiographic changes: Soft tissue swelling, periosteal reaction, juxta-articular demineralization. Later changes include joint-space loss, articular surface erosions, subchondral cyst formation, sclerosis, joint fusion
- If orthopnea ECG to rule-out pericarditis
- Radionuclide scans: For infection, malignancy
- MRI can assess synovial hypertrophy, cartilage degeneration. Also used to monitor clinical responsiveness to treatment in peripheral joints

Follow-Up Tests & Special Considerations
- RF and ANA present in mixed connective tissue disease (7)
- In interpreting results of dual energy x-ray photon absorptiometry scans, it is important to use pediatric, not adult, controls as normative data.

Diagnostic Procedures/Other
- Synovial biopsy: Indicated if the synovial fluid cannot be aspirated or if infection is suspected in spite of negative synovial fluid culture
- Arthrocentesis

Test Interpretation
Synovial Biopsy: Synovial cells hyperplasia, hyperemia, infiltration of small lymphocytes and mononuclear cells

 TREATMENT

GENERAL MEASURES
- Goal: Control active disease and extra-articular manifestations to achieve clinical remission
- All patients require regular (every 3–4 months for oligo-JIA and in ANA-positive patients) ophthalmic exams to uncover asymptomatic eye disease, at least for first 3 years
- Moist heat, sleeping bag, or electric blanket to relieve morning stiffness
- Splints for contractures
- Aerobic exercise: Weight bearing or aquatic to improve vital capacity (8)

MEDICATION
First Line
- ≤4 Joints:
  - NSAIDs: Adequate in ~50%, symptoms often improve within days, full efficacy 2–3 months
  - Drugs for children include:
    - Ibuprofen (Motrin, Advil, Nuprin): 30–50 mg/kg/d, divided q.i.d., max 800 mg t.i.d.

○ Naproxen (Naprosyn, Aleve): 10 mg/kg/d divided b.i.d., max dose of 500 mg b.i.d.
○ Tolmetin sodium: 20 mg/kg/d; t.i.d. or q.i.d., max dose 600 mg t.i.d.
○ Diclofenac: 2–3 mg/kg, divided t.i.d., max of 50 mg t.i.d.
○ Indomethacin: 1–2 mg/kg/d, divided b.i.d. to q.i.d., max of 4 mg/kg/day
○ Contraindications to NSAIDs: Known allergies
○ Precautions: May worsen bleeding diatheses; use caution with all NSAIDs in renal insufficiency and hypovolemic states; take with food
○ Significant possible interactions: NSAIDs may lower serum levels of digitalis and anticonvulsants and blunt the effect of loop diuretics. NSAIDs may increase serum methotrexate levels.

- Intra-articular long-acting corticosteroids: Immediately effective, local treatment. Improve synovitis, joint damage, contractures, prevent leg length discrepancy (7)[B]: Triamcinolone hexacetonide
  – Intra-articular glucocorticoids: Patients with oligoarthritis who have failed a 2-month NSAID trial or with poor prognosis factors (9)[C]
- ≥5 Joints:
  – If high disease activity or a failed 1–2 month NSAID trial→ methotrexate (9)[C]

Second Line
- 30–40% of patients will require addition of disease-modifying antirheumatic drugs (DMARDs), including methotrexate, sulfasalazine, leflunomide, and tumor necrosis factor (TNF) antagonists (etanercept, infliximab, adalimumab). Newer biologic therapies, including IL-1 and IL-6 receptor antagonists, currently under investigation
- Methotrexate: 10 mg/m^2/wk PO or SC. 10 mg/m^2/wk is most frequently used (7)[B]:
  – Plateau of efficacy reached with 15 mg/m^2/wk; further increase in dosage is not associated with therapeutic benefit (10)
- Sulfasalazine: Oligoarticular and HLA B27 spondyloarthritis (7)[B]
- Etanercept (Enbrel): 0.8 mg/kg given SC q1wk or 0.4 mg/kg SC twice a week, max of 50 mg
- Infliximab: 5 mg/kg q6–8wk
- Adalimumab: If weight <30 kg, 20 mg SC q2wk; if weight >30 kg, 40 mg SC q2wk
- Tocilizumab: IL-6 antibody demonstrating efficacy in phase III open label trials; ongoing studies to evaluate efficacy and appropriate dosing regimen (7)[B]
- Anakinra: IL-1 receptor antibody under investigation with phase II and III clinical trials for systemic JIA (7)[B]
- Begin treatment with TNF-α inhibitors in children with a history of arthritis in ≤4 joints and significant active arthritis despite treatment with methotrexate, or arthritis in ≥5 joints and any active arthritis following an adequate trial of methotrexate (9)
- Begin treatment with anakinra in children with systemic arthritis and active fever whose treatment requires a 2nd medication in addition to systemic glucocorticoids (9)
- Analgesics for pain control, including narcotics

ISSUES FOR REFERRAL
- Pediatric rheumatologist is best suited to manage JIA.
- Orthopedic surgeon if needed

- Ophthalmologist: Uveitis
- Physical therapist for joint protection, to maintain range of motion, improve muscle strength, prevent deformities
- Occupational therapist to maintain and improve the normal life function
- Psychologists to aid in coping

SURGERY/OTHER PROCEDURES
- Total hip and/or knee replacement may be needed for severe disease.
- Soft-tissue release, if splinting/traction unsuccessful
- Limb length or angular deformity corrections
- Synovectomy is rarely performed.

IN-PATIENT CONSIDERATIONS
Admission Criteria/Initial Stabilization
- Patient loses ambulatory ability
- Signs/Symptoms of pericarditis
- Persistent fever

Discharge Criteria
Resolution of fever and swelling or serositis

 ONGOING CARE

FOLLOW-UP RECOMMENDATIONS
Patient Monitoring
Determined by medication:
- NSAIDs: Periodic CBC, urinalysis, liver function tests (LFTs), renal function tests
- Aspirin and/or other salicylates: Transaminase and salicylate levels, weekly for 1st month, then every 3–4 months
- Methotrexate: Monthly LFTs, CBC, BUN, creatinine

DIET
Regular diet with special attention to adequate calcium, iron, protein, and caloric intake

PATIENT EDUCATION
- Ongoing education of patients and families with attention to: Psychosocial needs; school issues, educational needs; behavioral strategies for dealing with pain and noncompliance; use of healthcare resources; support groups
- Printed and audiovisual information available from local arthritis foundation

PROGNOSIS
- 50–60% ultimately remit, but functional ability depends on adequacy of long-term therapy (disease control, maintaining muscle and joint function).
- Poor prognosis: Active disease at 6 months, polyarticular disease, extended pauciarticular disease course, female gender, RF(+), ANA(+), persistent morning stiffness, rapid appearance of erosions, hip involvement

COMPLICATIONS
- Blindness, band keratopathy, glaucoma, short stature, micrognathia if temporomandibular joint involvement, debilitating joint disease, disseminated intravascular coagulation, hemolytic anemia
- On NSAIDs: Peptic ulcer, GI hemorrhage, CNS reactions, renal disease, leukopenia
- On DMARDs: Bone marrow suppression, hepatitis, renal disease, dermatitis, mouth ulcers, retinal toxicity (antimalarials, rare)
- On TNF antagonists: Higher risk of infection
- Osteoporosis, avascular necrosis
- Macrophage activation syndrome: Decreased blood cell precursors secondary to histiocyte degradation of marrow

REFERENCES

1. Restrepo R, Lee EY. Epidemiology, pathogenesis, and imaging of arthritis in children. *Orthop Clin N Am.* 2012;43:213–225.
2. Prince FH, Otten MH, van Suijlekom-Smit LW. Diagnosis and management of juvenile idiopathic arthritis. *BMJ.* 2010;341:c6434. Epub 2010 Dec 3.
3. Behren EM, Beukelman T, et al. Evaluation of the presentation of systemic onset juvenile rheumatoid arthritis: data from the Pennsylvania Systemic Onset Juvenile Arthritis Registry. *J Rheumatol.* 2008;35:343–348.
4. Beukelman T, Haynes K, Curtis JR, et al. Rates of malignancy associated with juvenile idiopathic arthritis and its treatment. *Arthritis Rheum.* 2012;64(4):1263–1271. Epub 2012 Feb 10.
5. Weiss JE, Ilowite NT. Juvenile idiopathic arthritis. *Rheum Dis Clin N Am.* 2007;33:441–470.
6. McKay GM, Cox LA, Long BW, et al. Imaging juvenile idiopathic arthritis: Assessing the modalities. *Radiol Technol.* 2010;81:318–327.
7. Kahn P. Juvenile idiopathic arthritis—current & future therapies. *Bull NYU Hosp Jt Dis.* 2009;67: 291–302.
8. Klepper S. Making the case for exercise in children with juvenile idiopathic arthritis: What we know and where we go from here. *Arthritis Rheum.* 2007;57(6):887–890.
9. Beukelman T, Patkar N, Saag K, et al. 2011 American College of Rheumatology recommendation for the treatment of juvenile idiopathic arthritis: Initiation and safety monitoring of therapeutic agents for the treatment of arthritis and systemic features. *Arthritis Care Res.* 2011;63:465–482.
10. Takken T, van der Net J, Helders P. Methotrexate for treating juvenile idiopathic arthritis. *Cochrane Database Syst Rev.* 2001;4:CD003129.
11. Kemper AR, Van Mater HA, Coeytaux RR, et al. Systematic review of disease-modifying antirheumatic drugs for juvenile idiopathic arthritis. *BMC Pediatr.* 2012;12:29. Epub 2012 Mar 15.

ADDITIONAL READING
Chang HJ, Burke AE, Glass RM. JAMA patient page. Juvenile idiopathic arthritis. *JAMA.* 2010;303(13): 1328.

 CODES

ICD10
- M08.00 Unsp juvenile rheumatoid arthritis of unspecified site
- M08.90 Juvenile arthritis, unspecified, unspecified site
- M08.99 Juvenile arthritis, unspecified, multiple sites

CLINICAL PEARLS
- High-titer RF correlates with severity, and positive titers confer poorer prognosis.
- Moderate strength evidence exists to support that DMARDs improve JIA-associated symptoms (11)[A].

ARTHRITIS, OSTEO

LCDR Patrick Wakefield Joyner, MD, MS

BASICS

DESCRIPTION
- A common joint disease that involves progressive loss of articular cartilage and reactive changes at joint margins and in subchondral bone
- Primary:
  - Idiopathic: Divided into subsets by clinical features (localized, generalized, erosive)
- Secondary:
  - Posttraumatic
  - Childhood anatomic abnormalities (e.g., congenital hip dysplasia, SCFE, Legg-Calvé-Perthes disease)
  - Inheritable metabolic disorders (e.g., Wilson disease, alkaptonuria, hemochromatosis)
  - Neuropathic arthropathy (Charcot joints)
  - Hemophilic arthropathy
  - Endocrinopathies: Acromegalic arthropathy, hyperparathyroidism, hypothyroidism
  - Paget disease
  - Noninfectious inflammatory arthritis (e.g., rheumatoid arthritis [RA], spondyloarthropathies)
  - Gout, calcium pyrophosphate deposition disease (pseudogout)
  - Septic or tuberculous arthritis
- System(s) affected: Musculoskeletal
- Synonym(s):Osteoarthrosis; Degenerative joint disease

EPIDEMIOLOGY
- Symptomatic disease: >40 years old
- Leading cause of disability in those >65
- Radiographic evidence (estimates): 33% to ~90% in those >65
- Predominant sex: Male = Female
- 90% of hip osteoarthritis is primary and predominantly found in Caucasians.

Prevalence
- ~60 million patients
- Increases with age, almost universal >65 (by x-ray study but not clinically)
- Moderate to severe hip osteoarthritis is 3–6% in Caucasians; <1% in East Indians, blacks, Chinese, and Native Americans

ETIOLOGY AND PATHOPHYSIOLOGY
- Failure of chondrocytes to maintain the balance between degradation and synthesis of extracellular matrix
- Biomechanical, biochemical, inflammatory, and immunologic factors all implicated in pathogenesis

Genetics
- Up to 65% of OA may occur on a genetic basis.
- The heritability of end-stage hip OA has been estimated by one study to be 27%.
- Twin studies in women show heritability rates of OA: Knee, 49%; hand, 65%; hip, 50%.
- The genetic contribution may involve a combination of effects on structure (collagen), cartilage, or bone metabolism or inflammation.

RISK FACTORS
- Increasing age: >50
- The effect of age as a risk factor is greatest for hip and knee OA, especially after 70
- Hand OA has his greatest prevalence in women after menopause.
- Obesity (weight-bearing joints)
- Prolonged occupational or sports stress

- Injury to a joint from trauma, infection, or pre-existing inflammatory arthritis
- Female gender (knee and hand osteoarthritis [OA])

DIAGNOSIS

HISTORY
- Slowly developing joint pain that typically follows use of a joint
- Transient stiffness (especially after awakening in morning and after sitting) that tends to lessen 10–15 minutes after some movement and mobility of the joint

PHYSICAL EXAM
- Joint bony enlargement (Heberden nodules of distal interphalangeal joints; osteophytes can be palpated in many joints with severe OA)
- Decreased range of motion with pain at the end of the range
- Tenderness usually absent; may occur along joint margin associated with synovitis
- Crepitation is a late sign.
- Weakness and wasting of muscles around the joint
- Local pain and stiffness with OA of spine, with radicular pain (if compression of nerve roots)
- Changes in overall joint alignment (i.e., genu varus [bow-legged] and genu valgum [knock-kneed])

DIFFERENTIAL DIAGNOSIS
- Distinguish from other types of arthritis by:
  - Absence of systemic findings
  - Minimal articular inflammation
  - Distribution of involved joints (e.g., distal and proximal interphalangeal joints, not wrist and metacarpophalangeal joints)
- In spine, distinguish from osteoporosis, metastatic disease, multiple myeloma, or other bone diseases.

DIAGNOSTIC TESTS & INTERPRETATION
Initial Tests (lab, imaging)
- Usually not helpful in diagnosis (sedimentation rate not increased)
- X-ray films usually normal early
- Later often show:
  - Narrowed, asymmetric joint space
  - Osteophyte formation
  - Subchondral bony sclerosis
  - Subchondral cyst formation
  - In the hip, may appreciate changes in anatomical shape of the femoral head, especially in later stages of avascular necrosis
- Erosions may occur on surface of distal and proximal interphalangeal joints when OA is associated with inflammation (erosive OA).

Follow-Up Tests & Special Considerations
- May be useful in monitoring treatment with NSAIDs (renal insufficiency and GI bleeding)
- In secondary OA, underlying disorder may have abnormal lab results (e.g., hemochromatosis [abnormal iron studies]).

Diagnostic Procedures/Other
- Joint aspiration:
  - May be helpful in distinguishing from chronic inflammatory arthritis
  - OA: Cell count usually <500 cells/mm^3, predominantly mononuclear
  - Inflammatory: Cell count usually >2,000 cells/mm^3, predominantly neutrophils

- Calcium pyrophosphate dihydrate and/or apatite crystals may be seen in effusions.

Test Interpretation
- Characterized macroscopically by patchy cartilage damage and bony hypertrophy
- Histological phases:
  - Edema of the extracellular matrix and cartilage microcracks
  - Fissuring and pitting of the subchondral bone
  - Erosion and osteocartilaginous loose bodies
- Subchondral bone trabecular microfractures and sclerosis with osteophyte formation
- Degradation response produced by release of proteolytic enzymes, collagenolytic enzymes, prostaglandins, and immune responses

TREATMENT

GENERAL MEASURES
- Weight reduction with a fitness program if overweight is essential (1,2,3)[A].
- Walking aids and proper footwear (1)[A]
- Heat (e.g., local, tub baths) or cold applications
- Physical therapy to maintain or regain joint motion and muscle strength:
  - Quadriceps-strengthening exercises can relieve knee pain and disability.
- Muscle strengthening exercises are specific for impairment-related outcomes (i.e., pain).
- Aerobic exercise contributes to better long-term functional outcomes.
- Maintain exercise; all benefits gained are lost 6 months after cessation of the program.
- Protect joints from overuse; ambulatory aides are beneficial (e.g., cane, crutches, walker).
- Assessment for bracing, joint supports, or insoles in those with biomechanical joint pain or instability:
  - Bracing is more beneficial in patients with unicompartmental disease of the knee, and in higher-demand patients.
  - Knee OA:

- *Nonpharmacologic modalities strongly recommended*: Aerobic, aquatic and/or resistance exercise and weight loss (3)[A]
- *Nonpharmacologic modalities conditionally recommended*: Medial wedge insoles for valgus knee OA, subtalar strapped lateral insoles for varus knee OA, medially directed patellar taping, manual therapy, walking aids, thermal agents, tai chi, self-management programs, and psychosocial intervention (3)[A]

MEDICATION
First Line
- Management of pain and inflammation:

  - Acetaminophen up to 1,000 mg q.i.d.: Good evidence as most effective for pain relief in OA of knee and hip (1)[A]

  - A number of studies, mainly of OA of knee, have shown short-term (<4 weeks) benefits from topical NSAID gels, creams, and ointments when compared with placebo. Topical NSAIDs should be a core treatment for knee and hand OA.

- If acetaminophen or topical NSAIDs are insufficient, then the addition or substitution by an PO NSAID/COX-2 inhibitor should be considered. Use at the lowest effective dose for the shortest time possible. Prolonged use is associated with renal insufficiency, hypertension, leg edema, and GI bleeding.
- May use nonacetylated salicylates (e.g., salsalate, choline-magnesium salicylate) or low-dose ibuprofen ≤1,600 mg/d.
- Topical NSAIDs and capsaicin can be effective as adjunctives and alternatives to PO analgesic/anti-inflammatory agents in knee OA (1)[A].
- Other NSAIDs have similar efficacy.
- Contraindications:
  - All PO NSAIDs/COX-2 inhibitors have analgesic effects of a similar magnitude but vary in their potential GI and cardio-renal toxicity.
  - NSAIDs are contraindicated in patients with renal disease, CHF, HTN, active peptic ulcer disease, and previous hypersensitivity to an NSAID or aspirin (asthma, nasal polyps, hypotension, urticaria/angioedema).
  - Combinations of NSAIDs or concomitant aspirin are contraindicated due to risk of adverse reactions.
  - If cardiovascular risk: Combination of a nonselective NSAID and low-dose aspirin is recommended.
  - Oral or parenteral corticosteroids are contraindicated.
- Precautions:
  - If PO NSAID/COX-2 inhibitor is necessary for a patient aged >65 or a patient <65 with any increased GI risk factors, offer a proton-pump inhibitor.
  - Significant possible interactions:
    o NSAIDs reduce effectiveness of ACE inhibitors and diuretics.
    o Aspirin and NSAIDs (except COX-2 inhibitors) may increase effects of anticoagulants.
    o Increased hypoglycemic effects of oral hypoglycemics with aspirin
    o Salicylates reduce effectiveness of spironolactone (Aldactone) and uricosurics.
    o Corticosteroids and some antacids increase salicylate excretion, whereas ascorbic acid and ammonium chloride reduce salicylate excretion and may cause toxicity.

Pregnancy Considerations
- ASA and NSAIDs: Some risk to fetus during 1st and 3rd trimesters of pregnancy
- Compatible with breastfeeding

Second Line
- Topical capsaicin should be considered as an adjunct therapy for knee and hand OA; may cause local burning.
- Topical NSAIDs: Volteran gel, not likely to help in obese patients; however, can eliminate the gastric and renal risks associated with oral NSAIDs.
- Rubefacients are not recommended.
- Physical therapy: Strengthening the core for hip OA, and strengthening the muscles about the knee for knee OA can greatly decrease joint reactive forces on the affected joint.
- Bracing: Medial unloader brace for lateral knee arthritis and lateral unloader bracing for medial knee arthritis can decrease joint reactive forces and possibly eliminate need for pharmaceutical treatment of OA.

Third Line
- Judiciously use intra-articular injections of corticosteroids (CS) for selected acute flare-ups of joints and for people who fail 1st- and 2nd-line treatments (no more than 4 per year up to a maximum of 12 injections per joint).
- Intra-articular viscosupplementation with hyaluronic acid (HA) preparations into a painful knee may provide relief of pain and improve function at earlier stages.
- HA injections are permitted every 6 months and frequently can be alternated with CS injections.
- Recent literature demonstrates no difference in clinical effects of CS vs. HA injections. However, HA injections are thought be more protective of the cartilage in affected joint.
- Additionally, recent literature demonstrates that TENS unit may be more effective than HA injection at 2-week and 3-month follow-ups. This has the benefit of not being as invasive or painful, but requires strict patience compliance.
- Ultrasound may allow for proper placement of an injection, vs. use of anatomic landmarks alone.

ADDITIONAL THERAPIES
Address psychosocial factors (i.e., self-efficacy, coping skills). Prevent or treat anxiety and depression. Improve social support.

SURGERY/OTHER PROCEDURES
May be indicated in advanced disease (e.g., osteotomy, debridement, removal of loose bodies, joint replacement, fusion)

COMPLEMENTARY AND ALTERNATIVE MEDICINE
- Nutritional supplements such as glucosamine and chondroitin sulfate may symptomatically benefit some patients and have low toxicity, but studies lack standardized case definition and outcome assessments. *If no response is apparent within 6 months, treatment should be discontinued.*
- A 2010 meta-analysis shows glucosamine, chondroitin, and their combination do not reduce joint pain or have an impact on narrowing of joint space compared with placebo.
- TENS units and acupuncture may be beneficial (1)[A].

 ONGOING CARE

FOLLOW-UP RECOMMENDATIONS
Patient Monitoring
- Follow range of motion and functional status at regular intervals.
- Watch for GI blood loss and follow cardiac, renal, and mental status in older patients on NSAIDs or aspirin.
- Periodic CBC, renal function tests, stool for occult blood

PATIENT EDUCATION
- American College of Rheumatology patient education overviews: Http://www.rheumatology.org/public/factsheets/index.asp?aud = pat
- Arthritis Foundation: Http://www.arthritis.org

PROGNOSIS
- Progressive disease: Early in course, pain relieved by rest; later, pain may occur at rest and at night.
- Joint effusions and enlargement may occur, especially in knees.
- Osteophyte (spur) formation, especially at joint margins

- Advanced stage with full-thickness loss of cartilage down to bone

COMPLICATIONS
- Leading causes of pain and disability
- Decompensated CHF, GI bleeding, decreased renal function on NSAIDs or aspirin

REFERENCES
1. Zhang W, Moskowitz RW, Nuki G, et al. OARSI recommendations for the management of hip and knee osteoarthritis, Part II: OARSI evidence-based, expert consensus guidelines. *Osteoarthr Cartil*. 2008;16:137–162.
2. Jiang L, Tian W, Wang Y, et al. Body mass index and susceptibility to knee osteoarthritis: A systematic review and meta-analysis. *Joint Bone Spine*. 2011.
3. Hochberg MC, Altman RD, April KT, et al. American College of Rheumatology 2012 recommendations for the use of nonpharmacologic and pharmacologic therapies in osteoarthritis of the hand, hip, and knee. *Arthritis Care Res (Hoboken)*. 2012;64(4):455–474.

ADDITIONAL READING
- Altman R, Barkin RL. Topical therapy for osteoarthritis: Clinical and pharmacologic perspectives. *Postgrad Med*. 2009;121:139–147.
- Atchia I, Kane D, Isaacs JD, et al. Efficacy of a single ultrasound-guided injection for the treatment of hip osteoarthritis. *Ann Rheum Dis*. 2011;70(1):110–116.
- Chen WL, Hsu WC, Lin YJ, et al. Comparison of intra-articular hyaluronic acid injections with transcutaneous electric nerve stimulation for the management of knee osteoarthritis: A randomized controlled trial. *Arch Phys Med Rehabil*. 2013;94(8):1482–1489.
- Prieto-Alhambra D, Judge A, Javaid MK, et al. Incidence and risk factors for clinically diagnosed knee, hip and hand osteoarthritis: Influences of age, gender and osteoarthritis affecting other joints. *Ann Rheum Dis*. Epub 2013 Jun.
- Shimizu M, Higuchi H, Takagishi K, et al. Clinical and biochemical characteristics after intra-articular injection for the treatment of osteoarthritis of the knee: Prospective randomized study of sodium hyaluronate and corticosteroid. *J Orthop Sci*. 2010;15(1):51–56.
- Walsh NE, Hurley MV. Evidence based guidelines and current practice for physiotherapy management of knee osteoarthritis. *Musculoskeletal Care*. 2009;7(1):45–56.

CODES

ICD10
- M19.90 Unspecified osteoarthritis, unspecified site
- M19.91 Primary osteoarthritis, unspecified site
- M19.93 Secondary osteoarthritis, unspecified site

CLINICAL PEARLS
- Morning stiffness lasts <15 minutes (vs. 1 hour in rheumatoid arthritis).
- Distal predominance in hands
- Limit intra-articular steroid injections to 4 per year; may benefit from alternating with HA injections.

ARTHRITIS, PSORIATIC

Andrew Kim, MD • Nikki A. Levin, MD, PhD

BASICS

Psoriatic arthritis (PsA) is a chronic, destructive, seronegative arthropathy seen most commonly in patients with long-standing psoriasis.

DESCRIPTION
PsA is a seronegative spondyloarthropathy characterized by inflammatory arthritis and enthesitis.
- 5 patterns of arthritis in PsA:
  - Asymmetric oligoarthritis: Involves <5 small or large joints
  - Distal interphalangeal (DIP) joint predominant: Osteoarthritis-like, often associated with nail psoriasis
  - Symmetric polyarthritis: May be indistinguishable from rheumatoid arthritis (RA), but typically milder clinical course
  - Spondyloarthritis: Asymmetric and discontinuous, unlike ankylosing spondylitis (AS)
  - Arthritis mutilans: Destructive, resorptive arthritis; produces so-called opera-glass or telescoping digit
- Although psoriasis generally is present, it may be limited in extent:
  - Course of arthritis and extent of psoriasis do not appear to correlate.
  - Other extra-articular features, such as iritis, are less common.
  - Damaging joint disease may occur in 40–57%. Characteristic radiologic changes include joint erosions that begin marginally and move centrally ("pencil-in-cup deformity") and periostitis.
- Rheumatoid factor (RF) and cyclic citrullinated peptide (anti-CCP) antibody are usually negative. HLA-B27 may be positive.

EPIDEMIOLOGY
- Peak onset age: 30–50 years
- Predominant gender: Female = Male
- Polyarthritis is more common in women
- Spondylitis in up to 25%, more common in males
- Psoriasis precedes arthritis in the majority by an average of 12 years. Arthritis may precede psoriasis in up to 15%, and this occurs more often in children. Arthritis and psoriasis also may present simultaneously.
- Psoriasis occurs in 2–3% of the US population; 6–42% of these individuals develop PsA (1).

Prevalence
Prevalence: 1–2/1,000 population (1)

ETIOLOGY AND PATHOPHYSIOLOGY
- CD4+/CD8+ T cells; tumor necrosis factor-α (TNF-α); interleukins (IL) 1, 6, 8, and 10; and matrix metalloproteases present in synovial fluid (2)
- Osteoclast precursor cell upregulation
- Unknown: Probably multifactorial: Immunologic, genetic, environmental factors

Genetics
- 30–40% concordance in identical twins
- HLA-B27 in 15–50% with PsA (spondylitis pattern) vs. 90% in AS
- Other HLA associations in psoriatic arthritis: HLA-B7, HLA-B38, HLA-B39, HLA-Cw6

RISK FACTORS
- Psoriasis
- Family history of PsA

GENERAL PREVENTION
There are no currently available prevention strategies. It is unknown if early systemic treatment of psoriasis prevents the onset of PsA.

COMMONLY ASSOCIATED CONDITIONS
Psoriasis

DIAGNOSIS

- Establishing a history of inflammatory arthritis, dactylitis, or enthesitis in a patient with existing psoriasis is usually adequate to establish the diagnosis. Nonetheless, differentiation from other inflammatory arthropathies, such as RA, can be difficult.
- The CASPAR (**ClAS**sification criteria for **P**soriatic **AR**thritis) criteria comprise a validated instrument that may be used to screen patients for the presence of PsA. The sensitivity and specificity of the CASPAR criteria are 91.4% and 98.7%, respectively. To establish the presence of PsA, a patient must have inflammatory articular disease (joint, spine, or entheseal) with ≥3 points from the following 5 categories (3):
  - Evidence of current psoriasis, a personal history of psoriasis, or family history of psoriasis (2 points)
  - Typical psoriatic nail dystrophy, including onycholysis, pitting, and hyperkeratosis (1 point)
  - A negative RF, preferentially analyzed by ELISA (1 point)
  - Current dactylitis or a history of dactylitis (1 point)
  - Radiologic evidence of new bone formation (excluding osteophyte formation) on plain radiographs of the hand or foot (1 point)

HISTORY
- Long-standing (most often) psoriasis
- Morning stiffness of hands, feet, or low back for >30 minutes
- Discomfort or pain of involved joints
- Swelling or redness of peripheral joints
- Low back or buttock pain
- Ankle or heel pain
- Dactylitis, or uniform swelling of an entire digit

PHYSICAL EXAM
- Affected peripheral joints may have overlying erythema, warmth, and swelling:
  - Synovitis
  - Dactylitis
  - Swelling of tendons (e.g., Achilles' tendon) and tenderness at insertion sites (e.g., calcaneus)
  - Limited range of motion of axial skeleton
  - Pain with stress on the sacroiliac joint
- Well-demarcated pink-to-red erythematous plaques with a white silvery scale; common locations include scalp, ears, trunk, buttocks, elbows and forearms, knees and legs, and palms and soles
- Nails may be dystrophic with pits, oil spots, crumbling, leukonychia, and red lunulae.

DIFFERENTIAL DIAGNOSIS
- Reactive arthritis
- Psoriasis and RA
- Psoriasis and osteoarthritis
- Psoriasis and polyarticular gout
- Psoriasis and AS

DIAGNOSTIC TESTS & INTERPRETATION
History and physical exam may provide adequate data to establish the diagnosis of PsA. Plain radiographs may demonstrate characteristic changes and aid in the diagnosis of PsA. Imaging allows assessment of current damage, disease progression, and response to therapy.

Initial Tests (lab, imaging)
- Serum RF is usually negative.
- Anti-CCP is usually negative.
- Antinuclear antibodies are usually negative.
- Acute-phase reactants (ESR and C-reactive protein) may be elevated.
- HLA-B27 is noted in 50–70% with axial disease and <15% with peripheral disease.
- Juxta-articular new bone formation (periostitis) and marginal joint erosions that may progress centrally to form the "pencil-in-cup" erosions are the most characteristic plain radiographic features.
- Baseline plain radiographs of affected joints

Follow-Up Tests & Special Considerations
Follow-up radiographs; interval based on severity

Diagnostic Procedures/Other
Diagnosis is clinical.

Test Interpretation
Diagnosis is clinical, and biopsy of either skin or synovium is not usually required.

TREATMENT

GENERAL MEASURES
Physical therapy and/or occupational therapy may be beneficial in all stages of disease.

- Treatment algorithms in PsA are based on severity of joint symptoms, extent of structural damage, and extent and severity of psoriasis (4)[A].
- NSAIDs may be considered for control of symptoms with mild disease. Intra-articular glucocorticoid injections may be given judiciously to control symptoms for persistent mono- or oligoarthritis.
- *There are no systematic trials of NSAIDs for PsA treatment.* NSAIDs doses are typically directed toward suppressing mild inflammation and selection should consider patient preference and dosing schedule.
- Monotherapy is as effective as combination therapy (≥2 drugs from the following: Analgesics, NSAIDs, opioids, opioid-like drugs, and neuromodulators [antidepressants, anticonvulsants, and muscle relaxants]) for adults (5)[A].
- All patients with moderate to severe peripheral arthritis should be started on disease-modifying antirheumatic drugs (DMARDs). DMARDs have the potential to reduce or prevent joint damage and preserve joint integrity and function.
- First-line DMARDs recommended for therapy are sulfasalazine, leflunomide, methotrexate, and cyclosporine. No evidence supports the use of combination DMARD therapy.
- Patients who fail to respond to at least 1 standard DMARD drug should be considered for anti-TNF-α therapy. Patients with poor prognosis could be considered for anti-TNF-α therapy even if they have not failed a standard DMARD (6)[A].

- With the exception of the TNF-α inhibitors, all medications discussed here are currently not FDA-approved for psoriatic arthritis and are being used off-label.

MEDICATION
First Line
NSAIDs (7)[A]: Sample doses of select NSAIDs:
- Ibuprofen 400–800 mg PO t.i.d.–q.i.d.
- Naproxen 250–500 mg PO b.i.d.–t.i.d.
- Meloxicam 7.5–15 mg/d PO

Second Line
Initial dosing regimens for DMARDs:
- Sulfasalazine (2 g/d PO divided in b.i.d. dosing) (8)[A]
- Leflunomide (loading dose of 100 mg/d PO for 3 days, then 20 mg/d PO) (7)[A]
- Methotrexate (1 test dose of 2.5–5 mg PO to assess for significant bone marrow suppression, then 7.5–25 mg once weekly) (8)[B]
- Cyclosporine (2.5–5 mg/kg/d PO divided in b.i.d. dosing) (8)[B]
- Azathioprine (0.5 mg/kg/d, with a max dose of 2.5 mg/kg/d if no signs of cytopenia at lower doses) (7,8)[B].

TNF-α inhibitors: Dosing regimens for biologics:
- Adalimumab (40 mg SC q2wk) (7)[A]
- Etanercept (50 mg SC weekly) (8)[A]
- Golimumab (50 mg SC monthly) (6)[A]
- Infliximab (5 mg/kg at 0, 2, and 6 weeks, q8wk afterward) (8)[A]

IL-12/23 inhibitor:
- Ustekinumab is currently dosed at 45 or 90 mg (depending on weight) at 0 and 4 weeks, q12wk thereafter (9)[A].

ALERT
- Anti-TNF agents should not be used in the setting of active infection, including in patients with TB and hepatitis B infection, with concurrent live vaccinations, with New York Heart Association (NYHA) class III–IV congestive heart failure, with malignancy, or with history of demyelinating disease.
- Ustekinumab should not be used in patients with active infection, especially mycobacterial or *Salmonella* infection, with concurrent live vaccinations, including bacillus Calmette-Guérin vaccination, or with history of malignancy.

Pregnancy Considerations
- Avoid teratogenic medications (e.g., category X medications such as methotrexate, leflunomide) during pregnancy.
- Adalimumab, etanercept, golimumab, infliximab, and ustekinumab are currently listed as Category B medications.

ISSUES FOR REFERRAL
- Rheumatology
- Dermatology

SURGERY/OTHER PROCEDURES
Joint fusion or replacement for advanced destruction

 ## ONGOING CARE

FOLLOW-UP RECOMMENDATIONS
Epidemiologic evidence suggests a relation between psoriasis, metabolic syndrome, myocardial infarction, and stroke. Periodic measurement of BP, fasting lipids and glucose, cholesterol, and body mass index is recommended (10).

PATIENT EDUCATION
- Stress noncontagious nature of condition
- For a listing of sources for patient education materials favorably reviewed on this topic, physicians may contact:
  – National Psoriasis Foundation, 6600 SW 92nd Ave., Suite 300, Portland, OR 97223. Also see www.psoriasis.org/i-have-psoriatic-arthritis
  – Arthritis Foundation, 2970 Peachtree Road NW, Suite 200, Atlanta, GA 30305, 404-237-8771. Also see www.arthritis.org/conditions-treatments/disease-center/psoriatic-arthritis/
  – American College of Rheumatology, 2200 Lake Boulevard NE, Atlanta, GA 30319, 404-633-3777. Also see www.rheumatology.org/practice/clinical/patients/diseases_and_conditions/psoriaticarthritis.asp

PROGNOSIS
- Course: Insidious and chronic joint disease and recurring and remitting chronic skin disease
- More favorable than for RA (except for patients who develop arthritis mutilans)

COMPLICATIONS
- Chronicity
- Disability
- Psychosocial impact of psoriasis

REFERENCES
1. American Academy of Dermatology Work Group, Menter A, Korman NJ, et al. Guidelines of care for the management of psoriasis and psoriatic arthritis: Section 6. Guidelines of care for the treatment of psoriasis and psoriatic arthritis: Case-based presentations and evidence-based conclusions. *J Am Acad Dermatol*. 2011;65: 137–174.
2. Gottlieb A, Korman NJ, Gordon KB, et al. Guidelines of care for the management of psoriasis and psoriatic arthritis: Section 2. Psoriatic arthritis: Overview and guidelines of care for treatment with an emphasis on the biologics. *J Am Acad Dermatol*. 2008;58:851–864.
3. Taylor W, Gladman D, Helliwell P, et al. Classification criteria for psoriatic arthritis: Development of new criteria from a large international study. *Arthritis Rheum*. 2006;54: 2665–2673.
4. Menter A, Korman NJ, Elmets CA, et al. Guidelines of care for the management of psoriasis and psoriatic arthritis. Section 3. Guidelines of care for the management and treatment of psoriasis with topical therapies. *J Am Acad Dermatol*. 2009;60:643–659.
5. Ramiro S, Radner H, van der Heijde D, et al. Combination therapy for pain management in inflammatory arthritis (rheumatoid arthritis, ankylosing spondylitis, psoriatic arthritis, other spondyloarthritis). *Cochrane Database Syst Rev*. 2011;10:CD008886.
6. Ash Z, Gaujoux-Viala C, Gossec L, et al. A systematic literature review of drug therapies for the treatment of psoriatic arthritis: Current evidence and meta-analysis informing the EULAR recommendations for the management of psoriatic arthritis. *Ann Rheum Dis*. 2012;71: 319–326.
7. Menter A, Korman NJ, Elmets CA, et al. Guidelines of care for the management of psoriasis and psoriatic arthritis: Section 4. Guidelines of care for the management and treatment of psoriasis with traditional systemic agents. *J Am Acad Dermatol*. 2009;61:451–485.
8. Ritchlin CT, Kavanaugh A, Gladman DD, et al. Treatment recommendations for psoriatic arthritis. *Ann Rheum Dis*. 2009;68:1387–1394.
9. McInnes I, Kavanaugh A, Gottlieb A, et al. Efficacy and safety of ustekinumab in patients with active psoriatic arthritis: 1 year results of the phase 3, multicentre, double-blind, placebo-controlled PSUMMIT 1 trial. *Lancet*. 2013;382:780–789.
10. Gottlieb AB, Dann F. Comorbidities in patients with psoriasis. *Am J Med*. 2009;122:1150.e1–e9.
11. Prey S, Paul C, Bronsard V, et al. Assessment of risk of psoriatic arthritis in patients with plaque psoriasis: A systematic review of the literature. *J Eur Acad Dermatol Venereol*. 2010;24(Suppl 2): 31–35.

ADDITIONAL READING
- Donahue KE, Jonas D, Hansen RA, et al. Drug therapy for psoriatic arthritis in adults: Update of a 2007 report [Internet]. 2012 April. Report No.: 12-EHC024-EF.
- Tillett W, McHugh N. Treatment algorithms for early psoriatic arthritis: do they depend on disease phenotype? *Curr Rheumatol Rep*. 2012;14(4): 334–342.
- Winchester R, Minevich G, Steshenko V, et al. HLA associations reveal genetic heterogeneity in psoriatic arthritis and in the psoriasis phenotype. *Arthritis Rheum*. 2012;64:1134–1144.

 ## CODES

ICD10
- L40.50 Arthropathic psoriasis, unspecified
- L40.51 Distal interphalangeal psoriatic arthropathy
- L40.53 Psoriatic spondylitis

CLINICAL PEARLS
- Severity of psoriasis may correlate with the likelihood of developing arthritis; however, severity of psoriasis does not correlate with severity of arthritis; 24% of psoriasis patients develop PsA (11)[A].
- Often overlooked locations of psoriasis include scalp, ears, umbilicus, and gluteal cleft.
- Other conditions may mimic or coexist with PsA, such as osteoarthritis and polyarticular gout.
- The polyarticular pattern of PsA may mimic RA; however, the presence of enthesitis and recognition of psoriasis characterize PsA.
- Axial skeleton involvement in PsA is asymmetric and discontinuous, in contrast to axial involvement in AS.

ARTHRITIS, RHEUMATOID (RA)
Dan Sepdham, MD • Kevin Ko, MD

BASICS

DESCRIPTION
- Chronic systemic autoimmune inflammatory disease with symmetric polyarthritis and synovitis of multifactorial etiology
- Progressive chronic inflammation leads to large and small joint destruction, deformity, and decline in functional status.
- System(s) affected: Musculoskeletal; Skin; Hematologic; Lymphatic; Immunologic; Muscular; Renal; Cardiovascular; Neurologic; Pulmonary

Geriatric Considerations
- Increased contribution/interaction of age-related comorbidities; pericarditis, septic arthritis, Sjögren syndrome are more common
- Less tolerance to drugs; increased incidence of hydroxychloroquine-associated maculopathy, D-penicillamine rash, and sulfasalazine-induced nausea/vomiting

Pregnancy Considerations
- Use effective contraception with disease-modifying antirheumatic drugs (DMARDs) Modify regimen with pregnancy or breastfeeding.
- >75% improve during pregnancy because of immunologic tolerance, but relapse in 6 months. First episodes may occur in pregnancy.

EPIDEMIOLOGY
Incidence
- Incidence of RA is 25–30/100,00 cases.
- Women are affected ~3–5× more than males.
- Peak age is 35–50 years (1).

Prevalence
US population: 1.0%. Affects all populations with increased prevalence in Native Americans

ETIOLOGY AND PATHOPHYSIOLOGY
- Pathogenesis is not completely known, but is postulated to be triggered by an insult, such as infection, that precipitates an initial autoimmune reaction. Systemic disorder primarily affecting synovial tissues whereby antibody-complement complex activation leads to synovial hypertrophy and joint inflammation. Pathogenesis mediated by abnormal B- and T-cell interactions.
- Multifactorial based on genetic, host (hormonal, immunologic), environmental (socioeconomic, smoking) factors

Genetics
- Genetic factors account for ~50% of development of RA.
- Monozygotic twin concordance 15–20%, implying nongenetic roles contributing to development of RA
- 1st-degree relatives have 1.5-fold higher risk than the general population of developing RA.
- HLA-DR4+ persons have increased relative risk of 4–5×.

RISK FACTORS
- HLA genes contribute to 30–50% genetic risk.
- Family history: 1st-degree relative has 2–3-fold increased risk
- Native American ethnicity
- History of smoking has shown an increased prevalence of RA.

COMMONLY ASSOCIATED CONDITIONS
Accelerated atherosclerosis, pericarditis, amyloidosis, felty syndrome (RA, splenomegaly, neutropenia), interstitial lung disease, pulmonary nodules, rheumatoid nodules, vasculitis, lymphomas

DIAGNOSIS

HISTORY
- Constitutional symptoms: Fatigue, malaise, weight loss, low-grade fevers
- Articular symptoms: Tender/swollen joints, early morning stiffness (at least 30 min), difficulty with ADLs
- Extra-articular involvement: Skin, heart, lungs, and eye symptoms. Onset is typically insidious; rarely, patients can present with abrupt onset of symptoms and extra-articular manifestations.

PHYSICAL EXAM
- Evaluate for swollen or tender joints, especially in the following:
  - Small joints: MCP, PIP, wrist, 2nd–5th MTP, and thumb IP joints. Pain and decreased ROM. Joint involvement is typically symmetric and involves smaller joints first.
  - Large joints: Shoulders, elbows, hips, knees, and ankles
  - Flexor tenosynovitis of fingers is common and suggests poor prognosis. Nerve entrapment may ensue.
  - Swan-neck deformity of the fingers may occur. Phalanges may shorten over time and become unstable.
- Extra-articular: Splenomegaly, lymphadenopathy, subcutaneous nodules, peripheral neuropathy, and atlantoaxial joint involvement may lead to cervical spine instability. Axial migration of dens into foramen magnum may contribute to occipital headaches.

DIFFERENTIAL DIAGNOSIS
- Sjögren syndrome, SLE, systemic sclerosis, adult Still disease
- Seronegative polyarthritis, erosive osteoarthritis, psoriatic arthritis, crystal arthropathy, septic arthritis, rheumatic fever, chronic Lyme disease, viral-induced arthritis (parvovirus B19, hepatitis C [with cryoglobulinemia]), occult malignancy, vasculitis (Behçet syndrome)

DIAGNOSTIC TESTS & INTERPRETATION
Initial Tests (lab, imaging)
- CBC: Mild anemia; thrombocytosis is common and associated with disease activity.
- ESR: Usually elevated marker of inflammation, used to assess disease activity
- CRP: Unspecific, direct measure of impact of IL-6 on liver cells; used to assess disease activity
- Rheumatoid factor (RF): >1:80 in 70–80% of patients with RA (most commonly IgM Ab)
- *Anticyclic citrullinated peptide antibodies (anti-CCP antibodies). Specificity >90%*
- Antinuclear antibody: Present in 20–30%
- Electrolytes, creatinine, liver function, and urinalysis to assess comorbid states

- Radiographic abnormalities are very useful in diagnosis and treatment.
- Plain film radiographs are the first choice in imaging RA:
  - Radiographs of the hands, wrists, and feet are generally initially assessed.
  - Hallmark is a lack of bony remodeling and symmetric joint space narrowing.
  - Earliest pattern of erosions is loss of cortical distinctness, followed by dot-dash pattern of cortical loss. Marginal erosions at cortical bone within joint capsule not covered by cartilage are called "mouse-ear" erosions.
- Periarticular osteopenia is an early finding in affected joints.

Follow-Up Tests & Special Considerations
- The 2010 American College of Rheumatology/ European League Against Rheumatism (ACR/EULAR) classification criteria: *Who should be screened?* (2)
- Patients with at least 1 joint and definite clinical synovitis which is not explained by another disease
- A score of ≥6 is needed for the classification of definite RA:
  - Score:
    - 1 large joint: 0
    - 2–10 large joints: 1
    - 1–3 small joints (with or without large joints. DIP, 1st MCP, and 1st MTP joints are excluded from assessment.): 2
    - 4–10 small joints (with or without large joints): 3
    - >10 joints (at least 1 small joint): 5
- Serology: At least 1 test is needed: Negative RF (rheumatoid factor) and negative ACPA (anticitrullinated protein antibody): 0; low positive RF or low positive ACPA: 2; high positive RF or high positive ACPA: 3
- Acute phase reactants: At least 1 result is needed. Normal CRP (C-reactive protein) and normal ESR: 0; abnormal CRP or ESR: 1
- Duration of symptoms: (self-reported) <6 weeks: 0; ≥6 weeks: 1
- Although patients with a score <6/10 are not classifiable as having RA, their status can be reassessed and the criteria might be fulfilled cumulatively over time.

Diagnostic Procedures/Other
- Joint aspiration can be performed to exclude crystal arthropathy and septic arthritis.
- Synovial fluid:
  - Typical analysis should include Gram stain, cell count, culture, crystal analysis, and overall appearance.
  - Yellowish-white, turbid, poor viscosity
  - WBC increased (3,500–50,000)
  - Protein: ~4.2 g/dL (42 g/L)
  - Serum-synovial glucose difference ≥30 mg/dL (≥1.67 mmol/L)

Test Interpretation
Synovial tissue is expanded by recruitment and retention of inflammatory cells, with formation of villous projections and pannus that invade and destroy cartilage and bone.

TREATMENT

Goals: Controlling disease activity, relieving pain, maintaining or improving function, preventing or correcting impairments, and promoting self-management

GENERAL MEASURES
- Early, aggressive treatment is desirable to prevent structural damage and disability.
- Key elements include periodical evaluation of disease activity and extent of synovitis.
- Arthritis self-management education is a proven effective intervention.

MEDICATION
- Early therapy with DMARDs is the standard of care as these agents slow disease progression and may induce more remissions.
- History of hepatitis, malignancy, CHF may alter 1st line therapy (3)[C].
- Recommend Tb testing prior to starting DMARDs (3)[C]
- Initial symptomatic therapy
  - NSAIDs naproxen (500 mg BID) or Motrin (800 mg TID) for symptomatic control. If poor response to initial NSAID after 2 weeks, try alternative NSAID.
  - If still poor response, can try prednisone (5–15 mg/d). Should taper off NSAID or prednisone as soon as effective control of disease activity with DMARD is achieved (1).
- DMARDS
  - Nonbiologic DMARDs:
    ○ Most experts agree that DMARD should be started when the diagnosis of RA is made (3).
    ○ Due to their greater convenience, lower toxicity profiles, and quicker onset of action, initial therapy is a nonbiologic DMARD: Methotrexate, sulfasalazine, and leflunomide have shown evidence of comparable efficacy.
    ○ Methotrexate (MTX) (Rheumatrex): 7.5–25 mg/wk PO. DMARD with the most predictable benefit; many significant side effects, but the addition of folate reduces toxicity. 3–6-month trial. Monitor CBC every month ×3 months, renal, and liver function every 8–12 weeks. Contraindicated in renal and hepatic diseases.
    ○ Sulfasalazine (SSZ): 500 mg/d, increase to 2 g/d over 1 month; max: 2–3 g/d; 6-month trial. Monotherapy for low disease activity. Monitor CBC, liver enzymes every 2 weeks ×3 mo, then every month ×3 mo, then every 3 mo. Screen for G6PD deficiency.
    ○ Leflunomide (Arava): Loading dose 100 mg/d ×3 days, then 10–20 mg/d. GI side effects and potentially teratogenic; contraindicated in pregnancy. Monitor CBC, LFTs, phosphate monthly first 6 months. Stop use if ALT > 3× upper limit normal.
    ○ Antimalarials: Hydroxychloroquine (HCQ) (Plaquenil) 400 mg qhs for 2–3 months, then 200 mg at bedtime; 6-month trial is usual. Usually used to treat milder forms or in combination with other DMARDs. Ophthalmologic exam every 3 months due to potential maculopathy. Adjust dose in renal insufficiency.

- Biological DMARDs:
  ○ Tumor necrosis factor (TNF) inhibitors: IV infliximab (Remicade), SC adalimumab (Humira), and SC etanercept (Enbrel). No evidence that one is superior. The combination with MTX appears to be the most effective. Optimal dosage and duration of treatment unclear. Low toxicity; costly. Check PPD prior to treatment and periodic CBC. Risk of lymphoma, CHF.
  ○ Anakinra (Kineret), an IL-1 receptor antagonist: Fewer clinical benefits than TNF inhibitors.
  ○ Abatacept (Orencia) and rituximab (Rituxan) approved for active moderate-to-severe RA with inadequate response to other DMARDs or failed anti-TNF agent
  ○ 2 long-acting anti-TNF agents, certolizumab pegol (Cimzia) and golimumab (Simponi), have been also approved in moderate to severe disease.
  - For guidelines on biologics, refer to 2012 update of 2008 American College of Rheumatology Recommendations for the Use of Disease Modifying Antirheumatic Drugs and Biologic Agents in the Treatment of Rheumatoid Arthritis (3).
- Flare ups:
  - Intra-articular steroids: If disease is well controlled except for a single joint or 2, after establishing that the joint is not infected

ADDITIONAL THERAPIES
- Capscasin Cream: apply 3–4 times per day. Best results seen after 2–4 weeks of continuous use (4)
- Interdisciplinary care and management including physical therapy to minimize the consequences of loss of function, joint damage, maladaptive coping, and social isolation
- RECOMMENDED VACCINATIONS
  - Pneumovax, HPV, Hep B, influenza (3)[C]

SURGERY/OTHER PROCEDURES
Surgical treatment, including synovectomy, tendon reconstruction, joint fusion, and joint replacement may be considered to prevent disability in advanced RA.

COMPLEMENTARY AND ALTERNATIVE MEDICINE
- Omega 3 shown to be beneficial in one small trial (4).
- Gamma linolenic acid and tripterygium wilfordi may have potential benefits.

ONGOING CARE

The goals of comprehensive, interdisciplinary care are to stop the disease process, reduce pain, manage symptoms such as fatigue and stiffness, preserve joint integrity and function, and maintain social and occupational roles and quality of life.

FOLLOW-UP RECOMMENDATIONS
- Encourage full activity, but avoid heavy work or exercise during active phases. Emphasize exercise, mobility, and reduction of joint stress.
- Promote general health care and psychosocial functional status.

Patient Monitoring
Address risk factors and evaluate for cardiovascular disease and osteoporosis.

DIET
Low-fat and low-sodium diet recommended as these patients are at increased risk for cardiovascular disease.

PATIENT EDUCATION
American College of Rheumatology patient education overviews: http://www.rheumatology.org/practice/clinical/patients/diseases_and_conditions/ra.asp

PROGNOSIS
- Poor prognostic findings:
  - Persistent moderate-to-severe disease; early or advanced age at disease onset
- 50% cannot function in their primary jobs within 10 years of onset.

REFERENCES
1. Wasserman, Amy. Diagnosis and Management of Rheumatoid Arthritis. *Am Fam Physician*. 2011;84 (11):1245–1252.
2. Aletaha D. 2010 Rheumatoid arthritis classification criteria: An American College of Rheumatology/ European League Against Rheumatism collaborative initiative. *Arthritis Rheum*. 2010; 62(9):2569–2581.
3. Singh JA, Furst DE, Bharat A, et al. 2012 Update of the 2008 American College of Rheumatology Recommendations for the use of Disease Modifying Antirheumatic Drugs and Biologic Agents in the Treatment of Rheumatoid Arthritis. *Arthritis Care Res (Hoboken)*. 2012;64(5):625–639.
4. Geusens P, Wouters. Long-term effect of omega-3 fatty acid supplementation in active rheumatoid arthritis. *Arthritis Rheum*. 1994;37(6):824.

ADDITIONAL READING
Richards BL. Neuromodulators for pain management in rheumatoid arthritis. *Cochrane Database Syst Rev*. 2012;1:CD008921.

CODES

ICD10
- M05.60 Rheu arthritis of unsp site w involv of organs and systems
- M06.80 Other specified rheumatoid arthritis, unspecified site
- M06.9 Rheumatoid arthritis, unspecified

CLINICAL PEARLS
- Females have more articular disease and males have more systemic presentations.
- RA is a chronic systemic inflammatory disease characterized by symmetric polyarthritis and synovitis of unknown cause.
- >75% improve during pregnancy because of immunologic tolerance, but relapse in 6 months
- Plain film radiographs are the first choice in imaging RA
- Early therapy with DMARDs is the standard of care as these agents slow disease progression and may induce more remissions

ARTHROPOD BITES AND STINGS

James E. Powers, DO, FACEP

 BASICS

DESCRIPTION

Arthropods make up the largest division of the animal kingdom; 2 classes, insects and arachnids, have the greatest medical impact on humans. Arthropods affect humans by inoculating poison or irritative substances through a bite or sting, by invading tissue, or by contact allergy to their skin, hairs, or secretions. The greatest medical importance is transmission of infectious micro-organisms that may occur during insect feeding. Sequelae to arthropod bites, stings, or contact may include:

- Local redness with itch, pain, and swelling: Common, usually immediate and transient
- Large local reactions increasing over 24–48 hours
- Systemic reactions with anaphylaxis, neurotoxicity, organ damage, or other systemic toxin effects
- Tissue necrosis or secondary infection
- Infectious disease transmission: Presentation may be delayed weeks to years

EPIDEMIOLOGY

Incidence
- Difficult to estimate, as most encounters unreported
- ~50 deaths per year in the US from fatal anaphylactic reaction to *Hymenoptera* stings
- Unrecognized anaphylactic reactions to *Hymenoptera* stings may be cause of 1/4 of sudden and unexpected deaths outdoors (1).

Prevalence
Widespread, with regional and seasonal variations

ETIOLOGY AND PATHOPHYSIOLOGY

- Arthropods: 4 medically important classes:
  – Insects: *Hymenoptera* (bees, wasps, hornets, fire ants), mosquitoes, bed bugs, flies, lice, fleas, beetles, caterpillars, and moths
  – Arachnids: Spiders, scorpions, mites, and ticks
  – Chilopods (centipedes)
  – Diplopods (millipedes)
- 4 general categories of pathophysiologic effects: toxic, allergic, infectious, traumatic:
  – Toxic effects of venom: Local (tissue inflammation or destruction) vs. systemic (neurotoxic or organ damage)
  – Allergic: Antigens in saliva may cause local inflammation. Exaggerated immune responses may result in anaphylaxis, serum sickness.
  – Trauma: Mechanical injury from biting or stinging causes pain, swelling, and portal of entry for bacteria and secondary infection. Retention of arthropod parts can cause a granulomatous reaction.
  – Infection: Arthropods are vectors and can transmit bacterial, viral, and protozoal diseases.

Genetics
Family history of atopy may be a factor in the development of more severe allergic reactions.

RISK FACTORS

- Previous sensitization is key to most severe allergic reactions, but exposure history may not be recalled.
- Although most arthropod contact is inadvertent, certain activities, occupations, and travel increase risk.
- Greater risk for adverse outcome in young, elderly, immune compromised, or those with unstable cardiac or respiratory status

GENERAL PREVENTION

- Avoidance of common arthropod habitats, where possible
- Insect repellents (not effective for bees, spiders, scorpions, caterpillars, bed bugs, fleas, ants):
  – DEET:
    ○ Most effective broad-spectrum repellent against biting arthropods (2)
    ○ Formulations with higher concentrations (20–50%) are first-line choice when visiting areas where arthropod-borne diseases are endemic (2)
    ○ Concentrations >30% give longer duration of effect
    ○ Safe for children >6 months of age and pregnant and lactating women (2)
  – Icaridin (formerly known as picaridin):
    ○ Use of concentrations <20% may require more frequent application to maintain effectiveness.
  – PMD: Component of lemon eucalyptus extract:
    ○ Recommended alternative repellent to DEET at concentrations >20% (2)
    ○ May be used in children > 6 months
  – IR3535: Less effective in most studies
  – Other botanical oils (citronella etc.): Less effective than DEET. Not for disease-endemic areas (2)
  – Barrier methods: Clothing, bed nets:
    ○ Use of light-colored pants, long-sleeved shirts, and hats may reduce arthropod impact.
    ○ Permethrin: Synthetic insecticide derived from chrysanthemum plant. Should not be applied to skin, but permethrin-impregnated clothing provides good protection against arthropods.
    ○ Mosquito nets: Insecticide-treated nets advised for all travelers to disease-endemic areas at risk from biting arthropods (2)
    ○ WHO-recommended nets are Permanet 2.0 (Vestergaard), Olyset (Sumitomo), and Interceptor (BASF) (2)
- Desensitization 75–95% effective for *Hymenoptera*-specific venom:
  – Skin tests are needed to determine sensitivity.
  – Refer to allergist/immunologist if candidate
- Fire ant control (but not elimination) possible:
  – Baits; sprays, dusts, aerosols; biologic agents
- Tick-borne diseases prevented by prompt removal of ticks within 24 hours of attachment

℞ DIAGNOSIS

HISTORY

- Sudden onset of pain or itching with visualization of arthropod
- Many cases unknown to patient or asymptomatic initially (bed bugs, lice, scabies, ticks). Consider in patients presenting with localized erythema, urticaria, wheals, papules, pruritus, or bullae.
- May identify insect by its habitat or by remnants brought by patient
- History of prior exposure useful, but not always available or reliable
- Travel, occupational, social, and recreational history important

PHYSICAL EXAM

- If stinger is still present in skin, remove by flicking or scraping away from skin.

- Anaphylaxis is a clinical diagnosis. Essential to examine for signs and symptoms of anaphylaxis:
  – Erythema, urticaria, angioedema
  – Itching/Edema of lips, tongue, uvula; drooling
  – Persistent vomiting
  – Respiratory distress, wheeze, repetitive cough, stridor, dysphonia
  – Hypotension, dysrhythmia, syncope, chest pain
- If anaphylaxis not present, exam focuses on the sting or bite itself. Common findings include local erythema, swelling, wheals, urticaria, papules, or bullae; excoriations from scratching.
- Thorough exam to look for arthropod infestation (lice, scabies) or attached ticks. Body lice usually found in seams of clothing. Skin scraping to identify scabies.
- Signs of secondary bacterial infection after 24–48 hours: Increasing erythema, pain, fever, lymphangitis, or abscess
- Delayed manifestations of insect-borne diseases

DIFFERENTIAL DIAGNOSIS

- Urticaria and localized dermatologic manifestations:
  – Contact dermatitis, drug eruption, mastocytosis, bullous diseases, dermatitis herpetiformis, tinea, eczema, vasculitis, pityriasis, erythema multiforme, viral exanthem, cellulitis, abscess, impetigo, folliculitis, erysipelas, necrotizing fasciitis
- Anaphylactic-type reactions:
  – Cardiac, hemorrhagic, or septic shock; acute respiratory failure, asthma; angioedema, urticarial vasculitis; flushing syndromes (catecholamines, vasoactive peptides); panic attacks, syncope
  – Differential diagnosis of the acute abdomen should include black widow spider bite.

DIAGNOSTIC TESTS & INTERPRETATION

Initial Tests (lab, imaging)
Seldom needed; basic lab parameters usually normal. Some findings may help confirm diagnosis of anaphylaxis:

- Plasma histamine levels elevated briefly (5–60 minutes) after mast cell activation
- Metabolite *N*-methyl-histamine elevated in urine for a number of hours (do 24-hour collection)
- Serum tryptase levels peak in 1 hour after anaphylaxis and stay up for 6 hours

Follow-Up Tests & Special Considerations
- Severe envenomations may affect organ function and require monitoring of lab values (CBC, comprehensive metabolic panel, prothrombin time/international normalized ratio)
- Labs for arthropod-borne diseases, as indicated:
  – Ticks: Lyme disease, Rocky Mountain spotted fever, relapsing fever, ehrlichiosis, babesiosis, tularemia
  – Flies: Tularemia, leishmaniasis, African trypanosomiasis, bartonellosis, loiasis
  – Chigger mites: Scrub typhus
  – Body lice: Epidemic typhus, relapsing fever
  – Kissing bugs: Chagas disease
  – Mosquitoes: Malaria, yellow fever, dengue fever, West Nile virus, equine encephalitis, chikungunya
- Refer to allergist for formal testing with history of anaphylaxis, significant systemic symptoms, progressively severe reactions

Diagnostic Procedures/Other
Various skin tests and immunologic tests available to try to predict anaphylactic risk

TREATMENT

ALERT
- The more rapidly anaphylaxis develops, the more likely the reaction is to be severe and potentially life-threatening (3). Most deaths due to anaphylaxis occur within 30–60 minutes of sting.
- Epinephrine should be given as soon as diagnosis of anaphylaxis is suspected (3). Delayed injection of epinephrine is associated with fatal anaphylaxis (4).
- Antihistamines do not replace epinephrine in anaphylaxis, and no direct outcome data regarding their effectiveness in anaphylaxis are available (3).
- Airway management critical if angioedema

GENERAL MEASURES
Local wound cleansing, ice, compress, elevation, analgesics

MEDICATION
First Line
- For arthropod bites/stings with anaphylaxis:
  - Order of treatment importance: Epinephrine, patient position, oxygen, IV fluids, nebulized therapy, vasopressors, antihistamines, corticosteroids (3)
  - Epinephrine: Most important: IM injection in midanterolateral thigh (vastus lateralis muscle):
    - IM injection: Epinephrine 1:1,000: Give 0.01 mg/kg of a 1 mg/mL (1:1,000) dilution to a maximum dose of 0.5 mg in an adult and 0.3 mg in a child. Can repeat every 5–15 minutes (4)[A].
    - IV infusion of epinephrine: For patients poorly responsive to IM epinephrine. No clear dosing regimen in anaphylaxis recognized (3). 1 regimen suggests adding 1 mg (1 mL) of 1:1,000 epinephrine to a 250-cc bag of D5W to produce 4 μg/mL concentration. Infuse at 2–10 μm/min (3)[C].
  - Positioning: Supine with legs elevated (3)
  - Oxygen 6–8 L/min to 100%, as needed
  - IV fluids: Establish 1–2 large-bore IV lines. Normal saline rapid bolus 1–2 L IV; repeat as needed (pediatrics 20–30 mL/kg)
  - H_1 antihistamines: Diphenhydramine 25–50 mg IV (pediatrics 1–2 mg/kg)
  - B_2 agonists: Albuterol for bronchospasm nebulized 2.5–5 mg in 3 mL
  - Emergency treatment of refractory cases: Consider epinephrine infusion, dopamine, glucagon, vasopressin, large-volume crystalloids
- Arthropod bites/stings without anaphylaxis:
  - Tetanus booster, as indicated
  - Oral antihistamines:
    - Diphenhydramine 25–75 mg q6h (pediatrics 5 mg/kg/d divided q4–6h)
    - Cetirizine 5–10 mg/d age >6 years; 2.5 mg/d if 6 months–2 years; 2.5–5 mg/d if 2–6 years
    - H_2 blockers: Ranitidine 150 mg PO b.i.d.; pediatrics 2–4 mg/kg PO b.i.d. no more than 300 mg/d
  - Oral steroids: Consider short course for severe pruritus. Prednisone or prednisolone 1–2 mg/kg once daily
  - Topical intermediate-potency steroid cream or ointment × 3–5 days:
    - Desoximetasone 0.05%
    - Triamcinolone 0.1%
    - Fluocinolone 0.025%
  - Wound care: Antibiotics *only* if infected
- Other specific therapies:
  - Scorpion stings: Treat excess catecholamine release (nitroprusside, prazosin, β-blockers). Diazepam for muscle spasms. Atropine for hypersalivation. Anascorp is equine-derived antivenom for scorpion envenomation. Approved by FDA in 2011 and only FDA-approved scorpion antivenom in US.
  - Black widow bites: Treat muscle spasms with diazepam, opioid analgesics PO or IV. Antivenom: Available for black widow, but should be administered in conjunction with toxicologist. Poison control 1-800-222-1222.
  - Fire ants: Characteristically cause sterile pustules. Leave intact: Do not open or drain.
  - Brown recluse spider: Pain control, supportive treatment. Surgical consult if debridement needed (5)[C]
  - Ticks: Early removal. Review guidelines for disease prophylaxis.
  - Pediculosis: Head, pubic, and body lice:
    - 1st line: Permethrin 1% (Nix) topical lotion. Apply to affected area, wash off in 10 minutes.
    - Alternatives: Pyrethrin or malathion 0.5% lotion, ivermectin (not FDA approved for pediculosis) orally
    - Repeat above treatment in 7–10 days
    - For eyelash infestation: Apply ophthalmic-grade petroleum jelly 2 × day for 10 days.
  - *Sarcoptes scabii* scabies:
    - Permethrin 5% cream: Apply to entire body. Wash off after 8–14 hours. Repeat in 1 week.
    - Ivermectin: 200 μg/kg PO once; repeat in 2 weeks (not FDA approved for this use)
    - Crotamiton 10% cream or lotion less efficacious; apply daily for 2 days after bathing

Second Line
2nd-line options for anaphylaxis:
- Ranitidine 150 mg IV (pediatrics 1–2 mg/kg)
- Methylprednisolone 125 mg IV (pediatrics 2 mg/kg)

ISSUES FOR REFERRAL
Refer to allergist with history of anaphylaxis, severe systemic symptoms, or progressively severe reactions

SURGERY/OTHER PROCEDURES
Debridement and delayed skin grafting may be needed for brown recluse spider and other bites.

COMPLEMENTARY AND ALTERNATIVE MEDICINE
- Some stings may be treated with a paste of 3 tsp of baking soda and 1 tsp water.
- None well tested

IN-PATIENT CONSIDERATIONS
Admission Criteria/Initial Stabilization
Anaphylaxis, vascular instability, neuromuscular events, pain, GI symptoms, renal damage/failure

ONGOING CARE

FOLLOW-UP RECOMMENDATIONS
- Immunotherapy as recommended by allergist/consultant for anaphylaxis or serious reactions; venom immunotherapy cornerstone of treatment for *Hymenoptera*.
- Patient-administered epinephrine must be provided to patients with anaphylaxis. Consider "med-alert" identifiers.

Patient Monitoring
- Monitor for delayed effects, including infectious diseases from arthropod vectors.
- Serum sickness reactions, vasculitis (rare)

PATIENT EDUCATION
Avoidance and prevention

PROGNOSIS
- Excellent for local reactions
- For systemic reactions, best response with early intervention to prevent cardiorespiratory collapse

COMPLICATIONS
- Scarring
- Secondary bacterial infection
- Arthropod-associated diseases as above
- Psychological effects, phobias

REFERENCES
1. Diaz JH. Recognition, management, and prevention of hymenopteran stings and allergic reactions in travelers. *J Travel Med.* 2009;16:357–364.
2. Moore SJ, Mordue AJ. Logan JG. insect bite prevention. *Infect Dis Clin North Am.* 2012;26: 655–673.
3. Lieberman P, Nicklas RA, Oppenheimer J, et al. The diagnosis and management of anaphylaxis practice parameter: 2010 update. *J Allergy Clin Immunol.* 2010;126:477–480.
4. Simons FE. Anaphylaxis. *J Allergy Clin Immunol.* 2010;125(2 Suppl 2):S161–S181.
5. Swanson DL, Vetter RS. Bites of brown recluse spiders and suspected necrotic arachnidism. *N Engl J Med.* 2005;352:700–707.

ADDITIONAL READING
- Centers for Disease Control and Prevention. http://cdc.gov/travel/yellowBookCh2-Insects_Arthropods.
- Centers for Disease Control and Prevention. Insect repellent use. Available at: www.cdc.gov/ncidod/dvbid/westnile/qa/insect_repellent.htm
- Demain JG, Minaei AA, Tracy JM. Anaphylaxis and Insect Allergy. *Curr Opin Allergy Clin Immunol.* 2010;10:318–322.
- Sicherer, SH. Leung DY. Advances in allergic skin disease, anaphylaxis, and hypersensitivity reactions to foods, drugs and insects in 2012. *J Allergy Clin Immunol.* 2013;131:55–66.
- Studdiford JS, Conniff KM, Trayes KP, et al. Bedbug infestation. *Am Fam Physician.* 2012;86:653–658.

 CODES

ICD10
- T63.301A Toxic effect of unsp spider venom, accidental, init
- T63.481A Toxic effect of venom of arthropod, accidental, init
- T63.484A Toxic effect of venom of oth arthropod, undetermined, init

CLINICAL PEARLS
- Urgent administration of epinephrine is key to anaphylaxis treatment.
- Local treatment and symptom management are sufficient in most insect bites and stings.

ASBESTOSIS
Ruben Peralta, MD, FACS

 BASICS

DESCRIPTION
- Slowly progressive lung disease caused by inhalation of dust from fibrous silicate asbestos used in insulation, cement, and other building and construction materials
- Nodular interstitial fibrotic lung disease caused by cascade of inflammatory responses to inhaled asbestos fibers:
  – Pleural fibrosis, pleural plaques, and interstitial fibrosis develop.
  – Lung cancer risk is increased.
- Synonym(s): Asbestos pneumoconiosis

EPIDEMIOLOGY
- In the US, an estimated 1.3 million people who work in maintenance and construction are at risk for exposure.
- In most of the world, data on mesothelioma are not available.
- Predominant age: Middle age (40–75 years)
- Predominant sex: Male > Female, due to exposure pattern

ETIOLOGY AND PATHOPHYSIOLOGY
- Asbestos fibers are inhaled. Macrophages engulf the fibers and release inflammatory mediators. Inflammatory mediators cause fibroblast proliferation, leading to fibrosis and remodeling of interstitial lung tissue, including intra-alveolar fibrosis and loss of alveolar capillary units.
- Disease continues to progress slowly over the course of years, even if exposure is not ongoing (1)[C].
- Symptoms may be related to impaired gas exchange and/or a pattern of restrictive lung disease.

Genetics
- Genetic polymorphisms have been implicated (2)[C].
- Familial mesothelioma has been reported.

RISK FACTORS
- Asbestos increases lung cancer mortality among nonsmokers (3)[B].
- Professional exposure most common in construction workers; those who mine, mill, or remove asbestos; ship builders; textile workers; railroad workers
- Office workers, teachers, and students in buildings with asbestos in place have exposure significantly lower than those of construction workers.
- Dose–response phenomenon: Higher amounts of asbestos exposure are associated with higher risk of asbestosis.
- Cigarette smoking markedly increases risk of radiographic changes and eventual lung cancer risk:
  – Likely mechanism: Decreased clearance of asbestos fibers

GENERAL PREVENTION
- In the US, asbestos is federally regulated by the Occupational Health and Safety Administration.
- Primary responsibility of employers is to provide safe work environment (2)[C].
- Exposure control: Substitution of safer materials or adoption of control technologies
- During high-exposure periods, such as building repair, use fit-tested personal respirators for workers.
- To limit exposure to others in their household, those who work with asbestos should leave their clothing at work, if possible. Work clothes should be washed and stored separately from other clothing.

COMMONLY ASSOCIATED CONDITIONS
In addition to asbestosis, inhalation of asbestos is associated with several lung problems (4)[C], including:
- Benign plaques
- Benign pleural effusions
- Lung cancer
- Malignant mesothelioma

 DIAGNOSIS

HISTORY
- Credible history of exposure (usually occupational) to asbestos fibers (3)[B],(5)[C],(6)[B]:
  – Ask about intensity and duration of exposure
  – Aircraft or electrical maintenance
  – Shipyard workers
  – Those exposed to cement or building materials
  – Asbestos mining
  – People exposed to asbestos when it is disrupted during building maintenance
  – Family members of those who work around asbestos
- In addition to job type and activities and length of exposure, ask patients whether there was visible dust in air or on surfaces, visible dust in sputum, personal protective equipment used, and whether the workplace was cleaned during or after a shift.
- Common symptoms include:
  – Dyspnea upon exertion
  – Nonproductive cough
- Delay from exposure to detection typically becomes clinically apparent 10–15 years after exposure.

PHYSICAL EXAM
- Insidious onset
- Progressive dyspnea is the most common symptom.
- Dry cough
- Progressive exercise intolerance
- Pleuritic chest pain
- Inspiratory crackles (may be best heard laterally)
- Wheeze with forced exhalation
- Digital clubbing and cyanosis in advanced disease
- Right-sided heart failure

DIFFERENTIAL DIAGNOSIS
Other pneumoconioses:
- Idiopathic pulmonary fibrosis
- Hypersensitivity pneumonitis
- Sarcoidosis
- Other pneumoconiosis, including mixed exposures

DIAGNOSTIC TESTS & INTERPRETATION
Pulmonary function testing:
- Not diagnostically specific
- *Mainly restrictive pattern unless a smoker* (7)[B].
- Decreased total lung capacity and vital capacity
- Reduction in diffusing capacity to carbon monoxide
- Useful for following level of impairment

Initial Tests (lab, imaging)
No pathognomonic lab findings:
- Chest x-ray (CXR) (sensitivity 90%, specificity 93%):
  – Most common findings are bilateral pleural thickening and circumscribed calcified pleural plaques
  – Pleural plaques usually posterior-lateral, may also involve diaphragm
  – As disease progresses, small, irregular, linear opacities with a fine reticular pattern are seen.
  – Less common: Rounded atelectasis (Blesovsky syndrome) when fibrosis of visceral pleura extends into parenchyma
- Classification scheme available through International Labour Office (www.ilo.org)
- High-resolution CT may increase sensitivity to near 100%:
  – Improves detection of interstitial fibrosis
  – May show honeycombing in later stages of the disease
- Gallium scan with higher uptake even if the CXR and CT are normal

Test Interpretation
- Lung biopsy or bronchoalveolar lavage (BAL) can reveal asbestos fibers or asbestos bodies:
  – May help diagnostically in cases with history of minimal exposure or with atypical clinical or radiographic features
  – Transbronchial biopsy is less reliable than BAL or open-lung biopsy in establishing diagnosis.
- Pleural plaques are found in parietal pleura; made up of collagen bundles with rare inflammatory cells. Pleural thickening involves the visceral pleura.
- Asbestos bodies may be seen with iron staining in intra-alveolar macrophages.

TREATMENT

GENERAL MEASURES
- No effective treatment is currently known to reverse the course of the disease.
- Clinical approach is directed at amelioration of symptoms, elimination of progression, and reduction of risk of associated disorders.
- Withdrawal from exposure:
  – Workers with no symptoms and only radiographic changes may make an informed choice to continue employment using maximum environmental and personal protection.
- Smoking cessation:
  – Cigarette smokers have more radiographic signs of disease and have a significantly increased risk for lung cancer.
- Pneumococcal and influenza vaccines
- Chest physiotherapy, as needed
- Home oxygen, as needed

MEDICATION
First Line
- No specific pharmacologic treatment
- Oxygen
- Bronchodilators for pulmonary toilet

Second Line
- Antibiotics for respiratory infections
- Diuretics if cor pulmonale develops

ISSUES FOR REFERRAL
All new cases must be reported to health authorities.

ONGOING CARE

Follow World Health Organization (WHO) recommendations for regular health screening of exposed workers:
- CXR film at baseline
- For workers with <10 years since 1st exposure: CXR every 3–5 years
- >10 years: CXR every 1–2 years
- >20 years: CXR annually
- All workers: Annual respiratory symptom questionnaire, physical exam, and spirometry (alternatively, can be done on CXR schedule)

FOLLOW-UP RECOMMENDATIONS
Patient Monitoring
- CXR
- Occasional pulmonary function tests
- Prompt treatment of infections

DIET
High-calorie, high-protein with advanced disease

PATIENT EDUCATION
- Smoking cessation counseling, as needed
- In the US, asbestos has been federally regulated by the Occupational Health and Safety Administration since 1972 (www.osha.gov).
- Printed patient information available from the National Cancer Institute (www.cancer.gov/cancertopics/factsheet/Risk/asbestos)
- Agency for Toxic Substances and Disease Registry (www.atsdr.cdc.gov)

PROGNOSIS
- *Severity depends on duration and intensity of exposure* (5)[B].
- Lung disease is irreversible.
- Increased risk for lung cancer (synergistic increase with cigarette smoking) (7)[C] and mesothelioma

COMPLICATIONS
- Mesothelioma:
  – Related to dose, time elapsed from exposure (usually 25–40 years after exposure)
  – Risk is higher with exposure to amphibole fibers rather than chrysotile fibers.
  – Pleural effusion in 80–95%
  – Insidious but progressive; median survival for mesothelioma is 8–18 months.
- Lung cancer risk is associated with asbestos exposure, whether asbestosis is present or not; synergistically increased risk in asbestos workers who smoke.
- GI cancer risk may also be increased with asbestos exposure.

REFERENCES

1. Centers for Disease Control and Prevention (CDC). Asbestosis-related years of potential life lost before age 65 years—United States, 1968–2005. *MMWR Morb Mortal Wkly Rep*. 2008;57:1321–1325.
2. Helmig S, Belwe A, Schneider J. Association of transforming growth factor beta1 gene polymorphisms and asbestos-induced fibrosis and tumors. *J Investig Med*. 2009;57:655–661.
3. Markowitz SB, Levin SM, Miller A, et al. Asbestos, asbestosis, smoking, and lung cancer. New findings from the North American insulator cohort. *Am J Respir Crit Care Med*. 2013;188:90–96.
4. Toyokuni S. Mechanisms of asbestos-induced carcinogenesis. *Nagoya J Med Sci*. 2009;71:1–10.
5. Banks DE, Shi R, McLarty J, et al. American College of Chest Physicians consensus statement on the respiratory health effects of asbestos. Results of a Delphi study. *Chest*. 2009;135:1619–1627.
6. Deng Q, Wang X, Wang M, et al. Exposure-response relationship between chrysotile exposure and mortality from lung cancer and asbestosis. *Occup Environ Med*. 2012;69:81–86.
7. Abejie BA, Wang X, Kales SN, et al. Patterns of pulmonary dysfunction in asbestos workers: A cross-sectional study. *J Occup Med Toxicol*. 2010;5:12.

ADDITIONAL READING

- Antonescu-Turcu AL, Schapira RM. Parenchymal and airway diseases caused by asbestos. *Curr Opin Pulm Med*. 2010;16:155–161.
- Brody AR. Asbestos and lung disease. *Am J Respir Cell Mol Biol*. 2010;42:131–132.
- Kamp DW. Asbestos-induced lung diseases: An update. *Transl Res*. 2009;153:143–152.
- Park EK, Takahashi K, Jiang Y, et al. Elimination of asbestos use and asbestos-related diseases: An unfinished story. *Cancer Sci*. 2012;103:1751–1755.
- Prazakova S, Thomas PS, Sandrini A, et al. Asbestos and the lung in the 21st century: An update. *Clin Respir J*. 2013, in press.
- Wang X, Yano E, Qiu H, et al. A 37-year observation of mortality in Chinese chrysotile asbestos workers. *Thorax*. 2012;67:106–110.

 CODES

ICD10
- J61 Pneumoconiosis due to asbestos and other mineral fibers
- J84.10 Pulmonary fibrosis, unspecified

CLINICAL PEARLS
- Associations between asbestos and all histologic subtypes of lung cancer have been observed.
- Detection of asbestosis due to asbestos exposure does not typically become clinically apparent until 10–15 years after exposure.
- Higher amounts of asbestos exposure are associated with higher risk of asbestosis.
- Smoking cessation is particularly important, because cigarette smokers have more radiographic signs of asbestosis and are at a synergistically increased risk for lung cancer.
- Those who work with asbestos should limit exposure to others in their household; clothing should either be left at work or be washed and stored separately from other clothing.

ASCITES

Hayden Tran, DO, MS • Athena Vuong, DO • Juan Sanabria, MD, MSc, FRCSC, FACS

 BASICS

DESCRIPTION

Accumulation of fluid in the peritoneal cavity; may occur in conditions that cause generalized edema

EPIDEMIOLOGY

- Children: Nephrotic syndrome and malignancy most common
- Adults: Cirrhosis, heart failure, nephrotic syndrome, peritonitis most common
- ~85% of all cases of ascites are caused by liver disease and cirrhosis.

Incidence

~50–60% of patients with cirrhosis will develop ascites within 10 years.

Prevalence

10% of patients with liver cirrhosis have ascites.

ETIOLOGY AND PATHOPHYSIOLOGY

- Acute liver failure
- Hepatitis (alcoholic, viral, autoimmune, drugs)
- Peritoneal infection and inflammation:
  - Bacterial infection (foreign body, fistula), tuberculosis, fungal disease, parasitic infection
  - Perforated viscus
  - Granulomatous peritonitis (e.g., sarcoidosis)
- Metabolic diseases:
  - Cirrhosis or prehepatic and posthepatic portal hypertension
  - Nephrotic syndrome
  - Myxedema
  - Protein malnutrition (hypoalbuminemia <2 g/dL)
- Cardiac congestion:
  - Congestive heart failure (CHF), constrictive pericarditis
- Trauma:
  - Pancreatic or biliary fistula
  - Lymphatic tear (chylous ascites), hemoperitoneum (trauma, ectopic pregnancy, tumor)
- Malignancy:
  - Peritoneal seeding: Ovarian, colon, pancreas, others
  - Primary peritoneal carcinoma, leukemia, or lymphoma
- Mixed (>1 of the above causes, e.g., cirrhosis and cancer)
- May develop as a consequence of sustained portal hypertension (portal pressure >12 mm Hg) Interactions of biochemical mediators (e.g., nitric oxide) lead to decreased systemic vascular resistance, splanchnic arterial vasodilation, reduced effective circulating arterial blood volume, and reduced renal perfusion.
- Renal hypoperfusion contributes to activation of systemic vasoconstrictors and antinatriuretic mechanisms, stimulating the sympathetic nervous system and renin-angiotensin-aldosterone system, ultimately culminating in sodium and water retention causing development of ascites and edema.

 DIAGNOSIS

HISTORY

Abdominal or flank pain, dyspnea/orthopnea, anorexia, nausea, early satiety, heartburn, edema, weight gain

PHYSICAL EXAM

- Abdominal distention, bulging flanks, abdominal fluid wave, umbilical/inguinal herniae
- Shifting dullness (most sensitive exam finding) or "puddle sign" (dullness over dependent abdomen)
- Edema (penile/scrotal, pedal), pleural effusion, rales
- Peripheral stigmata of cirrhosis/liver disease (palmar erythema, spider angiomata, gynecomastia)

DIAGNOSTIC TESTS & INTERPRETATION
Initial Tests (lab, imaging)

- Diagnostic paracentesis for ascitic fluid analysis should be obtained in all new-onset, new-to-treat, or hospitalized cases (1)[B] to access fluid infection and presence of portal hypertension:
  - Paracentesis has a complication rate of 1% despite high prevalence of abnormal coagulation parameters:
    ○ Cell count and differential:
      ▪ Polymorphonuclear leukocytes: $\geq$250 cells/mm³ suggests infection
    ○ Albumin in both serum and ascites: Calculate serum-to-ascites albumin gradient (SAAG):
      ▪ <1.1 g indicates exudate (i.e., inflammatory, biliary/pancreatic, carcinomatosis):
        □ Etiologies include neoplasms, myxedema, tuberculosis, pancreatitis, biliary pathology
      ▪ $\geq$1.1 g indicates transudate/portal hypertension:
        □ Etiologies include cirrhosis, CHF, constrictive pericarditis, Budd-Chiari syndrome, nephrotic syndrome, protein malnutrition/hypoalbuminemia
    ○ Fluid culture, if diagnostic paracentesis (not necessary in therapeutic paracentesis) or:
      ▪ If infection suspected (*cirrhotic patients with ascites can sometimes fail to mount adequate fever or significant leukocytosis, instead can produce acutely elevated PT/INR, serum creatinine, and bilirubin in setting of infection*)
      ▪ Fluid cultures are positive in 50–90% of cases.
    ○ Amylase, especially if suspecting bowel perforations, choledocholithiasis, or pancreatitis
    ○ Triglyceride if fluid appears milky
    ○ Lactate dehydrogenase (LDH) from fluid and serum: An ascitic fluid-to-serum LDH ratio >1.0 can indicate infection or tumor.
    ○ Gram stain, acid-fast stain, fungal cultures/smears, and cytology to evaluate for peritoneal infection or carcinomatosis
- Blood tests:
  - BUN/creatinine, electrolytes, and other labs as indicated by underlying condition (e.g., liver enzymes, tumor markers)
- Abdominal ultrasound: To confirm presence of ascites; highly sensitive, cost-effective, involves no radiation, and available at bedside
- CT scan to rule out intra-abdominal pathology (e.g., portal vein thrombosis, especially in setting of markedly elevated aminotransferases)
- MRI best for evaluation of liver disease or confirmation of portal vein thrombosis

Diagnostic Procedures/Other

Laparoscopy: Preferred when CT and fluid cytology are nondiagnostic:

- Important to evaluate ascites due to causes unrelated to portal hypertension (SAAG <1.1) and direct visualization of the peritoneal cavity
- Allows for biopsy of peritoneum, liver, and intra-abdominal lymph nodes
- Preferred for evaluating suspected peritoneal tuberculosis or malignancies

Test Interpretation

Cytology may reveal malignant cells: Typically, adenocarcinoma (ovary, breast, GI tract); rarely, primary peritoneal carcinoma

TREATMENT

For all patients:

- Daily record of weight to monitor gains and losses
- Restrict dietary sodium to 2 g/d (1)[A].
- Water restriction (1–1.5 L/d) generally not helpful; only necessary if serum sodium <120–125 mEq/L (1)[C]
- Creatinine >2.0 mg/dL: Decrease diuretic doses, peritoneal paracentesis
- Avoid NSAIDs.
- Complete abstinence from alcohol and adequate nutrition if liver disease (1)[A]

MEDICATION

ALERT

Carefully approach diuresis; too aggressive diuresis can induce prerenal acute kidney injury, encephalopathy, and hyponatremia. Monitor creatinine and electrolytes closely. Serum creatinine >2 mg/dL or serum sodium <120 mmol/L should prompt withdrawal of diuretics.

First Line

- Diuretics: Mainstay of treatment are sodium restriction and diuretics, with the goal of inducing a negative sodium balance:
  - Spironolactone 100–400 mg daily PO; typical initial dose is 100–200 mg given in A.M:
    ○ Diuretic of choice due to its antialdosterone effects on the underlying pathophysiology. Can be used as single agent in minimal ascites.
  - Furosemide 40–160 mg daily PO; typical initial dose is 40 mg given in A.M:
    ○ Antinatriuretic effect helps to achieve negative sodium balance. (*where sodium goes, water follows*). Not a first-line diuretic, but is an effective adjunct to potentiate maximum effects of spironolactone and better sodium excretion
  - May use spironolactone and furosemide together (maintaining a 10:4 ratio) for maximum efficacy. Most patients will require combination therapy eventually.
    ○ Doses should be sufficient to obtain net sodium loss in urine:
      ▪ Spot urine sodium (Na) in mEq/L × estimated urine output (1 L if no information) should equal estimated dietary Na. Increase diuretics daily until this goal is attained. Measure serum electrolytes before each dose change.
      ▪ Follow body weight daily. Emphasize sodium restriction.

- Diuretic-intractable ascites (10% of patients): Persistent or worsening ascites despite maximum doses of spironolactone (400 mg/d) and furosemide (160 mg/d) and sodium restriction OR progressive rise in creatinine to 2.0:
  - *Exclude compliance with dietary sodium restriction* with 24-hour urine sodium excretion: If <78 mEq/d, patient is compliant with 2 g dietary sodium restriction.
  - Therapeutic paracentesis or serial large volume paracentesis (LVP):
    - Complications: Infection, hemodynamic collapse, acute renal failure
    - Replace albumin when removing >5 L of ascites: 5.5–8 g albumin for each liter removed has been shown to decrease renal dysfunction, hyponatremia post paracentesis, and overall morbidity (2)[A], although limited studies directly compare albumin doses.
    - Continue diuretics at 1/2 previous doses.
- Precautions:
  - NSAIDs may worsen or initiate oliguria or azotemia.

Second Line
- Most commonly used in cases of GI intolerance or allergic reactions
- Alternatives to spironolactone: amiloride up to 10 mg/d; triamterene up to 200 mg/d in divided doses
- Alternatives to furosemide: torsemide up to 100 mg/d; ethacrynic acid 50 mg IV (may be effective when oral drugs cannot be used)
- Vaptans may have a beneficial effect on hyponatremia and ascites, but the data do not support their routine use in ascites (3)[A].

ISSUES FOR REFERRAL
Referral for liver transplant should be considered in patients with decompensated liver disease, whether or not ascites is present/controlled. Liver transplant is the definitive treatment of portal hypertension (HTN) (1)[B].

SURGERY/OTHER PROCEDURES
- Transjugular intrahepatic portosystemic shunt (TIPS):
  - Transjugular conduit from the liver to the hepatic vein used for intractable ascites; placed by interventional radiologists under fluoroscopy (4)[A]:
    - At time of placement, measure portal pressure; should drop ≥20 mm Hg or to <12 mm Hg, and ascites should be readily controlled with diuretics. Conduct yearly US study to confirm functional shunt.
    - Within 4 weeks after TIPS, urinary sodium and serum creatinine improve significantly, and can normalize after 6–12 months in combination with diuretics (4).
    - Dilation/replacement may be required after >2 years.
    - Encephalopathy is a complication. Superior to paracentesis to control ascites, but no difference in mortality (4)[A]
- Peritoneovenous shunt (Leveen or Denver shunt): Popularized in the 1970s as a physiologic method of treating refractory ascites, where a shunt is created to drain ascites directly into the inferior vena cava.
  - Clinical trials show poor long-term shunt patency, no survival advantage compared with medical therapy, and numerous complications, including:

- Bacteremia, bowel obstruction, and variceal bleed as a result of rapid volume overload from ascitic fluid into systemic circulation
  - Limited indications usually reserved for patients with refractory ascites who are not candidates for TIPS or liver transplant, and have numerous abdominal scars making repeated paracentesis unsafe (1)[A].
- Pleurodesis is sometimes performed in patients with recurrent pleural effusion due to chronic ascites resistant to treatments.

COMPLEMENTARY AND ALTERNATIVE MEDICINE
Caution patients to avoid herbs and other supplements (risk drug interactions, hepatotoxicity, coagulopathy).

 ONGOING CARE

PROGNOSIS
- Prognosis varies depending on underlying cause. Ascites is rarely life-threatening in itself, but can be a sign of life-threatening disease (e.g., cancer, end-stage liver disease).
- Conservative therapy usually successful if cause is reversible or treatable (e.g., infection).

COMPLICATIONS
- Spontaneous bacterial peritonitis (SBP):
  - Ascitic fluid polymorphonuclear (PMN) leukocyte count ≥250 cells/mm^3, positive cell cultures, and without evidence of infection source
    - Broad-spectrum antibiotic coverage with cefotaxime 2 g q8h or similar 3rd-generation cephalosporin is treatment of choice for suspected SBP. Covers 95% of flora (including *Escherichia coli, Klebsiella,* pneumococci) (1)[A].
    - Lifetime antibiotic prophylaxis with norfloxacin or trimethoprim-sulfamethoxazole (TMP-SMX) is indicated in some patients who survive an episode of SBP (1)[A]. Reduced incidence of SBP, delayed development of hepatorenal syndrome, and improved survival in patients who were administered daily, long-term norfloxacin (5)[C].
    - Suspect primary bacterial peritonitis (PBP) due to bowel perforations causing peritonitis when ascitic fluid yields >250 cells/mm^3 (often >5,000 cells/mm^3), and any 2 of the following:
    - Ascitic fluid total protein >1 g/dL (often >3 g/dL)
    - Ascitic fluid glucose <50 mg/dL (or 2.8 mmol/L)
    - Ascitic fluid LDH that is 3-fold greater than serum LDH
- Hepatorenal syndrome: Diagnosed when possible causes of acute renal failure are excluded, and at least 2 days of diuretic withdrawal and maximal intravascular volume expansion with albumin:
  - Urine volume <500 mL/d, rising BUN, and creatinine >1.5 mg/dL, fractional excretion of sodium <1%, and decreased urine sodium excretion (<20 mEq/L), indicates significant sodium avidity
    - Stop diuretics and begin intravascular volume expansion, preferably with colloid (5–20 g IV albumin/d) (6)[B].
    - Consider vasoactive drugs, such as octreotide 200 mcg SC t.i.d. and midodrine 12.5 mg PO t.i.d., either alone or together, in addition to colloid volume expanders rapidly progressive (type I) renal failure (1)[B].

- Liver transplant is definitive treatment.
  - May need hemodialysis to control azotemia and correct electrolyte imbalance while awaiting transplant.

REFERENCES
1. Runyon BA, Practice Guidelines Committee, American Association for the Study of Liver Diseases (AASLD). Management of adult patients with ascites due to cirrhosis. *Hepatology.* 2009;49: 2087–2107.
2. Bernardi M, Caraceni P, Navickis RJ, et al. Albumin infusion in patients undergoing large-volume paracentesis: A meta-analysis of randomized trials. *Hepatology.* 2012;55(4):1172–1181.
3. Watson H, Jepsen P, Wong F, et al. Satavaptan treatment for ascites in patients with cirrhosis: A meta-analysis of effect on hepatic encephalopathy development. *Metab Brain Dis.* 2013;28(2): 301–305.
4. Rössle M, Gerbes AL. TIPS for the treatment of refractory ascites, hepatorenal syndrome and hepatic hydrothorax: A critical update. *Gut.* 2010;59(7):988–1000.
5. Fernández J, Navasa M, Planas R, et al. Primary prophylaxis of spontaneous bacterial peritonitis delays hepatorenal syndrome and improves survival in cirrhosis. *Gastroenterology.* 2007;133(3): 818–824. Epub 2007 Jul 3.
6. Sussman AN, Boyer TD. Management of refractory ascites and hepatorenal syndrome. *Curr Gastroenterol Rep.* 2011;13(1):17–25.

ADDITIONAL READING
- Dahl E, Gluud LL, Kimer N, et al. Meta-analysis: The safety and efficacy of vaptans (tolvaptan, satavaptan and lixivaptan) in cirrhosis with ascites or hyponatraemia. *Aliment Pharmacol Ther.* 2012; 36(7):619–626. doi: 10.1111/apt.12025. Epub 2012 Aug
- Perumalswami PV, Schiano TD. The management of hospitalized patients with cirrhosis: The Mount Sinai experience and a guide for hospitalists. *Dig Dis Sci.* 2011;56(5):1266–1281. Epub 2011 Mar 18.

 SEE ALSO

- Cirrhosis of the Liver; Congestive Heart Failure; Nephrotic Syndrome; Hepatorenal Syndrome
- Algorithm: Cirrhosis

 CODES

ICD10
- R18 Ascites
- R18.0 Malignant ascites
- R18.8 Other ascites

CLINICAL PEARLS
Most common cause of "diuretic-intractable ascites" is noncompliance with dietary sodium restriction.

ASTHMA
Urooj Najm, MBBS • Najm Hasan Siddiqui, MD

BASICS

DESCRIPTION
- Chronic, reversible inflammatory airway disease characterized by recurrent attacks of breathlessness and wheezing
- 4 major classifications of asthma severity used primarily to initiate therapy (1,2):
  - Intermittent: Symptoms ≤2 d/wk, nighttime awakenings ≤2 ×/month, short-acting β-agonist use ≤2 d/wk, no interference with normal activity, and normal forced expiratory volume in 1 second (FEV_1) between exacerbations with FEV_1 (predicted) >80% and FEV_1/forced vital capacity (FVC) >80%
  - Mild persistent: Symptoms >2 d/wk, but not daily, nighttime awakenings 3–4 ×/month, short-acting β-agonist use >2 d/wk, but not daily, minor limitations in normal activity, and FEV_1 (predicted) >80% and FEV_1/FVC >80%
  - Moderate persistent: Daily symptoms, nighttime awakenings ≥1 ×/wk but not nightly, daily use of short-acting β-agonist, some limitation in normal activity, and FEV1 (predicted) 60–80% and FEV1/FVC 75–80%
  - Severe persistent: Symptoms throughout the day, nighttime awakenings often 7 ×/wk, short-acting β-agonist use several times a day, extremely limited normal activity, and FEV_1 (predicted) <60% and FEV_1/FVC <75%

EPIDEMIOLOGY
Prevalence
- Affects 5–10% of population
- One of the most common chronic diseases of childhood, affecting 7 million children
- In children, more common in boys than girls
- In adults, more common in women than men, African Americans than Caucasians

Pregnancy Considerations
In the US, maternal asthma complicates approximately 4–8% of all pregnancies.

Geriatric Considerations
Prevalence of asthma in seniors (>age 65) is 5.3%

ETIOLOGY AND PATHOPHYSIOLOGY
- Airway inflammation begins with inflammatory cell infiltration, sub-basement fibrosis, mucus hypersecretion, epithelial injury, smooth muscle hypertrophy, angiogenesis that then leads to intermittent airflow obstruction, and bronchial hyperresponsiveness
- Remodeling of airways may occur (1).

Genetics
- Inheritable component with complex genetics and environment interaction
- A gene-by-environment interaction occurs in which the susceptible host is exposed to environmental factors that are capable of generating immunoglobulin (Ig) E and sensitization occurs.

RISK FACTORS
- Host factors: Genetic predisposition, gender, race, BMI
- Environmental: Viral infections, animal and airborne allergens, tobacco smoke, etc.
- Exercise, obesity, and emotional stress

- Aspirin or NSAIDs hypersensitivity or β-blockers
- Food allergies and asthma → increased risk for fatal anaphylaxis from those foods.

GENERAL PREVENTION
- Eliminate or modify exposure to asthma triggers (e.g., allergens, smoking, aspirin, NSAIDs)
- Consider allergen immunotherapy.
- Treat comorbidities such as allergic rhinitis
- Annual influenza vaccine (inactivated influenza vaccine) for age <6 months
- Patients at risk for anaphylaxis should carry an EpiPen.

COMMONLY ASSOCIATED CONDITIONS
- Atopy: Eczema, allergic conjunctivitis, allergic rhinitis
- Obesity (associated with higher asthma rates)
- Sinusitis
- Gastroesophageal reflux disease (GERD)
- Obstructive sleep apnea (OSA)
- Allergic bronchopulmonary aspergillosis (rare)
- Stress/Depression

DIAGNOSIS

It is important to classify asthma severity

HISTORY
- Question frequency of symptoms and rescue inhaler use
- Symptoms include:
  - Cough (particularly if worse at night)
  - Wheeze
  - Chest tightness/difficulty breathing

PHYSICAL EXAM
- May be normal
- Focus on:
  - General appearance: Signs of respiratory distress, such as use of accessory muscles
  - Upper respiratory tract: Rhinitis, nasal polyps, swollen nasal turbinates
  - Lower respiratory tract: Wheezing, prolonged expiratory phase
  - Skin: Eczema

DIFFERENTIAL DIAGNOSIS
- In children:
  - Upper airway diseases (allergic rhinitis or sinusitis)
  - Large airway obstruction (foreign-body aspiration, vocal cord dysfunction, vascular ring or laryngeal web, laryngotracheomalacia, lymph nodes or tumor)
  - Small airway obstruction (viral bronchiolitis, cystic fibrosis, bronchopulmonary dysplasia, heart disease)
  - Other causes (recurrent cough *not* due to asthma, aspiration/GERD)
- In adults:
  - Chronic obstructive pulmonary disease, congestive heart failure, pulmonary embolism, benign or malignant tumor, pulmonary infiltration with eosinophilia, Churg-Strauss syndrome, drugs such as an ACE inhibitor, vocal cord dysfunction

DIAGNOSTIC TESTS & INTERPRETATION
Initial Tests (lab, imaging)
- Blood tests not required, but may find eosinophilia or elevated serum IgE levels
- Spirometry: Normal test does not rule out asthma. It measures the FVC and the FEV_1. A reduced predicted ratio of FEV_1/FVC with reversibility

(increase of 200 mL or 12% of FEV_1/FVC) after using a short-acting bronchodilator establishes the diagnosis.
- Bronchoprovocation (methacholine, histamine, cold air, or exercise) is used to simulate bronchoconstriction, very useful in atypical presentation/normal baseline spirometry. Abnormal test not entirely specific for asthma but normal test exclude asthma.
- Peak expiratory flow rates are inappropriate for diagnosis. Typically use for monitoring of symptoms in diagnosed asthma patients.
- Chest x-ray is used to exclude alternative diagnoses and to evaluate patients for complicating cardiopulmonary processes.

Follow-Up Tests & Special Considerations
Asthma action plan: Patients monitor their own symptoms and/or peak flow measurements.

Diagnostic Procedures/Other
- Allergy skin testing is not useful for diagnosis of asthma but may be considered to evaluate atopic triggers.
- Sweat testing if diagnosis of cystic fibrosis
- Arterial blood gases is indicated for patients with respiratory distress and hypoxia.

Test Interpretation
Inflammatory cell infiltration, edema, goblet cell hyperplasia, smooth muscle hyperplasia, thickened basement membrane

TREATMENT

GENERAL MEASURES
- Identify triggers and control exposures.
- Identify patients at risk for reactions to aspirin and NSAIDs, and avoid exposure.

MEDICATION
First Line
- Short-acting β-agonist (SABA) for quick relief of acute symptoms and to prevent exercise-induced bronchospasm (1):
  - SABA include albuterol, levalbuterol (Xopenex), metaproterenol (Alupent) Pirbuterol (Maxair) (3)
- Anticholinergic agent:
  - Ipratropium bromide: Used in combination with SABA for acute treatment, mainly in the ED
- Systemic corticosteroids can be used:
  - In all patients with acute asthma exacerbations (4)[A]
  - In moderate to severe asthma as adjunct
  - Prednisolone 1–2 mg/kg/d or equivalent for up to 7 days in adults and for 3 days in children with no need for tapering (4)[B]

ALERT
- Delivery of SABA and other inhaled agents via "spacer" or holding chamber (AeroChamber, OptiChamber, others) provides increased efficacy with decreased side effects when compared with nebulized delivery. Reserve nebulized delivery of medication for those unable to use spacer (e.g., infants, those intubated).
- All short-acting agents are pregnancy Category C.

Second Line

For long-term control (3):

- Inhaled corticosteroids (ICS):
  - Preferred long-term controller therapy for children and adults with persistent asthma and persistent asthma during pregnancy
  - Long-acting β_2-agonists (LABA):
    - Salmeterol or formoterol
    - Should not be used as monotherapy; doing so leads to an increased risk of severe outcomes, including death
  - Combination products, including an LABA and ICS, are available and are indicated if ICS alone do not provide control; preferred in moderate and severe persistent disease (3)[A].
  - Leukotriene receptor agonists: Alternative, preferable for mild and moderate persistent asthma (1)[A]
    - Montelukast or zafirlukast (patients ≥7 years)
  - Lipoxygenase pathway inhibitor: Alternative not preferred for adjunctive treatment in adults: Zileuton (patients ≥12 years)
  - Theophylline: Not preferred as adjunctive therapy with inhaled corticosteroids
  - Cromolyn sodium and nedocromil are also alternatives, but not preferred options
  - Immunomodulators:
    - Omalizumab: Adjunctive not preferred therapy for patients ≥12 years with allergies and severe persistent asthma (1)[B]

ISSUES FOR REFERRAL

Referral to an asthma specialist (either a pulmonologist or an allergist) should be considered:

- Diagnosis unclear
- Additional asthma education needed
- Comorbidities: Rhinitis, GERD, sinusitis, OSA
- Specialized testing (e.g., bronchoprovocation, skin testing)
- Specialized treatments (e.g., immunotherapy, anti-IgE therapy)
- Poorly controlled moderate to severe persistent asthma in adults
- Moderate to persistent asthma in children
- Poorly controlled asthma: Multiple emergency room visits for asthma

Pregnancy Considerations

- Poorly controlled asthma results in low birth weight, increased prematurity, and perinatal mortality.
- Most ICS agents are pregnancy Category C, except budesonide, montelukast, and zafirlukast, which are Category B.

ADDITIONAL THERAPIES

- Allergen immunotherapy when clear relationship between symptoms and exposure to an unavoidable allergen
- Omalizumab (Xolair): Anti-IgE therapy, approved for patients >12 years with moderate to severe asthma

IN-PATIENT CONSIDERATIONS

Admission Criteria/Initial Stabilization

No single measure is predictive:

- Dyspnea/Hypoxia
- Poor or no response to SABA
- Peak expiratory flow (PEF) or FEV$_1$ <40%

- Decision for admission should be based on duration and severity of symptoms, severity of airflow obstruction, response to ED treatment, course and severity of prior exacerbations, access to medical care and medication, and adequacy of home condition (1).
- Supplemental oxygen to correct hypoxemia

- Repeated doses or continuous administration of SABA (1)[A]
- Ipratropium bromide may be used in the ED, but is not for inpatient treatment (1)[B].
- Systemic corticosteroids for acute exacerbations (1)[A]
- Adjunctive therapy with MgSO$_4$ or heliox may be considered in severe cases (1)[B].

IV Fluids

- Avoid aggressive hydration in older children and adults
- Monitor electrolytes

Nursing

- Careful respiratory monitoring, including vital signs, pulse oximetry, response and duration of response to SABA, and, when possible, an objective measure of lung function such as PEF or FEV$_1$
- Asthma education

Discharge Criteria

- Minimal or absent asthma symptoms
- Hypoxia has resolved
- FEV$_1$ or PEF ≥70% predicted or personal best
- Bronchodilator response sustained ≥60 minutes

 ONGOING CARE

FOLLOW-UP RECOMMENDATIONS

Smoking cessation counseling or elimination of secondhand smoke, if applicable

Patient Monitoring

- Quality-of-life measures: Impact on activities, sleep, ED visits/hospitalizations, and so forth
- Pharmacotherapy: Efficacy, compliance, side effects, technique
- Peak flow to evaluate if cough is due to exacerbation in those with known asthma

DIET

Food allergies and sulfites (in food and wine) can precipitate symptoms for some patients.

PATIENT EDUCATION

- Patients' care plan and inhaled medication technique at every visit.
- American Academy of Allergy, Asthma and Immunology: 800-822-2762 or www.aaaai.org
- American Lung Association: www.lungusa.org
- Asthma and Allergy Foundation of America: 800-727-8462 or www.aafa.org

PROGNOSIS

- Prognosis is good for male patients, nonsmokers, children with mild disease.
- Asthma worsens in 1/3 of women during pregnancy and improves in another 1/3.

COMPLICATIONS

- Atelectasis
- Pneumonia

- Air leak syndromes: Pneumomediastinum, pneumothorax
- Medication-specific side effects/adverse effects/interactions
- Respiratory failure
- Death: ~50% of asthma deaths occur in the elderly (age >65 years), and mortality is increasing in that population (5).

REFERENCES

1. National Asthma Education and Prevention Program Expert Panel Report 3, Guidelines for the Diagnosis and Management of Asthma. No. 08-5846 Washington, DC: NIH, 2007.
2. Reddel HK, Taylor DR, Bateman ED, et al. An official American Thoracic Society/European Respiratory Society statement: Asthma control and exacerbations: Standardizing endpoints for clinical asthma trials and clinical practice. Am J Respir Crit Care Med. 2009;180:59–99.
3. Fanta CH. Asthma. N Engl J Med. 2009;360: 1002–1014.
4. Doherty S. Prescribe systemic corticosteroids in acute asthma. BMJ. 2009;338:b1234.
5. Stupka E, deShazo R. Asthma in seniors: Part 1 evidence for underdiagnosis, undertreatment and increasing morbidity and mortality. Am J Med. 2009;122:6–11.

ADDITIONAL READING

Dombrowski MP, Schatz M, ACOG Committee on Practice Bulletins-Obstetrics. ACOG practice bulletin: Clinical management guidelines for obstetrician-gynecologists number 90, February 2008: Asthma in pregnancy. Obstet Gynecol. 2008;111(2 Pt 1): 457–464.

 SEE ALSO

Algorithm: Asthma Exacerbation, Pediatric Acute

 CODES

ICD10

- J45.20 Mild intermittent asthma, uncomplicated
- J45.901 Unspecified asthma with (acute) exacerbation
- J45.909 Unspecified asthma, uncomplicated

CLINICAL PEARLS ✳ Triggers

- Asthma is a chronic, reversible inflammatory airway disease whose exacerbations are characterized by reversible bronchoconstriction, airway hyperresponsiveness, and airway edema.
- SABA is the most effective rescue therapy for acute asthma symptoms.
- ICSs are the preferred long-term control therapy for patients of all ages.
- Peak flow is an inexpensive and easily available monitoring device once the diagnosis of asthma has been established.

ATELECTASIS

Mary Lauren Worthen, MD • Adrian Worthen • David Worthen

 BASICS

DESCRIPTION
- Atelectasis is defined as incomplete expansion of lung tissue.
- The collapse of lung tissue and resultant loss of lung volume and function are due to various causes broadly defined in two groups:
  - Obstructive: Blockage of an airway
  - Nonobstructive: Loss of contact between the parietal and visceral pleurae, replacement of lung tissue by scarring or infiltrative disease, surfactant dysfunction, and parenchymal compression
- Symptoms and signs are determined by the rapidity with which the bronchial occlusion occurs, the size of the lung area affected, and the presence or absence of lung disease and comorbidities.
- Reduced respiratory gas exchange, leading to hypoxemia if severe

EPIDEMIOLOGY
- Affects all ages; mean age of presentation is 60 years.
- Male = Female. No racial predilection.

Incidence
- Round atelectasis (see "Imaging") is high in asbestos workers (65–70%)
- Incidence of lobar atelectasis depends on the collateral ventilation within each individual lung lobe.

Prevalence
Postoperative atelectasis is extremely common, affecting up to 90% of patients.

ETIOLOGY AND PATHOPHYSIOLOGY
- Obstructive (resorptive) atelectasis (most common); causes intrinsic respiratory blockage:
  - Due to luminal blockage (foreign body, mucous plug, asthma, cystic fibrosis, trauma, tumor) or airway wall abnormality (congenital malformation, emphysema)
  - Distal to the obstruction, air is reabsorbed from the alveoli into the deoxygenated venous system causing complete collapse of the alveolar tissue.
- Nonobstructive atelectasis:
  - Passive atelectasis: Results from pleural membrane separation of the visceral and parietal layers:
    ○ Pleural effusion, pneumothorax
  - Compression atelectasis: Alveoli compression leading to diminished resting volume (FRC):
    ○ Space-occupying lesions, lymphadenopathy, cardiomegaly, abscess, chest-wall pressure
  - Adhesive atelectasis: Surfactant dysfunction, resulting in increased surface tension and alveoli collapse:
    ○ Respiratory distress syndrome, acute respiratory distress syndrome (ARDS), radiation exposure, smoke inhalation, uremia
  - Cicatrization: Pleural or parenchymal scarring:
    ○ Granulomatous disease, toxic inhalation, drug-induced fibrosis (e.g., Amiodarone), radiation exposure
  - Replacement atelectasis: Diffuse tumor manifestation resulting in complete lobar collapse:
    ○ Bronchioalveolar cell carcinoma
  - Rounded atelectasis: Distinct form of atelectasis following asbestosis exposure
- Other:
  - Hypoxemia due to pulmonary embolus
  - Muscular weakness (anesthesia, neuromuscular disease)

- Obstructive atelectasis:
  - There are 3 collateral ventilation systems in each lobe, the pores of Kohn, canals of Lambert, and fenestrations of Boren. The patency and formation of the systems depends on multiple factors including age, lung disease, and FiO_2.
  - Age: Due to the late development of collaterals in children, atelectasis is frequently diagnosed after foreign-body aspiration.
  - Emphysema: The fenestra of Boren in emphysematous patients often become enlarged; this enlargement can lead to a delay in atelectasis despite an obstructing lesion or mass.
  - FiO_2: Oxygen rapidly dissociates from the alveoli to deoxygenated vessels in a obstructed airway. The 79% nitrogen in atmospheric air has a much slower rate of dissociation from the alveoli and thereby prevents collapse by maintaining a positive pressure inside the alveoli. With increased FiO_2, the concentration of nitrogen is decreased, predisposing the patient to a rapid development of atelectasis at the onset of obstruction.

RISK FACTORS
- General anesthesia (1):
  - Positive fluid balance, ≥4 units blood transfusion, use of nasogastric tube, long-acting muscle relaxants, hypothermia, postoperative epidural anesthesia, ventilator settings with high tidal volume and plateau pressure
- Common postoperatively, particularly following thoracic or upper abdominal surgery, neurosurgery, orofacial and neck surgery, surgery >3 hours in duration, emergency surgery, and vascular surgery (1,2)
- Risk factors for developing atelectasis after surgery:
  - Age >60 and <6, COPD, obstructive sleep apnea, CHF, alcohol abuse, pulmonary hypertension, albumin <3.5 g/dL, hemoglobin <10 g/dL, BMI >27 kg/m^2, ASA class II+ functional dependence in activities of daily living (ADL), heart failure, smoking (1)
- Intensive care and prolonged immobilization (3)
- Brock syndrome: Recurrent right-middle lobe collapse secondary to airway disease, infection, or a combination thereof. The right-middle lobe airway is long and thin and has the poorest drainage and clearance of all the lobes, resulting in trapped mucus.

GENERAL PREVENTION
- Encourage activity; breathing exercises, frequent changes in body position, coughing, and early mobilization. However, further large randomized controlled trials are needed before conclusions can be made regarding the effect of chest physiotherapy and incentive spirometry on postoperative pulmonary complications and mortality (4)[A].
- Ventilator settings during anesthesia with high tidal volumes (Vt >10 mL/kg), high plateau pressures (>30 cm H_2O) and without positive end-expiratory pressure (PEEP) are associated with postoperative pulmonary complications such as pneumonia and respiratory failure:
  - Ventilator-induced lung injury can be minimized by using low Vt and plateau pressures at sufficient PEEP, while maintaining lower FiO_2 during anesthetic induction and intraoperatively (5)[A].

- Application of CPAP during anesthesia induction and reversal of anesthesia-induced atelectasis after intubation by a recruitment maneuver may decrease postoperative pulmonary complications (5)[A].

COMMONLY ASSOCIATED CONDITIONS
- Chronic obstructive pulmonary disease and asthma
- Trauma
- ARDS, neonatal respiratory distress syndrome, pulmonary edema, pulmonary embolism
- Neuromuscular disorders (muscular dystrophy, spinal muscular atrophy, spinal cord injury), cystic fibrosis
- Respiratory syncytial virus (RSV), bronchiolitis
- Bronchial stenosis, pulmonic valve disease, pulmonary hypertension
- Pneumonia, pleural effusion, pneumothorax

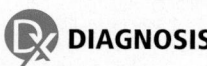 **DIAGNOSIS**

HISTORY
- Frequently asymptomatic
- Tachypnea and sudden-onset dyspnea
- Nonproductive cough
- Pleuritic pain on affected side
- History of smoking, radiation, asbestos, or other air pollutants

PHYSICAL EXAM
- Hypoxia, cyanosis
- Tracheal or precordial impulse displacement toward the affected side
- Bronchial breathing if airway is patent or absent breath sounds if airway is occluded
- Diminished chest expansion
- Wheezing may be heard with focal obstruction, dullness to percussion over the involved area.

DIFFERENTIAL DIAGNOSIS
The differential is found under "Etiology."

DIAGNOSTIC TESTS & INTERPRETATION
Initial Tests (lab, imaging)
- CBC and sputum culture if infection is suspected
- ABG: Despite hypoxemia, the partial pressure of carbon dioxide in ($PaCO_2$) level is usually normal or low.

Chest x-ray (CXR), posterior-anterior and lateral:
- Raised diaphragm, flattened chest wall, movement of fissures and mediastinal structures toward the atelectatic region
- Unaffected lung may show compensatory hyperinflation.
- Wedge-shaped densities: Obstructive atelectasis
- Small, linear bands (Fleischner lines) often at lung bases: Discoid (subsegmental or plate) atelectasis
- Lobar collapse:
  - Direct signs: Displacement of fissures and opacification of the collapsed lobe
  - Indirect signs: Displacement of the hilum, mediastinal shift toward the side of collapse, loss of volume on ipsilateral hemithorax, elevation of ipsilateral diaphragm, crowding of the ribs, compensatory hyperlucency of the remaining lobes, and silhouetting of the diaphragm or the heart border
  - Right upper lobe collapse may display the Golden inverted S sign, suggesting neoplastic shift of the minor fissure.

- Air bronchograms: Evidence of pleural fluid or air may indicate compressive atelectasis.
- Adhesive atelectasis may present as a diffuse reticular granular pattern progressing to a pulmonary edema pattern and finally to bilateral opacification in severe cases.
- Pleural-based round density on CXR: Round atelectasis
- Complete atelectasis of an entire lung: Opacification of the entire hemithorax and an ipsilateral shift of the mediastinum

Follow-Up Tests & Special Considerations
Albumin level: Low serum albumin level (<3.5 g/L) is a powerful marker of increased risk for postoperative pulmonary complications, including atelectasis (1)[A].

- Chest CT or MRI may be indicated to visualize airway and mediastinal structures and to identify cause of atelectasis.
- Pulmonary function tests (PFTs) may detect restrictive disease, decreased respiratory muscle pressures, or airflow obstruction.

Diagnostic Procedures/Other
Bronchoscopy to assess airway patency in unexplained or refractory cases

 TREATMENT

GENERAL MEASURES
- If known, treat the underlying cause.
- Ensure patient is lying on the unaffected side to promote drainage:
  - Maximize patient mobility and encourage frequent coughing and deep breathing every hour.
- Incentive spirometry:
  - Evidence has not shown that incentive spirometry prevents postoperative pulmonary complications in CABG (6)[A].
- Initiate intubation and mechanical ventilation with PEEP in severe respiratory distress or hypoxemia:
  - Lower tidal volume (6 mL/kg) and lower end-inspiratory values (<30 mm Hg) are associated with reduced mortality (7)[B].
  - PEEP 15–20 mL may be necessary to maintain arterial O_2 saturation in surfactant-impaired states (7)[B].
- Postsurgical measures include positive airway pressure, continuous or intermittent.

MEDICATION
First Line
Therapies directed at basic cause:
- Antibiotics for infection
- Chemo/Radiation therapy for tumor
- Steroids for asthma
- Analgesia for pain control to permit deep inspiration and coughing

Pediatric Considerations
- RhDNase may be effective in clearing mucinous secretions in persistent atelectasis in children (8)[C].
- Chest physiotherapy including percussion, drainage, deep insufflation, and saline lavage is a common treatment in the prevention and treatment of atelectasis in the hospital setting. However, caution is required when interpreting the possible positive effects of chest physiotherapy as the numbers of babies studied are small, the results are not consistent across trials, data on safety are insufficient, and applicability to current practice may be limited (9)[C].

- The application of continuous distending pressure has been shown to have some benefits in the treatment of preterm infants with respiratory distress syndrome. Continuous distending pressure has the potential to reduce lung damage particularly if applied early, before atelectasis has occurred (10)[A].

Second Line
Bronchofibroscopy in aspiration of inspissated secretions in atelectasis has been efficacious in several studies. However, counter-evidence continues to question its efficacy in the treatment of atelectasis.

Pediatric Considerations
In obstructive atelectasis, bronchoscopy remains controversial (11)[B]. In the presence of a mucus plug or cast, bronchoscopy may be beneficial (12)[C].

SURGERY/OTHER PROCEDURES
Only for resectable underlying disease (e.g., tumor, severe lymphadenopathy), bronchoscopy

IN-PATIENT CONSIDERATIONS
Admission Criteria/Initial Stabilization
Ensure adequate oxygenation (may start with 100% FiO_2 then taper) and humidification

 ONGOING CARE

FOLLOW-UP RECOMMENDATIONS
Patient Monitoring
- Varies with cause and patient status
- In simple atelectasis associated with asthma or infection, outpatient visits are adequate.

PATIENT EDUCATION
Maximize patient mobility and encourage frequent coughing and deep breathing every hour.

PROGNOSIS
- Spontaneous resolution usually occurs within 24 hours but can persist for days after surgery.
- The prognosis of lobar atelectasis secondary to endobronchial obstruction depends on treatment of the underlying malignancy.
- Surgical therapy is needed only for resectable causes or if chronic infection and bronchiectasis supervene.

COMPLICATIONS
- Pneumonia
- Acute atelectasis:
  - Hypoxemia and respiratory failure
  - Postobstructive drowning of the lung
- Chronic atelectasis:
  - Bronchiectasis
  - Pleural effusion and empyema

REFERENCES

1. Qaseem A, Snow V, Fitterman N, et al. Risk assessment for and strategies to reduce perioperative pulmonary complications for patients undergoing noncardiothoracic surgery: A guideline from the American College of Physicians. *Ann Intern Med.* 2006;144(8):575–580.
2. Ferreyra G, Long Y, Ranieri VM, et al. Respiratory complications after major surgery. *Curr Opin Crit Care.* 2009;15:342–348.
3. Brower RG. Consequences of bed rest. *Crit Care Med.* 2009;37:S422–S428.
4. Guimarães MM, El Dib R, Smith AF, et al. Incentive spirometry for prevention of postoperative pulmonary complications in upper abdominal surgery. *Cochrane Database Syst Rev.* 2009;(3):CD006058. Epub 2009 Jul 8.
5. Tusman G, Böhm SH, Warner DO, et al. Atelectasis and perioperative pulmonary complications in high-risk patients. *Curr Opin Anaesthesiol.* 2012;25(1):1–10.
6. Freitas ER, Soares BG, Cardoso JR, et al. Incentive spirometry for preventing pulmonary complications after coronary artery bypass graft. *Cochrane Database Syst Rev.* 2007;(3):CD004466. Epub 2007 Jul 18.
7. McCunn M, Sutcliffe AJ, Mauritz W, et al. Guidelines for management of mechanical ventilation in critically injured patients. *Trauma Care.* 2004;14(4):147–151.
8. Hendriks T, de Hoog M, Lequin MH, et al. DNase and atelectasis in non-cystic fibrosis pediatric patients. *Crit Care.* 2005;9(4):R351–6. Epub 2005 May 20.
9. Flenady V, Gray PH. Chest physiotherapy for preventing morbidity in babies being extubated from mechanical ventilation. *Cochrane Database Syst Rev.* 2002;(2):CD000283.
10. Ho JJ, Henderson-Smart DJ, Davis PG. Early versus delayed initiation of continuous distending pressure for respiratory distress syndrome in preterm infants. *Cochrane Database Syst Rev.* 2002;(2):CD002975.
11. Wu KH, Lin CF, Huang CJ, et al. Rigid ventilation bronchoscopy under general anesthesia for treatment of pediatric pulmonary atelectasis caused by pneumonia: A review of 33 cases. *Int Surg.* 2006;91:291–294.
12. Deng J, Zheng Y, Li C, et al. Plastic bronchitis in three children associated with 2009 influenza A(H1N1) virus infection. *Chest.* 2010;138:1486–1488.

 CODES

ICD10
J98.11 Atelectasis

CLINICAL PEARLS
- Bronchogenic carcinoma, which may present with atelectasis, must be excluded in all patients >35.
- In complete atelectasis of an entire lung, the mediastinal ipsilateral shift separates atelectasis from massive pleural effusion.
- Low serum albumin is a powerful predictor of postoperative pulmonary complications, including atelectasis.
- Anesthesia-induced atelectasis occurs in almost all anesthetized patients.

ATRIAL FIBRILLATION AND ATRIAL FLUTTER

Youhua Zhang, MD, PhD • Bianca Lee

 BASICS

This topic covers both atrial fibrillation (AFib) and atrial flutter (AFlut).

DESCRIPTION
- AFib: Paroxysmal or continuous supraventricular tachyarrhythmia characterized by rapid, uncoordinated atrial electrical activity and an irregularly irregular ventricular response. In most patients, the ventricular rate is usually rapid because the AV node is bombarded with very frequent atrial electrical impulses (400–600 bpm).
- AFlut: Paroxysmal or continuous supraventricular tachyarrhythmia with rapid but organized atrial electrical activity. The atrial rate is typically between 250 and 350 bpm and is often manifested as "saw-tooth" flutter (F) waves on the ECG, particularly in the inferior leads and V_1. AFlut commonly occurs with 2:1 or 3:1 AV block, so the ventricular response may be regular and typically at a rate of ~150 bpm.
- AFib and AFlut are related arrhythmias, sometimes seen in the same patient. Distinguishing the two is important as it may have implications for management.
- Clinical classifications:
  - Paroxysmal: Self-terminating episodes, usually <7 days
  - Persistent: Sustained >7 days, usually requiring pharmacologic or DC cardioversion to restore sinus rhythm
  - Permanent: Sinus rhythm cannot be restored.
- Lone Afib occurs in patients <60 (with possible genetic predisposition) who have no clinical or echocardiographic evidence of cardiovascular disease, including hypertension (HTN).

EPIDEMIOLOGY
- Incidence/Prevalence increases significantly with age.
- Young patients with AFib, particularly lone AFib, are most commonly male.

Incidence
- AFib: from <0.1%/yr <40 to >1.5%/yr >80
- Lifetime risk: 25% for those ≥40
- AFlut is less common.

Prevalence
- Estimated at 0.4–1% in general population, with 2.2 million patients in America.
- Increase with age, up to 8% in those ≥80.

ETIOLOGY AND PATHOPHYSIOLOGY
- Cardiac: Hypertension, ischemic heart disease, heart failure, valvular heart disease, cardiomyopathy, pericarditis, and infiltrative heart disease
- Pulmonary: Pulmonary embolism, chronic obstructive pulmonary disease (COPD), obstructive sleep apnea, pneumonia
- Ingestion: Ethanol, caffeine
- Endocrine: Hyperthyroidism, diabetes
- Obesity
- Postoperative: Cardiac, pulmonary, or esophageal
- Idiopathic: Lone AFib
- Patients with paroxysmal episodes are usually associated with premature atrial beats and/or bursts of tachycardia originating in pulmonary vein ostia or other sites (1).
- Many patients with AFib are thought to have some degree of atrial fibrosis or scarring. This is often subclinical and usually not detectable with current cardiac imaging techniques but plays an important role in the pathogenesis of the arrhythmia (1).
- Autonomic (vagal and sympathetic) tone may play a role in triggering the arrhythmia.
- The presence of AFib is associated with electrical and structural remodeling processes that promote arrhythmia maintenance in the atria, termed "AFib begets AFib."

Genetics
Familial forms are rare but do exist. There are ongoing efforts to identify the genetic underpinnings of such cases.

RISK FACTORS
Age, HTN, and obesity are the most important risk factors for both AFib and AFlut.

GENERAL PREVENTION
Adequate control of HTN may prevent development of AFib due to hypertensive heart disease and is the most significant modifiable risk factor for AFib. Weight reduction may decrease the risk of AFib in obese patients. Ethanol consumption may trigger AFib in some.

COMMONLY ASSOCIATED CONDITIONS
HTN and other cardiac diseases

 DIAGNOSIS

HISTORY
Symptoms vary from none to mild (palpitations, lightheadedness, fatigue, poor exercise capacity) to severe (angina, dyspnea, syncope).

PHYSICAL EXAM
- AFib: Irregularly irregular heart rate and pulse, frequently tachycardiac.
- AFlut: Similar to AFib, but may have regular pulse.

DIFFERENTIAL DIAGNOSIS
- Multifocal atrial tachycardia
- Sinus tachycardia with frequent atrial premature beats
- Paroxysmal supraventricular tachycardia (WPW, AVNRT)

DIAGNOSTIC TESTS & INTERPRETATION
- AFib: The ECG is diagnostic, with findings of low-amplitude fibrillatory waves without discrete P waves and an irregularly irregular pattern of QRS complexes. There is often tachycardia in the absence of heart rate–controlling medications (1).
- AFlut: The ECG is again diagnostic. Saw-tooth flutter waves are the classic sign, generally best seen in the inferior leads, although ventricular rate may need to be slowed to see the waves. QRS complexes may be regular or irregular; there is usually tachycardia (1).
- Holter monitor and event monitor are helpful in diagnosing paroxysmal AFib or AFlut and monitoring for recurrence (1).

Initial Tests (lab, imaging)
TSH, electrolytes, CBC, PT/INR (if anticoagulation is contemplated); digoxin level (if appropriate).

Follow-Up Tests & Special Considerations
- Occasional Holter monitoring and/or exercise stress testing to assess for adequacy of rate and/or rhythm control
- Chest x-ray (CXR) for cardiopulmonary disease
- ECG for signs of cardiac hypertrophy, ischemia and/or other arrhythmias.
- Transesophageal echocardiogram to detect left atrial appendage thrombus if cardioversion is planned.

Test Interpretation
- Atrial dilatation and fibrosis
- Atrial thrombus, especially in atrial appendage
- Valvular/rheumatic disease
- Cardiomyopathy

 TREATMENT

MEDICATION
- 2 primary issues in the management of AFib and/or AFlut:
  - Decisions on heart rate control (control ventricular rate while allowing AFib to continue) or rhythm control (terminate AFib and restore normal sinus rhythm).
  - Anticoagulation therapy to prevent thromboembolism (primarily stroke).
- Anticoagulation guidelines (the same for AFib and AFlut) (2)[C]:
  - Unless contraindicated, patients with AFib or AFlut with any high-risk factors for stroke (prior transient ischemic attack [TIA]/cerebrovascular accident [CVA]/thromboembolism) should receive long-term warfarin therapy to maintain an INR of 2.0–3.0 (3)[A]. Patients with mechanical valves should maintain an INR >2.5 (1)[B]. For patients with AFib and mitral stenosis, a target INR range of 2.0–3.0 is recommended (2)[B].
  - Dabigatran (Pradaxa), a direct thrombin inhibitor, apixaban (Eliquis) and rivaroxaban (Xarelto), Factor Xa inhibitors, have recently been approved as alternatives to warfarin for the prevention of 1st and recurrent stroke in patients with nonvalvular AFib (3). The selection of an antithrombotic should be individualized; consider the risks of each agent, cost, patient preference, and tolerability.
  - $CHADS_2$ scoring (**C**HF (1 point), **H**TN (1 point), **A**ge ≥75 (1 point), **D**M (1 point), prior **S**troke or TIA) (2 points):
    - Patients with a score ≥2 (high risk) should receive anticoagulation unless contraindicated (2,3)[A]. In patients with a prior history of stroke or TIA who are unable to take anticoagulants, aspirin alone is recommended (3)[A].
    - Patients with a score of 1 (intermediate risk) should be treated with anticoagulation or aspirin (81–325 mg/d) (1,3)[A].
    - Patients with a score of 0 (low risk) (including most patients with lone AFib) aspirin (81–325 mg/d) or no treatment is recommended (3)[A]. Anticoagulation is not recommended as risk likely exceeds benefit (1)[A].
  - Combination therapy of clopidogrel and aspirin is not recommended for patients with a hemorrhagic contraindication to warfarin (3)[B].
  - CHA_2DS_2VASc index further refines the risk calculation of $CHADS_2$ with the addition of **V**ascular disease (defined as history of MI, PAD, or complex aortic plaque), **A**ge 65–74 (1 point; 2 points for age ≥75), female **S**ex **c**ategory (1 point) (2,3). Anticoagulation generally recommended for score ≥2.
  - Anticoagulation recommendations are independent of AFib pattern (paroxysmal, persistent, and permanent) (1,2)[B].

- 4 classes of medications are available to achieve ventricular rate control: β-blockers (i.e., metoprolol), nondihydropyridine calcium channel blockers (i.e., verapamil, diltiazem), digoxin, and amiodarone. Optimal target for ventricular rate has not been firmly established, but there is evidence that aggressive control of the ventricular rate offers no benefit beyond more modest rate control (i.e., resting heart rate <110 bpm) (4)[B].

- Preventing rapid ventricular response rates using AV nodal blocking medications is also often effective at controlling a patient's symptoms associated with AFib or AFlut. Patients in whom rate control cannot be achieved or who continue to have persistent symptoms despite reasonable heart rate control may require attempts at restoration of sinus rhythm.

- Of note, ventricular rate control can often be difficult to achieve in AFlut due to the more organized nature of the atrial electrical activity. For this reason, conversion to sinus rhythm is often the preferred strategy, and catheter ablation is also considered as a first-line treatment in recurrent AFlut.

- Restoration of sinus rhythm using electrical or pharmacologic cardioversion may significantly reduce the symptom burden of AFib or AFlut in many patients and may also be useful for controlling ventricular rate. Cardioversion does not impact the long-term risk/benefit ratio of anticoagulation:
  - Cardioversion is most often performed electrically, but may also be achieved using antiarrhythmic drug therapy in some instances, by experienced clinicians (1).
  - If duration of AF is >24–48 hours or unknown, anticoagulate for ≥3 weeks before cardioversion to reduce the risk of stroke. Alternatively, once anticoagulation is established, a transesophageal echo may be performed to exclude the presence of left atrial thrombus, allowing cardioversion to proceed. After cardioversion, anticoagulation should be continued for ≥4 weeks in all patients in whom duration of AFib/AFlut is >24–48 hours, as the postcardioversion period is a time of increased stroke risk (2)[B].

- Randomized clinical trials (AFFIRM and RACE) comparing the outcomes of rate vs. rhythm control found no difference in morbidity, mortality, and stroke rates in patients assigned to one therapy or the other (1).

- Chronic PO antiarrhythmic therapy to suppress AFib recurrence is available for appropriately selected patients. Expert consultation is recommended owing to the complexities of safe antiarrhythmic drug selection.

ISSUES FOR REFERRAL
Management of AFib or AFlut refractory to standard medical therapy (i.e., unable to achieve adequate rate control with medication or development of significant bradycardia with treatment) may require the use of more aggressive treatments. These may include pacemaker implantation (to allow for more intensive pharmacologic blocking of the AV node) or an ablation procedure. AFlut in particular is often very amenable to ablation; thus, consideration should be given to early expert referral in appropriate patients. Antiarrhythmic drug therapy can often be very effective but should be prescribed by experienced practitioners.

SURGERY/OTHER PROCEDURES
- Electrophysiologic study and ablation may be considered for patients with either AFib or AFlut. In the case of AFlut, ablation is often a relatively straightforward procedure generally viewed as a

1st-line therapy due to its high rate of success in appropriate candidates. Ablation of AFib is a much more complex procedure with a more variable success rate; it continues to evolve. Thus, it is typically reserved for drug refractory patients.

- Cardiac surgery (e.g., the maze procedure, ligation of the left atrial appendage) may be considered in patients planning to undergo cardiac surgery for other reasons. Surgical therapy in isolation is rarely indicated for AFib or AFlut.

IN-PATIENT CONSIDERATIONS
Admission Criteria/Initial Stabilization
- Patients with any of the following features likely require admission to the hospital for a period of stabilization:
  - Significant symptoms
  - Rapid ventricular rate
  - Initiating antiarrhythmic therapy
  - AFib/AFlut triggered by an acute process (acute MI, CHF, pulmonary embolus)
- Outpatient management is reasonable for low-risk patients with controlled ventricular rates.
- Acute therapy for symptomatic or hemodynamically compromised patients with AFib or AFlut:
  - IV β- or calcium channel blocker for control of ventricular rate if BP is adequate. If successful, it is essential to follow this treatment with prompt administration of PO medication, as the duration of IV drugs is generally short (1)[C].
- Commonly utilized therapies in the acute setting include (5):
  - Metoprolol: 5 mg IV boluses q5min up to 15 mg, followed by PO metoprolol (1)[C].
  - Diltiazem: Initially 0.25 mg/kg IV over 2 minutes. If inadequate, may be followed by 0.35 mg/kg over 2 minutes after 15 minutes of the initial dose. If there is an appropriate response to diltiazem, PO administration or an IV infusion (5–15 mg/hr) may be initiated (1)[B].
  - Some patients will be far more responsive to 1 class of agents than another. For this reason, if rate control is difficult to achieve, switching drug classes may be useful.
- Urgent cardioversion should be performed in hemodynamically unstable patients. It is somewhat unusual for AFib or AFlut alone to cause marked hemodynamic insult; thus, the possibility of a concurrent process should be considered in this setting (1)[B].
- Consider the initiation of PO anticoagulation therapy. Inpatients may be "bridged" with IV or SC heparin while waiting for warfarin to become effective.

Discharge Criteria
Adequate rate or rhythm control without symptoms; long-term plan for anticoagulation established.

 ONGOING CARE

Given the increasing array of therapies available to manage AFib and AFlut, many patients may benefit from elective expert consultation. Alternatively, in patients with no significant symptoms, if ventricular rate control or sinus rhythm is easily achieved and the choice of thromboembolic prevention is clear, management in a primary care setting may be appropriate.

FOLLOW-UP RECOMMENDATIONS
Patient Monitoring
Adequate anticoagulation levels (if warfarin is employed) and ventricular rate control should be assessed on a regular basis.

DIET
Patients on warfarin should attempt to consume a stable amount of vitamin K to help keep the effect of the drug stable.

PROGNOSIS
Anticoagulation reduces the annual embolic stroke rate from ~5–6% per year to 1–2% for most patients. AFib and AFlut may increase morbidity and mortality, but the overall prognosis is a function of underlying heart disease and adherence with therapy. Reported risk of anticoagulation varies, but lies between 1% and 4% per year for major hemorrhage.

COMPLICATIONS
- Embolic stroke
- Peripheral arterial embolization
- Bleeding with anticoagulation
- Tachycardia-induced cardiomyopathy with prolonged periods of inadequate rate control

REFERENCES

1. Fuster V, Rydén LE, Cannom DS, et al. ACC/AHA/ESC 2006 guidelines for the management of patients with atrial fibrillation. *Circulation*. 2006; 114:700–752.
2. You JJ, Singer DE, Howard PA, et al. Antithrombotic therapy for atrial fibrillation: Antithrombotic therapy and prevention of thrombosis: American College of Chest Physicians Evidence-Based Clinical Practice Guidelines (9th edition). *Chest*. 2012;141 (2_suppl): e531S–e575S.
3. Furie KL, Goldstein LB, Albers GW, et al. Oral antithrombotic agents for the prevention of stroke in nonvalvular atrial fibrillation: a science advisory for healthcare professionals from the American Heart Association/American Stroke Association. *Stroke*. 2012;43:3442–3453.
4. Wann L, Curtis A, January C, et al. 2011 ACCF/AHA/HRS focused update on the management of patients with atrial fibrillation. *J Am Coll Cardiology*. 2011;123:104–123.
5. Neumar RW, Otto CW, Link MS, et al. Part 8: Adult advanced cardiovascular life support: 2010 American Heart Association Guidelines for Cardiopulmonary Resuscitation and Emergency Cardiovascular Care. *Circulation*. 2010; 122(18 Suppl 3):S746–S756.

 CODES

ICD10
- I48.0 Paroxysmal atrial fibrillation
- I48.1 Persistent atrial fibrillation
- I48.3 Typical atrial flutter

CLINICAL PEARLS
- Primary decision in persistent afib is whether to strive for rate control or rhythm control. Younger patients often do better with a rhythm control strategy, whereas older patients often do well with rate control. Decision is complex.
- Anticoagulate most patients with paroxysmal or persistent afib/flut without contraindication.

ATRIAL SEPTAL DEFECT (ASD)

Daniel Stein, MD, MPH • Stephen K. Lane, MD, FAAFP

BASICS

DESCRIPTION
- Anatomy:
  - Opening in the atrial septum allowing flow of blood between the two atria
  - Patent foramen ovale is similar, but is not open most of the time, causes no hemodynamic disturbance, and is not considered an atrial septal defect (ASD) (no tissue defect)
- Types (by location in the interatrial septum) (1):
  - 75%: Ostium secundum defect occurs in the fossa ovalis region.
  - 15%: Ostium primum defect occurs in the inferior septum; often associated with cleft mitral valve and failure of endocardial cushion development.
  - 10%: Sinus venosus defect occurs in the superior-posterior septum near the orifice of the superior vena cava; usually associated with partial anomalous right upper pulmonary venous return.
- Hemodynamic effects:
  - Left-to-right shunting in late ventricular systole and early diastole
  - Degree depends on size of the defect and relative pressures of the 2 ventricles.
  - Causes excessive blood flow through the right-sided circulation, ultimately leading to reactive pulmonary hypertension and heart failure
- Systems affected: Cardiovascular; Pulmonary

Pediatric Considerations
- Most cases of ASD are detected and corrected in the pediatric population.
- The smaller the defect and the younger the child, the greater the chance of spontaneous closure.

EPIDEMIOLOGY
Incidence
- Predominant age: present from birth, may be diagnosed at any age
- Predominant sex: Female > Male (2:1)
- No race predilection
- 4/10,000 births

Prevalence
Accounts for 10% of congenital heart defects, and 25–30% of congenital heart defects detected in adulthood

ETIOLOGY AND PATHOPHYSIOLOGY
- Flow across ASD usually left-to-right shunt because of higher left-sided pressures:
  - Minimal right-to-left shunting in early ventricular systole, especially during inspiration
  - Increased right-sided pressure/pulmonary hypertension can cause reversal of shunt flow (Eisenmenger syndrome) with resulting cyanosis and clubbing.
- Symptoms typically occur due to right ventricular and pulmonary vascular volume overload and right-sided heart failure.

Genetics
- Most cases are spontaneous.
- 5% with chromosomal abnormalities; other rare mutations exist
- ~25% prevalence in Down syndrome

RISK FACTORS
- Other congenital heart defects
- Family history (~7–10% recurrence)
- Thalidomide, alcohol exposure in utero

COMMONLY ASSOCIATED CONDITIONS
- ASDs may occur as a component of other complex cardiac structural defects.
- Important to exclude anomalous pulmonary venous return
- Occasionally can indicate underlying genetic syndromes, for example:
  - Holt-Oram syndrome: Secundum defect with bony abnormalities of forearms + hands
  - Ellis-von-Creveld syndrome: Chondroectodermal dysplasia + ASD
  - VACTERL (vertebral, anorectal, cardiac, tracheoesophageal, renal/urinary and limb defects)

DIAGNOSIS

HISTORY
- Initially, may be asymptomatic
- Infants/children may be small for age, even in the absence of other symptoms. Will generally improve with surgical treatment.
- Most common symptoms are dyspnea on exertion, palpitations, and easy fatigability.
- Consider if history of right-sided heart failure (more advanced, only 10% at diagnosis), frequent respiratory tract infections, stroke, or unexplained end-organ infarcts due to paradoxical emboli.

PHYSICAL EXAM
- Signs vary according to extent of shunting.
- Cardiac auscultation:
  - *Fixed, widely split S_2 (key physical finding)*
  - May also have:
    - Systolic ejection murmur (pulmonic flow murmur)
    - Low-pitched diastolic rumble (tricuspid flow murmur)
    - Diastolic murmur (pulmonic regurgitation)
    - Systolic murmur (mitral regurgitation)
- Right ventricular heave
- Palpable pulmonary artery pulse at left upper sternal border
- If heart failure has developed, may hear a 4th heart sound (right-sided).
- Signs of Eisenmenger syndrome:
  - Cyanosis and clubbing
  - Jugular venous distention and edema

DIFFERENTIAL DIAGNOSIS
- Other congenital heart disease
- Right bundle branch block (for widely split S_2)

DIAGNOSTIC TESTS & INTERPRETATION
Initial Tests (lab, imaging)
- Oximetry: Cyanosis may suggest Eisenmenger syndrome (right-to-left shunting).
- ECG findings may include:
  - Right axis deviation
  - Right atrial enlargement
  - Right ventricular conduction delay
  - Q wave in lead V1
  - Mild PR prolongation
  - Leftward axis, inverted P wave in lead III (sinus venosus)
  - Leftward axis (ostium primum)

- Echocardiography: First-line is transthoracic color Doppler imaging of the entire atrial septum
- Sensitivity is ~89% of secundum, ~100% of primum, and ~44% of sinus venosus ASDs.
- Patients with right ventricular overload by transthoracic echocardiography (TTE), but an otherwise negative study should have further testing.

Follow-Up Tests & Special Considerations
- "Bubble" contrast enhancement may be helpful.
- Transesophageal echocardiography (TEE) may be required to define ASD morphology and to locate the pulmonary veins; often used prior to percutaneous closure. TEE has excellent sensitivity and specificity.

Diagnostic Procedures/Other
- Cardiac catheterization:
  - Demonstrates right ventricle enlargement, location/fraction of the shunt, size of the ASD, any valvular disease, and overall anatomy
  - Used to assess pulmonary vascular resistance if pulmonary hypertension is suspected, particularly if surgery is planned
  - Generally not used in young patients for initial diagnosis, more often reserved for use when:
    - Part of a planned interventional (device) closure
    - Evaluating other disease simultaneously (e.g., coronary artery disease in older individuals)
    - Visualization by other methods insufficient
- Cardiac magnetic resonance: A noninvasive follow-up to echo that allows viewing the defect/pulmonary veins and measurement of shunt fraction and right ventricular (RV) function
- Exercise testing: Useful to quantify symptoms not consistent with clinical findings or to document change over time
- Chest x-ray: May demonstrate right ventricular and pulmonary artery enlargement, increased pulmonary vascular markings
- Ultrafast CT scans can also define ASDs, but with significant radiation exposure.

TREATMENT

GENERAL MEASURES
- 75% of small ASDs (<8 mm) will close spontaneously by 18 months of age; however, close follow-up is warranted (2).
- The likelihood of spontaneous closure is mainly determined by defect diameter: >10 mm at time of diagnosis is unlikely to spontaneously close (3).

MEDICATION
First Line
- Treatment of secondary atrial fibrillation/supraventricular tachycardia with anticoagulation and cardioversion, followed by anticoagulation with maintenance of sinus rhythm if possible, or rate control if this fails (1)[A]
- Respiratory tract infections should be treated promptly.
- Treatment of heart failure (diuretics, oxygen, digoxin, etc.)

Second Line

- No antibiotic prophylaxis is recommended for unrepaired ASDs.

- Antibiotic prophylaxis against infective endocarditis during dental or other oral procedures is recommended for 6 months by the American Heart Association (AHA) after a device or patch is placed (4)[B]:
  – In patients with repaired ASD who have a residual defect at or adjacent to the device, prophylaxis is recommended indefinitely.
  – If prophylaxis is indicated, for dental procedures, amoxicillin 2 g (adults) or 50 mg/kg (children). Other options include cephalosporins (e.g., ceftriaxone 1 g [adults] or 50 mg/kg [children] IM or IV) or clindamycin 600 mg PO (adults) or 20 mg/kg PO (children) in patients who are penicillin-sensitive (5).

- To prevent thrombus formation after device deployment, aspirin 325 mg daily for 6 months and clopidogrel 75 mg for at least 1 month

ISSUES FOR REFERRAL

Appropriate health care: Referral to a cardiologist for evaluation

SURGERY/OTHER PROCEDURES

- In adults, closure via percutaneous transcatheter device or surgery to reduce subsequent morbidity and mortality, if (6):
  – Right side heart enlargement regardless of symptoms
  – Pulmonary systemic flow ratio is ≥2:1 (or >1.5:1 and <21 years old according to the AHA)
  – Symptoms, such as documented orthodeoxia/platypnea, or paradoxical embolism (1)[C]

- Flow ratio can be measured with Doppler echo (lab-specific) or cardiac catheterization.

- Surgical repair is standard for a sinus venosus, coronary sinus, or primum ASD (1)[B].

- Percutaneous transcatheter device closure of secundum ASDs is standard and has largely replaced surgery except when other interventions are planned or anatomy is not favorable (6)[A]. Secundum ASDs that are suitable for percutaneous closure should be ≤35 mm in stretched balloon diameter and should have a sufficient rim of surrounding atrial tissue.

- Closure is not indicated for patients who have developed irreversible severe pulmonary hypertension without continued shunting or those who never develop symptoms and have an ASD <5 mm.

- In children, closure is usually delayed until preschool age (2–4 years), except for symptomatic defects (poor growth or exercise intolerance) because of the high rate of spontaneous closure.

- Closing small asymptomatic ASDs is controversial and not often done.

- Radiofrequency ablation, either before or after closure, can be considered for patients with refractory atrial fibrillation (7).

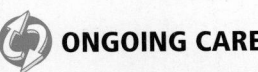 ONGOING CARE

FOLLOW-UP RECOMMENDATIONS

Echocardiography can be used to monitor both repaired and unrepaired ASDs.

Patient Monitoring

- In otherwise asymptomatic healthy children, follow until defect has closed or become negligible in size.
- Appropriate evaluation and management for atrial tachyarrhythmias in patients with long-term follow-up (1)
- If ASD repaired as an adult, periodic long-term follow-up indicated (1).
- ASDs repaired in childhood generally do not have late complications.
- In female patients with unrepaired ASD and Eisenmenger syndrome, pregnancy is not recommended due to increased risk of maternal and fetal mortality (1)[A].
- Pregnancy is well tolerated in patients with repaired ASD and small unrepaired ASDs.

PATIENT EDUCATION

For patient education materials on this topic, consult:
- American Heart Association: http://www.heart.org
- Mayo Clinic information: http://www.mayoclinic.com/health/atrial-septal-defect/DS00628

PROGNOSIS

- ASD closure in asymptomatic or minimally symptomatic adults reduces morbidity, but not mortality (8)[A].
- ASD closure before age 25 in symptomatic adults reduces morbidity and likely also mortality.
- ASD repair deferred until after adolescence may not decrease long-term risk of future atrial arrhythmias.
- Up to 50% mortality by age 50 in untreated symptomatic patients with large defects

COMPLICATIONS

- Unrepaired: Congestive heart failure, stroke, pulmonary hypertension/Eisenmenger syndrome, atrial arrhythmias, increased infection risk (pulmonary, cerebral abscess, infective endocarditis)
- Surgically repaired: Late-onset arrhythmias 10–20 years after surgery (5%), perioperative atrial tachyarrhythmias in 10–13% of patients
- Device closure: Device embolization (1%), cardiac perforation, thrombus formation, endocarditis, supraventricular arrhythmias

REFERENCES

1. Warnes CA, Williams RG, Bashore TM, et al. ACC/AHA 2008 guidelines for the management of adults with congenital heart disease. *J Am Coll Cardiol.* 2008;52(23):e143–263.
2. McMahon CJ, Feltes TF, Fraley JK, et al. Natural history of growth of secundum atrial septal defects and implications for transcatheter closure. *Heart.* 2002;87(3):256–259.
3. Hanslik A, Pospisil U, Salzer-Muhar U, et al. Predictors of spontaneous closure of isolated secundum atrial septal defect in children: A longitudinal study. *Pediatrics.* 2006;118: 1560–1565.
4. Nishimura RA, Carabello BA, Faxon DP, et al. ACC/AHA 2008 guideline update on valvular heart disease: Focused update on infective endocarditis. *Circulation.* 2008;118(8):887–896. Epub 2008 Jul 28.
5. Wilson W, Taubert KA, Gewitz M, et al. Prevention of infective endocarditis: Guidelines from the American Heart Association: A guideline from the American Heart Association Rheumatic Fever, Endocarditis, and Kawasaki Disease Committee, Council on Cardiovascular Disease in the Young, and the Council on Clinical Cardiology, Council on Cardiovascular Surgery and Anesthesia, and the Quality of Care and Outcomes Research Interdisciplinary Working Group. *Circulation.* 2007;116(15):1736–1754. Epub 2007 Apr 19.
6. Holzer R, Hijazi ZM. Interventional approach to congenital heart disease. *Curr Opin Cardiol.* 2004; 19:84–90.
7. Crandall M, Daoud E, Daniels C, et al. Percutaneous radiofrequency catheter ablation for atrial fibrillation prior to atrial septal defect closure. *J Cardiovasc Electrophysiol.* 2012;23(1):102–104.
8. Attie F, Rosas M, Granados N, et al. Surgical treatment for secundum atrial septal defects in patients >40 years old. A randomized clinical trial. *J Am Coll Cardiol.* 2001;38(7):2035–2042.

ADDITIONAL READING

- Furie KL, Kasner SE, Adams RJ, et al. Guidelines for the prevention of stroke in patients with stroke or transient ischemic attack: A guideline for healthcare professionals from the American Heart Association/American Stroke Association. *Stroke.* 2011;42(1):227–276. Epub 2010 Oct 21.
- Lindsey JB, Hillis LD. Clinical update: Atrial septal defect in adults. *Lancet.* 2007;369(9569): 1244–1246.

 SEE ALSO

Aortic Valvular Stenosis; Coarctation of the Aorta; Patent Ductus Arteriosus; Pulmonary Valvular Stenosis; Tetralogy of Fallot; Ventricular Septal Defect

 CODES

ICD10
- Q21.1 Atrial septal defect
- Q21.2 Atrioventricular septal defect

CLINICAL PEARLS

- ASD is often missed due to subtle clinical presentation.
- Ideally, hemodynamically significant ASDs should be closed in early childhood, although some benefit from closure is present in older patients.
- Many ASDs can be treated by catheter-directed percutaneous closure, rather than open-heart surgery.
- Routine endocarditis prophylaxis is not recommended for unrepaired ASDs.
- Patent foramen ovales, unlike large ASDs, are very common and generally require no treatment in asymptomatic individuals.

Wynne Morgan, MD • Frank J. Domino, MD

BASICS

- Adult attention-deficit/hyperactivity disorder (adult ADHD) is a psychiatric condition resulting in inattention and/or hyperactivity or impulsivity. It is associated with low self-esteem and challenges in interpersonal relationships, often impacting work environments.
- Adult ADHD has been shown to affect a significant portion of the adult population; >30% of patients diagnosed with this disorder as a child will meet criteria for this disorder into adulthood and many more will have symptoms related to the disorder (1).
- Young adults aging out of pediatric services and into adult services often lose access to ADHD medications in the transition period, leaving them at risk for disruption in their daily functioning.

DESCRIPTION

- ADHD is one of the most common pediatric disorders that also affects patients into adulthood who have symptoms as a child.
- Symptoms include difficulty concentrating, difficulty controlling behaviors, and hyperactivity/overactivity.
- The 3 main types of ADHD are: (i) Primary symptoms include hyperactivity-impulsivity; (ii) Primary symptoms include inattentiveness; and (iii) Combined symptoms of inattention and hyperactivity
- Cost to society in 2010 US dollars estimated to be $105–194 billion, with most of this cost from productivity and income losses, with "spillover" costs paid by families ranging from $33 to $43 billion (1)[A]

EPIDEMIOLOGY

Prevalence

- General population prevalence for adult ADHD 2.5% but population prevalence declines with age (2).

Genetics

ADHD has substantial heritability, 1st-degree biological relatives with ADHD are found more often in patients with ADHD (3). Some genes have been correlated with ADHD, although not necessary or sufficient causal factors (4). Some areas of study include the implicate duplications at 15q13.3, a possible novel risk factor for ADHD (5), as well as other links between genetic similarities of ADHD and substance abuse (6).

RISK FACTORS

History of childhood and adolescent ADHD diagnosis, particularly symptoms of hyperactivity and/or impulsivity, persisting into adulthood. ADHD is more frequent in males than females (7).

COMMONLY ASSOCIATED CONDITIONS

- Substance use and substance abuse disorders
- Mood disorders
- Anxiety disorders
- Intellectual disabilities
- Obsessive-compulsive disorder (OCD)
- Tic disorders

DIAGNOSIS

- Diagnosis is made from patient's history, and detailing patient's current level of functioning.
- It is particularly important to gather history of patient's childhood and school performance. Several ADHD symptoms should be present before age 12 years (8). If no diagnosis or concern for ADHD as a child, it is unlikely to be diagnosed as an adult.
- *DSM-V* criteria are used for adults as well children.

HISTORY

- History of childhood ADHD symptoms before age 12 years.
- *DSM-V* criteria include ≥5 hyperactivity/impulsivity symptoms and/or ≥5 inattentive symptoms. These symptoms must be present for ≥6 months.
- Symptoms must result in maladaptive behavior that impairs the patient's function.
- There also must be some impairment in ≥2 settings, such as work and home.
- Clear evidence must exist of impairment of function in work, home life, and education secondary to these symptoms of inattention/hyperactivity.
- These symptoms must happen outside an episode of psychosis, mood disorder, or related to pervasive developmental disorder (PDD) and may not be better explained by another *DSM* diagnosis (9).
- CAGE and substance abuse questions will help identify substance abuse issues, but will not determine if the substance abuse is the primary diagnosis or if the patient has this in addition to adult ADHD.
- History of cardiac disease and family history of cardiac disease and sudden death should be documented.
- History of lead exposure or other toxins.

PHYSICAL EXAM

- Physical exam is key to rule out other medical conditions.
- Exam should focus on the thyroid and neurologic exam. Examine the body for any sequelae of substance abuse.
- BP and baseline weight are also important to record and monitor when considering starting medication treatment (10).

DIFFERENTIAL DIAGNOSIS

Hearing impairment; hyperthyroid/hypothyroid; sleep deprivation; sleep apnea; phenylketonuria; OCD; lead toxicity; substance abuse (11)

DIAGNOSTIC TESTS & INTERPRETATION

- Adult ADHD screening tools. There are retrospective tools like the Childhood Symptom Scale and the Wender Utah Rating Scale; also current symptom scales, such as the Adult ADHD Rating Scale IV, Adult Self Report Scale Symptom Checklist, and the Connor Adult Rating Scale. These scales can take 5–20 minutes to complete.
- Provider/Patient screening checklist:
  – http://help4adhd.org/documents/ AdultADHDSelfReportScale-ASRS-v1-1.pdf
  – http://webdoc.nyumc.org/nyumc_d6/files/ psych_adhd_screener.pdf
- ECG with concerns for cardiac disease in patient or family history

Initial Tests (lab, imaging)

- Thyroid-stimulating hormone (TSH)
- Liver function test monitoring (with atomoxetine)
- Rapid plasma reagin (RPR) or VDRL (Venereal Disease Research Laboratory) test
- Serum lead levels (pending history)

Follow-Up Tests & Special Considerations

- A history of childhood behaviors is helpful to make the diagnosis, but adult patients often don't accurately recall childhood symptomology.
- Consider speaking with patient's parents or obtaining old school records and a developmental history as well as any family history of ADHD, substance abuse, or tic disorder to ensure accurate diagnosis.

ALERT

Mood disorders, generalized anxiety disorders, and substance abuse can also co-occur with adult ADHD; treating both the ADHD and co-morbid condition will provide the greatest prognosis for the patient.

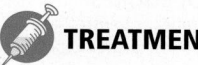

TREATMENT

- Most of the research and medication trials have been performed in children.
- Medications used with children are also effective to treat ADHD symptoms in adults (11).

ALERT

Stimulant medication prescriptions risk inducing dependency, substance abuse, and diversion. Perform pill counts and urine drug testing, as well as screening for signs of prescription drug abuse. Misuse of amphetamines may cause sudden death and serious cardiovascular adverse events.

GENERAL MEASURES

When prescribing stimulant medications for adults with ADHD, watch for misuse, abuse, and diversion of prescription medications. When substance abuse is not present, stimulants are first line treatment for ADHD and highly efficacious. There are multiple formulations of stimulants, and patients may require multiple trials of different preparations for effective response.

MEDICATION

- Psychotropic medications play a large part in the treatment of ADHD symptoms. Medications should be titrated slowly to effective dose to avoid side effects.
- Stimulants are more effective than antidepressants, but up to 30% discontinue medications because of side effects.
- Antidepressants studied for ADHD include bupropion, which has been shown to have a medium effect compared with stimulants (12)[A].

First Line

- Atomoxetine (Strattera) may be given as a single dose or split dose and has low abuse potential, making it a better choice over a stimulant medication for patients with substance abuse history. Atomoxetine should also be used with caution with those patients taking medications that inhibit cytochrome P2D6 (e.g., Paxil or Prozac). Also, there are rare cases of liver damage associated with these medications. Monitor for increased suicidal thinking (13)[B].

- Stimulants: Methylphenidate (Concerta, Ritalin), dexmethylphenidate (Focalin), dextroamphetamine/amphetamine (Adderall), dextroamphetamine (Dexedrine), lisdexamfetamine (Vyvanse)
  - Short-acting stimulants may be used for ADHD without co-occurring substance abuse; given the short half-life, they may require multiple dosing thought the day. Dextroamphetamine is commonly used with a half-life of 4–6 hours with an initial dose of 5 mg. Caution: Immediate release preparations have high abuse potential.
  - Dextroamphetamine/amphetamine (Adderall) is a 75%/25% mix that also comes in an extended-release form.
  - The extended-release form of methylphenidate (Concerta) has an oral osmotic release to decrease this abuse potential.
  - Patients may be transitioned to extended-release forms when they have no adverse effects from immediate-release stimulants.
  - Lisdexamfetamine (Vyvanse) is an extended-release stimulant that is a prodrug requiring metabolization to active component, dextroamphetamine.
  - Common side effects of stimulants include hypertension (HTN), tachycardia, insomnia, weight loss, stomach upset, increased anxiety/irritability, or worsening of tics (14).

- Antidepressants: Best used for those at risk or have history of substance abuse disorder:
  - Bupropion (Wellbutrin) is an antidepressant effective in adults with ADHD symptoms (14)[A].

ISSUES FOR REFERRAL

Patients with co-morbid conditions may need specialist evaluation to diagnosis and treat, and to manage complex ADHD symptomatology cases.

ADDITIONAL THERAPIES

Cognitive-behavioral therapy can be useful in conjunction with medication to help patient modify and cope with symptoms (15).

COMPLEMENTARY AND ALTERNATIVE MEDICINE

No data effective (16)

 ONGOING CARE

Often times, young adults transitioning from pediatrics to adult care will discontinue their ADHD medication, leading to issues with school, work, and personal life and also makes them at greater risk of substance abuse and criminal activities.

FOLLOW-UP RECOMMENDATIONS

- Close follow up of medication as dose is titrated
- Repeat screening checklists to quantify benefit of interventions
- Reinforce behavioral change (e.g., self-initiated, through cognitive-behavioral therapy), which is the cornerstone of long-term management.

REFERENCES

1. Doshi JA, Hodgkins P, Kahle J, et al. Economic impact of childhood and adult attention-deficit/hyperactivity disorder in the United States. *J Am Acad Child Adolesc Psychiatry.* 2012;51: 990–1002.
2. Simon V, Czobor P, Bálint S, et al: Prevalence and correlates of adult attention-deficit hyperactivity disorder: a meta-analysis. *Br J Psychiatry.* 2009; 194:204–211.
3. Stawicki JA, Nigg JT, von Eye A: Family psychiatric history evidence on the nosological relations of DSM-IV ADHD combined and inattentive subtypes: New data and meta-analysis. *J Child Psychol Psychiatry.* 2006;47:935–945.
4. Gizer IR, Ficks C, Waldman ID: Candidate gene studies of ADHD: A meta-analytic review. *Hum Genet.* 2009;126:51–90.
5. Williams NM, Franke B, Mick E, et al. Genome-wide analysis of copy number variants in attention deficit hyperactivity disorder: The role of rare variants and duplications at 15q13.3. *Am J Psychiatry.* 2012;169:195–204.
6. Carpentier PJ, Arias Vasquez A, Hoogman M, et al. Shared and unique genetic contributions to attention deficit/hyperactivity disorder and substance use disorders: A pilot study of six candidate genes. *Eur Neuropsychopharmacol.* 2013;23:448–457.
7. Kessler RC, Adler L, Barkley R, et al. The prevalence and correlates of adult ADHD in the United States: Results from the National Comorbidity Survey Replication. *Am J Psychiatry.* 2006;163:716–723.
8. Kieling C, Kieling RR, Rohde LA, et al. The age of onset of attention deficit hyperactivity disorder. *Am J Psychiatry.* 2010;167:14–16.
9. American Psychiatric Association. *Diagnostic and statistical manual of mental disorders*, 5th ed. Arlington, VA: American Psychiatric Association, 2013.
10. Post RE, Kurlansik SL. Diagnosis and management of adult attention-deficit/hyperactivity disorder. *Am Fam Physician.* 2012;85:890–896.
11. Castells X, Ramos-Quiroga JA, Bosch R, et al. Amphetamines for attention deficit hyperactivity disorder (ADHD) in adults. *Cochrane Database Syst Rev.* 2011;6:CD007813.
12. Verbeeck W, Tuinier S, Bekkering GE. Antidepressants in the treatment of adult attention-deficit hyperactivity disorder: A systematic review. *Adv Ther.* 2009;26:170–184.
13. Garnock-Jones KP, Keating GM. Atomoxetine: A review of its use in attention-deficit hyperactivity disorder in children and adolescents. *Paediatr Drugs.* 2009;11:203–226.
14. Maneeton N, Maneeton B, Srisurapanont M, et al. Bupropion for adults with attention-deficit hyperactivity disorder: Meta-analysis of randomized, placebo-controlled trials. *Psychiatry Clin Neurosci.* 2011;65:611–617.
15. Mongia M, Hechtman L. Cognitive behavior therapy for adults with attention-deficit/hyperactivity disorder: A review of recent randomized controlled trials. *Curr Psychiatry Rep.* 2012;14:561–567.
16. Bader A, Adesman A. Complementary and alternative therapies for children and adolescents with ADHD. *Curr Opin Pediatr.* 2012;24:760–769.

ADDITIONAL READING

Diagnostic Checklist: www.webdoc.nyumc.org/nyumc_d6/files/psych_adhd_screener.pdf

 CODES

ICD10

- F90.0 Attn-defct hyperactivity disorder, predom inattentive type
- F90.1 Attn-defct hyperactivity disorder, predom hyperactive type
- F90.9 Attention-deficit hyperactivity disorder, unspecified type

CLINICAL PEARLS

- Adult ADHD results in inattention, hyperactivity, and impulsive behavior; it is associated with low self-esteem and challenges in interpersonal relationships, including work environments.
- Psychotropic medications plus cognitive-behavioral treatments are the cornerstone of management.
- Substance abuse is a common co-morbidity; recommend not to use stimulant medication in those at risk.

ATTENTION DEFICIT/HYPERACTIVITY DISORDER, PEDIATRIC

Laura Novak, MD • Pramesh Patel, MD

 BASICS

DESCRIPTION

- Attention deficit hyperactivity disorder (ADHD) is a neurodevelopmental problem characterized by a short attention span, distractibility, low frustration tolerance, impulsivity, and hyperactivity. 3 subsets:
- Predominantly hyperactivity-impulsive (ADHD-HI), predominantly inattentive (ADHD-I), or combined (ADHD-C)
- System(s) affected: Nervous
- Synonym(s): Attention deficit disorder; Hyperactivity

EPIDEMIOLOGY

- Predominant age: Onset <12 years; lasts into adolescence and adulthood; 50% meet diagnostic criteria by age 4 years
- Predominant sex: Male > Female (2:1); predominantly inattentive type may be more common in girls

Prevalence
- 5% of school-aged children
- 2.5% of adult population

Genetics
Familial pattern

RISK FACTORS

- Family history
- Medical causes (especially affecting brain development)
- Environmental causes (toxins such as lead, fetal alcohol, and nutritional deficiencies)

GENERAL PREVENTION

- Children are at risk for abuse, depression, and social isolation.
- Parents need regular support and advice.
- Parents should establish contact with teacher each school year.

COMMONLY ASSOCIATED CONDITIONS

- Learning disabilities
- Mood disorders, oppositional defiant disorder, conduct disorder

 DIAGNOSIS

- American Academy of Pediatrics (AAP) guidelines recommend *DSM-IV* criteria to establish the diagnosis (1)[C],(2)[C]. (Note new DSM-5.)
- Children undergoing extreme stress (divorce, illness, homelessness, abuse) may demonstrate ADHD behaviors secondary to stress. This can be assessed using the American Academy of Child and Adolescent Psychiatry (AACAP) screening tool, if needed.
- If diagnostic behaviors are noted in only 1 setting, explore the stressors in that setting.
- The diagnostic behaviors are more noticeable in tasks that require concentration or boredom tolerance than in free play or office situations.
- *DSM-5* criteria: ≥6 inattention criteria and/or ≥6 hyperactivity/impulsivity criteria. Symptoms must begin by age 7 years, be present for >6 months, and be noticed in 2 settings (e.g., home and school). In addition to parents, teachers and caretakers also should fill out assessments.

- Inattention:
  - Careless mistakes in tasks; difficulty in sustaining attention or in organizing tasks; does not seem to listen, follow through, or finish tasks; avoids tasks that require sustained mental effort; loses things; easily distracted; forgetful in daily activities
- Hyperactivity/Impulsivity:
  - Fidgets or squirms; difficulty remaining seated; runs or climbs excessively, inappropriately; difficulty playing quietly; acts as if "driven by a motor"; talks excessively; blurts out answers before question is complete; has difficulty waiting turn; interrupts others

HISTORY

- Birth and development history
- Comprehensive psychosocial evaluation of home environment
- School performance history
- Psychiatric history or comorbid disorder

PHYSICAL EXAM

- Baseline weight for future monitoring
- Focus on soft neurologic signs, such as tics, clumsiness, mixed handedness

DIFFERENTIAL DIAGNOSIS

- Activity level appropriate for age
- Hearing/vision disorder
- Dysfunctional family situation
- Learning disability (e.g., dyslexia)
- Autism spectrum
- Oppositional/defiant disorder or conduct disorder
- Tourette syndrome: Motor and verbal tics
- Absence seizures (inattentive type ADHD only)
- Lead poisoning
- Medication reaction (decongestant, antihistamine, theophylline, phenobarbital)

DIAGNOSTIC TESTS & INTERPRETATION
Behavioral testing:

- Behavior rating scales (Connors, others) should be completed by parents and teachers. They are repeated after therapy is started to gauge differences (*DSM-5* criteria can be used in place of a rating scale)
- An ADHD toolkit with forms is available from www.nichq.org/adhd.html.
- Testing for learning disability (e.g., dyslexia) through the school may be needed

Initial Tests (lab, imaging)
Lead level if high risk

Diagnostic Procedures/Other
Electroencephalogram not needed unless symptoms are highly suggestive of seizure disorder (e.g., absence seizures)

 TREATMENT

GENERAL MEASURES
- Parent/school/patient education.
- Work closely with teacher.

MEDICATION
First Line
The 2011 AAP guideline recommends (1)[C] stimulant medications as first-line treatment. A 2nd type of stimulant should be tried if the 1st treatment fails. Titrate doses over 1–2 months to achieve maximum benefit with minimum adverse effects.

ALERT
The FDA recommends that patients with a personal or family history of congenital heart disease or sudden death be screened with an ECG and possible cardiology consultation before beginning stimulant medication.

- Stimulant:
  - Methylphenidate (Ritalin, Concerta, Metadate CD, Ritalin LA, Focalin XR, Daytrana, others):
    ○ Short-acting: Ritalin 5–20 mg in the morning, at noon, and at 4 P.M.; maximum dose, 60 mg/d
    ○ Long-acting: Concerta 18, 27, 36, 54 mg in the morning; Metadate CD 40 mg in the morning; Ritalin LA 20, 30, 40 mg in the morning
    ○ Methylphenidate patch (Daytrana): Apply to hip for up to 9 hours daily. Begin at 10 mg and titrate upward weekly as needed. Available as 10, 15, 20, and 30 mg.
    ○ Methylphenidate hydrochloride (Methylin): Available as liquid or chewable tab
    ○ Dexmethylphenidate XR (Focalin XR): 5–20 mg once daily
  - Dextroamphetamine:
    ○ Lisdexamfetamine (Vyvanse) 20–70 mg every morning, pediatric (ages 6–17 years) and adult
    ○ Dextroamphetamine: Short-acting 5–20 mg b.i.d.; long-acting, 40 mg/d
  - Mixed amphetamine salts:
    ○ Adderall: 2.5–20 mg q4–6h
    ○ Adderall XR: 5–30 mg every morning; ≥6 years
- Precautions:
  - If not responding, check compliance and consider another diagnosis.
  - Some children experience withdrawal (tearfulness, agitation) after a missed dose or when medication wears off. A small, short-acting dose at 4 P.M. may help to prevent this
  - Stimulants are drugs of abuse and should be monitored carefully. In many states a yearly reporting database must be accessed yearly to monitor patient.
  - Drug holidays should be given only if family/peer relationships are not harmed.
- Common adverse effects:
  - Anorexia, gastrointestinal effects, headache, and insomnia
- Significant possible interactions:
  - Stimulants may increase levels of anticonvulsants, SSRIs, tricyclics, and warfarin.

Pregnancy Considerations
Medications are Category C: Caution in pregnancy.

Second Line
Nonstimulant:

ALERT
Atomoxetine carries a "black box" warning regarding potential exacerbation of suicidality (similar to SSRIs). Close follow-up recommended: Weekly visits for 1st month, then every-other-week visits for 4 sessions, then visits every 12 weeks:
- Atomoxetine is associated with hepatic injury in a small number of cases; check liver enzymes if symptoms (jaundice, fatigue, malaise) develop.
- Atomoxetine (Strattera): Selective norepinephrine reuptake inhibitor; 0.5–2 mg/kg/d every morning (10, 18, 25, 40, 60 mg). Maximum dose, 1.4 mg/kg/d or 100 mg/d, whichever is less:
  – Slower onset of efficacy; GI side effects and sedation; not addictive.
  – Atomoxetine interacts with paroxetine (Paxil), fluoxetine (Prozac), and quinidine.
- Only 2 medications have evidence to support their use as adjunctive therapy with stimulant medications sufficient to achieve FDA approval: extended-release guanfacine and extended-release clonidine α_2-agonists:
  – Guanfacine (Intuiv): 1–4 mg once daily; very sedating, expensive
  – Clonidine (Kapvay): 0.1–0.4 mg divided; very sedating, expensive
- Other nonstimulant drugs (e.g., clonidine, tricyclic antidepressants, SSRIs): Mixed efficacy and high side effects. Consider consultation before use.

ISSUES FOR REFERRAL
Specialist referral should be considered for children <6, for psychological or medical complications, or poor response to medication (1)[C].

ADDITIONAL THERAPIES
- Medication alone or combined with behavioral therapy produced better results than therapy alone.
- Behavioral therapy may be useful when parents object to medication (3)[C].
- For preschool-aged children (4–5 years), prescribe evidence-based parent and/or teacher-administered behavior therapy as the first line of treatment.

COMPLEMENTARY AND ALTERNATIVE MEDICINE
- Surveys have shown that parents of children with ADHD use herbals and complementary treatments frequently (20–60%) (4,5).
- Many herbals studies are small and brief; therefore, difficult to translate into clinical recommendations.
- Omega-3 fatty acids (found in fish oil and some supplements) showed improvement in rating scales in 2 double-blind, placebo-controlled studies of 116 and 130 patients (6).
- Rapid eye training and biofeedback have contradictory results and can be costly.
- Insufficient evidence to assess the benefits of meditation, yoga, acupuncture, and homeopathy.

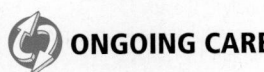 ONGOING CARE

Toolkit for physicians: http://www.nichq.org/adhd.html

FOLLOW-UP RECOMMENDATIONS
Patient Monitoring
- Parent/teacher rating scales initially, 2 weeks after an intervention and regularly
- Office visits to monitor side effects and efficacy: Endpoints are improved grades, improved rating scales, acceptable family interactions, and improved peer interactions.
- Monitor growth (especially weight) and BP.

DIET
- "Insufficient evidence exists to suggest that dietary interventions reduce the symptoms of ADHD in children" (6)[B].
- The AAP recommends that "For a child without a medical, emotional, or environmental etiology of ADHD behaviors, a trial of a preservative-free food coloring-free diet is a reasonable intervention" (1)[C].

PATIENT EDUCATION
- Excellent reference: www.parentsmedguide.org
- Key points for parents:
  – Behavioral interventions, such as token systems, may be helpful.
  – Find things child is good at and emphasize these.
  – Reinforce good behavior (with rewards and attention).
  – Make eye contact with each request.
  – Give 1 task at a time.
  – Stop behavior with quiet discipline before it escalates.
  – Coordinate homework with teachers using a daily assignment notebook.
  – Encourage parents to subtract 2 years from their child's chronological age when allowing privileges (e.g., treat a 16-year-old like a 14-year-old, delay driving until age 18).
- Support groups:
  – Children and Adults with Attention Deficit Disorder (CHADD): chadd.org
  – Attention Deficit Disorder Warehouse: addwarehouse.com
  – National Information Center for Children and Youth with Disabilities: www.nichcy.org

PROGNOSIS
- May last into adulthood; hyperactivity may become easier to control with increasing age.
- Relative deficits in academic and social functioning may persist into late adolescence and adulthood.
- Encourage career choices that allow autonomy and mobility.

COMPLICATIONS
- Untreated ADHD can lead to failing in school, parental abuse, social isolation, and poor self-esteem.
- Some children experience withdrawal (tearfulness, agitation) after a missed medication dose or when medication wears off.
- Monitor growth with stimulant use. If appetite is poor, as a side effect of stimulant medication, eat before the medication is given and after it wears off.
- Increased risk of substance abuse is controversial and may be related to comorbid conditions (conduct disorder).
- 2–4 times increase in automobile accidents and injuries; decreases with medication

REFERENCES
1. ADHD: Clinical Practice Guideline fort the Diagnosis, Evaluation, and Treatment of Attention Deficit/Hyperactivity Disorder in Children and Adolescents. *Pediatrics*. 2012;128:1007–1022.
2. American Psychiatric Association. *Diagnostic and Statistical Manual of Mental Disorders*, 5th ed. Washington, DC: American Psychiatric Association; 2013.
3. Laforett DR, Murray DW, Kollins SH. Psychosocial treatments for preschool-aged children with attention-deficit hyperactivity disorder. *Dev Disabil Res Rev*. 2008;14:300–310.
4. Sawni A. Attention-deficit/hyperactivity disorder and complementary/alternative medicine. *Adolesc Med State Art Rev*. 2008;19:313–326, xi.
5. Weber W, Newmark S. Complementary and alternative medical therapies for attention-deficit/hyperactivity disorder and autism. *Pediatr Clin North Am*. 2007;54:983–1006; xii.
6. Sinn N. Nutritional and dietary influences on attention deficit hyperactivity disorder. *Nutr Rev*. 2008;66:558–568.

ADDITIONAL READING
- Ghuman JK, Arnold LE, Anthony BJ. Psychophar-macological and other treatments in preschool children with attention-deficit/hyperactivity disorder: Current evidence and practice. *J Child Adolesc Psychopharmacol*. 2008;18(5):413–447.
- Millichap JG, Yee MM. The diet factor in attention-deficit/hyperactivity disorder. *Pediatrics*. 2012;129(2):330–337. Epub 2012 Jan 9.
- Post RE, Kurlansik SL. Diagnosis and management of adult attention-deficit/hyperactivity disorder. *Am Fam Physician*. 2012;85(9):890–896.
- Rader R, McCauley L, Callen EC. Current strategies in the diagnosis and treatment of childhood attention-deficit/hyperactivity disorder. *Am Fam Physician*. 2009;79(8):657–665.
- Soileau EJ. Medications for adolescents with attention-deficit/hyperactivity disorder. *Adolesc Med State Art Rev*. 2008;19(2):254–267, viii-ix.

 CODES

ICD10
- F90.0 Attn-defct hyperactivity disorder, predom inattentive type
- F90.1 Attn-defct hyperactivity disorder, predom hyperactive type
- F90.9 Attention-deficit hyperactivity disorder, unspecified type

CLINICAL PEARLS
- Children undergoing extreme stress (divorce, illness, homelessness, abuse) may demonstrate ADHD behaviors secondary to stress.
- 50% of children with ADHD have a parent with ADHD.
- AAP recommends the use of stimulant medications as the first-line treatment.

AUTISM SPECTRUM DISORDERS

Macario C. Corpuz, Jr., MD, FAAFP • Jennifer Luo Powell, DO

 BASICS

DESCRIPTION
Group of neurodevelopmental disorders of early childhood:

- By DSM-IV-TR, autism disorder includes autistic disorder, Rett syndrome, childhood disintegrative disorder, Asperger disorder, and pervasive developmental disorder not otherwise specified (PDD-NOS); DSM-V may eliminate the diagnosis of Asperger disorder.
- Autistic disorder includes classic autism and childhood autism.
- Rett syndrome involves mutations in the *MECP2* gene, mostly in females with initial normal development until ~18 months of age with microcephaly and dementia.
- Childhood disintegrative disorder: Regression after at least 2 years of normal development.
- Asperger disorder: Better development with mechanics of verbal expression, higher levels of cognition and interest in social activity.
- PDD-NOS: Meets some, but not all of *Diagnostic and Statistical Manual of Mental Disorders-Fourth Edition (Text Revision) DSM-IV-TR* criteria for autistic disorder.
- Characterized by:
  - Impairment of effective social skills
  - Absent or impaired communication skills
  - Repetitive and/or stereotyped behaviors and interests, especially in inanimate objects
  - System(s) affected: Nervous
- NOTE: Proposed measurement changes in DSM-5, anticipated to come out in May 2013, extending the ASD diagnosis criteria which involve increased sensitivity to early childhood age of onset, as long as the "social demands exceed limited capacities."

EPIDEMIOLOGY
- Predominant age: Onset in early childhood
- Predominant sex: Male > Female (5:1) except for Rett syndrome (1).

Pediatric Considerations
Symptom onset seen in children <3 years (except for childhood disintegrative disorder)

Prevalence
- Estimated 1/100 to 1/500 children
- Among 6-17 aged children within in United States, in 2011–2012, there is found to be a 2% (1 in 50) parent-reported prevalence compared to 1.16% (1 in 86) as reported in 2007 (2).

ETIOLOGY AND PATHOPHYSIOLOGY
- No single cause has been identified.
- General consensus: A genetic abnormality leads to altered neurologic development.
- No scientific evidence relating vaccines, such as vaccines for measles, mumps, or rubella (MMR) (3), or thimerosal causing ASDs.
- Pathophysiology is incompletely understood.

Genetics
- High concordance in monozygotic twins
- Increased recurrence risk (3–7%) in subsequent siblings

RISK FACTORS
Siblings of affected children have a 5-times greater risk of developing autism. Prevalence ranging from 2–8%.

GENERAL PREVENTION
- Early screening for early treatment means a better prognosis.
- Some autism spectrum disorders (ASDs) like Rett syndrome are caused by genetic mutations.

COMMONLY ASSOCIATED CONDITIONS
- Mental retardation
- ADHD
- Phenylketonuria (PKU), tuberous sclerosis, fragile X syndrome, Angelman syndrome, and fetal alcohol syndrome (rare)
- Anxiety
- Depression
- Obsessive behavior
- Seizures (increased risk if severe mental retardation)
- Maternal use of SSRIs during pregnancy

 DIAGNOSIS

HISTORY
- Impairment in social interaction:
  - Impairment in nonverbal behaviors such as eye-to-eye gaze, facial expression
  - Unable to develop peer relationships
  - Does not smile nor share emotions
  - Loss of social or emotional reciprocity
- Communication impairment:
  - Delay or lack of development in language skills
  - Inability to initiate or sustain conversation
  - Stereotyped and repetitive use of language
  - Preoccupation with parts of toys or body parts
- Repetitive and stereotyped patterns of behavior:
  - Excessively lines up toys or other objects
  - Unusually attached to one particular toy or object
  - Repetitive odd movements (toe walking, hand flapping)
  - Adherence to specific routines or rituals
- Asperger disorder does not have significant delays in cognitive development, language acquisitions, or learning/adaptive skills.
- Rett syndrome is predominantly in females with mcirocephaly.
- Childhood disintegrative disorder with normal development until 2 years of age
- PDD-NOS does not meet DSM-IV-TR criteria for autism.
- Prenatal, neonatal, and developmental history
- Seizure disorder
- Family history of autism, genetic disorders, learning disabilities, psychiatric illness, neurological disorders, genetic disorders, or mental retardation
- Commonly associated with sleep disorders (4)

PHYSICAL EXAM
- Macrocephaly in 25% (except in Rett syndrome); head circumference growth peaks at age 6 months and begins to decline by 1 year.
- Dysmorphic features consistent with genetic disorder (fragile X syndrome)
- Hypotonia occurs in autism, but should prompt imaging.
- Wood lamp skin exam to rule out tuberous sclerosis

DIFFERENTIAL DIAGNOSIS
Other mental and CNS disorders:
- Obsessive–compulsive disorder
- Elective mutism
- Language disorder/hearing impairment
- Intellectual disability/global developmental delay
- Stereotyped movement disorder
- Severe early deprivation/reactive attachment disorder
- Anxiety disorder
- Developmental language disorder

DIAGNOSTIC TESTS & INTERPRETATION
- Checklist for Autism in Toddlers (CHAT) to screen for ASDs at 18 months of age. (To order: http://www.autism.org.uk/working-with/health/screening-and-diagnosis/checklist-for-autism-in-toddlers-chat.aspx)
- The Pervasive Developmental Disorders Screening Test-II (PDDST-II) to screen for ASDs beginning at 18 months
- Modified Checklist for Autism in Toddlers (M-CHAT) to screen for ASDs at 16–30 months
- Social Communication Questionnaire (SCQ) (formerly Autism Screening Questionnaire)—used with children age 4 years and older—the gold standard diagnostic interview used in research studies

Initial Tests (lab, imaging)
- Lead screening
- PKU screening
- Karyotype and DNA analysis (fragile X, PKU, tuberous sclerosis, and others)
- Metabolic testing if signs of:
  - Lethargy, limited endurance
  - Hypotonia
  - Recurrent vomiting and dehydration
  - Developmental regression
  - Unusual habits
  - Specific food intolerance
- MRI is useful only if focal neurologic symptoms

Follow-Up Tests & Special Considerations
- Hearing tests: Audiometry and brainstem auditory evoked response (BAERS)
- Comprehensive speech and language evaluation
- Evaluation by multidisciplinary team: Includes a psychiatrist, neurologist, psychologist, speech therapist, and other autism specialists
- Intellectual level needs to be established and monitored, as it is one of the best measures of prognosis.
- Test used to follow autism are:
  - Autism Behavior Checklist (ABC)
  - Gilliam Autism Rating Scale (GARS)
  - Childhood Autism Rating Scale (CARS)
  - Autism Diagnosis Interview-Revised (ADI-R)
  - Autism Diagnostic Observation Schedule-Generic (ADOS-G) Imaging

Diagnostic Procedures/Other
EEG if history of seizures or spells

 TREATMENT

GENERAL MEASURES
- Comprehensive structured educational programming of a sustained and intensive design, most commonly applied behavioral analysis therapy
- Core features of a successful education program:
  - High staff–student ratio 1:2, or less
  - Individualized programming
  - Specialized teacher training with ongoing evaluation of teachers and programs
  - 25 hours a week minimum of specialized services

– A structured routine environment that emphasizes attention, imitation, communication, socialization, and play interactions

– Functional analysis of behavioral problems

– Transition planning and involvement of the family

• Currently no cure for ASDs. Early diagnosis and initiation of multidisciplinary intervention help enhance functioning in later life.

• Early intervention for ages 3 and under

• School-based special education for older children

• Some evidence indicates social skills groups can improve social competence for some children and adolescents with ASD (5).

• Find alternative methods of communication: Sign language; picture exchange communication system

MEDICATION

• Autistism behavior issues should be managed with maximal behavioral management prior to medication, as efficacy data is lacking.

• Medication directed at managing symptoms

First Line

• No true first-line medical therapy

• Stimulants (such as methylphenidate): Efficacious in treating concomitant symptoms of attention deficit disorder, such as impulsiveness, hyperactivity, and inattention; however, the magnitude of response is less than in typically developing children, and adverse effects are more frequent.

• SSRIs have shown some help in reducing ritualistic behavior and improving mood and language skills. Initial choice for anxiety and depressive mood. Also administered for dysregulated mood (6).

• Risperidone (an atypical antipsychotic) has been shown some benefits for treatment for irritability, repetitious behaviors, and social withdrawal for short-term efficacy. Aripriazole (an atypical antipscyhotic) has been shown that short-term treatment may be effective in treating short-term irritability, hyperactivity, and repetitive movements (7)[A]. Precautions: Causes weight gain as an adverse effect. Associated with sedation, dry mouth, agitation enuresis, dyspepsia, diarrhea, constipation, and tremor.

• Melatonin used for patients with concomitant sleep disorders.

Second Line

• Vitamin B6 and magnesium: Inconclusive evidence in improving behavior, speech, and language of children with autism spectrum disorder.

• Tricyclic antidepressants have limited and conflicting evidence of effect

ISSUES FOR REFERRAL

• Refer early to:

– Early learning for evaluation of behavior and language

– Genetic counseling

– Audiology

• Consider referrals to psychiatry, ophthalmology, otolaryngology, neurology, and nutrition

• Refer family members to parent support groups and respite programs

ADDITIONAL THERAPIES

COMPLEMENTARY AND ALTERNATIVE MEDICINE

• Parent Mediated early intervention for young children with autism spectrum has sufficient evidence of benefit in child outcomes related to

language understanding and severity of autism characteristics (8).

• Music therapy has been shown to improve communication skills in autistic patients; however, more research is needed to examine the effects of the therapy in a typical clinical practice and whether this therapy is enduring.

• No evidence to support use of auditory integration therapy or other sound therapies as an effective treatment for autism spectrum disorder (9).

• No evidence to support acupuncture for treatment of ASD.

• IV secretin has shown no evidence of efficacy and is not currently recommended as a treatment for ASD (10).

• Osteopathic manipulative treatment (OMT) has been used to improve sensory and motor performance with neurological problems

 ONGOING CARE

FOLLOW-UP RECOMMENDATIONS

Patient Monitoring

• Constant monitoring by caregivers

• Re-evaluation every 6–12 months by physician for seizures, sleep and nutritional problems, and prescribed medical management

• Intellectual and language testing every 2 years in childhood

DIET

• Gluten- and casein-free diets: Current evidence for efficacy is poor (11).

• Omega-3 fatty acids supplementation has not been found to improve outcomes

PATIENT EDUCATION

• Autism Society of America: http://www.autism-society.org

• Autism and vaccines: http://www.aap.org/immunization/families/faq/VaccineStudies.pdf

PROGNOSIS

• Beginning treatment at a young age (2–4 years) have significantly better outcomes.

• Prognosis is closely related to initial intellectual abilities, with only 20% functioning above the mentally retarded level.

• Communicative language development before 5 years is also associated with a better outcome.

• The general expected course is for a lifelong need for supervised structured care.

COMPLICATIONS

• Increasing incidents of seizure disorders in up to 1 in 4 children.

• Increased risk for physical and sexual abuse

• With pica, increased risk of lead poisoning

• Limited variety of food consumed due to dietary obsessions

• Increased risk for GI symptoms, including weight abnormalities and abnormal stool patterns

REFERENCES

1. Baio J, et al. Autism and Developmental Disabilities Monitoring Network Surveillance Year 2008 Principal Investigators. *MMWR Surveil Summ*. 2012:61(SS03):1–19.

2. Blumberg SJ, et al. Changes in Prevalence of Parent-reported Autism Spectrum Disorder in School-aged U.S. Children: 2007 to 2011–2012. *National Health Statistics Reports*. 2013; 65.

3. Demicheli V, Rivetti A, Debalini MG, et al. Vaccines for measles, mumps and rubella in children. *Cochrane Database Syst Rev*. 2012;2:CD004407. Epub 2012 Feb 15.

4. Vriend JL, Corkum PV, Moon EC, et al. Behavioral interventions for sleep problems in children with autism spectrum disorders: Current findings and future directions. *J Pediatr Psychol*. 2011;36(9):1017–1029.

5. Reichow B, Steiner AM, Volkmar F. Social skills groups for people aged 6 to 21 with autism spectrum disorders (ASD). *Cochrane Database Syst Rev*. 2012;7:CD008511. Epub 2012 Jul 11.

6. Williams K, Wheeler DM, Silove N, et al. Selective serotonin reuptake inhibitors (SSRIs) for autism spectrum disorders (ASD). *Cochrane Database Syst Rev*. 2010;(8):CD004677.

7. Ching H, Pringsheim T. Aripiprazole for autism spectrum disorders (ASD). *Cochrane Database Syst Rev*. 2012;5:CD009043. Epub 2012 May 16.

8. Oono IP, Honey EJ, McConachie H. Parent-mediated early intervention for young children with autism spectrum disorders (ASD). *Cochrane Database Syst Rev*. 2013;4:CD009774.

9. Sinha Y, Silove N, Hayen A, Williams K. Auditory integration training and other sound therapies for autism spectrum disorders (ASD). *Cochrane Database Syst Rev*. 2011;12:CD003681. Epub 2011 Sept 7.

10. Williams K, Wray JA, Wheeler DM. Intravenous secretin for autism spectrum disorders (ASD). *Cochrane Database Syst Rev*. 2012;4:CD003495. Epub 2012 Apr 18.

11. Millward C, Ferriter M, Calver S, et al. Gluten- and casein-free diets for autistic spectrum disorder. *Cochrane Database Syst Rev*. 2013;(2):CD003498. Epub 2009 Jan 21.

 SEE ALSO

Algorithm: Mental Retardation

CODES

ICD10

• F84.2 Rett's syndrome

• F84.3 Other childhood disintegrative disorder

• F84.0 Autistic disorder

CLINICAL PEARLS

ALARM mnemonic from the American Academy of Pediatrics (AAP):

• **A**utism spectrum disorder is prevalent (screen ALL children between 18 and 24 months).

• **L**isten to parents when they feel something is wrong.

• **A**ct early: Screen all children who fall behind in language and social developmental milestones (use early learning to help with evaluation).

• **R**efer to multidisciplinary teams (speech and language evaluation, genetic screening, social support groups).

• **M**onitor support for patient and families

BACK PAIN, LOW

Tyler Cymet, DO, FACP, FACOFP

 BASICS

DESCRIPTION

- Low back pain (LBP) includes a wide range of symptomatic conditions that can be divided into categories based on duration:
  - Acute (<6 weeks)
  - Subacute (>6 weeks, but <3 months)
  - Chronic (>3 months)
- A specific cause of most patients' low back pain will not be found. Even without a known cause for the LBP, most cases resolve regardless of therapy within 4–6 weeks after onset.
- It is important to rule out "red" flag symptoms that may be indicative of trauma-/nerve-related issues, infection, or cancer.
- The primary goal is to provide supportive care and encourage tolerable activity, but educate the patient about symptoms that should cause alarm and prompt a return visit to their physician.
- System(s) affected: Musculoskeletal, Neurologic
- Synonym(s): Lumbago, Lumbar sprain/strain, Low back syndrome

EPIDEMIOLOGY

Incidence

LBP is one of the most common primary care complaints.

Prevalence

- Lifetime prevalence: 80%
- Predominant sex: Male = Female
- Age: There is a bimodal distribution, with the first peak of people with low back pain symptoms occurring between 25 and 29 years and the second peak after 65 years for women and older for men.

ETIOLOGY AND PATHOPHYSIOLOGY

Age-related degenerative changes of the lumbosacral spine and atrophy of supporting musculature

RISK FACTORS

- Increasing age
- Activity (lifting, sudden twisting, bending)
- Obesity
- Sedentary lifestyle
- Physically strenuous work
- Psychosocial factors, such as anxiety, depression, and stress
- Smoking

GENERAL PREVENTION

- Maintain normal weight
- Maintain physical fitness and activity
- Stress reduction
- Proper lifting technique
- Good posture
- Smoking cessation
- USPSTF states there is insufficient evidence to recommend for or against preventative intervention in adults (strength of recommendation A)

 DIAGNOSIS

HISTORY

- Red flags:
  - Age >50 years
  - Recent trauma
  - Bowel incontinence or bladder retention
  - Neurologic deficits
  - History of cancer
  - Night pain, sweats, fever, weight loss
  - Osteoporosis
  - Immunosuppression, prolonged glucocorticoid use
- Onset of pain may be sudden or gradual
- Provoked with motion: flexion–extension, side-bending rotation, sitting, standing, and lifting; relieved with rest
- Radicular pain may radiate into buttocks, thighs, upper back.
- Patient may note improvement with NSAID use.

PHYSICAL EXAM

- Observe patient ambulation, position on examination table, and facial expressions
- Test lumbar spine range of motion:
  - Flexion: 60°
  - Extension: 30°
  - Side-bending: 30°
  - Rotation: 30°
- Can palpate point tenderness or muscle spasm
- Neurologic examination:
  - Visual examination: Signs of pallor or muscle atrophy
  - Bilateral lower extremity reflexes, strength, pulses, sensation
  - Straight leg test

DIFFERENTIAL DIAGNOSIS

- Musculoskeletal:
  - Lumbar strain/sprain
  - Herniated lumbar intervertebral disk
  - Degenerative disk disease
  - Spinal stenosis
  - Spondylolisthesis
  - Severe kyphosis or scoliosis
  - Fractures
- Inflammatory:
  - Ankylosing spondylitis and related inflammatory spondylopathies
  - Rheumatoid arthritis
- Infectious: Vertebral osteomyelitis
- Neoplastic:
  - Primary bone tumors
  - Metastatic disease
- Referred pain:
  - Cardiovascular: Abdominal aortic aneurysm, peripheral vascular disease/claudication
  - GI: Duodenal ulcer, chronic pancreatitis, cholecystitis, irritable bowel syndrome, diverticulitis
  - Genitourinary: Pyelonephritis, nephrolithiasis, prostatitis
  - Gynecologic: Pregnancy, endometriosis, ovarian cystic disease, pelvic inflammatory disease

DIAGNOSTIC TESTS & INTERPRETATION

Initial Tests (lab, imaging)

- Labs are unnecessary if this is the initial presentation and no red flag signs or symptoms present
- If suspecting malignancy or acute inflammatory/infectious process:
  - ESR
  - Serum alkaline phosphatase
  - CBC
- Imaging studies are unnecessary if this is the initial presentation and there are no red flag signs or symptoms (1):
  - Limited need for imaging during first 6 weeks of symptoms unless red flags present (2)[A]
- X-ray:
  - Not recommended for initial presentation or without red flags
  - Defer plain films for 6 weeks unless there is a high risk of disease
- MRI:
  - If patient presents with neurologic deficits, fails to improve within 6 weeks of conservative treatment, or with a strong suspicion of cancer or cauda equina syndrome

Diagnostic Procedures/Other

Surgical consult is necessary if patient presents with acute neurologic deficits or suspect cauda equina syndrome.

TREATMENT

MEDICATION

First Line

- Patients should be assured the pain is self-limited; treatment should be aimed at relieving pain and improving function.
- First-line therapy:
  - Osteopathic manipulative treatments: Myofascial, counter-strain, bilateral ligamentous techniques, as well as muscle energy, if tolerated
  - Spinal manipulation, acupuncture (3)
  - Encouraging activity as tolerated by LBP leads to quicker recovery than bed rest or specifically back mobilizing exercises
  - Traction, either alone or in combination with other treatments, has little or no impact on pain intensity, functional status, global improvement and return to work among people with LBP (4)[A].
- Medications: NSAIDs (5)[A]:
  - Ibuprofen 800 mg PO t.i.d. × 7–14 days (max 2,400 mg/d)
  - Naproxen 250–500 mg PO q12h (max 1,500 mg/d)
  - Aspirin 300–600 mg PO q4–6h (max 4 g/d)
  - Acetaminophen 325–1,000 mg PO q4–6h PRN pain (max 4 g/d)

Second Line
- Second-line therapy for moderate to severe pain:
  – Cyclobenzaprine 5–10 mg PO daily (max 30 mg/d) (6)
  – Hydrocodone 2.5–10 mg PO q4–6h PRN pain (max 1 g/4 h) (7)
  – Methadone 2.5–10 mg PO or 2.5–5 mg SC/IM/IV q8–12h PRN pain
- Alternate methods:
  – Epidural corticosteroid injections
  – Botulinum toxin A
- Lumbar facet joint interventions (8)[A]:
  – Good evidence for the use of conventional radiofrequency neurotomy
  – Fair to good evidence for lumbar facet joint nerve blocks for the treatment of chronic lumbar facet joint pain
- Antidepressants:
  – No clear evidence that antidepressants are more effective than placebo in the management of cases of chronic LBP (9)[A]

COMPLEMENTARY AND ALTERNATIVE MEDICINE
- Harpagophytum procumbens, Salix alba, and Capsicum frutescens may reduce pain more than placebo, but studies are lacking vs. standard therapy with NSAIDs (10)[A].
- Acupuncture is more effective than no treatment, but evidence is conflicting regarding effectiveness over other treatment modalities (11)[A].

 ONGOING CARE

FOLLOW-UP RECOMMENDATIONS
- Exercise
- Education

Patient Monitoring
- Reassurance is key. Follow up within 2–4 weeks of initial presentation is necessary to monitor patient progress:
  – Assess severity and quality of pain and range of motion
- Re-evaluate for possible underlying causes if improvement does not occur.

COMPLICATIONS
Regular NSAID use is associated with erectile dysfunction beyond what would be expected due to age and comorbidity (12).

REFERENCES
1. Flynn TW, Smith B, Chou R. Appropriate use of diagnostic imaging in low back pain: A reminder that unnecessary imaging may do as much harm as good. *J Orthop Sports Phys Ther*. 2011;41: 838–846.
2. Srinivas SV, Deyo RA, Berger ZD. Application of "less is more" to low back pain. *Arch Intern Med*. 2012;172:1016–1020.
3. Walker BF, French SD, Grant W, et al. A Cochrane review of combined chiropractic interventions for low-back pain. *Spine*. 2011;36:230–242.
4. Wegner I, Widyahening IS, van Tulder MW, et al. Traction for low-back pain with or without sciatica. *Cochrane Database Syst Rev*. 2013;8:CD003010.
5. Roelofs PD, Deyo RA, Koes BW, et al. Non-steroidal anti-inflammatory drugs for low back pain. *Cochrane Database Syst Rev*. 2008;1: CD000396.
6. van Tulder MW, Touray T, Furlan AD, et al. Muscle relaxants for non-specific low back pain. *Cochrane Database Syst Rev*. 2008;2:CD004252.
7. Furlan A, Deshpande A, Mailis-Gagnon A, et al. Opioids for chronic low-back pain. *Cochrane Database Syst Rev*. 2013;3:CD004959.
8. Falco FJ, Manchikanti L, Datta S, et al. An update of the effectiveness of therapeutic lumbar facet joint interventions. *Pain Physician*. 2012;15: E909–E953.
9. Urquhart DM, Hoving JL, Assendelft WW, et al. Antidepressants for non-specific low back pain. *Cochrane Database Syst Rev*. 2010;1:CD001703.
10. Gagnier JJ, van Tulder MW, Berman B, et al. Herbal medicine for low back pain: A Cochrane review. *Spine*. 2007;321:82–92.
11. Hutchinson AJ, Ball S, Andrews JC, et al. The effectiveness of acupuncture in treating chronic non-specific low-back pain: A systematic review of the literature. *J Orthop Surg Res*. 2012;71:36.
12. Gleason JM, Slézak JM, Jung H, et al. Regular nonsteroidal anti-inflammatory drug use and erectile dysfunction. *J Urol*. 2011;1854: 1388–1393.

ADDITIONAL READING
- Chou R, Huffman LH, American Pain Society, et al. Medications for acute and chronic low back pain: A review of the evidence for an American Pain Society/American College of Physicians clinical practice guideline. *Ann Intern Med*. 2007;1477: 505–514.

- Dahm KT, Brurberg KG, Jamtvedt G, et al. Advice to rest in bed versus advice to stay active for acute low-back pain and sciatica. *Cochrane Database Syst Rev*. 2010;6:CD007612.
- de Leon-Casasola OA. Opioids for chronic pain: new evidence, new strategies, safe prescribing. *Am J Med*. 2013;126(3 Suppl 1):S3–S11.
- Engers A, Jellema P, Wensing M, et al. Individual patient education for low back pain. *Cochrane Database Syst Rev*. 2011;1:CD004057.
- Henschke N, Ostelo RW, van Tulder MW, et al. Behavioural treatment for chronic low-back pain. *Cochrane Database Syst Rev*. 2010;7:CD002014.
- Kuijpers T, van Middelkoop M, Rubinstein SM, et al. A systematic review on the effectiveness of pharmacological interventions for chronic non-specific low-back pain. *Eur Spine J*. 2011;20: 40–50.
- Waterman BR, Belmont PJ, Shoenfeld AJ. Low back pain in the United States: Incidence and risk factors for presentation in the emergency setting. *Spine J*. 2012;1:63–70.

 SEE ALSO
- Lumbar (Intervertebral) Disc Disorders
- Algorithm: Low Back Pain, Acute

 CODES

ICD10
- G89.29 Other chronic pain
- M54.5 Low back pain

CLINICAL PEARLS
- Most patients have an unidentifiable cause to their LBP, and most cases resolve within 4–6 weeks of onset.
- It is important to rule out red flag symptoms that may be indicative of neurologic issues, infection, or cancer.
- The primary goal is to provide supportive care and encourage tolerable activity, but educate the patient of symptoms that should cause alarm and prompt a return visit to a physician.
- Labs and imaging studies are unnecessary unless the patient presents with red flag symptoms.

BACTERURIA, ASYMPTOMATIC
Mony Fraer, MD, FACP, FASN • Kantima Phisitkul, MD

 BASICS

DESCRIPTION
- Asymptomatic bacteriuria (AB) is diagnosed when significant bacteriuria is not accompanied by symptoms.
- Infectious Disease Society of America definition (1)[A]:
  - Significant bacteriuria is defined based on type of urine specimen, sex, and the amount of bacteria.
  - By midstream clean catch specimen
  - Male: > 100,000 CFU/mL of single bacteria species
  - Female: the same criteria as male, but needs 2 positive consecutive specimens
  - By catheterized specimen
  - Male & female: > 100 CFU/mL of 1 bacterial species. Required only 1 time collection

EPIDEMIOLOGY
Prevalence
- 5–10% of all pregnancies
- 14–22% and 6–10% of elderly women and men (>80 years), respectively
- 23–89% with self-catheterization
- 45–100% of patients with indwelling catheters
- 19–57% of residents of long-term care facilities

ETIOLOGY AND PATHOPHYSIOLOGY
- Women: *Escherichia coli* is isolated in 80% of cases.
- Other frequent organisms: *Klebsiella pneumoniae*, *Enterococcus* species, and coagulase-negative staphylococci
- Men >65 years: Coagulase-negative staphylococci followed by *E. coli* and *Enterococcus* species
- Patients with long-term urologic devices or those institutionalized usually have polymicrobial bacteriuria: *Pseudomonas aeruginosa*, *Proteus mirabilis*, *Morganella morganii*, *Providencia stuartii*
- Institutionalized patients have more resistant organisms: *P. aeruginosa*, *P. mirabilis*
- Microbiology is similar to that of other UTIs with bacteria originating from periurethral area, vagina, or gut. Host factors facilitate bacterial persistence.
- Patients frequently harbor organisms that are less virulent than those causing symptomatic infections.

RISK FACTORS
Similar to those described for other UTIs:
- Pregnant women
- Older persons
- Persistent genitourinary abnormalities
- Chronic indwelling devices (catheters, ureteric stents, or nephrostomy tubes)
- Patients with spinal cord injury and those with functional impairment
- Other: DM, immunocompromised, institutionalized residents, sexual activity and spermicide use

GENERAL PREVENTION
Screening for asymptomatic bacteriuria is indicated in only 2 conditions:
- Pregnancy during the first prenatal visit or at 12–16 weeks' gestation. Periodic screening following bacteriuria treatment is recommended. Rationale: to prevent acute pyelonephritis in pregnant mother and fetal complication such as premature delivery.
- Before urologic intervention in which mucosal bleeding is anticipated, especially TUPR and prostate biopsy
  Rationale: to decrease postintervention infectious complications

COMMONLY ASSOCIATED CONDITIONS
- Increased incidence of symptomatic UTIs (not attributable to bacteriuria)
- Pyuria is common and is not an indication for antimicrobial treatment on its own.

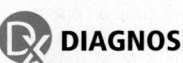 **DIAGNOSIS**

HISTORY
Asymptomatic

PHYSICAL EXAM
No specific abnormalities

DIAGNOSTIC TESTS & INTERPRETATION
Reagent test strips and direct microscopy have poor predictive value for detecting AB.
Initial Tests (lab, imaging)
Urine culture (collected in manner that minimizes contamination) screening in the populations listed above. Recommended thresholds:
- Men (single clean-catch voided urine specimen with isolation of a single organism with counts of $\geq 10^5$ CFU/mL)
- Women (2 consecutive clean-catch urine specimens with isolation of the same organism with counts of $\geq 10^5$ CFU/mL)
- Catheterized specimens (isolation of a single organism with counts of $\geq 10^2$ CFU/mL)

Follow-Up Tests & Special Considerations
Pyuria accompanies bacteriuria in most patients, but its frequency varies in different populations; screening for it is not a reliable method to rule out bacteriuria.

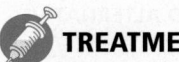 **TREATMENT**

ALERT
Treatment of AB with antibiotics is only indicated in pregnancy (2)[A], and prior to urologic procedures or hip arthroplasty (3)[C].
- Treatment of AB does not decrease the frequency of symptomatic infections or improve other outcomes in all patients, but it does increase cost, risk of potential drug side effects, and risk of antibiotic resistance.
- After treatment, relapse and reinfections are common.
- Asymptomatic candiduria is not an indication for antifungal therapy.

MEDICATION

- Urologic intervention should be initiated shortly before the procedure. Antibiotics should be continued only if an indwelling catheter remains in place post procedure if indwelling catheter is not removed.
- Women with catheter-acquired bacteriuria that persists 48 hours after indwelling catheter removal may be treated with short-course therapy.
- 3–7 days of antibiotics directed at the cultured organism is recommended in pregnancy. If infection recurs, prophylactic antimicrobials should be continued for the duration of the pregnancy.

First Line

- Treatment should be based on culture and sensitivity. Generally, recommendation for antibiotic use in pregnancy includes:
  - Nitrofurantoin 100 mg b.i.d. × 5 days.
  - Amoxicillin/Amoxicillin-clavulanate 500 mg b.i.d. × 3–7 days.
  - Cephalexin 500 mg b.i.d. × 3–7 days.
  - Fosfomycin 3 g po as a single dose
  - Consider suppressive treatment if bacteriuria recurs after 2 treatments.
  - Avoid trimethoprim in 1st trimester, and nitrofurantoin in closed term.
  - Contraindicated: Fluoroquinolones (FDA–C) & tetracyclines (FDA-D)
- Pregnancy Category C (no adequate well-controlled studies in women; only use if potential benefit justifies potential risk to fetus)

ADDITIONAL THERAPIES

Antibiotic impregnated indwelling catheters may reduce AB in short-term catheterized hospitalized adults (4).

 ONGOING CARE

FOLLOW-UP RECOMMENDATIONS

Monthly screening if treatment is required in pregnant women with previous episode of AB

PATIENT EDUCATION

Teaching for the care of chronic indwelling urinary catheters (see "Additional Reading")

COMPLICATIONS

- Late pregnancy pyelonephritis occurs in 20–35% of women with untreated bacteriuria (20–30-fold higher than among women with negative initial screening urine cultures or in whom bacteriuria was treated). Pyelonephritis is associated with premature delivery and worse fetal outcomes (infant with group B streptococcal infections, low-birth-weight infant). Antimicrobial treatment will decrease the risk of subsequent pyelonephritis from 20–35% to 1–4% and the risk of having a low-birth-weight baby from 15% to 5%.
- If bacteriuria remains untreated in patients who undergo traumatic urologic procedures, up to 60% develop bacteremia after the procedure and 5–10% progress to severe sepsis/septic shock.

REFERENCES

1. Nicolle LE, Bradley S, Colgan R, et al. Infectious Diseases Society of America guidelines for the diagnosis and treatment of asymptomatic bacteriuria in adults. *Clin Infect Dis*. 2005;40(5): 643–654. Epub 2005 Feb 4.
2. Smaill F, Vazquez JC. Antibiotics for asymptomatic bacteriuria in pregnancy. *Cochrane Database Syst Rev*. 2007;(2):CD000490. Epub 2007 Apr 18.
3. Gross PA, Patel B. Reducing antibiotic overuse: A call for a national performance measure for not treating asymptomatic bacteriuria. *Clin Infect Dis*. 2007;45(10):1335–1337. Epub 2007 Oct 8.
4. Schumm K, Lam TB. Types of urethral catheters for management of short-term voiding problems in hospitalised adults. *Cochrane Database Syst Rev*. 2008;(2).

ADDITIONAL READING

Lin K, Fajardo K, U.S. Preventive Services Task Force. Screening for asymptomatic bacteriuria in adults: Evidence for the U.S. Preventive Services Task Force reaffirmation recommendation statement. *Ann Intern Med*. 2008;149(1):W20–W24.

 SEE ALSO

- http://www.ahrq.gov/clinic/uspstf/uspsbact.htm
- http://www.webmd.com/a-to-z-guides/care-for-an-indwelling-urinary-catheter-topic-overview
- http://www.uroweb.org/gls/pdf/15_Urological_Infections.pdf

 CODES

ICD10

- B96.1 Klebsiella pneumoniae as the cause of diseases classd elswhr
- B96.20 Unsp Escherichia coli as the cause of diseases classd elswhr
- N39.0 Urinary tract infection, site not specified

CLINICAL PEARLS

Screening for and treatment of AB is appropriate only for pregnant women and for patients undergoing urologic procedures in which mucosal bleeding is anticipated.

BAKER CYST

Chris Wheelock, MD

 BASICS

DESCRIPTION
- A fluid-filled synovial sac arising in the popliteal fossa
- Distention of the gastrocnemial-semimembranous bursa
- Can be unilateral or bilateral
- Most frequent cystic mass around the knee (1)
- Primary cysts are a distention of the bursa arising independently without an intra-articular disorder.
- Secondary cysts occur if a communication exists between the bursa and knee joint, allowing articular fluid to fill the cyst. Pathologic joint processes can also be transmitted in this manner.
- Associated with synovial inflammation
- Synonym(s): Popliteal cyst

EPIDEMIOLOGY
Incidence
- Bimodal distribution:
  – Children ages 4–7
  – Adults increasing with age
- Primary cysts usually seen in children <15 years of age
- Secondary cysts seen in the adult population

Prevalence
- Varies by study
- Studies report a prevalence of 19–47% in symptomatic knees, 2–5% in asymptomatic knees.
- In children: 6.3% in symptomatic knees, 2.4% in asymptomatic knees

ETIOLOGY AND PATHOPHYSIOLOGY
Associated intra-articular pathologic findings include:
- Meniscal tears, posterior horn
- Anterior cruciate ligament (ACL) insufficiency
- Degenerative articular cartilage lesions
- Rheumatoid arthritis (20%)
- Osteoarthritis (50%)
- Osteochondritis
- Gout (14%)
- Other potential factors:
  – Infectious arthritis
  – Polyarthritis
  – Villonodular synovitis
  – Lymphoma
  – Sarcoidosis
  – Connective tissue diseases (2)
- Extension or herniation of synovial membrane of the knee joint capsule or connection of normal bursa with the joint capsule
- May be the result of increased intra-articular pressure
- Commonly seen with knee effusions
- Direct trauma to the bursa is likely the primary cause in children because of no communication between the bursa and the joint in children.
- A valvelike mechanism allowing 1-way passage of fluid from the joint to the bursal connection has been described.

RISK FACTORS
- Osteoarthritis of knee (most common) (3)[B]
- Rheumatoid arthritis
- Meniscal degeneration or tear
- Advancing age
- Ligamentous insufficiency

COMMONLY ASSOCIATED CONDITIONS
Any condition causing knee joint effusion

 DIAGNOSIS

HISTORY
- Painless mass arising in the popliteal fossa
- Most cysts are asymptomatic.
- Dull ache can be present if cyst is sizeable enough to hinder joint motion
- Painful if cyst ruptures
- May report restricted range of motion or tightness with knee flexion
- Large cysts may cause entrapment neuropathy of the tibial nerve.
- Vascular compression, most commonly of the popliteal vein, may produce claudication or thrombophlebitis.
- Activity will alter the cyst size.

PHYSICAL EXAM
- Examine in full extension and 90° of flexion.
- Foucher sign: Mass increases with extension and disappears with flexion.
- Most commonly found in medial aspect of popliteal fossa lateral to the head of the gastrocnemius and medial to the neurovascular bundle
- Mass may be fluctuant or tender.
- Transillumination can distinguish cyst from solid mass.
- Ruptured cyst typically painful with associated swelling over calf and medial malleolus, pseudothrombophlebitis, and, rarely, compartment syndrome (4)

DIFFERENTIAL DIAGNOSIS
- Infection/abscess
- Lipoma
- Liposarcoma
- Fibroma
- Fibrosarcoma
- Hematoma
- Deep venous thrombosis
- Vascular tumor
- Popliteal vein varices
- Xanthoma
- Aneurysm (rare)
- Ganglion cyst
- Any condition causing synovitis
- Thrombophlebitis
- Muscular herniation (rare, related to trauma)

DIAGNOSTIC TESTS & INTERPRETATION
Initial Tests (lab, imaging)
- CBC, sedimentation rate if suspecting septic arthritis
- Send aspirate for cell count to determine nature of effusion: Infectious, inflammatory, or mechanical

Follow-Up Tests & Special Considerations
- In children, consider observation before invasive testing.
- Ultrasound confirms presence and size; with Doppler, can differentiate Baker cysts from popliteal vessel aneurysms or soft tissue tumors (5)[B].
- MRI is useful to assess for causal derangements of internal joint structures and to identify cyst leakage or rupture.
- Radiographs may show soft tissue density posteriorly.
- Arthrography may demonstrate communication with joint capsule or rupture.
- CT–arthrography together is superior in visualizing cystic details and can help separate lipomas, aneurysms, and malignancies from cysts.

 TREATMENT

GENERAL MEASURES
- No treatment if cyst is asymptomatic
- Treat underlying conditions.
- Compressive wrap or sleeve may be used for comfort.

MEDICATION
Once etiology is identified from cellular fluid examination, treat the underlying condition.

First Line
Analgesics, NSAIDs for symptomatic relief

ADDITIONAL THERAPIES
- Physical therapy improves knee ROM and strength, particularly with coexisting pathology.
- Temporary relief with needle aspiration; recurrence common
- Improvement in joint ROM, knee pain, swelling, accompanied reduction in bursa size has been shown after intra-articular or intracystic corticosteroid injection (5,6)[B].
- Sclerotherapy injections of ethanol or dextrose/ sodium morrhuate shown to have good results in studies with small sample sizes (7)[B].

SURGERY/OTHER PROCEDURES

- Consider excision when symptoms persist despite treatment or no etiology is found.
- Surgery usually not required in children
- Recurrence after standard surgery is common and is highest when chondral lesions are present (8)[B]. Arthroscopic surgery, when the valvular mechanism is identified and intra-articular pathology is treated, is highly successful (9)[B].
- A modified surgical technique in children has proved effective without recurrence (10)[B].
- Excision via arthroscopy or open procedure often requires concomitant treatment of underlying pathology (11)[B].

ONGOING CARE

PROGNOSIS

- Variable
- Many cysts remain asymptomatic.
- Some cysts will regress or resolve with treatment of underlying etiology.
- In children, most cysts resolve without treatment because there is rarely internal derangement.

COMPLICATIONS

- Compartment syndrome in ruptured cyst
- Thrombophlebitis from compression of the popliteal vein
- Infection of popliteal cyst
- Hemorrhage into cyst if on anticoagulants

REFERENCES

1. Marra MD, Crema MD, Chung M, et al. MRI features of cystic lesions around the knee. *Knee*. 2008;15:423–438.
2. Liao ST, Chiou CS, Chang CC. Pathology associated to the Baker's cysts: A musculoskeletal ultrasound study. *Clin Rheumatol*. 2010;29(9): 1043–1047. Epub 2010 Jun 10.
3. Chatzopoulos D, Moralidis E, Markou P, et al. Baker's cysts in knees with chronic osteoarthritic pain: A clinical, ultrasonographic, radiographic and scintigraphic evaluation. *Rheumatol Int*. 2008;29(2):141–146.
4. Sanchez JE, Conkling N, Labropoulos N. Compression syndromes of the popliteal neurovascular bundle due to Baker cyst. *J Vasc Surg*. 2011;54(6):1821–1829. Epub 2011 Sep 29.
5. Acebes JC, Sanchez-Pernaute O, Diaz-Oca A, et al. Ultrasonographic assessment of Baker's cysts after intra-articular corticosteroid injection in knee osteoarthritis. *J Clin Ultrasound*. 2006;34: 113–117.
6. Di Sante L, Paoloni M, Ioppolo F, et al. Ultrasound-guided aspiration and corticosteroid injection of Baker's cysts in knee osteoarthritis: A prospective observational study. *Am J Phys Med Rehabil*. 2010;89(12):970–975.
7. Centeno CJ, Schultz J, Freeman M, et al. Sclerotherapy of Baker's cyst with imaging confirmation of resolution. *Pain Physician*. 2008;11:257–261.
8. Rupp S, Seil R, Jochum P, et al. Popliteal cysts in adults. Prevalence, associated intraarticular lesions, and results after arthroscopic treatment. *Am J Sports Med*. 2002;30(1):112–115.
9. Lie CW, Ng TP. Arthroscopic treatment of popliteal cyst. *Hong Kong Med J*. 2011;17(3):180–183.
10. Chen J-C, Cheng-Chang L, Lu Y-M, et al. A modified surgical method for treating Baker's cyst in children. *The Knee*. 2008;15:9–14.
11. Handy JR. Popliteal cysts in adults: A review. *Semin Arthritis Rheu*. 2001;31(2):108–118.

ADDITIONAL READING

Chatzopoulos D, Moralidis E, Markou P, et al. Baker's cysts in knees with chronic osteoarthritic pain: A clinical, ultrasonographic, radiographic and scintigraphic evaluation. *Rheumatol Int*. 2008;29(2): 141–146. Epub 2008 Jun 27.

SEE ALSO

Algorithm: Knee Pain

CODES

ICD10

- M71.20 Synovial cyst of popliteal space [Baker], unspecified knee
- M71.21 Synovial cyst of popliteal space [Baker], right knee
- M71.22 Synovial cyst of popliteal space [Baker], left knee

CLINICAL PEARLS

- In children, it is acceptable to wait and observe Baker cysts.
- Treat underlying cause.
- Pain and swelling over the medial malleolus is classic for cyst rupture, also known as pseudothrombophlebitis.
- Inflammatory etiologies were more likely to be associated with a ruptured Baker cyst.
- Presence of a Baker cyst is not associated with the severity of osteoarthritis.

BALANITIS, PHIMOSIS, AND PARAPHIMOSIS
James P. Miller, MD

 BASICS

DESCRIPTION
- Balanitis:
  - An inflammation of the glans penis
  - Posthitis is an inflammation of the foreskin.
  - Balanitis xerotica obliterans (BXO) is lichen sclerosis of the glans penis (uncommon).
- Phimosis and paraphimosis:
  - Phimosis: Tightness of the distal penile foreskin that prevents it from being drawn back from over the glans
  - Paraphimosis: Constriction by foreskin of an uncircumcised penis, preventing the foreskin from returning to its position over the glans; occurs after the retracted foreskin becomes swollen and engorged; a urologic emergency
- System(s) affected: Renal/Urologic; Reproductive; Skin/Exocrine

ALERT
- Recurrent infection and irritations (condom catheters) can lead to phimosis.
- Recurrent balanitis, either chemical or infectious, can lead to an acquired phimosis.
- Inappropriate forced reduction of a physiologic foreskin can lead to chronic scarring and acquired phimosis.

EPIDEMIOLOGY
- Balanitis: Predominant age: Adult; predominant gender: Male only
- Phimosis/Paraphimosis: Predominant age: Infancy and adolescence; unusual in adults; risk returns in geriatrics; predominant sex: Men only

Incidence
Balanitis: Will affect 3–11% of males

Prevalence
Phimosis: In the US: 1% of men >16 years of age

ETIOLOGY AND PATHOPHYSIOLOGY
- Balanitis:
  - Allergic reaction (condom latex, contraceptive jelly)
  - Infections (*Candida albicans, Borrelia vincentii,* streptococci, *Trichomonas,* HPV)
  - Fixed-drug eruption (sulfa, tetracycline)
  - Plasma cell infiltration (Zoon balanitis)
  - Autodigestion by activated pancreatic transplant exocrine enzymes
- Phimosis:
  - Physiologic: Present at birth; resolves spontaneously during the first 2–3 years of life through nocturnal erections, which slowly dilate the phimotic ring.
  - Acquired: Recurrent inflammation, trauma, or infections of the foreskin.
- Paraphimosis:
  - Often iatrogenically or inadvertently induced by the foreskin not being pulled back over the glans after voiding, cleaning, cystoscopy, or catheter insertion

Geriatric Considerations
Condom catheters can predispose to balanitis.

Pediatric Considerations
Oral antibiotics predispose male infants to *Candida balanitis.* Inappropriate care of physiologic phimosis can lead to acquired phimosis by repeated forced reduction of the foreskin.

RISK FACTORS
- Balanitis:
  - Presence of foreskin
  - Morbid obesity
  - Poor hygiene
  - Diabetes; probably most common
  - Nursing home environment
  - Condom catheters
  - Chemical irritants
  - Edematous conditions: CHF, nephrosis
- Phimosis:
  - Poor hygiene
  - Diabetes by repeated balanitis
  - Frequent diaper rash in infants
- Paraphimosis:
  - Presence of foreskin
  - Inexperienced health care provider (leaving foreskin retracted after catheter placement)
  - Poor education about care of the foreskin

GENERAL PREVENTION
- Balanitis:
  - Proper hygiene and avoidance of allergens
  - Circumcision
- Phimosis/Paraphimosis:
  - If the patient is uncircumcised, appropriate hygiene and care of the foreskin are necessary to prevent phimosis and paraphimosis.

DIAGNOSIS

HISTORY
- Balanitis:
  - Pain
  - Drainage
  - Dysuria
  - Odor
  - Ballooning of foreskin with voiding
  - Redness
- Phimosis:
  - Painful erections
  - Recurrent balanitis
  - Foreskin balloons when voiding
- Paraphimosis:
  - Uncircumcised
  - Pain
  - Drainage
  - Voiding difficulty

PHYSICAL EXAM
- Balanitis:
  - Erythema
  - Edema
  - Discharge
  - Ulceration
  - Plaque
- Phimosis
  - Foreskin will not retract
  - Secondary balanitis
- Paraphimosis
  - Edema
  - Drainage
  - Ulceration

DIFFERENTIAL DIAGNOSIS
- Balanitis:
  - Leukoplakia
  - Lichen planus
  - Psoriasis
  - Reiter syndrome
  - Lichen sclerosus et atrophicus
  - Erythroplasia of Queyrat
  - BXO: Atrophic changes at end of foreskin; can form band that prevents retraction
- Phimosis/Paraphimosis:
  - Penile lymphedema, which can be related to insect bites, trauma, or allergic reactions
  - Penile tourniquet syndrome: Foreign body around penis, most commonly a hair

DIAGNOSTIC TESTS & INTERPRETATION
Initial Tests (lab, imaging)
- Microbiology culture
- Wet mount
- Serology for syphilis
- Serum glucose; ESR (if concerns about Reiter syndrome)
- STD testing
- HIV testing
- Gram stain

Diagnostic Procedures/Other
Biopsy, if persistent

Pathological Findings
Plasma cells infiltration with Zoon balanitis

TREATMENT

GENERAL MEASURES
- Consider circumcision for recurrent balanitis and paraphimosis.
- Warm compresses or sitz baths
- Local hygiene

MEDICATION
- Balanitis:
  – Antifungal:
    ○ Clotrimazole (Lotrimin) 1% b.i.d.
    ○ Nystatin (Mycostatin) b.i.d.–q.i.d.
    ○ Fluconazole: 150 mg single dose (1)[B]
  - Antibacterial:
    – Bacitracin q.i.d.
    – Neomycin-polymyxin B-bacitracin (Neosporin) q.i.d.
    – If cellulitis, Cephalosporin or sulfa drug PO or parenteral:
      ○ Dermatitis: Topical steroids q.i.d.
      ○ Zoon balanitis: Topical steroids q.i.d.
- Phimosis:
  – 0.05% Fluticasone propionate daily for 4–8 weeks with gradual traction placed on foreskin
  – 1% pimecrolimus b.i.d. for 4–6 weeks. Not for use in children <2 years.
- Paraphimosis:
  – Manual reduction, if possible (should be done with the patient sedated). Place the middle and index fingers of both hands on the engorged skin proximal to the glans. Place both thumbs on glans and, with gentle pressure, push on the glans and pull on the foreskin to attempt reduction. If unsuccessful, a dorsal slit will be necessary, with eventual circumcision after the edema resolves.
  – Osmotic agents: Granulated sugar placed on edematous tissue for several hours to reduce edema (2)[C]
  – Puncture technique: Multiple punctures of foreskin with a 21-gauge needle will allow edematous fluid to escape and thus allow reduction (3)[C].
- BXO:
  – 0.05% betamethasone b.i.d. (2)[B]
  – 0.1% tacrolimus b.i.d. (3)[C]

ISSUES FOR REFERRAL
Recurrent infections or development of meatal stenosis

SURGERY/OTHER PROCEDURES
- Balanitis and phimosis: Consider circumcision as preventive measure.
- For paraphimosis:
  – Represents a true surgical emergency to avoid necrosis of glans
  – Dorsal slit with delayed circumcision, if reduction is not possible
  – Operative exploration if the possibility of penile tourniquet syndrome cannot be eliminated. Hair removal cream can be applied if a hair is thought to be the cause of the tourniquet.

IN-PATIENT CONSIDERATIONS
Admission Criteria
- Uncontrolled diabetes
- Sepsis

Nursing
Appropriate hygiene if condom catheters are used

Discharge Criteria
Resolution of problem

 ONGOING CARE

FOLLOW-UP RECOMMENDATIONS
Patient Monitoring
Balanitis:
- Every 1–2 weeks until etiology has been established
- Persistent balanitis may require biopsy to rule out malignancy or BXO.
- Evaluation for resolution of phimosis

DIET
Weight reduction, if obese

PATIENT EDUCATION
- Need for appropriate hygiene
- Appropriate foreskin care
- Avoidance of known allergens
- No sexual activity for 2–3 week after circumcision

PROGNOSIS
Should resolve with appropriate treatment

COMPLICATIONS
- Meatal stenosis
- Premalignant changes from chronic irritation
- UTIs
- Acquired phimosis
- Unreducible paraphimosis can lead to gangrene.
- Posthitis (inflammation of the prepuce)

REFERENCES
1. Stary A, Soeltz-Szoets J, Ziegler C, et al. Comparison of the efficacy and safety of oral fluconazole and topical clotrimazole in patients with candida balanitis. Genitourin Med. 1996;72:98–102.
2. Kiss A, Csontai A, Pirót L, et al. The response of balanitis xerotica obliterans to local steroid application compared with placebo in children. J Urol. 2001;165:219–220.
3. Pandher BS, Rustin MH, Kaisary AV. Treatment of balanitis xerotica obliterans with topical tacrolimus. J Urol. 2003;170:923.

ADDITIONAL READING
- Georgala S, Gregoriou S, Georgala C, et al. Pimecrolimus 1% cream in non-specific inflammatory recurrent balanitis. Dermatology. 2007;215(3):209–212.
- Palmer LS, Palmer JS. The efficacy of topical betamethasone for treating phimosis: A comparison of two treatment regimens. Urology. 2008;72(1):68–71. Epub 2008 May 2.
- Zavras N, Christianakis E, Mpourikas D, et al. Conservative treatment of phimosis with fluticasone proprionate 0.05%: A clinical study in 1185 boys. J Pediatr Urol. 2009;5(3):181–185. Epub 2008 Dec 20.

 SEE ALSO

Reiter Syndrome

CODES

ICD10
- N47.1 Phimosis
- N47.2 Paraphimosis
- N48.1 Balanitis

CLINICAL PEARLS
- Balanitis is an inflammation of the glans penis. Posthitis is an inflammation of the foreskin. BXO is lichen sclerosis of the glans penis.
- With recurrent infections and a plaque, a biopsy should be done to rule out BXO or malignancy.
- If there is a true phimosis that interferes with appropriate hygiene, treat the phimosis with steroids or circumcision to help with hygiene.

BAROTRAUMA OF THE MIDDLE EAR, SINUSES, AND LUNG

Mary Lauren Worthen, MD • Adrian Worthen • David Worthen

 BASICS

DESCRIPTION
- Barotrauma is tissue damage resulting from the direct effects of pressure. Extreme changes or imbalances between ambient pressure and pressure within an enclosed body cavity can cause physical damage to tissue lining the cavity.
- Body cavities at greatest risk for barotrauma:
  – Middle ear (otic barotrauma)
  – Paranasal sinuses (sinus barotrauma)
  – Lungs (pulmonary barotrauma)
- Dental barotrauma:
  – Dental work can create small pockets of air, which can cause rupture of teeth in scuba divers.
- Synonym(s): Dysbarism; Aerotitis; Otitic barotrauma; Middle ear barotrauma

ALERT
- Dizziness and sensorineural hearing loss warrant immediate ENT referral for inner ear involvement.
- Valsalva maneuver can spread nasopharyngeal infection into the middle ear.
- Vertigo and hearing loss may cause disorientation.

EPIDEMIOLOGY
Incidence
- Pulmonary barotrauma is the second leading cause of death among divers.
- Pulmonary barotrauma is noted in 3% of mechanically ventilated patients.
- Otic barotrauma is common in air travel. This is especially high among flight personnel (1).

Pediatric Considerations
- Children have difficulty opening the eustachian tube and commonly develop upper respiratory infections. This combination results in higher risk for otic and sinus barotraumas at smaller pressure changes, as compared with adults.
- Mechanical ventilation of neonates is associated with barotrauma and contributes to bronchopulmonary dysplasia.

ALERT
Increased nasal congestion in pregnancy increases risk of barotitis media.

ETIOLOGY AND PATHOPHYSIOLOGY
- Boyle's law relates to all forms of barotrauma. The volume of a gas varies inversely with pressure if temperature is held constant. When gas is trapped in a confined space, such as the middle ear, paranasal sinus, or lungs, a sudden decrease in ambient pressure causes expansion of the gas within the cavity.
- Otalgia (earache) and hearing loss occur as a result of stretching and deformation of the tympanic membrane.
- Sudden pressure differentials between middle and inner ear may lead to rupture of the round or oval window. This can create a labyrinthine fistula, which consequently can allow leakage of perilymph. Damage to inner ear may be permanent.
- When the transalveolar pressure disrupts the structural integrity of the alveolus, the alveolar wall can rupture, leading to interstitial emphysema, pneumothorax, or pneumomediastinum.

- Otic and sinus barotrauma:
  – Associated with rapid or extreme changes in environmental pressure: Air travel, mountain climbing, scuba diving:
    ○ Presence of nasal congestion or eustachian tube dysfunction of any etiology can lead to a higher incidence of damage.
    ○ Failure of eustachian tube to equilibrate pressure may distort the tympanic membrane, causing discomfort and injury.
    ○ Rupture of round or oval membrane may cause inner ear barotrauma, vertigo, and sensorineural hearing loss.
- Pulmonary barotrauma:
  – Iatrogenic complication of mechanical ventilation or complication of scuba diving.

RISK FACTORS
- Otic or sinus:
  – Participation in high-risk activities without adequate pressure equilibration:
    ○ Scuba diving, especially with rapid ascent or breath-holding
    ○ Airplane flight
    ○ Sky diving
    ○ High-altitude travel
    ○ High-impact sports: Boxing, soccer, water skiing
  – Recurrent upper respiratory infections
  – Nasal congestion or allergic rhinitis
  – Eustachian tube dysfunction of any kind
  – Exposure to blasting or explosions
  – The most common complication of hyperbaric oxygen (HBO) treatment is middle ear barotrauma, which can lead to permanent hearing loss and vertigo (2)[B].
  – Pregnancy (associated nasal congestion)
  – Anatomic obstruction in the nasopharynx:
    ○ Deviated nasal septum
    ○ Nasal polyps
    ○ Congenital anomalies, including cleft palate
  – Previous history of ear trauma
- Pulmonary:
  – Iatrogenic:
    ○ Mechanical ventilation, especially in the presence of asthma, chronic interstitial lung disease, acute respiratory distress syndrome
    ○ Hyperbaric oxygen therapy
  – Scuba diving or other underwater activities
  – Air travel with pre-existing pulmonary pathology

GENERAL PREVENTION
- Pulmonary barotrauma:
  – Cautious use of mechanical ventilation and hyperbaric oxygen therapy
  – Avoidance of breath-holding during ascent while scuba diving
- Otic barotrauma:
  – Avoidance of altitude changes or scuba diving with history of eustachian tube dysfunction
  – Treatment of upper respiratory congestion
- Equilibration of pressure: Valsalva maneuver, yawning, swallowing, drinking, or chewing gum

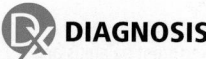 DIAGNOSIS

HISTORY
- Otic barotrauma: History of high-risk activity
- Otic (middle ear) barotrauma:
  – Otalgia, sensation of fullness or pressure in the ear
  – Hearing loss
  – Vertigo
  – Transient facial paralysis
  – Discharge of fluid from the ear
- All patients with middle ear barotrauma should be further evaluated for inner ear barotrauma:
  – Hearing loss
  – Tinnitus
  – Vertigo
  – Disorientation
- Sinus barotrauma:
  – Facial pain, sensation of fullness or pressure
- Pulmonary barotrauma: Recent history is vital. Ask about scuba diving, mechanical ventilation, air travel with pre-existing lung disease and if:
  – Chest pain, dyspnea

PHYSICAL EXAM
- Otic barotrauma:
  – Otoscopic exam
  – Assess patient's balance and hearing
  – Palpate eustachian tube for tenderness
- Otic (middle ear) barotrauma:
  – Conductive hearing loss with Weber and Rinne tests
  – Transient facial paralysis
- All patients with middle ear barotrauma should be evaluated for inner ear barotrauma:
  – Sensorineural hearing loss with Weber and Rinne tests
- Sinus barotrauma:
  – Facial tenderness
- Pulmonary barotrauma:
  – Hypoxia, hypotension
  – Auscultation, percussion
  – Assessment of respiratory distress

DIFFERENTIAL DIAGNOSIS
- Acute and chronic otitis media
- Otitis externa
- Temporomandibular joint syndrome
- Pulmonary: Other causes of decompensation on mechanical ventilation

DIAGNOSTIC TESTS & INTERPRETATION
Initial Tests (lab, imaging)
- Otic or sinus:
  – Imaging to rule out nasopharyngeal tumor or sinusitis, if indicated
- Pulmonary:
  – Chest radiograph
  – Chest CT if chest x-ray (CXR) not informative
  – Arterial blood gases (ABG)
- Other: Ultrasound

Diagnostic Procedures/Other
- Otic barotrauma:
  – Tympanometry
  – Audiometry: Conductive (middle ear) vs. sensorineural (inner ear) hearing loss
  – Surgical exploration to rule out inner ear involvement, if suspected
- Pulmonary barotrauma: Chest tube insertion, if indicated, for pneumothorax

Test Interpretation
- Tympanic membrane (TM) retraction or bulging:
  - Teed 0: No visible damage
  - Teed 1: Congestion around umbo
  - Teed 2: Congestion of entire TM
  - Teed 3: Hemorrhage into middle ear
  - Teed 4: Extensive middle ear hemorrhage; TM may rupture
  - Teed 5: Entire middle ear filled with deoxygenated blood
- Inner ear involvement with rupture of the round or oval windows, perilymphatic fistula, and leakage of perilymph into the middle ear
- Pulmonary barotrauma:
  - Alveolar rupture may progress to interstitial emphysema, pneumoperitoneum, pneumothorax.
- Petechial hemorrhages in area covered by diver's mask, as well as subconjunctival hemorrhages

 TREATMENT

GENERAL MEASURES
- Prevention/Avoidance is best: Avoid flying or diving when risk factors are present.
- Autoinflate the eustachian tube during pressure changes:
  - Valsalva method (3)[B] during ascent and descent in air travel
  - Infants: Breast-feeding or sucking on pacifier or bottle
  - ≥4 years: Chewing gum
  - ≥8 years: Blowing up a balloon
  - Adults: Chewing gum, swallowing, or yawning
- The nasal balloon is effective for prevention (3,4)[B].
- Pressure-equalizing earplugs are not recommended in air travel and do not prevent ear barotrauma (5)[B].
- For inner ear barotrauma:
  - Bed rest with head elevated to avoid leakage of perilymph
  - Tympanotomy and repair of round or oval window may be necessary.
  - Sudden or progressive sensorineural hearing loss accompanied by dizziness following barotrauma should prompt consideration of a perilymph fistula. Early surgical exploration is recommended to improve hearing and vestibular symptoms (6).
- Treatment of pneumothorax:
  - Removal of air from pleural space
- Adjustment of iatrogenic cause (e.g., adjustment of mechanical ventilation).

MEDICATION
- Treatment of predisposing conditions, upper respiratory congestion prior to air travel:
  - Oral decongestants
  - Nasal decongestants
  - Antihistamines
- Antibiotics are not indicated for middle ear effusion secondary to barotrauma.
- Hyperbaric oxygen therapy is the treatment of choice for patients with inner ear decompression sickness, but is contraindicated in patients with inner ear barotrauma (7)[B].
- Analgesics for pain control
- Tinnitus can be treated with high-dose steroids if given within 3 weeks of onset (8)[C].

ISSUES FOR REFERRAL
- Refer to otolaryngology if inner ear is exposed, perilymphatic fistula is present, or sensorineural hearing loss experienced.
- Chest tube placement

SURGERY/OTHER PROCEDURES
- If necessary, myringotomy or tympanoplasty
- Tympanotomy and repair of round or oval window may be necessary for inner ear barotrauma.
- Tube thoracostomy for persistent pneumothorax

IN-PATIENT CONSIDERATIONS
Admission Criteria/Initial Stabilization
- Patients with complicating emergencies (e.g., incapacitating pain requiring myringotomy, large tympanic perforation requiring tympanoplasty)
- Inner ear barotrauma with hearing loss
- Management of pneumothorax

 ONGOING CARE

FOLLOW-UP RECOMMENDATIONS
- No flying or diving until complete resolution of all signs and symptoms and Valsalva maneuver succeeds in equalizing pressure.
- Complete bed rest for inner ear barotrauma.
- No high-risk activities or air travel until pneumothorax is completely resolved.

Patient Monitoring
- Otoscopic exams until symptoms clear.
- In severe cases, audiograms may be used.

PATIENT EDUCATION
- Teach Valsalva maneuver.
- Avoid allergens.
- Controlling sinus infections.
- American Academy of Pediatrics Travel Safety Tips: http://www.aap.org
- Divers Alert Network of Duke University Medical Center information line: (919) 684-2948

PROGNOSIS
- Mild barotitis media may resolve spontaneously.
- Tympanic rupture recovery is within weeks to months.
- Hearing loss may be permanent in barotitis externa.
- Prognosis of pulmonary barotrauma depends on the extent of underlying pathology.

COMPLICATIONS
- Permanent hearing loss
- Ruptured tympanic membrane
- Chronic tinnitus, vertigo
- Fluid exudate in middle ear
- Perilymphatic fistula
- Sensorineural hearing loss

REFERENCES
1. Morgagni F, Autore A, Landolfi A, et al. Predictors of ear barotrauma in aircrews exposed to simulated high altitude. *Aviat Space Environ Med*. 2012; 83(6):594–597.
2. Capes JP, Tomaszewski C. Prophylaxis against middle ear barotrauma in US hyperbaric oxygen therapy centers. *Am J Emerg Med*. 1996;14(7): 645–648.
3. Stangerup SE. Point prevalence of barotitis and its prevention and treatment with nasal balloon inflation: A prospective, controlled study. *Otol Neurol*. 2004;25(2):89–94.
4. Landolfi A, Autore A, Torchia F, et al. Ear pain after breathing oxygen at altitude: Prevalence and prevention of delayed barotrauma. *Aviat Space Environ Med*. 2010;81(2):130–132.
5. Klokker M, Vesterhauge S, Jansen EC. Pressure-equalizing earplugs do not prevent barotrauma on descent from 8000 ft cabin altitude. *Aviat Space Environ Med*. 2005;76(11): 1079–1082.
6. Park GY, Byun H, Moon IJ, et al. Effects of early surgical exploration in suspected barotraumatic perilymph fistulas. *Clin Exp Otorhinolaryngol*. 2012;5(2):74–80. Epub 2012 Jun 12.
7. Klingmann C. Treatment of acute cochleovestibular damage after diving. *HNO*. 2004;52(10):891–896.
8. Duplessis C, Hoffer M. Tinnitus in an active duty navy diver: A review of inner ear barotrauma, tinnitus, and its treatment. *Undersea Hyperbaric Med*. 2006;33(4):223–230.

ADDITIONAL READING
- Mirza S, Richardson H. Otic barotrauma from air travel. *J Laryngol Otol*. 2005;119(5):366–370.
- Zadik Y, Drucker S. Diving dentistry: A review of the dental implications of scuba diving. *Aust Dent J*. 2011;56(3):265–271. Epub 2011 Jul 10.

 SEE ALSO

Algorithm: Ear Pain

 CODES

ICD10
- T70.0XXA Otitic barotrauma, initial encounter
- T70.1XXA Sinus barotrauma, initial encounter
- T70.29XA Other effects of high altitude, initial encounter

CLINICAL PEARLS
- Small children can equalize eustachian tube pressure by sucking on bottles or pacifiers. Crying also serves as autoinflation.
- Pulmonary barotrauma is the 2nd leading cause of death among divers.
- Otic barotrauma is common in air travel, especially among flight personnel.
- Pulmonary barotrauma is noted in 3% of mechanically ventilated patients.
- Sudden or progressive sensorineural hearing loss accompanied by dizziness following barotrauma should prompt consideration of a perilymphatic fistula. Early surgical exploration is recommended to improve hearing and vestibular symptoms.

BARRETT'S ESOPHAGUS
Jonathan True Lin, MD • Harlan G. Rich, MD

 BASICS

DESCRIPTION
- Metaplasia of the distal esophageal mucosa from the normal stratified squamous epithelium to abnormal columnar (intestinalized) epithelium, likely as a consequence of chronic GERD
- Predisposes to the development of adenocarcinoma of the esophagus

EPIDEMIOLOGY
- Predominant age: >50 years
- May occur in children (rare <5 years)

Incidence
- 10–15% of patients undergoing endoscopy for evaluation of reflux symptoms (1)
- Esophageal adenocarcinoma incidence is one of the fastest rising malignancies in the US (1):
  - From 1975 to 2001, nearly a 6-fold increase from 4 to 23 cases per million person-years
  - Attributed to trends in smoking and obesity rather than reclassification or overdiagnosis

Prevalence
- Difficult to ascertain because of cases commonly being asymptomatic, different populations studied, and varying definitions used
- As many as 1.5–2.0 million adults in the US, based on a 1.6% prevalence of the general population in Sweden (1)

ETIOLOGY AND PATHOPHYSIOLOGY
Caused by chronic GERD
- Gastric reflux injures the esophageal mucosa, triggering the development of columnar metaplasia from a progenitor cell that has not yet been fully described.
- Columnar cells in the esophagus have higher malignant potential than squamous cells.
- Elevated levels of COX-2, a mediator of inflammation and regulator of epithelial cell growth, have been associated with Barrett's esophagus (2).
- Classic progression: Normal epithelium → esophagitis → metaplasia (Barrett's esophagus) → Dysplasia (low- or high-grade) → Adenocarcinoma

Genetics
- Familial predisposition to GERD and Barrett's esophagus have been described, along with multiple genetic markers.
- Acquired genetic changes in the genome lead to progression to adenocarcinoma; many are being investigated for use as biomarkers for risk stratification and early detection (1).

RISK FACTORS
- Chronic reflux (>5 years)
- Hiatal hernia
- Age >50 years
- Male gender
- White ethnicity
- Smoking history
- Intra-abdominal obesity

GENERAL PREVENTION
Weight loss, smoking cessation, eating fruits and vegetables, and wine consumption may decrease risk of both Barrett's esophagus and progression to cancer (3,4)[C].

COMMONLY ASSOCIATED CONDITIONS
GERD, obesity, hiatal hernia

 DIAGNOSIS

HISTORY
- GERD symptoms common: Heartburn, regurgitation, or dysphagia
- Less common: Chest pain, odynophagia, chronic cough, water brash, globus sensation, laryngitis, or asthma
- Suggestive of complicated GERD or cancer: Weight loss, anorexia, dysphagia, odynophagia, or bleeding

ALERT
Up to 25% of patients with Barrett's esophagus are asymptomatic (2)[B].

PHYSICAL EXAM
No specific abnormal findings

DIFFERENTIAL DIAGNOSIS
- Erosive esophagitis: Should be treated prior to endoscopy (3)[B].
- Gastric fundic-type epithelium: May be found on pathology, but does not have clear malignant potential and may reflect sampling error (4)[B].
- Specialized intestinal metaplasia at the gastroesophageal junction (GEJ): Carries risk of cancer, but difficult to characterize due to varying definitions of the GEJ landmarks (4)[B]

DIAGNOSTIC TESTS & INTERPRETATION
Endoscopy with multiple biopsies for histologic examination are required to diagnose Barrett's esophagus. See "Diagnostic Procedures/Other" below.

ALERT
Screening for Barrett's esophagus in the general population with GERD (nonchronic) is **not** recommended because of the lack of demonstrated impact on mortality. The 2011 American Gastroenterological Association (AGA) guidelines suggest individualized screening for patients with multiple risk factors (4)[C].

Initial Tests (lab, imaging)
None:
- *Helicobacter pylori* testing is not indicated. In fact, meta-analyses have revealed an inverse relationship between *H. pylori* infections and Barrett's esophagus, which may be related to decreased acid production (5)[A].
- No biomarkers are currently effective for diagnosis, but many are under active investigation for risk stratification (1,4)[B].

Diagnostic Procedures/Other
- Endoscopy: Visual identification of columnar epithelium (reddish, velvety appearance) replacing the squamous lining of the distal esophagus:
  - Extent of disease may be characterized with:
    - Long-segment (≥3 cm) vs. short-segment (<3 cm)
    - Prague C (circumference) and M (maximum extent) criteria (1,4)[B]
  - White light endoscopy remains the standard of care (4)[C]:
    - Advanced imaging techniques, such as narrow band imaging (NBI), may help identify dysplasia, but are still under preliminary evaluation (1,3,4)[A].

- Systematic biopsies of columnar epithelium taken at endoscopy confirms the diagnosis:
  - Seattle Protocol: 4-quadrant biopsies at regular intervals with additional biopsies of visible mucosal irregularities:
    - More time-consuming, but higher diagnostic yield than random biopsies (4)[A]
- Capsule endoscopy is still under development and currently has poor sensitivity compared with conventional endoscopy (3)[B].

Test Interpretation
Specialized intestinal metaplasia (also called specialized columnar epithelium) is diagnostic:
- Dysplasia (low- or high-grade) should be confirmed by an expert pathologist before treatment (3,4)[B].
- Cardia-type columnar epithelium may predispose to malignancy, but with an unclear magnitude of risk; the AGA currently recommends against including this type of epithelium in the definition of Barrett's esophagus (4)[B].

TREATMENT

MEDICATION
- The goal of medical therapy is to control GERD to reduce esophagitis and maintain a healed mucosa (1,3)[A].
- Therapy usually does **not** result in reversal of Barrett's esophagus or risk of progression to cancer (1,2,4)[B].

ALERT
Neither suppression of gastric acid production via high-dose proton pump inhibitors (PPIs), nor reduction in esophageal acid exposure via antireflux surgery, has been shown to decrease cancer risk (1,3)[A].

First Line
- Unlike the stepwise management of GERD without evidence of Barrett's esophagus, patients with Barrett's esophagus and GERD symptoms should be treated initially with a once-daily PPI (1,3,4)[A]:
  - PPIs should be dosed 30 minutes before a meal (ideally, the 1st meal of the day).

ALERT
PPI therapy should be titrated to symptoms; pH monitoring is **not** recommended (1,4)[C].

- Chemoprevention of neoplastic progression is under active investigation.
- Case-controlled studies have shown that aspirin and NSAIDs may prevent progression to esophageal cancer due to the inhibition of COX-2 (6)[A]:
  - Administration of the COX-2 selective inhibitor celecoxib was not shown to affect progression of Barrett's dysplasia to adenocarcinoma (5)[A].
  - The use of aspirin and a PPI for chemoprevention of esophageal cancer is being investigated in a randomized, controlled trial (1,5).
  - Low-dose aspirin may be considered in patients with Barrett's esophagus who also have risk factors for cardiovascular disease (5,6).

- Statins, alone or in combination with aspirin or NSAIDs, appear to be effective in chemoprevention, but are not yet generally recommended.

Second Line
If once-daily PPI does not control symptoms, twice-daily dosing is recommended (3)[A].

ISSUES FOR REFERRAL
- PPI therapy should be initiated prior to endoscopy to reduce reactive esophagitis/atypia, which may be confused with low-grade dysplasia on biopsy (3)[C].
- Patients considering esophagectomy should be referred to a high-volume institution. See "Surgery/Other Procedures" below.

ADDITIONAL THERAPIES
- Low-grade dysplasia: Additional treatment controversial:
  - Endoscopic eradication therapy may be offered with shared decision making; a long-term benefit has not been clearly established (4)[B].
- High-grade dysplasia, without or with very limited submucosal invasion (Stage T1SM1 or lower by endoscopic ultrasound): Endoscopic eradication therapy is recommended (1,2,4)[B]. Methods include:
  - Photodynamic therapy (PDT): Eradication rate 77–100%, but with strictures in ~40%
  - Radiofrequency ablation (RFA): Eradication rate 54–90%, comparable efficacy to PDT, fewer adverse effects
  - Endoscopic mucosal resection (EMR): Eradication rate 86–100%, involves excision to submucosa, allows staging, preferred for visible irregularities:
  - Combination therapy:
    ○ EMR may be coupled with RFA or PDT to attempt to eliminate all Barrett's epithelium.
    ○ Focal EMR combined with RFA of other areas is considered the most effective eradication therapy (4)[B].
  - Cryotherapy and other ablative procedures: Additional studies still required before they can be recommended

ALERT
Endoscopic eradication therapy is **not** recommended for Barrett's esophagus in the absence of dysplasia, but surveillance should be continued.

SURGERY/OTHER PROCEDURES
- Fundoplication may control GERD symptoms, but it has not been convincingly shown to reverse Barrett's esophagus, decrease risk of cancer, or be more effective than medical therapy (1)[A].

COMPLEMENTARY AND ALTERNATIVE MEDICINE
A prospective study of 339 men and women with Barrett's esophagus found those taking either a multivitamin, vitamin C, or vitamin E once a day were less likely to develop esophageal adenocarcinoma (7)[B].

ALERT
Available data suggest that antireflux surgery does **not** decrease risk of esophageal cancer.
- Esophagectomy is definitive therapy and should be offered as an alternative to endoscopic eradication therapy to patients with high-grade dysplasia (1,4)[B]:

- Preferred for patients with evidence of submucosal invasion (Stage T1SM2 or higher)
- Added benefit of removing lymph nodes with potential metastases
- Mortality rate: 8–23%, but <5% among patients with high-grade dysplasia who are otherwise healthy
- Serious postoperative complications: 30–50%
- Ideally should be performed by an experienced surgeon in a high-volume medical center; mortality and morbidity rates are inversely related to volume (3,4)[A].

Geriatric Considerations
- If the patient is a poor operative candidate for endoscopic eradication therapy or esophagectomy, surveillance or no treatment may be preferable.
- Treatment must be individualized.

ONGOING CARE

FOLLOW-UP RECOMMENDATIONS
- Surveillance (to detect high-grade dysplasia or early carcinoma) remains controversial due to the lack of high-quality prospective studies.
- Recommended surveillance intervals depend on the grade of dysplasia (3,4)[B].

Patient Monitoring
2011 AGA guidelines for surveillance intervals in Barrett's esophagus (4)[C]:
- No dysplasia: 3–5 years
- Low-grade dysplasia: 6–12 months
- High-grade dysplasia without eradication therapy: 3 months

ALERT
- Adherence to recommended surveillance protocols may improve the rate of dysplasia and cancer detection.
- Surveillance should continue even if the patient has had endoscopic ablation therapy, antireflux surgery, or esophagectomy. Follow-up care and outcomes are still being characterized.

DIET
Patients should avoid foods that can trigger reflux: Caffeine, alcohol, chocolate, peppermint, carbonated drinks, garlic, onions, spicy foods, fatty foods, citrus, and tomato-based products.

PATIENT EDUCATION
- Lifestyle modifications:
  - Smoking cessation
  - Weight loss
  - Avoiding supine position after eating
  - Avoiding tight-fitting clothes
  - Head of bed elevation
- *No evidence suggests that treating GERD will reverse Barrett's esophagus or prevent esophageal cancer.*

PROGNOSIS
Annual incidence of esophageal cancer in patients with Barrett's esophagus is 0.5% per year or less (3,4)[B]:
- Low-grade dysplasia: May be transient; cancer risk 0.6% per year
- High-grade dysplasia: Cancer risk 5–7% per year

COMPLICATIONS
Same as GERD: Stricture, bleeding, ulceration (6)[C]

REFERENCES
1. Sharma P. Clinical practice. Barrett's esophagus. *N Engl J Med.* 2009;361(26):2548–2556.
2. Spechler SJ, Sharma P, Souza RF, et al. American Gastroenterological Association technical review on the management of Barrett's esophagus. *Gastroenterology.* 2011;140:e18–52; quiz e13.
3. Wang KK, Sampliner RE, Practice Parameters Committee of the American College of Gastroenterology. Updated guidelines 2008 for the diagnosis, surveillance and therapy of Barrett's esophagus. *Am J Gastroenterol.* 2008;103: 788–797.
4. American Gastroenterological Association, Spechler SJ, Sharma P, et al. American Gastroenterological Association medical position statement on the management of Barrett's esophagus. *Gastroenterology.* 2011;140:1084–1091.
5. Fischbach LA, Nordenstedt H, Kramer JR, et al. The association between Barrett's esophagus and *Helicobacter pylori* infection: A meta-analysis. *Helicobacter.* 2012;17(3):163–175. Epub 2012 Mar 20.
6. Bennett C, Vakil N, Bergman J, et al. Consensus statements for management of Barrett's dysplasia and early-stage esophageal adenocarcinoma, based on a Delphi process. *Gastroenterology.* 2012;143(2):336–346. Epub 2012 Apr 24.
7. Dong LM, Kristal AR, Peters U, et al. Dietary supplement use and risk of neoplastic progression in esophageal adenocarcinoma: A prospective study. *Nutr Cancer.* 2008;60(1):39–48.

ADDITIONAL READING
Corley DA, Kerlikowske K, Verma R, et al. Protective association of aspirin/NSAIDs and esophageal cancer: A systematic review and meta-analysis. *Gastroenterology.* 2003;124:47–56.

CODES

ICD10
- K22.70 Barrett's esophagus without dysplasia
- K22.710 Barrett's esophagus with low grade dysplasia
- K22.719 Barrett's esophagus with dysplasia, unspecified

CLINICAL PEARLS
- The incidence of esophageal carcinoma is rising faster than any other major malignancy. Barrett's esophagus is a known precursor.
- Highest incidence is among white males >50 years.
- Medical or surgical treatment of GERD in patients with Barrett's esophagus does **not** decrease cancer rates or mortality.
- Endoscopic eradication therapy is the preferred treatment for high-grade dysplasia without or with very limited submucosal invasion.
- Esophagectomy offers definitive therapy: Consider for all patients with high-grade dysplasia; preferred for patients with submucosal invasion.
- Promising areas of research include:
  - Biomarkers for risk stratification
  - Chemoprevention of neoplastic progression
  - Capsule endoscopy for screening
  - Advances in endoscopic imaging and endoscopic eradication therapy
  - Benefit of vitamins and antioxidants

BASAL CELL CARCINOMA

K. John Burhan, MD

 BASICS

DESCRIPTION

Basal cell carcinoma (BCC) is the most common cancer, originating from the basal cell layer of the skin appendages:

- Rarely metastasizes, but capable of local tissue destruction

Geriatric Considerations

- Greater frequency in geriatric patients (ages 55–75 years have 100 × incidence compared with those aged <20)
- The incidence is rapidly increasing in those 20–40 years.

Pediatric Considerations

Rare in children, but childhood sun exposure is important in adult disease.

EPIDEMIOLOGY

Worldwide, the most common form of cancer

Incidence

- Incidence in the US: 1 million cases per year; increasing about 10% each year
- Predominant age: Generally >40; incidence increasing in younger populations
- Predominant sex: Male > Female (although incidence is increasing in females)
- Lifetime risk of white North Americans: 30%

ETIOLOGY AND PATHOPHYSIOLOGY

- UV-induced inflammation and cyclooxygenase activation in skin
- Mutation of *PTCH1* (patched homolog 1), a tumor-suppressor gene that inhibits the hedgehog signaling pathway
- Mutation of the *SMO* (smoothened homolog) gene, which is also involved in the hedgehog signaling pathway
- UV-induced mutations of the *TP53* (tumor protein 53), a tumor-suppressor gene
- Activation of *BCL2*, an antiapoptosis proto-oncogene

Genetics

Several genetic conditions increase the risk of developing BCC:

- Albinism (recessive alleles)
- Xeroderma pigmentosum (autosomal recessive)
- Bazex syndrome (rare, x-linked dominant)
- Nevoid BCC syndrome/Gorlin syndrome (rare, autosomal-dominant)
- Cytochrome P-450 CYP2D6 and glutathione S-transferase detoxifying enzyme gene mutations (especially in truncal BCC, marked by clusters of basal cell carcinomas and a younger age of onset)

RISK FACTORS

- Chronic sun exposure (UV radiation)
- Most common in the following phenotypes:
  - Light complexion: Skin type I (burns, but does not tan) and skin type II (usually burns, sometimes tans)
  - Red or blond hair
  - Blue or green eyes
- Tendency to sunburn

- Male sex, although increasing risk in women due to lifestyle changes, such as tanning beds
- History of nonmelanoma skin cancer:
  - After initial diagnosis of skin cancer, 35% risk of new nonmelanoma skin cancer at 3 years and 50% at 5 years
- Family history of skin cancer
- 3–4 decades after chronic arsenic exposure
- 2 decades after therapeutic radiation
- Chronic immunosuppression: Transplant recipients (10 × higher incidence), patients with HIV or lymphomas

GENERAL PREVENTION

- Use broad-spectrum sunscreens of at least SPF 30 daily and reapply after swimming or sweating.
- Avoid overexposure to the sun by seeking shade between 10 AM and 4 PM and wearing wide-brimmed hats and long-sleeved shirts.
- Avoid tanning and sunburns (including tanning salons).

COMMONLY ASSOCIATED CONDITIONS

- Cosmetic disfigurement since head and neck most often affected
- Loss of vision with orbital involvement
- Loss of nerve function due to perineural spread or extensive and deep invasion
- Ulcerating neoplasms are prone to infections.

 DIAGNOSIS

HISTORY

Exposure to risk factors, family history

PHYSICAL EXAM

- 80% on face and neck, 20% on trunk and lower limbs (mostly women) (1)[B]

- Nodular: Most common (60%); presents as pinkish, pearly papule, plaque, or nodule often with telangiectatic vessels, ulceration, and a rolled periphery usually on face:
  - Pigmented: Presents as a translucent papule with "floating pigment"; more commonly seen in darker skin types
- Superficial: (30%); light red, scaly papule or plaque with atrophic center, ringed by translucent micropapules, usually on trunk or extremities; more common in men
- Morpheaform: (5–10%); firm, smooth, flesh-colored, scarlike papule or plaque with ill-defined borders

DIFFERENTIAL DIAGNOSIS

- Sebaceous hyperplasia
- Epidermal inclusion cyst
- Intradermal nevi (pigmented and nonpigmented)
- Molluscum contagiosum
- Squamous cell carcinoma
- Nummular dermatitis
- Psoriasis
- Melanoma (pigmented lesions)
- Atypical fibroxanthoma
- Rare adnexal neoplasms

DIAGNOSTIC TESTS & INTERPRETATION

Diagnostic Procedures/Other

- Clinical diagnosis and histological subtype are confirmed through skin biopsy and pathological examination.
- Shave biopsy is typically sufficient; however, punch biopsy is more useful to assess depth of tumor and perineural invasion.
- If a genetic disorder is suspected, additional tests may be needed to confirm it.

Test Interpretation

- Nodular BCC:
  - Extending from the epidermis are nodular aggregates of basaloid cells.
  - Tumor cells are uniform; rarely have mitotic figures; large, oval, hyperchromatic nuclei with little cytoplasm, surrounded by a peripheral palisade.
  - Early lesions are usually connected to the epidermis, unlike late lesions.
  - Increased mucin in dermal stroma:
    ○ Cleft formation (retraction artifact) common between BCC "nests" and stroma due to mucin shrinkage during fixation and staining
- Superficial BCC:
  - Appear as buds of basaloid cells attached to undersurface of epidermis
  - Peripheral palisading
- Morpheaform BCC:
  - Thin cords and strands of basaloid cells, embedded in dense, fibrous, "scarlike" stroma
  - Less peripheral palisading and retraction, greater subclinical involvement
- Infiltrating BCC:
  - Like morpheaform BCC, but no "scarlike" stroma and thicker, more spiky, irregular strands
  - Less peripheral palisading and retraction, greater subclinical involvement
- Micronodular BCC:
  - Small, nodular aggregates of tumor cells
  - Less retraction artifact and higher subclinical involvement than nodular BCC

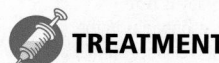 **TREATMENT**

MEDICATION

- May be especially useful in those who cannot tolerate surgical procedures and in those who refuse to have surgery
- 5-fluorouracil cream inhibits thymidylate synthetase, interrupting DNA synthesis for superficial lesions in low-risk areas; primary treatment only 5% applied b.i.d. for 3–10 weeks.
- Imiquimod (Aldara) cream approved for treatment of low-risk superficial BCC; daily dosing for 6–12 weeks; 90% histologic cure

ADDITIONAL THERAPIES

- Radiation therapy:
  - Useful for patients who cannot or will not undergo surgery
  - Used following surgery, particularly if margins of tumor were not cleared
  - Cure rate is ~90%.
  - Tumors that recur in areas previously treated with radiation are harder to treat, and the area is more difficult to reconstruct.
- Photodynamic therapy (PDT) (2)[A]:
  - 5-aminolevulinic acid, a photosensitizer, is activated by specific wavelengths of light, creating singlet oxygen radicals that destroy local tissue (no damage to surrounding or deep tissues).
  - Useful in areas where tissue preservation is cosmetically or functionally important

SURGERY/OTHER PROCEDURES

- Generally first choice; specific treatment selection varies with extent and location of lesion as well as tumor border demarcation (3)[A]
- High-risk areas:
  - Inner canthus, nasolabial sulcus, philtrum, preauricular area, retroauricular sulcus, lip, temple
- Curettage and electrodesiccation:
  - If nodular lesion <1 cm, in low-risk area, not deeply invasive
- Excision:
  - Useful for lesions in high-risk areas
  - Not as dependent on lesion size
- Cryosurgery:
  - Reserved for small lesions in low-risk areas
  - May want pre- and posttreatment biopsies
- Mohs surgery:
  - Preferred microsurgically controlled surgical treatment for lesions in high-risk areas, recurrent lesions, and lesions exhibiting an aggressive growth pattern
  - Requires referral to appropriately trained dermatologic surgeon

IN-PATIENT CONSIDERATIONS

Outpatient, unless extensive lesion

 ## ONGOING CARE

FOLLOW-UP RECOMMENDATIONS

- Avoid sun exposure.
- Oral retinoids may prevent the development of new BCCs in patients with Gorlin syndrome, renal transplant recipients, and patients with severe actinic damage.

Patient Monitoring

- Every month for 3 months, then twice yearly for 5 years; yearly thereafter
- Increased risk of other skin cancers (4)[C]

PATIENT EDUCATION

- Teach patient appropriate sun-avoidance techniques, sunscreens, and so forth.
- Monthly skin self-exam
- Educate patients concerning adequate vitamin D intake.

PROGNOSIS

- Proper treatment yields 90–95% cure.
- Most recurrences happen within 5 years.
- Development of new BCCs: Patients (36%) will develop a new lesion within 5 years.

COMPLICATIONS

- Local recurrence and spread
- Usually, recurrences will appear within 5 years.
- Metastasis: Rare (<0.1%), but metastatic disease usually fatal within 8 months

REFERENCES

1. Wong CS, Strange RC, Lear JT. Basal cell carcinoma. *BMJ*. 2003;327:794–798.
2. Soler AM, Angell-Petersen E, Warloe T, et al. Photodynamic therapy of superficial basal cell carcinoma with 5-aminolevulinic acid with dimethylsulfoxide and ethylenediaminetetraacetic acid: A comparison of two light sources. *Photochem Photobiol*. 2000;71:724–729.
3. Bath-Hextall FJ, Bong J, Perkins W, et al. Interventions for basal cell carcinoma of the skin. *Cochrane Database Syst Rev*. 2003;1:CD003412.
4. Friedman GD, Tekawa IS. Association of basal cell skin cancers with other cancers (United States). *Cancer Causes Control*. 2000;11:891–897.

 ## CODES

ICD10

- C44.31 Basal cell carcinoma of skin of other and unspecified parts of face
- C44.41 Basal cell carcinoma of skin of scalp and neck
- C44.91 Basal cell carcinoma of skin, unspecified

CLINICAL PEARLS

- Nodular: Pearly papule, plaque, or nodule often with telangiectatic vessels, ulceration, and a rolled periphery, usually on face.
- Pigmented: Presents as a translucent papule with "floating pigment"; more commonly seen in darker skin types.
- Superficial: Scaly papule or plaque with atrophic center, ringed by translucent micropapules, usually on trunk or extremities; more common in men.
- Morpheaform: Firm, smooth, flesh-colored, scarlike papule or plaque with ill-defined borders.
- Use diagnostic keys above to differentiate between BCC and cutaneous squamous cell carcinoma (SCC). SCC arises from actinic keratosis in 60% of cases and generally presents as an asymptomatic hyperkeratotic lesion. If unsure, biopsy or refer to a specialist.
- Some hyperpigmented BCCs may appear similar to melanoma. Remember the ABCDEs of melanoma recognition: **A**symmetry, **B**order irregularities, **C**olor variability, **D**iameter >6 mm, **E**nlargement. If unsure, refer to a specialist.
- The USPSTF concludes insufficient evidence and recommends for or against routine total body skin exams for melanoma, BCC, or SCC. Exams should be based on risk factors, including exposure and family and prior medical history. All patients should receive education about risks and self-exam.

BED BUGS

Fawn Winkelman, DO

BASICS

DESCRIPTION
- Nocturnal obligate blood parasites that take refuge on furniture and bedding
- 5–7 mm oval, reddish brown, flat, wingless (1)

EPIDEMIOLOGY
Incidence
- According to the 2013 "Bugs Without Borders" survey, bed bug infestations are increasing and continue to remain the most difficult pest to treat, more difficult than cockroaches, termites, and ants (2).
- Resurgence is due to the use of less toxic, less persistent insecticides as well as increased travel, use of secondhand furniture, and a high turnover rate of residents in hotels (3).

Prevalence
- Infestations are increasing across the US
- Sharp increase in prevalence, as only 11% of survey respondents reported bed bug calls more than 10 years ago (1).
- Bed bug encounters have become more common in public places (schools, hospitals, hotels/motels, aircrafts) than in previous years, increasing by 10–30% (1).

ETIOLOGY AND PATHOPHYSIOLOGY
- Insect family *Cimicidae*
- 3 species that bite humans: *Cimex letularius, Cimex hemipterus,* and *Leptocimex boueti* (1,2,3,4)
- Most prevalent special is *C. letularius*
- Found in tropical or temperate climates

- Hide in crevices of mattresses, box springs, headboards, and baseboards
- Infestations occur in hotels/motels, hospitals, cinemas, transportation vehicles, aircrafts, and homes
- Reactions range from an absent or minimal response to a more typical reaction presenting as pruritic, erythematous macules and papules, or a less-common urticarial and anaphylactic response (2)
- Skin reactions are due to host immunologic response to the parasite salivary proteins
- Papular urticarial reactions are mediated via immunoglobulin (Ig) G antibody response to salivary proteins
- Bullous reactions are caused by an IgE-mediated hypersensitivity to nitrophorin, the substance that transports nitric oxide in bed bug saliva (4)

GENERAL PREVENTION
- Avoidance of bed bugs: Vacuum regularly, reduce clutter, seal cracks in walls, inspect luggage and clothing
- Launder all bedding and cloth items in 130°F (50°C) or hotter for 2 hours or 20°F (-5°C) or cooler for 5 days (4)
- If present in the home, eradication is essential via professional extermination

RISK FACTORS
- Immunologically weak or compromised
- Recent travel
- High turnover environment
- Secondhand furniture in home

DIAGNOSIS

HISTORY
- Recent travel
- Blood specks on sheets
- Bed bug sighting
- New skin lesions in the morning
- Intense pruritus, pain, or burning

PHYSICAL EXAM
- Characteristic lesions are erythematous pruritic papules in an irregular linear pattern
- Found on body surfaces exposed during sleeping such as face, neck, arms, legs, and shoulders
- May appear hours to days after being bitten
- Patients are usually asymptomatic but may be anaphylactic and present with papular urticaria, diffuse urticaria, and/or bullous lesions (4)

DIFFERENTIAL DIAGNOSIS
- Urticaria
- Insect or spider bite
- Scabies
- Dermatitis herpetiformis

DIAGNOSTIC TESTS & INTERPRETATION
Initial Tests (lab, imaging)
- Skin scraping with mineral oil preparation (4)
- Skin biopsy (4)

Test Interpretation
- Skin scraping is negative with mineral oil, which helps to exclude scabies
- Skin biopsy shows nonspecific perivascular eosinophilic infiltrate consistent with arthropod bite reaction

TREATMENT

GENERAL MEASURES
- Self-limited and resolves within 1–2 weeks
- Treat symptomatically
- Avoidance of the bed bugs by inspection
- Prevention by laundering bedding and cloth

MEDICATION
First Line
- Disease is self-limited; treat symptoms
- Oral antihistamines (i.e., diphenhydramine, hydroxyzine)
- Topical antipruritics (i.e., pramoxine/calamine ointment or doxepin cream)
- Topical low to midpotency corticosteroids for 2 weeks (i.e., hydrocortisone, triamcinolone)
- Systemic corticosteroids (severe cases)

ADDITIONAL THERAPIES
- If secondarily infected, use topical or oral antibiotics against *Staphylococcal* and *Streptococcal* sp. (i.e., cephalexin, tetracycline, doxycycline, clindamycin, topical mupirocin) (1,2)
- Epinephrine for anaphylaxis
- Professional extermination may be necessary

 ONGOING CARE

FOLLOW-UP RECOMMENDATIONS
- Not necessary as disease is self-limited
- Recommended in extreme cases or if anaphylaxis ensues

PATIENT EDUCATION
- Avoid scratching to prevent superinfection
- Inspect bedding, furniture, luggage regularly
- CDC: www.cdc.gov/parasites/bedbugs/
- EPA: www.epa.gov/bedbugs/

COMPLICATIONS
- Bed bug dermatitis, allergic reactions, asthma exacerbations, anaphylaxis
- Significant psychological distress (insomnia, depression, anxiety, delusional parasitosis)[1]
- Secondary bacterial infections
- Transmission of blood-borne diseases (rare)

REFERENCES

1. Studdiford JS, Conniff KM, Trayes KP, et al. Bedbug infestation. *Am Fam Physician*. 2012;86:653–658.
2. Goddard J, deShazo R. Bedbugs (Cimex lectularius) and clinical consequences of their bites. *JAMA*. 2009;301:1358–1366.
3. Kolb A, Needham GR, Neyman KM, et al. Bedbugs. *Dermatol Ther*. 2009:347–352.
4. Thomas I, Kihiczak GG, Schwartz RA, et al. Bedbug bites: A review. *Int J Dermatol*. 2004;43:430–433.

CODES

ICD10
- S00.96XA Insect bite (nonvenomous) of unspecified part of head, initial encounter
- S10.96XA Insect bite of unspecified part of neck, initial encounter
- S40.269A Insect bite (nonvenomous) of unspecified shoulder, initial encounter

CLINICAL PEARLS
- 90% of infestations occur within 3 feet of beds.
- Wash bedding/clothing regularly in hot water.
- Vacuum carpet daily or steam clean daily.
- Inspect furniture, bedding, luggage regularly.
- Utilize professional services if necessary.
- Patient education and vigilance is paramount for bed bug prevention and avoidance.

BEHAVIORAL PROBLEMS, PEDIATRIC

William Elder, PhD

 BASICS

DESCRIPTION
Behavior that disrupts at least 1 area of psychosocial functioning. Commonly reported behavioral problems are:
- Noncompliance: Active or passive refusal to do as requested by parent or other authority figure
- Temper tantrums: Loss of internal control provoked by overtiredness, physical discomfort, or fear that leads to crying, whining, breath-holding, or in extreme cases, acts of aggression
- Sleep problems: Sleep patterns that are distressing to caregivers or child; difficulty going to sleep or staying asleep at night, nightmares, night terrors
- Nocturnal enuresis: Enuresis that occurs only at night in children >5 years of age with no medical problems:
  - Primary: Children who have never been dry at night
  - Secondary: Children dry at night for at least 6 months
- Functional encopresis: Repeated involuntary fecal soiling that is not caused by organic defect or illness
- Problem eating: "Picky eating," difficult mealtime behaviors
- Normative sexual behaviors: Developmentally appropriate behaviors in children in the absence of abuse
- Thumb sucking: An innate reflex that is self-soothing. May be protective against sudden infant death. If persists past eruption of primary teeth, can affect teeth alignment and mouth shape.

EPIDEMIOLOGY
- Noncompliance: May manifest as children develop autonomy; males have a modestly greater likelihood of being noncompliant. Decreases with age.
- Temper tantrums: 70% of 18–24-month-old children; 7% of 3–5-year-old children; in children with severe tantrums, 52% have other behavioral/emotional problems (1).
- Sleep problems:
  - Night waking in 25–50% of infants 6–12 months; bedtime refusal in 10–30% of toddlers
  - Nightmares in 10–30% of preschoolers; peaks between ages 6–10 years
  - Night terrors in 1–6.5% early childhood; peaks between ages 4–12 years
  - Sleepwalking frequently in 3–5%; peaks between ages 5–8 years (2)
- Nocturnal enuresis:
  - At least 20% of children in the 1st grade wet the bed occasionally; 4% wet ≥2 times per week.
  - At 10 years of age, 9% in boys, 3% in girls (3)
- Functional encopresis:
  - Rare before age 3, most common in 5–10-year-olds; more common in boys (4)
- Problem eating:
  - Prevalence peaks at 50% at 24 months of age; no relation to sex/ethnicity/income (5)
- Normative sexual behaviors:
  - Rare in infancy, except hand to genital contact
  - Increased in 3–5-year-olds; less observed in >5-year-olds because more covert (6)
- Thumb sucking: Decreases with age; most children spontaneously stop between 2 and 4 years.

COMMONLY ASSOCIATED CONDITIONS
- Temper tantrums: Difficult child temperament, stress
- Noncompliance: If exceeds what seems normative, rule out depression, adjustment disorder, inappropriate discipline.
- Sleep problems: Often with inconsistent bedtime routine or sleep schedule, stimulating bedtime environment; can be associated with hyperactive behavior, poor impulse control, and poor attention in young children (2)
- Enuresis: Secondary often with medical problems, especially constipation, and frequent behavior problems, especially ADHD
- Functional encopresis: Enuresis, UTIs, ADHD (4)
- Normative sexual behaviors: Family stressors such as separation or divorce (6)

 DIAGNOSIS

HISTORY
- Noncompliance: Complete history from caregivers and teachers, if applicable; direct observation of child or child–caregiver interaction:
  - Criteria: Is problematic for at least some adults, leading to difficult interactions for at least 6 months
  - Reduces child's ability to take part in structured activities
  - Creates stressful relationships with compliant children
  - Disrupts academic progress; places child at risk for physical injury
- Temper tantrums: History, with focus on development, family functioning, or violence: May consist of stiffening limbs and arching back, dropping to the floor, shouting, screaming, crying, pushing/pulling, stamping, hitting, kicking, throwing, or running away (1)
- Sleep disorders: Screening questions about sleep during well-child visit, such as the BEARS screen (Bedtime problems, Excessive daytime sleepiness, Awakenings during the night, Regularity and duration of sleep, and Snoring); bedtime routine (2)[C]
- Nocturnal enuresis: Severity, onset, and duration; daytime wetting or any associated genitourinary symptoms, family history of enuresis, medical and psychosocial history, constipation, child and caregiver's motivation for treatment (7)[C]
- Functional encopresis: Was fecal continence ever attained? Triggering event; frequency, location of defecation; nature of stools; pain with defecation or blood on stools; awareness of urge to defecate; how much stool passed accidentally; history of trauma or abuse (4)
- Problem eating: Review of child's diet, growth curves, nutritional needs, and caregiver's response to behavior (5)[C].
- Normative sexual behaviors: When was behavior first noticed? Any recent changes or stressors in family? Behavior solitary or with another; if with another, what age? Changes in frequency or nature of behaviors; occurs at home, daycare, school? Is behavior disruptive, intrusive, coercive? (6) See Child Sexual Behavior Inventory below.

PHYSICAL EXAM
- Nocturnal enuresis:
  - Physical exam of abdomen for enlarged bladder, kidneys, or fecal masses; rectal exam if history of constipation; back for spinal dysraphism seen in dimpling or hair tufts
  - Neurologic exam: Focus on lower extremities
  - Genital urinary exam:
    - Males: Meatal stenosis, hypospadias, epispadias, phimosis
    - Females: Vulvitis, vaginitis, labial adhesions, ureterocele at introitus; wide vaginal orifice with scar or healed laceration may be evidence of abuse.
- Functional encopresis:
  - Height and weight; abdominal exam for masses or tenderness; rectal exam for tone, size of rectal vault, fecal impaction, masses, fissures, hemorrhoids; back for signs of spinal dysraphism seen in dimpling or hair tufts (4)

DIAGNOSTIC TESTS & INTERPRETATION
Initial Tests (lab, imaging)
- For nocturnal enuresis: Urinalysis (dipstick test OK); if abnormal, consider urine culture
  - For secondary enuresis: Serum glucose, creatinine, thyrotropin (8)[C]
  - Urinary tract imaging and urodynamic studies if significant daytime symptoms with history or diagnosis of UTI, or history of structural renal abnormalities (8)[C]
- For functional encopresis: Tests for hypothyroidism or celiac disease if poor growth or family history; UA and culture if enuresis or features of UTI (4)
  - Spine imaging if evidence of spinal dysraphism or if both encopresis and daytime enuresis; barium enema if suspect Hirschsprung disease (4)

Follow-Up Tests & Special Considerations
Sleep disorders: Sleep studies may be performed in children if there is a history of snoring and daytime ADHD–type symptoms (2).

Diagnostic Procedures/Other
- Pediatric Symptom Checklist: www.brightfutures.org/mentalhealth/pdf/professionals/ped_symptom_chklst.pdf
- National Initiative for Children's Healthcare Quality (NICHQ) Vanderbilt Assessment (ADHD screen): www.myadhd.com/vanderbiltparent6175.html
- Child Sexual Behavior Inventory. Completed by female caregiver to assist with differentiation of normative vs. abnormal behaviors particularly those related to sexual abuse: www.nctsnet.org/content/child-sexual-behavior-inventory-csbi

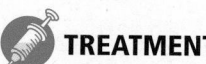 **TREATMENT**

- General: Educate caregiver about specific behavioral problem (3).
- Noncompliance: In the case of extreme child disobedience, consider parent training programs. Child may need to be formally screened for ADHD, oppositional defiant disorder (ODD), or conduct disorder (CD).
- Temper tantrums: Remind caregiver this is a normal aspect of childhood:
  - If tantrum is set off by external factors, such as hunger or overtiredness, then correct.
  - Other methods for dealing with a tantrum include one of the following:
    - Ignore the tantrum; remove the child and place him or her in time-out (1 minute for each year of age); hold/restrain child until calmed down; provide child with clear, firm, and consistent instructions, as well as enough time to obey

- Sleep problems: Intervention consists largely of education of the caregiver who may need a roadmap for dealing with this difficult and distressing problem. Developmental stages; environmental factors and cues; caregiver emotions and reactions; and child fears, stress, and habits are all important factors in sleep onset and maintenance that should be explored and explained to caregiver.
- Specific recommendations may also consist of other interventions including (2)[A]:
  - Graduated extinction: Caregiver ignores cries/tantrums for specified period. Can check at a fixed time or increasing intervals.
  - "Fading": Gradual decrease in direct contact with the child as child falls asleep; goal is for caregiver to exit the room and allow child to fall asleep independently.
  - Consider the "5S Intervention" for settling problems in toddlers (used to comfort infants in nurseries): Swaddling, sucking, shushing, stomach/side position, and swinging.
  - If fearful, preferred routines or inert sprays or glitter spread by the child (while avoiding the eyes) may help the child feel more secure.
- Nocturnal enuresis:
  - Bedwetting alarm: First-line therapy for caregivers who can overcome objection of having their sleep disturbed; about 2/3 of children respond while using the alarm; if enuresis recurs after use, it will often resolve with a 2nd trial (7)[A].
  - Decrease fluids an hour before bedtime
  - Little evidence from clinical trials, but good empirical evidence for behavioral training, including positive reinforcement (small reward for each dry night) or responsibility training (if old enough, child is responsible for changing or washing sheets), encouraging daily bowel movements, and frequent bladder emptying during the day (3)
- Functional encopresis:
  - First disimpaction: PO with Polyethylene glycol (PEG) solution or mineral oil; if unsuccessful, manual, mineral oil enemas,
  - Maintenance therapy:
    ○ Medical: Osmotics, such as polyethylene glycol, fiber, lactulose, magnesium citrate, magnesium hydroxide; lubricants—mineral oil; stimulants, such as senna or bisacodyl
    ○ Behavior modification: Toileting after meals for 10 minutes 2–3 times a day, star charts and rewards (4)[C]
- Problem eating:
  - Avoid punishment, prodding, or rewards. Offer a variety of healthy foods at every meal; limit milk to 24 oz/d and decrease juice (5)[C].
- Normative sexual behavior: No treatment needed; caregivers may need encouragement not to punish or admonish child and to use gentle distraction to redirect behavior when in public setting.
- Thumb sucking: Recommendations to caregivers include to praise children when not sucking their thumb, offer alternatives that are soothing (e.g., stuffed toys), provide reminders or negative reinforcement in the form of a bandage around or bitters on the thumb (5).

MEDICATION
Most pediatric behavioral issues respond well to nonpharmacologic therapy:

- Sleep disorders:
  - For certain delayed sleep-onset disorders, after behavioral methods are exhausted, melatonin 0.5–10 mg PO can be tried while behavior modification is continued (9). However, this is not approved by the FDA for children. Daytime exposure to bright or sun light should be assured before treatment.
- Nocturnal enuresis:
  - Desmopressin can decrease urine output to reduce enuresis episodes. Not before age 6; begin with 0.2 mg tablet at bedtime; titrate to 0.6 mg (8)[B]. However, use is questionable because effects of desmopressin do not persist once treatment is discontinued (10)[A]. Intranasal formulations can cause severe hyponatremia resulting in seizures and death in children. Behavioral interventions should be 1st-line treatment.

ISSUES FOR REFERRAL
- A patient who exhibits self-injurious behaviors, slow recovery time from tantrums, more tantrums in the home than outside the home, or more aggressive behaviors toward others may require referral to a child psychologist or psychiatrist.
- A child with loud nightly snoring, with observed apnea spells, daytime excessive sleeping, and neurobehavioral signs such as mood changes, ADHD-like symptoms, or academic problems, should be referred for sleep studies (2).
- With enuresis and obstructive sleep apnea symptoms, refer for sleep studies because surgical correction of airway obstruction often improves or cures enuresis and daytime wetting (9).
- Must distinguish sexual behavior problems: Developmentally inappropriate behaviors—greater frequency or much earlier age than expected, becomes a preoccupation, recurs after adult intervention/corrective efforts. If abuse not suspected, consider referral to a child psychologist. If abuse is suspected, must report to child protective services (6).
- If disimpaction by either manual or medical methods is unsuccessful, consult gastroenterology or general surgery. Patients who show no improvement after 6 months of maintenance medical therapy should be referred to gastroenterology (4).

 ONGOING CARE

DIET
Nutrition is very important in behavioral issues. Avoiding high-sugar foods and caffeine and providing balanced meals has been shown to decrease aggressive and noncompliant behaviors in children.

PATIENT EDUCATION
- See "Parent Training Programs: Insight for Practitioners" at: www.cdc.gov/violenceprevention/pdf/Parent_Training_Brief-a.pdf
- *The Happiest Baby Guide to Great Sleep: Simple Solutions for Kids from Birth to 5 Years.* Harvey Karp, MD New York, HarperCollins Publishers 2012, 384 pp.
- Products:
  - Monsters Away (bubble gum scented inert aerosol spray) by order to: helde2@uky.edu
  - Nytone Bed Wetting Alarms: by order to: http://www.nytone.com/products/nytone-enuresis-alarm?gclid=CM7Cm97i5rcCFSJ MgodW1wAgg

REFERENCES
1. Potegal M, Davidson RJ. Temper tantrums in young children: 1. Behavioral composition. *J Dev Behav Pediatr.* 2003;24:140–147.
2. Bhargava S. Diagnosis and management of common sleep problems in children. *Pediatr Rev.* 2011;32:91–98.
3. Robson WL. Clinical practice. Evaluation and management of enuresis. *N Engl J Med.* 2009;360:1429–1436.
4. Har AF, Croffie JM. Encopresis. *Pediatr Rev.* 2010;31(9):368–374; quiz 374.
5. Tseng AG, Biagioli FE. Counseling on early childhood concerns: Sleep issues, thumb sucking, picky eating, and school readiness. *Am Fam Physician.* 2009;80(2):139–142.
6. Kellogg ND. Sexual behaviors in children: Evaluation and management. *Am Fam Physician.* 2010;82(10):1233–1238.
7. Neveus T. Nocturnal enuresis-theoretical background and practical guidelines. *Pediatr Nephrol.* 2011;26:1207–1214.
8. Ramakrishnan K. Evaluation and treatment of enuresis. *Am Fam Physician.* 2008;78(4):489–496.
9. Gringras P. When to use drugs to help sleep. *Arch Dis Child.* 2008;93(11):976–981.
10. Glazener CMA, Evans JHC. Desmopressin for nocturnal enuresis in children. *Cochrane Database Syst Rev.* 2002;3:CD002112.

ADDITIONAL READING
- Miller JW. Screening children for developmental behavioral problems: Principles for the practitioner. *Prim Care Clin Office Pract.* 2007;34:177–201.
- Strachan E, Staples B. Masturbation. *Pediatr Rev.* 2012;33(4):190–191.
- Zahrt DM, Melzer-Lange MD. Aggressive behavior in children and adolescents. *Pediatr Rev.* 2011;32(8):325–332.

 SEE ALSO

Enuresis

CODES

ICD10
- F91.1 Conduct disorder, childhood-onset type
- F91.2 Conduct disorder, adolescent-onset type
- F91.9 Conduct disorder, unspecified

CLINICAL PEARLS
- Well-child visits provide opportunities for systematic screening for these common conditions.
- Parental education, including a review of age-appropriate discipline, is a key component of treatment.

BEHÇET SYNDROME

Mary Lauren Worthen, MD • Adrian Worthen • David Worthen

BASICS

DESCRIPTION
- Behçet syndrome is a systemic inflammatory disease of unknown etiology. It presents as a vasculitis of vessels of any size in both arterial and venous systems. It is a chronic disease, and, due to its involvement in all types of vessels, it can present in various parts of the body: Oral and genital mucocutaneous ulcerations, skin rashes, arthritis, thrombophlebitis, uveitis, colitis, and neurologic symptoms.
- Synonym(s): Mucocutaneous ocular syndrome; Franceschetti-Valero syndrome, Adamantiades' syndrome, Morbus Behçet, or Silk Road disease

Pregnancy Considerations
- Thalidomide for treatment contraindicated in pregnancy
- Possible increase in thrombosis and fetal demise

EPIDEMIOLOGY
- Predominant age: 3rd–4th decades; rare in pediatric and geriatric populations
- Predominant gender: Male = Female, with males affected more severely, especially in the Middle East and Central Asia

Prevalence
- Rare in the US and northern Europe; endemic in Japan, the Middle East, and the Mediterranean region. The disease is more prevalent in the region of the Silk Road linking China to Italy (1).
- 1/100,000 population in the US
- In other countries, per 100,000:
  – Turkey: 20–420
  – Islamic Republic of Iran: 16–100
  – Kingdom of Saudi Arabia: 20
  – Japan: 10
  – Northern Europe: 3

ETIOLOGY AND PATHOPHYSIOLOGY
Unknown: Classified as systemic vasculitis; associated with HLA-B51; possible immune response to ubiquitous heat-shock protein. Possible infectious causes: Herpes simplex virus (HSV), streptococcus; reportedly associated with HIV infection; possible environmental toxin (heavy metals, pesticides, possibly English walnuts or ginkgo nuts)

RISK FACTORS
HLA-B51/B5 carriage predominates in males; it is associated with moderately higher prevalences of genital ulcers, ocular and skin manifestations, and a decreased prevalence of GI involvement.

COMMONLY ASSOCIATED CONDITIONS
- Amyloid
- Myelodysplastic syndrome and trisomy 8

DIAGNOSIS

HISTORY
- Patient presents with exacerbations and remissions; often the disease is silent between events.
- GI: Recurrent painful stomatitis or aphthous ulcers (nearly all cases); at least 3 crops in 12 months; spontaneous healing without scar, abdominal pain, melena, anorexia, dyspepsia, vomiting
- Genital: Recurrent, painful ulcers with scarring; no urethritis or dysuria
- Musculoskeletal: Myositis (rare), morning stiffness (1/3 of patients), arthralgias
- Ocular: Painful, red eyes
- Neurologic: Headache, weakness, numbness, cranial nerve palsy, seizures

PHYSICAL EXAM
- GI: Painful, shallow, or deep oral ulcers with central yellowish necrotic base and punched-out, clean margin; commonly on tongue, lips, buccal mucosa, and gingivae; ulceration in terminal ileum, cecum, ascending colon
- Genital: Painful, scarring ulcers
- Dermal: Papulopustular (acneiform) lesions, erythema nodosum, pyoderma
- Musculoskeletal: Self-limited, nonerosive arthritis mostly mono- or oligoarthritis predominantly affecting lower extremities, rarely polyarthritis
- Ocular: Chronic, relapsing bilateral uveitis affecting the anterior and posterior chambers. Anterior uveitis with hypopyon, iridocyclitis, chorioretinitis, retinal vasculitis, vitreous hemorrhage, papilledema, secondary glaucoma, optic atrophy
- Thrombophlebitis: Peripheral, pulmonary, cerebral, Budd-Chiari syndrome
- Neurologic: Parenchymal involvement, common in brain stem; cranial nerve palsy, hemiplegia, intracranial hypertension, meningoencephalitis and recurrent meningitis, cerebral venous sinus thrombosis, confusional state (2)
- Pulmonary infiltrates, possibly related to thrombosis, noncavitating mass lesion
- Vascular: Peripheral gangrene, aneurysms
- Renal: Glomerulonephritis, epididymitis (rare)

DIFFERENTIAL DIAGNOSIS
- Reactive arthritis and other forms of seronegative spondyloarthropathy
- Inflammatory bowel disease (Crohn disease and ulcerative colitis)
- Syphilis and other venereal diseases
- Multiple sclerosis
- Aphthous stomatitis
- Herpes simplex
- Stevens-Johnson syndrome
- Other systemic vasculitides
- Relapsing polychondritis (mouth and genital ulcers with inflamed cartilage [MAGIC] syndrome)
- Coxsackievirus and echovirus infection
- Mollaret meningitis
- Sarcoidosis

DIAGNOSTIC TESTS & INTERPRETATION
Pathergy phenomenon: Hallmark of this condition: Nonspecific cutaneous hypersensitivity reaction—formation of sterile pustules and/or papules along sites of puncture or needle track

Initial Tests (lab, imaging)
- Normal to mildly elevated ESR and C-reactive protein (CRP)
- If elevated or high clinical suspicion, order follow-up tests as noted

Follow-Up Tests & Special Considerations
- Circulating immune complexes detected by Raji cell and C1q solid-phase assays and elevated interleukin 1 (IL-1), IL-8, and tumor necrosis factor α (TNF-α), but not clinically useful
- Hypergammaglobulinemia
- Depression of plasma antithrombin III levels with active disease
- Increased fibrinolytic activity during attacks; demyelinating antibodies in neurologic Behçet syndrome
- Anticardiolipin antibodies (rare), lupus anticoagulants
- Antiendothelial antibodies

Diagnostic Procedures/Other
- Careful history and physical examination, with frequent re-evaluations
- Synovial fluid: Inflammatory effusion
- Arteriography: For aneurysms or thrombosis
- Colonoscopy

Test Interpretation
- May be no recognizable changes; neutrophilic perivascular infiltration $\pm$ fibrinoid necrosis
- Picture of leukocytoclastic vasculitis in older lesions
- Neutrophilic dermatitis (Sweet syndrome) (rarely)

TREATMENT

MEDICATION
First Line
- Colchicine: 0.6 mg b.i.d. for mucocutaneous and joint symptoms, genital ulcers
- Topical steroids for ocular and genital lesions. Prednisone: 1 mg/kg for severe involvement, especially CNS
- Dapsone: 50–150 mg/d (3)[B]
- Azathioprine: 2–3 mg/kg/d PO
- Infliximab: A single infliximab infusion should be considered for the control of acute panuveitis, whereas repeated long-term infliximab infusions proved to be more effective in reducing the number of episodes in refractory uveoretinitis with faster regression and complete remission of cystoid macular edema (4)[B].
- Methotrexate: Use lowest possible dose; perhaps 7.5 mg/wk. Monitor liver function.
- Cyclosporine: 1–4 mg/kg, but monitor liver function, creatinine, magnesium, and lipids every 2 weeks for 3 months, then every month
- Sulfasalazine 2–6 g/d for GI involvement

- Resistant cases may require:
  - Tacrolimus (FK 506) 0.09–0.15 mg/kg/d
  - Thalidomide: 100 mg/d or 300 mg/d (5)[A]; regulated prescription, teratogenic; refer to manufacturer's literature.
  - Interferon-α for severe ocular and mucocutaneous syndrome (6)[A] and GI manifestations
  - Anticoagulants for patients with anticardiolipin antibodies: Warfarin (Coumadin) to establish PT international normalized ratio 3.0–3.5
  - Precautions: Absorption of drugs such as amitriptyline, diazepam, carbamazepine, and acetaminophen may be reduced in Behçet syndrome.

Second Line

- Cyclophosphamide: 2–2.5 mg/kg/d PO for severe cutaneous, arterial, pulmonary vasculitic or aneurysmal manifestations; risk of hemorrhagic cystitis with drug
- TNF inhibitors: Infliximab (7)[B], etanercept (8)[A]
- Topical sucralfate suspension
- Topical Pimecrolimus (9)[A]

ISSUES FOR REFERRAL
Ophthalmologic, neurological, GI, surgery, as appropriate

IN-PATIENT CONSIDERATIONS
Admission Criteria/Initial Stabilization
- Usually outpatient
- Inpatient usually required for neurologic complication or GI perforation

ONGOING CARE

FOLLOW-UP RECOMMENDATIONS
Patient Monitoring
- Depends on severity of system involvement and medication monitoring
- Periodic ophthalmologic examinations

DIET
No special diet

PATIENT EDUCATION
American Behçet's Association, 421 21st Avenue SW, Rochester, MN 55902; (507) 281-3059

PROGNOSIS
- Normal life expectancy, except with neurologic involvement, ruptured aneurysms, and catastrophic GI involvement. Most serious morbidity is blindness (posterior chamber or retinal nerve involvement)
- Remissions and exacerbations of disease activity, with severity abating over time

COMPLICATIONS
- Death
- Blindness (most serious morbidity)
- Paralysis
- Embolism/Thrombosis (pulmonary, vena cava, peripheral, intracardiac [rare])
- Aneurysms
- Amyloidosis
- Thrombotic events, especially when anticardiolipin antibodies present
- Intestinal perforation

REFERENCES

1. Kobayashi T, Kishimoto M, Swearingen CJ, et al. Differences in clinical manifestations, treatment, and concordance rates with two major sets of criteria for Behçet's syndrome for patients in the US and Japan: Data from a large, three-center cohort study. *Modern Rheumatology/Japan Rheumatism Association*. 2012. Epub 2012 Jun 30.
2. Al-Araji A, Kidd DP. Neuro-Behçet's disease: Epidemiology, clinical characteristics, and management. *Lancet Neurol*. 2009;8(2):192–204.
3. Lin P, Liang G. Behçet disease: Recommendation for clinical management of mucocutaneous lesions. *J Clin Rheumatol*. 2006;12(6):282–286.
4. Evereklioglu C. Ocular Behçet disease: Current therapeutic approaches. *Curr Opin Ophthalmol*. 2011;22(6):508–516.
5. Hamuryudan V, Mat C, Saip S, et al. Thalidomide in the treatment of the mucocutaneous lesions of the Behçet syndrome. A randomized, double-blind, placebo-controlled trial. *Ann Intern Med*. 1998; 128:443–450.
6. Alpsoy E, Durusoy C, Yilmaz E, et al. Interferon alfa-2a in the treatment of Behçet disease: A randomized placebo-controlled and double-blind study. *Arch Dermatol*. 2002;138:467–471.
7. Tugal-Tutkun I, Mudun A, Urgancioglu M, et al. Efficacy of infliximab in the treatment of uveitis that is resistant to treatment with the combination of azathioprine, cyclosporine, and corticosteroids in Behçet's disease: An open-label trial. *Arthritis Rheum*. 2005;52:2478–2484.
8. Melikoglu M, Fresko I, Mat C, et al. Short-term trial of etanercept in Behçet's disease: A double blind, placebo controlled study. *J Rheumatol*. 2005;32: 98–105.
9. Chams-Davatchi C, Barikbin B, Shahram F, et al. Pimecrolimus versus placebo in genital aphthous ulcers of Behçet's disease: A randomized double-blind controlled trial. *Int J Rheum Dis*. 2010;13(3):253–258.

ADDITIONAL READING

- Alpsoy E, Akman A. Behçet's disease: An algorithmic approach to its treatment. *Arch Dermatol Res*. 2009;301(10):693–702. Epub 2009 Aug 21.
- Maldini C, Lavalley MP, Cheminant M, et al. Relationships of HLA-B51 or B5 genotype with Behçet's disease clinical characteristics: Systematic review and meta-analyses of observational studies. *Rheumatology (Oxford)*. 2012;51(5):887–900. Epub 2012 Jan 11.
- Saadoun D, Wechsler B. Behçet's disease. *Orphanet Journal of Rare Diseases*. 2012;7(1):20. Epub 2012 Apr 12.

 CODES

ICD10
M35.2 Behçet's disease

CLINICAL PEARLS
- Nonsuperficial oral or genital ulcers suggest Behçet syndrome rather than reactive arthritis (previously called *Reiter syndrome*). The combination of oral and genital ulcers is especially suggestive.
- The pathergy phenomenon (a cutaneous hypersensitivity reaction—formation of sterile pustules and/or papules along sites of puncture or needle track) is helpful, if present, but cannot rule out Behçet syndrome, if absent.
- Colchicine is the first line of therapy for Behçet syndrome.
- IgG, IgM, and IgA assays for anticardiolipin antibody tests are indicated for vascular complications in Behçet syndrome.

BELL PALSY

Dylan C. Kwait, MD

 BASICS

DESCRIPTION
A peripheral lower motor neuron facial palsy, usually unilateral, which arises secondary to inflammation and subsequent swelling and compression of cranial nerve VII (facial) and the associated vasa nervorum

EPIDEMIOLOGY
- Affects 0.02% of the population annually
- Predominant sex: Male = Female
- Median age of onset is 40 years, but affects all ages
- Accounts for 60–75% of all cases of unilateral facial paralysis
- Occurs with equal frequency on the left and right sides of the face
- Most patients recover, but as many as 30% are left with facial disfigurement and pain

Incidence
- 20–30 cases per 100,000 people in the US per year
- Lowest in children ≤10 years of age; highest in adults ≥70 years of age
- Higher among pregnant women

Prevalence
Affects 40,000 Americans every year

ETIOLOGY AND PATHOPHYSIOLOGY
- Results from damage to the facial cranial nerve (VII)
- Inflammation of cranial nerve VII causes swelling and subsequent compression of both the nerve and the associated vasa nervorum
- May arise secondary to reactivation of latent herpes virus (herpes simplex virus [HSV] type 1 and herpes zoster virus) in cranial nerve ganglia or due to ischemia from arteriosclerosis associated with diabetes mellitus

Genetics
May be associated with a genetic predisposition, but it remains unclear which factors are inherited

RISK FACTORS
- Pregnancy
- Diabetes mellitus
- Age >30 years
- Exposure to cold temperatures
- Upper respiratory infection (e.g., coryza, influenza)

COMMONLY ASSOCIATED CONDITIONS
- HSV
- Lyme disease
- Diabetes mellitus
- Hypertension
- Herpes zoster virus
- Ramsay-Hunt syndrome
- Sjögren syndrome
- Sarcoidosis
- Eclampsia
- Amyloidosis

DIAGNOSIS

HISTORY
- Time course of the illness (rapid onset)
- Predisposing factors: Recent viral infection, trauma, new medications, hypertension, diabetes mellitus
- Presence of hyperacusis or history of recurrent Bell palsy (both associated with poor prognosis)

- Any associated rash (suggestive of herpes zoster, Lyme disease, or sarcoid)
- Weakness on affected side of face, often sudden in onset
- Pain in or behind the ear in 50% of cases, which may precede the palsy in 25% of cases (1)
- Subjective numbness on the ipsilateral side of the face
- Alteration of taste on the ipsilateral anterior 2/3 of the tongue (chorda tympani branch of the facial nerve)
- Hyperacusis (nerve to the stapedius muscle)
- Decreased tear production

PHYSICAL EXAM
- Neurologic:
  – Determine if the weakness is caused by a problem in either the central or peripheral nervous systems
  – Flaccid paralysis of muscles on the affected side, *including the forehead:*
    ○ Impaired ability to raise the ipsilateral eyebrow
    ○ Impaired closure of the ipsilateral eye
    ○ Impaired ability to smile, grin, or purse the lips
    ○ Bell phenomenon: Upward diversion of the eye with attempted closure of the lid
  – Patients may complain of numbness, but no deficit is present on sensory testing
  – Examine for involvement of other cranial nerves
- Head, ears, eyes, nose, and throat:
  – Carefully examine to exclude a space occupying lesion
  – Perform pneumatic otoscopic exam
- Skin: Examine for erythema migrans (Lyme disease) and vesicular rash (herpes zoster virus)

DIFFERENTIAL DIAGNOSIS
Etiologies include:
- Infectious:
  – Acute or chronic otitis media
  – Malignant otitis externa
  – Osteomyelitis of the skull base
- Cerebrovascular:
  – Brainstem stroke involving anteroinferior cerebellar artery
  – Aneurysm involving carotid, vertebral, or basilar arteries
- Neoplastic (onset of palsy is usually slow and progressive and accompanied by additional cranial nerve deficits and/or headache) (2):
  – Tumors of the parotid gland
  – Cholesteatoma
  – Skull-base tumor
  – Carcinomatous meningitis
  – Leukemic meningitis
- Traumatic:
  – Temporal bone fracture
  – Mandibular bone fracture
- Other:
  – Multiple sclerosis
  – Myasthenia gravis (should be considered in cases of recurrent or bilateral facial palsy) (1)
  – Guillain-Barré syndrome (may also present with bilateral facial palsy) (1)
  – Sjögren syndrome
  – Sarcoidosis
  – Amyloidosis
  – Melkersson-Rosenthal syndrome
  – Mononeuritis or polyneuritis

DIAGNOSTIC TESTS & INTERPRETATION
Initial Tests (lab, imaging)
- Blood glucose level (if diabetes a consideration)
- Lyme titer ELISA and Western blot for immunoglobulin (Ig) M, IgG for *Borrelia burgdorferi*
- ESR
- Consider CBC
- Consider rapid plasma reagin test
- Consider HIV test
- In appropriate clinical circumstances, consider titers for varicella zoster virus, cytomegalovirus, rubella, hepatitis A, hepatitis B, and hepatitis C

Follow-Up Tests & Special Considerations
- CSF analysis:
  – CSF protein is elevated in 1/3 of cases
  – CSF cells show mild elevation in 10% of cases with a mononuclear cell predominance
  – Not routinely indicated
- Salivary polymerase chain reaction for HSV1 or herpes zoster virus (largely reserved for research purposes)
- Facial radiographs:
  – In the setting of trauma, evaluate for fracture
- IV contrast-enhanced head CT:
  – Evaluate for fracture
  – Evaluate for stroke, if stroke is in the differential
- IV contrast-enhanced brain MRI:
  – Evaluate for central pontine, temporal bone, and parotid neoplasms (1)[A]
  – Not routinely indicated

Diagnostic Procedures/Other
- Electromyograph: Nerve conduction on affected and nonaffected sides can be compared to determine the extent of nerve injury, especially if there is dense palsy or no recovery after several weeks.
- Electroneurography: Evoked potentials of affected and nonaffected sides can be compared.

Test Interpretation
Invasive diagnostic procedures are not indicated because biopsy could further damage cranial nerve XII.

 TREATMENT

GENERAL MEASURES
- Artificial tears should be used to lubricate the cornea.
- The ipsilateral eye should be patched and taped shut at night to avoid drying and infection.

MEDICATION
- Corticosteroids decrease inflammation and limit nerve damage, thereby reducing the number of patients with residual facial weakness (3,4)[A].
- Routine use of antiviral medication is not recommended. Antiviral agents targeting herpes simplex, when administered concurrently with corticosteroids, may further reduce the risk of unfavorable outcomes in patients with a dense Bell palsy (3,5,6)[A]:
  – Antivirals alone are less likely to produce full recovery than corticosteroids (3)[A].
  – A combination of valacyclovir and steroids provides only minimal added benefit over steroid use alone (7)[B].

- Corticosteroids:
  - Prednisolone (8)[B]: Total of 500 mg over 10 days, 25 mg PO b.i.d.:
    - Treatment with prednisolone within 48 hours of palsy onset has shown higher complete recovery rates and less synkinesis compared with no prednisolone (8)[B]
    - Antivirals in combination with corticosteroids:
      - Valacyclovir (7)[B]: 1,000 mg × 5 days plus prednisolone 60 mg/d × 5 days; then 30 mg/d × 3 days, then 10 mg/d × 2 days
- Contraindications:
  - Documented hypersensitivity
  - Pre-existing infections, including tuberculosis (TB) and systemic mycosis
- Precautions: Use with discretion in pregnant patients and those with peptic ulcer disease and diabetes
- Significant possible interactions: Measles-mumps-rubella, oral polio virus vaccine, and other live vaccines

Pregnancy Considerations
Steroids should be used cautiously during pregnancy; consult with an obstetrician.

ISSUES FOR REFERRAL
Patients may need to be referred to an ear, nose, and throat specialist or a neurologist

ADDITIONAL THERAPIES
- Physical therapy: No evidence of significant benefit or harm, but facial exercises may reduce time to recover and/or sequelae (9)[C],(10).
- Electrostimulation (11)[C] and mirror biofeedback rehabilitation have limited evidence of effect.
- Acupuncture with strong stimulation has shown some therapeutic promise (12)[C].

SURGERY/OTHER PROCEDURES
- Surgical treatment of Bell palsy remains controversial and is reserved for intractable cases (13)[A].
- There is insufficient evidence to decide whether surgical intervention is beneficial or harmful in the management of Bell palsy (9)[B].
- In those cases where surgical intervention is performed, cranial nerve XII is surgically decompressed at the entrance to the meatal foramen where the labyrinthine segment and geniculate ganglion reside (1)[A].
- Decompression surgery should not be performed >14 days after the onset of paralysis because severe degeneration of the facial nerve is likely irreversible after 2–3 weeks (1)[A].

ONGOING CARE

FOLLOW-UP RECOMMENDATIONS
Patient Monitoring
- Patients should start steroid treatment immediately and be followed for 12 months.
- Patients who do not recover complete facial nerve function should be referred to an ophthalmologist for tarsorrhaphy.

PATIENT EDUCATION
American Academy of Family Physicians: www.aafp.org/afp/2007/1001/p1004.html

PROGNOSIS
- Most patients achieve complete spontaneous recovery within 2 weeks. More than 80% recover within 3 months.
- 85% of untreated patients will experience the first signs of recovery within 3 weeks of onset.
- 16% are left with a partial palsy, motor synkinesis, and autonomic synkinesis (2).
- 5% experience severe sequelae, and a small number of patients experience permanent facial weakness and dysfunction (2).
- Poor prognostic factors include:
  - Age >60 years
  - Complete facial weakness
  - Hypertension
  - Ramsay-Hunt syndrome
- The Sunnybrook and House-Brackmann facial grading systems are clinical prognostic models that identify Bell palsy patients at risk for nonrecovery at 12 months (14).
- Treatment with prednisolone or no prednisolone and the Sunnybrook score are significant factors for predicting nonrecovery at 1 month (14).

COMPLICATIONS
- Corneal abrasion or ulceration
- Steroid-induced psychological disturbances; avascular necrosis of the hips, knees, and/or shoulders
- Steroid use can unmask subclinical infection (e.g., TB)

REFERENCES
1. Gilden DH. Clinical practice. Bell's Palsy. *N Engl J Med*. 2004;351:1323–1331.
2. Holland NJ, Weiner GM. Recent developments in Bell's palsy. *BMJ*. 2004;329:553–557.
3. Gronseth GS, Paduqa R. Evidence-based guideline update: Steroids and antivirals for Bell palsy: Report of the Guideline Development Subcommittee of the American Academy of Neurology. *Neurology*. 2012;79:2209–2213.
4. Salinas RA, Alvarez G, Daly F, et al. Corticosteroids for Bell's palsy (idiopathic facial paralysis). *Cochrane Database Syst Rev*. 2010;3:CD001942.
5. Lockhart P, Daly F, Pitkethly M, et al. Antiviral treatment for Bell's palsy (idiopathic facial paralysis). *Cochrane Database Syst Rev*. 2009;4: CD001869.
6. Thaera GM, Wellik KE, Barrs DM, et al. Are corticosteroid and antiviral treatments effective for bell palsy? A critically appraised topic. *Neurologist*. 2010;16:138–140.
7. Worster A, Keim SM, Sahsi R, et al. Do either corticosteroids or antiviral agents reduce the risk of long-term facial paresis in patients with new-onset Bell's palsy? *J Emerg Med*. 2010;38: 518–523.
8. Madhok V, Falk G, Fahey T, et al. Prescribe prednisolone alone for Bell's palsy diagnosed within 72 hours of symptom onset. *BMJ*. 2009;338:b255.
9. Axelsson S, Berg T, Jonsson L, et al. Prednisolone in Bell's palsy related to treatment start and age. *Otol Neurotol*. 2011;32:141–146.
10. Teixeira LJ, Valbuza JS, Prado GF. Physical therapy for Bell's palsy (idiopathic facial paralysis). *Cochrane Database Syst Rev*. 2011;12: CD006283.
11. Alakram P, Puckree T. Effects of electrical stimulation on House-Brackmann scores in early Bell's palsy. *Physiother Theory Pract*. 2010;26: 160–166.
12. Xu SB, Huang B, Zhang C, et al. Effectiveness of strengthened stimulation during acupuncture for the treatment of Bell palsy: A randomized control trial. *CMAJ*. 2013;24:e286–e289.
13. McAllister K, Walker D, Donnan PT, et al. Surgical interventions for the early management of Bell's palsy. *Cochrane Database Syst Rev*. 2011;2: CD007468.
14. Marsk E, Bylund N, Jonsson L, et al. Prediction of nonrecovery in Bell's palsy using Sunnybrook grading. *Laryngoscope*. 2012;122:901–906.

 SEE ALSO

Amyloidosis; Diabetes Mellitus Type 1; Diabetes Mellitus Type 2; Herpes Simplex; Herpes Zoster; Lyme Disease; Melkersson-Rosenthal Syndrome; Ramsay-Hunt Syndrome; Sarcoidosis; Sjögren Syndrome

 CODES

ICD10
G51.0 Bell's palsy

CLINICAL PEARLS
- Initiate steroids immediately following the onset of symptoms.
- Look closely at the voluntary movement on the upper part of the face on the affected side; in Bell palsy, all of the muscles are involved (weak or paralyzed), whereas in a stroke, the upper muscles are spared (because of bilateral innervation).
- Protect the affected eye with lubrication and taping.
- In areas with endemic Lyme disease, Bell palsy should be considered to be Lyme disease until proven otherwise.

BIPOLAR I DISORDER

Laurie Carrier, MD

BASICS

DESCRIPTION
- Bipolar I (BP-I) is a mood disorder characterized by at least 1 manic or mixed episode, often alternating with episodes of major depression, that causes marked impairment and/or hospitalization.
- Symptoms are not caused by a substance (e.g., drug), a general medical condition, or a medication.

Geriatric Considerations
New onset in older patients (>50 years of age) requires a workup for organic or chemically induced pathology.

Pediatric Considerations
There is overlap with symptoms of attention-deficit/hyperactivity disorder (ADHD) and oppositional defiant disorder (ODD). Children and adolescents experience more rapid cycling and mixed states. Depression often presents as irritable mood.

Pregnancy Considerations
- Potential teratogenic effects of commonly used medications (e.g., lithium, valproic acid)
- Symptoms may be exacerbated in the postpartum period.

EPIDEMIOLOGY
- Onset usually between 15 and 30 years of age
- More common in single and divorced persons
- Less common in college graduates
- Increased incidence in higher socioeconomic groups

Prevalence
- 1.0–1.6% lifetime prevalence
- Equal among men and women (manic episodes more common in men; depressive episodes more common in women)
- Equal among races; however, clinicians tend to misdiagnose schizophrenia in African Americans with BP-I

ETIOLOGY AND PATHOPHYSIOLOGY
Genetic predisposition and major life stressors can trigger initial and subsequent episodes:
- Dysregulation of biogenic amines or neurotransmitters (particularly serotonin, norepinephrine, and dopamine)
- MRI findings suggest abnormalities in prefrontal cortical areas, striatum, and amygdala that predate illness onset (1).

Genetics
- Monozygotic twin concordance 40–70%
- Dizygotic twin concordance 5–25%
- 50% have at least 1 parent with a mood disorder
- 1st-degree relatives are 7 × more likely to develop BP-I than the general population.

RISK FACTORS
Genetics, major life stressors (especially loss of parent or spouse), or substance abuse

GENERAL PREVENTION
Treatment adherence and education can help to prevent relapses.

COMMONLY ASSOCIATED CONDITIONS
Substance abuse (60%), ADHD, anxiety disorders, and eating disorders

DIAGNOSIS

- The diagnosis of BP-I requires at least 1 manic or mixed episode (simultaneous mania and depression). Although a depressive episode is not necessary for the diagnosis, 80–90% of people with BP-I also experience depression.
- Manic episode, *DSM-5* criteria:
  – Distinct period of abnormally and persistently elevated, expansive, or irritable mood lasting at least 1 week (or any duration if hospitalization is necessary)
  – During the period of mood disturbance, 3 or more of the "DIG FAST" symptoms must persist (4 if the mood is only irritable) and must be present to a significant degree:
    ○ Distractibility
    ○ Insomnia, decreased need for sleep
    ○ Grandiosity or inflated self-esteem
    ○ Flight of ideas or racing thoughts
    ○ Agitation or increase in goal-directed activity
    ○ Speech pressured/more talkative than usual
    ○ Taking risks: Excessive involvement in pleasurable activities that have a high potential for painful consequences (e.g., financial or sexual)
  – Mixed episode: Criteria are met for both a manic and major depressive episode nearly every day during at least a 1-week period, and the mood disturbance causes significant impairment in functioning.
  – Signs and symptoms more likely in bipolar than in unipolar depression (2): Agitation/Restlessness, suicidal ideation/planning, increased frequency of depressive episodes, melancholia, psychomotor retardation, younger age of onset, hyperphagia, hypersomnia, family history of bipolar disorder, subsyndromal hypomanic symptoms (particularly increased goal-directed activity).

HISTORY
- Collateral information makes diagnostics more complete and is often necessary for a clear history.
- History: Safety concerns (e.g., Suicidal/Homicidal ideation? Safety plan? Psychosis present?); Physical well-being (e.g., Number of hours of sleep? Appetite? Substance abuse?); Personal history (e.g., Told life of the party? Talkative? Speeding? Spending sprees or donations? Credit-card or gambling debt? Promiscuous? Other risk-taking behavior? Legal trouble? Religious infatuation?)

PHYSICAL EXAM
- Mental status exam in acute mania:
  – General appearance: Bright clothing, excessive makeup, disorganized or discombobulated, psychomotor agitation
  – Speech: Pressured, difficult to interrupt
  – Mood/Affect: Euphoria, irritability/expansive, labile
  – Thought process: Flight of ideas (streams of thought occur to patient at rapid rate), easily distracted
  – Thought content: Grandiosity, paranoia, hyperreligious
  – Perceptual abnormalities: 3/4 of manic patients experience delusions, grandiose or paranoid
  – Suicidal/Homicidal ideation: Irritability or delusions may lead to aggression toward self or others; suicidal ideation (SI) is common with mixed episode.
  – Insight/Judgment: Poor/impaired

- See "Bipolar II Disorder" for an example of a mental status exam in depression.
- With mixed episodes, patients may exhibit a combination of manic and depressive mental states.

DIFFERENTIAL DIAGNOSIS
- Other psychiatric considerations: Unipolar depression ± psychotic features, schizophrenia, schizoaffective disorder, personality disorders (particularly antisocial, borderline, histrionic, and narcissistic), ADD ± hyperactivity, substance-induced mood disorder
- Medical considerations: Epilepsy (e.g., temporal lobe), brain tumor, infection (e.g., AIDS, syphilis), stroke, endocrine (e.g., thyroid disease), multiple sclerosis
- In children, consider ADHD and ODD.

DIAGNOSTIC TESTS & INTERPRETATION
- BP-I is a clinical diagnosis.
- The Mood Disorder Questionnaire is a self-assessment screen for bipolar disorders (sensitivity 73%, specificity 90%) (3)[B].
- Patient Health Questionnaire-9 helps to determine the presence and severity of a depressive episode.

Initial Tests (lab, imaging)
- TSH, CBC, BMP, LFTs, ANA, RPR, HIV, ESR
- Drug/Alcohol screen with each presentation
- Dementia workup if new onset in seniors
- Consider brain imaging (CT, MRI) with initial onset of mania to rule out organic cause (e.g., tumor, infection, or stroke), especially with onset in elderly and if psychosis is present.

Diagnostic Procedures/Other
Consider EEG if presentation suggests temporal lobe epilepsy (hyperreligiosity, hypergraphia).

TREATMENT

- Ensure safety.
- Psychotherapy (e.g., cognitive-behavioral therapy, social rhythm therapy)
- Stress reduction
- Patient and family education

GENERAL MEASURES
- Psychotherapy (e.g., cognitive-behavioral therapy, social rhythm, interpersonal) in conjunction with medications (4)[B]
- Regular exercise, a healthy diet, and sobriety have been shown to help prevent worsening of symptoms.

MEDICATION
First Line
- Treatment may consist of 1–4 mood stabilizers or other psychotropic medications. When combining these agents, add different classes (e.g., an atypical antipsychotic and/or an antiseizure medication and/or lithium) (5,6)[B].

- Lithium (Lithobid, Eskalith, generic): Dosing: 600–1,200 mg/d divided b.i.d.–q.i.d.; start 600–900 mg/d divided b.i.d.–t.i.d., titrate based on blood levels. *Warning:* Caution in kidney and heart disease; use can lead to diabetes insipidus, thyroid disease. Caution with diuretics or ACE inhibitors; dehydration can lead to toxicity (seizures, encephalopathy, arrhythmias). Pregnancy Category D (Ebstein anomaly). *Monitor:* Check ECG >40 years, TSH, BUN, creatine, electrolytes at baseline and every 6 months; check level 5 days after initiation or dose change, then every 2 weeks × 3, then every 3 months (goal: 0.8–1.2 mmol/L).
- Antiseizure medications:
  - Divalproex sodium, valproic acid (Depakote, Depakene, generic): Dosing: Start 250–500 mg b.i.d.–t.i.d.; maximum 60 mg/kg/d. *Black box warnings:* Hepatotoxicity, pancreatitis, thrombocytopenia, pregnancy Category D. *Monitor:* CBC, LFTs at baseline and every 6 months; check level 5 days after initiation and dose changes (goal: 50–125 μg/mL).
  - Carbamazepine (Equetro, Tegretol, generic): Dosing: 800–1,200 mg/d PO divided b.i.d.–q.i.d.; start 100–200 mg PO b.i.d. and titrate to lowest effective dose. *Warning:* Do not use with TCA or within 14 days of an MOAI. Caution in kidney/heart disease; risk of aplastic anemia/agranulocytosis, enzyme inducer; pregnancy Category D. *Monitor:* CBC, LFTs at baseline and every 3–6 months; check level 4–5 days after initiation and dose changes (goal: 4–12 μg/mL).
  - Lamotrigine (Lamictal, generic): Dosing: 200 mg/d; start 25 mg/d × 2 weeks, then 50 mg/d × 2 weeks, then 100 mg/d × 1 week, then 150 mg/d. (*Note:* Use different dosing if adjunct to valproate). *Warning:* Titrate slowly (risk of Stevens-Johnson syndrome); caution with kidney/liver/heart disease; pregnancy Category C.
  - Oxcarbazepine (Trileptal), gabapentin (Neurontin), and topiramate (Topamax) are also used in BP-I, but are not approved by the FDA.
- Atypical antipsychotics (AAs):
  - Side effects: Orthostatic hypotension, metabolic side effects (glucose and lipid dysregulation, weight gain), tardive dyskinesia, neuroleptic malignant syndrome (NMS), prolactinemia (except Abilify), increased risk of death in elderly with dementia-related psychosis, pregnancy Category C
  - Monitor: LFTs, lipids, glucose at baseline, 3 months, and annually; check for extrapyramidal symptoms (EPS) with Abnormal Involuntary Movement Scale (AIMS) and assess weight (with abdominal circumference) at baseline, at 4, 8, and 12 weeks, and then every 3–6 months; monitor for orthostatic hypotension 3–5 days after starting or changing dose.
  - Risperidone (Risperdal, Risperdal Consta, generic): Dosing: 1–6 mg/d divided q.d.–q.i.d. IM preparation available (q2wk)
  - Olanzapine (Zyprexa, Zydis, generic): *Dosing:* 5–20 mg/d; most likely to cause metabolic side effects (weight gain, diabetes)
  - Symbyax (olanzapine + fluoxetine): *Dosing:* 6/25 mg
  - Quetiapine (Seroquel, Seroquel XR, generic): Dosing: In mania, 200–400 mg b.i.d.; in bipolar depression, 50–300 mg qhs. XR dosing 50–400 mg qhs. *Caution:* Cataracts

  - Aripiprazole (Abilify): Dosing: 15–30 mg/d; less likely to cause metabolic side effects
  - Ziprasidone (Geodon): Dosing: 40–80 mg b.i.d.; less likely to cause metabolic side effects. *Caution:* QTc prolongation (>500 ms) has been associated with use (0.06%). Consider ECG at baseline.
  - Asenapine (Saphris): Dosing: 5–10 mg b.i.d.; comes in sublingual tab

Second Line
- Antidepressants (in addition to mood stabilizers) have mixed evidence to support use.
- Benzodiazepines (for acute agitation with mania, associated anxiety)
- Sleep medications

ISSUES FOR REFERRAL
- Depends on comfort level of the doctor, stability of patient
- Patients benefit from a multidisciplinary team, including a primary care physician, psychiatrist, and therapist.

ADDITIONAL THERAPIES
- Electroconvulsive therapy can be helpful in acute mania and depression.
- Light therapy for seasonal component to depressive episodes (use with caution because it can precipitate manic episode)
- Modest evidence supports transcranial magnetic stimulation, vagus nerve stimulation, ketamine infusion, sleep deprivation, hormone therapy (e.g., thyroid) in bipolar depression.

IN-PATIENT CONSIDERATIONS
Admit if dangerous to self or others.

Admission Criteria/Initial Stabilization
To admit involuntarily, the patient must have a psychiatric diagnosis (e.g., BP-I) and present a danger to self or others, or the mental disease must be inhibiting the person from obtaining basic needs (e.g., food, clothing).

Nursing
Alert staff to potentially dangerous or agitated patients. Acute suicidal threats need continuous observation.

Discharge Criteria
Determined by safety

 ONGOING CARE

FOLLOW-UP RECOMMENDATIONS
- Regularly scheduled visits support adherence with treatment.
- Frequent communication among primary care doctor, psychiatrist, and therapist

Patient Monitoring
Mood charts are helpful to monitor symptoms.

PATIENT EDUCATION
- National Alliance on Mental Illness (NAMI): www.nami.org/
- National Institutes of Mental Health (NIMH): www.nimh.nih.gov

PROGNOSIS
- Frequency and severity of episodes are related to medication adherence, consistency with therapy, quality of sleep, and support systems.
- 40–50% of patients experience another manic episode within 2 years of 1st episode.
- 25–50% attempt suicide, and 15% die by suicide.
- Substance abuse, unemployment, psychosis, depression, and male gender are associated with a worse prognosis.

REFERENCES

1. Fornito A, Yücel M, Wood SJ, et al. Anterior cingulate cortex abnormalities associated with a first psychotic episode in bipolar disorder. *Br J Psychiatry.* 2009;194:426–433.
2. Perlis RH, Brown E, Baker RW, et al. Clinical features of bipolar depression versus major depressive disorder in large multicenter trials. *Am J Psychiatry.* 2006;163:225–231.
3. Hirschfeld RM, Holzer C, Calabrese JR, et al. Validity of the mood disorder questionnaire: A general population study. *Am J Psychiatry.* 2003;160:178–180.
4. Depp CA, Moore DJ, Patterson TL, et al. Psychosocial interventions and medication adherence in bipolar disorder. *Dialogues Clin Neurosci.* 2008;10:239–250.
5. Licht RW. A new BALANCE in bipolar I disorder. *Lancet.* 2010;375(9712):350–352. Epub 2010 Jan 19.
6. American Psychiatric Association. Practice guideline for the treatment of patients with bipolar disorder (revision). *Am J Psychiatry.* 2002;159:1–50.

 SEE ALSO

Algorithm: Depressive Episode, Major

 CODES

ICD10
- F31.9 Bipolar disorder, unspecified
- F31.10 Bipolar disorder, current episode manic without psychotic features, unspecified
- F31.30 Bipolar disord, crnt epsd depress, mild or mod severt, unsp

CLINICAL PEARLS
- Bipolar I is characterized by at least 1 manic or mixed episode, often alternating with episodes of major depression, that causes marked impairment.
- 25–50% of BP-I patients attempt suicide, and 15% die by suicide.
- There is no way to prevent the onset of BP-I, but treatment adherence and education can help to prevent further episodes.
- Goal of treatment is to decrease the intensity, length, and number of episodes as well as greater mood stability between episodes.

BIPOLAR II DISORDER
Laurie Carrier, MD

BASICS

DESCRIPTION
Bipolar II (BP-II) is a mood disorder characterized by at least 1 episode of major depression and at least 1 episode of hypomania, a milder form of mania.

Geriatric Considerations
New onset in older patients (>50 years) requires a workup for organic or chemically induced pathology.

Pediatric Considerations
- Large overlap with symptoms of attention-deficit hyperactivity disorder (ADHD) and oppositional defiant disorder (ODD)
- Depression often presents as irritable mood.

Pregnancy Considerations
- Counsel women of childbearing age about potentially teratogenic effects of commonly used medications (e.g., lithium, valproic acid).
- Symptoms may be exacerbated in the postpartum period.

EPIDEMIOLOGY
More common in women

Prevalence
0.5–1.1% lifetime prevalence

ETIOLOGY AND PATHOPHYSIOLOGY
- Dysregulation of biogenic amines or neurotransmitters (particularly serotonin, norepinephrine, and dopamine)
- Genetics
- Major life stressors (especially loss of parent or spouse)

Genetics
Heritability estimate: >77%

GENERAL PREVENTION
No way to prevent the onset of BP-II, but treatment adherence and education can help to prevent further episodes.

COMMONLY ASSOCIATED CONDITIONS
Substance abuse or dependence, ADHD, anxiety disorders, and eating disorders

DIAGNOSIS

- *DSM-5 criteria*: Patient must experience at least 1 hypomanic episode and at least 1 major depressive episode. The symptoms have caused *some* distress or impairment in social, occupational, or other areas of functioning. There can be no history of full manic or mixed episodes.

- Hypomania is a distinct period of persistently elevated, expansive, or irritable mood, different from usual nondepressed mood, lasting at least 4 days:
  – The episode must include at least 3 of the "DIG FAST" symptoms below (4 if the mood is only irritable):
    ○ Distractibility
    ○ Insomnia, decreased need for sleep
    ○ Grandiosity or inflated self-esteem
    ○ Flight of ideas or racing thoughts
    ○ Agitation or increase in goal-directed activity (socially, at work or school, or sexually)
    ○ Speech pressured/more talkative than usual
    ○ Taking risks: Excessive involvement in pleasurable activities that have high potential for painful consequences (e.g., sexual or financial)
  – The symptoms are not severe enough to cause *marked* impairment in functioning or hospitalization, and there is no associated psychosis as with BP-I.
- Major depression:
  – Depressed mood or diminished interest and 4 or more of the "SIG E CAPS" symptoms are present during the same 2-week period:
    ○ **S**leep disturbance (e.g., trouble falling asleep, early morning awakening)
    ○ **I**nterest: Loss or anhedonia
    ○ **G**uilt (or feelings of worthlessness)
    ○ **E**nergy, loss of
    ○ **C**oncentration, loss of
    ○ **A**ppetite changes, increase or decrease
    ○ **P**sychomotor changes (retardation or agitation)
    ○ **S**uicidal/Homicidal thoughts
  – BP-II with rapid cycling is diagnosed when a patient experiences at least 4 episodes of a mood disturbance in a 12-month period (either major depression or hypomania).

- Signs, symptoms, and history seen more often in BP-II than in unipolar depression (1)[B]:
  – Agitation, hyperphagia, hypersomnia, melancholia, psychomotor retardation, suicidal ideation/planning, increased frequency of depressive episodes, younger age of onset, family history of bipolar disorder, subsyndromal hypomanic symptoms (especially overactivity) (2)[B]

- Note: If symptoms have *ever* met criteria for a full manic episode or hospitalization was necessary secondary to manic/mixed symptoms or psychosis was present, then the diagnosis changes to BP-I.

HISTORY
Collateral information makes diagnostics more complete and is often necessary for a clear history.

PHYSICAL EXAM
- Mental status exam in hypomania:
  – General appearance: Usually appropriately dressed, with psychomotor agitation
  – Speech: May be pressured, talkative, difficult to interrupt
  – Mood/Affect: Euphoria, irritability/congruent, or expansive
  – Thought process: May be easily distracted, difficulty concentrating on 1 task
  – Thought content: Usually positive, with "big" plans
  – Perceptual abnormalities: None
  – Suicidal/Homicidal ideation: Low incidence of homicidal or suicidal ideation
  – Insight/Judgment: Usually stable/may be impaired by their distractibility

- Mental status exam in acute depression:
  – General appearance: Unkempt, psychomotor retardation, poor eye contact
  – Speech: Low, soft, monotone
  – Mood/Affect: Sad, depressed/congruent, flat
  – Thought process: Ruminating thoughts, generalized slowing
  – Thought content: Preoccupied with negative or nihilistic ideas
  – Perceptual abnormalities: 15% of depressed patients experience hallucinations or delusions.
  – Suicidal/Homicidal ideation: Suicidal ideation is very common.
  – Insight/Judgment: Often impaired

DIFFERENTIAL DIAGNOSIS
- Other psychiatric considerations:
  – BP-I disorder, unipolar depression, personality disorders (particularly borderline, antisocial, and narcissistic), ADD with hyperactivity, substance-induced mood disorder
- Medical considerations:
  – Epilepsy (e.g., temporal lobe), brain tumor, infection (e.g., AIDS, syphilis), stroke, endocrine (e.g., thyroid disease), multiple sclerosis
- In children, consider ADHD and ODD.

DIAGNOSTIC TESTS & INTERPRETATION
- BP-II is a clinical diagnosis.
- Mood Disorder Questionnaire, self-assessment screen for BP, sensitivity 73%, specificity 90% (3)[B]
- Hypomania Checklist-32 distinguishes between BP-II and unipolar depression (sensitivity 80%, specificity 51%) (4)[B]
- Patient Health Questionnaire-9 helps to determine the presence and severity of depression.

Initial Tests (lab, imaging)
- Rule out organic causes of mood disorder during initial episode.
- Drug/Alcohol screen is prudent with each presentation.
- Dementia workup if new onset in seniors
- With initial presentation: Consider CBC, chem 7, TSH, LFTs, ANA, RPR, HIV, ESR
- Consider brain imaging (CT, MRI) with initial onset of hypomania to rule out organic cause, especially with onset in the elderly.

TREATMENT

- Ensure safety
- Medication management
- Psychotherapy (e.g., cognitive-behavioral therapy [CBT], social rhythm therapy, interpersonal therapy)
- Stress reduction
- Patient and family education

GENERAL MEASURES
- Psychotherapy (e.g., CBT, social rhythm, interpersonal, family focused) in conjunction with medications is key.
- Regular exercise, a healthy diet, and sobriety have been shown to help prevent worsening of symptoms.

MEDICATION

- Less research has been conducted on the appropriate treatment of BP-II, but current consensus is to treat with the same medications as BP-I.
- Antidepressant medications must be used with caution during depressive episodes, as they may precipitate hypomanic episodes (less common than with BP-I).

First Line

- American Psychological Association guidelines state lithium or lamotrigine as first-line treatment for bipolar depression.
- Treatment may be a combination of 1–4 different agents. When combining mood stabilizers, consider adding different classes (e.g., an atypical antipsychotic and/or an antiseizure medication and/or lithium) (5)[B].
- Lithium (Lithobid, Eskalith, generic): Dosing 600–1,200 mg/d divided b.i.d.–q.i.d., titrate based on blood levels:
  – Caution in kidney or heart disease; use can lead to diabetes insipidus, thyroid disease; caution in sodium-depleted patients (diuretics, ACE inhibitors); dehydration can lead to toxicity, which may cause seizures, encephalopathic syndrome, arrhythmias, pregnancy Category D (Ebstein anomaly with 1st-trimeter use)
  – Monitor electrocardiogram in patients >40 years, TSH, BUN, creatinine, electrolytes at baseline and q6mo; check level 5 days after initiation or dose change, then q1–2wk × 3, then q3mo (goal: 0.8–1.2 mmol/L)
- Anticonvulsants:
  – Valproic acid, divalproex sodium: Dosing: Start 250–500 mg b.i.d.–t.i.d., max 60 mg/kg/d. *Warning*: Hepatotoxicity, pancreatitis, thrombocytopenia, pregnancy Category D (neural tube defects). *Monitor*: CBC, LFTs at baseline and q6mo; check valproic acid level 5 days after initiation and dose changes (goal: 50–125 μm/mL).
  – Carbamazepine: Dosing: 800–1,200 mg/d PO divided b.i.d.–q.i.d., start 100–200 mg PO b.i.d. and titrate to lowest effective dose. Do not use with tricyclic antidepressants or within 14 days of monoamine oxidase inhibitor; caution with kidney or heart disease, may cause aplastic anemia/agranulocytosis, pregnancy Category D. Monitor: CBC, LFTs at baseline and q3–6mo; check level 4–5 days after initiation and dose changes (goal: 4–12 μm/mL).
  – Lamotrigine: Dosing: 200 mg/d start 25 mg × 2 weeks, then 50 mg × 2 weeks, then 100 mg × 1 week. (Note: Different dosing if adjunct to valproate.) Selected warnings: Titrate slowly (risk of Stevens-Johnson syndrome); caution with kidney, liver, or heart impairment; pregnancy Category C. Monitor: Patient to monitor for rash.
  – Oxcarbazepine, gabapentin, and topiramate are also used in bipolar depression, but are not FDA approved.
- Atypical antipsychotics (AAs):
  – Side effects of AAs: Orthostatic hypotension, negative metabolic side effects (effect glucose and lipid regulation, weight gain), tardive dyskinesia, neuroleptic malignant syndrome, prolactinemia (except Abilify), increased risk of mortality in elderly with dementia-related psychosis, pregnancy Category C

– Monitor: LFTs, lipids, glucose at baseline, 3 months and annually; check for extrapyramidal symptoms with Abnormal Involuntary Movement Scale (AIMS) and assess weight (with abdominal circumference) at baseline, then 4, 8, and 12 weeks, then q3–6mo; monitor for orthostatic hypotension 3–5 days after starting or changing dose.
– Aripiprazole: Dosing: 15 mg/d, max 30 mg/d, less likely to cause metabolic side effects
– Olanzapine: Dosing: 5–20 mg/d, most likely AA to cause metabolic side effects (weight gain, diabetes mellitus)
– Symbyax (olanzapine + fluoxetine): Dosing: 6/25 mg, FDA approved for bipolar depression
– Quetiapine: Dosing: Hypomania 200–400 mg b.i.d. Depression 50–300 mg qh. *Caution*: Cataracts, sedation.
– Risperidone: Dosing: 1–6 mg/d every day–b.i.d. Generic and q2wk IM preparations available.
– Ziprasidone: Dosing: 40–80 mg b.i.d. Less likely to cause metabolic side effects. *Warning*: QTc prolongation (>500 ms) has been associated with use (0.06%); consider ECG at baseline.
– Asenapine (Saphris): Dosing: 5–10 mg b.i.d.; comes in sublingual tab, FDA approved for acute and maintenance treatment

Second Line

- Antidepressants (in addition to mood stabilizers) have better data in BP-II than BP-I.
- Benzodiazepines (for acute agitation, anxiety)
- Sleep medications

ISSUES FOR REFERRAL

Patients benefit from care by a multidisciplinary team, including a primary care physician, therapist, and psychiatrist.

ADDITIONAL THERAPIES

- Electroconvulsive therapy with severe depression (may precipitate hypomania)
- Light therapy if there is a seasonal component to depressive episodes (may precipitate hypomania)
- Modest evidence exists to support transcranial magnetic stimulation, vagal nerve stimulation, ketamine infusion, sleep deprivation, hormone therapy (e.g., thyroid) in bipolar depression

IN-PATIENT CONSIDERATIONS

If hypomanic symptoms are severe enough to necessitate hospitalization, the patient automatically meets criteria for mania and BP-I.

Admission Criteria/Initial Stabilization

To admit patients (>18 years) to a psychiatric unit involuntarily, they must have a psychiatric diagnosis (e.g., major depression) and present a danger to themselves or others, or their mental disease must be inhibiting them from providing their basic needs (e.g., food, clothing, shelter).

Nursing

Acute suicidal threats need closer observation.

Discharge Criteria

Determined by safety

ONGOING CARE

FOLLOW-UP RECOMMENDATIONS

- Regularly scheduled visits support treatment adherence.
- Frequent communication between primary care doctor, psychiatrist, and therapist ensures comprehensive care.

Patient Monitoring

Mood charts are helpful adjuncts to care.

PATIENT EDUCATION

- Support groups for patients and families are recommended.
- National Alliance on Mental Illness: www.nami.org/

PROGNOSIS

- Frequency and severity of problematic episodes are related to medication adherence, consistency with psychotherapy, sleep, support systems, regularity of daily activities, and social history.
- Substance abuse, unemployment, persistent depression, and male gender are associated with a worse prognosis.
- Although data are limited, evidence indicates that patients with BP-II may be at greater risk of both attempting and completing suicide than with BP-I and unipolar depression.

REFERENCES

1. Perlis RH, Brown E, Baker RW, et al. Clinical features of bipolar depression versus major depressive disorder in large multicenter trials. *Am J Psychiatry*. 2006;163:225–231.
2. Benazzi F. A prediction rule for diagnosing hypomania. *Prog Neuropsychopharmacol Biol Psychiatry*. 2009;33:317–322.
3. Hirshfeld RM. Validation of the mood disorder questionnaire. *Bipolar Depression Bulletin*. 2004.
4. Angst J, Adolfsson R, Benazzi F, et al. The HCL-32: Towards a self-assessment tool for hypomanic symptoms in outpatients. *J Affect Disord*. 2005;88:217–233.
5. Licht RW. A new BALANCE in bipolar I disorder. *Lancet*. 2010;375:350–352.

ADDITIONAL READING

Benazzi F. Bipolar disorder—focus on bipolar II disorder and mixed depression. *Lancet*. 2007;369: 935–945.

 SEE ALSO

Algorithm: Depressive Episode, Major

 CODES

ICD10

F31.81 Bipolar II disorder

CLINICAL PEARLS

- BP-II is characterized by at least 1 episode of major depression and 1 episode of hypomania.
- Patients are often resistant to treatment during a hypomanic episode, as they enjoy the elevated mood and productivity.
- Evidence indicates that patients with BP-II may be at greater risk of both attempting and completing suicide than with BP-I and unipolar depression.

BITES, ANIMAL AND HUMAN
Kathryn Samai, PharmD, BCPS • Brian Kimbrell, MD, FACS

BASICS

DESCRIPTION
- Animal bites to humans from dogs (60–90%), cats (5–20%), rodents (2–3%), humans (2–3%), and rarely other animals, including snakes
- System(s) affected: Potentially any

Pediatric Considerations
Young children are more likely to sustain bites, and have bites that include the face, upper extremity or trunk.

EPIDEMIOLOGY
- Predominant age: All ages, but children > adults
- Predominant gender: Dog bites, Male > Female; cat bites, Female > Male

Incidence
- 2–5 million animal bites per year in the US
- Account for 1% of all emergency room visits
- 1–2% will require hospital admission, and 10–20 victims will die from bites annually (1).

ETIOLOGY AND PATHOPHYSIOLOGY
- Most dog bite wounds are from a domestic pet known to the victim.
- 89% of cat bites are provoked.
- Males, pit bull terriers, and German shepherds are most commonly associated with dog bites (2).
- Human bites are often the result of 1 person striking another in the mouth with a clenched fist.
- Bites can also occur incidentally in the case of paronychia due to nail biting, or thumb sucking, or "love nips" to the face, breasts, or genital areas.
- Animal bites can cause tears, punctures, scratches, avulsions, or crush injuries.
- Contamination of wound with flora from the mouth of the biting animal or from the broken skin of the victim can lead to infection.

RISK FACTORS
- Male dogs and older dogs are more likely to bite.
- Clenched-fist human bites are frequently associated with the use of alcohol.
- Patients presenting >8 hours following the bite are at greater risk of infection.

GENERAL PREVENTION
- Instruct children and adults about animal hazards and strongly enforce animal control laws.
- Educate dog owners.

DIAGNOSIS

HISTORY
- Obtain detailed history of the incident (provoked or unprovoked).
- Type of animal
- Vaccine status
- Site of the bite
- Geographic setting

PHYSICAL EXAM
- Dog bites (60–90% of bites):
  - Hands and face most common site of injury in adults and children, respectively
  - More likely to have associated crush injury
- Cat bites (5–20% of bites):
  - Predominantly involve the hands, followed by lower extremities, face, and trunk
- Human bites (2–3% of bites):
  - Intentional bite: Semicircular or oval area of erythema and bruising, with or without break in skin
  - Clenched-fist injury: Small wounds over the metacarpophalangeal joints from striking the fist against another's teeth
- Signs of wound infection include fever, erythema, swelling, tenderness, purulent drainage, and lymphangitis.

ALERT
Cat bites (often puncture wounds) are twice as likely to cause infection as dog bites, with higher risks of osteomyelitis, tenosynovitis, and septic arthritis.

Pediatric Considerations
If human bite mark on child has intercanine distance >3 cm, bite probably came from an adult and should raise concerns about child abuse.

DIAGNOSTIC TESTS & INTERPRETATION
Initial Tests (lab, imaging)
- Drainage from infected wounds should be Gram-stained and cultured (3)[A]:
  - If wound fails to heal, perform cultures for atypical pathogens (fungi, Nocardia, and mycobacteria) and ask lab to keep bacterial cultures for 7–10 days (some pathogens are slow-growing).
- 85% of bite wounds will yield a positive culture, with an average of 5 pathogens.
- Aerobic and anaerobic blood cultures should be obtained before starting antibiotics if bacteremia suspected (e.g., fever or chills).
- Previous antibiotic therapy may alter culture results.
- If bite wound is near a bone or joint, a plain radiograph is needed to check for bone injury and to use for comparison later if osteomyelitis is subsequently suspected (3)[B].
- Radiographs are needed to check for fractures in clenched-fist injuries.

Follow-Up Tests & Special Considerations
Subsequent suspicion of osteomyelitis warrants comparison plain radiograph or MRI severe skull bites warrant a CT scan and ultrasound can be useful for detection of abscess.

Diagnostic Procedures/Other
Surgical exploration may be needed to ascertain extent of injuries or to drain deep infections (such as tendon sheath infections), especially in serious hand wounds.

Test Interpretation
- Dog bites (4,5):
  - Pasteurella sp. is present in 50% of bites.
  - Also found: Viridans streptococci, Staphylococcus aureus, Staphylococcus intermedius, Bacteroides, Capnocytophaga canimorsus, Fusobacterium
- Cat bites:
  - Pasteurella sp. is present in 75% of bites.
  - Also found: Streptococcus spp. (including Streptococcus pyogenes), Staphylococcus spp. (including methicillin-resistant Staphylococcus aureus [MRSA]), Fusobacterium spp., Bacteroides spp., Porphyromonas spp., Moraxella spp.
- Human bites:
  - Streptococcus spp., S. aureus, Eikenella corrodens (29%), and various anaerobic bacteria (e.g., Fusobacterium, Peptostreptococcus, Prevotella, and Porphyromonas spp.)
  - Although rare, case reports have suggested transmission of viruses such as hepatitis, HIV, and herpes simplex.
- Reptile bites:
  - If from a venomous snake, use antivenom. Bacteria: P. aeruginosa, Proteus spp., Salmonella, Bacteroides fragilis, and Clostridium spp.
- Rodent bites:
  - Streptobacillus moniliformis or Spirillum minor, which cause rat-bite fever
- Monkey bites:
  - All monkey bites can transmit rabies, and bites of a macaque monkey may transmit herpes B virus, which is potentially fatal. Providers should contact CDC and administer an antiviral, such as valacyclovir, active against herpes B virus.

ALERT
Asplenic patients and those with underlying hepatic disease are at risk of bacteremia and fatal sepsis after dog bites infected with Capnocytophaga canimorsus (gram-negative rod).

TREATMENT

GENERAL MEASURES
- Elevation of the injured extremity to prevent swelling
- Contact the local health department regarding the prevalence of rabies in the species of animal involved (highest in bats).
- Snake bite: If venomous, patient needs rapid transport to facility capable of definitive evaluation. If envenomation has occurred, patient should receive antivenom. Be sure patient is stable for transport; consider measuring and/or treating coagulation and renal status along with any anaphylactic reactions before transport.

MEDICATION
- Consider need for antirabies therapy: Rabies immunoglobulin and human diploid cell rabies vaccine for those bitten by wild animals (in the US, primary vector is bat bite), rabid pets, or unvaccinated pets, or if animal cannot be quarantined for 10 days (3)[A].
- Tetanus toxoid for those previously immunized, but >5 years since their last dose; tetanus immunoglobulin and tetanus vaccination in patients without a full primary series of immunizations (6)[A]

- A patient negative for anti-HBs antibodies and bitten by an HBsAg-positive individual should receive both hepatitis B immunoglobulin (HBIG) and hepatitis B vaccine.
- HIV postexposure prophylaxis is generally not recommended for human bites, given the extremely low risk for transmission.

- Prophylactic antibiotics are only recommended for human bites and high risk wounds (deep puncture, crush injury, venous or lymphatic compromise, hands or near joint, face or genital area, immunocompromised hosts, requiring surgical repair) (3,7)[A].
- For prophylaxis and for empiric treatment of established infection, amoxicillin-clavulanate is first-line (3)[B]:
  – Adults: 875 mg PO b.i.d.
  – Children: <3 months: 30 mg/kg/d PO q12h; ≥3 months and <40 kg: 45 mg/kg/d q12h; >40 kg, use adult dosing
    ○ Adverse reaction: Amoxicillin-clavulanate should be given with food to decrease GI side effects.
    ○ Precautions: Dose antibiotics by body weight and renal function.
    ○ Significant possible interactions: Antibiotics may decrease efficacy of oral contraceptives.
  – Duration of therapy: Prophylaxis, 3–5 days; treatment of cellulitis/skin abscess, 5–10 days; bacteremia, 10–14 days:
    ○ Adults: Clindamycin (300–450 mg PO t.i.d.) plus either:
    ○ Trimethoprim-sulfamethoxazole (TMP-SMX; 1 DS tablet PO b.i.d.–t.i.d.) or
    ○ Ciprofloxacin (500 mg PO b.i.d.) (3)[B] for 7–21 days
    ○ Children: Clindamycin (5–10 mg/kg IV [to a maximum of 600 mg] followed by 10–30 mg/kg/d in 3–4 divided doses to a maximum of 300 mg per dose) plus
    ○ TMP-SMX (8–10 mg/kg/d of trimethoprim) in 2 divided doses
- Avoid 1st-generation cephalosporins (e.g., cephalexin), penicillinase-resistant penicillins (e.g., dicloxacillin), macrolides (e.g., erythromycin), and clindamycin (when not administered with another agent) as they lack activity against *P. multocida* (dog/cat bites) and *Eikenella corrodens* (human bites) (3)[B].

Pregnancy Considerations
- Penicillin-allergic pregnant women:
  – Azithromycin 250–500 mg PO every day (3)[B]
- Observe closely and note potential increased risk of failure.

ALERT
Consider community-acquired MRSA as possible pathogen (from human skin or colonized pet). If high suspicion, doxycycline or TMP-SMX provide good coverage (6)[A].

ISSUES FOR REFERRAL
- Deep wounds to the hand and face should be referred to a hand surgeon or plastic surgeon, respectively.
- Bites from primates or unusual species of animals should be referred to infectious disease specialist.

SURGERY/OTHER PROCEDURES
- Copious irrigation of the wound with normal saline via a catheter tip is needed to reduce risk of infection.

- Devitalized tissue needs débridement.
- Débridement of puncture wounds is not advised.
- Primary closure can be considered if the wound is clean after irrigation and bite is <12 hours old, and in bites to the face (cosmesis).
- Infected wounds and those at risk of infection (cat bites, human bites, bites to the hand, crush injuries, presentation >12 hours from injury) should be left open (8)[B].
- Delayed primary closure in 3–5 days is an option for infected wounds.
- Splint hand if it is injured.
- Large, gaping wounds should be reapproximated with widely spaced sutures or Steri-Strips.

IN-PATIENT CONSIDERATIONS
Admission Criteria/Initial Stabilization
- Patients with deep or severe wound infections, systemic infections requiring IV antibiotics, those requiring surgery, and the immunocompromised ABCs for associated trauma or severe infection
  – Adults: Ampicillin/Sulbactam 3 g IV q6h or piperacillin/tazobactam 3.375 g q6h or 4.5 g IV q8h or ticarcillin/clavulanate 3.1 g IV q4h (3)[B]
- If hospitalized with established infection (animal or human bite) (3)[B]:
  – Alternative: Ciprofloxacin 400 mg IV q12h or levofloxacin 500 mg IV every day with metronidazole 500 mg IV q8h
  – Children: Ampicillin/Sulbactam 200 mg/kg/d IV given in 4 divided doses to maximum of 3 g per dose

Discharge Criteria
Pending clinical improvement

 ## ONGOING CARE

FOLLOW-UP RECOMMENDATIONS
Patient Monitoring
- Patient should be rechecked in 24–48 hours if not infected at time of 1st encounter (9)[B].
- Daily follow-up is warranted for infections.
- Subsequent revisions of empiric antibiotic therapy should be based on culture results and clinical response.

PATIENT EDUCATION
- Educate parents at well-child checks about how to avoid animal bites.
- AAFP: http://familydoctor.org/online/famdocen/home/healthy/safety/kids-family/668.html
- CDC: http://www.cdc.gov/HomeandRecreational Safety/Dog-Bites/index.html

PROGNOSIS
Wounds should steadily improve and close over by 7–10 days.

COMPLICATIONS
- Septic arthritis
- Osteomyelitis
- Extensive soft tissue injuries with scarring
- Hemorrhage
- Gas gangrene
- Sepsis
- Meningitis
- Endocarditis
- Posttraumatic stress disorder
- Death

REFERENCES

1. Goldstein EJ. New horizons in the bacteriology, antimicrobial suseptability and therapy of animal bite wounds. *J Med Microbiol*. 1998;47–95.
2. Wiley JF. Mammalian bites. Review of evaluation and management. *Clin Pediatr (Phila)*. 1990;29(5): 283–287.
3. Stevens DL, Bisno AL, Chambers HF, et al. Practice guidelines for the diagnosis and management of skin and soft-tissue infections. *Clin Infect Dis*. 2005;41:1373–1406.
4. Bini JK, Cohn SM, Acosta SM, et al. Mortality, mauling, and maiming by vicious dogs. *Ann Surg*. 2011;253:791–797.
5. Abrahamian FM, Goldstein EJ. Microbiology of animal bite wound infections. *Clin Microbiol Rev*. 2011;24:231–246.
6. Oehler RL, Velez AP, Mizrachi M, et al. Bite-related and septic syndromes caused by cats and dogs. *Lancet Infect Dis*. 2009;9:439–447.
7. Medeiros I. Antibiotic prophylaxis for mammalian bites. *Cochrane Database Syst Rev*. 2008;2: CD001738.
8. Benson LS, Edwards SL, Schiff AP, et al. Dog and cat bites to the hand: Treatment and cost assessment. *J Hand Surg [Am]*. 2006;31:468–473.
9. Okonkwo U. Animal bites: Practical tips for effective management. *J Emerg Nursing*. 2008;34(3): 225–226.

ADDITIONAL READING

Rittner AV, Fitzpatrick K, Corfield A. Best evidence topic report. Are antibiotics indicated following human bites? *Emerg Med J*. 2005;22:654.

 ## SEE ALSO

Cellulitis; Rabies; Snake Envenomations; Bartonella Infections

 ## CODES

ICD10
- S01.85XA Open bite of other part of head, initial encounter
- S20.97XA Other superficial bite of unspecified parts of thorax, initial encounter
- S61.459A Open bite of unspecified hand, initial encounter

CLINICAL PEARLS

- Wound cleansing, débridement, and culture are essential. Most wounds should be left open.
- Prophylaxis is recommended for human bites and high risk wounds.
- Consider rabies and tetanus vaccination.
- Antibiotic and duration of therapy should be adjusted based on culture results and clinical improvement.
- Patients bitten by animals or humans require close follow-up to monitor for infection.

BLADDER CANCER

Margaret E. Thompson, MD

 BASICS

DESCRIPTION
- Primary malignant neoplasms arising in the urinary bladder
- Most common type is transitional cell carcinoma (90%)
- Other types include adenocarcinoma, small cell carcinoma, squamous cell carcinoma.
- Rhabdomyosarcoma of the bladder may occur in children.

EPIDEMIOLOGY
Incidence
- Increases with age (median age at diagnosis is 73 years)
- More common in Caucasians than in Asians or African Americans
- Male > Female (4:1), but in smokers, risk is 1:1
- 36.60/100,000 men per year (1)
- 8.9/100,000 women per year (1)
- 20.7/100,000 men and women per year (1)

Prevalence
As of January 1, 2010, 563,640 cases in the US (1)

ETIOLOGY AND PATHOPHYSIOLOGY
Unknown, other than related to risk factors:
- 70–80% is superficial (in lamina propria or mucosa):
  - Usually highly differentiated with long survival
  - Initial event seems to be activation of an oncogene on chromosome 9 in superficial cancers.
- 20% of tumors are invasive (deeper than lamina propria) at presentation:
  - Tend to be high grade with worse prognosis
  - Associated with other chromosome deletions

Genetics
Hereditary transmission is unlikely, although transitional cell carcinoma pathophysiology is related to oncogenes.

RISK FACTORS
- Smoking is the single greatest risk factor (increases risk 4-fold) and increases risk equally for men and women (2).
- Recent studies have demonstrated an increased risk of bladder cancer in patients with type 2 diabetes who take pioglitazone for >1 year. The risk seems to increase with duration of therapy, and may also be present with other thiazolidinediones (3).
- Other risk factors:
  - Occupational carcinogens in dye, rubber, paint, plastics, metal, and automotive exhaust
  - Schistosomiasis in Mediterranean (squamous cell) cancer
  - Arsenic in well water
  - History of pelvic irradiation
  - Chronic lower UTI
  - Chronic indwelling urinary catheter
  - Cyclophosphamide exposure
  - High-fat diet
  - Chronic low fluid intake
  - Slight increase in risk with prostate cancer

ALERT
Any patient who smokes and presents with microscopic or gross hematuria, or irritative voiding symptoms such as urgency and frequency not clearly due to UTI, should be evaluated by cystoscopy for the presence of a bladder neoplasm.

GENERAL PREVENTION
- Avoid smoking and other risk factors.
- The US Preventive Services Task Force has concluded there is insufficient evidence to determine the balance between risk and harm of screening for bladder cancer.

 DIAGNOSIS

HISTORY
- Painless hematuria is most common symptom.
- Urinary symptoms (frequency, urgency)
- Abdominal or pelvic pain in advanced disease
- Exposures (see "Risk Factors")

PHYSICAL EXAM
Normal in early cases, pelvic or abdominal mass in advanced disease, wasting in systemic disease

DIFFERENTIAL DIAGNOSIS
- Other urinary tract neoplasms
- UTI
- Prostatism
- Bladder instability
- Interstitial cystitis
- Urolithiasis
- Interstitial nephritis
- Papillary urothelial hyperplasia

DIAGNOSTIC TESTS & INTERPRETATION
Initial Tests (lab, imaging)
- Urinalysis is the initial test in patients presenting with gross hematuria or urinary symptoms such as frequency, urgency, and dysuria.
- Cystoscopy with biopsy is the gold standard for at-risk patients with painless hematuria.
- Macroscopic hematuria (55% sensitivity, positive predictive value [PPV] 0.22 for urologic cancer) (4)[C]

Follow-Up Tests & Special Considerations
- Urine cytology: 54% sensitivity overall (lower in less advanced tumors), 94% specific (5)[A]
- Other urine markers:

  - NMP22: 67% sensitive, 78% specific (5)[A]
  - Bladder tumor-associated antigen stat: 70% sensitive, 75% specific (5)[A]
  - Fluorescent in situ hybridization assay: 69% sensitive, 78% specific (PPV 27.1, negative predictive value 95.3) for all tumors, more sensitive and specific for higher grade (6)[B]
  - Circulating tumor cell (CTC) assays are more likely to detect advanced bladder cancer than superficial disease (sensitivity 35.1%, specificity 89.4%, LR+ 3.77, LR- 0.72), but not valuable as a screening test (7)[A].

- *Bottom line: None of the urine markers is sensitive enough to rule out bladder cancer on its own.*
- Liver function tests, alkaline phosphatase if metastasis suspected
- Done for staging and to evaluate extent of disease, but not for diagnosis itself:
  - CT urogram replacing IVP to image upper tracts if there is suspicion of disease there
  - Diffusion-weighted MRI and multidimensional CT scan are undergoing study for use in diagnosis and staging of bladder tumors.

- For invasive disease, metastatic workup should include chest x-ray.

- Bone scan should be performed if the patient has bone pain or if alkaline phosphatase is elevated (8)[B].
- Urologic CT scan (abdomen, pelvis, with and without contrast) or MRI (40–98% accurate), with MRI slightly more accurate (8)[B], is recommended if metastasis is suspected.
- Regular cystoscopy (initiated at 3 months postprocedure) is indicated after transurethral resection of superficial tumor (TURBT) and intravesical chemotherapy for superficial bladder cancers.

Diagnostic Procedures/Other
- Cystoscopy with biopsy is the gold standard for diagnosis, but 1 study showed that 33% of patients had residual tumor after TURBT (8)[B].
- Using photodynamic diagnosis (PDD; employing a photosensitizing agent in the bladder that is taken up by tumor cells and visualized using a particular wavelength of light, which is changed to a different wavelength by the photosensitizing agent) has been shown to increase detection and identification of cancerous superficial tumors when compared with plain white-light cystoscopy. A recent meta-analysis shows that this increases the likelihood of total resection (9)[A].
- TURBT with bladder washings: Sensitivity of cytology on bladder washings for carcinoma in situ is nearly 100%.

Test Interpretation
- Characterized as superficial or invasive
- 70–80% present as superficial lesion
- Superficial lesions:
  - Carcinoma in situ: Flat lesion, high grade
  - Ta: Noninvasive papillary carcinoma
  - T1: Extends into submucosa, lamina propria
- Invasive cancer:
  - T2: Invasion into muscle:
    - pT2a: Invasion into superficial muscle
    - pT2b: Invasion into deep muscle
  - T3: Invasion into perivesical fat:
    - pT3a: Microscopic
    - pT3b: Macroscopic
  - T4: Invasion into adjacent organs:
    - aT4a: Invades prostate, uterus, or vagina
    - aT4b: Invades abdominal or pelvic wall
  - N1–N3: Invades lymph nodes
- M: Metastasis to bone or soft tissue

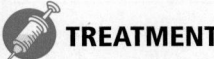 **TREATMENT**

For superficial bladder cancer, the treatment is generally removal via cystoscopic surgery (see above, re: PDD). For muscle-invasive cancer, a radical cystectomy is preferred.

MEDICATION
First Line
- A recent meta-analysis demonstrated neoadjuvant chemotherapy using platinum-based combination chemotherapy (with ≥1 of doxorubicin/epirubicin, methotrexate, or vinblastine), but not platinum alone, confers a significant survival advantage in patients with invasive bladder cancer, with an increase in survival at 5 years from 45% (without neoadjuvant treatment) to 50% (with treatment) (combined hazard ratio 0.86, 95% CI 0.77–0.95) (10)[A].
- Intravesical bacillus Calmette-Guérin (BCG) after TURBT in high-grade lesions has been shown to decrease recurrence in Ta and T1 tumors (11)[A].
- Intravesical BCG has been shown to be superior in efficacy to intravesical epirubicin in preventing recurrence of tumor in Ta and T1 tumors (12)[B].

Second Line
- Chemotherapy is the 1st-line treatment for metastatic bladder cancer:
  - Methotrexate-vinblastine-doxorubicin-cisplatin (MVAC) is the preferred regimen.
- A recent review showed that gemcitabine plus cisplatin may be better tolerated and result in equivalent survival to MVAC, making it a possible 1st choice in metastatic bladder cancer.

ISSUES FOR REFERRAL
Patients with microscopic or gross hematuria not otherwise explained or resolving should be referred to a urologist for cystoscopy.

ADDITIONAL THERAPIES
Radiotherapy:
- In the US, used for patients with muscle-invasive cancer who are not surgical candidates
- Preoperative (radical cystectomy) radiotherapy also an option
- Treatment of choice for muscle-invasive cancer in some European and Canadian centers:
  - 65–70 Gy over 6–7 weeks is standard.

SURGERY/OTHER PROCEDURES
- Surgery is definitive therapy for superficial and invasive cancer:
  - Superficial cancer: TURBT sometimes followed by intravesical therapy
- Invasive cancer:
  - Radical cystectomy for invasive disease that is confined to the bladder is more effective than radical radiotherapy. Urine is diverted via an ileal loop with ostomy or neobladder constructed with intestine.

IN-PATIENT CONSIDERATIONS
Admission Criteria/Initial Stabilization
Need for surgery or intensive therapy

 ONGOING CARE

FOLLOW-UP RECOMMENDATIONS
- Superficial cancers:
  - Urine cytology alone has not been shown to be sufficient for follow-up.
  - Cystoscopy every 3 months for 18–24 months, every 6 months for the next 2 years, then annually
- Follow-up for invasive cancers depends on the approach to treatment.
- Patients treated with BCG require lifelong follow-up.

DIET
Continue adequate fluid intake.

PATIENT EDUCATION
Smoking cessation

PROGNOSIS
- 5-year relative survival rates:
  - Overall survival: 77.7%
    - Localized: 93.7%
    - Regional metastasis: 46.0%
    - Distant metastasis: 6.2%
- Superficial bladder cancer:
  - BCG treatment prevents recurrence vs. TURBT alone; difference 30%, NNT 3.3
  - BCG prevents progression vs. TURBT alone, difference 8%
- Invasive cancer:
  - T2 disease: Radical cystectomy results in 60–75% 5-year survival.
  - T3 or T4 disease: Radical cystectomy results in 20–40% 5-year survival.
  - Neoadjuvant chemotherapy with cystectomy has led to varying degrees of increased survival.
  - Radiation with chemotherapy has led to varying degrees of increased survival.
- Metastatic cancer:
  - MVAC resulted in mean survival of 12.5 months.

COMPLICATIONS
- Superficial bladder cancer:
  - Local symptoms:
    - Dysuria, frequency, nocturia, pain, passing debris in urine
    - Bacterial cystitis
    - Perforation
  - General symptoms:
    - Flulike symptoms
    - Systemic infection
- Invasive cancer:
  - Symptoms related to definitive treatment, including incontinence, bleeding
  - Patients with neobladder at risk for azotemia and metabolic acidosis

REFERENCES

1. Howlander N, Noone AM, Krapcho M, et al. (eds.). SEER Cancer Statistics Review, 1975–2010, National Cancer Institute. Bethesda, MD. http://seer.cancer.gov/csr/1975_2010/, based on November 2012 SEER data submission, posted to the SEER web site, 2013.
2. Freedman N. Association between smoking and risk of bladder cancer among men and women. JAMA. 2011;306(7):737–745.
3. Zhu Z, Shen Z, Lu Y, et al. Increased risk of bladder cancer with pioglitazone therapy in patients with diabetes: a meta-analysis. Diabetes Res Clin Pract. 2012;98:159–163.
4. Buntinx F, Wauters H. The diagnostic value of macroscopic haematuria in diagnosing urological cancers: A meta-analysis. Fam Pract. 1997;14: 63–68.
5. Glas AS, Roos D, Deutekom M, et al. Tumor markers in the diagnosis of primary bladder cancer. A systematic review. J Urol. 2003;169: 1975–1982.
6. Sarosdy MF, Kahn PR, Ziffer MD, et al. Use of a multitarget fluorescence in situ hybridization assay to diagnose bladder cancer in patients with hematuria. J Urol. 2006;176:44–47.
7. Msaouel P, Koutsilieris M. Diagnostic value of circulating tumor cell detection in bladder and urothelial cancer: Systematic review and meta-analysis. BMC Cancer. 2011;11:336. Epub 2011 Aug 4.
8. Kirkali Z, Chan T, Manoharan M, et al. Bladder cancer: Epidemiology, staging and grading, and diagnosis. Urology. 2005;66:4–34.
9. Mowatt G, N'Dow J, Vale L, et al. Photodynamic diagnosis of bladder cancer compared with white light cystoscopy: Systematic review and meta-analysis. Int J Technol Assess Health Care. 2011;27:3–10.
10. Advanced Bladder Cancer Meta-analysis Collaboration. Neoadjuvant chemotherapy for advanced bladder cancer (Cochrane Review). In: Cochrane Library Issue 2, 2012. Chichester, UK: John Wiley and Sons, Ltd.
11. Shelley M, Court JB, Kynaston H, et al. Intravesical Bacillus Calmette-Guerin in Ta and T1 bladder cancer (Cochrane Review). In: Cochrane Library, Issue 3, 2010. Chichester, UK: John Wiley and Sons, Ltd.
12. Shang PF, Kwong J, Chang CP, et al. Intravesical Bacillus Calmette-Guerin versus epirubicin for Ta and T1 bladder cancer. Cochrane Database Syst Rev. 2011;11:5.

ADDITIONAL READING
Sharma S, Ksheersagar P, Sharma P. Diagnosis and treatment of bladder cancer. Am Fam Physician. 2009;80(7):717–723.

 SEE ALSO
- Hematuria
- Algorithm: Hematuria

 CODES

ICD10
- C67.3 Malignant neoplasm of anterior wall of bladder
- C67.4 Malignant neoplasm of posterior wall of bladder
- C67.9 Malignant neoplasm of bladder, unspecified

CLINICAL PEARLS
- Painless hematuria in smokers should be evaluated with cystoscopy.
- Be aware of potential link between pioglitazone treatment and risk for bladder cancer
- The US Preventive Services Task Force recommends against routine screening for bladder cancer.

BLADDER INJURY

Jeffrey Villaneuva, MD • Krishnan Venkatesan, MD

 BASICS

DESCRIPTION
- Bladder injury results from:
  - Blunt or penetrating trauma
  - Surgical iatrogenic injury
- Rupture is classified as intraperitoneal (urine leak into the peritoneal cavity) or extraperitoneal (urine leak outside of the peritoneal space), or both.
- May be associated with ureter/urethral injury
- Spontaneous rupture is extremely rare (1)

EPIDEMIOLOGY
Incidence
- ~0.5% of civilian trauma patients
- Often secondary to blunt trauma (usually in the context of an overdistended bladder)
- 10% of pelvic fractures can be associated with bladder injury (2).
- 90% of bladder injuries in the context of pelvic fracture have concomitant gross hematuria, the other 10% can exhibit clinically significant microscopic hematuria (3).
- During pelvic surgery, the bladder is a commonly injured organ (4).

ETIOLOGY AND PATHOPHYSIOLOGY
- Bladder rupture is usually caused either by blunt force pelvic injury during high-energy trauma (MVAs, falls), penetrating pelvic trauma, or penetrating objects (gunshot wound, knife, other projectile).
- Surgical iatrogenic injury also occurs during gynecology, general surgery, urology, and other procedures.
- Bladder overdistention in the context of blunt abdominal pressure can lead to an intraperitoneal rupture at the bladder dome (4).
- Pelvic bone fracture can lead to an extraperitoneal bladder wall tear (5).
- Penetrating trauma can result in either intraperitoneal or extraperitoneal bladder injury.
- After a major intraperitoneal bladder rupture, urine and blood can be reabsorbed from the peritoneal cavity, leading to metabolic abnormalities, including metabolic acidosis, low bicarbonate, uremia, and elevated chloride.

RISK FACTORS
- High-energy mechanism (fall, MVA)
- Pelvic fracture
- Penetrating wound (abdomen/pelvis)
- Prior bladder/pelvic surgery
- Prior pelvic radiotherapy

GENERAL PREVENTION
- Seat belts
- Voiding prior to driving

COMMONLY ASSOCIATED CONDITIONS
- Pelvic fracture
- Ureteral injury
- Urethral injury

DIAGNOSIS

HISTORY
- Isolated bladder injury in the context of blunt or penetrating trauma is rare. Typically, the patient has other serious traumatic injuries such as injured bowel or fractured pelvis.
- High-mechanism deceleration injury (fall, MVA)
- Penetrating trauma
- Abdominal/pelvic surgery
- Urinary retention
- Pre-existing bladder outlet obstruction or bladder atony
- Pelvic anatomical abnormalities:
  - Gross hematuria in context of clinical scenario consistent with bladder injury (mechanism) should always prompt an investigation for bladder rupture.
  - Clinician should consider the possibility of associated urethral injury in appropriate clinical context such as pelvic fracture.

PHYSICAL EXAM
- Abdominal exam: Suprapubic tenderness and/or distention, guarding or other signs of peritonitis, abdominal ecchymosis, decreased bowel sounds
- Genitourinary exam: Blood at the urethral meatus, gross hematuria, scrotal or perineal ecchymosis/hematoma, free-floating/high-riding/absent prostate on digital rectal examination, unstable pelvis

ALERT
Peritonitis is unusual in bladder injury, but may occur in the context of intraperitoneal bladder rupture.

DIFFERENTIAL DIAGNOSIS
- Urethral injury
- Ureteral injury
- Renal injury
- Other visceral trauma

DIAGNOSTIC TESTS & INTERPRETATION
Initial Tests (lab, imaging)
- Urinalysis generally demonstrates blood
- Basic metabolic profile, CBC, coagulation panel, beta-HCG pregnancy test (age-appropriate females)
- Serum BUN, creatinine, chloride, and potassium levels may be elevated, and sodium and bicarbonate may be decreased in intraperitoneal ruptures secondary to peritoneal absorption of urine. An increase in the BUN to creatinine ratio may be observed secondary to postrenal azotemia (3).

Follow-Up Tests & Special Considerations
- If blood is found at the urethral meatus, a high-riding or absent prostate gland is found on digital rectal examination (DRE), or if there is a mechanism of trauma that suggests urethral injury (i.e., pelvic fracture), the clinician should consider retrograde urethrography as a critical component of the initial evaluation (3).

- 2 types of imaging are acceptable:
  - CT cystogram or gravity cystogram: Bladder should be filled to physiologic capacity. For gravity cystogram, use 3-film technique: (i) Before contrast; (ii) after contrast instillation; and (iii) after bladder drainage (2).
    - Contusion: No extravasation, but with possible distortion of the bladder outline with contrast
    - Intraperitoneal: Contrast may be seen in cul-de-sac and paracolic gutters. Bowel loops may also be outlined.
    - Extraperitoneal: Flame-shaped perivesical stranding of contrast
  - CT cystography should be performed if the patient is undergoing a CT scan for other injuries (3).

ALERT
- Absolute indication for immediate cystography: Gross hematuria with a pelvic fracture, penetrating pelvic trauma or other mechanism of bladder injury
- Relative indications: Microhematuria with a pelvic fracture, penetrating pelvic trauma or other mechanism of bladder injury (1)

ALERT
During plain film cystography, a drainage view is mandatory as contrast in the bladder may mask extravasation (2).

- Retrograde urethrography *must* be performed before placing a Foley catheter when urethral injury is suspected (3).
- Other indicators of potential bladder injury can include free intraperitoneal fluid on CT scan or ultrasound.

Test Interpretation
- Pelvic hematoma
- Perforation at dome of bladder (blunt force bladder trauma with full bladder)
- Jagged tear in bladder (pelvic fracture, penetrating trauma)
- Intraoperative clues (4):
  - Appearance of Foley catheter/balloon or urine in the operative field
  - Presence of gas in the catheter bag (during laparoscopy)

TREATMENT

- Contusion: Observation; consider indwelling Foley catheter for several days
- Intraperitoneal rupture:
  - Immediate surgical repair
  - Indwelling catheter (20–24 French Foley catheter) for 7–14 days (variable based on clinical decision making)
  - Suprapubic tube may also be used, based on intraoperative decision making, such as concomitant urethral injury (1)
  - Iatrogenic intraoperative bladder injury falls under this heading and should be repaired immediately.
- Extraperitoneal rupture:
  - Indwelling catheter (20–24 French Foley catheter) for 7–14 days (variable based on clinical decision making) only after evaluation for a urethral injury has been performed (3).
  - In some cases, extraperitoneal bladder injury may be repaired immediately if patient is to go to the *or* for management of other associated injuries, particularly if there are bone fragments in bladder, open pelvic fracture, or associated rectal perforations (1):
    - Foley catheter times are variable and dependent on degree of bladder injury, the management of other concomitant injuries and comorbidities, and physician clinical judgment.

MEDICATION
- Analgesics
- Antibiotics
- Antispasmodics

First Line
- Narcotic pain control titrated to effect
- Antibiotics: Consider anaerobic and other coverage, depending on mechanism of trauma and associated injuries.
- Antispasmodics for bladder spasm

Pediatric Considerations
Bladders are intra-abdominal organs in children and are not protected by the bony pelvis as are bladders in adults.

ISSUES FOR REFERRAL
A urologist or trauma surgeon should be involved with all bladder injury management.

ADDITIONAL THERAPIES
- Exception: In pediatric patients, consider placing a suprapubic catheter because small catheters through the urethra may drain poorly or become obstructed and larger catheters through the urethra increase the risk for urethral stricture development (2):
  - A catheter should remain in place for 1–2 weeks (variable)
- Complicated extraperitoneal bladder rupture:
  - Should be managed with an open repair if the patient is hemodynamically stable enough for the *or*
  - Complicated rupture is considered when there is coexisting bladder neck injury, vaginal injury, rectal injury, or open pelvic fracture/bone fragments are present within the bladder lumen.
  - Consider open repair if the patient is scheduled for an exploratory laparotomy or internal fixation of an associated pelvic fracture (2).

- During pelvic surgery, iatrogenic full-thickness bladder injury can be fixed immediately with a 2-layer (mucosa and muscularis) closure using absorbable sutures:
  - Prior to repair, be sure to confirm ureters were not damaged concomitantly either with IV indigo carmine administration and visualization of blue dye expulsion from the ureteral orifices (UO) or by confirming easy placement of ureteral catheters through the UO (4).
  - In some instances, "on table" IV pyelography or retrograde pyelography may be considered to evaluate the ureters for associated injury.
- Cystography should be considered after operative bladder repair:
  - Cystography is necessary prior to removal of the Foley catheter to document bladder healing and the stability of any associated repair.

IN-PATIENT CONSIDERATIONS
Admission Criteria/Initial Stabilization
All patients with bladder injuries require admission for monitoring of renal function and other laboratory values (i.e., hematocrit), the assessment and of other associated injuries, and the maintenance of hemodynamic stability:
- Cervical spine precautions:
  - Stabilize respiratory status and hemodynamics
  - Stabilize pelvis
  - Follow Advanced Trauma Life Support protocols

Nursing
- Foley to gravity/management of hematuria
- Hourly urine output recorded

 ONGOING CARE

COMPLICATIONS
- Infection
- Urine leak and/or urinoma formation
- Abscess formation
- Peritonitis or sepsis
- Fistula formation
- Stricture: Rare complication of isolated bladder rupture
- Death; cited as 10–34%, most commonly from polytrauma (1)

REFERENCES

1. Matlock KA, Tyroch AH, Kronfol ZN, et al. Blunt traumatic bladder rupture: A 10-year perspective. *Am Surg.* 2013;79:589–593.
2. Kessler DO, Francis DL, Esernio-Jenssen D. Bladder rupture after minor accidental trauma: Case reports and a review of the literature. *Pediatr Emerg Care.* 2010;26:43–45.
3. Nakamura LY, Ferrigni RG, Stone WM, et al. Urinary bladder injuries during vascular surgery. *J Vasc Surg.* 2010;52:453–455.

4. Sharp HT, Swenson C. Hollow viscus injury during surgery. *Obstet Gynecol Clin North Am.* 2010;37:461–467.
5. Melo EL, de Menezes MR, Cerri GG. Abdominal gunshot wounds: Multi-detector-row CT findings compared with laparotomy: A prospective study. *Emerg Radiol.* 2012;19:35–41.

ADDITIONAL READING

Tonkin JB, Tisdale BE, Jordan GH. Assessment and initial management of urologic trauma. *Med Clin North Am.* 2011;95:245–251.

 SEE ALSO

Algorithm: Hematuria

CODES

ICD10
- S37.20XA Unspecified injury of bladder, initial encounter
- S37.22XA Contusion of bladder, initial encounter
- S37.29XA Other injury of bladder, initial encounter

CLINICAL PEARLS
- The Foley should remain in place for at least 7–14 days after bladder repair. After this point, ~85% of patients will have healed bladder injuries.
- A cystogram must be performed before Foley removal to verify no extravasation of fluid. If extravasation continues, recheck periodically until extravasation has resolved prior to catheter or suprapubic tube removal.
- An immediate intraoperative urology consult is indicated if an inadvertent bladder perforation occurs during another procedure. The bladder should be examined intravesically to evaluate for other associated injuries (i.e., ureteral orifices, bladder neck). Repair should not be delayed.
- Repair bladder injuries in 2 layers with absorbable sutures and place a Foley catheter. Consider suprapubic tube and pelvic drain placement after repair of the primary injury, as clinically indicated.

BLEPHARITIS
Mary Lauren Worthen, MD • Adrian Worthen • David Worthen

 BASICS

DESCRIPTION
- An inflammatory reaction of the eyelid margin:
  - Usually occurs as seborrheic or staphylococcal blepharitis
  - Multiple types may coexist
  - Itchiness, redness, flaking, and crusting of the eyelids
  - Categorization:
    ○ Based on the length of disease process: Acute or chronic
    ○ Anatomical location of disease: anterior (e.g., staphylococcal and seborrheic blepharitis), posterior (e.g., meibomian gland dysfunction), parasitic, or mixed
- System(s) affected: Skin/Exocrine
- Synonym(s): Granulated eyelids

EPIDEMIOLOGY
Incidence
- Very common
- All ethnic groups
- Predominant age: Adult
- Predominant sex: Male = Female

RISK FACTORS
- Seborrheic dermatitis
- Contact dermatitis
- Herpes simplex dermatitis
- Varicella-zoster dermatitis
- Acne rosacea
- Diabetes mellitus
- Immunocompromised state (e.g., AIDS, chemotherapy)
- Isotretinoin use
- Dry eye syndromes

ETIOLOGY AND PATHOPHYSIOLOGY
- Seborrheic:
  - Accelerated shedding of skin cells with associated sebaceous gland dysfunction
  - *Malassezia furfur* (formerly *Pityrosporum ovale*)
- Staphylococcal:
  - Superinfection of Zeis glands of lid margin and meibomian glands posterior to lashes with *Staphylococcus aureus*
  - Usually part of mixed blepharitis
- Meibomian gland dysfunction: Obstruction and inflammation of the meibomian glands; associated with acne rosacea, acne vulgaris, and oral retinoid therapy

- Other types of blepharitis:
  - Ulcerative blepharitis: More severe blepharitis with small marginal ulceration and destruction of the hair follicles
  - Contact dermatitis/blepharitis:
    ○ Develops from type IV hypersensitivity; common causes include ocular medications, topical anesthetics, antivirals, and cosmetics
    ○ May occur with secondary *Staphylococcus* infection
  - Eczematoid blepharitis:
    ○ Caused by type I hypersensitivity reaction to exotoxins and antigens from local flora
    ○ Strong association with eczema, asthma
    ○ Staphylococcal infection common
  - Angular blepharitis: Often caused by *Staphylococcus* or *Moraxella* infection
- The exact etiopathogenesis is unknown.
- Suspected to be multifactorial:
  - Chronic low-grade infections of the ocular surface with bacteria
  - Infestations with certain parasites such as the mite, *Demodex*
  - Inflammatory skin conditions such as atopy and seborrhea

COMMONLY ASSOCIATED CONDITIONS
See "Risk Factors" and "Differential Diagnosis."

 DIAGNOSIS

HISTORY
- Duration of symptoms
- Unilateral or bilateral presentation
- Note any exacerbating conditions (e.g., smoke, allergens, wind, contact lenses).
- Symptoms related to systemic diseases
- Current and recent medication use
- Recent exposure to infected individuals
- Frequently reported in all types of blepharitis:
  - Burning
  - Itching
  - Eyelid erythema
  - Conjunctival infection (red eyes)
  - Lacrimation, tearing
  - Tear deficiency
  - Foreign-body sensation
  - Photophobia (light sensitivity)
  - Impaired vision

PHYSICAL EXAM
- Test of visual acuity
- External exam (skin and eyelids):
  - Staphylococcal:
    ○ Recurrent stye (external or internal hordeolum)
    ○ Missing, broken, or misdirected eyelashes (trichiasis)
    ○ Eyelid deposits: Matted, hard scales; collarettes (ringlike formation around the lash shaft)
    ○ Ulcerations at base of eyelashes (rare)
    ○ Eyelid scarring may occur
  - Seborrheic blepharitis:
    ○ Eyelid deposits: Dry flakes; oily or greasy secretions on lid margins and/or lashes
    ○ Associated dandruff of scalp, eyebrows
  - Meibomian gland dysfunction:
    ○ Eyelash misdirection may occur with long-standing disease.
    ○ Eyelid deposits: Fatty deposits; may be foamy
    ○ Eyelid margin thickening
    ○ Plugged meibomian gland orifices
    ○ Chalazion (sometimes multiple)
    ○ Eyelid scarring with long-term disease
    ○ Association with ocular rosacea
  - Mixed blepharitis: Signs and symptoms of >1 type of blepharitis may be present.

DIFFERENTIAL DIAGNOSIS
Masquerade syndrome:
- Persistent inflammation and thickening of eyelid margin may indicate squamous cell, basal cell, or sebaceous cell carcinoma masquerading as blepharitis. These carcinomas also may mimic styes or chalazia.
- Sebaceous carcinoma of the eyelid has a 22% fatality rate. Up to 1/2 of these potentially fatal sebaceous cell carcinomas may resemble benign inflammatory diseases, particularly chalazia and chronic blepharoconjunctivitis.
- Consider masquerade syndrome in all cases of recurrent, persistent, or atypical chalazion; chronic unilateral unresponsive blepharoconjunctivitis; diffuse or nodular tumors of the eyelid; orbital mass developing after removal of an eyelid or caruncular tumor; and any tumor developing in a person with a history of ocular radiotherapy (1)[C].

DIAGNOSTIC TESTS & INTERPRETATION
Follow-Up Tests & Special Considerations
- Cultures in atypical blepharitis
- Biopsy in atypical cases for carcinoma
- Slit-lamp biomicroscopy:
  - Examine tear film, eyelid margins, eyelashes, tarsal and bulbar conjunctivae, and cornea.
  - Reveals loss of lashes (madarosis), whitening of the lashes (poliosis), trichiasis, crusting, eyelid margin ulcers, and lid irregularities

TREATMENT

GENERAL MEASURES
- Promote proper eyelid hygiene (2,3)[C]:
  - Apply warm compresses for several minutes once a day to soften adherent encrustations.
  - The eyelid margins then are scrubbed gently with eyelid cleanser or diluted baby shampoo twice a day to remove adherent material and clean the meibomian gland orifices (4)[C].
- Brief, gentle massage of the eyelids can help to express meibomian secretions in patients with meibomian gland dysfunction (2)[C].
- Discontinue soft contact lenses use during an acute case of blepharitis (3)[B].

MEDICATION
First Line
- According to Cochrane 2012, topical antibiotics provided some symptomatic relief and were effective in eradicating bacteria from the eyelid margin for anterior blepharitis. Lid hygiene may provide symptomatic relief for anterior and posterior blepharitis. The effectiveness of other treatments for blepharitis, such as topical steroids and PO antibiotics, was inconclusive (5)[A].
- No strong evidence supports any of the treatments in terms of curing chronic blepharitis (5)[A].
- Topical treatment to lid, if *Staphylococcus* likely:
  - Bacitracin: 500 μg/g or (2nd choice)
  - Erythromycin: 0.5% ophthalmic ointment:
    - Apply with a cotton-tipped applicator.
    - The frequency and duration of treatment are guided by the severity (2)[C].
- Topical corticosteroids (short term) may be useful for eyelid or ocular surface inflammation. The minimum effective dose should be used; long-term use should be avoided if possible (2,6)[C].
- For patients with meibomian gland dysfunction inadequately controlled with eyelid hygiene, consider doxycycline 100 mg/d or tetracycline 1,000 mg/d in divided doses, tapered after clinical improvement (2–4 weeks) to doxycycline 50 mg/d or tetracycline 250–500 mg/d (2)[C].
- Because aqueous tear deficiency is common in blepharitis, use twice-daily artificial tears in addition to eyelid hygiene and medications.
- Contraindications: Allergy to medication; tetracyclines are not for use in pregnancy, nursing women, or children <8 years of age.
- Precautions: Tetracyclines may cause photosensitivity; sunscreen is recommended. Corticosteroids may increase intraocular pressure and risk of cataract.

Second Line
- Topical fluoroquinolones (e.g., gatifloxacin 0.3%, levofloxacin 0.5%, or moxifloxacin 0.5%) may be helpful for persistent or recurrent staphylococcal blepharitis or for those patients who prefer a solution.
- Seborrheic blepharitis may respond to antifungal agents, such as a short course of itraconazole (7)[C].

ISSUES FOR REFERRAL
Chronic recurrent blepharitis requires referral to an ophthalmologist for evaluation as to whether patient should continue soft lens use.

ADDITIONAL THERAPIES
Various commercial products are marketed to consumers and prescribed to patients; however, there is no substantial evidence of effectiveness (5)[A].

 ONGOING CARE

FOLLOW-UP RECOMMENDATIONS
Patient Monitoring
- Patients should schedule a return visit if their condition worsens despite treatment.
- Return visit intervals for patients with severe disease vary.
- If corticosteroid is prescribed, re-evaluate within a few weeks to measure intraocular pressure and determine response to therapy.

PATIENT EDUCATION
- "Blepharitis Fact Sheet" from the American Academy of Ophthalmology
- Advise patient that blepharitis is a chronic condition, likely to recur if eyelid hygiene is not maintained after antibiotic treatment is discontinued (3)[C].

PROGNOSIS
- Symptoms frequently can be lessened, but rarely are eliminated.
- Long-term eyelid hygiene is required for control.

COMPLICATIONS
- Stye and chalazion
- Scarring of eyelid margin
- Corneal infection
- Superficial keratopathy
- Corneal neovascularization and ulceration
- Ectropion/Entropion

REFERENCES
1. Tsai T, O'Brien JM. Masquerade syndromes: Malignancies mimicking inflammation in the eye. *Int Ophthalmol Clin*. 2002;41:115–131.
2. American Academy of Ophthalmology Cornea/External Disease Panel, Preferred Practice Patterns Committee. Preferred practice pattern: *Blepharitis*. San Francisco: AAO. 2003.
3. Eyelid hygiene for blepharitis. *Insight*. 2011;36(1): 24.
4. McCulley JP, Shine WE. Changing concepts in the diagnosis and management of blepharitis. *Cornea*. 2000;19:650–658.
5. Lindsley K, Matsumura S, Hatef E, et al. Interventions for chronic blepharitis. *Cochrane Database Syst Rev*. 2012;5:CD005556. Epub 2012 May 16.
6. Abelson MB, Cohane K, Fink K. Blepharitis: Hiding in plain sight. *Review of Ophthalmology®*. 2004.
7. Ninomiya J, Nakabayashi A, Higuchi R, et al. A case of seborrheic blepharitis: Treatment with itraconazole. *Nippon Ishinkin Gakkai Zasshi*. 2002;43:189–191.

ADDITIONAL READING
- Bernardes TF, Bonfioli AA. Blepharitis. *Semin Ophthalmol*. 2010;25(3):79–83.
- Lemp MA, Bielory L. Contact lenses and associated anterior segment disorders: Dry eye disease, blepharitis, and allergy. *Immunol Allergy Clin North Am*. 2008;28:105–117, vi–vii.

 SEE ALSO

Conjunctivitis, Acute; Dry Eye Syndrome (Keratoconjunctivitis Sicca)

CODES

ICD10
- H01.009 Unspecified blepharitis unspecified eye, unspecified eyelid
- H01.019 Ulcerative blepharitis unspecified eye, unspecified eyelid
- H01.029 Squamous blepharitis unspecified eye, unspecified eyelid

CLINICAL PEARLS
- Blepharitis is often a chronic condition; symptoms frequently can be lessened, but rarely are eliminated.
- Promote proper eyelid hygiene.
- Bacitracin ophthalmic ointment is the first-line treatment if *Staphylococcus* is suspected.

BORDERLINE PERSONALITY DISORDER

Daniel E. Melville, MD • William G. Elder, Jr., PhD

 BASICS

DESCRIPTION

Beginning no later than adolescence or early adulthood, borderline personality disorder (BPD) is a consistent and pervasive pattern of labile affect and sense of self, impulsivity, and volatile interpersonal relationships (1):

- Common behaviors and variations:
  - Self-mutilation: Pinching, scratching, cutting
  - Suicide: Ideation, history of attempts, plans
  - Splitting: Idealizing then devaluing others
  - Presentation of helplessness or victimization
  - High utilization of emergency department and resultant inpatient hospitalizations for psychiatric treatment (2)
  - Patients with BPD are frequent users of primary care (3).
- High rate of associated mental disorders
- Typically display little insight into behavior

Geriatric Considerations
Illness (both acute and chronic) may exacerbate BPD and may lead to intense feelings of fear and helplessness.

Pediatric Considerations
Diagnosis is rarely made in children. Axis I disorders and general medical conditions are more probable.

Pregnancy Considerations
Physical, emotional, and social concerns may transiently mimic symptoms of BPD: Consider delay in diagnosis until pregnancy completed. Pregnancy may also induce stress or increased fears, resulting in escalation of borderline behaviors.

EPIDEMIOLOGY
Predominant age: Onset no later than adolescence or early adulthood (may go undiagnosed for years)

Prevalence
- General population: 0.5–5.9% of US population (3)
- Estimated lifetime prevalence: 10–13% (3)
- 10% of all psychiatric outpatients and between 15% and 25% of patients in psychiatry inpatient settings have BPD (3).
- 20–30% of patients in primary care outpatient settings have a personality disorder.

ETIOLOGY AND PATHOPHYSIOLOGY
Undetermined, but generally accepted that psychiatric disorders are due to a combination of the following:
- Hereditary temperamental traits
- Environment (i.e., history of childhood sexual and/or physical abuse, history of childhood neglect, ongoing conflict in home)
- Stress is theorized to exert damaging effects on the brain, specifically the hippocampus (3,4).
- Neurobiological research of BPD continues to increase the understanding of it cause:
  - Abnormalities of the frontolimbic circuitry in relation to poor emotional stability (3)
  - Potential alterations in the sensitivity of opioid receptors and/or deficiencies with endogenous opioids (5)
  - Heightened activity in brain circuits involved in the experience of negative emotions and reduced activation that normally suppresses negative emotion once it is generated (6).

Genetics
1st-degree relatives are at greater risk for this disorder (undetermined if due to genetic or psychosocial factors).

RISK FACTORS
- Genetic factors contribute; however, no specific genes have yet been identified as causative (3).
- Childhood sexual and/or physical abuse and neglect
- Disrupted family life
- Physical illness and external social factors may exacerbate borderline personality behaviors.

GENERAL PREVENTION
- Tends to be a multigenerational problem
- Children, caregivers, and significant others should have some time and activities away from the borderline individual, which may protect them.

COMMONLY ASSOCIATED CONDITIONS
Other psychiatric disorders, including:
- Co-occurring personality disorders, frequent
- Mood disorders, common
- Anxiety disorders, common
- Substance-related disorders, common
- Eating disorders, common
- Posttraumatic stress disorder, common
- BPD does not appear to be independently associated with increased risk of violence.

 DIAGNOSIS

- The comprehensive evaluation should focus on (7)[B]:
  - Comorbid conditions
  - Functional impairments
  - Adaptive/maladaptive coping styles
  - Psychosocial stressors
  - Patient strengths; needs/goals
- Initial assessment should focus on determining treatment setting (7)[B]:
  - Establish treatment agreement with patient and outline treatment goals.
  - Assess suicide ideation and self-harm behavior.
  - Assess for psychosis.
  - Hospitalization is necessary if patient presents a threat of harm to self or others.

HISTORY
- Clinic visits for problems that do not have biological findings
- Conflicts with medical staff members
- Idealizing or unexplained anger at physician
- History of unrealistic expectations of physician (e.g., "I know you can take care of me." "You're the best, unlike my last provider.")
- Obtain collateral information (i.e., from family, partner) about patient behaviors.

PHYSICAL EXAM
- Patients with BPD should have a thorough physical examination to help lower suspicion of organic disease, (especially thyroid disease) (1,3).
- Often physical examination reveals no gross abnormalities, other than related to scarring from self-mutilation.

DIFFERENTIAL DIAGNOSIS
- Mood disorders:
  - Look at baseline behaviors when considering BPD vs. mood disorders.
  - BPD symptoms increase the likelihood of misdiagnosing bipolar disorder.

- Psychotic disorder:
  - With BPD, typically only occurs under intense stress and is characterized as "micropsychotic"
- Other PD:
  - Thoughts, feelings, and behavior will differentiate BPD from other PDs.
- General medical condition (GMC):
  - Traits may emerge due to the effect of a GMC on the CNS.
- Substance use

DIAGNOSTIC TESTS & INTERPRETATION
- Consider age of onset. To meet criteria for BPD, borderline pattern will be present from adolescence or early adulthood.
- Formal psychological testing
- Rule out personality change due to a GMC (1)[C]:
  - Traits may emerge due to the effect of a GMC on the CNS.
- Rule out symptoms related to substance use.
- If symptoms begin later than early adulthood or are related to trauma (e.g., after a head injury), a GMC, or substance use, then consider other diagnoses.

Diagnostic Procedures/Other
According to DSM-5 criteria, patient must meet at least 5 of the following criteria (1)[C]:
- Attempt to avoid abandonment
- Volatile interpersonal relationships
- Identity disturbance
- Impulsive behavior:
  - In ≥2 areas
  - Impulsive behavior is self-damaging.
- Suicidal or self-mutilating behavior
- Mood instability
- Feeling empty
- Is unable to control anger, or finds it difficult to control
- Paranoid or dissociative when under stress
- With advent of DSM-5, an Alternative Model is being promulgated that may come to define the diagnosis as impairments in Personality Functioning AND the presence of Pathologic Traits. Attention to these features may ultimately enhance provider understanding, diagnosis, and treatment of patients with personality dysfunction.
  - Criteria regarding Personality Functioning refer to impairments of Self-Functioning (i.e., identity or self-direction) AND Interpersonal Functioning (i.e., empathy or intimacy).
  - Criteria regarding Personality Functioning refer to impairments of Self-Functioning (i.e., identity or self-direction) AND Interpersonal Functioning (i.e., empathy or intimacy).
  - Pathologic Personality Traits refer to characteristics in the domains of Negative Affectivity (i.e., emotional liability, anxiousness, separation insecurity, depressivity); disinhibition (i.e., impulsivity, risk taking); OR antagonism (1).

 TREATMENT

- Outpatient psychotherapy for BPD is the preferred treatment (3,7)[B]:
  - Dialectical behavior therapy (DBT) combines cognitive-behavioral techniques for emotional regulation and reality-testing with concepts of distress tolerance, acceptance, and self-awareness.

○ Following a dialectal process, therapists are tough-minded allies, who validate feelings and are unconditionally accepting, while also reminding patients to accept their dire level of emotional dysfunction and to apply better alternative behaviors.

○ DBT may be done individually and in groups.

- Consider transference-focused psychotherapy.
- Patient may need to be placed on suicide watch.
- Brief inpatient hospitalizations are ineffective in changing Axis II disorder behaviors:
  – Hospitalizations should be limited, and of short duration, to adjust medications, implement psychotherapy for crisis intervention, and to stabilize patients from psychosocial stressors.

- Extended inpatient hospitalization should be considered for the following reasons (7)[B]:
  – Persistent/severe suicidal ideation or risk to others
  – Comorbid substance use and/or nonadherence to outpatient or partial hospitalization treatments
  – Comorbid Axis I disorders that may increase threat to life for the patient (i.e., eating disorders, mood disorders)

GENERAL MEASURES
Focus on patient management rather than on "fixing" behaviors:
- Schedule consistent appointment follow-ups to relieve patient anxiety.
- Meet with and rely on treatment team to avoid splitting of team by patient, and to provide opportunity to discuss patient issues.
- Treatment is usually most effective when both medications and psychotherapy are used simultaneously.

MEDICATION
- Although no specific medications are approved by the FDA to treat BPD, American Psychiatric Association (APA) guidelines recommend pharmacotherapy to manage symptoms (3)[A],(7)[B].
- Treat Axis I disorders (8)[B].
- Consider high rate of self-harm and suicidal behavior when prescribing (3)[A].
- APA guideline recommendations (7)[B]:
  – Affective dysregulation: Mood stabilizers, SSRIs, and monoamine oxidase inhibitors (MAOIs)
  – Impulsive-behavioral control: SSRIs and mood stabilizers
  – Cognitive-perceptual symptoms: Antipsychotics
- With more neurobiological causes considered in relation to BPD, there is more emphasis on mood stabilizers and atypical antipsychotics, but research is uncertain and inconclusive (8)[B].
- Antipsychotics have short-lived benefit and offer no value other than transient treatment of cognitive perceptual symptoms (8)[B].

ISSUES FOR REFERRAL
- If hospitalized, consider for suicide risk, mood or anxiety disorders, or substance-related disorders.
- Urgency for scheduled follow-up depends on community resources (e.g., outpatient day programs for suicidal patients, substance abuse programs):
  – With increased risk for self-harm or self-defeating behaviors and low community resources, the patient can/will have increased need for frequent visits.

ADDITIONAL THERAPIES
Consider referring patient for specialty mental health behavioral services, including partial hospital therapy.

COMPLEMENTARY AND ALTERNATIVE MEDICINE
Omega-3 fatty acid dietary supplementation has shown beneficial effects (3)[B].

IN-PATIENT CONSIDERATIONS
Admission Criteria/Initial Stabilization
Admit for inpatient services immediately in presence of psychosis or threat of injury to self or others; include police, as necessary, for safety measures.
- Assess suicidal ideation.
- Consider trial of antipsychotic medications for psychosis.

Nursing
Nurses can be instrumental in managing and calling patients, potentially relieving patient stress.

Discharge Criteria
- Patient should not present risk of harm to self or others and have a safety plan.
- Follow-up should be scheduled with a mental health specialist and primary care provider.

 ## ONGOING CARE

FOLLOW-UP RECOMMENDATIONS
- Schedule visits that are short, more frequent, and focused to relieve patients' anxiety about relationships with their physician/provider and to help reduce risk of provider burnout.
- Maintain open lines of communication with mental health professionals providing psychological support.
- Emphasize importance of healthy lifestyle modifications (i.e., exercise, rest, diet).

Patient Monitoring
Monitor for suicidal or other self-harm behaviors.

PATIENT EDUCATION
Include patients in the diagnosis so they can make sense of their disease process and participate in the treatment strategy (7,9)[C].

PROGNOSIS
- Borderline behaviors may decrease with age and over time.
- Patients in treatment improve at a rate of 7 times compared with following natural course (10).
- Treatment is complex and takes time.
- Medical focus includes patient management and caring for medical and Axis I disorders.

REFERENCES
1. American Psychiatric Association (2013). *Diagnostic and Statistical Manual of Mental Disorders* (5th ed.). Arlington, VA: American Psychiatric Publishing.
2. Foti ME, Geller J, Guy LS, et al. Borderline personality disorder: Considerations for inclusion in the Massachusetts parity list of "biologically-based" disorders. *Psychiatr Q.* 2011;82(2):95–112.
3. Leichsenring F, Leibing E, Kruse J, et al. Borderline personality disorder. *Lancet.* 2011;377(9759): 74–84.
4. Ruocco AC, Amirthavasagam S, Zakzanis KK. Amygdala and hippocampal volume reductions as candidate endophenotypes for borderline personality disorder: A meta-analysis of magnetic resonance imaging studies. *Psychiatry Res.* 2012;201(3):245–252. Epub 2012 Apr 15.
5. Bandelow B, Schmahl C, Falkai P, et al. Borderline personality disorder: A dysregulation of the endogenous opioid system? *Psychol Rev.* 2010;117(2):623–636.
6. Ruocco A, Amirthavasagam S, Choi-Kain LW, et al. Neural correlates of negative emotionality in borderline personality disorder: An activation-likelihood-estimation meta-analysis. *Biologic Psychiatry.* 2013;73(2):153.
7. Oldham JA. *Guideline Watch: Practice Guideline for the Treatment of Patients with Borderline Personality Disorder.* Arlington, VA: American Psychiatric Association; 2005.
8. Feurino L, Silk KR. State of the art in the pharmacologic treatment of borderline personality disorder. *Curr Psychiatry Rep.* 2011;13(1):69–75.
9. Sanislow CA, Marcus KL, Reagan EM. Long-term outcomes in borderline psychopathology: Old assumptions, current findings, and new directions. *Curr Psychiatry Rep.* 2012;14(1):54–61.
10. Elder W, Walsh E. Personality disorders. In South-Paul J, Matheny S, Lewis E (eds.): *Current Diagnosis & Treatment: Family Medicine.* McGraw-Hill, 2011.

 ## CODES

ICD10
F60.3 Borderline personality disorder

CLINICAL PEARLS
- View BPD as a chronic condition with waxing and waning features. It is important to adjust medications/treatments as clinically appropriate when symptoms change.
- If there are problems with the patient disrespecting the physician or support staff, clear guidelines should be established with the treatment team and then with the patient.
- When considering terminating care, the patient may improve if empathetically confronted about certain behaviors and is given clear guidelines on how to behave in the clinic. It is the patient's job to follow the guidelines, and it is you and your team's job to enforce the guidelines. Designate a case management nurse or well-trained support staff person who can be the primary contact person for the patient.
- Have an agenda when you visit with patients with BPD. Be cordial—they deserve the same professionalism given any patient. Have and identify 1–2 issues to be discussed per clinic visit. Frequently scheduled visits can help with this.
- Regularly scheduled psychotherapy treatment helps physician performance by becoming the "home" for mental health treatment, leaving the physician to focus on the patient's immediate medical issues.
- Stay informed of neurobiological research: Input may change pharmacotherapy as more is understood regarding pathophysiology of BPD.
- Given the special needs of patients with BPD, consider limiting the number of patients with this diagnosis in your practice.

BOTULISM
Brian Yokers, DO • Mark S. Rosenberg, DO, MBA, FACEP

 BASICS

DESCRIPTION
- Botulism is a muscle-paralyzing illness caused by a neurotoxin made by the bacterium *Clostridium botulinum*.
- Characterized by acute onset of cranial nerve involvement (diplopia, difficulty swallowing or speaking), symmetric descending weakness and flaccid paralysis; retains normal mental state, but no fever or sensory dysfunction
- 7 types of *C. botulinum* (A–G) are distinguished by their antigenic characteristics. Types A, B, E, and, in rare cases, F, cause disease in humans.
- Forms include:
  - Foodborne: Caused by ingestion of preformed toxin
  - Infant botulism: Caused by ingestion of *C. botulinum* that produces toxin in the GI tract
  - Wound: Caused by wound infection with *C. botulinum* that secretes the toxin
  - Aerosolized/Inhalational botulinum: Bioterrorism attack potential because of high toxicity; <1 μg is lethal human dose. Does not occur naturally.
  - Adult intestinal toxemia: Like infant botulism, but occurring in adults (rare)
  - Iatrogenic: From injection of toxin.
- Diagnosis is made through history and clinical exam and confirmed by laboratory identification of toxin and/or positive cultures.
- Purified and diluted forms of botulinum toxin are used therapeutically (i.e., spastic neuromuscular disorders, glandular hypersecretion, pain) and for cosmesis.
- System(s) affected: Neuromuscular; Respiratory; GI
- Synonym(s): Sausage poisoning; Kerner disease

EPIDEMIOLOGY
Incidence
- Average of 110 cases of botulism reported annually in the U.S.
- ~20% of cases are foodborne; 30–40% wound-related; 65% infant botulism.
- Foodborne incidence highest among Alaska Natives. More than 1/2 of cases came from 5 western states (California, Washington, Colorado, Oregon, Alaska).
- Adult intestinal toxemia: More common in disorders of the GI tract (prior surgery, Crohn disease, recent antibiotic use)
- Inhalation: Only a single incident involving 3 laboratory workers has been described.

Prevalence
- Predominant age:
  - Foodborne: Mean age is 46 years; range of 3–78 years
  - Infantile: Mean age of onset 13 weeks, range of 1–63 weeks
  - Wound: Median age is 41 years, range of 23–58 years
- Predominant gender:
  - Foodborne and infantile: Male = Female
  - Wound: Female > Male

ETIOLOGY AND PATHOPHYSIOLOGY
- Disease results from hematogenous spread of toxin from mucosal surface (stomach, small intestine) or from an infected wound.
- The toxin permanently prevents acetylcholine release at presynaptic membranes, blocking neuromuscular transmission in cholinergic nerve fibers.

- Toxin produced by *C. botulinum*, an encapsulated, anaerobic, gram-positive, spore-forming, rod-shaped bacillus
- Ingestion of *C. botulinum* neurotoxins (A, B, and E most common)
- Foodborne: Usually from home-canned vegetables, prepared foods, or foods incubated in anaerobic conditions
- Infantile from ingestion of spores in environment or, occasionally, in honey
- Wound due to contamination with toxin-producing *C. botulinum*
- Iatrogenic: IM injections of botulinum toxin

RISK FACTORS
- Foodborne: Ingestion of home-canned or prepared contaminated foods
- Infantile: Ingestion of spores floating on dust particles in the environment; ingestion of honey (minor but preventable source) Immunocompromised state
- Wound: IV drug use (black tar heroin; IM/SC), "skin popping," snorting cocaine

GENERAL PREVENTION
- Foodborne: Proper handling, processing, preparation (heating), and storage of food; avoid eating food from bulging cans and food that smells/looks spoiled.
- Infant: Caretaker handwashing. Avoid honey <1 year of age.
- Wound: Abstaining from injection drugs or snorting of cocaine; proper wound care
- Health care providers: Standard precautions
- If meningitis is suspected in patients with flaccid paralysis, medical personnel should use droplet precautions.
- Heat potentially contaminated food or drink to an internal temperature of 85°C for at least 5 minutes.
- After exposure to *C. botulinum* toxin, clothing and skin should be cleaned with soap and water.
- Contaminated objects or surfaces should be cleaned with 0.1% bleach solution. All food suspected of contamination should be promptly removed from potential consumers.
- Vaccination has been discontinued (1).

DIAGNOSIS

HISTORY
- Adults:
  - Acute onset of symmetric neuropathies. Difficulty in swallowing or speaking, dry mouth. Diplopia, blurred vision, dilated or nonrelated ptosis. Dyspnea or progressive weakness
  - IV drug use, skin-popping, or cocaine use (wound botulism)
- Infant botulism: Disease presentation and severity variable:
  - Constipation, shortly followed by weakness, feeding difficulties, descending or global hypotonia, drooling, anorexia, irritability, and weak cry
- Ask about diet, travel, drug use, and contact with other persons with same symptoms over past 10 days (incubation for adult type is 12–36 hours to 10 days after ingestion; infant variable).

PHYSICAL EXAM
- General appearance: Oriented, flaccid; may complain of malaise, dizziness, nausea, vomiting
- Vital signs: Afebrile (fever may occur in wound botulism due to secondary infection), normal BP
- Head, eyes, ears, nose, throat: Dry mouth
- Chest/Lungs: Respiratory muscle weakness, respiratory dysfunction, paralysis
- Heart: Normal or slow rate
- Abdomen: Distention, constipation (early sign in infant form); may be absent in wound form
- Genitourinary: Urinary retention
- Neurologic:
  - Symmetric descending weakness beginning with the cranial nerves
  - Ptosis; extraocular muscle paresis; fixed, dilated pupils; dysphagia
  - Infant botulism: Poor muscle tone (loss of head control and facial expression), poor feeding (loss of suck), drooling, feeding difficulties, weak cry
  - Diminished or absent deep tendon reflexes

DIFFERENTIAL DIAGNOSIS
- Adult botulisms:
  - Guillain-Barré syndrome
  - Encephalitis, meningitis
  - Tick paralysis
  - Myasthenia gravis
  - Eaton Lambert myasthenic syndrome
  - Cerebrovascular accident: Basilar artery stroke
  - Congenital neuropathy or myopathy
  - Sepsis
  - Hypokalemic periodic paralysis
  - Poliomyelitis
  - Other poisonings (organophosphate, shellfish, *Amanita* mushrooms, atropine, and aminoglycosides)
  - Miller-Fisher variant of Guillain-Barré syndrome
  - Diphtheritic neuropathy
  - Carbon monoxide intoxication
  - Hypermagnesemia
- Infant botulism:
  - Sepsis
  - Meningitis
  - Electrolyte–mineral imbalance
  - Reye syndrome
  - Congenital myopathy
  - Leigh disease
  - Werdnig-Hoffman disease
  - SIDS (botulism suggested as a cause in some cases)

DIAGNOSTIC TESTS & INTERPRETATION
Initial Tests (lab, imaging)
- Laboratory confirmation is done by demonstrating the presence of toxin in serum or stool, or by culturing *C. botulinum* from stool, wounds, or food.
- Mouse neutralization assay confirmation:
  - Standard method of diagnosis (2)[B]
  - Available from CDC and some state laboratories; takes ~4 days for results
  - Found to be only 68% sensitive in wound botulism, emphasizing importance of clinical evaluation in diagnosis (3)[B]
- Routine tests (CBC, electrolytes, LFTs, U/A): Generally not helpful/show no characteristic abnormalities
- CSF testing: Normal helps differentiate from Guillain-Barré syndrome. Occasionally a borderline elevation in protein is seen.

- A normal Tensilon test helps to differentiate botulism from myasthenia gravis; borderline can occur in botulism.
- CT or MRI to rule out neurologic pathology

Diagnostic Procedures/Other
Electrophysiology testing is sensitive and specific in confirming botulism, but less reliable in assessing severity of intoxication (4)[B].

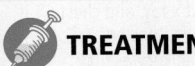

TREATMENT

MEDICATION
First Line
- Antitoxin therapy with trivalent A-B-E antitoxin:
  – Call CDC Assistance: (770) 488–7100.
  – Initiating botulinum antitoxin therapy is primarily based on symptoms and physical examination findings that are consistent with botulism (5)[B].
  – Early administration is important (5)[B].
  – Horse serum derived: Up to 9% develop hypersensitivity, but few are severe (6). Pretest with a small dose (follow package instructions). Consider pretreatment with steroids or antihistamines; have epinephrine available.
  – Supportive care, including mechanical ventilation (7)[C]
  – Antibiotics unproven by clinical trial, but widely used
- Infantile:
  – Treatment with human botulism immunoglobulin (BIG-IV or Baby BIG) for botulism types A and B (8)[A]
  – Available only through the California Infant Botulism Treatment and Prevention Program: (510) 231—7600
  – Antibiotics not recommended. Avoid use of anti-clostridial (lysis of bacteria with toxin release), or aminoglycosides (potentiation of neuromuscular weakness) (9)[C]

Second Line
May consider equine antitoxin for infant botulism if human immunoglobulin unavailable and benefit outweighs risk of anaphylaxis (6)[B].

Pregnancy Considerations
Safety of botulism antitoxin during pregnancy and breastfeeding unknown or controversial

ISSUES FOR REFERRAL
- Nutrition: For hyperalimentation, and later, tube feeding
- Physical/Occupational therapy: Including swallow evaluation

ADDITIONAL THERAPIES
- Stress ulcer and deep vein thrombosis prophylaxis
- Pulmonary and physical rehabilitation

SURGERY/OTHER PROCEDURES
Wound excision/débridement for wound botulism

IN-PATIENT CONSIDERATIONS
Admission Criteria/Initial Stabilization
All suspected cases must be admitted.
    Hospital admission with meticulous airway management

IV Fluids
Keep patient well hydrated.

Nursing
- Prevent decubitus ulcer, IV line infections, other nosocomial infections.
- Before administration of antitoxin, skin testing should be performed for sensitivity.

ONGOING CARE

FOLLOW-UP RECOMMENDATIONS
Outpatient follow-up with physical/occupational therapy, nutrition specialist, and psychiatry, as needed

Patient Monitoring
- Pulmonary function testing
- Cardiorespiratory monitoring

DIET
Nasogastric feedings, if needed

PATIENT EDUCATION
- Spores destroyed by pressure cooking at 250°F (120°C) for 30 minutes
- Toxin destroyed by boiling for 10 minutes or cooking at 175°F (80°C) for 30 minutes
- Avoid honey in 1st year of life.
- Avoid IV drug use.
- Do not eat/sample foods that look and smell rotten or come from bulging cans.

PROGNOSIS
- Delay in administering antitoxin: Most important factor affecting clinical course and outcome (5)[B]
- Mortality: Overall, 3–5%; reduced from a near 50% mortality, usually from respiratory failure (7)
- Some may have significant health, functional, and social limitations several years after infection (10)[C]:
  – Recovery follows the regeneration of new neuromuscular connections.
  – 2–8 weeks of ventilator support may be required in more severe cases.
- Patients who survive generally have a good prognosis, with most attaining full recovery, although it may take many months, depending on the severity of toxic insult.
- Dyspnea with severe ptosis and pupil abnormality has been shown to correlate with severe illness and respiratory failure (11)[C].
- Increased incubation time has been shown to correlate with better outcomes (11)[C].

COMPLICATIONS
- Complications of prolonged paralysis (i.e., aspiration and ventilator-associated pneumonia, pressure ulcers, muscle wasting)
- Hypoxic tissue damage if presenting late
- Death

REFERENCES

1. Centers for Disease Control and Prevention (CDC). Notice of CDC's discontinuation of investigational pentavalent (ABCDE) botulinum toxoid vaccine for workers at risk for occupational exposure to botulinum toxins. *MMWR Morb Mortal Wkly Rep.* 2011;60(42):1454–1455.
2. Lindström M, Korkeala H. Laboratory diagnostics of botulism. *Clin Microbiol Rev.* 2006;19: 298–314.
3. Wheeler C, Inami G, Mohle-Boetani J, et al. Sensitivity of mouse bioassay in clinical wound botulism. *Clin Infect Dis.* 2009;48(12): 1669–1673.
4. Witoonpanich R, Vichayanrat E, Tantisiriwit K, et al. Electrodiagnosis of botulism and clinico-electrophysiological correlation. *Clin Neurophysiol.* 2009;120(6):1135–1138. Epub 2009 May 1.
5. Dembek ZF, Smith LA, Rusnak JM. Botulism: Cause, effects, diagnosis, clinical and laboratory identification, and treatment modalities. *Disaster Med Public Health Prep.* 2007;1:122–134.
6. Vanella de Cuetos EE, Fernandez RA, Bianco MI, et al. Equine botulinum antitoxin for the treatment of infant botulism. *Clin Vaccine Immunol.* 2011;18(11):1845–1849. Epub 2011 Sep 14.
7. Botulism Facts for Healthcare Providers. Accessed 09/11/2012 at http://emergency.cdc.gov/agent/botulism/hcpfacts.asp.
8. Chalk C, Benstead TJ, Keezer M. Medical treatment for botulism. *Cochrane Database Syst Rev.* 2011;3:CD008123.
9. Infant Botulism Treatment and Prevention Program; Patient Management. Accessed 09/14/2012 at infantbotulism.org
10. Gottlieb SL, Kretsinger K, Tarkhashvili N, et al. Long-term outcomes of 217 botulism cases in the Republic of Georgia. *Clin Infect Dis.* 2007;45: 174–180.
11. Witoonpanich R, Vichayanrat E, Tantisiriwit K, et al. Survival analysis for respiratory failure in patients with food-borne botulism. *Clin Toxicol (Phila).* 2010;48:177–183.

ADDITIONAL READING

Hill SE, Iqbal R, Cadiz CL, Le J. Foodborne botulism treated with heptavalent botulism antitoxin. *Ann Pharmacother.* 2013;47(2):e12. doi: 10.1345/aph. 1R646. Epub 2013 Jan 29.

SEE ALSO

Food Poisoning, Bacterial

CODES

ICD10
- A05.1 Botulism food poisoning
- A48.51 Infant botulism
- A48.52 Wound botulism

CLINICAL PEARLS

- Botulinum antitoxin should be administered as soon as possible, based on clinical suspicion.
- Medical care providers who suspect botulism in a patient should immediately call their state health department's emergency 24-hour telephone number.
- A helpful mnemonic to recall progression of symptoms is the "dozen D's": Dry mouth, diplopia, dilated pupils, droopy eyes, droopy face, diminished gag reflex, dysphagia, dysarthria, dysphonia, difficulty lifting head, descending paralysis, and diaphragmatic paralysis.

BRAIN ABSCESS
Nathan Weldon, MD

 BASICS

DESCRIPTION
- Single or multiple abscesses within the brain, usually occurring secondary to a focus of infection outside the CNS
- May mimic brain tumor but generally evolves more rapidly (over days to weeks)
- Starts as a cerebritis, becomes necrotic, and subsequently becomes encapsulated
- Synonym(s): Cerebral abscess

Geriatric Considerations
Age does not affect outcome as much as the abscess size and state of neurologic dysfunction at presentation.

Pediatric Considerations
- ~1/3 of total cases occur in the pediatric age group.
- Rarely found in infants <1 year of age
- Cyanotic congenital heart disease frequently associated

EPIDEMIOLOGY
- Predominant age: Median age 30–40 years, although brain abscess occurs at all ages
- Predominant sex: Male > Female (2:1)

Incidence
Infrequent, but increasing due to increase in immune-suppressed individuals, opportunistic pathogens, and resistance to antibiotics

ETIOLOGY AND PATHOPHYSIOLOGY
- Hematogenous source is most common overall for single or multiple cerebral abscesses.
- Direct extension from otitis, mastoiditis, sinusitis, or dental infection
- Cranial osteomyelitis
- Penetrating skull trauma
- Prior craniotomy
- Bacteremia from lung abscess, pneumonia
- Bacterial endocarditis
- Fungal infection of the nasopharynx
- *Toxoplasma gondii* (in AIDS patients)
- Cyanotic congenital heart disease
- IV drug use
- No source found in 20%.
- Most common infective organisms: Streptococci, staphylococci (especially after neurosurgery), enteric gram-negative bacilli and anaerobes (usually same as source of infection), *Nocardia*
- Most common fungal sources include *Aspergillus* spp., *Candida* spp., and zygomycetes (1)
- Risk factors for fungal infection include immunocompromise, penetrating CNS trauma, immunocompetent hosts in fungal endemic areas
- Amebic brain abscess, amebiasis, amebic dysentery
- The frontal lobe of the brain is the most common site for an abscess.

Genetics
No known genetic pattern

RISK FACTORS
- HIV/AIDS
- Immunocompromised state
- IV drug abuse

GENERAL PREVENTION
- Adequate treatment of otitis media, mastoiditis, sinusitis, dental abscess, other ear/nose/throat (ENT) infections
- Prophylactic antibiotics after compound skull fracture or penetrating head wound

COMMONLY ASSOCIATED CONDITIONS
- AIDS
- Congenital heart disease
- Cardiac vegetations
- Diabetes
- Cirrhosis

 DIAGNOSIS

HISTORY
- Recent onset of headache becoming severe
- New focal neurological deficit
- Altered mental status progressing to stupor and coma
- Nausea and vomiting
- Seizures

PHYSICAL EXAM
- Afebrile or low-grade fever
- Papilledema
- Neck stiffness
- Focal neurologic signs, depending on location

DIFFERENTIAL DIAGNOSIS
- Brain tumors
- Cysticercosis
- Stroke
- Resolving intracranial hemorrhage
- Subdural empyema
- Extradural abscess
- Encephalitis

DIAGNOSTIC TESTS & INTERPRETATION
Abscess culture: Predominant organisms include *Toxoplasma* (AIDS), *Staphylococcus* (trauma), aerobic or anaerobic bacteria, fungi (rare).

ALERT
- Lumbar puncture often contraindicated
- Prior administration of antibiotics may alter lab results.

Initial Tests (lab, imaging)
- WBC count may be normal or mildly elevated.
- Blood studies: Mild polymorphonuclear (PMN) leukocytosis; elevated ESR
- Culture and susceptibilities of the abscess material
- If available, consider broad-range bacterial rDNA polymerase chain reaction with DNA sequencing (2)[C].
- Search for primary source of infection, depending on suspected source.
- Solitary intracerebral abscess suggests a direct contiguous source, such as sinus or ear infection.
- Multiple cerebral abscesses suggest hematological spread.

- Head CT and MRI are the diagnostic methods of choice. Specific findings depend on stages of the abscess (3)[B].
- CT provides sufficient diagnostic information in most cases (4)[B], including skull fracture, sinus infection, or otic source.
- Consider cardiac echo, chest x-ray, and chest CT if cardiac or pulmonary source suspected.
- Radionuclide [117]In-labeled leukocytes may distinguish abscess from neoplasm.

Diagnostic Procedures/Other
- Lumbar puncture often contraindicated
- Surgical burr hole with aspiration to make a specific bacteriologic diagnosis

Test Interpretation
- Suppuration, liquefaction, or encapsulation, depending on stage of evolution
- Fibrosis

 TREATMENT

Immediate neurosurgical consult is indicated for suspected CNS abscess.

GENERAL MEASURES
- Palliative and supportive

- Treatment of brain abscess requires a combination of antimicrobial agents, surgical intervention, and eradication of the primary foci of infection (5)[A].
- Initial medical therapy includes broad-spectrum antibiotics pending determination of the causative organism.
- Determination of point of entry and source of infection is critical to effective treatment (6)[C].
- Medical therapy only may be indicated:
  - For surgically inaccessible lesions or multiple abscesses
  - For abscesses in early cerebritis stage
  - For small (<2.5-cm) abscesses
- Antibiotic therapy may be directed toward most likely organism if no specific organism is identified.
- Monitor clinical response to antibiotic therapy.

MEDICATION
- Antibiotics according to organism and sensitivities, if known
- Initial empiric treatment according to suspected source
- Antifungal treatment, including amphotericin B, azoles, echinocandins, or flucytosine, in suspected or confirmed fungal cases, as appropriate
- Hematogenous sources should cover MRSA initially, and should include vancomycin, and may be broadened to include metronidazole and a 3rd-generation cephalosporin.
- For dental source, penicillin G and metronidazole are reasonable initial choices.
- For otogenic or sinus source, coverage should include metronidazole and either ceftriaxone or cefotaxime.

- For GI or genitourinary source, consider a 3rd-generation cephalosporin, such as cefotaxime, to cover gram negatives.
- For traumatic source, consider vancomycin plus either ceftriaxone or cefotaxime.
- Hospital-acquired sources, including postsurgical abscess, consider vancomycin and cefepime or ceftazidime
- If MSSA is isolated, change vancomycin to oxacillin or nafcillin.
- Use vancomycin in penicillin-sensitive patients.
- Generally a 6–8-week course of parenteral antibiotics is required.
- If brain abscess is associated with HIV/AIDS:
  – Daily doses of sulfadiazine and pyrimethamine
  – Lifelong therapy in AIDS patients
- Anticonvulsants:
  – Phenytoin until abscess resolves or perhaps longer
  – Monitor anticonvulsant levels.
- Following a neurosurgical procedure, use corticosteroids, such as dexamethasone, to reduce edema. Taper rapidly. Use is usually limited to 1 week.
- Contraindications: Sensitivity or allergy to any prescribed medications
- Precautions:
  – Sulfadiazine is poorly water-soluble. Patients must maintain adequate hydration or risk developing crystalluria.
  – Decrease dosage of penicillin in patients with renal dysfunction.
  – Monitor serum levels of anticonvulsants.
  – A dose of pyrimethamine is required for the treatment of toxoplasmosis, which may approach toxic levels. The patient should be observed for folic acid deficiency and treated with folinic acid (leucovorin) 5–15 mg (PO, IM, IV), if necessary.

ISSUES FOR REFERRAL
Neurosurgical referral for all patients. Consider infectious disease and neurology consultations if available.

SURGERY/OTHER PROCEDURES
- Surgery is mandatory when neurologic deficits are severe or progressive
- Surgery is often used when the abscess is in the posterior fossa or is the result of trauma
- Type of surgical treatment used depends on the patient's clinical status, the neuroradiographic characteristics of the abscess, and the experience of the surgeon(s) carrying out the procedure (5)[C].
- Abscess drainage via a needle under stereotactic CT guidance through a burr hole under local anesthesia is the most rapid and effective surgical method of treatment and may be repeated if needed.
- Craniotomy: If abscess is large or multilocular
- In general, similar outcomes for stereotactic-guided drainage or craniotomy (7)[B]

IN-PATIENT CONSIDERATIONS
Admission Criteria/Initial Stabilization
- On diagnosis for close monitoring, IV antibiotics, and possible surgery. A brain abscess often requires admission to an ICU, or may be a complication of ICU patients with neurologic injury, contributing significantly to morbidity and mortality (8)[B].
- Inpatient care for close observation, diagnostic evaluation, and specialty consultation (neurology, neurosurgery, or infectious disease)

IV Fluids
IV fluids if nausea and vomiting present

Discharge Criteria
When patient is asymptomatic, afebrile, and responding to therapy as determined by serial imaging studies

 ONGOING CARE

FOLLOW-UP RECOMMENDATIONS
- Bed rest until infection controlled and abscess evacuated or resolving, then as tolerated
- May need long-term rehabilitative care

Patient Monitoring
- Postsurgical monitoring, as needed
- Serial CT or MRI for at least 3 months to evaluate the therapeutic response, confirm progressive resolution, detect new lesions, and manage complications

DIET
IV fluids if significant nausea and vomiting

PATIENT EDUCATION
Brain Research Foundation, 208 S. LaSalle Street, Suite 1426, Chicago, IL 60604; (312) 782-4311.

PROGNOSIS
- The route of spread, the type and virulence of the organism, thickness of the capsule, location and number of abscesses in the brain, and immune status of the host are important determinants of outcome.
- Survival: >80% with early diagnosis and treatment
- In 1 retrospective analysis, 80% of patients recovered fully or had minimal incapacity and 10% died (4)[B].
- Patients with underlying cranial neoplasms or medical conditions have worse outcomes than those with a contiguous focus of infection or posttraumatic abscess (4)[B].

COMPLICATIONS
- Permanent neurologic deficits
- Surgical complications
- ICU-related complications
- Recurrent abscess
- Seizures
- Death

REFERENCES
1. Scully EP, Baden LR, Katz JT. Fungal brain infections. Curr Opin Neurol. 2008;21:347–352.
2. Al Masalma M, Armougom F, Scheld WM, et al. The expansion of the microbiological spectrum of brain abscesses with the use of multiple 16S ribosomal DNA sequencing. Clin Infect Dis. 2009;48(9):1169–1178.
3. Foerster BR, Thurnher MM, Malani PN. Intracranial infections: Clinical and imaging characteristics. Acta Radiol. 2007;48:875–893.
4. Carpenter J, Stapleton S, Holliman R. Retrospective analysis of 49 cases of brain abscess and review of the literature. Eur J Clin Microbiol Infect Dis. 2007;26:1–11.
5. Lu CH. Strategies for the management of bacterial brain abscess. J Clin Neurosci. 2006;13(10): 979–985. Epub 2006 Oct 23.
6. Bernardini GL. Diagnosis and management of brain abscess and subdural empyema. Curr Neurol Neurosci Rep. 2004;4:448–456.
7. Smith SJ, Ughratdar I, MacArthur DC. Never go to sleep on undrained pus: A retrospective review of surgery for intraparenchymal cerebral abscess. Br J Neurosurg. 2009;23:412–417.
8. Ziai WC, Lewin JJ. Update in the diagnosis and management of central nervous system infections. Neurol Clin. 2008;26:427–468, viii.

ADDITIONAL READING
Kao PT, Tseng HK, Liu CP, Su CP, Lee CM. Brain abscess: clinical analysis of 53 cases. J Microbiol Immunol Infect. 2003;36(2):129–136.

 CODES

ICD10
G06.0 Intracranial abscess and granuloma

CLINICAL PEARLS
- Headache and altered mental status are common presenting symptoms of a brain abscess.
- Determination of point of entry and source of infection is essential for adequate treatment.
- Treatment of a brain abscess may require a combination of antimicrobial agents for 6–8 weeks, surgical intervention, and eradication of the primary focus of infection.
- Serial head CTs for at least 3 months can help to evaluate a patient's response to therapies.

BRAIN INJURY, TRAUMATIC
Dana Collaguazo, MD

BASICS

DESCRIPTION
- A dynamic process with penetrating or blunt injury to the brain with initial bleeding followed by secondary injury due to cerebral edema and/or continued bleeding
- Frequently related to rapid deceleration, as in motor vehicle or diving accidents, or blunt trauma
- System(s) affected: Cardiovascular, Endocrine/Metabolic, Nervous
- Synonym(s): Head injury

EPIDEMIOLOGY
Incidence
- 1,365,000 hospital emergency room visits per year
- 275,000 hospitalizations/year
- 52,000 deaths/year

Prevalence
- Predominant age: 0–4, 15–19, and >65 years
- Predominant gender: Male > Female

ETIOLOGY AND PATHOPHYSIOLOGY
- Motor vehicle accidents (17%)
- Falls (35%)
- Assault
- Initial brain dysfunction from direct trauma (bleeding, laceration) followed by secondary injury due to cerebral edema, continued bleeding, decreased blood flow

RISK FACTORS
Alcohol, prior head injury, contact sports

Geriatric Considerations
Subdural hematomas are common after a fall or blow in elderly; symptoms may be subtle.

GENERAL PREVENTION
- Safety education
- Seat belts; bicycle and motorcycle helmets
- Protective headgear for contact sports

Pediatric Considerations
Child abuse: Consider if dropped or fell <4 feet (e.g., off bed, couch) and significant injury present or any retinal hemorrhages

COMMONLY ASSOCIATED CONDITIONS
Alcohol and drug abuse

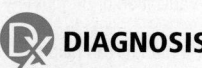

DIAGNOSIS

HISTORY
- Loss of consciousness (LOC)
- Headache
- Vomiting
- Amnesia
- Epidural hemorrhage from blunt trauma is generally acute, 30% with a "lucid interval" (initial LOC followed by recovery of consciousness, then LOC recurs and persists).

Geriatric Considerations
Subdural hemorrhage usually has a slower onset and may present weeks after the initial injury, especially in the elderly.

PHYSICAL EXAM
- Focal neurologic signs and symptoms
- Evidence of increased intracranial pressure (ICP) (elevated BP, decreased pulse rate, or slow/irregular breathing [Cushing triad]—only 30% have all 3)
- Decorticate or decerebrate posturing (bad prognostic signs)
- Seizures
- Signs of basilar skull fracture: Raccoon eyes, battle sign, hemotympanum, CSF rhinorrhea or otorrhea (see "Diagnostic Procedures")
- Unilateral dilated pupil in an alert patient is not consistent with impending herniation, as these patients are always unconscious.

DIFFERENTIAL DIAGNOSIS
Other causes of altered mental status (e.g., toxicologic, infectious, metabolic, vascular)

DIAGNOSTIC TESTS & INTERPRETATION
Initial Tests (lab, imaging)
- Evaluate for coagulopathy.
- Type and screen for possible surgical intervention.
- Perform drug and alcohol screening.
- CT, noncontrast, is study of choice to review bone windows, tissue windows, and subdural space:
- NEXUS II study (1)[B] demonstrated that if all 8 clinical criteria are absent, there is a low likelihood of significant traumatic brain injury (TBI):
  - Evidence of significant skull fracture (depressed, basilar, or diastatic)
  - Altered level of alertness
  - Neurologic deficit
  - Persistent vomiting
  - Presence of scalp hematoma
  - Abnormal behavior
  - Coagulopathy
  - Age >65 years

Pediatric Considerations
Skull radiographs are not helpful in most cases, but can be done to document child abuse.

Diagnostic Procedures/Other
- CSF rhinorrhea:
  - Contains glucose; nasal mucus does not
  - Check for the double-halo sign: If nasal discharge contains CSF and blood, 2 rings appear when placed on filter paper—a central ring followed by a paler ring.
- Placement of ICP monitor, when indicated
- Serial neurologic exams
- Neuropsychometric testing when able

Test Interpretation
- Epidural, subdural, or intraparenchymal hemorrhage
- Coup or contrecoup injury
- Evolving, diffuse axonal injury is a principal cause of neurologic sequelae with mild head trauma.

TREATMENT

GENERAL MEASURES
- Acute management depends on injury severity. Most patients need no interventions.
- Immediate goal: Determine who needs further therapy, imaging studies (CT), and hospitalization to prevent further injury.
- For the severely injured patient:
  - Avoid hypotension or hypoxia. Head injury causes increased ICP secondary to edema, and perfusion pressure must be maintained.
  - 30-degree head elevation decreases ICP and improves cerebral perfusion pressure (2)[B].
  - Hyperventilation (hypocapnia) use should be limited to patients with impending herniation while preparing for definitive treatment or intraoperatively. It should never be used prophylactically or accidentally because it can cause and/or worsen cerebral ischemia and injure other organs (3)[B].
  - Seizure prophylaxis does not change outcomes (such as death rates), but may prevent seizures. Consider phenytoin or levetiracetam for 1 week postinjury.
- Manage breakthrough seizures with lorazepam.
- Brain tissue oxygen monitors measure brain tissue hypoxia associated with mortality and poor outcome. Combined use with ICP monitoring is associated with better outcome than ICP monitors alone (4)[B].

MEDICATION
First Line
- Pain: Morphine: 1–2 mg IV PRN, with caution, because can depress mental status, further altering serial neurologic evaluations; bolus doses may increase ICP and decrease cerebral perfusion pressure (5)
- Increased ICP:
  - Mannitol: 0.25–2 g/kg (0.25–1 g/kg in children) given over 30–60 minutes in patients with adequate renal function; should not be used without evidence of increased ICP; prophylactic use is associated with worse outcomes.
  - Lasix: 20–40 mg IV to promote diuresis:
    - Neither furosemide nor mannitol should be given to a hypotensive patient.
  - Hypertonic saline: 2 mL/kg IV decreases ICP without adverse hemodynamic status and may have beneficial effects on immune system and excitatory neurotransmitters (6)[B].
  - Progesterone: Likely beneficial to reduce edema and free radical production thereby reducing mortality; multicentered studies in progress (7)[A]
- Sedation:
  - Propofol: Preferred due to short duration of action, which allows serial neurologic exams

- Seizures:
  – Phenytoin (Dilantin): 15 mg/kg IV (1 mg/kg/min IV, not to exceed 50 mg/min). Stop infusion if QT interval increases by >50%.
  – Lorazepam (Ativan): 1–2 mg (0.1 mg/kg in children) IV
  – Fosphenytoin (Cerebyx): 15 mg/kg IV, not to exceed 150 mg/min. May give IM.
  – Levetiracetam (Keppra): May be desirable; lower complication rates, but prospective studies are needed. Use at neurosurgeon's instruction.
- Contraindications: Allergy

Second Line
- Diuretics and IV β-blockers (e.g., esmolol or labetalol) can be used to maintain central cerebral pressure (CCP = mean arterial pressure [MAP] – ICP) between 50 and 70 mm Hg.
- Nitrates may be helpful; however, may increase ICP
- Antibiotics (e.g., cefazolin): Given if penetrating trauma is present; prophylactic antibiotics are not useful in basilar skull fractures.

ISSUES FOR REFERRAL
Consult neurosurgery for:
- All penetrating head trauma
- All abnormal head CTs

IN-PATIENT CONSIDERATIONS
Admission Criteria/Initial Stabilization
- Abnormal CT
- Abnormal GCS
- Clinical evidence of basilar skull fracture
- Persistent neurologic deficits (e.g., confusion, somnolence)
- Patient with no competent adult at home for observation
- Possibly admit: LOC, amnesia, patients on anticoagulants with negative CT
- ABCs take priority over head injury.
- C-spine immobilization should be considered in all head trauma.

IV Fluids
Use normal saline for resuscitation fluid.

Discharge Criteria
Normal CT with return-to-normal mental status and responsible adult to observe patient at home (see "Patient Monitoring")

 ONGOING CARE

FOLLOW-UP RECOMMENDATIONS
- Schedule regular follow-up within a week to determine return to activities.
- Rehabilitation indicated following a significant acute injury. Set realistic goals.

Patient Monitoring
Any patient discharged should have head-injury instructions to use to watch for symptoms indicating need for further intervention (e.g., changing mental status, worsening headache, focal findings). Give to a competent adult who will observe the patient. A patient whose condition deteriorates is not likely to remember or act on any instructions.

DIET
As tolerated

PATIENT EDUCATION
Proper counseling, symptomatic management, and gradual return to normal activities are essential to prevent a posttraumatic neurosis that can become refractory to treatment.

PROGNOSIS
- Gradual improvement for many
- 30–50% of severe head injuries may be fatal.
- Prolonged coma may be followed by satisfactory outcome.
- Predicting outcome is difficult, and patients may improve for years.

Geriatric Considerations
Poorer prognosis with increasing age. Patients ≥75 have the highest rate of TBI hospitalizations and death.

Pediatric Considerations
Outcome is more positive in pediatric patients, except in severe TBI.

COMPLICATIONS
- Delayed hematomas
- Chronic subdural hematoma, which may follow even "mild" head injury, especially in the elderly. Often presents with headache and decreased mentation.
- Delayed hydrocephalus
- Emotional disturbances and psychiatric disorders resulting from head injury may be refractory to treatment.
- Seizure disorders: In 50% of penetrating head injuries, in 20% of severe closed head injuries, and in <5% of head injuries overall. Hematomas significantly increase risk of epilepsy.
- Postconcussion syndrome can follow mild head injury without LOC and includes headaches, dizziness, fatigue, and subtle cognitive or affective changes.
- Second-impact syndrome occurs when the CNS loses autoregulation. An individual with a minor head injury is returned to a contact sport and, following even minor trauma (e.g., whiplash), the patient loses consciousness and may quickly herniate, with a 50% mortality. A similar syndrome of malignant edema can occur in children with even a single injury.
- Increased risk for Alzheimer disease, Parkinson disease, and other brain disorders whose prevalence increases with age

REFERENCES
1. Mower WR, Hoffman JR, Herbert M, et al. Developing a decision instrument to guide computed tomographic imaging of blunt head injury patients. *J Trauma*. 2005;59:954–959.
2. Meyer MJ, Megyesi J, Meythaler J, et al. Acute management of acquired brain injury part I: An evidence-based review of non-pharmacological interventions. *Brain Inj*. 2010;24:694–705.
3. Curley G, Kavanagh BP, Laffey JG, et al. Hypocapnia and the injured brain: More harm than benefit. *Crit Care Med*. 2010;38:1348–1359.
4. Nangunoori R, Maloney-Wilensky E, Stiefel M, et al. Brain tissue oxygen-based therapy and outcome after severe traumatic brain injury: A systematic literature review. *Neurocrit Care*. 2012;17(1):131–138.
5. Roberts DJ, Hall RI, Kramer AH, et al. Sedation for critically ill adults with severe traumatic brain injury: A systematic review of randomized controlled trials. *Crit Care Med*. 2011;39:2743–2751.
6. Meyer MJ, Megyesi J, Meythaler J, et al. Acute management of acquired brain injury part II: An evidence-based review of pharmacological interventions. *Brain Inj*. 2010;24:706–721.
7. Ma J, Huang S, Qin S, You C. Progesterone for acute traumatic brain injury. *Cochrane Database Syst Rev*. 2012;10:CD008409. doi: 10.1002/14651858.CD008409.pub3.

ADDITIONAL READING
Wahid Bouida, Soudani Marghli, Sami Souissi, et al. Prediction value of the Canadian CT head rule and the New Orleans criteria for positive head CT scan and acute neurosurgical procedures in minor head trauma: A multicenter external validation study. *Ann Emerg Med*. 2013;61(5):521–527.

 SEE ALSO

Brain Injury–Post Acute Care Issues; Postconcussive Syndrome; Seizure Disorders

 CODES

ICD10
- S06.5X0A Traum subdr hem w/o loss of consciousness, init
- S06.6X0A Traum subrac hem w/o loss of consciousness, init
- S06.9X0A Unsp intracranial injury w/o loss of consciousness, init

CLINICAL PEARLS
- Head injury is a dynamic process: Initial bleeding followed by secondary injury due to cerebral edema, continued bleeding, etc.
- Patients with history of head injury should have imaging if any of the following are present: Evidence of skull fracture, altered consciousness, neurologic deficit, persistent vomiting, scalp hematoma, abnormal behavior, coagulopathy, age >65 years.
- Patient with normal head CT who has returned to normal mental status may be discharged to home with a competent adult observer for 24 hours.
- Strict criteria exist for patients to return to normal sport activity following head injury to avoid the second-impact syndrome, which has 50% mortality.
- Predicting outcome is difficult, and patients may improve for years.

BRAIN INJURY—POST ACUTE CARE ISSUES
Maria I. Aguilar, MD

 BASICS

DESCRIPTION
Traumatic brain injury (TBI) is caused by externally inflicted trauma that may result in significant impairment of an individual's physical, cognitive, and psychosocial functioning. The management of acute TBI is outside the scope of this topic.

EPIDEMIOLOGY
- Predominant age: Highest incidence in the very young (0–4), in persons 15–24 years of age, and those >75
- Predominant sex: Male > Female (2:1)

Incidence
- 1.2–1.7 million in US sustain a TBI per year
- 50,000 deaths per year
- 80,000–90,000 sustain long-term disabilities

Prevalence
5.3 million in US have TBI-related disabilities

ETIOLOGY AND PATHOPHYSIOLOGY
- Falls and motor vehicle accidents (MVAs) are most common causes
- Violence-related TBI increasing (10% of all cases)
- Sports and recreation injuries (especially in teenagers and young adults)
- Cortical contusions due to coup-contrecoup injuries. Although axonal rupture from shear and tensile forces can occur at the time of severe head injury, milder degrees of axonal damage may play a role in mild TBI.
- Disruption of axonal neurofilament organization impairs axonal transport, leading to axonal swelling, Wallerian degeneration, and transection.
- Release of excitatory neurotransmitters acetylcholine, glutamate, and aspartate and generation of free radicals may contribute to secondary injury.

RISK FACTORS
- High risk: Male, age 15–34
- Moderate risk <5 years and >60 years
- Lower socioeconomic status (head injury)

GENERAL PREVENTION
Improved safety standards and programs designed to minimize injury from vehicular-related events (motor vehicle, motorcycle, bicycle, pedestrian), falls, violence, sports, and recreation provide best prevention against TBI (1)[C].

COMMONLY ASSOCIATED CONDITIONS
- Psychosis
- Suicide attempts
- Substance abuse
- Attention deficit disorder

 DIAGNOSIS

HISTORY
- Nonneurologic complications: Pulmonary, metabolic and endocrinologic, nutritional, GI, musculoskeletal, genitourinary, dermatologic, chronic pain
- Most neurologic complications are apparent within the 1st days following injury; long-term sequelae include seizures, headache, hydrocephalus, visual defects, neuroendocrine abnormalities, and movement and sleep disorders.

- Cognitive consequences: Memory impairment, difficulties in attention and concentration, language deficits, visual perception problems, and poor problem solving, reasoning, insight, judgment, and information processing
- Behavioral problems: Decreased ability to initiate responses, verbal and physical aggression, agitation, learning difficulties, shallow self-awareness, altered sexual functioning, impulsivity, social disinhibition
- Psychological consequences: Mood disorders, personality changes, altered emotional control, depression, anxiety
- Disruption of normal sleep
- Social consequences: Risk of suicide, divorce, unemployment, economic strain, alcohol/substance abuse

Pediatric Considerations
Interactions of physical, cognitive, and behavioral sequelae interfere with new learning. Effects of early TBI may not become apparent until later in the child's development.

PHYSICAL EXAM
TBI's degree (mild, moderate, severe) is classified based on the Glasgow coma scale (GCS), a point scoring system based on verbal response, eye opening response, and motor response to voice or pain following an injury.

DIFFERENTIAL DIAGNOSIS
- The diagnosis of pain following TBI can be difficult in light of limitations imposed by cognitive, language, and behavioral deficits:
  - Dysautonomia: Tachypnea, hypertension, painful posturing/contractions, diaphoresis
  - Neuropathic pain: Burning, shock-like, or pins and needles; allodynia/hyperpathia. 3 most common: Complex regional pain syndrome, central pain syndrome, and peripheral neuropathy
  - Spasticity or spastic dystonia
  - Headache: Posttraumatic headache, hydrocephalus, increased intracranial pressure
  - Myofascial pain syndrome
  - Neurogenic heterotopic ossification: Bone formation in soft tissue
  - Deep vein thrombosis
  - Constipation and urinary retention
  - Trauma: Fractures, musculoskeletal injuries
  - Shoulder: Subluxation, acromioclavicular separation, rotator cuff tendonitis/tear
- Chronic infection, depression, hypothyroidism, hydrocephalus, intracerebral hemorrhage, seizures, fractures, tracheal stricture, pain, alcohol, drugs, polypharmacy, and/or CNS depressant

DIAGNOSTIC TESTS & INTERPRETATION
- Evoked potentials (auditory, visual, somatosensory)
- Behavioral assessment, neuropsychologic testing, vocational assessment
- Cognitive test for orientation and arousal; use Western Neurosensory Stimulation Profile or Galveston Orientation Amnesia Test
- EEG

Initial Tests (lab, imaging)
As needed for suspected metabolic complications:
- Bone scan: Heterotopic ossification
- CT: Hydrocephalus, atrophy, hematoma

- Video fluoroscopic swallowing study
- MRI: To evaluate diffuse axonal injury
- EEG: To evaluate subclinical seizure activity; limited predictive value in the setting of acute TBI

Test Interpretation
- Evidence of microscopic axonal injury, axon retraction bulbs, and microglial clusters
- Hydrocephalus with periventricular edema
- Joint contractures result in collagen cross-linking: Decreased range of motion
- Heterotopic ossification: Disorganized osteoid calcification in soft tissue

 TREATMENT

GENERAL MEASURES
- Diminished level of arousal: Identify best modality for communication, assess functional skills (proper seating, hand function) with behaviorist/neuropsychologist.
- Social work (family education and long-term planning) and nursing
- Reduce sedatives
- Neurogenic bladder: Treat UTI:
  - If postvoid residual <50 mL, then try regular voiding routine q2h
  - If still incontinent, add oxybutynin
  - If still incontinent, try condom catheter during the day; incontinence pads at night
  - If high postvoid residuals or high-pressure bladder or dyssynergic bladder on urodynamics: Intermittent catheter q4–6h
- Neurogenic bowel: Regular bowel routine
- Contractures and spasticity; stretching:
  - If no progress after 4 weeks, consider serial casting or custom-made orthotic
  - Contractures >45 degrees: Consider tendon release
- Heterotopic ossification: Stretch soft tissue to decrease maturation of osteoid, consider orthotics/splinting, bone scan at baseline
- Skin: Turn patient q2h; avoid sitting, such as in bed, at 45 degrees, observe for erythema around tube sites, and rule out latex allergy
- Respiratory: Night humidification for tracheotomy
- Endocrine: Monitor fluid balance
- Rehabilitative practices: Rehabilitative programs should be interdisciplinary, comprehensive, and include cognitive and behavioral assessment and intervention (1)[C].

MEDICATION
- Psychostimulants may affect speed of cognitive processing, mood, and behavior. May also improve memory, attention, concentration, and mental processing in children/adults (2)[C]:
  - Methylphenidate 20–40 mg/d in 2 divided doses; dextroamphetamine 5–40 mg/d divided q.d.–t.i.d.
  - Modafinil had no clinically significant effect when compared with placebo for the treatment of fatigue and excessive daytime sleepiness (3)[B].

- Agitation:
  - Treat epilepsy or depression first:
  - Minimize the use of antipsychotics and benzodiazepines, as they worsen cognition
  - β-blockers have best evidence for efficacy in agitation/aggression (4)[A]
  - Antidepressants (selective serotonin reuptake inhibitors [SSRIs]) and antiepileptic drugs (AEDs) in the context of an affective disorder or epilepsy, respectively, may help agitation/aggression (5)[B]
  - If necessary, use antipsychotics of the atypical class (clozapine, olanzapine, quetiapine, risperidone, and ziprasidone) (6)[B]
- Abulia (lack of initiative): Amantadine (Symmetrel), bromocriptine, methylphenidate, levodopa (6)[C]
- Epilepsy: American Academy of Physical Medicine and Rehabilitation does not recommend AEDs for preventing late (>7 days post-TBI) posttraumatic seizures (7)[B]. If epilepsy occurs, avoid phenobarbital; too sedating (7)
- Spasticity caution: Be aware of potential negative consequences of all agents:
  - Use dantrolene sodium 25–200 mg/d divided t.i.d.; baclofen; intrathecal baclofen; diazepam, clonidine, tizanidine, and gabapentin; botulinum toxin injections for focal spasticity (8)[B]
- Neurogenic bladder: Oxybutynin 2.5 mg t.i.d.:
  - 10 mg q.i.d. if bladder pressures low and/or postvoid residuals low (1)[B]
- Bowel routine: Stool softener such as docusate sodium (daily) combined with laxative (night before suppository), high-fiber diet, and suppository (every other day) (1)[C]
- Heterotopic ossification: Indomethacin 25–50 mg t.i.d. If severe, progressive, or history of GI ulceration, then etidronate (Didronel) 20 mg/kg for 6 months or alendronate 20 mg/d (1)[C]
- Neurobehavioral problems: Weak evidence supports psychostimulants as effective in treatment of inattention, apathy, and slowness; high-dose β-blockers in treatment of agitation and aggression; and anticonvulsants and antidepressants in treatment of agitation and aggression with an affective disorder (5)[B]. Rivastigmine showed promising results when used at least 12 months after TBI in the subgroup of patients with moderate to severe memory deficits (9)[C].
- Precautions: Medications may have significant adverse effects in persons with TBI and can impede rehabilitation progress.
- Insomnia: Nonpharmacologic interventions (relaxation, cognitive-behavioral therapy, sleep hygiene education); pharmacologic interventions (zopiclone, lorazepam, melatonin, tricyclic antidepressants) (10)

ISSUES FOR REFERRAL
- Refer to multidisciplinary rehabilitation programs
- Suicide attempts and ideation (SI) are more prevalent in people with TBI, even after controlling for psychiatric disorders (11)[C]. Assess hopelessness and SI proactively.

COMPLEMENTARY AND ALTERNATIVE MEDICINE
- Cognitive exercises (including computer-assisted strategies), compensatory devices (memory books, paging systems), psychotherapy, behavior modification, vocational rehabilitation, school rehabilitation, nutritional support, music and art therapy, therapeutic recreation
- Hyperbaric oxygen therapy (HBOT) cannot be routinely recommended for patients with TBI because of few trials, methodologic shortcomings, and poor reporting (12)[A].

 ONGOING CARE

FOLLOW-UP RECOMMENDATIONS
Patient Monitoring
Patients make slow, steady gains; review medical status monthly

DIET
- Ensure adequate hydration; 2–2.5 L/d of water
- Bolus feeds preferred if fed by gastrostomy
- Upright and quiet for 30 minutes following feeds, as aspiration can occur even with a g-tube
- Early feeding is associated with trend toward better survival and disability outcomes (13)[A].

PATIENT EDUCATION
- Brain Injury Information Network: www.tbinet.org
- Brain Injury Association of America: www.biausa.org

PROGNOSIS
- Most rapid return of function occurs during first 2 years, but some improve slowly for 5–10 years
- Highly variable (80% of individuals with severe injuries become independent in dressing and self-care at 1 year)
- Negative prognostic factors:
  - Age >40 years old
  - Abnormal pupillary responses or extraocular eye movements
  - Prolonged coma
  - Abnormal evoked potentials
- Accurate prediction of return to work is not feasible, with rates in the 12–70% range.
- The Oxford Handicap Scale at hospital discharge is a good tool to predict disability at 6 months (14)[A].

COMPLICATIONS
Major affective disorder (depression, psychosis) in up to 50% of patients, family and caregiver burnout, substance abuse, social isolation, dental caries, osteoporosis, aspiration pneumonia, pressure ulcers, dysphagia, esophagitis, bladder incontinence, contractures/spasticity

REFERENCES

1. Consensus conference. Rehabilitation of persons with traumatic brain injury. NIH Consensus Development Panel on Rehabilitation of Persons With Traumatic Brain Injury. *JAMA.* 1999;282: 974–983.
2. Siddall OM. Use of methylphenidate in traumatic brain injury. *Ann Pharmacother.* 2005;39: 1309–1313.
3. Jha A, Weintraub A, Allshouse A, et al. A randomized trial of modafinil for the treatment of fatigue and excessive daytime sleepiness in individuals with chronic traumatic brain injury. *J Head Trauma Rehabil.* 2008;23:52–63.
4. Fleminger S. Pharmacological management for agitation and aggression in people with acquired brain injury. *Cochrane Database Syst Rev.* 2003/2006;1:CD003299.
5. Deb S, Crownshaw T. The role of pharmacotherapy in the management of behaviour disorders in traumatic brain injury patients. *Brain Inj.* 2004;18:1–31.
6. Elovic EP. The use of atypical antipsychotics in traumatic brain injury. *J Head Trauma Rehab.* 2003;18:177–195.
7. Bushnik T. Medical and social issues related to posttraumatic seizures in persons with traumatic brain injury. *J Head Trauma Rehab.* 2004;19: 296–304.
8. Zafonte R. Acute care management of post-TBI spasticity. *J Head Trauma Rehab.* 2004;19: 89–100.
9. Silver J, Koumaras B, Chen M. Effects of rivastigmine on cognitive function in patients with traumatic brain injury. *Neurology.* 2006;67: 748–755.
10. Zeiter JM, Friedman L, O'Hara R. Insomnia in the context of traumatic brain injury. *J Rehabil Res Dev.* 2009;6:827–836.
11. Simpson G, Tate R. Suicidality in people surviving a traumatic brain injury: Prevalence, risk factors and implications for clinical management. *Brain Inj.* 2007;21:1335–1351.
12. Bennett M, Heard R. Hyperbaric oxygen therapy for multiple sclerosis. *Cochrane Database Syst Rev.* 2004;1:CD003057.
13. Perel P, Yanagawa T, Bunn F, et al. Nutritional support for head-injured patients. *Cochrane Database Syst Rev.* 2006;4:CD001530.
14. Perel P, Edwards P, Shakur H, et al. Use of the Oxford Handicap Scale at hospital discharge to predict Glasgow Outcome Scale at 6 months in patients with traumatic brain injury. *BMC Med Res Methodol.* 2008;8:72.

 CODES

ICD10
- S06.9X9S Unsp intracranial injury w LOC of unsp duration, sequela
- S06.9X0S Unsp intracranial injury w/o loss of consciousness, sequela
- S06.9X9A Unsp intracranial injury w LOC of unsp duration, init

CLINICAL PEARLS
- TBI can cause both neurologic and nonneurologic manifestations.
- Best approach to treatment includes multi- and interdisciplinary team member participation.
- TBI can lead to devastating sequelae; prevention is key.

BRANCHIAL CLEFT FISTULA

Varun K. Bhalla, MD • Caleb J. Mentzer, DO • E. James Kruse, DO

 BASICS

DESCRIPTION
- A congenital, abnormal tract connecting the skin of the neck with an internal structure.
- Results from the incomplete closure or development of the branchial arches or associated clefts.
- Involves branchial clefts I–IV, which develop in the 4th week of gestation.
- System(s) affected: Skin/Exocrine

Pediatric Considerations
Most occur in the pediatric age group

EPIDEMIOLOGY
- Predominant age: By definition, all branchial cleft fistulae are present at birth; however, they may remain unnoticed for some time.
- Branchial cleft cysts may not present until adulthood, and are commonly diagnosed in the 3rd and 5th decades of life.
- Predominant sex: Male = Female

Incidence
Unknown

Prevalence
Unknown

ETIOLOGY AND PATHOPHYSIOLOGY
- Branchial anomalies result from the incomplete obliteration of pharyngeal clefts and pouches during embryogenesis.
- Both respiratory and squamous epithelium (alone or together) may line branchial anomalies.
- Squamous epithelium is found more commonly in cysts.
- Ciliated, columnar epithelium is found more commonly in sinuses and fistulae.
- The 1st branchial cleft contributes to the external auditory canal, middle ear cavity, mastoid air cells, and eustachian tube. Related fistulae are very rare and tend to be infra- or retroauricular. Preauricular cysts and sinuses are not thought to be of branchial cleft origin:
  – 1st branchial cleft anomalies enter the external auditory canal and/or occasionally the middle ear.
  – They represent 1–4% of all branchial cleft malformations.
  – Type I anomalies contain ectodermal elements only and course lateral to the facial nerve.
  – Type II anomalies contain ectoderm and mesoderm, coursing medial to the facial nerve.

- The 2nd branchial cleft forms the hyoid bone and tonsillar fossa. Related fistulae (most common variant) course between the internal and external carotid arteries:
  – 2nd branchial anomalies represent 90–95% of all branchial cleft lesions.
  – They course close to the glossopharyngeal and hypoglossal nerves, entering the pharynx at the level of supratonsillar fossa.
  – The external opening runs along anterior border of sternocleidomastoid muscle.
  – 2nd branchial cleft anomalies are subdivided into 4 subtypes:
    ○ Type I lesions are anterior to the SCM and do not involve the carotid sheath.
    ○ Type II lesions are the most common second arch anomalies, deep to the SCM, and anterior or posterior to the carotid artery.
    ○ Type III lesions pass between the internal and external carotid arteries and are adjacent to the pharynx.
    ○ Type IV lesions are medial to the sheath, adjacent to the tonsillar fossa.
- The 3rd and 4th branchial clefts form the parathyroid glands, thymus, and portions of thyroid gland (parafollicular cells):
  – 3rd branchial cleft anomalies represent 5% of all branchial anomalies.
  – Sinus tracts (also called pyriform sinuses) originate in the pyriform sinus and course adjacent to the thyroid cartilage.
  – Fistulae are rare, usually resulting from recurrent infections and/or repeated surgery.
  – Both 3rd and 4th fistulas should have external ostia on the lower anterior neck. Left-sided lesions are more common that right-sided ones.
  – They are often called pyriform sinus "fistulae," despite the frequent lack of an external opening to the skin.
  – Those from the 3rd branchial cleft course posterior to carotid artery.
  – Differentiated from 2nd branchial cleft anomalies by the location of their internal opening (external openings should be the same).
  – Presence of thymic tissue does not differentiate between 3rd and 4th branchial cleft anomalies, as accessory thymic tissue has been described in the latter (1).

Genetics
10% have family history.

RISK FACTORS
Positive family history

COMMONLY ASSOCIATED CONDITIONS
Microtia and aural atresia occur with failure of development of the 1st branchial cleft.

 DIAGNOSIS

HISTORY
- History of drainage from the cervical area
- Neck abscess or suppurative thyroiditis

PHYSICAL EXAM
- Presence of a tiny external opening usually on mid to lower neck along anterior border of sternocleido-mastoid muscle.
- Spontaneous mucoid drainage
- External openings may be marked by a skin tag or cartilage.
- Infection may be the presenting sign: Erythema, swelling, pain, or fever may also be present.
- Thyroid abscesses in children often represent an underlying branchial remnant, especially with (+) mixed-flora cultures (2).
- 10% are bilateral.
- Small orifices located in the mid-neck, most commonly along the anterior border of the sternocleidomastoid muscle (less commonly in the lower neck or postauricular).
- 3rd and 4th branchial cleft anomalies are predominantly left-sided (89%) (1).

DIFFERENTIAL DIAGNOSIS
- External sinuses
- Cystic hygroma
- Dermoid cysts
- Lymphadenopathy

DIAGNOSTIC TESTS & INTERPRETATION
Culture if signs of infection
- CT of neck with IV contrast is occasionally beneficial in 3rd and 4th branchial cleft fistulas/sinus (2)[C].
- CT may demonstrate the fistula tract in up to 64% of cases (3).
- MRI and US may also be useful to define the tract.
- A barium esophagogram may demonstrate the fistula tract and location; sensitivity rate of 50–80% when used to evaluate 3rd and 4th branchial anomalies (3)[C].
- An incisional biopsy should not be performed in children, as this may make subsequent resection more difficult.
- Contrast diagnostic modalities are more accurate in the noninfected state due to reduced edema and improved contrast penetration into the fistula tract.

Diagnostic Procedures/Other
- Sinogram or fistulogram may be done, but are usually of little value.
- Upper airway endoscopy may be useful to visualize the opening into the pharynx.

Test Interpretation
- Cysts are more commonly lined by stratified squamous epithelium and may contain hair follicles, sweat glands, sebaceous glands, or cartilage.
- Sinuses and fistulae are more commonly lined by ciliated, columnar epithelium.

TREATMENT

- Complete surgical excision is required to prevent recurrence.
- Outpatient status is usually appropriate.
- Acute infections should be treated with antibiotics first; if this fails to resolve, incision and drainage may be required (3). Typical offending organisms include *Streptococcus* and *Klebsiella,* although infections may be polymicrobial.
- If possible, an elective resection should be scheduled weeks after the acute infection.

SURGERY/OTHER PROCEDURES
- Stepladder incisions may be needed to visualize the upper portion of the tract.
- 1st branchial cleft lesions may require larger incisions.
- Methylene blue injection into fistula may be useful, although spillage complicates the dissection.
- Cannulation of the tract or fistula with a 2-0 or 3-0 monofilament suture may aid in establishing the course of the tract.
- Drains are not routinely used.
- For 3rd and 4th arch anomalies, fiberoptic endoscopy may assist in locating the opening into the pyriform sinus.
- 4th arch fistulas require an ipsilateral hemithyroidectomy to remove the tract; partial resection of the thyroid cartilage may be required to gain exposure to the tract as it enters the pyriform sinus (3).
- Antibiotics are used only for infection.

- Patients with abscesses related to 3rd branchial cleft anomalies frequently require initial incision and drainage (1)[B]:
  - Incision and drainage failure rates is ~94% on the 1st attempt.
  - Virtually all will require resection.
  - Those with acute suppurative thyroiditis may require partial thyroidectomy and removal of the fistula tract. Partial thyroidectomy is rarely curative (1)[B].
- Endoscopic cauterization of the internal orifice has been successfully used in some cases, especially in children <8 years (1)[B].

ONGOING CARE

FOLLOW-UP RECOMMENDATIONS
Patient Monitoring
- If infected, follow at weekly intervals until resolution of abscess and inflammatory reaction; then excise.
- Postoperative visit at 2–3 weeks
- Lack of epithelium in the fistula tract pathology specimen may indicate incomplete resection; have a high index of suspicion for future recurrence.

PROGNOSIS
Good

COMPLICATIONS
- Facial nerve injury (1st arch anomalies)
- Hypoglossal nerve injury
- Spinal accessory nerve injury
- Vagus nerve injury
- Infection
- Carotid artery injury
- Recurrence (full excision of tract epithelium required) – common with 1st arch anomalies due to incomplete excision.
- Neoplastic degeneration of branchial remnants (~250 reported cases) if not resected.

REFERENCES

1. Nicoucar K, Giger R, Jaecklin T, et al. Management of congenital third branchial arch anomalies: A systematic review. *Otolaryngol Head Neck Surg.* 2010;142:21–28.e2.
2. Liberman M, Kay S, Emil S, et al. Ten years of experience with third and fourth branchial remnants. *J Ped Surg.* 2002;37:685–690.
3. Waldhausen JH. Branchial cleft and arch anomalies in children. *Semin Pediatr Surg.* 2006;15:64–69.

 CODES

ICD10
Q18.0 Sinus, fistula and cyst of branchial cleft

CLINICAL PEARLS
- Most common: 2nd branchial cleft anomalies: An opening in the mid-neck at the anterior border of the sternocleidomastoid muscle with a history of an occasional discharge is diagnostic
- Radiographic confirmation is not needed; complete surgical excision as an outpatient is both diagnostic and therapeutic.
- Branchial cleft remnants, sinuses, and cysts result from the failure of branchial arches to close and/or complete their normal development.

BREAST ABSCESS
Shumaila Athar, MD • Tamara McGregor, MD

BASICS

DESCRIPTION
- Collection of pus, usually localized
- Can be associated with lactation or fistulous tracts secondary to squamous epithelial neoplasm or duct occlusion
- System(s) affected: Skin/Exocrine
- Synonym(s): Mammary abscess; Peripheral breast abscess; Subareolar abscess; Puerperal abscess

Pregnancy Considerations
Most commonly associated with postpartum lactation

EPIDEMIOLOGY
- Predominant age:
  – Puerperal abscess: Lactational
  – Subareolar abscess: Postmenopausal
- Predominant sex: Female
- African American higher incidence

Incidence
- 0.1–0.5% of breastfeeding women
- Puerperal abscess rare after first 6 weeks of lactation

ETIOLOGY AND PATHOPHYSIOLOGY
- Delayed treatment of mastitis
- Puerperal abscesses: Blocked lactiferous duct
- Subareolar abscess: Squamous epithelial neoplasm with keratin plugs or ductal extension with associated inflammation
- Peripheral abscess: Stasis of the duct
- Microbiology:
  – Most common cause:
    ○ *Staphylococcus aureus*
  – Less common causes:
    ○ *Streptococcus pyogenes*
    ○ *Escherichia coli*
    ○ Bacteroide
    ○ Corneybacterium
    ○ Pseudomonas
    ○ Proteus
- MRSA is an increasingly important pathogen in postpartum women; risk factors for post partum SA breast abscess have not changed with the advent of community-associated MRSA (1)[A].

RISK FACTORS
- Puerperal mastitis:
  – 5–11% go on to abscess:
    ○ Most often due to inadequate therapy
  – Risk factors for mastitis are those that result in milk stasis:
    ○ Infrequent or missing feeds
    ○ Poor latch
    ○ Damaged nipple
    ○ Illness in mother or baby
    ○ Rapid weaning
    ○ Breast pressure
    ○ Blocked nipple pore or duct
    ○ Maternal stress or fatigue
    ○ Maternal malnutrition

- General factors:
  – Smoking
  – Diabetes
  – Rheumatoid arthritis
  – Obesity
- Medically induced factors:
  – Steroids
  – Silicone/Paraffin implant
  – Lumpectomy with radiation
- Nipple retraction
- Nipple piercing for mastitis (2)
- Higher recurrence rate if multiorganism abscess

GENERAL PREVENTION
- Prevention of mastitis
- Early treatment of mastitis with milk expression and cold compresses
- Early treatment with antibiotics

COMMONLY ASSOCIATED CONDITIONS
Lactation

DIAGNOSIS

- Tender breast lump, fluctuant, usually unilateral
- Systemic malaise (although usually less malaise than with mastitis)
- Fever

HISTORY
Tender breast lump, usually unilateral

PHYSICAL EXAM
- Erythema
- Draining pus
- Local edema
- Nipple and skin retraction
- Proximal lymphadenopathy

DIFFERENTIAL DIAGNOSIS
- Carcinoma (inflammatory or primary squamous cell)
- Engorgement
- Galactocele
- Tuberculosis (may be associated with HIV infection)
- Actinomycosis
- Typhoid
- Sarcoid
- Granulomatous disease
- Syphilis
- Foreign body reactions (e.g., to silicone and paraffin)
- Mammary duct ectasia
- Hydatid cyst
- Sebaceous cyst

DIAGNOSTIC TESTS & INTERPRETATION
- CBC showing leukocytosis
- Elevated ESR
- Culture and sensitivity of drainage to identify pathogen, usually staphylococci or streptococci
- MRSA is a recent increasingly important pathogen in both lactational and nonlactational abscesses.
- Other bacteria:
  – Nonlactational abscess and recurrent abscesses associated with anaerobic bacteria:
    ○ *E. coli, proteus*; mixed bacteria less common
- Ultrasound
- Mammogram

Diagnostic Procedures/Other
- Aspiration for culture
- Fine-needle aspiration is not accurate to exclude carcinoma.

Test Interpretation
- Squamous metaplasia of the ducts
- Intraductal hyperplasia
- Epithelial overgrowth
- Fat necrosis
- Duct ectasia

TREATMENT

GENERAL MEASURES
- Cold compresses for pain control
- *Important to continue to breastfeed or express milk*

MEDICATION
Combine antibiotics (along with drainage) for cure.
- Culture midstream sample of milk for mastitis
- Culture abscess fluid for breast abscess

- There is insufficient evidence regarding the effectiveness of antibiotic therapies for lactational mastitis alone (3)[A].

First Line
- NSAIDs
- Dicloxacillin 500 mg q.i.d. for 10–14 days (4)[A]
- If no response in 24–48 hours, switch to cephalexin 500 mg q.i.d. for 10–14 days:
  – Or amoxicillin-clavulanate (Augmentin) 250 mg t.i.d.
- Clindamycin 300 mg t.i.d. if anaerobes suspected
- If MRSA a concern, TMP-SMZ 2 PO bid for 10–14 days, or clindamycin
- *Contraindications*: Allergy to the antibiotic
- Precautions: Refer to manufacturer's profile for each drug
- In severe infections, vancomycin may be necessary for inpatient treatment:
  – Dose (30 mg/kg) IV in 2 divided doses every 24 hours may be necessary until culture results are available.
  – A third-generation or a combination of a beta-lactam and beta-lactamase agent may need to be added as well.
- Subareolar abscess may need addition of metronidazole for anaerobic coverage.
- New techniques include percutaneous intracavitary urokinase irrigation for large abscesses in nonlactating women (5)[C].

SURGERY/OTHER PROCEDURES

- Aspiration under US (5,6)[B],(7)[C]
- Serial aspirations under US may be necessary (q2–3d) (8)[C].
- Needle aspiration alone (without antibiotics) may be effective for small breast abscesses (9)[A].
- If aspiration and antibiotics fail, incision and drainage with removal of loculations
- Biopsy of all nonpuerperal abscesses to rule out carcinoma
- Open all fistulous tracts, especially in nonlactating abscesses.
- US-guided aspiration of breast abscess with judicious use of antibiotics is better modality than incision and drainage (10)[A].

COMPLEMENTARY AND ALTERNATIVE MEDICINE

- Lecithin supplementation
- Acupuncture may help with breast engorgement, and possibly with breast abscess prevention (11)[A].

IN-PATIENT CONSIDERATIONS
Admission Criteria/Initial Stabilization
- Outpatient, unless systemically immunocompromised or septic
- Aggressive glycemic control important (7)[B]

 ONGOING CARE

FOLLOW-UP RECOMMENDATIONS
Patient Monitoring
Ensure resolution to exclude carcinoma.

PATIENT EDUCATION
- Care of wound
- Breastfeeding precautions

PROGNOSIS
- Complete healing expected in 8–10 days
- Subareolar abscesses frequently recur, even after incision and drainage (I&D) and antibiotics; may require surgical removal of ducts.

COMPLICATIONS
- Fistula: Mammary duct or milk fistula
- Poor cosmetic outcome

REFERENCES

1. Branch-Ellinman W, et al. Risk factors for *Staphylococcus aureus* post partum breast abscess. *Clin Infect Disease*. 2012;54(1):71–77
2. Gollapalli V, Liao J, Dudkavic A, et al. Risk factors for development and recurrence of primary breast abscess. *J Am Coll Surg*. 2010;211:41–48.
3. Jahanfar S. et al. Antibiotics for mastitis in breastfeeding women. *Cochrane Database Syst Review2*. 2013;CD005458
4. Cusack L, Brennan M. Lactational mastitis and breast abscess—diagnosis and management in general practice. *Aust Fam Physician*. 2011; 40(12):976–979.
5. Schwarz RJ, Shrestha R. Needle aspiration of breast abscesses. *Am J Surgery*. 2001;182:117.
6. Dener C, Inan A. Breast abscesses in lactating women. *World J Surgery*. 2003;27:130.
7. Christensen AF, Al-Suliman N, Nielsen KR, et al. Ultrasound-guided drainage of breast abscesses: Results in 151 patients. *Br J Radiol*. 2005;78: 186–188.
8. Elder E, Brennan M. Nonsurgical management should be first-line therapy for breast abscess. *World J Surg*. 2010;34:2257–2258.
9. Thirumalaikumar S, Kommu S. Best evidence topic reports. Aspiration of breast abscesses. *Emerg Med J*. 2004;21:333–334.
10. Naeem M, et al. Comparison of incision and drainage against needle aspiration for treatment of breast abscess *Am Surg* 2012;78(11): 1224–1227.
11. Mangesi L, Dowswell T. Treatments for breast engorgement during lactation. *Cochrane Database Syst Rev*. 2010;CD006946.

ADDITIONAL READING

- Berná-Serna JD, Berná-Mestre JD, Galindo PJ, et al. Use of urokinase in percutaneous drainage of large breast abscesses. *J Ultrasound Med*. 2009;28: 449–454.
- Dabbas N, Chand M, Pallett A, et al. Have the organisms that cause breast abscess changed with time?—Implications for appropriate antibiotic usage in primary and secondary care. *Breast J*. 2010;16:412–415.
- Rizzo M, Gabram S, Staley C, et al. Management of breast abscesses in nonlactating women. *Am Surg*. 2010;76:292–295.
- Trop I, Dugas A, David J, et al. Breast abscesses: Evidence-based algorithms for diagnosis, management, and follow-up. *Radiographics*. 2011;31(6):1683–1699.

 CODES

ICD10
- N61 Inflammatory disorders of breast
- O91.12 Abscess of breast associated with the puerperium
- O91.13 Abscess of breast associated with lactation

CLINICAL PEARLS

- 5–11% of cases of puerperal mastitis go on to abscess (most often due to inadequate therapy for mastitis). Risk factors for mastitis are those that result in milk stasis (infrequent feeds, missing feeds).
- Abscess not associated with lactation should prompt coverage with antibiotics that cover anaerobic bacteria.
- Treatment is antibiotic and aspiration, with I&D, with breakup of loculations reserved for those failing more conservative management.
- US-guided aspiration of breast abscess with judicious use of antibiotics is a better modality than incision and drainage (11)[A].
- Breastfeeding is suggested to be continued during the presence of lactation-associated breast infection. Hand expression or hand pumping may be done as well.

BREAST CANCER

Bethany Gentilesco, MD • Aaron Kofman, MD • Komal Talati, MD

BASICS

DESCRIPTION
- Malignant tumor originating from breast epithelial cells, glandular cells, or connective tissue (rare)
- Types: Ductal carcinoma in situ (DCIS—a precursor to invasive disease), invasive infiltrating ductal carcinoma, invasive lobular carcinoma, inflammatory breast cancer, Paget disease of the nipple, phyllodes tumor, angiosarcoma

EPIDEMIOLOGY
Incidence
- 122 cases per 100,000 women per year, 2005–09
- New invasive cancer 2013 (est.): Women: 232,340
- New in situ cancer 2013 (est.): 64,640 (85% ductal carcinoma in situ)
- Breast cancer (BC) deaths 2013 (est.): 39,620; lifetime risk BC: 1 in 8 (12.2%); lifetime risk BC death (2007–09): 2.76% (1 in 36)
- Most common malignancy in U.S. women, second only to lung cancer (CA) as cause of CA death

Prevalence
2.8 million women in the US (2010 est.)

ETIOLOGY AND PATHOPHYSIOLOGY
- Genetic mutations, such as *BRCA1* and *BRCA2*, can cause hereditary breast and ovarian cancer. These genes function as tumor suppressor genes, and a mutation leads to cell cycle progression and limitations in DNA repair.
- Mutations in estrogen/progesterone receptors through genetic changes can cause BC by inducing cyclin D1 and *c-myc* expression downstream, leading to cell cycle progression.
- ~1/3 of BCs do not express estrogen receptor (ER) mutations; however, many of these tumors may display cross-talk with ER receptor and epidermal growth factors receptors (EGFR).

Genetics
- Criteria for additional risk evaluation/gene testing in *affected individual* (1):
  - BC at age ≤50 years
  - BC at any age and ≥1 family member with BC ≤50 years or ovarian/fallopian tube/primary peritoneal CA any age or ≥2 family members with BC or pancreatic CA any age or population at increased risk (e.g., Ashkenazi Jew with BC or ovarian CA at any age)
  - Triple-negative BC (ER-, PR-, HER2-)
  - 2 BC primaries in single patient
  - Ovarian/Fallopian tube/primary peritoneal CA
  - 1+ family member with BC and CA of thyroid, adrenal cortex, endometrium, pancreas, CNS, diffuse gastric, aggressive prostate (Gleason >7), leukemia, lymphoma, sarcoma, dermatologic manifestations and/or macrocephaly, GI hamartomas
  - Male BC
  - Known BC *susceptibility gene* mutation in family
- Criteria for additional risk evaluation/gene testing in *unaffected BC individual* (1):
  - 1st- or 2nd-degree relative with BC ≤45 years
  - ≥2 breast primaries in one individual or ≥1 ovarian/fallopian tube/primary peritoneal CA from same side of family or ≥2 w/breast primaries on same side of family
  - 1+ family member with BC and CA of thyroid, adrenal cortex, endometrium, pancreas, CNS, diffuse gastric, aggressive prostate (Gleason >7),

leukemia, lymphoma, sarcoma, dermatologic manifestations, and/or macrocephaly, GI hamartomas
  - Ashkenazi Jewish with breast/ovary cancer at any age
  - Male BC (1)
  - Known BC *susceptibility gene* mutation in family
- *BRCA1* and *BRCA2*
- Other genes: *AR, ATM, BARD1, BRIP1, CDH1, PTEN, STK11, CHEK2, p53, ERBB2, DIRAS3, NBN, RAD50, RAD51*
- Cowden syndrome (PTEN): Autosomal dominant, BC, hamartomas of skin, intestine, oral mucosa (trichilemmoma), microencephaly, endometrial CA, nonmedullary thyroid CA, benign thyroid lesions
- Li-Fraumeni syndrome (*TP53*): Autosomal dominant, BC and CA in CNS, leukemia, sarcoma, osteosarcoma, adrenal cortex
- Ataxia-telangiectasia (*ATM*): Autosomal recessive, ataxia, telangiectasia, lymphoma, leukemia, CA of breast, stomach, ovary
- Peutz-Jeghers (*STK11*): Autosomal dominance, hamartomatous polyps of GI tract, mucocutaneous melanin in lips, buccal mucosa, fingers, toes, CA in GI, lung, breast, uterus, ovary

RISK FACTORS
- Female, race (e.g., Ashkenazi Jewish), family history (FH), genetics, nulliparity or older age at first live birth, early menarche, delayed menopause, increasing age, personal history of BC or ovarian cancer, prolonged hormone replacement therapy, obesity/high body mass index, heavy alcohol intake, physical inactivity, mammographic breast density, active oral contraceptive use (disappears once discontinued)
- Benign/at-risk breast disease: Atypical hyperplasia (ductal/lobular); lobular carcinoma in situ (LCIS) increases risk for bilateral BC
- Prior chest radiation (lymphoma), DES (diethylstilbestrol) exposure
- Number of prior breast biopsies of different lesions
- Men less at risk for BC, but at increased risk with Klinefelter syndrome, testicular pathology, FH, or *BRCA2* mutations
- Prior radiation therapy (RT) between ages 10 and 30
- Strong family history of hereditary breast and/or ovarian CA OR genetic predisposition (*high risk*):
  - Women: CCBE 6–12 months starting at age 30; mammogram and MRI yearly or individualized to earliest age of onset in family; At age 30: Semiannual transvaginal US
- Risk-modifying agents:
  - Premenopausal: Consider Tamoxifen if history of LCIS, DCIS, or atypical atypical ductal or lobular hyperplasia or if Gail modeling finds >1.66% over 5 years
  - Postmenopausal: Aromatase inhibitors or selective estrogen receptor modulator, Raloxifene. Tamoxifen use dependent on comorbid conditions, uterus status, age. Discuss risk-reducing mastectomy and salpingo-oophorectomy (limited to *BRCA1* or *BRCA2*) done after age 35 or after child-bearing
- Men: CBE 6–12 months starting at age 35; baseline mammogram at age 40; annual mammogram if gynecomastia or parenchymal/glandular breast

GENERAL PREVENTION
- General population screening (normal risk):
  - Risk assessment tool at http://www.cancer.gov/bcrisktool/
  - Clinical breast examination (CBE) if age 25–39 years: Every 1–3 years (controversial; no evidence CBE improves outcomes, but may decrease patient anxiety); age ≥40: Every year
  - Mammography: NCCN recommends every other year starting at age 40; USPSTF recommends every other year starting at age 50

DIAGNOSIS

PHYSICAL EXAM
- Visualize breasts with patient sitting for skin dimpling, peau d'orange, asymmetry
- Palpation of breast and regional lymph node exam: Supraclavicular, infraclavicular, axillary

DIFFERENTIAL DIAGNOSIS
- Benign breast disease: Fibrocystic disease, fibroadenoma, intraductal papilloma (bloody nipple discharge), duct ectasia, cyst, sclerosing adenosis, fat necrosis (s/p breast trauma)
- Infection: Abscess, cellulitis, mastitis

DIAGNOSTIC TESTS & INTERPRETATION
Initial Tests (lab, imaging)
- Mammography BI-RADS: Breast Imaging–Reporting and Data System is a quality assurance (QA) method published by the American Radiology Society.
- BI-RADS interpretation: 0: Incomplete (need additional imaging); 1: Negative; 2: Benign finding(s); 3: Probably benign; 4: Suspicious abnormality; 5: Highly suggestive of malignancy; 6: Known biopsy—proven malignancy
- All newly diagnosed BC: History and physical, CBC, LFTs, ALP, pathology review, ER/PR and HER2 status determination, genetic counseling if high risk, fertility counseling if indicated
- Clinical sign:
- Palpable mass ≥30 years: Obtain diagnostic mammography:
  - If BI-RADS 1–3, then get ultrasound ± biopsy.
  - If BI-RADS 4–6, then get core needle biopsy ± surgical excision.
- Palpable mass <30 years: Obtain ultrasound ± mammogram ± biopsy; if low clinical suspicion, observe for 1–2 menstrual cycles for resolution.
- Spontaneous, reproducible nipple discharge: Obtain mammogram, ± ultrasound:
  - If BI-RADS 1–3, then get ductogram ± MRI.
  - If BI-RADS 4–5, then surgical excision.
- Asymmetric thickening/nodularity ≥30 years: Obtain mammogram + ultrasound ± biopsy
- Asymmetric thickening/nodularity <30 years: Obtain ultrasound ± mammogram ± biopsy.
- Skin changes, peau d'orange: Obtain mammogram ± ultrasound ± biopsy.

Follow-Up Tests & Special Considerations
- Early disease (clinical stage I and IIB):
- Consider additional studies only if signs and symptoms warrant.
- Advanced disease (stage IIIA or higher):
- Chest diagnostic CT, abdominal ± pelvis CT, FDG positron emission tomography (PET)/CT scan, bone scan or sodium fluoride PET/CT if FDG-PET/CT indeterminate

- Most common metastasis: Lungs, liver, bone, brain
- Bone scan: Localized pain, elevated alkaline phosphate
- Abdominal ± pelvis CT: Abdominal symptoms, elevated alkaline phosphate, abnormal LFTs
- Chest imaging: Pulmonary symptoms
- MRI: CNS/Spinal cord symptoms

Diagnostic Procedures/Other
- Primary tumor: Fine-needle aspiration, ultrasound-guided core needle biopsy, stereotactic-guided core needle biopsy ± wire localization, sentinel lymph node, surgical excision, sentinel lymph node biopsy, post biopsy may get inflammatory changes/hematoma
- Genomic assay on formalin-fixed tissue for select +ER, −HER2, node negative tumor to assess chemotherapy responsiveness

Test Interpretation
- Ductal/Lobular/Other: Tumor size, inflammatory component, invasive/noninvasive, margins, nodal involvement
- Nodal micrometastases: Increased risk of disease recurrence
- ER, PR, HER2 assay

 TREATMENT

MEDICATION
- Secondary prevention:
- Chemoprevention/Hormone therapy for patients ages ≥35:
  – Risk reduction for ER-positive tumors
- Hormone therapy for ER-positive tumors:
- Tamoxifen: Premenopausal at diagnosis: 5-year treatment and consider for additional 5 years; avoid during lactation, pregnancy, or in patients with history of deep venous thrombosis/pulmonary embolism; routine CYP2D6 (tamoxifen metabolizing enzyme) testing not recommended; use strong CYP2D6-inhibiting medications with caution in conjunction with tamoxifen
- Aromatase inhibitors: Postmenopausal women, 5-year treatment following tamoxifen for 4.5–6 years, or tamoxifen for up to 10 years
- Ovarian ablation or suppression with luteinizing hormone-releasing hormone agonists: Premenopausal women
- Anti-HER2/neu antibody (e.g. trastuzumab) in select HER2/neu-positive patients:
- Monitor cardiac toxicity via ECG, especially with anthracycline.
- Neoadjuvant chemotherapy (preop): Premenopausal women should be counseled on potential effect of chemotherapy on fertility refer to fertility expert
- Locally advanced, inoperable advanced BC (stage III)
- Early operable BC for breast conservation surgery
- Triple negative BC
- Cytotoxic therapy: Anthracyclines, taxanes, alkylating agents, antimetabolites
- Higher-risk patients with nonmetastatic operable tumors
- Patients with high risk of recurrence after local treatment (serial/parallel [s/p] surgery ± radiation)
- Online tool to estimate recurrence risk and benefits of adjuvant chemotherapy (http://www.adjuvantonline.com/online.jsp)
- Cytotoxic therapy: Anthracyclines, alkylating agents, taxanes, antimetabolites

- Dose-dense chemotherapy demonstrates overall survival advantage in early BC (2).
- Advanced disease:
- Hormone therapy
- Cytotoxic therapy
- Bisphosphonates to decrease skeletal complications
- Antivascular endothelial growth factor antibody
- Anti-HER2/neu antibody in select HER2/neu-positive patients
- Metastatic disease:
- Monitoring metastatic disease: System assessment, physical examination, performance status, weight, LFT/CBC, CT scan/chest/abdomen/pelvis, bone scan, PET/CT, tumor markers

SURGERY/OTHER PROCEDURES
- Secondary prevention:
- Risk-reducing mastectomy and bilateral salpingo-oophorectomy for breast and ovary CA syndromes
- Breast-conserving partial mastectomy/lumpectomy, if possible:
- Negative margins; tumor usually <5 cm
- No prior breast radiation, relative contraindication: connective tissue disease (lupus, scleroderma)
- Modified radical mastectomy:
- Large tumors; multicentric disease; young women with known BRCA; consider immediate or delayed reconstruction.
- Radiation therapy should be initiated without delay:
- After breast-conserving therapy (BCT), stage I, IIA, IIB treatable with BCT + radiation
- Postmastectomy in select high-risk patients; palliation of metastatic disease; cord compression
- Pregnancy (treatment varies on trimester):
- Surgical: Mastectomy or breast conservation: Mastectomy preferred due to limitations of radiation during pregnancy.
- Sentinel lymph node biopsy: Safe to use with lymphoscintigraphy
- Chemotherapy: Appropriate in 2nd and 3rd trimesters, trastuzumab contraindicated
- Radiation therapy: Avoid until after delivery.

IN-PATIENT CONSIDERATIONS
Discharge Criteria
Postmastectomy:
- Complications: Seroma, phantom breast syndrome, cellulitis, chest wall/axilla/arm pain, long thoracic nerve damage leading to winged scapula sign
- Lymphedema; avoid having BP taken on side of surgery

 ONGOING CARE

FOLLOW-UP RECOMMENDATIONS
- Every 4–6 months × 5 years, then annually
- No evidence to support the use of routine CBC, LFTs, "tumor markers," bone scan, CXR, liver ultrasound, CT scans, MRI, PET
- Mammogram/imaging 1 year after initial mammogram, but 6–12 months postradiation, then annually
- Annual gynecologic exam for women on tamoxifen; bone mineral density at baseline and follow-up for women on aromatase inhibitors or with ovarian failure secondary to treatment

PROGNOSIS

Stage	5-year Survival Rate
0	93%
I	88%
IIA	81%
IIB	74%
IIIA	67%
IIIB	41%*
IIIC	49%*
IV	15%

COMPLICATIONS
- Hypercalcemia, metastatic disease, lymphedema
- Emotional issues, especially depression and body-image alteration

REFERENCES

1. NCCN Guidelines: Breast and/or Ovarian Cancer Genetic Assessment (Version1. 2012) © 2012 Breast Cancer National Comprehensive Cancer Network, Inc. Accessed 5/26/2013 at http://www.nccn.org.
2. Lyman GH, Barron RL, Natoli JL, et al. Systematic review of efficacy of dose-dense versus non-dose-dense chemotherapy in breast cancer, non-Hodgkin lymphoma, and non-small cell lung cancer. Crit Rev Oncol Hematol. 2012;81(3): 296–308.

ADDITIONAL READING

American Cancer Society: Facts & Figures 2013. Accessed 5/26/2013 at http://www.cancer.org.

 CODES

ICD10
- C50.911 Malignant neoplasm of unsp site of right female breast
- C50.912 Malignant neoplasm of unspecified site of left female breast
- C50.919 Malignant neoplasm of unsp site of unspecified female breast

CLINICAL PEARLS
- BC is most common malignancy in women in the U.S., with lifetime risk of 1 in 8.
- High alcohol use, high body mass index (BMI), and physical inactivity are modifiable risk factors.
- Pursue/Refer all abnormal breast physical examination/imaging findings.
- If patient ≥30 years with palpable mass, obtain mammogram, if <30 years obtain ultrasound.
- Normal mammography does not exclude possibility of CA with a palpable mass.

BREASTFEEDING

Zaiba Jetpuri, DO, MBA • Amimi Osayande, MD

BASICS

- Breastfeeding is the natural process of feeding infant human milk directly from the breast.
- Breast milk is the preferred nutritional source for all newborns and infants.
- The American Academy of Pediatrics (AAP), the American Academy of Family Physicians (AAFP), WHO, and other medical organizations recommend exclusive breastfeeding for 6 months, with continuation of breastfeeding for ≥1 year as desired by mother and infant (1).

DESCRIPTION
- Maternal benefits (as compared with mothers who do not breastfeed) include:
  - Decreased postpartum bleeding (due to oxytocin release)
  - Decreased risk of postpartum depression
  - Easier postpartum weight loss
  - Delayed postpartum fertility
  - Decreased risk of breast and ovarian cancer
  - Decreased risk of type 2 diabetes
  - Increased bonding
  - Convenience and cost
- Infant benefits (as compared with children who are formula-fed) include:
  - Ideal food: Easily digestible, nutrients well absorbed, less constipation
  - Lower rates of virtually all infections via maternal antibody protection:
    ○ Fewer respiratory and GI infections
    ○ Decreased incidence of otitis media
    ○ Decreased risk of bacterial meningitis and sepsis
    ○ Decreased incidence of necrotizing enterocolitis
  - Decreased incidence of obesity, type 1 and 2 diabetes
  - Decreased incidence of allergies and atopic dermatitis in childhood
  - Decreased risk of developing celiac disease and inflammatory bowel disease
  - Decreased risk of childhood leukemia
  - Decreased risk of sudden infant death syndrome (SIDS) and decreased mortality
  - Higher intelligence scores and better neurodevelopmental outcomes
  - Increased attachment between mother and baby

EPIDEMIOLOGY
Incidence
- According to the most recent breastfeeding scorecard, US breastfeeding rates are on the rise. Based on the CDC, in 2012 (2): Any breastfeeding: 76.9.0% (however, differs among different sociodemographic and culture).
- Breastfeeding at 6 months: 47.2%
- Breastfeeding at 12 months: 25.5%
- Exclusive breastfeeding at 3 months: 36%
- Exclusive breastfeeding at 6 months: 16.3%

ETIOLOGY AND PATHOPHYSIOLOGY
The overarching mechanism of milk production is based on supply and demand:
- Stimulation of areola causes secretion of oxytocin.
- Oxytocin is responsible for let-down reflex when milk is ejected into milk ducts.
- Sucking stimulates secretion of prolactin, which triggers milk production.
- Endocrine/metabolic: Thyroid dysfunction may cause delayed lactation or decreased milk.

GENERAL PREVENTION
- Most vaccinations can be given to breastfeeding mothers. The CDC recommends that the diphtheria-tetanus-acellular pertussis, hepatitis B, inactivated influenza virus (as opposed to live attenuated), measles-mumps-rubella (MMR), inactivated polio and varicella vaccines can be given. The CDC recommends avoiding the yellow fever or smallpox vaccine in breastfeeding mothers.
- The inactivated influenza virus is preferred to the live attenuated virus in women with infants' age 6–23 months, regardless of whether these infants are being breastfed.

DIAGNOSIS

PHYSICAL EXAM
- Examine breasts, ideally during pregnancy, looking for scars or inverted nipples.
- Breast cancer incidence low, but possible in premenopausal women

TREATMENT

GENERAL MEASURES
Flat or inverted nipples:
- When stimulated, inverted nipples will retract inward, flat nipples remain flat; check for this on initial prenatal physical.
- Nipple shells, a doughnut-shaped insert, can be worn inside the bra during the last month of pregnancy to force the nipple gently through the center opening of the shell.
- Babies can nurse successfully even if the shell does not correct the problem before birth.
- Contraindications:
  - Contraindications to breastfeeding are few (WHO; 1):
    ○ Maternal HIV (in industrialized world) or human T-cell leukemia virus (HTLV) infection
    ○ Active untreated tuberculosis
    ○ Active herpes simplex virus (HSV) lesions on the breast*
    ○ Substances of abuse and some medications that will pass into human milk
    ○ Infants with galactosemia or maple syrup urine disease should not be fed with breast milk. Infants with phenylketonuria may be fed breast milk under close observation.
    ○ Mothers who develop varicella 5 days before through 2 days after delivery*
    ○ Mothers acutely infected with influenza H1N1 until afebrile*
    ○ Maternal hepatitis is NOT a contraindication.

*Expressed milk can be used

ISSUES FOR REFERRAL
- Refer to trained physician, nurse, or lactation consultant for inpatient and/or outpatient teaching.
- Frequent follow-up if having problems with latching, sore nipples, or inadequate milk production

COMPLEMENTARY AND ALTERNATIVE MEDICINE
- Galactagogues:
  - Metoclopramide, oxytocin, fenugreek, and milk thistle have mixed results in improving milk production but efficacy and safety data are lacking in literature (3).
- Breastfeeding initiation:
  - Initiate breastfeeding immediately after birth, ideally placing the infant on mother's chest skin-to-skin.
  - Get mother in a comfortable position, usually sitting or reclining with the baby's head in crook of her arm.
  - Baby's belly and mother's belly should face each other or touch ("belly to belly"). Initiate the rooting reflex by tickling baby's lips with nipple or finger. As baby's mouth opens wide, mother guides her nipple to back of her baby's mouth while pulling the baby closer. This will ensure that the baby's gums are sucking on the areola, not the nipple (4)[C].
  - Feed every 2–3 hours, 10–15 minutes/side
  - Rooming-in to encourage on-demand feeding (4)
  - Observation of a nursing session by an experienced physician, nurse, or lactation consultant
  - Avoid supplementation with formula or water.
- Risk factors for suboptimal initiation
  - Breast surgery, especially reduction surgery, prior to pregnancy may disrupt breast milk production in the future.
  - Severe postpartum hemorrhage may lead to Sheehan syndrome, which is associated with difficulty breastfeeding due to poor milk production.
  - Parity
  - Delivery mode and duration of labor
  - Use of nonbreast milk fluids or pacifiers
  - Maternal infection
  - Culture

ONGOING CARE

FOLLOW-UP RECOMMENDATIONS
See mother and baby within a few days of hospital discharge, especially if 1st-time breastfeeding

Patient Monitoring
- Monitor infant's weight and output closely.
- Supplementation with infant formula recommended only if infant has lost ≥7% of birth weight, shows signs of dehydration such as decreased urine output, or has <3 small stools a day.
- Supplementation without persistent breast stimulation with frequent feedings or breast pump use will decrease milk production and decrease breastfeeding success.

DIET
FOR MOTHERS:
- Drink plenty of fluids: 8 glasses of liquid a day.
- Breastfeeding mothers require ~500 more calories a day than pre-pregnancy needs.
- Gassy foods, such as cabbage, may cause baby to have colic.
- Limit caffeine to 300 mg/d.

- Alcohol should be avoided. 1–2 drinks/wk of alcohol may be okay, but mothers should avoid nursing 2–3 hours after a drink. <2% of alcohol is passed to baby via breast milk.
- Continue prenatal vitamin supplements (1)

FOR INFANTS:

- In 2008, the AAP increased its recommended daily intake of vitamin D in infants from 200 to 400 IU. For exclusively breastfed babies, this will require taking a vitamin supplement, such as Poly-Vi-Sol or Vi-Daylin vitamin drops, 0.5 mL/d, beginning in the 1st few days of life (5).
- In 2010, the AAP recommended adding supplementation for breastfed infants with oral iron 1 mg/kg/d beginning at age 4 months (6):
  – Preterm infants fed human milk should receive an iron supplement of 2 mg/kg/d by 1 month of age, and this should be continued until the infant is weaned to iron-fortified formula or begins eating complementary foods that supply the 2 mg/kg of iron.
  – Fluoride supplement is unnecessary until 6 months of age.

PATIENT EDUCATION

- Primary care-initiated interventions to promote breastfeeding have been shown to be successful with respect to child and maternal health outcomes (7,8):
  – US Preventive Services Task Force (USPSTF) recommends structured breastfeeding education and behavioral counseling programs to promote breastfeeding:
    ○ Regular promotion of the advantages of breastfeeding/risks of not breastfeeding
    ○ Emphasize importance of exclusive breastfeeding for first 4 weeks of life to allow adequate buildup of sufficient milk supply.
- Milk usually comes in about postpartum day 3.
- Frequent nursing (feedings 8–12/24 hours)
- Baby should have ∼6 wet diapers/d and 3–4 bowel movements/d.
- Signs of adequate nursing:
  – Hard breasts become soft after feeding.
  – Baby satisfied; appropriate weight gain (average 1 oz/d in first few months)
- Weaning:
  – Solid food may be introduced at 6 months.
  – For mothers going to work, start switching the baby to breast milk feeding (or formula feeding) during hours mother will be gone about a week ahead of time
- Family planning:
  – Lactational amenorrhea method (LAM): Breastfeeding may be used as effective birth control option if (i) infant is <6 months old, (ii) infant is exclusively breastfeeding, and (iii) mother is amenorrheic.
  – Other options include barrier methods, implants, Depo-Provera, PO contraception, and intrauterine devices (IUDs). ACOG recommends that progesterone-only pills be used 2–3 weeks postpartum, and that Depo-Provera, IUDs, combined OCPs and Implanon can be used 6 weeks postpartum. However, ACOG recommends delaying use of combined OCPs until after 6 weeks postpartum when lactation is well-established.

- The Academy of Breastfeeding Medicine (ABM), a worldwide organization of physicians dedicated to the promotion, protection, and support of breastfeeding and human lactation: www.bfmed.org
- La Leche League at www.llli.org
- Protecting, Promoting and Supporting Breastfeeding: The Special Role of Maternity Services, a joint World Health Organization/United Nations Children's Fund (WHO/UNICEF) statement published by the World Health Organization: http://www.unicef.org/newsline/tenstps.htm
- Thomas Hale's *Medications and Mother's Milk: A Manual of Lactational Pharmacology*

COMPLICATIONS

- Breast milk jaundice should be considered if jaundice persists for >1 week in an otherwise healthy, well-hydrated newborn. It peaks at 10–14 days.
- Plugged duct:
  – Mother is well except for sore lump in 1 or both breasts without fever
  – Use moist, hot packs on lump prior to, and during, nursing; More frequent nursing on affected side
- Mastitis (see topic "Mastitis"):
  – Sore lump in 1 or both breasts plus fever and/or redness on skin overlying lump
  – Use moist, hot packs on lump prior to, and during, nursing
  – Antibiotics covering for *Staphylococcus aureus* (most common organism)
  – Other possible sources of fever should be ruled out; i.e., endometritis and pyelonephritis
  – Mother should get increased rest; use acetaminophen (Tylenol), p.r.n.
  – Fever should resolve within 48 hours or consider changing antibiotics. Lump should resolve. If it continues, an abscess may be present, requiring surgical drainage.
- Milk supply inadequate:
  – Check infant weight gain.
  – Review signs of adequate supply; technique, frequency, and duration of nursing.
  – Check to see if mother has been supplementing with formula, thereby decreasing her own milk production.
- Sore nipples:
  – Check technique and improve latch-on
  – Baby should be taken off the breast by breaking the suction with a finger in the mouth.
  – Air-dry nipples after each nursing and/or coat with expressed breast milk.
  – Use lanolin cream to help healing.
  – Do not wash nipples with soap and water.
  – Check for signs of thrush in baby and on mother's nipple. If affected, treat both.
  – Check for evidence of ankyloglossia (tongue tie) in the infant. Correction of ankyloglossia leads to decreased nipple soreness and improved breastfeeding.
- Engorgement:
  – Develops after milk first comes in (day 3 or 4 postpartum), resolves within a day or 2
  – Signs are warm, hard, sore breasts:
    ○ To resolve, offer baby more frequent nursing; breastfeed long enough to empty breasts.

REFERENCES

1. Breastfeeding and the Use of Human Milk. Policy statement from the American Academy of Pediatrics. *Pediatrics*. 2012;129(3):e827–841. http://pediatrics.aappublications.org/content/129/3/e827.full#content-block
2. Centers for Disease Control and Prevention, Breastfeeding Report Card – United States 2012. http://www.cdc.gov/breastfeeding/data/reportcard2.htm
3. Foranish AB, Yancey AM, Barnes KN, Myles TD. The use of galactogogues in the breastfeeding mother. *Ann Pharmacother*. 2012;46(10):1392–1404.
4. Sinusas K, Gagliardi A. Initial management of breastfeeding. *Am Fam Physician*. 2001;64(6):981–988.
5. Wagner CL, Greer FR, American Academy of Pediatrics Section on Breastfeeding and Committee on Nutrition. Prevention of rickets and vitamin D deficiency in infants, children, and adolescents. *Pediatrics*. 2008;122(5):1142–1152.
6. Baker RD, Greer FR, Committee on Nutrition American Academy of Pediatrics. Diagnosis and prevention of iron deficiency and iron-deficiency anemia in infants and young children (0–3 years of age). *Pediatrics*. 2010;126(5):1040–1050. Epub 2010 Oct 5.
7. Chung M, Raman G, Trikalinos T, et al. Interventions in primary care to promote breastfeeding: An evidence review for the U.S. Preventive Services Task Force. *Ann Intern Med*. 2008;149(8):565–582.
8. Breastfeeding: Maternal and infant aspects. *ACOG Clin Rev*. 2007;12(1):1S–16S. http://www.urmc.rochester.edu/flrpp/breast-feeding-hospital-policy/documents/ACOGBreastfeeding ClinicalReview.pdf

ADDITIONAL READING

Casey CF, Slawson DC, Neal LR. VItamin D supplementation in infants, children, and adolescents. *Am Fam Physician*. 2010;81(6):745–748.

 ## CODES

ICD10
Z39.1 Encounter for care and examination of lactating mother

CLINICAL PEARLS

- Breast milk is the optimal food for infants, with myriad health benefits for mothers and children.
- USPSTF recommends regular, structured education during pregnancy to promote breastfeeding.
- Vitamin D and iron supplementation should begin at birth and 4 months of age, respectively, for exclusively breastfed infants.

BRONCHIECTASIS

Sumera Ahmad, MD • Scott E. Kopec, MD

BASICS

DESCRIPTION
- Bronchiectasis is an irreversible dilation of ≥1 airways accompanied by recurrent transmural bronchial infection/inflammation and chronic mucopurulent sputum production.
- Generally classified into cystic fibrosis (CF) and noncystic fibrosis (non-CF) bronchiectasis.

EPIDEMIOLOGY
- Predominant age: Most commonly presents in 6th decade of life.
- Predominant sex: Female > Male

Incidence
Incidence has decreased in the US for 2 reasons:
- Widespread childhood vaccination against pertussis
- Effective treatment of childhood respiratory infections with antibiotics

Prevalence
- Prevalence in adult US population estimated to be >110,000 affected individuals
- Internationally, prevalence increases with age from 4.2/100,000 persons aged 18–34 years to 271.8/100,000 among those aged ≥75 years (1).

ETIOLOGY AND PATHOPHYSIOLOGY
- CF bronchiectasis: Bronchiectasis due to CF
- Non-CF bronchiectasis:
  - Most cases are idiopathic.
  - Most commonly associated with non-CF bronchiectasis is childhood infection.
- Vicious circle hypothesis: Transmural infection, generally by bacterial organisms, causes inflammation and obstruction of airways. Damaged airways and dysfunctional cilia foster bacterial colonization, which leads to further inflammation and obstruction.

RISK FACTORS
- Nontuberculous mycobacterial infection is both a cause and a complication of non-CF bronchiectasis.
- Severe respiratory infection in childhood (measles, adenovirus, influenza, pertussis, or bronchiolitis)
- Systemic diseases (e.g., rheumatoid arthritis and inflammatory bowel disease)
- Chronic rhinosinusitis
- Recurrent pneumonia
- Aspirated foreign body
- Immunodeficiency
- Congenital abnormalities

GENERAL PREVENTION
- Routine immunizations against pertussis, measles, *Haemophilus influenza* type B, influenza, and pneumococcal pneumonia
- Genetic counseling if congenital condition is etiology
- Smoking cessation

COMMONLY ASSOCIATED CONDITIONS
- Mucociliary clearance defects:
  - Primary ciliary dyskinesia
  - Young syndrome (secondary ciliary dyskinesia)
  - Kartagener syndrome
- Other congenital conditions:
  - α_1-Antitrypsin deficiency
  - Marfan syndrome
  - Cartilage deficiency (Williams-Campbell syndrome)
- Chronic obstructive pulmonary disease

- Pulmonary fibrosis, causing traction bronchiectasis
- Postinfectious conditions:
  - Bacteria (*H. influenzae* and *Pseudomonas aeruginosa*)
  - Mycobacterial infections (tuberculosis [TB] and *Mycobacterium avium* complex [MAC])
  - Whooping cough
  - *Aspergillus* species
  - Viral (HIV, adenovirus, measles, influenza virus)
- Immunodeficient conditions:
  - Primary: Hypogammaglobulinemia
  - Secondary: Allergic bronchopulmonary aspergillosis [ABPA], posttransplantation
- Sequelae of toxic inhalation or aspiration (e.g., chlorine, luminal foreign body)
- Rheumatic/Chronic inflammatory conditions:
  - Rheumatoid arthritis
  - Sjögren syndrome
  - Systemic lupus erythematosus
  - Inflammatory bowel disease
- Miscellaneous:
  - Yellow nail syndrome

DIAGNOSIS

- Typical symptoms include chronic productive cough, wheezing, and dyspnea.
- Symptoms are often accompanied by repeated respiratory infections (2).
- Once diagnosed, investigate etiology.

HISTORY
- Any predisposing factors (congenital, infectious, and/or exposure-related)
- Immunization history

PHYSICAL EXAM
Symptoms are commonly present for many years and include the following:
- Chronic cough (90%)
- Sputum: May be copious and purulent (90%)
- Rhinosinusitis (60–70%)
- Fatigue: May be a dominant symptom (70%)
- Dyspnea (75%)
- Chest pain: May be pleuritic (20–30%)
- Hemoptysis (20–30%)
- Wheezing (20%)
- Bibasilar crackles (60%)
- Rhonchi (44%)
- Digital clubbing (3%)

DIFFERENTIAL DIAGNOSIS
- CF
- Chronic obstructive pulmonary disease
- Asthma
- Chronic bronchitis
- Pulmonary TB
- ABPA

DIAGNOSTIC TESTS & INTERPRETATION
- Spirometry:
  - Moderate airflow obstruction and hyperresponsive airways
  - Forced expiratory volume in the 1st second of expiration (FEV_1): <80% predicted and FEV_1/FVC <0.7
- Special tests:
  - Ciliary biopsy by electron microscopy
- Sputum culture:
  - *H. influenzae*, nontypeable form (42%)

- *P. aeruginosa* (18%)
- Cultures may also be positive for *Streptococcus pneumoniae*, *Moraxella catarrhalis*, MAC, and *Aspergillus*.
- Of all isolates, 30–40% will show no growth.
- Special tests:
  - Sweat test for CF
  - Purified protein derivative (PPD) test for tuberculosis (TB)
  - Skin test for *Aspergillus*
  - HIV
  - Serum immunoglobulins to test for humoral immunodeficiency
  - Protein electrophoresis to test for α-1-antitrypsin deficiency
  - Barium swallow to look for abnormalities of deglutition, achalasia, esophageal hypomotility
  - pH probe to characterize reflux
  - Screening tests for rheumatologic diseases
- Chest radiograph:
  - Nonspecific; increased lung markings or may appear normal
- Chest CT:
  - Noncontrast high-resolution chest CT is the most important diagnostic tool.
  - Bronchi are dilated and do not taper, resulting in "tram track sign"; parallel opacities seen on scan.
  - Varicose constrictions and balloon cysts may be seen.
  - For focal bronchiectasis, rule out endobronchial obstruction.
  - For exclusively upper lobe bronchiectasis, consider CF and ABPA.

Diagnostic Procedures/Other
- Bronchoscopy may be used to obtain cultures and evacuate sputum.
- Bronchoscopy for hemoptysis
- Bronchoscopy may be useful to rule out airway obstructing lesions with focal bronchiectasis.

Test Interpretation
Bronchoscopy findings include the following:
- Dilation of airways and purulent secretions
- Thickened bronchial walls with necrosis of bronchial mucosa
- Peribronchial scarring

TREATMENT

- Treat underlying conditions.
- Recognize an acute exacerbation with 4 out of 9 criteria:
  - Change in sputum production
  - Increased dyspnea
  - Increased cough
  - Fever
  - Increased wheezing
  - Malaise, fatigue, lethargy
  - Reduced pulmonary function
  - Radiographic changes
  - Changes in chest sounds
- Non-CF bronchiectasis: Determine cause of exacerbations, promote good bronchopulmonary hygiene via daily airway clearance.
- Consider surgical resection of damaged lung for focal disease that is refractory to medical management.
- Medical management: Reduce morbidity by controlling symptoms and preventing disease progression.

- Patients with non-CF bronchiectasis may not respond to CF treatment regimens in the same way as patients with CF do.

GENERAL MEASURES

- Maintain hydration (nebulized hypertonic saline, 3% or 7% may be used to help increase mucus clearance) (3)[A].
- Noninvasive positive-pressure ventilation

MEDICATION

- Insufficient evidence exists to support efficacy of short-course antibiotics in adults and children with bronchiectasis (4)[A].
- Frequent exacerbations may be treated with prolonged and aerosolized antibiotics (2)[A].
- Role of mucolytics, anti-inflammatory agents, and bronchodilators is still unclear (2)[A].

First Line

- Antibiotics:
  - Potentially useful in acute exacerbations
  - Chronic therapy decreases sputum volume and purulence, but it does not diminish the frequency of exacerbations (5)[A].
  - Patients may require twice the usual dose and longer treatment for 14 days.
  - Sputum culture and sensitivity should direct therapy; antibiotic selection is complicated by a wide range of pathogens and resistant organisms.
  - Should be administered IV in cases of severe infection:
    - Augmentin: 500 mg PO q8–12h Pediatric: Base dosing on amoxicillin content.
    - Trimethoprim (TMP)/sulfamethoxazole (SMX): 160 mg TMP/800 mg SMX PO q12h Pediatric: ≥2 months, 8 mg/kg TMP and 40 mg/kg SMX PO/24 hours, administered in 2 divided doses q12h
    - Doxycycline and cefaclor given PO are also effective.
    - Nebulized aminoglycosides (tobramycin): 300 mg by aerosol b.i.d. (6)[B]
    - Ciprofloxacin: 750 mg PO q12h for adults for susceptible strain of *Pseudomonas*
    - Macrolides: Appear to have immunomodulatory benefits
- Bronchodilators:
  - Chronic use of β_2–agonists (e.g., albuterol) reverses airflow obstruction.
- Inhaled corticosteroids:
  - Insufficient evidence exists to recommend use of inhaled steroids with stable bronchiectasis (7)[A].
  - A therapeutic trial of inhaled steroids may be justified in adults with difficult-to-control symptoms (7)[A].
  - Decrease sputum and tend to improve lung function:
    - Fluticasone: 110–220 μg inhaled b.i.d.
  - Potential synergistic effect of long-acting β_2–agonists with inhaled corticosteroids, allowing for lower steroid dose (8):
    - Budesonide 640 μg/Formoterol 18 μg inhaled b.i.d.

Second Line

Other broad-spectrum antimicrobials, including antipseudomonals

ADDITIONAL THERAPIES

Sputum clearance techniques, including physiotherapy (percussion and postural drainage) and pulmonary rehabilitation (improves exercise tolerance)

SURGERY/OTHER PROCEDURES

- Surgery if area of bronchiectasis is localized and symptoms remain intolerable despite medical therapy or if disease is life threatening (2)[A]
- Surgery effectively improves symptoms in 80% of these cases.

IN-PATIENT CONSIDERATIONS

Admission Criteria/Initial Stabilization

Hemoptysis, although rare, may occur and can be life-threatening.

 ONGOING CARE

Long-term outpatient treatment recommendations for bronchiectasis in children (9)[B]:

- Children with CF- and non–CF-related bronchiectasis should be treated by comprehensive interdisciplinary chronic disease management programs.
- Pathogen-directed aerosolized tobramycin treatment should be used long term on a regular basis to improve the course of CF-related bronchiectasis.
- PO macrolide antibiotic use short term (up to 6 months) improves lung function among children with CF-related bronchiectasis.
- Chronic use of azithromycin as an oral macrolide in non-CF bronchiectasis has been shown to reduce exacerbations. Needs caution with respect to cardiovascular deaths, where it is a QTc prolonging medication.
- Long-term antibiotic use (PO or aerosolized) in children with non–CF-related bronchiectasis has not been studied enough to warrant routine use.
- Hypertonic saline administered by inhalation used long term (48 weeks) improves lung function and is safer when used with pretreatment bronchodilator therapy among children who have CF.
- Nebulized dornase improves multiple pulmonary outcomes of children who have CF and is indicated for long-term use.
- Risks for long-term oral corticosteroid use outweigh pulmonary benefits in the treatment of CF-related bronchiectasis.
- High-dose ibuprofen therapy reduces the rate of decline among children with mild CF-related bronchiectasis and is indicated for long-term use.
- Mucolytic agents, airway hydrating treatments, anti-inflammatory therapy, CPT, and bronchodilator therapy have not been studied sufficiently long term in children with non–CF-related bronchiectasis to merit their routine use.

FOLLOW-UP RECOMMENDATIONS

Regular exercise is recommended.

Patient Monitoring

- Serial spirometry, every 2–5 years, to monitor the course of the disease
- Routine microbiological sputum analysis

PATIENT EDUCATION

http://www.lungusa.org

PROGNOSIS

- Mortality rate (death due directly to bronchiectasis) is 13%.
- *Pseudomonas* infection is associated with poorer prognosis.

COMPLICATIONS

- Hemoptysis
- Recurrent pulmonary infections
- Pulmonary hypertension
- Cor pulmonale
- Lung abscess

REFERENCES

1. Pappalettera M, Aliberti S, Castellotti P, et al. Bronchiectasis: An update. *Clin Respir J.* 2009;3:126–134.
2. ten Hacken NH, Wijkstra PJ, Kerstjens HA. Treatment of bronchiectasis in adults. *BMJ.* 2007;335:1089–1093.
3. Kellett F, Niven RM. Nebulised 7% hypertonic saline improves lung function and quality of life in bronchiectasis. *Resp Med.* 2011;105:1831–1835.
4. Wurzel D, Marchant JM, Yerkovich ST, et al. Short courses of antibiotics for children and adults with bronchiectasis. *Cochrane Database Sys Rev.* 2011;CD008695.
5. Evans DJ, Bara AI, Greenstone M. Prolonged antibiotics for purulent bronchiectasis. *Cochrane Database Sys Rev.* 2006;4:CD00284.
6. Lobue PA. Inhaled tobramycin: Not just for cystic fibrosis anymore? *Chest.* 2005;127:1098–1101.
7. Kapur N, Bell S, Kolbe J. Inhaled steroids for bronchiectasis. *Cochrane Database Sys Rev.* 2009:CD000996.
8. Martinez-Garcia MA, Soler-Cataluna JJ, Catalan-Serra P, et al. Clinical efficacy and safety of budesonide-formoterol in non-cystic fibrosis bronchiectasis. *Chest.* 2012;141:461–468.
9. Redding GJ. Bronchiectasis in children. *Pediatr Clin North Am.* 2009;56:157–171, xi.

 SEE ALSO

Cystic Fibrosis; Chronic Obstructive Pulmonary Disease and Emphysema; Asthma; Tuberculosis; Aspergillosis; Kartagener Syndrome

CODES

ICD10

- J47.0 Bronchiectasis with acute lower respiratory infection
- J47.1 Bronchiectasis with (acute) exacerbation
- J47.9 Bronchiectasis, uncomplicated

CLINICAL PEARLS

- Symptoms of bronchiectasis include chronic productive cough, wheezing, and dyspnea, often accompanied by repeated respiratory infections.
- A chest x-ray has poor sensitivity and specificity for the diagnosis; a noncontrast high-resolution chest CT is the most important diagnostic tool.
- Current practice guidelines recommend treating acute exacerbations with short courses of antibiotics, even though the evidence is currently insufficient to support this strategy; frequent exacerbations may be treated with prolonged and aerosolized antibiotics.

BRONCHIOLITIS

Dennis E. Hughes, DO, FAAFP, FACEP

 BASICS

DESCRIPTION
- Inflammation and obstruction of small airways and reactive airways generally affecting infants and young children
- May be seasonal (November–April) and often occurs in epidemics
- Usual course: Insidious, acute, progressive
- Leading cause of hospitalizations in infants and children
- Predominant age: Newborn–2 years (peak age <6 months). Neonates are not protected despite transfer of maternal antibody.
- Predominant sex: Male > Female

EPIDEMIOLOGY
Incidence
- 21% in North America
- 18.8% (90,000 annually) of all pediatric hospitalizations (excluding live births) in children <2 years
- Incidence increasing since 1980 (with concomitant increase in relative rate of hospitalization from 2002 to 2007) (1)

ETIOLOGY AND PATHOPHYSIOLOGY
RSV accounts for 70–85% of all cases, but parainfluenza virus, adenovirus, rhinovirus, influenza virus, *Mycoplasma pneumoniae*, and *Chlamydophila pneumoniae* have all been implicated:
- Infection results in necrosis and lysis of epithelial cells and subsequent release of inflammatory mediators.
- Edema and mucus secretion which, combined with accumulating necrotic debris and loss of cilia clearance, results in luminal obstruction.
- Ventilation-perfusion mismatching resulting in hypoxia
- Air trapping is caused by dynamic airways narrowing during expiration, which increases work of breathing.
- Bronchospasm appears to play little or no role.

RISK FACTORS
- Smoking exposure
- Low birthweight
- Immunodeficiency
- Formula feeding (not breastfed)
- Contact with infected person (primary mode of spread)
- Children in daycare environment
- Heart–lung transplantation patient (immune compromise)
- Adults: Exposure to toxic fumes, connective tissue disease (respiratory epithelial damage)

GENERAL PREVENTION
- Hand washing
- Contact isolation of infected babies
- Persons with colds should keep contact with infants to a minimum.
- Palivizumab (Synagis), a monoclonal product, administered monthly, October–May, 15 mg/kg IM; used for respiratory syncytial virus (RSV) prevention ONLY in high-risk patients (2)
- High risk:
  – 32–35 weeks' gestation and <3 months of age at the start of RSV season with at least 1 risk factor: Either attending daycare or with a sibling <5 years at home
  – 28–32 weeks' gestation and age <6 months
  – <28 weeks' gestation and age <12 months
  – Moderately severe bronchopulmonary dysplasia and up to 2 years of age
  – Hemodynamically significant congenital heart disease (until age 6 months)
  – Once begun, continue through end of season regardless of age attained.
- RSV immunoglobulin, a human blood product, can also be used in at-risk patients. Monthly infusions of 750 mg/kg, October–May

Pediatric Considerations
Prior infection does not seem to confer subsequent immunity.

COMMONLY ASSOCIATED CONDITIONS
- Upper respiratory congestion
- Conjunctivitis
- Pharyngitis
- Otitis media
- Diarrhea

 DIAGNOSIS

History and physical examination should be the basis for the diagnosis of bronchiolitis.

HISTORY
- Irritability
- Anorexia
- Fever
- Noisy breathing (due to rhinorrhea)
- Cough
- Grunting
- Cyanosis
- Apnea
- Vomiting

PHYSICAL EXAM
- Tachypnea
- Retractions
- Rhinorrhea
- Wheezing
- Upper respiratory findings: Pharyngitis, conjunctivitis, otitis

DIFFERENTIAL DIAGNOSIS
- Other pulmonary infections such as pertussis, croup, or bacterial pneumonia
- Aspiration
- Vascular ring
- Foreign body
- Asthma
- Heart failure
- Gastroesophageal reflux
- Cystic fibrosis

DIAGNOSTIC TESTS & INTERPRETATION
Laboratory and other ancillary testing (including chest xray) not required.

Initial Tests (lab, imaging)
- Arterial oxygen saturation by pulse oximetry (<94% significant)
- Rapid respiratory viral antigen testing (not necessary during RSV season because the disease is managed symptomatically, but may be useful for epidemiologic, hospital cohorting, or in the very young to reduce unnecessary other workup.
- The American Association of Pediatrics (AAP) does not recommend routine RSV testing in infants and children with bronchiolitis:
  – Sensitivity 87–91%; specificity 96–100% (2)
    Chest x-ray (CXR):
- Increased anteroposterior diameter
- Flattened diaphragm
- Air trapping
- Patchy infiltrates
- Focal atelectasis: Right upper lobe common
- Peribronchial cuffing

Test Interpretation
- Mucosal: Hyperemia, edema
- Submucosal lymphocytic infiltrate, monocytic infiltrate, plasmacytic infiltrate
- Small airway debris, fibrin, inflammatory exudate, fibrosis
- Peribronchiolar mononuclear infiltrate

 TREATMENT

Mainstay of therapy is supportive to include upper airway suctioning, prevention of significant and prolonged hypoxia, and dehydration. The other interventions noted have historically varying affect on the course of the illness despite numerous studies.

MEDICATION
First Line

- Humidified oxygen (3)[A]
- Nebulized albuterol (0.15 mg/kg) is often tried for acute symptoms; a trial of therapy may be reasonable in the presence of a suspected bronchospastic component (or with a family history of asthma) (3)[B].
- Epinephrine aerosols (0.5 mL of 2.25% solution in 3 mL NS) some studies support short-term improvement in outpatient settings (used in combination with oral steroids) (4)[B].
- Corticosteroids:
  - Oral dexamethasone (1 mg/kg loading dose, then 0.6 mg/kg daily for 5 days) reduced subsequent hospitalization (5)[B].
  - Nebulized dexamethasone (2–4 mg in 3 mL NS) may have anecdotal benefit; studies show mixed results.
  - Neblized hypertonic (3%) saline has proven useful.

Second Line

- Antibiotics only if secondary bacterial infection present (rare)
- Heliox therapy (70% helium–30% oxygen) may be of benefit early in moderate-to-severe bronchiolitis to reduce degree of respiratory distress, but Cochrane review found little evidence of sustained benefit at 24 hours (6).
- Ribavirin (palivizumab) for patients at high risk:
  - Inhaled antiviral agent active against RSV
  - Nebulize via small-particle aerosol generator
  - Pregnant women should not be exposed.
- High-risk criteria:
  - 32–35 weeks' gestation and age <3 months at the start of RSV season with at least 1 risk factor: Either attending daycare or with a sibling <5 years of age at home
  - 28–32 weeks' gestation and age <6 months
  - <28 weeks' gestation and age <12 months
  - Moderately severe bronchopulmonary dysplasia and up to 2 years of age
  - Hemodynamically significant congenital heart disease (until age 6 months)
  - Once begun, continue through end of season regardless of age attained.

ADDITIONAL THERAPIES

- Positive-pressure ventilation (PPV) in the form of continuous positive airway pressure (CPAP) can be used in cases of respiratory failure. There is limited clinical evidence other than observational studies (4).
- Leukotriene receptor antagonists currently show no sustained benefit (4).

IN-PATIENT CONSIDERATIONS

Bronchiolitis can be associated with apnea in children <6 weeks of age.

Admission Criteria/Initial Stabilization

- Respiratory rate >45/min with respiratory distress or apnea
- Hypoxia is common; evidence-based cut-off requiring admission is not available (only D-level expert opinion), so clinical criteria are more helpful (pulse oximetry <94% used by many as cutoff).
- Ill or toxic appearance
- Underlying heart, respiratory condition, or immune suppression
- High risk for apnea (age <30 days, preterm birth [<37 weeks])
- Dehydrated or unable to feed
- Uncertain home care
- Use of Respiratory Distress Assessment Instrument may aid in determining admission. The five best predictors of admission: Age, respiratory rate, heart rate, oxygen saturation, and duration of symptoms were recently incorporated into a scoring instrument.
- Supplemental oxygen for pulse oximetry <94% on room air

IV Fluids

Indicated only if tachypnea precludes oral feeding. Weight-based maintenance rate plus insensible losses.

Discharge Criteria

Normal respiratory rate and no oxygen requirement. Recent small studies suggest that after a period of observation, children can be safely discharged on home oxygen.

ONGOING CARE

FOLLOW-UP RECOMMENDATIONS
Patient Monitoring

- Hospitalization is usually required only if oxygen is a requirement or unable to feed/drink.
- For a hospitalized patient, monitor as needed depending on the severity of the infection.
- If the patient is receiving home care, follow daily by telephone for 2–4 days; the patient may need frequent office visits.

PATIENT EDUCATION

- American Academy of Pediatrics: http://www.aap.org
- American Academy of Family Physicians: http://www.familydoctor.org

PROGNOSIS

- In most cases, recovery is complete within 7–14 days.
- Mortality statistics differ, but probably <1%
- High-risk infants (bronchopulmonary dysplasia, congenital heart disease) may have a prolonged course.

COMPLICATIONS

- Bacterial superinfection
- Bronchiolitis obliterans
- Apnea
- Respiratory failure
- Death
- Increased incidence of development of reactive airway disease (asthma)

REFERENCES

1. García CG, Bhore R, Soriano-Fallas A, et al. Risk factors in children hospitalized with RSV bronchiolitis versus non-RSV bronchiolitis. *Pediatrics*. 2010;126(6):e1453–1460. Epub 2010 Nov 22.
2. *REDBOOK: Report of the Committee on Infectious Disease*. Elk Grove Village, IL: American Academy of Pediatrics; 2009.
3. Umoren R, Odey F, Meremikwu MM. Steam Inhalation or Humidified oxygen for acute bronchiolitis in children up to 3 years of age. *Cochran Database Syst Rev*. 2011;1:CD006435.
4. Petruzella FD, Gorelick MH. Current therapies in bronchiolitis. *Pediatr Emerg Care*. 2010;26(4): 302–307; quiz 308–311.
5. Corneli HM, Zorc JJ, Majahan P, et al. A multicenter, randomized, controlled trial of dexamethasone for bronchiolitis. *N Engl J Med*. 2007;357:331–339.
6. Liet JM, Ducruet T, Gupta V, et al. Heliox inhalation therapy for bronchiolitis in infants. *Cochrane Database Syst Rev*. 2010;4:CD006915.

ADDITIONAL READING

- Fernandes RM, et al. Glucocorticoids for acute viral bronchiolitis in infants and young children. *Cochrane Database Syst Rev*. 2013;6:CD004878.
- Zorc JJ, Hall CB, Bronchiolitis: recent evidence on diagnosis and management. *Pediactrics*. 2010;125(2):342–349.

CODES

ICD10

- J21.0 Acute bronchiolitis due to respiratory syncytial virus
- J21.8 Acute bronchiolitis due to other specified organisms
- J21.9 Acute bronchiolitis, unspecified

CLINICAL PEARLS

- Bronchiolitis is the leading cause of hospitalizations in infants and children-esp < 3 months of age.
- Treatment is primarily supportive.
- Antibiotics are not helpful in most cases.
- Parental education of expected course of illness is most important.
- Be aware of new Synagis treatment guidelines for premature infants.

BRONCHIOLITIS OBLITERANS AND ORGANIZING PNEUMONIA

Gretchen M. Dickson, MD, MBA, FAAFP

BASICS

DESCRIPTION
- A primary or secondary process of the lungs characterized by granulation-like tissue involving the distal airways and alveoli
- Bronchiolitis obliterans and organizing pneumonia (BOOP) is a restrictive problem that is completely reversible, whereas bronchiolitis obliterans is an obstructive problem that causes permanent lung damage.
- A specific reaction of lung tissue to a variety of injuries
- It may occur as patchy infiltrates, or it may be nodular or secondary to another lung disease.
- May also appear to be a migrating process.
- May have a gradual or sudden onset.
- Lungs show a pattern of multiple patchy pneumonia, which are seen on the chest x-ray (CXR) as patchy alveolar or ground-glass opacifications, with or without interstitial infiltrates; there may be air bronchograms as well.
- Most cases will respond to corticosteroids, which may have to be given for a year or more.
- Synonym(s): Intraluminal fibrosis of distal airways; Idiopathic bronchiolitis obliterans and organizing pneumonitis (BOOP); Cryptogenic organizing pneumonia; Obliterative bronchiolitis

Geriatric Considerations
More common than originally thought and may be sudden and very severe

Pediatric Considerations
Rare, but has been reported after viral pneumonia (adenovirus influenza):
- Characteristics include delayed recovery, persistent cough, crackles, or wheezing after pneumonia.
- Laboratory findings generally not helpful.
- Imaging shows: Ventilation-perfusion ratio-matched defects; high-resolution CT, bronchiectasis, bronchogram, pruned tree appearance
- Diagnosis is confirmed by biopsy.

EPIDEMIOLOGY
- Incidence/Prevalence in the US: Estimated at 0.01%, but may be underdiagnosed.
- Predominant age: Reported cases range age 0–70; most commonly seen in ages 40–60s.

Prevalence
Unknown

ETIOLOGY AND PATHOPHYSIOLOGY
Idiopathic: A complex response to a variety of injuries, such as toxic inhalation, postmycoplasma, viral and bacterial infection, aspiration, immunologic factors, drugs

Genetics
No known genetic component

RISK FACTORS
- AIDS
- Immunocompromised patients, including transplant recipients
- Smoking

GENERAL PREVENTION
Except for prevention of relapse, none known

Pediatric Considerations
In the pediatric nontransplant recipient population, adenovirus infection is the most common cause of bronchiolitis obliterans (1).

COMMONLY ASSOCIATED CONDITIONS
- Drug-induced pneumonitis:
  - Paraquat poisoning
  - Amiodarone toxicity
  - Acebutolol toxicity
  - Amphotericin B
  - Bleomycin
  - Carbamazepine
  - Cephalosporins
  - Gold
  - Minocycline
  - Nitrofurantoin
  - Phenytoin
  - Sulfamethoxypyridazine
  - Sulfasalazine
  - Ticlopidine
  - Freebase cocaine pulmonary toxicity
  - Overdose of L-tryptophan
- Infections:
  - Chronic infectious pneumonia
  - Malaria
  - Chlamydia
  - *Legionella*
  - *Mycoplasma*
  - *Pneumocystis*
  - *Cryptococcus*
- Immunocompromise: Bone marrow, lung, renal, transplantation
- Connective tissue diseases:
  - Rheumatic lung
  - Sjögren syndrome
  - Polymyositis
  - Scleroderma
  - Essential mixed cryoglobulinemia
- Miscellaneous:
  - Cystic fibrosis
  - Bronchopulmonary dysplasia
  - Renal failure
  - Congestive heart failure (CHF)
  - Adult respiratory distress syndrome
  - Chronic eosinophilic pneumonia
  - Hypersensitivity pneumonitis
  - Histiocytosis X
  - Sarcoidosis
  - Pneumoconioses
- Radiation pneumonitis

DIAGNOSIS

Think of the possibility in patients presenting with (2):
- Flulike illness that lasts 4–10 weeks or longer. Most have been treated with antibiotics without success.
- Fatigue, fever, and weight loss
- Dry cough
- Dyspnea may be severe.
- Bilateral crackles

HISTORY
- Fatigue
- Fever
- Weight loss
- Dry cough
- Dyspnea may be severe.

PHYSICAL EXAM
- Hypoxia
- Respiratory distress
- Bilateral crackles

DIFFERENTIAL DIAGNOSIS
- Usual interstitial pneumonitis
- Noninfectious diseases
- Tuberculosis
- Sarcoidosis
- Histoplasmosis
- Berylliosis
- Goodpasture syndrome
- Neoplasm
- Polyarteritis nodosa
- Systemic lupus erythematosus
- Wegener granulomatosis
- Sjögren syndrome
- Chronic eosinophilic pneumonia
- Cryptogenic bronchiolitis

DIAGNOSTIC TESTS & INTERPRETATION
- May have normal or nonspecific laboratory findings
- Leukocytosis with a normal differential
- Elevated ESR
- Negative cultures
- Negative serology for mycoplasma, *Coxiella*, *Legionella*, psittacosis, and fungus
- Negative viral studies
- CXR: Often appears more normal than the physical examination
- CXR may show bilateral patchy alveolar opacities, often in the middle or upper lung area, a ground-glass pattern that may have air bronchograms.
- Throughout the disease, new infiltrates may appear or may seem to migrate.
- Effusions and cavitary lesions are rare on x-ray.
- Patients with linear opacities at lung bases may have a poorer prognosis.
- CT scans more accurately define the distribution and extent of the patchy alveolar opacities with areas of hyperlucency (3).
- Up to 90% of CT scans may show airspace consolidation with air bronchograms.
- Pulmonary function shows a restrictive/obstructive pattern.
- Flow-volume loop shows terminal airway obstruction.
- The involved area may seem to migrate.
- Ventilation-perfusion ratio scan: Matched patchy defects

Diagnostic Procedures/Other
- Open lung biopsy
- Transbronchial biopsy
- It may be wise to use a trial of steroids as a diagnostic trial, although not all would agree.
- If a diagnostic trial is successful, be prepared to treat the patient for at least 1 year.

Test Interpretation
- Intraluminal fibrosis of distal airspaces is the major pathologic feature.
- Fibroblasts and plugs of inflammatory cells and loose connective tissue fill these distal airways.
- Inflammatory cells are mainly lymphocytes and plasma cells.
- Interstitial fibrosis is present.
- Plugs of edematous granulation tissue in the terminal and respiratory bronchioles and alveolar ducts do not cause permanent damage.

 TREATMENT

Inpatient care may be required.

GENERAL MEASURES
- Monitor blood gases or pulse oximetry.
- Oxygen, as necessary

MEDICATION
First Line
Prednisone:
- 1 mg/kg (up to 60 mg/d) for 1–3 months, then 40 mg/d for 3 months, then 10–20 mg/d for up to 1 year
- May consider a 6-month-only taper or alternate day dosing for 1 year to limit steroid exposure
- Increase length of taper for patients on long-term therapy to avoid precipitating addisonian crisis.
- Treatment may be needed for ≥1 year.
- Contraindications: Refer to the manufacturer's literature.
- Precautions: Be aware of the patient's Mantoux status and history of peptic ulcer disease. Long-term steroid treatment is associated with significant adverse effects, including Cushing syndrome, fluid retention, osteoporosis, hyperkalemia, and poor wound healing.

Pediatric Considerations
Prednisone: 1 mg/kg q24h for 1 month, followed by weaning over several months

Second Line
- Steroids other than prednisone may be used.
- 1 paper reported the use of erythromycin 600 mg/d for 3–4 months after initial control with prednisone.
- Prescribe antimicrobials if the original infection is persistent. The proper choice depends on the pathogen.
- Anecdotal use of inhaled triamcinolone and cyclophosphamide has been reported.

ISSUES FOR REFERRAL
Patients should be followed by a pulmonologist.

 ONGOING CARE

FOLLOW-UP RECOMMENDATIONS
Patient Monitoring
- Frequent visits, weekly at first
- Prednisone must be continued because of the chance of relapse.
- Monitor the lung disease and the side effects of prednisone therapy:
  - Annual Mantoux/purified protein derivative
  - Monthly CBC
  - Funduscopic examination every 3–6 months
  - Serial dual-energy x-ray absorptiometry (DEXA) scans for osteoporosis

DIET
No special diet

PATIENT EDUCATION
- Compliance: Emphasize the need to continue prednisone because of the chance of a relapse.
- Recurrence in up to 1/3 who do not complete full steroid treatment.

PROGNOSIS
Typically complete recovery, but individual case management is mandatory.

COMPLICATIONS
- Bronchiectasis
- Most people recover completely without permanent sequelae if full course of steroids completed.
- Death occurs in up to 7%, but usually in individuals who are elderly or have pre-existing comorbid conditions.

REFERENCES
1. Moonnumakal SP, Fan LL. Bronchiolitis obliterans in children. *Curr Opin Pediatr*. 2008;20:272–278.
2. Cordier JF, Loire R, Brune J. Idiopathic bronchiolitis obliterans organizing pneumonia. Definition of characteristic clinical profiles in a series of 16 patients. *Chest*. 1989;96:999–1004.
3. Müller NL, Staples CA, Miller RR. Bronchiolitis obliterans organizing pneumonia: CT features in 14 patients. *AJR Am J Roentgenol*. 1990;154:983–987.

ADDITIONAL READING
- Drakopanagiotakis F, Polychronopoulos V, Judson MA. Organizing pneumonia. *Am J Med Sci*. 2008;335:34–39.
- Ruth-Sahd LA, White KA. Bronchiolitis obliterans organizing pneumonia. *Dimens Crit Care Nurs*. 2009;28(5):204–208.
- Schlesinger C, Koss MN. The organizing pneumonias: An update and review. *Curr Opin Pulm Med*. 2005;11(5):422–430.
- White KA, Ruth-Sahd LA. Bronchiolitis obliterans organizing pneumonia. *Crit Care Nurse*. 2007;27(3):53–66; quiz 67.

 SEE ALSO

Sjögren Syndrome

 CODES

ICD10
- J44.9 Chronic obstructive pulmonary disease, unspecified
- J84.89 Other specified interstitial pulmonary diseases

CLINICAL PEARLS
- BOOP and bronchiolitis obliterans are very different.
- BOOP are restrictive problems that are completely reversible, whereas bronchiolitis obliterans is an obstructive problem that causes permanent lung damage. BOOP treatment is a prolonged course of corticosteroids.

BRONCHITIS, ACUTE

Alan J. Cropp, MD • Ghazaleh Bigdeli, MD

 BASICS

DESCRIPTION
- Inflammation of trachea, bronchi, and bronchioles resulting from a respiratory tract infection or chemical irritant (1)
- Cough, the predominant symptom, may last as long as 10–20 days (1,2).
- Generally self-limited, with complete healing and full return of function (2)
- Most infections are viral if no underlying cardiopulmonary disease is present (2).
- Synonym(s): Tracheobronchitis; Chest cold

Geriatric Considerations
Can be serious, particularly if part of influenza, with underlying chronic obstructive pulmonary disease (COPD) or congestive heart failure (CHF) (3)

Pediatric Considerations
- Usually occurs in association with other conditions of upper and lower respiratory tract (trachea usually involved) (4).
- If repeated attacks occur, child should be evaluated for anomalies of the respiratory tract, immune deficiencies, or for chronic asthma.
- When acute bronchitis is caused by respiratory syncytial virus (RSV), it may be fatal.

EPIDEMIOLOGY
- Predominant age: All ages
- Predominant gender: Male = Female

Incidence
- ~5% of adults per year (3)
- Common cause of infection in children (4)

Prevalence
Results in 10–12 million office visits per year (3)

ETIOLOGY AND PATHOPHYSIOLOGY
- Viral infections, such as adenovirus, influenza A and B, parainfluenza virus, coxsackievirus, RSV, rhinovirus, coronavirus (types 1–3), herpes simplex virus (2)
- Bacterial infections, such as *Chlamydia pneumoniae* (Taiwan acute respiratory [TWAR] agent), *Mycoplasma, Bordetella pertussis, Haemophilus influenzae, Streptococcus pneumoniae, Moraxella catarrhalis,* and *Mycobacterium tuberculosis* (2)
- Secondary bacterial infection as part of an acute upper respiratory infection
- Possibly fungal infections
- Chemical irritants
- Acute bronchitis causes an injury to the epithelial surfaces, resulting in an increase in mucous production and thickening of the bronchiole wall (1).

Genetics
No known genetic pattern

RISK FACTORS
- Infants
- Elderly
- Air pollutants
- Smoking
- 2nd-hand smoke
- Environmental changes
- Chronic bronchopulmonary diseases
- Chronic sinusitis
- Tracheostomy
- Bronchopulmonary allergy
- Hypertrophied tonsils and adenoids in children
- Immunosuppression:
  – Immunoglobulin deficiency
  – HIV infection
  – Alcoholism
- Gastroesophageal reflux disease (GERD)

GENERAL PREVENTION
- Avoid smoking and 2nd-hand smoke.
- Control underlying risk factors (i.e., asthma, sinusitis, and reflux).
- Avoid exposure, especially daycare.
- Pneumovax, influenza immunization

COMMONLY ASSOCIATED CONDITIONS
- Allergic rhinitis
- Sinusitis
- Pharyngitis
- Epiglottitis (rare, but can be rapidly fatal)
- Coryza
- Croup
- Influenza
- Pneumonia
- Asthma
- COPD/Emphysema
- GERD

 DIAGNOSIS

HISTORY
- Sudden onset of cough and no evidence of pneumonia, asthma, exacerbation of COPD, or the common cold (3)
- Cough is initially dry and unproductive, then productive; later, mucopurulent sputum, which may indicate secondary infection
- Dyspnea, wheeze, fever, and fatigue may occur.
- Possible contact with others who have respiratory infections (1)

PHYSICAL EXAM
- Fever
- Tachypnea
- Pharynx injected
- Rales, rhonchi, wheezing
- No evidence of pulmonary consolidation

DIFFERENTIAL DIAGNOSIS
- Common cold
- Acute sinusitis
- Bronchopneumonia
- Influenza
- Bacterial tracheitis
- Bronchiectasis
- Asthma
- Reactive airways dysfunction syndrome (RADS)
- Allergy
- Eosinophilic pneumonitis
- Aspiration
- Retained foreign body
- Inhalation injury
- Cystic fibrosis
- Bronchogenic carcinoma
- Heart failure
- GERD

DIAGNOSTIC TESTS & INTERPRETATION
Initial Tests (lab, imaging)
- None normally needed; diagnosis is based on history and physical exam showing no post nasal drip or rales.
- If you consider a complicated picture, consider:
  – WBC with differential
  – Sputum culture/sensitivity if CXR is abnormal (3)
  – Influenza titers (if appropriate for time of year)
  – Viral panel
- No testing needed unless concerned about pneumonia
- Chest radiograph (CXR):
  – Lungs normal, if uncomplicated
  – Helps to rule out other diseases (pneumonia) or complications

Follow-Up Tests & Special Considerations
- Arterial blood gases: Hypoxemia (rarely)
- Pulmonary function tests (seldom needed during acute stages): Increased residual volume, decreased maximal expiratory rate (2)

 TREATMENT

GENERAL MEASURES
- Rest
- Stop smoking or avoid smoke.
- Steam inhalations
- Vaporizers
- Adequate hydration
- Antitussives
- Antibiotics are usually not recommended (1,3,5)[A].
- Treat associated illnesses (e.g., GERD).

MEDICATION

ALERT

Antibiotics are not recommended (1,3,5)[A] unless a treatable pathogen has been identified or significant comorbidities are present.

First Line

- Supportive; increased fluids (cough results in increased fluid loss)
- Antipyretic analgesic, such as aspirin, acetaminophen, or ibuprofen
- Decongestants if accompanied by sinus condition (1)
- Cough suppressant for troublesome cough (not with COPD); benzonatate (Tessalon), guaifenesin with codeine or dextromethorphan (3)[A]
- Mucolytic agents are not recommended (3)[B].
- Inhaled β-agonist (e.g., albuterol) or in combination with PO steroids for cough with bronchospasm (3,6)[B]
- Amantadine or rimantadine therapy if influenza A is suspected; most effective if started within 24–48 hours of development of symptoms (also consider oseltamivir [Tamiflu] or zanamivir [Relenza])
- Antibiotics if a treatable cause (i.e., pertussis) is identified (2)[A]:
  – Amoxicillin: 500 mg q8h or trimethoprim-sulfamethoxazole DS q12h for routine infection (6)[A]:
    ○ Penicillins and trimethoprim-based regimens seem to be equivalent in terms of effectiveness and toxicity for acute bacterial exacerbations of chronic bronchitis (ABECB) (5)[B].
    ○ Clarithromycin (Biaxin): 500 mg q12h or azithromycin (Zithromax) Z-pack for penicillin allergy or Mycoplasma infection
    ○ In patients with acute bronchitis of a suspected bacterial cause, azithromycin tends to be more effective in terms of lower incidence of treatment failure and adverse events than amoxicillin or amoxicillin-clavulanic acid (7)[B].
  – Doxycycline: 100 mg/d × 10 days if Moraxella, Chlamydia, or Mycoplasma suspected
  – Quinolone for more serious infections or other antibiotic failure or in elderly or patients with multiple comorbidities
  – Macrolide for pertussis (1)[A]
- Contraindication(s): Doxycycline and quinolones should not be used during pregnancy or in children.
- Precautions:
  – Watch for theophylline toxicity with macrolides and quinolones.
  – Multiple antibiotics have the potential to interfere with the effectiveness of PO contraceptives.
  – Cough and cold preparations should not be used in children <6.

Second Line

- Other antibiotics if indicated by sputum culture (Moraxella needs a different set of antibiotics)
- Antivirals
- Other macrolides or quinolones based on pathogen and sensitivity

ISSUES FOR REFERRAL

- Complications, such as pneumonia or respiratory failure
- Comorbidities, such as COPD
- Cough lasting >3 months

ADDITIONAL THERAPIES

- Antipyretic for fever (e.g., acetaminophen, aspirin, or ibuprofen)
- Systemic (PO) steroids if necessary for bronchospasm (e.g., Prednisone)

COMPLEMENTARY AND ALTERNATIVE MEDICINE

Throat lozenges for pharyngitis

IN-PATIENT CONSIDERATIONS

Admission Criteria/Initial Stabilization

- Hypoxia
- Severe bronchospasm
- Exacerbation of underlying disease
- Outpatient, unless elderly or complicated by severe underlying disease
- May require supplemental oxygen in selected patients
- Bronchodilators if patient is bronchospastic

IV Fluids

May be helpful if patient is dehydrated

Nursing

- Ensure patient comfort and monitor for signs of deterioration, especially if underlying lung disease exists.
- May need to follow oxygen saturation in patients with underlying lung disease

Discharge Criteria

Improvement in symptoms and comorbidities

 ## ONGOING CARE

FOLLOW-UP RECOMMENDATIONS

- Usually a self-limited disease not requiring follow-up
- Cough may linger for several weeks.
- In children, if recurrent, need to consider other diagnoses, such as asthma (4)

Patient Monitoring

- Oximetry until no longer hypoxemic
- Recheck for chronicity.

DIET

Increased fluids (3–4 L/d) while febrile

PATIENT EDUCATION

- For patient education materials favorably reviewed on this topic, contact the American Lung Association, 1740 Broadway, New York, NY 10019 (212) 315-8700; www.lungusa.org.
- American Academy of Family Physicians: www.familydoctor.org

PROGNOSIS

- Usual: Complete resolution
- Can be serious in the elderly or debilitated
- Cough may persist for several weeks after an initial improvement (1).
- Postbronchitic reactive airways disease (rare)
- Bronchiolitis obliterans and organizing pneumonia (rare)

COMPLICATIONS

- Superinfection, such as bronchopneumonia
- Bronchiectasis
- Hemoptysis
- Acute respiratory failure
- Chronic cough

REFERENCES

1. Wenzel RP, Fowler AA. Clinical practice. Acute bronchitis. N Engl J Med. 2006;355:2125–2130.
2. Albert RH. Diagnosis and treatment of acute bronchitis. Am Fam Physician. 2010;82(11): 1345–1350.
3. Braman SS. Chronic cough due to acute bronchitis: ACCP evidence-based clinical practice guidelines. Chest. 2006;129:95S–103S.
4. Fleming DM, Elliot AJ. The management of acute bronchitis in children. Expert Opin Pharmacother. 2007;8:415–426.
5. Gonzales R, Anderer T, McCulloch C, et al. A cluster randomized trial of decision support for reducing antibiotic use in acute bronchitis. JAMA Intern Med. 2013;173(4):267–273.
6. Korbila IP, Manta KG, Siempos II, et al. Penicillins vs trimethoprim-based regimens for acute bacterial exacerbations of chronic bronchitis: Meta-analysis of randomized controlled trials. Can Fam Physician. 2009;55:60–67.
7. Panpanich R, Lerttrakarnnon P, Laopaiboon M. Azithromycin for acute lower respiratory tract infections. Cochrane Database Syst Rev. 2008; CD001954.

 ## SEE ALSO

- Asthma; Chronic Obstructive Pulmonary Disease and Emphysema
- Algorithm: Cough, Chronic

 ## CODES

ICD10

- J20.4 Acute bronchitis due to parainfluenza virus
- J20.8 Acute bronchitis due to other specified organisms
- J20.9 Acute bronchitis, unspecified

CLINICAL PEARLS

- Acute bronchitis is a common and generally self-limited disease.
- It usually does not require treatment with antibiotics.
- Cough may linger for several weeks.
- Recurrent or seasonal episodes may suggest another disease process, such as asthma.

BULIMIA NERVOSA

Umer Farooq, MD/MBBS • Najm Hasan Siddiqui, MD

 BASICS

DESCRIPTION
- A pattern of discrete periods of uncontrolled eating, followed by compensatory behaviors (at least 2 times per week for 3 months)
- *DSM* classifies bulimia nervosa as purging and non-purging subtypes:
  - Purging: Often by self-induced vomiting, laxatives, diuretics
  - Nonpurging: Binges followed by sharply restricted diet and/or vigorous exercise
- System(s) affected: Oropharyngeal; Endocrine/metabolic; Gastrointestinal; Dermatologic; Cardiovascular; Nervous

EPIDEMIOLOGY
- Predominant age: Adolescents and young adults
- Mean age of onset: 18–21 years
- Predominant sex: Female > Male (10–20:1)

Incidence
28.8 women, 0.8 men per 100,000 per year

Prevalence
- More prevalent than anorexia nervosa
- 1–3% in women age 16–35 years
- 0.5% in young men (higher among gay and bisexual men)

ETIOLOGY AND PATHOPHYSIOLOGY
- Combination of biological, psychological, environmental, and social factors. Unique contribution of any specific factor remains unclear
- Evidence of serotonergic dysregulation in bulimia nervosa
- Substantial literature shows that bulimia nervosa is familial (1)

RISK FACTORS
- Female gender
- History of obesity and dieting
- Body dissatisfaction
- Critical comments by family or others about weight, body shape, or eating
- Severe life stressor
- Low self-esteem
- Perceived pressure to be thin
- Perfectionist or obsessive thinking
- Poor impulse control, alcohol misuse
- Environment stressing high achievement, physical fitness (e.g., armed forces, ballet, cheerleading, gymnastics, or modeling)
- Family history of substance abuse, affective disorders, eating disorder, or obesity
- Type 1 diabetes
- Sexual abuse is not causally related to bulimia.

GENERAL PREVENTION
- Prevention programs can reduce risk factors and future onset of eating disorders (2)[C].
- Target adolescents and young women ≥15 years
- Realistic and healthy weight management strategies and attitudes
- Decrease body dissatisfaction and promote self-esteem
- Reduce focus on thin as ideal
- Decrease anxiety/depressive symptoms and improve stress management

COMMONLY ASSOCIATED CONDITIONS
- Major depression and dysthymia
- Anxiety disorders
- Substance abuse/dependence
- Bipolar disorder
- Obsessive-compulsive disorder
- Borderline personality disorder

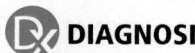 **DIAGNOSIS**

HISTORY
- Patients unlikely to self-identify binge eating or purging behaviors; corroborate with parent/relative
- Unhappiness and/or preoccupation with weight and diet attempts
- Pattern of restricting diet, binge eating, and purging behaviors:
  - Binge is context specific (usually within 2-hour period, they will eat what would be an unusually large amount for most people)
  - Vomiting (often with little effort)
  - Vigorous aerobic exercise
  - Distress/Shame related to loss of control
- Depressed mood and self-depreciation following the binges
- Relief and increased ability to concentrate following the purges
- Other possible signs and symptoms:
  - Requesting weight loss help and mildly underweight to overweight
  - Diet pill, diuretic, laxative, ipecac, and thyroid medication use/abuse
  - Menstrual disturbance
  - Fatigue and lethargy
  - Abdominal pain, bloating, constipation, diarrhea, rectal prolapse
  - Sore throat
  - Thermal tooth sensitivity
  - Frequent fluctuations in weight
  - Omission/Underdosing insulin in diabetes patients

PHYSICAL EXAM
- Often normal
- Bradycardia
- Eroded tooth enamel
- Perimylolysis
- Cheilosis
- Gingivitis
- Sialadenosis
- Asymptomatic, noninflammatory parotid gland enlargement
- Epigastric tenderness to palpation
- Calluses, abrasions, bruising on hand, thumb (Russell's sign)
- Peripheral edema

DIFFERENTIAL DIAGNOSIS
- Anorexia, binge eating/purging type
- Major depressive disorder
- Anxiety disorders
- Malabsorption
- Addison disease
- Celiac disease
- Diabetes mellitus

- Hyperthyroidism, hypothyroidism
- Hyperpituitarism
- Hypothalamic brain tumor
- Kleine-Levin syndrome
- Body dysmorphic disorder
- Borderline personality disorder

DIAGNOSTIC TESTS & INTERPRETATION
All lab results may be within normal limits and are not necessary for diagnosis.
- Psychological self-report screening tests:
  - Eating Attitudes Test
  - Eating Disorder Inventory
  - Eating Disorder Screen for Primary Care
  - Bulimia Test (revised)
  - Bulimia Investigatory Test Edinburgh
  - SCOFF (sick, control, one, fat, food)

Initial Tests (lab, imaging)
- Blood work:
  - Hypokalemia, hypochloremia
  - Hypomagnesaemia, hyponatremia, hypocalcemia, hypophosphatemia
  - Serum amylase levels
  - Alkalosis
  - Elevated BUN
  - Hypoglycemia
- Urinalysis:
  - Increased urine-specific gravity

Diagnostic Procedures/Other
Electrocardiogram:
- Bradycardia or arrhythmias
- Conduction defects
- Depressed ST segment due to hypokalemia

Test Interpretation
- Esophagitis
- Acute pancreatitis
- Cardiomyopathy and muscle weakness due to ipecac abuse
- Melanosis coli
- Cathartic colon syndrome
- Delayed or arrested skeletal growth
- Stress fracture
- Irreversible dental erosions
- Osteopenia/Osteoporosis

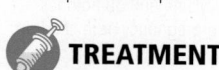 **TREATMENT**

- Cognitive-behavioral therapy (CBT) should be considered as first-line treatment (3,4,5)[A].
- Guided self-help therapies may be effective (4,5)[B].
- Interpersonal therapies and group therapies have been found to be helpful

GENERAL MEASURES
- Psychotherapies should be employed as first-line treatments.
- Multidisciplinary team:
  - Primary care physician, behavioral health provider, nutritionist

- Build trust; increase motivation for change
- Assess psychological and nutritional status
- Consider evidence-based self-help program
- CBT for bulimia nervosa (3,4,5,6)[A]:
  – 16–20 50-minute appointments
  – Involve patient in establishing goals
  – Self-monitoring of food intake, frequency of binges/purges, related antecedents, consequences, thoughts, and emotions
  – Self-monitoring of weight once per week
  – Educate about ineffectiveness of purging for weight control and adverse outcomes
  – Establish prescribed eating plan to develop regular eating habits and realistic weight goal
  – Gradually introduce feared foods into diet
  – Problem-solve how to cope with triggers
  – Decrease ruminations about calories, weight, and purging
  – Challenge fear of loss of control
  – Establish relapse prevention plan
  – Gradual laxative withdrawal
- Interpersonal therapy (3,4)[B]:
  – May act more slowly than CBT
- Transdiagnostic CBT
- Dialectical behavior therapy
- Family therapy for adolescents
- Nutritional education, relaxation techniques
- Educate patient to brush teeth and use baking soda to rinse mouth after vomiting.

MEDICATION
First Line
- Selective serotonin reuptake inhibitors (SSRIs), particularly fluoxetine (Prozac) at 60 mg, are effective in reducing symptoms with relatively few side effects. Higher doses than standard doses for depression are often needed (4,6,7)[B]:
  – Combination of medication and CBT has been shown to have added benefit over medication or therapy alone (7)
- To prevent relapse, maintain antidepressant at full therapeutic dose for at least 1 year.
- Bupropion not recommended due to its association with seizures in patients who purge.
- Misrepresentation and nonadherence may be more likely in this population
- Precautions:
  – Serious toxicity following overdose is common
  – Patients may vomit medications

Second Line
- Ondansetron (Zofran) 4–8 mg t.i.d. between meals can help prevent vomiting.
- Psyllium (Metamucil) preparations, 1 tbs q.h.s. with glass of water, can prevent constipation during laxative withdrawal

ISSUES FOR REFERRAL
Patients with bulimia require a multidisciplinary team, including a primary care physician, behavioral health provider, and a nutritionist. Important part of treatment is to arrange mental health therapist for psychotherapy.

ADDITIONAL THERAPIES
Most patients can be treated as outpatients.

COMPLEMENTARY AND ALTERNATIVE MEDICINE
Bright light therapy may help (4).

IN-PATIENT CONSIDERATIONS
- If possible, admit to a specialized eating disorders unit

- Supervised meals and bathroom privileges
- Monitor weight and physical activity
- Monitor electrolytes
- Gradually shift control to patients as they demonstrate responsibility

Admission Criteria/Initial Stabilization
Hospitalize if severe malnutrition, dehydration, electrolyte disturbances, cardiac dysrhythmia, uncontrolled binging and purging, psychiatric emergency (threat to self/others), or if outpatient treatment failed.

 ## ONGOING CARE

FOLLOW-UP RECOMMENDATIONS
Patient Monitoring
- Binge–purge activity, including antecedents and consequences
- Level of exercise activity
- Self-esteem, comfort with body and self
- Ruminations and depressive symptoms
- Repeat any abnormal lab values weekly or monthly until stable.

DIET
- Balanced diet, normal eating pattern
- Reintroduce feared foods.

PATIENT EDUCATION
Guided self-help treatment programs:
- Astrachan-Fletcher E, Maslar M. *The dialectical behavior therapy skills workbook for bulimia: Using DBT to break the cycle and regain control of your life.* Oakland, CA: New Harbinger; 2009.
- Fairburn CG. *Overcoming binge eating.* New York: Guilford Press; 1995.
- McCabe RE, McFarlane TL, Olmstead MP. *Overcoming bulimia: Your comprehensive, step-by-step guide to recovery.* Oakland, CA: New Harbinger; 2003.

PROGNOSIS
- After effective CBT:
  – In the short term, 50% of treated individuals do not meet criteria for diagnosis
  – In the long term (2–10 years), 70% may be asymptomatic
  – Symptomatic individuals may demonstrate remissions, relapses, subclinical, or other eating disorder–related behaviors.
- Untreated:
  – Likely to remain chronic/relapsing problem
- Greater weight fluctuations, other impulsive behaviors, childhood obesity, low self-esteem, family history of alcohol abuse, psychiatric comorbidity, and personality disorder diagnoses (e.g., avoidant personality disorder) may predict poor prognosis
- Mortality rate: 0.4%

COMPLICATIONS
- Drug and alcohol abuse
- Osteopenia/Osteoporosis
- Stress fracture
- Gastric dilatation
- Boerhaave syndrome
- Mallory-Weiss tears
- Pseudo-Bartter syndrome
- Spontaneous pneumomediastinum
- Potassium depletion, cardiac arrhythmia, cardiac arrest
- Suicide

Pregnancy Considerations
Maternal and fetal problems if pregnant:
- Binging/purging behaviors may persist, increase, or decrease with pregnancy
- Increased risk for preterm delivery, operative delivery, and infants with low birth weight, should be managed as high risk

REFERENCES

1. Lilenfeld LR, Kaye WH, Greeno CG, et al. A controlled family study of anorexia nervosa and bulimia nervosa: psychiatric disorders in first-degree relatives and effects of proband comorbidity. *Arch Gen Psychiatry.* 1998;55:603–610.
2. Stice E, Shaw H, Marti CN. A meta-analytic review of eating disorder prevention programs: Encouraging findings. *Annu Rev Clin Psychol.* 2007;3:207–231.
3. Hay PP, Bacaltchuk J, Stefano S, et al. Psychological treatments for bulimia nervosa and binging. *Cochrane Database Syst Rev.* 2009;4:CD000562.
4. Shapiro JR, Berkman ND, Brownley KA, et al. Bulimia nervosa treatment: A systematic review of randomized controlled trials. *Int J Eat Disord.* 2007;40:321–336.
5. NICE. *Eating disorders—Core interventions in the treatment of anorexia nervosa, bulimia nervosa, and related eating disorders.* NICE Clinical Guideline no. 9. London: NICE, 2004: Available at: www.nice.org.uk
6. *Practice guideline for the treatment of patients with eating disorders,* 3rd ed. American Psychiatric Association. Available at www.psych.org
7. Bacaltchuk J, Hay P, Trefiglio R. Antidepressants versus psychological treatments and their combination for bulimia nervosa. *Cochrane Database Sys Rev.* 2001;4:CD003385.

 ## SEE ALSO

- Anorexia Nervosa; Hyperkalemia; Laxative Abuse; Salivary Gland Tumors
- Algorithm: Weight Loss

 ## CODES

ICD10
F50.2 Bulimia nervosa

CLINICAL PEARLS
- Asking "Are you satisfied with your eating patterns?" and/or "Do you worry that you have lost control over how much you eat?" may help to screen for an eating problem.
- Binging and purging behaviors can be seen in anorexia nervosa as well.
- Weight is not severely lowered as in anorexia nervosa.
- Consider using a stepped-care approach. Start with a guided self-help program using instructional aids; next, begin CBT (e.g., 16–20 sessions over 4–5 months).
- SSRIs, particularly fluoxetine (60 mg daily), may be helpful as a 1st step or as an adjunctive treatment with CBT.

BUNION

Randolph Taylor II, MD • Yogi Patel, MD

BASICS

DESCRIPTION
- Hallux valgus (Latin for "big toe askew"), commonly known as a bunion. The 1st toe (hallux), is laterally deviated.
- This lateral deviation of the great toe, also described as a medial deviation of the 1st metatarsal, leads to a medial prominence of the 1st metatarsophalangeal (MTP) joint and a potentially painful and/or debilitating deformity.
- Progressive subluxation of the 1st MTP joint is common.
- System(s) affected: Musculoskeletal/Skin

EPIDEMIOLOGY
- Predominant age: More common in adults (1)[A]:
  – Estimated 23% in adults aged 18–65 years
  – Estimated 35.7% in elderly >65 years
- Predominant sex: Female > Male by ~50%

Prevalence
- Prevalence increases with age and is higher by 30% in females.
- Juvenile hallux valgus:
  – More common in girls, who account for >80% of the cases
- Bilaterality is common.
- Pain is not usually the presenting symptom.

ETIOLOGY AND PATHOPHYSIOLOGY
The disease is thought to be multifactorial. The risk factors listed here may all contribute to the development of the disease.
- Valgus deviation of the hallux promotes varus position of metatarsal
- Medial MTP joint capsule stretches and attenuates while the lateral capsule contracts.
- Metatarsal head moves medially, causing the sesamoid bones to lay lateral to it.
- Extensor hallucis longus deviates laterally.
- Lateral and plantar migration of abductor hallucis causes the toe to plantar flex and pronate laterally.
- Medial collateral ligament strains and eventually ruptures due to this deviation, decreasing stability and causing progressive subluxation of the 1st MTP joint.

RISK FACTORS
- Familial predisposition
- Abnormal mechanics (i.e., flexible flat feet)
- Joint laxity
- Pronation of hindfoot
- Achilles tendon contracture
- Pes planus (fallen arches)
- Metatarsus primus varus
- Amputation of 2nd toe
- Inflammatory joint disease
- Neuromuscular disorders
- Improper footwear, narrow toe box

GENERAL PREVENTION
Although the condition is known to be familial, proper foot wear has shown to decrease the progression of the disease.

COMMONLY ASSOCIATED CONDITIONS
- Medial bursitis of the 1st MTP joint (most common)
- Hammertoe deformity of the 2nd phalanx
- Plantar callus
- Central metatarsalgia
- Metatarsalgia of MTP joint
- Degeneration of 1st metatarsal head cartilage
- Pronated feet
- Ankle equinus
- Ingrown toenail
- Entrapment of the medial dorsal cutaneous nerve
- Synovitis of the MTP joint

DIAGNOSIS
- Clinical exam
- Radiographs are used for staging

HISTORY
- Painful MTP joint (mostly in adults)
- Abnormal turning of great toe
- Enlargement of the MTP joint medially
- Shoes don't fit appropriately

PHYSICAL EXAM
- Increased distal metatarsal articular angle (DMAA)
- Medial prominence at the MTP joint
- Inflammation and ulceration at the MTP joint medially
- Painful callus in the surrounding area due to over compensation as a result of the valgus deformity
- Great toe over- or underriding the 2nd toe
- Impaired gait due to pain
- Physician should examine the entire first ray for:
  – 1st MTP range of motion
  – 1st tarsometatarsal mobility
  – Neurovascular assessment of the foot
  – Degenerative osteoarthritis
  – Evaluate associated deformities as described in Risk Factors

DIFFERENTIAL DIAGNOSIS
- Trauma:
  – Turf toe
  – Sesamoiditis
  – Stress fracture
- Infection:
  – Osteomyelitis
  – Septic arthritis
- Joint disorder:
  – Osteoarthritis
  – Rheumatoid arthritis
  – Pseudogout
  – Gout
- Tendon disorder:
  – Tendinosis
  – Tenosynovitis
  – Tendon rupture
- Other:
  – Bursitis
  – Ganglia
  – Foreign-body granuloma

DIAGNOSTIC TESTS & INTERPRETATION
- Weight-bearing AP and lateral radiographs with sesamoid view optional:
  – Look for joint congruency and degenerative changes.
  – Displacement of the sesamoid bones laterally
- Radiographic parameters:
  – Hallux valgus angle: Long axis of the 1st MT and proximal phalanx is normally <15 degrees
  – Intermetatarsal angle: Between long axis of 1st and 2nd MT is normally <9 degrees
  – DMAA: Between 1st MT long axis and line through base of distal articular cap is normally <15 degrees
  – Hallux valgus interphalangeus: Between long axis of distal phalanx and proximal phalanx is normally <10 degrees

TREATMENT
- Primary indication for treatment is pain.
- There are both conservative and surgical approaches for treatment.
- Studies show that surgical treatment is more effective in improving patient concerns for pain; however, surgery also has its risk.

GENERAL MEASURES
Several nonoperative treatment options can improve symptoms and delay the degree of hallux valgus deformity:
- Proper fitting footwear: Low-heeled, wide-toe shoes to decrease stress on MTP joint (i.e., wide toe box)
- Orthoses: Shoe inserts correct alignment of the feet such as pes planus and overpronation. Improving gait may prevent bunion formation, as well diminish pressure on the MTP.
- Night splinting: There are limited randomized controlled trials studying the use of splints. In theory, they function to stabilize and balance soft tissue structures around the MTP. The minimal evidence that does exist shows improvement in degree of angulation in mild hallux valgus.
- Manual and manipulative therapy (MMT): Stretches contracted soft tissue
- Foot exercises and stretching: To improve intrinsic foot muscle strength and increase range of motion
- Pads/spacers: To decrease friction on the MTP joint. Placement of a toe spacer in the 1st interdigital space can straighten the hallux and friction between 1st and 2nd metatarsal.

MEDICATION
- Topical and PO medications such as NSAIDs can be used to relieve pain and swelling. Other topical options include capsaicin cream.
- Corticosteroid injections have also been proven to improve the pain associated with bunions.

ADDITIONAL THERAPIES

- Evidence suggests that custom-made orthoses are a safe intervention that may slightly decrease pain at 6 and 12 months (but no continued decrease in pain after 12 months) compared with no treatment; however, this improvement is less than that seen with surgical interventions (see below).

SURGERY/OTHER PROCEDURES

- Surgery is indicated if patient has severe pain, dysfunction, or symptoms that do not abate with conservative therapy.
- Surgery is shown to be more beneficial than conservative therapy, and patient should be referred to a foot and ankle surgeon:
  – >150 different surgical techniques to treat hallux valgus; however, none has been proven to be superior, and no universally accepted standard exists for selecting 1 procedure over another.
  – Choice of surgical technique will depend on the severity of disease, the HA and IM angles, congruency and subluxation of the MTP joint, patient-specific factors, and the pathologic element the surgeon determines needs correcting. Examples include:
    ○ Arthrodesis: Fusion of the 1st MTP joint; reserved for severe and/or recurrent hallux valgus
    ○ Arthroplasty: Removing the joint or replacing it with a prosthesis
    ○ Exostectomy/Bunionectomy: Removing the medial bony prominence of the MTP joint
    ○ Soft tissue realignment: Alters the function of surrounding ligaments and tendons; used for minor, flexible deformities
    ○ Osteotomy and realignment: Can correct large deformities, but evidence of long-term outcome is lacking
    ○ Mini-tight rope procedure: Use of a Fiberwire to correct the misalignment of the deformity. Reportedly allows for faster recover and earlier weight bearing.
- These options decrease pain and increase foot alignment in patients. However, ~25–30% have moderate to no improvement of symptoms despite interventions.

COMPLEMENTARY AND ALTERNATIVE MEDICINE

Marigold ointment may reduce pain and soft tissue swelling over an 8-week period (2)[C].

ONGOING CARE

FOLLOW-UP RECOMMENDATIONS

- Activity after surgery is indicated to decrease joint stiffness.
- Postoperative treatment may include physical therapy, physiotherapy, use of supportive shoe, continuous passive motion, or manual manipulation.
- Time until full weightbearing will depend on surgical procedure undergone. Recommend following the instructions of the surgeon.

PROGNOSIS

Patient outcome varies depending on individual factors, severity, and treatment modality used. The radiologic HA angle is a predictor of surgical correction; patients with an HA angle <37° have a higher chance of having the deformity corrected with surgery compared with patients with an HA angle >37° (3)[B].

COMPLICATIONS

- There is always risk associated with surgery, such as of infection, lack of improvement in pain, and poor cosmetic result.
- In addition, each surgical option listed has risk associated with it.
- Additional complications may include:
  – Early swelling
  – Hallux varus
  – Recurrence of bunion
  – Decreased sensation over the 1st metatarsal or phalanx

REFERENCES

1. Nix S. Prevalence of hallux valgus in the general population: A systemic review and meta-analysis. *J Foot Ankle Res.* 2010;3:21.
2. Khan MT. The podiatric treatment of hallux abductor valgus and its associated condition, bunion, with Tagetes patula. *J Pharm Pharmacol.* 1996;48:768–770.
3. Deenik AR, de Visser E, Louwerens JW, et al. Hallux valgus angle as main predictor for correction of hallux valgus. *BMC Musculoskelet Disord.* 2008; 9:70.

ADDITIONAL READING

- Choi JH, Zide JR, Coleman SC, et al. Prospective study of treatment of adult primary hallux valgus with scarf osteotomy and soft tissue realignment. *Foot Ankle Int.* 2013;684–690.
- Glasoe WM, Nuckley DJ, Ludewig PM, et al. Hallux valgus and the first metatarsal arch segment: A theoretical biomechanical perspective. *Phys Ther.* 2010;90:110–120.
- Holmes GB, Hsu AR. Correction of intermetatarsal angle in hallux valgus using small suture button device. *Foot Ankle Int.* 2013;543–549.
- Mafulli NI, Longo UM, Marinozzi AN, et al. Hallux Valgus: Effectiveness and safety of minimally invasive surgery. A systematic review. *Brit Med Bull.* 2010;1–19.
- Mann RA, Juvenile hallux valgus: Etiology and treatment. *Foot Ankle Int.* 1995;11:682–697.
- Schuh R, Hofstaetter SG, Adams SB, et al. Rehabilitation after hallux valgus surgery: Importance of physical therapy to restore weight bearing of the first day during the stance phase. *Phys Ther.* 2009;89:934–945.
- Smith SE, Landorf KB, Butterworth PA, et al. Scarf versus chevron osteotomy for the correction of 1–2 intermetatarsal angle in hallux valgus: A systematic review and meta-analysis. *J Foot Ankle Surg.* 2012;51(4):437–444. Epub 2012 Apr 8.

 CODES

ICD10

- M20.10 Hallux valgus (acquired), unspecified foot
- M20.11 Hallux valgus (acquired), right foot
- M20.12 Hallux valgus (acquired), left foot

CLINICAL PEARLS

- Pediatric bunions are commonly not painful.
- Patients should avoid any footwear with high heels, pointed toe boxes, or inadequate space for the toes to reduce the risk of bunions.
- No particular surgical method has shown to be superior in long-term pain relief.
- ~25–30% of patients have moderate to no improvement of symptoms despite surgical interventions.

BURNS

James R. Yon, MD • James E. Kruse, MD

BASICS

DESCRIPTION
- Tissue injuries caused by application of heat, chemicals, electricity, or irradiation
- Extent of injury (depth of burn) is result of intensity and duration of exposure:
  - 1st-degree involves superficial layers of epidermis
  - 2nd-degree involves varying amounts of epidermis (with blister formation) and part of the dermis
  - 3rd-degree involves destruction of all skin elements (full thickness) with coagulation of subdermal plexus
- System(s) affected: Endocrine/Metabolic; Pulmonary; Skin/Exocrine

Geriatric Considerations
- Prognosis is poorer for severe burns
- Patients >60 years of age account for 11% of burns

Pediatric Considerations
Consider child abuse or neglect when dealing with hot-water burns in children; abuse accounts for 15% of pediatric burns. Special concerns are sharply demarcated wounds, immersion injuries, suspect stories. Involve child welfare services early.

EPIDEMIOLOGY
- Predominant age: 30 years; 13% infants; 11% >60 years of age
- Predominant gender: Males account for 70%

Incidence
Per year in the US:
- 1.2–2 million burns; 700,000 emergency room visits; 45,000–50,000 hospitalizations; 3,900 deaths owing to burn-related complications
- In children: 250,000 burns; 15,000 hospitalizations; 1,100 deaths
- Estimated total cost of $2 billion annually for burn care
- House fires cause 75% of deaths
- Burn deaths decreasing nationally due to improved prevention and treatment

ETIOLOGY AND PATHOPHYSIOLOGY
- Open flame and hot liquid are the most common causes of burns (heat usually ≥45°C): Flame burns more common in adults; scald burns more common in children.
- Caustic chemicals or acids (may show little signs or symptoms for the 1st few days)
- Electricity (may have significant injury with very little damage to overlying skin)
- Excess sun exposure

RISK FACTORS
- Water heaters set too high
- Workplace exposure to chemicals, electricity, or irradiation
- Young children and older adults with thin skin are more susceptible to injury
- Carelessness with burning cigarettes: Related to 18% of fatal fires in 2006
- Inadequate or faulty electrical wiring
- Lack of smoke detectors: Lacking or nonfunctioning smoke alarms are implicated in 63% of residential fires.
- Arson: Cause of 27% of fires that resulted in fatalities in 2006

GENERAL PREVENTION
Home safety education should be a key mechanism for injury prevention:
- Families educated on home safety were more likely to have safe hot water temperatures.
- Safety education results in more families having functioning smoke alarms and increased use of fireguards.
- There is no evidence that home safety education results in increasing the chance of possessing a fire extinguisher.
- Home safety education did not improve the odds of keeping hot drinks or food out of reach of children and did not increase the safe storage of matches.
- There is a lack of evidence that home safety education (with or without the provision of safety equipment) results in a reduction of thermal injuries.

COMMONLY ASSOCIATED CONDITIONS
Smoke inhalation syndrome:
- May involve thermal burn to respiratory mucosa (e.g., trachea, bronchi), as well as carbon monoxide inhalation
- Occurs within 72 hours of burn
- Should be suspected in all burns occurring in an enclosed space or exposure to explosions

DIAGNOSIS

HISTORY
- History of source of burn
- In children or elderly: Check for consistency between the history and the burn's physical characteristics

PHYSICAL EXAM
- 1st-degree:
  - Erythema of involved tissue
  - Skin blanches with pressure
  - Skin may be tender
- 2nd-degree:
  - Skin is red and blistered
  - Skin is very tender
- 3rd-degree:
  - Burned skin is tough and leathery
  - Skin non-tender
- Rule of 9s (1)[C]:
  - Each upper extremity: Adult and child 9%
  - Each lower extremity: Adult 18%; child 14%
  - Anterior trunk: Adult and child 18%
  - Posterior trunk: Adult and child 18%
  - Head and neck: Adult 10%; child 18%
- Quick estimate: The surface area of the patient's hand (palmar surface plus fingers) is ~1% of the BSA.
- Carefully document of extent of burn and the estimated depth of burn.
- Check for any signs suggestive of potential airway involvement: Singed nasal hair, facial burns, carbonaceous sputum, progressive hoarseness, inflamed oropharynx, circumferential burns around the neck, tachypnea.

DIAGNOSTIC TESTS & INTERPRETATION
- Children: Glucose (hypoglycemia may occur in children because of limited glycogen storage)
- Smoke inhalation: ABG, carboxyhemoglobin
- Electrical burns: ECG, urine myoglobin, creatine kinase isoenzymes

Initial Tests (lab, imaging)
- Hematocrit
- Type and cross
- Electrolytes, including BUN and creatinine
- Urinalysis
- Chest radiograph
- Xenon scan useful in suspected smoke inhalation

Diagnostic Procedures/Other
Bronchoscopy may be necessary in smoke inhalation to evaluate lower respiratory tract.

TREATMENT

- Prehospital care (1)[C]:
  - Remove the patient from the source of burn.
  - Extinguish and remove all burning clothing.
  - Room-temperature water may be poured onto burn, but only in the first 15 minutes following burn exposure.
  - Wrap patient to prevent hypothermia.
  - All patients to receive 100% O_2 via face mask
- Hospitalization for all serious burns:
  - 2nd-degree burns >10% of body surface area (BSA)
  - Any 3rd-degree burn
  - Burns of hands, feet, face, or perineum
  - Electrical or lightning burns
  - Inhalation injury
  - Chemical burns
  - Circumferential burn
- Transfer to burn center for (2)[C]:
  - 2nd and 3rd-degree burns >10% of BSA in patients <10 years and >50 years of age
  - 2nd-degree burns >20% of BSA and full-thickness burns >5% BSA in any age range
  - 3rd-degree burns in any age group
  - Burns of hands, feet, face, or perineum
  - Electrical or lightning burns
  - Inhalation injury
  - Chemical burns
  - Circumferential burn
  - Burns in patients with additional trauma (fractures, etc.) in which the burn is the more severe injury. Otherwise, send to trauma center for stabilization.
  - Burn injuries in patients with preexisting medical conditions that could affect management, mortality, or recovery

GENERAL MEASURES
- Based on depth of burns and accurate estimate of total BSA involved (rule of 9s)
- Tetanus prophylaxis (if not current)
- Remove all rings, watches, and other items from injured extremities to avoid tourniquet effect.
- Remove clothing and cover all burned areas with dry sheets.
- Flush area of chemical burn (for ~2 hours).
- For all major burns, use 100% oxygen administration; consider early intubation.
- Do not apply ice to burn site.
- Nasogastric tube (high risk of paralytic ileus)
- Foley catheter
- Analgesia
- ECG monitoring in first 24 hours following electrical burn

- Whirlpool hydrotherapy followed by silver sulfadiazine (Silvadene) occlusive dressings in severe burns
- Daily or b.i.d. cleansing with dressing changes
- Burn fluid resuscitation (1)[C]:
  - Calculate fluid resuscitation from time of burn, not from time treatment begins.
  - 2–4 mL lactated Ringer's × body weight (kg) × % BSA burn (1/2 given in first 8 hours, in second 8 hours, and in third 8 hours); in children, this is given in addition to maintenance fluids and is adjusted according to urine output and vital signs. Protocol-based resuscitation leads to superior outcomes.
  - Colloid solutions are not recommended during the first 12–24 hours of resuscitation (1)[C], (3)[A].
- Other: Use of biologic membranes or skin substitutes may be indicated for burn coverage
- Inhalation injury:
  - Intubation, ventilation with positive end-expiratory pressure assistance
  - Hyperbaric oxygen treatment may be useful in patients with carbon monoxide levels >25%, patients with coma, focal neurologic deficit, ischemic ECG changes, and pregnant patients (1)[C].

MEDICATION
First Line
- IV meperidine (Demerol), morphine, or hydromorphone (Dilaudid) for severe pain
- PO analgesics, such as acetaminophen (Tylenol) with codeine, acetaminophen with oxycodone (Percocet), or acetaminophen with hydrocodone (Lortab) for moderate pain
- Silver sulfadiazine (Silvadene): Apply topically to burn site (can cause leukopenia). Do not use in sulfa-allergic patients.
- Neosporin or bacitracin ointment: Apply to facial burns.
- Mupirocin: Has potent inhibitory activity against methicillin-resistant *Staphylococcus aureus* (MRSA) (4)[B].
- Acticote A.B: A dressing consisting of 2 sheets of high-density polyethylene mesh coated with nanocrystalline silver; has a more controlled, prolonged release of silver, allowing less frequent dressing changes (4)[B].
- Electrical burn with myoglobinuria will require alkalinization of urine and mannitol.
- Consider H_2 blockers or proton-pump inhibitors (e.g., cimetidine, ranitidine, famotidine, lansoprazole, or nizatidine) for stress ulcer prophylaxis in severely burned patients.
- Tetanus toxoid/tetanus immunoglobulin
- There is no clear indication for prophylactic systemic antibiotics (4)[B].
- Use of VAC system may result in a low-protease environment with higher levels of angiogenic factor (vascular endothelial growth factor [VEGF]) during wound healing, leading to more chaotic, hyperkeratinized, thickened epidermis when compared with a standard hydrocolloid dressing (5)[C].

Second Line
- Mafenide (Sulfamylon) for full-thickness burn, best against *Pseudomonas* (*Caution:* Metabolic acidosis, painful)

- Silver nitrate 0.5% (messy, leaches electrolytes from burn, causes water toxicity)
- Povidone–iodine (Betadine) may result in iodine absorption from burn and "tan eschar," makes debridement more difficult.
- Travase (enzymatic debridement)

SURGERY/OTHER PROCEDURES
- Escharotomy may be necessary in constricting circumferential burns of extremities or chest, due to compartment syndrome.
- Tangential excision with split-thickness skin grafts
- Early excision of burns results in a significant reduction in mortality (excluding patients with inhalational injury) and a significant decrease in hospital length of stay (6)[B].

 ## ONGOING CARE

FOLLOW-UP RECOMMENDATIONS
Early mobilization is the goal

DIET
- High-protein, high-calorie diet when bowel function resumes
- Nasogastric tube feedings may be required in early postburn period.
- Total parenteral nutrition if NPO expected for >5 days
- Early initiation of enteral nutrition in first 24 hours of admission results in shorter ICU stay and lower wound infection rates.

PATIENT EDUCATION
- Use of sunscreen: Skin grafts or newly epithelialized skin is highly sensitive to sun exposure and thermal extremes.
- Prevent access to electrical cords/outlets.
- Isolate household chemicals.
- Use low-temperature setting for water heater (below 54°C).
- Household smoke detectors with special emphasis on maintenance
- Family/Household evacuation plan
- Proper storage and use of flammable substances
- Burn management: www.aafp.org/afp/20001101/2029ph.html
- Burn prevention: www.aafp.org/afp/20001101/2032ph.html

PROGNOSIS
- 1st-degree burn: Complete resolution
- 2nd-degree burn: Epithelialization in 10–14 days (deep 2nd-degree burns probably will require skin graft)
- 3rd-degree burn: No potential for re-epithelialization; skin graft required
- Length of hospital stay and need for ICU care depend on extent of burn, smoke inhalation, and age.
- A 50% survival rate can be expected with a 62% burn in patients aged 0–14 years, 63% burn in patients aged 15–40 years, 38% burn in patients aged 40–65 years, and 25% burn in patients >65 years of age (1)[C].
- 90% of survivors can be expected to return to an occupation comparable to their preburn employment.

COMPLICATIONS
- Gastroduodenal ulceration (Curling's ulcer)
- Marjolin's ulcer: Malignant squamous cell carcinoma developing in old burn site
- Signs of infection: Discoloration, green fat, edema, eschar separation, and conversion of 2nd- into 3rd-degree wound
- *Wound biopsy best way to diagnose.
- Burn wound sepsis: Most commonly *S. aureus* (including MRSA), vancomycin-resistant enterococci, and gram-negative organisms (4)[B]
- Pneumonia
- Decreased mobility with possibility of future flexion contractures
- Hypertrophic scarring common with burns

REFERENCES
1. Teague H, Sweneki SA, Tang A. The burned patient: Assessment, diagnosis, and management in the ED. *Trauma Reports.* 2005;6:1–12.
2. Bezuhly M, Fish JS. Acute Burn Care (Review). *Plast Reconstr Surg.* 2012;130:349E–358E.
3. Roberts I, Alderson P, Bunn F. Colloids versus crystalloids for fluid resuscitation in critically ill patients (Review). *Cochrane Database Syst Rev.* 2007;4:CD000567.
4. Church D, Elsayed S, Reid O, et al. Burn wound infections. *Clin Microbiol Rev.* 2006;19:403–434.
5. Caulfield RH, Tyler MP, Austyn JM. The relationship between protease/anti-protease profile, angiogenesis and re-epithelialisation in acute burn wounds. *Burns.* 2008;34:474–486.
6. Ong YS, Samuel M, Song C. Meta-analysis of early excision of burns. *Burns.* 2006;32:145–150.

ADDITIONAL READING
- Endorf FW, Ahrenholz D. Burn management (review). *Curr Opin Crit Care.* 2011;17:601–605.
- Fernandes de Carvalho V, Paggiaro AO, Isaac C, et al. Clinical trial comparing 3 different wound dressings for the management of partial-thickness skin graft donor sites. *J Wound Ostomy Continence Nurs.* 2011;38(6):643–647.

 ## CODES

ICD10
- T30.0 Burn of unspecified body region, unspecified degree
- T30.4 Corrosion of unspecified body region, unspecified degree

CLINICAL PEARLS
- 1st-degree: Erythema of involved tissue, Skin blanches with pressure. Skin may be tender.
- 2nd-degree: Skin is red and blistered. Skin is very tender.
- 3rd-degree: Burned skin is tough and leathery. Skin is not tender.

BURSITIS
Kylee Eagles, DO • J. Herbert Stevenson, MD

BASICS

DESCRIPTION
- A *bursa* is a sac that is formed or found in areas subject to friction, such as locations where tendons pass over bony landmarks.
- Most common sites are:
  - Subdeltoid/Subacromial
  - Olecranon
  - Prepatellar
  - Trochanteric
  - Radiohumeral
- Bursae essentially lubricate the region with synovial fluid.
- Large bursae usually communicate with joints and are responsible for retaining synovial fluid in place.
- Bursae are fluid-filled sacs that serve as a cushion between tendons and bones.
- E.G. Bywaters, an English rheumatologist, found at least 78 bursae symmetrically placed on each side of the body.
- System(s) affected: Musculoskeletal

Pediatric Considerations
Bursitis is less common in the pediatric population.

EPIDEMIOLOGY
Predominant age:
- 15–50 years (most common in skeletally mature)
- Traumatic bursitis more likely in patients <35 years of age

Incidence
- Common
- Trochanteric pain: 1.8/1,000 per year (1)

ETIOLOGY AND PATHOPHYSIOLOGY
- Bursitis may be acute or chronic.
- Many types of bursitis, including infectious, traumatic, and inflammatory
- Less often rheumatoid disease or tuberculosis, as well as gout and pseudogout

RISK FACTORS
- Individuals who engage in repetitive and vigorous training or others who suddenly increase their level of activity (e.g., "weekend warriors")
- Leg length discrepancy and a Trendelenburg gait increase risk for trochanteric bursitis.

GENERAL PREVENTION
- Appropriate warm-up and cool-down maneuvers, avoidance of overuse, or inadequate rest between workouts
- Range-of-motion (ROM) exercises
- Maintain high level of fitness and general good health.

COMMONLY ASSOCIATED CONDITIONS
- Tendinitis
- Sprains, strains
- Associated stress fractures
- Tight or deconditioned muscles

DIAGNOSIS

HISTORY
- Pain in the affected region, usually gradual in onset but can be rapid if due to trauma
- Decreased ROM in affected region
- Ask about physical activity at work and for pleasure.
- Have they injured the joint before?
- Subacromial bursitis: Recent repetitive activities involving the shoulder, pain with overhead activity
- Trochanteric bursitis: Recent ramp-up of running or other lower extremity exercise, associated knee pain, painful running, biking
- Prepatellar bursitis: Fall on patella, prolonged kneeling
- Olecranon bursitis: Leaning on elbows, trauma, decreased ROM at the elbow
- Radiohumeral bursitis: Repetitive forearm pronation (medial epicondylitis/golfer's elbow) or supination (lateral epicondylitis/tennis elbow), pain with opening jars, wringing out hair, opening doors

PHYSICAL EXAM
- Pain/Tenderness
- Decreased ROM of affected region (rare except at shoulder)
- Erythema if infection present
- Swelling
- Crepitus sometimes found
- Trochanteric bursitis is often seen in conjunction with tight ITB (i.e., positive Ober test and pain along ITB)
- Radiohumeral bursitis will often have forearm pain.
- Prepatellar bursitis does not usually cause decreased ROM in the knee.

DIFFERENTIAL DIAGNOSIS
- Septic arthritis
- Gout, pseudogout
- Rheumatic disorders
- Osteoarthritis
- Tendinitis, strains, and sprains
- Lyme arthritis

DIAGNOSTIC TESTS & INTERPRETATION
Consider ECG (if left shoulder pain mimics cardiac pain).

Initial Tests (lab, imaging)
Drugs that may alter lab results:
- ESR may be increased with coexistent use of methyldopa, methysergide, penicillamine, theophylline, vitamin A.
- ESR may be decreased with coexistent use of quinine, salicylates, and drugs that cause a high glucose level.
- The following may help in differentiating soft-tissue disease from rheumatic and connective tissue disease but are not usually necessary for routine evaluation:
  - CBC
  - ESR
  - Serum protein electrophoresis
  - Rheumatoid factor
  - Serum uric acid
  - Phosphorus
  - Alkaline phosphatase
  - Blood testing for syphilis
  - Joint fluid analysis and culture (when indicated)
  - Send joint fluid for: Gram stain, culture, cell count, crystal analysis
- Calcific deposits may be seen on plain radiograph.
- MRI may prove beneficial if diagnosis is unclear.
- US (2)[B]

Diagnostic Procedures/Other
- Aspiration of swollen bursa and evaluation of synovial fluid; the clinician must differentiate infected from inflammatory bursitis:
  - Fluid white blood cell (WBC) 2,000–5,000/μL imply inflammatory, whereas >5,000 imply infectious cause
  - Fluid analysis, Gram stain, culture, and crystal analysis are required to make the diagnosis.
- If the Gram stain and culture yield an infective cause, treat with appropriate antibiotics. If the etiology is inflammatory, give local care.

Test Interpretation
- Acute with early inflammation: Bursa is distended with watery or mucoid fluid.
- Infection: Purulent fluid on aspiration
- Chronic:
  - Bursal wall is thickened, and inner surface is shaggy and trabeculated.
  - The space is filled with granular, brown, inspissated blood admixed with gritty, calcific precipitations.
  - Upper extremity tendinitis and bursitis are usually the result of repetitive microtrauma, probably resulting in disruption of fibers, leading to pain, spasm, and disability.

TREATMENT

Outpatient; refer only difficult cases

GENERAL MEASURES
- Conservative therapy consists of rest, ice, and local care; elevation, gentle compression (often referred to as RICE therapy [rest-ice-compression-elevation]).
- Compression with Ace wrap or neoprene sleeve
- Bursa aspiration
- Corticosteroid injection if infectious etiology ruled out
- Treat any underlying infection.
- Treat underlying causes such as overtraining, poor body mechanics, repetitive trauma, or tight or deconditioned muscles.
- For prepatellar bursitis resulting from trauma, have patient wear knee pads during any prolonged kneeling.

MEDICATION
First Line
- NSAIDs or aspirin (3)[C]
- Antibiotic therapy if infection present; cover for staph and strep species (most common)

Second Line
- Injectable corticosteroids once infectious etiology ruled out (1)[C],(3)[C],(4)[B]
- Systemic steroids provide limited short-term benefit (5)[B].
- A recent study showed local corticosteroid injection may be used in the management of prepatellar and olecranon bursitis; however, steroid injection into the retrocalcaneal bursa may adversely affect the biomechanical properties of the Achilles tendon (6)[C].
- US guidance for bursa injections may increase effectiveness of therapy

ADDITIONAL THERAPIES
For trochanteric bursitis, low-energy shock-wave therapy (SWT) may be superior to other nonoperative modalities (7)[A].

SURGERY/OTHER PROCEDURES
- Surgical excision in severe cases unresponsive to conservative treatments
- Outpatient arthroscopic bursectomy under local anaesthesia is an effective procedure for the treatment of posttraumatic prepatellar bursitis after failed conservative treatments.

 ONGOING CARE

FOLLOW-UP RECOMMENDATIONS
Rest and elevation of affected extremity

Patient Monitoring
- Discontinue NSAIDs as soon as possible to avoid side effects.
- Some patients may require repeated injections (usually no more than 3) of a corticosteroid and lidocaine (1,3)[C].

DIET
Consider dietary changes if bursitis is directly related to obesity/crystalline deposition.

PROGNOSIS
- Most bouts of bursitis heal without sequelae.
- Repetitive acute bouts may lead to chronic bursitis, necessitating repeated joint/bursal aspirations or, eventually, surgical excision of involved bursa.
- Although multiple aspirations may not be curative, they can provide significant symptom relief while awaiting a more definitive treatment (i.e., surgery).

COMPLICATIONS
- Septic bursitis may extend to the nearby joint.
- Acute bursitis may progress to chronic.
- Severe long-range limitation of motion

REFERENCES

1. Williams BS, Cohen SP. Greater trochanteric pain syndrome: A review of anatomy, diagnosis and treatment. *Anesth Analg.* 2009;108(5):1662–1670.
2. Finlay K, Friedman L. Ultrasonography of the lower extremity. *Orthop Clin North Am.* 2006;37:245–275, v.
3. Talia AH, Cardone D. Diagnostic and therapeutic injection of the shoulder region. *Am Fam Phys.* 2003;67(6):1271–1278.
4. Gasparre G, Fusaro I, Galletti S, et al. Effectiveness of ultrasound-guided injections combined with shoulder exercises in the treatment of subacromial adhesive bursitis. *Musculoskelet Surg.* 2012;96(Suppl 1):S57–S61. Epub 2012 Apr 18.
5. Buchbinder R, Hoving JL, Green S, et al. Short course prednisolone for adhesive capsulitis (frozen shoulder or stiff painful shoulder): A randomised, double blind, placebo controlled trial. *Ann Rheum Dis.* 2004;63:1460–1469.
6. Aaron DL, Patel A, Kayiaros S, et al. Four common types of bursitis: Diagnosis and management. *J Am Acad Orthop Surg.* 2011;19:359–367.
7. Lustenberger DP, Ng VY, Best TM, et al. Efficacy of treatment of trochanteric bursitis: A systematic review. *Clin J Sport Med.* 2011;21(5):447–453.

ADDITIONAL READING

- Cardone D, Tallia AH. Diagnostic and therapeutic injection of the hip and knee. *Am Fam Phys.* 2003;67(10):2147–2153.
- Hsieh LF, Hsu WC, Lin YJ, Shih-Huiwu, Chang KC, Chang HL. Is Ultrasound-guided injection more effective in chronic subacromial bursitis? *Med Sci Sports Exerc.* 2013 May 21. Epub 2013 May 21.
- McFarland EG, Gill HS, Laporte DM, et al. Miscellaneous conditions about the elbow in athletes. *Clin Sports Med.* 2004;23(4):743–763, xi–xii.
- Wiegerinck JI, Kok AC, van Dijk CN. Surgical treatment of chronic retrocalcaneal bursitis. *Arthroscopy.* 2012;28(2):283–293. doi: 10.1016/j.arthro.2011.09.019

 SEE ALSO

- Tendinitis
- Video: Olecranon Bursitis Aspiration

 CODES

ICD10
- M70.20 Olecranon bursitis, unspecified elbow
- M71.9 Bursopathy, unspecified
- M75.50 Bursitis of unspecified shoulder

CLINICAL PEARLS
- Remember RICE acronym for conservative therapy:
  – Rest affected area.
  – Ice inflamed bursa.
  – Compress (with Ace wrap or neoprene sleeve)
  – Elevate joint.
- Treat any underlying cause of the bursitis.

BURSITIS, PES ANSERINE
Jennifer Schwartz, MD

 BASICS

DESCRIPTION

- The pes anserinus ("goosefoot") is formed by the combined insertion of the gracilis, sartorius, and semitendinosus tendons on the anteromedial tibia.
- The involved muscles help flex the knee and resist valgus stress.
- The pes bursa lies deep to the tendons and superficial to the tibial attachment of the medial collateral ligament.
- *Pes anserine syndrome* is due to bursitis and/or tendonitis in this area.

EPIDEMIOLOGY

Incidence
Common

ETIOLOGY AND PATHOPHYSIOLOGY
Pes anserine bursitis occurs secondary to:
- Overuse injury
- Excessive valgus and rotary stresses
- Direct trauma

RISK FACTORS
- Obesity
- Female
- Pes planus
- Genu valgum
- Knee joint laxity/ligamentous injury
- Long distance running, hill running
- Swimming (breaststroke)
- Cycling

COMMONLY ASSOCIATED CONDITIONS
- Osteoarthritis
  - Knee pain due to osteoarthritis often associated with pes bursitis, both of which may need treatment (1)[C].
- Valgus knee deformity
- Obesity
- Diabetes mellitus (questionable association)

 DIAGNOSIS

HISTORY
- Medial-sided knee pain is the most common complaint.
- Pain is located 4–6 cm distal to the medial joint line on the anteromedial aspect of the tibia.
- Pain exacerbated by knee flexion:
  - Going up or down stairs
  - Getting out of a chair

PHYSICAL EXAM
- Common findings:
  - Tenderness to palpation at the area of insertion:
    ○ 30% of asymptomatic patients also have tenderness to deep palpation in this area.
  - Pain worsens with flexion of the knee against resistance.
  - Possible localized swelling over the pes anserine insertion
- Findings that should prompt investigation of alternate diagnosis:
  - Joint effusion
  - Tenderness directly over the joint line
  - Locking of the knee
  - Erythema or warmth
  - Systemic signs, such as fever

DIFFERENTIAL DIAGNOSIS
- Medial collateral ligament injury
- Medial meniscal injury
- Medial plica syndrome
- Medial compartment osteoarthritis
- Semimembranosus bursitis
- Popliteal/Meniscal cyst
- Tibial stress fracture

DIAGNOSTIC TESTS & INTERPRETATION
Initial Tests (lab, imaging)
Lab work not indicated unless suspecting infection, in which case consider a:
- CBC
- ESR
- C-reactive protein (CRP)
- Aspirate fluid analysis
- Primarily a clinical diagnosis
- Imaging is not indicated unless there is concern for:
  - Bony injury/fracture
  - Ligamentous injury
  - Meniscal injury

Follow-Up Tests & Special Considerations
- Ultrasound (US):
  - Can demonstrate focal edema within the pes anserine bursa, but has poor correlation to clinical findings
  - Many patients diagnosed with pes anserine bursitis have no morphologic changes on US (2)[C].
- MRI: Can demonstrate inflammation of the bursa, delineate the pes anserine bursa from other structures, rule out other etiologies:
- T2W axial images best to see (3)[C].
  - No large studies evaluating correlation between clinical diagnosis and radiographic evidence on MRI
  - May see fluid in the pes bursa on MRI in 5% of asymptomatic patients (4)[C]

TREATMENT

Conservative therapy is the most common approach to treating pes anserine bursitis:

- Relative rest, avoiding offending activities (especially knee flexion)
- Ice
- Physical therapy
- NSAIDs
- Corticosteroid injection
- Weight loss

MEDICATION
First Line
NSAIDs, such as ibuprofen, (800 mg PO t.i.d.) or naproxen (500 mg PO b.i.d.) are considered the first-line therapy.

Second Line
- Corticosteroid injection combined with local anesthetic has been shown to provide relief in many patients (5)[C].
- US-guided injection appears to be superior to blind injection (6)[C].
- The injection is usually performed at the point of maximal tenderness:
  - The area is prepared with standard aseptic practices.
  - ~2 mL of anesthetic (i.e., 1% lidocaine) and 1 mL of steroid (i.e., 40 mg of methylprednisolone) is injected into the bursa using a small (e.g., 25-gauge 1-inch needle).
  - Care should be taken to avoid injecting directly into the tendon (7)[C].

ADDITIONAL THERAPIES
Physical therapy:
- Hamstring and Achilles stretching
- Quadriceps strengthening
- Adductor strengthening

SURGERY/OTHER PROCEDURES
- No role for surgery in routine isolated pes anserine syndrome
- Drainage or removal of bursa may be used in severe/refractory cases.

 ONGOING CARE

Home exercise program focusing on flexibility and strength

DIET
Consider dietary changes as part of a comprehensive weight-loss program if obesity is a contributing factor.

PROGNOSIS
Most cases of pes anserine syndrome respond to conservative therapy. Recurrence is common, and multiple treatments may be required.

REFERENCES

1. Esen S, Akarirmak U, Aydin F, et al. Clinical evaluation during the acute exacerbation of knee osteoarthritis: The impact of diagnostic ultrasonography. *Rheumatol Int*. 2013(33):711–117
2. Helfenstein M, Kuromoto J. Anserine syndrome. *Rev Bras Reumatol [online]*. 2010;50(3):313–327.
3. Chatra, P. Bursae around the knee joints. *Indian J Radiol Imaging*. 2012(22):27–30
4. Rennie WJ, Saifuddin A. Pes anserine bursitis: Incidence in symptomatic knees and clinical presentation. *Skeletal Radiol*. 2005;34:395–398.
5. Yoon HS, Kim SE, Suh YR, et al. Correlation between ultrasonographic findings and the response to corticosteroid injection in pes anserinus tendinobursitis syndrome in knee osteoarthritis patients. *J Korean Med Sci*. 2005;20:109–112.
6. Finnoff JT, Nutz DJ, Henning PT, et al. Accuracy of ultrasound-guided versus unguided pes anserinus bursa injections. *PMR*. 2010;2(8):732–739. Epub 2010 Jul 3.
7. Stephens MB, Beutler AI, O'Connor FG, et al. Musculoskeletal injections: A review of the evidence. *Am Fam Physician*. 2008;78:971–976.

ADDITIONAL READING

- Alvarez-Nemegyei J. Risk factors for pes anserine tendinitis/bursitis syndrome: A case control study. *J Clin Rheumatol*. 2007;13–20:63–65.
- Wittich CM, Ficalora RD, Mason TG, et al. Musculoskeletal injection. *Mayo Clin Proc*. 2009;84(9):831–836; quiz 837.

 CODES

ICD10
- M65.869 Other synovitis and tenosynovitis, unspecified lower leg
- M71.561 Other bursitis, not elsewhere classified, right knee
- M71.569 Other bursitis, not elsewhere classified, unspecified knee

CLINICAL PEARLS
- Consider pes anserine syndrome in patients presenting with medial-sided knee pain.
- Physical examination reveals tenderness over the insertion of the pes anserine tendon on the medial aspect of the tibia 4–6 cm distal to the joint line:
  - Remember that patients without pes anserine syndrome may have tenderness to palpation in this area. Correlate physical examination with history and clinical picture.
- Look for pes anserine syndrome in patients with persistent medial-sided osteoarthritis symptoms. This can be confounding the pain, and an injection may help.

CANDIDIASIS, MUCOCUTANEOUS

Hugh J. Silk, MD, MPH • Sheila O'Grady Stille, DMD, MAGD

 BASICS

DESCRIPTION
- A mucocutaneous disorder caused by infection with various *Candida* spp.
- >20 *Candida* species cause infection in humans. *Candida albicans* is the most common.
- Areas include:
  - GI:
    - Oropharyngeal candidiasis: Mouth, pharynx
    - Angular cheilitis: Fissures at mouth corners
    - Candida esophagitis: Esophagus
    - GI candidiasis: Gastritis and/or ulcers, associated with thrush; in tract or perianal
  - Non-GI:
    - Candida vulvovaginitis: Vaginal mucosa and/or cutaneous aspects of the vulva
    - Candidal balanitis: Glans penis
    - Candidal paronychia: Nail bed of a digit
    - Folliculitis: Hair follicles
    - Interdigital candidiasis: Webs of the digits
- System(s) affected: Oropharynx; GI; Skin/Exocrine; Genitourinary
- Synonym(s): Monilia; Thrush; Yeast

ALERT
Vaginal antifungal creams and suppositories can weaken condoms and diaphragms.

Pregnancy Considerations
No known fetal complications of maternal *Candida*

EPIDEMIOLOGY
- Common in the US; very common with immunodeficiency and/or uncontrolled diabetes
- Predominant age: None:
  - Infants and seniors: Thrush and cutaneous infections (infant diaper rash)
  - Women of childbearing age: Vaginitis
  - Prepubertal or postmenopausal: Yeast vaginitis uncommon
  - Predominant sex: Female > Male

Incidence
Not well studied, estimate 50/100,000 annually

Prevalence
Candida species are normal inhabitants of the oral cavity, pharynx, esophagus, and rest of the GI tract; present in >50% of US population.

ETIOLOGY AND PATHOPHYSIOLOGY
C. albicans predominant (responsible for 80–92% vulvovaginal and 70–80% oral isolates)

Genetics
Chronic mucocutaneous candidiasis is a heterogeneous, genetic syndrome with infection of the skin, nails, hair, and mucous membranes; presents in infancy or childhood, onset over age 30 is rare. Uncertain mode of inheritance

RISK FACTORS
- Immunosuppression, including HIV
- Hormonal fluctuations in women
- Antibacterial therapy, especially broad-spectrum antibiotics
- Douches, chemical irritants, and other vaginitides can predispose to yeast vaginitis.
- Denture wearers
- Birth control pills
- Hyperglycemia; diabetes

- Uncircumcised men (increased risk for Candida balanitis)

GENERAL PREVENTION
- Minimize antibiotic use.
- Minimize inhaled and systemic steroid use; rinse mouth after inhaled steroid use (1)[A].
- Avoid douching.
- Treat other vaginitides.
- Minimize moist environments (e.g., wear cotton underwear).
- Clean dentures often; use well-fitting dentures.
- Remove dentures while sleeping.
- Control diabetes (if present).
- Follow prevention guidelines during cancer treatments (2).
- Fluconazole prophylaxis against oral candidiasis in HIV-infected adults (3)[A].

COMMONLY ASSOCIATED CONDITIONS
- HIV and other leukopenias
- Diabetes mellitus
- Cancer and other immunosuppressive disorders
- Disorders requiring corticosteroids or other immunosuppressive chemotherapy

 DIAGNOSIS

HISTORY
- Infants/Children:
  - Oral: White patches in mouth and on the tongue
  - Perineal: Erythematous rash; can be painful if eroding skin layers
  - Angular cheilitis: Painful fissures in mouth corners, often cracked and bleeding
- Adults:
  - Vulvovaginal lesions; thin to thick, whitish, discharge; some have pruritus/burning
- Immunocompromised hosts:
  - Oral: White, raised, painless, distinct patches; red, slightly raised patches
  - Esophagitis: Dysphagia, odynophagia, retrosternal pain; usually with thrush
  - GI symptoms: Abdominal pain
  - Balanitis: Erythema, erosions, scaling; possible dysuria
  - Folliculitis: Follicular pustules
  - Interdigital: Redness, itchiness at base of fingers and/or toes, possible maceration

PHYSICAL EXAM
- Infants/Children:
  - Oral: White, raised, distinct patches within the mouth; can be wiped off to reveal red base
  - Perineal: Erythematous maculopapular rash with satellite pustules or papules
  - Angular cheilitis: Tender fissures in mouth corners, often cracked and bleeding
- Adults:
  - Vulvovaginal: Thick, whitish, cottage cheese-like discharge; vagina or perineum erythema
- Immunocompromised hosts:
  - Oral: White, raised, nontender, distinct patches; red, slightly raised patches; thick, dark-brownish coating; deep fissures
  - Esophagitis: Often oral thrush is visible.
  - Balanitis: Erythema, linear erosions, scaling
  - Folliculitis: Follicular pustules
  - Interdigital: Redness, excoriations at base of fingers and/or toes, often maceration

DIFFERENTIAL DIAGNOSIS
- For oral candidiasis:
  - Leukoplakia
  - Lichen planus
  - Geographic tongue
  - Herpes simplex
  - Erythema multiforme
  - Pemphigus
- Baby formula or breast milk can mimic thrush.
- Hairy leukoplakia: Does not rub off to erythematous base; usually on lateral tongue
- Angular cheilitis from vitamin B or iron deficiency, staphylococcus infection, or edentulous over closure
- *Bacterial vaginosis* and *Trichomonas vaginalis* tend to have more odor and itch, and have a different discharge, but symptoms similar to those of *C. vaginalis* include:
  - Marked vulvar irritation; labial erythema; external dysuria; vaginal tenderness

DIAGNOSTIC TESTS & INTERPRETATION
Initial Tests (lab, imaging)
- Slide preparation: Mycelia (hyphae) or pseudomycelia (pseudohyphae) yeast forms; *Candida* does not induce an increased polymorphonuclear leukocyte response.
- pH paper <4
- Barium swallow: Esophageal candidiasis may reveal a cobblestone appearance, fistulas, or esophageal dilatation (from denervation).

Diagnostic Procedures/Other
- If first-line treatment fails, perform culture for type and sensitivity, alternative infection.
- Esophagitis may require endoscopy with biopsy.
- Oral hyperplastic candidiasis should be biopsied to rule out carcinoma.
- HIV seropositivity plus thrush with dysphagia relieved by antifungal treatment are acceptable criteria for diagnosis of *Candida* esophagitis.

Test Interpretation
Biopsy: Epithelial parakeratosis with polymorphonuclear (PMN) leukocytes in superficial layers; periodic acid Schiff staining reveals presence of candidal hyphae.

 TREATMENT

GENERAL MEASURES
Screen severely immunodeficient patients routinely.

MEDICATION
First Line
- Vaginal (choose 1):
  - Miconazole (Monistat) 2% cream: 1 applicator or 100–200 mg (1 suppository), intravaginally qhs for 7 days
  - Clotrimazole (Gyne-Lotrimin, Mycelex): Intravaginal tablets (100 mg qhs for 6–7 days; 200 mg qhs for 3 days; 500 mg daily for 1 day) or 1% cream (1 applicator qhs for 6–7 days)
  - Fluconazole 150 mg PO in 1 dose
  - Nystatin (Mycostatin, Nilstat): 100,000 U/g cream (1 applicator) or 100,000-U tablets (1 tablet) intravaginally daily for 7–14 days

- Oropharyngeal:
  - Mild disease:
    - Clotrimazole (Mycelex): 10 mg troche, suck on 20 minutes 5 times a day for 7–14 days, or
    - Nystatin suspension: 100,000 U/mL given 4–6 times daily, or
    - Nystatin pastilles: 200,000 U each, administered q.i.d. daily for 7–14 days (4)[B]
    - Denture wearers:
      - Nystatin ointment: 100,000 U/g under denture and corners of mouth for 3 weeks
      - Remove dentures at night; clean twice weekly with diluted (1:20) bleach.
      - Moderate to severe disease:
    - Fluconazole: 100–200 mg (3 mg/kg) daily for 7–14 days
- Esophagitis:
  - Fluconazole: 100 mg/d for 14–21 days, load with 200 mg
  - Itraconazole (Sporanox):
    - Solution: 1–200 mg daily for 7–14 days
    - Capsules: 200 mg/d (with food) for 2–3 weeks

Pregnancy Considerations
Miconazole is usually the drug of choice.

Second Line
- Vaginal:
  - Terconazole (Terazol): Recurrent cases: 0.4% cream (1 applicator qhs for 10–14 days of induction therapy); 0.8% cream/80-mg suppositories (1 applicator or 1 suppository qhs for 3 days)
  - Prophylaxis: Fluconazole, 150 mg once per week for 6 months to prevent recurrence
    - In HIV patients: Concerns with this regimen include emergence of drug resistance (5)[A].
- Oropharyngeal:
  - Clotrimazole troches 10 mg 5 times daily
  - Nystatin oral suspension (100,000 U/mL):
    - Children: 5–10 mL q.i.d. daily for 10 days
    - Infants: 0.5 mL in each cheek q.i.d. daily for 10 days
    - Adults: Swish and swallow 5–10 mL q.i.d. daily for 14 days; prophylaxis is achieved with the same dosages 2–5 times a day.
  - Fluconazole: 100 mg/d for 7–14 days (load immunocompromised patient with 200 mg)
  - Itraconazole (Sporanox) suspension: 200 mg (20 mL) daily; swish and swallow for 7–14 days; capsules: 200 mg/d (with food) for 2–4 weeks
  - Miconazole oral gel (20 mg/mL): q.i.d., swish and swallow
  - Amphotericin B (Fungizone) oral suspension (100 mg/mL): 1 mL q.i.d. daily, swish and swallow; use between meals
  - Ketoconazole: 200–400 mg PO daily, 14–21 days
- Esophagitis:
  - Oral fluconazole at a dosage of 200–400 mg (3–6 mg/kg) daily for 14–21 days
  - Amphotericin B (variable dosing) IV dose of 0.3–0.7 mg/kg daily; an echinocandin should be used for patients who cannot tolerate oral therapy.
- Continue all treatments until 2 days after infection disappears:
  - Contraindications:
    - Ketoconazole, itraconazole, or nystatin (if swallowed): Severe hepatotoxicity
    - Amphotericin B: Renal failure
  - Precautions:
    - Miconazole: Can potentiate the effect of warfarin, but drug of choice in pregnancy

- Fluconazole: Renal excretion; rare hepatotoxicity; resistance frequent
- Itraconazole: Doubling the dosage results in ~3-fold increase in itraconazole plasma concentrations.
- Possible interactions (rarely seen with creams, lotions, or suppositories):
  - Fluconazole:
    - Rifampin: Decreased fluconazole concentrations
    - Tolbutamide: Decreased tolbutamide concentrations
    - Warfarin, phenytoin, cyclosporine: Altered metabolism; check levels
  - Itraconazole: Potent CYP 3A4 inhibitor. Carefully assess all coadministered medications.

ISSUES FOR REFERRAL
- Patients without obvious reasons for recurrent superficial candidal infections
- GI candidiasis

ADDITIONAL THERAPIES
- For infants with thrush: Boil pacifiers and bottle nipples; assess mother's breasts/nipples for candida infections as well.
- For denture-related candidiasis, disinfection of the denture (using soak solution containing benzoic acid, 0.12% chlorhexidine gluconate, or alkalize proteases), in addition to oral antifungal therapy.

COMPLEMENTARY AND ALTERNATIVE MEDICINE
Probiotics: *Lactobacillus* and *Bifidobacterium* may inhibit *Candida* spp (6).

IN-PATIENT CONSIDERATIONS
Nursing
Staff caring for elderly patients should be properly trained in oral hygiene. Protocols for brushing, proper denture care, and moistening the oral cavity can reduce incidence of candidal infections.

 ## ONGOING CARE

FOLLOW-UP RECOMMENDATIONS
Patient Monitoring
Immunocompromised persons may benefit from regular symptom evaluation.

DIET
Active-culture yogurt or other live lactobacillus may decrease colonization; indeterminate evidence.

PATIENT EDUCATION
- Advise patients at risk for recurrence about antibacterial therapy overgrowth.
- "Zole-type" medications are pregnancy Category C.

PROGNOSIS
- For immunocompetent individuals: Benign course, excellent prognosis
- For immunosuppressed persons: *Candida* may become an AIDS-defining illness, and chronicity may cause much morbidity.

COMPLICATIONS
In immunosuppressed persons, complications depend on the severity of immune status. In HIV infection, moderate immunosuppression (e.g., CD4 200–500 cells/mm^3) may be associated with chronic candidiasis. In severe immunosuppression (e.g., CD4 <100 cells/mm^3), thrush may lead to esophagitis, then systemic infection involving other organ systems.

REFERENCES
1. Yang IA, Clarke MS, Sim EH, et al. Inhaled corticosteroids for stable chronic obstructive pulmonary disease. *Cochrane Database Syst Rev.* 2012;7:CD002991. Epub 2012 Jul 11.
2. Glenny AM, Gibson F, Auld E, et al. The development of evidence-based guidelines on mouth care for children, teenagers and young adults treated for caner. *Eur J Cancer.* 2010;46(8): 1399–412. Epub 2010 Mar 11.
3. Pienaar ED, Young T, Holmes H. Interventions for the prevention and management of oropharyngeal candidiasis associated with HIV infection in adults and children. *Cochrane Database Syst Rev.* 2010;(11):CD003940. Epub 2010 Nov 10.
4. Pappas PG, Kauffman CA, Andes D, et al. Clinical practice guidelines for the management of candidiasis: 2009 update by the Infectious Diseases Society of America. *Clin Infect Dis.* 2009;48: 503–535.
5. Ray A, Ray S, George AT, et al. Interventions for prevention and treatment of vulvovaginal candidiasis in women with HIV infection. *Cochrane Database Syst Rev.* 2011;CD008739.
6. Strus M, Kucharska A, Kukla G, et al. The in vitro activity of vaginal Lactobacillus with probiotic properties against Candida. *Infect Dis Obstet Gynecol.* 2005;13:69–75.

ADDITIONAL READING
- Nyirjesy P, Sobel JD. Genital mycotic infections in patients with diabetes *Postgrad Med.* 2013;125(3): 33–46. doi: 10.3810/pgm.2013.05.2650.
- Terai H, Shimahara M. Tongue pain: Burning mouth syndrome vs Candida-associated lesion. *Oral Dis.* 2007;13:440–442.

 ## SEE ALSO

Candidiasis, Invasive; Candidiasis, Mucocutaneous; HIV Infection and AIDS

 ## CODES

ICD10
- B37.0 Candidal stomatitis
- B37.9 Candidiasis, unspecified
- B37.49 Other urogenital candidiasis

CLINICAL PEARLS
- The diagnosis of candidiasis is generally made clinically, but may include KOH. Rarely, a culture of skin scrapings or even a biopsy is needed for resistant strains or to explore the differential.
- Person-to-person transmission is rare. Rarely, *Candida* vaginitis may be sexually transmitted.
- If tongue pain continues after treatment, consider burning mouth syndrome.
- Topical antifungals rarely cause problems, but oral medications may have hepatic side effects.
- Amphotericin B can cause nephrotoxicity.

CARBON MONOXIDE POISONING

Deborah Lardner, DO, DTM&H • Jonathan Giordano, DO, BS • Michael Passafaro, DO, DTM&H, FACEP, FACOEP

BASICS

DESCRIPTION
- Carbon monoxide (CO) is an odorless, tasteless, colorless gas that can cause sudden illness and even death if inhaled; it is a leading cause of poisoning death in the US.
- CO is produced by combustion of carbon-containing compounds (wood, charcoal, oil, gas):
  - CO inhalation leads to displacement of oxygen from binding sites on hemoglobin.
  - Detrimental effects are related to tissue hypoxia from decreased oxygen content and a shift of the oxyhemoglobin dissociation curve to the left.
  - CO also binds to mitochondrial cytochrome oxidase, impairing adenosine triphosphate (ATP) production, and to myoglobin, affecting muscle function.
- System(s) affected: Cardiovascular; Pulmonary; Musculoskeletal; Nervous

Pregnancy Considerations
Tissue hypoxia includes the fetus. CO poisoning may cause significant fetal abnormalities, depending on the developmental stage. CO has a greater affinity for, and longer half-life when bound to fetal hemoglobin. Therefore, a pregnant mother potentially may be unaffected while the fetus is affected.

EPIDEMIOLOGY
Incidence
- ~50,000 emergency department visits annually (1)
- 5,000–6,000 deaths annually in the US
- Unintentional CO poisoning likely causes ~500 deaths annually.
- Unintentional poisoning is most common during winter months in cold climates, but can also occur in warm climates with use of generators, boats, etc.
- Intentional CO poisoning is ~10 times higher than unintentional poisonings.
- Likely markedly underdiagnosed because of vague symptoms.

ETIOLOGY AND PATHOPHYSIOLOGY
- CO is rapidly absorbed in lungs.
- CO has ~240 times the affinity for hemoglobin that oxygen has.
- CO binds to hemoglobin to form carboxyhemoglobin (COHb), resulting in impaired oxygen-carrying capacity, utilization, and delivery:
  - Leftward shift of the oxyhemoglobin dissociation curve occurs.
  - CO interferes with peripheral oxygen utilization by inactivating cytochrome oxidase.
- Delayed neurologic sequelae, probably due to lipid peroxidation by toxic oxygen species generated by xanthine oxidase.
- The half-life of CO while the patient is breathing room air is ~320 minutes, while breathing 100% oxygen via a tight-fitting, nonrebreathing face mask is ~74 minutes, and with 100% hyperbaric oxygen is ~30 minutes.

- CO exposure also causes inflammation through separate pathways than those that cause cardiac and neurologic sequelae (2).
- Inhaled or ingested methylene chloride (from paint remover [dichloromethane]) is metabolized to CO by the liver, causing CO toxicity in the absence of ambient CO.

RISK FACTORS
- Smoke inhalation
- Being in a closed or improperly ventilated space with a faulty furnace, stove, running engine, or any fuel-burning device
- Cigarette smoking
- Post-natural disaster power outages
- Extremes of age
- Predisposing cardiovascular disease, anemia, chronic respiratory conditions
- Exposure to exhaust (riding in the back of enclosed pickup trucks or swimming near a motor boat)
- Employment in a coal mine, as an auto mechanic, paint stripper, or in the solvent industry

GENERAL PREVENTION
- Appropriate ventilation, especially where there are fuel-burning devices
- Use of CO monitors
- Public education
- Determining the mechanism of exposure is critical in cases of accidental poisoning in order to limit future risk.
- Victims must not be discharged back to a contaminated environment.

COMMONLY ASSOCIATED CONDITIONS
- CO and cyanide poisoning can occur simultaneously following smoke inhalation (synergistic effect).
- Consider CO poisoning in a burn victim who has been in an enclosed space.

DIAGNOSIS

- Acute CO poisoning is suggested by history, physical exam, and an elevated COHb.
- Chronic CO intoxication is difficult to diagnose.
- The newest pulse CO-oximeters can screen for CO exposure using different wavelengths of light.
- Older pulse oximeters do not differentiate carboxyhemoglobin from oxyhemoglobin, causing normal pulse oximeter readings in hypoxic patients.
- A level >3% in a nonsmoker and >10% in a smoker confirms exposure, but the level does not correlate well with the clinical picture or the long-term prognosis (2)

HISTORY
- No single symptom is sensitive or specific, but may include the following:
  - Headaches
  - Dizziness
  - Nausea, vomiting, diarrhea
  - Weakness or fatigue
  - Confusion or impaired judgment
  - Chest pain
  - Shortness of breath
  - Loss of consciousness
  - Visual disturbances

PHYSICAL EXAM
- "Cherry red" appearance of the lips and skin (rare)
- Respiratory depression or tachypnea
- Cyanosis
- Visual-field defects, papilledema, or nystagmus
- CNS depression or coma, ataxia, seizure
- Tachycardia, hypotension, cardiac dysrhythmias, or even arrest

DIFFERENTIAL DIAGNOSIS
- Cyanide toxicity
- Viral syndromes
- Other causes of mental status changes:
  - Infections such as meningitis or encephalitis
  - Metabolic causes such as hypoglycemia
  - Drugs: Alcohol (ETOH) intoxication, opiates, acetylsalicylic acid (ASA) overdose
  - Trauma
  - CNS lesions

DIAGNOSTIC TESTS & INTERPRETATION
Initial Tests (lab, imaging)
- Measurement of COHb (may be low despite significant poisoning if patient has had O_2 or has been breathing room air for a time before the level is drawn)
- ABG (looking for metabolic acidosis)
  - Blood PO_2 tends to be normal as O_2 dissolved in blood is not affected by CO.
- Blood glucose
- Chemistries
- Anion gap $= ([Na^+] + [K^+]) - ([Cl^-] + [HCO_3^-])$ (HCO_3 decreased reflecting metabolic acidosis; anion gap >16)
- Pregnancy test in all women of child-bearing age
- Toxicology screen
- ECG in all patients
- Hemoglobin/Hematocrit
- Cardiac enzymes in:
  - ≥65 years
  - Patient with cardiac risk factors or anemia
  - Patients with symptoms suggestive of cardiac ischemia
- Head CT/MRI scan is helpful to rule out other causes of neurologic decompensation. May also show infarction due to hypoxia/ischemia.

Follow-Up Tests & Special Considerations

- Think of CO poisoning in younger patients with chest pain or symptoms suggestive of ischemia.
- Consider the diagnosis and inquire about exposure in afebrile patients with "flu-like" symptoms, especially in the winter when flu and CO poisoning are both more common.
- Look for clusters of patients (co-workers, family members, school children) with similar symptoms.
- Patients with intentional poisoning require psychiatric evaluation when medically stable.

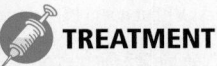 TREATMENT

GENERAL MEASURES

- Prompt removal from the CO source
- Supportive care as necessary
- Intubation and mechanical ventilation may be necessary for severe intoxication, if patient is not able to protect airway, or has significant respiratory depression.

MEDICATION

Rapid reduction in tissue hypoxia with 100% oxygen via nonrebreathing face mask (3)[A] until COHb is normal (<3%) and patient is asymptomatic

ADDITIONAL THERAPIES

- Hyperbaric oxygen has been somewhat controversial (3,4)[A]. Existing randomized trials do not establish whether the administration of hyperbaric oxygen to patients with CO poisoning reduces the incidence of adverse neurologic outcomes (4)[A].
- Hyperbaric oxygen recommended for levels >25–30%, evidence of cardiac involvement, severe acidosis, LOC, neurologic impairment, abnormal neuropsychiatric testing, age >36 (5)[C].
- Hyperbaric oxygen has been shown to be safe in pregnant woman, but there have been no prospective studies of efficacy (3)[A]. International consensus favors it as part of a more aggressive role in treating pregnant women (5)[C].
- If no improvement occurs in cardiovascular or neurologic function within 4 hours, transport the patient to the nearest facility with hyperbaric oxygen, regardless of distance.

IN-PATIENT CONSIDERATIONS

Admission Criteria/Initial Stabilization

Patients whose symptoms do not improve after 4–5 hours of 100% O2 should be transported to the nearest facility with hyperbaric oxygen. Those who demonstrate ECG or laboratory evidence of severe poisoning, who have evidence of end-organ damage, who require hyperbaric treatment, or who have another medical or social cause of concern should be hospitalized.

Discharge Criteria

Patients with mild symptoms from accidental poisoning can be managed in the ED and safely discharged.

 ONGOING CARE

FOLLOW-UP RECOMMENDATIONS

All patients treated for acute CO poisoning should be seen for clinical follow-up in 1–2 months after they are safely discharged (3).

Patient Monitoring

- Measurement of carboxyhemoglobin levels
- Arterial blood gasses

PATIENT EDUCATION

- Professional installation and maintenance of combustion devices: 1-800-638-2772; Consumer Products Safety Commission hotline
- Some states require CO detector installation in homes, especially near bedrooms and potential sources.
- Annual furnace inspections (6)[B]

PROGNOSIS

Most survivors recover completely, with only a minority developing chronic neuropsychiatric impairment.

COMPLICATIONS

- Cardiac:
  - Myocardial Infarction
  - Dysrhythmia
- Pulmonary:
  - Pulmonary edema
  - Pneumonia (aspiration)
- Neurologic:
  - Anoxic encephalopathy
  - Intellectual deterioration
  - Memory impairment
- Behavioral:
  - Irritability
  - Aggressiveness
  - Violence
  - Moodiness

Geriatric Considerations

- Higher incidence of cardiovascular and neurologic disease, increasing complications

REFERENCES

1. Hampson NB, Weaver LK. Carbon monoxide poisoning: A new incidence for an old disease. *Undersea Hyperb Med.* 2007;34:163–168.
2. Weaver LK. Carbon monoxide poisoning. *NEJM.* 2009;360:1217–1225.
3. Hampson NB, Piantadosi CA, Thom SR, et al. Practice recommendations in the diagnosis, management, and prevention of carbon monoxide poisoning. *Am J Respir Crit Care Med.* 2012; 186(11):1095–101.
4. Buckley NA, Juurlink DN, Isbister G, et al. Hyperbaric oxygen for carbon monoxide poisoning. *Cochrane Database Syst Rev.* 2011;4:CD002041. doi: 10.1002/14651858.CD002041.pub3
5. CDC. Clinical Guidance for Carbon Monoxide Poisoning After a Disaster. http://emergency.cdc.gov/disaters/co_guidance.asp.
6. Rupert DJ, Poehlman JA, Damon SA, et al. Risk and protective behaviours for residential carbon monoxide poisoning. *Inj Prev.* 2012. Epub 2012 May 31.

ADDITIONAL READING

- Internet resources available at: http://www.cpsc.gov, http://www.cdc.gov/co, and http://www.epa.gov/iaq/co.html.
- Iqbal S, Clower JH, Hernandez SA, Damon SA, Yip FY. A review of disaster-related carbon monoxide poisoning: surveillance, epidemiology, and opportunities for prevention. *Am J Public Health.* 2012;102(10):1957–1963.
- Satran D, Henry CR, Adkinson C, et al. Cardiovascular manifestations of moderate to severe carbon monoxide poisoning. *J Am Coll Cardiol.* 2005;45:1513–1516.
- World Health Organization's World Directory of Poison Centers: http://www.who.int/gho/phe/chemical_safety/poisons_centres/en/index.html.

 CODES

ICD10

- T58.94XA Toxic effect of carb monx from unsp source, undet, init
- T58.94XD Toxic effect of carb monx from unsp source, undet, subs
- T58.94XS Toxic effect of carb monx from unsp source, undet, sequela

CLINICAL PEARLS

- The most appropriate intervention in the management of a CO-poisoned patient is a prompt removal from the source of CO and institution of 100% oxygen by high-flow face mask or endotracheal tube.
- A pregnant woman may appear normal while her fetus is severely affected.
- Consider CO poisoning in younger patients with chest pain or ischemia or in patients who present in clusters.
- COHb levels do not correlate well with symptoms, severity of illness, or outcome, so manage the patient, not the level.

CARDIAC ARREST

Brent J. Levy, MD • Ryan R. Knapp, MD, MS

 BASICS

DESCRIPTION
- The absence of effective mechanical cardiac activity
- This section is not a substitute for an AHA-approved Advanced Cardiac Life Support (ACLS) course and is intended only as a quick reference.
- Synonym(s): "Code" or "Code Blue" in many institutions

Geriatric Considerations
This condition has a low rate of survival and a poor long-term outcome. Discuss Do Not Resuscitate orders with patients at risk.

Pediatric Considerations
Bradycardia is linked to hypoxia. Bradycardia is the most common initial form of cardiac arrest in children and is often the response to hypoxia. Adequate oxygenation and ventilation are critical.

Pregnancy Considerations
- Displace the uterus to the left, either manually or by placing a rolled towel under the right hip. If the patient cannot be resuscitated within 5–15 minutes, consider an emergency C-section to relieve uterine obstruction and increase blood return to the heart. This may also be done to save the fetus if the fetus has reached gestational age of viability.
- Consider amniotic fluid embolism or eclampsia-related seizures as precipitating factors.

EPIDEMIOLOGY
- Predominant age: Risk increases with age.
- Predominant sex: Male > Female

Incidence
0.5–1.5/1,000 persons per year

ETIOLOGY AND PATHOPHYSIOLOGY
- Asystole (confirm in 2 leads)
- Ventricular fibrillation (VF)
- Pulseless ventricular tachycardia (VT)
- Pulseless electrical activity (PEA)
- Consider possible reversible causes (6 Hs and 5 Ts):
  - Hypoxia, hypovolemia, hyper- and hypokalemia, [H^+] (acidosis), hypothermia, hypoglycemia
  - Cardiac tamponade, tension pneumothorax, thrombosis (pulmonary embolism, myocardial infarction [MI]), toxins (medications and overdoses), trauma

RISK FACTORS
- Male gender
- Advanced age
- Hypercholesterolemia
- HTN
- Cigarette smoking
- Family history of atherosclerosis
- Diabetes
- Cardiomyopathy
- Prolonged QT

COMMONLY ASSOCIATED CONDITIONS
- Coronary artery disease/acute coronary syndrome (ACS) (cardiac arrest may be presenting symptom)
- Valvular heart disease
- HTN
- Pulmonary embolism

DIAGNOSIS

- Loss of consciousness secondary to CNS hypoperfusion
- Absence of pulses in large arteries
- Apnea or agonal breathing
- Cyanosis or pallor

HISTORY
- Witnessed vs. unwitnessed
- Approximate downtime
- Initial resuscitation efforts and response
- History or risk factors
- Associated trauma
- Do Not Resuscitate (DNR)/Do Not Intubate (DNI) status

PHYSICAL EXAM
- Check for pulses.
- Check lungs (i.e., did patient have respiratory decline prior to cardiac decline?).
- Check for signs suggesting possible reversible causes:
  - Check for dialysis shunt: Patients on dialysis are at increased risk for an electrolyte imbalance that can cause arrest (especially hyperkalemia).
  - Check pupils: May indicate drug overdose (cannot interpret if patient has received atropine).
  - Check for obvious signs of trauma.

DIAGNOSTIC TESTS & INTERPRETATION
Laboratory results have limited value during initial resuscitation.

Initial Tests (lab, imaging)
- Fingerstick glucose
- ABG/VBG
- Chemistry and/or electrolyte panel
- Blood type and cross, if indicated
- Cardiac enzymes (troponin, CK, CK-MB)
- CBC with platelets
- Drug levels, if indicated (toxicology screen, acetaminophen/aspirin levels, history of specific medication (e.g., digoxin, antiepileptics)
- Consider:
  - RUSH (Rapid Ultrasound in SHock) exam to evaluate "the pump, tank, and pipes" to guide resuscitation (1)[C].
  - Perform emergency echocardiogram for pericardial effusion, assessment of cardiac motion, presence of intraventricular clot.
  - Chest x-ray for endotracheal tube (ET) placement, pneumothorax
  - Once stabilized, consider a CT scan of the brain.

Diagnostic Procedures/Other
- Obtain access:
  - Peripheral IV as close to central circulation as possible (preferred)
  - Intraosseous if no venous access.
  - Consider central venous acces if unable to achieve alternative access; femoral approach preferred to minimize interruptions in CPR
  - Many medications may be administered by endotracheal tube if access is otherwise unobtainable (double dose and flush with saline).
- Airway management/intubation
- Needle decompression/chest tube for pneumothorax
- Pericardiocentesis for cardiac tamponade
- ECG

TREATMENT

- C-A-B (Circulation, Airway, Breathing). Use compressions 1st, then check airway and breathing.
- Prompt initiation of high-quality CPR, particularly chest compressions (at least 100 per minute, depth 2 inches in adults, allowing recoil after each compression), and immediate defibrillation (in witnessed VF and pulseless VT but not in PEA) are 1st priority (2)[A]:
  - In unwitnessed arrest, complete 2 minutes of CPR before attempting defibrillation (3)[A].
  - Capnography should be used to evaluate the efficacy of chest compressions (2)[A].
  - Avoid excessive ventilation (2)[A].
- Establishing IV access, intubation, and medications are 2nd priority.
- Continue CPR for 1–2 minutes following the return of a potentially perfusing rhythm before stopping for a pulse check, except for witnessed arrest with a prompt return of rhythm following defibrillation.
- Patients with a return of spontaneous circulation (ROSC) should have an ECG and be strongly considered for primary coronary intervention. If not available in your facility, then consider transfer to a hospital with this capacity. Early 12-lead ECG may not demonstrate MI, but this may develop late. Intervention should not be delayed in the appropriate setting.

GENERAL MEASURES
- Perform CPR: 100/min, allowing for chest wall recoil, with minimal interruptions (4)[B]
- Sequence should be:
  - CPR
  - Rhythm check
  - Resume CPR
  - Shock/Meds (charge defibrillator and administer drugs during CPR)
  - Continue CPR (after shocking) for 5 cycles before rechecking rhythm (repeat as needed) (4)[B]
- In VF/pulseless VT, 1 shock should be delivered, then continue sequence above (4)[B]:
  - Monophasic automatic external defibrillators (AEDs) initial and subsequent shocks at 360 J
  - Biphasic AEDs:
    - 150–200 J for biphasic truncated exponential waveform
    - 120 J for rectilinear biphasic waveform
    - If not specified on the biphasic defibrillator, use default of 200 J.
  - Subsequent shocks should be the same or higher energy.
  - Pediatric manual defibrillation energy should be initial dose of 2 J/kg for the 1st attempt, followed by 4 J/kg for the next attempt. Increase energy with subsequent attempts, but do not exceed 10 J/kg or maximum adult dose.
- Consider possible causes of VT/VF, including hypoxia, hyperkalemia, hypokalemia, preexisting acidosis, drug overdose, and hypothermia.
- Administer 100% oxygen by bag-valve-mask or ETT.
- IV and IO are the preferred methods of medication administration, followed by ET.
- Start IV lines as close to the heart as possible. Large-bore peripheral lines can deliver fluid more quickly than a triple-lumen catheter.

- Use an end-tidal CO_2 monitor to assess gas exchange, if available. Capnography is the test of choice to assess ET tube placement, as esophageal intubation will produce a very low end-tidal CO_2 and requires proper reintubation (2). The use of sodium bicarbonate will increase ET-CO_2 levels.
- Consider a termination of efforts if no reversible underlying cause is found. Consider patient's age, comorbid conditions, and length of downtime to help guide decision making.

MEDICATION
First Line
- Vascular access for medications: IV or intraosseous
- Consider medications after initiation of CPR and defibrillation attempt; medications should be administered during CPR as soon as possible following a rhythm check.
- Epinephrine: 1 mg IV q3–5min (4)[B] or vasopressin 40 U IV single dose (4)[B] (can be used once in lieu of the 1st or 2nd dose of epinephrine in VT or VF, but not in PEA):
  – Vasopressin is not recommended in children.
  – Pediatric dose of epinephrine: 0.01 mg/kg
- Magnesium sulfate: 1–2 g diluted in 10 mL D_5W IV push in suspected torsades de pointes (4)[B]:
  – Magnesium is relatively contraindicated in renal failure, but given the consequences of not correcting this rhythm, contraindication is only relative in this setting.
- Antiarrhythmics:
  – Consider if VT/VF is unresponsive to 2–3 shocks and the 1st dose of vasopressor.
  – Amiodarone is the drug preferred by the AHA. Dosing: 300 mg IV push followed by 2nd dose of 150 mg IV (4)[B]
  – Amiodarone for perfusing tachyarrhythmias: 150 mg over 10 minutes; repeat as needed followed by a maintenance infusion of 1 mg/min for the first 6 hours.
  – Lidocaine: Initial dose, 1–1.5 mg/kg IV; a repeat loading dose of 1–1.5 mg/kg can be given at 5–10-minute intervals if VT/VF persist to maximum dose of 3 mg/kg (4)[C], then followed by drip if perfusing rhythm is recovered.
- Endotracheal medications (NAVEL): Narcan, atropine, vasopressin (and Valium), epinephrine, or lidocaine. Each may be placed in 5–10 mL of normal saline or sterile water and given by ET followed by bagging. Dosage should be 2–2.5× recommended IV dose. IV or IO is preferred.

Second Line
- Dopamine: 2–10 mcg/kg/min IV for bradycardia
- Procainamide: 30 mg/min IV in refractory VF/VT (maximum dose: 17 mg/kg) is permissible. However, because the time to a useful level by infusion is so long, it is unlikely to be of benefit in cardiac arrest, but may be useful in perfusing tachycardias (4)[C].
- Calcium: May be useful in hyperkalemia, ionized hypokalemia secondary multiple transfusions, and Ca^+ channel blocker toxicity; otherwise, no clear benefit is shown.
- High-dose epinephrine: No survival benefit is seen with a high dose (0.1 mg/kg), but it should be considered in exceptional situations, such as β-blocker or calcium channel blocker overdoses.

- Bicarbonate: 1 mEq/kg IV only in known preexisting bicarbonate-responsive acidosis, hyperkalemia, or to correct widened QRS complex in known responsive overdoses (i.e., tricyclics). Also may be considered in patients with prolonged or unknown downtime (4)[C].

ISSUES FOR REFERRAL
- Consider communication with the medical examiner's office.
- Consider communication with an organ/tissue bank.

ADDITIONAL THERAPIES
Therapeutic hypothermia after resuscitation (to 32–34°C within 6 hours of collapse for 12–24 hours) should be performed if possible. The greatest benefit is seen in VF as initial rhythm and short downtime (<25 minutes), but it should be considered with any patient who has ROSC and coma state (5).

IN-PATIENT CONSIDERATIONS
Admission Criteria/Initial Stabilization
- Decreasing the EMS response interval increases survival (4)[A].
- The home use of automatic external defibrillators does not improve survival (6).

 ## ONGOING CARE

FOLLOW-UP RECOMMENDATIONS
Patient Monitoring
- Admit to ICU or CCU on continuous monitoring.
- Consider EEG to assess for nonconvulsive status epilepticus.

PROGNOSIS
- The outcome is related to underlying disease, age, duration of arrest, and other factors.
- The outcome is poor with the following indicators:
  – >4 minutes to CPR or >8 minutes to ACLS
  – Arrest occurs out of hospital
  – Resuscitation effort >30 minutes
- ~17% survive in-hospital arrest.
- ~1–10% survive to leave the hospital in out-of-hospital arrest, varying by geographic region.
- ~10–15% of those with VF survive.
- If the arrest is out of hospital without a return of vital signs from ALS prehospital care, the patient is unlikely to respond to ED resuscitation efforts.
- If the patient has an ROSC with coma, strongly consider induced hypothermia to improve the neurologic outcome (number needed to treat in VF = 6).

COMPLICATIONS
- Significant neurologic, hepatic, renal, or cardiac ischemic injury or multiorgan systems failure
- Rib fractures, hemopneumothorax, abdominal organ injury from CPR

REFERENCES
1. Perera P, Mailhot T, Riley D, et al. The RUSH exam: Rapid Ultrasound in SHock in the evaluation of the critically ill. *Emerg Med Clin North Am*. 2010;28(1): 29–56, vii.
2. 2010 American Heart Association Guidelines for Cardiopulmonary Resuscitation and Emergency Cardiovascular Care. *Circulation*. 2010;122 (Suppl 3):S685–S767.
3. Stiell IG, Nichol G, Leroux BG, et al. Early versus later rhythm analysis in patients with out-of-hospital cardiac arrest. *N Engl J Med*. 2011;365(9):787–797.
4. Hypothermia after Cardiac Arrest Study Group. Mild therapeutic hypothermia to improve the neurologic outcome after cardiac arrest. *N Engl J Med*. 2002;346:549–556.
5. Testori C, Sterz F, Behringer W, et al. Mild therapeutic hypothermia is associated with favourable outcome in patients after cardiac arrest with non-shockable rhythms. *Resuscitation*. 2011;82(9):1162–1167. Epub 2011 Jun 12.
6. Bardy GH, Lee KL, Mark DB. Home use of automated external defibrillators for sudden cardiac arrest. *N Engl J Med*. 2008;358:1793–1804.

ADDITIONAL READING
- Holzer M. Targeted temperature management for comatose survivors of cardiac arrest. *N Engl J Med*. 2010;363(13):1256–1264.
- Wik L, Hansen TB, Fylling F. Delaying defibrillation to give basic cardiopulmonary resuscitation to patients with out-of-hospital ventricular fibrillation: A randomized trial. *JAMA*. 2003;289:1389–1395.

 ## SEE ALSO

Algorithm: Coronary Syndrome, Acute

 ## CODES

ICD10
- I46.2 Cardiac arrest due to underlying cardiac condition
- I46.8 Cardiac arrest due to other underlying condition
- I46.9 Cardiac arrest, cause unspecified

CLINICAL PEARLS
- C-A-B replaces ABCs for the priority of approach to a patient with a suspected cardiac arrest.
- Prompt initiation of CPR, particularly chest compressions (push hard, push fast, and don't interrupt!), and immediate defibrillation (in witnessed VF and pulseless VT but not in PEA) are 1st priority.
- For an unwitnessed arrest, complete 2 minutes of CPR before attempting defibrillation.
- Epinephrine is the 1st drug to give in any case requiring CPR: Intraosseous and endotracheal routes are preferred if peripheral access is not attainable. Central line may be considered if unable to achieve access and if performed femoral approach is preferred.
- Therapeutic hypothermia has significantly improved neurologic outcomes in cardiac arrest and should be initiated as soon as possible in any patient with ROSC and coma state.

CARDIOMYOPATHY, END STAGE

Timothy P. Fitzgibbons, MD, PhD • Theo E. Meyer, MD, DPhil

BASICS

DESCRIPTION

- Cardiomyopathy encompasses a large group of diseases of the myocardium that commonly result in mechanical and/or electrical pump dysfunction. The current classification scheme attempts to differentiate between myocardial diseases confined to the myocardium (primary) and those due to systemic disorders (secondary) (1). Specific causes of myocardial dysfunction due to other cardiovascular disorders are considered a third, separate category (1).
- Classification of cardiomyopathy:
  - Primary:
    - Genetic:
    - Hypertrophic (HCM)
    - Arrhythmogenic right ventricular cardiomyopathy/dysplasia (ARVC/D)
    - Left ventricular (LV) noncompaction (LVNC)
    - Glycogen storage (Danon type, PRKAG2)
    - Conduction defects
    - Mitochondrial myopathies
    - Ion channel disorders: Long QT syndrome, Brugada, short QT syndrome, catecholaminergic ventricular tachycardia (CVPT), Asian SUNDS
    - Mixed:
    - Dilated (DCM) (genetic or nongenetic)
    - Restrictive
    - Acquired:
    - Myocarditis, stress cardiomyopathy, peripartum, tachycardia-induced, infants of type 1 diabetic mothers
  - Secondary (see list below)
  - Specific:
    - Ischemic
    - Valvular
    - Hypertensive
    - Congenital heart disease
- Patients with end-stage cardiomyopathy have stage D heart failure or severe symptoms at rest refractory to standard medical therapy.
- System(s) affected: Cardiovascular; Renal

Pediatric Considerations
Etiology: Idiopathic, viral, congenital heart disease, and familial

Pregnancy Considerations
May occur in women postpartum

EPIDEMIOLOGY
Predominant age: Ischemic cardiomyopathy is the most common etiology; predominantly in patients aged >50 years. Consider uncommon causes in young.

Incidence
- 60,000 patients <65 years die each year from end-stage heart disease.
- 35,000–70,000 people might benefit from cardiac transplant or chronic support.

Prevalence
Most rapidly growing form of heart disease

ETIOLOGY AND PATHOPHYSIOLOGY
The most frequent causes are in bold:
- Ischemic heart disease: Most common etiology; up to 66% of patients
- Hypertension
- Valvular heart disease

- Primary genetic causes
- Congenital heart disease
- Peripartum/Postpartum
- Endocrine:
  - Diabetes mellitus
  - Hyperthyroidism
  - Hypothyroidism
  - Hyperparathyroidism
  - Pheochromocytoma
  - Acromegaly
- Nutritional deficiencies:
  - Beriberi, pellagra, scurvy, selenium, carnitine, kwashiorkor
- Autoimmune/Collagen:
  - Systemic lupus erythematosus
  - Dermatomyositis
  - Rheumatoid arthritis
  - Scleroderma
  - Polyarteritis nodosa
- Infectious causes:
  - Viral (e.g., HIV, Coxsackie virus, adenovirus)
  - Bacterial and mycobacterial (e.g., diphtheria, rheumatic fever)
  - Parasitic (e.g., toxoplasmosis, *Trypanosoma cruzi*)
- Infiltrative:
  - Amyloidosis
  - Gaucher disease
  - Hurler disease
  - Hunter disease
  - Fabry disease
- Storage:
  - Hemochromatosis
  - Fabry disease
  - Glycogen storage disease (type II, Pompe)
  - Niemann-Pick disease
- Neuromuscular/Neurologic:
  - Duchenne and Emery-Dreifuss muscular dystrophies
  - Friedreich's ataxia
  - Myotonic dystrophy
  - Neurofibromatosis
  - Tuberous sclerosis
- Toxic:
  - Alcohol
  - Drugs and chemotherapy: Anthracyclines, cyclophosphamide, Herceptin
  - Radiation
  - Heavy metal, chemical agents
- Inflammatory (granulomatous):
  - Sarcoidosis
- Idiopathic
- Endomyocardial:
  - Endomyocardial fibrosis
  - Hypereosinophilic syndrome (Loeffler's endocarditis)

Genetics
Autosomal dominant HCM is the most common form of primary genetic cardiomyopathy (1/500 in the general population). Genetic causes of DCM are less common, accounting for 1/3 cases, with mostly autosomal dominant inheritance. ARVC is also inherited in autosomal dominant fashion, in addition to LQTS and other ion-channel disorders.

RISK FACTORS
- Hypertension
- Hyperlipidemia
- Obesity

- Diabetes mellitus
- Smoking
- Physical inactivity
- Excessive alcohol intake
- Dietary sodium
- Obstructive sleep apnea
- Chemotherapy

GENERAL PREVENTION
Reduce salt and water intake; home BP and daily weight measurement

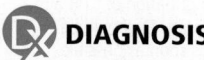

DIAGNOSIS

HISTORY
- Dyspnea at rest or with exertion
- Paroxysmal nocturnal dyspnea
- Orthopnea
- Postprandial dyspnea
- Right upper quadrant pain or bloating
- Fatigue
- Syncope
- Edema

PHYSICAL EXAM
- Tachypnea
- Low pulse pressure
- Cool extremities
- Jugular venous distention
- Bibasilar rales
- Tachycardia
- Displaced point of maximal impulse (PMI)
- S_3 gallop
- Blowing systolic murmur
- Hepatosplenomegaly
- Ascites
- Edema

DIFFERENTIAL DIAGNOSIS
- Severe pulmonary disease
- Primary pulmonary hypertension
- Recurrent pulmonary embolism
- Constrictive pericarditis
- Some advanced forms of malignancy
- Anemia

DIAGNOSTIC TESTS & INTERPRETATION
- ECG: LV hypertrophy, interventricular conduction delay, atrial fibrillation, evidence of prior Q-wave infarction
- Cardiopulmonary exercise testing: Maximal oxygen consumption <10 mL/kg/min correlates with 50% 1-year mortality, and >18 mL/kg/mm correlates with >90% 1-year survival. Used in stable outpatients to estimate prognosis and prior to cardiac transplant referral.
- Hyponatremia
- Prerenal azotemia
- Anemia
- Mild elevation in troponin
- Elevated B-type natriuretic peptide (BNP) or pro-BNP
- Mild hyperbilirubinemia
- Elevated liver function tests
- Elevated uric acid

Initial Tests (lab, imaging)
- Chest radiograph:
  - Cardiomegaly
  - Increased vascular markings to the upper lobes
  - Pleural effusions may or may not be present.
- Echocardiography:
  - In dilated cardiomyopathy, 4-chamber enlargement and global hypokinesis are present.
  - In hypertrophic cardiomyopathy, severe LV hypertrophy is present.
  - Segmental contraction abnormalities of the LV are indicative of previous localized myocardial infarction.
- Cardiac MRI:
  - May be useful to characterize certain nonischemic cardiomyopathies
- Myocardial stress perfusion imaging (MPI):
  - Recommended in those with new-onset LV dysfunction or when ischemia is suspected

Diagnostic Procedures/Other
Cardiac catheterization:
- Helpful to rule out ischemic heart disease
- Characterize hemodynamic severity
- Pulmonary artery catheters may be reasonable in patients with refractory heart failure (HF) to help guide management (2)[C].

TREATMENT

See "Congestive Heart Failure" for detailed treatment protocols.

GENERAL MEASURES
- Reduction of filling pressures
- Treatment of electrolyte disturbances

MEDICATION
First Line
- Systolic failure syndromes:
  - ACE inhibitors: Lisinopril, 5–40 mg/d or captopril, 6.25–50 mg t.i.d. (2)[A]
  - Loop diuretics:
    - May need to be given IV initially and then orally as patient stabilizes
    - Furosemide, 40–120 mg/d or t.i.d. (2)[A]
  - β-blockers:
    - Use with caution in acutely decompensated or low cardiac output states.
    - Metoprolol succinate, 12.5–200 mg/d; carvedilol, 3.125–25 mg b.i.d.; or bisoprolol, 1.25–10 mg/d (2)[A]
  - Aldosterone antagonists:
    - Patients with New York Heart Association (NYHA) II–IV congestive heart failure (CHF), ejection fraction (EF) <35%, on standard therapy; spironolactone, 12.5–25 mg/d (2)[A]
  - Digoxin, 0.125–0.250 mg/d for symptomatic patients on standard therapy (2)[A]
  - Combination hydralazine/isosorbide dinitrate is first-line treatment in African American patients with class III–IV symptoms (2)[A] already on standard therapy, and for all patients with reduced EF and symptoms incompletely responsive to ACE inhibitor and β-blocker.

- Diastolic failure:
  - Few evidence-based therapies for diastolic heart failure. Empiric management goals include:
    - Management of hypertension
    - Reduction of congestive states (i.e., diuretics)
    - Prevention of progression of LV hypertrophy (i.e., renin-angiotensin-aldosterone system blockade)
    - Maintenance of sinus rhythm
- Contraindications:
  - β-blockers: Low cardiac output, 1st- or 2nd-degree heart block
  - Ca-blockers (nondihydropyridine): Low cardiac output, heart block
  - Aldosterone antagonists: Oliguria, anuria, renal dysfunction
  - Loop diuretics: Hypokalemia, hypomagnesemia
  - ACE inhibitors: Pregnancy, angioedema
- Precautions:
  - In patients with chronic kidney disease, digoxin dosage should be ≤0.125 mg/d and drug levels followed carefully to avoid toxicity.
  - Closely monitor electrolytes.
  - ACE inhibitors: Initiate with care if BP is low. Begin with low-dose captopril, such as 6.25 mg t.i.d.
  - β-blockers: Avoid in patients with evidence of poor tissue perfusion; they may further depress systolic function.
  - Milrinone, amrinone: Contraindicated for long-term use due to increased mortality

Second Line
- Angiotensin receptor blockers as an alternative to, or (rarely) in addition to, ACE inhibitors
- Inotropic therapy (e.g., dobutamine or milrinone) for cardiogenic shock and support prior to surgery or cardiac transplantation (2)[C]
- Continuous inotrope infusion in stage D outpatients for symptom control in those who are not eligible for transplantation or mechanical circulatory support (2)[B]

ISSUES FOR REFERRAL
Management by a heart failure team improves outcomes and facilitates early transplant referral.

ADDITIONAL THERAPIES
- Prophylactic implantable cardioverter defibrillator (ICD) should be considered for patients with an LVEF <35% and mild to moderate symptoms (2)[A].
- Cardiac resynchronization therapy (CRT) is recommended for patients in sinus rhythm with a QRS >150 msec, LVEF<35%, and persistent symptoms despite optimal medical therapy (2)[A].
- Patients with severe, refractory HF with no reasonable expectation of improvement should not be considered for an ICD (2)[C].
- Consideration of an LV assist device as "permanent" or destination therapy is reasonable in selected stage D patients.

ONGOING CARE

DIET
Low-fat, low-salt, fluid restriction

PROGNOSIS
~20–40% of patients in NYHA functional class IV die within 1 year. With a transplant, 1-year survival is as high as 94%.

COMPLICATIONS
Worsening CHF, syncope, renal failure, arrhythmias, or sudden death

REFERENCES
1. Maron BJ, Towbin JA, Thiene G, et al. Contemporary definitions and classification of the cardiomyopathies: An American Heart Association Scientific Statement from the Council on Clinical Cardiology, Heart Failure and Transplantation Committee; Quality of Care and Outcomes Research and Functional Genomics and Translational Biology Interdisciplinary Working Groups; and Council on Epidemiology and Prevention. *Circulation*. 2006;113(14):1807–1816. Epub 2006 Mar 27.
2. Yancy CW, Jessup M, Bozkurt B, et al. 2013 ACCF/AHA guideline for the management of heart failure: A report of the American College of Cardiology Foundation/American Heart Association Task Force on Practice Guidelines. *Circulation*. 2013;128:1–375.

SEE ALSO

Alcohol Abuse and Dependence; Alcohol Withdrawal; Amyloidosis; Congestive Heart Failure; Diabetes Mellitus, Type 1; Diabetes Mellitus, Type 2; Hypertension, Essential; Hypothyroidism, Adult; Idiopathic Hypertrophic Subaortic Stenosis; Protein Energy Malnutrition; Rheumatic Fever; Sarcoidosis

CODES

ICD10
- I42.8 Other cardiomyopathies
- I42.9 Cardiomyopathy, unspecified
- I43 Cardiomyopathy in diseases classified elsewhere

CLINICAL PEARLS
- Cardiomyopathy represents the end-stage of a large number of disease processes involving the heart muscle.
- Ischemic, hypertensive, postviral, familial, alcoholic, and incessant tachycardia-induced are the most common cardiomyopathy varieties seen in the US.
- Core therapy for HF applies: Salt-restriction, diuretics, ACE inhibitors, β-blockers, digoxin, and electrical treatments, such as cardiac resynchronization and implantable defibrillators, as appropriate.

CAROTID STENOSIS

Edlira Yzeiraj, DO • Maria M. Plummer, MD

BASICS

Carotid stenosis may be caused by atherosclerosis, intimal fibroplasia, vasculitis, adventitial cysts, or vascular tumors; atherosclerosis is the most common etiology.

DESCRIPTION
- Narrowing of carotid artery lumen is typically due to atherosclerotic changes in the vessel wall. Atherosclerotic plaques are responsible for 90% of extracranial carotid lesions and up to 30% of all ischemic strokes.
- A "hemodynamically significant" carotid stenosis produces a drop in pressure, reduction in flow, or both and corresponds approximately to a 60% diameter-reducing stenosis (1).
- Carotid lesions are classified by:
  – Symptom status:
    ○ Asymptomatic: Tend to be homogenous and stable
    ○ Symptomatic (stroke, transient cerebral ischemic event): Tend to be heterogeneous and unstable
  – Degree of stenosis:
    ○ High grade: 80–99% stenosis
    ○ Moderate grade: 50–79% stenosis
    ○ Low grade: <50% stenosis

EPIDEMIOLOGY
More common in men and with increasing age (see "Risk Factors")

Incidence
Unclear (asymptomatic patients often go undiagnosed)

Prevalence
- Moderate stenosis (2):
  – Age <50 years: men 0.2%, women 0%
  – Age ≥80 years: men 7.5%, women 5%
- Severe stenosis (2):
  – Age <50 years: men 0.1%, women 0%
  – Age ≥80 years: men 3.1%, women 0.9%

ETIOLOGY AND PATHOPHYSIOLOGY
- Atherosclerosis formation begins during adolescence, consistently at carotid bifurcation. The carotid bulb has unique blood-flow dynamics. Hemodynamic disturbances cause endothelial injury and dysfunction. Plaque formation in vessel wall results, and stenosis then ensues.
- Initial cause not well understood, but certain risk factors are frequently present (see "Risk Factors"). Tensile stress on the vessel wall, turbulence, and arterial wall shear stress seem to be involved.

Genetics
- Increased incidence among family members
- Genetically linked factors:
  – Diabetes mellitus (DM), race, hypertension (HTN), family history, obesity
  – In a recent single nucleotide polymorphism study, the following genes were strongly associated with worse carotid plaque: TNFSF4, PPARA, TLR4, ITGA2, and HABP2

RISK FACTORS
- Nonmodifiable factors: Advanced age, male sex, family history, cardiac disease, congenital arteriopathies (1)
- Modifiable factors: Smoking, diet, dyslipidemia, physical inactivity, obesity, HTN, DM

GENERAL PREVENTION
- Antihypertensive treatment to maintain BP <140/90 mm Hg (systolic BP between 140 and 150 is target in elderly)
- Smoking cessation to reduce the risk of atherosclerosis progression and stroke.
- Lipid control: Regression of carotid atherosclerotic lesions seen with statin therapy.

COMMONLY ASSOCIATED CONDITIONS
- Transient ischemic attack (TIA)/Stroke
- Coronary artery disease (CAD)/Myocardial infarction (MI)
- Peripheral vascular disease (PVD)
- HTN
- DM
- Hyperlipidemia

DIAGNOSIS

Screening for carotid stenosis is not recommended. However, in the setting of symptoms suggestive of stroke or TIA, workup for this condition may be indicated.

HISTORY
- Identification of modifiable and nonmodifiable comorbidities (see "Risk Factors")
- History of cerebral ischemic event
- Stroke, TIA, amaurosis fugax (monocular blindness), aphasia
- Coronary artery disease/MI
- Peripheral arterial disease
- Full review of systems, with focus on risk factors for:
  – Cardiovascular disease
  – Stroke (HTN and arrhythmia)

PHYSICAL EXAM
- Lateralizing neurologic deficits: Contralateral motor and/or sensory deficit
- Amaurosis fugax: Ipsilateral transient visual obscuration from retinal ischemia
- Visual field defect
- Dysarthria and, in the case of dominant (usually left) hemisphere involvement, aphasia
- Carotid bruit (low sensitivity and specificity)

DIFFERENTIAL DIAGNOSIS
- Aortic valve stenosis
- Aortic arch atherosclerosis
- Arrhythmia with cardiogenic embolization
- Migraine
- Brain tumor
- Metabolic disturbances
- Functional/psychological deficit
- Seizure

DIAGNOSTIC TESTS & INTERPRETATION
Initial Tests (lab, imaging)
Workup for suspected TIA/stroke may include:
- CBC with differential
- Basic metabolic panel
- ESR (if temporal arteritis a consideration)
- Glucose/HbA1c
- Fasting lipid profile

- Duplex US identifies ≥50% stenosis, with 98% sensitivity and 88% specificity. Doppler US determines degree of stenosis by assessing velocity of blood flow through stenotic vessel. Although findings should be confirmed by angiogram (MR or CT), US is increasingly used to screen prior to surgical assessment.

Follow-Up Tests & Special Considerations
- Proceed to imaging if there is suggestion of stenosis from history or physical exam.
- Other noninvasive imaging techniques can add detail to duplex results:
  – CT angiography:
    ○ 88% sensitivity and 100% specificity
    ○ Requires contrast load with risk for subsequent renal morbidity
  – MR angiography:
    ○ 95% sensitivity and 90% specificity
    ○ Evaluates cerebral circulation (extracranial and intracranial), as well as aortic arch and common carotid artery
    ○ The presence of unstable plaque can be determined if the following characteristics are seen:
      ■ Presence of thin/ruptured fibrous cap
      ■ Presence of lipid-rich necrotic core
    ○ Tends to overestimate degree of stenosis

Diagnostic Procedures/Other
Cerebral (catheter) angiography is the traditional gold standard for diagnosis:
- Delineates anatomy pertaining to aortic arch and proximal vessels
- However, procedure is invasive and has multiple risks:
  – Contrast-induced renal dysfunction (1–5% complication rate)
  – Thromboembolic-related complications (1–2.6% complication rate) and neurologic complications
  – Should be used only when other tests are not conclusive

Test Interpretation
- Stenosis consistently occurs at carotid bifurcation, with plaque formation most often at proximal internal carotid artery:
  – Plaque is thickest at the carotid bifurcation.
  – Plaque occupies the intima and inner media and avoids outer media and adventitia.
- Plaque histology:
  – Homogenous (stable) plaques seldom hemorrhage or ulcerate:
    ○ Fatty streak and fibrous tissue deposition
    ○ Diffuse intimal thickening
  – Heterogenous (unstable) plaques may hemorrhage or ulcerate:
    ○ Presence of lipid-laden macrophages, necrotic debris, cholesterol crystals
    ○ Ulcerated plaques
  – Soft and gelatinous clots with platelets, fibrin, and red and white blood cells

C

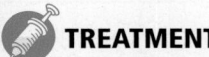

TREATMENT

Smoking cessation, BP control, use of antiplatelet medication, and statin medication are the primary treatments for both asymptomatic and symptomatic carotid stenosis.

GENERAL MEASURES
- Lifestyle modifications: Dietary control and weight loss, exercise of 30 min/d at least 5 d/wk.
- Patients should be advised to quit smoking and offered smoking cessation intervention to reduce the risk of atherosclerotic progression and stoke.
- Control of HTN with antihypertensive agents to maintain BP <140/90 (3)[A].

MEDICATION
- Antihypertensive treatment
- Statin initiation is recommended to reduce low-density lipoprotein (LDL) cholesterol <100 mg/dL (3)[A]
- Aspirin: 75–325 mg/d
- If patient has sustained ischemic stroke or transient ischemic attack (TIA), antiplatelet therapy with:
  – Aspirin alone (75–325 mg/d) (3)[A]
  – Clopidogrel alone (75 mg/d) (3)[A], or
  – Aspirin plus extended-release dipyridamole (25 and 200 mg b.i.d., respectively) (3)[A]

ISSUES FOR REFERRAL
- For acute symptomatic stroke, order imaging and contact neurology.
- For known carotid stenosis, some suggest duplex imaging every 6 months if stenosis is >50% and patient is a surgical candidate.

SURGERY/OTHER PROCEDURES
- Symptomatic carotid stenosis:
  – Carotid endarterectomy (CEA) is recommended in symptomatic patients with a carotid stenosis of 70–99% without near occlusion. Benefit in patients with carotid near-occlusion is uncertain in the long term (4)[A].
  – CEA is recommended for patients with a life expectancy of at least 5 years. The anticipated rate of perioperative stroke or mortality must be <6% (3)[A].
  – Treatment with aspirin (81–325 mg/d) is recommended for all patients who are having CEA. Aspirin should be started prior to surgery and continued for at least 3 months postsurgery, but may be continued indefinitely (5)[B].
  – Carotid artery stenting (CAS) provides similar long-term outcomes as CEA. However, CAS is associated with an increased risk of periprocedural stroke or death compared to CEA in older patients (6)[A]:
    ○ CAS is suggested in select patients with neck anatomy unfavorable for arterial surgery and those with comorbid conditions that greatly increase the risk of anesthesia and surgery (3)[A].

- Asymptomatic patients:
  – Some recommend CEA for asymptomatic men who have 60–99% stenosis, have a life expectancy of at least 5 years and the perioperative risk of stroke and death is <3% (6)[B]. The advantage of surgical compared with medical therapy has decreased with contemporary medical management. It is not possible to make an evidence-based recommendation for or against surgical therapy with current literature (7) [A].

IN-PATIENT CONSIDERATIONS
Admission Criteria/Initial Stabilization
Any patient with presentation of acute symptomatic carotid stenosis should be hospitalized for further diagnostic workup and appropriate therapy. Rapid evaluation for symptoms compatible with TIA should be obtained in the ED or inpatient setting.

Discharge Criteria
24–48 hours post-CEA, if ambulating, taking adequate PO intake, and neurologically intact

ONGOING CARE

FOLLOW-UP RECOMMENDATIONS
Patient Monitoring
After CEA, overnight in postanesthesia care unit or step-down:
- Duplex at 2–6 weeks postop
- Duplex every 6–12 months
- Reoperative CEA or CAS is reasonable if there is rapidly progressive restenosis (3)[A].

DIET
Low-fat, low-cholesterol, low-salt diet at discharge

PATIENT EDUCATION
- Signs and symptoms of TIA/stroke:
  – Lateralizing neurologic deficits, monocular blindness, aphasia
- Diet and lifestyle modification

COMPLICATIONS
- Untreated: TIA/Stroke (risk of ipsilateral stroke approximately 1.68% per year (7))
- Postoperative (s/p CEA):
  – Perioperative (within 30 days):
    ○ Stroke/Death, cranial nerve injury, hemorrhage, hemodynamic instability, MI
  – Late (>30 days postop):
    ○ Recurrent stenosis, false aneurysm at surgical site

REFERENCES

1. Goldstein LB, Bushnell CD, Adams RJ, et al. Guidelines for the primary prevention of stroke: A guideline for healthcare professionals from the American Heart Association/American Stroke Association. Stroke. 2011;42(2):517–584.
2. de Weerd M, Greving JP, Hedblad B, et al. Prevalence of asymptomatic carotid artery stenosis in the general population: An individual participant data meta-analysis. Stroke. 2010;41(6): 1294–1297.
3. Brott TG, Halperin JL. 2011 ASA/ACCF/AHA/AANN/ AANS/ACR/ASNR/CNS/SAIP/SCAI/SIR/SNIS/SVM/SVS guideline on the management of patients with extracranial carotid and vertebral artery disease: Executive summary. J Am Coll Cardiol. 2011;57(8): 1002–1044.
4. Rerkasem K, Rothwel PM. Carotid endarterectomy for symptomatic carotid stenosis. Cochrane Database Syst Rev. 2011;(3):CD000515.
5. Chaturvedi S, Bruno A, Feasby T. Carotid endarterectomy—an evidenced–based review: Report of the Therapeutics and Technology Assessment Subcommittee of the American Academy of Neurology. Neurology. 2005 65(6): 794–801.
6. Bonati LH, Lyrer P, Featherstone R. Percutaneous transluminal balloon angioplasty and stenting for carotid artery stenosis. Cochrane Database Syst Rev. 2012;(9):CD001081.
7. Raman G, Moorthy D, Hadar N, et al. Management strategies for asymptomatic carotid stenosis: A systematic review and meta-analysis. Ann Int Med. 2013;158(9):676–685.

ADDITIONAL READING

- Jahromi AS, Cinà CS, Liu Y, et al. Sensitivity and specificity of color duplex ultrasound measurement in the estimation of internal carotid artery stenosis: A systematic review and meta-analysis. J Vasc Surg. 2005;41:962–972.
- Lovrencic-Huzjan A, Rundek T, Katsnelson M. Recommendations for management of patients with carotid stenosis. Stroke Res Treat. 2012;2012: 175869.
- Murad MH, Shahrour A, Shah ND, et al. A systematic review and meta-analysis of randomized trials of carotid endarterectomy vs stenting. J Vasc Surg. 2011;53(3):792–797.
- Paraskevas KI, Mikhailidis DP, Veith FJ. Comparison of the five 2011 guidelines treatment of carotid stenosis. J Vasc Surg. 2012(55):1504–1508.

 SEE ALSO

Algorithms: Transient ischemic attack; Stroke; Hypercholesterolemia

 CODES

ICD10
- I65.21 Occlusion and stenosis of right carotid artery
- I65.22 Occlusion and stenosis of left carotid artery
- I65.29 Occlusion and stenosis of unspecified carotid artery

CLINICAL PEARLS
- Atherosclerosis is responsible for 90% of all cases of carotid artery stenosis.
- Duplex US is the best initial imaging modality.
- Antiplatelet therapy and aggressive treatment of vascular risk factors are the mainstays of medical therapy.
- Compared with CEA, CAS increases the risk of any stroke and decreases the risk of MI. For every 1,000 patients opting for stenting rather than endarterectomy:
  – 19 more patients would have strokes
  – 10 fewer would have MIs

CARPAL TUNNEL SYNDROME
Philip H. Aurigemma, MD • Marci D. Jones, MD

 BASICS

DESCRIPTION
- Carpal tunnel syndrome (CTS) is the most common cause of peripheral nerve compression.
- Increased pressure within the carpal tunnel leads to entrapment and compression of the median nerve.
- The tunnel is composed of the carpal bones dorsally and the transverse carpal ligament palmarly:
  - The tunnel contains flexor tendons and the median nerve.
- Symptoms tend to affect the dominant hand, but >50% of patients experience bilateral symptoms.
- System(s) affected: Musculoskeletal; Nervous

ALERT
Pregnancy: Increased incidence during pregnancy; incidence estimates vary

EPIDEMIOLOGY
- Predominant age: 40–60
- Predominant sex: Female > Male (3:1–10:1)

Incidence
- 2 peaks: Late 50s in women, and late 70s when the sex ratio is more equal
- Incidence rates of up to 276/100,000 have been reported.

Prevalence
- Incidence of 9.2% in women and 6% in men.
- Diabetic patients have a prevalence rate of 14% and 30% without and with diabetic neuropathy, respectively.
- Increasing prevalence may be due to increased lifespan of population, as well as increasing prevalence of diabetes.

ETIOLOGY AND PATHOPHYSIOLOGY
- Combination of mechanical trauma, inflammation, increased pressure, and ischemic injury to the median nerve within the carpal tunnel.
- Disorders affecting the musculoskeletal system in the region of the wrist, including the following:
  - Trauma or distal radius fracture
  - Degenerative joint disease
  - Rheumatoid arthritis
  - Ganglion cyst
  - Scleroderma
- Hypothyroidism and diabetes are frequently associated with this condition, which also occurs with increased frequency during pregnancy.
- Other miscellaneous causes include the following:
  - Acromegaly
  - Lupus erythematosus
  - Leukemia
  - Pyogenic infections
  - Sarcoidosis
  - Primary amyloidosis
  - Paget disease
  - Hormone replacement therapy
- Hyperparathyroidism, hypocalcemia

Genetics
Unknown; however, a familial type has been reported.

RISK FACTORS
- Prolonged postures in extremes of wrist flexion or extension and exposure to vibration are primary reported exposures for development of carpal tunnel syndrome.

- Conditions that alter the fluid balance in the body, including pregnancy, menopause, obesity, renal failure, hypothyroidism, congestive heart failure (CHF), and oral contraceptive use
- Neuropathic factors, such as diabetes, alcoholism, vitamin deficiency, or exposure to toxins, can play a role in eliciting CTS symptoms.
- No universal agreement that CTS is job-related

GENERAL PREVENTION
There is no known prevention for CTS. It is recommended to take a break once an hour when doing repetitive work involving hands.

COMMONLY ASSOCIATED CONDITIONS
- Diabetes
- Obesity
- Pregnancy

 DIAGNOSIS

HISTORY
- Burning pain and/or tingling in the fingers, particularly at night (acroparesthesias):
  - The altered sensation (tingling or prickling) is characteristically confined to the thumb, index, long, and radial 1/2 of the ring fingers, but many patients do not distinguish this localization and feel the entire hand is affected.
  - Occasional ascending, sometimes up to the shoulder, or descending irradiating pain
- Symptoms characteristically are relieved by shaking or rubbing the hands.
- During waking hours, symptoms occur when driving the car, reading the newspaper, talking on the phone, and occasionally when using the hands for repetitive maneuvers.
- Presence of predisposing factors, such as diabetes, adiposity, acromegaly, pregnancy

PHYSICAL EXAM
- Positive Tinel sign: Tapping over the palmar surface of the wrist proximal to the carpal tunnel may produce an electric sensation perceived by the patient, a sign of nerve compression (50% sensitivity; 77% specificity).
- Positive Phalen sign: Holding the wrist flexed for 60 seconds may precipitate the paresthesias experienced by the patient (68% sensitivity; 73% specificity) (1).
- Positive carpal compression test: Moderate pressure applied over the area of the carpal tunnel elicits paresthesias in the median nerve distribution within 30 seconds. (87% sensitivity; 95% specificity)
- Numbness and tingling in median nerve distribution
- Wasting of the thenar muscles is a late sign.
- Weakness of the hand for such tasks as opening jars is often noted by the patient early in the disorder.
- Loss of 2-point discrimination

DIFFERENTIAL DIAGNOSIS
- Cervical spondylosis (carpal tunnel may also occur with cervical spine disease; so-called double crush)
- Generalized peripheral neuropathy
- Brachial plexus lesion, in particular upper trunk
- CNS disorders (multiple sclerosis, small cerebral infarction)
- Thoracic outlet syndrome
- Pronator syndrome
- Anterior interosseous syndrome

DIAGNOSTIC TESTS & INTERPRETATION
- No laboratory test is diagnostic.
- Normal serum thyrotropin (thyroid-stimulating hormone [TSH]) and normal serum glucose may be helpful in excluding conditions associated with CTS.

Initial Tests (lab, imaging)
- Special tests:
  - Electrodiagnostic studies:
    - Sensitivity 85%; specificity 95%
    - Nerve conduction studies compare latency and amplitude of median nerve segment across the carpal tunnel to another nerve segment such as the radial or ulnar nerve.
    - Prolonged distal latency of the median motor and/or sensory nerves may be seen. Axon loss is suggested when amplitudes are decreased.
    - The most sensitive indicator is the median sensory distal latency, which is prolonged. Further, the sensory nerve action potential may be reduced or unobtainable.
    - Electromyographic changes are indicative of more longstanding or severe nerve dysfunction.
- Stimulation of the ulnar nerve should be done as well to exclude generalized polyneuropathy.
- Standard radiographs of the wrist to evaluate bony anatomy and degenerative joint disease
- Special radiographic views of the carpal tunnel may be obtained. These are of limited usefulness unless heterotopic calcification can be identified.
- Magnetic resonance neurography may be used to confirm compression of the median nerve in the carpal tunnel and to assess the success of surgical decompression:
  - MRI can detect rare pathological causes of CTS, such as ganglion cyst, hemangioma, or bony deformity.
- US may be used to help diagnose CTS by measuring cross-sectional area of median nerve. Roughly, 78% sensitive and 87% specific (2)[A]

 TREATMENT

GENERAL MEASURES
- Splinting of the wrist in a neutral position while sleeping may provide significant relief of symptoms:
  - Limited evidence indicates that splints worn at night are more effective than no treatment in the short term, but also insufficient evidence regarding effectiveness and safety of 1 splint design or wearing regimen over others (3)[A].
- Prolonged use of splinting, if possible, may allow some symptoms to resolve.
- Injection of the carpal tunnel with a steroid may provide significant temporary relief. This is particularly useful during pregnancy. This can be expected to provide relief for ≥1 month.
- Strong evidence indicates that corticosteroid injections are effective for short-term relief when compared with placebo (4)[A].

MEDICATION

First Line

NSAIDs, such as ibuprofen, 800 mg b.i.d. or t.i.d., or naproxen sodium, 500 mg b.i.d., are commonly used; however, insufficient evidence exists to determine the efficacy of this approach:

- Contraindications: GI intolerance
- Precautions: GI side effects of NSAIDs may preclude their use in selected patients.

Second Line

- Local steroids: Injections have been shown be more effective than systemic steroids or placebo at 1 and 3 months, and more effective than splinting at 6 months (5):
  - Possible side effects include reduction of collagen and proteoglycan synthesis, limiting tenocytes, and reducing mechanical strength of tendon, leading to further degeneration
- Oral steroids may provide a short term improvement (2–8 weeks) in symptoms:
  - The long-term risks of even a short course of steroids should be balanced with the limited potential benefit of symptom improvement.

ISSUES FOR REFERRAL

Most surgeons do not perform operative release of the carpal tunnel without preoperative nerve conduction studies.

SURGERY/OTHER PROCEDURES

- Surgical decompression of the carpal tunnel by dividing the transverse carpal ligament completely provides almost total relief of symptoms in >95% of patients.
- Surgical decompression is almost exclusively done as an outpatient procedure under regional anesthesia.
- Healing of the incision generally takes 2 weeks; an additional 2 weeks of recuperation may be required before the hand can be fully used for tasks requiring strength.
- Long-term results of open carpal tunnel release are excellent, with patients experiencing consistent pain relief over 10–15 years.
- Recent randomized, controlled studies indicate that surgery is more effective than splinting at 6 and 12 months (6)[A].
- Open vs. endoscopic procedures produce similar outcomes at 1 year, and the approach should be driven based on surgeon and patient preference (7)[A].
- Therapeutic US is an intervention that works by delivering sound waves that are absorbed by underlying connective tissue, such as ligaments and tendons:
  - Poor quality evidence from limited data that therapeutic US may be more effective than placebo for either short- or long-term symptom improvement in people with CTS (8)[A].
- Exercise and mobilization interventions, including chiropractic and osteopathic manual interventions, nervous system mobilization techniques (e.g., nerve and tendon gliding exercises), or mobilization techniques targeting the carpal bones, have limited benefit compared with other nonsurgical interventions for CTS (9)[A].

COMPLEMENTARY AND ALTERNATIVE MEDICINE

Despite studies, no data exist to support the use of vitamin B6 in the prevention or treatment of carpal tunnel syndrome.

IN-PATIENT CONSIDERATIONS

Admission Criteria/Initial Stabilization

- Outpatient
- Outpatient surgery

 ## ONGOING CARE

FOLLOW-UP RECOMMENDATIONS

Patient Monitoring

- Patients treated with wrist splints or other nonoperative measures, such as steroid injections, will require follow-up in the ensuing 4–12 weeks to assess the success of treatment modalities.
- There is only limited, low-quality evidence that rehabilitation exercises such as wrist immobilization, ice therapy, and multimodal hand rehabilitation are beneficial (10)[A].
- Patients treated surgically rarely experience recurrence of the disorder. Routine follow-up once healing of the incision has occurred is not necessary.

PATIENT EDUCATION

- Free online and printable patient information from the American Society for Surgery of the Hand: http://www.assh.org/Public/HandConditions/Pages/CarpalTunnelSyndrome.aspx
- Carpal Tunnel Syndrome Foundation. For patient education materials favorably reviewed on this topic, contact: American Academy of Family Physicians Foundation, P.O. Box 8418, Kansas City, MO 64114 (800) 274-2237, Ext. 4400.

PROGNOSIS

- Patients with severe CTS may not recover completely even following surgical release. Although paresthesias and weakness may persist, night symptoms are generally resolved.
- Untreated, more severe cases of the condition can be expected to lead to numbness and weakness in the hand, with atrophy of the thenar muscles and permanent loss of median nerve function.

COMPLICATIONS

- Postoperative infection (rare)
- Injury to recurrent branch of the nerve

REFERENCES

1. Jordan R, Carter T, Cummins C. A systematic review of the utility of electrodiagnostic testing in carpal tunnel syndrome. *Br J Gen Pract*. 2002;52: 670–673.
2. Fowler JR, Gaughan JP, Ilyas AM. The sensitivity and specificity of ultrasound for the diagnosis of carpal tunnel syndrome: A meta-analysis. *Clin Orthop Relat Res*. 2011;469(4):1089–1094. Epub 2010 Oct 21.
3. Page MJ, Massy-Westropp N, O'Connor D, et al. Splinting for carpal tunnel syndrome. *Cochrane Database Syst Rev*. 2012;7:CD010003. Epub 2012 Jul 11.
4. Huisstede BM, Hoogvliet P, Randsdorp MS, et al. Carpal tunnel syndrome. Part I: Effectiveness of nonsurgical treatments: A systematic review. *Arch Phys Med Rehabil*. 2010;91(7):981–1004.
5. Graham B. Nonsurgical treatment of carpal tunnel syndrome. *J Hand Surg Am*. 2009;34(3):531–534.
6. Shi Q, MacDermid JC. Is surgical intervention more effective than non-surgical treatment for carpal tunnel syndrome? A systematic review. *J Orthop Surg Res*. 2011;6:17. Epub 2011 Apr 11.
7. Ashworth NL. Carpal tunnel syndrome. *Clin Evid (Online)*. 2010;2010. Epub 2010 Mar 23.
8. Page MJ, O'Connor D, Pitt V, et al. Therapeutic ultrasound for carpal tunnel syndrome. *Cochrane Database Syst Rev*. 2013;3:CD009601. Epub 2013 Mar 28.
9. Page MJ, O'Connor D, Pitt V, et al. Exercise and mobilisation interventions for carpal tunnel syndrome. *Cochrane Database Syst Rev*. 2012;6:CD009899. Epub 2012 Jun 13.
10. Peters S, Page MJ, Coppieters MW, et al. Rehabilitation following carpal tunnel release. *Cochrane Database Syst Rev*. 2013;6:CD004158.

ADDITIONAL READING

- French C, Cartwright MS, Hobson-Webb LD, et al. Evidence-based guideline: Neuromuscular ultrasound for the diagnosis of carpal tunnel syndrome. *Muscle Nerve*. 2012;46(2):287–293.
- Louie DL, Earp BE, Collins JE, et al. Outcomes of open carpal tunnel release at a minimum of ten years. *J Bone Joint Surg*. 2013;95(12):1067–1073.
- Marshall S, Tardif G, Ashworth N. Local corticosteroid injection for carpal tunnel syndrome. *Cochrane Database Syst Rev*. 2007;CD001554.
- Sanati KA, Mansouri M, Macdonald D, et al. Surgical techniques and return to work following carpal tunnel release: A systematic review and meta-analysis. *J Occup Rehabil*. 2011;21(4): 474–481.
- Tai TW, Wu CY, Su FC, et al. Ultrasonography for diagnosing carpal tunnel syndrome: A meta-analysis of diagnostic test accuracy. *Ultrasound Med Biol*. 2012;38(7):1121–1128. Epub 2012 Apr 27.

 ## SEE ALSO

- Arthritis, Rheumatoid; Hypoparathyroidism; Scleroderma; Systemic Lupus Erythematosus (SLE)
- Algorithms: Carpal Tunnel Syndrome; Pain in Upper Extremity

CODES

ICD10

- G56.00 Carpal tunnel syndrome, unspecified upper limb
- G56.01 Carpal tunnel syndrome, right upper limb
- G56.02 Carpal tunnel syndrome, left upper limb

CLINICAL PEARLS

- The altered sensation (tingling or prickling) in CTS is characteristically confined to the thumb, index, long, and radial 1/2 of the ring fingers, but many patients do not distinguish this localization and feel that the entire hand is affected.
- Tinel and Phalen signs have poor sensitivity and specificity.
- Normal serum TSH and normal serum glucose may be helpful in excluding conditions associated with carpal tunnel syndrome.
- Strongly consider surgical treatment for moderate and severe cases. Atrophy is a late finding, indicating severe disease.

CATARACT
Yasir Ahmed, MD • Ingrid U. Scott, MD, MPH

 BASICS

DESCRIPTION
- A cataract is any opacity or discoloration of the lens, localized or generalized; the term is usually reserved for changes that affect visual acuity
- Etymology: From Latin *cataractes*, for "waterfall"; named after foamy appearance of opacity
- Leading cause of blindness worldwide, an estimated 20 million people
- Types include:
  - Age-related: 90% of total
  - Metabolic (diabetes via accelerated sorbitol pathway, hypocalcemia, Wilson disease)
  - Congenital (1/250 newborns; 10–38% of childhood blindness)
  - Systemic disease–associated (myotonic dystrophy, atopic dermatitis)
  - Secondary to associated eye disease, so-called complicated (e.g., uveitis associated with juvenile rheumatoid arthritis or sarcoid, tumor such as melanoma or retinoblastoma)
  - Traumatic (e.g., heat, electric shock, radiation, concussion, perforating eye injuries, intraocular foreign body)
  - Toxic/Nutritional (e.g., corticosteroids)
- Morphologic classification:
  - Nuclear: Exaggeration of normal aging changes of *central* lens nucleus, often associated with myopia due to increased refractive index of lens (some elderly patients consequently may be able to read again *without spectacles*, so-called 2nd sight of the aged)
  - Cortical: Outer portion of lens; may involve anterior, posterior, or equatorial cortex; radial, spoke-like opacities
  - Subcapsular: Posterior subcapsular cataract has more profound effect on vision than nuclear or cortical cataract; patients particularly troubled under conditions of miosis; near vision frequently impaired more than distance vision
- System(s) affected: Nervous

Geriatric Considerations
Some degree of cataract formation is expected in all people >70 years of age

Pediatric Considerations
See "Congenital Cataract"; may present as leukocoria

Pregnancy Considerations
See "Congenital Cataract" (i.e., medications, metabolic dysfunction, intrauterine infection, and malnutrition)

EPIDEMIOLOGY
Incidence
- ~48% of the 37 million cases of blindness worldwide result from cataracts
- Leading cause of treatable blindness and vision loss in developing countries
- Predominant age: Depends on type of cataract
- Predominant sex: Male > Female

Prevalence
- Cataract type and prevalence highly variable based on population demographic
- An estimated 50% of people 65–74 years of age and 70% of people >75 years of age have age-related cataract

ETIOLOGY AND PATHOPHYSIOLOGY
- Age-related cataract:
  - Continual addition of layers of lens fibers throughout life creates hard, dehydrated lens nucleus that impairs vision (nuclear cataract)
  - Aging alters biochemical and osmotic balance required for lens clarity; outer lens layers hydrate and become opaque, adversely affecting vision
- Congenital:
  - Usually unknown etiology
  - Drugs (corticosteroids in 1st trimester, sulfonamides)
  - Metabolic (diabetes in mother, galactosemia in fetus)
  - Intrauterine infection during 1st trimester (e.g., rubella, herpes, mumps)
  - Maternal malnutrition
- Other cataract types:
  - Common feature is a biochemical/osmotic imbalance that disrupts lens clarity
  - Local changes in lens protein distribution lead to light scattering (lens opacity)

Genetics
- Congenital (e.g., chromosomal disorders [Down syndrome])
- Genetics of age-related cataract not yet established, but likely multifactorial contribution (1,2)

RISK FACTORS
- Aging
- Cigarette smoking
- Ultraviolet (UV) sunlight exposure
- Diabetes
- Prolonged high-dose steroids
- Positive family history
- Alcohol

GENERAL PREVENTION
- Use of UV protective glasses (1,2)[A]
- Avoidance of tobacco products (1,2)[A]
- Effective control of diabetes (1,2)[A]
- Care with high-dose, long-term steroid use (systemic therapy > inhaled treatment) (2)[B]
- Protective methods using pharmaceutical intervention (e.g., antioxidants, acetylsalicylic acid [ASA], hormone replacement therapy [HRT]) show no proven benefit to date (1,2)[C]

COMMONLY ASSOCIATED CONDITIONS
- Diabetes (especially with poor glucose control)
- Myotonic dystrophy (90% of patients develop visually innocuous change in 3rd decade; becomes disabling in 5th decade)
- Atopic dermatitis (AD) (10% of patients with severe AD develop cataracts in 2nd–4th decades, often bilateral)
- Neurofibromatosis type 2
- Associated ocular disease or "secondary cataract" (e.g., chronic anterior uveitis, acute [or repetitive] angle-closure glaucoma or high myopia)
- Drug-induced (e.g., steroids, chlorpromazine)
- Trauma

 DIAGNOSIS

HISTORY
- Age-related cataract:
  - Decreased visual acuity, blurred vision, distortion, or "ghosting" of images
  - Problems with visual acuity in any lighting condition
  - Falls or accidents; injuries (e.g., hip fracture)
- Congenital: Often asymptomatic, leukocoria, parents notice child's visual inattention or strabismus
- Other types of cataract:
  - May also present with decreased visual acuity
  - Appropriate clinical history or signs to help with diagnosis

PHYSICAL EXAM
- Visual acuity assessment for all cataracts
- Age-related cataract: Lens opacity on eye examination
- Congenital:
  - Lens opacity present at birth or within 3 months of birth
  - Leukocoria (white pupil), strabismus, nystagmus, signs of associated syndrome (as with Down or rubella syndrome)
  - *Note:* Must always rule out ocular tumor; early diagnosis and treatment of retinoblastoma may be life saving
- Other types of cataract: May present with decreased visual acuity associated with characteristic physical findings (e.g., metabolic, trauma)

DIFFERENTIAL DIAGNOSIS
- An opaque-appearing eye may be due to opacities of the cornea (e.g., scarring, edema, calcification), lens opacities, tumor, or retinal detachment. Biomicroscopic examination (slit lamp) or careful ophthalmoscopic exam should provide diagnosis.
- In the elderly, visual impairment is often due to multiple factors, such as cataract and macular degeneration, both contributing to visual loss.
- Age-related cataract is significant if symptoms and ophthalmic exam support cataract as a major cause of vision impairment.
- Congenital lens opacity in the absence of other ocular pathology may cause severe amblyopia.
- *Note:* Cataract *does not* produce a relative afferent pupillary reaction defect. Abnormal pupillary reactions mandate further evaluation for other pathology.

DIAGNOSTIC TESTS & INTERPRETATION
- Visual quality assessment: Glare testing, contrast sensitivity sometimes indicated
- Retinal/Macular function assessment: Potential acuity meter testing
- Workup of underlying process

Test Interpretation
Consistent with lens changes found in the type of cataract; however, diagnosis is made by clinical examination

TREATMENT

- Outpatient (usually) (3)
- ~1.64 million cataract extractions in the US yearly

GENERAL MEASURES
Eye protection from UV light

MEDICATION
There are currently no medications to prevent or slow the progression of cataracts.

ISSUES FOR REFERRAL
If patient has cataract and symptoms do not seem to support recommended surgery, a 2nd opinion by another ophthalmologist may be indicated

SURGERY/OTHER PROCEDURES
- Age-related cataract:
  - Surgical removal is indicated if visual impairment–producing symptoms are distressing to the patient, interfering with lifestyle or occupation, or posing a risk for fall or injury
  - Because significant cataract may develop gradually, the patient may not be aware of how it has changed his or her lifestyle. Physician may note a significant cataract, and patient reports "no problems." Thus, evaluation requires effective physician–patient exchange of information.
  - Surgical technique: Cataract extraction via small incisions, followed by implantation of a prosthetic intraocular lens; lenses have power calculated based on size of the eye and curvature of cornea usually to correct for distance vision; surgery performed on 1 (worse) eye, with contralateral surgery only after recovery and if deemed necessary; generally takes <1 hour depending on surgical technique
  - Anesthesia: Usually regional injection or topical with sedation and monitoring of vital signs
  - Preoperative evaluation: By the primary care physician:
    ○ Patients on anticoagulants may need to be temporarily discontinued 1–2 weeks before surgery if possible (but not always necessary; thus, need to discuss with ophthalmologist)
    ○ Patients who have ever taken an α-blocker such as tamsulosin (Flomax) should alert their ophthalmologist (increased risk of intraoperative floppy iris syndrome [IFIS] even in patients who no longer use these drugs)
  - Postoperative care: Usually protective eye shield as directed, topical antibiotic, and steroid ophthalmic medications; avoid lifting or bending over for a few weeks
- Congenital cataract:
  - Treatment is surgical removal of cataract. Newborns may require surgery within days to reduce risk of severe amblyopia. Use of lens implants is controversial
  - Postoperative care: Long-term patching program for good eye to combat amblyopia; refractive correction of operative eye, with multiple repeat examinations; challenging for physician and parents

ONGOING CARE

FOLLOW-UP RECOMMENDATIONS
Patient Monitoring
- As cataract progresses, an ophthalmologist may change spectacle correction to maintain vision. When this is no longer successful and interferes with patient's activities of daily living, surgery is indicated.
- Following surgery, spectacle correction may be required to maximize near and/or far visual acuity. Refraction is usually prescribed several weeks after surgery.

PATIENT EDUCATION
Medline Plus on Cataracts at: www.nlm.nih.gov/medlineplus/cataract.html

PROGNOSIS
- Ocular prognosis good after cataract removal if no prior or co-existing ocular disease: 94.3% of otherwise healthy eyes achieve best corrected visual acuity of 20/40 or better. Success rates are lower with comorbidities such as diabetes and glaucoma (4).
- In congenital cataracts, prognosis often is poorer because of the high risk of amblyopia.

COMPLICATIONS
- Vary widely from delay in visual recovery or protracted visual discomfort to blindness and loss of eye
- Nearly all reported complications occur rarely (<2% of eyes) except for posterior capsule opacification (14.7–42.7% of eyes, usually treated with Nd-YAG laser capsulotomy in office with a rate of 4–25.3%) (5,6)[A].

REFERENCES

1. Asbell PA, Dualan I, Mindel J, et al. Age-related cataract. *Lancet*. 2005;365:599–609.
2. Abraham AG, Condon NG, Gower EW. The new epidemiology of cataract. *Ophthalmol Clin North Am*. 2006;19:415–425.
3. Fedorowicz Z, Lawrence D, Gutierrez P. Day care versus in-patient surgery for age-related cataract. *Cochrane Database Syst Rev*. 2005;1:CD004242.
4. Lundström M, Barry P, Henry Y, et al. Visual outcome of cataract surgery; study from the European Registry of Quality Outcomes for Cataract and Refractive Surgery. *J Cataract Refract Surg*. 2013;39:679.
5. Findl O, Buehl W, Bauer P, et al. Interventions for preventing posterior capsule opacification. *Cochrane Database Syst Rev*. 2010;2:CD003738.
6. Biber JM, Sandoval HP, Trivedi RH, et al. Comparison of the incidence and visual significance of posterior capsule opacification between multifocal spherical, monofocal spherical, and monofocal aspheric intraocular lenses. *J Cataract Refract Surg*. 2009;35:1234–1238.

ADDITIONAL READING

Riaz Y, Mehta JS, Wormald R, et al. Surgical interventions for age-related cataract. *Cochrane Database Syst Rev*. 2006;4:CD001323.

SEE ALSO

- Algorithm: Cataracts
- Floppy Iris Syndrome

CODES

ICD10
- E13.36 Other specified diabetes mellitus with diabetic cataract
- H25.9 Unspecified age-related cataract
- H26.9 Unspecified cataract

CLINICAL PEARLS

- Cataracts are the leading cause of blindness worldwide; 90% are age-related.
- Primary indication for cataract surgery is visual impairment leading to significant lifestyle changes for the patient.
- For congenital cataracts, must always rule out ocular tumor, since early diagnosis and treatment of retinoblastoma may be life saving.
- Before prescribing an α-blocker for an older adult with hypertension or a prostate or urinary retention problem, consider whether the patient has cataracts (due to increased risk of IFIS).

C

CELIAC DISEASE

Suma Chennubhotla, MD • Amaninderapal Singh Ghotra, MD • Thomas L. Abell, MD

BASICS

DESCRIPTION
- An autoimmune disease characterized by an immune-based reaction to dietary gluten (found in wheat, barley, rye), primarily affecting the small intestine in genetically predisposed individuals:
  - Seen primarily in people of Northern European ancestry.
- NOT a food allergy.
- Celiac presentations:
  - Typical:
    ○ Classically a diarrheal illness characterized by villous atrophy with symptoms of malabsorption (steatorrhea, weight loss, vitamin deficiencies, anemia) with resolution of symptoms with a gluten-free diet.
  - Atypical:
    ○ Only minor GI symptoms, but a myriad of extraintestinal symptoms (e.g., anemia, dental enamel defects, neurologic symptoms, infertility)
  - Asymptomatic (silent) disease:
    ○ Found when screening 1st-degree relatives
  - Latent:
    ○ Positive laboratory tests and genetics, without signs/symptoms
- System(s) affected: Gastrointestinal
- Synonym(s): Celiac sprue; Gluten enteropathy; Sprue

EPIDEMIOLOGY
Incidence
- Disease primarily of individuals of Northern European ancestry
- Predominant sex: Female > Male (3:2)

Prevalence
- ~1/133–160 persons in the US (1)
- An estimated 3 million Americans have celiac disease.
- Prevalence is increasing worldwide.

ETIOLOGY AND PATHOPHYSIOLOGY
Sensitivity to gluten, specifically gliadin fraction. Damage to villi when exposed to gluten due to autoimmune reaction. Subsequent malabsorption.

Genetics
Homogenicity for *HLA-DQ2* increases the risk of celiac disease and enteropathy associated T-cell lymphoma.

RISK FACTORS
- 1st-degree relatives: 5–10% incidence (2)
- Monozygotic twins: 70% incidence
- 25% in family member with an autoimmune disease

GENERAL PREVENTION
Avoid all gluten-containing products (wheat, barley, rye, and possibly oat products).

COMMONLY ASSOCIATED CONDITIONS
- *Dermatitis herpetiformis*: Very strong association with celiac disease (3); 85% of patients have celiac disease. All patients should follow gluten-free diet.
- Secondary lactase deficiency
- Marked decrease in bone density
- Thyroid disease: Hashimoto's thyroiditis
- Diabetes, type 1: 3–10% of patients have celiac disease.
- Elevated AST and ALT (with no direct cause)
- Recurrent fetal loss/infertility
- Irritable bowel syndrome (IBS)
- Restless leg syndrome

- GI lymphoma: Celiac disease is associated with both Hodgkin and non-Hodgkin lymphomas:
  - Particular increase in prevalence of T-cell non-Hodgkin lymphoma (4)
  - Recent studies show the risk of lymphoproliferative malignancies in celiac disease is dependent on small intestinal histopathology.
  - There appears to be little to no increased risk in latent celiac disease (seropositive, but normal biopsy) (5)[C].
- Migraine (more prevalent in patients with celiac disease) (6).
- Addison's disease, Turner's syndrome, Reynaud's syndrome
- Autoimmune disorders: SLE, RA, scleroderma, Sjögren's syndrome

Pregnancy Considerations
- Celiac disease may be an under appreciated cause of male and female infertility.
- Consider celiac disease in pregnant women with severe anemia.

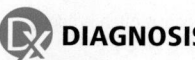

DIAGNOSIS

HISTORY
- Diarrhea, cramping, gas pains
- Steatorrhea (fatty stools)
- Muscle cramps
- Iron-deficiency anemia
- Nervousness, depression
- Weight loss
- Failure to thrive (slowing velocity of weight gain)
- Weakness, fatigue, lassitude
- Explosive flatulence
- Abdominal pain, nausea, vomiting
- Recurrent aphthous stomatitis
- Abdominal distention
- Delayed puberty
- Tingling numbness in hands, feet
- Bone or joint pain
- Migraines

Pediatric Considerations
Failure to thrive and delayed growth with short stature may be early manifestations. A few children may outgrow intolerance to wheat after prolonged gluten-free diets, but should be cautioned to watch for signs of recurrence in middle age.

PHYSICAL EXAM
Often normal, but look for:
- Oropharynx: Aphthous stomatitis
- Skin: *Dermatitis herpetiformis* (excoriations, symmetric erythematous papules and blisters on elbows, knees, buttocks, and back)
- Abdomen: Distention

DIFFERENTIAL DIAGNOSIS
- Short bowel syndrome
- Dyspepsia, GERD
- Pancreatic insufficiency
- Crohn disease
- Whipple disease
- Hypogammaglobulinemia
- Tropical sprue
- Lymphoma
- AIDS
- Acute enteritis

- Giardiasis
- Eosinophilic gastroenteritis
- Pancreatic disease

DIAGNOSTIC TESTS & INTERPRETATION
Initial Tests (lab, imaging)
In general, diagnosis should not be made based on serology alone.
- IgA antiendomysial antibodies (IgA EmA)
- IgA antitissue transglutaminase (IgA- anti-TTG)
- Total serum IgA

ALERT
Positive IgA anti-endomysial antibodies and IgA tissue transglutaminase have high sensitivity and specificity (sensitivity, 90–98%; specificity, 98%) when on normal (non–gluten-free) diet for at least 4 weeks:
- IgA-deficient patients have false–negative IgA anti-endomysial and IgA antitransglutaminase antibodies.
- Selective IgA deficiency is 10–15× more prevalent in patients with celiac (vs. the general population):
  - This can delay diagnosis due to "negative" IgA anti-endomysial antibody testing.
- The TTG antibody test is the preferred test (over the deamidated gliadin peptide [DGP] antibody) (7,8)[A].
- Assessment of symptoms, risk, predisposition, then antibody tests (anti-TTG antibody is gold standard)

Follow-Up Tests & Special Considerations
- If patient is IgA deficient OR if IgA EMA and IgA anti-TTG are negative, follow up blood tests:
  - Anti-deaminated gliadin peptide (DGP – IgA and IgG):
    ○ Sensitivity, 94%; specificity, 99% (similar to anti-TTG) (9)
- Antigliadin antibody (AgA – IgG and IgA):
  - Not considered sufficiently sensitive/specific for adults

Pediatric Considerations
- Antigliadin antibody (AgA–IgG and IgA) may be used for children age <2 because TTG and EMA antibodies may be absent.
- Anti-DGP test is sensitive in this group.
- 72-hour fecal fat showing >7% fat malabsorption
- Elevated LFT results
- d-Xylose test showing malabsorption
- Decreased calcium
- Increased prothrombin time (PT)
- Decreased neutral fats
- Decreased cholesterol
- Decreased vitamin A
- Decreased vitamin B$_{12}$ (rare)
- Decreased vitamin D
- Decreased vitamin C
- Decreased folic acid
- Decreased iron (common)
- Decreased total protein
- Decreased hemoglobin (common)

Follow-Up Tests & Special Considerations
Evaluate for osteoporosis.

C

Diagnostic Procedures/Other
- *Endoscopy with multiple diagnostic biopsies of the duodenal mucosa with repeat endoscopy and normal biopsy on a gluten-free diet is necessary before a firm diagnosis can be made (2).*
- Although endoscopy with small bowel biopsy is the gold standard for confirmation, recent studies suggest that video capsule endoscopy is an alternative, particularly when antibody screening and the clinical picture are consistent with celiac disease, even if duodenal biopsies are nondiagnostic (10)[A].

Test Interpretation
Small bowel biopsy:
- Flattened villi/villous atrophy, hyperplasia and lengthening of crypts, infiltration of plasma cells, and intraepithelial lymphocytosis in lamina propria

TREATMENT

GENERAL MEASURES
- Removal of gluten from the diet:
  – Rice, corn, and soybean flour are safe, palatable substitutes.
- Levels of IgA antigliadin normalize with gluten abstinence.
- LIFELONG abstinence is required; immune response to gluten will recur with resumption of gluten consumption.

MEDICATION
First Line
Usually no medications: Gluten-free diet is the treatment.

Second Line
- In refractory disease, consider:
  – Steroids (prednisone, 40–60 mg/d PO in cases of refractory sprue)
  – Azathioprine (immunosuppressants should be used with caution; use may lead to lymphoma in celiac disease).
  – Cyclosporine
  – Infliximab
  – Cladribine
- Patients may require supplemental calcium, calcium carbonate, 500 mg PO b.i.d., and vitamin D (ergocalciferol).

ISSUES FOR REFERRAL
- Additional nutritional support
- Refractory disease

ONGOING CARE

FOLLOW-UP RECOMMENDATIONS
- Consultation with registered dietitian
- Screening for osteoporosis

Patient Monitoring
- Repeat EGD in 1 year on a gluten-free diet to document normalization of villi.
- Increased intraepithelial lymphocytes may persist for up to 5 years after initial diagnosis, in some cases may persist indefinitely even with symptom resolution.
- Follow anti-TTG IgA or deaminated antigliadin antibodies as a measure of response/compliance with diet (vs. antigliadin IgA or IgG).

DIET
- Removal of gluten: Wheat, rye, barley, and those with gluten additives.

- This can be a challenging diet (especially learning sources of "hidden" gluten) and should be coordinated with a skilled registered dietitian.

PATIENT EDUCATION
- Discuss importance of recognizing gluten in various products.
- Highlight potential complications and outcomes of failing to follow a gluten-free diet.

PROGNOSIS
- Good prognosis with correct diagnosis and adherence to gluten-free diet.
- Patient should feel better within 7 days of compliance with diet.
- All symptoms usually disappear in 4–6 weeks.
- It is unknown whether strict dietary adherence decreases cancer risk.

COMPLICATIONS
- Malignancy: <10% of patients (50% of whom develop small bowel lymphoma)
- Refractory sprue:
  – May respond to prednisone 40–60 mg/d PO
  – Refractory sprue unresponsive to corticosteroid therapy raises the specter of adult-onset autoimmune enteropathy or cryptic T-cell lymphoma. In this circumstance, screening for anti-enterocyte autoantibodies and careful scrutiny of the small intestine, including retroperitoneal lymph node biopsy with full-thickness small bowel biopsy, may be needed.
- Chronic ulcerative jejunoileitis:
  – Associated with multiple ulcers, intestinal bleeding, strictures, perforation, obstruction, and peritonitis
  – 7% mortality
- Osteoporosis secondary to decreased vitamin D and calcium absorption
- Dehydration
- Electrolyte depletion
- Refractory cases may need total parenteral nutrition.

REFERENCES

1. Biagi F, Klersy C, Balduzzi D, et al. Are we not over-estimating the prevalence of coeliac disease in the general population? *Ann Med.* 2010;42: 557–561.
2. Rubio-Tapia A, Hill I, Kelly C, et al. ACG Clinical Guidelines: Diagnosis and management of celiac disease. *Am J Gastroenterol.* 2013;108:656–676; published online 16 April 2013.
3. Bolotin D, Petronic-Rosic V. Dermatitis herpetiformis. Part II. Diagnosis, management, and prognosis. *J Am Acad Dermatol.* 2011;64: 1027–1033.
4. Tio M, Cox MR, Eslick GD. Meta-analysis: Coeliac disease and the risk of all-cause mortality, any malignancy and lymphoid malignancy. *Aliment Pharmacol Ther.* 2012;84(5):540–551. Epub 2012 Jan 13.
5. Elfström P, Granath F, Ekström Smedby K, et al. Risk of lymphoproliferative malignancy in relation to small intestinal histopathology among patients with celiac disease. *J Natl Cancer Inst.* 2011;103: 436–444.
6. Dimitrova AK, Ungaro RC, Lebwohl B, et al. Prevalence of migraine in patients with celiac disease and inflammatory bowel disease. *Headache.* 2012;Nov 5. Epub 2012 Nov 5.
7. Lewis NR, Scott BB. Meta-analysis: Deaminated gliadin peptide antibody and tissue

transglutaminase antibody compared as screening tests for coeliac disease. *Aliment Pharmacol Ther.* 2010;31:73–81.
8. van der Windt DA, Jellema P, Mulder CJ, et al. Diagnostic testing for celiac disease among patients with abdominal symptoms: A systematic review. *JAMA.* 2010;303:1738–1746.
9. Sugai E, Vázquez H, Nachman F, et al. Accuracy of testing for antibodies to synthetic gliadin-related peptides in celiac disease. *Clin Gastroenterol Hepatol.* 2006;84(9):1112–1117. Epub 2006 Jul 24.
10. Rokkas T, Niv Y. The role of video capsule endoscopy in the diagnosis of celiac disease: A meta-analysis. *Eur J Gastroenterol Hepatol.* 2012;84(3):303–308.

ADDITIONAL READING
- AGA Institute. AGA Institute Medical Position Statement on the Diagnosis and Management of Celiac Disease. *Gastroenterology.* 2006;131: 1977–1980.
- Celiac Disease Foundation. Guidelines for a Gluten-free Lifestyle, 3rd ed. http://www.celiac.org.
- Celiac Sprue Association (CSA) http://www.csaceliacs.org.
- Giersiepen K, Lelgemann M, Stuhldreher N, et al. Accuracy of diagnostic antibody tests for coeliac disease in children: Summary of an evidence report. *J Pediatr Gastroenterol Nutr.* 2012;84(2):229–241.
- Green PHR, Jones R. *Celiac Disease: A Hidden Epidemic.* New York: HarperCollins; 2006.
- Prince HE. Evaluation of the INOVA diagnostics enzyme-linked immunosorbent assay kits for measuring serum immunoglobulin G (IgG) and IgA to deamidated gliadin peptides. *Clin Vaccine Immunol.* 2006;13(1):150–151.
- Quick Start Diet Guide: Celiac Disease Foundation (CDF) & Gluten Intolerance Group (GIG): http://www.celiac.org,http://www.gluten.net.
- Rozenberg O, Lerner A, Pacht A, et al. A novel algorithm for the diagnosis of celiac disease and a comprehensive review of celiac disease diagnostics. *Clin Rev Allergy Immunol.* 2012;42(3):331–341.

 SEE ALSO

Algorithms: Diarrhea, Chronic; Malabsorption Syndrome

 CODES

ICD10
K90.0 Celiac disease

CLINICAL PEARLS
- Increasingly common condition; may not be associated with diarrhea
- Definitive treatment is gluten-free diet, and patient should improve within 7 days if fully compliant with GF diet.
- Test for celiac disease in patients with presumed IBS or *Dermatitis herpetiformis*.
- Test IgA levels along with IgA anti-endomysial antibodies and anti-TTG antibodies.
- Positive serology alone is not sufficient to ascertain diagnosis; must have multiple small bowel biopsies via endoscopy.

CELLULITIS

Jowhara Al-Qahtani, MD • Amer Homsi, MD • Bakr Nour, MD, FACS

BASICS

DESCRIPTION
- An acute bacterial skin and skin-structure infection (ABSSI) of the dermis and subcutaneous tissue; commonly characterized by pain, erythema, warmth, and swelling:
  - Periorbital cellulitis: Bacterial infection of the eyelid and surrounding tissues (anterior compartment)
  - Orbital cellulitis: Infection of the eye posterior to the septum; sinusitis is the most common risk factor.
  - Facial cellulitis: Preceded by upper respiratory infection or otitis media
  - Buccal cellulitis: Infection of cheek in children associated with bacteremia (common before *Haemophilus influenzae* type B vaccine)
  - Peritonsillar cellulitis: Common in children associated with fever, sore throat, and "hot potato" speech
  - Abdominal wall cellulitis: Common in morbidly obese
  - Perianal cellulitis: Sharply demarcated, bright, perianal erythema
  - Necrotizing cellulitis: Gas-producing bacteria in the lower extremities; common in diabetics
- System(s) affected: Skin/Exocrine

EPIDEMIOLOGY
Predominant sex: Male = Female (common in elderly and adults, except perianal cellulitis which is common in children)

Incidence
200/100,000 patient-years

Prevalence
Unknown

ETIOLOGY AND PATHOPHYSIOLOGY
Cellulitis is caused by bacterial penetration through a break in the skin. Hyaluronidase mediates subcutaneous (SC) spread.
Microbiology:

- β-hemolytic streptococci (groups A, B, C, G, and F), *Staphylococcus aureus*, including MRSA and gram-negative aerobic bacilli (accounts for 27% and 51%, respectively) (1)[A]

- *S. aureus*: Periorbital and orbital cellulitis and IV drug users
- *Pseudomonas aeruginosa*: Diabetics and other immunocompromised patients
- *Aeromonas hydrophila* and *Vibrio vulnificus*: Cellulitis caused by waterborne pathogens
- *Haemophilus influenzae*: Buccal cellulitis
- Clostridia and non–spore-forming anaerobes: Necrotizing cellulitis (crepitant/gangrenous)
- *Streptococcus agalactiae*: Cellulitis following lymph node dissection
- *Pasteurella multocida* and *Capnocytophaga canimorsus*: Cellulitis preceded by bites
- *Streptococcus iniae*: Immunocompromised hosts
- Rare causes: Mycobacterium, fungal (mucormycosis, aspergillosis, syphilis)

Genetics
No genetic pattern

RISK FACTORS
- Disruption to skin barrier: Trauma, infection, insect bites, and injection drug use

- Inflammation: Eczema or radiation therapy
- Edema due to venous insufficiency, and lymphatic obstruction due to surgical procedures
- Increased risk factor: Elderly, diabetes, hypertension, obesity (1)
- Recurrent cellulitis: Immunocompromised, diabetes, hypertension, cancer, peripheral arterial or venous diseases, chronic kidney disease, dialysis, IV or SC drug use

GENERAL PREVENTION
- Maintain good skin hygiene
- Wear support stockings to decrease edema
- Maintain tight glycemic control and proper foot care for diabetics

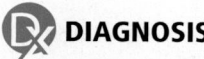

DIAGNOSIS

Mostly clinical diagnosis; high index of suspicion

HISTORY
- Previous trauma, surgery, or animal/human bites, dermatitis, fungal infection, all may serve as a portal of entry for bacterial pathogens
- Patient will often complain of pain, itching and/or burning
- Fever, chills, and malaise

PHYSICAL EXAM
- Localized pain and tenderness to touch with notable erythema, induration, swelling, and warmth
- Peau d'orange appearance
- Regional lymphadenopathy of the face, periorbital region, neck, or extremities
- Purulent drainage from abscesses
- Orbital cellulitis: Proptosis, globe displacement, limitation of ocular movements, vision loss, diplopia
- Facial cellulitis: Malaise, anorexia, vomiting, pruritus, burning, anterior neck swelling

DIFFERENTIAL DIAGNOSIS
Toxic shock syndrome, venous stasis dermatitis (commonly mistaken as cellulitis), bursitis, acute dermatitis or intertrigo, herpes zoster or herpetic Whitlow, deep vein thrombosis or thrombophlebitis, acute gout or pseudogout, necrotizing fasciitis or myositis, gas gangrene, osteomyelitis, erythema chronicum migrans or malignancy, drug reaction, sunburn, or insect stings

DIAGNOSTIC TESTS & INTERPRETATION
Initial Tests (lab, imaging)
- For signs of systemic disease (fever, heart rate >100 bpm, or systolic blood pressure <90 mm Hg): Blood cultures, CPK, CRP (2)[C]. Consider serum lactate levels.

- WBC has 84.5% specificity and 43.0% sensitivity whereas CRP had a sensitivity of 67.1% and specificity of 94.8% (PPV 94.65 and NPV 67.9%) (1)[A]

- Aspirates from point of maximum inflammation yield 45% positive culture compared with 5% from leading edge
- Blood cultures: Pathogens isolated in <5% of patients. Blood cultures in children are more likely to show a contaminant than true positive.

- CREST guidelines recommend wound swabs on open cellulitis wound (1)[A].

- Plain radiographs, CT, or MRI useful if osteomyelitis, fracture, necrotizing fasciitis, or retained foreign body is suspected or underlying abscess
- Gallium[67] scintillography is helpful for detecting cellulitis superimposed on recently increasing chronic lymphedema of a limb

Diagnostic Procedures/Other
Lumbar puncture should be considered for children with *H. influenzae* type B or if meningeal signs and facial cellulitis.

TREATMENT

GENERAL MEASURES
- Immobilization and elevation of the involved limb to reduce swelling
- Sterile saline dressings or cool aluminum acetate compresses for pain relief
- Edema: Compression stocking, pneumatic pumps, and diuretic therapy
- Steroids (prednisone 0.5 mg/kg/d for 5–8 days) if partial response to antibiotics in hemorrhagic or bullous cellulitis
- Mark the area of cellulitis to monitor its progress and assist the efficacy of the antibiotics regimen
- Tetanus immunization if needed

MEDICATION
First Line
- Treatment should be modified as indicated in the setting of known pathogens, underlying conditions such as diseases, or certain exposure like animal bites.
- Antibiotics selection relies on clinical presentation of purulent vs. nonpurulent:
  - Nonpurulent cellulitis
    - With nonpurulent drainage, treatment should be targeted towards β-hemolytic streptococci and methicillin-sensitive *S. aureus* (MSSA)
    - Outpatient: Cover for β-hemolytic streptococci and MSSA (3)[A],(4)[A]:
      - Oral: For mild cellulitis
        - Cephalexin 500 mg PO q6h 25–50 mg/kg/d in 3–4 doses
        - Dicloxacillin 500 mg PO q6h 25–50 mg/kg/d in 4 doses
        - Clindamycin 300–450 mg PO q6–8h 20–30 mg/kg/d in 4 doses
      - IV: For rapidly progressing cellulitis:
        - Cefazolin 1–2 g q8h 100 mg/kg/d
        - Oxacillin 2 g q4h 150–200 mg/kg/d in 4–6 doses
        - Nafcillin 2 g q4h 150–200 mg/kg/d in 4–6 doses
        - Clindamycin 600–900 mg q8h 25–40 mg/kg/d in 3–4 doses
  - Purulent cellulitis (probable community-acquired (CA)-MRSA):
    - Culture should be taken of all purulent wounds and followed up in 48 hours
    - If suspected CA-MRSA is a concern, management entails: Incision and drainage of abscess, empiric antibiotic therapy followed by culture-based therapy (5–10 days); duration should be individualized to patient outcome:
      - Oral:
        - Clindamycin 300–450 mg PO; 40 mg/kg/d in 3–4 doses

□ Trimethoprim-sulfamethoxazole (TMP-SMZ) 1 DS tab PO b.i.d. (TMP at 8–12 mg/kg/d)
□ Doxycycline 100 mg PO b.i.d.; ≤45 kg: 4 mg/kg/d; 100 mg PO b.i.d. PO
□ Minocycline 200 mg PO once, then 100 mg PO; 4 mg/kg PO once, then 4 mg/kg b.i.d.
□ Linezolid 600 mg PO b.i.d.; <12 years: 30 mg/kg/d PO t.i.d.; ≥12 years: 600 mg PO b.i.d.
▪ IV:
  □ Vancomycin 30 mg/kg IV q24h in 2 equally divided doses; not to exceed 2 g/24 hours unless therapeutic concentration in serum are low
  □ Daptomycin 4 mg/kg IV once daily if bacteremia is present or suspected 6 mg/kg IV once daily
  □ Linezolid 600 mg IV b.i.d.
  □ Ceftaroline 600 mg IV q12h
  □ Tigecycline 100 mg IV once, thereafter 50 mg IV q12h
– Necrotizing cellulitis: Clostridial and anaerobic, requires broad-spectrum coverage: Ampicillin-sulbactam 1.5–3.0 g q6–8h IV or piperacillin-tazobactam 3.37 g q6–8h IV plus ciprofloxacin 400 mg q12h IV plus clindamycin 600–900 mg/kg q8h IV
– In patients with recurrent infection underlying predisposing conditions, previous episode of proven MRSA infection, or systemic toxicity. Patients should be educated on personal hygiene and proper wound care. Use agents with activity against MRSA as outlined above.
– Uncomplicated, MSSA or streptococcal etiology: Penicillinase-resistant semisynthetic penicillin or a 1st-generation cephalosporin should be selected as recommended by the Infectious Diseases Society of America (2)[A]. 5-day therapy is as effective as 10 days (5)[B]:
  ○ Oral:
    ▪ Dicloxacillin 500 mg q.i.d. PO 25 mg/kg/d in 4 divided doses
  ○ IV:
    ▪ Nafcillin or oxacillin 1–2 g q4h IV 100–150 mg/kg/d in 4 divided doses
  ○ For penicillin-allergic patients, except those with immediate hypersensitivity reactions:
    ▪ Oral: Cephalexin 500 mg q.i.d. PO 25 mg/kg/d in 4 divided doses
    ▪ IV: Cefazolin 1 g q8h IV 50 mg/kg/d in 3 divided doses
– Freshwater exposure: Penicillinase-resistant: Penicillin plus gentamicin or fluoroquinolone. In salt water exposure: Doxycycline 200 mg IV in divided doses.
– Bites: The combination of amoxicillin and clavulanic acid has been shown to be effective in treating human bites and dog bites. Cefoxitin or the combination of penicillin or a 1st-generation cephalosporin plus a β-lactamase-resistant penicillin or the combination of ticarcillin and clavulanic acid will provide adequate parenteral therapy for animal or human bites (6)[B]. If mild allergy to penicillin, use cefoxitin or carbapenems. For severe penicillin reactions, use doxycycline, TMP/SMX, or a fluoroquinolone plus clindamycin.
– Facial cellulitis in adults: Cefotaxime IV

– Diabetic foot infection: Ampicillin/Sulbactam 3 g IV q6h or imipenem/cilastatin, or meropenem. Alternative: Combinations of targeting anaerobes as well as gram-positive and gram-negative aerobes
– Severe infection, toxicity, immunocompromised patients, or worsening infection despite empirical therapy. Patient should be admitted, and empiric antibiotic therapy covering MRSA as listed above should be started immediately.
– Recurrent streptococcal cellulitis: Penicillin IV 250 mg b.i.d., or if penicillin-allergic, use erythromycin 250 mg b.i.d.

Pediatric Considerations
• Avoid doxycycline in children ≤8 years old and during pregnancy.

• Nonpurulent: Stable without ongoing bacteremia or intravascular infection, empirical therapy with clindamycin 10–13 mg/kg/dose IV q6–8h (to administer 40 mg/kg/d) is an option if the clindamycin resistance rate is low (<10%) with transition to oral therapy if the strain is susceptibilized. Linezolid 600 mg PO/IV b.i.d. for children ≥12 years of age and 10 mg/kg/dose PO/IV q8h for children <12 years of age is an alternative (4)[A]

Second Line
Mild infection:
• Penicillin allergy: Erythromycin 500 mg PO q6h
• Cephalexin remains a cost-effective therapy for outpatient management of cellulitis at current estimated MRSA levels.

SURGERY/OTHER PROCEDURES
• Debridement for gas and purulent matter
• Intubation or tracheotomy may be needed for cellulitis of the head or neck.

IN-PATIENT CONSIDERATIONS
Admission Criteria/Initial Stabilization
• Severe infection, suspicion of deeper or rapidly spreading infection, tissue necrosis, or severe pain
• Marked systemic toxicity or worsening symptoms that do not resolve after 24–48 hours of therapy
• Patients with underlying risk factors or severe comorbidities

 ## ONGOING CARE
FOLLOW-UP RECOMMENDATIONS
Patient Monitoring
• Repeat blood count if patient is toxic
• Repeat lumbar puncture in case of meningitis
• Consider prophylaxis of deep vein thrombosis
• Cutaneous inflammation may worsen in 1st 24 hours due to release of bacterial antigens. Symptomatic improvement usually occurs in 24–48 hours, but visible improvement may take up to 72 hours.

DIET
Strict glucose control in diabetics

PATIENT EDUCATION
Practice good skin hygiene, especially with minor cuts, and report skin changes early.

PROGNOSIS
With adequate antibiotic treatment, prognosis is good.

COMPLICATIONS
• Local abscess or bacteremia
• Superinfection with gram-negative organisms
• Lymphangitis, especially if recurrent
• Thrombophlebitis or venous thrombosis
• Bacterial meningitis
• Gangrenous disorder

REFERENCES
1. Phoenix G, Das S, Joshi M. Diagnosis and management of cellulitis. BMJ. 2012;345:e4955.
2. Stevens DL, Bisno AL, Chambers HF, et al. Practice guidelines for the diagnosis and management of skin and soft-tissue infections. Clin Infect Dis. 2005;41:1373–1406.
3. Gunderson CG. Cellulitis: Definition, etiology, and clinical features. Am J Med. 2011;124:1113–1122.
4. Liu C, Bayer A, Cosgrove SE, et al. Clinical practice guidelines by the Infectious Diseases Society of America for the treatment of methicillin-resistant staphylococcus aureus infections in adults and children. Clin Infect Dis. 2011;52:1–38.
5. Hepburn MJ, Skidmore PJ, Starnes WF. Comparison of short-course (5 days) and standard (10 days) treatment for uncomplicated cellulitis. Arch Intern Med. 2004;164:1669–1674.
6. Brook I. Management of human and animal bite wounds: An overview. Adv Skin Wound Care. 2005;84:197–203.

ADDITIONAL READING
• Kilburn SA, Featherstone P, Higgins B, et al. Interventions for cellulitis and erysipelas. Cochrane Database Syst Rev. 2010;6:CD004299.
• Quirke M, O'Sullivan R, McCabe A, et al. Are two penicillins better than one? A systematic review of oral flucloxacillin and penicillin V versus oral flucloxacillin alone for the emergency department treatment of cellulitis. Eur J Emerg Med. 2013, in press.
• Swartz MN. Cellulitis. N Engl J Med. 2004;350:9.

CODES
CODE ICD-9 301

ICD10
• H05.019 Cellulitis of unspecified orbit
• L03.90 Cellulitis, unspecified
• L03.211 Cellulitis of face

CLINICAL PEARLS
• Staphylococcus aureus and group A Streptococcus cause most cases of cellulitis.
• Consider MRSA if cellulitis is not responding to antibiotics in the 1st 48 hours.
• Rapid expansion of infected area with red/purple discoloration and severe pain may suggest necrotizing fasciitis, requiring urgent surgical evaluation.

CELLULITIS, ORBITAL

Ellen Anderson Penno, MD, MS, Diplomate ABO, FRCSC

BASICS

DESCRIPTION
- Acute infection of orbital contents posterior to orbital septum, with edema and erythema of conjunctiva and eyelids
- Synonym(s): Postseptal cellulitis

ALERT
- Differentiating orbital from preseptal cellulitis is the critical diagnostic step.
- Diplopia, proptosis, vision loss, and fever suggest orbital involvement.
- Contrast CT is imaging method of choice.
- Treat with immediate IV antibiotics; ophthalmology referral; monitor frequently for vision loss, cavernous sinus thrombosis, abscess, and meningitis.
- Intraorbital foreign body (FB) may cause delayed orbital cellulitis.
- Metastatic tumors and autoimmune inflammation may masquerade as orbital cellulitis in rare cases.

EPIDEMIOLOGY
- More common in winter due to sinusitis incidence (1)[C].
- No frequency difference between the sexes in adults.
- More common in children; mean age of surgical pediatric cases: 10.1 years; medical pediatric cases: 6.1 years (2).
- *Haemophilus influenzae* type B (Hib) most common organism prior to Hib vaccine; *Staphylococcus* and *Streptococcus* spp. also common; >30% of cases culture negative
- Incidence of *Streptococcus anginosis* and methicillin-resistant *S. aureus* (MRSA) may be rising (3).

Incidence
Orbital cellulitis declined since Hib vaccine introduced in 1985. In 2000, incidence per 100,000 in California was 3.5 in whites, 6.1 in blacks, and 3.2 in Hispanics, compared to 6.5 in whites, 10.2 in blacks, and 5.5 in Hispanics in 1990.

ETIOLOGY AND PATHOPHYSIOLOGY
- Sinusitis is major risk factor due to thin medial orbital wall; upper respiratory infections, orbital trauma, orbital FB, orbital and periorbital surgery, bacteremia, and dental infections are risks.
- Cellulitis in closed bony orbit causes proptosis, globe displacement, orbital apex syndrome, optic nerve compression, and vision loss.
- Orbital abscess (medial wall common), meningitis, and cavernous sinus fibrosis may occur.
- Cultures in adults often grow multiple organisms, but >1/3 of cases have no pathogen recovered (3).
- Most common organisms (1,4)[C]:
  – *S. aureus, Streptococcus pneumoniae, Streptococcus anginosis*
- Less common organisms/precursor causes:
  – *Moraxella catarrhalis, H. influenza,* Group A β-hemolytic streptococcus, *Pseudomonas aeruginosa,* anaerobes, phycomycosis (mucormycosis), aspergillosis, *Mycobacterium tuberculosis, Mycobacterium avium* complex, trichinosis, echinococcus

- Since routine vaccination, *H. influenzae* B is no longer leading cause of orbital cellulitis (1,4)[B].

Genetics
No known genetic predisposition

RISK FACTORS
- Sinusitis present in 80–90% of cases (4)[C]
- Orbital trauma, retained orbital FB, ophthalmic surgery
- Dental, periorbital, skin, or intracranial infection; acute dacryocystitis and acute dacryoadenitis

GENERAL PREVENTION
- Appropriate treatment of bacterial sinusitis
- Proper wound care and perioperative monitoring of orbital surgery and trauma
- Hib vaccine
- High index of suspicion if fever present with eyelid and conjunctival erythema

COMMONLY ASSOCIATED CONDITIONS
- >80% of orbital cellulitis cases result from contiguous sinusitis.
- Trauma and intraorbital FB
- Preseptal cellulitis
- Diplopia
- Orbital apex syndrome, vision loss, abscess, meningitis, or cavernous sinus thrombosis
- Neutropenia and asthma are associated, but relationship is unclear.

DIAGNOSIS

- Differentiating preseptal cellulitis and orbital cellulitis on exam and imaging is key to management, with frequent monitoring for signs of abscess, meningitis, orbital apex syndrome, or cavernous sinus thrombosis.

- N. K. Chadha has proposed a new evidence-based staging in cases resulting from acute sinusitis (4)[A]:
  – Stage I: No abscess
  – Stage II a, b, c: Small, large, or extending medial subperiosteal abscess
  – Stage III: orbital abscess

- *Chandler staging is less widely used due to availability of imaging but remains most accepted method (5)[C]:*

  – Stage I: Periorbital cellulitis (considered different entity) (4)[B]

  – Stage II: Orbital lining edema, chemosis, proptosis, limitation of extraocular movement, fever
  – Stage III: Includes stage II with subperiosteal abscess and occasional vision loss
  – Stage IV: Orbital abscess, ophthalmoplegia with vision loss
  – Stage V: Extension to cavernous sinus, subdural space, meninges, or brain

HISTORY
- History of surgery, trauma, sinus or upper respiratory infection, dental infection
- Malaise, fever, stiff neck, vision loss, double vision, pain with eye movement, mental status changes
- Systemic immunosuppression or diabetes

ALERT
- Ophthalmoplegia, mental status changes, contralateral cranial nerve palsy, or bilateral orbital cellulitis may indicate CNS involvement.
- MRSA orbital cellulitis may present without associated upper respiratory infection.

PHYSICAL EXAM
- Exam should include:
  – Vital signs
  – Vision (with glasses if required)
  – Lid exam and palpation of the orbit
  – Pupil check for afferent pupillary defect
  – Extraocular movements
  – Red desaturation: Patient views red object with 1 eye and compares to the other; reduced red color may indicate optic nerve involvement.
  – Confrontation visual field
  – Critically ill may have limited abilities for testing.
  – Consult ophthalmology for slit lamp and dilated funduscopic exam; exophthalmometry measurement for proptosis, color vision, and automated visual field.
- Signs of orbital cellulitis include:
  – Proptosis, double vision, vision loss (or decreased field of vision), pain with eye movement, decreased color vision

DIFFERENTIAL DIAGNOSIS
- Preseptal cellulitis:
  – Eyelid erythema with or without conjunctival erythema, afebrile, no pain on eye movement, no diplopia, normal eye exam
- Idiopathic orbital inflammatory disease (orbital pseudotumor) (4)[C]:
  – Afebrile, normal WBCs; can be acute, may have pain, responds to steroids
- Orbital FB
- Arteriovenous fistula (carotid-cavernous fistula):
  – Spontaneous or due to trauma; bruit may be present
- Cavernous sinus thrombosis:
  – Signs of orbital cellulitis with cranial nerve 3, 4, 5, and 6 signs; often bilateral and acute
- Acute thyroid orbitopathy:
  – Afebrile; possible signs of thyroid disease
- Orbital tumor:
  – Acute rhabdomyosarcoma in children; acute lymphoblastic leukemia, or metastatic
- Trauma, insect bite, ruptured dermoid cyst

DIAGNOSTIC TESTS & INTERPRETATION
- CBC with differential, C-reactive protein, ESR
- Cultures from sinus aspirates and abscesses may grow multiple organisms.
- Cultures of eye secretions or nasopharyngeal aspirates often contaminated by normal flora, but may identify antibiotic-resistant organisms.
- Cultures from orbital and sinus abscesses more often yield positive results, but should be limited to cases where invasive procedures are indicated.
- Blood cultures should be obtained prior to initiation of antibiotic (4)[C] and lumbar puncture when indicated.

Initial Tests (lab, imaging)
Modality of choice is CT scan of orbits and sinuses with axial and coronal views, with and without contrast, to diagnose and screen for sinus disease, orbital FB, and abscess. To limit radiation exposure, bedside US imaging and MRI have been reported as alternatives (6)[B].

- Contrast CT is most widely used for evaluating orbital cellulitis (6)[B]:
  - Consider CT imaging if concern for Chandler Stage III or IV disease (6)[B].
  - Thin section (2 mm) CT, coronal and axial views with bone windows to differentiate periorbital from orbital cellulitis, confirm extension of inflammation into orbit, detect coexisting sinus disease, and identify orbital or subperiosteal abscesses
  - Deviation of medial rectus indicates intraorbital involvement.
- MRI offers superior resolution of soft-tissue infections for identification of cavernous sinus thrombosis but is less effective for bone imaging.
- US is used to rule out orbital myositis, locate FCBs or abscesses, and follow progression of drained abscess.

Follow-Up Tests & Special Considerations
- A full septic evaluation with lumbar puncture should be considered before antibiotic administration in toxic patients or if meningitis is suspected (5)[C].
- Frequent eye exam and vitals q4h is essential for early diagnosis and treatment of associated conditions, such as meningitis or abscess.

Diagnostic Procedures/Other
Neurology consult is needed in cases of suspected meningitis; otolaryngology consult for surgical management of sinus involvement.

 TREATMENT

Orbital cellulitis patients should be admitted for treatment and careful monitoring of ocular status, vitals, and signs of CNS involvement and IV broad-spectrum antibiotic treatment for gram-positive/-negative and anaerobic organisms for at least 1 week followed by PO antibiotics. Shorter duration for IV antibiotics may be effective.

MEDICATION
- Empiric antibiotic therapy at all ages should provide coverage for pathogens associated with acute sinusitis (S. pneumoniae, H. influenzae, M. catarrhalis, S. pyogenes), as well as for S. aureus, S. anginosis, and anaerobes.
- Modify IV antibiotic treatment when microbiological sensitivities return. Duration of IV therapy is usually a week, based on clinical picture.
- PO antibiotic therapy for 2–3 weeks or longer (3–6 weeks) is recommended for patients with severe sinusitis and bony destruction.

First Line
- Mainstay of therapy is broad-spectrum IV antibiotics for at least 1 week: Ampicillin/Sulbactam (Unasyn) or ceftriaxone plus metronidazole or clindamycin if anaerobic infection is suspected:
  - Ampicillin/Sulbactam: 3 g IV q6h for adult; 200–300 mg/kg/d divided q6h for children
  - Ceftriaxone: 1–2 g IV q12h for adults or 100 mg/kg/d divided b.i.d. in children with maximum 4 g/d
  - Clindamycin: 300 mg IV q6h for adults; 20–40 mg/kg/d IV q6–8h for children
  - Metronidazole: 30–35 mg/kg/d divided q8h
- In severe, culture-proven MRSA infection, vancomycin remains parenteral drug of choice:
  - Vancomycin: 1 g IV q12h for adults; 40 mg/kg/d IV divided q8–12h, max daily dose 2 g for children

ADDITIONAL THERAPIES
- *Steroid use is controversial* but may be recommended for orbital cellulitis secondary to sinusitis (4)[C].
- PO steroids as an adjunct to IV antibiotic therapy for orbital cellulitis may hasten resolution of inflammation with a low risk of exacerbating infection (7)[C].
- Topical erythromycin or nonmedicated ophthalmic ointment is needed to protect against exposure in cases with severe proptosis. Nasal decongestants may be indicated.
- PO antibiotics for ≥2 weeks are recommended following IV treatment although more recent studies report shorter durations may be effective. Children may be treated with amoxicillin/clavulanate 20–40 mg/kg/d divided t.i.d. or in adults 250–500 mg t.i.d. Cefaclor may be used 20–40 mg/kg/d, divided t.i.d. in children or 250–500 mg t.i.d. in adults.

ISSUES FOR REFERRAL
- Consultation with ophthalmologist, ID, ENT for orbital cellulitis; Neurology/Neurosurg. if intracranial spread is suspected (5)[B]

SURGERY/OTHER PROCEDURES
- IV antibiotic therapy is the best initial therapy.
- Surgical intervention warranted for visual loss, complete ophthalmoplegia, or well-defined large abscess (>10 mm) on presentation or no clinical improvement after 24 hours of antibiotic therapy.
- Trauma cases may need debridement or FB removal.
- Orbital abscess may need surgical drainage, and treatment of choice for brain abscess is surgical excision or drainage with 4–8 weeks of antibiotics.
- Surgical interventions may include external ethmoidectomy, endoscopic ethmoidectomy, uncinectomy, antrostomy, subperiosteal drainage.

IN-PATIENT CONSIDERATIONS
Patients with orbital cellulitis should be admitted for IV antibiotics and eye exam to evaluate progression of infection or involvement of optic nerve (1,4)[A]:
- Careful monitoring with temperature, WBC, visual acuity, papillary reflex, ocular motility, and proptosis measurement should be ≥q4h in severe/progressive cases.
- Repeat CT, surgical intervention, neurology consult with lumbar puncture may be required for worsening orbital cellulitis cases.

 ONGOING CARE

FOLLOW-UP RECOMMENDATIONS
Patient Monitoring
Visual acuity testing and slit lamp exam daily

ALERT
Bedside exam q4h is indicated, as complications can develop rapidly.

PATIENT EDUCATION
- Maintain proper hand washing and good skin hygiene.
- Avoid skin or lid trauma.

COMPLICATIONS
- Vision loss, CNS involvement, and death.
- Permanent vision loss:
  - Corneal exposure
  - Optic neuritis
  - Endophthalmitis
  - Septic uveitis or retinitis
  - Exudative retinal detachment
  - Retinal artery or vein occlusions
  - Globe rupture due to significantly increased intraocular pressure
  - Orbital compartment syndrome, compression of orbital soft tissues and optic nerve
- CNS complications:
  - Intracranial abscess, meningitis, cavernous sinus thrombosis (1,4)[B]

REFERENCES
1. Hauser A, Fogarasi S. Periorbital and orbital cellulitis. *Pediatr Rev.* 2010;31(6):242–249.
2. Mahalingam-Dhingra A, Lander L, Preciado DA, et al. Orbital and periorbital infections: A national perspective. *Arch Otolaryngol Head Neck Surg.* 2011;137(8):769–773.
3. Seltz LB, Smith J, Durairaj VD, et al. Microbiology and antibiotic management of orbital cellulitis. *Pediatrics.* 2011;127(3):e566–e572. Epub 2011 Feb 14.
4. Chadha NK. An evidence-based staging system for orbital infections from acute rhinosinusitis. *Laryngoscope.* 2012;122:S95–S96.
5. Kloek CE, Rubin PA. Role of inflammation in orbital cellulitis. *Int Ophthalmol Clin.* 2006;46:57–68.
6. Rudloe TF, Harper MB, Prabhu SP, et al. Acute periorbital infections: Who needs emergent imaging? *Pediatrics.* 2010;125:e719–e726.
7. Pushker N, Tejwani LK, Bajaj MS, et al. Role of oral corticosteroids in orbital cellulitis *Am J Ophthalmol.* 2013;156(1):178–183.e1. doi: 10.1016/j.ajo. 2013.01.031. Epub 2013 Apr 24.

ADDITIONAL READING
Bedwell J, Bauman NM. Management of pediatric orbital cellulitis and abscess. *Curr Opin Otolaryngol Head Neck Surg.* 2011;19(6):467–473.

CODES

ICD10
- H05.011 Cellulitis of right orbit
- H05.012 Cellulitis of left orbit
- H05.019 Cellulitis of unspecified orbit

CLINICAL PEARLS
- Most orbital cellulitis cases result from sinusitis.
- MRSA orbital cellulitis may present without associated upper respiratory infection.
- Older age (>10) and diplopia may predict need for surgical intervention in children.
- Patients should be admitted for monitoring and IV antibiotic treatment if orbital cellulitis is diagnosed.
- Ophthalmoplegia, mental status changes, contralateral cranial nerve palsy, or bilateral orbital cellulitis may herald intracranial involvement.
- Recommended diagnostic imaging is CT scan of orbits and sinuses with axial and coronal views, with and without contrast.

CELLULITIS, PERIORBITAL

Connie Chung, MD • Ryan Pearson, MD

 BASICS

DESCRIPTION
- An acute bacterial infection of the skin and SC tissue anterior to the orbital septum; does not involve orbital structures (globe, fat, and ocular muscles)
- Synonym(s): Preseptal cellulitis

ALERT
It is important to distinguish periorbital cellulitis from orbital cellulitis, which is a potentially life-threatening condition. *Orbital cellulitis is posterior to the orbital septum; symptoms include restricted eye movement, pain with eye movement, proptosis, and vision changes.*

EPIDEMIOLOGY
- Occurs more commonly in children; mean age 21 months.
- 3 times more common than orbital cellulitis (1)

Incidence
Increased incidence in the winter months (due to increased number of cases of sinusitis) (1)

ETIOLOGY AND PATHOPHYSIOLOGY
- An understanding of the anatomy of the eyelid is important in distinguishing preseptal from orbital cellulitis:
  - The orbital septum is a sheet of connective tissue that extends from the orbital bones to the margins of the upper and lower eyelids; it acts as a barrier to infection deep in the orbital structures.
  - Infection of tissues anterior to the orbital septum is called periorbital (preseptal) cellulitis.
  - Infection deep to the orbital septum is termed orbital (postseptal) cellulitis.
- Periorbital cellulitis classically arises from a contiguous infection of soft tissues of the face, secondary to:
  - Sinusitis (via lamina papyracea) extension
  - Local trauma
  - Insect or animal bites
  - Foreign bodies
  - Dental abscess extension
  - Hematogenous seeding
- Common organisms (1):
  - *Staphylococcus aureus,* typically MSSA (although increasing incidence of MRSA)
  - *Staphylococcus epidermidis*
  - *Streptococcus pyogenes*
- Atypical organisms:
  - *Acinetobacter* sp.
  - *Nocardia brasiliensis*
  - *Bacillus anthracis*
  - *Pseudomonas aeruginosa*
  - *Neisseria gonorrhoeae*
  - *Proteus* sp.
  - *Pasteurella multocida*
  - *Mycobacterium tuberculosis*
  - *Trichophyton* sp. (ringworm)
- Since the introduction of the *Hib* vaccine, the incidence of *Haemophilus influenzae* has decreased; however, this organism should be suspected in the unimmunized or partially immunized.

Genetics
No known genetic predisposition

RISK FACTORS
- Contiguous spread from upper respiratory infection
- Sinusitis
- Local skin trauma/puncture wound
- Insect bite
- Bacteremia

GENERAL PREVENTION
- Avoid dermatologic trauma.
- Avoid swimming in fresh or salt water with skin abrasion.
- Routine vaccination: The incidences of *H. influenzae B* and *Streptococcus pneumoniae* as potential etiologies for periorbital cellulitis have decreased.

 DIAGNOSIS

HISTORY
- Induration, erythema, warmth, and/or tenderness of periorbital soft tissue, usually with normal vision and eye movements.
- Chemosis (conjunctival swelling), proptosis; pain with extraocular eye movements can occur in severe cases of periorbital cellulitis, although these symptoms are more common with orbital cellulitis.
- Fever (although not necessary for diagnosis)

ALERT
Pain with eye movement and conjunctival swelling can occur in severe cases, although both should raise the suspicion for orbital cellulitis.

PHYSICAL EXAM
- Thorough inspection of the eye and surrounding structures is a key part of the physical exam.
- Erythema, swelling, and tenderness of lids without orbital congestion:
  - Violaceous discoloration of eyelid is more commonly associated with *H. influenza*.
- Evaluate for any skin break.
- Look for vesicle to rule out herpetic infection.
- Inspect nasal vaults and sinus palpation for signs of acute sinusitis.
- Exam oral cavity looking for dental abscesses.
- Test ocular motility and visual acuity to rule out orbital cellulitis.

DIFFERENTIAL DIAGNOSIS
- Orbital cellulitis:
  - Orbital cellulitis may have the same signs and symptoms as periorbital tissue, but also have proptosis, chemosis, ophthalmoplegia, pain with eye movement, decreased visual acuity, or fever.
- Abscess
- Dacryocystitis
- Hordeolum (stye)
- Allergic inflammation

- Orbital or periorbital trauma
- Idiopathic inflammation from orbital pseudotumor
- Orbital myositis
- Rapidly progressive tumors:
  - Rhabdomyosarcoma
  - Retinoblastoma
  - Lymphoma
- Leukemia

DIAGNOSTIC TESTS & INTERPRETATION
Initial Tests (lab, imaging)
- CBC with differential
- Blood cultures (low yield) (2)
- Wound culture of purulent drainage (if available)
- If doubt or suspicious for orbital involvement, then consider imaging studies.
- Also indicated in individuals who exhibit marked eyelid swelling, fever, and leukocytosis or fail to show improvement to appropriate antibiotics in 24–48 hours.
- CT can be used to evaluate the extent of infection and detect orbital inflammation or abscess (3)[B]:
  - The classic sign of orbital cellulitis on CT scan is bulging of the medial rectus.
  - CT should be performed with contrast, thin sections (2 mm), coronal and axial views with bone windows.

Follow-Up Tests & Special Considerations
- Children with periorbital or orbital cellulitis often have underlying sinusitis.
- If the child is febrile, <15 months old, and appears toxic, blood cultures should be performed and lumbar puncture considered.

 TREATMENT

MEDICATION
- Empiric antibiotic treatment regimens are based on coverage of the most likely organisms (*Staphylococcus* and *Streptococcus*).
- Pay attention to local prevalence and characteristics of MRSA to determine therapy.
- No evidence that IV antibiotics are more effective than PO in reducing recovery time or preventing secondary complications in the management of simple periorbital cellulitis (1).
- No evidence that use of steroids is indicated.

212

First Line
- Uncomplicated posttraumatic:
  - Usually due to skin flora, including *Staphylococcus* and *Streptococcus*
  - Cephalexin or dicloxacillin
  - Clindamycin, doxycycline, or trimethoprim-sulfamethoxazole (TMP-SMX) if MRSA is suspected.
- Extension from sinusitis:
  - Amoxicillin-clavulanate
  - 3rd-generation cephalosporin
- Dental abscess:
  - Amoxicillin-clavulanate or clindamycin
- Bacteremic cellulitis:
  - May be associated with meningitis
  - Ceftriaxone plus vancomycin or clindamycin to cover methicillin-resistant *S. aureus*
- Duration of therapy should be 7–10 days:
  - If symptoms do not improve within 24 hours, IV antibiotic therapy is indicated (4)[B].

ISSUES FOR REFERRAL
Management should include consultation with otolaryngologists and ophthalmologists when there is concern of orbital cellulitis or when first line treatment has failed (5).

SURGERY/OTHER PROCEDURES
- Usually not indicated in uncomplicated periorbital cellulitis
- If there is an abscess or potential compromise of critical structures, such as the brain or eye seen on imaging, orbital surgery is indicated (6).
- Diplopia is the strongest clinical predictor of surgery.

IN-PATIENT CONSIDERATIONS
Mild cases in adults and children >1 year can be managed on an outpatient basis, provided the patient is stable and without systemic signs of toxicity.

Admission Criteria/Initial Stabilization
Consider hospitalization and IV antibiotics:
- For children <1 year
- Patients who have not been immunized for *S. pneumoniae* or *H. influenza*
- If no signs of clinical improvement are apparent after 24 hours of oral antibiotics
- Cases where high suspicion of orbital cellulitis (eyelid swelling with reduced vision, diplopia, abnormal light reflexes, or proptosis)

Discharge Criteria
- No strict guidelines indicate when to switch therapy from parenteral to PO agents.
- Generally, switch to PO therapy after the patient is afebrile and the skin findings have begun to resolve, which usually takes 2–3 days.
- Therapy is typically for 10–14 days for orbital cellulitis or complicated periorbital cellulitis.

 ## ONGOING CARE

FOLLOW-UP RECOMMENDATIONS
Patient Monitoring
The patient should be monitored for signs of orbital involvement, including decreased visual acuity or painful/limited ocular motility.

PATIENT EDUCATION
- Maintain good skin hygiene.
- Avoid skin trauma.
- Report early skin changes to health care professional.

PROGNOSIS
- With timely treatment, patients do well.
- 10-day course of antibiotic treatment generally is sufficient.
- Recurrent periorbital cellulitis is a clinical entity in which a patient has ≥3 periorbital infections in the span of 1 year with at least 1 month of convalescence; must be differentiated from treatment failure due to antibiotic resistance (1).

COMPLICATIONS
- Orbital cellulitis
- Abscess formation
- Scarring
- Delay in diagnosis and adequate treatment may result in serious complications, including blindness.

REFERENCES

1. Hauser A, Fogarasi S. Periorbital and orbital cellulitis. *Pediatr Rev*. 2010;31:242.
2. Baring DE, Hilmi OJ. An evidence based review of periorbital cellulitis. *Clin Otolaryngol*. 2011;36(1):57–64.
3. Beech T, Robinson A, McDermott AL, et al. Paediatric periorbital cellulitis and its management. *Rhinology*. 2007;45:47–49.
4. Hennemann S, Crawford P, Nguyen L, et al. Clinical inquiries. What is the best initial treatment for orbital cellulitis in children? *J Fam Pract*. 2007;56(8):662–664.
5. Upile NS, Munir N, Leong SC, et al. Who should manage acute periorbital cellulitis in children? *Int J Pediatr Otorhinolaryngol*. 2012;76(8):1073–1077.
6. Mahalingam-Dhingra A, Lander L, Preciado DA, et al. Orbital and periorbital infections: A national perspective. *Arch Otolaryngol Head Neck Surg*. 2011;137(8):769–773.
7. Georgakopoulos CD, Eliopoulou MI, Stasinos S, et al. Periorbital and orbital cellulitis: A 10-year review of hospitalized children. *Eur J Ophthalmol*. 2010;20(6):1066–1072.

ADDITIONAL READING
- Chaudhry IA, Shamsi FA, Elzaridi E, et al. Inpatient preseptal cellulitis: Experience from a tertiary eye care centre. *Br J Ophthalmol*. 2008;92:1337–1341. doi:10.1136/bjo.2007.128975.
- Goldstein SM, Shelsta HN. Community-acquired methicillin-resistant *Staphylococcus aureus* periorbital cellulitis: A problem here to stay. *Ophthal Plast Reconstr Surg*. 2009;25:77.
- Yeilding RH, O'Day DM, Li C, et al. Periorbital infections after Dermabond closure of traumatic lacerations in three children. *JAAPOS*. 2012;16(2):168–172.

 ## CODES

ICD10
- H05.011 Cellulitis of right orbit
- H05.013 Cellulitis of bilateral orbits
- H05.019 Cellulitis of unspecified orbit

CLINICAL PEARLS
- Periorbital (preseptal) and orbital (postseptal) cellulitis occur most commonly in children.
- It is critical to differentiate between periorbital cellulitis and orbital cellulitis; the latter is more dangerous and can be life threatening.
- CT scan of the patient's sinuses and orbits can be utilized to differentiate periorbital cellulitis from orbital cellulitis.
- Early detection and treatment of periorbital cellulitis is important to prevent complications.
- The 2 most important predisposing factors for periorbital cellulitis are upper respiratory infections and eyelid trauma; sinusitis is more typically associated with orbital cellulitis (7)[C].

CEREBRAL PALSY

Michael J. Terzella, DO • Angela D. Hart, DO

BASICS

DESCRIPTION
Cerebral palsy (CP) is a group of clinically diagnosed disorders in the development of movement and posture due to permanent and nonprogressive disruptions in the developing fetal brain. Motor impairment resulting in activity limitation is necessary for this diagnosis. CP is classified by the nature of the movement disorder and its functional severity. Individuals with this disorder are affected with secondary musculoskeletal and neurologic problems (intellectual, sensory, speech and language impairment, and seizures).

EPIDEMIOLOGY
Incidence
- Overall, 1.5–2.5/1,000 live births
- Incidence increases as gestational age (GA) at birth decreases (1):
  - 146/1,000 for GA of 22–27 weeks
  - 62/1,000 for GA of 28–31 weeks
  - 7/1,000 for GA of 32–36 weeks
  - 1/1,000 for GA of 37+ weeks

Prevalence
3–4/1,000 of the population

ETIOLOGY AND PATHOPHYSIOLOGY
- Multifactorial; CP results from static injury or lesions in the developing brain, occurring prenatally, perinatally, or postnatally.
- Neuropathology linked to gestational age at time of brain insult
- Cytokines, free radicals, and inflammatory response are likely contributing factors.
- Etiology is most likely multifactorial and depends on timing of brain insult: Prenatally, perinatally, or postnatally (see "Risk Factors")
- Spastic CP is most common, usually related to premature birth, with either periventricular leukomalacia or germinal matrix hemorrhage.
- Dystonic or athetotic CP, often resulting from kernicterus, is now rare due to improved management of hyperbilirubinemia.

Genetics
There are reports of associations between CP and candidate genes: Thrombophilic, cytokines, and apolipoprotein E

RISK FACTORS
- Prenatal: Congenital anomalies, multiple gestation, in utero stroke, intrauterine infection (cytomegalovirus [CMV], varicella), intrauterine growth retardation (IUGR), clinical and histological chorioamnionitis, antepartum bleeding, maternal factors (cognitive impairment, seizure disorders, hyperthyroidism), abnormal fetal position (e.g., breech)
- Perinatal: Preterm birth, low birth weight, periventricular leukomalacia, perinatal hypoxia/asphyxia, intracranial hemorrhage/intraventricular hemorrhage, neonatal seizure or stroke, hyperbilirubinemia
- Postnatal: Traumatic brain injury or stroke, sepsis, meningitis, encephalitis, asphyxia, and progressive hydrocephalus

GENERAL PREVENTION
- Treating mothers with magnesium sulfate during preterm delivery is neuroprotective for fetus. Effect on term fetus is unknown (2)[B].
- Improved management of hyperbilirubinemia with decrease in kernicterus has greatly reduced dyskinetic CP.
- Prevention or reduction of chorioamnionitis and premature births

COMMONLY ASSOCIATED CONDITIONS
- Seizure disorder (22–40%)
- Intellectual impairment (23–44%)
- Behavioral problems
- Speech and language impairment (42–81%):
  - May have an impact on expressive and/or receptive language
  - May be nonverbal
- Sensory impairments:
  - Hearing deficits
  - Visual (62–71%): Poor visual acuity, strabismus (50%), or hemianopsia
- Feeding impairment, swallowing dysfunction, and aspiration: When severe, may require gastrostomy feedings
- Poor dentition, excessive drooling
- GI conditions: Constipation (59%), vomiting (22%), gastroesophageal reflux
- Decreased linear growth and weight abnormalities (under- and overweight)
- Osteopenia
- Bowel and bladder incontinence
- Orthopedic: Contractures, hip subluxation/dislocation, scoliosis (60%)

DIAGNOSIS

- A clinical diagnosis including:
  - Delayed motor milestones
  - Abnormal tone
  - Abnormal neurological exam suggesting a cerebral etiology for motor dysfunction
  - Absence of regression (not losing function)
  - Absence of underlying syndromes or alternative explanation for etiology
- Although the pathologic lesion is static, clinical presentation may change as the infant grows and develops.
- Accurate early diagnosis remains difficult. Neurologic abnormalities observed in the first 1–2 years of life may resolve; be cautious of diagnosing CP before age 2.

HISTORY
- Presentation: Concerns over movements or delayed motor development
- Ask about:
  - Prenatal, perinatal, and postnatal risk factors
  - Neurobehavioral signs:
    - Poor feeding/frequent vomiting
    - Irritability
  - Timing of motor milestones: Delay in milestones is not sensitive or specific until after 6 months of age.
  - Abnormal spontaneous general movements
  - Asymmetry of movements, such as early hand preference
- Regression of motor skills does not occur with CP

PHYSICAL EXAM
- Assess for ≥1 types of neurologic impairment:
  - Spasticity: Increased tone/reflexes/clonus
  - Dyskinesia: Abnormal movements
  - Hypotonia: Decreased tone
  - Ataxia: Abnormal balance/coordination
- Areas of exam:
  - Tone: May be increased or decreased
  - Trunk and head control: Often poor, but may be advanced due to high tone
  - Reduced strength and motor control
  - Persistence of primitive reflexes
  - Asymmetry of movement or reflexes
  - Decreased joint range of motion and contractures
  - Brisk deep tendon reflexes
  - Clonus
  - Delayed motor milestones: Serial exams most effective
  - Gait abnormalities: Scissoring, toe-walking
- CP is classified by (3):
  - Muscle tone or movement disorder:
    - Spasticity:
      - Unilateral: Hemiplegic
      - Bilateral: Diplegic (lower extremity [LE] > upper extremity [UE] involvement) or quadriplegic (UE ≥ LE involvement)
    - Dystonia: Hypertonia and reduced movement
    - Choreoathetosis: Irregular spasmodic involuntary movements of the limbs or facial muscles
    - Ataxia: Loss of orderly muscular coordination
  - Motor function severity:
    - The Gross Motor Function Classification System (GMFCS) scored I–IV:
      - Score of I: Ambulates without limitation
      - Score of II: Ambulates without assistive devices, but some limitation
      - Score of III: Ambulates with assistive mobility devices
      - Score of IV: Self-mobility limited, but technology can help
      - Score of V: Self-mobility severely limited, even with technology
    - The Manual Ability Classification System (MACS) can be used to assess upper extremity and fine motor function.

DIFFERENTIAL DIAGNOSIS
Benign congenital hypotonia, brachial plexus injury, familial spastic paraplegia, dopa-responsive dystonia, transient toe-walking, muscular dystrophy, metabolic disorders (e.g., glutaric aciduria type 1), mitochondrial disorders, genetic disorders (e.g., Rett syndrome)

DIAGNOSTIC TESTS & INTERPRETATION
CP is a clinical diagnosis based on history, physical, and risk factors. Laboratory testing is not needed to make diagnosis, but can help exclude other etiologies.
- Testing for metabolic and genetic syndromes (4)[C]:
  - Not routinely obtained in the evaluation for CP
  - Considered if no specific etiology is identified by neuroimaging or there are atypical features in clinical presentation.
  - Detection of certain brain malformations may warrant genetic or metabolic testing to identify syndromes.
- Screening for coagulopathies: Diagnostic testing for coagulopathies should be considered in children with hemiplegic CP with cerebral infarction identified on neuroimaging (4)[C].

Initial Tests (lab, imaging)
- Neuroimaging is not essential, but it is recommended in children with CP for whom the etiology has not been established (4)[C].
- MRI is preferred for determining etiology and timing of a brain insult (4)[C].
- Abnormalities in 80–90% of patients: Brain malformation, cerebral infarction, intraventricular or other intracranial hemorrhage, periventricular leukomalacia, ventricular enlargement, or other CSF space abnormalities

Diagnostic Procedures/Other
- The Communication Function Classification System has recently been developed as another means of assessing function.
- Screening for comorbid conditions: Developmental delay/intellectual impairment, vision/hearing impairments, speech and language disorders, feeding/swallowing dysfunction, or seizures
- EEGs should only be obtained if there is a history of suspected seizures.

Test Interpretation
Perinatal brain injury may include:
- White matter damage:
  - Most common in premature infants
  - Periventricular leukomalacia: Gliosis with or without focal necrosis with resulting cysts and scarring. May be multiple lesions of various ages. Necrosis can lead to cysts/scarring.
  - Germinal matrix hemorrhage: May lead to intraventricular hemorrhage
- Gray matter damage: More common in term infants. Cortical infarcts, focal neuronal damage, myelination abnormalities

TREATMENT

Focuses on control of symptoms; treatments reduce spasticity to prevent painful contractures, manage comorbid conditions, and optimize functionality and quality of life.

GENERAL MEASURES
- Early intervention programs for preterm infants influences motor and cognitive outcomes (5)[A]
- Referral to early intervention for children ages 0–3 years is essential.
- Various therapy modalities enhance functioning:
  - Physical therapy to improve posture stability and gait, motor strength and control, and prevent contractures
  - Occupational therapy to increase functional activities of daily living and other fine motor skills
  - Speech therapy for verbal and nonverbal speech and to aid in feeding
- Equipment optimizes participation in activities:
  - Orthotic splinting (ankle-foot orthosis) maintains functional positioning and prevents contractures
  - Spinal bracing (body jacket) may slow scoliosis
  - Augmentative communication with pictures, switches, or computer systems for nonverbal individuals
  - Therapeutic and functional electrical stimulation decreases activity limitation in gait
  - Use of adaptive equipment such as crutches, walkers, gait trainers, and wheelchairs for mobility and standers for weight bearing

MEDICATION
First Line
- Diazepam (6)[A]:
  - Short-term treatment for generalized spasticity; insufficient evidence on motor function
  - A γ-aminobutyric acid-A (GABA$_A$) agonist that facilitates CNS inhibition at spinal and supraspinal levels to reduce spasticity
  - Adverse effects: Ataxia and drowsiness
  - Adult dose: 2–12 mg/dose PO q6–12h
  - Pediatric dose (<12 years): 0.12–0.8 mg/kg/d PO, divided q6–8h
- Botulinum toxin type A (6)[A]:
  - Injected directly into muscles of interest for localized spasticity; insufficient evidence on motor function
  - Higher functional benefit when combined with occupational therapy
  - Acts at neuromuscular junction to inhibit the release of acetylcholine to reduce tone
  - Lasts for 12–16 weeks following injection

Second Line
- Baclofen (6)[A]:
  - GABA$_B$ agonist, facilitates presynaptic inhibition of mono- and polysynaptic reflexes
  - Adverse effects: Drowsiness and sedation
  - Abrupt withdrawal symptoms: Spasticity, hallucinations, seizures, confusion, hyperthermia
  - Adults: Initial dose is 5 mg t.i.d.; increase dosage every 3 days to an average maintenance dose of 20 mg t.i.d. 80 mg/d maximum
  - Pediatric dose (>2 years): Initial 10–15 mg/d. Titrate to effective dose. <8 years old = 40 mg/d maximum. >8 years old 60 mg/d maximum.
- Intrathecal baclofen (baclofen pump) (7)[A]:
  - Continuous intrathecal route allows greater maximal response with smaller dosage to reduce spasticity.
  - May help ambulatory individuals with gait, but no improvement seen in nonambulatory patients
  - Adverse effects: Infection, catheter malfunction, CSF leakage

ADDITIONAL THERAPIES
- Multidisciplinary care including ophthalmology, neurology, orthopedics, physiatry along with physical, occupational, and speech therapists.
- A primary care "medical home" that coordinates medical and community services, provides support for the patient and the patient's family (3)[C]

SURGERY/OTHER PROCEDURES
- Dorsal root rhizotomy selectively cuts dorsal rootlets from L1–S2. Best for patients with normal intelligence with spastic diplegia. Decreases spasticity in lower limbs when done in conjunction with physiotherapy, but associated with adverse effects. Evidence lacking as to long-term outcomes.
- Surgical treatment of joint dislocations/subluxation, scoliosis management, tendon lengthening, gastrostomy

COMPLEMENTARY AND ALTERNATIVE MEDICINE
Hyperbaric oxygen is controversial and not recommended in those who do not suffer hypoxic ischemic encephalopathy (8)[B]. Therapeutic horse riding or hippotherapy improves postural control and balance.

 ## ONGOING CARE

PROGNOSIS
Reduced lifespan strongly associated with level of functional impairment and intellectual disability.

REFERENCES
1. Himpens E, Van den Broeck C, Oostra A, et al. Prevalence, type, distribution, and severity of cerebral palsy in relation to gestational age: A meta-analytic review. Dev Med Child Neurol. 2008;50:334–340.
2. Nguyen TM, Crowther CA. Magnesium sulphate for women at term for neuroprotection of the fetus. Cochrane Database Syst Rev. 2013;2:CD009395.
3. O'Shea TM. Diagnosis, treatment, and prevention of cerebral palsy. Clin Obstet Gynecol. 2008;51:816–828.
4. Ashwal S, Russman BS, Blasco PA, et al. Practice parameter: Diagnostic assessment of the child with cerebral palsy: Report of the Quality Standards Subcommittee of the American Academy of Neurology and the Practice Committee of the Child Neurology Society. Neurology. 2004;62:851–863.
5. Spittle A, Orton J. Early developmental intervention programmes post-hospital discharge to prevent motor and cognitive impairments in preterm infants. Cochrane Database Syst Rev. 2012;12:CD005495.
6. Quality Standards Subcommittee of the American Academy of Neurology and the Practice Committee of the Child Neurology Society, Delgado MR, et al. Practice parameter: Pharmacologic treatment of spasticity in children and adolescents with cerebral palsy (an evidence-based review): Report of the Quality Standards Subcommittee of the American Academy of Neurology and the Practice Committee of the Child Neurology Society. Neurology. 2010;74:336–343.
7. Pin TW, McCartney L, Lewis J, et al. Use of intrathecal baclofen therapy in ambulant children and adolescents with spasticity and dystonia of cerebral origin: A systematic review. Dev Med Child Neurol. 2011;53:885–895.
8. Lacey DJ, Stolfi A, Pilati LE. Effects of hyperbaric oxygen on motor function in children with cerebral palsy. Ann Neurol. 2012;72:695–703.

 ## CODES

ICD10
- G80.0 Spastic quadriplegic cerebral palsy
- G80.2 Spastic hemiplegic cerebral palsy
- G80.9 Cerebral palsy, unspecified

CLINICAL PEARLS
- Management should focus on maximizing functioning and quality of life using multidisciplinary team approach.
- Regression of motor skills does not occur with CP.

C

CERVICAL HYPEREXTENSION INJURIES

Francesca L. Beaudoin, MD, MS • Sarah Lauren Harkness, MD

BASICS

DESCRIPTION
- Group of injuries involving the neck that result from a rapid, forceful, backwards motion
- May involve:
  - Injury to vertebral and paravertebral structures: Fractures, dislocations, ligamentous tears, and disc disruption/subluxation
  - Spinal cord injury: Traumatic central cord syndrome (CCS) secondary to cord compression or vascular insult
  - Blunt cerebrovascular injury (BCVI): Vertebral artery or carotid artery dissection
  - Soft-tissue injury around cervical spine: Cervical strain/sprain

EPIDEMIOLOGY
- Predominant age: Trauma and sports injuries more common in young adults (average age 29.4); however, CCS mostly seen in older population (average age 53)
- Predominant sex: Male > Female

Incidence
In the US:
- Cervical fractures: 2–5/100 blunt trauma patients
- Central cord syndrome: 3.6/100,000 people/yr
- BCVI: Estimated 1/1,000 of hospitalized trauma patients; incidence increased with cervical spine or thoracic injury (1,2)
- Cervical strain: 3–4/1,000 people/yr

ETIOLOGY AND PATHOPHYSIOLOGY
Blunt trauma due to motor vehicle accidents, sports injuries, falls, and assaults

RISK FACTORS
- Fractures: Osteoporosis, conditions predisposing to spinal rigidity, such as ankylosing spondylitis
- CCS: Preexisting spinal stenosis is present in >50% of cases, which may be:
  - Acquired: Prior trauma, spondylosis
  - Congenital: Klippel-Feil syndrome (congenital fusion of any 2 cervical vertebra) with cervical stenosis

GENERAL PREVENTION
Seat belts and use of proper safety equipment in sports activities can prevent/minimize injury.

COMMONLY ASSOCIATED CONDITIONS
Closed head injuries (concussion, cerebral contusions, intracranial hemorrhage), facial fractures, thoracic/lumbar spinal injury

DIAGNOSIS

HISTORY
Usually acute presentation with mechanism of cervical hyperextension (see "Etiology") and complaints of neck pain, stiffness, or headaches ± neurologic symptoms

PHYSICAL EXAM
- External signs of trauma on the head and neck such as abrasions, lacerations, ecchymoses, or contusions are clues to mechanism.
- Presence, severity, and location of neck tenderness localize involved structure(s):
  - Posterior midline, bony point tenderness concerning for bony injury
  - Paraspinal or lateral soft tissue tenderness suggestive of muscular/ligamentous injury
  - Anterior tenderness concerning for carotid injury
- Carotid bruit suggestive of carotid dissection
- Neurologic exam: Paresthesias/Numbness, weakness suggests spinal cord injury or stroke secondary to BCVI:
  - CCS often presents as:
    - Distal > proximal symptom distribution, upper extremity > lower extremity
    - Extremity weakness/paralysis predominates
    - Variable sensory changes below level of lesion (including paresthesias and dysesthesia)
    - Bladder/Bowel dysfunction may occur.

DIFFERENTIAL DIAGNOSIS
- Acute or chronic disc pathology (including herniation or internal disruption)
- Osteoarthritis
- Cervical radiculopathy
- For CCS:
  - Bell cruciate palsy
  - Bilateral brachial plexus injuries
  - Carotid or vertebral artery dissection

DIAGNOSTIC TESTS & INTERPRETATION
Initial Tests (lab, imaging)
- Low-risk patients can be cleared clinically (without radiographic evaluation) using either the Canadian C-Spine Rule (CCR) or the National Emergency X-ray Utilization Study (NEXUS) Criteria:
  - CCR: Clinically clear a stable, adult patient with no history of cervical spine disease/surgery if all of the following conditions are met:
    - Glasgow Coma Scale (GCS) ≥15
    - Nonintoxicated patients without a distracting injury
    - No dangerous mechanism or extremity paresthesias
    - Age <65 years
    - At least 1 "low-risk factor" (i.e., simple rear-end motor vehicle accident [MVA], ambulation at the accident scene, no midline cervical tenderness, delayed onset of neck pain, or sitting position at the time of exam)
  - NEXUS: Clinically clear if all of the following are met:
    - No alteration of mental status or intoxication
    - No focal/neuro deficits
    - No distracting injury
    - No posterior, midline C-spine tenderness
  - Reported sensitivity/specificity: CCR (99.4%/45.1%), NEXUS (90.7%/36.8%) (3)[A]
- In patients with high-risk mechanism or any concerning historical/physical exam elements, imaging should strongly be considered. Choose from the following options based on the suspected injury and level of clinical suspicion:
  - Plain radiographs: Recommended by some in patients who cannot be cleared clinically but still are in low-suspicion category: Sensitivity for C-spine injury as low as 39% (4)[B]:
    - Static: Lateral, anterior-posterior (A-P), and odontoid views; in addition to bony abnormalities, may show prevertebral soft tissue swelling
    - Dynamic: Flexion/Extension; only if asymptomatic and no neurologic deficits or mental impairment, may help identify ligamentous injury although limited utility in acute setting when compared to CT/MRI (5)
  - CT: Axial CT from occiput to T1 with coronal and sagittal reconstructions; rapidly replacing plain radiography as the test of choice for cases with moderate-to-high clinical suspicion of C-spine injury, given high sensitivity (90–100%) (4)[B]
  - MRI: Diagnostic test of choice in CCS with direct visualization of traumatic cord lesions (edema or hematomyelia), soft tissue compressing cord, and/or stenosis of canal. Also detects ligamentous injury and abnormalities of intervertebral discs and soft tissues, but modality is poor with fractures and is prone to false-positive results due to nonspecific findings. Some authors suggest that MRI is required to screen for occult injury in obtunded/noncommunicative patients with a negative CT scan; however, this recommendation is controversial, and evidence is limited (6)[B].
  - CT angiography: Visualization of cervical and cerebral vascular structures to detect BCVI, with reported sensitivity approaching 100% when a ≥16-slice CT scanner is used. MR angiography is an alternative modality, although reported sensitivities of 47–50% limit its utility (1)[B].

Test Interpretation
- Vertebral fractures: See "General Measures."
- CCS: Currently thought to be due to axonal disruption within the white matter of the lateral column, particularly the corticospinal tracts
- BCVI: Intimal disruption, leading to thrombosis and embolization
- Acute cervical strain/sprain: Models based on animal, cadaver, and postmortem studies show myofascial tearing, edema, and inflammation, but facet joint capsular pain may also play a role.

Geriatric Considerations
- Degenerative disease of the C-spine may be confused with acute traumatic change, and osteopenia may limit visualization of fractures, particularly on plain radiographs; CT imaging is more helpful to distinguish the two.
- Degenerative disease increases the risk of upper cervical spine injuries despite low speed trauma (7)

Pediatric Considerations
Consider spinal cord injury without radiographic abnormality (SCIWORA), which has a high incidence at <9 years and accounts for up to 50% of all pediatric cervical spine injuries. MRI may help detect the injury.

TREATMENT

GENERAL MEASURES
- Fractures:
  - Stability determined by imaging; decompression and stabilization are indicated in:
    - Incomplete spinal cord injuries (SCIs) with spinal canal compromise
    - Clinical deterioration or failure to improve despite conservative management
  - Hangman fracture: Traumatic spondylolisthesis of C2 (the "axis") with bilateral fractures through C2 pedicles, often with anterior subluxation of C2 over C3; can be unstable:
    - Managed with halo vest immobilization for 12 weeks until repeated flexion/extension films normalize

- Odontoid (dens) fractures: Treated according to type:
  - I: Through apex; usually stable; external immobilization with a cervical collar (less often halo vest) for up to 12 weeks
  - II: Most common, at base of dens, usually unstable; nonunion rates of up to 67% with halo immobilization alone, especially with dens displacement >6 mm or age >50
  - III: Through C2 body, usually stable; immobilization in halo or cervical collar for 12–20 weeks
- Hyperextension teardrop fractures:
  - If stable, rigid collar or cervicothoracic brace for 8–14 weeks
  - If unstable, halo brace for up to 3 months
- CCS: Neck immobilization with cervical collar, physical therapy/occupational therapy (PT/OT)
- Cervical strain: No evidence of different outcomes with active (PT) vs. passive (immobilization, rest) treatment (8)[A], but may use soft cervical collar for up to 10 days for symptomatic relief, then mobilization and activity as tolerated

MEDICATION
- Fractures: Pain control as needed with opiate analgesics
- CCS: Within 8 hours of injury, methylprednisolone 30 mg/kg IV over 15 minutes, then continuous infusion 5.4 mg/kg/h IV for 24 hours. Further improvement in motor function recovery may be seen if infusion is continued for 48 hours, especially if initial bolus administration is delayed by 3–8 hours after injury (9).
- BCVI: Anticoagulation with IV heparin, followed by warfarin therapy for 3–6 months, then long-term antiplatelet therapy is common practice. However, an antiplatelet agent is used as the sole initial therapy in patients with contraindications to anticoagulation (1)[B]. To date, no randomized controlled trials compare the efficacy of antiplatelets vs. anticoagulant therapy, so evidence-based recommendations are not available (10)[A].
- Cervical strain: Muscle relaxants, acetaminophen/NSAIDs ± opiate analgesics are commonly used

ISSUES FOR REFERRAL
- When cervical spine injury is suspected, the patient should be immobilized and sent to the ED for evaluation.
- Emergent consultation from a spinal surgeon (neurosurgery and/or orthopedics) is indicated if there is any concern for unstable fracture or spinal cord injury.

SURGERY/OTHER PROCEDURES
- Fractures:
  - Hangman's fracture: Consider surgical fixation in cases of excessive angulation or subluxation, disruption of intervertebral disc space, or failure to obtain alignment with external orthosis.
  - Odontoid fractures:
    - Type II: Early surgical stabilization recommended in setting of age >50, dens displacement >5 mm, and in certain fracture patterns
    - Type III: Surgical intervention often reserved for cases of nonunion/malunion after trial of external immobilization
  - Hyperextension teardrop fractures: Consider surgical repair if unstable with neurologic deficit

- CCS: Surgical decompression/fixation is indicated in setting of unstable injury and/or herniated disc, or when neurologic function plateaus/deteriorates
- BCVI: Surgical and/or angiographic intervention may be required if there is evidence of pseudoaneurysm, total occlusion, or transection of the vessel (1)[B].

IN-PATIENT CONSIDERATIONS
Admission Criteria/Initial Stabilization
- Varies by injury; clinical judgment, radiographic findings, concomitant injuries, and need for operative intervention influence decision
- Advanced Trauma Life Support (ATLS) protocol with backboard and collar

ONGOING CARE

FOLLOW-UP RECOMMENDATIONS
Patient Monitoring
Patients with known injuries will often be followed with serial radiographs under the care of a specialist.

PATIENT EDUCATION
For patient instruction on prevention: THINK FIRST Foundation at: http://www.thinkfirst.org

PROGNOSIS
- Overall, the most important prognostic factor is the initial neurologic status.
- Fractures:
  - Hangman fracture: 93–100% fusion rate after 8–14 weeks external immobilization
  - Odontoid fracture, fusion rate by type: Type I ~100% with external immobilization alone; type III, 85% with external immobilization, 100% with surgical fixation
- BCVI: With early diagnosis and initiation of antithrombotic therapy, patients may have fewer neurologic sequelae.
- CCS:
  - Spontaneous recovery of motor function in >50% of cases over several weeks, with younger patients more likely to regain function
  - Leg, bowel, and bladder functions return first, followed by upper extremities.
- Cervical strain: Up to 50% of patients continue to have neck pain at 1 year:
  - Prognostic factors for development of late whiplash syndrome (>6 months of symptoms affecting normal activity) include increased initial pain intensity, pain-related disability, and cold hyperalgesia.

COMPLICATIONS
- Fractures: Nonunion/Malunion of fractures or persistent instability requiring 2nd procedure, reactions, and infection related to orthosis
- BCVI: Embolic ischemic events and pseudoaneurysm formation

REFERENCES

1. Bromberg WJ. Blunt cerebrovascular injury practice management guidelines: The Eastern Association for the Surgery of Trauma. *J Trauma*. 2010;68(2):471–477.
2. Franz RW, Willette PA, Wood MJ, et al. A systematic review and meta-analysis of diagnostic screening criteria for blunt cerebrovascular injuries. *J Am Coll Surg*. 2012;214(3):313–327. Epub 2012 Jan 11.
3. Stiell IG, Clement CM, McKnight RD, et al. The Canadian C-spine rule versus the NEXUS low-risk criteria in patients with trauma. *N Engl J Med*. 2003;349:2510–2518.
4. Cain G. Imaging suspected cervical spine injury: Plain radiography or computed tomography? Systematic review (Structured abstract). *Radiography*. 2010;68–77.
5. Sierink JC, van Lieshout WAM, Beenen LF, et al. Systemic review of flexion/extension radiography of the cervical spine in trauma patients. *Eur J Radiol*. 2013;86(6):974–981.
6. Schoenfeld AJ. Computed tomography alone versus computed tomography and magnetic resonance imaging in the identification of occult injuries to the cervical spine: A meta-analysis (Structured abstract). *J Trauma*. 2010;109–114.
7. Watanabe M, Sakai D, Yamamoto Y, et al. Upper cervical spine injuries: Age-specific clinical features. *J Orthop Sci*. 2010;15(4):485–492.
8. Verhagen AP, Scholten-Peeters GGGM, van Wijngaarden S, et al. Conservative treatments for whiplash. *Cochrane Database Syst Rev*. 2007;2:CD003338.
9. Bracken MB. Steroids for acute spinal cord injury. *Cochrane Database Syst Rev*. 2012;1:CD001046. Epub 2012 Jan 18.
10. Lyrer P, Engelter S. Antithrombotic drugs for carotid artery dissection. *Cochrane Database Syst Rev*. 2010;(10):CD000255. Epub 2010 Oct 6.

ADDITIONAL READING
Pryputniewicz DM, Hadley MN. Axis fractures. *Neurosurgery*. 2010;66:68–82.

SEE ALSO
Cervical Spine Injury

CODES
ICD10
- S13.4XXA Sprain of ligaments of cervical spine, initial encounter
- S13.101A Dislocation of unspecified cervical vertebrae, init encntr
- S14.109A Unsp injury at unsp level of cervical spinal cord, init

CLINICAL PEARLS
- Follow NEXUS or Canadian Cervical Spine rules on every patient with potential neck injury to determine imaging needs, but use clinical judgment!
- Inquire about preexisting cervical spine injuries or conditions, especially in the elderly, as they may increase risk of injury or alter radiographic interpretation.
- Suspect SCI until exam and imaging suggest otherwise.
- Consider BCVI when neurologic deficits are inconsistent with level of known injury or significant mechanism exists.

CERVICAL MALIGNANCY
Benjamin P. Brown, MD • Meaghan Tenney, MD

BASICS

DESCRIPTION
- Invasive cancer of the uterine cervix
- Commonly involves the vagina, parametria, and pelvic side walls
- Invasion of bladder, rectum, and other pelvic sites in advanced disease

EPIDEMIOLOGY
Incidence
- Worldwide, cervical cancer is the 2nd most common malignancy among women (1).
- There is a higher incidence of cervical cancer in developing countries, contributing up to 83% of reported cases annually.
- In the US, it is the 3rd most common gynecologic cancer and the 6th most common solid malignant neoplasm among women.
- The disease has a bimodal distribution, with the highest risk among women ages 40–59 and >70.

Prevalence
- In 2013, the American Cancer Society (ACS) estimated there were 12,340 new cases in the US, with 4,030 deaths from the malignancy.
- African Americans and women in lower socioeconomic groups have the highest age-standardized cervical cancer death rates.
- Hispanic and Latina women have the highest incidence of the malignancy.

ETIOLOGY AND PATHOPHYSIOLOGY
- Arises from pre-existing dysplastic lesions, usually following persistent human papillomavirus (HPV) infection.
- Pattern of local growth may be exophytic or endophytic
- Lymphatic spread, typically through cervical lymphatic drainage
- Local tumor extension involving the bladder, ureters, rectum, and distant metastasis from hematogenous spread
- Epidemiologic and experimental evidence supports HPV strains 16 and 18 as etiologic agents in ~70% of cervical cancers.
- Association with E6 and E7 oncogenic proteins responsible for malignant cell transformation by inactivation of p53 and Rb tumor suppressor genes.
- Slow progression from dysplasia to invasive cancer allows sufficient time for effective screening and treatment of preinvasive disease.

Genetics
Not an inherited disease, except in very rare cases of Peutz-Jeghers syndrome

RISK FACTORS
- Causative agent in the majority of cases is persistent HPV infection.
- Other risk factors include:
  - Lack of regular Pap smears
  - Early coitarche
  - Multiple sexual partners
  - Unprotected sex
  - A history of sexually transmitted diseases (STDs)
  - Low socioeconomic status
  - High parity
  - Cigarette smoking
  - Immunosuppression
  - Diethylstilbestrol (DES) exposure in utero

GENERAL PREVENTION
- Patient education regarding safer sex, decreasing number of sexual partners
- Smoking cessation
- HPV vaccines
  - Gardasil vaccine: Quadrivalent vaccine containing proteins from HPV strains 6, 11, 16, and 18. FDA-approved in females and in males (for prevention of genital warts and anal cancer).
  - Cervarix vaccine: Bivalent vaccine against oncogenic HPV strains 16 and 18.
  - Neither vaccine yet conclusively shown to prevent cancer.
  - Recommended age of vaccination is 11–12 years (prior to coitarche), but Gardasil is approved from 9 to 26 and Cervarix from 10–25.
- Regular Pap smears and pelvic exams at appropriate intervals. In patients with no history of abnormal Paps, current guidelines from the American College of Obstetricians and Gynecologists (ACOG) are:
  - Cytology alone every 3 years between 21–30
  - Cytology plus HPV testing every 5 years after 30
- The International Federation of Gynecology and Obstetrics (FIGO) recommends visual inspection with acetic acid (VIA) or Lugol's iodine (VILI) as reasonable alternatives to Pap smear screening in resource-poor settings. A 3–5-year screening interval is currently recommended (2)[B].
- Despite HPV vaccination, cervical cancer screening will remain the main preventive measure for both vaccinated and nonvaccinated women.

COMMONLY ASSOCIATED CONDITIONS
- Condyloma acuminata
- Preinvasive/Invasive lesions of the vulva and vagina

DIAGNOSIS

HISTORY
- May be asymptomatic
- Most common symptom is vaginal bleeding, often postcoital
- Other gynecologic symptoms include intermenstrual or postmenopausal bleeding and vaginal discharge
- Other less common symptoms include low back pain with radiation down posterior leg, lower extremity edema, vesicovaginal and rectovaginal fistula, and urinary symptoms

PHYSICAL EXAM
- Disease is staged clinically, not surgically.
- Thorough internal and external pelvic exam is needed to look for lesions:
  - Most patients have a normal exam, especially with microinvasive disease.
  - Lesions may be exophytic, endophytic, polypoid, papillary, ulcerative, or necrotic.
  - Watery, purulent, or bloody discharge
- Bimanual and rectovaginal examination for uterine size, vaginal wall, rectovaginal septum, parametrial, uterosacral, and pelvic sidewall involvement
- Enlarged supraclavicular or inguinal lymphadenopathy, lower extremity edema, ascites, or decreased breath sounds with lung auscultation may indicate metastases.

DIFFERENTIAL DIAGNOSIS
- Marked cervicitis and erosion
- Glandular hyperplasia
- Sexually transmitted infection
- Cervical condyloma, leiomyoma, or polyp
- Metastasis from endometrial carcinoma or gestational trophoblastic disease

DIAGNOSTIC TESTS & INTERPRETATION
Initial Tests (lab, imaging)
- Biopsy of gross lesions and colposcopically directed biopsies are the definitive means of diagnosis.
- CBC may show anemia
- Urinalysis may show hematuria
- In advanced disease, BUN, creatinine, and liver function tests (LFTs) may be helpful.
- Initially, a CT scan of the chest, abdomen, and pelvis and/or a PET scan.
- Apart from chest x-ray (CXR) and intravenous pyelogram (IVP), imaging does not alter tumor stage.
- MRI may be helpful in evaluating parametrial involvement in patients who are surgical candidates.

Follow-Up Tests & Special Considerations
- Prompt multidisciplinary plan of care

Diagnostic Procedures/Other
- Exam under anesthesia may help in determining clinical stage and disease extent.
- Endocervical curettage and cervical conization as indicated to determine depth of invasion and presence of lymphovascular involvement
- Cystoscopy to evaluate bladder invasion
- Proctoscopy for invasion into rectum

Test Interpretation
- Majority of cases (80%) are invasive squamous cell types usually arising from the ectocervix.
- Adenocarcinomas comprise 10–15% of cervical cancer arising from endocervical mucus-producing glandular cells.
- Other cell types that may be present include rare mixed cell types, neuroendocrine tumors, sarcomas, lymphomas, and melanomas.

TREATMENT

GENERAL MEASURES
Improve nutritional state, correct any anemia, and treat any vaginal and/or pelvic infections.

MEDICATION
- Chemoradiation with cisplatin-containing regimen has superior survival rates over pelvic and extended-field radiation alone (3)[A].
- Neoadjuvant chemotherapy followed by surgery has not been shown to have a survival benefit for patients who are not initially surgical candidates due to tumor stage (4)[A].
- Adjuvant chemotherapy may improve progression-free survival in patients who receive primary chemoradiation for stage IIB–IVA tumors (5)[B]. The OUTBACK trial will further investigate these findings.

ISSUES FOR REFERRAL
Multidisciplinary management of patients as needed and in a timely fashion.

ADDITIONAL THERAPIES

- Chemoradiation (without surgery) is the first-line therapy for tumors stage IIB and higher (gross lesions with obvious parametrial involvement) and for most bulky stage IB2 tumors (6)[B].
- Combination of external beam pelvic radiation and brachytherapy is usually employed.
- If para-aortic lymph node metastases are suspected, extended-field radiation or lymph node dissection prior to radiation therapy may be performed.

SURGERY/OTHER PROCEDURES

- Surgical management is an option for patients with early-stage tumors.
- Removal of precursor lesions (cervical intraepithelial neoplasia [CIN]) by loop electrosurgical excision procedure (LEEP), cold knife conization, laser ablation, or cryotherapy (7)[A]
- Stage IA1 (lesions with <3-mm invasion from basement membrane) without lymphovascular space invasion: Option of conization or simple extrafascial hysterectomy (6)[B]
- Stage IA2 (lesions with >3-mm but <5-mm invasion from basement membrane): Option of radical hysterectomy with lymph node dissection or radiation, depending on clinical setting (6)[B]
- Stage IA2–IB1: Fertility-sparing radical trachelectomy may be considered in selected patients (6)[C]
- Stages IB1–IIA (gross lesions without obvious parametrial involvement): Option of radical hysterectomy with lymph node sampling or primary chemoradiation with brachytherapy and teletherapy (6)[A]
- Stage IVA (lesions limited to central metastasis to the bladder and/or rectum): Pelvic exenteration may be feasible.
- Stage IVB disease is treated with goal of palliation.

Pregnancy Considerations

- Management is guided by consideration of stage of lesion, gestational age, and maternal assessment of risks and benefits from treatment (6)[C].
- Abnormal cytology is best followed up by colposcopy with directed biopsies.
- CIN1 or less: Postpartum follow up
- CIN2–3: Management per established guidelines
- Microinvasive carcinoma: Conization or wedge biopsy. If depth of invasion ≤3 mm, follow up at the 6-week postpartum visit.
- Invasive carcinoma: Definitive therapy, with timing determined by maternal preference

IN-PATIENT CONSIDERATIONS

Admission Criteria/Initial Stabilization

- Signs of active bleeding
- Urinary symptoms
- Dehydration
- Complications from surgery, chemotherapy, or radiation
- Active vaginal bleeding can be controlled with timely vaginal packing and radiation therapy.
- Recognition of ureteral blockage, hydronephrosis, urosepsis, and timely intervention

Discharge Criteria

Discharge criteria based on multidisciplinary assessment

ONGOING CARE

FOLLOW-UP RECOMMENDATIONS

Patient Monitoring

- With completion of definitive therapy and based on individual risk factors, patients are evaluated with physical/pelvic examinations:
    - Every 3–6 months for 2 years
    - Every 6–12 months until the 5th year
    - Yearly thereafter (8)[B]
- Pap smears may be performed yearly but have a low sensitivity for detecting recurrence (8)[B].
- CT and PET scan are useful in locating metastases when recurrence is suspected (8)[B].
- Signs of recurrence include vaginal bleeding, unexplained weight loss, leg edema, and pelvic or thigh pain.

PATIENT EDUCATION

Patient education material available through the American College of Obstetricians and Gynecologists at www.acog.org, the Society of Gynecologic Oncology at www.sgo.org, the Foundation for Women's Cancer at www.foundationforwomenscancer.org, the American Cancer Society at www.cancer.org, and the National Cancer Institute at www.cancer.gov.

PROGNOSIS

Stage	5-yr Survival (%)
1	76–98
2	66–73
3	40–42
4	9–22

COMPLICATIONS

- Loss of ovarian function from radiotherapy or indication for bilateral oophorectomy
- Hemorrhage
- Pelvic infection
- Genitourinary fistula
- Bladder dysfunction
- Sexual dysfunction
- Ureteral obstruction with renal failure
- Bowel obstruction
- Pulmonary embolism
- Lower extremity lymphedema

REFERENCES

1. Scarinci IC, Garcia FA, Kobetz E, et al. Cervical cancer prevention: New tools and old barriers. *Cancer*. 2010;116:2531–2542.
2. International Federation of Obstetrics and Gynecology. Global Guidance for Cervical Cancer Prevention and Control. Available at: www.rho.org/files/FIGO_cervical_cancer_guidelines_2009.pdf
3. Chemoradiotherapy for Cervical Cancer Meta-analysis Collaboration (CCCMAC). Reducing uncertainties about the effects of chemoradiotherapy for cervical cancer: individual patient data meta-analysis. *Cochrane Database Syst Rev*. 2010;1:CD008285.
4. Rydzewska L, Tierney J, Vale CL, et al. Neoadjuvant chemotherapy plus surgery versus surgery for cervical cancer. *Cochrane Database Syst Rev*. 2010;1:CD007406.
5. Dueñas-González A, Zarbá JJ, Patel F, et al. Phase III, open-label, randomized study comparing concurrent gemcitabine plus cisplatin and radiation followed by adjuvant gemcitabine and cisplatin versus concurrent cisplatin and radiation in patients with stage IIB to IVA carcinoma of the cervix. *J Clin Oncol*. 2011;29:1678–1685.
6. National Comprehensive Cancer Network. NCCN Clinical Practice Guidelines in Oncology: Cervical Cancer. Available at: www.nccn.org/professionals/physician_gls/pdf/cervical.pdf
7. Martin-Hirsch PP, Paraskevaidis E, Bryant A, et al. Surgery for cervical intraepithelial neoplasia. *Cochrane Database Syst Rev*. 2010;6:CD001318.
8. Salani R, Backes FJ, Fung MFK, et al. Posttreatment surveillance and diagnosis of recurrence in women with gynecologic malignancies: Society of Gynecologic Oncologists recommendations. *Am J Obstet Gynecol*. 2011;204:466–478.

ADDITIONAL READING

- ACOG Committee on Practice Bulletins—Gynecology. ACOG Practice Bulletin no. 131: Screening for Cervical Cancer. *Obstet Gynecol*. 2012;120:1222–1238.
- American Society for Colposcopy and Cervical Pathology (ASCCP). Algorithms: Updated consensus guidelines for managing abnormal cervical cancer screening tests and cancer precursors. Available at: www.asccp.org/Portals/9/docs/Updated%20ASCCP%20Algorithms%204%2011%2013%20-%20PDF.pdf

SEE ALSO

Abnormal Pap and Cervical Dysplasia

CODES

ICD10

- C53.0 Malignant neoplasm of endocervix
- C53.1 Malignant neoplasm of exocervix
- C53.9 Malignant neoplasm of cervix uteri, unspecified

CLINICAL PEARLS

- Worldwide, cervical cancer is the 2nd most common malignancy among women. Improving access to screening is likely to have the greatest impact in reduction of burden of disease.
- Women with cervical cancer may be asymptomatic and have a normal physical exam.
- Surgical management is an option for patients with early-stage tumors.
- Chemoradiation is the first-line therapy for higher-stage tumors.

CERVICITIS, ECTROPION, AND TRUE EROSION
Kristina Duarte, MD • Marina MacNamara, MD, MPH

BASICS

DESCRIPTION
- Cervicitis refers to any inflammatory changes of the cervix; can result from infectious, noninfectious etiologies.
- Ectropion, often confused for cervicitis, is defined by the presence of cervical columnar cells on the vaginal portion of the cervix (portio); often seen during adolescence and during pregnancy.
- True erosion occurs with the loss of overlying cervical epithelium due to trauma (e.g., forceful insertion of vaginal speculum in patient with atrophic mucosa).
- System(s) affected: Reproductive

Geriatric Considerations
- Chronic cervicitis in postmenopausal women may be related to low levels of estrogen.
- The possibility of infectious cervicitis should not be overlooked in geriatric patients because many remain sexually active.

Pregnancy Considerations
Screen all pregnant women for infectious cervicitis because of risk of pregnancy complications and potential for transmission to the fetus.

Pediatric Considerations
Infectious cervicitis in children should lead to an investigation of possible sexual abuse.

EPIDEMIOLOGY
Incidence
- Cervicitis: Most commonly due to infectious etiologies, including:
  - Chlamydia: 1,412,791 cases were reported to the CDC in 2011, although it is estimated that as many as 2.86 million new cases of chlamydia occur in the US annually.
  - Gonorrhea: Next to chlamydia, gonorrhea is the 2nd most commonly reported notifiable disease in the US, with 321,849 cases reported to the CDC in 2011. It is estimated that there are 820,000 new infections annually.
  - Trichomoniasis: Case reporting data are not available. National Health and Nutrition Examination Survey (NHANES) data estimate an overall prevalence in the US of 3.1% (1).
  - *Mycoplasma genitalium* is becoming recognized as an important sexually transmitted pathogen that may be as common as chlamydia among high-risk, sexually active women (2,3).
- Ectropion: Typically related to higher levels of estrogen, ectropion is common among adolescents, women using oral contraceptive pills (OCP), and pregnant women.
- True erosion: Can be seen in women who have undergone cervical trauma.

ETIOLOGY AND PATHOPHYSIOLOGY
- Cervicitis: Often, no specific etiology is identified.
  - Infectious: *C. trachomatis, N. gonorrhoeae, T. vaginalis,* herpes simplex virus (HSV; especially primary infections of HSV-2), mycoplasmas (e.g., *M. genitalium*), *Ureaplasma,* cytomegalovirus. Nonsexually transmitted infectious cervicitis can be caused by overgrowth of β-hemolytic streptococcus or *E. coli.*
  - Noninfectious: Physical or chemical irritation (e.g., from douching or latex exposure or from vaginal foreign bodies), malignancy.

- Ectropion:
  - Hormonal changes with puberty, oral contraceptive use, or pregnancy
  - Resulting from cervical laceration during childbirth
- True erosion: Injury to atrophic epithelium: Estrogen-deficient states such as menopause

RISK FACTORS
- Infectious cervicitis:
  - Multiple sexual partners
  - Adolescence and young adulthood
  - Unprotected sex
  - History of STI
  - Smoking
  - Other reproductive tract infections: Vaginitis, pelvic inflammatory disease (PID)
- Noninfectious cervicitis
  - Foreign objects: Pessary, diaphragm, cervical cap, etc.
- Ectropion: Adolescence, pregnancy, use of OCP
- True erosion: Estrogen deficiency, trauma from foreign body.

GENERAL PREVENTION
- Sexually transmitted infections (chlamydia, gonorrhea, trichomonas):
  - Follow CDC-recommended screening measures: Annual screening for chlamydial infection in all sexually active nonpregnant young women ≤24 years and for older nonpregnant women who are at increased risk (1)[A] but not women ≥25 years who are not at increased risk (4)[C]. Screen among all pregnant women.
  - Annual screening for gonorrhea infection among all at-risk sexually active women (new partners, multiple partners, from communities with high prevalence). Screen among pregnant women at risk.
  - At least annual screening of trichomoniasis among HIV+ women.
  - Treat sexual partners of infected women.
  - Advise use of condoms and safer sexual practices.
- Estrogen deficiency: Estrogen replacement therapy

DIAGNOSIS

HISTORY
- May be asymptomatic
- Vaginal discharge
- Dyspareunia
- Bleeding/Spotting following intercourse

PHYSICAL EXAM
- Cervicitis: Purulent vaginal discharge, cervical friability, erythema, ulceration (HSV); punctate hemorrhage causes "strawberry" cervix appearance in trichomoniasis. Cervical motion tenderness may be appreciated on bimanual pelvic exam (suggests PID).
- Ectropion: Cervix appears red due to the color of the columnar epithelium.
- True erosion: Vaginal bleeding, sharply defined ulcers of cervix

DIFFERENTIAL DIAGNOSIS
- Cervical dysplasia
- Carcinoma of the cervix
- Bacterial vaginosis (discharge is noninflammatory)

DIAGNOSTIC TESTS & INTERPRETATION
- Saline and KOH preparation of cervical and vaginal smears may show leukorrhea (endocervical sample with >10 WBC/hpf suggests infectious cervicitis).
- Nucleic acid amplification tests: More sensitive and also be used on urine, self-obtained vaginal swabs, and endocervical specimens (5)[A]. This is also the most sensitive test for *M. genitalium,* although testing for this is not widely available.
- Vaginal wet mount for *T. vaginalis:*
  - Sensitivity for microscopy is low (~50%).
  - Culture, antigen assays, and nucleic acid amplification tests are available and have higher sensitivity for the detection of trichomoniasis. These should be considered in cases where microscopy is unavailable or inconclusive.
  - Pap smears should not be used to diagnose trichomoniasis as the sensitivity is low.
- If ulcerations are present, culture for HSV.

Diagnostic Procedures/Other
Colposcopy may be helpful in cases of chronic inflammation, with biopsy of suspicious areas.

Test Interpretation
- Cervicitis: Acute and chronic inflammatory changes, presence of infective organisms
- Ectropion: None/Squamous metaplasia
- True erosion: Sharply defined ulcer borders, loss of epithelium

TREATMENT

MEDICATION
First Line

- If infectious cervicitis suspected, treat without awaiting culture results: Ceftriaxone (Rocephin) 250 mg single dose IM, followed by either doxycycline (Vibramycin) 100 mg PO b.i.d. × 7 days or azithromycin (Zithromax) 1 g single dose (6)[A]. Option of ceftriaxone and azithromycin removes patient-compliance factor because they are 1-time doses.
- Chlamydia: For nonpregnant women, azithromycin 1 g PO once or doxycycline 100 mg b.i.d. PO × 7 days; for pregnant women, azithromycin 1 g once or erythromycin base 500 mg q.i.d. PO × 7 days or erythromycin ethylsuccinate 800 mg q.i.d. × 7 days.
- Gonorrhea: Due to increased resistance to antibiotics, the CDC currently recommends Ceftriaxone (Rocephin) 250 mg single dose IM, followed by either doxycycline (Vibramycin) 100 mg PO b.i.d. × 7 days or azithromycin (Zithromax) 1 g single dose.
- Trichomoniasis: Metronidazole 2 g once or 500 mg b.i.d. × 7 days or 1 g b.i.d. × 2 doses. A single oral dose of 2 g of tinidazole is also effective and may be better tolerated than metronidazole, although it is more expensive.
- *M. genitalium:* Azithromycin 1 g PO or 500 mg PO once followed by 250 mg PO daily × 4 days.
- Ectropion: None, unless patient is extremely symptomatic with copious discharge. In that case, acid-buffered vaginal jelly can be used to decrease discharge. Cautery can be used, but generally is considered overly invasive.

- True erosion: Conjugated estrogen cream applied vaginally daily for 1–2 weeks, followed by maintenance dosing twice weekly or oral hormone replacement therapy (HRT)
- Contraindications:
  – Metronidazole: Older references state that metronidazole is relatively contraindicated during 1st trimester of pregnancy. More recent meta-analyses suggest absence of teratogenicity. Treatment of trichomoniasis may be deferred until 2nd trimester if clinician remains concerned by product labeling.
  – Doxycycline: Pregnancy or lactation
  – Estrogen: See extended list of contraindications to estrogen use in standard texts.
- Precautions:
  – Metronidazole: See above; disulfiram reaction with ethanol ingestion
  – Doxycycline: Possible fetal harm if used during pregnancy; staining of the infant's teeth if used during breastfeeding; allergy; photosensitization
  – Erythromycin: Nausea or vomiting
  – Estrogens: History of estrogen-dependent neoplasms; history of thromboembolic diseases. See extended list of contraindications to estrogen therapy in standard texts.
- Significant possible interactions:
  – Metronidazole: Ethanol
  – Doxycycline: Dairy products, iron preparations, warfarin, and oral contraceptives (advise use of alternative contraceptive method)
  – Erythromycin: Theophylline (elevated theophylline level)
  – Estrogen: N/A

Pregnancy Considerations
- Doxycycline should be avoided in pregnancy.

Second Line
- Chlamydia:
  – Levofloxacin (Levaquin): 500 mg PO daily × 7 days
  – Ofloxacin (Floxin): 300 mg PO b.i.d. × 7 days
- Gonorrhea:
  – Cefixime: 400 mg PO single dose is an acceptable alternative to ceftriaxone, however, necessitates that the patient return in 1 week for a test-of-cure.
  – In the case of a true penicillin allergy, alternative regimens include:
    o Azithromycin (Zithromax): 2 g PO as a single dose, however, due to evidence of increasing resistance to macrolides, use should be limited.
    o Due to increasing resistance to quinolones, the following antibiotics should be prescribed with follow-up testing to ensure eradication (6):
    o Ofloxacin (Floxin): 400 mg PO single dose
    o Ciprofloxacin (Cipro): 500 mg PO single dose
    o Levofloxacin (Levaquin): 250 mg PO single dose
- M. genitalium: Moxifloxacin: 400 mg PO daily × 7–10 days
- Estrogen deficiency: A number of estrogen vaginal preparations are available commercially.

Pregnancy Considerations
Quinolones are also contraindicated in pregnancy.

SURGERY/OTHER PROCEDURES
- Chronic cervicitis with negative cultures that does not respond to empirical medical treatment may be treated with cryosurgery, electrocautery, or loop excision.
- Adverse effects of cautery or cryosurgery can include cervical stenosis, which may affect fertility.

 ## ONGOING CARE

FOLLOW-UP RECOMMENDATIONS
Patient Monitoring
- Test of cure is recommended in pregnant patients to document eradication of infection and should be performed approximately at least 3 weeks following treatment.
- Reinfection with gonorrhea and chlamydia is common, and repeat screening should be performed routinely for all patients 3–4 months following treatment.
- Estrogen deficiency: Re-examine in 1 month to confirm healing.

ALERT
Test of cure with nucleic acid amplification tests should not be done <3 weeks after treatment because of false-positive results due to dead organisms.

PATIENT EDUCATION
If the etiology of cervicitis is confirmed to be an STI, educate patient on the necessity of treating her sexual partners to avoid reinfection. To avoid reinfection, patient should abstain from sexual intercourse for 7 days after a single-dose regimen or after completion of a 7-day regi-men. Expedited partner therapy (EPT) is allowed in some states.

PROGNOSIS
- Cervicitis: Excellent after bacterial infection is eradicated.
- Ectropion: Spontaneous regression postpartum and with cessation of use of oral contraceptives.
- True erosion: Spontaneous healing.

COMPLICATIONS
- Cervicitis due to C. trachomatis or N. gonorrhoeae is associated with an 8–10% risk of developing subsequent PID. Adolescents are a high-risk group for reinfection with sexually transmitted organisms, and screening frequency should be at least once yearly in this population.
- M. genitalium may be associated with PID.
- Among women who are positive for HIV, the presence of cervicitis increases the risk of viral shedding and transmission to sexual partners (6).

REFERENCES
1. Sutton M, Sternberg M, Koumans EH, et al. The prevalence of Trichomonas vaginalis infection among reproductive-age women in the United States, 2001–2004. *Clin Infect Dis*. 2007;45: 1319–1326.
2. Haggerty CL, Taylor BD. Mycoplasma genitalium: An emerging cause of pelvic inflammatory disease. *Infect Dis Obstet Gynecol*. 2011;2011:959816. Epub 2011 Dec 25.
3. Cazanave C, Manhart LE, Bébéar C. Mycoplasma genitalium, an emerging sexually transmitted pathogen. *Med Mal Infect*. 2012;42(9):381–392. Epub 2012 Sep 10.
4. US Preventive Services Task Force. Screening for chlamydial infection: U.S. Preventive Services Task Force recommendation statement. *Ann Intern Med*. 2007;147:128–134.
5. Cook RL, Hutchison SL, Østergaard L, et al. Systematic review: Noninvasive testing for Chlamydia trachomatis and Neisseria gonorrhoeae. *Ann Intern Med*. 2005;142:914–925.
6. Workowski KA, Berman S, Centers for Disease Control and Prevention (CDC). Sexually transmitted diseases treatment guidelines, 2010. *MMWR Recomm Rep*. 2010;59(RR-12):1–110.

ADDITIONAL READING
- Gülmezoglu AM, Azhar M. Interventions for trichomoniasis in pregnancy. *Cochrane Database Syst Rev*. 2011;(5):CD000220. Epub 2011 May 11.
- Johnson LF, Lewis DA. The effect of genital tract infections on HIV-1 shedding in the genital tract: A systematic review and meta-analysis. *Sex Transm Dis*. 2008;35(11):946–959.
- Wilson JF. In the clinic. Vaginitis and cervicitis. *Ann Intern Med*. 2009;151(5):ITC3-1–ITC3-15; Quiz ITC3-16.

 ## CODES

ICD10
- N72 Inflammatory disease of cervix uteri
- N86 Erosion and ectropion of cervix uteri

CLINICAL PEARLS
- If infectious cervicitis is suspected, treatment of choice is ceftriaxone 250 mg IM plus azithromycin 1 g PO × 1 dose. Do not wait for test results.
- Encourage patient to have sexual partner(s) treated.
- Quinolones are no longer recommended to treat gonorrhea.
- Lubricants (e.g., KY Jelly) do not alter Pap smear results, so small quantities may be used when performing Pap smears.
- Positive results for N. gonorrhoeae or chlamydia should be reported to local or state health department.

CHANCROID

Jeffery T. Kirchner, DO, FAAFP, AAHIVS

 BASICS

DESCRIPTION
- A rare American STD characterized by painful genital ulcerations and inflammatory inguinal adenopathy.
- Although uncommon in the US, it is found worldwide.
- Chancroid is endemic in developing countries, especially sub-Saharan Africa, and is a cofactor for HIV transmission.

EPIDEMIOLOGY
Incidence
- <50 cases reported to CDC in 2004–2012
- Actual numbers are considered higher due to lack of testing and thus underreporting.

Prevalence
- Endemic in developing countries; annual estimated global prevalence of 4–6 million, but actual prevalence is unknown due to lack of testing
- Thought to be extremely common in:
  – Sub-Saharan Africa
  – Southeast Asia
  – Latin America

ETIOLOGY AND PATHOPHYSIOLOGY
- Involves entry of the bacteria through abraded skin, followed by attachment of the bacteria to susceptible cells
- Cytotoxin is secreted, which may play a role in epithelial injury and ulcer formation.
- The bacterium contains a fimbrialike protein (*flp*) operon that encodes proteins that contribute to adherence and pathogenesis.
- Dendritic cells and natural killer cells respond to *Haemophilus ducreyi,* and this innate host response determines bacterial clearance vs. disease progression.

Haemophilus ducreyi (gram-negative rod) thought to be strictly a human pathogen

RISK FACTORS
- Multiple sexual partners
- Uncircumcised men
- Prostitutes may be carriers.
- Patients presenting with other genital ulcerative diseases
- HIV

GENERAL PREVENTION
Condom use should be demonstrated and promoted.

COMMONLY ASSOCIATED CONDITIONS
- Syphilis: Concurrent in 10% of patients
- Herpes simplex virus (HSV) or HIV infection

 DIAGNOSIS

HISTORY
- Exposure to infected individual, but often not helpful or obtained
- Incubation period typically lasts 4–10 days.

PHYSICAL EXAM
- Tender erythematous genital papule that progresses into a pustule that erodes into an ulcer:
  – Infected persons commonly have 1–3 ulcers.
- Typical ulcer is 1–2 cm, but size is variable.
- Ulcers are painful, with erythematous base and ragged edges, which are sometimes undermined:
  – Common sites for ulcers in men include the penile shaft, glans, and meatus.
  – Common sites for ulcers in women include labia, introitus, and perianal areas.
- Inguinal lymphadenitis with abscess (bubo) formation occurs in ~50% of men, but less common in women.
- Buboes arise 1–2 weeks after ulceration and are typically painful.
- Buboes may spontaneously rupture if the primary disease is untreated.
- Atypical presentations include folliculitis and foreskin abscess.

DIFFERENTIAL DIAGNOSIS
- Syphilis (*Treponema pallidum*)
- Genital herpes (HSV-1 and -2)
- Lymphogranuloma venereum (*Chlamydia trachomatis*)
- Granuloma inguinale (donovanosis)
- Drug eruption; Behçet disease

DIAGNOSTIC TESTS & INTERPRETATION
CDC criteria for presumptive diagnosis:
- Definite: Isolation of *H. ducreyi* from a lesion
- Probable: Clinical findings, including genital ulcer and regional adenopathy, *plus* negative dark field exam, negative serologic test for syphilis, negative cultures for HSV, or a clinical presentation not typical for HSV.

Initial Tests (lab, imaging)
- "School of fish" pattern on Gram stain, with organisms clumped in long parallel strands
- Serologic testing for antibody to *H. ducreyi* with ELISA (although may not be diagnostic of acute infection)
- Culture of the organism on Mueller-Hinton agar with incorporated vancomycin, but sensitivity is <80%
- Multiplex polymerase chain reaction (PCR) has sensitivity of 95–98%, but no FDA-approved tests in the US; available from some commercial labs

Follow-Up Tests & Special Considerations
- All patients should also concurrently be tested for syphilis and HIV.

- Test of cure is not recommended (1)[A]

Diagnostic Procedures/Other
Gram stain and culture of exudate (2):
- Aspiration of inguinal bubo (lymph node); can also obtain culture material from base of cleansed ulcer
- PCR testing of ulcer exudate for *H. ducreyi* DNA
- Darkfield examination of exudate to rule out *T. pallidum* infection
- Culture or PCR testing for HSV

TREATMENT

GENERAL MEASURES
- Outpatient treatment
- Saline or Burrow's solution to soak ulcers
- Aspiration of buboes if >5 cm; approached through adjacent skin. Also consider incision and drainage for larger lesions.

ALERT
HIV may affect treatment response.

MEDICATION
First Line
- Azithromycin: 1 g PO single dose (3,4,5)[A], *OR*
- Ceftriaxone 250 mg IM single dose

Second Line
- Ciprofloxacin 500 mg PO b.i.d. for 3 days (3,4,5,6)[A]
- Erythromycin base 500 mg t.i.d. for 7 days (3,4,5,6)[A]
- Contraindications:
  - Allergy to the medication
  - Ciprofloxacin during pregnancy and lactation and in patients <18 years

ONGOING CARE

FOLLOW-UP RECOMMENDATIONS
Patient Monitoring
- Avoid sexual activity until ulcers are resolved.
- Clinical improvement usually occurs within 48 hours.
- Patients should be reexamined 3–7 days after initiation of therapy and followed closely until all clinical signs of infection are resolved.
- Baseline syphilis serology and at 3 months
- Baseline HIV testing and at 3 months posttreatment

PATIENT EDUCATION
- Sexual counseling
- Use of condoms
- Local wound care
- Treatment of all sexual partners with same regimen as index
- HIV testing

PROGNOSIS
- Full clinical resolution with appropriate treatment
- Failure to respond may be due to:
  - Incorrect diagnosis
  - Coinfection with syphilis
  - Coinfection with HIV
  - Medication nonadherence
  - Resistant *H. ducreyi*.
- *5% relapse after treatment*

COMPLICATIONS
- Phimosis
- Balanoposthitis
- Rupture of buboes with fistula formation and scarring

REFERENCES
1. Lewis DA, Ison CA. Chancroid. *Sex Transm Infect*. 2006;82(Suppl 4):iv19–20.
2. Alfa M. The laboratory diagnosis of *Haemophilus ducreyi*. *Can J Infect Dis Med Microbiol*. 2005; 16(1):31–34.
3. Lewis DA. Chancroid: Clinical manifestations, diagnosis, and management. *Sex Transm Inf*. 2003;79:68–71.
4. Kemp M, Christensen JJ, Lautenschlager S, et al. European guideline for the management of chancroid, 2011. *Int J STD AIDS*. 2011;22: 241–244.
5. Roett MA, Mayor MT, Uduhiri KA. Diagnosis and management of genital ulcers. *Am Fam Physician*. 2012;85(3):254–262.
6. Centers for Disease Control and Prevention. Sexually transmitted diseases treatment guidelines—2010. *MMWR*. 2010;59:19–20.

ADDITIONAL READING
- Centers for Disease Control and Prevention. *Morbidity and Mortality Weekly Report*. February 15, 2013/62(06); ND-7-ND-85.
- Janowicz DM, Li W, Bauer ME. Host-pathogen interplay of *Haemophilus ducreyi*. *Curr Opin Infect Dis*. 2010;23(1):64–69.
- Janowicz DM, Ofner S, Katz BP, et al. Experimental infection of human volunteers with *Haemophilus ducreyi*: Fifteen years of clinical data and experience. *J Infect Dis*. 2009;199(11):1671–1679.
- Mutua FM, Mimunya JM, Wiysonge CS. Genital ulcer disease treatment for reducing sexual acquisition of HIV. *Cochrane Database Syst Rev*. 2012 Aug 15;8: CD007933. doi: 10.1002/14651858.
- Kemp M, Christensen JJ, Lautenschlager S, et al. European guideline for the management of chancroid, 2011. *Int J STD AIDS*. 2011;22(5): 241–244. doi: 10.1258/ijsa.2010.010432.

CODES

ICD10
A57 Chancroid

CLINICAL PEARLS
- Chancroid is a rare disorder in the US, but more common elsewhere.
- Characterized by genital papules that progress to pustules that open, producing painful ulcers
- Treatment of choice is azithromycin 1 g, once.
- Treat sexual partners (from prior 3 months) even in the absence of signs or symptoms of disease.
- All patients should also concurrently be tested for syphilis and HIV.

CHICKENPOX (VARICELLA ZOSTER)

Kay A. Bauman, MD, MPH

 BASICS

DESCRIPTION
- Common, highly contagious generalized exanthem characterized by the development of crops of pruritic vesicles on the skin and mucous membranes
- Fever in up to 70% of persons
- Virus is spread by respiratory (airborne) droplets, direct contact with varicella vesicles, or, rarely, zoster lesions.
- Virus establishes latency in the dorsal root ganglia; reactivation results in herpes zoster or "shingles."
- Outbreaks tend to occur late winter to early spring in temperate climates.
- Usual incubation period is 14–16 days (range, 10–21). Patients are infectious from ~48 hours before appearance of the rash until the final lesions have crusted. Historically, most people acquire chickenpox during childhood and develop lifelong immunity:
  - *Now it is an immunizable disease.*
- System(s) affected: Nervous; Skin/Exocrine
- Synonym(s): Varicella

EPIDEMIOLOGY
- Predominant age: Peak incidence preschoolers to 9 years, but may occur at any age
- Predominant gender: Male = Female

Incidence
- Decreasing incidence since vaccine available: Estimated at 3.5 million cases annually prior to vaccine introduction, with an incidence rate of 8–9% in children age 1–9 years. Reported US varicella cases 1991: 147,076; reported for 2011: 14,513, provisionally reported for 2012: 11,477 cases (1,2,3)
- Prior to vaccine availability, ~100 deaths/year were reported in the US; for 2010, only 4 deaths were reported (1).
- US rates: 1994, prior to vaccine: 135.76/100,000 persons; 2009: 8.71/100,000 persons (1)
- Rates in the US had dropped continuously after vaccine development until mid-2000s when they evened out; 2nd dose of vaccine recommended in 2006, and rates again have declined year by year (1).

ETIOLOGY AND PATHOPHYSIOLOGY
- Skin lesions identical histologically to those of herpes simplex virus
- In fatal cases, intranuclear inclusions can be found in the endothelium of blood vessels and most organs.
- Varicella-zoster virus is a member of the α-Herpesviridae subfamily; a double-stranded DNA virus.
- Reservoir is humans.

RISK FACTORS
- No prior history of varicella infection
- Immunosuppressed patients (especially children with leukemia/lymphoma in remission or receiving high-dose corticosteroids)

Geriatric Considerations
- Infection more severe in adults than in children
- Latent varicella infection may reactivate and cause the exanthem known as shingles or zoster.
- Herpes zoster vaccine, a live attenuated vaccine licensed in 2006, is now recommended for persons ≥60 years to prevent zoster (shingles): FDA-approved for those ≥50 years:
  - 1-time dose. Recommended for those previously infected with varicella (chickenpox); those never infected should receive regular varicella vaccine. Dose: 0.65 mL SQ, available as single-dose vial.
  - Advisory Committee on Immunization Practices (ACIP) recommends routine vaccination of all persons aged >60 years with 1 dose of zoster vaccine. It is not necessary to ask patients about their history of varicella (chickenpox) or to conduct serologic testing for varicella immunity.
  - Most common cause of death: Primary viral pneumonia

Pediatric Considerations
- Neonates born to mothers who develop chickenpox from 5 days before to 2 days after delivery are at risk for serious disease. Must give varicella-zoster immune globulin.
- Varicella bullosa seen mainly in children <2 years. Lesions appear as bullae instead of vesicles. The clinical course does not change.
- Most common cause of death: Septic complications and encephalitis
- Avoid aspirin/acetylsalicylic acid in children because of link to Reye syndrome.

Pregnancy Considerations
- 25% risk of transplacental infection after maternal infection
- Congenital malformations are seen in 2% of patients when the fetus is infected during the 1st or 2nd trimesters, characterized by limb atrophy and scarring of the skin of the extremities and occasional CNS and eye manifestations.
- Morbidity is increased in women infected during pregnancy (e.g., pneumonia).

GENERAL PREVENTION
- Exposed, susceptible people should be considered at risk and potentially infectious for 21 days.
- Isolate hospitalized patients.
- Passive immunization with IM varicella-zoster immune globulin given within 96 hours of exposure, but recently approved for 10 days after exposure (4):
  - Recommended for people exposed to chickenpox or shingles who are immunocompromised; newborns of mothers with onset of chickenpox <5 days before delivery or <2 days after delivery; premature infants (<28 weeks) exposed in neonatal period, either whose mothers are not immune, or babies who weigh <1,000 g regardless of mom's immunity (4).

- Active immunization after exposure: Shown to prevent or reduce significantly the severity of varicella if given within 72 hours postexposure
- Active immunization: Varicella virus vaccine (Varivax): Live attenuated vaccine approved by FDA in 1995 for pediatrics immunization and recommended by ACIP for immunization of healthy patients ≥12 months who have not had chickenpox:
  - 12 months–12 years: Initial dose 0.5 mL SC at age 12–15 months; 2nd dose age 4–6 years. Prelicensure studies showed efficacy rates: 70–90% against any disease and 95% against severe disease 7–10 years after vaccination. Other studies showed 100% efficacy at 1 year and 98% at 2 years after vaccination. More recent studies show rates of 85–94% effectiveness, the higher end for the prevention of severe disease. The 2-dose regimen is even more effective, with rates of 96–98% effectiveness. Breakthrough disease generally has <50 lesions, shorter duration of illness, and lower incidence of fever (5)[A].
  - ≥13 years: Two 0.5 mL SC doses 4–8 weeks apart, seroconversion rates 78–82% after 1 dose, 99% after 2 doses. Adults have efficacy rates in the lower end of this range.
  - Estimated 2-dose vaccine coverage in the US for 2009 in children ages 19–35 months: 89.6%
  - Vaccine side effects are pain and redness at vaccine site.
  - Vaccine contraindications (6):
    - Severe allergic reaction (e.g., anaphylaxis) to a previous dose or vaccine component
    - Severe immunodeficiency (e.g., severely immunocompromised HIV patients, on chemotherapy, congenital immunodeficiency, or long-term immunosuppressive therapy)
    - Pregnancy
- Newly approved MMRV vaccine, which combines the measles, mumps, and rubella vaccine with varicella, is equally effective. There are rare reports of an increased risk of febrile seizures 5–12 days after vaccination in 1/2,300–2,600 patients (7)[A].
- May be considered for a subset of HIV-positive children in CDC class I with CD4 >25%:
  - Vaccine recipients should avoid contact with immunocompromised people and pregnant women who have never had chickenpox and their newborns, for up to 6 weeks after vaccination.
  - Children needing catch-up vaccination need at least 3 months between doses 1 and 2.

 DIAGNOSIS

HISTORY
- Prodromal symptoms: Fever, malaise, anorexia, mild headache
- Malaise, muscle aches, arthralgias, and headache more common in adults
- Subclinical in ~4% of cases

PHYSICAL EXAM
- Characteristic rash: Crops of "teardrop" vesicles on erythematous bases
- Lesions erupt in successive crops.
- Progress from macule to papule to vesicle, then begin to crust
- Pruritic rash is present in various stages of development.
- Lesions may be present on mucous membranes, both oral and vaginal.

DIFFERENTIAL DIAGNOSIS
- Herpes simplex virus infection
- Herpes zoster
- Impetigo
- Coxsackievirus infection
- Scabies
- Dermatitis herpetiformis
- Drug rash
- Rickettsial pox infection

DIAGNOSTIC TESTS & INTERPRETATION
Generally used for complicated cases and epidemiologic studies

Initial Tests (lab, imaging)
- Leukocyte count may be normal, low, or mildly increased.
- Marked leukocytosis suggests secondary infection.
- Multinucleated giant cells visible on Tzanck smear from scrapings of vesicles
- Isolated virus from human tissue culture

Follow-Up Tests & Special Considerations
- Visualization of the virus by electron microscopy, tissue culture (costly), and various methods of acute and convalescent sera collection: Latex agglutination (most available), enzyme immunoassay, indirect immunofluorescence antibody, fluorescent antibody to membrane assay, or polymerase chain reaction (PCR) assay, which can detect wild from vaccine viral strains
- Vaccine-modified cases can be more difficult to diagnose; consider PCR testing of skin lesions (8)[B].

TREATMENT

Outpatient, except for complicating emergencies

GENERAL MEASURES
- Supportive/symptomatic treatment
- Antihistamines and/or Aveeno or oatmeal baths, as needed, for itch
- Acetaminophen and/or ibuprofen, as needed
- Nail clipping in children to prevent scarring or secondary infection from itching

MEDICATION
First Line
- Supportive: Antipyretics for fever; avoid aspirin in children.
- Local and/or systemic antipruritic agents for itching
- In immunocompromised patients: Varicella-zoster immunoglobulin available for passive immunization. Varicella-zoster immunoglobulin must be given within 96 hours after exposure to be beneficial. After 4th day postexposure, wait for rash to develop, then give acyclovir 500 mg/m^2/d q8h for 7 days.

- Acyclovir: Decreases duration of fever and shortens time of viral shedding. Recommended for adolescents, adults, and high-risk patients. Most beneficial if initiated early in the disease ($\leq$24 hours):
  – 2–16-year-old patients: 20 mg/kg/dose (max. 800 mg/dose), q.i.d. for 5 days
  – Adults: 800 mg, 5 times daily
- Contraindications:
  – Hypersensitivity to the drug
- Precautions:
  – Possible renal insufficiency with acyclovir
  – Significant possible interactions
  – Concurrent administration of probenecid increases half-life; increased effects with zidovudine (e.g., drowsiness, lethargy)

Second Line
- Famciclovir: 500 mg t.i.d. for 7–10 days (adults)
- Valacyclovir: 1 g t.i.d. for 7–10 days (adults)

ONGOING CARE

FOLLOW-UP RECOMMENDATIONS
Patient Monitoring
- Usually none needed in mild cases. If complications occur, intensive supportive care may be required.
- Activity, as tolerated. Children may return to school when lesions have scabbed.

DIET
No special diet

PATIENT EDUCATION
- In the healthy child, chickenpox is rarely serious and recovery is complete.
- Confers lifelong immunity
- 2nd attack rare, but subclinical infection can occur; happens occasionally after vaccination in children
- Infection latent and may recur years later as herpes zoster in adults (and sometimes in children)
- Fatalities rarely occur from complications.

COMPLICATIONS
- Although only 2% of cases are reported after 2nd decade, 35% of deaths occur in this age group.
- Secondary bacterial infection: Cellulitis, abscess, erysipelas, sepsis, septic arthritis/osteomyelitis, or staphylococcal pyomyositis
- Pneumonia: 20–30% of adults with chickenpox have lung involvement; 1/400 is hospitalized.
- Encephalitis (the most common CNS complication)
- Meningitis
- Reye syndrome
- Purpura
- Thrombocytopenia
- Glomerulonephritis
- Arthritis
- Hepatitis

REFERENCES

1. Centers for Disease Control and Prevention. Summary of notifiable diseases, US, 2009. *MMWR*. 2011;58(53):1–100.
2. Provisional Cases of Notifiable Diseases. *MMWR*. 2012;60:1174.
3. Center for Disease Control and Prevention. *MMWR*, 2013;61:731.
4. Centers for Disease Control and Prevention (CDC). FDA approval of an extended period for administering VariZIG for postexposure prophylaxis of varicella. *MMWR Morb Mortal Wkly Rep*. 2012;61(12):212.
5. Marin M, Güris D, Chaves SS, et al. Prevention of varicella: Recommendations of the Advisory Committee on Immunization Practices (ACIP). *MMWR Recomm Rep*. 2007;56: 1–40.
6. National Center for Immunization and Respiratory Diseases. General recommendations on immunization—recommendations of the Advisory Committee on Immunization Practices (ACIP). *MMWR Recomm Rep*. 2011;60(2):1–64.
7. Marin M, Broder KR, Temte JL, et al. Use of combination measles, mumps, rubella, and varicella vaccine: Recommendations of the Advisory Committee on Immunization Practices (ACIP). *MMWR Recomm Rep*. 2010;59:1–12.
8. Leung J, Harpaz R, Baughman AL, et al. Evaluation of laboratory methods for diagnosis of varicella. *Clin Infect Dis*. 2010;51:23–32.

ADDITIONAL READING
- Centers for Disease Control and Prevention (CDC). Varicella-related deaths—United States, January 2003-June 2004. *MMWR*. 2005;54:272–274.
- Centers for Disease Control and Prevention. Summary of Notifiable Diseases, US, 1991. *MMWR*. 1992;40(53).
- Galea SA, Sweet A, Beninger P, et al. The safety profile of varicella vaccine: A 10-year review. *J Infect Dis*. 2008;197(Suppl 2):S165–S169.

SEE ALSO

Herpes Zoster

CODES

ICD10
- B01.9 Varicella without complication
- B01.89 Other varicella complications
- B02.9 Zoster without complications

CLINICAL PEARLS
- Infection is more likely to produce serious illness in adults than in children.
- All people being immunized should receive 2 doses of vaccine, preferably at least 3 months but no fewer than 28 days apart.
- Herpes zoster vaccine (Zostavax) recommended for persons $\geq$60 years of age to prevent shingles (zoster).

CHILD ABUSE
Karen A. Hulbert, MD

BASICS

DESCRIPTION
- Types of abuse: Neglect (most common and highest mortality), physical abuse, emotional/psychological abuse, sexual abuse
- System(s) affected: Gastrointestinal (GI); Endocrine/Metabolic; Musculoskeletal; Nervous; Renal; Reproductive; Skin/Exocrine; Psychiatric
- Synonym(s): Suspected nonaccidental trauma; Child maltreatment; Child neglect

EPIDEMIOLOGY
Incidence
- The National Incidence Study (NIS) estimates the incidence of neglect in the US using estimates from child protective service (CPS) statistics and other sources. Most recent NIS-4 (2010) looked at data from 2005 to 2006 (1).
- Using the stringent "Harm Standard" definition, >1.25 million children experience maltreatment (1 in 58).
- Using the "Endangerment Standard," 3 million children experienced maltreatment (1 child in 25).

Prevalence
- In 2011, there were an estimated 3.4 million referrals to CPS agencies involving the alleged maltreatment of ~6.2 million children (2).
- Nearly 2 million reports were screened for a CPS response, putting the victimization rate in 2011 at 9.1 for every 1,000 children; those aged <1 year had the highest rate (21.2 per 1,000 children) (2).
- The greatest percentage of children were neglected (78.5%) compared to 17.6% suffering physical abuse and 9.1% suffering sexual abuse (2).
- The overall rate of child fatalities was 2.1 deaths per 100,000 children; 81.6% were in children <4, and 78% of fatalities were caused by ≥1 parent. Boys had a higher fatality rate (2).

RISK FACTORS
- All ages; Male = Female:
  - Risk of physical abuse increases with age.
  - Risk of fatal abuse more common in those <2 years
  - Physical abuse 2.1× higher among children with disabilities (3)
- Poverty, drug abuse, lower educational status, parental history of abuse, mentally ill parent/maternal depression, poor support network, and domestic violence:
  - Child abuse 4.9× more likely in family with spouse abuse (3).
  - Children in households with unrelated adults, 50× more likely to die of inflicted injuries (3)
  - Adults who were abused as children are at higher risk of becoming abusers than those not abused.

GENERAL PREVENTION
- Know your patients and document their family situations; have increased suspicion to screen for risk factors at prenatal, postnatal, pediatric visits.
- Physicians can educate parents on range of normal behaviors to expect in infants and children:
  - Anticipatory guidance on ways to handle crying infants; methods of discipline for toddlers
- Train 1st responders—teachers, childcare workers—to look for signs of abuse.

- Some studies suggest developing screening tools to identify high-risk families early and offer interventions, such as early childhood home visitation programs (4)[A].

COMMONLY ASSOCIATED CONDITIONS
- Failure to thrive
- Prematurity
- Developmental deficits
- Poor school performance
- Poor social skills
- Low self-esteem, depression

DIAGNOSIS

- Relatively minor injuries, frenulum tears or bruising in precruising infants, may be the 1st indication of child physical abuse; these minor, suspicious injuries have been termed "sentinel injuries" (5).

- In a retrospective study of infants who were definitely abused, 27.5% had a sentinel injury (80% had a bruise), and, in 41.9% of those cases, the parent reported that a medical provider was aware of the injury (5)[B].

- Documentation:
  - The medical record is an important piece of evidence for investigation and litigation (6)[C].
  - Critical elements include (6)[C]:
    - Brief statement of child's disclosure or caregiver's explanation, including any alternate explanations offered
    - Time the incident occurred and date/time of disclosure
    - Whether witnesses were present
    - Developmental abilities of child
    - Objective medical findings
    - Interpretation of the findings
- DO NOT use terms such as "rule out," "R/O," and "alleged." They may cause ambiguity; clearly state physician opinion (6)[C].
- Documentation should include disposition of patient and record any report made to CPS (6)[C].

HISTORY
- History of a sentinel injury should prompt consideration of abuse; it may be the 1st and only abusive injury; there may be escalating and repeated violence instead of a single event of momentary loss of control (5)[B].

- Use nonjudgmental, open-ended questions (ask: Who, what, when, and where; NEVER why).
- Use quotes whenever possible.
- Document past medical and developmental history, child's temperament, and interactions among family members.
- Suggestive of intentional trauma:
  - No explanation or vague explanation (3)
  - Important detail of explanation changes dramatically (3)
  - Explanation is inconsistent with pattern, age, or severity (3)
  - Explanation is inconsistent with child's physical or developmental abilities (3)
  - Different witnesses provide markedly different history (3).
  - Considerable delay in seeking treatment
- Nonspecific symptoms of abuse:
  - Behavior changes; self-destructive behavior
  - Anxiety and/or depression

  - Sleep disturbances, night terrors
  - School problems

PHYSICAL EXAM
- Explain what the exam will involve and why procedures are needed.
- Examine child in a comfortable setting.
- Allow child to choose who will be in the room.
- Use appropriate positions to examine the anal and genital areas of children (7)[C].
- General assessment for signs of physical abuse, neglect, self-injurious behaviors (7)[C]
- Thorough physical exam:
  - Skin, head, eyes, ears, nose, and mouth
  - Chest/Abdomen
  - Genital (consider exam under sedation) or refer to emergency department (ED)
  - Extremities, with focus on inner arms and legs
  - Growth data
- Maintain high index of suspicion for occult head, chest, and abdominal trauma.
- Physical abuse (8):
  - Skin markings (e.g., lacerations, burns, ecchymoses, linear/shaped contusions, bites)
  - Immersion injuries with clearly distinguished outlines (e.g., from boiling water)
  - Oral trauma (e.g., torn frenulum, loose teeth)
  - Ear trauma (e.g., signs of ear pulling)
  - Eye trauma (e.g., hyphema, hemorrhage)
  - Head/Abdominal blunt trauma
  - Fractures
- Sexual abuse:
  - Unexplained penile, vaginal, hymenal, perianal, or anal injuries/bleeding/discharge
  - Pregnancy or STIs
  - Sperm is a definitive finding of child abuse.
- Neglect:
  - Child may be low weight for height, unclean, or unkempt.
  - Rashes
  - Fearful or too trusting
  - Clinging to or avoiding caregiver
  - Flat or balding occiput
  - Abnormal development or growth parameters
- Measurements, photographs, and careful descriptions are critical for accurate diagnosis.
- Collaboration with specialist and child abuse assessment team (3)[C]

DIFFERENTIAL DIAGNOSIS
- Physical trauma:
  - Accidental injury; toxic ingestion
  - Bleeding disorders (e.g., classic hemophilia)
  - Metabolic or congenital conditions
  - Conditions with skin manifestations (e.g., mongolian spots, Henoch-Schönlein purpura, meningococcemia, erythema multiforme, hypersensitivity, car seat burns, staphylococcal scalded skin syndrome, chickenpox, impetigo)
  - Cultural practices (e.g., cupping, coining)
- Neglect:
  - Endocrinopathies (e.g., diabetes mellitus)
  - Constitutional
  - GI (clefts, malabsorption, irritable bowel)
  - Seizure disorder
  - Sudden infant death syndrome (SIDS)
- Skeletal trauma:
  - Obstetrical trauma
  - Nutritional (scurvy, rickets)
  - Infection (congenital syphilis, osteomyelitis)
  - Osteogenesis imperfecta

DIAGNOSTIC TESTS & INTERPRETATION
Initial Tests (lab, imaging)
- Directed by history and physical exam:
  - Urinalysis (e.g., abdominal/flank/back/genital trauma), urine DNA probe for STIs
  - Complete blood chemistry. Consideration of coagulation studies and platelet count (e.g., rule out bleeding disorder, abdominal trauma) as appropriate.
  - Electrolytes, creatinine, BUN, glucose
  - Liver and pancreatic function tests (e.g., abdominal trauma)
  - Guaiac stool (abdominal trauma)
- In cases of suspected neglect:
  - Stool exam, calorie count, purified protein derivative and anergy panel, sweat test, lead and zinc levels
- In cases of suspected sexual abuse:
  - STI testing: Gonorrhea, chlamydia, trichomonas; also consider HIV, herpes simplex virus (HSV), hepatitis panel, syphilis (7)[C]
  - Serum pregnancy test (7)[C]
- A skeletal survey for abusive fractures, especially if <6 months. Obtain follow-up survey even if initial is negative in cases with significant concern (9).
- In 1 retrospective analysis, 79% of detected cases of abuse had healing fractures due to victims being abused on >1 occasion (9).
- All children with fractures and children with suspicious injuries <2 years:
  - Skeletal survey (3)[B]: X-rays include 2 views of each extremity; skull, anteroposterior (AP) and lateral; spine, AP and lateral, chest x-ray, and/or rib (posterior), abdomen, pelvis, hands, and feet
  - Consider bone scan for acute rib fractures and subtle long-bone fractures (3)[B].
- Intracranial and extracranial injury:
  - CT scan of head (3)[B]
  - Consider MRI of head/neck for better dating of injuries, looking at subtle findings, intercerebral edema, or hemorrhage (3)[B].
- Intra-abdominal injuries:
  - CT scan of abdomen

Follow-Up Tests & Special Considerations
- Bruising is a common presenting feature:
  - Bruising in babies who are not independently mobile is very uncommon (<1%) (8)[A].
- Patterns suggestive of abuse (8)[A]:
  - Bruises seen away from bony prominences
  - Bruises to face, back, abdomen, arms, buttocks, ears, hands
  - Multiple bruises in clusters or uniform shape
  - Patterned injuries (such as bite marks or the imprint of an object like a belt or cord) should be considered inflicted until proven otherwise.
- Red flags (3)[B]:
  - History that is inconsistent with the injury
  - No explanation offered for the injury, or injury blamed on sibling or another child
  - History that is inconsistent with the child's developmental level

Diagnostic Procedures/Surgery
Sexual abuse:
- Consider photocolposcopy.
- <72 hours from time of abuse: Collect samples for the forensic laboratory (contact authorities for appropriate protocol) (7)[C].

Test Interpretation
- Spiral fractures in nonambulatory patients (children who are not walking or cruising should not have bruising or fractures from "falls")
- Chip or bucket-handle fractures
- Epiphyseal/Metaphyseal rib fractures in infants
- Rupture of liver/spleen in abdominal blunt trauma
- Retinal hemorrhages in shaken baby syndrome
- Recent literature notes a greater risk of abuse with skull and femur fractures, unexplained injuries, and a delay in seeking care (9).

 TREATMENT

GENERAL MEASURES
Test for STIs before treatment (7)[C].

MEDICATION
First Line
Antibiotics as indicated for STIs

Second Line
Consider antidepressants if needed.

> **ALERT**
> Emergency contraception reduces rate of pregnancy after sexual assault if given within 5 days:
> Levonorgestrel: 1.5 mg as a single dose is as effective as 2 split doses (0.75 mg each) 12 hours apart (3,10)[A].

ISSUES FOR REFERRAL
- Consider managing in ED to collect forensic specimens and maintain chain of evidence.
- Mandatory reporting to child protective authorities

IN-PATIENT CONSIDERATIONS
Admission Criteria/Initial Stabilization
- Moderate-to-severe injuries or unstable
- Acute psychological trauma
- If safety of child outside the hospital cannot be guaranteed

Discharge Criteria
- Child should be sent to another relative or into foster care if the suspected abuser lives with the child.
- Counseling for individual and family
- After initial evaluation, consider referral to sexual assault center.

 ONGOING CARE

FOLLOW-UP RECOMMENDATIONS
As clinically indicated

Patient Monitoring
- Refer to the state protective services.
- Monitor injury healing over time.
- Follow-up assessment for STIs that may not present acutely (e.g., HPV)

PROGNOSIS
Without intervention, child abuse is often a chronic and escalating phenomenon.

COMPLICATIONS
Growing evidence that sexual, physical, and emotional abuse in childhood are risk factors for poorer adult mental and physical health

REFERENCES
1. Sedlak AJ, Mettenburg J, Basena M, et al. (2010) Fourth National Incidence Study of Child Abuse and Neglect (NIS-4): Report to Congress, Executive Summary. Washington DC: U.S. Department of Health and Human Services, Administration for Children and Families.
2. Department of Health & Human Services. Administration on Children, Youth & Families. Children's Bureau. Child Maltreatment 2011 Report. www.acf.hhs.gov/programs/cb/resource/child-maltreatment-2011.
3. Kellogg ND, American Academy of Pediatrics Committee on Child Abuse and Neglect. Evaluation of suspected child physical abuse. Pediatrics. 2007;119(6):1232–1241.
4. Hahn RA, Bilukha OO, Crosby A, et al. First reports evaluating the effectiveness of strategies for preventing violence: Early childhood home visitation. Findings from the Task Force on Community Preventive Services. MMWR Recomm Rep. 2003;52(RR-14):1–9.
5. Sheets LK, Leach ME, Koszewski AM, et al. Sentinel injuries in infants evaluated for child physical abuse. Pediatrics. 2013;131:701–707.
6. Jackson AM, Rucker A, Hinds T, et al. Let the record speak: Medicolegal documentation in cases of child maltreatment. Clin Ped Emerg Med. 2006;7(3):181–185.
7. Kellogg N, American Academy of Pediatrics Committee on Child Abuse and Neglect. The evaluation of sexual abuse in children. Pediatrics. 2005;116(2):506–512.
8. Maguire S, Mann MK, Sibert J, et al. Are there patterns of bruising in childhood which are diagnostic or suggestive of abuse? A systematic review. Arch Dis Child. 2005;90(2):182–186.
9. Preer G, Sorrentino D, Newton AW. Child abuse pediatrics: Prevention, evaluation, and treatment. Curr Opin Pediatr. 2012;24(2):266–273.
10. Cheng L, Gülmezoglu AM, Oel CJ, et al. Interventions for emergency contraception. Cochrane Database Syst Rev. 2004;(3):CD001324.

ADDITIONAL READING
Harris T. Bruises in children: Normal or child abuse? J Pediatr Health Care. 2010;24(4):216–221.

 CODES

ICD10
- T74.02XA Child neglect or abandonment, confirmed, initial encounter
- T74.12XA Child physical abuse, confirmed, initial encounter
- T74.22XA Child sexual abuse, confirmed, initial encounter

CLINICAL PEARLS
- When a bruise is present, it should be considered as potentially sentinel for physical abuse if no plausible explanation is given (5).
- High index of suspicion is important for prevention and recognition of abuse.
- Neglect is the most common and lethal form of abuse and should be aggressively reported.
- Detailed exam with documentation is key.
- Mandated reporting is required for suspected child abuse and neglect; the physician does not have to prove abuse before reporting.
- Child Abuse Hotline by state: http://www.childwelfare.gov/responding/reporting.cfm

CHLAMYDIAL SEXUALLY TRANSMITTED DISEASES

Casandra Cashman, MD

 BASICS

DESCRIPTION

- An intracellular membrane-bound prokaryotic organism, *Chlamydia trachomatis* is the most common bacterial STI in the US.
- Transmitted through vaginal, anal, or oral sex; may also occur vertically from mother to infant during vaginal birth
- Most common bacterial sexually transmitted disease reported to the CDC (1).
- Majority of cases are asymptomatic, especially in females. Untreated disease can lead to pelvic inflammatory disease (PID), ectopic pregnancy, infertility.
- System(s) affected: Reproductive

Pregnancy Considerations
Perinatal acquisition may result in neonatal pneumonia and/or conjunctivitis.

EPIDEMIOLOGY
Incidence
- Mandatory reporting started in 1985, with data showing steady increase in incidence since.
- 1.4 million *reported* cases in 2011. Increasing incidence reflects greater screening, improved testing modalities, and better reporting rather than a large increase in disease burden.
- Swedish new variant chlamydia (nvCT) was first reported in 2006; often produces false-negative tests; largely confined to Nordic countries (2). Sensitive testing of 473 samples from around the US found none of the variants.

Prevalence
- 457.6 /100,000 people in the US in 2011
- Populations most affected: Young females, particularly those of ethnic minority groups
- Peak incidence: Age 18–20
- Predominant sex: Females > Males. Females have >2.5 × higher reported incidence and prevalence than males, but this likely reflects increased testing in females. Increasing use of urine screening may increase screening in males.
- Minorities bear the highest burden, with infection rates among blacks in >7 × that of whites. Rates higher in larger, more metropolitan areas.
- Highest prevalence for males is in heterosexual adolescents

ETIOLOGY AND PATHOPHYSIOLOGY
C. trachomatis serotypes D–K

RISK FACTORS
Risk correlates with:
- Number of lifetime sexual partners and number of concurrent sexual partners
- Lack of barrier contraception during sexual intercourse
- Younger age (highest in females 15–19 years, males 20–24 years)
- Black/Hispanic/Native American and Alaskan Native ethnicity

GENERAL PREVENTION
- Populations with prevalence >5% should be screened at least annually (1). Screen if: New or >1 sex partner in past 6 months, attending an adolescent or family-planning clinic or STD or abortion clinic, attending a jail or other detention-center clinic, rectal pain, discharge or tenesmus, testicular pain; test any individual with urethral or cervical discharge.
- All sexually active women ≤25 years of age should be screened at least yearly, and repeat testing in ~3 months is recommended for those who screen positive, because reinfection rate is high regardless of whether the sexual partner is treated (3)[A].
- Screening sexually active men ≤25 years is controversial but should be strongly considered in high-risk populations.
- Annual screening is recommended for men who have sex with men; this may include, as appropriate, rectal nucleic acid amplification test (NAAT) and/or urethral (urine) testing.

COMMONLY ASSOCIATED CONDITIONS
- Females:
  – Pelvic inflammatory disease (PID): ~10% of women with positive chlamydia screen developed PID within 12 months (4).
  – Infertility and ectopic pregnancies
  – Chronic pelvic pain
  – Mucopurulent cervicitis with cervical edema and propensity to bleed during speculum exam
  – Urethral syndrome (dysuria, frequency, and pyuria in the absence of infection with uropathogen)
  – Arthritis (rare)
  – Spontaneous abortion (5)
- Males:
  – Epididymitis and nongonococcal urethritis
  – Reiter syndrome (HLA-B27)
  – Proctitis
- Neonates:
  – Inclusion conjunctivitis (occurs in ~40% of exposed neonates) (3)
  – Otitis media
  – Pneumonia
  – Pharyngitis
- Diseases caused by other chlamydial species:
  – Lymphogranuloma venereum: *C. trachomatis* serotypes L1–L3
  – Trachoma: *C. trachomatis* serotypes A–C

 DIAGNOSIS

- *Majority of patients are asymptomatic*. Of those with symptoms, the most common are:
  – In females: Mucopurulent vaginal discharge, dysuria (urethral syndrome), bartholinitis, abdominopelvic pain (endometritis, salpingitis/PID), right-upper-quadrant pain (Fitz-Hugh-Curtis perihepatitis syndrome)
  – In males: Dysuria, urethral discharge (urethritis), scrotal pain (epididymitis), rectal pain or discharge (proctitis), acute arthritis (Reiter syndrome)
  – In infants: Conjunctivitis, pneumonitis, carriage in pharynx/GI tract

- Lymphogranuloma venereum (LGV) (*C. trachomatis* serovars L1, L2, or L3): Primary lesion is a small papule that may ulcerate at the site of transmission after an incubation period of 3–30 days. May manifest as unilateral tender lymphadenopathy. With rectal transmission, LGV causes an invasive proctocolitis.

HISTORY
- Complete sexual history, including number of sex partners lifetime and past year, prior history of STIs, use of barrier protection, exchange of money or drugs for sex, oral or anal receptive intercourse, partner fidelity
- Symptom history, with onset dates

PHYSICAL EXAM
- Men and women: External genitalia (rash? lesions?), urethra (discharge? dysuria?), inguinal lymph nodes, pharynx and perianal area, if history indicates
- In addition, for women: Cervix (discharge? motion tenderness?), uterus, ovaries, adnexa

DIFFERENTIAL DIAGNOSIS
- *Neisseria gonorrhoeae*: Urethritis, proctitis, epididymitis, cervicitis, PID, Bartholin abscess
- *Mycoplasma* or *Ureaplasma urealyticum*: Urethritis, epididymitis, Reiter disease, PID
- *C. trachomatis* (serotypes L1–L3): LGV, proctitis
- Trichomoniasis

DIAGNOSTIC TESTS & INTERPRETATION
Initial Tests (lab, imaging)
- *Test of choice is NAAT*: Sensitivity >95%; specificity >99%.
- Urine is equally as sensitive as cervical swab.
- Patient self-collected vaginal swabs have also been shown to be effective.
- Lab tests may remain positive for as long as 3 weeks after successful treatment.
- Offer testing for other STDs, including gonorrhea, HIV, syphilis; perform Pap if appropriate; suggest barrier contraception.

Follow-Up Tests & Special Considerations
See "Patient Monitoring."

💉 **TREATMENT**

GENERAL MEASURES
- All patients with known or suspected chlamydia should be tested for gonorrhea, HIV (the latter requires individual counseling and consent), and possibly syphilis (3)[C]. Also, ensure females are up to date with Pap smears.
- Some experts recommend that all patients treated for chlamydia should be treated empirically for gonorrhea.
- All partners (most recent partner and all partners within the past 60 days) of patients treated for chlamydia should be tested, if possible. They should be treated empirically rather than waiting for test results. They should also be treated empirically even if they were not tested.
- Doxycycline shortages in the US may prompt increasing use of azithromycin; recent reports of increased rates of sudden death with azithromycin were associated with 5-day courses rather than the single dose used for chlamydial treatment.

MEDICATION

First Line

Treatment of chlamydial urethritis, cervicitis (including sexual partners of infected persons) (3)[A]:

- Azithromycin 1 g PO single dose, *or*
- Doxycycline 100 mg PO b.i.d. × 7 days
- First-line PID treatment (outpatient) (3):
  - Ceftriaxone 250 mg IM × 1 *PLUS* doxycycline 100 mg PO × 14 days with or without metronidazole 500 mg PO b.i.d. × 14 days, *or*
  - Cefoxitin 2 g IM × 1 with probenecid 1 g PO × 1 *PLUS* doxycycline 100 mg PO × 14 days with or without metronidazole 500 mg PO b.i.d. × 14 days
- First-line PID treatment parenteral therapy
- Practitioners may elect to give azithromycin and ceftriaxone together to the patient in the office to reduce patient noncompliance.
- Asymptomatic rectal chlamydia can be treated with doxycycline 100 mg b.i.d. × 7 days. Azithromycin 1 g × 1 is slightly less effective but can also be used, especially when compliance or medication availability is an issue 4,5[B].

ALERT

- Use with caution in patients with known QT prolongation, hypokalemia, hypomagnesemia, bradycardia, or who are currently treated with antiarrythmics.

Pregnancy Considerations

- Tetracyclines (e.g., doxycycline) and quinolones (e.g., ofloxacin, levofloxacin) are contraindicated in pregnant women.
- Consider azithromycin or amoxicillin:
  - Azithromycin as above, OR
  - Amoxicillin 500 mg PO t.i.d. × 7 days

ALERT

Tetracyclines and quinolones are contraindicated in children:

- <45 kg: Erythromycin base or ethinyl succinate 500 mg/kg/d PO q.i.d × 14 days
- >45 kg but <8 years: Azithromycin 1 g PO × 1
- >8 years: Adult regimen
- Rule out sexual abuse in children with *chlamydia* infection

Second Line

For chlamydial urethritis/cervicitis:

- Erythromycin base 500 mg PO q.i.d. × 7 days *OR* erythromycin ethylsuccinate 800 mg PO q.i.d. × 7 days
- Levofloxacin 500 mg PO daily × 7 days *or* ofloxacin 300 mg PO b.i.d. × 7 days

ADDITIONAL THERAPIES

Expedited partner therapy (EPT) is the practice of physicians delivering medications or prescriptions to sexual partners of persons infected with STIs without clinical assessment of the partners:

- EPT has been shown to be more effective than traditional partner referral in reducing recurrence rates.
- EPT is currently permissible in 33 states, "potentially allowable" in 11 states, and illegal in 6.
- For an updated review on the legal status of EPT, refer to the CDC website on this subject: www.cdc.gov/std/ept/legal/default.htm.

IN-PATIENT CONSIDERATIONS

Treatment of PID: Often outpatient treatment. Those falling into the following categories are recommended for inpatient treatment: Pregnancy, lack of response or intolerance to oral meds, suspicion of poor compliance, severe clinical illness, pelvic abscess, possible need for surgical intervention.

Admission Criteria/Initial Stabilization

- As outlined above
- Outpatient treatment, unless patient is moderately or severely ill.

 ONGOING CARE

FOLLOW-UP RECOMMENDATIONS

Patient and all partners should abstain from sexual contact until at least 7 days after treatment is complete.

Patient Monitoring

- Test of cure: It is not routine to test the patient to see if a cure has been obtained, except in pregnancy (3)[A].
- Sexual partners must be evaluated and treated empirically, if necessary, to prevent passing the disease back and forth between partners.
- Lack of resolution or recurrence of symptoms must be reported immediately to the physician.

PATIENT EDUCATION

- Suggest risk-reduction counseling, barrier protection, and encourage delay of initiation of sexual activity.
- Stress the need for both patient and partner to finish entire course of antibiotics.

PROGNOSIS

Prognosis is good with early and compliant therapy; however, because of the asymptomatic nature of the early disease and the population affected, symptomatic PID still accounts annually for 2.5 million outpatient visits and >250,000 hospitalizations.

COMPLICATIONS

- Both sexes: Enhancement of transmission of and susceptibility to HIV.
- Females: Tubal infertility (most common cause of acquired infertility), tubal (ectopic) pregnancy, chronic pelvic pain
  - Annual screening of sexually active women would prevent 61% of chlamydia-related pelvic inflammatory disease (6)[A]
- Males: Transient oligospermia and postepididymitis urethral stricture (rare).

REFERENCES

1. Centers for Disease Control and Prevention. 2011 Sexually transmitted disease surveillance. Available at: www.cdc.gov/std/stats11/chlamydia.htm
2. Unemo M, Clarke IN. The Swedish new variant of Chlamydia trachomatis. *Curr Opin Infect Dis*. 2011;24:62–69.
3. Workowski KA, Berman S, Centers for Disease Control and Prevention (CDC). Sexually transmitted diseases treatment guidelines, 2010. *MMWR*. 2010;59(RR12):1–110.
4. Elgalib A, Alexander S, Tong CY, et al. Seven days of doxycycline is an effective treatment for asymptomatic rectal Chlamydia trachomatis infection. *Int J STD AIDS*. 2011;22:474–477.
5. Drummond F, Ryder N, Wand H, et al. Is azithromycin adequate treatment for asymptomatic rectal chlamydia? *Int J STD AIDS*. 2011;22:478–480.
6. Price MJ, Ades AE, De Angelis D, et al. Risk of pelvic inflammatory disease following Chlamydia trachomatis infection: Analysis of prospective studies with a multistate model. *Am J Epidemiol*. 2013;178:484–492.

ADDITIONAL READING

- Baud D, Goy G, Jaton K, et al. Role of Chlamydia trachomatis in miscarriage. *Emerging Infect Dis*. 2011;17:1630–1635.
- Ray WA, Murray KT, Hall K, et al. Azithromycin and the risk of cardiovascular death. *N Engl J Med*. 2012;366:1881–1890.
- Won H, Ramachandran P, Steece R, et al. Is there evidence of the new variant Chlamydia trachomatis in the United States? *Sex Transm Dis*. 2013;40:352–353.

 SEE ALSO

Cervicitis, Ectropion, and True Erosion; Epididymitis; Gonococcal Infections; HIV Infection and AIDS; Pelvic Inflammatory Disease; Syphilis; Urethritis

CODES

ICD10

- A56.09 Other chlamydial infection of lower genitourinary tract
- A56.8 Sexually transmitted chlamydial infection of other sites
- A56.11 Chlamydial female pelvic inflammatory disease

CLINICAL PEARLS

- *C. trachomatis* is common in sexually active teens and young adults. To prevent recurrence, treat patients and their partners concurrently.
- Screen all sexually active women who are at high risk (remembering that simply having a new partner puts people at "high risk").
- Test of cure for pregnant patients treated for chlamydia at 3 months.

CHLAMYDOPHILA PNEUMONIAE

Fozia Akhtar Ali, MD • Teny Philip, MD

 BASICS

DESCRIPTION

- Chlamydophila pneumonia, formerly known as Chlamydia pneumonia, is an obligate intracellular gram-negative bacteria that causes mild atypical pneumonia or bronchitis in adolescents and young adults.
- In older adults, it can cause a more severe persistent latent infection.
- Humans are the only known reservoir.

EPIDEMIOLOGY

- The pathogen causes 10–20% of CAP among adults, ranking 2nd to mycoplasma as an agent of atypical pneumonia.
- Although infections occur every year, epidemiologic studies suggest 4-year cycle
- The incubation period is ~3–4 weeks.
- Most infected persons are asymptomatic.
- Of those who are symptomatic, relatively mild URI symptoms are present, but symptoms of bronchitis and pneumonia may follow in 1–4 weeks.
- Primary infection more common in persons 7–40 years; reinfection pneumonia more common in elderly
- Serologic evidence of previous infection is found in 50% of adults and 75% of elderly.
- Male > Female (60–90%); possibly due to cigarette smoking

Incidence

- Arnold et al., in a worldwide study that included 4,337 patients aiming to assess incidence of different atypical pathogens as a cause for CAP showed that *C. pneumonia* was responsible for 8% of cases in North America, 7% in Europe, 6% in Latin America, and 5% in Asia.
- Outbreaks have occurred among military recruits, university students, and nursing home residents, with incidence highest in elderly.

Prevalence

- Estimated 300,000 cases per year in US

ETIOLOGY AND PATHOPHYSIOLOGY

- The elementary body is the infectious form:
  – Metabolically inactive with rigid cell wall that allows it to live outside the host cell for a limited time
- The elementary body infects the host cell by receptor-mediated endocytosis and then becomes a reticulate body.
- Reticulate bodies divide in the cell, forming intracytoplasmic inclusions. As they divide, chlamydial antigens are released, eliciting a host immune response that leads to mucus production in the nasal passages, sinuses, bronchial tree, and alveoli, along with nasopharyngeal and airway inflammation and bronchospasm.
- After 48–72 hours, the reticulate bodies become elementary bodies again and are released by cell lysis.

RISK FACTORS

Close quarters such as classrooms, military recruits, shelters, nursing homes

GENERAL PREVENTION

- As transmission is via contact with respiratory secretions, advise hand washing and avoid exposure to infected persons.
- Incidence high among military recruits during basic training; weekly azithromycin prophylaxis was 58% effective.

COMMONLY ASSOCIATED CONDITIONS

- COPD
- Asthma
- HIV infection
- Cystic fibrosis
- Diabetes mellitus

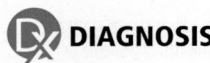 **DIAGNOSIS**

HISTORY

- Spectrum of illness may vary from mild and self-limited to severe pneumonia.
- Onset is often gradual with delayed presentation.
- Sore throat and hoarseness may precede cough by a week or more, giving biphasic appearance to illness (uncommon in *Legionella*, less common with *Mycoplasma*, *Streptococcus pneumoniae*, and *Haemophilus influenzae*).
- Dry cough
- Low-grade fever (usually early in illness)
- Chills
- Rhinitis
- Headache
- Malaise
- Myalgias
- Sinus congestion
- Nausea
- Altered mental status

PHYSICAL EXAM

- General appearance usually nontoxic
- Fever
- Tachypnea
- Tachycardia
- Crackles or wheezing
- Bronchial breath sounds
- Sinus percussion tenderness (more common *with C. pneumonia* than other pneumonias)
- Percussion dullness and egophony less sensitive but more specific for pneumonia
- Pharyngeal erythema without exudate
- Usually more severe disease in older adults
- Elderly patients are less likely to exhibit respiratory symptoms with pneumonia and may present with altered mental status or history of falls.

DIFFERENTIAL DIAGNOSIS

- Other causes of atypical pneumonia, including *M. pneumoniae* and *L. pneumophila*
- Other bacterial causes of pneumonia, including *S. pneumoniae. H. influenzae, Moraxella catarrhalis,* and *Staphylococcus aureus*
- Respiratory viruses: Adenovirus, influenza A, influenza B, parainfluenza virus, and respiratory syncytial virus
- Endemic fungal pathogens: Coccidioidomycosis, histoplasmosis
- Opportunistic fungal pathogens: *Candida* species, *Aspergillus* species, *Mucor* species, *Cryptococcus neoformans*
- Other: Psittacosis, Q fever, TB, tularemia
- Conditions that mimic CAP: Acute respiratory disease syndrome, idiopathic pulmonary fibrosis, neoplasm, pulmonary embolus, sarcoidosis, congestive heart failure

DIAGNOSTIC TESTS & INTERPRETATION

Initial Tests (lab, imaging)

- White blood count is usually not elevated but alkaline phosphate levels may be elevated.
- Blood cultures are recommended to rule out pyogenic bacterial etiology if toxic and requiring ICU admission; otherwise not likely to be helpful.
- Culture with oropharyngeal swab is the gold standard diagnostic method although it is not widely available:
  – Specificity 100%
  – Sensitivity 50–70% (1)
  – Samples should be obtained using nasopharyngeal swab
  – Specimen should be kept at melting ice temperature in specialized transport media
  – Most easily cultured in HL or HEp2 cells (2)
- PCR from pharyngeal swab or bronchioalveolar lavage specimen (30–95% sensitivity, >95% specificity) (2)
- Most commonly used test and test of choice is the microimmunofluorescence (MIF) test per CDC recommendations:
  – Sensitivity of 50–90% if using paired sera
  – IgM 1:16 or higher
  – IgG 1:512 or higher
  – IgM may not be detectable early in the disease
- Complement fixation for *Chlamydia* is available but cannot distinguish *C. pneumonia* from *C. psittaci*.
- Note: During an outbreak of *C. pneumoniae*, 1 study showed PCR was less sensitive (68% vs 79%) but more specific (93% vs 86%) than MIF IgM (3).

C

- Patients with suspected CAP should be evaluated with a chest x-ray (CXR) (2)[A].
- No characteristic radiograph findings
- CXR most commonly shows a single subsegmental infiltrate that is mainly located in the lower lobes.
- Extensive consolidation is rare, although cases of ARDS have been reported.
- Pleural effusion seen in 20–25% of cases.
- Histologically, intra-alveolar inflammation with mild interstitial reaction is characteristic of chlamydial pneumonias. Alveolar-lining cells contain intracytoplasmic inclusions.

Diagnostic Procedures/Other
Although serology is 95% specific, definitive diagnosis requires a positive culture or PCR testing (2)[A].

 TREATMENT

MEDICATION
- Administer empiric treatment when mixed infections are present because rapid testing is not readily available.
- An advantage in clinical efficacy or mortality by empiric coverage of atypical pathogens in patients with CAP has not been shown (4)[A].

First Line
- Doxycycline: 100 mg IV b.i.d. in inpatient setting *OR* doxycycline, 100 mg PO b.i.d. or tetracycline, 500 mg PO q.i.d. in outpatient setting
- Azithromycin: 500 mg on day 1, then 250 mg on days 2–5 *OR*
- Clarithromycin: 500 mg q12h for 10–14 days *OR*
- Doxycycline: 100 mg q12h for 10–14 days:
  – Tetracycline not for use during pregnancy or in children <8 years
  – Tetracycline may cause photosensitivity; sunscreen is recommended
  – Tetracyclines may increase the anticoagulant effect of warfarin.

Second Line
Alternative drugs:
- Levofloxacin: 250–500 mg/d (PO or IV) or other respiratory fluoroquinolones have good bioavailability and the convenience of once-daily dosing, but are recommended for use only when patients have failed treatment with a 1st-line drug or have had recent antibiotics, significant comorbidities, or allergies to alternatives.

Pregnancy Considerations
Tetracyclines and fluoroquinolones are contraindicated

IN-PATIENT CONSIDERATIONS
- Usually outpatient care for most. Those with severe pneumonia or coexisting illness may require hospitalization.
- Pneumonia severity index or other validated prediction rule can assist in predicting those patients with CAP with higher morbidity and those requiring hospitalization (5)[A].

Admission Criteria/Initial Stabilization
Infection in debilitated or hospitalized patients can be severe. Stabilize respiratory distress as per advanced cardiac life support protocol.

Discharge Criteria
Reversal of any respiratory distress, with the patient tolerating PO medications, otherwise stable medically, and stable for discharge per the clinical judgment of the physician

 ONGOING CARE

FOLLOW-UP RECOMMENDATIONS
Patient Monitoring
- Weekly patient monitoring until well
- Follow-up CXR for resolution
- Reinfection is possible

PROGNOSIS
- Pneumonia is especially life-threatening in older adults and patients with other underlying disease that affect the lungs (e.g., asthma, COPD) or the immune system (e.g., diabetes), with an overall 0.5–29% mortality rate.
- Estimated mortality rate from *C. pneumoniae* is 10%, but this may be an overestimate due to the number of subclinical cases.
- Death usually from secondary infection or underlying comorbidity

COMPLICATIONS
- Reactive airway disease
- Erythema nodosum
- Otitis media
- Endocarditis
- Pericarditis or myocarditis
- Meningoencephalitis
- Possible association with atherosclerotic disease: *C. pneumoniae* has been cultured from atherosclerotic plaque in patients with coronary artery disease and stroke, but treatment has not been shown to affect mortality.
- *C. pneumoniae* infection is associated with an increased risk for lung cancer (6)[A].

REFERENCES

1. Kumar S, Hammerschlag MR. Acute respiratory infection due to *Chlamydia pneumoniae*: Current status of diagnostic methods. *Clin Infect Dis*. 2007;44:568–576.
2. Lutfiyya MN. Diagnosis and treatment of community-acquired pneumonia. *AFP*. 2006;73(3): 442–450.
3. Hvidsten D, Halvorsen DS, Berdal BP, Gutteberg TJ. Chlamydophila pneumoniae diagnostics: Importance of methodology in relation to timing of sampling. *Clin Microbiol Infect*. 2009;15(1):42–49.
4. Shefet D. Empiric antibiotic coverage of atypical pathogens for community acquired pneumonia in hospitalized adults. *Cochrane Database Sys Rev*. 2006;1:CD004418.
5. Fine MJ, Auble TE, Yealy DM. A prediction rule to identify low-risk patients with community-acquired pneumonia. *N Engl J Med*. 1997;336:243–250.
6. Zhan P, Suo LJ, Qian Q, et al. Chlamydia pneumoniae infection and lung cancer risk: a meta-analysis. *Eur J Cancer*. 2011;47(5):742–747. doi: 10.1016/j.ejca.2010.11.003. Epub 2010 Dec 29.

ADDITIONAL READING

- Blasi F, Tarsia P, Aliberti S. *Chlamydophila pneumoniae*. *Clin Microbiol Infect*. 2009;15:29–35.
- Burillo A, Bouza E. Chlamydophila pneumoniae. *Infect Dis Clin North Am*. 2010;24(1):61–71.
- Conklin L, Adjemian J, Loo J, et al. Investigation of a Chlamydia pneumoniae outbreak in a federal correctional facility in Texas. *Clin Infect Dis*. 2013 Jul 9. [Epub ahead of print]
- Miyashita N, Fukano H, Okimoto N, et al. Clinical presentation of community-acquired Chlamydia pneumoniae pneumonia in adults. *Chest*. 2002; 121(6):1776–1781.
- Noll DR, Shores JH, Gamber RG, et al. Benefits of osteopathic manipulative treatment for hospitalized elderly patients with pneumonia. *J Am Osteopath Assoc*. 2000;100(12):776–782.
- Thibodeau KP, Viera AJ. Atypical pathogens and challenges in community-acquired pneumonia. *Am Fam Physician*. 2004;69(7):1699–1706.

 SEE ALSO

Algorithm: Cough, Chronic

 CODES

ICD10
- J16.0 Chlamydial pneumonia
- P23.1 Congenital pneumonia due to Chlamydia

CLINICAL PEARLS
- *C. pneumoniae* is a significant cause of adult and pediatric pneumonias. Think "walking pneumonia." Young patient who overall looks fine but has a pneumonia.
- Formal and accurate diagnosis of *C. pneumoniae* is difficult. Culture remains the gold standard. Serodiagnosis is used for acute infection (helpful if tests are paired).
- Initial treatment may be tetracyclines, macrolides, or quinolones. Do not use tetracyclines or quinolones in pregnant patients.

CHOLELITHIASIS

Hongyi Cui, MD, PhD, FACS, FICS

 BASICS

DESCRIPTION

- Cholelithiasis manifests in cholesterol, pigment, or mixed stones formed and contained in the gallbladder.
- Synonym(s): Gallstones

Pediatric Considerations

- Uncommon at <10 years
- Most gallstones in the pediatric population are pigment stones associated with blood dyscrasia.

EPIDEMIOLOGY

Incidence

- Increased in Native Americans and Hispanics
- Increases with age by 1–3% per year; peaks at 7th decade; 2% of the US population develops gallstones annually.

Prevalence

- Population: 8–10% of the US
- Predominant sex: Female > Male (2–3:1)

ETIOLOGY AND PATHOPHYSIOLOGY

Gallstone formation is a complex process mediated by genetic, metabolic, immune, and environmental factors. Gallbladder sludge (a mixture of cholesterol crystals, calcium bilirubinate granules, and mucin gel matrix) serves as the nidus for gallstone formation.

- Production of bile supersaturated with cholesterol (cholesterol stones)
- Decrease in bile content of either phospholipid (lecithin) or bile salts
- Biliary stasis or impaired gallbladder motility
- Generation of excess unconjugated bilirubin in patients with hemolytic diseases; passage of excess bile salt into the colon with subsequent absorption of excess unconjugated bilirubin in patients with inflammatory bowel disease (IBD) or after distal ileal resection (black or pigment stones)
- Hydrolysis of conjugated bilirubin or phospholipid by bacteria in patients with biliary tract infection or stricture (brown stones or primary bile duct stones; rare in the Western world and common in Asia)

RISK FACTORS

- Age (peak in 60–70s)
- Female gender, pregnancy, and multiparity
- Caucasian, Hispanic, or Native American descent
- High-fat diet rich in cholesterol
- Cholestasis or impaired gallbladder motility in association with prolonged fasting, long-term total parenteral nutrition, and rapid weight loss
- Hereditary (e.g., patients carrying the p.D19H variant for the hepatocanalicular cholesterol transporter ABCG5/ABG8 have an increased risk for gallstones)
- Metabolic syndrome (i.e., obesity, dyslipidemia, and type 2 diabetes) and metabolic changes in association with short gut syndrome, terminal ileal resection, and IBD
- Hemolytic disorders (e.g., hereditary spherocytosis and sickle cell anemia) and cirrhosis (for black or pigment stones)
- Medications (e.g., early use of birth control pills, estrogen replacement therapy at high doses, and long-term corticosteroid or cytostatic therapy)
- Viral hepatitis, biliary tract infection and stricture (for intraductal formation of brown pigment stones)

GENERAL PREVENTION

- Ursodiol (Actigall) taken during rapid weight loss prevents gallstone formation (1)[A].
- Regular exercise and dietary modification may reduce the incidence of gallstone formation.
- Lipid-lowering drugs (statins) may prevent cholesterol stone formation by reducing bile cholesterol saturation.

COMMONLY ASSOCIATED CONDITIONS

90% of people with gallbladder carcinoma have gallstones.

 DIAGNOSIS

HISTORY

- Mostly asymptomatic (80%): 5–10% become symptomatic each year. Over their lifetime, <1/2 of patients with gallstones develop symptoms.
- Episodic right upper quadrant or epigastric pain lasting >15 minutes and sometimes radiating to the back (biliary colic), usually postprandially; most patients will develop recurrent symptoms after the first episode.
- Nausea, vomiting; indigestion or bloating sensation; fatty food intolerance

PHYSICAL EXAM

- Physical exam is *usually normal* in patients with cholelithiasis without acute attack.
- Epigastric and/or right upper quadrant tenderness (Murphy sign) when in association with cholecystitis
- Fever and jaundice in patients with choledocholithiasis and cholangitis; jaundice can also be caused by extrinsic compression of the bile duct by a stone in the gallbladder or cystic duct (Mirizzi syndrome)
- Flank and periumbilical ecchymoses (Cullen sign and Grey-Turner sign) in patients with acute hemorrhagic pancreatitis
- In patients with concomitant acute calculus cholecystitis and gallbladder cancer, a mass in the right upper quadrant may be palpated.

DIFFERENTIAL DIAGNOSIS

- Peptic ulcer diseases and gastritis
- Hepatitis
- Pancreatitis
- Cholangitis
- Gallbladder cancer
- Gallbladder polyps
- Acalculous cholecystitis
- Biliary dyskinesia
- Choledocholithiasis

DIAGNOSTIC TESTS & INTERPRETATION

No lab study is specific for cholelithiasis.

Initial Tests (lab, imaging)

- Leukocytosis and elevated C-reactive protein level are associated with acute calculus cholecystitis.
- US (best technique to diagnose gallstones and differentiate from cholecystitis) can detect gallstones in 97–98% of patients.
- Thickening of the gallbladder wall (≥5 mm), pericholecystic fluid, and direct tenderness when the probe is pushed against the gallbladder (sonographic Murphy sign) are all radiographic signs of acute calculus cholecystitis.

Follow-Up Tests & Special Considerations

- CT scan (no advantage over US except in detecting distal common bile duct stones)
- MR cholangiopancreatography is reserved for cases of suspected common bile duct stones due to high cost.
- Endoscopic US has been shown to be as sensitive as endoscopic retrograde cholangiopancreatography (ERCP) for detection of common bile duct stones in patients with gallstone pancreatitis.
- Hepatobiliary iminodiacetic acid (HIDA) scan is useful in differentiating acalculous cholecystitis from other causes of abdominal pain. False–positive results can arise from fasting status, insufficient resistance of the sphincter of Oddi, and gallbladder agenesis:
  – Cholecystokinin (CCK)-HIDA is specifically used to diagnose gallbladder dysmotility disorder (i.e., biliary dyskinesia).
- 10–30% of gallstones, which are radiopaque calcium or pigment-containing gallstones, are more likely to be visible on plain x-ray. A "porcelain gallbladder" is a calcified gallbladder, visible by x-ray; associated with gallbladder cancer.

Test Interpretation

- Pure cholesterol stones have a white or slightly yellow color.
- Pigment stones may be black or brown. Black stones contain polymerized calcium bilirubinate, most often secondary to cirrhosis or hemolysis; these almost always form in the gallbladder.
- Brown stones are associated with biliary tract infection, caused by bile stasis, and as such may form either in the bile ducts or gallbladder.

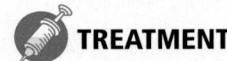 **TREATMENT**

GENERAL MEASURES

- Treat only symptomatic gallstones and observe asymptomatic stones.
- Attempt conservative therapy during pregnancy. If necessary, perform surgery preferentially in the 2nd trimester.
- Prophylactic cholecystectomy for patients with calcified (porcelain) gallbladder (risk for gallbladder cancer), patients with sickle cell disease, and patients with recurrent pancreatitis due to microlithiasis
- In morbidly obese patients, simultaneous cholecystectomy may be performed in combination with bariatric procedures (2) in an effort to reduce later stone-related complications.

Geriatric Considerations

Age alone should not alter the therapy plan.

MEDICATION

First Line

- Analgesics for pain relief:
  – NSAIDs may have a role in pain relief, given that prostaglandins are important in the development of pain.
  – A recent meta-analysis shows NSAIDs are the 1st-choice treatments as they control pain with the same efficacy as opioids (3)[A].
- Antibiotics are indicated in patients with signs of acute cholecystitis.

- Prophylactic antibiotics in low-risk patients do not prevent infections for laparoscopic cholecystectomies (4)[A].

ISSUES FOR REFERRAL

Patients with retained or recurrent bile duct stones following cholecystectomy should be referred to gastroenterology for ERCP.

SURGERY/OTHER PROCEDURES

- Surgical intervention should be considered for patients who have symptomatic cholelithiasis or gallstone-related complications, such as cholecystitis, or in asymptomatic patients with immune suppression, calcified gallbladder, or family history of gallbladder cancer (5)[A].
- Open, small incision, or laparoscopic cholecystectomy (LC) has similar mortality and complication rates (6)[A]. The minimally invasive techniques offer quicker recovery. In well-selected patients, single-incision LC (SILC) and robotic LC are novel methods for the treatment of symptomatic cholelithiasis. Natural orifice transluminal endoscopic surgery (NOTES) is still at an experimental stage, and NOTES cholecystectomy is only available in a limited number of specialized centers:
  - Surgery-related complications include common bile duct injury (0.5%), right hepatic duct/artery injury, retained stones, cystic duct or duct of Luschka leak, biloma formation, or bile duct stricture in the long term.
  - Conversion to open procedure based on judgment of the operating surgeon
  - In 10–15% patients with symptomatic cholelithiasis, common bile duct (CBD) stones are detected during LC with intraoperative cholangiogram (IOC). CBD stone(s) can be removed via either laparoscopic CBD exploration or postoperative ERCP, depending on surgeon expertise and GI availability.
  - IOC may help delineate bile duct anatomy when dissection proves difficult. Selective or routine use of IOC is a topic of debate, but may be associated with earlier recognition and decreased incidence of bile duct injury (7)[B].
- Percutaneous cholecystostomy (PC) used in high-risk patients with cholecystitis or gallbladder empyema. PC may also be used in patients with symptoms of cholecystitis for >72 hours in which altered anatomy might significantly increase the surgical risk. Interval cholecystectomy is usually advisable after the resolution of cholecystitis and optimization of associated medical conditions to prevent recurrent cholecystitis.

IN-PATIENT CONSIDERATIONS

For patients with symptomatic cholelithiasis, laparoscopic cholecystectomy has become an outpatient procedure; for patients who developed gallstone-related complications (i.e., cholecystitis, cholangitis, and pancreatitis), inpatient care is necessary.

Admission Criteria/Initial Stabilization

- Acute phase: NPO, IV fluids, and antibiotics
- Adequate pain control with narcotics and/or NSAIDs

 ONGOING CARE

FOLLOW-UP RECOMMENDATIONS
Patient Monitoring

- Medical attention if asymptomatic stones become symptomatic
- Patients on oral dissolution agents should be followed up with liver enzyme, serum cholesterol, and imaging studies.

DIET

A low-fat diet may be helpful.

PATIENT EDUCATION

- Change in lifestyle (e.g., regular exercise) and dietary modification (low-fat diet and reduction of total calorie intake) may reduce gallstone-related hospitalizations.
- Patients with asymptomatic gallstones should be educated about the typical symptoms of biliary colic and gallstone-related complications.

PROGNOSIS

- <1/2 of patients with gallstones become symptomatic.
- Cholecystectomy: Mortality <0.5% elective, 3–5% emergency; morbidity <10% elective, 30–40% emergency
- ~10–15% of the patients will have associated choledocholithiasis.
- After cholecystectomy, stones may recur in the bile duct.

COMPLICATIONS

- Acute cholecystitis (90–95% secondary to gallstones)
- Gallstone pancreatitis
- Common bile duct stones with obstructive jaundice and acute cholangitis
- Biliary-enteric fistula and gallstone ileus; Bouveret syndrome is a variant of gallstone ileus where the gallstone lodges in the duodenum or pylorus causing a gastric outlet obstruction.
- Gallbladder cancer
- Mirizzi syndrome (bile duct obstruction caused by gallstones lodged in gallbladder or cystic duct)

REFERENCES

1. Uy MC, Talingdan-Te MC, Espinosa WZ, et al. Ursodeoxycholic acid in the prevention of gallstone formation after bariatric surgery: A meta-analysis. *Obes Surg.* 2008;18(12):1532–1538. Epub 2008 Jun 24.
2. Sakcak I, Avsar FM, Cosgun E, et al. Management of concurrent cholelithiasis in gastric banding for morbid obesity. *Eur J Gastroenterol Hepatol.* 2011; 23(9):766–769.
3. Colli A, Conte D, Valle SD, et al. Meta-analysis: Nonsteroidal anti-inflammatory drugs in biliary colic. *Aliment Pharmacol Ther.* 2012;35(12):1370–1378. Epub 2012 Apr 29.
4. Zhou H, Zhang J, Wang Q, et al. Meta-analysis: Antibiotic prophylaxis in elective laparoscopic cholecystectomy. *Aliment Pharmacol Ther.* 2009; 29:1086–1095.
5. Society for Surgery of the Alimentary Tract. SSAT patient care guidelines. Treatment of gallstone and gallbladder disease. *J Gastrointest Surg.* 2007; 11(9):1222–1224.
6. Keus F, Gooszen HG, van Laarhoven CJ, et al. Open, small-incision, or laparoscopic cholecystectomy for patients with symptomatic cholecystolithiasis. An overview of Cochrane Hepato-Biliary Group reviews. *Cochrane Database Syst Rev.* 2010;CD008318.
7. Connor S, Garden OJ. Bile duct injury in the era of laparoscopic cholecystectomy. *Br J Surg.* 2006;93:158–168.

ADDITIONAL READING

- Bogue CO, Murphy AJ, Gerstle JT, et al. Risk factors, complications, and outcomes of gallstones in children: A single-center review. *J Pediatr Gastroenterol Nutr.* 2010;50:303–308.
- Brown LM, Rogers SJ, Cello JP, et al. Cost-effective treatments of patients with symptomatic cholelithiasis and possible common bile duct stones. *J Am Coll Surg.* 2011;212(6):1049–1060.
- Gurusamy KS, Samraj K. Cholecystectomy versus no cholecystectomy in patients with silent gallstones. *Cochrane Database Syst Rev.* 2007;CD006230.
- Zehetner J, Pelipad D, Darehzereshki A, et al. Single-access laparoscopic cholecystectomy versus classic laparoscopic cholecystectomy: A systematic review and meta-analysis of randomized controlled trials. *Surg Laparosc Endosc Percutan Tech.* 2013; 23(3):235–243.
- Warschkow R, Tarantino I, Ukegjini K, et al. Concomitant cholecystectomy during laparoscopic Roux-en-Y gastric bypass in obese patients is not justified: A meta-analysis. *Obes Surg.* 2013;23(3):397–407.

 SEE ALSO

Cholangitis, Acute; Choledocholithiasis

 CODES

ICD10

- K80.01 Calculus of gallbladder w acute cholecystitis w obstruction
- K80.20 Calculus of gallbladder w/o cholecystitis w/o obstruction
- K80.21 Calculus of gallbladder w/o cholecystitis with obstruction

CLINICAL PEARLS

- Laparoscopic cholecystectomy has become the most frequently used procedure; lithotripsy and oral dissolution therapy may be considered in rare circumstances.
- Acute acalculous cholecystitis is associated with bile stasis and gallbladder ischemia.
- Prophylactic cholecystectomy is not indicated in patients with diabetes and asymptomatic gallstones. No evidence suggests that asymptomatic diabetics are at increased risk of developing complications of gallstone disease.
- The best imaging modality for the diagnosis of gallstones is transabdominal US (sensitivity, 97%; specificity, 95%); not sensitive for occult gallstones or microlithiasis (stones <5 mm).
- Think of gallstones in patients complaining of "gas pains" after bariatric surgery as they adjust to their new diet.

CHRONIC COUGH

Jacqueline L. Olin, MS, PharmD, BCPS, CPP • Brian Hertz, MD

BASICS

DESCRIPTION
- Chronic cough is defined as a cough that persists for >8 weeks in adults.
- In children, chronic cough is often defined as a cough of >4 weeks in duration.
- Subacute cough describes a cough lasting 3–8 weeks.
- Patients present because of fear of the causative illness (e.g., cancer), as well as annoyance, self-consciousness, and hoarseness.
- At the primary care level, chronic obstructive pulmonary disease (COPD) and smoking-related cough are common causes of chronic cough.
- System(s) affected: Gastrointestinal; Pulmonary

EPIDEMIOLOGY
- Predominant age: All age groups
- Predominant sex: Male = Female, with females more likely to seek out medical attention

Incidence
Recurrent cough has been reported at 3–40% by various population estimates.

Prevalence
Chronic cough is one of the most common reasons for primary care visits.

ETIOLOGY AND PATHOPHYSIOLOGY
Varies with findings and disorders implicated
- Often multiple etiologies, but most are related to bronchial irritation. Most frequent etiologies (account for >90% of cases) in nonsmokers include:
  - Upper airway cough syndrome (UACS) (formerly referred to as postnasal drip syndrome) and other upper airway abnormalities, including allergic and vasomotor rhinitis syndromes
  - Asthma
  - Gastroesophageal reflux disease (GERD)
- Other causes:
  - ACE inhibitors
  - Chronic smoking or exposure to smoke or pollutants
  - Aspiration
  - Bronchiectasis
  - Infections (e.g., pertussis, tuberculosis)
  - Nonasthmatic eosinophilic bronchitis (NAEB)
  - Cystic fibrosis
  - Sleep apnea
  - Restrictive lung diseases (e.g., chronic interstitial lung disease)
  - Neoplasms: Bronchogenic or laryngeal cancer, other
  - Psychogenic (habit cough)
- Cough reflex hypersensitivity or cough hypersensitivity syndrome are new labels attempting to define a syndrome of cough with characteristic trigger symptoms not adequately explained by other medical conditions (1).

RISK FACTORS
Although various conditions may contribute to chronic cough, the main causes include smoking and pulmonary disease.

COMMONLY ASSOCIATED CONDITIONS
Patients with UACS, asthma, and GERD may present with chronic cough as the only symptom and not the usual symptoms associated with the diagnoses.

DIAGNOSIS

HISTORY
- Patient age, associated signs/symptoms, medical history, medication history (i.e., ACE inhibitors), environmental and occupational exposures, potential for aspiration, and smoking history may make some causes more likely.
- The character of cough or description of sputum quality is rarely helpful in predicting the underlying cause.
- Cough diaries have not correlated well with objective measures.
- Various ambulatory systems for recording cough are under development.
- Hemoptysis or signs of systemic illness preclude empiric therapy.

PHYSICAL EXAM
- Signs and symptoms are variable and related to the underlying cause; usually, a nonproductive cough with no other signs or symptoms.
- Possible signs and symptoms of UACS, sinusitis, GERD, congestive heart failure, chronic stressors
- Absence of additional signs/symptoms of a particular condition not necessarily helpful:
  - For example, 5% of patients with GERD have no other signs or symptoms and sometimes have poor response to empiric proton pump inhibitor (PPI) trials.

DIAGNOSTIC TESTS & INTERPRETATION
- Evaluation often starts with empiric therapy directed at likely underlying etiology and/or simple testing such as a chest x-ray (CXR).
- Extensive testing only if indicated by the history and physical

Pediatric Considerations
Children with chronic cough not responsive to an inhaled β-agonist and without overt stressors should undergo spirometry (if age-appropriate) and foreign body evaluation (CXR).

Initial Tests (lab, imaging)
- Evaluation will be dictated by findings in the comprehensive history and physical.
- If considering neoplasm, heart failure, or infectious etiologies, CXR may be indicated.
- In cases of failure to respond to initial trial of empiric therapy, CXR may also be beneficial.

Follow-Up Tests & Special Considerations
- Examples:
  - If considering COPD, asthma, or restrictive lung disease: Spirometry
  - If suspicious of cystic fibrosis: Sweat chloride testing
  - If suspicious of hypereosinophilic syndrome, tuberculosis, or malignancy: Sputum for eosinophils and cytology
- If abnormal CXR, suspected neoplasm, or underlying pulmonary disorder, consider a chest CT.
- Consider pulmonary consultation.
- Refer to gastroenterologist for endoscopy.

Diagnostic Procedures/Other
If diagnosis suggested and inadequate response to initial measures, other procedures can be considered:
- Pulmonary function testing
- Purified protein derivative (PPD) skin testing
- Allergen testing
- 24-hour esophageal pH monitor
- Bronchoscopy, if history of hemoptysis or smoking with normal CXR
- Endoscopic or video fluoroscopic swallow evaluation or barium esophagram
- Sinus CT
- Ambulatory cough monitoring and cough challenge with citric acid, capsaicin or other bronchodilator (at specialized cough clinic)
- Echocardiogram

Test Interpretation
Specific to underlying cause

TREATMENT

- With chronic cough, empiric treatment should be directed at the most common causes as clinically indicated (UACS, asthma, GERD) (2)[C].
- Oral antihistamine/decongestant therapy with a 1st-generation antihistamine or nasal steroid spray can be used as initial empiric treatment (2)[C].
- In patients with cough associated with the common cold, nonsedating antihistamines were not found to be effective in reducing cough (2)[C].
- In stable patients with chronic bronchitis, therapy with ipratropium bromide may reduce chronic cough (3)[C].
- Centrally acting antitussive drugs (dextromethorphan, hydrocodone) may be used for short-term symptomatic relief of coughing in patients with chronic bronchitis (3)[C], but have limited efficacy in cough due to upper respiratory infections (3)[C].
- For cough associated with lung cancer, narcotic cough suppressants are recommended (3)[C].
- The American Academy of Pediatrics does not recommend central cough suppressants for treating any kind of cough (2)[B].
- In children <14 years, when pediatric recommendations are not available, adult recommendations should be used with caution (2)[C].
- Some children with recurrent cough and no evidence of airway obstruction may benefit from an inhaled β-agonist (4)[C].
- In infants and children with nonspecific chronic cough, trials of empiric PPI therapy were not effective (5)[C].

GENERAL MEASURES

- In patients with chronic cough, considerations for potential etiology should include asthma (2)[B] or UACS (2)[C].
- With concomitant complaints of heartburn and regurgitation, GERD should be considered as a potential etiology (2)[C].
- 90% of patients will have resolution of cough after smoking cessation (2)[A].
- When indicated, ACE inhibitor therapy should be switched in patients in whom intolerable cough occurs (2)[A].
- Empirically treat postnasal drip and GERD.
- Consider nonpharmacologic options, such as warm fluids, hard candy, or nasal drops. In infants and children, try clearing secretions with a bulb syringe.
- Attempt maximal therapy for single most likely cause for several weeks, then search for coexistent etiologies.

MEDICATION

- Treatments (nasal steroids, classic antihistamines, antacids, bronchodilators, inhaled corticosteroids, PPIs, antibiotics) should be directed at the specific cause of cough.
- A comparative effectiveness review of 48 studies with common antitussives stated that evidence is insufficient to draw firm conclusions (6).
- The FDA issued a public health advisory stating that OTC cough and cold medicines, including antitussives, expectorants, nasal decongestants, antihistamines, or combinations, should not be given to children <2 years. Subsequently, manufacturers have changed labeling to state "do not use" in children < 4 years.
- Routine empiric treatment of children with chronic cough with leukotriene receptor antagonists lacks evidence and cannot be recommended (7).

First Line

- In adults, oral antihistamine/decongestant therapy can be empiric treatment. Multiple formulations are available OTC in combination with other ingredients. Advise patients to review labels carefully or consult pharmacist:
  – Chlorpheniramine 2 mg/phenylephrine 5 mg/acetaminophen 325 mg (Tylenol Allergy Multi-Symptom) 2 caplets or gel caps PO q4h (maximum 12 caplets or gel caps in 24 hours; for patients >12 years)
  – Nasal steroids: Fluticasone, budesonide, others, 1 spray b.i.d.
- Central cough suppressants for short-term symptomatic relief of nonproductive cough:
  – Dextromethorphan 10–20 mg PO q4h, for patients >12 years; use 5–10 mg PO q4h for patients 6–12 years:
    ○ Concomitant use of dextromethorphan and agents with serotonergic activity (e.g., SSRIs) should be avoided due to risk of serotonin syndrome.
  – Narcotics: Codeine 15–30 mg PO q6h; hydrocodone (Vicodin) 5 mg PO q6h; hydrocodone (Tussionex Pennkinetic) 10 mg (5 mL) PO q12h for patients ≥12

Second Line

- A peripherally acting antitussive agent has been used:
  – In patients >10, benzonatate (Tessalon Perles) 100–200 mg PO t.i.d. as needed (maximum 600 mg/d)
- Results from a small randomized placebo-controlled trial (n = 27) demonstrated subjective cough score improvement in patients using slow-release morphine sulfate. Patients had failed with other antitussive therapies. Side effects included constipation and drowsiness, and there were no discontinuations due to adverse events (8)[C]:
  – Morphine was administered 5–10 mg PO b.i.d.

ISSUES FOR REFERRAL

- Refer as needed, based on specific suspected diagnosis for cough.
- Patients with chronic cough may benefit from evaluation by pulmonary, gastroenterology, ear-nose-and-throat (ENT), and/or allergy specialists.

SURGERY/OTHER PROCEDURES

Fundoplication may be effective for cough secondary to refractory GERD.

 ## ONGOING CARE

FOLLOW-UP RECOMMENDATIONS

Consider stepwise withdrawal of medications after resolution of cough.

Patient Monitoring

Frequent follow-up is necessary to assess the effectiveness of treatment and the addition of other medications as needed.

DIET

Dietary modification: Patients with GERD may benefit by avoiding ethanol, caffeine, nicotine, citrus, tomatoes, chocolate, and fatty foods.

PATIENT EDUCATION

- Reassure patient that most cases of chronic cough are not life-threatening and that the condition can usually be managed effectively.
- Counsel that several weeks to a month may be needed for significant reduction or total elimination of cough.
- Prepare the patient for the possibility of multiple diagnostic tests and therapeutic regimens, because the treatment is very often empiric.

PROGNOSIS

- >80% of patients can be effectively diagnosed and treated using a systematic approach.
- Cough from any cause may take weeks to months until resolution, and resolution depends greatly on efficacy of treatment directed at underlying etiology.

COMPLICATIONS

- Cardiovascular: Arrhythmias, syncope
- Stress urinary incontinence
- Abdominal and intercostal muscle strain
- GI: Emesis, hemorrhage, herniation
- Neurologic: Dizziness, headache, seizures
- Respiratory: Pneumothorax, laryngeal, or tracheobronchial trauma
- Skin: Petechiae, purpura, disruption of surgical wounds
- Medication side effects
- Other: Negative impact on quality of life

REFERENCES

1. Chung KF. Chronic "cough hypersensitivity syndrome": A more precise label for chronic cough. *Pulm Pharmacol Ther.* 2011;24:267–271.
2. Irwin RS, Baumann MH, Bolser DC, et al. Diagnosis and management of cough executive summary: ACCP evidence-based clinical practice guidelines. *Chest.* 2006;129:1S–23S.
3. Bolser DC. Cough suppressant and pharmacologic protussive therapy: ACCP evidence-based clinical practice guidelines. *Chest.* 2006;129:238S–249S.
4. Gupta A. Management of chronic non-specific cough in childhood: An evidence-based review. *Arch Dis Child Educ Pract Ed.* 2007;92:ep33–ep39.
5. Chang AB, Lasserson TJ, Gaffney J, et al. Gastro-oesophageal reflux treatment for prolonged non-specific cough in children and adults. *Cochrane Database Syst Rev.* 2011;CD004823.
6. McCrory DC, Coeyaux RR, Yancy WS Jr., et al. Assessment and management of chronic cough. Comparative effective review no. 100. AHRQ Publication No. 13-EHC032-EF. Rockville, MD. Agency for Healthcare Research and Quality; January 2013.
7. Chang AB, Winter D, Acworth JP. Leukotriene receptor antagonist for prolonged non-specific cough in children. *Cochrane Database Syst Rev.* 2006;(2):CD005602. Epub 2006 Apr 19.
8. Morice AH, Menon MS, Mulrennan SA, et al. Opiate therapy in chronic cough. *Am J Respir Crit Care Med.* 2007;175:312–315.

 ## SEE ALSO

- Asthma; Bronchiectasis; Congestive Heart Failure; Eosinophilic Pneumonias; Gastroesophageal Reflux Disease; Laryngeal Cancer; Lung, Primary Malignancies; Pertussis; Pulmonary Edema; Rhinitis, Allergic; Sinusitis; Tuberculosis
- Algorithm: Cough, Chronic

 ## CODES

ICD10

- J41.0 Simple chronic bronchitis
- J44.9 Chronic obstructive pulmonary disease, unspecified
- R05 Cough

CLINICAL PEARLS

- Chronic cough is defined as a cough that persists for >8 weeks in adults.
- In patients with chronic cough, most frequent etiologies include a history of smoking, asthma, UACS, and GERD.
- The FDA issued a public health advisory stating that OTC cough and cold medicines should not be given to children <2 years.
- Manufacturers have changed OTC cough expectorant and suppressant product labels to state "do not use" in children <4 years.

CHRONIC FATIGUE SYNDROME

Anthony F. Valdini, MD, MS, FACP, FAAFP

 BASICS

DESCRIPTION
- A condition characterized by (1) profound mental and physical exhaustion, (2) with at least 6 months presence of multiple systemic and neuropsychiatric symptoms, and (3) at least 4 of 8 associated conditions are required per CDC definition:
  – Impaired memory
  – Sore throat
  – Tender lymph nodes
  – Persistent muscle or joint pain
  – New headaches
  – Nonrefreshing sleep
  – Postexertional malaise
- Must have a new or definite onset (not lifelong). Fatigue is not relieved by rest and results in >50% reduction in previous activities (occupational, educational, social, and personal). Other potential medical causes must be ruled out.
- Exclusions: See "History."

EPIDEMIOLOGY
- Predominant age: 20–50 years
- Predominant sex: Male < Female
- All socioeconomic groups
- Various, and at times contradictory, associations between ethnicity and incidence have been reported. Higher rates found in ethnic minorities (Native Americans and African Americans) compared with white populations, based on a population study. Service-based studies (tertiary care) have reported higher rates among whites or no association between incidence and ethnicity (1).

Prevalence
Estimates vary widely and depend on case definition and population studied, but a reasonable estimate using a strict case definition is 100 cases per 100,000 population. Community-based studies have reported prevalence rates of 0.23% and 0.42%.

ETIOLOGY AND PATHOPHYSIOLOGY
- Unknown and likely multifactorial:
  – Possible interaction between genetic predisposition, environmental factors, an initiating stressor, and perpetuating factors
- Physiologic or environmental stressor could be precipitant.
- Many patients with chronic fatigue recall significant stressors (e.g., major medical procedure, loss of a loved one, loss of employment) in months before symptoms began.
- Systems hypothesized to contribute to physiology include:
  – Neuroendocrine (e.g., diminished cortisol response to increased corticotropin concentrations)
  – Immune (e.g., increased C-reactive protein and β-2 microglobulin) (4)
  – Neuromuscular (e.g., dysfunction of oxidative metabolism) (4)
  – Autonomic (orthostatic hypotension is reported in a proportion of CFS sufferers)
- Serotonergic (e.g., hyperserotonergic mechanisms or upregulation of serotonin receptors)

Genetics
Higher concordance among monozygotic twins compared with dizygotic twins

RISK FACTORS
Possible predisposing factors include (2,3):
- Personality characteristics (neuroticism and introversion)
- Lifestyle:
  – Childhood inactivity or overactivity
  – Inactivity in adulthood after infectious mononucleosis
  – Familial predisposition
  – Comorbid mood disorders of depression and anxiety
- Long-standing medical conditions in childhood
- Childhood trauma (emotional, physical, sexual abuse)
- Prolonged idiopathic chronic fatigue (5)

COMMONLY ASSOCIATED CONDITIONS
Common comorbidities include:
- Fibromyalgia (more common in women)
- Irritable bowel syndrome
- Temporomandibular joint disorder
- Anxiety disorders
- Major depression
- Posttraumatic stress disorder (including physical and/or sexual past abuse)
- Domestic violence
- Attention-deficit hyperactivity disorder (ADHD)
- Postural orthostatic tachycardia syndrome (POTS)

DIAGNOSIS

HISTORY
- Discrete onset
- Profound mental and physical exhaustion
- At least 6 months presence of multiple systemic and neuropsychiatric symptoms
- At least 4 of 8 associated conditions per CDC definition:
  – Impaired memory, sore throat, tender lymph nodes, persistent muscle or joint pain, new headaches, nonrefreshing sleep, postexertional malaise
- Exclusion criteria:
  – <2 years after recovery of substance/alcohol abuse
  – <5 years after resolution of anorexia nervosa or bulimia
  – BMI ≥45
  – Malignancy
  – Previously diagnosed medical condition, unresolved clinically, e.g., hepatitis B or C

PHYSICAL EXAM
Complete physical exam to rule out other medical causes for symptoms. Note: Tender adenopathy is one of the defining criteria.

ALERT
Detailed mental status examination (or referral to psychiatrist) to rule out other primary etiologies or comorbidities

DIFFERENTIAL DIAGNOSIS
- Idiopathic chronic fatigue (i.e., fatigue of unknown cause for >6 months without meeting criteria for CFS)
- Psychiatric disorders:
  – Major depression
  – Somatization disorder

- Physiologic fatigue (inadequate or disrupted sleep, menopause)
- Pregnancy until 3 months postpartum
- Insomnia: Primary (no clear etiology) vs. secondary (e.g., due to anxiety, depression, environmental factors, poor sleep hygiene)
- Endocrine disorder (hypothyroidism, Addison disease, Cushing syndrome, diabetes mellitus)
- Localized infection (e.g., occult abscess)
- Chronic or subacute bacterial disease (e.g., endocarditis)
- Lyme disease
- Fungal disease (e.g., histoplasmosis, coccidioidomycosis)
- Parasitic disease (e.g., amebiasis, giardiasis, helminth infestation)
- HIV or related disease
- Iatrogenic (e.g., medication side effects)
- Toxic agent exposure
- Other known or defined systemic disease
- Morbid obesity, BMI >40
- Malignancy
- Autoimmune disease
- Chronic inflammatory disease (sarcoidosis, Wegener granulomatosis)
- Neuromuscular disease (multiple sclerosis, myasthenia gravis)

DIAGNOSTIC TESTS & INTERPRETATION
- No single diagnostic test available and finding an abnormal result is not always the same as discovering the cause of fatigue. Be prepared to review the search for the cause if the problem is treated and the patient remains fatigued.
- Standard laboratory tests are recommended to rule out other causes for symptoms (6):
  – Chemistry panel
  – CBC
  – Urinalysis
  – Thyroid-stimulating hormone (TSH)
  – ESR or C-reactive protein
  – Liver function
  – Screen for drugs of abuse
  – Age-/Gender-appropriate cancer screening
- Additional studies, if clinical findings are suggestive or patient at risk (6):
  – Antinuclear antibodies and rheumatoid factor (if positive ESR)
  – Creatine kinase
  – Tuberculin skin test
  – Serum cortisol
  – HIV, VDRL or RPR
  – Lyme serology
  – IgA tissue transglutaminase

Initial Tests (lab, imaging)
No applicable imaging tests available; however, EEG and/or MRI may be useful if patient has CNS symptoms; polysomnography, if patient is sleepy

Follow-Up Tests & Special Considerations
- Assess for comorbid psychiatric disorders.
- Assess for personality and psychosocial factors and maladaptive coping styles.
- In patients with sleep disturbance, polysomnography may reveal a treatable comorbid disease.

TREATMENT

Focus on changes in lifestyle and insight, with a goal to avoid complicating treatments (e.g., addicting medications, invasive testing) or interventions that support secondary gain.

GENERAL MEASURES

ALERT

Treatment cornerstones include *both* cognitive-behavioral therapy (CBT) and graded exercise therapy. Medication is of little value. 2 treatments have been shown effective, often used in combination (7,8,9):

- Individual CBT: Challenge fatigue-related cognition; plan social and occupational rehabilitation.
- Graded exercise therapy (GET): Track amount of exercise patient can do without exacerbating symptoms and gradually increase the intensity and duration. Both involve a carefully planned balance between activity and rest.
- Patients learn how to gradually increase activity in a way that will not exacerbate their illness. Vigorous exercise can trigger relapse, perhaps related to immune dysregulation (8).
- Improves functional capacity and diminishes sense of fatigue (9)
- GET is more effective with educational interventions using telephone reminders (9).
- The duration of illness does not predict treatment outcome, so aggressive combined care is indicated for all.

MEDICATION

- No established pharmacologic treatment recommendations
- Studies have been conducted with antidepressants, immunoglobulins, hydrocortisone, and modafinil. None has shown clear benefit (6).
- If insomnia is present, use of nonaddicting sleep aids (hydroxyzine, trazodone, doxepin, etc.) may improve outcomes.

ISSUES FOR REFERRAL

- Psychiatrist to assist in managing comorbid disorders if needed
- Rehabilitative medicine

COMPLEMENTARY AND ALTERNATIVE MEDICINE

- Insufficient to recommend any CAM option for all (10)[A].
- Social support groups have not proven to be effective.

ONGOING CARE

FOLLOW-UP RECOMMENDATIONS

- Gradual increase in physical exercise with scheduled rest periods.
- Avoid extended periods of rest.

Patient Monitoring

Although no consensus exists, periodic reevaluation is appropriate for support, relief of symptoms, and assessment for other possible causes of symptoms.

DIET

- No diet has been shown to be effective for treatment of CFS.
- A BMI of 40 has been associated with fatigue in general, and BMI ≥45 is a CFS exclusion.
- Whether weight loss improves symptoms in obese CFS patients has yet to be tested.

PATIENT EDUCATION

- Patient education is an important part of treatment of CFS, such as education on the benefits of cognitive therapies, lifestyle changes, and pharmacologic therapy directed at specific associated symptoms.
- Chronic Fatigue and Immune Dysfunction Syndrome Association of America: www.cfids.org
- CDC, Chronic Fatigue Syndrome: http://www.cdc.gov/cfs/

PROGNOSIS

- Fluctuating course
- Generally, improvement is slow, with a course of months to years.
- An estimated 5% fully recover.
- Patients with poor social adjustment, a strong belief in an organic etiology, or financial secondary gain are less likely to improve

COMPLICATIONS

- Depression
- Unemployment: Although studies document improvement with treatment, <1/3 of patients in trials return to work (11).
- The US Social Security Administration lists CFS as a bona fide form of disability.
- Receipt of government payments (secondary gain) has been associated with treatment nonresponse.
- Polypharmacy
- Chronic immune activation or an infection associated with CFS may play a role in an increased risk for non-Hodgkins lymphoma in elderly (>80) CFS patients.

REFERENCES

1. Dinos S, Khoshaba B, Ashby D, et al. A systematic review of chronic fatigue, its syndromes and ethnicity: Prevalence, severity, co-morbidity and coping. *Int J Epidemiol*. 2009;38:1554–1570.
2. Viner R, Hotopf M. Childhood predictors of self reported chronic fatigue syndrome/myalgic encephalomyelitis in adults: National birth cohort study. *BMJ*. 2004;329:941.
3. Heim C, Wagner D, Maloney E, et al. Early adverse experience and risk for chronic fatigue syndrome: Results from a population-based study. *Arch Gen Psychiatry*. 2006;63:1258–1266.
4. Fulle S, Pietrangelo T, Mancinelli R, et al. Specific correlations between muscle oxidative stress and chronic fatigue syndrome: A working hypothesis. *J Muscle Res Cell Motil*. 2007;28:355–362.
5. Jason LA, Porter N, Hunnell J, et al. CFS prevalence and risk factors over time. *J Health Psychol*. 2011;16(3):445–456. Epub 2011 Jan 11.
6. Baker R, Shaw EJ. Diagnosis and management of chronic fatigue syndrome or myalgic encephalomyelitis (or encephalopathy): Summary of NICE guidance. *BMJ*. 2007;335:446–448.
7. White PD, Goldsmith KA, Johnson AL, et al. Comparison of adaptive pacing therapy, cognitive behaviour therapy, graded exercise therapy, and

specialist medical care for chronic fatigue syndrome (PACE): A randomised trial. *Lancet*. 2011;377:823–836.
8. Nijs J, Paul L, Wallman K. Chronic fatigue syndrome: An approach combining self-management with graded exercise to avoid exacerbations. *J Rehabil Med*. 2008;40:241–247.
9. Price JR, Mitchell E, Tidy E, et al. Cognitive behaviour therapy for chronic fatigue syndrome in adults. *Cochrane Database Syst Rev*. 2008; CD001027.
10. Adams D, Wu T, Yang X, et al. Traditional Chinese medicinal herbs for the treatment of idiopathic chronic fatigue and chronic fatigue syndrome. *Cochrane Database Syst Rev*. 2009;CD006348.
11. Cairns R, Hotopf M. A systematic review describing the prognosis of chronic fatigue syndrome. *Occup Med-Oxford*. 2005;55:20–31.

ADDITIONAL READING

- Corbin LW, Kamaroff AL, Natelson BH, Rowe PC. A Case-Based Approach to Chronic Fatigue Syndrome.
- Diagnosis and Management of Chronic Fatigue Syndrome, CDC course for clinicians. http://www.cdc.gov/cfs/education/diagnosis/idex.html
- Duffy FH, McAnulty GB, McCreary MC, et al. EEG spectral coherence data distinguish chronic fatigue syndrome patients from healthy controls and depressed patients—a case control study. *BMC Neurol*. 2011;11:82. Epub 2011 Jul 1.
- http://www.medscape.org/viewarticle/782106. Online CME. Includes definition/discussion of pediatric CFS
- Social Security Administration, CFS Fact Sheet: https://www.socialsecurity.gov/disability/professionals/cfs-pub063.htm

SEE ALSO

Algorithm: Fatigue

CODES

ICD10
R53.82 Chronic fatigue, unspecified

CLINICAL PEARLS

- CFS and depression can be comorbid. However, to differentiate between the 2, sore throat, tender lymph nodes, and postexercise fatigue are much more characteristic of CFS.
- No universal pharmacologic agents (e.g., antidepressants, immune modulators) have been shown to be consistently effective.
- ~70% of patients show improvement with CBT, compared to 55% with GET; in many cases, these 2 treatments can be undertaken in combination.
- There are many more patients with idiopathic chronic fatigue than true CFS. To diagnose CFS, CDC criteria need to be met; standardized instruments (SF-36, symptom index and Multidimensional Fatigue Inventory [MFI]) have been shown to be of use in the empirical diagnosis of CFS and may be helpful for following patients' progress.

CHRONIC KIDNEY DISEASE

Urooj Najm, MBBS • Najm Hasan Siddiqui, MD

BASICS

Chronic kidney disease (CKD) is defined as structural or functional abnormalities of the kidney for ≥3 months, as determined by either pathologic abnormalities or markers of damage, including abnormalities in blood or urine tests, histology, imaging studies, or history of kidney transplant; *or a* GFR <60 mL/min/1.73 m² for ≥3 months.

DESCRIPTION
- In 2012, Kidney Disease Improving Global Outcome (KDIGO) classified CKD in 6 categories by GFR estimation:
  - G1: Kidney damage with normal or increased GFR ≥90 mL/min/1.73 m²
  - G2: Mild ↓ GFR 60–89 mL/min/1.73 m²
  - G3a: Mild to moderate ↓ GFR 45–59 mL/min/1.73 m²
  - G3b: Moderate to severe ↓ GFR 30–44 mL/min/1.73 m²
  - G4: Severe ↓ GFR 15–29 mL/min/1.73 m²
  - G5: Kidney failure: GFR <15 mL/min/1.73 m² or dialysis
- CKD per albumin-to-creatinine ratio (ACR) category:
  - A1: Normal to mild increased: <30 mg/g or <3 mg/mmol
  - A2: Moderately increased: 30–300 mg/g or 3–30 mg/mmol (formerly called microalbuminiuria)
  - A3: Severely increased: >300 mg/g or >30 mg/mmol (formerly called macroalbuminuria)
- System(s) affected: Renal/Urinary; Cardiovascular; Skeletal; Endocrine; Metabolic; Hematologic; Lymphatic; Immune; Neurologic
- Synonym(s): Chronic renal failure; Chronic renal insufficiency

Geriatric Considerations
GFR normally decreases with age, despite normal creatinine (Cr). Adjust renally cleared drugs for GFR in the elderly.

Pediatric Considerations
CKD definition is not applicable for children <2 years because of lower GFR even when corrected for body surface area. Calculated GFR based on serum Cr is used in this age group.

Pregnancy Considerations
- Renal function in CKD may deteriorate during pregnancy. Cr >1.5 and hypertension (HTN) are major risk factors for worsening renal function.
- Increased risk of premature labor, preeclampsia, and/or fetal loss
- ACE inhibitors and angiotensin receptor blockers (ARBs) are contraindicated due to teratogenicity. Use diuretics with caution.

EPIDEMIOLOGY
- Majority of people with CKD in stages 1–3
- African Americans are 3.6 × more likely to develop chronic kidney disease than Caucasians.
- Predominant sex: Similar in both sexes; however, incidence rate of end-stage renal disease (ESRD) is 1.6 × higher in males than females.

Incidence
Estimated annual incidence of 1,700/1 million population

Prevalence
Overall prevalence of CKD is 14.2%. Unadjusted prevalence/incidence rates of ESRD (stage 5) are 1,752 and 362.4/1 million, respectively. Numbers do not reflect the burden of earlier stages of CKD (stages 1–4), which are estimated to affect 13.1% of the population nationwide, or 26.3 million in the US.

ETIOLOGY AND PATHOPHYSIOLOGY
Progressive destruction of kidney nephrons; GFR will drop gradually, and plasma Cr values will approximately double, with 50% reduction in GFR and 75% loss of functioning nephrons mass. Hyperkalemia usually develops when GFR falls to <20–25 mL/min. Anemia develops from decreased renal synthesis of erythropoietin:

- Renal parenchymal/glomerular:
  - Nephritic: Hematuria, RBC casts, HTN, variable proteinuria:
    ○ Focal proliferative: IgA nephropathy, SLE, Henoch-Schönlein purpura, Alport syndrome; proliferative glomerulonephritis; crescentic glomerulonephritis
    ○ Diffuse proliferative: Membranoproliferative glomerulonephritis, SLE, cryoglobulinemia, rapidly progressive glomerulonephritis (RPGN), Goodpasture syndrome
  - Nephrotic: Proteinuria (>3.5 g/d), hypoalbuminemia, hyperlipidemia, and edema:
    ○ Minimal change disease, membranous nephropathy, focal segmental glomerulosclerosis
    ○ Amyloidosis, diabetic nephropathy
- Vascular: HTN, thrombotic microangiopathies, vasculitis (Wegener), scleroderma
- Interstitial-tubular: Infections, obstruction, toxins, allergic interstitial nephritis, multiple myeloma, connective tissue disease, cystic disease
- Postrenal: Obstruction (benign prostatic hyperplasia), neoplasm, neurogenic bladder

Genetics
- Alport syndrome, Fabry disease, sickle cell anemia, SLE, and autosomal-dominant polycystic kidney disease can lead to CKD.
- Polymorphisms in gene that encodes for podocyte nommuscle myosin IIA are more common in African Americans than Caucasians and appear to increase risk for nondiabetic ESRD

RISK FACTORS
- Type 1 or 2 diabetes mellitus (DM); most common
- Age >60 years
- Cardiovascular disease (e.g., HTN [common], renal artery stenosis, atheroemboli)
- Previous kidney transplant
- Urinary tract obstruction (e.g., benign prostatic hyperplasia)
- Autoimmune disease, vasculitis/connective tissue disorder
- Family history of CKD
- Nephrotoxic drugs (lithium, salicylate, high-dose or chronic NSAIDs, sulfa)
- Congenital anomalies, obstructive uropathy, renal aplasia/hypoplasia/dysplasia, reflux nephropathy
- Hyperlipidemia
- Low income/education/ethnic minority status
- Obesity/Smoking/Heroin use
- Chronic infection (hepatitis B, hepatitis C, HIV)

GENERAL PREVENTION
- Treat reversible causes: Hypovolemia, infections, diuretics, drugs (NSAIDs, aminoglycosides, IV contrast).
- Treat risk factors: DM, HTN, hyperlipidemia, smoking, and obesity; adjust medication doses to prevent renal toxicity.

COMMONLY ASSOCIATED CONDITIONS
HTN, DM, cardiovascular disease

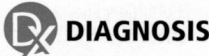

DIAGNOSIS

HISTORY
Patients with CKD stages 1–3 are usually asymptomatic; can present with:
- Oliguria, nocturia, polyuria, hematuria, change in urinary frequency
- Bone disease
- Edema, HTN, dyspnea
- Fatigue, depression, weakness
- Pruritus, ecchymosis
- Metallic taste in mouth, anorexia, nausea, vomiting
- Hyperlipidemia, claudication, restless legs
- Erectile dysfunction, decrease libido, amenorrhea

PHYSICAL EXAM
- Volume status (pallor, BP/orthostatics; edema; jugular venous distention; weight)
- Skin: Sallow complexion, uremic frost
- Ammonia-like odor (uremic fetor)
- Cardiovascular: Assess for murmurs, bruits, pericarditis.
- Chest: Pleural effusion
- Rectal: Enlarged prostate
- CNS: Asterixis, confusion, seizures, coma, peripheral neuropathy

DIAGNOSTIC TESTS & INTERPRETATION
Initial Tests (lab, imaging)
- GFR can be estimated by multiple equations (freely available in medical calculators) including MDRD equation:
  - GFR (mL/min/1.73 m²) = 175 × {[serum Cr μmol/1/88.4]$^{-1.154}$} × {age (years)$^{-0.203}$} × 0.742 for females *or* 1.21 for African American
- Cr clearance (CrCl) can be calculated using Cockroft-Gault formula:
  - CrCl (male) = ([140 – age] × weight(kg)/(serum Cr × 72)
  - CrCl (female) = CrCl (male) × 0.85
- Urine analysis:
  - Urine microscopy: WBC casts in pyelonephritis, RBC casts in glomerulonephritis/vasculitis, dysmorphic RBCs
  - Urine electrolytes: Sodium, Cr, urea (if on loop diuretics)
  - Proteinuria/Albuminuria:
    ○ 24-hour urine collection: >30–300 mg/24 h (20–200 μg/min) is micro- and >300 mg/24 h (>200 μg/min) is macroalbuminuria.
    ○ Albumin/Cr ratio (ACR): See "Description"
- Hematology: Normochromic, normocytic anemia, increased bleeding time
- Chemistry:
  - Elevated BUN, Cr, hyperkalemia, metabolic acidosis
  - Increased parathyroid hormone, decreased 25-(OH) vitamin D, hypocalcemia, hyperphosphatemia
  - Hyperlipidemia, decreased albumin

ALERT

Drugs that may alter lab result:
- Cimetidine: Inhibits Cr secretion
- Trimethoprim: Inhibits Cr and K^+ secretion and may cause/worsen hyperkalemia
- Cefoxitin and flucytosine: Increases serum Cr
- Diltiazem and verapamil (like ACE/ARBs) have significant antiproteinuric effects in patients with CKD.
- Ultrasound (initial test of choice): Small, echogenic kidneys; may see obstruction (e.g., hydronephrosis); cysts; kidneys may be enlarged with HIV and diabetic nephropathy
- Doppler ultrasound to assess for renovascular disease, thrombosis
- Noncontrast CT scan: Obstruction, calculi, cysts, neoplasm, renal artery stenosis
- MRI/MRA: Avoid gadolinium because of the risk of nephrogenic systemic fibrosis.
- Renal arteriogram for renal artery stenosis can be therapeutic (angioplasty or stenting).
- Renal scan to screen for differential function between kidneys
- Retrograde pyelogram: If strong suspicion for obstruction despite negative finding on ultrasound

Follow-Up Tests & Special Considerations
- Serology: ANA; double-stranded DNA, antineutrophil cytoplasmic antibody; complements (C3, C4, CH50); anti-GBM antibodies; hepatitis B, C; and HIV screening
- Serum and urine immunoelectrophoresis

Diagnostic Procedures/Other
Biopsy: Hematuria, proteinuria, acute/progressive renal failure, nephritic or nephrotic syndrome

TREATMENT

GENERAL MEASURES
- Lowering salt intake to < 2 g/d of sodium in adults, unless contraindicated (1)[C]
- Minimize radiocontrast exposure; prehydrate; N-acetylcysteine use is controversial. Avoid nephrotoxins (NSAIDs, aminoglycosides, etc.)
- Renal replacement: Prepare for dialysis or transplant when GFR <30 mL/min/1.73 m^2.
- Vaccines: Pneumococcal, influenza.
- Encourage smoking cessation, encourage weight loss (if applicable), and limit alcohol consumption

MEDICATION
- HTN: Goal is BP <130/80 (in nonhemodialysis patients) and <140/90 (in patients on hemodialysis) in the nephrology literature, but more recent analysis based on outcomes suggests a universal BP target of <140/90 (2).
- Antihypertensive agents should be selected based on the type of CKD and presence of cardiovascular disease.
- Long-acting (once daily) agents should be prescribed preferentially and given at bedtime.

- ACE inhibitors (drugs of choice) or ARBs for BP control and antiproteinuric effect:
  – Potential for hyperkalemia
  – Can tolerate up to 30% rise in serum Cr unless hyperkalemia develops
  – If goal not reached, add diuretic; thiazides are recommended for GFR ≥30 mL/min/1.73 m^2; loop diuretics are recommended for GFR <30 mL/min/1.73 m^2), followed by diltiazem or verapamil or a β-blocker.
- Secondary hyperparathyroidism:
  – Cinacalcet, paricalcitol (decrease PTH levels)
- Recommended serum phosphate maintenance levels for CKD patients:

Stage	mg/dL	mmol/L
Normal range *may vary by institution*	2.5–4.5	0.81–1.45
Stage 3 and 4 CKD (not on dialysis)	2.7–4.6	0.87–1.49
Stage 5 and ALL stages on dialysis	3.5–5.5	1.13–1.78

  – Stages 3–5 CKD (not on dialysis): Restrict dietary phosphate to 800–1,000 mg/d:
    ○ Calcium-containing phosphate binders (with meals): Calcium carbonate, calcium acetate (risk of hypercalcemia)
    ○ Non–calcium phosphate binders (with meals): Sevelamer, lanthanum
    ○ Vitamin D: Inactive vitamin D 25 (Ergocalciferol or Cholecalciferol), Calcitriol (active vitamin D 1,25 [OH]): Vitamin D may increase absorption of phosphate by intestines and should not be started until serum phosphate concentration is controlled.
  – Anemia: Ferrous sulfate, erythropoietin stimulating agents (ESAs): Before starting ESAs, nonrenal causes of anemia/iron stores should be checked. Start when Hgb <11 g/dL; goal range 11–12 g/dL, not to exceed 13 g/dL
  – Hyperlipidemia: Statins with low-density lipoprotein (LDL) goal is similar to coronary heart disease patients (LDL <70–100).
  – Glycemic control: Target HbA1c 7.0%, but it should be individualized based on life expectancy of patient, risk for adverse events related to glucose control, and patient preference (1). Tighter control may slow progression of microalbuminuria, but may not reduce progression to ESRD and death in patients with type 2 diabetes. Use of metformin is not advised with GFR <30 mL/min/1.73 m^2 because of possible risk of lactic acidosis. A reduction in metformin dosing is advisable if treatment is used for GFR between 30–44 mL/min/1.73 m^2 (1).
  – Metabolic acidosis: Start treatment when bicarb <20 mEq/L; goal >23 mEq/L:
    ○ Sodium bicarbonate: Daily dose of 0.5–1 mEq/kg/d or sodium citrate (should be avoided in patients taking aluminum-containing antacid)

ISSUES FOR REFERRAL
- Nephrology Consult:GFR <15: Immediate
- GFR 15–29: Urgent
- GFR 30–59: Non-Urgent Referral
- GFR 60–89: Not required unless co-morbidities

SURGERY/OTHER PROCEDURES
Placement of dialysis access or transplantation

IN-PATIENT CONSIDERATIONS
Admission Criteria/Initial Stabilization
Uremia: Nausea/vomiting, fluid overload, pericarditis, uremic encephalopathy, resistant HTN, hyperkalemia, metabolic acidosis, hyperphosphatemia

 ## ONGOING CARE

DIET
Nutrition consult for CKD diet: Protein restriction in early CKD is controversial but may be beneficial in ESRD; restricted intake of phosphates; sodium and water restriction to avoid volume overload; potassium restriction if hyperkalemic

PATIENT EDUCATION
National Kidney Federation patient Web site at: www.kidney.org/patients

PROGNOSIS
Patients with CKD gradually progress to ESRD, with bad prognoses. 5-year survival rate for US patients on dialysis is ~35%.

COMPLICATIONS
HTN, anemia, secondary hyperparathyroidism, renal osteodystrophy, sleep disturbances, infections, malnutrition, electrolyte imbalances, platelet dysfunction/bleeding, pseudogout, gout, metabolic calcification, sexual dysfunction

REFERENCES

1. KDIGO 2012 clinical practice guideline for the evaluation and management of chronic kidney disease. *Kidney International* Supplements. 2013. Available at: www.kdigo.org/clinical_practice_guidelines/pdf/CKD/KDIGO_2012_CKD_GL.pdf
2. 2013 ESH/ESC guidelines for the management of arterial hypertension. *J Hypertens*. 2013;31: 1281–1357.

 ## SEE ALSO

- Hydronephrosis; Nephrotic Syndrome; Polycystic Kidney Disease; Proteinuria
- Algorithm: Anuria or Oliguria

CODES

ICD10
- N18.1 Chronic kidney disease, stage 1
- N18.2 Chronic kidney disease, stage 2 (mild)
- N18.9 Chronic kidney disease, unspecified

CLINICAL PEARLS

- Maintaining BP <140/90 is imperative (in patients not on dialysis).
- Avoid nephrotoxins including ACE/ARB in AKI with or without CKD.
- CKD is a CHD risk equivalent.

CHRONIC OBSTRUCTIVE PULMONARY DISEASE AND EMPHYSEMA

Alan J. Cropp, MD • Bryon Veynovich, DO

 ## BASICS

DESCRIPTION
- Chronic obstructive pulmonary disease (COPD) usually describes a mixture of chronic bronchitis and emphysema. It is characterized by airflow limitation that is not fully reversible, inflammation, and is progressive (1,2).
- Chronic bronchitis is defined clinically by increased mucus production and recurrent cough present on most days for at least 3 months per year during at least 2 consecutive years.
- Emphysema, the destruction of interalveolar septa, occurs in the distal or terminal airways and involves both airways and lung parenchyma.

EPIDEMIOLOGY
Incidence
Affects more than 5% of adults in the US and is the 12th leading cause of morbidity (1)

Prevalence
- 3rd leading cause of death in the US (1)
- Projected to be the 3rd leading cause of death globally by 2020 (2)

ETIOLOGY AND PATHOPHYSIOLOGY
Cigarette and/or cannabis smoking, air pollution (including indoor), antiprotease deficiency (α_1-antitrypsin), occupational exposure (firefighters), infection (viral), occupational pollutants (cadmium, silica)
- Impaired gas (CO_2 and O_2) exchange
- Chronic bronchitis: Airway obstruction (3)
- Emphysema: Destruction of lung parenchyma

Genetics
- Chronic bronchitis is not a genetic disorder.
- Antiprotease deficiency (due to α_1-antitrypsin deficiency) is an inherited, rare disorder due to 2 autosomal-codominant alleles.

RISK FACTORS
- Smoking; passive smoking, especially adults whose parents smoked; cannabis use (1 joint is equivalent to 2.5–5 cigarettes) (1,2,3)
- Severe pneumonia early in life including viral (4)
- Aging
- Lower level of education and poverty (4)
- Airway hyperactivity
- Indoor pollution (open fire used for cooking) (4)
- Occupational organic or inorganic dusts (4)

GENERAL PREVENTION
- Avoidance of smoking is the most important preventive measure.
- Early detection through pulmonary function tests (PFTs) in high-risk patients may be useful in preserving remaining lung function.

COMMONLY ASSOCIATED CONDITIONS
- Pulmonary: Lung cancer, chronic respiratory failure, acute bronchitis, sleep apnea, pulmonary hypertension
- Cardiac: Coronary artery disease, arrhythmia
- Ear, nose, and throat (ENT): Chronic sinusitis, laryngeal carcinoma
- Miscellaneous: Malnutrition, osteoporosis, muscle dysfunction, depression

DIAGNOSIS

HISTORY
- Discuss patient's habits with regard to tobacco.
- Consider indoor pollution (coal furnace) (4).
- Review possible causes of exacerbation (e.g., recent infection) and history of cough, sputum, dyspnea
- Chronic bronchitis: Cough, sputum production, frequent infections, intermittent dyspnea, wheeze, hemoptysis, morning headache, pedal edema
- Emphysema: Minimal cough, scant sputum, dyspnea, weight loss, occasional infections

PHYSICAL EXAM
- Rarely diagnostic for COPD (2)
- Chronic bronchitis: Cyanosis, wheezing, weight gain, diminished breath sounds, distant heart sounds
- Emphysema: Barrel chest, minimal wheezing, accessory muscles used, pursed lip breathing, cyanosis slight or absent, breath sounds diminished

DIFFERENTIAL DIAGNOSIS
- Asthma (including occupational)
- Bronchiectasis
- Lung cancer
- Acute viral infection
- Normal aging of lungs
- Chronic pulmonary embolism
- Sleep apnea
- Primary alveolar hypoventilation
- Chronic sinusitis
- Reactive airways dysfunction syndrome (RADS)
- Congestive heart failure (CHF)
- Bronchiolitis obliterans
- Gastroesophageal reflux disease

DIAGNOSTIC TESTS & INTERPRETATION

- Spirometry (the most reliable/objective measurement of airflow obstruction) (1,2,3)[A]

Initial Tests (lab, imaging)
- Chronic bronchitis:
  - Arterial blood gases (ABGs) may show hypercapnia and hypoxia.
  - Hemoglobin may be increased.
- Emphysema:
  - Normal serum hemoglobin or polycythemia
  - Normal $PaCO_2$ on ABGs unless forced expiratory volume in 1 second (FEV_1) <1 L, in which case it can be elevated.
  - Mild hypoxia
- Spirometry (1,2,3)
- Chronic bronchitis CXR: Increased bronchovascular markings and cardiomegaly
- Emphysema CXR: Small heart, hyperinflation, flat diaphragms, and possibly bullous changes

Follow-Up Tests & Special Considerations
- Consider checking continuous overnight oximetry in selected patients.
- α_1-antitrypsin screening for those with COPD age <45 years or have a blood relative with this disease
- Chest CT may show diffuse bullous changes or upper lobe predominance. Also, small lung nodules may be identified (5)[B]

Diagnostic Procedures/Other
- Pulmonary function tests (PFTs) (1,2)[A]
  - Not indicated during acute exacerbation (3)
  - Decreased FEV_1 and resulting reduction in FEV_1:FVC (forced vital capacity) ratio
  - Poor or absent reversibility to bronchodilator
  - Normal or reduced FVC
  - Normal or increased total lung capacity
  - Increased residual volume and functional residual capacity
  - Diffusing capacity is normal or reduced.
- Staging: GOLD Criteria (3)
  - Mild COPD: FEV_1 $\geq$80% predicted
  - Moderate COPD: FEV_1 between 50% and 80% predicted
  - Severe COPD: FEV_1 between 30% and 50% predicted
  - Very severe COPD: FEV_1 <30% predicted or FEV_1 <50% predicted plus chronic respiratory failure

Test Interpretation
- Chronic bronchitis: Bronchial mucous gland enlargement, increased number of secretory cells in surface epithelium, thickened small airways from edema and inflammation, smooth muscle hyperplasia, mucus plugging, bacterial colonization of airways
- Emphysema: Entire lung affected, bronchi usually clear of secretions, anthracotic pigment, alveoli enlarged with loss of septa, cartilage atrophy, bullae

 ## TREATMENT

GENERAL MEASURES
- Smoking cessation: This is the most important intervention to decrease risk (1,2)[A].
- Aggressive treatment of infections (3)[B]
- Treat any reversible bronchospasm.
- Home oxygen: May improve survival; should be initiated PaO_2 $\leq$55 mm Hg or pulse oximetry trends $\leq$88% (1)[A]
- Influenza and pneumococcal immunizations (2)

MEDICATION
Medications help to reduce symptoms and exacerbations (1)

First Line
- Patients should have a short-acting β-agonist (Albuterol) to use as a rescue drug (1)
- Anticholinergics (2)[A]:
  - Ipratropium (Atrovent), tiotropium (Spiriva), aclidinium bromide (Turdoza) (2)[A] AND/OR
- Long-acting β-agonists:
  - Salmeterol (Serevent), formoterol (Foradil), 1 inhalation q12h; or arformoterol (Brovana), formoterol (Perforomist), nebulized q12h (1,2)[A]

ALERT
Acute exacerbation: Use oxygen, inhaled β-agonists, inhaled anticholinergic agents, and oral corticosteroids prednisone (up to 1 mg/kg/d commonly 40 mg/d for 5 days) (6)[A]. If bacterial infection is a concern, doxycycline or trimethoprim-sulfamethoxazole are considered 1st line (3)[B].

Second Line

- Trial of inhaled corticosteroids for moderate or severe disease (2)[A]:
  – May initiate earlier if suggestion of asthmatic component to disease
  – Systemic corticosteroids; prednisone (Deltasone) can be given orally 7.5–15 mg/d
  – Long-term monotherapy with steroids (oral or inhaled) is not recommended (2,3)[A].
  – Among patients with COPD, inhaled corticosteroid is associated with an increased risk of serious pneumonia (3).
- Theophylline if other long-term treatment is unavailable or unaffordable: 400 mg/d; increase by 100–200 mg in 1–2 weeks, if necessary (2)[B]:
  – Reduce dosage in patients with impaired renal or liver function, age >55, or CHF
  – Monitor serum level. Therapeutic range is 8–13 μg/mL
- Combination of inhaled corticosteroid, long-acting β-agonist, and anticholinergic indicated for severe disease (2)[A]
- Mucolytic agents may improve secretions, but do not improve outcomes.
- PDE4 inhibitor (Roflumilast) for patients with severe chronic bronchitis (2)[B]
- α1-antitrypsin, if deficient: 60 mg/kg/wk to maintain level >80 mg/dL
- Precautions:
  – Sympathomimetics: Excessive use may be dangerous. May need to reduce dosage or use levalbuterol (Xopenex) in patients with cardiovascular disease, hypertension (HTN), hyperthyroidism, diabetes, or convulsive disorders.
  – Anticholinergics: Narrow-angle glaucoma, benign prostatic hyperplasia, bladder-neck obstruction
  – Corticosteroids: Weight gain, diabetes, osteoporosis adrenal suppression
- Sympathomimetics may be aerosolized.
- Anticholinergics: Ipratropium (Atrovent) may be aerosolized or combined with albuterol (Combivent Respimat).

ISSUES FOR REFERRAL
Severe exacerbation, frequent hospitalizations, age <40, rapid progression, weight loss, severe disease, or surgical evaluation

ADDITIONAL THERAPIES
- Adequate hydration and pulmonary hygiene
- Consider postural drainage, flutter valve, or other devices to assist mucus clearance.
- Pulmonary rehabilitation (1,2,3)[A].
- Intermittent, noninvasive ventilation may help in severe chronic respiratory failure].
- Short course of antibiotics (5–10 days) for acute exacerbations (2)[B].

SURGERY/OTHER PROCEDURES
- Lung reduction surgery (selected cases)
- Lung transplantation (selected cases)

IN-PATIENT CONSIDERATIONS
Admission Criteria/Initial Stabilization
- Outpatient treatment is usually adequate.
- Exacerbation with acute decompensation (hypoxemia, hypercarbia)
- Serious comorbidities (i.e., decompensated CHF)
- Systemic steroids have been shown to reduce recovery time and improve hypoxia (2,6)[A]

- Supplemental oxygen and short-acting bronchodilators should be given (3)

ALERT
- If not already in place, have patient delineate an **A**dvance **D**irective, and if they have one, review patient's preferences
- www.agingwithdignity.org, www.putitinwriting.org
- Progressive nature of disease and severity of treatment methods (ventilation, etc.) make revisiting patient preferences beneficial
- Acute respiratory failure may require ICU and invasive or noninvasive (NIV) ventilation (2)[A]
- Systemic steroids (prednisone 40 mg/d for 5 days or equivalent) have been shown to reduce recovery time and improve hypoxia (6)[A]
- A short course of antibiotics for change in sputum volume, purulence, and increased dyspnea (2,3)[B]

Nursing
Teach proper inhaler use.

Discharge Criteria
- Ability to ambulate (3)
- Patient should have adequate gas exchange (3)
- Hypoxia can be treated with home O_2 (may only be temporary) (2)[A].
- Inhaled short-acting β-agonist therapy no more frequently than q4h (3)
- Ability to eat and sleep without interruption caused by dyspnea (3)

 ## ONGOING CARE

FOLLOW-UP RECOMMENDATIONS
- May taper or stop oral steroids as outpatient
- If pneumonia caused exacerbation, need to follow CXR or chest CT until clear.
- Pulmonary rehabilitation for exertional dyspnea (1)[A]

PATIENT MONITORING
- Severe or unstable patients should be seen monthly. When stable, see every 6 months.
- Check theophylline level with dose adjustment, then check every 6–12 months.
- On home O_2, check ABGs yearly or with change in condition. Frequently monitor O_2 saturation (pulse oximetry).
- Some patients only desaturate at night, thus only need nocturnal O_2
- Travel at high altitude with supplemental oxygen if necessary.
- Discuss advance directive and health care proxy.

DIET
A high-protein diet is suggested. Decreased carbohydrates may benefit those with hypercarbia.

PATIENT EDUCATION
American Lung Association: www.lung.org/lung-disease/copd/

PROGNOSIS
- Patient's age and postbronchodilator FEV$_1$ are the most important predictors of prognosis.
- Supplemental O_2, when indicated, is shown to increase survival (may only need at night) (1)[A]
- Smoking cessation improves prognosis (2)
- Malnutrition, cor pulmonale, hypercapnia, and pulse >100 indicate a poor prognosis.

COMPLICATIONS
- Malnutrition, poor sleep quality, infections, secondary polycythemia
- Acute or chronic respiratory failure, bullous lung disease, pneumothorax
- Arrhythmias, cor pulmonale, pulmonary HTN

REFERENCES

1. Amir Q, Wilt T, Weinberger S, et al. Diagnosis and management of stable chronic obstructive pulmonary disease: A clinical practice guideline update. *Ann Int Med.* 2011;55:179–191.
2. Vestbo J, Hurd S, Agusti A, et al. Global strategy for the diagnosis, management, and prevention of chronic obstructive pulmonary disease: GOLD executive summary. *Am J Respir Crit Care Med.* 2013;187:347–365.
3. Global strategy for the diagnosis, management, and prevention of COPD, Global Initiative for Chronic Obstructive Lung Disease. Revised 2013. Available at: www.goldcopd.org/
4. Lamprecht B, McBurnie M, Vollmer W, et al. COPD in never smokers: results from the population-based burden of obstructive lung disease study. *Chest.* 2011;139:752–763.
5. Detterbeck F, Mazzone P, Naidich D, Bach P. Screening for lung cancer: Diagnosis and management of lung cancer, 3rd ed.: ACCP evidence based guidelines. *Chest.* 2013;143:e78S–e92S.
6. Leuppi J, Schuetz P, Bingisser R, et al. Short-term vs conventional glucocorticoid therapy in acute exacerbations of chronic obstructive pulmonary disease. The REDUCE randomized clinical trial. *JAMA.* 2013;309:2223–2231.

ADDITIONAL READING
Maclay JD, Rabinovich RA, MacNee W. Update in chronic obstructive pulmonary disease 2008. *Am J Respir Crit Care Med.* 2009;179:533–541.

 ## SEE ALSO

- Bronchitis, Acute
- Algorithms: Clubbing; Cyanosis

 ## CODES

ICD10
- J42 Unspecified chronic bronchitis
- J43.9 Emphysema, unspecified
- J44.9 Chronic obstructive pulmonary disease, unspecified

CLINICAL PEARLS
- Consider screening PFTs on any high-risk patient.
- Overnight oximetry if daytime saturation is borderline.
- Influenza and pneumococcal vaccines should be current.
- Obtain advance directive before patient becomes seriously ill.
- Consider chest CT for patients age 55–74 plus a 30 pack-year smoking history for lung cancer screening.

CHRONIC PAIN MANAGEMENT: AN EVIDENCE-BASED APPROACH

Jennifer Reidy, MS, MD

 BASICS

- Chronic pain is pain persisting beyond the time of normal tissue healing, usually >3 months.
- Over time, neuroplastic changes in the CNS transform pain into a chronic disease itself. Pain levels can exceed observed pathology on exam or imaging.
- Pain experience is inherently related to emotional, psychological, and cognitive factors.
- An epidemic of undertreated pain coexists with an epidemic of prescription drug abuse in the US.
- Use a systems-based practice to safely and effectively prescribe opioids when indicated for chronic nonmalignant pain.

EPIDEMIOLOGY
Incidence
Incidence is rising, but exact rate is unclear. The annual economic cost of chronic pain in the US is estimated at $560–635 billion (1)[A].

Prevalence
In the US, an estimated 100 million adults live with chronic pain—more than the total affected by heart disease, cancer, and diabetes combined (1)[A].

ETIOLOGY AND PATHOPHYSIOLOGY
With intense, repeated, or prolonged stimulation of damaged or inflamed tissues, the threshold for activating primary afferent pain fibers is lowered, the frequency of firing is higher, and there is increased response to noxious and/or normal stimuli (peripheral and central sensitization). The amygdala, prefrontal cortex, and cortex are thought to relay emotions and thoughts that create the pain experience, and these areas may undergo structural and functional changes with chronic pain.

Many patients have an identifiable etiology (most commonly musculoskeletal problems or headache), but pain levels can be worse than observable tissue injury. A significant percentage of patients have no obvious cause of chronic pain.

Genetics
Current research suggests genetic polymorphism in opioid receptors, which may affect patient's response and/or side effects to individual opioids.

RISK FACTORS
- Traumatic: Motor vehicle accidents, repetitive-motion injuries, sports injuries, work-related injuries, falls
- Postsurgical: Any surgery, but especially back surgeries, amputations, thoracotomies
- Medical conditions: See "Commonly Associated Conditions" below.
- Psychiatric comorbidities: Substance abuse, depression, posttraumatic stress disorder (PTSD), personality disorders
- Aging: Increased incidence with age, but should not be considered a "normal" part of aging

GENERAL PREVENTION
- Avoidance of work-related injuries through the use of ergonomically correct workplace design
- Exercise and physical therapy to help prevent work-related low back pain

- Varicella vaccine and rapid treatment of shingles to lower risk of postherpetic neuralgia
- Tight glycemic control for diabetic patients, alcohol cessation for alcoholics, smoking cessation

COMMONLY ASSOCIATED CONDITIONS
Any chronic disease and/or its treatment can cause chronic pain, including diabetes, cardiovascular disease, HIV, progressive neurologic conditions, lung disease, cirrhosis, autoimmune disease, cancer, renal failure, depression, and mental illness.

 DIAGNOSIS

Chronic pain can be divided into 2 general categories:
- Nociceptive pain (2 types):
  - Somatic: Skin, bone, soft tissue disease; described as well localized, sharp, stabbing, aching
  - Visceral: Visceral inflammation/injury; described as poorly localized, dull, aching; may refer to sites remote from lesion
- Neuropathic pain: Damaged peripheral or central nerves; described as burning, tingling, and/or numbness:
  - Sympathetically mediated pain: Peripheral nerve injury can cause severe burning pain, swelling of the affected limb, and focal changes in sweat production and skin appearance. Example: Complex regional pain syndrome.

HISTORY
- Obtain pain history: Location, onset, intensity, duration, quality, temporal pattern, exacerbators, alleviators, prior treatments
- Assess and document how pain affects patient's functioning and quality of life, and what they expect from treatment.
- Screen for personal or family history of substance abuse (including tobacco addiction), mental health conditions, domestic violence, or sexual abuse.
- Use standardized tools: Pain severity—Brief Pain Inventory (short form); mood—Patient Health Questionnaire-9 (PHQ-9); substance abuse—Screener and Opioid Assessment for Patients with Pain (SOAPP), multiple versions
- Use this screening to risk stratify patients for risks of chronic opioid therapy and increased monitoring; a positive screen does not automatically exclude patients from opioid therapy.

PHYSICAL EXAM
Exam is guided by history and should include functional and mental assessments.

DIFFERENTIAL DIAGNOSIS
- The causes of pain are numerous, and clinic presentations are protean, depending on the individual patient.
- There is a spectrum of aberrant drug-taking behaviors, and differential diagnosis includes:
  - Inadequate analgesia ("pseudoaddiction"), disease progression, opioid-resistant pain, opioid-induced hyperalgesia, addiction, opioid tolerance, self-medication of nonpain symptoms, criminal intent (diversion)

DIAGNOSTIC TESTS & INTERPRETATION
Testing is based on differential diagnosis of pain syndrome to elucidate etiology.

Initial Tests (lab, imaging)
If substance abuse suspected, order urine drug screen. Most tests are immunoassays, which usually detect morphine and heroin but often not other opioids. Laboratory-based chromatography/spectrometry can identify specific drugs. Clinicians should be aware of uses and limitations of local laboratory testing (http://www.aafp.org/afp/2010/0301/p635.html).

Follow-Up Tests & Special Considerations
- If patient is taking chronic opioid therapy, order random urine drug screens as part of the "universal precautions" approach (see "Ongoing Care").
- Urine drug screen: Order qualitative analysis for drugs of abuse and quantitative analysis for the drug you are prescribing.

Diagnostic Procedures/Other
- Consider interventional pain clinic for complicated joint injections and nerve root blocks, which can be diagnostic.
- If complex regional pain syndrome is suspected, a sympathetic block can be diagnostic and possibly prevent chronic pain.

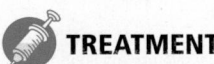 **TREATMENT**

- Goals of treatment are pain relief and restoring function, while balancing risks and benefits of therapies.
- Intradisciplinary teams offer most effective approach to chronic pain, including its physical, emotional, and psychological aspects. These teams may include the patient, family, primary care doctor, pain management specialist, psychologist, psychiatrist, physical and occupational therapists, physiatrist, complementary medicine practitioners, and (if needed) addiction medicine specialist (2)[B].
- Treatment should always include nonpharmacologic therapies such as exercise, cognitive-behavioral therapy (CBT), patient and family education, yoga, massage, relaxation techniques, support groups, meditation, and acupuncture.

GENERAL MEASURES
Keep a pain and function diary to record pain and activity levels and how much medication is taken.

MEDICATION
- Always begin with exercise, physical therapy, CBT, self-management skills before or with pain medications. Use sequential time-limited trials of medications, starting at low doses and gradually increasing until either effect or dose-limiting side effects are reached. Rational polypharmacy may be indicated (such as an opioid + neuropathic agent).
- For mild-to-moderate chronic pain:
  - Acetaminophen: Daily dose not to exceed total 4 g in healthy adults and 2 g in the elderly or those with hepatic disease or active or past history of alcohol use.

– NSAIDs: COX-2 selective inhibitors should be used with caution because of cardiac risks, but may have less gastric risk. If high cardiac risk, consider nonselective COX inhibitor (such as naproxen or ibuprofen) with or without gastric prophylaxis (depending on ulcer risk).

– "Weak" opioids, including tramadol. Caution: Opioid-analgesic combinations can lead to serious acetaminophen or NSAID toxicities if patients exceed safely prescribed doses.

– Avoid tramadol and propoxyphene in elderly or patients at risk for seizures.

– Topical agents: NSAIDs, lidocaine (gel less expensive than patch), ketamine, capsaicin

• For neuropathic pain:
– Classes of medications include: (i) tricyclic antidepressants (desipramine and nortriptyline have fewer side effects); (ii) selective serotonin-norepinephrine reuptake inhibitor (SSNRI) antidepressants (duloxetine); (iii) anticonvulsants (alpha 2-delta ligands, gabapentin and pregabalin); (iii) opioids, including tramadol. Example: Combination of nortriptyline + gabapentin.
– See "Neuropathic Pain" topic.

• For moderate-to-severe chronic pain:
– Strong opioids, including morphine, oxycodone, hydromorphone, oxymorphone, fentanyl. Check opioid equianalgesic tables for dosing by route of administration.
– No evidence supports any of these strong opioids as superior or having improved side-effect profile.
– In patients with chronic back pain, opioids may be efficacious for short-term use but long-term benefits and side effects are unclear; in addition, aberrant medication-taking behaviors range from 5–24% (3)[B]:
  ○ Morphine should be avoided in patients with significant renal insufficiency.
  ○ Methadone should only be prescribed by experienced providers. The only opioid that also acts as N-methyl-D-aspartate receptor antagonist, methadone has many drug interactions and can contribute to potentially fatal cardiac arrhythmias.
– Once stable dose of opioids is established, change to sustained-release formulations if pain constant or very frequent. Short-acting formulations are only for breakthrough or episodic pain.
– Common side effects: Constipation: Senna and docusate should be prescribed at time opioids are started. Also: Nausea, sedation, mental status changes, pruritus

ALERT
Patients on chronic opioid therapy must agree to monitoring. Clinicians should use "universal precautions" and systems-based practice, including written agreements, random urine drug screens, pill/patch counts, and other measures (see "Ongoing Care") (4,5) [B].

SURGERY/OTHER PROCEDURES
Consider interventional procedures, including joint injections, nerve blocks, spinal cord stimulation, and intrathecal medication among others, as needed.

COMPLEMENTARY AND ALTERNATIVE MEDICINE
• Acupuncture: Efficacy in chronic neck, back pain, and fibromyalgia
• Exercise: Efficacy in low back pain and fibromyalgia

• Improved mood and coping skills, decreased disability with CBT
• Mind–body interventions: Yoga, tai chi, hypnosis, progressive muscle relaxation, meditation

 ONGOING CARE

FOLLOW-UP RECOMMENDATIONS
Patient Monitoring
• It can be difficult to identify appropriate pain-relief seeking behavior from inappropriate drug-seeking, but consistent patient–clinician relationships over time can often discern the difference.
• Always maintain a risk–benefit stance and avoid judging a patient.
• Assess and document benefits, pain levels, functioning, and quality of life. In general, patients successfully taking opioids for pain become more engaged (better relationships and productive work).
• At each visit, assess and document harm, using "universal precautions" approach. This systems-based practice includes:
– Informed consent for opioid therapy
– Written or electronic agreement between patient and clinician
– 1 prescribing clinician (or designee) and 1 pharmacy
– No after-hours prescriptions or early refills
– Mandatory police reports for medication thefts
– Random urine drug tests, pill/patch counts
– Requirements for patient to continue with physical therapy, counseling, psychiatric medications, or other necessary treatments
– Participate in state's prescription drug monitoring program: See www.pmpalliance.org
– Taper and discontinue medications (10% dose reduction per week) if patient does not benefit, if side effects outweigh benefits, or if medications are abused or diverted. If addiction is suspected, always offer treatment for substance abuse (4,5) [A].

PATIENT EDUCATION
American Chronic Pain Association: http://theacpa.org

COMPLICATIONS
• Rate of addiction in chronic pain patients is unclear (3–19% in published literature), but it may reflect rate in the general population.
• Definitions:
– Addiction: Chronic biopsychologic disease characterized by impaired control over drug use, compulsive use, and continued use despite harm.
– Physical dependence: Withdrawal syndrome produced by abrupt cessation or rapid dose reduction; is not addiction but a physiologic phenomenon
– Tolerance: State of adaptation when a drug induces changes that diminish its effects over time
– Diversion: Selling drugs or giving them to persons other than for whom they are prescribed

ALERT
Caution: From 1999–2007, the rate of unintentional overdose death increased by 124%, largely due to prescription opioid overdoses (especially methadone); close monitoring is warranted.

REFERENCES
1. Institute of Medicine, Committee on Advancing Pain Research, Care and Education. *Relieving Pain in America: A Blueprint for Transforming Prevention, Care, Education and Research*. Washington, DC: The National Academies Press; 2011.
2. Dobscha SK, Corson K, Perrin NA, et al. Collaborative care for chronic pain in primary care: A cluster randomized trial. *JAMA*. 2009;301(12): 1242–1252.
3. American Society of Interventional Pain Physicians Guidelines for Responsible Opioid Prescribing in Chronic Non-Cancer Pain: Part 2 – Guidance. *Pain Physician*. 2012;15:S67–S116
4. Interagency Guideline on Opioid Dosing for Chronic Non-cancer Pain: An educational aid to improve care and safety with opioid therapy: Www.agencymeddirectors.wa.gov
5. American Society of Anesthesiologists Task Force on Chronic Pain Management, American Society of Regional Anesthesia and Pain Medicine. Practice guidelines for chronic pain management: An updated report by the American Society of Anesthesiologists Task Force on Chronic Pain Management and the American Society of Regional Anesthesia and Pain Medicine. *Anesthesiology*. 2010;112(4):810–833.

ADDITIONAL READING
• Bohnert AS, Valenstein M, Bair MJ, et al. Association between opioid prescribing patterns and opioid overdose-related deaths. *JAMA*. 2011; 305(13):1315–1321.
• Federation of State Medical Boards of the United States, Inc. Model Policy for the Use of Controlled Substances for the Treatment of Pain: www.painpolicy.wisc.edu/sites/www.painpolicy.wisc.edu/files/model04.pdf

 CODES

ICD10
• G89.21 Chronic pain due to trauma
• G89.28 Other chronic postprocedural pain
• G89.29 Other chronic pain

CLINICAL PEARLS
• Start with the presumption that the patient's pain is *real*, even if pathophysiological evidence for it cannot be found.
• Emphasize that being pain-free may not be possible, but that better function and quality of life can be shared goals.
• Use a multidisciplinary approach with nonpharmacologic therapies, exercise, patient self-management strategies, and thoughtful medication use with clear goals, expectations, and documentation of care plan.
• Use "universal precautions" and systems-based practice to safely and effectively prescribe opioids for chronic pain.

CIRRHOSIS OF THE LIVER
Urooj Najm, MBBS • Najm Hasan Siddiqui, MD

BASICS

DESCRIPTION
A chronic disease in which liver cell injury causes inflammation, necrosis, and stellate cell activation, leading to liver failure and/or cancer.

EPIDEMIOLOGY
- Predominant age: 40–50 years old
- Predominant sex: Male > Female; but more women get cirrhosis from alcohol abuse.
- 9th leading cause of death among all US adults

ETIOLOGY AND PATHOPHYSIOLOGY
- Chronic hepatitis C (26%)
- Alcohol abuse (21%)
- Hepatitis C with alcohol liver disease (15%)
- Nonalcoholic steatohepatitis/obesity (~10%)
- Hepatitis B plus hepatitis D infection (15%)
- Other: Hemochromatosis; autoimmune hepatitis; primary biliary cirrhosis; secondary biliary cirrhosis; primary sclerosing cholangitis; Wilson disease; α-1-antitrypsin deficiency; granulomatous disease (e.g., sarcoidosis); drug-induced liver disease (e.g., methotrexate, α-methyldopa, amiodarone); venous outflow obstruction (e.g., Budd-Chiari syndrome, veno-occlusive disease); chronic right-sided heart failure; tricuspid regurgitation; and rare genetic, metabolic, and infectious causes

Genetics
Hemochromatosis, Wilson disease, and α-1-antitrypsin deficiency in adults

RISK FACTORS
Alcohol abuse; IV drug abuse; obesity; blood transfusion

GENERAL PREVENTION
- Counsel patients to prevent risk factors for chronic liver disease (e.g., alcohol abuse); >80% of chronic liver disease is preventable.
- Limit alcohol consumption to <2 drinks/d and advise weight loss for obesity:
  - Raised BMI and alcohol both are linked to liver disease, with evidence of a supra-additive interaction between the 2 (1)[A].

COMMONLY ASSOCIATED CONDITIONS
Diabetes, alcoholism, drug abuse, depression, obesity

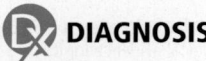
DIAGNOSIS

HISTORY
- Review risk factors (alcohol abuse, viral hepatitis; family history of primary liver cancer, other liver disease, or autoimmune disease)
- Symptoms:
  - Fatigue, malaise, weakness
  - Anorexia, weight loss (gain if ascites/edema)
  - Right upper abdominal pain
  - Absent/Irregular menses
  - Diminished libido, erectile dysfunction
  - Tea-colored urine, clay-colored stools
  - Edema, abdominal swelling/bloating
  - Bruising, bleeding, hematemesis, hematochezia, melena, pruritus
  - Night blindness

PHYSICAL EXAM
Physical exam may be normal until end-stage disease:
- Skin changes: Spider angiomata, palmar erythema, jaundice, scleral icterus, ecchymoses, caput medusa, hyperpigmentation
- Hepatomegaly (small liver in end-stage disease)
- Splenomegaly if portal hypertension
- Central obesity
- Abdominal fluid wave, shifting dullness if ascites
- Gynecomastia
- Dupuytren contractures
- Pretibial, presacral pitting edema and clubbing (especially in hepatopulmonary syndrome)
- Asterixis; mental status changes
- Muscle wasting, weakness

DIFFERENTIAL DIAGNOSIS
Diffuse hepatic parenchymal disease (e.g., fatty liver), other causes of portal hypertension (e.g., portal vein thrombosis, lymphoma), metastatic or multifocal cancer in the liver, vascular congestion (e.g., cardiac cirrhosis), reversible (e.g., acute alcoholic hepatitis)

DIAGNOSTIC TESTS & INTERPRETATION
Initial Tests (lab, imaging)
- Aspartate aminotransferase/alanine aminotransferase (AST/ALT): Mildly elevated; typically AST > ALT; enzymes normalize as cirrhosis progresses
- Elevated alkaline phosphatase (ALP), gamma-glutamyl transpeptidase (GGT), and total/direct bilirubin indicates cholestasis
- Anemia from hemolysis, folate deficiency, and splenomegaly
- Decreased platelet count from portal hypertension with splenomegaly
- Impaired synthetic liver function:
  - Low albumin and cholesterol
  - Prolonged prothrombin (PT), international normalized ratio (INR), partial thromboplastin time (PTT)
- Progressive cirrhosis:
  - Elevated ammonia level; decreased BUN, sodium, and potassium
- Alpha-fetoprotein level at diagnosis to screen for hepatocellular carcinoma (HCC)
- Abdominal ultrasound q6–12 mo to screen for hepatocellular carcinoma
- Doppler ultrasound of hepatic/portal veins
- MRI to clarify patency of blood vessels and collaterals; best follow-up test for HCC if α-fetoprotein elevated and/or liver mass found on ultrasound
- Noninvasive modalities, such as elastography, are being researched as an alternative to liver biopsy (2).

Follow-Up Tests & Special Considerations
To determine specific etiology, consider:
- Hepatitis B surface antigen (HBsAg), core antibody (HBcAb), and surface antibody (HBsAb)
- Hepatitis C antibody
- Serum ethanol and GGT if suspected ongoing alcohol abuse
- Antimitochondrial antibody to screen for primary biliary cirrhosis
- Antismooth muscle and antinuclear antibodies to screen for chronic active (autoimmune) hepatitis

- Iron saturation (>50%) and ferritin (markedly increased) to screen for hemochromatosis; if abnormal, check hemochromatosis (HFE) genetics/mutation analysis
- α-1-antitrypsin phenotype to screen for deficiency
- Ceruloplasmin level to screen for Wilson disease; if low, check copper excretion (serum copper plus 24-hour urine copper)

Diagnostic Procedures/Other
- Liver biopsy: Percutaneous if INR <1.5 and no ascites; otherwise, transjugular biopsy
- Liver–spleen scan to diagnose portal hypertension if patient cannot be biopsied
- Endoscopy if portal hypertension, rule out esophageal varices/portal hypertensive gastropathy (3)[C]

Test Interpretation
- Fibrosis and regenerative nodules are general features of cirrhosis on biopsy.
- Other histologic findings vary with etiology:
  - Alcoholic liver disease: Steatosis, polymorphonuclear (PMN) leukocyte infiltrate, ballooning degeneration of hepatocytes, Mallory bodies, giant mitochondria
  - Chronic hepatitis B and C: Periportal lymphocytic inflammation
  - Nonalcoholic steatohepatitis (NASH): Identical to alcoholic liver disease and confirmed by history. Steatosis may be absent in advanced disease ("burned-out NASH")
  - Biliary cirrhosis: PMN infiltrate in wall of bile ducts, inflammation increased in portal spaces, progressive loss of bile ducts in portal spaces
  - Hemochromatosis: Intrahepatic iron stores increased (iron stain or weighted biopsy tissue)
  - α-1-antitrypsin deficiency: Positive periodic acid-Schiff (PAS) bodies in hepatocytes

TREATMENT

Outpatient care except for major GI bleeding, altered mental status, sepsis/infection, rapidly progressing hepatic decompensation, renal failure

GENERAL MEASURES
- Patients *must* abstain from alcohol, drugs, and liver-toxic medications and herbs.
- Immunize for pneumococcal disease, hepatitis A and B, and influenza.
- NASH: Weight reduction, exercise, optimal control of lipids/glucose

MEDICATION
First Line
As indicated to treat the underlying cause (*note prescribing precautions in decompensated cirrhosis*):
- Hepatitis C: Goal of treatment is to eradicate hepatitis C virus (HCV) RNA in serum ≥6 months after completing antiviral treatment. Combination therapy of pegylated interferon (PEG-IFN) with ribavirin is the standard of care.
- Hepatitis B: Goal of treatment is to achieve HBeAg seroconversion. Adefovir 10 mg PO daily, entecavir 0.5–1 mg PO daily, telbivudine 600 mg PO daily, or lamivudine 100 mg PO daily for minimum of 1 year, or continue for at least 6 months after HBeAg seroconversion; alternatively, peginterferon-α 2a, 180 μg SC weekly for 48 weeks. Lamivudine is no longer recommended as first-line agent due to high rates of resistance.

- Biliary cirrhosis: Ursodeoxycholic acid (Ursodiol) 13–15 mg/kg PO divided b.i.d.–q.i.d., indefinitely (4)[A]; bile acid sequestrants (BAS) are 1st-line therapy for pruritus. Antihistamines, cholestyramine 4–8 g PO b.i.d., rifampicin 150–300 mg b.i.d. or PO opiate antagonists such as naltrexone 50 mg/d can be used for pruritus if ursodiol is ineffective.
- Wilson disease: Initial treatment with penicillamine 1,000–1,500 mg/d PO b.i.d.–q.i.d. or trientine 750–1,500 mg PO b.i.d.–t.i.d. Trientine (Syprine) is better tolerated. After 1 year, zinc acetate 75–300 mg PO b.i.d.–t.i.d. for maintenance. Zinc is a drug of choice for presymptomatic, pregnant, and pediatric populations.
- Autoimmune (chronic active) hepatitis: Prednisone 30–60 mg/d initially, maintenance 5–20 mg/d with or without azathioprine (Imuran) 0.5–1 mg/kg; adjust to keep transaminase levels normal. The combination regime is preferred. Maintenance therapy can be discontinued after at least 24 months of treatment and continued normal AST and ALT.
- Esophageal varices: Propranolol 40–160 mg or nadolol 40 mg daily, to lower portal pressure by 20 mm Hg, systolic pressure to 90–100 mm Hg, and pulse rate by 25% (3)[A].
- Ascites/Edema: Low-sodium (<2 g/d) diet and spironolactone 100–400 mg/d with or without furosemide 40–160 mg/d PO; torsemide may substitute for furosemide.
- Encephalopathy: Lactulose 15 mL b.i.d., titrate to induce 3 loose bowel movements daily. Combination therapy with rifaximin (550 mg PO b.i.d.) is superior to prevent recurrent hepatic encephalopathy (5).
- Pruritus: Ursodiol, cholestyramine, and antihistamines (e.g., hydroxyzine)
- Renal insufficiency: Stop diuretics and nephrotoxic drugs, normalize electrolytes, and hospitalize for plasma expansion or dialysis.
- Prophylactic antibiotics for invasive procedures, GI bleeding, or history of spontaneous bacterial peritonitis (3)[A]
- Proton pump inhibitor for esophageal varices requiring banding or portal hypertensive gastropathy (6)[A]
- Recombinant factor VIIa to correct bleeding shows no survival benefit (7).

ISSUES FOR REFERRAL
Liver transplant evaluation at first onset of complications (ascites, variceal bleed, encephalopathy), jaundice, or liver lesion suggestive of hepatocellular carcinoma and/or when evidence of hepatic dysfunction develops (Child-Turcotte-Pugh >7 and MELD >10).

SURGERY/OTHER PROCEDURES
- Varices: Endoscopic ligation, typically 4–6 treatments (if acute bleed, use pre-esophagogastroduodenoscopy [EGD] octreotide as vasoconstrictor); transjugular intrahepatic shunt (TIPS) 2nd-line or salvage therapy for acute bleed (3)
- Ascites: If tense, therapeutic paracentesis every 2 weeks PRN; caution if pedal edema absent.
- Fulminant hepatic failure: Liver transplantation
- Hepatocellular carcinoma: Curable if small with radiofrequency ablation or resection and transplant

COMPLEMENTARY AND ALTERNATIVE MEDICINE
- Zinc sulphate 220 mg b.i.d. may improve dysgeusia and appetite. It is also adjunctive therapy for hepatic encephalopathy.

- Milk thistle (silymarin) may lower transaminases and improve symptoms.
- Danshen and huangqi injections may promote improvement; further studies needed (8)[A]
- Hepatotoxicity and drug interactions are common with many herbal medications (9)[A].

IN-PATIENT CONSIDERATIONS
Admission Criteria/Initial Stabilization
Major GI bleeding, altered mental status, sepsis/infection, rapidly progressing hepatic decompensation, renal failure

 ## ONGOING CARE

FOLLOW-UP RECOMMENDATIONS
Regular conditioning may help fatigue.

Patient Monitoring
- Once stable, monitor liver enzymes, platelets, and PT q6–12 mo.
- Patients >55 years old with chronic hepatitis B or C, elevated INR or low platelets are at highest risk for HCC. Check α–fetoprotein and liver ultrasound q6–12 mo for screening in patients with cirrhotics (7)[A].
- Endoscopy at diagnosis and every 3 years in compensated and every 1 year in decompensated cirrhotic patients to screen for varices (3)[C]

DIET
- Protein (1–1.5 g/kg body weight), high fiber, daily multivitamin (without iron), and sodium (<2 g/d, essential if ascites/edema).
- A high-protein diet may precipitate encephalopathy, but protein restriction is no longer recommended (7).
- Coffee consumption has a graded and inverse association with liver cancer (10)[A].

PATIENT EDUCATION
- Educate caregivers about when to seek emergency care (e.g., hematemesis, altered mental status).
- Maintain sobriety/recovery/smoking cessation (includes no cannabis).
- Hepatitis A/B immunization and hepatitis C transmission precautions

PROGNOSIS
- At diagnosis of cirrhosis, expect 5–20 years of asymptomatic disease.
- At onset of complications, expect death within 5 years without transplant:
  – 5% per year develop HCC
  – 50% of cirrhotics develop ascites over 10 years; 50% 5-year survival if ascites develop
  – Acute variceal bleed most common fatal complication; carries 30% mortality
  – Median survival at onset decompensation (ascites, variceal bleed, encephalopathy) is 1.5 years (7).
  – With transplant, 85% survive 1 year; deaths after transplant, ~5% per year
- <25% of eligible patients receive a transplant because of donor organ shortage.

COMPLICATIONS
Ascites; edema; infections; encephalopathy; GI bleed; esophageal varices, gastropathy, colopathy; hepatorenal syndrome; hepatopulmonary syndrome; hepatocellular carcinoma; fulminant hepatic failure; complications after transplant (e.g., surgical, rejection, infections)

REFERENCES
1. Hart CL, Morrison DS, Batty GD, et al. Effect of body mass index and alcohol consumption on liver disease: Analysis of data from two prospective cohort studies. *BMJ.* 2010;340:c1240.
2. Tsochatzis EA, Gurusamy KS, Ntaoula S, et al. Elastography for the diagnosis of severity of fibrosis in chronic liver disease: A meta-analysis of diagnostic accuracy. *J Hepatol.* 2011;54:650–659.
3. Garcia-Tsao G, Sanyal AJ, Grace ND, et al. Prevention and management of gastroesophageal varices and variceal hemorrhage in cirrhosis. *Hepatology.* 2007;46:922–938.
4. Lindor KD, Gershwin ME, Poupon R, et al. Primary biliary cirrhosis. *Hepatology.* 2009;50:291–308.
5. Sharma P, Sharma BC. Rifaximin treatment in hepatic encephalopathy. *N Engl J Med.* 2010;362: 2423–2425.
6. Leontiadis GI, Sharma VK, Howden CW. Proton pump inhibitor therapy for peptic ulcer bleeding: Cochrane collaboration meta-analysis of randomized controlled trials. *Mayo Clin Proc.* 2007;82:286–296.
7. Garcia-Tsao G. Managing the complications of cirrhosis, hepatitis annual update 2008, clinical care options: Hepatitis. Available at: http://clinicaloptions.com/Hepatitis/Annual%20Updates/2008%20Annual%20Update.aspx
8. Zhu C, Cao H, Zhou X, et al. Meta-analysis of the clinical value of danshen injection and huangqi injection in liver cirrhosis. *Evid Based Complement Alternat Med.* 2013;2013:842824.
9. Verma S, Thuluvath PJ. Complementary and alternative medicine in hepatology: Review of the evidence of efficacy. *Clin Gastroenterol Hepatol.* 2007;5:408–416.
10. Bravi F, Bosetti C, Tavani A, et al. Coffee reduces risk for hepatocellular carcinoma: An updated meta-analysis. *Clin Gastroenterol Hepatol.* 2013;11:1413–1421.

ADDITIONAL READING
- Chou R, Wasson N. Blood tests to diagnose fibrosis or cirrhosis in patients with chronic hepatitis C virus infection: A systematic review. *Ann Intern Med.* 2013;158:807–820.
- Nierhoff J, Chávez Ortiz AA, Herrmann E, et al. The efficiency of acoustic radiation force impulse imaging for the staging of liver fibrosis: A meta-analysis. *Eur Radiol.* 2013;23:3040–3053.

 ## SEE ALSO
Algorithm: Cirrhosis

 ## CODES

ICD10
- K70.30 Alcoholic cirrhosis of liver without ascites
- K74.60 Unspecified cirrhosis of liver
- K74.69 Other cirrhosis of liver

CLINICAL PEARLS
- 80% of chronic liver disease that leads to cirrhosis is preventable (primarily alcoholic).
- Check abdominal ultrasound every 6 months for early detection of hepatocellular carcinoma.

CIRRHOSIS, PRIMARY BILIARY

Lauren Michal de Leon, MD • Edward Feller, MD

 BASICS

Primary biliary cirrhosis (PBC) should be suspected in women with unexplained pruritus or cholestatic pattern of liver enzymes.

DESCRIPTION
- PBC is a chronic T-cell–mediated liver disease characterized by destruction of small intrahepatic bile ducts.
- If untreated, PBC can lead to biliary cirrhosis, portal hypertension, and possibly liver transplantation.
- At diagnosis, 60% are asymptomatic.

EPIDEMIOLOGY
- PBC primarily affects women (95%) (1).
- Peak age: 40–60 years; can occur earlier, rarely in children

Prevalence
- Rare, present universally; more common in northern European countries and in the northern US
- Incidence: 0.33–5.8/100,000 (2)
- Prevalence: 1.91–40.2/100,000; depends on varied diagnostic criteria, physician awareness, quality of care, methods of detection, and case-finding (2)

ETIOLOGY AND PATHOPHYSIOLOGY
- PBC is caused by a T-cell–mediated attack on intralobular bile ducts.
- T cells are targeted against mitochondrial antigens responsible for oxidative phosphorylation.
- Autoimmune attack is isolated to small, intrahepatic bile ducts for unknown reasons.
- This destruction causes cholestasis, which can lead to cirrhosis and liver failure.
- Retained bile acids from bile duct destruction leads to foamy degeneration of hepatocytes.

Genetics
- PBC believed to occur in individuals with susceptible genetic makeup (multiple inherited defects in immune tolerance) exposed to specific environmental triggers.
- Monozygotic twins-concordance rate as high as 63%
- Family predisposition: 1–6% of individuals with PBC have at least 1 family member with the disease.
- Antimitochondrial antibody (AMA) positivity in sisters (20%), mothers (15%), daughters (10%)

RISK FACTORS
Smoking increases risk of disease development:
- Pregnancy may be a trigger for PBC; hormone replacement therapy is a possible, yet unproven precipitating factor. Increased PBC risk after pruritus or cholestasis after pregnancy
- Diverse autoimmune diseases associated with PBC

COMMONLY ASSOCIATED CONDITIONS
- PBC can be associated with diverse autoimmune diseases: Sjögren syndrome, scleroderma, rheumatoid arthritis, lupus erythematosus, autoimmune thyroiditis, celiac disease, and ulcerative colitis (2)[A].
- Overlap syndrome with autoimmune hepatitis exists in 5–15%. Diagnosis may be difficult and prognosis worse (3).
- Compared to the general population, PBC is associated with a relative risk of hepatocellular carcinoma as high as 18.8 (4).

DIAGNOSIS

HISTORY
- >60% are asymptomatic at diagnosis, identified by incidental finding of elevated serum alkaline phosphatase (ALP), γ-glutamyl transpeptidase (GGTP), total serum cholesterol, or investigation of an autoimmune disease, such as scleroderma.
- Unexpected hepatomegaly or cutaneous stigmata of chronic liver disease are present in some patients (3).

ALERT
Consider PBC in any middle-aged woman with unexplained pruritus or cholestasis.
- Common complaints include:
  - Fatigue (in 80%): Does not correlate with age, duration, or severity of disease.
  - Pruritus: Correlates with fatigue; may be severe and debilitating; precedes jaundice.
  - Hyperpigmentation of the skin (not jaundice)
  - Musculoskeletal complaints (often a peripheral arthropathy)
- If patient has a liver evaluation for other reasons, important information includes:
  - Medication history (cholestatic-causing drugs)
  - Family history of liver or autoimmune disease
  - Sexual history (assess risk of hepatitis, HIV)

PHYSICAL EXAM
Physical exam findings usually correlate with disease severity. Exam is often normal; in as many as 60% of asymptomatic patients:
- Skin: Hyperpigmentation, excoriations secondary to pruritus, xanthomas, jaundice (late finding)
- Abdomen: Hepatosplenomegaly (may be present in asymptomatic patients), spider nevi, and other cutaneous stigmata of portal hypertension (late)
- Evidence of decompensated portal hypertension in advanced cirrhosis (ascites, encephalopathy)
- Psychiatric: Fatigue, depression

DIFFERENTIAL DIAGNOSIS
Includes, but is not limited to:
- Cholestasis secondary to medications or pregnancy; nonalcoholic steatohepatitis; alcoholic liver disease
- Other autoimmune-related hepatobiliary conditions: Autoimmune hepatitis, primary sclerosing cholangitis.
- Pancreatic and other periampullary carcinomas
- Overlap syndrome exists: PBC: Autoimmune hepatitis

DIAGNOSTIC TESTS & INTERPRETATION
- Diagnostic evaluation is based on clinical suspicion or if liver enzymes are suspicious for cholestasis.
- Routine blood chemistries: Marked alkaline phosphatase increase in an asymptomatic woman
- The American Association for the Study of Liver Disease (AASLD) requires 2 of 3 of the following for diagnosis of PBC:
  - Serum antimitochondrial antibody (AMA) positive
  - Cholestasis based on lab results
  - Histologic evidence of bile duct destruction

Initial Tests (lab, imaging)
- Liver enzymes reflect a cholestatic picture: Disproportionate increase in cholestatic chemistries compared with hepatocellular markers (aminotransferases):
  - Marked elevation of alkaline phosphatase or γ-glutamyl transpeptidase
  - Elevated direct and indirect bilirubin (portends poor prognosis; usually late in disease)
  - Aminotransaminase elevations, if present, are mild. If they are, causes of cholestatic hepatitis may be considered (e.g., autoimmune hepatitis, drugs, viral hepatitis).
- Antimitochondrial antibodies: Positive in 95% of those with PBC (5):
  - AMA-positive and AMA-negative patients have similar natural history and have same response rates to treatment.
  - AMA titers do not correlate with disease progression nor with response to treatment.
- Antismooth muscle antibodies: Rule out autoimmune hepatitis or overlap syndrome.
- Lipid levels: Mild elevations in low-density lipoprotein (LDL) and very low-density lipoprotein (VLDL); marked elevation in high-density lipoprotein (HDL)
- Thrombocytopenia is common in advanced cirrhosis; is a sensitive marker for portal hypertension.
- Imaging of hepatobiliary system required to rule out obstruction; modalities include:
  - Right upper quadrant US; abdominal CT
  - MR cholangiopancreatography (MRCP) preferred to endoscopic retrograde cholangiopancreatography (ERCP) to visualize biliary system because it is noninvasive; ERCP useful if a therapeutic intervention is considered likely (stone removal, stent placement, biopsy)
  - Esophageal US (EUS)
- If any of these modalities are negative, proceed with serologic studies as above.

Follow-Up Tests & Special Considerations
- AMA-negative patients: Occurs in 5% with biopsy-proven PBC:
  – These patients commonly have antinuclear antibody (ANA) positivity (particularly anti-GB210 and anti-SP100) and/or antismooth muscle antibody (SMA) positivity.
- Drugs can cause a cholestatic picture that resembles PBC biochemically:
  – Phenothiazines, synthetic androgenic steroids, trimethoprim-sulfamethoxazole, among many others
- Women of childbearing age should have a pregnancy test, as symptoms can vary with pregnancy.

Diagnostic Procedures/Other
- Liver biopsy: Important if unclear diagnosis. Without biopsy, staging for features predicting clinical course, such as interface hepatitis and ductopenia, is unknown.
- MRCP or ERCP considered if serum AMA is negative or with suspicion of biliary obstruction (stricture, stone, bile duct or pancreatic carcinoma)

Test Interpretation
- Florid bile duct destruction is the pathognomonic finding for PBC, but is uncommon.
- Atypical bile duct hyperplasia with lymphocyte infiltration can be seen as well.

 ## TREATMENT

MEDICATION
First Line
- Ursodeoxycholic acid (UDCA) is the only FDA-approved treatment for PBC. 2013 reviews state that UDCA is associated with biochemical, histologic, and survival benefits (6,7).
- However, a December, 2012 Cochrane systemic review concluded that UDCA did not demonstrate any beneficial effects on all-cause mortality, liver transplantation, pruritus, or fatigue (8)[A].
- Dosing: 13–15 mg/kg/d for patients with abnormal liver enzymes, regardless of histologic stage.

ADDITIONAL THERAPIES
- Supplemental treatment includes symptomatic relief.
- Pruritus: Bile acid sequestrants (cholestyramine). Pruritus can be severe; this agent is very useful for symptomatic relief. If refractory, rifampicin 150–300 mg/d, opioid antagonist (e.g., naltrexone 50 mg/d), sertraline 75–100 mg/d can be tried.
- Fatigue: No suggested therapy. Can resolve with treatment of underlying condition or associated conditions (hypothyroidism).
- Although methotrexate may benefit other outcomes (pruritus score, serum alkaline phosphatase, IgM levels), insufficient evidence supports it for patients with primary biliary cirrhosis.
- Fibrates, Rituximab, tetrathiomolybdate therapy in unresponsive primary biliary cirrhosis show promise, but further studies are needed (5).

SURGERY/OTHER PROCEDURES
Liver transplantation is the only definitive treatment for patients with progressive or nonresponsive disease and decompensated cirrhosis:
- Posttransplant, 5-year survival is as high as 77%.
- Recurrent PBC posttransplant: 15% at 3 years, 30% at 5 years

 ## ONGOING CARE

FOLLOW-UP RECOMMENDATIONS
- Patients should be given the same counseling as patients with other liver disorders (e.g., decreased alcohol intake, weight management, smoking cessation, avoid hepatotoxic drugs).
- Complications of portal hypertension, such as esophageal varices or ascites, are treated in the same manner as for other cirrhotic patients.
- Pregnant women may need closer monitoring due to the increased incidence of symptoms and complications that can occur during pregnancy.

Patient Monitoring
- Liver tests every 3–6 months; monitor cholesterol
- Thyroid-stimulating hormone (TSH) annually
- Bone mineral density every 2–4 years
- Vitamin A, D, and K levels yearly
- If cirrhosis, thrombocytopenia or Mayo risk score >4.1, periodic endoscopic screening for esophageal varices.
- Periodic screening for liver cancer: US, with serum α-fetoprotein measurement, in patients with known cirrhosis

PROGNOSIS
- Varies widely. Prognostic factors include age, histologic stage, possibly UDCA therapy, bilirubin level, presence of thrombocytopenia, poor hepatic protein synthesis (albumin, prothrombin time).
- Median survival without liver transplantation is 10–15 years.
- Antibodies to the nuclear rim pore protein gp210 have shown promise as prognostic markers in PBC.

COMPLICATIONS
- Hepatocellular carcinoma (relative risk = 18.8) compared with general population (4)[A]
- Portal hypertension
- Varices, encephalopathy, ascites
- Osteopenia/Osteoporosis (in as many as 1/3 of patients)
- Intense pruritus, fatigue
- Malabsorption, steatorrhea, diarrhea

REFERENCES
1. Boonstra K, Beuers U, Ponsioen CY. Epidemiology of primary sclerosing cholangitis and primary biliary cirrhosis. J Hepatology. 2012;56:1181–1188.
2. Hirschfield GM, Gershwin ME. Immunobiology and pathophysiology of primary biliary cirrhosis. Ann Rev Path Mech Dis. 2013;8:303–330.
3. Mayo MJ. Cholestatic liver disease overlap syndromes. Clin Liver Dis. 2013;17:243–253.
4. Liang Y, Yang Z, Zhong R. Primary biliary cirrhosis and cancer risk: A systematic review and meta-analysis. Hepatology. 2012;56(4):1409–1417. Epub 2012 Aug 27.
5. Czaja AJ. Autoantibodies as prognostic markers in autoimmune liver disease. Dig Dis Sci. 2010;55: 2144–2161.
6. Czul F, Peyton A, Levy C. Primary biliary cirrhosis. Therapeutic advances. Clin Liver Dis. 2013;17: 229–242.
7. Boberg KM, Wisløff T, Kjøllesdal KS, et al. Cost and health consequences of treatment of primary biliary cirrhosis with ursodeoxycholic acid. Aliment Pharmacol Ther. 2013;38(7):794–803.
8. Rudic JS, Poropat G, Krstic MN, et al. Ursodeoxycholic acid for primary biliary cirrhosis. Cochrane Database Syst Rev. 2012;12:CD000551. DOI:10.1002/14651858.CD000551.pub3

ADDITIONAL READING
Selmi C, Bowlus FC, Gershwin ME, et al. Primary biliary cirrhosis. Lancet. 2011;377:1600–1609.

CODES

ICD10
K74.3 Primary biliary cirrhosis

CLINICAL PEARLS
Diagnostic algorithm:
- Consider PBC in middle-aged women with unexplained pruritus, especially with elevated serum alkaline phosphatase level.
- Exclude other causes of cholestatic liver disease; imaging to rule out obstruction if uncertainty persists.
- AMA, ANA, antismooth muscle antibody titers
- Consider liver biopsy if AMA negative or AST >5× normal.
- UDCA is associated with biochemical, histologic, and survival benefits.
- At diagnosis, 60% are asymptomatic.

CLOSTRIDIUM DIFFICILE INFECTION
Samuel Luke Brown, DO • Scott W. Rodi, MD, MPH

BASICS

DESCRIPTION
- *Clostridium difficile* is a gram-positive, spore-forming anaerobic bacillus.
- Infection caused by *C. difficile* is usually linked to broad-spectrum antibiotic use, hospitalization, and age.
- Severity of infection can range from diarrhea to colitis to perforation to death.
- System(s) affected: Gastrointestinal
- Synonyms(s): *C. difficile*–associated disease or diarrhea (CDAD); Antibiotic-associated diarrhea; *C. diff*

EPIDEMIOLOGY
Incidence
- In 1 study of hospitals between 1997 and 2005, the incidence rates were 3.4–8.4 cases/1,000 admissions.
- For outpatient setting, the rate is ~7.7 cases/ 100,000 person-years.

Prevalence
- *C. difficile* causes ~25% of all cases of antibiotic-associated diarrhea.
- Community-acquired *C. difficile* infection is increasing, which may make prevalence much higher than previously thought (1).

ETIOLOGY AND PATHOPHYSIOLOGY
- *C. difficile* exists in vegetative and spore forms. *C. difficile* spores can survive for months even in harsh conditions.
- *C. difficile* can thrive in the colon and cause infection if disruption of the normal flora and ingestion of *C. difficile* occur.
- Host factors, such as the presence of antibodies to *C. difficile* toxins, can reduce the severity and prevent recurrences of infection.
- *C. difficile* produces toxins that are essential for disease to occur:
  - Toxins A (enterotoxin) and B (cytotoxin) attract neutrophils and monocytes and degrade colonic epithelial cells, causing colitis, pseudomembrane colitis, and watery diarrhea.
- BI/NAP1/027 strain of *C. difficile* has been shown to produce more virulent characteristics (2).
- Binary toxin produces a virulent form of disease (different from toxin A or B); this may result in increased rates of colectomies and mortality.
- Altered colonic mucosa
- *C. difficile* spore ingestion
- Active toxin release

Genetics
No known genetic factors

RISK FACTORS
2 major categories of risk factors are associated with *C. difficile* infection:
- Host risk factors:
  - Age >65 years
  - Hospitalization or stay in long-term health care facility. The length of stay is directly correlated with the risk (3).
  - Comorbidities, including inflammatory bowel disease (IBD), immunosuppression, tube feeding, chronic liver disease, and end-stage renal disease
  - Previous *C. difficile* infection

- Recurrence from prior infection:
  - Recurrence rates are shown to be 15–35%. Patients who have 1 recurrence are 45% more likely to have a 2nd recurrence, and patients with a 2nd recurrences have up to a 65% chance of 3rd recurrence.
- Factors disrupting normal colonic microbiota:
  - Exposure to almost all antibiotics is associated with *C. difficile* infection (this includes perioperative prophylaxis).
  - Use of antacids, especially proton pump inhibitors (PPI) (3)
- Community-acquired *C. difficile* infections may affect patients without risk factors (e.g., younger, no recent antibiotic exposure).

Geriatric Considerations
C. difficile is the most common cause of acute diarrheal illness in long-term care facilities. As these patients tend to have multiple risk factors (older, more antibiotics, more antacids), it is difficult to isolate which is most contributory.

Pediatric Considerations
Neonates have a higher rate of *C. difficile* colonization (25–80%), but are generally less symptomatic than adults (possibly due to immature toxin receptors).

GENERAL PREVENTION
- Implementation of a comprehensive infection-control program can decrease in the incidence of *C. difficile* infection.
- The 2010 SHEA/IDSA guidelines make specific recommendations for *C. difficile* infection prevention:
  - Measures for health care workers, patients, and visitors:
    ○ Contact precautions, including gloves and gowns, on entry to room
    ○ Hand hygiene with soap and water before and after patient interaction:
      ■ Alcohol-based hand cleaners do not kill *C. difficile* spores.
    ○ Accommodate patients with *C. difficile* infection in private rooms, if possible.
  - Environmental cleaning and disinfection:
    ○ Disinfection with hypochlorite solution or other spore-killing solutions
    ○ Identification and reduction of environmental sources of *C. difficile,* including the use of nondisposable rectal thermometers
  - Antimicrobial use restrictions:
    ○ Minimize the frequency and duration of antibiotic therapy.

DIAGNOSIS

HISTORY
- Recent antibiotic use (especially broad-spectrum fluoroquinolones and cephalosporins)
- Diarrhea that is watery, foul-smelling, and sometimes bloody
- Fever (typically <10%)
- Recent hospitalization or stay at nursing facility

PHYSICAL EXAM
There is a wide range of physical exam findings, ranging from mild abdominal pain to peritoneal findings and shock:
- Mild or moderate disease: Mild lower abdominal pain, often cramping pain

- Severe disease: Fever, nausea/vomiting, dehydration
- Severe, complicated disease: Shock, peritonitis, ileus

DIFFERENTIAL DIAGNOSIS
- Antibiotic-associated diarrhea
- Inflammatory bowel disease
- Enteric infections
- Food poisoning

DIAGNOSTIC TESTS & INTERPRETATION
- Markers and lab abnormalities established by the SHEA/IDSA guidelines help classify the severity of disease:
  - Mild or moderate disease: Leukocytosis with WBC count <15,000 cells/μL and a serum creatinine level <1.5× the premorbid level
  - Severe, uncomplicated disease: Leukocytosis with a WBC count >15,000 cells/μL or a serum creatinine level >1.5× the premorbid level
  - Severe, complicated disease: Markers of severe or fulminant infection include hypotension, sepsis, markedly elevated WBC count, and bandemia
    ○ Other signs include obstruction, perforation, toxic megacolon, and colonic-wall thickening that can be seen on imaging.
- No single test is both sensitive and specific. Current recommendations are for a 2-step process using a sensitive initial screening test followed by a more specific confirmatory test if the screen is positive.
- General approach: Screen with the *C. difficile* common antigen test; if positive, confirm with either enzyme immunoassay test or cell cytotoxic assay.

Initial Tests (lab, imaging)
- Screening: *C. difficile* common antigen test: Tests for glutamate dehydrogenase (GDH), which is found on both toxic and nontoxic strains of *C. difficile* (sensitivity, 85–95%; specificity, 89–99%).
- Confirmatory: Enzyme immunoassay (EIA) for toxins (A/B or A). Rapid results, often used due to cost/ease of use (sensitivity 63–94%).
- Confirmatory: Cell cytotoxicity assay. Takes 24–48 hours for results; time and labor-intensive (sensitivity 67–100%).
- Stool culture is the most sensitive test; however, nontoxin-producing strains also detected. Generally used to evaluate epidemiology.
- Polymerase chain reaction (PCR)-based testing is rapidly becoming the preferred test for *C. difficile* based on the high test sensitivity.
- Repeat testing during the same episode of diarrhea is discouraged (2).
- Plain films may show thumbprinting and colonic distension.
- CT radiography may show mucosal wall thickening, thickened colonic wall, and pericolonic inflammation.

Diagnostic Procedures/Other
- Endoscopy can be used to evaluate for pseudomembranes and exclude other conditions:
  - Although not all patients with *C. difficile* infection have pseudomembranes, their presence is pathognomonic for *C. difficile* (3).
- Flexible sigmoidoscopy may miss 15–20% of pseudomembranes that may be more proximal in the colon.
- Colonoscopy evaluates the entire colon: Used when diagnosis is in doubt or severity demands rapid diagnosis.

Test Interpretation
Pseudomembranes consist of inflammatory and cellular debris that forms visible exudates that can obscure the underlying mucosa. These exudates have a yellow to grayish color.

TREATMENT

GENERAL MEASURES
- Avoid antimotility agents and opiates (4)[A].
- Avoid use of PPIs unless absolutely necessary, as they have been associated with a 42% increased risk of recurrence if used concurrently with treatment for *C. difficile* colitis (5).

MEDICATION
- 1st, it is important to discontinue the current antibiotic regimen, if at all possible.
- Treatment is based on antibiotics effective against *C. difficile*.

First Line
- Mild or moderate infection:
  - Metronidazole is the drug of choice for mild-to-moderate *C. difficile* infection due to low cost and to minimize the emergence of vancomycin-resistant organisms (2)[A]:
    ○ 500 mg PO t.i.d. for 10–14 days
    ○ If patient is unable to take oral medications, then IV metronidazole or intraluminal vancomycin can be used.
- Severe infection:
  - Vancomycin is 1st-line therapy in patients with severe or fulminant *C. difficile* infection:
    ○ 125 mg PO q.i.d. for 10–14 days
    ○ Vancomycin retention enema if unable to take PO or there is evidence of poor GI motility
- Severe, complicated infection:
  - Vancomycin: 500 mg PO q.i.d. *AND* metronidazole 500 mg PO t.i.d.
- 1st recurrence:
  - Treat the same as 1st episode.
- 2nd recurrence:
  - Vancomycin taper and/or pulse: Vancomycin 125 mg PO q.i.d. for 10–14 days, then 125 mg PO b.i.d. for 7 days, then 125 mg PO once daily for 7 days, then 125 mg PO every 2–3 days for 2–8 weeks:
    ○ The pulse dosing every 2–3 days allows spores to germinate and then be killed.

ALERT
When using vancomycin for treatment of *C. difficile* infection, oral or rectal formulations must be used because IV formulations are not excreted into the colonic lumen.

Second Line
- Vancomycin: Indicated for patients who cannot tolerate or have failed metronidazole therapy and for those who are pregnant
- Fidaxomicin is another drug option. It has been found to have similar cure rates to vancomycin, but had significantly lower recurrence rates:
  - It has been shown that fidaxomicin rapidly kills *C. difficile*, whereas vancomycin inhibits growth. It has also been shown to have a narrow antimicrobial spectrum and helps to preserve normal anaerobic flora.

SURGERY/OTHER PROCEDURES
If *C. difficile* infection progresses to toxic megacolon, peritonitis, or sepsis, other therapeutic options should be explored, including a surgical consult for colectomy.

COMPLEMENTARY AND ALTERNATIVE MEDICINE
- Fecal transplant has also been shown to be an effective treatment, especially against the virulent 027 strain. The reason for transplantation is that stool is biologically active and contains a mixture of living organisms that can help restore normal gut flora to the recipient (6).
- A recent meta-analysis of 11 studies showed a cure rate of 89% with no adverse events (7):
  - Donors are carefully selected, and donor stool is homogenized in water and then infused back into the patient via nasogastric tube or colonoscopy.
- There may be some benefit of probiotics in the future. A recent study showed that there was an inhibitory effect on *C. difficile*, but it appears to be strain specific, and more testing needs to be done before this is considered a standard of treatment. (8).
- Immunotherapy, including passive immunization and a humanized monoclonal antibody preparation of antitoxins, is also being researched currently.

IN-PATIENT CONSIDERATIONS
Admission Criteria/Initial Stabilization
- Hypovolemia
- Inability to keep up with enteric losses
- Hematochezia
- Electrolyte disturbances

- Institute supportive therapy with fluids and electrolytes, if needed (2)[A].
- Current nonessential antibiotic therapy should be discontinued, if possible (2)[A].

IV Fluids
Infuse to keep patient euvolemic.

Discharge Criteria
- Improved diarrhea severity and frequency
- Tolerating both medications and PO
- Do not test for toxins again as they may shed for weeks after acute infection.

ONGOING CARE

FOLLOW-UP RECOMMENDATIONS
Many patients can be treated as outpatients.

Patient Monitoring
- Relapses of colitis will occur in 15–30%.
- Relapses typically occur 2–10 days after discontinuation of antibiotics.

DIET
No restrictions; as tolerated

PATIENT EDUCATION
Patients should be kept informed of the progress of disease and taught to practice good hygiene (i.e., hand washing).

ALERT
It is important to remember that alcohol-based hand sanitizers are not effective against *C. difficile*. You must wash hands with soap and water.

PROGNOSIS
- Most patients will improve with conservative management and antibiotics.
- 1–3% of patients will develop severe colitis requiring emergency colectomy.

REFERENCES
1. Khanna S, Pardi DS, Aronson SL, et al. The epidemiology of community-acquired *Clostridium difficile* infection: A population-based study. *Am J Gastroenterol*. 2012;107(1):89–95. Epub 2011 Nov 22.
2. Cohen SH, Gerding DN, Johnson S, et al. Clinical practice guidelines for *Clostridium difficile* infection in adults: 2010 update by the Society for Healthcare Epidemiology of America (SHEA) and the Infectious Diseases Society of America (IDSA). *Infect Control Hosp Epidemiol*. 2010;31:431–455.
3. McCollum DL, Rodriguez JM. Detection, treatment, and prevention of *Clostridium difficile* infection. *Clin Gastroenterol Hepatol*. 2012;10(6):581–592. Epub 2012 Mar 17.
4. Koo HL, Koo DC, Musher DM, et al. Antimotility agents for the treatment of *Clostridium difficile* diarrhea and colitis. *Clin Infect Dis*. 2009;48: 598–605.
5. Linsky A, Gupta K, Lawler EV, et al. Proton pump inhibitors and risk for recurrent *Clostridium difficile* infection. *Arch Intern Med*. 2010;170:772–778.
6. Brandt LJ, Aronidias OC. An overview of fecal microbiota transplantation: techniques, indications, and outcomes. *Gastrointestinal Endoscopy*. 2013. Article in Press.
7. Kassam Z, Lee CH, Yuan Y, et al. Fecal microbiota transplantation for *Clostridium difficile* infection: Systematic review and meta-analysis. *Am J Gastroenterol*. 2013;108:500–508.
8. Schoster A. et al. In vitro inhibition of *Clostridium difficile* and *Clostridium perfringens* by commercial probiotic strains. *Anaerobe*. 2013;20:36–41.

CODES

ICD10
A04.7 Enterocolitis due to Clostridium difficile

CLINICAL PEARLS
- Testing and treatment of asymptomatic patients is not recommended.
- Therapeutic response should be based on clinical signs and symptoms. Patients may shed organism or toxin for weeks after treatment, so do not repeat tests for toxins to assess therapeutic response.

COLIC, INFANTILE
Daniel T. Lee, MD, MA • Arthur Ohannessian, MD

 BASICS

DESCRIPTION
- Colic is defined as excessive crying in an otherwise healthy baby.
- A commonly used criteria is the Wessel criteria, or the Rule of Three: Crying lasts for:
  - >3 hours a day
  - >3 days a week
  - Persists >3 weeks
- Many clinicians no longer use the criterion of persistence for >3 weeks because few parents or clinicians will wait that long before evaluation or intervention.
- Some clinicians feel that colic represents the extreme end of the spectrum of normal crying, whereas most feel that colic is a distinct clinical entity.

EPIDEMIOLOGY
Incidence
- Predominant age: Between 2 weeks and 4 months of age
- Predominant sex: Male = Female
Prevalence
- Probably between 10% and 25% of infants
- Range is somewhere between 8% and 40% of infants.
Pediatric Considerations
This is a problem during infancy.

ETIOLOGY AND PATHOPHYSIOLOGY
The cause is unknown. Factors that may play a role include:
- Infant gastroesophageal reflux disease
- Allergy to cow's milk, soy milk, or breast milk protein
- Fruit juice intolerance
- Swallowing air during the process of crying, feeding, or sucking
- Overfeeding or feeding too quickly; underfeeding also has been proposed
- Inadequate burping after feeding
- Family tension
- Parental anxiety, depression, and/or fatigue
- Parent–infant interaction mismatch
- Baby's inability to console him- or herself when dealing with stimuli
- Increased gut hormone motilin, causing hyperperistalsis
- Functional lactose overload (i.e., breast milk that has a lower lipid content can have faster transit time in the intestine, leading to more lactose fermentation in the gut and hence gas and distension) (1)[C]
- Tobacco smoke exposure
- Disorder of impaired synchronization between infant arousal and environment (2)[C]

RISK FACTORS
- Physiologic predisposition in infant, but no definitive risk factors have been established. However, emerging data suggest maternal smoking or exposure to nicotine replacement therapy during pregnancy is associated with higher incidence of infantile colic (3)[B].
- Infants with a maternal history of migraine headaches are twice as likely to have colic (4)[B].

GENERAL PREVENTION
Colic is generally not preventable.

 DIAGNOSIS

HISTORY
- Evaluation for Wessel criteria: Crying lasts for >3 hours per day, >3 days per week, and persists >3 weeks.
- The colicky episodes may have a clear beginning and end.
- The crying is generally spontaneous, without preceding events triggering the episodes.
- The crying is typically different from normal crying. Colicky crying may be louder, more turbulent, variable in pitch, and appear more like screaming.
- The infant may be difficult to soothe or console regardless of how the parents try to help.
- The infant acts normally when not colicky.
- Assess the support system of caregivers and families, including coping skills.

PHYSICAL EXAM
- A comprehensive physical exam is normal.
- Since excessive crying may be a risk factor for shaken baby syndrome or other forms of child abuse (5)[B], be sure to examine the child carefully for signs of shaken baby syndrome or other types of child abuse.

DIFFERENTIAL DIAGNOSIS
Any organic cause for excessive or qualitatively different crying in infants such as:
- Infections (e.g., meningitis, sepsis, otitis media, or UTI)
- GI issues, such as gastroesophageal reflux, intussusception, lactose intolerance, constipation, anal fissure, or strangulated hernia
- Trauma, which includes foreign bodies, corneal abrasion, occult fracture, digit or penile hair tourniquet syndrome, or child abuse

DIAGNOSTIC TESTS & INTERPRETATION
Diagnostic Procedures/Other
A thorough history and physical exam should be performed to rule out other causes. Otherwise, no diagnostic procedures or imaging is indicated.

 TREATMENT

GENERAL MEASURES
- Soothe by holding and rocking the baby.
- Use a pacifier.
- Use of gentle rhythmic motion (e.g., strollers, infant swings, car rides).
- Place near white noise (e.g., vacuum cleaner, clothes dryer, white-noise machine).
- Crib vibrators or car-ride simulators have not proven to be helpful (6)[B].
- Increased carrying or use of infant carrier has not been shown to improve colic (6)[B].
- Employ the 5-Ss (need to be done concurrently):
  - Swaddling: Tight wrapping with blanket; may be especially beneficial in infants <8 weeks old (7)[B]
  - Side: Laying baby on side
  - Shushing: Loud white noise
  - Swinging: Rhythmic, jiggly motion
  - Sucking: Sucking on anything (e.g., nipple, finger, pacifier)

MEDICATION
- Dicyclomine (Bentyl) has been proven beneficial, but the potential serious adverse effects (apnea, seizures, and syncope) have precluded its use. Further, the manufacturer has made the medication contraindicated for infants <6 months (8)[B].
- Simethicone has not been shown to be beneficial (8)[B].

ISSUES FOR REFERRAL
Excessive vomiting, poor weight gain, recurrent respiratory diseases, or bloody stools should prompt referral to a specialist.

COMPLEMENTARY AND ALTERNATIVE MEDICINE
- A recent RCT of 50 full-term infants diagnosed with colic evaluated the safety and effectiveness of *Lactobacillus reuteri* supplementation. Infants were exclusively breastfed, and mothers were instructed to avoid cow's milk during the 21-day study. Infants were randomized to receive *L. reuteri* or placebo 30 minutes before the 1st feed of each day. Crying times decreased in both groups, but infants in the *L. reuteri* group had significantly reduced median daily crying times throughout the study (370 to 35 min/d vs. 300 to 90 min/d in placebo group). Weight gain, stooling frequency, and incidence of regurgitation were similar in both groups (9)[B]:
  - *L. reuteri* is available as over-the-counter drops, but it is not regulated by the FDA.
- Herbal teas and supplements may help but are not recommended because of limited, inconclusive evidence. Examples:
  - One study concluded that herbal teas containing mixtures of chamomile, vervain, licorice, fennel, and balm-mint used up to t.i.d. may be beneficial (5)[C]. However, the study used high dosages, raising clinical concerns that this therapy may impair needed milk consumption in infants and be impractical to administer. In addition, preparations used in the study may not be commercially available in the US.
  - A 2nd double-blind, randomized trial of 0.1% fennel seed oil emulsion vs. placebo demonstrated a decrease in colic symptoms according to the Wessel criteria. However, this preparation of fennel seed oil is not commercially available in the US, and the long-term health effects are unknown (10).
- A home-based intervention focusing on reducing infant stimulation and synchronizing infant sleep–wake cycles with the environment, as well as parental support, has been shown to be effective (2)[B].
- Use of music may help (11,12)[C].
- Chiropractic treatment has shown no benefit over placebo.
- Infant massage has not been shown to be helpful.

ONGOING CARE

FOLLOW-UP RECOMMENDATIONS

Frequent outpatient visits as needed for parental reassurance, education, and monitoring and to ensure the health of the infant and parents.

Patient Monitoring

Follow for proper feeding, growth, and development

DIET

- If breastfeeding:
  - Continue breastfeeding. Switching to formula probably will not help.
  - Possible therapeutic benefit from eliminating milk products, eggs, wheat, and/or nuts from the diet of breastfeeding mothers (6)[B].
  - Along with eliminating the preceding foods from the maternal diet, removing soy, nuts, and fish may be beneficial.
- If formula feeding:
  - Feeding the infant in a vertical position using a curved bottle or bottle with collapsible bag may help to reduce air swallowing.
  - If no intervention or dietary change has improved the situation, consider a 1-week trial of hypoallergenic formulas, such as whey hydrolysate (e.g., Good Start) or casein hydrolysate (e.g., Alimentum, Nutramigen, Pregestimil) (6,8)[B].
  - The American Academy of Pediatrics concluded that there is no proven role for soy formula in the treatment of colic (13)[C].
  - Adding fiber to formula also has not been shown to be helpful (6,11)[B].
- Supplementing with sucrose solution may be helpful, but the effect may be short-lived (<1 hour) (6,8)[B].
- Despite the proposed mechanism of functional lactose overload, use of lactase enzymes in formula or breast milk or given directly to the infant has no therapeutic benefit (6)[B].

PATIENT EDUCATION

- Reassure parents that colic is not the result of bad parenting, and advise parents about having proper rest breaks, adequate sleep, and help in caring for the infant.
- Explain the spectrum of crying behavior.
- Avoid overfeeding or underfeeding.
- Instruct in better feeding techniques, such as improved bottles (low air, curved) and sufficient burping after feeding.
- Colic information at American Family Physician: www.aafp.org/afp/2004/0815/p741.html

PROGNOSIS

- Usually subsides by 3–6 months of age, often on its own.
- Despite apparent abdominal pain, colicky infants eat well and gain weight normally.
- A handful of studies indicate temper tantrums may be more common among formerly colicky infants, as studied in toddlers up to 4 years old (14,15).
- Colic has no bearing on the baby's intelligence or future development.

COMPLICATIONS

- Colic is self-limiting and does not result in lasting effects to infant or maternal mental health (16)[C].
- However, case-control studies have shown an increased incidence of diagnosing childhood migraine headaches in patients with a history of colic during infancy (17)[B].

REFERENCES

1. Douglas P, Hill P. Managing infants who cry excessively in the first few months of life. *BMJ*. 2011;343:d7772.
2. Keefe MR, Lobo ML, Froese-Fretz A, et al. Effectiveness of an intervention for colic. *Clin Pediatr (Phila)*. 2006;45:123–133.
3. Milidou I, Henriksen TB, Jensen MS, et al. Nicotine replacement therapy during pregnancy and infantile colic in the offspring. *Pediatrics*. 2012;129(3):e652–658.
4. Romanello S, Spiri D, Marcuzzi E, et al. Association between childhood migraine and history of infantile colic. *JAMA*. 2013;309(15):1607–1612.
5. Reijneveld SA, van der Wal MF, Brugman E, et al. Infant crying and abuse. *Lancet*. 2004;364: 1340–1342.
6. Garrison MM, Christakis DA. A systematic review of treatments for infant colic. *Pediatrics*. 2000; 106:184–190.
7. van Sleuwen BE, L'hoir MP, Engelberts AC, et al. Comparison of behavior modification with and without swaddling as interventions for excessive crying. *J Pediatr*. 2006;149:512–517.
8. Wade S, Kilgour T. Extracts from "clinical evidence": Infantile colic. *BMJ*. 2001;323: 437–440.
9. Savino F, Cordisco L, Tarasco V, et al. Lactobacillus reuteri DSM 17938 in infantile colic: A randomized double-blind placebo controlled trial. *Pediatrics*. 2010;126(3):e526–533.
10. Alexandrovich I, Rakovitskaya O, Kolmo E, et al. The effect of fennel (*Foeniculum vulgare*) seed oil emulsion in infantile colic: A randomized, placebo-controlled study. *Altern Ther Health Med*. 2003;9(4):58–61.
11. Clemons RM. Issues in newborn care. *Prim Care*. 2000;27:251–267.
12. McCollough M, Sharieff GQ. Common complaints in the first 30 days of life. *Emerg Med Clin North Am*. 2002;20:27–48, v.
13. O'Connor NR. Infant formula. *Am Fam Physician*. 2009;79:565–570.
14. Canivet C, Jakobsson I, Hagander B, et al. Infantile colic. Follow-up at four years of age: Still more "emotional." *Acta Paediatr*. 2000;89:13–17.
15. Rautava P, Lehtonen L, Helenius H, et al. Infantile colic: Child and family three years later. *Pediatrics*. 1995;96:43–47.
16. Clifford TJ, Campbell MK, Speechley KN, et al. Sequelae of infant colic: Evidence of transient infant distress and absence of lasting effects on maternal mental health. *Arch Pediatr Adolesc Med*. 2002;156:1183–1188.
17. Gelfand AA, Thomas KC, Goadsby PJ. Before the headache: Infant colic as an early life expression of migraine. *Neurology*. 2012;79(13):1392–1396.

ADDITIONAL READING

- Hill DJ, Roy N, Heine RG, et al. Effect of a low-allergen maternal diet on colic among breastfed infants: A randomized, controlled trial. *Pediatrics*. 2005;116:e709–715.
- Savino F, Pelle E, Palumeri E, et al. *Lactobacillus reuteri* (American Type Culture Collection Strain 55730) versus simethicone in the treatment of infantile colic: A prospective randomized study. *Pediatrics*. 2007;119:e124–130.

CODES

ICD10

R10.83 Colic

CLINICAL PEARLS

- Colic is defined as excessive crying in an otherwise healthy baby.
- Excessive crying may be a risk factor for shaken baby syndrome or other forms of child abuse.
- Usually subsides spontaneously by 3–6 months of age.
- Provide advice, support, and reassurance to parents.
- Prevent caregiver burnout by advising parents to get proper rest breaks, sleep, and help in caring for the infant.

COLITIS, ISCHEMIC

Neha Jakhete, MD • Pia Prakash, MD • Marie L. Borum, MD, EdD, MPH

BASICS

Ischemic colitis results from decreased blood flow to the colon and secondary inflammation from a variety of underlying etiologies.

DESCRIPTION
- Associated with the elderly, but can affect patients of all ages
- Patients can present with:
  - *Nonacute ischemic colitis* from a chronic process with irreversible ischemic injury
  - *Acute process* with self-limited transient mucosal ischemia
- Illness is self-limited and reversible in 80% of patients:
  - 20% of patients progress to full-thickness necrosis and require surgical intervention.
- Most commonly, ischemia is related to nonocclusive reduction in blood flow:
  - Occlusive events can occur, but are less common.
- Presentation may vary, but patients with acute ischemic colitis present with localized abdominal pain and tenderness. Additionally, frequent loose and bloody stool may be seen within 12–24 hours of onset.
- Laboratory and radiographic findings are nonspecific and must be correlated closely with clinical presentation.
- Colonoscopy is the gold standard diagnostic test in patients with suspected ischemic colitis.
- In the absence of complications, most patients require supportive care, including IV fluids, bowel rest, and close monitoring for clinical decompensation.
- Empiric broad-spectrum antibiotics should be considered in moderate-to-severe cases.

EPIDEMIOLOGY
- Data describing the incidence and prevalence of ischemic colitis are limited; it is uncommon in the general population.
- Females may be at increased risk.
- Patients with inflammatory bowel disease or COPD have an increased risk.

Geriatric Considerations
Rarely seen in those <60, with average age at diagnosis being 70.

Incidence
- 4.5–44 cases per 100,000 in the general population
- 1 case per 2,000 in hospitalized patients
- True incidence may be underestimated due to nonspecific clinical manifestations.

Prevalence
19 cases per 100,000 in the general population

ETIOLOGY AND PATHOPHYSIOLOGY
- Results from reduction in blood flow to the colon compromising ability of colonic tissue to meet metabolic demands
- Most commonly, an acute, self-limited process resulting in ischemia to segments of colon

- The colon is perfused by both the superior and inferior mesenteric arteries and branches of the internal iliac arteries. With extensive collateral circulation, occlusion of branches of the SMA or IMA rarely leads to ischemic consequences.
- Watershed areas of the colon (splenic flexure and rectosigmoid junction) are most susceptible to ischemic damage. Blood is carried by narrow branches of the SMA and IMA to these areas, putting them at increased risk for ischemia. The splenic flexure is supplied by the terminal branches of the SMA, and the rectosigmoid junction is supplied by the terminal branches of the IMA.
- The left colon is more commonly affected than the right.
- The rectum is often spared because of the additional blood supply from the internal iliac arteries.
- Poor perfusion may result from systemic etiologies, local vascular compromise, and anatomic or functional changes in the colon itself. An occluding lesion of the large vessels is usually not identified.
- Acute ischemic colitis is largely self-limited and often resolves without long-term complications.
- Repeated episodes of ischemia and inflammation may result in a chronic colonic ischemia, possibly resulting in stricture formation, recurrent bacteremia, and sepsis. These patients may have unresolving areas of colitis requiring segmental colonic resection.
- Hypoperfusion from shock
- Embolic occlusion of mesenteric vessels
- Hypercoagulable states
- Sickle cell disease
- Arterial thrombosis
- Venous thrombosis
- Vasculitis
- Mechanical colonic obstruction (e.g., tumor, adhesions, hernia, volvulus, prolapse, diverticulitis)
- Surgical complications (e.g., related to abdominal aortic aneurism repair)
- Trauma
- Medications (intestinally active vasoconstrictive substances, medications that induce hypotension and thus hypoperfusion)
- Cocaine abuse
- Aortic dissection
- Strenuous physical activity (e.g., long-distance running)

RISK FACTORS
- Age >60 (90% of patients)
- Hypertension
- Diabetes mellitus
- Rheumatologic disorders/vasculitis
- Cerebrovascular disease (history of stroke or heart attack)
- Ischemic heart disease
- Recent abdominal surgery
- Constipation-inducing medications
- History of vascular surgery
- Hypoalbuminemia
- Hemodialysis
- Smoking
- Hypercoagulable state

DIAGNOSIS

- Diagnosis is based on history, risk factors, and physical examination.
- Laboratory values and radiographic findings are usually nonspecific.
- Colonoscopy may reveal suggestive findings.

HISTORY
- Symptoms vary, depending on severity of ischemic colitis.
- Sudden-onset, mild-to-moderate abdominal pain with tenderness over the affected segment of bowel
- Loose, bloody bowel movements may occur, typically within 12–24 hours of abdominal pain onset. Hematochezia is rarely associated with hemodynamic compromise.
- Nausea, vomiting, and abdominal distention may develop if ileus or stricture is present:
  - This finding is more common in chronic ischemic colitis.
- It is important to differentiate ischemic colitis from mesenteric ischemia. Patient may describe lateral mild abdominal pain in ischemic colitis vs. intense periumbilical pain out of proportion to physical exam findings in mesenteric ischemia.

PHYSICAL EXAM
- In nonacute cases, physical exam may be relatively benign.
- Tenderness to palpation over the involved segment of bowel (21% sensitivity) (1)
- Abdominal distention
- Hypoactive or absent bowel sounds
- Peritoneal signs, including involuntary guarding and rebound tenderness, may suggest transmural ischemia or bowel perforation, which may require surgical intervention.

DIFFERENTIAL DIAGNOSIS
- Infectious colitis
- Inflammatory bowel disease (ulcerative colitis, Crohn disease)
- Colon cancer
- Diverticulitis
- Radiation enteritis
- Toxic megacolon

DIAGNOSTIC TESTS & INTERPRETATION
- Diagnosis is mostly clinical.
- Colonoscopy is the gold standard diagnostic test.
- Radiographic tests and laboratory values are nonspecific, but may increase clinical suspicion.

Initial Tests (lab, imaging)
- CBC for leukocytosis
- BMP to evaluate for metabolic acidosis
- Lactate
- CPK
- Alkaline phosphatase
- Lactate dehydrogenase (LDH)
- Amylase
  Imaging is nonspecific.

- Abdominal plain film should be obtained:
  - Nonspecific findings include generalized bowel distention, air-filled bowel loops, and mural thickening.
  - Thumbprinting of the colonic wall is a more specific finding; however, it is only seen in a small portion of patients.
  - Pneumatosis and pneumoperitoneum suggest advanced ischemia.
  - Abdominal plain film is necessary to rule out bowel perforation.
- Abdominal CT scan with contrast should also be obtained with abdominal pain in suspected ischemic colitis:
  - The most common CT finding is segmental circumferential thickening of the bowel wall, which is nonspecific, as it can be seen in other intestinal diseases.
  - Pneumatosis or pneumoperitoneum may also be seen, suggesting advanced ischemia.

Follow-Up Tests & Special Considerations
- Stool cultures, fecal leukocytes, stool ova, and parasites should be tested to rule out infectious etiologies.
- *Clostridium difficile* should also be excluded in patients with recent antibiotic use.
- Patients who have undergone aortic surgery should be closely monitored for postoperative ischemic colitis.

Diagnostic Procedures/Other
- Colonoscopy is gold standard; sigmoidoscopy may also be used:
  - Visualization of cyanotic hemorrhagic tissue and edematous mucosa is suggestive of ischemia.
  - Segmental distribution (watershed) and rectal sparing can be seen during colonoscopy in patients with ischemic colitis.
  - Biopsies should be obtained during colonoscopy.
- MRI may be used for diagnosis and staging of ischemic colitis to avoid invasive procedures, but data are limited (2).

Test Interpretation
Biopsies may reveal pathologic changes, including distorted crypt architecture, hemorrhage, intramural leukocyte infiltrates, capillary thrombosis, granulation tissue, and necrosis.

TREATMENT

- Treatment depends on the severity of disease.
- Continuous monitoring of clinical status, including vital signs and serial abdominal exams, is necessary.
- In the absence of colonic necrosis or perforation, most patients respond to supportive care, including (3)[A]:
  - Bowel rest
  - IV fluids
  - Oxygenation
  - Maintenance of hemodynamic stability
  - Broad-spectrum antibiotics covering aerobic and anaerobic bacteria to avoid bacterial translocation secondary to colonic mucosal damage

- Avoidance of intestinally active vasoconstrictive medications
- Avoidance of oral cathartics
- Avoidance of systemic corticosteroids, which may worsen ischemic damage
- If ileus is present, nasogastric tube should be placed.
- If radiographic findings are present, serial abdominal x-rays may be helpful.
- If signs of clinical deterioration are present despite supportive care, including increased abdominal pain, peritoneal signs, persistent diarrhea or bleeding, or sepsis, laparotomy or surgery must be considered.

MEDICATION
Broad-spectrum antibiotics as above

ADDITIONAL THERAPIES
Recent study found that implantation of adipose-derived stem cells in an ischemic colonic wall in a rat model enhanced tissue healing by promoting angiogenesis (4).

SURGERY/OTHER PROCEDURES
- 20% of patients progress to full-thickness necrosis and require surgical intervention.
- Surgery is indicated if patient has peritonitis and pneumoperitoneum (5)[A].
- Surgery may be indicated for patients with:
  - Development of peritoneal signs or increased abdominal tenderness
  - Persistent diarrhea
  - Persistent leukocytosis or fever, or clinical signs of sepsis
  - Bleeding for >2 weeks
- Most common surgical intervention is colectomy with end ileostomy (6):
  - If the margins appear ischemic, more bowel should be resected until well-perfused margins are achieved.
- Generally, the patient may undergo reversal of the ostomy after several months as clinical condition allows.
- Mortality ranges from 30–60% in patients who require surgery (3,7).

ONGOING CARE

DIET
- Bowel rest until symptoms resolve
- Parenteral nutrition can be considered for patients who have contraindications to surgery, therefore needing prolonged bowel rest (3).

PROGNOSIS
- In most patients, symptoms of ischemic colitis resolve within 24–48 hours.
- Radiographic or endoscopic resolution is seen within 2 weeks (3).
- Follow-up colonoscopy may be performed to ensure complete resolution.
- Right sided ischemic colitis appears to be the most significant predictor of outcome (8)[A].

COMPLICATIONS
20–30% of patients go on to develop chronic ischemic colitis with persistent diarrhea or stricture formation requiring surgical intervention (6).

REFERENCES
1. Huguier M, Barrier A, Boelle PY, et al. Ischemic colitis. *Am J Surg.* 2006;192:679–684.
2. Iacobellis F, Berritto D, Somma F, et al. Magnetic resonance imaging: A new tool for diagnosis of acute ischemic colitis? *World J Gastroenterol.* 2012;18:1496–1501.
3. Theodoropoulou A, Koutroubakis IE. Ischemic colitis: Clinical practice in diagnosis and treatment. *World J Gastroenterol.* 2008;14:7302–7308.
4. Joo HH, Jo HJ, Jung TD, et al. Adipose-derived stem cells on the healing of ischemic colitis: A therapeutic effect by angiogenesis. *Int J Colorectal Dis.* 2012;27(11):1437–1443. Epub 2012 May 16.
5. Paterno F, McGillicuddy EA, Schuster KM, et al. Ischemic colitis: Risk factors for eventual surgery. *Am J Surg.* 2010;200:646–650.
6. Sun MY, Maykel JA. Ischemic colitis. *Clin Colon Rectal Surg.* 2007;20:5–12.
7. Feuerstadt P, Brandt LJ. Colon ischemia: Recent insights and advances. *Curr Gastroenterol Rep.* 2010;12:383–390.
8. O'Neill S, Yalamarthi S. Systematic review of the management of ischaemic colitis. *Colorectal Dis.* 2012;14(11):e751–763. doi: 10.1111/j.1463-1318.2012.03171.x.

CODES

ICD10
- K55.0 Acute vascular disorders of intestine
- K55.1 Chronic vascular disorders of intestine
- K55.9 Vascular disorder of intestine, unspecified

CLINICAL PEARLS
- Ischemic colitis should be diagnosed promptly using clinical symptoms and examination, as surgical intervention may be required in 20% of cases.
- Suspicion for ischemic colitis should be high in patients with multiple risk factors and presenting with abdominal pain and loose bloody stools.
- Imaging yields nonspecific findings in most cases.
- Colonoscopy is the diagnostic modality of choice.
- Most often, ischemic colitis is a self-limited disease that responds to conservative management with IV fluids, bowel rest, and empiric broad-spectrum antibiotics.
- Peritoneal signs or lack of clinical improvement is suggestive of extensive ischemia and requires surgical intervention.

COLONIC POLYPS

Macario C. Corpuz, Jr., MD, MBA-HCM, FAAFP • Paul F Sahd, DO

 BASICS

DESCRIPTION
- A colonic polyp is a typically benign, intraluminal outgrowth arising from the large intestinal epithelial lining:
  - The potential for malignant transformation necessitates close evaluation and monitoring (see "Colorectal Malignancy").
- 3 types:
  - Adenomatous: May become malignant:
    ○ Villous: Polyps tend to be larger, most likely to become malignant (10%)
    ○ Tubular (75%)
    ○ Tubulovillous (15%)
  - Hyperplastic: Rarely become malignant
  - Inflammatory: No malignant potential

EPIDEMIOLOGY
- Varies considerably worldwide:
  - Industrialized countries are generally at greater risk compared with the rest of the world.
- Age is an important determinant in the US and in other high-risk countries.
- Adenomas more common in men than in women.

Incidence
- Estimated 5% of the US population
- ~20% of middle-aged and older adults
- 50% seen in ≥50 years

Prevalence
Average prevalence of 25% age <40 years to as high as 55% at age 80

ETIOLOGY AND PATHOPHYSIOLOGY
- Adenomatous polyps:
  - Formed from abnormal proliferation and from dysplasia
- Nonadenomatous polyps:
  - Result from abnormal mucosal maturation, inflammation, or architecture
Unknown. May be related to environmental and genetic factors.

Genetics
May occur in the setting of genetic syndromes that are associated with gene mutations

RISK FACTORS
- Advancing age
- Male
- Obesity
- Family history of polyposis, polyps, or colorectal cancer (CRC)
- Inflammatory bowel disease
- Current cigarette smoking
- Excessive alcohol intake: >8 drinks of beer or spirits a week (1)
- Sedentary lifestyle

GENERAL PREVENTION
- Diet: High-fiber diet has been a controversial risk; 2 recent studies stressed that doubling fiber intake can significantly reduce CRC risk (2,3).
- Avoid smoking.
- Limit alcohol intake.
- Calcium supplement: Shown reduction of colorectal adenoma recurrence (4)
- Vitamin D, folic acid, vitamin B_6
- Aspirin: 3 randomized, controlled trials revealed that ASA caused significant reduction in the recurrence of sporadic adenomatous polyps after 1–3 years, whereas short-term studies support regression of colorectal adenomas in familial adenomatous polyposis (FAP) (5).

COMMONLY ASSOCIATED CONDITIONS
Associated with several hereditary disorders:
- FAP
- Peutz-Jeghers syndrome
- Gardner syndrome
- Hereditary nonpolyposis colon cancer (HNPCC)

 DIAGNOSIS

HISTORY
- Asymptomatic
- Hematochezia
- Melena
- Diarrhea or constipation
- Anemia
- Fatigue
- Abdominal pain

PHYSICAL EXAM
- Usually normal
- Rectal lesions may be felt by digital examination.

DIAGNOSTIC TESTS & INTERPRETATION
Initial Tests (lab, imaging)
- CBC: Anemia
- Electrolyte abnormalities: In villous adenoma

Diagnostic Procedures/Other
- Colonoscopy (6): Gold standard:
  - Most sensitive test available, but its sensitivity is a concern.
  - Chromoscopy enhances the detection of neoplastic lesions in the colon and the rectum that could be missed with conventional colonoscopy (7).
  - Cap-assisted colonoscopy increased detection of polyps, with better success of cecal intubation compared with standard colonoscopy (8)[A].
- Magnetic resonance colonography accurately detects polyps >10 mm (9)[A].
- CT colonography may be a more suitable initial test than optical colonoscopy (10)[A].
- Chromoscopy: Studies are examining narrow-band imaging for histologic differentiation between adenomatous and hyperplastic polyps (11,12).
- Sigmoidoscopy
- Air-contrast barium enema:
  - Misses small lesions
- Fecal occult blood test (FOBT):
  - Many false–positive results
- Fecal DNA testing
- FIT (Fecal Immunochemical Test): Better detecting advanced adenomatous polyps over traditional FOBT (13). Patients are more likely to undergo a FIT screen than colonoscopy screen (14).
- Some polyps are more likely to become malignant; hence, they require histopathologic evaluation.

Test Interpretation
- Villous adenoma:
  - Gross: Velvety, multiple-frond projections
  - Micro: Glands proliferate in fingerlike projections, malignant degenerations
- Tubular adenoma:
  - Gross: Smooth, firm, pink surface; microlobulated; fissures; pedunculated
  - Glands proliferate in tubular fashion, nuclei elongated, hyperchromatic

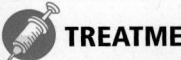

TREATMENT

SURGERY/OTHER PROCEDURES
- Endoscopic polypectomy: Major risks include perforation and bleeding
- Colonic resection: For multiple intestinal polyps associated with FAP

ONGOING CARE

FOLLOW-UP RECOMMENDATIONS
Benign polyps should have follow-up colonoscopy every 3–5 years.

Patient Monitoring
Offer CRC screening for average-risk patients beginning at age 50, earlier for at-risk patients:
- Most guidelines recommend to stop screening if life expectancy is <10 years.

DIET
Calcium supplementation might contribute a moderate degree to prevent colorectal adenomatous polyps (4).

PROGNOSIS
- Curable with polypectomy
- Projection estimates suggested that 50% of postpolypectomy patients will have a recurrence within 7.6 years; hence, need follow-up (15).
- Adenomatous polyps may undergo malignant transformation if not removed.
- Multiple polyps are particularly at increased risk of developing into CRC.

COMPLICATIONS
Perforation with colonoscopy is rare.

REFERENCES

1. Anderson JC, Alpern Z, Sethi G, et al. Prevalence and risk of colorectal neoplasia in consumers of alcohol in a screening population. *Am J Gastroenterol*. 2005;100:2049–2055.
2. Asano TK, McLeod RS. Dietary fibre for the prevention of colorectal adenomas and carcinomas. *Cochrane Database Syst Rev*. 2002;1:CD003430.
3. Peters U. Dietary fibre and colorectal adenoma in a colorectal cancer early detection programme. *Lancet*. 2003;361(9368):1491–1495.
4. Weingarten MA, Zalmanovici A, Yaphe J. Dietary calcium supplementation for preventing colorectal cancer and adenomatous polyps. *Cochrane Database Syst Rev*. 2008:CD003548.
5. Asano T, McLeod R. Nonsteroidal anti-inflammatory drugs (NSAID) and aspirin for preventing colorectal adenomas and carcinomas *Cochrane Database Syst Rev*. 2010;2:CD004079.
6. Kim DH, Pickhardt PJ, Taylor AJ, et al. CT colonography versus colonoscopy for the detection of advanced neoplasia. *N Engl J Med*. 2007;357:1403–1412.
7. Brown SR, Baraza W. Chromoscopy versus conventional endoscopy for the detection of polyps in the colon and rectum. *Cochrane Database Syst Rev*. 2010;(10):CD006439. Epub 2010 Oct 6.
8. Westwood DA, Alexakis N, Connor SJ. Transparent cap-assisted colonoscopy versus standard adult colonoscopy: A systematic review and meta-analysis. *Dis. Colon Rectum*. 2012;55(2):218–225.
9. Zijta FM, Bipat S, Stoker J. Magnetic resonance (MR) colonography in the detection of colorectal lesions: A systematic review of prospective studies. *Eur Radiol*. 2010;20(5):1031–1046.
10. Pickhardt PJ, Hassan C, Halligan S, et al. Colorectal cancer: CT colonography and colonoscopy for detection; systematic review and meta-analysis. *Radiology*. 2011;259(2):393–405.
11. Brown SR. Chromoscopy versus conventional endoscopy for the detection of polyps in the colon and rectum. *Cochrane Database Syst Rev*. 2007;4:CD006439.
12. Rastogi A. Recognition of surface mucosal and vascular patterns of colon polyps by using narrow-band imaging: Interobserver and intraobserver agreement and prediction of polyp histology. *Gastrointest Endosc*. 2009;69(Suppl 3):716–722.
13. Levi Z, Birkenfeld S, Vilkin A, et al. A higher detection rate for colorectal cancer and advanced adenomatous polyp for screening with immunochemical fecal occult blood test than guaiac fecal occult blood test, despite lower compliance rate. A prospective, controlled, feasibility study. *Cochrane Database Syst Rev*. 2011;128(10):2415–2424.
14. Quintero E, Castells A, Bujanda L, et al. Colonoscopy versus fecal immunochemical testing in colorectal-cancer screening. *Cochrane Database Syst Rev*. 2012: 336(8):697–706.
15. Yood MU. Colon polyp recurrence in a managed care population. *Arch Intern Med*. 2003;163(4):422–426.

ADDITIONAL READING

- Elwood PC, Gallagher AM, Duthie GG, et al. Aspirin, salicylates, and cancer. *Lancet*. 2009;373:1301–1309.
- Larsen IK, Grotmol T, Almendingen K, et al. Lifestyle as a predictor for colonic neoplasia in asymptomatic individuals. *BMC Gastroenterol*. 2006;6:5.
- Seong-Eun K. An association between obesity and the prevalence of colonic adenoma according to age and gender. *J Gastroenterol*. 2007;42(8). Epub.

SEE ALSO

Algorithm: Bleeding, Upper GI

CODES

ICD10
- D12.5 Benign neoplasm of sigmoid colon
- D12.6 Benign neoplasm of colon, unspecified
- K63.5 Polyp of colon

CLINICAL PEARLS
- Villous adenomatous polyps are the "villains" (most likely to become malignant).
- Hyperplastic polyps rarely become cancer.
- Up to 50% of patients who have polyps removed have recurrent polyps.
- Aspirin causes significant reduction in the recurrence of sporadic adenomatous polyps after 1–3 years.

C

COLORECTAL CANCER

Stephen M. Scott, MD, MPH

 BASICS

DESCRIPTION

- Colorectal cancer (CRC) denotes a neoplasm that develops in the colon or rectum.
- CRC is the 2nd leading cause of cancer deaths and is the 3rd most common cancer in men and women in the US.
- Screening for CRC reduces the incidence of, and mortality from, CRC.

EPIDEMIOLOGY

Incidence
102,480 new cases of colon cancer, 40,340 new cases of rectal cancer, and 50,830 deaths from colon and rectal cancer combined were estimated in the US in 2013 (1).

Prevalence
- The lifetime risk for developing CRC in the US is about 1 in 21 (4.82%).
- Death rates have been declining due to improved screening, prevention, and treatment.

ETIOLOGY AND PATHOPHYSIOLOGY

- Progression from the 1st abnormal cells to the appearance of CRC usually occurs over 10–15 years, a disease characteristic that contributes to the effectiveness of prevention.
- High-risk polyp findings include multiple polyps, villous polyps, and larger polyps; hyperplastic polyps are less likely to evolve into colorectal cancer.
- Multiple genetic and environmental factors have been linked to the development of CRC.

Genetics
- There does not seem to be a single genetic pathway to CRC.
- <10% of CRC cases are linked to an inherited gene:
  - APC, a tumor suppressor gene, is altered in FAP.
  - Genes encoding DNA mismatch repair (MMR) enzymes are implicated in HNPCC: MLH1, MSH2, MSH6, PMS1, PMS2, and others
  - STK11, a tumor suppressor gene, is altered in Peutz-Jeghers syndrome.
- Sporadic cases of CRC have been linked to oncogenes: ras, c-myc, src, HER2/neu, and others

RISK FACTORS

- Age: >90% of people diagnosed with CRC are >50 years of age.
- Personal history of colorectal polyps:
  - Risks increase with multiple polyps, villous polyps, and larger polyps.
- Personal history of cancer:
  - Rectal cancer has a higher incidence of local recurrence than proximal cancers (20–30% vs. 2–4%).
- History of inflammatory bowel disease:
  - Prevalence of CRC in ulcerative colitis and Crohn disease is ~3%, with a cumulative risk of CRC of 2% at 10 years, 8% at 20 years, and 18% at 30 years.
- Family history of CRC:
  - Having a single 1st-degree relative with a history of CRC increases risk 1.7-fold.
  - Risk is more than double for those who have a history of CRC or polyps in:
    - Any 1st-degree relative <60 years of age
    - ≥2 1st-degree relatives, regardless of age

- Inherited syndromes:
  - Hereditary nonpolyposis colon cancer (HNPCC, also called Lynch syndrome):
    - Often develops at younger age (average age at diagnosis of CRC is 44)
    - Lifetime risk of CRC 52–69%
    - Accounts for ~2% of all CRCs
  - Familial adenomatous polyposis (FAP):
    - Affected individuals develop hundreds to thousands of polyps in colon and rectum.
    - CRC usually present by age 40
    - Accounts for <1% of CRCs
  - Peutz-Jeghers syndrome:
    - Individuals may have freckles (mouth, hands, feet) and large polyps in GI tract.
    - Greatly increased risk for CRC and cancers
- Race and ethnicity:
  - African Americans have highest CRC incidence and mortality rates in the US.
  - Several different gene mutations have been identified among Ashkenazi Jews.
- Miscellaneous:
  - *Streptococcus bovis* bacteremia is associated with CRC.
  - Patients with acromegaly are at increased risk.

GENERAL PREVENTION

- Diets high in fruits and vegetables have been linked with decreased risk; those high in red and processed meats may increase CRC risk.
- Some studies suggest that vitamin D, calcium, folate, and fiber may lower CRC risk; more research is needed to understand how diet affects risks of CRC.
- People who are physically inactive are at higher risk for CRC.
- Long-term smokers are more likely than nonsmokers to develop and die from CRC.
- CRC has been linked to heavy alcohol consumption; may be related to low folic acid.
- NSAIDs may reduce risk in some groups; experts do not recommend NSAID use as a cancer prevention strategy in people at average risk for CRC.
- Colon cancer screening is one of the most powerful tools in preventing colon cancer.

ALERT

The US Preventive Services Task Force (USPSTF) strongly recommends that clinicians screen men and women between the ages of 50 and 75 for CRC using fecal occult blood testing, sigmoidoscopy, or colonoscopy (1)[A].

- American Cancer Society recommendations for screening include (2)[C]:
  - Fecal occult blood testing (FOBT) annually
  - Fecal immunochemical test (FIT) annually
  - Flexible sigmoidoscopy every 5 years
  - Colonoscopy every 10 years
  - CT colonography every 5 years (colonoscopy completed if positive)∗
  - Double-contrast barium enema every 5 years∗
  - Stool DNA test (sDNA) (none FDA approved; studies of next generation tests are ongoing)∗

  ∗The USPSTF does not recommend barium enema as a screening test and concludes the evidence is insufficient to assess the benefits and harms of CT colonography and stool DNA testing as screening modalities for CRC.

- Digital rectal exam (DRE), alone or in combination with a 1-sample FOBT or FIT test, is *not* an acceptable method for CRC screening.
- Screening in high-risk groups:
  - People with a personal history of polyps need more frequent colonoscopy screening, depending on risk (i.e., 1 or 2 <1 cm polyps with low-grade dysplasia is deemed low risk and may warrant repeat colonoscopy in 5–10 years; decision is influenced by family history, age, quality of initial colonoscopy, and patient comorbidities).
  - People who have a family history of CRC or adenomatous polyps before age 60 should begin colonoscopy at age 40 or 10 years younger than the age of relative at cancer diagnosis, whichever is earlier.
  - People with inflammatory bowel disease (IBD) should have regular surveillance colonoscopy with biopsies to detect dysplasia; guidelines for timing and location vary by professional society, but generally indicate starting surveillance by ~8 years of onset of disease followed by surveillance every 1–2 years.
  - Genetic testing may be appropriate for individuals with a strong family history of CRC or polyps:
    - Family members of a person affected by HNPCCC should start colonoscopy surveillance as early as age 20.
    - Individuals with suspected FAP should have yearly flexible sigmoidoscopy beginning at age 10–12; those who test positive for the gene linked to FAP may consider colectomy.

 DIAGNOSIS

HISTORY

- Many patients with CRC are asymptomatic.
- Common presenting symptoms and signs in symptomatic patients include:
  - Abdominal pain or cramping
  - Change in bowel habits (constipation, diarrhea, narrowing of stool)
  - Rectal bleeding, dark stools, or blood in stool
  - Weakness or fatigue
  - Anemia
  - Weight loss
- Other presentations may include symptoms due to the presence of metastatic lesions (lymph nodes, liver, lung, peritoneum), fever of unknown origin, and *S. bovis* or *Clostridium septicum* sepsis.

PHYSICAL EXAM

- Weight loss
- Signs of anemia (i.e., conjunctival pallor)
- Palpable abdominal mass

DIFFERENTIAL DIAGNOSIS

- >95% of CRCs are adenocarcinomas.
- Other colonic tumors include carcinoid tumors, lymphomas, and Kaposi sarcoma in HIV.
- Many conditions can mimic CRC, including other cancers, hemorrhoids, inflammatory bowel disease, infection, and extrinsic masses (i.e., cysts, abscesses).

DIAGNOSTIC TESTS & INTERPRETATION
Initial Tests (lab, imaging)
- CBC (to evaluate anemia)
- Liver function (CRC may spread to the liver)
- Colonoscopy
- CT colography if colonoscopy incomplete

Follow-Up Tests & Special Considerations
- CEA should be obtained preoperatively to assist with follow-up screening.
- CT to evaluate presence of metastatic disease
- Chest x-ray to evaluate presence of chest metastases
- Endoscopic US (EUS) may be used to evaluate the extent of rectal cancers; endorectal MRI may also provide further detail.
- Intraoperative US may be used to evaluate solid organs (e.g., the liver) after tumor resection.
- Positron emission tomography (PET) may be used in some cases to detect metastatic disease.

Diagnostic Procedures/Other
- Biopsy is usually performed (most often during colonoscopy) if CRC is suspected.
- CT needle-guided biopsy may be needed to evaluate a suspected tumor or metastasis.

Test Interpretation
The American Joint Committee on Cancer (AJCC) TNM staging is preferred:
- Stage 0: Limited to the mucosa (carcinoma in situ or intramucosal carcinoma, Tis, N0, M0)
- Stage I: Invades mucosa (T1) or muscularis propria (T2); no invasion of lymph nodes or distant sites (T1, N0, M0 or T2, N0, M0)
- Stage IIA: Invades pericolorectal tissues; no lymph nodes or distant sites (T3, N0, M0)
- Stage IIB: Penetrates to surface of visceral peritoneum; no lymph nodes or distant sites (T4a, N0, M0)
- Stage IIC: Directly invades or adherent to other organs or structures (T4b, N0, M0)
- Stage IIIA: Invades submucosa or muscularis propria with spread to 1–3 lymph nodes; no distant sites (T1, N1, M0 or T2, N1, M0)
- Stage IIIB: Invades pericolorectal tissues or surface of visceral peritoneum + spread to 1–3 lymph nodes; no distant sites (T3, N1, M0, or T4a, N1, M0)
- Stage IIIC: Invades pericolorectal tissues or peritoneum or other organs and to ≥4 nearby lymph nodes; no distant sites (any T3 or T4, N2, M0)
- Stage IVA: Any level of invasion with spread to one organ or site (any T, any N, M1a)
- Stage IVB: Any level of invasion with spread to more than one organ or site or peritoneum (any T, any N, M1b)

 TREATMENT

MEDICATION
Surgical resection is the primary treatment for CRC, as noted below. Adjuvant chemotherapy is most clearly beneficial for stage III (node-positive) disease, in which improvements of ~30% may be achieved in both disease recurrence and overall survival, compared with nontreated controls. Chemotherapeutic regimens for metastatic disease may extend overall survival from 6 months to ~2 years.

First Line
Combination chemotherapy is common and may include oxaliplatin, irinotecan, fluorouracil, leucovorin, and capecitabine.

Geriatric Considerations
Elderly patients tend to tolerate CRC chemotherapy and should be considered for treatment.

Second Line
Targeted therapies may be used alongside 1st-line agents or alone if 1st-line agents are ineffective:
- Bevacizumab (Avastin) is a monoclonal antibody that targets vascular endothelial growth factor (VEGF); inhibits angiogenesis.
- Cetuximab (Erbitux) and panitumumab (Vectibix) are monoclonal antibodies that target epidermal growth factor receptor (EGFR).
- Aflibercept and regorafenib are newer agents with actions on vascular endothelial growth factor (VEGF).

SURGERY/OTHER PROCEDURES
- Surgery is the primary treatment for localized CRC:
  – May involve segmental resection, hemicolectomy, or colectomy, as well as resection of nodes, depending on size and invasion
  – Laparoscopic-assisted colectomy is an emerging option for earlier-stage tumors.
  – Surgery for rectal cancer may include local transanal, low anterior, or abdominoperineal resection, or pelvic exenteration.
- Radiation therapy is most often used for peritoneal or rectal cancers; it may also be used to relieve symptoms.

COMPLEMENTARY AND ALTERNATIVE MEDICINE
- May serve as an adjunct to treatment for CRC
- 70–75% of cancer survivors report using at least 1 type of complementary and alternative medicine (CAM), and almost all report that the alternative therapy improved their well-being.

 ONGOING CARE

FOLLOW-UP RECOMMENDATIONS
Patient Monitoring
- People with a personal history of proximal cancer (nonrectal) should have follow-up colonoscopy in 1 year and, if normal, in 3 and 5 years subsequently.
- Carcinoembryonic antigen (CEA) and/or CA 19-9 are used to detect recurrence in people treated for CRC. (Note: CEA levels may be elevated in ulcerative colitis, nonmalignant GI tumors, liver disease, lung disease, and in smokers.)

PATIENT EDUCATION
- NCI: What You Need to Know About Cancer of the Colon and Rectum: http://www.cancer.gov/cancertopics/wyntk/colon-and-rectal
- AAFP: Colorectal Cancer Screening (includes Spanish): http://familydoctor.org/online/famdocen/home/common/cancer/risk/556.html

PROGNOSIS
5-year relative survival rate is determined by stage (adjusted for patients dying of other diseases): Stage I: 93%; stage II: 72–85%; stage III: 44–83%; stage IV: 8%

COMPLICATIONS
- Colorectal surgery: Pain, deep vein thrombosis, anastomotic leaks, infection, scarring, bowel obstruction
- Chemotherapy: Hair loss, nausea, vomiting, bruising, fatigue, increased risk for infections
- Radiation therapy: Skin irritation, nausea, rectal pain, incontinence, bladder irritation, fatigue, and sexual problems

REFERENCES
1. Screening for Colorectal Cancer, U.S. Preventive Services Task Force, http://www.uspreventiveservicestaskforce.org/uspstf/uspscolo.htm; accessed 07/03/2013.
2. American cancer society guidelines for the early detection of cancer. http://www.cancer.org/cancer/colonandrectumcancer/moreinformation/colonandrectumcancerearlydetection/colorectal-cancer-early-detection-acs-recommendations; Accessed 7/03/2013.

ADDITIONAL READING
- Colon Cancer Treatment (PDQ®), National Cancer Institute (Patient, Health Professional and Spanish versions): http://www.cancer.gov/cancertopics/pdq/treatment/colon/Patient
- Colon and Rectal Cancer, National Cancer Institute at the National Institutes of Health; http://www.cancer.gov/cancertopics/types/colon-and-rectal; accessed 07/03/2013.
- Howlader N, Noone AM, Krapcho M, et al. SEER Cancer Statistics Review, 1975–2010, National Cancer Institute. Bethesda, MD, http://seer.cancer.gov/csr/1975_2010/, based on November 2012 SEER data submission, posted to the SEER web site, April 2013.
- National Colorectal Cancer Roundtable: http://www.nccrt.org

 CODES

ICD10
- C18.9 Malignant neoplasm of colon, unspecified
- C19 Malignant neoplasm of rectosigmoid junction
- C20 Malignant neoplasm of rectum

CLINICAL PEARLS
- The USPSTF recommends screening beginning at age 50 and notes that evidence supports fecal occult blood testing (yearly), sigmoidoscopy, or colonoscopy (every 10 years).
- High-risk polyp findings include multiple polyps, villous polyps, and larger polyps; hyperplastic polyps are less likely to become cancerous.
- 10% of cases of CRC occur in people <50 years of age. People who have a family history of CRC without other risks (i.e., polyposis syndrome) should begin colonoscopy at age 40, or 10 years younger than the age of relative at cancer diagnosis, whichever is earlier.
- Iron deficiency anemia in the elderly should prompt a search for CRC and should not be attributed to normal aging.

COMPLEMENTARY AND ALTERNATIVE MEDICINE

Jennifer Caragol, MD • D. Matthew Ziegler, MD • Andrew Bentley, MS

 BASICS

- Complementary and alternative medicine (CAM) are medical and health care systems, practices, and products not presently considered part of conventional medicine.
- The National Center for Health Statistics (NCHS) 2007 survey reports 38% of adult Americans and 12% of children use some form of CAM, and this percentage is increasing.
- Medical professionals who incorporate CAM into their medical practice will often refer to their health care model as "integrative medicine."

DESCRIPTION

- Definitions and additional terms:
  - *Complementary medicine* is used with conventional medicine to address a health concern. For example, massage plus physical therapy to address low back pain, or medication plus osteopathic manipulation to address recurrent headaches.
  - *Alternative medicine* is used in place of conventional medicine to promote healing of conditions that cannot be explained by the conventional biomedical model or for which the effectiveness of therapy is not yet established by clinical research.
  - *Integrative medicine* is the combination of allopathic medicine with CAM and may be provided to the patient by a single licensed medical professional trained in CAM or by a group of diverse health care providers. E.g., a nurse on the oncology unit who integrates healing touch into the care of the patient.
  - *Holistic* is a descriptive term for a practitioner's approach to patient care. A holistic practitioner assesses the emotional, spiritual, mental, and physical state of wellness of the client, then works to provide comprehensive care. A holistic practice may include practitioners of different disciplines to best address all aspects of wellness or illness.
- *Biologically based therapies*: Diets, herbals, vitamins, supplements, flower essences
- *Manipulative and body-based methods*:
  - Massage therapy is the manipulation of the body's soft tissues, whereby the licensed practitioner uses knowledge of anatomy and physiology to restore function, promote relaxation, and relieve pain. There are several different types of massage.
  - Osteopathic manipulative medicine focuses on the musculoskeletal system. It includes indirect techniques (e.g., muscle energy, myofascial release, osteopathy in the cranial field, and strain-counterstrain approach), as well as direct action techniques (high-velocity thrusts).
  - Craniosacral therapy is a gentle manual treatment focusing on the release of bony and fascial restrictions in the craniosacral system, which includes the cranium, sacrum, spinal cord, meninges, and CSF.

- Chiropractic therapy focuses on the musculoskeletal and nervous systems and how imbalances in these systems can affect general health. It is used to treat back pain, neck pain, and joint pain. Doctors of chiropractic (DCs) complete 4–5 years of intensive training in anatomy, physiology, and manipulation.
- *Mind–body medicine*:
  - Meditation is a practice of detachment in which a person sits quietly, generally focusing on the breath, while releasing all thoughts from the mind with the intention to center the self, restore balance, and enhance well-being. Mindfulness meditation involves making oneself aware of the most immediate of activities in order to gain control over actions and anxiety
  - Spiritual practices; e.g., prayer
  - Yoga is an exercise of mindfulness, meditation, strength, and balance. It is composed of *asanas* (postures) and *pranayamas* (focused breathing).
  - Aromatherapy utilizes highly concentrated plant extracts to stimulate physical, emotional, and energetic healing processes. These aromatic oils are rubbed on the skin, aerosolized, or used in compresses.
  - Relaxation techniques such as breathing exercises, progressive muscle relaxation, and guided imagery
  - *Tai chi* and *qi gong* are Chinese exercise systems that combine meditation, regulated breathing, and flowing dance-like movements to enhance and balance chi (*qi*), or life force energy.
- *Alternative medical systems*:
  - Traditional Chinese medicine incorporates Chinese herbs and acupuncture. Acupuncture is the practice of regulating chi (*qi*) by inserting hair-thin needles at specific points along meridian pathways of the body. *Chi* movement is responsible for animating and protecting the body; relieving pain; and regulating blood, oxygen, and nourishment to every cell.
  - Ayurvedic medicine originated in India and is one of the world's oldest medical systems. It utilizes healing modalities and herbs to integrate and balance the body, mind, and spirit.
  - Homeopathy is a system of therapy based on the concept that very dilute quantities of an offending agent can stimulate the body's own immune system to produce a reaction against this offense, thereby healing itself. In general, homeopathic remedies are considered safe and unlikely to cause serious adverse reactions.
  - Naturopathy is based on providing natural and minimally invasive options for prevention and treatment of disease. Treatment regimens can include herbs, vitamins, supplements, dietary counseling, homeopathic remedies, manipulative therapies, acupuncture, and hydrotherapy. 4-year doctoral training programs are available; however, only 16 states have licensing laws for naturopathic practitioners.

- *Energy therapies*:
  - *Reiki*, which means "source energy," is a healing practice from Japan. Laying hands lightly on the patient or holding the hands just above the body, the *reiki* practitioner facilitates spiritual and physical healing by stimulating a patient's life force energy.
  - Healing touch was designed by a registered nurse. Practitioners use their hands to clear, energize, and balance a patient's energy field to enhance well-being.
- Common reasons patients choose CAM:
  - Additive therapy to address aspects not provided for in conventional medical treatment
  - Conventional medicine has been unsuccessful in fully addressing ailment
  - Preventative health care
  - Desire for a holistic and natural approach to well-being
  - Preference for noninvasive treatment options
  - Concern about side effects of medication
  - Desire for spiritual support to be incorporated into healing practice
  - Cultural or familial belief system may be more aligned with "natural" solutions not provided for or supported by the standard allopathic model of health care

EPIDEMIOLOGY

- All ages use CAM, but it is most prevalent among adults aged 30–69 years (1).
- Gender ratio: Female > Male (1)
- College graduates and residents from Western states are more likely to use CAM (1).
- Cancer survivors are more likely than the general population to use CAM.
- 11 most-utilized CAM therapies based on the NCHS 2007 survey; prayer is also reported. These CAM therapies were used by the indicated percentage of survey participants:
  - Prayer/Self (43%); prayer/others (24.4%); prayer group (9.6%)
  - Natural products (17.7%)
  - Deep breathing (12.7%)
  - Meditation (9.4%)
  - Chiropractic and osteopathic (8.6%)
  - Massage (8.3%)
  - Yoga (6.1%)
  - Diet-based therapies (3.6%)
  - Progressive relaxation (2.9%)
  - Guided imagery (2.2%)
  - Homeopathic treatment (1.8%)

C

 TREATMENT

- Variable evidence supports both safety and efficacy of:
  - Meditation for lowering BP (2)[A]
  - Acupuncture for chronic low back pain (3)[A]
  - Acupuncture may improve fertility
  - Spinal manipulative therapy for prophylactic treatment of headaches
  - Ginger for nausea, including that associated with chemotherapy
  - Manipulation, massage, and mobilization for acute low back and posterior neck pain
  - Massage therapy to promote weight gain in preterm infants
  - Acupuncture for nausea and vomiting
  - *Tai chi* for improving balance and decreasing the risk of and fear of falling in elderly
  - Aromatherapy massage for temporary relief of anxiety or depression in cancer patients (4)
  - Mind–body techniques for migraines, chronic pain, and insomnia
  - Homeopathic remedy for the treatment of chemotherapy-induced stomatitis in children
  - Riboflavin for migraine prophylaxis
  - Horse chestnut seed extract to improve lower leg venous tone, pain, and edema
  - Glucosamine and chondroitin sulfate for osteoarthritis and knee pain
  - Yoga and meditation appear to improve endothelial function in patients with CAD and can have potential beneficial effects on depressive disorders.
  - Oral probiotics may prevent URIs and shorten the duration of acute and antibiotic-associated diarrhea.
  - Omega-3 fatty acids may reduce inflammation and anxiety in young healthy adults (5).
  - Vitamin D 800 IU/d may reduce falls and fractures in the elderly (6).
- Evidence supports safety, but evidence regarding efficacy is inconclusive:
  - Acupuncture for recurrent headache
  - Homeopathy for induction and augmentation of labor
  - Dietary fat reduction for certain types of cancer
  - Mind–body techniques for metastatic cancer
  - Copper and magnetic bracelets for pain
  - Vitamin D levels >30 ng/mL correlate with lower risk of some cancers. Adequate vitamin D intake may decrease atopy and asthma symptoms (6).
- Evidence supports efficacy, but evidence regarding safety is inconclusive:
  - St. John's wort extract for short-term treatment of depression in adults
  - Licorice for gastritis
- Evidence indicates serious risk:
  - Delay in seeking medical care or replacement of curative conventional treatment
  - Use of toxic herbs or substances
  - Known herb–drug interactions

ONGOING CARE

PATIENT EDUCATION
The National Center for Complementary and Alternative Medicine (nccam.nih.gov)

COMPLICATIONS

ALERT
Ginkgo and St. John's wort account for most herb–drug interactions described in the medical literature.
- Herbs with possible adverse effects:
  - Serious adverse events from herbal remedies remain uncommon.
  - Some ethnic medicines, as those prescribed by practitioners of Ayurveda or traditional Chinese medicine, may intentionally contain heavy metals or other toxic substances. These are usually listed by their pharmacopeial names, e.g., Qian Dan = lead oxide.
  - Bitter orange (*Citrus sinensis*): Sympathomimetic; increases heart rate (HR), BP
  - California poppy (*Eschscholzia californica*): May cause respiratory depression, drowsiness; contains opioids
  - Cascara sagrada (*Frangula purshiana*): Depletes serum potassium
  - Chaparral (*Larrea tridentata*): Hepatotoxic
  - Ephedra (*Ephedra* spp.): Sympathomimetic; increases HR, BP; insomnia, gastric distress
  - Ginkgo (*Ginkgo biloba*): Extravasation, increased bleeding time
  - Guarana (*Paullinia cupana*): Tachycardia, hypertension; contains caffeine
  - Kava (*Piper methysticum*): Decreases utilization of niacin; possibly hepatotoxic
  - Licorice (*Glycyrrhiza* spp.): Long-term use depletes serum potassium.
  - Lily of the valley (*Convallaria majalis*): Contains cardiac glycosides
  - Poke root (*Phytolacca species*): Strong gastric irritant, may cause sedation
  - Senna (*Cassia* senna): Depletes serum potassium
  - Snakeroot (*Aristolochia* spp.): Nephrotoxic
  - St. John's wort (*Hypericum perforatum*): Numerous drug interactions; induces CYP(3a4) pathway, speeding metabolism of many drugs.
  - Wormwood (*Artemisia absinthium*): Elevates serotonin level, may raise BP
  - Yohimbe (*Pausinystalia yohimbe*): Elevates BP
- Important herbal–medication interactions
- Vitamins and minerals with potential toxicity

Pediatric Considerations

ALERT
Iron is a leading cause of accidental poisoning in children <6. Minerals (i.e., potassium, calcium, magnesium, zinc, copper, and selenium) may cause toxicity.
- Vitamin A is most common cause of hypervitaminosis.
- β-carotene may have a limited potential for overdose.

REFERENCES

1. Barnes PM, Bloom B, Nahin RL, et al. Complementary and alternative medicine use among adults and children: United States, 2007. *Natl Health Stat Report*. 2008;1–23.
2. Anderson JW, Liu C, Kryscio RJ. Blood pressure response to transcendental meditation: A meta-analysis. *Am J Hypertens*. 2008;21:310–316.
3. Manheimer E, White A, Berman B, et al. Meta-analysis: Acupuncture for low back pain. *Ann Intern Med*. 2005;142:651–663.
4. Wilkinson SM, Love SB, Westcombe AM, et al. Effectiveness of aromatherapy massage in the management of anxiety and depression in patients with cancer: A multicenter randomized controlled trial. *J Clin Oncol*. 2007;25:532–539.
5. Kiecolt-Glaser JK, Belury MA, Andridge R, et al. Omega-3 supplementation lowers inflammation and anxiety in medical students: A randomized controlled trial. *Brain Behav Immun*. 2011;25(8):1725–1734.
6. Makariou S, Liberopoulos EN, Elisaf M, et al. Novel roles of vitamin D in disease: What is new in 2011? *Eur J Intern Med*. 2011;22:355–362.

ADDITIONAL READING
- Bent S. Herbal medicine in the United States: Review of efficacy, safety, and regulation: Grand rounds at University of California, San Francisco Medical Center. *J Gen Intern Med*. 2008;23:854–859.
- Evidence-based Herbal Medicine. http://www.evidencebasedherbalmedicine.com.

CLINICAL PEARLS
- CAM are medical and health care systems, practices, and products not presently considered part of conventional medicine.
- Medical professionals who incorporate CAM into their medical practice will often refer to their health care model as "integrative medicine."

COMPLEX REGIONAL PAIN SYNDROME

Dennis E. Hughes, DO, FAAFP, FACEP

 BASICS

DESCRIPTION

- Complex regional pain syndrome (CRPS) is a pain syndrome after injury to bone and soft tissue; pathogenesis is obscure. Evidence suggests that these syndromes involve both the peripheral and central nervous system:
  - Type I: No nerve injury (reflex sympathetic dystrophy [RSD])
  - Type II: Associated with a demonstrable nerve injury (causalgia)
- System(s) affected: Nervous
- Synonym(s): Traumatic erythromelalgia; Weir Mitchell causalgia; Causalgia; Reflex sympathetic dystrophy; Posttraumatic neuralgia; Sympathetically maintained pain

EPIDEMIOLOGY

- Predominant age: Mean age 36–46 years
- Predominant gender: Female > Male (3:1, 60–81%)
- Extremely rare in children

Incidence

26.2/100,000 person-years, but may be higher due to misdiagnosis initially

Prevalence

~6 million in the US with estimates of 50,000 new cases annually

ETIOLOGY AND PATHOPHYSIOLOGY

- Poorly understood activation of abnormal sympathetic reflex that lowers pain threshold:
  - Increased excitability of nociceptive neurons in the spinal cord; "central sensitization"
  - Exaggerated responses to normally nonpainful stimuli (hyperalgesia, allodynia)
- Other than known nerve injury (type II or causalgia), no known definitive pathogenesis

Genetics

No known genetic pattern

RISK FACTORS

- Minor or severe trauma (upper extremity fracture noted in 44%)
- Surgery (particularly carpal tunnel release)
- Lacerations
- Burns
- Frostbite
- Casting/Immobilization after extremity injury
- Penetrating injury
- Polymyalgia rheumatica
- Myocardial infarction (MI)
- Cerebral vascular accident

GENERAL PREVENTION

- Early mobilization after fracture, stroke, and MI has proven benefit in reducing incidence of CRPS.
- 1 study of wrist fractures found that addition of 500 mg/d of vitamin C lowered rates of CRPS.
- There is evidence that limiting use of tourniquets, liberal regional anesthetic use, and ensuring adequate perioperative analgesia can reduce the incidence of CRPS-I (1)[A].

COMMONLY ASSOCIATED CONDITIONS

- Serious injury to bone and soft tissue
- Herpes zoster
- Postherpetic neuralgia results from partial or complete damage to afferent nerve pathways.
- Pain occurs in dermatomes as a sequela of herpes zoster.

 DIAGNOSIS

Unprovoked pain is the hallmark of the condition, and the diagnosis of CRPS is excluded by the existence of conditions that would otherwise account for the degree of symptoms.

HISTORY

- Inciting injury ranges from minor sprains to major trauma
- Hyperhidrosis
- Thermal hypersensitivity
- Hair loss
- Burning paroxysms of pain
- Increased symptoms during emotional stress
- Muscle spasms
- Hypersensitivity to light touch
- Mottled skin
- Partial motor paralysis

PHYSICAL EXAM

- Early: Area usually edematous; may be either hyper- or hypothermic; decreased hair; diminished nail growth
- Established: Skin is indurated, cool, hyperhydrotic; notable hair loss and nail changes; subcutaneous tissue atrophy
- Late: Skin appears thin and shiny; may see contractures of extremity

DIFFERENTIAL DIAGNOSIS

- Infection
- Hypertrophic scar
- Bone fragments
- Neuroma
- CNS tumor or syrinx
- Deep vein thrombosis or thrombophlebitis
- Thoracic outlet syndrome

DIAGNOSTIC TESTS & INTERPRETATION

Initial Tests (lab, imaging)

- CBC
- Erythrocyte sedimentation rate (ESR)
- Plain radiographs may show patchy demineralization within 3–6 weeks of onset of CRPS and more pronounced than would be see from disuse alone.
- 3-phase bone scanning has varying sensitivity but is most accurate for support of the diagnosis when there is diffuse activity (especially on phase 3).
- Bone density

Diagnostic Procedures/Other

- Electromyelography (EMG) shows nerve injury with type II CRPS.
- Sudomotor function testing (resting sweat testing, resting skin temperature, quantitative sudomotor axon reflex testing; all related to increased autonomic activity of the affected limb)

Test Interpretation

- Partial or complete damage to afferent nerve pathways and probably reorganized central pain pathways
- Nerves most commonly involved are median and sciatic.
- Atrophy in affected muscles
- Incomplete nerve plexus lesion

 TREATMENT

GENERAL MEASURES

Discourage maladaptive behaviors (pain-medication seeking, secondary gain).

MEDICATION

First Line

- No single drug or combination of drugs has produced consistent results; early therapy is crucial. There is no scientific support for the use of narcotic pain relievers, and this approach should be avoided.

- The following have literature support of either limited or suggestive benefit in treatment of CRPS-I (1)[A]:
  - Gabapentin 600–1,800 mg q24h for 8 weeks following diagnosis
  - 50% DMSO cream applied to affected extremity up to 5 times daily
  - N-acetylcysteine 600 mg t.i.d.
  - Bisphosphonates (alendronate) at 40 mg/d (however, optimal dose uncertain)
  - Nifedipine 20 mg/d showed benefit early in the course of the condition.
  - Corticosteroids seemed to be beneficial, but dosing is uncertain. Prednisone 30 mg/d for 2–3 weeks with a tapering dose over the following 2–4 weeks has been used.

- Although many have advocated the use of tricyclic antidepressants in the treatment of CRPS, there is no credible evidence of improvement of pain. They may be helpful in controlling depressive symptoms that develop with disease progression.
- No evidence currently exists that supports the use of oral muscle relaxants (1)[A].

Second Line
A number of small randomized controlled trials, clinical research, and observational studies show significant reduction in symptoms with the use of short courses (~1 week) of IV (and topical) ketamine (2)[B].

ISSUES FOR REFERRAL
- After 2 months of the illness, psychological evaluation generally is indicated to identify and treat any comorbid conditions.
- Identifying local resources and early referral for expert management give increased likelihood of long-term success in controlling condition.

ADDITIONAL THERAPIES
Type I:
- Physical and occupational therapy (beneficial to the overall prognosis for recovery):
  - Should be started early
  - "Mirror therapy" has shown good results (3)[A].
- Transcutaneous nerve stimulation
- Psychotherapy

SURGERY/OTHER PROCEDURES
- Type II responds more favorably to nerve-directed treatment:
  - Sympathetic blocks
  - Cervicothoracic or lumbar sympathectomies have little data to support their use and should be used judiciously and after all other therapies have failed (4)[A].
- Anesthetic blockade (chemical or surgical) of sympathetic nerve function:
  - Transient relief suggests that chemical or surgical sympathectomy will be helpful.
  - Little in the way of quality clinical trials exist to support local sympathetic blockage as the gold standard of therapy.
- IV regional sympathetic block with guanethidine or reserpine by pain specialist or anesthetist
- Transcutaneous electric nerve stimulation (controversial)

- Inject myofascial painful trigger points
- Spinal cord stimulation (quality of life improved only with implanted system)
- Intrathecal analgesia
- Amputation as a last resort in severe cases, with patients reporting improved quality of life

COMPLEMENTARY AND ALTERNATIVE MEDICINE
- Vitamin C (500 mg/d) may help to prevent CRPS in those with wrist fracture.
- Briskly rub the affected part several times per day
- Acupuncture
- Hypnosis can be suggested
- Relaxation training (alternate muscle relaxing and contracting)
- Biofeedback

IN-PATIENT CONSIDERATIONS
Admission Criteria/Initial Stabilization
Only for proposed surgical therapy

 ## ONGOING CARE

FOLLOW-UP RECOMMENDATIONS
Weekly, to monitor progress and initiate additional modalities as needed

PATIENT EDUCATION
- Stress need to remain active physically
- Instruct carefully about any prescribed medications
- Reflex Sympathetic Dystrophy Syndrome Association, www.rsds.org, 203-877-3790
- American RSD Hope Group, www.rsdhope.org, 207-583-4589

PROGNOSIS
Most improve with early treatment, but symptoms may be lifelong if there is limited response to initial treatments.

COMPLICATIONS
- Depression
- Disability
- Opioid dependence

REFERENCES
1. Perez RS, Zollinger PE, Dijkstra PU, et al. Evidence based guidelines for complex regional pain syndrome type I. *BMC Neurol*. 2010;10:20.
2. Azari P, Lindsay DR, Briones D, et al. Efficacy and safety of ketamine in patients with complex regional pain syndrome: A systematic review. *CNS Drugs*. 2012;26:215–228.
3. Ezendam D, Bongers RM, Jannink MJ, et al. Systematic review of the effectiveness of mirror therapy in upper extremity function. *Disabil Rehabil*. 2009;31:2135–2149.
4. Straube S, Derry S, Moore RA, et al. Cervical-thoracic or lumbar sympathectomy for neuropathic pain and complex regional pain syndrome. *Cochran Database Syst Rev*. 2010;7:CD002918.

ADDITIONAL READING
- Goebel A. Complex regional pain syndrome in adults. *Rheumatology*. 2011;50:1739–1750.
- Tran De QH, Duong S, Bertini P, et al. Treatment of complex regional pain syndrome: A review of the evidence. *Can J Anaesth*. 2010;57:149–166.

 ## SEE ALSO

Algorithm: Pain in Upper Extremity

 ## CODES

ICD10
- G90.50 Complex regional pain syndrome I, unspecified
- G90.519 Complex regional pain syndrome I of unspecified upper limb
- G90.529 Complex regional pain syndrome I of unspecified lower limb

CLINICAL PEARLS
- A pain syndrome after injury to bone and soft tissue.
- Pain control and early mobility are key to recovery.
- Avoid use of opiate analgesics.
- Use a multidisciplinary approach.

CONCUSSION (MILD TRAUMATIC BRAIN INJURY)

Christie Langenberg, MD • J. Herbert Stevenson, MD

BASICS

DESCRIPTION
- Concussion (or mild traumatic brain injury [mTBI]), is defined as a complex pathophysiologic process affecting the brain, induced by traumatic biomechanical forces. This can be caused by a direct blow to the head or indirectly anywhere on the body where impulsive force is then transmitted to the head (1)[C].
- Concussion may or may not involve loss of consciousness; headache, dizziness, and confusion are identified as the most common complaints. There is currently no widely accepted classification system for concussions.

Pediatric Considerations
Resolution of symptoms and return to neurocognitive baseline often take longer in pediatric and adolescent athletes (<18 years) (2)[C].

EPIDEMIOLOGY
- The CDC estimates 1.6–3.8 million concussions every year, although many go unreported (3)[C].
- >1 million ER visits every year are due to TBIs (falls, MVAs, assault, sports, other) (3)[C]:
  - >1/2 of these visits are by children 5–18 years
- High school and college athlete concussion rates have increased in the past 30 years, likely in part due to increased reporting (3)[C].
- American football is associated with the highest number of TBIs.
- Concussions occur more often in games than practices (3)[C].
- Female athletes have more reported concussions than male athletes and more frequently suffer cognitive impairment (3)[C].

Incidence
- The most common cause of TBI in the elderly (>65) is falls.
- Up to 1/3 of all sport-related concussions may go unreported or undiagnosed (4)[C]
- Sports:
  - Football: College 0.61 per 1,000 (0.39 per 1,000 in practice, 3.02 in games), high school 0.47 per 1,000 (0.21 per 1,000 in practice, 1.55 per 1,000 in games) (3)[C]
  - Basketball: College males 0.16 per 1,000; college females 0.22 per 1,000 (3)[C]
  - Hockey: Ice 3.9%, field 1.4%. college males 0.41 per 1,000, college females 0.91 per 1,
  - Lacrosse: College males 0.26 per 1,000, college females 0.25 per 1,000 (3)[C]
  - Soccer: College males 0.49 per 1,000, high school males 0.22 per 1,000, college females 0.63 per 1,000, high school females 0.36 per 1,000 (3)[C].
  - Skiing and snowboarding: 0.005 per 1,000 and 0.004 per 1,000, respectively. Snowboarders have a higher incidence of severe brain injuries than skiers (3)[C].

ETIOLOGY AND PATHOPHYSIOLOGY
- Structural abnormalities of the brain are typically absent based on imaging studies (5)[C].
- Identifiable metabolic changes include alterations in intra-/extracellular potassium, calcium, and glutamate with subsequent neuron dysfunction. Micro-tearing of cerebral blood vessels and a

relative decrease in cerebral blood flow also occurs. An increased requirement for glucose by the brain, coupled with decreased blood flow, may result in cellular dysfunction and increased susceptibility to subsequent brain insults (1)[C]. Other biochemical changes are currently being studied (6)[C].
- Direct or indirect injury to the head:
  - Falls
  - Sports-related injuries
  - Motor vehicle accidents

RISK FACTORS
- Patients at high risk for falls, elderly
- History of previous concussion
- Contact sports (particularly football) and activities such as bicycling, cheerleading, skiing, and snowboarding

GENERAL PREVENTION
- Educate athletes, coaches, parents, and officials about signs and symptoms of concussions
- Pre-participation exams to identify risk factors in athletes
- Strength and conditioning (athletes and elderly)
- Rule enforcement in sports (e.g., penalties for spearing or head-to-head contact) and teaching athletes correct sport-specific techniques
- Protective equipment, such as helmets and mouth guards, decrease injuries but have not been shown to decrease concussion rates.

DIAGNOSIS

HISTORY
- Cognitive signs and symptoms:
  - Confusion
  - Posttraumatic amnesia (PTA)
  - Retrograde amnesia (RGA)
  - Loss of consciousness (LOC)
  - Disorientation
  - Feeling "in a fog," "zoned out"
  - Inability to focus (i.e., difficulty at work or school)
  - Delayed verbal and motor responses
  - Slurred/Incoherent speech
  - Excessive drowsiness
- Physical signs and symptoms:
  - Headache
  - Fatigue
  - Disequilibrium, dizziness
  - Visual disturbances
  - Phonophobia
  - Nausea
- Emotional signs and symptoms:
  - Emotional lability
  - Irritability
  - Personality changes
- Sleep disturbance

PHYSICAL EXAM
Variable and dependent on acuteness of assessment, degree of injury:
- ABCs
- Evaluate for C-spine stability and possible serious head injury.
- Assess for focal neurologic signs and symptoms.
- Thorough neurologic exam, including:
  - State of alertness and orientation
  - Cranial nerves

  - 3- or 5-word recall at 5 minutes
  - Concentration/Attention (serial 3s or 7s)
  - Cerebellar function (finger-to-nose, gait assessment) and postural stability assessment (Romberg test, single leg balance)
  - Deep tendon reflexes
  - Extremity strength

DIFFERENTIAL DIAGNOSIS
- Subdural hematoma
- Epidural hematoma
- Cerebral contusion
- Facial or skull fracture
- Seizure

DIAGNOSTIC TESTS & INTERPRETATION
- Serial cognitive and neurologic evaluations should be done by an experienced healthcare provider. Other assessment tools, such as the sport concussion assessment tool (SCAT-3), can also be used. However, if baseline testing has not been done, assessment tools may not be helpful because a perfect baseline score cannot be assumed, particularly in adolescents (7,8)[C].
- SCAT-3 testing is appropriate for patients >13 (6)[C].
- The gold standard is a thorough evaluation and individualized treatment by a trained physician. Studies have not yet validated computerized testing as either improving outcomes or being cost effective.

Initial Tests (lab, imaging)
- C-spine with severe TBI. However, structural neuroimaging is usually normal in the setting of concussion (1,6)[C].
- MRI or CT is indicated with LOC, amnesia, focal neurologic deficit, >60–65, coagulopathy, GCS score <15, seizure, evidence of skull fracture, or overall worsening symptoms.

Diagnostic Procedures/Other
- Monitoring for several hours after injury is paramount, as signs and symptoms may worsen.
- EEG testing is not commonly used; however, in studies, electrophysiological abnormalities have been identified in concussed athletes for days after injury (5)[B].

TREATMENT

GENERAL MEASURES
- There are no specific treatments for concussion. Physical and cognitive rest are the most important factors in initial management (6)[C].
- Sunglasses, ear plugs if needed
- Consider no texting, video games, school, work, play, exercise, or sexual activity until symptoms begin to improve.
- A graded, individualized return to play plan can be initiated after complete resolution of all signs and symptoms (see "Follow-Up").

MEDICATION
- Ibuprofen or acetaminophen may be used for headache once structural brain injury ruled out.
- Prolonged symptoms such as sleep disturbance, depression, or anxiety may benefit from appropriate pharmacologic treatment for symptom relief (i.e., SSRIs, amitriptyline, etc.).

ISSUES FOR REFERRAL

- Most concussions can be managed by primary care physicians; referral to a specialist is not mandatory.
- Patients with prolonged signs and symptoms of concussion, or who have suffered recurrent concussions, should be referred to a sports medicine physician or neurologist for management and clearance prior to returning to sports activities.

SURGERY/OTHER PROCEDURES

Not indicated, unless signs of more severe TBI are present with increased intracranial pressure or large bleed.

IN-PATIENT CONSIDERATIONS

Admission Criteria/Initial Stabilization

- Progressive neurologic symptoms, including deterioration of mental status, seizures, and focal neurologic signs
- No competent adult at home
- ABCs take priority over head injury and concussion.
- C-spine immobilization should be considered in all head trauma.

Discharge Criteria

- Improving mental status at or near baseline
- Competent adult at home for patient observation

 ONGOING CARE

FOLLOW-UP RECOMMENDATIONS

- Any athlete with a suspected concussion should not be allowed to return to play on the same day.
- Return to play guidelines: Decisions for athletes should be individualized, graded, and not made without follow-up evaluation(s). This includes:
  – Complete rest until symptom-free
  – Gradual reintroduction of activity as long as symptom-free. Each step should generally be done 24 hours apart:
    ○ Light aerobic exercise
    ○ Sport-specific exercise
    ○ Noncontact training drills
    ○ Full-contact training
    ○ Game play (9)[C]
- If any signs or symptoms recur (i.e., exertional headache, visual disturbance, or disequilibrium), stop all activity until again asymptomatic for 24 hours. Restart return to play protocol at last step that the patient was asymptomatic.
- Athletes at high risk for prolonged recovery include pediatric athletes, athletes with mood disorders, learning disabilities, or migraine headaches. These athletes should have a slower return to play progression and may require more intensive evaluation (formal neuropsychologic, balance, symptom testing) (2)[C].
- Athletes with multiple concussions should have slower return to play and may benefit from sports medicine consultation or neurology referral.

Patient Monitoring

- Written instructions regarding postconcussion management should be given to a competent adult describing signs to watch for and when to bring the patient back for further evaluation.
- Have a follow-up plan prior to discharge to home, ideally to be seen within a few days.
- Instruct patients and families regarding postconcussive signs and symptoms.
- Ensure adequate cognitive and physical rest and symptom-free return to school, work, and sports-related activities.

DIET

As tolerated

COMPLICATIONS

- Delayed hematomas, including subdural hematomas, can present minutes to hours after initial injury, necessitating serial neurologic checks and close observation.
- 2nd-impact syndrome describes rare but life-threatening cerebral edema that occurs after repeated head injury, before the brain has had adequate time to completely recover (highest susceptibility within first 7–10 days of initial concussion). The etiology is thought to be due to loss of regulation of either cerebral circulation or glucose metabolism in the concussed brain.
- Postconcussion syndrome occurs when symptoms of concussion, such as headache, fatigue, memory changes, or emotional lability, are persistent and last at least 1–3 months or longer.
- Chronic traumatic encephalopathy (CTE), with chronic cognitive, mood, and potential Parkinson-type symptoms, is a distinct neurodegenerative disease that may be related to repeated concussions, although causality has not been proven (10)[C].
- Recovery can be prolonged or complicated by concussion history, persistent signs and symptoms, susceptibility, age (youths need more time to heal than adults), and pre-existing conditions (migraines, depression, ADHD, anxiety, learning disabilities) (1)[C].

REFERENCES

1. Herring SA, Cantu RC, Guskiewicz KM, et al. Concussion (mild traumatic brain injury) and the team physician: A consensus statement—2011 update. *Med Sci Sports Exerc*. 2011;43(12): 2412–2422.
2. Zuckerman SL, Odom M, Lee YM, et al. Sport-related concussion and age: Number of days to neurocognitive baseline. *Neurosurgery*. 2012;71(2):E558.
3. Daneshvar DH, Nowinski CJ, McKee AC, et al. The epidemiology of sport-related concussion. *Clin Sports Med*. 2011;30(1):1–17, vii.4,
4. Meehan WP 3rd, Mannix RC, O'Brien MJ, Collins MW. The prevalence of undiagnosed concussions in athletes. *Clin J Sport Med*. 2013 May 30. [Epub ahead of print]
5. Khurana VG, Kaye AH. An overview of concussion in sport. *J Clin Neurosci*. 2012;19(1):1–11. Epub 2011 Dec 5.
6. McCrory P, Meeuwisse W, Aubry M, et. al. Consensus statement on concussion in sport: the 4th International Conference on Concussion in Sport held in Zurich, November 2012. *Br J Sports Med*. 2013;47:250–258.
7. Jinguji TM, Bompadre V, Harmon KG, et al. Sport Concussion Assessment Tool-2: Baseline values for high school athletes. *Br J Sports Med*. 2012;46(5):365–370. Epub 2012 Jan 5.
8. Valovich McLeod TC, Bay RC, Lam KC, et al. Representative baseline values on the Sport Concussion Assessment Tool 2 (SCAT2) in adolescent athletes vary by gender, grade, and concussion history. *Am J Sports Med*. 2012;40(4):927–933. Epub 2012 Jan 11.
9. Scorza KA, Raleigh MF, O'Connor FG. Current concepts in concussion: Evaluation and management. *Am Fam Physician*. 2012;85(2): 123–132.
10. Guskiewicz KM, Marshall SW, Bailes J, et al. Association between recurrent concussion and late-life cognitive impairment in retired professional football players. *Neurosurgery*. 2005;57(4):719–726; discussion 719–726.

ADDITIONAL READING

- Almasi SJ, Wilson JJ. An update on the diagnosis and management of concussion. *WMJ*. 2012;111(1): 21–27; quiz 28.
- Grady MF. Concussion in the adolescent athlete. *Curr Probl Pediatr Adolesc Health Care*. 2010;40(7): 154–169.
- Halstead ME, Walter KD, Council on Sports Medicine and Fitness. American Academy of Pediatrics. Clinical report—sport-related concussion in children and adolescents. *Pediatrics*. 2010;126(3): 597–615. Epub 2010 Aug 30.

 SEE ALSO

Brain Injury, Post Acute Care Issues; Brain Injury, Traumatic; Postconcussive Syndrome; Seizure Disorders

 CODES

ICD10

- S06.0X0A Concussion without loss of consciousness, initial encounter
- S06.0X9A Concussion w loss of consciousness of unsp duration, init
- S06.9X0A Unsp intracranial injury w/o loss of consciousness, init

CLINICAL PEARLS

- Concussions occur from direct or indirect force to the head; loss of consciousness is not required.
- Monitor for several hours after concussion; frequent waking from sleep is controversial, and sleep deprivation can make symptoms worse (9)[C].
- Complete resolution of concussion symptoms most often spontaneously occurs within 7–10 days. Pediatric and adolescent populations, those with certain medical conditions, and those with a previous history of concussion, may take more time to fully recover.
- Complete cognitive and physical rest are paramount to the initial management of concussion.
- An individualized, graded return to play plan can be initiated after complete resolution of signs and symptoms of concussion. If symptoms recur during any step of the plan, the athlete should postpone activity until asymptomatic for 24 hours.

CONDYLOMATA ACUMINATA

Edward Onusko, MD

 BASICS

DESCRIPTION
- Condylomata acuminata are soft, skin-colored, fleshy lesions (commonly called genital warts) that are caused by human papillomavirus (HPV):
  – Warts appear singly or in groups (a single wart is a "condyloma"; multiple warts are "condylomas" or "condylomata"); small or large; typically appear on the anogenital skin (penis, scrotum, introitus, vulva, perianal area) but may occur in the anogenital tract (vagina, cervix, rectum, urethra, anus). Reports of conjunctival, nasal, oral, and laryngeal warts.
- System(s) affected: Skin/Exocrine; Reproductive; occasionally Respiratory

Pediatric Considerations
- Consider sexual abuse if seen in children, although children can be infected by other means (e.g., transfer from wart on another child's hand or prolonged latency period).
- American Academy of Pediatrics recommends all school-aged children who present with lesions be evaluated for abuse and screened for other STDs (1).

Pregnancy Considerations
- Warts often grow larger during pregnancy and regress spontaneously after delivery.
- Virus does not cross the placenta. Treatment during pregnancy is somewhat controversial. Cesarean section is not absolutely indicated for maternal condylomata.
- Cervical infection has been found to be a risk factor for preterm birth.
- There have been a few documented cases of laryngeal papillomas due to HPV transmission at the time of delivery. Although rare, the condition is life-threatening.
- HPV vaccination is contraindicated in pregnancy.

EPIDEMIOLOGY
- HPV types 6 and 11 associated with 90% of condylomata acuminata. Also types 16, 18, 31, 33, and 35 may be found in warts and may be associated with high-grade intraepithelial dysplasia in immunocompromised states such as HIV.
- Highly contagious; incubation period may be from 1–8 months. Initial infections may very well go unrecognized, so a "new" outbreak may be a relapse of an infection acquired years prior.
- Predominant age: 15–30 years
- Predominant sex: Male = Female
- Most infections are transient and clear spontaneously within 2 years.

Incidence
- One study population demonstrated that from 2007–2010, with the introduction of HPV vaccines, the incidence of genital warts decreased 35% (from 0.94% per year to 0.61% per year) in females <21 years, and decreased 19% in males <21 years (2).
- Increased size and number of warts in immunocompromised patients

Prevalence
- Most common viral sexually transmitted infection (STI) in the US. Most sexually active men and women will have acquired a genital HPV infection, usually asymptomatic, at some time.
- Peak prevalence in ages 17–33
- 10–20% of sexually active women may be actively infected with HPV. Studies in men suggest a similar prevalence.
- Pregnancy and immunosuppression favor recurrence and increased growth of lesions.

ETIOLOGY AND PATHOPHYSIOLOGY
HPV is a circular, double-stranded DNA molecule. There are >70 HPV subtypes. HPV types that cause genital warts do not cause anogenital cancers.

RISK FACTORS
- Usually acquired by sexual activity:
  – Young adults and adolescents
  – Multiple sexual partners; short interval between meeting new sex partner and first intercourse
  – Not using condoms
  – Young age of commencing sexual activity
  – History of other STI
- Immunosuppression (particularly HIV)

GENERAL PREVENTION
- Sexual abstinence or monogamy
- Quadrivalent HPV vaccine available against genital warts and cervical cancer. This vaccine is targeted to adolescents before the period of their greatest risk for exposure to HPV. The vaccine does not treat previous infections:
  – Immunity has been documented to last at least 5 years after HPV vaccination.
  – The HPV quadrivalent vaccine (Gardasil) protects against the 2 most common HPV serotypes (types 6 and 11, which cause most anogenital warts), and the 2 most cancer-promoting types (16 and 18) (3)[A].
  – Quadrivalent vaccine is indicated for females and males ages 9–26 (3): Vaccine is administered IM; 3 doses at 0, 2, and 6 months to achieve optimal seroconversion.
  – Vaccine efficacy for preventing external genital warts is related to age of administration of 1st dose: 76% if aged <20, 93% if <14 (4).
- Bivalent HPV vaccine is available, but does not cover the HPV types that cause most condyloma lesions (Cervarix).
- Quadrivalent vaccine has been proven effective in prevention of external lesions in males 16–26 years of age (5).
- Use of condoms is partially effective, although warts may be easily spread by lesions not covered by a condom (e.g., 40% of infected men have scrotal warts).
- Abstinence until treatment completed

COMMONLY ASSOCIATED CONDITIONS
- >90% of cervical cancer associated with HPV types 16, 18, 31, 33, and 35.
- 60% of oropharyngeal and anogenital squamous cell carcinomas are associated with HPV (6).
- STIs (e.g., gonorrhea, syphilis, chlamydia); AIDS

 DIAGNOSIS

HISTORY
- Explore sexual history, contraception use, and other lifestyle issues.
- Most warts are asymptomatic, but may cause:
  – Pruritus, burning, redness, pain, bleeding
  – Vaginal discharge
  – Large warts may cause obstructive symptoms in the anus (with defecation) or vaginal canal (with intercourse or childbirth)

PHYSICAL EXAM
- Lesions often have a typical rough, warty appearance with multiple finger-like projections; but may be soft, sessile, and smooth.
- Large lesions are cauliflower-like and may grow to >10 cm.
- Most common sites are penis, vaginal introitus, and perianal region.
- May be seen anywhere on the anogenital epithelium or in the anogenital tract.
- Warts often occur in clusters.
- Bleeding or irritation of the lesions may be noted.

DIFFERENTIAL DIAGNOSIS
- Condylomata lata (flat warts of syphilis)
- Lichen planus
- Normal sebaceous glands
- Seborrheic keratosis
- Molluscum contagiosum
- Keratomas, micropapillomatosis
- Scabies
- Crohn disease
- Skin tags
- Melanocytic nevi
- Vulvar intraepithelial neoplasia
- Squamous cell carcinoma

DIAGNOSTIC TESTS & INTERPRETATION
- Diagnosis is usually clinical, made by unaided visual examination of the lesions.
- Acetowhitening test: Subclinical lesions can be visualized by wrapping the penis with gauze soaked with 5% acetic acid (vinegar) for 5 minutes. Using a 10× hand lens or colposcope, warts appear as tiny white papules. A shiny white appearance of the skin represents foci of epithelial hyperplasia (subclinical infection), but because of low specificity, the CDC recommends against routine use of this test to screen for HPV mucosal infection (7).

Initial Tests (lab, imaging)
- Usually not required for diagnosis
- Serologic tests for syphilis may be helpful to rule out condylomata lata.
- Other testing for STIs, Pap smear may be indicated

Follow-Up Tests & Special Considerations
Because squamous cell carcinoma may resemble or coexist with condylomata, biopsy may be considered for lesions refractory to therapy.

Diagnostic Procedures/Other
- Biopsy with highly specialized identification techniques, such as HPV DNA detected through polymerase chain reaction, is rarely useful.
- Colposcopy, antroscopy, anoscopy, urethroscopy may be required to detect anogenital tract lesions.
- Screening men who have sex with men (MSM) with anal Pap smears is controversial. No generally accepted recommendation exists currently.

TREATMENT

GENERAL MEASURES
- May resolve spontaneously
- Change therapy if no improvement after 3 treatments, no complete clearance after 6 treatments, or therapy's duration or dosage exceeds manufacturer's recommendations.
- Appropriate screening/counseling of partners

MEDICATION

First Line
- No single therapy for genital warts is ideal for all patients or clearly superior to other therapies (7)[A].
- Recommendations for external genital warts, patient-applied (7):
  - Podofilox (Condylox): Antimitotic action; apply 0.5% solution or gel to warts q12h (allowing to dry) for 3 consecutive days at home. May repeat after 4 days, up to 4 total cycles. Max of 0.5 mL/d or area >10 cm
  - Imiquimod (Aldara): Immune enhancer; self-treatment with a 5% cream applied overnight 3 times weekly until warts resolve for up to 16 weeks. Wash off with soap and water 6–10 hours after application (1,7). Imiquimod has been noted to weaken condoms and diaphragms; therefore, patients should refrain from sexual contact while the cream is on the skin.
  - Sinecatechin (Veregen): Immune enhancer and antioxidant, extract from green tea; apply a 0.5 cm strand of ointment 3 times daily for up to 16 weeks. Do not wash off after use.
- Recommendations for external genital warts, provider-applied (7):
  - Cryotherapy: Liquid nitrogen applied to warts for two 10-second bursts with thawing in between; usually requires 2–3 weekly sessions
  - Podophyllin 25% in tincture of benzoin. Apply directly to warts, allow to air-dry in office before coming into contact with clothes. Wash off in 1–4 hours. Repeat every 7 days in office until gone (8)[A].
  - Trichloroacetic acid (TCA): 80% solution. Apply only to warts. Use powder/talc to remove unreacted acid. Repeat in office at weekly intervals. Ideal for isolated lesions in pregnancy.
- Recommendations for exophytic cervical warts: Biopsy to exclude high-grade SIL
- Recommendations for vaginal warts: Cryotherapy or TCA
- Recommendations for urethral meatus warts: Cryotherapy or podophyllin 10–25%
- Recommendations for anal warts: Cryotherapy, TCA or surgery. Specialty consultation for intra-anal warts

Pregnancy Considerations
Recommendations for pregnancy: Cryotherapy, surgery, or TCA. Medications contraindicated in pregnancy: Podophyllin, podophyllotoxin, and interferon. SAFETY NOT ESTABLISHED IN PREGNANCY: Imiquimod and sinecatechins

Second Line
Intralesional interferon, photodynamic therapy, topical cidofovir

SURGERY/OTHER PROCEDURES
- Larger warts may require surgical excision, laser treatment, or electrocoagulation (including infrared therapy):
  - Precaution: Laser treatment may create smoke plumes that contain HPV; it is recommended that masks be worn while performing this procedure.
- Intraurethral, external (penile and perianal), anal, and oral lesions can be treated with fulgurating CO_2 laser. Oral or external penile/perianal lesions can also be treated with electrocautery or surgery.

ONGOING CARE

FOLLOW-UP RECOMMENDATIONS
No restrictions, except for sexual contact

Patient Monitoring
- Patients should be seen every 1–2 weeks until lesions resolve.
- Patients should also follow up 3 months after completion of treatment.
- Persistent warts require biopsy.
- Sexual partners require monitoring.

PATIENT EDUCATION
- Provide information on HPV, STI prevention, and condom use.
- Explain to patients that it is difficult to know how or when a person acquired an HPV infection; a diagnosis in 1 partner does not prove sexual infidelity in the other partner.
- Emphasize the need for women to follow recommendations for regular Pap smears.

PROGNOSIS
- Asymptomatic infection persists indefinitely.
- Treatment has not clearly been shown to decrease transmissible infectivity.
- Warts may clear with treatment or resolve spontaneously, but recurrences are frequent, particularly in the first 3 months, and may necessitate repeated treatments.

COMPLICATIONS
- Cervical dysplasia (probably does not occur with types 6 or 11, which cause most warts)
- Malignant change: Progression of condylomata to cancer rarely, if ever, occurs, although squamous cell carcinoma may coexist in larger warts.
- Urethral, vaginal, or anal obstruction from treatment
- The prevalence of high-grade dysplasia and cancer in anal canal is higher in HIV-positive than in HIV-negative patients, probably because of increased HPV activity.

REFERENCES

1. Culton DA, Morrell DS, Burkhart CN, et al. The management of condyloma acuminata in the pediatric population. *Pediatr Ann*. 2009;38: 368–372.
2. Bauer HM, Wright G, Chow J. Evidence of human papillomavirus vaccine effectiveness in reducing genital warts: An analysis of California public family planning administrative claims data, 2007–2010. *Am J Public Health*. 2012;102(5): 833–835. Epub 2012 Mar 15.
3. Centers for Disease Control and Prevention (CDC). FDA licensure of quadrivalent human papillomavirus vaccine (HPV4, Gardasil) for use in males and guidance from the Advisory Committee on Immunization Practices (ACIP). *MMWR Morb Mortal Wkly Rep*. 2010;59(20):630–632.
4. Leval A, Herweijer E, Ploner A, et al. Quadrivalent human papillomavirus vaccine effectiveness: A Swedish national cohort study. *J Natl Cancer Inst*. 2013;105(7):469–474.
5. Giuliano AR, Palefsky JM, Goldstone S, et al. Efficacy of quadrivalent HPV vaccine against HPV Infection and disease in males. *N Engl J Med*. 2011;364:401–411.
6. van Monsjou HS, Balm AJ, van den Brekel MM, et al. Oropharyngeal squamous cell carcinoma: A unique disease on the rise? *Oral Oncol*. 2010;46: 780–785.
7. Workowski KA, Berman S, Centers for Disease Control and Prevention (CDC). Sexually transmitted diseases treatment guidelines, 2010. *MMWR Recomm Rep*. 2010;59(RR-12):1–110.
8. Lacey CJ, Goodall RL, Tennvall GR, et al. Randomised controlled trial and economic evaluation of podophyllotoxin solution, podophyllotoxin cream, and podophyllin in the treatment of genital warts. *Sex Transm Infect*. 2003;79(4):270–275.

ADDITIONAL READING
- Gormley RH, Kovarik CL. Human papillomavirus-related genital disease in the immunocompromised host: Part I. *J Am Acad Dermatol*. 2012;66(6):867. e1–14; quiz 881–882.
- Gormley RH, Kovarik CL. Human papillomavirus-related genital disease in the immunocompromised host: Part II. *J Am Acad Dermatol*. 2012;66(6):883. e1–17; quiz 899–900.

CODES

ICD10
A63.0 Anogenital (venereal) warts

CLINICAL PEARLS
- Condylomata acuminata are soft, skin-colored, fleshy lesions caused by human papillomavirus (HPV) subtypes 6, 11, 16, 18, 31, 33, and 35.
- Quadrivalent HPV vaccine is available against genital warts and cervical cancer.
- The use of 4 HPV-specific vaccine virion protein capsids addresses the 2 most common HPV serotypes to be contracted in types 6 and 11, and the 2 most cancer-promoting types in 16 and 18 (Gardasil).
- Vaccine: 0.5 mL IM first dose and at months 2 and 6
- The majority of sexually active men and women will have acquired a genital HPV infection, usually asymptomatic, at some time.
- No single therapy for genital warts is ideal for all patients or clearly superior to other therapies.
- Quadrivalent HPV vaccine is effective in preventing HPV infection, particularly if administered prior to the onset of engaging in sexual activity. Gardasil is approved and recommended for use in males and females aged 9–26.

CONJUNCTIVITIS, ACUTE
Frances Yung-tao Wu, MD

 BASICS

DESCRIPTION
- Inflammation of the bulbar and/or palpebral conjunctiva of <4 weeks' duration
- System(s) affected: Nervous, Skin/Exocrine
- Synonym(s): Pink eye

Geriatric Considerations
Suspect autoimmune, systemic, or irritative conditions

Pediatric Considerations
- Neonatal conjunctivitis may be gonococcal, chlamydial, irritative, or related to dacryocystitis.
- Pediatric ER study; 78% positive bacterial culture, mostly *Haemophilus influenzae*; 13% no growth; other studies showed >50% adenovirus
- Children <5 years were 7× more likely to be bacterial than were older children or adults.
- Daycare regulations sometimes require any child with presumed conjunctivitis to be treated with a topical antibiotic, despite lack of evidence.

EPIDEMIOLOGY
- Predominant age:
  - Pediatric: Viral, bacterial
  - Adult: Viral, bacterial, allergic
- Predominant sex: Male = Female

Incidence
In the US: Variable, but accounts for 1–2% of all ambulatory office visits

ETIOLOGY AND PATHOPHYSIOLOGY
- Viral:
  - Adenovirus (common cold) or coxsackie (implicated in recent hemorrhagic conjunctivitis epidemics in Asia and Mideast)
  - Enterovirus (acute hemorrhagic conjunctivitis)
  - Herpes simplex
  - Herpes zoster or varicella
  - Measles, mumps, or influenza
- Bacterial:
  - *Staphylococcus aureus* or *epidermidis*
  - *Streptococcus pneumoniae*
  - *H. influenzae* (children)
  - *Pseudomonas* spp. or anaerobes (in contact lens users)
  - *Acanthamoeba* from contaminated contact lens solution may cause keratitis.
  - *Neisseria gonorrhoeae* and *meningitidis*
  - *Chlamydia trachomatis*: Gradual onset >4 weeks
- Allergic:
  - Hay fever, seasonal allergies, atopy
- Nonspecific:
  - Irritative: Topical medications, wind, dry eye, UV light exposure, smoke
  - Autoimmune: Sjögren syndrome, pemphigoid, Wegener granulomatosis
  - Rare: Rickettsial, fungal, parasitic, tuberculosis, syphilis, Kawasaki disease, chikungunya, Graves, gout, carcinoid, sarcoid, psoriasis, Stevens-Johnson, Reiter syndrome

RISK FACTORS
- History of contact with infected persons
- STD contact: Gonococcal, chlamydial, syphilis, or herpes

- Contact lenses: Pseudomonal or acanthamoeba keratitis
- Epidemic bacterial (streptococcal) conjunctivitis reported in school settings

GENERAL PREVENTION
- Wash hands frequently.
- Demonstrate eye dropper technique: Eye is closed and head back, several drops at nasal margin; open eyes to allow liquid to enter. Never touch tip of dropper to skin or eye.

COMMONLY ASSOCIATED CONDITIONS
- Viral infection (e.g., common cold)
- Possible sexually transmitted disease

 DIAGNOSIS

HISTORY

ALERT
Red flag: Any decrease in visual acuity is not consistent with conjunctivitis alone; must document normal vision for diagnosis of isolated conjunctivitis.
- Viral: Contact or travel:
  - May start with 1 eye, then both
  - If herpetic, recurrences or vesicles on skin
- Bacterial: Difficult to distinguish from viral, unless contact lens user. Assume bacterial in contact lens wearer unless cultures negative. If recent STD, suspect chlamydia or GC.
- Allergic: Itching, atopy, seasonal, dander
- Irritative: Feels dry, exposure to wind, tear film deficit may persist 30 days after acute conjunctivitis, chemicals, or drug: Atropine, aminoglycosides, iodide, phenylephrine, antivirals, bisphosphonates, retinoids, topiramate, chamomile, COX-2 inhibitors
- Foreign body: Redness may persist 24 hours after removal.

PHYSICAL EXAM
- General: Common to all types of conjunctivitis:
  - Red eye, conjunctival injection
  - Foreign-body sensation
  - Eyelid sticking or crusting, discharge
  - Normal visual acuity and pupillary reactivity
- Viral:
  - Palpable preauricular lymphadenopathy may be present.
  - Hemorrhagic coxsackie related epidemics reported
  - Severe viral: Herpes simplex or zoster:
    - Burning sensation, rarely itching
    - Unilateral, herpetic skin vesicles in herpes zoster
    - Palpable preauricular edema
- Bacterial (non-STD): May be epidemic:
  - Mild pruritus, discharge mild to heavy
  - Conjunctival chemosis/edema
  - If contact lens user, must rule out pseudomonal (or other bacterial) keratitis
- Bacterial: Gonococcal (or meningococcal) hyperacute infection:
  - Rapid onset 12–24 hours
  - Severe purulent discharge
  - Chemosis/Conjunctival/Lid edema
  - Rapid growth of superior corneal ulceration
  - Preauricular adenopathy
  - Signs of STDs (chlamydia, GC, HIV, etc.)

- Allergic:
  - Itching predominant
  - Seasonal or dander allergies
  - Chemosis/Conjunctival/Eyelid edema
- Nonspecific irritative:
  - Dry eyes, intermittent redness, chemical/drug exposure
  - Foreign body: May have redness and discharge 24 hours after removal
- Must document normal visual acuity
- Cornea should be clear and without fluorescein uptake. Cloudy or ulcerated signifies keratitis; consult ophthalmologist.
- Recommend fluorescein exam: Evert lid to inspect for foreign bodies.
- Skin: Look for herpetic vesicles, nits on lashes (lice), scaliness (seborrhea), or styes.
- Limbal flush at corneal margin if uveitis
- If pupil is irregular (i.e., penetrating foreign body), emergent referral is warranted.
- Discharge but no conjunctival injection: Blepharitis

DIFFERENTIAL DIAGNOSIS
- Uveitis (iritis, iridocyclitis, choroiditis): Limbal flush (red band at corneal margin), hazy anterior chamber, and decreased visual acuity
- Penetrating ocular trauma: Emergently hospitalize
- Acute glaucoma (emergency): Headache, corneal clouding, poor visual acuity
- Corneal ulcer(s) or foreign body: Lesions on fluorescein exam
- Dacryocystitis: Tenderness and swelling over tear sac (below medial canthus)
- Scleritis and episcleritis: Red injected vessels radially oriented, sectoral (pie wedge), nodularity of sclera
- Pingueculitis: Inflammation of a yellow nodular or wedge-like area of chronic conjunctival degeneration (pinguecula)
- Ophthalmia neonatorum: Neonates in first 2 days of life (gonococcal; 5–12 days of life): Chlamydial, HSV, very rare *N. meningitidis*. Consider specialty consultation for required systemic therapy.
- Blepharitis: Lid margins inflamed and producing itching, scale, or discharge, but no conjunctival injection.

DIAGNOSTIC TESTS & INTERPRETATION
- Usually not needed initially for the most common causes
- Culture swab if STD suspected, very severe symptoms, or patient is a contact lens user.
- Viral swab for detection of adenovirus not yet in common use

Diagnostic Procedures/Other
- Fluorescein exam for ulcer or abrasion on cornea
- Small superficial foreign bodies may be removed with irrigation or moistened swab.

 TREATMENT

GENERAL MEASURES
- Appropriate health care: Outpatient
- Cleanse eyelid with wet cloth up to q.i.d.
- Stop use of contact lenses while red.
- Patching of eye is not beneficial.
- Avoid irritants such as smoke, wind, and sun.

MEDICATION
First Line
- Viral (nonherpetic):
  - Artificial tears for symptomatic relief
  - Vasoconstrictor/antihistamine (e.g., naphazoline/ pheniramine) q.i.d. for severe itching
  - May consider topical antibiotic (see bacterial below) if return to daycare requires treatment (1)[C]
  - Viral (herpetic) (by ophthalmologist): Ganciclovir gel: 0.15%, 5×/d for 7d (2)[C]
  - Acyclovir PO: 400 mg 5× day for herpes simplex virus (HSV) (800 mg for zoster) × 7 days
- Bacterial (non-STI):
  - Bacitracin ophthalmic ointment: Apply b.i.d. for 5 days
  - Erythromycin ophthalmic ointment: 1/2 inch b.i.d.–q.i.d. for 5 days
  - Sodium sulfacetamide (10% solution) (Bleph-10): 2 drops q4h (while awake) for 5 days
  - Tobramycin or gentamicin: 0.3% ophthalmic drops/ointment q4h (drops) to q8h (ointment)
  - Many others are approved (fluoroquinolones), but these are not recommended for children unless no alternative is available (3)[A].
- Bacterial (gonococcal): (Neonates: hospitalize for IV therapy):
  - Adults, ceftriaxone: 1 g IM as single dose and topical bacitracin ophthalmic ointment 1/2 inch q.i.d. Neonates 25–50 mg/kg IV or IM, not to exceed 125 mg, as a single dose. Chlamydia in neonates requires oral erythromycin ethyl-succinate: 50 mg/kg/d divided q6h PO × 14 d, max 3 g/d (4)[A].
- Allergic and atopic (listed by approximate, increasing cost, from lowest to highest): All are efficacious, but evidence favoring 1 over another is inconclusive:
  - Ketotifen (Zaditor; Alaway and other generics OTC): 0.25% 1 drop b.i.d.
  - Cromolyn (Opticrom) 4%: q.i.d.
  - Azelastine generic 0.05%: 1 gtt b.i.d.
  - Pemirolast (Alamast) 0.1%: 1 gtt q.i.d.
  - Alcaftadine (Lastacaft) 0.25%: 1 gtt q.d. (5)[A]
  - Emedastine 0.05%: 1 drop q.i.d.
  - Epinastine (Elestat) 0.05%: b.i.d.
  - Ketorolac (Acular) 0.1%: 1 drop q.i.d.
  - Olopatadine (Pataday, Patanol) 0.1%: 1 drop b.i.d. or 0.2% 1 drop daily
  - Pemirolast (Alamast) 0.1%: 1 gtt q.i.d.
  - Bepotastine (Bepreve) 1.5%: 1 gtt b.i.d.
  - Lodoxamide tromethamine (Alomide) 0.1%: 1 gtt q.i.d.
  - Nedocromil (Alocril) 2%: 1 gtt b.i.d. (5)[A]
  - Oral nonsedating antihistamines (Zyrtec [cetirizine] 10 mg/d, Allegra [fexofenadine] 60 mg b.i.d.), etc., may treat nasal symptoms but cause ocular drying (6)[A].
  - Oral antihistamine (e.g., diphenhydramine 25 mg t.i.d.) in severe cases
- Contraindications: Avoid topical steroids unless able to monitor intraocular pressure. Also case report of HSV keratitis presenting without distinguishing findings from viral conjunctivitis would discourage initial use of steroids.
- Precautions:
  - Do not allow dropper to touch the eye.
  - Vasoconstrictor/Antihistamine: Rebound vasodilation after prolonged use

Second Line
- Viral and allergic: Numerous over-the-counter products
- Bacterial: Polymyxin-gramicidin, ciprofloxacin, moxifloxacin, gatifloxin, besifloxin

ISSUES FOR REFERRAL
Any significantly decreased visual acuity, herpetic keratitis, or contact lens-related bacterial conjunctivitis warrants ophthalmologic consultation.

SURGERY/OTHER PROCEDURES
No surgery for this condition. Other eye surgeries may be delayed until resolution of this condition.

COMPLEMENTARY AND ALTERNATIVE MEDICINE
As condition is usually benign and self-limited, saline flushes and other placebos would be expected to appear to work.

IN-PATIENT CONSIDERATIONS
Acute gonococcal conjunctivitis (or very rare case of meningococcal conjunctivitis) requires inpatient treatment with ceftriaxone 50 mg/kg IV every day (pediatric), 1 g IM × 1 (adult) along with ophthalmologic consultation.

Admission Criteria/Initial Stabilization
Penetrating ocular trauma, gonococcal conjunctivitis

 ONGOING CARE

FOLLOW-UP RECOMMENDATIONS
- If not resolved within 5–7 days, alternate diagnoses should be considered or consultation obtained, although epidemic keratoconjunctivitis and other adenoviral conjunctivitis typically last 1–2 weeks.
- Children may be excluded from school until eye is no longer red, if viral or bacterial, depending on school policy. Allergic conjunctivitis should be able to return to school with doctor's note.

Patient Monitoring
Referral if worse in 24 hours

PATIENT EDUCATION
- Patients should not wear contacts until their eyes are fully healed (typically 1 week).
- Patients should discard current pair of contacts.
- Patients should discard any eye makeup that they have been using, especially mascara.
- Cool, moist compresses can ease irritation and itch.

PROGNOSIS
- Viral: 5–10 days for pharyngitis with conjunctivitis, 2 weeks with adenovirus
- Herpes simplex: 2–3 weeks
- Bacterial: Self-limited; 74–80% resolution within 7 days, whether treated or not

COMPLICATIONS
- Corneal scars with herpes simplex
- Lid scars or entropion with varicella zoster
- Corneal ulcers or perforation, very rapid with gonococcal
- Hypopyon: Pus in anterior chamber
- Chlamydial neonatal ophthalmia: Could have concomitant pneumonia
- Otitis media may follow *H. influenzae* conjunctivitis.
- The very rare *N. meningitidis* conjunctivitis may be followed by meningitis.

REFERENCES
1. Steeples L, Mercieca K. Acute conjunctivitis in primary care: Antibiotics and placebo associated with small increase in proportion cured by 7 days compared with no treatment. *Evid Based Med*. 2012;17(6):177–178.
2. Croxtall JD. Ganciclovir ophthalmic gel 0.15% in acute herpetic keratitis (dendritic ulcers). *Drugs*. 2011;71(5):603–610.
3. Bradley JS, Jackson MA. The use of systemic and topical fluoroquinolones. *Pediatrics*. 2011; 128(4):e1034–1042.
4. Mayor MT, Roett MA, Uhuhiri KA. Diagnosis and management of gonococcal infections. *Am Fam Physician*. 2012;86(10):931–938.
5. Drugs for Allergic Disorders. Treatment Guidelines. *Medl Lett*. 2013;11(129):43–52.
6. LaRosa M, Lionetti E, Reibaldi M, et al. Allergic conjunctivitis: A comprehensive review of the literature. *Ital J Pediatr*. 2013;39:18:e1–8. doi: 10.1186/1824-7288-39-18.

ADDITIONAL READING
- Chigbu DI. The management of allergic eye diseases in primary eye care. *Cont Lens Anterior Eye*. 2009;32(6):260–272.
- Jefferis J, Perera R, Everitt H, et al. Acute infective conjunctivitis in primary care: Who needs antibiotics? An individual patient data meta-analysis. *Br J Gen Pract*. 2011;61(590): e542–548.
- Richards A, Guzman-Cottrill JA. Conjunctivitis. *Pediatr Rev*. 2010;196–208.
- Sheikh A, Hurwitz B, van Schayck CP, et al. Antibiotics vs placebo for acute bacterial conjunctivitis. *Cochrane Database Syst Rev*. 2012.

 SEE ALSO

- Rhinitis, Allergic
- Algorithm: Eye Pain

 CODES

ICD10
- H10.30 Unspecified acute conjunctivitis, unspecified eye
- H10.32 Unspecified acute conjunctivitis, left eye
- H10.33 Unspecified acute conjunctivitis, bilateral

CLINICAL PEARLS
- Conjunctivitis does *not* alter visual acuity; decreased acuity or photophobia should prompt consideration of more serious ophthalmic disorders.
- Culture discharge in all *contact lens wearers*, consider referral, and remind patient to throw away current contacts and avoid contacts until eyes are fully healed.
- Antibiotic therapy is of no value in viral conjunctivitis (most cases of infectious conjunctivitis) and does not significantly alter the course of most types of bacterial conjunctivitis (therefore, it is optional in these cases).

CONSTIPATION

Robert A. Baldor, MD, FAAFP

BASICS

- A group of syndromes with similar findings that include unsatisfactory defecation characterized by infrequent stools, difficult stool passage, or both.
- Characteristics include <3 bowel movements a week, hard stools, excessive straining, prolonged time spent on the toilet, a sense of incomplete evacuation, and abdominal discomfort/bloating.

DESCRIPTION

- System(s) affected: Gastrointestinal (GI)
- Synonym(s): Obstipation

Geriatric Considerations

Increased incidence of colorectal neoplasms with age may be associated with constipation; thus, new onset of constipation after 50 years of age is considered a "red flag."

Pediatric Considerations

Consider Hirschsprung disease (absence of colonic ganglion cells): 25% of all newborn intestinal obstructions, milder cases diagnosed in older children with chronic constipation, abdominal distension, decreased growth. 5:1 Male:Female ratio. Associated with inherited conditions such as Down syndrome.

EPIDEMIOLOGY

- Predominant age: May affect all ages, but more pronounced in children and elderly
- Predominant sex: Female > Male (2:1)
- Nonwhites > Whites

Incidence

- 5 million office visits annually
- 100,000 hospitalizations

Prevalence

~15% of population affected

ETIOLOGY AND PATHOPHYSIOLOGY

- As food leaves the stomach, the ileocecal valve relaxes (gastroileal reflex) and chyme enters the colon (1–2 L/d) from the small intestine. In the colon, sodium is actively absorbed in exchange for potassium and bicarb. Water follows because of the generated osmotic gradient. Peristaltic contractions move the chyme through the colon into the rectum. The chyme is converted into feces (200–250 mL).
- Normal transit time for a meal to reach the cecum is 4 hours, and the pelvic colon 8 hours later. Transit then slows to the anus.
- Defecation follows as a reflex that can be inhibited by voluntarily contracting the external sphincter or facilitated by straining to contract the abdominal muscles while voluntarily relaxing the anal sphincter. Rectal distention initiates the defecation reflex. The urge to defecate occurs as rectal pressures increase. Distention of the stomach by food also initiates rectal contractions and a desire to defecate.
- Primary constipation:
  – Slow colonic transit time (13%)
  – Pelvic floor/anal sphincter dysfunction (25%)
  – Functional: Normal transit time and sphincter function, yet problems (bloating, abdominal discomfort, perceived difficulty going, presence of hard stools) (69%)
- Secondary constipation:
  – Irritable bowel syndrome (IBS)
  – Endocrine dysfunction (diabetes mellitus, hypothyroid)

– Metabolic disorder (increased calcium, decreased potassium)
  – Mechanical (obstruction, rectocele)
  – Pregnancy
  – Neurologic disorders (Hirschsprung, multiple sclerosis, spinal cord injuries)
- Medication effect:
  – Anticholinergic effects (antidepressants, narcotics, antipsychotics)
  – Antacids (calcium, aluminum)
  – Calcium channel blockers

Genetics

Unknown, but condition may be familial

RISK FACTORS

- Extremes of life (very young and very old)
- Polypharmacy
- Sedentary lifestyle or condition
- Improper diet and inadequate fluid intake

GENERAL PREVENTION

High-fiber diet, adequate fluids, exercise, and training to "obey the urge" to defecate are useful strategies.

COMMONLY ASSOCIATED CONDITIONS

- Debility, either general as in the aged or that imposed by specific underlying illness
- Dehydration
- Hypothyroidism
- Hypokalemia
- Hypercalcemia

DIAGNOSIS

A group of syndromes with similar findings that include unsatisfactory defecation characterized by infrequent stools, difficult stool passage, or both

ALERT

Red flags:
- New onset after age of 50
- Hematochezia/Melena
- Unintentional weight loss
- Anemia
- Neurologic defects

HISTORY

Ask about the Rome III criteria (1)[C]:
- At least 2 of the following, for 12 weeks, in the previous 6 months:
  – <3 stools/week
  – Straining at least a 1/4 of the time
  – Hard stools at least 1/4 of time
  – Need for manual assist at least 1/4 of time
  – Sense of incomplete evacuation at least 1/4 of time
  – Sense of anorectal blockade at least 1/4 of time
- Loose stools rarely seen without use of laxatives

PHYSICAL EXAM

- Digital rectal exam (masses, pain, stool, fissures, hemorrhoids, anal tone)
- Abdominal/Gynecologic exam (masses, pain)
- Neurologic exam

DIFFERENTIAL DIAGNOSIS

- Congenital:
  – Hirschsprung disease/syndrome
  – Hypoganglionosis
  – Congenital dilation of the colon
  – Small left colon syndrome

DIAGNOSTIC TESTS & INTERPRETATION

This is primarily a clinical diagnosis, as evidence to support the use of routine labs/x-rays/scoping is lacking in the workup of constipation (2)[B].

Initial Tests (lab, imaging)

Guidelines suggest CBC, glucose, TSH, calcium, and creatinine routinely and sigmoid/colonoscopy if red flags are present (3)[C].

Follow-Up Tests & Special Considerations

- If condition is refractory, pursue further testing:
  – Colonoscopy
  – Barium enema to look for obstruction and/or megarectum, megacolon, or Hirschsprung disease
- Consider further testing:
  – Measure colonic transit time by ingesting radiopaque (Sitz-Mark) markers:
  – Plain abdominal film obtained 5 days later (120 hours): Retention >20% markers indicates slow transit
  – Markers seen exclusively in distal colon/rectum suggests defecatory disorder.

Diagnostic Procedures/Other

Consider referral to evaluate defecation:
- Balloon expulsion
- Defecography using a barium paste
- Anorectal manometry with a rectal catheter

Test Interpretation

- None in common functional constipation
- Paucity or absence of intramural enteric ganglia in certain cases of congenital or acquired megacolon
- Neuromuscular abnormalities in certain cases of pseudo-obstruction

TREATMENT

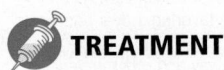

Address immediate concerns:
- If Bloating/Discomfort/Straining: Osmotic agents
- If Postop, childbirth, hemorrhoids, fissures: Stool softener to make defecation easier
- If impacted: Manual disimpaction, then treat the chronic condition

GENERAL MEASURES

- Attempt to eliminate medications that may cause or worsen constipation.
- Increase fluid intake.
- Increase fiber in diet.
- Enemas if other methods fail

MEDICATION

In patients with no known secondary causes of constipation, conservative nonpharmacologic treatment measures generally are recommended, including:
- Regular exercise
- Increased fluid intake
- Bowel habit training

First Line

Bulking agents (must be accompanied by adequate amounts of liquid to be useful):
- Hydrophilic colloids (bulk-forming agents):
  – Psyllium (Konsyl, Metamucil, Perdiem Fiber): 1 TBSP in 8 oz liquid PO daily up to t.i.d.
  – Bran methylcellulose (Citrucel): 1 TBSP in 8 oz liquid PO daily up to t.i.d.
  – Polycarbophil (Mitrolan, FiberCon): 1 g with 8 oz liquid PO up to q.i.d.

- Stool softeners:
  - Docusate sodium (Colace): 100 mg t.i.d.
- Osmotic laxatives:
  - Polyethylene glycol (MiraLax) (0.8 mg/kg/d) 17 g/d (current evidence shows PEG to be superior to lactulose) (4)[A]
  - Saccharines lactulose (Chronulac): 15–60 mL q.h.s. (flatulence, bloating, cramping)
  - Sorbitol: 15–60 mL q.h.s. (as effective as lactulose)
  - Magnesium salts (Milk of Magnesia) avoid in renal insufficiency

Second Line
- Stimulants (irritate bowel, causing muscle contraction; usually combined with a softener; work in 8–12 hours):
  - Senna/Docusate (Senokot-S, Ex-lax): 1–2 capsules or 15–30 mL at bedtime
  - Bisacodyl/Docusate (Dulcolax, Correctol): 2–3 tablets daily
  - Casanthranol/Docusate (Peri-Colace): Lubricants (contain mineral oil, coating the stool)
- Lubricants (soften stool and facilitate passage of the feces by its lubricating oily effects):
  - Mineral oil (15–45 mL/d)
  - Short-term use only. Can bind fat-soluble vitamins, with the potential for deficiencies; may similarly decrease absorption of some drugs
  - Avoid in those at risk for aspiration (lipid pneumonia).
- Suppositories:
  - Osmotic: Sodium phosphate
  - Lubricant: Glycerin
  - Stimulatory: Bisacodyl
  - Enemas: Sodium phosphate (Fleet enema)
- Lubiprostone (Amitiza): A selective chloride channel activator; 24 mcg b.i.d.:
  - Avoid in pregnancy and breastfeeding
- Methylnaltrexone (Relistor): A peripherally acting μ-opioid receptor (PAM-OR) antagonist; 12 mg SC every other day PRN:
  - Indicated for short-term(<4 months) palliative care use
  - Side effects: Abdominal pain and flatulence
- Prokinetic agents (partial 5-HT4 agonists) have been withdrawn due to cardiac side effects; only available via IND protocols: tegaserod (Zelnorm), cisapride (Propulsid).
- Other agents not approved by the FDA:
  - Misoprostol (Cytotec): A prostaglandin that increases colonic motility (5)[C]
  - Colchicine: Neurogenic stimulation to increase colonic motility (6)[C]

ADDITIONAL THERAPIES
Other nonpharmacologic therapies include (7)[C]:

- Biofeedback therapy
- Behavior therapy
- Electric stimulation

SURGERY/OTHER PROCEDURES
Surgery rarely indicated

IN-PATIENT CONSIDERATIONS
Toxic megacolon

Nursing
Manual disimpaction occasionally required in difficult chronic situations

 ## ONGOING CARE

FOLLOW-UP RECOMMENDATIONS
Encourage exercise and physical activity.

Patient Monitoring
If what seems to be simple, functional constipation persists, further investigate for a possible organic cause.

DIET
Increase fiber, but bloating and gas can be problematic:
- Gradually increase intake to 25 g/d over a 6-week period.
- Insoluble, less fermentable fiber, like wheat bran, tends to be better tolerated.
- Bran (hard outer layer of cereal grains)
- Vegetables and fruits
- Whole-grain foods
- Encourage liberal intake of fluids.

PATIENT EDUCATION
- Occasional mild constipation is normal.
- Instruction in consistent bowel training; the best time to move bowels is in the morning, after eating breakfast, when the normal bowel transit and defecation reflexes are typically functioning to move the bowels.

PROGNOSIS
- Constipation that is only occasional, brief, and responsive to simple measures is harmless.
- Habitual constipation can be a lifelong nuisance.
- Those with neurologic compromise can suffer from ill effects such as obstipation and impaction to toxic megacolon.
- No evidence for laxative dependence (8)[B]
- No evidence for harm from stimulant use; melanosis coli may develop, but it is a benign condition (8)[B].

COMPLICATIONS
- Volvulus
- Toxic megacolon
- Acquired megacolon: In severe, long-standing cases
- Fluid and electrolyte depletion: Laxative abuse
- Rectal ulceration (stercoral ulcer) related to recurrent fecal impaction
- Anal fissures

REFERENCES
1. Longstreth GF, Thompson WG, Chey WD, et al. Functional bowel disorders. *Gastroenterology*. 2006;130:1480–1491.
2. American College of Gastroenterology Chronic Constipation Task Force. An evidence-based approach to the management of chronic constipation in North America. *Am J Gastroenterol*. 2005;100(Suppl 1):S1–4.
3. Locke GR, Pemberton JH, Phillips SF. American Gastroenterological Association Medical Position Statement: Guidelines on constipation. *Gastroenterology*. 2000;119:1761–1766.
4. Lee-Robichaud H, Thomas K, Morgan J, et al. Lactulose versus polyethylene glycol for chronic constipation. *Cochrane Database Syst Rev*. 2010;7:CD007570.
5. Roarty TP, Weber F, Soykan I, et al. Misoprostol in the treatment of chronic refractory constipation: Results of a long-term open label trial. *Aliment Pharmacol Ther*. 1997;11:1059–1066.
6. Verne GN, Davis RH, Robinson ME, et al. Treatment of chronic constipation with colchicine: Randomized, double-blind, placebo-controlled, crossover trial. *Am J Gastroenterol*. 2003;98: 1112–1116.
7. van Dijk M, Benninga MA, Grootenhuis MA, et al. Chronic childhood constipation: A review of the literature and the introduction of a protocolized behavioral intervention program. *Patient Educ Couns*. 2007;67(1-2):63–77. Epub 2007 Mar 19.
8. Müller-Lissner SA, Kamm MA. Myths and misconceptions about chronic constipation. *Am J Gastroenterol*. 2005;100:232–242.

ADDITIONAL READING
- Basilisco G, Coletta M. Chronic constipation: A critical review. *Dig Liver Dis*. 2013 Apr 29. pii: S1590-8658(13)00116-3. doi: 10.1016/j.dld.2013.03.016. [Epub ahead of print]
- Bove A, Pucciani F, Bellini M, et al. Consensus statement AIGO/SICCR: Diagnosis and treatment of chronic constipation and obstructed defecation (part I: Diagnosis). *World J Gastroenterol*. 2012;18(14): 1555–1564.
- Spinzi G, Amato A, Imperiali G, et al. Constipation in the elderly: Management strategies. *Drugs Aging*. 2009;26(6):469–474.

 ## CODES

ICD10
- K59.00 Constipation, unspecified
- K59.01 Slow transit constipation
- K59.09 Other constipation

CLINICAL PEARLS
- Constipation can be characterized as unsatisfactory defecation, with infrequent stools, difficult stool passage, or both, for 3 months.
- Functional constipation (normal transit time and sphincter function) is seen most often.
- Workup is necessary in the presence of red flags: Onset >50 years, hematochezia/melena, unintentional weight loss, anemia, neurologic defects.
- Best evidence for effectiveness is for osmotic agents (polyethylene glycol [PEG]) (5)[A].

CONTRACEPTION

John Curington, MD

BASICS

DESCRIPTION
- Various methods to prevent pregnancy. These can be selected based on effectiveness, patient acceptability, STI prevention, and contraindications.
- The most effective methods of contraception are vasectomy, female sterilization, and the long-acting reversible contraceptive (LARC) methods, including the intrauterine devices and progesterone implant.

EPIDEMIOLOGY
Incidence
- 50% of all pregnancies in the US are unintended. 50% of these occur in women using a form of reversible contraception. 50% of all unintended pregnancies in the US result in termination.
- The most frequently used forms of contraception in the US (in order of prevalence) are oral contraceptive pills (OCPs), female sterilization, male condom, male sterilization, and depot injectables. Despite their proven safety, effectiveness, and cost-effectiveness, LARC methods (intrauterine devices [IUDs] and the subdermal implant) are underused in the US. Efforts to increase use of LARC remain a focus of family planning experts in the US (1).

RISK FACTORS
- Unintended pregnancy: Women ages 18–24, and 35–44 years, unmarried/cohabitating women, women with less than a college education, minority women, pregnancy ambivalence
- Contraception nonuse: Being dissatisfied with one's method of contraception, believing that contraceptive service providers were not available to answer method-related questions
- Risk of STI transmission: Reduced by condoms (both male and female), abstinence, and outercourse

DIAGNOSIS

HISTORY
Review contraindications for selected methods:
- Contraindications to estrogen-containing hormonal contraception (2):
  - History of coronary artery disease (CAD) or multiple risk factors (age >55, smoking, high BP, diabetes mellitus)
  - History of deep vein thrombosis (DVT)/pulmonary embolism (PE) or personal history of cerebrovascular accident (CVA)
  - History of migraines at age >35 or migraine at any age with aura
  - Current or past breast cancer, active liver disease, or hepatic tumor
  - Pregnancy, unexplained abnormal uterine bleeding without further investigation
  - Relative contraindication to estrogen-containing hormonal contraception: Smokers >35. Healthy nonsmokers may use oral contraceptives until menopause.
- Contraindications to IUDs (2):
  - Pregnancy, active uterine infection, malignancy in the uterus or cervix, an inability to place or retain the device, unexplained abnormal bleeding, and adverse reaction to product ingredients

DIAGNOSTIC TESTS & INTERPRETATION
- No routine testing is needed prior to initiating oral contraception except reassurance that the patient is not pregnant (by history or laboratory). Testing for gonorrhea and chlamydia may be performed, but is not required prior to IUD insertion. In high-risk populations, active infection should be ruled out prior to IUD insertion.
- If family history of thrombophilia, testing can be considered before initiation of estrogen-containing contraception, especially if specific defect is known (e.g., factor V Leiden or prothrombin 20210 mutation). In absence of known specific defect, current genetic testing not likely to be useful for patient in context of contraception.

Follow-Up Tests & Special Considerations
Routine 2–3 month follow up after initiation of all methods of contraception to assess patient tolerance and acceptability of contraceptive method. BP may be checked within 3 months of initiation in patients on combined OCPs due to the rare occurrence of hypertension in this population.

TREATMENT

The CDC issued comprehensive, highly useful guidelines in 2010 for contraception selection in patients with comorbid medical conditions (2).

GENERAL MEASURES
Nondrug methods:
- Barrier methods: Condoms (benefit: reduces risk of STIs), diaphragm (needs fitting), cervical cap (3 sizes, may cause vaginal irritation).
- Fertility awareness methods: Calendar method, cervical mucus method, temperature method. These methods are low cost, but generally not as effective as most other methods.
- Withdrawal method: Male partner withdraws from vagina before ejaculation. Failure occurs if withdrawal is not timed accurately or if the pre-ejaculatory fluid contains sperm.
- Lactational amenorrhea method: Breastfeeding is effective contraception only if (i) the infant is <6 months old, (ii) the infant is exclusively breastfeeding, and (iii) the mother has not resumed her regular menses.
- Abstinence or outercourse: Both methods avoid vaginal sex.

MEDICATION
- Oral contraceptive pills:
  - Combined estrogen/progestin pills (COCs) should be used for nonbreastfeeding patients without a contraindication to estrogen-containing contraception (see above):
    ○ Pills may be started at any time after pregnancy has been ruled out. Some providers prefer a "Sunday start" because they feel this is less confusing for patients. 1 study found better compliance at 3 months among patients assigned to start pills the day they were prescribed ("Quick start").
    ○ All COCs contain the same type of estrogen (ethinyl estradiol). COCs differ in the level of estrogen (range of 20–50 μg) and the type of progestin. Newer progestogens are less androgenic, but may have increased rate of venous thromboembolism (VTE).

○ Patient response to any 1 type of COC is unpredictable. A starting pill is one that is inexpensive (generic), contains an average amount of estrogen (30–35 μg), and contains a well-studied, lower-androgenicity progestin. Portia or Loestrin 1.5/30 are reasonable starting pills.
○ Patients should be instructed to take the pill every day and use backup birth control for the first 2 weeks after the initiation of pills. If a pill is missed, she should take 2 pills the following day. If 2 pills are missed, she should take 3 pills the following day and use a backup method for 7 days. If ≥3 pills are missed, the patient should be instructed to restart a new pack and use a backup for 2 weeks.
○ Most pills have a 21/7 regimen (21 active days and 7 placebo). Some new preparations have 24/4 combinations. It is reasonable for patients to skip the placebo pills and begin a new pack immediately on the active pill so as to avoid a period (continuous dosing). Most women require a withdrawal bleed at least 4 times a year to reduce breakthrough bleeding.
○ The most common side effects include nausea, bloating, headaches, and mastalgia. These symptoms tend to decrease over time. Nausea can be reduced by taking the pill at nighttime. Women who experience headaches can be counseled that these usually decrease over time.
  – Breastfeeding women desiring oral contraceptive medications should be prescribed progestin-only pills (e.g., Micronor), especially for the 1st months. Patients should be instructed to take these pills at the same time every day.
- Weekly hormonal patch (Ortho-Evra): The "patch" contains 20 μg ethinyl estradiol and 150 μg norelgestromin. It is applied transdermally and changed weekly. Produces higher serum estrogen levels than oral 20 μg pill and may be associated with a slightly increased risk of blood clot. Patch may cause local skin irritation. Not as reliable in women >90 kg.
- Vaginal contraceptive ring (NuvaRing): A flexible polymer ring containing 15 μg ethinyl estradiol and 120 μg etonogestrel; inserted into vagina for 3 weeks/cycle (also may be used for continuous cycling for 4 weeks, and replaced immediately with a fresh ring [off label])
- Medroxyprogesterone (Depo-Provera), also known as depot-medroxyprogesterone acetate (DMPA): 150 mg IM *or* 104 mg/0.65 mL SC, both are given every 3 months. Contraceptive levels of hormone persist for up to 4 months (2–4-week margin of safety). Major side effects include irregular bleeding and weight gain. Potential for decreased bone mineral density (BMD) if used for >2 years, so recommend that women take 1,300 mg of calcium and 400 IU of vitamin D when using DMPA (3). No evidence for increased fracture risk related to this method, and BMD recovers quickly upon discontinuation.
- IUDs: These are highly effective, long-acting reversible contraceptive methods with few side effects. 5-year failure rates are approximately 0.5%. IUD may be inserted anytime pregnancy is ruled out. May also be inserted immediately postpartum (within 10 minutes of removal of placenta) as well

as postabortion (4). IUDs are commonly used in adolescents and other nulliparous women. 3 types of IUDs are currently available in the US:

– ParaGard (Copper T): Interferes with sperm transport and ova fertilization; approved for up to 10 years, but likely remains effective for longer. May increase menstrual blood loss. Also effective as postcoital contraceptive up to 5 days from intercourse.

– Mirena (Levonorgestrel intrauterine system): A T-shaped IUD that releases 20 µg/d of levonorgestrel (very low serum levels). Approved for use up to 5 years; has been used off label for up to 7 years. Safe and effective for use in adolescents and nulliparous women. Side effects include irregular menstrual spotting for the first 3–6 months that usually resolves after 6 months of use.

– Skyla (Levonorgestrel intrauterine system): very similar to Mirena, but releases lower hormone dose (14 µg/d of levonorgestrel), is slightly smaller, and lasts 3 years. Smaller insertion tube might make this an easier IUD for nulliparous women.

• Etonogestrel implant (Nexplanon): A small, single, plastic rod that is implanted into the superficial SC tissue of the upper arm and provides continuous contraception via progestin hormone. This prevents ovulation and thickens cervical mucus to halt fertilization. Effective for up to 3 years. The device may be inserted only by trained and certified providers. Menstrual irregularities are common the first 6–12 months (and beyond); some will not have menses after 1 year, although others may have continuing irregular spotting for years.

• Spermicides: All contain nonoxynol-9; may alter vaginal flora and mucosal barrier.

• Sponge (Today Sponge): Soft foam disk contains nonoxynol-9. Moisten with water before use; effective for 24 hours; leave in for 6 hours after use; less effective in women who have given birth.

• Emergency contraception: Start within 72 hours for maximum effectiveness, but evidence supports up to 120 hours:

– Levonorgestrel: 1.5 mg taken as two 0.75-mg tablets (Plan B) or one 1.5-mg tablet (Plan B 1-Step). Less nausea and slightly more effective than the "Yuzpe regimen" (see below) (5)[A]: Available over the counter, but may be less expensive for many women if prescribed. Prescription is needed for women under age 17.

– Estradiol/Levonorgestrel (Preven, Ovral, Ogestrel): "Yuzpe regimen" 50 µg/0.25 mg, 2 tablets q12h (4 tablets total). Other OCs may be used as long as the dose of estrogen component ≥100 µg/dose. *Note:* Antinausea medication (e.g., Phenergan) should be given 1–2 hours before the doses.

– Copper-bearing IUD (Paragard): Insert up to 5 days after intercourse; >99% effective in preventing pregnancy and continues to provide contraception for up to 10 years.

– Ulipristal acetate (Ella): 30 mg; approved by FDA in 2010. Selective progesterone modulator, approved for use up to 5 days following unprotected intercourse.

SURGERY/OTHER PROCEDURES
Permanent sterilization. Female: Tubal ligation or Essure (fallopian tube inserts placed hysteroscopically). Essure requires confirmation with hysterosalpingogram 3 months after procedure. Male: Vasectomy. Male sterilization less complicated than female.

 ONGOING CARE

FOLLOW-UP RECOMMENDATIONS
Patient Monitoring
• Pelvic exam, Pap smear, and STI testing, per guidelines
• Check for IUD strings 1 month after insertion. Spontaneous expulsion rate highest in 1st month. The patient should monitor presence of the string monthly following menses.
• OC users: Monitor BP at least annually.

DIET
Some herbals, such as St. John's wort, may alter estrogen levels, reducing efficacy or causing breakthrough bleeding.

PATIENT EDUCATION
• Condoms: Water-based lubricants (inside and outside) reduce the risk of breakage. Withdraw penis before it becomes flaccid. New condom is required for each sex act. Male condoms available in both latex and nonlatex (if allergic to latex).
• IUD: Check string periodically.
• Diaphragm: Refit after childbirth or if weight changes by >10%. Before inserting, 1 tbs of water-soluble spermicidal jelly or cream should be placed in the dome. Leave in at least 6 hours after coitus. If coitus is repeated <6 hours, insert another teaspoon of spermicidal jelly into the vagina without removing the diaphragm.
• OCP: Pill should be taken at approximately the same time each day. If a pill is missed, see above instructions.
• Emergency contraception prevents pregnancy via several proposed mechanisms, including inhibition of sperm motility, alterations in tubal transport, unfavorable uterine receptivity, and/or fertilization inhibition. Emergency contraception does not affect an established pregnancy: 1-888-NOT-2-LATE or www.planbonestep.com/

COMPLICATIONS
• Hormonal contraceptives, serious: Stroke, thromboembolism, hypertension, myocardial infarction
• Hormonal contraceptives, minor: Nausea and vomiting: Take after eating. Breakthrough bleeding: Usually self-limiting after 3 months; if persists, change pill. Amenorrhea: Pregnancy must be ruled out. Cyclic weight gain: Use smallest dose of estrogen available. Breast tenderness: Rare with low-dose pill. Depression: Rare with low-dose pill. Chloasma: Stop pill or cover with makeup. Acne or hirsutism: Change to a less-androgenic progesterone. Cholestatic jaundice: Stop pill; do not restart. Weight gain throughout cycle: Use triphasic pill to minimize dose of progesterone or use newer progesterone.
• Injectable contraceptive (Depo-Provera): Irregular bleeding: No treatment needed; NSAID may help. Weight gain: Average of 5 lbs/yr of use. Amenorrhea: Common after 1 year of use. Possible ↑ bone resorption and ↓ bone mineral density, but rapid recovery following discontinuation. FDA recommends bone mineral density for use >2 years and to consider periodic estrogen.
• Progesterone implant: Irregular bleeding: Counsel patients extensively prior to insertion.
• Sponge and diaphragm: Associated with toxic shock syndrome (rare)

• IUD: Pelvic inflammatory disease (PID) or salpingitis: Device removal is not necessary for mild PID treated as outpatient. For infections requiring hospitalization: Remove device. For heavy bleeding and cramps: Trial of combined oral contraceptives, consider removing device. Although absolute risk less than without IUD, pregnancy, when it occurs, is more likely to be ectopic.

REFERENCES

1. Blumenthal PD, Voedisch A, Gemzell-Danielsson K, et al. Strategies to prevent unintended pregnancy: Increasing use of long-acting reversible contraception. *Hum Reprod Update.* 2011;17: 121–137.
2. Division of Reproductive Health, National Center for Chronic Disease Prevention and Health Promotion, Centers for Disease Control and Prevention (CDC), et al. US medical eligibility criteria for contraceptive use, 2010: Adapted from the WHO Medical Eligibility Criteria for Contraceptive Use, 4th ed. *MMWR Recomm Rep.* 2010;59:1–86. Available at: www.cdc.gov/mmwr/pdf/rr/rr59e0528.pdf.
3. Schrager SB. DMPA's effect on bone mineral density: A particular concern for adolescents. *J Fam Pract.* 2009;58:E1–E8.
4. Shimoni N. Intrauterine contraceptives: A review of uses, side effects and candidates. *Semin Reprod Med.* 2010;28:118–125.
5. Cheng L, Gülmezoglu AM, Piaggio G. Interventions for emergency contraception. *Cochrane Database Syst Rev.* 2008;3:CD001324.

ADDITIONAL READING
• For CDC summary chart of eligibility criteria for contraception, see www.cdc.gov/reproductivehealth/unintendedpregnancy/USMEC.htm
• For excellent chart to compare contraceptive methods, ARHP Method Match at www.arhp.org/methodmatch

 CODES

ICD10
• Z30.9 Encounter for contraceptive management, unspecified
• Z30.41 Encounter for surveillance of contraceptive pills
• Z30.431 Encounter for routine checking of intrauterine contracep dev

CLINICAL PEARLS
• Hormonal and IUD contraceptives may be initiated immediately ("Quick start") if the likelihood of pre-existing pregnancy is low.
• Clearly established noncontraceptive benefits of OCPs include reduction in ovarian cancer, endometrial cancer, ectopic pregnancies, and PID; less dysmenorrhea and anemia; reduced number of functional ovarian cysts, a regular menstrual cycle; improvement in acne.
• LARC methods provide high efficacy and convenience for patients.

COR PULMONALE
Parag Goyal, MD • Sergey Gurevich, MD • James Horowitz, MD

 BASICS

DESCRIPTION
- Enlargement and subsequent dysfunction and failure of the right ventricle (RV) in the presence of pulmonary hypertension secondary to abnormalities of the pulmonary system, including disorders of the lung parenchyma, pulmonary circulation, chest wall, and ventilatory mechanisms.
- For the purposes of this review, pulmonary arterial hypertension (WHO Group I) will not be considered as a cause of cor pulmonale.
- May occur in acute or chronic setting:
  - Acute: Rapid increase of pulmonary arterial pressure resulting in RV overload, dysfunction, and potential cardiovascular collapse.
  - Chronic: Progressive hypertrophy and dilation of the RV over months to years, leading to dysfunction and potentially failure

EPIDEMIOLOGY
- ~6–7% of all types of adult heart disease in US
- Estimated 10–30% of heart failure admissions in the US are the result of cor pulmonale, most commonly related to chronic obstructive pulmonary disease (COPD)

Incidence
Difficult to assess: Best estimate is 1/10,000–3/10,000/year (1).

Prevalence
Difficult to assess: Best estimate is 2/1,000–6/1,000 (1).

ETIOLOGY AND PATHOPHYSIOLOGY
- Acute: A sudden event, such as large pulmonary embolism (PE), increases resistance to blood flow in the pulmonary vasculature, causing a quick and significant increase of pressure proximally. The RV is unable to overcome this pressure, leading to low RV cardiac output, which ultimately leads to low left ventricle (LV) cardiac output. Increased RV pressures in conjunction with a low cardiac output may cause coronary ischemia, further impairing cardiac output and potentially causing complete cardiovascular collapse.
- Chronic: A disorder of the pulmonary system causing chronic hypoxia leads to vasoconstriction of the pulmonary vasculature. Over time, the pulmonary vasculature hypertrophies and the intrinsic vasodilatory mechanisms (mediated by nitric oxide) become dysregulated, leading to increases in pulmonary vasculature resistance. The resulting pulmonary hypertension (WHO Group III) transmits increased pressures and volumes to the thin-walled low-pressure RV, causing maladaptive remodeling (concentric hypertrophy, followed by eccentric dilation frequently with associated tricuspid regurgitation) and subsequent impairment in RV systolic and diastolic function.

 PD5-

- Pulmonary disorders:
  - Lung parenchymal disease: COPD (most common), interstitial lung disease
  - Pulmonary circulation: Thromboembolic disease (associated with pulmonary hypertension WHO Group IV)
  - Chest wall: Severe obesity, kyphoscoliosis

- Ventilation: Obstructive sleep apnea and obesity hypoventilatory syndrome, neuromuscular diseases such as Guillain-Barré syndrome, muscular dystrophy, myasthenia gravis, spinal cord injuries)
- LV failure is not considered a cause of cor pulmonale.

RISK FACTORS
- Acute cor pulmonale (most commonly caused by PE):
  - Risk factors associated with PE:
    - Vessel injury
    - Stasis
    - Hypercoagulable states
- Chronic cor pulmonale (most commonly caused by underlying pulmonary disorder):
  - Risk factors associated with pulmonary disorders:
    - Tobacco use (COPD)
    - Occupational exposures (interstitial lung disease)
    - Hypercoagulable state (chronic thrombo-embolic disease)
    - Obesity, age (chest wall abnormalities)

GENERAL PREVENTION
Management of underlying pulmonary disorder, including aggressive correction of hypoxia and acidosis, which may contribute to worsening pulmonary hypertension

COMMONLY ASSOCIATED CONDITIONS
Pulmonary hypertension, defined as the presence of a resting mean pulmonary artery pressure (PAP) >25 mm Hg.

 DIAGNOSIS

HISTORY
- Dyspnea is most common symptom, though nonspecific; may be present at rest, with exertion, or occur as paroxysmal nocturnal dyspnea
- Other pulmonary symptoms: Pleuritic chest pain, cough, hemoptysis
- General heart failure symptoms: Fatigue, lethargy, syncope, exertional angina less likely
- Right-sided heart failure symptoms: Anorexia, early satiety, right upper quadrant discomfort from hepatic congestion, lower extremity edema
- Hoarseness secondary to compression of the left recurrent laryngeal nerve by enlarged pulmonary vessels
- Cardiovascular collapse, shock, and/or cardiac arrest may occur in acute or advanced chronic setting.

PHYSICAL EXAM
- Peripheral edema is the most common sign of right-sided heart failure, although it is nonspecific.
- General: Pallor, diaphoresis, cyanosis, tachypnea
- Neck: Jugular venous distension, with prominent *a*-wave
- Lungs: tachypnea, wheezing
- Heart:
  - Increased intensity of pulmonic component of second heart sound (P_2)
  - Splitting of S_2 over the cardiac apex with inspiration
  - Audible right-sided S_3 or S_4
  - Jugular venous pressure (JVD), with prominent v-wave
  - RV heave

- Pansystolic murmur heard best at right midsternal border increasing with inspiration, consistent with tricuspid regurgitation (typically a late sign)
  - Early diastolic murmur heard best at left upper sternal border, consistent with pulmonary regurgitation
- Abdomen: Hepatomegaly
- Extremities: Clubbing, bilateral lower extremity edema, also signs of deep vein thrombosis (DVT) such as tenderness or unilateral swelling

DIFFERENTIAL DIAGNOSIS
- Other causes of right-sided failure:
  - Left-sided heart failure (WHO Group II)
  - WHO Groups I and V pulmonary hypertension
  - Right-sided cardiomyopathy

DIAGNOSTIC TESTS & INTERPRETATION
- 2D echocardiogram:
  - Initial diagnostic test of choice
  - Elevated pulmonary artery pressure (limited in the absence of tricuspid regurgitation)
  - Right ventricular hypertrophy
  - Bulging of the interventricular septum into the left ventricle with systole
  - Flattening of the interventricular or interatrial septum
  - Dilation and hypokinesis of the right ventricle
  - Tricuspid regurgitation
  - Dilation of the right atrium
  - Acute thromboembolic pulmonary disease as evidenced by right ventricular hypokinesis with sparing of the apex (McConnell sign)
  - Echocardiography can over- or underestimate the PAP depending on image quality, operator. PAP should therefore be verified by catheter.
- MRI:
  - If echocardiography is inconclusive or as a substitute
  - Most accurate modality for diagnosing emphysema and interstitial lung disease
  - Can assess pressures, size, function, myocardial mass and viability
  - Despite being superior to echocardiogram, diagnosis of cor pulmonale still requires assessment via catheterization.
- Right heart catheterization:
  - Gold standard for diagnosis of cor pulmonale
  - Elevated central venous pressure (CVP)
  - Mean pulmonary artery pressure >25 mm Hg at rest
  - Absence of left heart failure (pulmonary capillary wedge pressure <15 mm Hg)

Initial Tests (lab, imaging)
- CBC may show signs of polycythemia due to chronic hypoxia
- Basic metabolic panel (BMP) may demonstrate elevated creatinine secondary to poor cardiac output
- Liver function tests (LFTs) may be elevated due to hepatic congestion secondary to RV failure
- Brain-natriuretic peptide (BNP) and cardiac troponin can be elevated secondary to right ventricular strain
- D-dimer may be positive, as evidence of underlying thromboembolic pulmonary disease
- Arterial blood gas may show hypercapnea due to COPD

- ECG often shows signs of right-sided enlargement
  - Right axis deviation
  - An R/S wave ratio greater than 1 in V_1
  - Right ventricular hypertrophy (R wave in V_1 and V_2 with S waves in V_5 and V_6)
  - Right atrial enlargement as evidenced by P pulmonale (increased amplitude of P wave in lead II)
  - Incomplete or complete right bundle branch block
  - $S_1S_2S_3$ pattern, or $S_1Q_3T_3$, inverted pattern
- Chest x-ray:
  - Cardiomegaly
  - Enlargement of the central pulmonary arteries and reduced size of peripheral vessels (oligemia)
  - Reduced retrosternal space due to right ventricular enlargement on lateral views
  - Enlargement of the right atrium resulting in prominence of the right heart border
  - Evidence of COPD, interstitial lung disease (ILD), and structural disease (i.e., kyphosis)
  - Evidence of pulmonary embolism (Westermark sign and Hampton's hump)
- Spiral CT scan of chest:
  - Diagnosis of acute pulmonary embolism
  - Diagnosis of COPD and ILD
- Ventilation/perfusion scan (V/Q):
  - High specificity and sensitivity for acute and chronic thromboembolic disease
  - May be used for diagnosis of acute thromboembolic disease if contraindication to chest spiral CT
  - May be preferred to chest spiral CT for diagnosis of chronic thromboembolic pulmonary disease, given higher sensitivity (can detect peripheral pulmonary emboli otherwise missed by spiral CT)
  - Diagnosis of chronic thromboembolic disease may warrant confirmation by pulmonary angiography
- Pulmonary angiography:
  - Gold standard in diagnosis of chronic thromboembolic pulmonary disease
- Polysomnography:
  - Gold standard for diagnosis of obstructive sleep apnea (OSA)
- Pulmonary function tests (PFTs):
  - Impaired diffusion capacity
  - Obstructive and restrictive ventilatory defects (ILD, structural abnormalities, and COPD)

 TREATMENT

Reduce symptoms and improve quality of life and survival. Reduce disease burden via oxygenation, preservation of cardiac function, and attenuation of pulmonary hypertension.

GENERAL MEASURES
- Treat underlying disease:
  - For underlying pulmonary disease, bronchodilators and/or steroids may be beneficial
  - For underlying chronic thromboembolic disease, anticoagulation may be indicated
- Supportive therapy as necessary:
  - Continuous positive airway pressure/bilevel positive airway pressure may be used for hypoxia/sleep disorders.
  - Ventilation using positive-pressure masks, negative-pressure body suits, or mechanical ventilation is suggested for patients with neuromuscular disease.
  - Phlebotomy may be indicated for severe polycythemia (hematocrit >55%).

MEDICATION
- Oxygen:
  - Long-term continuous oxygen therapy improves the survival of hypoxemic patients with COPD and cor pulmonale.
  - All patients with pulmonary hypertension whose PaO_2 is consistently <55 mm Hg or saturation ≤88% at rest, during sleep, or with ambulation should be prescribed oxygen to keep O_2 >92 mm Hg (2)[A].
- Preservation of cardiac function:
  - Inotropes: dobutamine and milrinone may improve cardiac output
  - Diuretics: Decrease RV filling pressures; also reduces peripheral edema secondary to RHF:
    o Excessive volume depletion should be avoided.
    o Monitor closely for metabolic alkalosis, as this may suppress ventilatory drive and contribute to hypoxia.
- Amelioration pulmonary hypertension:
  - Treatment of underlying disease is hallmark of treatment
  - When refractory to traditional medical treatment, advanced therapies may be beneficial, though evidence is lacking
    o If "vasoreactive", calcium channel blockers (nifedipine, diltiazem, amlodipine) may be used; verapamil should be avoided
    o Other advanced therapies include: Phosphodiesterase inhibitors (sildenafil, tadalafil), endothelin receptor antagonists (bosentan, ambrisentan), prostanoids (iloprost, treprostinil, epoprostenol), and/or nitric oxide

ISSUES FOR REFERRAL
Patients with cor pulmonale should be referred to a specialized center for expert consultation.

SURGERY/OTHER PROCEDURES
- Endarterctomy for chronic thromboembolic disease (WHO Group IV)
- Moderate to severe disease refractory to medication may require lung and/or heart transplantation.

 ONGOING CARE

DIET
Salt and fluid restriction

PATIENT EDUCATION
- Smoking cessation and avoidance of exposure to secondary smoke is strongly recommended.
- Exertional activity should be limited.
- Pregnancy should be avoided.

PROGNOSIS
- Patients with cor pulmonale resulting from COPD have a greater likelihood of dying than do similar patients with COPD alone.
- Pulmonary arterial pressure is a reliable indicator of prognosis; higher pressure is associated with a worse prognosis.
- In patients with COPD and mild disease (PAP 20–35 mm Hg), 5-year survival is 50%.

REFERENCES
1. Naeije R. Pulmonary hypertension and right heart failure in chronic obstructive pulmonary disease. *Proc Am Thorac Soc.* 2005;2:20–22.
2. Barst RJ, Gibbs JS, Ghofrani HA, et al. Updated evidence-based treatment algorithm in pulmonary arterial hypertension. *J Am Coll Cardiol.* 2009;54: S78–S84.

ADDITIONAL READING
- Lee TM, Chen CC, Shen HN, et al. Effects of pravastatin on functional capacity in patients with chronic obstructive pulmonary disease and pulmonary hypertension. *Clin Sci* 2009;116: 497–505.
- McLaughlin VV, Archer SL, Badesch DB, et al. ACCF/AHA 2009 expert consensus document on pulmonary hypertension a report of the American College of Cardiology Foundation Task Force on Expert Consensus Documents and the American Heart Association developed in collaboration with the American College of Chest Physicians; American Thoracic Society, Inc.; and the Pulmonary Hypertension Association. *J Am Coll Cardiol.* 2009;53:1573–1619.
- Price LC, Wort SJ, Finney SJ, et al. Pulmonary vascular and right ventricular dysfunction in adult critical care: Current and emerging options for management: A systematic literature review. *Crit Care.* 2010;14:R169.
- Ryerson CJ, Nayar S, Swiston JR, et al. Pharmacotherapy in pulmonary arterial hypertension: A systematic review and meta-analysis. *Respir Res.* 2010;11:12.

 SEE ALSO

Chronic Obstructive Pulmonary Disease and Emphysema; Congestive Heart Failure; Pulmonary Arterial Hypertension; Pulmonary Embolism

 CODES

ICD10
- I26.09 Other pulmonary embolism with acute cor pulmonale
- I27.81 Cor pulmonale (chronic)

CLINICAL PEARLS
- Treatment of cor pulmonale requires treatment of an underlying disease.
- Continuous, long-term oxygen therapy improves life expectancy and quality of life in cor pulmonale.
- Referral of patients with cor pulmonale to a specialized center is strongly recommended.

CORNEAL ABRASION AND ULCERATION

John N. Dorsch, MD

 BASICS

DESCRIPTION

- Corneal abrasions result from scratching, denuding, abrading, or cutting of the epithelial layer of the cornea. They are usually traumatic and accidental, but can occur spontaneously as well.
- Corneal ulcers usually represent an infection deeper in the cornea by bacteria, viruses, or fungi as a result of breakdown in the protective epithelial barrier.
- Both corneal abrasions and ulcerations can result in scarring, which may impair vision.
- Both lesions can occur centrally or marginally.

EPIDEMIOLOGY

Incidence

- Corneal abrasion is the most common ophthalmologic visit to the emergency department and is a commonly seen problem in urgent care:
  - 64% of cases are caused by direct minor trauma to eye.
  - 12% of cases are due to contact lens-related problems.
- Ulceration is also common in the US.

ETIOLOGY AND PATHOPHYSIOLOGY

- Corneal abrasions most commonly result from accidental trauma (e.g., fingernail scratch, makeup brush):
  - Dirt, sand, sawdust, or other foreign body gets caught under eyelid.
- Corneal ulcers result from presence of an entryway to the external eye through dry eye; burns; abrasion; contact lenses; inappropriate use of topical anesthetics, antibiotics, or antiviral drops; immunosuppressant drugs; diabetes; or immunodeficiency: Causative of ulcerations include:
  - Infection with gram-positive organisms ~29–53% (*Staphylococcus aureus* and coagulation-negative streptococcus are common ones)
  - Infection with gram-negative organisms ~47–50% (*Pseudomonas* being most common, followed by *Serratia marcescens*, *Proteus mirabilis*, and gram-negative enteric bacilli)

ALERT

Patients with contact lenses may have colonization of the cornea with *Pseudomonas* and other gram-negative bacteria, and should be treated with ophthalmic quinolones or aminoglycosides to prevent corneal ulceration and infection.
- Viral infections, especially herpes
- Fungal infections (*Candida, Aspergillus, Fusarium, Acanthamoeba*) in agricultural workers or associated with ocular corticosteroid use
- Autoimmune disorders, such as rheumatoid arthritis (RA), systemic lupus erythematosus (SLE), and scleroderma, are the usual cause of peripheral ulcerative keratitis.
- Vitamin A deficiency may cause corneal necrosis or keratomalacia.

RISK FACTORS

- Any abrasive injury
- Foreign body in eye
- Contact lenses (especially soft lenses and extended-wear lenses)
- Blepharitis
- Dry eye syndrome
- Entropion (with lashes scratching cornea)
- Chronic topical steroid use
- Abuse of topical anesthetics
- Autoimmune disorders
- Vitamin A deficiency
- Chronic corneal exposure (e.g., Bell's palsy, exophthalmos)
- Recent eye surgery
- Immunosuppression and trigeminal nerve abnormalities
- Flash burn (welding burn or prolonged gazing directly at bright sunlight; symptoms often begin several hours after exposure)

GENERAL PREVENTION

- Eye protection to avoid injury during work, crafts, and sports
- Proper contact lens handling:
  - Do not sleep while wearing contact lens.
- Artificial tears for those with inability to blink or known dry eyes
- Lenses to block UV rays (e.g., welding helmets)

COMMONLY ASSOCIATED CONDITIONS

- Chronic ulcerations may be associated with neurotrophic keratitis due to lack of 5th nerve innervation of the cornea. Individuals with thyroid disease, diabetes, or immunosuppressive conditions are particularly at risk.
- Any cause of fat malabsorption may be associated with vitamin A deficiency.

 DIAGNOSIS

HISTORY

- Sudden onset of eye pain, photophobia, tearing, foreign-body sensation, blurring of vision, and/or conjunctival injection
- Abrasions and ulcerations are usually unilateral.
- History remarkable for contact lens use, dry eyes, rubbing eye, history of trauma from foreign body, or chemical burn
- History of connective tissue disorder

PHYSICAL EXAM

- Visual acuity may be decreased if abrasion or ulcer is centrally located.
- Conjunctival injection
- Increased lacrimation on affected side
- Photophobia
- Blepharospasm

- Lesion seen on slit lamp exam and area of damage shows fluorescein uptake; staining seen using Wood lamp or cobalt blue slit lamp:
  - "Dendritic" staining pattern with fluorescein indicative of viral keratitis
- Examine for foreign body under eyelids or in cornea ("rust ring")

DIFFERENTIAL DIAGNOSIS

- Foreign body in eye
- Unilateral iritis
- Acute or chronic glaucoma
- Keratitis
- Scleritis with corneal melting
- Herpes simplex or zoster
- Bilateral or true idiopathic lesions may suggest basement membrane dystrophy.

DIAGNOSTIC TESTS & INTERPRETATION

Initial Tests (lab, imaging)

- Culture ulcer and contact lens, if applicable.
- Pretreatment with topical antibiotics may alter culture results.

Diagnostic Procedures/Other

Scrapings of the corneal ulcer for culture and sensitivity ideally should be obtained before beginning local antibiotics. The sample should be plated directly onto the culture medium.

Test Interpretation

Scrapings for Gram and Giemsa stain may demonstrate bacteria, yeast, or intranuclear inclusions that may aid in the diagnosis.

TREATMENT

GENERAL MEASURES

- Simple corneal abrasions <4 mm in diameter can be managed by primary care physicians (1)[C]. See indications for referral below.
- All patients with corneal ulceration should be referred immediately to an ophthalmologist. Corneal cultures should be obtained before starting antibiotics. If immediate referral is not possible, it is reasonable to start antibiotics without delay.
- Flash burns from welding or prolonged exposure to sunlight may be treated like corneal abrasions.
- Topical ophthalmic steroids should be avoided: May delay healing of corneal abrasions.
- Use of topical anesthetics outside of clinical settings should be avoided: May develop corneal toxicity with prolonged use.

MEDICATION
First Line

- Eye patching does not reduce pain or speed the healing process (2)[A].
- Topical NSAIDs have been proven to reduce eye pain (2)[A],(3):
  - Ophthalmic NSAIDs: Diclofenac 0.1% q.i.d. helps relieve moderate pain:
    - Alternatives include ketorolac 0.5% and bromfenac 0.09%.
    - Caution: Ophthalmic NSAIDs may rarely cause corneal melting and perforation (3).
- Ophthalmic antibiotics may help prevent further infection and ulceration of corneal abrasions (4)[C](5).
- Some ophthalmic antibiotics include ciprofloxacin 0.3%, ofloxacin 0.3%, gentamicin 0.3%, erythromycin 0.5%, polymyxin B/Trimethoprim (Polytrim), tobramycin 0.3%:
  - Ointment preparations may be more soothing to the eye than solutions.
  - Topical antibiotics should be continued until eye pain is resolved.
  - Chloramphenicol should be avoided due to high risk of toxicity and Steven-Johnson syndrome.
- Large corneal abrasions (>4 mm) or very painful abrasions should be treated with combination of topical antibiotic and topical NSAID.
- Re-evaluate in 24 hours. If improving, no need for further follow up (4)[C].
- Fungal keratitis is treated with a protracted course of topical antifungal agents (by ophthalmologist).
- Herpetic keratitis should be referred promptly to ophthalmologist and treated initially with trifluridine:
  - Vidarabine and acyclovir are alternatives (6)[A]

Second Line
- Oral analgesic medication (hydrocodone and other opioids) if topical analgesia not adequate
- Supplemental topical cycloplegics (i.e., homatropine 5% and cyclopentolate 1%) have not been found to be beneficial (7)[B] in relieving pain in corneal abrasion.

ISSUES FOR REFERRAL
- Consultation with an ophthalmologist is recommended for all ulcers to help determine appropriate therapy (4)[C]. Moreover, ulcers need corneal cultures to be taken directly onto culture media.
- Also refer to ophthalmologist if there is history of (4)[C]:
  - Significant ocular trauma
  - Corneal infection is suspected (including viral keratitis)
  - Recurrent or nonhealing abrasion is encountered despite standard treatment.
  - Severe ocular pain not explained by apparent pathology (e.g., traumatic iritis)

 ONGOING CARE

FOLLOW-UP RECOMMENDATIONS
Patient Monitoring
- Contact lens wearer should be monitored daily with slit lamp for signs of secondary infection (4)[C].
- Minor abrasion should be re-evaluated only if becomes more painful (4)[C].
- Large abrasion (>4 mm) should be re-evaluated in 24 hours, and if improving, no need to follow further unless symptoms worsen again (4)[C].

PATIENT EDUCATION
Prevention of abrasions and proper handling of contact lenses can prevent recurrence of corneal ulcers.

PROGNOSIS
- Corneal abrasions and ulcerations should improve daily and heal with appropriate therapy.
- If healing does not occur within 24–48 hours or the lesion extends, obtain an ophthalmology consultation.

COMPLICATIONS
- Recurrence
- Scarring of the cornea
- Loss of vision
- Corneal perforation

REFERENCES
1. Wirbelauer C. Management of the red eye for the primary care physician. *Am J Med*. 2006;119: 302–306.
2. Turner A, Rabiu M. Patching for corneal abrasion. *Cochrane Database Syst Rev*. 2006;2:CD004764.
3. Vemuganti GK, Murthy SI, Dos S. Update on pathologic diagnosis of corneal infections and inflammations. *Middle East Afr J Ophthalmol*. 2011;18:277–284.
4. Fraser S. Corneal abrasion. *Clin Ophthalmol*. 2010;4:387–390.
5. Upadhyay MP, Karmacharya PC, Koirala S, et al. The Bhaktapur eye study: Ocular trauma and antibiotic prophylaxis for the prevention of corneal ulceration in Nepal. *Br J Ophthalmol*. 2001;85:388–392.
6. Wilhelmus KR. Therapeutic interventions for herpes simplex virus epithelial keratitis. *Cochrane Database Syst Rev*. 2008;1:CD002898.
7. Carley F, Carley S. Towards evidence based emergency medicine: Best BETs from the Manchester Royal Infirmary. Mydriatics in corneal abrasion. *Emerg Med J*. 2001;18:273.

ADDITIONAL READING
- Ehler JP, Shah CP, Fenton GL. *The Wills eye manual: Office and emergency room diagnosis and treatment of eye disease*. Baltimore: Lippincott Williams & Wilkins; 2008.
- Kaiser PK, Pineda R. A study of topical nonsteroidal anti-inflammatory drops and no pressure patching in the treatment of corneal abrasions. Corneal Abrasion Patching Study Group. *Ophthalmology*. 1997;104:1353–1359.
- Morden NE, Berke EM. Topical fluoroquinolones for eye and ear. *Am Fam Physician*. 2000;62: 1870–1876.
- Watson SL, Barker NH. Interventions for recurrent corneal erosions. *Cochrane Database Syst Rev*. 2007;4:CD001861, revised in *Cochrane Database Syst Rev*. 2012;9:CD001861.
- Wipperman JL, Dorsch JN. Evaluation and Management of Corneal Abrasions. *Am Fam Physician*. 2013;87:114–120.

 CODES

ICD10
- H16.009 Unspecified corneal ulcer, unspecified eye
- H16.049 Marginal corneal ulcer, unspecified eye
- S05.00XA Inj conjunctiva and corneal abrasion w/o fb, unsp eye, init

CLINICAL PEARLS
- Contact lens use should be discontinued until corneal abrasion or ulcer is healed and pain is fully resolved.
- Eye patching is not recommended.
- Prescribe topical and/or oral analgesic medication for symptom relief and consider ophthalmic antibiotics.
- Prompt referral to an ophthalmologist should be made with suspicion of an ulcer, recurrence of abrasion, retained foreign body, viral keratitis, significant visual loss, or lack of improvement despite therapy.

CORNS AND CALLUSES

Neil J. Feldman, DPM, DABPS

 BASICS

DESCRIPTION
- A callus (tyloma) is a diffuse area of hyperkeratosis, usually without a distinct border.
  - Typically the result of exposure to repetitive forces, including friction and mechanical pressure; tend to occur on the palms of hands and soles of feet (1)
- A corn (heloma) is a circumscribed hyperkeratotic lesion with a central conical core of keratin that causes pain and inflammation. The conical core in a corn is a thickening of the stratum corneum.
- Hard corn or heloma durum (more common): More often on toe surfaces, especially 5th toe (proximal interphalangeal [PIP]) joint
- Soft corn (heloma molle): Commonly in the interdigital space (1)
- Digital corns are also known as clavi.
- Intractable plantar keratosis is usually located under a metatarsal head (1st and 5th most common), is typically more difficult to resolve, and often is resistant to usual conservative treatments.

EPIDEMIOLOGY
Corns and calluses have the largest prevalence of all foot disorders.

Incidence
Incidence of corns and calluses increases with age. Less common in pediatric patients. Women affected more often than men. Blacks report corns and calluses 30% more often than whites.

Prevalence
- 9.2 million Americans
- ~38/1,000 people affected

ETIOLOGY AND PATHOPHYSIOLOGY
Increased activity of keratinocytes in superficial layer of skin leading to hyperkeratosis. This is a normal response to excess friction, pressure, or stress.
- Calluses typically arise from repetitive friction, motion, or pressure to skin.
- Soft corns arise from increased moisture from perspiration leading to skin maceration, along with mechanical irritation, especially between toes.
- Hard corns are an extreme form of callus with a keratin-based core. Often found on the digital surfaces and commonly linked to bony protrusions causing skin to rub against shoe surfaces.

Genetics
No true genetic basis identified because most corns and calluses are due to mechanical stressors on the foot/hands.

RISK FACTORS
- Extrinsic factors producing pressure, friction, and local stress:
  - Ill-fitting shoes
  - Not using socks, gloves
  - Manual labor
  - Walking barefoot
  - Activities that increase stress applied to skin of hands or feet (running, walking, sports)
- Intrinsic factors:
  - Bony prominences: Bunions, hammertoes
- Enlarged bursa or abnormal foot function/structure: Hammertoe, claw toe, or mallet toe deformity

GENERAL PREVENTION
External irritation is by far the most common cause of calluses and corns. General measures to reduce friction on the skin are recommended to reduce incidence of callus formation. Examples include wearing shoes that fit well and using socks and gloves.

Geriatric Considerations
In elderly patients, especially those with neurologic or vascular compromise, skin breakdown from calluses/corns may lead to increased risk of infection/ulceration. 30% of foot ulcers in the elderly arise from eroded hyperkeratosis. Regular foot exams are emphasized for these patients, as well as in diabetic patients (2).

COMMONLY ASSOCIATED CONDITIONS
- Foot ulcers, especially in diabetic patients or patients with neuropathy or vascular compromise
- Infection: Look for warning signs of:
  - Spreading or redness around sore
  - Puslike drainage
  - Increased pain/swelling
  - Fever
  - Change in color of fingers or toes
- Signs of gangrene

 DIAGNOSIS

- Most commonly a clinical diagnosis based on visualization of the lesion
- Examination of footwear may also provide clues.

HISTORY
- Careful history can usually pinpoint cause.
- Ask about neurologic and vascular history and diabetes. These may be risk factors for progression of corns/calluses to frank ulcerations and infection.

PHYSICAL EXAM
- Calluses:
  - Thickening of skin without distinct borders
  - Often on feet, hands; especially over palms of hands, soles of feet
  - Colors from white to gray-yellow, brown, red
  - May be painless or tender
  - May throb or burn
- Corns:
  - Hard corns: Commonly on dorsum of toes or dorsum of 5th PIP joint:
    - Varied texture: Dry, waxy, transparent to a hornlike mass
    - Distinct borders
    - More common on feet
    - Often painful
  - Soft corns:
    - Often between toes, especially between 4th and 5th digits at the base of the webspace
    - Often yellowed, macerated appearance
    - Often extremely painful

DIFFERENTIAL DIAGNOSIS
- Plantar warts (typically a loss of skin lines within the wart)
- Porokeratoses (blocked sweat gland)
- Underlying ulceration of skin, with or without infection (rule out especially with diabetic patients)

DIAGNOSTIC TESTS & INTERPRETATION
Initial Tests (lab, imaging)
- Radiographs may be warranted if no external cause found. Look for abnormalities in foot structure, bone spurs.
- Use of metallic radiographic marker and weightbearing films often highlight the relationship between the callus and bony prominence.

Diagnostic Procedures/Other
Biopsy with microscopic evaluation in rare cases

Test Interpretation
Abnormal accumulation of keratin in epidermis, stratum corneum

TREATMENT

GENERAL MEASURES
- Debridement of affected tissue and use of protective padding
- Low-heeled shoes; soft upper with deep and wide toebox
- Extra-width shoes for 5th-toe corns
- Avoidance of activities that contribute to painful lesions
- Prefabricated or custom orthotics

MEDICATION
- Most therapy for corns and calluses can be done as self-care in the home (1).
- Use bandages, soft foam padding, or silicone sleeve over the affected area to decrease friction on the skin and promote healing with digital clavi.
- Use socks or gloves regularly.
- Use lotion/moisturizers for dry calluses and corns.
- Keratolytic agents, such as urea or ammonium lactate, can be applied safely.
- Use sandpaper discs or pumice stones over hard, thickened areas of skin.

Geriatric Considerations
Use of salicylic acid corn plasters can cause skin breakdown and ulceration in patients with thin, atrophic skin; diabetes; and those with vascular compromise. The skin surrounding the callus will often turn white and can become quite painful.

ISSUES FOR REFERRAL
- May benefit from referral to podiatrist if use of topical agents and shoe changes are ineffective.
- Abnormalities in foot structure may require surgical treatment.
- Diabetic, vascular, and neuropathic patients may benefit from referral to podiatrist for regular foot exams to prevent infection or ulceration.

SURGERY/OTHER PROCEDURES
- Surgical treatment of areas of protruding bone where corns and calluses form
- Rebalancing of foot pressure through functional foot orthotics
- Shaving or cutting off hardened area of skin using a chisel or 15-blade scalpel. For corns, remove keratin core and place pad over area during healing.

COMPLEMENTARY AND ALTERNATIVE MEDICINE
- Many over-the-counter topical ointments and lotions are available for calluses (Keralac, CalleX, urea, Lac-Hydrin). Do not use on broken skin.
- Epsom salt soaks for 5–10 minutes at a time

IN-PATIENT CONSIDERATIONS
Admission Criteria/Initial Stabilization
- Admission usually not necessary, unless progression to ulcerated lesion with signs of severe infection, gangrene
- May require aggressive debridement in operating room should an abscess or deep-space infection be suspected.

Nursing
Wound care, dressing changes for infected lesions

ONGOING CARE

PATIENT EDUCATION
- General information available at: http://www.mayoclinic.com/health/corns-and-calluses/DS00033/DSECTION = 9
- American Podiatric Medical Association. Available at: http://www.apma.org

PROGNOSIS
Complete cure is possible once factors causing injury are eliminated.

COMPLICATIONS
Ulceration, infection

REFERENCES
1. Freeman DB. Corns and calluses resulting from mechanical hyperkeratosis. *Am Fam Physician*. 2002;65:2277–2280.
2. Pinzur MS, Slovenkai MP, Trepman E, et al. Guidelines for diabetic foot care: Recommendations endorsed by the Diabetes Committee of the American Orthopaedic Foot and Ankle Society. *Foot Ankle Int*. 2005;26:113–119.

ADDITIONAL READING
Theodosat A. Skin diseases of the lower extremities in the elderly. *Dermatol Clin*. 2004;22(1):13–21.

CODES

ICD10
L84 Corns and callosities

CLINICAL PEARLS
Most therapy for corns and calluses can be done as self-care in the home using padding over the affected area to decrease friction; however, if simple home care is not helpful, then removal of the lesions is often immediately curative.

CORONARY ARTERY DISEASE AND STABLE ANGINA

Edwin Q. Ravano, MD, MPH

BASICS

DESCRIPTION

- Predictable and reproducible chest discomfort occurring in a consistent pattern at a certain level of exertion or emotional stress and relieved with rest or sublingual nitroglycerin
- Definitions:
  - Typical angina: A sense of choking or of pressure or heaviness deep to the precordium, frequently radiating to the jaw, arms, or epigastrium; usually brought on by exertion or anxiety and relieved by rest. Discomfort may be described with a clenched fist over the sternum (Levine sign).
  - Atypical angina: Nonclassical symptoms and signs, such as absence of substernal localization and character, exertional trigger, or relief with nitroglycerin or rest
  - Anginal equivalent: Patients with angina may present without chest discomfort, but with nonspecific symptoms such as dyspnea, diaphoresis, fatigue, belching, nausea, lightheadedness, indigestion.
  - Unstable angina: Anginal symptoms that are new or are changed in character to become more frequent, more severe, or both. Considered an acute coronary syndrome in the same continuum as non–ST segment elevation myocardial infarction (NSTEMI) but without troponin leak.
- Low risk unstable angina (age <70, exertional pain lasting <20 minutes, pain not rapidly accelerating, normal or unchanged ECG, no elevation of cardiac markers) may be treated similarly to stable ischemic heart disease.
- Canadian Cardiovascular Society grading of chronic stable angina severity:
  - Class 1: Ordinary physical activity does not cause angina; angina with strenuous or rapid or prolonged exertion.
  - Class 2: Slight limitation of ordinary activity (walking rapidly or >2 blocks, climbing >1 flight of stairs, emotional stress).
  - Class 3: Marked limitation of ordinary physical activity.
  - Class 4: Inability to carry on any physical activity without discomfort. Angina may occur at rest.
- System(s) affected: Cardiovascular

Geriatric Considerations

Elderly patients may present with atypical anginal symptoms. Maintain a high degree of suspicion during evaluation. They may also be very sensitive to the side effects of medications.

EPIDEMIOLOGY

- Most common in middle-age and older men, postmenopausal women
- Predominant sex: Male > Female

Incidence

~785,000 new cases of stable angina occur yearly in patients aged ≥45 (1)

Prevalence

>16.3 million people aged ≥20 suffer from angina in the US (1)

ETIOLOGY AND PATHOPHYSIOLOGY

- In stable angina, a fixed reduction in the diameter of coronary arteries causes a reduction in coronary blood flow. Anginal symptoms occur during times of myocardial ischemia caused by a mismatch between coronary artery perfusion and myocardial oxygen demand. Sensory nerves travel up the sympathetic chain and enter the spinal cord at levels C7-T4, causing diffuse referred pain/discomfort in the associated dermatomes.
- Atherosclerotic narrowing of the coronary arteries is the most common pathology, with symptoms arising from stenosis of >70% in epicardial coronary arteries or >50% stenosis of the left main artery. Angina may occur in those with significant aortic valve disease or hypertrophic cardiomyopathy, even with normal coronary arteries.
- Atherosclerosis of the coronary arteries (most common)
- Aortic stenosis or aortic insufficiency
- Hypertrophic cardiomyopathy
- Primary pulmonary hypertension (HTN)

RISK FACTORS

Standard risk factors for coronary artery disease (CAD) include:

- Family history of premature CAD in 1st-degree relatives (in male relatives <55 or female relatives <65)
- Obesity, hypercholesterolemia
- Elevated BP
- Cigarette smoking
- Diabetes mellitus
- Male gender
- Advanced age

GENERAL PREVENTION

- Stop smoking.
- Low-fat/low-cholesterol diet, and statin medication if indicated by current Adult Treatment Panel (ATP) guidelines or a risk-based approach
- Regular aerobic exercise program, and weight loss (goal BMI <25)
- BP control (goal <140/90)

COMMONLY ASSOCIATED CONDITIONS

Hypercholesterolemia, peripheral vascular disease, HTN, obesity, diabetes mellitus

DIAGNOSIS

- Predictable and reproducible anginal symptoms lasting 3–15 minutes brought on by exertion, emotional stress, meals, cold air, or smoking; symptoms relieved by rest or nitrates. Careful history is important in eliciting symptoms of angina as listed above.
- Dyspnea on exertion may present as the only symptom. Atypical symptoms are more likely in women, elderly, and diabetic patients.

HISTORY

- Quality of any previous anginal episodes and pattern over time
- Underlying history of heart disease or valvular disease; assess risk factors
- Family history of myocardial infarction (MI), coronary artery disease (CAD), sudden death

PHYSICAL EXAM

- Measure vital signs: BP, heart rate, respiratory rate, and oxygen saturation
- Cardiac exam may reveal dysrhythmias, heart murmurs indicative of valvular disease, signs of ventricular hypertrophy, gallops, or signs of congestive heart failure.
- Vascular exam may show signs of peripheral vascular disease (diminished pulses, bruits, abdominal aneurysm).
- Pulmonary exam may reveal signs of obstructive or restrictive diseases, pulmonary edema.
- May see signs of dyslipidemia (xanthomas, xanthelasma)
- Normal physical exam should not exclude cardiac causes of anginal symptoms.

DIFFERENTIAL DIAGNOSIS

Pulmonary disease, gastroesophageal reflux (GERD), musculoskeletal etiologies (costochondritis, muscle strain)

DIAGNOSTIC TESTS & INTERPRETATION

- ECG:
  - May show evidence of prior MI. However, ECG is frequently unremarkable when asymptomatic. May show signs of myocardial ischemia during symptomatic episodes.
  - Bundle branch block, Wolff-Parkinson-White syndrome, or intraventricular conduction delay may make stress ECG interpretation unreliable.
- Stress testing (exercise testing preferable):
  - Exercise testing for those who can physically exercise (≥5 metabolic equivalents [METS]):
    ○ Standard exercise ECG for those with normal baseline ECG
    ○ Exercise stress testing with echo or perfusion imaging for those with abnormal baseline ECG or in premenopausal women
  - In patients who cannot tolerate exercise, pharmacologic stress testing with adenosine, Regadenoson, or dipyridamole. Dobutamine preferred if asthma or heart block (2nd or 3rd degree).
- Coronary angiography is the gold standard for confirmation and delineation of coronary disease and direction of interventional therapy or surgery.
- Total cholesterol and low-density lipoprotein (LDL) may be elevated, and high-density lipoprotein (HDL) cholesterol may be reduced.
- C-reactive protein (CRP): Most useful for those at intermediate risk of developing CAD (10–20% over 10 years by Framingham risk criteria) in whom an elevated CRP may suggest an increased likelihood of benefit from statin therapy

Initial Tests (lab, imaging)

- Hematocrit, fasting lipid profile, fasting blood sugar, basic metabolic panel; troponin for acute chest pain
- Consider echocardiogram if valvular disease or hypertrophic cardiomyopathy is suspected.
- Stress imaging with echocardiogram or perfusion imaging (see "Stress testing")
- Consider chest radiography if signs of pulmonary disease.
- Guideline directed medical therapy (GDMT): All patients should be started on aspirin (or clopidogrel if contraindicated). Lifestyle modifications, including weight loss, smoking cessation, and increased physical activity, are considered equally important as pharmacologic therapy. Start 1st-line antianginal agent, either β-blocker or calcium channel blocker (CCB). β-Blocker preferred if previous MI or left ventricle (LV) dysfunction. If angina persists, trial of the opposite class of anti-ischemic drug (CCB or β-blocker). If monotherapy ineffective, trial of combination β-blocker and CCB. Long-acting nitrates

may be tried when β-blockers and CCBs are ineffective. Short-acting nitrates can abort acute anginal attack. Seek immediate attention for angina unrelieved by 3 doses of nitroglycerin spaced 5 minutes apart.

Follow-Up Tests & Special Considerations
Titrate dosages to maximum dose tolerated, as limited by side effects. Re-evaluate effectiveness 2–4 weeks after starting or changing drug therapy.

Diagnostic Procedures/Other
All patients should have ECG performed. Stress testing should be performed to evaluate efficacy of treatment, for risk stratification, or to determine appropriateness of revascularization.

TREATMENT

GENERAL MEASURES
Lifestyle modifications are very important:
- BP control goal: <140/90 for most
- Smoking cessation goal: Complete cessation, no exposure to 2nd-hand smoke.
- Physical activity goal: 30–60 minutes of moderate aerobic activity, at least 5 and preferably 7 d/wk.
- Weight management. Goal: BMI 18.5–24.9 kg/m^2; waist circumference <35 inches (women) or <40 inches (men) (2)
- Lipid management goal: Treat with moderate or high-dose statin in all patients in the absence of contraindications or adverse effects.
- Glycemic control in diabetics. Individualize based on life expectancy, risk for adverse events related to glucose control, and patient preference. HgbA1c target generally <7–8.

MEDICATION
First Line
Anti-ischemic (antianginal) medications:
- β-Blockers decrease heart rate, BP, and myocardial contractility:
  – Atenolol (25–100 mg/d, taken daily or b.i.d.), metoprolol (25–200 mg daily [succinate] or divided b.i.d [tartrate]) (2)[A]. Adjust doses according to clinical response. Aim to maintain resting heart rate of 50–60 bpm.
  – CCBs cause arterial vasodilation, decrease myocardial oxygen demand, and improve coronary blood flow (2)[A]. Only long-acting CCBs should be used:
- Dihydropyridine CCBs such as nifedipine (30–90 mg/d), amlodipine (5–10 mg/d), or felodipine (2.5–10 mg/d) cause more vasodilation. Nondihydropyridine CCBs such as diltiazem (120–480 mg/d) or verapamil (120–480 mg/d). Amlodipine preferred in patients with low ejection fraction.
- Side effects include constipation and peripheral edema. The nondihydropyridine CCBs may also cause bradycardia, heart block, and precipitate heart failure in those with severe systolic dysfunction.
- Nitrates dilate systemic veins and arteries (including coronary vessels) and cause decreased preload; at higher doses, decreases BP and thus decreases afterload and increases myocardial flow:
  – Sublingual nitroglycerin 0.4 mg. For acute anginal episodes. Repeat 2–3 times over a 10–15-minute period; if no relief, immediate medical attention must be sought.
  – Long-acting nitrates: Should be used with a drug-free interval of 8–12 hours to prevent

tolerance. Side effects such as headaches and hypotension tend to clear with continued usage.
- Other therapies:
  – Antiplatelet therapy is indicated in all patients:
    ○ Clopidogrel (75 mg/d) may be used in patients with contraindications to aspirin.
    ○ Combination of aspirin and clopidogrel is indicated for those with stent placement to reduce rate of stent thrombosis (1 month for bare metal stents and ≥12 months for drug-eluting stents):
  – Statins (e.g., simvastatin, atorvastatin, pravastatin, lovastatin, rosuvastatin) for hypercholesterolemia (2)[A]:
    ○ Most beneficial as secondary prevention in those with CAD. Decrease incidence of symptomatic CAD and reduce both MI and death from MI. LDL target <100 mg/dL for established CAD. Consider target <70 in high-risk patients. NICE Guideline atorvastatin 40 mg for all (3).
    ○ Current ATP guidelines support using lipid-lowering drugs for those with suspected or documented CAD.
    ○ Side effects may include elevated transaminases, myalgias. May rarely cause myositis or rhabdomyolysis. Monitor labs with any changes in medication doses.
  – ACE inhibitors have been shown to reduce both cardiovascular death and MI. Indicated in patients with CAD or other vascular disease, particularly in those with diabetes or LV systolic dysfunction. Angiotensin receptor blockers may be used in patients intolerant of ACE inhibitors.

Second Line
Ranolazine (500–1,000 mg b.i.d.) inhibits late sodium channels, decreasing ischemia-associated calcium overload. Diastolic relaxation is normalized. Does not affect heart rate or BP. Use as adjunctive therapy in those who are still symptomatic on optimal doses of β-blockers, nitrates, or amlodipine. Side effects may include nausea, constipation, dizziness, and headache.

SURGERY/OTHER PROCEDURES
- Revascularization therapies: Consider if optimal medication management is inadequate in controlling symptoms: Percutaneous coronary intervention (PCI), balloon angioplasty, and/or stent placement (with drug eluting or bare metal stent). Although patients may become symptom-free faster, PCI does not decrease mortality or MI compared with optimal medical management in those with stable angina.
- Coronary artery bypass grafting (CABG)
- For refractory angina: Spinal cord stimulation, enhanced external counterpulsation, myocardial laser revascularization therapy

COMPLEMENTARY AND ALTERNATIVE MEDICINE
Relaxation/Stress reduction therapy may help reduce anginal episodes.

IN-PATIENT CONSIDERATIONS
Admission Criteria/Initial Stabilization
Inpatient evaluation for any patient with changes in angina symptoms, as this is classified as unstable angina in the continuum of acute coronary syndromes

Discharge Criteria
Without myonecrosis, discharge may be considered after appropriate risk stratification has been determined. Exercise stress testing or coronary CT angiogram may be useful tools.

ONGOING CARE
FOLLOW-UP RECOMMENDATIONS
Lifestyle modifications should be aggressively stressed at every visit.

Patient Monitoring
Frequent follow up after initial event: Every 4–6 months in 1st year, then 1–2 × per year.

DIET
Low-fat, low-cholesterol, low-salt diet

PROGNOSIS
Variable; depends on severity of symptoms, extent of CAD, and LV function

COMPLICATIONS
Unstable angina or MI, arrhythmia, cardiac arrest, heart failure

REFERENCES
1. Roger V, Go A, Lloyd-Jones D, et al. Heart disease and stroke statistics—2012 update: A report from the American Heart Association. *Circulation*. 2012;125:e2–e220.
2. Fihn SD, Gardin JM, Abrams J, et al. 2012 ACCF/AHA/ACP/AATS/PCNA/SCAI/STS guideline for the diagnosis and management of patients with stable ischemic heart disease. *J Am Coll Cardiol*. 2012;60:2564–2603.
3. O'Flynn N, Timmis A, Henderson R, et al. Management of stable angina: Summary of NICE guidance. *BMJ*. 2011;343:d4147.

ADDITIONAL READING
Fraker TD, Fihn SD, Gibbons RJ, et al. 2007 chronic angina focused update of the ACC/AHA 2002 guidelines for the management of patients with chronic stable angina. *Circulation*. 2007;116:2762–2772.

SEE ALSO
Algorithms: Chest Pain; Chest Pain/Acute Coronary Syndrome

CODES
ICD10
- I25.111 Athscl heart disease of native cor art w ang pctrs w spasm
- I25.118 Athscl heart disease of native cor art w oth ang pctrs
- I25.119 Athscl heart disease of native cor art w unsp ang pctrs

CLINICAL PEARLS
- Maximize antianginal therapy: Combine β-blockers, CCBs, and nitrates in those still symptomatic with monotherapy.
- Lifestyle changes and optimal medical therapy must be emphasized to control complicating factors that trigger ischemia and to prevent progression of the atherosclerotic process.

COSTOCHONDRITIS
Smriti Ohri, MD • Scott A. Fields, MD, MHA

BASICS

DESCRIPTION
- Anterior chest wall pain associated with pain and tenderness of the costochondral and costosternal regions
- System(s) affected: Musculoskeletal
- Synonym(s): Costosternal syndrome; Parasternal chondrodynia; Anterior chest wall syndrome; Chondrocostal junction syndrome

Pediatric Considerations
Pay special attention to psychogenic chest pain in children who perceive family discord.

EPIDEMIOLOGY
- Predominant age: 20–40 years
- Predominant gender: Female

Incidence
~30% of patients presenting to emergency room with chest pain; 15–20% of teenagers with chest pain may have costochondritis (1,2).

ETIOLOGY AND PATHOPHYSIOLOGY
- Not fully understood
- Trauma
- Overuse

RISK FACTORS
- Unusual physical activity or overuse
- Recent trauma (including motor vehicle accident, domestic violence) or new activity
- Recent upper respiratory infection (URI)

DIAGNOSIS

- Insidious onset
- Pain is usually sharp, achy, or pressurelike, sometimes pleuritic
- Pain involves multiple locations, the 2nd–5th costal cartilages most often involved (2).
- Pain is most often unilateral.
- Pain is exacerbated by upper body movements and exertional activities.
- Pain is reproduced by palpation of the affected cartilage segments (2).
- Chest tightness is often associated with the pain.
- Redness and warmth at sites of tenderness

HISTORY
- A complete and thorough history is mandatory for the diagnosis, with special emphasis on cardiac risk factor evaluation.
- Social history: Careful screening and evaluation for domestic violence and substance abuse

PHYSICAL EXAM
- A physical exam to exclude more serious conditions that may present with chest pain is necessary for the diagnosis.
- Tenderness elicited over the costochondral junctions is necessary to establish the diagnosis, but does not completely exclude other causes of chest pain.
- Various maneuvers (crowing rooster, horizontal arm flexion) can be used (3).
- Palpation of epigastric region to evaluate for gastroesophageal reflux disease (GERD) and deep palpation in right upper quadrant of abdomen to evaluate gall bladder.

Geriatric Considerations
Often presents with multiple problems capable of causing chest pain, making a thorough history and physical exam imperative.

DIFFERENTIAL DIAGNOSIS
- Cardiac:
  – CAD
  – Cardiac contusion from trauma
  – Aortic aneurysm
  – Mitral valve prolapse
  – Pericarditis
  – Myocarditis
- GI:
  – Gastroesophageal reflux
  – Peptic esophagitis
  – Esophageal spasm
- Musculoskeletal:
  – Tietze disease or syndrome (2,4)
  – Fibromyalgia
  – Slipping rib syndrome
  – Costovertebral arthritis
  – Painful xiphoid syndrome
  – Rib trauma with swelling
  – Ankylosing spondylitis
  – Precordial catch syndrome
- Psychogenic:
  – Anxiety disorder
  – Panic attacks
  – Hyperventilation
- Respiratory:
  – Asthma
  – Pulmonary embolism
  – Pneumonia
  – Chronic cough
  – Pneumothorax
- Other:
  – Domestic violence and abuse
  – Herpes zoster
  – Spinal tumor
  – Metastatic cancer
  – Substance abuse (cocaine)

DIAGNOSTIC TESTS & INTERPRETATION
- The diagnosis of costochondritis is primarily based on a thorough history and physical exam.
- Laboratory exams should be used only if concern exists regarding other elements of the differential diagnosis.
- ESR is inconsistently elevated.

Initial Tests (lab, imaging)
No imaging is indicated for the diagnosis of costochondritis; chest x-ray and rib films are often normal.

Diagnostic Procedures/Other
- None indicated for the diagnosis of costochondritis.
- Consider ECG in patients age >35 years, those with history or risk of coronary artery disease (CAD) (2).
- Consider chest x-ray in patients with clinical concern of pulmonary pathology.
- Consider spiral CT for pulmonary embolism and D-dimer if history or risk factors are present.

Test Interpretation
Costochondral joint inflammation

TREATMENT

Reassurance of benign nature of condition and potential for long, slow recovery from pain

GENERAL MEASURES
- Patient reassurance, rest, and heat (or ice massage, whichever makes the patient feel better)
- For ice massage, freeze a small paper cupful of water, then peel away a small amount of cup, massage should go from the patient's experience of cold, then burning, until numb, about 15 minutes 3×/d, until symptoms abate.
- Stretching exercises (4,5)

MEDICATION

First Line
NSAIDs (aspirin, ibuprofen, naproxen, or diclofenac); narcotics not indicated (6)

Second Line
Acetaminophen (6)

ISSUES FOR REFERRAL
Consider referral to osteopathy or physical therapy if any concern rib is partially dislocated.

COMPLEMENTARY AND ALTERNATIVE MEDICINE
Limited data on use of manipulation or ice massage, but may be safely tried if patient interested.

IN-PATIENT CONSIDERATIONS
Admission Criteria/Initial Stabilization
Only indicated if differential diagnosis is unclear and cardiac or other more serious etiology of chest pain is being considered.

 ONGOING CARE

FOLLOW-UP RECOMMENDATIONS
Follow-up within 1 week if diagnosis is unclear or symptoms do not abate with conservative treatment.

PATIENT EDUCATION
- Educate the patient in regard to the self-limited (although potentially recurrent) nature of the illness.
- Instruct patient on proper physical activity regimens to avoid overuse syndromes.
- Stress importance of avoiding sudden, significant changes in activity.

PROGNOSIS
- Self-limited illness, lasts for weeks to months, but usually abates by 1 year, although sometimes chronic especially in adolescents.
- Often recurs

COMPLICATIONS
Incomplete attention to differential diagnosis or overly aggressive interventions to ensure a more life-threatening diagnosis is not missed

REFERENCES

1. Verdon F, Herzig L, Burnand B, et al. Chest pain in daily practice: Occurrence, causes and management. *Swiss Med Wkly.* 2008;138: 340–347.
2. Proulx AM, Zryd TW. Costochondritis: Diagnosis and treatment. *Am Fam Physician.* 2009;80: 617–620.
3. Epstein SE, Gerber LH, Borer JS, et al. Chest wall syndrome. A common cause of unexplained cardiac pain. *JAMA.* 1979;241:2793–2797.
4. Stochkendahl MJ, Christensen HW. Chest pain in focal musculoskeletal disorders. *Med Clin North Am.* 2010;94:259–273.
5. Aspegren D, Hyde T, Miller M, et al. Conservative treatment of a female collegiate volleyball player with costochondritis. *J Manipulative Physiol Ther.* 2007;30:321–325.
6. Freeston J, Karim Z, Lindsay K, et al. Can early diagnosis and management of costochondritis reduce acute chest pain admissions? *J Rheumatol.* 2004;31:2269–2271.

ADDITIONAL READING
Rovetta G, Sessarego P, Monteforte P, et al. Stretching exercises for costochondritis pain. *G Ital Med Lav Ergon.* 2009;31:169–171.

 SEE ALSO

Algorithm: Chest Pain/Acute Coronary Syndrome

 CODES

ICD10
M94.0 Chondrocostal junction syndrome [Tietze]

CLINICAL PEARLS
- A very common disorder, accounting for perhaps 30% of all cases of chest pain
- Educate the patient in regard to the self-limited (although potentially recurrent) nature of the illness. Instruct patient on proper physical activity regimens to avoid overuse syndromes. Also stress importance of avoiding sudden, significant changes in activity.
- Consider an anxiety disorder as a contributor to all cases of persistent chest pain, whether musculoskeletal or cardiac.

C

COUNSELING TYPES

William T. Garrison, PhD

 BASICS

DESCRIPTION

- Psychotherapeutic and counseling interventions play an important role in the management of chronic and acute-onset diseases and disorders. They are typically the primary initial mode of evaluation and/or treatment for most mild-to-moderate psychiatric disorders that reach criteria using the DSM or ICD diagnostic classification systems. Treatment and successful control of either medical or psychological conditions requires some form of professional counseling experience. Best outcomes occur when they are employed by a skilled practitioner. However, psychotherapy differs from generic counseling, which can take many forms and is delivered commonly in nonmedical settings, with mixed results.
- Counseling approaches are usually tailored to the specific presenting problem or issue and serve educational and emotional support functions. Typically, such counseling in medical settings will be time-limited and problem-focused and often not intended to lead to major medical symptom relief or major behavioral changes.
- The goals of psychotherapy range from increasing individual psychological insight and motivation for change to reduction of interpersonal conflict in the marriage or family, reduction of chronic or acute emotional suffering, and reversal of dysfunctional or habitual behaviors. There are several general types of psychotherapy, starting with individual, marital, or family approaches. In addition, a number of psychological theories guide various methods and treatment philosophies. The following is a brief overview of commonly used psychotherapeutic and counseling methods.
- Psychodynamic therapy: Unconscious conflict manifests as patient's symptoms/problem behaviors:
  – Short-term (4–6 months) and long-term (≥1 year)
  – Focus is on increasing insight of underlying conflict or processes to initiate symptomatic change.
  – Therapist actively helps patient identify patterns of behavior stemming from existence of an unconscious conflict or motivations that may not be accurately perceived.
- Cognitive-behavioral therapy (CBT): Patterns of thoughts and behaviors can lead to development and/or maintenance of symptoms. Thought patterns may not accurately reflect reality and may lead to psychological distress:
  – Therapy aims at modifying thought patterns by increasing cognitive flexibility and changing dysfunctional behavioral patterns.
  – Encourages patient self-monitoring of symptoms and the precursors or results of maladaptive behavior
  – Uses therapist-assisted challenges to patient's basic beliefs/assumptions
  – May utilize *exposure,* a procedure derived from basic learning theories, which encourages gradual steps toward change.
  – Can be offered in group or individual formats
  – Therapist role is suggestive and supportive.

- Dialectical behavior therapy (DBT): Techniques such as social skills training, mindfulness, and problem solving are used to modulate impulse control and affect management:
  – Derivative of CBT
  – Originally used in treatment of patients with self-destructive behaviors (e.g., cutting, suicide attempts)
  – Seeks to change rigid patterns of cognitions and behaviors that have been maladaptive
  – Utilizes both individual and group treatment modalities
  – Therapist takes an active role in interpretation and support.
- Interpersonal psychotherapy: Interpersonal relationships in a patient's life are linked to symptoms. Therapy seeks to alleviate symptoms and improve social adjustment through exploration of patient's relationships and experiences. Focus is on 1 of 4 potential problem areas:
  – Grief
  – Interpersonal role disputes
  – Role transitions
  – Interpersonal deficits: Therapist works with the patient in resolving the problematic interpersonal issues to facilitate change in symptoms
- Family therapy: Focuses on the family as a unit of intervention:
  – Uses psychoeducation to increase patient's and family's insight
  – Teaches communication and problem-solving skills
- Motivational interviewing: Focuses on motivation as a key to successful change process:
  – Short-term and problem-focused
  – Focuses on identifying discrepancies between goals and behavior
  – "5 A's" model is a brief counseling framework developed specifically for physicians to effect behavioral change in patients:
    ○ Assess for a problem.
    ○ Advise making a change.
    ○ Agree on action to be taken.
    ○ Assist with self-care support to make the change.
    ○ Arrange follow-up to support the change.
- Counseling (heterogeneous treatment):
  – Often focuses on situational factors maintaining symptoms
  – Often encourages utilization of community resources
- Behavioral therapy: Relatively nontheoretical approach to behavioral change or symptom reduction/eradication through application of principles of stimulus and response

Pediatric Considerations

- Important distinctions are made between psychotherapy and counseling for children/teens compared to adults/couples.
- The focus of evaluation must include attention to parent and family processes and factors. Interventions typically include interactions and sessions with parents, as well as collateral work with teachers and other school personnel.

- Younger children will often be evaluated and diagnosed through behavioral descriptions provided by parents and other adults who know them well, as well as through direct observation and/or play techniques. Children of all ages should be screened using behavioral checklists that are norm-referenced for age.
- Any child or teenager who requests counseling should be interviewed initially by the primary care provider and referred appropriately. Most referrals will be in response to parental request, however.
- Psychotherapeutic interventions with the strongest empirical basis with children include behavior therapy/modification, CBT, and family/parenting therapy. Play therapy has the least empirical support, and insight-oriented therapies appear to be more effective with older children (>11 years).
- There is controversy regarding the efficacy of psychopharmacologic treatment in preadolescents, although clear benefits have been demonstrated in some studies. Treatment guidelines for mild-to-moderate depressed mood and/or anxiety disorders typically recommend pediatric CBT initially, and studies have typically supported this approach in preteen and milder cases.

EPIDEMIOLOGY

- ~18.8 million adults suffer from clinical depression, and 20 million suffer from a diagnosable anxiety disorder.
- 1 in 4 Americans report seeking some form of mental health treatment in their adult life. This includes generic counseling in nonmedical settings such as work, clergy, or school settings, but also includes visits to primary care providers. It is estimated that between 3.5% and 5% of adults in the US actually participate in formal mental health psychotherapy annually.
- Public health experts report that the majority of those adults with diagnosable psychiatric disorders, however, do not receive professional mental health services. This is due to multiple factors, including failure to identify, noncompliance with psychiatric referral, regional shortages of providers, economic barriers, and excessive time duration from referral to available service.
- A large study conducted between 1987 and 1997 concluded that the percentage of adults in psychotherapy remained relatively stable over that decade, the use of psychopharmacology doubled, and older adults (aged 55–64) increasingly sought psychotherapy services. In that same study, it was found that psychotherapy duration (number of sessions) decreased substantially, and about 1/3 of psychotherapy patients only attended 1 or 2 sessions.

RISK FACTORS

The need for psychotherapy or counseling services is directly and indirectly associated with a host of socioeconomic and biogenetic factors, including the general effects of poverty, family or marital dysfunction, life stressors, medical diseases or conditions, and individual biologic predisposition to mental health disorders.

GENERAL PREVENTION

It is generally assumed that early identification and intervention of child and adolescent psychopathology increases the likelihood of reducing the risk for adult psychopathology, but this has not been sufficiently validated in all categories of psychological disorders. Data support such claims in disorders such as childhood ADHD, anxiety disorders, and habit disorders of childhood, however.

 TREATMENT

GENERAL MEASURES

There is evidence of a "dose effect" in psychotherapy outcomes research, with some investigators suggesting that 6–8 sessions are necessary to yield positive initial effects, and upward of 15–20 sessions for longer term, sustainable therapeutic effects. This dose effect may not be applicable to counseling services with primarily informational or emotional/supportive functions. Also, long-term therapy should be evaluated at 6–12-month intervals to determine efficacy.

MEDICATION

- Psychotherapy is most likely to be accompanied by use of pharmaceutical adjuncts in moderate-to-severe cases of psychological dysfunction that do not respond to other therapies or in cases of extremely poor quality of life or high risk. The most common examples are in cases of clinical depression or anxiety that clearly incapacitates the patient or significantly reduces his or her quality of life. Patients at risk for suicide or who represent a danger to others are also candidates for acute psychopharmacotherapy. Studies suggest that verbal and behaviorally oriented therapies can add efficacy to medication treatment in both depression and anxiety.
- There is controversy in the research field regarding the efficacy of medication alone vs. psychotherapy alone vs. combined treatments. The most recent consensus has been that combined treatments in moderate-to-severe psychological dysfunction are most likely to render positive short-term results and increase the likelihood that such effects can be sustained over time.

ADDITIONAL THERAPIES

- Anxiety disorders:
  – Panic disorder with and without agoraphobia (1)[A]: CBT, psychodynamic therapy
  – Generalized anxiety disorder: CBT (2)[A]
  – Obsessive-compulsive disorder: CBT (3)[A]
  – Posttraumatic stress disorder: CBT
  – Specific phobia: CBT
  – Social phobia: CBT (4)[A]
- Mood disorders:
  – Unipolar depression: CBT, interpersonal therapy, psychodynamic therapy (1)[A], (5)[A]
  – Bipolar disorder: Family therapy, interpersonal therapy, CBT
  – Schizophrenia: Psychodynamic therapy, family therapy, CBT
- Eating disorders:
  – Binge eating disorder: CBT, interpersonal therapy
  – Bulimia nervosa: CBT, interpersonal therapy
- Personality disorders:
  – Borderline: DBT, CBT
- Substance-use disorders:
  – Alcohol: Counseling, CBT, motivational interviewing
  – Cocaine: CBT, counseling
  – Heroin: CBT, counseling
  – Smoking: 5 A's
- Somatoform disorders:
  – Hypochondriasis: CBT
  – Body dysmorphic disorder: CBT

COMPLEMENTARY AND ALTERNATIVE MEDICINE

A host of nonempirically based psychological and nutritional therapies can be found outside of mainstream medicine and psychological science. Very little or no evidence exists to support such experimental therapies, but all have the considerable power of the placebo effect fueling their anecdotal supports or claims. Placebo effects are also thought to be powerfully enhanced by the use of ingested or applied substances that create real physiologic, although not therapeutic, changes in the patient. If it makes them feel different, they are more likely to believe it helps.

REFERENCES

1. Furukawa TA, Watanabe N, Churchill R. Combined psychotherapy plus antidepressants for panic disorder with or without agoraphobia. *Cochrane Database Syst Rev*. 2007;(1):CD004364. Epub 2007 Jan 24.
2. Hunot V, Churchill R, Silva de Lima M, et al. Psychological therapies for generalised anxiety disorder. *Cochrane Database Syst Rev*. 2007;(1):CD001848. Epub 2007 Jan 24.
3. Eddy KT, Dutra L, Bradley R, et al. A multidimensional meta-analysis of psychotherapy and pharmacotherapy for obsessive-compulsive disorder. *Clin Psychol Rev*. 2004;24:1011–1030.
4. Rodebaugh TL, Holaway RM, Heimberg RG. The treatment of social anxiety disorder. *Clin Psychol Rev*. 2004;24:883–908.
5. Bortolotti B, Menchetti M, Bellini F, et al. Psychological interventions for major depression in primary care: A meta-analytic review of randomized controlled trials. *Gen Hosp Psychiatry*. 2008;30: 293–302.

 CODES

ICD10
- Z71.89 Other specified counseling
- Z71.9 Counseling, unspecified

CLINICAL PEARLS

- Combined medication and psychotherapeutic treatments in moderate-to-severe psychological dysfunction are most likely to render positive short-term results and increase the likelihood such effects can be sustained over time. Relapse is common over time and/or as treatments are discontinued. Children <10 may benefit significantly from counseling or psychotherapy alone for symptom relief. Older children and those with more severe symptoms typically require psychopharmacologic options in concert with counseling or verbal therapy approaches.
- There is evidence of a "dose effect" in psychotherapy outcomes research, with some investigators suggesting that 6–8 sessions are necessary to yield positive initial effects and upward of 15–20 sessions for longer term, sustainable therapeutic effects. This dose effect may not be applicable to counseling services with primarily informational or emotional/supportive functions. Since many patients cease attendance to psychotherapy sessions after 1 or a few sessions, most interventions of this type cannot be accurately evaluated by the referring provider. Long-term therapy should also be evaluated for effectiveness at regular periods.

CROHN DISEASE
Tracey G. Simon, MD • Edward Feller, MD, FACG • Samir A. Shah, MD, FACG, FASGE, AGAF

 BASICS

DESCRIPTION
Crohn disease (CD), a chronic, relapsing inflammatory GI tract disorder, most often of terminal ileum (80%):
- Hallmark features:
  - Transmural inflammation, which can result in fibrosis and stricture formation, as well as fissures leading to sinus tracts, abscesses, or fistulas
  - Noncaseating granulomas (50%), crypt abscesses
  - Skip lesions: Patchy, segmental distribution of disease; lesions may affect multiple bowel segments, interspersed with areas of normal mucosa; disease can also be continuous, potentially mimicking ulcerative colitis (UC)
  - Diverse presentations: Ileocolitis (50%); isolated colitis (20%); of these, 10% involve the rectum; anorectal (1/3); adult upper GI disease (<5%).
- Early disease:
  - Ulcerations: Initially focal with surrounding edema, resembling aphthous ulcers
  - Perianal disease (pain, anal fissures, perirectal abscess) may precede intestinal disease.
  - May present as wasting illness or anorexia
- Developed disease:
  - Mucosal cobblestoning; stenotic lumen; creeping fat; fissures develop between mucosal folds, resulting in strictures/adhesions and/or fistulae

EPIDEMIOLOGY
Incidence
- In the US, 8–10 cases/100,000 adult; incidence is rising in the US and Western Europe
- Bimodal age distribution: Predominant age is 15–25 years, with a 2nd smaller peak at 50–70 years
- Females slightly more affected than males; increased incidence among patients in northern climates
- Increased risk in whites vs. nonwhites: 2–5×
- Increased risk in Ashkenazi Jews: 3–5×

Prevalence
US adults: 100–200 cases/100,000

ETIOLOGY AND PATHOPHYSIOLOGY
- General: Clinical manifestations result from activation of inflammatory cells, whose by-products produce nonspecific tissue injury.
- Mechanism of diarrhea: Excess fluid secretion and impaired fluid absorption; bile salt malabsorption in inflamed ileum, with subsequent steatorrhea; bacterial overgrowth
- Multifactorial: Genetic, environmental triggers and immunological abnormalities result in inflammation and tissue injury in the genetically predisposed.

Genetics
Of CD patients, 15% have a 1st-degree relative with IBD; 1st-degree relative of an IBD patient has 3–30× the increased risk of developing IBD by age 28. As of May, 2012, 163 genes associated with IBD.
- Mutations in susceptibility loci:
  - Ileal CD: IBD1 gene (chromosome 16)
  - Early-onset CD (age <15): Mutations in 5q31-33 (IBD5), 21q22, and 20q13
  - North American white males with CD: 30% have HLA-DR7 and DQ4
  - Extra-intestinal manifestations of CD: Mutations in HLA-A2, HLA-DR1, HLA-DQw5
  - Others: IL-10, IL-23 receptors; ATG16L1; IRGM

- Genetic syndromes associated with IBD: Turner and Hermansky-Pudlak syndromes, glycogen storage disease, type 1b

RISK FACTORS
- Environmental factors:
  - Cigarette smoking doubles the risk of developing CD; cessation may reduce frequency of flares, relapse after surgery
  - Dietary factors: Higher incidence in diets high in refined sugars, protein (meat, fish)
  - *Salmonella* or *Campylobacter* confer increased risk of developing IBD (highest in 1 year).
  - *Clostridium difficile* infection may trigger a flare of IBD and make treatment more difficult.
- Immunological abnormalities: Not established whether immune responses in IBD are directed against self-antigens of intestinal epithelium or foreign, bacterial antigens:
  - Tumor necrosis factor (TNF): Up-regulation of inflammatory Th1 cytokines
  - Recent studies indicate that tissue inflammation may result from increased secretion of cytokine IL-17, by Th17 subset of CD4+ T cells.

COMMONLY ASSOCIATED CONDITIONS
- Extraintestinal manifestations:
  - Arthritis (20% of patients): Seronegative, primarily involving large joints; axial arthritis or ankylosing spondylitis (AS) and sacroiliitis (SI).
  - Skin disorders (10%): Erythema nodosum, pyoderma gangrenosum, psoriasis
  - Ocular disease (5%): Uveitis, iritis, episcleritis
  - Kidney stones: Calcium oxalate stones (from steatorrhea and diarrhea) or uric acid stones (from dehydration and metabolic acidosis)
  - Fat-soluble vitamin deficiency (A, D, E, K), B_{12}
  - Osteopenia and osteoporosis; hypocalcemia
  - Hypercoagulability: Venous thromboembolism prophylaxis critical in hospitalized patients
  - Gallstones: Cholesterol stones, resulting from impaired bile acid reabsorption
  - Primary sclerosing cholangitis (5%): More common with UC; asymptomatic, elevated alkaline phosphatase
  - Autoimmune hemolytic anemia
- Conditions that correlate with increased disease activity in the bowel:
  - Peripheral arthropathy (but not SI and AS)
  - Episcleritis (but not uveitis)
  - Oral aphthous ulcers and erythema nodosum
  - SI, AS, and uveitis are associated with HLA-B27.
- Potentially devastating complications: GI bleed, toxic megacolon, bowel perforation/peritonitis, malignancy, sclerosing cholangitis; recto-vaginal fistula

Rx DIAGNOSIS

HISTORY
Hallmarks: Fatigue, fever, weight loss, prolonged diarrhea; perianal disease, crampy abdominal pain, with or without gross bleeding. Children may present with growth failure:
- Factors that exacerbate CD: Concurrent infection, smoking, NSAIDs, and possibly stress

PHYSICAL EXAM
Presentation varies with location of disease:
- General: Signs of sepsis/disease activity (fever, tachycardia, hypotension) or wasting/malnutrition

- Abdominal: Focal or diffuse tenderness, distension, rebound/guarding
- Perianal: Fistulae, fissures
- Extraintestinal manifestations (see above)

DIFFERENTIAL DIAGNOSIS
- Acute, severe abdominal pain: Perforated viscus, pancreatitis, appendicitis, diverticulitis, bowel obstruction, kidney stones, gynecologic emergency
- Chronic diarrhea with crampy pain (colitis-like): UC, radiation colitis, infection, drugs, ischemia, microscopic colitis, IBD, celiac disease, malignancy (lymphoma, carcinoma), carcinoid
- Wasting illness: Malabsorption, malignancy, psychiatric illness

DIAGNOSTIC TESTS & INTERPRETATION
Initial Tests (lab, imaging)
- CBC; Chem10; LFTs; ESR/C-reactive protein (CRP); serum iron, vitamin B_{12}, vitamin D-25 OH
- If diarrhea, stool specimen for routine culture, fecal leukocytes, *C. difficile*, and ova and parasites
- In hospitalized patients with severe flare-ups, KUB to rule out toxic megacolon
- Colon: Colonoscopy with ileoscopy provides the greatest sensitivity and specificity.
  - Small bowel: Sensitivity of CT or MR enterography (MRE) surpasses SBFT and visualizes extraluminal disease. MR enterography: No radiation exposure (important in younger patients). Capsule endoscopy allows small bowel visualization but not biopsy:
  - Signs of small bowel disease: Narrowed lumen with nodularity and/or string sign; cobblestone appearance, fistula and abscess formation, bowel loop separation (from transmural inflammation with bowel-wall thickening)
- Gastroduodenal: Upper GI endoscopy:
  - Signs of gastroduodenal disease: Antral narrowing and segmental duodenal stricturing; inflammatory mucosal disease on endoscopy
- Perirectal complications: Optimal results from combination of endoscopic US (EUS) or MRI, with exam under anesthesia (EUA)
- Contraindications to endoscopy: Perforated viscus, recent myocardial infarction, severe diverticulitis, toxic megacolon, or inability to undergo appropriate bowel preparation; in most cases, unprepared limited sigmoidoscopy allows adequate visualization to assess severity, extent, and aspirate stool for *C. difficile*, obtain biopsies to assess histologic severity, exclude other disorders (e.g., cytomegalovirus)

Follow-Up Tests & Special Considerations
Evidence of complications:
- Stricture: Produces obstructive signs: Nausea, vomiting, pain, weight loss, diarrhea, or inability to pass gas or feces
- Abscess/Phlegmon: Localized abdominal peritonitis with fever and abdominal pain; diffuse peritonitis suggests intestinal perforation or abscess rupture (but may be masked by steroids, narcotics)
- Fistulae (seen in 33–50% of patients, after 10 and 20 years of disease, respectively):
  - Enteroenteric: Asymptomatic, or a palpable commonly indolent abdominal mass
  - Enterovesical: Pneumaturia, recurrent polymicrobial UTI

– Retroperitoneal: Psoas abscess, ureteral obstruction
– Enterovaginal: Vaginal passage of gas or feces; clear, nonfeculent drainage from ileal fistula may be misdiagnosed as primary vaginal infection

Diagnostic Procedures/Other
How to distinguish CD from UC:

- CD: Small bowel disease, rectal sparing; granulomas, perianal disease, and/or fistulae; no gross bleeding; focal gross/microscopic lesions:
  – Commercially available antibody tests (overall 70% sensitive): ASCA, Cbir-1, OmpC, I2
- UC: Diffuse, continuous involving the rectum; loss of normal vascularity, friable tissue; pANCA

ALERT
CD can mimic UC with continuous, not intermittent involvement; 10–15% of cases are difficult to differentiate; diagnosed as IBD undetermined.

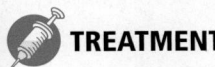

TREATMENT

- Assessment of disease severity: Clinical trials use formal grading systems, such as the Crohn's Disease Activity Index (CDAI). Others include HBI, IBDQ, CDEIS, and MAYO scores. Improved methods to assess disease severity, incorporating endoscopic findings, are currently in development including the Lemann Score:
  – Asymptomatic remission (CDAI <150)
  – Mild to moderate CD: Ambulatory patients able to tolerate PO intake without dehydration, obstruction or >10% weight loss. No abdominal tenderness, toxicity, or mass (CDAI 150–220)
  – Moderate to severe CD: Patients who have failed initial treatment or who continue to have mild symptoms such as fever, weight loss, and abdominal pain (CDAI 220–450)
  – Severe: Persistent symptoms despite outpatient therapy with glucocorticoids and/or biologics, or fulminant disease (peritonitis, cachexia, intestinal obstruction, abscess) (CDAI >450)
- General strategies:
  – Step-up approach: Begin treatment with milder therapy (5-ASA, antibiotics) followed by more aggressive agents (steroids, immunomodulators, anti-TNF agents), as needed (1)[A].
  – Top-down approach: Early management with immunomodulators and/or anti-TNF agents, before patients receive steroids, become steroid-dependent, or require surgery (1)[A]

GENERAL MEASURES
Additional therapies depend on location of disease:

- Oral lesions: Hydrocortisone and carboxymethyl-cellulose or topical sucralfate for aphthous ulcers, cheilitis, and/or granulomatous sialadenitis
- Gastroduodenal CD: No clinical trials, although slow-release mesalamine may be of benefit, as it is partially released in proximal small bowel. Case reports note success of anti-TNF therapies. Symptomatic relief possible from proton pump inhibitors, H_2-receptor blockers, and/or sucralfate.
- Ileitis: Patients often require supplementation of fat-soluble vitamins, as well as iron, B_{12}, and/or folate, and calcium to prevent bone loss.
- Treatment toxicity: Pancreatitis, bone marrow toxicity, lymphoma, nonmelanoma skin cancer, infections (TB, histoplasmosis, others), malignancy

MEDICATION
First Line
- Asymptomatic patients: Observation
- Mild CD:
  – Induction: Controversial: Slow-release oral 5-ASA agent (1.6–4.8 g/d). Evidence does not support this approach, but clinical practice suggests that some patients respond; therefore, it is commonly used as 1st-line therapy (2)[B].
  – Mesalamine preferred for ileitis. For ileocolitis, sulfasalazine (2–4 g/d) or mesalamine
  – Antibiotics use is also controversial.
  – Glucocorticoid therapy: Controlled ileal release budesonide (9 mg/d for 8–16 weeks, then discontinued over 2–4 week taper)
  – Consider adjunctive therapy: Antidiarrheals (loperamide); bile-acid binding resin (cholestyramine 4–12 g/d); probiotics (selected species either alone or in combination may prevent recurrent intestinal inflammation and reduce symptoms in acute CD) (1)[B].
  – Maintenance: 5-ASA 1.6–4.8 g/d. Controlled ileal release budesonide, 6 mg/d, effective for maintenance for up to 6 months (2)[A]
- Moderate-to-severe CD:
  – Induction: Prednisone 40–60 g/d, or controlled-release budesonide (for isolated, moderate ileitis), or anti-TNF agents (see below) (1)[A]
  – Maintenance: Little role for mesalamine. If steroids required for induction, then use immunomodulator biologic (anti-TNF agent) for maintenance. Except for budesonide, do not use steroids for maintenance (1,4,5)[A].
- Severe disease: Immunomodulators, anti-TNF agents ± steroids:
  – Azathioprine and 6-mercaptopurine: Thiopurine methyltransferase (TPMT) and LFTs, prior to initiation. Check CBC, LFTs every 2–3 months.
  – Methotrexate: Effective for steroid-dependent and steroid-refractory CD (1)[B]
    ○ Folic acid supplements 1 mg/d; follow LFTs
  – Anti-TNF therapies: Active disease, fistulae, steroid sparing, some extraintestinal disease. Infliximab, adalimumab, certolizumab pegol.
    ○ Prior to initiation: Check for TB, hepatitis B virus (3)[A].
    ○ Monitoring: Consider anti-drug Ab levels to assess for immunogenicity. Serum concentrations of anti-TNF agents may also correlate with disease activity (4)[B].
- Combination therapy:
  – Azathioprine + infliximab more effective than either alone in patients not previously treated with either
  – Rare: Hepatosplenic T-cell lymphoma (fatal)
- Antiadhesion molecules: Prevent inflammatory cells from entering GI tract. Reserved for patients who fail anti-TNF therapy:
  – Natalizumab: PML risk (1/1,000). Can minimize risk by testing for John Cunningham (JC) virus antibody. If negative, estimated PML risk 1/25,000 if treated × 3 years, with no further testing (after initial negative test). However, standard is to test every 6–12 months for JC virus on therapy to mitigate risk.

ADDITIONAL THERAPIES
Complications:
- Peritonitis: Bowel rest and antibiotic therapy (7–10 days parenteral antibiotics, followed by

2–4 week course of PO ciprofloxacin and metronidazole); surgery, as indicated:
– Consider holding steroids, which mask sepsis.
- Abscess: Antibiotics, percutaneous drainage, or surgery with resection of affected segments
- Small bowel obstruction: IV hydration, nasogastric (NG) suction, total parenteral nutrition (TPN) for malnutrition, with resolution typically in 24–48 hours. Surgery for nonresponders

 ONGOING CARE

FOLLOW-UP RECOMMENDATIONS
Patient Monitoring
Vaccinations in CD:
- Check titers; avoid live vaccines (MMR, varicella, zoster) in immunosuppression (steroids, 6MP, AZA, MTX, or anti-TNF)
- Regardless of immunosuppression: HPV, influenza, pneumococcal, meningococcal, hepatitis A, B; Tdap.

PATIENT EDUCATION
Crohn and Colitis Foundation of America (800) 343-3637; www.ccfa.org

REFERENCES
1. Lichtenstein GR, Hanauer SB, Sandborn WJ, et al. Management of Crohn's disease in adults. Am J Gastroenterol. 2009;104(2):465–483.
2. Talley NJ, Abreu MT, Achkar JP, et al. An evidence-based systematic review on medical therapies for inflammatory bowel disease. Am J Gastroenterol. 2011;106 (Suppl 1):S2–25.
3. Colombel JF, Sandborn WJ, Reinisch W, et al. Infliximab, azathioprine, or combination for Crohn's disease. N Engl J Med. 2010;362(15):1383–1395.
4. Vande CN, Ballet V, Van Assche G, et al. Early serial trough and antidrug antibody level measurements predict clinical outcome of infliximab and adalimumab treatment. Gut. 2012;61:321.

ADDITIONAL READING
- Louis E, Jean-Yves M, Vernier-Massouille G, et al. Maintenance of remission among patients with Crohn's disease on antimetabolite therapy after infliximab therapy is stopped. Gastroenterology. 2012;142:63–70.
- Baumgart DC, Sanborn WJ. Crohn's disease. Lancet. http://dx.doi.org/10.1016/50140-6736(12)60026-9.

 CODES

ICD10
- K50.00 Crohn's disease of small intestine without complications
- K50.10 Crohn's disease of large intestine without complications
- K50.919 Crohn's disease, unspecified, with unspecified complications

CLINICAL PEARLS
- MRE allows assessment of luminal and extraluminal CD without radiation exposure.
- Assess for TB and HBV prior to anti-TNF therapy.
- Cigarette smoking doubles the risk of developing CD; cessation may reduce frequency of flares.

CROUP (LARYNGOTRACHEOBRONCHITIS)

Garreth C Debiegun, MD

 BASICS

DESCRIPTION
- Croup is a subacute viral illness characterized by upper-airway symptoms such as barking cough, stridor, and fever. "Croup" is used to refer to viral laryngotracheitis or laryngotracheobronchitis (LTB), although it is sometimes used for LTB with pneumonitis, bacterial tracheitis, or spasmodic croup.
- Most common cause of upper-airway obstruction or stridor in children
- Spasmodic croup: Noninfectious form with sudden resolution:
  - No fever or radiographic changes
  - Initially treated as croup
  - Usually self-limiting and resolves with mist therapy at home
  - Often recurs on same night or in 2–3 nights
- System(s) affected: Pulmonary and respiratory
- Synonym(s): Croup; Infectious croup; Viral croup; LTB

EPIDEMIOLOGY
- Predominant age (1):
  - Common among children 7 months–3 years
  - Most common during the 2nd year of life
  - Rare among those >6 years
- Predominant sex: Male > Female (1.5:1) (1)
- Timing:
  - Possible during any time of year but is most common in autumn and winter (with parainfluenza 1 and respiratory syncytial virus [RSV])

Incidence
- 6 cases per year per 100 children <6 years old
- 1.5–6% of cases require hospitalization.
- 2–6% of those require intubation.
- Decreasing incidence in the US and Canada

ETIOLOGY AND PATHOPHYSIOLOGY
- Subglottic region/larynx is entirely encircled by the cricoid cartilage.
- Inflammatory edema and subglottic mucus production decrease airway radius.
- Small children have small airways with more compliant walls.
- Negative-pressure inspiration pulls airway walls closer together.
- Small decrease in airway radius causes significant increase in resistance (Poiseuille law: Resistance proportional to $1/\text{radius}^4$).
- Usually viruses that initially infect oropharyngeal mucosa and then migrate inferiorly
- Parainfluenza virus:
  - Most common pathogen: 75% of cases
  - Type 1 is most common, causing 18% of all cases of croup.
  - Types 2, 3, and 4 are also common.
  - Type 3 may cause a particularly severe illness.
- Other viruses: RSV, paramyxovirus, influenza virus type A or B, adenovirus, rhinovirus, enteroviruses (coxsackie and echo), reovirus, measles virus where vaccination not common, and meta-pneumovirus
- *Haemophilus influenzae* type B now rare with routine immunization (2)
- May have bacterial cause: *Mycoplasma pneumoniae* has been reported.

RISK FACTORS
- History of croup
- Recurrent upper respiratory infections
- Atopic disease increases the risk of spasmodic croup.

COMMONLY ASSOCIATED CONDITIONS
If recurrent (>2 episodes in a year) or during first 90 days of life, consider host factors:
- Underlying anatomic abnormality (e.g., subglottic stenosis):
  - In 1 study, found to be present in 59% children with recurrent croup (3)
- Paradoxical vocal cord dysfunction
- Gastroesophageal reflux disease
- Neonatal intubation

 DIAGNOSIS

- Most children who present with acute onset of barky cough, stridor, and chest-wall indrawing have croup.
- Croup is a clinical diagnosis; lab tests and imaging serve only ancillary purposes (4).
- Classic "seal-like" barking, spasmodic cough
- May have biphasic stridor
- Low-grade to moderate fever
- Upper respiratory infection prodrome lasting 1–7 days
- Severity usually is determined by clinical observation for signs of respiratory effort: Nasal flaring, retractions, tripoding, sniffing position, abdominal breathing, tachypnea. Later symptoms: Hypoxia/Cyanosis or fatigue.
- Westley Croup Scale (≤2 mild; 3–7 moderate; ≥8 severe), most useful for research purposes:
  - Level of consciousness: Normal, including sleep = 0; disoriented = 5
  - Cyanosis: None = 0; with agitation = 4; at rest = 5
  - Stridor: None = 0; with agitation = 1; at rest = 2
  - Air entry: Normal = 0; decreased = 1; markedly decreased = 2
  - Retractions: None = 0; mild = 1; moderate = 2; severe = 2
- No change in stridor with positioning
- Nontender larynx
- Inflamed subglottic region with normal-appearing supraglottic region
- Differentiate from epiglottitis: Nontoxic appearing, normal voice, no drooling, is coughing (5)

HISTORY
- 2–3 days of nonspecific prodromal syndrome with low-grade fever, coryza, and rhinorrhea
- Onset and recurrence at night when child is sleeping
- Symptoms often resolve en route to the hospital as the child is exposed to cool night air.
- Lack of prodrome indicates spasmodic croup.

PHYSICAL EXAM
- Pulse oximetry often is normal because there is no disturbance of alveolar gas exchange.
- Overall appearance: Is the child comfortable or struggling?
- Work of breathing: Labored or comfortable?
- Sound of breathing and voice: Hoarse, stridor, inspiratory wheezing, short sentences?
- Observed/Subjective tidal volume: Sufficient for child's size?

DIFFERENTIAL DIAGNOSIS
- Epiglottitis: Currently rare
- Foreign-body aspiration
- Subglottic stenosis (congenital or acquired)
- Bacterial tracheitis
- Simple upper respiratory infection
- Retropharyngeal or peritonsillar abscess
- Trauma
- Allergic reaction (acute angioneurotic edema)
- Airway anomalies (e.g., tracheo-/laryngomalacia)
- Other anatomic obstructions: Subglottic hemangioma, subglottic cyst

DIAGNOSTIC TESTS & INTERPRETATION
- No laboratory abnormality is diagnostic.
- WBCs may be low, normal, or elevated.
- Lymphocytosis is expected but not required.
- Rapid antigen or viral culture tests are available in some centers:
  - Guide isolation precautions, not management.

Initial Tests (lab, imaging)
- Posteroanterior and lateral neck films show funnel-shaped subglottic region with normal epiglottis: "Steeple," "hour-glass," or "pencil-point" sign (present in 40–60% of children with LTB).
- CT may be more sensitive for defining obstruction in a confusing clinical picture.
- Patient should be monitored during imaging; airway obstruction may occur rapidly.

Test Interpretation
- Inflammatory reaction of respiratory mucosa
- Loss of epithelial cells
- Thick mucoid secretions

 TREATMENT

GENERAL MEASURES
- Minimize lab tests, imaging, and procedures that upset the child; agitation worsens tachypnea and can be more detrimental than accepting a clinical diagnosis.
- ECG monitoring and pulse oximetry:
  - Frequent checks are more sensitive to worsening disease than is pulse oximetry.

MEDICATION
First Line
- Well established in the literature; cornerstones of treatment are immediate nebulized epinephrine and dexamethasone (6)[A].
- Racemic or L-epinephrine (equal efficacy and side-effect profiles (7); L-epinephrine is used for most other hospital purposes and is less expensive):
  - Racemic epinephrine: 0.05 mL/kg/dose (max, 0.5 mL) of 2.25% solution nebulized in normal saline to total volume of 3 mL
  - L-epinephrine: 0.5 mL/kg/dose (max, 5 mL) of a 1:1,000 dilution
  - Onset in 1–5 minutes, duration of 2 hours
  - Repeat as necessary if side effects are tolerated.
  - Must observe child for 3–4 hours

- Corticosteroids (8)[A]:
  - Dexamethasone (least expensive, easiest), 0.15–0.6 mg/kg; higher doses have been traditional care, but studies have shown 0.15 mg/kg has equal efficacy (9). Single dose; IV/IM/PO has proven equal efficacy. Recent randomized controlled trials show this begins to improve symptoms within 30 minutes (10).
  - Nebulized budesonide also has been proven effective (11)[B].
  - Other steroids (betamethasone and prednisolone) seem to be beneficial, but not as much as dexamethasone (7).
  - Onset by 6 hours
- Heliox: A helium-oxygen mixture:
  - Smaller, lower-mass helium molecule (compared with nitrogen) theoretically maintains laminar flow in narrower airways and serves as bridge therapy to steroids.
  - Minimum of 60% helium must be used; 70% is preferable; 79% if patient has no O_2 requirement
  - Limited data; anecdotal reports and 1 case series support its use, but 2 prospective studies showed no benefit (12). Also, a Cochrane review found insufficient evidence to support the use of Heliox in croup (13).
- Antibiotics not indicated in this viral illness:
  - Antecedent or subsequent bacterial infection is possible but uncommon.
- Oxygen as needed
- Humidified air shows no clinical benefit.

Second Line
Amantadine for influenza A: 100 mg PO b.i.d. for 3–5 days

SURGERY/OTHER PROCEDURES
- Intubation rarely is required; tube 0.5–1 mm smaller than normal:
  - After trial of medical management, intubation is for fatigue caused by work of breathing or beginning total obstruction; not secondary to low oxygen saturation.
  - Extubate in 3–5 days when there is an appropriate air leak around the endotracheal tube.
- Tracheotomy: Rarely; maintenance 3–7 days

COMPLEMENTARY AND ALTERNATIVE MEDICINE
- Although proven no benefit in hospital, may be helpful at home. Do not use high-temperature misters (e.g., teakettles) because of a risk of burns. A hot shower running in a bathroom is a good steam generator.
- Some children respond well to cold, dry air.
- Probiotics may decrease the incidence of upper respiratory tract infections (10),(14)[A].

IN-PATIENT CONSIDERATIONS
Admission Criteria/Initial Stabilization
Minor cases need no visit to a hospital or primary care physician (PCP):
- Outpatient care in mild cases
- Admit patients who do not respond to therapy or have recurrent stridor at rest after epinephrine wears off. Also admit those who have O_2 requirement, pneumonia, or congestive heart failure.
- In most cases, observation in the ED after medical management is sufficient.
- No stridor at rest, no difficulty breathing

- Child able to tolerate liquids PO
- No underlying medical condition
- Caretakers able to assess changes to clinical picture and reaccess medical care

Discharge Criteria
Patients who maintain a good response to medical therapy for 3–4 hours (after epinephrine dose) may be safely discharged as long as they have reliable caretakers and good access to medical services if symptoms return (13)[C].

 ONGOING CARE

FOLLOW-UP RECOMMENDATIONS
Patient Monitoring
Most patients will be seen in an ED or PCP office setting.

DIET
- NPO and IV fluids for severe cases
- Frequent small feedings with increased fluids for mild cases

PATIENT EDUCATION
- Must keep the patient quiet; crying may exacerbate symptoms.
- Educate parents about when to seek emergency care if mild cases progress.
- Provide emotional support and reassurance for the patient.

PROGNOSIS
- Up to 1/3 of patients will have a recurrence.
- Recovery is usually full and without lasting effects.
- If multiple recurrences, consider referral to ENT specialist to evaluate for possible anatomic etiology (3).

COMPLICATIONS
- Rare
- Subglottic stenosis in intubated patients
- Bacterial tracheitis
- Cardiopulmonary arrest
- Pneumonia

REFERENCES

1. Cherry JD. Clinical practice. Croup *N Engl J Med*. 2008;358:384–391.
2. Sobol SE, Zapata S. Epiglottitis and croup. *Otolaryngol Clin North Am*. 2008;41:551–566, ix.
3. Jabbour N, Parker NP, Finkelstein M, et al. Incidence of operative endoscopy findings in recurrent croup. *Otolaryngol Head Neck Surg*. 2011;144:596–601.
4. Everard ML. Acute bronchiolitis and croup. *Pediatr Clin North Am*. 2009;56:119–133, x–xi.
5. Tibballs J, Watson T. Symptoms and signs differentiating croup and epiglottitis. *J Paediatr Child Health*. 2011;47(3):77–82. Epub 2010 Nov 21.
6. Johnson DW, Jacobson S, Edney PC, et al. A comparison of nebulized budesonide, intramuscular dexamethasone, and placebo for moderately severe croup. *N Engl J Med*. 1998;339:498–503.
7. Bjornson C, Russell KF, Vandermeer B, et al. Nebulized epinephrine for croup in children. *Cochrane Database Syst Rev*. 2011;CD006619.
8. Russell KF, Liang Y, O'Gorman K, et al. Glucocorticoids for croup. *Cochrane Database Syst Rev*. 2011;CD001955.
9. Dobrovoljac M, Geelhoed GC. 27 years of croup: An update highlighting the effectiveness of 0.15 mg/kg of dexamethasone. *Emerg Med Australas*. 2009;21(4):309–314.
10. Dobrovoljac, Geelhoed. How fast does oral dexamethasone work in mild to moderately severe croup? A randomized double-blinded clinical trial. *Emerg Med Australas*. 2012;24:79–85.
11. Cetinkaya F, Tüfekçi BS, Kutluk G. A comparison of nebulized budesonide, and intramuscular, and oral dexamethasone for treatment of croup. *Int J Pediatr Otorhinolaryngol*. 2004;68:453–456.
12. Vorwerk C, Coats TJ. Use of helium-oxygen mixtures in the treatment of croup: A systematic review. *Emerg Med J*. 2008;25:547–550.
13. Vorwerk C, Coats T. Heliox for croup in children. *Cochrane Database Syst Rev*. 2010;(2): CD006822. Epub 2010 Feb 17.
14. Hao Q, Lu Z, Dong BR, et al. Probiotics for preventing acute upper respiratory tract infections. *Cochrane Database Syst Rev*. 2011;9:CD006895.

ADDITIONAL READING
Bjornson CL, Johnson DW. Croup. *Lancet*. 2008; 371(9609):329–339.

 SEE ALSO

Bronchiolitis; Epiglottitis; Tracheitis, Bacterial

 CODES

ICD10
- J05.0 Acute obstructive laryngitis [croup]
- J20.9 Acute bronchitis, unspecified

CLINICAL PEARLS
- Parainfluenza virus is the most common pathogen.
- Also caused by RSV, paramyxovirus, influenza virus type A or B, adenovirus, rhinovirus, enteroviruses (coxsackie and echo)
- Established efficacy of inhaled epinephrine and corticosteroids
- Lateral neck films show funnel-shaped subglottic region with normal epiglottis: "Steeple," "hour-glass," or "pencil-point" sign (present in 40–60% of children with laryngotracheobronchitis).

CRYPTORCHIDISM
Pamela Ellsworth, MD

 BASICS

DESCRIPTION
- Incomplete or improper descent of 1 or both testicles; also called undescended testes (UTD)
- Normally, descent is in the 7th–8th month of gestation. The cryptorchid testis may be palpable or nonpalpable.
- Types of cryptorchidism:
  - Abdominal: Located inside the internal ring
  - Canalicular: Located between the internal and external rings
  - Ectopic: Located outside the normal path of testicular descent from abdominal cavity to scrotum; may be ectopic to perineum, femoral canal, superficial inguinal pouch (most common), suprapubic area, or opposite hemiscrotum
  - Retractile: Fully descended testis that moves freely between the scrotum and the groin
  - Iatrogenic: Previously descended testis becomes undescended secondary to scar tissue after inguinal surgery, such as an inguinal hernia repair or hydrocelectomy.
  - Also may be referred to as *palpable* versus *nonpalpable*
- System(s) affected: Reproductive
- Synonym(s): Undescended testes (UDT)

EPIDEMIOLOGY
Incidence
- Predominant age: Premature newborns
- Predominant sex: Male only

Prevalence
- In the US, cryptorchidism occurs in 3% of full-term, and 33% of premature newborn males.
- Spontaneous testicular descent occurs by age 1–3 months in 50–70% of full-term males with cryptorchidism.
- Descent at 6–9 months of age is rare.

ETIOLOGY AND PATHOPHYSIOLOGY
- Not fully known
- May involve alterations in:
  - Mechanical factors (gubernaculum, length of vas deferens and testicular vessels, groin anatomy, epididymis, cremasteric muscles, and abdominal pressure), hormonal factors (gonadotropin, testosterone, dihydrotestosterone, and müllerian-inhibiting substance), and neural factors (ilioinguinal nerve and genitofemoral nerve)
  - Major regulators of testicular descent from intra-abdominal location into the bottom of the scrotum are the Leydig cell-derived hormones testosterone and insulin-like growth factor 3 (IGF-3).
  - Mutations in the gene for IGF-3 and in the androgen receptor gene have been recognized as causes of cryptorchidism as well as chromosomal alterations.
  - Environmental factors acting as endocrine disruptors of testicular descent also may contribute to the etiology of cryptorchidism (1).
- Risk of ascent may be as high as 50% in cases where 1 testis is significantly retractile (2).

Genetics
Occurrence of UDT in siblings, as well as fathers, suggests a genetic etiology.

RISK FACTORS
- Family history of cryptorchidism: Boys with UDTs: 4% of their fathers and 6.2–9.8% of their brothers have UDTs (3).
- Low birth weight, prematurity, and small for gestational age are associated with a substantial increase in incidence of cryptorchidism, which may reach 20–25% in infants with birth weight <2.5 kg (4).

COMMONLY ASSOCIATED CONDITIONS
- Inguinal hernia/hydrocele
- Abnormalities of vas deferens and epididymis
- Intersex abnormalities
- Hypogonadotropic hypogonadism
- Germinal cell aplasia
- Prune-belly syndrome
- Meningomyelocele
- Hypospadias
- Wilms' tumor
- Prader-Willi syndrome
- Kallmann syndrome
- Cystic fibrosis

℞ DIAGNOSIS

HISTORY
- ≥1 testicles in a site other than the scrotum
- May be an isolated defect or associated with other congenital anomalies

PHYSICAL EXAM
- Performed with warm hands, with child in sitting, standing, and squatting position
- A Valsalva maneuver and applied pressure to lower abdomen may help to identify the testes, especially a gliding testis.
- Failure to palpate a testis after repeated exams suggests an intra-abdominal or atrophic testis.
- An enlarged contralateral testis in the presence of a nonpalpable testis suggests testicular atrophy/absence.

DIFFERENTIAL DIAGNOSIS
- Retractile testis (hypermobile testis): A normally descended testis that ascends into the inguinal canal because of an active cremasteric reflex (more common in males 4–6 years of age)
- Atrophic testis: May occur as a result of neonatal torsion
- Vanished testis may be the result of a lack of development or in utero torsion.

DIAGNOSTIC TESTS & INTERPRETATION
Initial Tests (lab, imaging)
- In boys ≤3 months of age with bilateral, nonpalpable UDTs, hormone levels are helpful to determine whether the testes are present:
  - Luteinizing hormone (LH)
  - Follicle-stimulating hormone (FSH)
  - Testosterone
- >3 months of age, a human chorionic gonadotropin (hCG) stimulation test to determine presence or absence of testicular tissue (hCG 2,000 IU/d × 3 days, and check testosterone before and after stimulation)
- Ultrasound has a sensitivity of 45% (95% confidence interval [CI]: 29–61) and a specificity of 78% (95% CI: 43–94) (1):
  - Ultrasound does not reliably localize nonpalpable testes and does not rule out an intra-abdominal testis. A recent meta-analysis therefore concluded eliminating the use of ultrasound will not change management of nonpalpable cryptorchidism, but will decrease health care expenditures (1,5).
  - In earlier studies, ultrasonography had a sensitivity of 76%, a specificity of 100%, and an accuracy of 84% in the diagnosis of nonpalpable UDT (5).
- MRI has a sensitivity of 86%, a specificity of 79%, and an accuracy of 85% (5).
- CT scan findings in children are inconsistent.

Follow-Up Tests & Special Considerations
- In newborns and children <6–12 months of age, periodic examination to determine if testis is palpable and descended prior to considering further intervention
- In children with retractile testes, periodic examination is necessary to rule out subsequent ascent.

Diagnostic Procedures/Other
Laparoscopy is useful in a child with nonpalpable cryptorchidism to confirm testicular absence or presence accurately and to determine the feasibility of performing a standard orchiopexy (6)[C].

Test Interpretation
- Higher incidence of carcinoma in UDT and alterations in spermatogenesis
- Histologic changes occur by 1.5 years of age and include smaller seminiferous tubules, fewer spermatogonia, and more peritubular tissue.

C

 TREATMENT

GENERAL MEASURES
- Rule out retractile testis
- Appropriate health care: Outpatient until surgery performed
- Administration of chorionic gonadotropin may cause testicular descent in some boys. Reports of efficacy are inconsistent.

MEDICATION
- The International Health Foundation recommends biweekly hCG injections for 5 weeks: 250 IU for infants, 500 IU for children ≤6 years of age, and 1,000 IU for children ≥6 years of age. This is an off-label use of hCG.
- Success rates for descent into the scrotum range from 0–55% (7)[B]:
  - The more distal the testis, the more likely the descent
  - A systematic review with a meta-analysis of randomized clinical trials concluded that the evidence for the use of hCG vs. gonadotropin-releasing hormone (GnRH) shows advantages for hCG, but noted that the evidence was based on few trials (8)[B].
- Contraindications: hCG therapy is contraindicated in patients with a clinically apparent inguinal hernia, those with a history of previous ipsilateral groin surgery, or those with ectopic testicles. Also refer to manufacturer's literature.
- Precautions: (i) May induce precocious puberty; discontinue drug; effects should reverse in 4 weeks; (ii) premature epiphyseal closure
- Significant possible interactions: Refer to manufacturer's literature.
- GnRH is approved for use in Europe, and neoadjuvant GnRH therapy may improve fertility index in UDT (8)[C].

ISSUES FOR REFERRAL
- ≥1 testes not descended by 6 months to 1 year of age
- Bilateral nonpalpable UDTs

SURGERY/OTHER PROCEDURES
- Reasons to consider: Avoids torsion, averts trauma, decreases but does not eliminate risk of malignancy, and prevents further alterations in spermatogenesis
- Orchiopexy should be performed by age 1. Alterations in germ cell count in the cryptorchid testis have been identified by age 2.
- Surgery prior to 9 months of age has a beneficial effect on growth of previously undescended testis. (9)[B]
- Laparoscopy is performed first if testis is nonpalpable.
- If palpable, an inguinal approach is usually performed. Prepubertal approach is considered in select situations, but may increase the risk of hernia (10)[C].

 ONGOING CARE

FOLLOW-UP RECOMMENDATIONS
Initial follow-up within 1 month of surgery and periodically thereafter to assess testicular size/growth

Patient Monitoring
- Patients should be followed after surgery to evaluate testicular growth.
- Testicular tumors occur mainly during or after puberty; thus, these children should be taught self-examination when they are older.

DIET
No restrictions

PATIENT EDUCATION
Discuss with parents about causes, available treatments, and possible effects on patient's reproductive potential; also increased risk for testicular cancer and need for regular self-examination.

PROGNOSIS
- Disorder is usually corrected with medical or surgical therapy; however, possible lifelong consequences.
- If testicle is absent or orchiectomy is required, may consider placement of testicular prosthesis.
- Early orchidopexy may decrease risk of testicular damage and risk of malignancy.

COMPLICATIONS
- Progressive failure of spermatogenesis, if left untreated; even with orchiopexy, the fertility rate is still reduced, especially with bilateral UDTs.
- Spermatogenesis is related to the duration of cryptorchidism and the location of the testis.
- Formerly bilaterally cryptorchid men have a greater decrease in fertility compared with unilateral cryptorchid male and the general male population.
- Abnormalities also have been identified in the contralateral descended testis, although less severe.

REFERENCES

1. Tasian GE, Copp HL. Diagnostic performance of ultrasound in nonpalpable cryptorchidism: A systematic review and meta-analysis. *Pediatrics*. 2011;127:119–128.
2. Barthold JS. Undescended testis: Current theories of etiology. *Curr Opin Urol*. 2008;18:395–400.
3. Cortes D. Cryptorchidism: Aspects of pathogenesis, histology and treatment. *Scan J Nephrol*. 1998;9:54.
4. Foresta C, Zuccarello D, Garolla A, et al. Role of hormones, genes, and environment in human cryptorchidism. *Endocr Rev*. 2008;29:560–580.
5. Tasian GE, Yiee JH, Copp HL, et al. Imaging use and cryptorchidism: Determinants of practice patterns. *J Urol*. 2011;185:1882–1887.
6. Kanemoto K, Hayashi Y, Kojima Y, et al. Accuracy of ultrasonography and magnetic resonance imaging in the diagnosis of non-palpable testis. *Int J Urol*. 2005;12:668–672.
7. Patil KK. Laparoscopy for impalpable testis. *Br J Urol*. 2005;95:704–708.
8. Henna MR, Del Nero RG, Sampaio CZ, et al. Hormonal cryptorchidism therapy: Systematic review with metaanalysis of randomized clinical trials. *Pediatr Surg Int*. 2004;20:357–359.
9. Kollin C, Hesser U, Ritzen EM, Karpe B. Testicular growth from birth to 2 years of age, and the effect of orchidopexy at 9 months of age: A randomized, controlled study. *Acta Paediatr*. 2006;95: 318–234.
10. Schwentner C, Oswald J, Kreczy A, et al. Neoadjuvant gonadotropin-releasing hormone therapy before surgery may improve the fertility index in undescended testes: A prospective randomized trial. *J Urol*. 2005;173:974–977.

ADDITIONAL READING

- Al-Mandil M, Khoury AE, El-Hout Y, et al. Potential complications with the prescrotal approach for the palpable undescended testis? A comparison of single prescrotal incision to the traditional inguinal approach. *J Urol*. 2008;180:686–689.
- Cryptorchidism: A prospective study of 7500 consecutive male births, 1984–8. John Radcliffe Hospital Cryptorchidism Study Group. *Arch Dis Child*. 1992;67:892–899.
- Hutson JM, Balic A, Nation T, et al. *Cryptorchidism*. *Semin Pediatr Surg*. 2010;19:215–224.
- Lee PA. Fertility after cryptorchidism: Epidemiology and other outcome studies. *Urology*. 2005;66: 427–431.

CODES
ICD-9-
301.

ICD10
- Q53.9 Undescended testicle, unspecified
- Q53.10 Unspecified undescended testicle, unilateral
- Q53.20 Undescended testicle, unspecified, bilateral

CLINICAL PEARLS
- If testicular descent does not occur by 6–9 months of age, it is unlikely to occur. Therefore, refer patients to a urologist if a testis has not descended by 6 months to 1 year of age.
- Children with bilateral, nonpalpable UDTs require laboratory evaluation to determine if viable testicular tissue is present.
- Limiting the use of ultrasound may not change management of nonpalpable cryptorchidism.
- The risk of infertility is increased with bilateral UDTs.

CUBITAL TUNNEL SYNDROME
James Winger, MD

BASICS

DESCRIPTION
- Compression of the ulnar nerve on the medial aspect of the elbow where it enters the cubital tunnel. Often resulting in elbow pain and paresthesias of the forearm, wrist, 4th and 5th fingers.
- Synonym(s): Ulnar neuropathy

EPIDEMIOLOGY
- Predominant sex: Male > Female (3–8× more common in males)
- Elbow is most common site of compression of ulnar nerve:
  – Less common sites of entrapment include:
    ○ Arcade of Struthers
    ○ Medial intermuscular septum
    ○ Medial epicondyle
    ○ Deep flexor pronator aponeurosis (1)
- 2nd most common nerve compression of upper extremity (behind median nerve compression in carpal tunnel) (2)

ETIOLOGY AND PATHOPHYSIOLOGY
- The ulnar nerve is the terminal branch of the medial cord of the brachial plexus; it is composed of portions of the C8 and T1 nerve roots.
- The ulnar nerve becomes more superficial as it enters the ulnar sulcus ~3.5 cm proximal to the medial epicondyle. The nerve courses posterior to the medial epicondyle and medial to the olecranon, then enters the cubital tunnel (2).
- The cubital tunnel is a fibro-osseous canal. The roof is defined by the arcuate ligament of Osborne. The floor consists of the medial collateral ligament of the elbow, the joint capsule, and the olecranon.
- Elbow flexion increases distance from medial epicondyle to olecranon 5 mm for every 45 degrees.
- Elbow flexion places stress on medial (ulnar) collateral ligament, overlying retinaculum, and ulnar nerve.
- Shape of cubital tunnel changes from circular to ovoid, losing 2.5 mm of height with elbow flexion.
- Loss of height of cubital tunnel with elbow flexion decreases tunnel volume by 55%, which doubles intraneural pressure on the ulnar nerve.
- Maximal pressure on the ulnar nerve in cubital tunnel is created by shoulder abduction, elbow flexion, and wrist extension.
- Elbow flexion decreases volume of cubital tunnel, causing compression of ulnar nerve.
- Compression of ulnar nerve causes pain at medial aspect of elbow and symptoms at forearm and hand.
- Caused by constricting fascial bands, subluxation of ulnar nerve over medial epicondyle, cubitus valgus, bony spurs, hypertrophied synovium, tumors, ganglia, or direct compression of ulnar nerve as it crosses cubital tunnel

RISK FACTORS
- Patients who sleep or position themselves with their elbows bent, their arms overhead, or both
- Patients with occupations demanding prolonged time with elbows bent (3)[A]
- Athletes in throwing sports, racquet sports, weightlifting, and skiing
- Preexisting polyneuropathy
- Patients with end-stage renal disease on hemodialysis
- Patients placed in dependent positioning (surgery, ICU)

GENERAL PREVENTION
- Avoid long periods with elbows bent or pressure on elbows.
- Sleep with elbows straight and avoid sleeping with arms overhead.
- Keep proper posture when working at a desk.

COMMONLY ASSOCIATED CONDITIONS
- Ulnar nerve subluxation
- Ulnar collateral ligament laxity
- Osteoarthritis of elbow joint

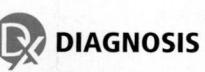

DIAGNOSIS

HISTORY
- Nocturnal elbow pain
- Medial elbow pain
- Paresthesias along medial forearm, wrist, and 4th and 5th digits
- Paresthesias may be intermittent at first and then become more constant.
- History of trauma over the area
- Repetitive elbow flexion and extension activities (e.g., hammering)
- Overhead throwing athlete with repetitive elbow motion
- Chronic symptoms: Loss of grip strength and loss of fine motor skills in hand

PHYSICAL EXAM
- Inspect carrying angle of both elbows.
- Palpate medial epicondyle and cubital tunnel for areas of tenderness or ulnar nerve subluxation.
- Assess elbow range of motion.
- Positive Hoffman-Tinel test (percussion at ulnar nerve) (2)
- Pain on palpating over ulnar nerve
- Atrophy of intrinsic hand muscles
- Loss of sensation at 5th digit and medial side of 4th digit
- Wasting of hypothenar muscles and flexion contracture of 4th and 5th digits (ulnar claw)
- Wartenberg sign is clawing or abduction of the 5th digit with extension.
- Assess ability to cross 2nd and 3rd digits.
- Evaluate grip and pinch strength for weakness.

- Froment's sign describes hyperflexion of thumb interphalangeal joint when trying to maintain a sheet of paper between the thumb and 1st finger as the examiner pulls the paper away (4).
- Assess vibration and light touch sensation.
- Recently, the scratch-collapse test has been described. Patient faces the examiner with arms adducted, elbows flexed, hands outstretched, and wrists at neutral. Patient resists bilateral shoulder adduction and internal rotation as examiner applies these forces to the forearm. Examiner "scratches" or swipes fingertips over course of compressed ulnar nerve. Force is then reapplied to the forearm. A positive result occurs when the patient has a temporary loss of external rotation resistance tone.
- Sensitivity for the scratch collapse was 69% compared with 54% and 46% for Tinel test and elbow flexion-compression test, respectively. Tinel test, however, had the highest negative predictive value (98%) of all tests for cubital tunnel (5).

DIFFERENTIAL DIAGNOSIS
- Cervical radiculopathy
- Thoracic outlet syndrome
- Carpal tunnel syndrome
- Medial Epicondylitis
- Ulnar collateral ligament injury
- Pancoast syndrome
- Metabolic disorders creating peripheral neuropathies
- Multiple sclerosis and other myelopathies

DIAGNOSTIC TESTS & INTERPRETATION
McGowan grades quantify the degree of physical exam findings and are specific for cubital tunnel syndrome:
- McGowan grade I: No wasting or weakness of intrinsic muscles, feeling of clumsiness in affected hand, mild paresthesias in ulnar nerve distribution
- McGowan grade II: Intermediate lesions with weak interossei and muscle wasting
- McGowan grade III: Severe lesions with paralysis of interossei and a marked weakness of the hand

Initial Tests (lab, imaging)
- X-ray study may reveal osteophyte impingement of cubital tunnel. Include anterior posterior (AP) lateral, and cubital tunnel views (1). Radiographs may also show signs of instability, deformity from old trauma, or presence of a supracondylar process (which can cause median nerve compression).
- Cubital tunnel view: Elbow is maximally flexed and x-ray beam is shot as an AP view of the distal humerus.

Follow-Up Tests & Special Considerations
- Chest x-ray if patient has history of smoking and ulnar nerve symptoms (to exclude Pancoast tumor in apical lung)
- MRI shows inflammation and irritation of ulnar nerve.
- High-resolution US

Diagnostic Procedures/Other
- Corticosteroid injection into ulnar groove
- Electromyogram (EMG) is not essential when diagnosis is obvious on clinical exam. Use to determine the efficacy of conservative treatment or when the diagnosis is unclear.
- EMG is considered positive if motor conduction delay across the elbow is <50 m/s or difference between motor velocity across elbow and below the elbow is >10 m/s.
- Nerve conduction studies

Test Interpretation
Inflammation and swelling of ulnar nerve

TREATMENT

- Mild cubital tunnel syndrome can often be treated without surgery.
- If provocative causes can be identified and avoided, there is trend toward recovery.
- In mild cases, nonoperative treatment is utilized for 3 months.
- Patients with constant symptoms and/or muscle atrophy typically require surgical intervention (1)[C].

GENERAL MEASURES
- Active rest
- Avoidance of aggravating activities
- Conservative treatment is initial approach if no motor weakness (6)[C]
- Instruct patient to avoid periods of prolonged elbow flexion.
- Instruct patient to avoid long periods of pressure and compression on ulnar nerve at elbow.
- Ice for symptom relief
- Splint or brace while sleeping to keep affected elbow in extension and take pressure off cubital tunnel (e.g., wrap towel around elbow and hold in place with tape; use a small size soft knee splint, but wear it backward on the elbow, tie a scarf around waist then around wrist)
- Physical therapy (nerve mobilization techniques and forearm and wrist stretching)
- Workplace/Ergonomic modifications (e.g., correct posture, avoid long periods with elbows bent)
- Otherwise activity, as tolerated

MEDICATION
First Line
NSAIDs and activity modification to limit elbow flexion

Second Line
Corticosteroid injection into the cubital tunnel (7)[B]

ISSUES FOR REFERRAL
Failure of 3–6 months of conservative treatment, loss of grip strength, flexion contracture of 4th and 5th digits, positive EMG for motor conduction delay (8)[C]

ADDITIONAL THERAPIES
- Use 1 mL lidocaine and 20–40 mg methylprednisolone injected into ulnar groove, parallel to ulnar nerve (7).
- Hand therapy and custom-splint prescription

SURGERY/OTHER PROCEDURES
- Goal of surgery is to create more space for the ulnar nerve (6).
- Many surgical treatments exist for the treatment of cubital tunnel syndrome. In situ decompression; transposition of the ulnar nerve into the SC, IM, or submuscular plane; or medial epicondylectomy have all been shown to be effective in the treatment of this disease process. Comparative studies have shown some short-term advantages to one or another technique, but overall results between the treatments have essentially been equivocal. The choice of surgical treatment is based on multiple factors, and a single surgical approach cannot be applied to all clinical situations (2)[A].

COMPLEMENTARY AND ALTERNATIVE MEDICINE
Vitamin B_6 (100 mg/d) not found to be effective in randomized trials

ONGOING CARE

FOLLOW-UP RECOMMENDATIONS
Patient Monitoring
- In severe cases, the nerve damage may be permanent and the patient may not recover.
- Patients with symptoms lasting >6 months have a worse prognosis.

DIET
No restrictions

PATIENT EDUCATION
- Use correct posture; avoid putting pressure on elbows, and place padding under elbows.
- Inability to straighten fingers is often a sign of severe ulnar nerve damage. Patients with this level of irritation usually do not recover, even with surgery.

PROGNOSIS
- Both conservative and surgical methods result in 85–90% good-to-excellent results.
- For McGowan grade III: Anterior IM transposition has best outcome (8)[C].

COMPLICATIONS
Anterior transposition and simple decompression may have recurrent subluxation of the ulnar nerve.

REFERENCES

1. Hariri S, McAdams TR. Nerve injuries about the elbow. *Clin Sports Med*. 2010;29:655–675.
2. Palmer BA, Hughes TB. Cubital tunnel syndrome. *J Hand Surg Am*. 2010;35:153–163.
3. van Rijn RM, Huisstede BM, Koes BW, et al. Associations between work-related factors and specific disorders at the elbow: A systematic literature review. *Rheumatology (Oxford)*. 2009;48(5):528–536.
4. Anderton M, Webb M. Cubital tunnel syndrome. *Br J Hosp Med (Lond)*. 2010;71:M167–169.
5. Cheng CJ, Mackinnon-Patterson B, Beck JL, et al. Scratch collapse test for evaluation of carpal and cubital tunnel syndrome. *J Hand Surg Am*. 2008;33: 1518–1524.
6. Mowlavi A, Andrews K, Lille S, et al. The management of cubital tunnel syndrome: A meta-analysis of clinical studies. *Plast Reconstr Surg*. 2000;106:327–334.
7. Rampen AJ, Wirtz PW, Tavy DL, et al. Ultrasound-guided steroid injection to treat mild ulnar neuropathy at the elbow. *Muscle Nerve*. 2011;44:128–130.
8. Mitsionis GI, Manoudis GN, Paschos NK, et al. Comparative study of surgical treatment of ulnar nerve compression at the elbow. *J Shoulder Elbow Surg*. 2010;19:513–519.

ADDITIONAL READING
- Assmus H, Antoniadis G, Bischoff C, et al. Cubital tunnel syndrome—a review and management guidelines. *Cent Eur Neurosurg*. 2011;72(2):90–98.
- Ehsan A, Hanel DP. Recurrent or persistent cubital tunnel syndrome. *J Hand Surg Am*. 2012;37(9): 1910–1912. Epub 2012 Feb 1.
- Shi Q, MacDermid J, Grewal R, et al. Predictors of functional outcome change 18 months after anterior ulnar nerve transposition. *Arch Phys Med Rehabil*. 2012;93(2):307–312.

 SEE ALSO

Epicondylitis

 CODES

ICD10
- G56.20 Lesion of ulnar nerve, unspecified upper limb
- G56.21 Lesion of ulnar nerve, right upper limb
- G56.22 Lesion of ulnar nerve, left upper limb

CLINICAL PEARLS
- Elbow flexion decreases depth of cubital tunnel, thus compressing the ulnar nerve.
- Sleeping with elbow bent and arm overhead can cause symptoms.
- Improper posture when working at a desk can cause symptoms.
- Conservative treatment consists of ice, rest, hand therapy, splint fabrication, and activity modifications for 3 months in selected patients.
- Both conservative and surgical methods result in good-to-excellent results 85–90% of the time.

CUSHING DISEASE AND CUSHING SYNDROME

Linda Paniagua, MD • Geetha Gopalakrishnan, MD

BASICS

DESCRIPTION
- Clinical abnormalities associated with chronic exposure to excessive amounts of cortisol (the major adrenocorticoid)
- Cushing syndrome is defined as excessive corticosteroid exposure from exogenous sources (medications) or endogenous sources (pituitary, adrenal, pulmonary, etc.), or tumor. Exogenous intake of steroids is the primary cause of Cushing syndrome.
- Cushing disease is defined as glucocorticoid excess due to excessive adrenocorticotropic hormone (ACTH) secretion from a pituitary tumor, the most common cause of primary Cushing syndrome.
- System(s) affected: Endocrine/Metabolic; Musculoskeletal; Skin/Exocrine; Cardiovascular; Neuropsychiatric

Pediatric Considerations
- Rare in infancy and childhood
- Cushing disease accounts for approximately 75% of all cases of Cushing syndrome in children >7 years.
- In children <7 years, adrenal causes of Cushing syndrome (adenoma, carcinoma, or bilateral hyperplasia) are more common.
- Most common presenting symptom is lack of growth consistent with the weight gain.

Pregnancy Considerations
- Pregnancy may exacerbate disease.
- Cortisol levels increase in normal pregnancy states.

EPIDEMIOLOGY
Incidence
Uncommon: 0.7–2.4/1 million per year
Prevalence
2–5% prevalence reported in difficult-to-control diabetics with obesity and hypertension (HTN)

ETIOLOGY AND PATHOPHYSIOLOGY
- Syndrome: Excessive corticosteroid exposure from exogenous sources (medications) or endogenous sources (pituitary, adrenal, pulmonary, etc.), or tumor
- Disease: Pituitary tumor causing excess ACTH (corticotropin)
- General population:
  - Exogenous glucocorticoids
  - Endogenous ACTH-dependent hypercortisolism: 80–85%:
    - ACTH-secreting pituitary tumor: 75%
    - Ectopic ACTH production (e.g., small-cell carcinoma of lung, bronchial carcinoid): 20%
  - Endogenous ACTH-independent hypercortisolism: 15–20%:
    - Adrenal adenoma
    - Adrenal carcinoma
    - Macronodular or micronodular hyperplasia
- Pediatric/Adolescent (1):
  - Adrenal hyperplasia secondary to McCune-Albright: Mean age 1.2 years
  - Adrenocortical tumors: Mean age 4.5 years
  - Ectopic ACTH syndrome: Mean age 10.1 years
  - Primary pigmented nodular adrenocortical disease: Mean age 13.0 years
  - Cushing disease: Mean age 14.1 years

- Pregnancy (2):
  - Pituitary-dependent Cushing syndrome: 33%
  - Adrenal causes: 40–50%
  - ACTH-independent adrenal hyperplasia: 3%

Genetics
- Multiple endocrine neoplasia
- Carney complex (an inherited multiple neoplasia syndrome)
- McCune-Albright syndrome (mutation of *GNAS1* gene)
- Familial isolated pituitary adenomas (mutations in the aryl hydrocarbon receptor interacting protein gene)

RISK FACTORS
- Prevalent sex: Female > Male (3:1)
- Most often occurs between the ages of 25 and 40
- Prolonged use of corticosteroids

GENERAL PREVENTION
Avoid corticosteroid exposure when possible.

DIAGNOSIS

HISTORY
- Weight gain: 95% (3)
- Decreased libido: 90%
- Menstrual irregularity: 80%
- Depression/Emotional lability: 50–80%
- Easy bruising: 65%
- Diabetes or glucose intolerance: 60%

PHYSICAL EXAM
- Obesity (usually central): 95%
- Facial plethora: 90%
- Moon face (facial adiposity): 90%
- Thin skin: 85%
- Hypertension: 75%
- Skeletal growth retardation in children (epiphyseal plates remain open): 70–80%
- Hirsutism: 75%
- Proximal muscle weakness: 60%
- Purple striae on the skin
- Increased adipose tissue in neck and trunk
- Acne

DIFFERENTIAL DIAGNOSIS
- Obesity
- Diabetes mellitus
- HTN
- Metabolic syndrome X
- Polycystic ovarian disease
- Pseudo-Cushing (e.g., alcoholism, physical stress, severe major depression)

DIAGNOSTIC TESTS & INTERPRETATION
Initial Tests (lab, imaging)
- Recent guidelines (4)[C]:
  - The 2008 Endocrine Society guidelines recommend against widespread testing for Cushing syndrome except in patients with:
    - Adrenal incidentaloma
    - Multiple progressive features suggestive of Cushing syndrome
    - Unusual features for their age, such as osteoporosis and HTN
    - Abnormal growth (children)

- Late-night salivary cortisol, 24-hour urinary-free cortisol, or low-dose dexamethasone suppression testing:
  - Elevated late-night salivary cortisol: Obtain at least 2 measurements. Cortisol secretion is highest in the morning and lowest between 11 PM and midnight. The nadir of serum cortisol is maintained in pseudo-Cushing (e.g., obesity, alcoholism, depression), but not in Cushing syndrome. Sensitivity and specificity are >90–95% (5,6)[B].
  - 24-hour urinary-free cortisol level: Obtain ≥2 samples to rule out intermittent hypercortisolism if results are normal and suspicion is high. Also measure 24-hour urinary creatinine excretion to verify adequacy of collection. Results may be falsely low if glomerular filtration rate <30 mL/min. Overall sensitivity and specificity varies, 90–97% and 85–96%, respectively (5)[B]. Avoid drinking excessive amounts of water due to risk of false-positive values. False-positive values can be seen in the presence of pseudo-Cushing states.
  - Low-dose dexamethasone suppression testing: Dexamethasone 1 mg is given between 11 PM and midnight, and fasting plasma cortisol is measured between 8–9 AM the following morning. A serum cortisol level below 1.89 μg/dL excludes Cushing syndrome, but specificity is limited. The presence of pseudo-Cushing states (depression, obesity, etc.), hepatic or renal disease, or any drug that induces cytochrome P-450 enzymes may cause a false result.
- High-dose dexamethasone suppression test may be useful when baseline ACTH levels are indeterminate:
  - 8 mg overnight dexamethasone suppression test: 8 mg of oral dexamethasone is given at 11 PM, with measurement of an 8 AM cortisol level the next day. A baseline 8 AM cortisol measurement is also obtained the morning prior to ingesting dexamethasone. Suppression of serum cortisol level to <50% of baseline is suggestive of a pituitary source of ACTH rather than ectopic ACTH or primary adrenal disease. Sensitivity and specificity are 95% and 100%, respectively (7)[B].
- If the initial results are positive or if clinical suspicion is high, perform additional studies to confirm diagnosis. Other tests to consider include:
  - Awake midnight plasma cortisol: Obtain samples on 3 consecutive nights. A late-evening serum cortisol >7.5 μg/dL has a sensitivity of 96% and specificity of 100% (8)[B]. Persistently elevated serum cortisol implies Cushing syndrome; nadir of serum cortisol is maintained in obese patients, but not in Cushing.
  - Corticotropin-releasing hormone (CRH) after dexamethasone: Used to distinguish Cushing syndrome from pseudo-Cushing syndrome. Dexamethasone 0.5 mg is given q6h for 48 hours starting at noon. CRH (1 μg/kg) is given 2 hours after the last dose of dexamethasone. Plasma cortisol is >1.4 μg/dL 15 minutes after CRH in patients with Cushing syndrome but not in those with pseudo-Cushing

- Pituitary MRI scan if pituitary tumor is suspected
- Abdominal CT scan if adrenal disease is suspected
- Chest CT scan if ectopic ACTH secretion is suspected (9)[C]
- Octreotide scintigraphy to look for occult ACTH-secreting tumor
- Dual-energy x-ray absorptiometry to evaluate for osteoporosis

ALERT
- Antiepileptic drugs, progesterone, oral contraceptives (withdraw estrogen-containing drugs 6 weeks before testing), rifampin, and spironolactone may cause a false-positive dexamethasone suppression test.
- Pregnancy (4)[C]: Urine-free cortisol is recommended instead of dexamethasone testing in the initial evaluation of pregnant women. Only urine-free cortisol in the 2nd or 3rd trimester $>3 \times$ the upper limit of normal can be taken to indicate Cushing syndrome.
- Epilepsy (4)[C]: Best to use measured cortisol from saliva and urine instead of serum cortisol after dexamethasone. No data to guide length of time needed after withdrawal of such medication to allow dexamethasone metabolism to return to normal; such medication change may not be clinically possible.

Follow-Up Tests & Special Considerations
- Once the diagnosis of Cushing syndrome is confirmed, localization is the next step:
  – ACTH level: Elevated in ACTH-dependent Cushing syndrome (e.g., pituitary and ectopic tumor) and low in ACTH-independent Cushing syndrome (e.g., adrenal tumors and exogenous glucocorticoids)
  – High-dose dexamethasone suppression testing: Used to distinguish between an ACTH-secreting pituitary tumor and ectopic ACTH-secreting tumors. 0.5 mg dexamethasone is given q6h for 8 doses, with serum cortisol measured at 2 and 6 hours after last dose (sensitivity 79%, specificity 74%).
- Diagnosis of Cushing syndrome is complicated by the nonspecificity and high prevalence of clinical symptoms in patients without the disorder and involves a variety of tests of variable sensitivity and specificity. Efficient screening and confirmatory procedures are essential before considering therapy.

Diagnostic Procedures/Other
Diagnostic procedure depends on clinical judgment. Inferior petrosal sinus sampling with CRH stimulation can be considered if ACTH-dependent tumor is suspected but not localized (9)[C].

Test Interpretation
- Thyroid function suppressed
- HTN
- Dyslipidemia
- Polycystic ovarian syndrome/hyperandrogenism
- Oligomenorrhea/hypogonadism
- Myopathy/cutaneous wasting
- Neuropsychiatric problems
- Ipsilateral adrenal gland hyperplasia and contralateral adrenal gland atrophy
- Hypercoagulable state
- Osteoporosis
- Nephrolithiasis
- Growth hormone reduced

 TREATMENT

MEDICATION
- Drugs usually not effective for primary long-term treatment; used in preparation for surgery or as adjunctive treatment after surgery, pituitary radiotherapy, or both.
- Metyrapone, ketoconazole, and mitotane all lower cortisol by directly inhibiting synthesis and secretion in the adrenal gland. As initial treatment, remission rates up to 85% (9)[C]
- Mifepristone is a potent antagonist of the glucocorticoid and progesterone receptors. It is FDA approved to control hyperglycemia in adults with endogenous Cushing syndrome who have type 2 diabetes or glucose intolerance secondary to hypercortisolism that has not responded to (or who are not candidates for) surgery.

SURGERY/OTHER PROCEDURES
- Tumor-specific surgery:
  – Transsphenoidal surgery for Cushing disease (remission rate 60–80%)
  – Resection of the ACTH-producing ectopic tumor
  – Adrenal surgery:
    ○ For unilateral adrenal adenomas, laparoscopic surgery is the treatment of choice.
    ○ For nodular hyperplasia, bilateral adrenalectomy is usually recommended.
    ○ For patients with Cushing disease, bilateral laparoscopic adrenalectomy can be considered if the patient has persistent disease even after pituitary surgery and radiotherapy.
- Pituitary radiotherapy can be used to treat persistent hypercortisolism after transsphenoidal surgery.
- Benefits of surgery have not been definitively established for mild or intermittent hypercortisolism.

 ONGOING CARE

PATIENT EDUCATION
- Teaching regarding diet and monitoring daily weight, early treatment of infections, emotional lability.
- National Adrenal Disease Foundation. Great Neck, NY 11021; 516-407-4992

PROGNOSIS
- Guardedly favorable prognosis with surgery for Cushing disease; generally chronic course with cyclic exacerbations and rare remissions
- Better prognosis following surgery for benign adrenal tumors; long-term recurrence rate is 20%.
- Poor with small-cell carcinoma of the lung producing ectopic hormone; neuroendocrine tumors (bronchial carcinoid) have much better prognosis (8)[C].

COMPLICATIONS
- Osteoporosis
- Increased susceptibility to infections
- Metastases of malignant tumors
- Increased cardiovascular risk even after treatment
- Lifelong glucocorticoid dependence following treatment with bilateral adrenalectomy
- Nelson syndrome (pituitary tumor) after treatment with bilateral adrenalectomy (can occur in 8–38% of patients)

REFERENCES
1. Storr HL, Chan LF, Grossman AB, et al. Pediatric Cushing's syndrome: Epidemiology, investigation and therapeutic advances. *Trends Endocrinol Met*. 2007;18:167–174.
2. Lindsay JR, Nieman LK. Adrenal disorders in pregnancy. *Endocrinol Metab Clin North Am*. 2006;35:1–20.
3. Newell-Price J, Bertagna X, Grossman AB, et al. Cushing's syndrome. *Lancet*. 2006;367: 1605–1617.
4. Nieman LK, Biller MK, Findling JW, et al. The diagnosis of Cushing's syndrome: An Endocrine Society clinical practice guideline. *J Clin Endocrinol Metab*. 2008;93:1526–1540.
5. Putignano P. Midnight salivary cortisol versus urinary free and midnight serum cortisol as screening tests for Cushing's syndrome. *J Clin Endocrinol Metabol*. 2003;88:4153–4157.
6. Yaneva M, Mosnier-Pudar H, Dugué MA, et al. Midnight salivary cortisol for the initial diagnosis of Cushing's syndrome of various causes. *J Clin Endocrinol Metab*. 2004;89:3345–3351.
7. Aytug S, Laws ER, Vance ML, et al. Assessment of the utility of the high-dose dexamethasone suppression test in confirming the diagnosis of Cushing disease. *Endocr Pract*. 2012;18:152–157.
8. Isidori AM. The ectopic adrenocorticotropin syndrome: Clinical features, diagnosis, management and long term follow up. *J Clin Endocrinol Metabol*. 2006;91:371–377.
9. Findling JF. Cushing's syndrome: Important issues in diagnosis and management. *J Clin Endocrinol Metabol*. 2006;10:3746–3753.

 SEE ALSO

Algorithm: Cushing Syndrome

 CODES

ICD10
- E24.0 Pituitary-dependent Cushing's disease
- E24.2 Drug-induced Cushing's syndrome
- E24.9 Cushing's syndrome, unspecified

CLINICAL PEARLS
- Cushing disease is due to excessive ACTH secretion from a pituitary tumor, resulting in corticosteroid excess.
- Cushing syndrome is due to excessive corticosteroid exposure from exogenous sources (medications) or endogenous sources (pituitary, adrenal, pulmonary, etc.), or tumor.
- Depression, alcoholism, medications, eating disorders, and other conditions can cause mild clinical and laboratory findings similar to those in Cushing syndrome (pseudo-Cushing syndrome).

C

CUTANEOUS DRUG REACTIONS
Sarah I. Jawed, MD • Sabrina Newman, MD

BASICS

DESCRIPTION
- An adverse cutaneous reaction in response to administration of a drug. Skin reactions are the most common adverse drug reactions.
- Severity can range from mild eruptions that resolve after the removal of the inciting agent to severe skin damage with multiorgan involvement.
- Morbilliform/Simple exanthem (75–95%) and urticarial (5–6%) eruptions are most common, but multiple morphologic types may occur.
- System(s) affected: Skin/Mucosa/Exocrine; Hematologic/Lymphatic/Immunologic

EPIDEMIOLOGY
- All ages affected
- Predominant sex: Female > Male
- Special consideration in the geriatric population who are on multiple medications: Increased likelihood of severe cutaneous and systemic reactions. Also consider in the pediatric group: Difficult to distinguish from viral exanthems

Incidence
In the US, prevalence of 2–3% in hospitalized patients; estimated 1/1,000 hospitalized patients has had a severe cutaneous reaction.

ETIOLOGY AND PATHOPHYSIOLOGY
- Predictable adverse reactions are due to overdose, side effect, or drug interaction.
- Unpredictable reactions include intolerance, drug idiosyncrasy secondary to abnormality in metabolism, or immune reaction. >700 drugs are known to cause a dermatologic reaction:
  - Immunologically mediated reaction: Immunoglobulin (Ig) E-mediated reaction (type I hypersensitivity), cytotoxic/IgG/IgM induced (type II), immune complex reactions (type III), and delayed-type hypersensitivity (type IV) with T cells, eosinophils, neutrophils, and monocytes
  - Acneiform: OCPs, corticosteroids, iodinated compounds, hydantoins, lithium
  - Erythema multiforme (EM)/Stevens-Johnson syndrome (SJS)/toxic epidermal necrolysis (TEN): Sulfonamides, penicillins, barbiturates, hydantoins, anticonvulsants, NSAIDs, cephalosporins, tetracycline, terbinafine
  - Fixed drug eruptions: NSAIDS, sulfonamides, tetracycline, barbiturates, salicylates, OCPs
  - Lichenoid: Thiazides, NSAIDS, gold, captopril, proton pump inhibitors, antimalarials, sildenafil
  - Photosensitivity: Doxycycline, thiazides, sulfonylureas, quinolones, sulfonamides
  - Vasculitis: Thiazides, gold, sulfonamides, NSAIDs, tetracycline
  - Drug rash with eosinophilia and systemic symptoms (DRESS) syndrome: Anticonvulsants, sulfonamides, dapsone, minocycline, allopurinol
  - Acute generalized exanthematous pustulosis (AGEP): Penicillins, cephalosporins, macrolides, calcium channel blockers, antimalarials, carbamazepine, acetaminophen, terbinafine, nystatin, vancomycin
  - Sweet syndrome (acute febrile neutrophilic dermatosis): Sulfa drugs, granulocyte colony-stimulating factor (G-CSF), granulocyte-macrophage colony-stimulating factor (GM-CSF)
  - Serum sickness-like reaction: Penicillins, propranolol, bupropion, minocycline

- Morbilliform/Urticarial/Exfoliative erythroderma: Numerous medications, including penicillins, cephalosporins, sulfonamides, tetracyclines, ibuprofen, naproxen, acetylsalicylic acid, radiocontrast media

Genetics
Genetics may play a role, as certain HLA antigens have been associated with increased predisposition to specific drug eruptions:
- HLA-B*5801 and HLA-B*1502 have been linked to allopurinol-induced and carbamazepine-induced SJS/TEN, respectively.
- HLA class I antigens, such as HLA-B12 and HLA-B22, have been linked to TEN and fixed drug eruptions, respectively.

RISK FACTORS
Previous drug reaction, multiple medications, concurrent infections, immunocompromised, disorders of metabolism, and certain genetic HLA haplotypes.

GENERAL PREVENTION
Always ask patients about prior adverse drug events. Be aware of medications with higher incidence of reactions as well as drug cross-reactions.

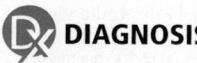

DIAGNOSIS

HISTORY
- New medications within the preceding 6 weeks: All oral, parenteral, and topical agents, including over the counter drugs, vitamins, and herbal remedies
- Consider other etiologies: Bacterial infections, viral exanthems, or underlying skin disease including cutaneous lymphoma

PHYSICAL EXAM
May present as a number of different eruption types, including, but not limited to:
- Morbilliform eruptions (exanthems):
  - Most frequent cutaneous reaction (75–95%); difficult to distinguish from viral exanthem; often secondary to antibiotic
  - Starts on trunk as pruritic red macules and papules and extends to extremities in confluent fashion, sparing face, palms, soles, and mucous membranes
  - Onset 7–21 days after drug initiation
- Urticaria:
  - Pruritic erythematous wheals distributed anywhere on the body, including mucous membranes; may progress to angioedema, appearing as nonpitting edema without erythema or margins
  - Individual lesions fade within 24 hours, but new lesions may develop.
- Acneiform eruptions:
  - Folliculocentric, monomorphous pustules typically involving the face, chest, and back distinguished from acne vulgaris by absence of comedones grossly and microscopically
  - Often become secondarily infected
- Fixed drug eruptions:
  - Single/Multiple, round, sharply demarcated, violaceous plaques with gray center that leave postinflammatory hyperpigmentation; occur on skin or mucous membrane.
  - Appear shortly after drug exposure and recur in identical location after re-exposure; some patients have a refractory period during which the drug fails to activate lesions.
  - Onset usually 48 hours after ingestion of drug

- AGEP:
  - Multiple sterile pinhead-sized nonfollicular pustules on erythematous background with desquamation after 7–10 days
  - Involves intertriginous areas, but can be generalized and involve the face
  - Appears similar to pustular psoriasis, but AGEP has fever and marked leukocytosis with neutrophilia and/or eosinophilia (1)
- DRESS syndrome:
  - Classic triad of fever, exanthem, and internal organ involvement with possible pharyngitis and lymphadenopathy
  - Can lead to exfoliative dermatitis, often accompanied by facial edema
  - Internal organ involvement: 80% hepatic, 40% renal, 33% pulmonary, and cardiac (2) lab tests show elevated liver transaminases and eosinophilia.
  - Onset 2–8 weeks after drug exposure; may develop 3 months or later into therapy
- EM:
  - Most commonly associated with herpes simplex virus and other viral/bacterial etiologies; less likely secondary to drug exposure
  - 3 zone target lesions and raised atypical 2-zone targets with localized erythema (2)
  - Lesions predominant on acral surfaces with limited mucosal involvement; <10% epidermal detachment
- SJS/TEN:
  - Classification and distinction between SJS and TEN determined by affected body surface area (BSA) (2)
    - SJS: <10% BSA; SJS-TEN overlap: 10–30% BSA; TEN: >30% BSA
  - Unlike EM, strong association with preceding drug exposure as opposed to infection except in children where infection is more common (e.g., mycoplasma)
  - Onset 1–3 weeks after starting offending agent: Flat atypical 2-zone target lesions and erythematous macules that are truncal and generalized with mucosal involvement (2)
  - May develop confluent areas of bullae, erosions, and necrosis; significant risk for infection and sepsis
  - SJS: 5–15% mortality; TEN: 30% mortality
- Lichenoid eruptions:
  - Flat-topped, violaceous, pruritic papules on extensor surfaces and involving oral mucosa
  - Reticular pattern: Lesions heal with hyperpigmentation
  - Chronic lesions: Persist for weeks/months after drug discontinued
- Photosensitivity reaction:
  - Phototoxic reactions within 24 hours of light exposure with exaggerated sunburn reaction; confined to sun-exposed areas
  - Photoallergic reactions: Caused by UVA exposure; more pruritic than painful; can involve non–sun-exposed areas
- Vasculitis:
  - Petechiae/Palpable purpura concentrated on lower extremities and dependent areas
  - Targetoid lesions with raised violaceous center and erythematous border
  - Possible renal, joint, and CNS involvement with fever, myalgias, arthritis, and abdominal pain

- Sweet syndrome:
  - Fever, neutrophilia, tender edematous violaceous papules, plaques, or nodules, with or without pustules/vesicles that spontaneously resolve
  - May have oral ulcers or ocular manifestations, such as conjunctivitis
  - Classically seen in young women after a mild respiratory illness, but 7–56% associated with malignancy
- Serum sickness-like reaction:
  - Fever, nonspecific cutaneous eruption with possible bullous lesions, arthralgias
  - Onset 7–14 days
- Exfoliative erythroderma:
  - Generalized erythema with exfoliation and/or fine desquamation over 90% of body surface
  - Difficult to distinguish between drug, primary cutaneous lymphoma, or inflammatory etiology
  - Lymphadenopathy, hepatosplenomegaly, leukocytosis, eosinophilia, or anemia may be present.
  - Increased risk of secondary infection, and insensible fluid and temperature loss with hemodynamic instability

DIFFERENTIAL DIAGNOSIS
- Viral exanthem: Presence of fever, lymphocytosis, and other systemic findings may help in the differential
- Primary dermatosis: Correlation of drug withdrawal to rash resolution may clarify diagnosis; skin biopsy is helpful.
- Bacterial infection: Cultures of pustules may distinguish primary infection from AGEP and acneiform eruptions.

DIAGNOSTIC TESTS & INTERPRETATION
Initial Tests (lab, imaging)
A minimum number of tests are useful in evaluating for internal organ involvement. CBC with differential; significant eosinophilia may be seen in DRESS and other drug-induced allergic reactions. LFT, urinalysis, and serum creatinine; chest x-ray if suspected vasculitis

Diagnostic Procedures/Other
- Special tests dependent on suspected mechanism:
  - Type I: Skin/Intradermal testing, radioallergosorbent (RAST)
  - Type II: Direct/Indirect Coombs test
  - Type III: ESR, C-reactive protein, ANA, antihistone antibody, tissue biopsy for immunofluorescence studies
  - Type IV: Patch testing, lymphocyte proliferation assay (investigational) (3)
  - Anaphylaxis/Nonimmunologic mast and basophil cell reaction: Serum tryptase levels
- Cultures useful in excluding infectious etiology; skin biopsy is nonspecific, but useful in characterizing an eruption and excluding primary skin pathologies.
- Develop a timeline documenting the onset and duration of all drugs, dosages, and onset of cutaneous eruption.

Test Interpretation
- Nonspecific histologic findings are superficial epidermal and dermal infiltrates composed variably of lymphocytes, neutrophils, and eosinophils.
- SJS/TEN: Partial or full-thickness necrosis of the epidermis; necrotic keratinocytes, vacuolization leading to subepidermal blister at basal membrane zone (4)

TREATMENT

GENERAL MEASURES
- Monitor for signs of impending cardiovascular collapse: Anaphylactic reactions, DRESS, SJS/TEN, extensive bullous reactions, and generalized erythroderma may require inpatient treatment.
- Do not rechallenge with drugs causing urticaria, bullae, angioedema, DRESS, anaphylaxis, or erythema multiforme.

MEDICATION
- Withdrawal of offending drug. Depending on the type of eruption, symptomatic treatment may be useful, but most require no additional therapy except cessation of offending agent.
- Anaphylaxis or widespread urticaria: Epinephrine 1:1,000, 0.01 mL/kg (max 0.3 mL) SC; prednisone may be given to prevent recurrence.
- Acute urticaria (<6 weeks) and chronic urticaria (>6 weeks): 1st-generation antihistamines: Diphenhydramine 10–25 mg q.h.s., hydroxyzine 10–25 mg t.i.d., doxepin 10–50 mg q.h.s. 2nd-generation antihistamines: Cetirizine 10–30 mg daily, loratadine 10–30 mg daily, fexofenadine 180 mg daily, levocetirizine 5 mg daily. H_2 antagonists: Cimetidine 400 mg b.i.d., ranitidine 150 mg b.i.d.
- Anaphylaxis, severe urticaria: Prednisone PO 1 mg/kg in tapering doses
- Erythema multiforme:
  - Treatment is generally supportive with management of suspected underlying infection.
  - Herpes simplex virus (HSV)-associated: Prophylaxis with acyclovir 10 mg/kg/d, valacyclovir 500–1,000 mg/d, or famciclovir 250 mg b.i.d.
  - "Magic mouthwash" b.i.d. or t.i.d. is helpful for mucosal erosions. Consider ophthalmology consult for severe ocular involvement.
- SJS/TEN: Treatment is supportive. Consult with a dermatologist and ophthalmologist. Systemic corticosteroids use remains controversial. Consider IVIG 2–3 g/kg for severe disease (2)[A]. In pediatric TEN patients, low-dose IVIG (0.05–0.1 g/kd/d) was effective (5)[A]. Varied success rates reported with use of anti-tumor necrosis factor-α agents, cyclosporine, cyclophosphamide, and plasmapheresis.
- DRESS: Needs prednisone with prolonged steroid taper (1–3 months) to prevent relapse. Transient hypothyroidism can occur 1–3 months following DRESS.

ONGOING CARE

FOLLOW-UP RECOMMENDATIONS
Patient Monitoring
- For urticarial, bullous, DRESS, or erythema multiforme spectrum lesions, close follow up is needed.
- Patients with anaphylaxis/angioedema should be given EpiPen for secondary prevention and a Med Alert bracelet; label the patient's medical record with the agent and reaction.
- If the patient needs to take the inciting drug (e.g., antibiotic) in the future, induction of drug tolerance or graded challenge procedures may be necessary.

PROGNOSIS
- Eruptions generally begin fading within days after removing offending agent. With morbilliform eruptions, eruption may spread distally even when agent is removed, resolving over time.
- Anaphylaxis, angioedema, DRESS, and bullous reactions are potentially fatal.

COMPLICATIONS
Anaphylaxis, bone marrow suppression, hepatitis (dapsone, hydantoin), renal failure, and pulmonary and thyroid toxicity

REFERENCES
1. Speeckaert MM, Speeckaert R, Lambert J, et al. Acute generalized exanthematous pustulosis: An overview of the clinical, immunological and diagnostic concepts. *Eur J Dermatol*. 2010;20: 425–433.
2. Chen YC, Chiu HC, Chu CY. Drug reaction with eosinophilia and systemic symptoms: A retrospective study of 60 cases. *Arch Dermatol*. 2010;146:1373–1379.
3. Barbaud A, Collet E, Milpied B, et al. A multicentre study to determine the value and safety of drug patch tests for the three main classes of severe cutaneous adverse drug reactions. *Br J Dermatol*. 2013;168:555–562.
4. Mockenhaupt M. The current understanding of Stevens-Johnson syndrome and toxic epidermal necrolysis. *Expert Rev Clin Immunol*. 2011;7: 803–815.
5. Huang YC, Li YC, Chen TJ. The efficacy of intravenous immunoglobulin for the treatment of toxic epidermal necrolysis: A systematic review and meta-analysis. *Br J Dermatol*. 2012;167:424–432.

ADDITIONAL READING
Worswick S, Cotliar J. Stevens-Johnson syndrome and toxic epidermal necrolysis: A review of treatment options. *Dermatol Ther*. 2011;24: 207–218.

CODES

ICD10
- L27.1 Loc skin eruption due to drugs and meds taken internally
- L50.0 Allergic urticaria
- R21 Rash and other nonspecific skin eruption

CLINICAL PEARLS
- Virtually any drug can cause a rash; antibiotics are the most common culprits that cause cutaneous drug reactions.
- Focus on drug history with new suspicious skin eruptions.
- Usually self-limited after withdrawal of offending agent.
- Symptoms such as tongue swelling/angioedema, skin necrosis, blisters, high fever, dyspnea, and mucous membrane erosions signify more severe drug reactions.

CUTANEOUS SQUAMOUS CELL CARCINOMA

Mercedes E. Gonzalez, MD • Herbert P. Goodheart, MD

BASICS

- Squamous cell carcinoma (SCC) is a malignant epithelial tumor arising from epidermal keratinocytes. Cutaneous (nonmucous membrane) SCC is the 2nd most common form of skin cancer.
- Lesions most frequently occur on sun-exposed sites of elderly, fair-skinned individuals. Most SCCs arise in actinic keratoses (solar keratoses). SCCs that develop from actinic keratoses are slow-growing, minimally invasive, unaggressive, and the prognosis is usually excellent because distant metastases are extremely rare.
- An SCC may also appear de novo without a preceding actinic keratosis or emerge from a preexisting human papilloma virus infection (verrucous carcinoma).
- SCCs may develop from causes other than sun exposure such as within an old burn scar or on sites previously exposed to ionizing radiation.
- Metastases are more likely occur in thicker tumors >6 mm deep (1)[A]. Other risk factors for metastases include: Lesions that arise on the ears, the vermilion border of the lips, or on mucous membranes. An SCC located on sites that received ionizing radiation, on the skin of organ transplant recipients, in chronic inflammatory lesions (e.g., discoid lupus erythematosus), or in long-standing scars or cutaneous ulcers (e.g., venous stasis ulcers) or other nonhealing wounds also have an increased rate of metastasis.
- System(s) affected: Skin/Exocrine
- Synonym(s): Squamous cell carcinoma of the skin; Epidermoid carcinoma; Prickle cell carcinoma

EPIDEMIOLOGY
- Predominant age: Elderly population
- Predominant sex: Males > Females
- In the US, 200,000 new cases each year.

Incidence
- The escalating incidence in the US is due to an increase in sun exposure in the general population, aging of the population, earlier and more frequent diagnosis of SCC, and the increase of immunosuppressed patients.
- The incidence is highest in Australia and in the Sun Belt of the US.

ALERT
Bowen disease (SCC in situ) and frank SCC are 2 of the few skin cancers that should be considered in African Americans. Such non–sun-related SCCs tend to arise on the extremities de novo, in an old scar, or in a lesion of discoid lupus erythematosus.

ETIOLOGY AND PATHOPHYSIOLOGY
- Exact mechanisms are not established; however, SCC is thought to arise from a multistep process that begins with a single mutated keratinocyte.
- UV radiation damages skin cell nucleic acids (DNA), resulting in a mutant clone of the tumor suppressor gene, p53. This leads to an uncontrolled growth of skin cells containing a mutated p53 gene. Additional mutations in genes controlling cellular proliferation and/or death lead to squamous cell dysplasia, which then progresses to SCC in situ and later invasive SCC that has the potential for metastasis.

- Cumulative UV radiation (including tanning salons, and psoralen-UV-A (PUVA) phototherapy (2)[A]) over a lifetime is the major etiologic factor in SCC.
- Epidemiologic and experimental evidence suggests other causative agents: Ionizing radiation exposure, inorganic arsenic exposure, coal tar, and other oil derivatives
- Immunosuppression by medications or disease such as HIV/AIDS

Genetics
- Persons of Irish or Scottish ancestry have the highest prevalence of SCC.
- Caucasians with the red hair/fair skin phenotype (associated with certain variant alleles of the human melanocortin-1 receptor [MC1R]) are predisposed to SCC.
- SCC is rare in people of African and Asian descent, although it is the most common form of skin cancer in these populations.

RISK FACTORS
- Older age
- Male sex: However, incidence is increasing in females due to lifestyle changes (e.g., suntan parlors, shorter dresses).
- Chronic sun exposure: SCC is noted more frequently in those with a greater degree of outdoor activity (e.g., farmers, sailors, gardeners).
- Patients with multiple actinic keratoses
- Personal or family history of skin cancer
- Northern European descent
- Fair complexion, fair hair, light eyes
- Poor tanning ability, with tendency to burn
- Organ transplant recipients, chronic immunosuppression
- Exposure to chemical carcinogens (e.g., arsenic, tar) or ionizing radiation
- Therapeutic UV and ionizing radiation exposure
- Defects in cell-mediated immunity related to lymphoproliferative disorders (chronic lymphocytic leukemia [CLL], lymphoma)
- Human papillomavirus (HPV) infection
- Chronic scarring and inflammatory conditions
- Specific genodermatoses (e.g., xeroderma pigmentosum, oculocutaneous albinism, and dystrophic epidermolysis bullosa)

GENERAL PREVENTION
Sun-avoidance measures: Sunscreens, hats, clothing and sunglasses with UV protection; tinted windshields and side windows in cars; sun-protective garments

COMMONLY ASSOCIATED CONDITIONS
- Some investigators consider an actinic keratosis to be an early SCC, although relatively few ultimately are found to develop into an SCC.
- Actinic cheilitis and leukoplakia of the mucous membranes of the lips
- Keratoacanthoma
- Cutaneous horn
- Actinic keratoses may be seen in association with:
- Xeroderma pigmentosum, albinism, and vitiligo
- Immunosuppression
- Chronic skin ulcers, preexisting scars, burns

DIAGNOSIS

PHYSICAL EXAM
Lesions occur chiefly on chronically sun-exposed areas:
- Face and backs of the forearms and hands
- Bald areas of the scalp and top of ears in men
- The sun-exposed "V" of the neck, as well as the posterior neck below the occipital hairline
- In elderly females, lesions tend to occur on the legs and other sun-exposed locations.
- In African Americans, equal frequency in sun-exposed and unexposed areas
- Clinical appearance:
  – Generally slow-growing, firm, hyperkeratotic papules, nodules, or plaques
  – Most SCCs are asymptomatic, although bleeding, pain, and tenderness may be noted.
  – Lesions may have a smooth, verrucous, or papillomatous surface.
  – Varying degrees of ulceration, erosion, crust, or scale
  – Color is often red to brown, tan, or pearly (indistinguishable from basal cell carcinoma).
- Clinical variants of SCC:
  – Bowen disease (SCC in situ): Solitary lesion that resembles a scaly psoriatic plaque
  – Invasive SCC: Often a raised, firm papule, nodule, or plaque. Lesions may be smooth, verrucous, or papillomatous, with varying degrees of ulceration, erosion, crust, or scale.
  – Cutaneous horn: SCC with an overlying cutaneous horn. A cutaneous horn represents a fingernail platelike keratinization produced by the SCC. Bowen disease may also produce a cutaneous horn on its surface.
  – Erythroplasia of Queyrat refers to Bowen disease of the glans penis, which manifests as one or more velvety red plaques.
  – Subungual SCC (3)[C] appear as hyperkeratotic lesions under the nail plate or on surrounding periungual skin, often mimicking warts.
  – Marjolin ulcer: An SCC evolving from a new area of ulceration or elevation at site of a scar or ulcer
  – HPV-associated SCC: Virally induced SCC most commonly as a new or enlarging warty growth on penis, vulva, perianal area, or periungual region
  – Verrucous carcinoma: Subtype of SCC that is extremely well differentiated, can be locally destructive, but rarely metastasizes. Lesions are "cauliflower-like" verrucous nodules or plaques.
  – Basaloid SCC: Less common than typical SCC; seen more often in men aged 40–70 years.

ALERT
Subungual SCC (3)[C]: Such lesions typically mimic warts.

DIFFERENTIAL DIAGNOSIS
- Solar keratosis: Early SCC lesions may be clinically difficult, if not impossible, to distinguish from a precursor actinic keratosis.
- Basal cell carcinoma may be indistinguishable from an SCC, particularly if the lesion is ulcerated.
- Keratoacanthoma: This lesion also may be clinically and histopathologically impossible to differentiate from an SCC; considered by some to be a low-grade variant of an SCC.
- Verruca vulgaris: The appearance of common warts is often similar to that of SCC lesions.

- Seborrheic keratosis
- Pyoderma gangrenosum
- Venous stasis ulcer
- Chemical or thermal burn

DIAGNOSTIC TESTS & INTERPRETATION
Initial Tests (lab, imaging)
Patients with lymphadenopathy should be evaluated for metastases with CT scanning, MRI, US, or PET.

Diagnostic Procedures/Other
- Surgical biopsy to ensure diagnosis: Shave, punch, excisional, incisional biopsy
- Sentinel lymph node biopsy rarely is used to identify micrometastases in patients with high-risk SCC and clinically negative nodes. Whether the early detection of lymph node metastasis leads to enhanced survival in SCC is unknown.

Test Interpretation
- Noninvasive SCC is characterized by an intraepidermal proliferation of atypical keratinocytes. Hyperkeratosis, acanthosis, and confluent parakeratosis are seen within the epidermis. Cellular atypia, including pleomorphism, hyperchromatic nuclei, and mitoses, are prominent. Atypical keratinocytes may be found in the basal layer and often extend deeply down the hair follicles, but they do not invade the dermis.
- In the in situ type of SCC (Bowen disease), atypia involves the full thickness of the epidermis but the basement membrane remains intact.
- An invasive SCC penetrates through the basement membrane into the dermis. It has various levels of anaplasia and may manifest relatively few to multiple mitoses and display varying degrees of differentiation, such as keratinization.
- Poorly differentiated tumors are clinically more aggressive. SCCs proliferate 1st by local invasion. Metastases, when they do occur, spread via local lymph ducts to local lymph nodes.

ALERT
Melanoma: An amelanotic melanoma and ulcerated melanoma may also be impossible to distinguish from an SCC.

TREATMENT

MEDICATION
First Line
- Total excision: Preferred method for SCCs, permitting histologic diagnosis of the tumor margins
- Electrocautery (electrodesiccation) and curettage (ED&C)
  - Best for small lesions (generally <1 cm) on flat surfaces (e.g., forehead, cheek) and SCC in situ (Bowen disease). ED&C may be used to treat superficially invasive SCCs without high-risk characteristics, but it is not appropriate for certain high-risk anatomic locations.
- Cryosurgery with LN_2 in selected lesions, such as SCC in situ
- Micrographic (Mohs) surgery is a microscopically controlled method of removing skin cancers that allows for controlled excision and maximum preservation of normal tissue. It has the highest cure rate (94–99%) of all surgical treatments. Mohs surgery may be indicated for the following:
  - Large, recurrent or invasive SCCs (e.g., to bone or cartilage)
  - Lesions with a poorly delineated clinical border

- Locations where preservation of normal tissue is extremely important (e.g., tip of the nose, eyelids, ala nasi, ears, lips, and glans penis)
- Radiation therapy is a primary treatment option that is generally restricted to older patients who are physically debilitated or are unable to undergo, or refuse to undergo, excisional surgery.

Second Line
Immunotherapy with topical imiquimod (Aldara) (4)[A] 5% cream, has been successfully used for the treatment of SCC in situ (Bowen disease), actinic keratoses, genital warts, and superficial basal cell carcinomas

- Topical chemotherapy: Topical formulations of 5-fluorouracil (5-FU) (4)[A]

- Intralesional 5-FU and bleomycin has also been used successfully to treat SCCs.
- Photodynamic therapy (PDT): PDT involves application of a photosensitizer (given topically or systemically) followed by exposure to a light source. Used primarily to treat large numbers of solar keratoses not recommended for treatment of invasive SCCs.
- In patients with multiple or recurrent SCCs, or those at high risk, such as organ transplant recipients, chemoprevention with systemic retinoids (5)[C], such as acitretin, may be effective for reducing the number of new SCCs, treating existing SCCs, or at reducing the risk of recurrence after treatment.

ADDITIONAL THERAPIES
For metastatic SCC, oral 5-FU, has been used alone or in combination with SC interferon. More recently, epidermal growth factor receptor (EGFR) inhibitors, such as cetuximab, are used in combination with systemic chemotherapy for metastatic disease.

SURGERY/OTHER PROCEDURES
- Complete lymphadenectomy of the draining nodal basin for high-risk tumors
- Metastatic disease requires aggressive management by a multidisciplinary team, involving plastic, ENT/maxillofacial, and general surgeons, or a surgical oncologist.

ONGOING CARE

FOLLOW-UP RECOMMENDATIONS
Patient Monitoring
Skin exam every month for 3 months, 6 months after treatment, and then yearly

PATIENT EDUCATION
Skin self-exam: Encourage sun-avoidance techniques, protective clothing, sunscreens, etc. Artificial tanning devices should be avoided.

PROGNOSIS
- For low risk SCCs: A 90–95% cure rate with appropriate treatment
- Overall, head and neck lesions have better prognosis (6); however, lip and ear lesions metastasize more frequently when compared with other sites.
- The ability to produce scale (keratinization) indicates a tendency for a lesion to be more differentiated and less likely to metastasize.
- Softer, nonkeratinizing lesions are not as well differentiated and thus are more likely to spread.
- Lesions ≥2 cm are more likely to recur.
- SCCs that arise in areas of non–sun-exposed skin or have a greater tendency to metastasize.

- An SCC arising on a mucous membrane, chronic ulcer, or in an immunocompromised patient should be regarded as potentially metastatic.
- SCCs that are deeply invasive (≥6 mm in SC fat), or have perineural involvement are more likely to metastasize.
- When SCC does metastasize, it usually occurs within several years from the time of diagnosis and involves draining lymph nodes.
- Once nodal metastasis of cutaneous SCC has occurred, the overall 5-year survival rate has historically been in the range of 25–35%.

COMPLICATIONS
- Untreated, an SCC becomes indurated, with a tendency to ooze, ulcerate, or bleed.
- Local recurrence
- Metastatic disease

REFERENCES
1. Brantsch KD, Meisner C, Schönfisch B, et al. Analysis of risk factors determining prognosis of cutaneous squamous-cell carcinoma: A prospective study. *Lancet Oncol.* 2008;9:713–720.
2. Archier E, Devaux S, Castela E, et al. Carcinogenic risks of psoralen UV-A therapy and narrowband UV-B therapy in chronic plaque psoriasis: A systematic literature review. *J Eur Acad Dermatol Venereol.* 2012;26(Suppl 3):22–31.
3. Riddel C, Rashid R, Thomas V. Ungual and periungual human papillomavirus-associated squamous cell carcinoma: A review. *J Am Acad Dermatol.* 2011;64:1147–1153.
4. Love WE, Bernhard JD, Bordeaux JS. Topical imiquimod or fluorouracil therapy for basal and squamous cell carcinoma: A systematic review. *Arch Dermatol.* 2009;145(12):1431–1438.
5. Greenberg JN, Zwald FO. Management of skin cancer in solid-organ transplant recipients: A multidisciplinary approach. *Dermatol Clin.* 2011;29(2):231–241.
6. Clayman GL, Lee JJ, Holsinger FC. Mortality risk from squamous cell skin cancer. *J Clin Oncol.* 2005;23:759–765.

CODES

ICD10
- C44.82 Squamous cell carcinoma of overlapping sites of skin
- C44.92 Squamous cell carcinoma of skin, unspecified
- C44.320 Squamous cell carcinoma of skin of unspecified parts of face

CLINICAL PEARLS
- SCCs that develop from actinic keratoses are generally unaggressive.
- Unlike most basal cell carcinomas, SCCs of the skin are associated with a risk of metastasis, especially those arising on mucous membranes, chronic ulcers, or in immunocompromised patients.
- A subungual SCC can easily be mistaken for a wart.

CYBERBULLYING
Edward Feller, MD • Marie DeLuca

 BASICS

DESCRIPTION
- Bullying: Repetitive, intentional behavior to harm based on imbalance of power.
- Cyberbullying: Behavior via electronic or digital media that repeatedly communicates hostile or aggressive messages intended to harm or discomfort others:
  - May include threats, rumors, harassment, sending sexually explicit or embarrassing images, or impersonation carried out through social media, email, online forums, or instant messaging services.
  - May occur between peers or older child against a younger one or an adult against a child or adult; or among siblings
- Increase in accessibility and Internet use has drawn attention to cyberbullying, which has grown in popularity with the popularity of the Internet:
  - Teens using the Internet (93%); owning a cell phone (75%) (1)
- Popular media focuses on high-profile cases, but minor, common episodes are pervasive and corrosive and may have more significant effects on the mental health of victims.
- Commonly a pediatric or young adult issue, but cyberbullying can occur at any age or any locale, such as the workplace:
  - Adult-on-child cyberbullying occurs, but is uncommon.
- Microepidemics can occur in schools or sports teams; not a single bully, but a contagion of peer-group bullying piling on a single victim or group.
- Compared with traditional bullying, cyberbullying is anonymous, opportunistic, free from supervision, easily accessible. Power differential may be absent.
- Youth not engaged in traditional bullying may participate because of limited consequences and lack of perceived harm to the victim.
- Computer and phone ubiquity allow continuous online access; victimization occurs anywhere, anytime.
- Intervention is difficult because cyberbullying occurs in spaces not monitored by school staff or supervisory adults in nonschool settings
- Infrequently reported, usually to a friend (30%), parent (<10%), rarely to school personnel (<5%). Cyberbullying creates a permanent record that can cause lasting emotional and social harm.

EPIDEMIOLOGY
Incidence
- 1-year incidence ~15% for high school students and a 2-month incidence of 18% for middle school students.

Prevalence
- As many as 1/2 of all middle and high school students report being targeted; 1/3 cyberbullied others (2)
- Overlap between cyberbullying and school bullying: 60% of cyberbullying victims were also bullying victims; 1/3 of bullying victims were also cyberbullying victims (1).

RISK FACTORS
- For bully victims:
  - Frequent Internet or social media use
  - Previous offline harassment
  - More likely to have psychosomatic, emotional, peer problems, social anxiety
  - More likely to come from families with structures other than a 2 biological parent model.
  - Females more are likely to cyberbully and are more frequent victims of cyber bullying.
  - Minor incidents may precede major bullying incidents and take an additive toll on emotional health.
  - Youth perceived as different due to physical or mental disability, race/ethnicity socioeconomic class, gender expression, or sexual preference may be targeted.
    - In 1 year, >1/2 of lesbian, gay, bisexual, or transgender (LGBT) students reported experiencing cyberbullying. 17% of LGBT students reported frequent electronic harassment (3).
    - Being bullied for sexual orientation shows a higher association with depression and suicidality than bullying for other reasons.
- For cyberbullies:
  - Hyperactivity; conduct disorder
  - Frequent smoking, alcohol
  - Not feeling safe at school
  - Low prosocial behavior (limited empathy)
  - Engagement in relational aggression (spreading rumors, exclusion)
  - Poor emotional bond with caregiver
  - Previous victims of traditional bullying

GENERAL PREVENTION
Recommendations to parents/guardians:
- Communicate with children about online use
  - Discuss positive and negative aspects of social media, Internet usage.
  - Learn about technologies children use.
- Teach children they may overestimate their statements are being made in jest. When they poke fun or criticize, they may unwittingly offend.
- Form an online-use plan with children:
  - Reduce time online or on social media sites.
  - Negotiate policies that fit desires and needs of both parents and children.
- Check privacy settings and supervise online activities:
  - Understand limitations of software monitoring to assess Internet use.

COMMONLY ASSOCIATED CONDITIONS
- Traditional bullying
- Behavioral health consequences
- Internet addiction (5)
- Cyber immersion: Utilization of cyber technology and Internet as a central element of daily life, communication, and relationships
- Bullied victims are more likely to bring guns to school and engage in school violence (6).
- Victims of cyberbullying via phone may report more safety concerns than victims of Internet bullying.
- Cyberbullying victims report more depressive symptoms whereas cyberbullies report more problems with substance use.

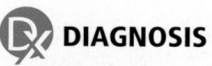 **DIAGNOSIS**

HISTORY
Unique technology-associated characteristics:
- Avoiding computers, cell phones, other devices
- Stress when receiving e-mail, instant message, or text
- Avoiding conversations about computer use
- Emotional, peer problems; not feeling safe at school. Fear of a particular person.
- Poor academic performance
- Physical complaints: Headache, abdominal pain, difficulty sleeping
- Withdrawal from family, friends, reluctance to attend school and social events
- See Risk Factors

PHYSICAL EXAM
- Symptoms consistent with depression: Sleep issues, anhedonia, fatigue, diminished school performance, flattened affect, diminished self-image, suicidal thoughts

DIFFERENTIAL DIAGNOSIS

- Traditional bullying: Physical abuse, sexual or verbal harassment (7)
- Child abuse or neglect
- Depression
- Conduct disorder
- Malingering; prevarication
- Cyberbullying as a feature of underlying psychiatric illnesses

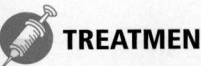 TREATMENT

GENERAL MEASURES

- Community-based approach: Parents, teachers, school officials should be aware of communications technology used by youth. Learn how technology is used and new trends in positive and negative social communications.
- Major incidents of cyberbullying should be addressed by the community.
- Encourage cyberbullying reporting to parents, teachers, and other supervising adults.
- School-wide programs addressing traditional bullying may also be effective in cyberbullying.
- Prepare parents to discuss online safety.
- In traditional bullying, mediation between bully and victim may be counterproductive; less evidence is available for cyberbullying.
- Gather information about the methods and context of cyberbullying:
  - Duration: Establish timeline, previous history as victim or bully.
  - When and where does the bullying occur?
  - How does bullying occur? Mediums of communication, traditional bullying
  - Content: Review printouts, text messages etc., look for themes.
  - Relationship between victim and bully: Power differential, age differences, previous conflicts
  - Check for external and internal consistency, malingering.
  - Bullies may view behavior as joking or not malicious.
  - Identify other participants since cyberbullying may occur with multiple offenders or onlookers.

ISSUES FOR REFERRAL

- Psychiatric sequelae such as depression, anxiety
- Suicidality or homicidal ideation should be referred urgently for psychiatric care.
- Any online sexual solicitations of minors by adults should be reported to law enforcement.
- Severe cases of cyberbullying may require referral for legal and criminal input.

 ONGOING CARE

FOLLOW-UP RECOMMENDATIONS

- Screen for cyberbullying at medical visits.
- Discuss efficacy of online privacy measures.
- Screen for traditional forms of bullying.
- Consider referral for ongoing psychiatric sequelae.

Patient Monitoring

- Screen for depression, substance and alcohol abuse, suicidality, homicidal ideation.
- Monitor technology use.

PATIENT EDUCATION

- Directed toward youth and parents
- See General Measures
- Efforts must be multidimensional, repeated, and involve school and health care personnel and community-wide involvement.
- http://www.stopbullying.gov/cyberbullying/
- http://kidshealth.org/parent/positive/talk/cyberbullying.html
- http://www.commonsensemedia.org/cyberbullying

PROGNOSIS

- Varies widely; lack of long-term demographic studies
- Bullying and cyberbullying may have chronic social, psychological, and medical sequelae that may not be evident during episodes.

COMPLICATIONS

- Linked with depression and suicidality
- Victims of both cyberbullying and traditional bullying show high rates of depressive symptoms and suicidality.
- Males: Cyberbullies are more likely to be suicidal.
- Females: Cyberbullying victimization linked with depression and suicidality

REFERENCES

1. Schneider SK, O'Donnell L, Stueve A, et al. Cyberbullying, school bullying, and psychological distress: A regional census of high school students. Am J Publ Health. 2012;102(1):171–177.
2. Bostic JQ, Brunt CC. Cornered: Approach to school bullying and cyberbullying, and forensic implications. Child Adolesc Clin N Am. 2011;20:447–465.
3. Kosciw JG, et al. The 2011 National School Climate Survey: The experiences of lesbian, gay, bisexual and transgender youth in our nation's schools. Gay, Lesbian, and Straight Education Network.
4. Freeman BW, Thompson C, Jacques C. Forensic aspects and assessment of school bullying. Psychiatr Clin N Am. 2012;35:877–900.
5. Englander EK. Spinning our wheels. Improving our ability to respond to bullying and cyberbullying. Child Adolesc Clin N Am. 2012;21:43–55.
6. Suzuki K, Asaga R, Sourander A, et al. Cyberbullying and adolescent mental health. Int J Adolesc Med Health. 2012;24:27–35.
7. Law DM, Shapka JD, Hymel S, et al. The changing face of bullying: An empiric comparison between traditional and internet bullying and victimization. Comp Hum Behav. 2012;28:226–232.

ADDITIONAL READING

- Donnerstein E. Internet bullying. Pediatr Clin N Am. 2012;59:623–633.
- Moreno MA, Kolb J. Social networking sites and adolescent health. Pediatr Clin N Am. 2012;59:601–612.
- Olweus D. School bullying: Development and some important challenges. Ann Revue Clin Psych. 2013;9:751–780.

CLINICAL PEARLS

- Cyberbullying is anonymous, occurs anywhere at any time, may not leave a permanent record, occurs in private without witnesses so more difficult to protect against; parents are unaware of extent.
- Cyberbullying can profoundly affect mental health.
- Rarely reported to adults; daily microaggressions may have a cumulative affect not perceived by parents, guardians, and school officials.
- Students perceived as different due to disability, socioeconomic status, gender identity, sexual orientation, race or ethnicity are more likely to be cyberbullied.
- Prevention requires awareness of this common issue and sustainable, community-wide interventions.

CYSTIC FIBROSIS

Emily Forbes, DO • Reem Abu-Sbaih, DO

BASICS

DESCRIPTION
- Cystic fibrosis (CF) is an autosomal-recessive genetic condition that most prominently affects the lungs and pancreas.
- The GI, endocrine, and reproductive systems, as well as the liver, sinuses, and skin can all be involved.
- Initially a pediatric disease, CF has become a chronic pediatric and adult medical condition as improvements in medical care have led to a dramatic increase in long-term survival.

EPIDEMIOLOGY
CF is the most common lethal inherited disease in Caucasians and is found in every racial group.

Incidence
Number of infants born with CF in relation to the total number of live births in the US:
- 1 in 3,000 Caucasians
- 1 in 4,000–10,000 Latin Americans
- 1 in 15,000–20,000 African Americans
- Uncommon in Africa and Asia, with reported frequency in Japan of 1 in 350,000 (1)[A]

Prevalence
- 30,000 patients with CF living in the US (2)[A]
- ~1,000 new diagnoses are made annually (2)[A].

ETIOLOGY AND PATHOPHYSIOLOGY
- Abnormal CFTR function leads to abnormally viscous secretions that alter organ function.
- The lungs: Obstruction, infection, and inflammation negatively affect lung growth, structure, and function:
  - Decreased mucociliary clearance
  - Infection is accompanied by an intense neutrophilic response.
  - Degradation of supporting tissues causes bronchiectasis and eventual failure.

Genetics
CFTR gene (cystic fibrosis transmembrane conductance regulator). >1,500 mutations exist that can cause phenotypic CF, all of which are recessively inherited. Most common is loss of the phenylalanine residue at 508th position (deltaF508), which accounts for 88.5% of affected alleles in the CF population in the US (1,2)[A]. G551D mutation accounts for 4.4% of affected alleles (2)[A].

RISK FACTORS
CF is a single-gene disorder. The severity of the phenotype can be affected by the specific CFTR mutation (most predictive of pancreatic disease), other modifier genes (CFTM1 for meconium ileus), gastroesophageal reflux disease (GERD), severe respiratory virus infection, and environmental factors, such as tobacco smoke exposure.

GENERAL PREVENTION
- ACOG recommends genetic analysis for all North American couples planning a pregnancy, with appropriate counseling to identified carriers and genetic analysis of siblings of known CF patients.
- Newborn screening for CF is offered throughout the US. Identification of affected newborns has resulted in a reduction of new cases.

- Amelioration of complications of CF can be accomplished through early diagnosis (by newborn screening) followed by referral to an accredited regional CF center.

COMMONLY ASSOCIATED CONDITIONS
- Upper respiratory:
  - Rhinosinusitis is seen in up to 100% of patients with CF.
  - Nasal polyps are seen in up to 86% of patients.
- The GI tract:
  - Pancreatic exocrine insufficiency (85–90%) (1)[A]
  - Malabsorption of fat, protein, and fat-soluble vitamins (A, D, E, and K)
  - Hepatobiliary disease (10.8%):
    - Focal biliary cirrhosis
    - Cholelithiasis
  - Meconium ileus at birth (10–15%) (1)[A]
  - Distal intestinal obstruction syndrome (DIOS): Intestinal blockage that typically occurs in older children and adults (4.7%) (2)[A]
  - GERD (28.9%) (2)[A]
- Endocrine:
  - CF-related diabetes (CFRD):
    - May present as steady decline in weight, lung function, or increased frequency of exacerbation
    - Leading comorbid complication (30.5% in patients age >18 years) (2)[A]
    - Result of progressive insulin deficiency
    - Early screening and treatment may improve reduced survival found in CFRD (3)[A].
  - Bone mineral disease (10.9%) (2)[A]
  - Joint disease (2.75%) (2)[A]
  - Hypogonadism:
    - Frequent low testosterone levels in men
    - Menstrual irregularities are common.
- Reproductive organs:
  - Congenital bilateral absence of the vas deferens: Obstructive azoospermia in 98% of males
- Depression (11.8%) (2)[A]

Pregnancy Considerations
- Pulmonary disease may worsen during pregnancy.
- Originally considered too dangerous for women with CF, successful pregnancies occur more frequently. In 2011, 211 women with CF became pregnant (2)[A].
- Advances in fertility treatments now allow men with CF to father children (2)[A].

DIAGNOSIS

- Median age at diagnosis: 5 months (2)[A]
- General (any age):
  - Family history
  - Chronic/Recurrent respiratory symptoms, including airway obstruction and infections
  - Persistent infiltrates on chest x-rays (CXRs)
  - Hypochloremic metabolic acidosis
- Neonatal:
  - Meconium ileus
  - Prolonged jaundice
- Infancy:
  - Failure to thrive
  - Chronic diarrhea

- Anasarca/Hypoproteinemia
- Pseudotumor cerebri (vitamin A deficiency)
- Hemolytic anemia (vitamin E deficiency)
- Childhood:
  - Recurrent endobronchial infection
  - Bronchiectasis
  - Recurrent sinusitis
  - Steatorrhea
  - Poor growth
  - DIOS
  - Allergic bronchopulmonary aspergillosis
- Adolescence and adulthood:
  - Recurrent endobronchial infection
  - Bronchiectasis
  - Allergic bronchopulmonary aspergillosis
  - Chronic sinusitis
  - Hemoptysis
  - Pancreatitis
  - Portal hypertension
  - Azoospermia
  - Delayed puberty

HISTORY
Suspect with failure to thrive, steatorrhea, and recurrent respiratory problems

PHYSICAL EXAM
- Respiratory:
  - Rhonchi and/or crackles
  - Hyperresonance on percussion
  - Nasal polyps
- GI: Hepatosplenomegaly when cirrhosis present
- Other: Digital clubbing, growth retardation, and pubertal delay

DIFFERENTIAL DIAGNOSIS
- Pulmonary:
  - Difficult-to-manage asthma
  - Chronic bronchitis
  - Recurrent pneumonia
  - Chronic/Recurrent sinusitis
  - Primary ciliary dyskinesia
- GI:
  - Celiac disease
  - Protein-losing enteropathy
  - Pancreatitis of unknown etiology
  - Shwachman-Diamond syndrome

DIAGNOSTIC TESTS & INTERPRETATION
Initial Tests (lab, imaging)
- Newborn screening (~58% of new cases) (2)[A] tests blood levels of immunoreactive trypsin (IRT).
- Sweat test (gold standard):
  - Sweat chloride:
    - >60 mmol/L is positive for CF.
    - <40 mmol/L is normal.
- CFTR mutation analysis:
  - Limited panel testing: Allele-specific polymerase chain reaction (PCR) identifies >90% of mutations; finite chance of false-negative finding. Full-sequence testing is more costly and time-consuming.
- CXR:
  - Hyperinflation early in disease
  - Bronchial thickening and plugging
  - Nodular densities, patchy atelectasis, and confluent infiltrates
  - Bronchiectasis

Follow-Up Tests & Special Considerations
- Sputum culture (common CF organisms)
- PFTs
- 72-hour fecal fat
- Stool elastase
- Oral glucose tolerance test (OGTT)
- Head CT: Abnormal sinus CT findings are nearly universal in CF and may include mucosal thickening, intraluminal sinus polyps, and sinus effusions. Many children with CF never develop aerated frontal sinuses.
- Chest CT (not routine): Useful when unusual findings noted on CXR

Diagnostic Procedures/Other
- Flexible bronchoscopy
- Bronchoalveolar lavage

TREATMENT

GENERAL MEASURES
- Yearly influenza vaccination for all CF patients age >6 months (4)[A]
- Palivizumab for prophylaxis of respiratory syncytial virus (RSV) in infants with CF <2 years (5)[A]
- Avoidance of smoke

MEDICATION
- Pulmonary:
  - Antibiotics, oral:
    - *Staphylococcus aureus*: Bactrim or cephalexin
    - *Pseudomonas aeruginosa*: Fluoroquinolones
    - Azithromycin (anti-inflammatory properties)
  - Antibiotics, inhaled:
    - TOBI (tobramycin): 300 mg/dose via nebulizer)
    - Colistin (more commonly used in Europe)
    - Cayston (aerosolized aztreonam)
  - Antibiotics, IV:
    - *S. aureus*: Zosyn or nafcillin
    - Methicillin-resistant *S. aureus* (MRSA): Vancomycin or linezolid
    - *P. aeruginosa*: Zosyn or ceftazidime plus aminoglycoside (tobramycin)
    - *B. cepacia*: ≥3 drugs based on synergy studies
  - Inhalation therapy:
    - β-agonist in conjunction with chest physiotherapy
    - Recombinant human DNAse (Dornase alpha)
    - Hypertonic saline
  - Anti-inflammatory agents:
    - Oral steroids (useful in setting of ABPA)
    - Ibuprofen (high dose)
  - CFTR modulation therapy:
    - Ivacaftor (VX770): A small-molecule CFTR potentiator shown to improve lung function and improve risk of pulmonary exacerbations in patients with at least 1 copy of G551D mutation (5)[A].
- GI:
  - Pancreatic enzymes (87.4%) (2)[A]:
    - Use in pancreatic-insufficient patients.
  - Fat-soluble vitamin supplementation (A, D, E, K)
  - Liver disease (cholestasis):
    - Ursodeoxycholic acid

ISSUES FOR REFERRAL
All patients should be followed in a CF center (accredited sites are listed at www.cff.org).

ADDITIONAL THERAPIES
- Airway clearance techniques (6)[A]
- Routine chest physiotherapy with postural drainage is critical in prevention of pulmonary exacerbations:
  - VEST (airway clearance system)
- Endocrine:
  - CFRD: Insulin is the primary therapy, and dietary restrictions should be avoided (3)[A].
  - CF-related bone disease: Consider bisphosphonate therapy

SURGERY/OTHER PROCEDURES
- Lung transplantation reserved for patients with limited life expectancy (FEV$_1$ <30% predicted):
  - 220 patients with CF underwent lung transplantation during 2011 (2)[A].
  - 5-year posttransplant survival is up to 62%.
- Liver transplantation is reserved for progressive liver failure ± portal hypertension with GI bleeding; 7 patients received liver transplantation in 2011 (2)[A].
- Nasal polypectomy in 4% of CF patients (2)[A]

IN-PATIENT CONSIDERATIONS
Admission Criteria/Initial Stabilization
- Pulmonary exacerbation (most common reason for admission):
  - Increased cough, sputum production, and decreased pulmonary function
  - Change in lung examination (rales, retractions, tachypnea)
  - New abnormalities on CXR
  - Decreased energy level and appetite and weight loss
  - Fever, leukocytosis, elevation of acute-phase reactants
- Bowel obstruction (due to DIOS, previously known as meconium ileus equivalent [MIE])
- Pancreatitis (in pancreatic-sufficient patients)
- Nasal cannula oxygen when the patient is hypoxemic (SaO$_2$ <90%)

IV Fluids
- Increased salt loss increases risk of hyponatremic hypochloremic dehydration.
- Cautious use of IV fluids with worsening lung disease

Nursing
Nursing assignments should involve only 1 CF patient per nurse for isolation purposes.

 ## ONGOING CARE

FOLLOW-UP RECOMMENDATIONS
- Upon discharge for a pulmonary exacerbation, follow-up with CF provider within 2–4 weeks
- Routine clinic visits every 3 months, with airway cultures and pulmonary function testing
- Annual comprehensive nutritional evaluation
- Yearly oral glucose tolerance test (OGTT) after 10 years of age (3)[A]
- Bone densitometry after age 18

DIET
High-calorie, high-fat diet with added salt

PATIENT EDUCATION
Cystic Fibrosis Foundation: www.cff.org

PROGNOSIS
- Most recent median survival is 36.8 years, as of 2010 CF Foundation Patient Registry (2)[A].
- Progression of lung disease usually determines length of survival.

REFERENCES
1. O'Sullivan BP, Freedman SD. Cystic fibrosis. *Lancet.* 2009;373:1891–1904.
2. Cystic Fibrosis Foundation Patient Registry; 2011 Annual Data Report. Bethesda, MD: Cystic Fibrosis Foundation; 2012.
3. Moran A, Brunzell C, Cohen RC, et al. Clinical care guidelines for cystic fibrosis-related diabetes: A position statement of the American Diabetes Association and a clinical practice guideline of the Cystic Fibrosis Foundation, endorsed by the Pediatric Endocrine Society. *Diabetes Care.* 2010;33:2697–2708.
4. Cystic Fibrosis Foundation, Borowitz D, Robinson KA, et al. Cystic Fibrosis Foundation evidence-based guidelines for management of infants with cystic fibrosis. *J Pediatr.* 2009;155(6 Suppl):S73–93.
5. Ramsey BW, Davies J, McElvaney NG, et al. A CFTR potentiator in patients with cystic fibrosis and the G551D mutation. *N Engl J Med.* 2011;365(18): 1663–1672.
6. Flume PA, Robinson KA, O'Sullivan BP, et al. Cystic fibrosis pulmonary guidelines: Airway clearance therapies. *Respir Care.* 2009;54(4):522–537.

ADDITIONAL READING
Oomen KP, April MM. Sinonasal manifestations in cystic fibrosis. *Int J Otolaryngol.* 2012;2012: 789572. Epub 2012 Aug 5.

 ## CODES

ICD10
- E84.0 Cystic fibrosis with pulmonary manifestations
- E84.9 Cystic fibrosis, unspecified
- E84.11 Meconium ileus in cystic fibrosis

CLINICAL PEARLS
- CF must be considered in *any* child with chronic diarrhea, especially if associated with poor growth or failure to thrive.
- All children with nasal polyps, digital clubbing, or bronchiectasis should be evaluated.
- Children with CF may present with generalized edema due to protein/calorie malnutrition.
- A rapid decline in pulmonary function suggests the acquisition of resistant organisms (e.g., *B. cepacia*), CF-related diabetes, ABPA, or GERD.

CYTOMEGALOVIRUS INCLUSION DISEASE

Kiki Patel, PharmD • Dilip Patel, MD

BASICS

Cytomegalovirus (CMV) is a ubiquitous virus that commonly infects people across all ages, ethnic and socioeconomic groups, and geographic areas.

- Although most CMV infections are asymptomatic or cause mild disease, the virus can cause serious disease in neonates and immunocompromised people.
- Because of its ubiquity, it is often difficult to define the role of CMV in a disease process.

DESCRIPTION
- CMV is a DNA virus in the *Herpesvirus* family, also known as HHV-5. It is a member of the β-herpesvirus subfamily, which also includes HHV-6 and -7.
- Primary infection: Often asymptomatic; may remain latent throughout a person's life if not immunocompromised
- Wide spectrum of disorders that range from asymptomatic subclinical infection to a mononucleosis syndrome in healthy patients to disseminated disease in immunocompromised hosts
- Severe disease can result from primary infection of the fetus and newborn or reactivation in setting of immunocompromise or organ transplantation.
- Name derives from the infected cells, which are large and contain intranuclear inclusions, described as "owl's eye."
- Not highly contagious:
  - Spread via close contact with persons shedding virus from saliva, urine, blood, breast milk, feces, semen, or organ transplantation
  - Any organ can be affected.
- Categories of CMV infections:
  - Congenital
  - Perinatal
  - Acute infection in a normal host
  - Latent infection
  - Infection in immunocompromised hosts: Solid organ transplant; bone marrow transplant; AIDS patients
- System(s) affected: Ophthalmic; Pulmonary; GI; Neurologic; Renal; Skin/Exocrine, Hepatic, Cardiac
- Synonym(s): Giant cell inclusion disease; CID CMV, HHV-5

Pregnancy Considerations
- CMV infection in pregnancy may cause illness in the newborn ranging from asymptomatic infection to severe disease or even death.
- Infection may occur in utero, intrapartum, or postnatally.
- Preexisting maternal CMV seropositivity substantially decreases, but does not completely eliminate fetal infection.

Pediatric Considerations
Breastfeeding can transmit virus to high-risk preterm infants. However, there is low risk of symptomatic disease and no evidence of long-term sequelae from transmission from breastfeeding. Currently, there are no recommendations for avoidance or treated breast milk (1).

EPIDEMIOLOGY
Incidence
- Common, but frequently asymptomatic
- <2–3 cases of end-organ disease per 100 person-years in HIV patients

- CMV infection is even more prevalent in populations at higher risk for HIV infection (IV drug users, 75%; homosexual males, 90%).
- CMV reactivation frequently occurs in immunocompromised hosts such as organ transplant recipients and HIV patients.
- Predominant age: All ages, peaks at <3 months, 16–40 years, and 40–75 years
- Predominant sex: Male > Female

Prevalence
- Occurs worldwide; higher prevalence in underdeveloped countries
- 40–100% of the general US population is seropositive from prior exposure during childhood or early adulthood (2).
- 20% of children in the US are seropositive before reaching puberty (2).
- Most common perinatally transmitted infection: 0.2–2.2% of births in the US (1)

ETIOLOGY AND PATHOPHYSIOLOGY
- Primary infection
- Reinfection with different CMV strains
- Reactivation of latent virus in patients who are immunosuppressed

RISK FACTORS
- HIV infection with specific risks, including:
  - CD4 count <50 cells/μL (3)[B]
  - Absence of treatment with or failure to respond to ART (3)[B]
  - Previous opportunistic infections (3)[B]
  - HIV viral load >100,000 (3)[B]
- Organ transplantation
- Blood transfusion
- Immunocompromise
- Living in closed population
- Corticosteroid therapy
- Daycare environment, infant, or geriatric
- For congenital infection, maternal infection during pregnancy
- Low socioeconomic status (1)[C]
- Critically ill immunocompetent adults in ICU settings (up to 1/3 develop CMV, primarily between days 4 and 12 after admission) (4)[A]
- Inflammatory bowel disease (5)[A]

GENERAL PREVENTION
- Hand washing/basic hygiene
- Avoid immunosuppression; maintain CD4 count >100 cells/mm³ in HIV patients.
- Highly active antiretroviral therapy (HAART) is the best method for high-risk HIV patients (2)[A].
- Primary prophylaxis is not recommended (3).
- Chronic maintenance therapy for secondary prophylaxis in HIV patients (3)
- Options include:
  - Parenteral or PO ganciclovir (6)[A]
  - Parenteral foscarnet (6)[A]
  - Combined parenteral ganciclovir and foscarnet (6)[A]
  - Parenteral cidofovir (6)[A]
  - Ganciclovir via intraocular implant or repetitive intravitreous injection of fomivirsen (6)[A]
- CMV antibody+, HIV+ children who are severely immunosuppressed require PO ganciclovir 30 mg/kg t.i.d.

- Antiviral suppression of CMV reactivation in CMV+ transplant recipients or recipients of CMV+ organs:
  - Solid organ transplant: Prophylactic or preemptive treatment with PO ganciclovir, valganciclovir (7)[A]
  - Bone marrow transplant: IV ganciclovir
- CMV immunoglobulins decrease rate of severe disease after liver transplant (8)[A] and decrease incidence of disease after renal transplant.

COMMONLY ASSOCIATED CONDITIONS
AIDS, corticosteroid therapy, transplantation, or immunosuppression

DIAGNOSIS

HISTORY
- Congenital:
  - ~1% (0.2–2.5%) of newborns are congenitally infected with CMV.
  - Most infected newborns appear normal and are asymptomatic.
  - As many as 15% of these children may later develop progressive hearing loss, which is most often unilateral.
  - ~10% (5–15%) of congenitally infected newborns will be symptomatic at birth, with manifestations including small size for gestational age, hepatosplenomegaly, petechial or purpuric rash, and jaundice.
- Perinatal: Exposure to CMV in maternal cervicovaginal secretions, breast milk, or from blood product transfusions; often asymptomatic
- Acute infection in a normal host: Symptomatic infection commonly presents with acute mononucleosis syndrome (6).
- Latent infection: Higher IgG titers may contribute to development of atherosclerotic disease (9).
- Infection in bone marrow and solid organ transplant patients:
  - Heart transplant: Early myocarditis followed by late atherosclerosis
  - Lung and bone marrow transplant: Interstitial pneumonia
  - Liver transplant: Hepatitis and colitis
  - Kidney transplant: Graft loss
- Infection in patients with AIDS: Most commonly retinitis; 2nd most common is colitis, followed by esophagitis and neurologic disease (3)
- Infections in other immunocompromised patients: Pulmonary, GI, or renal disease

PHYSICAL EXAM
- Congenital:
  - Asymptomatic cytomegaloviremia
  - Symptomatic: Small for gestational age, purpura/ petechiae, jaundice, hepatosplenomegaly, chorioretinitis, microcephaly, intracranial calcifications, hearing impairment
  - 90% have late complications: Sensorineural hearing loss occurs in 14%; 3–5% moderate to severe (8)[A]
  - Mental retardation, chorioretinitis, optic atrophy, seizures, learning disabilities (1)
- Acquired: Acute infection in a normal host (6):
  - Usually asymptomatic
  - Mononucleosis syndrome: Fever, malaise, sore throat, headache, antibiotic rash
  - Less common: Exudative pharyngitis, splenomegaly, cervical adenopathy, rash

- Infections in AIDS patients (3):
  - Retinitis: Usually unilateral, floaters, scotomata, peripheral field defects. Diagnosis is made when characteristic retinal changes are noted by ophthalmologist on funduscopic exam.
  - Colitis: Fever, weight loss, anorexia, abdominal pain, diarrhea, malaise; hemorrhage or perforation rare but serious
  - Esophagitis: Fever, odynophagia, nausea, abdominal discomfort
  - Pneumonitis: Dyspnea with or without exertion, nonproductive cough, hypoxemia
  - Neurologic disease: Dementia, lethargy, confusion, fever, focal neurologic signs
- Infections in transplant recipients:
  - Persistent fever (most common)
  - Bone marrow transplant: Interstitial pneumonia (7)
  - Liver transplant: Hepatitis (7)
  - Kidney transplant: CMV syndrome (fever, leucopenia, atypical lymphocytes, hepatomegaly, myalgia, arthralgia)

DIFFERENTIAL DIAGNOSIS

- Congenital: Toxoplasmosis, rubella, syphilis, hepatitis B
- Early infancy: Chlamydia, human respiratory syncytial virus
- Acquired in immunocompetent: Epstein-Barr virus (EBV) mononucleosis, viral hepatitis
- Acquired immunocompromised: Other viral, bacterial, fungal opportunistic infections

DIAGNOSTIC TESTS & INTERPRETATION
Initial Tests (lab, imaging)

- Congenital:
  - Isolation of the virus in urine or saliva samples collected within the first 3 weeks of life
  - Direct hyperbilirubinemia >3 mg/dL
  - Thrombocytopenia (<75,000/mL) (1)
  - Elevated liver transaminases (1)
- Acute infection in a normal host:
  - Elevated liver transaminases in 92%, although transaminases rarely increase to >5× normal ranges (6)
  - Anemia (6)
  - Thrombocytopenia (6)
  - Positive cold agglutinins (6)
  - Lymphocytosis with >10% atypical (6)
  - Negative heterophil antibody test (rules out Epstein-Barr virus mononucleosis (6)
  - Positive CMV IgM antibodies; may not peak until 4–7 weeks after acute infection (6)
  - CMV IgG should increase 4-fold during acute infection (6).
- Immunocompromised:
  - Viremia: PCR, antigen assays (pp65 lower-matrix protein in leukocytes), blood culture; although viremia can be present without CMV disease (3)[A]
  - Serum CMV antibodies not useful; can be falsely negative due to immunosuppression (3)[C]
  - Neurologic disease: CMV detected in CSF or brain tissue clinches diagnosis; enhanced by PCR analysis (3)[A].
  - Recovery of virus from tissue in symptomatic patient (GI or pulmonary tissue) indicates infection, although 1–6 weeks are required for distinctive cytopathic events to occur.
  - Quantitative DNA polymerase chain reaction (PCR) evidences disease and can be used to monitor therapy.

- Head CT or MRI: Periventricular enhancement (CMV neurologic disease in neonate)
- Chest x-ray: Interstitial infiltrates (CMV pneumonitis)

Diagnostic Procedures/Other

- Bronchoscopy: Identification of CMV inclusion bodies in lung tissue in context of pulmonary infiltrates (pneumonitis)
- Endoscopic exam of GI tract: Mucosal ulcerations and colonoscopic, rectal, or esophageal biopsy (colitis, esophagitis) (3)[B]

Test Interpretation
Giant cells with basophilic inclusion bodies (owl's eye)

 TREATMENT

MEDICATION
First Line

- Congenital disease: Ganciclovir 12 mg/kg IV q12h for 6 weeks (1)[B]
- Pediatric disseminated disease: IV ganciclovir (6)[A]
- CMV mononucleosis/asymptomatic viremia: No treatment (3)
- Retinitis: Effective treatments include the following and should be chosen in consultation with a specialist:
  - PO valganciclovir (for peripheral lesions) (3)[A]
  - IV ganciclovir (3)[A]
  - IV ganciclovir followed by PO valganciclovir (3)[A]
  - IV foscarnet (3)[A]
  - IV cidofovir (3)[A]
  - Ganciclovir intraocular implant with PO or IV valganciclovir (3)[A]
  - Treat until CD4 >100 for 3–6 months (3)[A]
- Colitis or esophagitis: Treat 21–42 days or until symptom resolution IV ganciclovir or PO valganciclovir (3)[A]
- IV foscarnet (3)[A]
- Neurologic disease: Prompt treatment with IV ganciclovir and IV foscarnet (3)[A] Pneumonitis: IV ganciclovir or IV foscarnet (3)[A]
- CMV disease in transplant patients: IV ganciclovir for 2–4 weeks (7)[B]

Second Line

- Adult CMV retinitis: Fomivirsen (1)[A]
- Pediatric disseminated disease: Foscarnet 60 mg/kg q8h for 14–21 days (1)[A], combination ganciclovir and foscarnet (1)[B]
- CMV disease in transplant patients: Valganciclovir (7)[C]
- CMV in bone marrow transplant patients:
  - Prophylaxis: Valacyclovir (7)[B]
  - Preemptive: Foscarnet (7)[B]

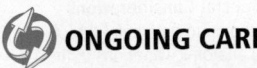 ONGOING CARE

FOLLOW-UP RECOMMENDATIONS
Bed rest

Patient Monitoring

- CMV urine culture at birth for all HIV-infected or -exposed and annual testing for CMV seronegative/HIV+ children
- Patients with CD4 counts <50 should have ophthalmologic screening every 3–6 months.
- Patients on therapy should be followed for neutropenia, anemia, and thrombocytopenia.

PROGNOSIS
Severe disease with primary infection in newborns and reactivation in immunocompromised

COMPLICATIONS

- Congenital: Hearing loss, mental retardation, optic atrophy, seizures, learning disabilities
- Colitis: Hemorrhage and perforation

REFERENCES

1. Mofenson LM, Oleske J, Serchuck L, et al. Treating opportunistic infections among HIV-exposed and infected children: Recommendations from CDC, the National Institutes of Health, and the Infectious Diseases Society of America. *MMWR Recomm Rep.* 2004;53:1–92.
2. Salzberger B, Hartmann P, Hanses F, et al. Incidence and prognosis of CMV disease in HIV-infected patients before and after introduction of combination antiretroviral therapy. *Infection.* 2005;33:345–349.
3. Guidelines for the Prevention and Treatment of Opportunistic Infections in HIV-Infected Adults and Adolescents: Recommendations from the CDC, the NIH, and IDSA. Available at http://aidsinfo.nih.gov/contentfiles/lvguidelines/adult_oi.pdf. Accessed 8/1/2013.
4. Osawa R, Singh N. Cytomegalovirus infection in critically ill patients: A systematic review. *Crit Care.* 2009;13:R68.
5. Cascio A, Iaria C, Ruggeri P, et al. Cytomegalovirus pneumonia in patients with inflammatory bowel disease: A systematic review. *Int J Infect Dis.* 2012;16(7):e474–479. Epub 2012 May 22.
6. Taylor GH. Cytomegalovirus. *Am Fam Phys.* 2003;67(3):519–524.
7. Razonable RR, Emery VC. 11th Annual Meeting of the IHMF (International Herpes Management Forum). Management of CMV infection and disease in transplant patients. 27–29 February 2004. *Herpes.* 2004;11:77–86.
8. Grosse SD, Ross DS, Dollard SC. Congenital cytomegalovirus (CMV) infection as a cause of permanent bilateral hearing loss: A quantitative assessment. *J Clin Virol.* 2008;41:57–62.
9. Kurath S, Halwachs-Baumann G, Müller W, et al. Transmission of cytomegalovirus via breast milk to the prematurely born infant: A systematic review. *Clin Microbiol Infect.* 2010;16:1172–1178.

ADDITIONAL READING

Kadambari S, Williams EJ, Luck S, et al. Evidence based management guidelines for the detection and treatment of congenital CMV. *Early Hum Dev.* 2011;87(11):723–728. Epub 2011 Sep 29.

 CODES

ICD10

- B25.8 Other cytomegaloviral diseases
- B25.9 Cytomegaloviral disease, unspecified
- P35.1 Congenital cytomegalovirus infection

CLINICAL PEARLS

- CMV mono has much less cervical adenopathy and/or splenomegaly than EBV mono in adults.
- CMV is a major cause of sensorineural hearing loss in young children.

DE QUERVAIN TENOSYNOVITIS

Christie Langenberg, MD • J. Herbert Stevenson, MD

 BASICS

DESCRIPTION
- First identified in 1895, de Quervain tenosynovitis is a painful condition of the radial aspect of the thumb and/or wrist due to tendon sheath stenosis in the 1st dorsal compartment of the wrist.
- Often caused by repetitive motion, gliding of the extensor pollicis brevis (EPB) and abductor pollicis longus (APL) over the radial styloid becomes painful due to motion resistance and thickening of the surrounding tendon sheath.

EPIDEMIOLOGY
The epidemiology of de Quervain tenosynovitis has not been well studied. However, it is known that the predominant age range is 30–50 years and women are up to 6 times more likely than men to have this diagnosis.

Incidence
- Based on a 2009 study, the overall incidence of de Quervain tenosynovitis is 0.93/1,000 person-years (with a denominator of 12 million person-years).
- For patients age >40 years, the incidence is 1.37/1,000 person-years compared with those age <20 years at 0.57/1,000 person-years.
- Women have an incidence rate ratio of 2.8/1,000 person-years compared with 0.6/1,000 person-years in men.
- The incidence ratio rate of de Quervain tenosynovitis is 1.31/1,000 person-years in blacks as opposed to 0.81 in whites (1)[B].

ETIOLOGY AND PATHOPHYSIOLOGY
- Repetitive motions of the wrist and/or thumb result in microtrauma and thickening of the tendons (EPB, APL) and surrounding tendon sheath.
- This thickening causes pain with movements of the thumb and wrist, as EPB and APL movement is resisted as they glide over the radial styloid.

RISK FACTORS
- Women age 30–50
- Pregnancy (primarily 3rd trimester and postpartum)
- African American race
- Systemic diseases (e.g., rheumatoid arthritis)
- Participation in activities that include repetitive motion or forceful grasping with thumb/wrist deviation such as golf, fly fishing, racquet sports, rowing, or bicycling
- Repetitive movements with the hand/thumb requiring forceful grasping with wrist ulna/radial deviation; seen in dental hygienists, musicians, carpenters, assembly workers, and machine operators

GENERAL PREVENTION
Avoid overuse or repetitive movements of the wrist and/or thumb associated with forceful grasping and ulnar/radial deviation.

 DIAGNOSIS

HISTORY
- Often involves repetitive motion activity or overuse of wrist or thumb
- Patients may complain of gradual worsening pain along the radial aspect of the thumb and wrist with certain movements, including ulnar deviation of the wrist.
- NSAIDs may or may not relieve pain.
- Rarely associated with trauma

PHYSICAL EXAM
- Pain is present over the radial styloid, which may be exacerbated when patients move the thumb or make a fist.
- Crepitus with movement of the thumb may be felt or heard.
- Swelling is often appreciated over the radial styloid.
- Occasionally slight swelling at the base of the thumb and wrist is also noted.
- Decreased range of motion of the thumb may be observed.
- Pain over the 1st dorsal compartment on resisted thumb abduction or extension
- Tenderness may extend proximally or distally along the tendons with palpation or stress.

DIFFERENTIAL DIAGNOSIS
- Scaphoid fracture
- Scapholunate ligament tear
- Dorsal wrist ganglion
- Osteoarthritis of the 1st carpometacarpal joint
- Flexor carpi radialis tendonitis
- Infectious tenosynovitis
- Tendonitis of the wrist extensors
- Intersection syndrome
- Trigger thumb

DIAGNOSTIC TESTS & INTERPRETATION
The Finkelstein test is useful for diagnosis: This test is positive if pain is elicited over the radial styloid when the patient's thumb is flexed into the palm of the hand and the examiner deviates the wrist in the ulnar direction.

Initial Tests (lab, imaging)
- No labs are indicated.
- This disease is primarily a clinical diagnosis, but if the diagnosis is questionable, radiographs of the wrist may be indicated to rule out other pathology.
- Radiographs may rule out carpometacarpal (CMC) arthritis, which can be misdiagnosed as de Quervain.
- MRI is the test of choice to rule out coexisting soft tissue injury or wrist joint pathology.

Follow-Up Tests & Special Considerations
Ultrasound has been shown to be a helpful tool, especially in detecting anatomic variations in the 1st dorsal extensor compartment of the wrist. Awareness of anatomic variations may aid in improving outcomes of corticosteroid injections (2,3)[C].

Test Interpretation
Inflamed and thickened retinacular sheath of the tendon

TREATMENT
- Rest and immobilization with a thumb spica splint
- NSAIDs may help if used with rest and splinting.
- Corticosteroid injection (preferably ultrasound guided)
- Surgery (if conservative measures fail >6 months)

GENERAL MEASURES
- If full relief is not being achieved, a corticosteroid injection of the tendon sheath has been shown to reduce symptoms (4)[C].
- Anatomic variants may complicate treatment, including 2 tendon sheaths in the 1st compartment or the EPB tendon may travel in a separate compartment. Ultrasound has been shown to be useful in helping distinguish these variants (2,3)[C].
- Surgical release may be indicated for cases not responding to 3–6 months of conservative treatment. Surgery has been found to be highly efficacious with low complication rates (4,5)[C].

MEDICATION
First Line
Splinting, rest, and NSAIDs

Second Line
- Corticosteroid injection of the tendon sheath has shown significant cure rates. An 83% success rate after single injection has been reported. Additional injections are sometimes required (4)[C].
- Corticosteroid injection plus immobilization has been shown to be more effective than immobilization alone (4)[C].
- A recent study has shown some evidence that a newer, 4-point injection technique may yield more favorable results compared with older, 1- and 2-point injection techniques in high-resistance training athletes (6)[B].

ISSUES FOR REFERRAL
Referral to a hand surgeon is indicated if no improvement is noted after conservative treatments.

ADDITIONAL THERAPIES
- Hand therapy, along with iontophoresis/phonophoresis, may help improve outcomes for moderate cases.
- Patients may incorporate thumb-stretching exercises into their rehabilitation.

SURGERY/OTHER PROCEDURES
- Only indicated for patients who have failed conservative treatment (7)[C].
- Endoscopic release may provide earlier and fewer superficial radial nerve complications, as well as greater scar satisfaction, when compared with open release (8)[C].

IN-PATIENT CONSIDERATIONS
Admission Criteria/Initial Stabilization
- Splinting of the thumb (thumb spica splint or dorsal hood splint)
- Rest
- Ice (15–20 minutes 5–6 times a day)
- Anti-inflammatory medications

ONGOING CARE

FOLLOW-UP RECOMMENDATIONS
- Additional corticosteroid injection may be performed at 4–6 weeks if symptoms are not significantly reduced.
- Avoid repetitive motions and activities that cause pain.

DIET
As tolerated

PATIENT EDUCATION
Modification of activities eliciting pain, such as repetitive movement of the wrist/thumb and forceful grasping

PROGNOSIS
Prognosis is extremely good with conservative treatments, with complete resolution taking up to 1 year (9)[C]. 95% success rates have been shown with conservative therapy over 1 year, although up to 1/3 of patients will have recurrence.

COMPLICATIONS
- Most complications are secondary to the treatment modalities. This includes GI, renal, and hepatic injury secondary to NSAIDs.
- Nerve damage may occur during surgery.
- Hypopigmentation, fat atrophy, bleeding, infection, and tendon rupture have been reported as potential adverse events from corticosteroid injection for de Quervain tenosynovitis.
- If not appropriately treated, thumb flexibility may be lost due to fibrosis.

REFERENCES

1. Wolf JM, Sturdivant RX, Owens BD. Incidence of de Quervain's tenosynovitis in a young, active population. *J Hand Surg Am*. 2009;34:112–115.
2. Choi SJ, Ahn JH, Lee YJ, et al. De Quervain disease: US identification of anatomic variations in the first extensor compartment with an emphasis on subcompartmentalization. *Radiology*. 2011;260: 480–486.
3. Kwon BC, Choi SJ, Shin DJ, et al. Sonographic identification of the intracompartmental septum in de Quervain's disease. *Clin Orthop Relat Res*. 2010;468:2129–2134.
4. Ashraf MO, Devadoss VG. Systematic review and meta-analysis on steroid injection therapy for de Quervain's tenosynovitis in adults. *Eur J Orthop Surg Traumatol*. 2013; in press
5. Scheller A, Schuh R, Hönle W, et al. Long-term results of surgical release of de Quervain's stenosing tenosynovitis. *Int Orthop*. 2009;33: 1301–1303.
6. Pagonis T, Ditsios K, Toli P, et al. Improved corticosteroid treatment of recalcitrant de Quervain's tenosynovitis with a novel 4-point injection technique. *Am J Sports Med*. 2011;39: 398–403.
7. Ilyas AM, Ast M, Schaffer AA, et al. De Quervain's tenosynovitis of the wrist. *J Am Acad Orthop Surg*. 2007;15:757–764.
8. Kang HJ, Koh IH, Jang JW, et al. Endoscopic versus open release in patients with de Quervain's tenosynovitis: A randomised trial. *Bone Joint J*. 2013;95-B:947–951.
9. Ilyas AM. Nonsurgical treatment for de Quervain's tenosynovitis. *J Hand Surg Am*. 2009;34:928–929.

ADDITIONAL READING

- Di Sante L, Martino M, Manganiello I, et al. Ultrasound-guided corticosteroid injection for the treatment of de Quervain's tenosynovitis. *Am J Phys Med Rehabil*. 2013;92:637–638.
- Peters-Veluthamaningal C, van der Windt DA, Winters JC, et al. Corticosteroid injection for de Quervain's tenosynovitis. *Cochrane Database Syst Rev*. 2009;3:CD005616.

SEE ALSO

Algorithm: Pain in Upper Extremity

CODES

ICD10
M65.4 Radial styloid tenosynovitis [de Quervain]

CLINICAL PEARLS

- Repetitive movements of the wrist and thumb and activities that require forceful grasping are the most common causes of de Quervain tenosynovitis.
- De Quervain tenosynovitis is a stenosis of the first dorsal compartment of the wrist, including the EPB and APL. It is due to thickening of the tendon sheath that surrounds the EPB and the APL, which leads to pain with certain movements of the thumb.
- The Finkelstein test is a useful diagnostic tool for de Quervain tenosynovitis. This test involves flexing the thumb into the palm while the examiner deviates the wrist in the ulnar direction. The test is positive if patient's symptoms are reproduced.
- Initial treatment includes rest, thumb immobilization, and NSAIDs. Corticosteroid injections are often helpful as well. Patients may return to activity, as tolerated, once pain free. However, most people need to modify their activities to assist with rehabilitation and to prevent pain recurrence.
- Risk factors include female sex, pregnancy or postpartum status, age $\geq$40, rheumatoid arthritis, African American race, and participation in jobs or sports with repetitive wrist and thumb movement.

D

DEEP VEIN THROMBOPHLEBITIS (DVT)

Alfonso J. Tafur, MD • Denisse Tafur

BASICS

DESCRIPTION
- Development of blood clot within the deep veins, usually accompanied by inflammation of the vessel wall
- Major clinical consequences are embolization (usually to the lung) and postphlebitic syndrome.
- System(s) affected: Cardiovascular

EPIDEMIOLOGY
- Age and gender adjusted incidence of venous thromboembolism (VTE) is 100× higher in the hospital than in the community.
- Of patients with VTE, 1/3 die within 30 days, 20% will have sudden death due to pulmonary embolism (PE). The 28-day DVT fatality rate is 9%.

Incidence
- In the US, VTE occurs for the 1st time in 100/100,000/year.
- ~2/3 of the new VTE cases are DVT alone.
- Higher incidence among Caucasians and African Americans relative to Hispanics and Asians
- Complicates ~1/1,000 pregnancies

Prevalence
Variable; depends on medical condition or procedure:
- 22–52% of the patients with PE have DVT.
- 25% of patients with superficial venous thrombosis (1)
- Present in 11% of patients with acquired brain injury entering to neurorehabilitation

ETIOLOGY AND PATHOPHYSIOLOGY
Factors involved may include venous stasis, endothelial injury, and abnormalities of coagulation.

Genetics
- Factor V Leiden is found in 5% of the population and in 20% of all VTE events. It is the most common thrombophilia. Homozygosity is found in 1/5,000 persons. It increases the risk of VTE 3–8-fold in heterozygous carriers and 50–80-fold in homozygous.
- Prothrombin (PT) 20210A is found in 3% of Caucasians. Increases the risk of thrombosis ~3-fold.

RISK FACTORS
- Acquired: Age, previous thrombosis, immobilization, major surgery, orthopedic surgery, malignancy, oral contraceptives, hormonal replacement therapy, antiphospholipid syndrome, polycythemia vera, paroxysmal nocturnal hemoglobinuria, prolonged travel, pregnancy/puerperium, diabetes who developed venous thromboembolism
- Inherited: Antithrombin deficiency, protein C deficiency, protein S deficiency, factor V Leiden R506Q, prothrombin G20210A, dysfibrinogenemia
- Mixed/Unknown: Hyperhomocysteinemia, high levels of factor VIII, activated protein C resistance not factor V Leiden, high levels of factor IX, high levels of thrombin activatable fibrinolysis inhibitor (TAFI), high levels of factor XI

GENERAL PREVENTION
- Mechanical thromboprophylaxis is recommended in patients with high bleeding risk and as adjunct to anticoagulant-based thromboprophylaxis. Mechanical measures include early ambulation, graduated compression stockings, venous foot pump, and intermittent pneumatic compression.
- For acutely ill and for critically ill hospitalized patients at increased risk of thrombosis; low-molecular-weight heparin [LMWH], low-dose unfractionate heparin [LDUH], or fondaparinux are recommended (2)[C].
- For surgical patients, the use of a prediction score for VTE is strongly recommended. If the risk is moderate or higher, LMWH is preferred.
- For most patients, prolonged prophylaxis is not recommended.

DIAGNOSIS

Wells criteria:
- Wells score/criteria (possible score −2–9):
  - Active cancer (treatment within last 6 months or palliative) +1 point. Calf swelling >3 cm compared with other calf (measured 10 cm below tibial tuberosity) +1 point. Collateral superficial veins (nonvaricose) +1 point. Pitting edema (confined to symptomatic leg) +1 point. Previous documented DVT +1 point. Swelling of entire leg +1 point. Localized pain along distribution of deep venous system +1 point. Paralysis, paresis, or recent cast immobilization of lower extremities +1 point. Recently bedridden >3 days, or major surgery requiring regional or general anesthetic in past 4 weeks +1 point. Alternative diagnosis at least as likely −2 points:
    ○ Interpretation: Score 0–1 DVT unlikely. Score ≥2: Moderate-to-high probability

HISTORY
- Establish pretest probability based on Wells criteria.
- Classify as "provoked" or "idiopathic." Determine the presence of risk factors, including family history.
- Clinical assessment of bleeding risk: Bleeding with previous history of anticoagulation, history of liver disease, recent interventions, history of GI bleed

PHYSICAL EXAM
- Physical exam is only 30% accurate for DVT.
- Resistance to dorsiflexion of the foot (Homan sign) is unreliable.
- Swelling of collateral veins. Massive edema with cyanosis is a medical emergency (phlegmasia cerulea dolens, rare).
- Thoracic outlet maneuvers in upper extremity DVT
- Attention to signs of possible malignancy

DIFFERENTIAL DIAGNOSIS
Cellulitis, fracture, ruptured synovial cyst (Baker cyst), lymphedema, muscle strain/tear, extrinsic compression of vein (e.g., by tumor/enlarged lymph nodes), compartment syndrome, localized allergic reaction, filariasis (in developing countries)

DIAGNOSTIC TESTS & INTERPRETATION
Initial Tests (lab, imaging)
- D-dimer (sensitive, but not specific; has a high negative predictive value [NPV]); most protocols are used to rule out DVT in low pretest probability cases: If D-dimer negative with a low pretest probability of disease, DVT is ruled out and no further testing is recommended.
- CBC, platelet count, activated partial thromboplastin time (aPTT), prothrombin time (PT)/INR
- In young patients with idiopathic/recurrent VTE, consider thrombophilia testing.
- Compression US (CUS): Noninvasive; sensitive, and specific for popliteal, femoral thrombi, but has poor ability to detect calf vein thrombi.
- Contrast venography: Gold standard, is technically difficult, risk of morbidity
- Impedance plethysmography: As accurate as duplex US, less operator dependency, but poor at detecting calf vein thrombi; not widely available
- MR venography: As accurate as contrast venography; may be useful for patients with contraindications to IV contrast
- ^{125}I-fibrinogen scan: Detects only active clot formation; very good at detecting ongoing calf thrombi; takes 4 hours for results
- In patients with suspected DVT, the choice of diagnostic test process should be guided by the assessment of the pretest probability:
  - Low pretest probability: D-dimer, proximal CUS
  - Moderate pretest probability: D-dimer, proximal CUS, whole leg US
  - High pretest probability: Proximal CUS, whole leg US
  - If risk stratification is not performed in patients with suspected 1st lower extremity DVT: Proximal CUS, whole leg US
- D-dimer (not useful in high-risk patients):
  - If negative, no further testing is recommended. If positive:
    ○ Low pretest probability, then CUS
    ○ Moderate pretest probability, then proximal CUS/whole leg US
- CUS: If positive, treat DVT; if negative:
  - Low pretest probability, then no further testing
  - Moderate pretest probability, then repeat proximal CUS in 1 week

Follow-Up Tests & Special Considerations
Risk of an underlying malignancy is more likely if: Recurrent VTE, risk: 3.2 (95% CI 2.0–4.8). Unprovoked VTE, 4.6× higher (vs. secondary); upper extremity DVT, not catheter associated; odds ratio (OR) 1.8 (3), abdominal DVT; OR 2.2 (3), bilateral lower extremity DVT, OR 2.1 (3)

TREATMENT

MEDICATION
All proximal DVTs should receive treatment. Consider starting therapy even before confirmation in patients with high pretest probability.

First Line
- UFH:
  - IV drip: Initial dose of 80 U/kg or 5,000 U followed by continuous infusion of 18 U/kg/hr. Target an aPTT ratio >1.5. The aPTT prolongation should correspond to a 0.3–0.7 anti-Xa level.
  - SC UFH: Monitored: 17,500 U or 250 U/kg b.i.d. with aPTT adjustment to an equivalent to 0.3–0.7 anti-Xa. Alternatively, fixed dose: 333 U/kg followed by b.i.d. dose 250 U/kg.
- Enoxaparin (Lovenox): 1 mg/kg/dose SC q12h or 1.5 mg/kg/dose/d
- Dalteparin (Fragmin): 200 U/kg SC q24h
- Fondaparinux (Arixtra): 5 mg (body weight <50 kg), 7.5 mg (body weight = 50–100 kg), or 10 mg (body weight >100 kg) SC once daily
- Rivaroxaban (Xarelto): 15 mg b.i.d. for the first 3 weeks.

- Maintenance therapy:
  - Warfarin (Coumadin): 5 mg/d for 3 days, then adjust to a target INR of 2–3
  - Rivaroxaban (Xarelto): 20 mg once daily after the first 3 weeks.
- Adverse effects:
  - Heparin or LMWH: Bleeding, edema, injection site irritation, skin eruptions, hematoma, thrombocytopenia
  - Fondaparinux: Bleeding, injection site irritation, rash, fever, anemia
  - Warfarin: Bleeding, skin necrosis, teratogenicity
- Contraindications:
  - Heparin or LMWH: Bleeding, heparin hypersensitivity, heparin-induced thrombocytopenia (HIT), idiopathic thrombocytopenic purpura (ITP), infants/neonates
  - Fondaparinux: Bleeding, endocarditis, renal failure, thrombocytopenia
  - Warfarin: Current bleeding, alcoholism, preeclampsia, pregnancy, surgery, high fall risk

Second Line
If warfarin is contraindicated, heparin can be given by intermittent SC self-injection.

Pregnancy Considerations
- Warfarin (Coumadin) is a teratogen; treat with full-dose heparin initially, followed by SC heparin starting at 15,000 U q12h.
- Warfarin is safe with breastfeeding.
- LMWH, dalteparin, and fondaparinux are pregnancy category B.

ADDITIONAL THERAPIES
- Dabigatran as a fixed PO dose is as effective as warfarin for the treatment of acute venous thromboembolism. However, this is not an approved indication in the US (4).
- Discharge with compression stockings 30–40 mm Hg; stress use to prevent postphlebitic syndrome.

SURGERY/OTHER PROCEDURES
- In selected patients with proximal DVT (iliofemoral DVT, <2 weeks of symptoms, good functional status, >1 year of life expectancy), consider catheter-directed thrombolysis/open thrombectomy.
- When anticoagulants have failed or are contraindicated, filtering devices are recommended.

IN-PATIENT CONSIDERATIONS
Admission Criteria/Initial Stabilization
Admission for respiratory distress, proximal VTE, candidate for thrombolysis, active bleeding, renal failure, phlegmasia cerulea dolens, history of heparin-induced thrombocytopenia

Nursing
Limb elevation

Discharge Criteria
Medically stable and properly anticoagulated; overlap of anticoagulation and warfarin monitoring may be done as an outpatient.

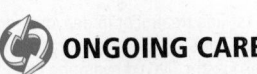 ONGOING CARE

FOLLOW-UP RECOMMENDATIONS
- Gradual resumption of normal activity, with avoidance of prolonged immobility

- Duration of warfarin treatment after DVT:
  - 3 months for treatment of a DVT secondary to a reversible risk factor
  - Patients with unprovoked DVT can be considered for prolonged secondary prophylaxis:
    - In patients who have completed 3 months of anticoagulation after an unprovoked VTE, a positive D-dimer 1 month after discontinuation of therapy correlates with the risk of VTE recurrence (5).
    - Tailoring the anticoagulation duration base on recanalization US evidence may reduce the rate of recurrent VTE (6).
  - Consider prolonged secondary prophylaxis (1 year or indefinitely): Recurrent DVT; PE; active cancer (LMWH preferred over warfarin); life-threatening event (large PE, limb-threatening DVT); cerebral/visceral vein thrombosis; antithrombin deficiency with event; homozygous for factor V Leiden; combined clotting disorders (e.g., combined heterozygous factor V Leiden and PT20210A); antiphospholipid syndrome

Patient Monitoring
- Monitor platelet count while on heparin, LMWH, fondaparinux.
- An anti-factor Xa activity level may help guide LMWH titration of therapy, but it is not usually needed.
- Investigate significant bleeding (e.g., hematuria or GI hemorrhage) because anticoagulant therapy may unmask a preexisting lesion (e.g., cancer, peptic ulcer disease, or arteriovenous malformation).

PATIENT EDUCATION
- Patients should wear compression stockings post-DVT.
- Dietary habits should be discussed when warfarin is initiated to ensure that intake of vitamin K-rich foods is monitored.

PROGNOSIS
- 20% of untreated proximal (e.g., above the calf) DVTs progress to pulmonary emboli, and 10–20% of those are fatal; with anticoagulant therapy, mortality is decreased 5–10-fold.
- DVT confined to the infrapopliteal veins has a small risk of embolization but can propagate into the proximal system. Best treatment is uncertain, but most recommend 6–12 weeks of anticoagulation.

COMPLICATIONS
PE (fatal in 10–20%), arterial embolism (paradoxical embolization) with arteriovenous (AV) shunting, chronic venous insufficiency, postphlebitic syndrome (pain and swelling in affected limb without new clot formation), treatment-induced hemorrhage, soft-tissue ischemia associated with massive clot and high venous pressures; phlegmasia cerulea dolens (rare, but a surgical emergency)

REFERENCES
1. Decousus H, Quéré I, Presles E, et al. Superficial venous thrombosis and venous thromboembolism: A large, prospective epidemiologic study. *Ann Intern Med*. 2010;152:218–224.
2. Holbrook A, Schulman S, Witt DM, et al. Evidence-based management of anticoagulant therapy: Antithrombotic Therapy and Prevention of Thrombosis, 9th ed.: American College of Chest Physicians Evidence-Based Clinical Practice Guidelines. *Chest*. 2012;141:e152S–184S.
3. Tafur AJ, Kalsi H, Wysokinski WE, et al. The association of active cancer with venous thromboembolism location: A population-based study. *Mayo Clin Proc*. 2011;86(1):25–30.
4. Schulman S, Kearon C, Kakkar AK, et al. Dabigatran versus warfarin in the treatment of acute venous thromboembolism. *N Engl J Med*. 2009;361(24):2342–2352.
5. Palareti G, Cosmi B, Legnani C, et al. D-dimer testing to determine the duration of anticoagulation therapy. *N Engl J Med*. 2006;355:1780–1789.
6. Prandoni P, Prins MH, Lensing AW, et al. Residual thrombosis on ultrasonography to guide the duration of anticoagulation in patients with deep venous thrombosis: A randomized trial. *Ann Intern Med*. 2009;150:577–585.

ADDITIONAL READING
- Einstein Investigators. Oral rivaroxaban for symptomatic venous thromboembolism. *N Eng J Med*. 2010;363:2499–2510.
- Kyrle PA, Rosendaal FR, Eichinger S, et al. Risk assessment for recurrent venous thrombosis. *Lancet*. 2010;376:2032–2039.
- Lyman GH, Khorana A, Kuderer N, et al. Venous thromboembolism prophylaxis and treatment in patients with cancer: American Society of Clinical Oncology Clinical practice guideline update. *J Clin Oncol*. 2013 Jun 10;31(17):2189–2204.

 SEE ALSO

Antithrombin Deficiency; Factor V Leiden; Protein C Deficiency; Protein S Deficiency; Prothrombin 20210 (Mutation); Pulmonary Embolism

 CODES

ICD10
- I80.3 Phlebitis and thrombophlebitis of lower extremities, unsp
- I80.9 Phlebitis and thrombophlebitis of unspecified site
- I80.209 Phlbts and thombophlb of unsp deep vessels of unsp low extrm

CLINICAL PEARLS
- Many cases are asymptomatic and are diagnosed after embolization.
- Of the patients with superficial thrombophlebitis, 25% will have DVT at presentation.
- Heparin and warfarin should overlap for a minimum of ≥5 days to achieve target INR.
- Use of anticoagulation must be personalized to the specific scenario, including prophylactic therapy.
- A LMWH dose reduction after the 1st month is recommended in patients with active cancer.
- The current American Society of Clinical Oncology guidelines acknowledge the value of primary prophylaxis in selected patients wit] active cancer receiving outpatient chemotherapy (8)[C].

DEHYDRATION
Jerin Mathew, MD • Mony Fraer, MD, FACP, FASN

BASICS

DESCRIPTION
- Dehydration is a state of negative fluid balance; strictly defined as free water deficiency.
- The 2 types of dehydration:
  - Water loss dehydration (hyperosmolar hyperglycemic state and diabetic ketosis)
  - Salt and water loss dehydration (combination of dehydration and hypovolemia)

EPIDEMIOLOGY
- Cause of 10% of all pediatric hospitalizations in the US
- Gastroenteritis, 1 of its leading causes, accounts to 13/1,000 children <5 years annually in the US.

Incidence
- More than a half-million hospital admissions annually in the US for dehydration
- Of hospitalized older persons, 7.8% have the diagnosis of dehydration (1).
- Worldwide, ~3–5 billion cases of acute gastroenteritis occur each year in children <5 years, resulting in nearly 2 million deaths.

ETIOLOGY AND PATHOPHYSIOLOGY
- Negative fluid balance occurs when ongoing fluid losses exceed fluid intake.
- Fluid losses can be insensible (sweat, respiration), obligate (urine, stool), or abnormal (diarrhea, vomiting, osmotic diuresis in diabetic ketoacidosis).
- Negative fluid balance can ultimately lead to severe intravascular volume depletion (hypovolemia) and ultimately end-organ damage from inadequate perfusion.
- The elderly are at increased risk as kidney function, urine concentration, thirst sensation, aldosterone secretion, release of vasopressin, and renin activity are all significantly lowered with age.
- Decreased intake
- Increased output: Vomiting, diarrheal illnesses, sweating, frequent urination
- Third-spacing of fluids: Effusions, ascites, capillary leaks from burns or sepsis

Genetics
Some underlying causes of dehydration have a genetic component (diabetes), whereas others do not (gastroenteritis).

RISK FACTORS
- Children <5 years of age at highest risk
- Elderly
- Decreased cognition
- Lack of access to water such as in critically sick intubated patients

GENERAL PREVENTION
- Patient/Parent education on the early signs of dehydration
- Observing universal precautions (including hand hygiene)

Geriatric Considerations
A systematic approach in assessing risk factors is necessary for early prevention and management of dehydration in the elderly, especially those in long-term care facilities.

COMMONLY ASSOCIATED CONDITIONS
- Hypo-/Hypernatremia
- Hypokalemia
- Hypovolemic shock
- Renal failure

DIAGNOSIS

Calculate % dehydration = (preillness weight – illness weight)/preillness weight × 100. Supplement this along with the ongoing fluid loss.

Clinical Finding (2)	Mild	Moderate	Severe
Dehydration: Children	5–10%	10–15%	>15%
Dehydration: Adults	3–5%	5–10%	>10%
General condition: Infants	Thirsty, alert, restless	Lethargic/Drowsy	Limp, cold, cyanotic extremities, may be comatose
General condition: Older children	Thirsty, alert, restless	Alert, postural dizziness	Apprehensive, cold, cyanotic extremities, muscle cramps
Quality of radial pulse	Normal	Thready/Weak	Feeble or impalpable
Quality of respiration	Normal	Deep	Deep and rapid/tachypnea
BP	Normal	Normal to low	Low (shock)
Skin turgor	Normal skin turgor	Reduced skin turgor, cool skin	Skin tenting, cool, mottled, acrocyanotic skin
Eyes	Normal	Sunken	Very sunken
Tears	Present	Absent	Absent
Mucous membranes	Moist	Dry	Very dry
Urine output	Normal	Reduced	None passed in many hours
Anterior fontanelle	Normal	Sunken	Markedly sunken

HISTORY
- Fever
- Intake (including description and amount)
- Diarrhea (including duration, frequency, consistency, ± mucus/blood)
- Vomiting (including duration, frequency, consistency, ± bilious/nonbilious)
- Urination pattern
- Sick contacts
- Medication history (e.g., diuretics, laxatives)

PHYSICAL EXAM
- The most useful individual signs for identifying dehydration in children are prolonged capillary refill time, abnormal skin turgor, and abnormal respiratory pattern (3).
- Vitals: Pulse, BP, temperature
- Orthostatic vital signs: Take BP and heart rate (HR) while supine, sitting, and standing:
  - Systolic BP decrease by 20, diastolic BP decrease by 10, or HR increase by 20 highly suggestive of hypovolemia (4)
- Weight loss: <5%, 10%, or >15%
- Mental status
- Head: Sunken anterior fontanelle (for infants)
- Eyes: Sunken, ± tear production
- Mucous membranes: Tacky, dry, or parched
- Capillary refill: Ranges from brisk to >3 seconds

DIFFERENTIAL DIAGNOSIS
- Decreased intake: Ineffective breastfeeding, inadequate thirst response, anorexia, malabsorption, metabolic disorder, obtunded state
- Excessive losses: Gastroenteritis, diarrhea, febrile illness, diabetic ketoacidosis, hyperglycemia, hyperosmolar hyperglycemic state, diabetes insipidus, intestinal obstruction, sepsis

DIAGNOSTIC TESTS & INTERPRETATION
Initial Tests (lab, imaging)
- For mild dehydration: Generally not necessary
- For moderate to severe dehydration:
  - Blood work, including electrolytes, BUN, creatinine, and glucose
  - Urinalysis (specific gravity, hematuria, glucosuria)
- Imaging does not play a role in the diagnosis of dehydration, unless diagnosis of the specific medical condition causing the dehydration requires imaging.
- In adults there is evidence to support the use of inferior vena cava collapsibility as a surrogate marker for volume status.

Pediatric Considerations
Infants and the elderly may not concentrate urine maximally, so a nonelevated specific gravity should *not* be reassuring.

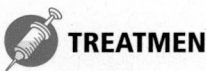 TREATMENT

MEDICATION
First Line
- Oral rehydration is 1st-line treatment in dehydrated children. If this is unsuccessful, use IV rehydration. If IV unobtainable, nasogastric (NG) rehydration can be considered (5).
- Oral rehydration is 1st-line treatment in dehydrated adults as long as they can tolerate fluids. Have a lower threshold for IV rehydration if needed.

- If the patient is experiencing excessive vomiting, consider using an antiemetic.
- Ondansetron (PO/IV) may be effective in decreasing the rate of vomiting, improving the success rate of oral hydration, preventing the need for IV hydration, and preventing the need for hospital admission (6,7).
- Antiemetic medications that are currently available include ondansetron, granisetron, tropisetron, dolasetron, ramosetron, promethazine, dimenhydrinate, metoclopramide, domperidone, droperidol, prochlorperazine, and trimethobenzamide.

Second Line
- Loperamide may reduce the duration of diarrhea compared with placebo in children with mild to moderate dehydration (2 randomized controlled trials [RCTs] yes, 1 RCT no).
- In children ages 3–12 with mild diarrhea and minimal dehydration, loperamide decreases diarrhea duration and frequency when used with oral rehydration.

Pediatric Considerations
Given a higher risk for serious adverse events, loperamide is not indicated for children <3 years of age with acute diarrhea.

ISSUES FOR REFERRAL
- For severe dehydration, critical care referral and ICU-level care may be warranted.
- Surgical consultation for acute abdominal issues

SURGERY/OTHER PROCEDURES
For specific underlying causes of dehydration, such as intestinal obstruction or appendicitis

IN-PATIENT CONSIDERATIONS
Admission Criteria/Initial Stabilization
- Intractable vomiting/diarrhea
- Electrolyte abnormalities
- Hemodynamic instability
- Inability to tolerate oral rehydration therapy (ORT)
- Stabilize ABCs.
- If mild dehydration, try ORT
- If excessive vomiting/severe dehydration with shock, start IV access and IV fluids immediately.

IV Fluids
- Stage I:
  – For moderate to severe dehydration in children: Isotonic saline or Ringer's lactate solution bolus of 10–20 mL/kg. May repeat up to 60 mL/kg; if still hemodynamically unstable, consider colloid replacement (blood, albumin, fresh frozen plasma) and address other causes for shock.
  – For moderate to severe hypovolemia in adults: Isotonic saline or Ringer's lactate 20 mL/kg/h until normal state of consciousness returns/vital signs stabilize. Also consider colloid replacement if continued fluids required beyond 3 L.
- Stage II: Replace fluid deficit along with maintenance over 48 hours. Fluid deficit = preillness weight − illness weight.
- An alternative IV treatment option for moderate (10%) dehydration in children:
  – Bolus with NS/LR at 20 mL/kg for 1 hour
  – Replete fluid deficit with D5 1/2 NS + 20 mEq KCl/L at 10 mL/kg for 8 hours (hours 2–9)
  – Replete 1.5 × maintenance fluids with D5 1/4 NS + 20 mEq/L of KCl for 16 hours (hours 10–24)

- An alternative to IV fluids is hypodermoclysis, the SC infusion of fluids into the body:
  – Indications: Hydration of patients with mild to moderate dehydration who do not tolerate oral intake because of cognitive impairment, severe dysphagia, advanced terminal illness, or intractable vomiting. It is also indicated to prevent dehydration, especially in frail elderly residents living in long-term care settings who reject the oral route for any reason. Useful technique for patients with difficult IV access.
  – Contraindications: Severe dehydration or shock, patients with coagulopathy or receiving full anticoagulation, patients with severe generalized edema (anasarca) or congestive heart failure, and those with fluid overload (8).

Nursing
Strict intake and outputs: Oral and IV intake and output of urine and stool, which may include weighing wet diapers

Discharge Criteria
- Intake > Output
- Underlying etiology treated and improving

 ONGOING CARE

FOLLOW-UP RECOMMENDATIONS
Activity as tolerated:
- If mild to moderate dehydration, the patient may be mobile without restrictions, although watch for orthostasis/falls.
- If moderate to severe dehydration, bed rest.

Patient Monitoring
Ongoing surveillance for recurrence

DIET
- Bland food such as a BRAT diet (bananas, rice, apples, toast)
- If diarrhea, avoid dairy for 48 hours after symptoms resolve. One review of weak RCTs and 3 of 5 subsequent RCTs found that lactose-free feeds reduced the duration of diarrhea in children with mild to severe dehydration, compared with lactose-containing feeds. However, 2 subsequent RCTs found no difference between lactose-free and lactose-containing feeds in duration of diarrhea.
- Small frequent sips of room-temperature liquids
- For children, Pedialyte (liquid or Popsicles)
- Continue breastfeeding ad lib.

PATIENT EDUCATION
- Patients should go to the nearest emergency facility or call 911 if they or their child feels faint or dizzy when rising from a sitting or lying position, becomes lethargic and/or confused, or complains of a rapid heart rate.
- Patients should call their physician if they are unable to keep down any fluids, vomiting has been going on >24 hours in an adult or >12 hours in a child, diarrhea has lasted >2 days in an adult/child, or an infant/child is much less active than usual or is very irritable.
- Patient information on dehydration: www.mayoclinic.com/health/dehydration/DS00561
- Additional patient information: http://familydoctor.org/online/famdocen/home/children/parents/common/stomach/196.html

PROGNOSIS
Self-limited if treated early; potentially fatal

COMPLICATIONS
- Seizures
- Renal failure
- Cardiovascular arrest

REFERENCES
1. Thomas DR, Cote TR, Lawhorne L, et al. Understanding clinical dehydration and its treatment. *J Am Med Dir Assoc*. 2008;9:292–301.
2. Gorelick MH, Shaw KN, Murphy KO. Validity and reliability of clinical signs in the diagnosis of dehydration in children. *Pediatrics*. 1997;99:E6.
3. Steiner MJ, DeWalt DA, Byerley JS. Is this child dehydrated? *JAMA*. 2004;291:2746–2754.
4. Lanier JB, Mote MB, Clay EC. Evaluation and management of orthostatic hypotension. *Am Fam Physician*. 2011;84:527–536.
5. Rouhani S, Meloney L, Ahn R, et al. Alternative rehydration methods: A systematic review and lessons for resource-limited care. *Pediatrics*. 2011;127:e748–e757.
6. Colletti JE, Brown KM, Sharieff GQ, et al. The management of children with gastroenteritis and dehydration in the emergency department. *J Emerg Med*. 2010;38:686–698.
7. Carter B, Fedorowic Z. Antiemetic treatment for acute gastroenteritis in children: An updated Cochrane systematic review with meta-analysis and mixed treatment comparison in a Bayesian framework. *BMJ Open*. 2012;2:e000622.
8. Lopez JH, Reyes-Ortiz CA. Subcutaneous hydration by hypodermoclysis. *Rev Clin Gerontol*. 2010;20:105–113.

 SEE ALSO

Oral Rehydration

 CODES

ICD10
- E86.0 Dehydration
- E87.1 Hypo-osmolality and hyponatremia

CLINICAL PEARLS
- Dehydration is the result of a negative fluid balance and is a common cause of hospitalization in both children and the elderly.
- Begin by assessing the level of dehydration and determining the underlying cause.
- Treatment is directed at restoring fluid balance via oral rehydration (first-line) therapy or IV fluids and treating underlying causes.

DELIRIUM
Jonathan M. Flacker, MD, AGSF

 BASICS

DESCRIPTION
- A neurologic complication of illness and/or medication(s), especially common in older patients, manifested by new confusion and impaired attention
- A medical emergency requiring immediate evaluation to decrease morbidity and mortality
- System(s) affected: Nervous
- Synonym(s): Acute confusional state; Altered mental status; Organic brain syndrome; Acute mental status change

EPIDEMIOLOGY
- Predominant age: Older persons
- Predominant sex: Male = Female

Incidence
- >50% in high-risk older patients

Prevalence
- 10% in older ER patients
- 10–40% in hospitalized older patients
- 25% in older post-acute care patients
- Highest rates (>50%) in ICU, post-hip fracture repair, post-cardiothoracic surgery

ETIOLOGY AND PATHOPHYSIOLOGY
- Believed to result from a decline in physiologic reserves with aging, resulting in a vulnerability to new stressors.
- Neuropathophysiology is not clearly defined; cholinergic deficiency, kynurenine pathway, and resolvins are leading hypotheses.
- Multicomponent approach addressing contributing factors can reduce incidence and complications.
- Usually multifactorial
- Often interaction between predisposing and precipitating risk factors
- With more predisposing factors (i.e., frail patients), fewer precipitating factors are needed to produce delirium.
- If few predisposing factors (e.g., very robust patients), more precipitating factors are needed to manifest delirium.

RISK FACTORS
- Predisposing risk factors:
  - Advanced age
  - Prior cognitive impairment
  - Functional impairment
  - High BUN:creatinine ratio
  - Dehydration
  - Malnutrition
  - Hearing or vision impairment
  - Frailty
- Precipitating risk factors:
  - Severe illness in any organ system(s)
  - Need for a urinary catheter
  - >3 medications
  - Specific medications, especially long-acting sedative hypnotics (e.g., diazepam and flurazepam), narcotics (especially meperidine), and anticholinergics (especially diphenhydramine)
  - Pain
  - Any adverse iatrogenic event

GENERAL PREVENTION
Follow treatment approach.

COMMONLY ASSOCIATED CONDITIONS
Multiple, but most common are:
- New medicine or medicine changes
- Infections (especially lung and urine, but consider meningitis as well)
- Toxic-metabolic (especially low sodium, elevated calcium, renal failure, and hepatic failure)
- Heart attack
- Stroke
- Alcohol or drug withdrawal
- Pre-existing cognitive impairment increases risk.

 DIAGNOSIS

The Confusion Assessment Method (CAM) is the most well-validated and tested tool and has been adapted for ICU setting in adults (CAM-ICU) and children (pCAM-ICU) (1)[B].

ALERT
- Key diagnostic features of the CAM:
  - Acute change in mental status that fluctuates
  - Abnormal attention and either disorganized thinking or altered level of consciousness
- Any of the following nondiagnostic symptoms may be present:
  - Short- and long-term memory problems
  - Sleep–wake cycle disturbances
  - Hallucinations and/or delusions
  - Emotional lability
  - Tremors and asterixis
- Subtypes based on level of consciousness:
  - Hyperactive delirium (15%): Patients are loud, rambunctious, and disruptive.
  - Hypoactive delirium (20%): Quietly confused; may sit and not eat, drink, or move
  - Mixed delirium (50%): Features of both hyperactive and hypoactive delirium
  - Normal consciousness delirium (15%): Still displays disorganized thinking, along with acute onset, inattention, and fluctuation

HISTORY
- Time course of mental status changes
- Recent medication changes
- Symptoms of infection
- New neurologic signs

PHYSICAL EXAM
- Comprehensive cardiorespiratory exam is essential.
- Focal neurologic signs are usually absent.
- Formal mini mental state exam is not diagnostic, but is helpful as a structured interview and followed serially over time.

DIFFERENTIAL DIAGNOSIS
- Depression (slow onset, disturbance of mood, normal level of consciousness, and fluctuates over weeks to months)
- Dementia (insidious onset, memory problems, normal level of consciousness, and fluctuates over days to weeks)
- Psychosis (rarely sudden onset in older adults)

DIAGNOSTIC TESTS & INTERPRETATION
Initial Tests (lab, imaging)
- Guided by history and physical exam
  - CBC
  - Electrolytes, BUN, and creatinine
  - Urinalysis, urine culture
  - Medication levels (digoxin, theophylline where applicable)
- Guided by history and physical exam
- Chest radiograph for most
- ECG as necessary
- Other if indicated by history and exam

Follow-Up Tests & Special Considerations
- If lab tests listed above do not indicate a precipitator of delirium, consider:
  - Arterial blood gases
  - Troponin
  - Toxicology screen
  - Liver panel
  - Thyroid-stimulating hormone
- Noncontrast-enhanced head CT scan if:
  - Unclear diagnosis
  - Recent fall
  - Receiving anticoagulants
  - New focal neurologic signs
  - Need to rule out increased intracranial pressure before lumbar puncture

Diagnostic Procedures/Other
- Lumbar puncture (rarely necessary):
  - Perform if clinical suspicion of a CNS bleed or infection is high.
- EEG (rarely necessary):
  - Consider after above evaluation if diagnosis remains unclear or suspicion of seizure activity.

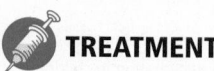 **TREATMENT**

- Stabilize vital signs if needed.
- Ensure immediate evaluation. Addressing 6 risk factors (i.e., cognitive impairment, sleep deprivation, dehydration, immobility, vision impairment, and hearing impairment) in at-risk hospitalized patients can reduce the incidence of delirium by 33%.

GENERAL MEASURES
- Postoperative patients should be monitored and treated for:
  - Myocardial infarction/ischemia
  - Pulmonary complications/pneumonia
  - Pulmonary embolism
  - Urinary or stool retention (attempt catheter removal by postoperative day 2)
- Anesthesia route (general epidural) does not affect the risk of delirium.

- Multifactorial treatment: Identify contributing factors and provide preemptive care to avoid iatrogenic problems (2)[A], with special attention to:
  - CNS oxygen delivery (attempt to attain the following):
    - SaO_2 >90% with goal of SaO_2 >95%
    - Systolic BP <2/3 of baseline or >90 mm Hg
    - Hematocrit >30%
- Fluid/electrolyte balance:
  - Sodium, potassium, and glucose normal (glucose <300 mg/dL in diabetics)
  - Treat fluid overload or dehydration.
- Treat pain:
  - Schedule acetaminophen (1 g q.i.d.) if daily pain
  - Morphine or oxycodone for breakthrough pain if acetaminophen ineffective

ALERT
- Avoid meperidine (Demerol).
- Eliminate unnecessary medications:
  - Investigate new symptoms as potential medication side effects.
- Regulate bowel/bladder function:
  - Bowel movement at least every 48 hours
  - Screen for urinary retention or incontinence, especially after catheter removal.
- Prevent major hospital-acquired problems:
  - 6-inch-thick foam mattress overlay or a pressure-reducing mattress
  - Avoid urinary catheter.
  - Incentive spirometry, if bed-bound
  - SC heparin 5,000 U b.i.d., if bed-fast
  - Environmental stimulation:
    - Glasses and hearing aids
    - Clock and calendar
    - Soft lighting
    - Radio, tapes, and television, if desired
  - Sleep:
    - Quiet environment
    - Soft music
    - Therapeutic massage
- Restraints do not reduce risk of falls/injury:
  - Use only in the most difficult-to-manage patients, as briefly as possible.

MEDICATION
- Nonpharmacologic approaches are preferred for initial treatment, but medication may be needed for behavioral management, especially in the ICU setting.
- Medications often treat only the symptoms and do not address the underlying cause.

First Line
- Neuroleptics:
  - Haloperidol (Haldol): Initially, 0.25–0.5 mg PO/IM/IV unless urgent sedation needed; re-evaluate and potentially redose hourly. Some evidence also suggests low-dose neuroleptics may protect against the development of delirium (3).
  - Quetiapine (Seroquel) 25–50 mg PO b.i.d.
  - Risperidone (Risperdal) 0.25–0.5 mg/d PO
- Short-acting benzodiazepines if neuroleptics do not work or should be avoided:
  - Lorazepam (Ativan): Initially, 0.25–0.5 mg PO/IM/IV q6–8h; may need to adjust to effect (caution in patients with impaired liver function)
- Contraindications: Avoid neuroleptics in patients with parkinsonism or Parkinson disease.

- Precautions: Neuroleptics may cause extrapyramidal effects; benzodiazepines may cause sedation. Both increase fall risk.

Second Line
- Olanzapine (Zyprexa) 2.5–5.0 mg/d PO
- Despite multiple trials, evidence does not support using cholinesterase inhibitors in the prevention or treatment of delirium.

ISSUES FOR REFERRAL
Psychiatric and/or neurologic assessment is helpful if delirium is not easily explainable after full evaluation.

ADDITIONAL THERAPIES
Early mobilization critical:
- Out of bed on hospital day 2 (or postoperative day 1) if no contraindications
- Out of bed several hours daily if able
- Daily therapy if not ambulating independently
- Daily therapy if not functionally independent

IN-PATIENT CONSIDERATIONS
General measures described above are also applicable to delirium prevention.

Admission Criteria/Initial Stabilization
New delirium is a medical emergency and requires admission, except in the setting of palliative home care.

IV Fluids
As needed for dehydration

Nursing
- Institute skin care program for patients with established incontinence.
- Turning regimen if at risk of pressure ulcers
- Soft restraints are acceptable for a short time only, if needed for protection of patient and others.

Discharge Criteria
- Resolution of precipitating factor(s)
- Safe discharge site if still delirious

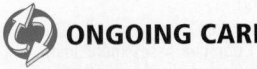
ONGOING CARE

FOLLOW-UP RECOMMENDATIONS
- If delirium at discharge, will usually be followed in postacute facility
- If no delirium at discharge, follow-up with primary care physician in 1–2 weeks.
- As tolerated
- Early physical therapy consultation to prevent deconditioning

Patient Monitoring
- Evaluate and assess mental status daily.
- Depends on specific conditions present

DIET
- Nutritional supplements (1–3 cans daily) if intake is poor
- Consider temporary nasogastric tube if unable to eat and bowels working.

PROGNOSIS
- Usually improves with treatment of underlying condition, but may become chronic
- Delirium complicating medical illness significantly increases a person's chance of dying from that illness.

COMPLICATIONS
- Falls
- Pressure ulcers
- Malnutrition
- Functional decline
- Oversedation
- Polypharmacy

REFERENCES
1. van Eijk MM, van Marum RJ, Klijn IA, et al. Comparison of delirium assessment tools in a mixed intensive care unit. *Crit Care Med*. 2009;37:1881–1885.
2. Fong TG, Tulebave SR, Inouye SK. Delirium in elderly adults: Diagnosis, prevention, and treatment. *Nat Rev Neurol*. 2009;5:210–220.
3. Wang W, Li HL, Wang DX, et al. Haloperidol prophylaxis decreases delirium incidence in elderly patients after noncardiac surgery: A randomized controlled trial. *Crit Care Med*. 2012;40(3): 731–739.

ADDITIONAL READING
- Jones RN, Fong TG, Metzger E, et al. Aging, brain disease, and reserve: Implications for delirium. *Am J Geriatr Psychiatry*. 2010;18(2):117–127.
- Quinlan N, Marcantonio ER, Inouye SK, et al. Vulnerability: The crossroads of frailty and delirium. *J Am Geriatr Soc*. 2011;59:S262–S268.
- Schiemann A, Hadzidiakos D, Spies C. Managing ICU delirium. *Curr Opin Crit Care*. 2011;17(2):131–140.

SEE ALSO
- Dementia; Depression; Substance Use Disorders
- Algorithm: Delirium

CODES

ICD10
- F10.231 Alcohol dependence with withdrawal delirium
- F19.931 Oth psychoactive substance use, unsp w withdrawal delirium
- R41.0 Disorientation, unspecified

CLINICAL PEARLS
- The Confusion Assessment Method (CAM) criteria for delirium are acute onset of fluctuating mental status, inattention, disorganized thinking, and either disorganized thinking or altered level of consciousness.
- In the absence of active monitoring, the hypoactive subtype of delirium can easily be missed.
- Addressing 6 risk factors (i.e., cognitive impairment, sleep deprivation, dehydration, immobility, vision impairment, and hearing impairment) in at-risk hospitalized patients can reduce the incidence of delirium by 33%.
- Delirium may not resolve as soon as the treatable contributors are fixed; resolution may take weeks or months. Rarely will become chronic.
- Avoid diphenhydramine in older patients. Nonpharmacologic measures are preferable as a sleep aid, if needed, zolpidem (5 mg at bedtime) or trazodone (25 mg at bedtime) are reasonable alternatives.

DEMENTIA
Umer Farooq, MD, MBBS • Najm Hasan Siddiqui, MD

BASICS

DESCRIPTION
A decline in <u>cognitive function</u>, which includes memory deficits and/either of <u>apraxia</u>, <u>agnosia</u>, <u>aphasia</u>, or disturbance in executive functioning:
- Alzheimer dementia (AD):
  - Progressive cognitive decline. Most common above age 65
- Vascular dementia (VaD):
  - Usually correlated with a cerebrovascular event and/or cerebrovascular disease
  - Stepwise deterioration with periods of clinical plateaus
- Lewy body dementia:
  - <u>Fluctuating</u> cognition associated with parkinsonism, hallucinations and delusions, gait difficulties, and falls
- Frontotemporal dementia:
  - Language difficulties, personality changes, and behavioral disturbances
- Creutzfeldt-Jacob disease (CJD):
  - Very rare; rapid onset
- HIV dementia

EPIDEMIOLOGY
Prevalence
- In patients age ≥71 years:
  - AD: 70%
  - VaD: 17%
  - Other: 13%
- Estimated 5.4 million Americans had AD in 2010:
  - 5 million >65 years of age; 200,000 <65 years
  - Prevalence expected to double by 2030

ETIOLOGY AND PATHOPHYSIOLOGY
- AD: Unknown, but involves β-amyloid protein accumulation and/or neurofibrillary tangles (NFTs), synaptic dysfunction, neurodegeneration, and eventual neuronal loss: Age, genetics, systemic disease, behaviors (smoking), and other host factors may influence the response to amyloid-β and/or the pace of progression toward the clinical manifestations of AD.
- VaD: Cerebral atherosclerosis/emboli with clinical/subclinical infarcts

Genetics
- AD: Positive family history in 50%, but 90% AD is sporadic; *APOE4* increases risk, but full role unclear
- Familial/Autosomal-dominant AD accounts for <5% AD: Amyloid precursor protein (APP), presenilin-1 (PSEN-1), and presenilin-2 (PSEN-2)

RISK FACTORS
- Age; sex: Female > Male
- Genetic predisposition
- Hypertension: AD; VaD
- Hypercholesterolemia: AD; VaD
- Diabetes: VaD
- Cigarette smoking: VaD
- Endocrine/Metabolic abnormalities: Hypothyroidism, Cushing syndrome; thiamine and vitamin B_{12} deficiency
- Chronic alcoholism, other drugs
- Lower educational status
- Head injury early in life
- Sedentary lifestyle

GENERAL PREVENTION
- Treat reversible causes of dementia, such as drug induced, alcohol induced, and vitamin deficiencies
- Treat hypertension, hypercholesterolemia, and diabetes
- No evidence for statins (or any other specific medication) to prevent onset of dementia (1)[A]
- BP control and low-dose aspirin may prevent or lessen cognitive decline in Vad
- Vitamin E is no longer recommended for the treatment of cognitive symptoms of dementia

COMMONLY ASSOCIATED CONDITIONS
- Anxiety and depression
- Psychosis (delusions; delusions of persecution are common)
- Delirium
- Behavioral disturbances (agitation, aggression)
- Sleep disturbances

DIAGNOSIS
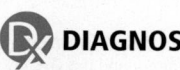

HISTORY
Probable diagnosis AD (2)[A]:
- Age between 40 and 90 (usually >65)
- Progressive cognitive decline of insidious onset
- No disturbances of consciousness
- Deficits in >2 areas of cognition
- No other explainable cause of symptoms
- Specifically rule out thyroid disease, vitamin deficiency (B_{12}), grief reaction, and depression
- Supportive factors: Family history of dementia

PHYSICAL EXAM
- No disturbances of consciousness
- Cognitive decline demonstrated by standardized instruments, including:
  - Mini-Mental Status Exam
  - MOCA (Montreal Cognitive Assessment Test)
  - ADAS-Cog
  - Clock draw test
  - Use caution in relying solely on cognition scores, especially in those with learning difficulty, language barriers, or similar limitations (3)

DIFFERENTIAL DIAGNOSIS
- Mild cognitive impairment
- Major depression
- Medication side effect
- Chronic alcohol use
- Delirium
- Subdural hematoma
- Normal pressure hydrocephalus
- Brain tumor
- Thyroid disease
- Parkinson disease
- Vitamin B_{12} deficiency
- Toxins (aromatic hydrocarbons, solvents, heavy metals, marijuana, opiates, sedative-hypnotics)

DIAGNOSTIC TESTS & INTERPRETATION
Initial Tests (lab, imaging)
- Used to rule out other causes (2)[A]:
  - CBC, comprehensive metabolic profile
  - Thyroid-stimulating hormone
  - Vitamin B_{12} level

- Select patients:
  - HIV, rapid plasma regain (RPR)
  - Erythrocyte sedimentation rate (ESR)
  - Folate
  - Heavy metal and toxicology screen
- Research studies with cerebrospinal fluid (CSF) biomarkers in patient with confirmed AD have shown decreased A beta (1–42) and increased tau and p-tau levels, which are specific features of AD, and CSF tau proteins are increased in CJD (4)[A].
- Neuroimaging (CT/MRI of brain): Cerebral atrophy
  - Early age of onset (<65 years), rapid progression, focal neurologic deficits, cerebrovascular disease risk, or atypical symptoms: Neuroimaging (MRI/CT) to rule out other causes (2)[A]
  - Important findings:
    - AD: Diffuse cerebral atrophy starting in association areas, hippocampus, amygdala
    - VaD: Old infarcts, including lacunar

Diagnostic Procedures/Other
PET scan not routinely recommended; has been approved to differentiate between Alzheimer disease and frontotemporal dementia (5)[A]

Test Interpretation
AD:
- Neurofibrillary tangles: Abnormally phosphorylated tau protein
- Senile plaques: Amyloid precursor protein derivatives
- Microvascular amyloid

TREATMENT

GENERAL MEASURES
- Daily schedules and written directions
- Emphasis on nutrition, personal hygiene, accident-proofing the home, safety issues, sleep hygiene, and supervision
- Socialization (adult day care)
- Sensory stimulation (display of clocks and calendars) in the early to middle stages
- Discussion with the family concerning support and advance directives
- High proportion of patients with dementia require placement in a long-term care facility

MEDICATION
- Cognitive dysfunction:
  - Medications for AD show a small, statistically significant improvement in some cognitive measures, but it remains unclear if the improvement is clinically significant (6)[A]:
  - Cognitive dysfunction, mild (5)[A]:
    - Cholinesterase inhibitors: Donepezil (Aricept), 5–10 mg/d; rivastigmine (Exelon), 1.5–6 mg b.i.d., transdermal system 4.6 mg/24 hours and 9.5 mg/24 hours; galantamine (Razadyne), 4–12 mg b.i.d., extended release 8–24 mg/d:
      - Adverse events: Nausea, vomiting, diarrhea, anorexia, nightmares
      - Galantamine warning: Associated with mortality in patients with mild cognitive impairment in clinical trial
      - Start drug with lowest acquisition cost; also consider adverse event profile, adherence, medical comorbidity, drug interactions, and dosing profiles (3).

- Cognitive dysfunction, moderate to severe (5)[A]:
  o Cholinesterase inhibitors OR
  o Memantine (Namenda), 5–20 mg/d:
    ■ Adverse events: Dizziness, confusion, headache, constipation
    ■ OR combination cholinesterase inhibitor and memantine
- Commonly associated conditions:
  o Psychosis and agitation/aggressive behavior:
    ■ Antipsychotics: Initiate low doses, risperidone 0.25–1 mg/d; olanzapine 1.25–5 mg/d; quetiapine 12.5–50 mg/d; aripiprazole 5 mg/d; ziprasidone 20 mg/d (5)[A]
    ■ Atypical antipsychotics associated with a better side effect profile: Quetiapine and aripiprazole often 1st line due to decreased extrapyramidal side effect

ALERT
Black box warning on atypical antipsychotics due to increased mortality in elderly with dementia

- Depression and insomnia
  o Depression:
    ■ Selective serotonin reuptake inhibitors (SSRIs): Initiate low doses, citalopram (Celexa) 10 mg/d; escitalopram (Lexapro) 5 mg/d; sertraline (Zoloft) 25 mg/d (5)[A].
    ■ Adverse events: Nausea, vomiting, agitation, parkinsonian effects, sexual dysfunction, hyponatremia
    ■ Fluoxetine (Prozac) and paroxetine (Paxil) should be avoided in elderly patients.
    ■ Venlafaxine, mirtazapine, and bupropion are also useful (5)[A]
  o Sleep disturbances:
    ■ Low-dose antidepressants (e.g., Remeron) have significant sedative properties at 7.5 or 15 mg.
    ■ Trazodone 25–100 mg is frequently used because of better side-effect profile
    ■ Zolpidem 5–10 mg; zaleplon 5–10 mg (5)[A]
    ■ Benzodiazepines only for short term, if anxiety/PRN: Lorazepam 0.5–1.0 mg; oxazepam 7.5–15 mg (5)[A]
  o Psychosis and agitation/aggressive behavior:
    ■ Some data for SSRIs (5)[A]
    ■ Benzodiazepines if agitation with anxiety; in elderly, use PRN (5)[A]

Geriatric Considerations
Initiate pharmacotherapy at low doses and titrate slowly up if necessary.
- If benzodiazepines indicated for anxiety, choose drug with short half-life.

ALERT
Benzodiazepine use is associated with increased fall risk.
- Watch decreased renal function and hepatic metabolism.

ISSUES FOR REFERRAL
Neuropsychiatric evaluation particularly helpful in early stages or mild cognitive impairment

ADDITIONAL THERAPIES
Behavioral modification:
- Socialization, such as adult day care, to prevent isolation and depression
- Sleep hygiene program as alternative to pharmaceuticals for sleep disturbance
- Scheduled toileting to prevent incontinence

COMPLEMENTARY AND ALTERNATIVE MEDICINE
- Vitamin E no longer recommended due to lack of evidence and possible association with an increase in mortality (5)[A].
- Ginkgo biloba not recommended due to lack of evidence (5)
- NSAIDs, selegiline, and estrogen lack efficacy and safety data (5)[A].
- Huperzine A: Clinical evidence lacking to recommend

IN-PATIENT CONSIDERATIONS
Admission Criteria/Initial Stabilization
- Worsening physical health issues
- Psychiatry admission may be required because of safety concerns (self-harm/harm to others), self-neglect, aggressive behaviors, or others behavioral issues

 ONGOING CARE

FOLLOW-UP RECOMMENDATIONS
Patient Monitoring
- Progression of cognitive impairment by use of standardized tool (e.g., MMSE, ADAS-Cog)
- Development of behavioral problems: Sleep, depression, psychosis
- Adverse events of pharmacotherapy
- Nutritional status
- Caregiver evaluation of stress
- Evaluate issues that may affect quality of life

PATIENT EDUCATION
- Safety concerns
- Long-term issues: Management of finances, medical decision making, possible placement when appropriate. Legal guardianship, if necessary, to avoid capacity and competency issues
- Advance directives
- National Institute on Aging. About Alzheimer's Disease: Other Dementias. www.nia.nih.gov/alzheimers/topics/other-dementias

PROGNOSIS
- AD: Usually steady progression leading to profound cognitive impairment:
  - Average survival of AD is about 8 years.
- VaD: Incrementally worsening dementia, but cognitive improvement is unlikely
- Secondary dementias: Treatment of the underlying condition may lead to improvement. Commonly seen with normal pressure hydrocephalus, hypothyroidism, and brain tumors.

COMPLICATIONS
- Wandering
- Delirium
- Sundowner syndrome: It is frequently common in older people (who are sedated) and also in people who have dementia (adverse reaction to small dose of psychoactive substances).
- Falls with injury:
  - Hip fracture
  - Head trauma
  - Subdural hematoma
- Aspiration pneumonia in end stage
- Neglect and abuse
- Caregiver burnout

REFERENCES
1. McGuinness B, Craig D, Bullock R, et al. Statins for the prevention of dementia. *Cochrane Database Syst Rev.* 2009;2:CD003160.
2. Blass DM, Rabins PV. In the clinic. *Dementia. Ann Intern Med.* 2008;148:ITC4-1–ITC4-16.
3. National Collaborating Centre for Mental Health. Dementia: The NICE-SCIE guideline on supporting people with dementia and their carers in health and social care [Internet] London: British Psychological Society, Royal College of Psychiatrists; 2007. (National clinical practice guideline number 42). Available from: http://www.nice.org.uk/nicemedia/live/10998/30320/30320/pdf
4. van Harten AC, Kester MI, Visser PJ, et al. Tau and p-tau as CSF biomarkers in dementia: A meta-analysis. *Clin Chem Lab Med.* 2011;49:353–366.
5. APA Work Group on Alzheimer's Disease and Other Dementias, Rabins PV, Blacker D. American Psychiatric Association practice guideline for the treatment of patients with Alzheimer's disease and other dementias, 2nd ed. *Am J Psychiatry.* 2007; 164:5–56.
6. Birks J. Cholinesterase inhibitors for Alzheimer's disease. *Cochrane Database Syst Rev.* 2006;1: CD005593.

 SEE ALSO

Algorithm: Dementia

 CODES

ICD10
- F01.50 Vascular dementia without behavioral disturbance
- F03 Unspecified dementia
- G30.9 Alzheimer's disease, unspecified

CLINICAL PEARLS
- Medications for AD show a small, statistically significant improvement in some cognitive measures, but it remains unclear if the improvement is clinically significant.
- Do not forget the role of adult protective services in case of elderly abuse.
- A particular concern in nursing homes relates to the use of physical restraints and antipsychotic medication, which are regulated by Omnibus Reconciliation Act of 1987.

DEMENTIA, VASCULAR

Birju B. Patel, MD, FACP, AGSF • N. Wilson Holland, MD, FACP

 BASICS

Vascular dementia is a heterogeneous disorder caused by the sequel of cerebrovascular disease that manifests in cognitive impairment affecting memory, thinking, language, behavior, and judgment.

DESCRIPTION
- Vascular dementia (previously known as multi-infarct dementia) was first mentioned by Thomas Willis in 1672. Later, it was further described in the late 19th century by Binswanger and Alzheimer as a separate entity from dementia paralytica caused by neurosyphillis. This concept has evolved tremendously since the advent of neuroimaging modalities.
- Synonym(s): Vascular cognitive impairment (VCI); Vascular cognitive disorder (VCD); Arteriosclerotic dementia; Post-stroke dementia; Senile dementia due to hardening of the arteries; Binswanger disease

EPIDEMIOLOGY
Second most common cause of dementia after Alzheimer dementia in the elderly

Incidence
About 6–12 cases/1,000/person age >70 years

Prevalence
- ~1.2–4.2% in those age >65 years
- 14–32% prevalence of dementia after a stroke

ETIOLOGY AND PATHOPHYSIOLOGY
Upon autopsy of those with dementia, many have significant vascular pathology present, but this is not necessarily correlated clinically with vascular dementia (1)[C]. No set pathologic criteria exist for the diagnosis of vascular dementia such as those that exist for Alzheimer dementia. Pathology includes:
- Large vessel disease: Cognitive impairment that follows a stroke
- Small vessel disease: Includes white matter changes (leukoaraiosis), subcortical infarcts, and incomplete infarction. This is usually the most common cause of multi-infarct dementia.
- Subcortical ischemic vascular disease: Due to small vessel involvement within cerebral white matter, brain stem, and basal ganglia. Lacunar infarcts and deep white matter changes are typically included in this category (2)[C].
- Noninfarct ischemic changes and atrophy
- Transient ischemic attack (TIA)/stroke
- Vascular, demographic, genetic factors
- Vascular disease (i.e., hypertension, PVD, atrial fibrillation, hyperlipidemia, diabetes)

Genetics
- Cerebral autosomal dominant arteriopathy with subcortical infarcts (CADASIL) is caused by a mutation in the *NOTCH3* gene on chromosome 19 that results in leukoencephalopathy and subcortical infarcts. This is clinically manifested in recurrent strokes and associated cognitive decline (3)[C].
- Apolipoprotein E gene type: Those with ApoE4 subtypes are at higher risk of developing both vascular and Alzheimer dementia.
- Amyloid precursor protein (APP) gene: Leads to a form of vascular dementia called heritable cerebral hemorrhage with amyloidosis (4)[B].

RISK FACTORS
- Age
- Previous stroke
- Smoking
- Diabetes
- Hypertension (HTN)
- Atrial fibrillation
- Peripheral vascular disease (PVD)
- Hyperlipidemia
- Metabolic syndrome
- Coronary atherosclerotic heart disease

GENERAL PREVENTION
- Optimization and aggressive treatment of vascular risk factors, such as HTN, diabetes, and hyperlipidemia
- HTN is the single most modifiable risk factor and treatment for it must be optimized.
- Lifestyle modification: Weight loss, physical activity, smoking cessation
- Medication management for vascular risk reduction: Aspirin usage, statin therapy for hyperlipidemia, antihypertensive therapy

COMMONLY ASSOCIATED CONDITIONS
- CADASIL
- Cerebral amyloid angiopathy (CAA): Accumulation of amyloid in cerebral vasculature resulting in infarctions and hemorrhages

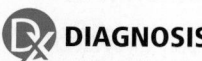 **DIAGNOSIS**

Differentiation between Alzheimer dementia and vascular dementia can be difficult, and significant overlap is seen in the clinical presentation of these two dementias. The diagnosis of vascular dementia is a clinical diagnosis.

HISTORY
- Gradual, stepwise progression is typical.
- Ask about onset and progression of cognitive impairment and the specific cognitive domains involved.
- Ask about vascular risk factors and previous attempts to control these risk factors.
- Ask about medication compliance.
- Ask about urinary incontinence and gait disturbances. Abnormal gait and falls are strong predictors of development of vascular dementia, particularly unsteady, frontal, and hemiparetic types of gait (5,6)[A].
- Look for early symptoms, including difficulty performing cognitive tasks, memory, mood, and assessment of instrumental activities of daily living (IADLs).
- Past history may include TIAs, cerebrovascular accidents (CVAs), coronary atherosclerotic heart disease, atrial fibrillation, hyperlipidemia, and/or peripheral vascular disease.

PHYSICAL EXAM
- Screen for HTN. Average daily BP and not office BP is associated with progression of cerebrovascular disease and cognitive decline in the elderly (7)[B].
- Focal neurologic deficits may be present.
- Gait assessment is important, especially looking at gait initiation, gait speed, and balance.
- Check for carotid bruits as well as abdominal bruits and assess for presence of peripheral vascular disease.
- Check body mass index and waist circumference.
- Do a thorough cardiac evaluation that includes looking for arrhythmias (i.e., atrial fibrillation).

DIFFERENTIAL DIAGNOSIS
- Alzheimer dementia
- Depression
- Drug intoxication
- CNS tumors
- Hypothyroidism
- Vitamin B$_{12}$ deficiency

DIAGNOSTIC TESTS & INTERPRETATION
- Cognitive testing, such as mini-mental status exam (MMSE), Saint Louis University Mental Status (SLUMS), and Montreal Cognitive Assessment (MOCA), provides more definitive information in terms of cognitive deficits, especially executive function, which may be lost earlier in vascular dementia.
- Neuropsychological testing may also be beneficial, especially in evaluating multiple cognitive domains and their specific involvements and deficits.

Initial Tests (lab, imaging)
As appropriate, consider: CBC, comprehensive metabolic profile, lipid panel, thyroid function, hemoglobin A1C, and vitamin B$_{12}$.
- Imaging is used in conjunction with history and physical examination to support a clinical diagnosis of vascular dementia.
- Cognitive deficits observed clinically do not always have to correlate with findings found on neuroimaging studies.
- MRI is best in terms of evaluation of subtle subcortical deficits.
- White matter changes and specific location of these changes can be associated with executive dysfunction and episodic memory impairment (8)[C].

 TREATMENT

Prevention is the real key to treatment:
- Control of risk factors, including HTN, hyperlipidemia, and diabetes
- Avoidance of tobacco and smoking cessation
- Healthy, low-cholesterol diet

MEDICATION

- Acetylcholinesterase inhibitors may be used, but are of limited benefit in vascular dementia (9)[B].
- Clinical evidence for use of memantine is not as strong as for acetylcholinesterase inhibitors and, therefore, the clinical benefit is likely modest.
- Controlling BP with any antihypertensive medications, treatment of dyslipidemia (e.g., statins), and treatment of diabetes are very important.
- Nicardipine has been studied and has been found to have some neuroprotective effects for vascular dementia (10)[C].
- Selective serotonin receptor inhibitors (SSRIs) may be of benefit for agitation and psychosis in vascular dementia (11)[B].

ADDITIONAL THERAPIES

- Limit alcohol drink intake to ≤1/d in women and 2/d in men.
- Heavy sustained alcohol use contributes to HTN.
- Aspirin and/or clopidogrel may be useful in some cases.

SURGERY/OTHER PROCEDURES

Carotid endarterectomy/stenting should be considered if evidence of significant internal carotid artery stenosis (i.e., >70–80%).

COMPLEMENTARY AND ALTERNATIVE MEDICINE

Ginkgo biloba should be avoided due to increased risk of bleeding, especially in cerebral amyloid angiopathy.

IN-PATIENT CONSIDERATIONS

- Remain sensitive to functional assessment and avoidance of pressure ulcers after CVAs.
- Avoid Foley catheter usage unless absolutely necessary due to increased risk of infection.

Nursing

- Nonpharmacologic approaches to behavior management should be attempted prior to medication usage.
- Providing optimal sensory input to patients with cognitive impairment is important during hospitalizations to avoid delirium and confusion. Patients should be given frequent cues to keep them oriented to place and time. They should be informed of any changes in the daily schedule of activities and evaluations. Family and caregivers should be encouraged to be with patients with dementia as much as possible to further help them from becoming confused during hospitalization. Recreational, physical, occupational, and music therapy can be beneficial during hospitalization in avoiding delirium and preventing functional decline.
- Particular emphasis has to be placed on screening for, and optimizing, the mood of the patient. Depression is very common in older patients, especially those who have had strokes and have become hospitalized. Depression in itself can present as "pseudodementia" with worsening confusion during hospitalization and is a treatable condition.

 ONGOING CARE

Vascular dementia is a condition that should be followed with multiple visits in the office setting with goals of optimizing cardiovascular risk profiles for patients. Future planning and advanced directives should be addressed early. Family and caregiver evaluation and burden should also be evaluated.

FOLLOW-UP RECOMMENDATIONS

Perform regular follow-up with a primary care provider or geriatrician for risk-factor modification and education on importance of regular physical and mental exercises as tolerated.

Patient Monitoring

Appropriate evaluation and diagnosis of this condition, need for future planning, optimizing vascular risk factors, lifestyle modification counseling, therapeutic interventions

DIET

- The American Heart Association diet and dietary approaches to stop hypertension (DASH) diet is recommended for optimal BP and cardiovascular risk factor control.
- Low-fat, decreased concentrated sweets and carbohydrates, especially in those with metabolic syndrome

PATIENT EDUCATION

- Lifestyle modification is important in vascular risk reduction (smoking cessation, exercise counseling, dietary counseling, weight-loss counseling).
- Optimizing vascular risk factors via medications (i.e., HTN, diabetes, atrial fibrillation, PVD, heart disease)
- Avoiding smoking, including second-hand smoke
- Home BP monitoring and glucometer testing of blood sugars if HTN, impaired glucose tolerance and/or diabetes is present

PROGNOSIS

- Lost cognitive abilities that persist after initial recovery of deficits from stroke do not usually return. Some individuals can have intermittent periods of self-reported improvement in cognitive function.
- Risk factors for progression of cognitive and functional impairment poststroke include age, prestroke cognitive abilities, depression, polypharmacy, and decreased cerebral perfusion during acute stroke.

COMPLICATIONS

- Physical disability from stroke
- Severe cognitive impairment
- Death

REFERENCES

1. OBrien RJ. Vascular dementia: Atherosclerosis, cognition and Alzheimer disease. *Curr Alzheimer Res*. 2011;8(4):341–344.
2. Arvanitakis Z, Leurgans SE, Barnes LL, et al. Microinfarct pathology, dementia, and cognitive systems. *Stroke*. 2011;42:722–727.
3. Kalimo H, Ruchoux MM, Viitanen M, et al. CADASIL: A common form of hereditary arteriopathy causing brain infarcts and dementia. *Brain Pathol*. 2002;12(3):371–384.
4. Russell MB. Genetics of dementia. *Acta Neurol Scand Suppl*. 2010:58–61.
5. Montero-Odasso M, Verghese J, Beauchet O, et al. Gait and cognition: A complementary approach to understanding brain function and the risk of falling. *J Am Geriatr Soc*. 2012;60(11):2127–2136.
6. Verghese J, Lipton RB, Hall CB, et al. Abnormality of gait as a predictor of non-Alzheimer's dementia. *N Engl J Med*. 2002;347(22):1761–1768.
7. White WB, Wolfson L, Wakefield DB, et al. Average daily blood pressure, not office blood pressure, is associated with progression of cerebrovascular disease and cognitive decline in older people. *Circulation*. 2011;124(21):2312–2319.
8. Smith EE, Salat DH, Jeng J, et al. Correlations between MRI white matter lesion location and executive function and episodic memory. *Neurology*. 2011;76:1492–1499.
9. Kavirajan H, Schneider LS. Efficacy and adverse effects of cholinesterase inhibitors and memantine in vascular dementia: A meta-analysis of randomised controlled trials. *Lancet Neurol*. 2007;6:782–792.
10. Amenta F, Lanari A, Mignini F, et al. Nicardipine use in cerebrovascular disease: A review of controlled clinical studies. *J Neurol Sci*. 2009;283(1-2):219–223. Epub 2009 Mar 20.
11. Seitz DP, Adunuri N, Gill SS, et al. Antidepressants for agitation and psychosis in dementia. *Cochrane Database Syst Rev*. 2011;(2):CD008191. Epub 2011 Feb 16.

ADDITIONAL READING

Gorelick PB. Vascular contributions to cognitive impairment and dementia: A statement for healthcare professionals from the American Heart Association/American Stroke Association. *Stroke*. 2011;42(9):2672–2713.

 SEE ALSO

Alzheimer Disease; Depression; Mild Cognitive Impairment

 CODES

ICD10

- F01.50 Vascular dementia without behavioral disturbance
- F01.51 Vascular dementia with behavioral disturbance

CLINICAL PEARLS

- Executive dysfunction and gait abnormalities are often seen early and are more pronounced in vascular dementia as opposed to Alzheimer dementia.
- Memory is relatively preserved in vascular dementia when compared with Alzheimer dementia in the early stages of this disease.
- Stepwise progression, as opposed to progressive decline in Alzheimer dementia, is typical.
- Considerable overlap exists between vascular dementia and Alzheimer dementia in clinical practice and classification into one of these categories is often difficult.

DENTAL INFECTION

Hugh J. Silk, MD, MPH • Sheila O'Grady Stille, DMD, MAGD

 BASICS

DESCRIPTION
- Very painful area ± swelling in the head and neck region arising from the teeth and supporting structures; if left untreated, can lead to serious and potentially life-threatening illnesses
- Assume any head and neck infection or swelling to be odontogenic in origin until proven otherwise.

EPIDEMIOLOGY
Incidence
- Caries is a contagious bacterial infection that is transmitted vertically from caregivers.
- The introduction of fluoride has dramatically decreased dental caries.

Prevalence
- >25% of 2–5-year-olds have caries (1)[A].
- Percent of children 6–19 years with untreated dental caries: 16.2% (2005–2008) (2)[A]
- 92% of adults 20–64 have had dental caries; 23% have untreated dental caries (2005–2008) (2)[A]
- 25% of children 5–17 years account for 80% of caries in the US.

ETIOLOGY AND PATHOPHYSIOLOGY
Caries or trauma can lead to pulpal death, which in turn leads to infection of pulp and/or abscess of adjacent tissues via direct or hematogenous bacterial colonization.
- *Streptococcus mutans* vertically transmitted to newly dentate infants from caregivers
- Acidic secretions from *S. mutans* are implicated in early caries.
- Often polymicrobial mix of strict anaerobes and facultative anaerobes in dental abscess:
  – Anaerobes, including *Pepto streptococci*, *Bacteroides*, *Prevotella*, and *Fusobacterium*, have been implicated. *Lactobacilli* not seen in healthy subjects, but seen in rampant caries subjects (3)[B]

RISK FACTORS
- Low socioeconomic status
- Parent and/or sibling with history of caries or existing untreated dental caries
- Previous caries
- Poor access to dental and health care
- Fear of dentist
- Poor oral hygiene
- Poor nutrition, including high level of sugary foods and drinks
- Trauma to the teeth or jaws
- Inadequate access to and use of fluoride
- Gingival recession (increased risk of root caries)
- Physical and mental disabilities
- Decreased salivary flow (e.g., use of anticholinergic medications, immunologic diseases)

GENERAL PREVENTION
- Prevent caries and contagious bacterial infection (*Streptococcus mutans*).
- Majority of dental problems can be avoided through flossing, brushing with fluoride toothpaste, systemic fluoride (water; supplements for high-risk patients in nonfluoridated areas), fluoride varnish for moderate-high risk patients, and regular cleaning (4)[B].
- Consider prevention of transmission of *S. mutans* from mother to infant by improving mother's dentition and decreasing mother's bacterial load through proper dental care, chlorhexidine gluconate rinses, and use of xylitol products (5)[B].
- Avoid smoking, which is linked to severe periodontal disease.
- Good control of systemic diseases (e.g., diabetes)
- Fluoride varnish provided by primary care providers twice per year (6)[B]

COMMONLY ASSOCIATED CONDITIONS
- Rampant caries throughout dentition; faulty restorations; extractions and multiple missing teeth
- Periapical abscesses associated with necrotic teeth
- Periodontal abscess
- Soft-tissue cellulitis
- Periodontitis (deep inflammation ± infection of gingiva and ligaments)

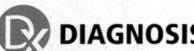 DIAGNOSIS

HISTORY
- Pain at infected site or referred pain to ears, jaw, cheek, or sinuses
- Sensitivity to hot or cold stimuli
- Unprovoked, intermittent, or constant throb along nerve pathway
- Pain on biting or chewing
- Trismus (inability to open mouth)
- Bleeding or purulent drainage from gingival tissues
- When severe infection (systemic):
  – Fever
  – Difficulty breathing or swallowing
  – Death
- Children <4 years with stiff neck, sore throat, and dysphagia should be worked up for retropharyngeal abscess secondary to primary molar infection.

PHYSICAL EXAM
- Gingival edema and erythema
- Cheek or intraoral swelling
- Presence of fluctuant mass
- Suppuration of gingival margin or from tooth
- Submandibular or cervical lymphadenopathy on side of complaint.
- Severe (systemic) infection may present with dysphagia, fever, and signs of airway compromise.

DIFFERENTIAL DIAGNOSIS
- Bacterial or viral throat infection
- Pericoronitis (inflamed ± infection of gum flap over mandibular last molar, typically 3rd molars)
- Otitis media
- Sinusitis
- Viral or aphthous stomatitis
- Temporomandibular joint (TMJ) dysfunction (myofascial pain)
- Parotitis
- Cyst
- Jaw pain can be anginal equivalent, especially in women, and especially lower-left portion of the jaw.

DIAGNOSTIC TESTS & INTERPRETATION
Initial Tests (lab, imaging)
- No initial labs needed, unless patient looks acutely ill
- If acutely ill:
  – Consider CBC with differential.

  – Culture and sensitivity; if abscess present, aspirate pus and culture for aerobes and anaerobes (3)[A].
  – Multiple organisms involved, most likely anaerobic gram-negative rods and anaerobic gram-positive cocci (4)[B]

- Individual dental films of suspected teeth, including root apices; test with palpation, percussion, and cold test to diagnose correct tooth.
- Panoramic film of the teeth and jaw for evaluation of the extent of infection

Follow-Up Tests & Special Considerations
CT scan can be used to determine the extent and density of the swelling, locating the abscess within the soft tissue and bone. This aids in determining treatment course and planning need for and location of external drainage.

 TREATMENT

- Place patient on appropriate antibiotic, if indicated (if systemic).
- If localized infection, incision and drainage may be warranted.
- Appropriate pain control: Anti-inflammatory agents are 1st line; short-course opioids in some cases (7)[A].
- Refer to dentist as soon as possible for definitive treatment: Root canal or extraction (8)[B]
- If infection is severe (systemic symptoms), consider hospitalization with IV antibiotics until stabilized. Patient may need intraoral or extraoral incision and drainage of abscess as well.

GENERAL MEASURES
- Ibuprofen 600–800 mg (or 10 mg/kg) q6h *or* acetaminophen 650–1,000 mg (10–15 mg/kg) q4–6h PRN pain
- For more severe pain, consider acetaminophen or ibuprofen + opioids.
- Can consider local anesthetic nerve block with long-acting anesthetic (bupivacaine) as adjunct; avoid penetrating infection with needle to avoid tracking infection.

MEDICATION

First Line

- Penicillin VK: Loading dose of 1,000 mg, followed by 500 mg q.i.d. for 7–10 days; in children, 40–60 mg/kg/d divided q.i.d. (9)[B]
- Amoxicillin: Loading dose of 1,000 mg, followed by 500 mg t.i.d. for 7–10 days; in children, 40–60 mg/kg/d divided t.i.d.
- If penicillin-allergic, use erythromycin or clindamycin (8)[B]

Second Line

If long-standing infection or previously treated infection that does not respond to 1st-line treatment:

- Clindamycin: Loading dose of 600 mg, followed by 300 mg PO t.i.d. for 7–10 days
- If severe infection, load with clindamycin 600 mg, 900 mg IV, then 300 mg q6h; consider double coverage with metronidazole for better bone penetration. Do not use metronidazole alone. Will increase development of resistant strains.

ISSUES FOR REFERRAL

A dentist should be consulted and follow-up definitive care appointment should be secured prior to discharge from medical office, emergency room, or hospital unit.

SURGERY/OTHER PROCEDURES

- Incision and drainage of abscess should be performed if abscess is large and fluctuant.
- Root canal or extraction should be performed as definitive treatment.

IN-PATIENT CONSIDERATIONS

Admission Criteria/Initial Stabilization

Criteria for hospital admission include swelling involving deep spaces of the neck, unstable vital signs, fever, chills, confusion or delirium, or evidence of invasive infection or cellulitis.

- Secure airway, if compromised, with either endotracheal intubation or tracheotomy.
- IV fluid resuscitation with normal saline may be indicated in acutely ill patients.

Nursing

- Ensure good oral hygiene.
- Rinse mouth with chlorhexidine gluconate b.i.d.
- Use warm salt water rinses several times per day to encourage drainage, especially after incision and drainage. In conjunction, use ice packs on outside of face to decrease swelling and help encourage drainage into mouth.

Discharge Criteria

Discharge patient if:

- Airway not compromised
- Abscess and sepsis eliminated
- Able to take PO intake and ambulate

 ONGOING CARE

Educate patient in need for proper oral hygiene, need for follow-up dental care, need for routine dental care, and stress medical complications that can and have occurred due to lack of dental care.

FOLLOW-UP RECOMMENDATIONS

- Follow-up with dentist within 24 hours.
- Ensure adequate PO intake, including protein.

DIET

- Maintain a healthful diet; bacteria thrive on refined sugar and starch.
- Avoid sugary foods that stick between the teeth.
- Avoid continuous sugary/carbonated drinks throughout day; encourage water as beverage of choice between meals.

Pediatric Considerations

In children, limit the frequency of sugary drinks and advise against sleeping with a bottle to decrease the chance of dental caries.

PATIENT EDUCATION

- Minimally, biannual dental visits
- Nutritional education:
  – Limit the frequency of sugar/carbonated drinks and sugary or sticky foods.
- In young children, avoid sleeping with a bottle to decrease the chance of dental caries.
- Brush twice daily and floss daily.
- Caretakers should tend to their personal oral hygiene, ± chlorhexidine rinses in first 3 years of the child's life to decrease the risk of transmission of the caries-causing microorganisms.

PROGNOSIS

Prognosis is excellent with proper treatment.

COMPLICATIONS

- Ludwig angina
- Retropharyngeal and mediastinal infection
- Osteomyelitis
- Endocarditis
- Submental infection
- Submandibular infection
- Can cause unstable diabetes in diabetics/worsen pre-existing heart disease
- Brain abscess/death

REFERENCES

1. CDC Chronic Disease Prevention and Health Promotion. Oral Health. Preventing cavities, gum disease, tooth loss, and other cancers. At a Glance, 2011.
2. National Center for Health Statistics. Health, United States, 2011: With Special Feature on Socioeconomic Status and Health. Table 76. Hyattsville, MD. 2012. Available at: http://www.cdc.gov/nchs/data/hus/hus11.pdf/
3. Robertson D, Smith AJ. The microbiology of the acute dental abscess. *J Med Microbiol*. 2009;58 (Pt 2):155–162.
4. Marinho VCC. Topical fluoride (toothpastes, mouthrinses, gels or varnishes) for preventing dental caries in children and adolescents. Cochrane Oral Health Group. *Cochrane Database Syst Rev*. 2007;(4):CD002781.
5. Mickenautsch S, Yengopal V. Anticariogenic effect of xylitol versus fluoride—a quantitative systematic review of clinical trials. *Int Dent J*. 2012;62:6–20.
6. U.S. Preventive Services Task Force. *Prevention of dental caries in children from birth through age 5 years: Draft recommendation statement*. AHRQ Publication No. 12-05170-EF-2. http://www.uspreventiveservicestaskforce.org/draftrec.htm
7. Cliff K. An evidence-based update of the use of analgesics in dentistry. *Periodontology*. 2008;46(1):143–164.
8. Douglass AB, Douglass JM. Common dental emergencies. *Am Fam Physician*. 2003;67:511–516.
9. Matijevi S, Lazi Z, Kulji-Kapulica N, et al. Empirical antimicrobial therapy of acute dentoalveolar abscess. *Vojnosanit Pregl*. 2009;66:544–550.

ADDITIONAL READING

- Clark MB, Douglass AB, Maier R, et al. *Smiles for life: A national oral health curriculum*. 3rd edition. Society of Teachers of Family Medicine. 2010; Course 4 Acute Dental Problems: www.smilesforlifeoralhealth.com.
- Lockhart PB, ed. *Dental care of the medically complex patient*, 5th ed. New York: Elsevier; 2004.
- Stefanopoulos PK, Kolokotronis AE. Controversies in antibiotic choices for odontogenic infections. *Oral Surg Oral Med Oral Pathol Oral Radiol Endod*. 2006;101:697–698.
- Stefanopoulos PK, Kolokotronis AE. The clinical significance of anaerobic bacteria in acute orofacial odontogenic infections. *Oral Surg Oral Med Oral Pathol Oral Radiol Endod*. 2004;98:398–408.

 CODES

ICD10

- K02.9 Dental caries, unspecified
- K04.7 Periapical abscess without sinus
- K12.2 Cellulitis and abscess of mouth

CLINICAL PEARLS

- Do not ignore toothache pain.
- Treat patients with facial swelling aggressively, as infections can spread quickly, leading to significant morbidity or death.
- Promote prevention (oral hygiene, fluoride, dental visits) to avoid infections.

DENTAL TRAUMA

Hugh J. Silk, MD, MPH • Sheila O'Grady Stille, DMD, MAGD

BASICS

DESCRIPTION
Loss or fracture of a tooth and/or supporting bone and tissue due to trauma. Can result in shifting of remaining teeth, loss of teeth, loss of alveolar bone, and displaced or nonunion of maxilla and/or mandible, resulting in functional and aesthetic deformities difficult to correct.

EPIDEMIOLOGY
- Dental injuries of the teeth, supporting bone, and surrounding soft tissue constitute 5% of all physical injuries and as high as 18% in preschool children (1)[A],(2)[B].
- Causes: Falls/Sports, 63%; assault, 17%; auto or motorcycle accidents, 2%
- Male > Female (2–3:1)

Prevalence
- Prevalence: 5% of all school-age children; 7–13% in primary dentition, 1–16% in permanent dentition
- Affects 13% of population <12 years

ETIOLOGY AND PATHOPHYSIOLOGY
Direct force sufficient to overcome the bond between the tooth and periodontal ligament within the alveolar socket or disruption of enamel and dentin; force against maxilla or mandibular arch great enough to cause fracture

RISK FACTORS
- Physical and mental disabilities
- Contact sports without wearing proper protective equipment (i.e., helmets, mouth guards)
- High-risk sports include football, boxing, wrestling, soccer, baseball, hockey, bicycling, and skateboarding
- Age: Youth <12 years (2)[B]
- Tongue/Mouth piercings
- Prior dental trauma
- Male gender (3)[B]

GENERAL PREVENTION
- Mouth guards and helmets. Custom mouth guards are better than boil and bite, which are better than stock guards.
- Avoid tongue and orofacial piercings.
- Wear seat belts while in the car.
- Monitor home for slippery areas.
- Childproof house with gates, and pad sharp table edges.

COMMONLY ASSOCIATED CONDITIONS
- Tooth loss can cause loss of space in dental arch.
- Malocclusion causing functional problems
- Trauma to dentition resulting in pulpitis, which causes necrosis of the pulp
- Child abuse: Be alert for history inconsistent with injuries (1)[A].

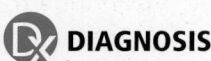

DIAGNOSIS

HISTORY
- Assess ABCs (airway, breathing, and circulation).
- Determine nature, time of injury; associated injuries

- Dental and alveolar fractures:
  - Ask patient if he or she has possession of missing tooth pieces or is aware of swallowed/aspirated teeth.
- Determine degree of injury: Concussion of teeth (mild injury to the periodontal ligament without tooth mobility or displacement); subluxation (significant injury to the periodontal ligament with some tooth mobility, tooth tender to percussion); intrusion (tooth pushed up); extrusion (partial displacement out of socket)
- Tooth avulsion:
  - Time out of socket (critical to management and prognosis)
  - Location of tooth when recovered
  - Type of tooth transfer medium (i.e., milk, saline, towel)
- Jaw or facial pain (maxilla or mandibular fracture)
- Other systemic injuries; neurologic status
- Consider child and domestic abuse in patients with dental fractures.
- Most recent tetanus vaccine

PHYSICAL EXAM
- Gently irrigate if blood, clots, or debris.
- Inspect for laceration, ecchymosis, embedded tooth fragments, or foreign bodies.
- Classify fracture by Ellis classification:
  - Ellis I fracture involves only the enamel.
  - Ellis II fracture includes enamel and dentin (pale yellow material underlying the enamel).
  - Ellis III fracture involves enamel, dentin, and pulp (red material under dentin).
- Check for sensitivity to hot/cold/percussion.
- Check if the tooth is mobile: Palpate tooth and surrounding bone.
- Check for mandibular fracture: Percuss/Twist with tongue blade to evaluate. Pain suggests possible fracture.
- Bimanual palpation for maxilla fracture/alveolar fracture
- If tooth is missing, investigate for intrusion of tooth or root fragment in socket or embedded in soft tissue.

DIFFERENTIAL DIAGNOSIS
- Crown fracture
- Root fracture
- Concussion, subluxation, or avulsion of tooth
- Extrusion/Intrusion of tooth
- Trismus
- If no history of trauma, consider infection, caries, pericoronitis, ulcer, stomatitis.

DIAGNOSTIC TESTS & INTERPRETATION
Initial Tests (lab, imaging)
No initial labs needed

- Multiple radiographic procedures for displacement of a tooth in its socket; occlusal film plus periapical films of teeth in region
- Panoramic radiograph of the teeth and jaw for evaluation of the extent of injury (note that there can be fractures of nonerupted teeth or jaw fractures that are not evident); CT scan is only needed if other associated head trauma is present.

Follow-Up Tests & Special Considerations
Chest x-ray may be needed for lost avulsed teeth: May be in trachea, lungs, esophagus, or stomach.

TREATMENT

Assess ABCs and neurologic exam for other problems associated with the traumatic injury.

GENERAL MEASURES
- Primary goal of reimplantation/repositioning is to protect periodontal ligament; tooth pulp may die, but tooth can be saved by root canal.
- Fractured teeth:
  - Ellis I: Smooth edges with emery board or dental drill; cosmetic repair can be done by dentist in follow-up.
  - Ellis II and III: Cover exposed area with calcium hydroxide paste (Dycal). Tooth must be dry before adding Dycal. If not available, Coe-Pak (zinc oxide preparation) can be used. Wrap preparation around fractured tooth edge. Follow-up with dentist within 24 hours, if other injuries permit. Use care not to cause occlusal interference, which could further traumatize the tooth.
- Subluxation (abnormal mobility) of teeth:
  - Patient should be referred to dentist ASAP for repositioning and splinting. Ensure no occlusal interference prior to referring.
  - Nonrigid splint should be placed ASAP.
- Intrusion (apical displacement of tooth into the alveolar bone):
  - Primary teeth should be left alone to allow for spontaneous re-eruption after dental follow-up.
  - For permanent teeth, do not reposition; refer to oral surgeon ASAP. Attempts to reposition may cause compromise of blood supply to supporting bone and nerve. Alveolar bone may have necrosis, causing bony defect. Tooth usually needs to be extracted when bone heals.

ALERT
- Avulsed teeth: Dental emergency:
  - Time is of the essence when reimplanting teeth.
  - If primary tooth: Do not reimplant. If unsure whether tooth is a primary or permanent tooth, consult dentist.
  - If permanent tooth: Avoid touching tooth root, handle only by the crown; rinse with normal saline. Minimize trauma to socket. If dirt or large clot in socket, perform gentle irrigation of the socket with normal saline and light aspiration of blood clot before implantation.
  - After implantation, have patient bite down on gauze while transporting to dentist.
  - If unable to implant at scene, transport in Hanks solution, milk, or saline (not water) or the buccal sulcus if patient is alert and age appropriate.
  - If tooth is outside of socket <20 minutes, attempt implantation of tooth and stabilize with resin/metal splint, or, if not available, zinc oxide (Coe-Pak) splint. Refer to dentist ASAP.
  - If tooth is outside of socket 20–60 minutes, soak tooth in Hanks solution for 30 minutes to preserve pH. If Hanks is not available, use saline. Attempt implantation and stabilization.
  - If tooth is outside of socket >60 minutes, soak tooth in citric acid and fluoride for 30 minutes; attempt reimplantation and stabilization. If citric acid/fluoride not available, use Hanks or saline.
  - Consult dentist for follow-up and for any questions.

- Soft foods only for 10–14 days, depending on injury (1)[A]
- Oral hygiene may be difficult: Brush with a soft brush after meals; apply chlorhexidine (0.1%) topically to the affected area(s) with cotton swabs b.i.d. × 1 week (1)[A]
- Jaw fracture:
  – Assess for displacement.
  – If nerve impingement, immediate surgery is needed. Contact oral surgeon ASAP.
  – If not displaced or no indication of nerve impingement, have patient see oral surgeon within 24 hours for fixation.

MEDICATION
First Line

- Acetaminophen, NSAIDs, and opioids all beneficial (4)[A]:
  – Ibuprofen: 600–800 mg (or 10 mg/kg) q6h, or acetaminophen 650–1,000 mg (10–15 mg/kg) q4–6h
  – For more severe pain, consider acetaminophen or ibuprofen + opioids.
  – Can consider local anesthetic nerve block with long-acting anesthetic (bupivacaine).
- Antibiotics for fractures or avulsions to prevent complications:
  – Penicillin VK: 500 mg q.i.d. for 7 days in adults; for children, 25–50 mg/kg/divided t.i.d.
  – Clindamycin: 150–300 mg t.i.d. (or 5–7.5 mg/kg/ dose) in penicillin-allergic patients
- Note: The evidence for benefit for antibiotics for avulsed teeth is equivocal but experts recommend antibiotics (5)[B].

Second Line
Clindamycin: 150–300 mg t.i.d. (or 5–7.5 mg/kg/ dose) in penicillin-allergic patients

ISSUES FOR REFERRAL
- All patients should be referred to a dentist for follow-up; x-rays to assess permanent noneruptee teeth for damage in children. Monitor q6mon.
- Splints are typically maintained in place for 7–10 days for subluxed teeth and 1–6 weeks for avulsed teeth. Alveolar fractures should be splinted for 3–4 weeks and can take up to 6 months to heal (6)[A].
- Avulsed teeth continue to deteriorate up to 36 months after injury and typically require root canal therapy. Warn patient of this possibility, which includes discoloration of tooth. Requires close evaluation by dentist.
- Oral surgeon should follow jaw fractures in consultation with general dentist.

ADDITIONAL THERAPIES
Tetanus booster should be considered if tetanus coverage is uncertain, if tooth has been in contact with soil, or if deep soft-tissue lacerations are present.

SURGERY/OTHER PROCEDURES
Oral surgeon consultation within 1 hour if patient has alveolar bone fracture or jaw fracture

COMPLEMENTARY AND ALTERNATIVE MEDICINE
Acupuncture for pain

IN-PATIENT CONSIDERATIONS
Admission Criteria/Initial Stabilization
Swelling compromising airway, mental status change due to concussion or hypoxia, aspiration of teeth, or unstable vital signs

IV Fluids
IV fluid resuscitation with normal saline may be indicated in septic patients.

Nursing
Ensure excellent oral hygiene. Rinse mouth with chlorhexidine gluconate.

Discharge Criteria
Discharge patient when:
- Abscess and sepsis have been eliminated.
- Patient is able to take in adequate PO and ambulate.
- Cleared from concussion

 ONGOING CARE

FOLLOW-UP RECOMMENDATIONS
Follow-up with dentist or oral surgeon within 24 hours after any dental trauma:
- Restrict use of pacifiers if dental injuries are involved.
- Ellis III fractures in children <12 years are likely to get infected; clinicians should consider antibiotic coverage.

Patient Monitoring
Biannual cleaning and follow-up. First 36 months are most critical to long-term prognosis.

PATIENT EDUCATION
- Use a soft toothbrush and soft diet for 10–14 days after dental trauma. Rinse with chlorhexidine 0.1% b.i.d. for 1 week to prevent plaque and debris accumulation (7)[A].
- If tooth avulsion occurs, handle tooth only by the crown, so as to not crush cells on root.
- Cold milk is the best transportation medium before coming to the emergency room; it maintains periodontal ligament for ~3 hours and has pH and osmolarity to maintain vitality of cells. Saline or saliva is a good substitute. Water is the least desirable transport medium.

PROGNOSIS
- <20 minutes of tooth separation from socket: Good prognosis
- >60 minutes of tooth separation: Poor prognosis for tooth reattachment
- Alveolar fracture: Poor prognosis for teeth involved
- Jaw fracture: Good prognosis with proper reduction/fixation

COMPLICATIONS
- Tooth loss
- Infection
- Cosmetic and/or functional deformity
- Anesthesia/Paraesthesia of nerve entrapment with fractured jaw, especially mandibular fracture

REFERENCES

1. Evidence-based review of clinical studies on trauma. *J Endod*. 2009;35:1160–1162.
2. Flores MT, Andersson L, Andreasen JO, et al. Guidelines for the management of traumatic dental injuries. I. Fractures and luxations of permanent teeth. *Dent Traumatol*. 2007;23:66–71.
3. Lieger O, Zix J, Kruse A, Iizuka T. Dental injuries in association with facial fractures. *J Oral Maxillofac Surg*. Aug 2009;67(8):1680–1604.
4. Ong CKS, Seymour RA. An evidence-based update of the use of analgesics in dentistry. *Periodontology*. 2008;46(1):143–164.
5. Evans D. Prescribing systemic antibiotics when replanting avulsed teeth. *Evid Based Dent*. 2009;10(4):103.
6. Kahler B, Heithersay GS. An evidence-based appraisal of splinting luxated, avulsed and root-fractured teeth. *Dent Traumatol*. 2008;24(1): 2–10.
7. Flores MT, Andersson L, Andreasen JO, et al. Guidelines for the management of traumatic dental injuries. II. Avulsion of permanent teeth. *Dent Traumatol*. 2007;23:130–136.

ADDITIONAL READING

- Andreasen JO, Bakland LK, Flores MT, Andreasen FM, Andersson L. *Traumatic dental injuries: A manual*. New York: Wiley & Sons, 2011.
- Berman LH, Blanco L, Cohen S. *A clinical guide to dental traumatology*. St. Louis: Mosby- Elsevier, 2007.
- Clark MB, Douglass AB, Maier R, et al. *Smiles for life: A national oral health curriculum*. 3rd edition. Society of Teachers of Family Medicine. 2010; Course 4 Acute Dental Problems: www.smilesforlifeoralhealth.com.

 CODES

ICD10
- K08.119 Complete loss of teeth due to trauma, unspecified class
- S02.5XXA Fracture of tooth (traumatic), init for clos fx
- S02.69XA Fracture of mandible of oth site, init for clos fx

CLINICAL PEARLS

- Do not reimplant primary teeth.
- Avulsed permanent teeth are a medical emergency. Reimplant permanent teeth ASAP.
- Milk is the best transportation medium before coming to emergency room; Hanks solution, saline, or saliva is a good substitute. Water is the least desirable.
- Consider child or domestic abuse in dental trauma cases.
- Young children are more likely to get infection after Ellis fractures; consider antibiotic coverage.
- Ensure tetanus vaccination is updated.

DEPRESSION

Rachel Bramson, MD • Michael L. Brown, MD • Robert E. Rogers

 ## BASICS

DESCRIPTION
- A primary mood disorder characterized by a sustained depressed mood and/or decreased interest in things that used to give pleasure (anhedonia), which represents a change from previous functioning.
- Synonym(s): Unipolar affective disorder, Major depressive disorder

EPIDEMIOLOGY
Incidence
6.6% from 2001 to 2002 in USA (1)

Prevalence
- 16.2% lifetime risk of having major depressive disorder (1)
- Patients can relapse; risk decreases with longer remission period but increases in patients with severe episodes, episodes at a younger age, and multiple episodes.
- Predominant age:
  – Low risk before early teens, but highest prevalence in teens and young adults (1)
- Predominant gender
  – Females > Males (2:1)

ETIOLOGY AND PATHOPHYSIOLOGY
Complex etiology with 2 major models in the literature (2):
- *Monoamine-deficiency hypothesis:* Symptoms related to decreased levels of norepinephrine (dullness and lethargy) and serotonin (irritability, hostility, and suicidal ideation) in multiple regions of the brain; other neurotransmitters involved include dopamine, acetylcholine, γ-aminobutyric acid (GABA), glutamate.
- *Stress/Hypothalamic-pituitary-adrenal axis:* Abnormalities in cortisol response lead to depression; elevated cortisol levels can be associated with depression, but cortisol tests are not indicated for diagnosis.
- Other areas of research interest: Inflammatory processes and abnormal circadian rhythms
- Impaired synthesis/metabolism of neurotransmitters
- Environmental factors and learned behavior may affect neurotransmitters and/or have an independent influence on depression.

Genetics
Multiple gene loci place a person at increased risk when faced with environmental stressor; twin studies suggest 37% concordance (2).

RISK FACTORS
- Female > Male (2:1)
- Severity of 1st episode
- Persistent sleep disturbances
- Presence of chronic disease(s), recent myocardial infarction (MI), cardiovascular accident (CVA)
- Strong family history (depression, bipolar, suicide, substance abuse), spouse with depression
- Substance abuse and dependence, domestic abuse/violence
- Losses, stressors, unemployment
- Single, divorced, or unhappily married

COMMONLY ASSOCIATED CONDITIONS
- Bipolar disorder, cyclothymic disorder, grief reaction, anxiety disorders, somatoform disorders, schizophrenia/schizoaffective disorders
- Medical comorbidity
- Substance abuse

 ## DIAGNOSIS

HISTORY
DSM V requires all of the following criteria:
- Criterion A: ≥ 5 of the following symptoms present nearly every day during the same 2-week period, with at least 1 of the 5 being either depressed mood or loss of interest or pleasure:
  – Depressed mood most of the day by subjective report or observation from other people
  – Diminished interest or pleasure in all activities most of the day by subjective report or observation from other people
  – Decreased or increased appetite or significant weight loss without dieting
  – Insomnia or hypersomnia
  – Fatigue or energy loss
  – Restlessness, irritability, or withdrawal observable by others
  – Worthlessness, excessive/inappropriate guilty feelings
  – Diminished thinking/concentration, poor memory, indecisiveness
  – Recurrent thoughts of death, suicidal ideations and may or may not have a specific plan
- Criterion B: Symptoms cause significant social, occupational, or functional distress or impairment
- Criterion C: Symptoms not attributable to substance effects or other medical conditions

Geriatric Considerations
- Difficult to diagnose due to medical comorbidity
- Can present with memory difficulties as chief complaint; treatment reverses memory difficulty
- Can be the initial presentation of irreversible dementia
- Geriatric Depression Scale 15 (GDS 15) improves rate of diagnosis in primary care setting (3)[A].

Pediatric Considerations
- Can present as irritable or angry rather than sad or dejected
- Failure to make expected weight gains can substitute weight loss symptom above.
- A sudden and remarkable drop in grades can indicate difficulty concentrating.
- Can present with separation anxiety

PHYSICAL EXAM
Complete physical with focus on: Endocrine, cardiac, neurologic and psychiatric (affect, attention, cognition, memory); look for evidence of contributing medical or neurologic disorder

DIFFERENTIAL DIAGNOSIS
- Psychiatric: Depressed phase of bipolar disorder, adjustment disorder, dysthymic disorder, bereavement
- Neurologic or degenerative CNS diseases, dementias
- Medical comorbidity: Adrenal disease, thyroid disorders, diabetes, metabolic abnormalities (hypercalcemia), liver/renal failure, malignancy, chronic fatigue syndrome, fibromyalgia, lupus
- Nutritional: Pernicious anemia, pellagra
- Medications/substances: Abuse, side effects, overdose, intoxication, dependence, withdrawal

DIAGNOSTIC TESTS & INTERPRETATION
- A clinical diagnosis made by eliciting personal, family, social, and psychosocial factors
- The Patient Health Questionnaire (PHQ-9) is a brief screening test valid for diagnosis of major depressive disorder in primary care settings (4)[A].
- Other validated standard rating scales include: Beck Depression Inventory, Zung, GDS 15, etc. Rating scales are also useful to track response to treatment over time.
- Rule out hypothyroidism, anemia, metabolic disorders with TSH, CBC, CMP.
- Order urine drug screen if symptoms suggest intoxication.

TREATMENT

American Psychiatric Association 2010 Guidelines recommend phasic approach: Acute phase (1st 3 months); Continuation phase (4–9 months); Maintenance (9 months until discontinuation) (5)[A].
- Acute phase:
  – Full evaluation, including risk to self and others, with selection of appropriate treatment setting (hospitalization for those at risk of harm to self or others, or so incapacitated as to be unable to take care of themselves and/or who have no support system to assist with treatment)
  – Goal should be symptom remission, with intervention based on clinical picture, including patient's preference, availability of services
  – For mild to moderate depression, psychotherapies (individual, interpersonal or cognitive–behavioral therapy [CBT]) and/or medication is recommended.
  – For refractory/severe depression, medication is indicated.
  – For patients not responding to medication alone, CBT should be initiated (6)[A].
  – Continue to increase dosage q3–4wks until symptoms in remission. Full medication effect is complete in 4–6 weeks. Augmentation with 2nd medication may be necessary.
  – See within 2 weeks of starting medication and q2wk until improvement, then monthly to monitor medication changes.
  – ≥ 6 visits recommended for monitoring (younger patients, those at high suicide risk, see within 1st week, and follow frequently).
- Continuation/Maintenance phase:
  – Regular visits to monitor for signs of relapse, q3–6mon if stable; depression rating scales should be used.
  – If medication has been started and produces remission, dosage should be continued for at least 4–9 months to reduce relapse; CBT is also effective in reducing relapse (visits typically q2wks) (5)[A].
  – If/when drug discontinuation is considered, medications should be tapered gradually (weeks to months).
- Primary care considerations:
  – Refer immediately for active suicidal ideations, psychosis, severe agitation, severe self-neglect, significant risk of self-harm.
  – Caution with personal or family history of bipolar disorder: Antidepressants can precipitate mania.
  – Refer to psychiatry for failed response to medication trials, suspected bipolar disorder, more persistent suicidal thoughts, self-neglect

MEDICATION

- Effectiveness of medications is comparable between/within classes; selection should be based on provider familiarity and patient characteristics/preferences (7,8)[A].
- SSRIs and tricyclic antidepressants (TCAs) are effective, but TCAs are 2nd-line due to side effects and lethality in overdose. Tolerability is much poorer than newer antidepressants (7)[A].
- First-line SSRIs* (starting dose; usual dose):
  - Fluoxetine (Prozac): 20 mg/d; 20–60 mg/d
  - Sertraline (Zoloft): 50 mg/d; 50–200 mg/d
  - Paroxetine (Paxil): 10 mg/d; 20–60 mg/d
  - Paroxetine CR (Paxil CR): 12.5 mg/d; 25–75 mg/d
  - Citalopram (Celexa): 20 mg/d; 20–40 mg/d (higher doses not advised; EKG monitoring for doses >40 mg/d due to increased risk of QTc prolongation)
  - Escitalopram (Lexapro): 10 mg/d; 10–30 mg/d
  - Precautions: Abrupt discontinuation may result in withdrawal symptoms (i.e., dizziness, nausea, headache, paresthesia)
  - Fluoxetine, Paroxetine may raise serum levels of other drugs; Escitalopram, Sertraline preferred for few to no drug interactions
  - Common side effects: Sexual dysfunction (20%), nausea, GI upset, dizziness, insomnia; headache: Typically resolve in the 1st week
  - Less common side effects: Drowsiness, weight gain, emotional blunting, dry mouth
  - *Lower starting doses for elderly, adolescents, those with comorbid conditions, panic disorder, significant anxiety or hepatic conditions
- Others (starting dose; usual dose):
  - Venlafaxine (Effexor, Effexor XR): 37.5 mg/d; 75–375 mg/d
  - Bupropion XL (Wellbutrin XL): 150 mg/d; 300–450 mg/d [Precautions: Lowers seizure threshold at doses >450 mg/d]
  - Duloxetine (Cymbalta): 30 mg/d; 60–120 mg/d
  - Desvenlafaxine (Pristiq): 50–100 mg/d

Second Line

- TCAs (starting dose; usual dose):
  - Amitriptyline (Elavil): 25–50 mg/d; 100–300 mg/d
  - Nortriptyline (Pamelor): 25 mg/d; 50–200 mg/d
  - Doxepin (Prudoxin, Zonalon): 25–50 mg/d; 100–300 mg/d
  - Imipramine (Tofranil, Tofranil-PM): 25–50 mg/d; 100–300 mg/d
  - Desipramine (Norpramin): 25–50 mg/d; 100–300 mg/d
  - Precautions: Advanced age, glaucoma, benign prostate hyperplasia, hyperthyroidism, cardiovascular disease, liver disease, monamine oxidase inhibitor (MAOI) treatment, potential for fatal overdose, arrhythmia, worsening glycemic control, *SSRIs recommended for patients with diabetes (5)[A]
  - Common side effects: Dry mouth, blurred vision, constipation, urinary retention, tachycardia, confusion/delirium, elderly particularly susceptible
- α_2-Antagonists (sedating) (starting dose; usual dose):
  - Mirtazapine (Remeron): 15 mg/d; 15–45 mg/d
- Atypical antipsychotics:
  - Adjunctive treatment: Aripiprazole or Quetiapine
  - Treatment resistant depression: Olanzapine
  - Significant side effects: Dyslipidemia, hyper-triglyceridemia, glucose dysregulation, diabetes mellitus, hyperprolactinemia, tardive dyskinesia, neuroleptic malignant syndrome, QTc prolongation

- Recommended for depression with psychotic features; consult with psychiatry and consider carefully before starting (5,9)[A].
- Significant potential interactions:
  - TCAs: Amphetamines, barbiturates, clonidine, epinephrine, ethanol, norepinephrine
  - ALL ANTIDEPRESSANTS: Allow 14-day washout period before starting MAOIs
  - MAOIs: Not recommended in primary care. Significant drug and food interactions limit use.

ALERT

Black box warning: Increased risk of suicidality in children, adolescents, and young adults up to age 25 who are treated with SSRIs. Although this has not been extended to adults, suicide risk assessments are warranted for all patients.

Pregnancy Considerations

SSRIs: Fluoxetine and sertraline considered safe in pregnancy. (Paroxetine Category D; other SSRIs Cat. C)

ADDITIONAL THERAPIES

- Electroconvulsive therapy (ECT) for refractory cases
- Transcranial magnetic stimulation may be more effective than pharmacotherapeutics but less effective than ECT.

COMPLEMENTARY AND ALTERNATIVE MEDICINE

Used in mild depression, but *not* regulated by FDA nor recommended by APA:

- Hypericum perforatum (St. John's wort): Multiple drug interactions; not safe in pregnancy.
- Data do not support S-adenosyl methionine (SAM-e) or acupuncture.

IN-PATIENT CONSIDERATIONS

Admission Criteria/Initial Stabilization

Inpatient care is indicated for severe depression, patients at risk of suicide/homicide, and for comorbid conditions.

Discharge Criteria

Depressive symptoms abating, no longer suicidal, appropriate outpatient follow-up in place

 ONGOING CARE

PATIENT EDUCATION

- Depression is a common medical illness, not a character defect.
- Emphasize the need for long-term treatment and follow-up, which includes lifestyle changes.
- Exercise, good sleep hygiene, good nutrition, and decreased use of tobacco and alcohol are recommended. The optimal regimen is one the patient prefers and will adhere to (4)[A].

PROGNOSIS

- 70% show significant improvement.
- Of patients with a single depressive episode, 50% will relapse over their lifetime.

COMPLICATIONS

- Suicide
- Lower quality of life

REFERENCES

1. Kessler RC, Berglund P, Demler O, et al. The epidemiology of Major Depressive Disorder: Results from the National Comorbidity Survey Replication (NCS-R). *JAMA*. 2003;289:3095–3105.
2. Belmaker RH, Agam G. Mechanisms of disease: Major depressive disorder. *N Engl J Med*. 2008;358:55–68.
3. Mitchell AJ, Bird V, Rizzo M, et al. Diagnostic validity and added value of the Geriatric Depression Scale for depression in primary care: A meta-analysis of GDS30 and GDS15. *J Affect Disord*. 2010;125:10–17.
4. Gilbody S, Richards D, Brealey S, et al. Screening for depression in medical settings with the Patient Health Questionnaire (PHQ): A diagnostic meta-analysis. *J Gen Intern Med*. 2007;22(11): 1596–1602.
5. American Psychiatric Association. *Practice guidelines for the treatment of patients with major depressive disorder*. 2010; http://www.psychiatryonline.com/pracGuide/pracGuideTopic_7.aspx
6. Wiles N, Thomas L, Abel A. Cognitive behavioural therapy as an adjunct to pharmacotherapy for primary care based patients with treatment resistant depression: Results of the CoBalT randomised controlled trial. *Lancet*. 2013;381: 375–384.
7. Arroll B, Elley CR, Fishman T, et al. Antidepressants versus placebo for depression in primary care. *Cochrane Database Syst Rev*. 2009;8(3): CD007954.
8. Gertlerner G, Hansen RA, Morgan LC. Comparative benefits and harms of second-generation antidepressants for treating major depressive disorder: An updated meta-analysis. *Ann Intern Med*. 2011;155:772–785.
9. Komossa K, Depping AM, Gaudchau A, et al. Second-generation antipsychotics for major depressive disorder and dysthymia. *Cochrane Database Syst Rev*. 2010;8(12):CD008121.

ADDITIONAL READING

American Psychiatric Association. *Diagnostic and statistical manual of mental disorders DSM-V*. 5th ed. Washington, DC: American Psychiatric Publishing; 2013.

 SEE ALSO

Algorithms: Depressed Mood Resulting from Medical Illness; Depressive Episode, Major

 CODES

ICD10

- F32.9 Major depressive disorder, single episode, unspecified
- F32.9 Major depressive disorder, single episode, unspecified
- F32.9 Major depressive disorder, single episode, unspecified

CLINICAL PEARLS

- Therapeutic alliance is important to treatment success.
- Given the high recurrence rates, long-term treatment is often necessary.

DEPRESSION, ADOLESCENT

Kenia Mansilla-Rivera, MD

 BASICS

DESCRIPTION
- DSM 5 Depressive disorders include disruptive mood dysregulations disorder (DMDD), major depressive disorder (MDD), dysthymia, premenstrual dysphoric disorder, substance/medication-induced depressive disorder and other non-specific depression (1). This chapter focuses on MDD.
- MDD is a primary mood disorder characterized by sadness and/or irritable mood with impairment of functioning, abnormal psychological development, and a loss of self-worth, energy, and interest in typically pleasurable activities.
- DMDD is characterized by a chronic, severe persistent irritability with frequent temper outbursts in response to frustration.
- Dysthymic disorder is differentiated from major depression by less intense symptoms that are more persistent, lasting at least 1 year.
- Treatment-resistant depression is a failure of treatment with 2 antidepressants administered in adequate dosage for at least 6 weeks.
- Adolescents with depression are likely to suffer broad functional impairment across social, academic, family, and occupational domains, along with a high incidence of relapse and a high risk for substance abuse and other psychiatric comorbidity.

EPIDEMIOLOGY
Incidence
During adolescence, 1–6%; many do not receive appropriate care.

Prevalence
- MDD: 6–12% of adolescents; twice as common in females (2)
- DMDD: 2–5%; more prominent in males (1)

ETIOLOGY AND PATHOPHYSIOLOGY
Unclear; low levels of neurotransmitters (serotonin, norepinephrine) may produce symptoms; decreased functioning of the dopamine system also contributes. External factors may affect neurotransmitters independently.

Genetics
A 76% concordance rate is found in monozygotic twins reared together and a 67% concordance rate among those reared apart, along with a 19% concordance rate in dizygotic twins reared together.

RISK FACTORS
- Increased 3–6× if 1st-degree relative has a major affective disorder; 3–4× in offspring of parents with depression
- Prior depressive episodes
- History of low self-esteem, anxiety disorders, attention deficit hyperactivity disorder (ADHD), and/or learning disabilities
- Hormonal changes during puberty
- Female gender
- Low socioeconomic status
- General stressors: Adverse life events, difficulties with peers, loss of a loved one, academic difficulties, abuse, chronic illness, and tobacco abuse

GENERAL PREVENTION
Insufficient evidence for universal depression prevention programs (psychological and social) (3)[B]; small benefit to regular exercise in preventing episodes of depression (4)[B]:
- Some evidence indicates that child and adolescent mental health can be improved by successfully treating maternal depression (5).
- Agency for Healthcare Research and Quality (AHRQ) recommends the screening of adolescents (12–18 years of age) for major depressive disorder when systems are in place to ensure accurate diagnosis, psychotherapy (cognitive-behavioral or interpersonal), and follow-up (6)[B].

COMMONLY ASSOCIATED CONDITIONS
- Eating disorders (especially bulimia)
- Alcohol and substance abuse
- Anxiety and somatization disorders
- Behavioral disorders (i.e., ADHD, oppositional-defiant disorder, conduct disorder)
- Learning disorders
- Headaches

 DIAGNOSIS

HISTORY
Based on DSM-5 criteria, ≥5 of the following symptoms have been present during the same 2-week period and represent a change from previous functioning: At least 1 of the symptoms is either depressed mood or loss of interest or pleasure (1); Criterion A:
- Depressed mood most of the day, nearly every day by either subjective report or observation by others. (feelings of sadness, emptiness, hopelessness; in children can be irritability)
- Markedly diminished interest or pleasure in all activities most of the day, nearly every day
- Significant weight loss when not dieting or weight gain (>5% body weight in 1 month)
- Insomnia or hypersomnia
- Psychomotor agitation or retardation nearly every day
- Fatigue or loss of energy
- Feelings of worthlessness or excessive or inappropriate feelings of guilt nearly every day
- Diminished ability to think or concentrate, or indecisiveness, nearly every day
- Recurrent thoughts of death, recurrent suicidal ideation, or attempt
- Criterion B. Symptoms cause clinically significant distress or impairment in social, occupational, or other important areas of functioning
- Criterion C. Episode is not attributable to substances effects or other medical conditions
- Criterion D. Episode not better explained by a schizoaffective, schizophreniform, or delusional disorder
- Criterion E. There has never been a manic or hypomanic episode.

PHYSICAL EXAM
- Psychomotor retardation/agitation may be present.
- Clinicians should carefully assess patients for signs of self-injury (wrist lacerations) or abuse.

DIFFERENTIAL DIAGNOSIS
- Normal bereavement
- Substance-induced mood disorder
- Bipolar disorder
- Mood disorder secondary to a medical condition (thyroid, anemia, vitamin deficiency, diabetes)
- Organic CNS diseases
- Malignancy
- Infectious mononucleosis or other viral diseases
- ADHD, posttraumatic stress disorder (PTSD), eating disorders, and anxiety disorders
- Sleep disorder

DIAGNOSTIC TESTS & INTERPRETATION
Initial Tests (lab, imaging)
May be used to rule out other diagnoses (i.e., CBC, TSH, glucose, mono spot, and urine drug)
Follow-Up Tests & Special Considerations
None with sufficient sensitivity/specificity for diagnosis

Diagnostic Procedures/Other
- Depression is primarily diagnosed after a formal interview, with supporting information from caregivers and teachers.
- Standardized tests useful as screening tools and to monitor response to treatment, but should not be used as the sole basis for diagnosis:
  - Beck Depression Inventory (BDI): 12–18 (2)
  - Child Depression Inventory (CDI): Ages 7–17
  - Reynolds Adolescent Depression Scale (RADS): Teenagers in grades 7–12
  - Mood and Feelings Questionnaire (MFQ) (5)
  - Patient Health Questionnaire-9 (PHQ-9): Ages 13–17 with ideal cut point of 11 or higher (instead of 10 used for adults) (7)
- Suicide risk assessment should be performed.

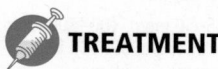 **TREATMENT**

- Psychotherapy, active support, and monitoring is recommended for mild cases (3)[B].
- In moderate to severe cases, starting medication with/without psychotherapy is recommended (3)[A].

GENERAL MEASURES
- Evidence for the effectiveness of cognitive–behavioral therapy (CBT) alone is mixed, but may be effective for mild to moderate depression and useful adjunct to SSRIs, although overall may be most effective for decreasing impairment in the short term with limited evidence for long-term benefit (2,5,8)[A]. Goal is to alter thoughts and behaviors to increase coping and communication skills, problem solving, to regulate emotions, improve mood and decrease negative thinking.
- Interpersonal psychotherapy (IPT) has been shown to be effective for adolescent depression. The treatment targets interpersonal problems to improve both interpersonal functioning and mood (5).
- Regular exercise may help reduce depressive symptoms (4)[B].

MEDICATION

First Line

- Fluoxetine: FDA approved for depression in age >8. Starting dose 10 mg/d; may increase after 1 week. Effective dose 20–40 mg/d. The most studied SSRI and with the most favorable effectiveness and safety data (2,9)[B]
- Escitalopram: Starting dose 10 mg/d. Effective dose 10–20 mg/d. May increase after 3 weeks. FDA approved for depression age >12 (2,10)[C]
- Citalopram: Starting dose 20 mg/d. May increase up to 40 mg after 2 weeks. FDA approved for depression in age >12 (2)[C]
- Sertraline: Starting dose 25 mg/d. Effective dose 50–200 mg/d. May titrate every 1 week. FDA approved for depression in age >12 (2)[C]
- Monitor for suicidal thoughts and behavior, given the possible increased risk while taking any antidepressant. However, no evidence proving causality, and there may be a decrease in suicidal ideation; completed suicide rates are higher in areas where SSRIs are not prescribed to adolescents (2,9)[C].

Second Line

Other antidepressants (less studied, but reasonable if failed 2 SSRIs) (10):

- Venlafaxine: 37.5–225 mg/d (consider if comorbid anxiety/if failed 2 SSRIs)
- Desvenlafaxine: 50–400 mg/d
- Bupropion: 37.5–400 mg/d (consider if comorbid ADHD)
- Duloxetine: 20–60 mg/d (although no randomized controlled trials in minors)

Pediatric Considerations

- Tricyclic antidepressants (TCAs) have not been proven to be effective in adolescents and should NOT be used (2)[A].
- Mirtazapine has not been shown to be effective in adolescents (10).
- Paroxetine (SSRI): Contraindicated due to short half-life, associated withdrawal symptoms, and higher association with suicidal ideation (10).

ISSUES FOR REFERRAL

Pediatric depression is often managed by primary care providers: Refer to a child psychiatrist for severe, recurrent, or treatment-resistant depression; if the patient has comorbidities or if clinician is uncomfortable prescribing complex therapies (11).

COMPLEMENTARY AND ALTERNATIVE MEDICINE

No evidence supports the use of St. John's wort or acupuncture.

IN-PATIENT CONSIDERATIONS

Admission Criteria/Initial Stabilization

If severely depressed, psychotic, suicidal, or homicidal; 1-on-1 supervision may be needed.

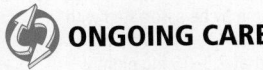 ONGOING CARE

Treatment for at least 6 months reduced the likelihood of suicide attempts, compared with treatment for <8 weeks (10)[B].

FOLLOW-UP RECOMMENDATIONS

- Systematic and regular tracking of goals and outcomes from treatment should be performed, including assessment of depressive symptoms and functioning in home, school, and peer settings (11).
- Diagnosis and initial treatment should be reassessed if no improvement is noted after 6–8 weeks of treatment (11).

Patient Monitoring

- Once started on antidepressants, patients are seen weekly for 1st month, biweekly for the 2nd month, and at least 12-week intervals thereafter. Monitor for suicidal thoughts/behavior, particularly in the first 2 months after initiation or dose increase. Monitor for signs of antidepressant-induced mania, especially between 1st and 4th weeks (10).
- Length of medication treatment:
  - 1st episode: Minimum 6–9 months followed by a slow taper over 6–8 weeks (risk of discontinuation syndrome highest with paroxetine)
  - 2nd episode: At least 1 year
  - 3rd episode: 1–3 years
  - >3 episodes: Lifelong
- Adverse effects (e.g., nausea, headaches, behavioral activation) occur in up to 93% treated with SSRIs and occur earlier than therapeutic response. Routine monitoring and discussion of possible side effects is critical for those treated with antidepressants. While it is rare, serotonin syndrome can occur with multiple medications or high doses of SSRIs (10).

PATIENT EDUCATION

Educate patients and parents about mental health and the fact that depression is a medical illness, not a character defect.

PROGNOSIS

- If left untreated, major depressive episode in adolescents typically lasts 7–9 months, with 90% resolving within 2 years.
- Recurrence is 40% by 2 years and 50–70% by 5 years.
- Persistent and severe depression in adulthood is more likely with an earlier onset of disease (5).
- Patients with family conflict, drug and alcohol use, and anxiety disorders are less likely to achieve remission (12).
- Psychological depression prevention programs were effective in preventing recurrent episodes of illness (1).

COMPLICATIONS

- Treatment-induced mania, aggression, or lack of improvement in symptoms
- School failure/refusal
- Suicide
- Low self-esteem, substance abuse (e.g., nicotine)

REFERENCES

1. American Psychiatric Association. *Diagnostic and statistical manual of mental disorders*. Fifth Ed. DSM-5. June 2013.
2. Clark MS, Jansen KL, Cloy A. Treatment of childhood and adolescent depression. *AAFP* Sept 1, 2012;86(5):442–448.
3. Merry SN, Hetrick SE, Cox GR, et al. Psychological and educational interventions for preventing depression in children and adolescents. *Cochrane Database Syst Rev*. 2011;(12):CD003380. Epub 2011 Dec 7.
4. Larun L, Nordheim LV, Ekeland E, et al. Exercise in prevention and treatment of anxiety and depression among children and young people. *Cochrane Database Syst Rev*. 2006;(3): CD004691.
5. Thapar A. Managing and preventing depression in adolescents. *BMJ*. 2010;340:c209.
6. US Preventive Services Task Force. Screening and treatment for major depressive disorder in children and adolescents: US Preventive Services Task Force Recommendation Statement. *Pediatrics*. 2009;123(4):1223–1228.
7. Richardson LP. Evaluation of the Patient Health Questionnaire-9 item for detecting major depression among adolescents. *Pediatrics*. 2010;126:1117–1123.
8. Dubicka B. Combined treatment with cognitive behavioral therapy in adolescent depression. *Br J Psychiatry*. 2010;197:433–440.
9. Hetrick SE, McKenzie JE, Cox JR, et al. Newer generation antidepressants for depressive disorders in children and adolescents. *Cochrane Database Syst Rev*. 2012;11:CD004851
10. Smiga SM, Elliott GR. Psychopharmacology of depression in children and adolescents. *Pediatr Clin N Am*. 2011;58:155–171.
11. Cheung AH, Zuckerbrot RA, Jensen PS, et al. Guidelines for Adolescent Depression in Primary Care (GLAD-PC): II. Treatment and ongoing management. *Pediatrics*. 2007;120(5): e1313–e1326.
12. Emslie GJ. Treatment of resistant depression in adolescents (TORDIA): Week 24 outcomes. *Am J Psychiatry*. 2010;167:782–791.

 CODES

ICD10

- F32.9 Major depressive disorder, single episode, unspecified
- F33.8 Other recurrent depressive disorders
- F33.9 Major depressive disorder, recurrent, unspecified

CLINICAL PEARLS

- Adolescent depression is underdiagnosed and often presents with irritability and anhedonia.
- Fluoxetine and escitalopram are the most studied FDA approved for treatment of adolescent depression.
- Citalopram and Sertraline are also FDA approved antidepressants.
- CBT combined with fluoxetine is efficacious for adolescents with major depression.
- Paroxetine, TCAs, and mirtazapine should not be used to treat adolescent depression. Referral to a child psychiatrist is appropriate for complex cases or treatment-resistant depression.
- Monitor all adolescents with depression for suicidality, especially during the 1st month of treatment with an antidepressant.

DEPRESSION, GERIATRIC
Abhijeet Patil, MD

BASICS

DESCRIPTION
- Depression is a primary mood disorder characterized by a depressed mood and/or a markedly decreased interest or pleasure in normally enjoyable activities for at least 2 weeks and causing significant distress or impairment in daily functioning.
- It is not considered a part of normal aging.

EPIDEMIOLOGY
Prevalence rates among the elderly vary, largely depending on the specific diagnostic instruments used and their current health and/or home environment:
- 1–3% of community-dwelling elderly
- 7.5% seen in primary care clinics
- 10–21% of hospitalized elderly patients
- 12–27% of nursing home residents

ETIOLOGY AND PATHOPHYSIOLOGY
- Significant gaps exist in the understanding of the underlying pathophysiology.
- Ongoing research has identified several possible mechanisms, including:
  - Monoamine transmission and associated transcriptional and translational activity
  - Epigenetic mechanisms and resilience factors
  - Neurotrophins, neurogenesis, neuroimmune systems, and neuroendocrine systems
- Depression appears to be a complex interaction between heritable and environmental factors.

RISK FACTORS
- General:
  - Chronic physical health condition(s)
  - History of mental health problems
  - Death of a loved one
  - Care giving
  - Social isolation
  - Lack/Loss of social support
  - Significant loss of independence
  - Uncontrolled pain
  - Insomnia/Sleep disturbance
- Prevalence of depression in medical illness:
  - Stroke (22–50%)
  - Cancer (18–50%)
  - Myocardial infarction (15–45%)
  - Parkinson disease (10–39%)
  - Rheumatoid arthritis (13%)
  - Diabetes mellitus (5–11%)
  - Alzheimer dementia (5–15%)
- Suicide:
  - Suicide is the 11th leading cause of death in the US for all ages.
  - Suicide rates are higher for Americans age >65 compared with the general population (~15/100,000 people).
  - Suicide rates are highest for males aged >75 (rate 38.5/100,000).

DIAGNOSIS

HISTORY
- Depressed mood most of the day, nearly every day, and/or loss of interest/pleasure in life for at least 2 weeks
- Other common symptoms include:
  - Feeling hopeless, helpless, or worthless
  - Insomnia and loss of appetite/weight (alternatively, hypersomnia with increased appetite/weight in atypical depression)
  - Fatigue and loss of energy
  - Somatic symptoms (headaches, chronic pain)
  - Neglect of personal responsibility or care
  - Psychomotor retardation or agitation
  - Diminished concentration, indecisiveness
  - Thoughts of death or suicide
- Screening with "SIGECAPS":
  - **S**leep: Changes in sleep habits from baseline, including excessive sleep, early waking, or inability to fall asleep
  - **I**nterest: Loss of interest in previously enjoyable activities
  - **G**uilt: Guilt that may or may not focus on a specific problem or circumstance
  - **E**nergy: Perceived lack of energy
  - **C**oncentration: Inability to concentrate on specific tasks
  - **A**ppetite: Increase/Decrease in appetite
  - **P**sychomotor: Restlessness and agitation, or the perception that everyday activities are too strenuous to manage
  - **S**uicidality: Desire to end life or hurt oneself, harmful thoughts directed internally or thoughts of homicidality

PHYSICAL EXAM
Mental status exam

DIFFERENTIAL DIAGNOSIS
Concurrent medical conditions, cognitive disorders, and medications may produce neurovegetative symptoms that may mimic depression:
- Medical conditions: Hypothyroidism, vitamin B_{12} deficiency, liver or renal failure, cancers, stroke
- Medication-induced: Interferon-α, β_2-blockers, isotretinoin
- Dementia and neurodegenerative disorders
- Delirium
- Psychiatric disorders: Bipolar disorder, dysthymic disorder, anxiety disorders, substance abuse-related mood disorders, psychotic disorders

DIAGNOSTIC TESTS & INTERPRETATION
Initial Tests (lab, imaging)
Initial laboratory evaluation is done primarily to rule out potential medical factors that could be causing symptoms.
- Thyroid-stimulating hormone (TSH)
- CBC with differential
- Comprehensive metabolic panel, including liver function
- Urine drug screen
- Vitamin B_{12}

Follow-Up Tests & Special Considerations
Additional testing for possible confounding medical and cognitive disorders, as warranted

Diagnostic Procedures/Other
Validated screening tools and rating scales:
- Geriatric Depression Scale: 15- or 30-point scales
- Patient Health Questionnaire (PHQ-2 or PHQ-9)
- Hamilton Depression Rating Scale
- Beck Depression Inventory
- Cornell Scale for Depression in Dementia (1)

TREATMENT

Although response alone, usually interpreted as a 50% reduction in symptoms, can be clinically meaningful, the goal is to treat patients to the point of remission (i.e., essentially the absence of depressive symptoms).

GENERAL MEASURES
Psychotherapy: Studies do show some benefit in depressed elderly patients (2)[B]:
- Cognitive-behavioral therapy
- Problem-solving therapy
- Interpersonal therapy
- Psychodynamic psychotherapy

MEDICATION
- Typically more conservative initial dosing and titration of antidepressants in the elderly, starting with 1/2 of the usual initiation dose and increasing within a couple of weeks, if tolerated
- Continue titrating dose every 2–4 weeks, as appropriate. It is important to reach an adequate treatment dose.

First Line
- SSRIs have been found to be effective in treating depression in the elderly (3)[A].
- No single SSRI clearly outperforms others in the class; choice of medication often reflects side-effect profile or practitioner familiarity:
  - Citalopram: Start at 10 mg/d. Treatment range 20–40 mg/d.
  - Sertraline: Start at 25 mg/d. Treatment range 50–200 mg/d.
  - Escitalopram: Start at 5–10 mg/d. Treatment range 10–20 mg/d.
  - Fluoxetine: Start at 10 mg/d. Treatment range 20–60 mg/d.
  - Paroxetine: Start at 10 mg/d. Treatment range 20–60 mg/d.
- SSRIs should not be used concomitantly with monoamine oxidase inhibitors (MAOIs).

Second Line
- Atypical antidepressants: More effective than placebo in treatment of depression in the elderly, although additional studies are needed to better delineate patient factors that determine response (4)[A]:
  - Bupropion (immediate, sustained/twice a day, and extended/once daily available): Start at 100 mg/d. Increase dose in 3 days. Treatment range 200–300 mg/d. Avoid in patients with elevated seizure risk.
  - Venlafaxine (immediate and sustained release available): Start at 37.5 mg and titrate weekly. Treatment range 75–300 mg/d. May be associated with elevated BP at higher doses.
  - Duloxetine: Start at 30 mg/d. Treatment range 30–60 mg/d. Also may be associated with elevated BP.
  - Mirtazapine: Start at 7.5–15 mg nightly. Treatment range 15–45 mg/d. Can produce problems with weight gain, sedation, and cognitive dysfunction.

- For patients who have not responded to initial SSRI trial:
  - Switch to a different SSRI medication, switch to an atypical antidepressant, or augment initial antidepressant with bupropion (5,6,7)[B].

ISSUES FOR REFERRAL
Depression with suicidal ideation, psychotic depression, bipolar disorder, comorbid substance-abuse issues, severe or refractory illness

ADDITIONAL THERAPIES
- Tricyclic antidepressants (TCAs) have been shown to be effective in treating depression in the elderly (3)[A]. However, they are difficult for elderly patients to tolerate due to side-effect profile and are potentially lethal in overdose, limiting their use as initial treatment agents.
- Although not FDA approved, buspirone, lithium, or triiodothyronine are sometimes used off-label to augment a primary antidepressant (5)[B].
- MAOIs also appear more effective than placebo in the treatment of depression in the elderly (3)[A]. They are not used frequently in clinical practice due to potential side effects and necessary dietary restrictions.
- Evidence for benefit of antidepressants in the treatment of depression in patients with dementia is equivocal. Consideration should be made for a limited trial with follow up for improvement and side effects or use only in patients with severe symptoms (8,9)[A].
- Electroconvulsive therapy (ECT): Has been shown to produce remission of depressive symptoms in the elderly (10)[B]. It should be considered as an initial option for patients with severe or psychotic depression.
- Exercise: May be beneficial for depression in the elderly population (11,12)[B].
- Acupuncture: Equally beneficial as counseling (13)[A]

COMPLEMENTARY AND ALTERNATIVE MEDICINE
- St. John's wort may have minimal benefit (14)[A].
- Tryptophan and hydroxytryptophan: 150–300 mg/d; possible efficacy, additional investigation required (15)[B],(16)[C].

IN-PATIENT CONSIDERATIONS
Inpatient care indicated for imminent safety risk (e.g., acutely suicidal patients) or for those patients unable to care adequately for themselves due to depression.

 ## ONGOING CARE

FOLLOW-UP RECOMMENDATIONS
Due to the delay of benefit following initiation of antidepressant therapy (2–4 weeks), it is necessary to ensure open communication with the patient to prevent premature discontinuation of therapy. An adequate explanation of potential side effects with instructions to call the office before discontinuing therapy is imperative.

Patient Monitoring
- A patient with severe depression who exhibits suicidality may require admission to an appropriate facility.
- Monitor for worsening anxiety symptoms or increase in suicidality.

DIET
No dietary restrictions are necessary, except for patients taking MAOIs, which necessitates dietary restriction of foods high in tyramine.

PATIENT EDUCATION
- Depression is a treatable illness.
- Medications may need to be taken for at least 2–4 weeks before any beneficial effect is noted.
- Depression is often a recurring illness.
- National Suicide Prevention Lifeline at 1-800-273-TALK (8255) is a free, 24-hour hotline available to anyone in suicidal crisis or emotional distress. Calls will be routed to the nearest crisis center.

PROGNOSIS
- Treatment outcomes in the elderly may be worse than in the general population, possibly mediated by physical comorbidities and other factors.
- Depending on the population studied and specific clinical measures used, estimates vary for initial clinical response and remission (between 30% and 70%).

COMPLICATIONS
- Impairment in social, occupational, or interpersonal functioning
- Difficulty performing activities of daily living and self-care
- Increase in medical services utilization and increased costs of care
- Suicide

REFERENCES
1. Alexopoulos GS, Abrams RC, Young RC, et al. Scale for depression in dementia. *Biol Psychiatry.* 1988;23:271.
2. Wilson KC, Mottram PG, Vassilas CA. Psychotherapeutic treatments for older depressed people. *Cochrane Database Syst Rev.* 2008;1: CD004853.
3. Wilson K, Mottram P, Sivanranthan A, et al. Antidepressant versus placebo for depressed elderly. *Cochrane Database Syst Rev.* 2001;2: CD000561.
4. Nelson JC, Delucchi K, Schneider LS, et al. Efficacy of second generation antidepressants in late-life depression: A meta-analysis of the evidence. *Am J Geriatr Psychiatry.* 2008;16:558–567.
5. Ruhe HG, Huyser J. Switching antidepressants after a first selective serotonin reuptake inhibitor in major depressive disorder: A systematic review. *J Clin Psychiatry* 2006;67:1836–1855.
6. Rush AJ, Trivedi MH. Bupropion-SR, sertraline, or venlafaxine-XR after failure of SSRIs for depression. *N Engl J Med.* 2006;354:1231–1242.
7. Trivedi MH, Fava M. Medication augmentation after the failure of SSRIs for depression. *N Engl J Med.* 2006;354:1243–1252.
8. Nelson JC, Devanand DP. A systematic review and meta-analysis of placebo-controlled antidepressant studies in people with depression and dementia. *J AM Geriatr Soc.* 2011;49: 577–585.
9. Banerjee S, Hellier J, Dewey M, et al. Sertraline or mirtazapine for depression in dementia (HTA-SADD): A randomised, multicentre, double-blind, placebo-controlled trial. *Lancet.* 2011;378:403–411.
10. Van der Wurff FB. Electroconvulsive therapy for the depressed elderly. *Cochrane Database Syst Rev.* 2003;2:CD003593.
11. Blake H, Mo P, Malik S, et al. How effective are physical activity interventions for alleviating depressive symptoms in older people? A systematic review. *Clin Rehabil.* 2009;23: 873–887.
12. Sjösten N, Kivelä SL. The effects of physical exercise on depressive symptoms among the aged: A systematic review. *Int J Geriatr Psychiatry.* 2006;21:410–418.
13. MacPherson H, Richmond S, Bland M, et al. Acupuncture and counselling for depression in primary care: A randomised controlled trial. *PLoS Med.* 2013;10:e1001518.
14. Linde K. St. John's wort for depression. *Cochrane Database Syst Rev.* 2005;2:CD000448.
15. Shaw K, Turner J, DelMar C. Tryptophan and 5-hydroxytryptophan for depression. *Cochrane Database Syst Rev.* 2002;1:CD003198.
16. Sarris J, Schoendorfer N, Kavanagh DJ. Major depressive disorder and nutritional medicine: A review of monotherapies and adjuvant treatments. *Nutr Rev.* 2009;67:125–131.

 ## SEE ALSO

Algorithms: Depressed Mood Resulting from Medical Illness; Depressive Episode, Major

 ## CODES

ICD10
- F03 Unspecified dementia
- F32.9 Major depressive disorder, single episode, unspecified

CLINICAL PEARLS
- Depression is not a normal part of aging.
- Depression in the elderly may be difficult to diagnose precisely due to medical and cognitive comorbidities.
- Depression may present primarily with cognitive dysfunction. Cognitive function may improve with treatment of the depression.
- A multidisciplinary approach to the treatment of depression is often most efficacious.
- SSRIs are considered first-line therapy for safety and tolerability. A full remission may take upward of 12 weeks of treatment. Long-term treatment may be needed to prevent recurrence.

D

DEPRESSION, POSTPARTUM
Isheeta Zalpuri, MD • Nancy Byatt, DO, MBA

 BASICS

DESCRIPTION
- Major depressive disorder (MDD) that recurs or has its onset in the postpartum period. May also occur in mothers adopting a baby or in fathers.
- Postpartum depression (PPD) is similar to nonpregnancy depression (sleep disorders, anhedonia, psychomotor changes, etc.); has its onset within the first 12 weeks postpartum.
- Different than postpartum "blues" (sadness and emotional lability), which is experienced by 30–70% of women and has an onset and resolution within first 10 days postpartum.

EPIDEMIOLOGY
Incidence
14.5% of women have a new episode of major or minor depression during postpartum period (1).

Prevalence
As many as 19.2% women suffer from depression in postpartum period (1).

ETIOLOGY AND PATHOPHYSIOLOGY
- May be related to sensitivity in hormonal fluctuations, including estrogen, progesterone, and other gonadal hormones, as well as neuroactive steroids; cytokines; HPA axis hormones; altered fatty acid, oxytocin, and arginine vasopressin levels; genetic and epigenetic factors.
- Multifactorial; including biologic–genetic predisposition in terms of neurobiologic deficit, destabilizing effects of hormone withdrawal at birth, inflammation, and psychosocial stressors.

RISK FACTORS
- Previous episodes of PPD
- History of MDD
- MDD during pregnancy
- Anxiety during pregnancy
- History of premenstrual dysphoria
- Family history of depression
- Unwanted pregnancy
- Socioeconomic stress
- Low self-esteem
- Young maternal age
- Alcohol abuse
- Marital conflict
- Multiple births
- African Americans and Hispanics may have higher rates of PPD.
- Preterm and low-birth-weight baby
- Postpartum pain, sleep disturbance, and fatigue
- Recent immigrant status
- Increased stressful life events
- History of childhood sexual abuse
- Decision to decrease antidepressants during pregnancy
- Intimate partner violence (2)

GENERAL PREVENTION
- Universal screening during pregnancy to allow for detection and treatment
- Screening using Edinburgh Postnatal Depression Scale during the postpartum year: http://www.testandcalc.com/etc/tests/edin.asp
- For women with depression, continuation of antidepressants during pregnancy may prevent PPD.

- Postnatal visits, psychotherapy, and/or psychoeducation for high-risk women
- Depression care manager who provides education, routine telephone contact, and follow-up to engage women in treatment

COMMONLY ASSOCIATED CONDITIONS
- Bipolar mood disorder
- Depressive disorder not otherwise specified
- Dysthymic disorder
- Cyclothymic disorder
- MDD

 DIAGNOSIS

HISTORY
- Increased/Decreased sleep
- Decreased interest in formerly compelling or pleasurable activities
- Guilt, low self-esteem
- Decreased energy
- Decreased concentration
- Increased/Decreased appetite
- Psychomotor agitation or retardation
- Suicidal ideation

DIFFERENTIAL DIAGNOSIS
- Baby blues: Not a psychiatric disorder; mood lability, resolves within days
- Postpartum psychosis: a psychiatric emergency
- Postpartum anxiety/panic disorder
- Postpartum obsessive-compulsive disorder
- Hypothyroidism
- Postpartum thyroiditis: Can occur in up to 5.7% of patients in the US (3) and can present as depression

DIAGNOSTIC TESTS & INTERPRETATION
Initial Tests (lab, imaging)
Thyroid-stimulating hormone (TSH)

Diagnostic Procedures/Other
- Edinburgh Postnatal Depression Scale is the primary screening tool.
- Beck, Hamilton, and Zung depression inventories may provide information about the severity of the depression and suicidal risks.
- Edinburgh Postnatal Depression Scale (Partner Version): To be completed by mother's partner to obtain his/her view of mother's depression

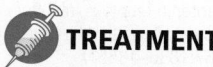 TREATMENT

GENERAL MEASURES
- Outpatient individual psychotherapy in combination with pharmacotherapy
- Support/psychotherapy groups may be helpful.
- Assess suicidal ideation.
- Assess homicidal ideation and thoughts of harming baby. Thoughts of harming baby require immediate hospitalization.
- Visiting nurse services can provide direct observations of the mother in regards to safety concerns and mother–child bonding.
- Peer support

MEDICATION
First Line
- SSRIs are generally effective and safe:
  - Fluoxetine (Prozac): 20–80 mg/d PO (most activating of all SSRIs)
  - Sertraline (Zoloft): 50–200 mg/d PO (mildly sedating)
  - Paroxetine (Paxil): 20–60 mg/d PO (sedating)
  - Citalopram (Celexa): 20–40 mg/d PO (FDA recommendation)
- Tricyclic antidepressants (TCAs) effective and less expensive; yet are lethal in overdose and have unfavorable side effects:
  - Avoid TCAs in mothers with a history of suicide attempts.
- Bupropion (Wellbutrin): 150–450 mg/d PO in patients with depression plus psychomotor retardation, hypersomnia, and with weight gain Bupropion is less likely to cause weight gain or sexual dysfunction and is highly activating.
- Mirtazapine (Remeron): 15–45 mg/d PO at bedtime; may assist with sleep restoration and weight gain; no sexual dysfunction
- Venlafaxine (Effexor XR): A dual-action antidepressant that blocks the reuptake of serotonin in doses of up to 150 mg/d and then blocks the reuptake of norepinephrine in doses of 150–450 mg/d PO.
- Bipolar disorder requires treatment with mood stabilizer.
- Among breastfeeding mothers:
  - Weigh potential efficacy of treatment with antidepressant, risks of exposure to infant, and negative effects of untreated PPD on child development.
  - All antidepressants are excreted in breast milk but are generally compatible with lactation.
  - Paroxetine and sertraline have lower translactal passage.
  - Selective serotonin reuptake inhibitors and nortriptyline have a better safety profile.
  - Translactal passage is greater with fluoxetine and citalopram (4)[B].
  - Start with low doses and increase slowly. Monitor infant for adverse side effects.
  - Continuing an efficacious medication is preferred over switching antidepressants to avoid exposing mother and infant to the risks of untreated PPD (4)[B].
  - Breastfeeding women need additional education and support regarding the risks and benefits of use of antidepressants during breastfeeding.
  - Discussions of the treatment options must be held with the patient and her partner. These include the patient's personal psychiatric history and previous response to treatment, the risks of no treatment or undertreatment, available data about the safety of medications during breastfeeding, and her individual expectations and treatment preferences (4)[B].
  - For further information: *Medications and Mother's Milk* by Thomas Hale, PhD

Second Line

Electroconvulsive therapy (ECT): This is an option for depressed postpartum women who do not respond to antidepressant medication, have severe or psychotic symptoms, cannot tolerate antidepressant medication, are actively engaged in suicidal self-destructive behaviors, or have a previous history of response to ECT (5)[B].

ISSUES FOR REFERRAL
- Obtain psychiatric consultation for patients with psychotic symptoms.
- Immediate hospitalization is mandatory if delusions or hallucinations are present.
- Hospitalization is indicated if mother's ability to care for self and/or infant is significantly compromised.

ADDITIONAL THERAPIES
- Psychoeducation, including providing reading material for the patient and family
- Psychotherapy: Interpersonal psychotherapy, cognitive-behavioral therapy, and psychodynamic psychotherapy shown to be effective (5)[B]

COMPLEMENTARY AND ALTERNATIVE MEDICINE
- Breastfeeding is effective in reducing stress and protecting maternal mood.
- Infant massage, infant sleep intervention, exercise, and bright light therapy may be beneficial (5)[B].

IN-PATIENT CONSIDERATIONS

ALERT
Obtain psychiatric consultation for patients with psychotic symptoms. If delusions or hallucinations are present, immediate hospitalization is mandatory. The psychotic mother should *not* be left alone with the baby.

Admission Criteria/Initial Stabilization
Presence of suicidal or homicidal ideation and/or psychotic symptoms and/or thoughts of harming baby and/or inability to care for self or infant, severe weight loss

Discharge Criteria
- Absence of suicidal or homicidal ideation and/or psychotic symptoms and/or thoughts of harming baby
- Mother must be able to care for self and infant.

 ONGOING CARE

FOLLOW-UP RECOMMENDATIONS
Patient Monitoring
- Collaborative care approach, including primary care visits and case manager follow-ups
- Consultation with the infant's doctor, particularly if mother is breastfeeding while taking psychotropic medications

DIET
- Good nutrition and hydration, especially when breastfeeding
- Mixed evidence to support the addition of multivitamin with minerals and omega-3 fatty acids

PATIENT EDUCATION
- *This Isn't What I Expected: Overcoming Postpartum Depression*, by Karen R. Kleinman and Valerie Davis Radkin
- *Down Came the Rain: My Journey Through Postpartum Depression*, by Brooke Shields, 2005
- *Behind the Smile: My Journey Out of Postpartum Depression*, by Marie Osmond, Marcie Wilkie, and Judith Morre, 2001
- *A Medication Guide for Breastfeeding Moms*, by Thomas Hale and Ghia Mcafee, 2008
- Web resources:
  - Postpartum support international: http://www.postpartum.net
  - http://www.4women.gov
  - La Leche League: http://www.lalecheleague.org
  - http://toxnet.nlm.nih.gov
  - www.mededppd.org
  - www.womensmentalhealth.org
  - www.motherrisk.org
  - www.step-ppd.com

PROGNOSIS
- Treatment of maternal depression to remission has been shown to have a positive impact on children's mental health.
- Some patients, particularly those with undertreated or undiagnosed depression, may develop chronic depression requiring long-term treatment.
- Untreated maternal depression is linked to impaired cognitive and language development delay (6).
- Postpartum psychosis is associated with tragic outcomes, such as maternal suicide and infanticide.

COMPLICATIONS
- Suicide
- Self-injurious behavior
- Psychosis
- Neglect of baby
- Harm to the baby

REFERENCES

1. Gavin NI, Gaynes BN, Lohr KN, et al. Perinatal depression: A systematic review of prevalence and incidence. *Obstet Gynecol.* 2005;106:1071–1083.
2. Cerulli C, Talbot NL, Tang W, et al. Co-occurring intimate partner violence and mental health diagnoses in perinatal women. *J Womens Health (Larchmt).* 2011;20:1797–1803.
3. Nicholson WK, Robinson KA, Smallridge RC, et al. Prevalence of postpartum thyroid dysfunction: A quantitative review. *Thyroid.* 2006;16:573–582.
4. Pearlstein T, Howard M, Salisbury A, et al. Postpartum depression. *Am J Obstet Gynecol.* 2009;200:357–364.
5. Fitelson E, Kim S, Baker AS, et al. Treatment of postpartum depression: Clinical, psychological and pharmacological options. *Int J Womens Health.* 2010;3:1–14.
6. Kingston D, Tough S, Whitfield H. Prenatal and postpartum maternal psychological distress and infant development: A systematic review. *Child Psychiatry Hum Dev.* 2012;43(5):683–714.

ADDITIONAL READING
- Edinburgh Postnatal depression scale: http://www.testandcalc.com/etc/tests/edin.asp
- Gjerdingen D, Katon W, Rich DE. Stepped care treatment of postpartum depression: A primary care-based management model. *Womens Health Issues.* 2008;18(1):44–52.
- Harrington AR, Greene-Harrington CC. Healthy Start screens for depression among urban pregnant, postpartum and interconceptional women. *J Natl Med Assoc.* 2007;99(3):226–231.
- Hirst KP, Moutier CY. Postpartum major depression. *Am Fam Physician.* 2010;82(8):926–933.
- Howard LM, Boath E, Henshaw C. Antidepressant prevention of postnatal depression. *PLoS Med.* 2006;3(10):e389.
- Kendall-Tackett K. A new paradigm for depression in new mothers: The central role of inflammation and how breastfeeding and anti-inflammatory treatments protect maternal mental health. *Int Breastfeed J.* 2007;2:6. Epub 2007 Mar 30.
- Musters C, McDonald E, Jones I. Management of postnatal depression. *BMJ.* 2008;337:a736. Epub 2008 Aug 8.
- Ng RC, Hirata CK, Yeung W, et al. Pharmacologic treatment for postpartum depression: A systematic review. *Pharmacotherapy.* 2010;30(9):928–941.
- Sit DK, Wisner KL. Identification of postpartum depression. *Clin Obstet Gynecol.* 2009;52(3):456–468.
- Tammentie T, Tarkka MT, Astedt-Kurki P, et al. Family dynamics and postnatal depression. *J Psychiatr Ment Health Nurs.* 2004;11(2):141–149.

 CODES

ICD10
F53 Puerperal psychosis

CLINICAL PEARLS
- PPD is a common, debilitating medical condition that impairs a mother's ability to function and interact with her infant and family.
- Universal screening for PPD is recommended during the 3rd trimester and at regular intervals during the postpartum period.
- Early diagnosis and treatment are vital, as untreated PPD can lead to developmental difficulties for the infant and prolonged disability and suffering for the mother.
- Breastfeeding is recommended for maternal and child health. Several medication options for treating depression in mothers are safe for breastfeeding infants.
- Treatment with antidepressants should be individualized for breastfeeding mothers (4)[B].

DEPRESSION, TREATMENT RESISTANT
Michelle Magid, MD • Roger Lowell McRoberts III, MD

 BASICS

DESCRIPTION
- Major depressive disorder (MDD) that has failed to respond to ≥2 adequate trials of antidepressant therapy in ≥2 different classes
- Antidepressant therapy must be given for 6 weeks at standard doses before being considered a failure.

EPIDEMIOLOGY
- Depression affects >18 million people in the US and >340 million people worldwide.
- 16% lifetime risk of MDD
- 40% of patients respond to the 1st choice of antidepressant medication.

ETIOLOGY AND PATHOPHYSIOLOGY
- Unclear. Low levels of neurotransmitters (serotonin, norepinephrine, dopamine) have been indicated.
- Serotonin has been linked to irritability, hostility, and suicidal ideation.
- Norepinephrine has been linked to low energy.
- Dopamine may play a role in low motivation and depression with psychotic features.
- Environmental stressors such as abuse and neglect may affect neurotransmission.

Genetics
Limited studies have shown that a genetic abnormality in the serotonin transporter gene (5-HTTLPR) may increase risk for treatment-resistant depression.

RISK FACTORS
- Severity of disease
- Mislabeling patients with depression who are bipolar
- Comorbid medical disease (including chronic pain)
- Comorbid personality disorder
- Comorbid anxiety disorder
- Comorbid substance abuse
- Familial predisposition to poor response to antidepressants

GENERAL PREVENTION
- Medication adherence in combination with psychotherapy
- Maintenance electroconvulsive therapy (ECT) may prevent relapse.

COMMONLY ASSOCIATED CONDITIONS
- Suicide
- Bipolar disorder
- Substance abuse
- Anxiety disorders
- Dysthymia
- Eating disorders
- Somatization disorders

DIAGNOSIS

HISTORY
- Symptoms are the same as in MDD. However, patients do not respond to standard form of treatment. Severity and duration are extreme.
- Especially important to screen for suicidality in treatment-resistant depression
- Screening with SIGECAPS:
  - Sleep: Too much or too little
  - Interest: Failure to enjoy activities
  - Guilt: Excessive and uncontrollable
  - Energy: Poor energy
  - Concentration: Inability to focus on tasks
  - Appetite: Too much or too little
  - Psychomotor changes: Restlessness/Agitation or slowing/lethargy
  - Suicidality: Desire to end life

PHYSICAL EXAM
Mental status exam may reveal poor hygiene, poor eye contact, blunted affect, tearfulness, weight loss or gain, psychomotor retardation, or agitation.

DIFFERENTIAL DIAGNOSIS
- Bipolar disorder
- Dysthymia
- Dementia
- Early-stage Parkinson disease
- Personality disorder
- Medical illness, such as malignancy, thyroid disease, HIV
- Substance abuse

DIAGNOSTIC TESTS & INTERPRETATION
Initial Tests (lab, imaging)
- Used to rule out medical factors that could be causing/contributing to treatment resistance:
  - CBC
  - Complete metabolic profile, including liver tests, calcium, and glucose
  - Urine drug screen
  - Thyroid-stimulating Hormone (TSH)
  - Vitamin D level (25 OH Vit D)
  - Testosterone
- CT or MRI of the brain if neurologic disease, tumor, or dementia is suspected.

Follow-Up Tests & Special Considerations
Delirium and dementia may often look like depression.

Diagnostic Procedures/Other
- Depression is a clinical diagnosis.
- Validated depression rating scales to assist:
  - Beck Depression Inventory
  - Hamilton Rating Scale for Depression
  - Patient Health Questionnaire 9 (PHQ-9)

 TREATMENT

MEDICATION
First Line
- Please see "Depression" topic. When those fail, augmentation and combination strategies are as follows:
  - Antidepressants in combination:
    - Citalopram (start 20 mg/d. Max dose 40 mg/d) + bupropion (start 100 mg b.i.d.; max dose 450 mg total) (1,2)[B]
    - TCAs and SSRIs may be used in combination. Proceed with caution, due to risk of serotonin syndrome. Citalopram (start 20 mg/d; max dose 40 mg/d) + nortriptyline (start 50 mg at bedtime; max dose 200 mg at bedtime)
  - Antidepressants + antipsychotics:
    - Citalopram (start 20 mg/d; max dose 40 mg/d) + aripiprazole (start 2–5 mg, titrate to 15–20 mg/d) OR + olanzapine (start 2.5 mg at bedtime; max dose 20 mg at bedtime) OR + quetiapine (start 25 mg at bedtime; titrate to 100–300 mg at bedtime. Maximum dose 600 mg at bedtime) (3,4)[B].
  - Antidepressant + lithium:
    - Tricyclic antidepressant (TCA): Nortriptyline (start 50 mg at bedtime; max dose 200 mg at bedtime) + lithium (start 300 mg at bedtime; max dose 900 mg b.i.d.) (3,5,6)[B]
    - SSRI: Citalopram (start 20 mg/d; max dose 40 mg q.d.) + lithium (start 300 mg at bedtime; max dose 900 mg b.i.d.) (1,3,5)[B]
  - Antidepressant + thyroid supplementation:
    - Citalopram (start 20 mg/d; max dose 40 mg/d) + triiodothyronine (T3) (12.5–50 μg/d) (1,3,7)[B]
- In above combinations, citalopram (Celexa) can be replaced with other SSRIs, such as fluoxetine (Prozac) 20–80 mg/d, sertraline (Zoloft) 50–200 mg/d, and escitalopram (Lexapro) 10–20 mg/d or with serotonin-norepinephrine reuptake inhibitor (SNRI) duloxetine (Cymbalta) 30–120 mg/d
- Maximum doses for medication in treatment-resistant cases are higher than in treatment-responsive cases.

Second Line
Monamine oxidase inhibitor (MAOI):
- Tranylcypromine (Parnate): Start 10 mg b.i.d. Increase 10 mg/d every 1–3 weeks; max dose 60 mg/d
- Selegiline transdermal (Emsam patch): Apply 6-mg patch daily, increase 3 mg/d; max dose 12 mg/d
- Side-effect profile (e.g., hypertensive crisis), drug–drug interactions, and dietary restrictions make MAOIs less appealing. Patch version does not require dietary restrictions at lower doses.
- High risk of serotonin syndrome, if combined with another antidepressant; 2-week washout period is advised.

ISSUES FOR REFERRAL
Treatment-resistant depression should be managed in consultation with a psychiatrist.

ADDITIONAL THERAPIES
- First line:
  - ECT: Safe and effective treatment for treatment-resistant and life-threatening depression, with a 50–80% success rate (8,9)[A]:
    - Known to rapidly relieve suicidality, psychotic depression, and catatonia
    - Controversy due to cognitive side effects during the treatment
    - 3 types of lead placements:
      - Bitemporal: Most effective, most cognitive side effects. Usually need 6–10 treatments at 1.5× seizure threshold
      - Right unilateral: May be slightly less effective, but fewer cognitive side effects. Usually need 8–12 treatments at 4–6× seizure threshold
      - Bifrontal lead placement is a newer technique that may offer similar efficacy to bilateral ECT with less cognitive side effects.
- Second line:
  - Deep brain stimulation (DBS): Surgical implantation of intracranial electrodes, connected to an impulse generator implanted in the chest wall (10,11)[C]:
    - Reserved for those who have failed medications, psychotherapy, and ECT
    - Preliminary data are promising, showing 53% response rate and 35% remission rate, but further trials are warranted.
  - Transmagnetic stimulation (TMS): Noninvasive brain stimulation technique that is generally safe. A few case reports on efficacy in treatment-resistant depression, but thus far is only FDA approved for less severe forms of the illness (11)[C].
  - Vagus nerve stimulation (VNS): Surgical implantation of electrodes onto left vagus nerve. Its use in treatment-resistant depression has become limited in recent years (11)[C].

IN-PATIENT CONSIDERATIONS
Admission Criteria/Initial Stabilization
Inpatient care is indicated for severely depressed, psychotic, catatonic, or suicidal patients.

Discharge Criteria
Symptoms improving, no longer suicidal, psychosocial stressors addressed

 ONGOING CARE

FOLLOW-UP RECOMMENDATIONS
- Frequent visits (i.e., every month)
- During follow-up, evaluate side effects, dosage, and effectiveness of medication, as well as need for referral to ECT.
- Patients who have responded to ECT may need maintenance treatments (q3–12wk) to prevent relapse.
- Combination of lithium/nortriptyline after ECT appears to be as effective as maintenance ECT in reducing relapse.

DIET
Patients on MAOIs need dietary restriction.

PATIENT EDUCATION
- Educate patients that depression is a medical illness, not a character defect.
- Review signs and symptoms of worsening depression and when patient needs to come in for further evaluation.
- Discuss safety plan to address suicidal thoughts.

PROGNOSIS
With medication adherence, close follow-up, improved social support, and psychotherapy, prognosis improves.

COMPLICATIONS
- Suicide
- Disability
- Poor quality of life

REFERENCES
1. Rush AJ. Acute and longer term outcomes in depressed patients who require one or several treatment steps: A STAR*D report. Am J Psych. 2006;163:1905–1917.
2. Zarrouf FA, Artz S, Griffith J, Sirbu C, Kommor MJ. Testosterone and depression: Systematic review and meta-analysis. J Psychiatr Pract. 2009;15(4):289–305.
3. Hicks P. How to best manage treatment-resistant depression? J Fam Pract. 2010;59:490–497.
4. Trivedi MH. Medication augmentation after the failure of SSRIs for depression. N Engl J Med. 2006;354:1243–1252.
5. Keller MB. Issues in treatment-resistant depression. J Clin Psychiatry. 2005;66(suppl 8):5–12.
6. Kellner CH. Continuation electroconvulsive therapy vs pharmacotherapy for relapse prevention in major depression: A multisite study from the Consortium for Research in Electroconvulsive Therapy (CORE). Arch Gen Psychiatry. 2006;63:1337–1344.
7. Nierenberg AA. A comparison of lithium and T3 augmentation following two failed medication treatments for depression: A STAR*D report. Am J Psych. 2006;163:1519–1530.
8. Chen J. Second-generation antipsychotics in major depressive disorder: Update and clinical perspective. Curr Opin in Psych. 2011;24:10–17.
9. Lisanby S. Electroconvulsive therapy for depression. N Engl J Med. 2007;357:1939–1945.
10. Fink M, Taylor MA. Electroconvulsive therapy evidences and challenges. JAMA. 2007;298:330–332.
11. Malone DA. Use of deep brain stimulation in treatment-resistant depression. Cleveland Clinic J Med. 2010;77(suppl 3):S77–S80.

ADDITIONAL READING
- American Psychiatric Association. Practice guideline for the treatment of patients with major depressive disorder, third edition. Am J Psychiatry. 2010;167(10):1–118.
- Holtzheimer PE, Mayberg HS. Deep brain stimulation for treatment-resistant depression. Am J Psychiatry. 2010;167:14377–14444.

CODES

ICD10
- F32.9 Major depressive disorder, single episode, unspecified
- F33.9 Major depressive disorder, recurrent, unspecified

CLINICAL PEARLS
- Treatment-resistant depression is common, affecting 1/3 of those with MDD.
- Combination and augmentation strategies with antidepressants, antipsychotics, and mood stabilizers can be helpful.
- ECT should be considered in severe and life-threatening cases.

DERMATITIS, ATOPIC
Dennis E. Hughes, DO, FAAFP, FACEP

 BASICS

DESCRIPTION
- A chronic, relapsing, pruritic eczematous condition affecting characteristic sites
- Although called atopic, most children with the typical clinical presentation will not have a measurable IgE-mediated sensitivity to allergens.
- System(s) affected: Skin/Exocrine

EPIDEMIOLOGY
Environmentally triggered in susceptible individuals

Incidence
- 45% of all cases begin in the first 6 months of life.
- 70% of affected children will have a spontaneous remission before adolescence.
- Incidence on the rise for the past 3 decades; overall, affects ~15% of children at some time (US).

Prevalence
- Also may have late-onset dermatitis in adults
- Asians and blacks affected more often than whites
- 60% if 1 parent affected; rises to 80% if both parents affected

ETIOLOGY AND PATHOPHYSIOLOGY
- Alteration in stratum corneum results in transepidermal water loss and defect in barrier function.
- Epidermal adhesion is reduced either as a result of: (a) Genetic mutation resulting in altered epidermal proteins or (b) defect in immune regulation causing an altered inflammatory response.
- Interleukin-31 (IL-31) upregulation is thought to be a major factor in pruritus mediated by cytokines and neuropeptides rather than histamine excess (1).

Genetics
- Arises from gene–gene and gene–environment interactions
- Both epidermal and immune coding likely involved

RISK FACTORS
- "Itch-scratch cycle" (stimulates histamine release)
- Skin infections
- Emotional stress
- Irritating clothes and chemicals
- Excessively hot or cold climate
- Food allergy in children (in some cases)
- Exposure to tobacco smoke
- Family history of atopy:
  – Asthma
  – Allergic rhinitis

COMMONLY ASSOCIATED CONDITIONS
- Food sensitivity/allergy in many cases
- Asthma
- Allergic rhinitis
- Hyper-IgE syndrome (Job syndrome):
  – Atopic dermatitis
  – Elevated IgE
  – Recurrent pyodermas
  – Decreased chemotaxis of mononuclear cells

 DIAGNOSIS

HISTORY
Presence of major symptoms, including relapsing of condition, family history, typical distribution, and morphology necessary to make diagnosis of AD.

PHYSICAL EXAM
- Distribution of lesions:
  – Infants: Trunk, face, and flexural surfaces; diaper-sparing
  – Children: Antecubital and popliteal fossae
  – Adults: Hands, feet, face, neck, upper chest, and genital areas
- Morphology of lesions:
  – Infants: Erythema and papules; may develop oozing, crusting vesicles
  – Children and adults: Lichenification and scaling are typical with chronic eczema as a result of persistent scratching and rubbing (lichenification rare in infants).
- Associated signs:
  – Facial erythema, mild to moderate
  – Perioral pallor
  – Infraorbital fold (Dennie sign/Morgan line)
  – Dry skin
  – Increased palmar linear markings
  – Pitiriasis alba (hypopigmented asymptomatic areas on face and shoulders)
  – Keratosis pilaris

DIFFERENTIAL DIAGNOSIS
- Photosensitivity rashes
- Contact dermatitis (especially if only the face is involved)
- Scabies
- Seborrheic dermatitis (especially in infants)
- Psoriasis or lichen simplex chronicus if only localized disease is present in adults
- Rare conditions of infancy:
  – Histiocytosis X
  – Wiskott-Aldrich syndrome
  – Ataxia-telangiectasia syndrome
- Ichthyosis vulgaris

DIAGNOSTIC TESTS & INTERPRETATION
Initial Tests (lab, imaging)
- No test is diagnostic.
- Serum IgE levels are elevated in as many as 80% of affected individuals, but test is not routinely ordered.
- Eosinophilia tends to correlate with disease severity.

Test Interpretation
- Epidermis thickened and hyperkeratotic
- Perivascular inflammation of dermis

TREATMENT

GENERAL MEASURES
- Decrease stress if possible.
- Avoid agents that may cause irritation (e.g., wool, perfumes).
- Minimize sweating.
- Lukewarm (not hot) baths
- Minimize use of soap (superfatted soaps best).
- Frequent systemic lubrication with thick emollient creams (e.g., Eucerin) over moist skin
- Sun exposure may be helpful.
- Humidify the house.
- Avoid excessive contact with water.
- Avoid lotions that contain alcohol.
- If very resistant to treatment, search for a coexisting contact dermatitis.

Pediatric Considerations
Chronic potent fluorinated corticosteroid use may cause striae, hypopigmentation, or atrophy, especially in children.

MEDICATION
First Line
- Frequent systemic lubrication with thick emollient creams (e.g., Eucerin, Vaseline) over moist skin is the mainstay of treatment before any other intervention is considered.
- Infants and children: 0.5–1% topical hydrocortisone creams or ointments (2)[C]
- Adults: Higher-potency topical corticosteroids in areas other than face and skin folds
- Short-course, higher-potency corticosteroids for flares; then return to the lowest potency (creams preferred) that will control dermatitis. Hypopigmentation can occur even with short-term use.
- Antihistamines for pruritus (e.g., hydroxyzine 10–25 mg at bedtime and as needed)

Second Line
- Topical immunomodulators (tacrolimus or pimecrolimus) for episodic use for children >2. There is a black box warning from the FDA regarding potential cancer risk (3).
- Plastic occlusion in combination with topical medication to promote absorption
- For severe atopic dermatitis, consider systemic steroids × 1–2 weeks (e.g., prednisone 2 mg/kg/d PO [maximum 80 mg/d] initially, tapered over 7–14 days).
- Topical tricyclic doxepin as a 5% cream may decrease pruritus.
- Modified Goeckerman regimen (tar and ultraviolet light)
- Immune modifiers (methotrexate, azathioprine, cyclosporine)

ISSUES FOR REFERRAL

- Ophthalmology evaluation for persistent vernal conjunctivitis
- If using topical steroids around eyes for extended periods, ophthalmology follow-up for cataract evaluation

ADDITIONAL THERAPIES

- Methods to reduce house mite allergens (micropore filters on heating, ventilation, and air-conditioning systems; impermeable mattress covers) (4)[C]
- Behavioral relaxation therapy to reduce scratching (4)[B]

COMPLEMENTARY AND ALTERNATIVE MEDICINE

- Evening primrose oil (includes high content of fatty acids):
  – May decrease prostaglandin synthesis
  – May promote conversion of linoleic acid to omega-6 fatty acid
- Probiotics may reduce the severity of the condition, thus reducing medication use (4)[C].

 ONGOING CARE

FOLLOW-UP RECOMMENDATIONS

Patient Monitoring

Evaluate to ensure that secondary bacterial or fungal infection does not develop as a result of disruption of the skin barrier. Most patients with atopic dermatitis are colonized by *Staphylococcus*. There is little evidence for the routine use of antimicrobial interventions to reduce skin bacteria, but treatment of clinical infection with coverage for Staphylococcus is recommended.

DIET

- Trials of elimination may find certain "triggers" in some patients.
- Breastfeeding in conjunction with maternal hypoallergenic diets may decrease the severity in some infants.

PATIENT EDUCATION

- http://www.aad.org/skin-conditions/dermatology-a-to-z/atopic-dermatitis
- National Eczema Association: www.nationaleczema.org

PROGNOSIS

- Chronic disease
- Declines with increasing age
- 90% of patients have spontaneous resolution by puberty.
- Localized eczema (e.g., chronic hand or foot dermatitis, eyelid dermatitis, or lichen simplex chronicus) may continue in some adults.

COMPLICATIONS

- Cataracts are more common in patients with atopic dermatitis.
- Skin infections (usually *Staphylococcus aureus*); sometimes subclinical
- Eczema herpeticum:
  – Generalized vesiculopustular eruption caused by infection with herpes simplex or vaccinia virus
  – Causes acute illness requiring hospitalization
- Atrophy and/or striae if fluorinated corticosteroids are used on face or skin folds
- Systemic absorption may occur if large areas of skin are treated, particularly if high-potency medications and occlusion are combined.

REFERENCES

1. Boguniewicz M, Leung D. Recent insights into atopic dermatitis and implications for management of infectious complications. *J Allergy Clin Immunol*. 2010;125(1):1–17.
2. Bieber T. Atopic dermatitis. *N Engl J Med*. 2008; 358:1483–1494.
3. Trammell S, Shakil A, Wilder L, et al. Clinical inquiries. What is the role of tacrolimus and pimecrolimus in atopic dermatitis? *J Fam Pract*. 2005;54:714–716.
4. Weston S. Effects of probiotics on atopic dermatitis: A randomized controlled trial. *Arch Disease Child*. 2005;90:892–897.

ADDITIONAL READING

Correa MCM, Nebus J, Management of patients with atopic dermatitis: The role of emollient therapy. *Dermatology Research and Practice*. 2012;2012:15pp.

 SEE ALSO

Algorithm: Rash, Focal

 CODES

ICD10

- L20.9 Atopic dermatitis, unspecified
- L20.89 Other atopic dermatitis

CLINICAL PEARLS

- Institute early and proactive treatment to reduce inflammation.
- Monitor for secondary bacterial infection.
- Frequent systemic lubrication with thick emollient creams (e.g., Eucerin, Vaseline) over moist skin is the mainstay of treatment before any other intervention is considered.
- Use the lowest-potency topical steroid that controls symptoms.

DERMATITIS, CONTACT
Aamir Siddiqi, MD

BASICS

DESCRIPTION
- A cutaneous reaction to an external substance
- Primary irritant dermatitis is due to direct injury of the skin. It affects individuals exposed to specific irritants and generally produces discomfort immediately after exposure (1).
- Allergic contact dermatitis (ACD) affects only individuals previously sensitized to a substance. It represents a delayed hypersensitivity reaction, requiring several hours for the cascade of cellular immunity to be completed to manifest itself.
- System(s) affected: Skin/Exocrine
- Synonym(s): Dermatitis venenata

EPIDEMIOLOGY
Common

Incidence
Occupational contact dermatitis: 20.5/100,000 workers/year in one Australian study

Prevalence
- Contact dermatitis represents >90% of all occupational skin disorders.
- Predominant sex: Male = Female:
  - Variations due to differences in exposure to offending agents, as well as normal cutaneous variations between males and females (eccrine and sebaceous gland function and hair distribution)

Geriatric Considerations
Increased incidence of irritant dermatitis secondary to skin dryness

Pediatric Considerations
Increased incidence of positive patch testing due to better delayed hypersensitivity reactions

ETIOLOGY AND PATHOPHYSIOLOGY
Hypersensitivity reaction to a substance generating cellular immunity response (2)
- Plants:
  - Urushiol (allergen): Poison ivy, poison oak, poison sumac
  - Primary contact: Plant (roots/stems/leaves)
  - Secondary contact: Clothes/fingernails (not blister fluid)
- Chemicals:
  - Nickel: Jewelry, zippers, hooks, and watches
  - Potassium dichromate: Tanning agent in leather
  - Paraphenylenediamine: Hair dyes, fur dyes, and industrial chemicals (3)
  - Turpentine: Cleaning agents, polishes, and waxes
  - Soaps and detergents
- Topical medicines:
  - Neomycin: Topical antibiotics
  - Thimerosal (Merthiolate): Preservative in topical medications
  - Anesthetics: Benzocaine
  - Parabens: Preservative in topical medications
  - Formalin: Cosmetics, shampoos, and nail enamel

Genetics
Increased frequency of ACD in families with allergies

RISK FACTORS
- Occupation
- Hobbies
- Travel
- Cosmetics
- Jewelry

GENERAL PREVENTION
- Avoid causative agents.
- Use of protective gloves (with cotton lining) may be helpful.

DIAGNOSIS

HISTORY
- Itchy rash
- Assess for prior exposure to irritating substance.

PHYSICAL EXAM
- Acute:
  - Papules, vesicles, bullae with surrounding erythema
  - Crusting and oozing
  - Pruritus
- Chronic:
  - Erythematous base
  - Thickening with lichenification
  - Scaling
  - Fissuring
- Distribution:
  - Where epidermis is thinner (eyelids, genitalia)
  - Areas of contact with offending agent (e.g., nail polish)
  - Palms and soles relatively more resistant, although hand dermatitis is common.
  - Deeper skin folds spared
  - Linear arrays of lesions
  - Lesions with sharp borders and sharp angles are pathognomonic.
- Well-demarcated area with a papulovesicular rash

DIFFERENTIAL DIAGNOSIS
- Based on clinical impression:
  - Appearance, periodicity, and localization
- Groups of vesicles:
  - Herpes simplex
- Diffuse bullous or vesicular lesions:
  - Bullous pemphigoid
- Photodistribution:
  - Phototoxic/allergic reaction to systemic allergen
- Eyelids:
  - Seborrheic dermatitis
- Scaly eczematous lesions:
  - Atopic dermatitis
  - Nummular eczema
  - Lichen simplex chronicus
  - Stasis dermatitis
  - Xerosis

DIAGNOSTIC TESTS & INTERPRETATION
Diagnostic Procedures/Other
Consider patch tests for suspected allergic trigger (systemic corticosteroids or recent, aggressive use of topical steroids may alter results).

Test Interpretation
- Intercellular edema
- Bullae

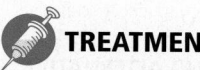

TREATMENT

GENERAL MEASURES
- Remove offending agent:
  - Avoidance
  - Work modification
  - Protective clothing
  - Barrier creams, especially high-lipid content moisturizing creams (e.g., Keri lotion, petrolatum, coconut oil)
- Topical soaks with cool tap water, Burow solution (1:40 dilution), saline (1 tsp/pint water), or silver nitrate solution (25.5%)
- Lukewarm water baths
- Aveeno oatmeal baths
- Emollients (white petrolatum, Eucerin)

MEDICATION
First Line
- Topical medications (4,5):
  - Lotion of zinc oxide, talc, menthol 0.25%, phenol 0.5% (Gold Bond, others)
  - Corticosteroids for allergic contact dermatitis as well as irritant dermatitis:
    ○ High-potency steroids: Fluocinonide (Lidex) 0.05% gel, cream, or ointment t.i.d.–q.i.d.
    ○ Use high-potency steroids only for a short time, then switch to low- or medium-potency steroid cream or ointment.
    ○ Caution regarding face/skin folds: Use lower-potency steroids and avoid prolonged usage. Switch to lower-potency topical steroid once the acute phase is resolved.
- Calamine lotion for symptomatic relief
- Topical antibiotics for secondary infection (bacitracin, erythromycin)
- Systemic:
  - Antihistamine:
    ○ Hydroxyzine: 25–50 mg PO q.i.d., especially useful for itching
    ○ Diphenhydramine: 25–50 mg PO q.i.d.
  - Corticosteroids:
    ○ Prednisone: Taper starting at 60–80 mg/d PO, over 10–14 days
    ○ Used for moderate-to-severe cases
    ○ May use burst dose of steroids for up to 5 days
  - Antibiotics for secondary skin infections:
    ○ Dicloxacillin: 250 mg PO q.i.d. for 7–10 days
    ○ Amoxicillin-clavulanate (Augmentin): 500 mg PO b.i.d. for 7–10 days
    ○ Erythromycin: 250 mg PO q.i.d. in penicillin-allergic patients
    ○ Trimethprim-Sulfamethoxazole (Bactrim DS) 160 mg (one tab) PO b.i.d. for 7–10 days (suspected resistant *Staphylococcus aureus*)

- Precautions:
  - Antihistamines may cause drowsiness.
  - Prolonged use of potent topical steroids may cause local skin effects (atrophy, stria, telangiectasia).
  - Use tapering dose of oral steroids if using >5 days.

Second Line
Other topical or systemic antibiotics, depending on organisms and sensitivity

Pregnancy Considerations
Usual caution with medications

ISSUES FOR REFERRAL
May need referral to a dermatologist or allergist if refractory to conventional treatment

COMPLEMENTARY AND ALTERNATIVE MEDICINE
The use of complementary and alternative treatment is a supplement and not an alternative to conventional treatment.

Admission Criteria/Initial Stabilization
Rarely needs hospital admission

 ## ONGOING CARE

FOLLOW-UP RECOMMENDATIONS
Stay active, but avoid overheating.

Patient Monitoring
- As necessary for recurrence
- Patch testing for etiology after resolved

DIET
No special diet

PATIENT EDUCATION
- Avoidance of irritating substance
- Cleaning of secondary sources (nails, clothes)
- Fallacy of blister fluid spreading disease

PROGNOSIS
- Self-limited
- Benign

COMPLICATIONS
- Generalized eruption secondary to autosensitization
- Secondary bacterial infection

REFERENCES

1. Ale IS, Maibacht HA. Diagnostic approach in allergic and irritant contact dermatitis. *Expert Rev Clin Immunol.* 2010;6:291–310.
2. Martin SF. Contact dermatitis: From pathomechanisms to immunotoxicology. *Exp Dermatol.* 2012;21:382–389.
3. Yazar K, Boman A, Lidén C, et al. p-Phenylenediamine and other hair dye sensitizers in Spain. *Contact Derm.* 2012;66:27–32.
4. Usatine RP, Riojas M. Diagnosis and management of contact dermatitis. *Am Fam Physician.* 2010;82:249–255.
5. Paller AS. Latest approaches to treating atopic dermatitis. *Chem Immunol Allergy.* 2012;96:132–140.

 ## SEE ALSO

Algorithm: Rash, Focal

 ## CODES

ICD10
- L23.9 Allergic contact dermatitis, unspecified cause
- L25.5 Unspecified contact dermatitis due to plants, except food
- L25.9 Unspecified contact dermatitis, unspecified cause

CLINICAL PEARLS

- Anyone exposed to irritants or allergic substances is predisposed to contact dermatitis, especially in occupations that have high exposure to chemicals.
- The most common allergens causing contact dermatitis are plants of the *Toxicodendron* genus (poison ivy, poison oak, poison sumac).
- The usual treatment for contact dermatitis is avoidance of the allergen or irritating substance and temporary use of topical steroids.
- A contact dermatitis eruption presents in a nondermatomal geographic fashion, due to the skin being in contact with an external source.

DERMATITIS, DIAPER
Dennis E. Hughes, DO, FAAFP, FACEP

 BASICS

DESCRIPTION
- Diaper dermatitis is a rash occurring under the covered area of a diaper. The rash may be a direct result of wearing the diaper, aggravated by the diaper, or coincidental with a rash that appears elsewhere on the body.
- System(s) affected: Skin/Exocrine
- Synonym(s): Diaper rash; Nappy rash, Napkin dermatitis.

Geriatric Considerations
Incontinence is a significant cofactor.

EPIDEMIOLOGY
Incidence
- The most common dermatitis found in infancy
- Peak incidence: 7–12 months of age, then decreases

Prevalence
Prevalence has been variably reported from 4–35% in the first 2 years of life.

ETIOLOGY AND PATHOPHYSIOLOGY
- Fecal proteases and lipases are irritants.
- Superhydrase urease enzyme found in the stratum corneum liberates ammonia from cutaneous bacteria.
- Fecal lipase and protease activity is increased by acceleration of GI transit; thus, a higher incidence of irritant diaper dermatitis is observed in babies who have had diarrhea in the previous 48 hours.
- Once the skin is compromised, secondary infection by *Candida albicans* is common. 40–75% of diaper rashes that last >3 days are colonized with *C. albicans*.
- Bacteria may play a role in diaper dermatitis through reduction of fecal pH and resulting activation of enzymes.
- Allergy is exceedingly rare as a cause in infants.
- Wet skin from prolonged contact with urine or feces resulting in susceptibility to chemical, enzymatic, and physical injury; wet skin is also penetrated more easily.
- Some have raised the possibility of contact allergy from the dye in disposable diapers.

RISK FACTORS
- Infrequent diaper changes
- Waterproof diapers
- Improper laundering (cloth diapers)
- Family history of dermatitis
- Hot, humid weather
- Recent treatment with oral antibiotics
- Diarrhea (>3 stools per day increases risk)
- Dye allergy
- Eczema may increase risk.

GENERAL PREVENTION
Attention to hygiene during bouts of diarrhea

COMMONLY ASSOCIATED CONDITIONS
- Contact (allergic or irritant) dermatitis
- Seborrheic dermatitis
- Psoriasis
- Candidiasis
- Atopic dermatitis

 DIAGNOSIS

HISTORY
- Onset, duration, and change in the nature of the rash
- Presence of rashes outside the diaper area
- Associated scratching or crying
- Contact with infants with a similar rash
- Recent illness, diarrhea, or antibiotic use
- Fever
- Pustular drainage
- Lymphangitis

PHYSICAL EXAM
- Mild forms consist of shiny erythema ± scale.
- Margins are not always evident.
- Moderate cases have areas of papules, vesicles, and small superficial erosions.
- It can progress to well-demarcated ulcerated nodules that measure ≥1 cm in diameter.
- It is found on the prominent parts of the buttocks, medial thighs, mons pubis, and scrotum.
- Skin folds are spared or involved last.
- *Tidemark dermatitis* refers to the bandlike form of erythema of irritated diaper margins.
- Diaper dermatitis can cause an id (autoeczematous) reaction outside the diaper area.

DIFFERENTIAL DIAGNOSIS
- Contact dermatitis
- Seborrheic dermatitis
- Candidiasis
- Atopic dermatitis
- Scabies
- Acrodermatitis enteropathica
- Letterer-Siwe disease
- Congenital syphilis
- Child abuse
- Streptococcal infection
- Kawasaki disease
- Biotin deficiency
- Psoriasis
- HIV infection

DIAGNOSTIC TESTS & INTERPRETATION
Initial Tests (lab, imaging)
Rarely needed

Follow-Up Tests & Special Considerations
- Consider a culture of lesions or a potassium hydroxide (KOH) preparation.
- The finding of anemia in association with hepatosplenomegaly and the appropriate rash may suggest a diagnosis of Langerhans cell histiocytosis or congenital syphilis.
- Finding mites, ova, or feces on a mineral oil preparation of a burrow scraping can confirm the diagnosis of scabies.

Test Interpretation
- Biopsy is rare.
- Histology may reveal acute, subacute, or chronic spongiotic dermatitis.

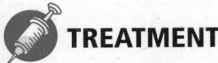

TREATMENT

See "General Measures" for first-line approach.

GENERAL MEASURES

- Expose the buttocks to air as much as possible (1)[B].
- Avoid waterproof pants during treatment (day or night); they keep the skin wet and subject to rash or infection.
- Change diapers frequently, even at night, if the rash is extensive. If using cloth diapers, change every q2hr regardless (2)[B].
- Superabsorbable diapers are beneficial (1,2)[B].
- Discontinue using baby lotion, powder, ointment, or baby oil (except zinc oxide).
- Disposable baby wipes may contain substances that induce or worsen contact or irritant dermatitis, such as fragrance, benzalkonium chloride, and isothiazolinone or alcohol.
- Apply zinc oxide ointment or other barrier cream to the rash at the earliest sign and b.i.d. or t.i.d. (e.g., Desitin or Balmex). Thereafter, apply to clean, thoroughly dry skin (1)[B].
- Use mild soap, and pat dry.
- Cornstarch can reduce friction. Talc powders that do not enhance the growth of yeast can provide protection against frictional injury in diaper dermatitis, but do not form a continuous lipid barrier layer over the skin and obstruct the skin pores. These treatments are not recommended.

MEDICATION
First Line

- For a pure contact dermatitis, a low-potency topical steroid (hydrocortisone 0.5–1% t.i.d.) and removal of the offending agent should suffice.
- If candidiasis is suspected or diaper rash persists, use an antifungal such as miconazole nitrate 2% cream, miconazole powder, econazole (Spectazole), clotrimazole (Lotrimin), or ketoconazole (Nizoral) cream at each diaper change (1)[B].
- If inflammation is prominent, consider a very low-potency steroid cream such as hydrocortisone 0.5–1% t.i.d. along with an antifungal cream ± a combination product such as clioquinol–hydrocortisone (Vioform–hydrocortisone) cream (1)[B].
- If a secondary bacterial infection is suspected, use an antistaphylococcal oral antibiotic or mupirocin (Bactroban) ointment topically.
- Precautions: Avoid high- or moderate-potency steroids often found in combination steroid antifungal mixtures (1)[B].

Second Line
Sucralfate paste for resistant cases

ISSUES FOR REFERRAL
Consider if a systemic disease such as Langerhans cell histiocytosis, acrodermatitis enteropathica, or HIV infection is suspected

IN-PATIENT CONSIDERATIONS
Admission Criteria/Initial Stabilization
- Febrile neonates
- Recalcitrant rash suggestive of immunodeficiency
- Toxic-appearing infants

Nursing
Assist 1st-time parents with hygiene education.

ONGOING CARE

FOLLOW-UP RECOMMENDATIONS
Patient Monitoring
Recheck weekly until clear; then at times of recurrence.

PATIENT EDUCATION
Patient education is vital to the treatment and prevention of recurrent cases.

PROGNOSIS
- Quick, complete clearing with appropriate treatment
- Secondary candidal infections may last a few weeks after treatment is begun.

COMPLICATIONS
- Secondary bacterial infection (consider community-acquired methicillin-resistant *Staphylococcus aureus* [MRSA] in pustular dermatitis that does not respond to normal therapy)
- Rare complication is inoculation with group A β-hemolytic *Streptococcus* resulting in necrotizing fasciitis.
- Secondary yeast infection

REFERENCES

1. Scheinfeld N. Diaper dermatitis: A review and brief survey of eruptions of the diaper area. *Am J Clin Derm*. 2005;6:273–281.
2. Serdaroglu S, Ustunbas TK. Diaper dermatitis (napkin dermatitis, nappy rash) *J Turk Acad Dermatol*. 2010;4(4):04401r.

ADDITIONAL READING

- Alberta L. Diaper dye dermatitis. *Pediatrics*. 2005;116(3):450–452.
- Kazaks EL. Diaper dermatitis. *Pediatr Clin North Am*. 2000;47(4):909–919.

SEE ALSO

Algorithm: Rash, Focal

CODES

ICD10
- B37.2 Candidiasis of skin and nail
- L22 Diaper dermatitis

CLINICAL PEARLS

- Hygiene is the main preventative measure.
- Look for secondary infection in persistent cases.

DERMATITIS HERPETIFORMIS

Cindy England Owen, MD • Jewell Gaulding, MD • Caroline Nyenke Robinson, MD

 BASICS

DESCRIPTION
- Dermatitis herpetiformis (DH) is a chronic, polymorphous, intensely pruritic, erythematous papulovesicular eruption with symmetrical distribution primarily involving extensor skin surfaces of the elbows, knees, buttocks, back, and scalp.
- DH is a multifactorial disease with genetic, environmental, and immunologic influences.
- DH is distinguished from other bullous diseases by characteristic histologic and immunologic findings, as well as associated gluten-sensitive enteropathy (GSE).
- System(s) affected: Skin
- Synonym(s): Duhring disease

EPIDEMIOLOGY
- Occurs most frequently in those of Northern European origin
- Rare in persons of Asian or African American origin
- Predominant age: Most common in 4th decade, but may present at any age
- Predominant sex: Male > Female (1.5:1 in the US, 2:1 worldwide)

Incidence
1/100,000 persons per year in the US

Prevalence
11/100,000 persons in the US population; as high as 39/100,000 persons worldwide

ETIOLOGY AND PATHOPHYSIOLOGY
- Evidence suggests that epidermal transglutaminase (eTG) 3, a keratinocyte enzyme involved in cell envelope formation and maintenance, is the autoantigen in DH.
- eTG is highly homologous with tissue transglutaminase (tTG), which is the antigenic target in celiac disease and gluten-sensitive enteropathy (GSE).
- The initiating event for DH is presumed to be the interaction of wheat peptides with tTGs, which results in the formation of an autoantigen with high affinity for particular class II major histocompatibility complex (MHC) molecules
- Presentation of the autoantigen leads to activation of T cells and the humoral immune system.
- IgA antibodies against tTG cross-react with eTG and result in IgA-eTG immune complexes that are deposited in the papillary dermis. Subsequent activation of complement and recruitment of neutrophils to the area result in inflammation and microabscesses.
- Skin eruption may be delayed 5–6 weeks after exposure to gluten.
- Gluten applied directly to the skin does not result in the eruption, whereas gluten taken by mouth or rectum does. This implies necessary processing by the GI system.
- Thought to be immune complex–mediated disease

Genetics
- High association with human leukocyte antigen DQ2 (95%), with remaining patients being positive for DQ8, DR4, or DR3
- Strong association with combination of alleles DQA1*0501 and DQB1*0201/0202, DRB1*03 and DRB1*05/07, *or* DQA1*0301 and DQB1*0302

RISK FACTORS
- GSE : >90% of those with DH will have GSE, which may be asymptomatic.
- Family history of DH or celiac disease

GENERAL PREVENTION
Gluten-free diet (GFD) results in improvement of DH and reduces dependence on medical therapy. GFD also may reduce the risk of lymphomas associated with DH.

COMMONLY ASSOCIATED CONDITIONS
- Gluten-sensitive enteropathy, gluten ataxia
- Gastric atrophy, hypochlorhydria, pernicious anemia
- GI lymphoma, non-Hodgkin lymphoma
- Hypothyroidism, hyperthyroidism, thyroid nodules, thyroid cancer
- Down syndrome, Turner syndrome
- IgA nephropathy
- Autoimmune disorders, including systemic lupus erythematosus, dermatomyositis, Sjögren syndrome, rheumatoid arthritis, sarcoidosis, Raynaud phenomenon, insulin-dependent diabetes mellitus, myasthenia gravis, Addison disease, vitiligo, alopecia areata, primary biliary cirrhosis and psoriasis

 DIAGNOSIS

Diagnosis of DH involves a clinicopathologic correlation among clinical presentation, histologic and direct immunofluorescence evaluation, serology, and response to therapy or dietary restriction.

HISTORY
- Waxing and waning, intensely pruritic eruption with papules and tiny vesicles
- Eruption may worsen with gluten intake.
- GI symptoms may be absent or may not be reported until prompted.

PHYSICAL EXAM
- Polymorphic presentation with symmetric, grouped, erythematous papules and vesicles
- May primarily present with erosions, excoriations, lichenification, hypopigmentation and/or hyperpigmentation secondary to scratching and healing of old lesions.
- Areas involved include extensor surfaces of elbows (90%), knees (30%), shoulders, buttocks, and sacrum. The scalp is also frequently affected. Oral lesions are rare (1,2).
- In children, purpura may be visible on digits and palmoplantar surfaces
- Adults with associated enteropathy are most often asymptomatic, with ~20% experiencing steatorrhea and <10% with findings of bloating, diarrhea, or malabsorption
- Children with associated enteropathy may present with abdominal pain, diarrhea, iron deficiency, and reduced growth rate (3).

DIFFERENTIAL DIAGNOSIS
- In adults (3):
  - Bullous pemphigoid: Linear deposition of C3 and IgG at the basement membrane zone
  - Linear IgA disease: Homogeneous and linear deposition of IgA at the basement membrane zone, absence of GSE
  - Nodular prurigo
  - Urticaria: Wheals, angioedema, dermal edema
  - Erythema multiforme

- In children (3):
  - Atopic dermatitis: Face and flexural areas
  - Scabies: Interdigital areas, axillae, genital region
  - Papular urticaria: Dermal edema
  - Impetigo

DIAGNOSTIC TESTS & INTERPRETATION
Initial Tests (lab, imaging)
- Serum IgA tTG antibodies: Detection of tTG antibodies was noted to be up to 95% sensitive and >90% specific for DH in patients on unrestricted diets.
- Serum IgA eTG antibodies: Antibodies to eTG, the primary autoantigen in DH, were shown to be more sensitive than antibodies to tTG in the diagnosis of patients with DH on unrestricted diets (95% vs. 79%).
- Serum IgA endomysial antibodies: Have a sensitivity between 50% and 100% and a specificity close to 100% in patients on unrestricted diets (3)

Follow-Up Tests & Special Considerations
Serologic assessment of anti-tTG and anti-eTG correlate with intestinal involvement of disease and in conjunction with antiendomysial antibodies (EMA) may be useful in monitoring major deviations from GFD (3,4).

Diagnostic Procedures/Other
The "gold standard" for diagnosing DH is a skin biopsy of perilesional skin evaluated via direct immunofluorescence, which demonstrates granular IgA deposited in dermal papillae and/or basement membrane (4,5).

Test Interpretation
- Direct immunofluorescence of perilesional skin reveals a granular pattern of IgA deposition in the dermal papillae (3).
- Histopathology of lesion with routine staining reveals neutrophilic microabscesses in the tips of the dermal papillae and may show subepidermal blistering (1).

 TREATMENT

MEDICATION
- Disease control is achieved with dietary modification and medication.
- Medication is useful for immediate symptom management but should be used as an adjunct to dietary modification (5).
- A GFD is necessary for long-term management of underlying gluten sensitivity.

First Line
- Dapsone is approved by the FDA for use in DH and is the most widely used medication (1)[A]. Adult doses range from 25–400 mg/d, which result in improvement of symptoms within 24–48 hours. Use minimum effective dose. Average maintenance dose is 1 mg/kg/d. Minor outbreaks on the face and scalp are common even with treatment. Not ideal for long-term use in DH.
- Dapsone works by inhibiting neutrophil recruitment and IL-8 release, inhibiting the respiratory burst of neutrophils, and protecting cells from neutrophil-mediated injury, thereby suppressing the skin reaction. It has no role in preventing IgA deposition or mitigating the immune reaction in the gut (1).

Precautions:
- Common side effects include nausea, vomiting, headache, dizziness, weakness and hemolysis.
- A drop in hemoglobin of 1–2 g is characteristic with dapsone 100 mg/d.
- G6PD deficiency increases severity of hemolytic stress. Dapsone should be avoided, if possible, in those who are G6PD-deficient.
- Dose-related methemoglobinemia may occur with doses >100 mg/d. Cimetidine may reduce the severity of this side effect.
- Risk of distal motor neuropathy

ALERT
- Monitor for potentially fatal dapsone-induced sulfone syndrome: Fever, jaundice and hepatic necrosis, exfoliative dermatitis, lymphadenopathy, methemoglobinemia, and hemolytic anemia
- Can occur 48 hours or 6 months after treatment, most often 5 weeks after initiation

Pediatric Considerations
- <2 years: Dosing not established
- >2 years: 0.5–1.0 mg/kg/d

Pregnancy Considerations
- Category C: Safety during pregnancy is not established.
- Secreted in breast milk and will produce hemolytic anemia in infants.
- Adherence to a strict GFD 6–12 months before conception should be considered with the hope of eliminating need for dapsone during pregnancy.

Second Line
Sulfapyridine (1–2 g/d) is FDA approved for use in DH and is thought to be the active metabolite in sulfasalazine (2–4 g/d) and sulfamethoxypyridazine (0.25–1.5 g/d) (6). Common side effects include nausea, vomiting, and anorexia. Enteric-coated form may reduce side effects. Other side effects include hypersensitivity reactions, hemolytic anemia, proteinuria, and crystalluria (3,6).

ISSUES FOR REFERRAL
Over time, interdisciplinary treatment may involve a dermatologist, gastroenterologist, and registered dietician. Genetic counseling and testing should be considered on diagnosis (5).

ADDITIONAL THERAPIES
GFD:
- Average of 2 years is often necessary for diet to completely eliminate skin eruptions, and lesions usually recur within 12 weeks of gluten reintroduction (3).
- Fundamentals of the GFD (7):
  - Grains that should be avoided: Wheat (includes spelt, kamut, semolina, and triticale), rye, and barley (including malt)
  - Safe grains (gluten-free): Rice, amaranth, buckwheat, corn, millet, quinoa, sorghum, teff (an Ethiopian cereal grain), oats
  - Sources of gluten-free starches that can be used as flour alternatives:
    ○ Cereal grains: Amaranth, buckwheat, corn, millet, quinoa, sorghum, teff, rice (white, brown, wild, basmati, jasmine), and montina
    ○ Tubers: Arrowroot, jicama, taro, potato, and tapioca

  ○ Legumes: Chickpeas, lentils, kidney beans, navy beans, pea beans, peanuts, and soybeans
  ○ Nuts: Almonds, walnuts, chestnuts, hazelnuts, and cashews
  ○ Seeds: Sunflower, flax, and pumpkin

 ONGOING CARE

FOLLOW-UP RECOMMENDATIONS
Patient Monitoring
If treating with dapsone, check a baseline CBC with differential, renal function test, liver function tests, and urinalysis and then follow safety monitoring protocol. If white blood cell count falls below 4,000 cells/mm^3 discontinue therapy. Screening for commonly associated autoimmune conditions is also indicated (5).

DIET
- 87% of patients showed complete remission of skin manifestations after 18 months of a GFD.
- Improvement in cutaneous disease and normalization of small bowel mucosa result from strict compliance with a GFD (3)[C].

PATIENT EDUCATION
- Patient should be made aware of potential hemolytic anemia and the signs associated with methemoglobinemia.
- American Academy of Dermatology, 930 N. Meacham Road, P.O. Box 4014, Schaumberg, IL 60168-4014; (708) 330-0230
- The University of Chicago Celiac Disease Center, 5841 S. Maryland Ave., Mail Code 4069, Chicago, IL 60637; (773) 702-7593; www.celiacdisease.net or www.cureceliacdisease.org
- Gluten Intolerance Group of North America, 31214-124 Ave. SE, Auburn, WA 98092; (206) 246-6652; fax (206) 246-6531; www.gluten.net
- The Celiac Disease Foundation, 13251 Ventura Blvd., #1, Studio City, CA 9160; (818) 990-2354; fax (818) 990-2379

PROGNOSIS
- Lifelong disease with favorable prognosis
- 10–15 year survival rates do not seem to differ from general population (5).
- Remission in 10–15% (8)
- Skin disease responds readily to dapsone. Occasional new lesions (2–3/wk) are to be expected and are not an indication for altering daily dosage.
- Strict adherence to a GFD improves clinical symptoms and decreases dapsone requirement. GFD is the only sustainable method of eliminating cutaneous and GI disease.
- Risk of lymphoma may be decreased in those who maintain a GFD.

COMPLICATIONS
- Malnutrition, weight loss, nutritional deficiencies (folate, B$_{12}$, iron)
- Abdominal pain, dyspepsia
- Osteoporosis, dental abnormalities
- Autoimmune diseases
- Lymphomas

REFERENCES
1. Kárpáti S. An exception within the group of autoimmune blistering diseases: Dermatitis herpetiformis, the gluten-sensitive dermopathy. *Immunol Allergy Clin North Am*. 2012;32(2): 255–262, vi. Epub 2012 Apr 17.
2. Bolotin D, Petronic-Rosic V. Dermatitis herpetiformis. Part I. Epidemiology, pathogenesis, and clinical presentation. *J Am Acad Dermatol*. 2011;64(6):1017–1024; quiz 1025–1026.
3. Caproni M, Antiga E, Melani L, et al. Guidelines for the diagnosis and treatment of dermatitis herpetiformis. *J Eur Acad Dermatol Venereol*. 2009;23(6):633–638. Epub 2009 Mar 10.
4. Kárpáti S. Dermatitis herpetiformis. *Clin Dermatol*. 2012 Jan-Feb;30(1):56–59.
5. Bolotin D, Petronic-Rosic V. Dermatitis herpetiformis. Part II. Diagnosis, management, and prognosis. *J Am Acad Dermatol*. 2011;64(6): 1027–1033; quiz 1033–1034.
6. Cardones AR, Hall RP 3rd. Management of dermatitis herpetiformis. *Immunol Allergy Clin North Am*. 2012 May;32(2):275–281. Epub 2012 Apr 18.
7. Green PH, Cellier C. Celiac disease. *N Engl J Med*. 2007;357:1731–1743.
8. Paek SY, Steinberg SM, Katz SI. Remission in dermatitis herpetiformis: A cohort study. *Arch Dermatol*. 2011;147(3):301–305. Epub 2010 Nov 15.

ADDITIONAL READING
- Bonciolini V, Bonciani D, Verdelli A, et al. Newly described clinical and immunopathological feature of dermatitis herpetiformis. *Clin Dev Immunol*. 2012;2012:967974. doi: 10.1155/2012/967974. Epub 2012 Jun 3.
- Cardones AR, Hall RP 3rd. Pathophysiology of dermatitis herpetiformis: A model for cutaneous manifestations of gastrointestinal inflammation. *Immunol Allergy Clin North Am*. 2012;32(2): 263–274.
- Karell K, Korponay-Szabo I, Szalai Z, et al. Genetic dissection between coeliac disease and dermatitis herpetiformis in sib pairs. *Ann Hum Genet*. 2002;66 (Pt 5–6):387–392.
- Nicolas ME, Krause PK, Gibson LE, et al. Dermatitis herpetiformis. *Int J Dermatol*. 2003;42:588–600.

 SEE ALSO

- Celiac Disease
- Algorithm: Rash, Focal

 CODES

ICD10
L13.0 Dermatitis herpetiformis

CLINICAL PEARLS
- DH is a chronic, intensely pruritic, papulovesicular eruption primarily involving extensor skin surfaces.
- Strong association with gluten-sensitive enteropathy
- Skin biopsy with direct immunofluorescence demonstrating granular IgA deposits in the dermal papillae is pathognomonic.
- Serologic levels of IgA transglutaminase aid in diagnosis and monitoring of deviations from GFD.
- Mainstay of treatment is a gluten-free diet with dapsone.

D

DERMATITIS, SEBORRHEIC

Juan Qiu, MD, PhD

 BASICS

DESCRIPTION
Chronic, superficial, recurrent inflammatory rash affecting sebum-rich, hairy regions of the body, especially scalp, eyebrows, and face

EPIDEMIOLOGY
Incidence
- Predominant age: Infancy, adolescence, and adulthood
- Predominant sex: Male > Female

Prevalence
Seborrheic dermatitis: 3–5%

ETIOLOGY AND PATHOPHYSIOLOGY
- Skin surface yeasts *Malassezia* (formerly *Plasmodium ovale*) may be a contributing factor (1,2,3)
- *Malassezia* spp. may have a role in T-cell suppression and complement activation.
- The mite *Demodex folliculorum* may have a direct/indirect role.
- Genetic and environmental factors: Flares are common with stress/illness.
- Parallels increased sebaceous gland activity in infancy and adolescence or as a result of some acnegenic drugs
- Helper T cells, phytohemagglutinin and concanavalin stimulation, and antibody titers are depressed compared with those of control subjects.

Genetics
Positive family history; no genetic marker identified to date

RISK FACTORS
- Parkinson disease
- AIDS (disease severity correlated with progression of immune deficiency)
- Emotional stress
- Medications may flare/induce seborrheic dermatitis: Auranofin, aurothioglucose, buspirone, chlorpromazine, cimetidine, ethionamide, gold, griseofulvin, haloperidol, interferon-α, lithium, methoxsalen, methyldopa, phenothiazine, psoralen, stanozolol, thiothixene, trioxsalen

GENERAL PREVENTION
Seborrheic skin should be washed more often than usual.

COMMONLY ASSOCIATED CONDITIONS
- Parkinson disease
- AIDS

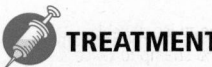 DIAGNOSIS

Diagnosis of seborrheic dermatitis usually can be made by history and physical exam.

HISTORY
- Intermittent active phases manifest with burning, scaling, and itching, alternating with inactive periods; activity is increased in winter and early spring, with remissions commonly occurring in summer.
- Infants:
  – Cradle cap: Greasy scaling of scalp, sometimes with associated mild erythema
  – Diaper and/or axillary rash
  – Age at onset typically ~1 month
  – Usually resolves by 8–12 months
- Adults:
  – Red, greasy, scaling rash in most locations consisting of patches and plaques with indistinct margins
  – Red, smooth, glazed appearance in skin folds
  – Minimal pruritus
  – Chronic waxing and waning course
  – Bilateral and symmetric
  – Most commonly located in hairy skin areas: Scalp and scalp margins, eyebrows and eyelid margins, nasolabial folds, ears and retroauricular folds, presternal area, middle to upper back, buttock crease, inguinal area, genitals, and armpits

PHYSICAL EXAM
- Scalp appearance varies from mild, patchy scaling to widespread, thick, adherent crusts. Plaques are rare.
- Seborrheic dermatitis can spread onto the forehead, the posterior part of the neck, and the postauricular skin, as in psoriasis.
- Skin lesions manifest as branny or greasy scaling over red, inflamed skin.
- Hypopigmentation is seen in African Americans.
- Infectious eczematoid dermatitis, with oozing and crusting, suggests secondary infection.
- Seborrheic blepharitis may occur independently.

DIFFERENTIAL DIAGNOSIS
- Atopic dermatitis: Distinction may be difficult in infants
- Psoriasis:
  – Usually knees, elbows, and nails are involved.
  – Scalp psoriasis will be more sharply demarcated than seborrhea, with crusted, infiltrated plaques rather than mild scaling and erythema.
- *Candida*
- Tinea cruris/capitis: Suspect these when usual medications fail/hair loss occurs.

- Eczema of auricle/otitis externa
- Rosacea
- Discoid lupus erythematosus: Skin biopsy will be beneficial.
- Histiocytosis X: May appear as seborrheic-type eruption
- Dandruff: Scalp only, noninflammatory

DIAGNOSTIC TESTS & INTERPRETATION
Diagnostic Procedures/Other
Consider biopsy if:
- Usual therapies fail
- Petechiae noted
- Histiocytosis X suspected
- Fungal cultures in refractory cases or when pustules and alopecia are present

Test Interpretation
Nonspecific changes:
- Hyperkeratosis, acanthosis, accentuated rete ridges, focal spongiosis, and parakeratosis are characteristic.
- Parakeratotic scale around hair follicles and mild superficial inflammatory lymphocytic infiltrate

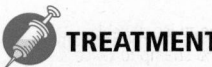 TREATMENT

GENERAL MEASURES
- Increase frequency of shampooing.
- Sunlight in moderate doses may be helpful.
- Cradle cap:
  – Frequent shampooing with a mild, nonmedicated shampoo
  – Remove thick scale by applying warm mineral oil, then wash off 1 hour later with a mild soap and a soft-bristle toothbrush or terrycloth washcloth (4).
- Adults: Wash all affected areas with antiseborrheic shampoos. Start with over-the-counter brands (Tegrin, Selsun Blue) and increase to more potent preparations (containing coal tar, sulfur, selenium, or salicylic acid) if no improvement is noted (4).
- For dense scalp scaling, 10% liquor carbonic detergens in Nivea oil may be used at bedtime, covering the head with a shower cap. This should be done nightly for 1–3 weeks.

MEDICATION

First Line

- Cradle cap: Use a coal tar shampoo or ketoconazole (Nizoral) shampoo if the nonmedicated shampoo is ineffective (4).
- Adults (5):
  - Topical antifungal agents:
    - Ketoconazole 2% foam/shampoo twice a week for clearance, then once a week or every other week for maintenance
    - Ketoconazole (Nizoral) and Sertaconazole 2% cream may be used to clear scales in other areas.
    - Ciclopirox 1% shampoo twice weekly (1)[B]
  - Topical corticosteroids:
    - Begin with 1% hydrocortisone and advance to more potent (fluorinated) steroid preparations, as needed.
    - Avoid continuous use of the more potent steroids to reduce the risk of skin atrophy, hypopigmentation, or systemic absorption (esp. in infants and children).
    - Precautions: Fluorinated corticosteroids and higher concentrations of hydrocortisone (e.g., 2.5%) may cause atrophy or striae if used on the face or on skin folds.
  - Other topical agents:
    - Coal tar 1% shampoo twice a week
    - Selenium sulfide 2.5% shampoo twice a week
    - Zinc pyrithione shampoo twice a week
    - Lithium succinate ointment twice a week
- Once controlled, washing with zinc soaps or selenium lotion with periodic use of steroid cream may help to maintain remission.

Second Line

- Calcineurin inhibitors:
  - Pimecrolimus 1% cream b.i.d. (6)[A]
  - Tacrolimus 0.1% ointment b.i.d.
- Systemic antifungal therapy:
  - Data are limited.
  - For moderate-to-severe seborrheic dermatitis:
    - Ketoconazole: 200 mg/d
    - Itraconazole: 200 mg/d
    - Daily regimen for 1–2 months followed by twice-weekly dosing for chronic treatment
    - Monitor potential hepatotoxic effects.
- Low-molecular weight hyaluronic acid:
  - Hyaluronic acid sodium salt gel0.2% b.i.d. (7)[B]

ISSUES FOR REFERRAL

No response to 1st-line therapy and concerns regarding systemic illness (e.g., HIV)

 ## ONGOING CARE

FOLLOW-UP RECOMMENDATIONS

Patient Monitoring

Every 2–12 weeks, as necessary, depending on disease severity and degree of patient sophistication

PATIENT EDUCATION

http://familydoctor.org/online/famdocen/home/common/skin/disorders/157.html

PROGNOSIS

- In infants, seborrheic dermatitis usually remits after 6–8 months.
- In adults, seborrheic dermatitis is usually chronic and unpredictable, with exacerbations and remissions. Disease is usually easily controlled with shampoos and topical steroids.

COMPLICATIONS

- Skin atrophy/striae is possible from fluorinated corticosteroids, especially if used on the face.
- Glaucoma can result from use of fluorinated steroids around the eyes.
- Photosensitivity is caused occasionally by tars.
- Herpes keratitis is a rare complication of herpes simplex: Instruct patient to stop eyelid steroids if herpes simplex develops.

 ## REFERENCES

1. Shuster S, Meynadier J, Kerl H, et al. Treatment and prophylaxis of seborrheic dermatitis of the scalp with antipityrosporal 1% ciclopirox shampoo. *Arch Dermatol*. 2005;141:47–52.
2. Darabi K, Hostetler SG, Bechtel MA, et al. The role of Malassezia in atopic dermatitis affecting the head and neck of adults. *J Am Acad Dermatol*. 2009;60(1):125–136.
3. Hay RJ. Malassezia, dandruff and seborrhoeic dermatitis: An overview. *Br J Dermatol*. 2011;165 (Suppl 2):2–8.
4. Johnson BA, Nunley JR. Treatment of seborrheic dermatitis. *Am Fam Physician*. 2000;61: 2703–2710, 2713–2714.
5. Stefanaki I, Katsambas A. Therapeutic update on seborrheic dermatitis. *Skin Therapy Lett*. 2010;15: 1–4.

6. Kim GK, Rosso JD. Topical pimecrolimus 1% cream in the treatment of seborrheic dermatitis. *Clin Aesthetic Dermatol*. 2013;6(2):29–34.
7. Schlesinger T, Powell CR. Efficacy and safety of a low-molecular weight hyaluronic acid topical gel in the treatment of facial seborrhoeic dermatitis. *Clil Aesthetic Dermatol*. 2012;5(10):20–23.

ADDITIONAL READING

- Bikowski J. Facial seborrheic dermatitis: A report on current status and therapeutic horizons. *J Drugs Dermatol*. 2009;8:125–133.
- Karincaoglu Y, Tepe B, Kalayci B, et al. Is *Demodex folliculorum* an aetiological factor in seborrhoeic dermatitis? *Clin Exp Dermatol*. 2009;34(8): e516–e520.
- Naldi L, Rebora A. Clinical practice. Seborrheic dermatitis. *N Engl J Med*. 2009;360(4):387–396.
- Shemer A, Kaplan B, Nathansohn N, et al. Treatment of moderate to severe facial seborrheic dermatitis with itraconazole: An open non-comparative study. *Isr Med Assoc J*. 2008;10(6):417–418.
- Shin H, Kwon OS, Won CH, et al. Clinical efficacies of topical agents for the treatment of seborrheic dermatitis of the scalp: A comparative study. *J Dermatol*. 2009;36(3):131–137.

 ## SEE ALSO

Algorithm: Rash, Focal

CODES

ICD10

- L21.0 Seborrhea capitis
- L21.1 Seborrheic infantile dermatitis
- L21.9 Seborrheic dermatitis, unspecified

CLINICAL PEARLS

- Search for an underlying systemic disease in a patient who is unresponsive to usual therapy.
- In adults, seborrheic dermatitis is usually chronic and unpredictable, with exacerbations and remissions. Disease is usually easily controlled with shampoos and topical steroids.

DERMATITIS, STASIS
Joseph A. Florence, MD • Fereshteh Gerayli, MD

BASICS

DESCRIPTION
- Chronic, eczematous, erythremic, scaling, and noninflammatory edema of the lower extremities accompanied by cycle of scratching, excoriations, weeping, crusting, and inflammation in patients with chronic venous insufficiency, due to impaired circulation and other factors (nutritional edema)
- Clinical skin manifestation of chronic venous insufficiency usually appears late in the disease.
- May present as a solitary lesion
- System(s) affected: Skin/Exocrine
- Synonym(s): Gravitational eczema; Varicose eczema; Venous dermatitis

EPIDEMIOLOGY
Incidence
- In the US: Common in patients age >50 years (6–7%)
- Predominant age: Adult, geriatric
- Predominant sex: Female > Male

Geriatric Considerations
Common in this age group:
- Estimated to affect 15–20 million patients age >50 years in the US

ETIOLOGY AND PATHOPHYSIOLOGY
- Incompetence of perforating veins causing blood to backflow to the superficial venous system leading to venous hypertension (HTN) and cutaneous inflammation
- Deposition of fibrin around capillaries
- Microvascular abnormalities
- Ischemia
- Continuous presence of edema in ankles, usually present because of venous valve incompetency (varicose veins)
- Weakness of venous walls in lower extremities
- Trauma to edematous, eczematized skin
- Itch may be caused by inflammatory mediators (from mast cells, monocytes, macrophages, or neutrophils) liberated in the microcirculation and endothelium.
- Abnormal leukocyte–endothelium interaction is proposed to be a major factor.
- A cascade of biochemical events leads to ulceration.

Genetics
Familial link probable

RISK FACTORS
- Atopy
- Superimposition of itch–scratch cycle
- Trauma
- Previous deep vein thrombosis (DVT)
- Previous pregnancy
- Prolonged medical illness
- Obesity
- Secondary infection
- Low-protein diet
- Old age
- Genetic propensity
- Chronic edema
- Tight garments that constrict the thigh
- Vein stripping
- Vein harvesting for coronary artery bypass graft surgery
- Previous cellulitis

GENERAL PREVENTION
- Use compression stockings to avoid recurrence of edema and to mobilize the interstitial lymphatic fluid from the region of stasis dermatitis and also following DVT.
- Topical lubricants twice a day to prevent fissuring and itching

COMMONLY ASSOCIATED CONDITIONS
- Varicose veins
- Venous insufficiency
- Other eczematous disease
- Hyperhomocysteinemia
- Venous hypertension (1)

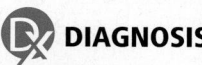

DIAGNOSIS

HISTORY
- Itching, pain, and burning may precede skin signs, which are aggravated during evening hours.
- Insidious onset
- Usually bilateral
- Description may include aching/heavy legs.
- Erythema, scaling, edema of lower extremities
- Noninflammatory edema preceded the skin eruption and ulceration.
- Edema initially develops around the ankle.

PHYSICAL EXAM
- Evaluation of the lower extremities characteristically reveals:
  - Bilateral scaly, eczematous patches, papules, and/or plaques
  - Violaceous (sometimes brown), erythematous-colored lesions due to deoxygenation of venous blood (postinflammatory hyperpigmentation and hemosiderin deposition within the cutaneous tissue)
- Distribution: Medial aspect of ankle, with frequent extension onto the foot and lower leg
- Brawny induration
- Stasis ulcers (frequently accompany stasis dermatitis) secondary to cuts, bruises, and excoriations to the weakened skin around the ankle
- Excoriations
- Weeping, crusting, inflammation of the skin
- Varicosities are often associated with ulcers.
- Clinical inspection reveals swelling, and warmth.
- Skin changes are more common in the lower 1/3 of the extremity and medially.
- Early signs include prominent superficial veins and pitting ankle edema.
- May present as a solitary lesion mimicking a neoplasm

DIFFERENTIAL DIAGNOSIS
- Other eczematous diseases:
  - Atopic dermatitis
  - Uremic dermatitis
  - Contact dermatitis (due to topical agents used to self-treat)
  - Neurodermatitis
  - Arterial insufficiency
  - Sickle cell disease causing skin ulceration
  - Cellulitis
  - Erysipelas
- Tinea dermatophyte infection
- Pretibial myxedema
- Nummular eczema
- Lichen simplex chronicus

- Xerosis
- Asteatotic eczema
- Amyopathic dermatomyositis

DIAGNOSTIC TESTS & INTERPRETATION
Initial Tests (lab, imaging)
Duplex ultrasound imaging is helpful in diagnosis (2).

Diagnostic Procedures/Other
Rule out arterial insufficiency (check peripheral pulses, leg BPs); ankle brachial pressure index (ABPI or ABI).

Test Interpretation
Chronic inflammation, characterized histologically by proliferation of small blood vessels in the papillary dermis

TREATMENT

GENERAL MEASURES
- Primary role of treatment is to reverse effects of venous HTN. Appropriate health care:
- Outpatient:
  - Reduce edema (3)[B]:
    - Leg elevation: Heels higher than knees; knees higher than hips
    - Compression therapy: Elastic bandage wraps: Ace bandages or Unna paste boot (zinc gelatin) if lesions are dry or compression stockings (Jobst or nonfitted type) (4,5)[A]
    - Multilayer or bilayer systems containing an elastic bandage or high compression stockings more effective than nonelastic or short stretch bandages for severe cases (6); avoid high compression in arterial insufficiency
    - Pneumatic compression devices
    - Diuretic therapy
  - Treat infection: Débride the ulcer base of necrotic tissue.
- Improvement of lipodermatosclerosis:
  - Activity:
    - Avoid standing still.
    - Stay active and exercise regularly.
    - Elevate foot of bed unless contraindicated.
- Inpatient, for endovascular radiofrequency ablation, vein stripping, sclerotherapy, or skin grafts:
  - Venous ulcer treatment includes autolytic, biologic, chemical, mechanical, and surgical:
    - Autolytic: Hydrogels, alginates, hydrocolloids, foams, and films
    - Biologic: Topical application of granulocyte macrophage colony-stimulating factor promotes healing of ulcers.
    - Chemical: Enzyme débriding agents
    - Mechanical: Wet to dry dressings, hydrotherapy, and irrigation
    - No specific type of topical dressing superior to another when used with compression therapy; maintain moist wound environment (7)
    - Surgical: Modifying cause of venous HTN (by venous ligation, valvuloplasty and endoscopic perforator vein surgery); treat ulcer by graft

MEDICATION

First Line

- Use of antibiotics topically or systemically is controversial, as stasis ulcer may not be infected.
- Antibiotics are indicated if bacterial infection is present or may be used empirically if bacterial infection is suspected.
- If ulcer is present, local povidone-iodine treatment is as effective as systemic antibiotics.
- If secondary infection, treat with PO antibiotics for *Staphylococcus* or *Streptococcus* organisms (e.g., dicloxacillin 250 mg q.i.d., cephalexin 250 mg q.i.d. or 500 mg b.i.d., or levofloxacin 250 mg daily.).
- Gram-negative colonization: Treat with topical antimicrobial agents (e.g., benzoyl peroxide, acetic acid, silver nitrate, or Hibiclens) or broad-spectrum topical antibiotics (e.g., neomycin or bacitracin-polymyxin B Polysporin]).
- 5% aluminum acetate (Burow solution) wet dressings and cooling pastes
- Topical triamcinolone 0.1% (Kenalog, Aristocort) cream/ointment t.i.d. or topical betamethasone
- Betamethasone valerate (Valisone) 0.1% cream/ointment/solution t.i.d.
- Topical antipruritic: Pramoxine, camphor, menthol, and doxepin
- Systemic steroids for severe cases
- Calcium dobesilate has been shown to be an effective adjuvant therapy.
- Evidence-based treatment options for associated venous ulcers include aspirin and pentoxifylline (3)[B].
- Insufficient evidence exists to either support or refute the routine use of silver sulfadiazine (SSD) for ambulatory patients with either partial-thickness burns or stasis dermatitis ulcers to decrease mortality, prevent infection, or augment wound healing.

Second Line

- Consider antibiotics on basis of culture results of exudate from ulcer craters.
- Lubricants when dermatitis is quiescent
- Chronic stasis dermatitis can be treated with topical emollients (e.g., white petroleum, lanolin, Eucerin).
- Antipruritic medications (e.g., diphenhydramine, cetirizine hydrochloride, desloratadine)

ISSUES FOR REFERRAL

Consider referral for:

- Nonhealing ulcer
- Uncertain diagnosis
- Associated disease (e.g., arterial insufficiency, symptomatic varicose veins)

ADDITIONAL THERAPIES

If the patient is on amlodipine therapy, consider discontinuing amlodipine.

SURGERY/OTHER PROCEDURES

Sclerotherapy and surgery may be required for associated disease.

 ONGOING CARE

FOLLOW-UP RECOMMENDATIONS

Patient Monitoring

If Unna boot compression is used: Cut off and reapply boot once a week. Unna boots reduce edema by compression and prevent scratching.

DIET

Lose weight, if overweight.

PATIENT EDUCATION

- Encourage staying active to keep circulation and leg muscles in good condition. Walking is ideal.
- Keep legs elevated while sitting or lying.
- Do not wear girdles, garters, or pantyhose with tight elastic tops.
- Do not scratch.
- Elevate foot of bed with 2–4-inch blocks.
- Apply compression stockings prior to getting out of bed when less edema is present.

PROGNOSIS

- Chronic course with intermittent exacerbations and remissions
- The healing process for ulceration is often prolonged and may take months.

COMPLICATIONS

- Sensations of itching, pain, and burning have negative impact on the quality of life.
- Secondary bacterial infection
- DVT
- Bleeding at dermatitis sites
- Squamous cell carcinoma in edges of long-standing stasis ulcers
- Scarring, which in turn leads to further compromise to blood flow and increased likelihood of minor trauma

REFERENCES

1. Sippel K, Mayer D, Ballmer B, et al. Evidence that venous hypertension causes stasis dermatitis. *Phlebology.* 2011;26:361–365.
2. Coleridge-Smith P, Labropoulos N, Partsch H, et al. Duplex ultrasound investigation of the veins in chronic venous disease of the lower limbs–UIP consensus document. Part I. Basic principles. *Eur J Vasc Endovasc Surg.* 2006;31:83–92.
3. Collins L, Seraj S. Diagnosis and treatment of venous ulcers. *Am Fam Physician.* 2010;81:989–996.
4. Partsch H, Flour M, Coleridge Smith P. Indications for compression therapy in venous and lymphatic disease consensus based on experimental data and scientific evidence. Under the auspices of the IUP. *Int Angiol.* 2008;27:193–219.
5. Coleridge-Smith PD. Leg ulcer treatment. *J Vasc Surg.* 2009;49:804–808.
6. *Cochrane Database Sysr Rev.* 2012 Nov 12 14; 11 CD000265
7. Dressings for healing venous leg ulcers - The Cochrane Library - Palfreyman - Wiley Online Library CD001103

 SEE ALSO

- Varicose Veins
- Algorithm: Rash, Focal

 CODES

ICD10

- I83.10 Varicose veins of unsp lower extremity with inflammation
- I83.11 Varicose veins of right lower extremity with inflammation
- I83.12 Varicose veins of left lower extremity with inflammation

CLINICAL PEARLS

- Treatment of edema associated with stasis dermatitis via elevation and/or compression stockings is essential for optimal results.
- Mild topical corticosteroids reduce inflammation and itching; however, these may potentiate infection; high-potency topical corticosteroids should be avoided due to increased risk of atrophy and ulceration.

DIABETES MELLITUS, TYPE 1

Robert A. Baldor, MD

 BASICS

DESCRIPTION
- Chronic disease caused by pancreatic insufficiency (deficiency) of insulin production
- Results in hyperglycemia and end-organ complications (e.g., accelerated atherosclerosis, neuropathy, nephropathy, and retinopathy)
- Features include:
  - Patients are insulinopenic and require insulin.
  - Ketosis
  - Usually rapid onset
  - Nutritional status: Normal or thin physique
- System(s) affected: Endocrine/Metabolic

Pregnancy Considerations
- During embryogenesis, hyperglycemia increases the incidence of congenital malformations. Tight control of blood sugar prior to conception is important.
- Women with microalbuminuria during the 1st trimester are at increased risk for preeclampsia and preterm delivery.
- A safe pregnancy is possible with vaginal delivery of a term baby. Close monitoring of blood sugar during labor is important.

EPIDEMIOLOGY
- Mean age of onset 8–12 years, peaking in adolescence
- Onset 1.5 years earlier in girls than boys
- Rapid decline in incidence after adolescence
- Overall incidence increasing worldwide
- Age of presentation has a bimodal distribution, being highest at ages 4–6 and 10–14 years.

Incidence
- 15/100,000 per year
- Racial predilection for whites
- African Americans have lowest overall incidence.

Pediatric Considerations
- Although onset is usually before the age of 19 years, true type 1 diabetes can occur for the 1st time in patients who are well into their 30s.
- Young children are more likely to present in diabetic ketoacidosis (DKA) due to atypical presentation and because they may not express thirst or obtain fluids as readily as older children or adults.

ETIOLOGY AND PATHOPHYSIOLOGY
- Alteration in immunologic integrity, placing the β cell at special risk for inflammatory damage, accounts for most cases.
- Autoantibodies to islet cells, glutamic acid decarboxylase (GAD), tyrosine phosphatase antibodies, and insulin identified in certain cases (type 1A diabetes)
- Some idiopathic cases (type 1B) have no evidence of autoimmune or other reason for β-cell damage.
- Inherited defect
- Associated environmental triggers (none has been verified):
  - Viruses (e.g., mumps, coxsackie, cytomegalovirus, and hepatitis viruses)
  - Diet high in nitrosamines
  - Environmental toxins
- Emotional and physical stress

Genetics
- Mode of genetic expression not clear
- Genes located on major histocompatibility complex on chromosome 6
- HLA DR3 and DR4 are individually associated with an increased risk; if a person is carrying both susceptibility genes, the relative risk is increased.
- HLA B8 and B15 also associated with increased risk

RISK FACTORS
- Certain human leukocyte antigen (HLA) types
- Presence of a specific 64,000 mw protein may be responsible for antibody formation.
- Family history: Insulin-dependent or noninsulin-dependent diabetes in any 1st-degree relatives
- Dietary factors: Breastfeeding may provide a degree of protection against the disease, whereas exposure to cow's milk at an early age is associated with an increased risk of the disease.
- Maternal age at birth may play a role (1).
- Slightly greater risk for a child if the father has type 1 diabetes

COMMONLY ASSOCIATED CONDITIONS
- Autoimmune diseases, such as celiac disease, hypothyroidism, and Addison disease:
  - Screening regularly for hypothyroidism is particularly important in females.
- Diabetes mellitus can also be seen as part of multiple endocrine adenomatosis.

 DIAGNOSIS

DIFFERENTIAL DIAGNOSIS
- Benign renal glycosuria
- Glucose intolerance
- Type 2 noninsulin-dependent diabetes:
  - Obese children might have maturity-onset diabetes of the young (MODY)
- Secondary diabetes:
  - Pancreatic disease (chronic pancreatitis, cystic fibrosis, hereditary hemochromatosis)
  - Hormonal disorders (pheochromocytoma, multiple endocrine adenomatosis)
  - Inborn errors of metabolism (glycogen storage disease, type 1)
  - Hereditary neuromuscular disease
  - Progeroid syndromes
  - Obesity (Prader-Willi syndrome)
  - Cytogenetic syndromes (trisomy 21, Klinefelter, and Turner syndromes)
  - Drug- or chemical-induced glucose intolerance: Glucocorticosteroids, HIV protease inhibitors, atypical antipsychotics, tacrolimus, cyclosporine
- Acute poisonings (salicylate poisoning can cause hyperglycemia and glycosuria, and may mimic DKA)

DIAGNOSTIC TESTS & INTERPRETATION
Initial Tests (lab, imaging)
- Criteria for the diagnosis of diabetes:
  - Fasting glucose >126 mg/dL (7.0 mmol/L) or
  - Random of >200 mg/dL (11.1 mmol/L) in a patient with classic symptoms of hyperglycemia or
  - Oral glucose tolerance test; plasma glucose ≥200 mg/dL 2 hours after a glucose load of 1.75 g/kg (max dose 75 g) or
  - Glycated hemoglobin (HbA1c) level ≥6.5% (2)[C]

- Other tests to consider:
  - Serum electrolytes, especially in sicker patients who may have ketoacidosis
  - Urinalysis for glucose and ketones and microalbuminuria
  - Pancreatic autoantibodies (to diagnose type 1A diabetes):
    - Islet cells, insulin, glutamic acid decarboxylase (GAD), tyrosine phosphatase antibodies
  - CBC (WBC count and hemoglobin may be elevated)
- C-peptide insulin level if needed to differentiate from type 2 diabetes

Test Interpretation
Inflammatory changes, lymphocytic infiltration around the islets of Langerhans, or islet cell loss

HISTORY
- Polyuria and polydipsia:
  - Polyuria may present as nocturia, bedwetting, or incontinence in a previously continent child.
  - Polyuria may be difficult to appreciate in diaper-clad children.
- Weight loss 10–30%:
  - Often almost devoid of body fat at diagnosis, due to hypovolemia and increased catabolism
- Prolonged or recurrent candidal infection, usually in the diaper area
- Increased fatigue, lethargy, muscle cramps
- Irritability and emotional lability, headaches, abdominal discomfort, nausea
- Vision changes, such as blurriness
- Altered school or work performance
- Anxiety attacks

TREATMENT

GENERAL MEASURES
- Overall control of carbohydrate metabolism for the very young child (3)[B]:
  - Normoglycemia (adjusted for age): Strive for blood glucose levels in range of 80–150 mg/dL (4.4–8.3 mmol/L) at all times (80–120 in older patients)
  - Very tight control might be dangerous in young children due to risk of repeated hypoglycemia
  - Hemoglobin A1c target levels:
    - Children <6 years: 7.5–8.5%
    - Children 6–12 years: <8.0%
    - Adolescents 13–19: <7.5% (<7.0% if achieved without excessive hypoglycemia)
    - Adults: <6.0%
- Normal growth and development and overall good health (asymptomatic):
  - Reach optimal height for genetic potential
  - Appropriate and timely pubertal maturation
  - Coping psychosocial development: Normal school or work attendance and performance; normal goals/career plans. Screen adolescents annually for depression.
- Prevent acute complications, including:
  - Hypoglycemic insulin reactions
  - Ketoacidosis
- Delay or prevent chronic complications.

MEDICATION

- All type 1 diabetes patients will require some form of insulin supplementation.
- Types of insulin:
  - Long-acting insulin analogues (insulin glargine Lantus] and insulin detemir Levemir]). These should not be mixed with other insulins in the same syringe.
  - Intermediate-acting insulin (NPH)—Humulin N or Novolin N—can be mixed with other insulins.
  - Short-acting (regular) insulin: Novolin R or Humulin R
  - Very rapid-acting insulin analogues (insulin lispro Humalog], insulin aspart Novolog], and insulin glulisine Apidra])

First Line

- Flexible intensive insulin therapy is the gold standard.
- Frequent daily injections (FDI) or continuous SC insulin infusion (CSII) have equal efficacy.
- Total initial dose is 0.2–0.4 units/gg/day for insulin-naïve patients.
- 40–60% of total dose given as basal insulin, with the rest as bolus insulin
- FDI regime:
  - Basal, long-acting insulin once or twice a day
  - Prandial, short-acting insulin based on number of carbohydrate portions (e.g., 1:10, meaning 1 unit of insulin for every 10 g of carbohydrate to be eaten)
  - Correctional short-acting mealtime insulin based on premeal blood glucose level (e.g., BS-100/50, meaning if the blood glucose is >150, subtract 100 from the blood glucose level, and divide that number by 50)
  - Administration of the mealtime insulin before a meal may be more efficacious than during or after the meal.
- CSII regime:
  - May use regular insulin or rapid-acting insulin analogues
  - Basal insulin is infused continuously at a preset rate, and bolus doses are given with meals as above.

Second Line

- Conventional insulin therapy
- Once- to twice-daily injections with NPH mixed with regular or rapid-acting insulin in the same syringe
- Not physiologic, but lower cost and fewer injections may improve compliance in the less motivated patient.
- Premixed insulin available as NPH/regular (Novolin or Humulin 70/30) or NPH/rapid-acting insulin (e.g., Novolog 75/25 Mix or Humulin 75/25 Mix)
- Pancreatic transplantation is usually reserved for patients with end-stage renal failure, who may receive kidney-pancreatic transplants at the same time.
- Oral hypoglycemics not indicated in type 1 diabetes (except in obese patients, who may have MODY, or a combination of type 1 and type 2): Metformin (Glucophage)

IN-PATIENT CONSIDERATIONS

Newly diagnosed type 1 diabetics may require hospitalization during initiation of insulin therapy.

 ONGOING CARE

FOLLOW-UP RECOMMENDATIONS

- Normal; full participation in sports activities
- Regular aerobic exercise is recommended.

Patient Monitoring

- BP monitoring at every office visit (4)[C]
- Monitor height, weight, and sexual maturation (in children).
- Daily home blood glucose monitoring with home blood glucose meter: Blood tests should be done at least 4–6 times daily (more frequently in pump patients) for optimal monitoring.
- Quarterly measurement of hemoglobin A1c
- Annual screenings after 5 years of diabetes, sooner if glycemic control is suboptimal:
  - Microalbuminuria for earliest signs of possible nephropathy
  - If elevated, depending on level, even if BP is normal, consider an ACE inhibitor (such as Vasotec [enalapril])
  - Ophthalmology exam (after 3–5 years of diabetes, also depending on glycemic control); annually thereafter
  - Annual lipid profile, thyroid levels, blood chemistries, CBC
  - Annual influenza vaccine

DIET

- American Diabetic Association diet: www.diabetes.org/food-and-fitness/food/
- Carbohydrate counting using insulin-to-carbohydrate ratio with all meals and snacks. Allows patient flexibility in eating and ability to eat almost anything.

PROGNOSIS

- Initial remission or honeymoon phase with decreased insulin needs and easier control, usually 3–6 months
- Progression to total diabetes when endogenous insulin is insignificant; usually is gradual, but stress or illness initiate it suddenly
- Current prognosis for reduced life expectancy:
  - Increasing longevity and quality of life with careful blood glucose monitoring and improvement in insulin delivery regimens

COMPLICATIONS

- Microvascular disease (retinopathy, nephropathy, neuropathy)
- Hyperlipidemia
- Macrovascular disease (coronary and cerebral artery disease)
- Chronic foot ulcers/amputations
- Hypoglycemia
- DKA
- Excessive weight gain
- Increased risk for preeclampsia and preterm delivery (5)
- Driving mishaps (6)
- Psychological problems of chronic disease

REFERENCES

1. Cardwell CR, Stene LC, Joner G, et al. Maternal age at birth and childhood type 1 diabetes: A pooled analysis of 30 observational studies. *Diabetes.* 2010;59:486–494.
2. Gillett MJ. International Expert Committee report on the role of the A1c assay in the diagnosis of diabetes: Diabetes Care 2009;32(7):1327–1334. *Clin Biochem Rev.* 2009;30:197–200.
3. Silverstein J, Klingensmith G, Copeland K, et al. Care of children and adolescents with type 1 diabetes: A statement of the American Diabetes Association. *Diabetes Care.* 2005;28:186–212.
4. American Diabetes Association (ADA). Standards of medical care in diabetes. V. Diabetes care. *Diabetes Care.* 2006;29(Suppl 1):S8–S17.
5. Jensen DM, Damm P, Ovesen P, et al. Microalbuminuria, preeclampsia, and preterm delivery in pregnant women with type 1 diabetes: Results from a nationwide Danish study. *Diabetes Care.* 2010;33:90–94.
6. Cox DJ, Ford D, Gonder-Frederick L, et al. Driving mishaps among individuals with type 1 diabetes: A prospective study. *Diabetes Care.* 2009;32:2177–2180.

 SEE ALSO

Diabetes Mellitus, Type 2; Diabetic Ketoacidosis

 CODES

ICD10

- E10.8 Type 1 diabetes mellitus with unspecified complications
- E10.9 Type 1 diabetes mellitus without complications
- E10.69 Type 1 diabetes mellitus with other specified complication

CLINICAL PEARLS

- Polyuria may present as nocturia, bedwetting, or incontinence in a previously continent child.
- Young children are more likely to present in DKA because they may not express thirst or obtain fluids as readily as older children or adults.
- Onset usually before the age of 19 years, but type 1 diabetes can present in patients who are well into their 30s.
- Obese children might have MODY.

DIABETES MELLITUS, TYPE 2

Swathi A. N. Rao, MD • Sathya S. Krishnasamy, MD

BASICS

DESCRIPTION
- Diabetes mellitus (DM) type 2 manifests as nonketotic hyperglycemia due to insulin resistance and relative impairment in insulin secretion.
- Significant contributing factor to blindness, renal failure, and lower limb amputations

Geriatric Considerations
Monitor elderly for hypoglycemia; adjust doses for renal/hepatic dysfunction.

Pediatric Considerations
Incidence is increasing and parallels weight gain.

Pregnancy Considerations
First-line drug is insulin (class B), but may consider glyburide after the 1st trimester. Metformin may be continued through 1st trimester (class B).

EPIDEMIOLOGY
Incidence
2 million new adult cases reported in 2010 within the US.

Prevalence
- 25.6 million adults in 2010
- Men and women equally affected
- 7% of non-Hispanic Caucasians, 12% of Hispanics and non-Hispanic African Americans, 8% of Asian Americans, and 33% of Native Americans

ETIOLOGY AND PATHOPHYSIOLOGY
- Peripheral insulin resistance
- Defective insulin secretion, especially in response to a glucose stimulus
- Increased gluconeogenesis
- Genetic factors: Monogenic (e.g., $PPAR\gamma$ mutations, insulin gene mutations) and polygenic (1)
- Obesity
- Hemochromatosis
- Drug- or chemical-induced (e.g., glucocorticoids, highly active antiretroviral therapy [HAART] medications, atypical antipsychotics, post-transplant immunosuppressants) (2)

Genetics
50% concordance in monozygotic twins.

RISK FACTORS
- Family history: 1st-degree relative
- Gestational diabetes (GDM) or history of baby with birth weight ≥4 kg (9 lbs)
- Polycystic ovary syndrome (PCOS)
- Obesity (body mass index [BMI] ≥25kg/M²) and visceral adiposity
- Hypertriglyceridemia or low high-density lipoprotein (HDL)
- Ethnicity: African American, Latino, Native American, Asian, and Pacific Islander
- Impaired fasting glucose (IFG)/impaired glucose tolerance (IGT)
- Sedentary lifestyle
- Genetic factors (3)

GENERAL PREVENTION
Weight loss of 5–10% body weight, exercise 150 min/wk, and decrease in fat and caloric intake (2)[A].

COMMONLY ASSOCIATED CONDITIONS
Hypertension, hyperlipidemia, metabolic syndrome, fatty liver disease, infertility, PCOS, acanthosis nigricans, genetic diabetic syndromes (Down syndrome, Klinefelter syndrome, Turner syndrome, Wolfram syndrome, Friedreich ataxia, Huntington chorea, Laurence-Moon-Biedl syndrome, myotonic dystrophy, porphyria, Prader-Willi syndrome) (2)

DIAGNOSIS

HISTORY
Polyuria, polydipsia, polyphagia, weight loss, weakness, fatigue, blurry vision, and frequent infections

PHYSICAL EXAM
BMI, funduscopic exam, oral exam, cardiopulmonary exam, abdominal exam for hepatomegaly, focused neurologic exam, and diabetic foot exam

DIFFERENTIAL DIAGNOSIS
- Type 1 DM
- Prediabetes
- Cushing syndrome, acromegaly, and glucagonoma

DIAGNOSTIC TESTS & INTERPRETATION
Initial Tests (lab, imaging)
Criteria for diagnosis:
- HbA1c ≥6.5% is diagnostic.
- Hyperglycemic crisis + random plasma glucose ≥200 mg/dL (11.1 mmol/L), or
- FPG ≥126 mg/dL (7.0 mmol/L) on 2 occasions, or
- 2-hour plasma glucose ≥200 mg/dL (11.1 mol/L) during oral glucose tolerance test (OGTT) with 75 g glucose load (2)[A]
- If equivocal, recommend repeat testing.

Follow-Up Tests & Special Considerations
Screen patients with history of gestational diabetes for persistent diabetes/prediabetes 6–12 weeks postpartum with OGTT and at least every 3 years thereafter (2)[A].

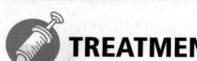

TREATMENT

- Use patient-centered approach (2)[A].
- A1C targets:
  - A1C <7.0 (or <6.5% if this can be achieved without significant hypoglycemia): For those with a long life expectancy and no cardiovascular disease, who have had DM for a short duration and no history of hypoglycemia
  - A1C <8.0%: For those with a limited life expectancy, advanced micro- or macrovascular complications, extensive comorbidities, and a history of hypoglycemia or long-standing DM in whom the general goal is difficult to attain (2)[A]
- FPG goal is <110 mg/dL (5.5 mmol/L) (3)[A]:
  - Use drugs from different classes to achieve adequate control and limit side effects.
  - Consider the addition of insulin if FPG is not controlled by oral agents.

GENERAL MEASURES
- Diabetic foot exam at every visit.
- Nephropathy: Annual urine microalbumin-to-creatinine ratio
- Retinopathy: Annual diabetic eye exam

- Low-density lipoprotein (LDL) goal <70 mg/dL in patients with existing cardiovascular disease (CVD) or risk factors for CVD per NCEP guidelines.
- If ≥40 years with ≥1 CV risk factor and suboptimal lipid profile, begin a statin.
- Low-dose aspirin for all adults with CVD risk unless contraindicated
- Hypertension: Goal BP <140/80 mm Hg (<130 preferred if tolerated)
- ACEI/ARB 1st-line hypertension drug. If contraindicated, consider calcium channel blocker (2)[A].
- Vaccination recommendation (CDC) update: Hep B

DIET
- Limit protein intake to 0.8–1 g/kg body weight/d for diabetic patients with early stages of chronic kidney disease (CKD).
- Limit protein intake to 1 g/kg body weight/d for diabetic patients with advanced CKD (2)[A].

PATIENT EDUCATION
- Diabetes self-management education and support by certified diabetes educator
- Regular aerobic exercise (150 min/wk) and resistance exercise can improve glucose tolerance and decrease medication requirements.
- Nutritional therapy by a registered dietician (2)[A]
- Lifestyle modifications with pharmacotherapy delays progression from prediabetes to diabetes (4)[A].

MEDICATION
First Line
- Biguanides:
  - Metformin (Glucophage, Fortamet, Riomet, Glumetza): Preferred 1st medication because it promotes weight loss and improves insulin resistance. Dosage: 500–2,000 mg in divided doses or ER 1,000–2,000 mg every evening. Maximum 2,550 mg/d except Glumetza 2,000 mg/d.
  - Avoid metformin and combination drugs containing metformin in renal insufficiency, prior to radiocontrast agent use, surgery, and severe acute illnesses (e.g., liver disease, cardiogenic shock, pancreatitis, hypoxia) due to increased risk of lactic acidosis.
  - Caution with congestive heart failure (CHF), alcohol abuse, elderly, or with tetracycline.
  - Associated with GI side effects, vitamin B_{12} deficiency (2)[A]
- Sulfonylureas:
  - Caution with renal or liver disease, sulfa allergy, creatinine clearance <50 mL/min, pregnancy.
  - Glipizide (Glucotrol): 2.5–40 mg/d. Dosage >10 mg/d given b.i.d. 30 minutes before meals
  - Glipizide extended-release: 5–20 mg/d
  - Glyburide (DiaBeta, Glynase, Micronase): 1.25–20 mg/d, Glynase 0.75–12 mg/d
  - Glimepiride (Amaryl): 1–8 mg/d
  - Chlorpropamide (Diabinese): 100–500 mg/d, max 750 mg/d
- Thiazolidinediones:
  - Pioglitazone (Actos): 15–45 mg/d. May increase risk of bladder cancer
  - Rosiglitazone (Avandia): Increased risk of myocardial infarction (MI), cardiovascular accident (CVA), pulmonary embolism (PE), CHF; use is restricted in the US.

- Monitor serum transaminases every 2 months for the 1st year. Contraindicated in patients with liver disease and symptomatic heart failure (2)[A].
- α-Glucosidase inhibitors:
  - Acarbose (Precose): 25–100 mg t.i.d.
  - Miglitol (Glyset): 25–100 mg t.i.d.
  - Take at beginning of meals to decrease postprandial hyperglycemia.
  - Poor patient compliance due to GI symptoms
  - Avoid in renal insufficiency, inflammatory bowel disease, colonic ulceration, or partial bowel obstruction (2)[A].
- Dipeptidyl peptidase-4 inhibitors:
  - Sitagliptin (Januvia): 100 mg/d
  - Sitagliptin/Simvastatin (Juvisync): 100 mg/40 mg/d
  - Sitagliptin/Metformin (Janumet): Start 50/500 mg b.i.d., max 100 mg/2,000 mg/d. Give with meals.
  - Saxagliptin (Onglyza): 2.5 mg/d, max 5 mg/d
  - Saxagliptin/Metformin XR (Kombiglyze XR): Start 5/500 mg/d, max 5/2,000 mg. Give with evening meal.
  - Linagliptin (Tradjenta): 5 mg/d
  - Renally excreted. Adjust dose for patients with renal failure.
  - Increased risk of acute pancreatitis (2)[A].
- Precautions: Warn patients of signs of hypo- and hyperglycemia:
  - Combination of metformin and sulfonylurea may increase relative risk of cardiovascular hospitalization or mortality.
- Significant interactions:
  - Drugs that may potentiate effects of sulfonylureas: Salicylates, clofibrate, warfarin (Coumadin), ethanol, and ACE inhibitors.
  - Thiazides can cause IGT.
  - Gatifloxacin can cause either severe hypo-/hyperglycemia.
  - Pioglitazone may decrease effectiveness of oral contraceptives.
  - Drug binders, such as cholestyramine resin, should be taken at least 2 hours apart from α-glucosidase inhibitors.

Second Line
- Insulin: Rapid (Aspart, Lispro, Glulisine), short (regular insulin), intermediate (NPH), and long-acting (Glargine and Detemir):
  - May be used in combination with certain oral agents or with an insulin of a different half-life.
  - Long-acting insulins have lower risk of hypoglycemia than short-acting insulin.
  - Insulindetemir (Levemir) or insulin glargine (Lantus): 0.5–1 U/kg/d. Onset of action 1 hour. No peak. Duration of action 6–23 hours. Given at bedtime or b.i.d. (2)[A].
- Amylinomimetic:
  - Pramlintide (Symlin): 60–120 μg SC before every meal
  - Prandial insulins (short-acting/rapid-acting) should be reduced by 50% if initiated on this drug to avoid hypoglycemia.
  - Contraindicated in patients with gastroparesis
  - Avoid anticholinergics that slow intestinal absorption of nutrients (2)[A].
- GLP-1 (glucagonlike peptide-1) receptor agonist:
  - Exenatide (Byetta): 5–10 μg SC b.i.d. within 60 minutes before meals and at least 6 hours apart
  - Bydureon (degludec): 2 mg/wk

- Liraglutide (Victoza): 0.6 mg/d SC for 1 week, then increase to 1.2, max 1.8 mg/d. Less expensive and better tolerated than exenatide; should not be used in patients with personal history/family history of medullary thyroid cancer or multiple endocrine neoplasia (MEN) type 2 (black box warning) (5)[A].
  - Increased risk of acute pancreatitis and kidney disease
  - Promotes weight loss, increases HDL, and decreases diastolic BP
  - Consider dose reduction of sulfonylureas due to risk of hypoglycemia (2)[A].
- Meglitinides:
  - Repaglinide (Prandin): 0.5–4 mg before meals. May be useful in patients with sulfa allergy or renal impairment.
- Diphenylalanine derivatives:
  - Nateglinide (Starlix): 60–120 mg before meals t.i.d.
- Bile acid sequestrants:
  - Colesevelam: 3.75 g/d or 1.875 g b.i.d.
- Dopamine-2-agonists:
  - Bromocriptine mesylate (Cycloset): 0.8–1.6 mg/d within 2 hours of awakening
  - Alters hypothalamic regulation of metabolism, reduces hepatic gluconeogenesis
  - May cause dizziness, nausea, fatigue, rhinitis (6)[C]
- SGLT2 Inhibitors:
  - Canagliflozin (Invokana) 100–300 mg single dose before breakfast. Adjust for GFR.
  - Inhibits glucose reabsorption by sodium glucose cotransporter-2 inhibition.
  - Hypotension, genital mycotic infections, UTI

SURGERY/OTHER PROCEDURES
For patients with BMI >35, consider bariatric surgery (7)[B].

COMPLEMENTARY AND ALTERNATIVE MEDICINE
Cinnamon has been shown to improve glycemic control, with improvements in A1C and FBG (8)[A].

 ## ONGOING CARE

FOLLOW-UP RECOMMENDATIONS
Patient Monitoring
- Frequency of office visits at physician's discretion
- Monitor glucose, HbA1c, BP, body weight, and renal and liver function.
- In most adults, measure fasting lipid profile at least annually. If lipid values are low-risk (LDL <100 mg/dL, HDL >50 mg/dL, triglycerides [TG] <150 mg/dL), check lipid profiles every 2 years.
- A1c twice a year for patients with well-controlled blood glucose and quarterly for patients with hyperglycemia or recent changes in therapy (2)[A]

PROGNOSIS
In susceptible individuals, complications begin to appear 10–15 years after onset, but can be present at time of diagnosis since disease may go undetected for years. There is evidence that intensive glycemic control in newly diagnosed diabetics may reduce long-term CVD rates (2)[A].

COMPLICATIONS
- Emergencies: Hyperosmolar coma, diabetic ketoacidosis (DKA), Charcot joints

- CVD: CAD, peripheral vascular disease, stroke
- Microvascular: Peripheral neuropathy, proliferative retinopathy, nephropathy, ED, and CKD
- Ophthalmic: Blindness, cataracts, glaucoma, retinopathy
- GI: NAFLD, gastroparesis, diarrhea.
- Neurologic: Autonomic dysfunction
- Foot ulcers and infections

REFERENCES
1. Moffett SP, Feingold E, Barmada MM, et al. The C161→T polymorphism in peroxisome proliferator-activated receptor gamma, but not P12A, is associated with insulin resistance in Hispanic and non-Hispanic white women: Evidence for another functional variant in peroxisome proliferator-activated receptor gamma. *Metab Clin Exp.* 2005;54:1552–1556.
2. American Diabetes Association. Standards of medical care in diabetes–2013. *Diabetes Care.* 2013;36(Suppl 1):S11–66.
3. Handelsman Y, Mechanick J, Blonde L, et. al. American Association of Clinical Endocrinologists Medical Guidelines for Clinical Practice for developing a diabetes mellitus comprehensive care plan. *Endocr Pract.* 2011;17(Suppl 2):1–53.
4. Blonde L. Current antihyperglycemic treatment guidelines and algorithms for patients with type 2 diabetes mellitus. *Am J Med.* 2010;123:S12–S18.
5. Fakhoury WK, Lereun C, Wright D, et al. A meta-analysis of placebo-controlled clinical trials assessing the efficacy and safety of incretin-based medications in patients with type 2 diabetes. *Pharmacology.* 2010;86:44–57.
6. Defronzo RA. Bromocriptine: A sympatholytic, d2-dopamine agonist for the treatment of type 2 diabetes. *Diabetes Care.* 2011;34:789–794.
7. Akilen R, Tsiami A, Devendra D, et al. Cinnamon in glycaemic control: Systematic review and meta analysis. *Clin Nutr.* 2012; 31(5):776; author reply 777.
8. Schauer PR, Kashyap SR, Wolski K, et al. Bariatric surgery versus intensive medical therapy in obese patients with diabetes. *N Engl J Med.* 2012; 366:1567–1576.

 ### SEE ALSO
- Diabetes Mellitus, Type 1; Diabetic Ketoacidosis (DKA); Hypertension, Essential
- Algorithm: Diabetes Mellitus, Type 2

 ## CODES

ICD10
- E11.8 Type 2 diabetes mellitus with unspecified complications
- E11.9 Type 2 diabetes mellitus without complications
- E11.319 Type 2 diabetes mellitus with unspecified diabetic retinopathy without macular edema

CLINICAL PEARLS
- Patient-centered care
- Target A1C <7.0 for those with a long life expectancy and no CVD, who have had DM for a short duration, and no history of hypoglycemia.

DIABETIC KETOACIDOSIS (DKA)

Charmiane Lieu, MD • Elizabeth Goldberg, MD

 BASICS

DESCRIPTION
- A true medical emergency secondary to severe insulin deficiency and characterized by hyperglycemia, ketosis, and metabolic acidosis.
- System(s) affected: Endocrine/Metabolic

EPIDEMIOLOGY
Incidence
- In the US: 46 episodes/10,000 diabetics; 2/100 patient-years of type 1 diabetes mellitus (DM) (1)
- Predominant age: 19–44 years (56%) and 45–65 years (24%); only 18% are <20.

ETIOLOGY AND PATHOPHYSIOLOGY
A deficiency of insulin, exacerbated by an increase in counterregulatory hormones (e.g., catecholamines, cortisol, glucagon, and growth hormone) leading to a hyperglycemic crisis, osmotic diuresis, and ketosis.
- Noncompliance/Insufficient insulin: 25%
- Infection: 30–40%
- 1st presentation of DM: 10–20%
- Myocardial infarction (MI): 5–7%
- No cause identified: 10–30%
- Cerebrovascular accident (CVA)
- Medications (corticosteroids, thiazides, SSRI, sympathomimetics)
- Drugs (cocaine)
- Trauma
- Surgery
- Emotional stress
- Pregnancy

RISK FACTORS
- Type 1 > type 2 DM
- Younger patients at higher risk

GENERAL PREVENTION
- Close monitoring of glucose during periods of stress, infection, and trauma
- Careful insulin control and monitoring of the blood glucose level
- "Sick day" management instructions

COMMONLY ASSOCIATED CONDITIONS
Complications of chronic DM such as nephropathy, neuropathy, and retinopathy

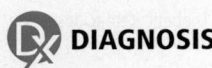 DIAGNOSIS

HISTORY
- Recent illness
- Changes in diet or medications
- Missed insulin doses/noncompliance
- Polyuria, nocturia
- Polydipsia, polyphagia
- Generalized weakness
- Malaise, lethargy
- Anorexia or increased appetite
- Nausea, vomiting
- Abdominal pain
- Decreased perspiration
- Fever
- Confusion
- Coma

PHYSICAL EXAM
- Hypotension
- Tachycardia
- Hypothermia or fever
- Tachypnea, Kussmaul respirations
- Fruity odor to breath (acetone smell)
- Decreased reflexes
- Abdominal tenderness, decreased bowel sounds
- Dry mucous membranes, poor skin turgor
- Decreased perspiration
- Confusion
- Coma

DIFFERENTIAL DIAGNOSIS
- Hyperosmolar hyperglycemic crisis
- Alcoholic ketoacidosis
- Starvation ketosis
- Toxic ingestions (e.g., salicylates)
- Lactic acidosis
- Acute hypoglycemic coma
- Uremia/Chronic renal failure

DIAGNOSTIC TESTS & INTERPRETATION
- ECG:
  – Usually shows sinus tachycardia
  – Changes consistent with electrolyte abnormalities
  – Ischemia/MI as a precipitating factor
- Urine and blood cultures
- Consider lumbar puncture (meningitis).

Initial Tests (lab, imaging)

> **ALERT**
> - Diagnostic criteria (1)[C]:
>   – Hyperglycemia (glucose usually 250–800 mg/dL)
>   – HCO_3 (usually $\leq$18 mEq/L)
>   – Metabolic acidosis on arterial blood gases (pH <7.3)
>   – Anion gap >10 mmol
> - Other pertinent labs:
>   – Serum ketosis: Check β-hydroxybutyrate (β-HB) instead of ketones to evaluate ketosis (2)[B].
>   – Urine ketosis (urinalysis [UA]) may only identify acetoacetate and not β-HB.
>   – Glycosuria
>   – Hyperamylasemia, hyperlipasemia
>   – Hypertriglyceridemia/Hypercholesterolemia
>   – Increased creatinine and BUN: Markedly increased serum ketones may cross-react and cause a falsely high serum creatinine.
>   – Pseudohyponatremia: Hyperglycemia or hypertriglyceridemia may cause an artificially low sodium concentration. The measured sodium is suppressed by 1.6 mg/dL for every 100 mg/dL of glucose over normal.
>   – Decreased calculated total-body K^+: Severe acidosis gives an artificially high K^+ level.
>   – Increased serum osmolality: [2 × Na + (plasma glucose)/18], if calculated osmolality <320 mOsm/kg, consider other etiologies than DKA.
>   – Elevated base deficit
>   – A1C helps determine history of diabetic control
> - CBC, electrolytes, BUN, creatinine
> - Serum β-HB or ketones
> - Arterial blood gases; venous blood gases (VBGs) also may be used (VBG pH $\leq$0.03)

- Chest x-ray to rule out pulmonary infection
- Head CT scan if suspected CVA or cerebral edema
- If necessary cardiac enzymes, blood cultures

Diagnostic Procedures/Other
Only if surgical problem is the underlying precipitant (e.g., appendicitis)

 TREATMENT

- Oxygen and airway management, as needed
- Establish IV access.
- Cardiac monitoring
- Start isotonic crystalloid solution (0.9% saline).
- Fingerstick glucose testing
- Empirical naloxone if altered mental status

GENERAL MEASURES
- All but mild cases require inpatient management; severe DKA requires an ICU setting.
- Goals:
  – Fluid resuscitation
  – Insulin therapy
  – Resolution of anion-gap acidosis
  – Correction of electrolytes
- Attempt to find precipitating cause (i.e., source of infection).
- Laboratory testing during management:
- Serum glucose q1–2h until stable
- Electrolytes, phosphorous, and venous pH q2–6h as needed

MEDICATION
First Line
- Insulin (1)[C]:
  – Bolus 0.1 U/kg IV then continuous infusion at 0.1 U/kg/hr
  – If without bolus, 0.14 U/kg/hr continuous infusion (3)[B]
  – When glucose 200 mg/dL, reduce infusion to 0.02–0.05 U/Kg/hr IV or give rapid-acting insulin at 0.1 U/Kg SC q2h; goal glucose is 150–200 mg/dL.
  – Overlap and continue IV insulin infusion for 1–2 hours after SC insulin initiated
- IV fluids: Start with 0.9% NaCl bolus, calculate corrected sodium; if serum Na^+ is high, consider 0.45% NaCl:
  – When glucose is 200 mg/dL, change to 5% dextrose with 0.45% NaCl at 150–250 mL/hr
- Potassium: Falsely elevated due to acidosis; when K^+ $\leq$5.2 mg/dL and if urine output is adequate, start replacement with 20–30 mEq/L of K^+ in 1 L IV fluids (1):
  – Hold insulin if K^+ $\leq$3.3 mg/dL; give IV potassium 20–30 mEq/hour with fluids until >3.3 mg/dL.
  – For each 0.1 unit of pH, serum K^+ will change by ~0.6 mEq in opposite direction.
- Phosphorus: Routine replacement may lead to hypocalcemia; if very low (<1.0), give 20–30 mEq/L of K-Phos in fluids.

- Sodium bicarbonate: No demonstrable benefit with a pH >7.0 (2,4)[B]; rehydration usually leads to resolution of acidosis. Guidelines recommend its use with pH <6.9 or in patients with life-threatening hyperkalemia; however, there is evidence that it may increase cerebral edema especially in children (5)[A].
- Magnesium: If Mg ≤1.8 mg/dL and the patient is symptomatic, consider replacement.
- Precautions:
  – If the patient is on an insulin pump, it should be stopped.
  – If glucose does not fall by 10% in 1st hour, give regular insulin 0.14 U/kg IV bolus, then continuous infusion at previous rate.
  – If using bicarbonate, add 100 mmol or 2 ampules of sodium bicarbonate to 400 mL isotonic solution with 20 mEq KCL over 200 mL/hr for 2 hours until venous pH is >7.0, then stop infusion (1).

Second Line
Insulin, SC or IM: Load with 0.3 U/kg SC, followed by 0.1 U/kg/h. Space dosing to q2h once glucose <250 mg/dL. In uncomplicated DKA, may be safe and cost effective (6)[B].

Pediatric Considerations
- Children with moderate-to-severe DKA should be transferred to the nearest pediatric critical-care hospital.
- Cerebral edema is a rare complication (~1%) but has mortality of 20–50% (7):
  – Diagnostic criteria exist for diagnosis, CT may rule out alternative diagnoses
  – Treat with IV bolus of mannitol 1 g/kg in 20% solution, reduce IV fluid rate, consider hypertonic 3% saline

Geriatric Considerations
Must be careful with impaired renal function or congestive heart failure when correcting fluid and electrolyte abnormalities

Pregnancy Considerations
- Pregnancy itself is diabetogenic. It also results in a compensated respiratory alkalosis (HCO_3 19–20 mEq/L) with theoretically reduced buffering capacity. Therefore, pregnant patients are more susceptible to DKA.
- Euglycemic DKA
- Increased risk of preeclampsia and fetal death
- β-tocolytics and corticosteroids can trigger DKA.
- Perinatal death: 9–35%

IN-PATIENT CONSIDERATIONS
Admission Criteria/Initial Stabilization
ADA admission guidelines: Blood glucose >250 mg/dL; pH <7.3; HCO_3 ≤15 mEq/L; ketones in urine; ICU setting for severe DKA (8)[C]

IV Fluids
- 1–1.5 L over the 1st hour, then, if serum corrected Na is high or normal, give 0.45% NaCl at 250–500 mL/hr depending on hydration state.

- Switch to 5% dextrose in 0.45% saline at maintenance rate when serum glucose <200 mg/dL. Maintain blood glucose between 150–250 mg/dL. Too rapid correction of fluid balance may precipitate cerebral edema (2)[C]. If the blood glucose level is falling too rapidly, consider using a 10% dextrose solution instead.

Pediatric Considerations
Bolus 10–20 mL/kg initially; 4-hour fluid total should be <50 mL/kg to reduce chance of cerebral edema.

Discharge Criteria
Discharge when DKA has resolved: anion gap <12, Glucose <200 mg/dL; pH >7.3; bicarbonate >18 mEq/L; additionally, patients must be tolerating PO intake and able to resume home medication regimen. Underlying precipitant (e.g., infection) must be identified and treated.

 ## ONGOING CARE

FOLLOW-UP RECOMMENDATIONS
Bed rest

Patient Monitoring
- Monitor mental status, vital signs, and urine output q30–60min until improved, then q2–4h.
- Monitor blood sugar q1h until <200 mg/dL, then q2–6h.
- Monitor electrolytes, BUN, venous pH, creatinine q2–4h.

DIET
- NPO initially
- Advance to preketotic diet when nausea and vomiting are controlled.
- Avoid foods with high glycemic index (e.g., soft drinks, fruit juice, white bread, etc.).

PROGNOSIS
- 16% of all diabetes-related fatalities
- Death 1–2%
- In children <10 years of age, DKA causes 70% of diabetes-related fatalities.

COMPLICATIONS
- Cerebral edema (most common cause of death in children)
- Pulmonary edema
- Vascular thrombosis
- Hypokalemia
- Hypophosphatemia
- Cardiac dysrhythmia
- MI
- Acute gastric dilatation
- Late hypoglycemia (secondary to treatment)
- Erosive gastritis
- Infection, mucormycosis
- Respiratory distress

REFERENCES

1. Kitabchi AE, Umpierrez GE, Miles JM, et al. Hyperglycemic crises in adult patients with diabetes. Diabetes Care. 2009;32:1335–1343.
2. Agus MS, Wolfsdorf JI. Diabetic ketoacidosis in children. Pediatr Clin North Am. 2005;52: 1147–1163, ix.
3. Kitabchi AE, Murphy MB, Spencer J, et al. Is a priming dose of insulin necessary in a low-dose insulin protocol for the treatment of diabetic ketoacidosis? Diabetes Care. 2008;31:2081–2085.
4. Kitabchi AE, Umpierrez GE, Murphy MB, et al. Hyperglycemic crises in diabetes. Diabetes Care. 2004;27(Suppl 1):S94–102.
5. Chua HR, Schneider A, Bellomo R. Bicarbonate in diabetic ketoacidosis - a systematic review. Ann Intensive Care. 2011;1(1):23. Epub 2011 Jul 6.
6. Umpierrez GE, Latif K, Stoever J, et al. Efficacy of subcutaneous insulin lispro versus continuous intravenous regular insulin for the treatment of patients with diabetic ketoacidosis. Am J Med. 2004;117(5):291–296.
7. Brown TB. Cerebral oedema in childhood diabetic ketoacidosis: Is treatment a factor? Emerg Med J. 2004;21:141–144.
8. American Diabetes Association. Hospital admission guidelines for diabetes. Diabetes Care. 2004;27(Suppl 1):S103.

ADDITIONAL READING

- American Diabetes Association. Standards of medical care in diabetes—2013. Diabetes Care. 2013;36(Suppl 1):S11–66.
- Carroll MA, Yeomans ER. Diabetic ketoacidosis in pregnancy. Crit Care Med. 2005;33(10 Suppl): S347–353.
- Sheikh-Ali M, Karon BS, Basu A, et al. Can serum beta-hydroxybutyrate be used to diagnose diabetic ketoacidosis? Diabetes Care. 2008;31(4):643–647. Epub 2008 Jan 9.
- Trachtenbarg DE. Diabetic ketoacidosis. Am Fam Physician. 2005;71:1705–1714.

 ## SEE ALSO

Diabetes Mellitus, Type 1

 ## CODES

ICD10
- E10.10 Type 1 diabetes mellitus with ketoacidosis without coma
- E10.11 Type 1 diabetes mellitus with ketoacidosis with coma
- E13.10 Oth diabetes mellitus with ketoacidosis without coma

CLINICAL PEARLS

- Admit if blood glucose >250 mg/dL, pH <7.3, HCO_3 ≤15 mEq/L, and ketones in urine.
- Potassium is falsely elevated due to acidosis; start replacement when K^+ ≤5.3 mg/dL and urine output is adequate.

DIARRHEA, ACUTE

Pia Prakash, MD • Marie L. Borum, MD, EdD, MPH

 BASICS

DESCRIPTION
- Acute diarrhea is an abnormal increase in stool frequency (≥3 in 24 hours) for <14 days duration
- Acute viral diarrhea (50–70%):
  - Most common form
  - Usually occurs for 1–3 days
  - Typically self-limited
- Bacterial diarrhea (15–20%):
  - Develops 6–24 hours after infected food ingested
  - Suspect if simultaneous illness is present in others who have shared contaminated food
  - Suspect *Clostridium difficile* in patients with recent antibiotic use or hospitalization.
- Protozoal infections (10–15%):
  - Cause prolonged, watery diarrhea (travelers from areas with contaminated water supply)
  - Consider if diarrhea lasts >7 days.
- Traveler's diarrhea typically begins 3–7 days after arrival in foreign location; often quite acute.

EPIDEMIOLOGY
- In developing countries, acute diarrhea is more common in children, whereas in developed countries it may be seen in people of all ages.
- Acute diarrhea accounts for >150,000 hospital admissions each year.

Prevalence
- 5th leading cause of death worldwide
- Affects 11% of the general population
- In developing countries, often seen in children age <5 years
- Rotavirus and adenovirus common in children age <2 years

ETIOLOGY AND PATHOPHYSIOLOGY
- Bacterial:
  - *Escherichia coli*
  - *Salmonella*
  - *Shigella*
  - *Campylobacter jejuni*
  - *Vibrio parahaemolyticus*
  - *Vibrio cholerae*
  - *Yersinia enterocolitica*
  - *Clostridium difficile*
  - *Staphylococcus aureus*
  - *Bacillus cereus*
  - *Clostridium perfringens*
  - *Listeria monocytogenes*
- Viral:
  - Rotavirus and norovirus (most common)
  - Adenovirus
  - Astrovirus
  - Cytomegalovirus (CMV) (HIV, immunocompromised)
- Protozoal:
  - *Giardia lamblia*
  - *Entamoeba histolytica*
  - *Cryptosporidium*
  - *Isospora belli*
  - *Cyclospora*
  - *Microspora*

RISK FACTORS
- Travel to developing countries
- Immunocompromised host
- Antibiotic use
- Daycare attendance
- Nursing home residency
- Pregnancy (20-fold increase for *Listeriosis*)

GENERAL PREVENTION
- Frequent handwashing; proper hygiene
- Strict food handling
- Special care during foreign travel to avoid contaminated water and uncooked vegetables
- Avoid undercooked meats.
- Probiotics may be used to help prevent traveler's diarrhea, although evidence is conflicting (1,2).
- Rotavirus vaccine for infants

COMMONLY ASSOCIATED CONDITIONS
- Inflammatory bowel disease
- Medications
- Ileal resection
- Gastrectomy
- Hyperthyroidism
- Diabetes mellitus
- Immunocompromise (HIV, malignancy, chemotherapy)

 DIAGNOSIS

HISTORY
- Duration of symptoms
- Stool characteristics (3)[A]:
  - Frequency
  - Quantity
  - Presence of mucus, blood, or fat;
  - consistency
- Weight loss
- Associated symptoms, such as change in appetite, abdominal pain or bloating, nausea/vomiting, or fever
- Recent hospitalization or antibiotic use
- Travel history
- Daycare attendance
- Ingestion of:
  - Raw or undercooked meat
  - Raw seafood
  - Unpasteurized milk
- Sick contacts
- Immunocompromise or pregnancy
- With *Giardia*: Cramping, pale, greasy stools; fatigue, weight loss

PHYSICAL EXAM
- General: Fever, volume status
- Cardiovascular: Tachycardia
- Abdominal: Bowel sounds, abdominal distention, abdominal tenderness, masses, hepatomegaly
- Rectal: Stool with blood or mucus

Geriatric Considerations
Watery diarrhea with chronic constipation may be caused by fecal impaction or obstructing neoplasm.

DIFFERENTIAL DIAGNOSIS
- Inflammatory bowel disease
- Malabsorption
- Medications (cholinergic agents, magnesium-containing antacids, chemotherapy)
- Pseudomembranous colitis secondary to antibiotic use
- Diverticulitis
- Spastic (irritable) colon
- Fecal impaction
- Ischemic colitis
- Endocrinopathies

DIAGNOSTIC TESTS & INTERPRETATION
Initial Tests (lab, imaging)
- CBC:
  - Leukocytosis may indicate an infectious process.
  - Anemia from blood loss
- Serum electrolytes
- BUN, creatinine may be elevated secondary to volume depletion.
- Non-anion gap metabolic acidosis
- Stool sample:
  - Occult blood present in inflammatory bowel disease, bowel ischemia, and certain bacterial infections
  - Fecal leukocytes
  - Stool ova and parasites
  - Stool culture:
    - For bloody diarrhea, consider *Salmonella*, *Shigella*, *Campylobacter*, *E. coli* O157:H7, *Y. enterocolitica*, *E. histolytica*.
  - *C. difficile* toxin (especially important if recent hospitalization or antibiotic use) (3)[B]
  - *Giardia* ELISA: >90% sensitive in at-risk population
  - Abdominal radiographs (flat plate and upright) indicated with severe abdominal pain or evidence of obstruction to rule out toxic megacolon and bowel ischemia

Diagnostic Procedures/Other
- Sigmoidoscopy or colonoscopy should be considered in patients with persistent diarrhea.
- Colonoscopy should be considered in patients with HIV to evaluate for CMV colitis.
- Colonoscopy may be helpful in distinguishing infectious diarrhea from inflammatory bowel disease.

Test Interpretation
- Viral diarrhea: Changes in small intestine cell morphology that include villous shortening, increased number of crypt cells, and increased cellularity of the lamina propria
- Bacterial diarrhea: Bacterial invasion of colonic wall leads to mucosal hyperemia; edema, and leukocytic infiltration.

TREATMENT

GENERAL MEASURES

- Oral rehydration and electrolyte management is the most important treatment in patients presenting with acute diarrhea (4)[A].
- Diet, as tolerated
- IV fluids if patient cannot tolerate oral rehydration

MEDICATION

First Line

- Empiric antibiotics (fluoroquinolones or macrolides) should be considered in patients with signs and symptoms of bacterial diarrhea, including (5):
  - Fever
  - Bloody diarrhea
  - Presence of fecal leukocytes
  - Immunocompromised host
  - Signs of volume depletion
  - Symptoms >1 week
- Antibiotic regimen should be tailored if organisms identified on stool culture:
  - *Giardia*: Metronidazole
  - *E. histolytica*: Metronidazole
  - *Shigella*: Trimethoprim-sulfamethoxazole (Bactrim DS) or ciprofloxacin
  - *Campylobacter*: Erythromycin or ciprofloxacin
  - *C. difficile*: Metronidazole, PO vancomycin, or fidaxomicin
  - Traveler's diarrhea: Ciprofloxacin or TMP/SMX (Bactrim DS) (4)[A] or rifaximin (6)[A]
- General considerations:
  - Antibiotics are not recommended in *Salmonella* infections unless caused by *S. typhosa*, patient is febrile, or immunocompromised.
  - Antibiotics should be avoided in patients with *E. coli* 0157:H7 due to increased risk of hemolytic-uremic syndrome.
  - Antibiotics are not indicated in foodborne toxigenic diarrhea.
  - Antimotility agents (e.g., loperamide) should be used with caution in patients suspected of having infectious diarrhea (especially, *E. coli* 0157:H7) or antibiotic-associated colitis.
  - Antimotility agents may speed recovery from traveler's diarrhea when used in combination with an antibiotic (7)[A].
- Significant possible interactions:
  - Salicylate absorption from bismuth subsalicylate can cause toxicity in patients already taking aspirin-containing compounds and may alter anticoagulation control in patients taking Coumadin.
  - Avoid alcoholic beverages with metronidazole due to the possibility of a disulfiram reaction.

COMPLEMENTARY AND ALTERNATIVE MEDICINE

- In patients being treated with antibiotics, administration of a probiotic at levels above 10^{10}/g may prevent diarrhea (8)(9)[A].
- Probiotics may be used to help prevent traveler's diarrhea (1).
- Zinc supplementation can decrease diarrhea-related morbidity and mortality (10)[A].

Admission Criteria/Initial Stabilization

Outpatient management, except for patients who are severely ill with signs of volume depletion.

 ONGOING CARE

DIET

- Early refeeding is encouraged.
- During periods of active diarrhea, avoid coffee, alcohol, dairy products, most fruits, vegetables, red meats, and heavily seasoned foods.
- Adequate nutrition is necessary. Patients can consider boiled starches and cereals with salt, if tolerated.
- The traditional bananas, rice, applesauce, toast diet (BRAT diet) has little evidence-based support, despite heavy clinical use, and may result in suboptimal nutrition.

PATIENT EDUCATION

See guidelines in "Prevention" section.

PROGNOSIS

Acute diarrhea is rarely life threatening if adequate hydration is maintained and causative agent can be identified.

COMPLICATIONS

- Volume depletion
- Sepsis
- Shock
- Anemia
- Hemolytic-uremic syndrome with *E. coli* 0157:H7
- Guillain-Barré with *C. jejuni*

REFERENCES

1. McFarland LV. Meta-analysis of probiotics for the prevention of traveler's diarrhea. *Travel Med Infect Dis*. 2007;5(2):97–105. Epub 2005 Dec 5.
2. Ritchie ML, Romanuk TN. A meta-analysis of probiotic efficacy for gastrointestinal diseases. *PLoS ONE*. 2012;7(4):e34938. Epub 2012 Apr 18.
3. Pawlowski SW, Warren CA, Guerrant R. Diagnosis and treatment of acute or persistent diarrhea. *Gastroenterology*. 2009;136(6):1874–1886.
4. DuPont HL. Clinical practice. Bacterial diarrhea. *N Engl J Med*. 2009;361(16):1560–1569.
5. Dryden MS, Gabb RJ, Wright SK. Empirical treatment of severe acute community-acquired gastroenteritis with ciprofloxacin. *Clin Infect Dis*. 1996;22(6):1019–1025.
6. Koo HL, DuPont HL. Rifaximin: A unique gastrointestinal-selective antibiotic for enteric diseases. *Curr Opin Gastroenterol*. 2010;26(1):17–25.
7. Riddle MS, Arnold S, Tribble DR. Effect of adjunctive loperamide in combination with antibiotics on treatment outcomes in traveler's diarrhea: A systematic review and meta-analysis. *Clin Infect Dis*. 2008;47(8):1007–1014.
8. McFarland LV. Evidence-based review of probiotics for antibiotic-associated diarrhea and *Clostridium difficile* infections. *Anaerobe*. 2009;15:274–280.
9. Johnston BC, Ma SS, Goldenberg JZ, et al. Probiotics for the prevention of Clostridium difficile-associated diarrhea: A systematic review and meta-analysis. *Ann Intern Med*. 2012; 157(12):878–888.
10. Walker CL, Black RE. Zinc for the treatment of diarrhoea: Effect on diarrhoea morbidity, mortality and incidence of future episodes. *Int J Epidemiol*. 2010;39(Suppl 1):i63–i69.

ADDITIONAL READING

- Chen CC, Kong MS, Lai MW, et al. Probiotics have clinical, microbiologic, and immunologic efficacy in acute infectious diarrhea. *Pediatr Infect Dis J*. 2010;29:135–138.
- DuPont HL. Systematic review: The epidemiology and clinical features of travellers' diarrhoea. *Aliment Pharmacol Ther*. 2009;30(3):187–196. Epub 2009 Apr 21.
- Goldenberg JZ, Ma SS, Saxton JD, et al. Probiotics for the prevention of Clostridium difficile-associated diarrhea in adults and children. *Cochrane Database Syst Rev*. 2013 May 31;5:CD006095. doi: 10.1002/14651858.CD006095.pub3

 SEE ALSO

Botulism; Cholera; Food Poisoning, Bacterial

CODES

ICD10

- A08.4 Viral intestinal infection, unspecified
- A09 Infectious gastroenteritis and colitis, unspecified
- R19.7 Diarrhea, unspecified

CLINICAL PEARLS

- Viruses, especially norovirus, are the most common causes of acute diarrheal illness in the US.
- Oral rehydration and correction of electrolyte imbalances are the most important in the treatment of acute diarrhea.
- Empiric antibiotics should be started in patients who are severely ill or immunocompromised.

DIARRHEA, CHRONIC

Neha Jakhete, MD • Marie L. Borum, MD, MPH, EdD

BASICS

DESCRIPTION
- Chronic diarrhea is defined as an increase in frequency of defecation or decrease in stool consistency (typically >3 loose stools per day) for >4 weeks:
  - Etiologies include: Osmotic, secretory, malabsorptive, inflammatory, and hypermotility
  - Infectious etiologies are possible, but less common in a chronic setting.
- System(s) affected: Gastrointestinal

EPIDEMIOLOGY
Prevalence
Variable depending on etiology, but overall ~5% of the US population is affected

ETIOLOGY AND PATHOPHYSIOLOGY
In most cases, chronic diarrhea is the result of disturbances in luminal water and electrolyte balance, but can vary depending on etiology.
- Osmotic (fecal osmotic gap >125 mOsm/kg):
  - Carbohydrate malabsorption:
    - Disaccharides including lactose
    - Monosaccharides including fructose
    - Polyols including sorbitol, xylotil, sucralose and saccharin are commonly used as a sugar substitutes.
    - These substances cannot be metabolized, thus creating an osmotic gradient.
  - Substances including magnesium, phosphate, sulfate
- Secretory (fecal osmotic gap <50 mOsm/kg):
  - Stimulant laxative ingestion
  - Postcholecystectomy:
    - Leads to excessive bile salts in intestinal lumen causing cholerheic diarrhea; often resolves in 6–12 months
  - Ileal bile acid malabsorption:
    - Ileal resection of <100 cm leads to cholerheic diarrhea due to excessive presentation of bile salts to colon.
  - Disordered motility (1):
    - Postvagotomy
    - Diabetic autonomic neuropathy
    - Hyperthyroidism
  - Neuroendocrine tumors:
    - VIPoma
    - Gastrinoma
    - Somatostatinoma
    - Carcinoid syndrome
  - Metastatic medullary carcinoma of the thyroid
  - Systemic mastocytosis
  - Protein-losing enteropathy
- Malabsorption:
  - Whipple disease
  - Giardiasis
  - Celiac disease
  - Short bowel syndrome:
    - Ileal resection of >100 cm leads to insufficient bile salt concentrations in the duodenum for optimal fat absorption, leading to fat and fat-soluble vitamin malabsorption.
  - Small intestinal bacterial overgrowth
  - Pancreatic exocrine insufficiency (CF, chronic pancreatitis)
  - Inadequate bile acid production/secretion

- Inflammatory:
  - Ulcerative colitis
  - Crohn disease
  - Microscopic colitis (lymphocytic or collagenous)
  - Vasculitis
  - Radiation enterocolitis
  - Eosinophilic enterocolitis
- Hypermotility (normal fecal osmotic gap):
  - Irritable bowel syndrome
  - Functional diarrhea
- Drugs: NSAIDs, colchicine, metformin, digoxin, SSRIs
- Herbal products: St. John's wort, echinacea, garlic, saw palmetto, ginseng, cranberry extract, aloe vera
- Infectious:
  - Bacterial: *Clostridium difficile, Mycobacterium avium intracellulare*
  - Viral: Cytomegalovirus
  - Parasites: *Giardia lamblia, Cryptosporidium, Isospora*
  - Helminths: *Strongyloides*

Genetics
- Celiac disease is associated with HLA-DQ2 and HLA-DQ8 haplotypes on MHC Class II antigen-presenting cells.
- IBD is polygenic, and new genome-wide association studies continue to demonstrate new polymorphisms.
- Cystic fibrosis (CF) is caused by a mutation in the CF transmembrane conductance regulator resulting in abnormal exocrine gland secretions.
- Familial diarrhea syndrome is linked to a missense mutation in GUCY2C resulting in hyperactivation of CFTR.

RISK FACTORS
- Osmotic:
  - Excessive ingestion of nonabsorbable carbohydrates
  - Lactose intolerance
  - Celiac disease
- Secretory:
  - Extensive small bowel resection/ileal surgery
  - History of neuroendocrine disease
  - History of stimulant laxative abuse (e.g., senna)
  - Dysmotility syndromes
- Malabsorptive (2):
  - CF
  - Chronic alcohol abuse
  - Chronic pancreatitis/pancreatic insufficiency
  - Celiac disease
  - Medications (e.g., Orlistat, Acarbose)
- Inflammatory:
  - Inflammatory bowel disease (IBD)
  - NSAID use
  - Thoracoabdominal radiation
  - HIV/AIDS
  - Antibiotic use
  - Immunosuppressant therapy
- Hypermotility:
  - Psychosocial stress
  - Preceding infection
- Genetic predisposition (3)

ALERT
Diabetes mellitus and history of cholecystectomy can cause both secretory and osmotic diarrhea.

GENERAL PREVENTION
- Variable depending on etiology of the diarrhea
- Treat the underlying disorder.

COMMONLY ASSOCIATED CONDITIONS
- Extraintestinal manifestations of IBD include arthralgias, aphthous stomatitis, uveitis/episcleritis, erythema nodosum, pyoderma gangrenosum, perianal fistulas, rectal fissures, ankylosing spondylitis, and primary sclerosing cholangitis.
- Celiac disease is associated with dermatitis herpetiformis.
- A significant number of patients with IBS have psychiatric comorbidities.

DIAGNOSIS

HISTORY
- Detailed history of symptoms, including:
  - Onset
  - Pattern and frequency
  - Stool volume and quality (including presence of blood or mucus)
  - Presence of nocturnal symptoms
  - Travel history
  - Antibiotic exposure
  - Dietary habits
  - Current medications
  - Family history
- Evaluate for aggravating or alleviating factors, including changes with oral intake or improvement with selective food avoidance (e.g., dairy products).
- Evaluate for recent unintentional weight loss.
- Complete review of systems, including rashes, arthritis, ocular problems, heat intolerance, polyuria/polydipsia, headache, fever, flushing, alcohol intake
- Evaluate for IBS or functional diarrhea by Rome III criteria:
  - IBS: Recurrent abdominal pain or discomfort and a change in bowel habits for 6 months with symptoms occurring on at least 3 days per week for at least 3 months. ≥2 of the following criteria must be met:
    - Pain relieved with defecation
    - Pain related to change in frequency of stool
    - Pain related to change in form of stool
  - Functional diarrhea: Loose or watery stools ≥75% of the time without pain for >3 months (symptoms >6 months)

PHYSICAL EXAM
- General: Assess for volume depletion, nutritional status
- Skin: Flushing (carcinoid), erythema nodosum (IBD), pyoderma gangrenosum (IBD), ecchymoses (vitamin K deficiency)
- HEENT: Iritis/Uveitis (IBD)
- Neck: Goiter (hyperthyroid), lymphadenopathy (Whipple disease)
- Cardiovascular: Tachycardia (hyperthyroid)
- Pulmonary: Wheezing (carcinoid)
- Abdomen: Hyperactive bowel sounds (IBD), abdominal distention (IBD/IBS), diffuse tenderness (IBD/IBS)
- Anorectal: Anorectal fistulas (IBD), anal fissures (IBD)
- Extremities: Arthritis (IBD)
- Neurologic: Tremor (hyperthyroid)

DIFFERENTIAL DIAGNOSIS
See above.

DIAGNOSTIC TESTS & INTERPRETATION
Initial Tests (lab, imaging)
- Blood: CBC with differential, electrolytes (Mg, P, Ca), total protein, albumin, thyroid-stimulating hormone (TSH), free T4
- Stool: WBCs, culture, ova and parasites, *Giardia* stool antigen, *C. difficile* toxin, stool electrolytes (fecal osmotic gap), fecal occult blood, qualitative fecal fat (Sudan stain)
- Plain film abdomen to evaluate for obstruction, toxic megacolon, bowel ischemia
- CT to rule out chronic pancreatitis if abnormal pancreatic enzymes or evidence of malabsorption

Follow-Up Tests & Special Considerations
- Celiac disease: Antiendomysial antibody IgA, antitissue transglutaminase (TTG) IgA, antigliadin (AGA) IgA, serum IgA (10% of celiac patients have IgA deficiency that may result in false-negative results)
- Chronic pancreatic insufficiency: Fecal elastase
- Protein-losing enteropathy: Fecal α-1 antitrypsin
- Carbohydrate malabsorption: Fecal pH
- Small bowel overgrowth: Hydrogen breath test
- Prior history of hospitalization or antibiotics: *C. difficile* toxin
- HIV ELISA, special stains for *Isospora* and *Cryptosporidium*
- Allergy testing
- Neuroendocrine tumor:
  - Serum: Chromogranin A, VIP, gastrin
  - Urine: 5-HIAA, histamine

Diagnostic Procedures/Other
- Colonoscopy with ileal intubation and biopsies: To diagnose IBD, microscopic colitis, CMV colitis, and colorectal neoplasia (4)[A]
- Flexible sigmoidoscopy: Especially if pregnant, with comorbidities, or if left-sided symptoms predominate (tenesmus and urgency) (4)[A]
- Esophagogastroduodenoscopy (EGD) with small bowel biopsies if malabsorption disorder suspected:
  - Celiac, *Giardia* infection, Crohn disease, eosinophilic gastroenteropathy, Whipple disease, intestinal amyloid, pancreatic insufficiency (4)[A]
- Capsule endoscopy if further evaluation of small bowel is needed
- Upper GI series with small bowel follow-through
- CT or magnetic resonance (MR) enterography

Test Interpretation
- Celiac disease: Marsh classification:
  - Intraepithelial lymphocytosis, increased ratio of crypt to villous height, villous blunting
- Crohn disease: Cobblestoning, linear ulcerations, skip lesions, noncaseating granulomas
- Ulcerative colitis: Crypt abscesses, superficial inflammation
- Lymphocytic colitis: increased intraepithelial infiltration of lymphocytes, increased inflammatory cells within the lamina propria, normal mucosal architecture
- Melanosis coli suggests laxative abuse.

 TREATMENT

GENERAL MEASURES
- First-line therapy is volume resuscitation with IV fluids if patient is volume depleted.
- Electrolyte replacement if indicated
- If the patient is stable, therapy is generally outpatient.

MEDICATION
First Line
- Based on underlying cause:
  - Lactose intolerance: Lactose-free diet and lactase supplementation
  - Cholecystectomy or ileal resection: Cholestyramine (Questran) or other bile acid resin 4–8 g q8h
  - Diabetes: Aggressive diabetes management and glucose control
  - Hyperthyroidism: Methimazole, propylthiouracil (PTU), thyroid ablation
  - *C. difficile*: Vancomycin PO or metronidazole (Flagyl) or Fidaxomicin (newer therapy)
  - *Giardia lamblia*: Metronidazole (Flagyl) or nitazoxanide
  - Whipple disease: Ceftriaxone IV or Bactrim PO
  - Small intestinal bacterial overgrowth: Rifaximin, fluoroquinolones, metronidazole, penicillins
  - Pancreatic insufficiency: Pancreatic enzyme replacement
  - HIV/AIDS: Antiretroviral therapy
  - Microscopic colitis: Budesonide, mesalamine, Pepto-Bismol
  - IBD: 5-ASA, corticosteroids (short-term only), antibiotics (short-term only), immunomodulators (6-MP, azathioprine, methotrexate), anti-TNF therapy (infliximab, adalimumab, certolizumab)
  - Neuroendocrine tumor: Octreotide
  - Celiac disease: Gluten-free diet (wheat/barley/rye avoidance)
  - IBS diarrhea predominant: Antidiarrheals
- Symptom relief:
  - Loperamide (Imodium) 2 mg after loose bowel movement; maximum 16 mg/d
  - Diphenoxylate-atropine (Lomotil) 5–20 mg/d

SURGERY/OTHER PROCEDURES
- Resection of neuroendocrine tumors
- Intestinal resection for medically refractory IBD

COMPLEMENTARY AND ALTERNATIVE MEDICINE
Many homeopathic and naturopathic formulations are available to treat diarrhea; however, most have not been evaluated by the FDA.

 ONGOING CARE

DIET
Abstain from gluten-containing foods, nonabsorbable carbohydrates, lactose-containing products, and food allergens depending on etiology of diarrhea.

PATIENT EDUCATION
- Reassure patient of wide variation in what is accepted as "normal" bowel habits.
- Restrict colon stimulants.
- Dietary changes as appropriate
- Etiology-specific education

PROGNOSIS
Depends on etiology

COMPLICATIONS
- Fluid and electrolyte abnormalities
- Malnutrition
- Anemia
- Malignancy (colon cancer in IBD, small bowel cancer in celiac disease and Crohn disease, lymphoma with IBD therapies)
- Infection with immunomodulator, biologic, and corticosteroid therapies for IBD

REFERENCES
1. Fan X, Sellin JH. Review article: Small intestinal bacterial overgrowth, bile acid malabsorption and gluten intolerance as possible causes of chronic watery diarrhea. *Aliment Pharmacol Ther*. 2009;29(10):1069–1077.
2. Fiskerstrand T, Arshad N, Haukanes BI, et al. Familial diarrhea syndrome caused by an activating GUCY2C mutation. *N Engl J Med*. 2012;366: 1586–1595.
3. Longstreth GF, Thomson WG, Chey WD, et al. Functional bowel disorders. *Gastroenterology*. 2006;130:1480–1491.
4. ASGE Standards of Practice Committee. The role of endoscopy in the management of patients with diarrhea. *Gastrointest Endosc*. 2010;71(6):887.

ADDITIONAL READING
El-Salhy M, Gundersen D, Hatlebakk JG, Hausken T. Clinical presentation, diagnosis, pathogenesis and treatment options for lymphocytic colitis. *Int J Mol Med*. 2013.

 SEE ALSO

Algorithm: Diarrhea, Chronic

 CODES

ICD10
K52.9 Noninfective gastroenteritis and colitis, unspecified

CLINICAL PEARLS
- In patients with chronic diarrhea, consider IBS, IBD, malabsorption syndromes (such as lactose intolerance), celiac disease, and chronic infections (particularly in patients who are immunocompromised).
- A thorough medical history should guide appropriate evaluation.
- The selection of specific tests should depend on the likelihood of specific diagnoses.
- Consider over-the-counter medications and herbal products as potential causative agents.

DIFFUSE INTERSTITIAL LUNG DISEASE

Jacqueline L. Olin, MS, PharmD, BCPS, CPP • Brian D. Hertz, MD • J. Andrew Woods, PharmD, BCPS

 BASICS

DESCRIPTION
- Interstitial lung diseases (ILDs) represent a diverse group of chronic progressive lung diseases associated with alveolar inflammation and/or potentially irreversible pulmonary fibrosis.
- >200 individual diseases may present with similar characteristics, making ILD difficult to classify.
- A classification scheme proposed by the American Thoracic Society and European Respiratory Society includes these subtypes:
  - Known causes (environmental, occupational, or drug-associated disease)
  - Systemic disorders (e.g., sarcoidosis, Wegener granulomatosis, collagen vascular disease)
  - Rare lung diseases (e.g., pulmonary histiocytosis, lymphangioleiomyomatosis)
  - Idiopathic interstitial pneumonias (IIPs)
- Based on clinical, radiologic, and histologic features, IIPs are further subclassified into the following diagnoses:
  - Idiopathic pulmonary fibrosis (IPF), characterized by progressive dyspnea, cough, restrictive lung disease, and a specific histopathologic pattern
  - IIPs other than IPF (including nonspecific interstitial pneumonia [NSIP], respiratory bronchiolitis-associated ILD [RBILD], acute interstitial pneumonia [AIP], cryptogenic organizing pneumonia [COP], etc.)
- Classification of IIPs and relationships between the subtypes continue to be areas of clinical controversy.

Pediatric Considerations
ILD in infants and children represents a heterogeneous group of respiratory disorders. Diseases result from a variety of processes involving genetic factors and inflammatory or fibrotic responses, and these processes are distinct from those that cause ILD in adults (1). Some diseases result from developmental disorders and growth abnormalities in infancy (1,2). After common causes are excluded, referral of infants to a subspecialist is recommended (1)

EPIDEMIOLOGY
Incidence
- Exact incidence is difficult to determine because of differences in case definitions and procedures used in diagnosis.
- Ranges cited for incidence of IPF: 4.6–10.7/100,000 (3) and pediatric ILD of 1.32/1,000,000 (2).

Prevalence
- Exact prevalence is difficult to determine because of differences in case definitions and procedures used in diagnosis.
- Ranges cited for prevalence of IPF: 2–29 cases/100,000 in the general population (3) and pediatric ILD of 3.6/1 million (2)

ETIOLOGY AND PATHOPHYSIOLOGY
- Alveolar inflammation may progress into irreversible fibrosis.
- Varying degrees of ventilatory dysfunction occur among the ILD subtypes.
- ILD associated with collagen vascular disease and systemic connective disorders can manifest involvement of skin, joints, muscular, and ocular systems.

Some types of ILD are associated with specific exposures:

- Medications (amiodarone, antibiotics [especially nitrofurantoin], chemotherapy agents, gold, illicit drugs)
- Inorganic dusts (silicates, asbestos, talc, mica, coal dust, graphite)
- Organic dusts (moldy hay, inhalation of fungi, bacteria, animal proteins)
- Metals (tin, aluminum, cobalt, iron, barium)
- Gases, fumes, vapors, aerosols

Genetics
Some subtypes of ILD may be associated with specific predisposing genes and environmental exposures; however, the role of genetic factors is unknown.

RISK FACTORS
- Environmental or occupational exposure to inorganic or organic dusts
- 66–75% of patients with ILD have a history of smoking.
- Due to diversity of diseases, age is not a reliable predictor of pathology:
  - Most patients with connective tissue disease-related pathology and inherited subtypes present between ages 20 and 40.
  - Median age of patients with IPF is 66 years. Studies of clinical predictors of survival including age, ethnicity, and smoking status have been inconsistent (4).

GENERAL PREVENTION
Avoiding environmental/occupational exposure to organic or inorganic dust and smoking cessation may reduce incidence or improve clinical course in patients with established ILD.

COMMONLY ASSOCIATED CONDITIONS
Many systemic disorders and primary diseases are associated with ILD. A partial list includes:
- Collagen vascular disease
- Sarcoidosis
- Amyloidosis
- Goodpasture syndrome
- Churg-Strauss syndrome
- Wegener granulomatosis

DIAGNOSIS

- Diagnosis should be based on clinical, radiologic, and histologic data.
- A multidisciplinary consensus is recommended for diagnosis, because even among experts, diagnostic criteria are subject to interpretation.
- Accurate diagnosis imperative as treatment choices and prognosis can vary with pathogenesis.
- Diagnosis of IPF requires exclusion of other known ILD causes, the presence of a UIP pattern on high-resolution computed tomography (HRCT), and/or surgical lung biopsy pattern (3).

HISTORY
- Symptoms may include progressive exertional dyspnea and nonproductive cough.
- Patients may also present with hemoptysis or fatigue.
- Obtaining a history of illness duration (acute vs. chronic), potential environmental/occupational exposures, travel, medical conditions (including systemic diseases), and medication reconciliation is important in assessing the cause of the ILD.

- Some cases of lung disease may occur weeks to years after discontinuation of an offending agent (e.g., carmustine.)

PHYSICAL EXAM
Physical findings are usually nonspecific. Some common features include:
- Crackles (typically present upon auscultation of lung bases on posterior axillary line)
- Rales
- Inspiratory "squeaks"
- Clubbing of the digits and cyanosis in advanced disease

DIFFERENTIAL DIAGNOSIS
- Acute pulmonary edema
- Diffuse hemorrhage
- Atypical pneumonia
- Diffuse bronchoalveolar cell carcinoma or lymphatic spread of tumor

DIAGNOSTIC TESTS & INTERPRETATION
Initial Tests (lab, imaging)
- O_2 saturation
- Peak expiratory flow rate
- CBC with differential, comprehensive metabolic profile
- CRP or sedimentation rate
- Chest x-ray (CXR): Most commonly reticular pattern, less commonly nodular or mixed patterns

Follow-Up Tests & Special Considerations
HRCT of the chest is the most useful tool for distinguishing among ILD subclasses, especially if normal CXRs.
- If indicated, arterial blood gas (ABG), hypersensitivity pneumonitis panel, plasma ACE inhibitor concentration (sarcoidosis).
- If a systemic disorder is suspected, consider antinuclear antibody (ANA), rheumatoid factor (RF), erythrocyte sedimentation rate (ESR), and antineutrophil cytoplasmic antibodies (ANCA).

Diagnostic Procedures/Other
- Pulmonary function testing (PFT; spirometry, lung volumes, carbon monoxide diffusing capacity):
  - Commonly demonstrates a restrictive defect (decreased vital capacity and total lung capacity)
  - Forced vital capacity (FVC) has been shown to decline 100–200 mL/yr in the placebo arm of IPF patients in clinical trials (4).
- Bronchoscopy:
  - Bronchoalveolar lavage (BAL) cellular analysis studies may be useful in distinguishing subtypes (including sarcoidosis, hypersensitivity pneumonitis, cancer). If performed, the BAL target site should be chosen based on the HRCT finding (5).
  - Bronchoscopic transbronchial lung biopsy may help diagnose sarcoidosis and, on occasion, is sufficiently supportive of other ILD diagnoses.
- Thoracoscopic surgery for lung biopsy has the greatest diagnostic specificity for ILDs, but is less frequently used given improved specificity of HRCT. May be indicated if a diagnosis cannot be determined from transbronchial biopsy or HRCT.

Test Interpretation
- Diagnostic classifications of IIPs are based on histopathologic patterns seen on lung biopsy.
- Major histologies include an inflammation and fibrotic and granulomatous patterns.

- Characteristic changes on HRCT may help to distinguish between subtypes:
  - Reticulonodular, ground-glass opacities, and, in later stages, honeycombing may be seen.
  - Associated hilar and mediastinal adenopathy are characteristic of stage I and II sarcoidosis.
- No specific test is the gold standard, which emphasizes the importance of a multidisciplinary consensus for diagnosis with clinical, radiologic, and pathologic findings.

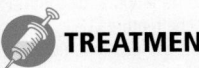 TREATMENT

- Evidence does not support the routine use of any specific therapy for ILD in general, and especially IPF (3).
- No survival benefit of home oxygen use in ILD (6)
- No evidence that any FDA-approved pharmacologic therapies improve survival or quality of life (3)[B]
- Small prospective trials with co-trimoxazole, thalidomide, and/or sildenafil have shown improvement in some quality of life parameters
- Corticosteroids have a role in some ILD subtypes (7)[A]
- Current evidence does not clearly support routine use of noncorticosteroid anti-inflammatory agents for IPF, including cyclosporine, azathioprine, colchicines, cyclophosphamide, cytokines, bosentan, etanercept, methotrexate, or interferon (3,8,9).
- Clinical trials have indicated that anticoagulation (warfarin) and endothelin receptor antagonists (ambrisentan, bosentan) are ineffective, potentially harmful, and therefore not recommended in the treatment of IPF (10,11,12,13)

GENERAL MEASURES
- Avoid/Minimize offending environmental/occupational exposures/medications
- Smoking cessation
- Supplemental oxygen, if indicated

MEDICATION
First Line
- Corticosteroids are most effective for certain ILDs, especially exacerbations of sarcoidosis, NSIP, COP, and hypersensitivity pneumonitis. However, response rates have been variable across and within subtypes. The optimal dose and duration of therapy are unknown.
- Common starting dose of prednisone is 0.5–1 mg/kg/d for 4–12 weeks, with potential up-titration to 0.5 mg/kg based on patient response.

Second Line
- 2nd-line agents have been used for IPF alone or in combination with steroids, with limited success rates:
  - Azathioprine was studied at 2–3 mg/kg/d (not to exceed 200 mg/d; adjusted to the nearest 25-mg dose increment) in combination with prednisone and, ultimately, as a steroid-sparing agent.
  - Interim analysis of a multicenter, three-arm trial comparing combination therapy (prednisone, azathioprine, N-acetylcysteine [NAC]), NAC alone, and placebo revealed that combination therapy was associated with increased mortality, hospitalization, and adverse events compared with placebo (14). The combination arm was terminated. Results from the NAC and placebo arms are expected at the end of 2013.
  - Pirfenidone, an orally active antifibroblast agent, available outside the US, demonstrated a

favorable risk-to-benefit profile in 2 randomized, placebo-controlled trials of patients with IPF (15). An additional phase III trial (ASCEND, Clinicaltrials.gov NCT01366209) is currently ongoing with results expected in 2014.
- An experimental tyrosine kinase inhibitor (BIBF 1120, nintedanib) was evaluated in a 12-month phase 2 trial in patients with IPF. Treatment resulted in a significant reduction in the annual rate of decline in FVC and fewer acute exacerbations (16). Results of phase 3 trials are expected in 2014.
- Several 2nd-line agents have been used in Wegener granulomatosis:
  - Cyclophosphamide is commonly used in treatment of Wegener granulomatosis. It is given 1.5–2 mg/kg/d PO for 3–6 months.
  - Methotrexate has been used in treatment of mild Wegener granulomatosis in combination with corticosteroids. A studied dosing regimen consisted of an initial methotrexate dose of 0.3 mg/kg (maximum dose of 15 mg) once weekly, with 2.5 mg titration each week (maximum dose of 25 mg/wk).
  - Other 2nd-line agents that have been studied include mycophenolate mofetil and rituximab.

SURGERY/OTHER PROCEDURES
Single- or double-lung transplantation may be a treatment of last resort. Some ILDs associated with systemic disease may recur in the recipient lung.

 ONGOING CARE

FOLLOW-UP RECOMMENDATIONS
Follow-up testing should include PFTs, cardiopulmonary stress test, pulse oximetry, and CXR.

PATIENT EDUCATION
National Heart, Lung, and Blood Institute at www.nhlbi.nih.gov/health/dci/Diseases/ipf/ipf_whatis.html

PROGNOSIS
IPF confers the worst prognosis (median survival of 2.5–3 years) (4). A clinical prediction model to estimate the risk of death from ILD has been described (17). Other subtypes, including hypersensitivity pneumonitis, nonspecific interstitial pneumonia, and cryptogenic organizing pneumonia, have a good prognosis.

COMPLICATIONS
- Cor pulmonale
- Pneumothorax
- Progressive respiratory failure

REFERENCES
1. Kurland G, Deterding RR, Hagood JS, et al. An official ATS clinical practice guideline: Classification, evaluation, and management of childhood interstitial lung disease in infancy. *Am J Respir Crit Care Med.* 2013;188:376–394.
2. Cazzato S, diPalmo E, Ragazzo V, et al. Interstitial lung disease in children. *Early Hum Dev.* 2013;S0378–S3782:00168-0.
3. Raghu G, Collard HR, Egan JJ, et al. An official ATS/ERS/JRS/ALAT statement: Idiopathic pulmonary fibrosis: Evidence-based guidelines for diagnosis and management. *Am J Respir Crit Care Med.* 2011;183:788–824.
4. Ley B, Collard HR, King TE, et al. Clinical course and prediction of survival in idiopathic pulmonary fibrosis. *Am J Respir Crit Care Med.* 2011;183: 431–440.
5. Meyer KC, Raghu G, Baughman RP, et al. An official ATS clinical practice guideline: The clinical utility of bronchoalveolar lavage cellular analysis in interstitial lung disease. *Am J Respir Crit Care Med.* 2012;185:1004–1014.
6. Crockett AJ, Cranston JM, Antic N, et al. Domiciliary oxygen for interstitial lung disease. *Cochrane Database Syst Rev.* 2001;3:CD002883.
7. Richeldi L, Davies HR, Ferrara G, et al. Corticosteroids for idiopathic pulmonary fibrosis. *Cochrane Database Syst Rev.* 2003;3:CD002880.
8. Spagnolo P, Del Giovane C, Luppi F, et al. Non-steroid agents for idiopathic pulmonary fibrosis. *Cochrane Database Syst Rev.* 2010;9:CD003134.
9. Davies HR, Richeldi L, Walters EH. Immunomodulatory agents for idiopathic pulmonary fibrosis. *Cochrane Database Syst Rev.* 2003;(3):CD003134.
10. Noth I, Anstrom KJ, Calvert SB, et al. A placebo-controlled randomized trial of warfarin in idiopathic pulmonary fibrosis. *Am J Respir Crit Care Med.* 2012;186:88–95.
11. Raghu G, Behr J, Brown JJ, et al. Treatment of idiopathic pulmonary fibrosis with ambrisentan: a parallel, randomized trial. *Ann Intern Med.* 2013;158:641–649.
12. King TE Jr, Behr J, Brown KK, et al. Build-1: A randomized placebo-controlled trial of bosentan in idiopathic pulmonary fibrosis. *Am J Respir Crit Care Med.* 2008;177:75–81.
13. King TE Jr, Brown KK, Raghu G, et al. Build-3: A randomized, controlled trial of bosentan in idiopathic pulmonary fibrosis. *Am J Respir Crit Care Med.* 2011;184:92–99.
14. Idiopathic Pulmonary Fibrosis Clinical Research Network, Raghu G, Anstrom KJ, et al. Prednisone, azathioprine, and N-acetylcysteine for pulmonary fibrosis. *N Engl J Med.* 2012;366:1968–1977.
15. Noble PW, Albera C, Bradford WZ, et al. Pirfenidone in patients with idiopathic pulmonary fibrosis: Two randomised trials. *Lancet.* 2011;377:1760–1769.
16. Richeldi L, Costabel U, Selman M, et al. Efficacy of a tyrosine kinase inhibitor in idiopathic pulmonary fibrosis. *N Engl J Med.* 2011;365:1079–1087.
17. Ryerson CJ, Vittinghoff E, Ley B, et al. Predicting survival across chronic interstitial lung disease: The ILD-GAP model. *Chest.* 2013, in press.

 CODES

ICD10
- J84.9 Interstitial pulmonary disease, unspecified
- J84.10 Pulmonary fibrosis, unspecified
- J84.111 Idiopathic interstitial pneumonia, not otherwise specified

CLINICAL PEARLS
- ILD differs from COPD; anatomically, ILD involves the lung parenchyma (i.e., alveoli) and COPD involves both airways and alveoli.
- In some cases, avoiding or minimizing offending environmental/occupational exposures, medications, and smoking may alter disease severity.
- A wide degree of prognostic variation occurs among different subtypes of ILD.

DISSECTION, CAROTID AND VERTEBRAL ARTERY
Robert A. Baldor, MD

 BASICS

DESCRIPTION
A cervical artery dissection occurs when the structural integrity is compromised in ≥1 of the 3 layers comprising the arterial walls of the internal carotid artery or vertebral artery. As a result, an intramural hematoma or pseudoaneurysm is formed. Together, carotid artery dissections (CAD) and vertebral artery dissections (VAD) make up a significant portion of ischemic strokes among young and middle-aged adults, although they can occur at any age.

EPIDEMIOLOGY
The incidence of cervical artery dissection in the general population is quite low (2.6 new cases in 100,000 per year; 95% CI 1.9–3.3) and likely underestimated due to the unknown number of asymptomatic cases only discovered anecdotally on imaging or autopsy (1). Of note, however, CAD occurs more frequently than VAD. CAD occurs 1.7 times per 100,000 per year (95% CI, 0.5–1.4) (1), whereas VAD occurs 1.0 times per 100,000 per year (95% CI, 1.1–2.3) (1). In fact, CAD and VAD even occur simultaneously in 13–16% of cases.

Incidence
- CAD was first described in 1959 in a case study of a spontaneous internal carotid artery dissection.
- Spontaneous CADs account for 14–20% of ischemic strokes in patients <50 years of age and 0.6–32% of ischemic strokes in all age groups (2). In total, nearly 1/4 of ischemic strokes affecting young adult patients can be attributed to CAD.
- Peak incidence occurs in the 5th decade of life, with women being affected on average 5 years earlier than men.

Prevalence
- Although cross-sectional North American studies have not shown any gender predominance (50–52% female), their European counterparts have demonstrated a male predominance (53–57% male).
- Seasonal patterns suggest higher rates of occurrence during the autumn and winter months, which may correlate with the incidence of weather-related confounding variables such as infection rates and seasonal sports (3).

ETIOLOGY AND PATHOPHYSIOLOGY
- Dissection can occur as a result of intimal tearing caused by traumatic shearing forces. Expansion of the intramural hematoma that develops eventually results in vascular lumen stenosis.
- Dissection can also occur through intramural bleeding directly from the rupture of penetrating vasa vasorum vessels. In this case, adventitial expansion results in an aneurysmal dilation of the injured artery.
- Extracranial arterial segments are more vulnerable than their intracranial counterparts. This is a result of neck mobility exceeding vascular elasticity:
  - The internal carotid artery is endangered by tethering at the carotid canal, its entry point into the skull.
  - The vertebral artery is at risk as it tortuously passes through the transverse foramina of C2 to C1.

- Embolism of intraluminal thrombi at the site of intimal tearing makes up 92% of the ischemic strokes following cervical artery dissection. Other mechanisms of CNS hypoperfusion include stenosis, occlusion, and pseudo-aneurysmal rupture.
- When arterial dissections extend intracranially, subarachnoid hemorrhages can occur. This is because intracranial arterial walls are thinner and less elastic than their cervical counterparts.
- Roughly classified as traumatic and spontaneous mechanisms:
  - Traumatic: Includes significant penetrating or blunt trauma. Occurs in 1–2% of trauma patients, in particular those with skull fractures. CAD is associated with major thoracic injuries, whereas VAD occurrence is more often related to cervical spine fractures.
  - Spontaneous: Unprovoked lesions associated with a wide variety of physical activities, otherwise presumed to be benign, involving sudden or sustained neck hyperextensions or rotations including, but not limited to, coughing, sneezing, vomiting, swimming, chiropractic manipulation, and yoga.

Genetics
- Concomitant occurrence with genetic disorders such as Ehlers-Danlos type IV (most common), Marfan syndrome, osteogenesis imperfecta type I, syphilis, autosomal-dominant polycystic kidney disease, α_1-antitrypsin deficiency, hereditary hemochromatosis, Turner syndrome, and Williams syndrome have all been published in case reports. Therefore, 20% of CAD and 25% of VAD are considered to be associated with these rare connective tissue disorders (4).
- Polymorphisms: ICAM-1 (intracellular adhesion molecule-1) and MTHFR (methylene-tetrahydrofolate reductase) have been implicated as well, but studies are underpowered (4).

RISK FACTORS
- Recent studies have proposed a number of potential risk factors, including infection, hyperhomocystein anemia, low folate levels, oral contraceptive use, migraines, and arterial hypertension, as potential predisposing risk factors. However, the literature on this topic is composed of isolated case studies and single-institution trials limited by small sample size, selection bias, and confounding variables.

GENERAL PREVENTION
No specific prevention measures are known.

COMMONLY ASSOCIATED CONDITIONS
- Retinal ischemia and ischemic optic neuropathy (CAD)
- Spinal cord ischemia and cervical radiculopathies (VAD)
- Horner syndrome (CAD more often than VAD)

 DIAGNOSIS

HISTORY
- Symptoms preceding cerebral ischemia:
  - Headaches: The most common finding. Gradual to sudden onset that precedes ischemic symptoms by minutes to days:
    ○ CAD: Ipsilateral and frontotemporal discomfort with stereotypic headache features.
    ○ VAD: Occipital and posterior location; more challenging to identify.
  - Neck pain: More common in VAD (46%) than in CAD (26%)
  - Horner syndrome (oculosympathetic palsy): Presents as ipsilateral miosis and ptosis without anhidrosis (the sympathetic innervation of facial sweat glands is located on the external carotid artery). More common in CAD (28–58%) than in VAD (27%).
  - Cranial nerve palsy: Relatively rare (7% incidence); most commonly affects the hypoglossal nerve (12%), presenting as taste impairment and pulsatile tinnitus, followed by the glossopharyngeal and the vagus nerves.
  - Transient monocular blindness may also precede an ischemic stroke.
- Manifestations of cerebral transient ischemic attacks: Occur in 67% of cervical artery dissections and can vary in onset from minutes to up to a month before the stroke itself (1). 20% of patients have no warning signs prior to their strokes.

PHYSICAL EXAM
- Horner syndrome: Ptosis and miosis without anhidrosis; innervation to the sweat glands is from the sympathetic plexus around the external carotid artery.
- Cerebral ischemia:
  - CAD: Most commonly affects the middle cerebral artery perfusion territory, which includes most of the outer cortex of the brain, the basal ganglia, and the posterior and anterior internal capsules. Therefore, sequelae of an ischemic injury include a wide range of motor and/or sensory deficits.
  - VAD: Typically affects the brainstem, cerebellum, and occipital lobes, resulting in a range of medullary syndromes, ataxias, and visual impairments.

DIFFERENTIAL DIAGNOSIS
- Migraine, cluster, or tension headaches
- Neck trauma and cervical spine fracture
- Ischemic stroke, hemorrhagic stroke
- Retinal artery or vein occlusion

DIAGNOSTIC TESTS & INTERPRETATION
Initial Tests (lab, imaging)
- No specific labs
- Imaging is crucial in the diagnosis and monitoring of CAD. Angiographic images facilitate high-resolution visualization of intramural and intraluminal hematoma development:
  - CT angiography is the test of choice ("string and pearl sign"), although digital subtraction arteriography is the gold standard.
  - CT angiography is a noninvasive method using contrast and providing useful information about the arterial lumen and the vessel wall, with a sensitivity approaching 100% and specificity approaching 96–98% when compared with conventional angiography (4)[C].
  - Conventional angiography is no longer recommended because of the associated risks of a more invasive procedure and poor visualization of intramural lesions.
  - MRI/MRA is rapidly replacing CT angiography in many centers as the image quality continues to improve. Benefits include no radiation exposure, renoprotective doses of contrast, better intramural visualization, and T_1-weighted fat-suppression techniques detect smaller lesions (5)[C].

Diagnostic Procedures/Other
Color duplex ultrasound is noninvasive and has a sensitivity of 96% and a specificity of 94% for patients with CAD who have symptoms of carotid territory ischemia. However, it is highly operator dependent, and findings always require confirmation by CT angiography or MRI/MRA.

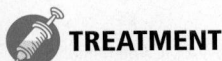

TREATMENT

MEDICATION
- Anticoagulation therapy, short-acting (acute phase)
- Antiplatelet therapy (acute phase)
- Anticoagulation therapy, long-acting (subacute phase)
- Antiplatelet therapy (chronic phase)

First Line
- Anticoagulation or antiplatelet therapy should be initiated in the acute phase of a CAD to reduce the incidence of primary or recurrent ischemic stroke. Despite being standard practice, a randomized control trial comparing the efficacy of each treatment modality is not yet available (6)[A].
- Anticoagulation is sometimes preferred over antiplatelet therapy with severe stenosis or evidence of a free-floating thrombus or a cerebral embolism.
- Antiplatelet therapy is favored when a large infarction or hemorrhage has occurred. In addition, antiplatelet therapy should be used when the dissection affects the intracranial portion of the vessels, which significantly increases the risk of subarachnoid hemorrhage.
- Patients who undergo antiplatelet therapy have a 1.8–3.8% risk of stroke, whereas anticoagulation has a 1.2% risk of stroke and a 0.5% risk of intracranial hemorrhage.

- Despite expressed concerns, available data show that IV thrombolysis (tPA) should not be withheld in cases where CAD is associated with acute ischemic stroke (6)[A].

Second Line
See "Surgery/Other Procedures."

SURGERY/OTHER PROCEDURES
- Surgical therapies include thrombectomy, vessel ligation, primary dissection, and repair. However, surgical interventions are often technically challenging and more risky than endovascular techniques.
- Endovascular therapy includes stenting, coiling, stent-assisted coiling, and embolization and occlusion of the vascular lesion along with the parent vessel:
  - Endovascular therapy is recommended in patients who fail medical therapy after 6 months of anticoagulation therapy or for whom anticoagulation is contraindicated.
  - Failure of medical therapy is defined as a new ischemic event, worsening neurologic findings, or enlargement of the pseudoaneurysm.

  - Data on endovascular interventions are limited and lacking homogeneity between surgical technique and equipment types; however, overall outcomes analysis suggests impressive results (98.4% technical success with only a 1.3% complication rate) (7)[A].

 ONGOING CARE

FOLLOW-UP RECOMMENDATIONS
- Follow up with a neurologist is highly recommended.
- After initiating a short course of anticoagulation or antiplatelet therapy, patients should be bridged to warfarin for 3 months.
- Repeat imaging is useful to guide further treatment decisions. Another 3 months of warfarin therapy may be considered if persistent stenosis is detected.
- Anticoagulants are usually maintained for no longer than 6 months. Following this period, anticoagulation is either stopped or substituted by antiplatelet therapy, which can be continued for 2 years.

Patient Monitoring
Closer follow up for an extended period of time is recommended in patients with underlying connective tissue disorders, as they are at a higher risk of recurrence.

PROGNOSIS
- Highest risk of death occurs during the acute phase (<5%); however, among patient subgroups symptomatic for ischemic stroke, risk of mortality can rise to 23%.
- Recurrence rates for ischemic events within the 1st year varied from 0% to 13.3%; however, most occurred in the initial weeks after dissection.
- Overall, good long-term prognosis with low rates of recurrence and complications and high rates of favorable outcome (4)

REFERENCES
1. Lee VH, Brown RD, Mandrekar JN, et al. Incidence and outcome of cervical artery dissection: A population-based study. Neurology. 2006;67: 1809–1812.
2. Chandra A, Suliman A, Angle N, et al. Spontaneous dissection of the carotid and vertebral arteries: The 10-year UCSD experience. Ann Vasc Surg. 2007; 21:178–185.
3. Paciaroni M, Georgiadis D, Arnold M, et al. Seasonal variability in spontaneous cervical artery dissection. J Neurol Neurosurg Psychiatr. 2006;77: 677–679.
4. Kim YK, Schulman S. Cervical artery dissection: Pathology, epidemiology and management. Thromb Res. 2009;123:810–821.
5. Provenzale JM. MRI and MRA for evaluation of dissection of craniocerebral arteries: Lessons from the medical literature. Emerg Radiol. 2009;16: 185–193.
6. Menon R, Kerry S, Norris JW, et al. Treatment of cervical artery dissection: A systematic review and meta-analysis. J Neurol Neurosurg Psychiatr. 2008;79:1122–1127.
7. Pham MH, Rahme RJ, Arnaout O, et al. Endovascular stenting of extracranial carotid and vertebral artery dissections: A systematic review of the literature. Neurosurgery. 2011;68:856–866.

CODES
ICD10
- I77.71 Dissection of carotid artery
- I77.74 Dissection of vertebral artery

CLINICAL PEARLS
- CAD and VAD are common causes of ischemic stroke in young and middle-aged adults.
- Neck pain, headache, and/or Horner syndrome followed by manifestations of cerebral ischemia should prompt evaluation for CAD.
- The mechanism of cerebral ischemia is, in most cases, embolic and, less commonly, thrombotic or hemorrhagic.
- CT angiography is the test of choice ("string and pearl sign").
- Anticoagulation and/or antiplatelet therapy is the mainstays of treatment. Patients refractory to conservative treatment after 6 months should be re-evaluated for invasive interventions, including angioplasty, stenting, surgical ligation, or primary vascular repair.

D

DISSEMINATED INTRAVASCULAR COAGULATION

Jan Cerny, MD, PhD • Mary Lopresti, DO

 BASICS

DESCRIPTION

- Disseminated intravascular coagulation (DIC) is an acquired syndrome characterized by diffuse activation of intravascular coagulation. It can originate from and cause damage to the microvasculature, which, if sufficiently severe, can produce organ dysfunction.
- Occurs as a complication of pregnancy (e.g., abruptio placentae, fetus retention, amniotic fluid embolism), infection (especially gram-negative), malignancy (uncontrolled, metastatic tumor or leukemia), trauma, and other severe illnesses
- System(s) affected: Hematologic/Lymphatic/Immunologic
- Synonym(s): Consumptive coagulopathy

EPIDEMIOLOGY

Incidence

>500,000 patients per year in the US

Prevalence

- Predominant age: None
- Predominant sex: Male = Female

ETIOLOGY AND PATHOPHYSIOLOGY

- Systemic formation of fibrin is the result of the simultaneous coexistence of:
  - Increased thrombin generation via tissue factor-/factor VII-mediated pathway
  - Suppression of the physiologic anticoagulant pathways:
    ○ Antithrombin due to consumption, degradation, and impaired synthesis
    ○ Proteins C and S due to decreased levels of thrombomodulin (TM)
  - Impaired fibrinolysis (early on):
    ○ Sustained increase in plasminogen activator inhibitor, type 1
- Increased fibrinolysis (late during the process) leads to bleeding.

Causes can be classified as acute or chronic, systemic or localized:

- Sepsis/Severe infection (any micro-organism)
- Trauma (polytrauma, neurotrauma)
- Obstetric complications (amniotic fluid embolism, abruptio placentae)
- Solid tumors and leukemias (especially acute promyelocytic leukemia)
- Vascular disorders, such as Kasabach-Merritt syndrome, large vascular aneurysms, and thrombosis
- Organ destruction (severe pancreatitis, severe liver failure)

- Severe toxic or immunologic reactions:
  - Snake bite
  - Recreational drugs
  - Transfusion reactions
  - Transplant rejection
  - Thermal injury
- Infant and adult respiratory distress syndrome
- Neonatal purpura fulminans

RISK FACTORS

See "Etiology and Pathophysiology."

GENERAL PREVENTION

Aggressive interventions aimed at early treatment of the underlying clinical conditions

COMMONLY ASSOCIATED CONDITIONS

Thromboembolic phenomena are associated with venous thrombosis, thrombotic vegetations on the aortic heart valve, arterial emboli, and neonatal purpura fulminans (homozygous protein C or protein S deficiency).

Pediatric Considerations

Neonatal purpura fulminans is associated with DIC and protein C or protein S deficiency (homozygous).

 DIAGNOSIS

Symptoms and signs are related to the underlying disease process and DIC.

HISTORY

Symptoms of microvascular thrombosis (e.g., renal failure), as well as diffuse bleeding

PHYSICAL EXAM

- Bleeding manifestations:
  - Skin (petechiae, purpura, ecchymosis, generalized oozing from venipuncture sites and wounds)
  - Renal (hematuria)
  - GI (mucous membranes and intestinal bleeding)
  - Neurologic (hemorrhagic infarction, massive intracerebral bleeding)
  - Respiratory (epistaxis, pulmonary hemorrhage)
- Microvascular thrombosis:
  - Skin (skin infarction, digital gangrene)
  - GI (mucosal ulcerations, bowel infarction)
  - Renal (oliguria, anuria, uremia)
  - Pulmonary (hypoxemia, acute respiratory distress syndrome)
  - Neurologic (convulsions, delirium, coma, multifocal cortical infarction)

DIFFERENTIAL DIAGNOSIS

- Fulminant liver failure or massive hepatic necrosis
- Vitamin K deficiency
- Thrombotic thrombocytopenic purpura
- Hemolytic–uremic syndrome
- Heparin-induced thrombocytopenia
- Primary fibrinolysis
- HELLP syndrome in pregnancy (hemolysis, elevated liver function, and low platelets)

DIAGNOSTIC TESTS & INTERPRETATION

No single laboratory test is sensitive and specific enough to allow a definitive diagnosis of DIC.

Initial Tests (lab, imaging)

- Thrombocytopenia
- Increased partial thromboplastin time (PTT)
- Increased prothrombin test (PT)
- Decreased fibrinogen (serial levels)
- Increased fibrin degradation product (FDP)
- Positive D-dimer
- Decreased antithrombin III, decreased protein C
- Other labs that may have prognostic significance:
  - Decreased Adams-13
  - Increase soluble TM, plasminogen activator inhibitor-1 (PAI-1), von Willebrand factor peptide
  - Decrease des-R-prothrombin activation peptide fragment 2 (1):
- Microangiopathic hemolytic anemia (schistocytes, increased lactate dehydrogenase levels, low hemoglobin)

ALERT

Diagnostic algorithm for overt DIC (International Society on Thrombosis and Haemostasis) (2):

- Assess if underlying disease is known to be associated with DIC:
  - YES: Proceed with this algorithm.
  - NO: Do not use this algorithm.
- Order global coagulation tests (PT, PTT, fibrinogen, soluble fibrin monomers, or FDPs)
- Score global coagulation test results:
  - Platelet count (>100 = 0, <100 = 1, <50 = 2)
  - Elevated fibrin-related markers (no increase = 0, moderate increase = 2, strong increase = 3)
  - Prolonged PT (<3 seconds = 0, >3 but <6 seconds = 1, >6 seconds = 2)
  - Fibrinogen level (>1 g/L = 0, <1 g/L = 1)
- Calculate score:
  - If ≥5: Compatible with DIC; repeat scoring daily. If <5: Suggestive of nonovert DIC; repeat in 1–2 days (3).

Follow-Up Tests & Special Considerations

Frequent follow up of initially abnormal laboratory tests to see effect of therapeutic interventions

TREATMENT

Heterogeneity of the underlying disorders and the clinical presentations makes the therapeutic approach to DIC difficult:

- Appropriate health care: Inpatient and intensive care unit (depending on underlying condition)
- Treat underlying condition (e.g., evacuation of uterus in abruptio placentae; broad-spectrum antibiotics for gram-negative sepsis)
- Supportive care with transfusions in patients who are bleeding, going for surgery, or at high risk of bleeding. Do not treat abnormal laboratory parameters:
  – Fresh frozen plasma
  – Platelet concentrates
  – Cryoprecipitate or fibrinogen concentrates (4)
- Anticoagulants remain very controversial. Therapeutic heparin may be considered in cases where thrombosis dominates. Deep venous thrombosis prophylaxis is recommended in patients who are not bleeding.
- Restoration of anticoagulant pathways:
  – Recombinant human-activated protein C once had a level of evidence for use only in selected high-risk patients in ICU setting (5)[A]. The drug was, however, removed from the market in 2012.
  – Activated factor VII, antithrombin, and recombinant human TM-α use remains controversial.
  – Antifibrinolytic treatment is generally not recommended but may be considered in those with severe bleeding and marked hyperfibrinolytic state (i.e., trauma and acute promyelocytic leukemia).

MEDICATION
Broad-spectrum antibiotics for sepsis

SURGERY/OTHER PROCEDURES
Surgical treatment or procedures should be considered, especially if they are treating the underlying condition (e.g., evacuation of uterus in abruptio placentae; some trauma or bleeding situations).

IN-PATIENT CONSIDERATIONS
Admission Criteria/Initial Stabilization
Usually dictated by severity of underlying condition. Some cases can be managed in a standard ward, but ICU care is typical.

- Treat underlying disorder
- Frequent monitoring of clinical and laboratory response

Discharge Criteria
Once clinical and laboratory criteria are significantly improved and underlying reason for DIC is under control

ONGOING CARE

FOLLOW-UP RECOMMENDATIONS
Patient Monitoring
- Monitor closely until much improved
- Serial platelet count, coagulation tests, and fibrinogen levels to see effect of therapeutic interventions

PROGNOSIS
- Related to the severity of cause
- Decreased antithrombin level is a poor prognostic factor in DIC.

COMPLICATIONS
- Acute renal failure
- Shock
- Cardiac tamponade
- Hemothorax
- Intracerebral hematoma
- Various thrombotic complications, including myocardial infarction, stroke, gangrene, and loss of digits

REFERENCES

1. Chung S, Kim JE, Kim HK, et al. Serum des-R prothrombin activation peptide fragment 2: A novel prognostic marker for disseminated intravascular coagulation. *Thromb Res.* 2013;131:547–553.
2. Voves C, Wuillemin WA, Zeerleder S, et al. International Society on Thrombosis and Haemostasis score for overt disseminated intravascular coagulation predicts organ dysfunction and fatality in sepsis patients. *Blood Coagul Fibrinolysis.* 2006;17:445–451.
3. Levi M, Toh CH, Thachil J, et al. Guidelines for the diagnosis and management of disseminated intravascular coagulation. British Committee for Standards in Haematology. *Br J Haematol.* 2009; 145:24–33.
4. Franchini M, Lippi G, Manzato F. Recent acquisitions in the pathophysiology, diagnosis and treatment of disseminated intravascular coagulation. *Thromb J.* 2006;4:4.
5. Vincent JL, Bernard GR, Beale R, et al. Drotrecogin alfa (activated) treatment in severe sepsis from the global open-label trial ENHANCE: Further evidence for survival and safety and implications for early treatment. *Crit Care Med.* 2005;33:2266–2277.

ADDITIONAL READING

- Levi M. Disseminated intravascular coagulation. *Crit Care Med.* 2007;35:2191–2195.
- Taylor FB, Toh CH, Hoots WK, et al. Towards definition, clinical and laboratory criteria, and a scoring system for disseminated intravascular coagulation. *Thromb Haemost.* 2001;86: 1327–1330.

CODES

ICD10
- D65 Disseminated intravascular coagulation
- P60 Disseminated intravascular coagulation of newborn

CLINICAL PEARLS

- Treat underlying condition(s); transfusions represent supportive measures.
- Transfusions are not indicated in patients with abnormal laboratory parameters without clinical bleeding.

D

DIVERTICULAR DISEASE

David M. Hardy, MD • Steven Holsten, MD

BASICS

DESCRIPTION
Diverticular disease includes asymptomatic diverticulosis, symptomatic uncomplicated diverticulitis, symptomatic complicated diverticulitis, and diverticular bleeding.
- Diverticula: Outpouchings of colonic mucosa and submucosa through weakened muscle layers in the colonic wall:
  - Diverticulosis has a higher prevalence in societies that consume a low-fiber diet.
  - In Western societies, 90–95% of diverticulosis is left-sided; Asian populations have more right-sided disease.
  - Prevalence of diverticulosis and number of diverticula increase with age.
- Diverticular hemorrhage: Occurs in 3–5% of patients with diverticular disease:
  - Accounts for >40% of lower GI bleeds and 17–40% of cases of hematochezia in general
  - Bleeding more common if right-sided.
- Uncomplicated diverticulitis: Typical presentation, affects 10–25% of patients with diverticulosis
- Symptomatic uncomplicated diverticular disease [SUDD]: Recurrent abdominal pain attributed to diverticula in the absence of macroscopically overt colitis or diverticulitis (1)
- Complicated diverticulitis includes associated abscess, perforation, fistula, or stricture.
- System(s) affected: Gastrointestinal

EPIDEMIOLOGY
Incidence
- Diverticulosis <5% in general population, diverticulitis 1–2% in the US (1)
- Diverticulitis: 2,400–3,800/100,000
- Yearly mortality rate: 2.5/100,000

Prevalence
- 5% by age 40; 30% by age 60; 65% by age 85
- Male = Female overall, but more male <65 and more female >65

ETIOLOGY AND PATHOPHYSIOLOGY
Diverticula form at the site of penetration of the mucosa by the vasa recta. Structural changes result in decreased resistance to intraluminal pressure. Diverticulitis occurs when perforation of the diverticulum occurs.
- Age-related degeneration of mucosal wall; increased intraluminal pressure from dense, fiber-depleted stools and abnormal colonic motility
- Occur at areas of weakness from junctures of penetrating arteries in the muscular wall
- Bleeding is caused by medial thinning of the vasa recta and weakening of the artery as it courses over the neck of the diverticula.
- Diverticulitis occurs when increased intraluminal pressure results in local inflammation and necrosis, leading to micro- or macroperforation.
- Chronic microscopic inflammation around diverticula is also a cause (1).
- Another hypothesis is shifting in intestinal microbiota, leading to chronic inflammation (1,2).
- Evidence for overlapping of diverticular disease and irritable bowel syndrome (IBS) (visceral hypersensitivity)

Genetics
- No known genetic pattern
- Asian and African populations have lower prevalence, but diverticular disease develops with adoption of a Western lifestyle.

RISK FACTORS
- Age >40
- Low-fiber diet
- Sedentary lifestyle, obesity
- Previous diverticulitis and number of diverticula
- Smoking increases the risk of perforation (1).
- NSAIDs, steroids, and opiate analgesics increase diverticular hemorrhage whereas calcium channel blockers and statins have protective effects.

GENERAL PREVENTION
High-fiber diet (>30 g/d of fiber) or add nonabsorbable fiber (psyllium)

COMMONLY ASSOCIATED CONDITIONS
Connective tissue diseases, colon cancer, and inflammatory bowel disease

DIAGNOSIS

HISTORY
Immunocompromised patients may not present with fever or leukocytosis; they are at higher risk for perforation and abscess formation (2):
- Diverticulosis:
  - 80–85% of patients remain asymptomatic. Of the 15–20% with symptoms, 1–2% will need hospitalization and 0.5% will need surgery.
  - Pain: Dull, colicky, mostly in left lower quadrant, can be worse after eating, some relief following bowel movement or passage of flatus
  - Diarrhea or constipation
- Diverticulitis: Uncomplicated (75%) and complicated (25%):
  - Pain: Acute onset, mostly localized in left lower quadrant; prominently associated with tenderness in same region
  - Fever with chills as severity increases
  - Anorexia, nausea (20–62%), or vomiting
  - Constipation (50%) or diarrhea (25–35%)
  - Dysuria, frequency if bladder involved
  - Pneumaturia, fecaluria if colovesical fistula develops
- Diverticular hemorrhage:
  - Melena, hematochezia
  - Painless rectal bleeding

PHYSICAL EXAM
- Diverticulosis:
  - May be completely normal
  - May have intermittent distension or tympany
  - No signs of peritoneal inflammation
- Diverticulitis:
  - Localized tenderness usually LLQ
  - Rebound tenderness, involuntary guarding, or rigidity
  - Palpable mass in LLQ (20%) that is tender, firm, or fixed
  - Abdominal distension and tympany
  - Bowel sounds hypoactive or could be high-pitched and intermittent if obstruction ensues
  - Rectal exam may reveal tenderness, induration, or mass in the cul-de-sac.

- Colovaginal, colovesical, and perirectal fistulae may be the initial manifestation (rarely).
- Important: If tenderness and guarding are generalized, have high suspicion for perforation.

DIFFERENTIAL DIAGNOSIS
IBS, lactose intolerance, carcinoma, inflammatory bowel disease, fecal impaction, incarcerated hernia, gallbladder disease, angiodysplasia, colitis, acute appendicitis, ectopic pregnancy

DIAGNOSTIC TESTS & INTERPRETATION
Initial Tests (lab, imaging)
- WBC normal in diverticulosis; usually elevated with immature polymorphs in diverticulitis (normal in up to 45% of diverticulitis patients)
- Hemoglobin normal (unless bleeding)
- ESR elevated in diverticulitis
- UA may be abnormal with microscopic pyuria, hematuria, pneumaturia, or fecaluria (if fistula)
- Urine culture: Persistent infection in colovesical fistula
- Blood culture: Positive in diverticulitis with generalized peritonitis
- Malnutrition, steroids, or immunosuppressive drugs may alter lab results.
- Diverticulosis:
  - Asymptomatic diverticulosis is commonly an incidental finding on colonoscopy.
- Diverticulitis:
  - Plain film abdomen, supine and upright; useful for urgent assessment of megacolon or free air
  - If suspected diverticulitis: CT scan with IV, oral, and rectal contrast (3)[A]
  - CT helps determine degree of acute perforation and assists in surgical planning.
  - US is effective in identifying diverticulitis in the acute setting.
  - Barium enema is not recommended due to risk of extravasation into the peritoneum.
- Diverticular bleeding/Hematochezia:
  - Endoscopy is the test of choice for the evaluation of lower GI bleeding (4).
  - Angiography is used if massive bleeding obscures endoscopy or when endoscopy cannot visualize a source (4).

Follow-Up Tests & Special Considerations
- After resolution of an initial episode of acute diverticulitis: Colonoscopy to exclude any associated malignancies, strictures, or inflammatory bowel disease (3).
- After an episode of lower GI bleeding, colonoscopy should be performed to exclude neoplasia.

Diagnostic Procedures/Other
- For evaluation of hematochezia in suspected diverticular hemorrhage:
  - A nasogastric tube should be placed to exclude upper GI sources of bleeding (4).
  - 99mTc-pertechnetate–labeled RBC scans can be used before angiography to evaluate if angiography can be effective in revealing a source (not studied in a comparison trial) (4).
- For diverticulitis, gallium- or indium-labeled leukocytes to localize abscess (rarely used)

Test Interpretation

- Most right-sided diverticula are true diverticula (all layers of the colonic wall).
- Most left-sided diverticula are actually pseudodiverticula (outpouchings of the mucosa and submucosa).
- Surgical and autopsy studies show mycosis, a constellation of thickened circular muscle (pseudohypertrophy due to increased elastin in the taeniae), short taeniae, and luminal narrowing.
- Diverticulitis: Inflammation with lymphocytic infiltrate, ulceration, mucin depletion necrosis, Paneth cell metaplasia, and cryptitis

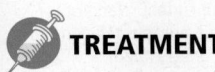 TREATMENT

GENERAL MEASURES

- Diverticulosis: Outpatient with fiber supplements to soften stools
- Outpatient diverticulitis: Pain, tenderness, leukocytosis, but no toxicity or peritoneal signs; use oral antibiotics. 1–2% of subjects require hospitalization for toxicity, septicemia, peritonitis, or failure of symptoms to be resolved in a few days. Up to 30% of patients may require surgery at 1st episode of diverticulitis. Up to 50% of patients with diverticulitis eventually may come to surgery.
- Toxic patients require hospitalization, bowel rest with clear liquids or NPO, and IV antibiotics at least until there is a positive response.
- Symptomatic improvement is expected within 2–3 days of initiating antibiotics, and antibiotics are continued for 7–10 days.
- 80% of diverticular hemorrhages will resolve spontaneously (4).

MEDICATION
First Line

- Diverticulosis:
  - High fiber intake is recommended (preferably >20–30 g/d) (3)[A].
- Symptomatic uncomplicated diverticular disease: Cyclical rifaximin or mesalamine continuously (3)[B]; mesalamine 400–800 mg b.i.d. decreases relapse and relieves symptoms (1)
- Uncomplicated diverticulitis:
  - Oral antibiotics for outpatient treatment of mild disease: Cover for anaerobes and gram-negative rods with:
  - A quinolone (ciprofloxacin or levofloxacin) *PLUS* metronidazole (Flagyl) (may use clindamycin if metronidazole intolerant) *OR*
    ○ Bactrim *PLUS* metronidazole
    ○ Treat for 7–10 days
  - New evidence shows no significant difference between antibiotics vs. no antibiotics in uncomplicated diverticulitis; further studies are needed (5)[A].
  - Inpatient: Use IV antibiotics:
    ○ Quinolone plus metronidazole
    ○ Monotherapy with a β-lactam/β-lactamase inhibitor: Zosyn or Unasyn or ertapenem
    ○ Unresponsive or severe disease: Imipenem or meropenem
  - Recurrences of acute diverticulitis may be decreased by using mesalamine ± rifaximin (6)[A] or probiotics.
- Diverticular bleeding:
  - Consider vasopressin 0.2–0.3 units/min through selective intra-arterial catheter.

- Precautions:
  - Avoid morphine and other opiates that may increase intraluminal pressure or promote ileus.
  - Increased fiber intake is not recommended in the acute management of diverticulitis.

Second Line
- Outpatient: Augmentin or Moxifloxacin
- Severely ill inpatients: Ampicillin + metronidazole + a quinolone *OR* ampicillin + metronidazole + an aminoglycoside

ISSUES FOR REFERRAL
Acutely suspected perforation, peritoneal signs, persistent bleeding requiring multiple transfusions

SURGERY/OTHER PROCEDURES
- Indication for emergent surgery: Peritonitis, uncontrolled sepsis, visceral perforation, colonic obstruction, or acute deterioration
- Surgery for nonemergent state is controversial, sometimes even in complicated cases.
- Elective surgery after acute diverticulitis: Decision for elective resection should be made on a case-by-case basis (3)[B]:
  - After 1st episode, there is a 33% chance of recurrence; if it does recur, there is a 66% chance of a 3rd bout.
  - Most complicated cases occur on the 1st presentation with subsequent presentations being uncomplicated.
  - Emergent surgery carries a 9-fold increase in mortality vs. elective.
  - Elective surgery recommendations should be based not on number of recurrences but on severity of complaints and complications.
  - Elective resection is typically advised after recovery from a complicated diverticulitis treated nonoperatively (3)[B].
  - Age: Younger patients more likely to have recurrence
  - Immunocompromised patients: More likely to present with acute complicated diverticulitis, fail medical management, and have complications from elective surgery.
- Large abscesses (>4 cm) are usually drained radiologically, and many of these patients can be acutely managed nonoperatively (3).
- In diverticular hemorrhage, if >4 units of RBC transfused, then 60% chance of requiring surgical intervention to stop bleeding (if <4 units, typically not) (4).

COMPLEMENTARY AND ALTERNATIVE MEDICINE
Probiotics such as *Lactobacillus casei* and *E. coli* Nissle 1917 may lengthen remission (2).

IN-PATIENT CONSIDERATIONS
Admission Criteria/Initial Stabilization
- ~1–2% need admit for toxicity, septicemia, peritonitis
- IV fluids, analgesics, antibiotics, NG suction

 ONGOING CARE

DIET
- NPO during acute diverticulitis; progress to fluids, then high-fiber diet as bowel function returns
- Patients with known diverticulosis or a history of diverticulitis should eat a high-fiber diet (>30 g/d) to prevent recurrence (7).
- Nuts, corn, and popcorn do not increase risk for diverticulosis or diverticular complications (8).

PROGNOSIS
- Good with early detection and treatment of complications
- Recurrence risk increases with each bout.
- If diverticular bleeding, rebleeding occurs in up to 6%.
- Diverticulitis recurs more often in younger patients, but severity is similar to elderly (9)[A].

COMPLICATIONS
Hemorrhage, perforation, peritonitis, obstruction, abscess, or fistula

REFERENCES
1. Strate LL, Modi R, Cohen E, et al. Diverticular disease as a chronic illness: Evolving epidemiologic and clinical insights. *Am J Gastroenterol*. 2012; 107(10):1486–1493.
2. Sheth AA, Longo W, Floch MH. Diverticular disease and diverticulitis. *Am J Gastroenterol*. 2008;103(6): 1550–1556.
3. Rafferty J, Shellito P, Hyman NH, et al. Practice parameters for sigmoid diverticulitis. *Dis Colon Rectum*. 2006;49(7):939–944.
4. Zuccaro G. Management of the adult patient with acute lower gastrointestinal bleeding. American College of Gastroenterology. *Practice Parameters Committee. Am J Gastroenterol*. 1998;93: 1202–1208.
5. Shabanzadeh DM, Wille-Jørgensen P. Antibiotics for uncomplicated diverticulitis. *Cochrane Database Syst Rev*. 2012;11:CD009092. Epub 2012 Nov 14.
6. Gatta L, Vakil N, Vaira D, et al. Efficacy of 5-ASA in the treatment of colonic diverticular disease. *J Clin Gastroenterol*. 2010;44:113–119.
7. Ravikoff JE, Korzenik JR. Presentations the role of fiber in diverticular disease. *J Clin Gastroenterol*. 2011;45:S7–11.
8. Strate LL, Liu YL, Syngal S, et al. Nut, corn, and popcorn consumption and the incidence of diverticular disease. *JAMA*. 2008;300:907–914.
9. Katz LH, Guy DD, Lahat A, et al. Diverticulitis in the young is not more aggressive than in the elderly, but it tends to recur more often: Systematic review and meta-analysis. *Gastroenterol Hepatol*. 2013 May 22. doi: 10.1111/jgh.12274. [Epub ahead of print]

CODES

ICD10
- K57.30 Dvrtclos of lg int w/o perforation or abscess w/o bleeding
- K57.90 Dvrtclos of intest, part unsp, w/o perf or abscess w/o bleed
- K57.92 Diverticulitis of intestine, part unspecified, without perforation or abscess without bleeding

CLINICAL PEARLS
- Diverticula occur in up to 20% of the general population, but increase progressively with age, reaching up to 2/3 of people by the 8th decade.
- Patients with known diverticulosis should eat a high-fiber diet; nuts, corn, and popcorn do not increase risk for diverticular complications.
- WBC are not elevated in up to 45% of cases.

DOMESTIC VIOLENCE

Rhonda A. Faulkner, PhD • Mary Segraves Lindholm, MD

 BASICS

DESCRIPTION

- Domestic violence (DV) is behavior in any relationship that is used to gain or maintain power and control over an intimate partner.
- May include physical, sexual, and/or emotional abuse, economic or psychological actions, or threats of actions that influence another person
- Although women are at greater risk of experiencing DV, it occurs among patients of any race, age, sexual orientation, religion, gender, socioeconomic background, and education level.
- Synonym(s): Intimate partner violence (IPV); Spousal abuse; Family violence

EPIDEMIOLOGY
Incidence
8% in the US; women are more likely to report partner violence than are men.

Prevalence
- DV occurs in 1 in 4 American families. Nearly 5.3 million incidents of DV occur each year among US women ≥18 years, and 3.2 million incidents among men.
- DV results in nearly 2 million injuries and up to 4,000 deaths annually in the US.
- 30% of women and 22% of men have experienced physical, sexual, or psychological IPV during their lifetime in the US.
- 14–35% of adult female patients in emergency departments report experiencing DV within the past year.
- Costs of DV are estimated to exceed $5.8 billion annually, of which $4.1 billion are for direct medical and mental health services.
- DV survivors have a 1.6–2.3-fold increase in health care use compared with the nonabused population.

Geriatric Considerations
- 4–6% of elderly are abused, with ~2 million elderly persons experiencing abuse and/or neglect each year. In 90% of cases, the perpetrator is a family member.
- Elder abuse is any form of mistreatment that results in harm or loss to an older person; may include physical, sexual, emotional, financial abuse, and/or neglect.

Pediatric Considerations
- >3 million children aged 3–17 years are at risk of witnessing acts of DV.
- ~1 million abused children are identified in the US each year.
- Children living in violent homes are at increased risk of physical, sexual, and/or emotional abuse; anxiety and depression; decreased self-esteem; emotional, behavioral, social, physical disturbances; and lifelong poor health.

Pregnancy Considerations
DV occurs during 7–20% of pregnancies. Women with unintended pregnancy are at 3 × greater risk of DV. 25% of abused women report exacerbation of abuse during pregnancy. There is a positive correlation between DV and postpartum depression (1).

RISK FACTORS
- Patient/Victim risk factors:
  – Substance abuse
  – Poverty/financial stressors/unemployment
  – Recent loss of social support
  – Family disruption and lifecycle changes
  – History of abusive relationships or witness to abuse as child
  – Mental or physical disability in family
  – Social isolation
  – Pregnancy
- Abuser risk factors:
  – Substance abuse (e.g., heavy drinking)
  – Young age
  – Unemployment
  – Low academic achievement
  – Witnessing or experiencing violence as child
  – Depression
  – Personality disorders
- Relational risk factors:
  – Marital conflict
  – Marital instability
  – Economic stress
  – Traditional gender role norms
  – Poor family functioning

Geriatric Considerations
Factors associated with the abuse of older adults include increasing age, nonwhite race, low-income status, functional impairment, cognitive disability, substance use, poor emotional state, low self-esteem, cohabitation, and lack of social support.

Pediatric Considerations
Factors associated with child abuse or neglect include low-income status, low maternal education, nonwhite race, large family size, young maternal age, single-parent household, parental psychiatric disturbances, and presence of a stepfather.

 DIAGNOSIS

- DV is often underdiagnosed, with only 10–12% of physicians conducting routine screening.
- Although prevalence of DV in primary care settings is 7–50%, <15% are screened.
- Pregnancy increases risk.
- Barriers to screening: Time constraints, discomfort with the subject, fear of offending the patient, and lack of perceived skills and resources to manage DV.
- Abused patients may refuse to disclose abuse for many reasons:
  – Not feeling emotionally ready to admit the reality of the situation
  – Shame and self-blame
  – Feelings of failure if abuse is admitted
  – Fear of rejection by the physician
  – Fear of retribution from abuser
  – Belief that abuse will not happen again
  – Belief that no alternatives or available resources exist

HISTORY
- Physicians should introduce the subject of DV in a general way (i.e., "I routinely ask all patients about domestic violence. Have you ever been in a relationship where you were afraid?").

- How to screen:
  – Screen patient alone, without partner or others present.
  – Ask screening questions in patient's primary language; do not use children or other family members as interpreters.
- Partner Violence Screen (sensitivity 35–71%; specificity 80–94%):
  – "Have you ever been hit, kicked, punched, or otherwise hurt by someone within the past year? If so, by whom?"
  – "Do you feel safe in your current relationship?"
  – "Is there a partner from a previous relationship who is making you feel unsafe now?"
- CDC-recommended RADAR system:
  – **R**: Routinely screen every patient; make screening a part of everyday practice in prenatal, postnatal, routine gynecologic visits, and annual health screenings.
  – **A**: Ask questions directly, kindly, and be nonjudgmental.
  – **D**: Document findings in the patient's chart using the patient's own words, with details. Use body maps and photographs as necessary.
  – **A**: Assess the patient's safety and see if the patient has a safety plan.
  – **R**: Review options for dealing with DV with the patient and provide referrals.
- SAFE Questions:
  – **S**tress/Safety: "Do you feel safe in your relationship?"
  – **A**fraid/Abused: "Have you ever been in a relationship where you were threatened, hurt, or afraid?"
  – **F**riends/Family: "Are your friends or family aware that you have been hurt? Could you tell them, and would they be able to give you support?"
  – **E**mergency Plan: "Do you have a safe place to go and the resources you need in an emergency?"
- "How often does your partner: Physically hurt you? Insult or talk down to you? Threaten you with harm? Scream or curse at you?"
- Assess pregnancy difficulties such as poor/late prenatal care, low-birth-weight babies, and perinatal deaths
- Pelvic and abdominal pain, chronic without demonstrable pathology
- Headaches, back pain
- Gynecologic disorders
- STIs including HIV/AIDS
- Depression, suicidal ideation, anxiety, fatigue
- Substance abuse
- Eating disorders
- Overuse of health services/frequent emergency room visits
- Noncompliance

PHYSICAL EXAM
- Clinical presentation/psychological signs and symptoms:
  – Delay in seeking treatment
  – Inconsistent explanation of injuries
  – Reluctance to undress
  – Signs of battered woman syndrome and/or PTSD (flat affect/avoidance of eye contact, evasiveness, heightened startle response, sleep disturbance, traumatic flashbacks)
  – Depression, anxiety, chronic fatigue, substance abuse

– Suspicious partner accompaniment at appointment; overly solicitous partner and/or refusal to leave exam room

• Physical signs and symptoms:
  – Tympanic membrane rupture
  – Rectal or genital injury (centrally located injuries with bathing-suit pattern of distribution—concealable by clothing)
  – Head and neck injuries (site of 50% of abusive injuries)
  – Facial scrapes, loose or broken tooth, bruises, cuts, or fractures to face or body
  – Knife wounds, cigarette burns, bite marks, welts with outline of weapon (such as belt buckle)
  – Broken bones
  – Defensive posture injuries
  – Injuries inconsistent with the explanation given
  – Injuries in various stages of healing

DIAGNOSTIC TESTS & INTERPRETATION

• The US Preventive Services Task Force (USPSTF) in 2013 issued guidelines recommending that clinicians screen all women of childbearing age (14 to 46 years old) for DV and provide or refer women to intervention services when appropriate (2)[A]

• Other recommendations:
  – American College of Physicians (ACOG) recommends routine screening for DV for all women in primary care settings at periodic intervals and when women present for emergency care with traumatic injuries.
  – The American Medical Association (AMA) recommends that all patients be routinely screened for DV with inquiry into history of family violence.
  – US Surgeon General and American Association of Family Practitioners recommend that physicians consider the possibility of DV as a cause of illness and injury.
  – The Partner Violence Screen is a 3-question screening tool with a high specificity.
  – There is no evidence of harm in screening for DV.

Pediatric Considerations
American Academy of Pediatrics (AAP) and American Medical Association (AMA) recommend that physicians remain alert for signs and symptoms of child physical and sexual abuse in the routine exam.

Pregnancy Considerations
ACOG and AMA guidelines on DV recommend that physicians routinely assess all pregnant women for DV. ACOG recommends periodic screening throughout obstetric care (at the first prenatal visit, at least once per trimester, at the postpartum checkup)

Initial Tests (lab, imaging)
LFTs, amylase, lipase if abdominal trauma is suspected

TREATMENT

• Treatment includes: Initial diagnosis; ongoing medical care; emotional support, counseling, and patient education regarding the DV cycle; referrals to community and supportive services as needed.
• On diagnosis, use the SOS-DoC intervention:
• **S:** Offer *S*upport and assess *S*afety:
  – Support: "You are not to blame. I am sorry this is happening to you. There is no excuse for DV."
  – Remind patient of your commitment to confidential communication.
  – Safety: Listen and respond to safety issues for the patient: "Do you feel safe going home?"; "Are your children safe?"

• **O:** Discuss *O*ptions, including safety planning and follow up:
  – Provide information about DV and help where needed. Make referrals to local resources:
    ◦ "Do you need or want to access a safety shelter or DV service agency?"
    ◦ "Do you want police intervention and if so, would you like me to call the police so they can make a report with you?"
    ◦ Offer numbers to local resources and National DV Hotline: 1-800-799-SAFE (open 24/7; can provide physicians in every state with information on local resources).
• **S:** Validate patient's *S*trengths:
  – "It took courage for you to talk with me today. You have shown great strength in very difficult circumstances."
• **Do:** *Do*cument *o*bservations, assessment, and plans:
  – Use patient's own words regarding injury and abuse.
  – Legibly document injuries: Use a body map.
  – If possible, take instant photographs of patient's injuries if given patient consent.
  – Make patient safety plan. Prepare patient to get away in an emergency:
    ◦ Encourage patient to keep the following items in a safe place: Keys (house and car); important papers (Social Security card, birth certificates, photo ID/driver's license, passport, green card); cash, food stamps, credit cards; medication for self and children; children's immunization records; important phone numbers/addresses (friends, family, local shelters); personal care items (e.g., extra glasses).
    ◦ Encourage patient to arrange a signal with someone to let that person know when she or he needs help.
• **C:** Offer *C*ontinuity:
  – Offer a follow-up appointment and assess barriers to access.

GENERAL MEASURES
• Reporting child and elder abuse to protective services is mandatory in most states. Several states have laws requiring mandatory reporting of IPV.
• Contact the local DV program to find out about laws and community resources before they are needed.
• Display resource materials (National DV Hotline: 1-800-799-SAFE) in the office, all exam rooms, and restrooms.

ADDITIONAL THERAPIES
• National DV Hotline: 1-800-799-SAFE (7233)
• Post in all exam rooms posters in both English and Spanish; available at www.thehotline.org/resources/resource-download-center/

 ONGOING CARE

FOLLOW-UP RECOMMENDATIONS
• Schedule prompt follow-up appointment.
• Inquire about what has happened since last visit.
• Review medical records and ask about past episodes to convey concern for the patient and a willingness to address this health issue openly.
• DV often requires multiple interventions over time before it is resolved.

PATIENT EDUCATION
• Counsel patients about nonviolent ways to resolve conflict.
• Educate patients about the cycle of violence.
• Counsel parents about developmentally appropriate ways to discipline their children.
• Educate parents about the negative consequences of arguments on children and each other.
• National Coalition Against Domestic Violence: www.ncadv.org
• CDC: www.cdc.gov/violenceprevention

PROGNOSIS
Most DV perpetrators do not voluntarily seek therapy unless pressured by partners or upon legal mandate. Current evidence is insufficient on effectiveness of therapy for perpetrators.

REFERENCES
1. Wu Q, Chen HL, Xu XJ. Violence as a risk factor for postpartum depression in mothers: A meta-analysis. *Arch Womens Ment Health*. 2012;15: 107–114.
2. Kottenstette JB, Stulberg D. PURLs: Time to routinely screed for intimate partner violence? *J Fam Pract*. 2013;62:90–92.

ADDITIONAL READING
• Cronholm PF, Fogarty CT, Ambuel B, et al. Intimate partner violence. *Am Fam Physician*. 2011;83: 1165–1172.
• Rhodes KV, Kothari CL, Ditcher M, et al. Intimate partner violence identification and response: Time for a change in strategy. *J Gen Intern Med*. 2011;26:294–899.
• Walton MA, Murray R, Cunningham RM, et al. Correlates of intimate partner violence among men and women in an inner city emergency department. *J Addict Dis*. 2009;28:366–381.

 CODES

ICD10
• T74.11XA Adult physical abuse, confirmed, initial encounter
• T74.31XA Adult psychological abuse, confirmed, initial encounter
• T74.91XA Unspecified adult maltreatment, confirmed, initial encounter

CLINICAL PEARLS
• Display resource materials in the office (e.g., posting abuse awareness posters/National DV Hotline, 1-800-799-SAFE, in both English and Spanish, in all exam rooms and restrooms).
• Despite lack of data, screen all women: "Have you ever been threatened, hit, kicked, or are you afraid of your partner?"
• For those who screen positive, offer resources, reassure confidentiality, and provide close follow up.

DOWN SYNDROME
Michele Roberts, MD, PhD • Brian G. Skotko, MD, MPP

 BASICS

DESCRIPTION
- Down syndrome (DS) is a congenital condition associated with intellectual disability and an increased risk of multisystem medical problems
- System(s) affected: Neurologic (100%); Cardiac (40–50%); GI (8–12%)
- Etiology: Presence of all or part of an extra chromosome 21
- Synonym(s): Trisomy 21

Pediatric Considerations
- Congenital heart disease is a common cause of infant mortality.
- Murmur may not be present at birth. Delay in recognition of heart condition may lead to irreversible pulmonary hypertension.

Geriatric Considerations
- Life expectancy has increased to ~60 years.
- Age-related health issues occur at earlier age than in the general population.
- Communication difficulties may interfere with prompt recognition of some medical issues.

Pregnancy Considerations
- The ACOG recommend all pregnant women be offered traditional prenatal screening and diagnostic testing for DS:
  - Maternal prenatal screening may be performed in the 1st or 2nd trimester.
  - Prenatal diagnosis includes chorionic villus sampling or amniocentesis.
- The ACOG and the Society for Maternal-Fetal Medicine (SMFM) recommend noninvasive prenatal screening (NIPS) for "high-risk" women.
- Most, but not all, men with DS are believed to be infertile.
- Most women with DS are subfertile, but can conceive children with and without DS.

EPIDEMIOLOGY
Incidence
In the US, 1/830 live births, ~4,700 births/year (1)
Prevalence
~250,000 persons in the US

ETIOLOGY AND PATHOPHYSIOLOGY
- Trisomy 21: 95% of DS, an extra chromosome 21 is found in all cells due to nondisjunction, usually in maternal meiosis.
- Translocation DS: 3–4% of DS, extra chromosome 21q material is translocated to another chromosome (usually 13, 14, or 21); ~25% have parental origin.
- Mosaic trisomy 21: 1–2% of DS, manifestations may be milder.

Genetics
- Online Mendelian Inheritance in Man (OMIM) 190685
- Inheritance: Most commonly sporadic nondisjunction resulting in trisomy 21

- Chance of having another child with DS is:
  - 1% (or age risk, whichever is greater) after conceiving a pregnancy with nondisjunction trisomy 21
  - 10–15% for mothers/sisters and 3–5% for fathers/brothers who carry balanced translocation with chromosome 21
  - 100% if the parental balanced translocation is 21:21 (45,t[21:21])
  - Unclear after child with mosaic DS, but ~1%

RISK FACTORS
- DS believed to occur in all races with equal frequency.
- Chance of having an infant with DS increases with mother's age.
- Relatively more infants with DS are born to younger mothers because younger women are more likely to become pregnant.
- Prenatal diagnosis of DS is more common in older women, and a high percentage of such pregnancies are terminated.

GENERAL PREVENTION
- No prevention for nondisjunction trisomy 21
- Preimplantation diagnosis with in vitro fertilization (IVF), prenatal diagnosis and termination, and adoption are current options for expectant parents who do not wish to raise a child with DS.

COMMONLY ASSOCIATED CONDITIONS
- Cardiac:
  - Congenital heart defects (40–50%)
- GI/Growth:
  - Feeding problems are common in infancy.
  - Structural defects (12%)
  - Gastroesophageal reflux
  - Constipation
  - Celiac disease (5%)
- Pulmonary:
  - Tracheal stenosis/tracheoesophageal fistula
  - Pulmonary hypertension
  - Obstructive sleep apnea (50–75%)
- Genitourinary:
  - Cryptorchidism, hypospadias
- Hematologic/Neoplastic:
  - Transient myeloproliferative disorder (10%): Generally resolves spontaneously; can be preleukemic (acute megakaryoblastic leukemia [AMKL]) in 20–30%
  - Leukemia (AMKL or acute lymphoblastic leukemia [ALL]) in 0.5–1%
  - Decreased risk of most solid tumors; increased risk of germ cell tumors
- Endocrine:
  - Hypothyroidism: Congenital or acquired (4–18%)
  - Diabetes
- Skeletal:
  - Atlantoaxial instability (15%): 2% symptomatic
  - Short stature is common
  - Scoliosis (some cases have adult onset)
  - Hip problems (1–4%)
- Immune/Rheumatologic:
  - Abnormal immune function with increased rate of respiratory infections
  - Increased risk of autoimmune disorders, including Hashimoto thyroiditis, celiac disease, alopecia

- Neurologic:
  - Intellectual ability ranging from near-normal to severe disability. Average is moderate intellectual disability.
  - Autism spectrum disorder (<18%); autism (<6%)
  - Seizures: (8%), typically occurring <1 year of age or >30 years of age
  - Alzheimer disease: At least 25% at age 35 develop signs of dementia; percentage increases with age
- Psychiatric:
  - ADHD, obsessive-compulsive disorder (OCD), oppositional-defiant disorder, autism spectrum disorder increased frequency in children
  - Generalized depression and anxiety with increased frequency in young adults/adults
- Sensory:
  - Hearing loss (75%): Mostly conductive due to high frequency of asymptomatic middle ear effusion; otitis media (50–70%)
  - Visual impairment (60%): Mostly strabismus (refractive errors, 15%), nystagmus, cataracts (15%)
- Dermatologic:
  - Xerosis, eczema, palmoplantar hyperkeratosis, atopic or seborrheic dermatitis, onychomycosis, syringomas, furunculosis/folliculitis

 DIAGNOSIS

HISTORY
~85% of mothers of infants with DS learn of the diagnosis postnatally.

PHYSICAL EXAM
- Typical growth curves should be used (2).
- Infants and children:
  - Brachycephaly (100%)
  - Hypotonia (80%)
  - Small ears, often low set and simplified
  - Up-slanting palpebral fissure (90%)
  - Epicanthic folds (90%)
  - Brushfield spots
  - Depressed nasal bridge
  - Short neck, often with increased nuchal folds
  - Single palmar crease, single flexion crease on 5th finger
  - Increased space between toes 1 and 2; 5th finger clinodactyly; brachydactyly

DIAGNOSTIC TESTS & INTERPRETATION
Initial Tests (lab, imaging)
- Maternal prenatal screening includes:
  - 1st trimester: Combined screen (maternal age, β-human chorionic gonadotropin (β-hCG), pregnancy-associated plasma protein A, and nuchal translucency)
  - 2nd trimester: Quad screen (α-fetoprotein, β-hCG, estriol, inhibin-A)
  - Sequential screen (combined screen in 1st trimester, if abnormal, obtain amniocentesis OR await 2nd trimester quad screening)
  - Integrated screen (combined screening in 1st trimester plus quad screen in 2nd trimester)
  - Noninvasive prenatal screening with cell-free DNA (beginning at 10 weeks' gestation)

- Prenatal diagnosis includes:
  - Chorionic villus sampling: 1st trimester, ~99% accurate, ~1% miscarriage
  - Amniocentesis: 2nd trimester, ~99% accurate, ~0.25% miscarriage rate
- Postnatal diagnosis:
  - Fluorescence in situ hybridization (FISH) can be performed at time of clinical suspicion, but karyotype should always be done to differentiate type of DS
  - Parental (and adult-aged sibling) chromosome study indicated only if translocation DS found in child.
- Echo, with or without murmur (2)
- CBC with differential (to look for transient myeloproliferative disorder) (2)
- Thyrotropin (TSH) (2)
- Audiogram (2)
- Ophthalmologic exam (look for red reflex) (2)
- Swallowing study for those with feeding difficulties (2)

Follow-Up Tests & Special Considerations
- After delivering a prenatal diagnosis, the physician should offer "Understanding a Down Syndrome Diagnosis" (www.lettercase.org).
- If the diagnosis is postnatal, the mother, and her partner, should be informed of the diagnosis promptly by a physician (preferably the obstetrician and pediatrician or family physician), on the basis of clinical observations and before the karyotype is available, but with consideration of extenuating circumstances (e.g., mother's medical condition). The spouse/partner and infant should be present unless this would cause undue delay. The meeting should be private. Refer to the baby by name (3).
- In the postnatal setting, the physician should be knowledgeable on the subject of DS and should conduct a discussion with content that is current, respectful, balanced, informative, and realistic, but not overly pessimistic, concentrating on what is relevant to the 1st year of life (3).
- Cardiac follow up, as indicated (2)

 TREATMENT

GENERAL MEASURES
Genetic evaluation and counseling

ISSUES FOR REFERRAL
- Infant stimulation programs (early intervention)
- Lactation consultant
- Physical/Occupational/Speech therapy
- Inclusion programs can be successful.
- Pediatric cardiologist, if indicated
- DS specialty clinics can improve medical outcomes.

SURGERY/OTHER PROCEDURES
Repair of congenital anomalies is appropriate. Plastic surgery for facial features not recommended.

COMPLEMENTARY AND ALTERNATIVE MEDICINE
- A 2008 randomized controlled trial provided no evidence to support the use of antioxidant or folinic acid supplements in children with DS (4).
- Craniosacral manipulation is dangerous due to potential atlantoaxial instability.
- Sicca is illegal in US, potentially dangerous, and without any evidence of benefit.
- Piracetam is much publicized, without scientific evidence of benefit.

IN-PATIENT CONSIDERATIONS
Discharge Criteria
If the social situation indicates adoption: The National Down Syndrome Adoption Network (NDSAN) (www.ndsan.org), national registry of families seeking to adopt a child with Down syndrome.

 ONGOING CARE

FOLLOW-UP RECOMMENDATIONS
Patient Monitoring
The American Academy of Pediatrics recommends ongoing assessment and review, at least annually, the following surveillance (2):

- Vision: Assess for strabismus, cataracts, and nystagmus by ophthalmologist by 6 months, annually between ages 1–5; every 2 years ages 5–13; every 3 years ages 13–21
- Hearing: Neonatal screen with ABR or OAE, then audiogram every 6 months until age 3 years, then annually
- Thyroid: Initial newborn screen. Repeat TSH at 6 months, 12 months, and then annually.
- Screening for celiac disease (total IgA and TTG-IgA) annually, if symptomatic
- 3-view C-spine films is patient symptomatic beginning at 3–5 years of age
- Hemoglobin annually to screen for iron-deficiency anemia
- Echocardiogram for all newborns, regardless of murmur. Repeat in teens if murmur, fatigue.

DIET
- No special diet, but caloric needs are lower in adolescents/adults with DS than their peers.
- Obesity is prevalent at all ages.
- No scientific evidence supports megavitamin therapy or dietary supplements.

PATIENT EDUCATION
- National Down Syndrome Congress 800-232-NDSC; www.ndsccenter.org
- National Down Syndrome Society 800-221-4602; www.ndss.org
- The Down Syndrome Research and Treatment Foundation provides information on the latest research for people with DS: www.dsrtf.org/
- www.lettercase.org provides peer-reviewed booklet for parents who have received a prenatal diagnosis of Down syndrome and have not yet made a decision about their pregnancy.
- http://Downsyndromepregnancy.org provides a free downloadable book for expectant mothers who have decided to continue their pregnancies after a prenatal diagnosis of DS.
- www.downsyndromdiagnosis.org

PROGNOSIS
- Associated congenital anomalies are the immediate concern during the newborn period.
- 99% of young adults/adults with DS report being happy with their lives.
- Life expectancy ~60 years.

REFERENCES

1. Parker SE, Mai CT, Canfield MA, et al. Updated national birth prevalence estimates for selected birth defects in the United States, 2004–2006. *Birth Defects Res Part A Clin Mol Teratol*. 2010;88:1008–1016.
2. Bull MJ, Committee on Genetics. Health supervision for children with Down syndrome. *Pediatrics*. 2011;128:393–406.
3. Sheets KB, Crissman BG, Feist CD, et al. Practice guidelines for communicating a prenatal or postnatal diagnosis of Down syndrome: Recommendations of the national society of genetic counselors. *J Genet Couns*. 2011;20:432–441.
4. Ellis JM, Tan HK, Gilbert RE, et al. Supplementation with antioxidants and folinic acid for children with Down's syndrome: Randomised controlled trial. *BMJ*. 2008;336:594–597.

ADDITIONAL READING
- Skotko BG, Capone GT, Kishnani PS, et al. Postnatal diagnosis of Down syndrome: Synthesis of the evidence on how best to deliver the news. *Pediatrics*. 2009;124:e751–e758.
- Skotko BG, Kishnani PS, Capone GT, et al. Prenatal diagnosis of Down syndrome: How best to deliver the news. *Am J Med Genet A*. 2009;149A:2361–2367.
- www.downsyndromediagnosis.org

 SEE ALSO

Algorithm: Mental Retardation

 CODES

ICD10
- Q90.0 Trisomy 21, nonmosaicism (meiotic nondisjunction)
- Q90.1 Trisomy 21, mosaicism (mitotic nondisjunction)
- Q90.9 Down syndrome, unspecified

CLINICAL PEARLS
- 99% of young adults/adults with DS report being happy with their lives.
- DS specialty clinics can improve medical outcomes.

DRUG ABUSE, PRESCRIPTION

Edward Han, PharmD • Matthew Silva, PharmD, RPh, BCPS • Jeffrey Baxter, MD

BASICS

DESCRIPTION
- Prescription drug abuse behaviors exist on a continuum and may include:
  – Using medication for nonmedical reasons such as to get high or enhance performance
  – Using medication for medical reasons other than what the prescriber intended
  – Using medication for any reason by someone other than the person for whom the medication was originally prescribed
- Commonly abused prescription medications include opioid analgesics (morphine, oxycodone, hydrocodone, oxymorphone, hydromorphone, fentanyl, methadone, buprenorphine), stimulants (amphetamine, methylphenidate), benzodiazepines (alprazolam, clonazepam), and barbiturates (secobarbital, amobarbital).
- *Diversion* is a term used to describe the rerouting of medications from prescriptions or other legitimate supplies for recreational use or criminal activity, such as selling prescription medication for personal profit.

EPIDEMIOLOGY
- In 2010, 49.6% of the 2.5 million drug-related ED visits attributed to drug misuse and abuse were due to pharmaceuticals (1.24 million) (1).
- A 2010 study found 62% of college students diverted ADHD medicine and 35% diverted prescription analgesics (1).

Incidence
- Predominant sex: Males > Females (2)
- Predominant age: Highest among adults 18–25, then adolescents and teens 12–17, followed by adults ≥26 (2)
- >20% of the 3.1 million persons who were 1st-time substance abusers in 2011 used prescription medications nonmedically (2).
- The average age of persons with the 1st reported instance of nonmedical prescription drug use is 22.4 years (2).

Prevalence
- Prescription opioids are the 2nd most commonly used class to initiate illicit drug use (1.9 million) (2).
- The number of persons with nonmedical opioid dependence increased from 936,000 in 2002 to 1.4 million in 2011 (2).
- Lifetime prevalence of prescription drug abuse are highest for opioids, benzodiazepines, and stimulants.

ETIOLOGY AND PATHOPHYSIOLOGY
- Prescription medications are now perceived by young adults to be more socially acceptable than other illicit drugs.
- Pharmacokinetics, compound purity, government approval, extensive media advertising, along with personal or family experiences with prescription medication, contribute to perceived advantages of prescription drug misuse over street drugs and other illicit substances.

Genetics
Variant alleles affecting the expression and function of opioid, dopamine, acetylcholine, serotonin, and GABA may explain susceptibility to all forms of prescription and nonprescription drug abuse behaviors.

RISK FACTORS
- Sociodemographic, psychosocial, pain- and drug-related factors
- Genetics and environment; family history

GENERAL PREVENTION
- Educate and raise awareness about the dangers of misuse and abuse of prescription drugs. Focus on individuals, then families, then communities.
- Educate and reinforce safe practices in evaluating patients and prescribing medications. Use office based peer-to-peer education and follow-up with pharmacies when abuse behaviors are suspected.
- Develop or adopt a standard practice agreement for prescribing and monitoring controlled substances with abuse potential (3,4,5).
- Prescription monitoring plans (PMP) show fair evidence in reducing doctor shopping but have not reliably shown reductions in ED visits for drug overdose and prescription drug-abuse–related deaths (3).
- Avoid prescribing benzodiazepines and hypnotics to elderly (6).
- Avoid using benzodiazepines >2–4 weeks.
- Minimize controlled substances when patients have a personal or family history of substance abuse or psychiatric disorders.
- Limit or avoid prescribing controlled medications on 1st visit and until a relationship can be established (7).
- Take a thorough history, contact family members and past prescribers, perform observed urine drug screens. Stop prescribing prescription analgesics for chronic pain when they are not working, if a patient is unable to take medications as prescribed, or if there are problems related to opioid and nonopioid analgesics. Identify and treat underlying substance abuse problems and involve behavioral health providers when possible

COMMONLY ASSOCIATED CONDITIONS
- Benzodiazepines: Withdrawal syndromes/delirium, psychosis, anxiety, sleep driving, blackout states, cognitive impairment, impaired driving while awake; increased fall risk and mortality in elderly patients
- Amphetamines: Hypertension, tachyarrhythmias, myocardial ischemia, seizures, hypothermia, psychosis, hallucinations, paranoia, anxiety
- Opioids: Respiratory depression and death with overdose, low testosterone, sexual dysfunction with chronic abuse. Methadone is associated with QT-prolongation, which increases risk for torsades de pointes.

DIAGNOSIS

Screening: "How many times in the past year have you used an illegal drug or used a prescription medication for nonmedical reasons?"; primary care setting sensitivity of 100% and specificity of ~75% (8)[C]

HISTORY
Consider aberrant behaviors found when taking a history. Patient may asks for dose escalations, early refills ("spilled the bottle, pharmacist shorted me...etc."), has strong preference for one drug, targets appointments at end of day and after hours, shows hostile/threatening behavior or overly flattering behavior

DIAGNOSTIC TESTS & INTERPRETATION
- Urine drug screens are recommended to identify patients who are noncompliant or abusing prescription drugs despite limited evidence of reliability and accuracy (3,9)[C].
- Urine drug screen (UDS): Order an expanded panel to detect commonly used opioids (ask specifically for semisynthetics (hydrocodone, hydromorphone oxycodone) and synthetics (methadone, fentanyl, propoxyphene, meperidine) along with tramadol and buprenorphine.
- Clonazepam and lorazepam rarely show up as benzodiazepines in routine UDS and should be ordered specifically.

Initial Tests (lab, imaging)
- Interpretation: Results are positive if drugs that are not prescribed are present; positive in presence of illicit drugs (marijuana, cocaine); can be negative for prescribed drug (suspect diversion).
- Be suspicious if patient refuses test.
- OxyContin will only be positive for oxycodone,
- Hydrocodone will be positive for hydrocodone and hydromorphone.
- Codeine will be positive for codeine plus morphine,
- Heroin will be positive for morphine.
- Thus, if UDS is positive for morphine, it could mean that a patient took morphine, codeine, heroin, or hydrocodone.

Diagnostic Procedures/Other
CAGE (Cut down, Anger at being questioned about use, Guilt about prior use, Eye-opener use early in day) or AUDIT to assess current alcohol use. DAST (drug abuse screening test) helps determine patient's involvement with drugs over the past year. Details: http://counsellingresource.com/lib/quizzes/drug-testing/drug-abuse/SOAPP (Screener and Opioid Assessment for Patients with Pain), ORT (Opioid Risk Tool), and DIRE (Diagnosis, Intractability, Risk, Efficacy) are tools used to assess risk of opioid misuse (10)[C].

Test Interpretation
See "History."

TREATMENT

- Whenever there is evidence of prescription opioid abuse, the controlled substance should be tapered to begin discontinuing drug therapy (3)[C].
- Benzodiazepines cannot be stopped abruptly for risk of seizures and death. A Cochrane Review supported a gradual benzodiazepine withdrawal over 10 weeks (11)[A].
- Amphetamines can be stopped abruptly without risk of severe withdrawal or death.
- The general approach to treatment includes inpatient, residential, or outpatient detoxification as required; counseling and intensive counseling as needed; ongoing medication assisted treatment.

GENERAL MEASURES

Alcoholics Anonymous/Narcotics Anonymous are helpful, as are Alanon/Alateen for family members. Nonjudgmental interactions and cognitive behavioral therapy focused on motivational interviewing, goal-setting, and brief interventions help manage anxiety, insomnia, and denial, and improve willingness to change.

MEDICATION

- Opioid detoxification programs use clonidine (12)[A], buprenorphine (12,13)[A], or methadone (14)[A] under the direction of an addiction specialist. Buprenorphine is as effective as methadone but safer (15)[A]. Both Buprenorphine and methadone are more effective than clonidine for detoxification.
- Buprenorphine and methadone have been found to be similarly effective when used in long-term opioid maintenance therapy. Long-term therapy supervised by an addiction specialist is preferable to short-term detoxification.
- Subutex (buprenorphine) lacks naloxone and is prone to diversion and abuse, since patients can crush, snort, or shoot to get high. Suboxone (buprenorphine and naloxone) discourages abuse and diversion because naloxone displaces buprenorphine binding to opioid receptors. Newer Suboxone sublingual film is preferred as the dosage form is difficult to adulterate.
- There is no support for using or converting to long half-life benzodiazepines before beginning a slow, gradual 10-week benzodiazepine tapers although diazepam is often preferred. Nor are there any benefits shown using propranolol, buspirone, progesterone, hydroxyzine, or dothiepin to manage withdrawal symptoms. Carbamazepine may be useful in patients who were dependent on ≥20 mg diazepam equivalents daily (11)[B], and antidepressants may be helpful for depression and anxiety linked to benzodiazepine withdrawal.
- Atomoxetine and bupropion SR can also be helpful in managing ADHD symptoms in select patients.

ISSUES FOR REFERRAL

Refer to chemical dependency groups/addiction specialists/pain management and psychiatry/psychology when patients have polysubstance abuse and to treat underlying mood and anxiety disorders, PTSD, ADHD. See related topic "Substance Abuse Disorders."

COMPLEMENTARY AND ALTERNATIVE MEDICINE

Acupuncture, yoga, meditation, or martial arts may aid in anxiety management and stress reduction.

IN-PATIENT CONSIDERATIONS
Admission Criteria/Initial Stabilization

Indications for inpatient detoxification are concomitant alcohol and benzodiazepine dependence (increased risk of seizures), mental confusion/delirium, history of seizures, psychosis, active suicidal ideation, serious comorbid medical issues, and absence of social support.

 ONGOING CARE

PATIENT EDUCATION

- Advise patients receiving controlled medication to keep them hidden and inaccessible to others. Inform patients that giving their medication to others may result in legal charges. Warn about potential addiction when starting controlled substances and about withdrawal symptoms when a medication is stopped abruptly. Warn of the dangers of respiratory depression and death when opioids are mixed with benzodiazepines. Advise patients on controlled substances avoid all alcohol and any illicit drugs.
- Tell patient to come to you if he or she begins to need medication in increasing amounts, uses it to feel high or overcome stress, or spends a lot of time craving it and thinking about the next dose. Emphasize that you will create a mutual plan to stop the medication and try something new. Inform spouse/family members when family dynamics are an important behavioral component.

REFERENCES

1. Substance Abuse and Mental Health Services Administration, *Drug Abuse Warning Network, 2011: National Estimates of Drug-Related Emergency Department Visits.* HHS Publication No. (SMA) 13-4760, DAWN Series D-39. Rockville, MD: Substance Abuse and Mental Health Services Administration, 2013.
2. Substance Abuse and Mental Health Services Administration, Results from the 2011 National Survey on Drug Use and health: Summary of National Findings, NSDUH Series H-44, HHS Publication No. (SMA) 12-4713. Rockville, MD: Substance Abuse and Mental Health Services Administration, 2012.
3. Manchikanti L, Abdi S, Atluri S, et al. American Society of Interventional Pain Physicians (ASIPP) guidelines for responsible opioid prescribing in chronic non-cancer pain: Part 2–guidance. *Pain Physician.* 2012;15(3 Suppl):S67–116.
4. Starrels JL, Becker WC, Alford DP, et al. Systematic review: Treatment agreements and urine drug testing to reduce opioid misuse in patients with chronic pain. *Ann Intern Med.* 2010;152(11):712–720.
5. Hariharan J, Lamb GC, Neuner JM. Long-term opioid contract use for chronic pain management in primary care practice. A five year experience. *J Gen Intern Med.* 2007;22(4):485–490.
6. American Geriatrics Society 2012 Beers Criteria Update Expert Panel. American Geriatrics Society updated Beers Criteria for potentially inappropriate medication use in older adults. *J Am Geriatr Soc.* 2012;60(4):616–631. Epub 2012 Feb 29.
7. Miotto K, Kaufman A, Kong A, et al. Managing co-occurring substance use and pain disorders. *Psychiatr Clin North Am.* 2012;35(2):393–409. Epub 2012 May 5.
8. Smith PC, Schmidt SM, Allensworth-Davies D, et al. A single-question screening test for drug use in primary care. *Arch Intern Med.* 2010;170(13):1155–1160.
9. Manchikanti L, Abdi S, Atluri S, et al. American Society of Interventional Pain Physicians (ASIPP) guidelines for responsible opioid prescribing in chronic non-cancer pain: Part I–evidence assessment. *Pain Physician.* 2012;15(3 Suppl):S1–65.
10. Chou R, Fanciullo GJ, Fine PG, et al. Clinical guidelines for the use of chronic opioid therapy in chronic noncancer pain. *J Pain.* 2009;10(2):113–130.
11. Denis C, Fatséas M, Lavie E, et al. Pharmacological interventions for benzodiazepine mono-dependence management in outpatient settings. *Cochrane Database Syst Rev.* 2006;(3):CD005194. Epub 2006 Jul 19.
12. Gowing L, Ali R, White JM, et al. Buprenorphine for the management of opioid withdrawal. *Cochrane Database Syst Rev.* 2009;CD002025.
13. Maremmani I, Gerra G. Buprenorphine-based regimens and methadone for the medical management of opioid dependence: Selecting the appropriate drug for treatment. *Am J Addictions.* 2010;19:557–568.
14. Mattick RP, Breen C, Kimber J, et al. Methadone maintenance therapy versus no opioid replacement therapy for opioid dependence. *Cochrane Database Syst Rev.* 2009;CD002209.
15. Mattick RP, Kimber J, Breen C, et al. Buprenorphine maintenance versus placebo or methadone maintenance for opioid dependence. *Cochrane Database Syst Rev.* 2008;(2):CD002207. Epub 2008 Apr 16.

 CODES

ICD10

- F11.10 Opioid abuse, uncomplicated
- F15.10 Other stimulant abuse, uncomplicated
- F19.10 Other psychoactive substance abuse, uncomplicated

CLINICAL PEARLS

- Education and prescription monitoring programs are important for preventing prescription drug abuse.
- Use a standardized office practice agreement when prescribing controlled substances.
- Screening: "How many times in the past year have you used an illegal drug or prescription medication for nonmedical reasons?"
- Avoid prescribing controlled substances and nonbenzodiazepine hypnotics to patients at risk for substance abuse or with an Axis 1 or Axis 2 diagnosis.
- Discontinue prescription opioid analgesics if pain or functionality does not improve and if there's evidence of prescription or illicit drug abuse (i.e., positive UDS, DWI, accidental or intentional overdose, early refills).
- Limit benzodiazepine use to 2–4 weeks.
- Do frequent, observed UDS.
- Addiction is a potentially fatal disease.

DUCTAL CARCINOMA IN SITU
Caitlin Bonney, MD • Mitchell A. Cahan, MD, FACS

 BASICS

DESCRIPTION
- Common, noninvasive precancerous lesion originating from epithelial cells. Malignant cells are bound by the basement membranes of breast ducts.
- Types are classified by histologic architecture (solid, cribriform, papillary, micropapillary), tumor grade (high, intermediate, low), and presence or absence of central (comedo) necrosis.

EPIDEMIOLOGY
Incidence
- Rarely diagnosed prior to 1980 (1)
- Incidence has been rising in the US since the 1970s from 1.87 to 32.5 cases/100,000 in 2004 (1).
- Represents 27% of all new breast cancer diagnoses or estimated 77,795 cases in 2011 (2)
- Ductal carcinoma in situ (DCIS) accounts for 84% of insitu disease (15% LCIS) (2).

ETIOLOGY AND PATHOPHYSIOLOGY
- DCIS is a precancerous lesion resulting from local malignant proliferation of epithelial cells, without invasion of the stroma.
- Presumed to be part of the spectrum of proliferative transformation from normal epithelium to hyperplasia without atypia to atypical ductal hyperplasia to DCIS and finally to microinvasive disease.
- A small number of those with DCIS will develop invasive breast cancer, but the determinants of progression remain unclear.
- Tumor grade is related to risk of recurrence and progression to invasive disease, with high-grade tumors sharing molecular characteristics with invasive lesions.

Genetics
- *BRCA1* and *BRCA2* gene mutations observed
- If patients are high risk, may recommend genetic counseling after diagnosis of DCIS.

RISK FACTORS
- Similar, but not identical to risk factors for invasive breast cancer
- Female gender, age (unusual before age 35 years, peaks 60–74), nulliparity/1st birth after age 30, early menarche, late menopause, family history of breast cancer, heavy alcohol consumption, sedentary lifestyle, prior breast biopsies
- Increased risk with higher breast density (1)
- No clear association with use of hormone replacement therapy or body mass index (BMI) (1)

GENERAL PREVENTION
- General screening guidelines: US Preventive Services Task Force (USPSTF)
  - USPSTF recommendations based on outcome data:
    - Biennial mammography for women aged 50–74 years
    - Decision to start biennial mammographic screening before age 50 based on patient's individual risks and preferences
    - Advises against teaching breast self-exam (BSE) and insufficient evidence for recommendation of clinical breast exam (CBE) in women after age 40
- General screening guidelines: National Comprehensive Cancer Network (NCCN) (3):
  - NCCN recommendations based on limited data
  - Ages 25–39:
    - Breast awareness with BSE
    - CBE at least every 3 years
  - Age ≥40:
    - Breast awareness/BSE
    - Yearly CBE
    - Mammography
- Risk reduction
  - Limit alcohol intake to <39 g/week or ∼3 drinks (4)
  - Increase physical activity to at least 4 hours/week (4)
  - Potential benefit of frequent ASA use (4)
  - Decreased DCIS with tamoxifen chemoprevention (1)
  - Modifying additional factors for breast cancer may provide some benefit in reducing risk of disease progression.

 DIAGNOSIS

HISTORY
- Most DCIS is now diagnosed by screening mammography; patients often asymptomatic with nonpalpable lesions
- More advanced lesions may present with a palpable mass, nipple discharge, or Paget disease.

PHYSICAL EXAM
- CBE with inspection of breasts with patient in upright and supine position, evaluating for asymmetry, skin changes (peau d'orange, erythema, scaling), nipple retraction/excoriation (Paget disease)
- Palpation of all breast quadrants with patient in upright and supine position and lymph node examination (axillary, supraclavicular, and internal mammary nodes)

DIFFERENTIAL DIAGNOSIS
Atypical ductal hyperplasia, lobular carcinoma in situ, microinvasive carcinoma

DIAGNOSTIC TESTS & INTERPRETATION
Initial Tests (lab, imaging)
- Mammography Breast Imaging Reporting and Data System (BI-RADS) developed by the American College of Radiology is used for uniform reporting of mammography results (3).
- BI-RADS interpretation:
  - Category 0: Incomplete/needs additional imaging
  - Category 1: Negative
  - Category 2: Benign finding
  - Category 3: Probably benign finding
  - Category 4: Suspicious abnormality
  - Category 5: Highly suggestive of malignancy
  - Category 6: Known biopsy-proven malignancy
- Similar to algorithm for suspected breast cancer (3)
- Palpable mass, age ≥30, obtain screening mammogram:
  - BI-RADS 1–3, proceed to US biopsy
  - BI-RADS 4–5, follow up after diagnostic mammogram
- Palpable mass, age <30:
  - Obtain ultrasound (US) ± mammogram
  - Observe for 1–2 menstrual cycles; if persists then US
- Spontaneous nipple discharge with no palpable mass, obtain US (age <30) and/or mammogram (age >30):
  - BI-RADS 1–3, ductogram/MRI followed by ductal excision
  - BI-RADS 4–5; proceed to biopsy
- DCIS commonly seen as clustered microcalcifications (5):
  - Calcifications usually pleomorphic, varying in size, shape, and density; may be arranged in segmental/linear patterns along ductal tracts

Follow-Up Tests & Special Considerations
- MRI has a higher detection rate for DCIS than mammography (85–92% vs. 50–56%) (6).
- MRI better at establishing tumor size and multi-centricity; can aid in surgical decision-making
- Up to 25% of core needle biopsies for suspected DCIS have invasive carcinoma. Treatment modified based on risk (6)

Diagnostic Procedures/Other
- Tissue is necessary for diagnosis: Obtain sample via needle biopsy, core needle biopsy (US-guided/stereotactic), or vacuum-assisted biopsy
- Fine-needle aspiration (FNA) is not adequate for diagnosis.

Test Interpretation
- Histologic classification (5):
  - Traditionally classified primarily by architectural pattern (cribriform, papillary, micropapillary, comedo, and solid types)
  - Morphology, nuclear grade, and presence of central necrosis
- In future, classification of DCIS may change to ductal intraepithelial neoplasia (DIN) (5)
- Determination of estrogen receptor (ER) status (7)
- Surgical margins <1 mm have significant risk of recurrence. Unclear benefit of margins >2 mm (5)

TREATMENT

MEDICATION

- Secondary chemoprevention following breast-conserving surgery (7):
  - Premenopausal at diagnosis: Tamoxifen for 5 years ± ovarian suppression or ablation
  - Postmenopausal at diagnosis: aromatase inhibitor for 5 years or tamoxifen for 5–10 years
    - While addition of tamoxifen reduces the risk of recurrence in both breasts, it has not been shown to affect overall mortality (8).
  - Consider in patients with lumpectomy alone.
  - Benefit in patients with ER-negative disease unclear
- Potential future utility of Oncotype DX in prediction of recurrence rate after BCT (5)

SURGERY/OTHER PROCEDURES

- Breast-conserving therapy/lumpectomy whole breast radiation therapy:
  - Radiation decreases recurrence rates by 50%; however, no proven survival advantage over lumpectomy alone (7).
- Mastectomy sentinel node biopsy reconstruction:
  - Option for patients with multifocal disease or with evidence of invasive disease, at which time sentinel node biopsy is necessary for staging:
    - Nodal metastases in DCIS <1–2%, likely secondary to unrecognized invasive disease (5)

ONGOING CARE

FOLLOW-UP RECOMMENDATIONS

- History of physical exam every 6 months for 1st 5 years, then annually (7)
- Mammography at 6 and 12 months after radiation, then annually (7)
- No evidence for routine testing, such as bone scan, chest x-ray (CXR), CT scan, CBC, or LFTs, in asymptomatic patients (5)

PROGNOSIS

- DCIS has good overall prognosis:
  - 10-year mortality from breast cancer after diagnosis of DCIS is <2% (1).
- Risk of local recurrence after mastectomy <1% (5)
- Higher risk of local recurrences after breast-conserving therapy in those of younger age (particularly before age 40), with larger tumor size, high nuclear grade, comedo necrosis, and positive surgical margins:
  - ER-positive tumors associated with lower recurrence risk (1)
  - HER2-positive tumors linked to increased recurrence risk (1):
    - Limited data, potential for tumor typing and trastuzumab currently being investigated
- Roughly half of recurrences are invasive cancer (5).

COMPLICATIONS

- Most prominent during 1st 6 months after surgery (5)
- Postoperatively:
  - Seromas, edema
- Postradiation:
  - Skin thickening
  - Discoloration may be permanent.

REFERENCES

1. Virnig BA, Tuttle TM, Shamliyan T, et al. Ductal carcinoma in situ of the breast: A systematic review of incidence, treatment, and outcomes. *J Natl Cancer Inst*. 2010;84(3):170–178. Epub 2010 Jan 13.
2. Kerlikowske K. Epidemiology of ductal carcinoma in situ. *J Natl Cancer Inst Monographs*. 2010;84(41):139–141.
3. NCCN Clinical Practice Guidelines in Oncology: Breast Cancer Screening and Diagnosis (Version 2.2013) 2013 National Comprehensive Cancer Network, Inc. Accessed 10/27/2013 at http://www.nccn.org.
4. Virnig BA, Shamliyan T, Tuttle TM, et al. Diagnosis and management of ductal carcinoma in situ (DCIS). *Evid Rep Technol Assess (Full Rep)*. 2009;(185):1–549.
5. Lee RJ, Vallow LA, McLaughlin SA, et al. Ductal carcinoma in situ of the breast. *Int J Surg Oncol*. 2012;2012:123549. Epub 2012 Jul 18.
6. Badruddoja M. Ductal carcinoma in situ of the breast: A surgical perspective. *Int J Surg Oncol*. 2012;2012:761364. Epub 2012 Sep 4.
7. NCCN Clinical Practice Guidelines in Oncology: Breast Cancer (Version 3.2013) 2013 National Comprehensive Cancer Network, Inc. Accessed 10/27/2013 at http://www.nccn.org.
8. Staley H, McCallum I, Bruce J. Postoperative tamoxifen for ductal carcinoma in situ. *Cochrane Database Syst Rev*. 2012;10:CD007847. Epub 2012 Oct 17.

ADDITIONAL READING

- Goodwin A, Parker S, Ghersi D, et al. Post-operative radiotherapy for ductal carcinoma in situ of the breast. *Cochrane Database Syst Rev*. 2009;(4):CD000563. Epub 2009 Oct 7.
- Wang SY, Chu H, Shamliyan T, et al. Network meta-analysis of margin threshold for women with ductal carcinoma in situ. *J Natl Cancer Inst*. 2012;84(7):507–516. Epub 2012 Mar 22.

 SEE ALSO

Breast Cancer

 CODES

ICD10

- D05.10 Intraductal carcinoma in situ of unspecified breast
- D05.11 Intraductal carcinoma in situ of right breast
- D05.12 Intraductal carcinoma in situ of left breast

CLINICAL PEARLS

- DCIS is a heterogeneous group of noninvasive neoplastic lesions arising from the breast ductal epithelial cells.
- The incidence of DCIS had been steadily rising until recently with the increase in screening mammography.
- The goal of DCIS treatment is to prevent invasive breast cancer.
- Current standard of care is breast-conserving therapy followed by postoperative radiation therapy, unless otherwise contraindicated.

DUMPING SYNDROME

Hongyi Cui, MD, PhD, FACS, FICS

BASICS

DESCRIPTION
GI and vasomotor symptoms resulting from rapid gastric emptying and delivery of large amounts of hyperosmolar content into the small intestine:
- Usually occurs following gastric and esophageal surgery (gastrectomy, vagotomy, pyloroplasty, esophagectomy, Nissen fundoplication, or gastric bypass procedures).

EPIDEMIOLOGY
- Overall, ~10% of patients following gastric surgery and up to 50% of patients who undergo esophagectomy develop dumping symptoms.
- Predominant age: Middle age to elderly
- Predominant sex: Female > Male

Incidence
- In the US, 0.9% of proximal gastric vagotomy without any drainage procedure; 10–22% truncal vagotomy and drainage:
  - After partial gastrectomy, 14–20% of patients develop symptoms of dumping.
- Prominent feature after bariatric surgery:
  - >70% of gastric bypass patients experience varying degrees of dumping symptoms.
  - Regarded as a beneficial feature of gastric bypass surgery, because patients learn to avoid calorie-rich foods and eat small meals

ETIOLOGY AND PATHOPHYSIOLOGY
The pathogenesis of dumping syndrome is multifactorial. It includes at least the following interplay of factors:
- Alterations in the storage function of the stomach and/or the pyloric emptying mechanism, leading to rapid delivery of hyperosmolar material into the intestine. This results in fluid shifts from the intravascular compartment into the bowel lumen, leading to rapid small-bowel distention and an increase in the frequency of bowel contractions (early dumping).
- Supraphysiologic release of various GI peptides/vasoactive mediators, leading to paradoxical vasodilation in a relatively volume-contracted state
- Reactive hypoglycemia secondary to hyperinsulinemia caused by high concentration of carbohydrates in the proximal small intestine and rapid absorption of glucose (late dumping)
- Pancreatic islet cell hyperplasia, rather than late dumping, is thought to be the underlying mechanism for hyperinsulinemic hypoglycemia with nesidioblastosis after gastric bypass. These patients do not respond to treatment for dumping syndrome, but the confirmation of such a rare condition is very cumbersome.

RISK FACTORS
Accelerated gastric emptying resulting from gastric surgery is a main risk factor for dumping syndrome. In fact, the severity of dumping syndrome is proportional to the rate of gastric emptying. The common gastric surgical procedures associated with dumping syndrome are:

- Bariatric surgery (i.e., Roux-en-Y gastric bypass):
  - A recent study showed that a significant proportion of patients after laparoscopic sleeve gastrectomy (LSG) for morbid obesity also experienced dumping syndrome upon provocation (with oral glucose challenge), suggesting that LSG might not be a pure restrictive procedure for weight loss (1)[B].
- Gastric drainage procedures (e.g., pyloroplasty)
- Partial gastrectomy
- Total gastrectomy: Those with pouch formation have significantly less dumping and heartburn (2)[A].
- Esophagectomy
- Antiulcer surgery (e.g., vagotomy)
- Antireflux surgery (e.g., Nissen fundoplication, especially in pediatric patients)

GENERAL PREVENTION
- Dietary modifications (e.g., eating frequent, small, dry meals that contain limited amount of refined carbohydrates; restrict fluids to between meals; avoid milk products and increase protein/fat intake and supplement dietary fibers)
- Postural changes (i.e., lying supine for 30 minutes after meals)
- New surgical techniques may reduce postoperative dumping syndrome in bariatric surgery (3)[B].

COMMONLY ASSOCIATED CONDITIONS
- Peptic ulcer disease
- Reactive hypoglycemia
- Gastrectomy/Vagotomy/Pyloroplasty
- Esophagectomy
- After Nissen fundoplication for reflux disease in pediatric population
- After gastric bypass or sleeve gastrectomy procedure for morbid obesity

DIAGNOSIS

A suggestive symptom profile in a patient who has undergone gastric (including bariatric) or esophageal surgery warrants the investigation for dumping syndrome.

HISTORY
- History of gastric procedures
- GI symptoms (in early dumping):
  - Cramping abdominal pain
  - Diarrhea (postprandial)
  - Borborygmi
  - Bloating or epigastric fullness
  - Nausea/Vomiting
- Systemic/Vasomotor symptoms (both early and late dumping):
  - Palpitations
  - Diaphoresis
  - Faintness, fatigue, and headache
  - Flushing
  - Lightheadedness and desire to lie down
  - Confusion and syncope
  - Malnutrition and weight loss
- Early dumping symptoms include GI (e.g., abdominal pain, nausea, bloating, borborygmi and diarrhea) and vasomotor (e.g., perspiration and facial flushing, a desire to lie down, palpitations, weakness and syncope) symptoms.

- Late dumping symptoms include perspiration, palpitations, hunger, weakness, confusion and syncope, and so forth.

PHYSICAL EXAM
- Diagnosis is mainly based on typical symptoms in patients with history of gastric procedures.
- A diagnostic scoring system has been developed by Sigstad based on various weighting factors allocated to the symptoms of dumping:
  - A score index >7 is suggestive of dumping syndrome.
  - The score index is very helpful in assessing a response to therapy.
    Sigstad's Scoring System (4):

Shock	+5
Fainting, Syncope, Unconscious	+4
Desire to lie or sit down	+4
Breathlessness, Dyspnea	+3
Weakness, exhaustion	+3
Sleepiness, drowsiness, apathy	+3
Palpitation	+3
Dizziness	+2
Restlessness	+2
Headaches	+1
Feeling of warmth, sweating, pallor, clammy	+1
Nausea	+1
Abdominal fullness	+1
Borborygmus	+1
Eructation	−1
Vomiting	−1

- No physical signs are specific for dumping syndrome.

DIFFERENTIAL DIAGNOSIS
- Abnormal contractions of the duct (tract spasms)
- Afferent loop syndromes
- Bile acid reflux after surgery
- Bowel obstruction
- Celiac disease
- Gastroenteric fistula
- Inflammation of the gallbladder (cholecystitis)
- Inflammatory bowel disease
- Low blood sugar (hypoglycemia)
- Pancreatic insufficiency

DIAGNOSTIC TESTS & INTERPRETATION
Initial Tests (lab, imaging)
- Postprandial hypoglycemia
- Anemia
- Hypoalbuminemia
- Drugs that may alter lab results: Insulin
- Disorders that may alter lab results: Diabetes mellitus
- Upper GI series: Barium rapidly emptying from stomach
- Nuclear medicine gastric emptying study
- Endoscopy (to define anatomy and exclude mechanical obstruction)

Diagnostic Procedures/Other
- Dumping syndrome is a clinical diagnosis based on typical symptoms in patients who have undergone gastric surgery.
- Oral glucose challenge test (i.e., oral intake of 50 g of glucose following 10-hour fasting) can elicit typical signs and symptoms in patients with dumping syndrome. A rise in heart rate by ≥ 10 beats/minute in the 1st hour is the best predictor for dumping syndrome.
- Hydrogen breath test after oral ingestion of glucose is also a sensitive test.

TREATMENT
- Dietary modifications are the mainstay of treatment in patients with dumping syndrome.
- Medical therapy is effective in patients with incapacitating symptoms who fail dietary modifications.
- Remedial surgery is only considered in patients refractory to medical management.

GENERAL MEASURES
Most patients can be managed conservatively with dietary modification and medical treatment. Only a small percentage of patients ultimately require surgical intervention.

MEDICATION
First Line
- Octreotide (Sandostatin, 100–500 μg SC b.i.d.) relieves dumping symptoms by delaying gastric emptying and inhibiting the release of GI hormones:
  – Can be very expensive (5)[B]
  – Patients may have increased steatorrhea during octreotide treatment, and pancreatic enzyme supplement is effective in relieving this symptom.
  – Gallstone formation is also associated with long-term use of octreotide.
- Late dumping symptoms can be ameliorated by the α-glucosidase inhibitor acarbose (100–200 mg PO t.i.d.), which lowers blood glucose by delaying GI absorption of carbohydrates:
  – Patients on acarbose treatment often develop symptoms of bloating diarrhea due to bacterial fermentation of unabsorbed carbohydrate in the intestine.
- Pectin/Guar gum (ingestion of up to 15 g with each meal) is effective by delaying glucose absorption and prolonging small-bowel transit time.

Second Line
Anticholinergics: Results generally are disappointing.

ADDITIONAL THERAPIES
- Continuous trophic enteral feeding via a jejunostomy has been reported to be an effective approach in patients refractory to all other treatment measures.
- Individual psychotherapy plus behavior modification and, in selective cases, hypnotherapy (3)
- Adjuncts: Group therapy, expressive art therapy, occupational and recreational therapy when not associated with dissociative amnesia or fugue

SURGERY/OTHER PROCEDURES
- Remedial surgery only if dietary and medical management unsuccessful and symptoms debilitating; the results are variable and unpredictable. A proper selection of the surgical intervention is very important. Most patients with dumping syndrome as a result of gastric bypass will find that the effects ameliorate with time (>2 years).
- Options of surgery include Roux-en-Y conversion (from Billroth I and II), pyloric reconstruction (for patients who have severe dumping following pyloroplasty), reversed jejunal segment (for patients who failed Roux-en-Y reconstruction), and conversion of Billroth II to Billroth I anastomosis.
- Patients with refractory dumping symptoms after loop gastrojejunostomy may benefit from simple takedown of the anastomosis; conversion to Roux-en-Y gastrojejunostomy is a reasonable option for patients with disabling dumping after distal gastrectomy. Other procedures have been attempted with limited success.
- The syndrome of hyperinsulinemic hypoglycemia with nesidioblastosis (a hyperplasia of islet cells) after Roux-en-Y gastric bypass (>1–2 years postop) can usually be managed with low-carbohydrate diet and α-glucosidase inhibitors. Subtotal or total pancreatectomy (as has been suggested in the literature) is usually unnecessary.

ONGOING CARE
FOLLOW-UP RECOMMENDATIONS
Lying supine for 30 minutes after eating or when symptoms occur may reduce the chance of syncope.
Patient Monitoring
Follow to be sure of adequate nutrition.
DIET
- Low-carbohydrate, high-protein diet
- Add dietary fiber.
- Milk or milk products should be avoided.
- Frequent small meals with minimal liquid
- Avoid hyperosmolar liquids.
PATIENT EDUCATION
National Digestive Diseases Information Clearinghouse, Box NDDIC, Bethesda, MD 20892, (301) 468-6344, digestive.niddk.nih.gov
PROGNOSIS
Favorable
COMPLICATIONS
- Hypoglycemia
- Malnutrition and weight loss
- Electrolyte disturbances, including hypokalemia

REFERENCES
1. Tzovaras G, Papamargaritis D, Sioka E, et al. Symptoms suggestive of dumping syndrome after provocation in patients after laparoscopic sleeve gastrectomy. *Obes Surg.* 2012;22(1):23–28.
2. Gertler R, Rosenberg R, Feith M, et al. Pouch vs. no pouch following total gastrectomy: Meta-analysis and systematic review. *Am J Gastroenterol.* 2009;104:2838–2851.

3. Dikic S, Randjelovic T, Dragojevic S, et al. Early dumping syndrome and reflux esophagitis prevention with pouch reconstruction. *J Surg Res.* 2012;175(1):56–61. Epub 2011 Mar 5.
4. Sigstad, H. A Clinical Diagnostic Index in the diagnosis of the dumping syndrome. Changes in plasma volume and blood sugar after a test meal. *Acta Med Scand.* 1970;188:479–486.
5. Ukleja A. Dumping syndrome: Pathophysiology and treatment. *Nutr Clin Pract.* 2005;20:517–525.
6. Gonzalez-Sánchez JA, Corujo-Vázquez O, Sahai-Hernández M. Bariatric surgery patients: Reasons to visit emergency department after surgery. *Bol Asoc Med P R.* 2007;99:279–283.
7. Penning C, Vecht J, Masclee AA. Efficacy of depot long-acting release octreotide therapy in severe dumping syndrome. *Aliment Pharmacol Ther.* 2005;22:963–969.

ADDITIONAL READING
- Banerjee A, Ding Y, Mikami DJ, et al. The role of dumping syndrome in weight loss after gastric bypass surgery. *Surg Endosc.* 2013;27(5):1573–1578. doi: 10.1007/s00464-012-2629-1. Epub 2012 Dec 12.
- Bouras EP, Scolapio JS. Gastric motility disorders: Management that optimizes nutritional status. *J Clin Gastroenterol.* 2004;38:549–557.
- Tack J, Arts J, Caenepeel P. Pathophysiology, diagnosis and management of postoperative dumping syndrome. *Nat Rev Gastroenterol Hepatol.* 2009;6:583–590.

SEE ALSO
- Diarrhea, Chronic; Hypoglycemia, Nondiabetic; Peptic Ulcer Disease
- Algorithm: Diarrhea, Chronic

CODES
ICD10
K91.1 Postgastric surgery syndromes

CLINICAL PEARLS
- Vagotomy affects gastric emptying through increased gastric tone and decreased receptive relaxation.
- Dumping syndrome is the most common cause for emergency room presentation after bariatric surgery (6)[B].
- An increase in heart rate of 10 BPM is noted after glucose challenge (50 g PO glucose) in patients with dumping syndrome.
- Depot octreotide has shown some promise as an alternative to standard SC octreotide (7)[B].
- Some side effects of octreotide are gallstones, steatorrhea, and diarrhea.

DUPUYTREN CONTRACTURE

Jeffrey F. Minteer, MD

BASICS

DESCRIPTION
- Palmar fibromatosis; caused by progressive fibrous proliferation and tightening of the fascia inside the palms, resulting in flexion deformities and loss of function
- Not the same as "trigger finger," which is caused by thickening of the distal flexor tendon
- Similar change may rarely occur in plantar fascia; it usually appears simultaneously.
- System(s) affected: Musculoskeletal

EPIDEMIOLOGY
Prevalence
- Unknown in the US
- Norway:
  – 9% males and 3% females

ETIOLOGY AND PATHOPHYSIOLOGY
Unknown; possibly a T-cell–mediated autoimmune disorder

Genetics
- Autosomal-dominant with incomplete penetrance:
  – Siblings with 3-fold risk
- 68% of male relatives of affected patients develop disease at some time.

RISK FACTORS
- Smoking (mean 16 pack-years, odds ratio 2.8)
- Increasing age
- Male/Caucasian; Male > Female (1.7:1)
- Workers exposed to vibration (1)
- Diabetes mellitus (affected, increases with time, usually mild; middle and ring finger involved)
- Epilepsy
- Chronic illness (e.g., pulmonary tuberculosis, liver disease, HIV)
- Hypercholesterolemia
- Alcohol consumption

GENERAL PREVENTION
Avoid risk factors, especially in those with a strong family history.

COMMONLY ASSOCIATED CONDITIONS
- Alcoholism
- Epilepsy
- Diabetes mellitus
- Chronic lung disease
- Occupational hand trauma (vibration white finger)
- Shoulder–hand syndrome
- Status postmyocardial infarction
- Hypercholesterolemia
- Carpal tunnel syndrome

DIAGNOSIS

HISTORY
- Caucasian male aged 50–60 years
- Family history
- Mild pain early:
  – Begins in palm then spread to digits
- Unilateral or bilateral (50%)
- Right hand more frequent
- Ring finger more frequent
- Ulnar digits more affected than radial digits
- Flexion contracture of metacarpophalangeal (MCP) before proximal interphalangeal (PIP) joint
- 3 stages
  – Nodules of the palm
  – Involves facia and digits
  – Spread to fingers

PHYSICAL EXAM
- Painless plaques or nodules in palmar fascia
- Extends into a cordlike band in the palmar fascia
- Skin adheres to fascia and becomes puckered.
- Nodules can be palpated under the skin.
- Digital fascia becomes involved as disease progresses.
- Reduced flexibility of MCP and PIP joints
- No sign of inflammation
- Web space contractures
- Dupuytren diathesis can involve plantar (Ledderhose—10%) and penile (Peyronie—2%) fascia:
  – Knuckle pads over PIP:
    ○ Garrod nodes commonly associated with severe disease
- Disease stages:
  – Early: Skin pits (can also be seen in nevoid basal cell cancer and palmar keratosis)
  – Intermediate: Nodules and cords
  – Late: Contractures

DIFFERENTIAL DIAGNOSIS
- Early for callosity
- Tendon abnormalities
- Camptodactyly: Early teens; tight fascial bands on ulnar side of small finger
- Diabetic cheiroarthropathy: All 4 fingers
- Volkmann ischemic contracture

DIAGNOSTIC TESTS & INTERPRETATION
Diagnostic Procedures/Other
MRI can assess cellularity of lesions that correlate with higher recurrence after surgery.

Test Interpretation
- Myofibroblasts
- Nodules: Lumps fixed to skin hypercellular masses
- Cords: Organized collagen type III arranged parallel and hypocellular
- 1st stage (proliferative): Increased myofibroblasts
- 2nd stage (residual): Dense fibroblast network
- 3rd stage (involutional): Myofibroblasts disappear

TREATMENT

GENERAL MEASURES
- Physiotherapy alone is ineffective:
  – Intermittent splinting is unlikely to be effective.
  – Continuous splinting may be helpful pre- and postoperative.
- Isolated involvement of palmar fascia can be followed.
- MCP joint involvement can be followed if flexion contracture is <30 degrees.

MEDICATION
First Line
- Steroid injection for an acute tender nodule, painful knuckle pad
- Clostridial collagenase injections (FDA approved 2010):
  – Degrades collagen to allow manual rupture of diseased cord
  – Best for isolated cord of MCP joint 77% and 40% with PIP
  – Recurrence rate at 8 years 67% in MCP joints, but less severe than initial contracture (2)[B]
  – Complications: Edema, pain
  – Can do 2 cords concurrently
  – Can be effective after recurrence post surgery

Second Line
- Topical high-potency steroids: Case report of improvement with clobetasol 0.1% b.i.d. and at bedtime for 2–4 weeks
- Surgery for contracture >30%

ISSUES FOR REFERRAL
- Any involvement of PIP joints
- MCP joints contracted >30 degrees
- Positive Hueston test

ADDITIONAL THERAPIES
- Continuous elongation technique is useful to prepare a severely contracted PIP joint for surgery.
  - The digit can frequently be completely extended; however, it will relapse if surgery is not performed.
- Prophylactic external beam radiation: 87% either no progression or improvement at 12 months; concern about local effects in a benign disease
- Intraoperative 5-fluorouracil ineffective
- Percutaneous and needle fasciotomy:
  - Best for MCP joint
  - Recurrence common
  - Not indicated in severe or recurrent disease

SURGERY/OTHER PROCEDURES
- Selective fascial ray release/partial fasciectomy (3)[B]:
  - No studies have yet compared collagenase injection with limited fasciectomy or percutaneous needle fasciotomy (4).
  - Night extension orthosis in combination with standard hand therapy has no greater effect on maintaining finger extension than hand therapy alone in the 3 months following surgical release of Dupuytren contracture (5)[C]
- Indications:
  - Any involvement of the PIP joints
  - MCP joints are contracted at least 30 degrees.
  - Positive Hueston tabletop test: When the palm is placed on a flat surface, the digits cannot be simultaneously placed fully on the same surface as the palm because of flexion contractures.
- May require skin grafts for wound closure with severe cutaneous shrinkage. Reports of clinical regression with continuous passive skeletal traction in extension and under a skin graft.
- 80% have full range of movement if operated on early.
- Amputation of little finger if severe and deforming
- MCP joints respond better than PIP joints, especially if contracted >45 degrees.
- Percutaneous needle aponeurotomy: Elderly with comorbid conditions may do better when used for MCP joints; has higher rate of recurrence

 ONGOING CARE

FOLLOW-UP RECOMMENDATIONS
Patient Monitoring
Regular follow-up by physician every 6 months–1 year

PATIENT EDUCATION
- Avoid risk factors, especially in those with a strong family history.
- Mild disease: Passively stretch digits twice a day and avoid recurrent gripping of tools.

PROGNOSIS
- Unpredictable, but usually slowly progressive
- 10% may regress spontaneously.
- Patients likely to have aggressive disease if ≥1 of the following present: Age <40 years at onset, knuckle pads, positive family history, bilateral disease involving radial side of hand
- Recurrence rate after surgery is high; more with aggressive features
- Prognosis better for MCP vs. PIP joint after surgery and collagenase injection

COMPLICATIONS
- Postsurgery development of reflex sympathetic dystrophy
- Postoperative recurrence or extension in 46–80%
- Postoperative hand edema and skin necrosis
- Digital infarction

REFERENCES
1. Descatha A, Jauffret P, Chastang JF, et al. Should we consider Dupuytren's contracture as work-related? A review and meta-analysis of an old debate. *BMC Musculoskelet Disord*. 2011;12:96. Epub 2011 May 16.
2. Watt AJ, Curtin CM, Hentz VR, et al. Collagenase injection as nonsurgical treatment of Dupuytren's disease: 8-year follow-up. *J Hand Surg Am*. 2010;35:534–539, 539.e1.
3. van Rijssen AL, Werker PM. [Treatment of Dupuytren's contracture; an overview of options] *Ned Tijdschr Geneeskd*. 2009;153:A129.
4. Stanbury SJ, Hammert WC. Dupuytren contracture. *J Hand Surg Am*. 2011;36(12):2038–2040. Epub 2011 Jun 11.
5. Collis J, Collocott S, Hing W, et al. The effect of night extension orthoses following surgical release of Dupuytren contracture: A single-center, randomized, controlled trial. *J Hand Surg Am*. 2013;38(7):1285–1294.e2. doi: 10.1016/j.jhsa.2013.04.012.
6. Rayan GM. Clinical presentation and types of Dupuytren's disease. *Hand Clin*. 1999;15:87–96, vii.

ADDITIONAL READING
- Ball C, Pratt AL, Nanchahal J. Optimal functional outcome measures for assessing treatment for Dupuytren's disease: A systematic review and recommendations for future practice. *BMC Musculoskelet Disord*. 2013;14:131. doi: 10.1186/1471-2474-14-131.
- Black E, Blazar P. Dupuytren disease: An evolving understanding of an age-old disease. *J Am Acad Orthop Surg*. 2011;19:746–757.
- Rayan GM. Dupuytren disease: Anatomy, pathology, presentation, and treatment. *J Bone Joint Surg Am*. 2007;89(1):189–198.

 CODES

ICD10
- M72.0 Palmar fascial fibromatosis [Dupuytren]
- M72.2 Plantar fascial fibromatosis

CLINICAL PEARLS
- 90% of cases are progressive.
- Refer those with any involvement of the PIP joints or MCP involvement >30 degrees.
- Neither surgical nor enzymatic fasciotomy offers a cure; both have high rate of recurrence (6).

DYSFUNCTIONAL UTERINE BLEEDING
Tracy L. Williams, MD

 BASICS

DESCRIPTION
- Dysfunctional uterine bleeding (DUB) is irregular menstrual bleeding (usually heavy, prolonged, or frequent); it is a diagnosis of exclusion after establishment of normal anatomy and the absence of other medical illnesses.
- Commonly associated with anovulation

EPIDEMIOLOGY
Adolescent and perimenopausal women are affected most often.

Incidence
5% of reproductive age women will see a doctor in any given year for DUB.

Prevalence
10–30% of reproductive age women have DUB.

ETIOLOGY AND PATHOPHYSIOLOGY
- Anovulation accounts for 90% of DUB:
  - Loss of cyclic endometrial stimulation
  - Elevated estrogen levels stimulate endometrial growth.
  - No organized progesterone withdrawal bleed
  - Endometrium eventually outgrows blood supply, breaks down, and sloughs from uterus.
- Adolescent DUB is usually due to an immature hypothalamic-pituitary-ovarian (HPO) axis that leads to anovulatory cycles.
- DUB can be broadly divided into anovulatory bleeding (usually irregular and unpredictable menses) or ovulatory bleeding (usually heavy regular menses) after pathologic causes of abnormal bleeding have been ruled out:
  - Pregnancy: Ectopic pregnancy, threatened or incomplete abortion, or hydatidiform mole
  - Reproductive pathology and structural disorders:
    ○ Uterus: Leiomyomas, endometritis, hyperplasia, polyps, trauma
    ○ Adnexa: Salpingitis, functional ovarian cysts
    ○ Cervix: Cervicitis, polyps, STIs, trauma
    ○ Vagina: Trauma, foreign body
    ○ Vulva: Lichen sclerosis, STIs
- Malignancy of the vagina, cervix, uterus, and ovaries
- Systemic diseases:
  - Inflammatory bowel disease
  - Hematologic disorders (e.g., Von Willebrand disease, thrombocytopenia)
  - Advanced or fulminant liver disease
  - Chronic renal disease
- Diseases causing anovulation:
  - Hyperthyroidism/Hypothyroidism
  - Adrenal disorders
  - Pituitary disease (prolactinoma)
  - Polycystic ovarian syndrome (PCOS)
  - Eating disorders
- Medications (iatrogenic causes):
  - Anticoagulants
  - Steroids
  - Tamoxifen
  - Hormonal medications: Intrauterine devices
  - SSRIs
  - Antipsychotic medications
- Other causes of abnormal uterine bleeding:
  - Excessive weight gain
  - Increased exercise
  - Stress

Genetics
Unclear, but can include inherited disorders of hemostasis

RISK FACTORS
Risk factors for endometrial cancer (which can cause DUB):
- Age >40
- Obesity
- Diabetes mellitus
- Nulliparity
- Early menarche or late menopause (>55 years)
- Hypertension
- Chronic anovulation or infertility
- Unopposed estrogen therapy
- History of breast cancer or endometrial hyperplasia
- Tamoxifen use
- Family history: Gynecologic, breast, or colon cancer

 DIAGNOSIS

HISTORY
- Menstrual history:
  - Onset, severity (quantified by pad/tampon use, presence and size of clots), timing of bleeding (unpredictable or episodic)
  - Menorrhagia with onset of menarche is suggestive of a coagulation disorder.
  - Menopausal status
  - Association with other factors (e.g., coitus, contraception, weight loss/gain)
- Gynecologic history: Gravidity and parity, STI history, previous pap smear results
- Review of systems (exclude symptoms of pregnancy and of bleeding disorders, bleeding from other orifices, stress, exercise, recent weight change, visual changes, headaches, galactorrhea)
- Medication history: Evaluate for use of aspirin, anticoagulants, hormones, herbal supplements.

ALERT
Postmenopausal bleeding is any bleeding that occurs >1 year after the last menstrual period; cancer must always be ruled out.

PHYSICAL EXAM
Discover anatomic or organic causes of DUB:
- Evaluate for:
  - Body mass index (obesity)
  - Pallor, vital signs (anemia)
  - Visual field defects (pituitary lesion)
  - Hirsutism or acne (hyperandrogenism)
  - Goiter (thyroid dysfunction)
  - Galactorrhea (hyperprolactinemia)
  - Purpura, ecchymosis (bleeding disorders)
- Pelvic exam:
  - Evaluate for uterine irregularities and Tanner stage.
  - Check for foreign bodies.
  - Rule out rectal or urinary tract bleeding.
  - Include Pap smear and tests for STIs.

Pediatric Considerations
Premenarchal children with vaginal bleeding should be evaluated for foreign bodies, physical/sexual abuse, possible infections, and signs of precocious puberty.

DIFFERENTIAL DIAGNOSIS
See "Etiology."

DIAGNOSTIC TESTS & INTERPRETATION
Initial Tests (lab, imaging)
- Everyone: Urine human chorionic gonadotropin (hCG; rule out pregnancy and/or hydatiform mole) and complete blood count (CBC) (1)
- If anovulation suspected: Thyroid stimulating hormone (TSH) level, prolactin level (1)
- Consider other tests based on differential diagnosis:
  - Follicle-stimulating hormone (FSH) level to evaluate for hypo- or hypergonadotropism
  - Coagulation studies and factors if coagulopathy is suspected
  - Electrolytes and LFT if renal or hepatic disease is suspected
  - 17-hydroxyprogesterone if congenital adrenal hyperplasia suspected
  - Testosterone and/or DHEA-S if PCOS
  - Screening for STI
- Transvaginal US (TVUS):
  - Indications: Postmenopausal patients, suspicion of pregnancy or anatomic abnormalities, PCOS
  - High sensitivity for endometrial carcinoma in postmenopausal women; if ≤5 mm, endometrial cancer is unlikely.
  - If endometrial thickness >5 mm, proceed to endometrial biopsy (EMB)
  - No clear consensus on upper limit of normal endometrial thickness for premenopausal women
- TVUS, sonohysterography, and hysteroscopy may be similarly effective in detection of intrauterine pathology in premenopausal women with DUB (2)[A].

Diagnostic Procedures/Other
- Pap smear to screen for cervical cancer if age >21
- EMB should be performed in:
  - Women age >35 years with DUB to rule out cancer or premalignancy
  - Postmenopausal women with endometrial thickness >5 mm
  - Women aged 18–35 with DUB and risk factors for endometrial cancer (see "Risk Factors")
  - Perform on or after day 18 of cycle, if known; secretory endometrium confirms ovulation occurred.
- Dilation and curettage (D&C):
  - Perform if bleeding is heavy, uncontrolled, or if emergent medical management has failed.
  - Perform if unable to perform EMB in office.
- Hysteroscopy if another intrauterine lesion is suspected

Test Interpretation
Pap smear could reveal carcinoma or inflammation indicative of cervicitis. Most EMBs show proliferative or dyssynchronous endometrium (suggesting anovulation). but can show simple or complex hyperplasia without atypia, hyperplasia with atypia, or endometrial adenocarcinoma.

TREATMENT

Attempt to rule out other causes of bleeding prior to instituting therapy.

GENERAL MEASURES
NSAIDs (naproxen sodium 500 mg b.i.d., mefenamic acid 500 mg t.i.d., ibuprofen 600–1,200 mg/d):
- Decreases amount of blood loss compared with placebo, with no one clearly superior NSAID
- Diminishes pain

MEDICATION
First Line
- Acute, emergent, nonovulatory bleeding:
  – Conjugated equine estrogen (Premarin): 25 mg IV q4h (max 6 doses) or 2.5 mg PO q6h should control bleeding in 12–24 hours (3)[A]
  – D&C if no response after 2–4 doses of Premarin or sooner if bleeding >1 pad/hour
  – Then change to oral contraceptive pill (OCP) or progestin for cycle regulation
- Acute, nonemergent, nonovulatory bleeding:
  – Combination OCP with ≥30 μg estrogen given as a taper. An example of a tapered dose: 4 pills/d for 4 days; 3 pills/d for 3 days; 2 pills/d for 2 days, daily for 3 weeks then 1 week off, then cycle on OCP for at least 3 months.
- Nonacute, nonovulatory bleeding:
  – OCPs: 20–35 μg estrogen plus progesterone
  – Progestins: Medroxyprogesterone acetate (Provera) 10 mg/d for 5–10 days each month. Daily progesterone for 21 days/cycle results in significantly less blood loss (4)[A].
  – Levonorgestrel intrauterine device (Mirena) is most effective form of progesterone delivery (5)[A] and is not inferior to surgical management (6)[A].
- Do not use estrogen if contraindications, such as suspicion for endometrial hyperplasia or carcinoma, history of deep vein thrombosis (DVT), or the presence of smoking in women >35 years of age (relative contraindication), are present.
- Precautions:
  – Failed medical treatment requires further workup.
  – Consider DVT prophylaxis when treating with high-dose estrogens.

Second Line
- Leuprolide (varying doses and duration of action); gonadotropin-releasing hormone (GnRH) agonist.
- Danazol (200–400 mg/d for a maximum of 9 months) is more effective than NSAIDs, but is limited by androgenic side effects and cost. It has been essentially replaced by GnRH agonists.
- Antifibrinolytics like tranexamic acid (Lysteda, 650 mg, 2 tablets t.i.d. (max 5 days during menstruation)

ISSUES FOR REFERRAL
- If an obvious cause for vaginal bleeding is not found in a pediatric patient, refer to a pediatric endocrinologist.
- Patients with persistent bleeding despite medical treatment require re-evaluation and referral to a gynecologist.

ADDITIONAL THERAPIES
- Antiemetics if treating with high-dose estrogen or progesterone
- Iron supplementation if anemia (usually iron deficiency) is identified

SURGERY/OTHER PROCEDURES
- Hysterectomy in cases of endometrial cancer, if medical therapy fails, or if uterine pathology found
- Endometrial ablation is less expensive than hysterectomy and is associated with high patient satisfaction; failure of primary medical treatment is not necessary (7)[A].

IN-PATIENT CONSIDERATIONS
Admission Criteria/Initial Stabilization
Significant hemorrhage causing acute anemia with signs of hemodynamic instability; with acute bleeding, replace volume with crystalloid and blood, as necessary.

Nursing
Pad counts and clot size can be helpful to determine and monitor amount of bleeding.

Discharge Criteria
- Hemodynamic stability
- Control of vaginal bleeding

 ONGOING CARE

FOLLOW-UP RECOMMENDATIONS
Routine follow-up with a primary care or OB/GYN provider

Patient Monitoring
Women treated with estrogen or OCPs should keep a menstrual diary to document bleeding patterns and their relation to therapy.

DIET
No restrictions

PATIENT EDUCATION
- Explain possible/likely etiologies.
- Answer all questions, especially those related to cancer and fertility.
- http://www.acog.org/For_Patients

PROGNOSIS
- Varies with pathophysiologic process
- Most anovulatory cycles can be treated with medical therapy and do not require surgical intervention.

COMPLICATIONS
- Iron-deficiency anemia
- Uterine cancer in cases of prolonged unopposed estrogen stimulation

REFERENCES
1. Sweet MG, Schmidt-Dalton TA, Weiss PM, et al. Evaluation and management of abnormal uterine bleeding in premenopausal women. *Am Fam Physician*. 2012;85(1):35–43.
2. Farquhar C, Ekeroma A, Furness S, et al. A systematic review of transvaginal ultrasonography, sonohysterography and hysteroscopy for the investigation of abnormal uterine bleeding in premenopausal women. *Acta Obstet Gynecol Scand*. 2003;82(6):493–504.
3. DeVore GR. Use of intravenous Premarin in the treatment of dysfunctional uterine bleeding: A double-blind randomized control study. *Obstet Gynecol*. 1982;59(3):285–291.
4. Lethaby A. Cyclical progestogens for heavy menstrual bleeding. *Cochrane Database Syst Rev*. 2008;(1):CD001016.
5. Lethaby AE, Cooke I, Rees M, et al. Progesterone or progestogen-releasing intrauterine systems for heavy menstrual bleeding. *Cochrane Database Syst Rev*. 2005;CD002126.
6. Marjoribanks J, Lethaby A, Farquhar C, et al. Surgery versus medical therapy for heavy menstrual bleeding. *Cochrane Database Syst Rev*. 2006; CD003855.
7. Lethaby A, Shepperd S, Cooke I, et al. Endometrial resection and ablation versus hysterectomy for heavy menstrual bleeding. *Cochrane Database Syst Rev*. 2000;CD000329.

ADDITIONAL READING
- Diagnosis of abnormal uterine bleeding in reproductive-aged woman. ACOG Committee Opinion No. 128. American College Obstetricians and Gynecologists. *Obstet Gynecol*. 2012;120: 197–206.
- Dijkhuizen FP. The accuracy of transvaginal ultrasonography in the diagnosis of endometrial abnormalities. *Obstet Gynecol*. 1996;87(3): 345–349.
- Ely JW, Kennedy CM, Clark EC, et al. Abnormal uterine bleeding: A management algorithm. *J Am Board Fam Med*. 2006.;19(6):590–602.
- Kouides PA, Conard J, Peyvandi F, et al. Hemostasis and menstruation: Appropriate investigation for underlying disorders of hemostasis in women with excessive menstrual bleeding. *Fertil Steril*. 2005; 84(5):1345–1351.
- Lethaby A, Farquhar C, Cooke I. Antifibrinolytics for heavy menstrual bleeding. *Cochrane Database Syst Rev*. 2000;(4):CD000249.

 SEE ALSO

- Dysmenorrhea; Menorrhagia
- Algorithm: Menorrhagia

 CODES

ICD10
- N93.0 Postcoital and contact bleeding
- N93.8 Other specified abnormal uterine and vaginal bleeding
- N97.0 Female infertility associated with anovulation

CLINICAL PEARLS
- DUB is irregular bleeding that occurs in the absence of pathology, making it a diagnosis of exclusion.
- Anovulation accounts for 90% of DUB.
- An EMB should be performed in all women >35 years of age with DUB to rule out cancer or premalignancy, and it should be considered in women aged 18–35 with DUB and risk factors for endometrial cancer.

DYSHIDROSIS
Cara Marshall, MD

 BASICS

DESCRIPTION
- A skin rash (dermatitis) within the "dyshidrosis" family. Literature supports the presence of several different classes within the family "dyshidrosis," but no general agreement about a strict definition of these classes.
- Dyshidrotic eczema:
  - Common, chronic, or recurrent; nonerythematous; symmetric vesicular eruption primarily of the palms, soles, and interdigital areas
  - Associated with burning, itching, and pain
- Pompholyx (from Greek, "bubble"):
  - Rare condition characterized by abrupt onset of large bullae
  - Sometimes used interchangeably with dyshidrotic eczema (small vesicles). Some believe these to be discrete entities.
- Lamellar dyshidrosis:
  - Fine, spreading exfoliation of the superficial epidermis in the same distribution as described above
- System(s) affected: Dermatologic; Exocrine; Immunologic
- Synonym(s): Cheiropompholyx; Keratolysis exfoliativa; Vesicular palmoplantar eczema; Desquamation of interdigital spaces; Palmar pompholyx reaction; Acute and recurrent hand dermatitis (1)

EPIDEMIOLOGY
Incidence
- Mean age of onset is <40 years
- Male = Female
- Comprises 5–20% of hand eczema cases

Prevalence
20 cases/100,000 population

ETIOLOGY AND PATHOPHYSIOLOGY
- Exact mechanism unknown; thought to be multifactorial
- Dermatopathology: Spongiosis with intraepidermal vesicles
- Despite the name, sweat glands are not altered/affected (2).
- Vesicles remain intact due to thickness of stratum corneum of palmar/plantar skin (1).
- Exact cause not known
- Aggravating factors (debated):
  - Hyperhidrosis (in 40% of patients with the condition)
  - Climate: Hot/cold weather; humidity
  - Contact sensitivity (in 30–67% of patients with the condition) (2)
  - Nickel, cobalt, and chromate sensitivity (may include implanted orthopedic or orthodontic metals) (1)
  - Irritating compounds and solutions
  - Stress
  - Dermatophyte infection (present in 10% of patients with the condition) (2)
  - Prolonged wear of occlusive gloves
  - IV immunoglobulin therapy
  - Smoking

Genetics
- Atopy: 50% of patients with dyshidrotic eczema have atopic dermatitis (1).
- Rare autosomal-dominant form of pompholyx found in Chinese population maps to chromosome 18q22.1–18q22.3 (2).

RISK FACTORS
- Many risk factors are disputed in the literature, with none being consistently associated.
- Atopy
- Other dermatologic conditions:
  - Atopic dermatitis (early in life)
  - Contact dermatitis (later in life)
  - Dermatophytosis
- Sensitivity to:
  - Foods
  - Drugs: Neomycin, quinolones, acetaminophen, and oral contraceptives
  - Contact and dietary: Nickel (more common in young women), chromate (more common in men) and cobalt (1)
  - Smoking in males

GENERAL PREVENTION
- Control emotional stress.
- Avoid excessive sweating.
- Avoid exposure to irritants.
- Avoid diet high in metal salts (chromium, cobalt, nickel).
- Avoid smoking.

COMMONLY ASSOCIATED CONDITIONS
- Atopic dermatitis
- Allergic contact dermatitis
- Parkinson's disease
- HIV (2)

 DIAGNOSIS

HISTORY
- Episodes of pruritic rash
- Recent emotional stress
- Familial or personal history of atopy
- Exposure to allergens or irritants (3):
  - Occupational, dietary, or household
  - Cosmetic and personal hygiene products
  - Vesicular eruption typically occurs 24 hours after allergen challenge (1).
- Costume jewelry use
- IV immunoglobulin therapy
- HIV
- Smoking

PHYSICAL EXAM
- Symmetric distribution on the palms and soles; also may affect the dorsal aspects of hands and feet
- Lesions may not heal completely between flares (1).
- Early findings:
  - 1–2 mm, clear, nonerythematous, deep-seated vesicles
- Late findings:
  - Unroofed vesicles with inflamed bases
  - Desquamation
  - Peeling, rings of scale, or lichenification common

DIFFERENTIAL DIAGNOSIS
- Vesicular tinea pedis/manuum
- Vesicular id reaction
- Contact dermatitis (allergic or irritant)
- Scabies
- Chronic vesicular hand dermatitis
- Drug reaction
- Dermatophytid
- Bullous disorders: Dyshidrosiform bullous pemphigoid, pemphigus, bullous impetigo, epidermolysis bullosa
- Pustular psoriasis
- Acrodermatitis continua
- Erythema multiforme
- Herpes infection
- Pityriasis rubra pilaris
- Vesicular mycosis fungoides

DIAGNOSTIC TESTS & INTERPRETATION
Follow-Up Tests & Special Considerations
- Skin culture in suspected secondary infection (most commonly, *Staphylococcus aureus*) (4)
- Consider antibiotics based on culture results and severity of symptoms.

Diagnostic Procedures/Other
- Diagnosis is based on clinical exam.
- KOH wet mount (if concerned about dermatophyte infection)
- Patch test (if suspecting allergic cause)

Test Interpretation
- Fine, 1–2-mm spongiotic vesicles intraepidermally with little to no inflammatory change
- No eccrine glandular involvement
- Thickened stratum corneum

 TREATMENT

Identification and avoidance of aggravating factors

GENERAL MEASURES
- Avoid possible causative factors: Stress, direct skin contact with irritants, nickel, occlusive gloves, household cleaning products, smoking, sweating
- Moisturizers/Emollients for symptomatic relief and to maintain effective skin barrier
- Skin care:
  - Wear shoes with leather rather than rubber soles (e.g., sneakers).
  - Wear socks and gloves made of cotton and change frequently.
  - Wash infrequently, carefully dry, then apply emollient.
  - Avoid direct contact with fresh fruit (5)[C].

MEDICATION

First Line

- Mild cases: Topical steroids (high potency) (2)[B]:
  - Considered cornerstone of therapy, but limited published evidence
- Moderate-to-severe cases:
  - Ultrahigh-potency topical steroids with occlusion over treated area (4)[B]
  - Oral steroids 40–100 mg/d tapered after blister formation ceases (2)[B]
  - Psoralens plus ultraviolet (UV)-A therapy (PUVA), either systemic/topical *or* immersion in psoralens (2)[B]
- Recurrent cases (4)[B]:
  - Systemic steroids at onset of itching prodrome
  - Prednisone 60 mg PO × 3–4 days

Second Line

- Topical calcineurin inhibitors (mitigate the long-term risks of topical steroid use):
  - Topical tacrolimus (6)[B]
  - Topical pimecrolimus (6)[B]
  - May not be as effective on plantar surface
- Other therapies (typically with dermatology consultation):
  - Oral cyclosporine (4)[B]
  - Injections of botulinum toxin type A (BTXA) (6)[B]:
    - Newer topical forms of BTXA currently being developed show promise.
    - Painful, requires nerve block
  - Systemic alitretinoin (teratogenic) (5)[B]
  - Topical bexarotene (a teratogenic retinoid X receptor agonist approved for use in cutaneous T-cell lymphoma) (6)[B]
  - Methotrexate (6)[C]
  - Azathioprine (1)[C]
  - Disulfiram or sodium cromoglycate in nickel-allergic patients (1)[C]
  - Mycophenolate mofetil (2)(C)
  - Tapwater ionotophoresis (2)[C]

ISSUES FOR REFERRAL

- Allergist (if allergen testing required)
- Psychologist (if stress modification needed)

ADDITIONAL THERAPIES

- Radiation therapy (1)[C]
- UV-free phototherapy (5)[C]
- Treat underlying dermatopytosis (1)

COMPLEMENTARY AND ALTERNATIVE MEDICINE

- Topical treatments to minimize pruritus (not curative) (4)[C]: Burow's solution (aluminum acetate) or vinegar compress
- Exposure to sunlight as maintenance therapy, 12 minutes every other day, 10–15 exposures (5)[C]
- Dandelion juice (avoid in atopic patients) (6)[C]

 ONGOING CARE

FOLLOW-UP RECOMMENDATIONS

Patient Monitoring

- Dyshidrotic Eczema Area and Severity Index (DASI) (1)
- Parameters used in the DASI score:
  - Number of vesicles per square centimeter
  - Erythema
  - Desquamation
  - Severity of itching
  - Surface area affected
- Grading: Mild (0–15), moderate (16–30), severe (31–60)
- Monitor BP and glucose in patients receiving systemic corticosteroids.
- Monitor for adverse effects of medications.

DIET

- Consider diet low in metal salts if there is history of nickel sensitivity (4)[B].
- Updated recommendations for low-cobalt diet are available (1).

PATIENT EDUCATION

- Instructions on self-care, complications, and avoidance of triggers/aggravating factors
- PubMed Health: Dyshidrotic Eczema at: http://www.ncbi.nlm.nih.gov/pubmedhealth/PMH0001835/

PROGNOSIS

- Condition is benign.
- Usually heals without scarring.
- Lesions may spontaneously resolve.
- Recurrence is common.

COMPLICATIONS

- Secondary bacterial infections (*S. aureus* most common)
- Dystrophic nail changes
- Fissures
- Skin tightening/discomfort
- Psychological distress

REFERENCES

1. Veien NK. Acute and recurrent vesicular hand dermatitis. *Dermatol Clin*. 2009;27:337–353.
2. Wollina U. Pompholyx: A review of clinical features, differential diagnosis, and management. *Am J Clin Dermatol*. 2010;11(5):305–314.
3. Guillet MH, Wierzbicka E, Guillet S, et al. A 3-year causative study of pompholyx in 120 patients. *Arch Dermatol*. 2007;143:1504–1508.
4. Lofgren SM. Dyshidrosis: Epidemiology, clinical characteristics, and therapy. *Dermatitis*. 2006;17: 165–181.
5. Letic M. Use of sunlight to treat dyshidrotic eczema. *JAMA Dermatol*. 2013 May1;149(5):634–635.
6. Wollina U. Pompholyx: What's new? *Expert Opin Investig Drugs*. 2008;17:897–904.

ADDITIONAL READING

- Chen J. The gene for a rare autosomal dominant form of pompholyx maps to chromosome 18q22.1–18q22.3. *J Invest Dermatol*. 2006;126: 300–304.
- Molin S, Diepgen TL, Ruzicka T, et al. Diagnosing chronic hand eczema by an algorithm: A tool for classification in clinical practice. *Clin Exp Dermatol*. 2011;36(6):595–601.
- Rashid RM, Salah W, Keuer EJ. Vexing vesicles. *Am J Med*. 2007;120(7):589–590.
- Stuckert J, Nedorost S. Low-cobalt diet for dyshidrotic eczema patients. *Contact Derm*. 2008;59(6):361–365.
- Sumila M, Notter M, Itin P, et al. Long-term results of radiotherapy in patients with chronic palmoplantar eczema or psoriasis. *Strahlenther Onkol*. 2008;184(4):218–223.
- Thiers BH. What's new in dermatologic therapy. *Dermatol Ther*. 2008;21(2):142–149.
- Tzaneva S, Kittler H, Thallinger C, et al. Oral vs. bath PUVA using 8-methoxypsoralen for chronic palmoplantar eczema. *Photodermatol Photoimmunol Photomed*. 2009;25(2):101–105.

 SEE ALSO

Algorithm: Rash, Focal

 CODES

ICD10

L30.1 Dyshidrosis [pompholyx]

CLINICAL PEARLS

- Dyshidrosis is a transient, recurrent vesicular eruption most commonly of the palms, soles, and interdigital areas.
- Etiology and pathophysiology are unknown, but are most likely related to a combination of genetic and environmental factors.
- Best prevention is effective skin care and limiting exposure to irritating agents.
- Treatments are based on disease severity; preferred treatments include topical steroids, oral steroids, and calcineurin inhibitors.
- Condition is benign and usually heals spontaneously and without scarring. Medical treatment decreases healing time and risk for progression to secondary bacterial infection.

D

DYSMENORRHEA
Jessica Kim, MD • Clara Keegan, MD

BASICS

DESCRIPTION
- Pelvic pain occurring at/around the time of menses; a leading cause of absenteeism for women <30 years of age
- Primary dysmenorrhea: Without pathologic physical findings
- Secondary dysmenorrhea: Often more severe than primary, having a secondary pathologic (structural) cause
- Classified by severity:
  – Mild: Pelvic discomfort, cramping, or heaviness on 1st day of bleeding, with no associated symptoms
  – Moderate: Discomfort occurring during 1st 2–3 days of menses, accompanied by mild malaise, diarrhea, and headache
  – Severe: Intense, cramp-like pain lasting 2–7 days, often with nausea, diarrhea, back pain, thigh pain, and headache
- System affected: Reproductive
- Synonym(s): Menstrual cramps

EPIDEMIOLOGY
- Predominant age:
  – Primary: Teens to early 20s
  – Secondary: 20s–30s
- Predominant sex: Women only

Prevalence
- 43–91% of adolescent females have primary dysmenorrhea (1).
- 16–67% prevalence in women >18 years of age (1)
- 10–30% of women who work/study lose 1–2 work/school days/month in the US (1).

ETIOLOGY AND PATHOPHYSIOLOGY
See "Etiology."
- Primary: Elevated production of prostaglandins (PGF$_{2\alpha}$) through indirect hormonal control (stimulation of production by estrogen) which causes hypercontractility and increased uterine muscle tone with resultant uterine ischemia. Ischemia results in type C pain neuron stimulation through buildup of anaerobic metabolites.
- Secondary:
  – Congenital abnormalities of uterine/vaginal anatomy
  – Cervical stenosis
  – Pelvic infection
  – Adenomyosis
  – Endometriosis
  – Pelvic tumors, especially leiomyomata (fibroids)
  – Uterine polyps
  – Use of IUD

Genetics
Not well studied

RISK FACTORS
- Primary:
  – Cigarette smoking
  – Alcohol use
  – Depression
  – Weight Loss
  – Early menarche
  – Irregular/heavy menstrual flow
- Secondary:
  – Pelvic infection
  – Use of IUD
  – Structural pelvic malformations

GENERAL PREVENTION
- Primary: Choose a diet low in animal fats.
- Secondary: Reduce risk of STIs

Pediatric Considerations
Onset with 1st menses raises probability of genital tract anatomic abnormality, such as transverse vaginal septum, imperforate or minimally perforated hymen, and uterine anomalies.

COMMONLY ASSOCIATED CONDITIONS
- Irregular/Heavy menstrual periods
- Longer menstrual cycle length/duration of bleeding

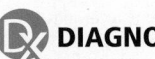 DIAGNOSIS

- Primary: History is characteristic.
- Based on characteristic history of cramping pain felt in suprapubic/low back
- Patients may have associated diarrhea, headache, fatigue, or pain radiating into the inner thighs.

HISTORY
- Onset once ovulatory cycles are established in adolescents; 2 years after menarche on average
- Recurrence at or just before the onset of the menstrual flow:
  – Pelvic pain occurring between menstrual periods is not likely to be dysmenorrhea.
  – Present with most menstrual periods
- Relief associated with:
  – Continued bleeding for the usual duration
  – Use of analgesics, especially NSAIDs
  – Orgasm
  – Local heat application
- Response to NSAIDs helps confirm diagnosis.

PHYSICAL EXAM
- Primary: Physical exam typically is normal. Examine to rule out secondary dysmenorrhea.
- Secondary: Exam may show evidence of uterine enlargement, tenderness, irregularity, or fixation.

DIFFERENTIAL DIAGNOSIS
- Primary: History is characteristic.
- Secondary:
  – Pelvic/Genital infection
  – Complication of pregnancy
  – Missed/Incomplete abortion
  – Ectopic pregnancy
  – Uterine/Ovarian neoplasm
  – Endometriosis
  – UTI
  – Complication with IUD use

DIAGNOSTIC TESTS & INTERPRETATION
Initial Tests (lab, imaging)
- Pregnancy test
- Gonorrhea/Chlamydia cervical testing, especially in women age <25 years and in high prevalence areas
- Primary: Consider pelvic ultrasound to rule out secondary abnormalities if history is not characteristic.
- Secondary: Ultrasound/Laparoscopy to define anatomy for severe/refractory cases

Follow-Up Tests & Special Considerations
Counsel regarding appropriate preventive measures for STI and pregnancy.

Diagnostic Procedures/Other
Laparoscopy is rarely needed.

Test Interpretation
- Primary:
  – None
- Secondary:
  – Uterine enlargement
  – Leiomyomata
  – Ligamentous thickening
  – Fixation of pelvic structures
  – Endometritis
  – Salpingitis
  – Adenomyosis

Pregnancy Considerations
Consider ectopic pregnancy when pelvic pain occurs with vaginal bleeding.

TREATMENT

- Reassure the patient that treatment success is very likely with adherence to recommendations.
- Relief may require the use of several treatment modalities at the same time.

GENERAL MEASURES
- Exercise and local heat are noninvasive general measures to relieve pain.
- High-frequency transcutaneous electrical nerve stimulation (TENS) was found to be effective for the treatment of dysmenorrhea. Conflicting evidence for low-frequency TENS was found.
- Secondary dysmenorrhea: Treatment of infections; suppression of endometrium if endometriosis suspected; remove IUD if contributing factor.

MEDICATION
First Line
- NSAIDs (1)[A]: No NSAID has been found to be better than another for treatment of pelvic pain in primary dysmenorrhea. In theory, COX-2 inhibitors are more selective for the endometrium, although they have not been FDA approved for use in primary dysmenorrhea. Preferred duration of treatment is ≤3 days (2) beginning just before/at onset of menses:
  – Ibuprofen 400 mg q8h
  – Naproxen sodium 500 mg b.i.d.
- Combination oral contraceptives (COCs) (1)[A]: In women who wish to use a contraceptive, the preferred method of treatment; NNT = 6. COCs containing 0.02 mg of ethinyl estradiol used in 2 randomized, controlled trials were shown to relieve pain of primary dysmenorrhea. Continuous rather than cyclic administration may be more effective for reducing pain (3)[A].
- Depo medroxyprogesterone acetate (DMPA) 150 mg IM every 12 weeks (4)
- Potential contraindications to NSAIDs and COCs:
  – Platelet disorders
  – Gastric ulceration or gastritis
  – Thromboembolic disorders
  – Vascular disease
  – Migraine with aura
- Precautions:
  – GI irritation
  – Lactation
  – Coagulation disorders
  – Impaired renal function
  – Congestive heart failure
  – Liver dysfunction

- Significant possible interactions:
  – Coumadin-type anticoagulants
  – Aspirin with other NSAIDs

Second Line
- Local heat can help relieve pain.
- Exercise may have beneficial effects in relieving pain (5)[A].
- Behavioral interventions, such as relaxation exercises, may help alleviate pain in primary dysmenorrhea.
- β_2-adrenoceptor agonists have not definitively been shown to relieve pain in dysmenorrhea (6)[A].
- Levonorgestrel IUDs can decrease primary dysmenorrhea. Copper IUDs have not been shown to be helpful.

SURGERY/OTHER PROCEDURES
Laparoscopic uterosacral nerve ablation has been shown to relieve pain at >12 months postoperatively.

COMPLEMENTARY AND ALTERNATIVE MEDICINE
- Spinal manipulation for primary/secondary dysmenorrhea has not been shown to be effective in treating pain (7)[A].
- Chinese herbal medicine shows promising evidence of decreasing pain, but more evidence is needed (8)[A].
- Acupuncture treatments have been shown to decrease pain in dysmenorrhea, but further randomized, well-designed studies are needed.
- Acupoint stimulation, particularly noninvasive stimulation (acupressure, moxibustion, and acupoint herbal patches), can relieve pain.
- Aromatherapy abdominal massage performed daily for 10 minutes 7 days prior to onset of menses can decrease primary dysmenorrhea (9)[A].

IN-PATIENT CONSIDERATIONS
Both primary and secondary dysmenorrhea usually are managed in the outpatient setting.

Admission Criteria/Initial Stabilization
- Primary: Outpatient care
- Secondary: Usually outpatient care

 ONGOING CARE

FOLLOW-UP RECOMMENDATIONS
Normal

DIET
- Vitamin B_1 100 mg daily been shown to be helpful in relieving dysmenorrhea (10)[A].
- Magnesium has been shown to be useful, but the correct dosage has not been determined (10)[A].
- Insufficient evidence to show usefulness of fish oil, zinc, and vitamin E at this time (10)[A].
- Low-fat vegetarian diet can be helpful in some patients.

PATIENT EDUCATION
Reassure the patient that primary dysmenorrhea is treatable with use of NSAIDs, COCs, or local heat and that it will usually abate with age and parity.

PROGNOSIS
- Primary: Reduced with age and parity
- Secondary: Likely to require therapy based on underlying cause

COMPLICATIONS
- Primary: Anxiety and/or depression
- Secondary: Infertility from underlying pathology

REFERENCES
1. Zahradnik HP, Hanjalic-Beck A, Groth K. Nonsteroidal anti-inflammatory drugs and hormonal contraceptives for pain relief from dysmenorrhea: A review. *Contraception*. 2010;81(3):185–196. Epub 2009 Nov 6.
2. Marjoribanks J, Proctor M, Farquhar C, et al. Nonsteroidal anti-inflammatory drugs for dysmenorrhoea. *Cochrane Database Syst Rev*. 2010;(1):CD001751. Epub 2010 Jan 20.
3. Edelman A., et al. Continuous or extended cycle vs. cyclic use of combined hormonal contraceptives for contraception. *Cochrane Database Syst Rev* 2010;
4. French L. Dysmenorrhea. *Am Fam Physician*. 2005 Jan 15;71(2):285–291.
5. Brown J, Brown S. Exercise for dysmenorrhoea. *Cochrane Database Syst Rev*. 2010;(2): CD004142. Epub 2010 Feb 17.
6. Fedorowicz Z, Nasser M, Jagannath VA, et al. Beta2-adrenoceptor agonists for dysmenorrhoea. *Cochrane Database Syst Rev*. 2012;5:CD008585. Epub 2012 May 16.
7. Proctor ML, Hing W, Johnson TC, et al. Spinal manipulation for primary and secondary dysmenorrhoea. *Cochrane Database Syst Rev*. 2006;(3):CD002119. Epub 2006 Jul 19.
8. Zhu X, Proctor M, Bensoussan A, et al. Chinese herbal medicine for primary dysmenorrhoea. *Cochrane Database Syst Rev*. 2008;CD005288.
9. Marzouk TMF, El-Nemer AMR, Baraka HN. The effect of aromatherapy abdominal massage on alleviating menstrual pain in nursing students: A prospective randomized cross-over study. *Evidence-Based Complementary and Alternative Medicine*. 2013; Epub 2013 Apr 11.
10. Proctor ML, Murphy PA. Herbal and dietary therapies for primary and secondary dysmenorrhoea. *Cochrane Database Syst Rev*. 2001;CD002124.

ADDITIONAL READING
- Akin MD, Weingand KW, Hengehold DA, et al. Continuous low-level topical heat in the treatment of dysmenorrhea. *Obstet Gynecol*. 2001;97(3): 343–349.
- Allen LM, Lam AC. Premenstrual syndrome and dysmenorrhea in adolescents. *Adolesc Med State Art Rev*. 2012;23(1):139–163.
- Cho SH, Hwang EW. Acupuncture for primary dysmenorrhoea: A systematic review. *B J Obstet Gynaecol*. 2010;117:509–521.
- Eby G. Zinc treatment prevents dysmenorrhea. *Med Hypoth*. 2007;69.2:297–301.
- Khan KS, Champaneria R, Latthe PM. How effective are non-drug, non-surgical treatments for primary dysmenorrhoea? *BMJ*. 2012;344:e3011. Epub 2012 May 14.
- Latthe P, Mignini L, Gray R, et al. Factors predisposing women to chronic pelvic pain: Systematic review. *BMJ*. 2006;332(7544):749–755. Epub 2006 Feb 16.
- Sanfilippo J, Erb T. Evaluation and management of dysmenorrhea in adolescents. *Clin Obstet Gynecol*. 2008;51:257–267.
- Yang H, Liu CZ, Chen X, et al. Systematic review of clinical trials of acupuncture-related therapies for primary dysmenorrhea. *Acta Obstet Gynecol Scand*. 2008:1–9.
- Zhao L, Li P. A survey of acupuncture treatment for primary dysmenorrhea. *J Tradit Chin Med*. 2009;29: 71–76.

 ### SEE ALSO
- Endometriosis
- Algorithm: Pelvic Girdle Pain

 ### CODES

ICD10
- N94.4 Primary dysmenorrhea
- N94.5 Secondary dysmenorrhea
- N94.6 Dysmenorrhea, unspecified

CLINICAL PEARLS
- Dysmenorrhea is a leading cause of absenteeism for women age <30 years.
- In women who desire contraception, combined oral contraceptives are preferred treatment.
- All NSAIDs studied have been found to be equally effective in the relief of dysmenorrhea.

DYSPAREUNIA

Scott T. Henderson, MD

BASICS

DESCRIPTION
- Recurrent and persistent genital pain associated with sexual activity, which is not exclusively due to lack of lubrication or vaginismus.
- May be the result of organic, emotional, or psychogenic causes:
  - Primary: Present throughout one's sexual history
  - Secondary: Arising from some specific event or condition (e.g., menopause, drugs)
  - Superficial: Pain at, or near, the introitus or vaginal barrel associated with penetration
  - Deep: Pain after penetration located at the cervix or lower abdominal area
  - Complete: Present under all circumstances
  - Situational: Occurring selectively with specific situations
- System(s) affected: Reproductive

EPIDEMIOLOGY
- Predominant age: All ages
- Predominant sex: Female > Male

Incidence
>50% of all sexually active women will report dyspareunia at some time.

Geriatric Considerations
Incidence increases dramatically in postmenopausal women primarily because of vaginal atrophy.

Prevalence
- Most sexually active women will experience dyspareunia at some time in their lives:
  - ~15% (4–40%) of adult women will have dyspareunia on a few occasions during a year.
  - ~1–2% of women will have painful intercourse on a more-than-occasional basis.
- Male prevalence is ~1%.

ETIOLOGY AND PATHOPHYSIOLOGY
- Disorders of vaginal outlet:
  - Adhesions
  - Clitoral irritation
  - Episiotomy scars
  - Fissures
  - Hymeneal ring abnormalities
  - Inadequate lubrication
  - Infections
  - Lichen planus
  - Lichen sclerosus
  - Postmenopausal atrophy
  - Trauma
  - Vulvar papillomatosis
  - Vulvar vestibulitis/vulvodynia
- Disorders of vagina:
  - Abnormality of vault owing to surgery or radiation
  - Congenital malformations
  - Inadequate lubrication
  - Infections
  - Inflammatory or allergic response to foreign substance
  - Masses or tumors
  - Pelvic relaxation resulting in rectocele, uterine prolapse, or cystocele
- Disorders of pelvic structures:
  - Endometriosis
  - Levator ani myalgia/spasm
  - Malignant or benign tumors of the uterus
  - Ovarian pathology
  - Pelvic adhesions
  - Pelvic inflammatory disease (PID)
  - Pelvic venous congestion
  - Prior pelvic fracture
- Disorders of the GI tract:
  - Constipation
  - Crohn disease
  - Diverticular disease
  - Fistulas
  - Hemorrhoids
  - Inflammatory bowel disease
- Disorders of the urinary tract:
  - Interstitial cystitis
  - Ureteral or vesical lesions
- Chronic disease:
  - Behçet syndrome
  - Diabetes
  - Sjögren syndrome
- Male:
  - Cancer of penis
  - Genital muscle spasm
  - Infection or irritation of penile skin
  - Infection of seminal vesicles
  - Lichen sclerosus
  - Musculoskeletal disorders of pelvis and lower back
  - Penile anatomy disorders
  - Phimosis
  - Prostate infections and enlargement
  - Testicular disease
  - Torsion of spermatic cord
  - Urethritis
- Psychological disorders:
  - Anxiety
  - Conversion reactions
  - Depression
  - Fear
  - Hostility toward partner
  - Phobic reactions
  - Psychological trauma

RISK FACTORS
- Fatigue
- Stress
- Depression
- Diabetes
- Estrogen deficiency:
  - Menopause
  - Lactation
- Previous PID
- Vaginal surgery
- Alcohol/marijuana consumption
- Medication side effects (antihistamines, tamoxifen, bromocriptine, low-estrogen oral contraceptives, depo-medroxyprogesterone, desipramine)

Pregnancy Considerations
Pregnancy is a potent influence on sexuality; dyspareunia is common.

COMMONLY ASSOCIATED CONDITIONS
Vaginismus

Pregnancy Considerations
Episiotomies do not have a protective effect (1)[A].

DIAGNOSIS

HISTORY
- Identify pain characteristics:
  - Onset
  - Duration
  - Location: Entry vs. deep; single vs. multiple sites; positional
  - Intensity/Quality: Varying degrees of pelvic/genital pressure, aching, tearing, and/or burning
  - Pattern (precipitating or aggravating factors): When pain occurs (at entry, during, or after intercourse)
  - Relief measures: Avoid intercourse, change positions, have intercourse only at certain times of the month
- Include menstrual, obstetric, reproductive, sexual, domestic violence, and rape histories with medical and psychosocial history.

PHYSICAL EXAM
- A complete exam, including a focused pelvic exam, to identify pathology and provide patient education
- Because examination often reproduces the pain, examiner should be cautious and sensitive to patient's anxiety. Exam must include inspection and palpation of vulva and vaginal areas; palpation of the uterine and adnexal structures; and a rectovaginal exam. Sensory mapping with a cotton-tipped applicator to identify sensitive and painful areas.
- Inspect and palpate urethra and base of the bladder

DIFFERENTIAL DIAGNOSIS
Vaginismus

DIAGNOSTIC TESTS & INTERPRETATION
Initial Tests (lab, imaging)
Based on history and exam findings:
- Wet mount
- Gonorrhea and chlamydia cultures
- Herpes culture
- Urinalysis and urine culture
- Pap smear

Follow-Up Tests & Special Considerations
- Serum estradiol if vulvodynia or atrophic vaginitis
- Voiding cystourethrogram if urinary tract involvement
- GI contrast studies if GI symptoms
- Ultrasound and CT scan are of limited value; perform if clinically indicated

Diagnostic Procedures/Other
Based on history and exam findings:
- Colposcopy and biopsy if vaginal/vulvar lesions
- Laparoscopy if complex deep-penetration pain
- Cystoscopy if urinary tract involvement
- Endoscopy if GI involvement

Test Interpretation
Depends on etiology

TREATMENT

- Potential relationships exists between primary dyspareunia and vaginismus, low libido, and arousal disorders.
- Endocrine factors, such as primary amenorrhea, might reduce the biologic basis of sexual response.
- If pain prevents penetration, severe vaginismus may be present.

GENERAL MEASURES
- Educate the patient and partner as to the nature of the problem. Reassure both there are solutions to the problem.
- Initiate specific treatment when initial evaluation identifies an organic cause.
- Once organic causes are ruled out, treatment is a multidimensional and multidisciplinary approach (2)[C]:
  – Individual behavioral therapy:
    ○ Indicated to help the patient deal with intrapersonal issues and assess the role of the partner
  – Couple behavioral therapy:
    ○ Indicated to help resolve interpersonal problems
    ○ May involve short-term structured intervention or sexual counseling
    ○ Designed to desensitize systemically uncomfortable sexual responses and intercourse through a series of interventions over a period of weeks
    ○ Interventions range from muscle relaxation and mutual body massage to sexual fantasies and erotic massage

MEDICATION
First Line
Depends on the etiology:
- Antibiotics, antifungals, or antivirals, as indicated, for infection
- Lubricants for dryness
- Analgesics and topical anesthetics for pain
- Topical estrogen for vaginal and vulvar atrophy
- Neuropathic pain associated with vulvar vestibulitis/vulvodynia may respond to tricyclic antidepressants (amitriptyline or nortriptyline) or gabapentin.

Second Line
- Ospemifene for vulvar and vaginal atrophy due to menopause

ISSUES FOR REFERRAL
Referral for long-term therapy may be necessary.
ADDITIONAL THERAPIES
- Physical therapy for pelvic floor muscle pain (3)[C]
SURGERY/OTHER PROCEDURES
- Laparoscopic excision of endometriotic lesions has shown benefit (4)[B].
- Surgical vestibulectomy can be considered if medical measures fail with vulvar vestibulitis (3)[C].
COMPLEMENTARY AND ALTERNATIVE MEDICINE
- Sitz baths may relieve painful inflammation.
- Perineal massage

 ONGOING CARE

FOLLOW-UP RECOMMENDATIONS
Patient Monitoring
- Outpatient follow up depends on therapy
- Every 6–12 months once resolved
DIET
A high-fiber diet may help if constipation is a contributing cause.
PATIENT EDUCATION
- Boston Women's Health Book Collective. Our bodies, ourselves: A new edition for a new era. New York: Simon & Schuster; 2005.
- Kegel exercise information
- Provide couples with information about sexual arousal techniques.
PROGNOSIS
Depends on underlying cause, but most patients will respond to treatment.

REFERENCES
1. Carroli G, Mignini L. Episiotomy for vaginal birth. Cochrane Database Syst Rev. 2009;1:CD000081.
2. Crowley T, Richardson D, Goldmeier D, et al. Recommendations for the management of vaginismus: BASHH Special Interest Group for Sexual Dysfunction. Int J STD AIDS. 2006;17:14–18.
3. Steege JF, Zolnoun DA. Evaluation and treatment of dyspareunia. Obstet Gynecol. 2009;113:1124–1136.
4. Ferrero S, Abbamonte LH, Giordano M, et al. Deep dyspareunia and sex life after laparoscopic excision of endometriosis. Hum Reprod. 2007;22:1142–1148.

ADDITIONAL READING
- Boardman LA, Stockdale CK. Sexual pain. Clin Obstet Gynecol. 2009;52:682–690.
- Frank JE, Mistretta P, Will J. Diagnosis and treatment of female sexual dysfunction. Am Fam Physician. 2008;77:635–642.
- Sung SC, Jeng CJ, Lin YC. Sexual health care for women with dyspareunia. Taiwan J Obstet Gynecol. 2011;50:268–274.

 SEE ALSO

- Balanitis; Endometriosis; Pelvic Inflammatory Disease (PID); Sexual Dysfunction in Women; Vaginismus; Vulvovaginitis, Estrogen Deficient; Vulvovaginitis, Prepubescent
- Algorithms: Dyspareunia; Discharge, Vaginal

CODES
ICD10
- F52.6 Dyspareunia not due to a substance or known physiol cond
- N94.1 Dyspareunia

CLINICAL PEARLS
- Careful history to determine if patient feels pain before, during, or after intercourse will help identify cause:
  – Pain before intercourse suggests a phobic attitude toward penetration and/or the presence of vestibulitis.
  – Pain during intercourse combined with the location of the pain is most predictive of the causes of pain.
  – Introital pain after intercourse suggests vestibulitis in women of childbearing age, hypertonic pelvic floor, or vulvovaginal dystrophia.
- Potential relationship exists between primary dyspareunia and vaginismus, low libido, and arousal disorders.
- Episiotomy does not offer any benefit in the prevention of dyspareunia; a mediolateral episiotomy in fact may cause more future discomfort.

DYSPEPSIA, FUNCTIONAL
Marco Cornelio, MD • Macario C. Corpuz, Jr., MD, FAAFP

 BASICS

DESCRIPTION
- A condition characterized by the presence of chronic intermittent symptoms without mucosal lesions or other structural abnormalities of the GI tract (1)[A] for at least 3 months:
  - Symptoms include:
    - Epigastric pain
    - Postprandial fullness
    - Early satiety
    - Epigastric burning
- Analogous to irritable bowel syndrome (IBS) of the upper GI tract
- System(s) affected: GI
- Synonym(s): Nonulcer dyspepsia; Moynihan dyspepsia; Pseudoulcer dyspepsia; Phantom ulcer; Nonorganic dyspepsia; Nervous dyspepsia

EPIDEMIOLOGY
Incidence
- 1–3%/year incidence of dyspepsia
- Accounts for 70% of patients with dyspepsia
- Accounts for ~5% of primary care visits
Prevalence
- 15–30% prevalence in developed countries
- Predominant age: Adults, but can be seen in children
- Predominant gender: Female > Male

ETIOLOGY AND PATHOPHYSIOLOGY
- Not well understood
- Motility disorder
- Visceral hypersensitivity
- Inflammation after Helicobacter pylori infection
- Psychosocial factors
- Often unknown; may be of several different etiologies
- Evanescent ulcers (20–30% go on to develop ulcers)
- Gastric motility disorder (delayed/accelerated)
- Visceral hypersensitivity to gastric distention, lipids, and acids (2)[B]
- Impaired gastric accommodation (2)[B]
- Association with *H. pylori* infection
- Adverse drug effects (NSAIDs, bisphosphonate, corticosteroids)
- Carbohydrate malabsorption
- Food intolerance
- Psychosocial factors
Genetics
Possible link to G-protein β-3 subunit 825 CC genotype and serotonin transport genes

RISK FACTORS
- Other functional disorders
- Anxiety
- Depression

GENERAL PREVENTION
Avoid foods and habits known to exacerbate symptoms (see "Diet").

COMMONLY ASSOCIATED CONDITIONS
Other functional bowel disorders

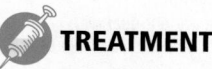 **DIAGNOSIS**

HISTORY
- Belching
- Aerophagia, gaseousness, abdominal distension
- Borborygmus
- Epigastric pain:
  - Gnawing/Burning
  - Eating may improve or worsen symptoms.
- Substernal pain: Gnawing/Burning
- Early satiety
- Anorexia, nausea, or vomiting
- Change in bowel habits
- Abdominal tenderness
- Stress, anxiety, depression
- Exclude disorders in differential diagnosis (see below).

Pediatric Considerations
Look for family system dysfunction.

Pregnancy Considerations
Pregnancy may exacerbate condition.

Geriatric Considerations
Cancer risk is higher.

PHYSICAL EXAM
To rule out other disorders:
- Murphy sign for cholelithiasis
- Rebound and guarding for ulcer perforation

DIFFERENTIAL DIAGNOSIS
- Gastroesophageal reflux disease (GERD)
- Cholecystitis
- Peptic ulcer disease
- Gastric cancer
- Esophageal spasm
- Malabsorption syndromes
- Pancreatic disease
- IBS
- Intestinal parasites
- Ischemic heart disease
- Diabetes mellitus
- Thyroid disease
- Connective tissue disorders
- Conversion disorder

DIAGNOSTIC TESTS & INTERPRETATION
Initial Tests (lab, imaging)
- CBC
- Chemistry panel
- *H. pylori* serology
- Stool for occult blood
- LFTs (if high suspicion of gallbladder disease present)
- Usual:
  - Endoscopy (3)[A]:
    - Recommended for
    - Patients with alarm symptoms
    - Patients who failed antisecretory medications
    - Patients who failed *H. pylori* test and treat strategy

- Alarm symptoms:
  - Onset of symptoms >45–55 years
  - Unexplained weight loss
  - Signs of a GI bleed
  - Family history of GI cancer
  - Progressive dysphagia
  - Persistent vomiting
- Sometimes:
  - Kidney, ureter, and bladder (KUB) x-ray for ulcer perforation
  - Right upper quadrant ultrasound for cholelithiasis

Diagnostic Procedures/Other
- Esophageal manometry (rarely needed)
- 24-hour intraesophageal pH monitoring (rarely needed unless dysphagia is present)

Test Interpretation
None (by definition)

TREATMENT

GENERAL MEASURES
- Appropriate health care: Outpatient
- Supportive measures:
  - Reassurance
  - Do not investigate excessively.
  - Dietary changes (see "Diet")
  - Elevate head of bed (where applicable).
  - Remain upright 30–60 minutes after eating.
  - Maintain ideal body weight.
  - Explore psychological issues.

MEDICATION
First Line
- 40% of patients improve with placebo.
- Acid reduction drugs:
  - H_2 antagonists: Ranitidine, famotidine (4)[A]
  - Over-the-counter omeprazole (5,6)[A]
- *H. pylori* eradication (test and treat strategy) (6,7)[A]
- Significant possible interactions:
  - H_2 blockers interact with drugs metabolized by and affecting the liver.

Second Line
- Gastric motility drugs (4)[B]:
  - Metoclopramide (Reglan)
  - Erythromycin
- Amitriptyline: 50 mg at bedtime
- SSRIs
- Antacids
- Sucralfate
- Misoprostol
- Contraindications:
  - Avoid magnesium-containing antacids in patients with significant renal dysfunction.
- Precautions:
  - Calcium-containing antacids may precipitate the kidney stone formation.
  - Metoclopramide can cause tardive dyskinesia and parkinsonian symptoms in older people.

ADDITIONAL THERAPIES

- Stress reduction:
  – Relaxation techniques
  – Physical exercise
  – Reflux precautions where applicable

- Psychological therapy (1)[B]:
  – Cognitive–behavioral therapy
  – Hypnotherapy
  – Psychotherapy

COMPLEMENTARY AND ALTERNATIVE MEDICINE

- Peppermint oil
- Iberogast: Mixture of 9 plant extracts

- Modified chaihu shugan powder (MCSP) may be more effective than prokinetic drugs, but studies show high risk of bias (8)[A].

ONGOING CARE

FOLLOW-UP RECOMMENDATIONS

Patient Monitoring

- Usual duration of medication is 4 weeks, then 2 weeks intermittently for exacerbations:
  – If chronic medication use is needed, endoscopy evaluation is indicated.
- Continue observation to provide support and reassurance.
- Minimize diagnostic studies unless disabling symptoms persist/new problems arise.

DIET

- Symptoms are frequently triggered/exacerbated by fatty foods (2)[B].

- Eat frequent small meals.
- Avoid:
  – Foods known to exacerbate symptoms
  – Peppers, spices, citrus fruit
  – Regular and decaffeinated coffee
  – Tea, cocoa, and chocolate
  – Heavy alcohol use
  – Cigarette smoking
  – Aspirin-containing compounds and NSAIDs
  – Late evening meals

PATIENT EDUCATION

Prevention: Continue healthy habits listed under "Treatment" and "Diet" (i.e., avoid activities known to exacerbate problems, maintain healthy lifestyle, continue stress-reduction techniques).

PROGNOSIS

Long-term/Chronic symptoms with symptom-free periods

COMPLICATIONS

Iatrogenic, from evaluation to rule out serious pathology

REFERENCES

1. Drossman DA. The functional gastrointestinal disorders and the Rome III process. *Gastroenterol.* 2006;130:1377–1390.
2. Oustamanolakis P, Tack J. Dyspepsia: Organic versus functional. *J Clin Gastroenterol.* 2012;46: 175–190.
3. Delaney B, Ford AC, Forman D, et al. Initial management strategies for dyspepsia. *Cochrane Database Syst Rev.* 2005:CD001961.
4. Loyd R, McClellan D. Update on the evaluation and management of functional dyspepsia. *Am Fam Phys.* 2011;83(5):547–552.
5. Lacy B, Cash B. A 32 year old woman with chronic abdominal pain. *JAMA.* 2008;299(5):555–565.
6. Lacy BE, Talley NJ, Locke GR 3rd, et al. Review article: Current treatment options and management of functional dyspepsia. *Aliment Pharmacol Ther.* 2012;36(1):3–15.
7. Mazzoleni LE, Sander GB, Francesconi CF, et al. Helicobacter pylori eradication in functional dyspepsia: HEROES trial. *Arch Intern Med.* 2011; 171:1929–1936.
8. Yang N, Jiang X, Qiu X, Hu Z, Wang L, Song M. Modified chaihu shugan powder for functional dyspepsia: Meta-analysis for randomized controlled trial. *Evid Based Complement Alternat Med.* 2013;2013:791724. doi: 10.1155/2013/791724. Epub 2013 May 13.

ADDITIONAL READING

- Amini M, Ghamar Chehreh ME, Khedmat H, et al. Famotidine in the treatment of functional dyspepsia: A placebo-controlled double-blind, placebo-controlled trial. *J Egypt Public Health Assoc.* 2012;87:29–33.
- Camilleri M, Stanghellini V. Current management strategies and emerging treatments for functional dyspepsia. *Nat Rev Gastroenterol Hepatol.* 2013 Apr 23. doi: 10.1038/nrgastro.2013.79. [Epub ahead of print]
- Farre R, Vanheel H, Masaoka T, et al. In functional dyspepsia, hypersensitivity to postprandial distention correlates with meal-related symptom severity. *Gastroenterology.* 2013 May 20. pii: S0016-5085(13)00750-6. doi: 10.1053/j.gastro.2013.05.018. [Epub ahead of print]

- Feinle-Bisset C, Azpiroz F. Dietary and lifestyle factors in functional dyspepsia. *Nat Rev Gastroenterol Hepatol.* 2013;10(3):150–157.
- Graham D, Rugge M. Clinical practice: Diagnosis & evaluation of dyspepsia. *J Clin Gastroenterol.* 2010;44:167–172.
- Tack J, Masaoka T, Janssen P, et al. Functional dyspepsia. *Curr Opin Gastroenterol.* 2011;27: 549–557.
- Tack J, Talley NJ. Functional dyspepsia—symptoms, definitions and validity of the Rome III criteria. *Nat Rev Gastroenterol Hepatol.* 2013;10(3):134–141.

SEE ALSO

- Dyspepsia, Endoscopic-Negative Reflux Disease, Gastritis; Irritable Bowel Syndrome
- Algorithms: Dyspepsia; Epigastric Pain; Esophageal Regurgitation

CODES

ICD10

K30 Functional dyspepsia

CLINICAL PEARLS

- When no organic cause for dyspepsia is found, it is considered functional or idiopathic.
- Extensive diagnostic testing is not recommended unless the patient presents with alarm symptoms (vomiting, early satiety, weight loss, or anemia).
- Consider empiric treatment with acid suppressants or *H. pylori* eradication if serology is positive.

DYSPHAGIA

Jennifer N. Smith, MD • Felix B. Chang, MD

BASICS

Difficulty during the progression of the alimentary bolus from the mouth to the stomach

DESCRIPTION
- Oropharyngeal: Difficulty transferring food bolus from oropharynx to proximal esophagus
- Esophageal dysphagia: Difficulty moving food bolus through esophagus

EPIDEMIOLOGY
10% of individuals >50 years of age

Prevalence
- 23% of dysphagia reported in family medicine patients
- Impaired swallowing common in nursing home residents 29–32%

ETIOLOGY AND PATHOPHYSIOLOGY
- Oropharyngeal (Transfer dysphagia):
  – *Mechanical causes:* Pharyngeal and laryngeal cancer, acute epiglottitis, carotid body tumor, pharyngitis, tonsillitis, strep throat, lymphoid hyperplasia of lingual tonsil, lateral pharyngeal pouch, hypopharyngeal diverticulum
- Esophageal:
  – *Esophageal mechanical lesions:* Carcinomas, esophageal diverticula, esophageal webs, Schatzki's ring, structures (peptic, chemical, trauma, radiation), foreign body
  – *Extrinsic mechanical lesions:* Peritonsillar abscess, thyroid disorders, tumors, mediastinal compression, vascular compression (enlarged left atrium, aberrant subclavius, aortic aneurysm), osteoarthritis cervical spine, adenopathy, esophageal duplication cyst
- Neuromuscular: Achalasia, diffuse esophageal spasm, hypertensive lower esophageal sphincter, scleroderma, nutcracker esophagus, CVA, Alzheimer's disease, Huntington chorea, Parkinson disease, multiple sclerosis, skeletal muscle disease (polymyositis, dermatomyositis), neuromuscular junction disease (myasthenia gravis, Eaton-Lambert syndrome, botulism), hyper/hypothyroidism, Guillain-Barré syndrome, systemic lupus erythematosus, acute lymphoblastic leukemia, amyloidosis, diabetic neuropathy, brain stem tumors, Chagas disease
- Infection: Diphtheria, chronic meningitis, tertiary syphilis, Lyme disease, rabies, poliomyelitis, CMV, esophagitis (Candida, Herpetic)

RISK FACTORS
- Children: Hereditary and/or congenital malformations
- Adults: Age >50 years. Elderly: GERD, stroke, COPD, chronic pain
- Smoking, excess alcohol intake, obesity
- Infection: Diphtheria, chronic meningitis, tertiary syphilis, Lyme disease, rabies, poliomyelitis, CMV), HIV
- Medications: quinine, potassium chloride, vitamin C, tetracycline, Bactrim, clindamycin, NSAIDs, procainamide, anticholinergics, bisphosphates
- Neurologic events or diseases: CVA, myasthenia gravis, multiple sclerosis, Parkinson disease, amyotrophic lateral sclerosis (ALS), Huntington chorea
- HIV patients with CD4 cell count <100 cells/mm^3.

- Trauma or irradiation of head, neck, and chest; mechanical lesions
- Extrinsic mechanical lesions: Lung, thyroid tumors, lymphoma, metastasis
- Iron deficiency
- Anterior cervical spine surgery (Up to 71% first 2 weeks postop; 12–14% 1 year postop) (1)[A]

GENERAL PREVENTION
- Correct poorly fitting dentures in older patients.
- Education on prolonged chewing, drinking large amounts of water with meals, and diet consisting of liquids and soft foods
- Avoid drinking alcohol with meals.
- Swallowing evaluation:
  – Observe level of consciousness, postural control-upright position, oral hygiene, mobilization of oral secretions.
- Prophylactic swallowing exercises in patients with head and neck cancer undergoing chemoradiation

COMMONLY ASSOCIATED CONDITIONS
Peptic structure, esophageal webs and rings, carcinoma; history of stroke, dementia, pneumonia

DIAGNOSIS

HISTORY
- Dysphagia to both solids and liquids from the onset of symptoms is probably a motility disorder of the esophagus.
- Oropharyngeal dysphagia presents as difficulty in initiating swallow.
- Dysphagia for solids that later progresses to involve liquids is more likely to reflect mechanical obstruction.
- Progressive dysphagia is usually caused by cancer or a peptic stricture, whereas intermittent dysphagia is most often related to a lower esophageal ring.
- Inquire about heartburn, weight loss, hematemesis, coffee ground emesis, anemia, regurgitation of food particles, and respiratory symptoms.
- Is there regurgitation, aspiration, or drooling, immediately after swallowing?
  – May represent oropharyngeal dysphagia
- Does the food bolus feel stuck?
  – Upper sternum or back of throat: May represent oropharyngeal dysphagia, whereas sensation over the lower sternum is typical of esophageal dysphagia.
- Is odynophagia present?
  – May represent inflammation, achalasia, diffuse esophageal spasm, esophagitis, pharyngitis, pill-induced esophagitis, cancer.
- Globus sensation?
  – Indicates cricopharyngeal or laryngeal disorders.
- History of sour taste in the back of the throat, or history of chronic heartburn?
  – GERD
- How much alcohol and/or tobacco used?
- Are there associated symptoms such as weight loss or chest pain?
  – Double aortic arch, right aortic arch with retroesophageal left subclavian artery and left ligamentum arteriosum
  – Anticholinergics, antihistamines, and some antihypertensives can decrease salivary production.
- Halitosis: Rule out diverticulitis.

- Connective tissue disorder?
- Changes in speech, hoarseness, weak cough, dysphonia? Rule out neuromuscular dysfunction.

PHYSICAL EXAM
- General: History of fever
- Skin:
  – Telangiectasia, sclerodactyly, calcinosis (r/o autoimmune), Reynaud's phenomenon, sclerodactyly may be found in CREST syndrome or systemic scleroderma.
- HEENT:
  – Oropharyngeal:
    ○ Pharyngeal erythema/edema, tonsillitis, pharyngeal ulcers or thrush, odynophagia (bacterial, viral, fungal infections)
    ○ Tongue fasciculations (ALS)
  – Neck:
    ○ Neck masses, lymphadenopathy, neck tenderness, goiter
    ○ Neck tenderness: Acute thyroiditis
- Neurological:
  – Cranial nerve exam:
    ○ Sensory testing of cranial nerves V, IX, and X
    ○ Motor examination of cranial nerves V, VII, X, XI and XII
  – CNS, mental status exam, strength testing, Horner's syndrome, ataxia, cog wheel rigidity (CVA, dementia, Parkinson disease, Alzheimer disease)
    ○ Eye position, extraocular motility: Stroke

DIFFERENTIAL DIAGNOSIS
Cardiac chest pain, globus hystericus, functional heartburn

DIAGNOSTIC TESTS & INTERPRETATION
Adults:
- Barium swallow
- Fiberoptic endoscopic examination of swallowing (FEES)
- Gastroesophageal endoscopy
- Barium cine/video esophagogram
- Ambulatory 24-hour pH testing
- Esophageal manometry
- Videofluoroscopic swallowing study (VFSS): Oropharyngeal dysphagia

Initial Tests (lab, imaging)
- As suggested by specific differential diagnosis under consideration
  – CBC to screen for infectious and inflammatory condition
  – Serum protein and albumin levels for nutritional assessment
  – Thyroid function studies to detect dysphagia associated with hypothyroidism or hyperthyroidism, cobalamin levels
  – Antiacetylcholine antibodies in selected patients
- Barium swallow: Detect mild strictures, evaluation of stenosis

Follow-Up Tests & Special Considerations
- CT scan of chest
- MRI of brain and cervical spine
- Videofluoroscopic swallowing function study (VSFS) (lips, tongue, palate, pharynx, larynx, proximal esophagus)
- No significant difference regarding the diagnostic efficacy of fiberoptic endoscopic evaluation of swallowing compared to videofluoroscopy (2)[A]

Diagnostic Procedures/Other

Endoscopy with biopsy; esophageal manometry; esophageal pH monitoring

Test Interpretation

- Squamous cell or adenocarcinoma
- Barrett metaplasia
- Fibrous tissue of a ring, web, or stricture
- Loss of smooth muscle (scleroderma)
- Acute or chronic inflammatory changes
- Oropharyngeal lesions

TREATMENT

GENERAL MEASURES

Exclude cardiac disease. Ensure airway and pulmonary function. Assess nutritional status. Speech therapy evaluation is helpful.

MEDICATION

First Line

- For spasms: Calcium channel blockers: Nifedipine 10–30 mg t.i.d.; amitriptyline 0.5–2 mg/kg at bedtime; dicyclomine 20 mg q.i.d.
- For esophagitis:
  – Antacids: Tums, Mylanta, Maalox
  – H_2 blockers: Cimetidine, ranitidine, nizatidine, famotidine
  – Proton pump inhibitors: Omeprazole, lansoprazole, rabeprazole, esomeprazole, pantoprazole
  – Prokinetic agents: Metoclopramide, erythromycin (rarely used due to contraindications)
- Anticholinergics: Obstructive uropathy, glaucoma, myasthenia gravis, achalasia, dementia/delirium, advanced age
- Nitrates: Early myocardial infarction (MI), severe anemia, increased intracranial pressure (ICP), hypertension (HTN)
- Precautions: May need to use liquid forms of medications because patients might have difficulty swallowing pills.

ISSUES FOR REFERRAL

- Gastroenterology: Endoscopy, refractory
- Surgery: Dilation, esophageal myotomy, biopsy

ADDITIONAL THERAPIES

Speech therapy for swallowing assessment, dietary and positioning recommendations, and muscle-strengthening exercise; no eating at bedtime; remaining upright after eating (3,4)[A]

SURGERY/OTHER PROCEDURES

- Esophageal dilatation (pneumatic or bougie)
- Esophageal stent; laser for cancer palliation
- Treatment for underlying problem (e.g., thyroid goiter, vascular ring, esophageal atresia)
- Nd:YAG laser incision of lower esophageal rings refractory to dilation
- Photodynamic therapy (cancer)
- Cricopharyngeal myotomy (for oropharyngeal dysphagia)
- Surgery for Zenker diverticulum, refractory strictures, or myotomy (for achalasia)
- Percutaneous gastrostomy (PEG) decreases risk of dysphagia when compared with nasogastric tube (5)[A].

COMPLEMENTARY AND ALTERNATIVE MEDICINE

- Acupuncture for neurogenic dysphagia (6)[A]
- Electroacupuncture combined with dilating granule in the treatment of GERD

IN-PATIENT CONSIDERATIONS

Admission Criteria/Initial Stabilization

- Complete or partial esophageal obstruction with malnutrition or hypovolemia/dehydration
- Comorbid conditions complicating etiology of dysphagia
- Enteral feeding requirement
- Outpatient for conditions where patient is able to maintain nutrition and has little risk of complications
- Hospitalization may be required for adults when dysphagia is associated with total or near-total obstruction of esophageal lumen.
- Endoscopy and/or esophageal dilation; surgery diagnostic or therapeutic

IV Fluids

For dehydrated, hypovolemic patients and patients, impaired consciousness

Discharge Criteria

Correction of dysphagia. Tolerating adequate diet without nausea/pain. Adequate nutritional intake. (4)[A]

ONGOING CARE

DIET

See "Prevention."

PATIENT EDUCATION

Dietary modification, no eating at bedtime, remaining upright after eating, pharmacologic therapy, smoking cessation

PROGNOSIS

Course and prognosis vary with specific diagnosis

COMPLICATIONS

- Oropharyngeal: Pneumonia, lung abscess, aspiration, airway obstruction
- Malnutrition and dehydration

REFERENCES

1. Cho SK, Lu Y, Lee DH. Dysphagia following anterior cervical spinal surgery: A systematic review. *Bone Joint J*. 2013 Jul;95-B(7):868–873. doi: 10.1302/0301-620X.95B7.31029.
2. Al-Hussaini A, Latif EH, Singh V. 12-minute consultation: an evidence-based approach to the management of dysphagia. *Clin Otolaryngol*. 2013 Jun;38(3):237–243. doi: 10.1111/coa.12116.
3. Anderson U, Beck A, et al. Systematic review and evidence based recommendations on texture modified foods and thickened fluids for adults with oropharyngeal dysphagia. *E-SPEN Journal*. 31 May 2013. http://dx.doi.org/10.1016/j.clnme.2013.05
4. Geeganage C, Ellender S, et al. Interventions for dysphagia and nutritional support in acute and subacute stroke. *Cochrane Database Syst Rev*. Stroke Group. 2012: DOI: 10.1002/14651858.CD000323.
5. Gomes CA JR, Lustosa SA, Matos D, et al. Percutaneous endoscopic gastrostomy versus nasogastric tube feeding for adults with swallowing disturbances. *Cochrane Database Syst Rev*. 2012;3:CD008096.Epub 2012 Mar 14.
6. Chan SL, Or KH, Sun WZ, et al. Therapeutic effects of acupuncture for neurogenic dysphagia—a randomized controlled trial. *J Tradit Chin Med*. 2012;32(1):25–30.

ADDITIONAL READING

Park Y, Han H, et al. Prevalence and associated factors of dysphagia in nursing home residents. *Geriatric Nursing*. 2013 34(3):212–217.

SEE ALSO

Gastroesophageal Reflux Disease

CODES

ICD10

- R13.10 Dysphagia, unspecified
- R13.12 Dysphagia, oropharyngeal phase
- R13.14 Dysphagia, pharyngoesophageal phase

CLINICAL PEARLS

- Weight loss is usually associated with malignancy or achalasia.
- Dysphagia should be considered an alarm symptom, indicating need for immediate evaluation.

DYSPLASTIC NEVUS SYNDROME

Andrew Kim, MD • Dori Goldberg, MD

BASICS

Dysplastic nevus syndrome (DNS), also known as atypical mole syndrome (AMS), is a sporadic or hereditary disorder resulting in numerous clinically atypical nevi and an increased risk for developing malignant melanoma.

DESCRIPTION
- Condition resulting in elevated total body nevi count, including clinically atypical nevi:
  - Usually >50, although often >100
  - Larger number in hereditary DNS vs. sporadic DN (as few as <10 in sporadic, although high numbers also possible)
- Increased risk of melanoma (1):
  - Up to 90% occurrence by age 80 in certain high-risk individuals
  - Earlier onset than sporadic melanoma cases
  - Most arise out of healthy skin as opposed to a preexisting atypical nevus
  - Higher risk for appearance at unusual sites (e.g., scalp)
- DNS terminology often used interchangeably with AMS, familial atypical multiple-mole melanoma (FAMMM) syndrome, and B-K mole syndrome
- Median age of diagnosis for melanoma is 10–20 years earlier than the general population, with documented cases of melanoma as early as in the early teens and 20s (2).
- Melanomas in the setting of DNS are most often superficial spreading or nodular type.

EPIDEMIOLOGY
Incidence
Uncertain due to phenotype variability and limited data, but ~10% of melanoma cases are diagnosed as familial.

Prevalence
At least 32,000 cases in the US per NIH calculations (3)

ETIOLOGY AND PATHOPHYSIOLOGY
CDKN2A mutations have been observed in kindreds with familial DNS and multiple melanomas. The *CDKN2A* (cyclin-dependent kinase inhibitor 2A) gene on 9p21 encodes for the proteins p16 and p14. p16 binds to CDK4 and 6 and is a negative cell-cycle regulator via inhibition of the CDK-cyclin D interaction needed for cell-cycle progression from G_1 to S. Similarly, p14 functions by stabilizing the tumor-suppressor protein p53 in the G_1 phase of the cell cycle.
- Unclear for sporadic cases, although somatic p16 inactivation noted in 40% of familial melanoma
- Familial cases of germline *CDKN2A* mutations considered to be transmitted genetically in an autosomal–dominant fashion

Genetics
- Autosomal–dominant inheritance in hereditary cases, but variable expressivity and incomplete penetrance
- *CDKN2A* mutation observed in 25–40% of hereditary cases

RISK FACTORS
Family history DN, DNS, and/or melanoma

GENERAL PREVENTION
- No currently available prevention strategies
- Treatment is directed toward secondary prevention of melanoma complications with routine skin exams, biopsy of suspect lesions, and environmental risk mitigation (e.g., sun protection and sun avoidance).
- Experimental early detection protocols for pancreatic cancer in use with some high-risk individuals

COMMONLY ASSOCIATED CONDITIONS
- Malignant melanoma, including ocular melanoma
- Ocular nevi
- Pancreatic cancer in *CDKN2A* mutation

DIAGNOSIS

DNS is a clinical diagnosis with various classifications schemes proposed in the past. Although not widely accepted, diagnostic criteria as defined by the NIH require the 3 features of (i) malignant melanoma in ≥1 1st- or 2nd-degree relatives; (ii) numerous melanocytic nevi (frequently >50), some of which are clinically atypical; and (iii) nevi that have certain histologic features on pathologic examination (4).

HISTORY
- Changing lesions: Bleeding, scaling, size, texture, nonhealing, hyper- or hypopigmentation
- Prior skin biopsies
- Prior melanoma
- Pancreatic cancer
- In 1st- or 2nd-degree relatives:
  - DNS
  - Melanoma
  - Pancreatic cancer

PHYSICAL EXAM
- ABCDE mnemonic for pigmented lesions: Asymmetry, Border irregularity, Color variegation, Diameter >6 mm, Evolving lesion:
  - Melanoma typically with several characteristics of ABCDEs on gross exam (dysplastic nevi often defined as ≥5 mm + at least 2 other features)
  - Difficult differentiating dysplastic nevi from melanoma using these criteria

- Most common features of dysplastic nevi on dermatoscopy magnification per the pattern analysis method include (5):
  - Atypical pigment network
  - Irregular/peripheral depigmentation areas
  - Irregular distribution of brown globules
  - Pigmentation with central heterogeneity and abrupt termination
- Some dermatoscopic features more suggestive of melanoma include (5):
  - Depigmented areas
  - Whitish veil
  - Homogenous areas distributed irregularly, in multiple areas, or >25% of total lesion
  - ≥4 colors

DIFFERENTIAL DIAGNOSIS
- Acquired melanocytic nevi
- Sporadic atypical nevi
- Melanoma
- Seborrheic keratosis
- Dermatofibroma
- Lentigo
- Pigmented actinic keratosis

DIAGNOSTIC TESTS & INTERPRETATION
Initial Tests (lab, imaging)
Genetic testing is available for *CDKN2A* mutations, but the sensitivity and specificity are not yet secure and, thus, the results cannot be adequately utilized for management or surveillance.
- When the total nevus count is high and individually following each nevus impractical, total-body photography may aid in the evaluation of evolving nevi, as well as in documenting new nevi.
- Further exam of nevi with a dermatoscope may help in distinguishing between benign and malignant pigmented lesions. Although no pathognomonic findings for melanoma exist, dermoscopy aids in the diagnostic accuracy, with reported sensitivities ranging as high as 94%.

Diagnostic Procedures/Other
- Biopsy is recommended of any new lesion where melanoma cannot be excluded or for any existing evolving lesion concerning for melanoma.
- Acceptable methods include full-thickness excisional biopsy of the entire lesion with a 2-mm margin of normal skin or a sampling of a smaller portion with either a shave or punch biopsy:
  - Excisional biopsy provides the most accurate diagnosis and should be performed when possible.
  - Take care to provide a sufficiently deep sample to allow assessment of the depth of any melanomas.

Test Interpretation
Dysplastic nevi: Possible features include melanocyte proliferation in the dermo-epidermal junction, bridging of rete ridges by melanocytic nests, dermal fibrosis, and interstitial lymphocytic inflammation.

TREATMENT

MEDICATION
No medications are available at this time to treat atypical nevi.

ISSUES FOR REFERRAL
- Referral to a dermatologist for routine skin exam
- Consider referral to a specialty pigmented lesion clinic.
- Ophthalmologic exams for ocular nevi/melanoma screening
- Oncology or specialized genetics study group involvement if strong family predisposition to pancreatic cancer
- Possible cosmetic surgery consultation for cosmetically poor excision outcomes

ADDITIONAL THERAPIES
- Topical chemo- and immunotherapies therapies have been unsuccessfully attempted to treat atypical nevi.
- Laser treatment should be avoided because it is both unsafe and ineffective for melanocytic nevi.

SURGERY/OTHER PROCEDURES
Surgical excision of all atypical nevi is not recommended as most melanomas in DNS appear *de novo* on healthy skin and the procedure leads to both poor cosmetic outcomes and a false sense of security. Lesions suspicious for melanoma should be biopsied or removed surgically (6).

ONGOING CARE

FOLLOW-UP RECOMMENDATIONS
Close follow-up with a dermatologist and sun avoidance/protection is highly advised.

Patient Monitoring
- Total body skin exam (including nails, scalp, genital area, and oral mucosa) every 3–6 months initially, starting at puberty; may be reduced to annually once nevi are stable.
- Dermatoscopic evaluation for suspect lesions
- Ocular exam for those with familial DNS
- Excision of suspect lesions
- Total body photography at baseline
- Monthly self-exams of skin
- Sun avoidance and sun protection

PATIENT EDUCATION
- Teach patients the ABCDE mnemonic for assessing nevi and identifying potential melanomas.
- Encourage adequate sun protection/minimization of sun exposure.
- Educate on proper application of sunscreen, use of protective clothing (e.g., hats), and avoidance of tanning booths.
- Provide instruction on skin self-exam techniques.

- A sample listing of patient-centric review sources on this topic are as follows:
  - American Academy of Dermatology (http://www.aad.org/skin-conditions/dermatology-a-to-z/atypical-mole)
  - Skin Cancer Foundation (http://www.skincancer.org/skin-cancer-information/dysplastic-nevi)
  - Melanoma Research Foundation (http://www.melanoma.org/learn-more/melanoma-101/what-melanoma)

PROGNOSIS
- Multiple classification schemes have been developed over the years to delineate risk of melanoma in patients with DNS. Individuals with a family history of melanoma are at greatest risk. A classification system developed by Rigel is simply and readily applied in the clinical setting. Points are assigned based on incidence of melanoma, with 1 point given for a personal history with melanoma, and 2 points for each family member with melanoma (modified nuclear family consisting of 1st-degree relatives + grandparents and uncles/aunts) and stratified as follows (7):
  - Score = 0, Rigel Group 0, 6% 25-year accumulated risk for melanoma
  - Score = 1, Rigel Group 1, 10% risk
  - Score = 2, Rigel Group 2, 15% risk
  - Score ≥ 3, Rigel Group 3, 50% risk
- The *CDKN2A* mutation has also been associated with a 60–90% risk of melanoma by age 80 and a 17% risk for pancreatic cancer by age 75.

COMPLICATIONS
- Malignant melanoma
- Poor cosmetic outcomes from biopsy

REFERENCES

1. Newton JA, Bataille V, Griffiths K, et al. How common is the atypical mole syndrome phenotype in apparently sporadic melanoma? *J Am Acad Dermatol*. 1993;29(6):989–996.
2. Silva JH, Sá BC, Avila AL, et al. Atypical mole syndrome and dysplastic nevi: Identification of populations at risk for developing melanoma - review article. *Clinics (Sao Paulo)*. 2011;66: 493–499.
3. Familial atypical multiple mole melanoma syndrome. In: Riegert-Johnson DL, Boardman LA, Hefferon T, et al., eds. *Cancer Syndromes*. Bethesda, MD: National Center for Biotechnology Information, 2009.
4. NIH Consensus conference. Diagnosis and treatment of early melanoma. *JAMA*. 1992;268: 1314–1319.
5. Salopek TG, Kopf AW, Stefanato CM, et al. Differentiation of atypical moles (dysplastic nevi) from early melanomas by dermoscopy. *Dermatol Clin*. 2001;19:337–345.
6. Duffy K, Grossman D. The dysplastic nevus: from historical perspective to management in the modern era: part II. Molecular aspects and clinical management. *J Am Acad Dermatol*. 2012;67(1): 19.e1–12; quiz 31–32.
7. Rigel DS, Rivers JK, Friedman RJ, Kopf AW. Risk gradient for malignant melanoma in individuals with dysplastic naevi. *Lancet*. 1988;1:352–353. 10.1016/S0140-6736(88)91139-7.

ADDITIONAL READING

- American Society of Clinical Oncology. American Society of Clinical Oncology policy statement update: Genetic testing for cancer susceptibility. *J Clin Oncol*. 2003;21(12):2397–2406. Epub 2003 Apr 11.
- Czajkowski R, Placek W, Drewa G, et al. FAMMM syndrome: Pathogenesis and management. *Dermatol Surg*. 2004;30(2 Pt 2):291–296.
- Duffy K, Grossman D. The dysplastic nevus: From historical perspective to management in the modern era: part I. Historical, histologic, and clinical aspects. *J Am Acad Dermatol*. 2012;67(1):1.e1–16; quiz 17–18.
- Farber MJ, Heilman ER, Friedman RJ. Dysplastic nevi. *Dermatol Clin*. 2012;30(3):389–404.
- Friedman RJ, Farber MJ, Warycha MA, et al. The "dysplastic" nevus. *Clin Dermatol*. 2009;27(1): 103–115.
- Hocker TL, Alikhan A, Comfere NI, Peters MS. Favorable long-term outcomes in patients with histologically dysplastic nevi that approach a specimen border. *J Am Acad Dermatol*. 2013;68(4): 545–551.
- Naeyaert JM, Brochez L. Clinical practice. Dysplastic nevi. *N Engl J Med*. 2003;349(23):2233–2240.
- Slade J, Marghoob AA, Salopek TG, et al. Atypical mole syndrome: Risk factor for cutaneous malignant melanoma and implications for management. *J Am Acad Dermatol*. 1995;32(3):479–494.

 CODES

ICD10
D23.9 Other benign neoplasm of skin, unspecified

CLINICAL PEARLS
- Melanoma in DNS tends to arise from healthy skin despite a large number of atypical nevi.
- ~20% of individuals with familial DNS will develop pancreatic cancer by age 75.
- Patients with DNS tend to produce neoplasms in unusual sites such as the scalp, eyes, and double sun-protected areas (e.g., gluteal folds).
- ~10% of melanomas are featureless on dermatoscopy.

D

ECTOPIC PREGNANCY

Dawn S. Tasillo, MD • Julie M. Tabroff, MD • Katherine Quayle, MD

BASICS

DESCRIPTION
Ectopic: Pregnancy implanted outside the confines of the uterine cavity. Subtypes include:
- Tubal: Pregnancy implanted in any portion of the fallopian tube
- Abdominal: Pregnancy implanted intra-abdominally, most commonly after tubal abortion or rupture of tubal ectopic pregnancy
- Heterotopic: Pregnancy implanted intrauterine and a separate pregnancy implanted outside uterine cavity
- Ovarian: Implantation of pregnancy in ovarian tissue
- Cervical: Implantation of pregnancy in cervix
- Intraligamentary: Implantation of pregnancy within the broad ligament

EPIDEMIOLOGY
Incidence
- 108,800 cases in 1992 in the US, according to CDC census (most recent data available) meaning that 1.5–2.0% of all pregnancies were ectopic. The true incidence is difficult to estimate because many patients are treated in the outpatient setting.
- In the US, ectopic pregnancy is the leading cause of 1st trimester maternal deaths and accounts for 6% of all pregnancy-related deaths (1)
- Heterotopic pregnancy, although rare (1:30,000), occurs with greater frequency in women undergoing in vitro fertilization (IVF) (1/1,000) (1).

Prevalence
~33% recurrence rate if prior ectopic pregnancy (1)

ETIOLOGY AND PATHOPHYSIOLOGY
- 97% of ectopic pregnancies occur in the fallopian tube (1), of which, 55% in the ampullary portion of the tube, 25% in the isthmus, and 17% in the fimbria.
- Of the remaining 3%, most are ovarian, cervical, abdominal pregnancies, or heterotopic.
- For a tubal pregnancy, impaired movement of the fertilized ovum to the uterine cavity due to dysfunction of the tubal cilia, scarring, or narrowing of the tubal lumen
- Other locations are rare, but may occur from reimplantation of an aborted tubal pregnancy or from uterine structural abnormalities (mainly cervical pregnancy).

RISK FACTORS
- History of pelvic inflammatory disease (PID), endometritis, or current gonorrhea/chlamydia infection
- Previous ectopic pregnancy
- History of tubal surgery (~33% of pregnancies after tubal ligation will be ectopic) (1)[A]
- Pelvic adhesive disease (infection or prior surgery)
- Use of an IUD: Overall chance of pregnancy of any type with an IUD is low; however, there is an increased likelihood of ectopic location if pregnancy occurs. IUDs reduce absolute risk of ectopic pregnancy.
- Use of assisted reproductive technologies
- Diethylstilbestrol exposure in utero (DES was last used in 1972)
- Tobacco use
- Patients with disorders that affect ciliary motility may be at increased risk (e.g., endometriosis, Kartagener's).

GENERAL PREVENTION
- Reliable contraception or abstinence
- Screening and treatment of STIs (i.e., gonorrhea, chlamydia) that can cause PID and tubal scarring

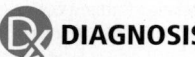

DIAGNOSIS

HISTORY
In >50% of presenting cases, patients have sudden-onset abdominal pain coupled with cessation of/or irregular menses. Other common symptoms include nausea and/or vomiting, vaginal bleeding, and pain referred to the shoulder (from hemoperitoneum).

PHYSICAL EXAM
- Abdominal tenderness ± rebound tenderness
- Vaginal bleeding
- Palpable mass on pelvic exam (adnexal or cul-de-sac fullness)
- Cervical motion tenderness
- In cervical cases, an hourglass-shaped cervix might be noted.
- In cases of rupture and significant intraperitoneal bleeding, signs of shock such as pallor, tachycardia, and hypotension may be present.

DIFFERENTIAL DIAGNOSIS
- Missed, threatened, inevitable, or completed abortion
- Gestational trophoblastic neoplasia ("molar pregnancy")
- Appendicitis
- Salpingitis, PID
- Ruptured corpus luteum or hemorrhagic cyst
- Ovarian tumor, benign or malignant
- Ovarian torsion
- Cervical polyp, cancer, trauma, or cervicitis

DIAGNOSTIC TESTS & INTERPRETATION
Initial Tests (lab, imaging)
- Human chorionic gonadotropin (hCG): Serial quantitative serum levels normally increase by at least 66% every 48 hours in the first 8 weeks of gestation (1)[A]: Abnormal rise should prompt workup for gestational abnormalities. Clinical impression of acute abdomen/intraperitoneal bleeding concurrent with a positive hCG level is indicative of ectopic pregnancy until proven otherwise.
- CBC and ABO type and antibody screen
- Serum progesterone level (>20 mg/mL associated with lower risk of ectopic pregnancy). In women with pain and/or bleeding who have an inconclusive US, serum progesterone level <3.2 ng/mL ruled out a viable pregnancy in 99.2% of women (2)[A].
- Under investigation: evaluation of serum progesterone levels in conjunction with vascular endothelial growth factor, inhibin A, and activin A using an algorithm. This diagnosed patients with ectopic pregnancy with 99% accuracy (3)[B].
- Transvaginal US (TVUS) is the gold standard for diagnosis (1)[A]:
  – Failure to visualize a normal intrauterine gestational sac when serum hCG is above the discriminatory level (>1,500–2,000 IU/L) suggests an abnormal pregnancy.

– Some evidence suggests the discriminatory level is not always reliable for excluding an intrauterine pregnancy; additional scans on patients with hCG levels above the discriminatory level and no intrauterine pregnancy on initial US are occasionally found to have normal IUP on subsequent scans.

- MRI is also useful, but costly, and rarely used if TVUS is available.

Diagnostic Procedures/Other
- In the setting of an undesired pregnancy, sampling of the uterine cavity with endometrial biopsy or D&C can identify the presence/absence of intrauterine chorionic villi.
- Historically, culdocentesis was performed to confirm suspected hemoperitoneum prior to surgical management. Currently, TVUS quantification of pelvic fluid is sufficient.

Test Interpretation
Products of conception (POC; especially chorionic villi) outside the uterine cavity

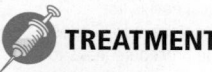

TREATMENT

MEDICATION
- Methotrexate (MTX): Treatment for unruptured tubal pregnancy or for remaining POCs after laparoscopic salpingostomy (2)[A]. MTX inhibits DNA synthesis via folic acid antagonism by inactivating dihydrofolate reductase. Most effective when pregnancy is <3 cm diameter, hCG <5,000 mIU/mL, and no fetal heart movement is seen. (1)[A]. Success rate is 88% if hCG <1,000, 71% if hCG <2,000. (4)[B]:
  – Dosage:
    ○ Single (1)[A]: IM methotrexate: 50 mg/m² of body surface area; may repeat once (preferred method) if <15% decline in hCG by day 7
    ○ Two dose (1)[A]: Methotrexate 50 mg/m² of body surface area once and then repeated on day 4; if <15% decline in hCG on day 7, may repeat dose on days 7 and 11
    ○ Multidose (1)[A]: Methotrexate 1 mg/kg IM/IV every other day, with leucovorin 0.1 mg/kg IM in between. Maximum 4 doses; course may be repeated 7 days after last dose if necessary.
  – Contraindications (5)[A]:
    ○ Hemodynamic instability or any evidence of rupture
    ○ Moderate to severe anemia
    ○ Severe hepatic or renal dysfunction
    ○ Immunodeficiency
  – Relative contraindications (5)[A]:
    ○ Fetal heart rate seen
    ○ Large gestational sac
    ○ Noncompliance or limited access to hospital or transportation
    ○ Recurrent ectopic pregnancies
    ○ Patients who desire permanent sterilization
    ○ High hCG count >6,000
- Precautions: Immunologic, hematologic, renal, GI, hepatic, and pulmonary disease, or interacting medications
- Pretreatment testing: Serum hCG, CBC, liver and renal function tests, blood type, and screen

- Patient counseling: During therapy, refrain from use of alcohol, aspirin, NSAIDs, and folate supplements (decreases efficacy of MTX); avoid excessive sun exposure:
  - Adherence to scheduled follow-up appointments is critical.
  - Increased abdominal pain may occur during treatment; however, severe pain, nausea, vomiting, bleeding, dizziness, or lightheadedness may indicate treatment failure and require urgent evaluation.
- Rupture of ectopic pregnancy during MTX treatment ranges from 7% to 14%. (5)[A].
- Side effects include stomatitis, conjunctivitis, abdominal cramping, and rarely neutropenia, pneumonitis, or alopecia. (5)[A].

ISSUES FOR REFERRAL
- Consult a gynecologist for medical treatment.
- Refer to a gynecologist for surgical care.

ADDITIONAL THERAPIES
- Physician or patient may elect for surgical treatment as primary method, then post-op hCG should guide need for MTX
- After evidence of medical failure or tubal rupture, surgery is necessary.
- Surgery may either be salpingostomy (with preservation of tube) or salpingectomy (tubal removal). Abdominal entry is typically laparoscopic.
- Treatment of cervical, ovarian, abdominal, or other ectopic pregnancy is complicated and requires immediate specialist referral.
- Follow all patients treated medically to an hCG of 0 to prevent surgical intervention.
- Offer anti-D RH prophylaxis at a dose of 50 μg to all RH-negative women who have a surgical procedure to manage an ectopic pregnancy (6)[A].
- Expectant management to allow for spontaneous resolution of ectopic pregnancy is acceptable in asymptomatic patients with no evidence of rupture or hemodynamic instability coupled with an appropriately low hCG (<200 mU/mL) and no evidence of fetal cardiac activity (1)[A]. Ruptured tubal pregnancies may occur even with extremely low hCG levels (<100).

SURGERY/OTHER PROCEDURES
- Indications include ruptured ectopic pregnancy, inability to comply with medical follow-up, previous tubal ligation, known tubal disease, current heterotopic pregnancy, desire for permanent sterilization at time of diagnosis.
- Laparoscopy is 1st-line surgical management (7)[A].
- Salpingostomy preferred in patients who wish to maintain fertility (7)[A]:
  - Slightly higher recurrence rate than with salpingectomy
  - Persistent trophoblastic tissue with salpingostomy remains in the fallopian tube in 5–20% of cases.
- Salpingectomy indicated for uncontrolled bleeding, recurrent ectopic pregnancy, severely damaged tube, gestational sac >4 cm, or patient desire for sterilization

IN-PATIENT CONSIDERATIONS
Admission Criteria/Initial Stabilization
- Fails criteria for methotrexate management, suspicion of rupture, orthostatic, shock, and severe abdominal pain requiring IV narcotics

- Inpatient observation in the setting of an uncertain diagnosis, particularly with an unreliable patient, may be appropriate.

Surgical emergency:
- 2 IV access lines should be placed immediately if suspicion of rupture; aggressive resuscitation as needed
- Blood product transfusion if necessary en route to OR
- In cases of shock, pressors and cardiac support may be necessary.

IV Fluids
- Unnecessary for a stable ectopic pregnancy being medically treated
- Critical for a surgical patient who is bleeding

Nursing
Strict input/output, hourly vitals, orthostatics if mobile, frequent abdominal exams, serial hematocrit, pad counts if heavy vaginal bleeding

Discharge Criteria
Afebrile, abdominal pain resolving or resolved, diagnosis established, surgical treatment, and recovery complete

 ## ONGOING CARE

FOLLOW-UP RECOMMENDATIONS
Patient Monitoring
- Serial serum quantitative hCG until level drops to zero:
  - After methotrexate administration, a strict monitoring protocol should be followed.
  - Following salpingostomy, weekly levels are appropriate.
  - Following salpingectomy, further follow-up may be unnecessary.
- Pelvic US for persistent or recurrent masses
- Pain control: Brief course of narcotics usually necessary
- Liver and renal function tests following methotrexate administration if repeat dosing is required
- Delay of subsequent pregnancy for at least 3 months after treatment with methotrexate due to teratogenicity (folate deficiency)

DIET
- During treatment, avoid foods and vitamins high in folate (leafy greens, liver, edamame) due to interaction with methotrexate efficacy.
- Maintain excellent hydration.

PATIENT EDUCATION
- Signs and symptoms of ectopic pregnancy should be reviewed.
- Patients should be encouraged to plan subsequent pregnancies and seek early medical care on discovery of future pregnancies.

PROGNOSIS
- Chronic ectopic pregnancies are rare and treated with surgical removal of the fallopian tube.
- Future fertility depends on fertility prior to ectopic pregnancy and degree of tubal compromise.
- ~66% of women with a history of ectopic pregnancy will have a future intrauterine pregnancy if they are able to conceive (1).
- If infertility persists beyond 12 months, the fallopian tubes should be evaluated.

COMPLICATIONS
- Hemorrhage and hypovolemic shock
- Persistent trophoblastic tissue after medical or surgical management
- Infection
- Infertility
- Blood transfusions with associated infections/transfusion reaction
- Disseminated intravascular coagulation in the setting of massive hemorrhage

REFERENCES

1. Medical management of ectopic pregnancy. ACOG Practice Bulletin. No. 94. American College of Obstetricians and Gynecologists. *Obstet Gynecol.* 2008;111:1479–1485.
2. Verhaegen J, Gallos ID, van Mello NM, et al. Accuracy of single progesterone test to predict early pregnancy outcome in women with pain or bleeding: Meta-analysis of cohort studies. *BMJ.* 2012;345:e6077. Epub 2012 Sep 27.
3. Rausch ME, Sammel MD, Takacs P, et al. Development of a multiple marker test for ectopic pregnancy. *Obstet Gynecol.* 2011;117(3):573–582.
4. Sagiv R, Debby A, Feit H, et al. The optimal cutoff level of human chorionic gonadotropin for efficacy of methotrexate treatment in women with extrauterine pregnancy. *Int J Gynecol Obstet.* 2012;116(2):101–104.
5. Bachman EA, Barnhart KT. Medical management of ectopic pregnancy: A comparison of regimens. *Clin Obstet Gynecol.* 2012;55(2):440–447.
6. National Institute for Clinical Excellence. *Diagnosis and Initial Management in Early Pregnancy of Ectopic Pregnancy and Miscarriage.* London: National Institute for Clinical Excellence, 2012.
7. Barnhart KT. Clinical practice. Ectopic pregnancy. *N Engl J Med.* 2009;361(4):379–387.

ADDITIONAL READING

Hajenius PJ, Mol F, Mol BW, et al. Interventions for tubal ectopic pregnancy. *Cochrane Database Syst Rev.* 2009;CD000324.

 ## CODES

ICD10
- O00.0 Abdominal pregnancy
- O00.1 Tubal pregnancy
- O00.9 Ectopic pregnancy, unspecified

CLINICAL PEARLS

- Ectopic pregnancy is the leading cause of 1st-trimester maternal death and accounts for 6% of US pregnancy deaths.
- 97% of ectopic pregnancies occur in the fallopian tube.
- Diagnosis requires high clinical suspicion in the setting of abdominal pain and a positive pregnancy test.

EJACULATORY DISORDERS

Tanya E. Anim, MD

 BASICS

DESCRIPTION

- Premature/rapid ejaculation: Inability to control ejaculatory reflex; most common type of sexual dysfunction affecting all age groups:
  - American Urological Association (AUA) 2004 Guidelines definition: Ejaculation occurs sooner than desired, either before or shortly after penetration, causing distress to either one or both partners (1).
  - Natural biologic response is to ejaculate within 2–5 minutes after vaginal penetration.
  - Ejaculatory control is an acquired behavior that increases with experience.
- Delayed (retarded) ejaculation: Prolonged time to ejaculate (>30 minutes) despite desire, stimulation, and erection.
- Aspermia (lack of sperm in the ejaculate):
  - Anejaculation: Lack of emission or contractions of bulbospongiosus muscle
  - Retrograde ejaculation: Partial or complete ejaculation of semen into the bladder
  - Obstruction: Ejaculatory duct obstruction or urethral obstruction
- Painful ejaculation: Genital or perineal pain during or after ejaculation
- Ejaculatory anhedonia: Normal ejaculation lacking orgasm or pleasure
- Hematospermia: Presence of blood in the ejaculate
- Ejaculatory duct obstruction
- System(s) affected: Nervous; Reproductive
- Synonym(s): Premature ejaculation; Rapid ejaculation; Retarded ejaculation; Retrograde ejaculation; Anejaculation; Inhibited orgasm in males; Ejaculatory dysfunction

EPIDEMIOLOGY

- Premature ejaculation is common. Reported prevalence in US males ages 18–59: 21%
- Retarded ejaculation is reported in ~5–8% of men between age 18 and 59, but <3% experience the problem for >6 months.
- Predominant age: All sexually mature age groups
- Predominant sex: Male only

Prevalence
20% of men affected

ETIOLOGY AND PATHOPHYSIOLOGY
Male sexual response:

- Erection mediated by parasympathetic nervous system
- Ejaculation consists of 2 phases:
  - Emission phase: Semen is deposited into urethra by contraction of prostate, seminal vesicles, and vas deferens; under autonomic sympathetic control.
  - Ejaculation phase: Semen is forcibly propelled out of urethra by rhythmic contractions of the bulbospongiosus and ischiocavernosus muscles. This is mediated by the somatic nervous system on the motor branches of the pudendal nerve.
- Bladder neck contracture occurs during the above process and is induced by α-adrenergic receptors to ensure anterograde ejaculation.
- Orgasm: The pleasurable sensation associated with ejaculation (cerebral cortex)

- Premature ejaculation (many theoretical causes):
  - Penile hypersensitivity
  - 5-hydroxytryptamine (5-HT)-receptor sensitivity
  - Sexual inexperience
  - High level of sexual arousal and/or long interval since last ejaculation
  - Fear of sexual transmitted infections (STIs)
  - Anxiety or guilty feelings about sex
  - Lack of privacy
  - Interpersonal maladaptation (e.g., marital problems, unresponsiveness of partner)
- Retarded ejaculation (2)[B]:
  - Rarely due to underlying painful disorder (e.g., prostatitis, seminal vesiculitis)
  - Psychogenic
  - Sexual performance anxiety and other psychosocial factors
  - Medications may impair ejaculation (e.g., monoamine oxidase inhibitors [MAOIs], SSRIs, α- and β-blockers, thiazides, antipsychotics, tricyclic and quadricyclic antidepressants, NSAIDs, opiates, or alcohol).
- Never any ejaculate:
  - Congenital structural disorder (Müllerian duct cyst, Wolffian abnormality)
  - Acquired (radical prostatectomy, postinfectious, posttraumatic, T10–12 neuropathy)
- Anejaculation:
  - Medications (α- and β-blockers, benzodiazepines, SSRIs, MAOIs, TCAs, antipsychotics, aminocaproic acid)
  - Diabetes mellitus (DM) (neuropathy)
  - Retroperitoneal lymph node dissection
  - Sympathetic nerve injury (spinal cord injury, intraoperative injury)
  - Radical prostatectomy
- Retrograde ejaculation:
  - Transurethral resection of the prostate (25%) or other prostate resection procedures
  - Surgery on the neck of the bladder
  - Extensive pelvic surgery
  - Retroperitoneal lymph node dissection for testicular cancer (also may produce failure of emission)
  - Neurologic disorders (MS, DM)
  - Medications (α-blockers, in particular tamsulosin, ganglion blockers, antipsychotics)
  - Urethral stricture
  - Trauma
- Painful ejaculation:
  - Infection or inflammation (orchitis, epididymitis, prostatitis, urethritis)
  - Ejaculatory duct obstruction
  - Seminal vesicle calculi
  - Obstruction of the vas deferens
  - Psychological
- Ejaculatory anhedonia:
  - Medications
  - Psychological
  - Hormonal imbalances
  - Decreased libido
- Hematospermia (often unable to diagnose cause):
  - Inflammation/infection
  - Calculi: Bladder, seminal vesicle, prostate, urethra
  - Trauma to genital area (i.e., cycling or constipation)

  - Obstruction
  - Cyst
  - Tumor (prostate cancer [1–3% present with hematospermia])
  - Arteriovenous malformations
  - Iatrogenic
  - Hypertension

COMMONLY ASSOCIATED CONDITIONS

- Neurologic disorders (e.g., multiple sclerosis [MS])
- Diabetes mellitus
- Prostatitis
- Ejaculatory duct obstruction
- Urethral stricture
- Psychological disorders
- Endocrinopathies
- Relationship/Interpersonal difficulties

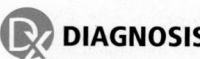 **DIAGNOSIS**

- Ejaculation occurs before individual wishes.
- Ejaculation does not occur following normal stimulation (including masturbation).

HISTORY

- Detailed sexual history, including:
  - Time frame of the problem
  - Evaluation of the quality of patient's sexual response
  - Sense of ejaculatory control and sexual distress
  - Overall assessment of the relationship
- Detailed history of recent and current medications
- History of past trauma or recent infections
- Past surgical history with particular attention to genitourinary (GU) surgeries
- Inquire about home remedies attempted.
- Many men do not distinguish initially between problems related to erection and ejaculation.
- Some men have unrealistic expectations of ejaculatory response and frequency.
- Include the sexual partner in the interview, especially if the patient expresses a belief that he is not meeting his partner's needs.
- In review of systems, elicit any evidence of testosterone deficiency or prolactin excess for diagnosis of anhedonia.

PHYSICAL EXAM

- Look for MS, spinal cord injury, and emotional disorders.
- Thorough GU exam, including (3):
  - Size and texture of testes and epididymis
  - Verification of the presence of the vas deferens
  - Location and patency of urethral meatus
  - Digital rectal examination to evaluate prostate consistency and size and possible midline lesions

DIAGNOSTIC TESTS & INTERPRETATION

- Laboratory test results may be normal.
- Fasting blood sugar or HgbA1c to rule out diabetes
- Postorgasmic urinalysis will confirm retrograde ejaculation. Sperm, fructose level, and viscosity can be measured.

- Anejaculation will have fructose negative, sperm negative, nonviscous postorgasmic urinalysis.
- In painful ejaculation, urinalysis and urine culture
- If prostate cancer is considered, check prostate-specific antigen (PSA).
- In anhedonia, consider checking testosterone, prolactin, and thyroid levels.
- In hematospermia, painful ejaculation, or if ejaculatory duct obstruction is considered, transrectal ultrasound (TRUS) may be helpful.
- TRUS-guided seminal vesicle aspiration; if ejaculatory duct obstruction is present, then the aspirate will contain sperm.
- If suspicious of anatomic abnormality, can use US and/or MRI.

 TREATMENT

GENERAL MEASURES
- Identifying any medical cause (even if not reversible) helps patient accept condition.
- Improve partner communication.
- Psychological counseling
- Reduce performance pressure through reassurance.
- Use of a variety of resources may be necessary (e.g., psychiatrist, psychologist, sex therapist, vascular surgeon, urologist, endocrinologist, neurologist).
- Premature ejaculation (4)[A]:
  – Use sensate focus therapy (gradual progression of nonsexual contact to sexual contact)
  – Quiet vagina: Female partner stops moving just prior to ejaculation
  – Techniques to learn ejaculatory control (e.g., coronal squeeze technique [squeezing the glans penis until ejaculatory urge ceases] or start-and-stop technique [cessation of penile stimulation when ejaculation approaches and resumption of stimulation when ejaculatory feeling ends])
- Delayed ejaculation:
  – Change to antidepressant less likely to cause delayed ejaculation (citalopram, fluvoxamine, nefazodone).
  – Penile vibratory stimulation (not frequently used)
- Anejaculation/Retrograde ejaculation:
  – Discontinue offending medication(s).
  – Diabetic control
  – If urethral obstruction present, refer to urology.
  – Retrograde ejaculation may be helped if intercourse occurs when bladder is full.
  – Consider penile vibratory stimulation (effective in spinal cord injuries >T10) or electroejaculation (place on monitor if lesions above T6 because autonomic dysreflexia may result) to collect sperm in anejaculation cases.
- Painful ejaculation:
  – Counseling may be beneficial.
  – If seminal vesicle stones are possible, refer to urology.
- Hematospermia:
  – Often resolves spontaneously, without known cause.
  – May try empiric antibiotic, but little evidence to support.
  – If persistent or high degree of suspicion for abnormality, refer to urologist.

MEDICATION
- Premature ejaculation:
  – Treating underlying erectile dysfunction (if identified)
  – Behavioral/Sex therapy
  – Topical anesthetic gel applied (2.5% prilocaine ± 2.5% lidocaine [EMLA]) 2.5 g under a condom for 30 minutes prior to intercourse
  – Experimental PSD502 topical aerosol preparation of lidocaine/prilocaine effective in phase III trials (5)
  – Clomipramine 20–50 mg/d or sertraline 25–200 mg/d, fluoxetine 5–20 mg/d, or paroxetine 10–40 mg/d have been shown to delay ejaculation (6)[B].
  – Clomipramine shown to be the most effective, but has higher rate of side effects
  – On-demand use of clomipramine 20–40 mg 4–24 hours before intercourse, or sertraline 50 mg 4–8 hours before intercourse, or paroxetine 20 mg 3–4 hours before intercourse
  – Switching antidepressants to bupropion, nefazodone, mirtazapine, or possibly trazodone may eliminate drug-induced ejaculatory disturbance.
  – Dapoxetine, a short-acting SSRI for on-demand use, was effective in phase III trials (7).
- Delayed (retarded) ejaculation:
  – Retarded orgasm and ejaculation in patients who must continue SSRIs may respond to bupropion, buspirone, cyproheptadine, or yohimbine supplementation before intercourse.
  – Some evidence that cyproheptadine and amantadine may be helpful (8)
- Anejaculation/retrograde ejaculation:
  – α-Agonists and antihistamines can be helpful but are not approved by the FDA:
    ○ Pseudoephedrine 60 mg PO every day to q.i.d.
    ○ Imipramine 25 mg PO b.i.d.
    ○ Ephedrine sulfate 10–15 mg PO q.i.d. (9)
- Painful ejaculation:
  – Treat underlying infection/inflammatory process.
  – α-Blockers may have some benefit.

ISSUES FOR REFERRAL
The following conditions, when suspected, should be referred to a urologist:
- Ejaculatory duct obstruction
- Seminal vesicle or prostatic stones
- Urethral obstruction
- Vas deferens obstruction
- Calculi
- Persistent or severe hematospermia

SURGERY/OTHER PROCEDURES
Surgical treatment of ejaculatory duct obstruction:
- Transurethral resection of the ejaculatory ducts

 ONGOING CARE

PATIENT EDUCATION
See "General Measures."

PROGNOSIS
Often improves with therapy and counseling

COMPLICATIONS
Psychological impact on some males: Signs of severe inadequacy, self-doubt, additional anxiety, and guilt

REFERENCES
1. Montague DK, Jarow J, Broderick GA, et al. AUA guideline on the pharmacologic management of premature ejaculation. J Urol. 2004;172:290–294.
2. Richardson D, Goldmeier D, BASHH Special Interest Group for Sexual Dysfunction. Recommendations for the management of retarded ejaculation: BASHH Special Interest Group for Sexual Dysfunction. Int J STD AIDS. 2006;17:7–13.
3. Schuster TG, Ohl DA. Diagnosis and treatment of ejaculatory dysfunction. Urol Clin North Am. 2002;29:939–948.
4. McCarty E, Dinsmore W. Dapoxetine: An evidence-based review of its effectiveness in treatment of premature ejaculation. Core Evid. 2012;7:1–14. Epub 2012 Jan 19.
5. Dinsmore WW, Wyllie MG. PSD502 improves ejaculatory latency, control and sexual satisfaction when applied topically 5 min before intercourse in men with premature ejaculation: Results of a phase III, multicentre, double-blind, placebo-controlled study. Br J Urol Int. 2009;103(7):940–949. Epub 2009 Feb 23.
6. Porst H. An overview of pharmacotherapy in premature ejaculation. J Sex Med. 2011;8(Suppl 4):335–341.
7. Hellstrom WJ. Emerging treatments for premature ejaculation: Focus on dapoxetine. Neuropsychiatr Dis Treat. 2009;5:37–46. Epub 2009 Apr 8.
8. McMahon CG, Abdo C, Incrocci L, et al. Disorders of orgasm and ejaculation in men. J Sex Med. 2004;1:58–65.
9. Colpi G, Weidner W, Jungwirth A, et al. EAU guidelines on ejaculatory dysfunction. Eur Urol. 2004;46(5):555–558.

ADDITIONAL READING
Heidelbaugh JJ. Management of erectile dysfunction. Am Fam Physician. 2010;81(3):305–312.

 CODES

ICD10
- F52.4 Premature ejaculation
- N53.11 Retarded ejaculation
- N53.14 Retrograde ejaculation

CLINICAL PEARLS
- If erectile dysfunction is contributing to ejaculatory difficulty, management of erectile dysfunction should precede attempted management of ejaculatory disorders.
- Medications should always be thoroughly reviewed, as they may be the primary cause of ejaculatory disorders.
- A multidisciplinary approach, including the primary care physician, urologists, psychologists, and other appropriate health care professionals, is essential to the proper treatment of ejaculatory disorders.

ELDER ABUSE

Nitin Budhwar, MD • Philip Silva, MD

 BASICS

DESCRIPTION
- The National Center of Elder Abuse divides abuse in to 3 categories (older than age 60):
  - **Domestic:** Abuse from someone who has a special relationship with the elderly individual (spouse, child, friend, or in-home caregiver) that occurs in the home of the elderly or caregiver
  - **Institutional:** Occurs in the setting of a facility that is responsible for caring for the elderly, such as a nursing home or long-term care facility
  - **Self-neglect:** The behavior of the elderly individual leads to harm
- Types of abuse:
  - Physical
  - Sexual
  - Financial
  - Neglect
  - Psychological or emotional
  - Self-neglect: The most common form of abuse (1)
  - Taken advantage of: Misinformation and unregulated online pharmaceutical, financial companies, etc. that specifically target the elderly leading to deleterious outcomes (2).

EPIDEMIOLOGY
Incidence
Estimate is that as many as 1:10 have been victims of abuse (3), placing a conservative number at 50,000 cases per year.

Prevalence
A recent national survey measuring prevalence of abuse in individuals of at least 60 years and older found that 11.9% of the surveyed population suffered some form of abuse:
- 5.2% encountered financial mistreatment by family members.
- 5.1% suffered potential neglect.
- 4.6% encountered emotional mistreatment, mostly by humiliation or verbal abuse.
- 1.6% encountered physical mistreatment, mostly through battery.
- 0.6% sexually mistreated, mostly through forced intercourse (4).

ETIOLOGY AND PATHOPHYSIOLOGY
The etiology of elder abuse is a complex biopsychosocial combination of increased dependence on the caregiver by the abuser in a suboptimal environment with poor behavioral coping methods, which is compounded by increased stress.

Genetics
Not contributory

RISK FACTORS
- The victim:
  - Advanced age
  - Dementia or other cognitive impairment
  - Female gender
  - Disability in caring for him/herself
  - Depression
  - Social isolation
  - Stress: Health, financial, or situational

- The abuser:
  - Mental illness
  - Financial dependency
  - Substance abuse
  - History of violence
  - Other antisocial behavior (5)

GENERAL PREVENTION
- Improve patient social contact and support.
- Identify and correct potential risk factors for elder abuse:
  - Home visit to identify for potential risks of fall hazards and barriers to ambulation that could lead to fractures and functional decline that could leave the individual vulnerable to abuse.
  - Evaluate for assist devices that help the patient independently complete his/her ADLs and prevent caregiver dependence.
  - Screen for depression using validated tools like the Geriatric Depression Scale.
  - Early identification and treatment of cognitive impairment
- Identify caregiver stress and burden, refer to community programs that aid with emotional assistance.
- Advance life directives planning, including identifying possible caregivers, choosing a MPOA, estate and will planning, and so forth.

COMMONLY ASSOCIATED CONDITIONS
Most common associated conditions with elder abuse are also identified as risk factors, social isolation, increased dependence for ADL/IADLs, depression, cognitive impairment, and aggressive behavior (4,5).

 DIAGNOSIS

A high index of suspicion when risk factors are present is important; types of abuse should be kept in mind as some types might not be obvious. It can be difficult to diagnose elder abuse in a single clinic visit, so it is important to get social services involved and to do home visits when abuse is suspected (5).

HISTORY
It is important to take a detailed history with focus on the living arrangements, degree of functionality, who the caregivers are, and other risk factors listed above.

PHYSICAL EXAM
- It is important objectively to document positive and negative findings in your physical exam and to be very detailed because it can be admissible in court if abuse is suspected.
- Vital signs: Check weight and assess for progressive loss in weight; BP can be an indicator of dehydration that could be secondary to neglect.
- General overall appearance:
  - Wasting or cachexia
  - Poor hygiene, unkempt clothing
  - If the patient is bedbound, it is important to assess the integrity of the mattress and sheets. Look for excessive skin flakes, hair, or urine-soiled mattresses.

- Oral exam:
  - Assess for poor dentition, oral ulcers, or abscesses.
- Skin exam:
  - Most bruises from elder abuse are large (>5 cm) and located on the face, lateral arm, or back.
  - Bite marks
  - It is important to check for pressure ulcers on the bony prominences of the patient, elbows, sacrum, heels, and scapula.
- Mental/psychiatric:
  - Withdrawn, anxious, fearful, blunted
- Genital/rectal exam if sexual abuse is suspected

DIFFERENTIAL DIAGNOSIS
- Advanced dementia can present with individuals appearing withdrawn and they are often malnourished.
- Elderly with advanced dementia of Alzheimer type or Lewy body dementia can present with delusions of persecution and aggression that can be confused for elder abuse.
- Patients with Parkinson disease often fall and may exhibit fractures and bruises on a frequent basis that may mimic recurrent physical abuse.
- Coagulopathy seen in patients in advanced malignancy with bone marrow suppression or invasion, and those on chronic antiplatelet therapy can appear with bruising that can be easily confused with elder abuse.
- Wasting from malignancy, infections, chronic disease
- Thyroid disorder can present with AMS, depression, or anxiety.
- Chronic lung disease can present with decreased weight.
- Delirium from acute electrolyte disturbances, infectious etiology, or cardiovascular compromise can all present similar to elder abuse.
- Impaired financial status can also be confused with self-neglect.

DIAGNOSTIC TESTS & INTERPRETATION
The following workup is recommended:
- Nutritional Assessment iron, B_{12}, folate, thiamine, albumin, prealbumin, CBC, LFTs, electrolytes
- Malignancy workup, as per current guidelines
- If bruising is noted, check for coagulopathies (e.g., platelets, bleeding times, PT/INR, and PTT).
- If cognitive impairment is observed, check thyroid-stimulating hormone, vitamin B_{12} level; consider syphilis and HIV testing if indicated.
- Assessment of infection: may include urinalysis and culture, chest radiograph, blood count, and cultures.
- Radiographic imaging of areas below soft tissue injury is indicated if there is evidence of infection (osteomyelitis) at a pressure ulcer site or bruising of a limb (fracture).
- If physical abuse is suspected and cognitive impairment present, then cranial imaging to look for hemorrhage (e.g., subdural) is indicated using CT scan or MRI.

Diagnostic Procedures/Other

- Pulse test: Check BP and pulse in presence and absence of suspected abuser. Elevation of either in the presence of the suspected abuser should raise suspicion. Useful in patients with dementia or other condition that makes history-taking difficult.
- Folstein MMSE, MOCA, or other validated tools to assess for cognitive impairment if suspected
- Geriatric Depression Screen if suspected
- Documentation: Practitioners may make statements of "suspected mistreatment," but should avoid making definitive diagnosis of abuse in their initial assessment, unless it is very obvious.

 TREATMENT

Most states require all health care providers to report suspected elder abuse to a local agency such as the Adult Protective Services. (http://www.nccafv.org/state_elder_abuse_hotlines.htm)

MEDICATION
None

IN-PATIENT CONSIDERATIONS
Admission Criteria/Initial Stabilization
- Victims of elder abuse should be admitted to the hospital if there are no safe discharge alternatives.
- Management of uncontrolled chronic conditions due to neglect (i.e. wound care from ulcers, or infections).
- Cases of suspected abuse *must be reported* to the state's Adult Protective Services agency or a designated alternative (e.g., if patient resides in nursing home, then report to that state's regulatory entity). Social services may help. If physical harm has occurred, consider reporting to local law enforcement for investigation.
- Hospital security may need to be notified if restricted visitor access to a patient is required, and the patient's name may be hidden from the public hospital census.
- If the patient is a victim of elder abuse he/she must be relocated to a safer alternative and may need admission for sequelae caused by the abuse.

Discharge Criteria
Victims should not be discharged to a potentially abusive environment. Alternatives to discharge to the unsafe environment may include:
- Friend or family member
- Nursing home
- Personal care home
- Assisted living facility
- Local victims' rescue or sheltering program if available

 ONGOING CARE

FOLLOW-UP RECOMMENDATIONS
Victims of abuse should not be discharged without adequate follow-up, including:
- Primary care physician visit within 1 week
- Follow-up with Adult Protective Services or other agency; a home visit should be scheduled prior to discharge if the patient is going back home.
- Home Health Agency for assessment of safety (physical therapy)
- Follow-up with appropriate mental health care

Patient Monitoring
The patient should have frequent visits and be followed through the appropriate agencies to reduce continuation of abuse and to identify recurring abuse.

PATIENT EDUCATION
- For Elder Abuse Resources in your state you can go to the National Center of Elder Abuse at www.ncea.aoa.gov.
- Or your local representative by calling 1-800-677-1166

PROGNOSIS
Elder abuse and self-neglect are associated with an overall increased risk in mortality (6).

COMPLICATIONS
Complications of elder abuse can lead to worsening depression, increased mortality, and overall poor quality of life (1).

REFERENCES

1. Mosqueda L, Dong X. Elder abuse and self-neglect: "I don't care anything about going to the doctor, to be honest . . ." *JAMA*. 2011;306:532–540.
2. Liang BA, Lovett KM, Mackey TK, et al. Elder abuse. *J Am Geriatr Soc*. 2012;60:398–400.
3. ACOG Committee on Health Care and Womens Health Opinion Statement Number 568: July 2013.
4. Acierno R, Hernandez MA, Amstadter AB, et al. Prevalence and correlates of emotional, physical, sexual, and financial abuse and potential neglect in the United States: The National Elder Mistreatment Study. *Am J Public Health*. 2010;100:292–297.
5. Halphen JM, Varas GM, Sadowsky JM, et al. Recognizing and reporting elder abuse and neglect. *Geriatrics*. 2009;64:13–18.
6. Dong X, Simon M, Mendes de Leon C, et al. Elder self-neglect and abuse and mortality risk in a community-dwelling population. *JAMA*. 2009;302:517–526.

ADDITIONAL READING

- Cooper C, Katona C, Finne-Soveri H, et al. Indicators of elder abuse: A crossnational comparison of psychiatric morbidity and other determinants in the Ad-HOC study. *Am J Geriatr Psychiatry*. 2006;14:489–497.
- Lachs MS, Pillemer K. Elder abuse. *Lancet*. 364(9441):1263–1272.
- Lachs MS, Williams CS, O'Brien S, et al. Adult protective service use and nursing home placement. *Gerontologist*. 2002;42(6):734–739.
- Lachs MS, Williams CS, O'Brien S, et al. The mortality of elder mistreatment. *JAMA*. 1998;280(5):428–432.
- Widera E, Steenpass V, Marson D, et al. Finances in the older patient with cognitive impairment: "He didn't want me to take over." *JAMA*. 2011;305(7):698–706.
- Wiglesworth A, Austin R, Corona M, et al. Bruising as a marker of physical elder abuse. *J Am Geriatr Soc*. 2009;57(7):1191–1196. Epub 2009 Jun 3.
- Wiglesworth A, Mosqueda L, Mulnard R, et al. Screening for abuse and neglect of people with dementia. *J Am Geriatr Soc*. 2010;58(3):493–500.

 CODES

ICD10
- T74.01XA Adult neglect or abandonment, confirmed, initial encounter
- T74.11XA Adult physical abuse, confirmed, initial encounter
- T74.21XA Adult sexual abuse, confirmed, initial encounter

CLINICAL PEARLS

- Elder abuse, or elder mistreatment, is a condition in which the physical, psychological, or financial well-being of an older adult is infringed upon through intentional acts or lack of action, even if harm is not intended.
- It is important to identify vulnerable individuals through proper evaluation of potential risk factors for abuse (social isolation, depression, cognitive impairment, disability requiring assistance, and financial dependence by the caregiver).
- Correction of risk factors is important to reduce the incidence of elder abuse (strengthen the patients' social support, treat depression, provide the patient with assist devices, screen for cognitive impairment with a trial of medication if possible, and identify caregiver burn out).
- Clearly document your physical exam with only specific objective findings.
- Contact APS or your local resources if elder abuse is suspected; it is unlawful not to report suspected elder abuse.

ENCEPHALITIS, VIRAL

Aditya Chandrasekhar, MD, MPH • Sarah H. Cheeseman, MD

BASICS

DESCRIPTION
- Inflammatory process of the brain associated with clinical evidence of neurologic dysfunction
- System(s) affected: Nervous
- Synonym(s): Meningoencephalitis

EPIDEMIOLOGY
Incidence
3.5–7.4/100,000 persons/year
Prevalence
- Seasonal variation (e.g., arboviruses, enteroviruses)
- Nonseasonal: Most others (e.g., herpes simplex virus [HSV])
- Vaccines have altered prevalence and seasonality (e.g., mumps is no longer common and not seasonal)

ETIOLOGY AND PATHOPHYSIOLOGY
- Most common entry site is through the respiratory or GI tract, followed by hematogenous spread.
- Rarer modes of entry include neurotropic spread (e.g., rabies)
- Specific cell lines may be infected and are associated with specific symptom complexes:
  - Neurons: Associated with seizures
  - Oligodendroglia: May cause demyelination alone, cortical infection, or reactive parenchymal swelling; changes in state of consciousness
  - Brainstem neurons: Coma, respiratory failure
  - Microglia, macrophages: Neurologic dysfunction
- Pathologic changes seen with postinfectious and postvaccinal encephalomyelitis include perivascular infiltration of mononuclear inflammatory cells.
- Most commonly identified etiologies in the US: HSV, West Nile virus, enteroviruses
- Despite extensive evaluations, the etiologic agent frequently has not been identified.

RISK FACTORS
- Age: Increased incidence among infants and elderly
- Contact with animals or insect vectors
- Impaired immune status
- Occupation (e.g., lab or animal-care workers)
- Recreational activities (e.g., camping, hunting)
- Transfusion and transplantation
- Travel to endemic areas
- Recent vaccinations/unvaccinated status

GENERAL PREVENTION
- Appropriate clothing to protect against mosquitos
- Use of mosquito repellants (DEET, Picaridin)
- Avoidance and removal of ticks
- Elimination of mosquito breeding sources
- Vaccines, when available (e.g., mumps, measles, polio, rabies, Japanese encephalitis)

COMMONLY ASSOCIATED CONDITIONS
- Seizures
- Hyperthermia
- Increased intracranial pressure (ICP)
- Inappropriate antidiuretic hormone (ADH) secretion

DIAGNOSIS

- Seek epidemiologic clues and assess risk factors in all patients with encephalitis.
- Consider acute disseminated encephalomyelitis (ADEM) with history of recent infectious illness or vaccination associated with clinical presentation of encephalitis (1)[B].
- Specific diagnostic studies should be done in most patients (see "Diagnostic Tests & Interpretation" section) (1)[A].

HISTORY
- The classic triad includes:
  - Fever
  - Headache
  - Altered mental status
- Focal neurologic deficits can be present and may correlate to areas affected by individual viruses (e.g., personality changes with frontal lobe involvement or speech deficits with temporal lobe involvement in HSV)
- Important to assess travel, animal exposure, occupation, and immune status

PHYSICAL EXAM
- General signs:
  - Fever
  - Rash
  - Parotitis
- Neurologic findings:
  - Altered level of consciousness
  - Acute cognitive dysfunction
  - Behavioral changes
  - Neck stiffness
  - Focal neurologic signs
  - Cranial nerve palsies
  - Paresthesias
- Other:
  - Loss of temperature or vasomotor control

DIFFERENTIAL DIAGNOSIS
- Autoimmune (e.g., Anti-NMDA)
- Meningitis
- Intracranial space-occupying lesions
- Nonviral encephalitis (e.g., rickettsia)
- Noninfectious encephalopathies (e.g., poisoning)
- Infectious encephalopathies (e.g., progressive multifocal leucoencephalopathy)
- Infectious endocarditis with CNS involvement
- Vasculitis
- Paraneoplastic syndromes
- Postinfectious encephalitis
- Postimmunization encephalitis
- ADEM

DIAGNOSTIC TESTS & INTERPRETATION
- Recommended general diagnostic studies (outside CNS) for all suspected encephalitis patients:
  - Blood cultures (1)[B]
  - Serum samples: At time of initial presentation and stored for future studies
  - HIV testing (2)[C]

- Additional studies based on risk factors and clinical findings:
  - Nucleic acid amplification tests (polymerase chain reaction [PCR]) e.g., *Borrelia burgdoferi* (1)[B]
  - Cultures of stool, nasopharynx, sputum (1)[B]
  - Skin scrapings of active vesicles (direct fluorescent antibody [DFA] testing to identify viral antigen)
  - Tissue biopsies with culture, antigen detection, nucleic acid amplification testing, and histology (1)[A]
  - Serologic testing: IgM antibodies (1)[A], IgM and IgG capture ELISAs
  - Serum cryptococcal antigen testing is valuable in suspected cases.
  - Acute and convalescent phase serum to show seroconversion: Not helpful to initiate therapy, but may be helpful for the retrospective diagnosis of a specific pathogen (1)[B]
  - Serum IgG antibodies should be considered in patients where the encephalitis may be the result of reactivation of a previously acquired infection.

Initial Tests (lab, imaging)
- Lumbar puncture is essential (unless specific contraindication) (1)[A]:
  - CSF shows pleocytosis (10–2,000 cells/mm^3). Mononuclear cells usually predominate. Finding of CSF eosinophils may suggest certain pathogens (e.g., highest with helminths, but can also be seen with other pathogens).
  - CSF glucose normal or mildly depressed
  - CSF protein usually mild or moderately increased
  - Direct examination of CSF fluid with Gram stain for bacteria and acid–fast stain for *Mycobacteria*
  - CSF culture for bacteria, mycobacteria, fungi, amoeba, and viruses
  - CSF culture for viruses has limited value; not routinely recommended
  - CSF nucleic acid amplification tests (e.g., PCR) (1)[A]; herpes simplex PCR should be performed on all specimens (1)[A]; if negative, consider repeat in 3–7 days for those with compatible clinical syndrome or temporal lobe localization on neuroimaging (1)[B]
  - Viral-specific IgM (1)[A]
  - CSF testing for cryptococcal antigen is superior to India ink preparations.
- In up to 10% of cases with viral encephalitis, CSF findings are normal.
- MRI is imaging of choice and must be obtained in all cases, unless contraindicated (or diagnosis is already certain) (2)[C].
- MRI is most sensitive for HSV encephalitis where T$_2$-weighted and fluid attenuated inversion recovery (FLAIR) images show temporal lobe and limbic involvement.
- Diffusion-weighted imaging is superior to conventional MRI in encephalitis caused by HSV, enterovirus, and West Nile virus.
- FLAIR imaging may be helpful with enterovirus 71 encephalitis, flaviviruses, and eastern equine encephalitis.
- CT, with and without contrast enhancement, is less sensitive and slower at showing changes, but can be used if MRI is not an option (1)[B].

Follow-Up Tests & Special Considerations
- PCR may be negative early on; repeat in 48–72 hours.
- Follow-up imaging is not indicated unless initial imaging was done in early stages when it may have been unrevealing and later show abnormalities.

Diagnostic Procedures/Other
- CSF culture is not routinely used to diagnose encephalitis.
- Electroencephalogram (EEG) is nondiagnostic, but may be useful in early herpes simplex encephalitis and, less commonly, in other herpes viruses (varicella zoster virus [VZV], Epstein–Barr virus [EBV], human herpesvirus 6 [HHV6])
- Serologic testing
- Brain biopsy: *Rarely used and not routinely recommended.* Consider if unknown etiology and condition is deteriorating despite treatment with acyclovir (1)[B].

Test Interpretation
- Prominent inflammatory reaction in meninges and in a perivascular distribution
- Swelling and degenerative changes

 TREATMENT

- Most will require intensive care
- In general, empiric therapy with acyclovir is appropriate in most cases of suspected encephalitis while diagnosis is awaited (1)[A].
- When appropriate, combine with therapy for bacterial, rickettsial, or ehrlichia infection.
- Once an etiologic agent has been identified, therapeutic intervention should be re-evaluated, focusing on pathogen-specific therapy and discontinuing therapy if no available therapy exists for the specific etiologic agent.

GENERAL MEASURES
- Supportive therapy
- Monitoring for drug-related toxicities

MEDICATION
- No specific drug therapy is available for most types of viral encephalitis.
- HSV is the most important exception: Acyclovir therapy is effective.
- Acyclovir is also effective against VZV encephalitis.
- Foscarnet and ganciclovir are effective against cytomegalovirus (CMV) or acyclovir-resistant HSV.
- Appropriate antiviral therapy (i.e., oseltamivir or zanamivir) should be started as soon as possible for hospitalized patients with neurologic symptoms and suspected seasonal or 2009 H1N1 influenza infection (3)[C].
- Use of corticosteroids in viral encephalitis continues to remain an area of active investigation (2)[C], (4)[A]
- Doxycycline should be added to an empiric regimen when clinical clues suggest rickettsial or ehrlichia infection (1)[A].

ISSUES FOR REFERRAL
- Monitoring and management of ICP
- Evaluation and treatment of seizures
- Multidisciplinary teams often provide care

ADDITIONAL THERAPIES
- Very limited data for most adjunctive therapies, not to be used without consulting infectious diseases specialists (e.g., interferon-α or IVIG in West Nile virus encephalitis)
- In particular, various treatments have been tried for rabies encephalitis, with reported success using induced coma by the Milwaukee protocol.

SURGERY/OTHER PROCEDURES
- No surgical modality of treatment routinely indicated
- Central line placement, intubation, and other procedures as needed for support

IN-PATIENT CONSIDERATIONS
- Admit suspected cases of encephalitis to hospital for evaluation, supportive care, and treatment. Most will require intensive care services.
- Although standard isolation precautions are appropriate for most viral encephalitides, exceptions exist (e.g., rabies, influenza).

Admission Criteria/Initial Stabilization
All suspected cases of encephalitis warrant admission due to high risk from not detecting and treating reversible causes:
- Protect airway, when appropriate, and, when indicated, provide:
  – Supplemental oxygen
  – Intubation and mechanical ventilatory support
- Assessment and management of circulatory status, fluids, glucose, and electrolytes

IV Fluids
- Monitor labs as needed for support and drug therapy
- Monitor for syndrome of inappropriate ADH hypersecretion

Nursing
- Isolation, when indicated (e.g., rabies, influenza)
- Precautions for seizure and altered mental status
- Routine nursing care for skin care, patient comfort, monitoring, and family support
- Educate families about the importance of vaccines when available

Discharge Criteria
Resolution of acute symptoms:
- No longer need hospital-level care

 ONGOING CARE

Patients with suspected or proven encephalitis are best cared for in hospitals and many need intensive care.

FOLLOW-UP RECOMMENDATIONS
- Postencephalitis sequelae are primarily neurologic, and follow up should be guided by patient's condition (e.g., anticonvulsants for seizures).
- Physical therapy may be necessary.

PATIENT EDUCATION
- DEET-containing mosquito repellants
- Avoidance of outdoor activities during periods of peak mosquito activity
- Use of protective clothing
- Adequate vector control and environmental sanitation
- Vaccines when available
- Prompt treatment of animal bites or bat exposure

PROGNOSIS
- Often difficult to predict; anticipate slow, but often complete, recovery from deficits in most cases.
- Outcomes worse in elderly and infants
- Some agents have high mortality (rabies, herpes B virus, untreated HSV, eastern equine encephalitis), whereas others are less likely to be lethal (West Nile virus, enteroviruses).

COMPLICATIONS
Vary with age, etiologic agent, and clinical course

REFERENCES

1. Tunkel AR, Glaser CA, Bloch KC, et al. The management of encephalitis: Clinical practice guidelines by the Infectious Diseases Society of America. *Clin Infect Dis*. 2008;47:303–326.
2. Solomon T, Michael BD, Smith PE, et al. Management of suspected viral encephalitis in adults—Association of British Neurologists and British Infection Association National Guidelines. *J Infect*. 2012;64:347–373.
3. Centers for Disease Control and Prevention. Neurologic complications associated with novel influenza A (H1N1) virus infection in children—Dallas, Texas, May 2009. *MMWR*. 2009;58:773–778.
4. Ciro R-E, Lizarraga KJ, Merenda A. A systematic review on the role of adjunctive corticosteroids in herpes simplex virus encephalitis: Is timing critical for safety and efficacy? *Antivir Ther*. 2013, in press.

ADDITIONAL READING

- Kneen R, Michael BD, Menson E, et al. Management of suspected viral encephalitis in children—Association of British Neurologists and British Paediatric Allergy, Immunology and Infection Group national guidelines. *J Infect*. 2012;64:449–477.
- Long SS. Encephalitis diagnosis and management in the real world. *Adv Exp Med Biol*. 2011;697: 153–173.

 CODES

ICD10
- A83.9 Mosquito-borne viral encephalitis, unspecified
- A85.2 Arthropod-borne viral encephalitis, unspecified
- A86 Unspecified viral encephalitis

CLINICAL PEARLS

- Routine treatment is only available for HSV encephalitis, and empiric treatment with acyclovir is warranted in most cases of suspected viral encephalitis.
- All patients suspected of having encephalitis must have MRI and CSF analysis, unless contraindicated.
- Vaccines are very important in preventing infections with viruses for which effective immunization is available.

ENCOPRESIS

Jay Fong, MD • William T. Garrison, PhD

BASICS

DESCRIPTION
- The involuntary or intentional passage of feces into clothing or other inappropriate places by a child 4–18 years of age:
  - Age may be chronologic or developmental.
  - Absence of underlying organic process
  - At least 1 event per month for 3 months
  - Classified into functional constipation (retentive encopresis) and functional nonretentive fecal incontinence (FNRFI): Both cause fecal incontinence, but no constipation in FNRFI. *Functional constipation is more common.*
- System(s) affected: GI; Psychological
- Synonyms(s): Fecal incontinence, Soiling

EPIDEMIOLOGY
Incidence
Predominant sex: Male > Female (3:1). Constipation accounts for 3% of general pediatric referrals; up to 84% of constipated children have fecal incontinence at some point.

Prevalence
Occurs in 1–3% of children >4 years of age

ETIOLOGY AND PATHOPHYSIOLOGY
- In 90% of cases, encopresis develops as a consequence of chronic constipation, with resulting overflow incontinence, which typically is termed *retentive encopresis*. The other 10% are caused by specific organic etiologies.
- Chronic constipation due to irregular and incomplete evacuation results in progressive rectal distension and stretching of both the internal and external anal sphincters.
- As the child habituates to chronic rectal distension, he or she may no longer sense the normal urge to defecate. Eventually, soft or liquid stool begins to leak around the retained fecal mass.
- Many children voluntarily withhold stool in response to the urge to defecate for fear of pain or due to a preoccupation with not interrupting social activities.
- Psychological:
  - Stool withholding, fear, anxiety
  - Difficulty with toilet training, including unusual anxiety or conflict with parent
  - Resistance to using public toilet facilities, such as school bathrooms or outdoor toilets
  - Known association with sexual abuse in boys; likely similar association in girls as well
  - Developmental delay
- Anatomic:
  - Rectal distension and desensitization
  - Anal fissure or painful defecation
  - Muscle hypotonia
  - Slow intestinal motility
  - Hirschsprung disease
  - Cystic fibrosis
  - Spinal cord defects (e.g., spina bifida)
  - Congenital anorectal malformations
  - Anal stenosis
  - Anterior displacement of the anus
  - Postoperative stricture of anus or rectum
  - Pelvic mass
  - Neurofibromatosis
- Dietary or metabolic:
  - Lack of fiber
  - Excessive protein or milk intake
  - Inadequate water intake
  - Hypothyroidism
  - Hypercalcemia
  - Hypokalemia
  - DI or DM
  - Food allergy
  - Gluten enteropathy
- Medication side effects

Genetics
None known, although incidence may be higher in children with family history of constipation

RISK FACTORS
- Male gender
- Constipation
- Very low birth weight
- Painful defecation
- Difficulty with bowel training, including pressure related to early daycare placement
- Organic/Anatomic causes
- Anxiety and depression
- Insufficient fluid intake
- Refusal to use public restrooms
- Attention deficit

GENERAL PREVENTION
Family education: Avoid toilet training prior to readiness, optimal feeding, early detection of problems. Look for signs of relapse: Large-caliber stools, decrease in stool frequency, and soiling

COMMONLY ASSOCIATED CONDITIONS
- Common: Constipation, Hirschsprung disease
- Intermediate: Cerebral palsy, cystic fibrosis
- Less: Developmental and behavioral diagnoses, urinary incontinence

DIAGNOSIS

HISTORY
- Look for signs/symptoms of constipation:
  - Hard, large-caliber stools
  - <3 defecations/week
  - Pain or discomfort with stool passage, withholding of stool
  - Blood on stools
  - Decreased appetite
  - Abdominal pain improving with stool passage
  - Hiding while defecating before child is toilet trained; avoiding use of the toilet
  - Diet low in fiber or fluids, high in dairy
  - Passed stool within first 48 hours of life
  - Pasty stool found on underclothes
  - Recurrent UTIs
- Abrupt onset after age 5 years more likely to be associated with psychological trauma
- Overlap with ADD common in children >5 years
- Medications, such as opiates, phenobarbital, and tricyclic antidepressants (TCAs)
- Family history of constipation

PHYSICAL EXAM
- Detailed history and physical exam usually make the diagnosis without need for lab testing.
- Neurologic exam of lower extremities and perineal area, with attention to S1–S4 distribution, perineal sensation, cremasteric reflex, and anal sphincter tone
- Genital area
- Digital rectal exam: Assess for anal fissures, sphincter tone, rectal distension/impaction, presence of occult or visible blood
- Abdominal exam: Mild abdominal distension; palpable stool in left lower quadrant

DIAGNOSTIC TESTS & INTERPRETATION
Most cases of fecal incontinence do not require extensive lab work.

Initial Tests (lab, imaging)
- Done to rule out organic causes when conventional treatment fails: UA/Urine culture: UTI/glucosuria; thyroid function tests: hypothyroidism; electrolyte panel, including calcium, may show hypokalemia, hypercalcemia, or hyperglycemia
- Abdominal plain films may be useful if an impaction is suspected but not detected by abdominal or rectal exam.
- Comprehensive history and physical exam. Management includes education, disimpaction if necessary, prevention, and follow-up.

Follow-Up Tests & Special Considerations
Failure to pass meconium within 48 hours of birth, failure to thrive, bloody diarrhea, or bilious vomiting in a neonate is almost always associated with aganglionic megacolon, and that history would warrant a barium enema and/or rectal biopsy. Constipation and diarrhea, rash, failure to thrive, or recurrent pneumonia should prompt evaluation for cystic fibrosis. Celiac disease should also be a consideration. Patients with abdominal distension or ileus should be evaluated for possible obstruction.

Diagnostic Procedures/Other
Manometric studies may be useful in patients who have constipation that does not respond to treatment.

TREATMENT

A treatment approach that integrates both laxative treatment and behavioral therapy improves continence in children with fecal incontinence over laxative treatment alone (1).

GENERAL MEASURES
- Anticipatory guidance relative to toilet training beginning at 18 months, with special attention to when children should reduce reliance on diapers or pull-ups during the daytime hours
- Eliminate impaction prior to maintenance Rx.
- Avoid frequent and repeated rectal exams, enemas, and suppositories, especially in infants.
- Once stools seem regular in frequency, child should sit on toilet b.i.d. at the same time each day for 10–15 minutes and for 10–15 minutes after meals. Incorporate positive reinforcement for successfully produced bowel movements.
- Reassurance to school-going children to utilize the toilet with the full cooperation of school staff.

MEDICATION
- Remove stool impaction, then start maintenance treatment program.
- No randomized, controlled studies have compared methods of disimpaction: Can use oral agents, enemas, and rectal suppositories; oral agents are least traumatic. Glycerin suppositories best option for infants.

First Line

- Disimpaction with PEG has been shown to be more effective than lactulose in 1 study (2)[B]:
  - Give 17 g (240 mL) water or juice: 1–1.5 g/kg/d × 3 days for disimpaction
  - 0.26–0.084 g/kg/d for maintenance
- Disimpaction with mineral oil for child >1 year also effective; give 15–30 mL/yr of age to max 240 mL:
  - Maintenance: 1–3 mL/kg/d or divided b.i.d.
  - May mix with orange juice to make palatable; *avoid in infants to avoid aspiration and lipoid pneumonia*
- Other maintenance regimens include:
  - Milk of magnesia (MOM) 400 mg (5 mL): 103 mL/kg/d b.i.d. (3)[A]
  - Lactulose 10 g (15 mL): 1–3 mL/kg/d b.i.d.
  - Senna syrup 8.8 g sennoside (5 mL): Age 2–6 years: 2.5–7.5 mL/d b.i.d.; age 6–12 years: 5–15 mL/d b.i.d.
  - Bisacodyl suppository 10 mg: 0.5–1 suppository once or twice per day

Second Line

Another disimpaction protocol is as follows:

- Give 1 oz (28.4 g) of mineral oil the 1st day.
- On the next day, give 1–3 enemas until clear; this may be repeated over the next 1–2 days.
- Give an oil-retention enema.
- Follow the oil-retention enema with hypophosphate enemas (e.g., sodium phosphate Fleet] 1 oz [28.4 g] per 20 lb [9.1 kg]) of body weight *or*
- Normal saline enemas: 2 tsp table salt/qt (946 mL) of warm water, and give 2 oz (60 mL)/yr of age to a maximum of 16 oz (480 mL)

ISSUES FOR REFERRAL

If symptoms do not improve after 6 months of good compliance with a multifactorial treatment model, refer to pediatric GI for further evaluation.

ADDITIONAL THERAPIES

Behavioral treatment and counseling

COMPLEMENTARY AND ALTERNATIVE MEDICINE

- Children who receive behavioral treatment in addition to medications are more likely to have resolution of encopresis at 3 and 6 months than children who get medication alone.
- No evidence that biofeedback training adds any benefit to conventional treatment for functional fecal incontinence in children (1)[A].
- Some evidence that behavioral interventions plus laxative therapy (rather than laxative therapy alone) improves continence in children with functional fecal incontinence associated with constipation (1)[A].

SURGERY/OTHER PROCEDURES

If ongoing constipation refractory to a combination of medical and behavioral therapy, consider anorectal manometry to evaluate for internal anal sphincter achalasia (or ultrashort-segment Hirschsprung disease). If present, this condition can be treated successfully in most patients with an internal sphincter myectomy.

IN-PATIENT CONSIDERATIONS

Admission Criteria/Initial Stabilization

Admission criteria should include:

- Continued soiling and recurrent impaction on outpatient medical therapy, whether from lack of medication efficacy or patient medication nonadherence
- Decreased PO intake for fluid and food
- Vomiting or obstructive-type symptoms

Hospital admission and abdominal films may be necessary to ensure complete removal of impaction. This may include gastric administration of balanced electrolyte–polyethylene glycol solutions if the patient cannot tolerate the medication by mouth. Serial abdominal films as well as careful observation of the rectal effluent can help to determine when the patient is adequately treated.

IV Fluids

IV fluids should be considered when the pediatric patient is heading toward dehydration while undergoing bowel cleanout.

Nursing

Nursing is essential to observing and documenting the stool consistency and clarity.

Discharge Criteria

- Stools becoming more loose in consistency and clear in appearance would signify a successful in-patient endpoint.
- Abdominal radiograph showing much less fecal loading (compared with a pretreatment radiograph) plus improving serial abdominal exams

 ONGOING CARE

FOLLOW-UP RECOMMENDATIONS

Patient Monitoring

- Continue the maintenance treatment program for at least 6 months, possibly 1–2 years.
- Visits every 4–10 weeks for support and to ensure compliance; more often with oppositional or anxious children
- Telephone availability to adjust doses and to provide continued encouragement to caregivers
- Treat redevelopment of impaction promptly.
- Chief target behaviors in a behavior plan for such children include compliance with medication, compliance with sits, and self-initiation of bathroom visits.
- Children who do not progress with a well-designed behavior plan should be referred for more in-depth mental health evaluation and counseling.

DIET

Hydration, high fiber; decrease or avoid cow's milk products if a trial shows this to be helpful. Avoid excessive consumption of bananas, rice, apples, and gelatin.

PATIENT EDUCATION

- Education and demystifying of the process
- Careful and full explanation of the treatment plan and dietary changes
- Avoid punishment for soiling.
- In children >4 years of age, explain to parents how overreliance on diapers and pull-ups, while convenient, can prolong the problem.
- Always attempt to use positive reinforcement first for successful toilet sits and medication compliance.

- If positive approach is unsuccessful, consider removing daily desired privileges (e.g., TV, video games, time with friends) for noncompliance with behavioral plan. Some children respond better to use of a token economy (chips or tickets to earn privileges the child desires).

PROGNOSIS

- Initial good response with a high relapse rate due to noncompliance by parents and/or child
- Depending on the study, anywhere from 30–50% of children still may have encopresis after 5 years of treatment.
- Children with psychosocial or emotional problems that preceded the encopresis are more recalcitrant to treatment.

COMPLICATIONS

- Colitis due to excessive enema/suppository
- Perianal dermatitis
- Anal fissure

REFERENCES

1. Brazzelli M, Griffiths PV, Cody JD, et al. Behavioural and cognitive interventions with or without other treatments for the management of faecal incontinence in children. *Cochrane Database Syst Rev.* 2011;7(12):CD002240.
2. Loening-Baucke V, Pashankar DS. A randomized, prospective, comparison study of polyethylene glycol 3350 without electrolytes and milk of magnesia for children with constipation and fecal incontinence. *Pediatrics.* 2006;118:528–535.
3. Constipation Guideline Committee of the North American Society for Pediatric Gastroenterology, Hepatology and Nutrition. Evaluation and treatment of constipation in infants and children: Recommendations of the North American Society for Pediatric Gastroenterology, Hepatology and Nutrition. *J Pediatr Gastroenterol Nutr.* 2006;43(3): e1–e13.

ADDITIONAL READING

- Borowitz SM, Cox DJ, Tam A, et al. Precipitants of constipation during early childhood. *J Am Board Fam Pract.* 2003;16(3):213–218.
- Levitt M, Peña A. Update on pediatric faecal incontinence. *Eur J Pediatr Surg.* 2009;19(1):1–9. Epub 2009 Feb 16.

 CODES

ICD10

- F98.1 Encopresis not due to a substance or known physiol condition
- R15.1 Fecal smearing
- R15.9 Full incontinence of feces

CLINICAL PEARLS

- Remove any impaction before embarking on a treatment regimen
- 90% of encopresis results from chronic constipation.
- Address toddler constipation early (decrease excessive milk intake, increase fruits/vegetables).

ENDOCARDITIS, INFECTIVE
Mariya Milko, DO • Theodore B. Flaum, DO, FACOFP

 BASICS

DESCRIPTION
- An infection primarily of the valvular endocardium and, occasionally, the mural endocardium
- System(s) affected: Cardiovascular; Endocrine/ Metabolic; Hematologic/Lymphatic; Immunologic; Pulmonary; Renal/Urologic; Skin/Exocrine; Neurologic
- Synonym(s): Bacterial endocarditis; Subacute bacterial endocarditis; Acute bacterial endocarditis

EPIDEMIOLOGY
Incidence
- In industrialized countries: 3–9/100,000 (1)[A]
- 1.5-3.0% at 1 year after prosthetic valve replacement; at 5 years, 3–6%.
- Incidence is increased in the elderly.

ETIOLOGY AND PATHOPHYSIOLOGY
- Acute endocarditis: *Staphylococcus aureus*; *Streptococcus* groups A, B, C, G; *S. pneumoniae*; *S. lugdunensis*; *Enterococcus* spp. (gram-positive); *Haemophilus influenzae* or *parainfluenzae*; *Neisseria gonorrhoeae* (gram-negative)
- *Subacute endocarditis*: α-Hemolytic streptococci (Viridans group strep), *S. bovis, Enterococcus* spp., *S. aureus, S. epidermidis* (gram-positive); HACEK organisms: *H. aphrophilus* or *paraphrophilus*, *Actinobacillus (aggregatibacter) actinomycetemcomitans, Cardiobacterium hominis, Eikenella corrodens, Kingella kingae*
- Endocarditis in IV drug abusers (tricuspid valve): *S. aureus, Enterococcus* spp. (gram-positive); *Pseudomonas aeruginosa, Burkholderia cepacia*, other bacilli (gram-negative); *Candida* spp.
- Early prosthetic-valve endocarditis (<60 days after valve implantation): *S. aureus, S. epidermidis* (gram-positive); gram-negative bacilli; fungi: *Candida* spp., *Aspergillus* spp.
- Late prosthetic-valve endocarditis (>60 days after valve implantation): α-Hemolytic streptococci, *Enterococcus* spp., *S. epidermidis* (gram-positive); *Candida* spp., *Aspergillus* spp.
- Culture-negative endocarditis: 10% of cases (1)[A]; *Bartonella quintana* (homeless); *Brucella* spp., fungi, *Coxiella burnetii* (Q fever), *Chlamydia trachomatis, C. psittaci*, HACEK organisms; abiotrophia (formerly B₆-deficient streptococci); use of antibiotics prior to blood cultures

RISK FACTORS
- Injection drug use, IV catheterization, certain malignancies (colon cancer)
- High-risk cardiac conditions:
  - Prosthetic cardiac valve
  - Previous infective endocarditis (IE)
  - Congenital heart disease (CHD), such as unrepaired cyanotic CHD, including palliative shunts and conduits, repaired CHD with prosthetic device during the prior 6 months, repaired CHD with residual defects at or near the site of prosthetic material, cardiac transplantation recipients who develop valvulopathy (2)[B]

GENERAL PREVENTION
- Maintain good oral hygiene.
- Antibiotic prophylaxis is only recommended for high-risk cardiac conditions (2)[C] (see "Risk Factors")
- *Procedures requiring prophylaxis:*
  - Oral/Upper respiratory tract: any manipulation of gingival tissue or periapical region of teeth or perforation of the oral mucosa (2)[C], invasive respiratory procedures involving incision, or biopsy of the respiratory mucosa, use amoxicillin 2 g PO (if penicillin-allergic, clindamycin 600 mg PO) 30–60 minutes before procedure or ampicillin 2 g IV/IM. For penicillin-allergic patients use clindamycin 600 mg IV, *or* cephalexin 2 g PO, *or* azithromycin/clarithromycin 500 mg PO, *or* cefazolin/ceftriaxone 1 g IV/IM 30 minutes before procedure. For pediatric doses, use amoxicillin 50 mg/kg PO; cephalexin 50 mg/kg PO; clindamycin 20 mg/kg PO; and ampicillin or ceftriaxone 50 mg/kg IM/IV.
  - GI/GU: Only consider coverage for enterococcus (with penicillin, ampicillin, piperacillin, or vancomycin) for patients with an established infection undergoing procedures (2)[B].
  - Cardiac valvular surgery or placement of prosthetic intracardiac/intravascular materials: Perioperative cefazolin 1–2 g IV 30 minutes pre-op, or vancomycin 15 mg/kg 60 minutes pre-op in the penicillin-allergic patient (2)[B]
  - Skin: Incision and drainage of infected tissue; use agents active against skin pathogens (e.g., cefazolin 1–2 g IV q8h or vancomycin 15 mg/kg q12h) if penicillin-allergic or if methicillin-resistant MRSA suspected.

 DIAGNOSIS

- Modified Duke Criteria for Diagnosis of IE (3)[B] (definite: 2 major criteria, or 1 major and 3 minor criteria, or 5 minor criteria; possible: 1 major and 1 minor criteria, or 3 minor criteria)
- Major clinical criteria:
  - Positive blood culture: Isolation of typical microorganism for IE from 2 separate blood cultures, *or* persistently positive blood culture
  - Single positive blood culture for *C. burnetii* or anti–phase-1 IgG antibody titer >1:800
  - Positive echocardiogram: Presence of vegetation, abscess, or new partial dehiscence of prosthetic valve; must be performed rapidly if IE is suspected (4)[A]
  - New valvular regurgitation (change in pre-existing murmur not sufficient)
- Minor criteria:
  - Predisposing heart condition or IV drug use
  - Fever ≥38.0°C (100.4°F)
  - Vascular phenomena: Major arterial emboli, septic pulmonary infarcts, mycotic aneurysm, intracranial hemorrhage, conjunctival hemorrhage, Janeway lesions
  - Immunologic phenomena: Glomerulonephritis, Osler nodes, Roth spots, rheumatoid factor
  - Microbiologic evidence: Positive blood culture, but not a major criterion (excluding single positive cultures for coagulase-negative staphylococci and organisms that do not cause endocarditis) or serologic evidence of infection likely to cause IE

HISTORY
- Fever (>38°C), chills, cough, dyspnea, orthopnea; especially in subacute endocarditis: night sweats, weight loss, fatigue
- Predisposition to IE (see "Risk Factors")
- Symptoms of transient ischemic attack, cerebrovascular accident (CVA), or myocardial infarction on presentation

PHYSICAL EXAM
- New heart murmur in most patients with IE: Change in heart murmur is suggestive of IE, but rare; rales, edema
- Splinter hemorrhages in fingernail beds, Osler nodes on fleshy portions of extremities, "Roth spot" retinal hemorrhages, Janeway lesions (cutaneous evidence of septic emboli), palatal or conjunctival petechiae, splenomegaly, hematuria (due to emboli or glomerulonephritis)
- Neurologic findings consistent with CVA, such as visual loss, motors weakness, and aphasia

DIFFERENTIAL DIAGNOSIS
Fever of unknown origin; infected central venous catheter; marantec endocarditis; connective tissue diseases; intra-abdominal infections; rheumatic fever; salmonellosis; brucellosis; malignancy; tuberculosis; atrial myxoma; septic thrombophlebitis

DIAGNOSTIC TESTS & INTERPRETATION
- 3 sets of blood cultures drawn >2 hours apart *before administration of antibiotics*
- Leukocytosis in acute endocarditis
- Anemia, decreased C3, C4, CH50, and rheumatoid factor (RF) in subacute endocarditis
- Elevated ESR, C-reactive protein (CRP)
- Hematuria, microscopic or macroscopic
- Consider serologies for *Chlamydia*, Q fever, and *Bartonella* in "culture-negative" endocarditis.
- Transthoracic or transesophageal echocardiogram: Should be performed rapidly as soon as IE is suspected.
- CT scan may be useful in locating abscesses (e.g., splenic abscess).

Pathological Findings
- Vegetations are composed of platelets, fibrin, and colonies of microorganisms. Destruction of valvular endocardium, perforation of valve leaflets, rupture of chordae tendineae, abscesses of myocardium, rupture of sinus of Valsalva, and pericarditis may occur.
- Emboli, abscesses, and/or infarction may be found in any organ.
- Immune-complex glomerulonephritis

TREATMENT

MEDICATION
First Line
- Initial empirical treatment: Should be started after 3 sets of blood cultures have been drawn, while waiting for a causative organism to be identified:
  - Native valves: Ampicillin-sulbactam 12 g/d IV or amoxicillin-clavulanate 12 g/d IV both in 4 doses with gentamicin 3 mg/kg/d IV/IM in 2 or 3 doses. If PCN allergic, use vancomycin 30 mg/kg/d IV in 2 doses with gentamicin 3 mg/kg/d IV/IM in 2 or 3 doses and ciprofloxacin 1,000 mg/d PO or 800 mg/d IV, both in 2 doses (4)[A].

– Prosthetic valves: Vancomycin 30 mg/kg/d IV in 2 doses with gentamicin 3 mg/kg/d IV/IM in 2 or 3 doses and rifampin 1,200 mg/d PO in 2 doses, if <12 months post surgery. If >12 months, use native valve regimen (4)[A].

- PCN-susceptible viridans group streptococci or *S. bovis*:
  – Native valve: Pen G 12–18 million U/d IV continuously or in 4–6 doses *or* ceftriaxone 2 g/d IV/IM in 1 dose, both for 4 weeks (3)[A].
  – Prosthetic valve: Pen G 24 million U/d IV continuously or 4–6 doses for 6 weeks *or* ceftriaxone 2 g/d IV/IM in 1 dose ± gentamicin 3 mg/kg IV/IM q24h for 2 weeks (peak gentamicin level 3 μg/mL and trough <1 μg/mL).

- PCN-resistant viridans group streptococci or *S. bovis*
  – Native valve: Pen G 24 million U/d IV, either continuously or in 6 equally divided doses, *or* ceftriaxone 2 g/d IV/IM in 1 dose for 4 weeks + gentamicin 3 mg/kg IV/IM q24h for 2 weeks (peak gentamicin level 3 μg/mL and trough <1 μg/mL) (3)[B].
  – Prosthetic valve: Regimen is equivalent, but length of therapy is 6 weeks for all antibiotics.

- *Staphylococcus*:
  – Native valve: Oxacillin or nafcillin 2 g IV q4h for 4–6 weeks. Use of gentamicin 1 mg/kg q8h IV/IM for the first 3–5 days does not improve survival and increases the chance of nephrotoxicity. For oxacillin-resistant strains use vancomycin 15 mg/kg/d IV q12h for 6 weeks for goal trough of 15–20 μg/mL (3)[B].
  – Prosthetic valve: Oxacillin or nafcillin 12 g/d IV in 6 doses + rifampin 300 mg IV/PO q8h, for 6 weeks, + gentamicin 1 mg/kg q8h IV/IM for first 2 weeks (peak gentamicin level 3 μg/mL and trough <1 μg/mL) (3)[B]. For oxacillin-resistant strains, use vancomycin 15 mg/kg IV q12h, + rifampin 300 mg IV/PO q8h, both for 6 weeks, + gentamicin 3 mg/kg/d IV/IM in 2–3 doses for the first 2 weeks (peak gentamicin level 3 μg/mL and trough <1 μg/mL) (3)[B].

- Penicillin-sensitive *Enterococcus*, native or prosthetic valve: Ampicillin 2g IV q4h *or* Pen G 18–30 million U/d IV continuously or in 6 doses + gentamicin 1 mg/kg IV q8h for 4–6 weeks (peak gentamicin level 3 μg/mL and trough <1 μg/mL) (3)[A]. Consider expert consultation for penicillin-resistant enterococci.

- *HACEK* organisms: Ceftriaxone 2 g IM or IV q24h for 4 weeks (3)[B] *or* ampicillin-sulbactam 2 g IV q6h for 4 weeks (2)[B] *or* ciprofloxacin 1 g/d PO or 800 mg/d IV in 2 equally divided doses for 4 weeks (3)[C]

- Precautions: In patients with renal impairment, dosage adjustment should be made for penicillin G, gentamicin, cefazolin, ampicillin, ampicillin/sulbactam, ciprofloxacin, and vancomycin. Rapid infusion of vancomycin <1 hour may cause "red-man syndrome" due to histamine release, not an allergic reaction. Treat with antihistamines and decrease infusion rate.

- Interactions: Vancomycin + gentamicin increases renal toxicity. Rifampin increases the requirement for Coumadin and oral hypoglycemic agents.

Second Line
For patients allergic to penicillin:

- Penicillin-susceptible or resistant viridans group streptococci or *S. bovis*: Vancomycin 30 mg/kg (not to exceed 2 g/d) IV for 4 weeks (6 weeks for prosthetic valve endocarditis) for goal trough of 10–15 μg/mL (3)[B]

- *Enterococcus*, native or prosthetic valve: Desensitization to penicillin should be considered. Vancomycin 15 mg/kg (usual dose, 1 g) IV q12h, + gentamicin or streptomycin (peak gentamicin level 3 μg/mL and trough <1 μg/mL) for 4–6 weeks (6 weeks for prosthetic valve endocarditis) (3)[B]

- *Staphylococcus* of native valve: Cefazolin 2 g IV q8h (not to be used in patients with immediate-type hypersensitivity to penicillin) for 4–6 weeks (3)[B] *or* vancomycin 30 mg/kg (usual dose, 1 g) IV q12h for a goal trough of 15–20 μg/mL, for 6 weeks (3)[B]

SURGERY/OTHER PROCEDURES
Surgical therapy is required in 50% of IE cases. Indications for surgery include (4)[A]:

- Heart failure due to involvement of aortic or mitral valve
- Prevention of embolism: Aortic or mitral valve vegetations >10 mm with prior embolic episodes; isolated very large vegetation >15 mm; in patients with major ischemic stroke, surgery is delayed for at least 4 weeks, if possible (5)[C].
- Uncontrolled infection: Persistent fever and positive cultures >7–10 days; infection caused by fungi or resistant organism; presence of abscess, fistula, false aneurysm, or enlarging vegetations
- Early prosthetic valve IE (6)[B]

 ## ONGOING CARE

FOLLOW-UP RECOMMENDATIONS
Patient Monitoring
- Check gentamicin peak (~3 μg/mL) and trough (<1 μg/mL) levels if used for >5 days, and with renal dysfunction. Perform twice-weekly BUN and serum creatinine while on gentamicin. Consider audiometry baseline and follow up during long-term aminoglycoside therapy.
- Check vancomycin trough (15–20 μg/mL) levels in all patients (3)[B].
- Baseline ECG, and monitor ECG for conduction disturbances/myocardial infarction (MI) in initial weeks.
- TTE at the end of therapy
- Blood cultures q48h until negative

PROGNOSIS
Late complications occurring after the initial infection contribute to the poor prognosis of IE. The main complications are heart failure, reinfection, cerebral emboli. Long-term survival is 60–90% at 10 years (4)[A].

COMPLICATIONS
- Cerebral complications are the most severe and most frequent complications, occurring in 15–20% of patients (1)[A].
- Emboli: Arterial (e.g., MI, mesenteric, splenic, cerebral infarct); infectious (e.g., abscesses of heart, lung, brain, meninges, bone, pericardium):
  – Neurologic events are the most frequent complications in patients with IE requiring ICU admission. Ischemic stroke is the presenting symptom of IE in 20% of cases (7)[A].
- Inflammatory/immune disorders (e.g., arthritis, myositis, glomerulonephritis)
- Other complications: Congestive heart failure (CHF), ruptured valve cusp, sinus of valsalva aneurysm, arrhythmia, and mycotic aneurysms

REFERENCES

1. Bruno H, Duval X. "Infective endocarditis." *New Engl J Med*. 2013;368.15:1425–1433. Print.
2. Wilson W. Prevention of infective endocarditis. Guidelines from the American Heart Association. A Guideline from the American Heart Association Rheumatic Fever, Endocarditis, and Kawasaki Disease Committee, Council on Cardiovascular Disease in the Young, and the Council on Cardiology, Council on Cardiovascular Surgery and Anesthesia, and the Quality of Care and Outcomes Research Interdisciplinary Working Group. *Circulation*. 2007;116:1736–1754.
3. Baddour LM, Wilson WR, Bayer AS, et al. Infective endocarditis: Diagnosis, antimicrobial therapy, and management of complications: A statement for healthcare professionals from the Committee on Rheumatic Fever, Endocarditis, and Kawasaki Disease, Council on Cardiovascular Disease in the Young, and the Councils on Clinical Cardiology, Stroke, and Cardiovascular Surgery and Anesthesia, American Heart Association: Endorsed by the Infectious Diseases Society of America. *Circulation*. 2005;111:e394–e434.
4. Habib G, Hoen B, Tornos P, et al. Guidelines on the prevention, diagnosis, and treatment of infective endocarditis (new version 2009): The Task Force on the Prevention, Diagnosis, and Treatment of Infective Endocarditis of the European Society of Cardiology (ESC). Endorsed by the European Society of Clinical Microbiology and Infectious Diseases (ESCMID) and the International Society of Chemotherapy (ISC) for Infection and Cancer. *Eur Heart J*. 2009;30(19):2369–2413. Epub 2009 Aug 27.
5. Byrne JG, Rezai K, Sanchez JA, et al. Surgical management of endocarditis: The society of thoracic surgeons clinical practice guideline. *Ann Thorac Surg*. 2011;91(6):2012–2019.
6. Head SJ, Mokhles MM, Osnabrugge RL, et al. Surgery in current therapy for infective endocarditis. *Vasc Health Risk Manag*. 2011;7:255–263.
7. Sonneville R, Mirabel M, Hajage D, et al. Neurologic complications and outcomes of infective endocarditis in critically ill patients: The ENDOcardite en REAnimation prospective multicenter study. *Crit Care Med*. 2011;39(6): 1474–1481.

 ## CODES

ICD10
- A54.83 Gonococcal heart infection
- I33.0 Acute and subacute infective endocarditis
- I39 Endocarditis and heart valve disord in dis classd elswhr

CLINICAL PEARLS

- Antibiotic prophylaxis is recommended for people with artificial heart valves, history of IE, congenital heart diseases, and cardiac transplants with valvulopathy.
- TEE/TTE and blood cultures are the cornerstone of diagnosis of IE.
- Most common organisms involved in IE include viridians *Streptococcus* spp. and staphylococcus.

ENDOMETRIAL CANCER AND UTERINE SARCOMA

Benjamin Hilliker, MD • Michael P. Hopkins, MD, MEd

 BASICS

DESCRIPTION
- Endometrial cancer: Malignancy of the endometrial lining of the uterus:
  - 2 types:
    - I: Estrogen dependent, lower grade, better prognosis
    - II: Estrogen independent, higher grade, more aggressive
- Cell types: Adenocarcinoma, adenosquamous (malignant squamous elements), clear cell, and papillary serous
- Sarcomas: Malignancy of the uterine mesenchyme and mixed tumors:
  - Mixed müllerian sarcoma (carcinosarcoma): Heterologous sarcoma elements are not native to the müllerian system (e.g., cartilage or bone); homologous sarcoma elements are native to the müllerian system (40–50% prevalence of all sarcomas).
  - Leiomyosarcoma develops in the myometrium or, rarely, in a myoma (fibroid) (30% prevalence of all sarcomas).
  - Endometrial stromal sarcoma develops from the stromal component of the endometrium (15% prevalence of all sarcomas).
  - Poorer prognosis
- Predominant age:
  - Endometrial cancer: Most patients are postmenopausal:
    - Median age: 66 years
  - Sarcomas: Age 40–69 years
- System(s) affected: Reproductive
- Synonym(s): Uterine cancer; Endometrial cancer; Corpus cancer

Pregnancy Considerations
This malignancy is not associated with pregnancy.

EPIDEMIOLOGY
Incidence
- Endometrial cancer is the most common gynecologic malignancy, 4th most common cancer in women, and 8th leading cause of cancer-related death in women worldwide.
- In the US, it is estimated that endometrial cancer will account for 49,560 new cases and 8,190 deaths in 2013.

Prevalence
500,000 women in the US

ETIOLOGY AND PATHOPHYSIOLOGY
Continuous estrogen stimulation unopposed by progesterone
- Endometrial: Unopposed estrogen:
  - Estrogen replacement therapy without concomitant progesterone increases the risk. Addition of progesterone decreases risk to that of general population.
- Sarcomas: Etiology unknown

Genetics
- Endometrial: Lynch syndrome (hereditary nonpolyposis colorectal cancer)
- Sarcoma: African American

RISK FACTORS
- Early menarche/late menopause
- Nulliparity
- Personal or family history of colon or reproductive system cancer
- Obesity
- Diabetes mellitus
- Hypertension
- Polycystic ovarian syndrome
- Menstrual irregularities
- Endometrial hyperplasia
- Unopposed estrogens
- Tamoxifen use
- Age
- Prior pelvic irradiation (sarcoma)

GENERAL PREVENTION
- In young women who are obese or anovulatory, the risk of endometrial cancer can be reduced by taking oral contraceptive pills, permanently losing weight, or taking cyclic progesterone to prevent unopposed estrogen's effects on the uterus.
- Estrogen replacement therapy should always include progesterone unless the woman has had a hysterectomy.
- Cigarette smoking has been associated with a lower risk of endometrial cancer; however, it is not recommended secondary to its many health risks.

COMMONLY ASSOCIATED CONDITIONS
- Endometrial hyperplasia: 1–25% will progress to endometria adenocarcinoma:
  - Simple without atypia
  - Complex without atypia
  - Simple with atypia
  - Complex with atypia:
    - 43% with complex hyperplasia with atypia have concurrent endometrial cancer.
- Endometrial cancer patients should be screened regularly for breast and colon cancer because of an increased risk of these cancers.
- Patients who have breast or colon cancer are at increased risk for endometrial cancer.
- Granulosa cell tumors of the ovary produce estrogen; these patients will have an increased risk of endometrial cancer.

⨁ DIAGNOSIS

HISTORY
- Endometrial cancer:
  - Postmenopausal bleeding is the most frequent sign. Any spotting or abnormal discharge mandates evaluation.
  - Premenopausal patients with history of anovulation, heavy, irregular, or prolonged periods that fail multiple medical managements mandate evaluation.
- Sarcoma:
  - Mixed müllerian sarcoma: Bleeding and prolapsing tissue, pain
  - Leiomyosarcoma: Increasing size of presumed uterine myomas, pain

PHYSICAL EXAM
Pelvic exam: Enlarged uterus

DIFFERENTIAL DIAGNOSIS
- Atypical complex hyperplasia: A premalignant lesion of the endometrium
- Cervical cancer
- Ovarian cancer invading the uterus
- Endometriosis
- Adenomyosis
- Leiomyoma

DIAGNOSTIC TESTS & INTERPRETATION
Initial Tests (lab, imaging)
- Liver and renal function tests
- Transvaginal ultrasound usually shows increased endometrial thickness (>5 mm in postmenopausal patients, or >5 mm in patients with irregular or heavy periods if >35 years of age)
- Levels of cancer antigen 125 (CA-125) may be elevated when intra-abdominal disease is present.
- Chest x-ray (CXR): Most common site of metastases is the lungs.
- Mammogram and colonoscopy: Endometrial cancer is associated with breast and colon cancer.

Follow-Up Tests & Special Considerations
- A biopsy of a pregnant uterus can produce tissue that looks hyperplastic or premalignant.
- Pap smear is rarely positive.
- CT scan, bone scan, liver spleen scan: Not part of the routine evaluation, but may be needed if metastasis is suspected.
- MRI has been reported to show the depth of myometrial penetration accurately, but is not always cost-effective.

Diagnostic Procedures/Other
- Office endometrial biopsy (90% accurate): If negative with high suspicion for cancer, a dilation and curettage (D&C) is necessary. Endometrial stromal sarcoma and leiomyosarcoma rarely are diagnosed preoperatively. Any patient with history of irregular, heavy, or prolonged periods should undergo endometrial biopsy prior to endometrial ablation procedures.
- Fractional D&C is 99% accurate except in cases of sarcoma.
- Hysteroscopy, which may be associated with higher risk of positive washings/cytology, is controversial.

Test Interpretation
- Federation of Gynecology and Obstetrics Staging System: Revised 2009 (1)
  - Stage I (confined to corpus uteri):
    - A: No or <1/2 myometrial invasion
    - B: Invasion ≥1/2 the myometrium
  - Stage II: Tumor invades cervical stroma but does not extend beyond the uterus
  - Stage III: Local and/or regional spread:
    - A: Uterine serosal and or adnexal invasion
    - B: Vaginal and/or parametrial involvement
    - C: Metastases to pelvic and/or para-aortic lymph nodes:
    - IIIC1: +Pelvic nodes
    - IIIC2: +Para-aortic lymph nodes positive pelvic lymph nodes
  - Stage IV: Tumor invades bladder and/or bowel mucosa and/or distant metastases:
    - A: Tumor invades bladder and/or bowel mucosa
    - B: Distant metastases, including intra-abdominal metastases and/or inguinal lymph nodes
- Uterine sarcoma criteria for diagnosis: Mitotic index, cellular atypia, and areas of coagulative necrosis separated from tumor

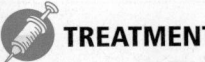

TREATMENT

GENERAL MEASURES
- Main treatment for uterine cancer is surgery.
- Radiation is used to prevent tumor recurrence at the vaginal cuff.

MEDICATION
First Line
- Endometrial:
  – Chemotherapy for advanced or recurrent disease incurable with surgery and radiation (2,3)[A]:
  o Doxorubicin + cisplatin + paclitaxel
  o Paclitaxel + carboplatin
  – Hormonal therapy:
  o Medroxyprogesterone acetate: For recurrence or metastases (2)[A]
  o Megestrol (Megace) 160 mg/d for 3 months for women with premalignant lesions, atypical complex hyperplasia, or well-differentiated endometrial cancer in patients desiring fertility. Follow with D&C to determine cancer resolution.
  o Levonorgestrel-containing intrauterine device: As above for patients who desire future fertility
- Sarcoma:
  – Chemotherapy:
  o Doxorubicin as single agent or in combination (4)[A]
  – Hormonal:
  o Tamoxifen or aromatase inhibitors; not fully studied
  o Progesterones

Second Line
Ondansetron (Zofran), dronabinol (Marinol), metoclopramide (Reglan), and others to control nausea from chemotherapy

ADDITIONAL THERAPIES
Radiation therapy:
- Nonoperative candidates: Radiation therapy alone (5)[A]
- Low risk: No adjuvant radiation therapy (5)[A]
- Intermediate risk: Consider adjuvant vaginal brachytherapy. Reduces local recurrences, but has no effect on overall survival (5)[A].
- High risk: Chemotherapy and radiation therapy in some cases (6)[A]

SURGERY/OTHER PROCEDURES
Surgical staging:
- Extrafascial hysterectomy and bilateral salpingo-oophorectomy
- Cytologic washings
- Pelvic and para-aortic lymph node dissection
- Omental sampling, as indicated
- Optimal tumor debulking

Geriatric Considerations
Older (and obese) patients may be at high risk for surgery. Alternative radiation therapy can be considered.

IN-PATIENT CONSIDERATIONS
Admission Criteria/Initial Stabilization
- Excessive vaginal bleeding
- Preoperative stabilization

Nursing
Routine; ensure postoperative pain is controlled

Discharge Criteria
Postsurgical criteria: Pain controlled, tolerating diet, ambulating, and voiding

ONGOING CARE

FOLLOW-UP RECOMMENDATIONS
Speculum and rectovaginal exam every 3–4 months for 2–3 years, then every 6 months for 3 years, and then annually for life

Patient Monitoring
Annual CXR

DIET
As tolerated and according to comorbidities

PATIENT EDUCATION
After surgery:
- No intercourse for ~6 weeks
- No lifting >10–15 lb
- No driving until pain free
- Do not expect resumption of full activity for 6 weeks.

PROGNOSIS
5-year survival rates:
- Uterine adenocarcinoma

Stage	Survival (%)
IA	88
IB	75
II	69
IIIA	58
IIIB	50
IIIC	47
IVA	17
IVB	15

- Uterine sarcoma

Stage	Survival (%)
I	70
II	45
III	30
IV	15

COMPLICATIONS
- Surgical: Excessive bleeding, wound infection, lymphedema, deep vein thrombosis (DVT), and damage to the urinary or intestinal systems
- Radiation: Diarrhea, ileus, bowel obstruction or fistula, radiation cystitis, proctitis, vaginal stenosis, DVT
- Chemotherapy: Per the drug given

REFERENCES
1. Creasman W. Revised FIGO staging for carcinoma of the endometrium. *Int J Gynaecol Obstet*. 2009; 105:109.
2. Polyzos NP, Pavlidis N, Paraskevaidis E, et al. Randomized evidence on chemotherapy and hormonal therapy regimens for advanced endometrial cancer: An overview of survival data. *Eur J Cancer*. 2006;42:319–326.
3. Fleming GF, Brunetto VL, Cella D, et al. Phase III trial of doxorubicin plus cisplatin with or without paclitaxel plus filgrastim in advanced endometrial carcinoma: A Gynecologic Oncology Group Study. *J Clin Oncol*. 2004;22:2159–2166.
4. Bramwell VH, Anderson D, Charette ML, et al. Doxorubicin-based chemotherapy for the palliative treatment of adult patients with locally advanced or metastatic soft tissue sarcoma. *Cochrane Database Syst Rev*. 2003;3:CD003293.
5. Einhorn N, Tropé C, Ridderheim M, et al. A systematic overview of radiation therapy effects in uterine cancer (corpus uteri). *Acta Oncol*. 2003;42: 557–561.
6. Humber C. Chemotherapy for advanced, recurrent or metastatic endometrial carcinoma. *Cochrane Database Syst Rev*. 2005;4:CD003915.

ADDITIONAL READING
- American College of Obstetricians and Gynecologists. ACOG practice bulletin, clinical management guidelines for obstetrician-gynecologists, number 65, August 2005: Management of endometrial cancer. *Obstet Gynecol*. 2005;106:413–425.
- Gadducci A, Cosio S, Romanini A, et al. The management of patients with uterine sarcoma: A debated clinical challenge. *Crit Rev Oncol Hematol*. 2008;65:129–142.

SEE ALSO
- Cervical Malignancy
- Algorithm: Pelvic Pain

CODES
ICD10
- C54.1 Malignant neoplasm of endometrium
- C54.2 Malignant neoplasm of myometrium
- C55 Malignant neoplasm of uterus, part unspecified

CLINICAL PEARLS
- Most common presenting symptom is abnormal uterine bleeding.
- Any patient with history of irregular, heavy, or prolonged periods should undergo endometrial biopsy.
- Primary cause is unopposed estrogen.
- Endometrial thickness on transvaginal ultrasound of <5 mm makes endometrial cancer very unlikely.
- Primary treatment is with surgery, with possible chemotherapy ± radiation.

E

ENDOMETRIOSIS

Katherine L. Ball, MD • Jeanne M. Cawse-Lucas, MD

 BASICS

DESCRIPTION

- Endometriosis is a common, recurring disease in women of reproductive age that may persist into early menopause (1).
- Generally associated with pain and infertility
- Heterotopic islands of endometrial glands and stroma found outside the uterus:
  - Pelvic sites: Peritoneal surfaces (bladder, cul-de-sac, pelvic walls, ligaments, and fallopian tubes), vagina, cervix, lymph nodes, ovaries, bowel
  - Distant sites: Abdominal wall, spleen, gallbladder, stomach, nasal mucosa, spinal canal, lungs, breasts, diaphragm, pleura, pericardium
- Classified as peritoneal, ovarian, or deep endometriosis
- Staged according to the American Society for Reproductive Medicine surgical scoring system:
  - Based on disease severity: Extent and characteristics of endometrial implants and adhesions
  - Stage I (minimal) to IV (severe)
- System(s) affected: Reproductive
- Synonym(s): Endometriosis externa

ALERT
Staging is useful in therapeutic planning, but does not correlate with pain severity or predict response to treatment for symptoms or infertility.

EPIDEMIOLOGY
Incidence
- Affects 0.5–5% of fertile women
- Found in 30–50% of infertile women (2)
- Found in 50–60% of women and adolescent women with pelvic pain (3)

Prevalence
- Predominant sex: Female only
- Difficult to assess true prevalence as some women are asymptomatic
- Estimated to affect 6–10% of reproductive-age women

Pediatric Considerations
Endometriosis may begin with puberty, causing debilitating pelvic pain and severe dysmenorrhea associated with missed school, social, and family activities.

Pregnancy Considerations
Pelvic endometriosis generally is ameliorated with pregnancy, but infertility is significantly associated with the disease itself.

Geriatric Considerations
Although menopause often results in a resolution of symptoms, pelvic endometriosis may extend into menopause and is exacerbated by hormone replacement therapy (HRT).

ETIOLOGY AND PATHOPHYSIOLOGY
- Not fully understood; tendency for abnormal endometrial tissue to implant and proliferate, causing chronic peritoneal inflammation
- Endometrial-associated infertility is multifactorial:
  - Pelvic inflammation
  - Anatomic disruption of pelvic structures (involvement of the fallopian tube may cause isthmic tubal obstruction)
  - Proliferation and activation of peritoneal macrophages (may predispose to gamete phagocytosis)
  - Alteration in eutopic endometrium
- Not fully understood; theories include:
  - Sampson theory: Retrograde menstruation results in peritoneal implantation and disease. Affected women have an immune dysfunction that prevents clearing of implants.
  - Halban theory: Distant disease probably caused by hematogenous/lymphatic dissemination or metaplastic transformation.
  - Coelomic metaplasia: Coelomic epithelium undergoes metaplasia, forming functioning endometrium.

Genetics
Genetic predisposition is common.

RISK FACTORS
- Diethylstilbestrol exposure in utero
- Low birth weight
- Obstruction of menstrual flow (Müllerian anomalies)
- Prolonged exposure to endogenous estrogen:
  - Early menarche
  - Short menstrual cycles
  - Late menopause
  - Delayed childbearing
  - Obesity
- Hereditary/genetic predisposition
- Exposure to endocrine-disrupting chemicals
- Increased dietary intake of red meat and trans fats

GENERAL PREVENTION
- Prevention is not possible, but some factors are considered protective:
  - Fruits, green vegetables, n-3 long-chain fatty acids
  - Multiple pregnancies
  - Prolonged lactation
- Early diagnosis and treatment might help prevent the possible sequelae.

COMMONLY ASSOCIATED CONDITIONS
Associated with increased risk of other autoimmune diseases (3); increased risk of ovarian, endometrioid, and clear-cell cancers as well as other cancers (e.g., non-Hodgkin lymphoma)

 DIAGNOSIS

- Diagnosis can be challenging because symptoms overlap with many other gynecologic and nongynecologic conditions.
- Collect a complete medical, surgical, social, and family history from patients.
- Perform a complete physical exam, including a pelvic exam.

HISTORY
- Dysmenorrhea (50–90% of cases)
- Dyspareunia
- Chronic pelvic pain (≥6 months) that worsens with time and activity:
  - Intermittent/Continuous
  - Dull/Throbbing/Sharp
- Premenstrual spotting
- Dyschezia, painful defecation, hematochezia
- Cyclic nausea, abdominal distention, and early satiety
- Hematuria
- Infertility

- Spontaneous abortion (theoretical)
- History of pelvic pain, infertility, and hysterectomy in 1st- or 2nd-degree relative

PHYSICAL EXAM
- Focal pain/tenderness on pelvic exam (associated with endometriosis in 66% of patients) (3)
- Pelvic mass
- Immobile pelvic organs (frozen pelvis)
- Rectovaginal exam revealing uterosacral nodules, beading, or tenderness

DIFFERENTIAL DIAGNOSIS
Differential diagnosis of pelvic pain includes all causes of acute abdomen and:
- Complications of intrauterine/ectopic pregnancy
- Pelvic adhesions
- Acute salpingitis/pelvic inflammatory disease
- Ruptured ovarian cyst
- Uterine leiomyomas
- Adenomyosis
- Irritable bowel syndrome
- Inflammatory bowel disease
- Intussusception
- UTI/cystitis
- Interstitial cystitis
- Malignancies
- Depression
- History of sexual abuse
- Myofascial pain

DIAGNOSTIC TESTS & INTERPRETATION
Initial Tests (lab, imaging)
- No special labs; CA-125 levels are not recommended (poor sensitivity and specificity) and may be falsely elevated due to peritoneal irritation.
- Current research is underway to diagnose and stage ultrasound-negative endometriosis using peptide and protein analysis of plasma and urine.
- Routine imaging is not recommended.
- If history and physical exam reveal adnexal pain or tenderness with/without fullness on pelvic exam:
  - Transvaginal ultrasound (US) and MRI are equally effective in detecting ovarian endometriomas: Sensitivity, 80–90%; specificity, 60–98% for both (3)
  - US is preferred (less costly).
  - Both modalities are poor in detecting peritoneal implants and adhesions.

Diagnostic Procedures/Other
- Definitive diagnosis is made via visualization of lesions during surgery (laparoscopy or laparotomy).
- Hysterosalpingography for tubal occlusion (proximal or distal) and periadnexal adhesions

Test Interpretation
- Red and blue-black lesions described as "powder-burns," adhesions, and "chocolate cysts."
- Endometrial glands and stroma on histologic analysis of biopsied lesions

 TREATMENT

GENERAL MEASURES
Endometriosis should be considered a chronic disease with the goal of optimizing medical management to avoid repeat surgical procedures (4).

MEDICATION

Medications may be helpful in treating symptoms of pain and dysmenorrhea, but symptoms frequently recur.

First Line

Empirical medical treatment is indicated for symptom management, but has not been shown to improve fertility (5):

- NSAIDs initiated at the beginning or just before menses
- Cyclic combined oral contraceptive pills (OCPs)

Second Line

- Continuous combined OCPs. Switch from cyclic to continuous OCPs for 3–6 months if symptoms persist or if there is chronic, noncyclic pelvic pain
- Progestins:
  - Levonorgestrel IUD (Mirena), especially for symptomatic rectovaginal endometriosis (although not FDA approved) or instead of continuous OCPs in pain that persists despite first-line treatment
  - Medroxyprogesterone acetate 150 mg IM or 104 mg SC every 3 months. Prolonged use may lead to loss of bone mineral density of uncertain clinical significance.
- GnRH agonists inhibit pituitary gonadotropin synthesis and induce a hypoestrogenic state (3):
  - Leuprolide acetate (Depo-Lupron) 3.75 mg IM each month or 11.25 mg IM every 3 months (gluteal)
  - Nafarelin (Synarel) intranasal spray 400 μg/d divided into 2 inhalations/d, 1 in each nostril (start between days 2 and 4 of menstrual cycle)
  - Goserelin (Zoladex) implant 3.6 mg SC in upper abdominal wall every 28 days for 6 months
- GnRH agonists should be given with estrogen-progestogen add-back therapy to minimize effects of hypoestrogenism (most importantly, reduced bone mineral density) (3)[A]:
  - Norethindrone acetate 5 mg PO once daily
  - Conjugated equine estrogen 0.635 mg PO once daily
- Danazol was an early treatment (now second or third line). Use is limited by androgenic side effects.
- Aromatase inhibitors (anastrozole and letrozole) reduce local estrogen production and endometriotic growth. Risk with long-term use is reduction in bone mineral density.

ALERT

Calcium (1,000–1,500 mg/d) with vitamin D 1,000–2,000 IU daily is recommended when using GnRH agonists to prevent calcium loss.

ISSUES FOR REFERRAL

- Refer early to a board-certified reproductive endocrinologist or gynecologist with expertise in infertility if the patient has difficulty conceiving.
- Other indications for referral to a gynecologist include:
  - Need for definitive diagnosis (failure to respond to a conservative first-line therapy)
  - Chronic pelvic pain
  - Adolescent with severe dysmenorrhea/dyspareunia

ADDITIONAL THERAPIES

Regular exercise and counseling for pain-management strategies (avoidance of narcotics is ideal)

SURGERY/OTHER PROCEDURES

Surgery (laparoscopy or laparotomy) is both diagnostic and therapeutic (first line or when conservative measures fail):

- Peritoneal endometriosis: Laser ablation/excision/fulguration
- Ovarian endometriosis (endometriomas) >3 cm: Ablation, excision, drainage

ALERT

Surgery for endometriomas may decrease ovarian reserve in advanced disease.

- Lysis of adhesions (LOA)
- Hysterectomy with bilateral salpingo-oophorectomy for debilitating symptoms refractory to other medical or surgical treatments (3)[C]:
  - Relieves pain in 80–90%, but pain recurs in 10% within 1–2 years after surgery.
  - Postoperative HRT should include estrogen and progestogen (3)[C].
- Interruption of nerve pathways: Laparoscopic ablations and presacral neurectomy improve dysmenorrhea (3)[A].
- Fertility procedures: Ablation of lesions with LOA is recommended to treat infertility in stage I–II disease (3)[A]:
  - Spontaneous conception should be attempted for 1 year prior to assisted reproduction techniques.
  - Disease does not endanger in vitro fertilization (IVF) pregnancies.

COMPLEMENTARY AND ALTERNATIVE MEDICINE

- Physical therapy (3)[C]
- Acupuncture may be more effective than danazol to decrease pain, irregular menstruation, back pain, and perineal swelling (3)[C].
- Osteopathic manipulation (6)[B]
- Post surgical use of Chinese herbal medicine (oral and enema administration) is more effective than danazol at improving dysmenorrhea and reducing size of adnexal masses and has fewer side effects (7)[B].

 ONGOING CARE

FOLLOW-UP RECOMMENDATIONS

Routine gynecologic care

Patient Monitoring

- Symptomatic and asymptomatic pelvic masses <5 cm may be followed with serial US.
- Patients receiving GnRH agonist therapy should have serum estradiol levels monitored to assess degree of hypoestrogenemia and efficacy of add-back therapy: Estradiol between 30–45 pg/mL (109–164 pmol/L) prevents bone loss without stimulating disease.
- Endometriosis likely is an independent risk factor for the development of epithelial ovarian cancer.

DIET

No restrictions

PATIENT EDUCATION

American College of Obstetrics and Gynecology at www.acog.org

PROGNOSIS

- Excellent, especially if diagnosis and treatment plans are initiated early in disease course
- Poor for recovery of fertility if the disease has progressed to stage III/IV

COMPLICATIONS

Possible sequelae include chronic pelvic pain, repetitive surgical intervention, costs, and infertility.

REFERENCES

1. Ozkan S, Murk W, Arici A. Endometriosis and infertility: Epidemiology and evidence-based treatments. *Ann N Y Acad Sci*. 2008;1127:92–100.
2. Härkki P, Tiitinen A, Ylikorkala O, et al. Endometriosis and assisted reproduction techniques. *Ann N Y Acad Sci*. 2010;1205: 207–213.
3. Giudice LC. Clinical practice. Endometriosis. *N Engl J Med*. 2010;362:2389–2398.
4. *Treatment of pelvic pain associated with endometriosis*. AU Practice Committee of American Society for Reproductive Medicine. SO Fertil Steril. 2008;90(5 Suppl):S260.
5. Rodgers AK. Treatment strategies for endometriosis. *Exp Opin Pharmacother*. 2008;9(2): 243–255.
6. Chadwick K, Morgan A. The efficacy of osteopathic treatment for primary dysmenorrhea in young women. *The AAO Journal: A Publication of the American Academy of Osteopathy*. 1996;6(3): 15–17, 29–31.
7. Flower A, Liu JP, Leweth G, et al. Chinese herbal medicine for endometriosis. *Cochrane Database Syst Rev*. 2012, issue 5; CD006568.

ADDITIONAL READING

- Brown J, Pan A, Hart RJ, et al. Gonadotrophin-releasing hormone analogues for pain associated with endometriosis. *Cochrane Database Syst Rev*. 2010;CD008475.
- Davis L, Kennedy SS, Moore J, et al. Modern combined oral contraceptives for pain associated with endometriosis. *Cochrane Database Syst Rev*. 2007:CD001019.
- de Ziegler D, Borghese B, Chapron C, et al. Endometriosis and infertility: Pathophysiology and management. *Lancet*. 2010;376:730–738.
- Hughes E, Brown J, Collins JJ, et al. Ovulation suppression for endometriosis. *Cochrane Database Syst Rev*. 2007:CD000155.
- Jacobson TZ, Duffy JM, Barlow D, et al. Laparoscopic surgery for pelvic pain associated with endometriosis. *Cochrane Database Syst Rev*. 2009;CD001300.

 SEE ALSO

Algorithm: Pelvic Pain

 CODES

ICD10

- N80.2 Endometriosis of fallopian tube
- N80.3 Endometriosis of pelvic peritoneum
- N80.9 Endometriosis, unspecified

CLINICAL PEARLS

- Severe dysmenorrhea and dyspareunia are never normal. Failure to respond to NSAIDs and/or OCPs warrants further investigation.
- A rectovaginal exam can be useful in patients suspected of having endometriosis.

ENDOMETRITIS AND OTHER POSTPARTUM INFECTIONS

Justin P. Lavin, Jr., MD, FACOG • Jacoby Spittler, DO

 BASICS

DESCRIPTION
- Endometritis (infection of the endometrium) is the most common postpartum infection.
- Bacterial infection of the genital tract, usually within the 1st week after delivery, but can occur 1–6 weeks postpartum
- Less common are postpartum infections of the myometrium and parametrial tissues, vaginal and cervical infections, perineal cellulitis, pelvic cellulitis, septic pelvic vein thrombophlebitis, and parametrial phlegmon.
- System(s) affected: Reproductive
- Synonym(s): Postpartum infection; Endometritis; Endoparametritis; Endomyometritis; Myometritis; Endomyoparametritis; Metritis; Metritis with pelvic cellulitis

EPIDEMIOLOGY
Incidence
- Predominant age: Women of childbearing years
- Predominant sex: Female only

Prevalence
- Occurs in 1–3% of all births
- 10 times more likely with cesarean section:
  - 2–15% prior to labor
  - 30–35% after labor without prophylaxis
  - 2–15% after labor with prophylaxis
  - 5th leading cause of maternal mortality, accounting for 11% of maternal deaths

ETIOLOGY AND PATHOPHYSIOLOGY
- Endometritis commonly follows chorioamnionitis.
- Other infections follow trauma to the perineum, vagina, cervix, and uterus.
- Infection is nearly always polymicrobial and involves organisms that have ascended from the lower genital tract:
  - Aerobic isolates in 70%: *Streptococcus faecalis, S. agalactiae, S. viridans, Staphylococcus aureus, Escherichia coli*
  - Anaerobic isolates in 80%: *Peptococcus* sp., *Peptostreptococcus* sp., *Clostridium* sp., *Bacteroides bivius, B. fragilis, Fusobacterium* sp.
- Other genital mycoplasmata: Very common
- Herpes simplex virus and cytomegalovirus should be considered in immunocompromised patients if antibiotics fail.

RISK FACTORS
- Cesarean delivery is the most important risk factor.
- Chorioamnionitis
- Bacterial vaginosis
- Group B streptococcal colonization of genital tract
- HIV infection
- Prolonged labor
- Prolonged rupture of membranes
- Multiple vaginal examinations
- Internal fetal monitoring during labor
- Operative vaginal delivery
- Manual extraction of the placenta
- Low socioeconomic status
- Obesity
- Anemia

GENERAL PREVENTION
- Vaginal delivery:
  - Avoid unnecessary vaginal examinations
  - Treat chorioamnionitis during labor
  - Spontaneous placental extraction
  - Avoid retained placental fragments or membranes
  - Antibiotic prophylaxis for 3rd- and 4th-degree laceration (1)[B]
  - Use of aseptic technique during operative vaginal delivery
  - No data to support antibiotic prophylaxis for operative vaginal delivery (2)[A]
- Cesarean delivery:
  - Preoperative preparation using a paint and scrub technique with a 10% povidone-iodine scrub and topical solution has been shown to decrease puerperal infection by 38% (3)[B].
  - Administering prophylactic antibiotics before both emergency and scheduled cesarean reduces the prevalence of postpartum infection after cesarean (4)[A]:
    - Administering the antibiotics prior to skin incision in cesarean delivery (as opposed to the prior practice of waiting for cord clamping) is considered the standard of care.
    - Antibiotics should be administered within 1 hour of the surgery start time.
    - There is a 40% reduction in postpartum maternal infections without any increase in neonatal infectious outcomes or difficulty in evaluating the neonate (5)[A].
  - Extending the spectrum of coverage to include both a cephalosporin and azithromycin decreases the incidence of infections (6)[A],(7)[B].
  - Vaginal preparation with povidone-iodine solution reduces the risk of postoperative endometritis (8)[A].
  - Antibiotic dosage should be increased in obese patients to ensure appropriate tissue concentrations prior to skin incision (9)[B].

COMMONLY ASSOCIATED CONDITIONS
- Chorioamnionitis
- Wound infection

DIAGNOSIS

HISTORY
- Fever and chills
- Malaise
- Headache
- Anorexia
- Abdominal pain
- Heavy vaginal bleeding or foul smelling vaginal discharge

PHYSICAL EXAM
- Oral temperature >38.7°C (101.6°F) in first 24 hours postpartum or >38°C (100.4°F) in 2 of first 10 days postpartum (excluding first 24 hours)
- Tachycardia
- Uterine tenderness on exam
- Other localized tenderness on exam
- Purulent or malodorous lochia
- Heavy vaginal bleeding
- Ileus
- Group A or B streptococcal bacteremia may have no localizing signs.

DIFFERENTIAL DIAGNOSIS
- UTI
- Viral syndrome
- Dehydration
- Pneumonia
- Wound infection
- Thrombophlebitis
- Thyroid storm
- Mastitis

DIAGNOSTIC TESTS & INTERPRETATION
Initial Tests (lab, imaging)
- CBC: Interpret with care, because *physiologic leukocytosis may be as high as 20,000 WBCs.*
- 2 sets of blood cultures (especially if sepsis is suspected)
- Note: Diagnosis is usually made clinically, but consider additional testing, including:
  - Genital tract cultures and rapid test for group B streptococci, which may be done while patient is in labor
  - Amniotic fluid Gram stain: Usually polymicrobial
  - Uterine tissue cultures: Prep the cervix with Betadine and use a shielded specimen collector or Pipelle. Difficult to obtain without contamination.
- If patient is not responsive to antibiotics in 24–48 hours:
  - Ultrasound for retained products of conception, pelvic abscess, or mass
  - CT or MRI looking for pelvic vein thrombophlebitis, abscess, or deep-seated wound infection

Diagnostic Procedures/Other
Paracentesis or culdocentesis with culture rarely is necessary.

Test Interpretation
- Superficial layer of infected necrotic tissue in microscopic sections of uterine lining
- >5 neutrophils per high-power field in superficial endometrium; ≥1 plasma cell in endometrial stroma
- Thrombosis of any of the pelvic veins, including the vena cava
- Phlegmon on leaves of the broad ligament
- Abscess

TREATMENT

MEDICATION

First Line

- Clindamycin 900 mg IV q8h + gentamicin 5 mg/kg IV q24h (10)[A]
- Potential side effects include nephrotoxicity, ototoxicity, pseudomembranous colitis, or diarrhea (in up to 6%)

Second Line

- Clindamycin 900 mg IV q8h + aztreonam 1–2 g q8h (10)[A]
- Metronidazole 500 mg q12h + penicillin 5 million units q6h, OR
- Ampicillin 2 g q6h + gentamicin 5 mg/kg q24h (10)[A]
- Cefoxitin 2 g IV q6h. Add ampicillin 2 g IV q6h, if clinical failure after 48 hours (10)[A]
- Cefotetan 2 g IV q12h. Add ampicillin 2 g IV q6h, if clinical failure after 48 hours (10)[A]
- Note: Base therapy on cultures, sensitivities, and clinical response.
- Contraindications:
  – Drug allergy
  – Renal failure (aminoglycosides)
  – Avoid sulfa, tetracyclines, and fluoroquinolones before delivery and if breastfeeding. Metronidazole is relatively contraindicated if breastfeeding; however, consider clinical scenario.
- Precautions:
  – Clindamycin and other antibiotics occasionally cause pseudomembranous colitis.
- Significant possible interactions: Refer to the manufacturer's literature for each drug.
- Note: Consider adding a macrolide antibiotic (for chlamydia coverage) for infections occurring after 48 hours.
- Note: Heparin may be indicated for septic pelvic vein thrombophlebitis; requires 10 days of full anticoagulation.

SURGERY/OTHER PROCEDURES

- Curettage of retained products of conception
- Surgery to drain an abscess
- Surgery to decompress the bowel
- Surgical drainage of a phlegmon is not advised unless it is suppurative.

IN-PATIENT CONSIDERATIONS

Admission Criteria/Initial Stabilization

- Inpatient care for postpartum infections
- Most infections (94%) occur after hospital discharge.
- IV antibiotics and close observation for severe infections
- Open and drain infected wounds
- Normalize fluid status

 ONGOING CARE

FOLLOW-UP RECOMMENDATIONS

Patient Monitoring

- Individualize according to severity
- IV antibiotics can be stopped when the patient is afebrile for 24–48 hours.
- Oral antibiotics on discharge are not necessary, except in cases of bacteremia; then continue oral antibiotics to complete a 7-day course.

DIET

As tolerated, although may be limited by ileus

PATIENT EDUCATION

- Advise patient to call her doctor if she has fever >38°C (100.4°F) postpartum, heavy vaginal bleeding, foul-smelling lochia, or other symptoms of infection.
- Information available at: www.healthline.com/yodocontent/pregnancy/infections-postpartum-endometritis.html

PROGNOSIS

- With supportive therapy and appropriate antibiotics, most patients improve within a few days.
- If no improvement occurs on antibiotics, consider retained placental fragments or membranes, abscess, wound infection, hematoma, cellulitis, phlegmon, or septic pelvic vein thrombosis.

COMPLICATIONS

- Resistant organisms
- Peritonitis
- Pelvic abscess
- Septic pelvic thrombophlebitis
- Ovarian vein thrombosis
- Sepsis
- Death

REFERENCES

1. Duggal N, Mercado C, Daniels K, et al. Antibiotic prophylaxis for prevention of postpartum perineal wound complications: A randomized controlled trial. Obstet Gynecol. 2008;111:1268–1273.
2. Liabsuetrakul T. Antibiotic prophylaxis for operative vaginal delivery. Cochrane Databse Sys Rev. 2009;1:CD004455.
3. Weed S, Bastek JA, Sammel MD, et al. Comparing postcesarean infectious complication rates using two different skin preparations. Obstet Gynecol. 2011;117:1123–1129.
4. Smaill FM, Gyte GM. Antibiotic prophylaxis versus no prophylaxis for preventing infection after cesarean section. Cochrane Database of Sys Rev. 2010;1:CD007482.
5. Baaqeel H, Baaqeel R. Timing of administration of prophylactic antibiotics for caesarean section: A systematic review and meta-analysis. BJOG. 2013;120:661–669.
6. Costantine MM, Rahman M, Ghulmiyah L, et al. Timing of perioperative antibiotics for cesarean delivery: A metaanalysis. Am J Obstet Gynecol. 2008;199:301.e1–e6.
7. Tita AT, Owen J, Stamm AM, et al. Impact of extended-spectrum antibiotic prophylaxis on incidence of postcesarean surgical wound infection. Am J Obstet Gynecol. 2008;199:303.e1–e3.
8. Haas DM, Morgan S, Contreras K. Vaginal preparation with antiseptic solution before cesarean section for preventing postoperative infections. Cochrane Database Syst Rev. 2013;1:CD007892.
9. Pevzner L, Swank M, Krepel C, et al. Effects of maternal obesity on tissue concentrations of prophylactic cefazolin during cesarean delivery. Obstet Gynecol. 2011;117:877–882.
10. French LM, Smaill F. Antibiotic regimens for endometritis after delivery. Cochrane Database Sys Rev. 2009;1:CD001067.

ADDITIONAL READING

- American College of Obstetricians and Gynecologist. Use of Prophylactic Antibiotics in Labor. ACOG practice bulletin no. 120. Obstet Gynecol. 2011;117:1472–1483.
- Belfort MA, Clark SL, Saade GR, et al. Hospital readmission after delivery: Evidence for an increased incidence of nonurogenital infection in the immediate postpartum period. Am J Obstet Gynecol. 2010;202:35.e1–e7.
- Mackeen AD, Seibel-Seamon J, Grimes-Dennis J, et al. Tocolytics for preterm premature rupture of membranes. Cochrane Database Syst Rev. 2011;10: CD007062.
- Maharaj D. Puerperal pyrexia: A review. Part I. Obstet Gynecol Surv. 2007;62:393–399.
- Maharaj D. Puerperal pyrexia: A review. Part II. Obstet Gynecol Surv. 2007;62:400–406.

 SEE ALSO

Algorithm: Pelvic Pain

 CODES

ICD10

- O86.4 Pyrexia of unknown origin following delivery
- O86.12 Endometritis following delivery
- O86.13 Vaginitis following delivery

CLINICAL PEARLS

- Endometritis, a postpartum complication, causes fever and uterine tenderness in 1–3% of all births.
- Infection is nearly always polymicrobial and involves organisms that have ascended from the lower genital tract.
- Evidence supports antibiotic prophylaxis prior to skin incision for all cesarean deliveries, but not for operative vaginal deliveries.
- Recommended treatment of endometritis is clindamycin 900 mg IV q8h and gentamicin 5 mg/kg q24h until the patient is afebrile for 24–48 hours.
- Antibiotics can be stopped completely when the patient has been afebrile for 24–48 hours, except in cases of documented bacteremia, which require a 7-day course of therapy.

E

ENURESIS
Melanie J.S. Malec, MD

BASICS

DESCRIPTION
- Nocturnal enuresis (NE): Repeated spontaneous voiding of urine during sleep after the anticipated age of bladder control (age 5)
- Daytime incontinence: Uncontrollable leakage of urine while awake
- Bladder dysfunction: NE with daytime symptoms
- Classification:
  - Primary NE: 1% of adult population; 80% of all cases; child/adult who has never established urinary continence on consecutive nights for a period of ≥6 months
  - Secondary NE: 20% of cases; resumption of enuresis after at least 6 months of urinary continence
- Also categorized as:
  - Monosymptomatic NE (uncomplicated): Bed wetting without lower urinary tract (LUT) symptoms other than nocturia and no history of bladder dysfunction
  - Nonmonosymptomatic NE: Bed wetting with LUT symptoms, such as frequency, urgency, daytime wetting, hesitancy, straining, weak or intermittent stream, posturination dribbling, lower abdominal or genital discomfort, sensation of incomplete emptying
  - Daytime LUT condition: Bed wetting with LUT daytime symptoms

ALERT
Adult-onset NE with absent daytime incontinence is a serious symptom; complete urologic evaluation and therapy are warranted.
- System(s) affected: Nervous; Renal/Urologic
- Synonym(s): Bed wetting; Sleep enuresis; Nocturnal incontinence; Primary nocturnal enuresis

EPIDEMIOLOGY
Incidence
- Depends on family history
- Spontaneous resolution: 15% per year, 99% children are dry by age 15
Prevalence
- Very common. Affects 5–7 million children in the US.
- 40% of 3-year-olds; 10% of 6-year-olds; 3% of 12-year-olds; 1% of adults
- Male > Female (3:1)
- Nocturnal > Day (3:1)
Geriatric Considerations
Infrequent; often associated with daytime incontinence (formerly referred to as diurnal enuresis)

ETIOLOGY AND PATHOPHYSIOLOGY
- A disorder of sleep arousal, a low nocturnal bladder capacity, and nocturnal polyuria are the 3 factors that interrelate to cause nocturnal enuresis (1).
- Both functional and organic causes (below); many theories, none absolutely confirmed
- Detrusor instability
- Deficiency of arginine vasopressin (AVP); decreased nocturnal AVP or decreased AVP stimulation secondary to an empty bladder (bladder distension stimulates AVP)
- Maturational delay of CNS
- Severe NE with some evidence of interaction between bladder overactivity and brain arousability: Association with children with severe NE and frequent cortical arousals in sleep

- Organic urologic causes in 1–4% of enuresis in children: UTI, occult spina bifida, ectopic ureter, lazy bladder syndrome, irritable bladder with wide bladder neck, posterior urethral valves
- Organic nonurologic causes: Epilepsy, diabetes mellitus, food allergies, obstructive sleep apnea, chronic renal failure, hyperthyroidism, pinworm infection, sickle-cell disease
- NE occurs in all stages of sleep.

Genetics
Most commonly, NE is an autosomal-dominant inheritance pattern with high penetrance (90%):
- 1/3 of all cases are sporadic.
- 75% of children with enuresis have a 1st-degree relative with the condition.
- Higher rates in monozygotic vs. dizygotic twins (68% vs. 36%)
- If both parents had NE, risk in child is 77%; 44% if 1 parent affected. Parental age of resolution often predicts when child's enuresis should resolve.

RISK FACTORS
- Family history
- Stressors (emotional, environmental) common in secondary enuresis (e.g., divorce, death)
- Constipation
- Encopresis
- Organic disease: 1% of monosymptomatic NE (e.g., urologic and nonurologic causes)
- Psychological disorders:
  - Comorbid disorders are highest with secondary NE: Depression, anxiety, social phobias, conduct disorder, hyperkinetic syndrome, internalizing disorders
  - Association with ADHD; more pronounced in ages 9–12 years
  - Abuse; 11% sexually abused girls
- Altered mental status or impaired mobility

GENERAL PREVENTION
No known measures

COMMONLY ASSOCIATED CONDITIONS
- Obstructive sleep apnea syndrome; ↑ atrial natriuretic factor → inhibits renin-angiotensin-aldosterone pathway → ↑ diuresis
- Constipation (1/3 of patients with NE)
- Behavioral problems (specifically ADHD)

DIAGNOSIS

HISTORY
- Age of onset, duration, severity
- LUT tract symptoms
- Constipation and encopresis (15% with comorbid encopresis)
- Daily intake patterns
- Voiding and elimination patterns (voiding diary)
- Psychosocial history
- Family history of enuresis
- Investigation and previous treatment history

PHYSICAL EXAM
- ENT: Evaluation for adenotonsillar hypertrophy
- Abdomen: Enlarged bladder, kidneys, fecal masses, or impaction
- Back: Look for dimpling or tufts of hair on sacrum.
- Genital urinary exam:
  - Males: Meatal stenosis, hypospadias, epispadias, phimosis

- Females: Vulvitis, vaginitis, labial adhesions, ureterocele at introitus; evidence of abuse
- Rectal exam: Tone and constipation
- Neurologic exam, especially lower extremities

DIFFERENTIAL DIAGNOSIS
- Primary NE:
  - Delayed physiologic urinary control
  - UTI (both)
  - Spina bifida occulta
  - Obstructive sleep apnea (both)
  - Idiopathic detrusor instability
  - Previously unrecognized myelopathy or neuropathy (e.g., multiple sclerosis, tethered cord, epilepsy)
  - Anatomic urinary tract abnormally (e.g., ectopic ureter)
- Secondary NE:
  - Bladder outlet obstruction
  - Neurologic disease, neurogenic bladder (e.g., spinal cord injury)

DIAGNOSTIC TESTS & INTERPRETATION
Initial Tests (lab, imaging)
- Only obligatory test in children is urinalysis.
- Urinalysis and urine culture: UTI, pyuria, hematuria, proteinuria, glycosuria, and poor concentrating ability (low specific gravity) may suggest organic etiology, especially in adults.
- Urinary tract imaging is usually not necessary.
- If abnormal clinical findings or adult onset: Renal and bladder US
- IV pyelogram, voiding cystourethrogram (VCUG) or retrograde pyelogram as indicated
- Spine radiographs for spina bifida occulta
Follow-Up Tests & Special Considerations
- Secondary enuresis: Serum glucose, BUN, creatinine, thyroid-stimulating hormone (TSH), urine C/S
- In children, imaging and urodynamic studies are helpful for significant daytime symptoms, history of UTIs, suspected structural abnormalities, and in refractory cases.

Diagnostic Procedures/Other
Urodynamic studies may be beneficial in adults and nonmonosymptomatic NE.

Test Interpretation
- Dysfunctional voiding
- Detrusor instability and/or reduced bladder capacity most common findings

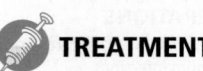

TREATMENT

- Prior to either alarm or pharmacologic treatment, supportive treatment measures should be attempted:
  - Counseling and information provision, such as explanation of the 3 pathophysiologic factors
  - Review of eating and drinking habits, with emphasis on normal drinking patterns during daytime hours and reduction of intake in the hours prior to sleep.
  - Positive reinforcement of the child should also be encouraged.

- If supportive measures have no success, combined therapy (e.g., enuresis alarm, bladder training, motivational therapy, and pelvic floor muscle training) is more effective than each component alone or than pharmacotherapy (2)[A].

GENERAL MEASURES

- Use nonpharmacologic approaches as first line before prescribing medications (3)[A].
- Simple behavioral interventions (e.g., scheduled wakening, positive reinforcement, bladder training, diet changes)
- Enuresis alarms (bells or buzzers):
  - 66–70% success rate; must be used nightly for 3–4 months; offers cure; significant parental involvement; disruption of sleep for entire family
  - In children, NNT = 2 (4)[A]
  - See Patient Education for options

MEDICATION
First Line

- Desmopressin (DDAVP): Synthetic analogue of vasopressin that decreases nocturnal urine output (5)[A]:
  - Adults only: 20 μg intranasally at bedtime
  - FDA recommends against use in children due to reports of severe hyponatremia resulting in seizures and deaths in children using intranasal formulations of desmopressin.
  - Oral DDAVP: Dose dependent: Begin at 0.2 mg tablet taken at bedtime on empty stomach; may titrate to 0.6 mg:
    - Maximally effective in 1 hour; cleared within 9 hours
    - Trial nightly for 6 months, then stop for 2 weeks for test of dryness
    - Suspend dose in children who experience acute condition affecting fluid/electrolyte balances (fever, vomiting, diarrhea, vigorous exercise)
  - 10–70% success; safe even when used for >12 months; high relapse rate after discontinuation without a structured withdrawal program
  - In children, NNT = 6 (6)[A]

- Anticholinergics:
  - Oxybutynin (Ditropan, Ditropan XL, Oxytrol patch): Anticholinergic; smooth muscle relaxant, antispasmodic; may increase functional bladder capacity and aids in timed voiding:
    - Ditropan: Adults and children >5 years of age: 5 mg PO t.i.d.–q.i.d.; children 1–5 years of age: 0.02 mg/kg/dose b.i.d.–q.i.d. (syrup 5 mg/5 mL)
    - Ditropan XL: Adults: 5 mg/d PO; increase to 30 mg/d PO (5-, 10-mg tabs)
    - Oxytrol patch: 1 patch every 3–4 days (3.9 mg/patch) (periodic trials off the medication, i.e., weekends or weeks at a time, will help determine efficacy and resolution of primary disturbance)
    - Ditropan: 5–10 mg at night; 30–50% success; 50% relapse after stopped
  - Tolterodine (Detrol, Detrol LA): Anticholinergic; fewer side effects than Ditropan:
    - Detrol: 1–2 mg PO b.i.d.
    - Detrol LA: 2–4 mg/d

Pediatric Considerations

FDA recommends against using intranasal formulations of desmopressin in children due to reports of severe hyponatremia resulting in seizures and deaths (7,8)[A].

Second Line

- Imipramine (Tofranil): Tricyclic antidepressant, anticholinergic effects; increases bladder capacity, antispasmodic properties:
  - Primarily in adults; use in children is reserved for resistant cases.

- Dose: Adults, 25–75 mg and children >6 years, 10–25 mg PO at bedtime; increase by 10–25 mg at 1–2-week intervals; treat for 2–3 months; then taper.
  - 25–30% success when used >3 months.
  - Pretreatment ECG recommended identifying underlying rhythm disorders.
- Precautions:
  - Oxybutynin: Glaucoma, myasthenia gravis, GI or genitourinary obstruction, ulcerative colitis, megacolon; use a decreased dose in the elderly.
  - Tolterodine: Urinary retention, gastric retention, or uncontrolled narrow-angle glaucoma; significant drug interactions with CYP2D6, CYP3A3/4 substrates
  - DDAVP: Avoid in patients at risk for electrolyte changes or fluid retention (congestive heart failure [CHF], renal insufficiency).
  - Imipramine: Do not use with monoamine oxidase inhibitors (MAOIs), hypotension, and arrhythmias; low toxic therapeutic ratio.
- Combination therapy with DDAVP and oxybutynin has better results than individual use.
- Prostaglandin inhibitors (e.g., indomethacin) have been studied; may increase bladder capacity; not as effective as DDAVP and ↑ adverse effects.

ALERT
Imipramine: Cardiotoxicity and death with overdose have been described.

ISSUES FOR REFERRAL
- Primary NE: Persistent enuresis despite nonpharmacologic and pharmacologic therapies
- Diurnal incontinence or nonmonosymptomatic enuresis with voiding dysfunction or underlying medical condition

ADDITIONAL THERAPIES
Individual psychotherapy, crisis intervention, and family therapy

SURGERY/OTHER PROCEDURES
Only for surgically correctable causes (e.g., tethered cord, ectopic ureter, benign prostatic hypertrophy, obstructive sleep apnea)

COMPLEMENTARY AND ALTERNATIVE MEDICINE
Acupuncture and hypnosis are other treatments offered; few data support their use (9,10)[B].

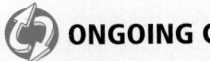 ## ONGOING CARE

FOLLOW-UP RECOMMENDATIONS
Patient Monitoring
Follow patient until condition resolves. Monitor therapy.

DIET
- Limit fluid and caffeine intake 2 hours prior to bedtime.
- Limit dairy products 4 hours prior to bedtime (decrease osmotic diuresis).

PATIENT EDUCATION
Web resources for alarms and supplies:
- www.bedwettingstore.com/index.htm; www.dri-sleeper.com; www.enurad.com; www.mitetrain-r.com; www.sleepydryalarm.com; www.wetstop.com; www.pottypager.com/

PROGNOSIS
In children, NE is usually self-limiting; 1% will persist as adult; evaluate for organic causes.

COMPLICATIONS
UTI, perineal excoriation, psychological disturbance (especially in children)

REFERENCES
1. Robson WL. Current management of nocturnal enuresis. Curr Opin Urol. 2008;18:425–430.
2. Zaffanello M, Giacomello L, Brugnara M, et al. Therapeutic options in childhood nocturnal enuresis. Minerva Urol Nefrol. 2007;59:199–205.
3. Robson WL. Clinical practice. Evaluation and management of enuresis. N Engl J Med. 2009; 360:1429–1436.
4. Glazener CM, Evans JH, Peto RE. Alarm interventions for nocturnal enuresis in children. Cochrane Database Syst Rev. 2005; CD002911.
5. Vande Walle J, Stockner M, Raes A, et al. Desmopressin 30 years in clinical use: A safety review. Curr Drug Saf. 2007;2:232–238.
6. Glazener CM, Evans JH. Desmopressin for nocturnal enuresis in children. Cochrane Database Syst Rev. 2002;CD002112.
7. Graham KM, Levy JB. Enuresis. Pediatr Rev. 2009;30:165–172; quiz 173.
8. www.fda.gov/Drugs/DrugSafety/PostmarketDrugSafetyInformationforPatientsandProviders/ucm107924.htm
9. Neveus T, Eggert P, Evans J, et al. Evaluation of and treatment for monosymptomatic enuresis: A standardization document from the International Children's Continence Society. J Urol. 2010;183: 441–447.
10. Libonate J, Evans S, Tsao JC, et al. Efficacy of acupuncture for health conditions in children: A review. Sci World J. 2008;8:670–682.

ADDITIONAL READING
Vande Walle J, Rittig S, Bauer S, et al. Practical consensus guidelines for the management of enuresis. Eur J Pediatr. 2012;171(6):971–983. Epub 2012 Feb 24.

 ### SEE ALSO
- Incontinence, Urinary Adult Female; Incontinence, Urinary Adult Male
- Algorithm: Enuresis

 ## CODES

ICD10
- F98.0 Enuresis not due to a substance or known physiol condition
- N39.44 Nocturnal enuresis
- R32 Unspecified urinary incontinence

CLINICAL PEARLS
- Diagnosis is usually made based on history, physical examination, and urinalysis.
- If the condition is not distressing to child and caretakers, treatment is unnecessary.
- Dryness is possible for most children.

E

EOSINOPHILIC ESOPHAGITIS

Benjamin Hyatt, MD

 BASICS

Eosinophilic esophagitis (EoE) is a chronic, immune-mediated, inflammatory esophageal disease characterized clinically in adults by dysphagia, food impaction, and heartburn and in children with nonspecific abdominal complaints abdominal pain and failure to thrive. Histologically EoE is characterized by eosinophilic predominate inflammation (1)[A].

EPIDEMIOLOGY
- All ages, most common in 20s–30s
- Predominant sex: Male > Female (3:1)

Incidence
- Incidence in general population is 0.03% (2)[A]
- Incidence in those with gastroesophageal reflux disease (GERD)/dysphagia symptoms: 2.8% (2)[A]

Prevalence
- Gradually increasing, perhaps due to better case finding, understanding of EoE in multiple clinical guises; 45–55/100,000
- Increased prevalence in those with celiac disease

ETIOLOGY AND PATHOPHYSIOLOGY
- Believed to be an atopic inflammatory disease of which pathogenesis is an aberrant immune response to antigenic stimulation
- Like eczema and asthma, T-helper 2 (T_H2) lymphocytes play a role, as do mixed IgE and non-IgE-mediated allergic responses to food and environmental allergens.
- Although not well understood, the pathophysiology of EoE is postulated to be due to increased recruitment and activation of eosinophils in the esophagus. Eosinophil chemoattractants include eotaxin-3, IL-5, and IL-13.

Genetics
- EoE susceptibility may be caused by polymorphisms in thymic stromal lymphopoietin protein (TSLP) (2)[A].
- Potential new subphenotype of EoE (may also overlap with GERD): Proton pump inhibitor (PPI)-responsive esophageal eosinophilia, where PPIs may act to decrease the inflammatory response in EoE (2)[A].

RISK FACTORS
- >50% with EoE have a personal history of atopy/allergic disorders, such as asthma, hay fever, or eczema (1)[A].
- High rate of associated food antigen allergies/anaphylaxis

 DIAGNOSIS

There are no pathognomonic findings for EoE. A definitive diagnosis is made by esophageal endoscopy and biopsy.

HISTORY
- Solid-food dysphagia and food impaction are the most common symptoms and are usually present for 3–4 years prior to the diagnosis.
- Patients may also have reflux symptoms. Often, the diagnosis is entertained after patients fail a trial of antireflux medications. Other common complaints include nausea or vomiting, regurgitation, chest pain, upper abdominal pain, or decreased appetite.
- Patients may also have a history of food or environmental allergies, as well as asthma or atopic conditions (e.g., dermatitis).

PHYSICAL EXAM
No specific physical exam findings are associated with the diagnosis. However, signs and symptoms of allergies or asthma with symptoms of ongoing dysphagia or GERD-like symptoms should raise suspicion; some patients will have signs indicating weight loss or malnutrition.

DIFFERENTIAL DIAGNOSIS
- GERD:
  - Associated with EoE; diseases may coexist in individual patients
- PPI-responsive esophageal eosinophilia (PPI-REE):
  - Characteristics of PPI-REE:
    ○ Shows classic EoE symptoms
    ○ Diagnosis of GERD has been excluded
    ○ Responds to PPIs clinically and histologically
- Secondary causes of esophageal eosinophilia including celiac disease, Crohn esophagitis, infection, vasculitis, PPIs, achalasia, connective tissue disease, eosinophilic gastrointestinal diseases
- Functional dyspepsia
- Congenital rings
- Esophageal carcinoma
- Esophageal motility disorders

DIAGNOSTIC TESTS & INTERPRETATION
- To exclude PPI-REE, patients with suspected EoE should be given a 2-month course of PPI followed by endoscopy with biopsies.
- Solid-food dysphagia is an indication for esophagogastroduodenoscopy (EGD), as are other concerning or "red-flag" symptoms, many of which occur in patients with EoE; they include:
  - Odynophagia
  - Weight loss
  - Early satiety or vomiting
  - Aspiration/Wheezing or cough
  - GI bleeding
  - Unexplained iron-deficiency anemia
  - Male >45 with long-standing symptoms
- GERD patients who show no symptomatic improvement after 8–12 weeks of a PPI should also be considered for EGD and biopsy.
- Serum IgE levels are elevated in 70% of patients.
- Peripheral eosinophilia occurs in 10–50% of patients.

Follow-Up Tests & Special Considerations
Testing for asthma and IgE-mediated food/inhalant allergies, if clinically relevant, can help manage coexisting atopic conditions:
- Serum IgE, skin prick test, or atopy patch test

Diagnostic Procedures/Other
- EGD: 17% of biopsy proven cases of EoE had an endoscopically normal exam (3)[A].
  - Endoscopic findings: Esophageal rings (trachealization), strictures, white plaques or exudates, linear furrows, narrow-caliber esophagus and pallor or decreased vasculature.
  - Esophageal biopsies are required for diagnosis, 2–4 biopsies from both proximal and distal esophagus. At initial diagnosis, biopsies should be obtained from antrum and/or duodenum to rule out other causes of esophageal eosinophilia in all children and adults with gastric or small intestinal symptoms or endoscopic abnormalities (1)[A].
    ○ Biopsy specimen: Pathological findings may include surface layering of eosinophils, eosinophilic microabscesses, subepithelial lamina propria fibrosis, or basal cell hyperplasia.
- Barium contrast radiography:
  - Can help to identify anatomic abnormalities in EoE but has a low sensitivity for diagnosis
  - May be an alternative to repeated endoscopies in previously treated patients who have changing symptoms
- pH monitoring: May be helpful in differentiating EoE from GERD
- Consensus American Gastroenterologic Association guidelines for diagnosis of EoE (1)[A]:
  - Clinical symptoms of esophageal dysfunction
  - ≥15 eosinophils in 1 high-power field on biopsy
  - Mucosal eosinophilia is isolated to esophagus and persists after PPI use
  - Secondary causes of esophageal eosinophilia are excluded

TREATMENT

Endpoints of therapy of EoE include improvements in clinical symptoms and esophageal eosinophilic inflammation. Defining evidence-based endpoints in EoE is still an area of active research (1)[A].

MEDICATION
First Line
- Corticosteroids: Topical steroids (swallowed, not inhaled) are 1st-line pharmacologic treatment:
  - Initial dosing for treatment of EoE: Swallowed fluticasone dose in adults is 880–1,760 μg/d in a divided dose and in children is determined based on age or weight. Swallowed budesonide dose in adults is 2 mg/d, typically in divided doses; in children determined based on age or weight. Initial duration of treatment is 8 weeks. Medication should be discontinued if patient develops side effects or other intolerances. Patients have relapsed after withdrawal of the medication. Inhaled topical steroid trials are ongoing.

- Systemic steroids: Prednisone can be helpful if topical steroids are not effective or for patients who require a more rapid improvement to symptoms, such as those with refractory dysphagia and in patients who are hospitalized. Long-term toxicity limits use (1)[A].

- Diet:
  - Dietary elimination is considered initial therapy in both children and adults.
  - 3 dietary regimens have been shown to be effective in treatment of EoE: (i) Elemental amino-acid based diet, (ii) Elimination diet based on various food allergy tests, and (iii) 6-food elimination diet of the most common food groups known to trigger EoE: wheat, soy, cow's milk, eggs, nuts, and seafood. All 3 methods have been shown to be effective in children for both clinical and histologic improvement, with the elemental diet being most effective:
    - In children, success rates of 77–98% have been reported for clinical and histologic remission using an elemental amino acid formula. A retrospective chart review comparing the 3 diets showed that the elemental diet was superior, with 96% remission (4)[B]. Yet this treatment has not gained popularity because of its high cost, impaired quality of life, and overall practicality.
  - In adults, food allergy may play an important role in EoE and a single food elimination diet (SFED) is an effective therapy (5)[B]:
    - Gonsalves et al. evaluated SFED in adult patients with EoE and demonstrated clinical, endoscopic, and histologic improvement. Symptoms improved in 94% of patients. Reintroduction of eliminated food caused reactivation of EoE, with wheat (60%) and cow's milk (50%) as the leading causative agents. Skin-prick allergy testing was only 13% predictive in identifying food triggers (5)[B].

Second Line

Endoscopic esophageal dilation:

- May be used effectively in symptomatic patients with strictures that are resistant to medical or dietary treatments and initially in patients with severe and symptomatic esophageal stenosis (1)[A].

- A systematic review showed that 92% of patients treated with dilation had improvement in dysphagia symptoms for up to 1–2 years.

- Patients should be informed of the risks of esophageal dilation, with the most common risk being postprocedure chest pain, which occurs in 75% of patients. The perforation rate for dilation is 0.3%, contrary to early reports that showed higher rates of perforation. Bleeding requiring endoscopic intervention or blood products is very rare, with only 1 incidence reported to date (6)[A],(1)[A].

ISSUES FOR REFERRAL

Refer to an allergist and/or nutritionist to help identify/manage allergic disorders and diet regimens

ADDITIONAL THERAPIES

Other pharmacologic therapies:

- Montelukast, mepolizumab (IL-5 monoclonal antibody), purine analogues, anti-TNF therapy. Biologic agents have been well tolerated with low after effects, yet no studies have shown prolonged symptomatic relief 1[A].

- Antihistamines: Case studies showed no benefit

 ONGOING CARE

FOLLOW-UP RECOMMENDATIONS

- EoE is a chronic disease with symptom recurrence after discontinuing treatment the rule rather than the exception. Prevention of progression of esophageal dysfunction is primary. Maintenance therapy with swallowed topical corticosteroid therapy and/or dietary restriction should be considered in all patients after clinicopathologic remission indefinitely or PRN (1)[A]. This is not yet standardized; only 1 randomized controlled maintenance study has been done using low-dose budesonide (0.25 mg b.i.d.) vs. placebo after remission for 50 weeks. Those maintained on budesonide had modest reduction in eosinophilia and fewer symptom recurrences, but there was still significant recurrence (7)[A]. As such, ongoing therapy needs to be tailored to individual patient cases.

- Patient should be counseled on the high likelihood of symptom recurrence after discontinuing treatment

Patient Monitoring

- No guidelines have yet been established. It is reasonable to order periodic endoscopy based on symptoms or after completing a recent therapeutic regimen.

- There is no evidence to date of esophageal malignancy or hypereosinophilic syndromes associated with EoE.

- Esophageal candidiasis is a common side effect of chronic corticosteroid therapy.

PROGNOSIS

EoE does not seem to affect life expectancy. Quality of life is affected to some extent due to the chronic nature of the disease and difficulty in adhering to a restrictive diet. Nutritional status can be maintained with appropriate care and diligence.

COMPLICATIONS

- Food impaction
- Esophageal stricture/ring/narrowing
- Nutritional deficiencies
- Subglottic stenosis or laryngeal edema is very rare.

REFERENCES

1. Dellon ES, Gonsalves N, Hirano I, et al. ACG clinical guidelines: Evidenced based approach to diagnosis and management of esophageal eosinophilia and eosinophilic esophagitis. *Am J Gastroentergol*. 2013;108:679–692.

2. Liacouras CA, Furuta GT, Hirano I, et al. Eosinophilic esophagitis: Updated consensus recommendations for children and adults. *J Allergy Clin Immunol*. 2011;128:3–20.e6.

3. Kim HP, Vance RB, Shaheen NJ, et al. The prevalence and diagnostic utility of endoscopic features of eosinophilic esophagitis: A meta-analysis. *Clin Gastroenterol Hepatol*. 2012;10:988–996.

4. Henderson CJ, Abonia JP, King EC, et al. Comparative dietary therapy effectiveness in remission of pediatric eosinophilic esophagitis. *J Allergy Clin Immunol*. 2012;129:1570–1578.

5. Gonsalves N, Yang GY, Doerfler B, et al. Elimination diet effectively treats eosinophilic esophagitis in adults; food reintroduction identifies causative factors. *Gastroenterology*. 2012;142:1451–1459.e1.

6. Bohm ME, Richter JE. Review article: Oesophageal dilation in adults with eosinophilic oesophagitis. *Aliment Pharmacol Ther*. 2011;33:748–757.

7. Straumann A, Conus S, Degen L, et al. Long-term budesonide maintenance treatment is partially effective for patients with eosinophilic esophagitis. *Clin Gastroenterol Hepatol*. 2011;9:400–409.e1.

ADDITIONAL READING

- Dellon ES, Jensen ET, Martin CF, et al. The Prevalence of eosinophilic esophagitis in the United States. *Clin Gastroenterol Hepatol*. 2013; S1542–S3565:01304-9.

- Stewart MJ, Shaffer E, Urbankski SJ. The association between celiac disease and eosinophilic esophagitis in children and adults. *BMC Gastroenterol*. 2013;1:96.

 ## CODES

ICD10

K20.0 Eosinophilic esophagitis

CLINICAL PEARLS

- Food impaction or recurrent solid-food dysphagia in a young, adult male: Think EoE.
- EoE commonly mimics disorders like GERD and PPI-REE.
- A PPI trial is now required prior to the diagnosis of EoE.
- Remember "red flags" in patients with empiric GERD: Dysphagia, odynophagia, weight loss, early satiety or vomiting, aspiration/wheezing/cough, GI bleed, unexplained iron-deficiency anemia, age >50. Each "red flag" justifies EGD.

EPICONDYLITIS
Kevin Heaton, DO

BASICS

DESCRIPTION
- Tendon injury characterized by pain and tenderness at the tendinous origins of the wrist flexors/extensors on the epicondyles of the humerus
- May be acute (traumatic) or chronic (overuse)
- 2 types:
  - Medial epicondylitis or "golfer's elbow":
    - Involvement of the wrist flexors and pronators on the medial epicondyle
  - Lateral epicondylitis or "tennis elbow":
    - Involvement of the wrist extensors and supinators on the lateral epicondyle
- May be caused by many different athletic or occupational activities
- Common in carpenters, plumbers, gardeners, and politicians
- Usually occurs unilaterally on the epicondyles of the dominant arm
- Lateral epicondyle involvement is more common than medial.

EPIDEMIOLOGY
- Predominant age: >40
- Predominant sex: Male = Female

Incidence
- Very common site of overuse injury
- Lateral > Medial
- Estimated between 1% and 3%

Prevalence
- Lateral epicondylitis: 1.3%
- Medial epicondylitis: 0.4%

ETIOLOGY AND PATHOPHYSIOLOGY
- Acute (tendonitis):
  - Inflammatory response to injury
- Chronic (tendinosis):
  - Overuse injury
  - Tendon degeneration, fibroblast proliferation, microvascular proliferation, lack of inflammatory response
- Repetitive wrist motions
- Tool/racquet gripping
- Shaking hands
- Sudden maximal muscle contraction
- Direct blow

RISK FACTORS
- Repetitive wrist motions:
  - Flexion/Pronation: Medial
  - Extension/Supination: Lateral
- Smoking
- Obesity
- Upper extremity forceful activities

GENERAL PREVENTION
- Limit overuse of the wrist flexors, extensors, pronators, and supinators.
- Use proper techniques when working or playing racquet sports.
- Use lighter tools and smaller grips.

DIAGNOSIS

HISTORY
- Occupational activities
- Sport participation
- Direct trauma
- Duration of symptoms
- Treatments or medication use
- Pain with gripping
- Sensation of mild forearm weakness

PHYSICAL EXAM
- Localized pain just distal to the affected epicondyle
- Increased pain with wrist flexion/pronation (medial)
- Increased pain with wrist extension/supination (lateral)
- Medial epicondylitis:
  - Tenderness at origin of wrist flexor tendons
  - Increased pain with resisted wrist flexion and pronation
  - Normal elbow range of motion
  - Increased pain with gripping
- Lateral epicondylitis:
  - Tenderness at origin of wrist extensors
  - Increased pain with resisted wrist extension/supination
  - Normal elbow range of motion
  - Increased pain with gripping

DIFFERENTIAL DIAGNOSIS
- Elbow osteoarthritis
- Fractures of the epicondyles
- Posterior interosseous nerve entrapment (lateral)
- Ulnar neuropathy (medial)
- Synovitis
- Medial collateral ligament injury
- Referred pain from shoulder or neck

DIAGNOSTIC TESTS & INTERPRETATION
Initial Tests (lab, imaging)
No imaging is required for initial evaluation and treatment of a classic overuse injury.
Follow-Up Tests & Special Considerations
- Anterior-posterior/lateral radiographs if decreased range of motion, trauma, or no improvement with initial conservative therapy. Assess for fractures or signs of arthritis.
- For recalcitrant cases:
  - Musculoskeletal US can show abnormal tendon appearance (e.g., tendon thickening, partial tear at tendon origin, calcifications) and neovascularity when color flow Doppler is used. It can also be used to guide steroid or other alternative injections.
  - MRI can show intermediate or high T2 signal intensity within the common flexor or extensor tendon or the presence of peritendinous soft tissue edema.

Diagnostic Procedures/Other
A local anesthetic could be injected to document resolution of symptoms if the diagnosis is in doubt.

TREATMENT

GENERAL MEASURES
Initial treatment consists of activity modification, counterforce bracing, oral or topical NSAIDs, ice, and physical therapy:
- Observation: If left untreated, symptoms typically last between 6 months and 2 years. For patients with good function and minimal pain, conservative management with a "wait and see" policy may be considered.
- Activity modification, relative rest, and correction of faulty biomechanics
- Counterforce bracing with a forearm "tennis elbow" strap is easy to use and inexpensive. Systematic reviews have been unable to provide a solid conclusion about overall efficacy, but initial bracing may improve a patient's ability to perform daily activities in the first 6 weeks.
- Nighttime wrist splinting can also be effective. Consider for repetitive daily activities if counterforce bracing fails.
- Frequent ice application after activities
- Physical therapy:
  - Begin once acute pain is resolved.
  - Eccentric strength training regimen and stretching program
  - US therapy
  - Corticosteroid iontophoresis

MEDICATION
First Line
- Topical NSAIDs: Significantly more effective than placebo with respect to pain and participant satisfaction in the short term (≤6 weeks) with minimal adverse effects (1)[A]
- Oral NSAIDs: Some evidence for short-term (≤6 weeks) benefit with respect to pain and function, but this benefit is not sustained. Associated with GI adverse effects (1)[A].

Second Line
Corticosteroid injections: Short-term (≤6 weeks) reduction in pain, global improvement, and grip strength compared to placebo, local anesthetic, and conservative treatments. No benefits found for intermediate or long-term outcomes (1)[A].

ISSUES FOR REFERRAL
Failure of conservative therapy

ADDITIONAL THERAPIES

- Platelet-rich plasma injections (2)[B]:
  – Involves the injection of a concentrated portion of the patient's platelet-rich plasma. The localized injection leads to a local inflammatory response causing the platelets to degranulate, releasing growth factors, which then stimulates the physiologic healing cascade.
- US-guided percutaneous needle tenotomy (3)[C]:
  – Involves the injection of a local anesthetic followed by US-guided tendon fenestration, calcification fragmentation and aspiration, and abrading the underlying bone. The procedure is thought to break apart scar tissue and stimulate an inflammatory and healing response.
- Prolotherapy (4)[B]:
  – Involves the injection of a dextrose solution into and around the tendon attachment. This stimulates a localized inflammatory response, leading to increased blood supply to the area, which increases the flow of nutrients and healing mediators to stimulate tendon healing.
- Glyceryl trinitrate (GTN) transdermal patch (5)[B]:
  – Nitric oxide (NO) is a small, free radical generated by 3 isoenzymes called nitric oxide synthases. NO is expressed by fibroblasts and is postulated to aid in collagen synthesis. Topical application of glyceryl trinitrate theoretically improves healing by this mechanism. 1/4 of a 5-mg/24-hour GTN transdermal patch is applied once daily for up to 24 weeks.
- Botulinum toxin A for chronic lateral epicondylitis:
  – Injections into the forearm extensor muscles (60 units) can be performed in the outpatient setting.

SURGERY/OTHER PROCEDURES

- Elbow surgery may be indicated in refractory cases:
  – Fair evidence for treatment (6)[A]
  – Involves débridement and release of the involved tendons
  – Can be performed open or arthroscopically
- Denervation of the lateral humeral epicondyle
  – Transection of the posterior cutaneous nerve of the forearm with implantation into the triceps may help with chronic symptoms and pain.

COMPLEMENTARY AND ALTERNATIVE MEDICINE

Acupuncture (1)[A]: Effective for short-term pain relief for lateral epicondyle pain

 ## ONGOING CARE

PROGNOSIS
Good: Majority resolve with conservative care.

REFERENCES

1. Coombes BK, Bisset L, Vicenzino B. Efficacy and safety of corticosteroid injections and other injections for management of tendinopathy: A systematic review of randomised controlled trials. *Lancet.* 2010;376(9754):1751–1767.
2. Taylor DW, Petrera M, Hendry M, et al. A systematic review of the use of platelet-rich plasma in sports medicine as a new treatment for tendon and ligament injuries. *Clin J Sport Med.* 2011;21(4):344–352.
3. McShane JM, Shah VN, Nazarian LN. Sonographically guided needle tenotomy for treatment of common extensor tendinosis in the elbow: Is a corticosteroid necessary? *J Ultrasound Med.* 2008;27(8):1137–1144.
4. Rabago D, Best TM, Zgierska A, et al. A systematic review of four injection therapies for lateral epicondylosis: Prolotherapy, polidocanol, whole blood and platelet-rich plasma. *Br J Sports Med.* 2009;43:471–481.
5. Paoloni JA, Murrell GAC, Burch RM, et al. Randomised, double-blind, placebo-controlled clinical trial of a new topical glyceryl trinitrate patch for chronic lateral epicondylosis. *Br J Sports Med.* 2009;43:299–302.
6. Yeoh KM, King GJ, Faber KJ, et al. Evidence-based indications for elbow arthroscopy. *Arthroscopy.* 2012;28(2):272–282.

ADDITIONAL READING

- Cullinane FL, Boocock MG, Trevelyan FC. Is eccentric exercise an effective treatment for lateral epicondylitis? A systematic review. *Clin Rehabil.* 2013 Jul 23. [Epub ahead of print].
- Dingemanse R, Randsdorp M, Koes BW, et al. Evidence for the effectiveness of electrophysical modalities for treatment of medial and lateral epicondylitis: a systematic review. *Br J Sports Med.* 2013; Jan 18. [Epub ahead of print].

- Kalichman L, Bannuru RR, Severin M, et al. Injection of botulinum toxin for treatment of chronic lateral epicondylitis: Systematic review and meta-analysis. *Semin Arthritis Rheum.* 2011;40(6):532–538. Epub 2010 Sep 6.
- Rose NE, Forman SK, Dellon AL. Denervation of the lateral humeral epicondyle for treatment of chronic lateral epicondylitis. *J Hand Surg Am.* 2013;38(2):344–349.

 ## SEE ALSO

Algorithm: Pain in Upper Extremity

 ## CODES

ICD10
- M77.00 Medial epicondylitis, unspecified elbow
- M77.01 Medial epicondylitis, right elbow
- M77.10 Lateral epicondylitis, unspecified elbow

CLINICAL PEARLS

- Tendon injury characterized by pain and tenderness at the tendinous origins of the wrist flexors/extensors on the epicondyles of the humerus
- 2 types:
- Medial epicondylitis or "golfer's elbow" involves wrist flexors and pronators on the medial epicondyle.
- Lateral epicondylitis or "tennis elbow" involves wrist extensors and supinators on the lateral epicondyle.
- If left untreated, symptoms typically last between 6 months and 2 years.
- Most patients will improve with conservative treatment.
- NSAIDs first line; steroid injection second line
- Frequent ice application after activities
- Elbow straps during activity (counterforce bracing)
- Physical therapy as symptoms improve

E

EPIDIDYMITIS

Katherine Vlasica, DO

BASICS

- Acute epididymitis: Pain for <6 weeks
- Chronic epididymitis: Pain for >3 months

DESCRIPTION

- Inflammation (infectious or noninfectious) of epididymis resulting in scrotal pain and swelling, induration of the posterior epididymis, and eventual scrotal wall edema, involvement of the adjacent testicle, and hydrocele formation
- Classification: Infectious (bacterial, viral, fungal, parasitic) versus sterile (chemical, traumatic, autoimmune, idiopathic, industrial, noninfectious, vasoepididymal reflux syndrome, vasal reflux syndrome); chronic versus acute
- System(s) affected: Reproductive
- Synonym(s): Epididymo-orchitis

EPIDEMIOLOGY

- Predominant age: Usually younger, sexually active men or older men with UTIs; in older men, usually secondary to bladder outlet obstruction
- Predominant sex: Male only

Pediatric Considerations

In prepubertal boys: Epididymitis is found to be the most common cause of acute scrotum—more common than testicular torsion.

Incidence

- Common (600,000 cases annually in the US) (1)
- 1 in 1,000 males per year

Prevalence

Common

ETIOLOGY AND PATHOPHYSIOLOGY

- Infectious epididymitis:
  - Retrograde passage of urine or urinary bacteria from the prostate or urethra to the epididymis via the ejaculatory ducts and the vas deferens; rarely, hematogenous spread
  - Causative organism is identified in 80% of patients, and varies according to patient age.
- Sterile epididymitis:
  - Can develop as a sequelae of strenuous exercise with a full bladder when urine is pushed through internal urethral sphincter (located at proximal end of prostatic urethra).
  - Reflux of urine through orifice of ejaculatory ducts at verumontanum may occur with history of urethritis/prostatitis, as inflammation may produce rigidity in musculature surrounding orifice to ejaculatory ducts, holding them open.
  - Exposure of epididymis to foreign fluid may produce inflammatory reaction within 24 hours.
- <35 years and sexually active:
  - Usually *Chlamydia trachomatis* or *Neisseria gonorrhoeae*
  - Look for serous urethral discharge (chlamydia) or purulent discharge (gonorrhea).
  - With anal intercourse, likely *Escherichia coli* or *Haemophilus influenzae*

- >35 years:
  - Coliform bacteria usually, but sometimes *Staphylococcus aureus* or *S. epidermidis*
  - In elderly men, often with distal urinary tract obstruction, BPH, UTI, or catheterization
  - Tuberculosis, if sterile pyuria and nodularity of vas deferens (hematogenous spread)
  - Sterile urine reflux after transurethral prostatectomy
  - Granulomatous reaction following BCG intravesical therapy for bladder cancer
- Prepubertal boys:
  - Usually coliform bacteria
  - Evaluate for underlying congenital abnormalities, such as vesicoureteral reflux, ectopic ureter, or anorectal malformation (rectourethral fistula).
- Amiodarone may cause noninfectious epididymitis; resolves with decreasing drug dosage.
- Syphilis, blastomycosis, coccidioidomycosis, and cryptococcosis are rare causes, but brucellosis can be a common cause in endemic areas (2).

RISK FACTORS

- UTI, prostatitis
- Indwelling urethral catheter
- Urethral instrumentation or transurethral surgery
- Urethral or meatal stricture
- Transrectal prostate biopsy
- Prostate brachytherapy (seeds) for prostate cancer
- Anal intercourse
- High-risk sexual activity
- Strenuous physical activity
- Prolonged sedentary periods
- Bladder obstruction (benign prostatic hyperplasia, prostate cancer)
- HIV-immunosuppressed patient
- Severe Behçet disease
- Presence of foreskin (3)
- Constipation
- Sterile epididymitis:
  - Increased intra-abdominal pressure (due to frequent physical strain):
    ○ Military recruits, especially who begin physically unprepared
    ○ Laborers; restaurant kitchen workers
    ○ Full bladder during intense physical exertion

GENERAL PREVENTION

- Vasectomy or vasoligation during transurethral surgery
- Safer sexual practices
- Mumps vaccination
- Antibiotic prophylaxis for urethral manipulation
- Early treatment of prostatitis/benign prostatic hyperplasia (BPH)
- Avoid vigorous rectal exam with acute prostatitis.
- Sterile epididymitis:
  - Emptying the bladder prior to physical exertion
  - Physically conditioning the body prior to engaging in regular intense physical exertion (4)
  - Treat constipation

COMMONLY ASSOCIATED CONDITIONS

- Prostatitis/Urethritis/Orchitis
- Hemospermia
- Constipation
- UTI

DIAGNOSIS

- Scrotal pain, sometimes radiating to the groin region, may begin acutely over several hours.
- Urethral discharge or symptoms of UTI, such as frequency of urination, dysuria, cloudy urine, or hematuria (5)
- Initially, only the posterior-lying epididymis, usually the lowermost tail section, is very tender and indurated; will eventually progress to involvement of body and head of epididymis.
- Elevation of the testes/epididymis reduces the discomfort (Prehn sign).
- Entire hemiscrotum becomes swollen and red; the testis becomes indistinguishable from the epididymis; the scrotal wall becomes thick and indurated; and reactive hydrocele may occur.
- Sterile epididymitis:
  - Unilateral scrotal pain and swelling preceded by several hours of intense physical exertion. Patient may recall full bladder prior to exertion.
  - No symptoms of infection

Pediatric Considerations

- In prepubertal patients, may be postinfectious inflammatory condition; treat with anti-inflammatories, analgesics, and usually no antibiotics (6).
- Bacteremia from *Haemophilus influenzae* infection may produce acute epididymitis.
- In adolescent males, particularly age >13 years, must rule out testicular torsion
- History not helpful in distinguishing epididymitis from testicular torsion.

Geriatric Considerations

Diabetics with sensory neuropathy may have no pain despite severe infection/abscess.

PHYSICAL EXAM

- The tail of the epididymis is larger in comparison with the contralateral side.
- Epididymis is markedly tender to palpation.
- Absence of a cremasteric reflex should raise suspicion for testicular torsion.

DIFFERENTIAL DIAGNOSIS

- Epidymal congestion following vasectomy
- Testicular torsion
- Torsion of testicular appendages
- Orchitis
- Testicular malignancy
- Testicular trauma
- Epididymal cyst
- Inguinal hernia
- Urethritis
- Spermatocele
- Hydrocele
- Hematocele
- Varicocele
- Epididymal adenomatoid tumor
- Epididymal rhabdomyosarcoma
- Vasculitis (Henoch-Schönlein purpura)

DIAGNOSTIC TESTS & INTERPRETATION
Initial Tests (lab, imaging)
- Urinalysis and urine culture, preferably on first void urine
- GC/Chlamydia testing (urethral swab or urine testing)
- Gram stain urethral discharge
- WBC count may be elevated.
- Urinalysis clear and culture-negative suggest sterile epididymitis
- If testicular torsion cannot be excluded (especially in pediatrics), Doppler ultrasound is test of choice (1)
- In adult men, Doppler ultrasound: Sensitivity and specificity of 100% in evaluation of acute scrotum (7)

Pediatric Considerations
Further radiographic imaging in children should be done to rule out anatomic abnormalities.

Diagnostic Procedures/Other
This is a clinical diagnosis.

Test Interpretation
- Epididymis:
  - Surrounding tissue fibrosis and scarring
  - Interstitial, nonspecific acute infiltration, edema, congestion, PMNs, and lymphocytes
  - Fine inflammatory adhesions
  - Can progress to abscess or necrosis (4)
- Vas deferens:
  - Possible fibrosis of this structure

TREATMENT

- Bed rest or restriction on activity
- Athletic scrotal supporter
- Scrotal elevation
- Ice pack/warm compress
- If chemical epididymitis:
  - No strenuous physical activity and avoidance of any Valsalva maneuvers for several weeks
  - Empty bladder prior to strenuous exercises.

GENERAL MEASURES
Spermatic cord block with local anesthesia in severe cases

MEDICATION
First Line
- <35 years, for chlamydia: Doxycycline 100 mg PO b.i.d. for 10 days PO ceftriaxone 250 mg IM × 1. Treat sexual partner(s) (8).
- If penicillin-allergic or participates in insertive anal intercourse: Ciprofloxacin (Cipro) 500 mg PO b.i.d. or ofloxacin (Floxin) 200 mg PO b.i.d. for 10 days
- Older men with bacteriuria:
  - Levofloxacin (Levaquin) 500 mg/d PO for 7–10 days (8)
  - Ofloxacin 300 mg PO b.i.d. for 10 days (8)
  - Ciprofloxacin (Cipro) 500 mg PO b.i.d. or ciprofloxacin (Cipro XL) 1,000 mg/d for 10–14 days
- Analgesia (infectious and chemical epididymitis):
  - NSAIDs (e.g., naproxen or ibuprofen) for mild to moderate pain
  - Consider corticosteroid if patient cannot tolerate NSAID.
  - Acetaminophen-codeine or acetaminophen-oxycodone for moderate-to-severe pain

- Septic or toxic patient:
  - 3rd-generation cephalosporin or aminoglycoside
- For Beçhet, sarcoid, Henoch-Schönlein purpura:
  - Corticosteroids, such as methylprednisolone, 40 mg/d recommended

Second Line
- Trimethoprim-sulfamethoxazole (Bactrim, Septra) double-strength PO b.i.d. for 10–14 days; increasing bacterial resistance may limit effectiveness.
- Add rifampin (rifampicin) or vancomycin, as required.

ISSUES FOR REFERRAL
- If suspicion is high for testicular torsion or cancer, consult a urologist.
- Epididymitis in prepubertal boys requires a urology referral due to high incidence of associated urogenital abnormalities.
- If medical management fails, should be referred to urologist to rule out anatomic abnormality or chemical epididymitis.

SURGERY/OTHER PROCEDURES
- Vasostomy to drain infected material if severe or refractory case
- Scrotal exploration if unable clinically to distinguish between epididymitis or testicular torsion
- Drainage of abscesses, epididymectomy (acute suppurative), or epididymo-orchiectomy in severe cases refractory to antibiotics
- Surgery to correct underlying anatomic abnormality or obstruction

IN-PATIENT CONSIDERATIONS
Admission Criteria/Initial Stabilization
- Intractable pain
- Sepsis
- Abscess
- Persistent vomiting
- Scheduled surgery
- Purulent drainage
- Most cases can be managed with outpatient care.

ONGOING CARE

FOLLOW-UP RECOMMENDATIONS
Patient Monitoring
- Office visits until all signs of infection have cleared
- In chemical epididymitis, follow up in 4 weeks to assess efficacy of NSAIDs and lifestyle changes.

DIET
If constipation is contributing to chemical epididymitis, consider a high-fiber diet.

PATIENT EDUCATION
- Stress completing course of antibiotics, even when asymptomatic.
- Early recognition and treatment of UTI or prostatitis
- Safer sexual practices
- If chemical epididymitis, then educate on noninfectious etiology and proper lifestyle changes.

PROGNOSIS
- Pain improves within 1–3 days, but induration may take several weeks/months to completely resolve.
- If bilateral involvement, sterility may result
- In chemical epididymitis, symptoms usually resolve in <1 week.

COMPLICATIONS
- Recurrent epididymitis
- Infertility
- Oligospermia
- Testicular necrosis or atrophy
- Secondary abscess formation
- Fournier gangrene (necrotizing synergistic infection)

REFERENCES
1. Trojian TH, Lishnak TS, Heiman D. Epididymitis and orchitis: An overview. *Am Fam Physician*. 2009;79: 583–587.
2. Akinci E, Bodur H, Cevik MA, et al. A complication of brucellosis: Epididymoorchitis. *Int J Infect Dis*. 2006;10:171–177.
3. Bennett RT, Gill B, Kogan SJ. Epididymitis in children: The circumcision factor? *J Urol*. 1998;160: 1842–1844.
4. Wolin LH. On the etiology of epididymitis. *J Urol*. 1971;105:531–533.
5. Tracy CR, Steers WD, Costabile R. Diagnosis and management of epididymitis. *Urol Clin North Am*. 2008;35:101–108; vii.
6. Somekh E, Gorenstein A, Serour F. Acute epididymitis in boys: Evidence of a post-infectious etiology. *J Urol*. 2004;171:391–394; discussion 394.
7. Rizvi SA, Ahmad I, Siddiqui MA, et al. Role of color Doppler ultrasonography in evaluation of scrotal swellings: Pattern of disease in 120 patients with review of literature. *Urol J*. 2011;8(1):60–65.
8. US Centers for Disease Control and Prevention. Drugs for sexually transmitted infections. *Treat Guidel Med Lett*. 2007;5(61):81–88.

CODES

ICD10
- N45.1 Epididymitis
- N45.3 Epididymo-orchitis

CLINICAL PEARLS
- With epididymitis, the pain is gradual in onset, and the tenderness is mostly posterior to the testis. With testicular torsion, the symptoms are quite rapid in onset, the testis will be higher in the scrotum and may have a transverse lie, and the cremasteric reflex will be absent. The absence of leukocytes on urine analysis and decreased blood flow on scrotal ultrasound with Doppler will suggest torsion.
- Prostatic massage is contraindicated in epididymitis because the risk for worsening local infection and potential for sepsis are increased with acute prostatitis.
- Chemical epididymitis is a clinical diagnosis of exclusion, and infectious causes are much more common, but certain occupations, such as soldiers and laborers, must be considered.

EPISCLERITIS

Robert A. Baldor, MD

BASICS

- Episcleritis is inflammation of the vascular connective tissue located superficial to the sclera.
- It is usually a self-limited condition, typically lasting ~21 days (1).
- Most cases resolve without treatment.
- Recommended treatment is topical and is aimed at relieving symptoms.

DESCRIPTION
- Defined as edema and injection confined to the episcleral tissue
- 2 types: Simple or nodular

EPIDEMIOLOGY
Occurs equally in men and women

Incidence
- Condition is typically not seen in childhood.
- Men: Usually in their 30s and 60s, with peak incidence occurring in the 40s
- Women: Peak incidence in their 40s and 50s
- Nodular episcleritis has a peak incidence in the 5th decade.
- Simple episcleritis is more common in the 4th decade

Prevalence
1 study found all cases of rheumatoid-associated episcleritis in females, consistent with the higher incidence of rheumatoid arthritis in women (2)

ETIOLOGY AND PATHOPHYSIOLOGY
Pathogenesis can be either immune or nonimmune:
- One example of a nonimmune mechanism is dry eye syndrome:
  - Histologic examination of this syndrome reveals widespread vasodilation, edema, and lymphocytic infiltration.

COMMONLY ASSOCIATED CONDITIONS
- Rheumatoid arthritis
- Inflammatory bowel disease
- Gout
- Herpes zoster
- Hypersensitivity disorders:
  - Rosacea
  - Contact dermatitis
  - Penicillin sensitivity
  - Erythema multiforme

DIAGNOSIS

Episcleritis is a clinical diagnosis (3)[C].

HISTORY
- A detailed history should be taken, including family history.
- Ask questions about any contact with chemical irritants/solvents, as well as if there is any history of rheumatic, connective tissue or skin disease, gout, venereal disease, tuberculosis, or sarcoidosis
- Discomfort occurs in 51% of patients and is equally common in simple and nodular types. The pain or discomfort is localized to the eye in 1/4 of patients with simple episcleritis and 1/3 of patients with nodular type.

PHYSICAL EXAM
- Check for visual acuity
- Simple episcleritis:
  - Diffuse edema of the episcleral tissue, sometimes infiltrated by grayish deposits appearing yellowish in red-free light
  - Vessels retained their normal position and architecture
  - Slit-lamp examination shows how deep the edema is with the narrow beam
  - Eyes are tender to touch (1/3 of patients).
- Nodular episcleritis:
  - Edema and infiltration were localized to 1 part of the globe.
  - Nodules are usually single, but can be multiple, reaching the size of a large pea.
  - Eyes are tender to touch (40% of patients).

- It is important to exclude other complications, such as glaucoma, uveitis, pars planitis, choroiditis, secondary retinal detachment, and optic neuritis.
- Complete physical exam (particularly the skin, joints, heart, and lung) should be done to assess for any associated conditions.

ALERT
Limitation of extraocular muscles and proptosis should lead to suspicion of involvement of posterior sclera.

DIFFERENTIAL DIAGNOSIS
- Scleritis that presents with intense pain, photophobia, and a deep red or purplish scleral hue:
  - Slit-lamp exam is used to detect scleral edema and involvement of the scleral vessels.
- Bacterial conjunctivitis
- Viral conjunctivitis
- Herpes keratitis

DIAGNOSTIC TESTS & INTERPRETATION
- Most patients with episcleritis do not require any further lab work or diagnostic studies.
- Studies would be indicated in patients with persistent or recurrent episcleritis attacks (3)[C].
- Evaluation can also be considered for patients whose history and physical exam suggest a systemic cause.
- CBC
- Rheumatoid arthritis latex agglutination test (typically used as the confirmatory test for rheumatoid factor)
- Serum uric acid
- Erythrocyte sedimentation rate (ESR)
- C-reactive protein (CRP)

TREATMENT

MEDICATION
Treatment for episcleritis typically consists of symptomatic relief. The goal is to suppress the inflammation, which, in turn, will relieve the discomfort and prevent any destructive changes from occurring. Most of the time, treatment is not needed.

First Line
- Topical lubricants are typically used for initial management of episcleritis, such as artificial tear preparations (e.g., Refresh Plus or Bion Tears) (3)[B].
- Topical glucocorticoids are useful for severe cases (3)[B].
  - Prednisolone 0.5% eye drops hourly until 24 hours after inflammation has subsided. Then reduce to t.i.d. for 4 days
  - Betamethasone 1% (Betnesol) eye ointment q.i.d.

ISSUES FOR REFERRAL
Rarely, an episode of episcleritis at the initial presentation can progress to scleritis. At this time, an ophthalmology referral may be needed.

ADDITIONAL THERAPIES
- Topical NSAIDs have not been shown to have a significant benefit (4)[B]
- Only 16.7% of patients with episcleritis required more than topical corticosteroids for treatment, and these patients required oral NSAIDs (5). Typically recommended is oral indomethacin, and it is usually prescribed 25 mg PO t.i.d. (2)[C].

IN-PATIENT CONSIDERATIONS
Episcleritis rarely requires inpatient management.

 # ONGOING CARE

FOLLOW-UP RECOMMENDATIONS
In 1 of the largest studies of episcleritis, it was found that episodes of episcleritis were usually self-limited and did not require any treatment.

PROGNOSIS
- Most of the patients have no ocular complications.
- Prognosis for episcleritis is excellent, with most patients making a full recovery.

COMPLICATIONS
Associated complications, such as anterior uveitis, keratitis, glaucoma, or secondary cataract, are uncommon and are never severe (5):
- Minimal corneal changes were seen in 15% of the patients with simple episcleritis and in 15% of patients with nodular disease, but none of these changes were severe.
- Keratitis is the most common complication in both simple and nodular disease.
- Low-grade anterior uveitis is seen with severe attacks of episcleritis: Onset of photophobia, pain, and decreased vision. This is best diagnosed by slit-lamp exam by an ophthalmologist.
- Anterior uveitis was present in 11% of patients with episcleritis and was mild. It is more commonly associated with scleritis (42%) than with episcleritis (11%) (6).

REFERENCES
1. Williams CP, Browning AC, Sleep TJ, et al. A randomised, double-blind trial of topical ketorolac vs artificial tears for the treatment of episcleritis. *Eye (Lond)*. 2005;19:739–742.
2. McGavin DD, Williamson J, Forrester JV, et al. Episcleritis and scleritis. A study of their clinical manifestations and association with rheumatoid arthritis. *Br J Ophthalmol*. 1976;60:192–226.
3. Cronau H, Kankanala RR, Mauger T. Diagnosis and management of red eye in primary care. *Am Fam Physician*. 2010;81:137–144.
4. Williams CP, Browning AC, Sleep TJ, et al. A randomised, double-blind trial of topical ketorolac vs artificial tears for the treatment of episcleritis. *Eye*. 2005;19:739–742.
5. Jabs DA, Mudun A, Dunn JP, et al. Episcleritis and scleritis: Clinical features and treatment results. *Am J Ophthalmol*. 2000;130:469–476.
6. Sainz de la Maza M, Jabbur NS, Foster CS, et al. Severity of scleritis and episcleritis. *Ophthalmology*. 1994;101:389–396.

 # CODES

ICD10
- H15.101 Unspecified episcleritis, right eye
- H15.102 Unspecified episcleritis, left eye
- H15.109 Unspecified episcleritis, unspecified eye

CLINICAL PEARLS
- Episcleritis typically is a benign disorder, and the associated complications, such as anterior uveitis, keratitis, secondary cataract, and glaucoma, are uncommon and never severe.
- Does not present with any decrease in visual acuity and is often not painful.
- Treatment is aimed at symptomatic relief and attacks usually resolve quickly.
- Episcleritis can be an early presentation of scleritis, which is more severe. Accurate diagnosis of episcleritis is important.

EPISTAXIS
William Valencia, MD • Ryan Pearson, MD

 BASICS

DESCRIPTION
- Hemorrhage from the nose involving either the anterior or posterior mucosal surfaces
- Synonym(s): Nosebleed

EPIDEMIOLOGY
Incidence
- In the US: Common
- Estimated lifetime incidence ~60%
- Bimodal, with peaks in children up to 15 and in adults >50 years
- Rare in children younger than age 2

ETIOLOGY AND PATHOPHYSIOLOGY
- Local vs. systemic disease. Most are due to local causes.
- Anterior: 90–95% of all cases (Kiesselbach plexus)
- Posterior: Usually branches of sphenopalatine arteries: May be asymptomatic or may present with other symptoms
- Idiopathic
- Local inflammation/irritation:
  – Infection
  – Irritant inhalation
  – Topical steroid use
  – Septal deviation (more air movement on 1 side)
  – Low humidity
- Trauma:
  – Epistaxis digitorum (nose picking)
  – Foreign bodies
  – Septal perforation
  – Sinus fracture

RISK FACTORS
- Local irritation from multiple causes (see "Etiology and Pathophysiology")
- Medications/Supplements, including aspirin and clopidogrel

GENERAL PREVENTION
- Humidification at night
- Cut fingernails to minimize picking.

COMMONLY ASSOCIATED CONDITIONS
- Vascular malformation/telangiectasia
- Neoplasm (rare, but consider in persistent unilateral cases)
- Systemic:
  – Coagulopathy: Primary or iatrogenic
  – Thrombocytopenia
  – Cirrhosis
  – Renal failure
  – Alcoholism
- No proven association with hypertension (HTN), but may make control of bleeding more difficult.

 DIAGNOSIS

HISTORY
- Initial presentation, including detail on which side bleeding began
- Trauma, including nose picking
- Previous episodes
- Comorbid conditions
- Current medications, including over-the-counter and supplements

PHYSICAL EXAM
- Blood loss through 1 or both nostrils in most cases is due to anterior nasal septal bleeding and can often be directly visualized.
- Focus on localizing site of bleeding to anterior vs. posterior nasal cavity.
- Patient seated, head forward, to avoid blood going down the posterior pharynx

DIFFERENTIAL DIAGNOSIS
- Diagnosis usually apparent; the differential for the etiology is key.
- Posterior bleeding must be included in the differential for any chronic blood loss.

DIAGNOSTIC TESTS & INTERPRETATION
- Indicated only in complicated cases
- Lab testing is not indicated in most uncomplicated cases in which bleeding is reasonably easily controlled and is not truly hemorrhagic.

Initial Tests (lab, imaging)
- Mild cases, responsive to pressure: No labs
- For recurrent or intractable cases
- CBC, platelet count, PT
- PT/PTT if on warfarin or other medications affecting coagulation
- Cross-match, when appropriate
- Toxicology screen when nasal use of illicit drugs is suspected

For most cases, imaging not indicated

Follow-Up Tests & Special Considerations
If recurrent unilateral epistaxis, especially if not responding to treatment measures, consider evaluation for neoplasm.

Diagnostic Procedures/Other
Nasal endoscopy

Pediatric Considerations
More likely anterior, idiopathic, and recurrent

Geriatric Considerations
More likely to be posterior bleed

 TREATMENT

- Most cases managed as outpatient (1)[B]
- Patient applies direct pressure by pinching the lower part of the nose for 5–20 minutes without a break. This will stop active bleeding in most patients.
- An ice pack placed over the dorsum of the nose may help with hemostasis.
- Inspect the nasal septum for the bleeding site.

GENERAL MEASURES
Resuscitation, as indicated. Use universal "ABC" approach.

MEDICATION
First Line
If general measures fail, affected naris may be sprayed with topical vasoconstrictor, such as phenylephrine or oxymetazoline.

Second Line
NosebleedQR: A nonprescription powder of hydrophilic polymer with potassium salt; induces scab formation

ISSUES FOR REFERRAL
- Posterior bleeding frequently requires an otolaryngology consultation.
- Intractable bleeding may require more specialized measures:
  – Endoscopic laser or electrocauterization
  – Angiography with arteriolar embolization

ADDITIONAL THERAPIES
- Nasal packing: Either with ribbon gauze or preformed nasal tampons. Systemic prophylactic antibiotics are unnecessary in the majority of patients with nasal packs; topical antibiotics may be as effective and cheaper (2)[B].
- FloSeal: A biodegradable hemostatic sealant (a thrombin-type gel) in 1 study more effective and better tolerated than packing (3)[B]
- If an actively bleeding anterior septal site is visualized, this may be treated with gentle and specific silver nitrate cautery for ~10 seconds for definitive treatment.

- Limit cautery (silver nitrate) to 1 side of septum, or wait 4–6 weeks in between treatments to reduce risk of perforation.
- Posterior: Posterior packing or tamponade with balloon devices (Foley catheter has been used)
- Recurrent epistaxis: Cochrane Review in children shows no difference in effectiveness between antiseptic nasal cream, petroleum jelly, silver nitrate cautery, or no treatment (4)[A]:
  – When using silver nitrate cautery, 75% is more effective and less painful than 95%
  – Silver nitrate cautery followed by 4 weeks of antiseptic cream may be better than antiseptic cream alone (5)[B].

SURGERY/OTHER PROCEDURES
- Packing:
  – Layering of Vaseline ribbon gauze:
    o For gauze packing, be certain both ends of the ribbon gauze protrude from the nostril.
    o Packing is layered from the floor upward.
    o Secure packing with gauze across the outside of the nostril.
  – Nasal tampon may be used after lubricating the tip with KY Jelly or antibiotic cream or ointment.
  – Additional saline may be needed to expand the tampon if the bleeding has slowed.
  – Merocel and Rapid Rhino packs are easier to use than gauze packing and are usually well tolerated.
- Posterior bleed:
  – In the emergent setting, this may be attempted utilizing a Foley catheter or a specific posterior packing balloon.
  – With both methods, the tubing is introduced through the nose similar to the passage of a nasogastric tube. Once it reaches the posterior oral pharynx, the balloon is inflated and the tubing is pulled back outward to tamponade the posterior bleeding source:
    o If using a Foley catheter (10–14 French), the balloon can be inflated with 10 mL of saline.
    o Traction is maintained with an umbilical cord clamp with adequate padding between the clip and the nose to avoid injury.

IN-PATIENT CONSIDERATIONS
Consider hospitalization for elderly or for patients with posterior bleeding or coagulopathy. May also consider if significant comorbidities.

Admission Criteria/Initial Stabilization
- Posterior bleed
- Hemodynamic changes
- Clotting dysfunction
- Universal "airway/breathing/circulation" (ABC) approach. Stop blood loss.

 ONGOING CARE

FOLLOW-UP RECOMMENDATIONS
Patient Monitoring
- When significant blood loss, hemodynamic monitoring
- 24-hour minimum of packing in place; some authors recommend 3–5 days. The latter recommendation carries the risk of mucosal injury and toxic shock syndrome. The former has the risk of rebleed, which usually occurs between 24 and 48 hours.

PATIENT EDUCATION
- Demonstrate proper pinching pressure techniques.
- Avoidance of trauma or irritants is key.
- Management of systemic illness and proper use of medication

PROGNOSIS
- Most are self-limited.
- Good results with proper treatment

COMPLICATIONS
- Septal perforation
- Pressure-induced tissue necrosis of the nasal mucosa
- Toxic shock syndrome with packing
- Arrhythmias triggered by packing

REFERENCES
1. Melia L, McGarry GW. Epistaxis: Update on management. *Curr Opin Otolaryngol Head Neck Surg.* 2011;19:30–35.
2. Biggs TC, Nghtingale K, Patel NN, et al. Should prophylactic antibiotics be used routinely in epistaxis patients with nasal packs? *Ann R Coll Surg Engl.* 2013; 95(1):40–42.
3. Mathiasen RA, Cruz RM. Prospective randomized, controlled clinical trial of a novel matrix hemostatic sealant in patients with acute anterior epistaxis. *Laryngoscope.* 2005;115:899–902.
4. Qureishi A, Burton MJ. Interventions for recurrent idiopathic epistaxis in children. *Cochrane Database Syst Rev.* 2012: CD004461
5. Calder N, Kang S, Fraser L, et al. A double-blind randomized controlled trial of management of recurrent nosebleeds in children. *Otolaryngol Head Neck Surg.* 2009;140:670–674.

ADDITIONAL READING
- Manes RP. Evaluating and managing the patient with nosebleeds. *Med Clin N Am.* 2010:903–912.
- Schlosser RJ. Epistaxis. *N Engl J Med.* 2009:360: 784–789.

 CODES

ICD10
R04.0 Epistaxis

CLINICAL PEARLS
- Most episodes are anterior in etiology and respond to timed pressure over the anterior nares for 5–20 minutes.
- Most are idiopathic or as a result of nose picking.
- Posterior nosebleeds can be asymptomatic or present with nausea, hematemesis, or heme-positive stool.
- Consider evaluation for neoplasm if recurrent unilateral episodes.

E

ERECTILE DYSFUNCTION

Michael Barros, PharmD, BCPS, BCACP • Neela Bhajandas, PharmD • Vishnu Kulasekaran, MD

 BASICS

DESCRIPTION
- Erectile dysfunction (ED): The consistent or recurrent inability to acquire or sustain an erection of sufficient rigidity and duration for sexual intercourse.
- In the past, ED was assumed to be a symptom of the aging process in men, but it can result from concurrent medical conditions of the patient or from medications that patients may be taking to treat those conditions.
- Sexual problems are frequent among older men and have a detrimental effect on their quality of life but are infrequently discussed with their physicians (1).
- Synonym(s): Impotence

ALERT
When ED occurs in a younger man, it is associated with a significantly increased risk of future cardiac events (2).

EPIDEMIOLOGY
Incidence
It is estimated that >600,000 new cases of ED will be diagnosed annually in the US, although this may be an underestimation of the true incidence, as ED is vastly underreported.

Prevalence
Overall prevalence for ED:
- 52% in men age 40–70 years
- Age-related increase ranging from 12.4% in men age 40–49 years up to 46.6% in men age 50–69 years

ETIOLOGY AND PATHOPHYSIOLOGY
- ED is a neurovascular event:
  - With stimulation, there is release of nitrous oxide, which increases production of cGMP.
  - This leads to relaxation of cavernous smooth muscle, leading to increased blood flow to penis.
  - As cavernosal sinusoids distend with blood, there is passive compression of subtunical veins, which decreases venous outflow and this leads to an erection.
- Alterations in any of these events leads to ED.
- ED may result from problems with systems required for normal penile erection:
  - Vascular: Diseases that compromise blood flow:
    ○ Peripheral vascular disease, arteriosclerosis, essential hypertension
  - Neurologic: Diseases that impair nerve conduction to brain or penile vasculature:
    ○ Spinal cord injury, stroke, diabetes
  - Endocrine: Diseases associated with changes in testosterone, luteinizing hormone, prolactin levels
  - Psychological: Patients suffering from malaise, depression, performance anxiety
- Social habits such as smoking or excessive alcohol intake
- Medications may cause ED.
- Structural injury or trauma (bicycling accident)

Genetics
Rarely related to chromosomal disorders

RISK FACTORS
- Advancing age
- Cardiovascular disease
- Diabetes mellitus
- Metabolic syndrome
- Cigarette smoking
- Urologic surgery, radiation, trauma/injury to pelvic area or spinal cord
- Medications that induce ED
- Central neurologic and endocrinologic conditions
- Substance abuse
- Psychological conditions: Stress, anxiety, or depression

GENERAL PREVENTION
The 2 best ways to prevent ED are by:
- Making healthy lifestyle choices by exercising regularly, eating well-balanced meals, limiting alcohol, and avoiding smoking
- Treating existing health problems and working with your patients to manage diabetes, heart disease, and other chronic problems

ALERT
Aging alone is not a cause.

COMMONLY ASSOCIATED CONDITIONS
- Cardiovascular disease:
  - Men with ED have a greater likelihood of having angina, myocardial infarction, stroke, transient ischemic attack, congestive heart failure, or cardiac arrhythmia compared to men without ED (3).
- Diabetes
- Psychiatric disorders

 DIAGNOSIS

Inability to achieve or maintain erection satisfactory for intercourse

HISTORY
- Identify concurrent medical illnesses or surgical procedures, history of trauma, and a list of current medications
- Psychosocial history: Smoking, ethanol intake, recreational drug use, anxiety and depression, satisfaction with current relationship
- Presence or absence of morning erections
- Detailed sexual history important to rule out premature ejaculation, as this is frequently confused with ED

PHYSICAL EXAM
- Signs and symptoms of hypogonadism: Gynecomastia, small testicles, decreased body hair
- Penile plaques (Peyronie disease)
- Detailed examination of the cardiovascular, neurologic, and genitourinary systems:
  - Check femoral and lower extremity pulses to assess vascular supply to genitals.
  - Check anal sphincter tone and genital reflexes, including cremasterics and bulbocavernosus.

DIFFERENTIAL DIAGNOSIS
- Premature ejaculation
- Decreased libido
- Anorgasmia
- Sudden versus chronic ED

DIAGNOSTIC TESTS & INTERPRETATION
Vascular and/or neurologic assessment, and monitoring of nocturnal erections may be indicated in select patients but not for routine workup (4)[C].

Initial Tests (lab, imaging)
- Fasting serum glucose level, lipid panel, TSH, and morning total testosterone level (3)[C]
- Doppler, angiogram, and cavernosogram are available radiologic modalities, but not recommended in routine practice for the diagnosis of ED (4)[C].

Follow-Up Tests & Special Considerations
Other hormonal tests, such as prolactin, should only be ordered when there is suspicion for a specific endocrinopathy.

Diagnostic Procedures/Other
Questionnaires can be offered to assess the severity of ED, including the International Index of Erectile Function (IEFF) and its validated and more easily administered abridged version, the Sexual Health Inventory for Men (SHIM) (4)[C].

 TREATMENT

- Lifestyle modifications and managing medications contributing to ED is first-line therapy for ED (5)[C]. Use least invasive therapy first; reserve more invasive therapies for nonresponders.
- Phosphodiesterase type 5 (PDE-5) inhibitor choice should be based on patient's preference (cost, ease of use, and adverse effects)

GENERAL MEASURES
- Psychotherapy alone or in combination with psychoactive drugs may be helpful in men whose ED is caused by depression or anxiety.
- Weight loss and increased physical activity for obese men with ED

MEDICATION
First Line
Phosphodiesterase type 5 (PDE-5) inhibitors are effective in the treatment of ED in many men, including those with diabetes mellitus and spinal cord injury, and sexual dysfunction associated with antidepressants (3)[A]. There is insufficient evidence to support the superiority of 1 agent over the others (5)[A]:
- Sildenafil (Viagra): Usual daily dose: 50–100 mg within at least 60 minutes of sexual intercourse.
- Vardenafil (Levitra): Usual daily dose 5–20 mg within at least 60 minutes of sexual intercourse.
- Vardenafil (Staxyn): ODT: Usual dose 10 mg within 60 minutes of sexual intercourse.

- Tadalafil (Cialis): Usual daily dose 5–20 mg within at least 30 minutes of sexual intercourse or 2.5 mg once daily without regard to sexual activity.
  - Adverse effects of PDE-5 inhibitors: Headache, facial flushing, dyspepsia, nasal congestion, dizziness, hypotension, increased sensitivity to light (sildenafil and vardenafil), vision changes, lower back pain (tadalafil), and priapism (with excessive doses)
  - Sildenafil and vardenafil should be taken on an empty stomach for maximum effectiveness

Geriatric Considerations
Use doses at the lower end of the dosing range for elderly patients:
- Sildenafil 25 mg daily
- Vardenafil 5 mg daily

Second Line

- Intraurethral and intracavernosal injectables are second-line therapies shown to be effective and should be administered based on patient preference (3)[B]. Intraurethral suppositories are a less invasive treatment option than intracavernosal injections; however, they are not as effective (5)[C]. Alprostadil, also known as prostaglandin E1, causes smooth muscle relaxation of the arterial blood vessels and sinusoidal tissues in the corpora:
  - Intraurethral alprostadil (Muse):
    - Urethral suppository: 125-, 250-, 500-, and 1,000-mcg pellets. Administer 5–50 minutes before intercourse. No more than 2 doses in 24 hours are recommended.
  - Intracavernosal alprostadil (available in 2 formulations):
    - Alprostadil (Caverject): Usual dose: 10–20 mcg, with max dose of 60 mcg. Injection should be made at right angles into one of the lateral surfaces of the proximal third of the penis using a 0.5-inch 27- or 30-gauge needle. Do not use >3 times a week or more than once in 24 hours.
    - Alprostadil may also be combined with papaverine (Bimix) plus phentolamine (Tri-Mix).

ALERT
- Initial trial dose should be administered under supervision of a specialist or primary care physician with expertise in these therapies.
- Patient should notify physician if erection lasts >4 hours for immediate attention.
- Vacuum pump devices are a noninvasive second-line option and are available over the counter. Do not use vacuum devices in men with sickle cell anemia or blood dyscrasias.
- Testosterone supplementation in men with hypogonadism improves ED and libido (3)[B]. Available formulations include injectable depots, transdermal patches and gels, SC pellets, and oral therapy.
- Contraindications:
  - Nitroglycerin (or other nitrates) and phosphodiesterase inhibitors: Potential for severe, potentially fatal hypotension

- Precautions/Side effects:
  - Testosterone: *Precautions*: Exogenous testosterone reduces sperm count and thus do not use in patients wishing to keep fertility; *side effects*: Acne, sodium retention
  - Intraurethral suppository: Local penile pain, urethral bleeding, dizziness, and dysuria
  - Intracavernosal injection: Penile pain, edema and hematoma, palpable nodules or plaques, and priapism
  - Sildenafil: Hypotension (caution for patients on nitrates)
  - PDE-5 inhibitors: Use caution with congenital prolonged QT syndrome, class Ia or II antiarrhythmics, nitroglycerin, α-blockers (e.g., terazosin, tamsulosin), retinal disease, unstable cardiac disease, liver and renal failure
  - Significant possible interactions:
  - PDE-5 inhibitor concentration is affected by CYP3A4 inhibitors (e.g., erythromycin, indinavir, ketoconazole, ritonavir, amiodarone, cimetidine, clarithromycin, delavirdine, diltiazem, fluoxetine, fluvoxamine, grapefruit juice, itraconazole, nefazodone, nevirapine, ritonavir, saquinavir, and verapamil). Serum concentrations and/or toxicity may be increased. Lower starting doses should be used in these patients.
  - PDE-5 inhibitor concentration may be reduced by rifampin and phenytoin.

ADDITIONAL THERAPIES

Behavioral therapy: Couples therapy aimed at improving relationship difficulties found that men who received this therapy plus sildenafil had more successful intercourse than those who received only sildenafil (6)[A].

SURGERY/OTHER PROCEDURES

Penile prosthesis should be reserved for patients who have failed or are ineligible first- or second-line therapies (3)[B].

COMPLEMENTARY AND ALTERNATIVE MEDICINE

Trazodone, yohimbine, and herbal therapies are not recommended for the treatment of ED, as they have not proven to be efficacious (5)[C].

 ONGOING CARE

FOLLOW-UP RECOMMENDATIONS
Patient Monitoring
Treatment should be assessed at baseline and after the patient has completed at least 1–3 weeks of a specific treatment: Monitor the quality and quantity of penile erections, and monitor the level of satisfaction patient achieves.

DIET
Diet and exercise recommended to achieve a normal body mass index; limit alcohol

PROGNOSIS

- All commercially available PDE-5 inhibitors are equally effective. In the presence of sexual stimulation, they are 55–80% effective (5)[A]:
  - Lower success rates with diabetes mellitus and radical prostatectomy patients who suffer from ED
- Overall effectiveness is 70–90% for intracavernosal alprostadil and 43–60% for intraurethral alprostadil (4)[B].
- Penile prostheses are associated with an 85–90% patient satisfaction rate (4)[C].

REFERENCES

1. Lindau ST, Schumm LP, Laumann EO, et al. A study of sexuality and health among older adults in the United States. *N Engl J Med*. 2007;357(8):762–774.
2. Inman BA, Sauver JL, Jacobson DJ, et al. A population-based, longitudinal study of erectile dysfunction and future coronary artery disease. *Mayo Clin Proc*. 2009;84(2):108–113.
3. Heidelbaugh JJ. Management of erectile dysfunction. *Am Fam Physician*. 2010;81:305–312.
4. McVary KT. Clinical practice. Erectile dysfunction. *N Engl J Med*. 2007;357:2472–2481.
5. The American Urological Association (AUA). Guideline on the management of erectile dysfunction: Diagnosis and treatment recommendations. Reviewed and Validitiy Confirmed in 2011.
6. Melnik T, Soares BGO, Nasselo AG. Psychosocial interventions for erectile dysfunction. *Cochrane Database Syst Rev*. 2007;(3):CD004825.

CODES

ICD10
- N52.1 Erectile dysfunction due to diseases classified elsewhere
- N52.9 Male erectile dysfunction, unspecified
- F52.21 Male erectile disorder

CLINICAL PEARLS

- Nitrates should be withheld for 24 hours after sildenafil or vardenafil administration and for 48 hours after use of tadalafil. PDE-5 inhibitors are contraindicated in patients taking concurrent nitrates of any form (regular or intermittent nitrate therapy) as it can lead to severe hypotension and syncope.
- Reserve surgical treatment for patients who do not respond to drug treatment.
- The use of PDE-5 inhibitors with alpha-adrenergic antagonists may increase the risk of hypotension. Tamsulosin is the least likely to cause orthostatic hypotension.
- ED serves as a predictor for future cardiovascular events; thus, these patients should be followed vigilantly.

ERYSIPELAS
Khasha Touloei, DO, MBS • Alissa Craft, DO, MBA

BASICS

DESCRIPTION
- Distinct form of cellulitis notable for acute, well-demarcated, superficial bacterial skin infection with lymphatic involvement almost always caused by *Streptococcus pyogenes*
- Usually acute, but a chronic recurrent form also exists (1)
- System(s) affected: Skin; Exocrine
- Synonym(s): Saint Anthony's Fire

EPIDEMIOLOGY
- Predominant age: Infants, children, and adults >40 years.
- Greatest in elderly (>75 years)
- No gender/racial predilection
- Affects all races

Incidence
- Erysipelas occurs in ~1/1,000 persons/year (2).
- Incidence on the rise since the 1980s (3)

Prevalence
Unknown

ETIOLOGY AND PATHOPHYSIOLOGY
- Group A streptococci induce inflammation and activation of the contact system, a proinflammatory pathway with antithrombotic activity, releasing proteinases and proinflammatory cytokines
- The generation of antibacterial peptides and the release of bradykinin, a proinflammatory peptide, increase vascular permeability and induce fever and pain.
- The M proteins from the group A streptococcal cell wall interact with neutrophils, leading to the secretion of heparin-binding protein, an inflammatory mediator that also induces vascular leakage.
- This cascade of reactions leads to the symptoms seen in erysipelas: Fever, pain, erythema, and edema.
- Group A β-hemolytic streptococci primarily; occasionally, other streptococcus groups C/G
- Rarely, group B streptococci/*Staphylococcus aureus* may be involved.

RISK FACTORS
- Disruption in the skin barrier (surgical incisions, insect bites, eczematous lesions, local trauma, abrasions, dermatophytic infections)
- Chronic diseases (diabetes, malnutrition, nephrotic syndrome, heart failure)
- Immunocompromised (HIV)/debilitated
- Fissured skin (especially at the nose and ears)
- Toe-web intertrigo and lymphedema (2)
- Leg ulcers/Stasis dermatitis
- Venous/Lymphatic insufficiency (saphenectomy, varicose veins of leg, phlebitis, radiotherapy, mastectomy, lymphadenectomy)
- Alcohol abuse
- Morbid obesity
- Recent streptococcal pharyngitis

GENERAL PREVENTION
- Good skin hygiene.
- It is recommended that predisposing medical conditions, such as tinea pedis and stasis dermatitis, be appropriately managed first.
- Men who shave within 5 days of facial erysipelas are more likely to have a recurrence.
- With recurrences, search for other possible sources of streptococcal infection (e.g., tonsils, sinuses).
- Compression stockings should be encouraged for patients with lower extremity edema.
- Consider suppressive prophylactic antibiotic therapy, such as penicillin, in patients with >2 episodes in a 12-month period.

Pediatric Considerations
Group B streptococcus may be a cause of erysipelas in neonates/infants.

DIAGNOSIS

Prodromal symptoms before the skin eruption of erysipelas may include:
- Moderate- to high-grade fever
- Chills
- Headache
- Malaise
- Anorexia, usually in the 1st 48 hours (4)[B]
- Vomiting
- Arthralgias

ALERT
It is important to differentiate erysipelas from a methicillin-resistant *S. aureus* (MRSA) infection, which usually presents with an indurated center, significant pain, and later evidence of abscess formation.

PHYSICAL EXAM
- Vital signs: Moderate- to high-grade fever with resultant tachycardia. Hypotension may occur.
- The presence of a fever in erysipelas can be considered a differentiating factor from other skin infections.
- Headache and vomiting may be prominent.
- Acute onset of erythematous plaque that is sharply demarcated, raised, fiery-red, tender, and spreads circumferentially over hours/days with marked swelling
- Peau d'orange appearance
- Vesicles and bullae may form, but are not uniformly present.
- Desquamation may occur later.
- Location:
  - Lower extremity 70–80% of cases
  - Face involvement is less common (5–20%), especially nose and ears
  - Chronic form usually recurs at site of the previous infection and may recur years after initial episode.
- Patients on systemic steroids may be more difficult to diagnose because signs and symptoms of the infection may be masked by anti-inflammatory action of the steroids.

- Systemic toxicity resolves rapidly with treatment; skin lesions desquamate on days 5–10, but usually heal without scarring.
- In geriatric patients, facial involvement presents in a butterfly pattern. Pustules characteristically absent, and regional lymphadenopathy with lymphangitic streaking is seen.

Pediatric Considerations
- Abdominal involvement more common in infants, especially around umbilical stump
- Face, scalp, and leg involvement common in older children due to the excoriations of anterior rhinitis sicca allowing an easy port of entry

Geriatric Considerations
- Fever may not be as prominent.
- Face and lower extremity are the most common areas.
- High-output cardiac failure may occur in debilitated patients with underlying cardiac disease.
- More susceptible to complications

DIFFERENTIAL DIAGNOSIS
- Cellulitis (margins are less clear)
- Necrotizing fasciitis (systemic illness and more pain)
- Dermatophytes
- Impetigo (blistered/crusted appearance; superficial)
- Ecthyma (ulcerative impetigo)
- Herpes zoster (dermatomal distribution)
- Erythema annulare centrifugum (raised pink-red ring/bulls-eye marks)
- Contact dermatitis (no fever, pruritic)
- Giant cell urticaria (transient, wheal-appearance, severe itching)
- Angioneurotic edema (no fever)
- Scarlet fever (widespread rash with indistinct borders and without edema; rash is most common early in skin folds; develops generalized "sandpaper" feeling as it progresses)
- Toxic shock syndrome (diffuse erythema with evidence of multiorgan involvement)
- Lupus (of the face; less fever, positive antinuclear antibodies)
- Polychondritis (common site is the ear)
- Other bacterial infections to consider:
  - Meat, shellfish, fish, and poultry workers: *Erysipelothrix rhusiopathiae* (known as erysipeloid)
  - Human bite: *Eikenella corrodens*
  - Cat/Dog bite: *Pasteurella multocida/Capnocytophaga canimorsus*
  - Salt water exposure: *Vibrio vulnificus*
  - Fresh/brackish water exposure: *Aeromonas hydrophilia*

DIAGNOSTIC TESTS & INTERPRETATION
Reserve diagnostic tests for severely ill, toxic patients, or those who are immunosuppressed.

Initial Tests (lab, imaging)
- Leukocytosis
- Blood culture (<5% positive)
- Elevated erythrocyte sedimentation rate (ESR) and C-reactive protein (CRP)
- Streptococci may be cultured from exudate/noninvolved sites.

Test Interpretation
Biopsy is not needed. However, skin findings would show:
- Dermal and epidermal edema, extending into the SC tissues
- Peau d'orange appearance caused by edema in the superficial tissue surrounding the hair follicles
- Vasodilation and enlarged lymphatics
- Mixed interstitial infiltrate mainly consisting of neutrophils and mononuclear cells
- Endothelial cell swelling
- Gram-positive cocci in lymphatics and tissue with rare invasion of local blood vessels
- Fibrotic thickening of lymphatic vessel walls with possible luminal occlusion may be seen in recurrent erysipelas.

 TREATMENT

GENERAL MEASURES
- Symptomatic treatment of myalgias and fever
- Adequate fluid intake
- Local treatment with cold compresses
- Elevation of affected extremity
- Appropriate therapy for any underlying predisposing condition

MEDICATION
First Line
- Adults:
  - Extremities, nondiabetic:
    - Primary:
    - Penicillin G: 1–2 million U IV q6h or (nafcillin or oxacillin 2 g IV q4h)
    - If not severe, dicloxacillin 500 mg PO q6h or cefazolin 1 g IV q8h
    - Alternative:
    - Erythromycin, cefazolin, azithromycin, clarithromycin, tigecycline
    - Ceftobiprole (CFB): 500 mg IV q12h
  - Diabetics:
    - Early-mild:
    - Trimethoprim-sulfamethoxazole (TMP-SMX)-DS: 1–2 tabs PO b.i.d. and penicillin VK 500 mg PO q.i.d. or cephalexin 500 mg PO q.i.d.
  - Severe disease:
    - IMP or MER or ERTA IV and linezolid 600 mg IV/PO b.i.d. or vancomycin IV
  - Facial:
    - Primary:
    - Vancomycin: 1 g IV q12h
    - If the patient is >100 kg, give 1.5 g IV q12h
    - Alternative:
    - Linezolid: 600 mg IV q12h
- Children:
  - Mild:
    - Penicillin VK:
    - <12 years: 25–50 mg/kg/d PO divided q6–8h max 3 g/d
    - >12 years: Adult dose
    - Penicillin G procaine:
    - <30 kg: 300,000 U/d IM
    - >30 kg: Adult dose
  - Severe:
    - Nafcillin or oxacillin 2 g IV q4h or penicillin G parenterally is recommended for severe/complicated cases (1–2 million U q4–6h).
- No reported group A streptococci resistance to β-lactam antibiotics

- In chronic recurrent infections, prophylactic treatment after the acute infection resolves:
  - Penicillin G benzathine: 1.2 million U IM every month or penicillin VK 250 mg PO b.i.d.
- If staphylococcal infection is suspected or patient is acutely ill, consider a β-lactamase-stable antibiotic.
- Consider community-acquired MRSA and, depending on regional sensitivity, may treat MRSA with TMP-SMX, clindamycin, or tetracycline. If resistance is a concern or patient is clinically unstable, treat with vancomycin, daptomycin, or linezolid.

ISSUES FOR REFERRAL
Recurrent infection, treatment failure

ADDITIONAL THERAPIES
Some patients may notice a deepening of erythema after initiating antimicrobial therapy. This may be due to the destruction of pathogens that release enzymes, increasing local inflammation. In this case, treatment with corticosteroids in addition to antimicrobials can mildly reduce healing time and antibiotic duration in patients with erysipelas. Consider prednisolone 30 mg/d with taper over 8 days (5).

IN-PATIENT CONSIDERATIONS
Admission Criteria/Initial Stabilization
- Patient with systemic toxicity
- Patient with high-risk factors (e.g., elderly, lymphedema, postsplenectomy, diabetes)
- Outpatient care

IV Fluids
IV therapy if systemic toxicity/unable to tolerate PO

Discharge Criteria
No evidence of systemic toxicity with resolution of erythema and swelling

 ONGOING CARE

FOLLOW-UP RECOMMENDATIONS
Bed rest with elevation of extremity during acute infection, then activity as tolerated

Patient Monitoring
Patients should be treated until all symptoms and skin manifestations have resolved.

PATIENT EDUCATION
Stress importance of completing prescribed medication regimen.

PROGNOSIS
- Patients should recover fully if adequately treated.
- Mortality is <1% in patients receiving appropriate treatment.
- Bullae formation suggests longer disease course, and often indicates a concomitant S. aureus infection that may require antibiotic coverage for MRSA.
- Chronic edema/scarring may result from chronic recurrent cases.
- Rarely, obstructive lymphadenitis may result from chronic recurrent cases.

COMPLICATIONS
- Recurrent infection
- Abscess (suggests staphylococcal infection)
- Necrotizing fasciitis
- Lymphedema
- Bacteremia (which may lead to sepsis/involvement of other organ systems)

- Sepsis
- Pneumonia (due to sepsis/toxin-producing organism)
- Meningitis (due to sepsis/toxin-producing organism)
- Embolism
- Gangrene
- Bursitis, septic arthritis, tendinitis, or osteitis

REFERENCES
1. Gabillot-Carré M, Roujeau JC. Acute bacterial skin infections and cellulitis. *Curr Opin Infect Dis*. 2007;20:118–123.
2. Bernard P. Management of common bacterial infections of the skin. *Curr Opin Infect Dis*. 2008;21:122–128.
3. Celestin R, Brown J, Kihiczak G, et al. Erysipelas: A common potentially dangerous infection. *Acta Dermatovenerol Alp Panonica Adriat*. 2007;16: 123–127.
4. Stevens DL. Practice guidelines for the diagnosis and management of skin and soft tissue infections. *Clin Infect Dis*. 2005;41:1973.
5. Bergkvist PI, Sjöbeck K. Antibiotic and prednisolone therapy of erysipelas: A randomized, double blind, placebo-controlled study. *Scand J Infect Dis*. 1997;29:377–382.

ADDITIONAL READING
- Breen JO. Skin and soft tissue infections in immunocompetent patients. *Am Fam Physician*. 2010;81:893–899.
- Gilbert D, Moellering RC, Eliopoulos GM, eds. *The Sanford guide to antimicrobial therapy 2010*. Sperryville, VA: Sanford Guides; 2010.

 CODES

ICD10
A46 Erysipelas

CLINICAL PEARLS
- Athlete's foot is the most common portal of entry for this superficial bacterial skin infection caused by *Streptococcus pyogenes*.
- Erysipelas is distinguished from cellulitis by its sharp, shiny, fiery-red, raised border.
- In recurrent cases, search for other possible source of streptococcal infection (e.g., tonsils, sinuses, intertrigo).
- Most erysipelas infections now occur on the legs, rather than the face.

ERYTHEMA MULTIFORME

Eric C. Wilkerson, MD • M. Tye Haeberle, MD • Cindy England Owen, MD

BASICS

- Erythema multiforme (EM) is an acute, self-limited hypersensitivity reaction:
  - Mostly (~90% of cases) triggered by infectious agents (up to 50% by herpes simplex virus [HSV]-1 or -2) or, less commonly, by drugs (1,2)
  - Involving the skin and the mucous membrane, most commonly the mouth (60–70% of all patients with EM have oral lesions) (3)
  - Skin lesions include raised typical target or "iris" lesions or raised atypical lesions predominantly involving the extremities; flat, atypical lesions and macules with or without blisters are more suggestive of Stevens-Johnson (SJS) or toxic epidermal necrolysis (TEN) (4).
- Currently, there are no universal diagnostic criteria for EM. It was previously considered a spectrum of disease, consisting of EM, EM major, SJS, and TEN; however, a growing consensus believes EM is a condition distinct from SJS and TEN due to the differences in clinical presentation, histopathologic features, patient demographics, possible etiology and pathogenesis, and treatment plan (1,2,4–6).

DESCRIPTION

- 2 subtypes, erythema multiforme minor (EMm) and erythema multiforme major (EMM), with the former involving none or 1 mucous membrane, and the latter involving at least 2 mucous membrane sites (1)
- Recurrent EM is defined as >3 attacks, but has a mean number of 6 attacks (range 2–24) per year and a mean duration of 6–9.5 years (range 2–36) (1,7).

EPIDEMIOLOGY

Incidence
Annual US incidence is estimated at 0.01–1% (6).

Prevalence
- Peak incidence in 20s and 40s; rare <3 and >50
- Male > Female (3:2–2:1) (1,2)

ETIOLOGY AND PATHOPHYSIOLOGY

- The exact pathophysiology of EM is unknown.
- Possible immunologically mediated lymphocytic reaction to an infectious agent or a drug at the dermal–epidermal junction
- HSV-triggered EM seems to involve CD4+ T-cell infiltration and associated IFN-γ activation.
- Drug-triggered EM (<10% of cases) involves CD8+ T-cells and associated TNF-α activation (6).
- Most cases appear to be due to a preceding infection (~90% of cases).
- Viral infections, particularly HSV (up to 50% of cases); also Epstein-Barr, coxsackie, echovirus, varicella, mumps, poliovirus, hepatitis C, cytomegalovirus, HIV, molluscum contagiosum virus
- Bacterial infections, particularly *Mycoplasma pneumoniae;* other reported bacterial infections include *Treponema pallidum,* and *Gardnerella vaginalis*
- Fungal infection, including *Histoplasma capsulatum* and *Coccidioides immitis*

- Medications, including sulfonamides, penicillins, anticonvulsants (carbamazepine, phenytoin, phenylbutazone, phenothiazines, barbiturates), hydantoins, NSAIDs (including rofecoxib, valdecoxib), oral contraceptives, and statins. Other sparsely reported medications include cimetidine, salicylic acid, angiotensin receptor blockers (ARBs; candesartan, metformin, bupropion, ciprofloxacin, sorafenib, gemfibrozil, risperidone, paclitaxel, metoprolol, tumor necrosis factor (TNF) inhibitors (adalimumab, etanercept, infliximab), and methotrexate (3)
- Vaccines: Tetanus/Diphtheria, bacillus Calmette-Guérin, oral polio, hepatitis B, human papillomavirus, H1N1 influenza
- Occupational exposures: Herbicides (alachlor and butachlor), iodoacetonitrile
- Protozoan infections
- Radiation therapy
- Premenstrual hormone changes
- Sarcoidosis
- Cannabis-induced EM-like drug eruption
- Rowell's syndrome: lupus erythematosus (specifically, chronic cutaneous LE) with EM-like lesions

Genetics
Strong association with HLA-DQ3 in herpes-related cases; possible association in recurrent cases with HLA-B15, -B35, -A33, -DR53, DQB1*0301, and DQW3 (1)

RISK FACTORS
Previous history of EM

GENERAL PREVENTION
- Known or suspected etiologic agents should be avoided.
- Acyclovir or valacyclovir may help prevent herpes-related recurrent EM (1,2,7)[B].

COMMONLY ASSOCIATED CONDITIONS
See "Etiology" above.

DIAGNOSIS

Clinical

HISTORY
- Absent or mild prodromal symptoms
- Preceding HSV infection (up to >50% of cases) 10–15 days before the skin eruptions (1,2)
- Rash involving the skin and sometimes the mucous membrane, most commonly the mouth

PHYSICAL EXAM
- Skin pleomorphic eruption with a mixture of papules of various sizes, and target lesions:
  - Typical target lesions: Raised and cyanotic center, edematous light intermediate ring and bright erythematous border (3 zones)
  - Raised atypical target lesions: 2 zones only (center and intermediate ring) with poorly defined border
  - Symmetrically distributed eruption, mainly on the palms, soles, dorsum of the hands, and extensor surface of the extremities and the face

- Mucosal involvement:
  - Minimal involvement in EM minor; if present, most commonly involves the mouth (usually cutaneous or mucosal lips) (3)
  - At least 2 mucosal sites involved in EM major, including eyes (conjunctivitis, keratitis), mouth (stomatitis, cheilitis, characteristic blood-stained crusted erosions on lips) (3), and probable trachea, bronchi, GI tract, or genital tract (balanitis and vulvitis)
  - Multiple papules and vesicles, superficial irregular erosions, shallow painful ulcers with erythematous margin (1)

DIFFERENTIAL DIAGNOSIS
- SJS (4,5,7):
  - Generalized distribution of lesions; concentrated on the trunk
  - No raised typical target lesion
  - Atypical flat target lesions or macules with coalescence of lesions
  - Blisters and skin detachment <10% of the total body surface area
  - Usually with systemic complications (i.e., CNS, lung, GI system, kidney); 1–5% mortality rate
  - Presence of high fever (>38.5°C) more likely with SJS than EM
  - More likely to have mucosal involvement at ≥2 sites, lymphadenopathy, high C-reactive protein levels (>10 mg/dL), and hepatic dysfunction
- TEN (1,5):
  - Full-thickness skin necrosis and skin detachment >30% of the total body surface area
  - 10–30% mortality rate
  - Otherwise similar to SJS
- Urticaria
- Pemphigus vulgaris
- Pemphigoid
- Paraneoplastic pemphigoid
- Mucocutaneous lymph node syndrome
- Erythema annulare centrifugum
- Acute hemorrhagic edema of infancy
- Subacute cutaneous lupus erythematosus
- Necrotizing vasculitis
- Drug eruptions
- Contact dermatitis
- Pityriasis rosea
- HSV
- Secondary syphilis
- Tinea corporis
- Dermatitis herpetiformis
- Herpes gestationis
- Septicemia
- Serum sickness
- Viral exanthem
- Rocky Mountain spotted fever
- Meningococcemia
- Lichen planus
- Behçet syndrome
- Recurrent aphthous ulcers
- Herpetic gingivostomatitis
- Granuloma annulare

DIAGNOSTIC TESTS & INTERPRETATION
- No lab test is indicated to make the diagnosis of EM (1,2,5,6).
- Skin biopsy of lesional and perilesional tissue in equivocal conditions (1,2,5,6)
- Direct and indirect immunofluorescence (DIF and IIF) to differentiate EM from other vesiculobullous diseases (1)[C]. DIF is detected on a biopsy of perilesional skin, and IIF is detected from a blood sample.
- HSV tests in recurrent EM (serologic tests, swab culture, or tests using skin biopsy sample to check HSV antigens or DNA in keratinocytes by direct immunofluorescence [DFA] or polymerase chain reaction [PCR]) (6)
- Antibody staining to IFN-γ and TNF-α to differentiate HSV- from drug-associated EM (6)
- Elevated *M. pneumonia* antibody titer in *M. pneumonia*–associated EM (1)

Initial Tests (lab, imaging)
No imaging studies are indicated in most cases unless there is suspicion for *M. pneumonia.*

Follow-Up Tests & Special Considerations
Chest x-ray may be necessary if an underlying pulmonary infection (*M. pneumonia*) is suspected.

Test Interpretation
- Vacuolar interface dermatitis with CD4$^+$ T lymphocytes and histiocytes in papillary dermis and the dermal–epidermal junction
- Superficial perivascular lymphocytic inflammation
- Satellite cell necrosis
- Necrotic keratinocytes mainly in the basal layer
- Papillary dermal edema (1,2,6)

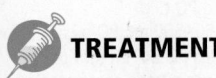

TREATMENT

GENERAL MEASURES
- Meticulous wound care and Burow solution or Domeboro solution dressings for severe cases with epidermal detachment followed by Vaseline gauze and curlex
- Mouth washes with warm saline or a solution of diphenhydramine, lidocaine (Xylocaine), and Kaopectate for oral lesions to provide symptomatic relief and oral hygiene, and to facilitate oral intake

MEDICATION
First Line
- Treatment of any underlying or causative disease (1,2)[B]
- Withdrawal of any drugs that might be the cause (1,2)[B]
- Symptomatic treatment with oral antihistamines and topical corticosteroids for mild cases (1,2)[B]
- Early treatment with acyclovir may lessen the number and duration of cutaneous lesions for patients with coexisting or recent HSV infection (2)[B]:
  – Acyclovir for adults: 200 mg, 5× a day for 7–10 days in the onset of EM
  – For pediatric patients: 10 mg/kg or t.i.d. for 7–10 days
- Recurrent EM: Oral acyclovir (400 mg b.i.d.), even if HSV infection has not been confirmed (2)[B]
- Valacyclovir (Valtrex, 500–1,000 mg/d) and famciclovir (Famvir, 125–250 mg/d) may be tried (2)[C]: Reduce dosage once the patient is recurrence-free for 4 months and eventually discontinue.

Second Line
- Recurrent EM cases nonresponsive to antiviral therapy: Dapsone (100–150 mg/d), azathioprine (Imuran, 100–150 mg/d), thalidomide (100–200 mg/d), tacrolimus (0.1% ointment daily), mycophenolate mofetil (CellCept <3 g/d), hydroxychloroquine (<400 mg/d), colchicine (<1.2 mg/d) (2,7)[C]
- Cyclosporine given intermittently (4 mg/kg/d for a week) may also be used for recurrent EM (2).
- Systemic steroid use is controversial: May decrease the patient's resistance to HSV and increase EM eruptions (1,2)[C].

IN-PATIENT CONSIDERATIONS
Admission Criteria/Initial Stabilization
- Care at home
- Hospitalization needed for fluid, electrolyte management if patient with severe mucous membrane involvement, impaired oral intake, and dehydration
- IV antibiotics if secondary infection develops

 ONGOING CARE

FOLLOW-UP RECOMMENDATIONS
Patient Monitoring
- The disease is self-limiting.
- Complications are rare, with no mortality.

DIET
As tolerated, with increased fluid intake

PATIENT EDUCATION
- The disease is self-limiting. However, the recurrence risk may be 30%.
- Antiviral therapy with acyclovir may reduce the duration and frequency of outbreaks.
- Avoid any identified etiological agents.

PROGNOSIS
- Rash evolves over 1–2 weeks and subsequently resolves within 2–6 weeks, generally without scarring or sequelae.
- Following resolution, there may be some postinflammatory hyper- or hypopigmentation.

COMPLICATIONS
Secondary infection

REFERENCES
1. Al-Johani KA, Fedele S, Porter SR. Erythema multiforme and related disorders. *Oral Surg Oral Med Oral Pathol Oral Radiol Endod*. 2007;103(5):642–654. Epub 2007 Mar 6.
2. Lamoreux MR, Sternbach MR, Hsu WT. Erythema multiforme. *Am Fam Physician*. 2006;74:1883–1888.
3. Sanchis JM, Bagán JV, Gavaldá C, et al. Erythema multiforme: Diagnosis, clinical manifestations and treatment in a retrospective study of 22 patients. *J Oral Pathol Med*. 2010;39(10):747–752.
4. Wolf R, Wolf D, Davidovici B, et al. In the pursuit of classifying severe cutaneous adverse reactions. *Clin Dermatol*. 2007;25:348–349.
5. Auquier-Dunant A, Mockenhaupt M, Naldi L, et al. Correlations between clinical patterns and causes of erythema multiforme majus, Stevens-Johnson syndrome, and toxic epidermal necrolysis: Results of an international prospective study. *Arch Dermatol*. 2002;138:1019–1024.
6. Aurelian L, Ono F, Burnett J. Herpes simplex virus (HSV)-associated erythema multiforme (HAEM): A viral disease with an autoimmune component. *Dermatol Online J*. 2003;9:1.
7. Wetter DA, Davis MD. Recurrent erythema multiforme: Clinical characteristics, etiologic associations, and treatment in a series of 48 patients at Mayo Clinic, 2000 to 2007. *J Am Acad Dermatol*. 2010;62:45–53.

ADDITIONAL READING
- Chen M, Doherty SD, Hsu S, et al. Innovative uses of thalidomide. *Dermatol Clin*. 2010;28:577–586.
- Higgins E, Collins P. Recurrent bullous erythema multiforme treated with topical tacrolimus 0.1% ointment. *Br J Dermatol*. 2011;164(4):884–886.
- Sokumbi O, Wetter D. Clinical features, diagnosis, and treatment of erythema multiforme: A review for the practicing dermatologist. *Int J Dermatol*. 2012;51:889–902.
- Torchia D, Romanelli P, Kerdel FA. Erythema multiforme and Stevens-Johnson syndrome/toxic epidermal necrolysis associated with lupus erythematosus. *J Am Acad Dermatol*. 2012;67(3):417–421

 SEE ALSO

Cutaneous Drug Reactions; Dermatitis Herpetiformis; Herpes Gestationalis; Stevens-Johnson Syndrome; Toxic Epidermic Necrotisis; Urticaria

CODES
ICD10
- L51.0 Nonbullous erythema multiforme
- L51.8 Other erythema multiforme
- L51.9 Erythema multiforme, unspecified

CLINICAL PEARLS
- EM is diagnosed clinically by careful review of the history, thorough detailed physical exam, and by excluding other similar disorders. No lab tests are required for the diagnosis.
- Typical lesions are characteristic target or "iris" lesions, but can include raised atypical (2-zone) targets.
- Lesions are symmetrically distributed on palms, soles, dorsum of the hands, and extensor surfaces of extremities and face. The oral mucosa is the most affected mucosal region in EM.
- Management of EM involves determining the etiology when possible. The 1st step is to treat the suspected infection or discontinue the causative drug.
- Complications are rare. Most cases are self-limited. However, the recurrence risk may be as high as 30%.
- Recurrent cases often are secondary to HSV infection. Antiviral therapy may be beneficial.

ERYTHEMA NODOSUM

Sophia L. Delano, MD, MPP • Nikki A. Levin, MD, PhD

BASICS

DESCRIPTION
- A delayed-type hypersensitivity reaction to infectious agents, medications, or malignancies, or in the setting of autoimmune disorders, presenting as an SC panniculitis.
- Clinical pattern of multiple, bilateral, erythematous, tender SC nodules that undergo a characteristic pattern of color changes, similar to that seen in bruises. Unlike erythema induratum, the lesions of erythema nodosum (EN) do not typically ulcerate.
- Occurs most commonly on the shins, less commonly on the thighs and forearms
- May be accompanied by fever and arthralgias
- Often idiopathic but may be associated with a number of clinical entities
- Usually remits spontaneously in weeks to months without scarring or atrophy
- Synonym(s): Dermatitis contusiformis

Pregnancy Considerations
May have repeat outbreaks during pregnancy

EPIDEMIOLOGY
Incidence
- 1–5/100,000/year
- Predominant age: 20–30 years
- Predominant sex: Female > Male (3:1).

Prevalence
Varies geographically depending on the prevalence of disorders associated with EN

ETIOLOGY AND PATHOPHYSIOLOGY
- Idiopathic: 37–60%
- Bacterial: Streptococcal infections (most common cause in children), tuberculosis, leprosy, tularemia, gonorrhea, *Yersinia enterocolitica*, *Campylobacter*, *Salmonella*, *Shigella*
- Sarcoid
- Drugs: Sulfonamides, amoxicillin, oral contraceptives, bromides, azathioprine (1), vemurafenib
- Pregnancy, progesterone injection during 1st trimester as part of assisted reproductive therapy
- Fungal: Dermatophytes, coccidioidomycosis, histoplasmosis, blastomycosis
- Viral/Chlamydial: Infectious mononucleosis, lymphogranuloma venereum, paravaccinia, HIV
- Enteropathies: Ulcerative colitis, Crohn disease, Behçet disease (2), celiac disease, diverticulitis
- Malignancies: Lymphoma/Leukemia, sarcoma, myelodysplastic syndrome, after radiation therapy
- Sweet syndrome

RISK FACTORS
See "Etiology and Pathophysiology."

COMMONLY ASSOCIATED CONDITIONS
See "Etiology and Pathophysiology."

DIAGNOSIS

HISTORY
- Increasingly tender and aching nodules on the legs, usually over the shins
- Fever, malaise, chills, fatigue
- Eruptions often preceded by symptoms of pharyngitis or upper respiratory infection
- Headache
- Arthralgias

PHYSICAL EXAM
- Initially warm, tender, brightly erythematous nodules, which may be raised, on anterior shins; lesions become bluish and fluctuant, gradually fading to yellowish, resembling a bruise.
- May occur on any area with SC fat
- Diameter usually 2–6 cm, but may rarely be larger

DIFFERENTIAL DIAGNOSIS
- Nodular vasculitis or erythema induratum (warm ulcerating calf nodules)
- Superficial thrombophlebitis
- Cellulitis
- Septic emboli
- Weber-Christian disease (violaceous, scarring nodules)
- Lupus panniculitis
- Cutaneous polyarteritis nodosa
- Sarcoidal granulomas
- Cutaneous T-cell lymphoma
- Erythema nodosum leprosum (clinically similar to EN but shows vasculitis on histopathology)
- Vasculitis

DIAGNOSTIC TESTS & INTERPRETATION
Diagnosis is usually clinical.
- ESR: May be elevated or normal
- CBC: Mild leukocytosis
- Antistreptolysin titers may be elevated.
- Throat culture (usually negative because the infection typically resolves before lesions appear)
- Stool culture and leukocytes, if indicated
- Skin testing for mycobacteria, if indicated
- Drugs that may alter lab results: Antecedent antibiotics may affect cultures.

Initial Tests (lab, imaging)
CXR for hilar adenopathy or infiltrates related to sarcoidosis or tuberculosis

Diagnostic Procedures/Other
Deep-incisional skin biopsy including SC fat; rarely necessary except in atypical cases with ulceration, duration >12 weeks

Test Interpretation
- Septal panniculitis without vasculitis
- Neutrophilic infiltrate in septa of fat tissue early in course
- Actinic radial (Miescher's) granulomas, consisting of collections of histocytes around a central stellate cleft, may be seen (3).
- Fibrosis, paraseptal granulation tissue, lymphocytes, and multinucleated giant cells predominate late in course.

TREATMENT

- Medication usually more effective in acute than in chronic disease
- Condition often self-limited
- All medications listed as treatment for erythema nodosum are off-label uses of the medications. There are no FDA-approved medications for EN.

GENERAL MEASURES
- Mild compression bandages and leg elevation may reduce pain. (Wet dressings, hot soaks, and topical medications are not useful.)
- Discontinue potentially causative drugs
- Treat underlying disease

MEDICATION
First Line
- NSAIDs:
  – Ibuprofen 400 mg PO q4–6h (not to exceed 3,200 mg/d)
  – Indomethacin 25–50 mg PO t.i.d.
  – Naproxen (Naprosyn) 250–500 mg PO b.i.d.
- Aspirin 325 mg, 1–2 tablets PO q4–6h (not to exceed 12 tablets a day); use enteric-coated tablets to decrease GI upset.
- Precautions:
  – GI upset/bleeding
  – Fluid retention
  – Dose reduction in elderly, especially those with renal disease, diabetes, or heart failure
  – May mask fever
  – NSAIDs may elevate liver function tests
- Significant possible interactions:
  – May blunt antihypertensive effects of diuretics and β-blockers
  – NSAIDs can elevate plasma lithium levels.
  – Caution is advised with naproxen or any highly protein-bound drug because it may compete for albumin binding and elevate levels.
  – NSAIDs can cause significant elevation and prolongation of methotrexate levels.

Second Line

- Potassium iodide 400–900 mg/d divided b.i.d. or t.i.d. × 3–4 weeks (for persistent lesions). Need to monitor for hypothyroidism with prolonged use. Pregnancy Class D.
- Corticosteroids for severe, refractory cases in which an infectious workup is negative. Prednisone 1 mg/kg/d for 1–2 weeks often helps resolve the lesions (4). Potential side effects include hyperglycemia, hypertension, weight gain, worsening GERD, mood changes, bone loss, osteonecrosis, myopathy.
- Recent reports of improvement with colchicine 0.6–1.2 mg b.i.d. Potential side effects include GI upset and diarrhea.
- Hydroxychloroquine, thalidomide, and cyclosporine may also be used.
- In a case of refractory erythema nodosum, minocycline 100 mg b.i.d. has been successfully used.

COMPLEMENTARY AND ALTERNATIVE MEDICINE

Vitamin B_{12} replacement. A single case report of resolution of lesions with B_{12} replacement in a patient who had B_{12} deficiency and EN.

IN-PATIENT CONSIDERATIONS

Admission Criteria/Initial Stabilization

Occasionally, admission may be needed for the antecedent illness (e.g., tuberculosis).

ONGOING CARE

FOLLOW-UP RECOMMENDATIONS

- Keep legs elevated
- Elastic wraps or support stockings may be helpful when patients are ambulating.

Patient Monitoring

Monthly follow-up or as dictated by underlying disorder

DIET

No restrictions

PATIENT EDUCATION

- Lesions will resolve over a few weeks to months.
- No scarring is anticipated.
- Joint aches and pains may persist.
- <20% recur

PROGNOSIS

- Individual lesions resolve generally within 2 weeks.
- Total time course of 6–12 weeks but may vary with underlying disease.
- Joint aches and pains may persist for years.
- Lesions do not scar.
- Recurrences in 12–14% of patients: Occurs over variable periods, averaging several years; seen most often in sarcoid, streptococcal infection, pregnancy, and oral contraceptive use

COMPLICATIONS

- Vary according to underlying disease
- None expected from lesions of erythema nodosum

REFERENCES

1. de Fonclare AL, Khosrotehrani K, Aractingi S, et al. Erythema nodosum-like eruption as a manifestation of azathioprine hypersensitivity in patients with inflammatory bowel disease. *Arch Dermatol*. 2007;143:744–748.
2. Psychos DN, Voulgari PV, Skopouli FN, et al. Erythema nodosum: The underlying conditions. *Clin Rheumatol*. 2000;19:212–216.
3. Schwartz RA, Nervi SJ. Erythema nodosum: A sign of systemic disease. *Am Fam Physician*. 2007;75:695–700.
4. Requena L, Yus ES. Erythema nodosum. *Dermatol Clin*. 2008;26:425–438.

ADDITIONAL READING

- Bartyik K, Várkonyi A, Kirschner A, et al. Erythema nodosum in association with celiac disease. *Pediatr Dermatol*. 2004;21:227–230.
- Chong TA, Hansra NK, Ruben BS, et al. Diverticulitis: An inciting factor in erythema nodosum. *J Am Acad Dermatol*. 2012;67:e60–e62.
- Davis MD. Response of recalcitrant erythema nodosum to tetracyclines. *J Am Acad Dermatol*. 2011;64:1211–1212.
- González-Gay MA, García-Porría C, Pujol RM, et al. Erythema nodosum: A clinical approach. *Clin Exp Rheumatol*. 2001;19:365–368.
- Harris T, Henderson MC. Concurrent Sweet's syndrome and erythema nodosum. *J Gen Intern Med*. 2011;26:214–215.
- Jeon HC, Choi M, Paik SH, et al. A case of assisted reproductive therapy-induced erythema nodosum. *Ann Dermatol*. 2011;23:362–364.
- Louthrenoo W, Lertprasertsuke N, Kasitanon N, et al. Erythema nodosum as a manifestation of HIV infection. *Asian Pac J Allergy Immunol*. 2002;20:175–178.
- Then C, Langer A, Adam C, et al. Erythema nodosum associated with myelodysplastic syndrome: A case report. *Onkologie*. 2011;34:126–128.
- Volkov I, Rudoy I, Press Y. Successful treatment of chronic erythema nodosum with vitamin B12. *J Am Board Fam Pract*. 2005;18:567–569.

 ## CODES

ICD10

- A18.4 Tuberculosis of skin and subcutaneous tissue
- L52 Erythema nodosum

CLINICAL PEARLS

- Lesions of EN appear to be erythematous patches, but when palpated, their underlying nodularity is appreciated.
- EN in the setting of hilar adenopathy may be seen with multiple etiologies and does not exclusively indicate sarcoidosis.
- In patients with a history of Hodgkin lymphoma, EN may be an early sign of recurrence.

ESOPHAGEAL VARICES
Avani Sinha, MD • Edward Feller, MD

 BASICS

DESCRIPTION
- Dilated veins in the distal esophagus that connect the portal and systemic circulations
- Result from resistance to portal blood flow and increased portal venous blood inflow as a direct consequence of portal hypertension
- Cirrhosis leads to increased pressure and turbulent flow; superficial location of distal esophageal veins makes them susceptible to rupture, producing major GI bleeding with high morbidity, mortality.

EPIDEMIOLOGY
Incidence
1-year rate of 1st variceal bleeding is ~5% for small varices, 15% for large varices (1).

Pediatric Considerations
Portal hypertension commonly complicates chronic liver disease in children. Incomplete data on screening, endoscopic treatment, β-blockers use (2)

Prevalence
- Esophageal varices in patients with cirrhosis (correlating with disease severity): 50%
- Patients with esophageal varices who bleed during their lifetime: 50%
- Bleeding from esophageal varices is associated with 15–20% mortality at 6 weeks.
- Predominant gender: Male > Female

ETIOLOGY AND PATHOPHYSIOLOGY
- Portal hypertension: Due to splanchnic arteriolar vasodilatation, increased portal inflow, and increased resistance to outflow due to fibrous tissue and regenerative nodules (3)
- Increased production of endothelin-1 and decreased production of nitrous oxide causing intrahepatic vasoconstriction
- Portal hypertension: Defined as a pressure gradient >10 mm Hg between the portal vein and inferior vena cava. Collateral vessels (varices) form to decompress portal circulation.
- Cirrhotic portal hypertension:
  - >90% of cases (4)
  - Alcohol and hepatitis C: Most common
  - Less common: Hemochromatosis, hepatitis B, nonalcoholic fatty liver disease
  - Uncommon: Biliary cirrhosis, autoimmune cirrhosis
- Noncirrhotic portal hypertension (5):
  - Extrahepatic portal/splenic vein thrombosis from umbilical vein infection, trauma, chronic pancreatitis, thrombotic disease, polycythemia
  - Malignant invasion of liver sinusoids/portal vein; in lymphoma, leukemia, hepatocellular, or other carcinomas
  - Metabolic disease altering liver sinusoids: Amyloidosis, Gaucher disease, Budd-Chiari syndrome, veno-occlusive disease

Genetics
Rare hereditary causes of cirrhosis

RISK FACTORS
- Cirrhosis: Can result from alcohol abuse, viral hepatitis, autoimmune inflammation, hemochromatosis, Wilson disease, primary biliary cirrhosis, primary sclerosing cholangitis, nonalcoholic fatty liver disease, or medications.
- In cirrhotic patients, thrombocytopenia and splenomegaly, correlated with portal hypertension, are independent predictors of esophageal varices.
- Noncirrhotic portal hypertension

GENERAL PREVENTION
- Prevention and treatment of causes of cirrhosis, including alcohol cessation, hepatitis B vaccine, clean needles, or detox in IV drug use (IVDU) to avoid hepatitis C exposure; specific therapy for hepatitis B and C, hemochromatosis
- See "Treatment" section for prevention of 1st and 2nd bleeds.

COMMONLY ASSOCIATED CONDITIONS
- Portal hypertensive gastropathy; varices in stomach, duodenum, colon, rectum (causes massive bleeding, unlike hemorrhoids); rarely at umbilicus (caput medusa) or ostomy sites
- Other complications of cirrhosis: Hepatic encephalopathy, ascites, hepatorenal syndrome, spontaneous bacterial peritonitis
- Gastric varices: Isolated gastric varices can occur due to splenic vein thrombosis/stenosis from hypercoagulability/contiguous inflammation (most commonly, chronic pancreatitis). Tumors can compress/infiltrate the splenic vein leading to pressure increase in short gastric veins. Signs of portal hypertension may be absent (6).

DIAGNOSIS

- First indication of varices can be GI bleeding (generally severe): Painless hematemesis, hematochezia, and/or melena
- Occult bleeding with anemia: Uncommon
- Signs of cirrhosis/portal hypertension
- Endoscopic screening with known cirrhosis every 2–3 years; yearly in decompensated cirrhosis (1)[C]

HISTORY
- Generally, a history of cirrhosis/liver disease
- Painless hematemesis, melena, or hematochezia
- Rapid upper GI bleed can also present as rectal bleeding.

PHYSICAL EXAM
- Assess hemodynamic stability: Possible hypotension/tachycardia (if bleeding)
- Small, hard liver; hepatomegaly possible
- Splenomegaly, ascites
- Visible abdominal periumbilical collateral circulation (caput medusae)
- Spider angiomata on chest/back; palmar erythema
- Testicular atrophy; gynecomastia
- Anal varices (which collapse with digital pressure, whereas hemorrhoids do not)
- Hepatic encephalopathy; assess for asterixis
- Blood on rectal exam

DIFFERENTIAL DIAGNOSIS
- Upper GI bleeding:
  - In patients with known varices, as many as 50% bleed from nonvariceal sources.
  - Peptic ulcer disease; gastritis
  - Gastric/Esophageal malignancy
  - Congestive gastropathy of portal hypertension
  - Arteriovenous malformation
  - Mallory-Weiss tears
  - Hemoptysis; nosebleed
- Lower GI bleeding:
  - Rectal varices; hemorrhoids
  - Colonic neoplasia
  - Diverticulosis
  - Arteriovenous malformation
  - Rapidly bleeding upper GI site
- Continued/Recurrent bleeding risk: Actively bleeding/large varix, high Childs-Pugh severity score, infection, renal failure

DIAGNOSTIC TESTS & INTERPRETATION
Initial Tests (lab, imaging)
- Anemia from blood loss; hemoglobin may be normal despite active bleed; may require 6–24 hours to equilibrate; other causes of anemia are common in cirrhotics.
- Thrombocytopenia: Most sensitive and specific lab parameter to indicate portal hypertension, large esophageal varices
- Possibly abnormal aspartate aminotransferase (AST), alanine aminotransferase (ALT), alkaline phosphatase, bilirubin, prolonged PT, or low albumin-reflecting cirrhosis
- BUN, creatinine to assess hydration
- Esophagogastroduodenoscopy:
  - Identify and treat nonbleeding varices appearing as protruding submucosal veins in the distal third of the esophagus (4)[C].
  - Can identify actively bleeding varices as well large varices and stigmata of recent hemorrhage
  - Can treat active bleeding with esophageal band ligation (preferred to sclerotherapy); prevent rebleeding. Can detect gastric varices, portal hypertensive gastropathy; diagnose alternative bleeding site, such as ulcer.

Diagnostic Procedures/Other
- Video capsule endoscopy screening: In early trials, has lower sensitivity and specificity for detection; not for treating varices; alternative for those unwilling to undergo screening endoscopy
- Doppler sonography (second-line): Demonstrates patency, diameter, and flow in portal and splenic veins, and intra-abdominal collaterals; very sensitive for gastric varices and in surveillance to document patency after ligation or transjugular intrahepatic portosystemic shunt (TIPS)
- MRI (second-line, not routine): Demonstrates large vascular channels in abdomen, mediastinum:
  - Can demonstrate patency of intrahepatic portal vein and splenic vein. Venous-phase celiac arteriography: Demonstrates portal vein and collaterals; can diagnose hepatic vein occlusion.
  - Portal pressure measurement using retrograde catheter in hepatic vein

Test Interpretation
- Extensive collateral circulation in the mediastinum and abdomen in addition to large vessels in the esophageal submucosa
- When bleeding occurs, large veins protrude into esophageal submucosa and rupture into the lumen.

TREATMENT

GENERAL MEASURES
- Treat comorbid conditions, generally related to cirrhosis.
- Variceal bleeding is complicated commonly by hepatic encephalopathy and infection.
- Refer for liver transplantation where appropriate.
- Active bleeding:
  - IV access; assess breathing, circulation; monitor intake and output.
  - Type and cross-match packed RBCs.
  - Appropriate resuscitation and maintenance of blood volume; transfuse. Overtransfusion increases portal pressure and increases rebleeding risk.
  - Treat coagulopathy, if necessary. Be aware that fresh frozen plasma may increase blood volume and increase rebleeding risk.
  - Avoid sedation, monitor mental state, avoid nephrotoxic drugs.
  - Inject thiamine as indicated, monitor blood glucose, delirium tremens.
  - IV octreotide to lower portal venous pressure as adjuvant to endoscopic management. IV bolus of 50 mg followed by drip of 50 mg/h.
  - Urgent upper endoscopy for diagnosis and treatment:
    - Variceal band ligation/sclerotherapy for bleeding varices/nonbleeding medium-to-large varices to decrease bleeding risk
    - Variceal band ligation is preferred due to improved bleeding cessation, fewer complications (4).
  - Repeat ligation/sclerosant if bleeding recurs.
  - If endoscopic treatment fails to stop bleeding, may need Sengstaken Blakemore or Minnesota tube as emergency rescue therapy to stabilize patient for TIPS (4)[B].
  - During bleeding, antibiotic prophylaxis for spontaneous peritonitis, other infections with IV ciprofloxacin, or oral norfloxacin for 7–10 days (4)[A]
  - In active bleeding, avoid β-blockers, which decrease BP and blunt the physiologic increase in heart rate during acute hemorrhage.
- Preventing recurrence of acute bleeding:
  - Vasoconstrictors: Terlipressin, octreotide (reduce portal pressure) (1,4)[A]
  - Endoscopic band ligation (EBL): If bleeding recurs/portal pressure measurement shows portal pressure remains >12 mm Hg
  - Endoscopic sclerotherapy: Second-line and uncommonly used (if EBL cannot be performed)
  - TIPS: Second-line therapy if above methods fail TIPS decreases portal pressure by creating communication between hepatic vein and an intrahepatic portal vein branch.

MEDICATION
Primary prevention of variceal bleeding:
- Endoscopy: Assesses variceal size, presence of red wale sign (varix with a weak wall), to determine risk stratification:

- Endoscope every 2–3 years if cirrhosis, but no varices; every 1–2 years if small varices and not receiving β-blockers

First Line
- Nonselective β-blockers reduce portal pressure and decrease risk of first bleed from 25% to 15% in primary prophylaxis. Used in cirrhosis with small varices and increased hemorrhage risk, as well as cirrhosis + medium-to-large varices (1,7)[A]:
  - Propranolol: 40 mg b.i.d. increase until heart rate decreased by 25% from baseline
  - Nadolol 80 mg daily; increase as above
  - Contraindications: Severe asthma with β-blockers
- Nitrates should not be used in the primary prophylaxis of variceal bleed.

Second Line
Obliteration of varices with esophageal banding for those intolerant of medication prophylaxis:
- During ligation: Proton pump inhibitors, such as lansoprazole 30 mg/d, until varices obliterated

ISSUES FOR REFERRAL
Primarily, those associated with endoscopy, liver transplantation, interventional radiology for TIPS procedure

ADDITIONAL THERAPIES
Cirrhotic patients should receive pneumococcal vaccine and hepatitis A/B virus (HAV/HBV) vaccine as indicated.

SURGERY/OTHER PROCEDURES
- Esophageal transection: In uncontrollable, exsanguinating bleeding
- Liver transplantation: Referral after diagnosis

IN-PATIENT CONSIDERATIONS
Admission Criteria/Initial Stabilization
Inpatient for acute bleeding

Discharge Criteria
Cessation of bleeding, stability of comorbidities, complications

ONGOING CARE

FOLLOW-UP RECOMMENDATIONS
Patient Monitoring
- Close monitoring of vital signs if actively bleeding
- Endoscopic variceal ligation, repeated every 1–4 weeks until varices eradicated
- If TIPS, repeat endoscopy only if clinically bleeding
- Post-TIPS, follow-up recommended: Doppler sonogram every 6 months to assess shunt patency

PATIENT EDUCATION
National Digestive Information Clearinghouse, 2 Information Way, Bethesda, MD 20892 (digestive.niddk.nih.gov/) or American Liver Foundation, 1425 Pompton Way, Cedar Grove, NJ 07009 (www.liverfoundation.org)

PROGNOSIS
- Depends on prognosis of underlying condition
- With cirrhosis: 1-year survival for those who are alive 2 weeks after variceal bleed is 50%.
- Prognosis in noncirrhotic portal fibrosis is better than that of cirrhotics.

COMPLICATIONS
- Gastric: Other uncommon varices may occur following eradication of esophageal varices.
- Esophageal varices can recur after obliteration.

- Encephalopathy; renal dysfunction
- Infections after banding/ligation of varices

REFERENCES

1. Garcia-Tsao G, Bosch J. Management of varices and variceal hemorrhage in cirrhosis. *N Engl J Med*. 2010;362:823–832.
2. D'Antiga L. Medical management of esophageal varices and portal hypertension in children. *Semin Pediatr Surg*. 2012;21:211–218.
3. Maruyama H, Yokosuka O. Pathophysiology of portal hypertension and esophageal varices. *Int J Hepatol*. 2012;2012:895787. Epub 2012 May 15.
4. Cordon JP, Torres CF, Garcia AB, et al. Endoscopic management of esophageal varices. *World J Gastrointest Endosc*. 2012;4:312–322.
5. Sarin SK, Kumar A. Noncirrhotic portal hypertension. *Clin Liver Dis*. 2006;10:627–651.
6. Shayan I, Kowdley K, Kozarek R. Gastric varices: An updated review of management. *J Clin Gastroenterol*. 2011;45:133–148.
7. Asrani SK, Kamath PS. Natural history of cirrhosis. *Curr Gastroenterol Rep*. 2013;15:8–13.

ADDITIONAL READING

- Bințințan A, Chira RI, Mircea PA. Non-invasive ultrasound-based diagnosis and staging of esophageal varices in liver cirrhosis. A systematic review of the literature published in the third millennium. *Med Ultrason*. 2013;15(2):116–124.
- Boyer TD, Haskal ZJ, American Association for the Study of Liver Diseases. The Role of Transjugular Intrahepatic Portosystemic Shunt (TIPS) in the Management of Portal Hypertension: Update 2009. *Hepatology*. 2010;51(1):306.
- D'Amico G, Pagliarol L, Pietrosi G. Emergency sclerotherapy vs vasoactive drugs for bleeding esophageal varices in cirrhotics. *Cochrane Database Syst Rev*. 2010;CD002233.

 SEE ALSO

Cirrhosis of the Liver; Portal Hypertension

 CODES

ICD10
- I85.00 Esophageal varices without bleeding
- I85.01 Esophageal varices with bleeding
- I85.10 Secondary esophageal varices without bleeding

CLINICAL PEARLS

- Rapid upper GI bleeds, as from varices, can present as isolated rectal bleeding.
- In acute bleeding, avoid β-blockers, which decrease BP and blunt the physiologic increase in heart rate.
- In acute bleeding, overtransfusion can elevate portal pressure, which increases bleeding risk.
- Thrombocytopenia: Sensitive marker of increased portal pressure, large esophageal varices
- During bleeding, consider antibiotic prophylaxis for spontaneous peritonitis and other infections with IV ciprofloxacin or oral norfloxacin for 7–10 days.

ESSENTIAL TREMOR SYNDROME

Jonathon M. Firnhaber, MD

 BASICS

DESCRIPTION

- A postural (occurring with voluntary maintenance of a position against gravity) or kinetic (occurring during voluntary movement) flexion–extension tremor that is slow and rhythmic and primarily affects the hands and forearms, head, and voice with a frequency of 4–12 Hz.
- Older patients tend to have lower-frequency tremors, whereas younger patients exhibit frequencies in the higher range.
- May be familial, sporadic, or associated with other movement disorders
- Can begin at any age, but the incidence and prevalence increase with age
- The tremor can be exacerbated by emotional or physical stresses, fatigue, and caffeine.
- System(s) affected: Neurologic; Musculoskeletal; Ear/Nose/Throat (ENT) (voice)

EPIDEMIOLOGY

Essential tremor is the most common pathologic tremor in humans.

Incidence

- Can occur at any age, but bimodal peaks exist in the 2nd and 6th decades.
- Incidence rises significantly after age 49.

Prevalence

0.4–5% of the general population

ETIOLOGY AND PATHOPHYSIOLOGY

- Suspected to originate from an abnormal oscillation within thalamocortical and cerebello-olivary loops, as lesions in these areas tend to reduce essential tremor.
- Essential tremor is not a homogenous disorder; many patients have other motor manifestations and nonmotor features, including cognitive and psychiatric symptoms.

Genetics

- Positive family history in 50–70% of patients; autosomal-dominant inheritance is demonstrated in many families, but twin studies suggest that environmental factors are also involved.
- A link to genetic loci exists on chromosomes 2p22–25, 3q13, and 6p23. In addition, a Ser9Gly variant in the dopamine D_3 receptor gene on 3q13 has been suggested as a risk factor.

COMMONLY ASSOCIATED CONDITIONS

- Can be present in 10% of patients with Parkinson disease (PD); characteristics of PD that distinguish it from essential tremor include 3–5-Hz resting tremor; accompanying rigidity, bradykinesia, or postural instability; and no change with alcohol consumption.
- Resting tremor, typically of the arm, may be seen in up to 20 to 30% of patients with essential tremor. Although action tremor is the hallmark feature of essential tremor, it is commonly found in patients with PD as well.

 DIAGNOSIS

HISTORY

- Core criteria for diagnosis:
  - Bilateral (less likely unilateral) action (postural or kinetic) tremor of the hands and forearms that is most commonly asymmetric
  - Absence of other neurologic signs, with the exception of cogwheel phenomenon
  - May have isolated head tremor with no signs of dystonia
- Secondary criteria include long duration (>3 years), positive family history, and beneficial response to alcohol (1)[C].

PHYSICAL EXAM

- Tremor can affect upper limbs (~95% of patients).
- Less commonly, the tremor affects head (~34%), lower limbs (~30%), voice (~12%), tongue (~7%), face (~5%), and trunk (~5%).

DIFFERENTIAL DIAGNOSIS

- Parkinson disease
- Wilson disease
- Hyperthyroidism
- Multiple sclerosis
- Dystonic tremor
- Cerebellar tremor
- Asterixis
- Psychogenic tremor
- Orthostatic tremor
- Drug-induced or enhanced physiologic tremor (valproic acid, SSRIs, steroids, lithium, cyclosporine, β-adrenergic agonists, ephedrine, theophylline, tricyclic antidepressants [TCAs], antipsychotics)

DIAGNOSTIC TESTS & INTERPRETATION

Initial Tests (lab, imaging)

- No specific biological marker or diagnostic test is available.
- Ceruloplasmin and serum copper to rule out Wilson disease
- Thyroid-stimulating hormone to rule out thyroid dysfunction
- Serum electrolytes, BUN, creatinine
- Brain MRI usually is not necessary or indicated unless Wilson disease is found or exam findings imply central lesion.

Diagnostic Procedures/Other

- Accelerometry evaluates tremor frequency and amplitude; more than 95% of PD cases exhibit frequencies in the 4–6-Hz range, and 95% of essential tremor cases exhibit frequencies in the 5–8-Hz range.
- Surface electromyography is less helpful in distinguishing essential tremor from PD (2).

Test Interpretation

Posture-related tremor

 TREATMENT

MEDICATION

Pharmacologic treatment should be considered when tremor interferes with ADLs or causes psychological distress.

First Line

- Propranolol 60–320 mg/d in divided doses or in long-acting formulation reduces limb-tremor magnitude by ~50%, and almost 70% of patients experience improvement in clinical rating scales. There is insufficient evidence to recommend propranolol for vocal tremor. Single doses of propranolol, taken before social situations that are likely to exacerbate tremor, are useful for some patients.
- Primidone 25 mg at bedtime, gradually titrated to 150–300 mg at bedtime, improves tremor amplitude by 40–50%. Maximum dose is 750 mg/d, with doses >250 mg/d typically divided to b.i.d. or t.i.d. Low-dose therapy (<250 mg/d) is just as effective as high-dose (750 mg/d) therapy.
- Propranolol and primidone have similar efficacy when used as initial therapy for limb tremor; both carry a level A recommendation.
- 30–50% of patients will not respond to either propranolol or primidone (3)[C].

Second Line

- Topiramate at a mean dose of 292 mg/d demonstrated significantly greater reduction in tremor rating scale (TRS) compared with placebo (7.7 vs. 0.08; p <.005; baseline TRS = 37.0) in a small study combining results of 3 double-blind, randomized, controlled trials following a common protocol (4)[B]. Use is limited by dropout rates as high as 40% due to appetite suppression, weight loss, paresthesias, and concentration difficulties.
- Gabapentin up to 400 mg t.i.d.
- Sotalol, nadolol, and atenolol are alternative β-blockers; each has less evidence than propranolol to support use.
- Clonazepam and alprazolam should be used with caution because of abuse potential.
- Clozapine has shown efficacy at doses of 6–75 mg/d, but is recommended only for refractory cases of limb tremor because of a 1% risk of agranulocytosis. The American Academy of Neurology (AAN) indicates that insufficient evidence exists to support or refute the efficacy of clozapine for chronic use (5).
- Memantine, in a pilot study using doses up to 40 mg/d, showed significant benefit in a small subset of the study group. Adverse events at this dose included dizziness, somnolence, and poor energy (6).
- Levetiracetam and 3,4-diaminopyridine are probably ineffective at reducing limb tremor and should not be considered, according to the AAN (7)[C].

- Other medications that have been evaluated for treatment of essential tremor, with limited data to support their use, include acetazolamide, clonidine, flunarizine, methazolamide, nimodipine, olanzapine, phenobarbital, pregabalin, quetiapine, sodium oxybate, and zonisamide.
- Alcohol may provide transient improvement in symptoms, but its brief duration of action, subsequent rebound, and associated risk of developing alcohol addiction make it an inappropriate treatment.
- Botulinum toxin A injections should be offered as a treatment option for cervical dystonia (Level A recommendation from AAN), and may be offered for blepharospasm, focal upper extremity dystonia, adductor laryngeal dystonia, and upper extremity essential tremor (8)[B]. Limited data support its use for head and voice tremor (4).

ISSUES FOR REFERRAL
Referral to a neurologist can help to differentiate those with dystonia, neuropathic tremor, PD, or drug-induced tremor.

SURGERY/OTHER PROCEDURES
- Deep brain stimulation provides a magnitude of benefit that is superior to all available medications and may be used to treat medically refractory limb tremor; it has fewer adverse effects than thalamotomy (9)[A].
- Bilateral thalamic stimulation is effective in reducing tremor and functional disability; however, dysarthria is a possible complication.
- Unilateral thalamotomy may be used to treat limb tremor that is refractory to medical management.
- Bilateral thalamotomy is not recommended because of adverse side effects.

ONGOING CARE

DIET
Avoid caffeine.

PROGNOSIS
Tremor tends to worsen with age, increasing in amplitude.

REFERENCES

1. Bain P, Brin M, Deuschl G, et al. Criteria for the diagnosis of essential tremor. *Neurology.* 2000; 54:S7.
2. Thenganatt MA, Louis ED. Distinguishing essential tremor from Parkinson's disease: Bedside tests and laboratory evaluations. *Expert Rev Neurother.* 2012;12(6):687–696.
3. Koller WC, Vetere-Overfield B. Acute and chronic effects of propranolol and primidone in essential tremor. *Neurology.* 1989;39(12):1587–1588.
4. Connor GS, Edwards K, Tarsy D. Topiramate in essential tremor: Findings from double-blind, placebo-controlled, crossover trials. *Clin Neuropharmacol.* 2008;31:97–103.
5. Zesiewicz TA. Practice parameter: Therapies for essential tremor: Report of the Quality Standards Subcommittee of the American Academy of Neurology. 2005;28;64(12):2008–2020.
6. Handforth A, Bordelon Y, Frucht SJ, et al. A pilot efficacy and tolerability trial of memantine for essential tremor. *Clin Neuropharm.* 2010;33: 223–226.
7. Zesiewicz TA, Elble RJ, Louis ED, et al. Evidence-based guideline update: Treatment of essential tremor: Report of the Quality Standards subcommittee of the American Academy of Neurology. *Neurology.* 2011;77(19):1752–1755. Epub 2011 Oct 19.
8. Simpson DM. Therapeutics and Technology Assessment Subcommittee of the American Academy of Neurology. Assessment: Botulinum neurotoxin for the treatment of movement disorders (an evidence-based review): Report of the Therapeutics and Technology Assessment Subcommittee of the American Academy of Neurology. *Neurology.* 2008;70(19):1699–1706.
9. Flora ED, Perera CL, Cameron AL, et al. Deep brain stimulation for essential tremor: A systematic review. *Mov Disord.* 2010;25:1550–1559.

ADDITIONAL READING
- Buijink AW, Contarino MF, Koelman JH, et al. How to tackle tremor—systematic review of the literature and diagnostic work-up. *Front Neurol.* 2012;3:146.
- Deuschl G, Raethjen J, Hellriegel H, et al. Treatment of patients with essential tremor. *Lancet Neurol.* 2011;10:148–161.
- Sullivan KL, Hauser RA, Zesiewicz TA. Essential tremor: Epidemiology, diagnosis, and treatment. *Neurologist.* 2004;10(5):250–258.

CODES

ICD10
G25.0 Essential tremor

CLINICAL PEARLS
- Core criteria for diagnosis of essential tremor include bilateral action (intention) tremor of the hands, forearm, and/or head without resting component.
- Beneficial response to alcohol and positive family history help to differentiate essential tremor from PD (PD is characterized by tremor at rest, bradykinesia, and rigidity, and it does not improve with alcohol use).
- 10% of patients with PD will have both resting tremors of PD and essential (intention) tremors.
- Wilson disease, thyroid disease, and medication effect should be ruled out.
- Brain MRI is usually not necessary or indicated.
- First-line treatments include propranolol and primidone.

E

EUSTACHIAN TUBE DYSFUNCTION

Shumaila Athar, MD • Amimi S. Osayande, MD

 BASICS

DESCRIPTION

- Eustachian tube dysfunction (ETD) is a functional or structural obstruction of the eustachian tube. It occurs due to improper opening in response to atmospheric pressure changes and negative pressure in the middle ear.
- May occur in the setting of pressure changes (e.g., scuba diving or plane travel) or acute upper airway inflammation (e.g., allergic or infectious rhinosinusitis)
- Chronic ETD may lead to a retracted tympanic membrane, recurrent serous effusions, recurrent otitis media (OM), adhesive OM, chronic mastoiditis, or cholesteatoma.
- ETD can be classified as *patulous dysfunction*, in which the eustachian tube is excessively open, or *dilatory dysfunction*, in which there is failure of the tubes to dilate appropriately.
- System(s) affected: Auditory
- Synonym(s): Auditory tube dysfunction; Eustachian tube disorder; Blocked eustachian tube; Patulous eustachian tube

ALERT

- Sudden single-sided deafness (SSNHL) can be misdiagnosed as ETD.
- A simple 512-Hz tuning fork test lateralizes to the opposite ear in sudden sensorineural hearing loss and to the affected ear in ETD with conductive hearing loss.
- Any sudden sensorineural hearing loss is a medical emergency and should be referred to an otolaryngologist immediately.

EPIDEMIOLOGY

- Most common in children <5 years (1)
- Usually decreases with age

Incidence
70% of children by age 7 have experienced ETD.

Prevalence
- Males > Females
- Highest prevalence among Native Americans, Inuits, Australian Aborigines, Hispanics, Africans

ETIOLOGY AND PATHOPHYSIOLOGY

- Under normal circumstances, the eustachian tube is closed, but it can open to let a small amount of air through to equalize pressure between the middle ear and the atmosphere.
- ETD is failure of the system at the proximal end (ET, palate, nasal cavities, and nasopharynx) to regulate the middle ear and mastoid.
- Eustachian tube functions:
  - Ventilation/Regulation of middle ear pressure
  - Protection from nasopharyngeal secretions
  - Drainage of middle ear fluid
  - ET is closed at rest and opens with yawning, swallowing, chewing.

- Cycle of dysfunction: Structural or functional obstruction of the ET compromises 3 functions of this system:
  - Negative pressure develops in middle ear.
  - Serous exudate is drawn from the middle ear mucosa by negative pressure or refluxed into the middle ear if the ET opens momentarily.
  - Infection of static fluid causes edema and release of inflammatory mediators, which exacerbates cycle of inflammation and obstruction.
- In children, a horizontal and shorter ET predisposes to difficulties with ventilation and drainage (1).
- Adenoid hypertrophy can block the torus tubarius (proximal opening of the ET) (1).
- In adults, paradoxical closing with swallowing has been noted in a majority of patients (1).

Genetics
Twin studies show a genetic component (1). Specific genetic cause is still undefined.

RISK FACTORS

- Adult and pediatric:
  - Allergic rhinitis, tobacco exposure, GERD, chronic sinusitis, adenoid hypertrophy or nasopharyngeal mass, neuromuscular disease, altered immunity
- Pediatric:
  - In addition to those listed above, prematurity and low birth weight, young age, daycare, exposure to many other children, crowded living conditions, low socioeconomic status, prone sleeping position, prolonged bottle use, craniofacial abnormalities (e.g., cleft palate, Down syndrome)

Pregnancy Considerations
ETD may be exacerbated by rhinitis of pregnancy; symptoms resolve postpartum.

GENERAL PREVENTION

- Control sources of upper airway inflammation: Allergies, infectious rhinosinusitis, GERD.
- Autoinsufflation of middle ear (i.e., blow gently against pinched nostril and closed mouth)
- Avoid atmospheric pressure changes (e.g., plane flight, scuba diving) in the setting of acute allergy exacerbation or URI.
- Avoid exposure to environmental irritants: Tobacco smoke, pollutants.

COMMONLY ASSOCIATED CONDITIONS

- Hearing loss
- Middle ear effusion
- Recurrent OM
- Chronic mastoiditis
- Cholesteatoma
- Allergic rhinitis
- Chronic sinusitis/URI
- Adenoid hypertrophy
- GERD
- Cleft palate
- Down syndrome
- Obesity
- Nasopharyngeal carcinoma or other tumor

 DIAGNOSIS

HISTORY

- ETDQ-7 is a reliable and disease-specific symptom score for adult patients with ETD:
  - Pressure in ears in past 1 month?
  - Pain in ears in past 1 month?
  - A feeling that ears are clogged or "under water"?
  - Ear symptoms when you have cold or sinusitis?
  - Crackling or popping sounds in the ears?
  - Ringing in ears?
  - A feeling that your hearing is muffled?

- Questions are answered based on the presence and intensity of symptoms in the past 1 month. Severity of each symptom is rated on an ascending scale of 1–7, with 1 indicating no problem and 7 indicating severe problems. A total score cutoff point >14.5 categorizes the patient as having the diagnosis of ETD (2)[B].

- Other important things to remember:
  - Determine unilateral or bilateral involvement. If an adult presents with persistent unilateral symptoms, work up for nasopharyngeal process such as tumor.
  - History of previous ear infections, surgeries, head trauma, recent flying or diving
  - Voice change (hypo- or hypernasal voice, consider NP mass or palatal dysfunction)
  - Differentiate patulous dysfunction, in which patient complains of hearing his own voice and breath sounds are amplified (autophony), from dilatory dysfunction, in which patient complains more of ear pain, "plugged" ear, hearing loss, and tinnitus.

PHYSICAL EXAM

- Pneumatic otoscopy: Retracted tympanic membrane, effusion, decreased drum movement
- Toynbee maneuver: View changes of the drum while patient autoinsufflates against closed lips and pinched nostrils. May show various degrees of retraction:
  - Entire drum may be retracted and "lateralize" with insufflation.
  - Posterosuperior quadrant (pars flaccida) may form a retraction pocket.
- Tuning fork tests: 512-Hz fork placed on the forehead lateralizes to affected ear (Weber test); the fork will be louder behind the ear on the mastoid than in front of the ear (bone conduction > air conduction, Rinne test) in conductive hearing loss
- Nasopharyngoscopy: Adenoid hypertrophy or nasopharyngeal mass
- Anterior rhinoscopy: Deviated nasal septum, polyps, mucosal hypertrophy, turbinate hypertrophy

DIFFERENTIAL DIAGNOSIS

- SSNHL (a medical emergency)
- Tympanic membrane perforation
- Barotrauma
- TMJ disorder
- Ménière disease
- Superior semicircular canal dehiscence

DIAGNOSTIC TESTS & INTERPRETATION
None

Initial Tests (lab, imaging)
- Radiologic studies are not performed routinely if clinical signs/symptoms suggest ETD.
- CT scan may show changes related to OM or middle ear/mastoid opacification.
- Functional MRI might determine cause of ETD as the ET opening can be visualized during Valsalva, as well as lesions hampering tubal opening.

Diagnostic Procedures/Other
- Audiogram may show conductive hearing loss.
- Tympanometry: Type B or C tympanograms indicate fluid or retraction, respectively. Negative middle ear peak pressures seen even with normal (type A) tympanograms.

TREATMENT

- Reduce cycle of infection/inflammation.
- Tympanostomy tubes ± adenoidectomy when indicated for recurrent ear infections or severe progressive retractions

MEDICATION

- Few data support pharmacologic treatments for ETD. Multiple retrospective Cochrane Reviews argue against use of decongestants, nasal steroids, or antihistamines for ETD (3)[A].
- Medication options here are for treatment of comorbid conditions; treat based on symptoms and possible etiology.
- Decongestants, topical, oral (1)[C]:
  – Avoid prolonged use (>3 days); can cause rhinitis medicamentosa.
  – Decongestants are most useful for acute ETD related to a resolving URI.
  – Decongestants are not typically employed for relief of chronic ETD in children:
    ○ Phenylephrine (Dimetapp Cold Drops, PediaCare Children's Decongestant, others): Adults and children >12, 1 (10 mg) tablet q4h PRN; children 6–11, 5 mg q4h PRN; children <4, 2.5 mg q4h PRN
    ○ Pseudoephedrine (Sudafed): Adults, 60 mg q4–6h PRN; children <12, 30 mg q4–6h PRN
    ○ Oxymetazoline (Afrin Nasal Spray): Adults and children >6 years, 1–2 sprays each nostril q12h PRN. Limit use to ≤3 days.
    ○ Phenylephrine (Neo-synephrine Nasal Spray): Adults, 1–2 sprays each nostril q4h PRN. Limit use to ≤3 days.
- Nasal steroids (may be beneficial for those with allergic rhinitis) (1)[B]:
  – Beclomethasone (Beconase, Vancenase): Adults and children >12, 1–2 sprays each nostril b.i.d.; children 6–12, 1 spray each nostril b.i.d. Not recommended for children <6.
  – Budesonide (Rhinocort): Adults and children >6, 1 spray each nostril daily
  – Ciclesonide (Omnaris) (a prodrug activated on nasal mucosa): Adults and children >6, 2 sprays each nostril daily
  – Flunisolide (Nasarel, Nasalide): Adults and children >6, 2 sprays each nostril b.i.d.
  – Fluticasone furoate (Veramyst): Adults and children >12, 2 sprays each nostril daily; children 2–11, 1 spray each nostril daily

  – Fluticasone propionate (Flonase): Adults 1–2 sprays each nostril daily; children >4, 1 spray each nostril daily
  – Mometasone (Nasonex): Adults and children >12, 2 sprays each nostril daily; children 2–12, 1 spray each nostril daily. Only steroid nasal spray with indication for use in children ≥2.
  – Triamcinolone (Nasacort): Adults and children >6, 1–2 sprays each nostril daily; children 2–5, 1 spray each nostril daily
- 2nd-generation H$_1$ antihistamines (may be beneficial for those with ETD and chronic rhinitis) (1)[B]:
  – Cetirizine (Zyrtec) (tablets, chewable tablets, liquid): Adults and children >6, 5–10 mg/d PO; children 6 months–5 years: 2.5–5 mg/d PO or divided b.i.d.
  – Desloratadine (Clarinex) (tablets, Redi-tabs, liquid): Adults and children >12, 5 mg/d PO; children 6–11 years, 2.5 mg/d PO; children 12 months–5 years, 1.25 mg/d PO; children 6–11 months, 1 mg/d PO
  – Fexofenadine (Allegra) (tablets, Redi-tabs, liquid): Adults and children >12, 60 mg PO b.i.d. or 180 mg/d PO; children 6–11, 30 mg PO b.i.d.
  – Levocetirizine (Xyzal) (tablets, liquid): Adults and children >12, 2.5–5 mg PO every evening; children 6–11, 2.5 mg PO every evening; children 6 months–5 years, 1.25 mg PO every evening
- Antihistamine nasal sprays (may be beneficial for those with ETD and chronic rhinitis):
  – Azelastine (Astepro or Astelin): Adults and children >12, 1–2 sprays each nostril b.i.d.; children 6–11, 1 spray each nostril b.i.d.
  – Olopatadine (Patanase): Adults and children >12, 2 sprays each nostril b.i.d.; children 6–11, 1 spray each nostril b.i.d.
- If ETD leads to OM associated with tympanic membrane perforation or if ventilation tube present, topical antibiotic drops are more efficacious than PO antibiotics (1)[A]:
  – Neomycin–polymyxin–hydrocortisone suspension (Cortisporin): 4 drops q.i.d. × 10 days
  – Ciprofloxacin–hydrocortisone suspension (Cipro HC): 5 drops b.i.d. × 7 days
  – Ofloxacin (Floxin): 5–10 drops b.i.d. × 10 days for acute OM

SURGERY/OTHER PROCEDURES

- Myringotomy and pressure equalization tube placement to ventilate middle ear, relieve pressure, and prevent sequelae of chronically retracted drum (1)[A]
- Patients with ETD during pressure changes may benefit from minimally invasive laser eustachian tuboplasty (4)[B].
- Adenoidectomy if hypertrophied tissue is present:
  – In children, 1st set of tubes are typically placed alone. Adenoidectomy is performed with 2nd set of tubes if problems recur (1)[A].
  – Some advocate adenoidectomy even in absence of excess tissue; reduces frequency and number of subsequent tubes.

 # ONGOING CARE

FOLLOW-UP RECOMMENDATIONS
- Monitor pressure equalization tubes every 6–8 months in children and every 6–12 months in adults.

- Monitor tympanic membrane retraction pocket for progression every 6–12 months to allow for early intervention for progression in hearing loss, obvious ossicular erosion, or cholesteatoma.

DIET
In newborns, breastfeeding has been associated with lower incidence of ETD and OM (1)[A].

PROGNOSIS
If symptoms of ETD persist beyond age 7, patient is more likely to have long-term problems and require regular monitoring.

COMPLICATIONS
Morbidity related to hearing compromise or associated sequela of chronic ear infections

REFERENCES
1. Bluestone CD. Studies in otitis media: Children's Hospital of Pittsburgh-University of Pittsburgh progress report—2004. *Laryngoscope.* 2004;114: 1–26.
2. McCoul ED, Anand VK, Christos PJ. Validating the clinical assessment of eustachian tube dysfunction: The Eustachian Tube Dysfunction Questionnaire (ETDQ-7). *Laryngoscope.* 2012;122(5):1137–1141. Epub 2012 Feb 28.
3. Simpson SA, Lewis R, van der Voort J, et al. Oral or topical nasal steroids for hearing loss associated with otitis media with effusion in children. *Cochrane Database Syst Rev.* 2011;5.
4. Jumah MD, Jumah M, Pazen D, et al. Laser Eustachian tuboplasty: Efficiency evaluation in the pressure chamber. *Otol Neurotol.* 2012;33: 406–412.

ADDITIONAL READING
- Gluth MB, McDonald DR, Weaver AL, et al. Management of eustachian tube dysfunction with nasal steroid spray: a prospective, randomized, placebo-controlled trial. *Arch Otolaryngol Head Neck Surg.* 2011;137(5):449–455. doi: 10.1001/archoto.2011.56.
- Seibert JW, Danner CJ. Eustachian tube dysfunction and the middle ear. *Otolaryngol Clin North Am.* 2006;39(6):1221–1235.

 ## SEE ALSO
Algorithm: Ear Pain

 ## CODES

ICD10
- H69.00 Patulous Eustachian tube, unspecified ear
- H69.90 Unspecified Eustachian tube disorder, unspecified ear
- H68.109 Unspecified obstruction of Eustachian tube, unspecified ear

CLINICAL PEARLS
- ETD can be an acute or chronic problem, and treatment should base on underlying etiology.
- SSNHL (medical emergency) can be misdiagnosed as ETD and should always be ruled out, especially in patients with unilateral symptoms.

E

FACTOR V LEIDEN

Samuel B. Carli, MD • Parminder Singh, MD

 BASICS

DESCRIPTION
- Factor V Leiden is a genetic mutation in the coagulation pathway that results in the most common thrombophilic disease.
- System(s) affected: Cardiovascular; Gastrointestinal; Hemo-/Lymphatic/Immunologic; Nervous; Pulmonary; Reproductive.
- Synonym(s): Factor V Leiden thrombophilia; Factor V Leiden mutation, Hereditary APC Resistance

Pediatric Considerations
Increased thrombosis risk in patients with factor V Leiden

Pregnancy Considerations
Recurrent late pregnancy loss is a possible complication.

EPIDEMIOLOGY
- Predominant age: Thrombosis typically occurs after the second decade.
- Predominant sex: Male = Female

Prevalence
- Most common in Caucasians: Studies estimate ~5–8% occurance in Caucasians, with Asian Americans affected the least at ~0.45%

ETIOLOGY AND PATHOPHYSIOLOGY
- In the 'checks and balances' of the coagulation pathway, the clotting cascade and ultimately thrombin, will create activated protein C (APC) in an effort to establish a negative feedback loop.
- APC and its cofactor, protein S, lead to inactivation of factors V and VIII.
- Point mutation causing substitution of arginine for glutamine in location 506 of factor V gene, rendering it less susceptible to inactivation by activated protein C (APC)
- This, in turn, reduces the anticoagulant role of factor V and increases the *procoagulant* role of activated factor V, as there is now 20-fold slower degradation of activated factor V Leiden.

RISK FACTORS
- Risk for venous thromboembolism (VTE) is ~7-fold in heterozygous and ~80-fold in homozygous factor V Leiden individuals, compared with individuals without the mutation (1).
- Having non-O blood type (A, B or AB) can increase the risk VTE in both heterozygotes and homozytoes by 2- to 4-fold.
- Increased estrogen states may cause an acquired resistance to APC, thus:
  - Oral contraceptives in homozygotes may increase the risk 100-fold; in heterozygotes, 35-fold.
  - The increased risk is halved when the patient uses desogestrel-containing oral contraceptives.
- Hormone replacement therapy (HRT) and selective estrogen receptor modulators (SERMs) both increase the risk of thrombosis; in patients with factor V Leiden, that risk is increased substantially.

- Pregnancy and *homozygous* factor V Leiden increase the risk of thrombosis 7–16-fold during pregnancy and the puerperium. Other complications of pregnancy may be increased in patients with factor V Leiden.
- Data are conflicting with regard to risk for recurrent VTE for patients with FVL, but trend toward an increased risk (2,3).

GENERAL PREVENTION
Patients with factor V Leiden without thrombosis do not require prophylactic anticoagulation.

COMMONLY ASSOCIATED CONDITIONS
Venous thrombosis

 DIAGNOSIS

HISTORY
- Previous thrombosis
- Family history of thrombosis

PHYSICAL EXAM
- Family history of factor V Leiden mutation
- Findings suggestive of VTE, which can include deep venous thrombosis (DVT), pulmonary embolus (PE), and cerebral vein thrombosis: 10–26% of patients with VTE are carriers of the FVL mutation.
- Thrombosis in unusual locations, such as the sagittal sinus, mesentery, and portal systems, is less common in patients with factor V Leiden than in patients with deficiency of protein C or S.
- Obstetric complications and venous thrombosis are increased in patients with factor V Leiden and especially in those taking oral contraceptives.
- There is a weak, however significant, association between procoagulant states (including FVL) and coronary events in younger patients (4).

DIFFERENTIAL DIAGNOSIS
- Protein C deficiency
- Protein S deficiency
- Antithrombin deficiency
- Other causes of activated protein C resistance (e.g., antiphospholipid antibodies)
- Dysfibrinogenemia
- Dysplasminogenemia
- Homocystinemia
- Prothrombin 20210 mutation
- Elevated factor VIII levels

DIAGNOSTIC TESTS & INTERPRETATION
Initial Tests (lab, imaging)
- For evaluation of a new clot in patient at risk: CBC with peripheral smear, PT/INR, aPTT, thrombin time, lupus anticoagulant, antiphospholipid antibodies, factor VIII, anticardiolipin antibody, anti-B2 glycoprotein I antibody, activated protein C resistance, protein S antigen and resistance, antithrombin III assay, fibrinogen, factor V Leiden, prothrombin G20210A

- Genetic test: DNA-based test for factor V mutation; will be unaffected by anticoagulation and other drugs
- Functional test: Plasma-based coagulation assay using factor V–deficient plasma to which patient plasma is added along with purified activated protein C. The relative prolongation of the activated partial thromboplastin time (aPTT) is used to assay for the defect. Heparin, direct thrombin inhibitors and factor Xa inhibitor may cause false–negative results.
- Extremity US for DVT
- V/Q scan of spiral CT for PE

Follow-Up Tests & Special Considerations
- US may not show DVT acutely; repeat in 5–7days if strong suspicion.
- V/Q scan may be difficult to interpret in patients with other lung disease.

Diagnostic Procedures/Other
Magnetic resonance angiography (MRA), venography, or arteriography to detect thrombosis

 TREATMENT

Indicated if thrombotic event

GENERAL MEASURES
- Like general VTE treatment, patients with factor V Leiden and a 1st thrombosis should be anticoagulated initially with heparin or LMWH and warfarin for at least 3 months.
- Treatment with low-molecular-weight heparin (LMWH) is recommended over unfractionated heparin, unless the patient has severe renal failure (5)[A].
- Treat as outpatient, if possible (5)[A].
- Initiate warfarin with heparin on the 1st treatment day, and discontinue heparin after 5 days and when INR >2 (5)[A].
- Patients should be maintained on warfarin with an INR of 2–3 for at least 3–6 months (5)[A].
- For those patients with recurrence, the risks and benefits of indefinite anticoagulation need to be assessed.

MEDICATION
First Line
- Low-molecular-weight heparin (LMWH):
  - Enoxaparin (Lovenox): 1 mg/kg SC b.i.d., start warfarin simultaneously, continue Lovenox for at least 5 days and until INR is >2, at which time it can be stopped.
  - Fondaparinux (Arixtra): 5–10 mg(weight based) SC daily
  - Tinzaparin (Innohep): 175 anti-Xa IU/kg SC daily for 6 days and patient is adequately anticoagulated with warfarin (INR of at least 2 for 2 consecutive days)
  - Dalteparin (Fragmin): 200 IU/kg SC daily
- Oral anticoagulant:
  - Warfarin (Coumadin) PO with dose adjusted to an INR of 2–3 (3)[A]

- Contraindications:
  - Active bleeding precludes anticoagulation.
  - Risk of bleeding is a relative contraindication to long-term anticoagulation.
  - Warfarin is contraindicated in patients with history of warfarin skin necrosis (5)[A].
  - Warfarin is contraindicated in pregnancy.
- Precautions:
  - Observe patient for signs of embolization, further thrombosis, or bleeding.
  - Avoid IM injections. Periodically check stool and urine for occult blood; monitor CBCs, including platelets.
  - Heparin: Thrombocytopenia and/or paradoxic thrombosis with thrombocytopenia
  - Warfarin: Necrotic skin lesions (typically breasts, thighs, or buttocks)
  - LMWH: Adjust dosage in renal insufficiency. May also need dose adjustment in pregnancy.
- Significant possible interactions:
  - Agents that intensify the response to oral anticoagulants: Alcohol, allopurinol, amiodarone, anabolic steroids, androgens, many antimicrobials, cimetidine, chloral hydrate, disulfiram, all NSAIDs, sulfinpyrazone, tamoxifen, thyroid hormone, vitamin E, ranitidine, salicylates, acetaminophen
  - Agents that diminish the response to anticoagulants: Aminoglutethimide, antacids, barbiturates, carbamazepine, cholestyramine, diuretics, griseofulvin, rifampin, oral contraceptives

Second Line
- Heparin 80 mg/kg IV bolus followed by 18 g/kg/h continuous infusion
- Adjust dose depending on aPTT.
- In patients requiring large daily doses of heparin, measure an anti-Xa level for dose guidance.
- Alternatively, for outpatients, weight-adjusted sub-cutaneous unfractionated heparin with 333 U/kg first, then 250 U/kg, without monitoring (5)[A].
- Consider deficiency of antithrombin as a co-mutation in patients with significant elevated heparin requirements.

ISSUES FOR REFERRAL
- Recurrent thrombosis on anticoagulation
- Difficulty anticoagulating
- Genetic counseling

SURGERY/OTHER PROCEDURES
- Anticoagulation must be held for surgical interventions.
- For most patients with DVT, recommendations are against routine use of vena cava filter in addition to anticoagulation except when there is contraindication for anticoagulation (5)[A].
- Thrombectomy may be necessary in some cases.

IN-PATIENT CONSIDERATIONS
Admission Criteria/Initial Stabilization
Complicated thrombosis, such as PE
Nursing
- Teach LMWH and warfarin use.
- See above for drug interactions.
Discharge Criteria
Stable on anticoagulation

 ONGOING CARE

FOLLOW-UP RECOMMENDATIONS
Patient Monitoring
Warfarin use requires periodic (~monthly after initial stabilization) INR measurements, with a goal of 2–3 (5)[A].

DIET
- No restrictions
- Large amounts of foods rich in vitamin K may interfere with anticoagulation with warfarin.

PATIENT EDUCATION
- Patients should be educated about:
  - Use of oral anticoagulant therapy
  - Avoidance of NSAIDs while on warfarin
- The role of family screening is unclear, as most patients with this mutation do not have thrombosis. In a patient with a family history of factor V Leiden, consider screening during pregnancy or if considering oral contraceptive use.

PROGNOSIS
- Most patients heterozygous for factor V Leiden do not have thrombosis.
- Homozygotes have about a 50% lifetime incidence of thrombosis.
- Recurrence rates after a 1st thrombosis are not clear, with some investigators finding rates as high as 5% and others finding rates similar to the general population.
- Despite the increased risk for thrombosis, factor V Leiden does not increase overall mortality.

COMPLICATIONS
- Recurrent thrombosis
- Bleeding on anticoagulation

REFERENCES

1. Rosendaal FR, Koster T, Vandenbroucke JP, et al. High risk of thrombosis in patients homozygous for factor V Leiden (activated protein C resistance). *Blood*. 1995;85(6):1504.
2. Lijfering WM, Middeldorp S, Veeger NJ, et al. Risk of recurrent venous thrombosis in homozygous carriers and double heterozygous carriers of factor V Leiden and prothrombin G20210A. *Circulation*. 2010;121:1706–1712.
3. Ho WK, Hankey GJ, Quinlan DJ, et al. Risk of recurrent venous thromboembolism in patients with common thrombophilia: A systematic review. *Arch Intern Med*. 2006;166(7):729.
4. Ye Z, Liu EH, Higgins JP, et al. Seven haemostatic gene polymorphisms in coronary disease: Meta-analysis of 66,155 cases and 91,307 controls. *Lancet*. 2006;367(9511):651–658.
5. Guyatt GH, Akl EA, Crowther M, et al. Executive summary: Antithrombotic Therapy and Prevention of Thrombosis, 9th ed: American College of Chest Physicians Evidence-Based Clinical Practice Guidelines. *Chest*. 2012;141(2 Suppl):7S–47S.

ADDITIONAL READING

Seligsohn U, Lubetsky A. Genetic susceptibility to venous thrombosis. *N Engl J Med*. 2001;344: 1222–1231.

 SEE ALSO

Deep Vein Thrombophlebitis (DVT)

 CODES

ICD10
D68.51 Activated protein C resistance

CLINICAL PEARLS
- Extremely rare in Asian and African populations
- Asymptomatic patients with factor V Leiden do not need anticoagulation.
- For pregnant women homozygous for factor V Leiden but no prior history of VTE, postpartum prophylaxis with prophylactic or intermediate-dose LMWH or vitamin K antagonists with target INR 2–3 for 6 weeks is recommended. Antepartum prophylaxis is added if there is positive family of VTE (3)[B].

F

FAILURE TO THRIVE

Durr-e-Shahwaar Sayed, DO

 BASICS

DESCRIPTION

- Failure to thrive (FTT) is not a diagnosis but a sign of inadequate nutrition in young children manifested by a failure of physical growth, usually affecting weight. In severe cases, decreased length and/or head circumference may develop.
- Various parameters are used to define FTT:
  - Weight for age <5th percentile on >1 occasion
  - Weight that drops ≥2 major percentile lines on standard growth charts
  - Weight <80% median weight for length
  - Weight <75% median weight for age
  - Weight for length <5th percentile
  - Height for age <5th percentile
- Weight for length may be the simplest method to identify FTT, but verify with other parameters.

Pediatric Considerations

- Children with genetic syndromes, intrauterine growth restriction (IUGR), or prematurity follow different growth curves.
- 25% of children will decrease their weight or height crossing ≥2 major percentile lines in the 1st 2 years of life. These children are failing to reach their genetic potential or demonstrating constitutional growth delay (slow growth with a bone age < chronologic age). After shifting down, these infants grow at a normal rate along their new percentile and do not have FTT.

EPIDEMIOLOGY

Incidence

- Predominant age: 6–12 months; 80% <18 months
- Predominant sex: Male = Female

Prevalence

- As many as 10% of children seen in primary care have signs of growth failure.
- 1–5% of pediatric inpatient admissions are for FTT.
- Occurs more frequently in children living in poverty (1).

ETIOLOGY AND PATHOPHYSIOLOGY

- Mismatch between caloric intake and caloric expenditure
- Often grouped into 4 major categories:
  - Inadequate caloric intake (most frequent)
  - Inadequate caloric absorption
  - Excessive caloric expenditure
  - Defective utilization
- Traditionally, FTT was classified as organic or nonorganic, but most cases are multifactorial
- FTT often begins with a specific event and may lead to persistent difficulties.
- Causes of FTT can be grouped by pathophysiology (including examples):
  - Inadequate intake: Breastfeeding difficulty, incorrect formula preparation, poor transition to food (6–12 months), poor feeding habits (e.g., excessive juice, restrictive diets), mechanical problems (e.g., oromotor dysfunction, congenital anomalies, GERD, CNS or PNS anomalies), oral aversion, poverty, neglect, poor parent–child interaction
  - Inadequate absorption: Necrotizing enterocolitis, short gut syndrome, biliary atresia, liver disease, cystic fibrosis, celiac disease, milk protein allergy, vitamin/mineral deficiency

- Increased expenditure: Hyperthyroidism, congenital/chronic cardiopulmonary disease, HIV, immunodeficiencies, malignancy, renal disease
- Defective utilization: Metabolic disorders, congenital infections (TORCH: Toxoplasmosis, Other Agents, Rubella, Cytomegalovirus, Herpes simplex)

Genetics

Multiple genetic disorders can cause FTT.

RISK FACTORS

- Psychosocial risks:
  - Poverty, parent(s) with mental health disorder or cognitive impairment, poor parenting skills or hypervigilant parents, families with unique health/nutritional beliefs, physical or emotional abuse, substance abuse, and social isolation
- Medical risks:
  - Intrauterine exposures, history of IUGR (symmetric or asymmetric), congenital abnormalities, oromotor dysfunction, premature or sick newborn, infant with physical deformity, acute or chronic medical conditions, developmental delay, lead poisoning, anemia

Pregnancy Considerations

FTT is linked to intrauterine exposures, IUGR, and prematurity.

GENERAL PREVENTION

- Educate parents on normal feeding and parenting skills
- Access to supplemental feeding programs (WIC)

 DIAGNOSIS

HISTORY

- Prenatal and developmental history
- Past medical history: Acute/Chronic disease affecting caloric intake, digestion, absorption, or causing increased energy need or defective utilization
- Medication history, including complementary and alternative medications
- Family history: Stature of parents and growth trajectories of siblings, chronic diseases, genetic disorders, developmental delay
- Diet history from birth: Breastfeeding or formula feeding; timing and introduction of solids; who feeds the child, when, and how often; placement of child during feeds; amounts consumed/caloric intake; beverages consumed; snacking; vomiting or stooling associated with feeds; oral aversions or unusual behaviors during feeding
- Social history: Family composition: socioeconomic status, child-rearing beliefs, stressors, parental depression, parental substance abuse, caretaker personal history of abuse/neglect
- Review of systems: Anorexia, activity level, mental status, fevers, dysphagia, vomiting, gastroesophageal reflux, stooling pattern/consistency, dysuria, urinary frequency

PHYSICAL EXAM

- *Accurate* measurement of height, weight, and head circumference on National Center for Health Statistics (NCHS) growth charts (www.cdc.gov/growthcharts)

- The World Health Organization (WHO) growth charts may be more appropriate for breastfed infants (www.who.int/childgrowth/standards/en/), and growth charts exist for many other syndromes/conditions such as Down syndrome, Turner syndrome, and premature infant.
- Exam should assess for the following:
  - Signs of dehydration or severe malnutrition:
    - Severity of malnutrition estimated via Gomez classification: Compare current weight for age with expected weight for age (50th percentile): Severe, <60% of expected; Moderate, 61–75%; Mild, 76–90%
  - Underlying medical disease
  - Dysmorphic features
  - Mental status (alert, responsive to stimuli)
  - Any signs of physical abuse and/or neglect
- Observe interaction with caregivers and feeding techniques, specifically bonding and social/psychological cues.

DIFFERENTIAL DIAGNOSIS

Differentiate based on growth patterns:

- FTT classically presents as low weight for age, normal linear growth, normocephalic *or* low weight for age, followed by decreased linear growth *or* low weight for age, leading to decreased linear growth and decreased head circumference (without neurologic signs):
  - In this situation, consider differential diagnosis as outlined in "Etiology and Pathophysiology."
- If low linear growth with normal weight for length *or* low linear growth and proportionately low weight and decreased head circumference:
  - Consider genetic potential (constitutional short stature or growth delay), genetic syndromes, teratogens, endocrine disorders
- If microcephaly with prominent neurologic signs, with poor growth secondary to presumed neurologic disorder:
  - Consider TORCH infections, genetic syndromes, teratogens, brain injury (i.e., hypoxic/ischemic)

DIAGNOSTIC TESTS & INTERPRETATION

- Labs useful only in ~1% of cases, usually those cases where underlying disease is suspected.
- A period of renutrition is preferable prior to extensive labs and other workup.

Initial Tests (lab, imaging)

Labs should be ordered based on history and physical exam findings and the age of the patient.

- Tests often considered in initial evaluation:
  - CBC, ESR
  - Electrolytes, BUN/creatinine, liver function tests
  - Urinalysis and urine culture
  - Lead level
- Other tests as dictated by the history and exam:
  - TSH, amylase/lipase, serum zinc level, iron studies, karyotype, genetic testing, sweat chloride test, stool for ova and parasite or fat/reducing substances, guaiac, α-1-antitrypsin and elastase, radioallergosorbent test testing for IgE food allergies, tissue transglutaminase and total IgA (celiac sprue), P-ANCA and anti-Saccharomyces cerevisiae antibodies for *IBD*), TB test, *HIV*, ELISA, hepatitis A, B, other infections

Follow-Up Tests & Special Considerations
- Home visit by a clinician to observe infant feeding, interaction with caretakers, and home environment (2).
- Observe breastfeeding and/or formula preparation to ensure adequacy and offer instruction.
- Prospective 3-day food diary for accurate record of caloric intake should be obtained.
- Additional indicated evaluations may be performed by dietitians, occupational, physical and speech therapists, social workers, developmental specialists, psychiatrists, psychologists, visiting nurses, lactation consultants, and/or child protection services.

Can consider:
- Skeletal survey if suspicion of physical abuse
- Bone age if possible endocrine disorder
- Swallowing studies, small bowel follow through if possible oromotor dysfunction, GERD, structural abnormalities
- Brain imaging if microcephalic and/or neurologic findings on examination

TREATMENT

GENERAL MEASURES
- Treat underlying conditions.
- Caregiver and infant interaction should be evaluated in infants and children with FTT.
- The goal is to improve nutrition to allow catch-up growth (weight gain 2–3 times > average for age).
- Calculate energy needs based on recommended energy intake for age, increased by 50%:
  – Recommended energy intake (use *expected*, not actual weight, to calculate needs):
    ○ 0–1 month: 120 kcal/kg/d
    ○ 1–2 months: 115 kcal/kg/d
    ○ 2–3 months: 105 kcal/kg/d
    ○ 3–6 months: 95 kcal/kg/d
    ○ 6 months to 3 years: 90 kcal/kg/d (3)[C]
- Alternatively, may calculate caloric requirements for infants to achieve catch-up growth:
  – kcal/kg/d required = [RDA for age (kcal/kg) × Ideal weight for height/Actual weight, where ideal weight for height is the median weight for the patient's height.
- Try various strategies to increase caloric intake:
  – Optimize breastfeeding support, consider supplementation
  – Higher calorie formulas
  – Addition of rice cereal or fats to current foods
  – Limit intake of milk to 24–32 oz/d
  – Avoid juice and soda
  – Vitamin and/or nutritional supplements
  – Assist with social and family problems (WIC, food stamps, and other transitional assistance).
- Rapid high-calorie intake can cause diarrhea, malabsorption, hypokalemia, hypophosphatemia. Therefore, increasing formulas above 24 kcal/oz is not recommended.
- The target energy intake should be slowly increased to goal over 5–7 days.
- Catch-up growth should be seen in 2–7 days.
- Accelerated growth should be continued for 4–9 months to restore weight and height.

MEDICATION
Use only for identified underlying conditions

ISSUES FOR REFERRAL
- Refer as indicated for underlying conditions.
- Multidisciplinary care is beneficial (1)[B]. Specialized multidisciplinary clinics may be of benefit for children with complicated situations, failure to respond to initial treatment, or when the PCP does not have access to specialized services such as nutrition, psychology, PT/OT, speech therapy (4).

ADDITIONAL THERAPIES
In severe cases, nasogastric tube feedings or gastrostomy may be considered.

IN-PATIENT CONSIDERATIONS
Most cases of FTT can be managed as outpatients.

Admission Criteria/Initial Stabilization
Hospitalization should be considered if:
- Outpatient management fails.
- There is evidence of severe dehydration or malnutrition.
- There are signs of abuse or neglect.
- There are concerns that the psychosocial situation presents harm to child.
- During catch-up growth, some children will develop nutritional recovery syndrome:
  – Symptoms include sweating, increased body temperature, hepatomegaly (increased glycogen deposits), widening of cranial sutures (brain growth > bone growth), increased periods of sleep, fidgeteness, and mild hyperactivity.
- There may also be an initial period of malabsorption with resultant diarrhea.

Discharge Criteria
Catch-up growth should be seen in 2–7 days. If this is not seen, re-evaluation of causes is needed.

ONGOING CARE

FOLLOW-UP RECOMMENDATIONS
- If specific disease identified, follow-up as indicated.
- Close long-term follow up with frequent visits is important to create and maintain a healthy, supportive environment (2).
- Children with history of FTT are at increased risk of recurrent FTT, and growth should be monitored closely (1).
- If the family fails to comply, child protection authorities must be notified.

DIET
Nutritional requirements for a "normal" child:
- Infant:
  – 120 kcal/kg/d, decreased to 95 kcal/kg/d at 6 months; if breastfed, ensure appropriate frequency and duration of feeding.
  – Between 6–12 months, continue breast milk and/or formula, but pureed foods should be consumed several times a day during this period.
- Toddler:
  – 3 meals plus 2 nutritional snacks, 16–32 oz milk/d; avoid juice and soda, and feed in a social environment.
  – Do not restrict fat and cholesterol in children <2 years.
- Rate of weight gain expected for age:
  – 0–3 months: 26–31 g/d
  – 3–6 months: 17–18 g/d
  – 6–9 months: 12–13 g/d
  – 9–12 months: 9 g/d
  – 1–3 years: 7–9 g/d

PATIENT EDUCATION
- Counsel parents regarding the need to avoid "food battles," which worsen the problem.
- Educate parents regarding infant social and physiological cues, formula/food preparation, proper feeding techniques, and importance of relaxed and social mealtimes.
- When environmental deprivation is identified, educating in a nonpunitive way is essential.
- "Failure to thrive: What this means for your child," available from AAFP at: www.aafp.org/afp/2011/0401/p837.html
- WIC provides grants to states for supplemental foods, health care referrals, and nutrition education for low-income pregnant, breastfeeding, and non-breastfeeding postpartum women, and to infants and children up to age 5 at nutritional risk: www.fns.usda.gov/wic/

PROGNOSIS
- Many children with FTT show adequate improvement in dietary intake with intervention.
- Some studies looking at children with FTT have demonstrated an association with later problems with cognitive development, behavioral issues, and growth, but there is no consensus on these long-term outcomes or their clinical significance (5).
- Children with FTT are at increased risk for future undernutrition, overnutrition, and eating disorders.

REFERENCES

1. Cole SZ, Lanham JS. Failure to thrive: An update. *Am Fam Physician*. 2011;83:829–834.
2. Shields B, Wacogne I, Wright CM, et al. Weight faltering and failure to thrive in infancy and early childhood. *BMJ*. 2012;345:e5931.
3. Krugman SD, Dubowitz H. Failure to thrive. *Am Fam Physician*. 2003;68:879–884.
4. Atalay A, McCord M. Characteristics of failure to thrive in a referral population: Implications for treatment. *Clin Pediatr (Phila)*. 2012;51:219–225.
5. Jaffe AC. Failure to thrive: Current clinical concepts. *Pediatr Rev*. 2011;32:100–107.

 SEE ALSO

Down Syndrome; Irritable Bowel Syndrome; Turner Syndrome

 CODES

ICD10
- P92.6 Failure to thrive in newborn
- R62.51 Failure to thrive (child)

CLINICAL PEARLS
- FTT is a sign of inadequate nutrition.
- Underlying medical and/or social issues are generally suggested by history and physical exam, and extensive laboratory or imaging tests are rarely needed.
- A multidisciplinary team approach to diagnosis and treatment is critical to help children with FTT and their families.

FATTY LIVER SYNDROME

Alisha Lakhani, MD, MPH • Edward Feller, MD

 BASICS

Nonalcoholic fatty liver disease (NAFLD): A spectrum of fatty liver disease ranging from nonalcoholic fatty liver (NAFL), hepatic steatosis without hepatocellular injury by imaging or histology, to nonalcoholic steatohepatitis (NASH) and cirrhosis with hepatocyte injury with/without fibrosis. May be implicated in up to 90% of patients with asymptomatic, mild aminotransferase elevation not caused by alcohol, viral hepatitis, or medications.

DESCRIPTION
- Fatty liver:
  - Reversible condition in which large vacuoles of triglyceride fat accumulate in hepatocytes; liver biopsy usually shows fatty deposits in >30% of liver cells; no necrosis, no fibrosis
  - Alanine aminotransferase/aspartate aminotransferase (ALT/AST) enzymes usually normal, but may be elevated, rarely >3–4× the upper limit of normal
- NAFLD:
  - Fatty liver not due to excess alcohol consumption (see definition)
  - Risk factors: Obesity, metabolic syndrome, dyslipidemia, insulin resistance, and type 2 diabetes (T2DM)
  - Emerging associations: Polycystic ovary, hypothyroidism, obstructive sleep apnea, hypopituitarism, hypogonadism, pancreatic resection
- NASH:
  - Progressive form of NAFLD; liver biopsy: Fatty deposits in >50% of liver cells with acute and chronic inflammation, fibrosis
  - Asymptomatic; ALT and AST elevated, generally <3–4× upper limit of normal
  - Disease may progress to cirrhosis and/or liver cancer; incomplete data to assess natural history, although some evidence indicates that 30% with NASH have progression of fibrosis over 5 years.
- Both diseases usually identified in the 4th and 5th decade; may occur at any age
- Associated with obesity, T2DM, dyslipidemia, and metabolic syndrome.
- Synonym(s): Steatosis; Steatonecrosis; NAFLD; Steatohepatitis; NASH

Pregnancy Considerations
- Acute fatty liver of pregnancy: Severe complication of 3rd trimester. May be associated with pre-eclampsia
- Abrupt onset of confusion and restlessness with possible jaundice and right upper quadrant pain
- ALT, AST always elevated, >300 IU/L, but usually <1,000 IU/L
- Emergency liver biopsy confirms diagnosis.
- Prompt delivery corrects the liver disease.
- Recurrence rare in subsequent pregnancies

EPIDEMIOLOGY
NAFLD: Most common chronic liver disease globally; usually benign, asymptomatic fatty liver. NASH may be symptomatic with progressive inflammation and fibrosis; increases with age, slight male predominance (1)

Incidence
- Present in up to 50% obese (body mass index [BMI] >30) and 90% of morbidly obese (BMI >39) persons
- Present in 5–10% patients with T2DM
- Predominant age: 40s–50s; does occur in children
- Predominant sex: Male = Female

Prevalence
US prevalence: Estimated at 6–24%. NAFLD: Worldwide: 6.3–33%; increases to 58–74% in obesity (2), to 69–87% in T2DM, and 50% of individuals with dyslipidemia (1).

ETIOLOGY AND PATHOPHYSIOLOGY
Primary derangement is *insulin resistance*, which leads to increased lipolysis, triglyceride synthesis, and increased hepatic uptake of fatty acids (3).
- NAFLD: Most commonly an impaired ability of the liver to remove fatty acids
- NASH: "2-hit" hypothesis involving macrovesicular steatosis due to increased hepatic lipid synthesis, reduced hepatic transfer of lipids, increasing insulin resistance with increased hepatic oxidative stress (3). Mitochondrial damage leading to impaired restoration of ADT stores, lipid peroxidation, and increased iron stores each are found in 25–40% of NASH patients.

Genetics
Largely unknown: Data suggest familial clustering, slight increased heritability. NAFL: More 1st-degree relatives with cirrhosis than matched controls; NASH: 18% had an affected 1st-degree relative (1). Carriers of hemochromatosis gene are more likely to be affected; possible genetic variants in apolipoprotein C3 gene may play a role in fatty liver, insulin resistance, hypertriglyceridemia.

RISK FACTORS
- Obesity: BMI >30 and visceral obesity, T2DM, dyslipidemia; high serum triglycerides and low serum high-density lipoprotein (HDL) levels, metabolic syndrome
- New data suggest hypothyroidism, hypopituitarism, hypogonadism, sleep apnea, and polycystic ovary syndrome are risk factors for NAFLD.
- Protein–calorie malnutrition; total parenteral nutrition (TPN) >6 weeks
- Increasing age associated with increased prevalence, severity, advanced fibrosis, or mortality
- Severe acute weight loss (starvation, bariatric surgery)
- Organic solvent (e.g., chlorinated hydrocarbons, toluene) exposure; vinyl chloride; hypoglycin A
- Gene for hemochromatosis/other conditions with increased iron stores
- Drugs: Tetracycline, glucocorticoids, tamoxifen, methotrexate, valproic acid, fialuridine, many chemotherapy regimens, and nucleoside analogues

Pediatric Considerations
- Reye syndrome: Fatty liver with encephalopathy:
  - Vomiting with dehydration; usually postviral URI
  - Progressive CNS damage
  - Signs of hepatic injury: Extensive fatty vacuolization
  - Hypoglycemia
- Etiology unknown; viral agents and drugs, especially salicylates, are implicated.
- Mortality rate: 50%
- Treat with mannitol, IV glucose, and FFP

GENERAL PREVENTION
- Avoid excess alcohol: >30 g/d (men); >20 g/d (women).
- Maintain/Attain appropriate BMI.
- Optimize prevention and management of diabetes.
- Avoid hepatotoxic medications.
- HAV and HBV vaccination if not immune.
- Pneumovax and yearly influenza vaccination.

COMMONLY ASSOCIATED CONDITIONS
Preeclampsia in pregnancy, central obesity, T2DM, insulin resistance, hyperlipidemia, hypertension; possible increased risk in hypothyroidism, hypogonadism, sleep apnea

 DIAGNOSIS

- Consider hepatic steatosis in any patient with asymptomatic aminotransferase elevation.
- Can occur with normal/fluctuating AST and ALT.
- NASH has no distinguishing historical/laboratory features from other chronic liver disorders.
- Index of suspicion is higher with risk factors such as metabolic syndrome, insulin resistance, or obesity.
- May present as cryptogenic cirrhosis
- Noninvasive biomarkers of steatosis/fibrosis are not sufficiently reliable. Liver biopsy is the definitive diagnostic test. Biopsy should be considered only when results are likely to change management (4).

HISTORY
- Typically asymptomatic
- Possible fatigue and/or abdominal fullness
- History of medication and alcohol use, family history

PHYSICAL EXAM
Hepatomegaly: Incidentally observed enlarged liver/spleen on physical exam or imaging:
- Most common signs (all are infrequent):
  - Liver pain/tenderness
  - Mild to marked hepatomegaly
  - Splenomegaly
  - In advanced cases: Cutaneous stigmata of chronic liver disease or portal hypertension, variceal bleed, ascites, encephalopathy, edema

DIFFERENTIAL DIAGNOSIS
- Viral hepatitis
- Alcoholic fatty liver (history of alcoholism may be difficult to document/exclude)
- Drug- or toxin-induced hepatitis
- Occupational exposure
- Metabolic liver disease
- Autoimmune hepatitis
- Celiac disease
- Muscle disease, if nonhepatic cause of elevated enzymes are possible

DIAGNOSTIC TESTS & INTERPRETATION
Initial Tests (lab, imaging)
- Both ALT and AST may be elevated:
  - Nonalcoholic, usually ALT:AST >1
  - If alcohol-induced, usually AST:ALT ≥2; serum alkaline phosphatase and direct bilirubin may be mildly elevated.
  - If advanced cirrhosis is present, marked, nonspecific enzyme abnormalities may exist.
- Level of enzyme elevation does not correlate with degree of fibrosis (5)[C]. Normal blood chemistries are common in cirrhosis.

- Severity in acute liver disease is marked by defects in ability to produce plasma proteins (serum albumin, PT), which are also clues to chronicity.
- Thrombocytopenia may indicate chronicity and portal hypertension.
- Lipids commonly abnormal with elevated cholesterol, low-density lipoprotein (LDL), triglyceride, and decreased HDL
- Biomarkers of inflammation, increased oxidative stress, or hepatocyte apoptosis such as leptin, adiponectin, CRP, serum caspase, and cytokeratin 18 are investigational; may help differentiate NASH from NAFLD.
- Serologic studies to exclude viral hepatitis are vital: Serum ALT and AST, alkaline phosphatase, direct and total bilirubin, albumin and globulin, CBC, serum electrolytes, BUN, and creatinine
- Fatty liver identified as hyperechoic liver on US, the 1st-line imaging modality for assessment of liver chemistry abnormalities; MRI/CT may also be used.

Follow-Up Tests & Special Considerations
Patients require evaluation of other causes of asymptomatic aminotransferase elevations, such as celiac disease and hemochromatosis.

- Imaging modalities such as FibroScan, which detects tissue elasticity in cases of suspected hepatic fibrosis, and MR spectroscopy are currently being evaluated (5)[B]. Newer contrast agents, particularly for MRI, are being evaluated to help characterize NAFLD (6).
- No imaging modality can distinguish simple steatosis from steatohepatitis.

Diagnostic Procedures/Other
- Liver biopsy is the only reliable diagnostic method; however, it is invasive. Liver biopsy must have reasonable likelihood of changing management as a precondition.
- Predictors associated with increased risk of fibrosis are BMI >30, age >50 years, insulin resistance/diabetes mellitus, and elevated serum ALT, AST.

Test Interpretation
- Liver biopsy is the gold standard to differentiate fatty liver with good prognosis from NASH (1)[B].
- In NASH, steatosis, ballooning, and lobular inflammation are minimal criteria for diagnosis; other common, but not necessary, findings include mild–moderate portal inflammation, acidophil bodies, perisinusoidal zone 3 fibrosis, megamitochondria, and Mallory hyaline in hepatocytes.
- Staging is based largely on the extent of fibrosis.

 ## TREATMENT

- Sustained weight loss: Primary successful intervention in NASH.
- Most cited recommendation is lifestyle modification through improved diet and regular exercise. Studies show a reduction in liver fat, improved glucose control and insulin sensitivity (7).
- Promising early results reported with weight loss pharmacotherapy and bariatric surgery. Studies assessing insulin-sensitizing and hepatoprotective agents are inconclusive.
- Currently, no proven medication treatment regimen

GENERAL MEASURES
- Aerobic exercise 3× weekly for 20–45 minutes; reduce energy intake, modify diet.
- Diabetes should be tightly regulated.
- Components of metabolic syndrome (hypertension, dyslipidemia, and obesity) should be treated.
- Discontinue alcohol; avoid hepatotoxic medications.

MEDICATION
No specific therapy currently exists, but several promising agents are under investigation:

- Drugs improving insulin resistance may decrease aminotransferase levels and histologic damage, but they are not definitive. These include metformin (controversial) and pioglitazone.
- Vitamins E and C have shown mild improvement in treating hepatic steatosis and inflammation; results do not support widespread use (5)[B].
- Other drugs studied in small pilot trials and animal studies include fibrates, gemfibrozil, statins, omega-3 fatty acids, betaine, angiotensin-receptor blockers, and ursodeoxycholic acid. However, large randomized controlled studies are needed.

ISSUES FOR REFERRAL
Persistent liver enzyme elevation 2–3× above upper limit of normal without diagnosis or those with fibrosis on biopsy benefit from hepatologist evaluation.

COMPLEMENTARY AND ALTERNATIVE MEDICINE
Be wary of potential hepatotoxicity of complementary medications, which may also contain impurities.

SURGERY/OTHER PROCEDURES
Bariatric procedures: Not yet established as treatment option (1)[B]. Bariatric surgery is not contraindicated with morbid obesity (BMI >40).

 ## ONGOING CARE

FOLLOW-UP RECOMMENDATIONS
Patient Monitoring
- Repeat LFTs yearly.
- Perform yearly US/CT scan to document diminution in fat.
- Changes toward normal provide major motivation to continue lifestyle changes.
- Routine liver biopsy is not recommended.

DIET
Diet low in fat; low in simple carbohydrates; low in high-fructose corn syrup; devoid of trans fats; replete with vitamins, minerals, and natural antioxidants; avoid alcohol.

PATIENT EDUCATION
Life-long change in eating, exercise, and alcohol use

PROGNOSIS
Within the spectrum of NALFD, only NASH has been shown to be progressive, potentially leading to cirrhosis, hepatocellular carcinoma, cholangiocarcinoma, or liver failure:
- Cirrhosis develops in up to 25% of patients with NASH within 10 years of diagnosis; liver failure from cirrhosis occurs in 1–5%.
- Transplantation is effective, but NASH may recur after transplantation.

COMPLICATIONS
Progressive disease may be complicated by decompensated cirrhosis and portal hypertension, such as ascites, encephalopathy, bleeding varices, hepatorenal, or hepatopulmonary syndromes.

REFERENCES

1. Chalasani N, Younossi Z, Lavine JE, et al. Diagnosis and management of non-alcoholic fatty liver disease: Practice guideline by the AASLD, ACG, and the AGA. *Amer J Gastroenterol.* 2012;107: 811–826.
2. Foxx-Orenstein AE. Gastrointestinal symptoms and diseases related to obesity: An overview. *Gastroenterol Clin North Am.* 2010;39:23–37.
3. Edmison J, McCullough AJ. Pathogenesis of non-alcoholic steatohepatitis: Human data. *Clin Liver Dis.* 2007;11:75–104, ix.
4. Festi D, Schiumerini R, DiBiase AR, et al. Review article: The diagnosis of non-alcoholic fatty liver disease—availability and accuracy of non-invasive methods. *Aliment Pharmacol Ther.* 2013;37: 392–400.
5. Kleiner DE, Brunt EM. NAFLD: Pathologic patterns and biopsy evaluation in clinical research. *Semin Liver Dis.* 2012;32:3–13.
6. Browning JD. New imaging techniques for non-alcoholic steatohepatitis. *Clin Liver Dis.* 2009;13:607–619.
7. Thoma C, Day CP, Trenell MI. Lifestyle interventions for the treatment of non-alcoholic fatty liver disease in adults: A systematic review. *J Hepatol.* 2012;56:255–256.
8. Schwimmer JB, Pardee PE, Lavine JE, et al. Cardiovascular risk factors and the metabolic syndrome in pediatric nonalcoholic fatty liver disease. *Circulation.* 2008;118:277–283.

 ## SEE ALSO

Alcohol Abuse and Dependence; Cirrhosis of the Liver; Diabetes Mellitus, Type 2; Metabolic Syndrome

 ## CODES

ICD10
- K74.60 Unspecified cirrhosis of liver
- K75.81 Nonalcoholic steatohepatitis (NASH)
- K76.0 Fatty (change of) liver, not elsewhere classified

CLINICAL PEARLS
- NAFLD: Major cause of liver disease. Spectrum ranges from simple steatosis to NASH, advanced fibrosis, and, rarely, progression to cirrhosis.
- NAFLD: Most common chronic liver disease in children. Overweight children with NAFLD are more likely to have metabolic syndrome, central obesity; elevated total cholesterol, LDL, triglycerides; low HDL; impaired fasting glucose (8)[B].
- NAFLD: Common cause of asymptomatic mild serum aminotransferase elevation

FECAL IMPACTION

Pia Prakash, MD • Marie L. Borum, MD, EdD, MPH

 BASICS

DESCRIPTION
Incomplete evacuation of feces leading to the formation of a large, firm, immovable mass of stool typically in the rectum or distal sigmoid colon

EPIDEMIOLOGY
Incidence
Incidence increases with age:
- Predominant age: >70 years

Geriatric Considerations
42% of patients in a geriatric ward found to have fecal impaction

Prevalence
- 60% of patients with fecal impaction have a history of chronic constipation.
- In North America, the prevalence of constipation among the general population is between 1.9% and 27.2% (1).
- 78% of all children with encopresis were found to have fecal impaction (2).
- In children, encopresis is 3× more common in boys than girls (2).

ETIOLOGY AND PATHOPHYSIOLOGY
- Age-related degenerative changes of the enteric nervous system, colonic hypomotility, and age-related anatomic changes of the lower GI tract may contribute to delayed gut transit time and decreased stool water content (3).
- The rectosigmoid colon dilates to accommodate mass of fecal material, which, in turn, is not pliable enough to pass through the disproportionately small anal canal as a result of the patient's weak defecation effort.
- Impacted stool may exist as a single mass (stercolith) or as a composite of small, rounded fecal particles (scybalum).
- Poor diet:
  – Lacking in fiber
  – Inadequate water intake
  – Low calorie
- Medication side effect (1,4):
  – Stimulant laxatives
  – Opiate analgesics
  – Anticholinergics
  – Diuretics
  – Calcium channel blockers
  – Aluminum (sucralfate, antacids)
  – Iron
  – NSAIDs
- Neurogenic disorders:
  – Hirschsprung disease
  – Chagas disease
  – Autonomic neuropathy
  – Multiple sclerosis
  – Spinal cord injury
  – Cauda equina
  – Parkinson disease
- Metabolic derangements:
  – Hypothyroidism
  – Hyperparathyroidism
  – Diabetes mellitus
- Electrolyte disturbances:
  – Hypokalemia
  – Hypercalcemia
  – Hypermagnesemia
- Anatomic:
  – Anorectal stenosis
  – Neoplasm
  – Megarectum
  – Painful rectal conditions inhibiting voluntary defecation (e.g., anal fissure, hemorrhoids, fistulas)
- Psychological:
  – Depression
  – Anxiety
  – Anorexia nervosa
- Immobility
- Rectal bezoars
- Pelvic floor dysfunction or dyssynergia
- Irritable bowel syndrome, constipation predominant
- Idiopathic

Genetics
Fecal impaction of the cecum may be seen in cystic fibrosis.

RISK FACTORS
- Institutionalization
- Constipation
- Psychogenic illness
- Immobility, inactivity
- Pica
- Chronic renal failure
- Urinary incontinence
- Cognitive decline, disability
- Heavy metal ingestion or exposure
- Poor toileting habits
- Excessive seed consumption (common in Middle East cultures), leading to rectal seed bezoars

Pediatric Considerations
Habitual neglect of defecation urge may promote impaction.

GENERAL PREVENTION
- Maintain adequate hydration.
- Maintain high-fiber diet (5)[C].
- Regular exercise and ambulation (5)[B]
- Establish regular, consistent toilet time using gastrocolic reflex (5)[C].
- Psyllium (6)[B]
- Periodic enemas, if indicated
- Periodic polyethylene glycol powder (MiraLax) (6)[A]
- Lactulose (6)[A]

 DIAGNOSIS

HISTORY
- Abdominal pain and bloating
- Constipation
- Rectal discomfort
- Fecal incontinence, paradoxical diarrhea
- Nausea
- Vomiting
- Anorexia
- General malaise
- Agitation and confusion in elderly
- Urinary frequency
- Urinary incontinence

PHYSICAL EXAM
May be unremarkable, but the following are possible:
- Vital signs:
  – Tachycardia
  – Tachypnea
  – Low-grade fever
- General:
  – Agitated
  – Confused
  – Poor hydration status
- Abdominal:
  – Distention
  – Palpable, tubular mass in lower quadrant
- Rectal:
  – Copious amount of stool in rectal vault. If impaction is in sigmoid colon however, rectal exam will be nondiagnostic.
  – Fissures
  – Hemorrhoids
  – Loss of sphincter tone

DIFFERENTIAL DIAGNOSIS
- Colitis
- Diverticulitis
- Appendicitis
- Colorectal cancer

DIAGNOSTIC TESTS & INTERPRETATION
Initial Tests (lab, imaging)
- Laboratory testing is often unremarkable, but the following are possible:
  – Leukocytosis
  – Hyponatremia
  – Hypokalemia
  – Hypercalcemia
  – Hypermagnesemia
  – Hypothyroidism
  – Stool may be positive for occult blood.
- Plain abdominal radiography may reveal stool or signs of obstruction, including dilated colon or small bowel, and air-fluid levels.

Geriatric Considerations
Attempts to identify underlying cause should be carried out in all patients. Thyroid and electrolyte disturbances are common in elderly patients presenting with impaction.

Follow-Up Tests & Special Considerations
Pediatrics:
- Celiac antibodies (antigliadin and antiendomysial)
- Lead levels

Diagnostic Procedures/Other
Sigmoidoscopy may be used to clarify the nature of a rectosigmoid mass.

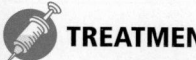 TREATMENT

GENERAL MEASURES
- Manual disimpaction and extraction of fecal mass often required.
- For stool located higher in the rectum, a rigid proctoscope may be used to disimpact stool or to pass enema solution to soften stool (4).

MEDICATION
First Line
- Enemas to soften stool and stimulate defecation:
  – Mineral oil enema or warm water enema to aid passage of stool
- Osmotic laxatives, such as polyethylene glycol solutions and magnesium citrate, may soften stool.
- Enemas and polyethylene glycol-electrolyte are equally effective in treating fecal impaction in children (7)[B].
- Precautions:
  – Use of osmotic laxatives is contraindicated with bowel obstruction (4).
  – Use magnesium citrate with caution in patients with renal insufficiency.
  – Lactulose may result in colonic distension due to bacterial fermentation.
  – Avoid soap, hot water, hydrogen peroxide enemas as they may result in rectal mucosal irritation.

COMPLEMENTARY AND ALTERNATIVE MEDICINE
Biofeedback improves constipation in patients with dyssynergic defecation, which may decrease incidence of impaction (8).

SURGERY/OTHER PROCEDURES
- Surgery may be necessary with intestinal perforation
- After disimpaction, colonoscopy or barium enema can be considered to evaluate for anatomic abnormalities contributing to impaction.

IN-PATIENT CONSIDERATIONS
Admission Criteria/Initial Stabilization
- Disimpaction usually performed in outpatient setting.
- Hospitalization is necessary if several attempts at outpatient management have failed.
- Signs and symptoms of obstruction, intestinal perforation, or peritonitis
- Hemodynamic instability or poor hydration status

 ONGOING CARE

FOLLOW-UP RECOMMENDATIONS
Patient Monitoring
Attempt at maintaining >3 bowel movements/week

DIET
High fiber (30 g/d) with adequate hydration (minimum 2 L/d)

PATIENT EDUCATION
- Increased activity
- Comprehensive program, including use of osmotic laxatives, bulking agents, behavioral changes, dietary changes
- Effective education with regard to constipation is crucial in changing chronic behavior patterns.
- Regular toileting using gastrocolic reflex
- Attempt defecation when urge for bowel movement is sensed.

PROGNOSIS
- Reimpaction is likely if program is not followed.
- Prognosis is poor if complicated by intestinal perforation or peritonitis.
- Mortality with impaction and obstruction is highest in the very young and the very old (up to 16%).

COMPLICATIONS
- Intestinal obstruction
- Urinary tract obstruction
- Recurrent UTIs
- Spontaneous perforation of colon
- Stercoral ulceration
- Incarcerated hernia
- Volvulus
- Megacolon
- Rectal prolapse
- Rectovaginal fistula
- Dystocia in pregnancy

REFERENCES
1. Leung L, Riutta T, Kotecha J, et al. Chronic constipation: An evidence-based review. *J Am Board Fam Med*. 2011;24(4):436–451.
2. Constipation Guideline Committee of the North American Society for Pediatric Gastroenterology, Hepatology and Nutrition. Evaluation and treatment of constipation in infants and children: Recommendations of the North American Society for Pediatric Gastroenterology, Hepatology and Nutrition. *J Pediatr Gastroenterol Nutr*. 2006;43: e1–e13.
3. McCrea GL, Miaskowski C, Stotts NA, et al. Pathophysiology of constipation in the older adult. *World J Gastroenterol*. 2008;14(17):2631–2638.
4. Araghizadeh, F. Constipation and functional bowel disease: Fecal impaction. *Clin Colon Rectal Surg*. 2005;18(2):116–119.
5. Hsieh C. Treatment of constipation in older adults. *Am Fam Physician*. 2005;72:2277–2284.
6. Brandt LJ, Prather CM, Quigley EM, et al. Systematic review on the management of chronic constipation in North America. *Am J Gastroenterol*. 2005;100(Suppl 1):S5–S21.
7. Bekkali N, van den Berg M, Dijkgraaf M, et al. Rectal fecal impaction treatment in childhood constipation: Enemas versus high doses oral PEG. *Pediatrics*. 2009;124;e1108–1115.
8. Rao SS, Seaton K, Miller M, et al. Randomized controlled trial of biofeedback, sham feedback, and standard therapy for dyssynergic defecation. *Clin Gastroenterol Hepatol*. 2007;5:331–338.

ADDITIONAL READING
- Biggs WS, Dery WH. Evaluation and treatment of constipation in infants and children. *Am Fam Physician*. 2006;73(3):469–477.
- Candy D, Belsey J. Macrogol (polyethylene glycol) laxatives in children with functional constipation and faecal impaction: A systematic review. *Arch Dis Child*. 2009;94(2):156–160. Epub 2008 Nov 19.
- Enck RE. An overview of constipation and newer therapies. *Am J Hosp Palliat Care*. 2009;26(3): 157–158.
- Hosia-Randell H, Suominen M, Muurinen S, et al. Use of laxatives among older nursing home residents in Helsinki, Finland. *Drugs Aging*. 2007;24(2):147–154.
- Lee-Robichaud H, Thomas K, Morgan J, et al. Lactulose versus polyethylene glycol for chronic constipation. *Cochrane Database Syst Rev*. 2010;7:CD007570. Epub 2010 Jul 7.

 SEE ALSO

Constipation; Diarrhea, Chronic; Encopresis

 CODES

ICD10
- K56.41 Fecal impaction
- K59.00 Constipation, unspecified

CLINICAL PEARLS
- Constipation and resulting fecal impaction are often seen in elderly patients and hospitalized patients.
- When treating chronic pain patients with opioid preparations, be sure to supplement with stool softeners or osmotic laxatives.
- Prevent recurrent fecal impaction with increased fiber intake, adequate hydration, exercise, osmotic laxatives, and bulking agents.

F

FEMALE ATHLETE TRIAD/TETRAD

Jennifer L. Hopp, MD • Rahul Kapur, MD, CAQSM

 BASICS

Syndrome composed of 3 interrelated clinical entities: Low energy availability (EA), menstrual dysfunction (MD), low bone mineral density (BMD). Recent research has alluded to a 4th component: Endothelial dysfunction.

DESCRIPTION
- Female athlete triad terminology 1st used in 1992: Athletes may meet criteria for only 1 or 2 components of the triad.
- 2007 American College of Sports Medicine (ACSM) Position Stand:
  - Highlights that each component of the triad represents a continuous spectrum ranging from health to dysfunction
  - Underscores the importance of energy availability as fundamental to the propagation of the triad
  - Emphasizes that without correction of low energy availability, full recovery is not possible (1)[C]
- Energy availability (EA):
  - Dietary energy intake minus exercise energy expenditure and considered to be the core component of the tetrad/triad.
  - Represents the amount of dietary energy remaining for bodily functions after exercise training
  - Low EA results in reducing mechanisms of cellular maintenance, thermoregulation, growth, and reproduction.
  - Low EA occurs either intentionally or inadvertently. Examples include: Increasing training disproportionately to energy intake; disordered eating, reducing energy intake by restricting, fasting, binging and purging, or by using diet pills, laxatives, diuretics, or enemas. Only some athletes will meet the diagnostic criteria from *Diagnostic and Statistical Manual* (DSM)-V for feeding and eating disorders.
- Menstrual dysfunction (MD):
  - Low EA alters the hypothalamic-pituitary axis, resulting in decreased estrogen levels.
  - Represents a spectrum ranging from eumenorrhea to amenorrhea and includes athletes who have low estrogen levels, but still experience menstruation
  - Energy deficit resulting in menstrual dysfunction occurs at ~30 kcal/kg lean body mass per day threshold (1)[C].
  - Includes luteal suppression (shortened luteal phase, prolonged follicular phase, and decreased estradiol level), anovulation, oligomenorrhea (menstrual cycle >35 days), and primary and secondary hypothalamic amenorrhea
  - Primary amenorrhea, although less common, can occur in young athletes. Secondary amenorrhea is defined as the absence of menstrual cycles for >3 months after menarche has occurred.
  - Hypothalamic suppression is the most common cause of secondary amenorrhea in these athletes, although other causes must be ruled out prior to attributing the problem to low EA.
- BMD:
  - Ranges from optimal bone health to osteoporosis, a skeletal disorder characterized by compromised bone strength predisposing a person to an increased fracture risk
  - Bone health refers to bone strength, as well as bone quality. Current technology allows for the measurement of bone density but not quality, which helps to account for the fact that 2 athletes

with the same BMD may have very different bone fracture histories:
  ○ ACSM Position Stand recommends using the International Society of Clinical Densitometry (ISCD) guidelines for BMD which refers to Z-scores below −2.0 in premenopausal women as "low bone density below the expected range for age" and in children "low bone density for chronological age" (1)[C].
  ○ Since most athletes have a higher BMD than nonathletes, ACSM recommends further workup for any athlete with a Z-score <−1, even in the absence of fracture.
  - Endothelial dysfunction:
    ○ Emerging evidence that the female athlete triad is associated with endothelial dysfunction. Reduced levels of estrogen directly reduces vasodilation at the level of gene transcription. Athletic amenorrhea is associated with reduced brachial artery flow-mediated dilation. Abnormal brachial dilation has a 95% positive predictive value for coronary endothelial dysfunction. Long-term consequences include decreased blood flow to critical muscles during exercise and, chronically, to accelerated atherosclerosis and earlier cardiovascular events. In the future, this clinical syndrome may be best considered as a tetrad (2)[B].

EPIDEMIOLOGY
Unknown, as patients often avoid physicians and hide symptoms

Prevalence
- Overall prevalence: 0–15.9% of all female athletes. Prevalence of 2 criteria varied depending on which 2 criteria were seen: MD + BMD 0–7.5% (n = 460), MD + LE 17.5% (n = 80), and BMD + LE 3.75% (n = 80)
- Disordered eating: 0–48% vs. 3.8–8% in the general population
- Menstrual dysfunction: Prevalence of secondary amenorrhea found to be as high as 60% in female athletes compared to 2–5% in the general population. Most patients exhibit a luteal deficiency or anovulatory cycle in 1 out of 3 menstrual cycles.
- Bone health: Using the World Health Organization (WHO) criteria for low BMD, prevalence of osteopenia (T-score between −1 and −2) ranges from 0–39.8% in female athletes, as compared to 12% in the normal population.

ETIOLOGY AND PATHOPHYSIOLOGY
- A baseline caloric deficit or low EA causes a disruption in the hypothalamic-pituitary-ovarian axis, decreasing the pulsatile release of gonadotropin-releasing hormone (GnRH).
- Low EA alters the levels of various metabolic hormones, some of which are thought to play a role in the regulation of GnRH secretion. Low GnRH levels subsequently decrease luteinizing hormone (LH) and follicle-stimulating hormone (FSH) levels, causing a decrease in estrogen production, resulting in varying degrees of menstrual dysfunction.
- Estrogen deficiency also negatively affects bone density, and a chronic state of malnutrition reduces the rate of bone formation and increases the rate of bone resorption. This change in increased bone resorption and declined rate of bone formation begins within 5 days of a reduction in EA.

- Endothelial dysfunction resulting from low estrogen levels has also been implicated in increased cardiovascular dysfunction among female athletes.

RISK FACTORS
- Lean physique sports, sports with an aesthetic component (e.g., ballet, figure skating, gymnastics, distance running, diving, and swimming) or sports with weight classifications (e.g., martial arts and wrestling). Frequent weigh-ins, consequences for weight gain, domineering coaches or parents, and a win-at-all-cost attitude increase the risk of developing the triad.
- Presence of 1 component of the triad.
- A lack of family or social support, either secondary to intense training hours causing social isolation or entering a new environment (boarding school or college). An athlete with comorbid psychological conditions (e.g., anxiety, depression, and/or obsessive–compulsive disorder) is more likely to develop the triad (3)[C].

GENERAL PREVENTION
- Education of athletes (middle school through college), coaches, trainers, parents, and physicians about the triad is crucial. Young athletes are extremely impressionable and may turn negative comments and unhealthy advice from adults into maladaptive eating and exercising habits.
- General screening during pre-participation exam (PPE) and annual physicals is endorsed by AAP, AAFP, ACSM, AAOSM, and AMSSM.
- Female Athlete Triad Coalition developed 12-question screening that should be included in PPE.
- Athletes presenting with "red flag" conditions such as fractures, weight changes, fatigue, amenorrhea, bradycardia, orthostatic hypotension, syncope, arrhythmia, electrolyte abnormalities, or depression should also be screened for the triad.

COMMONLY ASSOCIATED CONDITIONS
- Anorexia nervosa, bulimia nervosa, avoidant/restrictive food intake disorder, rumination disorder and other psychological disorders, including low self-esteem, depression, and anxiety. In 1 study, 5.4% of athletes with eating disorders reported suicide attempts.
- Low BMD predisposes athletes to stress fractures and may not be fully reversible. This may lead to an even higher rate of fractures as these athletes reach postmenopausal status.

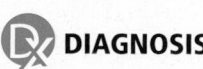 **DIAGNOSIS**

The female athlete triad is a clinical diagnosis based mainly on patient history. Screening for the female athlete triad should occur at annual sports physicals, routine exams, and acute visits for any concerning complaints or components of the triad (1,4)[C].

HISTORY
Athletes should be assessed for menstrual history (including oral contraceptive use), fracture history, and symptoms of depression (1)[C]. Special dietary practices, eating behaviors, and weight changes should also be collected. Body image; fear of weight gain; fluctuations in weight; history of disordered eating; and use of laxatives, diet pills, or enemas are crucial to understanding the extent of the disease.

PHYSICAL EXAM
- Height, weight, and vital signs
- Common findings in patients with disordered eating include bradycardia, orthostatic hypotension, hypothermia, cold or cyanotic extremities, lanugo, hypercarotenemia, parotid gland enlargement or tenderness, epigastric tenderness, eroded tooth enamel, and knuckle or hand calluses (Russell sign).
- Patients with primary amenorrhea should undergo a pelvic exam to determine the presence of a uterus. A pelvic exam in patients with secondary amenorrhea is warranted to rule out anomalies. Vaginal atrophy may be present in the hypoestrogenic state (1)[C].

DIFFERENTIAL DIAGNOSIS
Patients must be screened for anorexia nervosa, bulimia nervosa, avoidant/restrictive food intake disorder, and rumination disorder using the DSM-V criteria. Similarly, before presuming a diagnosis of hypothalamic amenorrhea secondary to energy deficit, the following diagnoses must be ruled out:
- Pregnancy and endocrine abnormalities: Thyroid dysfunction, Cushing syndrome (3)[B]
- Hypothalamic dysfunction: Psychological stress-induced amenorrhea, medication-induced amenorrhea, Kallmann syndrome
- Pituitary dysfunction: Prolactinoma or other pituitary neoplasm, Sheehan syndrome, sarcoidosis, empty-sella syndrome
- Ovarian dysfunction: Polycystic ovarian syndrome, premature ovarian failure, menopause, gonadal dysgenesis, Turner syndrome, ovarian neoplasm, autoimmune disease
- Uterine dysfunction: Asherman syndrome, absence of uterus

DIAGNOSTIC TESTS & INTERPRETATION
Initial Tests (lab, imaging)
- Basic metabolic panel, magnesium, phosphorus, albumin, CBC with differential, ESR, thyroid-stimulating hormone (TSH), 25-OH vitamin D, and urinalysis.
- Primary evaluation for secondary amenorrhea includes a urine pregnancy test, FSH, LH, prolactin, and TSH (1)[B].
- ECG to rule out a prolonged QT interval. The QT interval may be prolonged even in the absence of electrolyte abnormalities.

Follow-Up Tests & Special Considerations
Recommendation for BMD testing by dual-energy x-ray absorptiometry (DEXA) remains controversial. ACSM current guidelines recommend DEXA studies for patients with disordered eating, eating disorders >6 months, hypoestrogenism, amenorrhea, oligomenorrhea, and/or in patients with a history of stress fractures or fractures from minimal impact. In patients with persistent components of the triad, re-evaluation by the same DEXA machine is recommended in 12 months from initial scan (1)[C].

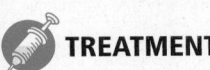 TREATMENT

- The treatment goal is to optimize nutritional status by establishing healthy eating behaviors and treating any associated maladaptive thought processes or psychological disorders.
- A multidisciplinary team, including a physician (or other health care provider), registered dietitian, and a mental health provider is crucial for treatment (1)[C]. Communication with team coaches, trainers, and family is also a critical intervention.

- Studies have shown a positive EA of >30 kcal/kg of fat-free muscle mass/day is sufficient to restore menstrual cycling, whereas an EA of >45 kcal/kg of fat-free muscle mass/day is likely needed for BMD improvement (1)[C].

MEDICATION

First Line
The use of oral contraceptive pills (OCPs), hormone replacement therapy (HRT), and/or bisphosphonates has not been clearly shown to increase BMD or aid in the restoration of normal menstrual cycling. OCPs can be considered to minimize further bone loss in patients >16 who, despite adequate nutrition and body weight gain, continue to have decreasing BMD and functional hypothalamic amenorrhea (1)[C]. New evidence is emerging for the use of folic acid (10 mg/d) can improve endothelial dysfunction and improve vasodilation (3)[C].

IN-PATIENT CONSIDERATIONS
Patients with disordered eating or clinically diagnosable eating disorders must be evaluated for potentially life-threatening conditions requiring hospital admission, including bradycardia, severe orthostatic hypotension, significant electrolyte imbalances, hypothermia, arrhythmias, or prolonged QT interval on ECG (3)[C].

 ONGOING CARE

- Patients with components of the triad should undergo frequent monitoring by all members of the multidisciplinary treatment team.
- To continue training and competing, athletes with disordered eating or clinically diagnosable eating disorders must agree to the following stipulations in the form of a behavior contract: To comply with all treatment strategies; to be closely monitored by health care providers; to place treatment goals over training goals; and to modify the type, duration, and intensity of training or competition if necessary.
- Athletes with disordered eating behaviors who do not comply with this agreement may need to be restricted from training (1)[C].

PATIENT EDUCATION
All young female patients should be counseled on the importance of proper nutrition, calcium, and vitamin D intake and the benefits of regular weightbearing exercise. Patients presenting with ≥1 components of the triad should be educated about the short- and long-term effects of low BMD.

PROGNOSIS
- The short- and long-term prognosis for patients with female athlete triad depends on time to diagnosis and response to treatment.
- Assuming early intervention with a multidisciplinary team, prognosis is very good. With adequate treatment and an increase in EA, patients will regain normal menstrual cycling and fertility, and begin to increase BMD.
- Since the triad often occurs within the age window of optimal bone strengthening, patients with a prolonged disease course may suffer from complications of decreased BMD throughout their adolescent and adult life.
- In addition, patients with disordered eating behaviors may require long-term ongoing therapy to manage their disease (3)[C].

- The emerging association of the female athlete triad with endothelial dysfunction raises significant concerns for long-term cardiac endothelial implications in these athletes. It remains to be seen whether the endothelial dysfunction is reversible with intervention (2)[B].

REFERENCES
1. Nattiv A, Loucks AB, Manore MM, et al. American College of Sports Medicine position stand. The female athlete triad. *Med Sci Sports Exerc*. 2007; 39:1867–1882.
2. Lanser EM, Zach KN, Hoch AZ, et al. The female athlete triad and endothelial dysfunction. *PM R*. 2011;3:458–465.
3. Hoch AZ, Temme KE. American College of Sports Medicine. Recognition and rehabilitation of the female athlete triad/tetrad: A multidisciplinary approach. *Curr Sports Med Reports*. 2013;12(3): 190–199.
4. Deimel JF, Dunlap BJ. The female athlete triad. *Clin Sports Med*. 2012;31(2):247–254.

ADDITIONAL READING
Barrack MT, Ackerman KE, Gibbs JC. Update on the female athlete triad. *Musculoskeletal Med*. 2013; 195–204.

 SEE ALSO

Algorithms: Amenorrhea, Primary (Absence of Menarche by Age 16); Amenorrhea, Secondary; Weight Loss

CODES

ICD10
- M85.9 Disorder of bone density and structure, unspecified
- N92.6 Irregular menstruation, unspecified
- R53.83 Other fatigue

CLINICAL PEARLS
- The female athlete triad consists of pathology in 3 clinical areas: EA, menstrual dysfunction, and BMD. Athletes may exhibit varying degrees of dysfunction along each of the 3 spectra forming the triad. Endothelial dysfunction is emerging as a 4th component of concern (1,2).
- Regular screening of adolescent and adult females at PPE, annual visits and relevant acute visits is critical to early diagnosis and intervention.
- Immediate intervention by a multidisciplinary team, including physicians, registered dietitians, mental health professionals, coaches, trainers, and parents, is crucial to minimize further bone loss, recover BMD, and regain menstrual cycling.
- ACSM current guidelines recommend DEXA studies for patients with disordered eating, eating disorders >6 months, hypoestrogenism, amenorrhea, oligomenorrhea, and/or in patients with a history of stress fractures or fractures from minimal impact.

F

FEVER OF UNKNOWN ORIGIN
Scott T. Henderson, MD

 BASICS

DESCRIPTION
- Classic definition by Petersdorf and Beeson (2)[B]:
  - Fever >38.3°C on several occasions
  - Fever duration at least 3 weeks
  - Uncertain diagnosis after 1 week of study in the hospital
- Modifications to the definition have evolved, including eliminating the in-hospital evaluation and shortening the exam time.
- Some have suggested expansion of the definition to include nosocomial, neutropenic, and HIV-associated fevers that may not be prolonged.

EPIDEMIOLOGY
Incidence
No data on actual incidence

ETIOLOGY AND PATHOPHYSIOLOGY
- >200 causes; each with prevalence of ≤5%
- *Most commonly an atypical presentation of a common condition*
- Infection:
  - Abdominal abscesses
  - Amebic hepatitis
  - Catheter infections
  - Cytomegalovirus
  - Endocarditis/Pericarditis
  - HIV (advanced stage)
  - Mycobacterial infection (often with advanced HIV)
  - Osteomyelitis
  - Renal
  - Sinusitis
  - Wound infections
  - Other miscellaneous infections
- Neoplasms:
  - Atrial myxoma
  - Colon cancer
  - Hepatoma
  - Lymphoma
  - Leukemia
  - Solid tumors (hypernephroma)
- Collagen vascular disease:
  - Giant cell arteritis
  - Polyarteritis nodosa
  - Polymyalgia rheumatica
  - Systemic lupus erythematosus
  - Rheumatic fever
  - Rheumatoid arthritis
- Other causes:
  - Alcoholic hepatitis
  - Cerebrovascular accident
  - Cirrhosis
  - Drug fever/medication induced:
    - Allopurinol, captopril, carbamazepine, cephalosporins, cimetidine, clofibrate, erythromycin, heparin, hydralazine, hydrochlorothiazide, isoniazid, meperidine, methyldopa, nifedipine, nitrofurantoin, penicillin, phenytoin, procainamide, quinidine, sulfonamides
  - Endocrinologic diseases
  - Factitious/fraudulent fever
  - Granulomatous diseases
  - Occupational causes
  - Periodic fever
  - Pulmonary emboli/deep vein thrombosis
  - Thermoregulatory disorders

- In up to 20% of cases, the cause of the fever will not be identified despite thorough workup.

RISK FACTORS
- Recent travel
- Exposure to biologic or chemical agents
- HIV-infected patients with advanced disease
- Persons in AIDS risk group
- Elderly
- Drug abuse
- Immigrants
- Young female health care workers; consider factitious fever

Geriatric Considerations
Most common causes are acute leukemia, Hodgkin lymphoma, intra-abdominal infections, tuberculosis (TB), and temporal arteritis.

- Infections account for over half of causes, with collagen-vascular diseases the 2nd most likely etiology.

Pediatric Considerations
- ~50% of fevers of unknown origin (FUO) in published pediatric case series are ultimately shown to be due to infections; collagen vascular disease and malignancy also being common diagnoses (1)[A].
- Inflammatory bowel disease is a common etiology in older children and adolescents.

 DIAGNOSIS

HISTORY
- History should focus on relevant symptoms:
  - Constitutional symptoms almost always accompany a fever:
    - Chills, night sweats, myalgias, weight loss with an intact appetite (infectious)
    - Arthralgias, myalgias, fatigue (inflammatory)
    - Fatigue, night sweats, weight loss with loss of appetite (neoplasms)
- Past medical history should include information about previously treated chronic infections and any prior diagnosis of cancer.
- Past surgical history should include specific information about type of surgery performed, postoperative complications, and any indwelling foreign materials.
- Obtain a comprehensive list of all medications, including over-the-counter and herbal remedies.
- Family history to identify prior illnesses in family members that may have a genetic link, such as periodic fever syndromes, and recent illnesses in family members to which the patient may have been exposed

ALERT
Special attention should be paid to travel and occupational, sexual, and drug exposure.

PHYSICAL EXAM
- Physical exam should focus on areas that have high diagnostic yield:
  - Funduscopic exam for choroid tubercles or Roth spots
  - Temporal artery palpation
  - Gums and oral cavity
  - Auscultation for bruits and murmurs
  - Abdominal palpation for organomegaly
  - Rectal examination
  - Testicular examination
  - Palpate for adenopathy
  - Skin and nail bed exam for clubbing, nodules, lesions, and rashes
  - Focal neurologic signs of bony tenderness joint effusion
  - Repeated exams are essential to determine cause.

DIFFERENTIAL DIAGNOSIS
See "Etiology and Pathophysiology."

DIAGNOSTIC TESTS & INTERPRETATION
Initial Tests (lab, imaging)
- CBC
- Peripheral blood smear
- LFTs
- C-reactive protein
- ESR
- HIV antibody test
- Blood cultures (not to exceed 6 sets)
- Urinalysis and urine culture
- Chest x-ray
- CT or MRI of abdomen and pelvis (plus directed biopsy, if indicated) (2)[C]

Follow-Up Tests & Special Considerations
- Rheumatoid factor and antinuclear antibody test
- Serologic tests: Epstein-Barr, hepatitis, syphilis, Lyme disease, Q fever, cytomegalovirus, amebiasis, coccidioidomycosis
- Serum ferritin
- Serum protein electrophoresis
- Sputum and urine cultures for tuberculosis
- Thyroid function tests
- Tuberculin skin test:
  - May not be helpful if anergic or acute infection
  - If test negative, repeat in 2 weeks
- Technetium-based scan, if infectious process or tumor suspected (2)[B]
- PET scan using the radiolabeled glucose analogue 18F-fluorodeoxyglucose if infectious process, inflammatory process, or tumor suspected; PET scans have a high negative predictive value and good sensitivity (but may have false positives) (3,4)[A].
- Ultrasound of abdomen and pelvis (plus directed biopsy, if indicated) if mass lesions, renal obstruction, or gallbladder/biliary tree pathology suspected

- ECG if cardiac valve lesions (endocarditis), atrial myxomas, or pericardial effusion suspected (transthoracic vs. transesophageal)
- Lower extremity Doppler if deep vein thrombosis/pulmonary embolism suspected
- CT scan of chest if pulmonary emboli suspected
- Indium-labeled leukocyte scanning if inflammatory process suspected
- Bone scan if osteomyelitis or metastatic disease suspected

Diagnostic Procedures/Other
- Liver biopsy if granulomatous disease suspected (2)[C]
- Temporal artery biopsy, particularly in the elderly (2)[B]
- Lymph node, muscle, or skin biopsy, if clinically indicated
- Bone marrow biopsy, if clinically indicated
- Spinal tap, if clinically indicated

Test Interpretation
Depends on etiology

TREATMENT

GENERAL MEASURES
- Attempt to determine the etiology before initiating the therapy.
- Avoid therapeutic trials unless as a last resort and only if therapy is reasonably specific.
- "Shotgun" approaches are condemned because they obscure the clinical picture, have untoward effects, and do not solve the problem (2)[C].

MEDICATION
First Line
- First-line drugs depend on the diagnosis.
- Evidence does not support treatment of fever (5)[C].

Second Line
If the patient has symptoms with the fever or continues to decline, consider a therapeutic trial:
- Antibiotic trial based on patient's history
- Antituberculous therapy if there is a high risk for granulomatous disease pending culture results
- Steroid trial based on patient's history (once occult malignancy is ruled out)

ALERT
If a steroid trial is initiated, patient may have a relapse after treatment or if certain conditions (e.g., TB) have been undiagnosed.

ADDITIONAL THERAPIES
With temperature elevations, patients will have increased caloric and fluid demands.

SURGERY/OTHER PROCEDURES
Need for exploratory laparotomy has been largely eliminated with the advent of more sophisticated tests and imaging modalities.

IN-PATIENT CONSIDERATIONS
Admission Criteria/Initial Stabilization
- Reserved for the ill and debilitated
- Consider if factitious fever has been ruled out or an invasive procedure is indicated.

 ONGOING CARE

FOLLOW-UP RECOMMENDATIONS
Patient Monitoring
If the etiology of the fever remains unknown, repeat the history and physical exam along with screening lab studies.

DIET
With temperature elevations, patients will have increased caloric and fluid demands.

PATIENT EDUCATION
Maintain an open line of communication between physician and patient/family as the workup progresses:
- The extended time required in establishing a diagnosis can be frustrating.

PROGNOSIS
- Depends on etiology and age:
  - Patients with HIV have the highest mortality.
- 1-year survival rates reflecting deaths due to all causes

Age	Survival
<35	91%
35–64	82%
>64	67%

COMPLICATIONS
Dependent on etiology

Pregnancy Considerations
Fever increases the risk of neural tube defects and trigger preterm labor.

REFERENCES

1. Chow A, Robinson JL. Fever of unknown origin in children: A systematic review. *World J Pediatr*. 2011;7:5–10.
2. Mourad O, Palda V, Detsky AS. A comprehensive evidence-based approach to fever of unknown origin. *Arch Intern Med*. 2003;163:545–551.
3. Dong MJ, Zhao K, Liu ZF, et al. A meta-analysis of the value of fluorodeoxyglucose-PET/PET-CT in the evaluation of fever of unknown origin. *Eur J Radiol*. 2011;80:834–844.
4. Hao R, Yuan L, Kan Y, et al. Diagnostic performance of 18F-FDG PET/CT in patients with fever of unknown origin: a meta-analysis. *Nucl Med Commun*. 2013l;34:682–688.
5. Plaisance KI, Mackowiak PA. Antipyretic therapy: Physiologic rationale, diagnostic implications, and clinical consequences. *Arch Intern Med*. 2000;160: 449–456.

ADDITIONAL READING
- Ben-Baruch S, Canaani J, Braunstein R, et al. Predictive parameters for a diagnostic bone marrow biopsy specimen in the work-up of fever of unknown origin. *Mayo Clin Proc*. 2012;87:136–142.
- Cunha BA. Fever of unknown origin: Focused diagnostic approach based on clinical clues from the history, physical examination, and laboratory tests. *Infect Dis Clin North Am*. 2007;21:1137–1187.
- Hayakawa K, Ramasamy B, Chandrasekar PH. Fever of unknown origin: An evidence-based review. *Am J Med Sci*. 2012;344:307–316.
- Varghese GM, Trowbridge P, Doherty T. Investigating and managing pyrexia of unknown origin in adults. *BMJ*. 2010;341:C5470.

 SEE ALSO

- Arthritis, Juvenile Idiopathic; Colorectal Cancer; Cytomegalovirus Inclusion Disease; Endocarditis, Infective; Hepatoma; HIV Infection and AIDS; Leukemia; Lupus Erythematosus, Discoid; Osteomyelitis; Polyarteritis Nodosa; Polymyalgia Rheumatica; Pulmonary Embolism; Rheumatic Fever; Sinusitis; Stroke, Acute; Temporal Arteritis
- Algorithms: Fever, Acute; Fever in the First 3 Months of Life; Fever of Unknown Origin

 CODES

ICD10
R50.9 Fever, unspecified

CLINICAL PEARLS

- History, exam, diagnostic tests, and imaging should focus on the relevant causes of FUO:
- A sequential approach leads to a rational sequential diagnosis or rules out causes of FUO.
- Avoid a "shotgun" approach to treatment; use empiric therapy only in carefully defined circumstances.
- FUO cases that defy precise diagnosis after intensive investigation and prolonged observation generally carry a favorable prognosis.
- In many cases, FUO in older persons may represent atypical, nonclassic presentations of common infectious and noninfectious diseases.

F

FIBROCYSTIC CHANGES OF THE BREAST
Katherine M. Callaghan, MD • Dawn S. Tasillo, MD

 BASICS

DESCRIPTION
- Fibrocystic changes (FCC) of the breast is a generalized term for a heterogeneous group of changes affecting the stromal and glandular tissues of the breast.
- It is the most common of all benign breast conditions.
- Commonly presents as mastalgia, engorgement, increased breast nodularity, and/or cysts:
  - Mastalgia (breast pain) is usually in upper outer quadrants of breast, bilateral, and may radiate to shoulders or upper arms.
  - Localized pain may occur with a rapidly enlarging cyst.
  - Nodules are usually small (2–10 mm), diffuse, and bilateral, with a rubbery consistency.
  - Cysts are more common in women in their 40s.
  - Larger cysts may have consistency of a water-filled balloon.
- Symptoms are most prominent in premenstrual (luteal) phase.
- System(s) affected: Endocrine/Metabolic; Reproductive
- Synonym(s): Fibrocystic breast disease; Mammary dysplasia; Chronic cystic mastitis

EPIDEMIOLOGY
Most common in women of reproductive years; occasionally seen after menopause with hormone replacement

Incidence
Unknown but very frequent

Prevalence
50–60% of women without breast disease are found to have this pattern of fibrous change and cyst formation (1).

ETIOLOGY AND PATHOPHYSIOLOGY
- Estrogen likely a causative factor for many (2).
- May be the result of an exaggerated response of breast tissue to cycling hormones or a subtle imbalance in the ratio of estrogen to progesterone.
- Cystic disease is caused by dilation of ducts and acini, proliferation and metaplasia of epithelial lining, and multiplication of ducts and acini, resulting in obstruction of the terminal ductal lobular unit.

RISK FACTORS
- The effect of consumption of methylxanthine-containing substances (e.g., coffee, tea, cola, and chocolate) has not been found to be a contributing factor (3)[A].
- Diet high in fruits and vegetables and high parity independently decrease risk of FCC.
- Diet high in saturated fats may increase risk of FCC.

COMMONLY ASSOCIATED CONDITIONS
Fibrocystic change found clinically confers no increased risk of breast cancer (1).

 DIAGNOSIS

HISTORY
- May present in 3 overlapping, indistinct stages:
  - Mastoplasia (breast enlargement) and mastalgia, which may subside after menses; common in women in their 20s
  - Adenosis: Appearance of multiple small breast nodules; common in women in their 30s
  - Cystic phase: Tender cysts, usually small, but up to 5 cm in diameter; common in women in their 40s
- Obtain personal history of breast biopsy and family history of breast disease (benign or malignant).

PHYSICAL EXAM
- With patient first upright, then supine, turn rotated on to contralateral hip, evaluate all breast tissue from sternum to midaxillary line, from clavicle to mammary ridge.
- Using fingertip, proceed in a linear fashion from top of sternum past breast tissue using 3 different depths of pressure at each palpation. Continue superiorly again to clavicle in a "lawnmower" fashion.
- Quantitate size, consistency, mobility, location, and skin changes.
- Findings in FCC may include:
  - Smooth, tense, or fluctuant masses
  - Bilateral masses
  - Breast thickening
  - Nipple discharge
- Palpate for axillary lymph nodes.

DIFFERENTIAL DIAGNOSIS
- Pain:
  - Mastitis
  - Costochondritis
  - Pectoralis muscle strain
  - Neuralgia
  - Breast cancer
  - Angina pectoris
  - Gastroesophageal reflux (GERD)
  - Superficial phlebitis of the thoracoepigastric vein (Mondor disease)
- Masses:
  - Breast cancer
  - Sebaceous cyst
  - Fibroadenoma
  - Lipoma
  - Fat necrosis
- Skin changes:
  - Breast cancer (peau d'orange: Thickened skin similar to peel of an orange)
  - Eczema

DIAGNOSTIC TESTS & INTERPRETATION
- Evaluation should focus on excluding breast cancer.
- Testing may be conducted based on a level of clinical suspicion.

Initial Tests (lab, imaging)
- Ultrasound (US): Signs of malignancy include irregular mass, clustered masses, calcifications, architectural distortion, dilated duct; US is useful for differentiating cystic from solid lesions.
- Mammography may reveal mass or dense tissue ± calcifications.

Follow-Up Tests & Special Considerations
- Mammogram may be normal in presence of malignancy and difficult to interpret in women <35 years of age due to dense breast tissue; US may be more helpful, particularly in the presence of a palpable mass.
- MRI is indicated in patients with BRCA1 or BRCA2 mutation or in any woman with ≥25% lifetime risk for breast cancer (4).

Diagnostic Procedures/Other
- Fine-needle aspiration (FNA) and biopsy:
  - Allows differentiation of cystic and solid lesions
  - Aspirate may be straw-colored, dark brown, or green
  - Cells sent for cytology can reveal cancer with high accuracy
  - Low morbidity
- If mass disappears, no further evaluation is necessary (including cytologic evaluation of aspirated fluid).

Test Interpretation
Certain histologic changes in the setting of fibrocystic change confer an increased risk for breast cancer:
- Atypia: Relative risk of 4.24
- Proliferative changes without atypia: Relative risk of 1.88
- Nonproliferative changes: Relative risk of 1.27 (5)

TREATMENT

- After ruling out malignancy by means of examination, and/or imaging and diagnostic procedures, FCC may not require treatment and often resolves with time.
- Cool compresses, avoiding trauma, and around-the-clock wearing of a well-fitting, supportive brassiere may be useful for symptom relief.

MEDICATION
First Line
For cyclic pain and swelling: NSAIDs:
- Ibuprofen 400 mg q.i.d./PRN
- Naproxen 500 mg b.i.d./PRN

Second Line

- Oral contraceptives may be useful in modulating symptoms or in preventing the development of new changes.
- For severe pain, consider (6,7):
  - Danazol (Danocrine) 100–400 mg/d divided in 2 doses × 4–6 months
  - Bromocriptine 2.5 mg b.i.d. × 3 months
  - Tamoxifen 10 mg/d × 3–6 months
  - These medications are not without serious side effects and thorough counseling is required. Consultation with a breast specialist may be considered.

ISSUES FOR REFERRAL

- If discrete palpable lesion in a woman ≤35 years: US, then refer to a surgeon.
- If discrete palpable lesion in a woman >35 years: Diagnostic mammography ± US, then refer to surgeon.

SURGERY/OTHER PROCEDURES

Breast cyst aspiration can be both diagnostic and therapeutic.

COMPLEMENTARY AND ALTERNATIVE MEDICINE

Evidence supporting evening primrose oil, vitamin E, or pyridoxine as treatment for the discomforts of FCC is insufficient to draw conclusions about effectiveness (3).

 ## ONGOING CARE

FOLLOW-UP RECOMMENDATIONS

Condition is benign, chronic, and recurrent.

Patient Monitoring

- The patient needs to be assessed with clinical examination, radiologic studies, and sometimes biopsy to be certain a lump is not malignant.
- Follow-up times are variable, depending on the clinical situation.
- US is useful to differentiate cysts from solid lesions and in evaluating women <35 years of age for FCC, but is not useful for screening.
- Screening mammograms should be obtained after age 40–50. Refer to the US PSTF, ACOG, or ACS recommendations for screening schedules.
- Aspiration cytology is useful to differentiate cysts from solid lesions. The sensitivity and specificity of cyst aspirate cytology for cancer diagnosis depends on the skill of the clinician and cytopathologist and may be as high as 98%.
- When physical examination, mammography, and FNA are used in combination, detection rates for breast cancer range from 93–100%.

DIET

There is insufficient evidence that changes in diet (e.g., caffeine intake) effect symptoms from FCC. Individual patient response will vary.

PATIENT EDUCATION

- Patient information on fibrocystic breasts from the Mayo Foundation for Medical Education and Research: www.mayoclinic.com/health/fibrocystic-breasts/DS01070
- Information on breast cancer prevention from the National Cancer Institute: www.cancer.gov
- Information on fibrocystic breasts from the American Cancer Society: www.cancer.org/Healthy/FindCancerEarly/WomensHealth/Non-CancerousBreastConditions/non-cancerous-breast-conditions-fibrocystic-changes

REFERENCES

1. Santen RJ, Mansel R. Benign breast disorders. *N Engl J Med*. 2005;353:275–285.
2. Meisner AL, Fekrazad MH, Royce ME. Breast disease: Benign and malignant. *Med Clin North Am*. 2008;92:1115–1141.
3. Horner NK, Lampe JW. Potential mechanisms of diet therapy for fibrocystic breast conditions show inadequate evidence of effectiveness. *J Am Diet Assoc*. 2000;100:1368–1380.
4. Morris E. Diagnostic breast MR imaging: Current status and future directions. *Magn Reson Imaging Clin North Am*. 2010;18:57–74.
5. Hartmann LC, Sellers TA, Frost MH, et al. Benign breast disease and the risk of breast cancer. *N Engl J Med*. 2005;353:229–237.
6. Srivastava A, Mansel RE, Arvind N, et al. Evidence-based management of Mastalgia: A meta-analysis of randomised trials. *Breast*. 2007;16:503–512.
7. Mousavi SR, Mousavi SM, Samsami M, et al. Comparison of tamoxifen with danazol in the management of fibrocystic disease. *Int J Med Med Sci*. 2011;2:329–331.

ADDITIONAL READING

- Amin AL, Purdy AC, Mattingly JD, et al. Benign breast disease. *Surg Clin North Am*. 2013;93:299–308.
- Griffin JL, Pearlman MD. Breast cancer screening in women at average risk and high risk. *Obstet Gynecol*. 2010;116:1410–1421.
- Rinaldi P, Ierardi C, Costantini M, et al. Cystic breast lesions: Sonographic findings and clinical management. *J Ultrasound Med*. 2010;29:1617–1626.
- Saslow D. American Cancer Society guidelines for breast screening with MRI as an adjunct to mammography. *CA J Clin*. 2007;57:75–89.

 ## CODES

ICD10

- N60.09 Solitary cyst of unspecified breast
- N60.19 Diffuse cystic mastopathy of unspecified breast
- N60.29 Fibroadenosis of unspecified breast

CLINICAL PEARLS

- Fibrocystic breast change is a common finding in reproductive aged women and generally does not confer an increased cancer risk.
- Symptoms can be managed expectantly, with NSAIDs or oral contraceptives.
- Palpable breast lesions should be evaluated as clinically indicated.

F

FIBROMYALGIA
F. Stuart Leeds, MS, MD

BASICS

DESCRIPTION
- Chronic, widespread noninflammatory musculoskeletal pain syndrome with multisystem manifestations. Although the specific pathophysiology has not been elucidated, it is generally thought to be a disorder of altered central pain regulation.
- Synonym(s): FMS; fibrositis, psychogenic rheumatism (archaic and inaccurate)

EPIDEMIOLOGY
Incidence
- Predominant sex: Female > Male (~90% are females)
- Predominant age range: 20–65 years

Prevalence
2–5% of adult US population (1)

ETIOLOGY AND PATHOPHYSIOLOGY
- Idiopathic, but appears to be a primary disorder of central pain processing, often described as *central sensitization*
- Decrease in blood flow to the thalamus and caudate nucleus
- Afferent augmentation of peripheral nociceptive stimuli
- Alterations in neuroendocrine, neuromodulation, neurotransmitter, neurotransporter, biochemical, and neuroreceptor function/physiology (2)
- May be triggered or exacerbated by a situational stressor, physical injury, or illness

Genetics
- Genetics:
  - High familial aggregation
  - Inheritance is unknown, but likely polygenic
  - Odds ratio may be as high as 8.5 for a 1st-degree relative of a familial proband
  - Commonly comorbid with mood or anxiety disorders in families
- Environmental:
  - Physical trauma or injury, or severe illness
  - Stressors (e.g., work, family, life events, and abuse)
  - Some studies report correlations to certain infections (e.g., Lyme disease and hepatitis C).

RISK FACTORS
- Female gender
- Poor functional status
- Negative/stressful life events
- Low socioeconomic status

GENERAL PREVENTION
No specific prevention known

COMMONLY ASSOCIATED CONDITIONS
Fibromyalgia frequently occurs as a concomitant to other rheumatologic disorders, both inflammatory and noninflammatory and may, in fact, be triggered by same. As previously noted, it often presents with one or more regional/functional syndromes.

DIAGNOSIS

- Per the 2010 revised ACR criteria (1):
  - Based on Widespread Pain Index (WPI) and Symptom Score (SS):
  - Must have WPI $\geq$ 7 + SS $\geq$ 5, or WPI 3–6 and SS $\geq$ 9; *and*
  - Symptoms for >3 months; *and*
  - No other explanation for these symptoms
- Note: the 1990 ACR criteria relied on the presence of *tender points* (generally, 11/18 present). These are still used for diagnosis by some clinicians.
- A questionnaire tool to facilitate WPI/SS patient scoring and diagnosis may be found at: www.fmnetnews.com/docs/NewFibroCriteriaSurvey.pdf
- This tool assesses the following:
  - WPI counts the number of sites of regional pain occurring over past week (score 0–19):
    - Above the waist:
      - Jaw, right and left
      - Neck
      - Shoulder girdle, right and left
      - Upper back
      - Upper arm, right and left
      - Lower arm, right and left
      - Chest
      - Abdomen
      - Lower back
    - Below the waist:
      - Hip (buttock, trochanter), right and left
      - Upper leg, right and left
      - Lower leg, right and left
  - The SS scale score is the sum of two parts. Part (1) grades and adds together the severity of three key complaints (fatigue, waking unrefreshed, cognitive symptoms) on a 0–3 scale, yielding a summed score of 0–9. Part (2) counts the presence or absence of >40 associated symptoms, and grades them as a group, giving a single score of 0–3, corresponding to none, few, moderate, or many symptoms. Parts 1 and 2 are added together to give a total SS of 0–12.
  - The Visual Analogue Scale Fibromyalgia Impact Questionnaire (VASFIQ), an updated questionnaire taking <2 minutes, is easy to score. This can be a useful assessment of the functional impact of symptoms (3). It is available here: www.fmmgmt.com/pdf/Quiz/mVASFIQ.pdf

HISTORY
- Universal symptoms include:
  - Chronic widespread pain $\geq$3 months: bilateral limbs and in the axial skeleton
  - Generalized fatigue and sleep disturbances
- Often present:
  - Mood disorders, including depression, anxiety, and panic symptoms
  - Cognitive impairment: qualitatively different from that seen in isolated mood disorders ("fibrofog";4)
  - Headaches: typically, tension and migraine types
  - Other regional pain syndromes, such as irritable bowel syndrome, chronic pelvic pain, vulvodynia, and interstitial cystitis
  - Paresthesias, often "nonanatomic"
  - Exercise intolerance, dyspnea, and palpitations
  - Sexual dysfunction
  - Ocular dryness

- "Multiple chemical sensitivity" and an increased tendency to report drug reactions
- Impaired social/occupational functioning
- Symptoms can wax and wane on a day-to-day basis, varying in quality, intensity, and location.

PHYSICAL EXAM
- Classic fibromyalgia tender points: 9 symmetric pairs (5 anterior, 4 posterior) located at: anterior sternocleidomastoids, upper-mid trapezius, medial 2nd intercostals spaces, lateral epicondyles, medial fat pad of knees; and, posteriorly, at occipital insertions, upper medial scapular insertions, upper outer quadrants of gluteals, and posterior greater trochanters. Note: These are no longer considered diagnostic criteria for fibromyalgia, but have a sensitivity of 88.4% and specificity 81.1% for the disease (5).
- Generalized hyperalgesia and allodynia may be present.
- Joints examined for swelling, tenderness, erythema, range of motion, crepitus, cystic or mass lesions
- Document absence of inflammatory musculoskeletal disease features (e.g., no synovitis, enthesopathy, dermatologic/ocular findings).
- Neurologic exam: Typically unremarkable

DIFFERENTIAL DIAGNOSIS
- RA, SLE, sarcoidosis, and other inflammatory connective tissue disorders
- Diffuse/Advanced OA
- Seronegative spondyloarthopathies (AS, psoriatic arthritis, etc.)
- Polymyalgia rheumatica
- Inherited myopathies
- Drug-induced and endocrine myopathies
- Viral/postviral polyarthralgia
- Anemia and iron deficiency
- Electrolyte disturbances: Mg, Na, K, Ca
- Primary sleep disorders, including obstructive sleep apnea
- Osteomalacia/vitamin D deficiency
- Opioid-induced hyperalgesia
- Hypothyroidism
- Multiple sclerosis
- Lyme disease
- Hepatis B and C (chronic)
- Inclusion-body myositis
- Spinal stenosis/neuropathies
- Peripheral vascular disease
- Somatoform disorder
- Overlap syndromes:
  - Chronic fatigue syndrome
  - Myofascial pain syndromes (more anatomically localized than fibromyalgia)

DIAGNOSTIC TESTS & INTERPRETATION
Initial Tests (lab, imaging)
- CBC with differential, ESR or CRP, CPK, TSH, comprehensive metabolic profile; also consider 25-OH vitamin D level, Mg, B_{12}, folate, urine drug screen.
- ANA, RF, and other rheumatologic labs unnecessary, unless there is evidence of an inflammatory connective tissue disorder.
- Imaging generally not indicated, except to exclude other diagnoses.

Diagnostic Procedures/Other

- Sleep studies may be indicated to rule out obstructive sleep apnea or narcolepsy.
- Consider psychiatric or neuropsychiatric evaluation for mood disorders and cognitive disturbances.

 TREATMENT

According to the HHS National Guideline Summary (6):

- Nonpharmacologic:
  - Educate the patient about the diagnosis, signs, symptoms, and treatment options (6)[A]
  - Provide Internet education resources (6)[A] via well-established sites, including:
    - www.fmaware.org
    - www.nfra.net
    - www.fmnetnews.com
  - Use the Fibromyalgia Impact Questionnaire (FIQ) for initial assessment and interval evaluation during treatment (6)[A].
  - Cognitive-Behavioral Therapy: Improves mood, energy, pain and functional status (6)[A]
  - Aerobic exercise: Moderately intense, with gradual progression to avoid symptom exacerbation. Once-daily regimens, with titration to patient's tolerance, are recommended (7)[A]
  - Mild strength training (6)[A], acupuncture (8)[B], biofeedback (8)[B]
  - Hypnotherapy (8)[B]
  - Balneotherapy (mineral-rich baths): Hot or cold, with or without massage (8)[B]
  - Treatments likely to be *ineffective*: Chiropractic treatment, massage, electrotherapy, ultrasound, trigger point injections, flexibility exercise (6)[A]
- Pharmacologic:
  - The 3 FDA-approved drugs are: Pregabalin, Duloxetine, and Milnacipran (9); others are used off-label.

MEDICATION
First Line

- Amitriptyline: 10–50 mg PO at bedtime, to treat for pain, fatigue, and sleep disturbances (9,10)[B]
- Duloxetine: Initially 30 mg/d × 1 week, then titrated to max tolerated dosage (120 mg/d) (10)[B]
- Milnacipran: Day 1: 12.5 mg/d; days 2–3, *begin dividing doses*: 12.5 mg b.i.d.; days 4–7: 25 mg BID; after day 7: 50 mg b.i.d.; max dose 100–200 mg b.i.d. (10). Should be tapered, if discontinued (10)[B]
- Pregabalin: Start with 75 mg b.i.d., titrate over 1 week to 150 b.i.d.; max dose 450 mg/d divided b.i.d.–t.i.d. (10)[B]
- Cyclobenzaprine 5 mg HS; titrate up to 10 mg b.i.d.–t.i.d. (6)[A]

Second Line

- Gabapentin start at 300 mg HS, titrate to 1,200–2,400 mg/d divided b.i.d.–t.i.d. (6)[A]
- Fluoxetine 10–80 mg/d PO (higher doses may be more effective) (6)[A]
- Paroxetine CR 12.5–62.5 mg/d (6)[A]
- Tramadol 50–100 mg q6h; likely more effective in combination with acetaminophen (6)[A]
- Medications likely to be *ineffective* include NSAIDs, opioids, benzodiazepines, magnesium, guaifenesin, thyroxine, corticosteroids, DHEA, melatonin, calcitonin (6)[A].

ISSUES FOR REFERRAL

In the case of unclear diagnosis or poor response to therapy, may refer to rheumatology, neurology,, and/or pain management.

COMPLEMENTARY AND ALTERNATIVE MEDICINE

- Acupuncture, biofeedback, hypnotherapy, and balneotherapy, as previously noted
- Limited double-blind trials have shown effectiveness of supplementation with 5-HTP(may not be safe), SAMe, and Acetyl-L-Carnitine
- Transcranial direct current stimulation and repetitive transcranial magnetic stimulation may be considered for those with adequate symptom relief with other therapies (11).

 ONGOING CARE

FOLLOW-UP RECOMMENDATIONS
Patient Monitoring

- For efficacy of therapy at 2–4 week intervals
- Patient follow-up required if intolerant to exercise; reduce intensity and duration until tolerated.

DIET

No proven efficacy of any specific diet. A nutrient-rich, varied diet with avoidance of processed foods is generally recommended.

PROGNOSIS

- 50% with partial remission after 2–3 years of therapy
- Typically has fluctuating, chronic course
- Poorer outcome with:
  - Longer illness duration, more severe symptoms, depression, advanced age, lack of social support

REFERENCES

1. Wolfe F, Clauw DJ, Fitzcharles MA, et al. The American College of Rheumatology preliminary diagnostic criteria for fibromyalgia and measurement of symptom severity. *Arthritis Care Res (Hoboken)*. 2010;62:600–610.
2. Smith HS, Barkin RL. Fibromyalgia syndrome: A discussion of the syndrome and pharmacotherapy. *Dis Mon*. 2011;57:248–285.
3. Boomershine CS, Emir B, Wang Y, et al. Simplifying fibromyalgia assessment: The VASFIQ Brief Symptom Scale. *Ther Adv Musculoskelet Dis*. 2011;3(5):215–226.
4. Glass JM. Cognitive dysfunction in fibromyalgia and chronic fatigue syndrome: new trends and future directions. *Curr Rheumatol Rep*. 2006; 8(6):425–429.
5. Wolfe F, Häuser W. Fibromyalgia diagnosis and diagnostic criteria. *Ann Med*. 2011;43(7): 495–502. Epub 2011 Jul 19.
6. National Guideline Clearinghouse, Guideline Summary NCG-7367; Management of Fibromyalgia Syndrome in Adults.
7. Häuser W, Klose P, Langhorst J, et al. Efficacy of different types of aerobic exercise in fibromyalgia syndrome: A systematic review and meta-analysis of randomised controlled trials. *Arthritis Res Ther*. 2010;12(3):R79. Epub 2010 May 10.
8. Hauser W, Bernhard M, Schiltenwolf M. Efficacy of multicomponent treatment in fibromyalgia syndrome: A meta-analysis of randomized controlled clinical trials. *Arth Rheum*. 2009;61(2): 216–224.
9. Smith HS, Harris R, Clauw D. Fibromyalgia: An afferent processing disorder leading to a complex pain generalized syndrome. *Pain Physician*. 14(2): E217–E245.
10. Häuser W, Petzke F, Üceyler N, et al. Comparative efficacy and acceptability of amitriptyline, duloxetine and milnacipran in fibromyalgia syndrome: A systematic review with meta-analysis. *Rheumatology (Oxford)*. 2011;50: 532–543.
11. Marlow NM, Bonilha HS, Short EB. Efficacy of transcranial direct current stimulation and repetitive transcranial magnetic stimulation for treating fibromyalgia syndrome: A systematic review. *Pain Pract*. 2012. Epub 2012 May 28.

ADDITIONAL READING

- American College of Rheumatology. Practice guidelines, patient education. Available at: www.rheumatology.org.
- Gamber RG, Shores JH, Russo DP, et al. Osteopathic manipulative treatment in conjunction with medication relieves pain associated with fibromyalgia syndrome: Results of a randomized clinical pilot project. *J Am Osteopath Assoc*. 2002;102(6):321–325.
- Hassett AL, Williams DA. Non-pharmacological treatment of chronic widespread musculoskeletal pain. *Best Pract Res Clin Rheumatol*. 2011;25(2): 299–309.
- Websites with fibromyalgia resources, including www.nfra.net, www.fmaware.org, www.fmmgmt. com, and www.fmnetnews.com

 SEE ALSO

Algorithm: Fatigue

 CODES

ICD10
M79.7 Fibromyalgia

CLINICAL PEARLS

- Suspect fibromyalgia when a patient describes severe symptoms of chronic pain, fatigue, and multiple regional complaints in the *absence* of laboratory or physical exam findings.
- Use rigorous ACR criteria to make the diagnosis.
- Fibromyalgia is not a somatoform disorder, and is not merely a manifestation of depression or anxiety, although, as with all chronic pain syndromes, it is frequently associated with mood disturbances.
- The pathophysiology is still unclear, but the disease is considered a disorder of pain regulation, sometimes described as central sensitization.
- Best outcomes occur in patients who understand their illness and are willing to actively engage in a multimodal treatment plan, including exercise, medication, CBT, and lifestyle modifications.

FOLLICULITIS

Rosanne Marie Paul, DO • Jenifer Lloyd, DO

BASICS

DESCRIPTION
- Inflammation of the upper part (superficial) or lower (deep) part of the hair follicle caused by infection, physical injury (traction), or chemical irritation (1)
- Can occur anywhere on the body that hair is found.
- Most frequent symptom is pruritus.
- Clinically manifests as painless or tender pustules, vesicles or pink/red papulopustules ~1–5 mm in size.
- Most commonly infectious in etiology
  - Most frequently caused by *Staphylococcus aureus* bacteria:
    - Bacterial sycosis is a chronic staph infection involving the entire hair follicle; commonly affects males in their 3rd or 4th decade.
  - *Pseudomonas aeruginosa* usually involves the trunk following exposure to poorly chlorinated hot tubs, pools, or contaminated water.
  - Fungal (dermatophytic, *Pityrosporum, Candida*), viral (HSV) or parasitic (*Demodex* spp.) causes
- Noninfectious types:
  - Acneiform folliculitis
  - Actinic superficial folliculitis
  - Acne vulgaris
  - Keloidal folliculitis
  - Folliculitis decalvans
  - Perioral dermatitis
  - Rosacea
  - Fox-Fordyce disease
  - Pruritus folliculitis of pregnancy
  - Eosinophilic pustular folliculitis (3 variants: Ofuji disease in patients of Asian descent, HIV positive/immunocompromised, infantile)
  - Toxic erythema of the newborn
  - Eosinophilic folliculitis (seen in HIV-positive/immunocompromised)
  - Follicular mucinosis
- Skin disorders may produce a follicular eruption that includes:
  - Pseudofolliculitis: Similar in appearance; occurs after shaving; affects the face, scalp, pubis, and legs
  - Atopic dermatitis
  - Follicular psoriasis

EPIDEMIOLOGY
- Many people have been affected at some point in their lifetime.
- Affects persons of all ages, gender, and race

ETIOLOGY AND PATHOPHYSIOLOGY
Predisposing factors to folliculitis:
- Chronic *Staphylococcal* carrier
- Diabetes mellitus
- Malnutrition
- Pruritic skin disease (e.g., scabies, eczema, etc.)
- Exposure to poorly chlorinated swimming pools/hot tubs or water contaminated with *P. aeruginosa*
- Occlusive corticosteroid use (for multiple hours)
- Bacteria:
  - Superficial or deep
  - Most frequently due to *S. aureus* (increasing number of MRSA cases)
  - Also due to *Streptococcus* species, *Pseudomonas* (following exposure to water contaminated with the species), *Proteus*.

- May progress to furunculosis (painful pustular nodule with central necrosis that leaves a permanent scar after healing)
- Fungal:
  - Dermatophytic (tinea capitis, corporis, pedis)
  - Pityrosporum (Pityrosporum orbiculare) commonly affecting teenagers and men, predominantly on upper chest and back
  - *Candida albicans,* although rare, has been reported in those who abuse heroin, resulting in candidemia that leads to pustules and nodules in hair-bearing areas.
- Viral:
  - Herpes simplex virus
  - May be due to molluscum contagiosum, which is usually a sign of immunosuppression
- Parasitic:
  - *Demodex* spp. mites
  - *D. folliculorum* is most commonly implicated.
- Acneiform type commonly drug-induced (systemic and topical corticosteroids, lithium, isoniazid, rifampin)
- Severe vitamin C deficiency
- Actinic superficial type occurs within 24–48 hours of exposure to the sun, resulting in multiple follicular pustules on the shoulders, trunk, and arms.
- Acne vulgaris
- Keloidal folliculitis is chronic condition affecting mostly black patients; involves the neck and occipital scalp, resulting in hypertrophic scars and hair loss.
- Folliculitis decalvans is a chronic folliculitis that leads to progressive scarring and alopecia of the scalp.
- Rosacea consists of papules, pustules, and/or telangiectasias of the face; individuals are genetically predisposed. *H. pylori* and *D. folliculorum* have also been implicated.
- Perioral dermatitis seen most commonly in children and young women; restricted to the perioral region as well as the lower eyelids. May be due to cosmetics, hyperandrogenemia, or use of fluorinated topical corticosteroids.
- Fox-Fordyce disease affects the skin containing apocrine sweat glands, resulting in chronic pruritic, annular, follicular papules.
- Eosinophilic pustular folliculitis (EPF) has 3 variants: Classic (Ofuji disease), associated with HIV infection, and infantile
- Toxic erythema of the newborn is a self-limiting pustular eruption usually appearing during the first 3–4 days of life and subsequently fading in the following 2 weeks.

RISK FACTORS
- Hair removal (shaving, plucking, waxing)
- Other pruritic skin conditions: Eczema, scabies
- Occlusive dressing/clothing
- Personal carrier or contact with methicillin-resistant *S. aureus* (MRSA)-infected persons
- Diabetes mellitus
- Immunosuppression (medications, chemotherapy, HIV)
- Use of hot tubs or saunas
- Use of EGFR Inhibitors (2)

GENERAL PREVENTION
- Good hygiene practices:
  - Frequent hand washing
  - Antibacterial soaps
  - Frequent washing in hot water of towels/linens to avoid reinfection from contaminated clothing and washcloths, etc.
- Good hair removal practices:
  - Exfoliate beforehand.
  - Use witch hazel, alcohol, or TendSkin afterward.
  - Shave in direction of hair growth; use moisturizer/warm water
  - Decrease frequency of shaving.

COMMONLY ASSOCIATED CONDITIONS
- Impetigo
- Acne
- Eczema
- Scabies
- Follicular psoriasis
- Furunculosis

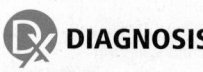 DIAGNOSIS

HISTORY
- Inquire about use of hot tubs, swimming pools, topical corticosteroid use, hair styling and shaving practices, recent antibiotics or systemic steroid use, HIV status, history of sexually transmitted diseases (specifically syphilis).
- MRSA exposures/carrier status, home and work environment (risk/exposure potential)
- Pityrosporum folliculitis occurs more often in warm, moist climates.
- Inquire about the timeline in which the lesions have occurred, including previous similar episodes.

PHYSICAL EXAM
- Characteristic lesions are 1–5 mm-wide vesicles, pustules, or papulopustules with surrounding erythema.
- Rash occurs on hair-bearing skin, especially the face (beard), proximal limbs, scalp, and pubis.
- Pseudomonal folliculitis appears as a widespread rash, mainly on the trunk and limbs.
- In pseudofolliculitis, the growing hair curls around and penetrates the skin at shaved areas.

DIFFERENTIAL DIAGNOSIS
- Acne vulgaris/Acneiform eruptions
- Cutaneous candidiasis
- Contact dermatitis
- Atopic dermatitis
- Follicular psoriasis
- Hidradenitis suppurativa
- Milia
- Arthropod bite

DIAGNOSTIC TESTS & INTERPRETATION
Initial Tests (lab, imaging)
- Diagnosis usually made clinically, taking risk factors, history, and location of lesion into account
- Swab and Gram stain of the pustule by scraping the pustule with a No. 15 blade and not directly swabbing the skin to identify infectious agent and sensitivities to antibiotics
- KOH preparation as well as Wood's lamp fluorescence to identify candida or yeast
- Tzanck smear where suspicion of herpetic simplex viral folliculitis is high

Follow-Up Tests & Special Considerations
- If risk factors or clinical suspicion exist, consider serologies for HIV or syphilis.
- If recurrent, consider HIV testing and A1C/fasting blood sugar testing to evaluate for diabetes.
- Punch biopsy may be considered if lesions persist despite treatment.

Test Interpretation
- Treat positive bacterial culture according to sensitivities.
- Positive HIV serology: Follow-up with CD4 count and punch biopsy to rule out eosinophilic folliculitis.
- Eosinophilic folliculitis: Collect eosinophils within superficial follicle.

 TREATMENT

GENERAL MEASURES
- Lesions often resolve spontaneously.
- Warm compresses may be applied to areas of concern up to t.i.d.
- Topical mupirocin may be used in presumed S. aureus infection.
- Topical antifungals for fungal folliculitis
- Preventive measures are key to avoidance of recurrence:
  – Antibacterial soaps (Dial soap, chlorhexidine or benzyl peroxide wash when showering/bathing)
  – Bleach baths (1/2 cup of 6% bleach per standard bathtub and soak for 5–15 minutes followed by water rinse 1–2 times a week)
  – Keep skin intact; daily skin care with noncomedogenic moisturizers; avoid scratching.
  – Clean shaving instruments daily or use disposable razor, disposing after 1 use.
  – Change washcloths, towels, and sheets daily.

MEDICATION
For most occurrences, antiseptic and supportive care is enough. Systemic antibiotics may be used, but their efficacy is questionable.

First Line
- Staphylococcal folliculitis:
  – Mupirocin ointment applied t.i.d.
  – Cephalosporin (Cephalexin): 250–500 mg PO q.i.d. for 7–10 days
  – Dicloxacillin: 250 mg PO q.i.d. for 7–10 days
- For MRSA:
  – Bactrim DS: 1 tablet (160 mg/800 mg) b.i.d. PO for 7–10 days
  – Clindamycin: 300 mg PO t.i.d. for 10–14 days
  – Minocycline or doxycycline: 100 mg PO b.i.d. for 10–14 days
- Pseudomonal folliculitis:
  – Topical dilute acetic acid baths
  – Ciprofloxacin: 500 mg PO b.i.d. for 7–14 days only if patient is immunocompromised or lesions are persistent
- Eosinophilic folliculitis/eosinophilic pustular folliculitis:
  – HAART treatment for HIV positive-related causes
  – Topical corticosteroids: Betamethasone 0.1% b.i.d. for 3–24 weeks or
  – Tacrolimus: Topically b.i.d. for 3–24 weeks or
  – Isotretinoin: 0.5 mg/kg/d PO for 4–8 weeks or
  – Indomethacin: 25–50 mg/d PO for 1–8 weeks or
  – Itraconazole or metronidazole or cetirizine: 20–40 mg PO b.i.d. for pruritus

- Fungal folliculitis:
  – Topical antifungals: Ketoconazole 2% cream or shampoo or selenium sulfide shampoo daily or
  – Econazole cream applied to affected area b.i.d. for 2–3 weeks
    ○ Systemic antifungals for relapses: Fluconazole (100–200 mg/d for 3 weeks) or Itraconazole (200 mg/d for 1–3 weeks)
    ○ Griseofulvin (tinea capitis in children; 10–20 mg/kg/d for 6 weeks minimum)
- Parasitic folliculitis:
  – 5% permethrin: Apply to affected area, leave on for 8 hours and wash off
  – Ivermectin: 200 g 1× dose
- Herpetic folliculitis:
  – Valacyclovir: 500 mg PO t.i.d. for 5–10 days or
  – Famciclovir: 500 mg PO t.i.d. for 5–10 days or
  – Acyclovir: 200 mg PO 5× daily for 5–10 days

ISSUES FOR REFERRAL
Unusual or persistent cases should be biopsied and then referred to dermatology.

ADDITIONAL THERAPIES
Public Health Measures:
- Outbreaks of culture-positive Pseudomonas hot tub folliculitis should be reported so that source identification can be determined and superchlorination (14 parts/million) can occur.

SURGERY/OTHER PROCEDURES
Incision and drainage is unlikely to be necessary and typically not preferred due to potential for scar formation.

 ONGOING CARE

FOLLOW-UP RECOMMENDATIONS
Patient Monitoring
- Resistant cases should be followed every 2 weeks until cleared.
- 1 return visit in 2 weeks if symptoms abate

DIET
For obese and type 2 diabetic individuals, weight reduction may be helpful as skin-to-skin friction will be lessened.

PATIENT EDUCATION
Avoid shaving in involved areas.

PROGNOSIS
- Usually resolves with treatment; however, S. aureus carriers may experience recurrences.
- Mupirocin nasal treatment for carrier status and for family/household members may be required.
- Resistant or severe cases may warrant testing for diabetes mellitus or immunodeficiency (HIV).

COMPLICATIONS
- Primary complication is recurrent folliculitis.
- Extensive scarring with hyperpigmentation
- Progression to furunculosis or abscesses

REFERENCES
1. Luelmo-Aguilar J, Santandreu MS. Folliculitis: Recognition and management. Am J Clin Dermatol. 2004;5(5):301–310.
2. Bachet JB, et al. Folliculitis induced by EGFR inhibitors, preventive and curative. Oncologist. 2012;17:555–568.

ADDITIONAL READING
- Böer A, Herder N, Winter K, et al. Herpes folliculitis: Clinical, histopathological, and molecular pathologic observations. Br J Dermatol. 2006;154:743–746.
- Brooke RCC, Griffiths CEM. Folliculitis decalvans. Clin Exp Dermatol. 2001;26:120–122.
- Ellis E, Scheinfeld N. Eosinophilic pustular folliculitis: A comprehensive review of treatment options. Am J Clin Dermatol. 2004;5(3):189–197.
- Fiorillo L, Zucker M, Sawyer D, et al. The pseudomonas hot-foot syndrome. N Engl J Med. 2001;345(5):335–338.
- Fridkin SK, Hageman JC, Morrison M, et al. Methicillin-resistant Staphylococcus aureus disease in three communities. N Engl J Med. 2005;352(14):1436–1444.
- James WD. Clinical practice. Acne. N Engl J Med. 2005;352(14):1463–1472.
- Nervi SJ, Schwartz RA, Dmochowski M. Eosinophilic pustular folliculitis: A 40 year retrospect. J Am Acad Dermatol. 2006;55(2):285–289.

SEE ALSO
Algorithm: Rash, Focal

CODES
ICD10
- L66.2 Folliculitis decalvans
- L73.8 Other specified follicular disorders
- L73.9 Follicular disorder, unspecified

CLINICAL PEARLS
- The lesions of folliculitis measure 1–5 mm in size, are clustered in groups, and are pustular, erythematous, and pruritic in nature.
- Most commonly due to S. aureus; with increasing incidence of MRSA in the community consider:
  – Double-strength trimethoprim-sulfamethoxazole (TMP-SMP) (Bactrim DS): 1 tablet b.i.d. PO for 7–10 days
- It is extremely important to educate patients on proper hygiene and skin care techniques in order to prevent chronic or recurrent cases.
- Consider underlying immunocompromised state or punch biopsy for difficult cases.
- Consider intranasal mupirocin treatment for chronic MRSA carrier state.

FOOD ALLERGY

Stanley Fineman, MD

 BASICS

DESCRIPTION
- Hypersensitivity reaction caused by certain foods
- System(s) affected: Gastrointestinal; Hemic/Lymphatic/Immunologic; Pulmonary; Skin/Exocrine
- Synonym(s): Allergic bowel disease; Dietary protein-sensitivity syndrome

EPIDEMIOLOGY
- Predominant age: All ages, but more common in infants and children
- Predominant sex: Male > Female (2:1)

Incidence
Prospective studies indicate ~2.5% of infants experience hypersensitivity reactions to cow's milk in their 1st year of life (1)[B].

Prevalence
- The prevalence of IgE-mediated food allergy is likely 1–2% in the US (2,3)[A].
- In young children, the most common food allergies are cow's milk (2.5%), egg (1.3%), peanut (0.8%), and wheat (0.4%).
- Adults tend to have allergies to shellfish (2%), peanut (0.6%), tree nuts (0.5%), and fish (0.4%) (3)[B].
- In general, only 3–4% of children >4 years have persisting food allergy; it is frequently a transient phenomenon.
- 20% of children with peanut-protein allergy outgrow their sensitivity by school age (3,4)[B].

ETIOLOGY AND PATHOPHYSIOLOGY
Allergic response owing to immunologic mechanisms, such as the classic IgE-allergic response or nonimmunologic-mediated mechanisms
- Any food or ingested substance can cause allergic reactions:
  - Most commonly implicated foods include cow's milk, egg whites, wheat, soy, peanuts, fish, tree nuts (walnut and pecan), and shellfish
- Several food dyes and additives may elicit allergic-like reactions.

Genetics
In family members with a history of food hypersensitivity, the probability of food allergy in subsequent siblings may be as high as 50%.

RISK FACTORS
- Persons with allergic or atopic predisposition have increased risk of hypersensitivity reaction to food.
- Family history of food hypersensitivity

GENERAL PREVENTION
- Avoidance of offending food
- In patients at risk for anaphylaxis, epinephrine auto-injectors should be readily available

 DIAGNOSIS

PHYSICAL EXAM
- GI (system usually affected):
  - More common: Nausea, vomiting, diarrhea, abdominal pain, occult bleeding, flatulence, and bloating
  - Less common: Malabsorption, protein-losing enteropathy, eosinophilic-enteritis, colitis
- Dermatologic:
  - More common: Urticaria/Angioedema, atopic dermatitis, pallor, or flushing
  - Less common: Contact rashes
- Respiratory:
  - More common: Allergic rhinitis, asthma and bronchospasm, cough, serous otitis media
  - Less common: Pulmonary infiltrates (Heiner syndrome), pulmonary hemosiderosis
- Neurologic:
  - Less common: Migraine headaches
- Other symptoms:
  - Systemic anaphylaxis, vasculitis

DIFFERENTIAL DIAGNOSIS
- A careful history is necessary to document a temporal relationship with the manifestations of suspected food hypersensitivity.
- GI, dermatologic, respiratory, neurologic, or other systemic manifestations may mimic a variety of clinical entities.

DIAGNOSTIC TESTS & INTERPRETATION
Initial Tests (lab, imaging)
- Eosinophilia in blood or tissue suggests atopy
- Epicutaneous (prick or puncture) allergy skin tests are used to document IgE-mediated immunologic hypersensitivity and can be done using commercially available extracts (variable sensitivities) or fresh-food skin testing.
- Pretest probability, based on history, has a greater sensitivity than skin testing or serum IgG.
- Skin testing using the suspect food is helpful. If positive on skin test, an oral challenge may aid in diagnosis. The overall correlation between commercially available allergy skin testing and oral food challenge is 60%, but increases to 90% when fresh-food skin testing is done (i.e., a positive skin test correlates with a positive challenge to a particular food) (4)[A]:
  - Skin testing has a high sensitivity (low false-negative rate) *but* a low specificity (high false-positive rate) so *only* skin test against antigens found on history
- Food-specific IgE assays (radioallergosorbent [RAST] and fluorescent enzyme immunoassay [FEI]) detect specific IgE antibodies to offending foods and are less sensitive to skin testing:
  - In certain laboratories, the ImmunoCap food-specific IgE was almost as accurate as a skin test in predicting positive oral challenges (5)[B].
  - Using a serum assay alone to diagnose food allergy has been shown to result in misdiagnosis of true clinical food allergic sensitivity, particularly in children with atopic dermatitis (6)[A]. Do not test using a panel, but rather for specific IgE to foods based on patient history.

- Periodic monitoring of the peanut-specific IgE levels every 2 years may be helpful. If the level of peanut-specific IgE falls to <0.5 kU/L, then a cautious oral challenge under the supervision of an allergist may be considered. A fresh-food skin test with peanut protein should be considered prior to the oral challenge.
- Patch testing for foods for determining delayed-sensitivity immunologic reactions, in patients with eosinophilic esophagitis and atopic dermatitis, is considered of marginal benefit (7)[B].
- Widespread allergy skin testing or serum IgE tests are *not* recommended because of their poor predictive value without a clinical correlating history (8)[B].
- Leukocyte histamine release and assays for circulating immune complexes are predominantly research procedures and are of limited use in clinical practices:
  - Assays for IgG and IgG 4 subclass antibodies are commercially available.
  - No convincing data suggest that these tests are reliable for the diagnosis of food allergy.
- The provocative injection and sublingual provocative tests are highly controversial and have been proven useless for diagnosis of food allergy.
- The leukocytotoxic assay is an unproven diagnostic procedure and is not useful for the diagnosis of allergy (7)[A].
- Other unproven diagnostic procedures that are not recommended include: Provocative neutralization, lymphocyte stimulation, hair analysis, and applied kinesiology (8)[B].

Diagnostic Procedures/Other
Elimination and challenge test is the best procedure for confirming food allergy:
- The suspected food is eliminated from the diet for 1–2 weeks.
- The patient's symptoms are monitored. If they disappear or substantially improve, an oral challenge with the suspected food should be performed under medical supervision.
- Optimally, this challenge should be performed in a double-blind, placebo-controlled manner.
- Patients with history of anaphylaxis should not have an oral challenge unless lack of IgE sensitivity can be documented.
- Most allergic reactions will occur within 30 minutes to 2 hours after challenge, although late reactions have also been described that may occur from 12–24 hours.

Test Interpretation
Pathologic findings are not common in food allergies; however, inflammatory changes can sometimes be seen in the GI tract. The diagnosis of eosinophilic esophagitis is defined by the finding of >15–20 eosinophils per high-power field on esophageal biopsy (9)[B].

TREATMENT

GENERAL MEASURES
- Avoiding the offending food is the most effective mode of treatment for patients with food allergies.
- Those patients with exquisite and severe allergy hypersensitivity to a food should be more cautious in their avoidance of that food. They should carry epinephrine for self-administration in the event that the offending food is ingested unknowingly and a subsequent immediate reaction develops.
- Immunotherapy or hyposensitization with food extracts by various routes, including SC immunotherapy or sublingual neutralization, are not recommended. Research studies are in progress, but immunotherapy is considered experimental at this time.

MEDICATION
- Patients with significant type 1, IgE-mediated hypersensitivity should have epinephrine for autoinjection available in case of accidental ingestion and resulting severe anaphylactic reaction.
- After receiving epinephrine for a systemic anaphylactic reaction to a food, the patient should be monitored in a medical facility, since 15–20% of patients may require >1 dose of epinephrine.
- Symptomatic treatment for milder reactions (e.g., antihistamine)
- The use of cromolyn has been suggested but is not recommended for use in most patients with food allergy.

COMPLEMENTARY AND ALTERNATIVE MEDICINE
There are reports of benefit using various Chinese herbal medicines in laboratory animals with induced food allergy. Benefits have not been reported in humans at this time.

ONGOING CARE

FOLLOW-UP RECOMMENDATIONS
Patient Monitoring
As needed

DIET
- As determined by tests and clinical evaluation
- Strict avoidance of offending food

PATIENT EDUCATION
- Patients should be counseled by a dietitian to maintain a nutritionally sound diet despite avoiding those foods to which the patient is sensitive.
- Patient support: Food Allergy Research & Education, Inc.: 7925 Jones Branch Drive Suite 1100 McLean, VA 22102 Toll-Free: 800-929-4040; Web site www.foodallergy.org
- Other information available at www.aanma.org, www.acaai.org and www.aaaai.org

PROGNOSIS
- Most infants will outgrow their food hypersensitivity by 2–4 years:
  – It may be possible to reintroduce the offending food cautiously into the diet (particularly helpful when the food is one that is difficult to avoid). It is critical that a specific IgE to the offending food is checked, optimally by fresh-food allergy skin test, and is negative prior to an oral challenge.
  – 20% of young children with peanut allergy experience resolution by the age of 5 (10)[B].
  – 42% of children with egg allergy and 48% of children with milk allergy develop clinical tolerance and lose their sensitivity over time (8)[B].
- Adults with food hypersensitivity (particularly to milk, fish, shellfish, or nuts) tend to maintain their allergy for many years.

COMPLICATIONS
- Anaphylaxis
- Angioedema
- Bronchial asthma
- Enterocolitis
- Eosinophilic esophagitis
- Eczematoid lesions

REFERENCES
1. Hst A, Halken S. A prospective study of cow milk allergy in Danish infants during the first 3 years of life. Clinical course in relation to clinical and immunological type of hypersensitivity reaction. *Allergy*. 1990;45:587–596.
2. Chafen JJ, Newberry SJ, Riedl MA, et al. Diagnosing and managing common food allergies: A systematic review. *JAMA*. 2010;303: 1848–1856.
3. Sicherer SH, Sampson HA. Food allergy. *J Allergy Clin Immunol*. 2010;125:S116–S125.
4. Sampson HA. Utility of food-specific IgE concentrations in predicting symptomatic food allergy. *J Allergy Clin Immunol*. 2001;107: 891–896.
5. Maloney JM, Rudengren M, Ahlstedt S, et al. The use of serum-specific IgE measurements for the diagnosis of peanut, tree nut, and seed allergy. *J Allergy Clin Immunol*. 2008;122(1):145–151. Epub 2008 May 27.
6. Fleischer DM, Bock SA, Spears GC, et al. Oral food challenges in children with a diagnosis of food allergy. *J Pediatr*. 2011;158(4):578–583.e1. Epub 2010 Oct 28.
7. Spergel JM, Brown-Whitehorn T, Beausoleil JL, et al. Predictive values for skin prick test and atopy patch test for eosinophilic esophagitis. *J Allergy Clin Immunol*. 2007;119:509–511.
8. Boyce JA, Assa'ad A, Burks AW, et al. Guidelines for the diagnosis and management of food allergy in the United States: Report of the NIAID-Sponsored Expert Panel. *J Allergy Clin Immunol*. 2010;126:S1–58.
9. Furuta GT, Lacouras CA. Eosinophilic esophagitis in children and adult: A systematic review and consensus recommendations for diagnosis and treatment. *Gastroenterology*. 2007;133: 1342–1363.
10. Sicherer SH, Sampson HA. Peanut allergy: Emerging concepts and approaches for an apparent epidemic. *J Allergy Clin Immunol*. 2007;120.
11. Bernstein IL, Li JT, Bernstein DI, et al. Allergy diagnostic testing: An updated practice parameter. *Ann Allergy Asthma Immunol*. 2008; 100:S1–148.
12. Greer FR, Sicherer SH, Burks AW, et al. Effects of early nutritional interventions on the development of atopic disease in infants and children: The role of maternal dietary restriction, breastfeeding, timing of introduction of complementary foods, and hydrolyzed formulas. *Pediatrics*. 2008;121: 183–191.

ADDITIONAL READING
Burks AW, Tang M, Sicherer S, et al. ICON: Food allergy. *J Allergy Clin Immunol*. 2012;129(4): 906–920. Epub 2012 Feb 23.

SEE ALSO

Anaphylaxis; Celiac Disease; Irritable Bowel Syndrome

CODES

ICD10
- L27.2 Dermatitis due to ingested food
- T78.1XXA Oth adverse food reactions, not elsewhere classified, init
- T78.00XA Anaphylactic reaction due to unspecified food, init encntr

CLINICAL PEARLS
- Recent studies suggest that up to 20% of children with peanut allergy may outgrow their sensitivity:
  – Periodic monitoring of the peanut-specific IgE levels every 2 years may be helpful. If the level of peanut-specific IgE falls to <0.5 kU/L, then a cautious oral challenge under the supervision of an allergist may be considered. A fresh-food skin test with peanut protein should be considered prior to the oral challenge.
- Oral itching following ingestion of fresh fruit may be a warning of risk for anaphylaxis but may also represent oral allergy syndrome:
  – This syndrome is the result of cross-reacting proteins in pollens (e.g., patients sensitive to birch tree pollen frequently have cross-reactivity to fresh apples and pears. Cooked fruits are usually tolerated) (11)[B].
- Current evidence does not support a major role for maternal dietary restrictions during pregnancy or lactation in the prevention of atopic disease in infants. It is generally recommended to exclusively breast-feed for the first 6 months of life, particularly when there is a family history of atopy and food allergy. Although solid foods should not be introduced before 4–6 months of age, there is no convincing evidence that delaying their introduction beyond this period has a significant protective effect on the development of allergies (12)[B].

F

FOOD POISONING, BACTERIAL

Frank J. Domino, MD

 BASICS

DESCRIPTION
- Food poisoning (aka foodborne infection) is an illness resulting from the consumption of contaminated food.
- The illness may be produced by bacterial infection or by toxins produced by the bacteria.
- The most commonly recognized foodborne infections acquired in the US are those caused by the bacteria *Salmonella, Campylobacter,* and *Clostridium perfringens.* In traveler's diarrhea, *Escherichia coli* enters this group.
- *Vibrio* incidence is rare, but increasing substantially in last 10 years.

EPIDEMIOLOGY
Incidence
- In the US, an estimated 48 million cases of foodborne poisoning annually (most due to viral etiology), resulting in 128,000 hospitalizations and 3,000 deaths. ~1 of 6 Americans will have an episode.
- >1/2 of water-borne bacterial food poisoning in the US occurs in water not intended for drinking—untreated or inadequately treated ground water.

ETIOLOGY AND PATHOPHYSIOLOGY
- Short incubation period (1–6 hours): Likely pre-formed toxin-induced:
  - *Bacillus cereus*:
    - Food sources: Improperly cooked rice/fried rice and red meats
    - Causes sudden onset of severe nausea and vomiting. Diarrhea may be present.
  - *Staphylococcus aureus*:
    - Food sources: Nonrefrigerated or improperly refrigerated meats and potato and egg salads
    - Causes sudden onset of severe nausea and vomiting. Abdominal cramps and fever may be present.
- Medium incubation period (8–16 hours):
  - *Bacillus cereus* (toxin):
    - Food sources: Meat, stew gravy, vanilla sauce
    - Causes watery diarrhea, abdominal cramps, nausea
  - *C. perfringens*:
    - Food sources: Dry/precooked meats and poultry
    - Causes watery diarrhea, nausea, abdominal cramps
- Long incubation period (>16 hours):
  - Toxin-producing organisms:
    - *Clostridium botulinum*: Source is commercially canned or improperly home-canned foods. Causes vomiting, diarrhea, slurred speech, diplopia, dysphagia, and descending muscle weakness/flaccid paralysis.
    - Enterohemorrhagic *E. coli* (e.g., 0157:H7): Food sources are undercooked beef, especially hamburger, unpasteurized milk, raw fruits and vegetables, and contaminated water. Causes severe diarrhea that often becomes bloody, abdominal pain, vomiting. More common in children <4 years of age.
    - Enterotoxigenic *E. coli*: Food sources are foods or water contaminated by human feces. Causes watery diarrhea, abdominal cramps, and vomiting.

- *Vibrio cholerae*: Food sources are contaminated water, fish, and shellfish, especially food sold by street vendors. Causes profuse watery diarrhea and vomiting, which can lead to severe dehydration and death within hours.
- Invasive organisms: Often bloody stool and fever:
  - *Salmonella:* Food sources are contaminated eggs, poultry, unpasteurized milk or juice, cheese, contaminated raw fruits and vegetables, contaminated peanut butter. Causes watery diarrhea, fever, abdominal cramps, vomiting.
  - *Campylobacter jejuni:* Food sources are raw and undercooked poultry, unpasteurized milk, contaminated meats. Causes diarrhea (may be bloody), cramps, vomiting, fever.
  - *Shigella*: Food sources are food or water contaminated by human fecal material. Causes abdominal cramps, fever, diarrhea.
  - *Vibrio parahaemolyticus*: Food source is raw shellfish. Causes nausea, vomiting, diarrhea, abdominal pain.
  - *Vibrio vulnificus:* Food source is undercooked and raw seafood; wounds exposed to sea water. Causes vomiting, diarrhea, abdominal pain, bacteremia, wound infections. Can be fatal in patients with liver disease or those who are immunocompromised.
  - *Yersinia enterocolitica* and *Y. pseudotuber-culosis*: Food sources are undercooked pork, unpasteurized milk, tofu, contaminated water. Causes appendicitislike symptoms: Abdominal pain, fever, diarrhea, vomiting; occurs primarily in older children and younger adults.
  - *Listeria*: Sources include unpasteurized/contaminated milk, soft cheese, processed/delicatessen meats. Causes nausea, vomiting, fever, watery diarrhea.

RISK FACTORS
- Travel to developing countries
- Improper food storage/handling
- Cross-contamination during preparation of food
- Weakened immune system, pregnancy, very young, elderly, and those with chronic diseases
- Underlying GI disorders
- Patients taking antacids, H_2 blockers, and proton pump inhibitors

GENERAL PREVENTION
- When preparing food at home:
  - Clean:
    - Wash hands, cutting boards, and surfaces before food preparation and after preparing each food item.
    - Wash fresh produce thoroughly before eating.
  - Separate:
    - Keep raw meat, poultry, fish, and their juices away from other food that will not be cooked (e.g., salad).
    - Place cooked meat on a clean platter.
  - Cook: Thoroughly cook meat to the following internal temperature:
    - Fresh beef, veal, pork, and lamb: 145°F
    - Ground meats and egg dishes: 160°F
    - Poultry: 165°F. Cook chicken eggs thoroughly until the yolk is firm.
  - Chill:
    - Refrigerate leftovers within 2–3 hours in clean, shallow, covered containers. If the temperature is >90°F, refrigerate within 1 hour.

- When traveling to underdeveloped countries:
  - Eat only freshly prepared foods.
  - Avoid beverages diluted with nonpotable water, such as ice and milk.
  - Avoid food washed in nonpotable water, like salads.
  - Other risky foods include raw or undercooked meat and seafood, unpeeled raw fruits and vegetables.
  - In developing nations: "Boil it, Cook it, Peel it, or Forget it."
  - Bottled, carbonated, and boiled beverages are generally safe to drink.
- Bismuth subsalicylate (Pepto-Bismol), two 262-mg tablets q.i.d. has been shown to protect travelers to developing countries ~60% of the time. However, it is not recommended for persons taking anticoagulants or other salicylates.

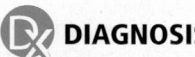 **DIAGNOSIS**

HISTORY
- Food poisoning most often presents as gastroenteritis.
- Most cases of gastroenteritis have a viral etiology. Suspect bacterial food poisoning when multiple persons have rapid onset of symptoms after eating the same meal; have high fever, blood or mucus in stool; severe abdominal pain or neurologic involvement.
- Suspect bacterial gastroenteritis if traveling in, or recent travel to, an underdeveloped country.
- Timing and presentation can aid in establishing an etiology.
- Any of the following should prompt further evaluation, and possible supportive treatment: High fever (≥101.5°F); blood in the stools; prolonged vomiting; signs of dehydration (decrease in urination, a dry mouth and throat, and feeling dizzy when standing up); diarrheal illness that lasts >3 days (1)[C].

PHYSICAL EXAM
- Focus on signs of dehydration: Skin turgor, mucous membranes, and orthostatic changes.
- Abdominal exam: Distension with tenderness (suggestive of bowel obstruction). Auscultation may demonstrate increased bowel sound in obstruction or decreased bowel sounds with an ileus.
- Neurologic: Weakness, paresthesias, diplopia.

DIFFERENTIAL DIAGNOSIS
- Infectious gastroenteritis of any kind (i.e., viral)
- *Clostridium difficile* colitis
- Inflammatory bowel disease
- Appendicitis and other acute abdominal surgical processes
- Hepatitis
- Malabsorption

DIAGNOSTIC TESTS & INTERPRETATION
Initial Tests (lab, imaging)
- Culture of stool and sensitivity, fecal leukocytes, and hemoccult testing; consider ova and parasites if history of foreign travel or symptoms lasting >2 weeks.
- May need to specify to lab if concerns for *Vibrio, E. coli* 0157:H7: Require special cultures

- BMP and WBC count if diarrhea is severe, temperature >101.5°F (38.5°C), persistently bloody stools, severe abdominal pain, or if patient is immunocompromised, elderly, or very young

Follow-Up Tests & Special Considerations
Epidemiologic investigation may be warranted.

 TREATMENT

Most cases of food poisoning are self-limiting and do not require medication.

MEDICATION
First Line

- Children, the elderly, and pregnant patients with signs of mild diarrhea should be started on oral rehydration solution to prevent dehydration (2)[B].
- Oral rehydration options can be purchased or mixed simply from common home ingredients: 6 tsp sugar, 1/2 tsp salt in 1 L of clean, potable water; may add 1/2 cup orange juice or mashed banana for taste and potassium (3)[A].
- Travelers may consider empiric treatment for diarrhea with a single dose of ciprofloxacin 750 mg together with loperamide (see "Additional Treatment").

Second Line

For severe cases of food poisoning (up to 8% have bacteremia) or if the patient has a prosthetic valve, the following medications are recommended (1)[B]:

- *Bacillus cereus:*
  – Supportive care only
- *Campylobacter jejuni:*
  – Mild: Supportive care only
  – Severe: Children: Azithromycin 10 mg/kg/d for 3 days
  – Severe: Adults: Azithromycin 500 mg/d for 3 days
- *Clostridium botulinum:*
  – Supportive care. Antitoxin can be helpful if administered early in the course of the illness.
- *Clostridium perfringens:*
  – Supportive care only
- *Clostridium difficile:*
  – Metronidazole 500 mg t.i.d. for 10–14 days or vancomycin 125 mg PO q.i.d. for 10 days or rifaximin 400 mg q.i.d. for 10–14 days
- Enterohemorrhagic *E. coli* (e.g., 0157:H7):
  – Supportive care only. Closely monitor renal function, hemoglobin, and platelets. Infection associated with hemolytic uremic syndrome (HUS). Antibiotics may increase this risk.
- Enterotoxigenic *E. coli* (common cause of traveler's diarrhea):
  – Generally self-limited. Antibiotics shorten course of illness.
  – Children: Azithromycin 10 mg/kg/d for 3 days or ceftriaxone 50 mg/kg/d for 3 days
  – Adults: Ciprofloxacin 750 mg/d for 3 days or azithromycin 1 g × single dose. Rifaximin rising as an alternate.
- *Salmonella:*
  – Children: Ceftriaxone 100 mg/kg/d divided b.i.d. for 7–10 days or azithromycin 20 mg/kg/d for 7 days
  – Adults: Levofloxacin 500 mg/d for 7–10 days or azithromycin 500 mg daily for 7 days Either can be given for 14 days for immunosuppressed patients. Quinolone resistance has been reported.

- *Shigella:*
  – Children: Azithromycin 10 mg/kg/d for 3 days or ceftriaxone 50 mg/kg/d for 3 days
  – Adults: Ciprofloxacin 750 mg/d for 3 days or azithromycin 500 mg/d for 3 days
- *S. aureus:*
  – Supportive care only
- *Vibrio cholerae:*
  – Children: Erythromycin 30 mg/kg/d given t.i.d. for 3 days or azithromycin 10 mg/kg/d for 3 days
  – Adults: Doxycycline 300 mg 1-time dose or tetracycline 500 mg q.i.d. for 3 days or erythromycin 250 mg t.i.d. for 3 days or azithromycin 500 mg/d for 3 days
- *Vibrio parahaemolyticus:*
  – Supportive care only
  – May use doxycycline 300 mg 1 dose if severe
- *Vibrio vulnificus:*
  – Adults: Minocycline or doxycycline 100 mg b.i.d. + either cefotaxime 2 g IV q8h or ceftriaxone 1 g IV daily with doses appropriately adjusted for underlying renal or hepatic disease
- *Yersinia:*
  – Usually supportive care only
  – Quinolones or 3rd-generation cephalosporin if severe

ADDITIONAL THERAPIES
- Loperamide 4 mg initially, then 2 mg after each loose stool to a maximum of 16 mg in a 24-hour period may be used *unless* high fever, bloody diarrhea, and/or severe abdominal pain present (signs of enteroinvasion). Among travelers with mild–moderate diarrhea and cramping, a single dose of ciprofloxacin 750 mg together with loperamide may eliminate the diarrhea. If symptoms persist after 24 hours, treat with antibiotics for an additional 1–2 days.
- Probiotics (i.e., *Lactobacillus* sp.) have shown decrease in duration of diarrhea by ~25 hours; more research is needed (4)[A].
- Diligent handwashing during course will decrease spread.

 ONGOING CARE

DIET
- Avoid food while nausea is present, but drink plenty of fluids in frequent sips.
- As the nausea subsides, drink adequate fluids, add in bland, low-fat meals and rest. Avoid alcohol, coffee, nicotine, spicy foods.
- Nursing infants should continue to be breast-fed on demand, and infants and older children should be offered their usual food.

PROGNOSIS
Most infections are self-limited and will resolve over the course of 4–5 days.

COMPLICATIONS
- Dehydration
- Hemolytic uremic syndrome (3–5% *E. coli* 0157:H7)
- Guillain-Barré syndrome after *Campylobacter* enteritis
- Reiter syndrome after *Salmonella* enteritis
- *C. difficile* colitis after antibiotic use
- Postinfectious irritable bowel

REFERENCES
1. Dupont HL. Bacterial diarrhea. *NEJM*. 2009; 361:1560–1569.
2. Ang JY, Mathur A. Traveler's diarrhea: Updates for pediatricians. *Pediatric Ann*. 2008;37:814–820.
3. Reduced osmolarity oral rehydration solution. *Cochrane Database Syst Rev*. 2007;3.
4. Allen SJ, Martinez EG, Gregorio GV, et al. Probiotics for treating acute infectious diarrhoea. *Cochrane Database Syst Rev*. 2010;(11): CD003048. Epub 2010 Nov 10.

ADDITIONAL READING
- Centers for Disease Control and Prevention. Trends in foodborne illness in the United States, 1996–2010. Available at: www.cdc.gov/foodborneburden/trends-infoodborne-illness.html.
- CDC. 2011 Estimates. www.cdc.gov/ncidod/dbmd/diseaseinfo/foodborneinfections_g.htm.
- Diagnosis and management of foodborne illnesses: A primer for physicians. *MMWR Recomm Rep*. 2004;53(RR04):1–33.
- Rehydration Project. http://rehydrate.org/ors/made-at-home.
- Scorza K, Williams A, Phillips JD, et al. Evaluation of nausea and vomiting. *Am Fam Physician*. 2007; 76:76–84.
- www.cdc.gov/ncidod/dbmd/diseaseinfo/foodborneinfections_g.htm#howtreated.

 SEE ALSO

Appendicitis, Acute; Botulism; Brucellosis; Dehydration; Diarrhea, Acute; Guillain-Barré Syndrome; Hypokalemia; Intestinal Parasites; Salmonella Infection; Typhoid Fever

 CODES

ICD10
- A02.0 Salmonella enteritis
- A04.5 Campylobacter enteritis
- A05.9 Bacterial foodborne intoxication, unspecified

CLINICAL PEARLS
- Consider bacterial food poisoning when multiple people present after ingesting the same food with fevers and blood/mucus in stool, or have recently returned from a developing nation.
- In developing nations: "Boil it, Cook it, Peel it, or Forget it."
- Consider culture and antibiotics in a prolonged febrile state with blood/mucus in stool, septicemic states, and traveler's diarrhea.
- With signs of enteroinvasion (high prolonged fever, bloody diarrhea, severe pain, septicemia) consider withholding antispasmodics (e.g., Imodium).
- Reintroduce food as soon as tolerated; use oral rehydration, limit high-fat foods and foods high in simple sugars. Lactose limitation is controversial.

FRAGILE X SYNDROME

Thomas J. Hansen, MD

BASICS

DESCRIPTION
- Fragile X syndrome (FXS) is the most common inherited form of mental retardation (also referred to as mental impairment) and is one of the leading known causes of autism (1).
- Among the genetic causes of mental impairment, FXS is the 2nd most common cause following Down syndrome.
- In addition to mental impairment, FXS is characterized by a group of symptoms that may include specific physical features, distinctive behavior patterns, defective speech and language, seizure disorder, and cognitive deficits (2).
- Synonym(s): Marker X syndrome; Martin-Bell syndrome; Escalante syndrome

EPIDEMIOLOGY
- Although this condition is seen in both sexes, males are usually more severely affected than females.
- Affected males almost always have mental impairment, mostly of moderate severity.
- Only 1/3–1/2 of affected females have mental impairment, usually in the mild-to-moderate range (2).

Prevalence
- FXS with full mutation is seen in 1:4,000 males and 1:8,000 females (3).
- FXS with premutation is seen in 1:800 males and 1:200 females (2).

Genetics
- This is an X-linked dominant disorder with variable penetrance.
- The syndrome is caused by an abnormal expansion of cytosine-guanine-guanine (CGG) on the fragile X mental retardation 1 (FMR1) gene. FMR1 normally synthesizes the fragile X protein (FMRP), but mutations in FMR1 lead to a lack of FMRP synthesis, which is important for normal brain development (4).
- The number of CGG repeats in the FMR1 gene are classified as:
  – Full mutation (>200 CGG repeats)
  – Premutation (~6–200 CGG repeats)
- Most males with full mutation have mental impairment in addition to some form of the physical and behavioral features.
- Males with premutation have normal intelligence but have an increased risk for tremor-ataxia syndrome between age 50 and 60.
- Females with full mutation have an ~50% chance of mental impairment in addition to some form of physical and behavioral features.
- Females with premutation have normal intelligence but have a 20% risk for premature ovarian failure.
- Since a male has only 1 X chromosome, it is never passed on to his son. He will pass the affected chromosome to all of his daughters.
- An affected female has a 50% chance of passing her affected chromosome to all of her children.

COMMONLY ASSOCIATED CONDITIONS
- Autistic spectrum disorder (3)
- Connective tissue manifestations, including flat feet and inguinal hernias (3)
- Mitral valve prolapse (develops during adolescence and adulthood) (3)
- Recurrent otitis media and sinusitis in childhood (3)
- Seizure disorder (15–20% for boys and 5% for girls) (4)
- Social phobias and other anxiety disorders (4)

DIAGNOSIS

HISTORY
- Family history of mental impairment, particularly with multiple male relatives
- Family history of premature ovarian failure or fragile X-related tremor ataxia syndrome
- Delay of ≥1 developmental milestones, especially when there is mental impairment in the family (2)
- After the 1st year of life, delay in speech and language along with impaired fine motor skills

Pediatric Considerations
Average age at the time of diagnosis is 8 years, reflecting the subtlety of features in young children (2).

PHYSICAL EXAM
- Physical characteristics become more prominent with advancing age (1).
- Birth–1 month:
  – Examine for orthopedic abnormalities, especially congenital hip dysplasia and clubfoot.
  – Evaluate occipitofrontal circumference, which may be increased.
  – Monitor for feeding difficulties and gastroesophageal reflux (GERD).
- 1 month–1 year:
  – Monitor for hypotonia that frequently results in mild motor delay.
  – Monitor for irritability secondary to sensory problems.
  – Evaluate for feeding problems and the presence of vomiting secondary to GERD.
- 1–5 years:
  – Perform an ophthalmologic evaluation to check for strabismus and refractory errors.
  – Monitor for ptosis and nystagmus.
  – Evaluate for orthopedic problems related to connective tissue dysplasia, such as pes planus, hypermobile joints, and scoliosis.
  – Examine for inguinal hernias.
  – Monitor for recurrent otitis media, conductive hearing loss, and recurrent sinusitis.
  – Monitor for language delay.
  – Monitor for emotional and behavioral status closely, especially tantrums and hyperactivity, and signs of autism.

- 5–12 years:
  – Evaluate for macroorchidism and hernias in boys and precocious puberty in females.
  – Monitor for the child's developmental status.
  – Assess for hyperactivity, obsessive-compulsive behaviors, and anxiety.
  – Assess for cognitive impairments.
- 13–21 years:
  – Assess for seizures, especially atypical seizures.
  – Monitor for cardiac murmur or click.
- Adulthood:
  – Assess for mitral valve prolapse.
  – Evaluate for premature menopause (up to 20% before age 40).
  – Assess for fragile X-associated tremor/ataxia syndrome as patients approach the age of 50.

DIFFERENTIAL DIAGNOSIS
- Pervasive developmental disorder
- Learning disability
- Autism
- Attention deficit hyperactivity disorder (ADHD)
- Other causes of mental impairment

DIAGNOSTIC TESTS & INTERPRETATION
Diagnosis of FXS is made by DNA-based molecular tests, such as Southern blot test and PCR, to isolate the FMR1 gene mutation. Indications for testing include (1):
- Patients with a family history of mental impairment or FXS
- Any child with developmental delay of uncertain etiology or autism
- Individual with mental impairment of unknown etiology
- Women with premature ovarian failure of unknown cause
- Individuals with late-onset intentional tremor or ataxia, especially with a family history of movement disorders, FXS, or undiagnosed mental impairment
- Prenatal testing is offered only if maternal premutation or full mutation is present:
  – Chorionic villus sampling or amniocentesis is used for prenatal diagnosis.
  – Preimplantation genetic diagnosis may be another option for women with a premutation FXS; however, there are several limitations to this approach.

Initial Tests (lab, imaging)
Newborn screening for FXS is not routine at present (5)[B].

TREATMENT

- Treatment is usually supportive and includes the use of stimulants, selective serotonin reuptake inhibitors, atypical antipsychotics, and α-agonists.
- However, there currently is no robust evidence to support recommendations on pharmacologic treatments in patients with FXS in general or in those with an additional diagnosis of ADHD or autism (6).

MEDICATION
Depending on the clinical presentation, pharmacotherapy may include (7)[B]:
- Atypical antipsychotics
- SSRIs
- L-acetyl carnitine in patients with Fragile X and ADHD
- Minocycline
- Antiepileptics
- Methylphenidate
- Dextroamphetamines
- Clonidine
- Guanfacine

Second Line
Cochrane systematic review found insufficient quality data to support use of folic acid on FXS (8)[A].

ISSUES FOR REFERRAL
- The proband and family should be referred for genetic counseling and tested for the FMR1 gene.
- Also see "Additional Treatment" section.

ADDITIONAL THERAPIES
Nonpharmacologic therapies are of tremendous value (9)[B] and include:
- Behavior therapy
- Speech and language therapy
- Psychotherapy and counseling
- Occupational and physical therapy
- Social skill training, support group
- Special education and preschool intervention programs (9)

 ONGOING CARE

PATIENT EDUCATION
- In young females with FXS who are planning for future pregnancies, review the reproductive options, such as egg donation, prenatal diagnosis, adoption, and preimplantation genetic diagnosis.
- Useful Web sites:
  - The National Fragile X Foundation (www.fragilex.org)
  - FRAXA Research Foundation (http://www.fraxa.org)
  - Gene Tests (www.genetests.org, www.geneclinics.org)
  - American College of Medical Genetics (www.acmg.net)
  - Dolan DNA Learning Center: Your Genes, Your Health (www.ygyh.org)
  - National Institute of Child Health and Human Development (www.nichd.nih.gov)

PROGNOSIS
- Patients with FXS have a normal lifespan.
- About 20–33% of women carrying a premutation for FXS are at increased risk for premature ovarian failure.
- 1/3 of males and, to a lesser extent, females carrying the premutation are at increased risk for late-onset (>50) progressive neurodegenerative disorder. It is characterized by intentional tremor and ataxia, called fragile X-associated tremor/ataxia syndrome (FXTAS). Other associated findings include parkinsonism, autonomic dysfunction, peripheral neuropathy, and dementia.

REFERENCES

1. Santoro MR, Bray SM, Warren ST. Molecular mechanisms of fragile X syndrome: A twenty-year perspective. *Annu Rev Pathol*. 2012;7:219–245. Epub 2011 Oct 10.
2. Wattendorf DJ, Muenke M. Diagnosis and management of fragile X syndrome. *Am Fam Physician*. 2005;72:111–113.
3. Visootsak J, Warren ST, Anido A, et al. Fragile X syndrome: An update and review for the primary pediatrician. *Clin Pediatr (Phila)*. 2005;44: 371–381.
4. Tsiouris JA, Brown WT. Neuropsychiatric symptoms of fragile X syndrome: Pathophysiology and pharmacotherapy. *CNS Drugs*. 2004;18:687–703.
5. Bailey DB, Skinner D, Davis AM, et al. Ethical, legal, and social concerns about expanded newborn screening: Fragile X syndrome as a prototype for emerging issues. *Pediatrics*. 2008;121:e693–e704.
6. Rueda JR, Ballesteros J, Tejada MI, et al. Systematic review of pharmacological treatments in fragile X syndrome. *BMC Neurol*. 2009;9:53.
7. Hagerman RJ, Berry-Kravis E, Kaufmann WE, et al. Advances in the treatment of fragile X syndrome. *Pediatrics*. 2009;123:378–390.
8. Rueda JR, Ballesteros J, Guillen V, et al. Folic acid for fragile X syndrome. *Cochrane Database Syst Rev*. 2011;CD008476.
9. Solomon M, Hessl D, Chiu S, et al. A genetic etiology of pervasive developmental disorder guides treatment. *Am J Psychiatry*. 2007;164:575–580.

ADDITIONAL READING

- American College of Obstetricians and Gynecologists Committee on Genetics. ACOG committee opinion. No. 338: Screening for fragile X syndrome. *Obstet Gynecol*. 2006;107:1483–1485.
- Cornish KM, Gray KM, Rinehart NJ, et al. Fragile X syndrome and associated disorders. *Adv Child Dev Behav*. 2010;39:211–235.
- Hersh JH, Saul RA, Committee on Genetics, et al. Health supervision for children with fragile X syndrome. *Pediatrics*. 2011;127:994–1006.
- McConkie-Rosell A, Finucane B, Cronister A, et al. Genetic counseling for fragile x syndrome: Updated recommendations of the national society of genetic counselors. *J Genet Couns*. 2005;14:249–270.
- McLennan Y, Polussa J, Tassone F, et al. Fragile x syndrome. *Curr Genomics*. 2011;12(3):216–224.
- Orr HT, Zoghbi HY. Trinucleotide repeat disorders. *Annu Rev Neurosci*. 2007;30:575–621.

 SEE ALSO

Algorithm: Mental Retardation

CODES

ICD10
Q99.2 Fragile X chromosome

CLINICAL PEARLS
- FXS is the most common inherited form of mental retardation.
- FXS is an X-linked dominant disorder with variable penetrance. Therefore, although this condition is seen in both sexes, males are usually more severely affected than females.
- Newborn screening for FXS is not routine.
- The average age at the time of diagnosis is 8 years.

F

FROSTBITE
Alan M. Ehrlich, MD

BASICS

DESCRIPTION
- A localized complication of exposure to cold, causing tissue to freeze, resulting in diminished blood flow to the affected part (especially hands, face, or feet)
- System(s) affected: Endocrine/Metabolic; Skin/Exocrine
- Synonym(s): Dermatitis congelationis; Frostnip; Environmental injuries

EPIDEMIOLOGY
- Predominant age: All ages
- Predominant sex: Male = Female

ETIOLOGY AND PATHOPHYSIOLOGY
- Ice crystals form intracellularly.
- Vasoconstriction reduces blood flow and microclotting leads to ischemia.
- Dehydration, enzymatic destruction, and ultimately cell death occur.
- In severe cases, deep-tissue freezing may occur with damage to underlying blood vessels, muscles, and nerve tissue.
- Prolonged exposure to cold
- Refreezing thawed extremities

RISK FACTORS
- Previous cold-related injury
- Decreased caloric intake (<1,500 calories/d)
- Dehydration or hypovolemia
- Impaired cerebral function
- Under the effects of alcohol or drug abuse
- Underlying psychiatric disturbance
- Ambient temperature ≤−17.8°C (0°F)
- Smoker
- Elderly
- Lean body mass
- Low level of fitness
- Lack of proper clothing or shelter
- Raynaud phenomenon
- Peripheral vascular disease
- Diabetes mellitus
- Constriction from excessively tight clothing (including too many layers of socks)
- Vehicular failure leading to prolonged cold exposure

GENERAL PREVENTION
- Dress in layers with appropriate cold-weather gear.
- Avoid clothing (including footwear) that is too constricting.
- Cover exposed areas and extremities appropriately.
- Prepare properly for trips to cold climates.
- Minimize wind exposure.
- Stay dry.
- Avoid alcohol.
- Ensure adequate hydration and caloric intake.
- Supplemental oxygen at very high altitudes (>7,500 m).

COMMONLY ASSOCIATED CONDITIONS
Alcohol and/or drug abuse

DIAGNOSIS

HISTORY
- Throbbing pain
- Paresthesia
- Excessive sweating
- Joint pain
- Determine duration and severity of cold exposure.

PHYSICAL EXAM
- Feet, hands, and face most commonly affected
- Injured area appears cold, hard, and white and is anesthetic to touch. It progresses to blotchy-red, swollen, and painful regions after rewarming.
- 1st degree: Redness and edema without blister formation
- 2nd degree: Redness, edema, and blister formation
- 3rd degree: Same as above, with addition of hemorrhagic vesicles
- 4th degree: Necrosis and gangrene
- Pallor
- Loss of cutaneous sensation
- Numbness
- Limited movement of affected joints
- SC edema
- Hyperemia
- Blistering
- Blue discoloration
- Skin necrosis
- Gangrene

DIFFERENTIAL DIAGNOSIS
- Frostnip: A superficial cold injury that does not cause permanent damage
- Chilblains (pernio): An inflammatory reaction to short-term cold, wet exposure without tissue freezing
- Immersion syndrome (trench foot): Inflammatory reaction to prolonged cold, wet exposure, typically socks or footwear

DIAGNOSTIC TESTS & INTERPRETATION
ECG in hypothermia may show bradycardia, atrial fibrillation, atrial flutter, ventricular fibrillation, diffuse T-wave inversion, Osborn waves (upward-going "hump" following S wave in the RS–T segment).

Initial Tests (lab, imaging)
- May show signs of hemoconcentration, such as elevated hemoglobin or high BUN:creatinine ratio
- LFTs for decreased hepatic function
- Triple-phase bone scan can identify tissue viability at early stage and facilitate early debridement.
- Other imaging techniques sometimes used include MRI/MRA, infrared thermography, angiography, digital plethysmography, and laser Doppler studies.

Test Interpretation
- Ice crystallization in the intravascular extracellular space
- Atrophy
- Fibroblastic proliferation
- Skin necrosis

TREATMENT

Geriatric Considerations
- Associated disease states increase mortality.
- Periarticular osteoporosis complicates
- More prone to hypothermia

Pediatric Considerations
Loss of epithelial growth centers

ALERT
Acidosis

GENERAL MEASURES
- If transport time will be short (1–2 hours at most), the risks posed by improper rewarming or refreezing outweigh the risks of delaying treatment for deep frostbite (1)[C].
- If transport will be prolonged (>1–2 hours), frostbite will often thaw spontaneously. It is more important to prevent hypothermia than to rewarm frostbite rapidly in warm water. This does not mean that a frostbitten extremity should be kept in the cold to prevent spontaneous rewarming. Anticipate that frostbitten areas will rewarm as a consequence of keeping the patient warm; protect the patient from refreezing at all costs (1)[C].
- Frozen extremity should not be used for walking or climbing, if at all possible, until definitive care is available (2)[C].

- Moderate or severe hypothermia should be treated before specifically treating frostbite injury (2)[B].
- Rapid rewarming (3)[B]:
  - Immerse frozen body part in warm water (40–41°C [104–106°F]) whirlpool bath for at least 30 minutes and until thawing is complete.
  - Do not let affected part touch sides of whirlpool unit.
  - Continue rewarming until a red/purple color appears and the affected part becomes pliable.
  - It is critical not to allow refreezing after thawing has occurred.
  - Repeat treatment for 30 minutes b.i.d. until distinction of viable from nonviable tissue is clear or evidence of clear healing is present.

- After rewarming, injured parts should be covered with nonadhesive dressings, splinted, and elevated.
- Remove jewelry and clothing, if present, from the affected area.
- Apply topical aloe vera q6h.
- Sterile cotton between fingers or toes, if applicable, to prevent maceration
- Keep the patient dry.
- If conscious, give the patient warm fluids with high sugar content.
- Prevent infection once treatment begins.
- Institute ongoing whirlpool therapy for cleansing and debridement.
- Prevent damage to other body parts.
- Prohibit use of nicotine-containing products (including cigarettes) or other vasoconstrictive agents.
- Maintenance: Gastric lavage, peritoneal dialysis, hemodialysis, and mediastinal lavage if needed (using warmed fluids)

MEDICATION

First Line

- tPA administered within 24 hours of injury may prevent damage from thrombosis and may reduce amputation rate (4,5)[B].
- Low molecular weight dextran should be considered in patients not given other systemic treatments (e.g., thrombolysis) (2)[C].
- Aspirin 250 mg plus buflomedil 400 mg IV followed by 8 days of iloprost 0.5–2 ng/kg/min for 6 hr/d may prevent amputation in patients with frostbite extending to the proximal phalanx (6)[B].
- Tetanus toxoid
- Penicillin G 500,000 U q6h for 48–72 hours prophylactically (7)[B]
- Ibuprofen 400 mg q12h to inhibit prostaglandins (7)[C].
- NSAIDs for mild to moderate pain. For severe pain, narcotic analgesia.
- Precautions: tPA should not be used with history of recent bleeding, stroke, ulcer, etc.

Second Line

Pentoxifylline has been tried with some success (7)[C].

ADDITIONAL THERAPIES

- Heated oxygen
- Warm IV fluids via central venous pressure line.

SURGERY/OTHER PROCEDURES

- Urgent surgery rarely needed except fasciotomy for compartment syndrome
- Suspect compartment syndrome if tissue swollen and compartment pressures >37–40 mm Hg
- Fasciotomy indicated if elevated compartment pressures (2)[B]
- Surgical debridement, as needed, to remove necrotic tissue
- Amputation should not be considered until tissues are definitively dead: May take ~3 weeks to know whether the tissue is permanently injured.

IN-PATIENT CONSIDERATIONS

Admission Criteria/Initial Stabilization

Hospitalization generally recommended (5)

- Institute emergency measures for hypothermic patient without pulse or respiration. Such measures may include CPR and internal warming with warm IV fluids and warm oxygen (see topic "Hypothermia").
- Prevent refreezing.
- It may be necessary to keep the frostbitten part frozen until the patient can be transported to a care facility. Prolonged freezing is preferable to warming and refreezing (8)[C].
- Remove nonadherent wet clothing.
- Treat for hypothermia.
- Treat for pain:
  – NSAIDs and/or narcotics, if needed
- Do not rub areas to warm them; increased tissue damage may occur (4)[C].
- Do not allow patient with frostbitten feet to walk, except when the life of the patient or rescuer is in danger (1)[C].

IV Fluids

If patient cannot tolerate oral fluids or has altered mental status, give warmed normal saline (2)[C].

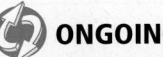 ONGOING CARE

FOLLOW-UP RECOMMENDATIONS

Outpatient or inpatient, depending on severity:

- As tolerated; protect injured body parts.
- Initiate physical therapy once healing progresses sufficiently.

Patient Monitoring

- Preferably, electronic probe for temperature monitoring (rectal or vascular)
- Follow-up for physical therapy progress, infection, other complications

DIET

- As tolerated
- Warm oral fluids

PATIENT EDUCATION

- Refer to local library for information.
- Provide education on:
- Exposure protection
- Early signs and symptoms of frostbite

PROGNOSIS

- Anesthesia and bullae may occur.
- The affected areas will heal or mummify without surgery; the process may take 6–12 months for healing.
- Patient may be sensitive to cold and experience burning and tingling.
- Cyanotic nonblanching skin and blisters with dark fluid suggest worse prognosis (8)[C].

COMPLICATIONS

- Hyperglycemia
- Acidosis
- Refractory arrhythmias
- Tissue loss: Distal parts of an extremity may undergo spontaneous amputation.
- Gangrene
- Death

REFERENCES

1. State of Alaska Cold Injury Guideline: Alaska Multi-level 2003 Version. http://www.hypothermia.org/Hypothermia_Ed_pdf/Alaska-Cold-Injuries.pdf.
2. McIntosh SE, Hamonko M, Freer L, et al. Wilderness Medical Society practice guidelines for the prevention and treatment of frostbite. *Wilderness Environ Med*. 2011;22:156–166.
3. Hallam MJ, Cubison T, Dheansa B, et al. Managing frostbite. *BMJ*. 2010;341:c5864.
4. Bruen KJ, Ballard JR, Morris SE, et al. Reduction of the incidence of amputation in frostbite injury with thrombolytic therapy. *Arch Surg*. 2007;142:546–551; discussion 551–553.
5. Jurkovich GJ. Environmental cold-induced injury. *Surg Clin North Am*. 2007;87:247–267, viii.
6. Cauchy E, Cheguillaume B, Chetaille E, et al. A controlled trial of a prostacyclin and rt-PA in the treatment of severe frostbite. *N Engl J Med*. 2011;364:189–190.
7. Imray C, Grieve A, Dhillon S, et al. Cold damage to the extremities: Frostbite and non-freezing cold injuries. *Postgrad Med J*. 2009;85:481–488.
8. Biem J, Koehncke N, Classen D, et al. Out of the cold: Management of hypothermia and frostbite. *CMAJ*. 2003;168:305–311.

ADDITIONAL READING

- Cappaert TA, Stone JA, Castellani JW, et al. National Athletic Trainers' Association position statement: Environmental cold injuries. *J Athl Train*. 2008;43:640–658.
- Murphy JV, Banwell PE, Roberts AH, et al. Frostbite: Pathogenesis and treatment. *J Trauma*. 2000;48:171–178.
- Twomey JA, Peltier GL, Zera RT. An open-label study to evaluate the safety and efficacy of tissue plasminogen activator in treatment of severe frostbite. *J Trauma*. 2005;59:1350–1354; discussion 1354–1355.

 SEE ALSO

- Hypothermia
- Algorithm: Hypothermia

 CODES

ICD10

- T33.829A Superficial frostbite of unspecified foot, initial encounter
- T33.90XA Superficial frostbite of unspecified sites, init encntr
- T34.90XA Frostbite with tissue necrosis of unsp sites, init encntr

CLINICAL PEARLS

- Frostbite is considered a tetanus-prone injury. Treat as any injury involving tissue destruction.
- Avoid rewarming en route to the hospital if there is a chance of refreezing. Avoid burns to affected areas, which may be numb and insensitive to heat.

F

FROZEN SHOULDER

Crystal L. Hnatko, DO

 BASICS

DESCRIPTION
- A poorly understood condition marked by the painful, gradual loss of both active and passive glenohumeral (GH) motion in >1 plane, due to a progressive fibrosis/contracture of the GH joint capsule.
- Most agree that the clinical course of adhesive capsulitis (AC) follows a somewhat predictable progression:
  - Stage 1, Freeze/Pain: The subacute onset of diffuse vague pain, lasting 2–9 months
  - Stage 2, Frozen/Adhesive: The insidious onset of stiffness, lasting 4–12 months
  - Stage 3, Thaw/Recovery: Gradual resolution, lasting 5–24+ months
- Resolution may be protracted (symptoms lasting >36 months) and incomplete but rarely results in a functional limitation.
- AC may also be categorized as primary (idiopathic) and secondary (underlying cause or associated condition).
- System(s) affected: Musculoskeletal
- Synonym(s): Adhesive capsulitis; Pericapsulitis; Scapulohumeral periarthritis

EPIDEMIOLOGY
- Predominant age: 40–60 years
- Predominant sex: Female > Male

Prevalence
- General population: 2–5% (1)
- Diabetics type I and type II: 10–20%

ETIOLOGY AND PATHOPHYSIOLOGY
- Synovial inflammation and capsular fibrosis resulting in contracture of the rotator interval, coracohumeral ligament, and anterior shoulder capsule restricting movement of the shoulder (2,3).
- A poorly understood chronic inflammatory response with fibroblastic proliferation, possibly immunomodulated (2).

Genetics
No known genetic predispositions

RISK FACTORS
- Sedentary vocation
- Age >40 years
- History of AC: 20–30% will develop the condition in the other shoulder (2)
- Minor injury: 20–30% of those with AC will report recent minor trauma to the shoulder
- Systemic diseases: Endocrinopathies, autoimmune disorders, atherosclerotic disease (see "Commonly Associated Conditions")

GENERAL PREVENTION
No current evidence regarding prevention

COMMONLY ASSOCIATED CONDITIONS
- Idiopathic AC can be associated with a history of Dupuytren contractures.
- Secondary AC is associated with: Diabetes type I and II, thyroid disease, autoimmune diseases, rotator cuff injury or minor shoulder trauma, surgery or immobilization of shoulder, prior cerebrovascular accident, or myocardial infarction (3,4)

 DIAGNOSIS

HISTORY
- Insidious onset of progressive, diffuse shoulder pain followed by the complaint of gradual onset of stiffness
- Pain (Stage 1, early Stage 2) predominates early in the course of the disease:
  - Night pain often interrupts sleep
  - Debilitating pain: Achy at rest and sharper with movement, poorly localized
  - Muscle spasm/pain in the neck, shoulder, acromial clavicular joint and posterior thorax due to scapular overcompensation (can also cause shoulder impingement)
- Stiffness (Stage 2 and 3) predominates later as pain wanes:
  - Manifests as difficulties with activities of daily living (ADLs):
    ○ Inability to reach overhead or into back pocket
  - Patient may complain of weakness (subjective).
- Preceding injury, illness, or immobilization (secondary AC)

PHYSICAL EXAM
- Limited active and passive shoulder ROM in >1 plane of motion: Document ROM for forward flexion, abduction, external and internal rotation on every patient with shoulder complaints, every visit.
- Diffuse shoulder tenderness with deep palpation
- Loss of natural arm swing with gait
- Normal 5/5 strength ("pseudo" weakness may be present if pain inhibits effort)
- Special tests (Neer, Hawkins etc.) may be positive and difficult to perform; none is diagnostic of AC.
- No neurovascular deficits should be present.

DIFFERENTIAL DIAGNOSIS
- Rotator cuff strain/tear/impingement syndrome
- GH or acromioclavicular joint osteoarthritis (OA)
- Cervical strain/radiculopathy/OA
- Myofascial pain syndromes
- Calcific tendonitis
- Fracture, dislocation
- Bony neoplasm/metastases

DIAGNOSTIC TESTS & INTERPRETATION
Initial Tests (lab, imaging)
No lab is diagnostic for primary (idiopathic) AC. If suspected, labs may be indicated to rule out any underlying systemic diseases associated with secondary AC: Hbg A1C, TSH, etc. (5).
- Plain radiograph (anteroposterior [AP], axillary, supraspinatus outlet views) to rule out osteoarthritis, calcific tendinitis, avascular necrosis, osteomyelitis, fracture, dislocation, and tumor
- Radiographs should be normal but may demonstrate disuse osteopenia of the proximal humerus late in the course.
- If suspicious for secondary AC, consider MRI to evaluate for a characteristic thickening of the axillary pouch and to rule out other shoulder disorders (3).

Follow-Up Tests & Special Considerations
- Serial exam is advised in patients who present with nonspecific shoulder pain and normal radiographs eluding a specific diagnosis. At follow-up visits, the diagnosis is supported if progressive motion restriction is identified in >1 plane of motion.

- Early in stage 1, pain is the predominant feature and restriction of motion may be difficult to identify. At 8-week follow-up, the patient may not have a complaint of stiffness but the loss of passive ROM may be easier to identify on exam.
- *Early on, AC is almost indistinguishable from subacromial bursitis. The loss of passive external rotation may be the only finding on exam to differentiate early AC from the myriad of conditions that can cause subacromial bursitis. The only other condition that may cause insidious loss of passive external rotation is GH arthritis (3).*

Diagnostic Procedures/Other
Diagnostic subacromial injection of anesthetic may be used to differentiate AC from rotator cuff pathologies in some cases:
- Resolution of pain and restored ROM after subacromial injection suggests rotator cuff pathology or other cause of subacromial bursitis.
- Intact muscle strength and persistent active and passive ROM deficits with a firm mechanical, tethered end point are consistent with AC.

Test Interpretation
If performed, surgical arthroscopy classically demonstrates capsular thickening and synovial inflammation with adhesions to the humerus.

TREATMENT

- There is no agreed-upon approach to treatment as no therapy or combination of therapies has definitively altered the long-term outcome of AC.
- Typical conservative therapy consists of any combination of physical therapy, oral medications, and joint or bursal injections.
- Most sources suggest a minimum of 4–6 months of conservative therapies before more invasive surgical options are considered, such as manipulation under anesthesia (MUA) or capsular release.
- Once the diagnosis is suspected, education and expectations should be discussed to include:
  - Protracted recovery (months to years) characterized by resolution of pain prior to the return of function
  - Full ROM may never be recovered; however, functional limitations are uncommon.
- Optimizing treatment depends on recognition of the clinical stage at presentation in order to target the predominating process (pain vs. stiffness) with hopes of limiting the symptom severity (4)[C].

GENERAL MEASURES
- Goal of all therapies: Control pain, preserve mobility, and allow for restful sleep.
- Heat and/or ice: May temporarily improve pain and secondary spasm
- Address underlying causes of secondary adhesive capsulitis (see "Associated Conditions").
- Patient reassessment must be ongoing to reinforce expectations and determine patient's goals.

MEDICATION

First Line

- NSAIDs: Widely used in the treatment of AC and thought to be most beneficial in stage 1 when pain is the predominant feature. If contraindicated, reasonable alternatives include acetaminophen or opioid analgesics. Concomitant use of NSAIDs with oral or injectable corticosteroids has no added benefit (1)[A].
- Oral corticosteroids: Rarely used in clinical practice, but evidence demonstrates short-term improvement in pain and ROM (up to 6 weeks) most likely beneficial early in the course of the disease (stage 1 and early stage 2) (1,6)[A]:
  - Prednisolone: 30 mg/d for 3 weeks (alternatively 10 mg × 4 weeks, then 5 mg × 2 weeks)
- Subacromial (SA) corticosteroid injection: At any stage, SA injection in conjunction with PT provides short-term (16 weeks) benefit in pain and ROM (3)[B].
- Intra-articular (IA) corticosteroid injection: Like SA injections, IA injections have demonstrated short-term (16 weeks) improvement in pain and ROM if used in conjunction with physical therapy (1,6,7)[A].
  - May require serial injection and requires technical expertise.

Second Line

Tricyclic antidepressants (amitriptyline) have been used as neuromodulators. No evidence exists to support use in AC.

ISSUES FOR REFERRAL

- The majority of cases are managed by primary care physicians.
- 7–12% of cases will not respond to nonoperative treatment (4).
- Orthopedic surgical referral should be considered if patient is considering a more invasive treatment option and the patient has not responded adequately to conservative treatment within 4–6 months.

ADDITIONAL THERAPIES

- Physical therapy: No known benefit to aggressive physical therapy vs. gentle stretching and active motion within the pain-free range (4)[A]. Additive effect when used in conjunction with other treatments (injections, MUA, surgical release) but there is no evidence to support the use of physical therapy alone in the treatment of AC (4)[A].
- Iontophoresis (electromotive drug administration) is generally not recommended in this condition.
- Although not commonly used, supervised neglect is a plausible treatment option for some patients (5).
- Capsular hydrodilation (arthrography distention): Intra-articular injection of large volume saline/steroid has demonstrated some short-term improvements (12 weeks) in pain and function (2,3,4)[C].
- Suprascapular Nerve Block: Early evidence suggests short-term improvement in pain (4)[C].
- Low-power laser therapy: Superior to placebo (4)[C]
- Botox and hyaluronic acid: Evidence suggests no benefit.

ALERT

Indications for more invasive options remain highly subjective and need to be individualized to each patient.

SURGERY/OTHER PROCEDURES

- MUA: Recent evidence questions the advantages of this procedure (3)[B]. Contraindicated in posttraumatic or postsurgical AC.
- Arthroscopic capsular release: Most common surgical method for treating recalcitrant AC:
  - Short-term benefits: Improved pain and function
  - Long-term benefits: Mixed findings (similar vs. superior to conservative therapy) (3,4,6)[C]

COMPLEMENTARY AND ALTERNATIVE MEDICINE

- Acupuncture: Unable to draw a conclusion on available evidence (4)
- Osteopathic manipulative technique: Evidence is lacking.

IN-PATIENT CONSIDERATIONS

Initial Stabilization

Outpatient care

 ONGOING CARE

FOLLOW-UP RECOMMENDATIONS

Reinforce the natural course of the disease and discuss the various treatment options as the patient progresses through different stages of the disease. Many patients are more likely to request invasive procedures (injections, capsular distension, MUA, surgery) when the stiffness starts to affect ADLs.

Patient Monitoring

Close monitoring and frequent encouragement are usually needed for successful recovery.

DIET

No restrictions

PATIENT EDUCATION

Long-term course of treatment until resolution of symptoms; stretching and ROM exercises daily during and after improvement:

- Codman pendulum exercises: Lean forward onto table or chair with unaffected arm bending at the waist; let the affected arm dangle. Now, swing the affected arm slowly by moving the torso. Try smaller and then bigger circles (clockwise and counterclockwise).
- Climbing the wall: Put the hand flat on a wall in front of you; use the fingers to "climb" the wall; pause 30 seconds every few inches. Repeat the exercise after turning 90 degrees to wall (abduction).

PROGNOSIS

- AC is considered self-limiting, yet up to 50% have permanent restrictions of ROM (usually external rotation) (1,2).
- Rare functional disability results (3,6)

COMPLICATIONS

Surgical complications and complications due to MUA can be disabling, but are uncommon.

REFERENCES

1. Favejee MM, Huisstede BM, Koes BW. Frozen shoulder: The effectiveness of conservative and surgical interventions—systematic review. Br J Sports Med. 2011;45:49–56. Epub 2010 Jul 20.
2. Robinson CM, Seah KT, Chee YH, et al. Frozen shoulder. J Bone Joint Surg Br. 2012;94:1–9.
3. Hsu J, Anakqenze O, Warrender W, et al. Current review of adhesive capsulitis. J Shoulder Elbow Surg. 2011;20:502–514.
4. Neviaser AS, Neviaser RJ. Adhesive capsulitis of the shoulder. J Am Acad Orthop Surg. 2011;19:536–542.
5. Maund E, Craig D, Suekarran S, et al. Management of frozen shoulder: A systematic review and cost-effectiveness analysis. Health Technol Assess. 2012;16:1–264.
6. Rill BK, Fleckenstein CM, Levy MS, et al. Predictors of outcome after nonoperative and operative treatment of adhesive capsulitis. Am J Sports Med. 2011;39:567–574. Epub 2010 Dec 15.
7. Shin S, Lee S. Efficacies of corticosteroid injection at different sites of the shoulder for the treatment of adhesive capsulitis. J Shoulder Elbow Surg. 2013; 22:521–527.

ADDITIONAL READING

Ewald A. Adhesive capsulitis: A review. Am Fam Physician. 2011;83(4):417–422.

 CODES

ICD10

- M75.00 Adhesive capsulitis of unspecified shoulder
- M75.01 Adhesive capsulitis of right shoulder
- M75.02 Adhesive capsulitis of left shoulder

CLINICAL PEARLS

- Early on in the course, AC is nearly indistinguishable from rotator cuff pathology, but restriction of external ROM is highly suggestive of adhesive capsulitis.
- Diagnostic subacromial bursa injection may assist in differentiating early AC from impingement syndrome. (In AC, ROM deficits persist and strength is intact after injection.)
- Normal radiographs in the setting of progressive restriction of motion in >1 plane confirm the diagnosis.
- Initial treatment by primary care mainly consists of conservative measures: NSAIDs; oral, bursal, or intra-articular corticosteroids; coupled with physical therapy and appropriate patient education.
- Although highly variable depending on the individual, invasive treatment options can generally be considered after 4–6 months: Capsular distention, MUA, and arthroscopy (about 10% of those affected)

FURUNCULOSIS

Zoltan Trizna, MD, PhD

BASICS

DESCRIPTION
- Acute bacterial abscess of a hair follicle (often *Staphylococcus aureus*)
- System(s) affected: Skin/Exocrine
- Synonym(s): Boils

EPIDEMIOLOGY
Incidence
- Predominant age:
  - Adolescents and young adults
  - Clusters have been reported in teenagers living in crowded quarters, within families, or in high school athletes.
- Predominant sex: Male = Female

Prevalence
Exact data are not available.

ETIOLOGY AND PATHOPHYSIOLOGY
- Infection spreads away from hair follicle into surrounding dermis.
- Pathogenic strain of *S. aureus* (usually); most cases in US are now due to community-acquired methicillin-resistant *S. aureus* (CA-MRSA), whereas methicillin sensitive *S. aureus* (MSSA) most common elsewhere (1).

Genetics
Unknown

RISK FACTORS
- Carriage of pathogenic strain of *Staphylococcus* sp. in nares, skin, axilla, and perineum
- Rarely, polymorphonuclear leukocyte defect or hyperimmunoglobulin E–*Staphylococcus* sp. abscess syndrome
- Diabetes mellitus, malnutrition, alcoholism, obesity, atopic dermatitis
- Primary immunodeficiency disease and AIDS (common variable immunodeficiency, chronic granulomatous disease, Chediak-Higashi syndrome, C3 deficiency, C3 hypercatabolism, transient hypogammaglobulinemia of infancy, immunodeficiency with thymoma, Wiskott-Aldrich syndrome)
- Secondary immunodeficiency (e.g., leukemia, leukopenia, neutropenia, therapeutic immunosuppression)
- Medication impairing neutrophil function (e.g., omeprazole)
- The most important independent predictor of recurrence is a positive family history (2).

GENERAL PREVENTION
Patient education regarding self-care (see "General Measures"); treatment and prevention are interrelated.

COMMONLY ASSOCIATED CONDITIONS
- Usually normal immune system
- Diabetes mellitus
- Polymorphonuclear leukocyte defect (rare)
- Hyperimmunoglobulin E–*Staphylococcus* sp. abscess syndrome (rare)
- See "Risk Factors."

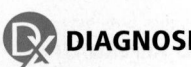

DIAGNOSIS

HISTORY
- Located on hair-bearing sites, especially areas prone to friction or repeated minor traumas (e.g., underneath belt, anterior aspects of thighs, nape, buttocks)
- No initial fever or systemic symptoms
- The folliculocentric nodule may enlarge, become painful, and develop into an abscess (frequently with spontaneous drainage).

PHYSICAL EXAM
- Painful erythematous papules/nodules (1–5 cm) with central pustules
- Tender, red, perifollicular swelling, terminating in discharge of pus and necrotic plug
- Lesions may be solitary or clustered.

DIFFERENTIAL DIAGNOSIS
- Folliculitis
- Pseudofolliculitis
- Carbuncles
- Ruptured epidermal cyst
- Myiasis (larva of botfly/tumba fly)
- Hidradenitis suppurativa
- Atypical bacterial or fungal infections

DIAGNOSTIC TESTS & INTERPRETATION
Initial Tests (lab, imaging)
Obtain culture if multiple abscesses marked by surrounding inflammation, cellulitis, systemic symptoms, such as fever, or if immunocompromised.

Follow-Up Tests & Special Considerations
- Immunoglobulin levels in rare (e.g., recurrent or otherwise inexplicable) cases
- If culture grows gram-negative bacteria or fungus, consider polymorphonuclear neutrophil leukocyte functional defect.

Test Interpretation
Histopathology (although a biopsy is rarely needed):
- Perifollicular necrosis containing fibrinoid material and neutrophils
- At deep end of necrotic plug, in SC tissue, is a large abscess with a Gram stain positive for small collections of *S. aureus*.

TREATMENT

GENERAL MEASURES
- Moist, warm compresses (provide comfort, encourage localization/pointing/drainage) 30 minutes q.i.d.
- If pointing or large, incise and drain: Consider packing.
- Routine culture is not necessary for localized abscess in nondiabetic patients with normal immune system.
- Sanitary practices: Change towels, washcloths, and sheets daily; clean shaving instruments; avoid nose picking; change wound dressings frequently; do not share items of personal hygiene.

MEDICATION
First Line
- Systemic antibiotics usually *unnecessary*, unless extensive surrounding cellulitis or fever
- If suspecting MRSA, see "Second Line" (3).
- If multiple abscesses, lesions with marked surrounding inflammation, cellulitis, systemic symptoms, such as fever, or if immunocompromised: Place on antibiotics directed at *S. aureus* × 10–14 days:
  - Dicloxacillin (Dynapen, Pathocil) 500 mg PO q.i.d. *or* cephalexin 250–500 mg PO q.i.d. *or* clindamycin 150 mg q.i.d. if penicillin-allergic
- Suppression of pathogenic strain (if topical treatment fails):
  - Dicloxacillin/Cloxacillin: 500 mg b.i.d. × 10–14 days
  - Cephalexin or clindamycin (if penicillin-allergic)
  - If preceding fails: Dicloxacillin/cloxacillin 500 mg b.i.d. + rifampin 600 mg PO daily × 7–10 days *or* clindamycin 150 mg/d × 3 months

Second Line
- Resistant strains of *S. aureus* (MRSA): Clindamycin 300 mg q6h or doxycycline 100 mg q12h or trimethoprim-sulfamethoxazole (TMP-SMX DS) 1 tab q8–12h or minocycline 100 mg q12h
- If known or suspected impaired neutrophil function (e.g., impaired chemotaxis, phagocytosis, superoxide generation), add vitamin C 1,000 mg/d × 4–6 weeks (prevents oxidation of neutrophils).
- If antibiotic regimens fail:
  - May try PO pentoxifylline 400 mg t.i.d. × 2–6 months (4)[C]
  - Contraindications: Recent cerebral and/or retinal hemorrhage; intolerance to methylxanthines (e.g., caffeine, theophylline); allergy to the particular drug selected
  - Precautions: Prolonged prothrombin time (PT) and/or bleeding; if on warfarin, frequent monitoring of PT

 ## ONGOING CARE

FOLLOW-UP RECOMMENDATIONS
Patient Monitoring
Instruct patient to see physician if compresses unsuccessful.

DIET
Unrestricted

PROGNOSIS
- Self-limited: Usually drains pus spontaneously and will heal with or without scarring within several days.
- Recurrent/Chronic: May last for months or years.
- If recurrent, usually related to chronic skin carriage of *Staphylococci* (nares or on skin). Treatment goals are to decrease or eliminate pathogenic strain *or* suppress pathogenic strain:
  - Culture nares, skin, axilla, and perineum (culture nares of family members).
  - Apply mupirocin ointment to anterior nares b.i.d. × 5 days (patient and family members/carriers).
  - Culture anterior nares every 3 months. If failure, retreat with mupirocin or consider oral antibiotics.
  - See "Medications," "First Line," "Suppression of Pathogenic Strain."
- Especially in recurrent cases, wash entire body and fingernails (with nailbrush) daily for 1–3 weeks with povidone–iodine (Betadine), chlorhexidine (Hibiclens), or hexachlorophene (pHisoHex soap), although all can cause dry skin (5).

COMPLICATIONS
- Scarring
- Bacteremia
- Seeding (e.g., septal/valve defect, arthritic joint)

REFERENCES
1. Demos M, McLeod MP, Nouri K. Recurrent furunculosis: A review of the literature. *Br J Dermatol*. 2012;167(4):725–732.
2. El-Gilany AH, Fathy H. Risk factors of recurrent furunculosis. *Dermatol Online J*. 2009;15:16.
3. Rivera AM, Boucher HW. Current concepts in antimicrobial therapy against select gram-positive organisms: Methicillin-resistant *Staphylococcus aureus*, penicillin-resistant pneumococci, and vancomycin-resistant enterococci. *Mayo Clin Proc*. 2011;86:1230–1243.
4. Wahba-Yahav AV. Intractable chronic furunculosis: Prevention of recurrences with pentoxifylline. *Acta Derm Venereol*. 1992;72:461–462.
5. Fritz SA, Camins BC, Eisenstein KA, et al. Effectiveness of measures to eradicate Staphylococcus aureus carriage in patients with community-associated skin and soft-tissue infections: A randomized trial. *Infect Control Hosp Epidemiol*. 2011;32:872–880.
6. Winthropp KL. An outbreak of mycobacterium furunculosis associated with footbaths at a nail salon. *N Engl J Med*. 2002;346(18):1366–1371.
7. McConeghy KW, Mikolich DJ, LaPlante KL, et al. Agents for the decolonization of methicillin-resistant *Staphylococcus aureus*. *Pharmacotherapy*. 2009;29:263–280.

 ## SEE ALSO

Folliculitis; Hidradenitis Suppurativa

 ## CODES

ICD10
- L02.12 Furuncle of neck
- L02.92 Furuncle, unspecified
- L02.421 Furuncle of right axilla

CLINICAL PEARLS
- Pathogens may be different in different localities. Keep up-to-date with the locality-specific epidemiology.
- If few, furuncles/furunculosis do not need antibiotic treatment. If systemic symptoms (e.g., fever), cellulitis, or multiple lesions occur, oral antibiotic therapy is used.
- Other treatments for MRSA include linezolid PO or IV and IV vancomycin.
- Folliculitis, furunculosis, and carbuncles are parts of a spectrum of pyodermas.
- Other causative organisms include anaerobic (e.g., *Escherichia coli, Pseudomonas aeruginosa,* and *Streptococcus faecalis*), anaerobic (e.g., *Bacteroides, Lactobacillus, Peptobacillius,* and *Peptostreptococcus*), and *Mycobacteria* (6).
- Decolonization (treatment of the nares with topical antibiotic) is only recommended if the colonization was confirmed by cultures because resistance is common and treatment is of uncertain efficacy (7).

F

GALACTORRHEA

Katherine M. Callaghan, MD • Dawn S. Tasillo, MD

BASICS

DESCRIPTION
- Milky nipple discharge not associated with gestation or present >1 year after weaning. Galactorrhea does not include serous, purulent, or bloody nipple discharge.
- System(s) affected: Endocrine/Metabolic, Nervous, Reproductive
- Synonym(s): Disordered lactation; Nipple discharge

Pregnancy Considerations
Most cases of galactorrhea during pregnancy are physiologic.

EPIDEMIOLOGY
- Predominant age: 15–50 years (reproductive age)
- Predominant sex: Female > Male (rare, for example, in patients with multiple endocrine neoplasia type 1 [MEN1], the most common anterior pituitary tumors are prolactinomas)

Incidence
Common

Prevalence
6.8% of women referred to physicians with a breast complaint have nipple discharge.

ETIOLOGY AND PATHOPHYSIOLOGY
Disorders of lactation are associated with elevated prolactin levels, either from overproduction or loss of inhibitory regulation by dopamine.
- Nipple stimulation
- Pituitary gland overproduction:
  - Prolactinoma
- Loss of dopamine via hypothalamic dysregulation:
  - Craniopharyngiomas
  - Meningiomas or other tumors
  - Sarcoid
  - Irradiation
  - Vascular insult
  - Stalk disruption
  - Traumatic injury
- Medications that suppress dopamine:
  - Typical and atypical antipsychotics
  - SSRIs
  - Tricyclic antidepressants
  - Butyrophenones
  - Cimetidine
  - Ranitidine
  - Reserpine
  - α-methyldopa
  - Verapamil
  - Estrogens
  - Isoniazid
  - Opioids
  - Stimulants
  - Neuroleptics
  - Metoclopramide
  - Domperidone
  - Protease inhibitors (1)

- Chest wall injury:
  - Zoster, surgical or other trauma
- Postoperative condition, especially oophorectomy
- Renal failure
- Other causes:
  - Primary hypothyroidism
  - Cirrhosis
  - Cushing disease
  - Ectopic prolactin secretion
  - Renal failure
  - Sarcoid
  - Lupus
  - Multiple sclerosis
  - Polycystic ovary syndrome
- Idiopathic:
  - Normal prolactin levels

GENERAL PREVENTION
Frequent nipple stimulation can cause galactorrhea.

COMMONLY ASSOCIATED CONDITIONS
See "Etiology and Pathophysiology."

DIAGNOSIS

- Findings vary with causes.
- Look for signs/symptoms of associated conditions:
  - Adrenal insufficiency
  - Acromegaly
  - Hypothyroidism
  - Chest wall conditions

HISTORY
- Usually bilateral milky nipple discharge; may be spontaneous or induced by stimulation
- Determine possibility of pregnancy or recent discontinuation of lactation.
- Signs of hypogonadism from hyperprolactinemia:
  - Oligomenorrhea, amenorrhea
  - Inadequate luteal phase, anovulation, infertility
  - Decreased libido (especially in affected males)
- Mass effects from pituitary enlargement:
  - Headache, cranial neuropathies
  - Bitemporal hemianopsia, amaurosis, scotomata

PHYSICAL EXAM
Breast examination should be performed with attention to the presence of spontaneous or induced nipple discharge.

DIFFERENTIAL DIAGNOSIS
- Pregnancy-induced lactation or recent weaning
- Nonmilky nipple discharge:
  - Intraductal papilloma
  - Fibrocystic disease
- Purulent breast discharge:
  - Mastitis
  - Breast abscess
  - Impetigo
  - Eczema
- Bloody breast discharge: Consider malignancy (Paget disease, breast cancer)

DIAGNOSTIC TESTS & INTERPRETATION
Perform formal visual field testing if pituitary adenoma suspected.

Initial Tests (lab, imaging)
- Prolactin level, thyroid-stimulating hormone, pregnancy test, liver, and renal functions
- Drugs that may alter lab results: Medications that can cause hyperprolactinemia
- Situations that may alter lab results:
  - Lab evaluation of prolactin may be falsely elevated by a recent breast examination
  - Vigorous exercise
  - Sexual activity
  - High-carbohydrate diet
  - Consider repeating the test under different circumstances if the value is borderline (30–40) elevated.
- Prolactin levels may fluctuate. Elevated prolactin levels should be confirmed with at least 1 additional level drawn in a fasting, nonexercised state, with no breast stimulation (2)[C].
- Prolactin levels >250 ng/mL are highly suggestive of a pituitary adenoma (3)[B].
- If a breast mass is palpated in the setting of nipple discharge, evaluation of that mass is indicated with mammogram and/or ultrasound.
- Pituitary MRI with gadolinium enhancement if the serum prolactin level is significantly elevated (>200 ng/mL) or if a pituitary tumor is otherwise suspected

Follow-Up Tests & Special Considerations
- Consider evaluation of follicle-stimulating hormone and luteinizing hormone if amenorrheic.
- Consider evaluation of growth hormone levels if acromegaly suspected.
- Measure adrenal steroids if signs of Cushing disease present.

Diagnostic Procedures/Other
If diagnosis is in question, confirm by microscopic evaluation that nipple secretions are lipid.

Test Interpretation
None unless pituitary resection required

TREATMENT

- Avoid excess nipple stimulation.
- Idiopathic galactorrhea (normal prolactin levels) does not require treatment.
- Discontinue causative medications, if possible.
- Treat to manage symptoms, reduce patient anxiety, and restore fertility.
- Treat tumors >10 mm (even if asymptomatic) to reduce pituitary tumor size or prevent progression to avoid neurologic sequelae.
- If microadenoma, watchful waiting can be appropriate, because 95% do not enlarge.

MEDICATION
- Dopamine agonists work to reduce prolactin levels and shrink tumor size. Therapy is suppressive, not curative.
- Treatment is discontinued when tumor size has reduced or regressed completely or after pregnancy has been achieved.
- Cabergoline (Dostinex):
  - Start at 0.25 mg PO weekly and increase by 0.25 mg monthly until prolactin levels normalize. Usual dose ranges from 0.25–1 mg PO once or twice weekly.
  - More effective (4)[A] and better tolerated than bromocriptine (3)[B]
  - Convenient dosing
  - Although cabergoline has been associated with valvular heart disease in patients treated for Parkinson disease, the lower doses used in treatment of prolactinomas have not been adequately studied (5)[C].
- Bromocriptine:
  - Start at 1.25 mg/d PO with food and increase weekly by 1.25 mg/d until therapeutic response achieved (usually 2.5–15 mg/d, divided once daily/t.i.d.)
  - More expensive and more frequent dosing; however, most providers have experience with this effective drug.
  - Long-term treatment can cause woody fibrosis of the pituitary gland.
- Contraindications are similar for all and include:
  - Uncontrolled hypertension
  - Sensitivity to ergot alkaloids
- Precautions:
  - Nausea, vomiting, and drowsiness are common.
  - Orthostasis, lightheadedness, or syncope
  - Hypertension, seizures, acute psychosis, and digital vasospasm are rare.
- Significant possible interactions:
  - Phenothiazines, butyrophenones, other drugs listed under "Etiology and Pathophysiology"

SURGERY/OTHER PROCEDURES
- Surgery:
  - Macroadenomas need surgery if (i) medical management does not halt growth, (ii) neurologic symptoms persist, (iii) size >10 mm, or (iv) patient cannot tolerate medications. Also considered in young patients with microadenomas to avoid long-term medical therapy (6).
  - Transsphenoidal pituitary resection
  - 50% recurrence after surgery
- Radiotherapy:
  - Radiation is an alternate tumor therapy for macroprolactinomas not responsive to other modes of treatment:
    ○ 20–30% success rate
    ○ 50% risk of panhypopituitarism after radiation
    ○ Risk of optic nerve damage, hypopituitarism, neurologic dysfunction, and increased risk for stroke and secondary brain tumors (6).

 ONGOING CARE

FOLLOW-UP RECOMMENDATIONS
- Outpatient care unless pituitary resection required
- Bromocriptine patients need adequate hydration.
- Dopamine agonist therapy should be discontinued in pregnancy (3).

Patient Monitoring
- Varies with cause
- Check prolactin levels every 6 weeks until normalized, then every 6–12 months
- Monitor visual fields and/or MRI at least yearly until stable

DIET
No restrictions

PATIENT EDUCATION
- Warn about symptoms of mass enlargement in pituitary
- Discuss treatment rationale, risks of treating, and expectant management
- Patient education material available from American Family Physician: www.aafp.org/afp/20040801/553ph.html

PROGNOSIS
- Depends on underlying cause
- Symptoms can recur after discontinuation of a dopamine agonist.
- Surgery can have 50% recurrence (7)
- Prolactinomas <10 mm can resolve spontaneously

COMPLICATIONS
- If enlarging pituitary adenoma, risk of permanent visual field loss
- Panhypopituitarism can complicate radiation or surgical therapy.
- Osteoporosis if amenorrhea persists without estrogen replacement

REFERENCES
1. Molitch ME. Drugs and prolactin. *Pituitary*. 2008;11:209–218.
2. Huang W, Molitch ME. Evaluation and management of galactorrhea. *Am Fam Physician*. 2012;85:1073–1080.
3. Melmed S, Casanueva FF, Hoffman AR, et al. Diagnosis and treatment of hyperprolactinemia: An Endocrine Society clinical practice guideline. *J Clin Endocrinol Metab*. 2011;96:273–288.
4. Wang AT, Mullan RJ, Lane MA, et al. Treatment of hyperprolactinemia: A systematic review and meta-analysis. *Syst Rev*. 2012;1:33.
5. Córdoba-Soriano JG, Lamas-Oliveira C, Hidalgo-Olivares VM, et al. Valvular heart disease in hyperprolactinemic patients treated with low doses of cabergoline. *Rev Esp Cardiol*. 2013;66:410–412.
6. Mancini T, Casanueva FF, Giustina A. Hyperprolactinemia and prolactinomas. *Endocrinol Metab Clin North Am*. 2008;37:67–99.
7. Schlechte JA. Long-term management of prolactinomas. *J Clin Endocrinol Metab*. 2007;92:2861–2865.

 SEE ALSO

Hyperprolactinemia

CODES

ICD10
N64.3 Galactorrhea not associated with childbirth

CLINICAL PEARLS
- Galactorrhea is a common disorder, affecting up to 50% of reproductive-age women.
- Common causes include idiopathic, from excess nipple stimulation, dopamine-suppressing medications, or pituitary prolactinoma.
- Most cases may be adequately evaluated by thyroid-stimulating hormone, prolactin, and human chorionic gonadotropin measurement, with additional testing as suggested by the presence of other symptoms or signs.
- Lab evaluation of prolactin may be falsely elevated due to recent sexual activity, breast examination, exercise, or a high-carbohydrate diet. Repeat any borderline elevation before continuing evaluation or initiating treatment.
- Evaluate prolactin >200 ng/mL (or suspicion of pituitary macroadenoma) with a gadolinium-enhanced MRI.

G

GAMBLING ADDICTION

Robert A. Baldor, MD

 ## BASICS

DESCRIPTION
Gambling is the act of placing something of value at risk in the hopes of gaining something of greater value. Gambling addiction is an impulse-control disorder ranging in severity from problem gambling to the more severe pathologic gambling (PG). Disordered gambling is a dynamic behavior, and patients frequently move in both directions along the continuum of normal and PG behavior over relatively short time periods. Gambling addiction is further categorized into levels:

- Level 0: Nongamblers
- Level 1: Gambled without adverse consequences
- Level 2: Experienced negative consequences from gambling behavior but do not meet criteria for PG
- Level 3: Gambling meets *DSM* criteria for PG: Persistent and recurrent maladaptive gambling behavior indicated by ≥5 *DSM* criteria
- Level 4: Seeking help for gambling addiction regardless of degree of gambling addiction

EPIDEMIOLOGY
- Predominant sex: Male > Female
- The younger a person starts gambling, the more likely he or she is to become a pathologic gambler.

Prevalence
- Lifetime pathologic gambling prevalence is 2.3% in the US.
- 2.5% of the population of the US and Canada meet criteria for problem gambling.

GENERAL PREVENTION
Focus on treatment, patient education, and awareness of risk factors, associated conditions, and warning signs of pathologic or problematic gambling behaviors

ETIOLOGY AND PATHOPHYSIOLOGY
- The brains of pathologic gamblers may have some predisposition to illness. Functional MRI studies indicate that the ventromedial prefrontal cortex is less activated when gambling stimuli are presented to pathologic gamblers.
- Abnormalities in the neurotransmitters serotonin, norepinephrine, dopamine, and glutamate may be implicated in PG.
  - Norepinephrine: Low levels seem to help a patient avoid gambling, whereas high levels may lead to poor decision making.
  - Serotonin: Involved in impulse control by helping a patient weigh the risks of gambling.
  - Dopamine: High levels in the nucleus accumbens while gambling lead to a pleasurable rush. May induce reversible PG in Parkinson patients who take dopamine agonists.
- Gambling addiction can be classified as an addiction as well as an impulse control disorder, and medicine classes for each category have been used to treat it.

Genetics
- *SLC6A4* serotonin transporter gene has been associated with PG in males but not females.
- Dopamine receptor genes *DRD1, DRD2, DRD3, DRD4* have been correlated with pathologic gambling.

RISK FACTORS
- Some types of gambling present a greater risk to cause PG than other types: Pull tabs, casino gambling, bingo, and card games outside a casino
- Being involved with several gaming modalities is related to PG and suggests that the gambler is very captivated with risking money for excitement as opposed to risking money for social pleasure or for an interest in sports.
- Alcohol abuse and dependence are correlated with problem gambling.
- Lower socioeconomic status positively correlates with increased gambling pathology because these persons have few financial resources and cannot recover as easily from losses. Persons even may believe that gambling is a way to ease their financial burden.
- A higher likelihood exists if parents have PG or if there is a family history of substance abuse and mental disorders

COMMONLY ASSOCIATED CONDITIONS
- Poor nutrition
- Stress-related medical conditions (e.g., peptic ulcer disease [PUD], hypertension, migraine)
- Suicidal ideation and attempts
- Substance abuse disorder
- Attention-deficit/hyperactivity disorder (ADHD)
- Bipolar disorder and other mood disorders
- Impulse-control disorders
- Personality disorders
- Incarceration
- Financial problems

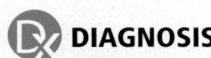 ## DIAGNOSIS

DSM criteria for PG:
- Persistent and recurrent maladaptive gambling behavior, as indicated by ≥5 of the following:
  - Preoccupation with gambling
  - Need to gamble with increasing amounts of money to achieve the desired excitement
  - Repeated unsuccessful efforts to control, cut back, or stop gambling
  - Restless or irritable when attempting to cut down or stop gambling
  - Gambles as a way of escaping from problems or of relieving a dysphoric mood
  - After losing money gambling, often returns another day to get even
  - Lies to family members, therapist, or others to conceal the extent of involvement with gambling
  - Has committed illegal acts such as forgery, fraud, theft, or embezzlement to finance gambling
  - Has jeopardized or lost a significant relationship, job, or educational or career opportunity because of gambling
  - Relies on others to provide money to relieve a desperate financial situation caused by gambling
  - The gambling behavior is not better accounted for by a manic episode.

HISTORY
- Preoccupation with gambling
- Preoccupation with money
- Unexplained new financial problems
- New participation in illegal or dishonest money-making endeavors or activities
- Disruptions in personal life or career
- Patient may ask his or her family and friends to pay off his or her debts ("bailing them out")

DIFFERENTIAL DIAGNOSIS
- Social gambling
- Professional gambling
- Bipolar disorder, manic episode
- Substance use disorder
- Personality disorder

DIAGNOSTIC TESTS & INTERPRETATION
- Lie/Bet method: "Have you ever had to lie to people important to you about how much you gambled?" "Have you ever felt a need to bet more money?":
  - A patient who answers at least 1 question with a "Yes" screens positively for PG.
  - This test has been shown to have >85% specificity and >95% sensitivity (1)[B].
- South Oaks Gambling Screen (SOGS):
  - 20-question screen for PG
  - Score of 3–4 suggests problem gambling.
  - Score of ≥5 indicates probable PG.
  - Criticized as overestimating the number of pathologic gamblers and being too lengthy to administer (2)[B]
- Gamblers Anonymous 20 questions:
  - Easily obtainable from Gamblers Anonymous website
  - Scores of >7 are indicative of problem/PG.

Initial Tests (lab, imaging)
None usually indicated

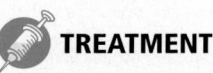 ## TREATMENT

To treat PG, treat comorbidities first. The usual comorbid disorders are substance abuse, bipolar disorder, ADHD, and other impulse-control disorders (3,4). Nonpharmacologic therapies are more effective than pharmacologic therapies. Some data suggest that gambling abstinence is not necessary for treatment; patients can still exhibit controlled gambling.

GENERAL MEASURES
- Get a sense of the patient's readiness for change
- Provide intervention/patient education. Although there are no FDA-approved drug treatments for PG, make clinically based medication recommendations.
- Screen for and treat comorbid conditions
- Provide referrals:
  - Addiction psychiatrist/counselor
  - Gamblers Anonymous
  - Consumer credit organizations
  - Bankruptcy lawyers
  - Gam-Anon for family members

MEDICATION

- There are no FDA-approved medicines for gambling addiction.
- SSRIs:
  - Currently seen as beneficial for treating comorbid impulse-control disorders, although their efficacy has been under question for PG.
  - Used to treat gambling addiction because of link with serotonergic dysfunction: Some studies show that low levels of serotonin cause a suppression of inhibitory responses.
  - Citalopram (Celexa) was noted to be helpful in past literature. Celexa does carry the possibility of life-threatening prolonged QT interval, especially at doses >40 mg/d, and should be used with caution. See medication package information for complete warnings.
  - Fluvoxamine (Luvox) has been shown to be effective in multiple studies.
  - Use of paroxetine (Paxil) or sertraline (Zoloft) in PG has not been found effective in limited studies.
- Modafinil helps pathologic gamblers with high impulsivity but increases gambling behavior in low-impulsivity pathologic gamblers. Modafinil shows decreases in motivation to gamble, risky decision making, and impulsivity in high-impulsivity pathologic gamblers (5)[B].
- Valproate and carbamazepine, as well as lithium carbonate, are effective treatments (5)[A].
- Opiate antagonists have the ability to decrease dopamine release in the dopamine reward pathway. Naltrexone and nalmefene are efficacious for PG and reduce urges to gamble. Positive family history of alcoholism predicted a positive response to opiate antagonist treatment (5). These medicines may be effective because gambling itself causes a release of endogenous opioids through release of dopamine.
- Selected antipsychotics have been shown to be ineffective in PG (i.e., olanzapine is not efficacious for the treatment of PG, and haloperidol may increase the desire to gamble in pathological gamblers) (5)[B].
- N-acetylcysteine (NAC), a glutamate-modulating agent, causes significant improvements in gambling thoughts and behaviors.
- Single case report indicated that disulfiram (Antabuse) was helpful (6)[C].
- Acamprosate (Campral) and baclofen were not found to be effective according to a single case report (7)[B].
- D-amphetamine increased the urge to gamble in problem gamblers (8)[B].

ADDITIONAL THERAPIES

- Patients are often forced to come in for treatment and patients' personal characteristics (i.e., pride, denial, or impatience) can hinder therapy.
- Mental health workers must avoid negative transference.
- Because of increased suicide rates, patients may need to be hospitalized acutely for safety and to prevent gambling.
- Because patients are at increased risk from mental and physical illness, they benefit from relaxation exercises to reduce stress, identify triggers, substitute gambling with other activities, and a complete physical and lab work with nutrition evaluation.

- Cognitive-behavioral therapy (CBT) (9)[C]:
  - The main effective interventions for CBT are psychoeducation, cognitive restructuring, problem solving, social skills training, and relapse prevention. Studies indicated that CBT resulted in significant improvement as short-term therapy.
  - CBT may be done in several formats: Individual, group, brief group, and dual diagnosis. All these formats have been shown to be effective. Group therapy is favored because patients are often extroverted. Couple or family therapy also may be used.
- Gamblers Anonymous:
  - A 12-step program similar to Alcoholics Anonymous for a person suffering from a gambling addiction
  - Dropout rate is high if this is the only means of therapy (1)[B].
  - Patients may deny need to attend in the 1st place, and for that reason, Gamblers Anonymous may not be appropriate for patients who are in the precontemplation stage.
- Motivational enhancement therapy (MET):
  - Provides nonargumentative exploration of patient's stage of change
  - Patient receives positive reinforcement from clinician
  - Motivational enhancement strategies support self-efficacy
  - Improves patient rapport; aids in removing barriers to treatment
  - In 1 study, MET alone did not show any improvement, but MET and CBT together improved outcome measures (5)[B].

ONGOING CARE

FOLLOW-UP RECOMMENDATIONS

Patients seeking treatment for gambling addiction should be followed routinely to monitor the response to treatment, tolerance to medications, and possibility of relapse.

PATIENT EDUCATION

- Gamblers Anonymous:
  - www.gamblersanonymous.org
  - National hotline 1-888-GA-HELPS (888-424-3577)
- Gam-Anon: Support group for spouses, family, or close friends: www.gam-anon.org
- Responsible Gambling Council: www.responsiblegambling.org
- Humphrey H. This must be hell: A look at pathological gambling. Bloomington, IN: iUniverse; 2000.
- Lee B. Born to lose: Memoirs of a compulsive gambler. Center City, MN: Hazelden; 2005.

PROGNOSIS

- Patients with gambling addiction can be treated, but many relapse.
- 36–39% of patients did not experience any gambling-related problems according to 1 study, and only 7–12% sought formal treatment or Gamblers Anonymous meetings.
- Roughly 1/3 of patients who have a gambling addiction recover without any intervention.

REFERENCES

1. Potenza MN, Fiellin DA, Heninger GR, et al. Gambling: An addictive behavior with health and primary care implications. *J Gen Intern Med*. 2002;17:721–732.
2. Rossow I, Molde H. Chasing the criteria: Comparing SOGS-RA and the Lie/Bet screen to assess prevalence of problem gambling and "at-risk" gambling among adolescents. *J Gambling Issues*. 2006;18:57–71.
3. Potenza MN. Review. The neurobiology of pathological gambling and drug addiction: An overview and new findings. *Philos Trans R Soc Lond B Biol Sci*. 2008;363:3181–3189.
4. Chou K, Afifi TO. Disordered (pathologic or problem) gambling and axis I psychiatric disorders: Results from the national epidemiologic survey on alcohol and related conditions. *Am J Epidemiol*. 2011;173:1289–1297.
5. Leung KS, Cottler LB. Treatment of pathological gambling. *Curr Opin Psychiatry*. 2009;22:69–74.
6. Mutschler J, Buhler M, Grosshans M, et al. Disulfiram, an option for treatment of pathological gambling? *Alcohol Alcohol*. 2010;45:214–216.
7. Dannon PN, Rosenberg O, Schoenfeld N, et al. Acamprosate and baclofen were not effective in the treatment of pathological gambling: Preliminary blind rater comparison study. *Front Psychiatry*. 2011;2:1–4.
8. Nussbaum D, Honarmand K, Govoni R, et al. An eight component decision-making model for problem gambling: A systems approach to stimulate integrative research. *J Gambl Stud*. 2011;27:523–563.
9. Okuda M, Balan I, Petry NM, et al. Cognitive-behavioral therapy for pathological gambling: Cultural considerations. *Am J Psych*. 2009;166:1325–1330.

CODES

ICD10

- F63.0 Pathological gambling
- Z72.6 Gambling and betting

CLINICAL PEARLS

- Several brief screening strategies can be used to identify PG, including the lie/bet method, the SOGS, and the Gamblers Anonymous 20 questions.
- To treat PG, 1st treat comorbidities such as substance abuse, bipolar disorder, ADHD, and other impulse-control disorders.
- Nonpharmacologic therapies are more effective than pharmacologic therapies. There is no FDA-approved therapy for PG.
- Patients seeking treatment for gambling addiction should be followed routinely by physicians and counselors to monitor the response to treatment, tolerance to medications, and possibility of relapse.

GANGLION CYST

Mary S. Lindholm, MD

 BASICS

- Ganglions are common benign tumors that are not related to nerve tissue (as implied incorrectly by the name).
- Can be located throughout the body, usually adjacent to or within joints and tendons, mostly on wrist, foot, and ankle
- Average size is 3 cm.
- Most are asymptomatic except for changing size, but local nerve compression can result in pain or activity limitation.

EPIDEMIOLOGY

- Can affect all age groups, but unusual in children
- Most common in young adults and can occur 3× more commonly in women
- Mucous cysts are usually seen in older patients.
- Hand and wrist ganglions are commonly seen in dorsal wrist, radial wrist, and dorsum of the distal interphalangeal (DIP) joint (which is referred to as a mucous cyst).
- 60–70% of hand and wrist ganglions are in dorsal wrist, 15–20% are at the volar wrist.

Prevalence

- Prevalence of wrist ganglia in patients presenting with wrist pain has been reported as 19%.
- Prevalence of ganglia in patients with a palpable mass in the wrist has been reported as 27%.
- Reported prevalence in ankles is 5.6%.

ETIOLOGY AND PATHOPHYSIOLOGY

Pathogenesis is unclear. Several theories:

- Mucoid degeneration of connective tissue results in formation of hyaluronic acid, leading to cystic space formation.
- Herniation of synovial lining creates a 1-way valve:
  - This is supported by dye studies that show communication of fluid from the wrist joint into the cyst, but not from the cyst to the joint.
  - This is disputed by lack of epithelial lining of the cyst wall.
- A rent in the joint capsule or tendon sheath allows synovial fluid to leak into surrounding tissue. Local irritation leads to production of a pseudocapsule and ganglion. This would explain why no lining is seen on pathology.
- Recurrent stress and microtrauma at the synovial–capsular interface may stimulate mucin production by mesenchymal cells or fibroblasts.
- Etiology is unknown.
- May be associated with trauma, but most patients cannot recall specific trauma.

Genetics

No specific genetic links have been found.

RISK FACTORS

- Female > Male
- Osteoarthritis for mucoid cysts
- No known occupational risk factors

COMMONLY ASSOCIATED CONDITIONS

Mucous cysts are usually associated with some level of osteoarthritis of DIP joint.

 DIAGNOSIS

- Usually made on basis of history and physical examination
- Patients usually present when there is pain, increased size, interference with activities, or weakness.

HISTORY

- Patients usually present with asymptomatic mass present for months or years, decreasing and increasing in size.
- Mostly asymptomatic, but can be associated with pain and limitations in activity

PHYSICAL EXAM

- Mass:
  - Compressible
  - Subcutaneous
  - Transilluminating
  - Slightly mobile
  - Without overlying skin changes
- Extension or flexion of wrist can cause pain through nerve compression.
- Small ganglions may only be palpable in full wrist flexion or extension.
- Occult ganglions are not palpable, but can be quite painful.

DIFFERENTIAL DIAGNOSIS

- A mobile mass of extensor tendons of wrist may be a ganglion or tendon sheath, giant cell tumor, or tenosynovitis from infection or inflammation.
- Other tumors include lipoma, sarcoma, hamartoma, and interosseous neuroma.
- Firm mass may represent osteophyte.
- Overlying skin changes suggest an alternate diagnosis.

DIAGNOSTIC TESTS & INTERPRETATION

Unless diagnosis is unclear, most ganglions do not require imaging for confirmation.

Initial Tests (lab, imaging)

- Several options:
  - US
  - MRI
  - Bone scintigraphy, arthroscopy
- US and MRI have similar rates of sensitivity and specificity.
- Scintigraphy is less specific and not useful for this making this diagnosis.
- US is less expensive than MRI, but more operator-dependent.
- Arthroscopy is used for both diagnostic and therapeutic purposes and should be considered when initial workup is nondiagnostic and conservative treatment is not effective.
- Most are apparent clinically and do not need imaging.

Test Interpretation

- Gross pathologic evaluation shows that cysts are often multilobulated.
- Microscopic exam reveals outer wall with several layers of randomly oriented collagen fibers, relatively acellular with a few fibroblasts, and mesenchymal cells in the collagen fibers.
- As pathology does not show an epithelial lining, it is therefore not a true cyst.
- Viscous fluid contains glucosamine, albumin, globulin, and hyaluronic acid.
- Ganglions are histopathologically identical regardless of anatomic location.

TREATMENT

4 primary treatment options (1):

- Reassurance and observation: Ganglia are not likely to be malignant or to cause damage:
  - 33% dorsal ganglions and 45% volar ganglions resolve spontaneously by 6 years; up to 80% of ganglion in children resolve.
- Closed rupture: Historically done by hitting cyst with a book:
  - Results in initial decreased clinical symptoms by 22–66%, but often leads to recurrence
- Aspiration: Can be done in an office under local anesthesia with a 16-guage needle at base of cyst:
  - Studies demonstrate mixed results on aspirations of a ganglion; evidence supporting injecting steroids is weak; splinting after the procedure may help cure rate, but recurrence may be as high as 80% after a single aspiration. This can be reduced to 20% with multiple aspirations.
  - Aspirations are more frequently being done with US guidance, allowing direct visualization of the ganglion and perhaps more successful conservative treatment, although no studies to date have prospectively evaluated this (2).
  - Volar ganglia should not be aspirated without US guidance due to risk of damage to neurovascular structures from blind aspiration attempts.
  - Mucous cysts can be aspirated, but recurrence is >50% and pain may not resolve if it is due to underlying osteoarthritis.
- Surgical excision:
  - 1/3 of patients presenting with ganglion cyst elect for surgical intervention (3).

MEDICATION

First Line

- Although evidence for steroid injection after aspiration is weak, this is still not an uncommon practice.
- No other medications have been shown to be effective.

SURGERY/OTHER PROCEDURES

- 6-year study comparing blind aspiration to surgery to watchful waiting found:
  - Recurrence rates: 58% after aspiration, 39% after surgery, and 58% in untreated patients
  - Satisfaction: 81% aspiration, 83% surgery, and 53% who were reassured, a significant difference
  - Persistent pain: 23% of patients who were satisfied vs. 45% who were unsatisfied
  - No significant difference seen in pain, weakness, or stiffness between groups.
  - Significant reduction in pain was seen in all groups.
  - Authors conclude that neither aspiration nor surgical excision provides a clear long-term benefit over the natural history of wrist ganglion, and the only benefit of surgery is early resolution of the appearance of the ganglia (4)[C].
- Bottom line:
  - Surgical excision yields less risk of recurrence, but similar rates of pain, weakness, and stiffness as aspiration or reassurance.
  - Patient satisfaction is higher with excision or aspiration; however, longer time out of work is seen with excision compared with aspiration and reassurance.
- 2 methods:
  - Arthroscopic compared to open excision: After 1 year, ~10% had recurrence; no significant difference in surgical approaches (5)[C].

 ONGOING CARE

May require supervised hand therapy after surgical repair to aid in pain reduction, improve stiffness and function

FOLLOW-UP RECOMMENDATIONS

- Hand therapy may be helpful if ganglion symptoms persist despite rest.
- Improved resolution rates with multiple aspirations
- Splinting is often used after surgical repair, and follow-up with orthopedics occurs for several weeks; hand therapy may be indicated for residual symptoms.

PROGNOSIS

- Very good
- Up to 50% will resolve with watchful waiting.
- Higher rate of resolution in children

COMPLICATIONS

- Risk of recurrence is present regardless of treatment; no specific recommendations to minimize this risk.
- Risks of surgical excision include:
  - Residual pain
  - Poor cosmesis
  - Neuropathy
  - Stiffness and instability of the wrist, especially scapholunate ligament instability; also may require open excision if arthroscopic treatment fails to resolve symptoms

REFERENCES

1. Thommasen HV. Management of the occasional wrist ganglion. *Can J Rural Med*. 2006;11:51–53.
2. Jose J, Fourzali R, Lesniak B, et al. Ultrasound-guided aspiration of symptomatic intraneural ganglion cyst within the tibial nerve. *Skeletal Radiol*. 2011;40(11):1473–1478.
3. Wong AS, Jebson PJ, Murray PM, et al. The use of routine wrist radiography is not useful in the evaluation of patients with a ganglion cyst of the wrist. *Hand*. 2007;2:117–119.
4. Dias JJ, Dhukaram V, Kumar P. The natural history of untreated dorsal wrist ganglia and patient reported outcome 6 years after intervention. *J Hand Surg Eur*. 2007;32:502–508.
5. Kang L, Akelman E, Weiss AP. Arthroscopic versus open dorsal ganglion excision: A prospective, randomized comparison of rates of recurrence and of residual pain. *J Hand Surg [Am]*. 2008;33: 471–475.

ADDITIONAL READING

- Dias J, Buch K. Palmar wrist ganglion: Does intervention improve outcome? A prospective study of the natural history and patient-reported treatment outcomes. *J Hand Surg [Br]*. 2003;28:172–176.
- Kang HJ, Koh IH, Kim JS, et al. Coexisting intraarticular disorders are unrelated to outcomes after arthroscopic resection of dorsal wrist ganglions *Clin Orthop Relat Res*. 2013;471(7):2212–2218. Epub 2013 Feb 21.

- Lee SW, Kim SG, Oh-Park M. Ganglion cyst of radiocapitellar joint mimicking lateral epicondylitis: Role of ultrasonography. *Am J Phys Med Rehabil*. 2013;92(5):459–460.
- Lowden CM, Attiah M, Garvin G, et al. The prevalence of wrist ganglia in an asymptomatic population: Magnetic resonance evaluation. *J Hand Surg [Br]*. 2005;30:302–306.
- Sawyer GA, DaSilva MF, Akelman E. Volar wrist ganglion excision through the flexor carpi radialis sheath. *Tech Hand Up Extrem Surg*. 2012;16(3): 145–147.

 SEE ALSO

Algorithm: Pain in Upper Extremity

 CODES

ICD10

- M67.40 Ganglion, unspecified site
- M67.48 Ganglion, other site
- M67.439 Ganglion, unspecified wrist

CLINICAL PEARLS

- Ganglia, the most common masses in the wrist, are not true cysts.
- Typical history and examination will make the diagnosis in most cases; plain films are nondiagnostic and usually not necessary.
- Can consider MRI or US if occult ganglion is suspected.
- Surgical excision may yield lower recurrence rates than aspiration, although recurrence rates with a series of 3 aspirations have been reported as low as 20%.
- Volar wrist ganglia should not be aspirated without US guidance by an experienced provider due to the risk of damage to neurovascular structures from blind aspiration.

G

GASTRIC MALIGNANCY

Scott T. Henderson, MD

 BASICS

DESCRIPTION
- May occur anywhere in the stomach
- Infiltration to lymph nodes, omentum, lungs, and liver is rapid.
- Uncommon in US natives
- Synonym(s): Linitis plastica

Pediatric Considerations
Rare

Pregnancy Considerations
- Rarely diagnosed during pregnancy
- Prognosis is poor if diagnosed.

EPIDEMIOLOGY
- Predominant age: >55 (2/3 >65)
- Predominant gender: Male > Female (1.7:1)
- Incidence is decreasing globally, but it remains the 2nd-leading cause of cancer death.

Incidence
- 5.9/100,000 males (North America)
- 2.5/100,000 females (North America)
- 21,130 new cases per year (US)

ETIOLOGY AND PATHOPHYSIOLOGY
Unknown

Genetics
- More common in people with blood group A
- 2–4 times more common in 1st-degree relatives
- 1–3% of gastric cancers are associated with inherited gastric cancer predisposition syndromes, known as hereditary diffuse gastric cancer.
- Amplification or overexpression of the HER2 protein is associated with some gastric cancers:
  – May play a role in pathogenesis and progression

RISK FACTORS
- *Helicobacter pylori* infection
- Achlorhydria
- Atrophic gastritis/intestinal metaplasia
- Pernicious anemia
- Prior gastric resection
- Polyps or dysplasia anywhere in alimentary canal
- Familial polyposis
- Barrett esophagus
- Smoking/Tobacco abuse
- Patients in lower socioeconomic classes are at greater risk of developing gastric tumors.
- Diet rich in additives (e.g., smoked, pickled, or salted foods; highly spiced Asian foods)
- Low consumption of fruits and vegetables
- Overweight and obesity: Strength of association increases with increasing body mass index (BMI)
- Ethnic background: Hispanic, Japanese, Chilean, Costa Rican:
  – Migrants from high-incidence areas (e.g., Iceland, Chile, or Japan) to low-incidence areas maintain an increased risk, whereas their offspring have an occurrence rate that corresponds to that of the new location.

GENERAL PREVENTION
- A healthy lifestyle (not smoking, not consuming excess alcohol, avoiding obesity, and maintaining a good diet) is associated with reduced risk of gastric cancer:
  – Diets including 5–20 servings of both fruits and vegetables each week reduce the risk of gastric malignancy by ~50%.
- Insufficient data to establish that screening would decrease mortality in US population
- Screening may be of benefit in high-prevalence areas.

COMMONLY ASSOCIATED CONDITIONS
- Giant hypertrophic gastritis (Ménétrier disease)
- Intestinal metaplasia of the stomach
- Atrophic gastritis
- *H. pylori* infection

 DIAGNOSIS

HISTORY

ALERT
- Symptoms present late in the course.
- Anorexia/Weight loss (70–80%)
- Cachexia
- Early satiety
- Nausea and vomiting
- Change in bowel habits
- Chronic noncolicky abdominal pain (especially in epigastrium):
  – Ranges from postprandial fullness to severe steady pain (70%)
  – Unrelieved by antacids
  – Exacerbated by food
  – Relieved by fasting
- Gross GI bleeding (10%)
- Dysphagia (rare)

PHYSICAL EXAM
- Abdominal palpation for masses and/or ascites
- Palpation for lymph nodes:
  – Left supraclavicular node (Virchow)
  – Sister Mary Joseph nodule at umbilicus
- Assess for jaundice

DIFFERENTIAL DIAGNOSIS
- Angiodysplasia of the colon
- Carcinoma of body or tail of the pancreas
- Carcinoma of the colon
- Crohn disease
- Eosinophilic gastroenteritis
- Functional dyspepsia
- Gastric lymphoma
- Giant hypertrophic gastritis
- GI sarcoidosis
- Peptic ulcer with or without hemorrhage
- Small intestinal lymphoma

DIAGNOSTIC TESTS & INTERPRETATION
Initial Tests (lab, imaging)
- CBC and platelet count:
  – Hemoglobin <12 g/dL (1.86 mmol/L)
  – Hematocrit <35 (0.35)
- Serum chemistry analysis:
  – Albumin <3 g/dL
- Coagulation studies
- *H. pylori* testing
- Stool guaiac
- Upper endoscopy for direct visualization, biopsy, and cytology:
  – Minimum of 6 biopsies should be done to achieve a diagnosis of malignancy (1)[C].
- CT scan of chest, abdomen, and pelvis with contrast and gastric distension should be done for staging (1)[C].

Follow-Up Tests & Special Considerations
- Pentagastrin test (stomach pH <6):
  – Pernicious anemia may cause a false-positive pentagastrin test.
- Consider pelvic US in females.

Diagnostic Procedures/Other
- Endoscopic US is most accurate preoperative staging tool to identify proximal and distal extent of tumor (2)[C].
- Laparoscopy may be useful in select patients for staging (3)[C].

Test Interpretation
- Adenocarcinomas: 90% (intestinal [well-differentiated] and diffuse [undifferentiated/linitis plastica])
- Gastric lymphomas, sarcomas, and other rare types: 10%

 TREATMENT

GENERAL MEASURES
- Multidisciplinary treatment is mandatory.
- Surgical excision of the tumor is the only potentially curative option:
  – Extent of lymph nodes resection is controversial.
  – Endoscopic mucosal resection for early gastric mucosal cancers (≤2 cm in size, histologically differentiated, and nonulcerated) and high-grade dysplasia may be curative (2)[B].
  – Even patients with incurable lesions should be offered an attempt at surgical reduction of the tumor:
    ○ Surgical reduction offers the best form of palliation and improves the likelihood of benefit if chemotherapy and/or radiation therapy is administered.
- Adjuvant chemotherapy may provide benefit compared to surgery alone (4)[A].
- Patients with inoperable, locally advanced disease should be offered chemotherapy and reassessed for surgery if response is favorable (2)[A].
- Patients with stage IV disease should be offered chemotherapy, which improves survival compared with the best supportive care (2)[A].

- Radiation therapy:
  - Used in combination with surgery and/or chemotherapy
  - Little benefit when used alone because of the radiation resistance of gastric tumors
  - Does have use in the palliation of pain, bleeding, and obstruction

MEDICATION

First Line

Combination chemotherapy improves survival compared to single-agent 5-FU (4)[A]:

- Among the combination chemotherapy regimens studied, best survival results are achieved with regimens containing 5-FU, anthracyclines, and cisplatin.
- In this category, epirubicin, cisplatin, and continuous-infusion 5-FU are tolerated best.

Second Line

- Ondansetron (Zofran), dronabinol (Marinol), metoclopramide (Reglan), and others for nausea control
- Pain control with opioids

ISSUES FOR REFERRAL

Referral to a high-volume surgery center is usually indicated.

ADDITIONAL THERAPIES

- Trastuzumab in combination with cisplatin or 5-FU should be considered in patients with HER2-positive tumors (1)[A].
- The neoadjuvant use of radiotherapy is not recommended outside clinical trials.

SURGERY/OTHER PROCEDURES

- Radical subtotal gastrectomy with gastrojejunostomy or gastroduodenostomy is the usual treatment of choice:
  - Removal of a large part of the stomach along with the greater and lesser omentum en bloc
  - Splenectomy or distal pancreatectomy done in certain situations
  - Excision of direct extensions
- Total gastrectomy indicated only if necessary to remove the local lesion
- Local excision, endoscopic laser therapy, or electrocautery for palliation of incurable lesion by resection of bleeding area or area of obstruction

COMPLEMENTARY AND ALTERNATIVE MEDICINE

Commonly used but with little supportive evidence

IN-PATIENT CONSIDERATIONS

Admission Criteria/Initial Stabilization

- Inpatient care is common, but depends on stage at time of diagnosis.
- Most of the follow-up treatment is outpatient.

 ONGOING CARE

FOLLOW-UP RECOMMENDATIONS

Symptom-driven follow-up visits to monitor disease state, assess treatments, monitor for recurrence/metastasis, and assess nutritional status (2)[B]

Patient Monitoring

Monitor vitamin B_{12} and iron levels following surgical resection; supplement if indicated.

DIET

- Consider preoperative nutritional support in patients at high nutritional risk.
- All patients undergoing surgery should be considered for early postoperative nutritional support:
  - Enteral route preferred
  - Consider placement of jejunostomy feeding tube.

PATIENT EDUCATION

- Contact local American Cancer Society: www.cancer.org
- Cancer Research Institute Helpbook: What to Do If Cancer Strikes. FDR Station, Box 5199, New York, NY 10150-5199.

PROGNOSIS

- Because most lesions do not produce symptoms until late in course, gastric carcinomas are usually advanced at the time of diagnosis.
- Overall 5-year relative survival rate is 24% (if local disease 61%, regional spread 24%, distant spread 3%).
- Detection of early gastric cancers usually occurs when performing screening endoscopy in endemic areas or as an incidental finding.
- Primary gastric lymphoma is more treatable than gastric adenocarcinoma:
  - 5-year survival rate is 40–60% with subtotal gastrectomy followed by combination chemotherapy.

COMPLICATIONS

- Early lymphatic spread
- Aggressive metastatic disease (especially hepatic, cerebral, peritoneum, and pulmonary)
- Anemia (especially pernicious)
- Pyloric stenosis
- Dumping syndrome may occur following gastric surgery.

REFERENCES

1. Allum WH, Blazeby JM, Griffin SM, et al. Guidelines for the management of oesophageal and gastric cancer. *Gut.* 2011;60(11):1449–1472. Epub 2011 Jun 24.
2. Okines A, Verheij M, Allum W, et al. Gastric cancer: ESMO Clinical Practice Guidelines for diagnosis, treatment and follow-up. *Ann Oncol.* 2010; 21(Suppl 5):v50–54.
3. Sarela AI, Lefkowitz R, Brennan MF, et al. Selection of patients with gastric adenocarcinoma for laparoscopic staging. *Am J Surg.* 2006;191: 134–138.
4. Wagner AD, Unverzagt S, Grothe W, et al. Chemotherapy for advanced gastric cancer. *Cochrane Database Syst Rev.* 2010;3:CD004064.

ADDITIONAL READING

- Khushalani N. Cancer of the esophagus and stomach. *Mayo Clin Proc.* 2008;83:712–722.
- Karpeh MS Jr. Palliative treatment and the role of surgical resection in gastric cancer. *Dig Surg.* 2013;30(2):174–180. Epub 2013 Jul 18.
- Chen WW, Wang F, Xu RH. Platinum-based versus non-platinum-based chemotherapy as first line treatment of inoperable, advanced gastric adenocarcinoma: a meta-analysis. *PLoS One.* 2013; 8(7):e68974. Epub 2013 Jul 11.

 SEE ALSO

Multiple Endocrine Neoplasia (MEN)

 CODES

ICD10

- C16.2 Malignant neoplasm of body of stomach
- C16.8 Malignant neoplasm of overlapping sites of stomach
- C16.9 Malignant neoplasm of stomach, unspecified

CLINICAL PEARLS

- Accurate preoperative staging is necessary to enhance survival.
- Endoscopic US is the most accurate preoperative staging tool.
- To enhance survival, therapy with surgery, combination chemotherapy, and radiation is necessary.

G

GASTRITIS
Jill A. Grimes, MD, FAAFP

 BASICS

DESCRIPTION
- Inflammatory reaction in the stomach:
  - Typically involves the mucosa; seldom the full thickness of the stomach wall
- Patchy erythema of gastric mucosa:
  - A common endoscopic finding; usually insignificant
- Erosive gastritis:
  - A reaction to mucosal injury by a noxious chemical agent (e.g., drugs especially NSAIDs or alcohol)
- Reflux gastritis:
  - A reaction to protracted reflux exposure to bile and pancreatic juice, usually associated with a defective pylorus
  - Typically limited to the prepyloric antrum
- Hemorrhagic gastritis (stress ulceration):
  - A reaction to hemodynamic disorder (e.g., hypovolemia or hypoxia [as in shock])
  - Also common in ICUs
  - Seen after severe burns
  - Seen after significant physical trauma
  - Seen rarely with dabigatran, the 1st oral thrombin inhibitor
- Infectious gastritis:
  - Commonly associated with *Helicobacter pylori* (possibly causative, maybe opportunistic)
  - Viral infection, usually as a component of systemic infection, is common.
  - Significant infection by other specific microbes is rare.
- Atrophic gastritis:
  - Frequent, in varying degrees, in the elderly
  - Primarily from long-standing *H. pylori* infections (1)[A]
  - May be caused by prolonged PPI use (2)[A]
  - Major risk factor for onset of gastric cancer (1)[A]
  - Invariable in primary (pernicious) anemia
  - Autoimmune disease
  - Neutrophil cellular infiltration in acute gastritis
  - Patches of lymphoid follicles noted in chronic gastritis, along with plasma cells and macrophages; antibodies to parietal cells and intrinsic factor
  - >50% of humans are colonized with *H. pylori*.
- Synonym(s): Erosive gastritis; Reflux gastritis; Hemorrhagic gastritis; Acute gastritis

Geriatric Considerations
Persons age >60 years often harbor *H. pylori* infection.

Pediatric Considerations
Gastritis rarely occurs in infants or children.

EPIDEMIOLOGY
- Predominant age: All ages
- Predominant sex: Male = Female

ETIOLOGY AND PATHOPHYSIOLOGY
- Noxious agents cause a breakdown in the gastric mucosal barrier, leaving the epithelial cells unprotected.
- Bacterial infection (e.g., *H. pylori*) most common cause
- Alcohol
- Aspirin and other NSAIDs
- Bile reflux
- Pancreatic enzyme reflux
- Stress (hypovolemia or hypoxia)
- Radiation
- *Staphylococcus aureus* exotoxins
- Viral infection
- Pernicious anemia
- Gastric mucosal atrophy
- Portal hypertensive (HTN) gastropathy
- Emotional stress

Genetics
Unknown, but observational studies show that 10% of a given population is never colonized with *H. pylori*, regardless of exposure. Genetic variations in *TLR1* may help explain some of this observed variation in individual risk for *H. pylori* infection (3)[A].

RISK FACTORS
- Age >60 years
- Exposure to potentially noxious drugs or chemical agents, including alcohol or NSAIDs
- Hypovolemia, hypoxia (shock)
- Autoimmune diseases (thyroid and diabetes mellitus 1)
- Family history of *H. pylori* and/or gastric cancer

GENERAL PREVENTION
- Patients should be warned of known or potentially injurious drugs or chemical agents.
- Patient with hypovolemia or hypoxia (especially patients confined to an intensive care ward) should receive prophylactic therapy with antacids.
- H₂ receptor antagonists, prostaglandins, or sucralfate used frequently in the ICU for burn and trauma victims
- Consider testing for *H. pylori* (and eradicating if present) in patients facing long-term NSAID therapy (4)[A].

COMMONLY ASSOCIATED CONDITIONS
- Gastric or duodenal peptic ulcer
- Primary (pernicious) anemia
- Portal HTN
- Development of gastric lymphoma linked to the lymphoid follicles

 DIAGNOSIS

HISTORY
- Nondescript epigastric distress, often aggravated by eating, often severe, burning
- Anorexia
- Nausea, with or without vomiting
- Significant bleeding is unusual except in hemorrhagic gastritis.
- Hiccups
- Bloating or abdominal fullness

PHYSICAL EXAM
- Mild epigastric tenderness
- May have heme-positive stool
- Stool may be black in color

DIFFERENTIAL DIAGNOSIS
- Functional GI disorder
- Peptic ulcer disease
- Linitis plastica
- Viral gastroenteritis
- Pancreatic disease
- Gastric cancer (elderly)
- Cholecystitis
- Pancreatic disease (inflammation vs. tumor)

DIAGNOSTIC TESTS & INTERPRETATION
Initial Tests (lab, imaging)
- Usually unremarkable, except when blood loss results in anemia
- Drugs that may alter lab results: Antibiotics or omeprazole may affect urea breath test for *H. pylori*.
- ¹³C-urea breath test for *H. pylori*
- Serologic test available for *H. pylori*, serum IgG (office and clinical laboratory):
  - Inexpensive
  - Cannot be used to assess eradication
- Gastric acid analysis may be abnormal, but is not a reliable indicator of gastritis.
- Stool analysis for *H. pylori* antigen
- Nuclear scintigraphy is not done clinically.

Follow-Up Tests & Special Considerations
Endoscopic tests:
- Culture
- Polymerase chain reaction (PCR)
- Histology
- Rapid urease testing

Diagnostic Procedures/Other
- Gastroscopy, usually with biopsy, is essential for a precise diagnosis.
- Biopsies recommended if there is a poor response to the initial treatment. *Patient must discontinue PPIs for 2 weeks prior to endoscopy to improve accuracy of result* (5)[C]

Test Interpretation
Acute or chronic inflammatory infiltrate in gastric mucosa, often with distortion or erosion of adjacent epithelium. Presence of *H. pylori* may be confirmed.

TREATMENT

GENERAL MEASURES
- Treatment of *H. pylori* is required to relieve symptoms; no specific therapy for the gastritis
- Parenteral fluid and electrolyte supplements required if vomiting prevents food intake.
- Consider discontinuing NSAIDs or adding misoprostol.
- Encourage alcohol and smoking cessation.
- Endoscopy indicated for patients not responsive to treatment

MEDICATION
First Line
- Antacids: Best given in liquid form, 30 mL 1 hour after meals and at bedtime; useful mainly as an emollient
- H_2 receptor antagonists (e.g., cimetidine [Tagamet]): Oral cimetidine 300 mg q6h (or ranitidine [Zantac] or famotidine [Pepcid] or nizatidine [Axid]). Not shown to be clearly superior to antacids (6)[C]:
  - For severely ill patients: Priming dose of 300 mg IV, then a steady infusion of 37.5–75 mg/h, dissolved in the running fluid
- Sucralfate (Carafate): 1 g q4–6h on an empty stomach; rationale uncertain, but empirically helpful
- Prostaglandins (misoprostol [Cytotec]): Can help allay gastric mucosal injury; suggested dosage 100–200 μg q.i.d.
- PPIs can be used if there is no response to antacids or H_2 receptor blockers.
- *H. pylori* eradication:
  - Bismuth quadruple therapy (BQT):
    ○ PPI (omeprazole 20 mg) b.i.d. plus bismuth (Pepto-Bismol) 30 mL liquid or 2 tablets q.i.d. plus metronidazole 250–500 mg t.i.d. plus tetracycline 500 mg q.i.d. for 7–10 days (7)[A]
  - Clarithromycin triple therapy (CTT) (7)[A]:
    ○ A short-course therapy (7–10 days) of amoxicillin 1 g b.i.d., omeprazole 20 mg b.i.d., and clarithromycin 500 mg b.i.d.
      ■ Optimal treatment regimens continue to be debated and tested.
      ■ 2013 meta-analysis shows compliance and side-effect rates are similar for short-course triple and quadruple therapy, and that BQT overcomes clarithromycin resistance and is not affected by metronidazole resistance. Overall eradication rates were 77.6% for BQT and 68.9% for CTT (7)[A].
- With treatment failure, utilize a different regimen, substitute metronidazole for clarithromycin:
  - Consider sequential antibiotic therapy with omeprazole 20 mg and amoxicillin 1 g b.i.d. for 5 days followed by clarithromycin 500 mg and tinidazole mg b.i.d. with omeprazole 20 mg for 5 days. Some studies show it works just as well or better than triple therapy (8)[B],(9)[A]
- New regimens utilizing a PPI + amoxicillin 1 g b.i.d., levofloxacin 500 mg b.i.d. is recommended as 3rd-line or rescue therapy; it works well but easily develops resistance (8)[A]
- Contraindications: Hypersensitivity to the drug(s)

- Precautions:
  - If bismuth is prescribed, warn the patient about the side effect of stool becoming black.
  - Refer to the manufacturer's profile of each drug.
  - Significant possible interactions: Refer to the manufacturer's profile of each drug.

IN-PATIENT CONSIDERATIONS
Gastritis may occur in ICU patients.

Admission Criteria/Initial Stabilization
Outpatient, except for severe hemorrhagic gastritis

ONGOING CARE

FOLLOW-UP RECOMMENDATIONS
Usually no restrictions

Patient Monitoring
- Gastroscopy should be repeated after 6 weeks if gastritis has been severe or if symptomatic response to treatment has not been achieved.
- Patients with chronic gastritis are at increased risk for gastric carcinoma (lymphoma or adenocarcinoma).

DIET
Restrictions, if any, depend on symptom severity (e.g., bland, light, soft foods); it is wise to avoid caffeine and spicy foods, as well as alcohol.

PATIENT EDUCATION
- Explanation, reassurance
- Smoking cessation
- Dietary changes
- Relaxation therapy

PROGNOSIS
- Most cases clear spontaneously when the cause has been identified and treated.
- Recurrence of *H. pylori* infection requires a repeated course of treatment.

COMPLICATIONS
- Bleeding from extensive mucosal erosion or ulceration
- Clearing *H. pylori* before chronic gastritis develops may prevent development of gastric cancer.

REFERENCES
1. Rugge M, Pennelli G, Pilozzi E, et al. Gastritis: The histology report. *Dig Liver Dis*. 2011;43(Suppl 4): S373–S384.
2. Eslami L, Nasseri-Moghaddam S. Meta-analyses: Does long-term PPI use increase the risk of gastric premalignant lesions? *Arch Iran Med*. 2013;16: 449–458.
3. Mayerle J, den Hoed CM, Schurmann C, et al. Identification of genetic loci associated with Helicobacter pylori serologic status. *JAMA*. 2013; 309:1912–1920.
4. Lanza FL, Chan FK, Quigley EM, et al. Guidelines for prevention of NSAID-related ulcer complications. *Am J Gastroenterol*. 2009;104:728–738.
5. El-Zimaity H, Serra S, Szentgyorgyi E, et al. Gastric biopsies: The gap between evidence-based medicine and daily practice in the management of gastric Helicobacter pylori infection. *Can J Gastroenterol*. 2013;27:e25–e30.
6. Nazareno J, Driman DK, Adams P. Is Helicobacter pylori being treated appropriately? A study of inpatients and outpatients in a tertiary care centre. *Can J Gastroenterol*. 2007;21:285–288.
7. Venerito M, Krieger T, Ecker T, et al. Meta-analysis of bismuth quadruple therapy versus clarithromycin triple therapy for empiric primary treatment of Helicobacter pylori infection. *Digestion*. 2013;88: 33–45.
8. Graham DY, Rimbara E. Understanding and appreciating sequential therapy for Helicobacter pylori eradication. *J Clin Gastroenterol*. 2011;45: 309–313.
9. Yoon H, Lee DH, Kim N, et al. Meta-analysis: Is sequential therapy superior to standard triple therapy for Helicobacter pylori infection in Asian adults? *J Gastroenterol Hepatol*. 2013, in press.

ADDITIONAL READING
- Fellows SE, Rosini JM, Curtis JA, et al. Hemorrhagic gastritis with dabigatran in a patient with renal insufficiency. *J Emerg Med*. 2013;44:e221–225.
- Gisbert JP. Rescue therapy for Helicobacter pylori infection 2012. *Gastroenterol Res Pract*. 2012; 2012:974594.
- Lahner E, Annibale B, Delle Fave G. Systematic review: Helicobacter pylori infection and impaired drug absorption. *Aliment Pharmacol Ther*. 2009;29:379–386.
- McColl KE. Clinical practice. Helicobacter pylori infection. *N Engl J Med*. 2010;362:1597–1604.

CODES

ICD10
- K29.00 Acute gastritis without bleeding
- K29.70 Gastritis, unspecified, without bleeding
- K29.71 Gastritis, unspecified, with bleeding

CLINICAL PEARLS
- >50% the population is colonized with *H. pylori*.
- *H. pylori* is the most common cause of gastritis.
- *H. pylori* antibodies decline in the year after treatment, but should not be used to determine eradication.
- *H. pylori* stool antigen tests can be used both before and after therapy.
- *H. pylori* antibody titers rise significantly with reinfection.
- Several rescue therapies may be necessary to eradicate *H. pylori* successfully.
- Discontinue PPIs 2 weeks prior to endoscopy to improve diagnostic accuracy.

G

GASTROESOPHAGEAL REFLUX DISEASE
Ruben Peralta, MD, FACS

 BASICS

DESCRIPTION
Reflux of gastroduodenal contents into the esophagus, larynx, or lungs, with or without resultant esophageal inflammation

Pediatric Considerations
Symptoms (vomiting, weight loss, failure to thrive) usually resolve by 18 months.

EPIDEMIOLOGY
Incidence
Children affected: 1/300–1,000
Prevalence
- Prevalence of gastroesophageal reflux disease (GERD): 10–20% in the US
- Prevalence of Barrett esophagus: 1.5%
- 65% adults have had heartburn
- 15% have weekly symptoms
- In a European population-based study, reflux symptoms were found only in 40% of subjects with Barrett esophagus, and in 1/3 of patients with documented esophagitis.

ETIOLOGY AND PATHOPHYSIOLOGY
- Occurs with loss of the normal pressure gradient between the lower esophageal sphincter (LES) and the stomach
- Most commonly due to inappropriate relaxation of LES:
  – Foods (high fat, spicy, citrus, chocolate, peppermint, onions)
  – Medications (anticholinergic, smooth muscle relaxants, i.e., calcium channel blockers, nitrates)
- Other contributing factors include:
  – Pregnancy (progestational hormones decrease LES pressure)
  – Ineffective peristalsis
  – Scleroderma
  – Delayed gastric emptying
  – Positional: Recumbency, bending
- Obesity (1)[B]

Genetics
Gene polymorphism identified

RISK FACTORS
- Obesity
- Alcohol use
- Smoking
- Caffeine use
- Position of the acid pocket above the diaphragm in patients with hiatal hernia (see below) (2,3)

GENERAL PREVENTION
Positional treatment: Use infant seat for 2–3 hours after meals; thickened feedings:
- Avoid alcohol, nicotine, and caffeine.
- Avoid lying down immediately after a meal.
- Elevate head of bed.

COMMONLY ASSOCIATED CONDITIONS
- Reflux esophagitis: Due to exposure to acid, pepsin; classified as erosive (mucosal damage apparent, ulcers, friability) or nonerosive

- Extraesophageal reflux:
  – Aspiration
  – Chronic cough
  – Laryngitis, vocal cord granuloma
  – Sinusitis
  – Otitis media
- Halitosis
- Hiatal hernia: The position of the acid pocket (the zone of high acidity detected in the proximal stomach after a meal) above the diaphragm in patients with hiatal hernia is a major risk factor (1,2,3).
- Peptic stricture: In 10% with GERD
- Barrett esophagus
- Esophageal adenocarcinoma

 DIAGNOSIS

- Heartburn (70–85%)
- Regurgitation of digested food (60%)
- Anginalike chest pain (33%)
- Abdominal pain (29%)
- Hoarseness (21%)
- Dysphagia (for solids; if solids and liquids, consider another cause) (20%)
- Bronchospasm (asthma) (15–20%)
- Aspiration (14%)
- Chronic cough
- Loss of dental enamel

HISTORY
- Heartburn: Retrosternal burning
- Regurgitation; sour or acid taste in mouth
- Symptoms with bending or recumbency
- Extraesophageal symptoms (e.g., cough)
- Diet, alcohol, smoking, and caffeine
- Diagnosis often made based on history alone, followed by a 1-week empiric trial with an antacid regimen

PHYSICAL EXAM
Typically unremarkable:
- May have weight loss or palpable epigastric mass

DIFFERENTIAL DIAGNOSIS
- Infectious esophagitis (*Candida*, herpes, HIV, cytomegalovirus)
- Chemical esophagitis (lye ingestion)
- Pill-induced esophagitis
- Radiation injury
- Crohn disease
- Angina
- Stricture
- Esophageal carcinoma
- Achalasia
- Scleroderma
- Peptic ulcer disease

DIAGNOSTIC TESTS & INTERPRETATION
- Treat empirically if no red flags (dysphagia odynophagia, weight loss, early satiety, anemia, new onset, male >45 years) suggesting need to screen for more serious disease.
- 24-hour pH monitoring: Gold standard for diagnosis; records number of reflux episodes and number that occur supine or upright; can be correlated with symptom diary
- Esophageal manometry records pressure of LES and effectiveness of peristalsis

Initial Tests (lab, imaging)
- Check for anemia due to bleeding esophageal erosions or due to poor B_{12} absorption on proton pump inhibitor (PPI).
- Barium swallow:
  – Presence of a sliding hiatal hernia appears to be a predictor of reflux esophagitis
  – Mucosal irregularity due to inflammation and edema

Diagnostic Procedures/Other
- Endoscopy:
  – Not part of initial workup, unless anemia, unintentional weight loss, progressive dysphagia, GI bleeding, persistent vomiting, palpable epigastric mass, suspicion based on imaging study
  – Recommended for patients age >55 years who continue with symptoms after 4 weeks of treatment
  – Confirm mucosal injury; look for Barrett esophagus; biopsy for adenocarcinoma
  – ~50–70% of patients with heartburn have negative findings on endoscopy (nonerosive or endoscopy-negative reflux disease).
- Savary-Miller classification:
  – For grading esophagitis based on endoscopic findings:
    ○ Grade I: ≥1 nonconfluent reddish spots, with or without exudate
    ○ Grade II: Erosive and exudative lesions in the distal esophagus; may be confluent, but not circumferential
    ○ Grade III: Circumferential erosions in the distal esophagus
    ○ Grade IV: Chronic complications, such as deep ulcers, stenosis, or scarring with Barrett metaplasia

Test Interpretation
- Acute inflammation (especially eosinophils)
- Hyperplasia of the basal zone of the epithelium seen in 85%
- Barrett epithelial change: Gastric columnar epithelium replaces squamous epithelium in distal esophagus.

 TREATMENT

GENERAL MEASURES
Lifestyle changes are 1st intervention:
- Elevate head of bed and avoid lying down soon after meals.
- Avoid stooping, bending, tight-fitting garments.
- Avoid medications that relax the LES (anticholinergic, calcium channel blockers).
- Lose weight.
- Stop smoking.
- Avoid alcohol.
- Decrease caffeine.

MEDICATION
First Line
- Stepped therapy:
  – Phase I: Lifestyle and diet modifications, antacids plus H_2 blockers or PPIs
  – Phase II: Symptoms persist, consider endoscopic evaluation
  – Phase III: Surgery

- H₂ blockers in equipotent oral doses (e.g., cimetidine 800 mg b.i.d. or 400 mg q.i.d., or ranitidine 150 mg b.i.d., or famotidine 20 mg b.i.d., or nizatidine 150 mg b.i.d.)
- PPIs: Irreversibly bind proton pump, onset of effect 4 days. Include omeprazole 20 mg/d, lansoprazole 30 mg/d, pantoprazole 40 mg/d, rabeprazole 20 mg/d, esomeprazole 40 mg/d.
- Erosive esophagitis: PPI given for 8 weeks will be effective for healing in 90%:
  – PPI more effective than H₂ blocker for healing erosive esophagitis.
  – 2013 Meta-analysis showed rabeprazole demonstrates a clinical advantage over omeprazole in symptomatic relief but no significant difference in endoscopic relief of erosive GERD for treatment up to 8 weeks (4)[A]

Pediatric Considerations
Antacids or liquid histamine type 2 blockers, omeprazole, metoclopramide

Second Line
- Antacids and agents like sucralfate may relieve breakthrough symptoms.
- Metoclopramide: 5–10 mg before meals
- Precautions:
  – Blood dyscrasias with PPIs and H₂ blockers
  – H₂ blockers must be renally dosed.
  – Metoclopramide is a dopamine blocker; risk of dystonia and tardive dyskinesia
  – On PPI, monitor B₁₂; B₁₂ and iron absorption and calcium absorption compromised on PPI
- Significant possible interactions:
  – PPIs and H₂ blockers: Multiple cytochrome P450 drug interactions; examples include warfarin, phenytoin, antifungals

SURGERY/OTHER PROCEDURES
Open or laparoscopic Nissen fundoplication to increase pressure gradient between stomach and esophagus by wrapping gastric fundus around distal esophagus, often circumferential (360° fundoplication)

- Indications: Evidence of severe esophageal injury, incomplete response to medical treatment, medication treatment that has been or is expected to be prolonged
- Rule out esophageal dysmotility prior to surgery. If motility problems, consider a partial (270°, Toupet) wrap.
- Open and laparoscopic procedures both produce >90% response, equally effective for symptom reduction, quality of life, and decreased need for medications (3)[A].
- Cost analysis has indicated that if patient requires >10 years of PPI treatment, surgery may be more cost-effective.

Pediatric Considerations
Surgery for severe symptoms (apnea, choking, persistent vomiting)

 ## ONGOING CARE

FOLLOW-UP RECOMMENDATIONS
Patient Monitoring
- Follow symptomatically.
- Repeat endoscopy at 4–8 weeks for poor symptomatic response to medical therapy, especially in older patients.
- Current guideline is endoscopic surveillance every 2–5 years in patients with Barrett esophagus, assuming treatment if cancer is detected.

DIET
Avoid foods that make symptoms worse.

PATIENT EDUCATION
- Chocolate, peppermint, citrus, onions, spicy foods, and foods high in fat can make GERD symptoms worse.
- Eat small meals.
- Avoid lying down soon after meals.
- Elevate head of bed.
- Lifestyle changes, such as losing weight, smoking cessation, and avoiding alcohol and caffeine, help.

PROGNOSIS
- Symptoms and esophageal inflammation often return promptly when treatment is withdrawn; to prevent relapse of symptoms, patients should be treated with continued antisecretory therapy:
  – PPI maintenance therapy may improve quality of life better than H₂ blocker maintenance.
  – Full-dose PPIs more effective than 1/2 dose for maintenance (5)[A]
  – In erosive esophagitis, daily maintenance therapy with a PPI has been proven to prevent relapse; intermittent PPI therapy has not been proven effective (6)[A].
- In terms of symptom reduction, medical and surgical therapy are equally effective (5)[A].
- Antireflux surgery:
  – 90–94% symptom response
  – 5% continued symptoms: Should have anatomy evaluated by esophagram
  – Long-term follow-up shows some surgically treated patients may eventually require medical therapy.
- Regression of Barrett epithelium does not routinely occur, despite aggressive medical or surgical therapy.

COMPLICATIONS
- Peptic stricture: 10–15%
- Barrett esophagus: 10%:
  – Adenocarcinoma from Barrett epithelium (rate of cancer development 0.5% annually)
  – Primary treatment for Barrett esophagus with high-grade dysplasia is endoscopic radiofrequency ablation (7)[B].
- Extraesophageal symptoms: 5–10%, including hoarseness, aspiration, including aspiration pneumonia
- Bleeding due to mucosal injury
- Noncardiac chest pain

Geriatric Considerations
Complications more likely (e.g., aspiration pneumonia)

REFERENCES

1. Lee YY, Wirz AA, Whiting JG, et al. Waist belt and central obesity cause partial hiatus hernia and short segment acid reflux in asymptomatic volunteers. *Gut.* 2013 Sep 24. doi.1136/gutjnl-2013-305803.
2. Beaumont H, Bennink RJ, de Jong J, et al. The position of the acid pocket as a major risk factor for acidic reflux in healthy subjects and patients with GORD. *Gut.* 2010;59:441–451.
3. McColl KE, Clarke A, Seenan J, et al. Acid pocket, hiatus hernia and acid reflux. *Gut.* 2010;59:430–431.
4. Xia XM, Wang H. Gastroesophageal reflux disease relief in patients treated with rabeprazole 20 mg versus omeprazole 20 mg: A meta-analysis. *Gastroenterol Res Pract.* 2013;2013:327571. Epub 2013 Sep
5. Agency for Healthcare Research and Quality. Comparing effectiveness of management strategies for gastroesophageal reflux disease. An update to the 2005 report. Available at: http://effectivehealthcare.ahrq.gov. Accessed July 7, 2010.
6. Zacny J, Zamakhshary M, Sketris I, et al. Systematic review: The efficacy of intermittent and on-demand therapy with histamine H2-receptor antagonists or proton pump inhibitors for gastro-oesophageal reflux disease patients. *Aliment Pharmacol Ther.* 2005;21:1299–1312.
7. Hur C, Choi SE, Rubenstein JH, et al. The cost effectiveness of radiofrequency ablation for Barrett's esophagus. *Gastroenterology.* 2012;143(3):567–575. Epub 2012 May 21.
8. Chang AB, Lasserson TJ, Kiljander TO, et al. Systematic review and meta-analysis of randomised controlled trials of gastro-oesophageal reflux interventions for chronic cough associated with gastrooesophageal reflux. *BMJ.* 2006;332:11–17.

ADDITIONAL READING

- Leggett CL, Gorospe EC, Calvin AD, et al. Obstructive sleep apnea is a risk factor for Barrett's esophagus. *Clin Gastroenterol Hepatol.* 2013:pii: S1542-3565(13)01300-1.
- Martigne L, Delaage PH, Thomas-Delecourt F, et al. Prevalence and management of gastroesophageal reflux disease in children and adolescents: A nationwide cross-sectional observational study. *Eur J Pediatr.* 2012;171(12):1767–1773.
- Quartarone G. Gastroesophageal reflux in pregnancy: a systematic review on the benefit of raft forming agents. *Minerva Ginecol.* 2013;65(5):541–549.

 ## SEE ALSO

Algorithms: Dyspepsia; Epigastric Pain

 ## CODES

ICD10
- K21 Gastro-esophageal reflux disease
- K21.0 Gastro-esophageal reflux disease with esophagitis
- K21.9 Gastro-esophageal reflux disease without esophagitis

CLINICAL PEARLS

- No evidence supports that treatment with PPI causes regression of Barrett esophagus or inhibits progression of esophageal dysplasia beyond benefits of symptomatic relief.
- Primary treatment for Barrett esophagus with high-grade dysplasia is endoscopic radiofrequency ablation (7)[B].
- GERD treatments are used to treat chronic cough. Meta-analysis of randomized clinical trials suggest PPIs help with cough resolution in some adults (8)[A].
- The role of *Helicobacter pylori* as an etiologic agent in GERD remains controversial.

G

GENITO-PELVIC PAIN/PENETRATION DISORDER VAGINISMUS

Adriana C. Linares, MD, MPH, DrPH

 BASICS

Genito-pelvic pain/penetration disorder is the new name of the conditions formally known as vaginismus and dyspareunia. It has overlapping elements of hypertonic pelvic floor muscles (recurrent or persistent involuntary contractions), pain, and avoidance of sexual intercourse leading to difficulty in vaginal penetration.

DESCRIPTION
- Persistent or recurrent difficulties for 6 months or more with at least 1 of the following:
  - Inability to have vaginal intercourse/penetration on at least 50% of attempts
  - Marked genito-pelvic pain during at least 50% of vaginal intercourse/penetration attempts
  - Marked fear of vaginal intercourse/penetration or of genito-pelvic pain during intercourse/penetration on at least 50% of vaginal intercourse/penetration attempts
  - Marked tensing or tightening of the pelvic floor muscles during attempted vaginal intercourse/penetration on at least 50% of occasions.
- The disturbance causes marked distress or interpersonal difficulty
- Specify if with a general medical condition (e.g. lichen sclerosis, endometriosis)

Pregnancy Considerations
- Pregnancy can occur in patients with genito-pelvic pain/penetration disorder when ejaculation occurs on the perineum.
- Vaginismus may be an independent risk factor for cesarean delivery.

EPIDEMIOLOGY
Incidence
The incidence of vaginismus is thought to be about 1–17% per year worldwide (1).

Prevalence
- True prevalence is unknown due to limited data/reporting.
- Population-based studies report prevalence rates of 0.5–30% (1).
- Affects women in all age groups

ETIOLOGY AND PATHOPHYSIOLOGY
Most often multifactorial in both primary and secondary vaginismus:
- Primary:
  - Psychologic and psychosocial issues:
    - Negative messages about sex and sexual relations in upbringing may cause phobic reaction.
    - Poor body image and limited understanding of genital area
    - History of sexual trauma
  - Abnormalities of the hymen

- Secondary:
  - Vaginal infection
  - Inflammatory dermatitis
  - Surgical or postdelivery scarring
  - Endometriosis
  - Inadequate vaginal lubrication
  - Pelvic radiation
  - Estrogen deficiency
  - Conditioned response to pain from physical issues previously listed

RISK FACTORS
- Although the exact role in the condition is unclear, many women report a history of abuse or sexual trauma (2).
- Often associated with other sexual dysfunctions

COMMONLY ASSOCIATED CONDITIONS
- Marital stress, family dysfunction
- Anxiety
- Vulvodynia/Vestibulodynia

 DIAGNOSIS

DSM-5 has combined vaginismus and dyspareunia in a condition called genito-pelvic pain/penetration disorder

HISTORY
- Complete medical history
- Full psychosocial and sexual history, including:
  - Relationship difficulty
  - Inability to allow vaginal entry for different purposes:
    - Sexual (penis, digit, object)
    - Hygiene (tampon use)
    - Health care (pelvic examination)
  - Infertility
  - Past traumatic experiences
  - Religious beliefs
  - Views on sexuality

PHYSICAL EXAM
- Pelvic examination is necessary to exclude structural abnormalities or organic pathology.
- Educating the patient about the examination and giving her control over the progression of the examination is essential, as genital/pelvic examination may induce varying degrees of anxiety in patients.
- Referral to a gynecologist, family physician, or other provider specializing in the treatment of sexual disorders may be appropriate.

- Lamont classification system aids in the assessment of severity:
  - 1st degree: Perineal and levator spasm relieved with reassurance
  - 2nd degree: Perineal spasm maintained throughout the pelvic exam
  - 3rd degree: Levator spasm and elevation of buttocks
  - 4th degree: Levator and perineal spasm and elevation with adduction and retreat

DIFFERENTIAL DIAGNOSIS
- Vaginal infection
- Vulvodynia/Vestibulodynia
- Vulvovaginal atrophy
- Urogenital structural abnormalities
- Interstitial cystitis

DIAGNOSTIC TESTS & INTERPRETATION
No laboratory tests indicated

Test Interpretation
- Not available, may be needed to check for secondary causes

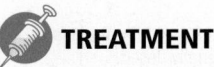 **TREATMENT**

- Genito-pelvic pain penetration disorder may be successfully treated.
- Outpatient care is appropriate.
- Treatment of physical conditions, if present, is 1st line (see "Secondary" under "Etiology and Pathophysiology").
- Role for pelvic floor physical therapy and myofascial release
- Some evidence suggests that cognitive-behavioral therapy may be effective (3)[C]: Includes desensitization techniques, such as gradual exposure, aimed at decreasing avoidance behavior and fear of vaginal penetration
- Based on a Cochrane review (4), a clinically relevant effect of systematic desensitization cannot be ruled out.

- Evidence suggests that Masters and Johnson's sex therapy may be effective (5)[C]:
  - Involves Kegel exercises to increase control over perineal muscles
  - Stepwise vaginal desensitization exercises:
    - With vaginal dilators that the patient inserts and controls
    - With woman's own finger(s) to promote sexual self-awareness
    - Advancement to partner's fingers with patient's control
    - Coitus after achieving largest vaginal dilator or 3 fingers; important to begin with sensate-focused exercises/sensual caressing without necessarily a demand for coitus
    - Female superior at first; passive (nonthrusting); female directed
    - Later, thrusting may be allowed.
- Topical anesthetic with desensitization exercises may be considered.
- Patient education is an essential component of treatment (see "Patient Education" section).

MEDICATION
Botulinum neurotoxin type A injections may improve vaginismus in patients who do not respond to standard cognitive-behavioral and medical treatment for vaginismus (6):
- Dosage: 20, 50, and 100–400 U of botulinum toxin type A injected in the levator ani muscle have been shown to improve vaginismus.

ISSUES FOR REFERRAL
For diagnosis and treatment recommendations, the following resources may be consulted:
- Obstetrics/Gynecology
- Pelvic floor physical therapy
- Psychiatry
- Sex therapy
- Hypnotherapy

SURGERY/OTHER PROCEDURES
Contraindicated

COMPLEMENTARY AND ALTERNATIVE MEDICINE
- Biofeedback
- Functional electrical stimulation

ONGOING CARE

FOLLOW-UP RECOMMENDATIONS
Desensitization techniques of gentle, progressive, patient-controlled vaginal dilation

Patient Monitoring
General preventive health care

DIET
No special diet

PATIENT EDUCATION
- Education about pelvic anatomy, nature of vaginal spasms, normal adult sexual function
- Handheld mirror can help the woman to learn visually to tighten and loosen perineal muscles
- Important to teach the partner that spasms are not under conscious control and are not a reflection on the relationship or a woman's feelings about her partner
- Instruction in techniques for vaginal dilation
- Resources:
  - American College of Obstetricians & Gynecologists (ACOG), 409 12th St., SW, Washington, DC 20024-2188; 800-762-ACOG. www.acog.org
  - Valins L. *When a woman's body says no to sex: Understanding and overcoming vaginismus*. New York: Penguin; 1992.

PROGNOSIS
Favorable, with early recognition of the condition and initiation of treatment

REFERENCES
1. Wimons JS, Carey MP. Prevalence of sexual dysfunctions: Results form a decade of research. *Arch Sex Behav*. 2001;30:177–217.
2. Reissing E, Binik Y, Khalife S, et al. Etiological correlates of vaginismus: Sexual and physical abuse, sexual knowledge, sexual self-schema, and relationship adjustment. *J Sex Marital Ther*. 2003;29:47–59.
3. ter Kuile MM, van Lankveld JJDM, de Groot E, et al. Cognitive behavioral therapy for women with lifelong vaginismus: Process and prognostic factors. *Behav Res Therapy*. 2008;45:359–373.
4. Melnik T. Hawton K, McGuirre H. Interventions for vaginismus. *Cochrane Database Syst Rev*. 2012; 12:CD001760.
5. Jeng CJ, Wang LR, Chou CS. Management and outcome of primary vaginismus. *J Sex Marital Ther*. 2006;32:379–387.
6. Pacik PT. Vaginismus: Review of current concepts and treatment using botox injections, bupivacaine injections, and progressive dilation with the patient under anesthesia. *Aesthetic Plast Surg*. 2011; 35:1160–1164.

ADDITIONAL READING
- American Psychiatric Association. *The diagnostic and statistical manual of mental disorders*, 5th ed. Washington, DC. American Psychiatric Association, 2013.
- Basson R, Wierman ME, van Lankveld J. Summary of the recommendations on sexual dysfunctions in women. *J Sex Med*. 2010;7:314–326.
- Crowley T, Goldmeier D, Hiller J. Diagnosing and managing vaginismus. *BMJ*. 2009;338:b2284.
- Lahaie MA, Boyer SC, Amsel R, et al. Vaginismus: A review of the literature on the classification/diagnosis, etiology and treatment. *Womens Health (Lond Engl)*. 2010;6:705–719.

 SEE ALSO

Dyspareunia; Sexual Dysfunction in Women

 CODES

ICD10
- F52.6 Dyspareunia not due to a substance or known physiol cond
- N53.12 Painful ejaculation
- N94.1 Dyspareunia

CLINICAL PEARLS
- In a patient with suspected genito-pelvic pain penetration disorder, a complete medical history, including a comprehensive psychosocial and sexual history, and a patient-centric, patient-controlled educational pelvic exam should be conducted.
- This condition can be treated effectively.
- Cognitive-behavioral therapy may be effective for the treatment of this condition.
- Botox injection therapy is in the experimental stages, but looks promising for the treatment of vaginismus. Bupivacaine and dilation under general anesthesia has also been tried as a treatment for vaginismus.

G

GIARDIASIS

Kristyn T. Fagerberg, MD

BASICS

DESCRIPTION
- Intestinal infection caused by the protozoan parasite *Giardia lamblia*:
  - *G. lamblia* is also called *G. duodenalis* and *G. intestinalis*.
- Infection results from ingestion of the cysts, which excyst into trophozoites:
  - Trophozoites colonize the small intestine and cause symptoms.
  - Cycle is continued when the trophozoites encyst in the small intestine and, subsequently, water, food, or hands are contaminated by feces of the infected person.
- Most infections result from fecal–oral transmission or ingestion of contaminated water (e.g., while swimming).
- Less commonly, giardiasis is the result of contaminated food.

EPIDEMIOLOGY
- Predominant age:
  - All ages, but most common in early childhood ages 1–9 and adults 35–44 (1)[A]
- Predominant gender:
  - Male > Female (slightly)
- There is minimal seasonal variability; however, a slight increase in cases is noted in the summer months (2).

Pediatric Considerations
Common in early childhood

Prevalence
- 5% of patients with stools submitted for ova and parasite exams
- >19,000 cases/year in reportable US states:
  - Giardia is not reportable in Indiana, Kentucky, Mississippi, North Carolina, and Texas.

ETIOLOGY AND PATHOPHYSIOLOGY
- *Giardia* trophozoites colonize the surface of the proximal small intestine: The mechanism by which they cause diarrhea is unknown.
- Protozoan parasite (*G. lamblia*) infection acquired through fecal–oral transmission or ingestion of contaminated water, less commonly from contaminated food

Genetics
No known genetic risk factors

RISK FACTORS
- Daycare centers
- Anal intercourse
- Wilderness camping
- Travel to developing countries
- Children adopted from developing countries
- Public swimming pools

GENERAL PREVENTION
- Good hand washing when caring for diapered children
- Water purification when camping and when traveling to developing countries
- Cooking all foods

COMMONLY ASSOCIATED CONDITIONS
Hypogammaglobulinemia and possibly IgA deficiency: Diarrhea more severe and prolonged in these patients

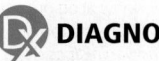

DIAGNOSIS

HISTORY
- 25–50% of infected persons are symptomatic.
- Symptoms usually appear 1–2 weeks after an exposure.
- Chronic diarrhea (lasting >5–7 days and frequently weeks)
- Abdominal bloating
- Flatulence
- Loose, greasy, foul-smelling stools
- Weight loss
- Nausea
- Lactose intolerance

PHYSICAL EXAM
Nonspecific; abdominal bloating and afebrile

DIFFERENTIAL DIAGNOSIS
- Includes other etiologies of small-intestine diarrhea
- Infectious causes include cryptosporidiosis, isosporiasis, and cyclosporiasis.
- Other causes of malabsorption include celiac sprue, tropical sprue, bacterial overgrowth syndromes, and Crohn ileitis.
- Irritable bowel is suspected when diarrhea is not accompanied by weight loss.

DIAGNOSTIC TESTS & INTERPRETATION
Initial Tests (lab, imaging)
- Stool for ova and parasites:
  - Repeated 3× if necessary
  - Cysts are seen in fixed or fresh stools and, occasionally, trophozoites are found in fresh diarrheal stools.
- Fluorescent antibody (FA) and ELISA tests of fecal specimens are available:
  - *A single FA or ELISA is at least as sensitive as 3 stools for ova and parasites.*
- Polymerase chain reaction (PCR) techniques have been found to be more sensitive than microscopy, but have not been widely adopted secondary to cost (3).

Follow-Up Tests & Special Considerations
String test (Enterotest):
- A gelatin capsule on a string is swallowed and left in the duodenum for several hours or overnight.
- The end of the string is then visualized microscopically.

Diagnostic Procedures/Other
Esophagogastroduodenoscopy (EGD) with biopsy and sample of small intestinal fluid

Test Interpretation
Intestinal biopsy shows flattened, mild lymphocytic infiltration and trophozoites on the surface.

TREATMENT

Outpatient for mild cases; inpatient if symptoms are severe enough to cause dehydration

GENERAL MEASURES
- Medical therapy for all infected individuals
- Fluid replacement if dehydrated

MEDICATION
First Line
- Metronidazole (Flagyl): 250 mg t.i.d. for 5–7 days (4)[B]
- Tinidazole: 2 g single dose (50 mg/kg up to 2 g for children) (4)[B]
- Albendazole: 400 mg/d for 5 days:
  - Albendazole has comparable effectiveness to metronidazole with fewer side effects and low cost (5)[A],(6)
- Precautions:
  - Theoretical risk of carcinogenesis with metronidazole
- Significant possible interactions: Occasional disulfiram reaction with metronidazole or tinidazole

Pregnancy Considerations
- Concern for potential teratogenicity of medications; consult infectious disease specialist or gastroenterologist for symptomatic disease.
- Medications to treat giardiasis are relatively contraindicated during pregnancy; use caution.

Second Line
- Furazolidone: 8 mg/kg/d t.i.d. for 10 days (slightly less effective, but commonly used in pediatrics because it is well tolerated)
- Paromomycin (Humatin): A nonabsorbable aminoglycoside that is probably less effective but commonly recommended in pregnancy because of theoretical risk of teratogenicity of other agents
- Quinacrine: 100 mg t.i.d. for 5–7 days; was the treatment of choice for giardiasis, but has been withdrawn from the U.S. market
- Nitazoxanide suspension was approved by the FDA in 2003 for treatment of giardiasis in children 1–11. Children 1–4 receive 100 mg b.i.d. and 5–11 receive 200 mg b.i.d. for 3 days
- 2 other nitroimidazole antibiotics, omidazole and secnidazole, are effective against *Giardia* but are not available in the US (7).

ADDITIONAL THERAPIES
- Lactose intolerance may follow *Giardia* infection and be a cause of persistent diarrhea post treatment.
- There have been anecdotal reports of herbal products containing *Mentha crispa* being effective in the treatment of *Giardia*. However, when studied, it was shown to be only 47.8% effective when compared to 84% for secnidazole (a metronidazole analog) (8).
- A recent study showed tetrahydrolipstatin (Orlistat) had activity against *Giardia* and may be investigated as a potential treatment option in the future for patients who are resistant to metronidazole (9)

ONGOING CARE

FOLLOW-UP RECOMMENDATIONS
Patient Monitoring
Symptoms, weight, stool exams

DIET
Good nutrition, low lactose, low fat, monitor for dehydration

PATIENT EDUCATION
- Hand washing may be more important than water purification to prevent transmission in outdoor recreationalists.
- CDC Facts about *Giardia* and Swimming Pools: www.cdc.gov/healthywater/pdf/swimming/resources/giardia-factsheet.pdf:
  – Don't swim when you have diarrhea.
  – Wash hands with soap after changing diapers before you return to the pool.
  – Do not put pool, lake, or river water in your mouth when you swim.

PROGNOSIS
- Untreated giardiasis lasts for weeks.
- Patients usually (90%) respond to treatment within a few days:
  – Most nonresponders or relapses respond to a 2nd course with the same or a different agent.

COMPLICATIONS
Malabsorption and weight loss

REFERENCES

1. Yoder JS, Harral C, Beach MJ, et al. Giardiasis surveillance—United States, 2006–2008. *MMWR Surveill Summ.* 2010;59:15–25.
2. Lal A, Hales S, French N, et al. Seasonality in human zoonotic enteric diseases: A systematic review. *PLoS ONE.* 2012;7(4):e31883. Epub 2012 Apr 2.
3. Haque R, Roy S, Siddique A, et al. Multiplex real-time PCR assay for detection of *Entamoeba histolytica, Giardia intestinalis,* and *Cryptosporidium* spp. *Am J Trop Med Hyg.* 2007;76:713–717.
4. Fallah M, Rabiee S, Moshtaghi AA. Comparison between efficacy of a single dose of tinidazole with a 7-day standard dose course of metronidazole in giardiasis. *Pak J Med Sci.* 2007;23(1):43–46.
5. Solaymani-Mohammadi S, Genkinger JM, Loffredo CA, et al. A meta-analysis of the effectiveness of albendazole compared with metronidazole as treatments for infections with *Giardia duodenalis*. *PLoS Negl Trop Dis.* 2010;4:e682.
6. Cañete R, Rodríguez P, Mesa L, et al. Albendazole versus metronidazole in the treatment of adult giardiasis: A randomized, double-blind, clinical trial. *Curr Med Res Opin.* 2012;28(1):149–154. Epub 2011 Dec 12.
7. Almirall P, Escobedo AA, Ayala I, et al. Mebendazole compared with secnidazole in the treatment of adult giardiasis: A randomised, no-inferiority, open clinical trial. *J Parasitol Res.* 2011;2011:636857. Epub 2011 Nov 20.
8. Teles NS, Fechine FV, Viana FA, et al. Evaluation of the therapeutic efficacy of *Mentha crispa* in the treatment of giardiasis. *Contemp Clin Trials.* 2011;32(6):809–813.
9. Hahn J, Seeber F, Kolodziej H, et al. High sensitivity of Giardia duodenalis to tetrahydolipstatin (Orlistat) in vitro. *PLoS One.* 2013;8(8):e71597. doi: 10.1371/journal.pone.0071597.

ADDITIONAL READING

- Shields JM, Gleim ER, Beach MJ. Prevalence of *Cryptosporidium* spp. and *Giardia intestinalis* in swimming pools, Atlanta, Georgia. *Emerg Infect Dis.* 2008;14:948–950.
- L Alexander C, Niebel M, Jones B. The rapid detection of Cryptosporidium and *Giardia* species in clinical stools using the Quik Chek immunoassay *Parasitol Int.* 2013;62(6):552–553.

 SEE ALSO

Algorithm: Diarrhea, Chronic

 CODES

ICD10
A07.1 Giardiasis [lambliasis]

CLINICAL PEARLS
- Daycare facilities and public swimming pools are common sources of *Giardia* (don't assume camping or travel is required).
- Treatment with metronidazole is often poorly tolerated, but has higher cure rates.
- Most treatment failures respond to a 2nd course of antibiotics (whether or not you switch drugs).
- A single fluorescent antibody (FA) or ELISA is at least as sensitive as 3 stool samples for ova and parasites.

G

GILBERT DISEASE

Robert A. Marlow, MD, MA

 BASICS

DESCRIPTION
Mild chronic or intermittent unconjugated hyperbilirubinemia (not due to hemolysis) with otherwise normal liver function (1)

Pediatric Considerations
Rare for the disorder to be diagnosed before puberty (2)

Pregnancy Considerations
The relative fasting that may occur with morning sickness can elevate bilirubin level.

EPIDEMIOLOGY
- Predominant age: Present from birth, but most often presents in the 2nd or 3rd decade of life; heterozygous for single abnormal gene (3)
- Predominant sex: Male > Female (2–7:1)

Prevalence
Prevalence in the US: ~7% of the population (4) ~1 in 3 of those affected are not aware that they have the disorder.

ETIOLOGY AND PATHOPHYSIOLOGY
The hyperbilirubinemia results from impaired hepatic bilirubin clearance (~30% of normal). Hepatic bilirubin conjugation (glucuronidation) is reduced, although this is likely not the only defect (3).

Genetics
A gene defect resulting in reduced bilirubin uridine diphosphate–glucuronosyltransferase-1 appears to be necessary but not sufficient for Gilbert syndrome (5).

RISK FACTORS
Male gender

COMMONLY ASSOCIATED CONDITIONS
Gilbert disease may be part of a spectrum of hereditary disorders that includes types I and II Crigler-Najjar syndrome.

 DIAGNOSIS

HISTORY
No significant symptoms, although a variety of nonspecific symptoms have been described. An episode of nonpruritic jaundice can be triggered by stressors such as fasting, dehydration, infections, physical exertion, lack of sleep, and surgery. Some medications may also trigger episodes of jaundice, such as drugs that inhibit glucuronyl transferase, such as gemfibrozil and the protease inhibitors atazanavir and indinavir. Any symptoms present during an episode of jaundice, including fatigue, are caused by the triggering factor and are not directly a result of the Gilbert disease (6).

PHYSICAL EXAM
No abnormal physical findings other than occasional mild jaundice that can be precipitated by the above-mentioned triggers (fasting, dehydration, infections, physical exertion, lack of sleep, and surgery).

DIFFERENTIAL DIAGNOSIS
- Hemolysis
- Ineffective erythropoiesis (megaloblastic anemias, certain porphyrias, thalassemia major, sideroblastic anemia, severe lead poisoning, congenital dyserythropoietic anemias)
- Cirrhosis
- Chronic persistent hepatitis
- Pancreatitis
- Biliary tract disease

DIAGNOSTIC TESTS & INTERPRETATION
Initial Tests (lab, imaging)
- Bilirubin: Elevated but <6 mg/dL (103 μmol/L) and usually <3 mg/dL (51 μmol/L), virtually all unconjugated (indirect), with conjugated bilirubin within the normal range and/or <20% of the total bilirubin (6).
- CBC with peripheral smear is normal.
- Reticulocyte count is normal.
- Liver function tests (aspartate aminotransferase [AST], alanine transaminase [ALT], alkaline phosphatase, and glutamyl transpeptidase [GGT]) are normal.
- Fasting and postprandial serum bile acids are normal.
- Up to 60% of patients have clinically insignificant mild hemolysis that frequently can only be detected with sophisticated red cell survival studies.
- Drugs that may alter lab results: Bilirubin level may be raised by nicotinic acid and lowered by phenobarbital.
- Disorders that may alter lab results: Bilirubin levels increase during fasting and may increase during a febrile illness.

Follow-Up Tests & Special Considerations
If history, physical exam, and laboratory tests are normal, see the patient on 2–3 further occasions during the ensuing 12–18 months. If the patient develops no symptoms, reticulocytosis, or new liver function abnormalities, make the diagnosis of Gilbert disease.

Diagnostic Procedures/Other

ALERT
A liver biopsy is not usually needed to exclude other diagnoses (4).
- Some clinicians recommend confirming the diagnosis by reducing daily caloric intake to 400 kcal for 48 hours, which results in a 2–3-fold increase in unconjugated bilirubin, but other clinicians consider this impractical and nonspecific for Gilbert disease.
- After 12 hours of fasting, an increase of total bilirubin to >1.9 mg/dL 2 hours after an oral dose of rifampin 900 mg distinguishes patients with Gilbert disease with a sensitivity of 100% and a specificity of 100% (7).

TREATMENT

- Outpatient
- The most important treatment is to make a positive diagnosis of Gilbert disease to reassure the patient and prevent further unnecessary procedures.

ONGOING CARE

FOLLOW-UP RECOMMENDATIONS
Patient Monitoring
If history, physical exam, and laboratory tests are normal, see the patient on 2–3 further occasions during the ensuing 12–18 months. If the patient develops no symptoms, reticulocytosis, or new liver function abnormalities, make the diagnosis of Gilbert disease.

PATIENT EDUCATION
Reassure the patient that the condition is benign with no known sequelae.

PROGNOSIS
- The disorder is benign with an excellent prognosis.
- There is some preliminary evidence that patients with Gilbert disease may have a lower incidence of cardiovascular disease (8,9). Elevated levels of bilirubin may exert an antioxidation effect (9).
- Patients with Gilbert syndrome are able to serve as donors for right lobe of liver for transplantation (10).

COMPLICATIONS
No known complications

REFERENCES

1. Bosma PJ. Inherited disorders of bilirubin metabolism. *J Hepatol*. 2003;38:107–117.
2. Fretzayas A, Moustaki M, Liapi O, et al. Gilbert syndrome. *Eur J Pediatr*. 2012;171(1):11–15. Epub 2011 Dec 9.
3. Strassburg CP. Pharmacogenetics of Gilbert's syndrome. *Pharmacogenomics*. 2008;9:703–715.
4. Radu P, Atsmon J. Gilbert's syndrome—clinical and pharmacological implications. *Isr Med Assoc J*. 2001;3:593–598.
5. Bosma PJ, Chowdhury JR, Bakker C, et al. The genetic basis of the reduced expression of bilirubin UDP-glucuronosyltransferase 1 in Gilbert's syndrome. *N Engl J Med*. 1995;333:1171–1175.
6. Claridge LC, Armstrong MJ, Booth C, et al. Gilbert's syndrome. *BMJ*. 2011;342:d2293.
7. Murthy GD, Byron D, Shoemaker D, et al. The utility of rifampin in diagnosing Gilbert's syndrome. *Am J Gastroenterol*. 2001;96:1150–1154.
8. Inoguchi T, Sasaki S, Kobayashi K, et al. Relationship between Gilbert syndrome and prevalence of vascular complications in patients with diabetes. *JAMA*. 2007;298:1398–1400.
9. Bulmer AC, Blanchfield JT, Toth I, et al. Improved resistance to serum oxidation in Gilbert's syndrome: A mechanism for cardiovascular protection. *Atherosclerosis*. 2008;199:390–396.
10. Demirbas T, Piskin T, Dayangac M, et al. Right-lobe liver transplant from donors with Gilbert syndrome. *Exp Clin Transplant*. 2012;10(1):39–42.

CODES

ICD10
- E80.4 Gilbert syndrome
- E80.6 Other disorders of bilirubin metabolism
- E80.7 Disorder of bilirubin metabolism, unspecified

CLINICAL PEARLS

- Gilbert disease: A mild chronic or intermittent unconjugated hyperbilirubinemia (not due to hemolysis) with otherwise normal liver function
- The hyperbilirubinemia results from impaired hepatic bilirubin clearance (~30% of normal). Hepatic bilirubin conjugation (glucuronidation) is reduced, although this is likely not the only defect.
- The most important reason to make the diagnosis of Gilbert disease is to reassure the patient that this is a benign condition with no known sequelae and to prevent unnecessary procedures.
- To diagnosis Gilbert disease: History, physical exam, and laboratory tests (LFTs, reticulocytosis, etc.) are normal on visits every 6 months over 18 months.
- A liver biopsy is not usually needed to rule out other liver diseases. The diagnosis can be confirmed by otherwise normal liver function tests, no evidence of hemolysis, and the response to fasting or a dose of rifampin.
- The etiology of Gilbert disease can result when the patient has a gene defect resulting in reduced conjugation of bilirubin. The gene defect is necessary but not sufficient to produce Gilbert disease.

G

GINGIVITIS

Hugh J. Silk, MD, MPH • Sheila O'Grady Stille, DMD, MAGD

BASICS

DESCRIPTION
Gingivitis is a reversible form of inflammation of the gingiva. It is a mild form of periodontal disease. Classification includes:
- Plaque-induced
- Not plaque-induced (bacterial, viral, or fungal; e.g., acute necrotizing gingivitis, Vincent disease, denture-related)
- Modified by systemic factors (e.g., pregnancy, puberty, HIV, diabetes, leukemia)
- Modified by medications (antihypertensives, antipsychotics, antiepileptics, hormones)
- Modified by malnutrition (vitamin deficiencies)
- System(s) affected: Gastrointestinal; Ears, Nose, Throat; Dental
- Synonym(s): Mild periodontal disease; Gum disease

Geriatric Considerations
More frequent in this age group (due more to additive effects than to increased susceptibility)

Pediatric Considerations
Mild cases common in children (most common form of pediatric periodontal disease) and usually require no specific interventions than improved oral hygiene

Pregnancy Considerations
- Very common in pregnant women; hormonal effect
- Hyperplasia
- Common; self-limited

EPIDEMIOLOGY
- Predominant age: >35 years (but as young as 5)
- Predominant sex: Male = Female

Prevalence
- ~50% of children
- ~90% of adolescents and adult population
- ~30–75% of pregnant women

ETIOLOGY AND PATHOPHYSIOLOGY
Inflammation of gingiva. This can progress to deeper, destructive inflammation
- Usually noncontagious
- Inadequate plaque removal
- Blood dyscrasias (pregnancy)
- Oral contraceptives
- Allergic reactions
- Nutritional deficiencies
- Vasoconstriction (nicotine, methamphetamine)
- Endocrine/Hormonal variations:
  – Pregnancy
  – Menses
  – Menarche
- Chronic debilitating disease
- Vincent disease:
  – Synergistic infection with fusiform bacillus (*Fusobacterium* spp.) and spirochete (*Borrelia vincentii*)

Genetics
Possible genetic link (up to 30% of population). Rare condition called hereditary gingival fibromatosis associated with hirsutism

RISK FACTORS
- Poor dental hygiene/plaque formation
- Pregnancy
- Uncontrolled diabetes mellitus
- Malocclusion or dental crowding
- Smoking
- Mouth breathing
- Faulty dental restoration
- HIV-positive; AIDS
- Stress
- Hospitalization (1)[A]
- Vitamin C deficiency; coenzyme Q10 deficiency
- Dental appliances (dentures, braces)
- Eruption of primary or secondary teeth
- Necrotizing ulcerative gingivitis:
  – Stress
  – Lack of sleep
  – Malnutrition
  – Viral illness
  – Typically younger patients/teens and young adults
- Bronchial asthma (2)[B]
- Rheumatoid arthritis (3)[B]

GENERAL PREVENTION
- Good oral hygiene:
  – Adults:
    ○ Regular twice-daily brushing with fluoride toothpaste and increased benefit of using circular oscillating electric brush rather than regular brush (4)[A]
    ○ Daily "high-quality" flossing (many studies show that flossing does not help because it is often done incorrectly) (5)[A]
    ○ Chlorhexidine with oral hygiene better than other oral rinse agents (6)[A]
  – Pediatrics:
    ○ Regular twice-daily brushing with fluoride toothpaste under parental supervision until full manual dexterity (~8 years of age)
    ○ Regular flossing if no spaces between teeth
- Cleaning by a dentist or hygienist every 6 months or more frequently, if indicated
- Mouth rinse with essential oils (menthol, thymol, eucalyptol; e.g., Listerine) combined with brushing reduces gingivitis more than brushing alone (7)[B].
  – Caution: Long-term use of alcohol-based mouth rinse may be associated with an increase risk of oral cancer (8)[A].

COMMONLY ASSOCIATED CONDITIONS
- Periodontitis
- Glossitis
- Pedunculated growths (pyogenic granulomata)

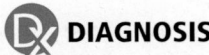

DIAGNOSIS

HISTORY
- Gum swelling and edema
- Gums are tender when touched but otherwise painless.
- Gum erythema: Bright red or red-purple appearance of gums
- Bleeding of gums when brushing, flossing, or eating
- Inquire about HIV risk, pregnancy, nutritional deficiencies, diabetes, and other risk factors as indicated (see "Risk Factors").
- Smoking history
- Oral hygiene, dental visit history

PHYSICAL EXAM
- Normal gums should appear pink, firm, and shiny.
- Gum swelling, red and edema (usually painless, except to touch)
- Erythema
- Bleeding with manipulation of gums
- Change of normal gum contours
- Plaque and calculus (not easily removed)
- Edema of interdental papillae
- HIV gingivitis:
  – Also called linear gingival erythema
  – Narrow band of bright red inflamed gum surrounding neck of tooth
  – Painful
  – Bleeds easily
  – Rapid destruction of gingival tissue and underlying support tissues (periodontal ligament, supporting alveolar bone)
- Vincent disease:
  – Ulcers
  – Fever
  – Malaise
  – Regional lymphadenopathy
  – Pain
  – Mouth odor

DIFFERENTIAL DIAGNOSIS
- Periodontitis (deeper inflammation, causing destruction to connective tissue, ligaments, and alveolar bone)
- Glossitis
- Desquamative gingivitis (painful, persistent, usually middle-aged women)
- Pericoronitis (gum flap traps food and plaque over partially erupted molar), common in adolescence
- Gingival ulcers (aphthous, herpetic, malignancy, TB, syphilis)
- Specific forms of gingivitis: See "Description," including acute necrotizing ulcerative gingivitis (Vincent disease) and HIV gingivitis (linear gingival erythema).

DIAGNOSTIC TESTS & INTERPRETATION
Initial Tests (lab, imaging)
- Possible smear or culture to identify causative agent (HIV gingivitis includes gram-negative anaerobes, enteric strains, and candida)
- Labs for contributing conditions (HIV, pregnancy, diabetes, nutritional deficiencies)
- No tests usually needed

Test Interpretation
- Acute or chronic inflammation
- Hyperemic capillaries
- Polymorphonuclear infiltration
- Papillary projections in subepithelial tissue
- Fibroblasts

TREATMENT

GENERAL MEASURES
- Stop any contributing medications
- Remove irritating factors (plaque, calculus, faulty dental restorations, or partial dentures)
- Good oral hygiene (see "General Prevention")
- Regular dental checkups (for scaling and polishing if plaque and/or tartar are present)
- Smoking cessation
- Warm saline rinses b.i.d.
- Special care needs patients: Use of tray-applied 10% carbamide peroxide gels (9)[C]

MEDICATION
First Line
- Chlorhexidine rinses or varnishes may be used (10)[B].
- Mouth rinses with essential oils (EOMW) may be equally effective to chlorhexidine for reduction of gingival inflammation (while EOMW is not as effective for plaque control) (11)[A].
- Both chlorhexidine and essential oil mouth rinses are as clinically effective as oral prophylaxis and oral hygiene instruction at 6-month recall (12)[B].
- Antibiotics indicated only for acute necrotizing ulcerative gingivitis (Vincent disease)
- Antibiotics:
  – Penicillin V: Pediatric dose, 25–50 mg/kg/d divided q6h; adult dose, 250–500 mg q6h, OR
  – Erythromycin: Pediatric dose 30–40 mg/kg/d divided q6h; adult dose, 250 mg q6h
  – Doxycycline: Adult dose, 100 mg b.i.d. first day, then q.d. × 10 days.
- Topical corticosteroids:
  – Triamcinolone (0.147 mg/g) in Orabase (spray or ointment), applied locally t.i.d., q.i.d.
- Contraindications:
  – Allergy to specific medication
- Precautions:
  – Erythromycin frequently causes significant GI issues.

Second Line
- Acetaminophen or ibuprofen for any pain (rare)
- Other antibiotics or antifungal rinses or systemics according to culture or smear
- Decapinol oral rinse (surfactant that acts as a physical barrier, making it harder for bacteria to stick to tooth and mucosal surfaces) to reduce bacteria (not recommended for pregnant women or children <12 years). Should be used in conjunction with other oral hygiene practices when those practices alone are not enough.

ISSUES FOR REFERRAL
- Dental referral for cleanings and further treatment, as needed
- If gingivitis becomes periodontitis, deep root scaling and planing may be indicated.

SURGERY/OTHER PROCEDURES
- Debridement for acute necrotizing gingivitis
- Minor surgery may be necessary to correct tissue overgrowth for gingivitis caused by medicines.

COMPLEMENTARY AND ALTERNATIVE MEDICINE
- Bilberry: Potentially helpful in reducing inflammation and stabilizing collagen tissue
- Coenzyme Q10: Topically, to restore coenzyme Q10 deficiency
- Replace any other deficiencies (e.g., vitamin C).

 ONGOING CARE

FOLLOW-UP RECOMMENDATIONS
- Outpatient
- No restrictions

Patient Monitoring
Until clear; dental follow up for continued cleanings and secondary prevention

DIET
- Well-balanced diet that includes fruits, vegetables, vitamin C; avoid sugary snacks and drinks, which contribute to plaque formation.
- Soft foods during flare, if significant inflammation/bleeding

PATIENT EDUCATION
- Good oral hygiene, including twice-daily brushing with fluoridated toothpaste and daily flossing; regular dental visits
- Printable and viewable patient information available under "periodontal diseases" from the American Dental Association at www.ada.org; and the American Academy of Periodontology at www.perio.org

PROGNOSIS
- Usual course: Acute, relapsing, intermittent, chronic
- Prognosis: Generally favorable, responds well to appropriate treatment
- Left untreated, may progress to periodontitis (controversial), which is a major cause of tooth loss

COMPLICATIONS
Severe periodontal disease (which is associated with heart disease, diabetes, and preterm birth)

REFERENCES
1. Terezakis E, Needleman I, Kumar N, et al. The impact of hospitalization on oral health: A systematic review. J Clin Periodontol. 2011;38:628–636.
2. Mehta A, Sequeira PS, Sahoo RC, et al. Is bronchial asthma a risk factor for gingival diseases? A control study. N Y State Dent J. 2009;75:44–46.
3. Nilsson M, Kopp S. Gingivitis and periodontitis are related to repeated high levels of circulating tumor necrosis factor-alpha in patients with rheumatoid arthritis. J Periodontol. 2008;79:1689–1696.
4. Robinson PG, Deacon SA, Deery C, et al. Manual versus powered toothbrushing for oral health. Cochrane Database Syst Rev. 2005;2:CD002281.
5. Sambunjak D, Nickerson JW, Poklepovic T, et al. Flossing for the management of periodontal diseases and dental caries in adults. Cochrane Database Syst Rev. 2011;12:CD008829.
6. Van Strydonck DA, Slot DE, Van der Velden U, et al. Effect of a chlorhexidine mouthrinse on plaque, gingival inflammation and staining in gingivitis patients: a systematic review. J Clin Periodontol. 2012;39:1042–1055.
7. Stoeken JE, Paraskevas S, van der Weijden GA. The long-term effect of a mouthrinse containing essential oils on dental plaque and gingivitis: A systematic review. J Periodontol. 2007;78:1218–1228.
8. McCullough M, Farah CS. The role of alcohol in oral carcinogenesis with particular reference to alcohol-containing mouthwashes. Aust Dent J. 2008;53:302–305.
9. Lazarchik DA, Haywood VB. Use of tray-applied 10 percent carbamide peroxide gels for improving oral health in patients with special-care needs. J Am Dent Assoc. 2010;141:639–646.
10. Puig-Silla M, Montiel-Company JM, Almerich-Silla JM. Use of chlorhexidine varnishes in preventing and treating periodontal disease. A review of the literature. Med Oral Patol Oral Cir Bucal. 2008;13:E257–E260.
11. Van Leeuwen MP, Slot DE, Van der Weijden GA, et al. Essential oils compared to chlorhexidine with respect to plaque and parameters of gingival inflammation: A systematic review. J Periodontol. 2011;82:174–194.
12. Gunsolley JC. Clinical efficacy of antimicrobial mouthrinses. J Dent. 2010;38(Suppl 1):S6–S10.

 SEE ALSO

- Dental Infection; Glossitis
- Algorithm: Bleeding Gums

 CODES

ICD10
- K05.00 Acute gingivitis, plaque induced
- K05.10 Chronic gingivitis, plaque induced
- K05.11 Chronic gingivitis, non-plaque induced

CLINICAL PEARLS
- Gingivitis may be prevented and treated with regular dental cleanings, good oral hygiene, and use of certain mouth rinses including chlorhexidine.
- Untreated, gingivitis may progress to periodontitis, a possible contributor to systemic inflammation and its consequences (e.g., coronary artery disease and preterm labor).
- New-onset or difficult-to-treat gingivitis, consider differential of etiology: Pregnancy, HIV, diabetes, medications, vitamin deficiencies.

G

GLAUCOMA, PRIMARY CLOSED-ANGLE

Ryan B. Feeney, PharmD • Michael C. Barros, PharmD, BCPS, BCACP • J. Michael O'Connell, Jr., MD

BASICS

DESCRIPTION
- Acute-angle closure (the term *glaucoma* is added when glaucomatous optic neuropathy is present):
  - At least 2 of the following symptoms: Ocular pain, nausea/vomiting, intermittent blurred vision with halos, *plus*
  - At least 3 of the following signs: Intraocular pressure (IOP) >21 mm Hg, conjunctival injection, corneal epithelial edema, mid-dilated nonreactive pupil, shallower chamber in the presence of occlusion
- Primary-angle closure (the term *glaucoma* is added when glaucomatous optic neuropathy is present):
  - Occludable drainage angle *plus* signs that the peripheral iris has obstructed the trabecular meshwork (e.g., elevated IOP, lens opacities)
- Chronic angle-closure glaucoma: Refers to an eye with permanent closure of areas of the anterior chamber angle by peripheral anterior synechiae

Geriatric Considerations
Increased risk with age and prior history of cataract, hyperopia, and/or uveitis

Pregnancy Considerations
Medications used may cross the placenta and be excreted into breast milk.

EPIDEMIOLOGY
- Leading cause of blindness is glaucoma of this type
- Age >40
- Female > Male
- Inuit and Asian > African and European
- Most common form of glaucoma worldwide, but only 10% of glaucoma in the US

Prevalence
Acute-angle closure glaucoma occurs in 1 in 1,000 Caucasians; 1 in 100 Asians; 2–4 in 100 Eskimos (lifetime).

ETIOLOGY AND PATHOPHYSIOLOGY
- Peripheral iris apposition to the trabecular meshwork obstructs the outflow of aqueous humor through the trabecular meshwork, which causes elevation in IOP.
- The underlying mechanism is anterior lens displacement or other anatomic abnormality, leading to pupillary block in which aqueous humor egress through the pupil is limited. This causes pressure to build posterior to the iris, leading to anterior iris displacement.
- Predisposing ocular anatomy

Genetics
Polygenic inheritance: 1st-degree relatives have a 2–5% lifetime risk.

RISK FACTORS
- Hyperopia
- Age >40
- Shallow anterior chamber
- Female gender
- Family history of angle closure
- Asian or Inuit descent
- Pseudoexfoliation
- Short axial length
- Thick crystalline lens

- Medications that may induce angle-closure glaucoma:
  - ACE inhibitors (rare), adrenergic agonists (albuterol), anticholinergics, antihistamines, antidepressants including SSRIs and TCAs, cholinergic agents (pilocarpine), noncatecholamine adrenergic agonists, sulfa-based drugs, topiramate, warfarin (rare)

GENERAL PREVENTION
- Routine eye exam with gonioscopy for high-risk populations
- US Preventive Services Task Force: Insufficient evidence to recommend for or against screening adults for glaucoma

COMMONLY ASSOCIATED CONDITIONS
- Cataract
- Hyperopia
- Microphthalmos
- Systemic hypertension

DIAGNOSIS

HISTORY
- Patient's previous medical and ophthalmologic history
- Family history of glaucoma
- Obtain history of prescription, over-the-counter, and herbal medications
- Precipitating factors (dim light, meds)
- Review of symptoms
- Acute:
  - Severe unilateral ocular pain
  - Blurred vision
  - Lacrimation
  - Photophobia
  - Halos around lights/objects
  - Frontal, ipsilateral, headache
  - Nausea and vomiting
- Chronic:
  - May have subacute symptoms (intermittent subacute attacks)
  - Compromised peripheral, then central vision
  - May be asymptomatic

PHYSICAL EXAM
- Includes, but is not limited to, the following in the undilated eye (1)[C]:
  - Visual acuity
  - Visual field testing and ocular motility
  - Pupil size and reactivity (mid-dilated, minimally reactive)
  - External examination
  - Undilated fundus exam (congestion, cupping, atrophy of optic nerve)
  - Slit-lamp biomicroscopy (anterior segments)
  - Tonometry (determination of IOP)
  - Gonioscopy (visualization of the angle)
- Acute:
  - Elevated intraocular pressure (40–80 mm Hg)
  - Corneal microcystic edema (haze)
  - Lid edema, conjunctival hyperemia, and circumcorneal injection (ciliary flush)
  - Fixed mid-dilated pupil (often oval) and firm globe
  - Shallow anterior chamber, often with inflammatory reaction (cell and flare)
  - Blepharospasm (severe cases)
  - Pain with eye movement
  - Closed angle by gonioscopy

- Chronic:
  - Multiple peripheral anterior synechiae
  - Normal or elevated intraocular pressure
  - Increased cup-to-disc ratio or excavation of disc
  - Glaucoma flecks (lens) and iris atrophy (previous acute attacks)

DIFFERENTIAL DIAGNOSIS
- Acute orbital compartment syndrome
- Traumatic hyphema
- Conjunctivitis, episcleritis
- Corneal abrasion
- Glaucoma, malignant or neovascular
- Herpes zoster ophthalmicus
- Iritis and uveitis
- Orbital/Periorbital infection
- Plateau iris syndrome
- Vitreous or subconjunctival hemorrhage
- Tight necktie, causing increased IOP
- Lens-induced angle closure

DIAGNOSTIC TESTS & INTERPRETATION
Initial Tests (lab, imaging)
US biomicroscopy

Diagnostic Procedures/Other
Careful ophthalmic examination, including gonioscopy and tonometry (1,2,3)[C]

Test Interpretation
- Corneal stromal and epithelial edema
- Endothelial cell loss (guttata)
- Iris stromal necrosis
- Anterior subcapsular cataract (*glaukomflecken*)
- Optic disc congestion, cupping, excavation
- Optic nerve atrophy

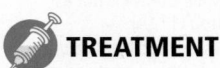

TREATMENT

Goals of treatment:
- Reverse or prevent angle-closure process
- Control IOP
- Prevent damage to the optic nerve

GENERAL MEASURES
- For acute form:
  - Manage nausea and pain.
  - Immediate ophthalmology consultation
- Ocular goals of therapy through medical and surgical treatment:

  - Reduce IOP to <35 mm Hg or by >25% of presenting IOP (4)[B].

MEDICATION

- Acute angle glaucoma is managed with PO mannitol or glycerin for a rapid decrease in IOP; after the cornea clears, a peripheral iridotomy is done.
- Initiate medical therapy first, using some or all of the following (1)[C],(4)[B]:
  - Topical/Systemic carbonic anhydrase inhibitor:
    - Acetazolamide (Diamox): 500 mg IV/PO; may repeat in 2–4 hours to a maximum of 1 g/d:
      - When used acutely, give with a topical β-blocker and topical steroid, such as prednisolone (Predsol) 0.5% solution, followed by further topical therapy to achieve IOP goals.
    - Dorzolamide (Trusopt) 2% eyedrops: 1 drop in affected eye(s) t.i.d.
    - Brinzolamide (Azopt) 1% suspension: 1 drop in affected eye(s) t.i.d.:
      - Contraindications/Precautions: Sulfa allergy (risk of cross-sensitivity)
  - β-Blockers:
    - Timolol (Timoptic) 0.5% solution: 1 drop in affected eye(s) b.i.d.
    - Timolol (Istalol) 0.5% solution: 1 drop daily in the morning
    - Timolol (Timolol GFS, Timoptic-XE) 0.25–0.5% gel-forming solution: 1 drop daily
    - Levobunolol (Betagan) 0.25–0.5% solution: 1 drop in affected eye(s) 1–2 times daily
    - Betaxolol (Betoptic) 0.5% solution: 1–2 drops in affected eye(s) b.i.d.
    - Carteolol (generic) 1% solution: 1 drop in affected eye(s) b.i.d.
    - Metipranolol (OptiPranolol) 0.3% solution: 1 drop in affected eye(s) b.i.d.:
      - Contraindications/Precautions: Decompensated heart failure, sinus bradycardia, heart block, severe COPD/asthma; increased risk of bradycardia or heart block with digoxin, verapamil, diltiazem, or clonidine; effect on IOP may be lessened in patients taking oral β-blockers
  - α₂-Agonists:
    - Apraclonidine (Iopidine) 0.5% solution: 1–2 drops in affected eye(s) t.i.d.
    - Brimonidine (Alphagan P) 0.15–0.2% solution: 1 drop in affected eye(s) t.i.d.:
      - Contraindications/Precautions: MAO inhibitor therapy, CNS depression
  - Prostaglandin analogs:
    - Latanoprost (Xalatan) 0.005% solution, Travoprost (Travatan Z) 0.004% solution, Bimatoprost (Lumigan) 0.01–0.03% solution: 1 drop in affected eye(s) nightly:
      - Precautions: Irreversible changes to iris, eyelid and eyelash pigmentation, eyelash growth, itching, redness, edema
      - Bimatoprost (Latisse) 0.03% topical solution: Indicated for hypotrichosis of the eyelashes
  - Cholinergic agonists:
    - Pilocarpine (IsoptoCarpine) (1%, 2%, 4% solution): 1–2 drops up to 6 times daily; per ophthalmologist
    - Carbachol (IsoptoCarbachol) 3% solution: 1–2 drops up to t.i.d.
    - Echothiophate iodide (phospholine iodide) 0.125% solution: 1 drop b.i.d.:
      - Precautions: May worsen the condition due to anterior rotation of the lens–iris diaphragm, impaired night vision

  - Combination products:
    - Timolol-dorzolamide (Cosopt) 0.5/2% solution: 1 drop in affected eye(s) b.i.d.
    - Timolol-brimonidine (Combigan) 0.5/0.2% solution: 1 drop in affected eye(s) b.i.d.
    - Brinzolamide-brimonidine (Simbrinza) 1/0.2% solution: 1 drop in affected eye(s) t.i.d.

ADDITIONAL THERAPIES

Keep patient supine.

SURGERY/OTHER PROCEDURES

- Acute (1,5)[B]:
  - Laser peripheral iridotomy per ophthalmology (1,5)[B]
  - Perform surgical iridectomy if laser is not possible.
- Chronic:
  - Goniosynechialysis
  - Phacoemulsification

IN-PATIENT CONSIDERATIONS

Admission Criteria/Initial Stabilization

- Patient requires metabolic ± electrolyte and volume status monitoring (with osmotic agents).
- Maintain ophthalmology follow-up.

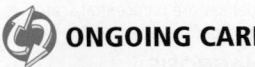 ONGOING CARE

FOLLOW-UP RECOMMENDATIONS

Schedule an immediate ophthalmologic follow-up.

Patient Monitoring

- Postsurgical follow-up
- Fellow eye evaluation
- Chronic monitoring post–acute attack per ophthalmology

DIET

Regular as tolerated

PATIENT EDUCATION

- Advise patient to seek emergency medical attention if experiencing a change in visual acuity, blurred vision, eye pain, or headache.
- If narrow angles but no peripheral iridotomy performed: Avoid decongestants, motion sickness medications, adrenergic agents, antipsychotics, antidepressants, and anticholinergic agents.
- Correct eyedrop administration technique, including:
  - Remove contact lenses before administration and wait 15 minutes before reinserting.
  - Allow at least 5 minutes between administration of multiple ophthalmic products.
- Patients with significant visual impairment should be referred to vision rehab and social services.
- Patient education materials:
  - Glaucoma Research Foundation: www.glaucoma.org
  - National Eye Institute: www.nei.nih.gov
  - Glaucoma handout from American Academy of Family Physicians
  - Handout on using glaucoma eyedrops in *Am Fam Physician* 1999;59(7):1882

PROGNOSIS

- With timely treatment, most patients do not have permanent vision loss.
- Prognosis depends on ethnicity, underlying eye disease, and time-to-treatment.

COMPLICATIONS

- Chronic corneal edema
- Corneal fibrosis and vascularization
- Iris atrophy

- Cataract
- Optic atrophy
- Malignant glaucoma
- Central retinal artery/vein occlusion
- Permanent decrease in visual acuity
- Repeat episode
- Fellow eye attack

REFERENCES

1. American Academy of Ophthalmology. *Primary Angle Closure Preferred Practice Pattern*. San Francisco: American Academy of Ophthalmology; 2010. Available at: www.aao.org.
2. Asrani S, Sarunic M, Santiago C, et al. Detailed visualization of the anterior segment using Fourier-domain optical coherence tomography. *Arch Ophthalmol.* 2008;126:765–771.
3. Barkana Y, Dorairaj SK, Gerber Y, et al. Agreement between gonioscopy and ultrasound biomicroscopy in detecting iridotrabecular apposition. *Arch Ophthalmol.* 2007;125:1331–1335.
4. Choong YF, Irfan S, Menage MJ. Acute angle closure glaucoma: An evaluation of a protocol for acute treatment. *Eye.* 1999;13(Pt 5):613–616.
5. Saw SM, Gazzard G, Friedman DS. Interventions for angle-closure glaucoma: An evidence-based update. *Ophthalmology.* 2003;110:1869–1878; quiz 1878–1879, 1930.

 SEE ALSO

Glaucoma, Primary Open-Angle

 CODES

ICD10

- H40.20X0 Unsp primary angle-closure glaucoma, stage unspecified
- H40.20X1 Unspecified primary angle-closure glaucoma, mild stage
- H40.20X2 Unspecified primary angle-closure glaucoma, moderate stage

CLINICAL PEARLS

- Examiner can determine if patient is hyperopic by observing the magnification of the patient's face through his or her glasses (myopic lenses minify).
- A careful history may reveal similar episodes of angle closure that resolved spontaneously.
- Miotics are ineffective in the setting of high IOP (due to iris sphincter ischemia) and potentially can worsen angle closure by causing anterior rotation of the lens–iris diaphragm.
- Latanoprost, a prostaglandin analog, has recently become available generically. This agent has shown greater reductions in IOP compared to β-blockers and CAIs (5)[B]. Although all of these agents can still be used as 1st-line treatment, an increase in the use of prostaglandin analogs may be seen in the future as other agents in this class become generically available and the cost of their therapy becomes comparable with these other agents. Generic latanoprost availability provides the option of once-daily medication administration, helping to improve patient adherence.

G

GLAUCOMA, PRIMARY OPEN-ANGLE

Richard W. Allinson, MD

 BASICS

DESCRIPTION
- Primary open-angle glaucoma (POAG) is an optic neuropathy resulting in visual field loss frequently associated with increased intraocular pressure (IOP).
- Normal IOP is 10–22 mm Hg. However, glaucomatous optic nerve damage also can occur with normal IOP and as a secondary manifestation of other disorders, such as corticosteroid-induced glaucoma.
- System(s) affected: Nervous
- Synonym(s): Chronic open-angle glaucoma

Pregnancy Considerations
Prostaglandins should be avoided during pregnancy in the treatment of POAG.

EPIDEMIOLOGY
Incidence
- Predominant age: Usually >40 years
- Increases with age
- Predominant gender: Male = Female

Prevalence
Prevalence of POAG in persons >40 years of age is ~1.8%.

Geriatric Considerations
Increasing prevalence with increasing age

ETIOLOGY AND PATHOPHYSIOLOGY
- Abnormal aqueous outflow resulting in increased IOP
- Normally, aqueous is produced by the ciliary epithelium of the ciliary body and is secreted into the posterior chamber of the eye.
- Aqueous then flows through the pupil and enters the anterior chamber to be drained by the trabecular meshwork in the iridocorneal angle of the eye into the Schlemm canal and into the venous system of the episclera.
- 5–10% of the total aqueous outflow leaves via the uveoscleral pathway.
- Impaired aqueous outflow through the trabecular meshwork
- Increased resistance within the aqueous drainage system

Genetics
A family history of glaucoma increases the risk for developing glaucoma.

RISK FACTORS
- Increased IOP
- Myopia
- Diabetes mellitus (DM)
- African American
- Elderly
- Hypothyroidism
- Positive family history
- Central corneal thickness <550 μm
- Larger vertical cup-to-disc ratio (CDR)
- Larger horizontal CDR
- CDR asymmetry
- Disc hemorrhage
- Prolonged use of topical, periocular, inhaled, or systemic corticosteroids
- Obstructive sleep apnea (1)[B]

GENERAL PREVENTION
Possible reduced risk of open-angle glaucoma with long-term use of oral statins among persons with hyperlipidemia (2)[C]

COMMONLY ASSOCIATED CONDITIONS
Diabetes mellitus

 DIAGNOSIS

HISTORY
Painless, slowly progressive visual loss; patients are generally unaware of the visual loss until late in the disease. Central visual acuity remains unaffected until late in the disease.

PHYSICAL EXAM
- Visual acuity and visual field assessment
- Ophthalmoscopy to assess optic nerve for glaucomatous damage
- Increased IOP
- CDR >0.5: Normal eyes show a characteristic configuration for disc rim thickness of inferior ≥ superior ≥ nasal ≥ temporal (ISNT rule).
- Earliest visual field defects are paracentral scotomas and peripheral nasal steps.

DIFFERENTIAL DIAGNOSIS
- Normal-tension glaucoma
- Optic nerve pits
- Anterior ischemic optic neuropathy
- Compressive lesions of the optic nerve or chiasm
- Posthemorrhagic (shock optic neuropathy)

DIAGNOSTIC TESTS & INTERPRETATION
Initial Tests (lab, imaging)
- Optical coherence tomography can be useful in the detection of glaucoma by measuring the thickness of the retinal nerve fiber layer (RNFL).
- RNFL is thinner in patients with glaucoma.
- RNFL thickness is affected by age, ethnicity, axial length, and optic disc area. RNFL tends to be thinner with older age, in Caucasians, greater axial length, and smaller optic disc area.
- Factors associated with variability in RNFL thickness measurements include signal-strength variability, low analysis confidence, and low RNFL thickness.

Diagnostic Procedures/Other
- Visual field testing: Perimetry
  - A multifocal intraocular lens may reduce visual sensitivity on standard automated perimetry (3)[C]
- Tonometry to measure IOP

Test Interpretation
- Atrophy and cupping of optic nerve
- Loss of retinal ganglion cells and their axons produces defects in the retinal nerve fiber layer.

 TREATMENT

GENERAL MEASURES
- Early Manifest Glaucoma Trial:
  - Early treatment delays progression.
  - The magnitude of initial IOP reduction influences disease progression (4)[A].
- Ocular Hypertension Treatment Study:
  - Patients who only had increased IOP in the range of 24–32 mm Hg were treated with topical ocular hypotensive medication.
  - Treatment produced ~20% reduction in IOP.

- At 5 years, treatment reduced the incidence of POAG by >50%: 9.5% in the observation group vs. 4.4% in the medication-treated group (5)[A].
- The Advanced Glaucoma Intervention Study:
  - Eyes were randomized to laser trabeculoplasty or filtering surgery when medical therapy failed.
  - In follow-up, if the IOP was always <18 mm Hg, the visual fields tended to stabilize. When IOP was >17 mm Hg, more than 1/2 the time, patients tended to have worsening of their visual fields (6)[A].
  - Whites did better with trabeculectomy first, whereas African Americans did better with argon laser trabeculoplasty as the initial procedure.
- Collaborative Initial Glaucoma Treatment Study:
  - Both initial medical and surgical treatment achieved significant IOP reduction, and both had little visual field loss over time (7)[A].
  - There was a 5-year risk of endophthalmitis of 1.1% after trabeculectomy (8)[A].

MEDICATION
- >1 medication, with different mechanisms of action, may be needed.
- When ≥3 medications are required, compliance is difficult, and surgery may be needed. Ocular hypotensive agent categories:
  - β-adrenergic antagonists (nonselective and selective): Decrease aqueous formation: Timolol 0.5% 1 drop in affected eye q12h
  - Parasympathomimetics (miotic), including cholinergic (direct-acting) and anticholinesterase agents (indirect-acting parasympathomimetic): Increase aqueous outflow:
    - Pilocarpine 1–4%: 1 drop in affected eye b.i.d.–q.i.d. (cholinergic)
    - Demecarium bromide 0.125%: 1 drop in affected eye b.i.d. (anticholinesterase)
- Carbonic anhydrase inhibitors (oral, topical): Decrease aqueous formation:
  - Acetazolamide: 250 mg PO q.i.d.
  - Dorzolamide 2%: 1 drop t.i.d.
- Adrenergic agonists (nonselective and selective α_2-adrenergic agonists):
  - Epinephrine 0.5–2%: 1 drop b.i.d. and Propine (dipivefrin) 0.1% 1 drop b.i.d. are both nonselective agents that increase aqueous outflow through the trabecular meshwork and increase uveoscleral outflow.
  - Brimonidine tartrate 0.1%: 1 drop t.i.d. (α_2-adrenergic agonist) decreases aqueous formation and increases uveoscleral outflow.
- Prostaglandin analogues: Enhance uveoscleral outflow and increase aqueous outflow through the trabecular meshwork: Latanoprost 0.005% 1 drop at bedtime
- Hyperosmotic agents: Increase blood osmolality, drawing water from the vitreous cavity:
  - Mannitol 20% solution: Administered IV at 2 g/kg of body weight
  - Glycerin 50% solution: Administered PO; dosage is usually 4–7 oz
- Contraindications:
  - Nonselective β-adrenergic antagonists: Avoid in asthma, chronic obstructive pulmonary disease (COPD), 2nd- and 3rd-degree atrioventricular (A-V) block, and decompensated heart failure. Betaxolol is a selective β-adrenergic antagonist and is safer in pulmonary disease.

– Parasympathomimetics (miotic): Indirect-acting parasympathomimetic agents increase risk of ocular and systemic side effects and are used rarely.
– Carbonic anhydrase inhibitors:
  ○ Do not use with sulfa drug allergies.
  ○ Do not use with cirrhosis because of the risk of hepatic encephalopathy.
– Adrenergic agonists: Caution recommended when using brimonidine and monoamine oxidase (MAO) inhibitor or tricyclic antidepressant (TCA) and in patients with vascular insufficiency. Brimonidine can cause excessive sleepiness and lethargy in children.
– Prostaglandin analogues: Caution with uveitis and avoided during pregnancy
– Hyperosmotic agents:
  ○ Glycerin can produce hyperglycemia or ketoacidosis in diabetic patients.
  ○ Can cause congestive heart failure
  ○ Do not use in patients with anuria.
• Precautions:
  – β-adrenergic antagonists: Caution with obstructive pulmonary disease, heart failure, and DM
  – Parasympathomimetics (miotic): Cause pupillary constriction and may cause decreased vision in patients with a cataract; may cause an eye ache or myopia due to increased accommodation. All miotics break down the blood–aqueous barrier and may induce chronic iridocyclitis.
  – Adrenergic agonists (e.g., brimonidine): Caution with vascular insufficiency
  – Prostaglandin analogues may cause increased pigmentation of the iris and periorbital tissue (eyelid):
    ○ Increased pigmentation and growth of eyelashes
    ○ Should be used with caution in active intraocular inflammation (iritis/uveitis)
    ○ Caution is also advised in eyes with risk factors for herpes simplex, iritis, and cystoid macular edema.
    ○ Macular edema may be a complication associated with treatment.
  – Hyperosmotic agents: Caution in diabetics; dehydrated patients; and those with cardiac, renal, and hepatic disease
• Significant possible interactions: β-adrenergic antagonists: Caution in patients taking calcium antagonists because of possible A-V conduction disturbances, left ventricular failure, or hypotension
• Parasympathomimetics (miotic): Indirect-acting parasympathomimetic agents, anticholinesterase eye drops, can reduce serum pseudocholinesterase levels. If succinylcholine is used for induction of general anesthesia, prolonged apnea may result.

SURGERY/OTHER PROCEDURES
• Argon laser trabeculoplasty (ALT):
  – Applied to 180 degrees of the trabecular meshwork
  – Improves aqueous outflow
  – The Glaucoma Laser Trial Research Group showed in newly diagnosed, previously untreated patients with POAG that ALT was as effective as topical glaucoma medication within the first 2 years of follow-up.
  – Usually reserved for patients needing better IOP control while taking topical glaucoma drops
• Trabeculectomy (glaucoma filtering surgery):
  – Usually reserved for patients needing better IOP control after maximal medical therapy and who may have previously undergone an ALT

– Mitomycin C can be applied at the time of surgery to increase the chances of a surgical success.
– Subconjunctival bevacizumab may be a beneficial adjunctive therapy for reducing late surgical failure after trabeculectomy (9)[C].
• Shunt (tube) surgery:
  – For example, Molteno and Ahmed devices
  – Generally reserved for difficult glaucoma cases in which conventional filtering surgery has failed or is likely to fail
• Tube Versus Trabeculectomy (TVT) Study:
  – After 5 years of follow-up, both procedures were associated with similar IOP reduction and the number of glaucoma medications needed (10)[A].
• Ciliary body ablation: Indicated to lower IOP in patients with poor visual potential or those who are poor candidates for filtering or shunt procedures
• Canaloplasty can control IOP in patients with POAG. Canaloplasty involves the placement of a microcatheter circumferentially through Schlemm canal, viscodilation of the canal, and placement of a nylon tensioning suture (11)[C].
• Cataract extraction can decrease IOP in patients with ocular hypertension (12)[C].

 ## ONGOING CARE

FOLLOW-UP RECOMMENDATIONS
Patient Monitoring
• Monitor vision and IOP every 3–6 months.
• Visual field testing every 6–18 months
• Optic nerve evaluation every 3–18 months, depending on POAG control
• A worsening of the mean deviation by 2 dB on the Humphrey field analyzer and confirmed by a single test after 6 months had a 72% probability of progression.
• The IOP response to ocular hypotensive agents tends to be reduced in persons with thicker corneas.

PATIENT EDUCATION
POAG is a silent robber of vision, and patients may not appreciate the significance of their disease until much of their visual field is lost.

PROGNOSIS
• With standard glaucoma therapy, the rate of visual field loss in POAG is slow.
• Patients still may lose vision and develop blindness, even when treated appropriately.
• The rate of legal blindness from POAG over a follow-up of 22 years is 19%.
• The rate of progression of visual field loss increases with older age.

COMPLICATIONS
Blindness

REFERENCES

1. Lin CC, Hu CC, Ho JD, et al. Obstructive sleep apnea and increased risk of glaucoma: A population-based matched-cohort study. Ophthalmology. 2013;120(8):1559–1564.
2. Stein JD, Newman-Casey PA, Talwar N, et al. Relationship between statin use and open-angle glaucoma. Ophthalmology. 2012;119(10): 2074–2081.
3. Aychoua N, Junoy Montolio FG, Jansonius NM. Influence of multifocal intraocular lenses on standard automated perimetry test results. JAMA Ophthalmol. 2013;131:481–485.
4. Heijl A, Leske MC, Bengtsson B, et al. Reduction of intraocular pressure and glaucoma progression: Results from the Early Manifest Glaucoma Trial. Arch Ophthalmol. 2002;120:1268–1279.
5. Kass MA, Heuer DK, Higginbotham EJ, et al. The Ocular Hypertension Treatment Study: A randomized trial determines that topical ocular hypotensive medication delays or prevents the onset of primary open-angle glaucoma. Arch Ophthalmol. 2002;120:701–713; discussion 829–830.
6. The Advanced Glaucoma Intervention Study (AGIS): The relationship between control of intraocular pressure and visual field deterioration. The AGIS Investigators. Am J Ophthalmol. 2000;130:429–440.
7. Lichter PR. CIGTS Study Group. Interim clinical outcomes in the Collaborative Initial Glaucoma Treatment Study comparing initial treatment randomized to medications or surgery. Ophthalmology. 2001;108:1943–1953.
8. Zahid S, Musch DC, Nizol LM, et al. Risk of endophthalmitis and other long-term complications of trabeculectomy in the Collaborative Initial Glaucoma Treatment Study (CIGTS). Am J Ophthalmol. 2013;155:674–680.
9. Nilforushan N, Yadgari M, Kish SK, et al. Subconjunctival bevacizumab versus mitomycin C adjunctive to trabeculectomy. Am J Ophthalmol. 2012;153:352–357.e1.
10. Gedde SJ, Schiffman JC, Feuer WJ, et al. Treatment outcomes in the tube versus trabeculectomy (TVT) study after five years of follow-up. Am J Ophthalmol. 2012;153:789–803.
11. Ayyala RS, Chaudhry AL, Okogbaa CB, et al. Comparison of surgical outcomes between canaloplasty and trabeculectomy at 12 months' follow-up. Ophthalmology. 2011;118: 2427–2433.
12. Mansberger SSL, Gordon MO, Jampel H, et al. Reduction in intraocular pressure after cataract extraction: The Ocular Hypertension Treatment Study. Ophthalmology. 2012;119:1826–1831.

 ## CODES

ICD10
• H40.11X0 Primary open-angle glaucoma, stage unspecified
• H40.11X1 Primary open-angle glaucoma, mild stage
• H40.11X2 Primary open-angle glaucoma, moderate stage

CLINICAL PEARLS
• Topical or systemic steroids can cause the IOP to increase.
• Pain is not a frequent symptom of POAG.
• Painless, slowly progressive visual loss; patients generally are unaware of the visual loss until late in the disease. Central visual acuity remains unaffected until late in the disease.
• Patients still may lose vision and develop blindness, even when treated appropriately.

G

GLOMERULONEPHRITIS, ACUTE

Carla M. Nester, MD, MSA

BASICS

DESCRIPTION

- Acute glomerulonephritis (GN) is an inflammatory process involving the glomerulus of the kidney, resulting in a clinical syndrome consisting of hematuria, proteinuria, hypertension, and renal insufficiency.
- Acute GN may be 1 of many primary diseases, or it may present as part of a systemic disease:
  - Postinfectious GN
  - IgA nephropathy–Henoch Schönlein purpura
  - Antiglomerular basement membrane disease (anti-GBM disease)
  - Antineutrophil cytoplasmic antibody (ANCA)-associated GN
  - Membranoproliferative GN (MPGN)
  - Lupus nephritis
  - Cryoglobulin-associated GN
- Clinical severity ranges from asymptomatic microscopic or gross hematuria to a rapid loss of kidney function (rapidly progressive GN [RPGN]).

ALERT
Urgent investigation and treatment are required to avoid irreversible loss of kidney function.

EPIDEMIOLOGY

- Postinfectious GN:
  - Most commonly follows group A β-hemolytic *Streptococcus* infection, but can occur as a result of other infections
  - Onset occurs 1–3 weeks after an infectious process (throat or skin).
  - Accounts for 80% of acute GN in children
- IgA nephropathy:
  - Most common form of primary acute GN
  - Occurs mainly in the 2nd and 3rd decades
  - Male > Female (3:1)
  - Incidence differs geographically: Asia > US
- Anti-GBM disease:
  - Also known as Goodpasture disease
  - A noted cause of the pulmonary–renal syndrome
  - Occurs most commonly in the 2nd or 3rd decade
  - Male > Female (6:1)
- ANCA-associated GN:
  - Uncommon: Often has a relapsing and remitting course
  - 3 disease presentations:
    - Granulomatosis with polyangiitis (formerly Wegener's granulomatosis)
    - Churg-Strauss disease
    - Microscopic polyangiitis
  - Older patients are more commonly affected, although this GN can affect any age group.
- MPGN:
  - May be primary or secondary
  - May present in the setting of a systemic viral or rheumatic illness
- Lupus nephritis:
  - 30–70% of systemic lupus patients will have renal involvement.
- Cryoglobulin-associated vasculitis:
  - 80% of cases are associated with hepatitis C infection.

ETIOLOGY AND PATHOPHYSIOLOGY

- In general, an immunologic mechanism triggers inflammation and proliferation of glomerular tissue.
- Postinfectious GN: Host immune reaction to nephritogenic strains of streptococci as a trigger.
- IgA nephropathy: Relates to an abnormal glycosylation of IgA
- Anti-GBM disease: Caused by autoantibodies that target type IV collagen of basement membranes
- ANCA-associated GN: Autoantibodies against neutrophil granules are involved in the pathogenesis.
- MPGN: An immune or genetic etiology is presumed, which triggers renal deposits and inflammation.
- Lupus nephritis: An immune complex-mediated glomerular disease
- Cryoglobulin-associated GN: An immune etiology is presumed, but not clearly defined.

Genetics
Genetic factors are likely to play a role in susceptibility to many of the acute GNs, although these have not been sufficiently defined to be useful clinically in most circumstances.

RISK FACTORS
- Epidemics of nephritogenic strains of streptococci are triggers for postinfectious GN.
- Hepatic cirrhosis and celiac disease place patients at risk for IgA nephropathy.
- Anti-GBM disease has been associated with influenza A infection and inhaled hydrocarbon solvent exposure.
- ANCA-associated GN is increased in settings where there is increased silica exposure (i.e., earthquakes and farming).
- Infection with hepatitis B and/or C are known to be associated with MPGN.
- Infection with hepatitis C is a risk factor for developing cryoglobulinemic GN.
- Mutations in alternate complement pathway genes are associated with MPGN.

GENERAL PREVENTION
Early detection is paramount.

DIAGNOSIS

HISTORY
- Patients may complain of cola- or tea-colored urine and decreased urine volume.
- Edema occurs in many patients, typically face and lower extremities.
- Shortness of breath may occur with significant fluid overload.
- Generalized malaise
- Patients may also present with complaints more specific to the associated disease:
  - Joint pain or rash in lupus nephritis
  - Hemoptysis in anti-GBM disease
  - Sinusitis and pulmonary infiltrates in ANCA-associated GN
  - Abdominal or joint pain and purpura in IgA-Henoch Schönlein purpura
  - Purpura and skin vasculitis in cryoglobulinemia-associated GN

PHYSICAL EXAM
- A complete physical exam may discover clues to systemic disease as a potential cause.
- Sinus disease: ANCA-associated GN
- Pharyngitis or impetigo: Postinfectious GN
- Pulmonary abnormality: Anti-GBM disease or lupus nephritis
- Hepatomegaly or liver tenderness could point to cryoglobulinemia-associated GN or IgA nephropathy.
- Purpura may point to ANCA-associated GN or Henoch Schönlein purpura GN.

DIFFERENTIAL DIAGNOSIS
- The differential for hematuria (without clear indication that it is of glomerular origin) should include trauma, prostate diseases, urologic cancer, or renal stone disease.
- If the urine blood is felt to be of glomerular origin, the differential should include each of the glomerular diseases that can present as an acute GN.

DIAGNOSTIC TESTS & INTERPRETATION
Initial Tests (lab, imaging)
- Urinalysis with examination of sediment: Dysmorphic RBCs or RBC casts on urine microscopy indicate glomerular hematuria and suggest the diagnosis of an acute GN.
- Electrolytes, BUN, creatinine, CBC
- Antistreptolysin O titer, Streptozyme
- Complement levels (C3 and C4):
  - C3 complement levels are abnormal in postinfectious GN; C3 and C4 are abnormal in lupus nephritis and MPGN; C4 can be low in cryoglobulinemia.
- Proteinuria: 24-hour collection or random urine protein/creatinine ratio
- Antinuclear antibody to rule out lupus nephritis
- ANCA antibody screen: MPO and PR3 antibodies
- Anti-GBM antibody
- Hepatitis B antigen
- Hepatitis C antibody
- A chest x-ray may be useful to define the significance of hemoptysis or a suspected infiltrate on exam.

Test Interpretation
Renal biopsy:
- If clinical picture is consistent with postinfectious GN in a child, a biopsy may not be required.
- If there is clinical suspicion for other causes of acute GN, renal biopsy should be done.
- Light microscopy: Diffuse hypercellularity suggests a proliferative disease, such as IgA nephropathy, lupus nephritis, or postinfectious GN.
- Immunofluorescence: IgA staining is pathognomonic for IgA nephropathy, with the absence of staining suggesting ANCA-associated GN.
- Electron microscopy: The location of immunoglobulin deposits is useful in pointing to a particular diagnosis.

TREATMENT

Supportive in postinfectious

MEDICATION
First Line
- Hypertension:
  – Diuretics are useful, given that salt retention and edema are often present.
  – Calcium channel blockers
  – Avoid ACE inhibitors if significant renal dysfunction is present.
- Peripheral edema: Loop diuretics are often required due to the degree of edema.
- Pulmonary edema: Oxygen and diuretic
- Hyperkalemia: Sodium polystyrene sulfonate (Kayexalate) resin: 15 g PO every day to q.i.d.
- Acidosis: Sodium bicarbonate 1–2 mEq/kg per dose (1–2 mmol/kg per dose) IV or PO

Second Line
- Each of the glomerular diseases often requires a specific treatment plan based on renal biopsy results; therefore, a nephrologist is often guiding care at this point.
- Pulse methylprednisolone has been reported to be useful in rapidly progressive forms of GN (1,2)[A].
- Crescents noted on renal biopsy are treated with the alkylating agent cyclophosphamide (1,2)[A].
- ANCA-associated renal disease, anti-GBM disease, and proliferative forms of lupus are treated with steroids, plus either cyclophosphamide, rituximab, or mycophenolate (1,2,3,4,5)[A].
- Plasmapheresis has been shown to be effective in cases of pulmonary hemorrhage and in some patients who present in renal failure (2)[A].
- Dialysis may be needed for uremia, hyperkalemia refractory to medical management, intractable acidosis, and diuretic-resistant pulmonary edema.

ISSUES FOR REFERRAL
Consultation with a nephrologist is usually required to assist with renal biopsy to confirm diagnosis and assist with management.

IN-PATIENT CONSIDERATIONS
Admission Criteria/Initial Stabilization
Consider admission for patients with no urine output, significant hypertension, and suspicion of pulmonary hemorrhage or fluid overload that is compromising heart or respiratory function.

Discharge Criteria
Hemodynamically stable patients without complications may be managed as outpatients.

 ## ONGOING CARE

FOLLOW-UP RECOMMENDATIONS
Patient Monitoring
Depends on type of GN:
- Regular BP checks and urinalysis to detect recurrence; assessment of renal function to detect acute or follow chronic renal disease as a result of the primary event; and regular clinical assessment to detect suspicious symptoms that may herald a recurrence (i.e., rash, joint complaint, hemoptysis)
- Periodic reassessment of serology tests to detect asymptomatic individuals

DIET
- No-added-salt diet and fluid restriction until edema and hypertension clear
- Avoid high-potassium foods if significant renal dysfunction is present.

PATIENT EDUCATION
- National Kidney Foundation, 30 E. 33rd Street, Suite 1100, New York, NY 10016; 212-889-2210
- Web site: http://vsearch.nlm.nih.gov/vivisimo/cgi-bin/query-meta?v%3Aproject=medlineplus&query=glomerulonephritis&x=48&y=10 (search under the individual disease)

PROGNOSIS
- In general, the prognosis depends on the cause of the GN.
- The GN may be self-limited (i.e., postinfectious GN) or part of a chronic disease that makes the possibility of recurrence of acute disease likely, with the potential for progressive loss of renal function over time.

COMPLICATIONS
- Hypertensive retinopathy and encephalopathy
- Rapidly progressive GN
- Microscopic hematuria may persist for years.
- Chronic kidney disease
- Nephrotic syndrome (~10%)

REFERENCES

1. Flanc RS, Roberts MA, Strippoli GF, et al. Treatment for lupus nephritis. *Cochrane Database Syst Rev.* 2004;1:CD002922.
2. Smith RM, Jones RB, Guerry MJ, et al. Rituximab for remission maintenance in relapsing antineutrophil cytoplasmic antibody-associated vasculitis. *Arthritis Rheum.* 2012;64:3760–3769.
3. Hu W, Liu C, Xie H, et al. Mycophenolate mofetil versus cyclophosphamide for inducing remission of ANCA vasculitis with moderate renal involvement. *Nephrol Dial Transplant.* 2008;23:1307–1312.
4. Walsh M, James M, Jayne D, et al. Mycophenolate mofetil for induction therapy of lupus nephritis: A systematic review and meta-analysis. *Clin J Am Soc Nephrol.* 2007;2:968–975.
5. Isenberg D, Appel GB, Contreras G, et al. Influence of race/ethnicity on response to lupus nephritis treatment: The ALMS study. *Rheumatology (Oxford).* 2010;49:128–140.

ADDITIONAL READING

Kaplan AA. The use of apheresis in immune renal disorders. *Ther Apher Dial.* 2003;7:165–172.

 ## SEE ALSO

- Hyperkalemia; Hypertensive Emergencies; Renal Failure, Acute
- Algorithm: Hematuria

 ## CODES

ICD10
- N00.9 Acute nephritic syndrome with unsp morphologic changes
- N02.8 Recurrent and persistent hematuria w oth morphologic changes

CLINICAL PEARLS
- Dysmorphic RBCs and RBC casts are a key component of the urinalysis in GN.
- Postinfectious GN in children is typically a self-limited disease.
- Searching for other organ involvement is useful in establishing a definitive diagnosis.
- With discovery of a GN, monitor the initial renal function labs frequently to identify a rapidly progressive GN.

G

GLOMERULONEPHRITIS, POSTINFECTIOUS

Kelly H. Beers, DO • Theodore B. Flaum, DO, FACOFP

BASICS

DESCRIPTION
Postinfectious glomerulonephritis (PIGN) is an immune complex disease preceded by infection with certain strains of bacteria, most commonly streptococcus and staphylococcus. The most common form of PIGN, poststreptococcal glomerulonephritis (PSGN), predominantly affects children. The clinical presentation varies from asymptomatic to the acute nephritic syndrome, characterized by gross hematuria, proteinuria, edema, hypertension (HTN), and acute kidney injury.

EPIDEMIOLOGY
A global decline in incidence, especially in developed countries, is attributed to better hygiene and a decreased incidence of streptococcal skin infections. Of cases, 97% occur in developing countries. PSGN is primarily a pediatric disease, but a recent increase has been seen in nonstreptococcal GN in the older population (>65) (1).

Incidence
- Pediatrics: 24.3 cases/100,000 persons per year in developing countries, 6 cases/100,000 persons per year in developed countries
- Adults: 2 cases/100,000 persons in developing countries, 0.3 cases/100,000 persons in developed countries (2)
- Male > Female (2:1)

Prevalence
Unknown

ETIOLOGY AND PATHOPHYSIOLOGY
- Glomerular immune complex disease induced by specific nephritogenic strains of bacteria, commonly group A β-hemolytic streptococcus (GAS) or staphylococcus
- Proposed mechanisms for the glomerular injury (3):
  - Deposition of circulating immune complexes with streptococcal antigens (4)
  - In situ immune complex formation from deposition of streptococcal antigens within the glomerular basement membrane (GBM) and subsequent antibody binding
  - In situ glomerular immune complex formation promoted by antibodies to streptococcal antigens
  - Alteration of normal renal antigen leading to molecular mimicry that elicits an autoimmune response
- Glomerular immune complex causing complement activation and inflammation:
  - Nephritis-associated plasmin receptor (NAPlr): Activates plasmin, contributes to activation of the alternative complement pathway
  - Streptococcal pyrogenic exotoxin B (SPE B): Binds plasmin and acts as a protease; promotes the release of inflammatory mediators
- Activation of the alternative complement pathway causes initial glomerular injury as evidenced by C3 deposition and decreased levels of serum C3. The lectin pathway of complement activation has also been recently implicated in glomerular injury (5).

RISK FACTORS
- Children 5–12 years of age
- Older patients (>65 years of age) (1):
  - Diabetics
  - Patients with immunocompromising comorbid conditions

GENERAL PREVENTION
- Early antibiotic treatment for streptococcal and staphylococcal infections, when indicated, although efficacy in preventing GN is uncertain.
- Improved hygiene
- Prophylactic penicillin treatment to be used in closed communities and household contacts of index cases in areas where PIGN is prevalent.

COMMONLY ASSOCIATED CONDITIONS
Streptococcal infection; staphylococcal infection

DIAGNOSIS

HISTORY
- Patients present with sudden onset of hematuria associated with edema and hypertension 1–2 weeks after an infection.
- A triad of edema, hematuria, and HTN is classic.
- PIGN in children usually follows group A β-hemolytic streptococcal (GAS) skin/throat infection.
- The latent period between GAS infection and PIGN depends on the site of infection: 1–3 weeks following GAS pharyngitis and 3–6 weeks following GAS skin infection.
- Adult PIGN most commonly follows staphylococcal infections (3× more common than streptococcal infections) of the upper respiratory tract, skin, heart, lung, bone, or urinary tract. Studies show 7–16% of cases of adult PIGN have no preceding evidence of infection and, in 24–59%, the offending microorganism cannot be identified (6).

PHYSICAL EXAM
- Edema: Present in ~2 of 3 patients due to sodium and water retention
- Gross hematuria: Present in 25–60% of patients. Urine described as "tea-colored" or "cola-colored"
- Hypertension: Present in 80–90% of patients and varies from mild to severe; secondary to fluid retention. Hypertensive encephalopathy is an uncommon, but serious complication.
- Microscopic hematuria: Subclinical cases of PIGN
- Respiratory distress: Due to pulmonary edema (rare)

DIFFERENTIAL DIAGNOSIS
The diagnosis of PIGN is generally by history once the diagnosis of acute nephritis is made, with documentation of a recent infection, with nephritis beginning to resolve 1–2 weeks after presentation. However, with progressive disease >2 weeks, persistent hematuria/HTN >4–6 weeks, or no adequate documentation of a GAS or other infection, the differential diagnosis of GN needs to be considered and renal biopsy ordered:
- Membranoproliferative glomerulonephritis (MPGN): The presentation of MPGN may be indistinguishable initially with hematuria, hypertension, proteinuria, and hypocomplementemia after an upper respiratory infection. However, patients with MPGN continue to have persistent nephritis and hypocomplementemia beyond 4–6 weeks and possibly also have a further elevation in serum creatinine. Patients with PIGN tend to have resolution of their disease and a return of normal C3 and CH50 levels within 2–4 weeks.

- Secondary causes of glomerulonephritis: Lupus nephritis and Henoch-Schönlein purpura nephritis have features similar to PIGN. Extrarenal manifestations and laboratory tests for these underlying systemic diseases help differentiate them from PIGN. Hypocomplementemia is not characteristic of Henoch-Schönlein purpura and the hypocomplementemia that occurs in lupus nephritis is with reductions in both C3 and C4, whereas C4 levels are normal in PIGN.
- IgA nephropathy often presents after an upper respiratory infection. It can be distinguished from PIGN based on a shorter time frame between the upper respiratory illness and hematuria, as well as history of gross hematuria, as PIGN recurrence is rare. IgA nephropathy is a chronic illness and will recur. Patients with IgA nephropathy have normal C3/C4 levels. Note: IgA-dominant PIGN is a newly recognized form of PIGN occurring in post-staphylococcal GN. This differs from primary IgA nephropathy in that these patients do not have a history of renal disease.
- Pauci-immune crescentic glomerulonephritis: In elderly patients with severe renal failure and active urine sediment, this is much more common, so ANCA testing should be done (1).

DIAGNOSTIC TESTS & INTERPRETATION
Initial Tests (lab, imaging)
Urinalysis with hematuria. Can be with/without RBC casts and pyuria. Proteinuria present, but nephrotic range proteinuria is uncommon in children (more likely in adults).

Follow-Up Tests & Special Considerations
- Culture: PSGN usually presents weeks after a GAS infection, only ~25% of patients will have either a positive throat or skin culture.
- Complement: 90% of patients will have depressed C3 and CH50 levels in the first 2 weeks of the disease, whereas C2 and C4 levels remain normal. C3 and CH50 levels return to normal within 4–8 weeks after presentation.
- Creatinine: Elevated to the point of renal insufficiency in 25–83% of cases, more commonly in adults (83%) (5)
- Serology: Elevated titers of antibodies support evidence of a recent GAS infection. Streptozyme test measuring antistreptolysin O (ASO), antihyaluronidase (AHase), antistreptokinase (ASKase), anti–nicotinamide-adenine dinucleotidase (anti-NAD), and anti-DNAse B antibodies: Positive in >95% of patients with PSGN due to pharyngitis and 80% with skin infections. In pharyngeal infection, ASO, anti-DNAse B, anti-NAD, and AHase titers elevated. In skin infection, only the anti-DNAse and AHase titers are typically elevated.

Diagnostic Procedures/Other
Renal biopsy rarely done in children. Recommended in most adults to confirm the diagnosis and rule out other glomerulopathies with similar clinical presentations that require immunosuppressive treatment.

Test Interpretation

- Light microscopy: Diffuse proliferative glomerulonephritis with prominent endocapillary proliferation and numerous neutrophils within the capillary lumen. Deposits may also be found in the mesangium ("starry sky"). Severity of involvement varies and correlates with clinical findings. Crescent formation is uncommon and is associated with a poor prognosis.
- Immunofluorescence microscopy: Deposits of C3 and IgG distributed in a diffuse granular pattern.
- Electron microscopy: Dome-shaped subepithelial electron-dense deposits that are referred to as "humps." These deposits are immune complexes and they correspond to the deposits of IgG and C3 found on immunofluorescence. Rate of clearance of these deposits affects recovery time.
- Renal biopsy: Usually not performed in most patients to confirm the diagnosis of PIGN as clinical history is highly suggestive and resolution of PIGN typically begins within 1 week of presentation. A biopsy is done when other glomerular disorders are being considered, such as in the case of persistently low C3 levels beyond 6 weeks for possible diagnosis of membranoproliferative glomerulonephritis, recurrent episodes of hematuria suggestive of IgA nephropathy, or a progressive increase in serum creatinine not characteristic of PIGN.

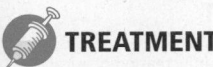

TREATMENT

MEDICATION

- No specific therapy exists for PIGN, and no evidence indicates that aggressive immunosuppressive therapy has a beneficial effect in patients with rapidly progressive crescentic disease. Despite this, patients with >30% crescents on renal biopsy are often treated with steroids (5)[B].
- Management is supportive, with focus on treating the clinical manifestations of PIGN. These include HTN and pulmonary edema:
  - General measures include salt and water restriction and loop diuretics.
  - Calcium channel blockers/ACE inhibitors may be used in cases of severe HTN (5)[B].
- Patients with evidence of persistent bacterial infection should be given a course of antibiotic therapy.

SURGERY/OTHER PROCEDURES

In patients with severe acute renal failure, dialysis may be required.

ONGOING CARE

FOLLOW-UP RECOMMENDATIONS

Patient Monitoring

- Repeat urinalysis to check for clearance of hematuria and/or proteinuria.
- Consider other diagnosis if no improvement within 2 weeks.
- Recurrence is rare.

DIET

Renal diet if requiring instances of dialysis

PROGNOSIS

- Most children with PIGN have an excellent outcome, with >90% of cases achieving full recovery of renal function.
- Elderly patients, especially adults, develop hypertension, recurrent proteinuria, and renal insufficiency long after the initial illness. Adults with multiple comorbid factors have the worst prognosis and highest incidence of chronic renal injury following PIGN.
- Complete remission in adult PIGN is only 26–56%. This has declined since the 1990s, suggesting prognosis is worsening (6).
- The presence of diabetes, higher creatinine levels, and more severe glomerular disease (e.g., crescents) on biopsy are all risk factors for developing end-stage renal disease (1).

REFERENCES

1. Nasr SH, Fidler ME, Valeri AM, et al. Postinfectious glomerulonephritis in the elderly. *J Am Soc Nephrol*. 2011;84(1):187–195. Epub 2010 Nov 4.
2. Nasr SH, Radhakrishnan J, D'Agati VD. Bacterial infection-related glomerulonephritis in adults. *Kidney Int*. 2013;83:792–803.
3. Nadasdy T, Hebert LA. Infection-related glomerulonephritis: Understanding mechanisms. *Semin Nephrol*. 2011;31(4):369–375.
4. Uchida T, Oda T, Watanabe A, et al. Clinical and histologic resolution of poststreptococcal glomerulonephritis with large subendothelial deposits and kidney failure. *Am J Kidney Dis*. 2011;58(1):113–117.
5. Ramdani B, Zamd M, Hachim K, et al. [Acute postinfectious glomerulonephritis]. *Nephrol Ther*. 2012;84(4):247–258. Epub 2012 Apr 6.
6. Wen YK. Clinicopathological study of infection-associated glomerulonephritis in adults. *Int Urol Nephrol*. 2010;84(2):477–485. Epub 2009 Aug 11.

ADDITIONAL READING

- Eison TM, Ault BH, Jones DP, et al. Post-streptococcal acute glomerulonephritis in children: Clinical features and pathogenesis. *Pediatr Nephrol*. 2011;84(2):165–180. Epub 2010 Jul 23.
- Nast CC. Infection-related glomerulonephritis: Changing demographics and outcomes. *Adv Chronic Kidney Dis*. 2012;84(2):68–75.
- Rodriguez-Iturbe B, Musser JM. The current state of poststreptococcal glomerulonephritis. *J Am Soc Nephrol*. 2008;19(10):1855–1864.
- Singh GR. Glomerulonephritis and managing the risks of chronic renal disease. *Pediatr Clin North Am*. 2009;56(6):1363–1382.

CODES

ICD10

- N00.9 Acute nephritic syndrome with unsp morphologic changes
- N05.9 Unsp nephritic syndrome with unspecified morphologic changes

CLINICAL PEARLS

- PIGN is an immune complex disease occurring after infection with certain strains of bacteria, most commonly group A *Streptococcus pyogenes*.
- The clinical presentation varies from asymptomatic to the acute nephritic syndrome, characterized by gross hematuria, proteinuria, edema, HTN, and acute kidney injury.
- Persistent nephritis and low C3 levels for >2 weeks should prompt evaluation for other causes of GN, such as membranoproliferative glomerulonephritis or systemic lupus erythematosus nephritis.

G

GLUCOSE INTOLERANCE
Nicolas Hernandez, MD • Felix B. Chang, MD

 BASICS

DESCRIPTION
- Glucose intolerance is defined as blood glucose higher than normal whose glucose levels do not meet criteria levels for diabetes
- Individuals with impaired fasting glucose (IFG) and/or impaired glucose intolerance (IGT) have been referred to as having prediabetes:
  - IFG: 100–125 mg/dL
  - IGT: 140–199 mg/dL 2 hours after ingestion of 75 g oral glucose load.
  - Hemoglobin A1C as a screening test 5.5–6.4%.

EPIDEMIOLOGY
- 1 of every 3 US adults had prediabetes in 2010.
- 79 million people in the US have prediabetes aged 20 years or older (1).
- Just 7% of people with prediabetes are aware of their condition.
- 9.3% prevalence of diabetes and 26% prevalence of IFG among adults >20 years old in the US
- 50% of all Americans aged 65 years and older have prediabetes.

INCIDENCE
- 15–30% of people with prediabetes will develop type 2 diabetes within 5 years.
- Prospective studies indicate that A1C range of 5.5–6.0% have a 5-year cumulative incidence from 12% to 25% for developing diabetes

ETIOLOGY AND PATHOPHYSIOLOGY
- Insulin resistance-increased insulin requirement
- Relative insufficient insulin secretion-beta cell dysfunction.

RISK FACTORS
- Body mass index (BMI) ≥25: Overweight.
- Obesity and metabolic syndrome
- 10-fold risk increase for future diabetes in A1C ranges 5.7–6.4%.
- HbA1c ≥6.5% at age 12–39 years associated with increased risk of death before age 55 years compared with HbA1c <5.7%

GENERAL PREVENTION
- Lifestyle modification
- Medical therapy
  - Phenteramine
  - Orlistat
  - Locaserin
  - Phentermine/topiramate ER
- Surgical therapy (BMI ≥35)
  - Lap band
  - Gastric sleeve
  - Gastric bypass
- A decrease in excess body fat provides the greatest risk reduction.
- Patients with IFG/IGT should be monitored for diabetes every 1–2 years (2)[C].
- Patients with other cardiovascular risk factors (e.g., dyslipidemia, hypertension, obesity, tobacco use) should receive appropriate counseling to modify diet and exercise. (3,4,5,6)

Pregnancy Considerations
- Screening for diabetes in pregnancy is based on risk factor analysis:
  - High risk: 1st prenatal visit
  - Average risk: 24–28 weeks' gestation
- Women with GDM should be screened for diabetes 6–12 weeks postpartum (2)[C].

COMMONLY ASSOCIATED CONDITIONS
- IFG and IGT are associated obesity (abdominal and visceral obesity)
- Dyslipidemia with high TG
- Metabolic syndrome
- PCOS
- GDM
- Low HDL
- Cholesterol
- HTN

 DIAGNOSIS

Who to screen:
- Having prediabetes, which may be called IGT and/or IFG
- Adults >45 years old
- 1st-degree relative
- Low HDL <35 mg/dL
- High TGs >250 mg/dL
- HTN: BP >140/90 mm Hg or on treatment
- Hx of GDM
- Physical inactivity
- Hx of cardiovascular disease
- Ethnic group at increased risk (African American, native American, Latino, Asian American, Pacific Islander)
- HgbA1c >5.7%, IGT, or IFG on previous testing
- Polycystic ovarian syndrome (PCOS)
- Conditions associated with insulin resistance, such as severe obesity or acanthosis nigricans

HISTORY
- No clear symptoms
- Polyuria
- Polydipsia
- Weight loss
- Blurred vision
- Polyphagia

PHYSICAL EXAM
General physical exam

DIFFERENTIAL DIAGNOSIS
- Acromegaly
- Cushing syndrome
- Glucagonoma
- Pheochromocytoma
- Hyperthyroidism
- Somatostatinoma
- Aldosteronoma

- Drug-induced hyperglycemia:
  - Thiazide diuretics (high doses)
  - Beta blockers
  - Corticosteroids (including inhaled corticosteroids)
  - Niacin
  - Thyroid hormone
  - Phenytoin
  - INF gamma
  - Pentamidine
  - Protease inhibitors
  - Atypical antipsychotics

DIAGNOSTIC TESTS & INTERPRETATION
Initial Tests (lab, imaging)
- Fasting glucose
- OGTT
- A1C
- A1C: 5–6.4% high risk for prediabetes and requires screening for glucose criteria (2)[C]

Follow-Up Tests & Special Considerations
- Fasting lipid profile
- Dcreatinine and GFR
- Urianalysis
- Thyroid-stimulating hormones

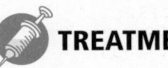 **TREATMENT**

- Structure lifestyle aimed at increasing physical activity and producing 5–10% loss of body weight, prevent or delay the development of diabetes in people with IGT.
- American Diabetes Association (ADA) recommends lifestyle modification as the primary intervention in subjects with IGT, IFG, or an A1C of 5.7–6.4%
- Specific goals include:
  - Modest weight loss (5–10% of body weight)
  - Moderate-intensity exercise (30 minutes daily)
  - Smoking cessation

- Diabetes Prevention program (DPP) participants: <60 years of age, BMI ≥35 kg/m2, women with a history of gestational diabetes. Because of its effectiveness, low cost, and long-term safety, the ADA recommends consideration of metformin for prevention of diabetes in individuals at highest risk for developing diabetes, such as those with IGT, IFG, or an A1C of 5.7–6.4%, particularly for those who benefited most from metformin (7)[A]
- Among individuals at high risk for developing type 2 diabetes, structured programs that emphasize lifestyle changes that include moderate weight loss (7% body weight) and regular physical activity (150 min/wk), with dietary strategies including reduced calories and reduced intake of dietary fat, can reduce the risk for developing diabetes and are therefore recommended (6)[A].
- For weight loss, either low-carbohydrate, low-fat calorie-restricted, or Mediterranean diets may be effective in the shortterm (up to 2 years) (6)[A].
- Individuals who have prediabetes or diabetes should receive individualized MNT (Medical nutrition therapy) as needed to achieve treatment goals, preferably provided by a registered dietitian familiar with the components of diabetes MNT (8)[A]

MEDICATION

- Metformin (drug of choice) 500 mg b.i.d. or 850 mg daily, may reduce incidence of new-onset diabetes and BMI (level 2)
- Consider metformin for prevention of type 2 diabetes in patients with IGT (6)[A]
- Consider metformin especially in patients with prediabetes if BMI >35 mg/m^2, age <60 years, or history of gestational diabetes mellitus (6)[A]
- Acarbose: Started as 50 mg PO once daily and titrated to 100 mg PO t.i.d., may reduce incidence of diabetes and might reduce incidence of myocardial infarction in patients with prediabetes (8)[B]
- Valsartan may reduce diabetes in patients with IGT but not associated with differences in cardiovascular outcomes (8)[B]

ISSUES FOR REFERRAL

- Nutritionist
- Diabetes educator/registered dietician
- Exercise physiologist

ADDITIONAL THERAPIES

Weight loss of 5–10% improves glycemic control, increases insulin sensitivity, improves lipids, and lowers BP.

ONGOING CARE

FOLLOW-UP RECOMMENDATIONS

- At least 150 min/wk of moderate-intensity aerobic exercise and/or at least 90 min/wk of vigorous aerobic exercise (2)[A]
- Resistance exercise improves insulin sensitivity to the same extent as aerobic exercise; resistance training 3×/wk is recommended for those with type 2 diabetes (2)[A].

Patient Monitoring

- Consider self-monitoring of blood glucose.
- The A1C should be measured at least twice a year in patients meeting treatment goals and quarterly in those whose therapy has changed or who are not meeting glycemic goals (2)[C].
- BP should be routinely measured.
- Annual testing for lipid abnormalities and microalbuminuria (for detection and therapy modification of incipient diabetic nephropathy)
- Annual dilated fundal exam
- Annual foot exam, including monofilament testing for distal polyneuropathy
- DIET
- Monitor carbohydrate intake.
- Low-carbohydrate diet
- Low-fat, calorie-restricted diet
- Mediterranean diet
- Maximize low-glycemic index foods,
- Low-fat (<25%) intake (3)[B]: Saturated fat intake should be <7% of total calories.
- Minimize *trans* fat intake.
- Low-sodium intake (3)[B]
- High-fiber (~50 g/d; 14 g/1,000 kcal) and whole-grain intake (3)[B]
- Drink ample quantities of water, minimum 10 glasses and strictly avoid carbonated drinks.
- Moderate alcohol intake.

PROGNOSIS

- Individuals with IFG and/or IGT have high risk for the future development of diabetes.
- Prediabetes increases the risk of developing type 2 diabetes, heart disease, and stroke.
- The potential impact of interventions to reduce mortality or the incidence of cardiovascular disease has not been demonstrated to date.
- Incidence of diabetes with A1C 6.0–6.5% is more than 10 times likely that of people with lower levels.
- A1C <6.5% range fails to identify a substantial number of patients who have IFG and/or IGT.
- A1C 5.5–6.0% has a 5-year cumulative indicidence from 12–25%. (4,5,6,8)
- HbA1c >6.5% at age 12–39 years associated with increased risk of death before age 55 years compared with HbA1c <5.7%.

COMPLICATIONS

- Cardiovascular disease
- PAD
- Stroke: 2–4 times higher risk
- Ketoacidosis
- Sexual dysfunction
- Gastroparesis
- Nephropathy and potential for renal failure
- Retinopathy and potential for loss of vision
- Peripheral and autonomic neuropathy

REFERENCES

1. Prediabetes Facts. Available at: http://www.cdc.gov/diabetes/prevention/factsheet.htm.
2. American Diabetes Association. Diagnosis and classification of diabetes mellitus. Position Statement. *Diabetes Care*. 2013;36(Suppl 1): S67–S74.
3. Pradham AD, Rifai N. Hemoglobin A1C predicts diabetes but not cardiovascular disease in nondiabetic women. *Am J Med*. 2007;120: 720–727.
4. Sato KK, Hayashi T. Combined measurement of fasting plasma glucose and A1C is effective for the prediction of type 2 diabetes: The Kansai Health Care study. *Diabetes Care*. 2009;32:644–646.
5. Shimazaki T, Kadowaki T. Hemoglobin A1c (HbA1c) predicts future drug treatment for diabetes mellitus: A follow up study using routine clinical data in a Japanese university hospital. *Translational Res*. 2007;149:196–204.
6. American Diabetes Association. Standards of Medical Care in Diabetes—2013. *Diabetes Care*. 2013;36(Suppl 1):S11–S66.
7. Maruthur NM, Ma Y, Delahanty LM, et al. Early response to preventive strategies in the Diabetes Prevention Program. *J Gen Intern Med*. 2013; 28(12):1629–1636.
8. Ramachandran A, Riddle MC, Kabali C, et al. Relationship between A1C and fasting plasma glucose in dysglycemia or type 2 diabetes: An analysis of baseline data from the ORIGIN trial. *Diabetes Care*. 2012;84(4):749–753. Epub 2012 Feb 8.

ADDITIONAL READING

- Centers for Disease Control and Prevention. National diabetes fact sheet: National estimates and general information on diabetes and prediabetes in the United States, 2011. Atlanta, GA: U.S. Department of Health and Human Services, Centers for Disease Control and Prevention, 2011.
- Diabetes risk test: http://www.diabetes.org/diabetes-basics/prevention/diabetes-risk-test/risk-test-flyer-2012.pdf
- Edelman D, Olsen MK. Utility of hemoglobin A1C in predicting diabetes risk. *J Gen Intern Med*. 2004;19:1175–1180.

 CODES

ICD10

- R73.01 Impaired fasting glucose
- R73.09 Other abnormal glucose
- E74.39 Other disorders of intestinal carbohydrate absorption

CLINICAL PEARLS

- Lifestyle optimization is essential for all patients with prediabetes.
- The potential impact of lifestyle intervention to reduce mortalitiy or the incidence of cardiovascular disease has not been demonstrated to date.
- Screening for prediabetes is part of type 2 diabetes screening.
- Research shows that you can lower your risk for type 2 diabetes by 58% by losing 7% of your body weight (or 15 lb. if you weigh 200 lb.).
- Exercising moderately (such as brisk walking) 30 minutes a day, 5 days a week

G

GONOCOCCAL INFECTIONS

Jill A. Grimes, MD, FAAFP

 BASICS

DESCRIPTION

Gonorrhea is a sexually or vertically transmitted bacterial infection caused by *Neisseria gonorrhoeae*:

- *N. gonorrhoeae* is a gram-negative intracellular diplococcus.
- Commonly presents as urethritis, salpingitis, cervicitis, pelvic inflammatory disease (PID), epididymitis, or proctitis
- Hematogenous dissemination may also occur and lead to fever, skin lesions, arthralgias, purulent or sterile arthritis, tenosynovitis, endocarditis, or, rarely, meningitis.
- Asymptomatic carrier state can occur in both sexes.
- In newborns, gonococcal ophthalmia neonatorum, a purulent conjunctivitis, may occur after vaginal delivery by an infected mother and may lead to blindness if not treated promptly.
- System(s) affected: Cardiovascular; Musculoskeletal; Nervous; Reproductive; Skin/Exocrine
- Synonym(s): Gonococcal infection (GC); Clap

EPIDEMIOLOGY

- Predominant age: 15–24 years
- Predominant sex: Prior to 1996, men > female; 2010: Women 105.5/100,000 vs. men 91.9/100,000

Incidence

CDC Stats: 2011: 321,849 reported cases (104.2/100,000 US population—a 4% increase over 2010, although a decline of 11.7% overall from 2007)

Prevalence

As a treatable disease, incidence and prevalence of diagnosed disease are approximately equal. The true prevalence is higher due to the asymptomatic nature of the disease.

- Rates peaked in mid-1970s and fell 74% over the next 20 years with national control program
- Highest rate: 20–24 year old women (584.2/100,000)
- Blacks (427.3/100,000) have 17 × greater rate than whites (25.2/100,000).
- The southern regions of the US have higher rates, with Louisiana having the highest rate by state (202.3/100,000).

ETIOLOGY AND PATHOPHYSIOLOGY

Infection requires 4 steps: (i) Mucosal attachment; (ii) Local penetration/invasion; (iii) Local proliferation; (iv) Inflammatory response or dissemination *N. gonorrhoeae* (gonococcus)

Genetics

Congenital deficiency of late components of complement cascade (C7,8,9) are prone to develop dissemination of local gonococcal infections.

RISK FACTORS

- History of previous gonorrhea infection or other STIs
- Sexual exposure to an infected individual without barrier protection (condom)
- New/Multiple sexual partners
- Inconsistent condom use
- Sex work or drug use
- Infants: Infected mother
- Children: Sexual abuse by infected individual
- Autoinoculation (finger to eye)
- For PID: Use of intrauterine devices

GENERAL PREVENTION

- Condoms offer partial protection, but must be used for oral, anal, and vaginal intercourse to be effective.
- Treat sexual contacts; consider expedited partner therapy (EPT) (1)

COMMONLY ASSOCIATED CONDITIONS

Other STIs: *Chlamydia*, syphilis, HIV, hepatitis B, herpes

 DIAGNOSIS

HISTORY

- Sexual history:
  - Number of partners and age of onset of sexual activity; STI history
  - New/Recent change in sexual partner
  - Contact with sex workers
  - Condom use
  - Menses and possibility of pregnancy
- *10% males and 20–40% of women are asymptomatic.*
- If symptoms: Onset, context, duration, timing, severity, associated symptoms, and modifying factors of symptoms:
  - Symptoms typically appear within 1–14 days after exposure (if present at all)
- Ocular symptoms: Discharge, itch, redness
- Pharyngeal symptoms: Asymptomatic infection (98%), sore throat
- GI symptoms: Acute diarrhea
- Urinary symptoms: Urinary frequency, urgency, dysuria
- Urethral symptoms: Copious urethral discharge:
  - Males: Scant to copious purulent urethral discharge (82%), dysuria (53%), testicular pain (1%), asymptomatic infection (10%), proctitis
  - Females: Asymptomatic cervical infection (20%), endocervical discharge (96%), vaginal discharge, Bartholin gland abscess, dysmenorrhea, menometrorrhagia, abdominal pain/tenderness, cervical motion tenderness, rebound, infertility, chronic pelvic pain
- Either sex, for receptive anal intercourse: Rectal discharge, tenesmus, rectal burning, asymptomatic
- Disseminated syndromes:
  - Fever, chills, malaise, dermatitis, polyarthralgia
  - Endocarditis: High fevers
  - Meningitis: Meningeal signs, headache, skin lesions, fever, altered mental status

PHYSICAL EXAM

- General: Fever, chills
- Ocular: Purulent discharge, conjunctivitis, chemosis, eyelid edema, corneal ulceration
- Pharyngeal infection: Exudative pharyngitis (<1%)
- GI: Acute diarrhea, hyperactive bowel sounds
- Genitourinary (GU):
  - Males: Scant to copious purulent urethral discharge (82%), testicular tenderness (1%), asymptomatic infection (10%), proctitis
  - Females: Asymptomatic cervical infection (20%), endocervical discharge (96%), vaginal discharge, Bartholin gland abscess, abdominal pain/tenderness, cervical motion tenderness, rebound
- Either sex, for receptive anal intercourse: Rectal discharge; may appear normal
- Disseminated syndromes:
  - Fever, chills, malaise, tenosynovitis, dermatitis, polyarthralgia, purulent arthritis

- Endocarditis: Rapid cardiac valve destruction, heart murmurs, high fevers
- Meningitis: Meningeal signs, headache, skin lesions, fever, altered mental status

DIFFERENTIAL DIAGNOSIS

Chlamydia trachomatis, UTIs, other vaginitis, or urethritis (bacterial, viral, or parasitic)

DIAGNOSTIC TESTS & INTERPRETATION

Initial Tests (lab, imaging)

The CDC recommends nucleic acid amplification (NAAT) as the most sensitive and specific test for *N. gonorrhoeae*. Other options include:

- Genital culture
- Add pharyngeal culture in adolescents (2).
- Gram stain (recommended for urethritis)
- Urethral smear, sensitivity in symptomatic male: ≥95%. Sensitivity of endocervical smear in infected woman: 40–60%. Specificity: 100%
- DNA probes and polymerase chain reaction (PCR) sensitivity: 92–99% dependent on population. Specificity: >97%; can replace culture
- Sensitivity of blood culture in disseminated disease: 50%. Sensitivity of joint fluid culture in septic arthritis: 50%
- Screen for additional STIs, especially chlamydia, syphilis, and HIV
- Imaging is not generally recommended

Follow-Up Tests & Special Considerations

- Test-of-cure testing is not generally recommended.
- Follow-up testing may be considered in cases of recurrent infection and/or in areas where significant antibiotic resistance exists.
- Pelvic ultrasound or CT scan may demonstrate thick, dilated fallopian tubes or abscess formation.

Diagnostic Procedures/Other

Culdocentesis may demonstrate free purulent exudate and provide material for Gram staining and culture. Gram staining material from unroofed skin lesions may show typical organisms.

Test Interpretation

- Exudate of polymorphonuclear leukocytes is typical.
- Gram-negative intracellular *diplococci*
- Nonpathologic gram-negative *diplococci* may be found in extragenital locations. For this reason, Gram stain of pharyngeal or rectal swabs is not recommended.

 TREATMENT

GENERAL MEASURES

- Counseling concerning risk reduction and condom use
- In children and adolescents, suspect sexual abuse.

MEDICATION

- *N. gonorrhoeae* multidrug antimicrobial resistance continues to increase: *CDC recommends dual therapy for all uncomplicated GC infections in US adults and adolescents* (both to treat for concomitant chlamydia and to increase efficacy against drug-resistant strains) (3).
- Quinolones not recommended since 2007
- *If treatment failure, check culture and sensitivities, and report to CDC through local health authorities.*
- Treat routinely with regimen that is also effective against uncomplicated genital chlamydial infection.

First Line
- Uncomplicated gonorrheal infection of the cervix, urethra, or rectum:
  – Ceftriaxone, 250 mg IM in a single dose (4)[A]
  – *PLUS* treatment for chlamydia (azithromycin 1 g PO single dose or doxycycline 100 mg PO b.i.d. for 7 days)
- Pharyngitis: Ceftriaxone, 250 mg IM once + chlamydia treatment above
- Conjunctivitis: Ceftriaxone, 1 g IM
- PID: Parenteral and oral treatments are equivalent for mild to moderate severity PID. If using IV therapy, switch to PO within 24 hours of clinical improvement:
  – Cefotetan 2 g IV q12h *OR* Cefoxitin 2 g IV q6h + doxycycline 100 mg PO or IV q12h *OR*
  – Clindamycin 900 mg IV q8h + gentamicin loading dose IV or IM (2 mg/kg of body weight), followed by a maintenance dose (1.5 mg/kg) q8h (may substitute single daily dosing)
  – Preferred "oral" regimen includes:
    ○ Ceftriaxone, 250 mg IM once + doxycycline, 100 mg PO b.i.d. for 14 days
    ○ *With or without* metronidazole, 500 mg PO b.i.d. for 14 days
- Disseminated infection in adults:
  – Ceftriaxone, 1 g IM or IV q24h until 24–48 hours after improvement begins, then switch to Cefixime 400 mg PO b.i.d. to complete at least 1 week of antibiotic treatment. *Also treat for chlamydial infection.*
- Meningitis and endocarditis:
  – Ceftriaxone, 1–2 g IV q12h 10–14 days for meningitis; 4 weeks for endocarditis
- *Contraindications:* Doxycycline *is contraindicated in pregnancy and young children.*

Pediatric Considerations
- Treatment of infants and children: <45 kg (patients >45 kg should receive full adult dose)
- Uncomplicated genital, pharyngeal, rectal, or conjunctival infection and infants born to mothers with untreated gonorrhea:
  – Ceftriaxone, 125 mg IM in single dose
  – Disseminated infections: Ceftriaxone, 50 mg/kg IV or IM daily (max dose 1 g) in single dose; bacteremia: 7 days; meningitis: 10–14 days; endocarditis: 4 weeks
- Ophthalmic neonatorum prophylaxis: Single application of erythromycin 0.5% ophthalmic ointment
- Neonatal conjunctivitis: Ceftriaxone 25–50 mg/kg IV or IM in a single dose (not to exceed 125 mg)
- Scalp abscesses (from scalp electrodes): Ceftriaxone 25–50 mg/kg/d IV or IM in a single daily dose for 7 days
- Asymptomatic infants born to mothers with untreated gonorrhea: Ceftriaxone 25–50 mg/kg IV or IM, not to exceed 125 mg, in a single dose

Second Line
- No 2nd-line agent available in the US for gonococcal infections:
  – Recent gonococcal isolates within the US have demonstrated significant rates of resistance to both azithromycin and quinolones. Neither is currently recommended as a single agent for treatment (5)[A].

– Progressive resistance to sulfonamides, penicillins, tetracyclines, and fluoroquinolones, now developing resistance in Asia, Australia, and elsewhere to 3rd-generation cephalosporins makes prevention critically important (6)[B].
– Gentamicin may become a useful alternative agent as cephalosporin resistance increases
- PID can be treated with clindamycin and gentamicin.
- For additional treatment options see the CDC report on STD treatment guidelines (including 2012 update) at: www.cdc.gov/std/treatment/2010/gonococcal-infections.htm

IN-PATIENT CONSIDERATIONS
Admission Criteria/Initial Stabilization
- Hematogenously disseminated infection
- Pneumonia or eye infection in infants
- PID: If unable to take oral medications, significant tubo-ovarian abscess, or patient is pregnant

 ## ONGOING CARE

FOLLOW-UP RECOMMENDATIONS
Patient Monitoring
US Preventive Services Task Force (USPSTF) *is being updated*, but now recommends (7)[A]:
- Screen all sexually active women if they are at increased risk of infection (*simply having a new partner is considered "increased risk"*).
- Insufficient evidence to recommend screening men at increased risk of infection
- Strongly recommend prophylactic ocular topical medication for all newborns
- Gonorrhea is a reportable disease:
  – Providers must contact both the state health department and the CDC.

PATIENT EDUCATION
- Counseling concerning risk reduction, condom use, future fertility, and full STI testing
- Encourage patient to notify partners (from past 60 days); consider *expedited partner therapy* (1).

PROGNOSIS
With adequate, early therapy, complete cure with return to normal function is the rule.

COMPLICATIONS
- Infertility
- Urethral stricture
- Corneal scarring
- Destruction of joint articular surfaces
- Cardiac valvular damage

Pediatric Considerations
Vertical transmission to newborn infants is a significant risk among patients with gonococcal infection at the time of delivery.

REFERENCES
1. Gift TL, Kissinger P, Mohammed H, et al. The cost and cost-effectiveness of expedited partner therapy compared with standard partner referral for the treatment of chlamydia or gonorrhea. *Sex Transm Dis*. 2011;38:1067–1073.

2. Giannini CM, Kim HK, Mortensen J, et al. Culture of non-genital sites increases the detection of gonorrhea in women. *J Pediatr Adolesc Gynecol*. 2010;23:246–252.
3. Campos-Outcalt D. CDC update on gonorrhea: Expand treatment to limit resistance. *J Fam Pract*. 2011;60:736–740.
4. Bai ZG, Bao XJ, Cheng WD, et al. Efficacy and safety of ceftriaxone for uncomplicated gonorrhoea: A meta-analysis of randomized controlled trials. *Int J STD AIDS*. 2012;23:126–132.
5. Centers for Disease Control and Prevention (CDC). Update to CDC's sexually transmitted diseases treatment guidelines, 2006: Fluoroquinolones no longer recommended for treatment of gonococcal infections. *MMWR Morb Mortal Wkly Rep*. 2007;56:332–336.
6. Barry PM, Klausner JD. The use of cephalosporins for gonorrhea: The impending problem of resistance. *Expert Opin Pharmacother*. 2009;10:555–577.
7. *Screening for Gonorrhea*, Topic Page. May 2005. U.S. Preventive Services Task Force. Available at: www.uspreventiveservicestaskforce.org/uspstf/uspsgono.htm

ADDITIONAL READING
- Centers for Disease Control and Prevention (CDC). Cephalosporin susceptibility among Neisseria gonorrhoeae isolates–United States, 2000–2010. *MMWR Morb Mortal Wkly Rep*. 2011;60:873–877.
- Dowell D, Kirkcaldy RD. Effectiveness of gentamicin for gonorrhea treatment: systematic review and meta-analysis. *Postgrad Med J*. 2013;89:142–147.
- Jamil MS, Hoking JS, Bauer HM, et al. Home-based chlamydia and gonorrhea screening: A systematic review of strategies and outcomes. *BMC Public Health*. 2013;12:189.

 ## SEE ALSO

Chlamydial Sexually Transmitted Diseases; HIV Infection and AIDS; Pelvic Inflammatory Disease; Syphilis

 ## CODES

ICD10
- A54.01 Gonococcal cystitis and urethritis, unspecified
- A54.9 Gonococcal infection, unspecified
- A54.24 Gonococcal female pelvic inflammatory disease

CLINICAL PEARLS
- Gonorrhea antibiotic resistance is a severe problem that continues to expand, and treatment recommendations have changed to include routine dual therapy.
- Patients testing positive for gonorrhea should also be considered for additional STI testing, including chlamydia, syphilis, HIV, and hepatitis.
- Treat also for chlamydia, unless chlamydia infection ruled out.

G

GOUT

Timothy D. Pelkowski, MD, MS, FAAFP

BASICS

DESCRIPTION
- Gout is an inflammatory arthritis related to a hyperuricemia (serum uric acid [SUA] level >6.8 mg/dL) (1).
- Acute gouty arthritis can affect ≥1 joints; the 1st metatarsophalangeal joint is most commonly involved at presentation (podagra).
- Although hyperuricemia is necessary for the development of gout, it is not the only determining factor.
- Characterized by deposition of monosodium urate (MSU) crystals that accumulate in joints and soft tissues; resulting in acute and chronic arthritis, soft-tissue masses called tophi, urate nephropathy, and uric acid nephrolithiasis.
- After an initial flare, a 2nd flare occurs in ~60% of patients within 1 year and 78% within 2 years of the initial attack (2).
- Management involves treating acute attacks and preventing recurrent disease by long-term reduction of SUA levels through pharmacology and lifestyle adjustments.

EPIDEMIOLOGY
Incidence
Annual incidence of gout (3):
- Uric acid 7–8.9 mg/dL is 0.5%
- Uric acid >9 mg/dL is 4.5%

Prevalence
- Increasing prevalence over the past decades (3).
- 2007–2008 prevalence of gout in the US (3):
  – Men 5.8% (6.1 million)
  – Women 2.0% (2.2 million)
- 2008 prevalence of hyperuricemia in the US (3):
  – Men 21.2% (SUA >7.0 mg/dL)
  – Women 21.6% (SUA >5.7 mg/dL)

ETIOLOGY AND PATHOPHYSIOLOGY
- Hyperuricemia results from urate overproduction, underexcretion, or often a combination of the 2.
- Gout occurs when monosodium urate, a product of purine metabolism, precipitates out of solution and accumulates in joints and soft tissues.
- Transient changes in urate solubility caused by local temperature decrease, trauma, or acidosis, may lead to an acute gouty attack.
- Urate crystals that precipitate trigger an immune response.
- Left untreated, this crystal deposition leads to permanent joint damage and tophus formation.

Genetics
- Phosphoribosyl pyrophosphate (PRPP) deficiency and hypoxanthine-guanine-phosphoribosyltransferase (HGPRT) deficiency (Lesch-Nyan syndrome) are inherited enzyme defects associated with overproduction of uric acid.
- Polymorphisms in the URAT1 and SLC 2A9 (GLUT9) renal transporters are hereditary enzyme defects resulting in primary underexcretion of uric acid.

RISK FACTORS
- Age >40
- Male gender
- Increased purine uptake (meats and seafood)
- Alcohol intake (especially beer)
- High fructose intake
- Obesity

- Hyperuricemia
- Congestive heart failure
- Coronary artery disease
- Dyslipidemia
- Renal disease
- Organ transplant
- Hypertension
- Hyperinsulinemia
- Metabolic syndrome
- Diabetes mellitus
- Urate-elevating medications:
  – Thiazide diuretics
  – Loop diuretics
  – Niacin
  – Calcineurin inhibitors (cyclosporine and tacrolimus)
  – Acetylsalicylic acid (not recommended to stop this medication in those with cardiac disease)

GENERAL PREVENTION
- Maintain optimal weight.
- Regular exercise
- Diet modification
- Reduce alcohol consumption (beer and liquor).
- Maintain fluid intake and avoid dehydration.

COMMONLY ASSOCIATED CONDITIONS
- Hypertension
- Dyslipidemia
- Nontraumatic joint disorders
- Heart disease
- Urinary tract disease
- Diabetes mellitus
- Metabolic syndrome
- Obesity
- Renal disease

DIAGNOSIS

HISTORY
- Classic presentation of acute gouty arthritis:
  – Intense pain and tenderness in the 1st metatarsophalangeal joint (podagra)
  – Can occur in the midtarsal, ankle, or knee joints
  – Joint may be swollen, warm, and red
  – Often awakes patients from sleep due to an intolerance to contact with clothing or bed sheets
  – There is a rapid onset of intense pain, often beginning in the early morning and progressing rapidly over 12–24 hours.
  – In the absence of treatment, flares can last up to 10 days.
- Fever can be seen.
- SC or intraosseous nodules, referred to as tophi
- Pain with urination secondary to uric acid renal stones

PHYSICAL EXAM
- Examine suspected joint(s) for tenderness, swelling, and range of motion (ROM).
- Assess for presence of firm nodules known as tophi.

DIFFERENTIAL DIAGNOSIS
Acute bursitis, tendonitis, septic arthritis, pseudogout (calcium pyrophosphate deposition disease), cellulitis, osteoarthritis

DIAGNOSTIC TESTS & INTERPRETATION
- Serum uric acid (may be normal during an acute flare).

- CBC (can see elevation of WBC during an acute gout flare).
- Synovial fluid analysis: Urate crystals (negatively birefringent under polarizing microscopy), cell count (WBC usually 2,000–50,000/mm³); culture to rule out infection. Some guidelines suggest that gout can be diagnosed clinically without synovial fluid analysis.
- Screen for uric acid overproduction 24-hour urine uric acid in those patients with gout onset before the age of 25 or a history of urolithiasis (1)[C].
- Radiograph is normal early in disease but can reveal:
  – Swelling in acute gout
  – Periarticular erosions with periosteum overgrowth in chronic gout
- Urate kidney stones are radiolucent and thus invisible on radiograph.

TREATMENT

GENERAL MEASURES
Topical ice as needed (4)[B]

MEDICATION
- Acute Treatment
  – General principles:
    ○ Acute gouty arthritis attacks should be treated with pharmacologic therapy (4)[C].
    ○ Pharmacologic treatment should be initiated within 24 hours of acute gout attack onset (4)[C].
    ○ Ongoing pharmacologic urate-lowering therapy should not be interrupted during an acute gout attack (4)[C].
    ○ Choice of agent is based on severity of pain and the number of joints involved (4).
  – Mild/moderate gout severity (≤6 of 10 on visual analog pain scale, particularly for an attack involving only 1 or a few small joints or 1–2 large joints).
    ○ NSAIDs:
      ▪ Naproxen: 750 mg followed by 250 mg q8h for 5–8 days (4)[A]
      ▪ Indomethacin: 50–150 mg/d for 2–7 days (4)[A].
      ▪ Sulindac: 200 mg b.i.d. for 7–10 days (4)[A]
      ▪ Celecoxib:
        □ Not FDA approved, but can be considered in selected patients with contraindications or intolerance to NSAIDs (4)[B].
        □ Dose at 800 mg once followed by 400 mg on day 1, then 400 mg b.i.d. for 1 week (4)[B].
    ○ Corticosteroids:
      ▪ Those with an acute flare involving 1–2 large joints can consider intra-articular corticosteroids; can consider using PO corticosteroids in combination.
      ▪ For other acute flares use PO corticosteroids:
        □ Prednisone: 0.5 mg/kg/d for 5–10 days (4)[A] or alternately 2–5 days at full dose followed by tapering for 7–10 days and then discontinuing (4)[C]
        □ Methylprednisolone dose pack (4)[C]
        □ Triamcinolone acetonide: 60 mg IM single dose followed by oral corticosteroids (4)[C]

○ Colchicine:
- Used for gout attacks where the onset was <36 hours prior to treatment initiation (4)[A]
- Begin a loading dose of 1.2 mg followed by 0.6 mg 1 hour later, followed by 0.6 mg once or twice daily 12 hours later, until the gout attack resolves (4)[C].
- Dose reduction recommended in moderate to severe kidney disease and in those on inhibitors of cytochrome P450 3A4 and P-glycoprotein (clarithromycin, erythromycin, cyclosporine, and disulfiram) (4)

– Severe gout (≥7 of 10 on visual analog pain scale, involving ≥4 joints with arthritis involving >1 region, or involving 3 separate large joints):
○ Initial combination therapy is an option and includes the use of full doses of (4)[C]:
- Colchicine and NSAIDs
- PO corticosteroids and colchicine
- Intra-articular steroids with all other modalities
– For patients not responding to initial pharmacologic monotherapy, add a 2nd agent (4)[C].

• Chronic Treatment
– Indications for pharmacologic urate-lowering therapy include any patient with:
○ Tophus or tophi by clinical exam or imaging study (1)[A]
○ Frequent attacks of acute gouty arthritis (≥2 attacks/year) (1)[A]
○ Chronic kidney disease stage 2 or worse (1)[C]
○ Past urolithiasis (1)[C]
– Treat to the serum urate:
○ Minimum serum urate target is <6 mg/dL (1)[A]
○ Serum urate target may need to be <5 mg/dL to improve gout signs and symptoms (1)[B].
– Urate-lowering agents can be prescribed during an acute attack (1)[C].
– Pharmacologic antiinflammatory prophylaxis recommended with or just prior to initiating urate lowering therapy
○ 1st line:
- Low-dose colchicine: 0.6 mg once or twice daily (4)[A]
- Low-dose NSAIDs with proton pump inhibitor where indicated: Naproxen 250 mg PO b.i.d. (4)[C]
○ 2nd line: Use if colchicines and NSAIDs both are not tolerated, contraindicated, or ineffective:
- Low dose prednisone or prednisolone at ≤10 mg/d (4)[C]
○ Treatment duration for the greater of:
- At least 6 months (4)[A] *or*
- 3 months after achieving serum urate appropriate for the patient with no tophi on exam (4)[B] or for 6 months after achieving serum urate appropriate for the patient with ≥1 tophi on exam (4)[C]

– Pharmacologic urate lowering agents:
○ Allopurinol: Xanthine oxidase inhibitor (1)[A]:
- Starting dose should be no higher than 100 mg/d (1)[B].
- Gradually titrate the dose upward q2–5wks to appropriate maximum dose (1)[C].
- Dose can be >300 mg/d, even with renal impairment, as long as accompanied by patient education and monitoring for drug toxicity; maximum FDA approved dosage is 800 mg/d (1)[B]

- Regularly monitor for allopurinol hypersensitivity syndrome (AHS), pruritus, rash, elevated hepatic transaminases, eosinophilia
- Screening for the HLA-B*5801 allele for AHS should be performed in those of Korean, Han Chinese, or Thai descent (1)[A].
○ Febuxostat: Selective xanthine oxidase inhibitor (1)[A]:
- No renal or hepatic adjustments needed for mild-to-moderate hepatic or renal impairment
- Starting dose 40 mg/d; may be titrated to 80 mg/d
- In select instances, may dose up to 120 mg/d (not FDA approved) (1)[A].
○ Probenecid: Uricosuric agent (1)[B]:
- Alternative 1st-line urate-lowering therapy; use if at least 1 xanthine oxidase inhibitor is contraindicated or not tolerated (1)[B]
- Multiple drug interactions exist, as well as risk of urolithiasis with this agent.
- Not recommended if CrCl is <50 or with patient history of urolithiasis (1)[C].
- Starting dose is 250 mg b.i.d.; gradually titrate to 2,000 mg/d

• Other Treatment
– Acute treatment: Adrenocorticotropic hormone (ACTH): 25–40 IU SC (4)[A]; especially in those NPO
– Pegloticase in select severe instances (1)

SURGERY/OTHER PROCEDURES
• Large tophi that are infected or interfering with joint motion may need to be surgically removed.

 ONGOING CARE

FOLLOW-UP RECOMMENDATIONS
Patient Monitoring
• SUA q2–5wks while titrating urate-lowering treatment to goal (1)[C]
• Regularly monitor CBC, renal, liver function test, and urinalysis.

DIET
• General lack of evidence regarding specific recommendations, although the American College of Rheumatology has outlined the following (1)[C]:
• General measures:
– Weight loss for obese patients
– Healthy overall diet
– Exercise
– Smoking cessation
– Stay well hydrated
• Avoid:
– Organ meats high in purine content (sweetbreads, liver, kidney) (1)[A]
– High-fructose corn syrup-sweetened sodas, other beverages, or foods
– Alcohol overuse (>2 servings per day for men and >1 serving per day for women) (1)[A]
– Any alcohol use in gout during periods of frequent gout attacks or advanced gout under poor control
• Limit:
– Serving sizes of beef, lamb, pork, seafood with high purine content such as sardines and shellfish (1)[B]
– Servings of naturally sweetened fruit juices

– Table sugar and sweetened beverages and desserts
– Table salt, including in sauces and gravies
– Alcohol (particularly beer) in all gout patients (1)[B]
• Encourage:
– Low-fat or nonfat dairy products (1)[B]
– Vegetables

PATIENT EDUCATION
• Dietary and lifestyle modifications (1)[B].
• Patient instructions on initiating treatment on signs and symptoms of an acute gout attack without the need to consult health care provider for each attack (1)[B]
• Discussion that gout is caused by excess uric acid and that effective urate-lowering therapy is essential treatment (1)[B].

PROGNOSIS
Gout can usually be successfully managed with proper treatment.

COMPLICATIONS
• Allopurinol hypersensitivity syndrome
• Increased susceptibility to infection
• Urate nephropathy
• Renal stones

REFERENCES
1. Khanna D, Fitzgerald JD, Khanna PP, et al. 2012 American College of Rheumatology guidelines for management of gout. Part 1: Systematic nonpharmacologic and pharmacologic therapeutic approaches to hyperuricemia. *Arthritis Care Res.* 2012;64:1431–1446.
2. Doghramji PP. Managing your patient with gout: a review of treatment options. *Postgrad Med.* 2011;123:56–71.
3. Zhu Y, Pandya BJ, Choi HK. Prevalence of gout and hyperuricemia in the US general population: The National Health and Nutrition Examination Survey 2007–2008. *Arthritis Rheum.* 2012;64: 3136–3141.
4. Khanna D, Khanna PP, Fitzgerald JD, et al. 2012 American College of Rheumatology guidelines for management of gout. Part 2: Therapy and antiinflammatory prophylaxis of acute gouty arthritis. *Arthritis Care Res.* 2012;64:1447–1461.

 CODES

ICD10
• M10.00 Idiopathic gout, unspecified site
• M10.079 Idiopathic gout, unspecified ankle and foot
• M10.9 Gout, unspecified

CLINICAL PEARLS
• MSU crystals found in synovial fluid aspirate are pathognomonic for gout.
• Acute gout and sepsis can coexist.
• Asymptomatic hyperuricemia does not require treatment.
• Pharmacologic urate-lowering therapy can be started during an acute gouty attack, provided that effective anti-inflammatory management is instituted.
• Reduce SUA level to <6 mg/dL to eliminate gout flares and tophi.

GRANULOMA ANNULARE
M. Tye Haeberle, MD • Peter J Hayes, MD • Timothy S. Brown, MD

 BASICS

DESCRIPTION
A benign skin condition characterized by grouped papules, which typically occur in an annular pattern. 5 variants have been described, the most common of which is localized granuloma annulare (GA). The other types are generalized, patch-type, SC (deep dermal), and perforating.

EPIDEMIOLOGY
Incidence
- GA is not common, although its occurrence in the general population is unknown.
- Predominant sex: Female > Male (2:1)
- Most lesions resolve in 2–24 months, but may last up to 5–10 years. 2/3 of patients are <30, and the age distribution varies by type, as follows:
  - Localized: Children and adults <30
  - Generalized: Bimodal: Children <10 and adults 30–60
  - Patch-type: Adults >30
  - SC: Children 2–10
  - Perforating: Typically children, but also young adults

Prevalence
Among cases of GA, the approximate distribution is as follows:
- Localized: 75%
- Generalized: 10–15%
- Patch-type: <5%
- SC: <5%
- Perforating: <5% (perhaps higher in Hawaii)

ETIOLOGY AND PATHOPHYSIOLOGY
The cause of GA remains unknown, although it is hypothesized to be a delayed-type hypersensitivity to an unknown antigen.

Genetics
There is some evidence for a possible hereditary component.

RISK FACTORS
No definite risk factors have been identified. There is weak evidence for possible associations with diabetes mellitus, TB, HIV, EBV and other viral infections, interferon-α therapy, trauma, insect bites, borreliosis, and malignancies (most commonly lymphoma).

GENERAL PREVENTION
There are no established strategies for preventing GA.

COMMONLY ASSOCIATED CONDITIONS
A recent case-control study found that those patients with granuloma annulare were more likely to have dyslipidemia, with the strongest association seen in patients with generalized subtype (1)

 DIAGNOSIS

HISTORY
Cutaneous lesions of GA are generally asymptomatic. They may persist for months or years; longer duration is more often seen in the generalized subtype. They typically resolve spontaneously, and they may recur.

PHYSICAL EXAM
- Localized: Small (1–2 mm) papules arranged in a ring, which may enlarge from 5 mm–5 cm. Color may range from skin-colored to red. The most common locations are the dorsal aspects of the distal extremities.
- Generalized: Similar to localized, but a higher number of lesions (>10), which are more diffuse distribution, often larger, and typically persist longer
- Patch-type: Erythematous macules and patches distributed symmetrically on the extremities and trunk. The typical annular configuration may not be present.
- SC: Firm, nontender, SC nodule, which tends to grow rapidly. Usually solitary, but may occur in groups. Most common location is lower extremities, especially pretibial; other sites include upper extremities, scalp, buttocks
- Perforating: Papules may be up to 4 mm and display umbilication, crusting, or scale. Lesions are often generalized and may occur anywhere.

DIFFERENTIAL DIAGNOSIS
- Localized: Tinea corporis, annular lichen planus, necrobiosis lipoidica, pityriasis rosea, erythema migrans of Lyme disease, leprosy
- Generalized: Sarcoidosis, lichen planus, cutaneous metastases, mycosis fungoides
- Patch-type: Erythema migrans
- SC: Rheumatoid nodule
- Perforating: Molluscum contagiosum, sarcoidosis, insect bites

DIAGNOSTIC TESTS & INTERPRETATION
Initial Tests (lab, imaging)
- Diagnosis is typically established by the history and physical, so lab investigations are rarely needed. Skin scraping/KOH test may be useful for excluding a fungal process.
- Consideration could be given to testing for dyslipidemia (1)[B].
- Rarely indicated, but may occasionally be useful in the workup of suspected SC subtype

Diagnostic Procedures/Other
Skin punch biopsy is useful to confirm the diagnosis and designate subtype. Immunohistochemical streptavidin-biotin-horseradish peroxidase (HRP) analysis for CD68/KP-1, which is a marker for histiocytic differentiation, may aid in the diagnosis.

Test Interpretation
Dermal granulomatous infiltrate demonstrating foci of degenerative collagen associated with palisading around an anuclear dermis with mucin deposition. Histologic variants include interstitial (histiocytic infiltrate between collagen fibers), classic (palisading dermal granulomas), and epithelioid (tuberculoid and sarcoidal granulomas) (2).

TREATMENT

GENERAL MEASURES
GA is a self-limited, asymptomatic condition that is likely to regress spontaneously (3)[C]. The clinician's primary role after diagnosis is to educate the patient regarding the anticipated natural history and to provide reassurance.

MEDICATION
- No strong evidence supports therapeutic intervention for GA. Reassurance with observation may be adequate treatment for localized, asymptomatic disease.
- The trauma induced by biopsy alone can cause involution of the lesions through an unknown mechanism (4).
- The following therapies have been tried with variable success, and the possible benefit of treatment must be weighed against the significant toxicities of these treatments.

First Line
Corticosteroids:
- High-potency topical, with or without occlusion
- Intralesional triamcinolone: 2.5–5 mg/mL (5)[B]

Second Line
- Methotrexate: 15 mg IM weekly
- Rifampin: 600 mg, ofloxacin 400 mg, minocycline 100 mg once-daily combination therapy
- Tacrolimus 0.1% ointment b.i.d.
- Pimecrolimus 1% cream b.i.d.
- Isotretinoin: 0.5–0.75 mg/kg/d
- Dapsone: 100 mg/d
- Chloroquine: 3 mg/kg/d
- Hydroxychloroquine: 6 mg/kg/d
- Cyclosporine: 3–4 mg/kg/d
- Niacinamide: 500 mg t.i.d.
- TNF-α inhibitors, such as Infliximab 5 mg/kg IV or adalimumab 80 mg SC × 1 for the 1st week then 40 SC × 1 for weeks 2–4

ADDITIONAL THERAPIES
- Fractional thermolysis (Er:YAG fractionated laser) (4)[B]
- Psoralen ultraviolet A (PUVA) (1)[B]
- Cryotherapy
- Surgical excision for SC GA

 ## ONGOING CARE

FOLLOW-UP RECOMMENDATIONS
Routine follow-up is not required unless treatment is initiated. Then follow-up may be important to monitor for possible adverse effects associated with treatment. Referral to a dermatologist is prudent in cases of generalized GA and in those cases that persist despite conservative therapy (5).

PATIENT EDUCATION
The patient should be educated that GA is a benign, self-limited condition that may persist a long time, resolve, and/or recur.

PROGNOSIS
>50% of cases resolve spontaneously within 2 months–2 years, although recurrence—typically at the original site—is common (>40%) (5). Patients <39 have been shown to have a shorter duration (3) of illness.

COMPLICATIONS
Complications of treatment are much more likely than complications from GA.

REFERENCES
1. Wu W, Robinson-Bostom L, Kokkotou E. Dyslipidemai in granuloma annulare. *Arch Dermatol*. 2012;148(10):1131–1136.
2. Marcus DV, Mahmoud BH, Hamzavi IH. Granuloma annulare treated with rifampin, ofloxacin, and minocycline combination therapy. *Arch Dermatol*. 2009;145(7):787–789.
3. Misago N, Narisawa Y. Subcutaneous granuloma annulare with overlying localized granuloma annulare. *J Dermatol*. 2010;37(8):755–757.
4. Liu A, Hexsel CL, Moy RL. Granuloma annulare successfully treated using fractional photothermolysis with a 1,550-nm erbium-doped yttrium aluminum garnet fractionated laser. *Dermatol Surg*. 2011;37(5):712–715.
5. Cyr PR. Diagnosis and management of granuloma annulare. *Am Fam Physician*. 2006;74(10):1729–1734.

ADDITIONAL READING
- Browne F, Turner D, Goulden V. Psoralen and ultraviolet A in the treatment of granuloma annulare. *Photodermatol Photoimmuno Photomed*. 2011;27(2):81–84.
- Duarte AF, Mota A. Generalized granuloma annulare—response to doxycycline. *J Eur Acad Dermat and Vener*. 2009;23:84–85.
- Mazzatenta C, Ghilardi A, Grazzini M. Treatment of disseminated granuloma annulare with allopurinol: Case report. *Dermatol Therapy*. 2010;23:S24–S27.
- Plotner AN, Mutasim DF. Successful treatment of disseminated granuloma annulare with methotrexate. *Br J Dermatol*. 2010;163(5):1123–1124.
- Shanmuga SC, Rai R, Laila A, et al. Generalized granuloma annulare with tuberculoid granulomas: A rare histiopathologic variant. *Indian J Dermatol Venereol Leprol*. 2010;76(1):73–75.
- Werchau S, Enk A, Hartmann M. Generalized interstitial granuloma annulare–response to adalimumab. *Int J Dermatol*. 2010;49:457–460.

 ## CODES

ICD10
L92.0 Granuloma annulare

CLINICAL PEARLS
- This condition is benign.
- In cases of suspected tinea that lack scaling, consider GA.
- Consider lipid testing, especially in those with generalized subtype.

G

BASICS

DESCRIPTION
- Pyogenic granuloma are benign, acquired, solitary vascular proliferations that involve exposed areas of the skin, such as the distal extremities (especially the hands) and face, the oral cavity (most frequently the gingiva), and subcutaneous tissue.
- Tendency to bleed easily due to the vascular nature of the lesion
- Smooth, red to purple, sessile or pedunculated, grow rapidly
- System(s) affected: Gastrointestinal; Skin (external ear canal)/Exocrine; Eye (i.e., eyelid, lacrimal sac)
- Synonym(s): Pregnancy tumor; granuloma gravidarum; granuloma telangiectaticum; lobular capillary hemangioma

EPIDEMIOLOGY
Mean age of patients with pyogenic granuloma is 40.5 years

Incidence
- In children, pyogenic granuloma accounts for <1% of all skin nodules.
- 5% of pregnant women in the US are affected.

Prevalence
Relatively common condition

ETIOLOGY AND PATHOPHYSIOLOGY
- Thought to be an aberrant healing response to minor trauma in many cases
- May be related to hormonal changes in pregnancy
- Not caused by bacterial infection, but associated with capillary proliferation
- Not considered a hemangioma or neoplasm
- Associated with acute and chronic trauma, peripheral nerve injury, inflammatory systemic diseases, infection, drugs (systemic steroids, antiretroviral therapy, epidermal growth factor receptor inhibitors) (1)

RISK FACTORS
- Pregnancy
- Trauma
- Intraoral trauma or surgery
- Inflammatory systemic diseases

GENERAL PREVENTION
Good oral hygiene

DIAGNOSIS

HISTORY
- Solitary lesion that develops rapidly from days to weeks after minor trauma
- Tends to bleed easily
- Grows early in pregnancy and partially regresses postpartum

PHYSICAL EXAM
- Most commonly located at head, neck, and upper extremities
- Among oral lesions, gingiva is the most common location
- Bright red, purple, yellow, or brown
- Moist and sometimes scaly-appearing surface
- Usually <1 cm, but ranges from a few millimeters to 2–3 cm in diameter
- Giant lesions may occur on areas such as the foot (rare)
- Soft; sessile or pedunculated
- Granular, smooth, or slightly nodular
- Solitary red papule, grows rapidly, forming a stalk, may bleed and ulcerate
- Red structureless areas surrounded by a white collarette intersected by white lines (2)
- Erythematous, soft compressible papule with serosanguineous crusting and sharp demarcation

DIFFERENTIAL DIAGNOSIS
- Peripheral ossifying granuloma
- Giant cell granuloma
- Odontogenic fibroma
- Kaposi sarcoma
- Malignant melanoma
- Angiolymphoid hyperplasia with eosinophilia
- Metastatic carcinoma
- Pilomatricoma
- In AIDS patients: Bacillary angiomatosis, deep mycoses
- Amelanotic/hypomelanotic melanoma (2)[C]

DIAGNOSTIC TESTS & INTERPRETATION
Initial Tests (lab, imaging)
No labs are necessary for the diagnosis.

Diagnostic Procedures/Other
- Excisional biopsy
- Send for pathology

Test Interpretation
Microscopic examination reveals:
- Small, endothelial-lined vascular spaces
- Loose/Dense connective tissue stroma
- Acute and chronic inflammatory cells
- No true granuloma formation
- Abundant mitotic activity
- Resembles granulation tissue in an edematous matrix, showing immature capillaries with interspersed tissue (3)

TREATMENT

MEDICATION
- Pyogenic granuloma that involve the nails may be treated with a 2–3-week course of a high-potency topical steroid under occlusion (clobetasol proprionate 0.05% ointment, betamethasone dipropionate 0.05% ointment, fluocinonide 0.1% cream) in the morning and topical antibiotic (2% mupirocin ointment) in the evening (4)[C].
- Small lesions can be cauterized without excision with topical silver nitrate:
  – Perform excisional biopsy, if recurrent.

SURGERY/OTHER PROCEDURES

- For smaller lesions in noncosmetically sensitive areas, surgical excision with simple closure gives the best result with least recurrence (4,5)[C].
- Liquid nitrogen may be nonsurgical option with the lowest recurrence rate (5).
- Shave excision with cautery may be optimal treatment for a lesion on fingertips.
- Topical 5% imiquimod cream may be useful for children.
- Electrosurgery (electrodesiccation and curettage)
- Topical 1.5% phenol solution may be used for periungual lesion (6)[C].
- CO_2 laser destruction
- Excision must be adequate to avoid recurrence. Even a small fragment of tissue left behind may lead to recurrence.
- Excisional biopsy should be tried in all situations, if possible, to ensure a proper diagnosis (i.e., not missing malignancies such as amelanotic melanoma or basal cell carcinoma).

ONGOING CARE

PATIENT EDUCATION
Patient should avoid trauma to area following excision

PROGNOSIS
- Some lesions spontaneously resolve on their own (usually within 6 months).
- Complete resolution is expected with adequate excision.

COMPLICATIONS
Recurrence: After removal or destruction of solitary lesion, multiple satellite lesions can form around original treatment site.

REFERENCES

1. Piraccini BM, Bellavista S, Misciali C, et al. Periungual and subungual pyogenic granuloma. *Br J Dermatol*. 2010;163:941–953.
2. Zalaudek I, Kreusch J, Giacomel J, et al. How to diagnose nonpigmented skin tumors: A review of vascular structures seen with dermoscopy: Part II. Nonmelanocytic skin tumors. *J Am Acad Dermatol*. 2010;63:377–386.
3. Greene AK. Management of hemangiomas and other vascular tumors. *Clin Plast Surg*. 2011;38:45–63.
4. Gilmore A, Kelsberg G, Safranek S, et al. Clinical inquiries. What's the best treatment for pyogenic granuloma? *J Fam Pract*. 2010;59:40–42.
5. Lee J, Sinno H, Tahiri Y, et al. Treatment options for cutaneous pyogenic granulomas: A review. *J Plast Reconstr Aesthet Surg*. 2011;64:1216–1220.
6. Losa Iglesias ME, Becerro de Bengoa Vallejo RB. Topical phenol as a conservative treatment for periungual pyogenic granuloma. *Dermatol Surg*. 2010;36:675–678.

CODES

ICD10
- K06.8 Oth disrd of gingiva and edentulous alveolar ridge
- K13.4 Granuloma and granuloma-like lesions of oral mucosa
- L98.0 Pyogenic granuloma

CLINICAL PEARLS

- Benign, acquired, usually rapidly growing, solitary vascular proliferation that involves exposed areas, such as distal extremities and face, as well as in the oral cavity.
- Excision must be adequate to avoid recurrence.
- Excisional biopsy recommended to ensure proper diagnosis (and to not miss a malignant lesion)
- Excision with primary closure or excision with cautery should be the 1st choice for treatment in most lesions.

G

GRAVES DISEASE

Mohita A. Patel, MD • Nora Gimpel, MD

BASICS

DESCRIPTION
Autoimmune disease in which thyroid-stimulating antibodies cause increased thyroid function; most common cause of hyperthyroidism. Classic findings are goiter, ophthalmopathy (orbitopathy), and occasionally dermopathy (pretibial or localized myxedema).

EPIDEMIOLOGY
Prevalence
- Overall prevalence of hyperthyroidism in US: ~2% for women and 0.2% for men
- More common in white and Hispanic populations in comparison to the black population
- Graves disease accounts for 60–80% of all cases of hyperthyroidism.
- Hyperthyroidism occurs in 0.2% of pregnancies, of which 95% is due to Graves disease
- Predominant age: 30–40 years
- Synonym(s): Basedow disease

ETIOLOGY AND PATHOPHYSIOLOGY
- Excessive production of TSH receptor antibodies from B cells primarily within the thyroid, likely due to genetic clonal lack of suppressor T cells
- Binding of these antibodies to TSH receptors in the thyroid activates the receptor, stimulating thyroid hormone synthesis and secretion, as well as thyroid growth (leading to goiter)
- Binding to similar antigen in retro-orbital connective tissue causes ocular symptoms.

Genetics
Higher risk with personal or family history of any autoimmune disease, especially Hashimoto thyroiditis

RISK FACTORS
- Female gender
- Postpartum period
- Stressful life events
- Medications: Iodine, amiodarone, lithium, highly active antiretroviral (HAART); rarely, immune-modulating medications (e.g., interferon therapy)
- Smoking (higher risk of developing ophthalmopathy)

GENERAL PREVENTION
Screening thyroid-stimulating hormone (TSH) in asymptomatic patients is not recommended. No data conclusively show that treatment of subclinical thyroid dysfunction improves quality of life or clinical outcome measures (1)[A].

COMMONLY ASSOCIATED CONDITIONS
- Mitral valve prolapse
- Type 1 diabetes mellitus
- Addison disease, hypokalemic periodic paralysis
- Vitiligo, alopecia areata
- Other autoimmune disorders (myasthenia gravis, celiac disease)

DIAGNOSIS

Hyperthyroid patients appear hypermetabolic with increased adrenergic tone.

HISTORY
- Tachycardia, palpitations
- Tremor, restlessness
- Hyperactivity, anxiety, emotional lability, insomnia
- Sweating, heat intolerance
- Pruritus, skin changes
- Weight loss with increased appetite
- Fatigue, dyspnea (due to muscle weakness)
- Oligo-/Amenorrhea (women), loss of libido, erectile dysfunction (men), gynecomastia
- Loose, frequent stools
- Blurred vision or diplopia, lacrimation, photophobia, gritty sensation in eyes (ocular dryness), retro-orbital discomfort, painful eye movement, loss of color vision or visual acuity
- Worsening of chronic medical conditions (anxiety or bipolar disorder, glucose intolerance, heart failure, or angina)

Geriatric Considerations
Elderly patients may not display classic symptoms; may present with atrial fibrillation, weight loss, or shortness of breath (2)[B].

PHYSICAL EXAM
- Ophthalmologic (present in 50% of cases): Grittiness/discomfort in the eyes, retrobulbar pressure/pain, lid lag/ retraction, proptosis, ophthalmoplegia; papilledema and loss of color vision may signify optic neuropathy
- Thyroid: Enlarged (goiter), nontender, and without nodules; possible bruit (increased blood flow)
- Integumentary: Fine hair, warm skin, onycholysis of nails, palmar erythema, possible pretibial myxedema (orange peel appearance), possible hyperpigmented plaques (dermopathy)
- Cardiac: Resting tachycardia, hyperdynamic circulation, possible atrial fibrillation
- Extremities: Fine tremor, hyperreflexia, proximal myopathy; rarely, soft-tissue edema of extremities and clubbing of digits (acropachy)

DIFFERENTIAL DIAGNOSIS
- Toxic multinodular goiter (multiple hormone-producing nodules)
- Toxic adenoma (single hormone-producing nodule)
- Thyroiditis (hormone leakage):
  - Subacute, usually postviral (thyroid will be tender)
  - Lymphocytic, including postpartum
  - Hashimoto thyroiditis (anti-thyroperoxidase [TPO] antibodies may stimulate TSH receptors)
- Iatrogenic (treatment-induced):
  - Iodine-induced (dietary, radiographic contrast, or medications)
  - Amiodarone
  - Thyroid hormone overreplacement (accidental or intentional)
- Tumor:
  - Pituitary adenoma producing TSH
  - Human chorionic gonadotropin (hCG)-producing tumors (stimulate TSH receptors)
  - Extraglandular thyroid hormone production (e.g., struma ovarii or metastatic thyroid cancer)

DIAGNOSTIC TESTS & INTERPRETATION
Initial Tests (lab, imaging)
- TSH is initial test: Suppressed (low or undetectable) TSH confirms hyperthyroidism.
- Free T_4 level will be high in Graves disease.
- After confirming suppressed TSH and high T_4, perform radioactive iodine uptake (RAIU) and scan. Patients with Graves disease will have diffuse, elevated RAIU (vs. localized/nodular elevated uptake in adenoma and multinodular goiter, and decreased uptake in thyroiditis or exogenous thyroid hormone).

Pregnancy Considerations
Increase in serum thyroxine binding globulin concentration and initial stimulation of TSH by hCG resulting in a total T4 and T3 rise during first ½ of pregnancy. The TSH level is decreased throughout pregnancy and should be compared to the trimester-specific ranges for pregnancy. Measurement of thyrotropin receptor antibody (TRAb) is positive in 95% of patient's with Graves and should be used if diagnosis is unclear in pregnancy.

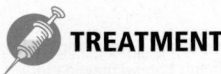

TREATMENT

MEDICATION
Goal is to correct hypermetabolic state with the fewest side effects and lowest incidence of posttreatment hypothyroidism.

First Line
- Radioactive iodine (RAI):
  - Concentrates in the thyroid gland and destroys thyroid tissue
  - Treatment of choice in the US for Graves disease (3)[C]
  - High cure rate with single treatment, especially with high-dose regimen
  - Risks: Side effects (neck soreness, flushing, decreased taste); worsening ophthalmopathy (15% incidence, higher in smokers); posttreatment hypothyroidism (80% incidence, not dosage-dependent); radiation thyroiditis (1% incidence); need to adhere to safety precautions until radiation is eliminated from the body.
  - May worsen Graves orbitopathy (GO): Symptoms are usually mild and transient in those patients with no or mild ophthalmopathy, however, treatment for patients with moderate-to-severe GO is still guided by expert opinion pending further study (4)[C].
  - Pretreatment with antithyroid medication should be considered in patients with severe disease and the elderly to reduce risk of posttreatment trans-ient hyperthyroidism and posttreatment radiation thyroiditis, as well as quicker return to normal thyroid function. Controversy remains regarding whether pretreatment results in treatment failure, and no definitive data support use (5)[C].
  - May be repeated in as soon as 3 months, but usually after 6 months if not euthyroid

Pregnancy Considerations
RAI is contraindicated in pregnancy and during breastfeeding:
- Antithyroid drugs: Methimazole (MMI) and propylthiouracil (PTU):
  - Compete with the thyroid for iodine, thereby decreasing the synthesis of thyroid hormone; PTU also blocks peripheral conversion of T_4 to T_3.
  - Treatment of choice for children and for adults who refuse radioactive iodine
  - May use as pretreatment for older or cardiac patients before radioactive iodine or surgery
  - MMI is usually first choice due to lower cost and once-daily dosing; additionally, the risk of hepatocellular inflammation (30%) and severe liver damage (0.1%) with PTU make it second-line to MMI for most patients (6)[C].

– No improvement in remission rates noted with higher-dose MMI; lowest effective dose should be used (7)[B]

– Minor side effects (<5% incidence): Controlled by switching from 1 agent to another: Rash, fever, arthralgias, GI side effects

– Major side effects necessitating change in treatment:
  ○ Polyarthritis (1–2%)
  ○ Agranulocytosis (<0.5%)
  ○ Cholestasis, jaundice (rare with MMI)

– Discontinue treatment after 1 year if patient is euthyroid and thyroid-stimulating antibody level is undetectable.

– 60% remission rate with 2 years of treatment (standard regimen); newer studies suggest no increased benefit to treatment beyond 18 months (3,8)[B].

– Relapse rates up to 50% in patients who respond initially; higher rates if smoker, large goiter, or positive thyroid-stimulating antibodies at end of treatment.

Pregnancy Considerations
PTU is preferred in 1st trimester of pregnancy due to teratogenic effects of MMI. Switch to MMI in 2nd and 3rd trimester due to risk of PTU-induced hepatotoxicity (9,10)[C].

Second Line
Plasmapheresis is under investigation as a treatment option (11)[C], as is rituximab (immune modulator) for thyroid eye disease (12)[C] and possibly dermatopathy (13)[C].

ISSUES FOR REFERRAL
- Endocrinologist for radioactive iodine therapy; if patient is pregnant or breastfeeding
- Graves ophthalmopathy
- Surgery if failed drug therapy or refusing RAI; obstruction or cosmesis

ADDITIONAL THERAPIES
- β-blockers provide prompt control of adrenergic symptoms; start while workup is in progress. Long-acting propranolol is used most commonly and titrated to symptom control (40–320 mg/d). Calcium channel blockers are an alternative for heart rate control in patients who cannot take β-blockers (11)[C].
- Symptom control may be achieved with iodides, which block conversion of T_4 to T_3 and inhibit TSH release. Use for pregnant patients who do not tolerate antithyroid medication or in conjunction with antithyroid medications. Should not be used long term (may cause paradoxical increase in TSH release) or in combination with radioactive iodine.
- For corneal protection: Tinted glasses when outdoors, artificial tears, patching or taping the lids at night
- For orbitopathy: Moderate-to-severe cases should be treated with pulse-dose IV glucocorticoid, if no contraindications (14)[C]. Alternative is PO steroid (prednisone 60–80 mg/d for 2–4 weeks, then taper off).
- For dermopathy, medium- to high-potency topical corticosteroid

SURGERY/OTHER PROCEDURES
Total thyroidectomy is the procedure of choice. A subtotal thyroidectomy preserves some thyroid function, but has a less predictable outcome (3)[C].

Minimal-incision thyroidectomy is also suggested as a safe and feasible option.

COMPLEMENTARY AND ALTERNATIVE MEDICINE
Nutritional supplementation with L-carnitine may act as an antagonist of thyroid hormone and reduce hyperthyroid symptoms as well as decrease bone demineralization.

IN-PATIENT CONSIDERATIONS
Indications for hospital admission:
- Thyroid storm (rare, but life-threatening complication): Admit to ICU.
- Ophthalmopathy with visual impairment: Admit with ophthalmology consult.
- Severe cardiac symptoms (congestive heart failure [CHF], rapid atrial fibrillation, angina)

 ONGOING CARE

FOLLOW-UP RECOMMENDATIONS
Patient Monitoring
- Monitoring is for resolution of hyperthyroidism and for development of hypothyroidism.
- Check TSH and T_4 levels every 1–2 months for first 6 months after treatment, then every 3 months for a year, then every 6–12 months thereafter. For patients on treatment with PTU and MMI, check anti-TSH receptor antibodies at 12 months of treatment to determine possibility of discontinuing medication.

Pregnancy Considerations
Postpartum exacerbation of hyperthyroidism is common for women not currently under treatment, so TSH and symptoms should be monitored.

PATIENT EDUCATION
Adherence to both follow-up surveillance and medication regimens is the most important way to achieve a good outcome and promote lifelong health.

PROGNOSIS
- Generally good with treatment
- May have irreversible ocular, cardiac, and psychiatric consequences
- Increased morbidity and mortality due to osteoporosis, atherosclerotic disease, insulin resistance and obesity, and endothelial cell dysfunction (thromboembolic risk)

COMPLICATIONS
Hypothyroidism is most common consequence of treatment (25–80%, depending on treatment modality). Patients should be monitored annually, even if asymptomatic.

REFERENCES
1. Helfand M. U.S. Preventive Services Task Force. Screening for subclinical thyroid dysfunction in nonpregnant adults: A summary of the evidence for the U.S. Preventive Services Task Force. *Ann Intern Med*. 2004;140:128–141.
2. Boelaert K, Torlinska B, Holder RL, et al. Older subjects with hyperthyroidism present with a paucity of symptoms and signs: A large cross-sectional study. *J Clin Endocrinol Metab*. 2010;95(6):2715–2726. Epub 2010 Apr 14.
3. Bahn RS, Burch HB, et al. Hyperthyroidism and other causes of thyrotoxicosis: Management guidelines of the American Thyroid Association and American Association of Clinical Endocrinologists. *Thyroid*. 2011;21(6):593–646.
4. Bartalena L. The dilemma of how to manage Graves' hyperthyroidism in patients with associated orbitopathy. *J Clin Endocrinol Metab*. 2011;96(3):592–599.
5. Oszukowska L, Knapska-Kucharska M, Lewiński A. Effects of drugs on the efficacy of radioiodine (131I) therapy in hyperthyroid patients. *Arch Med Sci*. 2010;6:4–10.
6. Cooper DS, Rivkees SA. Putting propylthiouracil in perspective. *J Clin Endocrinol Metab*. 2009;94(6): 1881–1882.
7. Benker G, Reinwein D. Is there a methimazole dose effect on remission rate in Graves disease? Results from a long-term prospective study. *Clin Endocrinol*. 2004;49(4):451–457.
8. Maugendre D, Gatel A. Antithyroid drugs and Graves disease—prospective randomized assessment of long-term treatment. *Clin Endocrinol*. 2004;50(1):127–132.
9. Yoshihara A, Noh J, Yamaguchi T, et al. Treatment of Graves' disease with antithyroid drugs in the first trimester of pregnancy and the prevalence of congenital malformation. *J Clin Endocrinol Metab*. 2012;97(7):2396–2403. Epub 2012 Apr 30.
10. Stagnaro-Green A, Abalovich M, Alexander E, et al. Guidelines of the American Thyroid Association for the diagnosis and management of thyroid disease during pregnancy and postpartum. *Thyroid*. 2011;21(10):1081–1125.
11. Reid JR, Wheeler SF. Hyperthyroidism: Diagnosis and treatment. *Am Fam Physician*. 2005;72: 623–630.
12. Hegedus L, Smith TJ, Douglas RS, Nielsen CH. Targeted biological therapies for Graves' disease and thyroid-associated ophthalmopathy. Focus on B-cell depletion with Rituximab. *Clin Endocrinol (Oxf)*. 2011;74:1–8.
13. Mitchell AL, Gan EH, Morris M, et al. The effect of B cell depletion therapy on anti-TSH receptor antibodies and clinical outcome in glucocorticoid-refractory Graves' orbitopathy. *Clin Endocrinol*. 2013;79(3):437–442.
14. Zang S, Ponto KA, Kahaly GJ. Clinical review: Intravenous glucocorticoids for Graves' orbitopathy: Efficacy and morbidity. *J Clin Endocrinol Metab*. 2011;96(2):320–322.

 SEE ALSO

See also topics: Anxiety; Cardiac Arrhythmias; Weight Loss

 CODES

ICD10
- E05.0 Thyrotoxicosis with diffuse goiter
- E05.00 Thyrotoxicosis w diffuse goiter w/o thyrotoxic crisis
- E05.01 Thyrotoxicosis w diffuse goiter w thyrotoxic crisis or storm

CLINICAL PEARLS
Thyroid hormone controls metabolic rate and affects many organ systems. Hyperthyroid patients appear hypermetabolic, with symptoms and signs of increased adrenergic tone.

G

GROWTH HORMONE DEFICIENCY

Abigail Hoffman, MD • Rod Pellenberg, MD • Edward Kruse, DO

BASICS

DESCRIPTION
- Insufficient production of growth hormone (GH) in adults or children caused by problems arising in the pituitary gland
- GH is produced by somatotroph cells of the anterior pituitary gland, which is stimulated by growth hormone-releasing hormone (GHRH) and inhibited by somatostatin from the hypothalamus.
- GH, also called *somatotropin*, is a polypeptide hormone that stimulates growth and cell reproduction.
- Hypopituitarism is GH deficiency (GHD) plus a deficiency in at least 1 other anterior pituitary hormone.
- Panhypopituitarism is a deficiency in all the hormones produced in the pituitary gland.
- System(s) affected: Endocrine; Musculoskeletal; Psychological
- Synonym(s) and Keywords: Hypopituitarism, familial short stature, short height, growth pattern, pituitary dwarfism, acquired GHD, isolated GHD, congenital GHD, panhypopituitarism

EPIDEMIOLOGY
Incidence
- Most common cause of GHD in children is idiopathic.
- Most common cause of GHD in adults is a pituitary adenoma or treatment of the adenoma with surgery or radiotherapy:
  - 76% of patients with GHD had a pituitary tumor.
  - 13% had an extrapituitary tumor.
  - 8% idiopathic cause
  - 1% had sarcoidosis.
  - 0.5% had Sheehan syndrome.

Prevalence
- In children, isolated GHD is reported to affect 1 in 5,000.
- Adult-onset idiopathic GHD is extremely rare.

ETIOLOGY AND PATHOPHYSIOLOGY
- GHD is caused by a genetic or acquired absence or decline in production of GH.
- Hypothalamus secretes GHRH, which stimulates the pituitary to secrete GH. Somatostatin is secreted by the hypothalamus to inhibit GH secretion. When GH pulses are secreted into the blood, then insulin-like growth factor (IGF)-1 is released. GHD may result from disruption of the GH axis—in the higher brain, the hypothalamus, or the pituitary gland.
- Congenital:
  - Genetic (see "Genetics")
  - Structural brain defects:
    - Agenesis of corpus callosum
    - Septo-optic dysplasia
    - Empty-sella syndrome
    - Encephalocele
    - Hydrocephalus
    - Arachnoid cyst
  - Associated midline facial defects:
    - Single central incisor
    - Cleft lip/palate

- Acquired:
  - Trauma
  - CNS infection
  - Tumors of hypothalamus or pituitary:
    - Pituitary adenoma
    - Craniopharyngioma
    - Rathke cleft cyst
    - Glioma/Astrocytoma
    - Germinoma
    - Metastatic
  - Cranial irradiation
  - Pituitary infarction
  - Surgery
  - Hemochromatosis (rare)

Genetics
A variety of congenital genetic causes of GHD:
- Transcription factor defects (POU1F1/PIT-1, PROP-1, LHX3/4, HESX-1, and PITX-2)
- GHRH receptor gene defects
- GH secretagogue receptor gene defects
- GH gene defects
- GH receptor/postreceptor defects
- Prader-Willi syndrome
- Deletion and mutation of GH-1

COMMONLY ASSOCIATED CONDITIONS
- Macroadenoma
- Sarcoidosis
- Sheehan syndrome

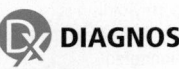

DIAGNOSIS

HISTORY
- Children:
  - Poor height velocity, slower muscular development, and delayed gross motor milestones, such as standing, walking, and jumping
  - Clinical questions:
    - Birth weight and length
    - Previous growth points
    - Nutritional history
    - General health of child
    - Height of parents
    - Timing of puberty in parents
- Adults: Always consider evaluation in patients with structural hypothalamic/pituitary disease, surgery or radiation to hypothalamic/pituitary region, head trauma, and evidence of other pituitary disorders:
  - Fatigue
  - Muscle weakness
  - Depression
  - Social withdrawal
  - Poor memory
  - Loss of strength and/or stamina
  - Reduced physical performance

PHYSICAL EXAM
- Children with GHD:
  - Most common presentation is short stature and drop off in height, then weight, then head circumference on the growth curve:
    - Strong suspicion if >2.5 SD below mean (corresponds to <0.5 percentile) for height (for chronological, age, sex, and background) and/or height velocity >2 SD below mean (corresponds to approximately <3rd percentile) (1)[B]
  - Newborns may present with hypoglycemia, prolonged jaundice, or micropenis.
  - Children with severe GHD have maxillary hypoplasia and forehead prominence.
  - Accurately measure height and weight.
  - Assess pubertal status using Tanner staging system.
- Adults:
  - Decreased lean body mass
  - Poor bone density
  - Abnormal labs:
    - Altered lipid metabolism
    - Increased insulin resistance

DIFFERENTIAL DIAGNOSIS
- Adrenal insufficiency
- Hypothyroidism
- Turner syndrome
- Renal failure
- Small size for gestational age in newborns
- Prader-Willi syndrome
- Idiopathic short stature
- Noonan syndrome
- Russell-Silver syndrome
- Down syndrome

DIAGNOSTIC TESTS & INTERPRETATION
Initial Tests (lab, imaging)
- Thyroid-stimulating hormone (TSH): Hypothyroidism should be excluded as a cause, and thyroxine should be adequately replaced prior to testing for deficiency.
- Serum electrolytes (low bicarbonate levels may indicate renal tubular acidosis)
- CBC and ESR
- Karyotype (in females to rule out Turner syndrome)
- Radiograph of hand and wrist to determine skeletal age in children
- GHD is effectively excluded in children with normal bone age and height velocity.

TREATMENT

GENERAL MEASURES

Pain: Both gabapentin and carbamazepine have been shown to decrease opiate requirements in patients with GBS. One study found gabapentin 300 mg t.i.d. superior to carbamazepine 100 mg t.i.d. in terms of pain control and need for supplementary analgesia. Opiates used with caution as risk of ileus already increased (3)[B].

MEDICATION
First Line
- Plasma exchange (PE):
  - Compared with supportive treatment, patients treated with PE fare significantly better in terms of time to recover walking, requirement for artificial ventilation, duration of artificial ventilation, full muscle strength recovery, and severe sequelae at 1 year (4)[A].
  - In mild GBS, 2 sessions of PE are superior to none. In moderate GBS, 4 sessions are superior to 2. In severe GBS, 6 sessions are not significantly better than 4 (4)[A].
  - More beneficial if started within 7 days of disease onset, but still beneficial at up to 30 days (4)[A].
  - Value of PE in children age <12 years is not known.
- IVIG 0.4 g/kg/d for 5 days:
  - In severe disease, IVIG started within 2 weeks from onset hastens recovery as much as PE (5)[A].
  - In children, IVIG probably hastens recovery compared with supportive care alone (5)[A].
  - IVIG and PE are equally effective and associated with similar rates of adverse events. IVIG may be preferred due to convenience of administration (5)[A].
  - Treatment with IVIG after PE does not confer additional benefit compared with either treatment alone (5)[A].

Second Line
Corticosteroids given alone do not significantly hasten recovery from GBS or affect the long-term outcome (6)[A].

COMPLEMENTARY AND ALTERNATIVE MEDICINE
A small trial showed that the Chinese herbal medicine Tripterygium polyglycoside hastened recovery significantly more than corticosteroids, but additional confirmatory studies are needed (7)[A].

IN-PATIENT CONSIDERATIONS
Admission Criteria/Initial Stabilization
- Admit any patient suspected of having GBS.
- Mildly affected patients who remain capable of walking unaided and are stable for >2 weeks are unlikely to experience disease progression and may be managed as outpatients.
- 25–30% of patients will require mechanical ventilation, yet classic signs of respiratory distress occur too late to serve as guidelines for management. Serial measurement of vital capacity (VC) and static inspiratory and expiratory pressures (PI_{max} and PE_{max}) are the most useful parameters for evaluating respiratory compromise.

- Predictors of respiratory failure include rapid disease progression (≥3 days between onset of weakness and hospital admission), the presence of facial and/or bulbar weakness, VC <20 mL/kg, VC decrease >30%, and Medical Research Council (MRC) sum score indicating muscle weakness (8)[B].
- Monitor closely for complications of autonomic dysfunction (e.g., hyper-/hypotension, tachy-/bradyarrhythmias, urinary retention, ileus).

Nursing
- Prevent complications of immobilization with graduated compression stockings and SC heparin.
- Respiratory care, aspiration precautions, and frequent turning
- Monitor bowel and bladder function for urinary retention and ileus.

 ONGOING CARE

FOLLOW-UP RECOMMENDATIONS
Patient Monitoring
- Pulmonary function testing (vital capacity, respiratory frequency) q2–6h in the progressive phase and q6–12h in the plateau phase (8)
- Monitor bulbar weakness and airway secretions.
- Telemetry in patients with severe disease

PATIENT EDUCATION
Important to emphasize expectation of full or significant recovery and explain phases of illness

PROGNOSIS
- If untreated, 3 phases of illness:
  - Initial progression phase up to 4 weeks; highest risk of death and complication during this phase
  - Variable plateau phase
  - Recovery phase (weeks–months): Return of proximal followed by distal strength
- Mortality estimates range from 4–15% in all patients and up to 20% in those requiring mechanical ventilation. Major causes of death include sepsis, acute respiratory distress syndrome (ARDS), pulmonary emboli, and arrhythmias.
- ~80% achieve functional recovery within 6–12 months. Recovery is maximal at 18 months past onset.
- Up to 20% have residual disability at 1 year; neurologic sequelae include bilateral footdrop, intrinsic hand muscle wasting, sensory ataxia, and dysesthesia.
- Factors associated with poor functional outcome include age >60 years, rapid disease progression, severe disease indicated by GBS disability score or MRC sum score, preceding diarrhea, positive *C. jejuni* or CMV serology, axonal degeneration, and need for mechanical ventilation (8).

REFERENCES

1. Salmon DA, Proschan M, Forshee R, et al. Association between Guillain-Barré syndrome and influenza A (H1N1) 2009 monovalent inactivated vaccines in the USA: a meta-analysis. *Lancet*. 2013;381(9876):1461–1468.
2. Kwong JC, Vasa PP, Campitelli MA, et al. Risk of Guillain-Barré syndrome after seasonal influenza vaccination and influenza health-care encounters: A self-controlled study. *Lancet Infect Dis*.2013; Epub ahead of print.
3. Pandey CK, Raza M, Tripathi M, et al. The comparative evaluation of gabapentin and carbamazepine for pain management in Guillain-Barré syndrome patients in the intensive care unit. *Anesth Analg*. 2005;101:220–225.
4. Raphael JC, Chevret S, Hughes RA, et al. Plasma exchange for Guillain-Barré syndrome. *Cochrane Database Syst Rev*. 2002;(2):CD001798.
5. Hughes RA, Swan AV, van Doorn PA. Intravenous immunoglobulin for Guillain-Barré syndrome. *Cochrane Database Syst Rev*. 2012;7:CD002063. Epub 2012 Jul 11.
6. Hughes RAC, van Doorn PA. Corticosteroids for Guillain-Barré syndrome. *Cochrane Database Syst Rev*. 2012;8:CD001446. doi:10.1002/14651858. CD00144pub4.6
7. Hughes RAC, Pritchard J, Hadden RDM. Pharmacological treatment other than corticosteroids, intravenous immunoglobulin and plasma exchange for Guillain-Barré syndrome. *Cochrane Database Syst Rev*. 2013;2:CD008630. doi:10.1002/14651858.CD008630.pub3.
8. Walgaard C, Lingsma HF, Ruts L, et al. Prediction of respiratory insufficiency in Guillain-Barré syndrome. *Ann Neurol*. 2010;67(6):781–787.

ADDITIONAL READING
- Rinaldi S. Update on Guillain-Barré syndrome. *J Peripher Nerv Syst*. 2013;18(2):99–112.
- Sejvar JJ, Baughman AL, Wise M, et al. Population incidence of Guillain-Barré syndrome: A systematic review and meta-analysis. *Neuroepidemiology*. 2011;36(2):123–133. Epub 2011 Mar 21.

CODES

ICD10
G61.0 Guillain-Barre syndrome

CLINICAL PEARLS
- Natural history of GBS is to resolve; treatment with IVIG or PE speeds rate of recovery and reduces disability.
- Most useful diagnostic tests are lumbar puncture and nerve conduction studies.
- If GBS is suspected, initial evaluation must include measurement of vital capacity and inspiratory force to evaluate respiratory compromise.
- Risk of GBS following influenza infection 40–70× greater than risk following seasonal influenza vaccine.

G

GYNECOMASTIA

Frank J. Domino, MD

BASICS

DESCRIPTION
- Benign glandular enlargement of male breast that is generally bilateral (may be asymmetric or unilateral):
  - Type 1: Benign adolescent hypertrophy; physiologic discoid subacute mass
  - Type 2: Physiologic gynecomastia; generalized enlargement to greater degree
  - Type 3: Stimulated by obesity
  - Type 4: Pectoral muscle hypertrophy
- System(s) affected: Endocrine/Metabolic; Skin/Exocrine
- Synonym(s): Male breast hypertrophy

EPIDEMIOLOGY
- Predominant age: Puberty; >65 years of age (especially with weight gain)
- Predominant sex: Male only

Pediatric Considerations
Transient gynecomastia is seen in neonatal boys.

Geriatric Considerations
Drug-induced form is more common in geriatric patients.

Prevalence
- 38–64% of pubertal males may have mild form. Usual onset is 11–12 years of age, with resolution by age 16–17 years.
- Nonpubertal forms are rare except when drug-induced.

ETIOLOGY AND PATHOPHYSIOLOGY
The cause of pubertal gynecomastia is not clear (1)[C]:
- May be related to transient imbalance of androgens and estrogens
- May be related to higher leptin levels (may result in altered local estrogen levels)
- Physiologic: Transient in neonatal boys and at puberty:
  - 60–90% of newborn males develop transient breast enlargement related to transplacental estrogen.
  - In pubertal boys, may require 1–3 years to regress or may not regress at all
  - Men age 60–90 years may develop gynecomastia related to declining levels of testosterone.
- Exposure to a high level of estrogen compared with testosterone concentration
- Identifiable syndrome/cause found in 12% of pubertal boys
- Tumors: Estrogen-secreting, gonadotropin-secreting, prolactin-secreting pituitary adenomas, hepatic fibrolamellar carcinoma
- Drugs (10–25% of gynecomastia) (2): Hormones, marijuana, digitalis, spironolactone, cimetidine, ketoconazole, phenytoin, furosemide, verapamil, cytotoxic drugs, antihypertensives, sedatives, antidepressants, amphetamines, heroin, methadone, anabolic steroids (1)[C]
- Systemic disorders: Cirrhosis, thyrotoxicosis, renal failure
- Androgen production deficiency
- Androgen-insensitivity syndromes
- Idiopathic (25% of gynecomastia)

Genetics
Some instances of familial gynecomastia may be inherited as a male-limited autosomal trait.

RISK FACTORS
- Obesity
- Liver disease
- Renal disease
- Recovery from prolonged severe illness associated with malnutrition and weight loss (refeeding gynecomastia)
- Multiple therapeutic as well as nontherapeutic drugs (e.g., spironolactone, cimetidine, ranitidine, omeprazole, isoniazid, ketoconazole, amlodipine, captopril, diltiazem, enalapril, nifedipine, verapamil, diazepam, haloperidol, digitalis, statin drugs, anabolic steroids, androgens, estrogens, growth hormone, amphetamines, heroin, methadone, marijuana, and ethanol, among others) (2)
- Family history
- Exposures: Marijuana, alcohol, some medications (see "Etiology")

GENERAL PREVENTION
In men taking estrogen for prostate cancer: Low-dose radiation prior to institution of diethylstilbestrol

COMMONLY ASSOCIATED CONDITIONS
- Peutz-Jeghers syndrome
- Male pseudohermaphroditism
- Hyperthyroidism
- Hypothyroidism
- Hepatic disease
- Prostate carcinoma
- Adrenal neoplasms (adenoma or carcinoma)
- Renal disease or dialysis
- True hermaphrodism
- Klinefelter syndrome
- Testicular failure (enzymatic defects of testosterone production, androgen insensitivity)
- Testicular neoplasms (germ cell, Leydig cell, Sertoli cell tumors)

DIAGNOSIS

HISTORY
- Determine onset and duration of symptoms.
- Investigate concurrent drug treatments.

PHYSICAL EXAM
- Careful breast exam to evaluate characteristics of breast:
  - May involve one or both breasts
  - Usually asymptomatic, but may be tender if it has developed rapidly
  - Usually located concentrically beneath the nipple and areola
- Abdominal exam
- Testicular exam
- Rectal exam

DIFFERENTIAL DIAGNOSIS
- Obesity with increase in adipose tissue
- Carcinoma of male breast
- Lipomas
- Neurofibromas
- Cystic hygroma

DIAGNOSTIC TESTS & INTERPRETATION
- Most cases in teenage boys are self-limiting and require reassurance alone.
- Full endocrine investigations may be indicated if symptoms of other disease states are indicated:
  - Thyroid function studies, testosterone, estradiol, β-human chorionic gonadotropin, luteinizing hormone (LH), liver functions tests (LFTs), GGT, prolactin, α-fetoprotein

Initial Tests (lab, imaging)
- Laboratory evaluation rarely indicated in teenage boys
- If worsening symptoms or clinical suspicion of nonexposure secondary cause, consider:
  - Human chorionic gonadotropin (hCG) levels: High levels may indicate choriocarcinoma or other hCG-secreting tumor.
  - Plasma testosterone and LH measurements: Help diagnose hypogonadism
  - Serum estradiol (E_2)
  - Serum prolactin
  - Prostate-specific antigen (PSA)
  - LFTs
  - Others if clinically indicated (e.g., thyroid function, chromosomal analysis)
  - CT scan of chest and abdomen if hepatic, adrenal, or extragonadal germ cell tumor is suspected
  - Testicular US if there is a palpable mass or abnormality of one or both testicles (rarely indicated)
  - MRI of pituitary fossa if prolactin levels are elevated (to exclude a prolactinoma)

Follow-Up Tests & Special Considerations
Disorders that may alter lab results:
- Cirrhosis
- Thyrotoxicosis
- Renal failure

Diagnostic Procedures/Other
Biopsy, if suspicious

Test Interpretation
- Dense, periductal, hyaline, collagenous connective tissue
- Hyperplastic ductal lining
- Plasma cell infiltrate

TREATMENT

- In teenage males, only reassurance and follow-up are usually indicated:
  - Spontaneous resolution in many within the first 1–2 years
  - Persistent idiopathic gynecomastia in 7–8% of teenage boys at 3 years following diagnosis (1)[C]
- Little evidence exists to recommend medical treatment of idiopathic gynecomastia in pediatric patients at this time (3):
  - Medical management is most likely to be effective in the early (proliferative) phase of gynecomastia (4)[C].
- Consider eliminating medication or illicit drug use in adult males before initiating treatment.

GENERAL MEASURES
- Correct underlying disorder.
- Withdraw causative drug (if feasible).
- Observe with reassurance that the problem is transient.

MEDICATION
- Danazol (100 mg b.i.d. × 1 week followed by 100 mg t.i.d. × 2–6 weeks) (5)[B]:
  - Effective in 80% of patients
  - Especially effective in reducing tenderness
  - Dose can be repeated for responders.
  - Drug is licensed for treatment of gynecomastia in the UK.
- Tamoxifen (20–40 mg/d) has been used (5)[B]:
  - May be effective in 78–83% of men with gynecomastia
  - Less effective in breasts with a large amount of fatty tissue
  - May have high relapse rate
  - Short-term tamoxifen treatment also has been used successfully in the treatment of pubertal gynecomastia (6)[C].
- Anastrazole has been studied in pediatric patients with idiopathic gynecomastia and is not effective (3).
- Timing of treatment with medications may influence patient response:
  - Treatment early in the course of developing gynecomastia may be more beneficial (1)[C].
- Testosterone may be of some benefit, but has not been well studied and is used infrequently.
- Clomiphene has been used infrequently.

ISSUES FOR REFERRAL
Refer to endocrinologist if abnormally elevated hormone levels are confirmed.

SURGERY/OTHER PROCEDURES
- Biopsy if suspicious for cancer:
  - Needle or excisional biopsy
  - Gynecomastia is believed to be a risk factor for the development of male breast cancer.
- SC mastectomy for severe, painful, or persistent cases or for patients with psychological concerns (7)[C]:
  - Usually performed as outpatient surgery
  - General anesthesia required
  - Liposuction of the SC tissue may be required as well as skin removal if the breast is pendulous (4)[C],(8).

 ONGOING CARE

FOLLOW-UP RECOMMENDATIONS
No restrictions

Patient Monitoring
- Every 3–6 months for physiologic gynecomastia
- Until well for nonphysiologic gynecomastia

DIET
- No special diet
- If obesity a problem, weight-loss diet

PATIENT EDUCATION
Surgical procedures for gynecomastia in pubertal boys are rarely covered by insurance because most insurance companies consider these procedures to be cosmetic.

PROGNOSIS
- Type 1: Resolves spontaneously
- Type 2: Clears without treatment (may take up to 2 years)
- Type 3: Little change without substantial weight loss
- Drug-induced: Drug withdrawal should result in resolution of gynecomastia in most cases.
- Other causes: Outcome depends on etiology.
- Good results with SC mastectomy: High degree of postoperative satisfaction (82%) (4)[C]

COMPLICATIONS
- Nipple inversion may occur following SC mastectomy.
- Asymmetry of breasts
- Postoperative fluid collection (seroma or hematoma)
- Withdrawal behavior related to drugs
- Depression
- Weight gain may be associated with danazol treatment.

REFERENCES

1. Nordt CA, Divasta AD. Gynecomastia in adolescents. *Curr Opin Pediatr*. 2008;20:375–382.
2. Eckman A, Dobs A. Drug-induced gynecomastia. *Expert Opin Drug Saf*. 2008;7:691–702.
3. Ma NS, Geffner ME. Gynecomastia in prepubertal and pubertal men. *Curr Opin Pediatr*. 2008;20:465–470.
4. Brafa A, Campana M, Grimaldi L, et al. Management of gynecomastia: An outcome analysis in a multicentric study. *Minerva Chir*. 2011;66:375–384.
5. Devalia HL, Layer GT. Current concepts in gynaecomastia. *Surgeon*. 2009;7:114–119.
6. Derman O, Kanbur NO, Kutluk T. Tamoxifen treatment for pubertal gynecomastia. *Int J Adolesc Med Health*. 2003;15:359–363.
7. Gabra H. Gynaecomastia in the adolescent: A surgically relevant condition. *Eur J Ped Surg*. 2004;14:3–6.
8. Cordova A, Moschella F. Algorithm for clinical evaluation and surgical treatment of gynaecomastia. *J Plast Reconstr Aesthet Surg*. 2008;61(1):41–49. Epub 2007 Nov 5.

ADDITIONAL READING
Johnson RE, Murad MH. Gynecomastia: Pathophysiology, evaluation, and management. *Mayo Clin Proc*. 2009;84:1010–1015.

 SEE ALSO

Algorithm: Gynecomastia

CODES

ICD10
N62 Hypertrophy of breast

CLINICAL PEARLS
- The initial workup of gynecomastia is history, physical exam, and fasting labs, including serum hCG, testosterone, LH, E_2, prolactin, PSA, and LFTs.
- Lab tests do not need to be done in boys with suspected pubertal gynecomastia, but they should be considered if the gynecomastia persists for >1 year.
- Screen all for alcohol, opioid or marijuana abuse

G

HAMMER TOES

Jill A. Grimes, MD, FAAFP

 BASICS

Hammer toes are classified as a form of lesser toe (digits 2–5) deformities.

DESCRIPTION
- Plantar flexion deformity of the proximal interphalangeal (PIP) joint with varying degrees of hyperextension of the metatarsophalangeal (MTP) and distal interphalangeal (DIP) joints (1). Occurs primarily in sagittal plane.
- Can be flexible, semirigid, or fixed:
  – Flexible: Passively correctable to neutral position
  – Semirigid: Partially correctable to neutral position
  – Fixed: Not passively correctable to neutral position

EPIDEMIOLOGY
Most common deformity of lesser toes, typically affecting only 1–2 digits:
- 2nd toe most commonly involved

Incidence
- Undefined, with limited data
- Increases with age, duration of deformity (from flexible to rigid)

Prevalence
- Predominant sex: Female > Male (2):
  – Female predominance from 2.5:1 to 9:1, depending on age group
- Can range from 1–20% of population studied
- Blacks more affected than whites (2)

ETIOLOGY AND PATHOPHYSIOLOGY
- Any biomechanical dysfunction that results in loss of function of extensor digitorum longus (EDL) tendon at PIP joint and the flexor digitorum longus (FDL) tendon at the MTP joint; the intrinsic muscles sublux dorsally as the MTP hyperextends. This results in plantar flexion of the PIP joint and hyperextension of the MTP joint (2).
- Specific pathomechanics vary by etiology:
  – Toe length discrepancy or narrow toe box induces PIP joint flexion by forcing digit to accommodate shoe wear.
    ○ May also lead to MTP joint synovitis secondary to overuse, with elongation of plantar plate and MTP joint hyperextension.
  – Rheumatoid arthritis (RA) causes MTP joint destruction and resultant subluxation
- Congenital
- Acquired:
  – Any condition that compromises intra-articular and periarticular tissues, such as 2nd ray longer than 1st, inflammatory joint disease, improper fitting shoes, and trauma (1).
  – Damage to joint capsule, collateral ligaments, or synovia leads to unstable PIP joint or MTP joint.

Genetics
- Specific genetic markers not identified
- Seen more frequently in families

RISK FACTORS
- Pes cavus and planus
- Hallux valgus
- Metatarsus adductus
- Ankle equinus
- Neuromuscular disease (rare)
- Trauma
- Improperly fitted shoes (e.g., with narrow toe box) and/or hosiery
- Abnormal metatarsal and/or digit length
- Inflammatory joint disease (e.g., RA)
- Connective tissue disease
- Diabetes mellitus

GENERAL PREVENTION
- No documented means of prevention
- Modification of shoe wear using pressure-dispersive devices reduces pain (1).
- Foot orthoses modulate biomechanical dysfunction and muscular imbalance, thereby preventing progression (2).
- Control of predisposing factors (e.g., inflammatory joint disease) may slow progression.

COMMONLY ASSOCIATED CONDITIONS
- Hallux valgus
- Cavus foot
- Metatarsus adductus
- Dorsal callus

 DIAGNOSIS

History and physical exam often sufficient for diagnosis of hammer toes. Additional testing available to exclude other conditions.

HISTORY
- Location, duration, severity, and rate of progression of foot deformity (3)[C]
- Type, location, duration of pain:
  – Patients often relate sensation of lump on plantar aspect of MTP joint.
- Degree of functional impairment
- Factors that improve and exacerbate the condition
- Type of footwear and hosiery worn
- Peripheral neurologic symptoms
- Any prior treatment rendered

PHYSICAL EXAM
- Note MTP joint hyperextension, PIP joint flexion, and DIP joint extension
- Observe any adjacent toe deformities (e.g., hallux valgus, flexion contractures)
- Assess degree of flexibility and reducibility of deformity in both weight-bearing and non–weight-bearing positions (2)[C]
- Note any hyperkeratosis over the joint, ulcers, clavi (dorsal PIP joint, metatarsal head), adventitious bursa, erythema, or skin breakdown (2)
- Palpate for pain over dorsal aspect of PIP joint or MTP joint
- Drawer test of MTP joint
- Palpate web spaces to exclude interdigital neuroma
- Neurovascular evaluation (e.g., pulses, sensation, muscle bulk)

DIFFERENTIAL DIAGNOSIS
- Hammer toe: Hyperextension of the MTP and DIP joints and plantar flexion of the PIP joint
- Claw toe: Dorsiflexion of MTP joint and plantar flexion of the DIP joint
- Mallet toe: Fixed or flexible deformity of the DIP joint of the toe
- Overlapping 5th toe
- Interdigital neuroma
- Plantar plate rupture
- Nonspecific synovitis of MTP joint
- Exostosis
- Arthritis (e.g., rheumatoid, psoriatic)
- Fracture

DIAGNOSTIC TESTS & INTERPRETATION
Initial Tests (lab, imaging)
- Not required unless clinically indicated to rule out suspected metabolic or inflammatory arthropathies (2)[C]: Rheumatoid factor, antinuclear antibodies (ANA), HLA-B27 serologies for inflammatory disease.
- Weight-bearing x-rays of affected foot in anterior–posterior (AP), lateral, and oblique views (2)[C]:
  – AP view superior for assessing MTP subluxation or dislocation
  – Lateral view best for evaluation of gross hammer toe deformity

Follow-Up Tests & Special Considerations
MRI or bone scan if suspect osteomyelitis

Diagnostic Procedures/Other
- Nerve conduction studies or EMG if neurologic disorder is suspected
- Doppler or plethysmography if impaired circulation and surgery is considered
- Computerized weight-bearing pressure testing is indicated only in setting of neuromuscular deficiencies of toes

Test Interpretation
Histologic evaluation typically not necessary before treatment

 TREATMENT

- Goal of treatment is to reduce or relieve symptoms so that patients may return to their normal activity level.
- Management includes surgical and nonsurgical interventions.
- Mild cases, however, may not require treatment.

GENERAL MEASURES
Nonsurgical (conservative) treatment includes:
- Shoe modifications, such as wider and/or deeper toe box, may be used to accommodate the deformity and decrease the pressure over osseous prominences. Avoid high-heeled shoes (2)[C].
- Toe sleeve or orthodigital padding of the hammer toe prominence (4)[C]
- Hammer toe–straightening orthotics or taping to reduce flexible deformities

- Debridement of hyperkeratotic lesions is effective in reducing symptoms. Topical keratolytics may be helpful (2)[C].
- Shoe orthotics may be used to control abnormal biomechanical influences.
- Physical therapy for stretching and strengthening of the toes may help to preserve flexibility.

MEDICATION
Indicated if adequate pain relief is achievable nonsurgically or patient is poor surgical candidate.

First Line
NSAIDs may be helpful in managing symptoms of pain, as well as soft tissue and joint inflammation.

Second Line
Anti-inflammatory (cortisone) injectables if local inflammation or bursitis exists (1)[C]

ISSUES FOR REFERRAL
If nonsurgical (conservative) treatment is unsuccessful and/or impractical or patient has combined deformity of MTP joint, PIP joint, and/or DIP joint, then patient may be referred to an orthopedic surgeon or surgical podiatrist for surgical interventions.

SURGERY/OTHER PROCEDURES
- Surgical procedures for the correction of hammer toes rely on the degree and flexibility of the contracture(s) and the related abnormalities that exist.
- Surgical interventions for *flexible* hammer toes include (1,4)[C]:
  – PIP joint arthroplasty (most common)
  – Flexor tendon lengthening/flexor tenotomy
  – Extensor tendon lengthening/tenotomy/MTP joint capsulotomy
  – Exostosectomy
  – Implant arthroplasty
- Surgical interventions for semirigid/rigid hammer toes include (1,4)[C]:
  – PIP joint resection arthroplasty or arthrodesis
  – Girdlestone-Taylor flexor-to-extensor transfer
  – Metatarsal shortening (Weil osteotomy)
  – Exostosectomy
  – Diaphysectomy of the proximal phalanx (less common)
  – Middle phalangectomy (less common)
  – Soft tissue releases/lengthening
- Procedures may be performed as isolated operations or in conjunction with other procedures.
- Contraindications for surgery: Active infection, inadequate vascular supply, and desire for cosmesis alone

ONGOING CARE

FOLLOW-UP RECOMMENDATIONS
- Radiographs should be taken immediately following surgery or at the 1st postoperative visit. Subsequent x-rays may be taken as needed.
- Full weight bearing in a postoperative (surgical) shoe or other device is indicated based on the procedure(s) performed and on the individual patient.

- Elevate the foot above nose to minimize swelling, which can lead to pain and delay wound healing.
- Return to regular shoe wear depends on the postoperative course.
- Role and efficacy of postoperative physical therapy (3 × a week for 2–3 weeks) unclear

Patient Monitoring
In the absence of complications, the patient should be seen initially within the 1st week following the procedure(s). Frequency of subsequent visits is determined based on the procedure(s) performed and the postoperative course.

PATIENT EDUCATION
- Patients should be aware of mild-to-moderate swelling and plantar foot discomfort that may persist for many (1–6) months after surgery and may limit footwear options until resolved.
- MTP joint and PIP joint may remain stiff for extended period.
- "Molding" of the operative toe (assumes shape of adjacent toes)
- Encourage patients to wear shoes of adequate size with rounded or squared toe box in future.

PROGNOSIS
- Nonoperative (conservative) treatment usually alleviates pain; however, the deformity may progress despite diligent care.
- Surgical treatment of flexible hammer toe deformity reliably corrects the deformity and alleviates pain. Recurrence and progression are common, especially if the patient resumes wearing improperly fitted shoes.
- Surgical treatment of fixed hammer toe deformity provides reliable deformity correction and pain relief. Recurrence is uncommon.

COMPLICATIONS
- Common complications specific to digital surgery include but are not limited to:
  – Persistent edema
  – Recurrence of deformity
  – Residual pain
  – Excessive stiffness
  – Metatarsalgia
- Less common complications include:
  – Numbness (e.g., digital nerve palsy)
  – Flail toe
  – Symptomatic osseous regrowth
  – Malposition of toe
  – Malunion/Nonunion
  – Infection
  – Vascular impairment (e.g., toe ischemia, gangrene)

REFERENCES

1. Academy of Ambulatory Foot and Ankle Surgery. *Hammertoe syndrome*. Philadelphia: Academy of Ambulatory Foot and Ankle Surgery; 2003.
2. Clinical Practice Guideline Forefoot Disorders Panel of the American College of Foot and Ankle Surgeons. Diagnosis and treatment of forefoot disorders. Section 1: Digital deformities. *J Foot Ankle Surg*. 2009;48:230–238.
3. Schrier JC, Verheyen CC, Louwerens JW. Definitions of hammer toe and claw toe: An evaluation of the literature. *J Am Podiatr Med Assoc*. 2009;99: 194–197.
4. Smith BW, Coughlin MJ. Disorders of the lesser toes. *Sports Med Arthrosc*. 2009;17:167–174.

ADDITIONAL READING

- Miller JM, Blacklidge DK, Ferdowsian V, et al. Chevron arthrodesis of the interphalangeal joint for hammertoe correction. *J Foot Ankle Surg*. 2010; 49:194–196.
- O'Kane C, Kilmartin T. Review of proximal interphalangeal joint excisional arthroplasty for the correction of second hammer toe deformity in 100 cases. *Foot Ankle Int*. 2005;26:320–325.
- Pietrzak WS, Lessek TP, Perns SV. A bioabsorbable fixation implant for use in proximal interphalangeal joint (hammer toe) arthrodesis: Biomechanical testing in a synthetic bone substrate. *J Foot Ankle Surg*. 2006;45:288–294.
- Shirzad K, Kiesau CD, DeOrio JK, et al. Lesser toe deformities. *J Am Acad Orthop Surg*. 2011;19: 505–514.

 SEE ALSO

Algorithm: Foot Pain

 CODES

ICD10
- M20.40 Other hammer toe(s) (acquired), unspecified foot
- M20.41 Other hammer toe(s) (acquired), right foot
- M20.42 Other hammer toe(s) (acquired), left foot

CLINICAL PEARLS
- Hammer toe is plantar flexion deformity of PIP joint.
- Patients may complain of pain at the PIP or MTP joint.
- Perform a careful inspection and examination of foot, especially PIP and MTP joints.
- Initial management of hammer toe deformity consists of conservative therapy; however, if unsuccessful, surgical interventions are indicated.
- Well-fitting shoe wear is vital to minimizing recurrence after treatment, and patients should be aware of mild-to-moderate swelling and plantar foot discomfort that may persist for many (1–6) months after surgery and may limit footwear options until resolved.

H

HAND-FOOT-AND-MOUTH DISEASE

Chris Wheelock, MD

 BASICS

DESCRIPTION

- Common acute viral illness affecting mostly children
- Characterized by vesicles on the buccal mucosa and tongue, and peripherally distributed small, tender cutaneous lesions on the hands, feet, buttocks, and (less commonly) genitalia
- Group A coxsackieviruses are the most common causative agent (1).
- Synonym(s): Herpangina

EPIDEMIOLOGY

- Self-limiting illness resolves in 7–10 days
- Moderately contagious
- Infection is spread by direct contact with nasal discharge, saliva, blister fluid, or stool.
- Infected individuals are most contagious during the 1st week of the illness.
- The viruses that cause hand-foot-and-mouth disease (HFM) can persist for weeks after symptoms have resolved, most commonly in stool, allowing transmission following resolution of symptoms.
- The incubation period is 3–5 days (2).

Incidence

- Children <10 years most commonly affected
- Can occur as isolated cases, outbreaks, or epidemics
- Occurs worldwide
- Mother to fetus transmission is possible.
- Most large outbreaks occur in Southeast Asia.

ETIOLOGY AND PATHOPHYSIOLOGY

Transmission by the fecal–oral route or contact with skin lesions or oral secretions

- Most commonly coxsackievirus A16
- Also coxsackieviruses A5, A7, A9, A10, B2, B5, and Enterovirus 71

GENERAL PREVENTION

- Handwashing, especially around food handling or stooling/diaper changes (3)[B]
- Exclusion of children from group settings during the 1st few days of the illness in the setting of open lesions in the mouth or on the skin may reduce the spread of infection (2)[C].
- Hand hygiene measures are effective in reducing transmission (3,4).
- Pregnant woman should avoid contact with infected individuals.

 DIAGNOSIS

HISTORY

- Rash on hands and feet
- Sore throat
- Painful mouth lesions
- 1-day prodrome of fever, anorexia, malaise, abdominal pain, upper respiratory symptoms
- Fever may last 3–4 days
- Often history of sick contacts

PHYSICAL EXAM

- Tender vesicles or ulcers on buccal mucosa, sides of tongue, and palate
- Begin as small red papules and evolve into vesicles and then ulcerations
- May persist for up to 1 week
- Cutaneous vesicles 3–5 mm in diameter start as maculopapular eruptions, occur typically on dorsal aspect of fingers and toes
- May also occur on the palms, soles, buttocks, and groin
- Adults are less likely to have cutaneous findings.

DIFFERENTIAL DIAGNOSIS

- Herpes simplex
- Herpes zoster
- Scarlet fever
- Roseola infantum
- Fifth disease
- Other enteroviral infections
- Kawasaki disease
- Viral pharyngitis
- Erythema multiforme
- Varicella (5)

DIAGNOSTIC TESTS & INTERPRETATION

Typically clinically diagnosed

Initial Tests (lab, imaging)

Culture for responsible virus (virus isolation) can be obtained from oral lesions, cutaneous vesicles, nasopharyngeal swabs, stool, and CSF, although not typically performed.

 TREATMENT

- Symptomatic
- Avoid spicy or acidic foods to limit oral pain.
- Numbing sprays or viscous lidocaine can be used for oral pain.
- IV fluids may be required in more severe cases of dehydration.

MEDICATION

- Symptomatic care using acetaminophen or ibuprofen for pain from oral ulcers or fever
- Soothing mouth washes can be compounded by the pharmacy containing equal amounts of viscous lidocaine, diphenhydramine, and Maalox. Instruct to swish and spit.

Pediatric Considerations

Avoid aspirin use in treating febrile illness in children.

IN-PATIENT CONSIDERATIONS

- Patients with CNS manifestations may require hospitalization.
- Admit those with dehydration unable to maintain adequate oral hydration.

ONGOING CARE

DIET
- Encourage cold liquids (e.g., milk products, popsicles) to prevent dehydration.
- Avoid acidic, salty, and spicy foods, as they will increase pain.

COMPLICATIONS
- Dehydration most common due to painful oral ulcerations
- Rarely, aseptic meningitis or other neurologic complications
- Concomitant CNS disease may occur when HFM syndrome is caused by enterovirus 71 (6).
- Cardiopulmonary complications include myocarditis, pneumonitis, and pulmonary edema.
- Fever >3 days and lethargy are associated with CSF pleocytosis (7).
- Usually resolves in 7–10 days without complications

REFERENCES

1. Frydenberg A, Starr M. Hand, foot and mouth disease. *Aust Fam Physician*. 2003;32(8):594–595.
2. Richardson M, Elliman D, Maguire H, et al. Evidence base of incubation periods, periods of infectiousness and exclusion policies for control of communicable diseases in schools and preschools. *Pediatr infect Dis J*. 2001;20(4):380–391.
3. Ruan F, Yang T, Jin Y, et al. Risk factors for hand, foot, and mouth disease and herpangina and the preventive effect of hand-washing. *Pediatrics*. 2011;127(4):e898–904. Epub 2011 Mar 21.
4. Ma E, Wong S, Wong C, et al. Effects of public health interventions in reducing transmission of hand, foot, and mouth disease. *Pediatr Infect Dis J*. 2011;30(5):432–435.
5. Quail G. The painful mouth. *Aust Fam Physician*. 2008;37(11):935–938.
6. Chang LY, Tsao KC, Hsia SH, et al. Transmission and clinical features of enterovirus 71 infections in household contacts in Taiwan. *JAMA*. 2004;291(2):222–227.
7. Ooi MH, Wong SC, Mohan A, et al. Identification and validation of clinical predictors for the risk of neurological involvement in children with hand, foot, and mouth disease in Sarawak. *BMC Infect Dis*. 2009;9:3.

ADDITIONAL READING

- Centers for Disease Control and Prevention. Notes from the field: severe hand, foot, and mouth disease associated with coxsackievirus A6. *MMWR Morb Mortal Wkly Rep*. 2012;61(12):213–214.
- Scott LA, Stone MS. Viral exanthems. *Dermatol Online J*. 2003;9(3):4.

 CODES

ICD10
B08.4 Enteroviral vesicular stomatitis with exanthem

CLINICAL PEARLS
- Most common May–October
- Children <5 tend to have worse symptoms than older children.
- Hand-foot-and-mouth disease is the most common cause of mouth sores in pediatric patients.
- Usually self-limiting, resolving in 7–10 days
- Careful handwashing to limit spread

H

HEADACHE, CLUSTER
Jeffrey W. Phillips, MD

BASICS

DESCRIPTION
- Primary headache disorder
- Multiple attacks of unilateral, excruciating, sharp, searing, or piercing pain. Typically localized in the periorbital area and temple accompanied by signs of ipsilateral autonomic features.
- Autonomic symptoms: Parasympathetic hyperactivity signs (ipsilateral lacrimation, eye redness, nasal congestion) and sympathetic hypoactivity (ipsilateral ptosis and miosis)
- Patients often pace, rub their head to try to alleviate the pain
- Symptoms usually remain on the same side during a single cluster attack.
- Individual attacks last 15–180 minutes if untreated and occur from once every other day to 8 times per day.
- Attacks usually occur in series (cluster periods) lasting for weeks or months separated by remission periods usually lasting months or years. However, about 10–15% of patients have chronic symptoms without remissions.

EPIDEMIOLOGY
Incidence
1-year incidence: 53/100,000
Prevalence
- Lifetime prevalence 124/100,000 (~0.1%)
- Predominant sex: Male > Female (4.3:1)
- Mean age of onset: Between 29.6 and 35.7 years
- Episodic/Chronic ratio 6:1

ETIOLOGY AND PATHOPHYSIOLOGY
- Complex and incompletely understood
- Proposed mechanisms include:
  - Activation of posterior hypothalamus may trigger an attack, causing activation of the trigeminal nerve, leading to intense pain symptoms
  - Autonomic symptoms: Activation of craniofacial parasympathetic nerve fibers secondary to pathologic activation of trigemino-autonomic brainstem reflex

Genetics
- Usually sporadic: Autosomal dominant in ~5% of cases, autosomal recessive or multifactorial in other families
- Evidence varies: 1st-degree relatives carry 5–8-fold; 2nd-degree 1–3-fold increased relative risk of disease

RISK FACTORS
- Male gender
- Age (70% onset before age 30)
- Cigarette smoking
- Family history of cluster headache (CH)
- Head trauma
- Alcohol induces attacks during a cluster, but not during remission.
- Small amounts of vasodilators (e.g., alcohol, nitroglycerine, sildenafil)
- Strong odors

COMMONLY ASSOCIATED CONDITIONS
- Depression (24%)
- Increased risk of suicide secondary to the extreme nature of the pain
- Medication overuse headache
- Asthma (9%)
- History of migraine, frequently in female patients
- Sleep apnea (14%)
- Increased prevalence of cardiac right-to-left shunt and patent foramen ovale (relationship unclear)

DIAGNOSIS

- Diagnosis is clinical.
- *International Classification of Headache Disorders* (2nd edition) criteria: At least 5 attacks of severe or very severe unilateral orbital, supraorbital, or temporal pain lasting 15–180 minutes if untreated
- At least 1 of the following:
  - Ipsilateral:
    - Conjunctival injection and/or lacrimation
    - Nasal congestion and/or rhinorrhea
    - Eyelid edema
    - Forehead and facial sweating
    - Miosis and/or ptosis
  - Sense of restlessness or agitation
- Attack frequency: 1 every other day to 8 per day
- Episodic CH: At least 2 cluster periods lasting 7 days–1 year, separated by a pain-free interval of >1 month (80–90% of cases)
- Chronic CH: Cluster-free interval of <1 month in a ≥12-month period

HISTORY
- Episodic periods of headache described as excruciating, unilateral, sharp, searing, or piercing pain, typically localized in the periorbital area
- Eye redness, tearing, nasal discharge, sweating
- Timing of headaches often circadian in nature.

PHYSICAL EXAM
- Usually patients seen between attacks
- Acute distress, crying, screaming, restless, and/or agitated during attacks
- Ipsilateral lacrimation, injected conjunctivae, ptosis, and miosis
- Nasal stuffiness or rhinorrhea
- Bradycardia or tachycardia

DIFFERENTIAL DIAGNOSIS
- Paroxysmal hemicrania, short-lasting unilateral neuralgiform headache attacks with conjunctival injection and tearing (SUNCT).
- Hemicrania continua, hypnic headaches, trigeminal and other facial neuralgias, migraine, temporal arteritis, herpes zoster
- Secondary cluster headache:
  - Vertebral or carotid artery dissection, brain arteriovenous malformations, intracranial artery aneurysms
  - Pituitary tumors
  - Nasopharyngeal carcinoma
  - Maxillary sinus foreign body/sinusitis
  - Cavernous hemangioma
  - Meningiomas/carcinomas/metastases

DIAGNOSTIC TESTS & INTERPRETATION
- Diagnosis is primarily clinical
- Diagnosis is often delayed (>40% report 5 year delay in diagnosis)
- Consider neuroimaging (MRI/CT head and vascular imaging of brain):
  - Abnormal neurologic exam
  - Suspect secondary CH

TREATMENT

Many of the medications discussed below are used off-label in the treatment of cluster headache.

GENERAL MEASURES
- Avoid major changes in sleep habits
- Stop smoking
- Avoid use of alcohol during cluster period
- Avoid extreme changes in altitude due to changes in oxygen levels
- Avoid exposure to chemical agents/solvents

MEDICATION
- Avoid pain therapy, especially narcotic analgesics, for acute attacks
- Goal is abortion of acute attack and prophylaxis for expected duration of the cluster
- Assess cardiovascular risk before instituting a vasoactive drug, such as triptans or ergot derivatives

First Line
- For acute attacks:
  - Oxygen:
    - 100% at 6–12 L/min for 15 minutes via nonrebreathing mask provides relief within 15 minutes.
    - Avoid in severe chronic obstructive pulmonary disease (COPD) as might affect hypoxic respiratory drive (1)[A].
  - Sumatriptan (Imitrex):
    - 6 mg SC, max 12 mg/24 h with at least 1 hour between injections is most effective medication for acute attacks. NNT (needed to treat) 2.4 for headache relief in 15 minutes. Sumatriptan nasal spray: 20 mg. May repeat in 2 hours, max dose 40 mg/24 h. NNT 3.2 for headache relief at 30 minutes (2)[A].
  - Zolmitriptan
    - Nasal spray: 5- and 10-mg dosage both effective. May repeat in 2 hours, max 10 mg/24 h. NNT 12 and 4.9 for headache relief in 15 minutes for 5 mg and 10 mg, respectively. Zolmitriptan tablet: 5- and 10-mg dosage both effective. May repeat in 2 hours, max dose 10 mg/24 h. NNT 6.7 and 4.5 for headache relief in 30 minutes for 5 and 10 mg, respectively (2)[A].

ALERT
Triptans are contraindicated in ischemic cardiac disease, stroke, uncontrolled hypertension, prinzmetal angina, basilar migraine, hemiplegic migraine, ischemic bowel disease, and peripheral vascular disease.
- Prophylaxis: Used at start of cluster period to prevent and shorten further attacks. Start as soon as possible:
  - Verapamil:
    - Can start at 80 mg t.i.d. and increase by 40 mg units. Short- or long-acting equivalent. Most patients respond to daily dose of 200–480 mg, but up to 960 mg/d may be needed. NNT = 1.2 (3)[A]
    - ECG monitoring required because of risk of bradycardia (q3m used as a guideline)
  - Similar efficacy to lithium, but fewer adverse effects and faster onset make it the preferred choice.

Second Line
- Acute attack:
  - Lidocaine/Cocaine: 10 mg (1 mL) of lidocaine or 40–50 mg of 10% cocaine intranasal. No well controlled randomized controlled trials (RCTs) done. Most common side effects are nasal congestion, unpleasant taste
  - Octreotide: SC 100 μg. Can be considered in patients when triptans are contraindicated. Main side effect is GI upset (4)[A]
  - Ergotamine/Dihydroergotamine (DHE): Original treatments for CH. Now rarely used because of significant side effects. No controlled trials done. Still used for transitional prophylaxis (see below).
- Prophylaxis:
  - Lithium: Start 300 mg b.i.d., titrate to therapeutic range of 0.8–1.1 mEq/L. Most patients benefit from 600–1,200 mg/d. Widely used without formal evidence of efficacy. Retrospective case series show that lithium led to >50% reduction in attack frequency within 2 weeks in 77% of the patients with episodic CH (5)[B]. Must monitor levels, liver, renal, and thyroid function. Caution with nephrotoxic drugs, diuretics. Inferior to verapamil.
  - Melatonin: 10 mg in the evening showed reduction in headache frequency vs. placebo in small RCT. No side effects were reported (6)[A].
  - Antiepileptics: Topiramate, sodium valproate, gabapentin: Open studies showed reduction of cluster duration and frequency of headache, but RCT did not show superiority to placebo. Significant adverse effects.
  - Civamide: 100 μL of 0.025% into each nostril daily. Only studied in episodic CH in 1 trial of 28 patients. Not available in the US. Most common side effects were nasal burning, lacrimation, pharyngitis, rhinorrhea.
  - Capsaicin: 0.025% ipsilateral nostril for 7 days shows benefit in small RCT.
  - Methysergide: No studies available to confirm efficacy. Has serious adverse effects, including pulmonary and retroperitoneal fibrosis. Cannot be given with triptans and ergots.

ADDITIONAL THERAPIES
Transitional preventive treatment:
- Used until longer-term preventive treatment becomes effective. Longer-term maintenance agents are started concurrently:
  - Steroids: Several open studies suggested benefit, but no rigorous trials to prove efficacy. Studies support at least 40 mg/d (up to 80 mg/d) prednisone with a 10–30-day taper provides benefit to 60–90% patients. Adverse effects for short-term use: Insomnia, psychosis, hyponatremia, edema, hyperglycemia, peptic ulcer.
  - Ergot derivatives: Dihydroergotamine (DHE): 1 mg IV/SC/IM, repeat hourly to max of 3 mg/24 h. A small, retrospective study showed that inpatient IV DHE may be beneficial in refractory cluster headache. Ergotamine tartrate: 1–2 mg/d or in divided doses. No trials to prove efficacy.

ALERT
Ergots are contraindicated in patients with cardiovascular disease and cannot be used with triptans.

Pregnancy Considerations
Collaboration between headache specialist, obstetrician, and pediatrician strongly encouraged. Patient should be informed of treatment benefits and risks as well as drug's potential teratogenic effect. For abortive treatment, oxygen is most appropriate first-line therapy. Nasal lidocaine (pregnancy Category B) can be used as second-line therapy. As preventive therapy, verapamil (pregnancy Category C) and steroids (pregnancy Category C) remain the preferred options. Use of SC or intranasal sumatriptan (pregnancy Category C) should be limited as much as possible. Avoid ergotamines (pregnancy Category X).

ISSUES FOR REFERRAL
Consider a neurology or headache center referral for refractory or complicated patients.

SURGERY/OTHER PROCEDURES
- Surgery may be considered only for patients who are refractory to, or have contraindications to, medical therapy.
- Various techniques focus on stimulation or ablation of segments of trigeminal nerve root and sphenopalatine ganglion. Other techniques are aimed at decreasing pain and inflammation surrounding the greater occipital nerve.
- Greater occipital nerve steroid injection: A retrospective analysis showed ~80% of patients with partial or complete response. Effect lasted 3.5 weeks; 21 mg of betamethasone and 2 mL of 2% lidocaine were used. One class I RCT showed benefit within 72 hours in 85% of lidocaine/betamethasone group compared with none in lidocaine/saline group. Cortivazol injection reduced severity and frequency of headache compared with placebo in another class I RCT.
- Neurostimulation:
  - Occipital nerve stimulation (ONS) was shown to reduce severity and attack frequency in chronic CH patients.
  - Deep brain stimulation (DBS) of the posterior inferior hypothalamus shows therapeutic effect possibly due to modulation of a local CH generator in hypothalamus or mesencephalic gray matter or through nonspecific antinociceptive mechanisms.

IN-PATIENT CONSIDERATIONS
Suicidal ideation, unwilling to contract for safety

 ONGOING CARE

FOLLOW-UP RECOMMENDATIONS
Patient Monitoring
- Anticipate cluster bouts and initiate early prophylaxis.
- Monitor for depression
- Watch for adverse medication response and side effects, such as unmasking of underlying cardiovascular disorder when using medications to treat CH.

PROGNOSIS
- Unpredictable course. With aging, attack frequency often decreases.
- Poor prognosis associated with older age of onset, male gender, disease duration of >20 years for episodic form
- Possibility of transformation of episodic cluster to chronic cluster and occasionally chronic cluster to episodic cluster

COMPLICATIONS
- Depression and suicide
- Side effects of medication, including unmasking of coronary artery disease
- Potential for drug abuse/misuse.

REFERENCES
1. Cohen AS, Burns B, Goadsby PJ, et al. High-flow oxygen for treatment of cluster headache: A randomized trial. *JAMA.* 2009;302:2451–2457.
2. Law S, Derry S, Moore RA. Triptans for acute cluster headache. *Cochrane Database Syst Rev.* 2010;4:CD008042.
3. Leone M, D'Amico D, Frediani F, et al. Verapamil in the prophylaxis of episodic cluster headache: A double-blind study versus placebo. *Neurology.* 2000;54:1382–1385.
4. Matharu MS, Levy MJ, Meeran K, et al. Subcutaneous octreotide in cluster headache: Randomized placebo-controlled double-blind crossover study. *Ann Neurol.* 2004;56:488–494.
5. Stochino ME, Deidda A, Asuni C, et al. Evaluation of lithium response in episodic cluster headache: A retrospective case series. *Headache.* 2012;52:1171–1175.
6. Leone M, D'Amico D, Moschiano F, et al. Melatonin versus placebo in the prophylaxis of cluster headache: a double blind pilot study with parallel groups. *Cephalgia.* 1996;7:494–496.

ADDITIONAL READING
- Askenazi A, Schwedt T. Cluster headache: Acute and prophylactic therapy. *Headache.* 2011;51:272–286
- Hainer B, Matheson E. Approach to acute headache in adults. *Am Fam Physician.* 2013;87:682–687.

 SEE ALSO

Algorithm: Headache, Chronic

 CODES

ICD10
- G44.009 Cluster headache syndrome, unspecified, not intractable
- G44.019 Episodic cluster headache, not intractable
- G44.029 Chronic cluster headache, not intractable

CLINICAL PEARLS
- CHs are rare, but disabling. Patients are often agitated and restless during the attack.
- Oxygen and triptans, not narcotics, are first-line therapy for acute attacks.
- Abortive, transitional, and prophylaxic treatment must all be considered.

HEADACHE, MIGRAINE
Jay H. Levin, MD • Michelle L. Mellion, MD

BASICS

DESCRIPTION
- Headache disorder with episodic manifestation characterized by recurrent painful paroxysms of moderate-to-severe, throbbing pain, typically unilateral, capable of altering daily function and lasting from 4–72 hours. Preheadache symptoms are nonspecific (e.g., neck stiffness, yawning, irritability) and may occur hours to days before headache onset. Most frequent subtypes of migraine are:
  - Without aura (common migraine): Defining >80% of attacks, often associated with nausea, vomiting, photophobia, and/or phonophobia
  - With aura (classic migraine): Visual or other types of neurologic phenomenon lasting 5–60 minutes before the headache
- Other subtypes:
  - Chronic (transformed) migraine: Chronic headache pattern evolving from episodic migraine. Migraine-like attacks are superimposed on a daily or near-daily headache pattern (e.g., tension headaches), >15 headache days/month for at least 3 months.
  - Medication overuse headache: Daily or near-daily use of acute medication perpetuating the headache pattern
  - Basilar-type migraine: Brain stem headache, with aura symptoms of dysarthria, vertigo, tinnitus, ataxia, and bilateral paresis or paresthesias
  - Hemiplegic migraine: Aura consisting of hemiplegia and/or hemiparesis
  - Ophthalmoplegic: Migraine-like neuralgia accompanied by palsy of an ocular cranial nerve during the headache phase
  - Retinal: Monocular symptoms of retinal vascular involvement during migraine
  - Menstrual-related (moliminal) migraine: Associated with onset of menstrual period
  - Childhood periodic syndromes (migraine equivalents): Recurrent, often cyclic, episodes of symptoms, such as vomiting, intense nausea, and/or abdominal pain
  - Status migrainosus: Debilitating migraine that lasts >72 hours
  - Migrainous infarction: Persistent or permanent neurologic deficits persisting beyond migraine attack, usually with neuroimaging changes

EPIDEMIOLOGY
Female > Male (3:1)

Prevalence
- Affects >28 million Americans
- Adults: Women 18%; Men 6%

ETIOLOGY AND PATHOPHYSIOLOGY
- No longer believed to be primarily vascular in etiology; rather, cortical spreading depolarization/depression
- Trigeminovascular hypothesis: Hyperexcitable trigeminal sensory neurons in brain stem are stimulated and release neuropeptides, such as substance P and calcitonin gene-related peptide (CGRP), leading to vasodilation and neurogenic inflammation (1).

Genetics
- >80% of patients have a positive family history.
- Familial hemiplegic migraine has been shown to be linked to both chromosomes 19 and 1.

RISK FACTORS
- Family history of migraine
- Female gender
- Stress
- Menstrual cycle, hormones
- Sleep pattern disruption
- Diet: Skipped meals (40–56%), alcohol (29–35%), chocolate (19–22%), cheese (9–18%), caffeine overuse (14%), monosodium glutamate (MSG) (12%), and artificial sweeteners (e.g., aspartame, sucralose)
- Medications: Estrogens, vasodilators

GENERAL PREVENTION
- Avoid precipitants of attacks.
- Biofeedback, education, and psychological intervention
- Preventative therapy if attacks frequent, interfere with lifestyle, or are not controlled by acute interventions
- Lifestyle modifications are the cornerstone of migraine prevention: Sleep hygiene, stress management, healthy diet, regular aerobic exercise.

COMMONLY ASSOCIATED CONDITIONS
- Depression, psychiatric disorders
- Sleep disturbance (e.g., sleep apnea)
- Cerebral vascular disease
- Peripheral vascular disease
- Seizure disorders
- Irritable bowel syndrome
- Obesity
- Patent foramen ovale (PFO)

DIAGNOSIS

A thorough history and neurologic examination are usually all that is necessary to make the diagnosis. Migraine is a clinical diagnosis.

HISTORY
- Screening mnemonic "POUND": **P**ulsating, duration of 4–72 h**O**urs, **U**nilateral, **N**ausea, **D**isabling):
  - LR = 24 for migraine diagnosis if 4 of 5 criteria present
  - LR = 0.41 for migraine diagnosis if ≤2 criteria present (2)
- Headache usually begins with mild pain that escalates into a unilateral (30–40% bilateral), throbbing (40% nonthrobbing) pain lasting 4–72 hours.
- Intensified by movement and associated with systemic manifestations: Nausea (87%), vomiting (56%), diarrhea (16%), photophobia (82%), phonophobia (78%), muscle tenderness (65%), lightheadedness (72%), vertigo (33%)
- May be preceded by aura:
  - Visual disruptions are most common, including scotoma, hemianopsia, fortification spectra, geometric visual patterns, and occasionally hallucinations.
  - Somatosensory disruption in face or arms
  - Speech difficulties
- Obtain adequate headache profile: Total number of headaches/month, number of days/month whereby headaches limit daily activities; frequency and amount of all headache medications used (3).
- Identify possible triggers (e.g., stress, sleep disturbance, food, caffeine, alcohol).

PHYSICAL EXAM
Full neurologic exam to exclude other etiologies.

DIFFERENTIAL DIAGNOSIS
- Other primary headache syndromes
- If focal neurologic signs/symptoms are present, consider transient ischemic attack (TIA), stroke.
- Secondary headaches: Tumor, infection, vascular pathology, prescription or illicit drug use
- Drug-seeking patients
- Psychiatric disease
- Rarely, atypical forms of epilepsy

DIAGNOSTIC TESTS & INTERPRETATION
Neuroimaging is appropriate ONLY with suspicious symptomatology and/or an abnormality on physical examination. Other red flags include:
- New onset in patient >50 years of age
- Change in established headache pattern
- Atypical pattern or unremitting/progressive neurologic symptoms
- Prolonged or bizarre aura

Pregnancy Considerations
- Migraine frequency may decrease in 2nd and 3rd trimesters.
- Nonpharmacologic methods are mainstay of treatment (see below).
- No treatment drug has FDA approval during pregnancy:
  - Acetaminophen, short-acting opioids, and antiemetics (e.g., prochlorperazine) can be considered for acute headaches during pregnancy.
  - Ergotamines are contraindicated.
  - Avoid herbal remedies.
  - Early data for sumatriptan and naratriptan suggest no increase in birth defects.
  - Sumatriptan by injection is ideal for breastfeeding women with disabling migraines.
  - Propranolol is safe, effective for migraine prevention during pregnancy/lactation.

TREATMENT

GENERAL MEASURES
- Most patients manage attacks with self-care.
- Cold compresses to area of pain
- Withdrawal from stressful surroundings
- Sleep is desirable.

MEDICATION
- First-line abortive treatments:
  - Paracetamol (acetaminophen 1,000 mg) or aspirin (975 mg) plus the addition of a dopamine antagonist (e.g., metoclopramide 10 mg) may be as effective as PO sumatriptan 100 mg for acute migraine headache; NNT = 5.2 for 2-hour headache relief (3)[A].
  - Aspirin 500 mg–acetaminophen 500 mg–caffeine 130 mg (AAC) combination (e.g., Excedrin Migraine) is an inexpensive, nonprescription, and FDA-approved treatment for acute migraine:
    - As early treatment for mild- to moderate-intensity migraines, AAC combination showed favorable results compared with PO sumatriptan 50 mg (4)[B].

- Triptans are commonly used when OTC agents fail for moderate to severe attacks (1,4):
  - Oral sumatriptan 100 mg; NNT = 3.4 for 2-hour headache relief; expense varies, only some triptan generics available:
    - 44–77% of patients taking triptans report complete pain relief within 2 hours.
    - All triptans have similar effectiveness and tolerability, but some patients may respond better to 1 triptan over another (4)[B].
    - Early intervention with triptans during the aura, prior to onset of pain, may prevent headache 89% of the time.
- Ergotamines (e.g., dihydroergotamine SC, Migranal intranasal): Drug of choice in status migrainosus and nonpregnant patients with high-degree disability
- NSAIDs, such as ibuprofen, naproxen, and diclofenac, are generally inexpensive and effective in up to 60% of cases (3,4)[A]:
  - Aspirin 1,000 mg plus the addition of a dopamine antagonist (e.g., metoclopramide 10 mg) may be as effective as PO sumatriptan 100 mg for acute migraine headache; NNT = 3.3 for 2-hour headache relief (3)[A].
- Antiemetics: Consider antinausea medications that antagonize dopamine receptors:
  - Metoclopramide, prochlorperazine
- IV dexamethasone: Use as adjunctive emergency therapy; 26% reduction of acute severe migraine recurrence, status migrainosus; NNT = 9 (4)[A].
- Contraindications to treatments:
  - Avoid 5-HT-1 agonists (triptans) and ergots in coronary artery disease, peripheral vascular disease, uncontrolled hypertension, complex migraine (e.g., basilar or hemiplegic migraine)
  - Triptans should not be used with ergot derivative, MAOI, or other triptans.
  - Avoid narcotics or butalbital in addiction-prone patients and patients with frequent migraines.
- Precautions:
  - Frequent use of acute-treatment drugs may lead to increase in migraine patterns and medication overuse headache.
- Second-line abortive treatment:
  - Opiates use is controversial:
    - Some advocate the use of long-acting opioids in patients with refractory migraine.
    - Opiates may contribute to medication overuse or chronic daily headache with use as few as 8 days per month (3)[C].
- First-line preventative treatment:
  - Lifestyle modifications: Sleep hygiene, stress management, healthy diet, regular aerobic exercise, medication overuse
  - ~38% of migraineurs need preventative therapy, but only 3–13% use it (5). Trial and error is needed to determine optimal therapy.
  - Consider starting preventative treatment when:
    - Quality of life is severely impaired (6)
    - ≥2 attacks/month
    - Migraine attacks do not respond to acute drug treatment
    - Frequent, very long, or uncomfortable auras occur

- For prevention of *episodic migraine*, effective treatments include: Valproate, topiramate, propranolol, timolol, and (off-label) metoprolol (5)[A]:
  - Topiramate 50–100 mg b.i.d. and (off-label) low-dose amitriptyline 25–75 mg daily are considered 1st-line migraine preventative treatments (6)[A].
  - Venlafaxine XR is probably effective (5)[B]. Calcium channel blockers (e.g., verapamil) (off-label) are effective for some patients. Other antidepressants and antihypertensives lack definitive data.
  - NSAIDs, such as fenoprofen, ibuprofen, ketoprofen, and naproxen, are probably effective for migraine prevention but pose a risk for medication overuse headache (7)[B].
- For treatment of *chronic migraine*, FDA has approved botulinum toxin A (Botox) as it significantly reduced the frequency of headache days in chronic migraineurs (1)[B].

ISSUES FOR REFERRAL
- Obscure diagnosis, concomitant medical conditions, significant psychopathology
- Unresponsive to usual treatment
- Analgesic-dependent headache patterns

COMPLEMENTARY AND ALTERNATIVE MEDICINE
- Butterbur (*Petasites hybridus*; Petadolex): 50–75 mg b.i.d. (7)[A]
- Riboflavin (vitamin B_2): 400 mg/d (7)[B]
- Magnesium: 400 mg/d (7)[B]
- MIG-99 (Feverfew): 6.25 mg t.i.d. (7)[B]
- Histamine SC: 1–10 ng twice weekly (7)[B]

IN-PATIENT CONSIDERATIONS
Admission Criteria/Initial Stabilization
Consider if diagnosis not clear; status migrainosus; may need to exclude intracranial bleeds, TIA, stroke; monitor vital signs, patient comfort

IV Fluids
Fluids are a necessary part of inpatient management. Keeping patients hydrated and on antiemetics around the clock may be helpful.

Discharge Criteria
Judgment based on patient's overall clinical status, patient's ability to tolerate PO medications

 ONGOING CARE

FOLLOW-UP RECOMMENDATIONS
- Early intervention is key at the onset of an attack.
- Preventative treatment should aim to decrease frequency and severity of acute attacks, make acute treatments more efficacious, and minimize adverse drug reactions (6).

Patient Monitoring
- Monitor frequency of attacks, pain behaviors, and medication usage via headache diary.
- Encourage lifestyle modifications. Counsel patients and manage expectations.

PATIENT EDUCATION
Educate patients about migraine triggers.

PROGNOSIS
- With increasing age, there may be a reduction in severity, frequency, and disability of attacks.
- Most attacks subside within 72 hours.

COMPLICATIONS
- Status migrainosus (>72 hours)
- Cerebral ischemic events (rare)
- Iatrogenic effects of treatment

REFERENCES
1. Marmura MJ, Silberstein SD. Current understanding and treatment of headache disorders: Five new things. *Neurology.* 2011;76:S31–36.
2. Detsky ME, McDonald DR, et al. Does this patient with headache have a migraine or need neuroimaging? *JAMA.* 2006;296(10):1274–1283.
3. Taylor FR, Kaniecki RG. Symptomatic treatment of migraine: When to use NSAIDs, triptans, or opiates. *Curr Treat Options Neurol.* 2011;13:15–27.
4. Gilmore B, Michael M. Treatment of acute migraine headache. *Am Fam Physician.* 2011;83(3): 271–280.
5. Silberstein SD, Holland S, Freitag F, et al. Evidence-based guideline update: Pharmacologic treatment for episodic migraine prevention in adults: Report of the Quality Standards Subcommittee of the American Academy of Neurology and the American Headache Society. *Neurology.* 2012;78:1337–1345.
6. Fenstermacher N, Levin M, Ward T. Pharmacological prevention of migraine. *BMJ.* 2011;342:540–543.
7. Holland S, Silberstein SD, Freitag F, et al. Evidence-based guideline update: NSAIDs and other complementary treatments for episodic migraine prevention in adults: Report of the Quality Standards Subcommittee of the American Academy of Neurology and the American Headache Society. *Neurology.* 2012;78:1346–1353.

 SEE ALSO

Algorithm: Headache, Chronic

 CODES

ICD10
- G43.109 Migraine with aura, not intractable, w/o status migrainosus
- G43.409 Hemiplegic migraine, not intractable, w/o status migrainosus
- G43.909 Migraine, unsp, not intractable, without status migrainosus

CLINICAL PEARLS
- Migraine is a chronic headache disorder of unclear etiology often characterized by unilateral, throbbing headaches that may be associated with additional neurologic symptoms.
- Accurate diagnosis of migraine is crucial.
- Consider nonspecific analgesics for milder attacks; migraine-specific treatments (triptans) for more severe attacks. Avoid opiates when possible. In frequent migraineurs, consider preventative treatments.

H

HEADACHE, TENSION

Kaelen C. Dunican, PharmD • Robert A. Baldor, MD

BASICS

DESCRIPTION
- Typically characterized by bilateral mild to moderate pain and pressure; may be associated with pericranial tenderness at the base of the occiput
- 2 types:
  - Episodic tension-type headache (ETTH) divided into:
    - Infrequent: <1 day per month
    - Frequent: ≥1 but <15 days per month
  - Chronic tension-type headache (CTTH): ≥15 days per month for >3 months
- Synonym(s): Muscle contraction headache; Stress headache

EPIDEMIOLOGY
Most common type of primary headache

Prevalence
- Lifetime prevalence is 79%.
- More prevalent among women
- Prevalence of CTTH is 3%.
- Prevalence of ETTH decreases with age, whereas the prevalence of CTTH increases with age.

ETIOLOGY AND PATHOPHYSIOLOGY
- Debatable: Peripheral and/or central mechanisms
- Activation of peripheral nociceptors leads to muscle tenderness in ETTH.
- Central sensitization is associated with CTTH:
  - Nitric oxide may play an important role in central sensitization.
  - Debatable: Low platelet serotonin
- Peripheral: May provoke the central mechanism leading from ETTH to CTTH
- Stress is the most frequently reported precipitating factor.

Genetics
An increased genetic risk has been suggested by studies, particularly for CTTH.

RISK FACTORS
Associated with triggers/precipitating factors:
- Stress (mental or physical)
- Change in sleep regimen
- Skipping meals
- Certain foods (caffeine, alcohol, chocolate)
- Dehydration
- Physical exertion
- Environmental factors (sun glare, odors, smoke, noise, lighting)
- Poor or sustained posture
- Female hormonal changes
- Medications (e.g., nitrates, SSRIs, antihypertensives)
- Overuse of abortive headache medication

GENERAL PREVENTION
- Identify and avoid triggers/precipitating factors.
- Minimize emotional stress.
- Encourage relaxation techniques:
  - Biofeedback, relaxation therapy, and physical therapy
  - Consider counseling/psychotherapy.

COMMONLY ASSOCIATED CONDITIONS
- 83% of patients with migraine headaches also suffer from tension-type headaches.
- Debatable: Increased prevalence of comorbid anxiety and depression

DIAGNOSIS

Diagnosis is based on clinical symptoms:
- Diagnostic criteria provided by the International Headache Society:
  - Headache lasting 30 minutes 7 days
  - At least 2 of the following:
    - Bilateral location
    - Pressing/Tightening (nonpulsating) quality
    - Mild or moderate intensity
    - Not aggravated by routine physical activity
  - Not associated with nausea or vomiting (chronic type may be associated with nausea)
  - No more than 1 of the following: Photophobia or phonophobia
- Headache not due to another disorder
- Fronto-occipital or generalized pain (dull, pressing, or bandlike)
- Associated symptoms:
  - Fatigue
  - Irritability
  - Difficulty concentrating
  - Muscular tightness, tenderness, or stiffness in neck, occipital, and frontal regions

HISTORY
Obtain a thorough headache history to rule out other headache disorders, including severity, symptoms, onset, location and radiation of pain; quality of pain; concurrent medical conditions and medications; and recent trauma or other procedures:
- Onset of new headache in patients >40 years of age is cause for careful study, including imaging.

PHYSICAL EXAM
- General physical exam: Vital signs, funduscopic and cardiovascular assessment, palpation of the head and neck
- Neurologic exam: Mental status, pupillary responses, motor-strength testing, deep tendon reflexes, sensation, cerebellar function, gait testing, signs of meningeal irritation

DIFFERENTIAL DIAGNOSIS
- Migraine headache
- Cluster headache
- Head trauma
- Subarachnoid hemorrhage
- Subdural hematoma
- Unruptured vascular malformation
- Ischemic cerebrovascular disease
- Temporal arteritis
- Arterial hypertension (HTN)
- Cerebral venous thrombosis
- Benign intracranial HTN
- Intracranial neoplasm, infection, or meningitis
- Low CSF pressure
- Medication (nonprescription analgesic dependency, nitrates)
- Caffeine dependency
- Metabolic disorders (hypoxia, hypercapnia, hypoglycemia)
- Toxic effects from drugs or fumes
- Temporomandibular joint syndrome
- Eyes: Glaucoma, refractive errors
- Sinusitis or middle-ear infection
- Cervical spondylosis

- Severe anemia or polycythemia
- Uremia and hepatic disorders
- Paget disease of bone

DIAGNOSTIC TESTS & INTERPRETATION
Labs and neuroimaging (CT or MRI) are only necessary when a secondary cause is suspected:
- Atypical pattern of headache (does not fit specific category, such as migraine, cluster, or tension) (1)[A]
- Focal neurologic findings
- New onset after age 40 years
- Sudden onset or worsening with exertion or Valsalva maneuver (1)[A]
- CT scan, with and without contrast, is as sensitive as MRI and is the test of choice.
- Use MRI when lesions of the posterior fossa or an aneurysm is suspected.

TREATMENT

- NSAIDs, acetaminophen (APAP), and aspirin (ASA) are effective for short-term pain relief of ETTH (2,3)[B].
- Amitriptyline should be considered first-line for prophylaxis of CTTH (2,3)[B].

GENERAL MEASURES
Relief measures: Relaxation routines; rest in quiet, dark room; hot bath or shower; massage of back of neck and temples

MEDICATION
Choice of simple analgesic is based on patient-specific parameters:
- NSAIDs may be more effective than APAP for ETTH (2)[C]:
  - Ibuprofen and naproxen may be preferred due to better GI tolerability.
- APAP should be considered for patients taking warfarin, unable to tolerate NSAIDs, or allergic to ASA or NSAIDs.

First Line
- For acute attack (ETTH): NSAIDs, APAP, or ASA:
  - NSAIDs:
    - Ibuprofen (Motrin, Advil): 400–800 mg; may repeat q8h PRN (max 3.2 g/d)
    - Naproxen (Naprosyn): 375–500 mg or naproxen sodium (Aleve, Anaprox) 440–550 mg; may repeat q8–12h PRN (max 1,250 mg naproxen base/d)
    - Ketoprofen (Orudis): 12.5–50 mg; may repeat q6–8h PRN (max 300 mg/d)
    - Diclofenac (Voltaren, Cataflam): 50–100 mg; may repeat q8h PRN (max 150 mg/d)
    - Contraindications: ASA or NSAID allergy or bronchospasm, renal disease, bleeding disorders, increased risk of cardiovascular events (myocardial infarction [MI], stroke, new onset, or worsening of HTN)
    - Drug interactions: Antihypertensives, anticoagulants, antiplatelet drugs, ASA, lithium, methotrexate
    - Adverse effects: Epigastric distress, peptic ulcer
  - APAP (Tylenol): 1,000 mg; may repeat q6h PRN (max 4 g/d):
    - Adverse effects (rare): Rash, pancytopenia, liver damage

○ Precaution: Hepatic impairment, consumption of ≥3/d alcoholic beverages
- Aspirin: 500–1,000 mg; may repeat q6h PRN (max 4 g/d):
  – Contraindication: ASA or NSAID allergy or bronchospasm, bleeding disorders
  – Drug interactions: Anticoagulants, antiplatelet drugs, ACE inhibitors, β-blockers, corticosteroids, NSAIDs, sulfonylureas
  – Adverse effects: GI irritation/bleeding, thrombocytopenia
- Prophylaxis for CTTH: Tricyclic antidepressants (TCAs) (amitriptyline [Elavil]) 10–75 mg/d:
  – Not FDA approved for CTTH.
  – Contraindications: Acute recovery phase of MI, use of monamine oxidase inhibitors (MAOIs) within 14 days
  – Drug interactions: Clonidine, MAOIs, quinolone antibiotics, SSRIs, sympathomimetics, azole antifungals, valproic acid
  – Adverse effects: Drowsiness, dry mouth, tachycardia, heart block, blurred vision, urinary retention, seizure

Second Line
- For acute attack (ETTH):
  – Caffeine combinations: 130 mg caffeine with 500 mg APAP and/or 500 mg ASA q6h PRN (2)[C]
  – Narcotic analgesics (rarely indicated; consider secondary causes of headache or secondary gain, such as drug-seeking behavior for personal use or diversion/sale)
  – Ketorolac: 60 mg IM, single dose
- For CTTH prophylaxis:
  – Mirtazapine: 15–30 mg/d (not FDA approved for CTTH) (2,3)[B]
  – Venlafaxine XR (Effexor XR): 37.5–300 mg/d (not FDA approved for CTTH) (2,3)[B]

ALERT
Use of abortive agents >2 d/wk may lead to *medication-overuse headaches*; must withdraw acute treatment to diagnose.

Pediatric Considerations
ASA and antidepressants are contraindicated.

ADDITIONAL THERAPIES
- The combination of stress management therapy and a TCA (amitriptyline) may be most effective for CTTH.
- Maprotiline: 75 mg/d (not FDA approved for CTTH) (2)[C]
- Topiramate: 100 mg/d (limited clinical evidence for prevention of CTTH; not FDA approved for CTTH)
- Alternative TCAs (although limited evidence of benefit, all are widely used for prophylaxis) (4)[B]:
  – Desipramine (Norpramin): 50–100 mg/d
  – Imipramine (Tofranil): 50–100 mg/d
  – Nortriptyline (Pamelor): 25–50 mg/d
  – Protriptyline (Vivactil): 25 mg/d
- Drugs with conflicting clinical evidence for CTTH (not FDA approved for CTTH):
  – Tizanidine: 2–6 mg t.i.d.
  – Memantine: 20–40 mg/d
- Botulinum toxin type A is not likely to be effective for ETTH or CTTH (5)[A].

COMPLEMENTARY AND ALTERNATIVE MEDICINE
- Electromyographic (EMG) biofeedback may be effective and is enhanced when combined with relaxation therapy (2,6)[C].
- Cognitive-behavioral therapy may be helpful (2,6)[C].
- Physical therapy, including positioning, ergonomic instruction, massage, transcutaneous electrical nerve simulation, and application of heat/cold may help.
- Alternative agents (not FDA approved for TTH):
  – Tiger Balm or peppermint oil applied topically to the forehead may be effective for ETTH.
  – Limited evidence for use of acupuncture and physical therapy (7,8)[B]
- Chiropractic spinal manipulation cannot be recommended for the management of ETTH; recommendations cannot be made for CTTH (8)[B].

IN-PATIENT CONSIDERATIONS
Admission Criteria/Initial Stabilization
Outpatient treatment

ONGOING CARE

FOLLOW-UP RECOMMENDATIONS
- Regulate sleep schedule.
- Regular exercise

DIET
- Identify and avoid dietary triggers.
- Regulate meal schedule.

PATIENT EDUCATION
For additional information, contact:
- National Headache Foundation: www.headaches.org
- American Council for Headache Education: www.achenet.org

PROGNOSIS
- Usually follows a chronic course when life stressors are not changed
- Most cases are intermittent.

COMPLICATIONS
- Lost days of work and productivity (more with CTTH)
- Cost to health system
- Dependence/Addiction to narcotic analgesics
- GI bleeding from NSAID use

REFERENCES
1. Detsky ME, McDonald DR, Baerlocher MO, et al. Does this patient with headache have a migraine or need neuroimaging? *JAMA.* 2006;296:1274–1283.
2. Bendtsen L, Jensen R. Treating tension-type headache—an expert opinion. *Expert Opin Pharmacother.* 2011;12(7):1099–1109. Epub 2011 Jan 20.
3. Bendtsen L, Evers S, Linde M, et al. EFNS guideline on the treatment of tension-type headache—report of an EFNS task force. *Eur J Neurol.* 2010;17:1318–1325.
4. Verhagen AP, Damen L, Berger MY, et al. Lack of benefit for prophylactic drugs of tension-type headache in adults: A systematic review. *Fam Pract.* 2010;27:151–165.
5. Jackson JL, Kuriyama A, Hayashino Y. Botulinum toxin A for prophylactic treatment of migraine and tension headaches in adults: A meta-analysis. *JAMA.* 2012;307(16):1736–1745.
6. Sun-Edelstein C, Mauskop A. Complementary and alternative approaches to the treatment of tension-type headache. *Curr Pain Headache Rep.* 2012;16:539–544.
7. Linde K, Allais G, Brinkhaus B, et al. Acupuncture for tension-type headache. *Cochrane Database Syst Rev.* 2009;CD007587.
8. Bryans R, Descarreaux M, Duranleau M, et al. Evidence-based guidelines for the chiropractic treatment of adults with headache. *J Manipulative Physiol Ther.* 2011;34:274–289.

 SEE ALSO

Algorithm: Headache, Chronic

 CODES

ICD10
- G44.209 Tension-type headache, unspecified, not intractable
- G44.219 Episodic tension-type headache, not intractable
- G44.229 Chronic tension-type headache, not intractable

CLINICAL PEARLS
- Tension-type headache may be difficult to distinguish from migraine without aura. A tension-type headache is typically described as bilateral, mild to moderate, dull pain, whereas a migraine is typically pulsating; unilateral; and associated with nausea, vomiting, and photophobia or phonophobia.
- Evidence suggests that NSAIDs may be more effective than APAP for ETTH. Consider APAP for patients who cannot tolerate, or have a contraindication, to NSAIDs. Initial dose of APAP should be 1,000 mg (500 mg may not be as effective).
- CTTH is difficult to treat, and these patients are more likely to develop medication-overuse headache. Clinical evidence supports the use of amitriptyline + stress-management therapy for CTTH.
- Medication-overuse headaches must be avoided by limiting use of abortive agents to no more than 2 d/wk.
- A headache diary may be useful to identify triggers, response to treatment, and medication-overuse headaches.

HEARING LOSS
Robert A. Baldor, MD

BASICS

DESCRIPTION
- Decrease in the ability to comprehend sound. It can be partial, complete, unilateral, or bilateral.
- Types of hearing loss include conductive hearing loss (CHL or air–bone gap), sensorineural hearing loss (SNHL), or mixed hearing loss.
- System(s) affected: Auditory; External and middle ear (CHL), or inner ear (SNHL)

EPIDEMIOLOGY
- All ages affected; common in children (CHL) and elderly (SNHL)
- Predominant sex: Male = Female

Incidence
- 3/10 people >60 years of age
- At least 1.4 million children (≤18 years)

Prevalence
Hearing loss rate has decreased from 12.2% (1992) to 8.1% (2000) in men, and 7% (1992) to 4.2% (2000) in women (1).

Geriatric Considerations
- ~50% of people age >85 years have hearing loss.
- Hearing aids are underutilized.
- Loss of communication is a source of emotional stress and a physical risk for the elderly.

Pediatric Considerations
- Congenital hearing loss:
  - 1–3/1,000 infants have hearing loss.
  - Mandatory newborn screening (OAE and ABR testing are ideal)
- Audiologic testing after major intracranial infection (meningitis)

Pregnancy Considerations
Otosclerosis (a CHL) can worsen during pregnancy.

ETIOLOGY AND PATHOPHYSIOLOGY
- CHL: Hearing loss can result from middle ear effusion, obstruction of canal (cerumen/foreign body, osteomas/exostoses, cholesteatoma, tumor), loss of continuity (ossicular discontinuity), stiffening of the components (myringosclerosis, tympanosclerosis, and otosclerosis), and loss of the pressure differential across the tympanic membrane (TM) (perforation).
- SNHL: Damage along the pathway from oval window, cochlea, auditory nerve, and brainstem. Examples include vascular/metabolic insult, mass effect, infection and inflammation, acoustic trauma:
  - Noise-induced hearing loss is caused by acoustic insult that affects outer hair cells in the organ of Corti, causing them to be less stiff. Over time, severe damage occurs with fusion and loss of stereocilia. Eventually may progress to inner hair cells and auditory nerve as well.
- Large vestibular aqueduct or superior canal dehiscence: Third mobile window shunts acoustic energy away from cochlea.

Genetics
- Connexin 26 (13q11–12): Most common cause of nonsyndromic genetic hearing loss
- Mitochondrial disorders (may predispose to aminoglycoside ototoxicity)
- Otosclerosis: Familial
- Most common congenital syndromes:
  - Hemifacial microsomia
  - Stickler syndrome
  - Congenital cytomegalovirus
  - Usher syndrome
  - Branchio-oto-renal syndrome
  - Pendred syndrome
  - CHARGE association
  - Neurofibromatosis type II
  - Waardenburg syndrome

RISK FACTORS
- Conductive:
  - Chronic sinusitis; allergy
  - Cigarette smoking
  - Sleep apnea with continuous positive airway pressure (CPAP) use
  - Adenoid hypertrophy; nasopharyngeal mass
  - Eustachian tube dysfunction
  - Neuromuscular disease
  - Family history/heredity
  - Prematurity and low birth weight
  - Craniofacial abnormalities (e.g., cleft palate, Down syndrome)
  - Third mobile window (superior canal dehiscence or large vestibular aqueduct)
- Sensorineural:
  - Aging/Older age
  - Loud noise/acoustic trauma
  - Dizziness/Vertigo: Especially Ménière disease or history of labyrinthitis
  - Medications (aminoglycosides, loop diuretics, quinine, aspirin, chemotherapeutic agents)
  - Bacterial meningitis
  - Head trauma
  - Atherosclerosis
  - Vestibular schwannoma/skull base neoplasm
  - Previous ear surgery
- Sensorineural, pediatric specific:
  - Postnatal asphyxia
  - Mechanical ventilation lasting ≥5 days
  - In utero infections (TORCH syndrome; Toxoplasmosis, Other Agents, Rubella, Cytomegalovirus, Herpes simplex)
  - Toxemia of pregnancy
  - Maternal diabetes
  - Rh incompatibility
  - Prematurity or birth weight <1,500 g
  - Hyperbilirubinemia; exchange transfusions
  - Anomalous temporal bone (Mondini or large vestibular aqueduct)
  - Infectious diseases: Chickenpox, measles, encephalitis, influenza, mumps

GENERAL PREVENTION
- Limit noise exposure; use hearing protection
- Avoid ear canal instrumentation (e.g., cotton swabs)
- Limit ototoxic medications

DIAGNOSIS

HISTORY
- Social problems and comments from friends and family members are often the 1st presentation of presbyacusis as patients are often unaware of the degree of hearing loss they experience and how it affects their life. Onset is gradual.
- Difficulty hearing:
  - Rapid vs. gradual decline: Rapid loss (<3 days) is a medical emergency. If suspicious of a sudden SNHL, refer to ENT ASAP.
  - Difficulty with discrimination
  - Difficulty hearing in crowds
  - Frequently having to ask speakers to repeat
  - Friends/Family complain of hearing loss
  - TV, phone volume increasing
- Tinnitus, bilateral or unilateral
- Otalgia
- Otorrhea, clear or purulent
- Dizziness or vertigo
- Ear fullness
- Autophony (hearing own voice louder or echoing)
- Facial nerve twitching or asymmetry
- Depression
- Anxiety
- History of ear infections or ear surgeries
- History of trauma or noise exposure
- Family history of hearing loss
- History of recent viral infection
- Nasal obstruction
- Frequent epistaxis

PHYSICAL EXAM
- Whispering screen: A whisper heard from ~2 ft away is a good screen for intact hearing. Patients with SNHL have difficulty with this because their hearing loss is usually in the high frequency range.
- 512-Hz tuning fork tests:
  - Sensorineural loss:
    ○ Placed on the forehead: Lateralizes to nonaffected ear (Weber test)
    ○ Base of tuning fork placed on the mastoid and then fork end placed next to ear; heard louder next to ear (Rinne test)
  - Conductive loss:
    ○ Placed on the forehead or teeth lateralizes to affected or symptomatic ear
    ○ Placed on the mastoid and then next to ear; heard louder behind the ear on the side of conductive deficit
- Otoscopy: Assess for deformity, canal patency, and otorrhea; TM integrity/retraction/mobility with insufflation; canal; or middle ear mass
- Facial symmetry
- Cranial nerve exam
- Nasopharyngoscopy: Adenoid hypertrophy or nasopharyngeal mass (mandatory in adult patient with new unilateral serous effusion)
- Pediatric: Survey for syndromic anomalies

DIFFERENTIAL DIAGNOSIS
- Conductive:
  - Cerumen impaction/foreign body
  - Perforation of tympanic membrane
  - Middle ear fluid (serous otitis media)
  - Acute otitis media/adhesive otitis media
  - Ossicular erosion (infection, cholesteatoma)

- Myringosclerosis/Tympanosclerosis
- Temporal bone fracture
- Otosclerosis
- Congenital malleus fixation
- Glomus tumor
- Congenital aural atresia
- Osteogenesis imperfecta
- Superior canal dehiscence
• Sensorineural:
  - Presbycusis (hearing loss related to aging)
  - Noise-induced (recreational, occupational)
  - Ménière disease
  - Ototoxicity (aspirin, aminoglycosides)
  - Viral labyrinthitis
  - Cerebellopontine angle tumor
  - Large vestibular aqueduct syndrome
  - Syndromic hearing loss
  - Congenital cochlear malformation
  - Labyrinthine artery infarct
  - Idiopathic
  - Syphilis
  - Cytomegalovirus (CMV)
  - Rubella
  - Temporal bone fracture
  - Metabolic (hyper-/hypothyroid)
  - Paget disease
  - Perilymphatic (inner ear) fistula
  - Autoimmune inner ear disease

DIAGNOSTIC TESTS & INTERPRETATION
Often labs are not needed. If indicated:
• Pendred syndrome (goiter, mental retardation + SNHL): Perchlorate test, thyroid function tests
• Alport syndrome (nephritis + SNHL): Urinalysis, renal function tests
• Jervell and Lange-Nielsen syndrome (syncope, family history of sudden death + profound SNHL): ECG
• Any pediatric patient with SNHL: Consider genetic testing for connexin 26, mitochondrial studies
• TORCH screening test
• Rapid Plasma Reagin (RPR) or Venereal Disease Research Laboratory (VDRL) confirmed with fluorescent treponemal antibody absorption (FTA-Abs)
• Lyme titer in endemic areas
• Antinuclear antibodies and sedimentation rate as a screen for autoimmune disease
• Fine-cut CT temporal bones without contrast may help in the evaluation of CHL.
• MRI of brain and brainstem with gadolinium to evaluate SNHL in congenital, early onset, and asymmetric hearing loss
• Any sudden SNHL (usually unilateral) is a medical emergency; obtain a hearing testing and start steroid therapy.
• Treatment with high-dose steroids (1 mg/kg/d prednisone for 7–14 days, followed by taper) should begin ASAP, ideally within 1–2 weeks of onset.
• For patients who cannot tolerate systematic steroids, intratympanic steroids are equally effective (2)[A].
• A simple 512-Hz tuning fork test lateralizes to unaffected ear in sudden SNHL (emergency) and lateralizes to the affected ear in CHL (not an emergency).

Diagnostic Procedures/Other
• Audiometry: Pure tone (air and bone), speech testing, and impedance (middle ear pressure) testing
• Tympanometry: Type B or C tympanograms indicate fluid or retraction, respectively. Negative middle ear peak pressures seen even with normal (type A) tympanograms.

• Other tests:
  - Auditory brainstem response
  - Otoacoustic emissions: "Echo" of the cochlea
  - Behavioral (visual reinforcement) audiometry; used in children 6 months–5 years
• Myringotomy and tubes can be considered for persistent fluid with hearing loss.

Test Interpretation
Varies depending on etiology

 ## TREATMENT

Hearing rehabilitation:
• Personal amplifiers, situation-specific amplification (e.g., amplified phone), or personal hearing aids can be considered for any individual who has significant communication difficulties due to hearing loss.
• Cochlear implants for patients with bilateral severe to profound hearing loss who no longer derive benefit from hearing aids

MEDICATION
• Depends on cause. Hearing loss is a broad topic with many possible etiologies.
• Sudden SNHL: High-dose oral steroids: 1 mg/kg or 60–100 mg/d prednisone or 12–16 mg/d dexamethasone for 7–14 days, followed by a taper:
  - Clinical practical guidelines for sudden hearing loss include (3)[C]:
    ○ Distinguishing SNHL from CHL; testing for bilateral sudden hearing loss in patients with unilateral sudden hearing loss; obtaining an MRI, auditory brainstem response or audiometric follow up to evaluate for retrocochlear pathology; offer intratympanic steroid perfusion for refractory cases after initial management fails to treat idiopathic SNHL (ISSNHL) and follow up within 6 month of diagnosis.
    ○ May offer corticosteroids as initial therapy to patients with ISSNHL and hyperbaric oxygen within 3 months of ISSNHL diagnosis
    ○ Recommended against prescribing antivirals, thrombolytics, vasodilators, vasoactive substances, or antioxidants to patients with ISSNHL
    ○ Also recommended against routine laboratory tests in patients with ISSNHL

ISSUES FOR REFERRAL
• Audiology: If hearing loss is suspected, referral to audiology is warranted. Audiologists also provide hearing aid options and maintenance.
• Genetics: If congenital syndrome or familial hearing loss is suspected
• Speech therapist: If speech delay or speech impediment is present
• Endocrinology: Pendred syndrome, other associated endocrine disorder (hypo-/hyperthyroidism)
• Cardiology: Jervell and Lange-Nielsen syndrome
• Ophthalmology: Usher syndrome
• Neurotology and neurosurgery: Cerebellopontine angle (CPA) lesion, intracranial complication of middle ear disease

SURGERY/OTHER PROCEDURES
• CHL often has surgical options for repair:
  - Tympanostomy and tube placement
  - Tympanoplasty
  - Mastoidectomy

- Ossicular chain reconstruction
- Stapedectomy/Stapedotomy
- Canaloplasty
• Those with profound bilateral SNHL may qualify for cochlear implantation.

 ## ONGOING CARE

FOLLOW-UP RECOMMENDATIONS
Patient Monitoring
Audiogram and clinical exam are primary means of monitoring patient.

DIET
Salt restriction to 2 g/d is helpful for patients with Ménière disease.

PATIENT EDUCATION
National Institute on Deafness and Other Communication Disorders: www.nidcd.nih.gov/health/hearing/

PROGNOSIS
SNHL is usually permanent and may be progressive. However, amplification devices (e.g., hearing aids) may help improve functionality.

COMPLICATIONS
Acute middle ear problems may become chronic (perforations, cholesteatoma).

REFERENCES
1. Ikeda N, Murray CJL, Salomon JA. Tracking population health based on self-reported impairments: Trends in the prevalence of hearing loss in US adults, 1976–2006. *Am J Epidemiol*. 2009;170:80–87.
2. Spear SA, Schwartz SR. Intratympanic steroids for sudden sensorineural hearing loss: A systematic review. *Otolaryngol Head Neck Surg*. 2011; 145:534–543.
3. Stachler RJ, Chandrasekhar SS, Archer SM, et al. Clinical practice guideline: Sudden hearing loss. *Otolaryngol Head Neck Surg*. 2012;146(3 Suppl): S1–S35.

 ## CODES

ICD10
• H90.2 Conductive hearing loss, unspecified
• H90.5 Unspecified sensorineural hearing loss
• H91.90 Unspecified hearing loss, unspecified ear

CLINICAL PEARLS
• In sudden hearing loss, if a 512-Hz tuning fork test (Weber test) lateralizes to the *unaffected ear*, suspect sensorineural causes (emergent evaluation needed), but if it lateralizes to the *affected* ear, the diagnosis is conductive hearing loss (not an emergency).
• ~50% of people age >85 years have hearing loss, so encourage screening and treatment, especially in patients with early dementia (to maximize sensory input and sort out confusion vs. lack of hearing).

HEART FAILURE, ACUTELY DECOMPENSATED
David Tegay, DO, FACMG, FACOI • Farzan Gorgani, MS

 BASICS

DESCRIPTION
Acute decompensated heart failure (ADHF) is a heterogeneous syndrome of acute impairment in cardiac pump function resulting in inefficient perfusion to bodily tissues. This may be due to structural or functional cardiac disorders and may represent a new diagnosis or worsening of pre-existing chronic HF.

EPIDEMIOLOGY
Incidence
- Medicare spends more to diagnose and treat HF than any other medical condition. In 2009, the total cost of HF approached $37 billion. In the US, there are 670,000 new cases annually. HF is the primary cause of >55,000 deaths each year and a contributing factor in >280,000 deaths
- 1 million admissions/year; 30% incident ADHF; 70% decompensated chronic HF
- About ½ of people who have heart failure die within 5 years of diagnosis.
Prevalence
- ~5.8 million people in the US carry a HF diagnosis; <1% in those <50, increasing to 10% of those >70.
- Primarily a disease of the elderly; 75% of hospital admissions for HF are in persons >65.

ETIOLOGY AND PATHOPHYSIOLOGY
2 physiologic components explain most of the clinical findings of ADHF:
- Systolic dysfunction: An *inotropic* abnormality, often due to MI or dilated or ischemic cardiomyopathy, resulting in diminished systolic emptying (ejection fraction <45%)
- Diastolic dysfunction: A *compliance* abnormality, often due to hypertensive cardiomyopathy, in which the ventricular relaxation is impaired (ejection fraction >45%)
- Exacerbation of chronic HF
- CAD, MI (especially new onset ADHF)
- Arrhythmia (afib or tachyarrhythmias, high-grade heart block)
- Valvular and vascular abnormalities: Aortic stenosis or regurgitation, rheumatic heart disease (mitral and aortic valvular disease)
- Severe hypertension (both systemic and pulmonary)
- High output states: Hyperthyroidism, anemia
- Medications: Cardiac depressants (β-blocker overdose), chemotherapeutic agents
- Other (infiltrative disease, Chagas disease, pericardial disease, postpartum cardiomyopathy, wet beri-beri, sepsis)

Genetics
Familial cardiomyopathy predisposes to development of HF (rare).

RISK FACTORS
- History of chronic HF
- Coronary artery disease (CAD) and myocardial infarction (MI)
- Hypertension (HTN), systemic or pulmonary
- Valvular heart disease
- Diabetes mellitus
- Cardiotoxic medications
- Renal insufficiency and renal failure
- Arrhythmia
- Infection

GENERAL PREVENTION
Control BP and other risk factors. Thiazide diuretics and ACE inhibitors are superior to other agents in preventing development of HF. Treat cardiovascular disease.

COMMONLY ASSOCIATED CONDITIONS
- Dysrhythmia followed by pump failure is the leading causes of death in ADHF. Most patients have >5 comorbid medical conditions (especially CAD, chronic kidney disease, and diabetes) and take >5 medications.
- Cardiogenic shock
- Hyponatremia and altered mental status, especially in the elderly

 DIAGNOSIS

Clinical diagnosis, no gold standard; ED diagnosis of ADHF is incorrect 10–20%.

HISTORY
- History of HF
- Dyspnea on exertion: *Cardinal sign of left-sided HF*. Deteriorating exercise capacity: Easy fatigue, general weakness, possibly chest pain/discomfort if acute coronary syndrome (ACS) is present
- Nocturnal nonproductive cough, orthopnea, and paroxysmal nocturnal dyspnea; sometimes frothy or pink sputum
- Wheezing, especially nocturnal, in absence of history of asthma or infection (cardiac asthma)
- Edema, often with cool extremities due to peripheral vasoconstriction; abdominal bloating (ascites) or anasarca; cyanosis

PHYSICAL EXAM
- S3 and/or JVD most useful positive finding, although no vital sign/PE finding has sensitivity >70%
- Peripheral edema, cool extremities, edema, cyanosis, hepatomegaly, hepatojugular reflex, hypotension, laterally displaced apical impulse
- Lung exam: Rales (crackles) and sometimes wheezing, Cheyne-Stokes respirations

DIFFERENTIAL DIAGNOSIS
Pulmonary embolism, exertional asthma, acute MI, cardiac ischemia with angina, chronic obstructive pulmonary disease (COPD), constrictive pericarditis, pneumonia, tamponade, tension pneumothorax, high-output states: Anemia, sepsis, hyperthyroidism

DIAGNOSTIC TESTS & INTERPRETATION
- Laboratory data are adjunctive and indicative of complications.
- Perform ECG to evaluate for ACS.

Initial Tests (lab, imaging)
- Cardiac troponins (to evaluate for ACS)
- B-type natriuretic peptide (BNP) and N-type pro-BNP (BT-BNP) may be helpful in:
  - ED setting to help differentiate the cause of dyspnea. BNP <100 essentially rules out HF as a cause of dyspnea with negative predictive value (NPV) of ~99%. Most dyspneic patients with ADHF have BNP >400. Elevation in BNP is not able to differentiate systolic vs. nonsystolic HF adequately.
  - BNP may be higher in obesity or if renal disease is present. BNP and N-type pro-BNP have been shown to have similar specificities and sensitivities in identifying ADHF (1).

- BNP values of 100–400 are more problematic, as they may indicate HF or may be due to conditions like pulmonary embolism, renal failure, ACS, and pulmonary HTN.
- Patients may have BNP elevated due to HF, but acute dyspnea may be from another cause (pneumonia or pulmonary embolism).
- Other lab findings in early and mild-to-moderately severe ADHF include respiratory alkalosis, mild azotemia, dilutional hyponatremia (poor prognosis).
- Chest x-ray (CXR) (changes lag clinical symptoms by up to 6 hours): Increased heart size, vascular redistribution (cephalization) with "butterfly" pattern of pulmonary edema, interstitial and alveolar edema, Kerley B lines, pleural effusions
- Bedside cardiac US (available in the ED) to assess pump function (identify systolic vs. diastolic dysfunction, tamponade, valvular abnormalities, etc.)

Follow-Up Tests & Special Considerations
Please see Chronic Heart Failure section.

Diagnostic Procedures/Other
Determining ejection fraction (EF) is critical to proper diagnosis and management: Formal echocardiographic study is most useful single test to determine EF and valvular abnormalities; may be repeated if change suspected in underlying cardiac status. Pulmonary artery catheterization may be performed to guide therapy in severe cases with cardiogenic shock.

Test Interpretation
Cardiac pathology depends on the etiology of HF. Please refer to Chronic Heart Failure section.

 TREATMENT

Approach is to improve symptoms, hemodynamics, and renal function, and to minimize myocardial damage and hospital length of stay.

MEDICATION

ALERT
Many medications have been shown to improve hemodynamics and symptoms in ADHF but do not decrease mortality. Diuretics are used initially in fluid-overload acute HF, with nitrates added if needed. Nitrates are primary therapy in ischemic acute HF (flash pulmonary edema) and hypertensive ADHF, with diuretics secondary. Once acute HF is stabilized, an ACE inhibitor or β-blocker should be started. Instruct patients not to use NSAIDs. Avoid use of diltiazem and verapamil in patients with systolic dysfunction.

First Line
- Loop diuretics initially for fluid-overloaded ADHF in hemodynamically stable patients (contraindicated if SBP <90, severe hyponatremia, acidosis). Be cautious of electrolyte abnormalities if kidney disease is present. Avoid if possible diagnosis of pneumonia. Continuous infusion is not better than bolus, and high dose is not significantly better than low dose (2)[B]:
  - Furosemide (Lasix): 20–320 mg IV/IM/PO
  - If on Lasix chronically, give double home dose as PO or give PO dose IV (max 180 mg). Monitor for appropriate urine output.
  - Metolazone (Zaroxolyn): 2.5–20 mg/d PO, more useful if reduced creatinine clearance

- Thiazides in combination with loop diuretics may be useful if resistant to diuresis (HCTZ 25 mg PO). Thiazides and spironolactone or eplerenone (25–50 mg PO) may be used in combination with loop diuretics if excessive volume overload.
- Vasodilators: First line if hypertensive (SBP >140–160); don't use if SBP <90, history of aortic stenosis, or phosphodiesterase inhibitor use:
  – IV nitroglycerin may be of short-term benefit to decrease preload, afterload, and systemic resistance (IV 10–20 mcg/min)
  – IV nitroprusside: Administer with caution, infusion rate 0.3 μg/kg/min. Consider an arterial line.
- Morphine: IV boluses 2.5–5 mg IV helps with chest pain and restlessness. Monitor respirations.

Second Line
- Tolvaptan (an oral vasopressin antagonist), in addition to normal treatment (including diuretics) may improve dyspnea and decrease body weight at 24 hours but confers no survival or morbidity benefit (3)[B].
- Inotropes: Consider adding if signs of hypoperfusion and in patients with dilated cardiomyopathy. Withdraw as soon as hemodynamic parameters improve, as these may increase short- and medium-term mortality:
  – Phosphodiesterase inhibitors (milrinone, enoximone) decrease pulmonary resistance; may be used for patients on β-blockers, but may increase medium-term mortality in CAD patients.
  – Levosimendan (calcium sensitizer) improves hemodynamic parameters but not survival compared to placebo while improving hemodynamic parameters and survival compared to dobutamine (4)[B].
  – Dobutamine infusion requires close BP monitoring; avoid in cardiogenic shock or with tachyarrhythmias.
- Nesiritide, a BNP analog, has not been shown to significantly improve symptoms (compared to nitroglycerin) or outcomes (death, rehospitalization rate) in a broad population of ADHF patients. May cause hypotension. Should not be used in the ED (5)[A].

ADDITIONAL THERAPIES
- Oxygen: Begin treatment early; ideally, arterial oxygen saturation >92% (90% if COPD). For acute cardiogenic pulmonary edema, noninvasive ventilation (BiPAP, CPAP) decreases early mortality compared to standard therapy (6)[A].
- No significant difference between continuous positive airway pressure (CPAP) and noninvasive positive pressure ventilation (NIPPV). If possible, avoid mechanical ventilation for patients with right-heart failure.
- Treat anemia with transfusion: Conservative trigger Hgb <8–9; target Hgb 10.
- For patients with new-onset arrhythmias, consider pacing and/or antiarrhythmics.
- For patients in severe cardiogenic shock, consider intra-aortic balloon pump or percutaneous or surgically implanted ventricular assist devices (VADs).
- Please refer to Chronic Heart Failure for maintenance treatments.

SURGERY/OTHER PROCEDURES
- Heart valve surgery if defective heart valve is responsible
- PCI/CABG for patients with CAD/MI if applicable

- Cardiac transplantation considered in patients <55 and without other disqualifying medical problems who are developing chronic decompensated HF unresponsive to other therapeutic maneuvers and who are considered to have a life expectancy of >1 year.

IN-PATIENT CONSIDERATIONS
Post-discharge appointment, left ventricular ejection fraction assessment, start on ACEi (or ARB) and β-blocker if left ventricular systolic dysfunction present (7)[A].

Admission Criteria/Initial Stabilization
See above.
- Acute change in HF, with pulmonary edema accompanied by decreased oxygenation, change in mental status, with acute renal insufficiency, or significant hyponatremia
- Consider observation unit stay for hemodynamically stable ED patients assuming pre-existing HF and:
  – No acute interventions needed for comorbid condition
  – SBP >120 mm Hg, BUN <40, creatinine <3.0, absence of elevated troponins/ischemic ECG changes
  – Respiratory rate <32 bpm without needing noninvasive ventilation
  – No actively titrated vasoactive IV infusions
  – Partial improvement in vital signs and/or increased urine output with initial treatment
  – Clinical impression that patient could be discharged in the next 24 hours and rapid outpatient follow-up is available.

IV Fluids
Restrict fluids if possible. Avoid sodium-containing fluids unless necessary to urgently correct hyponatremia.

Discharge Criteria
Subjective improvement, resting heart rate (HR) <100, systolic BP >80 mm Hg, HF outpatient education performed

ONGOING CARE

FOLLOW-UP RECOMMENDATIONS
Critical patient education performed at all outpatient and inpatient physician visits. Please see Chronic Heart Failure section.

Patient Monitoring
Rapid office follow-up after hospitalization and home health monitoring by specially trained nurses have both been shown to decrease frequency of hospitalizations.

DIET
Reduce sodium (2 g); maintain cardiac or diabetic diet if these comorbidities are present.

PATIENT EDUCATION
- Definition and etiology: Understand the cause of HF and why symptoms occur.
- Prognosis: Understand important prognostic factors and make realistic decisions.
- Symptom monitoring and self-care: Recognize signs/symptoms, record daily weight, know how and when to contact a healthcare provider; may increase diuretic dose with >1 kg in a day or >2 kg weight gain in 5 days or dyspnea/contact healthcare provider.
- Pharmacologic treatment: Understand indications, dosing, effects, and side effects of drugs.

- Adherence: Understand the importance of maintaining the treatment plan.
- Alcohol, smoking, and drugs: Modest intake/abstinence is recommended in patients with alcohol-induced cardiomyopathy. Otherwise, normal alcohol guidelines apply. Smoking and illicit drug cessation.
- Exercise: Understand the benefits of exercise, perform regularly, be comfortable about physical activity.

PROGNOSIS
- The ADHERE risk tree stratifies ADHF patients for inpatient mortality using systolic blood pressure, BUN, and creatinine.
- S3 on physical exam correlates with poor prognosis.
- After diagnosis, 1-year survival ~75%, 5-year survival <50%, 10-year <25%

COMPLICATIONS
Sudden death (arrhythmic), acute pulmonary edema, hyponatremia, death

REFERENCES
1. Worster A, Balion CM, Hill SA, et al. Diagnostic accuracy of BNP and NT-proBNP in patients presenting to acute care settings with dyspnea: A systematic review. Clin Biochem. 2008;41: 250–259.
2. Felker GM, Lee KL, Bull DA, et al. Diuretic strategies in patients with acute decompensated heart failure. N Engl J Med. 2011;364:797–805.
3. Konstam MA, Gheorghiade M, Burnett JC, et al. Effects of oral tolvaptan in patients hospitalized for worsening heart failure: The EVEREST Outcome Trial. JAMA. 2007;297:1319–1331.
4. Delaney A, Bradford C, McCaffrey J, et al. Levosimendan for the treatment of acute severe heart failure: A meta-analysis of randomised controlled trials. Int J Cardiol. 2010;138:281–289.
5. O'Connor CM, Starling RC, Hernandez AF, et al. Effect of nesiritide in patients with acute decompensated heart failure. N Engl J Med. 2011;365:32–43.
6. Mariani J, Macchia A, Belziti C, et al. Noninvasive ventilation in acute cardiogenic pulmonary edema: A meta-analysis of randomized controlled trials. J Card Fail. 2011;17:850–859.
7. McMurray JJV, Adamopoulos S, Anker SD, et al. ESC Guidelines for the diagnosis and treatment of acute and chronic heart failure 2012. Eur Heart J. 2012;33:1787–1847.

ADDITIONAL READING
http://www.cdc.gov/dhdsp/data_statistics/fact_sheets/docs/fs_heart_failure.pdf

CODES

ICD10
I50.9 Heart failure, unspecified

CLINICAL PEARLS
- IV diuretics are used initially in fluid-overload acute HF, with nitrates added if needed. Nitrates are primary therapy in ischemic acute HF.
- Evaluate for PDE inhibitor (Viagra, etc.) use before considering nitroglycerin.

HEART FAILURE, CHRONIC

Jeffrey Shih, MD • Jeremy Golding, MD

BASICS

DESCRIPTION
- Heart failure (HF) is the condition resulting from inability of the heart to fill and/or pump blood sufficiently to meet tissue metabolic needs. Alternatively, HF may occur when adequate cardiac output can be achieved only at the expense of elevated filling pressures. It is the principal complication of heart disease.
- HF is the preferred term over congestive heart failure (CHF) because patients are not always congested (fluid overloaded).
- HF may involve the left heart, the right heart, or be biventricular. The New York Heart Association (NYHA) Classification is a fundamental descriptive system used for classifying patients with HF: NYHA I: Asymptomatic; NYHA II: Symptomatic with moderate exertion; NYHA III: Symptomatic with mild exertion and may limit activities of daily living; NYHA IV: Symptomatic at rest. For acute heart failure see "Heart Failure (CHF), Acutely Decompensated."

EPIDEMIOLOGY
The annual cost of heart failure in the US is ~$34.4 billion.

Incidence
In the US, 550,000 new cases annually with >250,000 deaths per year

Prevalence
- ~5.7 million people in the US have HF; <1% in those <50, increasing to 10% of those >80
- Primarily a disease of the elderly; 75% of hospital admissions for HF are for persons >65

ETIOLOGY AND PATHOPHYSIOLOGY
2 physiologic components explain most of the clinical findings of HF and result in classifications of patients in 4 general categories:
- HF with reduced ejection fraction (HFrEF) or systolic HF: An *inotropic* abnormality, often due to myocardial infarction (MI) or dilated cardiomyopathy, resulting in diminished systolic emptying (ejection fraction (EF) ≤40%).
- HF with preserved ejection fraction (HFpEF) or diastolic HF: A *compliance* abnormality, often due to hypertensive cardiomyopathy, in which the ventricular relaxation is impaired (ejection fraction ≥50%).
- Borderline HFpEF (EF 41–49%): Mild systolic dysfunction but clinically behaves like HFpEF.
- Improved HFpEF (EF >40%): Previously HFrEF but with improvement in systolic function.
- Patients with systolic dysfunction may also have diastolic dysfunction.
- Most common etiologies: CAD/ischemia/MI and HTN.
- Myocarditis and cardiomyopathy (CM): Alcoholic, viral, long-standing HTN, drugs (e.g., chemotherapeutic agents), muscular dystrophy, amyloidosis (infiltrative), sarcoidosis (infiltrative), postpartum state, infectious (e.g., Chagas disease, HIV), hypertrophic CM.
- Valvular and vascular abnormalities: Aortic stenosis or regurgitation, rheumatic heart disease (mitral and aortic valvular disease); renal artery stenosis, usually bilateral, may cause recurrent "flash" pulmonary edema, especially in setting of severe chronic HTN

- Chronic lung disease and pulmonary HTN (cor pulmonale)
- Iatrogenic volume overload (requires extreme overload in patients with normal hearts and kidneys)
- Arrhythmias (atrial fibrillation and other tachyarrhythmias, high-grade heart block)
- Miscellaneous: High-output states: Hyperthyroidism, anemia; cardiac depressants (β-blocker overdose), stress-induced.
- Idiopathic: 20–50% of idiopathic dilated cardiomyopathies are familial.

Genetics
Multiple protein abnormalities responsible for a variety of phenotypes have been identified (hypertrophic cardiomyopathy, arrhythmogenic right ventricular [RV] dysplasia, left ventricular [LV] noncompaction, dilated cardiomyopathy).

RISK FACTORS
- For development of HF: Coronary artery disease (CAD) and MI, HTN (80% of cases of HF in the US caused by either CAD or HTN), valvular heart disease, diabetes mellitus, cardiotoxic medications, obesity, older age
- For HF exacerbation: Sodium intake and/or fluid excess; nonadherence to medication regimen; arrhythmia (e.g., atrial fibrillation); ischemic ventricular dysfunction; negative inotropic drugs (e.g., calcium blocker, introduction of β-blocker); excessive physical, emotional, or environmental stress; thyrotoxicosis; pregnancy; or increased metabolic demand

GENERAL PREVENTION
Control BP and other risk factors. Thiazide diuretics and ACE inhibitors are superior to other agents in preventing development of HF.

COMMONLY ASSOCIATED CONDITIONS
Dysrhythmia and pump failure are the leading causes of death. Most patients have >5 comorbid medical conditions and take >5 medications.

DIAGNOSIS

HISTORY
- Dyspnea on exertion: *Cardinal sign of left HF*. Deteriorating exercise capacity: Easy fatigue, general weakness
- Nocturnal nonproductive cough, orthopnea, and paroxysmal nocturnal dyspnea; sometimes frothy or pink sputum. Wheezing, especially nocturnal, in absence of history of asthma or infection (cardiac asthma); Cheyne-Stokes breathing.
- Anorexia and/or fullness or dull pain in right upper quadrant (hepatic congestion)
- Edema: Abdominal bloating (ascites) or anasarca

PHYSICAL EXAM
Enlarged or displaced point of maximal impulse indicating remodeling, rales (crackles) and sometimes wheezing, peripheral edema, S3 gallop, hepatomegaly, jugular venous distension, hepatojugular reflux, ascites, hypotension, pulsus alternans, tachycardia, narrow pulse pressure, cool extremities, cyanosis

DIFFERENTIAL DIAGNOSIS
Simple dependent edema, pulmonary embolism, exertional asthma, cardiac ischemia, asthma/COPD, constrictive pericarditis, nephrotic syndrome, cirrhosis, venous occlusive disease with subsequent peripheral edema, high-output states: Anemia, sepsis, hyperthyroidism

DIAGNOSTIC TESTS & INTERPRETATION
Diagnosis should be primarily clinical, with laboratory data as adjunctive and indicative of complications.

Initial Tests (lab, imaging)
- β-type natriuretic peptide (BNP) and N-type pro-BNP (NT-BNP) helpful in the acute setting to differentiate the cause of dyspnea (BNP <100 essentially rules out HF; most dyspneic patients with HF have a BNP >400). Other, non-HF conditions, such as pulmonary embolism, renal failure, and acute coronary syndromes, may cause elevated BNP. Obesity may lower BNP levels. The utility of BNP-guided therapy in chronic HF and acutely decompensated HF is not well-established, particularly in primary care settings.
- Lab findings in early and mild to moderately severe HF include respiratory alkalosis, mild azotemia, decreased ESR, proteinuria (usually <1 g/24 h), elevated creatinine (cardiorenal syndrome), dilutional hyponatremia (poor prognosis), hyperuricemia, and, rarely, hyperbilirubinemia.
- Chest x-ray (changes lag clinical symptoms by up to 6 hours): Increased heart size, vascular redistribution (cephalization) with "butterfly" pattern of pulmonary edema, interstitial and alveolar edema, Kerley B lines, pleural effusions

Diagnostic Procedures/Other
Determination of LV ejection fraction (LVEF) is critical to proper diagnosis and management:
- Echocardiogram is most useful test to determine ejection fraction, RV function, diastolic dysfunction, ventricular size, wall thickness and valvular abnormalities. May be repeated if change suspected in underlying cardiac status.
- Nuclear imaging to estimate ventricular sizes, perfusion, and systolic function
- Cardiac MRI can be considered in select circumstances: Suspicion of cardiac sarcoidosis, arrhythmogenic RV CM, acute myocarditis, and hemochromatosis. It is also useful for differentiating restrictive CM and constrictive pericarditis.
- Cardiac catheterization is important for excluding CAD as an etiology in the setting of risk factors.

Test Interpretation
- Cardiac pathology depends on underlying etiology.
- Noncardiac findings: Liver is engorged, firm, and fluid-filled. Microscopic analysis reveals dilated central hepatic veins and sinusoids. Late/Chronic findings include hemosiderin deposits in lungs and "nutmeg" liver with centrilobular necrosis.

TREATMENT

MEDICATION
Diuretics are used initially in fluid-overload acute HF, with nitrates added if needed. The addition of ACE inhibitors and aldosterone antagonists can be added at any time. Once acute HF is stabilized, a β-blocker should be started. Avoid NSAIDs, which markedly worsen HF. Avoid use of diltiazem and verapamil in patients with systolic dysfunction.

First Line

- ACE inhibitors: Used to decrease afterload. Shown to increase survival, improve general symptomatology and overall exercise capacity in patients in all NYHA classifications; benefit greatest for patients with systolic dysfunction and post-MI. Number needed to treat (NNT) ~25/year for mortality (1)[A].

- β-blockers used in systolic or diastolic HF (Note: Initiate in hospital or outpatient setting in hemodynamically stable patients at low dose and titrate upward slowly); NNT = 25 for mortality. Mortality decreased in systolic HF. Evidence mounting for titration to heart rate rather than specific dose:
  - Carvedilol: 3.125 mg PO b.i.d. to a maintenance of 25 mg PO b.i.d.; metoprolol succinate extended release: 12.5 mg/d PO to a maximum of 200 mg/d PO (metoprolol tartrate may be equivalent but is taken b.i.d.) or bisoprolol 1.25–10 mg once daily (currently not FDA approved for the treatment of HF).

- Digoxin reduces symptoms, but has not clearly shown any positive effect on mortality (1)[A]: In patients with preserved renal function (creatinine clearance >50 mL/min), the recommended dose is 0.125 mg/d. Levels lower than used for atrial fibrillation are effective and safer.

- Diuretics helpful to manage volume overload/reduce preload:
  - Furosemide (Lasix): 20–320 mg IV/IM/PO divided dose; bumetanide (Bumex): 0.5 mg–10 mg IV/PO divided; torsemide (Demadex): 10–200 mg PO divided
  - Metolazone (Zaroxolyn): 2.5–20 mg/d PO divided dose; hydrochlorothiazide: 12.5–100 mg PO divided; chlorothiazide (Diuril): 250–2,000 mg IV/PO divided
  - Spironolactone, eplerenone (improve mortality when added to standard therapy in NYHA Class II- IV+EF<35%) (1,2)[A]: Spironolactone 12.5–25 mg/d PO; maximum 50 mg/d PO; eplerenone 25–50 mg/d. Caution regarding hyperkalemia and CKD (1)[A].

- Angiotensin receptor blockers (ARBs) are indicated for those who are unable to take ACE inhibitors. They are equally or slightly less effective than ACE inhibitors.

- The combination of hydralazine (75 mg/d divided b.i.d. or t.i.d.) and isosorbide dinitrate (40 mg q.i.d.) is effective for African Americans (1)[A] or if unable to take ACE inhibitors or an ARB.

- Anticoagulation is not recommended in patients with HFrEF unless there are other indications such as atrial fibrillation, cardioembolism, or intracardiac thrombus.

ADDITIONAL THERAPIES

Device therapy including implantable cardioverter defibrillators (ICD) and cardiac resynchronization (CRT) shown to improve outcomes.

- CRT is recommended for patients in sinus rhythm with a QRS width ≥150 due to left bundle branch block (LBBB) and LVEF ≤35% and persistent mild-moderate HF (NYHA II–III) despite optimal medical therapy. CRT may be considered for ambulatory NYHA class IV patients in sinus rhythm with a QRS width ≥150 ms, LBBB and LVEF ≤35%.

- CRT may be considered for patients with LVEF ≤35%, sinus rhythm, QRS width ≥150, non-LBBB pattern, and NYHA III or ambulatory NYHA IV symptoms.

- CRT may also be considered for patients with a QRS width between 120–150 ms, LBBB, LVEF ≤35%, and persistent mild-severe HF (NYHA II–IV) despite optimal medical therapy (3,4,5)[A].

- ICDs are recommended for: Primary prevention in patients with *non-ischemic* CM and *ischemic* CM who are at least 40 days post-MI; LVEF ≤35%, NYHA class II or III HF or LVEF ≤30%, NYHA I HF; on optimal medical therapy, and >1 year estimated survival (1)[A]. Generally not indicated in AHA Stage D (end-stage) HF.

SURGERY/OTHER PROCEDURES

- Heart valve surgery if defective heart valve is responsible; mitral valve repair especially helpful if mitral regurgitation is aggravating condition.

- Advanced therapies such as cardiac transplantation and LV assist device (LVAD) implantation can be considered in patients with HF refractory to conventional medical/device therapies without other disqualifying medical and psychosocial conditions. Cardiac transplantation is generally considered for patients <65–70 years old with a predicted 1-year survival worse than that afforded by transplantation. Indications for LVAD implantation are generally similar to cardiac transplantation but are evolving.

IN-PATIENT CONSIDERATIONS

Admission Criteria/Initial Stabilization

- Sublingual nitroglycerin is rapid-onset and reduces primarily preload. Oxygen for symptoms. Diuretics to reduce preload. See "Heart Failure, Acutely Decompensated."

- Hemodynamic/Respiratory compromise, hypoxia/hypoxemia, change in mental status, acute renal insufficiency, significant volume overload, significant electrolyte abnormalities (e.g., hyponatremia)

Discharge Criteria

Subjective improvement, euvolemia on clinical assessment, resting heart rate (HR) <100, systolic BP >80 mm Hg, HF outpatient education performed

 ## ONGOING CARE

FOLLOW-UP RECOMMENDATIONS

Critical patient education performed at all outpatient and inpatient physician visits "MAWDS":

- **M**edications: Take every day; don't skip.
- **A**ctivity: A little every day; don't overdo.
- **W**eight: Daily. If gain >2 lb in a day or 5 lb above ideal, CALL.
- **D**iet: Eat <2,000 mg Na+ daily.
- **S**ymptoms: Know the signs of worsening HF (cough, weight gain, worsening or rest dyspnea, swelling) and call the doctor early! Quit smoking, if a smoker!

Patient Monitoring

Rapid office follow-up (1–2 weeks) after hospitalization and home health monitoring by specially trained nurses have both been shown to decrease frequency of hospitalizations.

DIET

Reduce sodium load (<2 g/d).

PATIENT EDUCATION

American Heart Association: www.americanheart.org

PROGNOSIS

After diagnosis: 1-year survival ~75%, 5-year survival <50%, 10 year <25%.

COMPLICATIONS

Sudden death (arrhythmic), acute pulmonary edema, death, progressive pump failure

REFERENCES

1. Yancy C, Jessup M, Bozkurt B, et al. 2013 ACCF/AHA Guideline for the Management of Heart Failure: A report of the American College of Cardiology Foundation/American Heart Association Task force on Practice Guidelines. *J Am Coll Cardiol*. 2013;62(16):e147–e239.
2. Zannad F. Eplerenone in patients with systolic heart failure and mild symptoms. *N Engl J Med*. 2011; 364:11–21.
3. Al-Majed NS. Meta-analysis: Cardiac resynchronization therapy for patients with less symptomatic heart failure. *Ann Intern Med*. 2011;84(6):401–412.
4. Wells G, Parkask R, Healey JS, et al. Cardiac resynchronization therapy: A meta-analysis of randomized controlled trials. *CMAJ*. 2011;183: 421–429.
5. Stevenson WG, Hernandez AF, Carson PE, et al. Indications for cardiac resynchronization therapy: 2011 update from the Heart Failure Society of America Guideline Committee. *JCF*. 2012;18: 94–106.

ADDITIONAL READING

Felker GM, Lee KL, Redfield MM, et al. Diuretic strategies in patients with acute decompensated heart failure. *N Engl J Med*. 2011;64:797.

 SEE ALSO

Algorithms: Congestive Heart Failure; Congestive Heart Failure, Treatment

CODES

ICD10

- I50.1 Left ventricular failure
- I50.9 Heart failure, unspecified
- I50.22 Chronic systolic (congestive) heart failure

CLINICAL PEARLS

- Have patients weigh themselves daily and report weight gains of >2 lb in a day or 5 lb above dry weight.
- β-Blockers, ACE inhibitors, and aldosterone antagonists are the core medications for management of this condition.
- Consider referral for biventricular pacing in patients with bundle branch block and ICD in those with low EF.

HEAT EXHAUSTION AND HEAT STROKE

Brian Frank, MD • Scott A. Fields, MD, MHA

 BASICS

DESCRIPTION
- A continuum of increasingly severe heat illnesses caused by dehydration, electrolyte losses, and failure of the body's thermoregulatory mechanisms:
  - Heat exhaustion is an acute heat injury with hyperthermia owing to dehydration.
  - Heat stroke is extreme hyperthermia with thermoregulatory failure and profound CNS dysfunction.
- System(s) affected: Endocrine/Metabolic; Nervous
- Synonym(s): Heat illness; Heat injury; Hyperthermia; Heat collapse; Heat prostration

Geriatric Considerations
Elderly persons are more susceptible.

Pediatric Considerations
Children are more susceptible.

Pregnancy Considerations
Pregnant women may be more susceptible to volume depletion with heat stress.

EPIDEMIOLOGY
- Predominant age: More likely in children or elderly
- Predominant sex: Male = Female

Incidence
Depends on intensity of heat; estimate of 20/100,000 persons per season

Prevalence
- Depends on predisposing conditions in combination with environmental factors
- Roughly 240 deaths/year in the US

ETIOLOGY AND PATHOPHYSIOLOGY
- Interplay between failure of heat-dissipating mechanisms, an overwhelming heat stress, and an exaggerated acute-phase inflammatory response
- Direct cellular toxicity of heat, imbalance between inflammatory and anti-inflammatory cytokines, and vascular endothelial damage causing end-organ dysfunction

RISK FACTORS
- Poor acclimatization to heat or poor physical conditioning
- Salt or water depletion
- Obesity
- Acute febrile or GI illnesses
- Chronic illnesses: Uncontrolled diabetes mellitus or hypertension, cardiac disease
- Alcohol and other substance abuse
- High heat and humidity, poor air circulation in environment
- Heavy, restrictive clothing
- Nutritional supplementation that includes ephedra

GENERAL PREVENTION
- The most important factor in preventing heat stress is adequate fluid replacement.
- Allow acclimatization to hot weather through proper conditioning and activity modification.
- Dress appropriately with loose-fitting, open-weave, light-colored clothing.

 DIAGNOSIS

- Heat exhaustion: Symptoms are milder than in heat stroke, with no severe CNS derangements:
  - Fatigue and lethargy
  - Weakness
  - Dizziness
  - Nausea, vomiting
  - Myalgias
  - Headache
  - Profuse sweating
  - Tachycardia
  - Hypotension
  - Lack of coordination
  - Agitation
  - Intense thirst
  - Hyperventilation
  - Paresthesias
  - Core temperature elevated but <103°F (<39.4°C)
- Heat stroke: Divided into 2 categories: Classic and exertional:
  - Classic: Caused by environmental exposure, primarily in elderly or chronically ill patients, and may develop gradually over days:
    o Delirium
    o Confusion
    o Coma
    o Core temperature >104°F (>40°C)
  - Exertional: Typically younger, very active patients; rapid onset:
    o Exhaustion
    o Confusion, disorientation
    o Delirium
    o Coma
    o Hot, flushed, and dry skin (sweating may continue in exertional heat stroke)
    o Core temperature >105°F (>40.5°C)

DIFFERENTIAL DIAGNOSIS
- Other causes of elevated temperature, dehydration, or circulatory collapse
- Febrile illnesses, sepsis
- Drug-induced fluid loss
- Cardiac arrhythmia or infarction
- Acute cocaine intoxication
- Neuroleptic malignant syndrome
- Malignant hyperthermia (an autosomally inherited disorder of skeletal and cardiac muscle in which patients have abnormal muscle metabolism on exposure to halothane or skeletal muscle reactants)

DIAGNOSTIC TESTS & INTERPRETATION
Used primarily to detect end-organ damage

Initial Tests (lab, imaging)
- Electrolytes, urinalysis
- Creatinine, BUN
- Liver enzymes, muscle enzymes (creatine phosphokinase)
- CBC
- Increased urine specific gravity
- Results of these studies may indicate hypernatremia, hyperchloremia, and hemoconcentration.
- Drugs that may alter lab results: Diuretics

Diagnostic Procedures/Other
Rectal temperature monitoring (do not rely on oral temp)

 TREATMENT

GENERAL MEASURES
- Fluid and electrolyte replacement with hypotonic PO fluids or IV 0.5–1 L normal saline initial bolus
- Consider central venous pressure (CVP) monitoring.
- Body immersion in ice water (1,2)[C]
- Evaporative cooling: Spraying water over the patient and facilitating evaporation and convection with the use of fans (1,2)[C]
- Immersing the hands and forearms in cold water (1,2)[C]
- Use of ice or cold packs on the neck, groin, and axillae (3)
- No clear superiority of any one method (4)

MEDICATION
First Line
No medications are required in the initial management. Use isotonic saline solution to rehydrate (1,2)[C].

Second Line
- Consider immunomodulators such as corticosteroids (2)[C].
- Iced gastric, bladder, or peritoneal lavage (1,2)[C]
- Dantrolene: 2–4 mg/kg for chemically assisted cooling (2)[C]
- In disseminated intravascular coagulopathy (DIC), consider appropriate replacement therapy.

IN-PATIENT CONSIDERATIONS
Admission Criteria/Initial Stabilization
- Emergency treatment; best in a hospital setting
- Rapid cooling: Remove clothing, wet patient down, and apply ice packs.

ONGOING CARE

FOLLOW-UP RECOMMENDATIONS
Rest with legs elevated (1,2)[C]

Patient Monitoring
- Rectal temperature monitoring: Cooling may be discontinued when the core temperature drops to 102°F (38.9°C) and stabilizes.
- Heat stroke patients may require airway management, hemodynamic monitoring, and careful fluid and electrolyte administration and monitoring.
- Consider CVP monitoring.

DIET
- Cool or cold clear liquids only (noncarbonated)
- Avoid caffeine.
- Unrestricted sodium

PATIENT EDUCATION
- The key to prevention is proper hydration.
- Stress the importance of proper conditioning and acclimatization.
- Instruct patients to recognize heat stress signs and symptoms.
- Maintain as much skin exposure as possible in hot, humid conditions while using proper sunblock protection.
- Avoid dehydration by consuming a proper amount of fluids during activity or exercise: 8 oz fluid intake for every 15 minutes of moderate exercise.
- Never leave children unattended in cars during hot weather.
- Try to gain access to air-conditioned environments during hot weather.

PROGNOSIS
- The prognosis is good when mental function is not altered and when serum enzymes are not elevated; recovery is within 24–48 hours in most cases.
- The mortality rate for heat stroke (10–80%) is directly related to the duration and intensity of hyperthermia, as well as to the speed and effectiveness of diagnosis and treatment.

COMPLICATIONS
- May involve failure of any major organ system
- Cardiac arrhythmias or infarction
- Pulmonary edema, acute respiratory distress syndrome
- Coma, seizures
- Acute renal failure
- Rhabdomyolysis
- DIC
- Hepatocellular necrosis

REFERENCES

1. Cleary M. Predisposing risk factors on susceptibility to exertional heat illness: Clinical decision-making considerations. *J Sport Rehabilitation*. 2007;16(3): 204–214.
2. Muldoon S. Identification of risk factors for exertional heat illness: A brief commentary on genetic testing. *J Sport Rehabilitation*. 2007;16(3): 222–226.
3. Gaffin SL, Gardner JW, Flinn SD. Cooling methods for heatstroke victims. *Ann Intern Med*. 2000;132: 678.
4. Bouchama A, Dehbi M, Chaves-Carballo E. Cooling and hemodynamic management in heatstroke: Practical recommendations. *Crit Care*. 2007;11(3): R54.

ADDITIONAL READING

- American College of Sports Medicine, Armstrong LE, Casa DJ, et al. American College of Sports Medicine position stand. Exertional heat illness during training and competition. *Med Sci Sports Exerc*. 2007;39: 556–572.
- Bouchama A, Knochel JP. Heat stroke. *N Engl J Med*. 2002;346:1978–1988.
- Charaton F. Ephedra supplement may have contributed to sportsman's death. *Br Med J*. 2003;326:464.

- Glazer JL. Management of heatstroke and heat exhaustion. *Am Fam Physician*. 2005;71(11): 2133–2140.
- Mazerolle S, Ganio M, Casa D, et al. Is oral temperature an accurate measurement of deep body temperature? A systematic review. *J Athl Train*. 2011;46(5):566–573. doi: PMCID:PMC3418963
- Smith JE. Cooling methods used in the treatment of exertional heat illness. *Br J Sports Med*. 2005;39:503–507; discussion 507.
- Yeo TP. Heat stroke: A comprehensive review. *AACN Clin Issues*. 2004;15:280–293.

 ## CODES

ICD10
- T67.0XXA Heatstroke and sunstroke, initial encounter
- T67.3XXA Heat exhaustion, anhydrotic, initial encounter
- T67.5XXA Heat exhaustion, unspecified, initial encounter

CLINICAL PEARLS

- The diagnosis of heat stroke relies on both hyperthermia and CNS dysfunction (e.g., irritability, ataxia, confusion, seizures, or coma).
- Start the cooling process immediately when heat exhaustion or heat stroke is recognized, beginning with wetting the skin with a cool mist and giving oral rehydration solutions containing saline, if the patient is alert and oriented.
- Do not rely on oral temperature.

HEMATURIA

Tracy O. Middleton, DO

 BASICS

DESCRIPTION
Blood or RBCs in the urine:
- Gross (visible) or microscopic (nonvisible)
- Symptomatic or asymptomatic

EPIDEMIOLOGY
Prevalence
- Microscopic hematuria in school-aged children: 0.5–2%
- Microscopic hematuria in asymptomatic adults varies from 0.19–21%, depending on population studied (1,2).

ETIOLOGY AND PATHOPHYSIOLOGY
- Trauma:
  - Exercise-induced (resolves with rest)
  - Abdominal trauma or pelvic fracture with renal, bladder, or ureteral injury
  - Iatrogenic from abdominal or pelvic surgery; chronic indwelling catheters
  - Foreign body, physical/sexual abuse
- Neoplasms:
  - Malignancies
  - Benign tumors
  - Endometriosis of the urinary tract (suspect in females with cyclic hematuria)
- Inflammatory causes:
  - UTI: Most common cause of hematuria in adults
  - Renal diseases: Radiation nephritis and cystitis, acute/chronic tubulointerstitial nephritis (due to drugs, infections, systemic disease)
  - Glomerular disease:
    - Goodpasture syndrome (antiglomerular basement membrane disease; autoimmune; associated pulmonary hemorrhage)
    - IgA nephropathy
    - Lupus nephritis
    - Henoch-Schönlein purpura
    - Membranoproliferative, poststreptococcal, or rapidly progressive glomerulonephritis (GN)
    - Wegener granulomatosis
  - Endocarditis/Visceral abscesses
  - Other infections: Schistosomiasis, TB, syphilis
- Metabolic causes:
  - Stones (85% have hematuria):
    - Hypercalciuria: A common cause of both gross and microscopic hematuria in children
    - Hyperuricosuria
- Congenital/Familial causes:
  - Cystic disease: Polycystic kidney disease, solitary renal cyst
  - Benign familial hematuria or thin basement membrane nephropathy (autosomal dominant)
  - Alport syndrome (X-linked in 85%; hematuria, proteinuria, hearing loss, corneal abnormalities)
  - Fabry disease (X-linked recessive inborn error of metabolism; vascular kidney disease)
  - Nail-patella syndrome (autosomal dominant; nail and patella hypoplasia; hematuria in 33%)
  - Renal tubular acidosis type 1 (autosomal dominant or autoimmune)
- Hematologic causes:
  - Bleeding dyscrasias (e.g., hemophilia)
  - Sickle cell anemia/trait (renal papillary necrosis)
- Vascular causes:
  - Hemangioma
  - Arteriovenous malformations (rare)
  - Nutcracker syndrome: Compression of left renal vein and subsequent renal parenchymal congestion
  - Renal artery/vein thrombosis
  - Arterial emboli to kidney
- Chemical causes:
  - Nephrotoxins: Aminoglycosides, cyclosporine
  - Other drugs: Analgesics, oral contraceptives, Chinese herbs
- Obstruction:
  - Strictures or posterior urethral valves
  - Hydronephrosis from any cause
  - Benign prostatic hyperplasia: Rule out other causes of hematuria.
- Other causes: Loin pain hematuria (most often in young women on oral contraceptives)

RISK FACTORS
- Smoking
- Occupational exposures (dyes, rubber or tire manufacturing)
- Analgesic abuse (e.g., phenacetin)
- Medications (e.g., cyclophosphamide)
- Pelvic irradiation
- Chronic infection, especially with calculi
- Recent upper respiratory tract infection
- Positive family history of renal diseases (stones, glomerulonephritis)
- Underlying primary renal disorder
- Chronic indwelling foreign body

 DIAGNOSIS

HISTORY
Considerations:
- Burning, urgency, frequency: UTI
- Dark cola-colored urine: Glomerular origin
- Clots: Extraglomerular bleeding
- Arthritis/Arthralgias/Rash: Lupus, vasculitis, Henoch-Schönlein purpura
- Flank pain: Stones, infarction, pyelonephritis
- Recent upper respiratory infection (URI): Poststreptococcal GN, membranoproliferative GN
- Concurrent URI: IgA nephropathy
- Excessive vitamin use: Stones
- Marathon runner: Traumatic, rhabdomyolysis
- Travel: Schistosomiasis, tuberculosis
- Painless hematuria and/or weight loss: Malignancy
- Family history: Alport disease (hereditary nephritis), sickle cell, polycystic, IgA nephropathy, thin basement membrane disease

PHYSICAL EXAM
Considerations:
- Elevated BP, edema, and weight gain: Glomerular disease
- Fever: Infection
- Palpable kidney: Neoplasm, polycystic
- Genitalia: Look for meatal erosion, lesions

DIAGNOSTIC TESTS & INTERPRETATION
- A hematuria risk index has been developed to assist in stratifying patients at risk for urothelial malignancies who require more intensive testing. High-risk indicators are gross hematuria, age >50, male gender, and smoking (3)[B].
- American Urological Association (AUA) suggests upper urinary tract imaging in all adults with unexplained hematuria, and cystoscopy in all unexplained hematuria patients ≥ 35 (4)[C].

Initial Tests (lab, imaging)
- Urine dipstick (sensitivity 91–100%; specificity 65–99%):
  - False negatives are rare, but can be caused by high-dose vitamin C.
  - False positives: Oxidizers (povidone, bacterial peroxidases, bleach), myoglobin, alkaline urine (>9), semen, food coloring, food (beets, blackberries, rhubarb, paprika) (5)
  - Phenazopyridine may discolor the dipstick, making interpretation difficult.
- Microscopic urinalysis should always be done to confirm dipstick findings and quantify RBCs:
  - AUA defines clinically significant microscopic hematuria as ≥3 RBCs/hpf on a properly collected urinary specimen when there is not an obvious benign cause (4)[C].
  - Positive dipstick but a negative microscopic exam should be followed by 3 repeat tests. If any 1 is positive, proceed with a workup (4)[C].
  - Exclude factitious or nonurinary causes, such as menstruation, mild trauma, exercise, poor collection technique, or chemical/drug causes, through cessation of activity/cause and a repeat urinalysis in 48 hours (1)[C].
- Voided urine cytology: Recommended if risk factors for transitional cell carcinoma; obtain 1st urine voided on 3 consecutive days; send for "urine cytology"; may require special fixative (Saccomanno, others)
- Renal function tests (eGFR, BUN, creatinine) to differentiate intrinsic renal disease and to evaluate for risks for imaging contrast dye or certain medications.
  - Indicators of renal disease are significant (>500 mg/d) proteinuria, red cell casts (pathognomonic of glomerular disease), dysmorphic RBCs, and increased creatinine (4)[C].
- Urine culture if suspected infection/pyuria (6)
- PT/INR for patients on warfarin or suspected of abusing warfarin
- Renal ultrasound:
  - Best 1st test in evaluation of microscopic hematuria and for those who are pregnant
  - Best for differentiating cystic from solid masses
  - Sensitive for hydronephrosis
  - No radiation or iodinated contrast exposure
  - Cost-efficient
  - Poor sensitivity for renal masses <3 cm
  - Main disadvantage is inability to thoroughly evaluate the urothelium for transitional cell cancer
- Multidetector CT urography (MDCTU); sensitivity 88–100%, specificity 93–100%:
  - The initial imaging of choice in nonpregnant adults with unexplained hematuria (5,7)[B]
  - Highly specific and relatively sensitive for the diagnosis of urinary tract neoplasms, especially when >1 cm (7)[B]

– Higher radiation dose; weigh risk of disease vs. risk of radiation exposure
– Does not obviate the need for cystoscopy, particularly in high-risk patients (7)[B]
– Presence of calculi on noncontrast does not exclude another diagnosis or need for contrast phase
– Visualization of ureters is discontinuous.
– Less cost-efficient
• CT:
– Perform unenhanced helical CT as 1st test for suspected stone disease (1)[B].
• Magnetic resonance urography (MRU):
– High sensitivity/specificity for renal parenchyma; less useful for collecting system
– Can be used in patients with contraindications to MDCTU (4)[C]
• IV urography (IVU):
– Limited sensitivity for small renal masses and for differentiating cystic from solid masses
– Addition of US or CT often necessary to evaluate renal parenchyma
– Potential reactions to IV iodine contrast media
• MRI:
– Similar to CT in sensitivity for renal masses
– No radiation exposure
– Least cost-efficient
– Limited ability to reliably detect urinary tract calcifications
– Can be combined with retrograde pyelogram (RPG) for patients who cannot tolerate MDCTU or MRU (4)[C]

Diagnostic Procedures/Other
• Flexible cystoscopy:
– Best for evaluation of bladder pathology, especially small urothelial lesions; negative predictive value for bladder tumors is 99% (1)[B].
– AUA recommends all patients with hematuria who are ≥35 with risk factors for bladder cancer receive cystoscopy (4)[C].
• Renal biopsy:
– Not routine, but may be necessary to diagnose glomerulonephritis or in the face of increasing renal insufficiency
• Retrograde pyelogram (RPG):
– Reserved for patients in which findings on MDCTU are equivocal or in addition to US or noncontrast studies in patients who are contraindicated for contrast or MRI (4)[C]
– Sensitive for small lesions of supravesicular collecting system
– Requires cystoscopy
• Ureteroscopy/Pyeloscopy:
– For visualization of suspected supravesical collecting system lesions
– Biopsy, excision, fulguration, or extraction of lesions/stones possible
– Requires anesthesia
– Requires cystoscopy
– Risk of injury to collecting system

Follow-Up Tests & Special Considerations
• Other tests depend on suspected etiology: STD) testing, antineutrophil cytoplasmic antibody (ANCA), C3, C4, antistreptolysin O (ASO) titer, hemoglobin electrophoresis (6).
• Urinary tumor markers are available but not routinely recommended.
• In the case of glomerulonephritis, consider CXR to rule out cardiac enlargement, effusions, or pulmonary bleeding (5)[C].

Pregnancy Considerations
Renal US is initial imaging choice for pregnant patients (5)[C]. MRU or RPG combined with either MRI or US are alternatives.

Pediatric Considerations
• Consider glomerulonephritis, Wilms tumor, child abuse
• Isolated asymptomatic microscopic hematuria may not need full workup; these patients rarely need cystoscopy; observe for development of hypertension, gross hematuria, or proteinuria (6)[C].
• Gross or symptomatic hematuria needs a full workup.
– If eumorphic RBCs, consider US (rule out stones, congenital abnormalities) and urinary Ca:Cr ratio. Urine Ca:Cr ratio >0.2 mg/mg is suggestive of hypercalciuria in children >6 years (6).
• If dysmorphic RBCs, consider renal consult
• Renal US identifies most congenital and malignant conditions; CT is reserved for cases of suspected trauma (with contrast) or stones (without contrast) (6,8)[C].

 ## TREATMENT

MEDICATION
None indicated for undiagnosed hematuria

ISSUES FOR REFERRAL
Prompt nephrology referral for proteinuria, red cell casts, and elevated serum creatinine (4)[C]

SURGERY/OTHER PROCEDURES
Gross hematuria: Clots may require continuous bladder irrigation with a large-bore Foley catheter (2- or 3-way catheter may be helpful) to prevent clot retention.

 ## ONGOING CARE

FOLLOW-UP RECOMMENDATIONS
After initial workup, 35% of patients remain without a diagnosis.

Patient Monitoring
• Some experts still recommend periodic urinalysis; recent literature suggests that, after thorough initial negative investigations (imaging, cystoscopy), no follow up is indicated for the asymptomatic patient with microscopic hematuria unless symptoms or frank hematuria develop (2)[B]. AUA recommends annual urinalyses in these patients, until 2 consecutive are negative, and the consideration for a repeat workup at 3–5 years if hematuria is persistent (4)[C].

DIET
Increased fluids for stones or clots, and decreased soda intake for stone prevention.

PROGNOSIS
• Generally excellent for common causes of hematuria
• Poorer for malignant tumors and certain types of nephritis

REFERENCES
1. McDonald MM, Swagerty D, Wetzel L. Assessment of microscopic hematuria in adults. Am Fam Physician. 2006;73:1748–1754.
2. Mishriki SF, Nabi G, Cohen NP. Diagnosis of urologic malignancies in patients with asymptomatic dipstick hematuria: Prospective study with 13 years' follow-up. Urology. 2008;71:13–16.
3. Loo RK, Lieberman SF, Slezak JM, et al. Stratifying risk of urinary tract malignant tumors in patients with asymptomatic microscopic hematuria. Mayo Clin Proc. 2013;88:129–138.
4. Davis R, Jones JS, Barocas DA, et al. Diagnosis, evaluation and follow-up of asymptomatic microhematuria (AMH) in adults: AUA guideline. J Urol. 2012;188:2473–2481.
5. Choyke PL. Radiologic evaluation of hematuria: Guidelines from the American College of Radiology's appropriateness criteria. Am Fam Physician. 2008;78:347–352.
6. Massengill SF. Hematuria. Pediatr Rev. 2008;29:342–348.
7. Sudakoff GS, Dunn DP, Guralnick ML, et al. Multidetector computerized tomography urography as the primary imaging modality for detecting urinary tract neoplasms in patients with asymptomatic hematuria. J Urol. 2008;179:862–867.
8. Dillman JR, Coley BD, Karmazyn B, et al. Expert Panel on Pediatric Imaging. ACR Appropriateness Criteria® hematuria—child. Reston, VA: American College of Radiology; 2012. Available at: www.guideline.gov/content.aspx?id=43874

 ## SEE ALSO
Algorithm: Hematuria

 ## CODES

ICD10
• R31.1 Benign essential microscopic hematuria
• R31.2 Other microscopic hematuria
• R31.9 Hematuria, unspecified

CLINICAL PEARLS
• Screening asymptomatic patients for microscopic hematuria is not recommended (1,6)[A].
• Asymptomatic hematuria and hematuria persisting after treatment of UTIs must be evaluated (1)[B].
• Patients with bladder cancer can have intermittent microscopic hematuria; a thorough evaluation in high-risk patients is needed after just 1 episode.
• Evaluation of upper and lower urinary tracts, including imaging and cystoscopy, must be performed in all patients with gross hematuria and in high-risk patients with microscopic hematuria (4)[C].
• After initial workup, 35% of patients remain without a diagnosis.
• Routine use of anticoagulants should not cause hematuria unless there is an underlying urologic abnormality (1)[B].
• Signs of underlying renal disease indicate the need for a nephrologic workup; but a urologic evaluation is still needed in the presence of persistent hematuria (4)[C].

HEMOCHROMATOSIS

Robert A. Marlow, MD, MA

 BASICS

DESCRIPTION
Hemochromatosis is a hereditary disorder in which the small intestine absorbs excessive iron (1,2):
- Early clinical features include arthralgia, fatigue, and decreased libido.
- Late effects include cirrhosis of the liver, diabetes, hypermelanotic pigmentation of the skin, and heart failure.
- Because there is no mechanism to excrete excess iron, the excess is stored in muscle and in organs, including the liver, pancreas, and heart, eventually resulting in severe damage to the affected organs.
- Liver damage ultimately may result in hepatocellular carcinoma.
- System(s) affected: Endocrine/Metabolic
- Synonym(s): Bronze diabetes; Troisier-Hanot-Chauffard syndrome

EPIDEMIOLOGY
Incidence
- Predominant age: Metabolic abnormality is congenital, but symptoms usually present in the 5th and 6th decades.
- Predominant sex: Gene frequency: Male = Female (8:1), although clinical signs are more frequent in men (3)

Prevalence
- 3/1,000 people (heterozygote frequency, 1/10) (4)
- The most common genetic abnormality in the US.

Pediatric Considerations
Rarely, iron overload may occur as early as 2 years of age. The disorder can be diagnosed before iron overload is clinically apparent.

ETIOLOGY AND PATHOPHYSIOLOGY
- Type 1 hemochromatosis is caused by mutations in the *HFE* gene; type 2 by mutations in either the *HFE2* gene or *HAMP* gene; type 3 by mutations in the *TFR2* gene; and type 4 by mutations in the *SLC40A1* gene. The cause of neonatal hemochromatosis is unknown.
- The mechanism for increased iron absorption in the face of excessive iron stores is not clear. Iron metabolism appears normal in this disease except for a higher level of circulating iron.
- Iron overload may be caused by thalassemia, sideroblastic anemia, liver disease, excess iron intake, or chronic transfusion.

Genetics
- Genetically heterogeneous disorder of iron overload; types 1, 2, and 3 are autosomal recessive; type 4 is autosomal dominant. Neonatal hemochromatosis is rare.
- Penetrance is incomplete; expressivity is variable.
- Factors contributing to variable expressivity include different mutations in the same gene, mitigating or exacerbating genes, and environmental factors.

RISK FACTORS
- The disease is a genetic disorder.
- Affected individuals should not ingest iron supplements, eat raw shellfish, or eat large quantities of iron-rich food, such as red meat.
- Alcohol increases the absorption of iron. (As many as 41% of patients with symptomatic disease are alcoholic.)
- Loss of blood, such as that which occurs during menstruation and pregnancy, delays the onset of symptoms.

GENERAL PREVENTION
- Family members of affected individuals should be screened.
- Pregnant women with the disorder should avoid iron supplements.

ALERT
Screening of population is *not* recommended because the vast majority of those with homozygous hemochromatosis will remain asymptomatic and have a normal life span (5,6)[A].

COMMONLY ASSOCIATED CONDITIONS
See "Complications."

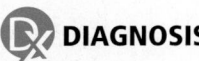 **DIAGNOSIS**

HISTORY
- Weakness (83%)
- Abdominal pain (58%)
- Arthralgia (43%)
- Loss of libido or potency (38%)
- Amenorrhea (22%)
- Dyspnea on exertion (15%)
- Neurologic symptoms (6%)
- Symptoms of diabetes

PHYSICAL EXAM
- Hepatomegaly (83%)
- Increased skin pigmentation (75%)
- Loss of body hair (20%)
- Splenomegaly (13%)
- Peripheral edema (12%)
- Jaundice (10%)
- Gynecomastia (8%)
- Ascites (6%)
- Testicular atrophy
- Hepatic tenderness

DIFFERENTIAL DIAGNOSIS
- Repeated transfusions
- Hereditary anemias with ineffective erythropoiesis
- Alcoholic cirrhosis
- Porphyria cutanea tarda
- Atransferrinemia
- Excessive ingestion of iron (rare)

DIAGNOSTIC TESTS & INTERPRETATION
- After the diagnosis is established, consider having the patient take an oral glucose tolerance test to rule out diabetes and undergo an echocardiogram to rule out cardiomyopathy:
  - Transferrin saturation (serum iron concentration ÷ total iron-binding capacity × 100): >70% is virtually diagnostic of iron overload; ≥45% warrants further evaluation. Iron supplements and transfusions may elevate serum iron.
  - Serum ferritin: >300 μg/L for men and postmenopausal women and 200 μg/L for premenopausal women (7); may be elevated by inflammatory reactions, other forms of liver disease, certain tumors (e.g., acute granulocytic leukemia), and rheumatoid arthritis
  - Urinary iron
  - Increased urine hemosiderin
  - Hyperglycemia
  - Decreased FSH
  - Decreased LH
  - Decreased testosterone
  - Increased serum glutamic-oxaloacetic transaminase
  - Hypoalbuminemia
- If the diagnosis is uncertain after laboratory testing, MRI may be helpful (1).

Diagnostic Procedures/Other
- Liver biopsy for stainable iron is the standard for diagnosis. Presence or absence of cirrhosis also can be ascertained. However, with the availability of genetic testing, liver biopsy is not frequently necessary to confirm the diagnosis (7)[C].
- DNA PCR testing for *HFE* gene mutations C282Y and H63D: Present in 85–90% of patients
- Homozygosity for the C282Y mutation with biochemical evidence for iron overload can confirm the diagnosis.

Test Interpretation
- Increased hepatic parenchymal iron stores
- Hepatic fibrosis and cirrhosis with hepatomegaly
- Pancreatic enlargement
- Excess hemosiderin in liver, pancreas, myocardium, thyroid, parathyroid, joints, skin
- Cardiomegaly
- Joint deposition of iron

TREATMENT

MEDICATION

- None. Only when phlebotomy is not feasible or in the presence of severe heart disease should the iron-chelating agent deferoxamine (Desferal) be considered.
- Hepatitis A and hepatitis B immunizations should be done if there is no evidence of previous exposure (6).

GENERAL MEASURES

- Remove excess iron by repeated phlebotomy once or twice weekly to establish and maintain a mild anemia (hematocrit of 35–39%) (7)[C].
- When the patient finally becomes iron deficient, a lifelong maintenance program of 2–6 phlebotomies a year to keep storage iron normal; maintain serum ferritin 50-100 μg/L

IN-PATIENT CONSIDERATIONS

Admission Criteria/Initial Stabilization
Outpatient treatment

ONGOING CARE

FOLLOW-UP RECOMMENDATIONS
Full activity unless there is significant heart disease

Patient Monitoring
- Measure hematocrit before each phlebotomy; skip phlebotomy if hematocrit <36%.
- Schedule an additional phlebotomy when hematocrit >40%.
- When anemia becomes refractory, repeat transferrin saturation and serum ferritin to confirm depletion of iron stores.
- When iron stores are depleted, 2–6 phlebotomies a year should keep iron stores normal; maintain serum ferritin 50-100 μg/L.
- During maintenance therapy, measure transferrin saturation and serum ferritin yearly.

DIET
- An iron-poor diet is not of significant benefit.
- Avoid alcohol, iron-fortified foods, iron-containing supplements, and uncooked shellfish (increased susceptibility to *Vibrio* sp.).
- Restrict vitamin C to small doses between meals.
- Tea chelates iron and may be drunk with meals.

PATIENT EDUCATION
- Iron Disorders Institute, PO Box 675, Taylors, SC 29687
- Iron Overload Diseases Association, Inc., 525 Mayflower Rd, West Palm Beach, FL 33405
- American Hemochromatosis Society, Inc., 4044 W. Lake Mary Blvd., Unit 104, Lake Mary, FL 32746-2012

PROGNOSIS

- Patients diagnosed before cirrhosis develops and treated with phlebotomy have a normal life expectancy.
- Life expectancy is reduced in patients with cirrhosis and DM and in those who require >18 months of phlebotomy therapy to return iron stores to normal.
- Patients with ferritin levels <1,000 μg/L are unlikely to have cirrhosis (2,3)

COMPLICATIONS

- Cirrhosis
- Hepatoma (only in patients with cirrhosis)
- Diabetes mellitus
- Cardiomyopathy
- Arthritis
- Hypogonadism

REFERENCES

1. van Bokhoven MA, van Deursen CT, Swinkels DW, et al. Diagnosis and management of hereditary haemochromatosis. *BMJ*. 2011;342:c7251.
2. Janssen MC, Swinkels DW. Hereditary haemochromatosis. *Best Pract Res Clin Gastroenterol*. 2009;23:171–183.
3. Allen KJ, Gurrin LC, Constantine CC, et al. Iron-overload-related disease in HFE hereditary hemochromatosis. *N Engl J Med*. 2008;358:221–230.
4. Brandhagen DJ, Fairbanks VF, Baldus W. Recognition and management of hereditary hemochromatosis. *Am Fam Phys*. 2002;65:853–860.
5. Bacon BR, Adams PC, Kowdley KV, et al. Diagnosis and management of hemochromatosis: 2011 practice guideline by the American Association for the Study of Liver Diseases. *Hepatology*. 2011;54(1):328–343.
6. Alexander J, Kowdley KV. Hereditary hemochromatosis: Genetics, pathogenesis, and clinical management. *Ann Hepatol*. 2005;4:240–247.
7. Qaseem A, Aronson M, Fitterman N, et al. Screening for hereditary hemochromatosis: A clinical practice guideline from the American College of Physicians. *Ann Intern Med*. 2005;143:517–521.

ADDITIONAL READING

- Crownover BK, Covey CJ. Hereditary hemochromatosis. *Am Fam Physician*. 2013;87(3):183–190.
- Fleming RE, Ponka P. Iron overload in human disease. *N Engl J Med*. 2012;366(4):348–359.
- U.S. Preventive Services Task Force. Screening for hemochromatosis: Recommendation statement. *Ann Intern Med*. 2006;145(3):204–208.

CODES

ICD10
E83.110 Hereditary hemochromatosis

CLINICAL PEARLS

- The best laboratory tests available to screen a patient initially for hemochromatosis are serum ferritin and transferrin saturation. An elevated transferrin saturation is the earliest abnormality in hemochromatosis. Ferritin is a sensitive measure of iron overload but can be elevated in a variety of infectious and inflammatory conditions without iron overload being present.
- Liver biopsy need not be done to confirm the diagnosis or to check for cirrhosis if the patient is homozygous for C282Y or is heterozygous for C282Y/H63D. If the patient's serum ferritin is <1,000 μg/L, LFTs are normal, and hepatomegaly is not present, cirrhosis is very unlikely, so liver biopsy is not needed.
- Initially, a patient with hemochromatosis should have a phlebotomy weekly until the serum ferritin is 50–100 μg/L and the transferrin saturation falls to <30%. Then, lifelong maintenance therapy of 2–6 phlebotomies a year is mandatory to keep the ferritin 50–100 μg/L and the transferrin saturation <50%.
- Most patients with hemochromatosis go undiagnosed. Because treatment with phlebotomy will prevent all complications when begun early, physicians should consider the diagnosis of hemochromatosis much more frequently. However, the US Preventive Services Task Force recommends against routine screening of asymptomatic average-risk populations.

H

HEMOPHILIA

Hayden T. Tran, DO, MS • Jason Donovan Klein, DO

 BASICS

DESCRIPTION
- Deficiency of factor VIII (hemophilia A) or factor IX (hemophilia B) coagulation proteins leading to bleeding tendencies in affected individuals. The majority of cases are due to inherited genetic mutations in factor VIII or factor IX coagulation proteins. However, an estimated 30% of all hemophilia cases result from spontaneous mutations.
- Hemophilia A and B are clinically indistinguishable, but can be differentiated by assays that detect levels of factors VIII and IX, respectively.
- Disease severity correlates with the relative levels of coagulation factors present in serum analysis (1,2):
  - Severe: Frequent spontaneous bleeding (factor activity <1%)
  - Moderate: Bleeding with mild-to-moderate trauma (factor activity 1–5%)
  - Mild: Bleeding with major trauma, tooth extraction, or surgery (factor activity 5–40%)
- Frequency of bleeding is similar when levels of severity are comparable in hemophilia A and B.
- Synonym(s): Christmas disease (hemophilia B)

EPIDEMIOLOGY
- Worldwide, an estimated 400,000 people are affected with hemophilia.
- Hemophilia A represents 80–85% of the total hemophilia population; hemophilia B comprises the remaining 15–20%.

ETIOLOGY AND PATHOPHYSIOLOGY
- Damage to vascular endothelium leads to exposure of subendothelial tissue factors, which interact with platelets, plasma proteins, and coagulation factors to produce a localized platelet plug contributing to hemostasis. Complexes involving factors VIII and IX participate in the intrinsic coagulation pathway to activate factor X, FXa. Downstream interactions involving FXa culminate in the conversion of prothrombin to thrombin, mediating platelet activation and fibrin deposition necessary for stabilization of the platelet plug.
- Deficiencies of factor VIII or factor IX result in decreased production of FXa, leading to an unstable platelet plug and impaired hemostasis.

Genetics
- Exhibits an X-chromosome linked inheritance pattern. Therefore, males are almost exclusively affected with hemophilia and females are asymptomatic carriers, unless their factor activity is <40% of normal.
- Carriers with symptomatically low clotting factor levels are treated similarly to patients with the trait:
  - Occasional female carrier will bleed at time of surgery.
- Males within the same family share similar deficiencies and level of severity owing to the same genetic defect.

GENERAL PREVENTION
- Hemophilia patients should carry medical ID tags listing their bleeding disorder or factor deficiency, inhibitor status, type of treatment products used, and initial treatment doses for mild, moderate, or severe bleeding.

- Immediate family members of affected patients should have factor VIII and IX levels checked prior to invasive procedures, childbirth, and if bleeding tendencies occur.
- Genetic testing should be offered to at-risk female family members of persons with hemophilia to facilitate genetic counseling or prenatal testing.

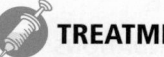 **DIAGNOSIS**

- History and initial presentation:
  - 2/3 of presenting hemophilic patients have a positive family history. All male infants born to known carriers should have factor level testing.
  - Prolonged bleeding with circumcision, dental work, surgery, or injury
  - Excessive or easy bruising in early childhood, hematomas, hemarthroses
  - Spontaneous bleeding, especially in joints, muscle, or soft tissue
- Life-threatening bleeds:
  - Intracranial hemorrhage: Generally resulting from trauma, incidence of 1:10, fatal in 30% of cases
  - Hematomas of bowel wall can cause obstruction or intussusception, as well as pain mimicking appendicitis.
  - Neck or throat bleeds: Can lead to airway obstruction
- Serious bleeds:
  - Hemarthrosis, most commonly of ankles, elbows, and knees:
    ○ Infants may present with irritability or decreased use of limb.
    ○ Adults may have prodromal stiffness, acute pain, and swelling of joint.
    ○ Arthropathy results from repeated bleeding into joints, damaging cartilage and subchondral bone:
      ▪ Can result in fixed joints, muscle wasting, and significantly impaired mobility
  - Muscular hematomas most commonly occur in quadriceps, iliopsoas, and forearm:
    ○ May result in compartment syndrome and ischemic nerve damage, such as femoral nerve neuropathy due to undetected retroperitoneal hemorrhage
  - Mucous membrane bleeding, such as in the genitourinary tract, leading to hematuria
  - Pseudotumor syndrome: Untreated hemorrhage causing a hematoma, which calcifies (named because it can be mistaken for cancer)

DIFFERENTIAL DIAGNOSIS
- Von Willebrand disease
- Vitamin K deficiency, warfarin (Coumadin) therapy (factor IX is vitamin K–dependent)
- Other factor deficiencies, afibrinogenemia, dysfibrinogenemia, fibrinolytic defects, platelet disorders
- Child abuse

DIAGNOSTIC TESTS & INTERPRETATION
Initial Tests (lab, imaging)
- CBC with platelet count, PT, aPTT, platelet function (preferred) or bleed time, vWF, factor VIII:C assay, factor IX assay. Prolonged aPTT: Corrected when mixed with pooled normal plasma in absence of inhibitors

- PT, platelet count, and platelet function are normal.
- Diagnosis based on factor VIII:C or IX activity:
  - Normal factor levels: 50–150 IU/dL
  - Mild 5–40 IU/dL,
  - Moderate 1–5 IU/dL
  - Severe <1 IU/dL

Follow-Up Tests & Special Considerations
Inhibitors to factor VIII and IX (see "Complications"):
- Should be periodically measured using the Nijmegen or Bethesda assay, which quantifies the alloantibody titer
- Screen before invasive procedures and at regular intervals.

Diagnostic Procedures/Other
Prenatal diagnosis: Genetic testing of a sample of chorionic villus or fluid obtained at amniocentesis

Test Interpretation
In affected joints: Synovial hemosiderosis, articular cartilage degeneration, thickening of periarticular tissues, bony hypertrophy

TREATMENT

GENERAL MEASURES
- Avoid aspirin or other NSAIDs.
- Treat early; symptoms may occur before bleeding is clinically apparent.
- For surgical prophylaxis:
  - If major surgery is undertaken, factor levels should be maintained at >50% for at least 2–3 weeks after the procedure:
    ○ Fibrin glue products may be beneficial for oozing at extensive incision sites.
  - Dental extractions: Antifibrinolytics (Amicar, tranexamic acid) may be used.
  - Minor procedures: May use desmopressin (DDAVP).
- Hepatitis A and B vaccinations are recommended.
- Encourage physical activity: Patients should avoid high-impact contact sports; restrict activities in proportion to degree of factor deficiency.

MEDICATION
First Line
- Principles of therapy:
  - Primary prophylaxis: Administration of specific factor replacement therapy in the absence of bleeding to maintain adequate baseline plasma levels sufficient for hemostasis in all categories of severity (3)[B]:
    ○ Lower frequency of acute bleeds and episodes of life-threatening hemorrhage compared to on-demand therapy
    ○ Standard of care for children with severe hemophilia A to prevent joint bleeds and joint degeneration
    ○ Dosing, frequency, duration of therapeutic regimens tailored to individual patient needs in clinical practice
    ○ Opinions differ about optimal age to initiate prophylaxis, optimal dosing and frequency, and if or when to transition from prophylaxis to on-demand therapy.

– On-demand therapy: Treatment administered in response to occurrence of bleeding:
  ○ Amount and duration of factor replacement depends on location and severity of bleeding:
    ▪ A target factor level of >30% is generally sufficient for mild bleeding episodes.
    ▪ Major hemorrhages and large muscle bleeds require correction to levels between 50% and 100%.
    ▪ Life-threatening bleeds require levels between 80% and 100%, which should be sustained with bolus dosing or continuous infusion.

• Specific agents: Consensus guidelines express no preference for recombinant vs. plasma-derived factor concentrates (4):
  – Hemophilia A: Replacement with factor VIII concentrates is treatment of choice (4)[A]:
    ○ 2 sources for the factor available:
      ▪ Purified plasma-derived factor VIII: Donor pool is screened and the plasma-derived factor is treated to inactivate viruses (HIV, hepatitis B, and hepatitis C). Theoretical risks still exist.
      ▪ Recombinant factor VIII
        □ Dosing: 1 IU of factor VIII (the amount in 1 mL of plasma)/kg body weight administered will raise the plasma level of the recipient by 2%.
  – Hemophilia B: Replacement with factor IX concentrates is treatment of choice (4)[A]:
    ○ Plasma-derived factor IX and recombinant factor IX (preferred) (2) are commercially available.
      ▪ Dosing: 1 IU/kg body weight administered will raise plasma factor IX levels 1%.

• Hemophilia patients with inhibitors (neutralizing alloantibodies to factors VIII or IX) (4)[A]:
  – Inhibitor formation should be suspected when replacement with the deficient factor fails to correct coagulopathy.
  – Low-titer (<5 BU/mL) patients: Replace with high doses of the deficient factor to overcome the circulating inhibitor concentration.
  – High-titer patients: Treat using products that *bypass* the factor neutralized by the alloantibody, or emergently with high doses of the specific deficient factor:
    ○ 2 bypassing agents available; both are efficacious at providing 80% of bleeding episodes (5)[B]:
      ▪ Anti-inhibitor coagulation complex (AICC)
      ▪ Recombinant activated factor VII (rFVIIa)
  – Immune tolerance induction (ITI): Protocols to promote immune tolerance through repeated exposure to high-dose factor VIII therapy over 12–18 months, with or without immunosuppressive therapy (corticosteroids, cyclophosphamide, rituximab). Success rate are 60–80% (6).

Second Line

• Cryoprecipitate and fresh frozen plasma (FFP): Can be used in instances where the specific factor concentrate is unavailable for *emergent hemostasis* (4)[B]:
  – FFP: Contains all coagulation factors, but generally difficult to attain high levels of factors VIII or IX:
    ○ Acceptable starting dose: 15–20 mL/kg
  – Cryoprecipitate: Derived from precipitates of cooled FFP; contains significant levels of factor VIII (up to 100 IU/bag), but *not* factor IX:
    ○ Dosing: 1 mL cryoprecipitate has ~3–5 IU factor VIII.
• Desmopressin (DDAVP): Synthetic vasopressin; stimulates endogenous release of factor VIII *(and vWF)* from endothelial stores; used in mild-moderate hemophilia (4)[B]:
  – IV or SC: 0.3 μg/kg infused 30 minutes prior to procedure; may repeat if needed
  – Intranasal (150 μg/spray): Adult dose, 1 spray to each nostril (300 μg total). Alternate dose if <50 kg: 150 μg once.
  – Adverse effect: Hyponatremic seizures, especially in children; restrict fluids and watch sodium levels and urine output.
• Antifibrinolytic agents: Inhibit plasminogen activation, thereby stabilizing the clot:
  – Effective in controlling mucosal bleeding, such as bleeding in oral cavity, epistaxis, and menorrhagia. Can also be used prophylactically (e.g., prior to tooth extractions) (4)[B]:
    ○ Tranexamic acid (25 mg/kg PO q6–8h or 10 mg/kg IV q6–8h)
    ○ Aminocaproic acid (Amicar) is less frequently used.

 ## ONGOING CARE

FOLLOW-UP RECOMMENDATIONS
Patient Monitoring
Regular evaluations every 6–12 months, including a musculoskeletal evaluation, an inhibitor screen, liver tests, and tests for antibodies to hepatitis viruses and HIV (4)

PATIENT EDUCATION
• National Hemophilia Foundation: www.hemophilia.org
• World Federation of Hemophilia: www.wfh.org

PROGNOSIS
• Survival is normal for those with mild disease; mortality is increased 2–6-fold in those with moderate to severe disease.
• Intracranial hemorrhage is a leading cause of death in hemophilia.
• Hemophilic arthropathy is the main cause of morbidity in patients with severe hemophilia.

COMPLICATIONS
• Hemophilic arthropathy: Symptoms include pain, limitation of motion, and contractures.
• Theoretical transmission of bloodborne infections, such as hepatitis A, B, C, D, and HIV; this risk has been greatly reduced with current testing of blood products.

• Development of inhibitor autoantibodies:
  – More common in hemophilia A (20–30% of patients compared to 5% in hemophilia B) (1), and in patients with severe disease requiring multiple transfusions
  – Risk factors for inhibitor development:
    ○ Specific genetic defect (family history); null mutations have higher inhibitor incidence.
    ○ Very low or no circulating factor, therefore requiring multiple transfusions
    ○ Age of 1st exogenous factor exposure; previous studies report a higher incidence of developing antibodies in those exposed to exogenous factor at <6 months of age, but new studies show this may be due to severity of disease.
    ○ Concurrent inflammation/infection when administering factor (e.g., surgical prophylaxis)
    ○ Duration of factor exposure
  – No increased risk of bleeding, but when bleeding occurs, it is more difficult to achieve hemostasis due to decreased response to factor replacement (6).

REFERENCES

1. Berntorp E, Shapiro AD. Modern haemophilia care. *Lancet*. 2012;379:1447–1456.
2. Gater A, Thomson TA, Strandberg-Larsen M. Haemophilia B: Impact on patients and economic burden of disease. *Thromb Haemost*. 2011;106:398–404.
3. Ragni MV, Fogarty PJ, Josephson NC, et al. Survey of current prophylaxis practices and bleeding characteristics of children with severe haemophilia A in US haemophilia treatment centres. *Haemophilia*. 2012;18:63–68.
4. Srivastava A, Brewer AK, Mauser-Bunschoten EP, et al. Guidelines for the management of hemophilia. *Haemophilia*. 2013;19:e1–e47.
5. Leissinger C, Gringeri A, Antmen B, et al. Anti-inhibitor coagulant complex prophylaxis in hemophilia with inhibitors. *N Engl J Med*. 2011;365:1684–1692.
6. Benson G, Auerswald G, Elezovi I, et al. Immune tolerance induction in patients with severe hemophilia with inhibitors: Expert panel views and recommendations for clinical practice. *Eur J Haematol*. 2012;88:371–379.

ADDITIONAL READING

• Fischer K. Prophylaxis for adults with haemophilia: One size does not fit all. *Blood Transfus*. 2012;10:169–173.
• Franchini M, Mannucci PM. Past, present and future of hemophilia: A narrative review. *Orphanet J Rare Dis*. 2012;7:24.

 ## CODES

ICD10
• D66 Hereditary factor VIII deficiency
• D67 Hereditary factor IX deficiency
• D68.1 Hereditary factor XI deficiency

H

HEMORRHOIDS

Juan Qiu, MD, PhD

BASICS

DESCRIPTION
- Varicosities of the hemorrhoidal venous plexus
- External hemorrhoids:
  - Located below the dentate line
  - Covered by squamous epithelium
- Internal hemorrhoids:
  - Located above the dentate line
- Both types of hemorrhoids often coexist.
- Classification of internal hemorrhoids:
  - 1st-degree: Hemorrhoids do not prolapse.
  - 2nd-degree: Prolapse through the anus on straining but reduce spontaneously
  - 3rd-degree: Protrude and require digital reduction
  - 4th-degree: Cannot be reduced
- Hemorrhoids often progress from itching, bleeding stage to protrusion with easy reduction, then difficult reduction, and finally rectal prolapse. Thrombosis may occur at any protrusion stage.

Geriatric Considerations
Common in elderly, along with rectal prolapse

Pediatric Considerations
- Uncommon in infants and children. Look for underlying cause (e.g., venacaval or mesenteric obstruction, cirrhosis, portal HTN).
- Occasionally, as in adults, hemorrhoids may result from chronic constipation, fecal impaction, and straining at stool. Surgery is rarely required in children.

Pregnancy Considerations
- Common in pregnancy
- Usually resolves after pregnancy
- No treatment required, unless extremely painful

EPIDEMIOLOGY
- Predominant age: Adults; peak between 45 and 65
- Predominant sex: Male = Female

Incidence
Common

Prevalence
~4–5% in general population in the US

ETIOLOGY AND PATHOPHYSIOLOGY
- Dilated veins of hemorrhoidal plexus
- Tight internal anal sphincter
- Abnormal distention of the arteriovenous anastomosis
- Prolapse of the cushions and the surrounding connective tissues

Genetics
No known genetic pattern

RISK FACTORS
- Pregnancy
- Pelvic space-occupying lesions
- Liver disease
- Portal HTN
- Constipation
- Occupations that require prolonged sitting
- Loss of muscle tone in old age, rectal surgery, episiotomy, anal intercourse
- Obesity
- Chronic diarrhea

GENERAL PREVENTION
- Avoid constipation with high-fiber diet and hydration.
- Lose weight, if overweight.
- Avoid prolonged sitting on the toilet.

COMMONLY ASSOCIATED CONDITIONS
- Liver disease
- Pregnancy
- Portal HTN
- Constipation

DIAGNOSIS

Diagnosis is usually made by history and inspection of the perineum, rectal exam, and anoscopy.

HISTORY
- All cases:
  - Classically, bright red blood per rectum:
    - May be scant blood on toilet paper *or*
    - Copious in the toilet bowl
  - Constipation or diarrhea
  - Straining with defecation
- Small or minimal external hemorrhoids:
  - Episodic bleeding on stool or toilet paper, pruritus
- More extensive internal hemorrhoids:
  - Feeling of incomplete evacuation

PHYSICAL EXAM
- Anorectal exam including anoscopy
- Inspection following straining at stool
- For protruding hemorrhoids: Mass, more prominent bleeding
- If not reducible, increased risk of strangulation and/or thrombosis with acute pain
- External hemorrhoids cause pain; internal hemorrhoids generally do not.
- Thrombosed hemorrhoids present as acute discomfort and the presence of a painful mass.

DIFFERENTIAL DIAGNOSIS
- Rectal or anal neoplasia
- Condyloma
- Skin tag
- Inflammatory bowel disease (1)
- Anal fistula, fissure, or abscess (2)

DIAGNOSTIC TESTS & INTERPRETATION
Diagnostic Procedures/Other
Sigmoidoscopy or colonoscopy depending on coexistent risk factors for malignancy in patients who present with bleeding.

TREATMENT

- All these treatments, except surgical, are outpatient with quick recovery time, usually <48 hours.
- Prevention:
  - Fiber supplements
  - Stool softeners

GENERAL MEASURES
- Hemorrhoids are a recurrent disease, even after surgical excision; measures for prevention should be taken.
- For mild symptoms or prevention:
  - Avoid prolonged sitting during bowel movements.
  - Avoid straining.
  - Avoid constipation by eating a high-fiber diet or by taking fiber supplements; if necessary, take regular stool softeners.
  - Regular exercise
- For pain, Sitz baths warm water or hypertonic Epsom salts (1 cup per 2 quarts of water)
- Mild and minimal hemorrhoids respond to changed diet, relief of constipation, and brief stooling.
- Pruritus or mild discomfort after stooling responds to hydrocortisone ointment, anesthetic ointments or sprays, and warm Sitz bath.
- Constipation relief, anal hygiene, local ointments, and Sitz baths are effective through the stage of easy reduction, but the more severe stages require rubber band ligation or rectal surgery.

MEDICATION
First Line
- Dietary modification with adequate fluid and fiber is the primary first-line, nonoperative therapy for symptomatic hemorrhoid disease (3)[A].
- Pain:
  - Hydrocortisone ointment (0.5–1%)
  - Analgesic sprays or ointments: Benzocaine, dibucaine (Nupercainal). Use sprays with caution as they may contain alcohol that can cause burning sensation when applied.
- Pruritus: Hydrocortisone (Anusol-HC, Cortifoam) ointment
- Bleeding:
  - Astringent suppositories (Preparation H)
  - Hydrocortisone (Anusol; Cortifoam) ointment

Second Line
Treatment for special cases:

- Thrombosed external hemorrhoids: Fairly common complication of hemorrhoidal disease. With conservative treatment, the thrombus will be absorbed over the course of weeks and pain improves within 2–3 days (1)[B].
- With severe acute pain, prompt excision should be performed under local anesthetic and the wound left open without packing. Use Sitz baths, topical anesthetics, and mild pain relievers for first 7–10 days after excision (1)[B].
- Strangulated hemorrhoid: From irreducible 3rd- or 4th-degree hemorrhoid. If untreated, can progress to ulceration and thrombosis. Treatment requires urgent or emergent hemorrhoidectomy.
- Acute hemorrhoidal bleeding associated with portal HTN: Bleeding can be life-threatening. Treatment should be suture of the bleeding site with incorporation of the mucosa, submucosa, and internal sphincter. Coagulopathy should be corrected.

SURGERY/OTHER PROCEDURES

- Indications: Failure of medical and nonoperative therapy, symptomatic 3rd- or 4th-degree symptoms in presence of a concomitant anorectal condition requiring surgery, or patient preference (2)[B] (4)
- Incision of thrombosed hemorrhoid: For severe pain
- Severe protruding hemorrhoids:
  – Rubber band ligation (internal hemorrhoids only)
  – Sclerotherapy: For symptomatic prolapsed stage I or II hemorrhoids; care must be (5) taken injecting near periprostatic parasympathetic nerves. Not for advanced disease or if evidence of infection, inflammation, ulceration is present (1)[B]:
    ○ Cryotherapy is no longer recommended due to high rate of complications (2)[B].
  – Prolapsed rectum:
    ○ Requires surgical correction
  – Surgical resection:
    ○ Gold standard: Conventional hemorrhoidectomy should be considered for grade III hemorrhoids not responding to banding (6)[A], mixed internal and external, grade IV hemorrhoids, or when complicated by fissures, fistula, or extensive skin tags.
- Newer techniques: Superior vs. traditional methods with reduced surgical time, early postop pain, urinary retention, and time to return to normal activity (7)[A]:
  – Stapled hemorrhoidopexy; less painful than traditional surgery, but higher incidence of skin tags and recurrent prolapse (7)[A]
  – LigaSure hemorrhoidectomy; reduces operating time, is superior in patient tolerance, and is equally effective as conventional hemorrhoidectomy in long-term symptom control (8)[B]

COMPLEMENTARY AND ALTERNATIVE MEDICINE

Aloe vera cream on the surgical site after hemorrhoidectomy is effective in reducing postoperative pain and decreasing both healing time and analgesic requirements (9)[B].

 ## ONGOING CARE

FOLLOW-UP RECOMMENDATIONS
- Encourage physical fitness.
- Avoid prolonged sitting and straining on the toilet.

Patient Monitoring
As needed, depending on treatment

DIET
High-fiber (25–30 g of insoluble fiber/d), adequate fluids (6–8 glasses of water/d); avoid excessive caffeine

PATIENT EDUCATION
High-fiber diet: Today's Dietitian Top Fiber-Rich Foods List: http://www.todaysdietitian.com/newarchives/063008p28.shtml (10)

PROGNOSIS
- Spontaneous resolution
- Recurrence

COMPLICATIONS
- Thrombosis
- Ulceration
- Anemia (rare)
- Incontinence
- Pelvic sepsis following hemorrhoidectomy

REFERENCES

1. Kaidar-Person O, Person B, Wexner SD. Hemorrhoidal disease: A comprehensive review. *J Am Coll Surg.* 2007;204:102–117.
2. Clinical Practice Committee, American Gastroenterological Association. American Gastroenterological Association medical position statement: Diagnosis and treatment of hemorrhoids. *Gastroenterology.* 2004;126: 1461–1462.
3. Rivadeneira DE, Steele SR, Ternent C, et al. Practice parameters for the management of hemorrhoids (revised 2010). *Dis Colon Rectum.* 2011;54:1059–1064.
4. Castellvi J, Sueira A, Espinosa J, et al. LigaSure versus diathermy hemorrhoidectomy under spinal anesthesia or pudendal block with ropivacaine: A randomized prospective clinical study with 1-year follow-up. *Int J Colorectal Dis.* 2009;24(9): 1011–1018.
5. Nienhuijs S, de Hingh I. Conventional versus LigaSure hemorrhoidectomy for patients with symptomatic Hemorrhoids. *Cochrane Database Syst Rev.* 2009;(1):CD006761. Epub 2009 Jan 21.
6. Shanmugam V, Hakeem A, Campbell KL, et al. Rubber band ligation versus excisional haemorrhoidectomy for haemorrhoids. *Cochrane Database Syst Rev.* 2005;1:CD005034. Updated 2011;3.
7. Chen JS, You JF. Current status of surgical treatment for hemorrhoids—systematic review and meta-analysis. *Chang Gung Med J.* 2010;33: 488–500.
8. Chen CW, Lai CW, et al. Results of 666 consecutive patients treated with LigaSure hemorrhoidectomy for symptomatic prolapsed hemorrhoids with a minimum follow-up of 2 years. *Surgery.* 2013;153(2):211–218.
9. Eshghi F, Hosseinimehr SJ, Rahmani N, et al. Effects of Aloe vera cream on posthemorrhoidectomy pain and wound healing: Results of a randomized, blind, placebo-control study. *J Altern Complement Med.* 2010;16(6): 647–650.
10. Palmer S, The Top Fiber-Rich Foods List. *Today's Dietitian.* 2008;10(7):28.

ADDITIONAL READING

- Giordano P, Gravante G, Sorge R, et al. Long-term Outcomes of stapled hemorrhoidopexy vs conventional hemorrhoidectomy. *Arch Surg.* 2009;144(3):266–272.
- Reese GE, von Roon AC, Tekkis PP. *Haemorrhoids. Clin Evid (Online).* 2009. Epub 2009 Jan 29.
- Rivadeneira DE, Steele SR, Ternent C, et al. Practice parameters for the management of hemorrhoids (revised 2010). *Dis Colon Rectum.* 2011;54(9): 1059–1064.

 ## SEE ALSO

Colorectal Cancer; Portal Hypertension

 ## CODES

ICD10
- K64.4 Residual hemorrhoidal skin tags
- K64.8 Other hemorrhoids
- K64.9 Unspecified hemorrhoids

CLINICAL PEARLS

- Hemorrhoids are uncommon in inflammatory bowel disease, and pain is most related to perianal inflammation, irritation, and swelling. Anal hygiene and symptomatic pain relief are the treatments of choice.
- No pain is associated with internal hemorrhoids. Pain occurs with external hemorrhoids only.
- For pain, Sitz baths warm water or hypertonic Epsom salts (1 cup per 2 quarts of water)

HENOCH-SCHÖNLEIN PURPURA

Shani I. Muhammad, MD

BASICS

DESCRIPTION
- Henoch-Schönlein purpura (HSP) is a nonthrombocytopenic, predominantly IgA-mediated, small vessel vasculitis that affects multiple organ systems and occurs in both children and adults (1).
- HSP is often self-limited, with the greatest morbidity and mortality attributable to long-term renal damage (2).
- Characterized by a tetrad of purpuric skin lesions, arthralgia, abdominal pain, and nephropathies (3).

EPIDEMIOLOGY
Incidence
- Annual incidence: 135/1 million children and 3.4–14.3/1 million adults (1,2)
- Mean age of patients affected is 6 years, 90% <10 years of age but has been reported in patients age 6 months to 75 years old (4)
- Gender: Male:Female ratio is 1.2:1 (5)
- Race/ethnicity: Most common in Caucasians and Asians, less common among African Americans (5)

Prevalence
- Annual prevalence: 10–22/100,000 persons (6)
- Year-round occurrence; more common in late fall to early spring (6)

ETIOLOGY AND PATHOPHYSIOLOGY
- Autoimmune disorder in which IgA production is increased in response to trigger(s), IgA1 immune complexes then activate the complement pathway, leading to production of inflammatory cytokines and chemokines (1).
- Immune complex deposition results in small vessel inflammation, fibrosis, and necrosis within skin, intestinal mucosa, joints, and kidneys (2).
- No single etiologic agent has been identified
- Known triggers include infection, drugs, vaccinations, and insect bites (7).
- Infectious antigens include (but are not limited to): Group A streptococcus (may be present in up to 30% of HSP-associated nephritis), parvovirus B19, *Bartonella henselae*, *Helicobacter pylori*, *Haemophilus parainfluenza*, Coxsackie virus, adenovirus, hepatitis A and B viruses, mycoplasma, Epstein-Barr virus, varicella, *Campylobacter*, methicillin-resistant *Staphylococcus aureus* (5,6).
- Drugs: Acetaminophen, quinolones, etanercept, codeine, clarithromycin (5)
- Vaccinations: MMR (measles, mumps, rubella), pneumococcal, meningococcal, influenza, hepatitis B (5)

Genetics
Associated with α_1-antitrypsin deficiency, familial Mediterranean fever, HLA-DRB1*01, HLA-B35 (5)

COMMONLY ASSOCIATED CONDITIONS
Malignancy (rare): Greatest association is with solid tumors, including lymphoma, prostate cancer, and non–small cell lung cancer, but also associated with multiple myeloma (5).

DIAGNOSIS

Palpable purpura and *at least 1* of the following (6,8)[C]:
- Diffuse abdominal pain
- Biopsy with predominant IgA deposition
- Arthralgia or arthritis
- Renal involvement (hematuria or proteinuria)

HISTORY
- History of exposure to known trigger, including recent infection (particularly upper respiratory infection), vaccination, or offending drug
- Rash (most common presenting symptom): Purpuric, palpable; distribution often symmetric on lower extremities and buttocks; may present on upper extremities, trunk, face; typical duration 3–10 days; no definitive temporal association with other symptoms (5,7)
- Fatigue (6)
- Low-grade fever (6)
- Nausea/vomiting
- Abdominal pain (diffuse, colicky, may be transient or constant) (7)
- Hematochezia/Melena
- Polyarthritis (often symmetric involvement of knees and ankles) (7)
- Gross hematuria
- Rare symptoms: Periorbital or scrotal swelling, headache, neuropathy, hemoptysis (2,7)

PHYSICAL EXAM
- Rash (96% of cases, 74% primary presenting symptom) (1,7,9):
  - May start as urticaria, develops into nonblanching purpura, with or without petechiae and ecchymoses, may also be bullous (5)
  - Distribution usually symmetric, most commonly involving the lower extremities, but may involve the face and trunk
- Abdominal tenderness (66% of cases, 12% primary presenting symptom) (1,7):
  - Evidence of GI hemorrhage (28% of cases) (1)
- Joint tenderness (64% of cases, 15% primary presenting symptom) (1,7):
  - Mainly affects knees or ankles; may have associated warmth and limited range of motion, less commonly effusion; erythema is absent (6,7)
  - Mostly nonmigratory, transient, and nondeforming (6)
- Orchitis (5%) (1):
  - Presents as scrotal swelling and tenderness, may have associated torsion
- Renal disease (<1% primary presenting symptom) (7):
  - Hypertension may be present.
- Rarely, patients present with CNS or pulmonary involvement, which may manifest as signs of cerebral hemorrhage or diffuse interstitial pneumonia, respectively (2).

DIFFERENTIAL DIAGNOSIS
- Infection:
  - Meningococcemia
  - Rocky Mountain spotted fever
  - Bacterial endocarditis
  - Rheumatic fever
- Immune mediated:
  - Polyarteritis nodosa
  - Wegener granulomatosis
  - Systemic lupus erythematosus
  - Kawasaki disease
- Other:
  - Inflammatory bowel disease
  - Idiopathic thrombocytopenic purpura
  - Juvenile rheumatoid arthritis
  - Leukemia
  - Acute surgical abdomen (6)
  - Child abuse (6)

DIAGNOSTIC TESTS & INTERPRETATION
- No single lab test confirms the diagnosis of HSP.
- Labs directed toward excluding other illnesses and assessing degree of renal involvement (6,10)

Initial Tests (lab, imaging)
The following are generally accepted as initial labs for HSP (1,6,9):
- CBC:
  - Leukocytosis and thrombocytosis may occur. Thrombocytopenia indicates an alternative cause of purpura.
  - Hemoglobin is variable, depending on whether GI hemorrhage occurs.
- Basic serum chemistry panel (electrolytes, BUN, creatinine:
  - Electrolyte imbalances or elevated creatinine indicate renal dysfunction.
- Urinalysis:
  - Gross or microscopic hematuria, proteinuria, red cell casts indicate renal dysfunction
- PT and PTT:
  - Normal in HSP
- Imaging is not part of the routine workup for HSP but may be performed to rule out alternative etiologies or for evaluation of suspected complications, particularly in cases of GI and renal involvement. Initial imaging modalities to consider include (1,6,11):
  - Abdominal radiographs, with or without barium enema: Evaluate for free abdominal air suggestive of bowel perforation.
  - Abdominal ultrasound: Sensitive for the detection of intramural bleeding in HSP and may also show thickened bowel wall, reduced peristalsis, intussusception
- Renal ultrasound: Evaluate for hydronephrosis in cases of renal failure.

Follow-Up Tests & Special Considerations
The following labs are also useful in diagnosing HSP (1,4,9):
- Blood culture:
  - To rule out sepsis/bacteremia when diagnosis unclear
- Acute phase reactants:
  - Expect mild elevation
- IgA level:
  - Often elevated, although nonspecific, nonsensitive
- Complement levels:
  - Normal; sometimes decreased
- Antinuclear antibody/antineutrophil cytoplasmic antibody:
  - Negative
- Antistreptolysin-O titer:
  - Evaluate for preceding streptococcal infection.
- Stool guaiac if suspected GI hemorrhage

- CT arteriography may be necessary to identify the location of bleeding in patients with GI hemorrhage (6).

Diagnostic Procedures/Other
- Renal biopsy: Obtain if diagnosis uncertain or if nephrotic range proteinuria. Shows mesangial IgA deposition, mesangial proliferation, or, in severe cases, crescentic glomerulonephritis (2).
- Skin biopsy of purpura: IgA deposition in the dermis on immunofluorescence (5).
- Endoscopy may be considered in cases of GI hemorrhage given symptomatic overlap of HSP with inflammatory bowel disease.
- Barium enema may be therapeutic in some instances of intussusception, although surgical correction is commonly needed (6).

TREATMENT

GENERAL MEASURES
Rest and elevation of affected areas may limit purpura (6).

MEDICATION
- In the absence of renal dysfunction or complication, HSP is usually self-limited and best managed with supportive care.
- NSAIDs are effective for symptomatic treatment of joint pain. Caution is advised in cases of GI hemorrhage; avoid use in cases of renal involvement and consider acetaminophen as an alternative (7,11)[B].
- Steroids given early in disease course using oral prednisone 1–2 mg/kg/d for 1–2 weeks decrease both duration of abdominal pain and severity of joint pain and may have benefit in preventing GI bleeding and causes of surgical abdomen, including intussusception (1,2,6)[A].
- Steroids have benefit in treatment of severe and/or bullous purpura (11,12)[B].
- Steroids given early in disease are effective for the acute treatment of crescentic nephritis, and may prevent chronic renal disease in such patients (2)[A].
- Early intervention with steroids has no effect on the prevention or development of renal involvement after 1 year (13)[A]
- High-dose IV pulse steroids (500 mg to 1 g) may be considered in cases of mesenteric vasculitis and severe renal impairment. Evidence is very limited to support use of cyclophosphamide, plasmapheresis, and intravenous immunoglobulin (IVIG) for severe renal and GI involvement, as well as colchicine for severe skin lesions (1,2,5)

ISSUES FOR REFERRAL
- Consider nephrology referral for renal biopsy if nephrotic range proteinuria at any time or proteinuria >100 mg/mmol for 3 months after diagnosis (11).
- Dermatology referral for skin biopsy

IN-PATIENT CONSIDERATIONS
Admission Criteria/Initial Stabilization
- Insufficient oral intake
- Renal insufficiency
- Severe abdominal pain
- Severe GI bleeding
- Altered mental status

- Mobility restriction due to arthritis
- Hypertension (HTN)
- Nephrotic syndrome (7)

IV Fluids
Hydration should be maintained

 ONGOING CARE

FOLLOW-UP RECOMMENDATIONS
Patient Monitoring
- Patients should be seen weekly during the acute illness. Visits should include history and physical exam to include BP measurement and urinalysis (11).
- Because ~100% of patients who develop renal involvement will do so within 6 months of HSP diagnosis, all patients should be followed at least monthly with BP and urinalysis for a duration of no less than 6 months (6,11)[C].
- Women with a history of HSP should be monitored for proteinuria and HTN during pregnancy.
- Consider workup for occult malignancy in patients with adult-onset HSP (2).

PATIENT EDUCATION
- American Family Physician handout on HSP available at: www.aafp.org/afp/980800ap/980800b.html
- National Kidney and Urologic Diseases Information Clearinghouse (NKUDIC): http://kidney.niddk.nih.gov/kudiseases/pubs/hsp/

PROGNOSIS
- Long-term prognosis heavily dependent on presence and severity of nephritis (4)
- HSP is self-limited in 94% of children and 89% of adults (5).
- Most cases of HSP resolve within 4 weeks of diagnosis. Recurrence rate within 6 months of diagnosis is 33% (6,7).
- Factors associated with poorer prognosis include age >8 years, fever at presentation, purpura above the waist, elevated ESR or IgA concentration, increasing severity of renal histology grade (5).
- Chronic renal disease occurs in up to 20% of children with nephritic and nephrotic syndrome compared with 50% of adults who had any renal involvement. Risk of long-term renal failure is ≤5% (2,7).

COMPLICATIONS
- Nephrotic/Nephritic syndrome and renal failure
- HTN
- Hemorrhagic cystitis
- Ureteral obstruction
- Intestinal infarction, perforation, obstruction, stricture
- GI hemorrhage
- Intussusception
- Alveolar hemorrhage
- CNS complications, including cerebral hemorrhage and seizure
- Anterior uveitis
- Myocarditis
- Orchitis
- Testicular torsion

REFERENCES

1. Batu ED, Ozen S. Pediatric vasculitis. *Curr Rheumatol Rep.* 2012;14:121–129.
2. Jithpratuck W, Elshenawy Y, Saleh H, et al. The clinical implications of adult-onset Henoch-Schonelin purpura. *Clin Mol Allergy.* 2011;9:9.
3. Boulis E, Majithia V, McMurray R. Adult onset Henoch-Schonlein purpura with positive c-ANCA (anti-protinease 3): Case report and review of literature. *Rheumatology International.* 2013; 33:493–496.
4. Saulsbury FT. Henoch-Schönlein purpura. *Curr Opin Rheumatol.* 2001;13:35–40.
5. Sohagia AB, Gunturu SG, Tong TR, et al. Henoch-Schonlein purpura—A case report and review of the literature. *Gastroenterol Res Pract.* 2010;2010:597648.
6. Reamy BV, Williams PM, Lindsay TJ. Henoch-Schönlein purpura. *Am Fam Physician.* 2009;80: 697–704.
7. Antoon JW, Keane MW. Migratory polyarthritis in a child. *Clin Pediatr (Phila).* 2012;51:401–403.
8. Dillon MJ, Ozen S. A new international classification of childhood vasculitis. *Pediatr Nephrol.* 2006;21:1219–1222.
9. Ozen S, Pistorio A, Iusan SM, et al. EULAR/PRINTO/PRES criteria for Henoch-Schönlein purpura, childhood polyarteritis nodosa, childhood Wegener granulomatosis and childhood Takayasu arteritis: Ankara 2008. Part II: Final classification criteria. *Ann Rheum Dis.* 2010;69:798–806.
10. Kawasaki Y. The pathogenesis and treatment of pediatric Henoch-Schonlein purpura nephritis. *Clin Exp Nephrol* 2011;5:648–657.
11. McCarthy HJ, Tizard EJ. Diagnosis and management of Henoch-Schönlein purpura. *Eur J Pediatr.* 2010;169:643–650.
12. Weiss PF, Klink AJ, Localio R, et al. Corticosteroids may improve clinical outcomes during hospitalization for Henoch-Schönlein purpura. *Pediatrics.* 2010;126:674–681.
13. Hoyer PF. Prevention of renal disease in Henoch-Schonlein purpura: Clear evidence against steroids. *Arch Dis Child.* 2013;98:750–751.

ADDITIONAL READING

González LM, Janniger CK, Schwartz RA. Pediatric Henoch-Schönlein purpura. *Int J Dermatol.* 2009; 48:1157–1165.

 CODES

ICD10
D69.0 Allergic purpura

CLINICAL PEARLS

- HSP is a systemic small vessel vasculitis characterized by clinical tetrad of palpable purpura, abdominal pain, arthralgia, and renal dysfunction.
- The main form of treatment is supportive care, but oral corticosteroids are beneficial in certain circumstances.
- In all patients with HSP, regardless of renal involvement at presentation, it is reasonable to check BP and urinalysis at weekly to monthly intervals for no less than 6 months after diagnosis to monitor for developing renal dysfunction.

H

HEPARIN-INDUCED THROMBOCYTOPENIA

Rami Farhat, DO • Tipsuda Junsanto-Bahri, MD, FCAP • Maria Antoinette Pino, PhD

BASICS

DESCRIPTION
- Unexplained decrease in platelet count in a patient treated with heparin:
  - Minimum platelet count falls between 30% and 50% from baseline.
- Antibody-mediated prothrombotic disorder initiated by heparin administration
- Unlike other thrombocytopenias, HIT produces thrombosis rather than bleeding.
- Idiosyncratic reaction
- 2 types: Nonimmune heparin-associated thrombocytopenia (previously called HIT type I) and HIT (immune-induced; previously called HIT type II):
  - Nonimmune heparin-associated thrombocytopenia: More common, onset 1–4 days after starting heparin, mild thrombocytopenia (>100,000), few complications
  - HIT: Less common, onset 5–14 days after primary exposure to heparin, thrombocytopenia often <100,000 but usually >20,000; high risk of thrombosis:
    - Presentation of thrombocytopenia can be immediate with recent heparin exposure (within past 100 days).

EPIDEMIOLOGY
Incidence
- 10–15% of heparin-treated patients will experience decrease in platelet count.
- 0.3–3% will develop HIT.

ETIOLOGY AND PATHOPHYSIOLOGY
- Nonimmune heparin-associated thrombocytopenia: Potentially a result of direct platelet membrane binding with heparin
- HIT: Heparin can cause an increase in the blood concentration of platelet factor 4 (PF4), a chemokine. PF4 will form a complex with heparin.
- This heparin/PF4 complex can, in turn, stimulate the production of specific antiheparin/PF4 complex antibodies. These antibodies cause platelet activation and a prothrombotic state. Ultimately, this hypercoagulable state leads to thromboembolic complications in many patients.

RISK FACTORS
- Postsurgical > Medical > Obstetric:
  - Postcardiopulmonary bypass is the most significant risk factor.
- Bovine unfractionated heparin (UFH) > porcine UFH > low-molecular-weight heparin (LMWH) (1)[A]
- Female > Male
- Heparin duration >4 days

GENERAL PREVENTION
- Inquire about recent heparin exposure and any history of HIT.
- Use of LMW heparin (vs. unfractionated) and for a shorter duration reduce the risk of developing HIT.
- Properly document past HIT reactions in patient's medical record.
- No form of heparin should be administered once the diagnosis of HIT is confirmed.

COMMONLY ASSOCIATED CONDITIONS
- Venous thrombosis: Deep venous thrombosis (DVT), pulmonary embolism, adrenal vein thrombosis with hemorrhagic infarction
- Arterial thrombosis
- Skin lesions (skin necrosis at site of injection)
- Acute systemic reactions

DIAGNOSIS

- Nonimmune heparin-associated thrombocytopenia: Asymptomatic drop in platelet count
- HIT: Thrombocytopenia or thrombosis with the presence of heparin-dependent antibodies:
  - A clinicopathologic syndrome, meaning the foundation for diagnosis is based on both clinical and serologic findings

HISTORY
- Duration of current heparin therapy
- Previous exposure to heparin, including heparin flushes and heparin-coated catheters
- In patients being treated with heparin for thrombosis, in which thrombosis recurs during therapy, consider HIT as a potential cause.
- Pretest probability for HIT can be calculated using the "4 Ts" methodology (2):
  - **T**hrombocytopenia of new onset
  - **T**iming of thrombocytopenia (5–10 days after exposure)
  - **T**hrombosis of new onset
  - **T**hrombocytopenia by other causes is ruled out
- The HIT Expert Probability score, although only validated once to date, may become an alternative pretest probability tool (3)[C].

PHYSICAL EXAM
- Signs of venous or arterial thrombosis
- Skin necrosis (begins with erythema, progresses to ecchymosis and necrosis)
- Ischemic changes (signs of limb, renal, splenic, mesenteric ischemia)
- Bleeding (less common)
- Acute systemic reactions after IV bolus of heparin
- (e.g., signs of anaphylaxis)

DIFFERENTIAL DIAGNOSIS
Other potential causes of thrombocytopenia include (list is not all-inclusive):
- Sepsis and other infections
- Drug reactions
- Autoimmune
- Transfusion reactions
- Physical destruction (e.g., during cardiopulmonary bypass)

DIAGNOSTIC TESTS & INTERPRETATION
- Serial platelet counts in patients receiving heparin who have a possible risk of HIT >1%: Check platelets at baseline and then every 2–3 days from day 4–14 of heparin therapy (3)[B]:
  - Withhold platelet monitoring for patients receiving heparin with risk of HIT <1%.
- Confirmatory lab tests needed for a clinical diagnosis can be divided into 2 major categories:
  - Antigen assay to detect presence of HIT antibodies:
    - ELISA: Up to 99% sensitive, poor specificity; thus, has an excellent negative predictive value for HIT
  - Functional assay to detect evidence of platelet activation in the presence of heparin:
    - Serotonin release assay (SRA), gold standard for diagnosis: High specificity and high sensitivity
    - Heparin-induced platelet activation (HIPA): High specificity and low sensitivity
- Either a functional assay or an antigenic assay alone may not be adequate for clinical diagnosis; their use in combination is usually recommended:
  - Antigenic assay should be the initial test.
- The diagnostic interpretation of these laboratory tests must be made in the context of the clinical estimation of the pretest probability because HIT is a clinicopathologic syndrome. Patients may form heparin-dependent antibodies and still not develop HIT (4).

TREATMENT

Treatment is by prompt withdrawal of heparin and replacement with a suitable alternative anticoagulant.

GENERAL MEASURES
- Discontinue all heparin products, including flushes and heparin-coated catheters.
- Nonimmune heparin-associated thrombocytopenia generally resolves when heparin is stopped:
  - Consider a nonheparin alternative such as fondaparinux if pharmacologic DVT prophylaxis is warranted.
- Give platelet transfusions only if bleeding or during the performance of an invasive procedure with a high risk of bleeding (3)[C].
- Adverse reaction to heparin should be clearly documented in the medical record with instruction to avoid all heparin products.
- For patients with a documented history of HIT, under special circumstances only (such as the need for cardiopulmonary bypass), the use of heparin for a short duration may be acceptable if the absence of heparin/PF4 complex antibodies can be documented (5)[C].
- All patients with a diagnosis of HIT should receive alternative anticoagulation as they are of high thrombotic risk.

MEDICATION

- Most patients require anticoagulation either because of:
  - Preexisting thrombosis *or*
  - Risk of thrombosis during 30 days after HIT diagnosis; consider anticoagulation for 30 days (6)[B]
- Dosing of anticoagulant depends on indication (prophylaxis vs. treatment):
  - In cases with a clinically low suspicion/pretest probability of HIT and laboratory confirmation is pending, it may be appropriate to continue antithrombotic prophylaxis using nonheparin anticoagulants.
  - In cases with high suspicion/pretest probability of HIT and laboratory confirmation is pending, it is appropriate to begin anticoagulation treatment with a nonheparin product.
- Direct thrombin inhibitors (DTIs) (argatroban and bivalirudin):
  - Reduce relative risk of thrombosis by 30% and are associated with a 5–10% risk of important bleeding (3)[B]
  - Can produce misleading elevation in international normalized ratio (INR) (most likely an in vitro reaction) (7):
    - ○ Argatroban > Bivalirudin
  - Argatroban:
    - ○ Initial dose, 2 μg/kg/min; decrease dose with reduced hepatic function or with critical illness
    - ○ Dose adjustments based to achieve aPTT 1.5 to 3× baseline.
  - Bivalirudin:
    - ○ Favorable pharmacologic profile; however, evidence for use is insufficient compared to argatroban (limited to case series)
    - ○ Reduced risk of bleeding in patients undergoing percutaneous artery interventions (PCIs) and other cardiac procedures (8)[B]
    - ○ Initial dose of 0.15 mg/k/hr followed by adjustments to keep aPTT 1.5–2.5× baseline. Reduced dose with renal insufficiency (CrCl <30 mL/min) (9)[B]
    - ○ Dose adjustments based on aPTT
- Factor Xa inhibitor (fondaparinux):
  - Reports of its use are theorized to be useful; however, minimal data support its efficacy for HIT, and an ideal dose has yet to be determined.
  - Association with the development of HIT has been reported (10)[C].
  - Optional agent for thromboembolic prophylaxis when practitioner wants to avoid heparin
  - Avoid in patients with renal dysfunction (CrCl <30 mL/min).
- Warfarin:
  - Must anticoagulate with an immediate-acting agent before starting warfarin.
  - Use of warfarin without other anticoagulants should be avoided because it can cause thrombosis (3)[A].
  - Begin warfarin after platelet count >150,000 (3)[B].
  - Discontinue other anticoagulant and continue only warfarin after INR is therapeutic (2–3) for at least 5 days (3)[A]. This management differs from the normal heparin-to-warfarin transition in other conditions requiring anticoagulation.

- LMWH:
  - Although LMWH has a lower risk of initiating a HIT reaction, it should *not* be used when antibodies are already present. These antibodies can cross-react with LMWH and induce thrombosis and thrombocytopenia (3)[A].

IN-PATIENT CONSIDERATIONS

Nursing
- Avoid heparin flushes.
- Avoid platelet transfusion.
- Clearly document reaction in all medical records to control the future use of heparin.

ONGOING CARE

FOLLOW-UP RECOMMENDATIONS
- The transition period of anticoagulation with a DTI and warfarin in patients with HIT can be problematic.
- The INR while administering both a DTI and warfarin should be therapeutic (2–3) for at least 5 days before discontinuing the DTI.
- Warfarin therapy should not be commenced until the platelet count has stabilized within a normal range.
- Warfarin therapy should continue for a minimum of 3 months.
- DTIs can prolong INR; therefore, if INR is >4 while on both warfarin and a DTI, temporarily hold the DTI for 4–6 hours and recheck INR; this second INR will represent only the anticoagulant effect of warfarin.

Patient Monitoring
- Serial platelet counts.
- Monitor PTT or INR as determined by the anticoagulation agent.

PATIENT EDUCATION
- Patient should inform all health care providers of any previous adverse reaction to heparin.
- HIT information available at: http://medlibrary.org/medwiki/Heparin-induced_thrombocytopenia

PROGNOSIS
- Thrombosis in HIT has 20–30% mortality, with additional morbidity from stroke and limb ischemia.
- Platelet counts normalize within weeks after stopping heparin.
- Risk of delayed thrombosis, especially in the first 30 days

REFERENCES

1. Martel N, Lee J, Wells PS. Risk for heparin-induced thrombocytopenia with unfractionated and low-molecular-weight heparin thromboprophylaxis: A meta-analysis. *Blood*. 2005;106:2710–2715.
2. Lo GK, Juhl D, Warkentin TE, et al. Evaluation of pretest clinical score (4 T's) for the diagnosis of heparin-induced thrombocytopenia in two clinical settings. *J Thromb Haemost*. 2006;4:759–765.
3. Cuker A, Arepally G, Crowther MA, et al. The HIT Expert Probability (HEP) Score: A novel pre-test probability model for heparin-induced thrombocytopenia based on broad expert opinion. *J Thromb Haemost*. 2010;8:2642–2650.

4. Shantsila E, Lip GY, Chong BH. Heparin-induced thrombocytopenia: A contemporary clinical approach to diagnosis and management. *Chest*. 2009;135:1651–1664.
5. Warkentin TE, Kelton JG. Temporal aspects of heparin-induced thrombocytopenia. *N Engl J Med*. 2001;344:1286–1292.
6. Dager WE, Dougherty JA, Nguyen PH, et al. Heparin-induced thrombocytopenia: Treatment options and special considerations. *Pharmacotherapy*. 2007;27:564–587.
7. Warkentin TE, Greinacher A, Craven S, et al. Differences in the clinically effective molar concentrations of four direct thrombin inhibitors explain their variable prothrombin time prolongation. *Thromb Haemost*. 2005;94: 958–964.
8. Stone GW, Ware JH, Bertrand ME, et al. Antithrombotic strategies in patients with acute coronary syndromes undergoing early invasive management: One-year results from the ACUITY trial. *JAMA*. 2007;298(21):2497–2506.
9. Bakchoul T, Greinacher A. Recent advances in the diagnosis and treatment of heparin-induced thrombocytopenia. *Ther Adv Hematol*. 2012;3(4): 237–251.
10. Warkentin TE, Maurer BT, Aster RH. Heparin-induced thrombocytopenia associated with fondaparinux. *N Engl J Med*. 2007;356: 2653–2655; discussion 2653–2655.

ADDITIONAL READING

Linkins LA, Dans AL, Moores LK, et al. Treatment and prevention of heparin-induced thrombocytopenia: Antithrombotic Therapy and Prevention of Thrombosis, 9th ed.: American College of Chest Physicians Evidence-Based Clinical Practice Guidelines. *Chest*. 2012;141(2 Suppl):e495S–530S.

 # CODES

ICD10
D75.82 Heparin induced thrombocytopenia (HIT)

CLINICAL PEARLS

- Heparin exposure through virtually any preparation (including LMWH), any dose, or any route can cause HIT.
- LMWH is contraindicated in HIT; although LMWH is less likely to cause HIT, once HIT is present, the antibodies will cross-react and continue to cause a HIT reaction.
- If a patient is suspected of HIT (with or without confirmatory testing), immediately discontinue all forms of heparin.
- Patients will require anticoagulation either because of pre-existing thrombosis or the risk of thrombosis in first 30 days after HIT.
- A DTI should be used until a patient's INR is therapeutic (2–3) on warfarin for at least 5 days.
- The key to avoiding sequelae from HIT is awareness, vigilance, and a high degree of suspicion.

HEPATIC ENCEPHALOPATHY

Walter M. Kim, MD, PhD • Jyoti Ramakrishna, MD

 BASICS

DESCRIPTION
- Hepatic encephalopathy (HE) is characterized by reversible altered mental and neuromotor functioning associated with acute or chronic liver disease and/or portal systemic shunting of blood.
- The prominent features are confusion, impaired arousability, and a "flapping tremor" (asterixis).
- System(s) affected: Gastrointestinal; Nervous
- Synonym(s): Portosystemic encephalopathy; Hepatic coma; Liver coma

EPIDEMIOLOGY
Predominant sex: Male = Female (reflecting underlying liver disease)

Prevalence
- Occurs in 1/3 of cirrhosis cases
- Occurs in all cases of fulminant hepatic failure
- Present in nearly 1/2 of patients who require liver transplantation
- Parallels the age predominance of fulminant liver disease: Peaks in the 40s; cirrhosis peaks in the late 50s; may occur at any age

ETIOLOGY AND PATHOPHYSIOLOGY
- Failure of liver to detoxify agents noxious to the CNS (e.g., ammonia, mercaptan, fatty acids)
- Increased aromatic and reduced branched-chain amino acids in blood; these act as false neurotransmitters, possibly interacting with the γ-aminobutyric acid (GABA) receptor
- Shunting of intestinal blood through the severely diseased liver without the intervention of viable liver cells
- Most common in long-standing cirrhosis of the liver with spontaneous shunting of intestinal blood through collateral vessels
- Shunting of such blood through collateral circulation or surgically constructed portacaval shunts
- Transjugular intrahepatic portosystemic shunt (TIPS), a widely used radiologically inserted shunt to lower portal pressure, produces HE
- Acute onset of HE: Search for risk factors

Genetics
- Unknown
- Conditions such as cystic fibrosis, α-1-antitrypsin deficiency, and Wilson disease can contribute to HE

RISK FACTORS
In patients with underlying liver disease, precipitating factors include:
- Infection (overt or occult, including spontaneous bacterial peritonitis)
- GI hemorrhage
- Use of sedative or opiate drugs
- Fluid or electrolyte disturbance (Na^+, K^+, Mg^{2+}, or other electrolyte depletion)
- TIPS

GENERAL PREVENTION
- Recognize early signs and seek prompt treatment
- Avoid nonessential medications, particularly opiates, benzodiazepines, and sedatives

COMMONLY ASSOCIATED CONDITIONS
- Occurs rarely with portacaval shunt with normal liver function
- May occur as a complication of acute fatty liver of pregnancy

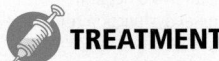 **DIAGNOSIS**

HISTORY
- Pre-existing liver disease
- Confusion
- Impaired arousability

PHYSICAL EXAM
- Age 10–60 years:
  - Prominent signs of underlying liver disease (50%); jaundice most common, ascites second most common
  - GI hemorrhage with hematemesis or melena: 20%
  - Systemic infection, urinary tract or pulmonary: 20%
  - 4 stages of confusion and degree of obtundation described:
    ○ Stage 1: Forgetfulness, disturbance in nocturnal sleep, daytime drowsiness
    ○ Stage 2: Mild confusion, drowsy but arousable
    ○ Stage 3: Patient arousable, markedly confused, with limited orientation and inability to follow commands
    ○ Stage 4: Patient is unable to be aroused and exhibits extensive posturing.
  - Handwriting and hand coordination deteriorate in stages 1 and 2
  - Asterixis prominent in stage 2
  - Reflexes symmetrically hyperactive in stage 3
  - Psychotic thoughts infrequent
  - Mental and neurologic signs change rapidly (over 6–12 hours)
- Age >60 years:
  - Signs of underlying liver disease diminish (25%)
  - Confusion more prominent
  - Precipitating GI hemorrhage or infection is less often identified.
  - Remains in stage 1 or 2 for many days
  - Progression is slower.
- Age <10 years:
  - Signs of underlying liver disease prominent; usually fulminant hepatic failure or extremely advanced cirrhosis
  - Progression through the stages is very rapid, often 6–12 hours
  - Wilson disease can imitate HE.
- Vital signs:
  - Bradycardia
  - Increased blood pressure suggestive of increased intracranial pressure
- Jaundice, ascites, and other correlates of liver disease
- CNS exam pertaining to stage of HE: Assess short-term memory and presence of asterixis

DIFFERENTIAL DIAGNOSIS
- Metabolic encephalopathy related to anoxia, hypoglycemia, hypokalemia, hypo- or hypercalcemia, or uremia
- Head trauma, concussion, subdural hematoma
- Transient ischemic attack (TIA), ischemic stroke
- Alcohol withdrawal syndrome
- Alcohol intoxication
- Toxic confusion due to medication or drugs
- Meningitis
- Wilson disease
- Reye syndrome

DIAGNOSTIC TESTS & INTERPRETATION
- The clinical setting and findings are adequate to establish diagnosis in 80% of the cases
- The treatment response often confirms the diagnosis.
- EEG: Shows symmetric slowing of basic (α) rhythm common with other forms of metabolic encephalopathy (1)[A]; useful to a limited extent
- Visual evoked potential: Specific in stages 2, 3, and 4
- Number connection test, line drawing test, clicker flicker frequency test, and other psychometric tests may be used to assess for minimal HE (2)[A]

Initial Tests (lab, imaging)
- Liver tests, including aspartate aminotransferase (AST), alanine aminotransferase (ALT), and serum albumin to evaluate severity of underlying liver disease
- Prothrombin time (PT) and international normalized ratio (INR) are elevated in liver failure due to impaired hepatic synthesis of coagulation factors
- Elevated ammonia often present (3)[A]; levels affected by infusion of amino acid solutions, opiate administration producing severe constipation, uremia, and rapid and severe tissue breakdown, massive burns, trauma, or infection
- Hematology to identify anemia and signs of infection
- Standard biochemistry profile to identify hypokalemia, hyperbilirubinemia, altered calcium concentration, hypomagnesemia, and hypoglycemia
- BUN: Creatine >20 suggestive of dehydration or GI bleeding
- Blood, urine, and ascitic fluid cultures to identify infection, if clinically indicated
- Consider arterial blood gas measurement
- Toxicology screen for illicit drugs
- Useful only to rule out other diagnoses
- CT scan of the head may be the most useful imaging modality to identify frontal cortical atrophy and mild general edema (4)[A].
- MRI may demonstrate increased T1 signal in globus pallidus.

Diagnostic Procedures/Other
EEG has typical rhythm (see above)

Test Interpretation
- Brain edema in 100% of fatal cases
- Glial hypertrophy in chronic encephalopathy

TREATMENT

GENERAL MEASURES
- Identify and vigorously treat precipitating causes: GI bleeding, infection, sedative drugs, and electrolyte imbalance are most common
- Stage 2 or higher: Ensure adequate fluid intake and at least 1,000 kcal (4.19 megajoules) daily; avoid hypoglycemia
- Give initial enema to all patients without diarrhea.
- If clumsiness and poor judgment are prominent, be sure the patient has the care needed to avoid falls, cuts on broken glass, smoking burns, and machinery/auto accidents

- Avoid sedative or opiate medications: Benzodiazepine sedatives and opiate derivatives, such as diphenoxylate/atropine, have caused liver coma.
- Stage 4: Protect the airway, as aspiration is common (tracheal intubation is often used); feed intravenously or with jejunal feeding tube

MEDICATION
First Line
- Lactulose syrup (nonabsorbable disaccharide whose laxative action decreases colonic transit time while bacterial digestion acidifies the colon thereby promoting excretion of ammonia): 30–60 mL of 50% solution PO up to every hour for goal of 3–6 bowel movements per day. Diminish to 15–30 mL b.i.d. when ≥ 3 bowel movements occur daily
- Lactulose enema (for patients who cannot tolerate oral lactulose or have suspected ileus): 300 mL lactulose plus 700 mL tap water, retained for 1 hour
- If worsening occurs acutely or no improvement in 2 days, add antibiotics:
  - Rifaximin: 400 mg PO t.i.d. (nonabsorbable antibiotic) (5)[A]; highly effective in reversing minimal HE (6)[A]
  - Neomycin: 1–2 g/d PO divided q6–8h, if renal function is within normal limits
  - Metronidazole and vancomycin are alternative antibiotics
- Antacids as needed
- Contraindications:
  - Total ileus
  - Hypersensitivity reaction
- Precautions:
  - Hypokalemia
  - Electrolyte imbalance
  - Renal failure
- For significant possible interactions, refer to manufacturer's profile of each drug

Second Line
Flumazenil

ISSUES FOR REFERRAL
Refer early to a transplant center

SURGERY/OTHER PROCEDURES
- Artificial liver perfusion devices have proven useful in fulminant hepatic failure to bridge the patient until a donor liver is available for transplantation.
- Stages 3 and 4 patients should be considered for liver transplantation.

COMPLEMENTARY AND ALTERNATIVE MEDICINE
Probiotics and prebiotics have been associated with improvement of HE through modulation of gut flora (7)[C] and reduced recurrence of HE in patients with underlying cirrhosis (8)[B].

IN-PATIENT CONSIDERATIONS
Admission Criteria/Initial Stabilization
- Monitor closely in stages 1 and 2 when diagnosis is clear, and watch for progression
- Inpatient management for stages 3 and 4
- Stage 3 or 4 in fulminant hepatic failure is a strong indication for evaluation for liver transplantation; transfer to a transplant center should be considered

ONGOING CARE

FOLLOW-UP RECOMMENDATIONS
- Activity as tolerated
- Avoid driving or operating machinery

Patient Monitoring
- To optimize treatment, a trail-making test should be followed (a pencil/paper connect-the-dots according to numbers). Apply to stages 1 and 2 patients to determine how much maintenance treatment is needed and what diet is appropriate. The test should be run daily at first and then at each visit when changes in drugs and diet are made.
- Patients with changed findings should be seen twice weekly.
- Stable patients should be seen monthly.
- Number connection test or line drawing test at each office visit
- In cirrhosis, evaluate for transplantation and periodically monitor Model for End-stage Liver Disease (MELD) score

DIET
- Integrate with needs of underlying liver disease
- Lower total protein (0.8–1.2 g/kg/d); vegetable protein diets are better tolerated than animal protein diets; special IV/enteral formulations with increased branched-chain amino acids are available
- Stages 3 and 4 patients need parenteral nutrition or jejunal feeds
- As coma improves, increase dietary protein as tolerated
- Have dietitian instruct patient in eating lower-protein diet

PATIENT EDUCATION
Pamphlets suitable for patient and family are available from the American Association for the Study of Liver Diseases, 1729 King Street, Suite 200, Alexandria, Virginia 22314; 703-299-9766; www.aasld.org

PROGNOSIS
- Acute or fulminant disease: With adequate aggressive treatment, disappears without residue or recurrence
- Chronic disease:
  - Coma returns
  - With each recurrence, becomes more and more difficult to treat
  - Plateau of maximum improvement shows a decrement over several years such that the degree of improvement with treatment is increasingly less; the mortality rate is 80%.

COMPLICATIONS
- Recurrence
- With many recurrences, permanent basal ganglion injury (non-Wilsonian hepatolenticular degeneration)
- Hepatorenal syndrome

REFERENCES

1. Saxena N, Bhatia M, Joshi YK, et al. Electrophysiological and neuropsychological tests for the diagnosis of subclinical hepatic encephalopathy and prediction of overt encephalopathy. Liver. 2002;22:190–197.
2. Weissenborn K, Ennen JC, Schomerus H, et al. Neuropsychological characterization of hepatic encephalopathy. J Hepatol. 2001;34:768–773.
3. Ong JP, Aggarwal A, Krieger D, et al. Correlation between ammonia levels and the severity of hepatic encephalopathy. Am J Med. 2003;114:188–193.
4. Quero Guillén JC, Herrerías Gutiérrez JM. Diagnostic methods in hepatic encephalopathy. Clin Chim Acta. 2006;365:1–8.
5. Bass NM, Mullen KD, Sanyal A, et al. Rifaximin treatment in hepatic encephalopathy. N Engl J Med. 2010;362:1071–1081.
6. Sidhu SS, Goyal O, Mishra BP, et al. Rifaximin improves psychometric performance and health-related quality of life in patients with minimal hepatic encephalopathy (the RIME Trial). Am J Gastroenterol. 2011;106:307–316.
7. Liu Q, Duan ZP, Ha DK, et al. Synbiotic modulation of gut flora: Effect on minimal hepatic encephalopathy in patients with cirrhosis. Hepatology. 2004;39:1441–1449.
8. Agrawal A, Sarma CB, et al. Secondary prophylaxis of hepatic encephalopathy in cirrhosis: an open-label, randomized controlled trial of lactulose, probiotics and no therapy. Am J. Gastroenterol. 2012:107:1043–1050.
9. Als-Nielsen B. Non-absorbable disaccharides for hepatic encephalopathy: Systematic review of randomised trials. Br Med J. 2004;328:1046–1511.

ADDITIONAL READING

- Blei AT, Córdoba J, Practice Parameters Committee of the American College of Gastroenterology. Hepatic encephalopathy. Am J Gastroenterol. 2001;96:1968–1976.
- Ferenci P, Lockwood A, Mullen K, et al. Hepatic encephalopathy–definition, nomenclature, diagnosis, and quantification: Final report of the working party at the 11th World Congresses of Gastroenterology, Vienna, 1998. Hepatology. 2002;35:716–721.
- Kircheis G, Fleig WE, Görtelmeyer R, et al. Assessment of low-grade hepatic encephalopathy: A critical analysis. J Hepatol. 2007;47:642–650.
- McGee RG, Bakens A, Wiley K, et al. Probiotics for patients with hepatic encephalopathy. Cochrane Database Syst Rev. 2011;11:CD008716.

 SEE ALSO

Algorithm: Delirium

 CODES

ICD10
- K72.9 Hepatic failure, unspecified
- K72.90 Hepatic failure, unspecified without coma
- K72.91 Hepatic failure, unspecified with coma

CLINICAL PEARLS
- Closely monitor the mental status of your patient for confusion/drowsiness and through psychometric testing to determine if your patient with liver disease is developing HE.
- Although questions regarding the superiority of lactulose over antibiotics have been raised (9), at present, there is not sufficient evidence to change current treatment recommendations.
- It is recommended that all patients with HE receive a liver transplantation evaluation.

HEPATITIS A
Edward Feller, MD

 BASICS

DESCRIPTION
Infection with the hepatitis A virus (HAV) primarily involving the liver. One of the world's most common viral diseases.

EPIDEMIOLOGY
Pediatric Considerations
- Disease is often milder or asymptomatic in pediatric population, severity increases with age.
- Infections are asymptomatic in 70% of children age <6 years.
- In 2009, <1/2 of 13–17-year-olds (in the US) had been vaccinated (1).
- As many as ½ of current HAV infections in the US acquired from travel to endemic countries.

Pregnancy Considerations
- Pregnant women with HAV have increased gestational complications, pre-term labor.

Incidence
- World-wide problem: 1.4 million cases globally.
- Since the hepatitis A vaccine has been in use (1995), incidence of HAV has decreased by >90% (2).
- Estimated cases: 22,000 HAV infections in 2009 (lowest ever recorded in the US)
- Incidence in the US: 0.6/100,000
- Predominant sex: Male = Female

Prevalence
Serologic evidence of prior HAV infection: 1/3 of US population. Anti-HAV prevalence related to age, ranging from 9% in children ages 6–11 to 75% of those >70. Related inversely to income

ETIOLOGY AND PATHOPHYSIOLOGY
- Hepatitis A is a single-stranded linear RNA enterovirus and a member of the *Picornaviridae* family.
- Humans are the only natural host.
- Incubation is 2–6 weeks:
  - Mean of 4 weeks
- Greatest infectivity is during the 2 weeks before the onset of clinical illness.
- Infection occurs after eating food or drinking water contaminated with HAV or direct contact with infected person who has poor personal hygiene.
- Food can become contaminated if handled by an infected individual with poor personal hygiene.
- Shellfish, such as clams and oysters, may be contaminated if harvested from waters contaminated with HAV.
- Bloodborne transmission occurs, but is rare.
- No chronicity in HAV

Genetics
Autoimmune hepatitis is associated with human leukocyte antigen class II; DR3 and DR4 after active infection with HAV, although rare.

RISK FACTORS
- Foreign travel to developing countries accounts for >50% of cases in North America and Europe.
- Employment in health care
- Household exposure
- Intimate exposure, especially men who have sex with men
- Childcare centers, schools
- Institutionalized individuals
- Clotting factor disorders, such as hemophilia
- Blood exposure/transfusion rare
- No identifiable risk factor in 50%

GENERAL PREVENTION
- HAV vaccines: Havrix and Vaqta; Twinrix-combination HAV and HBV vaccine for active immunization only
- Separate syringe site from immunoglobulin
- For travelers, daycare staff/children, custodial facility employees, sewage workers, military, men who have sex with men (MSM), food handlers, IVDUs
- For close contacts of children adopted from countries with HAV infection. Ideally ≥2 weeks before arrival
- HIV-infected patients who are negative for HAV IgG should receive HAV vaccine series, preferably early in course of HIV infection:
  - If CD4 count is <200 cells/mm³ or the patient has symptomatic HIV disease, it is preferable to defer vaccination until several months after initiation of antiretroviral (ARV) therapy to maximize the antibody response to the vaccine (2)[A].
  - Coadministration of the HAV vaccine with measles-mumps-rubella (MMR) and varicella vaccines had no impact on the immunogenicity of any of the vaccines and was well tolerated (3)[B].
- Passive immunization: Immunoglobulin is
  - effective for both pre- and postexposure prophylaxis of hepatitis A (4)[A]:
    - 0.02–0.06 mL/kg IM given within 2 weeks after exposure prevents illness in 80–90%.
    - HAV vaccine has similar efficacy to immunoglobulin in postexposure prophylaxis if given within 2 weeks.
    - Use immunoglobulin in cases where travelers need immediate protection, children age <1 year, and pregnant women who will be traveling.
    - Use 0.06 mL/kg q5mo for long-term travelers if they are unable to receive the vaccine.
    - Do not give immunoglobulin with MMR or varicella vaccines.
- Good sanitation; good hygiene, including handwashing, especially for food handlers, healthcare, and daycare workers
- HAV is *not* killed by freezing.
- HAV is killed by:
  - Heating to 185°F for 60 seconds
  - Chlorine
  - Iodine

DIAGNOSIS

HISTORY
- Fever
- Malaise
- Nausea and vomiting, headache
- Anorexia
- Dark urine:
- Right upper abdominal pain
- Fatigue; myalgias
- Pruritus; a sign of cholestasis
- Symptom severity has direct correlation to age.
- Pediatric cases frequently asymptomatic
- Incubation: 15–50 days (mean of 28 days)

PHYSICAL EXAM
- Hepatomegaly or splenomegaly are possible
- Fever
- Jaundice
- Right upper quadrant abdominal tenderness

DIFFERENTIAL DIAGNOSIS
- Hepatitis B, C, D, E
- Not clinically distinguishable from other forms of viral hepatitis; diagnosis may be suspected with typical symptoms during an outbreak.
- Infectious mononucleosis, CMV
- Primary or secondary hepatic malignancy
- Ischemic hepatitis
- Drug-induced hepatitis
- Alcoholic hepatitis
- Hemochromatosis in adults
- Autoimmune hepatitis; Wilson disease
- Nonhepatobiliary disease (elevated AST/ALT): Celiac disease, congestive heart failure, thyroid disease

DIAGNOSTIC TESTS & INTERPRETATION
Initial Tests (lab, imaging)
- AST and ALT elevated: ALT usually > AST
- Hepatocellular injury pattern
- Anti-HAV IgM: Positive at time of onset of symptoms with sensitivity and specificity > 95%
- Anti-HAV IgG: Appears soon after IgM and generally persists for years
- Alkaline phosphatase: Mildly elevated
- Bilirubin: Conjugated and unconjugated fractions usually increased. Usually follows rises in ALT/AST.
- Prothrombin time and partial thromboplastin time: Usually remain normal or near normal:
  - Significant rises should raise concern.

- CBC: Mild leukocytosis; aplasia and pancytopenia are rare:
  – Thrombocytopenia may predict illness severity.
- Albumin, electrolytes, and glucose
- Urinalysis: Bilirubinuria
- Usually not needed
- Consider US to rule out biliary obstruction only if lab pattern is cholestatic.

Follow-Up Tests & Special Considerations
Illness usually resolves within 4 weeks from onset of symptoms. Usually can be managed as outpatient

Diagnostic Procedures/Other
Liver biopsy usually not necessary

Test Interpretation
- Portal inflammation
- Immunofluorescent stains for HAV-antigen positive
- Positive serum markers in hepatitis A:
  – Acute disease: Anti-HAV IgM
  – Recent disease: Anti-HAV IgM and IgG positive
  – Previous disease: Anti-HAV IgM negative and IgG positive

TREATMENT

GENERAL MEASURES
- Monitor coagulation defects, fluid and electrolytes, acid–base imbalance, hypoglycemia, and impairment of renal function (5).
- Report acute cases to local public health department.
- Maintain bed rest and appropriate nutrition/hydration.

MEDICATION
Postexposure prophylaxis to persons within 2 weeks of exposure to HAV:
- Administer hepatitis A vaccine to persons between the ages of 1 and 40.
- Administer immunoglobulin to persons <1 and >40 years of age.

First Line
- No antiviral medications indicated; spontaneous resolution occurs in almost all patients
- Steroids not indicated unless patient has autoimmune hepatitis

Second Line
- Antiemetics
- IV fluids
- Pruritus: Diphenhydramine 50 mg PO/IM q6h and cholestyramine 4 g b.i.d.

ISSUES FOR REFERRAL
- Dictated by severity of illness
- Hepatic failure

SURGERY/OTHER PROCEDURES
Liver transplant in fulminant hepatic failure

COMPLEMENTARY AND ALTERNATIVE MEDICINE
Avoid botanicals with hepatotoxicity potential, including barberry, comfrey, golden ragwort, groundsel, huang qin, kava kava, pennyroyal, sassafras, senna, valerian, wall germander, wood sage.

IN-PATIENT CONSIDERATIONS
Admission Criteria/Initial Stabilization
Treatment is usually outpatient; dictated by severity of illness.

IV Fluids
Treat dehydration and electrolyte imbalances.

Nursing
Enteric isolation. Private rooms, gowns, and masks are not necessary. Frequent handwashing. Use gloves when handling material potentially contaminated with feces.

 ONGOING CARE

FOLLOW-UP RECOMMENDATIONS
Return to work/school 10–14 days after onset of symptoms with diligence to hygiene

Patient Monitoring
- Monitor coagulation defects, fluid and electrolytes, acid–base imbalance, hypoglycemia, and impairment of renal function.
- Report acute cases to local public health department.
- Usually infectious 4 weeks from initial symptoms

DIET
- Adequate balanced nutrition
- Avoid alcohol.
- Avoid medications that may accumulate in the liver.

PATIENT EDUCATION
- Segregate food handlers with HAV.
- HAV immunity after infection
- CDC Hepatitis A Fact Sheet Link: http://www.cdc.gov/hepatitis/A/PDFs/HepAGeneralFactSheet_BW.pdf

PROGNOSIS
- Excellent; mortality is 0.2%.
- Risk increased with underlying chronic liver disease and in the elderly

COMPLICATIONS
- Coagulopathy, encephalopathy, and renal failure
- Relapsing HAV: Usually milder than the initial case
- Positive anti-HAV IgM. Total duration is usually <9 months.
- Prolonged cholestasis: Characterized by protracted periods of jaundice and pruritus (>3 months)
- Resolves without intervention
- Autoimmune hepatitis: Good response to steroids
- Hepatic failure: Rare (1–2%)
- Postviral encephalitis, Guillain-Barré syndrome, aplastic or hemolytic anemia, agranulocytosis, thrombocytopenic purpura, pancytopenia, arthritis, vasculitis, and cryoglobulinemia (all rare)

REFERENCES

1. Dorrell Cg, Yankey D, Byrd KK, et al. Hepatitis A vaccination coverage among adolescents in the United States. *Pediatrics*. 2012;129:213–221.
2. Lu PJ, Euler GL, Hennessey KA, et al. Hepatitis A vaccination coverage among adults aged 18–49 years in the United States. *Vaccine*. 2009;27(9):1301–1305.
3. National Guideline Clearinghouse (NGC) Agency for Healthcare Research and Quality AHRQ). Prevention of secondary disease: Preventive medicine. *Viral Hepatitis*. 2011. www.guideline.gov.
4. Liu JP, Nikolova D, Fei Y. Immunoglobulins for preventing hepatitis A. *Cochrane Database Syst Rev*. 2009;(2):CD004181.
5. Matheny SC, Kingery JE. *Hepatitis A. Review. Am Fam Physician*. 2012;86:1027–1034.

ADDITIONAL READING

- American Academy of Pediatrics Committee on Infectious Diseases. Recommendations for administering hepatitis A vaccine to contacts of international adoptees. *Pediatrics*. 2011;128(4):803–804. Epub 2011 Sep 26.
- Lee TH, Kim WR, Poterucha JJ. Evaluation of elevated liver enzymes. *Clin Liver Dis*. 2012;16:183–188.
- Rowe IA. Hepatitis A vaccination in Hepatitis C infection: Consequence of quality measure implementation. *Hepatology*. 2012;56:501–506.
- Trofa AF, Klein NP, Paul IM, et al. Immunogenicity and safety of an inactivated hepatitis A vaccine when coadministered with diphtheria-tetanus-acellular pertussis and haemophilus influenzae type B vaccines in children 15 months of age. *Pediatr Infect Dis J*. 2011;30(9):e164–169.

 SEE ALSO

- Hepatitis B; Hepatitis C
- Algorithm: Hyperbilirubinemia

 CODES

ICD10
- B15.9 Hepatitis A without hepatic coma
- K75.4 Autoimmune hepatitis

CLINICAL PEARLS
- Acute HAV can occur in underlying chronic liver disease (HBV, HCV, alcohol). Clues may be evidence of portal hypertension on exam, poor hepatic synthesis (hypoalbuminemia, increased INR), thrombocytopenia.
- Vaccine is indicated for travelers, daycare staff/children, custodial facility employees, sewage workers, military, men who have sex with men (MSM), food handlers, IV drug users.
- HAV disease severity directly correlates with age; children are often asymptomatic.
- Check HAV IgG in all HIV patients; immunize all who are negative.

H

HEPATITIS B
Michael P. Curry, MD

 BASICS

DESCRIPTION
Systemic viral infection that may cause acute and chronic liver disease and hepatocellular carcinoma (HCC)

EPIDEMIOLOGY
Incidence
- Predominant age: All ages
- Predominant sex: Fulminant hepatitis B virus (HBV): Male > Female (2:1)
- In the US, estimated 38,000 new infections in 2009, 70% due to IV drug use
- African Americans: Highest rate of acute HBV infection in the US
- Overall rate of new infections down 82% since 1991 (due to national immunization strategy)
- US vaccine coverage increased from 68.6% in 2011 to 71.6% in 2012 for the birth dose of HepB (1)[A]

Prevalence
- In the US, 800,000–1.4 million people have chronic hepatitis B virus (HBV).
- Asia and the Pacific Islands have the largest populations at risk for HBV.
- Chronic HBV worldwide: 350–400 million persons:
  – Per year: 1 million deaths:
    ○ 2nd most important carcinogen (behind tobacco)
    ○ Of chronic carriers, 25% die of cirrhosis or HCC
    ○ Of chronic carriers, 75% are Asian

ETIOLOGY AND PATHOPHYSIOLOGY
HBV is a DNA virus of the family *Hepadnaviridae*.

Genetics
Family history of HBV and/or HCC to determine exposure and future HCC risk

RISK FACTORS
- Screen high-risk groups with HBsAg/sAb (1)[A]:
  – Persons born in endemic areas (45% of world)
  – Hemodialysis patients
  – IV drug users (IVDU), past or present
  – Men who have sex with men (MSM)
  – HIV- and HCV-positive patients
  – Household members of HBsAg carriers
  – Sexual contacts of HBsAg carriers
  – Inmates of correctional facilities
  – Patients with chronically elevated aspartate aminotransferase/alanine aminotransferase (ALT/AST)
- *Vaccinate all above groups if negative.*
- Additional risk factors:
  – Needle stick/occupational exposure
  – Recipients of blood/products; transplanted organ recipients
  – Intranasal drug users
  – Body piercing/tattoos

Marker	Acute infection	Chronic infection	Inactive carrier	Resolved infection
HBsAg	+	+	+	–
HBsAb	–	–	–	+
HBcAb	+IgM	–IgM; +total/IgG	+	+
HBeAg	+	±	–	–
HBeAb	–	±	+	±
HBV DNA	Present	Present	Low–negative	–
Negative ALT		Marked elevation	Transient mild elevation	Normal

Pediatric Considerations
- Shorter acute course; fewer complications
- 90% of vertical/perinatal infections become chronic

Pregnancy Considerations
- Screen all pregnant women for HBsAg (2)[A].
- High viral load at 28 weeks should prompt consideration for treatment with oral nucleos(t)ide medicines from 32 weeks to reduce perinatal transmission.
- Infant of HBV-infected mother needs HB immune globulin (HBIg) (0.5 mL) plus HBV vaccine within 12 hours of birth and HBV series at 0, 1, and 6 months (2)[A].
- Breastfeeding is safe if HBIg and HBV vaccine are administered and nipples are without fissures. Oral nucleos(t)ide medications are not recommended in lactating mothers. Risk and benefits must be assessed.
- HIV coinfection significantly increases risk of vertical transmission.
- Continue medications if pregnancy occurs while on an oral antiviral therapy to prevent acute flare.

GENERAL PREVENTION
Most effective: HBV vaccination series (3 doses):
- Vaccinate:
  – All infants at birth
  – All at-risk patients (see "Risk Factors")
  – Health care and public safety workers
  – Sexual contacts of HBsAg carriers
  – Household contacts of HBsAg carriers
- Proper hygiene/sanitation by health care workers, IVDU, and tattoo/piercing artists:
  – Barrier precautions, needle disposal, sterilization of equipment, cover open cuts
- Do not share personal items exposed to blood (e.g., nail clipper, razor, toothbrush).
- Safe sexual practices (condoms)
- HBsAg carriers cannot donate blood or tissue.
- Postexposure (e.g., needle stick): HBIg 0.06 mL/kg in <24 hours and vaccination

COMMONLY ASSOCIATED CONDITIONS
Arthritis, polyarteritis nodosa, membranous glomerulopathy, anemia (including aplastic anemia), dermatitis, cardiomyopathy, hepatitis D virus infection, metabolic syndrome

 DIAGNOSIS

HISTORY
- Exposure: Detailed family and social history
- Acute HBV:
  – Fever, malaise, fatigue, arthralgias, myalgias
  – Anorexia, nausea, vomiting
  – Jaundice, scleral icterus
  – Dark urine, pale stools
  – Right upper quadrant (RUQ) abdominal pain
- Chronic HBV: Typically asymptomatic

PHYSICAL EXAM
Acute: Ill; jaundice/scleral icterus; RUQ tenderness, hepatomegaly

DIFFERENTIAL DIAGNOSIS
- Epstein–Barr virus (EBV); cytomegalovirus (CMV); hepatitis A, C, or E
- Drug-induced, alcoholic, or autoimmune hepatitis
- Wilson disease or rheumatologic/immunologic disorders

DIAGNOSTIC TESTS & INTERPRETATION
Initial Tests (lab, imaging)
- AST/ALT: Marked elevation in acute HBV, particularly of ALT, 400 to several thousand IU/mL (may be normal or mildly elevated in chronic HBV):
  – Elevated before bilirubin elevates
- Bilirubin: Normal to markedly elevated in acute HBV, conjugated/unconjugated:
  – Last test to normalize as acute infection resolves
- Alkaline phosphatase: Mild elevation
- HBcAb IgM may be the only early finding ("window period," when HBsAg/sAb–).
- For acute hepatitis:
  – Monitor PT, albumin, electrolytes, glucose, CBC
  – If severe acute HBV, check for superinfection with hepatitis D (HDV Ag and HBDV Ab)
  – Hepatitis B serologic markers
- Hepatitis Be antigen (HBeAg+) indicates high replication/infectivity; confirmed with high HBV DNA ($\geq 10^5$ copies/mL); these patients benefit from medical therapy.
- HBV precore mutants have undetectable HBeAg despite active viral replication (confirm with HBV DNA level), as well as antibody to e antigen (HBeAb+).
- Screen for HDV, HIV, HCV, and immunity to hepatitis A virus (HAV Ab total/IgG).
- US to demonstrate ascites, splenomegaly, portal hypertension, rule out obstruction, screen for HCC
- Contrast CT or MRI if abnormal US or elevated α-fetoprotein (AFP)

Follow-Up Tests & Special Considerations
HBsAg+ persistence >6 months defines chronic HBV:
- Measure HBV DNA level and ALT every 3–6 months.
- If age >40 and ALT borderline or mildly elevated, consider liver biopsy.
- Measure baseline AFP
- Follow HBeAg for loss (every 6–12 months).
- Lifetime monitoring for progression, need for treatment, and screening for HCC

Diagnostic Procedures/Other
Liver biopsy, serum markers of fibrosis (Hepascore, Fibro test) or measurement of elastography (Fibroscan) determines extent of injury and excludes other liver disease.

Test Interpretation
Liver biopsy in chronic HBV may show interface hepatitis and inflammation, necrosis, cholestasis, fibrosis, cirrhosis, or chronic active hepatitis.

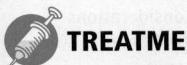

TREATMENT

GENERAL MEASURES
- Vaccinate for HAV if seronegative.
- Monitor CBC, coagulation, electrolytes, glucose, renal function, phosphate.
- Monitor ALT and HBV DNA; increased ALT and reduced DNA implies response to therapy.
- Screen for HCC even in those without cirrhosis.

MEDICATION
First Line
- Acute HBV:
  – Supportive care; antiviral therapy not indicated; spontaneously resolves in 95% of immunocompetent adults. Treatment for acute HBV resulting in acute liver failure.

Chronic hepatitis B therapy (2)

HBeAg	HBV DNA viral load	ALT*	Recommend
(+)	≥20,000 IU/mL	Elevated	
(−)	≥2,000 IU/mL	Elevated	Consider biopsy or serum fibrosis marker and treatment
(+)	≤20,000 IU/mL	Any	Monitor q6–12 mo
(−)	≥2,000 IU/mL	Normal	Biopsy; treat if disease
(+)	≥20,000 IU/mL	Normal	Observe, consider treatment if ALT elevated. Biopsy if age >40 or ALT is high normal to mild elevation
(−)	≤2,000 IU/mL	Any	Monitor q6–12 mo
Cirrhosis	Any	Any	Treat with mono or combination treatment (4)
Decomposition	Any	Any	Treat + refer for transplant

*ALT elevated if >2 × ULN; ULN for male = 30 IU/mL and for female = 19 IU/mL.

- Chronic HBV: Treatment based on HBeAg status:
  – FDA-approved drugs: Lamivudine 100 mg, adefovir 10 mg, entecavir 0.5–1 mg, telbivudine 600 mg, or tenofovir 300 mg, all given PO every day (dose based on renal function); pegylated interferon (peg-IFN) α2a SC weekly (2,3)[A]
- Lamivudine is no longer recommended as first-line therapy due to high rates of resistance.
- Entecavir, tenofovir, peg-IFN are preferred first-line agents (2)[A].
- Oral agents given for extended period:
  – If HBeAg+, treat 6–12 months postloss of HBeAg and gain of HBeAb, and monitor after cessation (2)[A].
  – If HBeAg−, treat indefinitely or until HBsAg clearance and HBsAb development (2)[A].
- Change/Add drug based on development of resistance:
  – Confirm patient compliance with medications before assuming resistance
  – Adherence to therapy lowers rate of resistance
- Dose adjustment made for elevated creatinine
- Standard interferon (Intron A) no longer used in favor of peg-IFN:
  – Peg-IFN (Pegasys) injections given weekly for 48 weeks
  – Best efficacy in genotype A
  – Contraindicated if decompensated cirrhosis
- Goals of therapy: Undetectable HBV DNA, normal ALT, loss of HBeAg, gain of HBeAb; loss of HBsAg and gain of HBsAb

- Precautions:
  – Oral drugs: Renal insufficiency
  – Peg-IFN: Coagulopathy, myelosuppression, depression/suicidal ideation

Second Line
Emtricitabine effective; pending FDA approval

ISSUES FOR REFERRAL
- Refer all HBsAg+ patients for consideration of antiviral therapy.
- Refer to liver transplant program ASAP if fulminant acute hepatitis, end-stage liver disease, or HCC.

SURGERY/OTHER PROCEDURES
Liver transplantation, operative resection, radiofrequency ablation

IN-PATIENT CONSIDERATIONS
Admission Criteria/Initial Stabilization
- Worsening course (marked increase in bilirubin, transaminases, or symptoms)
- Hepatic failure (high PT, low albumin)

ONGOING CARE

FOLLOW-UP RECOMMENDATIONS
Patient Monitoring
- Vaccinate for HAV if seronegative (2)[B].
- Monitor serial ALT and HBV DNA:
  – High ALT + low HBV DNA associated with favorable response to therapy
- Serologic markers: See chart
- Metabolic complications and renal function
- WBC/platelets with interferon therapy
- Monitor HBV DNA q3–6 mo during therapy:
  – Undetectable DNA at week 24 of oral drug therapy associated with low resistance at year 2.
- Monitor for complications (ascites, encephalopathy, variceal bleed) in cirrhosis.

DIET
Avoid alcohol

PATIENT EDUCATION
- Acute HBV:
  – Review transmission precautions (2)[A].
- Chronic HBV:
  – Alcohol/Smoking accelerates progression of liver disease.
  – Strict compliance with oral medication is critical to prevent flare.
- Patient education materials in English and Spanish available at www.cdc.gov/hepatitis/Resources/PatientEdMaterials.htm

PROGNOSIS
- Acute infection: 95% of adults recover
- Severity of encephalopathy predicts survival in fulminant hepatic failure.
- Acute HBV: Mortality 1%
- Acute HBV + HDV: Mortality 2–20%
- Chronic HBV:
  – Spontaneous resolution: 0.5% per year
  – Premature death from cirrhosis or HCC: 25%
  – Risk of HCC rises with rate of viral replication, even if no cirrhosis
  – US and AFP q6–12 mo for screening (patient-specific guidelines) (2,4)[B]

COMPLICATIONS
- Acute or subacute hepatic necrosis; cirrhosis; hepatic failure
- HCC (all chronic HBV patients are at risk)
- Severe flare of chronic HBV with corticosteroids: Avoid corticosteroids if possible.
- Reactivation of resolved infection if immunosuppressed (e.g., chemotherapy): Prophylactic premedication recommended if HBsAg+ (2,4) or if HBcAb+ and received systemic chemotherapy.

REFERENCES

1. National, state, and local area vaccination coverage among children aged 19–35 months—United States, 2012. *MMWR Morb Mortal Wkly Rep*. 2013;62:733–740.
2. Lok AS, McMahon BJ. Chronic hepatitis B: Update 2009. *Hepatology*. 2009;50:661–662.
3. Woo G, Tomlinson G, Nishikawa Y, et al. Tenofovir and entecavir are the most effective antiviral agents for chronic hepatitis B: A systematic review and Bayesian meta-analyses. *Gastroenterology*. 2010;139:1218–1229.
4. Weinmaum C. Recommendations for identification and public health management of persons with chronic hepatitis B infection. *MMWR Morb Mortal Wkly Rep*. 2008;57:1–20.

 SEE ALSO

- Cirrhosis of the Liver; Hepatitis A; Hepatitis C
- Algorithm: Hyperbilirubinemia

CODES

ICD10
- B16.9 Acute hepatitis B w/o delta-agent and without hepatic coma
- B18.1 Chronic viral hepatitis B without delta-agent
- B19.10 Unspecified viral hepatitis B without hepatic coma

CLINICAL PEARLS
- All patients born in endemic countries should be screened with HBsAg.
- Patients with chronic HBV need lifetime monitoring for progressive disease and HCC.

H

HEPATITIS C
Michael P. Curry, MD

 BASICS

DESCRIPTION
Acute/Chronic systemic viral infection primarily involving liver

EPIDEMIOLOGY
- Predominant age: Highest incidence in ages 20–39; highest prevalence ages 30–49 years
- Predominant sex: Male = Female

Geriatric Considerations
Age >60 less likely to respond; treat earlier if able

Pediatric Considerations
- Prevalence: 0.3%
- Fewer symptoms or abnormal liver tests; more likely to clear spontaneously; slower rate of progression

Pregnancy Considerations
- Vertical transmission 1–5% if HIV negative
- Breastfeeding safe if no fissures (1)
- Ribavirin is teratogenic; contraindicated in pregnancy and in male partners of pregnant/impregnable women without contraception

Incidence
- In the US, 17,000 new cases of *chronic* hepatitis C virus (HCV) in 2010: Reports of *acute* infections rare (asymptomatic); 2/3 of people with chronic HCV are undiagnosed.
- Rate of new infections reduced since 1992 when effective donor blood screening began.

Prevalence
- ~2.7–3.9 million in US (1–1.5%) HCV Ab+
- Prevalence is 3.25% in persons born between 1945 and 1965 ("baby boomers").
- ~3 million have chronic HCV (HCV RNA+)
- ~12,000 deaths annually
- Most common cause of chronic liver disease and liver transplants in the US
- Genotype 1 predominant (75% of cases)

ETIOLOGY AND PATHOPHYSIOLOGY
Single-stranded RNA virus of family *Flaviviridae*

RISK FACTORS
- Screen patients with persistently elevated alanine aminotransferase (ALT) or known risk factors (1)[B]:
  - Hemodialysis
  - Blood ± product transfusion before 1992
  - Hemophilia treatment before 1987
  - IV drug use: 60–70% of new infections
    - *High transmission 1st use; "once" is high risk*
  - Sexually active homosexual male
  - HIV/Hepatitis B infection
  - Household exposure to infected body fluids
  - Organ transplant recipients before 1992
  - Children of HCV+ mothers (test >18 months)
  - Current sexual partners of HCV+ persons
- Possible risk factors:
  - Inhaled cocaine use; body piercing/tattoos; needle sticks

GENERAL PREVENTION
- *CDC: Screen all adults born between 1945 and 1965 once for hepatitis C.*
- No vaccine/postexposure prophylaxis available
- HCV Ab+ does not confer immunity to reinfection.
- Do not share razors/toothbrushes/nail clippers.
- Use and dispose of needles properly.
- Sexual transmission rare in long-term partners (1.5%) if monogamous (1)[C]

COMMONLY ASSOCIATED CONDITIONS
Diabetes, metabolic syndrome, iron overload, depression, substance abuse/recovery, autoimmune and hematologic disease, HIV, and hepatitis B coinfections

 DIAGNOSIS

HISTORY
- Determine exposure: *Complete* social history
- Chronic HCV: Vast majority mildly symptomatic (nonspecific fatigue) or asymptomatic elevated ALT/aspartate aminotransferase (AST)
- Acute HCV: *If* symptoms develop (rare):
  - Onset ≥2 weeks postexposure and persist 2–12 weeks
  - Usually spontaneous clearance of fever; malaise/fatigue; arthralgias/myalgias; nausea/vomiting/anorexia; right upper quadrant (RUQ) pain; jaundice/icterus/pruritus/dark urine/pale stools

PHYSICAL EXAM
- Typically normal unless advanced fibrosis/cirrhosis
- May have RUQ tenderness/hepatomegaly

DIFFERENTIAL DIAGNOSIS
Hepatitis A or B; Epstein-Barr virus (EBV), cytomegalovirus (CMV); alcoholic hepatitis; nonalcoholic steatohepatitis (NASH); hemochromatosis, Wilson disease, α1–antitrypsin deficiency; ischemic, drug-induced, or autoimmune hepatitis

DIAGNOSTIC TESTS & INTERPRETATION
Initial Tests (lab, imaging)
- AST/ALT: Normal/Persistently elevated in chronic HCV; ALT usually 1–2 × upper limit of normal (ULN); AST may be normal/elevated, but < ALT
- AST/ALT ratio ≥1 associated with cirrhosis:
  - If ratio >2, rule out alcohol abuse
  - Marked elevation only in acute hepatitis (400 to several thousand U/L)
  - If acute, serial PT to monitor for liver failure (acute liver failure from HCV alone is exceedingly rare)
- Alkaline phosphatase and γ-glutamyltransferase: Usually normal; more likely abnormal if cirrhosis, alcohol/fatty liver, or biliary obstruction
- Bilirubin: Normal in chronic HCV unless end-stage disease; markedly elevated in acute HCV (both direct/indirect); occurs after ALT/AST increase, ≥6 weeks postexposure
- Albumin and PT normal until liver failure
- Anti-HCV negative until 8–9 weeks postexposure
- HCV RNA positive 1–3 weeks postexposure
- Persistent HCV RNA >6 months = chronic HCV
- False (+) antibody: Autoimmune disease; false (–): Immunosuppressed
- Screen for other liver disease (differential diagnosis):
  - Ferritin (moderately high levels typical in HCV), ceruloplasmin, antinuclear antibody (ANA), α1-antitrypsin phenotype, fasting glucose/lipid panel
- If chronic, baseline α-fetoprotein (AFP) serum markers in hepatitis C diagnosis
- Ultrasound (US): Hepatomegaly, fatty liver, rule out mass
- MRI with contrast if US/AFP abnormal; early cirrhosis not detectable by imaging

Follow-Up Tests & Special Considerations
Vaccinate if seronegative for hepatitis A/B (1)[C].

Diagnostic Procedures/Other
Liver biopsy/serum fibrosis marker (Hepascore, Fibrotest) or elastography recommended in chronic HCV to determine extent of injury, exclude other disease, guide treatment, and determine prognosis (2)[C].

Test Interpretation
- Periportal lymphocytic inflammation
- Inflammation: Grade 0–4; fibrosis: Stage 0–4 (Metavir scoring system)

Serum markers in hepatitis C diagnosis

Result	Marker (Lab test)
(+)	Anti-HCV (antibody):
	• ELISA III
	• RIBA (distinguishes false–positive HCV Ab from spontaneous clearance)
(+)	• HCV RNA (viral load):
	• Qualitative
	• Quantitative, confirms (+) qualitative (PCR or bDNA)
1, 2, 3, 4, or 6 (rare) (also >50 subtypes)	Genotype (1)[A]:
	• Indeterminate if RNA too low, spontaneous clearance, or false–positive anti-HCV
	• 2a, 2b, 3a: Duration of therapy with pegylated interferon and ribavirin is 24 weeks.
	• 1a, 1b: Duration of therapy is determined by response and includes pegylated interferon, ribavirin, and a protease inhibitor, such as telaprevir or boceprevir.

 TREATMENT

GENERAL MEASURES
- Report acute cases to the health department
- Pretreatment patient counseling is critical.
- Control all other medical conditions prior to treatment.
- Side effects of interferon/ribavirin:
  - Fatigue, weight loss, insomnia, headache, depression/irritability, cognitive changes, nausea, rash, cough, thyroiditis, alopecia (temporary)
  - Premedicate injections with acetaminophen or NSAIDs if not contraindicated; early and prophylactic treatment of somatic and psychiatric side effects is key to adherence (3).
- Side effects of protease inhibitors:
  - Skin rash (mild to moderate in 50%, severe in 5%, DRESS and Stevens-Johnson syndrome seen in <1%), anemia, anorectal pain, dysgeusia
- Growth factors help maintain dose and tolerability (erythropoietin for ribavirin-induced anemia, granulocyte colony-stimulating factor [G-CSF] for interferon-induced neutropenia); however, not associated with improved sustained virologic response (SVR) (4)[C].

- Team (PCP, GI/hepatologist/infectious disease physician, counselor, help line/support group, insurance disease management program, family, 12-step sponsor) improves outcomes (3).

MEDICATION

First Line

- Acute HCV: Antiviral therapy highly effective if given within 12 weeks of infection (2)[B]:
  – Pegylated interferon (peg-IFN) alone or with low-dose ribavirin, for 12–24 weeks
- Chronic HCV: Antiviral therapy variably effective peg-IFN/ribavirin (1)[A]:
  – Peg-IFN/ribavirin (RBV)/protease inhibitor combined therapy:
    ○ Peg-IFN α2b 1.5 μg/kg SC weekly *OR*
    ○ Peg-IFN α2a 180 μg SC weekly *WITH*
    ○ Ribavirin 800–1,400 mg PO, divided b.i.d. (weight-based)
    ○ Telaprevir (Incivek) 375 mg, 2 tablets q8h with a snack containing fatty foods for 12 weeks *OR*
    ○ Boceprevir 200 mg, 4 tablets q8h with a snack starting on day 1 of week 5 of therapy
  – Duration of therapy: 24–48 weeks based on genotype, cirrhosis, and response-guided therapy with assessment of HCV viral load (VL) at weeks 4 and 12 for IFN/RBV and telaprevir and at weeks 8 and 24 for IFN/RBV and boceprevir.
  – Treatment of HCV in the setting of HIV infection should be with IFN/RBV for 48 weeks regardless of HCV genotype.
  – Telaprevir and boceprevir are not FDA approved for acute HCV infection, HIV and HCV infection, and non–genotype 1 HCV infection.
  – For genotype 2 or 3, 24 weeks sufficient if early viral response (EVR):
    ○ Cirrhosis lowers sustained viral response (SVR) by 50% in all genotypes.
    ○ Dose-reduced ribavirin/therapy interruption, especially before RNA negative, reduces SVR (4)[B]
  – Contraindications: Mouse IG, egg, or neomycin allergy; pregnancy/breastfeeding; decompensated liver disease/renal failure; untreated psychiatric disease; corticosteroid use/uncontrolled autoimmune disease; DDI or D4T in HIV patients (substitute comparable agent)
  – Precautions: Disorders of coagulation, anemia, or myelosuppression; seizures; depression/suicidal ideation (psychiatric clearance and monitoring recommended); retinopathy (diabetic/hypertensive) needs ophthalmology clearance/monitoring
  – Antidepressant pretreatment with SSRI's lowers the incidence and severity of IFN-associated depression in chronic hepatitis C infection (5)[A]

ISSUES FOR REFERRAL

- Refer all patients to a specialist experienced with HCV therapy (2)[C] (clinical trial if uninsured)
- Refer to liver transplant program if fulminant acute hepatitis, at 1st complication of end-stage disease, or at diagnosis of HCC (2)[A].

ADDITIONAL THERAPIES

Interferon-alfacon-1 (consensus IFN, Infergen); up to 37% cure rate in nonresponders/relapsers (6)[C].

COMPLEMENTARY AND ALTERNATIVE MEDICINE

- No medical evidence exists for herbal/alternative therapy in HCV/cirrhosis/HCC (1)[C].

- Milk thistle (silymarin) safe; may reduce ALT, but does not eradicate virus or improve outcomes; avoid while on IFN.

 ## ONGOING CARE

FOLLOW-UP RECOMMENDATIONS

- If treatment is deferred, annual LFTs; monitor for complications; and maintain sobriety/recovery.
- No need to monitor serial VL unless on antiviral therapy; unrelated to disease severity or prognosis, and individual lab assays not well standardized.
- In cirrhosis, lifetime risk HCC 20%; screen with US/AFP every 6–12 months (2)[C].

Patient Monitoring

- Serial ALT/AST; serial fasting glucose
- Serial Hgb/Hct, WBCs, absolute neutrophil count, platelets
- Follow electrolytes, thyroid-stimulating hormone (TSH), renal function, PT
- HCV qualitative RNA negativity at week 4 is rapid viral response (RVR); confers ~90% chance of SVR in all genotypes (1)
- HCV quantitative RNA negativity (or drop of $\geq$2 log) at week 12 is EVR; confers good chance SVR
- SVR also more likely in patients with these factors (3): Age $\leq$40; female gender; white; absence of bridging fibrosis/cirrhosis; HCV RNA <400,000 IU/mL; genotypes 2 and 3; BMI <30 kg/m^2; absence of insulin resistance and steatosis; absence of HIV; recent infection (e.g., needle stick)
- HCV RNA >1,000 IU/mL at week 4 or week 12 for patients on IFN/RBV and telaprevir requires discontinuation of therapy
- HVCV RNA >100 IU/mL at week 12 for patients on IFN/RBV and boceprevir requires discontinuation of therapy.
- Monitor for decompensation (low albumin, ascites, encephalopathy, GI bleed) in cirrhotics.
- Goal of therapy is SVR: Eradication of HCV by negative qualitative RNA (TMA) 6 months posttreatment (relapse extremely rare after 6 months)

DIET

- Low-fat, high-fiber diet, and exercise to treat obesity/fatty liver
- Extra protein and fluids while on IFN therapy

PATIENT EDUCATION

- Avoid alcohol, tobacco, and drugs (including marijuana); refer to rehab/12-step program and monitor for relapse.
- Warn against claims of false cures
- Recommend avoidance of herbs, supplements, and hepatotoxic medications (may contain hepatotoxins and contaminants
- www.cdc.gov/knowmorehepatitis/

PROGNOSIS

- Of acute infections, 70–80% become chronic.
- Of chronic infections, 30% will progress to cirrhosis at a rate of 1–3% per year over 10–30 years.
- Cirrhosis progresses to liver failure and/or cancer (HCC) in 30%; more rapid if older age when infected; male gender; alcohol/substance abuse; HIV/HBV coinfection; insulin resistance/diabetes (7)
- Chronic HCV is *curable* in ~70% of cases; in noncirrhotic genotype 2 or 3, cure rate ~90%.

COMPLICATIONS

- Acute/Subacute hepatic necrosis, liver failure, transplant and complications, death
- HCC: Risk factors include cirrhosis, age >55, male, obesity/diabetes/fatty liver, and ongoing alcohol/tobacco/marijuana/drug use.

REFERENCES

1. Ghany M, Strader D. AASLD practice guidelines: Diagnosis, management, and treatment of Hepatitis C: An update. *Hepatology*. 2009;49:1335–1374.
2. Chronic hepatitis C: Current disease management, NIH Pub. no. 07-4230 Nov. 2006. Available at: http://digestive.niddk.nih.gov/ddiseases/pubs/chronichepc/
3. Agudelo E. Optimizing therapy in treatment-naïve genotype 1 patients. *Curr Hepatitis Rep.* 2008;7:64–71.
4. Shiffman ML. Optimizing the current therapy for chronic hepatitis C virus: Peginterferon and ribavirin dosing and the utility of growth factors. *Clin Liver Dis.* 2008;12:487–505.
5. Sarkar S, Schaefer M. Antidepressant pretreatment for the prevention of interferon alfa-associated depression: A systematic review and meta-analysis psychosomatics. *Psychosomatics.* 2013;S0033-3182:00130-8.
6. Leevy CB. Consensus interferon and ribavirin in patients with chronic hepatitis C who were nonresponders to pegylated interferon alfa-2b and ribavirin. *Dig Dis Sci.* 2008;53:1961–1966.
7. Zein N. Steatosis and metabolic syndrome: An emerging enigma in the natural history of chronic hepatitis C. *Curr Hepatitis Rep.* 2008;7:61–63.

ADDITIONAL READING

- Ghany MG, Nelson DR, Strader DB, et al. An update on treatment of genotype 1 chronic hepatitis C virus infection: 2011 practice guideline by the American Association for the Study of Liver Diseases. *Hepatology.* 2011;54:1433–1444.
- Smith BD, Morgan RL, Beckett GA, et al. Recommendations for the identification of chronic hepatitis C virus infection among persons born during 1945–1965. *MMWR Recomm Rep.* 2012; 61(RR-4):1–32.

 ## SEE ALSO

- Hepatitis A; Hepatitis B; Cirrhosis of the Liver
- Algorithm: Hyperbilirubinemia

 ## CODES

ICD10

- B17.10 Acute hepatitis C without hepatic coma
- B18.2 Chronic viral hepatitis C
- B19.20 Unspecified viral hepatitis C without hepatic coma

CLINICAL PEARLS

- 1 of 10 patients with hepatitis C have no identifiable risk factors.
- Of infected persons, 15–25% spontaneously resolve infection without treatment.

H

HEPATOMA

E. James Kruse, DO, FACS • David M. Hardy, MD • Ray King, MD

BASICS

DESCRIPTION
Hepatoma, also known as hepatocellular carcinoma (HCC), is the most common primary malignant tumor of the liver, arising from hepatic parenchymal cells (hepatocytes); 80% are associated with underlying liver disease, most commonly cirrhosis (exception: Rare fibrolamellar type).

EPIDEMIOLOGY
Incidence
- Most common cause of cancer death worldwide
- 6th most common malignancy worldwide, >700,000 new cases/yr worldwide (1)
- 3–4 new cases/100,000/yr of the US population; 120 new cases/100,000/yr in Asia and sub-Saharan Africa
- Among known cirrhotics, 2–5 cases/100 cirrhotics/yr
- Incidence increasing since 1980s in the US (due to increase in hepatitis C infection)
- In the US, estimate is 28,720 new cases of primary liver cancer will be diagnosed in 2012 and 20,550 deaths.
- Male > Female (~3:1 for incidence and 2:1 for deaths)

Prevalence
- Asians > Native American > Hispanics > African Americans > Caucasians
- Predominant age: Median age 65 in the West, 4th–5th decades in Asia and Africa
- Predominant sex: Male > Female (3–4:1)

ETIOLOGY AND PATHOPHYSIOLOGY
- Cirrhosis accounts for 80–90% of HCC. Alcoholic cirrhosis is most common in the Western world. Reported risk in patients with alcoholic cirrhosis is 3–10% with micronodular pattern.
- HBV and HCV are independent and synergistic risk factors for HCC:
  - Associated with >70% of cases worldwide
  - Most important factor in Africa and Asia
- Chronic alcohol use
- Chronic tobacco abuse
- ? Morbid obesity
- Mycotoxins (aflatoxins): Metabolite of the fungus *Aspergillus flavus* that contaminates foods
- Vinyl polymers associated with angiosarcoma and, less commonly, hepatocellular carcinoma

Genetics
No known genetic pattern

RISK FACTORS
- For HCC:
  - 80–90% of HCC associated with cirrhosis (2)[B]:
    ○ Cirrhosis can be from any etiology: Hepatitis B and C, alcoholism, hemochromatosis, nonalcoholic steatohepatitis, α_1–antitrypsin deficiency, biliary cirrhosis, autoimmune hepatitis, Wilson disease, glycogen storage disease
  - Fungal aflatoxins (contaminants of grain in Africa and Asia): Synergistic effect with other causes of liver disease
  - Vinyl chloride
  - Thorium dioxide
  - Anabolic steroids
  - Arsenic
  - Nonalcoholic fatty liver disease/nonalcoholic steatohepatitis (3)[C]

- For fibrolamellar type: No identified risk factors
- For angiosarcoma: Vinyl chloride

GENERAL PREVENTION
- The major risk factor for HCC is cirrhosis. Prevention of cirrhosis and tumor surveillance in patients with or at risk for cirrhosis are key.
- Prevent hepatitis B virus (HBV) and hepatitis C virus (HCV) infection through safe sexual practices; avoidance of shared IV drug paraphernalia; and HBV vaccination.
- Treat chronic HBV and HCV with lamivudine, adefovir, entecavir, tenofovir, or ribavirin/pegylated interferon, according to guidelines.
- Avoid excessive alcohol use.
- High-risk individuals:
  - Chronic hepatitis with HBV or HCV
  - Alcoholic cirrhosis
  - Genetic hemochromatosis
  - Exposure to vinyl chloride >10 years (screen every 6 months)
  - Primary biliary cirrhosis
  - Morbid obesity
- Screen high-risk patients by US and α-fetoprotein every 6–12 months (4)[B].
- HCC progresses from dysplastic nodules to vascular invasion (after tumor is >2 cm in diameter).

DIAGNOSIS

- In children:
  - Feminization, precocious puberty
  - Palpable liver mass, pain, asymmetrical hepatomegaly
- In adults:
  - Known cirrhosis or clinical signs of cirrhosis: 80%
  - Abdominal pain: 80%; right upper quadrant, dull to severe ache
  - Hepatomegaly: 80–90%; irregular, nodular, firm/hard, tender
  - Weight loss: 30%
  - Hepatic arterial bruit: 20%
  - Friction rub: Rare; more common in metastatic liver disease
  - Paraneoplastic syndromes: Hypertrophic osteoarthropathy, carcinoid syndrome, feminization, polycythemia
  - Unexplained deterioration of stable cirrhosis
  - Budd-Chiari syndrome (hepatic vein obstruction)
  - Portal vein thrombosis

DIFFERENTIAL DIAGNOSIS
- Small, asymptomatic tumors or underlying liver conditions:
  - Cirrhosis with regenerative nodules
  - Benign liver nodules
  - Hamartoma
  - Hemangioma
  - Metastatic adenocarcinoma
  - Cholangiocarcinoma
  - Adenomas
- Larger, symptomatic tumor with hepatomegaly:

  - Cirrhosis
  - Hepatic cyst
  - Adenoma
  - Hemangioma
  - Abscess

- Metastatic malignancy of liver
- Thrombosis of hepatic veins, portal vein, or inferior vena cava
- Active viral hepatitis or alcoholic hepatitis
- Ruptured tumor: All causes of acute abdomen
- Traumatic hemoperitoneum

DIAGNOSTIC TESTS & INTERPRETATION
Initial Tests (lab, imaging)
LFTs, alkaline phosphatase, BUN and creatinine, CBC, calcium, α-fetoprotein (AFP).

- US (1,4)[B]:
  - Detects tumors >1 cm; performance dependent on examiner, technology, and degree of cirrhosis (decreases sensitivity)
  - More sensitive than AFP level
  - May be useful to follow patients with cirrhosis to help identify hepatocellular cancer at an early tumor stage
  - If US is positive, CT or MRI is performed to confirm (4)[B].
  - May be used as image guidance during percutaneous liver biopsy or other therapy (injection or ablation)
- Helical 3-phase CT scan:
  - Detects 1 cm tumors
  - Valuable in determining extrahepatic spread (most commonly to lung, periportal lymph nodes, bone, brain)
  - Delineates vascular anatomy to guide treatment
- Positron emission tomography (PET)/PET-CT improves CT detection rates.
- MRI:
  - More sensitive than helical CT scan for early detection of HCC
  - Helps differentiate benign from malignant tumors
  - Helpful in delineating the tumor and invasion of vessels
- Arteriography: Used rarely because of the accuracy of MRI and CT
- 1–2 cm nodules with typical imaging features have specificities and positive predictive values nearing 100% and sensitivities up to 70%; can be used to identify HCC without tissue diagnosis (1,4).

Follow-Up Tests & Special Considerations
- LFT abnormalities (aspartate aminotransferase, alanine aminotransferase, alkaline phosphatase)
- AFP:
  - Most important lab test for diagnosis of HCC but *not* recommended as a sole screening test (60% sensitivity, 80% specificity) (2)[B]
  - Level of >400 ng/mL (>400 μg/L) is diagnostic. Level of >200 ng/mL is highly suggestive of HCC; level does not correlate with prognosis, but is useful in monitoring for recurrence.
  - Fibrolamellar carcinoma usually does not produce AFP.
- Some conditions, such as acute or chronic hepatitis, germ cell tumors, and pregnancy, may cause a slight elevation in AFP.
- Specific treatments will be determined by the degree of liver impairment, commonly utilizing the Child-Pugh classification and/or Model for End-Stage Liver Disease score.
- Rare paraneoplastic syndrome: Polycythemia, elevated calcium, low glucose

Diagnostic Procedures/Other

- Tissue diagnosis is used to confirm mass seen on imaging with atypical findings or in a noncirrhotic liver. Tissue confirmation is also useful to rule out liver metastases (4)[B].
- Liver biopsy: Performed using image guidance (US or CT) when nodules are not palpable. This is *not indicated* when a lesion has typical CT/MRI characteristics and an elevated AFP.
- Laparoscopy: To evaluate extent of cirrhosis and perform resection or ablation in skilled centers
- Preoperative workup: Evaluation of extrahepatic metastases
- *It is unnecessary to biopsy* a liver mass with typical radiographic features and elevated AFP in the setting of cirrhosis. These findings are diagnostic.

Test Interpretation

- Nodular: 75%; usually in cirrhotic liver
- Massive: Common in children and noncirrhotic livers; prone to rupture
- Diffuse: Rare; usually a large portion of liver is involved
- Hepatocellular: Most commonly multicentric and well differentiated; usually superimposed on underlying cirrhosis

 TREATMENT

MEDICATION

- Chemotherapy with sorafenib offers a small survival benefit in patients with disease not amenable to surgical intervention (5).
- Treatment of hepatoma in patients with active HCV with pegylated interferon-α and ribavirin prolongs survival and improves quality of life.

SURGERY/OTHER PROCEDURES

- Surgical resection and liver transplantation offer highest cure rate in HCC (2)[B]:
  - Resection should be considered in children and may include up to 1 lobe of the liver.
  - The resected specimen should contain a negative margin of normal liver tissue.
  - Intraoperative US should be performed to survey for additional lesions.
  - Resection is the preferred treatment in noncirrhotic patients with HCC if liver function is preserved and there is no evidence of portal hypertension (2)[B]:
    ○ Varies from segmental to trisegmental resection (up to 80% of the liver)
  - Transplantation is the preferred treatment for cirrhotic patients or unresectable tumors that meet transplantation criteria (2)[B]. This modality is limited due to lack of donors relative to number of patients currently awaiting transplant.
  - Advanced liver disease, medical comorbidities, and extrahepatic metastases are common; therefore, only 15–30% of HCC patients are eligible for resection (2)[B].
  - The cure rate is high for both surgical options with the presence of ≤3 nodules, each <5 cm.

- Tumor ablation:
  - Tumor ablation in patients not deemed candidates for resection or transplantation is often a safe alternative.
  - Ablation may be chemical with alcohol; cryotherapy with liquid nitrogen probes; or hyperthermic with radiofrequency, microwave, or laser.
  - Ablation may be performed surgically or percutaneously, depending on the location.
  - Radiofrequency ablation (RFA) is considered superior to alcohol injection for localized therapy (6)[B].
  - Recent trials show similar survival rates for RFA vs. surgical resection in small HCCs. Insufficient evidence exists to change recommendations favoring surgery at this time.
  - Irreversible electroporation is a newer ablation technique that is undergoing clinical trials.
- Percutaneous treatments are best for unresectable disease, as a bridge to surgical resection or transplantation, and for early-stage tumors that are not amenable to surgery:
  - Regional transarterial therapy (chemoembolization which delivers chemotherapy directly to the tumor via its immediate blood supply or selective internal radiation therapy) are used for intermediate-stage tumors or when primary surgery is not planned; these modalities may provide palliation or down-stage the tumor, making surgery possible (7)[B]. These 2 approaches can be used together and may yield a better outcome than either treatment alone (7)[B].
- Fibrolamellar variant should be treated by surgical resection; this has shown excellent survival rates.

 ONGOING CARE

FOLLOW-UP RECOMMENDATIONS
Patient Monitoring
Even after successful resection, there is a high risk of recurrence:
- AFP level q3mo
- US q4–6mo or contrast-enhanced CT/MRI scan, depending on local expertise

DIET
Attention to nutrition: High-calorie diet

PATIENT EDUCATION
Emphasize preventive measures and HBV vaccine.

PROGNOSIS
- Depends on amount of tumor replacing normal liver tissue and degree of hepatic impairment
- Unresectable, symptomatic tumors: Grave; patients seldom live >6 months
- Resectable, asymptomatic tumors:
  - Surgery curative in >70% of children, 40% of adults
  - Surgery curative in >80% of cirrhotic adults with tumors <3 cm
- Transplantation: Similar to tumor-free patients with tumors <2 cm; 5-year survival rate of >70% with 1 tumor <5 cm or maximum of 3 lesions <3 cm (United Network of Organ Sharing criteria) (4)[B]

COMPLICATIONS
- Rupture
- Hemoperitoneum
- Liver failure
- Cachexia
- Metastases
- Thrombosis of portal, hepatic, renal veins: Variceal bleeding

REFERENCES

1. Forner A, Llovet JM, Bruix J. Hepatocellular carcinoma. *The Lancet*. 2012;379:1245–1255.
2. Cha CH, Saif MW, Yamane BH, et al. Hepatocellular carcinoma: Current management. *Curr Probl Surg*. 2010;47:10–67.
3. Siegel AB, Zhu AX. Metabolic syndrome and hepatocellular carcinoma: Two growing epidemics with a potential link. *Cancer*. 2009;115:5651–5661.
4. El-Serag HB, Marrero JA, Rudolph L, et al. Diagnosis and treatment of hepatocellular carcinoma. *Gastroenterology*. 2008;134:1752–1763.
5. NCCN Clinical Practice Guidelines Version 2.2011. Hepatocellular Cancers. www.nccn.org.
6. Cho YK, Kim JK, Kim MY, et al. Systematic review of randomized trials for hepatocellular carcinoma treated with percutaneous ablation therapies. *Hepatology*. 2009;49:453–459.
7. Garrean S, Hering J, Helton WS, et al. A primer on transarterial, chemical, and thermal ablative therapies for hepatic tumors. *Am J Surg*. 2007;194(1):79–88.

ADDITIONAL READING
- Cancer Facts and Figures 2012. www.cancer.org
- European Association for the Study of the Liver, European Organisation for Research and Treatment of Cancer. EASL-EORTC clinical practice guidelines: Management of hepatocellular carcinoma. *J Hepatol*. 2012;56:908–943.

 CODES

ICD10
C22.0 Liver cell carcinoma

CLINICAL PEARLS
- With benign liver tumors, most patients will have normal LFTs; 97% with HCC will have >1 abnormal test.
- Hepatitis C is the greatest risk factor, especially if combined with alcohol abuse.
- Aggressive use of Hepatitis B vaccination
- Most common cause of cancer death worldwide; in the West, secondary to ethyl alcohol; in rest of world, secondary to hepatitis B and C

H

HEPATORENAL SYNDROME

Tomoki Tsukahara, MD • Mony Fraer, MD, FACP, FASN

 BASICS

DESCRIPTION

- Hepatorenal syndrome (HRS) is kidney failure in decompensated cirrhosis with ascites due to decreased effective arterial blood volume (EABV) caused by severe splanchnic vasodilatation.
- HRS has a poor prognosis with median survival of weeks (rapidly progressive disease, type 1) to months (slowly progressive disease, type 2) if untreated.
- Liver transplant is the 1st choice of treatment for type 1 HRS.
- Vasoconstrictors and albumin have been tried for both type 1 and type 2 with variable results.

EPIDEMIOLOGY
Incidence
- Few studies available; ~40% in cirrhotic patients with ascites after 5 years of follow-up.
- Differentiation between HRS and acute kidney injury of other causes is not universal.
- Higher incidence with progression of end-stage liver disease (ESLD).

ETIOLOGY AND PATHOPHYSIOLOGY
- Portal hypertension leads to splanchnic vasodilatation by increasing nitric oxide production, which reduces EABV.
- Inflammatory response involving mesenteric lymph nodes triggered by bacterial translocation is suspected as an important factor for vasodilatation.
- Reduced EABV, if mild, could be compensated by increase in cardiac output, activation of renin-angiotensin-aldosterone system, or secretion of vasopressin.
- However, compensatory mechanism cannot compensate marked reduction in EABV and can worsen the perfusion of kidneys by vasoconstriction.

Genetics
- Genetic liver diseases (e.g., Wilson disease, hereditary hemochromatosis, α1-antitrypsin deficiency) could lead to HRS.
- No genetic link to HRS by itself has been found.

RISK FACTORS
- Infections:
  – Spontaneous bacterial peritonitis (SBP); ~30% of patients with SBP develop HRS
  – Bacterial infection
- Reduction of EABV in cirrhosis:
  – Low mean arterial pressure
  – Excessive diuretics
  – Large-volume paracentesis
  – Diarrhea (e.g., lactulose induced)
  – Vomiting
  – GI bleeding
  – Low serum albumin level
  – Increased intra-abdominal pressure from ascites

GENERAL PREVENTION
- Early diagnosis and aggressive treatment of infections in cirrhotic patients is essential.
- Long-term PO norfloxacin (400 mg/d) reduces HRS in cirrhotic patients with ascites and elevated creatinine (1).
- Albumin replacement with large-volume paracentesis (8 g per liter of ascites removed) is controversial; AASLD guidelines suggest that it could be considered and EASL guideline recommends it should be performed (2,3).
- Pentoxifylline 400 mg PO t.i.d. reduced the incidence of HRS from 32% in the placebo group to 7% in the pentoxifylline group (4)[B].

COMMONLY ASSOCIATED CONDITIONS
SBP, ESLD with ascites, alcoholic liver disease, hepatitis B and C, GI bleed, and other infections

 DIAGNOSIS

- Cirrhosis with ascites
- Serum creatinine >1.5 mg/dL (>133 mmol/L)
- No improvement in serum creatinine level (decrease to <1.5 mg/dL [<133 mmol/L]) after >2 days with diuretic withdrawal and volume expansion with albumin (a single infusion of 1 g/kg of body weight, maximum of 100 g)
- Absence of shock
- No current or recent treatment with nephrotoxic drugs
- Absence of parenchymal kidney disease as indicated by proteinuria >500 mg/d, microhematuria (>50 RBC/hpf), and/or abnormal renal US

HISTORY
- Symptoms of decompensated cirrhosis
- Symptoms of renal failure

PHYSICAL EXAM
- Signs of renal failure:
  – Oliguria
  – Edema
  – Altered mental status
- Signs of reduced EABV:
  – Hypotension
  – Tachycardia
- Signs of decompensated cirrhosis:
  – Ascites
  – Splenomegaly
  – Jaundice
- Signs of infection:
  – Fever
  – Altered mental status
  – Abdominal tenderness

DIFFERENTIAL DIAGNOSIS
Other causes of AKI:
- Drug-induced nephrotoxicity (NSAIDs, gentamicin, etc.)
- Prerenal failure due to intravascular volume depletion
- Glomerulonephritis
- Postrenal (obstruction)

DIAGNOSTIC TESTS & INTERPRETATION
Other causes of AKI need to be ruled out.

Initial Tests (lab, imaging)
- Serum creatinine, BUN, electrolytes (Na, K, Cl, HCO_3)
- Urinalysis with microscopy
- Urine Na, creatinine, protein
- Other: LFTs, Prothrombin time
- Renal US to rule out chronic kidney disease, hydronephrosis, or obstruction
- Abdominal US to confirm ascites

Test Interpretation
- Elevated BUN and creatinine
- Hyponatremia
- Bland urine sediment
- No proteinuria
- Low urine Na (<20 mEq/L)
- Normal renal US

 TREATMENT

GENERAL MEASURES
- Discontinue diuretics.
- Avoid NSAIDs, aminoglycosides, or other nephrotoxins.
- Relieve urinary obstruction when present.

MEDICATION
First Line
- Albumin starts with priming dose of 1 g/kg body weight followed by 20–40 g/d.
- Vasoconstrictors:
  – Terlipressin (1 mg q4–6h IV; titrated up to 2 mg q4–6h after 3 days):
    ○ Cardiovascular or ischemic complications in ~12% of patients (5)[B]
    ○ Unavailable in the US; currently in a clinical trial
  – Midodrine (7.5–12.5 mg PO t.i.d.) and Octreotide (100–200 mg SC t.i.d.) (6)[B]
  – Norepinephrine (0.5–3 mg/h continuous IV; titrated to increase mean arterial pressure by >10 mm Hg) (7)[B]

ADDITIONAL THERAPIES

Dialysis is indicated only as a supportive measure for patients awaiting liver transplant or in patients with acute, potentially reversible liver failure.

- Not enough data available to determine the best dialysis modality.
- Liver dialysis (e.g., molecular absorbent recirculating systems) has been investigated.

SURGERY/OTHER PROCEDURES

- Liver transplant with a survival rate of 65% in type 1 HRS:
  - High mortality rate while on the waiting list
  - Simultaneous liver and kidney transplant is considered for patients with advanced CKD or on dialysis for >6–8 weeks.
- Transjugular intrahepatic portosystemic shunt (TIPS) has been proposed but very limited data are available.

IN-PATIENT CONSIDERATIONS

Early nephrology and hepatology consultation should be considered.

Admission Criteria/Initial Stabilization

- Type 1 HRS requires hospitalization.
- Type 2 HRS may be managed in outpatient setting.

Discharge Criteria

- Stable renal function
- Following liver transplant

 ONGOING CARE

FOLLOW-UP RECOMMENDATIONS

Patient Monitoring

- Monitor renal and hepatic function and serum electrolytes.
- Follow-up with a hepatologist and nephrologist.

DIET

Low-sodium diet

PATIENT EDUCATION

- Avoid NSAIDs and IV contrast exposure.
- Notify clinician about weight gain, lightheadedness, vomiting, diarrhea, GI bleed, or confusion.
- Alcohol abstinence in order to qualify for listing for liver transplantation.

PROGNOSIS

- Grave: Median survival if untreated is 2 weeks for type 1 HRS and 6 months for type 2 HRS.
- The time and degree of renal recovery after liver transplantation is variable, but a substantial number of patients do show significant renal improvement.

COMPLICATIONS

- Death
- Dialysis dependency/end-stage renal disease
- Fluid overload with congestive heart failure or pulmonary edema
- Hepatic coma
- Secondary infections

REFERENCES

1. Fagundes C, Ginès P. Hepatorenal syndrome: A severe, but treatable, cause of kidney failure in cirrhosis. *Am J Kid Dis*. 2012;59:874–885.
2. Salerno F, Gerbes A, Ginès P, Wong F, Arroyo V. Diagnosis, prevention and treatment of hepatorenal syndrome in cirrhosis. *Gut*. 2007;56:1310–1318.
3. Fernández J, Navasa M, Planas R, et al. Primary prophylaxis of spontaneous bacterial peritonitis delays hepatorenal syndrome and improves survival in cirrhosis. *Gastroenterology*. 2007;133:818–824.
4. Tyagi P, Sharma P, Sharma BC, et al. Prevention of hepatorenal syndrome in patients with cirrhosis and ascites: A pilot randomized control trial between pentoxifylline and placebo. *Eur J Gastroenterol Hepatol*. 2011;23:210–217.
5. Gluud LL, Kjaer MS, Christensen E, et al. Terlipressin for hepatorenal syndrome. *Cochrane Database Syst Rev*. 2012;9:CD005162.
6. Skagen C, Einstein M, Lucey MR, et al. Combination treatment with octreotide, midodrine, and albumin improves survival in patients with type 1 and type 2 hepatorenal syndrome. *J Clin Gastroenterol*. 2009;43:680–685.
7. Singh V, Ghosh S, Singh B, et al. Noradrenaline vs. terlipressin in the treatment of hepatorenal syndrome: A randomized study. *J Hepatol*. 2012;56: 1293–1298.

ADDITIONAL READING

- European Association for the Study of the Liver. EASL clinical practice guidelines on the management of ascites, spontaneous bacterial peritonitis, and hepatorenal syndrome in cirrhosis. *J Hepatology*. 2010;53:397–417.
- Runyon BA, AASLD Practice Guidelines Committee. Management of adult patients with ascites due to cirrhosis: an update. *Hepatology*. 2009;49: 2087–2107.

 SEE ALSO

Acetaminophen Poisoning; Cirrhosis of the Liver; Hepatitis A; Hepatitis B; Hepatitis C; Renal Failure, Acute

 CODES

ICD10
K76.7 Hepatorenal syndrome

CLINICAL PEARLS

- HRS is a diagnosis of exclusion, and other causes of acute renal failure must be ruled out.
- Liver transplantation is the treatment of choice.

H

HERNIA
Margaret Fairhurst, DO • Eric J. Csernyik, DO

 BASICS

DESCRIPTION
Hernias are areas of weakness or frank disruption of the fibromuscular tissues of the body wall through which intracavity structures pass:

- Types:
  - Inguinal:
    - Direct inguinal: Acquired; herniation through defect in transversalis fascia of abdominal wall medial to inferior epigastric vessels; increased frequency with age as fascia weakens
    - Indirect inguinal: Congenital; herniation lateral to the inferior epigastric vessels, through internal inguinal ring into inguinal canal. A "complete hernia" is one that descends into the scrotum, whereas an "incomplete hernia" remains within the inguinal canal.
  - Pantaloon: Combination of direct and indirect inguinal hernia with protrusion of abdominal wall on both sides of the epigastric vessels
  - Femoral: Herniation that descends through the femoral canal deep to the inguinal ligament. Because of the narrow neck of a femoral hernia, this type of hernia is especially prone to incarceration and strangulation.
  - Incisional or ventral: Herniation through a defect in the anterior abdominal wall at the site of a prior surgical incision
  - Congenital: Herniation through fascial defect in abdominal wall, secondary to collagen deficiency disease
  - Umbilical: Defect occurs at umbilical ring tissue. Epigastric: Protrusion through the linea alba above the level of the umbilicus. These may develop at exit points of small paramidline nerves and vessels, or through an area of congenital weakness in the linea alba. Interparietal (e.g., Spigelian hernia): Hernia sac insinuates itself between layers of the abdominal wall; strangulation common, often mistaken for tumor or abscess Other: Obturator, sciatic, perineal
- Definitions:
  - Reducible: Extruded sac and its contents can be returned to original intra-abdominal position, either spontaneously or with gentle manual manipulation.
  - Irreducible/incarcerated: Extruded sac and its contents cannot be returned to original intra-abdominal position.
  - Strangulated: Blood supply to hernia sac contents is compromised.
  - Richter: Partial circumference of the bowel is incarcerated or strangulated. Partial wall damage may occur, increasing potential for bowel rupture and peritonitis.
  - Sliding: Wall of a viscus forms part of the wall of the inguinal hernia sac (i.e., R-cecum, L-sigmoid colon).

Geriatric Considerations
Abdominal wall hernias increase with advancing age, with significant increase in risk during surgical repair.

Pregnancy Considerations
- Increased intra-abdominal pressure and hormone imbalances with pregnancy may contribute to increased risk of abdominal wall hernias.
- Umbilical hernias are associated with multiple, prolonged deliveries.

EPIDEMIOLOGY
Incidence
- 75–80% groin hernias: Inguinal and femoral
- 2–20% incisional/ventral, depending on whether a prior surgery was associated with infection or contamination
- 3–10% umbilical, considered congenital
- 1–3% other
- Groin:
  - 6–27% lifetime risk in adult men
  - 2-peak theory: Most inguinal hernias present before 1 year of age or after 55 years
  - ~50% of children under 2 will have a patent processus vaginalis, decreasing to 40% after age 2. Only between 25% and 50% will become clinically significant.
  - Inguinal hernia found in <5% of newborns, but M:F ratio is 10:1
  - Increased incidence in premature infants (1)[B]
  - Increased incidence in patients with abdominal aortic aneurysms
  - Femoral <10% of all groin hernias, 40% present as a surgical emergency
- Incisional/ventral: ~10–23% of abdominal surgeries complicated by an incisional hernia, most common in upper midline incisions.
- Incidence ratio: Male = Female
- Umbilical: 10–20% of newborns (2); most close by 5 years.

Prevalence
- Groin and inguinal hernias are more prevalent in men.
- Femoral and umbilical hernias more prevalent in women.
- Most inguinal hernias are indirect in both genders.
- Incisional/ventral hernias are more prevalent in obese persons, as well as in smokers. The opposite may be true for inguinal hernias (3)[C].

ETIOLOGY AND PATHOPHYSIOLOGY
Loss of tissue strength and elasticity, especially with aging or congenital defect in abdominal fascia resulting in a defect in the fascia of the abdominal wall. Most pediatric hernias are congenital defects (e.g., patent processus vaginalis), whereas most adult hernias are a result of acquired weakness in the tissues of the anterior abdominal wall.

Genetics
No known genetic pattern

RISK FACTORS
- Increased abdominal pressure, coughing, heavy lifting, constipation, pregnancy, ascites, prostatism, obesity, advancing age (loss of tissue turgor), smoking, steroid use, low birth weight, prematurity
- Age: Femoral and scrotal hernias, along with recurrent groin hernias, are associated with increased risk for acute hernia surgery (4).

COMMONLY ASSOCIATED CONDITIONS
Obesity, chronic obstructive pulmonary disease, multiple abdominal surgeries, pregnancy, advanced age, Ehlers-Danlos syndrome, Marfan syndrome, PKD, osteogenesis imperfecta, Down syndrome, abdominal aortic aneurysm

 DIAGNOSIS

HISTORY
- Pain, nausea, vomiting, bloating; relieved with reclining; many are asymptomatic.
- May observe protrusion through abdominal wall during increased intra-abdominal pressure (Valsalva maneuver or cough)

PHYSICAL EXAM
- Exam should initially occur with patient standing. During palpation, the patient should be instructed to cough, strain, or perform Valsalva maneuver so the extent of intracavitary content movement can be appreciated. Exam should also be performed with patient in supine position.
- Inguinal (superior to inguinal ligament):
  - Direct inguinal hernia: Finger in inguinal canal finds defect of the transversalis fascia as a deep (posterior to anterior) bulge palpated by pad of finger with increased intra-abdominal pressure.
  - Indirect inguinal hernia: Finger in inguinal canal finds a persistent process vaginalis as a bulge (lateral to medial) palpated by fingertip; it may extend down into scrotum.
- Femoral (inferior to inguinal ligament): Bulge in upper middle thigh; neck of the sac will protrude lateral to and below a finger placed on the pubic tubercle.
- Umbilical: Palpable protrusion at umbilicus
- Incisional/Ventral: Palpable protrusion at site of prior abdominal incision or midline superior to the umbilicus
- Epigastric: Palpable protrusion that occurs off midline above umbilicus

DIFFERENTIAL DIAGNOSIS
Lymphadenopathy, hydrocele, lipoma, varices, cryptorchidism, abscess, tumor, sports hernia (athletic pubalgia), pelvic fractures, adductor tears, omphalomesenteric duct, urachal cyst

DIAGNOSTIC TESTS & INTERPRETATION
Hernia evaluation rarely requires imaging; reserve for suspected abdominal hernia or unclear diagnosis. Plain radiographs to rule out obstruction:

- US can be used to assess inguinal hernias.
- CT or tangential radiography for incisional and abdominal wall hernias and postsurgical patients with complaints of abdominal pain
- Herniography is no longer recommended (5)[A].

Pediatric Considerations
There is insufficient evidence for contralateral exploration in pediatric patients, except using US.

Follow-Up Tests & Special Considerations
For occult hernias not well appreciated on exam or with imaging, diagnostic laparoscopy may be beneficial.

TREATMENT

- Elective setting:
  - Elective surgical repair is associated with significantly lower morbidity and mortality.
- Acute setting:
  - Pain management is recommended for symptomatic hernias.
  - Strangulated hernias should be surgically repaired as early as possible to prevent complications such as necrosis and viscus perforation.
  - Manual reduction of incarcerated hernia improves outcomes by allowing for elective repair after reduction of acute swelling and inflammation.
  - Complication rate is nearly 20× greater in emergent repair of pediatric inguinal hernias than elective procedures (6)[A].
  - Acute hernia repair carries a higher morbidity and lower survival rate (4).

MEDICATION

- Antibiotics: Antibiotic prophylaxis did not reduce wound infections after groin hernia repairs.
- Pain: Local anesthetic during surgical repair results in significant reduction of postoperative pain (6)[A]. Tension-free procedures, such as Lichtenstein, may be performed under local anesthesia.

ADDITIONAL THERAPIES
Geriatric Considerations
Use of a truss (external supportive device) for direct inguinal hernias is common; no data exist regarding efficacy.

ISSUES FOR REFERRAL
Warn patients of symptoms or signs of incarceration or strangulation (acute abdominal pain, fever, bloody bowel movements), which mandate immediate self-referral to emergency room.

SURGERY/OTHER PROCEDURES
All inguinal hernias should be surgically repaired, but watchful waiting in the asymptomatic patient is a safe option if significant comorbidities may compromise emergent repair (6)[A]:

- Incarceration and strangulation are absolute indications for hernia repair.
- Contraindications: Patients who are not surgical candidates based on cardiovascular risk factors:
  - Elective repair should be avoided in pregnant patients or those with active infections.
- Special considerations:
  - Umbilical hernias <0.5 cm usually obliterate and can be managed by observation (2).
  - Umbilical hernias in children age 2–4 years may be observed, as there is a high rate of spontaneous closure.
  - Laparoscopic repair of incisional/ventral hernias is associated with fewer complications and shorter hospital stays when compared with open repair. However, postoperative pain and recurrence rates are similar (7).
  - "Watchful waiting" is recommended in pregnancy. Elective postpartum hernia repair provided similar results to the nonpregnant population without increased risk of incarceration or strangulation before or during delivery (8).
  - Women had lower recurrence rates with laparoscopic methods than with Lichtenstein open method.

- Ascites is not a strict contraindication for surgical repair. There is a greater risk of strangulation and complication without repair than the increased risks associated with repair in the presence of ascites.
- The more emergent hernia operations can be performed using the same methods for nonacute situations. However, incarceration with strangulation may require laparotomy with partial bowel resection.
- Gold standard:
  - Inguinal hernia:
    - Open: Lichtenstein with mesh (37%) or mesh plug (34%): Decreased recurrence rates (6)[A]
    - Laparoscopic (14%) with mesh: Decreased hospital stay and postoperative pain (6)[A]:
      - Requires general anesthesia
      - Transabdominal preperitoneal (TAPP) vs. total extraperitoneal (TEP)
    - Pediatric: Recovery and outcome similar after open and laparoscopic repair. Laparoscopic hernia repair associated with increased operation/anesthesia time and postoperative pain
  - Incisional/Ventral:
    - Laparoscopic repair is effective for most patients with primary or recurrent ventral hernias; it is associated with a <10% recurrence rate.
  - Umbilical:
    - Pediatric: Open excision and closure with suture
    - Adult: Open repair with mesh or plug may reduce hernia recurrence.
- Newer techniques:
  - Prolene hernia system
  - Biologic wound closure system: Reduced recurrence in contaminated procedures
- Complications:
  - Recurrence
  - Seromas
  - Postoperative pain, temporary or chronic: Improved in laparoscopic approach vs. open
  - Wound infection
  - Injury to cord structures in inguinal herniorrhaphy; with nerve injury, most symptoms will resolve.

ONGOING CARE

PATIENT EDUCATION
- Cleveland Clinic: http://my.clevelandclinic.org/disorders/hernia/hic_hernia.aspx
- Umbilical hernias: Boston Children's Hospital: www.childrenshospital.org/az/Site1018/mainpageS1018P0.html

PROGNOSIS
- Groin (pediatric): Low recurrence rates (<3%) with surgical treatment; may spontaneously resolve in infants
- Groin (adult): ≥1%/year risk of bowel strangulation without surgical treatment; 0–10% postoperative recurrence rates, depending on surgeon's experience level and method
- Incisional/Ventral: 3–5% postoperative occurrence: 2–17% postrepair recurrence, increased to 20–46% in larger hernias
- Umbilical (pediatric):
  - High rate of spontaneous resolution
  - Hernia less likely to close further in older children and in children with larger defects

- Umbilical (adult): Up to 11% postoperative recurrence rate
- Epigastric: Most will ultimately become incarcerated and/or strangulated without surgical treatment. Recurrence is high due to frequency of missed defects during repair.

REFERENCES

1. Brandt ML. Pediatric hernias. *Surg Clin North Am.* 2008;88:27–43, vii–viii.
2. Snyder CL. Current management of umbilical abnormalities and related anomalies. *Semin Pediatr Surg.* 2007;16:41–49.
3. Rosemar A, Anger's U, Rosengren A. Body mass index and groin hernia: A 34-year follow-up study in Swedish men. *Ann Surg.* 2008;247:1064–1068.
4. Abi-Haidar Y, Sanchez V, Itani KM. Risk factors and outcomes of acute versus elective groin hernia surgery. *J Am Coll Surg.* 2011;213(3):363–369. Epub 2011 Jun 15.
5. Ng TT, Hamlin JA, Kahn AM, et al. Herniography: Analysis of its role and limitations. *Hernia.* 2009;13:7–11.
6. Matthews RD, Neumayer L. Inguinal hernia in the 21st century: An evidence-based review. *Curr Probl Surg.* 2008;45:261–312.
7. Sajid MS, Bokhari SA, Mallick AS, et al. Laparoscopic versus open repair of incisional/ventral hernia: A meta-analysis. *Am J Surg.* 2009;197(1):64–72. Epub 2008 Jul 9.
8. Buch KE, Tabrizian P, Divino CM. Management of hernias in pregnancy. *J Am Coll Surg.* 2008;207(4):539–542. Epub 2008 Jun 24.

SEE ALSO

Algorithms: Abdominal Pain, Lower; Intestinal Obstruction; Pelvic Pain

CODES

ICD10
- K40.90 Unil inguinal hernia, w/o obst or gangr, not spcf as recur
- K41.90 Unil femoral hernia, w/o obst or gangrene, not spcf as recur
- K46.9 Unspecified abdominal hernia without obstruction or gangrene

CLINICAL PEARLS

- Inguinal:
  - Direct inguinal: Acquired; herniation through defect in transversalis fascia of abdominal wall medial to inferior epigastric vessels
  - Indirect inguinal: Congenital; herniation lateral to the inferior epigastric vessels; a "complete hernia" descends into the scrotum; an "incomplete hernia" remains within the inguinal canal.
- Pantaloon: Combination of direct and indirect inguinal hernia
- Femoral: Descends through the femoral canal deep to the inguinal ligament
- Incisional or ventral: Iatrogenic, herniation through a defect at site of a prior surgical incision
- Umbilical: Defect occurs at umbilical ring tissue.

H

HERPES EYE INFECTIONS

Rachel A. Marinch, MD • Juliet McKee, MD

 BASICS

DESCRIPTION
- Eye infection (blepharitis, conjunctivitis, keratitis, stromal keratitis, uveitis, retinitis, glaucoma, or optic neuritis) caused by herpes simplex virus (HSV) types 1 or 2; or varicella-zoster virus (VZV, aka HHV3)
- Categories:
  - HSV: Can affect many parts of the eye, but most often affects the cornea (herpes keratoconjunctivitis); HSV1 > HSV2.
  - VZV: When VZV is reactivated and affects the ophthalmic division of the 5th cranial nerve, this is known as herpes zoster ophthalmicus (HZO), a type of shingles
- System(s) affected: Eye; Skin; Central Nervous System (CNS) (neonatal)

EPIDEMIOLOGY
- Predominant age: HSV-mean age of onset 37.4, but can occur at any age, including primary infection in newborns; VZV, usually advancing age (>50)
- Predominant sex: HSV: Male = Female; HZO: Female > Male

Incidence
- HSV: 11.8 new cases of eye infection due to HSV1 or 2 reported per 100,000 in the US annually (1)
- VZV: 1 million new cases of shingles per year; 25–40% develop ophthalmic complications. Temporary keratitis is most common.

Prevalence
- 90% of adults exhibit HSV1 exposure, and 25% exhibit HSV2 exposure. Lifetime prevalence of HSV ocular infection is 150/100,000.
- VZV: Prevalence of herpes zoster infection is 20–30%, with a 1% prevalence of resultant HZO.

ETIOLOGY AND PATHOPHYSIOLOGY
- HSV and VZV are *Herpesviridae* DNA viruses
- HSV: Primary infection from direct contact with infected person via saliva, genital contact, or birth canal exposure (neonates):
  - Primary infection may lead to severe disease in neonates, including eye, skin, CNS, and disseminated disease.
  - Recurrent infection is more common overall cause of herpetic eye infections.
- VZV: Primary infection from direct contact with infected person may cause varicella ("chickenpox") and/or lead to a latent state within trigeminal ganglia:
  - Reactivation of the virus may affect any dermatome (resulting in herpes zoster or "shingles"), including the ophthalmic branch (HZO).

RISK FACTORS
- HSV: History or close contact with HSV-infected person:
  - General risk factors for reactivation: Stress, trauma, fever, UV light exposure, other viral infections
  - Risk factors for HSV keratitis: UV laser eye treatment, some topical ocular medications such as prostaglandin analogues, and primary/secondary immunosuppression
- HZO: History of varicella infection:
  - Advancing age (>50), sex (female > male), trauma, stress, immunosuppression

GENERAL PREVENTION
- Contact precautions with active lesions
- VZV can be spread to those who have not had chickenpox and are not immunized.
- Antiviral prophylaxis necessary if started on topical steroids
- Varicella vaccination (Zostavax) (VZV only): Single 0.65 mL SC dose; no booster. There is no need to inquire about history of varicella or to perform testing for antibody. Can be given to those with prior zoster episode. Not used in treatment of acute zoster or postherpetic neuralgia (PHN).
- Acyclovir can be used prophylactically to prevent recurrence.

Pregnancy Considerations
- Pregnant women without history of chickenpox should avoid contact with persons with active zoster.
- Pregnancy increases risk of recurrence.
- Live vaccine (Zostavax) is contraindicated during pregnancy.

COMMONLY ASSOCIATED CONDITIONS
Primary and secondary immunocompromised states

 DIAGNOSIS

HISTORY
- Varies according to the virus and the ocular structures involved
- History of varicella or herpes simplex infection
- Acute onset, eye pain, headache, photophobia, tearing, ocular redness, decreased or blurry vision
- May present with a prodromal period of fever, malaise, headache, and eye pain before skin eruptions and eye lesions (HZO)

PHYSICAL EXAM
- Varies according to the virus and ocular structures involved:
  - HSV most commonly affects the corneal epithelium.
  - VZV most commonly affects corneal stroma and uvea.
- Typically unilateral in presentation:
  - HZO presents as early as 1–2 days after unilateral vesicular eruption in a dermatomal pattern.
- Decreased visual acuity
- Conjunctival injection near the limbus
- Decreased corneal sensation
- Slit-lamp exam:
  - Fluorescein and rose bengal stain: Dendritic corneal lesions most often seen in HSV, followed by stromal keratitis, corneal edema, or infiltrate (1)[C]
  - Stromal keratitis often seen in HZO, although dendritic lesions may form

DIFFERENTIAL DIAGNOSIS
- Any other cause of red, painful eye:
  - Bacterial, fungal, allergic, or other viral conjunctivitis
  - Acute angle closure glaucoma
- Corneal abrasion, recurrent corneal erosion, toxic conjunctivitis
- Temporal arteritis
- Trigeminal neuralgia

DIAGNOSTIC TESTS & INTERPRETATION
Initial Tests (lab, imaging)
- Typically none needed, as diagnosis is primarily based on history and physical exam
- Other:
  - Corneal swab for HSV DNA by polymerase chain reaction (PCR) (PPV = 96%)
  - If vesicle present, can perform a Tzanck smear for VZV or HSV (multinucleated giant cells)
  - Antibody titers to assess exposure only; DFA (direct fluorescent antibody); tissue culture

 TREATMENT

GENERAL MEASURES
- Avoid contact with nonimmune people.
- No contact lenses should be worn during treatment period.
- Cool compresses
- Artificial tears
- Oral pain medications

MEDICATION
First Line
- HSV corneal epithelial disease:
  - Trifluorothymidine 1% (Trifluridine, Viroptic): Apply 1 drop q2h while awake to a max of 9 drops daily until re-epithelialization occurs, then 1 drop q4h for another 7 days (2)[A]
  - Ganciclovir 0.15% gel (Zirgan): Apply 1 drop in eye q3h while awake, ~5× daily, until re-epithelialization occurs, then 1 drop q8h for 7 days (2)[A].
  - Vidarabine 3% ointment (Vira-A): Apply 0.5 inch into lower conjunctival sac 5× daily q3h, until re-epithelialization occurs (2)[A].
  - Acyclovir: Ophthalmic ointment is available internationally but not approved in the US.
  - Acyclovir: 400 mg PO 5× per day is equivalent to topical acyclovir (3)[B].
  - Epithelial débridement by an ophthalmologist: Removes virus quickly and may accelerate healing
  - Avoid topical steroids.

- HSV stromal keratitis or uveitis (without epithelial disease): Combination of antiviral and steroid treatment; requires ophthalmology evaluation:
  - Prednisolone acetate: 1% drops q.i.d. with slow taper
  - Consider systemic steroids in severe uveitis.
  - Trifluorothymidine: 1% drops q.i.d. for prophylaxis while on topical steroids
- HZO:
  - Acyclovir: 800 mg PO 5× a day for 7–10 days *or* valacyclovir (Valtrex) 1 g PO t.i.d. for 7–10 days *or* famciclovir (Famvir) 500 mg PO t.i.d. for 7–10 days (4,5)[A]. Note: Many studies indicate reduced incidence of long-term complications and PHN with the use of PO antivirals, but a consensus of data is lacking.
  - Topical antibiotic ophthalmic ointment to protect ocular surfaces (e.g., Bacitracin Polymyxin [0]): 0.5-inch ribbon b.i.d.–t.i.d. for 7–10 days (5)[C]
  - If immunocompromised: Acyclovir 10–15 mg/kg IV q8h for 10 days (4,5)[A]
  - Prednisolone acetate: 1% drops q.i.d. with slow taper with an ophthalmologist (5)[B]
- Cycloplegic agent if anterior uveitis present; intraocular pressure-lowering agent if necessary

ALERT
- HZO: Antiviral therapy is most effective within the first 72 hours of rash onset but should still be initiated >72 hours after onset because of the possible complications of HZO.
- Topical steroids:
  - Should only be prescribed by an ophthalmologist
  - Contraindicated with active corneal epithelial disease, which is best monitored with a slit lamp
  - Can increase intraocular pressure, cause corneal thinning, and, with long-term use, cause cataracts
- Topical antiviral agents:
  - Toxic to corneal epithelium, especially after 10–14 days of continuous use
- Acyclovir: Reduce dosage in renal insufficiency
- Prednisone: Contraindicated in immunocompromised patients

Second Line
- HSV: Acyclovir 2 g/d PO in divided doses over 10 days in patients intolerant of topical antivirals
- Topical idoxuridine, acyclovir, brivudine, although approved internationally, are not approved for use in the US.
- Concomitant treatment with interferon may also improve outcomes but is not currently available.

ISSUES FOR REFERRAL
Emergent or urgent ophthalmology referral, depending on severity of disease

ADDITIONAL THERAPIES
- Recurrent HSV requires suppressive therapy:
  - Acyclovir 800 mg/d PO or valacyclovir 500 mg/d PO
- HZO leading to PHN is very common and can be treated with gabapentin or pregabalin, TCAs, opioids, and lidocaine gel.

SURGERY/OTHER PROCEDURES
Corneal transplantation for severe scarring or perforation

IN-PATIENT CONSIDERATIONS
Admission Criteria/Initial Stabilization
- Severe systemic VZV disease
- Systemic HSV in neonates

Discharge Criteria
Resolution of systemic disease

 # ONGOING CARE

FOLLOW-UP RECOMMENDATIONS
Patient Monitoring
- Monitor with slit-lamp exam q1–2d until improvement, then q3–4d until epithelial defect resolves.
- Weekly after epithelial disease resolves until off topical antivirals

PATIENT EDUCATION
Educate patients about importance of early recognition of recurrent symptoms and need for prompt evaluation and treatment.

PROGNOSIS
- Many cases are self-limited but, depending on the ocular structure involved, can lead to permanent blindness, especially in the setting of recurrent disease.
- Recurrent ocular HSV:
  - HSV epithelial disease without treatment:
    - Without sequelae, 40% resolve.
    - With treatment, 90–95% resolve without complication.

Pediatric Considerations
- Neonatal primary HSV often disseminated, with high mortality rate; 37% develop vision worse than 20/200
- Pediatric cases more likely to be bilateral (26%); recurrent (48% in 15 months); and may cause amblyopia

COMPLICATIONS
- Recurrence
- Corneal neovascularization and scarring resulting in poor vision
- Neurotrophic ulcer with perforation
- Secondary bacterial or fungal infection
- Secondary glaucoma in 10%
- PHN in 20–40% with VZV, typically longer lasting in older patients
- Vision loss from optic neuritis or chorioretinitis

REFERENCES
1. Rowe AM, St Leger AJ, Jeon S, et al. Herpes keratitis. *Prog Retin Eye Res*. 2013;32:88–101. Epub 2012 Aug 27.
2. Wilhelmus KR. Antiviral treatment and other therapeutic interventions for herpes simplex virus epithelial keratitis. *Cochrane Database Syst Rev*. 2010;(12):CD002898.
3. Wilhelmus KR. Therapeutic interventions for herpes simplex virus epithelial keratitis. *Cochrane Database Syst Rev*. 2008;(1).
4. Carter WP, Germann CA, Baumann MR, et al. Ophthalmic diagnoses in the ED: Herpes zoster ophthalmicus. *Am J Emerg Med*. 2008;26: 612–617.
5. Dworkin RH, Johnson RW, Breuer J, et al. Recommendations for the management of herpes zoster. *Clin Infect Dis*. 2007;44(Suppl 1):S1–S26.

ADDITIONAL READING
- Ghaznawi N, Virdi A, Dayan A, et al. Herpes zoster opthalmicus: Comparison of disease in patient 60 years and older versus younger than 60 years. *Ophthalmology*. 2011;118(8):1524–1530.
- Knickelbein JE, Hendricks RL, Charukamnoetkanok P, et al. Management of herpes simplex virus stromal keratitis: An evidence-based review. *Surv Ophthalmol*. 2009;54:226–234.
- Liesegang TJ. Herpes zoster ophthalmicus natural history, risk factors, clinical presentation, and morbidity. *Ophthalmology*. 2008;115(2 Suppl): S3–S12.

 ## SEE ALSO

Algorithm: Eye Pain

 ## CODES

ICD10
- B00.50 Herpesviral ocular disease, unspecified
- B00.52 Herpesviral keratitis
- B02.30 Zoster ocular disease, unspecified

CLINICAL PEARLS
- HSV and VZV can lead to a wide array of ocular manifestations, ranging from self-limited disease to potentially vision-threatening disease and complications.
- A slit-lamp exam with fluorescein stain should be performed on all patients with possible HSV keratitis or HZO.
- Topical antiviral treatment is appropriate for HSV, but systemic PO antiviral treatment is necessary for HZO.
- An ophthalmologist should be consulted before prescribing topical steroids. All HZO patients should be referred to an ophthalmologist.
- Hutchinson sign (vesicular lesion on nose from VZV) is a strong indicator of HZO.
- Zostavax is effective at preventing zoster and decreasing the duration of PHN.

H

HERPES SIMPLEX
Sonia Rivera-Martinez, DO, FACOFP

 BASICS

DESCRIPTION
- Usually seen as an exanthem consisting of painful vesicles that occur often in clusters on skin, cornea, or mucous membranes
- Local skin lesions primarily located in oral and genital regions:
  – Herpes simplex virus (HSV)-1 primarily associated with blisters on lips, in mouth, face, eyes
  – HSV-2 is primary source of genital herpes, although cross-reactivity is common (with HSV-1 being a cause of genital sores as well due to oral–genital contact).
- Viral disease with a wide range of sequelae. Complexity and variation of presentation depends on whether disease is disseminated, the age and immune status of host, and whether the rash outbreak is primary or recurrence.
- HSV can lead to meningitis/encephalitis and pneumonia among its systemic manifestations.
- Amount of viral shedding varies, but is greatest in the 1st/primary infection and lessens with subsequent infections.

EPIDEMIOLOGY
- Predominant age: Affects all ages; however, most HSV-1 is acquired in childhood, and most HSV-2 is acquired in young–middle adulthood.
- Predominant sex: Male = Female

Incidence
- 29.2/100,000 office visits per year for herpes simplex-related codes
- HSV is never eliminated from the body but stays dormant and can reactivate, causing symptoms.

Prevalence
- Widespread; 0.65–25% of adults may be excreting HSV-1 or HSV-2 at any given time, many of whom are unaware of this infection status.
- Prevalence of antibodies to HSV-1 is 90% by adulthood in the general population, and 30% of adults have antibodies to HSV-2.

ETIOLOGY AND PATHOPHYSIOLOGY
HSV, a DNA virus of 2 major types: HSV-1 and HSV-2. Most often, HSV-1 is associated with oral lesions, and HSV-2 with genital lesions, but reverse also occurs.

RISK FACTORS
- Immunocompromised host, both acutely and chronic:
  – During presence of other illness or stress
  – Chemotherapy, malignancy/chronic disease states, such as diabetes or AIDS, older age
- Atopic eczema, especially in children
- Prior HSV infection
- Sexual intercourse with infected person (condoms help minimize HSV transmission, but location of lesions outside condom-protected areas limit their effectiveness)
- Occupational exposure:
  – Dental professionals at higher risk for HSV-1 and resulting herpetic whitlow
- Neonatal herpes simplex: Primary perinatal infection is life-threatening and usually acquired by vaginal birth via infected mother; fetal risk and neonatal risk are greater in mothers with primary genital herpes infection because shedding is more prolonged and the inoculum is greater; incubation is usually from

5–7 days (rarely 4 weeks); cutaneous, mucous membrane, or ocular signs seen in only 70%.

GENERAL PREVENTION
- Those with active disease should avoid direct contact with immunocompromised people, the elderly, and newborns.
- Wash hands often. Wash all linens with hot water immediately after lesions resolve.
- Kissing, sharing beverages from the same container, and sharing food utensils/toothbrushes can transmit HSV.
- Genital herpes: Avoid sexual contact while disease is active (recognizing herpes simplex is transmitted even when disease appears to be inactive), discuss condom benefits and limits, consider antiviral therapy to reduce viral shedding, and reinforce benefits of mutually monogamous sexual relations.
- Topical microbicides (gels) are showing promise (but not yet commercially available) to prevent acquisition of HSV-2 (1)[A].

COMMONLY ASSOCIATED CONDITIONS
- Erythema multiforme: 50% of associated cases are caused by HSV-1 or -2.
- All severe, unusual locations or treatment-resistant HSV cases should be screened for HIV.

 DIAGNOSIS

HISTORY
- Most patients admit no known exposure to herpes, as transmission is often distant in time or via asymptomatic contacts.
- Report of a prodrome of fatigue, low-grade fever, itching, tingling, or hot skin area for a few days immediately prior to the rash outbreak
- In herpes labialis: Precipitating events may be sunlight, fever, trauma, menses, stress; prodrome of pain, burning, itching may last 6–48 hours before vesicles appear.

PHYSICAL EXAM
- Vesicles: Usually cluster and open as painful ulcerated lesions, often with erythematous base
- Primary genital herpes: See "Herpes, Genital"
- Primary herpetic gingivostomatitis and pharyngitis: Usually in early childhood; incubation from 2–12 days, followed by fever, sore throat, pharyngeal edema, and erythema:
  – Small vesicles develop on pharyngeal and oral mucosa, rapidly ulcerate, and increase in number to involve soft palate, buccal mucosa, tongue, floor of mouth, and often lips and cheeks; tender gums may bleed; cervical adenopathy; fever, general toxicity, poor oral intake, and drooling contribute to dehydration; autoinoculation of other sites may occur; resolves in 10–14 days.
- Primary herpes keratoconjunctivitis: Unilateral conjunctivitis with regional adenopathy, as blepharitis with vesicles on lid margin, as keratitis with dendritic lesions, or with punctate opacities; lasts 2–3 weeks; systemic involvement prolongs process
- Eczema herpeticum: Diffuse poxlike eruption complicating atopic dermatitis; sudden appearance of lesions in typical atopic areas (upper trunk, neck, head); high fever, local edema, adenopathy
- Herpetic whitlow: Localized primary infection on a finger with intense itching and pain, followed by vesicles that may coalesce with swelling and

erythema, and may mimic pyogenic paronychia; neuralgia and axillary adenopathy sometime occur; heals over 2–3 weeks without incision
- Congenital infection via prenatal transplacental virus transfer may present with jaundice, hepatosplenomegaly, disseminated intravascular coagulation (DIC), encephalitis, seizures, temperature instability, chorioretinitis, and/or conjunctivitis with/without skin vesicles
- Recurrent diseases from endogenous reactivation include:
  – Herpes labialis: Recurrent lesions on lips with HSV-1; usually <1 recurrence/6 months, but 5–25% may have >1 attack/month; vesicles often at vermilion border, then ulcerate and crust within 48 hours; heal within 8–10 days generally; may have local adenopathy
  – Ocular herpes: May recur as keratitis, blepharitis, or keratoconjunctivitis; patients may have dendritic ulcers, decreased corneal sensation, less visual acuity; uveitis may cause permanent visual loss.

DIFFERENTIAL DIAGNOSIS
- Impetigo: Straw-colored vesicles that crust
- Aphthous stomatitis: Grayish, shallow erosions with ring of hyperemia, usually only anterior in mouth and lips
- Herpes zoster: Unilateral dermatome distribution
- Syphilitic chancre: Usually painless ulcer
- Folliculitis: Herpes may mimic "shave bumps" in the genital area.
- Herpangina: Vesicles predominate on anterior tonsillar pillars, soft palate, uvula, and oropharynx, but not more anteriorly on lips/gums (usually caused by group A coxsackievirus).
- Stevens-Johnson syndrome

DIAGNOSTIC TESTS & INTERPRETATION
- Screen for other sexually transmitted infections (STIs) in patients with primary genital herpes.
- Viral: HIV, hepatitis B and C, human papillomavirus (HPV) have crossover.
- Bacterial: Gonorrhea, chlamydia should be screened for in new primary genital outbreaks.

Initial Tests (lab, imaging)
- Tzanck smear shows multinucleated giant cells with 12–15 nuclei, often with eosinophilic intranuclear inclusions (scrape material from lesion onto slide, fix with ethanol/methanol, stain with Giemsa or Wright preparation); varicella (herpes zoster) has identical findings.
- HSV culture: On viral-specific media, swab and sample may need to be refrigerated; can take up to 6 days to be positive. Highly specific; hence, reliable if positive, but has 20% false–negative rate.
- HSV type-specific antibody tests distinguish between HSV-1 and HSV-2:
  – PCR (polymerase chain reaction), DFA (direct fluorescent antibody), ELISA, and Western blot
  – 3 weeks after infection, 50% of those infected test positive; 6 weeks after infection: 70%; >16 weeks: Nearly all infected test positive

Diagnostic Procedures/Other
Occasionally a biopsy is needed.

Test Interpretation
- See Tzanck prep above.
- Intraepithelial edema (ballooning degeneration) and intracellular edema

- Brain biopsy (in encephalitis) has hemorrhagic necrosis of gray and white matter with acute and chronic inflammation, thrombosis, fibrinoid necrosis of parenchymal vessels; intranuclear inclusions in astrocytes, oligodendroglia, and neurons.

 TREATMENT

GENERAL MEASURES

- Intermittent, cool, moist dressings with Domeboro or Burrow solution
- Painful urination and inability to void due to painful genital lesions is helped by pouring a cup of warm water over genitals while urinating or by sitting in a warm bath while urinating (Sitz baths).
- Children with gingivostomatitis who resist oral intake due to pain or extensive skin disease (eczema herpeticum) may require IV hydration and volume replacement.

MEDICATION
First Line

- In all cases, regardless of choice of agent, treatment should begin as early as possible, preferably in prodromal phase even before lesions develop.
- Acyclovir (generic):
  - Mucocutaneous (or genital) HSV:
    ○ Primary/1st infection: 400 mg t.i.d. × 7–10 days
    ○ If severe, start with IV q8h dosing for 1st few days, then complete 10-day course PO route.
    ○ Recurrence: 400 mg PO t.i.d. × 5 days *or* 800 mg b.i.d. × 5 days *or* 800 mg t.i.d. × 2 days
    ○ Suppression: 400 mg b.i.d. daily
  - Keratitis HSV: 400 mg PO 5×/d; however, topical treatment is preferred 1st line.
  - Pediatric dosing: Neonatal herpes simplex or encephalitis: 60 mg/kg/d IV divided q8h × 14–21 days:
    ○ Older (>3 months of age) immunocompetent is weight-based dosing (15 mg/kg/d divided q8h for 5–7 days)
  - Safe in pregnancy and lactation – category B
  - Recurrent herpes labialis: 800–1,600 mg/d for prevention (2)[A]
- Penciclovir (Denavir): 10 mg/g cream. Apply to oral lesions q2h × 4 days.
- Valacyclovir (Valtrex) (3):
  - Primary genital herpes: 1 g PO b.i.d. for 7–10 days Recurrent genital herpes: 500 mg PO b.i.d. for 3 days; suppression: 500–1,000 mg PO daily (depending on frequency of outbreaks); labialis HSV (cold sores/oral lesions): 2,000 mg PO q12h × 1 day
  - 500-mg daily dose if suppression is needed/desired
  - Recurrent herpes labialis: 500 mg/d for 4 months for prevention (2)[A]
- Precautions:
  - Renal dosing required in all oral antivirals
  - Significant possible interactions: Probenecid with IV acyclovir and possibly probenecid with valacyclovir may reduce renal clearance and elevate antiviral drug levels.

Second Line

- Foscarnet:
  - Drug of choice for acyclovir resistance in immunocompromised persons with systemic HSV
  - 40 mg/kg IV q8h (assume valacyclovir and famciclovir resistance also if acyclovir resistance occurs)

- Other topicals:
  - Ophthalmic preparations for herpes keratoconjunctivitis; acyclovir, vidarabine (Vira-A), ganciclovir, trifluridine
  - Topical acyclovir and penciclovir improve healing times for recurrent herpes labialis by ~10% (4)[A].
  - Topical analgesics: Lidocaine 2% or 5% helps reduce the pain sequelae associated with vulvar and penile herpes outbreaks.
- Over-the-counter topical antivirals: Abreva

ISSUES FOR REFERRAL
Recurrent cases of herpes keratoconjunctivitis should be referred to an ophthalmologist.

IN-PATIENT CONSIDERATIONS
Admission Criteria/Initial Stabilization

- Pregnancy considerations:
  - Caesarean section and/or acyclovir indicated if any active genital lesions (or prodrome) present at time of delivery; should be considered if primary genital herpes occurred within prior 4 weeks (5)[B]
  - Daily oral antivirals from 36 weeks onward in women with history of recurrent genital herpes to prevent outbreak near to/at time of delivery
  - Avoid fetal scalp electrodes, forceps, vacuum extractor, and artificial rupture of membranes if mother has history of genital HSV.
  - Risk of viral shedding at delivery from asymptomatic recurrent genital HSV is low (~1.6%); not predicted by monitoring cultures.
- Pediatric considerations:
  - Neonates with likely exposure (high index of suspicion) to HSV at birth or with signs of infection should have culture of all bodily fluid sources and immediate treatment with IV acyclovir.

 ONGOING CARE

FOLLOW-UP RECOMMENDATIONS

- For most typical cases, follow-up is not necessary. Lesions and symptoms resolve rapidly within 10 days. Extensive/Primary cases should be rechecked in 1 week; monitor for secondary bacterial infections.
- Consider long-term suppression treatment.

DIET
If oral lesions present, avoid salty, acidic, or sharp foods (e.g., chips and orange juice).

PATIENT EDUCATION

- Explain the natural history of this viral illness, that timing of exposure is difficult to determine, and that the virus will be in system forever. Try to minimize psychological impact of this diagnosis (reduce any stigma).
- Hygiene techniques to avoid self-spreading to other body areas (autoinoculation) or exposing others. Frequent hand washing; avoid scratching; cover any active, wet lesions.

PROGNOSIS

- Usual course of primary disease is 5 days–2 weeks.
- Antiviral treatment can limit length of disease state, reduce complicating sequelae, and nearly eliminate recurrences (if used daily).
- Viral shedding in recurrence is briefer than with primary disease; frequency of recurrence extremely variable, depends on individual patient factors.
- Newborns/Immunocompromised individuals are at risk for major morbidity/mortality.

- HSV is never eliminated from the body but stays dormant and can reactivate, causing symptoms.

COMPLICATIONS

- Herpes encephalitis: A brain biopsy may be needed for diagnosis.
- Herpes pneumonia

REFERENCES

1. Obiero J, Mwethera PG, Wiysonge CS. Topical microbicides for prevention of sexually transmitted infections. *Cochrane Database Syst Rev*. 2012;6:CD007961. Epub 2012 Jun 13.
2. Rahimi H, Mara T, Costella J, et al. Effectiveness of antiviral agents for the prevention of recurrent herpes labialis: A systematic review and meta-analysis. *Oral Surg Oral Med Oral Pathol Oral Radiol*. 2012;113(5):618–627. Epub 2012 Apr 12.
3. Cernik C, Gallina K, Brodell RT, et al. The treatment of herpes simplex infections: An evidence-based review. *Arch Intern Med*. 2008;168:1137–1144.
4. Harmenberg J, Oberg B, Spruance S, et al. Prevention of ulcerative lesions by episodic treatment of recurrent herpes labialis: A literature review. *Acta Derm Venereol*. 2010;90:122–130.
5. Gupta R, Warren T, Wald A. Genital herpes. *Lancet* 2007;370(9605):2127–2137.

ADDITIONAL READING

- Pinninti SG, Kimberlin DW. Neonatal herpes simplex virus infections. *Pediatr Clin North Am*. 2013;60(2): 351–365. doi: 10.1016/j.pcl.2012.12.005.
- Wang X, Zhou F, Zhao J, et al. Elevated risk of opportunistic viral infection in patients with Crohn's disease during biological therapies: A meta analysis of randomized controlled trials. *Eur J Clin Pharmacol*. 2013 Jul 25. [Epub ahead of print]

 SEE ALSO

- Herpes, Genital
- Algorithm: Genital Ulcers

CODES

ICD10

- B00.1 Herpesviral vesicular dermatitis
- B00.9 Herpesviral infection, unspecified
- A60.9 Anogenital herpesviral infection, unspecified

CLINICAL PEARLS

- 25–30% of the US population has genital herpes, and >80% of the US population is seropositive for herpesvirus exposure/antibody evidence of infection.
- Most individuals are unaware that they have been infected and pass on the virus during asymptomatic periods.
- Chronic suppression for those with frequent recurrences is effective at preventing transmission and decreases outbreak frequency; however recurrences naturally become less frequent over time.

H

HERPES ZOSTER
Robert J. Hyde, MD, MA

BASICS

DESCRIPTION
- Usually presents as a painful unilateral vesicular eruption within a dermatome
- Results from reactivation of varicella-zoster virus (human herpesvirus type 3)
- Postherpetic neuralgia (PHN) is usually defined as pain persisting at least 1 month after rash has healed. Because of variable definitions of PHN used in research, the term *zoster-associated pain* may be more clinically useful.
- System(s) affected: Nervous; Integumentary; Exocrine
- Synonym(s): Shingles

EPIDEMIOLOGY
Predominant sex: Male = Female

Incidence
- Incidence is increasing as population ages.
- Incidence increases with age: 2/3 of cases occur in adults age $\geq$50 years.
- Herpes zoster: 3.6/1,000 person-years (1)
- PHN: 18% in adult patients with herpes zoster; 33% $\geq$79 years of age

Prevalence
Nearly 1 million new herpes zoster cases yearly

Pregnancy Considerations
May occur during pregnancy

Geriatric Considerations
- Increased incidence of zoster outbreaks
- Increased incidence of PHN

Pediatric Considerations
- Occurs less frequently in children
- Has been reported in newborns primarily infected in utero

ETIOLOGY AND PATHOPHYSIOLOGY
Reactivation of varicella-zoster virus (human herpesvirus type 3) from dorsal root/cranial nerve ganglia

RISK FACTORS
- Most persons affected have no underlying illness.
- Increasing age
- Reduced immunity associated with some malignancies (e.g., lymphoma)
- Treatment of malignancy (chemotherapy/radiotherapy)
- HIV infection
- Use of immunosuppressant drugs after organ transplant surgery or for disease management
- Spinal surgery

GENERAL PREVENTION
- Herpes zoster vaccination was licensed by the US FDA May 25, 2006. Zostavax is available and ACIP recommended for patients $\geq$60 years of age (and in 2011, FDA approved for patients >50) (2,3,4):
  - Vaccine is proven to reduce cases of zoster and the incidence of PHN (5,6).
- Patients with zoster may transmit virus-causing varicella (chickenpox) to susceptible persons.

COMMONLY ASSOCIATED CONDITIONS
Immunocompromised individuals, including HIV infection, posttransplantation, immunosuppressive drugs, and malignancy

DIAGNOSIS

HISTORY
- Prodromal phase (sensations over involved dermatome prior to rash):
  - Tingling
  - Itching
  - Boring/Knifelike pain
- Acute phase:
  - Constitutional symptoms variable (e.g., fatigue, malaise, headache, low-grade fever)
  - Dermatomal rash

PHYSICAL EXAM
- Acute phase:
  - Weakness (1% may have weakness in distribution of rash)
  - Initially erythematous and maculopapular; evolves rapidly to grouped vesicles
  - Vesicles become pustular and/or hemorrhagic in 3–4 days.
  - Resolution of rash, with crusts separating by 14–21 days
- Possible sine herpete (zoster without rash) and other chronic disorders associated with varicella-zoster virus without the typical rash
- Chronic phase:
  - PHN (15% overall; increases with age)
  - A small percentage (1–5%) may affect the motor nerves, causing weakness (called *zoster motorius*), facial nerve (e.g., Ramsay Hunt syndrome), spinal motor radiculopathies

DIFFERENTIAL DIAGNOSIS
- Rash:
  - Herpes simplex virus
  - Coxsackievirus
  - Contact dermatitis
  - Superficial pyoderma
- Pain:
  - Cholecystitis
  - Appendicitis
  - Nephrolithiasis
  - Pleuritis
  - Myocardial infarction
  - Diabetic neuropathy

DIAGNOSTIC TESTS & INTERPRETATION
Initial Tests (lab, imaging)
Rarely necessary because clinical appearance is usually sufficiently distinctive

Follow-Up Tests & Special Considerations
- Viral culture
- Tzanck smear (does not distinguish from herpes simplex, and false-negative results occur)
- Polymerase chain reaction analysis
- Immunofluorescent antigen staining
- Varicella-zoster–specific IgM

Test Interpretation
- Multinucleated giant cells with intralesional inclusion
- Lymphatic infiltration of sensory ganglia with focal hemorrhage and nerve cell destruction

TREATMENT

GENERAL MEASURES
- Treatment should be directed to control acute symptoms and prevent complications.
- Antiviral therapy decreases viral replication, lessens nerve damage and inflammation, and reduces the severity and duration of long-term pain syndromes (7)[A].
- Prompt analgesic control of pain may shorten the duration of zoster-associated pain.
- Lotions, such as calamine and colloidal oatmeal, may reduce itching and burning sensation.

MEDICATION
First Line
- Acute treatment:
  - Antiviral agents initiated within 72 hours of rash may relieve symptoms, speed resolution of rash, and prevent and/or ameliorate PHN (7)[A]:
    ○ Evidence from quality trials have shown significant reduction in risk of pain with valacyclovir and famciclovir (8)[A].
  - Valacyclovir: 1,000 mg t.i.d. × 7 days
  - Famciclovir: 500 mg t.i.d. × 7 days
  - Acyclovir: 800 mg q4h (5 doses daily) × 7 days
- Analgesics (acetaminophen, NSAIDs, opioids)
- Corticosteroids given acutely during zoster infection are ineffective in preventing PHN (9).
- Treatment of complications:
  - Secondary bacterial skin infections: Silver sulfadiazine topically and/or systemic antibiotics
- PHN and zoster-associated pain (7):
  - Tricyclic antidepressants (TCAs; amitriptyline 25 mg at bedtime and other low-dose TCAs) relieve pain acutely and may reduce pain duration.
  - Lidocaine patch 5% (Lidoderm) applied after skin rash closure over painful areas (limit 3 patches simultaneously or trim a single patch) for up to 12 hours has been reported to be effective in 1 limited trial.
  - Gabapentin: 100–600 mg t.i.d. for pain and other quality-of-life indicators; limited by adverse effects
  - Opioids, capsaicin cream, and other analgesics may be useful adjuncts.
  - Pregabalin: 50–100 mg t.i.d. reduces pain, but usefulness is limited by side effects.
- Prevention of PHN and zoster-associated pain: No treatment has been shown to prevent PHN completely, but treatment may shorten duration and/or reduce severity of symptoms (10)[A]:
  - Antiviral therapy with valacyclovir, famciclovir, or acyclovir given during acute skin eruption may be effective in limiting the duration of pain.
  - Low-dose amitriptyline in the same dosage as for treatment of PHN but started within 72 hours of rash onset and continued for 90 days may reduce PHN incidence/duration.
  - Insufficient evidence suggests that corticosteroids reduce incidence, severity, or duration of PHN (9).

- Contraindications: Refer to the manufacturer's profile of each drug.
- Precautions:
  – Assess renal function prior to using valacyclovir, famciclovir, or acyclovir.
  – Valacyclovir, famciclovir, and acyclovir are pregnancy Category B.
  – Refer to the manufacturer's profile of each drug.
- Significant possible interactions: Refer to the manufacturer's profile of each drug.

Second Line
Numerous therapies have been advocated, but good supporting evidence is lacking.

COMPLEMENTARY AND ALTERNATIVE MEDICINE
Many studies on cupping therapy (traditional Chinese medicine) show potential effect, but evidence is conflicting (11)[A].

IN-PATIENT CONSIDERATIONS
Admission Criteria/Initial Stabilization
Outpatient treatment, unless disseminated or occurring as complication of serious underlying disease requiring hospitalization

 ## ONGOING CARE

FOLLOW-UP RECOMMENDATIONS
No restrictions

Patient Monitoring
Depends on symptoms

DIET
No special diet

PATIENT EDUCATION
- Inform patient that the duration of rash is 2–3 weeks.
- Encourage good hygiene and proper skin care.
- Warn of potential for dissemination (dissemination must be suspected with constitutional illness signs and/or spreading rash).
- Warn of potential PHN.
- Warn of potential risk of transmitting illness (chickenpox) to susceptible persons.

PROGNOSIS
- Immunocompetent individuals should experience spontaneous and complete recovery within a few weeks.
- Resolution of acute rash within 14–21 days
- PHN may occur in patients age ≥50 years despite treatment with antiviral medications.

COMPLICATIONS
- PHN
- Ophthalmic herpes zoster: 10–20%
- Superinfection of skin lesions:
  – Meningoencephalitis
  – Cutaneous dissemination
  – Hepatitis
  – Pneumonitis
  – Myelitis
  – Cranial and peripheral nerve palsies
  – Acute retinal necrosis

REFERENCES

1. Yawn BP, Saddier P, Wollan PC, et al. A population-based study of the incidence and complication rates of herpes zoster before zoster vaccine introduction. *Mayo Clin Proc.* 2007; 82(11):1341–1349.
2. Centers for Disease Control and Prevention (CDC). Adult vaccination coverage–United States, 2010. *MMWR Morb Mortal Wkly Rep.* 2012;61:66–72.
3. Schmader KE, Levin MJ, Gnann JW, et al. Efficacy, safety, and tolerability of herpes zoster vaccine in persons aged 50–59 years. *Clin Infect Dis.* 2012; 54:922–928.
4. Harpaz R, Ortega-Sanchez IR, Seward JF, et al. Prevention of herpes zoster: Recommendations of the Advisory Committee on Immunization Practices (ACIP). *MMWR Recomm Rep.* 2008;57: 1–30.
5. Chen N, Li Q, Zhang Y, et al. Vaccination for preventing postherpetic neuralgia. *Cochrane Database Syst Rev.* 2011;(3):CD007795.
6. Langan SM, Smeeth L, Margolis DJ, et al. Herpes zoster vaccine effectiveness against incident herpes zoster and post-herpetic neuralgia in an older US population: A cohort study. *PLoS Med.* 2013;10(4):e1001420.
7. Mounsey AL, Matthew LG, Slawson DC. Herpes zoster and postherpetic neuralgia: Prevention and management. *Am Fam Physician.* 2005;72: 1075–1080.
8. McDonald EM, de Kock J, Ram FS. Antivirals for management of herpes zoster including ophthalmicus: A systematic review of high-quality randomized controlled trials. *Antivir Ther (Lond).* 2012;17(2):255–264. Epub 2011 Dec 15.
9. Chen N, Yang M, He L, et al. Corticosteroids for preventing postherpetic neuralgia. *Cochrane Database Syst Rev.* 2010;(12):CD005582.
10. Li Q, Chen N, Yang J, et al. Antiviral treatment for preventing postherpetic neuralgia. *Cochrane Database Syst Rev.* 2009;(2):CD006866.
11. Cao H, Li X, Liu J. An updated review of the efficacy of cupping therapy. *PLoS ONE.* 2012;7(2): e31793. Epub 2012 Feb 28.

 ## SEE ALSO

- Bell Palsy; Chickenpox (Varicella Zoster); Herpes Eye Infections; Herpes Simplex
- Algorithm: Genital Ulcers

 ## CODES

ICD10
- B02.9 Zoster without complications
- B02.29 Other postherpetic nervous system involvement

CLINICAL PEARLS

- In herpes zoster ophthalmicus, Hutchinson sign is a vesicular rash at the nasal tip, indicating involvement of the external branch of cranial nerve V; associated with increased incidence of ocular zoster.
- Patients should be referred to an ophthalmologist for Hutchinson sign in the early phase of ophthalmic zoster or if they have visual complaints or an unexplained red eye.
- All patients should begin a course of antiviral therapy regardless of age. To be effective, therapy should be started within 72 hours of the onset of rash. After 72 hours, antiviral therapy is recommended for any immunocompromised patient who still has vesicles. However, no data examine the effect of antiviral medication after 72 hours.
- Zoster vaccine is ACIP recommended for patients ≥60 years of age (and since 2011, FDA approved for patients >50).

H

HERPES, GENITAL
Terri Warren, RN, MEd, MSN • Jill A. Grimes, MD, FAAFP

 BASICS

DESCRIPTION
- Herpes simplex virus (HSV) infection involving the genitals (anywhere within the boxer shorts area; innervation of the sacral ganglia)
- Primary, nonprimary 1st episode/recurrent
- Synonym(s): Herpes genitalis

EPIDEMIOLOGY
- Predominant age: 15–65 years, with increasing prevalence as ages increases (cumulative cases, no cure)
- Overall prevalence of HSV2 in the US: 16% of the population age >14 and <50 years
- Overall prevalence of HSV1 in the US: 57% of the population age >14 and <50 years
- Predominant sex: Female > Male; women are almost twice as likely as men to be infected due to receptive position with intercourse.
- African American 3× > Caucasian. ~50% of African Americans between the ages of 14 and 49 are infected with HSV2.
- HSV1: 10–50% (increasing incidence); now greater than HSV2 in some clinical settings. *~75% of new genital HSV among college students is HSV1.*
- HSV2: 60–90%; accounts for the significant majority of recurrent disease

Incidence
300,000–1,500,000 cases/year. Genital herpes was the 3rd most incident STI in the US in 2011.

Prevalence

ALERT
45–50 million. HSV2 was the most prevalent STI in the US in 2011; *this number does not take into account cases of genital herpes that are caused by HSV1.*

ETIOLOGY AND PATHOPHYSIOLOGY
HSV: A double-stranded DNA, *Alphaherpesvirinae* virus subfamily

RISK FACTORS
- Primary infection with HSV2:
  - Increasing age, black race, number of lifetime partners, and history of STIs
- Transmission of HSV2:
  - Incubation period for symptomatic disease: 1–10 days (mean, 5.5 days). *Most new cases are without symptoms.*
  - Annual risk: Susceptible female acquiring disease from an infected male partner, ~10–30%; for susceptible male from infected female, ~5%. These risks include no condom use, no daily antiviral therapy, no sex with recognized symptoms and both partners aware of infection being present and disclosed.
  - Those with prior HSV1 infection are those least likely to display symptoms of HSV2 when it is acquired.
  - >70% new cases result from transmission during asymptomatic (clinically unrecognized) shedding.
  - Risk of HSV2 asymptomatic shedding: 13% of days; highest within 6 months of new infection (42% of days)
  - Daily antiviral therapy (e.g., valacyclovir 500 mg) reduces viral shedding and reduces transmission of HSV2 by 48%. Transmission studies have not been done on the other antiviral medicines

(acyclovir and famciclovir), but they likely have similar results. Neither famciclovir nor valacyclovir shows a better reduction in viral shedding than b.i.d. acyclovir
- Genital transmission of HSV1:
  - Mostly due to receiving oral sex from someone who has oral HSV1 infection, with or without an active cold sore.
  - Distinguishing between canker sores and cold sores is important when speaking with patients: Canker sores are *not* caused by herpes virus.
  - Daily antiviral therapy is also effective against HSV1 shedding, although slightly less so than for HSV2.
- Recurrence triggers for genital herpes are unknown. Ultraviolet light is a known trigger for oral herpes.

Pediatric Considerations
Neonatal infection occurs in 20–50/100,000 live births. 80% of infections result from asymptomatic maternal viral shedding during an undiagnosed 1st infection in the 3rd trimester.

GENERAL PREVENTION
- Oral, vaginal, and anal sexual abstinence is only option to provide complete protection.
- Condoms reduce transmission by ~30–50%.
- Reducing the frequency and number of partner changes likely reduces the risk of infection.
- Pregnant women who test antibody negative for HSV1 and HSV2 should avoid unprotected intercourse and receptive oral sex in late pregnancy unless partner is known also to be negative for both.
- Screening with type-specific antibody in the general population and in pregnancy is not recommended by the USPSTF (although experts disagree about pregnancy):
  - Consider screening in asymptomatic patients with HIV infection and offer suppressive prescription if positive.
  - Consider HSV antibody testing as part of STI screening panel *or be certain patients know it is not included if it is not.*
  - Offer screening to discordant couples (1 partner with known HSV, the other without).
  - Use antibody testing for patients whose genital symptoms cannot be definitely diagnosed as some other problem.
- Avoid sex if lesions or prodromal symptoms are present. Transmission is possible even when no symptoms are present. See above for transmission reduction strategies.
- Infants with possible HSV infection should be isolated in the nursery; maternal separation is not necessary; breastfeeding is allowed.
- Vaccines not available yet, but clinical development has reached human trials (1)
- HIV disease: Prevalence of HSV-2 shedding and genital ulcer disease increases significantly after initiation of antiretroviral therapy; consider starting acyclovir to mitigate if co-infected (2)[A].

COMMONLY ASSOCIATED CONDITIONS
All STIs

 DIAGNOSIS

HISTORY
- At least 80% of patients with HSV2 are asymptomatic or do not recognize clinical manifestations of disease.

- Common presentations: Genital itching, pain, dysuria/visible blisters/sores; local symptoms can last 3–21 days.
- Constitutional symptoms are possible, mostly with 1st infection: Headache, photophobia, malaise, myalgia, fever

PHYSICAL EXAM
- Impossible to differentiate among primary, 1st-episode nonprimary, recurrent disease or type of virus (HSV1 or HSV2) on basis of symptoms and clinical findings
- Genital irritation, localized erythema, vulvar, penile, anal, perineal ulcers, sores, fissures, cracks, watery discharge from vagina/urethra, or pyuria without frequency and urgency:
  - Female: Pelvic examination of internal reproductive organs; external genitalia, vagina, cervix
  - Male: Penis and scrotum
  - Male and female: Rectum, thighs, buttocks, pubic hair area, mouth, inguinal lymph nodes
- Adenopathy, sacral paresthesias resulting in inability to urinate/defecate

Pediatric Considerations
Genital lesions in children suggest sexual abuse.

DIFFERENTIAL DIAGNOSIS
- Primary syphilis
- Chancroid
- Herpes zoster
- Trauma
- Behçet syndrome
- Ulcerative balanitis
- Granuloma inguinale
- Neoplasia

DIAGNOSTIC TESTS & INTERPRETATION
Initial Tests (lab, imaging)
- Viral detection from lesion:
  - Swab lesions; PCR (2–4× more sensitive than culture) preferred. Viral culture. Both should always include request for typing of virus.
  - Use Dacron or polyester-tipped swabs with plastic shafts, not cotton tips/wood shafts; both inhibit viral growth and/or replication.
- Type-specific serologic assays (TSST):
  - Western blot (gold standard), and type-specific IgG antibody (glycoprotein G) ELISA to discriminate between HSV1 and HSV2:
    - Seroconversion occurs 10 days to 4 months after infection. Use of daily herpes medicine may delay seroconversion. *Antibody testing is not necessary if a positive typed swab test has been obtained.*
    - Type-specific antibody tests have a 4–6% false-positive rate when index value is in low positive range. Anyone with a value of 1.1–3.5 on the type-specific IgG HSV2 antibody test needs confirmation with another test, preferably herpes Western blot. If a low positive has been obtained early after possible infection, it is also acceptable to redo the ELISA when 3–4 months have passed in lieu of ordering a Western blot.
    - IgM antibody testing is never appropriate: Cannot distinguish with accuracy new from old infection, is often present with recurrent disease, and has many false-positive findings.
- Commercially available ELISA tests include HerpesSelect-1 and 2 (ELISA), HerpesSelect 1/2 (immunoblot), Captia, and Biokit HSV-2 and

SureVue HSV-2 (fingerstick, point-of-care) and herpes Western blot. Western blot is done only at the University of Washington in the US. A test kit can also be ordered directly from the University of Washington and sent to the health care provider for collection and return to the lab. Other confirmatory tests are inferior.

Test Interpretation
Histopathology: Cytopathology is not a recommended method for diagnosing herpes because it cannot be typed and may be confused with other viruses in the herpes family.

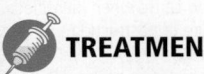

TREATMENT

GENERAL MEASURES
- Cool compresses of aluminum acetate (Burow solution) 4–6×/d
- Ice packs to perineum, sitz baths, spray-on topical anesthetic
- Analgesics, NSAIDs

MEDICATION
Antiviral medications should be started at the 1st sign/symptom of disease, preferably within 48 hours, even if not confirmatory diagnosis has been made yet.

First Line
- Acyclovir (3)[A]:
  - 1st infection: 400 mg PO t.i.d. for 7–10 days or 200 mg PO 5× a day for 7–10 days, longer if needed for incomplete healing
  - Episodic therapy: 400 mg t.i.d. for 5 days or 800 mg b.i.d. for 5 days or 800 mg t.i.d. for 2 days. Shorter course, better compliance
  - Daily suppression: 400 mg PO b.i.d. As effective as other treatment regimens in reducing viral shedding
  - Severe local/disseminated disease: 5–10 mg/kg IV q8h for 5–7 days
  - HIV infection: 400 mg PO 3–5×/d until clinical resolution is attained
  - Precautions:
    - Pregnancy: Not approved by FDA for routine use (Category B). Studies have demonstrated safety of use. 36 weeks on. Need b.i.d. therapy with valacyclovir or t.i.d. with acyclovir
    - Drug is excreted in breast milk.
    - Modify dose in patients with renal insufficiency or those who are taking nephrotoxic medicines.
    - Nephropathy and neuropathy are possible with high doses given IV.
    - Rate of resistance in immunocompetent populations: 0.3%
- Valacyclovir (Valtrex) (3)[A]: Pregnancy Category B, Pro-drug of acyclovir with better bioavailability, thus less frequent dosing possible:
  - 1st infection: 1 g PO b.i.d. for 7–10 days
  - Episodic therapy: 500 mg PO b.i.d. for 3–5 days or 1 g PO daily for 5 days
  - Daily suppression: 500 mg/d PO or 1,000 mg/d. If breaking through, attempt 500 mg b.i.d.
- Famciclovir (Famvir) (3)[A]: Pregnancy Category B:
  - 1st infection: 250 mg PO t.i.d. for 7–10 days
  - Episodic therapy: 125 mg PO b.i.d. for 5 days or 1 g PO b.i.d. × 1 day
  - Daily suppression: 250 mg PO b.i.d.

Pregnancy Considerations
ACOG Clinical Management Guidelines (4,5)[A]:
- Primary HSV during pregnancy/lesions near/at term: Consider antiviral therapy (reduces duration/severity and viral shedding)

- Women with a history of genital herpes at or beyond 36 weeks should be offered suppression; may reduce C-section rate by 70%, clinical HSV, and HSV shedding; continue through delivery; acyclovir 400 mg t.i.d. or valacyclovir 500 mg b.i.d.

Second Line
- Foscarnet: 40 mg/kg IV q8h in severe disease with proven/suspected acyclovir-resistant strains
- Vidarabine: 10 mg/kg/d infused over 10 hours; benefits HIV patients with HSV1 infection failing acyclovir and foscarnet therapy
- Cidofovir (Vistide) topical: 0.1–0.3% gel for 5 days for progressive/resistant lesions
- Trifluridine (Viroptic) ophthalmic solution for mucocutaneous lesions resistant to acyclovir

Pediatric Considerations
- High-risk infant: Acyclovir 30 mg/kg/d IV q9h for 10–14 days
- Low-risk infant, asymptomatic: Culture eyes, nose, and mouth at 24–36 hours and observe.

COMPLEMENTARY AND ALTERNATIVE MEDICINE
L-lysine, although popular, has not been shown to be beneficial in reducing outbreak duration or frequency.

ONGOING CARE

FOLLOW-UP RECOMMENDATIONS
- Avoid intercourse when symptomatic lesions are present.
- Make sex partners aware of herpes status prior to sexual activity.
- Use daily suppression therapy to reduce the risk of transmission by almost 1/2.
- Have potential/current partners antibody tested prior to sexual activity; they may be infected and not know it.
- Concordant couples (i.e., both have the same type of herpes [HSV1/HSV2]) may have sex without worry of triggering outbreaks.

Patient Monitoring
- Latent infection: Check pregnant women at prenatal visits and onset of labor for presence of lesions. If yes, C-section recommended.
- Test for all other STIs if initial HSV infection.

DIET
No benefits from diet change, despite popular recommendations re:↑ lysine and ↓ arginine.

PATIENT EDUCATION
- Herpes Resource Center: www.ashastd.org/herpes/herpes_overview.cfm.
- Warren T. The good news about the bad news: Herpes: Everything you need to know. Oakland, CA: New Harbinger Publications; 2009.

PROGNOSIS
- Resolution of signs/symptoms: 3–21 days
- Latent infection: Recurrences in 80% within 1 year of initial HSV2 infection; immunocompetent: 3–4/year for genital HSV2; 1/year for genital HSV1, 80% with HSV1 infection who do not experience a recurrence in the 1st year likely never will.
- HSV infection in immunocompromised patients: More severe, longer duration, resists treatment
- Antivirals do not eliminate virus from body, but reduce transmission, shedding, and outbreaks.

Pediatric Considerations
Neonatal infection survival rates: Localized, >95%; CNS, 85%; systemic, 30%

COMPLICATIONS
- Urinary and bowel: Temporary nonfunction
- Transient aseptic meningitis
- Transmission to infant w/new infection at 3rd trimester, prolonged ROM, scalp electrodes, prematurity, and cervical lesions
- Increased risk for HIV infection (2–3×) than in someone who does not have HSV2
- Lowered self-esteem, guilt, anger, depression, fear of rejection, fear of transmission to partner

REFERENCES
1. Tavares F, Cheuvart B, Heineman T, et al. Meta-analysis of pregnancy outcomes in pooled randomized trials on a prophylactic adjuvanted glycoprotein D subunit herpes simplex virus vaccine. Vaccine. 2013;31(13):1759–1764. doi: 10.1016/j.vaccine.2013.01.002. Epub 2013 Jan 10.
2. Tobian AA, Grabowski MK, Serwadda D, et al. Reactivation of herpes simplex virus type 2 after initiation of antiretroviral therapy. J Infect Dis. 2013;208(5):839–846. doi: 10.1093/infdis/jit252. Epub 2013 Jun 28.
3. CDC. 2010 STD treatment guidelines. Atlanta, GA: Author. www.cdc.gov/std/treatment/2010/.
4. Money D, Steben M, Society of Obstetricians and Gynaecologists of Canada. SOGC clinical practice guidelines: Guidelines for the management of herpes simplex virus in pregnancy. Number 208, June 2008. Int J Gynaecol Obstet. 2009;84(2): 167–171.
5. Sheffield JS, Hollier LM, Hill JB, et al. Acyclovir prophylaxis to prevent herpes simplex virus recurrence at delivery: A systematic review. Obstet Gynecol. 2003;102:1396–1403.

SEE ALSO

Algorithm: Genital Ulcers

CODES

ICD10
- A60.00 Herpesviral infection of urogenital system, unspecified
- A60.01 Herpesviral infection of penis
- A60.04 Herpesviral vulvovaginitis

CLINICAL PEARLS
- Genital herpes infections are frequently contracted from oral sex.
- Never use IgM testing: Many false-positive results; cannot differentiate HSV1 from HSV2.
- Condom use can decrease transmission by 30% and daily antiviral therapy by ~50%.
- Therapeutic vaccines for treatment of herpes are the wave of the future.

HICCUPS
James H. Lewis, MD, FACP, FACG, AGAF

BASICS

DESCRIPTION
- Hiccups are caused by a repetitive sudden involuntary contraction of the inspiratory muscles (predominantly the diaphragm) terminated by abrupt closure of the glottis, stopping the inflow of air and producing the characteristic sound.
- System(s) affected: Nervous; Pulmonary
- Synonym(s): Hiccoughs; Singultus

Geriatric Considerations
Can be a serious problem among the elderly

Pregnancy Considerations
- Fetal hiccups are noted as rhythmic fetal movements (confirmed sonographically) that can be confused with contractions.
- Fetal hiccups often recur in subsequent pregnancies.

EPIDEMIOLOGY
- Predominant age: All ages (including fetus)
- Predominant sex: Male > Female (4:1)

Prevalence
Self-limited hiccups are extremely common, as are intra- and postoperative hiccups.

ETIOLOGY AND PATHOPHYSIOLOGY
- Pathophysiologic significance is unknown; may be a vestigial reflex; hiccups have been associated with >100 underlying disorders (1). The latest theory suggests hiccups function to remove swallowed gas from the stomach as a burping reflex (2).
- Results from stimulation of ≥1 limbs of the hiccup reflux arc (vagus and phrenic nerves) with a "hiccup center" located in the upper spinal cord
- In men, >90% have an organic basis, whereas in women a psychogenic cause may be more likely.
- Specific underlying causes include:
  - Alcoholism
  - CNS lesions (brain stem tumors, vascular lesions, Parkinson disease) (3)
  - Diaphragmatic irritation (tumors, pericarditis, eventration, splenomegaly, hepatomegaly, peritonitis)
  - Hair, insect, or foreign body irritating tympanic membrane
  - Pharyngitis, laryngitis
  - Mediastinal and other thoracic lesions (pneumonia, aortic aneurysm, tuberculosis [TB], myocardial infarction [MI], lung cancer, rib exostoses)
  - Esophageal lesions (reflux esophagitis, achalasia, *Candida* esophagitis, carcinoma, obstruction)
  - Gastric lesions (ulcer, distention, cancer)
  - Hepatic lesions (hepatitis, hepatoma)
  - Pancreatic lesions (pancreatitis, pseudocysts, cancer)
  - Inflammatory bowel disease
  - Cholelithiasis, cholecystitis
  - Prostatic disorders
  - Appendicitis
  - Postoperative, abdominal procedures (4)
  - Toxic metabolic causes (uremia, hyponatremia, gout, diabetes)
  - Drug-induced (dexamethasone, methylprednisolone, anabolic steroids, benzodiazepines, α-methyldopa, propofol)
  - Psychogenic causes (hysterical neurosis, grief, malingering)
  - Idiopathic

RISK FACTORS
- General anesthesia; conscious sedation
- Postoperative state
- Genitourinary disorders
- Irritation of the vagus nerve branches
- Structural, vascular, infectious, neoplastic, or traumatic CNS lesions

GENERAL PREVENTION
- Identify and correct the underlying cause if possible.
- Avoid gastric distention.
- Seek medical attention for frequent bouts or persistent hiccups.
- Acupuncture appears to be as or more efficacious than chronic drug therapy to control hiccups.

COMMONLY ASSOCIATED CONDITIONS
See "Etiology."

DIAGNOSIS

- Hiccup attacks usually occur at brief intervals and last only a few seconds or minutes. Persistent bouts lasting >48 hours often imply an underlying physical or metabolic disorder.
- Intractable hiccups may occur continuously for months or years.
- Hiccups usually occur with a frequency of 4–60 per minute.

HISTORY
- Recent surgery (especially genitourinary)
- General anesthesia
- Medications
- Alcoholism
- GI, cardiac, or pulmonary disorders (see "Etiology")

PHYSICAL EXAM
- See "Etiology" for specific findings to look for.
- Examine the ear canal for foreign bodies.

DIFFERENTIAL DIAGNOSIS
See "Etiology"; burping (eructation) may be confused with hiccups.

DIAGNOSTIC TESTS & INTERPRETATION
Consider CBC, metabolic panel as suggested by history
Fluoroscopy is useful to determine whether 1 hemidiaphragm is dominant.

Diagnostic Procedures/Other
- Upper endoscopy, colonoscopy, CT scan (or other imaging) of brain, thorax, abdomen, and pelvis looking for etiological causes; exploratory laparoscopy or laparotomy for peritoneal lesions (carcinomatosis, etc.); GYN pathology; etc.
- The extent of the workup is often in proportion to the duration and severity of the hiccups.

TREATMENT

- Outpatient (usually)
- Inpatient (if elderly, debilitated, or intractable hiccups)
- Nearly all hiccup treatments are anecdotal; those with recorded success are listed below.

GENERAL MEASURES
- Treat any specific underlying cause when identified:
  - Dilate esophageal stricture or obstruction.
  - Treat ulcers or reflux disease.
  - Remove hair or foreign body from ear canal.
  - Angostura bitters for alcohol-induced hiccups
  - Catheter stimulation of pharynx for operative and postoperative hiccups
  - Antifungal treatment for *Candida* esophagitis
  - Correct electrolyte imbalance.
- Medical measures:
  - Relief of gastric distention (gastric lavage, nasogastric aspiration, induced vomiting)
  - Counterirritation of the vagus nerve (supraorbital pressure, carotid sinus massage, digital rectal massage) to be used with caution
  - Respiratory center stimulants (breathing 5% CO_2)
  - Psychiatric (hypnosis, behavioral modification)
  - Phrenic nerve block or electrical stimulation (5) (or pacing) of the dominant hemidiaphragm
  - acupuncture
  - Miscellaneous (cardioversion)

MEDICATION
First Line
Possible drug remedies:

- Baclofen, a GABA analog: 5–10 mg t.i.d. (best choice) (6)[A]
- Chlorpromazine: 25–50 mg IV (1)[B]
- Haloperidol: 2–12 mg IM
- Phenytoin: 200 mg IV, then 100 mg q.i.d.
- Metoclopramide: 5–10 mg q.i.d. (1)[B].
- Nifedipine: 10–20 mg/d to t.i.d.
- Amitriptyline: 10 mg t.i.d.
- Lidocaine: 1.5 mg/kg IV infusion followed by 0.75 mg/kg on subsequent days
- Gabapentin (Neurontin): up to 1,800 mg/d in divided doses (7)[B]
- Contraindications: Refer to manufacturer's literature:
  - Baclofen is not recommended in patients with stroke or other cerebral lesions, or in severe renal impairment (5).
- Precautions: Refer to manufacturer's literature:
  - Abrupt withdrawal of baclofen should be avoided.
- Maintenance drug therapy (e.g., baclofen, 5–10 mg t.i.d.; phenytoin, 100 mg q.i.d.; valproic acid, 15 mg/kg in divided doses; nifedipine, 10–20 mg daily to t.i.d.; metoclopramide, 10 mg q.i.d.); gabapentin, up to 1,800 mg in divided doses

Second Line
- Amantadine, carbidopa-levodopa in Parkinson disease
- Steroid replacement in Addison disease
- Antifungal agent in *Candida* esophagitis
- Ondansetron in carcinomatosis with vomiting
- Nefopam (a nonopioid analgesic with antishivering properties related to antihistamines and antiparkinsonian drugs) is available outside the US in both IV and oral formulations (8)[B].

ISSUES FOR REFERRAL
For acupuncture or phrenic nerve crush, block, or electrostimulation; cardioversion

SURGERY/OTHER PROCEDURES
- Phrenic nerve crush or transaction or electrostimulation of the dominant diaphragmatic leaflet (9)
- Resection of rib exostoses

COMPLEMENTARY AND ALTERNATIVE MEDICINE
- Acupuncture is increasingly being used to manage persistent or intractable hiccups (10,11)[B], especially in patients with cancer (12).
- Simple home remedies:
  - Swallowing a spoonful of sugar
  - Sucking on a hard candy or swallowing peanut butter
  - Holding breath and increasing pressure on diaphragm (Valsalva maneuver)
  - Tongue traction
  - Lifting the uvula with a cold spoon
  - Inducing fright
  - Smelling salts
  - Rebreathing into a paper (not plastic) bag
  - Sipping ice water
  - Rubbing a wet cotton-tipped applicator between hard and soft palate for 1 minute (13)[C]

IN-PATIENT CONSIDERATIONS
Admission Criteria/Initial Stabilization
Most patients can be managed as outpatients; those with severe intractable hiccups may require rehydration, pain control, IV medications, or surgery.

ONGOING CARE

FOLLOW-UP RECOMMENDATIONS
Patient Monitoring
Until hiccups cease

DIET
Avoid gastric distension from overeating, carbonated beverages, and aerophagia.

PATIENT EDUCATION
See "General Measures."

PROGNOSIS
- Hiccups often cease during sleep.
- Most acute benign hiccups resolve with home remedies or spontaneously.
- Intractable hiccups may last for years or decades.
- Hiccups have persisted despite bilateral phrenic nerve transection.

COMPLICATIONS
- Inability to eat
- Weight loss
- Exhaustion, debility
- Insomnia
- Cardiac arrhythmias
- Wound dehiscence
- Death (rare)

REFERENCES

1. Lewis JH. Hiccups and their cures. *Clin Perspect Gastroenterol*. 2000;3:277–283.
2. Howes D. Hiccups: A new explanation for the mysterious reflex. *Bioessays*. 2012;34(6):451–453. Epub 2012 Feb 29.
3. Miwa H, Kondo T. Hiccups in Parkinson's disease: An overlooked non-motor symptom? *Parkinsonism Relat. Disord*. 2010;16:249–251.
4. Kranke P, Eberhart LH, Morin AM. Treatment of hiccups during general anaesthesia or sedation: A qualitative systematic review. *Eur J Anaesthesiol*. 2003;20:239–244.
5. Chen KS, Bullard MJ, Chien YY, et al. Baclofen toxicity in patients with severely impaired renal function. *Ann Pharmacother*. 1997;31(11):1315–1320.
6. Ramírez FC, Graham DY. Treatment of intractable hiccup with baclofen: Results of a double-blind randomized, controlled, cross-over study. *Am J Gastroenterol*. 1992;87:1789–1791.
7. Thompson DF, Brooks KG. Gabapentin therapy of hiccups. *Ann Pharmacother*. 2013;47(6):897–903.
8. Bilotta F, Rosa G. Nefopam for severe hiccups. *N Engl J Med*. 2000;343:1973–1974.
9. Okuda Y, Kitajima T, Asai T. Use of a nerve stimulator for phrenic nerve block in treatment of hiccups. *Anesthesiology*. 1998;88:525–527.
10. Moretto EN, Wee B, Wiffen PJ, et al. Interventions for treating persistent and intractable hiccups in adults. *Cochrane Database Syst Rev*. 2013 Jan 31;1:CD008768 doi:10.1002/14651858.
11. Schiff E, River Y, Oliven A. Acupuncture therapy for persistent hiccups. *Am J Med Sci*. 2002;323:166–168.
12. Choi T-Y, Lee MS, Ernst E. Acupuncture for cancer patients suffering from hiccups: A systematic review and meta-analysis. *Complement Ther Med*. 2012;20(6):447–455.
13. Brostoff JM, Birns J, Benjamin E. The "cotton bud technique" as a cure for hiccups. *Eur Arch Otorhinolaryngol*. 2009;266(5):775–776.

ADDITIONAL READING

- Chang FY, Lu CL. Hiccup: Mystery, nature and treatment. *J Neurogastroenterol Motil*. 2012;18(2):123–130. Epub 2012 Apr 9.
- Landers C, Turner D, Makin C, et al. Propofol associated hiccups and treatment with lidocaine. *Anesth Analg*. 2008;107(5):1757–1758.
- Marinella MA. Diagnosis and management of hiccups in the patient with advanced cancer. *J Support Oncol*. 2009;7:122–127, 130.

 CODES

ICD10
- F45.8 Other somatoform disorders
- R06.6 Hiccough

CLINICAL PEARLS
- An organic cause for persistent hiccups is more likely to be found in men.
- Rule out a foreign body in the ear canal as a trigger.
- Baclofen remains the only pharmacologic therapy proven effective in a clinical trial setting.
- Acupuncture is proving very effective in persistent hiccups refractory to other therapies.

H

HIDRADENITIS SUPPURATIVA

Bridget E. McIlwee, DO • Jessica L. Borowicz, DO, FAOCD

 BASICS

DESCRIPTION
- Acute, tender, cystlike or nodular subcutaneous abscesses, commonly occurring in the skin of the axillae, perineum, areolae, and inframammary regions (rarely near umbilicus, scalp, trunk, or face)
- Chronic abscess formation with rupture and re-epithelialization causes sinus tracts to develop.
- Common from late puberty through age 40
- System affected: Skin
- Synonym(s): Acne inversa; Verneuil disease; Apocrinitis; Hidradenitis axillaris

Geriatric Considerations
Rare after menopause

Pediatric Considerations
Rarely occurs before puberty; occurrence in children associated with premature adrenarche

Pregnancy Considerations
No isotretinoin (Accutane) or tetracycline treatment during pregnancy. Disease may ease during pregnancy and rebound after parturition.

EPIDEMIOLOGY
- Predominant age of onset: 11–40 years
- Predominant sex: Female > Male (3:1)

Incidence
Peak onset during 2nd and 3rd decades of life

Prevalence
0.3–4%

ETIOLOGY AND PATHOPHYSIOLOGY
- Traditionally considered a disorder of apocrine glands, but now believed to be an inflammatory disorder of the hair follicle triggered by follicular plugging within apocrine gland–bearing skin.
- Lymphohisticytic and granulomatous inflammation of the terminal hair follicle, sinus tract formation, and scarring
- Bacterial involvement is a secondary event.
- Sebum excretion is not an important factor.
- Smoking is a major factor in disease onset and severity.
- Considered part of follicular occlusive tetrad: Acne conglobata, dissecting cellulitis of scalp, hidradenitis suppurativa, and pilonidal cysts
- A genetic component may exist.

Genetics
Unknown; some studies suggest single gene transmission (autosomal-dominant), but the condition may also be polygenic.

RISK FACTORS
- Obesity
- Smoking
- Hyperandrogenism
- Lithium may trigger onset of or exacerbate this condition.
- Androgenic progestins in oral contraceptive pills (OCPs) may trigger onset of this condition.

GENERAL PREVENTION
- Weight loss if overweight or obese.
- Smoking cessation (1)[A]
- Avoid constrictive clothing/synthetic fabrics, frictional trauma, heat exposure, excessive sweating, shaving, depilation, and deodorants.
- Use antiseptic soaps; apply tea tree oil topically.

COMMONLY ASSOCIATED CONDITIONS
- Acne conglobata (not acne vulgaris)
- Perifolliculitis capitis abscedens et suffodiens (dissecting cellulitis of scalp)
- Pilonidal disease
- Arthritis and spondyloarthritis (seronegative)
- Obesity with associated diabetes mellitus, atopy, or acanthosis nigricans
- Irritable bowel disease (notably Crohn disease)
- Squamous cell carcinoma

 DIAGNOSIS

HISTORY
Diagnostic criteria adopted by the 2nd International Conference on Hidradenitis Suppurativa, March 2009, San Francisco, CA. All 3 criteria must be present for diagnosis:
- Typical lesions (i.e., deep-seated painful nodules): "Blind boils" in early lesions; abscesses, draining sinus, bridged scars, and "tombstone" double-ended pseudocomedones in secondary lesions.
- Typical topography (i.e., axillae, groins, perineal and perianal region, buttocks, infra- and intermammary folds
- Chronicity and recurrences:
  – Other historical considerations:
    ○ Onset after puberty; flares associated with menstrual cycles
    ○ Poor response to conventional antibiotics
    ○ Personal or family history of acne or pilonidal sinuses and premenstrual exacerbation of boils
    ○ Early signs of pruritus, erythema, and local hyperhidrosis
    ○ Associated arthritis and arthropathy

PHYSICAL EXAM
- Tender nodules (dome-shaped) 0.5–3 cm in size are present:
  – Location corresponds with the distribution of apocrine-related mammary tissue and terminal hair follicles dependent on low androgen concentrations, with axillae and the groin being most common sites.
  – Sites ordered by frequency of occurrence: Axillary, inguinal, perianal and perineal, mammary and inframammary, buttock, pubic region, chest, scalp, retroauricular, eyelid (1)
  – Large lesions are often fluctuant; comedones may be present.
  – Possible malodorous discharge
- Staging: Commonly done with the Hurley staging system, although the Sartorius staging system may soon become more common:
  – Hurley staging system:
    ○ Stage I: Abscess formation (singular or multiple) without sinus tracts or scarring
    ○ Stage II: ≥1 widely separated, recurrent abscesses with tract formation and scars
    ○ Stage III: Multiple interconnected tracts and abscesses throughout an entire area

DIFFERENTIAL DIAGNOSIS
- Furunculosis/Carbuncles: Differentiate by specific culture, response to specific antibiotics.
- Infected Bartholin or sebaceous cysts
- Lymphadenopathy/Lymphadenitis
- Cutaneous Langerhans cell histiocytosis
- Actinomycosis

- Granuloma inguinale
- Lymphogranuloma venereum
- Apocrine nevus
- Crohn disease with anogenital fistula(s) (may coexist with hidradenitis suppurativa or be mistaken for it)
- Cutaneous tuberculosis
- Fox-Fordyce disease

DIAGNOSTIC TESTS & INTERPRETATION
Initial Tests (lab, imaging)
- Cultures of skin or aspirates of boils are most commonly negative. When positive, cultures are often polymicrobial and commonly grow *Staphylococci aureus* and *S. epidermidis*.
- Consider lesion biopsy to differentiate from, e.g., Crohn disease or squamous cell carcinoma.
- May note increased ESR, leukocytosis, decreased serum iron, normocytic anemia, or changes in serum electrophoresis pattern
- Consider additional studies at baseline:
  – CBC count with differential
  – Basic metabolic panel + magnesium
  – LFTs
  – Glucose-6-phosphate dehydrogenase level
  – Fasting lipids
- Purified protein derivative

Follow-Up Tests & Special Considerations
- Consider biopsy of concerning lesions due to increased risk of squamous cell carcinoma, other malignancies with chronic disease.
- If the patient is female, overweight, and/or hirsute, check:
  – Dehydroepiandrosterone sulfate
  – Testosterone: Total and free
  – Sex-hormone-binding globulin
  – Progesterone

Diagnostic Procedures/Other
- Incision and drainage of lesion(s) with culture and biopsy.
- US may be useful in planning an excision to identify the full extent of sinus tracts.

Test Interpretation
- Dermis shows granulomatous inflammation and inflammatory cells, giant cells, sinus tracts, subcutaneous abscesses, and, later, extensive fibrosis.
- Hair follicular dilatation and occlusion by keratinized stratified squamous epithelium is typically observed.

 TREATMENT

- Conservative treatment includes all items under general prevention, plus use of warm compresses, sitz baths, topical antiseptics for inflamed lesions, and nonopioid analgesics (2)[C].
- Weight loss and smoking cessation result in marked improvement (3).
- For stage I–II, attempt medical treatment first because of the extensive nature of surgical treatment. Short medical trial may be appropriate in stage III prior to moving on to surgical therapies. (1)[A]
- No medications are curative; relapse is almost inevitable, but the disease may be temporarily controlled.

GENERAL MEASURES
- Symptomatic treatment for acute lesions
- Frequent local cleansing with germicidal soap
- Improve environmental factors that cause follicular blockage (see "General Prevention").
- Smoking cessation and weight loss

MEDICATION
First Line
- Stage I disease: Consider either systemic or topical antibiotics:
  - Topical antibiotics: Select 1 of the following (clindamycin has the most evidence):
    - Clindamycin 1% solution b.i.d. (×12 weeks at a minimum) (1,2,4) [A]
    - Benzoyl peroxide 5–10% solution b.i.d. (4)[C]
    - Chlorhexidine 4% solution b.i.d. (4)[C]
  - Systemic antibiotics: Select 1 of the following:
    - Tetracycline: 500 mg b.i.d. (>12 weeks)
    - PO clindamycin: 300 mg b.i.d. and rifampin 300 mg b.i.d. for 12 weeks (5)[B]
- Stage II–III disease:
  - Address overlying bacterial infection with broad-spectrum coverage. Base antibiotic selection on disease location, characteristics (e.g., clindamycin/rifampin, rifampin/moxifloxacin/metronidazole) (1)[A]
  - More aggressive treatment (i.e., surgery) will likely be needed, but alternative medical management may lead to improvement:
    - Immunosuppressive therapies with infliximab, adalimumab, (1,2,4)[A,C], or etanercept (6)

Second Line
- Stage I:
  - Consider low-dose birth control pills for women (e.g., Norinyl, Ortho-Novum) (2)[C].
  - Sulfamethoxazole/trimethoprim DS b.i.d. (4).
  - Oral amoxicillin 250–500 mg b.i.d., tetracycline, minocycline 50–100 mg b.i.d., doxycycline 50–100 mg b.i.d., or erythromycin (2)[C]
  - Limited lesions or flares can be treated with intralesional or short-course PO corticosteroids: Triamcinolone (2)[C].
  - Dapsone topical, apply b.i.d. (2)[C]
  - Finasteride 5 mg/d (consider only after menopause) (2,4)[C]
- Stage II–III disease or recalcitrant Stage I:
  - Systemic retinoids: Isotretinoin 40–80 mg PO every day for 4 months (2)[C]
  - Cyproterone acetate (if available) (2)[B]

ISSUES FOR REFERRAL
- Lack of response to treatment, stage II–III disease, or concern for malignancy (such as squamous cell carcinoma) is a reason to refer for surgical excision or radiation/laser treatment (stage II).
- If significant psychosocial stress exists secondary to disease, referral for stress management and a support group is recommended.
- Suspicion of hyperandrogenic states (e.g., PCOS) should prompt referral to endocrinology (1)[A].
- Severe perianal/perivulvar disease or otherwise very extensive disease may prompt referral to plastic surgeon or reconstructive urologist (1)[A].

SURGERY/OTHER PROCEDURES
- Various surgical approaches have been used for stage II–III disease:
  - Incision and drainage is discouraged as it is rarely curative (2,7)[C].

- Deroofing and marsupialization of the sinus tracts may be of benefit primarily for Hurley stage I–II disease, as healing time is reduced. Recurrences are sometimes seen, but usually are smaller than the original lesions.
  - Wide full-thickness excision with healing by granulation or flap placement is the most definitive treatment and rarely has local recurrence if all sinus tracts are excised. Rates of local recurrence (within 3–72 months) are axillary (3%), perianal (0%), inguinoperineal (37%), and submammary (50%).
- Laser therapy for Hurley stage I–II disease:
  - Consider monthly treatments with Nd:YAG laser for 3–4 months (1)[A].
  - CO_2 laser ablation with healing by secondary intention has recent data with good results (1)[A].

ONGOING CARE

FOLLOW-UP RECOMMENDATIONS
Follow-up monthly or sooner to evaluate progress and to assist with symptom management.

DIET
No limitations; if overweight, weight loss should be encouraged.

PATIENT EDUCATION
- Severity can range from only 2–3 papules per year to extensive draining sinus tracts.
- Medications are temporizing measures; rarely curative. Smoking cessation and weight loss can improve symptoms significantly.
- Attempts at local surgical "cures" do not affect recurrence at other sites.
- Hidradenitis suppurativa is considered a misnomer; acne inversa may be a more accurate term.
- Hidradenitis Suppurativa Foundation: www.hs-foundation.org

PROGNOSIS
- Individual lesions (with or without drainage) heal slowly in 10–30 days.
- Recurrences may last for several years.
- Spontaneous resolution rarely occurs.
- Relentlessly progressive scarring and sinus tracts are likely with severe disease.
- Radical wide-area excision, with removal of all hair-bearing skin in the affected area, shows the greatest chance for cure.

COMPLICATIONS
- Contracture of skin after extensive abscess rupture, scarring, and healing; or at sites of surgical excisions.
- Rarely, squamous cell carcinoma may develop in indolent sinus tracts (usually anogenital).
- Disseminated infection or septicemia (unusual)
- Lymphedema
- Urethral/Rectal fistula
- Anemia, amyloidosis, and hypoproteinemia (due to chronic suppuration) (5)
- Interstitial keratitis
- Lumbosacral epidural abscess
- Sacral bacterial osteomyelitis
- Depression and/or suicide

REFERENCES
1. Rambhatla PV, Lim HW, Hamzavi I. A systematic review of treatments for hidradenitis suppurativa. Arch Dermatol. 2012;148(4):439–446.
2. Lam J, Krakowski AC, Friedlander SF. Hidradenitis suppurativa (acne inversa): Management of a recalcitrant disease. Pediatr Dermatol. 2007;24: 465–473.
3. Sartorius K, Emtestam L, Jemec GB, et al. Objective scoring of hidradenitis suppurativa reflecting the role of tobacco smoking and obesity. Br J Dermatol. 2009;161(4):831–839.
4. Lee RA, Yoon A, Kist J. Hidradenitis suppurativa: An update. Adv Dermatol. 2007;23:289–306.
5. Alikhan A, Lynch PJ, Eisen DB. Hidradenitis suppurativa: A comprehensive review. J Am Acad Dermatol. 2009;60(4):539–561.
6. Grant A, Gonzalez T, Montgomery MO, et al. Infliximab therapy for patients with moderate to severe hidradenitis suppurativa: A randomized, double-blind, placebo-controlled crossover trial. J Am Acad Dermatol. 2010;62:205–217.
7. Slade DE, Powell BW, Mortimer PS. Hidradenitis suppurativa: Pathogenesis and management. Br J Plast Surg. 2003;56:451–461.

ADDITIONAL READING
- Hazen PG, Hazen BP. Hidradenitis suppurativa: Successful treatment using carbon dioxide laser excision and marsupialization. Dermatol Surg. 2010;36:208–213.
- Jemec GB, Wendelboe P. Topical clindamycin versus systemic tetracycline in the treatment of hidradenitis suppurativa. J Am Acad Dermatol. 1998;39: 971–974.
- Kagan RJ, Yakuboff KP, Warner P, et al. Surgical treatment of hidradenitis suppurativa: A 10-year experience. Surgery. 2005;138(4):734–740; discussion 740–741.
- Mandal A, Watson J. Experience with different treatment modules in hidradenitis suppuritiva: A study of 106 cases. Surgeon. 2005;3(1):23–26.
- Mendonça CO, Griffiths CE. Clindamycin and rifampicin combination therapy for hidradenitis suppurativa. Br J Dermatol. 2006;154(5):977–978.
- Shuja F, Chan CS, Rosen T. Biologic drugs for the treatment of hidradenitis suppurativa: An evidence-based review. Dermatol Clin. 2010;28(3):511–521, 523–524; quiz 522–523.

CODES

ICD10
L73.2 Hidradenitis suppurativa

CLINICAL PEARLS
- Hidradenitis suppurativa is a chronic inflammatory disease of the skin, occurring most commonly in areas corresponding to apocrine-related mammary tissue, such as the axillae, perineum, and inframammary regions. The disease is often difficult to control with behavior changes and medication alone.
- For patients with refractory or severe disease, surgery (wide local excision with removal of all hair-bearing skin in the area) provides the only chance at a cure. Success rates depend on the location and extent of excision.

H

HIRSUTISM

Laura Novak, MD • Jigar Kadakia, MD

 BASICS

DESCRIPTION
- Presence of excessive body and facial hair, in a male pattern, in women of reproductive age
- May be present in normal adults as an ethnic characteristic, or may develop as a result of androgen excess
- Often seen in association with polycystic ovarian syndrome (PCOS); may be accompanied by menstrual irregularities, insulin resistance, obesity, or acne
- System(s) affected: Dermatologic; Endocrine/Metabolic; Reproductive

Pregnancy Considerations
- May have related infertility. Offer intervention, if desired.
- As hormone balance improves, fertility may increase; provide contraception, as needed.
- Several medications used for treatment are contraindicated in pregnancy.

EPIDEMIOLOGY
Prevalence
5–10% of adult women

ETIOLOGY AND PATHOPHYSIOLOGY
Hirsutism is due to increased androgenic (male) hormones, either from increased peripheral binding (idiopathic), which is most common, or increased production from the ovaries, adrenals, or fat. Exogenous medications can also be associated with hirsutism.

Genetics
Multifactorial

RISK FACTORS
- Family history, race, ethnicity
- Anovulation

GENERAL PREVENTION
- Women with late-onset congenital adrenal hyperplasia should be counseled that they may be carriers for the severe early-onset childhood disease.
- Avoid quackery and unlicensed electrolysis.

COMMONLY ASSOCIATED CONDITIONS
- PCOS: Most common cause of hirsutism. Variable presentation, but commonly presents with some combination of excess androgen and abnormal menses and insulin resistance. It is estimated that 75% of hirsute women have PCOS.
- Insulin resistance syndromes/metabolic syndrome:
  – Presence of associated insulin resistance or PCOS can increase the risk of heart disease.
- Prolonged amenorrhea and anovulation:
  – Prolonged amenorrhea may, over time, put the patient at risk for endometrial hyperplasia or carcinoma.

- Hypothyroidism or hyperprolactinemia
- Late-onset congenital adrenal hyperplasia (21-hydroxylase deficiency): A genetic enzyme deficiency associated with more severe and earlier onset hirsutism. Present in <2% of hirsute, amenorrheic patients
- Tumor: Rare (<0.2%); ovarian or adrenal; especially if associated with virilization (rapid onset, clitoromegaly, balding, deepening voice)
- Cushing syndrome: Rare; characterized by central obesity, moon facies, striae, hypertension

 DIAGNOSIS

HISTORY
- Age of onset (usually gradual), duration of symptoms
- Obtain a menstrual and fertility history: Irregular menses may indicate PCOS.
- Medication history: Look for use of valproic acid, testosterone, danazol, athletic performance drugs.
- If galactorrhea is present, workup for hyperprolactinemia

PHYSICAL EXAM
- The Ferriman-Gallwey scale (an instrument that rates hair growth in 9 areas on a scale of 0–4, with >8 being positive) may be used for diagnosis, but underrates patient's perception of hirsutism.
- Increased androgens may be associated with acne, obesity, insulin resistance, and hyperlipidemia.
- Increased hair growth on face, chest, and groin. May be hidden by plucking.
- Acanthosis nigricans: Velvety black skin in the axilla, neck, in insulin resistance
- Virilization: Deep voice, balding, clitoromegaly can indicate risk of tumor.

DIFFERENTIAL DIAGNOSIS
Hirsutism is associated with a number of different conditions (see "Etiology").

DIAGNOSTIC TESTS & INTERPRETATION
- Diagnosis is clinical.
- Empiric treatment without lab workup is an acceptable option in mild–moderate hirsutism (1)[C].
- Lab testing is performed to rule out underlying tumor and pituitary diseases, which are rare.

Initial Tests (lab, imaging)
Basic workup recommended by ACOG (2)[C]. Total testosterone, thyroid-stimulating hormone (TSH), and, if clinically suspicious, an insulin resistance workup:

- Testosterone: Random testosterone level is usually sufficient. A morning free testosterone is slightly more sensitive, but the difference is not clinically relevant (2,3)[A]: Level >150 ng/dL may indicate ovarian tumor.

- TSH elevation indicates hypothyroidism.
- Insulin resistance testing: Results vary with age and ethnicity:
  – Fasting insulin level >20 or fasting glucose-to-insulin ratio <4.5 may indicate resistance.
  – ACOG recommends fasting and 2-hour glucose after 75-g glucose load in PCOS, but this may not be necessary.
- If testosterone is >150, the patient may have a tumor. Testosterone is made by both the ovaries and adrenals, so both areas should be scanned. US is best for the ovaries, and CT is best for the adrenals.
- Ovarian US can help in the diagnosis of PCOS.

Follow-Up Tests & Special Considerations
- 17-hydroxyprogesterone (17-OHP):
  – Elevations of 17-OHP (>300) can indicate nonclassic congenital adrenal hyperplasia; rare (<2%).
  – Consider in patients with onset in early adolescence or high-risk group (Ashkenazi Jews).
  – Elevated levels require additional testing.
- Prolactin level, if galactorrhea
- Dehydroepiandrosterone sulfate (DHEA-S) is no longer recommended routinely (4,5)[A]:
  – Levels >700 may indicate adrenal tumor.

 TREATMENT

GENERAL MEASURES
- Treatment is slow and often lifelong.
- If patient desires pregnancy, induction of ovulation may be necessary.
- Provide contraception, as needed.
- Encourage patient to maintain ideal weight.
- Treat accompanying acne.

MEDICATION
First Line
- Treatment goal is to decrease new hair growth and improve metabolic disorders.
- Oral contraceptives will decrease androgens, improve metabolic syndrome, and slow but not resolve hair growth. Takes 6 months to show effect and is continued for years; any preparation is effective (2)(C).
- Eflornithine (Vaniqa) HCl cream: Apply b.i.d.; reduces facial hair in 40% of women (with long-term use). Only FDA-approved hirsutism treatment.

Second Line

- Insulin sensitizers (metformin, thioglitazones) are mildly effective, but less so than oral contraceptives. May be used in diabetes or if oral contraceptives are contraindicated. Metformin is more effective than thioglitazones (6)[B].
- Antiandrogenic drugs must be used in combination with oral contraceptives to prevent menorrhagia and potential fetal toxicity; will further reduce hirsutism 15–25% (7,8)[B]. Usually begun after 6 months of first-line therapy if results are suboptimal. All should be avoided in pregnancy:
  - Spironolactone, 50–200 mg/d: Onset of action is slow; use with oral contraceptives to prevent menorrhagia. Watch for hyperkalemia, especially with drospirenone-containing OCP (Yasmin); contraindicated in pregnancy.
  - Finasteride: 5 mg/d decreases androgen binding; not approved by FDA. Use with contraception (pregnancy Category X).
  - Cyproterone, not available in the US: 12.5–100 mg/d days 5–15 of cycle combined with ethinyl estradiol 20–50 mcg days 5–25 of cycle
  - Flutamide: Nonsteroidal androgen receptor antagonist. Has not been used in the past due to hepatotoxicity and side effects, but at lower doses (125 mg/d) and used with oral contraceptives and metformin, has significant clinical effect (1,9).
- Steroids: Used in nonclassic congenital adrenal hyperplasia (NCCAH):
  - Dexamethasone: 2 mg/d

COMPLEMENTARY AND ALTERNATIVE MEDICINE

- Saw palmetto (Serenoa repens): In small studies, decreases hair growth via blocking 5-α-reductase activity in the skin (3)[C]. Has similar peripheral action to finasteride (decreasing 5-α-reductase).
- Spearmint tea: 1 cup b.i.d.: In a study of 21 patients, 1 cup b.i.d. for 6 months led to decreased hirsutism (10)[C].
- Licorice: In a small study, 9 women using 3.5 g/d for 2 cycles had benefit. Excess licorice can lead to hypokalemic hypertension (3)[C].

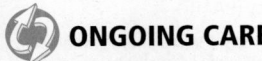

ONGOING CARE

FOLLOW-UP RECOMMENDATIONS
No special activity

Patient Monitoring
Monitor for known side effects of medications.

DIET
No special diet

PATIENT EDUCATION

- Hormonal treatment stops further hair growth, but will not usually reverse present hair.
- Treatment takes 6 months for effect and may be lifelong.
- Cosmetic measures include plucking, bleaching, shaving, electrolysis, laser hair removal, and cover-up cosmetics.
- If professional hair removal is chosen, laser/photoepilation is the preferred method, with the possible addition of eflornithine (Vaniqa) (1)[C].

PROGNOSIS

- Good (with long-term therapy) for halting further hair growth
- Moderate to poor for reversing current hair growth

COMPLICATIONS

- If PCOS is present, dysfunctional uterine bleeding may lead to anemia.
- If PCOS is present, anovulation may increase uterine cancer risk.
- Androgenic excess may adversely affect lipid status, cardiac risk, and bone density.
- Poor self-image/shame

REFERENCES

1. Martin KA, Chang RJ, Ehrmann DA, et al. Evaluation and treatment of hirsutism in premenopausal women: An endocrine society clinical practice guideline. *J Clin Endocrinol Metab*. 2008;93(4):1105–1120. Epub 2008 Feb 5.
2. ACOG Clinical Practice Guideline No. 44. *On the diagnosis and management of polycystic ovarian syndrome*. Washington, DC: American College of Obstetrics and Gynecology; 2002.
3. Meletis C, Zabriskis N. Natural approaches for treating polycystic ovarian syndrome. *Altern Complement Ther*. 2006;12(4):157–164.
4. Azziz R. The evaluation and management of hirsutism. *Obstet Gynecol*. 2003;101:995–1007.
5. Rosenfeld RL. Hirsutism. *N Eng J Med*. 2005; 353(24):2578–2588.
6. Harborne L, Fleming R, Lyall H, et al. Metformin or antiandrogen in the treatment of hirsutism in polycystic ovary syndrome. *J Clin Endocrinol Metab*. 2003;88:4116–4123.
7. Farquhar C, Lee O, Toomath R, et al. Spironolactone versus placebo or in combination with steroids for hirsutism and/or acne. *Cochrane Database Syst Rev*. 2003;CD000194.
8. Swiglo BA, Cosma M, Flynn DN, et al. Clinical review: Antiandrogens for the treatment of hirsutism: A systematic review and metaanalyses of randomized controlled trials. *J Clin Endocrinol Metab*. 2008;93:1153–1160.
9. Ong KK, de Zegher F, López-Bermejo A, et al. Flutamide metformin for post-menarcheal girls with preclinical ovarian androgen excess: Evidence for differential response by androgen receptor genotype. *Eur J Endocrinol*. 2007; 157(5):661–668.
10. Akdoan M, Tamer MN, Cüre E, et al. Effect of spearmint (*Mentha spicata*, Labiatae) teas on androgen levels in women with hirsutism. *Phytother Res*. 2007;21(5):444–447.

ADDITIONAL READING

- NIH- Evidence-based methodology workshop on PCOS. http://prevention.nih.gov/workshops/2012/pcos/docs/PCOS_Final_Statement.pdf.
- Radosh L. Drug treatments for polycystic ovary syndrome. *Am Fam Physician*. 2009;79:671–676.

 SEE ALSO

Acne Vulgaris; Infertility; Polycystic Ovarian Syndrome (PCOS)

 CODES

ICD10
- E28.2 Polycystic ovarian syndrome
- L68.0 Hirsutism

CLINICAL PEARLS

- PCOS is the most common cause of hirsutism.
- Treatment is long term and often lifelong.

H

HIV INFECTION AND AIDS
Adam Barta, MD

BASICS

DESCRIPTION
HIV is a retrovirus that integrates into CD4 T lymphocytes (a critical component of cell-mediated immunity), causing cell death and resulting in severe immunodeficiency, opportunistic infections, and malignancies:

- Because of treatment advances, HIV is now a classified a chronic disease.
- The natural history of untreated HIV infection includes viral transmission, acute retroviral syndrome, recovery and seroconversion, asymptomatic chronic HIV infection, and symptomatic HIV infection or AIDS.
- Without antiretroviral treatment, the average patient develops AIDS ~10 years after transmission.
- All HIV-infected persons with CD4 <200 cells/mm^3 or having AIDS-defining illnesses are categorized as having AIDS.

EPIDEMIOLOGY
Incidence
- At the end of 2008, 33.4 million people were estimated to be living with HIV/AIDS worldwide per UNAIDS and the World Health Organization. Yearly, 2.7 million new HIV infections and 2 million deaths are attributable to AIDS
- In the US, HIV incidence has remained relatively stable at about 50,000 infections per year since the mid-1990s.

Prevalence
- Estimated 1.2 million persons in the US are living with HIV/AIDS as of 2010 (1,2); 20% unaware of their status (2)
- HIV/AIDS cases are disproportionately high among racial/ethnic minority populations
- Transmission of a drug-resistant virus rising
- Younger females particularly vulnerable

ETIOLOGY AND PATHOPHYSIOLOGY
HIV, a retrovirus

Genetics
People who lack CCR5, a cell-surface chemokine coreceptor used by HIV to infect cells, are highly resistant to HIV infection

RISK FACTORS
- Sexual activity (70% of world transmission): Viral load strongest predictor of heterosexual transmission with ulcerative urogenital lesions (3)[B].
- Male-to-male sexual contact accounted for 61% of newly diagnosed HIV/AIDS cases in 2009.
- Injection drug use
- Children of HIV-infected women:
  - Maternal HIV-1 RNA level is the best predictor of transmission risk.
  - HIV testing and use of antiretroviral drugs in pregnant women and their newborns has reduced the incidence of perinatal HIV transmission by >70% (from 25–29% without treatment to 8% with treatment) (4)[B].
  - Pregnant women should be treated until viral load is undetectable.
  - Can be transmitted through breastfeeding
- Recipients of blood products between 1975 and March 1985
- Occupational exposure

GENERAL PREVENTION
Avoid unprotected sexual intercourse and injection drug abuse.

COMMONLY ASSOCIATED CONDITIONS
- Syphilis may be more aggressive if HIV-infected
- Tuberculosis (TB) is coepidemic with HIV; test all persons with HIV for TB. Dually infected patients: 100 × greater risk of developing active TB disease (compared with non-HIV) and higher rates of multidrug-resistant TB
- Patients coinfected with hepatitis C have a more rapid progression to cirrhosis.

DIAGNOSIS

- Acute retroviral syndrome: Precipitous decline in CD4 lymphocyte count and increased viremia ~1–4 weeks after transmission. Confirmed by demonstrating a high HIV RNA in the absence of HIV antibody.
- Mononucleosis-like syndrome, including:
  - Fever (97%)
  - Adenopathy
  - Pharyngitis (73%)
  - Rash (77%)
  - Myalgias/Arthralgia (58%)
  - Less common: Headache, diarrhea, nausea, vomiting, hepatosplenomegaly, weight loss, thrush, and neurologic symptoms (12%)
  - Seroconversion: Development of a positive HIV antibody test usually occurs within 4 weeks of acute infection and invariably by 6 months.
  - Asymptomatic infection: Variable duration (average 8–10 years) and is accompanied by a gradual decline in CD4 cell counts and a relatively stable HIV RNA levels (the viral "set point"). Persistent lymphadenopathy: >1 cm in ≥2 extrainguinal sites; persists >3 months
- Symptomatic conditions:
  - Fever or diarrhea >1 month, bacillary angiomatosis, thrush, persistent candidal vulvovaginitis, cervical dysplasia or carcinoma in situ, oral hairy leukoplakia, herpes zoster, idiopathic thrombocytopenic purpura, pelvic inflammatory disease, peripheral neuropathy or myelopathy
- AIDS: Defined by a CD4 cell count <200, a CD4 cell percentage of total lymphocytes <14%, or 1 of several AIDS-related opportunistic infections: *Pneumocystis jiroveci (carinii)* pneumonia, cryptococcal meningitis, recurrent bacterial pneumonia, candida esophagitis, CNS toxoplasmosis, tuberculosis and non-Hodgkin lymphoma (NHL), progressive multifocal encephalopathy, HIV nephropathy, Kaposi sarcoma, NHL, Hodgkin lymphoma, invasive cervical cancer
- Advanced HIV disease: CD4 cell count <50. Most AIDS-related deaths occur at this time. Common late opportunistic infections: Cytomegalovirus (CMV) disease (retinitis, colitis) or disseminated *Mycobacterium avium* complex as well as HIV wasting syndrome (>10% weight loss) and HIV encephalopathy/dementia/minor cognitive-motor disorder.

HISTORY
- Medical history, including STDs and TB
- Review of systems: Fever, chills, night sweats, diarrhea, weight loss, fatigue, adenopathy, oral sores, odynophagia (esophageal candidiasis), cough, shortness of breath and dyspnea on exertion (early *P. jiroveci* pneumonia), visual changes (CMV retinitis <200 CD4), skin rash, neurologic symptoms (CNS infection, malignancy, or dementia), sinusitis
- Social history, transmission risks, adherence
- Immunization review

PHYSICAL EXAM
Focus on weight, skin, retinal exam, oropharynx; lymph nodes; liver, spleen, mental status, sensation, genital and rectal examinations

DIFFERENTIAL DIAGNOSIS
Order other tests/serologies if HIV RNA test is negative. Order throat cultures for bacterial/viral respiratory pathogens, Epstein-Barr virus viral capsid antigen IgM/Igg, CMV IgM/IgG, human herpesvirus 6 IgM/IgG, and hepatitis serologies as appropriate to establish a diagnosis for patient's symptoms.

DIAGNOSTIC TESTS & INTERPRETATION
Initial Tests (lab, imaging)
- Screening: ELISA reported as reactive or nonreactive; sensitivity and specificity >98%. Obtain HIV RNA if acute HIV infection is suspected:
  - New rapid and oral test available (home test kit, OraSure, OraQuick Advance Rapid HIV test).
- Confirmatory: Western blot:
  - Results positive, negative, or indeterminate
  - Per the CDC: Positive test is reaction with 2 of these 3 bands: P24, gp 41, and gp 120/160. If indeterminate, repeat test in 3–6 months.
- CD4 cell count and percentage (5)[A]
- HIV RNA viral load (5)[A]
- CBC with differential
- Serum chemistry
- Serologies: Hepatitis A, B, and C; syphilis.
- Urine screen for STIs (*Neisseria gonorrhoeae, Chlamydia trachomatis*)
- Cervical cytology
- Purified protein derivative (PPD)
- Glucose-6-phosphate levels
- Lipids at baseline and during highly active antiretroviral therapy (HAART)
- Genotypic tests for resistance to antiretrovirals for patients who have pretreatment HIV RNA >1,000 copies/mL regardless of whether therapy will be initiated immediately (5)[A]
- Chest x-ray if pulmonary symptoms or positive PPD.

TREATMENT

- Antiretroviral therapy should be initiated in all patients with a history of an AIDS-defining illness or with a CD4 count <350 (5)[A]
- Antiretroviral therapy should be initiated regardless of CD4 count in patients with the following conditions: Pregnancy, HIV-associated nephropathy and HBV coinfections when treatment of hepatitis B virus is indicated (5)[A], rapidly declining CD4 counts (e.g., >100 cells/mm^3 decrease per year), higher viral load (e.g., >100,000 copies/mL) (5)[B]
- Antiretroviral therapy is recommended for all patients with CD4 count between 350 and 500 (5)[A].
- Consider for patients with CD4 count >500 (5)[B].

- Emtricitabine/tenofovir disoproxil fumarate (Truvada) FDA approved in July 2012 for pre-exposure prophylaxis (PrEP) in combination with safer sex practices to reduce the risk of sexually acquired HIV infection in adults at high risk.

GENERAL MEASURES
- Main goal of HAART: Reduce the viral load, ideally to <50 HIV-1 RNA copies/mL), and delay immune suppression. Viral load is the most important indicator of response to HAART.
- Check for transmitted drug resistance before starting HAART 5(A)
- An adequate CD4 response for most patients on therapy is defined as an increase in CD4 count in range of 50–150 cells/mm^3 per year with an accelerated response in the first 3 months (5).
- Prevent HIV-associated complications, short- and long-term adverse drug reactions, HIV transmission, HIV drug resistance, and preservation of HIV treatment options.
- Assess substance abuse, economic factors (e.g., unstable housing), social support, mental illness, comorbidities, high-risk behaviors, and other factors that are known to impair the ability to adhere to treatment and to promote HIV transmission.
- Occupational exposure: Treatment after exposure in conjunction with expert consultation
- Prophylactic antimicrobial agents and vaccines:
  – *P. jiroveci:* Trimethoprim/sulfamethoxazole (TMP-SMX) 1 DS daily or 1 SS daily indicated if CD4 <200/mm^3, prior *P. jiroveci*, thrush, or unexplained fever for >2 weeks
  – *Mycobacterium tuberculosis:* Treat if PPD >5 mm induration without prior prophylaxis or treatment, recent TB contact, or history of inadequately treated TB that healed. Confirmed by culture. Treatment is based on susceptibility.
  – *Toxoplasma gondii:* 33% per year risk of infection in untreated patients with CD4 <100/mm^3; prophylaxis: TMP-SMX DS daily.
  – *M. avium* complex: 20–40% risk with CD4 <50 and no HAART. Preferred prophylaxis is clarithromycin 500 mg PO b.i.d., or azithromycin 1,200 mg PO weekly.
  – Varicella: Seronegative and unexposed are at risk if exposed to chickenpox or shingles. Preferred regimen is VZIG 5 vials within 96 hours but preferably within 48 hours.
  – *Streptococcus pneumoniae:* 50–100 times increased risk of invasive infection compared with general population; Pneumovax every 5 years
  – Influenza vaccine each autumn
  – Hepatitis A and B vaccines for at-risk patients
  – Tetanus: dT vaccine in adults

MEDICATION
- Nucleoside reverse transcriptase inhibitors (NRTIs):
  – Abacavir (ABC, Ziagen), didanosine (DDL, Videx), emtricitabine (FTC, Emtriva), lamivudine (3TC, Epivir), stavudine (d4T, Zerit), tenofovir (Viread), zalcitabine (ddC, Hivid), zidovudine (AZT, Retrovir), zidovudine + lamivudine (Combivir), zidovudine ± lamivudine ± abacavir (Trizivir), tenofovir ± emtricitabine (Truvada), abacavir ± lamivudine (Epzicom)
- Nonnucleoside reverse transcriptase inhibitors (NNRTIs): Delavirdine (Rescriptor); efavirenz (Sustiva); nevirapine (Viramune); rilpivirine (6)[A] (Edurant); efavirenz ± Truvada (Atripla); rilpivirine ± Truvada (Complera)
- Protease inhibitors (PIs): Amprenavir (Agenerase), atazanavir (Reyataz), darunavir (Prezista),

fosamprenavir (Lexiva), indinavir (Crixivan), lopinavir-ritonavir (Kaletra), nelfinavir (Viracept), ritonavir (Norvir), saquinavir (Fortovase, Invirase), tipranavir (Aptivus)
- Fusion inhibitors: Enfuvirtide (Fuzeon)
- Entry inhibitors: Maraviroc (Selzentry)
- Integrase inhibitors: Raltegravir (Isentress) Stribild (elvitegravir ± cobicistat ± tenofovir ± emtricitabine)
- Drug failure: Before selecting regimen, review clinical symptoms, history of HAART, and adherence. Perform resistance testing.
- Protease inhibitors can cause metabolic syndrome (lipodystrophy, decreased high-density lipoprotein, increased triglycerides, high BP, and hyperglycemia).
- HAART, especially the protease inhibitors, have potentially life-threatening interactions.

First Line
- Nonnucleoside reverse-transcriptase inhibitors (NNRTI) + 2 NNRTI (5)[A]
- Efavirenz is a preferred NNRTI in 1st-line treatment regimen for HIV treatment, particularly in resource limited settings (7)[A]
- PIs (preferably boosted with ritonavir) + 2 NRTI (5)[A]
- Integrase inhibitor + 2 NRTI (5)[A]

ONGOING CARE

FOLLOW-UP RECOMMENDATIONS
Patient Monitoring
- If HIV RNA is detectable at 2–8 weeks, repeat every 4–8 weeks until suppression to less than level of detection, then every 3–6 months (5)
- Monitor HIV RNA, CD4, and CBC every 3–4 months (5).
- Test fasting lipids and fasting glucose annually if normal. Basic chemistry, aspartate aminotransferase, alanine aminotransferase, T/D bilirubin every 6–12 months (5)
- HLA-B 5701 if considering abacavir (5)
- Pregnancy test if starting efavirenz (5)

DIET
- Encourage good nutrition and multivitamin use
- Avoid raw eggs and unpasteurized milk. Severely immunocompromised patients should boil tap water to prevent *Cryptosporidium.*

PATIENT EDUCATION
- Provide nonjudgmental prevention counseling, reviewing routes and behaviors leading to transmission to others and acquisition of super infection with resistant strains.
- Counsel on importance of adherence to HAART and prevention of resistance.
- National AIDS Hotline: 800-342-2437 [Spanish 800-342-7432]
- National Institute of Health AIDS Clinical Trials Group: 800-874-2572
- American Foundation for AIDS Research: 212-719-0033 (new treatments and research)
- Information available at: www.aidsinfo.nih.gov

PROGNOSIS
- When untreated HIV infection leads to AIDS, the life expectancy is 3.7 years.
- AIDS-defining opportunistic infections usually do not develop until CD4 <200.
- In untreated HIV infection, CD4 counts decline at a rate of 50–80 per year, with more rapid decline as counts drop <200.

- Adherence failure—not drug resistance—is the most common cause of treatment failure (2)[B].

COMPLICATIONS
- Immunodeficiency
- Opportunistic infections
- Malignancy, including cervical or anal cancer

REFERENCES
1. Centers for Disease Control and Prevention: Diagnoses of HIV infection and AIDS in the United States and Dependent Areas, 2008 HIV Surveillance Report, Volume 2. Available at: www.cdc.gov/hiv/surveillance/resources/reports/2008report/
2. HIV in the United States: At a glance. Available at: www.cdc.gov/hiv/resources/factsheets/PDF/HIV_at_aa_glance.pdf
3. Quinn TC, Wawer MJ, Sewankambo N, et al. Viral load and heterosexual transmission of human immunodeficiency virus type 1. Rakai Project Study Group. *N Engl J Med.* 2000;342:921–929.
4. US Public Health Service Task Force recommendations for use of antiretroviral drugs in pregnant HIV-1 infected women for maternal health interventions to reduce perinatal HIV-1 transmission in the US. *MMWR.* 2002;51:1–38.
5. US Department of Health and Human Services. Guide for the use of antiretroviral agents in HIV-1 infected adults and adolescents. Available at: http://aidsinfo.nih.gov/contentfiles/HealthCare OccupExpoGL.pdf
6. Schafer JJ, Short WR. Rilpivirine, a novel non-nucleoside reverse transcriptase inhibitor for the management of HIV-1 infection: A systematic review. *Antivir Ther (Lond).* 2012;17:1495–1502.
7. Pillay P, Ford N, Shubber Z, et al. Outcomes for efavirenz versus nevirapine-containing regimens for treatment of HIV-1 infection: A systematic review and meta-analysis. *PLoS One.* 2013;8:e68995.

ADDITIONAL READING
Simon V, Ho DD, Abdool Karim Q. HIV/AIDS epidemiology, pathogenesis, prevention, and treatment. *Lancet.* 2006;368:489–504.

 CODES

ICD10
- B20 Human immunodeficiency virus [HIV] disease
- R75 Inconclusive laboratory evidence of human immunodef virus
- Z21 Asymptomatic human immunodeficiency virus infection status

CLINICAL PEARLS
- Acute HIV symptoms: Fever, sore throat, adenopathy, myalgias, and rash.
- Treatment guidelines are evolving to include earlier initiation of HAART in the course of the illness.
- Transmitted drug resistance is increasing so evaluate for resistant strains before starting HAART.
- The prophylactic measures strongly recommended for HIV-infected patients are vaccination and prophylactic antibiotics based on history and CD4 count.

H

HODGKIN LYMPHOMA
Jennifer Gao, MD • Fred J. Schiffman, MD

 BASICS

DESCRIPTION
Historical background:

- Described in 1832 by Thomas Hodgkin in *On some morbid appearance of the absorbent glands and spleen*
- First neoplasm to be: (i) Defined by cytologic grounds based on presence of Reed-Sternberg cells, (ii) clinically staged neoplastic disease, and (iii) treated with chemotherapy and/or radiotherapy
- Neoplastic Reed-Sternberg (RS) cells of monoclonal lymphoid B-cell origin within inflammatory background of lymphocytes (T-helper type 2 and regulatory T cells), eosinophils, histiocytes, and plasma cells
- 2 subtypes: Classic Hodgkin lymphoma (CHL, 95% of cases) and nodular lymphocyte predominant Hodgkin lymphoma (NLPHL, 5% of cases) (1):
  - NLPHL: B cells, neoplastic luteinizing hormone (LH) cells with multilobulated nuclei, small nucleoli, and popcorn-like appearance
  - CHL histologic subdivisions: Nodular sclerosing (60%), mixed cellularity (30%), lymphocyte depleted (<10%), lymphocyte rich (<10%)
  - Frequency of lymph node involvement: Cervical > Mediastinal > Axillary > Para-aortic

EPIDEMIOLOGY
Incidence: 2.8/100,000/year (2)

Geriatric Considerations
Poorer prognosis if present at ≥60 years (1):
- Less likely to tolerate intensive chemotherapy
- Less likely to be included in clinical trial

Pediatric Considerations
Young females (<30 years of age) treated with thoracic radiation are at high risk for breast cancer and early breast cancer screening is recommended (3).

Pregnancy Considerations
- Abdominal ultrasonography to detect subdiaphragmatic disease
- Treatment (3):
  - Delay until after delivery if asymptomatic and early-stage
  - ABVD safely used in 2nd and 3rd trimesters
  - Vinblastine monotherapy to control symptoms
  - 1st trimester: ABVD may or may not cause fetal malformations

Incidence
- ~9,000 new cases in the US annually (2)
- Mean age at diagnosis: 38 years (2)

Prevalence
~175,000 living with Hodgkin lymphoma in the US in 2009

ETIOLOGY AND PATHOPHYSIOLOGY
- RS cells likely derived from germinal center B cells with mutations in immunoglobulin variable chain
- Seasonal features and higher frequencies with EBV suggest environmental factors.
- T-lymphocyte defects persist even after successful treatment.

Genetics
- 1st-degree relative: 3–9 × risk
- Siblings of younger patients: 7 × risk
- Weak correlation between familial HL and HLA class I regions containing HLA A1, B5, B8, B18 alleles

RISK FACTORS
- Immunodeficiency (inherited or acquired)
- Autoimmune disorders
- EBV
- Seasonal factors

COMMONLY ASSOCIATED CONDITIONS
In HIV (3):
- AIDS-defining illness
- Predominantly mixed-cellularity or lymphocyte-depleted histologic subtypes
- At diagnosis: Widespread disease, extranodal involvement, systemic symptoms

 DIAGNOSIS

HISTORY
- Asymptomatic lymphadenopathy (cervical/supraclavicular)
- Pel-Ebstein fever
- Constitutional symptoms: Night sweats, weight loss, fatigue, anorexia
- Alcohol-induced pain
- Pruritus

PHYSICAL EXAM
Focus on lymph nodes, spleen, and liver

DIFFERENTIAL DIAGNOSIS
Non-Hodgkin lymphoma, infectious lymphadenopathy, solid tumor metastases, sarcoidosis, autoimmune disease, AIDS/HIV, drug reaction

DIAGNOSTIC TESTS & INTERPRETATION
Initial Tests (lab, imaging)
- CBC and electrolytes
- LFT, including hepatitis serologies
- HIV
- Pregnancy test
- Pulmonary function tests (diffusion capacity of the lung for carbon monoxide for ABVD or BEACOPP) (4)
- Chest x-ray (4)
- CT of chest, abdomen, and pelvis (4)
- PET: For initial staging, midtreatment decision making, and end-of-treatment evaluation
- Bone scan, gallium scan, abdominal ultrasound

Follow-Up Tests & Special Considerations
- Fertility considerations (4):
  - Semen cryopreservation if chemotherapy or pelvic radiation therapy
  - In vitro fertilization or ovarian tissue/oocyte cryopreservation
- Radiation therapy (RT) considerations (4):
  - Splenic RT: Pneumococcal, *Haemophilus influenzae*, meningococcal vaccine

Diagnostic Procedures/Other
- Excisional lymph node biopsy (4)
- Immunohistochemistry (4)
- Bone marrow biopsy
- Liver biopsy (in selected cases)

Test Interpretation
RS cell characteristics (4):
- Diameter: 20–50 μm
- Abundant acidophilic cytoplasm
- Bi- or polylobulated nucleus
- Acidophilic nucleoli
- CD30+, CD15+, CD45–, CD3–, CD20+ in 40% of cases
- RS cells necessary, but not sufficient, for diagnosis (need inflammatory background)

 TREATMENT

- Ann Arbor staging with Cotswold modification (4):
  - Stage I: Single lymph node or of a single extralymphatic organ or site
  - Stage II: ≥2 lymph node regions on the same side of diaphragm alone or with involvement of extralymphatic organ or tissue
  - Stage III: Node groups on both sides of the diaphragm
  - Stage IV: Dissemination involving extra-nodal organs (except the spleen, which is considered lymphoid tissue)
  - Subclasses: A = no systemic symptoms; B = systemic symptoms (fever, night sweats, weight loss >10% body weight); X = bulky disease (widened mediastinum, > intrathoracic diameter, or >10-cm nodal mass)
  - Pathologic stage at given site denoted by: M = bone marrow, H = liver, L = lung, O = bone, P = pleura, D = skin):
    ○ Splenectomy, liver biopsy, lymph node biopsy, bone marrow biopsy mandatory for pathological staging
- Goal: Aim for cure
- All subsequent treatment and follow-up care recommendations based on National Comprehensive Cancer Network (NCCN) consensus. Please refer to NCCN Practice Guidelines in Oncology for Hodgkin Lymphoma (4).

MEDICATION
First Line
- ABVD: Doxorubicin, bleomycin, vinblastine, dacarbazine (1):
  - Dacarbazine: Highly emetic, severe phlebitis
  - Monitor cardiac function on doxorubicin
- BEACOPP: Bleomycin, etoposide, doxorubicin, cyclophosphamide, vincristine, procarbazine, prednisone, G-CSF (1):
  - Bleomycin: Risk of pulmonary toxicity, death
- Stage I/II with no risk factors: 2 cycles ABVD followed by 20 Gy involved-field radiotherapy (IFRT)
- Stage I/II with risk factors (large mediastinal mass, unfavorable histology, age, extranodal disease, erythrocyte sedimentation rate (ESR), B symptoms, number of nodal areas): 4 cycles chemotherapy (BEACOPP and/or ABVD) followed by 30 Gy IFRT
- Stage III/IV: 4–6 cycles chemotherapy (BEACOPP and/or ABVD) and consider autologous stem cell transplant (SCT) or radiotherapy
- Relapsed and refractory: High-dose conditioning therapy (HDCT) followed by autologous SCT
  - Maintenance therapy: Trials with brentuximab vedotin (anti-CD30) and lenalidomide under way)
  - Brentuximab vedotin: Anti-CD30, use in relapsed HL) after 2 prior lines of treatment have been tried, side effects include peripheral neuropathy, nausea, fatigue, neutropenia, diarrhea.
  - Allogeneic SCT to be considered if failed autologous SCT (used in trials only)

Second Line
- Median survival < 3 years if fail 2nd-line therapy, including SCT (5)
- SCT in progressive disease or relapse (1)
  - High-dose therapy and autologous stem cell transplant (HDCT/ASCT): Improved event-free and progression-free survival compared with conventional chemotherapy, but not overall survival
- Rituximab: Excellent activity against lymphocyte-predominant variant due to CD20+ lymphocytes
- Brentuximab vedotin: Anti-CD30 chimeric antibody conjugated to synthetic anti-microtubule agent monomethyl auristatin E (5)
  - Approved by FDA in 2011 for patients who failed/not candidate for SCT or failure of 2 prior multiagent chemotherapy regimens
- Novel agents undergoing studies: NF-kB inhibitors (bortezomib), mTOR inhibitors (everolimus), immunomodulators (lenalidomide), cell signaling targets HDAC inhibitors (vorinostat, panobinostat, mocetinostat) (5,6)

 ## ONGOING CARE

FOLLOW-UP RECOMMENDATIONS
Patient Monitoring
- During therapy: CBC, nutrition, and hydration
- Restage with PET after 2–4 cycles of chemotherapy: Sensitive prognostic indicator (4)
- Posttreatment monitoring (4):
  - H&P: q2–4mo for first 2 years, then q3–6mo for next 3–5 years
  - Laboratory studies:
    - CBC, platelets, ESR, chemistry profile q2–4 mo for 1–2 years, then q3–6 mo for next 3–5 years
    - TSH annually if radiation to neck
  - Imaging:
    - Chest: Chest x-ray or CT q6–12 mo during first 2–5 years
    - Abdominal/pelvic: CT q6–12 mo during first 2–3 years
    - Annual breast mammogram or MRI beginning 8–10 years after therapy or at age 40 years if chest or axillary irradiation
    - Surveillance PET should not be done routinely due to risk of false-positive findings.

PATIENT EDUCATION
- Reproductive impact
- Risks of secondary malignancy
- Oral and dental care during therapy
- Leukemia Society of America (www.lls.org)

PROGNOSIS
- Cure rate for classic Hodgkin lymphoma: 80% (6)
- Relapse or progression of disease rate: 5–20%
- Overall survival rates (7):
  - 1-year survival: 92%
  - 5-year survival: 85%
  - 10-year survival: 81%
- International Prognostic Score for advanced disease (4):
  - Age $\geq$45 years
  - Male gender
  - Albumin <4 g/dL
  - Hemoglobin <10.5 g/dL
  - Lymphocytopenia: <600 lymphocyte cells/dL or lymphocytes <8% of WBC
  - WBC $\geq$15,000 cells/dL
  - Stage IV disease

- Main cause of death (7):
  - Initial 5 years: Hodgkin lymphoma
  - After 5–10 years: Leukemia, myelodysplastic syndrome
  - After 20 years: 2nd primary malignancy, cardiovascular disease

REFERENCES
1. Borchmann P, Eichenauer DA, Engert A. State of the art in the treatment of Hodgkin lymphoma. *Nat Rev Clin Oncol*. 2012;9:450–459.
2. SEER stat fact sheet. Hodgkin lymphoma. Available at: http://seer.cancer.gov/statfacts/html/hodg.html
3. Armitage JO. Early-stage Hodgkin's lymphoma. *N Engl J Med*. 2010;363:7.
4. NCCN clinical practice guidelines in oncology. Hodgkin lymphoma. Version 2.2013. Available at: www.nccn.org
5. Czuczman M, Straus D, Gribben J, et al. Management options, survivorship, and emerging treatment strategies for follicular and Hodgkin lymphomas. *Leuk Lymphoma*. 2010;51:41–49.
6. Dinner S, Advani R. Targeted therapy in relapsed classical Hodgkin lymphoma. *J Natl Compr Canc Netw*. 2013;11:968–976.
7. von Tresckow B, Engert A. Refractory Hodgkin lymphoma. *Curr Opin Oncol*. 2013;25:463–469.

 ## CODES

ICD10
- C81.90 Hodgkin lymphoma, unspecified, unspecified site
- C81.98 Hodgkin lymphoma, unspecified, lymph nodes of multiple sites
- C81.99 Hodgkin lymphoma, unsp, extranodal and solid organ sites

CLINICAL PEARLS
- Neoplastic disease of lymphatics
- Reed-Sternberg (RS) cells of monoclonal lymphoid B-cell origin within inflammatory background of lymphocytes
- 2 subtypes: Classic Hodgkin lymphoma (CHL, 95% of cases) and nodular lymphocyte predominant Hodgkin lymphoma (NLPHL, 5% of cases)
- Cure rate for classic Hodgkin lymphoma: 80%
- Relapse or progression of disease rate: 5–20%

H

HOMELESSNESS

Dana Sprute, MD, MPH, FAAFP • Margaret Gilmore, MD

BASICS

DESCRIPTION
"Homeless" or "homeless individual or homeless person" includes: (i) An individual who lacks a fixed, regular, and adequate nighttime residence; and (ii) an individual who has a primary nighttime residence that is: (a) A supervised publicly or privately operated shelter designed to provide temporary living accommodations (including welfare hotels, congregate shelters, and transitional housing for the mentally ill); (b) an institution that provides a temporary residence for individuals intended to be institutionalized; (c) a public or private place not designed for, or ordinarily used as, a regular sleeping accommodation for human beings.

EPIDEMIOLOGY
Prevalence
3.5 million people in the US experience homelessness each year; 37% are homeless families, 46% are not chronically homeless individuals, and 17% are chronically homeless individuals (1):
- 2010–2012: Chronic homelessness decreased by 1% due to $1.5 billion infused into communities for the Homelessness Prevention and Rapid Re-Housing Program (HPRP). The largest decrease was among veterans (11% decrease) (1).

RISK FACTORS
- Root cause of homelessness explained by economics: Insufficient financial resources to acquire or maintain housing; 83% of the homeless population experience temporary, transitional, or episodic periods of homelessness (1).
- Economic factors:
  - Poverty: Increase in US rates past 25 years until 2010; rate flat/unchanged 2010–2012.
    - 2013 federal poverty definition: $23,550 annual income for 4-person household.
    - In 2011, 15% of the US population fell below federal poverty definition. Children overrepresented in homeless population (2),
  - US unemployment rate: 7.6% in May 2013 (US Bureau of Labor Statistics, accessed 7/3/13)
  - Lack of affordable health care: In 2011, 46.6 million people in US without health insurance (3):
    - 40% of uninsured are disproportionately young (ages 18–34). Affordable Care Act allows children to remain on parental plans until age 26; led to a decrease in the uninsured rate for ages 18–24 starting in September 2010 (3).
  - Lack of affordable housing: Housing is considered affordable if ≤30% of household income:
    - Percentage of households defined by HUD as "severely housing cost burdened" (those who spend ≥50% of income on housing) increased by 6% between 2009 and 2011. 1 of 4 re-enter households is severely housing cost burdened (1).
  - Increase in home foreclosures:
    - 2008–2009: 32% increase in foreclosures; 10% become homeless as a result of foreclosure; 49% report medical problems played a role in foreclosure.

- At-risk populations: Domestic violence and victims of violence; youth (particularly those aging out of foster care); veterans; rural; addiction; psychiatric illness; disabled due to chronic medical disease, psychiatric illness or substance use disorder; re-entry after incarceration/prison:
  - Domestic violence: 63% of homeless women experience domestic violence and 13% of families report leaving last residence due to abuse or violence (4).
  - Youth: 2010 HUD point-in-time data estimated 8,153 homeless youth and 14,678 youth used the shelter system on any given night (1).
  - Veterans: 11% of the homeless population; homelessness rate decreased between 2009 and 2012 (2)
  - Addiction disorders: 46% of homeless individuals report alcohol and/or drug use as a major factor contributing to homelessness (4).
  - Psychiatric illness: 45% of homeless report indicators of a mental health issue in the past year; 25% of homeless adults suffer from chronic mental illness (4).
  - Re-entry after incarceration: 30–50% of parolees homeless at any given time (4)
- Fundamental issues in homelessness and health care that require ongoing consideration:
  - Unstable housing; limited access to nutritious food and water; lack of transportation
  - Higher risk for abuse and violence
  - Physical/Cognitive impairments; behavioral health problems
  - Developmental discrepancies for children: Speech delay, chronic ear infection, insufficient opportunity to practice gross and fine motor skills
  - Higher risk for communicable disease
  - Lack of health insurance/resources; discontinuous/inaccessible health care; lack of a medical home; barriers to disability assistance
  - Cultural/Linguistic barriers: Racial and ethnic groups overrepresented in homeless population
  - Limited education/literacy
  - Lack of social supports: Alienation from family and friends precipitates homelessness.
  - Criminalization of homelessness: Frequent arrests for loitering, sleeping in public places

GENERAL PREVENTION
- Policy & funding for community programs that provide emergency/rapid housing, housing stabilization & case management services to address risk factors
- Affordable Care Act (ACA): In 2010 increased Medicaid eligibility for homeless and expanded home and community-based services and case management to the homeless population (5).
- Social Justice Policy Recommendations: Permanent affordable housing, foreclosure and homelessness prevention, increased funds for HUD McKinney-Vento programs (emergency, transitional, and permanent housing), rural homeless assistance, universal health care, universal livable income, employment/workforce services, prevention of hate crimes against the homeless, decriminalization of homelessness

COMMONLY ASSOCIATED CONDITIONS
- Hunger
- Medical conditions:
  - Heart, lung, liver, renal disease, diabetes, HTN, cancer, pneumonia (6)
  - Infectious diseases:
    - Tuberculosis, HIV/AIDS, STI (6)
    - Skin/Nail infections (cellulitis, fungal infection) and infestation (lice and scabies)
    - Liver disease (e.g., hepatitis B or C, or alcohol-related)
  - Cognitive impairment: Traumatic brain injury, cardiovascular accident (CVA), substance use
  - Dental problems (e.g., caries, periodontal disease)
  - Exposure-related conditions (frostbite, heatstroke) (6)
- Psychiatric illness (6)
- Trauma: Increased risk of assault; victims of hate crimes
- Criminalization of homelessness

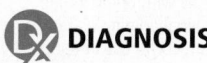

DIAGNOSIS

HISTORY
- Living conditions: Location, access to food, restrooms, place to store medicines, safety
- Prior homelessness: What precipitated it, first time, chronic
- Individual/Family history of reactive airway disease (RAD), chronic otitis media, anemia, diabetes, cardiovascular disease (CVD), TB, HIV/STIs, hospitalizations
- Family members, especially dependent children
- Medications: Include OTC meds, dietary supplements, meds "borrowed" from others
- Prior providers: Oral health, primary care, current medical home
- Mental health: Stress, anxiety, appetite, sleep, concentration, mood, speech, memory, thought process and content, suicidal/homicidal ideation, insight, judgment, impulse control, social interactions; symptoms of brain injury (headaches, seizures, memory loss, lability, irritability, dizziness, insomnia, poor organizational/decision-making skills)
- Alcohol/Nicotine/Drug use: Amount, frequency, duration
- Gender identity/orientation, behaviors, rape, pregnancies, hepatitis, HIV, other STIs
- History or current abuse: Emotional, physical, sexual; patient safety
- Legal problems/violence: History of incarceration
- Regular/Strenuous activities: Routines (treatment feasibility); level of strenuous activity
- Work: Previous types of jobs, length held, veteran status, occupational injuries/toxic exposures; vocational skills, interest
- Education: Highest level; ever in special education; assess ability to read/language skills/English fluency
- Nutrition/Hydration: Diet, food resources, preparation skills, liquid intake
- Cultural heritage/affiliations: Family, friends, faith community, other sources of support
- Strengths: Coping skills, resourcefulness, abilities, interests

PHYSICAL EXAM
- Comprehensive exam: Height/Weight, BMI, especially: Liver, dermatologic, oral, feet, neurologic, mental status
- Focused exams: For patients uncomfortable with full-body, unclothed exam at 1st visit
- Dental assessment: Age-appropriate teeth, obvious caries, dental/referred pain, diabetes, CVD

DIAGNOSTIC TESTS & INTERPRETATION
- Mental health: Patient Health Questionnaire (PHQ-9, PHQ-2), MHS-III, MDQ
- Cognitive assessment: Mini-Mental Status Exam (MMSE), Traumatic Brain Injury Questionnaire (TBIQ), Repeatable Battery for the Assessment of Neuro-Psychological Status (RBANS)
- Developmental assessment: Ages & Stages Questionnaires, Parents' Evaluation of Developmental Status (PEDS), Denver II or other standard screening tool
- Interpersonal violence: Domestic violence, rape, and so forth
- Forensic evaluation: If strong evidence of abuse
- Baseline labs: As needed, to address suspected medical concerns
- Tuberculosis screening: PPD
- STI screening: HIV, chlamydia, gonorrhea, syphilis, hepatitis B antigen, hepatitis C AB, trichomonas, bacterial vaginosis, monilia
- Substance abuse: SSI-AOD (Simple Screening Instrument for Alcohol and Other Drugs), urine drug screen

Follow-Up Tests & Special Considerations
- **Reproductive Health Care & STIs:** Obtain detailed sexual history (sexual identity, orientation, behaviors/sexual practices, number of partners). Consider possible exploitation of patient, especially if mental illness/developmental disability suspected. Communicate willingness to initiate contraception first visit without exam. Genital exam recommended, but be sensitive to patient needs if possible sexual abuse history. If pelvic exam refused, consider empiric treatment for STI (& possibility of multiple orifice infection). Dispense medications on site; ask if partner needs treatment.
- **Pediatric Care:** Complete exam every visit, use each visit to identify/address problems & provide vaccinations as homeless families may not see a medical provider unless child is sick. Vision and hearing screening at every visit and refer for abnormalities.

TREATMENT
- Establish rapport: Sensitivity to prior negative health care experiences
- Enlist resources: Mental health and substance abuse programs, free clinics, case management
- Health care maintenance: Vaccinations (hepatitis A and B, pneumovax, TdaP, influenza) cancer and chronic disease screening for adults; Early Periodic Screening, Diagnosis, and Treatment Program (EPSDT) screening and vaccinations for children
- Care plan:
  - Basic needs: Food, clothing, housing may be higher priorities than health care.
  - Patient goals and priorities: Immediate/Long-term health needs. Address patient wants first.
  - Action plan: Simple language, portable pocket card
  - After hours: Extended clinic hours
  - Safety plan: For violence and abuse suspected; mandatory reporting requirements
  - Emergency plan: Location of nearest ED, preparation for evacuation
  - Adherence plan: Use of interpreter, identification of potential barriers

MEDICATION
- Simple regimen: Low pill count, once-daily dosing.
- Dispensing: small amounts on-site to promote follow-up, decrease loss/theft/misuse risk. Determine resources for written prescriptions.
- Storage of medications: If no access to refrigeration, no prescription for meds requiring it
- Patient assistance: Free/Low-cost drugs if readily available for continuous use
- Aids to adherence: Harm reduction, outreach/case management, directly observed therapy
- Side effects: Primary reason for nonadherence (diarrhea, polyuria, nausea, disorientation)
- Analgesia/Symptomatic treatment: Contract, single provider for pain medication refills
- Dietary supplements: Multivitamins with minerals, nutritional supplements
- Managed care: Generics, if possible; assistance getting prescription filled
- Lab monitoring: Monitor patients on antipsychotic medications for metabolic disorders.

ADDITIONAL THERAPIES
- Associated problems/complications:
  - Fragmented care: Multiple providers. Use EMR; list prescribed meds on wallet-sized card.
  - Masked symptoms/misdiagnosis: For example, weight loss, dementia, edema, lactic acidosis
  - Focus on immediate concerns, not possible future consequences.
  - Integrated treatment for concurrent mental illness/substance use disorders
  - Support for parent of child abused by others and for abused parent
- Follow-up:
  - Reliable phone/email contact for patient/friend/family/case manager
  - Frequent follow-up, incentives, nonjudgmental care regardless of adherence
  - Anticipate/Accommodate unscheduled clinic visits.
  - Provide car fare, tokens, help with transportation services.
  - Monitor school attendance, address health/developmental problems with family/school.

IN-PATIENT CONSIDERATIONS
Admission Criteria/Initial Stabilization
Homeless likely to benefit from admission if living conditions are suboptimal to treat medical, psychiatric, and substance use disorders.

Discharge Criteria
- Bed rest, extended periods of elevation, rest, or icing are not feasible in most instances.
- Plans requiring multiple return visits likely to fail if no transportation.
- Admission to inpatient rehabilitation if appropriate and possible

ONGOING CARE

FOLLOW-UP RECOMMENDATIONS
- Patients with a history of nonadherence need additional support (e.g., case manager, outreach) to succeed in ongoing care after hospital discharge.
- Limited access to telephones to schedule appointments; may be unable to receive telephone messages with test results or rescheduled appointment times.
- Arrange appointments prior to discharge.
- Document the best way to contact the individual.
- Refer to health care agency designed to address needs of people who are homeless with integrated physical/mental health services & substance use treatment

PROGNOSIS
Mortality rates for chronically homeless adults are 4 times higher and average life expectancy is 42–52 years compared with 78 years for the general population.

REFERENCES

1. National Alliance to End Homelessness. The State of Homelessness in America, 2013. (accessed 7/3/13).
2. U.S. Dept of Housing & Urban Development, Office of Community Planning & Development. 2012 Point-in-Time Annual Homeless Assessment Report to Congress.
3. U.S. Department of Health and Human Services. Overview of the Uninsured in the United States: A Summary of the 2012 Current Population Survey Report. September 12, 2012.
4. National Alliance to End Homelessness, www.endhomelessness.org. (accessed 7/3/13)
5. United States Interagency Council on Homelessness. Opening Doors: Federal Strategic Plan to Prevent and End Homelessness, Update 2011.
6. Bonin E, Brehove T, Carlson T, et al. *Adapting your practice: General recommendations for the care of homeless patients*. Nashville (TN): Health Care for the Homeless Clinicians' Network, National Health Care for the Homeless Council, Inc.; 2010.

CODES

ICD10
- Z59.0 Homelessness
- Z59.1 Inadequate housing
- Z59.8 Other problems related to housing and economic circumstances

CLINICAL PEARLS
- Ending homelessness requires permanent housing, supportive services & implementing policies to prevent chronic homelessness. (www.endhomelessness.org/content/article/detail/1623). National Alliance to End Homelessness, January 2010.
- Assistance in gaining access to benefits or meeting basic needs may decrease stress, improve therapeutic relationship and allow individuals to direct attention to physical health.

H

HORDEOLUM (STYE)

Konstantinos E. Deligiannidis, MD, MPH

BASICS

DESCRIPTION
- An acute inflammation or infection of the eyelid margin involving the sebaceous gland of an eyelash (external hordeolum) or a meibomian gland (internal hordeolum)
- System(s) affected: Skin/Exocrine
- Synonym(s): Internal hordeolum; External hordeolum; Zeisian stye; Meibomian stye; Stye

EPIDEMIOLOGY
- Predominant age: None
- Predominant sex: Male = Female

Incidence
Unknown: Although external hordeolum is common, internal hordeolum is rare.

ETIOLOGY AND PATHOPHYSIOLOGY
- Bacterial infection of sebaceous or meibomian glands, causing an acute inflammatory reaction
- In an internal hordeolum, the meibomian gland may become obstructed, leading to a pustule on the conjunctival surface as opposed to the margin of the eyelid (1).
- Most commonly caused by *Staphylococcus aureus* (~90–95% of all cases) or by *S. epidermidis*.
- Seborrhea can predispose to infections of the eyelid.

Genetics
No known genetic pattern

RISK FACTORS
- Poor eyelid hygiene
- Previous hordeolum
- Contact lens wearers
- Application of makeup
- Predisposing blepharitis (low-grade infections of the eyelid margin)
- Ocular rosacea

GENERAL PREVENTION
Eyelid hygiene

COMMONLY ASSOCIATED CONDITIONS
- Acne
- Seborrhea
- An association may exist between hordeolum during childhood and developing rosacea in adulthood (2).

DIAGNOSIS

HISTORY
- Localized inflammation (vs. involvement of the entire eyelid or surrounding skin)
- Foreign-body sensation in the eye
- Prior episodes are common.

PHYSICAL EXAM
- Localized inflammation of the eyelashes or a small pustule at the margin of the eyelid
- Localized swelling and tenderness on the internal or external aspect of the eyelid with an opening to either side
- To determine if an internal hordeolum is obstructed, the eyelid should be gently everted to examine for a pustule on the tarsal conjunctiva (1).
- Itching or scaling of the eyelids; collection of discharge, redness, and irritation leading to localized tenderness and pain

DIFFERENTIAL DIAGNOSIS
- Chalazion
- Blepharitis
- Eyelid neoplasms
- Periorbital cellulitis
- Dacryocystitis

DIAGNOSTIC TESTS & INTERPRETATION
Culture of the eyelid margins usually is not necessary.

Diagnostic Procedures/Other
History and eye exam

Test Interpretation
Bacterial contamination and white cells in eyelid discharge

TREATMENT

GENERAL MEASURES
- The hordeolum should not be expressed.
- Warm compresses to the area of inflammation can help increase blood supply and encourage spontaneous drainage.
- Application of an antibiotic ointment (e.g., erythromycin) to the margin of the eyelid after proper cleansing (except in children age <12 years, in whom there is a risk of blurred vision and amblyopia) helps reduce bacterial proliferation.
- Good personal hygiene with attention to cleansing the eyelids on a daily basis helps to prevent recurrent infections.

MEDICATION
First Line
- A Cochrane review found no evidence for or against nonsurgical treatment of internal hordeolum (3)[A]. External hordeola were not considered.
- Usually, a hordeolum spontaneously drains, aided by warm compresses to the area.
- There is little evidence that any topical therapy is effective. Erythromycin ophthalmic 0.5% ointment may be applied up to 6×/d for 7–10 days.
- Treat underlying dry eye with artificial tears.

Second Line
- Occasionally, the use of an aminoglycoside ophthalmic ointment, such as gentamicin or tobramycin, may be necessary if condition is refractory to simpler treatment (case reports).
- Oral dicloxacillin or cephalexin for 2 weeks if refractory to topical antibiotics

ISSUES FOR REFERRAL
Consider referral if unresponsive to oral antibiotics.

SURGERY/OTHER PROCEDURES
- If the infection becomes localized to a single gland, incision, drainage, or curettage sometimes is necessary. This is an in-office procedure with a local anesthetic: Exercise caution because ocular perforation has been reported with the injection of an anesthetic to an infected lid (4)[C].
- Use of combined antibiotic ointment (neomycin sulfate, polymyxin B sulfate, and gramicidin) after surgery was not shown to have any statistically significant benefit compared with artificial tears (5)[B].

COMPLEMENTARY AND ALTERNATIVE MEDICINE
Broncasma berna is a polyvalent antigen vaccine that may be useful in the treatment of recurrent hordeolum (6).

IN-PATIENT CONSIDERATIONS
Admission Criteria/Initial Stabilization
Outpatient

ONGOING CARE

FOLLOW-UP RECOMMENDATIONS
No restrictions

Patient Monitoring
The patient should be seen within several weeks to assess the effectiveness of therapy or should at least call the physician's office with a progress report.

DIET
No special diet

PATIENT EDUCATION
- The patient should be instructed in proper cleansing of the eyelids using a solution of tap water and baby shampoo or a commercially prepared hypoallergenic cleanser.
- The stye should not be squeezed or incised.

PROGNOSIS
- Usually responds well to good hygiene and warm compresses
- Inflammation usually improves within a week.
- Hordeolum tends to recur in some patients.

COMPLICATIONS
An internal hordeolum, if untreated, may lead to chalazion, infections of adjacent glands, or generalized cellulitis of the lid.

REFERENCES

1. Wald ER. Periorbital and orbital infections. *Infect Dis Clin North Am.* 2007;21:393–408, vi.
2. Bamford JT, Gessert CE, Renier CM, et al. Childhood stye and adult rosacea. *J Am Acad Dermatol.* 2006;55:951–955.
3. Lindsley K, Nichols JJ, Dickersin K. Interventions for acute internal hordeolum. *Cochrane Database Syst Rev.* 2010;(9):CD007742. Epub 2010 Sep 8.
4. Kim JH, Yang SM, Kim HM, et al. Inadvertent ocular perforation during lid anesthesia for hordeolum removal. *Korean J Opththalmol.* 2006;20(3):199–200.
5. Hirunwiwatkul P, Wachirasereechai K. Effectiveness of combined antibiotic ophthalmic solution in the treatment of hordeolum after incision and curettage: A randomized, placebo-controlled trial: A pilot study. *J Med Assoc Thai.* 2005;88:647–650.
6. Nakatani M. Treatment of recurrent hordeolum with Broncasma Berna. *Eye.* 1999;13(Pt 5):692.

CODES

ICD10
- H00.019 Hordeolum externum unspecified eye, unspecified eyelid
- H00.029 Hordeolum internum unspecified eye, unspecified eyelid
- H00.039 Abscess of eyelid unspecified eye, unspecified eyelid

CLINICAL PEARLS
- A hordeolum should not be expressed.
- Warm compresses to the area of inflammation can encourage spontaneous drainage.
- Application of an antibiotic ointment (e.g., erythromycin) to the margin of the eyelid after proper cleansing (except in children age <12 years, in whom there is a risk of blurred vision and amblyopia) helps reduce bacterial proliferation, but may have no effect on healing of the stye.
- Good personal hygiene with attention to cleansing the eyelids on a daily basis can prevent recurrent infections.

H

HORNER SYNDROME

Jonathan Giordano, DO • Edlira Yzeiraj, DO • Deborah Lardner, DO

BASICS

DESCRIPTION
- Horner syndrome presents as a classic triad of ipsilateral miosis, eyelid ptosis, and/or anhidrosis of the face and neck (with iris heterochromia in children).
- It is caused by the interruption of sympathetic nerve supply to the head, neck, and eye:
  - Central or preganglionic lesion (complete syndrome): 1st- or 2nd-order neuron
  - Peripheral postganglionic lesion (incomplete syndrome, no anhidrosis): 3rd-order neuron
- System(s) affected: Nervous; Skin/Exocrine
- Synonym(s): Bernard-Horner syndrome; Bernard syndrome; Horner's syndrome; Cervical sympathetic syndrome; Oculosympathetic syndrome; Oculosympathetic paralysis; Oculosympathetic deficiency; Oculosympathetic paresis

EPIDEMIOLOGY
- Predominant age: None
- Predominant sex: Male = Female

Incidence
Unknown

Prevalence
Unknown

ETIOLOGY AND PATHOPHYSIOLOGY
- Constellation of signs produced when sympathetic innervation to the head, neck and eye is interrupted somewhere along the 3-neuron arc:
  - Absence of innervation of iris dilator and Müller muscles leads to miosis and slight ptosis, respectively.
  - Sympathetic innervation also controls sweat glands; interruption causes anhidrosis.
- Oculosympathetic pathway:
  - 1st-order neuron: Sympathetic nerve fibers originate in the hypothalamus, descend through the brainstem, and synapse at the ciliospinal center (of Budge) located at approximately the C8–T2 levels of the spinal cord.
  - 2nd-order neuron: Exits the spinal column at the T1 level primarily, arches over the apex of the lung and under the subclavian artery, ascending to the superior cervical ganglion at the level of the carotid bifurcation and angle of the jaw
  - 3rd-order neuron: Ascends along the adventitia of the internal carotid artery, through the cavernous sinus in proximity to cranial nerve [CN] VI, and joins CN V_1 to innervate the iris dilator muscle and Müller muscle in the eye.
- Sympathetic fibers innervating sweat glands and vasodilatory muscles branch off before the cervical sympathetic ganglion traveling along the external carotid artery, so distal lesions will not result in anhidrosis.
- Lesions anywhere along this pathway will lead to ipsilateral Horner syndrome.
- Idiopathic (40%), congenital, or acquired
- Best classified by which order neuron is affected and by age (pediatric vs. adult)

- 1st-order neuron (13%):
  - Arnold-Chiari malformation
  - Basal meningitis (e.g., syphilis)
  - Basal skull tumors
  - Cerebral vascular accident: Lateral medullary (Wallenberg) syndrome
  - Cervical cord trauma
  - Demyelinating disease (multiple sclerosis)
  - Intrapontine hemorrhage
  - Neck trauma
  - Pituitary tumor
  - Syringomyelia
  - Unintended subdural placement of lumbar epidural catheter
- 2nd-order neuron (44%):
  - Aneurysm/Dissection of aorta
  - Central venous catheterization
  - Chest tubes
  - First rib fracture
  - Lymphadenopathy (Hodgkin, leukemia, tuberculosis, mediastinal tumors, sarcoid)
  - Mandibular tooth abscess
  - Neurofibromatosis type I and II
  - Pancoast tumor or infection of lung apex
  - Proximal common carotid artery dissection
  - Trauma/Surgical injury
- 3rd-order neuron lesions (43%):
  - Carotid cavernous fistula or other pathology
  - Carotid endarterectomy or carotid artery stenting
  - Cluster headaches
  - Internal carotid artery dissection
  - Herpes zoster
  - Lesions of the middle ear (acute otitis media)
  - Nasopharyngeal cancer
  - Tonsillectomy
  - Raeder paratrigeminal syndrome
- Drugs: Acetophenazine, alseroxylon, bupivacaine, butaperazine, carphenazine, chloroprocaine, deserpidine, diacetylmorphine, diethazine, ethopropazine, etidocaine, guanethidine, influenza virus vaccine, levodopa, lidocaine, mepivacaine, mesoridazine, methdilazine, methotrimeprazine, oral contraceptives, perazine, prilocaine, procaine, prochlorperazine, promazine, propoxycaine, reserpine, thioproperazine, thioridazine, trifluoperazine

Genetics
Rare autosomal dominant inheritance

RISK FACTORS
- Most common: Apical bronchogenic carcinoma (Pancoast tumor) in smokers
- Aneurysm of the carotid or subclavian artery
- Injuries to the carotid artery high in the neck
- Dissection of the carotid arteries
- Carotid artery occlusion:
  - 15% of patients with carotid artery occlusion develop ipsilateral Horner syndrome.
  - May occur without evidence of cerebral ischemia, neck injuries, or operative procedures
- Cluster headaches:
  - 20% have an ipsilateral Horner syndrome

Pediatric Considerations
2nd-order neuron lesion is most common etiology: Birth trauma to neck and shoulder, chest surgery, neuroblastoma (paraspinal), and vascular anomalies of the carotid arteries

COMMONLY ASSOCIATED CONDITIONS
- Wallenberg syndrome
- Pancoast tumor
- C8 radiculopathy

DIAGNOSIS

HISTORY
- Ptosis (typically mild; 1–2 mm)
- Miosis (with an associated dilation lag)
- Anhidrosis or hypohidrosis (often not appreciated by patients or clinicians):
  - Ipsilateral side of the body: Central (1st-order neuron)
  - Ipsilateral face: Preganglionic (2nd-order neuron)
  - Medial portion of forehead and side of nose: Postganglionic (3rd-order neuron after vasomotor and sudomotor fiber have branched off)

Pediatric Considerations
In infants and children, loss of facial flushing is appreciated more than anhidrosis (harlequin sign).

ALERT
Horner syndrome in the presence of pain merits special consideration:
- Axial, shoulder, scapula, arm, or hand pain may be related to Pancoast tumor.
- Acute-onset, ipsilateral facial or neck pain: Consider carotid artery dissection until proven otherwise.
- Paratrigeminal syndromes:
  - Raeder paratrigeminal syndrome type I: Orbital pain, miosis, ptosis, with associated ipsilateral lesions of CN III–VI; suspect middle cranial fossa mass lesion.
  - Raeder paratrigeminal syndrome type II: Episodic retrobulbar or orbital pain, miosis, ptosis with no CN lesions; suspect migraine variant, syphilis, herpes zoster, hypertension.

PHYSICAL EXAM
- Measure pupillary diameter in dim and bright light and reactivity to light and accommodative response:
  - Anisocoria is greatest in dark, with affected pupil failing to dilate.
  - Redilation (after light is removed) may lag 15–20 seconds on the affected side.
- Examine the upper lids for ptosis (<2 mm).
- Examination of the lower lids for "upside-down ptosis": Elevation of lower lid due to Müller muscle weakness:
  - Illusion of enophthalmos secondary to narrowing of palpebral fissure

- Ipsilateral impaired flushing may be found.
- Loss of ciliospinal reflex. Pinching the skin on back of the neck normally produces ipsilateral pupil dilation (unreliable).
- Biomicroscopic exam of the papillary margin and iris structure and color:
  – In congenital Horner syndrome, long-standing Horner syndrome, or Horner syndrome that occurs in children <2 years: Iris shows reduced pigmentation, blue-gray, mottling of the affected eye (heterochromia iridis) because formation of iris pigment early in life is under sympathetic control.
- Observe for the presence of nystagmus, facial swelling, lymphadenopathy, or vesicular eruptions.
- Ophthalmoparesis, specifically CN VI palsy with Horner syndrome is suggestive of cavernous sinus lesion.
- Neurologic and chest exams for associated physical findings

DIFFERENTIAL DIAGNOSIS
- Neurologic diseases
- 3rd nerve palsy
- Unilateral use of miotics
- Unilateral use of mydriatics
- Adie tonic pupil
- Iris sphincter muscle damage

DIAGNOSTIC TESTS & INTERPRETATION
Initial Tests (lab, imaging)
CBC, fluorescent treponemal antibody absorption test, venereal disease research laboratory, purified protein derivative; vanillylmandelic acid, homovanillic acid to rule out neuroblastoma in pediatric patients

- Chest x-ray if patient is a smoker (apical bronchogenic carcinoma)
- CT/MRI/MRA of the brain, chest, and spinal cord:
  – If painful, order MRI/MRA to evaluate for carotid artery dissection emergently.

Pediatric Considerations
In a child of any age without contributory history, MRI brain, neck, and chest to exclude a mass lesion (1)[B]

Diagnostic Procedures/Other
- Confirmation of Horner syndrome:
  – 4–10% topical cocaine:
    ○ A normal pupil will dilate. The miotic pupil in Horner syndrome (regardless of location of lesion) will not dilate or will dilate poorly after 45 minutes because of the absence of norepinephrine at the nerve endings of the 3rd-order neuron (2)[A].
    ○ Positive test is anisocoria of ≥1 mm
    ○ Cocaine blocks the reuptake of norepinephrine by the neuron.
    ○ If the diagnosis is clear clinically, this test is not required.
    ○ Alternate test: Topical 0.5% apraclonidine (2)[A],(3)[B],(4)[B]

- Distinguishing a 3rd-order neuron disorder from a 1st- or 2nd-order neuron disorder:
  – Topical 1% hydroxyamphetamine (2)[A]:
    ○ If there is a 1st- or 2nd-order neuron lesion, dilation will take place 1 hour later.
    ○ Failure of the pupil to dilate, or poor dilation, indicates a 3rd-order neuron lesion (positive when anisocoria increases by ≥1 mm).
    ○ No pharmacologic test exists to differentiate between a 1st- or 2nd-order neuron lesion.
    ○ Hydroxyamphetamine causes release of endogenous norepinephrine stored in the postganglionic neuron.
    ○ Alternative test: 1% topical pholedrine
- Must wait >24 hours between the cocaine and hydroxyamphetamine tests

Pediatric Considerations
Due to transsynaptic degeneration in children, the hydroxyamphetamine test is not reliable.

Test Interpretation
- Brainstem lesion
- Massive hemisphere lesion
- Cervical cord lesion
- Root lesion
- Sympathetic chain lesion

TREATMENT

GENERAL MEASURES
- Horner syndrome in itself does not produce any disability or necessarily require treatment.
- Treat the underlying etiology.
- Search for a tumor or other compressive lesion.

MEDICATION
Carotid artery dissection: Pharmacologic treatment options include thrombolysis, antithrombotic therapy with anticoagulation or antiplatelet therapy. No randomized control trials have compared these treatment options (5)[C].

ISSUES FOR REFERRAL
- Neurologic, neuro-ophthalmic, oculoplastic
- Neurologic or vascular surgery: Interventional in cases of suspected carotid artery dissection or aneurysm
- Neurosurgery, surgical oncology, oncology, or radiotherapy consultation depends on the particular etiology.

SURGERY/OTHER PROCEDURES
- Surgical care depends on etiology.
- Consider ptosis repair surgery (oculoplastics).

ONGOING CARE

PROGNOSIS
- Postganglionic: Usually benign
- Central and preganglionic: Poorer prognosis

COMPLICATIONS
- Chronic pupillary constriction
- Cosmesis

REFERENCES

1. Al-Moosa A, Eggenberger E. Neuroimaging yield in isolated Horner syndrome. Curr Opin Ophthalmol. 2011;22(6):468–471.
2. Antonio-Santos AA, Santo RN, Eggenberger ER. Pharmacological testing of anisocoria. Expert Opin Pharmacother. 2005;6(12):2007–2013.
3. Koc F, Kavuncu S, Kansu T, et al. The sensitivity and specificity of 0.5% apraclonidine in the diagnosis of oculosympathetic paresis. Br J Ophthalmol. 2005; 89(11):1442–1444.
4. Chen PL, Chen JT, Lu DW, et al. Comparing efficacies of 0.5% apraclonidine with 4% cocaine in the diagnosis of Horner syndrome in pediatric patients. J Ocul Pharmacol Ther. 2006;22(3): 182–187.
5. Patel RR, Adam R, Maldjian C, et al. Cervical carotid artery dissection: Current review of diagnosis and treatment. Cardiol Rev. 2012;20(3):145–152.

ADDITIONAL READING

- Ahmadi O, Saxena P, Wilson BK et al. First rib fracture and Horner's syndrome: A rare clinical entity. Ann Thoracic Surg. 2013;95(1):355.
- Almog Y, Gepstein R, Kesler A. Diagnostic value of imaging in Horner syndrome in adults. J Neuro-ophthalmol. 2010;30(1):7–11.
- Bazari F, Hind M, Ong YE. Horner's syndrome—not to be sneezed at. Lancet. 2010;375(9716):776.
- Lee JH, Lee HK, Lee DH, et al. Neuroimaging strategies for three types of Horner syndrome with emphasis on anatomic location. AJR Am J Roentgenol. 2007;188(1):W74–81.
- Mahoney NR, Liu GT, Menacker SJ, et al. Pediatric Horner syndrome: Etiologies and roles of imaging and urine studies to detect neuroblastoma and other responsible mass lesions. Am J Ophthalmol. 2006;142(4):651–659.
- Martin TJ. Horner's syndrome, pseudo-Horner's syndrome, and simple anisocoria. Curr Neurol Neurosci Rep. 2007;7(5):397–406.
- Reede DL, Garcon E, Smoker WR, et al. Horner's syndrome: Clinical and radiographic evaluation. Neuroimaging Clin N Am. 2008;18(2):369–385, xi.

 CODES

ICD10
G90.2 Horner's syndrome

CLINICAL PEARLS
- Horner syndrome triad: Ipsilateral miosis, eyelid ptosis, and anhidrosis caused by a lesion of the sympathetic innervation to the neck, head, and eye
- Ptosis is mild, usually <2 mm.
- Red flags: If associated with pain, suspect central or preganglionic lesion.
- Confirm the diagnosis clinically with topical cocaine to the affected eye.
- Use hydroxyamphetamine to differentiate which order neuron is affected.
- Order imaging studies based on history and physical and hydroxyamphetamine testing.
- Horner syndrome in the presence of acute-onset, ipsilateral facial or neck pain: Consider carotid artery dissection until proven otherwise.

H

HYDROCELE

Varun K. Bhalla, MD • Mohamad Masoumy, MD • E. James Kruse, DO

 BASICS

DESCRIPTION
A collection of fluid within the scrotum:
- Communicating hydrocele:
  – Associated with a patent processus vaginalis
  – Has an associated indirect inguinal hernia
- Noncommunicating hydrocele (the processus vaginalis is not patent):
  – Infantile type: Often spontaneous resolution
  – Adult type: Infrequent resolution
- Hydrocele of the cord: Distal portion of the processus vaginalis has closed; midportion patent and fluid filled; proximal portion open or closed.
- Acute hydrocele: Fluid collection resulting from an acute process within the tunica vaginalis.
- System(s) affected: Reproductive

Pediatric Considerations
In a communicating hydrocele, consider contralateral inguinal exploration.

EPIDEMIOLOGY
Predominant age: Childhood

Incidence
Estimated at 0.7%-4.7% of male infants (1)

Prevalence
- 1,000/100,000
- Estimated at 1% of adult men

ETIOLOGY AND PATHOPHYSIOLOGY
- Closure of the processus vaginalis, resulting in trapped peritoneal fluid (noncommunicating).
- Closure of the distal processus, trapping fluid in midportion of the processus vaginalis (hydrocele of the cord).
- Failure of closure of the processus vaginalis (communicating hydrocele).
- Infection
- Tumors
- Trauma
- Ipsilateral renal transplantation

RISK FACTORS
- Ventriculoperitoneal shunt
- Exstrophy of the bladder
- Cloacal exstrophy
- Ehlers-Danlos syndrome
- Peritoneal dialysis

COMMONLY ASSOCIATED CONDITIONS
- Testicular tumors
- Trauma
- Ventriculoperitoneal shunt
- Nephrotic syndrome
- Renal failure with peritoneal dialysis

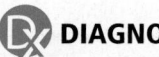 DIAGNOSIS

HISTORY
- Acute or subacute onset of scrotal swelling
- Frequent changes in size of the hydrocele (indicative of a communication)
- Swelling in the scrotum or inguinal canal
- Usually painless
- Sensation of heaviness in the scrotum
- Pain radiating to the flank/back (occasionally)

PHYSICAL EXAM
- Swelling in the scrotum or inguinal canal
- Scrotal mass, usually fluctuant
- Fluctuation in size (communicating hydrocele)
- Scrotal fluid collection that transilluminates

DIFFERENTIAL DIAGNOSIS
- Indirect inguinal hernia
- Orchitis
- Epididymitis
- Traumatic testicular injury
- Testicular torsion or torsion of appendix testes

DIAGNOSTIC TESTS & INTERPRETATION
Lab studies are rarely helpful.
- Inguinoscrotal US: Can demonstrate the presence of bowel (e.g., distinguish incarcerated hernia from a hydrocele of the cord) as well as the presence of testicular torsion (2)
- Testicular nuclear scan or Doppler US: Can distinguish testicular torsion
- Abdominal radiograph: May be useful to distinguish incarcerated hernias from hydroceles (rarely needed)

Diagnostic Procedures/Other

ALERT
Aspiration of a hydrocele for diagnosis should be discouraged.

Test Interpretation
Patent processus vaginalis in communicating hydroceles

 TREATMENT

ISSUES FOR REFERRAL
Recovery should be rapid and complete.

SURGERY/OTHER PROCEDURES
- In children, surgical treatment is generally deferred until 2 years of age, since many hydroceles will spontaneously resolve (1)[C].
  – Surgical: An inguinal approach with ligation of the processus vaginalis and excision, distal splitting, or drainage of hydrocele sac in children (in a hydrocele of cord, the sac can be completely removed) (3)[B]
  – Patients age <12 years should undergo an inguinal approach, whereas a scrotal approach can be considered in children age >12 years (4)[C].
- In adults, no therapy is needed unless the hydrocele causes discomfort or unless there is a significant underlying cause such as a tumor (5).
  – Surgical: A scrotal approach with internal drainage of the hydrocele in adults carries the highest recurrence rate (6)[C].
  – Surgical: A scrotal approach with resection of hydrocele sac has the highest complication rate, but lowest recurrence rate (6)[C].
- Jaboulay-Winkelmann procedure (for a thick hydrocele sac): The hydrocele sac is wrapped posteriorly around cord structures (6)[C], (7)[A].
- Lord procedure (for a thin hydrocele sac): Radial sutures are used to gather the hydrocele sac posterior to testis and epididymis (6)[C], (7)[A].
- Aspiration of the hydrocele with instillation of a sclerosing agent has been successfully used in adults (8)[B]:
  – Aspiration with instillation of sodium tetradecyl sulphate was compared prospectively with the Jaboulay procedure (30 patients each group) (9)[B]:
    ○ The aspiration instillation group had fewer complications with a lower hospital cost, but higher recurrence rates (34%) and more patient dissatisfaction.
  – Aspiration with instillation of 200–400 mg of doxycycline diluted in 10 mL of 0.5% bupivacaine has demonstrated an 84% success rate with a single treatment for nonseptated hydroceles (10)[B]:
    ○ Doxycycline is an inexpensive tetracycline derivative, leading to significantly lower patient hospital costs (11).
- Hydrocelectomy may be performed endoscopically via a transscrotal approach; it involves cauterization of the entire parietal surface of the tunical vaginalis (12)[A].

IN-PATIENT CONSIDERATIONS
Admission Criteria/Initial Stabilization
- Outpatient surgery
- Observation in early infancy until a definite communication is demonstrated or until 2 years of age

 ## ONGOING CARE

FOLLOW-UP RECOMMENDATIONS
Full activity after surgery
Patient Monitoring
- Follow at 3–6-month intervals until a decision is made for/against surgery.
- Postoperative follow-up at 2–4 weeks and subsequent 2–3 month intervals until resolution of any postoperative (traumatic) hydrocele.

COMPLICATIONS
- Complication rate for a scrotal approach may reach 30% (13)[C].
- Postoperative traumatic hydrocele is common and usually resolves spontaneously.
- Injury to vas deferens or spermatic vessels
- Suture granuloma
- Hematoma
- Wound infection: Preoperative antibiotics may be beneficial in reducing postoperative infections (13)[C].
- Recurrence
- Tense infantile abdominoscrotal hydrocele may have high complication rate (14)[C]:
  - May have significant rate of testicular dysmorphism (including hypoplasia)

REFERENCES

1. Hall NJ, Ron O, Eaton S, et al. Surgery for hydrocele in children-an avoidable excess? *J Ped Surg.* 2011;46:2401–2405.
2. Clarke S. Pediatric inguinal hernia and hydrocele: An evidence-based review in the era of minimal access surgery. *J Laparoendosc Adv Surg Tech A.* 2010;20:305–309.
3. Gahukamble DB, Khamage AS. Prospective randomized controlled study of excision vs. distal splitting of hernial sac and processus vaginalis in the repair of inguinal hernias and communicating hydroceles. *J Ped Surg.* 1995;30:624–625.
4. Wilson JM, Aaronson DS, Schrader R, et al. Hydrocele in the pediatric patient: Inguinal or scrotal approach? *J Urol.* 2008;180:1724–1727; discussion 1727–1728.
5. de Castilla-Ramírez B, López-Flores SY, del Rocío Rábago-Rodríguez M, et al. [A clinical guideline for diagnosis and treatment of hydrocele in childhood]. *Rev Med Inst Mex Seguro Soc.* 2011; 49:101–108.
6. Ku JH, Kim ME, Lee NK, et al. The excisional placation and internal drainage techniques: A comparison of the results for idiopathic hydrocele. *BJU.* 2001;87:82–84.
7. Miroglu C, Tokuc R, Saporta L. Comparison of an extrusion procedure and eversion procedures in the treatment of hydrocele. *Int Urol Nephrol.* 1994;26:673–679.
8. Yilmaz U, Ekmekcioglu O, Tatlisen A, et al. Does pleurodesis for pleural effusions give bright ideas about the agents for hydrocele sclerotherapy? *Int Urol Nephrology.* 2000;32:89–92.
9. Khaniya S, Agrawal CS, Koirala R, et al. Comparison of aspiration-sclerotherapy with hydrocelectomy in the management of hydrocele: A prospective randomized study. *Int J Surg (London).* 2009;7:392–395.
10. Francis JJ, Levine LA. Aspiration and sclerotherapy: A nonsurgical treatment option for hydroceles. *J Urol.* 2013;189:1725–1729.
11. Loughlin K. Scrotal pathology: An opportunity for innovative treatment and cost savings. *J Urol.* 2013;189:1624–1625.
12. Emir L, Sunay M, Dadali M, et al. Endoscopic versus open hydrocelectomy for the treatment of adult hydroceles: A randomized controlled clinical trial. *Int Urol Nephrol.* 2011;43:55–59.
13. Swartz MA, Morgan TM, Krieger JN. Complications of scrotal surgery for benign conditions. *Urology.* 2007;69:616–619.
14. Cozzi DA, Mele E, Ceccanti S, et al. Infantile abdominoscrotal hydrocele: A not so benign condition. *J Urol.* 2008;180:2611–2615; discussion 2615.

 ## CODES

ICD10
- N43.2 Other hydrocele
- N43.3 Hydrocele, unspecified

CLINICAL PEARLS
- A hydrocele can usually be diagnosed by physical exam and will transilluminate. Occasionally, US is needed, especially with any concern for an underlying process.
- Aspirating a hydrocele is not recommended as the primary treatment. If a presumed hydrocele is actually an incarcerated inguinal hernia, aspiration may result in significant complications. In addition, hydroceles tend to recur following aspiration unless a sclerosing agent is used.

H

HYDROCEPHALUS, NORMAL PRESSURE

Dennis E. Hughes, DO, FAAFP, FACEP

 BASICS

DESCRIPTION
- Normal pressure hydrocephalus (NPH) is a clinical triad of gait instability, incontinence, and dementia (mnemonic: *wet, wobbly, wacky*). Originally described by Hakim and Adams in 1965, it occurs rarely, but is potentially treatable.
- 2 forms of the disorder: Idiopathic and secondary (to traumatic brain injury, infection, mass lesions or aqueductal stenosis)
- Absence of papilledema on clinical exam and normal CSF pressures at lumbar puncture

Geriatric Considerations
Idiopathic NPH primarily affects persons >60; extremely rare before 40.

EPIDEMIOLOGY
Incidence
- No formal epidemiologic data exist regarding NPH because of the lack of consensus-derived diagnostic criteria. The natural history of untreated NPH has not been studied.
- Idiopathic (iNPH) form primarily affects elderly; at least >40 years of age.
- Secondary form can occur at any age.
- Male = Female

Prevalence
- 3.3/100,000 age 50–59 to 181.7/100,000 age 70–79 for iNPH (1)
- Estimated to be a contributing factor in ~6% of all cases of dementia (2)

ETIOLOGY AND PATHOPHYSIOLOGY
- This is a communicating hydrocephalus, a disorder of decreased CSF absorption (not overproduction). In iNPH, the leading theory suggests that poor venous compliance impairs the subarachnoid granulations' ability to maintain baseline removal of CSF. In secondary NPH, scarring is likely.
- The result is a pressure gradient between the subarachnoid space and ventricular system.
- CSF production decreases in the face of an increased pressure set-point (but still in excess of the amount of CSF absorbed).
- Elevated pressure distends ventricles and compresses the brain parenchyma.
- As a result of compression, ischemic changes occur in the parenchymal vasculature with subsequent tissue damage and loss.
- Some believe that the idiopathic form is a result of persistently insufficient removal of CSF by immature subarachnoid granulations from childhood.
- Secondary NPH may result from:
  – Subarachnoid hemorrhage
  – Head trauma
  – Resolved acute meningitis
  – Chronic meningitis (tuberculosis, syphilis)
  – Paget disease of the skull

RISK FACTORS
- Idiopathic risk is unknown (case reports suggest a possible genetic link, but unsubstantiated).
- Secondary form is due to head trauma, subarachnoid hemorrhage, meningitis, or encephalitis.

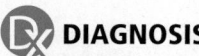 **DIAGNOSIS**

HISTORY
- Insidious and usually progressive; gait instability usually manifests initially, followed by changes in mentation, and eventually, urinary incontinence.
- Difficulty with initiation of movement: Feet appear "glued to the floor." Gait is wide-based, shuffling, and turning appears "en bloc."
- Inattention, forgetfulness, and lack of spontaneity often are seen with the subcortical dementia of NPH.
- Urinary urgency initially, followed by lack of inhibition and then frank incontinence.
- Behavioral changes noted in many cases: Depression, mania, and psychotic features
- A minimum duration of at least 3–6 months of symptoms and progression over time
- A remote trauma or infection suggests secondary vs. the idiopathic form.
- A lack of psychiatric, neurologic, or other medical conditions to explain the symptoms (including structural reasons for CSF flow restriction)
- Because memory impairment may be present, it is important to include a knowledgeable informant who is familiar with the patient's premorbid state.
- Frontal lobe function is affected disproportionately to the memory impairment (objective testing may lead to an early diagnosis).

PHYSICAL EXAM
- Decreased step height and length
- Reduced speed of walking (cadence)
- Widened standing base
- Swaying of trunk during walking
- Decreased fine motor speed and accuracy
- Recall impaired for recent events
- Impaired ability to do multistep tasks or interpret abstractions

DIFFERENTIAL DIAGNOSIS
- Alzheimer disease (may be a comorbid condition in as many as 75%)
- Parkinson disease
- Chronic alcoholism
- Intracranial infection
- Multi-infarct dementia
- Subdural hematoma
- Carcinomatous meningitis
- Collagen vascular disorders
- Depression
- Syphilis
- B_{12} deficiency
- Urologic disorders
- Other hydrocephalus disorders

DIAGNOSTIC TESTS & INTERPRETATION
Initial Tests (lab, imaging)
- Thyroid-stimulating hormone (TSH)
- Syphilis serology
- CBC
- Serum B_{12}, folate
- Metabolic profile
- Blood alcohol, analysis for drugs of abuse
- Urinalysis
- CSF analysis, including an opening pressure <245 mm H_2O (a value greater than this rules out iNPH by definition)
- Imaging is essential:
  – Either CT or MRI shows the ventriculomegaly (particularly lateral and 3rd ventricles) with preservation of the cerebral parenchyma (as opposed to ventricular enlargement seen in other forms of dementia where brain atrophy is present). A narrow subarachnoid space ("tight convexity") was recently shown to correlate to probable or definite iNPH (1)[C].
  – MRI can allow detection of other features, such as signs of altered brain water content and callosal angles. However, these supportive findings are not independently diagnostic of NPH.

Diagnostic Procedures/Other

CSF removal aids in the definitive diagnosis as well as predicting response to surgical treatment:

- High volume (30–70 mL) CSF removal via spinal tap on 3 successive days or continuous spinal drainage (150–200 mL/d) for 3 days
- Comparison of gait analysis before and after CSF removal (a ≥20% improvement indicates a positive test) (2)

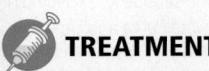

TREATMENT

MEDICATION

- No medication is significantly helpful (2)[C].
- Use of carbonic anhydrase inhibitors (acetazolamide) with repeat lumbar punctures has provided mild and transient relief.
- Use of levodopa to rule out Parkinson disease may be helpful (NPH will display little, if any, significant improvement to dopamine agonist).

ISSUES FOR REFERRAL

- Neurology or neurosurgical consultation is helpful in suspected cases when other reversible medical conditions are ruled out.
- Recent cohort studies have demonstrated clinical improvement after surgical shunts. Perimeters of urinary continence, gait stability, and cognitive scores all improved at 1 year post shunt (3)[B].

ADDITIONAL THERAPIES

Gait training and use of ambulation assist devices, as indicated

SURGERY/OTHER PROCEDURES

- Current therapy is limited to placement of ventriculoperitoneal or ventriculoatrial shunt from a lateral ventricle tunneled SC and drained into the peritoneal cavity (or right atrium). There is no compelling evidence (no RCT) that this therapy is effective (4)[A].
- Patients whose symptoms have been present for a shorter period (<2 years) have a greater chance of improvement with shunting. Also, patients with a known cause of NPH tend to respond more favorably. However, improvement has been seen in patients with symptoms present for a long time.

IN-PATIENT CONSIDERATIONS

Admission Criteria/Initial Stabilization

Usually only for planned surgical treatment

 ONGOING CARE

FOLLOW-UP RECOMMENDATIONS

- Assessment and modification of environment for fall risks
- Evaluation for ability to operate a motor vehicle safely (if driving)

Patient Monitoring

- Repeat neuropsychological testing to evaluate the status of the dementia after treatment
- Improvement in the incontinence and walking speed can also be objectively measured.

PATIENT EDUCATION

Information at: http://www.ninds.nih.gov/disorders/normal_pressure_hydrocephalus/normal_pressure_hydrocephalus.htm

PROGNOSIS

Natural history is progressive deterioration. Patient's axial skeletal stability worsens with inability to walk, stand, sit, or turn over in bed.

COMPLICATIONS

- In patients treated surgically, cerebral infarcts, hemorrhage, infection, and seizures (in addition to the usual surgical risks): All usual age-related illnesses (as NPH is a condition affecting those age >65 years)
- Shunt malfunction (especially when symptoms recur after successful shunt placement)
- Falls due to gait instability
- UTIs
- Skin breakdown, pressure ulcers, infections as movement dysfunction progresses

REFERENCES

1. Shprecher D, Schwalb J, Kurlan R. Normal Pressure Hydrocephalus: Diagnosis and Treatment. *Curr Neurol Neurosci Rep*. 2008;8(5):371–376.
2. Kiefer M, Unterberg A. The differential diagnosis and treatment of normal-pressure hydrocephalus. *Dtsch Arztebl Int*. 2012;109(1–2):15–26.
3. Hashimoto M, Ishikawa M, Mori E, et al. Diagnosis of idiopathic normal pressure hydrocephalus is supported by MRI-based scheme: A prospective cohort study. *Cerebrospinal Fluid Res*. 2010;7:18.
4. Esmonde T, Cooke S, Shunting for normal pressure hydrocephalus (NPH). *Cochran Database Syst Rev*. 2002;3:CD003157.

ADDITIONAL READING

- Pujari S, Kharkar S, Metellus P, et al. Normal pressure hydrocephalus long-term outcome after shunt surgery. *J Neuro Neurosurg Psychiatry*. 2008;79(11):1282–1286.
- Razay G, Vreughenhil A, Liddell J. A prospective study of ventriculo-peritoneal shunting for idiopathic normal pressure hydrocephalus. *J Clin Neurosci*. 2009;16(9):1180–1183.

 SEE ALSO

Algorithm: Ataxia

 CODES

ICD10

- G91.0 Communicating hydrocephalus
- G91.2 (Idiopathic) normal pressure hydrocephalus

CLINICAL PEARLS

- Consider in unexplained dementia.
- Poor prognosis without therapy

H

HYDRONEPHROSIS
Pang-Yen Fan, MD • Jayaprakash Dasari, MD

BASICS

DESCRIPTION
- Hydronephrosis refers to a structural finding—dilatation of the renal calyces and pelvis:
  - May occur with urinary tract infection (UTI), vesicoureteric reflux (VUR), high urine output, or physiologic changes in pregnancy
  - Sometimes accompanied with hydroureter
  - Presentation varies from incidental finding to discovery during workup for UTI or for flank or abdominal pain.
- Hydronephrosis should not be used interchangeably with obstructive uropathy, which refers to the damage to renal parenchyma resulting from urinary tract obstruction (UTO).

EPIDEMIOLOGY
- Hydronephrosis is found in 3% of autopsy specimens.
- Acute unilateral obstruction is more common than bilateral.

ETIOLOGY AND PATHOPHYSIOLOGY
- Hydronephrosis develops with increased pressure in the urinary collecting system.
- Increased pressure within the renal collecting system can cause calyceal fornix rupture and urinary extravasation.
- Over time, pressures return to normal, but kidney function declines from intense renal vasoconstriction.
- With concomitant urinary infection, bacteria can enter the renal vasculature, resulting in sepsis.
- UTO: May be acute/chronic, partial/complete, uni-/bilateral:
  - Intraluminal obstruction: Calculi, sloughed renal papillae, blood clot
  - Intrinsic abnormality of the urinary collecting system: Transitional cell carcinomas, benign prostatic hypertrophy, prostate cancer, congenital ureteropelvic junction (UPJ) obstruction, ureterocele, neurogenic bladder (functional obstruction), urethral stricture or tuberculosis (TB) (can cause ureteral narrowing)
  - Extrinsic compression of the urinary collecting system: Extraurinary malignancy (lymphoma, colon, cervix), aortic/iliac aneurysm, retroperitoneal fibrosis, uterine prolapse (15% affected), endometriosis, ovarian vein syndrome, IgG4 related disease (1)
  - Transplant hydronephrosis: Consider BK virus
- Vesicoureteric reflux (VUR) resulting in varying degrees of hydroureteronephrosis
- Physiologic hydronephrosis of pregnancy
- Hydronephrosis due to high urine output (e.g., diabetes insipidus, psychogenic polydipsia)
- Hydronephrosis of infection: Due to bacterial toxins inhibiting smooth muscle contraction of the renal pelvis and ureter

Pediatric Considerations
- Antenatal hydronephrosis is diagnosed in 1–5% of pregnancies, usually by US, as early as the 12th–14th week of gestation.
- Children with antenatal hydronephrosis are at greater risk of postnatal pathology.
- Postnatal evaluation begins with US exam; further studies, such as voiding cystourethrogram (VCUG), based on the severity of postnatal hydronephrosis

- In neonates, it is the most common cause of abdominal mass.
- Common etiologies in children are VUR, congenital UPJ obstruction, neurogenic bladder, and posterior urethral valves.
- Pediatric diagnostic algorithm differs from adult due to different differential diagnosis necessitating age-appropriate testing.

Pregnancy Considerations
- Physiologic hydronephrosis in pregnancy is more prominent on the right than left and can be seen up to 80% of pregnant women.
- Dilatation is caused by hormonal effects, external compression from expanding uterus, and intrinsic changes in the ureteral wall.
- Despite high incidence, most cases are asymptomatic.
- If symptomatic and refractory to medical management, ureteric calculus should be considered and urinary infection must be excluded.

DIAGNOSIS

Symptoms vary according to cause, chronicity, location, and degree of obstruction.

HISTORY
- Although often asymptomatic, hydronephrosis can be associated with pain ranging from vague, intermittent discomfort to severe renal colic.
- Nausea, vomiting may be associated with severe pain or infection.
- Fever, chills with coexisting infection
- Polyuria may occur due to impaired urinary concentration in partial obstruction, postobstructive diuresis.
- Anuria, if complete bilateral obstruction or complete obstruction of a solitary kidney
- Symptoms of chronic kidney disease: Anorexia, malaise, weight gain, edema, shortness of breath, mental state changes, tremors from longstanding bilateral obstruction.
- Dietl crisis: Sudden attack of flank pain due to distension of renal pelvis caused by rapid ingestion of large amount of liquid or kinking of a ureter producing temporary occlusion of urine flow
- Symptoms of bladder outlet obstruction: Weak urine stream, nocturia, straining to void, overflow incontinence, urgency, and frequency
- General medical and surgical history: Malignancy (extrinsic compression), radiotherapy (ureteric stricture/fibrosis), surgery (iatrogenic obstruction), trauma (hematoma or fibrosis), gynecologic disease (endometriosis, ovarian masses, uterine prolapse), smoking (urothelial cancer), drugs (methysergide-induced retroperitoneal fibrosis)

PHYSICAL EXAM
- General signs:
  - Volume overload (edema, rales, hypertension [HTN]) from renal failure
  - Diaphoresis, tachycardia, tachypnea with pain
  - High-grade fever, if infection
- Abdominal exam: CVA tenderness, palpable bladder, rarely palpable abdominal mass (may be visible, particularly in thin children)

- Pelvic exam: Pelvic mass, uterine prolapse, palpable enlarged prostate (cancer or benign), urethral meatal stenosis, phimosis

DIAGNOSTIC TESTS & INTERPRETATION
- Urinalysis with microscopy: Hematuria, proteinuria, crystalluria, pyuria
- Midstream urine culture and sensitivity: Exclude UTI
- Basic metabolic panel: Elevated urea and creatinine may indicate obstructive uropathy. Hyperkalemic nonanion gap metabolic acidosis may indicate type 4 distal RTA due to obstruction.
- CBC: Anemia of chronic kidney disease (CKD), leukocytosis, if infection; check platelet count prior to considering ureteral instrumentation.
- Prostate-specific antigen (PSA): Adult males age >50 or with abnormal digital rectal exam or bladder outlet obstruction signs or symptoms
- Urine cytology: For malignant cells in urothelial malignancies
- US and noncontrast CT scanning are effective in diagnosing presence and cause of obstruction in most cases.
- US: Screening test of choice for hydronephrosis:
  - Sensitivity 90%, specificity 84.5% compared with IVU. Does not assess function and rarely detects cause and level of obstruction. Degree of hydronephrosis does not correlate with duration or severity of the obstruction
  - Advantages: Detects renal parenchymal disease (decreased renal size, increased cortical echogenicity, cortical thinning, cysts). No exposure to radiation or contrast. Safe in pregnancy, contrast allergy, and renal dysfunction.
  - False–positive findings 15.5% (for UTO): Normal extrarenal pelvis, parapelvic cysts, VUR, excessive diuresis.
  - False–negative findings 10%: Dehydration, acute obstruction, calyceal dilatation misinterpreted as renal cortical cysts, and retroperitoneal fibrosis.

- Noncontrast helical CT (NHCT): Test of choice for suspected nephrolithiasis (2,3)[A]:
  - Reported sensitivity 94–96%, specificity 94–100% (3)[A]. Stone is most commonly found at levels of ureteric luminal narrowing: UPJ, pelvic brim, and the vesicoureteric junction.
  - Typical findings in acute obstruction are hydronephrosis with hydroureter proximal to the level of obstruction, perinephric stranding, and renal swelling. If chronic, renal atrophy may be noted.
  - Advantages: No contrast exposure, time-saving, cost-effective, identifies extraurinary pathology.
  - Disadvantages: Does not assess function or degree of obstruction; higher radiation exposure, although low radiation dose protocols have shown comparable accuracy.

- DTPA or MAG-3 radionuclide renal scan (diuretic renal scintigraphy):
  - Indicated only for evaluation of hydronephrosis without apparent obstruction
  - Determines presence of true obstruction, as well as total and split (R vs. L) renal function
  - Furosemide is given 20 minutes after the tracer and the t1/2 for the tracer's washout is measured. T1/2 <10 minutes is unobstructed, >20 minutes is obstructed, and 10–20 minutes is equivocal; some experts consider <15 minutes normal.
  - Advantages: No contrast exposure, safe in contrast allergy and renal dysfunction

- False–positive findings: Delayed excretion due to renal failure, massive dilatation causing a water-reservoir effect of delayed excretion without obstruction
  - False–negative findings: Dehydration or inadequate diuretic challenge
- Multiphase contrast-enhanced CT:
  - Nonenhanced phase detects stones and swelling.
  - Parenchymal phase demonstrates decreased enhancement of renal parenchyma with acute obstruction; can identify extrarurinary causes of obstruction and determine the relative glomerular filtration rage (GFR) of each kidney with accuracy equal to radionuclide renal scan.
  - Delayed phase allows visualization of the collecting system and soft-tissue filling defects (e.g., urothelial cancer).
- MR urography (MRU): Indicated when US and NHCT are nondiagnostic:
  - Provides anatomic, functional, and prognostic information. Sensitivity not superior to US or NHCT for nephrolithiasis (70%), but superior for soft-tissue causes including strictures.
  - Advantages: No radiation exposure, safe in young children and pregnant women.
  - Disadvantages: More expensive, less available, and time-consuming compared with CT (35 vs. 5 minutes). Gadolinium contraindicated in renal failure due to risk of nephrogenic systemic fibrosis.

Diagnostic Procedures/Other

Cystoscopy, retrograde pyelogram ± ureteroscopy and biopsy are occasionally used to determine the cause of obstruction (e.g., small urothelial cancer missed on imaging) or to confirm a normal distal ureter prior to pyeloplasty. In addition, such procedures are often needed to establish a definitive pathologic diagnosis for mass lesions.

 TREATMENT

GENERAL MEASURES

- Medical treatment: Correction of fluid and electrolyte abnormalities, pain control, antibiotics as an adjunct to drainage if infection present.
- Relief of obstruction: Prompt drainage indicated in the presence of UTI, compromised renal function, or uncontrollable/persistent pain:
  - Bladder outlet obstruction: Urethral or suprapubic catheter
  - Ureteric obstruction: Retrograde (cystoscopic) or antegrade (percutaneous) stenting
- VUR is often managed conservatively with antibiotics; surgical management required in severe cases in children or women of child-bearing age
- Medical expulsive therapy (MET) with α-blockersk or calcium-channel blockers indicated for urethral stones <10 mm in patients with controlled pain, no signs of sepsis, with good renal function (4)[A]

SURGERY/OTHER PROCEDURES

- Hydronephrosis due to obstruction:
  - Congenital UPJ obstruction: Pyeloplasty (open or laparoscopic) and minimally invasive stricture incision (endopyelotomy) are used with comparable results.
  - Nephrolithiasis: Extracorporeal shock wave lithotripsy (ESWL) is the initial treatment of choice for management of impacted upper urethral stones ≤2 cm (5,6)[A]. Ureteroscopy with or without intracorporeal lithotripsy has lower retreatment, but higher complication rates and longer hospital stay (6)[A]. Ureteral stenting pre-ESWL or post ureteroscopy associated with no additional benefit and more discomfort and morbidity (5,7)[A].
  - Transitional cell cancer: Nephroureterectomy
  - Idiopathic retroperitoneal fibrosis: Ureterolysis (frees ureters from inflammatory mass)
  - Prostate disorders: Various treatment modalities, including transurethral resection of the prostate (TURP) and radical prostatectomy
- Nonobstructed hydronephrosis:
  - VUR: Ureteric reimplantation, endoscopic suburethral injection

IN-PATIENT CONSIDERATIONS
Admission Criteria/Initial Stabilization

Obstruction coexisting with infection (pyonephrosis) is a true urologic emergency requiring urgent drainage. Typically, this requires placement of percutaneous nephrostomy tube(s) as retrograde (cystoscopic) stenting is often difficult, but both are equally effective (8)[A].

 ONGOING CARE

FOLLOW-UP RECOMMENDATIONS

- Serial monitoring of kidney function (electrolytes, BUN, and creatinine) and BP until renal function stabilizes. Frequency of monitoring depends on severity of renal dysfunction.
- Follow-up US after stabilization of renal function to assess for resolution of hydronephrosis. If hydronephrosis persists, consider diuretic radionuclide study to rule out persistent obstruction.

PROGNOSIS

- Recovery of renal function depends on etiology, presence or absence of UTI, and degree and duration of obstruction.
- Significant recovery can occur, despite days of complete obstruction, although some irreversible injury may develop within 24 hours. Delays in therapy can lead to irreversible renal damage.
- Diagnostic testing is of poor predictive value. Course of incomplete obstruction is highly unpredictable.

COMPLICATIONS

- Urine stasis: Increased risk of infection and stones formation
- Obstruction causes progressive atrophy of kidney with irreversible loss of function.
- Spontaneous rupture of a calyx may occur with urine extravasation in the perinephric space.

- Postobstructive diuresis: Marked polyuria after relief of obstruction:
  - Caused mostly by fluid and solute overload, but may be exacerbated by impaired renal tubular concentrating ability. Urine output may >500 mL/h.
  - Replace urine losses with hypotonic fluid (usually with 0.45% NaCl) and only enough to avoid volume depletion. Replacement of urine output with equal amounts of saline will perpetuate the diuresis.

REFERENCES

1. Stone JH, Zen Y, Deshpande V. IgG4 related disease. *N Engl J Med*. 20129;36(6):539–551.
2. Worster A, Preyra I, Weaver B, et al. The accuracy of noncontrast helical computed tomography versus intravenous pyelography in the diagnosis of suspected acute urolithiasis: A meta-analysis. *Ann Emerg Med*. 2002;40:280–286.
3. Pfister SA, Deckart A, Laschke S, et al. Unenhanced helical computed tomography vs intravenous urography in patients with acute flank pain: Accuracy and economic impact in a randomized prospective trial. *Eur Radiol*. 2003;13:2513–2520.
4. Seitz C, Liatsikos E, Porpiglia F, et al. Medical therapy to facilitate the passage of stones: What is the evidence? *Eur Urol*. 2009;56:455–471.
5. Ghoneim IA, El-Ghoneimy MN, El-Naggar AE, et al. Extracorporeal shock wave lithotripsy in impacted upper ureteral stones: A prospective randomized comparison between stented and non-stented techniques. *Urology*. 2010;75:45–50.
6. Aboumarzouk OM, Kata SG, Keeley FX, et al. Extracorporeal shock wave lithotripsy (ESWL) versus ureteroscopic management for ureteric calculi. *Cochrane Database Syst Rev*. 2011:CD006029.
7. Shen P, Jiang M, Yang J, et al. Use of ureteral stent in extracorporeal shock wave lithotripsy for upper urinary calculi: A systematic review and meta-analysis. *J Urol*. 2011;186:1328–1335.
8. Ramsey S, Robertson A, Ablett MJ, et al. Evidence-based drainage of infected hydronephrosis secondary to ureteric calculi. *J Endourol*. 2010;24:185–189.

 CODES

ICD10

- N13.2 Hydronephrosis with renal and ureteral calculous obstruction
- N13.30 Unspecified hydronephrosis
- N13.39 Other hydronephrosis

CLINICAL PEARLS

- US and non-contrast CT identify most causes of hydronephrosis.
- Relief of obstruction, when present, is the primary treatment.

H

HYPERCHOLESTEROLEMIA
Sebastian Tong, MD, MPH • Wendy Brooks Barr, MD, MPH, MSCE

BASICS

DESCRIPTION
- Serum cholesterol >200 mg/dL (5.18 mmol/L):
  - A function of lifestyle and genetic (familial) influences
  - Secondary causes exist and should be evaluated.
- Lipoprotein subtypes:
  - Low-density lipoproteins (LDL): Primary target of therapy, atherogenic
  - High-density lipoproteins (HDL): Atheroprotective
  - Triglycerides (TG)
- High cholesterol is a significant risk factor for cardiovascular (CV) disease.
- System(s) affected: CV; Endocrine/Metabolic

EPIDEMIOLOGY
Age: Increases with age (female onset delayed by 10–15 years compared with male)

Prevalence
- 54.9% of men and 46.5% of women in the US with cholesterol >200 mg/dL

ETIOLOGY AND PATHOPHYSIOLOGY
- Pathophysiology:
  - Deposition of cholesterol in vascular walls creating fatty streaks that become fibrous plaques
  - Inflammation causes plaque instability leading to plaque rupture
- Etiology:
  - Primary: Diet, lack of physical activity, obesity
  - Secondary: Hypothyroidism, diabetes, nephritic syndrome, liver disease, chronic renal failure, medications (thiazide diuretics, carbamazepine, cyclosporine, progestins, anabolic steroids, corticosteroids, protease inhibitors)

Genetics
- Type 2 familial hypercholesterolemia (FH):
  - Most severe familial form: autosomal dominant
  - Prevalence = 1/500 in the US
  - High cholesterol levels from birth; atherosclerotic disease in early adulthood and high coronary heart disease (CHD) risk in 40s–50s
  - Tendon xanthomas on Achilles and extensor tendons of hands common
  - Early lipid-lowering drug therapy shown to reduce CHD risk
- Other types: Mutation in apolipoprotein B-100 gene (APO-B) or proprotein convertase subtilisin/kexin type 9 gene (PCSK9)
- Early cholesterol testing of family members beneficial

RISK FACTORS
Diet rich in saturated fat and cholesterol, obesity (BMI >30 kg/m²), physical inactivity, heredity

GENERAL PREVENTION
- Reduced intakes of saturated fat and cholesterol
- Regular physical activity
- Weight control (see "Ongoing Care" section)

COMMONLY ASSOCIATED CONDITIONS
Hypertension, diabetes mellitus (DM), obesity

DIAGNOSIS

Screening recommendations:
- National Cholesterol Education Program (NCEP) Adult Treatment Panel (ATP) III: Fasting lipoprotein profile (total cholesterol, LDL-C, HDL-C, TG) (1)[C]: All adults ≥20 every 5 years
- US Preventive Services Task Force (USPSTF): Total cholesterol and HDL-C every 5 years:
  - All men ≥35 (2)[A]
  - Women ≥45 if at increased risk for CHD (2)[A]
  - Men aged 20–35 and women aged 20–45 if at increased risk for CHD (2)[A]
- American Diabetic Association: Yearly dyslipidemia screening for diabetics

Pediatric Considerations
- National Heart, Lung and Blood Institute (NHLBI): recommends lipid screening on all children between 9 and 11 years (3)[C]. However, these recommendations are quite controversial and not supported by most other organizations.

HISTORY
- Review possible secondary etiologies.
- Review medications that may change lipid levels.
- Assess other CHD risk factors.

PHYSICAL EXAM
Nonspecific findings and not important in diagnosis

DIAGNOSTIC TESTS & INTERPRETATION
Initial Tests (lab, imaging)
- Fasting lipid panel: Total cholesterol, LDL-C, HDL-C, triglycerides (TG) (1): LDL-C is usually a calculated value and is accurate if TG <350 mg/dL
- If elevated LDL-C or other form of hyperlipidemia, clinical/laboratory assessment to rule out secondary dyslipidemia before initiating lipid-lowering therapy: TSH, glucose, creatinine, liver enzymes, uric acid
- Consider genetic etiology in very high LDL (>190 mg/dL).

TREATMENT

- Inconsistent evidence for treatment of hypercholesterolemia for primary prevention: Some evidence to prevent CV disease, no clearly proven benefit in all cause mortality (4)[A]. Number needed to treat (statin therapy) likely ≥ 500/year in most populations to prevent 1 death, if effective.
- Substantial evidence for treatment if history of CV disease
- Many more patients treated and medications used in the US than elsewhere in the world without substantial evidence for improved outcomes.
- In the US, the primary target in hypercholesterolemia therapy is lowering LDL-C (1)[C]:

Risk Factors	LDL Goal
0–1	<160
2+	<130
CHD or CHD risk equivalent	<100

- Optimal goal of LDL <70 for very-high-risk patients although NNT is likely >40–50 people/year to prevent 1 vascular event in secondary prevention.
- Major risk factors that affect CHD risk:
  - Cigarette smoking
  - Hypertension (BP >140/90 mm Hg)
  - Low HDL cholesterol (<40 mg/dL) (if HDL >60 mg/dL, subtract 1 risk factor)
  - Family history of premature CHD (CHD in male 1st-degree relative <55; CHD in female 1st-degree relative <65)
  - Age (men >45, women >55)
- If ≥2 risk factors, assess 10-year risk for CHD
- CHD risk equivalents:
  - Atherosclerotic disease: Peripheral arterial disease, abdominal aortic aneurysm, symptomatic carotid artery disease
  - Diabetes
  - Multiple risk factors that confer a 10-year risk for CHD >20%
- In the UK, decision to initiate treatment is based on 10-year cardiovascular risk:
  - No history of CV disease: If 10 year risk >20%, start simvastatin 40 mg (old recommendation) or atorvastatin 40 mg (likely new recommendation), no further lipid monitoring (5)[A]
  - History of CV disease: Start simvastatin 40 mg (old recommendation) or atorvastatin 40 mg (likely new recommendation); higher intensity if do not attain target (5)[A].

ALERT
Elevated serum TG:
- If >500, TG lowering becomes primary target until TG <500 to prevent acute pancreatitis.
  - 1st line: Fibrate + therapeutic life changes; 2nd line, nicotinic acid

MEDICATION
- Therapeutic lifestyle changes are cornerstone therapies to be attempted before drug therapy (diet and regular exercise; see "Ongoing Care").
- Start meds when >30 mg/dL over LDL goal despite lifestyle modification (US) or 10-year risk >20% (UK).
- Check fasting lipoprotein profile 6 weeks after starting drug therapy to evaluate response (US).
- Once goal reached: Monitor q4–6mo (US).

First Line
HMG-CoA reductase inhibitors (statins):
- Types: Atorvastatin 10–80 mg/d; fluvastatin 20–80 mg/d; lovastatin 10–80 mg/d; pravastatin 10–80 mg/d; rosuvastatin (Crestor, no generic) 5–40 mg/d; simvastatin 5–40 mg/d
- To be taken in the evening or at bedtime for best effect
- Effect is greatest in lowering LDL-C; shown to decrease CHD incidence and all-cause mortality (secondary prevention)(1)[A].
- Contraindications: Pregnancy, lactation, or active liver disease
- Drug interactions: Cyclosporine, macrolide antibiotics, various antifungal agents, HIV protease inhibitors, fibrates/nicotinic acid (to be used with caution)

- Adverse reactions:
  - Liver transaminase elevations (up to 3% of patients): ALT/AST before therapy to establish baseline; subsequent monitoring no longer recommended
  - Myopathies (considered rare but not well studied):
    - ○ Creatine kinase (CK) monitoring not indicated
    - ○ More likely in patients with multiple comorbidities or taking concurrent medications that increase statin concentrations
    - ○ Instruct patients to report immediately any muscle pain, muscle weakness, or brown urine.
    - ○ If myopathy or rhabdomyolysis suspected, discontinue statin use and draw serum CK
    - ○ Can rechallenge statin at lower dose after resolution of symptoms

ALERT
FDA alert: Simvastatin should no longer be prescribed at 80 mg/d doses due to increased risk of myopathy. Patients who have been at this drug dosage for >1 year can continue if no signs of myopathy. Dose restrictions to reduce myopathy risk include:
- Do not exceed simvastatin 10 mg/d with amiodarone, verapamil, and diltiazem.
- Do not exceed simvastatin 20 mg/d with amlodipine and ranolazine.

ALERT
Avoid grapefruit juice.

Pregnancy Considerations
- Statins contraindicated during pregnancy: Class X
- Lactation: Possibly unsafe

Second Line
- Ezetimibe:
  - Can be taken by itself or in combination with a statin: Monotherapy (Zetia 10 mg/d) or ezetimibe/simvastatin (Vytorin 10/10, 10/20, 10/40, 10/80 mg/d)
  - Effect: Lowers LDL-C; no studies to date have shown CV benefit or decreased mortality/morbidity rates (6)[C]. Current indication for use of medication is not clear.
  - Adverse reactions: Generally well tolerated
- Fibrates:
  - Types: Gemfibrozil (Lopid) 600 mg b.i.d., fenofibrate (Antara, Lofibra, Tricor, Triglide) 200 mg/d.
  - Effect: Most effective in lowering TG with moderate effect in lowering LDL and raising HDL. More recent studies with statins fail to show benefit in most patients (6)[C].
  - Contraindications: Severe hepatic or renal insufficiency
  - Possible interactions: Potentiates effects of warfarin and oral hypoglycemic agents. Technically, should be avoided with statins due to increased risk of rhabdomyolysis.
  - Adverse reactions: GI complaints; increased likelihood of gallstones

- Nicotinic acid:
  - Types: Crystalline 1.5–4.5 g/d b.i.d. or t.i.d.; extended-release 1–2 g at bedtime
  - Effect: Most effective lipid-lowering agent for raising HDL levels, but little evidence for improved outcomes in statin era (6)[C]
  - Contraindications: Chronic liver disease, severe gout, hyperuricemia, severe peptic ulcer disease
  - Use with caution with high doses in type 2 diabetes
  - Adverse reactions: Cutaneous flushing, hyperglycemia, hyperuricemia/gout, upper GI distress, hepatotoxicity
- Bile acid sequestrant:
  - Types: Cholestyramine (Questran) 4–16 g/d; colestipol (Colestid) 5–30 g/d; colesevelam (Welchol) 2.6–3.6 g/d
  - Contraindications: Familial dysbetalipoproteinemia; TG >200 mg/dL (relative); TG >400 mg/dL (absolute); complete biliary obstruction; bowel obstruction
  - Possible interactions: Can decrease absorption of other drugs (separate from warfarin, digoxin, and amiodarone administration by at least 2 hours)
  - Adverse reactions: Constipation, nausea, bloating; rarely used now because poorly tolerated by patients

COMPLEMENTARY AND ALTERNATIVE MEDICINE
- Omega-3 fatty acids and fish oil intake: Sources are fish oil (salmon), plant sources (flaxseed, canola oil, soybean oil, nuts); mainly lower TG level, but has some benefit in lowering LDL and raising HDL although overall CV benefit and mortality reduction uncertain. AHA recommendation:
  - No history of CHD: Eat variety of oily fish twice a week
  - History of CHD: 1 g of combined eicosapentaenoic acid (EPA) and docosahexaenoic acid (DHA) daily; preferably from natural oily fish but can consider supplements with physician guidance
- β-Sitosterols and red yeast rice (contains natural lovastatin-analogue) can reduce total cholesterol and LDL.
- Garlic: Appears to have some lipid-lowering effect but more studies needed; effective dose not established but generally 1–2 cloves of raw garlic/d, 300 mg, dried garlic powder tablet b.i.d. or t.i.d., or 7.2 g of aged garlic extract/d

 ## ONGOING CARE

FOLLOW-UP RECOMMENDATIONS
Exercise: Sustained exercise for 30 minutes, 3–4 times per week: Increases HDL, lowers total cholesterol, and helps control weight

Patient Monitoring
Initially, lipid panel every 6 weeks until target goals reached, then q4–6mo to promote compliance and monitor continued response. If taking a statin, check LFTs at baseline, consider at 6 weeks. Subsequent monitoring unnecessary.

DIET
NCEP Therapeutic Lifestyle Changes Diet:
- Dietary fats, 25–35% of total calories: Saturated fat, <7% of total calories; polyunsaturated, <10% of total calories; monounsaturated, <20% of total calories
- Carbohydrates: 50–60% of total calories from whole grains, fruits, vegetables
- Fiber: 20–30 g/d
- Cholesterol: <200 mg/d
- Protein: ~15% of total calories

REFERENCES
1. National Cholesterol Education Program (NCEP) Expert Panel on Detection, Evaluation, and Treatment of High Blood Cholesterol in Adults (Adult Treatment Panel III). Third Report of the National Cholesterol Education Program (NCEP) Expert Panel on Detection, Evaluation, and Treatment of High Blood Cholesterol in Adults (Adult Treatment Panel III) final report. *Circulation.* 2002;84(25):3143–3421.
2. U.S. Preventive Services Task Force. Screening for Lipid Disorders in Adults. Recommendation Statement. June 2008. http://uspreventiveservicestaskforce.org/uspstf/uspschol.htm
3. Integrated Guidelines for Cardiovascular Health and Risk Reduction in Children and Adolescents. December 2011. http://www.nhlbi.nih.gov/guidelines/cvd_ped/index.htm
4. Taylor F, Ward K, Moore TH, et al. Statins for the primary prevention of cardiovascular disease. *Cochrane Database Syst Rev.* 2011;(1):CD004816. Epub 2011 Jan 19.
5. NICE Clinical Guideline 67 (2010) http://www.nice.org.uk/nicemedia/live/11982/40689/40689.pdf
6. Last AR, Ference JD, Falleroni J, et al. Pharmacologic treatment of hyperlipidemia. *Am Fam Physician.* 2011;84:551–558.

 ## SEE ALSO

- Atherosclerosis; Hypothyroidism, Adult
- Algorithm: Hypercholesterolemia

CODES

ICD10
E78.0 Pure hypercholesterolemia

CLINICAL PEARLS
- Hypercholesterolemia is a significant risk factor for CHD. Primary target of therapy is lowering LDL-C (US), treating high-risk patients with statin (UK).
- Diet and exercise should be tried before pharmaceutical interventions.
- Statins are considered 1st-line medications for hypercholesterolemia. Other medications show little evidence of benefit in modern era.

H

HYPEREMESIS GRAVIDARUM

Emma Brooks, MD • Scott A. Fields, MD, MHA

 BASICS

DESCRIPTION
- Hyperemesis gravidarum is persistent vomiting in a pregnant woman that interferes with fluid and electrolyte balance as well as nutrition:
  - Usually associated with the 1st 8–20 weeks of pregnancy
  - Believed to have biomedical and behavioral aspects
  - Associated with high estrogen and human chorionic gonadotropin (hCG) levels
  - Symptoms usually begin ~2 weeks after 1st missed period.
- System(s) affected: Endocrine/Metabolic; Gastrointestinal; Reproductive
- Synonym(s): Morning sickness

Pregnancy Considerations
Common condition during pregnancy, typically in the 1st and 2nd trimesters but may persist into the 3rd trimester.

EPIDEMIOLOGY
Incidence
Hyperemesis gravidarum occurs in 1–2% of pregnancies.

Prevalence
Hyperemesis gravidarum is the most common cause of hospitalization in the 1st half of pregnancy and the 2nd most common cause of hospitalization of pregnant women.

ETIOLOGY AND PATHOPHYSIOLOGY
- Unknown
- Possible psychologic factors
- Hyperthyroidism
- Hyperparathyroidism
- Gestational hormones
- Liver dysfunction
- Autonomic nervous system dysfunction
- CNS neoplasm

RISK FACTORS
- Obesity
- Nulliparity
- Multiple gestations
- Gestational trophoblastic disease
- Gonadotropin production stimulated
- Altered GI function
- Hyperthyroidism
- Hyperparathyroidism
- Liver dysfunction
- Female fetus
- Helicobacter pylori infection

GENERAL PREVENTION
Anticipatory guidance in 1st and 2nd trimesters regarding dietary habits in hopes of avoiding dehydration and nutritional depletion

Pregnancy Considerations
- 2% of pregnancies have electrolyte disturbances.
- 50% of pregnancies have at least some GI disturbance.

COMMONLY ASSOCIATED CONDITIONS
Hyperthyroidism

 DIAGNOSIS

HISTORY
- Hypersensitivity to smell
- Alteration in taste
- Excessive salivation
- Poor appetite
- Nausea
- Vomiting with retching
- Decreased urine output
- Fatigue
- Dizziness with standing

DIAGNOSTIC TESTS & INTERPRETATION
Initial Tests (lab, imaging)
- Urinalysis: May see glucosuria, albuminuria, granular casts, and hematuria (rare); ketosis more common
- Thyroid-stimulating hormone (TSH), T4
- Electrolytes, BUN, creatinine:
  - Electrolyte abnormalities due to nausea and vomiting and subsequent dehydration
  - Acidosis
- Calcium
- Increased uric acid
- Hypoalbuminemia
- No imaging is indicated for the diagnosis of hyperemesis gravidarum.

Follow-Up Tests & Special Considerations
- If hypercalcemia, consider checking parathyroid hormone (PTH) for hyperparathyroidism.
- Drugs are unlikely to alter lab results.
- Severe hyperemesis may be associated with increased hCG levels in genetic triple testing.

Diagnostic Procedures/Other
Indicated only if it is necessary to rule out other diagnoses, as listed below

DIFFERENTIAL DIAGNOSIS
Other common causes of vomiting must be considered:
- Gastroenteritis
- Gastritis
- Reflux esophagitis
- Peptic ulcer disease
- Cholelithiasis
- Cholecystitis
- Pyelonephritis
- Anxiety
- Hyperparathyroidism

 TREATMENT

Pyridoxine and metoclopramide (pregnancy Category A) are first-line treatments for hyperemesis gravidarum, followed by prochlorperazine (pregnancy Category C), prednisolone (pregnancy Category A), promethazine (pregnancy Category C), and ondansetron (pregnancy Category B1) (1).

GENERAL MEASURES
- Patient reassurance
- Bed rest
- If dehydrated, IV fluids, preferably normal saline with potassium supplementation as needed. Repeat if there is a recurrence of symptoms following initial improvement.
- For severe cases, consider PO thiamine 25–50 mg t.i.d. or IV 100 mg in 100 mL of normal saline over 30 minutes once weekly (2).
- Ondansetron carries an FDA warning regarding concerns for QT prolongation, but this is in the setting of high-dose IV administration and in patients with heart disease. It has unclear risk in the setting of pregnancy (3)[C]. The current studies appear to show no increased risk of fetal malformation with the use of ondansetron, but this is still an area of controversy (4,5)[B].

MEDICATION
- Pyridoxine (vitamin B_6) 10–30 mg/d PO or IV
- Antihistamines (e.g., diphenhydramine [25–50 mg q4–6h] or doxylamine [12.5 mg PO b.i.d.])
- Combination product Diclegis (sustained release pyridoxine 10 mg and doxylamine 10 mg) dosed 2 tabs daily-2 b.i.d. approved in 2013
- Phenothiazines (e.g., promethazine or prochlorperazine):
  - Precautions: Phenothiazines are associated with prolonged jaundice, extrapyramidal effects, hyper- or hyporeflexia in newborns
- Meclizine 25 mg PO q6h
- Methylprednisolone 16 mg/d PO for 3 days, then taper over 2 weeks if initial 3-day treatment effective (6)
- Ondansetron 4–8 mg PO q8h

Pregnancy Considerations
All medications taken during pregnancy should balance the risks and benefits both to the mother and the fetus.

COMPLEMENTARY AND ALTERNATIVE MEDICINE

- Ginger 350 mg PO t.i.d. may help (7)[B].
- Motion sickness wristbands are another nonpharmacologic intervention that may improve symptoms.
- Evidence is mixed regarding the impact of acupressure and acupuncture in treating hyperemesis gravidarum. but currently no convincing evidence for their use in this setting.
- Medical hypnosis may be a powerful adjunct to the typical medical treatment regimen.

IN-PATIENT CONSIDERATIONS
Admission Criteria/Initial Stabilization
- Typically outpatient therapy
- In some severe cases, parenteral therapy in the hospital or at home may be required.
- Enteral volume and nutrition repletion may be indicated.

ONGOING CARE

FOLLOW-UP RECOMMENDATIONS
Activity as tolerated after improvement (7,8)
Patient Monitoring
- In severe cases, follow up on a daily basis for weight monitoring.
- Special attention should be given to monitoring for ketosis, hypokalemia, or acid–base disturbances due to hyperemesis.

DIET
- NPO for first 24 hours if patient is ill enough to require hospitalization
- For outpatient: A diet rich in carbohydrates and protein, such as fruit, cheese, cottage cheese, eggs, beef, poultry, vegetables, toast, crackers, rice. Limit intake of butter. Patients should avoid spicy meals and high-fat foods. Consider cold foods.

PATIENT EDUCATION
- Attention should be given to psychosocial issues, such as possible ambivalence about the pregnancy.
- Patients should be instructed to take small amounts of fluid frequently to avoid volume depletion.
- Avoid individual foods known to be irritating to the patient.
- Wet-to-dry nutrients (sherbet, broth, gelatin to dry crackers, toast)

PROGNOSIS
- Self-limited illness with good prognosis if patient's weight is maintained at >95% of prepregnancy weight.
- With complication of hemorrhagic retinitis, mortality rate of pregnant patient is 50%.

COMPLICATIONS
- Patients with >5% weight loss are associated with intrauterine growth retardation and fetal anomalies.
- Poor weight gain is associated with slightly increased risk for small for gestational age infant <2,500 g and premature birth <37 weeks (9)[A].
- Hemorrhagic retinitis
- Liver damage
- CNS deterioration, Wernicke encephalopathy secondary to thiamine deficiency, coma

REFERENCES

1. Tan PC, Omar SZ. Contemporary approaches to hyperemesis during pregnancy. *Curr Opin Obstet Gynecol*. 2011;23:87–93.
2. Jarvis S, Nelson-Piercy C. Management of nausea and vomiting in pregnancy. *BMJ*. 2011;342:d3606.
3. Doggrell SA, Hancox JC. Cardiac safety concerns for ondansetron, an antiemetic commonly used for nausea linked to cancer treatment and following anesthesia. *Expert Opin Drug Saf*. 2013;12:421–431.
4. Pasternak B, Svanstrom H, Hviid A. Ondansetron in pregnancy and risk of adverse fetal outcomes. *N Engl J Med*. 2013;368:814–823.
5. Anderka M, Mitchell AA, Louik C, et al. Medications used to treat nausea and vomiting of pregnancy and the risk of selected birth defects. *Birth Defects Res A Clin Mol Teratol*. 2012;94:22–30.
6. Yost NP, McIntire DD, Wians FH, et al. A randomized, placebo-controlled trial of corticosteroids for hyperemesis due to pregnancy. *Obstet Gynecol*. 2003;102:1250–1254.
7. Borrelli F, Capasso R, Aviello G. Effectiveness and safety of ginger in the treatment of pregnancy-induced nausea and vomiting. *Obstet Gynecol*. 2005;105:849–856.
8. Cedergren M, Brynhildsen J, Josefsson A. Hyperemesis gravidarum that requires hospitalization and the use of antiemetic drugs in relation to maternal body composition. *Am J Obstet Gynecol*. 2008;198:412.e1–e5.
9. Veenendaal MV, van Abeelen AF, Painter RC, et al. Consequences of hyperemesis gravidarum for offspring: A systematic review and meta-analysis. *BJOG*. 2011;118:1302–1313.

ADDITIONAL READING

- Matthews A, Dowswell T, Haas DM, et al. Interventions for nausea and vomiting in early pregnancy. *Cochrane Database Syst Rev*. 2010;9:CD007575.
- Peled Y, Melamed N, Krissi H, et al. The impact of severe hyperemesis gravidarum on the triple test screening results. *J Matern Fetal Neonatal Med*. 2012;25:637–638.
- Poursharif B, Korst LM, Fejzo MS, et al. The psychosocial burden of hyperemesis gravidarum. *J Perinatol*. 2008;28:176–181.
- Rashid M, Rashid MH, Malik F, et al. Hyperemesis gravidarum and fetal gender: A retrospective study. *J Obstet Gynaecol*. 2012;32:475–478.
- Sheehan P. Hyperemesis gravidarum–assessment and management. *Aust Fam Physician*. 2007;36:698–701.
- Simon EP, Schwartz J. Medical hypnosis for hyperemesis gravidarum. *Birth*. 1999;26:248–254.
- Terry AR, Barker FG, Leffert L, et al. Outcomes of hospitalization in pregnant women with CNS neoplasms: A population-based study. *Neuro-oncology*. 2012;14:768–776.
- Trogstad LI, Stoltenberg C, Magnus P, et al. Recurrence risk in hyperemesis gravidarum. *BJOG*. 2005;112:1641–1645.
- Verberg MF, Gillott DJ, Al-Fardan N, et al. Hyperemesis gravidarum, a literature review. *Hum Reprod Update*. 2008;11:527–539.
- Xu J, MacKenzie IZ. The current use of acupuncture during pregnancy and childbirth. *Curr Opin Obstet Gynecol*. 2012;24:65–71.

 CODES

ICD10
- O21.0 Mild hyperemesis gravidarum
- O21.1 Hyperemesis gravidarum with metabolic disturbance
- O21.9 Vomiting of pregnancy, unspecified

CLINICAL PEARLS
- Do not allow patients to become volume depleted. Once this occurs, it is more difficult to interrupt the process.
- Do not be hesitant to use medications to assist the patient, as this may help avoid volume depletion.
- Consider secondary causes of hyperemesis if it develops after 12 weeks of gestation (2).

H

HYPEREOSINOPHILIC SYNDROME

Lacey Beth Elwyn, DO • Jenifer Rae Lloyd, DO

BASICS

DESCRIPTION

- Hypereosinophilic syndrome (HES): A group of disparate disorders that sustain an overproduction of eosinophils that subsequently infiltrate and damage multiple organs:
- Defining features (1,2):
  – Hypereosinophilia (HE); with eosinophilia-mediated organ damage
  – Hypereosinophilia:
    ○ A persistent blood eosinophilia >1.5 × 109 cells/L on two examinations separated by at least 1 month and/or tissue HE
    ○ Exclusion of all other causes of organ damage and eosinophilia (e.g., "MAAACP": **m**alignancy, **a**sthma, **a**llergy, **A**ddison disease (AD), **c**onnective tissue disease, **p**arasitic infection).
    ○ Tissue HE defined by:
      ▪ Eosinophils >20% of all nucleated cells on bone marrow section and/or
      ▪ Extensive tissue infiltration on histopathology and/or
      ▪ Marked deposition of eosinophil granular proteins in tissue
- System(s) affected: Hematologic; Cardiac; Cutaneous; Pulmonary; Neurologic; Gastrointestinal; Rheumatologic; Ocular
- Clinically relevant variants (3):
  – T-cell lymphocytic (L-HES): Benign polyclonal hypergammaglobulinemia, but may progress to T-cell lymphoma. CD3−/CD4+, interleukin (IL)-5–producing T cells. Prominent skin findings include erythroderma, plaques, and/or urticarial.
  – Myeloproliferative (F/P+HES): Almost exclusively in males with *FIP1L1-PDGFRa* fusion (Fip1-like-1 fused with platelet derived growth factor receptor alpha (F/P)[2] and increased serum B_{12}, bicytopenia, organomegaly, increased serum tryptase, and positive mast cell abnormalities)
  – Familial HES: AD asymptomatic eosinophilia present at birth
  – Benign HES: Hypereosinophilia without end organ damage
  – Complex HES: Multisystem organ involvement
  – Episodic HES: Periodic rise in IL-5 leads to angioedema and eosinophilia, resolves spontaneously. May progress to L-HES
  – Overlap HES: Restricted eosinophilia to a single organ (GI, pulmonary, cardiac, vascular)
  – Associated HES: Other clinical situations with hypereosinophilia:
    ○ Churg-Strauss syndrome (eosinophilic vasculitis that can affect skin, sinuses, heart, lungs, peripheral nerves), Gleich syndrome (episodic HES with pruritus, urticarial, fever, weight gain, increase serum IgM and leukocytosis)
    ○ Immunodysregulation conditions (collagen vascular disease, sarcoid, ulcerative colitis, autoimmune lymphoproliferative syndrome, HIV)
    ○ Hypereosinophilia of undetermined significance (no complications related to tissue eosinophilia)

EPIDEMIOLOGY

A rare condition, prevalence 0.36–6.3/100,000, typically seen between 20 and 50 years

Incidence

- Peak incidence in 4th decade of life
- Uncommon in children
- Incidence decreases in elderly
- Predominant sex: Male > Female (9:1)

ETIOLOGY AND PATHOPHYSIOLOGY

- Primary molecular defect resulting in clonal eosinophilic proliferation and/or overproduction or functional abnormalities of eosinophilopoietic cytokines and/or defects in normal suppressive regulation of eosinophilopoiesis
- Three hematopoietic cytokines: IL-3, IL-5, and granulocyte-macrophage colony-stimulating factor (GM-CSF) stimulate bone marrow myeloid progenitors to overproduce eosinophils; IL-5 is most specific for eosinophil differentiation.
- Pathogenesis:
  – HES: Eosinophils infiltrate organs and release toxic granules containing major basic protein, eosinophil peroxidase, eosinophil cationic protein (ECP), eosinophil-derived neurotoxin (EDN), Charcot Leyden crystals, VIP, and substance P. Neurotoxic, cytotoxic, and prothrombotic; creates oxidative burst, reactive oxygen species
  – EDN and ECP activate fibroblasts: Fibrosis and organ dysfunction

Genetics

- F/P+HES: Microdeletion at 4q12 causing gene fusion creates constitutively active tyrosine kinase.
- Other *PDGFRA* fusion partners besides *FIP1L1*; *PDGFRb* → translocation at 5q31-33 and *FGFR1* → translocation at 8p11-13
- L-HES: Clonal T-cell expansion; mutations such as 16q breakage, partial 6q or 10p deletions, trisomy 7
- Familial eosinophilia: Autosomal dominant, at 5q31-q33; eosinophilia at birth, often asymptomatic
- Cardiac disease more in males, carriers of HLA-Bw44

RISK FACTORS

Male gender (F/P+HES)

GENERAL PREVENTION

No documented measures

DIAGNOSIS

- A persistently elevated eosinophil count >1.5 × 10^9 cells/L on 2 examinations at least 1 month apart and/or tissue hypereosinophilia
- Eosinophil-medicated organ damage in which other potential causes for the damage have been excluded

PHYSICAL EXAM

- Dermatologic manifestations (37%) may cause pruritic lichenified eczematous rash with papules and nodules, plus dermatographism, and/or recurrent urticaria and angioedema. May also cause erythroderma. Mucosal ulcerations are more common in patients with *FIP1L1-PDGFRa* fusion (4)
- Pulmonary manifestations (25%) may cause dyspnea, wheezing, and nonproductive cough (4).
- GI manifestations (14%): Gastritis/enteritis: Diarrhea, vomiting, abdominal pain (embolic bowel infarction); hepatic manifestations of hepatitis, Budd-Chiari syndrome (4)

- Cardiac manifestations (5%) may cause endocarditis, myocarditis, shortness of breath, chest pain (4), ventricular failure, cardiomegaly, and/or restrictive cardiomyopathy. Eosinophilic myocarditis more common in patients with *FIP1L1-PDGFRα* fusion (4)
- Asymptomatic hypereosinophilia (6%) (4)
- Neurologic manifestations may result from thromboembolic disease: Behavioral changes, memory loss, confusion, neuropathy (4)
- Ocular manifestations: Blurry vision/blindness from microemboli (4)
- Other: Myalgias, arthralgias (4)

DIFFERENTIAL DIAGNOSIS

- Leukemias, lymphomas, paraneoplastic syndromes, *KIT* mutation-associated systemic mastocytosis with eosinophilia, drug hypersensitivity reactions, and helminth infections
- Chronic eosinophilic leukemia: Clonality like F/P+HES but differs by having 2–20% blasts peripherally or 5–20% blasts in the marrow
- Acute eosinophilic leukemia: A form of AML with 50–80% immature eosinophils, >10% blast in marrow; may cause cardiac and neurologic complications

DIAGNOSTIC TESTS & INTERPRETATION

- Hypereosinophilia >1.5 × 10^9 cells/L on 2 occasions; may be discovered incidentally on routine lab testing
- CBC with differential and peripheral smear:
  – Leukocytosis of 10,000–30,000 (>90,000 carries poor prognosis)
  – Mature eosinophils ≥1,500 cells/μL (nuclear hypersegmentation, hypo- and hypergranularity): Hypogranularity and vacuolization more common with cardiac disease
  – Often normal platelets, but may have thrombocytosis or thrombocytopenia in cases with features of MPD (plus tear drop cells)
  – Normocytic anemia (anemia of chronic disease)
- Genetics:
  – Fluorescent in situ hybridization (FISH) analysis or reverse transcription-polymerase chain reaction (RT-PCR): Assess *FIP1L1/PDGFRA* translocation/other TK mutations such as *PDGFRA* variants, *PDGFRB*, *FGFR1*
  – Rule our *c-KIT* mutation (mastocytosis)
  – RT-PCR or Southern blot: Assess IL-5-producing CD3−/CD4+ T lymphocytes
- Chemistries:
  – Increased IgE
  – Increased serum tryptase and B_{12} levels (F/P+myeloproliferative HES)
  – L-HES: Increased IL-5, IgG, IgM, thymus and activation-regulated chemokine (TARC) levels
- ECG: T-wave inversion, restrictive cardiomyopathy

Initial Tests (lab, imaging)

- Elevated serum tryptase
  – Peripheral blood screening for *FIP1L1-PDGFRA* first.
  – If negative, then bone marrow biopsy and cytogenetics for *FIP1L1/PDGFRA*, *BCR/ABL*, *c-KIT* translocations; T-lymphocyte phenotyping with flow cytometry and T-cell receptor (TCR) analysis (5)
- If all negative, consider idiopathic HES.
- Echocardiogram
- Abdominal/chest CT: Assess splenomegaly, end-organ involvement

Diagnostic Procedures/Other
- Tissue biopsy (organ-restricted disease); bone marrow aspirate and biopsy
- Histopathology:
  – Organ infiltration with eosinophils and lymphocytes, tissue necrosis, eosinophil degranulation, and microabscesses

 TREATMENT

- One must consider *FIP1L1/PDGFRA* (F/P) transcript status.
- Initial treatment involve a trial of glucocorticoids alone in all patients *EXCEPT* those with F/P+

MEDICATION
- F/P+HES:
  – Tyrosine kinase inhibitors (TKIs) in all patients with or without symptoms
  – Danger of heart failure with therapy initiation (rapid release of killed eosinophil contents): Obtain troponin, monitor carefully, treat with corticosteroids 1–2 mg/kg/d concurrently or prior to initiation of therapy if complications arise, cardiac enzymes elevated, abnormal echocardiogram.
  – TKIs shown to induce complete molecular response (no F/P transcript); not yet known to be curative
- F/P–HES:
  – Corticosteroids are the mainstay of treatment.
  – A corticosteroid-sparing agent (interferon-alfa, anti-CD52 agents in L-HES, IL-5 inhibitors, chemotherapeutic agents) may be used if steroids poorly tolerated or fail to manage disease.
  – May respond to TKI, suggesting non-F/P tyrosine kinase activity

First Line
- F/P+, PDGFRA/B, FGFR1 HES: Imatinib mesylate (Gleevec) at 100–400 mg/d:
  – 100 mg/d in *PDGFRA*
  – 400 mg/d in *PDGFRB* and *FGFR1*
  – Generally, lower doses needed to induce/maintain remission than with chronic myelogenous (or myeloid) leukemia (CML). Therapy is continued indefinitely.
  – Side effects: Thrombocytopenia, anemia, nausea, diarrhea, increased liver function tests (LFTs)
  – Resistance: T674I point mutation, similar to CML
- F/P–HES: Prednisone: Initial challenge of 60 mg once to determine responsiveness, followed by 1 mg/kg/d × 1–2 weeks. A taper should be initiated based on disease severity, persistent eosinophilia:
  – Intolerance should prompt decreasing dose, adding 2nd agent.
  – Once stable, may add corticosteroid-sparing agent

Second Line
- F/P+HES: Patients rarely have shown resistance to imatinib; initiate trial of other TKI such as nilotinib, sorafenib, or dasatinib.
- F/P–HES:
  – Imatinib:
    ○ Trial of 400 mg/d once stabilized on steroids or fail to respond/intolerant to steroids.
  – Interferon-alfa:
    ○ Effective dose 1–8 million U 3–7 times a week; start low, increase as tolerated.
    ○ Side effects: Flu-like symptoms, cytopenia, depression, elevated LFTs, GI disturbances
  – Hydroxyurea:
    ○ Start at 500–1,000 mg/d, increase to 2,000 mg/d

  ○ Side effects: Cytopenia, nausea, rash, alopecia, diffuse pulmonary infiltrates, elevated LFTs, teratogen
  – Mepolizumab (in clinical trials) (6):
    ○ Anti-IL5 antibody; administered 750 mg IV every 4 weeks. Decreases steroid use
    ○ FDA approved Orphan Drug Designation
    ○ Side effects: Fatigue, headaches, arthralgia, pruritus
  – Alemtuzumab (7):
    ○ Anti-CD52 antibody, IV administration
    ○ Effective for relapsed refractory idiopathic HES and chronic eosinophilic leukemia NOS
    ○ Side effects: Infusion reactions and hematologic toxicity with immunosuppression, leading to increased risk of opportunistic infections, especially CMV reactivation

ISSUES FOR REFERRAL
Refer to a hematologist and appropriate specialist for organ involved.

ADDITIONAL THERAPIES
Being studied:
- A European study of *PDGFR* fusion oncogenes shows that they proliferate autonomously and differentiate toward eosinophil lineage via nuclear factor (NF)-κB, suggesting possible treatment (8).
- JAK 1/2 inhibitor, ruxolitinib, may have a role in treatment (3).

SURGERY/OTHER PROCEDURES
- Allogeneic stem cell transplant:
  – Patients failing other treatment modalities and/or aggressive disease
  – Patients with L-HES progressing to T-cell lymphoma
  – Role has not been well established
- Cardiac surgery for complications of HES has been efficacious. If valve replacement is necessary, use porcine valve because of underlying hypercoagulable state.

IN-PATIENT CONSIDERATIONS
Admission Criteria/Initial Stabilization
- Emergency treatment for eosinophilia >100,000 includes high-dose corticosteroids (prednisone 1 mg/kg).
- If levels fail to decrease in 24 hours: Vincristine 1–2 mg/m^2, imatinib 400 mg, or plasmapheresis
- Heart failure, splenic rupture, organ failure; very high eosinophilia

 ONGOING CARE

FOLLOW-UP RECOMMENDATIONS
Depends on etiology of disease, response to treatment, and severity of end-organ damage

Patient Monitoring
- Weekly CBC on treatment; longer when stable
- L-HES: Increased risk of T-cell lymphoma; CBC every 3 months; flow cytometry biannually to monitor abnormal lymphocytosis
- Patients on imatinib: LFTs and CBC monthly; RT-PCR for the F/P transcript; echocardiogram every 3 months
- Screen for organ involvement every 6 months: Cardiac enzymes, pulmonary function tests, LFTs, renal function tests, ECG, echocardiogram
- Anticoagulation unnecessary unless thrombi present.

PROGNOSIS
- Better prognosis:
  – Absence heart disease
  – Presentation with angioedema
  – Corticosteroid responsive
  – Absent indicators of myeloproliferative disease (elevated B$_{12}$ or tryptase, splenomegaly, abnormal lymphocytes, cytogenetic abnormalities)
- Worse prognosis:
  – Concurrent myeloproliferative disorder
  – Male sex
  – Peripheral blood blasts
  – WBC count >100,000

REFERENCES
1. Chusid MJ, Dale DC, West BC, et al. The hypereosinophilic syndrome: analysis of fourteen cases with review of the literature. *Medicine (Baltimore)*. 1975;54:1.
2. Valent P, Klion AD, Horny HP, et al. Contemporary consensus proposal on criteria and classification of eosinophilic disorders and related syndromes. *J Allergy Clin Immunol*. 2012;130:607.
3. Simon HU, Rothenberg ME, Bochner BS, et al. Refining the definition of hypereosinophilic syndrome. *J Allergy Clin Immunol*. 2010;126:45.
4. Ogbogu PU, Bochner BS, Butterfield JH, et al. Hypereosinophilic syndrome: a multicenter, retrospective analysis of clinical characteristics and response to therapy. *J Allergy Clin Immunol*. 2009;124:1319.
5. Tefferi A, Gotlib J, Pardanani A, et al. Hypereosinophilic syndrome and clonal eosinophilia: Point-of-care diagnostic algorithm and treatment update. *Mayo Clin Proc*. 2010;85:158–164.
6. Gotlib J. World Health Organization-defined eosinophilic disorders: 2012 update on diagnosis, risk stratification, and management. *Am J Hematol*. 2012;87:903–914.
7. Verstovsek S, Tefferi A, Kantarjian H, et al. Alemtuzumab therapy for hypereosinophilic syndrome and chronic eosinophilic leukemia. *Clin Cancer Res*. 2009;15:368–373.
8. Montano-Almendras CP, Essaghir A, Schoemans H, et al. ETV6-PDGFRB and FIP1L1-PDGFRA stimulate human hematopoietic progenitor cell proliferation and differentiation into eosinophils: The role of nuclear factor-κB. *Haematologica*. 2012;97:1064–1072.

CODES

ICD10
D72.1 Eosinophilia

CLINICAL PEARLS
- HS encompasses a group of diseases with eosinophils >1,500/μL and end-organ damage without an identifiable secondary cause.
- F/P+ transcript should be determined early in the course of treatment.
- Prognosis and treatment depend on subtype.
- Cardiac disease is a dangerous complication of this condition and may not be reversible.

H

HYPERKALEMIA
Ruben Peralta, MD, FACS

 BASICS

DESCRIPTION
- Hyperkalemia is a common electrolyte disorder with a plasma potassium (K) concentration >5.5 mEq/L (>5 mmol/L).
- Hyperkalemia depresses cardiac conduction and can lead to fatal arrhythmias.
- Normal K regulation:
  - Ingested K enters portal circulation; pancreas releases insulin in response. Insulin facilitates K entry into cells.
  - K in renal circulation causes renin release from juxtaglomerular cells, leading to activation of angiotensin I, which is converted to angiotensin II in lungs. Angiotensin II acts in adrenal zona glomerulosa to stimulate aldosterone secretion. Aldosterone, at the renal collecting ducts, causes K to be excreted and sodium (Na) to be retained.
- 4 major causes:
  - Increased load: Either endogenous from tissue release or exogenous from a high intake, which is usually in association with impaired excretion
  - Decreased excretion: Due to decreased glomerular filtration rate
  - Cellular redistribution: Shifting of intracellular space (which is the major store of K) to extracellular space
  - Pseudohyperkalemia: Related to improper collection or transport of blood sample

Geriatric Considerations
Increased risk for hyperkalemia because of decreases in renin and aldosterone as well as increased number of comorbid conditions

EPIDEMIOLOGY
Prevalence
- 1–10% of hospitalized patients
- Predominant sex: Male = Female
- No age-related predilection

ETIOLOGY AND PATHOPHYSIOLOGY
- Pseudohyperkalemia:
  - Hemolysis of red cells in phlebotomy tube (spurious result is most common)
  - Thrombolysis
  - Leukocytosis
  - Thrombocytosis
  - Hereditary spherocytosis
  - Infectious mononucleosis
- Traumatic venipuncture or fist clenching during phlebotomy (spurious result)
- Transcellular shift (redistribution):
  - Metabolic acidosis
  - Insulin deficiency
  - Hyperglycemia
  - Tissue damage (rhabdomyolysis, burns, trauma) (1)
  - Tumor lysis syndrome (2)
  - Cocaine abuse
  - Exercise with heavy sweating
  - Mannitol

- Impaired K excretion:
  - Renal insufficiency/failure
  - Addison disease
  - Mineralocorticoid deficiency
  - Primary hyporeninemia, primary hypoaldosteronism
  - Type IV renal tubular acidosis
- Medication-induced:
  - Excess K supplementation
  - Lipid-lowering agents: Statins
  - ACE inhibitors (3)
  - Angiotensin receptor blockers
  - β-blockers
  - Cyclosporine
  - Digoxin toxicity
  - Ethinyl estradiol/drospirenone
  - Heparin
  - NSAIDs
  - Penicillin G potassium
  - Pentamidine
  - Spironolactone
  - Succinylcholine
  - Tacrolimus
  - Trimethoprim (3,4)

Genetics
Associated with some inherited diseases and conditions:
- Familial hyperkalemic periodic paralysis
- Congenital adrenal hyperplasia

RISK FACTORS
- Impaired renal excretion of K
- Acidemia
- Massive cell breakdown (rhabdomyolysis, burns, trauma)
- Use of K-sparing diuretics
- Excess K supplementation

GENERAL PREVENTION
Diet and oral supplement compliance

 DIAGNOSIS

HISTORY
- Neuromuscular cramps
- Diarrhea
- Abdominal pain
- Myalgias
- Numbness
- Weakness

PHYSICAL EXAM
- Decreased deep tendon reflexes
- Flaccid paralysis of extremities

DIAGNOSTIC TESTS & INTERPRETATION
- Serum electrolytes
- Renal function: BUN, creatinine
- Urinalysis: K, creatinine, osmoles (to calculate fractional excretion of K and transtubular K gradient; both assess renal handling of K)
- Disorders that may alter lab results:
  - Acidemia: K shifts from the intracellular to extracellular space in an effort to buffer the acid load.
  - Insulin deficiency
  - Hemolysis of sample
- Cortisol and aldosterone levels to check for mineralocorticoid deficiency when other causes are ruled out

Diagnostic Procedures/Other
ECG:
- Peaked T wave in precordial leads (most common, usually earliest ECG change) (5)
- Loss of P wave
- Widened QRS
- Sine wave at very high K

TREATMENT

MEDICATION
- After initial treatment with calcium gluconate IV to stabilize myocardial membranes (if life-threatening hyperkalemia is present), institute measures to decrease total body K:
  - Sodium polystyrene sulfonate (Kayexalate): 30–60 g PO or rectally
  - This is effective in 1–4 hours and is a definitive treatment. This may be repeated q6h, if necessary.
  - Enema form more quickly effective
- Little clinical evidence for the use of diuretics (loop and thiazides) (1)[B].
- Dextrose 50% 1 amp (if plasma glucose <250 mg/dL) and insulin 10 U IV may drive potassium intracellularly, but does not decrease total body potassium and may result in hypokalemia (close monitoring advised).
- Nebulized albuterol and other β-agonists also drive potassium inside cells, but do not lower total body potassium.
- Consider the use of recombinant urate oxidase (Rasburicase) in patients with tumor lysis syndrome.
- Hemodialysis is the definitive therapy when other measures are not effective. Conditions such as digitalis toxicity or rhabdomyolysis exist in patients with end-stage renal disease, severe chronic kidney disease, acute kidney injury, or comorbidity.

ALERT

- Kayexalate provides a sodium load that may exacerbate fluid overload in patients with cardiac or renal failure.
- Rapid administration of calcium in patients with suspected digitalis toxicity may result in a fatal dysrhythmia. Calcium should be administered slowly over 20–30 minutes in 5% dextrose with extreme caution.
- Calcium and dextrose/insulin are only temporizing measures and do not actually lower total body K levels.
- Sodium bicarbonate is no longer recommended to lower K, although it may be appropriate in patients with severe metabolic acidosis.

IN-PATIENT CONSIDERATIONS
Admission Criteria/Initial Stabilization

- If hyperkalemia is severe, treat first, and then do diagnostic investigations.
- IV calcium to stabilize myocardium (caution in setting of digoxin toxicity, when calcium may worsen effects of toxicity)
- Insulin (usually 10 U IV, given with 50 mL of 50% glucose to avoid hypoglycemia); consider repeating if elevation persists.
- Inhaled β_2-agonist (nebulized albuterol)
- Discontinue any medications that may increase K (e.g., K-sparing diuretics, exogenous K).
- Admit for cardiac monitoring if ECG changes are present or if K is >6 mEq/L (6 mmol/L).

 ONGOING CARE

FOLLOW-UP RECOMMENDATIONS
Patient Monitoring

- Reduction of plasma K should begin within the 1st hour of treatment initiation.
- Serum K levels should be rechecked every 2–4 hours until the patient has stabilized and recurrent hyperkalemia is no longer a threat.
- Identification and elimination of possible causes and risk factors for hyperkalemia are essential.

DIET
≤80 mEq (≤80 mmol) of K/24 hours

PATIENT EDUCATION
Consult with a dietitian about a low-K diet.

PROGNOSIS

- Associated with poor prognosis in patients with heart failure
- Associated with poor prognosis in disaster medicine, trauma (1)
- Associated with poor prognosis in hemodialysis patients with higher dietary K^+ intake (6)

COMPLICATIONS

- Life-threatening cardiac arrhythmias
- Hypokalemia
- Potential complications of the use of ion-exchange resins for the treatment of hyperkalemia include volume overload and intestinal necrosis (7).

REFERENCES

1. Zimmerman JL, Shen MD. Rhabdomyolysis. *Chest.* 2013;144:1058–1065.
2. Howard SC, Jones DP, Pui CH. The tumor lysis syndrome. *N Engl J Med.* 2011;364:1844–1854.
3. Antoniou T, Gomes T, Juurlink DN, et al. Trimethoprim-sulfamethoxazole-induced hyperkalemia in patients receiving inhibitors of the renin-angiotensin system: A population-based study. *Arch Intern Med.* 2010;170:1045–1049.
4. Weir MA, Juurlink DN, Gomes T, et al. Beta-blockers, trimethoprim-sulfamethoxazole, and the risk of hyperkalemia requiring hospitalization in the elderly: A nested case-control study. *Clin J Am Soc Nephrol.* 2010;5:1544–1551.
5. Wong R, Banker R, Aronowitz P, et al. Electrocardiographic changes of severe hyperkalemia. *J Hosp Med.* 2011;6:240.
6. Noori N, Kalantar-Zadeh K, Kovesdy CP, et al. Dietary potassium intake and mortality in long-term hemodialysis patients. *Am J Kidney Dis.* 2010;56:338–347.
7. Sterns RH, Rojas M, Bernstein P, et al. Ion-exchange resins for the treatment of hyperkalemia: Are they safe and effective? *J Am Soc Nephrol.* 2010;21:733–735.

ADDITIONAL READING

- Bosch X, Poch E, Grau JM. Rhabdomyolysis and acute kidney injury. *N Engl J Med.* 2009;361:62–72.
- Cross NB, Webster AC, Masson P, et al. Antihypertensives for kidney transplant recipients: Systematic review and meta-analysis of randomized controlled trials. *Transplantation.* 2009;88:7–18.
- Hall AB, Salazar M, Larison DJ. The sequencing of medication administration in the management of hyperkalemia. *J Emerg Nurs.* 2009;35:339–342.
- Hollander-Rodriguez JC, Calvert JF. Hyperkalemia. *Am Fam Physician.* 2006;73:283–290.
- Kim HJ, Han SW. Therapeutic approach to hyperkalemia. *Nephron.* 2002;92(Suppl 1):33–40.
- Pepin J, Shields C. Advances in diagnosis and management of hypokalemic and hyperkalemic emergencies. *Emerg Med Pract.* 2012;14:1–18.
- Putcha N, Allon M. Management of hyperkalemia in dialysis patients. *Semin Dial.* 2007;20:431–439.

- Riccardi A, Tasso F, Corti L, et al. The emergency physician and the prompt management of severe hyperkalemia. *Intern Emerg Med.* 2012;7(Suppl 2):S131–S133.
- Shapiro MI, Badea A, Luchette FA. Rhabdomyolysis in the intensive care unit. *J Int Care Med.* 2012;27:335–342.
- Stevens MS, Dunlay RW. Hyperkalemia in hospitalized patients. *Int Urol Nephrol.* 2000;32:177–180.

 SEE ALSO

- Addison Disease; Hypokalemia
- Algorithm: Hyperkalemia

 CODES

ICD10
E87.5 Hyperkalemia

CLINICAL PEARLS

- Emergency and urgent management of hyperkalemia takes precedent over a thorough diagnostic workup. Urgent treatment includes stabilization of the myocardium to protect against arrhythmias and mobilizing potassium from the extracellular (vascular) space into the cells.
- Multiple herbal medications can also increase K levels, including alfalfa, dandelion, horsetail nettle, milkweed, hawthorne berries, toad skin, oleander, foxglove, and ginseng.
- Many foods contain K. Those that are particularly high in K (>6.4 mEq per serving) include bananas, orange juice, other citrus fruits and their juices, tomatoes, tomato juice, cantaloupe, honeydew melon, peaches, potatoes, salt substitutes, and many herbal medications.
- To lower a patient's risk of developing hyperkalemia, have the patient follow a low-K diet, use selective β_1-blockers, such as metoprolol or atenolol, instead of nonselective β-blockers such as carvedilol. Avoid NSAIDs. Concomitant use of kaliuretic loop diuretics may be useful.

H

HYPERNATREMIA

Zahraa Hajjiri, MD • Pang-Yen Fan, MD

 BASICS

DESCRIPTION
- Serum sodium (Na) concentration >145 mEq/L
- Often represents a state of hyperosmolality.
- Sodium concentration reflects balance between total body water and total body sodium. Hypernatremia occurs from deficit of water relative to sodium.
- Hypernatremia results from net water loss or, more rarely, from primary Na gain.
- May exist with hypo-, hyper-, or euvolemia, although hypovolemia is by far most common type:
  - Hypovolemic: Occurs with a decrease in total body water (TBW) and a proportionately smaller decrease in total body Na.
  - Euvolemic: No change in TBW with a proportionate increase in total body Na
  - Hypervolemic: Increase in TBW and a proportionately greater increase in total body Na
- It has been shown to be an indicator for higher mortality in critically ill patients and patients with CKD (1,2).

EPIDEMIOLOGY
Incidence
- More common in elderly and young:
  - Occurs in 1% of hospitalized elderly patients (3)
- Gastroenteritis with diarrhea is the most common cause of hypernatremia in infants.
- Women are at an increased risk due to decreased TBW, as compared with men.

ETIOLOGY AND PATHOPHYSIOLOGY
- Pure water loss (total body Na normal) resulting from:
  - Adipsia/Hypodipsia (e.g., impaired thirst regulation, decreased access to water)
  - Nephrogenic diabetes insipidus (congenital or due to renal dysfunction, hypercalcemia, hypokalemia, medication-related, particularly lithium)
  - Central diabetes insipidus (due to head trauma, stroke, meningitis)
  - Increased insensible water loss (e.g., fever, hyperventilation, hypermetabolic state, heat exposure, newborns under radiant warmers)
- Hypotonic fluid loss (total body Na decreased) resulting from:
  - Loss of fluid containing relatively more water than Na (e.g., excessive sweating, severe burns)
  - Urinary loss:
    ○ Osmotic diuresis: Hyperglycemia, mannitol
    ○ Diuretics, especially loop diuretics
    ○ Diabetes mellitus, particularly new presentation/decompensated
    ○ Post-ATN or postobstructive diuresis
    ○ Intrinsic renal disease
  - Gastrointestinal loss:
    ○ Diarrhea, especially in children
    ○ Vomiting, nasogastric (NG) lavage
    ○ Enterocutaneous fistula

- Excess Na (increase in total body Na) resulting from (2):
  - IV NaCl or NaHCO$_3$ during cardiopulmonary resuscitation, metabolic acidosis, or hyperkalemia
  - Sea water ingestion
  - Excessive use of NaHCO$_3$ antacid
  - Incorrect infant formula preparation
  - Intrauterine NaCl for abortion
  - Excessive Na in dialysate solutions
  - Disorders of the adrenal axis (Cushing syndrome, Conn syndrome, congenital adrenal hyperplasia)
  - Tube feeds

Genetics
Some forms of diabetes insipidus may be hereditary.

RISK FACTORS
- Infants/Children
- Old age
- Patients who are intubated/have altered mental status
- Diabetes mellitus
- Prior brain injury
- Surgery
- Diuretic therapy, especially loop diuretics
- Lithium treatment

GENERAL PREVENTION
- Treatment/Prevention of underlying cause
- Properly prepare infant formula and never add salt to any commercial infant formula.
- Keep patients well hydrated.

COMMONLY ASSOCIATED CONDITIONS
- Gastroenteritis
- Altered mental status
- Burns
- Hypermetabolic conditions
- Head injury
- Renal dysfunction

 DIAGNOSIS

HISTORY
- Excessive thirst, nausea, vomiting, diarrhea, oliguria, polyuria
- Fever, myalgia, muscle weakness
- Neurologic symptoms common: Altered mental status, seizure (especially if rapid development of hypernatremia), lethargy, irritability, coma, anophthalmus
- Symptoms tend to develop when Na >160 mEq in adults.
- Obtain list of current and recent medications.
- Review recent illnesses and activities.

PHYSICAL EXAM
- Sinus tachycardia, hypotension, orthostatic hypotension, poor O$_2$ saturation
- Dry mucous membranes, cool/gray skin
- Neurologic abnormalities: Lethargy, weakness, focal deficits (in cases of intracerebral bleeding/lesion), confusion, coma, seizures

DIFFERENTIAL DIAGNOSIS
- Diabetes insipidus
- Hyperosmotic coma
- Salt ingestion
- Hypertonic dehydration
- Hypothyroidism
- Cushing syndrome

DIAGNOSTIC TESTS & INTERPRETATION
Initial Tests (lab, imaging)
- Serum Na, potassium, BUN, creatinine, calcium, and osmolality (serum lithium if appropriate) (4)
- Urine Na and osmolality:
  - Diabetes insipidus (DI): Urine osmolality < serum osmolality and urine Na usually low normal/slightly low (due to dilution)
  - Osmotic diuresis: Urine osmolality intermediate, urine sodium low/low-normal, total daily osmole excretion high
  - Salt ingestion: Increased urine osmolality and high urine Na
  - Hypertonic dehydration: Increased urine osmolality and decreased urine Na
- Serum glucose
- Special tests for DI:
  - Water deprivation test: In DI, urine osmolality does not increase as it normally should when hypernatremic.
  - Antidiuretic hormone (ADH) stimulation: Distinguishes central vs. nephrogenic DI:
    ○ Urine osmolality does not increase after ADH or DDAVP in nephrogenic DI
- Head CT/MRI in DI to rule out craniopharyngioma, other brain tumor or masses, or median cleft syndrome (4)[C]

Diagnostic Procedures/Other
History, physical, laboratory studies, family history for central DI

 TREATMENT

GENERAL MEASURES
- Goal Na is 145. Treat underlying cause.
- Speed of correction depends on symptom severity/rate of development of hypernatremia. Avoid rapid correction to prevent development of cerebral edema if chronic hypernatremia (>24 hrs):
  - Maximum of 0.5 mEq/L/hr or 10 mEq/L/d (5)[C]
  - May correct at up to 1 mEq/L/hr if acute hypernatremia (<24 hours)
- Treat volume depletion 1st, then hypernatremia:
  - Restore intravascular volume with IV fluids to normalize serum Na levels.
- Replace water orally if patient is conscious.
- Important formulas in determining rate of fluid administration:
  - Calculated free water deficit (liters) = [(0.5 × wt) × (Na − 140)] ÷ 140:
    ○ Note: wt = weight in kilograms; Na = current serum Na
  - Change in serum Na per 1 L infusate = [(infusate Na + infusate K) − serum Na]/(TBW + 1)
- Account for ongoing fluid losses during calculation of rate of fluid administration
- Dialysis: Especially with serum Na >200 mEq/L

MEDICATION
First Line
- See "General-Measures" below for overall approach.
- Dehydration: Use isotonic fluids initially if signs of hemodynamic compromise, then change to hypotonic fluids when stable:
  - Hypotonic fluids (0.45% NaCl or dextrose 5% in water) (3)[B]:
    - Important not to decrease serum Na by >0.5 mEq/L/hr or 10 mEq/L/d to prevent cerebral edema
- Hypervolemia: Give furosemide along with hypotonic fluids. Dose varies depending on desired urine output. Loop diuretics with fluid restriction worsens hypernatremia.
- Central DI:
  - Desmopressin (DDAVP) acetate: Use parenteral form for acute symptomatic patients, and use intranasal or oral form for chronic therapy.
  - Free water replacement: May use 2.5% dextrose in water if giving large volumes of water in DI to avoid glycosuria
  - May consider sulfonylureas/thiazide diuretics for chronic, but not acute, treatment
- Nephrogenic diabetes insipidus:
  - Treat with diuretics and NSAIDs
  - Lithium-induced nephrogenic DI: Hydrochlorothiazide 50 mg PO b.i.d. or indomethacin 50 mg PO t.i.d., or amiloride hydrochloride 5–10 mg PO b.i.d.
- Precautions:
  - Rapid correction of hypernatremia can cause cerebral edema, seizures, or death. Hypocalcemia and more rarely acidosis can occur during correction.
  - DI: High rates of dextrose 5% in water can cause hyperglycemia and glucose-induced diuresis.

Second Line
- Consider NSAIDs in nephrogenic DI (3)[A].
- Modalities requiring further investigations:
- CRRT: Multiple case reports and case series have shown success and safety in using CRRT to treat hypernatremia in critically ill patients with CHF and severe burns (6,7)[C].

ISSUES FOR REFERRAL
Underlying renal involvement associated with hypernatremia would benefit from a nephrology referral.

IN-PATIENT CONSIDERATIONS
Admission Criteria/Initial Stabilization
Symptomatic patient with serum Na >155 mEq/L requires IV fluid therapy.

IV Fluids
Refer to "Medication" section.

Nursing
Bed rest until stable or underlying condition resolved/controlled

Discharge Criteria
Stabilization of serum Na level and symptoms are minimal

 ## ONGOING CARE

FOLLOW-UP RECOMMENDATIONS
Patient Monitoring
- Frequent re-exams in an acute setting
- Frequent electrolytes: Initially q6–8h
- Urine osmolality and urine output in DI
- Ensure adequate ingestion of calories because patients may ingest so much water that they feel full and do not eat.
- Daily weights

DIET
- Ensure proper nutrition during acute phase.
- After resolution of acute phase, may want to consider Na-restricted diet for patient.
- Low-salt, low-protein diet in nephrogenic DI

PATIENT EDUCATION
Patients with nephrogenic DI must avoid salt and drink large amounts of water.

PROGNOSIS
Most recover, but neurologic impairment can occur.

COMPLICATIONS
- CNS thrombosis/hemorrhage
- Seizures
- Mental retardation
- Hyperactivity
- Chronic hypernatremia: >2 days duration has higher mortality
- Serum Na >180 mEq/L (>180 mmol/L): Often results in residual CNS damage
- More common if rapid development of hypernatremia

REFERENCES

1. Waite MD, Fuhrman SA. Intensive care unit–acquired hypernatremia is an independent predictor of increased mortality and length of stay. *JCC.* 2012;28 (4):405–412
2. Kovesdy CP, Lott EH. Hyponatremia, hypernatremia, and mortality in patients with Chronic kidney disease with or without congestive heart failure. *JAHA.* 2012;125:677–684.
3. Bagshaw SM, Townsend DR, McDermid RC. Disorders of sodium and water balance in hospitalized patients. *Can J Anaesth.* 2009;56:151–167.
4. Kraft MD, Btaichel F, Sachs GS, et al. Treatment of electrolyte disorders in adult patients in the intensive care unit. *Am J Health-System Pharm.* 2005;62:166382.
5. Mastrangelo S, Arlotta A, Cefalo MG, Maurizi P, Cianfoni A, Riccardi R. Central pontine and extrapontine myelinosis in a pediatric patient following a rapid correction of hypernatremia. *Neuropediatrics.* 2009;40(3):144–147. Epub 2009 Dec 17.
6. Park HS, Hong YA. Usefulness of continuous renal replacement therapy for correcting hypernatremia in a patient with severe congestive heart failure. *Hemodial Int.* 2012;16:559–563.
7. Huang C, Zhang P. Treatment of acute Hypernatremia in severely burned patients using continuous veno-venous hemofiltration with gradient sodium replacement fluid: A report of nine cases. *Intensive Care Med.* 2013;39:1495–1496.

ADDITIONAL READING
- Al-Absi A, Gosmanova EO, Wall BM. A clinical approach to the treatment of chronic hypernatremia. *Am J Kidney Disease.* 2012;60(6):1032–1038.
- Adrogue HJ, Madias NE. Hypernatremia. *N Engl J Med.* 2000;342:1493–1499.
- Hannon MJ, Finucane FM, Sherlock M, et al. Clinical review: Disorders of water homeostasis in neurosurgical patients. *J Clin Endocrinol Metab.* 2012;84(5):1423–1433. Epub 2012 Feb 22.

 ## SEE ALSO
- Diabetes Insipidus
- Algorithm: Hypernatremia

 ## CODES

ICD10
E87.0 Hyperosmolality and hypernatremia

CLINICAL PEARLS
- Occurs from water deficit in comparison to total body Na stores
- Common causes include dehydration, diabetes insipidus, impaired access to fluids
- Determine if the patient has hypervolemic, euvolemic, or hypovolemic hypernatremia in the differential diagnosis of etiology; most commonly hypovolemic; other entities rare.
- Avoid rapid correction of hypernatremia to prevent development of cerebral edema when hypernatremia is chronic (>24 hours).
- Use hypotonic fluids unless patient has hemodynamic compromise, which necessitates use of isotonic fluids.

H

HYPERPARATHYROIDISM
Diana Teplitsky, DO • Oleg Kotelskiy, DO

 BASICS

DESCRIPTION
A dysfunction of the body's normal regulatory feedback mechanisms for parathyroid hormone (PTH):

- Primary hyperparathyroidism (HPT): Intrinsic parathyroid gland dysfunction resulting in excessive secretions of PTH with a lack of response to feedback inhibition by elevated calcium
- Secondary HPT: Excessive secretion of PTH in response to hypocalcemia, which can be caused by vitamin D deficiency or renal failure
- Tertiary HPT: Autonomous hyperfunction of the parathyroid gland in the setting of long-standing secondary HPT

EPIDEMIOLOGY
Incidence
Predominant sex: Female > Male (2:1)

Prevalence
Primary HPT: 1/1000 in the U.S.

ETIOLOGY AND PATHOPHYSIOLOGY
- PTH is made in 4 parathyroid glands located behind the 4 poles of the thyroid gland (locations can vary).
- PTH releases calcium from bone by osteoclastic stimulation (bone resorption).
- PTH increases reabsorption of calcium in the distal tubules of the kidneys.
- PTH stimulates conversion of 25-hydroxycholecalciferol (25(OH)D) to 1,25-dihydroxycholecalciferol (1,25(OH)$_2$D or active vitamin D) in the kidneys:
  - 1,25(OH)$_2$D increases calcium absorption from the GI tract, increase calcium and phosphate reabsorption in the kidneys, and stimulates osteoclastic activity as well as bone resorption.
- Primary HPT: Unregulated PTH production and release, causing increase in serum calcium:
  - Solitary adenoma (89%)
  - Double adenomas (5%)
  - Diffuse hyperplasia (6%) caused by multiple adenomas, multiple endocrine neoplasia (MEN) types 1 and 2a, familial hypocalciuric hypercalcemia
  - Parathyroid carcinoma (<2%)
- Secondary HPT: Adaptive parathyroid gland hyperplasia and hyperfunction:
  - Dietary: Vitamin D or calcium deficiency
  - Chronic renal disease resulting in:
    o Renal parenchymal loss causing hyperphosphatemia
    o Impaired calcitriol production causing hypocalcemia
    o General skeletal and renal resistance to PTH
- Tertiary HPT: Autonomous oversecretion of PTH following prolonged parathyroid stimulation

Genetics
- MEN types 1 and 2a: Patients with multiple gland hyperplasia in the absence of renal disease should be screened for MEN-1 gene mutation.
- Neonatal severe primary HPT
- HPT–jaw tumor syndrome
- Familial hypocalciuric hypercalcemia (FHH): Autosomal dominant
- Familial isolated HPT

RISK FACTORS
Chronic kidney disease, increasing age, poor nutrition, radiation, and/or family history

GENERAL PREVENTION
Adequate intake of calcium and vitamin D may help prevent secondary HPT.

COMMONLY ASSOCIATED CONDITIONS
- MEN syndromes type 1 and 2a
- Chronic renal failure

 DIAGNOSIS

HISTORY
- History of present illness:
  - Bone, abdominal, and flank pain as well as psychosis, which are all classic complaints of hypercalcemia
- Past medical history:
  - The following conditions may be associated with HPT:

    o MEN syndrome (MEN-associated conditions include pancreatic cancer, pituitary adenomas, medullary thyroid cancer, pheochromocytoma), nephrolithiasis (in 20–30%) (1)[A], nephrocalcinosis, pancreatitis, gastroduodenal ulcer, hypertension, short QT interval, left ventricular hypertrophy, osteitis fibrosa cystica, cystic bone lesions, spontaneous fracture, vertebral collapse, osteoporosis, gout, pseudogout, periarticular calcification, anxiety, depression, psychosis, coma, conjunctivitis, band keratopathy, conjunctival calcium deposits, radiation to the neck
- Medications: Thiazides or lithium
- Review of systems:
  - Possible symptoms are polydipsia, polyuria, flank pain, abdominal pain, constipation, vomiting, anorexia, weight loss, muscle fatigue, pain, weakness, hypotonia, arthralgia, bone pain, fatigue, apathy, somnolence

PHYSICAL EXAM
- Limited usefulness; 70–80% of patients have no obvious symptoms or signs of disease (1)[A].
- Possible findings on physical exam:
  - Refer to HPI and ROS and to the physical exam findings that usually accompany the disease processes mentioned under PMHx

DIFFERENTIAL DIAGNOSIS
- Increased PTH: Ectopic HPT
- Nonparathyroid causes:
  - Malignancy: Lung (squamous cell) carcinoma, breast carcinoma, multiple myeloma, lymphoma, leukemia, prostate cancer, Paget disease
  - Granulomatous disease: Sarcoidosis, tuberculosis, berylliosis, histoplasmosis, coccidioidomycosis
  - Drugs: Thiazide diuretics, vitamin D intoxication, vitamin A excess, lithium, milk-alkali syndrome, exogenous calcium intake
  - Endocrine: Hyperthyroidism, acute adrenal insufficiency
  - Familial: Hypocalciuric hypercalcemia

DIAGNOSTIC TESTS & INTERPRETATION
Initial Tests (lab, imaging)
- Disease is often detected by an incidental finding of hypercalcemia.
- Order serum calcium level and albumin:
  - Calculate plasma albumin-adjusted calcium >2.65 mmol/L on 2 occasions (1)[A]
- If hypercalcemia is confirmed, follow with intact PTH level:
  - High PTH (>3.0 pmol/L) suggests primary HPT (1)[A].
  - Low PTH (<3.0 pmol/L) suggests non–PTH–mediated hypercalcemia (1)[A].
- If elevated calcium is inconsistent, elevated ionized serum calcium in the setting of high PTH confirms diagnosis. Other findings may include low serum phosphate, elevated serum chloride, decreased serum CO$_2$, and abnormal 24-hour urine calcium excretion.
- In secondary HPT, an elevated phosphorus means chronic renal failure; a low phosphorus suggests another cause, most commonly vitamin D deficiency.

Follow-Up Tests & Special Considerations
- A 24-hour urine calcium concentration to creatinine clearance ratio >0.02 suggests primary HPT; a ratio <0.01 may be normal or indicate FHH (1)[A]; important because FHH does not require surgery.
- Routine measurement of 25(OH)D levels is recommended in all patients with primary HPT. In case of vitamin D deficiency (<20 ng/mL or <50 nmol/L), defer management decisions until levels are maintained >20 ng/mL (50 nmol/L) (2)[A].
- Intraoperative measurement of intact PTH and/or γ-probe localization of abnormal glands with technetium-99m sestamibi scan has aided focused resections for patients with single-gland etiology (3)[A].
- Screening for kidney stones is not recommended in those without history of nephrolithiasis (3)[A].

Diagnostic Procedures/Other
- Consider EKG to assess for short QT interval.
- Imaging is not required for diagnosis. It is required for surgical planning, especially for minimally invasive parathyroidectomy (MIP) (1,4)[A].
  - It is also indicated to localize hyperplasia or an ectopic parathyroid gland in repeat surgery.
- Imaging options for presurgical localization:
  - Technetium-99m sestamibi with single-photon emission computed tomography (SPECT) (1,5)[A]:
    o Has had the greatest reported success in localizing single parathyroid adenomas (1)[A]
  - US (1)[A]:
    o Painless, noninvasive, inexpensive, and does not expose the patient to radiation; however, its accuracy is very operator-dependent (6)[A]
  - Positron emission tomography (PET) using C-methionine (MET-PET) is comparable to US and technetium 99-m sestamibi with SPECT in terms of diagnostic utility (4)[A].
  - Four-dimensional CT (4D-CT) may be more effective for primary localization than both US and sestamibi-SPECT (7)[A].
  - CT and MRI are mostly used to localize ectopic mediastinal glands (4)[A].

– Comprehensive cervical US (CCU) used for further localization following a negative sestamibi scan will reveal a single adenoma in most cases (8)[A]:
  ○ A negative sestamibi scan likely indicates parathyroid hyperplasia/multiglandular disease and thus requires open neck exploratory surgery (8)[A].
  ○ CCU after negative sestamibi result allows more patients who were previously excluded to be candidates for MIP (8)[A].

Test Interpretation
See "Etiology"

 TREATMENT

MEDICATION
- Primary HPT: Operative management is curative. For those awaiting or unable to have surgery:
  – Bisphosphonates (alendronate) (1)[A]: Reduces bone turnover and helps to maintain bone density; avoid in kidney disease
  – Calcimimetics (cinacalcet): Further studies needed to establish long-term benefit in primary HPT (9)[A]
  – Selective estrogen receptor modulator therapy (raloxifene) (1)[A]
  – Hormone replacement therapy with estrogens is not recommended as first-line treatment; must weigh benefit with risks of known systemic effects:
    ○ Can be used in postmenopausal women who do not undergo or refuse surgery
- Secondary HPT:
  – Calcium replacement
  – Vitamin D analogues (paricalcitol and calcitriol)
  – Phosphorus-binding agents (sevelamer)
  – Calcimimetic (cinacalcet) (1,9)[A]: Activates calcium-sensing receptor in parathyroid gland thereby inhibiting PTH secretion
- Tertiary HPT:
  – Medical treatment is not curative and generally not indicated

SURGERY/OTHER PROCEDURES
- Operative management is curative for patients with primary HPT in 95–98% of patients with 1–2% complications
- Indications for parathyroidectomy:
  – Symptomatic primary HPT:
    ○ Nephrolithiasis
    ○ Nephrocalcinosis
    ○ Osteitis fibrosa cystica
  – Asymptomatic primary HPT (3)[A]:
    ○ Serum Ca$^+$ level >1 mg/dL above normal
    ○ Age <50
    ○ GFR <60 mL/min/1.73 m^2 or creatinine clearance reduced to <60 mL/min
    ○ Bone density loss with a *T* score ≤−2.5 at the lumbar spine, femoral neck, total hip, or 33% radius
  – Tertiary hyperparathyroidism (1)[A]
- Surgical removal of diseased gland or tissue is only proven curative therapy for HPT.

- Surgical options include:
  – Bilateral open neck exploratory surgery
  – MIP using preoperative sestamibi scan with SPECT and intraoperative PTH levels result in decreased pain, smaller incisions, improved cosmetic results, lower morbidity, decreased length of hospital stay when compared with open neck exploratory surgery (1)[A]:
    ○ Refer to "Imaging" section
- Postoperative course needs special attention paid to serum calcium level (hypocalcemia in "hungry bone" syndrome), bleeding, and risk of airway compromise; injectable calcium and seizure precautions must be maintained at bedside.
- Monitor renal function closely.

IN-PATIENT CONSIDERATIONS
Admission Criteria/Initial Stabilization
Critical hypercalcemia requires IV fluid rehydration, IV bisphosphonate therapy, and SC calcitonin (4 U/kg q12h) for severe symptoms (1)[A].

 ONGOING CARE

FOLLOW-UP RECOMMENDATIONS
Asymptomatic patients with primary HPT require monitoring of calcium and PTH.

Patient Monitoring
In patients with primary HPT who are asymptomatic, measurements of serum calcium and creatinine annually and bone density scan every 1–2 years is sufficient (3)[A].

DIET
- In the presence of hypercalciuria or elevated 1,25(OH)$_2$D levels, dietary calcium restriction is recommended. Otherwise, daily calcium intake should be maintained at up to 1,000 mg (10)[C].
- Dietary phosphate restriction in secondary HPT (9)[A]

PATIENT EDUCATION
- Importance of periodic lab testing
- Signs of severe hypercalcemia

PROGNOSIS
Prognosis after surgery is excellent in primary HPT, with resolution of many of the preoperative symptoms

COMPLICATIONS
Related to high levels of PTH and/or elevated calcium.

REFERENCES

1. Fraser WD. Hyperparathyroidism. *Lancet*. 2009; 374(9684):145–158.
2. Eastell R, Arnold A, Brandi ML, et al. Diagnosis of asymptomatic primary hyperparathyroidism: Proceedings of the third international workshop. *J Clin Endocrinol Metab*. 2009;94:340–350.
3. Bilezikian JP, Khan AA, Potts JT, et al. Guidelines for the management of asymptomatic primary hyperparathyroidism: Summary statement from the third international workshop. *J Clin Endocrinol Metab*. 2009;94(2):335–339.
4. Caldarella C, Treglia G, Isgrò MA, et al. Diagnostic performance of positron emission tomography using (11)C-methionine in patients with suspected parathyroid adenoma: A meta-analysis. *Endocrine*. 2012. Epub 2012 Jul 18.

5. Caldarella C, Treglia G, Pontecorvi A, et al. Diagnostic performance of planar scintigraphy using (99m)Tc-MIBI in patients with secondary hyperparathyroidism: A meta-analysis. *Ann Nucl Med*. 2012;9. Epub 2012 Aug 9.
6. Udelsman R, Pasieka JL, Sturgeon C, et al. Surgery for asymptomatic primary hyperparathyroidism: Proceedings of the third international workshop. *J Clin Endocrinol Metab*. 2009;94(2):366–372.
7. Cheung K, Wang TS, Farrokhyar F, Roman SA, Sosa JA. A meta-analysis of preoperative localization techniques for patients with primary hyper-parathyroidism. *Ann Surg Oncol*. 2012; 19(2):577–583.
8. Kandil E, Malazai AJ, Alrasheedi S, et al. Minimally invasive/focused parathyroidectomy in patients with negative sestamibi scan results. *Arch Otolaryngol Head Neck Surg*. 2012; 138(3):223–225. Epub 2012 Feb 20.
9. Li D, Shao L, Zhou H, et al. The efficacy of cinacalcet combined with conventional therapy on bone and mineral metabolism in dialysis patients with secondary hyperparathyroidism: A meta-analysis. *Endocrine*. 2012. Epub 2012 Jun 6.
10. Bilezikian JP, Brandi ML, Rubin M, et al. Primary HPT: New concepts in clinical densitometric and biochemical features. *J Intern Med*. 2005; 257:6–17.

ADDITIONAL READING

Khan A, Grey A, Shoback D, et al. Medical management of asymptomatic primary hyperparathyroidism: Proceedings of the third international workshop. *J Clin Endocrinol Metab*. 2009;94:373–381.

 CODES

ICD10
- E21.0 Primary hyperparathyroidism
- E21.1 Secondary hyperparathyroidism, not elsewhere classified
- E21.3 Hyperparathyroidism, unspecified

CLINICAL PEARLS
- Many patients with primary HPT are asymptomatic.
- Disease is often detected by an incidental finding of hypercalcemia.
- HPT may cause malaise and fatigue before classic symptoms are seen.
- Classic complaints of hypercalcemia include painful bones, renal stones, abdominal groans, and psychic moans.
- A repeat calcium (elevated), serum albumin, and intact PTH tests are required to make an initial diagnosis.
- Surgical technique has changed in the past few years to include minimally invasive parathyroidectomy.
- The 2 most commonly used imaging modalities in HPT are technetium-99m sestamibi scan and US.
- A genetic etiology is increasingly recognized.

H

HYPERPROLACTINEMIA

Ruben Peralta, MD, FACS

 BASICS

DESCRIPTION
Hyperprolactinemia is an abnormal elevation in the serum prolactin level with multiple possible etiologies.

EPIDEMIOLOGY
Prevalence
- Predominant age: Reproductive age
- Predominant sex: Female > Male
- More readily detected in females because a slight elevation in prolactin causes changes in menstruation and galactorrhea.

ETIOLOGY AND PATHOPHYSIOLOGY
- Prolactin, which is produced by lactotrophs in the anterior pituitary, is regulated by:
  - Inhibitory factors, primarily dopamine, produced in the hypothalamus and delivered via the hypothalamic-pituitary vessels in the pituitary stalk
  - Stimulatory factors, primarily thyrotropin-releasing hormone (TRH)
- Causes of hyperprolactinemia include:
  - Physiologic:
    o Pregnancy
    o Breastfeeding
    o Nipple stimulation
    o Stress, including postoperative state
  - Medications:
    o Dopamine (D_2) blockers: Antipsychotics (1), metoclopramide
    o Dopamine depleters: α-methyldopa, reserpine
    o Opiates
    o Verapamil (but no other calcium-channel blockers; thought to decrease hypothalamic synthesis of dopamine)
    o Possibly antidepressants (minimal data)
  - Hypothyroidism (due to elevated TRH)
  - Chest wall conditions:
    o Herpes zoster
    o After thoracotomy
    o Trauma
  - Prolactin-secreting adenoma, categorized:
    o Microadenoma: $\leq$1 cm
    o Macroadenoma: >1 cm
  - Pituitary stalk compression/disruption:
    o Craniopharyngioma
    o Rathke cleft cyst
    o Meningioma
    o Astrocytoma
    o Metastases
    o Head trauma
    o Infiltrative/Inflammatory disorders
  - Diminished prolactin clearance:
    o Renal failure
    o Cirrhosis
- Cocaine

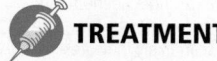 **DIAGNOSIS**

HISTORY
- Galactorrhea
- Amenorrhea
- Oligomenorrhea
- Infertility
- Osteoporosis/osteopenia
- Decreased libido, impotence
- Weight gain
- Also may have signs and symptoms of pituitary enlargement:
  - Headache
  - Visual field impairment (bitemporal hemianopsia)
  - Hypopituitarism (secondary to tumor pressure on surrounding structures)
- Also may have signs and symptoms of associated conditions:
  - Hypothyroidism
  - Cushing disease
  - Acromegaly
  - Multiple endocrine neoplasia (MEN)-1 syndrome

PHYSICAL EXAM
- Visual field testing
- Cranial nerve exam

DIFFERENTIAL DIAGNOSIS
Macroprolactinemia: Macroprolactin, a polymer of several units of prolactin, is detected by immunologically based lab tests but is not biologically active. If patient is asymptomatic but found to have elevated prolactin (PRL), consider this diagnosis and notify the lab. No treatment is required.

DIAGNOSTIC TESTS & INTERPRETATION
- Serum prolactin (most accurate results if checked fasting, in morning)
- Pregnancy test
- Thyroid-stimulating hormone (TSH)
- Luteinizing hormone (LH)/follicle-stimulating hormone (FSH) if amenorrheic
- Chemistry, renal function
- LFTs

Initial Tests (lab, imaging)
A single measurement of serum prolactin; a level above the upper limit of normal confirms the diagnosis (2)[C].

- Pituitary MRI
- CT scan if MRI is contraindicated

Follow-Up Tests & Special Considerations
Formal visual field testing if pituitary adenoma suspected

TREATMENT

GENERAL MEASURES
- Discontinue offending medications, if any
- Treat underlying causes
- For asymptomatic patients with mild PRL elevations, observation alone may be considered.
- Medications indicated for (3)[C]:
  - Symptoms of hypogonadism, such as decreased libido
  - Galactorrhea (if bothersome to patient)
  - Restoration of fertility
  - Pituitary adenoma
  - Prevention of osteoporosis

MEDICATION
Dopamine agonists:
- Bromocriptine (Parlodel): Often 1st-line treatment given. This has longest clinical history: Dosed b.i.d.; preferred by some clinicians when infertility is an indication for treatment (3)[C].
- Cabergoline (Dostinex): Has recently been reported to be associated with significant improvements in the body mass index, total HDL, and LDL-cholesterol levels and insulin sensitivity, decreased in pro-inflammatory markers and carotid intima media thickness (4)[B]. Dosed twice weekly; may be better tolerated; some consider this a 1st-line drug; indicated with bromocriptine failure or resistance
  - Both are effective for reducing tumor size and improving symptoms (5)[C].
- Cabergoline has been shown to reduce erectile dysfunction in hyperprolactinemic men.
  - Adverse effects (better tolerated if start with low dose, slow titration, given at night with food):
    o Nausea/vomiting
    o Headache
    o Dizziness
    o Fatigue
    o Lightheadedness
    o Postural hypotension
- Pergolide (Permax), also a dopamine agonist, is used less commonly.

ADDITIONAL THERAPIES
Radiation therapy and stereotactic radiosurgery sometimes are considered in medically unresponsive, surgically unresectable tumors; PRL normalizes in 20–30%, with a high risk of hypopituitarism.

SURGERY/OTHER PROCEDURES

- For adenomas, medical treatment will be successful in 80–90% of patients. In some cases, surgery is indicated.
- Indications (6)[C]:
  - Intolerance or resistance to medical treatment
  - Headache
  - Visual field loss
  - CSF leak due to tumor apoplexy or shrinkage
  - Cranial nerve deficit
- Risks:
  - High recurrence rate (up to 40%) (6)[C]
  - CSF leakage
  - Meningitis
- Pituitary insufficiency

 ONGOING CARE

FOLLOW-UP RECOMMENDATIONS
Patient Monitoring
- Depends on etiology
- Consider:
  - Prolactin level every 6–12 months
  - Formal visual field testing yearly
  - Serial MRIs if clinically indicated

Pregnancy Considerations
- If pregnancy is desired in a woman with hyperprolactinemia, dopamine agonists are not approved during pregnancy and should be discontinued once pregnancy is confirmed, but their use is recommended if neurologic findings are present (6)[C].
- With microprolactinoma: Treat with bromocriptine if symptomatic; monthly pregnancy tests; discontinue bromocriptine when pregnancy is confirmed.
- With macroprolactinomas: Treat with bromocriptine if neurologic findings (due to tumor enlargement) are present and at least until optic system is no longer compromised.
- Careful monitoring of visual fields in each trimester and PRL levels during pregnancy is advised.

PATIENT EDUCATION

- Discuss risks of untreated hyperprolactinemia:
  - Headache
  - Visual field loss
  - Decreased bone density
  - Infertility
- Patient guide to hyperprolactinemia diagnosis and treatment www.ncbi.nlm.nih.gov/pubmed/21296988

PROGNOSIS

- Tends to recur after discontinuation of medical therapy
- Over 10 years, 7% chance of progression of prolactin-secreting microadenoma

COMPLICATIONS

- Depends on underlying cause
- If pituitary adenoma, risk of permanent visual field loss

REFERENCES

1. Inder WJ, Castle D. Antipsychotic-induced hyperprolactinaemia. *Aust N Z J Psychiatry.* 2011;45:830–837.
2. Melmed S, Casanueva FF, Hoffman AR, et al. Diagnosis and treatment of hyperprolactinemia: An Endocrine Society clinical practice guideline. *J Clin Endocrinol Metab.* 2011;96:273–288.
3. Molitch ME. Prolactin-secreting tumors: What's new? *Expert Rev Anticancer Ther.* 2006;6(Suppl 9): S29–S35.
4. Inancli SS, Usluogullari A, Ustu Y, et al. Effect of cabergoline on insulin sensitivity, inflammation, and carotid intima media thickness in patients with prolactinoma. *Endocrine.* 2013;44:193–199.
5. Jackson J, Safranek S. What is the recommended evaluation and treatment for elevated serum prolactin? *JFP.* 2006;54:897–899.
6. Klibanski A. Clinical practice. Prolactinomas. *N Engl J Med.* 2010;362:1219–1226.
7. Bhasin S, Enzlin P, Coviello A, et al. Sexual dysfunction in men and women with endocrine disorders. *Lancet.* 2007;369:597–611.

ADDITIONAL READING

- Casanueva FF, Molitch ME, Schlechte JA, et al. Guidelines of the Pituitary Society for the diagnosis and management of prolactinomas. *Clin Endocrinol (Oxf).* 2006;65:265–273.
- Keil MF, Stratakis CA. Pituitary tumors in childhood: Update of diagnosis, treatment and molecular genetics. *Expert Rev Neurother.* 2008;8:563–574.
- Molitch ME. Pituitary gland: Can prolactinomas be cured medically? *Nat Rev Endocrinol.* 2010;6: 186–188.
- Wang AT, Mullan RJ, Lane MA, et al. Treatment of hyperprolactinemia: A systematic review and meta-analysis. *Syst Rev.* 2012;1:33.

 CODES

ICD10
E22.1 Hyperprolactinemia

CLINICAL PEARLS

- If a cause for hyperprolactinemia cannot be found by history, examination, and routine laboratory testing, an intracranial lesion might be the cause and brain MRI with specific pituitary cuts and intravenous contrast media should be performed.
- Treatment of hyperprolactinemia should be targeted at correcting the cause (hypothyroidism, discontinuation of offending medications, etc.).
- At the time of diagnosis, pituitary tumors in men are generally larger than tumors in women. Possible explanations are that women experience amenorrhea and galactorrhea when prolactin is only slightly elevated, whereas presenting symptoms in men—erectile dysfunction, diminished libido—tend to be more insidious and occur at higher levels of prolactin.
- There is a difference among antipsychotics in influencing prolactin levels. In general, those with the highest-potency D_2 antagonism are most likely to elevate prolactin levels. Among the newer atypical antipsychotics, risperidone has been identified as more likely to elevate prolactin.
- High prolactin levels decrease testosterone by inhibiting gonadotropin-releasing hormone (GnRH), LH, and FSH secretion and by decreasing central dopamine activity, both of which are important in mediating sexual arousal (7)[C].

H

HYPERSENSITIVITY PNEUMONITIS
Kenia Mansilla-Rivera, MD

BASICS

DESCRIPTION
- Hypersensitivity pneumonitis (HP) is also called extrinsic allergic alveolitis (EAA). A diffuse inflammatory disease of the lung caused by an immunologic reaction to aerosolized antigenic particles found in a variety of environments, occurring within the pulmonary parenchyma. Classification depends on time frame involved:
  - Acute: Fever, chills, diaphoresis, myalgias, nausea; cough and dyspnea common, but not necessarily present. Occurs 4–12 hours after heavy exposure to an inciting agent. Symptoms subside within 12 hours to several days after removal from exposure. Complete resolution occurs within weeks.
  - Subacute: Mainly caused by continual low-level antigen exposure, could have a low-grade fever 1st week, cough, dyspnea, fatigue, anorexia, weight loss—develops over days to weeks.
  - Chronic: From recurrent exposure either acute or subacute cases, prolonged and progressive cough, dyspnea, fatigue, weight loss, could lead to fibrosis and respiratory failure
- Farmer's lung is an old term of this disease, a type of HP, particular to the farmer population, where the causative agent is a bacterium found in moldy hay or straw. Farmer's lung now has new and different etiologies due to modernization of farming practices (1).

EPIDEMIOLOGY
Not well defined. Tends to occur in adults as a result of occupation-related exposure, but some home environmental exposures are also seen.

Incidence
0.9 per 100,000

Prevalence
- Farmers: 1–19% exposed farmers
- Bird fanciers: 6–20% exposed individuals
- Others: 1–8% exposed

ETIOLOGY AND PATHOPHYSIOLOGY
- Hypersensitivity reaction involving immune complexes: Inhaled antigens bind to IgG, triggering complement cascade.
- Cellular-mediated reaction: T-cell–mediated immune inflammatory response
- Farming, vegetable, or dairy cattle workers:
- Moldy hay, grain, silage: Thermophilic actinomycetes, such as *Faenia rectivirgula*
- Mold on pressed sugar cane: *Thermoactinomyces sacchari, T. vulgaris*
- Tobacco plants: *Aspergillus* sp., *Scopulariopsis brevicaulis*
- Mushroom worker's lung: Mushroom spores, thermophilic actinomycetes
- Potato riddler's lung: Thermophilic actinomycetes, *T. vulgaris, F. rectivirgula, Aspergillus* sp.
- Wine maker's lung: *Mucor stolonifer*
- Cheese washer's lung: *Penicillium casei, Aspergillus clavatus*
- Coffee worker's lung: Coffee-bean dust
- Tea grower's lung: Tea plants

- Ventilation and water-related contamination:
  - Humidifier fever: Thermoactinomyces, *Klebsiella oxytoca, Naegleria gruberi, Acanthamoeba polyphaga, Acanthamoeba castellani*
  - Unventilated shower: *Epicoccum nigrum*
  - Hot-tub lung: *Cladosporium* sp., *Mycobacterium avium* complex
  - Sauna taker's lung: *Aureobasidium* sp.
  - Summer-type pneumonitis: *Trichosporon cutaneum*
  - Lifeguard lung: Aerosolized endotoxin from pool-water sprays and fountains
  - Contaminated basement pneumonitis: *Cephalosporium*
- Bird and poultry handling:
  - Bird fancier's lung: Droppings, feathers, serum proteins
  - Poultry worker's lung: Serum proteins
  - Turkey-handling disease: Serum proteins
  - Canary fancier's lung: Serum proteins
  - Duck fever: Feathers, serum proteins
- Veterinary work and animal handling:
  - Laboratory worker's lung: Urine, serum, pelts, proteins
  - Pituitary snuff taker's disease: Dried, powdered neurohypophysis
  - Furrier's lung: Animal pelts
  - Bat lung: Bat serum protein
  - Fish meal worker's lung: Fish meal
  - Coptic lung: Cloth wrapping of mummies
  - Mollusc shell HP: Sea-snail shell
  - Pearl oyster shell pneumonitis: Oyster shells
- Grain and flour:
  - Grain measurer's lung: Cereal grain, grain dust
  - Miller's lung: *Sitophilus granarius*
  - Malt worker's disease: *Aspergillus fumigatus, A. clavatus*
- Lumber milling, construction, wood stripping, paper, wallboard manufacture:
  - Wood dust pneumonitis: *Alternaria* sp., *Bacillus subtilis*
  - Sequoiosis: *Graphium, Pullularia, Trichoderma* sp., *Aureobasidium pullulans*
  - Maple bark disease: *Cryptostroma corticale*
  - Wood trimmer's disease: *Rhizopus* sp., *Mucor* sp.
  - Wood pulp worker's disease: *Penicillium* sp.
  - Suberosis: *T. viridis, Penicillium glabrum*
- Plastic manufacturing, painting, electronics, chemicals:
  - Chemical HP: Diphenyl diisocyanate, toluene diisocyanate
  - Detergent worker's lung: *Bacillus subtilis* enzymes
  - Pauli's reagent alveolitis: Sodium diazobenzene sulfate
  - Vineyard sprayer's lung: Copper sulfate
  - Pyrethrum: Pyrethrum
  - Epoxy resin lung: Phthalic anhydride
  - Bible printer's lung: Moldy typesetting water
  - Machine operator's lung: *Pseudomona fluorescens*, aerosolized metal working fluid
- Textile workers:
  - Byssinosis: Cotton mill dust
  - Velvet worker's lung: Nylon, tannic acid, potato starch
  - Upholstery fabric: Aflatoxin-producing fungus, *Fusarium* sp.
  - Lycoperdonosis: Puffball spores

Genetics
No evidence of clear genetic susceptibility. Possible genetic predisposition involving tumor necrosis factor alpha (TNF-α) and major histocompatibility complex (MHC) class II genes (1,2)[B]

RISK FACTORS
- Contact with organic antigens increases the risk of developing HP. Viral infection at time of exposure could also increase risk (3).

- Nonsmokers have an increased incidence of HP compared with smokers (nicotine could have a protective effect) (2,3)[B]:
  - Smokers have a diminished antibody response to inhaled antigens.
  - However, smokers that develop disease tend to have the chronic form and mortality is higher.

GENERAL PREVENTION
Avoidance of offending antigen and/or use of protective equipment

COMMONLY ASSOCIATED CONDITIONS
Constrictive bronchiolitis

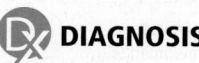

DIAGNOSIS

HISTORY
- Diagnosis criteria most widely used but not validated: (i) History, physical and pulmonary function tests (PFTs) indicating interstitial lung disease. (ii) Radiologic imaging consistent with HP. (iii) Exposure to a recognized cause. (iv) Antibody to that antigen (2).
- 6 significant predictors: Exposure to a known antigen, positive precipitating antibodies, recurrent episodes of symptoms, inspiratory crackles, symptoms 4–8 hours after exposure, weight loss (4)
- Acute form: Develops 4–12 hours following exposure. Cough, dyspnea without wheezing, fever, chills, diaphoresis, headache, nausea, malaise, chest tightness. Symptoms last hours to days.
- Sequela (prior subacute, chronic): Gradual or progressive productive cough, dyspnea, fatigue, anorexia, weight loss can lead to respiratory failure; develops over days, weeks to months.
- Known exposure to pets, hot tubs, areas with water damage, occupational exposures
- Symptomatic improvement when away from work or home

PHYSICAL EXAM
- Acute: Fever, tachypnea, diffuse fine rales
- Sequela or chronic: Inspiratory crackles, progressive hypoxia, weight loss, diffuse rales, clubbing, rarely wheezing

DIAGNOSTIC TESTS & INTERPRETATION

- Testing for antibodies (Ab): Not always identifiable. Positive serum Ab is a significant predictor of HP. Antigens that cover most cases: Pigeon and parakeet sera, dove feather, *Aspergillus sp*, *Penicillium*, *S. rectivirgula*, and *Thermoactinomyces viridans* (2).
- PFTs: Typical profile is a restrictive pattern with low diffusing capacity, could also have an obstructive pattern (4)
- Bronchoalveolar lavage (BAL) with lymphocytosis: Usually with low CD4-to-CD8 ratio. Findings not unique to HP (4).
- Positive inhalation challenge testing: Re-exposure to the environment, inhalation challenge to the suspected antigen in a hospital setting. Lacks standardization and can cause serious reactions (2,4)
- Chest x-ray (CXR): Used to rule out other diseases:
  – Acute: Ground-glass infiltrates, nodular or striated patchy opacities interstitial pattern in a variety of distributions in lung field. Up to 20% could be normal.
  – Sequela/Chronic: Upper lobe fibrosis, nodular or ground-glass opacities, volume loss, emphysematous changes
- CT scan of chest: Patterns not specific to HP:
  – Acute: Ground-glass opacities, poorly defined centrilobular nodules and ground-glass opacities and air trapping on expiratory images (5,6)
  – Chronic: Fibrosis, ground-glass attenuation, irregular opacities, bronchiectasis, loss of lung volume, honeycombing, emphysematous changes (6)
- High-resolution CT (HRCT) appearance is a mid-to-upper zone predominance of centrilobular ground glass or nodular opacities with signs of air trapping (6).
- Usually start with CXR; may progress to CT based on findings

Diagnostic Procedures/Other
Lung biopsy:

- Transbronchial: Reveals small, poorly formed noncaseating granulomas near respiratory or terminal bronchioles, large foam cells, peribronchial fibrosis.
- Open lung biopsy: Highest yield in advanced disease. Reveals varying patterns of organizing pneumonia, centrilobular and perilobular fibrosis, multinucleated giant cells with clefts.

DIFFERENTIAL DIAGNOSIS

- Acute: Acute infectious pneumonia: Influenza (or other viral pneumonia), mycoplasma, *Pneumocystis jiroveci* pneumonia, asthma
- Chronic: Sarcoidosis, chronic bronchitis, chronic obstructive pulmonary disease, tuberculosis, collagen vascular disease, idiopathic pulmonary fibrosis, lymphoma, fungal infections, *P. jiroveci* pneumonia

ALERT
HP in farmers must be distinguished from febrile, toxic reactions to inhaled dusts (organic dust toxic syndrome [ODTS]). Nonimmunologic reactions occur 30–50% more commonly than HP in farmers. ODTS is associated with intense exposure occurring on a single day.

 TREATMENT

GENERAL MEASURES
Outpatient, except for acute pneumonitis cases and admission for workup (BAL, lung biopsy)

MEDICATION
First Line
- Avoidance of offending antigen is primary therapy and results in disease regression (1,4)
- Corticosteroids: Help control the symptoms of exacerbations but do not improve long-term outcomes (2,4):
  – Prednisone: 20–50 mg daily (2,4)[C].
  – For severe symptomatic patients, initial course of 1–2 weeks with taper (1,4)

Second Line
- Bronchodilators and inhaled corticosteroids may symptomatically improve patients with wheeze and chest tightness (2,3,4)[B].
- Oxygen may be needed in advanced cases.
- Lung transplantation may be the last resort in severe cases unresponsive to therapy.

ISSUES FOR REFERRAL
Referral to pulmonologist/immunologist

IN-PATIENT CONSIDERATIONS
Admission Criteria/Initial Stabilization
Supportive management, as needed, to maintain oxygenation and ventilation:
- Unstable ventilation, oxygen requirement, mental status changes
- Need for invasive evaluation (lung biopsy)

 ONGOING CARE

FOLLOW-UP RECOMMENDATIONS
Patient Monitoring
- Initial follow-up should be weekly–monthly, depending on severity and course.
- Follow treatments with serial CXR, PFTs, circulating antibody levels.

DIET
No dietary restrictions

PATIENT EDUCATION
Note that chronic exposure may lead to a loss of acute symptoms with exposure (i.e., the patient may lose awareness of exposure–symptom relationship).

PROGNOSIS
- Presence of fibrosis is a poor prognosis factor (1).
- Acute: Good prognosis with reversal of pathologic findings if elimination of offending antigen early in disease (3).
- Sequela/Chronic: Corticosteroids have been found to improve lung function acutely, but offer no significant difference in long-term outcome (2,3,4)[C].

COMPLICATIONS
- Progressive interstitial fibrosis with eventual respiratory failure
- Cor pulmonale and right-sided heart failure

REFERENCES

1. Girard M, Cormier Y. Hypersensitivity pneumonitis. *Curr Opin Allergy Clin Immunol*. 2010;10(2): 99–103.
2. Girard M, Lacasse Y, Cormier Y. Hypersensitivity pneumonitis. *Allergy*. 2009;64(3):322–334.
3. Selman M, Buendia-Roldan I. Immunopathology, diagnosis and management of hypersensitivity pneumonitis. *Semin Respir Crit Care Med*. 2012;33:543–554.
4. Lacasse Y, Girard M, Cormier Y. Recent advances in hypersensitivity pneumonitis. *Chest*. 2012;142(1): 208–217.
5. Hirschmann JV, Pipavath SN, Godwin JD. Hypersensitivity pneumonitis: A historical, clinical, and radiologic review. *Radiographics*. 2009;29(7): 1921–1938.
6. Ohshimo S, Bonella F, Guzman J, et al. Hypersensitivity pneumonitis. *Immunol Allergy Clin North Am*. 2012;32(4):537–556.

 CODES

ICD10
- J67.0 Farmer's lung
- J67.8 Hypersensitivity pneumonitis due to other organic dusts
- J67.9 Hypersensitivity pneumonitis due to unspecified organic dust

CLINICAL PEARLS

- Skin testing is not useful for the diagnosis of HP.
- Once the disease is established, smoking does not appear to attenuate its severity, and it may predispose to more chronic and severe course.
- Use of protective gear on individual with high-risk exposure occupations can prevent HP.

H

HYPERSPLENISM

Jennifer C. Colvin, MD • Fred J. Schiffman, MD

 BASICS

DESCRIPTION
- Hypersplenism is defined as overactivity of the spleen and presents as:
  - Splenomegaly (commonly but not always)
  - Cytopenias with respective bone marrow hyperplasia of precursors
  - Resolution of cytopenias with splenectomy (1)
- Hypersplenism can usually be diagnosed without splenectomy.
- Splenomegaly is not synonymous with hypersplenism. Overactivity of the spleen can occur without enlargement, as is seen in immune thrombocytopenic purpura (ITP) and autoimmune hemolytic anemia.

EPIDEMIOLOGY
May be as common as 30–70% in patients with cirrhosis and portal hypertension (HTN).

ETIOLOGY AND PATHOPHYSIOLOGY
Enlargement of the spleen results in sequestration of formed blood elements, leading to peripheral cytopenias and concomitant bone marrow precursor hyperplasia. Many of the common etiologies are listed below. Almost any process involving the spleen or the hematologic system can result in hypersplenism:
- Infectious:
  - Tuberculosis
  - Malaria
  - Leishmaniasis
  - Candidiasis
  - Viral
  - Syphilis
  - Schistosomiasis
- Hematologic:
  - Myeloproliferative disorders
  - Polycythemia vera
  - Primary hypersplenism
  - ITP
  - Autoimmune hemolytic anemia
- Neoplastic:
  - Hematologic malignancies
  - Melanoma
  - Various carcinomas
- Storage diseases:
  - Gaucher disease
  - Niemann-Pick disease
  - Amyloidosis
  - Glycogen storage disease
- Inflammatory:
  - Sarcoidosis
  - Systemic lupus erythematosus
  - Felty syndrome
- Congestive

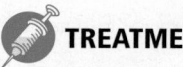 DIAGNOSIS

HISTORY
- Patients may complain of abdominal fullness or protrusion of the spleen through the abdominal wall; may complain of early satiety if the spleen is compressing stomach.
- Patients may complain of tenderness in the left upper quadrant, especially with viral infections. In lymphoproliferative disorders, spleen may be enlarged but asymptomatic unless there is splenic infarction. Given location of the spleen next to the diaphragm, a sense of fullness may be referred through the phrenic nerve to the C3–5 dermatomes in the left shoulder.

PHYSICAL EXAM
- Jaundice: If hemolytic anemia is present
- Splenomegaly:
  - The normal spleen is usually not palpable. A palpable spleen may indicate pathology such as splenomegaly—and, in turn, hypersplenism in the appropriate clinical context—or may indicate a wandering spleen.
  - Begin by percussing Traube semilunar space, demarcated laterally by left anterior axillary line, inferiorly by the left costal margin, and superiorly by the left 6th rib. This space is usually hollow. Splenic enlargement may cause dullness to percussion in this area. Other processes that may cause dullness include pleural or pericardial effusions. Additionally, if the patient recently ate a large meal, this area may be dull to percussion.
  - With patient supine, rest hand gently on the abdomen to prevent sudden tensing of the abdominal musculature, which may obscure palpation. As the spleen enlarges, it moves caudally and medially. Start by palpating in the right lower quadrant and moving toward the umbilicus, toward the left upper quadrant. If there is doubt about whether the spleen has moved beyond the costal margin, ask patient to take a large breath, which will push the diaphragm and, in turn, the spleen toward the examiner's hands.

DIAGNOSTIC TESTS & INTERPRETATION
On CBC, any and all cell lines may be decreased, resulting in:
- Anemia
- Leukopenia
- Thrombocytopenia

Initial Tests (lab, imaging)
- CBC
- Reticulocyte count if anemia
- If there is hemolysis, there should be an elevated reticulocyte count along with evidence of hyperbilirubinemia.
- US
- CT
- Tc-99m sulfur colloid scintigraphy
- PET
- MRI

Follow-Up Tests & Special Considerations
Based on other historical and exam findings, testing for specific infectious etiologies may be warranted:
- Blood parasite smear for malaria
- EBV serologies
- HIV ELISA with Western blot
- JAK2 mutation in polycythemia vera
- PPD for tuberculosis

Diagnostic Procedures/Other
Bone marrow biopsy

Test Interpretation
Hyperplasia of bone marrow precursors, especially those correlating with the patient's individual cytopenias

TREATMENT

MEDICATION
- No specific medication can be recommended for patients with hypersplenism. The most important intervention is to treat the underlying disorder.
- If ITP is the cause, the patient may benefit from:
  - Prednisone or methylprednisolone
  - IVIg
  - Rituximab
- If an infectious cause is discovered, treatment with appropriate antibiotic therapy may help to improve the cytopenias.

SURGERY/OTHER PROCEDURES
- Many patients undergo splenectomy to alleviate severe cytopenias resulting from hypersplenism.

ALERT

- Splenectomized patients should receive immunization to pneumococcus, meningococcus, *Haemophilus influenzae*, and influenza at least 14 days prior to splenectomy (2).
- If this cannot be done (i.e., in cases of emergent splenectomy), wait at least 14 days post splenectomy to immunize (3)[B]:
  - Pneumococcal vaccine:
    - Pneumococcal polyvalent-23 vaccine (PPSV23) for use in adults and fully immunized children ≥2 years
    - Pneumococcal polyvalent-13 vaccine (PCV13) for infants and young children ≥2 months
    - Current guidelines recommend single revaccination 5 years after the initial dose (4).
  - *Haemophilus influenzae* vaccine
  - Meningococcal vaccine:
    - Meningococcal conjugate vaccine (MCV4) for use in patients between 2 and 55 years
    - Meningococcal polysaccharide vaccine (MPSV4) for use in patients >55
    - Revaccination is recommended every 5 years (5).
  - Influenza vaccine should be administered yearly based on prevalent circulating strains. Although patients are not at higher risk from influenza itself, infection with influenza may place patients at higher risk for secondary bacterial infections.
- Radiofrequency ablation (RFA) is becoming more available and can be successful at preventing recurrence of hypersplenism. It is not currently known whether there are differences between RFA and splenectomy in terms of postprocedure infectious risks (6). Other alternatives to splenectomy include total and partial splenic embolization and shunting, although these techniques are evolving and additional studies are needed to evaluate efficacy and morbidity as compared to splenectomy (7).

IN-PATIENT CONSIDERATIONS
Admission Criteria/Initial Stabilization

- Hypersplenism alone generally does not warrant admission. However, all patients should be monitored closely for complications of the resulting cytopenias, including bleeding and infection, as well as complications of splenomegaly, including increased risk of splenic rupture. In some patients, the large spleen compresses the stomach and prevents adequate oral intake.
- Splenectomized patients are at increased risk of infection and postsplenectomy sepsis, especially with *Streptococcus pneumoniae*. Fevers, chills, or pain concerning for underlying infection warrant immediate attention as clinical decompensation can occur within hours. Empiric broad-spectrum antibiotics should not be delayed while evaluation is ongoing. Common empiric regimens include:
  - Ceftriaxone: 2g IV q24h and vancomycin 1 g IV q12h
  - Levofloxacin: 750 mg IV q24h and vancomycin 1 g IV q12h in β-lactam allergic patients

 ONGOING CARE

- Adult patients who are splenectomized should be advised to monitor closely for fever or rigors at home, which may be an early sign of bacteremia. They should be instructed to begin antibiotics immediately prior to proceeding to a medical facility for evaluation. Early antibiotics have been shown to reduce the mortality from overwhelming postsplenectomy sepsis.
- Controlled trials have not been performed, but some regimens include:
  - Amoxicillin-clavulanate: 875 mg PO
  - Cefuroxime axetil: 500 mg PO
- Patients allergic to β-lactam antibiotics can be given an extended-spectrum fluoroquinolone such as levofloxacin 750 mg PO *or* moxifloxacin 400 mg PO
- In children with splenectomy, daily antibiotic prophylaxis for overwhelming postsplenectomy sepsis with penicillin VK or amoxicillin is recommended until age 5 or at least 3 years after splenectomy (8)[C]:
  - Age 2 months to 5 years: 125 mg PO b.i.d.
  - >5 years old: 250 mg PO b.i.d.

PATIENT EDUCATION
Patients who are splenectomized should be counseled extensively about the risk of overwhelming postsplenectomy sepsis and the need to obtain prompt medical evaluation in the event of fevers, chills, or any other concerning symptoms.

REFERENCES

1. Jandl JH, Aster RH, Forkner CE, et al. Splenic pooling and the pathophysiology of hypersplenism. *Trans Am Clin Climatol Assoc.* 1967;78:9–27.
2. Mourtzoukou EG, Pappas G, Peppas G, et al. Vaccination of asplenic or hyposplenic adults. *Br J Surg.* 2008;95:273–280.
3. Shatz DV, Schinsky MF, Pais LB, et al. Immune responses of splenectomized trauma patients to the 23-valent pneumococcal polysaccharide vaccine at 1 versus 7 versus 14 days after splenectomy. *J Trauma.* 1998;44:(5):760–765; discussion 765–766.
4. Advisory Committee on Immunization Practices. Recommended adult immunization schedule: United States, 2012. *Ann Intern Med.* 2012;156(3):211–217. Epub 2012 Jan 31.
5. Centers for Disease Control and Prevention (CDC). Updated recommendations for use of meningococcal conjugate vaccines—Advisory Committee on Immunization Practices (ACIP), 2010. *MMWR Morb Mortal Wkly Rep.* 2011;60: 72–76.
6. Feng K, Ma K, Liu Q, et al. Randomized clinical trial of splenic radiofrequency ablation versus splenectomy for severe hypersplenism. *Br J Surg.* 2011;98:354–361.
7. Abdella HM, Abd-El-Moez AT, Abu El-Maaty ME, et al. Role of partial splenic arterial embolization for hypersplenism in patients with liver cirrhosis and thrombocytopenia. *Indian J Gastroenterol.* 2010; 29:59–61.
8. American Academy of Pediatrics. Children with asplenia or functional asplenia. In: Pickering LK, Baker CI, Kimberlin DW, et al., eds. *Red Book: 2009 Report of the Committee on Infectious Diseases,* 28th ed. Elk Grove Village, IL: American Academy of Pediatrics; 2009:72.

ADDITIONAL READING

- Di Sabatino A, Carsetti R, Corazza GR, et al. Post-splenectomy and hyposplenic states. *Lancet.* 2011;378:86–97.
- Iriyama N, Horikoshi A, Hatta Y, et al. Localized, splenic, diffuse large B-cell lymphoma presenting with hypersplenism: Risk and benefit of splenectomy. *Intern Med.* 2010;49(11):1027–1030. Epub 2010 Jun 1.
- Kapoor P, Singh E, Radhakrishnan P, et al. Splenectomy in plasma cell dyscrasias: A review of the clinical practice. *Am J Hematol.* 2006;81(12): 946–954.

 SEE ALSO

Anemia, Autoimmune Hemolytic; Immune Thrombocytopenic Purpura; Malaria; Polycythemia Vera; Tuberculosis

 CODES

ICD10
D73.1 Hypersplenism

CLINICAL PEARLS

- Splenectomy is not necessary to make the diagnosis.
- Avoid splenectomy in patients unless absolutely necessary. Splenectomized patients are at lifelong risk for overwhelming postsplenectomy infection and sepsis.
- If splenectomy is to be performed, give immunization for pneumococcus, meningococcus, *Haemophilus*, and influenza at least 14 days prior to surgery. Otherwise, wait until the 14th postop day to immunize.

H

HYPERTENSION, ESSENTIAL

Lisa M. Schroeder, MD • Kashif S. Anwar, MD

BASICS

DESCRIPTION
- Hypertension (HTN) is defined (as of JNC VIII) as ≥2 elevated BPs:
  - Age 60 or older: systolic BP (SBP) ≥150 mm Hg and/or diastolic BP (DBP) ≥90 mm Hg) at ≥2 visits
  - Age <60 years with chronic kidney disease or diabetes: SBP ≥150 mm Hg and/or (DBP) ≥90 mm Hg) at ≥2 visits
  - Operationally, any BP at which drug treatment results in a net benefit to a population (1)[A].
- HTN is a strong risk factor for cardiovascular disease.
- Synonym(s): Benign, Chronic, Idiopathic, Familial, or Genetic HTN; High BP

Geriatric Considerations
- Isolated systolic HTN is common.
- Therapy has been shown to be effective and beneficial at preventing stroke, although target SBP is higher than in younger patients (~150 mm Hg systolic), and adverse reactions to medications are more frequent. The benefit of therapy has been conclusively demonstrated in older patients for systolic blood pressure ≥ 160 mm Hg (2).

Pediatric Considerations
- Measure BP during routine exams for >3 years of age.
- Defined as SBP or DBP ≥95th percentile on repeated measurements.
- Pre-HTN: SBP or DBP between 90th and 95th percentile (3)

Pregnancy Considerations
- Elevated BP during pregnancy may be either chronic HTN or pregnancy-induced preeclampsia. ACE inhibitors and angiotensin II receptor blockers (ARBs) are contraindicated.
- Maternal and fetal mortality benefit from treatment of severe HTN. Evidence not clear for mild HTN (see topic "Preeclampsia").

EPIDEMIOLOGY
Incidence
- Lifetime risk for men and women aged 55–65 by age 80–85 is >90%.
- Predominant age: Essential (primary, benign, idiopathic) onset usually in the 20s–30s.
- Predominant sex: Male > Female; males tend to run higher than females and have a significantly higher risk of cardiovascular disease at any given pressure.

Prevalence
In 2009–2010, prevalence in adults was 28.6% (2009–2010 NHANES)

ETIOLOGY AND PATHOPHYSIOLOGY
- >90% of HTN has no identified cause.
- Secondary causes of HTN (see "Hypertension, Secondary and Resistant"): Renal parenchymal: Glomerulonephritis, pyelonephritis, polycystic kidneys; Endocrine: Primary hyperaldosteronism, pheochromocytoma, hyperthyroidism, Cushing syndrome; Vascular: Coarctation of aorta, renal artery stenosis; Chemical: Commonly, oral contraceptives, NSAIDs, decongestants, corticosteroids; sleep apnea

Genetics
BP levels are strongly familial, but no clear genetic pattern exists. Familial risk for cardiovascular diseases should be considered.

RISK FACTORS
Family history, obesity, alcohol use, excess dietary sodium, stress, physical inactivity, tobacco abuse, insulin resistance

DIAGNOSIS

HISTORY
- HTN is asymptomatic except in extreme cases or after related cardiovascular complications develop.
- Headache can be seen with higher BP, often present on awakening and occipital in nature.

PHYSICAL EXAM
- Retinopathy: Narrowed arteries, arteriovenous (AV) nicking, copper or silver wiring of retinal arterioles
- Increased S2 (Aortic component heart sound)
- Synchronous radial and femoral pulse can help to rule out coarctation of the aorta.

DIFFERENTIAL DIAGNOSIS
Secondary HTN: Because of the low incidence of reversible secondary HTN, special tests should be considered only if the history, physical exam, or basic laboratory evaluation indicate the possibility. (See "Hypertension, Secondary and Resistant.")

DIAGNOSTIC TESTS & INTERPRETATION
ECG to evaluate possible presence of left ventricular hypertrophy (LVH) or rhythm abnormalities affecting therapy

Initial Tests (lab, imaging)
- Hemoglobin and hematocrit or CBC
- Complete urinalysis (may reveal proteinuria)
- Potassium, calcium, and creatinine, uric acid
- Lipid Panel (total, HDL, LDL, TG)
- Fasting blood glucose, hemoglobin A1c
- Only if history or physical indicate (see "Hypertension, Secondary and Resistant")

Follow-Up Tests & Special Considerations
- Special tests (only if history, physical, or labs indicates). (See "Hypertension, Secondary and Resistant.")
- Ambulatory (24-hour) BP monitoring if "white coat" HTN is suspected
- Home BP monitoring is effective, especially if "white coat" HTN is a consideration (4); elevated home BPs correlate with adverse outcomes, possibly more so than office BPs, and normal readings are reassuring.

Diagnostic Procedures/Other
- Age 60 or older: systolic BP (SBP) ≥150 mm Hg and/or diastolic BP (DBP) ≥90 mm Hg) at ≥2 visits
- Age <60 years with chronic kidney disease or diabetes: SBP ≥150 mm Hg and/or (DBP) ≥90 mm Hg) at ≥2 visits
- Operationally, any BP at which drug treatment results in a net benefit to a population.
- Assuming proper resting conditions, cuff size, and application are maintained.
- The Joint National Committee (JNC) (5) recommends emphasis on:
  - Family or personal history of HTN, cardiovascular, cerebrovascular, renal disease, and diabetes
  - Previous elevated BPs
  - Previous treatments

- History of weight gain, exercise activities, sodium and fat intake, and alcohol use
- Symptoms suggesting secondary HTN
- Psychosocial and environmental factors affecting BP and risk for cardiovascular disease
- Other cardiovascular risk factors, such as obesity, smoking, hyperlipidemia, and diabetes
- Funduscopic exam for arteriolar narrowing, AV compression, hemorrhages, exudates, and papilledema
- Body mass index (BMI)
- Waist circumference
- BP in both arms
- Complete cardiac and peripheral pulse exam: Compare radial and femoral pulse for differences in volume and timing, auscultation for carotid and femoral bruits.
- Abdominal exam for masses and bruits: Listen high in the flanks over the kidneys.
- Neurologic assessment

TREATMENT

GENERAL MEASURES
- Treating patients to lower-than-standard BP targets, ≤140/90 mm Hg, does not further reduce mortality or morbidity (2,6)[A]. Individualize goal pressures based on risk factors; best target may be SBP at or just below 150 mm Hg in patients >75–80 years of age (2)[A].
- Primary focus is SBP goal; treatment should accommodate patient preferences (4).
- Aerobic exercise, (30 minutes of aerobics 4–5 days/week), weight reduction for obese patients
- Smoking cessation
- Risk stratification affects the treatment:
  - Pre-HTN (120–139/80–89 mm Hg): Drug therapy for chronic renal disease or diabetes. ACCORD trial did not support <140/90 for Type 2 diabetes mellitus (7)
  - Evidence for benefit in treatment of Stage 1 hypertension (140–159/90–99 mm Hg) is sparse. Assess overall risk and individualize decision to treat. Begin thiazide diuretics for many patients
  - Stage 2 HTN (>160/>100 mm Hg): Consider starting 2 drugs initially.

MEDICATION
- The amount of BP reduction is probably more important than the choice of antihypertensive.
- Multiple drugs at submaximal dose may achieve target BP with fewer side effects.
- Thiazide diuretics have the most proven benefits (cost, compliance, and effectiveness). Chlorthalidone and hydrochlorothiazide (HCTZ) equally effective, some data states rate of adverse events (hypokalemia, hyponatremia) are more common with chlorthalidone (8,9)[A].
- Sequential monotherapy attempts might be tried with different classes because individual responses vary.
- Most patients will require multiple medications.
- First line agents for uncomplicated essential HTN include thiazide diuretics. Angiotensin Converting Enzyme Inhibitors (ACEi) and long-acting dihydropyridine calcium channel blocker (amlodipine, felodipine, nifedipine).
- If concomitant conditions, choose first line agent based upon comorbidity (1).

- Combination first line agents: Benazepril combined with amlodipine may be superior to combination with HCTZ in high-risk patients). Some suggest that ACE/ARB + dihydropyridine calcium channel blocker is first choice after monotherapy.
- β-Blockers had been strongly recommended until recent meta-analyses. Atenolol may be particularly *ineffective* in reducing adverse outcomes of hypertension (except in patients with left ventricle hypertrophy undergoing dialysis).
- ACE inhibitors should be used in patients with diabetes, proteinuria, atrial fibrillation, or congestive heart failure (CHF), but not in pregnancy.
- α-Adrenergic blockers are not the 1st choice for monotherapy (7)[A]. Might benefit males with benign prostatic hypertrophy (BPH).
- β-Blockers might benefit patients with ischemic heart disease, CHF, or migraine post STEMI.
- Calcium channel blockers could be considered in patients with isolated systolic HTN, atherosclerosis, angina, migraine, or asthma; well documented to reduce risk of stroke (7).

First Line
- Thiazide diuretics:
  – Chlorthalidone: 12.5–50 mg/d
  – Hydrochlorothiazide: 6.25–50 mg/d
  – Indapamide: 1.25–5 mg/d
- ACE inhibitors:
  – Lisinopril: 5–40 mg/d
  – Enalapril: 2.5–40 mg/d
  – Ramipril: 2.5–20 mg/d
  – Benazepril: 10–40 mg/d
- Calcium channel blockers:
  – Diltiazem CD: 180–360 mg/d
  – Nifedipine (sustained release): 30–90 mg/d
  – Verapamil (sustained release): 120–480 mg/d
  – Amlodipine: 2.5–10 mg/d
- Contraindications:
  – Diuretics may worsen gout.
  – β-Blockers (relatively) in reactive airway disease, heart block, diabetes, and peripheral vascular disease; probably should be avoided in patients with metabolic syndrome or insulin-requiring diabetes
  – Diltiazem or verapamil: Do not use with systolic dysfunction heart failure or heart block
  – ACE inhibitors can worsen bilateral renovascular disease and are pregnancy Category D.

Second Line
- ARBs:
  – Losartan: 25–100 mg in 1 or 2 doses; has unique but modest uricosuric effect
  – Valsartan: 80–320 mg daily
  – Irbesartan: 75–300 mg daily
  – Candesartan: 4–32 mg daily
  – Renin inhibitor: Aliskiren 150–300 mg daily
- Many may be combined. Choose additional medications with complementary effects (i.e., ACEI/ARB with diuretic or a vasodilator with a diuretic or β-blocker).
- Centrally acting α-2 agonists: Clonidine: 0.1–1.2 mg b.i.d. or weekly patch 0.1–0.3 mg/d, guanfacine: 1–3 mg daily, or methyldopa: 250–2,000 mg b.i.d.

- α-Adrenergic antagonists: Prazosin: 1–10 mg b.i.d., terazosin: 1–20 mg/d, or doxazosin: 1–16 mg/d
- Peripherally acting adrenergic inhibitors: Rarely used: Reserpine: 0.1–0.25 mg/d
- Vasodilators:
  – Hydralazine: 25–150 mg b.i.d.; risk of tachycardia, so generally combined with β-blocker; also drug-induced systemic lupus erythematosus (SLE)
  – Minoxidil: Rarely used due to adverse effects. May be more effective than other medications in renal failure and refractory hypertension.
- Loop diuretics (for volume overload): Furosemide: 20–320 mg/d *or* bumetanide: 0.5–2 mg/d
- K⁺-sparing diuretics in patients with hypokalemia while taking thiazides, or with medication-refractory HTN or suspected aldosteronism: Amiloride: 5–10 mg/d, spironolactone: 25–100 mg/d, or triamterene: 50–150 mg/d

COMPLEMENTARY AND ALTERNATIVE MEDICINE
Biofeedback and relaxation exercise

ONGOING CARE

FOLLOW-UP RECOMMENDATIONS
Patient Monitoring
- Re-evaluate patients q3–6mo until stable, then q6–12mo. Consider use of home self-BP monitoring; quality-of-life issues, including sexual function should be considered.
- Poor medication adherence is a leading cause of apparent medication failure.
- Annual urinalysis, creatinine, and potassium

DIET
- ~20% of patients will respond to reduced-salt diet (<100 mmol/d; <6 g NaCl or <2.4 g Na).
- Consider Dietary Approaches to Stop Hypertension (DASH) diet: www.nhlbi.nih.gov/health/public/heart/hbp/dash/new_dash.pdf.
- Limit alcohol consumption to <1 oz/d.

PATIENT EDUCATION
- Emphasize the asymptomatic nature of HTN and importance of lifetime treatment.
- Printed aids for high BP education available: www.nhlbi.nih.gov/health/public/heart/index.htm#hbp

COMPLICATIONS
Heart failure, renal failure, LVH, myocardial infarction, retinal hemorrhage, stroke, hypertensive heart disease, drug side effects

REFERENCES

1. James PA, Oparil S, Carter BL, et al. Evidence-Based Guideline for the Management of High Blood Pressure in Adults. Report From the Panel Members Appointed to the Eighth Joint National Committee (JNC 8). *JAMA*. 2014 Published online December 18, 2013. doi:10.1001/jama.2013.284427.
2. Mancia G, Fagard R, Nariewicz K, et al. 2013 ESH/ESC guidelines for the management of arterial hypertension: the Task Force for the Management of Arterial Hypertension of the European Society of Hypertension (ESH) and of the European Society of Cardiology (ESC). *Eur Heart J*. 2013;34: 2159–2219.
3. National High Blood Pressure Education Program Working Group on High Blood Pressure in Children and Adolescents. The Fourth Report on the Diagnosis, Evaluation, and Treatment of High Blood Pressure in Children and Adolescents. *Pediatrics*. 2004;114(2)(suppl 4):555–576.
4. NICE Clinical Guideline 127. Hypertension: Clinical management of primary hypertension in adults. 2011;www.nice.org.uk/nicemedia/live/13561/56008/56008.pdf
5. Chobanian AV, Bakris GL, Black HR, et al. The Seventh Report of the Joint National Committee on Prevention, Detection, Evaluation, and Treatment of High Blood Pressure: The JNC 7 report. *JAMA*. 2003;289:2560–2572.
6. Arguedas JA, Perez MI, Wright JM. Treatment blood pressure targets for hypertension. *Cochrane Database Syst Rev*. 2009:CD004349.
7. The ACCORD Study Group. Effects of intensive blood-pressure control in type 2 diabetes mellitus. *N Engl J Med*. 2010;362(17):1575–1585. PubMed PMID: 20228401.
8. ALLHAT Officers and Coordinators for the ALLHAT Collaborative Research Group. The Antihypertensive and Lipid-Lowering Treatment to Prevent Heart Attack Trial. Major outcomes in high-risk hypertensive patients randomized to angiotensin-converting enzyme inhibitor or calcium channel blocker vs diuretic: The Antihypertensive and Lipid-Lowering Treatment to Prevent Heart Attack Trial (ALLHAT). *JAMA*. 2002;288: 2981–2997.
9. Dorsch MP, Gillespie BW, Erickson SR, et al. Chlorthalidone reduces cardiovascular events compared with hydrochlorothiazide. *Hypertension*. 2011;57:689–694.

 SEE ALSO

Hypertension, Secondary and Resistant; Hypertensive Emergencies; Polycystic Kidney Disease

 CODES

ICD10
I10 Essential (primary) hypertension

CLINICAL PEARLS
- Treatment of HTN reduces risk of many serious medical conditions with numbers needed to treat to prevent 1 serious event (e.g., stroke or myocardial infarction [MI]) ranging from ~20 patients/year for severe HTN to more than several hundred per year for mild HTN.
- Multiple submaximal doses are likely to have fewer side effects and more effectiveness than fewer maximum-dosed drugs.
- In older patients, measure BP standing to avoid overtreatment and syncope.

H

HYPERTENSION, SECONDARY AND RESISTANT

George H. Maxted, MD

BASICS

DESCRIPTION
Uncontrolled hypertension (HTN) is composed of the following entities:

- Resistant hypertension was not addressed by JNC-8, but it can be assumed the goal would be <150/90 for those 60 and older who are uncontrolled on 3 antihypertensives, including a diuretic and 140/90 for those with chronic kidney disease and diabetes (1,2,3)
- Secondary HTN: Elevated BP that results from an identifiable underlying mechanism (1,2)

Geriatric Considerations
- Onset of hypertension in adults >60 years of age is a strong indicator of secondary HTN.
- In patients >80, consider a higher target systolic blood pressure (SBP) of ≤150 (4).
- Elderly may be particularly responsive to diuretics and dihydropyridine calcium channel blockers (4).
- Systolic HTN is particularly problematic in the elderly.
- Secondary causes more common in the elderly; include sleep apnea, renal disease, renal artery stenosis, and primary aldosteronism (2).

ALERT
Pseudoresistance:
- Inaccurate measurement of BP:
  – Cuff too small
  – Patient not at rest; sitting quietly for 5 minutes
- Poor adherence: In primary care settings, this has been estimated to occur in 40–60% of patients with HTN (2).
- White-coat effect: Prevalence 20–40%. Do not make clinical decisions about HTN based solely on measurement in the clinic setting. Home BP monitoring and/or ambulatory BP monitoring is more reliable (5).
- Inadequate treatment (2)

EPIDEMIOLOGY
- Predominant age: In general, HTN has its onset between ages 30 and 50. Patients with resistant HTN are more likely to experience the combined outcomes of death, myocardial infarction, congestive heart failure (CHF), stroke, or chronic kidney disease (3).
- Depending on etiology, age of onset can vary. Age of onset <20 or >50 increases likelihood of a secondary cause for HTN.
- The strongest predictors for resistant HTN are age (>75), presence of left ventricular hypertrophy (LVH), obesity (body mass index [BMI] >30), and high baseline systolic BP. Other predictors include chronic kidney disease, diabetes, living in the southeastern US, African American race (especially women), and excessive salt intake (2).
- In the ACCOMPLISH, INVEST, CONVINCE, ALLHAT, and LIFE studies, percent of patients reaching JNC-7 BP goals ranged from 45–82% (1).

Prevalence
Prevalence of resistant HTN is unknown. NHANES analysis indicates only 53% of adults are controlled to a BP of <140/90.

ETIOLOGY AND PATHOPHYSIOLOGY
- Obstructive sleep apnea (OSA): 1 study diagnosed OSA in 83% of treatment-resistant hypertensives (2).
- Primary hyperaldosteronism (17–22% of resistant HTN cases) (2)
- Chronic renal disease (2–5% of hypertensives)
- Renovascular disease (0.2–0.7%, up to 35% of elderly, 20% of patients undergoing cardiac catheterization) (2)
- Cushing syndrome (0.1–0.6%)
- Pheochromocytoma (0.04–0.1% of hypertensives)
- Other rare causes: Hyperthyroidism, hyperparathyroidism, aortic coarctation, intracranial tumor
- Drug-related causes:
  – Medications, especially NSAIDs (may also blunt effectiveness of ACE-inhibitors), decongestants, stimulants (e.g., amphetamines, attention-deficit hyperactivity disorder [ADHD] medications), anorectic agents (e.g., modafinil, ephedra, guarana, ma huang, bitter orange), erythropoietin, natural licorice (in some chewing tobacco), yohimbine, glucocorticoids
  – Oral contraceptives: Unclear association; mainly epidemiologic and with higher estrogen pills
  – Cocaine, amphetamines, other illicit drugs; drug and alcohol withdrawal syndromes
- Lifestyle factors: Obesity, dietary salt may negate the beneficial effect of diuretics. Excessive alcohol, physical inactivity also contributors

Genetics
In some patients, there is a possible relationship to ENaC gene variants (Liddle syndrome) and a CYP3A5 allele (cortisol metabolism, especially African Americans) (2).

RISK FACTORS
A recent large cohort study revealed that those with resistant HTN (16.2%) were more likely to be male, Caucasian, older, and diabetic. They were also more likely to be taking β-blockers, calcium channel blockers, and α-adrenergic blockers compared with other drug classes (3). Factors predictive of resistant or secondary HTN: Female sex, African-American race, obesity, diabetes, worsening of control in previously stable hypertensive patient, onset in patients age <20 or >50, lack of family history of HTN, significant target end-organ damage, stage 2 HTN (systolic BP >160 mm Hg or diastolic BP >100 mm Hg), renal disease, and alcohol or drug use

GENERAL PREVENTION
The prevention of resistant and secondary HTN is thought to be the same as for primary or essential HTN: Adopting a DASH (Dietary Approaches to Stop Hypertension) diet, a low-sodium diet, weight loss in obese patients, exercise, limitation of alcohol intake, and smoking cessation may all be of benefit. Relaxation techniques may be of help, but data are limited.

DIAGNOSIS

HISTORY
- Ask or review at every visit: "The Big Four" SANS mnemonic: 1. Salt intake, 2. Alcohol intake, 3. NSAID use, 4. Sleep (author's suggestion, based on reference listed).
- Review home BP readings; consider ambulatory BP monitoring.
- History will vary with etiology of HTN:
  – Pheochromocytoma: Episodes of headache, palpitations, sweating
  – Cushing syndrome: Weight gain, fatigue, weakness, easy bruising, amenorrhea
  – OSA: Loud snoring while asleep, daytime somnolence
  – Increased intravascular volume: Swelling

PHYSICAL EXAM
- Ensure that the BP is measured correctly. The patient should be sitting quietly with back supported for 5 minutes before measurement. Proper cuff size: Bladder encircling at least 80% of the arm. Support arm at heart level. Minimum of 2 readings at least 1 minute apart. Check BP in both arms. Also check standing BP for orthostasis.
- Attention to findings related to possible etiologies: Renovascular HTN: Systolic/diastolic abdominal bruit. Pheochromocytoma: Diaphoresis, tachycardia. Cushing syndrome: Hirsutism, moon facies, dorsal hump, purple striae, truncal obesity. Thyroid disease: Enlarged thyroid, tremor, exophthalmos, tachycardia. Coarctation of the aorta: Upper limb HTN with decreased or delayed femoral pulses.
- Funduscopic exam

DIAGNOSTIC TESTS & INTERPRETATION
- ECG performed as part of the initial workup; LVH is an important marker of resistant HTN.
- Sleep study if history and physical indicate. Overnight oximetry is a good screen for nocturnal hypoxia. If positive, formal polysomnography may be indicated.

Initial Tests (lab, imaging)
Initial limited diagnostic testing should include (2)[A]: Urinalysis, CBC, potassium, sodium, glucose, creatinine, lipids, thyroid-stimulating hormone (TSH), calcium. 50% of patients with hyperaldosteronism may have normal potassium levels (1,2).

- Imaging tests listed are necessary only if history, physical, or lab data indicate.
- Abdominal US: If renal disease is suspected
- MR angiography (MRA) of renal vasculature: Preferred test for renovascular HTN. Sensitive, but low specificity. Conventional angiography or CT angiography 2nd-line after MRA to look at distal renal artery. Renal arteriography remains gold standard for renovascular disease.
- Adrenal "incidentaloma" frequently arises in this era of multiple CT studies. If present in the setting of resistant HTN, consider hyperaldosterone or hyperadrenalcorticoid states.
- Doppler or CT imaging of aorta along with chest x-ray looking for notched ribs (sign of coarctation)

Follow-Up Tests & Special Considerations

Further testing for primary aldosteronism (PA) may be considered:

- Empiric treatment with an aldosterone inhibitor may be preferable, and more clinically relevant: Spironolactone or eplerenone. Amiloride may be more effective in African Americans.
- Plasma aldosterone-to-renin ratio (ARR) is the preferred lab test, *but* the test is difficult to perform and interpret properly. Consult your reference lab and interpret results with caution:
  – Further testing for pheochromocytoma: Plasma metanephrine screening test of choice: Confirmed by a 24-hour urinary metanephrine-to-creatinine ratio
  – Other tests to consider for resistant or secondary hypertension: 24-hour urine for free cortisol, calcium, parathyroid hormone (PTH), overnight 1-mg dexamethasone suppression test, urine toxicology screen

Diagnostic Procedures/Other

Consider 24-hour ambulatory BP monitoring, especially if white-coat effect is suspected. Home BP monitor results predict mortality, stroke, and other target organ damage better than office BP (5). Optimal protocol involves 2 paired measurements morning and evening (4 measurements) over 4–7 days:

- Oscillometric, electronic, upper arm, fully automatic device with memory. Average multiple readings over several days.
- See www.dableducational.org for validated monitors.

TREATMENT

- Treatment modality depends on etiology of HTN. Please see each etiology listed for information on proper treatment.
- Emphasize: Adherence to interventions according to JNC-7 recommendations. Lack of, or underuse of, diuretic therapy is often found. Nonpharmacologic measures include weight loss, dietary salt restriction, moderation of alcohol intake, increased physical activity:
  – Obese patients, African Americans, elderly may be particularly responsive to diuretics (6).
  – Tolerance to diuretics may occur: Long-term adaptation to thiazides or the "braking effect." Consider increasing the dose of thiazide or adding an aldosterone inhibitor (6).
- Treatment specific to certain secondary etiologies:
  – Primary aldosteronism: Aldosterone receptor antagonist: Spironolactone or eplerenone
  – Cushing syndrome: Aldosterone receptor antagonist
  – OSA: Continuous positive airway pressure (CPAP) ± oxygen, surgery, weight loss
  – Nocturnal hypoxia: Oxygen supplementation
- Renal sympathetic denervation may be beneficial in refractory cases.

MEDICATION

- Diuretics, especially chlorthalidone, are 1st line (6). Additional benefit has been demonstrated with ACE inhibitors, angiotensin II receptor blocker (ARB) agents, calcium channel blockers (2)[C].
- β-Blockers are considered 1st-line only for patients with ischemic heart disease or CHF. Combined α-β antagonists (e.g., labetalol) may be more effective for HTN.

- Aldosterone antagonists may offer significant benefit (1)[C],(2,7).
- Central-acting agents (e.g., clonidine) are effective at reducing BP, but outcome data are lacking.

ALERT

- Agents specific for treatment of HTN emergencies should be initiated under a situation in which immediate BP reduction will prevent or limit end-organ damage (see topic "Hypertensive Emergencies").
- Renovascular HTN: Angioplasty is the treatment of choice for fibromuscular dysplasia of a renal artery. Endovascular treatment of atherosclerotic disease is controversial, with no clear benefit over medical management. Cardiovascular Outcomes in Renal Atherosclerotic Lesions (CORAL) study is pending and may help determine risk/benefit (2).
- Referral to an HTN specialist or clinic: Retrospective studies indicate improved control rates for patients with resistant HTN referred to special HTN clinics (2)[C].

First Line

See topic "Hypertension."

IN-PATIENT CONSIDERATIONS
Admission Criteria/Initial Stabilization

Hospitalization may be necessary for hypertensive urgency or emergency general measures.

 ONGOING CARE

FOLLOW-UP RECOMMENDATIONS

Encourage aerobic activity of 30 min/d, depending on patient condition.

DIET

- Reduced salt may lower BP.
- Recommend the Mediterranean Diet or DASH.

PATIENT EDUCATION

Home BP monitoring is recommended.

REFERENCES

1. Sarafidis PA, Bakris GL. Resistant hypertension: An overview of evaluation and treatment. *J Am Coll Cardiol*. 2008;52:1749–1757.
2. Calhoun DA. Resistant hypertension: Diagnosis, evaluation, and treatment. A scientific statement from the American Heart Association Professional Education Committee of the Council for High Blood Pressure Research. *Hypertension*. 2008;51(6):1403–1419.
3. Daugherty SL, Powers JD, Magid DJ, et al. Incidence and prognosis of resistant hypertension in hypertensive patients. *Circulation*. 2012;125(13):1635–1642. Epub 2012 Feb 29.
4. Aronow WS, Fleg JL, Pepine CJ, et al. ACCF/AHA 2011 expert consensus document on hypertension in the elderly: A report of the American College of Cardiology Foundation Task Force on Clinical Expert Consensus documents developed in collaboration with the American Academy of Neurology, American Geriatrics Society, American Society for Preventive Cardiology, American Society of Hypertension, American Society of Nephrology, Association of Black Cardiologists, and European Society of Hypertension. *J Am Coll Cardiol*. 2011;57:2037–2114.
5. Powers BJ, Olsen MK, Smith VA, et al. Measuring blood pressure for decision making and quality reporting: Where and how many measures? *Ann Intern Med*. 2011;154:781–788.
6. Ernst ME, Moser M. Use of diuretics in patients with hypertension. *N Engl J Med*. 2009;361:2153–2164.
7. Calhoun DA. Low-dose aldosterone blockade as a new treatment paradigm for controlling resistant hypertension. *J Clin Hypertens*. 2007;91(Suppl 1):19–24.
8. James PA, Oparil S, Carter BL, et al. Evidence-Based Guideline for the Management of High Blood Pressure in Adults. Report From the Panel Members Appointed to the Eighth Joint National Committee (JNC 8). *JAMA*. 2014 Published online December 18, 2013. doi:10.1001/jama.2013.284427.

ADDITIONAL READING

- Agarwal R, Bills JE, Hecht TJ, et al. Role of home blood pressure monitoring in overcoming therapeutic inertia and improving hypertension control: A systematic review and meta-analysis. *Hypertension*. 2011;57:29–38.
- Brandt MC, Mahfoud F, Reda S, et al. Renal sympathetic denervation reduces left ventricular hypertrophy and improves cardiac function in patients with resistant hypertension. *J Am Coll Cardiol*. 2012;59(10):901–909.
- Gaddam KK, Nishizaka MK, Pratt-Ubunama MN, et al. Characterization of resistant hypertension: Association between resistant hypertension, aldosterone, and persistent intravascular volume expansion. *Arch Intern Med*. 2008;168(11):1159–1164.
- Johansson JK, Niiranen TJ, Puukka PJ, et al. Optimal schedule for home blood pressure monitoring based on a clinical approach. *J Hypertens*. 2010;28(2):259–264.

 SEE ALSO

Aldosteronism, Primary; Coarctation of the Aorta; Cushing Disease and Cushing Syndrome; Hyperparathyroidism; Hypertension, Essential; Hyperthyroidism; Pheochromocytoma

 CODES

ICD10

- I15.0 Renovascular hypertension
- I15.8 Other secondary hypertension
- I15.9 Secondary hypertension, unspecified

CLINICAL PEARLS

- Onset of HTN in adults >60 years of age is a strong indicator of secondary HTN.
- Common causes of resistant HTN: Obstructive sleep apnea, excessive salt intake, medication nonadherence
- Common secondary causes include sleep apnea, renal disease, renal artery stenosis, and primary aldosteronism.
- Home BP monitoring predicts outcomes better than office monitoring of BP.

H

HYPERTENSIVE EMERGENCIES
John A. Guisto, MD, FACEP • Arthur B. Sanders, MD, MHA

BASICS

DESCRIPTION
- Numerous terms, often overlapping. Some definitions include a specific BP reading; others emphasize acute change in BP or presence of specific clinical syndromes.
- Severe HTN is defined as a diastolic BP of $\geq$115 mm Hg (15.3 kPa).
- A hypertensive emergency occurs only when an acute elevation of BP causes rapid and progressive end-organ damage, particularly in the cardiovascular, renal, and CNS.
- System(s) affected: Cardiovascular; Nervous; Pulmonary; Renal
- Synonym(s): Hypertensive crisis; Severe HTN; Malignant HTN; Accelerated HTN; Hypertensive emergency

EPIDEMIOLOGY
Incidence
Incidence of hypertensive emergency: 1% of patients with hypertension annually in the US

Prevalence
- Overall prevalence of HTN in the US: 29.3% based on a 2003–2004 survey data
- Predominant age: Elderly

ETIOLOGY AND PATHOPHYSIOLOGY
- Increased sympathetic tone leads to increased BP.
- Angiotensin II has multiple effects contributing to HTN and end-organ damage:
  – Stimulates sympathetic tone, aldosterone release, and antidiuretic hormone release
  – Chronic HTN induces vascular thickening and sclerosis.
  – Central effects include enhanced resorption of salt and water.
  – Chronic HTN shifts autoregulation of BP and cerebral blood flow.
- Renal disease
- Abrupt withdrawal from antihypertensives, especially clonidine (Catapres)
- Withdrawal from CNS depressants
- Medications: SSRIs, decongestants, appetite suppressants, steroids (including oral contraceptives), MAOI interaction with certain foods or drugs, drugs of abuse (cocaine, amphetamine)
- Eclampsia/Preeclampsia
- Thrombotic thrombocytopenic purpura
- Pheochromocytoma
- Severe burns
- Postoperative HTN

Genetics
- Genetics: Risk of hypertensive emergency is higher in African Americans.
- Predominant sex: Male > Female

RISK FACTORS
- History of poorly controlled HTN
- Drug abuse
- Noncompliance with medications; abruptly stopping antihypertensive medication without supervision

GENERAL PREVENTION
Treat HTN and counsel patients on importance of compliance with antihypertensive treatment and dangers of stopping medications abruptly.

COMMONLY ASSOCIATED CONDITIONS
- Chronic renal failure
- Renovascular HTN
- Acute glomerulonephritis
- Renal vasculitis

Geriatric Considerations
Elderly patients may experience isolated systolic HTN due to decreased baroreceptor sensitivity.

Pediatric Considerations
- Usually associated with renal disease
- May present with abdominal pain
- Preferred agents for children include labetalol, nicardipine, and nitroprusside.

Pregnancy Considerations
- Labetalol, nicardipine, or hydralazine are preferred. Nitroprusside decreases placental blood flow and cyanide metabolite crosses the placenta; may result in fetal toxicity with prolonged exposure.
- Treat preeclampsia.

DIAGNOSIS

Clinical presentation varies depending on organ system affected.

HISTORY
- Headache
- Altered mental status
- Nausea, vomiting
- Neurologic disturbance
- Shortness of breath, dyspnea, orthopnea
- Chest pain
- Abdominal pain
- Epistaxis

PHYSICAL EXAM
- HTN
- Focal neurologic deficits, stupor, coma
- Retinopathy: Funduscopic exam may reveal papilledema, exudates, or hemorrhages.
- Pulmonary edema
- Hemorrhage, thrombosis, embolus
- Renal or abdominal bruit
- Unequal BP or pulses in the extremities

DIFFERENTIAL DIAGNOSIS
- Myocardial infarction or angina pectoris
- Aortic dissection
- CHF
- Stroke
- Other CNS pathology (e.g., encephalopathy)
- Acute pulmonary edema
- Renal failure

DIAGNOSTIC TESTS & INTERPRETATION
Initial Tests (lab, imaging)
- Urinalysis and renal function tests (red cell casts, hematuria, proteinuria are common)
- Drug screen
- Blood count and smear may indicate microangiopathic hemolytic anemia or thrombocytopenia.

- Serum electrolytes, which may indicate hypokalemic alkalosis; calcium, glucose
- Cardiac enzymes if concerned for myocardial ischemia
- Chest radiograph:
- May show pulmonary edema and cardiomegaly due to CHF
- Mediastinal widening and blunting of the aortic knob consistent with aortic aneurysm (potential rupture)
- If CNS symptoms, order CT scan or MRI of the head.
- If chest, abdominal, or back pain, consider CT angiography or MRA for suspected aortic dissection.

Follow-Up Tests & Special Considerations
- Subsequent workup for pheochromocytoma in selected patients
- Workup for hyperaldosteronism (hypernatremia, hypokalemia, elevated HCO_3, and decreased Ca^{++}) and for renal artery stenosis may be indicated in selected patients, especially young patients who may have fibromuscular dysplasia.

Diagnostic Procedures/Other
- ECG may reveal ischemia or left ventricular hypertrophy.
- The BP should be measured with an appropriately sized cuff, with $\geq$2 readings from both arms; then average readings.

Test Interpretation
Extreme BP elevations can overwhelm autoregulatory mechanisms for organ blood flow, resulting in damage to arteriolar and capillary beds. This process produces organ hemorrhages and edema.

TREATMENT

GENERAL MEASURES
If ongoing end-organ damage is thought to be secondary to hypertensive state, prompt treatment with IV medication is indicated. Monitor patient closely so rapid fall in BP can be avoided.

MEDICATION
A 2008 Cochrane Review (1) noted no randomized clinical trials show reduction in mortality from recommended treatments and no clear basis for recommending 1 drug over another. These treatments do reduce BP in these circumstances, and evidence levels reflect their effectiveness. A single randomized trial and review article compared IV nicardipine with labetalol, suggesting nicardipine more reliably reaches target BP with similar rate of overshoot or need for additional rescue medication (2,3).

ALERT
- The general goal is to lower mean arterial pressure (MAP) by ~20% or reduce diastolic pressure to 100–110 mm Hg (13.3–14.6 kPa) over 1 hour.
- Lower BP </= 20% in the 1st hour; then, if stable, lower to 160/100–110 over the next 2–6 hours
- MAP is ~1/3 of the sum of twice the diastolic pressure plus the systolic pressure.

First Line
- IV unless otherwise indicated:
  - Nicardipine: 4–15 mg/h (4,5,6)[B]
  - Labetalol (Normodyne, Trandate): Bolus 20–80 mg q10–15min infusion 0.5–2 mg/min (4,5)[A]
  - Nitroglycerin (NTG): Infusion 5–100 μg/min (4,5,7)[A]
  - NTG 0.4 mg SL tablet: Repeat q5min if needed. Consider IV infusion after 3 doses (4)[B].
  - Phentolamine (Regitine): Bolus 5–10 mg q5–15min (4,5)[A]
  - Esmolol: 0.05–0.3 mg/kg/min (4,5,7)[A]
  - Enalapril: 0.625–1.25 mg (4,5)[B]
- Drug(s) used depends on end organs affected and patient's clinical status:
  - Hypertensive encephalopathy: Nicardipine, labetalol, esmolol, or enalaprilat (5,8)[A]
  - CNS events: Nicardipine, labetalol. In ischemic stroke, withhold treatment unless systolic >220 mm Hg or diastolic >120 mm Hg, except when needed for treating concomitant cardiovascular disease or pulmonary edema (4,5,7,8)[A]. In patients with intracerebral hemorrhage and systolic BP 150–220 mm Hg, acutely lowering to a systolic of 140 mm Hg is probably safe and may decrease additional bleeding (9)[B].
  - Subarachnoid hemorrhage: Nicardipine, labetalol, or esmolol (5,7,8)[A]
  - Myocardial ischemia: Nitroglycerin infusion, or labetalol, or esmolol (4,5,7)[A]
  - CHF: Nitroglycerin infusion, or enalaprilat or nicardipine with a loop diuretic (4,5,8)[A]
  - Aortic dissection: Nitroprusside plus β-blocker, labetalol, esmolol plus nicardipine/clevidipine, or nitroglycerin infusion (4,5,7,8)[A]
  - Renal failure: Labetalol, nicardipine, or fenoldopam; consider dialysis (4,7,8)[A].
  - Pheochromocytoma: Phentolamine, or labetalol, or nitroprusside infusion (4)[A]
  - Antihypertensive withdrawal: Labetalol or phentolamine (4)[A]
  - Interactions between MAOIs and foods or drugs: Phentolamine or labetalol (4)[B]
  - Eclampsia/Preeclampsia: Labetalol, nicardipine, or hydralazine (4,5,7,8)[A]

Second Line
- Nitroprusside (Nipride, Nitropress): Infusion 0.5–10 μg/kg/min; contraindicated in pregnancy (4,5)[A]
- Clevidipine: Start 1–2 mg/h, double q90sec until near goal, then smaller increases q5–10min. May be a good alternate choice for patients with signs/symptoms of acute heart failure
- Fenoldopam (Corlopam): 0.1 μg/kg/min IV initial dose. Increase by 0.1 μg/kg/min q15min to desired effect. Maximum dose, 1.6 μg/kg/min.
- Hydralazine: Bolus 5–15 mg; used frequently in pregnancy (4,5,7)[A]
- PO clonidine: PO loading dose 0.2 mg followed by 0.1 mg/h until BP has been lowered or a total dose of 0.8 mg has been administered (4,7)[B]
- Trimethaphan (Arfonad): Infusion 0.5–5 mg/min (4)[B]

SURGERY/OTHER PROCEDURES
An arterial catheter may be used to monitor BP; advantage over noninvasive monitoring not clearly proven (7)[C]

COMPLEMENTARY AND ALTERNATIVE MEDICINE
Comfortable environment, which may lower the BP

IN-PATIENT CONSIDERATIONS

Admission Criteria/Initial Stabilization
In general, lower the BP no more than 20% in the 1st hour; then, if stable, lower to 160/100–110 in the next 2–6 hours.
- All patients with true hypertensive emergencies should be hospitalized.
- Associated end-organ effects may require specific treatment (e.g., acute myocardial infarction).

IV Fluids
Fluid restriction may be appropriate for associated pathology, such as pulmonary edema.

Nursing
Bed rest

Discharge Criteria
Patient should be stabilized on PO antihypertensives as appropriate (6)[A].

 ## ONGOING CARE

FOLLOW-UP RECOMMENDATIONS
Close outpatient follow-up with primary care physician is recommended to ensure ongoing control of HTN.

Patient Monitoring
- Follow BP closely to avoid a rapid drop.
- Begin oral therapy as soon as possible after BP control has been achieved with IV medications.
- Ongoing BP control plus monitoring of affected organ system(s) (e.g., renal function) for evidence of continued morbidity

DIET
Low-sodium diet

PATIENT EDUCATION
- Avoid abrupt discontinuation of antihypertensive medicines.
- Stress importance of compliance.
- Emphasize the lack of symptoms with HTN until organ damage occurs.

PROGNOSIS
- BP should return to acceptable levels within 24 hours.
- Long-term prognosis depends on extent of secondary end-organ damage in addition to ongoing BP control.

COMPLICATIONS
- Complications depend on organ system(s) secondarily affected.
- Abrupt or excessive lowering of BP may result in inadequate cerebral or cardiac blood flow, leading to stroke or myocardial ischemia.
- The benefits of aggressive treatment may outweigh the risks in patients with severe HTN but no end-organ damage. No studies prove that aggressive treatment reduces the risk of long-term morbidity or mortality from hypertensive urgencies.

REFERENCES

1. Perez MI, Musini VM. Pharmacological interventions for hypertensive emergencies. *Cochrane Database Syst Rev.* 2008;(1):CD003653. Epub 2008 Jan 23.
2. Peacock WF, Varon J, Baumann BM, et al. CLUE: A randomized comparative effectiveness trial of IV nicardipine versus labetalol use in the emergency department. *Crit Care.* 2011;15(3):R157. Epub 2011 Jun 27.
3. Peacock WF, Hilleman DE, Levy PD, et al. A systematic review of nicardipine vs labetalol for the management of hypertensive crises. *Am J Emerg Med.* 2012;30(6):981–993. Epub 2011 Sep 9.
4. Flanigan JS, Vitberg D. Hypertensive emergency and severe hypertension: What to treat, who to treat, and how to treat. *Med Clin North Am.* 2006;90:439–451.
5. Shayne PH, Pitts SR. Severely increased blood pressure in the emergency department. *Ann Emerg Med.* 2003;41:513–529.
6. Chobanian AV, Bakris GL, Black HR, et al. The Seventh Report of the Joint National Committee on Prevention, Detection, Evaluation, and Treatment of High Blood Pressure: The JNC 7 report. *JAMA.* 2003;289:2560–2572.
7. Management of Hypertension and Hypertensive Emergencies in the Emergency Department: The EMCREG-International Consensus Panel Recommendations. 2008;51(3):S1–S38.
8. Marik PE, Rivera R. Hypertensive emergencies: An update. *Curr Opin Crit Care.* 2011;17(6):569–580.
9. Morgenstern LB. Guidelines for the management of spontaneous intracerebral hemorrhage: A guideline for healthcare professionals from the American Heart Association. *Stroke.* 2010;41:2108–2129.

 ## SEE ALSO

Aortic Dissection; Hypertension, Essential; Pheochromocytoma; Preeclampsia and Eclampsia (Toxemia of Pregnancy)

 ## CODES

ICD10
I10 Essential (primary) hypertension

CLINICAL PEARLS
- Treatment of severe HTN (hypertensive urgency) without evidence of acute end-organ damage is controversial. In this case, treatment is in the emergency department by initiation of oral medication, with close follow-up.
- If severe HTN and evidence of end organ damage, slowly initiated IV treatment with close inpatient monitoring is recommended.
- Avoid rapid prehospital lowering of BP.
- Treatment depends on the organ systems affected.
- Esmolol, nitroprusside, and ACE inhibitors are contraindicated in pregnancy.

HYPERTHYROIDISM

Anup Sabharwal, MD, MBA, FACE, CCD • Atil Y. Kargi, MD

BASICS

Hyperthyroidism or thyrotoxicosis is composed of a spectrum of clinical findings consistent with thyroid hormone excess. The former describes excess from the thyroid gland, whereas the latter can be produced from another source.

DESCRIPTION

- Graves disease (GD): The most common form; diffuse goiter and thyrotoxicosis are common characteristics. Infiltrative orbitopathy is seen in 50% of patients. Infiltrative dermopathy is rare. Autoantibodies are directed at the thyrotropin-stimulating hormone (TSH) receptors.
- Toxic multinodular goiter (TMNG): 2nd most common; a TSH receptor mutation has been found in 60% of patients; patients >40 years, insidious onset, frequent in iodine-deficient areas
- Toxic adenoma: Younger patients, autonomously functioning nodules
- Iodine-induced hyperthyroidism
- Thyroiditis: Transient autoimmune process:
  - Subacute thyroiditis/De Quervain: Granulomatous giant cell thyroiditis, benign course; viral infections have been involved.
  - Postpartum thyroiditis
  - Drug-induced thyroiditis: Amiodarone, interferon-α, interleukin 2, lithium
  - Miscellaneous: Thyrotoxicosis factitia, TSH-secreting pituitary tumors, and functioning trophoblastic tumors
- Subclinical hyperthyroidism: Suppressed TSH with normal thyroxine (T_4); may be associated with osteoporosis and atrial fibrillation (1).
- Thyroid storm: Rare hyperthyroidism; fever, tachycardia, systolic hypertension, CNS dysfunction (e.g., coma); up to 50% mortality

Geriatric Considerations
- Characteristic symptoms and signs may be absent.
- Atrial fibrillation is common when TSH <0.1 mU/L.

Pediatric Considerations
- Neonates and children are treated with antithyroids for 12–24 months.
- Radioactive iodine is controversial in patients <15–18 years.

Pregnancy Considerations
Propylthiouracil (PTU) is currently the drug of choice during pregnancy. Treat with lowest effective dose. Avoid treatment-induced hypothyroidism. Radioiodine therapy is contraindicated.

EPIDEMIOLOGY
- 1.3% of population
- Predominant sex: Female > Male (7–10:1).
- Predominant age: Autoimmune thyroid disease in 2nd and 3rd decades. TMNG presents in patients >40 years. GD is seen between 40 and 60 years of age.

Incidence
- Female 1/1,000
- Male: 1/3,000

ETIOLOGY AND PATHOPHYSIOLOGY
- GD: Autoimmune disease
- TMNG: 60% TSH receptor gene abnormality; 40% unknown
- Toxic adenoma: Point mutation in TSH receptor gene with increased hormone production
- Thyroiditis:
  - Hashitoxicosis: Autoimmune destruction of the thyroid; antimicrosomal antibodies present
  - Subacute/De Quervain thyroiditis: Granulomatous reaction; genetic predisposition in specific HLAs; viruses, such as coxsackievirus, adenovirus, echovirus, and influenza virus, have been implicated; self-limited course, 6–12 months
  - Suppurative: Infectious
  - Drug-induced thyroiditis: Amiodarone produces an autoimmune reaction and a destructive process. Lithium, interferon-α, and interleukin 2 cause an autoimmune thyroiditis.
  - Postpartum thyroiditis: Autoimmune thyroiditis that lasts up to 8 weeks and, in 60% of patients, hypothyroidism manifests in the future.

Genetics
Concordance rate for GD among monozygotic twins is 35%.

RISK FACTORS
- Positive family history, especially in maternal relatives
- Female
- Other autoimmune disorders
- Iodide repletion after iodide deprivation, especially in TMNG

COMMONLY ASSOCIATED CONDITIONS
- Autoimmune diseases
- Down syndrome
- Iodine deficiency

DIAGNOSIS

HISTORY
- Thyrotoxicosis is a hypermetabolic state in which energy production exceeds needs, causing increased heat production, diaphoresis, and even fever.
- Thyrotoxicosis affects several different systems:
  - Constitutional: Fatigue, weakness, increased appetite, weight loss
  - Neuropsychiatric: Agitation, anxiety, emotional lability, psychosis, coma, poor concentration and memory
  - GI: Increased appetite, hyperdefecation
  - Gynecologic: Oligomenorrhea, amenorrhea
  - Cardiovascular: Tachycardia (most common) and chest discomfort that mimics angina

Geriatric Considerations
Apathetic hyperthyroidism in the elderly

PHYSICAL EXAM
- Adults:
  - Skin: Warm, moist, pretibial myxedema (GD only)
  - Head, eye, ear, nose, throat (HEENT): Exophthalmos, lid lag
  - Endocrine: Hyperhidrosis, heat intolerance, goiter, gynecomastia, low libido, and spider angiomata (males)
  - Cardiovascular: Tachycardia, atrial fibrillation, cardiomegaly

  - Musculoskeletal: Skeletal demineralization, osteopenia, osteoporosis, fractures
  - Neurologic: Tremor, proximal muscle weakness, anxiety and lability, brisk deep tendon reflexes
  - Rarely: Thyroid acropathy (clubbing), localized dermopathy
- Children:
  - Linear growth acceleration
  - Ophthalmic abnormalities more common

DIFFERENTIAL DIAGNOSIS
- Anxiety
- Malignancy
- Diabetes mellitus
- Pregnancy
- Menopause
- Pheochromocytoma
- Depression
- Carcinoid syndrome

DIAGNOSTIC TESTS & INTERPRETATION
- 95% have suppressed TSH and elevated free T_4. Total T_4 and triiodothyronine (T_3) represent the bound hormone and can be affected by pregnancy and hepatitis.
- T_3: Elevated, especially in T_3 toxicosis or amiodarone-induced thyrotoxicosis
- T_4: Elevated; TSH autoantibodies rarely needed
- Free thyroxine index (FTI): Calculated from T_4 and thyroid hormone-binding ratio; corrects for misleading results caused by pregnancy and estrogens
- Inappropriately normal or elevated TSH with high T_4 suspicious for pituitary tumor or thyroid hormone resistance
- Drugs may alter lab results: Estrogens, heparin, iodine-containing compounds (including amiodarone and contrast agents), phenytoin, salicylates, steroids (e.g., androgens, corticosteroids)
- Drug precautions: Amiodarone and lithium may induce hyperthyroidism; MMI may cause warfarin resistance
- Other findings that can occur: Anemia, granulocytosis, lymphocytosis, hypercalcemia, transaminase, and alkaline phosphate elevations

Initial Tests (lab, imaging)
- TSH, free T_4, T_4, T_3, TSI
- TSH-receptor (-R) antibodies (Abs): The routine assay is the TSH-binding inhibitor immunoglobulin assay (TBII). TSH-R Abs are useful in the prediction of postpartum Graves thyrotoxicosis and neonatal thyrotoxicosis.
- Thyroxine/Triiodothyronine ratio: The T_4:T_3 ratio may be a useful tool when the iodine uptake testing is not available/contraindicated. ~2% of thyrotoxic patients have "T_3 toxicosis."
- Nuclear medicine scanning (^{123}I or ^{131}I): The reference-range values for 24-hour radioiodine uptake is between 5% and 25%.
- Increased thyroid iodine uptake is seen with TMNG, toxic solitary nodule, and GD.
- GD shows a diffuse uptake and can have a paradoxical finding of high uptake at 4–6 hours, but normal uptake at 24 hours because of the rapid clearance (2).
- TMNG will show a heterogeneous uptake, whereas solitary toxic nodule will show a warm or "hot" nodule.

- In iodine-deficient areas, an increased uptake is associated with low urine iodine levels.
- Hashimoto thyroiditis can have an increased uptake at an early stage, but no increased thyroid hormone production.
- Causes of thyrotoxicosis with low iodine uptake:
  – Acute thyroiditis, thyrotoxicosis factitia, and iodine intoxication with amiodarone or contrast material can cause low-uptake transient thyrotoxicosis. After thyroiditis resolves, the patient can become euthyroid or hypothyroid.
  – Iodine loading can cause iodine trapping and decreased iodine uptake (Wolff-Chaikoff effect).
  – Thyrotoxicosis factitia: Thyroglobulin levels are low in exogenous intake and high in endogenous production.
  – Other extrathyroidal causes include struma ovarii and metastatic thyroid carcinoma.
  – Technetium-99m scintigraphy: Controversial because it has a 33% discordance rate with radioactive iodine scanning.

Follow-Up Tests & Special Considerations
In severe cases, such as thyroid storm, hospitalize until stable, especially if >60 years of age, because of the risk of atrial fibrillation.

Diagnostic Procedures/Other
Neck US will show increased diffuse vascularity in GD.

Test Interpretation
- GD: Hyperplasia
- Toxic nodule: Nodule formation

 ## TREATMENT

- Radioactive iodine therapy (RAIT): Most common definitive treatment used in the US for GD and TMNG (2)[B]
- Pretreatment with antithyroid drugs is preferred to avoid worsening thyrotoxicosis. MMI is preferred over PTU as pretreatment because of decreased relapse, but it is held 3–5 days before therapy.
- There is concern for a slightly higher risk of lymphoma and leukemia in patients treated with RAIT.
- Usually patients become hypothyroid 2–3 months after therapy; therefore, antithyroid medications are continued after ablation.
- Glucocorticoids: Reduce the conversion of active T_4 to the more active T_3. In Graves ophthalmopathy, the use of prednisone before and after RAIT improves outcome.
- After RAIT, the release of antigens can worsen the inflammatory reaction and the ophthalmopathy.
- Smoking in GD patients is a risk factor for ophthalmopathy when treated with RAIT.
- For TMNG, the treatment of choice is RAIT. Medical therapy with antithyroid medications has shown a high recurrence rate. Surgery is considered only in special cases.
- Treatment for subacute thyroiditis is supportive with NSAIDs and β-blockers. Steroids can be used for 2–3 weeks.

- For amiodarone-induced thyrotoxicosis (AIT) type I, the treatment is antithyroid drugs and β-blockers. Potassium perchlorate also can be used as an iodine uptake inhibitor. Thyroidectomy is the last option. AIT type II is self-limited.
- Graves dermopathy: Difficult to treat in the chronic phase. Topical steroids with occlusive dressing may help in acute phase.

MEDICATION
First Line
- Antithyroid drugs: MMI and PTU are thionamides that inhibit iodine oxidation, organification, and iodotyrosine coupling. PTU can block peripheral conversion of T_4 to active T_3. Both can be used as primary treatment for GD and prior to RAIT or surgery (3)[A].
- Duration of treatment: 6 months to 2 years; 50–60% relapse after stopping; treatment beyond 18 months did not show any further benefit. The most serious side effects are hepatitis (0.1–0.2%), vasculitis, and agranulocytosis:
  – MMI: Adults: 10–15 mg q12h; children aged 6–10 years: 0.4 mg/kg/d PO once daily
  – PTU: Adults (preferred in thyroid storm and pregnant and lactating women): 100–150 mg PO q8h, not to exceed 200 mg/d during pregnancy
- β-Adrenergic blocker: Propranolol in high doses (>160 mg/d) inhibits T_3 activation by up to 30%. Atenolol, metoprolol, and nadolol can be used.
- Glucocorticoids: Reduce the conversion of active T_4 to the more active T_3
- Cholestyramine: Anion exchange resin that decreases thyroid hormone reabsorption in the enterohepatic circulation; dose: 20–30 g/d
- Other agents:
  – Lithium: Inhibits thyroid hormone secretion and iodotyrosine coupling; can be dosed at 300 mg q8h, with close monitoring of levels to avoid toxicity
  – Lugol solution: Saturated solution of potassium iodide (SSKI); blocks release of hormone from the gland, but should be administered at least 1 hour after thionamide was given; acts as a substrate for hormone production (Jod-Basedow effect)
  – Potassium perchlorate: Especially for amiodarone-induced thyrotoxicosis
  – RAIT: See "Treatment" section.

Second Line
Ipodate sodium (Oragrafin): 0.5 g PO q.i.d. most effectively prevents conversion of T_4 to T_3 and thyroid hormone release; also useful in thyroid storm

ISSUES FOR REFERRAL
Patients with Graves ophthalmopathy should be referred to an experienced ophthalmologist.

SURGERY/OTHER PROCEDURES
Thyroidectomy for compressive symptoms, masses, and thyroid malignancy may be performed in the 2nd trimester of pregnancy only.

 ## ONGOING CARE

FOLLOW-UP RECOMMENDATIONS
Patient Monitoring
- Repeat thyroid tests once a year, CBC and LFTs on thionamide therapy; continue therapy with thionamides for 12–18 months (3)[B].
- After RAIT, thyroid function tests at 6 weeks, 12 weeks, 6 months, and annually thereafter if euthyroid; TSH may remain undetectable for months if patient is euthyroid; follow T_3 and T_4.

DIET
Sufficient calories to prevent weight loss

PROGNOSIS
Good (with early diagnosis and treatment)

COMPLICATIONS
- Surgery: Hypoparathyroidism, recurrent laryngeal nerve damage, and hypothyroidism
- RAIT: Postablation hypothyroidism
- GD: High relapse rate with antithyroid drug as primary therapy
- Graves ophthalmopathy, worsening heart failure if cardiac condition, atrial fibrillation, muscle wasting, proximal muscle weakness, increased risk of cerebrovascular accident (CVA) and cardiovascular mortality

REFERENCES
1. Cappola AR, Fried LP, Arnold AM, et al. Thyroid status, cardiovascular risk, and mortality in older adults. *JAMA.* 2006;295:1033–1041.
2. Nayak B, Hodak SP. *Hyperthyroidism. Endocrinol Metab Clin North Am.* 2007;36:617–656.
3. Abraham P, Avenell A, Watson WA, et al. A systematic review of drug therapy for Graves' hyperthyroidism. *Cochrane Database Sys Rev.* 2005;153(4):489–498.

 ## CODES

ICD10
- E05.10 Thyrotxcosis w toxic sing thyroid nodule w/o thyrotxc crisis
- E05.90 Thyrotoxicosis, unspecified without thyrotoxic crisis or storm
- E06.1 Subacute thyroiditis

CLINICAL PEARLS
- Not all thyrotoxicoses are secondary to hyperthyroidism.
- GD presents with hyperthyroidism, ophthalmopathy, and goiter.
- Medical treatment for GD has a high relapse rate after stopping medications.
- Thyroid storm is a medical emergency that needs hospitalization and aggressive treatment.

HYPERTRIGLYCERIDEMIA

S. Lindsey Clarke, MD, FAAFP

BASICS

DESCRIPTION

- Hypertriglyceridemia is a common form of dyslipidemia characterized by an excess fasting plasma concentration of triglycerides (TGs):
  - TGs are fatty molecules made of glycerols that are esterified by fatty acids at all 3 hydroxyl groups.
  - They occur naturally in vegetable oils and animal fats.
  - In humans, TGs are major sources of dietary energy; they are packaged into chylomicrons and very low-density lipoproteins.
  - Hypertriglyceridemia is independently associated with cardiovascular disease risk, but the degree to which excess TGs cause atherosclerosis is uncertain and debatable.
- Hypertriglyceridemia is a biomarker of risk for premature coronary artery disease in both men and women at levels ≥200 mg/dL and for pancreatitis at levels ≥1,000 mg/dL.
- Classification of TG levels in adults after a 12-hour fast (1):
  - Normal: <150 mg/dL (1.7 mmol/L)
  - Borderline to high: 150–199 mg/dL
  - High: 200–499 mg/dL
  - Very high: ≥500 mg/dL
  - Divide by 88.5 to convert to millimoles per liter
- TGs are considered high in children who exceed the 95th percentiles for age and sex:
  - 143 mg/dL for adolescent boys, 126 mg/dL for adolescent girls
  - 111 mg/dL for preadolescent boys, 120 mg/dL for preadolescent girls

EPIDEMIOLOGY

- Predominant gender: Male > Female
- Predominant race: Hispanic, white > black

Prevalence

- 33% of US population has TG levels ≥150 mg/dL.
- 1.7% has TG levels ≥500 mg/dL.
- Highest prevalence at age 50–70 years
- The most common genetic syndromes with hypertriglyceridemia are:
  - Familial hypertriglyceridemia (5–10%)
  - Familial combined hyperlipidemia (1–2%)

ETIOLOGY AND PATHOPHYSIOLOGY

- Primary:
  - Familial
  - Acquired (sporadic)
- Secondary:
  - Obesity and overweight
  - Physical inactivity
  - Cigarette smoking
  - Excess alcohol intake
  - Very high-carbohydrate diets (>60% of total caloric intake)
  - Certain medications:
    - α-Interferon
    - Atypical antipsychotics
    - β-Blockers other than carvedilol
    - Bile acid sequestrants
    - Corticosteroids
    - Oral estrogens
    - Protease inhibitors
    - Raloxifene
    - Retinoic acid
    - Tamoxifen
    - Thiazides
  - Medical conditions:
    - Type 2 diabetes mellitus
    - Hypothyroidism
    - Chronic renal failure, nephrotic syndrome
    - Autoimmune disorders (e.g., systemic lupus erythematosus)
    - Paraproteinemias (e.g., macroglobulinemia, myeloma, lymphoma, lymphocytic leukemia)
    - Pregnancy (usually physiologic and transient)

Genetics

- Familial hypertriglyceridemia and familial combined hyperlipidemia: Likely polygenic
- Familial dysbetalipoproteinemia, lipoprotein lipase deficiency, Apo CII deficiency: Autosomal-recessive

RISK FACTORS

- Genetic susceptibility
- Obesity, overweight
- Diabetes
- Alcoholism
- Certain medications (see "Etiology")
- Medical conditions (see "Etiology")

GENERAL PREVENTION

- Weight reduction
- Moderation of dietary fat and carbohydrates
- Regular aerobic exercise

COMMONLY ASSOCIATED CONDITIONS

- Coronary artery disease
- Dyslipidemias:
  - Decreased high-density lipoprotein (HDL) cholesterol
  - Increased low-density lipoprotein (LDL), non-HDL, and total cholesterol
  - Small, dense LDL particles
- Nonalcoholic steatohepatitis (NASH)
- Insulin resistance and type 2 diabetes mellitus
- Metabolic syndrome (3 of following):
  - Abdominal obesity (waist circumference >40 inches in men, >35 inches in women)
  - TGs ≥150 mg/dL
  - Low HDL cholesterol (<40 mg/dL in men, <50 mg/dL in women)
  - BP ≥130/85 mm Hg
  - Fasting glucose ≥100 mg/dL
- Pancreatitis
- Polycystic ovary syndrome

DIAGNOSIS

HISTORY

- Usually asymptomatic
- Patients with chylomicronemia syndrome can have memory loss, headache, vertigo, dyspnea, and paresthesias.
- Pancreatitis: Epigastric pain, nausea, and vomiting
- Assess for other cardiac risk factors.
- Family history of coronary artery disease

PHYSICAL EXAM

- Obesity, overweight (body mass index ≥25 kg/m^2)
- Eruptive cutaneous, tuberous, and striate palmar xanthomas
- Lipemia retinalis
- Epigastric pain, nausea in pancreatitis
- Hepatomegaly in NASH and chylomicronemia

DIFFERENTIAL DIAGNOSIS

Primary and secondary hypertriglyceridemia

DIAGNOSTIC TESTS & INTERPRETATION

Initial Tests (lab, imaging)

- Serum: Turbid with milky supernatant
- Fasting lipid profile (12-hour fast):
  - Routine screening every 5 years beginning at age 35 for men and age 45 for women
  - Start screening at age 20 in men who have other cardiac risk factors.
  - For interpretation, see "Description."
- Secondary causes:
  - Glycosylated hemoglobin, fasting or postprandial glucose for type 2 diabetes mellitus
  - Creatinine, urinary protein measurement for nephrotic syndrome, renal failure
  - Thyroid-stimulating hormone for hypothyroidism
  - Human chorionic gonadotropin for pregnancy
- Atherosclerosis: Cardiac stress imaging, coronary angiography, CT arteriography
- Pancreatitis: CT scan, US of pancreas

Follow-Up Tests & Special Considerations

- Repeat lipid panel after 2 months of therapy.
- High levels of apolipoprotein (apo) B (≥90 mg/dL) are a strong predictor of coronary death in patients whose LDL cannot be calculated because of very high TGs. Measurement of nonfasting apo B can help to identify patients at highest risk of atherosclerosis, such as those with familial combined hyperlipidemia.

Test Interpretation

- Chylomicronemia syndrome: Lipid-laden macrophage (foam cell) infiltration of visceral organs, bone marrow, and skin
- Atherosclerosis
- Pancreatitis

TREATMENT

GENERAL MEASURES
- Therapeutic lifestyle changes, 1st-line interventions for all patients, can reduce TGs by as much as 50% (1)[C]:
  – Dietary modifications can reduce TGs by 20–50% (see "Diet").
  – Moderate-intensity physical activity can reduce TGs by 20–30%.
  – Weight loss of 5–10% can reduce TGs by 20%.
  – Persons with very high TGs should abstain from alcohol.
- Search for correctable secondary causes; treat underlying illness or remove offending drug.
- Improve glycemic control if diabetic.
- Control other cardiac risk factors such as hypertension, diabetes mellitus, and smoking.
- Primary hypertriglyceridemia: Screen other family members.
- According to current guidelines, getting LDL cholesterol to goal takes priority over correction of TGs, unless TGs ≥500 mg/dL (1)[A], [C] for lowering TGs]
- Usually outpatient; see "Admission Criteria."

MEDICATION
First Line
- Statins if TGs <500 mg/dL and LDL is not at goal (10–30% reduction in TGs) (1)[A]: Only statins have been shown to reduce cardiovascular mortality:
  – Atorvastatin (Lipitor): 10–80 mg/d
  – Pravastatin (Pravachol): 10–80 mg/d
  – Rosuvastatin (Crestor): 5–40 mg/d
  – Simvastatin (Zocor): 5–40 mg nightly
  – Adverse reactions: Hepatotoxicity, myalgias, myopathy, rhabdomyolysis (especially with simvastatin >40 mg); contraindicated in pregnancy and lactation
- Fibrates if TGs ≥500 mg/dL or if LDL is already at goal (30–50% reduction in TGs) (1)[C]: Fibrates have been shown in older studies to decrease nonfatal myocardial infarction, but not all-cause mortality (2)[B]:
  – Fenofibrate (Tricor, others): 35–200 mg daily
  – Gemfibrozil (Lopid): 600 mg b.i.d.
  – Adverse reactions: GI upset, hepatotoxicity, cholelithiasis, myalgias, rhabdomyolysis (when combined with a statin), gemfibrozil–warfarin interaction (enhanced anticoagulation)
  – Do not use gemfibrozil in combination with CYP3A4-dependent statins due to high risk of muscle injury. If combination therapy is needed, use fenofibrate or a non–CYP3A4-dependent statin (fluvastatin, pravastatin, or rosuvastatin 5–10 mg).
  – Combination of fibrate and statin does not seem to reduce cardiovascular risk better than statin alone (3)[B].

Second Line
- Niacin (20–50% reduction in TGs with immediate-release [IR] niacin, 10–30% with extended-release [ER] forms) (4)[C]:
  – 1,000–3,000 mg IR daily divided b.i.d.–t.i.d.; 500–2,000 mg ER nightly
  – Pretreatment with aspirin reduces flushing.
  – Adverse reactions: Flushing, pruritus, peptic ulcer disease, hepatotoxicity, fulminant hepatic necrosis (with ER forms), hyperuricemia and gout, hyperglycemia, and toxic amblyopia

- Omega-3 acid ethyl esters (20–50% reduction in TGs) (5,6)[C]:
  – Lovaza: 4 g daily or 2 g b.i.d.
  – USP-verified fish oil, 9–12 capsules daily in divided doses
  – Safe, well-tolerated, but scant outcomes data
  – Must be marine-derived to provide benefit; the content of eicosapentaenoic acid (EPA) and docosahexaenoic acid (DHA) in nonprescription omega-3 dietary supplements varies widely.

ISSUES FOR REFERRAL
- Hypertriglyceridemia refractory to treatment
- Familial hypertriglyceridemia syndromes

IN-PATIENT CONSIDERATIONS
Admission Criteria/Initial Stabilization
- Acute pancreatitis
- Acute coronary syndrome
- In medical emergencies such as hypertriglyceridemic pancreatitis with TG levels >1,000 mg/dL, TGs can be lowered rapidly and safely by apheresis.

Discharge Criteria
Stabilization of acute complicating illness

ONGOING CARE

FOLLOW-UP RECOMMENDATIONS
2 months after initiation or modification of therapy (repeat fasting lipid profile)

Patient Monitoring
- Fasting lipid profile q6–12mo
- Maintain TGs <1,000 mg/dL to reduce risk of acute pancreatitis (possibly effective, unproven).
- Hepatic transaminases
- Creatine phosphokinase if patient has myalgias

DIET
- Restrict dietary fat to 30% of total caloric intake; restrict further to 15% of caloric intake if TGs ≥1,000 mg/dL (1)[C].
- Limit carbohydrates (especially simple carbohydrates and sugars) to 60% of total caloric intake.
- Mediterranean-style diet reduces TGs 10–15% more than a low-fat diet.
- Increase marine-derived omega-3 polyunsaturated fatty acids (4 g/d reduces TGs by 25–30%, dose-response relationship).
- Eliminate trans-fatty acids.
- Increase dietary fiber.
- Avoid concentrated sugars such as fructose.
- Moderate alcohol intake (<1 oz/d or complete abstinence if TGs are very high)

PATIENT EDUCATION
Smoking cessation

PROGNOSIS
- Good with correction of triglyceride levels
- Patients with primary hypertriglyceridemia usually require lifelong treatment.

COMPLICATIONS
- Atherosclerosis
- Chylomicronemia syndrome
- Pancreatitis

REFERENCES

1. Miller M, Stone NJ, Ballantyne C, et al. Triglycerides and cardiovascular disease: A scientific statement from the American Heart Association. *Circulation*. 2011;123:2292–2333.
2. Abourbih S, Filion KB, Joseph L, et al. Effect of fibrates on lipid profiles and cardiovascular outcomes: A systematic review. *Am J Med*. 2009;122(10):962.e1–8.
3. ACCORD study group. Effects of combination lipid therapy in type 2 diabetes mellitus. *N Engl J Med*. 2010;362:1563–1574.
4. Wi J, Kim JY, Park S, et al. Optimal pharmacologic approach to patients with hypertriglyceridemia and low high-density lipoprotein-cholesterol: Randomized comparison of fenofibrate 160 mg and niacin 1500 mg. *Atherosclerosis*. 2010;213: 235–240.
5. Bays HE, McKenney J, Maki KC, et al. Effects of prescription omega-3-acid ethyl esters on non–high-density lipoprotein cholesterol when coadministered with escalating doses of atorvastatin. *Mayo Clin Proc*. 2010;85:122–128.
6. Hartweg J, Perera R, Montori V, et al. Omega-3 polyunsaturated fatty acids (PUFA) for type 2 diabetes mellitus. *Cochrane Database Syst Rev*. 2008;CD003205.

ADDITIONAL READING
- Berglund L, Brunzell JD, Goldberg AC, et al. Evaluation and treatment of hypertriglyceridemia: an Endocrine Society clinical practice guideline. *J Clin Endocrinol Metab*. 2012;97:2969–2989.
- PL Detail-Document, Strategies for lowering triglycerides. *Pharmacist's Letter /Prescriber's Letter*. June 2011.

SEE ALSO
- Atherosclerosis; Hypercholesterolemia; Pancreatitis
- Algorithm: Hypertriglyceridemia

CODES

ICD10
E78.1 Pure hyperglyceridemia

CLINICAL PEARLS
- Hypertriglyceridemia is a risk factor for coronary artery disease at levels ≥200 mg/dL and for pancreatitis at levels ≥1,000 mg/dL.
- Diet and exercise are first-line interventions for all patients who have hypertriglyceridemia.
- In patients with TG levels <500 mg/dL, the primary goal in cholesterol management is control of LDL, typically with statins.
- For patients with TG levels ≥500 mg/dL, the greatest amount of TG lowering is achieved with fibrates, although magnitude of clinical benefit is uncertain.

H

HYPERTROPHIC CARDIOMYOPATHY

Arka Chatterjee, MD • Nirmanmoh Bhatia, MD • Ihab Hamzeh, MD, FACC

BASICS

DESCRIPTION
- Hypertrophic cardiomyopathy (HCM) is a form of primary myocardial hypertrophy, with or without presence of left ventricular outflow tract (LVOT) obstruction; it is characterized by 4 cardinal features:
  - Idiopathic LV hypertrophy (LVH) in absence of other cardiac or systemic disease causing hypertrophy of such magnitude
  - Cardiac myocyte and myofibrillar disarray
  - Familial occurrence
  - Associated sudden cardiac death
- System(s) affected: Cardiovascular
- Synonym(s): Hypertrophic obstructive cardiomyopathy (HOCM); Muscular subaortic stenosis (MSS), Idiopathic Hypertrophic Subaortic Stenosis (IHSS)

EPIDEMIOLOGY
- The disorder may present at any age.
- It is seen in equal frequency in both sexes, although it is often underrecognized in females and African Americans.
- Apical HCM is a variant seen more often in China and Japan (Yamaguchi apical variant).

Incidence
~1% of patients with HCM die annually, but this is no different from the overall population.

Prevalence
- Prevalence of phenotypically expressed HCM in the adult general population is 1:500 (0.2%).
- ~600,000 people are affected with HCM in the US.
- HCM is the most common genetic cardiovascular disease.

ETIOLOGY AND PATHOPHYSIOLOGY
- LV hypertrophy:
  - ≥1 regions of LV wall are thickened: Classically at the basal anterior septum, but may involve posterior septum or LV free wall and apex
  - Hypertrophy develops usually in adolescence, with an average 100% increase in LV mass.
- Systolic anterior motion (SAM) of the mitral valve:
  - Mitral valve abnormalities are primary manifestations of HCM: 1 or both leaflets may be elongated.
  - SAM is the abrupt motion of the MV leaflet toward the septum, which creates dynamic LVOT obstruction on contact with the septum.
  - Caused by drag effect of the high-velocity jet caused by ejection through a narrowed LVOT and/or a Venturi phenomenon.
- Disorganized myocardial architecture:
  - Myocytes and myofilaments are laid down in disorganized pattern, with increased matrix components causing myocyte disarray.
  - Microvascular disease leads to ischemia and replacement fibrosis.
- Diastolic dysfunction:
  - Result of reduced ventricular compliance; contributes predominantly to the symptoms of heart failure, such as dyspnea

Genetics
- Inherited as a mendelian autosomal dominant trait with >50% penetrance and variable expressivity.
- 11 sarcomeric gene mutations are known, including, among others, β-myosin heavy chain, myosin-binding protein C, and troponin I and T.

RISK FACTORS
Risk factors for sudden cardiac death (SCD) in patients with IHSS include (1):
- A prior history of cardiac arrest or spontaneous sustained ventricular tachycardia (VT)
- Family history of premature SCD (especially in close relative or multiple)
- Unexplained syncope
- Extreme LVH measuring >30 mm
- Hypotensive response to exercise
- Nonsustained VT during Holter monitoring
- Other factors that may indicate increased risk are LVOT obstruction (resting gradient >30 mm Hg), LV apical aneurysm, high-risk mutation, delayed enhancement on cardiac MRI, intense physical exertion.

GENERAL PREVENTION
- Avoid strenuous exercise (particularly involving burst exertion) and heavy lifting (induces Valsalva maneuver).
- Maintain hydration to avoid volume depletion.
- Avoid alcohol.
- Certain drugs, such as nitrates, digoxin, β-agonists, vasodilators, and diuretics, are best avoided, particularly in presence of increased LVOT gradient.
- Implantable cardioverter defibrillator (ICD) is recommended for patients at high risk for sudden cardiac death (1,2)[C].

DIAGNOSIS

HISTORY
- Symptoms of heart failure: Dyspnea, paroxysmal nocturnal dyspnea, fatigue
- Angina pectoris
- Palpitations
- Exertional syncope or presyncope
- Symptoms may be worsened by anemia, hot and humid weather, a large meal, alcohol, or fever.
- Clinical symptoms correlate poorly with the severity of LVOT obstruction.
- 50% of these patients have positive family history for HCM (and 50% are sporadic).

PHYSICAL EXAM
- A systolic crescendo/decrescendo murmur from LVOT obstruction is best heard at left lower sternal border.
- Intensity of murmur is dynamic and changes with maneuvers that affect the degree of obstruction.
- Maneuvers that decrease venous return (e.g., Valsalva, standing position, amyl nitrite) increase intensity of the murmur.
- Maneuvers that increase LV afterload (e.g., handgrip) will soften the murmur.
- Bisferiens pulse
- Double or triple apical impulse
- Prominent S_4
- Holosystolic murmur of mitral regurgitation may be heard at the apex.

DIFFERENTIAL DIAGNOSIS
- Valvular aortic stenosis
- Hypertensive heart disease, especially in elderly
- Athlete's heart: Differentiated by normal/enlarged LV cavity, regression of LVH on deconditioning
- Cardiac amyloidosis
- Noonan syndrome, mitochondrial myopathy, and metabolic storage disorders (e.g., Anderson Fabry disease and Friedrich ataxia)

DIAGNOSTIC TESTS & INTERPRETATION
- ECG: Common findings (50–90%):
  - Nonspecific ST-T wave abnormalities
  - LVH
- ECG: Less common findings (<50%):
  - Prominent and abnormal Q waves in anterior precordial and lateral limbs lead
  - Left atrial enlargement
  - Diffuse, marked, symmetric giant negative T waves in lateral precordial leads seen in patients with apical HCM
- Holter findings may include supraventricular tachycardia (SVT), ventricular premature contractions (PVC), nonsustained ventricular tachycardia (VT), and atrial fibrillation
- Chest x-ray may show cardiomegaly and left atrial enlargement.
- Echocardiogram helps establish the diagnosis most easily and reliably. Typical echo findings:
  - Asymmetric septal hypertrophy with septal-to-free-wall ratio >1.3:1 classically
  - LV hypertrophy (especially LV wall thickness in diastole >15 mm)
  - Small LV chamber
  - In patients with apical IHSS, LV cavity looks like a spade.
  - Abnormal systolic anterior motion of mitral valve leaflet
  - Continuous-wave Doppler best measures significant dynamic outflow obstruction.
  - Evidence of diastolic dysfunction
  - Provocative measures, such as inhalation of amyl nitrate/ Valsalva/ dobutamine/ exercise, may be necessary to elicit significant LVOT gradients during echocardiography.
- 24-/48-hour Holter monitoring is recommended (2).
- Stress testing may be used to assess BP response with exercise (2).
- Cardiac MR is useful if echo images are suboptimal or LV segmental hypertrophy is seen in an unusual location; delayed gadolinium enhancement is increasingly being considered an independent risk factor for mortality (2,3); mitral valve morphology can be better defined and may have a novel role in assessment.

TREATMENT

- These patients must be counseled against competitive athletics, irrespective of LVOT obstruction, presence of ICD, previous septal reduction therapy, and associated symptoms (2).
- Adequate hydration should be maintained.
- Not a high-risk condition for endocarditis prophylaxis
- Genetic counseling may be appropriate.
- Only symptomatic patients will benefit from drug therapy.

MEDICATION
First Line
- β-blockers:
  - First-line drugs for patients with provocable gradient
  - Indicated for treatment of symptoms (angina/dyspnea) in adults with HCM (obstructive or nonobstructive) (2)
  - 1/3–2/3 of patients experience symptomatic improvement.
- Disopyramide:
  - Used as an adjunct with β-blockers or calcium channel blockers only, as it may accelerate AV conduction (2,4)[B]
- Verapamil:
  - Treatment of those who do not tolerate/respond to β-blockers
  - Caution in patients with high gradients/advanced heart failure, given the systemic vasodilatory effects (2)
- Dihydropyridine calcium channel blockers are potentially harmful in HCM patients with resting or provocable obstruction (2)[C].

Second Line
- Atrial fibrillation is common and should be controlled.
- Maintenance of sinus rhythm should be aggressively pursued because of association of atrial fibrillation (AF) with heart failure symptoms and embolic phenomena (5)[C].
- Amiodarone is most effective for sinus rhythm maintenance in IHSS-associated atrial fibrillation, disopyramide with concomitant β-blockers or verapamil is an alternative option.

ADDITIONAL THERAPIES
Pregnant patients with HCM:
- Patients who wish to become pregnant should be counseled prenatally regarding its autosomal dominant inheritance.
- In women with HCM who are asymptomatic or whose symptoms are controlled on β-blockers (2)[C]:
  - Pregnancy is reasonable.
  - β-Blockers should be continued, but increased fetal surveillance is warranted for bradycardia or related complications.
  - Expert maternal/fetal medical specialist care, including cardiovascular and prenatal monitoring, is recommended.
- Women with gradient >50 mm Hg or with uncontrolled symptoms have increased risk with pregnancy and referral to high-risk obstetrician is indicated.

- Pregnancy with HCM and advanced heart failure is associated with excess morbidity/mortality.
- Should be monitored closely in a tertiary care center during labor, as peripheral vasodilatation, fluid shift, and epidural analgesia pose a theoretical risk in presence of LVOT obstruction
- Spinal analgesia is contraindicated. Careful administration of epidural analgesia is controversial.

SURGERY/OTHER PROCEDURES
- Ventricular septal myotomy-myectomy (Morrow procedure):
  - The gold standard for drug-refractory symptomatic patients with obstructive IHSS (2,6)[B], and for relief of obstruction with outflow gradient >50 mm Hg at rest/with provocation
  - 5–10 g of tissue is removed from the proximal septum.
  - Most (about 70%) patients achieve subjective improvement in symptoms lasting ≥5 years following their surgery.
  - Postoperative complications may include left bundle branch block (LBBB), ventricular septal defect (VSD), and aortic regurgitation.
- Percutaneous alcohol septal ablation:
  - Controlled alcohol-induced septal myocardial infarction resulting in an akinetic septal segment with instantaneous obliteration of the outflow obstruction and gradient
  - Preferred in patients at high risk from septal myectomy, those who refuse surgical therapy, and those who have failed surgical myectomy
  - Better outcomes reported in patients >65 years, septal diameter <18 mm, and gradient <100 mm Hg (7)
- Implantable cardiac defibrillators for prevention of SCD in patient at high risk (1)[C]
- Ablation of refractory ventricular arrhythmia can be considered; combined endocardial and epicardial approach may be required (8)
- Heart transplant is advocated: For HCM patients not amenable to other treatment modalities (2)[B] and children with refractory symptoms due to restrictive physiology not responding to conventional treatment (2)[C]

 ONGOING CARE

FOLLOW-UP RECOMMENDATIONS
- Annual follow-up is recommended for stable patients.
- Among the 1st-degree relatives, screening with ECG and echo is recommended q12–24mo between ages 12 and 21 and every 5 years in adults, particularly if adverse IHSS-related events have occurred in the family.

PATIENT EDUCATION
Patients with characteristic phenotype of HCM (LVH) are excluded from all competitive sports except those with low static and dynamic intensity (e.g., golf) (2)[C].

PROGNOSIS
Annual mortality of 1% is no different from the general US population. Although HCM may be associated with important symptoms and premature SCD, these patients have no or relatively mild disability and normal life expectancy.

COMPLICATIONS
- Sudden death (1% per year), usually due to ventricular arrhythmia
- Atrial fibrillation
- Infective mitral endocarditis
- Progressive heart failure

REFERENCES
1. Maron BJ. Contemporary insights and strategies for risk stratification and prevention of sudden death in hypertrophic cardiomyopathy. *Circulation*. 2010;121:445–456.
2. Gersh BJ, Maron BJ, Bonow RO, et al. 2011 ACCF/AHA guideline for the diagnosis and treatment of hypertrophic cardiomyopathy: A report of the American College of Cardiology Foundation/American Heart Association Task Force on Practice Guidelines. *Circulation*. 2011;124(24):e783–831. Epub 2011 Nov 8.
3. Green JJ, Berger JS, Kramer CM, et al. Prognostic value of late gadolinium enhancement in clinical outcomes for hypertrophic cardiomyopathy. *JACC Cardiovasc Imaging*. 2012;5:370–377.
4. Sherrid MV, Barac I, McKenna WJ, et al. Multicenter study of the efficacy and safety of disopyramide in obstructive hypertrophic cardiomyopathy. *J Am Coll Cardiol*. 2005;45:1251–1258.
5. Maron BJ, Olivotto I, Bellone P, et al. Clinical profile of stroke in 900 patients with hypertrophic cardiomyopathy. *J Am Coll Cardiol*. 2002;39:301–307.
6. Maron BJ. Hypertrophic cardiomyopathy: A systematic review. *JAMA*. 2002;287:1308–1320.
7. Sorajja P, Binder J, Nishimura RA, et al. Predictors of an optimal clinical outcome with alcohol septal ablation for obstructive hypertrophic cardiomyopathy. *Catheter Cardiovasc Interv*. 2013;81(1):E58–67.
8. Dukkipati SR, d'Avila A, Soejima K, et al. Long-term outcomes of combined epicardial and endocardial ablation of monomorphic ventricular tachycardia related to hypertrophic cardiomyopathy. *Circ Arrhythm Electrophysiol*. 2011;4(2):185–194.

CODES

ICD10
- I42.1 Obstructive hypertrophic cardiomyopathy
- I42.2 Other hypertrophic cardiomyopathy

CLINICAL PEARLS
- HCM should be considered in all patients with a history of unexplained SCD. It is the most common cause of SCD in young athletes in the US.
- Delayed de novo onset of LVH may occur in midlife.
- Intense competitive sports, strenuous exercise, and heavy lifting should be restricted because of high risk of SCD.

H

HYPOGLYCEMIA, DIABETIC

Joseph A. Florence, MD • Emily K. Flores, PharmD, BCPS

 BASICS

DESCRIPTION
- Abnormally low concentration of glucose in circulating blood of a patient with diabetes; often referred to as an *insulin reaction*
- Classification includes:
  - Severe hypoglycemia: An event requiring assistance of another person to actively administer treatment
  - Documented symptomatic hypoglycemia: An event during which typical symptoms are accompanied by a measured plasma glucose of <70 mg/dL (3.9 mmol/L)
  - Asymptomatic hypoglycemia: An event not accompanied by symptoms, but a measured glucose of <70 mg/dL (3.9 mmol/L)
  - Probable symptomatic hypoglycemia: Event with symptoms, but glucose not tested
  - Relative hypoglycemia: An event with typical symptoms, but glucose ≥70 mg/dL (3.9 mmol/L)
- Hypoglycemia is the leading limiting factor in the glycemic management of type 1 and type 2 diabetes. Severe or frequent hypoglycemia requires modification of treatment regimens, including higher treatment goals.

ALERT
Hypoglycemic unawareness:
- Major risk factor for severe hypoglycemic reactions
- Most commonly found in patients with long-standing type 1 diabetes and children age <7 years

EPIDEMIOLOGY
Incidence
- From the Accord Study, the annual incidence of hypoglycemia was:
  - 3.14% in the intensive treatment group
  - 1.03% in the standard group
  - Increased risk among women, African Americans, those with less than a high school education, aged participants, and those who used insulin at trial entry
- From the RECAP-DM study: Hypoglycemia was reported in 38% of patients with type 2 diabetes who added a sulphonylurea or thiazolinedione to metformin therapy during the past year.

ETIOLOGY AND PATHOPHYSIOLOGY
- Loss of hormonal counter-regulatory mechanism in glucose metabolism
- Diet: Too little food (skipping meal), decreased carbohydrate intake
- Medication: Too much insulin or oral hypoglycemic agent (improper dose or timing)
- Erratic absorption of insulin or oral hypoglycemics
- Adverse reaction from other medications
- Exercise/physical activity: Unplanned or excessive
- Alcohol consumption
- Vomiting or diarrhea
- Gastroparesis

RISK FACTORS
- Nearly 3/4 of severe hypoglycemic episodes occur during sleep
- Autonomic neuropathy
- Illness, stress, and unplanned life events

- Duration of diabetes >5 years, advanced age, renal/liver disease, congestive heart failure (CHF), hypothyroidism, hypoadrenalism, gastroenteritis, gastroparesis (unpredictable CHO delivery)
- Starvation or prolonged fasting
- Alcoholism: Evening consumption of alcohol is associated with an increased risk of nocturnal and fasting hypoglycemia, especially in patients with type 1 diabetes.
- Current smokers with type 1 diabetes
- Oral hypoglycemics with long duration and high potency have greater hypoglycemic risks.
- Insulin secretagogues: Sulfonylureas (glipizide, glibenclamide, glibornuride, gliclazide, chlorpropamide, glimepiride) and glinide derivatives (repaglinide, Nateglinide) stimulate insulin secretion and can cause hypoglycemia. Hypoglycemia is rare in diabetics not treated with insulin or insulin secretagogues.
- Severe hypoglycemia is associated with comorbid conditions in patients age ≥65 years and in users of a long-acting sulphonylurea.
- Intensive insulin therapy (further lowering A1C from 7% to 6%) is associated with higher rate of hypoglycemia.
- Gastroparesis causing unpredictable carbohydrate delivery predisposes to hypoglycemia.

GENERAL PREVENTION
- Maintain routine schedule of diet, medication, and exercise.
- Stabilize daily carbohydrate intake.
- Regular blood glucose testing, if taking insulin or insulin secretagogue:
  - ≥3× daily testing if multiple injections of insulin, insulin pump therapy, or pregnant diabetic; frequency and timing dictated by needs and treatment goals
  - Particularly helpful for asymptomatic hypoglycemia
- Diabetes treatment and teaching programs (DTTPs) especially for high-risk type 1 patients, which teach flexible insulin therapy to enable dietary freedom
- Use of rapid-acting and long-acting insulin analogs is associated with less hypoglycemia (1)[C].
- Hypoglycemia rates are reduced by up to 70% using continuous SC insulin infusion pumps compared with multiple daily injections (1)[C].
- Continuous glucose monitoring may supplement self-glucose monitoring and is especially useful with hypoglycemic unawareness and/or frequent hypoglycemic episodes (1)[C].
- If pre-exercise glucose is <100 mg/dL and taking insulin or secretagogue, then carbohydrate consumption or reduction in medication may prevent hypoglycemia (1)[C].

COMMONLY ASSOCIATED CONDITIONS
- Autonomic dysfunction
- Neuropathies
- Cardiomyopathies
- Older type 2 diabetics with severe hypoglycemia have a higher risk of dementia (2).

 DIAGNOSIS

HISTORY
- Ask at-risk patients at each encounter about symptomatic and asymptomatic hypoglycemia (1)[C].
- Symptoms vary considerably between individuals.

- Adrenergic hypoglycemia symptoms:
  - Hunger, trembling, pallor
  - Sweating, shaking, pounding heart, anxiety
- Neuroglycopenic hypoglycemia symptoms:
  - Dizziness, poor concentration, drowsiness, weakness, confusion, lightheadedness, slurred speech, blurred vision, double vision, unsteadiness, poor coordination
- Behavioral hypoglycemia symptoms:
  - Tearfulness, confusion, fatigue, irritability, aggressiveness

- If low cognition and/or declining cognition is found in the diabetic, hypoglycemia should be considered as a possible cause (1)[B].

PHYSICAL EXAM
- General: Confusion, lethargy
- HEENT: Diplopia
- Coronary: Tachycardia
- Neurologic: Tremulousness, weakness, paresthesias, stupor, seizure, or coma
- Mental status: Irritability, inability to concentrate, or short-term memory loss
- Skin: Pale, diaphoresis
- End-organ damage: Microvascular, macrovascular, ophthalmologic, neurologic, renal

DIFFERENTIAL DIAGNOSIS
- Hypoglycemia may be seen in chronic alcoholics and binge drinkers.
- GI dysfunction causing postprandial hypoglycemia or alimentary reactive hypoglycemia
- Hormonal deficiency states (hormonal reactive hypoglycemia)
- Hypoglycemia of sepsis
- Islet cell tumors
- Factitious hypoglycemia from surreptitious injection of insulin
- Hypoglycemia may be found in early pregnancy, prolonged fasting, long periods of strenuous exercise, heart failure, malignancy, and renal or liver disease.

DIAGNOSTIC TESTS & INTERPRETATION
- Plasma, serum or whole-blood glucose <70 mg/dL
- Self-monitoring blood glucose and continuous glucose monitoring are especially useful for asymptomatic hypoglycemia
- A hypoglycemic reading from a continuous glucose monitoring sensor should be verified by fingerstick glucose testing prior to treatment.
- Suspect hypoglycemic unawareness in type 1 diabetics with low/normal HgbA1c.
- Chronic hypoglycemia is indicated by low HgbA1c level.
- Disorders that may alter lab results:
  - Conditions that affect erythrocyte turnover, such as hemolysis or blood loss, and hemoglobin variants may alter HbgA1c (1)[B].

 TREATMENT

GENERAL MEASURES
- Glucose: Preferred; any form of carbohydrate that contains glucose should be effective (1)[C].
  - Any sugar-containing food or beverage that can be rapidly absorbed: Juice or nondiet soda (4–5 oz) or candy (5–6 pieces of hard candy)

- Glucagon: People in close contact with people with diabetes should be instructed in using an emergency glucagon kit (1)[C].
- Glucagon should be prescribed to patients at significant risk of severe hypoglycemia (1)[C].
- If a patient using an α-glucosidase inhibitor, such as acarbose or Precose, experiences hypoglycemia, the patient should eat something containing monosaccharides, such as glucose tablets. Since α-glucosidase inhibitors prevent the digestion of complex carbohydrates, starchy foods will not effectively reverse a hypoglycemic episode in a patient taking it (1)[C].
- Patients with severe hypoglycemia combined with hypoglycemic unawareness should have glycemic targets raised to avoid hypoglycemia (1)[A].
- Continuous glucose monitoring can supplement self-glucose monitoring in those with hypoglycemia unawareness and/or frequent hypoglycemic episodes (1)[C].
- Insulin analogs should be used to reduce the risk of hypoglycemia in most type 1 patients (1)[A].

MEDICATION
- Conscious patients:
  - Glucose (15–20 g) is the preferred treatment, although any form of carbohydrate that contains glucose may be used (1)[C]:
    ○ Takes ~15 minutes for carbohydrates to be digested and enter bloodstream as glucose.
    ○ Blood glucose value may correct prior to symptoms resolving.
    ○ "Rule of 15": 15–20 g glucose (~60–80 calories simple carbohydrate) repeated q15min until blood sugar is ≥70 mg/dL
  - Once sugar has normalized, a meal or snack should be consumed to prevent recurrence of hypoglycemia (1)[C].
- Loss of consciousness at home (1)[C]:
  - Administer glucagon
  - IM or SC in the deltoid or anterior thigh:
    ○ Age <5 years: 0.25–0.50 mg
    ○ Age 5–10 years: 0.50–1 mg
    ○ Age >10 years: 1 mg
- In unconscious, if emergency medical personnel are present or patient hospitalized (1)[C]:
  - Give 1/2 ampule 50% dextrose every 5–10 minutes until patient awakens.
  - Then, feed orally and/or administer 5% dextrose IV at level that will maintain blood glucose >100 mg/dL.
  - Patients with hypoglycemia secondary to oral hypoglycemics should be monitored for 24–48 hours, because hypoglycemia may recur after apparent clinical recovery.
- Significant possible interactions:
  - Overtreatment may cause hyperglycemia (Somogyi effect/phenomenon).
  - Clearance of certain oral hypoglycemics from plasma may be prolonged in persons with renal or liver disease.

ISSUES FOR REFERRAL
- Frequent, recurring, or episodes that do not readily respond to treatment
- Consultant pharmacists in long-term care facilities

ADDITIONAL THERAPIES
Use of a continuous glucose monitoring system in the management of severe hypoglycemia decreases the number of hypoglycemic values (3)[B].

IN-PATIENT CONSIDERATIONS
Admission Criteria/Initial Stabilization
- Any doubt of cause
- Expectation of prolonged hypoglycemia (e.g., caused by sulfonylurea drug)
- Inability of patient to drink
- Treatment has not resulted in prompt recovery of sensorium
- Seizures, coma, or altered behavior (e.g., ataxia, disorientation, unstable motor coordination, dysphasia) secondary to documented or suspected hypoglycemia
- For critically ill hospitalized diabetic patients, an IV insulin protocol has demonstrated efficacy and safety in achieving desired glucose range without increasing risk for severe hypoglycemia (1)[C].

Discharge Criteria
Patient has normoglycemia and risk of severe hypoglycemia is negligible.

 ## ONGOING CARE

FOLLOW-UP RECOMMENDATIONS
Rest until glucose is normal

Patient Monitoring
Self-monitoring of blood glucose

DIET
- If alcohol consumed, combine with food to reduce risk of hypoglycemia (1)[C].
- Protein does not slow absorption of carbohydrates.
- Fats may slow absorption of carbohydrates and may retard and then prolong the acute glycemic response (4)[B].

PATIENT EDUCATION
- Always have access to quick-acting carbohydrate.
- For planned exercise, consider a reduced insulin dosage; additional carbohydrates are needed for unplanned exercise.
- For patients with hypoglycemia unawareness or ≥1 episodes of severe hypoglycemia, glycemic targets should be raised to avoid further hypoglycemia for at least several weeks.
- Educate patients and their relatives, close friends, teachers, and supervisors to be aware of diabetes diagnosis and signs/symptoms of hypoglycemia and treatment.
- Teach self-monitoring of blood glucose and self-adjustment for insulin therapy, diet control, and exercise regimen.
- Wear medical alert identification bracelet or necklace.
- The annual Diabetes Forecast Consumer Guide has a description and list of commercially available products for treating lows: http://forecast.diabetes.org/magazine/resource-guide/products-treating-low-blood-glucose

PROGNOSIS
Full recovery usually depends on rapidity of diagnosis and treatment.

COMPLICATIONS
- Coma, seizure, myocardial infarction (MI), stroke (especially in elderly)
- Prolonged or severe hypoglycemia may cause permanent neurologic damage and/or cognitive impairment.
- Children with type 1 diabetes have a greater vulnerability to neurologic manifestations of hypoglycemia.

ALERT
The ACCORD trial (adults with type 2 diabetes) demonstrated that intensively lowering blood glucose below current recommendations increased the risk of death vs. standard treatment strategy (5)[B].

REFERENCES
1. American Diabetes Association. Standards of medical care in diabetes–2013. *Diabetes Care.* 2013;36(Suppl 1):S11–S66.
2. Whitmer RA, Karter AJ, Yaffe K, et al. Hypoglycemic episodes and risk of dementia in older patients with type 2 diabetes mellitus. *JAMA.* 2009;301:1565–1572.
3. Alvarez Guisasola F, Tofé Povedano S, Krishnarajah G, et al. Hypoglycaemic symptoms, treatment satisfaction, adherence and their associations with glycaemic goal in patients with type 2 diabetes mellitus: Findings from the Real-Life Effectiveness and Care Patterns of Diabetes Management (RECAP-DM) Study. *Diabetes Obes Metab.* 2008;10(Suppl 1):25–32.
4. Franz MJ, Powers MA, Leontos C, et al. The evidence for medical nutrition therapy for type 1 and type 2 diabetes in adults. *J Am Diet Assoc.* 2010;110:1852–1889.
5. Action to Control Cardiovascular Risk in Diabetes Study Group, Gerstein HC, Miller ME, et al. Effects of intensive glucose lowering in type 2 diabetes. *N Engl J Med.* 2008;358:2545–2559.

ADDITIONAL READING
Ryan EA, Germsheid J. Use of continuous glucose monitoring system in the management of severe hypoglycemia. *Diabetes Technol Ther.* 2009;11:635–639.

 ## SEE ALSO
- Diabetes Mellitus, Type 1
- Algorithm: Hypoglycemia

 ## CODES

ICD10
- E10.649 Type 1 diabetes mellitus with hypoglycemia without coma
- E11.649 Type 2 diabetes mellitus with hypoglycemia without coma
- E13.649 Oth diabetes mellitus with hypoglycemia without coma

CLINICAL PEARLS
- Hypoglycemia unawareness is most common with tightly controlled, long-standing type 1 diabetes and children age <7 years.
- Any form of carbohydrate that contains glucose should be effective, such as sugar-containing food or beverage that can be rapidly absorbed:
  - 4–5 oz juice or nondiet soda; 5–6 pieces of hard candy; OTC glucose tablets, liquids, gels, or bits
- Diabetics who use insulin or secretagogues should be educated on how to recognize and manage hypoglycemia.

HYPOGLYCEMIA, NONDIABETIC

Matthew Silva, PharmD, RPh, BCPS • Pablo I. Hernandez Itriago, MD

BASICS

DESCRIPTION
- Hypoglycemia defined by Whipple triad:
  - Low plasma glucose level (≤60 mg/dL)
  - Hypoglycemic symptoms that are relieved when glucose level is corrected
  - Occurs commonly in patients with diabetes receiving sulfonylurea or insulins; less commonly in patients without diabetes
- Reactive hypoglycemia:
  - Occurs in response to a meal, drugs, herbal substances, or nutrients
  - May occur 2–3 hours postprandially or later
  - Symptoms generally observed with serum glucose ≤60 mg/dL, lower in patients with hypoglycemic unawareness
  - Also seen after GI surgery (in association with dumping syndrome in some patients)
- Spontaneous (fasting) hypoglycemia:
  - May be associated with a primary condition, including hypopituitarism, Addison disease, myxedema, or in disorders related to hepatic dysfunction or renal failure
  - If hypoglycemia presents as a primary disorder, consider hyperinsulinism and extrapancreatic tumors

EPIDEMIOLOGY
Incidence
- True incidence is unknown.
- 8.6% of hospitalized inpatients ≥65 years:
  - Asymptomatic in 25% of cases

Prevalence
True prevalence is unknown:
- Predominant age: Older adult
- Predominant sex: Female > Male

ETIOLOGY AND PATHOPHYSIOLOGY
- Reactive, postprandial:
  - Alimentary hyperinsulinism
  - Meals high in refined carbohydrate
  - Certain nutrients, including fructose, galactose, leucine
  - Glucose intolerance (prediabetes)
  - GI surgery
  - Idiopathic (unknown cause)
- Spontaneous:
  - Fasting
  - Alcohol or prescription medication (insulin, sulfonylureas, thiazolidinediones, incretin-mimetics, DPP-IV inhibitors, β-blockers, salicylates, quinine, hydroxychloroquine, fluoroquinones, doxycycline, sertraline, disopyramide, pentamidine)
  - Nonprescription over-the-counter (OTC) agents, including performance-enhancing agents. Adulterated versions of phosphodiesterase inhibitors and performance-enhancing agents are routinely imported and may contain sulfonylureas and other hypoglycemic agents.
  - Consider medication errors as a source of unexplained hypoglycemia even in patients without diabetes.
  - Surreptitious drug use (self-injection of insulin or ingestion of oral hypoglycemic medications in patients with diabetes)
  - Natural medicines or herbs (bitter melon, caffeine, cassia cinnamon, chromium, fenugreek, ginseng, guarana, mate, Stevia, vanadium)

- Postsurgical (e.g., gastrectomy, Roux-en-Y) hypoglycemia/dumping syndrome
- Islet cell hyperplasia or tumor (insulinoma)
- Extrapancreatic insulin secreting tumor
- Hepatic disease
- Glucagon deficiency
- Adrenal insufficiency
- Catecholamine deficiency
- Hypopituitarism
- Hypothyroidism
- Eating disorders
- Exercise
- Fever
- Pregnancy
- Renal glycosuria
- Large tumors
- Ketotic hypoglycemia of childhood
- Enzyme deficiencies or defects
- Severe malnutrition
- Sepsis
- Total parenteral nutrition therapy
- Hemodialysis

Genetics
Some aspects may involve genetics (e.g., hereditary fructose intolerance).

RISK FACTORS
Refer to "Etiology and Pathophysiology."

GENERAL PREVENTION
- Follow dietary and exercise guidelines
- Patient recognition of early symptoms and knowledge of corrective action

Pediatric Considerations
- Usually divided into 2 syndromes:
  - Transient neonatal hypoglycemia
  - Hypoglycemia of infancy and childhood
- Screening infants for hypoglycemia is appropriate when pregnancy was complicated by maternal diabetes.
- Cases of hypoglycemia observed in children taking propranolol for infantile hemangioma
- Associated with indomethacin when treating patent ductus arteriosus

Geriatric Considerations
- More likely to have underlying disorders or be caused by medications
- Iatrogenic hypoglycemia is common in the hospitalized elderly with renal insufficiency.

COMMONLY ASSOCIATED CONDITIONS
- Severe liver disease; alcoholism
- Addison disease; adrenocortical insufficiency
- Myxedema
- Malnutrition (patients with renal failure)
- GI surgery
- Panhypopituitarism
- Insulinoma

DIAGNOSIS

HISTORY
- CNS (neuroglycopenic) symptoms predominate with gradual glucose reduction:
  - Headache
  - Confusion
  - Lightheadedness
  - Fatigue and weakness
  - Visual disturbances
  - Changes in personality
- Adrenergic symptoms: More prominent in acute drop in glucose:
  - Anxiety
  - Tremulousness
  - Dizziness
  - Diaphoresis
  - Warmth/Flushing
  - Heart palpitations
- GI symptoms:
  - Hunger
  - Nausea
  - Belching

PHYSICAL EXAM
- CNS (neuroglycopenic) symptoms predominate with gradual glucose reduction:
  - Convulsions
  - Coma
  - Hypotension
- Adrenergic symptoms: More prominent in acute drop in glucose:
  - Tremulousness
  - Diaphoresis
  - Warmth/Flushing
  - Heart palpitations

DIFFERENTIAL DIAGNOSIS
CNS disorders:
- Psychogenic
- Pseudohypoglycemia: Symptoms of hypoglycemia or self-diagnosis in patients in whom low blood glucose may not be detectable and who may be impossible to convince that they do not suffer from hypoglycemia after all tests are found to be normal

DIAGNOSTIC TESTS & INTERPRETATION
Initial Tests (lab, imaging)
- Blood glucose ≤45 mg/dL (≤2.5 mmol/L) when symptomatic followed by symptom resolution with feeding (1,2)[C]:
- Plasma glucose overnight fasting: ≤60 mg/dL (≤3.33 mmol/L); confirm on ≥2 occasions (2)[C]
- Plasma glucose 72-hour fasting: ≤45 mg/dL (≤2.5 mmol/L) for females; ≤55 mg/dL (≤3.05 mmol/L) for males; fast may be ended when Whipple triad is achieved or hypoglycemia is demonstrated (2)[C].
- Abdominal CT to rule out abdominal tumor

Follow-Up Tests & Special Considerations
- Oral glucose tolerance: ≤50 mg/dL (≤2.78 mmol/L) (1,2,[C])
- Misinterpretation of glucose tolerance tests may lead to misdiagnosis of hypoglycemia; ≥1/3 of normal patients have hypoglycemia, with or without symptoms, during the 4-hour glucose tolerance test. These patients may be at future risk for type 2 diabetes.
- C-peptide measurement (2)[C]
- Check liver studies, serum insulin, adrenocorticotrophic hormone (ACTH), and cortisol. Serum insulin should be suppressed when glucose is <60 mg/dL (2)[C].
- Serum β-hydroxybutyrate
- Insulin radioimmunoassay: Elevated insulin levels suggest islet cell hyperplasia or tumor (2)[C].
- Drugs that may alter lab results: Many drugs can affect glucose levels; refer to drug or laboratory reference (2)[C].

Diagnostic Procedures/Other
- For definitive diagnosis, patient should have (2)[C]:
  - Documented low glucose levels
  - Symptoms when glucose levels are low
  - Evidence that symptoms are relieved specifically by ingestion of sugar or other food
  - Identification of the specific type of hypoglycemia
- Serum β-hydroxybutyrate <2.7 mg/dL in the presence of high serum insulin, C-peptide, and low serum glucose suggests excessive insulin production.

 TREATMENT

GENERAL MEASURES
- Outpatient except for severe cases; may also be inpatient for testing
- Oral carbohydrate for alert patient without drug overdose (2–3 tbsp of sugar in glass of water or fruit juice, 1–2 cups of milk, piece of fruit, or several soda crackers) (1)[C]
- If unable to swallow: Use glucagon IM or SC (1)[C]
- If caused by medication or nutrients: Avoid or control causative agents (1)[C]
- If triggered by meals: Try high-protein diet with carbohydrate restriction (1)[C]
- Nonhypoglycemic hypoglycemia or pseudohypoglycemia:
  - Many patients (often women aged 20–45) present with diagnosis of reactive hypoglycemia (self-diagnosed or misinterpretation of tests)
  - Symptoms may pertain to chronic fatigue and somatic complaints (stress often plays a role in these symptoms)
  - Management difficult; listening is important. Try 120-g carbohydrate diet (1)[C]
  - Counseling may be useful for stress and other problems.

MEDICATION
- Once diagnosis is established, begin therapy appropriate to underlying disorder.
- If unable to swallow: Glucagon 1 mg (1 unit) IM or SC. If no response, give IV bolus of 25–50 g of 50% glucose solution followed by continuous infusion until patient able to take by mouth (1)[C].
- Postsurgical gastrectomy patients unresponsive to dietary changes may benefit from propantheline, psyllium, fiber, or oat bran, which delays gastric emptying (1)[C].
- Insulinoma

SURGERY/OTHER PROCEDURES
If islet cell tumor (insulinoma) or other insulin-secreting tumor, surgery is treatment of choice; if inoperable, diazoxide may relieve symptoms.

IN-PATIENT CONSIDERATIONS
Admission Criteria/Initial Stabilization
Hypoglycemia unresponsive to oral intake

 ONGOING CARE

FOLLOW-UP RECOMMENDATIONS
- Exercise routine or daily activity may need to be re-evaluated.
- Patients with recurrent hypoglycemia should have glucose source at hand for immediate ingestion during symptoms.

Patient Monitoring
- Depends on type and severity of symptoms and treatment of underlying cause
- Hypoglycemia from sulfonylureas can last for hours to days depending on half-life and renal function.

DIET
- High protein, high fiber, complex carbohydrates from multigrain and whole foods in moderation
- Frequent small feedings (6 daily)
- Avoid fasting.

PATIENT EDUCATION
- Dietary instruction
- Counseling for stress, if appropriate
- Recognition of early symptoms of hypoglycemia and how to take corrective action

PROGNOSIS
- Favorable, with appropriate treatment

COMPLICATIONS
- Insulinoma: If tumor identified and removed, some surgical risk is involved.
- Organic brain syndrome: May occur with extensive, prolonged hypoglycemia

REFERENCES
1. Bharmal SV, Moyes V, Ahmed S, et al. Hypoglycaemia: Possible mediation by chromium salt medication. *Hormones (Athens)*. 2010;9: 181–183.
2. Cansu DU, Korkmaz C. Hypoglycaemia induced by hydroxychloroquine in a non-diabetic patient treated for RA. *Rheumatology (Oxford)*. 2008;47: 378–379.

ADDITIONAL READING
- Carroll MF, Burge MR, Schade DS. Severe hypoglycemia in adults. *Rev Endocr Meta Dis*. 2003;4:149–157.
- Chan TY. Outbreaks of severe hypoglycaemia due to illegal sexual enhancement products containing undeclared glibenclamide. *Pharmacoepidemiol Drug Saf*. 2009;18:1250–1251.
- Chaubey SK, Sangla KS, Suthaharan EN, et al. Severe hypoglycaemia associated with ingesting counterfeit medication. *Med J Aust*. 2010;192:716–717.
- Lawrence KR, Adra M, Keir C. Hypoglycemia-induced anoxic brain injury possibly associated with levofloxacin. *J Infect*. 2006;52:e177–e180.
- Murad MH, Coto-Yglesias F, Wang AT, et al. Clinical review: Drug-induced hypoglycemia: A systematic review. *J Clin Endocrinol Metab*. 2009;94:741–745.
- Pollak PT, Mukherjee SD, Fraser AD. Sertraline-induced hypoglycemia. *Ann Pharmacother*. 2001;35:1371–1374.
- Singh M, Jacob JJ, Kapoor R, et al. Fatal hypoglycemia with levofloxacin use in an elderly patient in the post-operative period. *Langenbecks Arch Surg*. 2008;393:235–238.
- Yamada C, Nagashima K, Takahashi A, et al. Gatifloxacin acutely stimulates insulin secretion and chronically suppresses insulin biosynthesis. *Eur J Pharmacol*. 2006;553:67–72.

 SEE ALSO

- Hypoglycemia, Diabetic; Insulinoma
- Algorithm: Hypoglycemia

 CODES

ICD10
- E16.1 Other hypoglycemia
- E16.2 Hypoglycemia, unspecified
- P70.4 Other neonatal hypoglycemia

CLINICAL PEARLS
- Symptoms coincide with low blood glucose levels.
- Symptoms resolve with PO/IV glucose or glucagon.
- Avoid known agents/nutrients that trigger hypoglycemia.
- Treat underlying cause.

HYPOKALEMIA

Ruben Peralta, MD, FACS

 BASICS

DESCRIPTION
Hypokalemia is defined as a serum potassium concentration <3.5 mEq/L (normal range, 3.5–5 mEq/L).
- Mild hypokalemia (serum potassium 3–3.5 mEq/L)
- Moderate hypokalemia (serum potassium 2.5–3 mEq/L).
- Severe hypokalemia (serum potassium <2.5 mEq/L).

EPIDEMIOLOGY
Predominant sex: Male = Female

Incidence
- Electrolyte abnormality is commonly encountered in clinical practice (1).
- Found in >20% of hospitalized patients (when defined as potassium <3.6 mEq/L).
- Higher incidence (5–20%) in individuals with eating disorders
- >10% of inpatients with alcoholism
- Higher incidence in patients with AIDS
- Higher incidence in patients receiving diuretics
- Associated risk after bariatric surgery

ETIOLOGY AND PATHOPHYSIOLOGY
Most common causes:
- Decreased intake: Deficient diet in alcoholics and elderly; anorexia nervosa
- GI loss: Vomiting, diarrhea, nasogastric tubes, laxative abuse, fistulas, villous adenoma, ureterosigmoidostomy, malabsorption, chemotherapy, radiation enteropathy, bulimia
- Intracellular shift of potassium: Metabolic alkalosis, insulin excess, β-adrenergic catecholamine excess (acute stress, B_2 agonists) (2), hypokalemic periodic paralysis, intoxications (theophylline, caffeine, barium, toluene)
- Renal potassium loss:
  - Drugs: Diuretics (especially loop and thiazides), amphotericin B, aminoglycosides (3,4)
  - Mineralocorticoid-excess states: Primary hyperaldosteronism; secondary hyperaldosteronism (congestive heart failure [CHF], cirrhosis, nephrotic syndrome, malignant hypertension, renin-producing tumors); renovascular hypertension; Bartter syndrome; Gitelman syndrome; congenital adrenogenital syndromes; exogenous mineralocorticoids (glycyrrhizic acid in licorice, carbenoxolone, steroids in nasal sprays); Liddle syndrome; vasculitis
- Glucocorticoid-excess states: Cushing syndrome, exogenous steroids, ectopic adrenocorticotrophic hormone (ACTH) production, II B hydroxysteroid dehydrogenase deficiency.
- Renal tubular acidosis (type I and II):
  - Leukemia
  - Magnesium depletion
  - Thyrotoxic hypokalemic paralysis
- Osmotic diuresis (e.g., poorly controlled diabetes)
- Refeeding syndrome

Genetics
Some rare, familial disorders cause hypokalemia:
- Familial hypokalemic periodic paralysis: Hypokalemia after a high-carbohydrate or high-sodium meal or after exercise
- Congenital adrenogenital syndromes
- Liddle syndrome: Increases K+ secretion
- Familial interstitial nephritis

GENERAL PREVENTION
When initiating a diuretic, especially loop and thiazide diuretics, advice patients to increase their dietary potassium intake (see "Diet").

COMMONLY ASSOCIATED CONDITIONS
Acute GI illnesses with severe vomiting or diarrhea increased the risk of cardiac arrhythmias; atrial fibrillation (5).

 DIAGNOSIS

- Patients with hypokalemia often have no symptoms, especially if the hypokalemia is mild (serum potassium 3–3.5 mEq/L).
- Neuromuscular (most prominent manifestations):
  - Skeletal muscle weakness (proximal > distal muscles, lower limbs > upper limbs) may range from mild weakness to total paralysis, including respiratory muscles; it may lead to rhabdomyolysis and/or respiratory arrest in severe cases.
  - Smooth-muscle involvement may lead to GI hypomotility, producing ileus and constipation
- Cardiovascular:
  - Ventricular arrhythmias; higher risk if underlying CHF, left ventricular failure (LVF), cardiac ischemia
  - Increased risk of atrial fibrillation (5)[B]
  - Hypotension
  - Cardiac arrest
- Renal: Polyuria, polydipsia, nocturia owing to impaired ability to concentrate, myoglobinuria
- Metabolic: Hyperglycemia

HISTORY
Muscle weakness, hypotension, vomiting, diarrhea, polyuria, polydipsia, dyspnea on exertion

PHYSICAL EXAM
Skin turgor, hypotension, orthostasis, pulmonary congestion/rales, peripheral edema

DIFFERENTIAL DIAGNOSIS
- Spurious hypokalemia: Occurs when blood with high WBC count (>100,000/mm^3) is allowed to stand at room temperature (WBCs extract potassium from plasma).
- Thyrotoxicosis

DIAGNOSTIC TESTS & INTERPRETATION
- Serum potassium <3.5 mEq/L (<3.5 mmol/L)
- Disorders that may alter lab results: Leukemia and other conditions with high WBCs

Initial Tests (lab, imaging)
- If source of potassium loss not likely to be medications or GI tract: Serum electrolytes, urinary potassium, ECG
- Calculate plasma anion gap normal (anion gap = Na − [Cl + HCO$_3$]); normal values, 12 ± 4 mEq/L. Must correct calculated anion gap for hypoalbuminemia. Increase calculated anion gap by 2.5 mEq/L for each 1 g/dL decrease in albumin <4 g/dL.
- CT scan of adrenal glands if there is evidence of mineralocorticoid excess

Follow-Up Tests & Special Considerations
- Excessive renal potassium loss: Urinary potassium is >20 mEq/d in the presence of hypokalemia: In patients with excessive renal potassium loss and hypertension, plasma renin and aldosterone levels should be determined to differentiate adrenal from nonadrenal causes of hyperaldosteronism.
- If hypertension is absent and the patient is acidotic, renal tubular acidosis should be considered.
- If hypertension is absent and serum pH is normal to alkalotic, high urine chloride (>10 mEq/d [>10 mmol/d]) suggests hypokalemia secondary to diuretics or Bartter syndrome; low urine chloride (<10 mEq/d [<10 mmol/d]) suggests vomiting as a probable cause.
- ECG:
  - Hypokalemia increases the myocyte resting potential, which increases the refractory period; this can lead to arrhythmias.
  - Flattening or inversion of T waves
  - Increased prominence of U waves (small, positive deflection after T wave, best seen in V$_2$ and V$_3$)
  - Depression of ST segment
  - Ventricular ectopia

Test Interpretation
In severe hypokalemia, necrosis of cardiac and skeletal muscle

TREATMENT

GENERAL MEASURES
- For asymptomatic patients treated with oral replacement, outpatient follow up is sufficient.
- Patients with cardiac manifestations require IV replacement with cardiac monitoring in an intensive care setting.

MEDICATION
- Nonemergent conditions (serum potassium >2.5 mEq/L [>2.5 mmol/L], no cardiac manifestations):
  - Oral therapy preferred: 40–120 mEq/d (40–120 mmol/d) in divided doses usually is adequate.
  - IV potassium should be given only when oral administration is not feasible (e.g., vomiting, postoperative state). Rate should not exceed 10 mEq/h, and concentration should not exceed 40 mEq/L. Up to 40 mEq in 100 mL over 1 hour can be given safely through a central venous line. The patient's cardiac rhythm should be closely monitored.
  - Potassium chloride is suitable for all forms of hypokalemia.
  - Other potassium salts may be indicated if a coexisting disorder is present: Potassium bicarbonate or bicarbonate precursor (gluconate, acetate, or citrate) in metabolic acidosis or phosphate in phosphate deficiency
- Emergent situations (serum potassium <2.5 mEq/L [<2.5 mmol/L], arrhythmias), IV replacement: Rate of administration should not exceed 20 mEq/h (20 mmol/h); maximum recommended concentration, 60 mEq/L (60 mmol/L) of saline for peripheral administration. Administration through central venous lines may allow for greater concentrations.
- Check serum magnesium and replace, if needed; cannot adequately replace potassium in a setting of low magnesium.
- Precautions:
  - Any form of potassium replacement carries the risk of hyperkalemia.
  - Serum potassium should be checked more frequently in groups at higher risk: The elderly, diabetic patients, and patients with renal insufficiency
  - Patients receiving digitalis and patients with diabetic ketoacidosis in whom intracellular shift in potassium is expected after insulin therapy is initiated must have more aggressive replacement.
- Significant possible interactions: Concomitant administration of potassium-sparing diuretics (spironolactone, triamterene, amiloride, ACE inhibitors) magnifies risk of hyperkalemia.

Geriatric Considerations
May need to correct magnesium depletion

 ONGOING CARE

FOLLOW-UP RECOMMENDATIONS
Patient Monitoring
- Patients receiving IV therapy should have cardiac monitoring and serum potassium level checked frequently (q4–6h).
- Patients requiring potassium supplements should have serum potassium studied at intervals dictated by clinical judgment and patient compliance.

DIET
In patients with mild hypokalemia (potassium, 3–3.5 mEq/L [3–3.5 mmol/L]) not caused by GI losses, dietary supplementation may be sufficient; potassium-rich foods include oranges, bananas, cantaloupes, prunes, raisins, dried beans, dried apricots, and squash.

PATIENT EDUCATION
- Instructions for appropriate diet
- If potassium supplementation is necessary, stress the need for compliance.

PROGNOSIS
- Associated with higher morbidity and mortality because of cardiac arrhythmias
- Ease of correction of hypokalemia and need for prolonged treatment rest on the primary cause; if it can be eliminated (e.g., resolution of diarrhea, discontinuation of diuretics, removal of adrenal tumor), hypokalemia can be expected to resolve and no further treatment is indicated.

COMPLICATIONS
- Hyperkalemia can occur during the course of treatment (1).
- Increased risk of digoxin toxicity
- Increased risk of atrial fibrillation (5)[B]

REFERENCES

1. Crop MJ, Hoorn EJ, Lindemans J, et al. Hypokalaemia and subsequent hyperkalaemia in hospitalized patients. *Nephrol Dial Transplant.* 2007;22:3471–3477.
2. Tran CT, Kjeldsen K. Protection against β adrenoceptor agonist reduction of plasma potassium in severe but not in moderate hypokalemia. *Fundam Clin Pharmacol.* 2011;25:452–461.
3. Ben Salem C, Hmouda H, Bouraoui K. Drug-induced hypokalaemia. *Curr Drug Saf.* 2009;4:55–61.
4. Ernst ME, Moser M. Use of diuretics in patients with hypertension. *N Engl J Med.* 2009;361:2153–2164.
5. Kritjthe BP, Heeringa J, Kors JA, et al. Serum potassium levels and the risk of atrial fibrillation: The Rotterdam study. *Int J Cardiol.* 2013;S0167-5273(13):01598-2.
6. Unwin RJ, Luft FC, Shirley DG, et al. Pathophysiology and management of hypokalemia: A clinical perspective. *Nat Rev Nephrol.* 2011;7:75–84.

ADDITIONAL READING

- Arsenault KA, Yusuf AM, Crystal E, et al. Interventions for preventing post-operative atrial fibrillation in patients undergoing heart surgery. *Cochrane Database Syst Rev.* 2013;1:CO003611.
- Asmar A, Mohandas R, Wingo CS. A physiologic-based approach to the treatment of a patient with hypokalemia. *Am J Kidney Dis.* 2012;60:492–497.
- Chan KE, Lazarus JM, Hakim RM. Digoxin associates with mortality in ESRD. *J Am Soc Nephrol.* 2010;21:1550–1559.
- Facchini M, Sala L, Malfatto G, et al. Low-K+ dependent QT prolongation and risk for ventricular arrhythmia in anorexia nervosa. *Int J Cardiol.* 2006;106:170–176.
- Jones E. Hypokalemia. *N Engl J Med.* 2004;350:1156.
- Osadchii OE. Mechanisms of hypokalemia-induced ventricular arrhythmogenicity. *Fundam Clin Pharmacol.* 2010;24:547–559.
- Palmer BF. A physiologic-based approach to the evaluation of a patient with hypokalemia. *Am J Kidney Dis.* 2010;56:1184–1190.
- Zietse R, Zoutendijk R, Hoorn EJ. Fluid, electrolyte and acid-base disorders associated with antibiotic therapy. *Nat Rev Nephrol.* 2009;5:193–202.

 SEE ALSO

- Hyperkalemia
- Algorithm: Hypokalemia

 CODES

ICD10
E87.6 Hypokalemia

CLINICAL PEARLS

- In patients without heart disease, a low potassium level will rarely cause cardiac disturbances. In an otherwise healthy patient, gentle repletion using oral potassium or an increase in potassium-rich foods should be adequate.
- In patients with cardiac ischemia, heart failure, or left ventricular hypertrophy, even mild to moderate hypokalemia can cause arrhythmias. These patients should receive potassium repletion as well as cardiac monitoring.
- To safely prevent hypokalemia in diabetic and renal insufficiency patients, ensure adequate dietary potassium intake with foods rich in potassium, including spinach, tomatoes, broccoli, squash, potatoes, bananas, cantaloupe, and oranges. Avoid potassium-sparing diuretics, if possible.
- Uncorrected hypomagnesemia can hinder the correction of hypokalemia. Check magnesium levels and replete as necessary (6).

H

HYPONATREMIA

Ruben Peralta, MD, FACS

BASICS

DESCRIPTION
- Hyponatremia is a plasma sodium concentration of <135 mEq/L. Hyponatremia itself does not provide information about the "total body water" state of the patient. Patients with hyponatremia may be fluid overloaded, hypovolemic, or euvolemic.
- System(s) affected: Endocrine/Metabolic

EPIDEMIOLOGY
Incidence
- Most common electrolyte disorder seen in the general hospital population (1)
- Predominant age: All ages
- Predominant sex: Male = Female

Prevalence
2.5% of hospitalized patients (1)

Geriatric Considerations
The elderly have lower total body water, a decreased thirst mechanism, and decreased urinary concentrating ability; their kidneys are less responsive to antidiuretic hormone (ADH), and they show decreased renal mass, renal blood flow, and glomerular filtration rate, making them at higher risk for hyponatremia.

ETIOLOGY AND PATHOPHYSIOLOGY
- Hypovolemic hyponatremia: Decrease in total body water and greater decrease in total body sodium; decreased extracellular fluid volume; orthostatic hypotension and other changes consistent with hypovolemia are present.
- Euvolemic hyponatremia: Increase in total body water with normal total body sodium; extracellular fluid volume is minimally to moderately increased but with no edema.
- Hypervolemic hyponatremia: Increase in total body sodium and greater increase in total body water; extracellular fluid increased markedly; edema is present.
- Redistributive hyponatremia: Shift of water from intracellular compartment to extracellular compartment with resulting dilution of sodium; total body water and total body sodium unchanged; occurs with hyperglycemia
- Pseudohyponatremia: Dilution of aqueous phase by excessive proteins, glucose, or lipids; total body water and total body sodium unchanged; occurs in hypertriglyceridemia or multiple myeloma
- Low sodium creates an osmotic gradient between plasma and cells and fluid shifts into cells, causing edema and increased intracranial pressure.
- Hypovolemic hyponatremia: Extrarenal loss of sodium (<30 mmol/L in urine):
  - GI loss: Vomiting, diarrhea
  - 3rd spacing: Peritonitis, pancreatitis, burns, rhabdomyolysis
  - Skin loss: Burns, sweating, cystic fibrosis
  - Heat-related illnesses

- Hypovolemic hyponatremia: Renal loss of sodium (>30 mmol/L in urine):
  - Cerebral salt wasting syndrome
  - Adrenal pathology (e.g., Addison disease, hemorrhage, tuberculosis)
  - Diuretics
  - Osmotic diuresis
- Euvolemic hyponatremia (>30 mmol/L in urine):
  - Hypothyroidism
  - Hypopituitarism or other cause of glucocorticoid deficiency
  - Medications (e.g., carbamazepine, clofibrate, cyclosporine, levetiracetam, opiates, oxcarbazepine, phenothiazines, citalopram, tricyclic antidepressants, thiazide diuretics, vincristine) (2).
  - Primary polydipsia
  - Syndrome of inappropriate antidiuretic hormone secretion (SIADH)
  - Iatrogenic (e.g., excess hypotonic IV fluids)
- Hypervolemic hyponatremia (<30 mmol/L in urine, except chronic renal failure):
  - Nephrotic syndrome
  - Cirrhosis
  - Congestive heart failure (CHF)
  - Chronic renal failure
- Redistributive hyponatremia:
  - Hyperglycemia
  - Mannitol infusion
  - Hypertriglyceridemia
- Multiple myeloma

Genetics
- Polymorphisms have been demonstrated.
- Mutations have been associated with nephrogenic syndrome of inappropriate antidiuresis (NSIAD, SIADH).

GENERAL PREVENTION
Depends on underlying condition

COMMONLY ASSOCIATED CONDITIONS
- Hypothyroidism
- Hypopituitarism
- Adrenocortical hormone deficiency
- HIV patients
- SIADH is associated with cancers, pneumonia, tuberculosis, encephalitis, meningitis, head trauma, cerebrovascular accident, HIV infection (3).
- Acute neurological patients, brain injury
- Marathon runners in hot environments

DIAGNOSIS

- Symptoms related to the rate of fall in serum sodium and the degree of hyponatremia (3)
- Mild (130–135 mEq/L): Usually asymptomatic
- Moderate (120–130 mEq/L): Nausea, vomiting, malaise
- Severe: (115–120 mEq/L): Headache, lethargy, restlessness, disorientation

- Severe/Rapid decreases can cause seizure, coma, and respiratory arrest and may be fatal.
- Other signs and symptoms: Weakness, muscle cramps, anorexia, hiccups, depressed deep tendon reflexes, hypothermia, positive Babinski responses, cranial nerve palsies, orthostatic hypotension

PHYSICAL EXAM
- Volume status: Skin turgor, jugular venous pressure, heart rate, orthostatic BP
- Exam for underlying illness: Signs of CHF, cirrhosis, hypothyroidism

DIFFERENTIAL DIAGNOSIS
See "Etiology and Pathophysiology."

DIAGNOSTIC TESTS & INTERPRETATION
Initial Tests (lab, imaging)
- Comprehensive metabolic profile (BUN, creatinine (Cr), glucose, electrolytes, liver function studies, etc.)
- Thyroid-stimulating hormone (TSH)
- Lipid panel
- Serum osmolality
- Urine sodium and osmolality
- CT scan of head if pituitary problem suspected or if SIADH from CNS problem suspected
- Chest x-ray to rule out pulmonary pathology if SIADH diagnosed

Follow-Up Tests & Special Considerations
- Serum sodium <135 mmol/L
- Plasma osmolality
- Urine sodium and osmolality
- Hypovolemic hyponatremia:
  - Plasma osmolality low
  - BUN:Cr ratio >20:1
  - If urine sodium >20 mEq/L (>20 mmol/L): Renal loss
  - If urine sodium <10 mEq/L (<10 mmol/L): Extrarenal loss
  - Serum potassium >5 mEq/L (>5 mmol/L): Consider mineralocorticoid deficiency.
- Euvolemic hyponatremia:
  - Plasma osmolality low
  - BUN:Cr ratio <20:1
  - Urine sodium >20 mEq/L (>20 mmol/L)
  - TSH test to rule out hypothyroidism
  - 1-hour cosyntropin-stimulation test to rule out adrenal insufficiency
- Hypervolemic hyponatremia:
  - Plasma osmolality low
  - Urine sodium <10 mEq/L (<10 mmol/L) in nephrotic syndrome, CHF, cirrhosis
  - Urine sodium >20 mEq/L (>20 mmol/L) in acute and chronic renal failure
- Redistributive hyponatremia:
  - Plasma osmolality normal or high
  - Glucose or mannitol levels elevated
- Pseudohyponatremia:
  - Plasma osmolality normal
  - Triglyceride, glucose, or protein levels elevated

TREATMENT

GENERAL MEASURES
- Assess all medications patient is taking.
- Institute seizure precautions.

MEDICATION

ALERT
Rapid correction of severe symptomatic hyponatremia has been associated with central pontine myelinolysis, a neurologic disorder in which loss of myelin and supportive structures in pons and occasionally in other areas of the brain occurs. This results in irreversible injury. Symptoms are apparent 2–6 days after injury and include seizure, coma, spastic paraparesis, dysarthria, and dysphagia.

- Treatment tailored to clinical situation: The degree of hyponatremia, how rapidly the hyponatremia developed, and whether the patient is symptomatic influence the urgency of correction. Some general principles apply (3)[B]:
  - Formula to determine correction available at www.mdcalc.com/sodium-correction-rate-inhyponatremia and www.medcalc.com/sodium.html
- Asymptomatic, euvolemic patients can be treated with fluid restriction; the underlying cause also must be addressed.
- For severely hyponatremic/symptomatic patients, it is generally considered safe to increase the serum sodium by 0.6–2 mEq/L each hour, not to exceed 8 mEq/24 h.
- For mild to moderate hyponatremia use isotonic saline solution (0.9%). For moderate to severe hyponatremia consider specialist consultation for use of hypertonic saline (3%) via central line access at a rate of 1–2 mL/kg body weight/h; increasing serum sodium levels by 0.5 mmol/L/h and monitoring frequently the plasma sodium level (~q2h).
- In patients with severe hyponatremia (euvolemic and hypervolemic state) who do not respond to the above-mentioned approach, consider the use of newly FDA-approved aquaretics (vaptans), such as tolvaptan, an oral vasopressin V_2-receptor antagonist, or conivaptan for IV treatment of moderate to severe euvolemic and hypervolemic hyponatremia (4)[A].
- Treat underlying condition: Heart failure, cirrhosis, etc.
- Chronic hyponatremia resulting from SIADH: Demeclocycline (inhibits ADH action at the collecting duct) if fluid restriction alone is not effective:
  - Contraindication: Can cause nephrotoxicity in patients with liver disease
  - In doses of 600–1,200 mg/d, the drug produces a nephrogenic diabetes insipidus.
  - Significant possible interactions: Oral anticoagulants, oral contraceptives, penicillin

ALERT
Caution: If severe, consider hypertonic saline (3% sodium chloride) with central line access; exercise extreme caution and monitor serum sodium as frequently as q1–2h.

IN-PATIENT CONSIDERATIONS
Admission Criteria/Initial Stabilization
- Admission is mandatory if the patient has acute hyponatremia or is symptomatic; acute hyponatremia (developing over <48 hours) carries the risk of cerebral edema.
- Admission is advised if patient is asymptomatic and has a serum sodium <125 mEq/dL.

ONGOING CARE

DIET
- Euvolemic hyponatremia: Restrict water to 1 L/d.
- Hypervolemic hyponatremia: Water and sodium restriction

PROGNOSIS
- In hospitalized patients, hyponatremia is associated with an elevated risk of adverse clinical outcomes and higher mortality (5).
- Recently, in community-dwelling, middle-aged, and elderly adults, mild hyponatremia has been shown to be an independent predictor of death.
- Associated with poor prognosis in patients with acute pulmonary embolism
- Associated with poor prognosis in patients with liver cirrhosis and those waiting for liver transplant; it is associated with significant postop risk and short-term graft loss (5).

COMPLICATIONS
- Occult tumor may present with SIADH.
- Hypervolemia if saline used
- Osmotic demyelination (central pontine and extrapontine irreversible myelinolysis) (6).
- Hyponatremia is the cause in 30% new-onset seizures in intensive care settings.
- Chronic hyponatremia is associated with increased odds of osteoporosis.

REFERENCES

1. Upadhyay A, Jaber BL, Madias NE. Epidemiology of hyponatremia. *Semin Nephrol*. 2009;29:227–238.
2. Meulendijks D, Mannesse CK, Jansen PA, et al. Antipsychotic-induced hyponatraemia: A systematic review of the published evidence. *Drug Saf*. 2010;33:101–114.
3. Ellison DH, Berl T. Clinical practice. The syndrome of inappropriate antidiuresis. *N Engl J Med*. 2007;356:2064–2072.
4. Rozen-Zvi B, Yahav D, Gheorghiade M, et al. Vasopressin receptor antagonists for the treatment of hyponatremia: Systematic review and meta-analysis. *Am J Kidney Dis*. 2010;56:325–337.
5. Cárdenas A, Ginès P. Predicting mortality in cirrhosis—serum sodium helps. *N Engl J Med*. 2008;359:1060–1062.
6. Esposito P, Piotti G, Bianzina S, et al. The syndrome of inappropriate antidiuresis: Pathophysiology, clinical management and new therapeutic options. *Nephron Clin Pract*. 2011;119:c62–c73.

ADDITIONAL READING

- Abraham WT, Hensen J, Gross PA, et al. Lixivaptan safely and effectively corrects serum sodium concentrations in hospitalized patients with euvolemic hyponatremia. *Kidney Int*. 2012;82:1223–1230.
- Callahan MA, Do HT, Caplan DW, et al. Economic impact of hyponatremia in hospitalized patients: A retrospective cohort study. *Postgrad Med*. 2009;121:186–191.
- Cowtan T. Thiazide diuretics. *N Engl J Med*. 2010;362:659–660.
- Ernst ME, Moser M. Use of diuretics in patients with hypertension. *N Engl J Med*. 2009;361:2153–2164.
- Friedman B, Cirulli J. Hyponatremia in critical care patients: Frequency, outcome, characteristics, and treatment with the vasopressin V(2)-receptor antagonist tolvaptan. *J Crit Care*. 2013;28:219e1–e12.
- Lim YJ, Park EK, Koh HC, et al. Syndrome of inappropriate secretion of antidiuretic hormone as a leading cause of hyponatremia in children who underwent chemotherapy or stem cell transplantation. *Pediatr Blood Cancer*. 2010;54:734–737.
- Sood L, Sterns RH, Hix JK, et al. Hypertonic saline and desmopressin: A simple strategy for safe correction of severe hyponatremia. *Am J Kidney Dis*. 2013;61:571–578.
- Sterns RH, Hix JK, Silver SM. Management of hyponatremia in the ICU. *Chest*. 2013;144:672–679.

SEE ALSO

Algorithm: Hyponatremia

CODES

ICD10
E87.1 Hypo-osmolality and hyponatremia

CLINICAL PEARLS

- Alcohol-dependent individuals with vitamin deficiencies, elderly women taking thiazide diuretics, and people with hypokalemia or burns are at increased risk of central pontine myelinolysis. A longer duration of hyponatremia is also a risk factor.
- Bronchogenic carcinoma, pancreas, duodenal, prostate, thymoma, lymphoma, and mesothelioma are neoplastic diseases associated with SIADH.
- Formulas have been developed for safe correction of hyponatremia and are available online (www.medcalc.com/sodium.html).

HYPOPARATHYROIDISM
Diana P. Vaca, MD • Felix B. Chang, MD

BASICS

DESCRIPTION
- Deficient secretion of parathyroid hormone (PTH)
- Usually asymptomatic
- Acute hypoparathyroidism: Tetany, muscle cramps, carpopedal spasm, irritability, altered mental status, convulsion, stridor, and tingling of the circumoral area, hands, and feet
- Chronic: Lethargy, personality changes, anxiety, blurry vision, parkinsonism, mental retardation
- System(s) affected: Endocrine/Metabolic; Musculoskeletal; Nervous; Bones; Kidneys; Parathyroid

Pediatric Considerations
- May occur in premature infants
- Neonates born to hypercalcemic mothers may experience suppression of developing parathyroid glands.
- Congenital absence of parathyroids
- May appear later in childhood as autoimmune or APS-1

Geriatric Considerations
Hypocalcemia is fairly common in elderly; however, rarely secondary to hypoparathyroidism.

Pregnancy Considerations
Use of magnesium as a tocolytic may induce functional hypoparathyroidism.

EPIDEMIOLOGY
More common in women. Affects all ages.

Incidence
Most common after surgical procedure of the anterior neck. Transient hyperparathyroidism is seen after 20% of thyroidectomies; whereas permanent hypoparathyroidism, 0.8–3.0%.

Prevalence
Wide variation. Autosomal-dominant hypocalcemia with hypercalciuria (ADHH): 1/70,000 typically in infancy with hypocalcemic seizures

ETIOLOGY AND PATHOPHYSIOLOGY
- PTH is involved in the control of serum ionized calcium levels:
  - Mobilizes calcium and phosphorus from bone stores
  - Stimulates formation of 1,25-dihydroxy-vitamin D
  - Stimulates reabsorption of calcium in the distal convoluted tubule and phosphate excretion in proximal tubule
- Loss of PTH action results in hypocalcemia, hyperphosphatemia, and hypercalciuria.
- Magnesium is crucial for PTH secretion and activation of the PTH receptor; hypo- or hypermagnesemia may result in functional hypoparathyroidism.

- Acquired hypoparathyroidism:
  - Surgical: Removal or damage to parathyroid glands or their blood supply. Thyroid, parathyroid, or radical neck surgery for head and neck cancers (1)
  - Autoimmune: Isolated or combined with other endocrine deficiencies in polyglandular autoimmune (PGA) syndrome
  - Deposition of heavy metals in gland: Copper (Wilson disease) or iron (hemochromatosis, thalassemias), radiation-induced destruction, and metastatic infiltration
  - Functional hypoparathyroidism: Associated with hypomagnesemia. Hypermagnesemia
  - Congenital:
    - Calcium-sensing receptor (CaSR) abnormalities. Hypocalcemia with hypercalciuria
    - HDR or Barakat syndrome: Deafness, renal dysplasia
    - Familial: Mutations of the *TBCE* gene. Abnormal PTH secretions
    - 22q11.2 deletion syndrome
- Autoimmune: Genetic gain-of-function mutation in calcium-sensing receptor
- Infiltrative: Metastatic carcinoma, hemochromatosis, Wilson disease, granulomas
- Hypo- (alcoholics) or hypermagnesemia: Chronic iron overloads

Genetics
- Genetic defects may result in X-linked or in autosomal-recessive hypoparathyroidism due to abnormal parathyroid gland development. Associated with mutations in the transcription factor glial-cell missing B (BCMB)
- Mutations in transcription factors or regulators of parathyroid gland development:
  - Component of a larger genetic syndrome (APS-1 or DiGeorge syndrome) or in isolation (X-linked hypoparathyroidism) (2)
  - May be autosomal–dominant (DiGeorge), autosomal recessive (APS-1), or X-linked recessive (X-linked hypoparathyroidism) (2)
  - Congenital syndromes:
    - 22q11.2 deletion syndrome, familial hypomagnesemia, hypoparathyroidism with lymphedema (2)
    - Hypoparathyroidism with sensorineural deafness
    - ADHH: Mutations gain-of-function of the CaSR gene suppressing the parathyroid gland, without elevation of PTH
  - PGA syndrome type 1: Mucocutaneous candidiasis, hypoparathyroidism, and Addison disease

RISK FACTORS
Neck surgery and neck trauma, neck malignancies, family history of hypocalcemia, PGA syndrome

GENERAL PREVENTION
Intraoperative identification and preservation of parathyroid tissue

COMMONLY ASSOCIATED CONDITIONS
- DiGeorge syndrome
- PGA syndrome type 1
- Multiple endocrine deficiency autoimmune candidiasis (MEDAC) syndrome
- Juvenile familial endocrinopathy
- Addison disease
- Moniliasis (HAM) syndrome: A polyglandular deficiency syndrome, possibly genetic, characterized by hypoparathyroidism

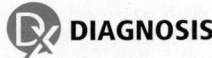

DIAGNOSIS

HISTORY
Often asymptomatic, ask about previous neck trauma or surgery, head or neck irradiation, family history of hypocalcemia, presence of other autoimmune endocrinopathies.
- Fatigue, circumoral or distal extremity paresthesias
- Muscle cramps, seizures, neuropsychiatric symptoms

PHYSICAL EXAM
- Surgical scar on neck
- Chvostek sign: Ipsilateral twitching of the upper lip upon tapping the facial nerve on the cheek. 10% normal people have positive Chvostek's sign.
- Trousseau sign: Painful carpal spasm after 3-minute occlusion of brachial artery with BP cuff. BP cuff inflated to > systolic BP for 3 minutes leads to carpal spasm (flexion of metacarpophalangeal [MCP] joints, extension of interphalangeal [IP] joints, adduction of fingers and thumb).
- Tetany, laryngeo- or bronchospasm, cataracts, cardiac arrhythmias or failure; dry hair, brittle nails
- Loss of deep tendon reflexes
- Dysrhythmias (secondary hypocalcemia)
- Cataracts
- Tooth enamel defects

DIFFERENTIAL DIAGNOSIS
- Vitamin D deficiency/resistance
- Pseudohypoparathyroidism, which presents in childhood, kidney and bone unresponsiveness to PTH; characterized by hypocalcemia, hyperphosphatemia, and, in contrast to hypoparathyroidism, elevated rather than reduced PTH concentrations
- Hypoalbuminemia, renal failure, malabsorption, familial hypocalcemia, hypomagnesemia

DIAGNOSTIC TESTS & INTERPRETATION
Initial Tests (lab, imaging)
- Calcium: Total and ionized (low) (correct serum calcium level for albumin):
  - Corrected serum calcium = total serum calcium + 0.8 (4 − serum albumin)
- Phosphorus (high)
- PTH (low or inappropriately normal)
- Magnesium (low or high may cause hypoparathyroidism; may also be normal)
- BUN, creatinine, 25 OH vitamin D level (especially in elderly)

- Urinary calcium (normal or high)
- Calcium should be monitored after thyroid or parathyroid surgery.
- Radiographs may show absent tooth roots, calcification of cerebellum, choroid plexus, or cerebral basal ganglia.

Follow-Up Tests & Special Considerations
- ECG: Prolongation of ST and QTc intervals nonspecific repolarization changes, dysrhythmias
- Urine calcium:creatinine ratio (normal 0.1–0.2) may be low before treatment, but should be monitored to prevent stones due to hypercalciuria.
- Gene sequencing: Evaluation of other hormone levels may be required to diagnose APS-1.
- Hungry bone syndrome (transient hypoparathyroidism after parathyroid surgery):
  – Hypocalcemia due to hungry bone syndrome may persist despite recovery of PTH secretion from the remaining normal glands. Thus, serum PTH concentrations may be low, normal, or even elevated.
- Infiltrative: Osteoblastic metastasis of prostate, breast or lung cancer
- Metabolic/nutritional: Renal failure neonatal hypocalcemia hypoalbuminemia malabsorption calcium (Ca^{++}) chelators hypomagnesemia
- Familial hypocalcemia acute hyperphosphatemia (rare) vitamin D deficiency
- Autoantibodies against NACHT leucine-rich-repeat protein 5(NALPS) found in 49% of 73 patients with APS-1 and hypoparathyroidisms.

Test Interpretation
Parathyroid gland parenchymal tissue completely or almost completely replaced by fat

TREATMENT

GENERAL MEASURES
- Monitor ECG during calcium repletion.
- Maintenance therapy: May require lifelong treatment with calcium and calcitriol (2):
  – Maintain serum calcium in low normal range: 8–8.5 mg/dL (2–2.12 mmol/L)
- If hypercalcemia occurs, hold therapy until calcium returns to normal. Treat magnesium deficiency if present.
- Phosphate binders required if high calcium-phosphate product
- Thiazide diuretics combined with a low-salt diet may be used to prevent hypercalciuria, nephrocalcinosis, and nephrolithiasis.
- Oral calcium administration and vitamin D supplementation after thyroidectomy may reduce the risk for symptomatic hypocalcemia after surgery.

MEDICATION
First Line
- Hypoparathyroid tetany, severe symptoms (tetany, seizures, cardiac failure, laryngospasm, bronchospasm):
  – IV calcium gluconate: 1 or 2 g, each infused over a period of 10 minutes. Central venous catheter preferred because calcium-containing solutions can irritate surrounding tissues. Follow with infusion 10 g calcium gluconate in 1 L 5% dextrose water at a rate of 1–3 mg calcium gluconate/kg of body weight/hr

- Maintenance:
  – Oral calcium: Calcium salts: 1–3 g/d PO
  – Calcitriol: (vitamin D 1,25-dihydroxycholecalciferol): 0.25 mcg/d. Doses 0.5–2 mcg/d are usually required.
- Hypomagnesemia: Acutely: 1–2 g IV q6h. Long-term magnesium oxide tablets (600 mg), once or twice per day

Second Line
Cholecalciferol 10,000–50,000 U duration of action 4–8 weeks

ISSUES FOR REFERRAL
Endocrinologist, Nephrologist, Ophthalmologist

ADDITIONAL THERAPIES
Parathyroid hormone 1–34 (SC) (3,4)[A]:
- May be as effective as calcitriol for maintaining growth and serum calcium levels in children with chronic hypoparathyroidism.

SURGERY/OTHER PROCEDURES
Autotransplantation of cryopreserved parathyroid tissue: Restores normocalcemia in 23% of cases

IN-PATIENT CONSIDERATIONS
Admission Criteria/Initial Stabilization
Laryngospasm, seizures, tetany, QT prolongation

Discharge Criteria
Resolution of hypocalcemic symptoms, patient educated on hypoparathyroidism and treatment

 ## ONGOING CARE

FOLLOW-UP RECOMMENDATIONS
Patient Monitoring
- Goal is a total corrected serum calcium level in low normal range (8–8.5 mg/dL or 2–2.12 mmol/L), 24-hour urine calcium <300 mg, and calcium-phosphate product <55.
- Outpatient measurement of serum calcium, phosphorus, and creatinine weekly to monthly during initial management; measure calcium, phosphate, and creatinine twice yearly when stable.
- Measure urine calcium and creatinine twice yearly.
- Annual slit-lamp and ophthalmologic evaluations are recommended.
- DEXA scan

DIET
Low-phosphate diet in patients with hyperphosphatemia

PATIENT EDUCATION
www.hypopara.org

PROGNOSIS
Hypoparathyroidism following neck surgery is often transient. Length of required treatment may vary depending on origin.

COMPLICATIONS
- Reversible: Due to low calcium levels; most likely to improve with adequate treatment:
  – Neuromuscular symptoms: Paresthesias (circumoral, fingers, toes), tetany, seizures, parkinsonian symptoms; pseudotumor cerebri has been described.
  – Renal: Hypercalciuria, nephrocalcinosis, nephrolithiasis
  – Cardiovascular: Heart failure; arrhythmias

- Irreversible: When condition starts early in childhood and will not improve with calcium and vitamin D treatment:
  – Stunting of growth
  – Enamel defects and hypoplasia of teeth
  – Atrophy, brittleness, and ridging of nails
  – Cataracts and basal ganglia calcifications

REFERENCES
1. Al-Azem, Khan A. Hypoparathyroidism. *Best Pract Res Clin Endocrinol Metab*. 2012;26(4):517–522.
2. de la Morena MT, Eitson JL, Dozmorov IM, et al. Signature MicroRNA expression patterns identified in humans with 22q11.2 deletion/DiGeorge syndrome. *Clin Immunol*. 2013;147(1):11–22.
3. Khan A, Fong J. Hypocalcemia: Updates in diagnosis and management for primary care. *Can Fam Physician*. 2012;58(2):158–162.
4. Winer KK, Zhang B, Shrader JA, et al. Synthetic human parathyroid hormone 1–34 replacement therapy: A randomized crossover trial comparing pump versus injections in the treatment of chronic hypoparathyroidism. *J Clin Endocrinol Metab*. 2012;97(2):391–399.

ADDITIONAL READING
Cusano NE, Rubin MR, McMahon DJ, et al. The effect of PTH(1-84) on quality of life in hypoparathyroidism. *J Clin Endocrinol Metab*. 2013;98(6):2356–2361.

 ## CODES

ICD10
- E89.2 Postprocedural hypoparathyroidism
- E20.8 Other hypoparathyroidism
- E20.9 Hypoparathyroidism, unspecified

CLINICAL PEARLS
Often asymptomatic; consider if hypocalcemic with fatigue and circumoral or distal extremity paresthesias
- Correct the serum calcium level for albumin level.
- Monitor calcium after thyroid or parathyroid surgery.
- Serum levels of magnesium and 25(OH) should be measured to rule out deficiency that could contribute to reduced serum calcium levels.

HYPOTENSION, ORTHOSTATIC

Nirmanmoh Bhatia, MD • Ziad Alnabki, MD • Marcus F. Stoddard, MD

 BASICS

Postural or orthostatic hypotension (OH) represents the failure of cardiovascular reflexes to maintain adequate BP on standing from a supine or sitting position.

DESCRIPTION

- OH is defined as a sustained and persistent drop in systolic BP (SBP) ≥20 mm Hg or diastolic BP (DBP) ≥10 mm Hg within 3 minutes of achieving a standing position, or head-up tilt to at least 60 degrees on tilt table. Delayed OH can infrequently occur with a slow decline in SBP beyond 3 minutes of standing, and may be revealed by extending the period of orthostatic stress (1).
- Characteristic symptoms of OH are recurrent dizziness, lightheadedness, presyncope, or syncope with assumption of an upright posture, typically relieved by achieving a recumbent position, and can be incapacitating. In the elderly, OH may be asymptomatic or present with nonspecific complaints of weakness.

EPIDEMIOLOGY

Asymptomatic OH is far more common than symptomatic OH and is an independent risk factor for mortality and cardiovascular disease. OH is also a manifestation of many underlying diseases and may be the initial sign of autonomic failure in many neurologic disorders. The prevalence increases with age, hypertension (HTN), diabetes, and use of antihypertensive medication (2).

Incidence
80,095 orthostatic-related hospitalizations occurred in the US in 2004; OH was the primary diagnosis in 35%.

Prevalence
~6% of middle-aged persons, and 18% of individuals ≥65 years of age; more common in those living in long-term care facilities (45% vs. 6% living in the community) (2). In those with HTN, prevalence is 13.4–32.1% (2)

ETIOLOGY AND PATHOPHYSIOLOGY

- During standing, 500–1,000 mL of blood pools in the lower extremities and the splanchnic vasculature. This reduces cardiac preload, but is opposed by an increase in sympathetic tone and vasopressin release that maintains cerebral perfusion pressure, by increasing peripheral vascular resistance. Impairment of these compensatory mechanisms by autonomic dysfunction, or nonneurogenic causes, such as medications, hypovolemia, or cardiac pump failure, leads to an inability to maintain effective cerebral perfusion pressure. Autonomic dysfunction also impairs proximal tubule renal sodium reabsorption, which contributes to OH through urinary sodium wasting and a consequent reduction in circulating plasma volume. In older people vascular stiffening and decreased baroreceptor sensitivity predispose to OH.
- Supine hypertension (SH), due to baroreflex dysfunction and fluid redistribution upon assuming a horizontal position, is common in patients with OH. Increased renal perfusion pressure in the recumbent position also leads to nocturnal natriuresis, which decreases circulating volume, worsening orthostatic tolerance in the morning.

- Medications (iatrogenic causes):
  – Anticholinergics: Benztropine, oxybutynin
  – Antidepressants: TCA, MAOIs, SSRIs, and SNRIs
  – Antihypertensives: Of classes including diuretics
  – Dopamine agonists: Levodopa, bromocriptine, ropinirole, pramipexole
  – Ethanol
  – Insulin (may exacerbate OH in the setting of diabetic neuropathy)
  – Narcotics/Sedatives: Morphine, benzodiazepines, barbiturates, promethazine
  – Neuroleptics: Chlorpromazine, quetiapine
  – Neurotoxic drugs: Amiodarone, vincristine, cisplatin
- Neurogenic causes:
  – Idiopathic OH (1/3 of cases of OH)
  – Central autonomic nervous system diseases: Familial dysautonomia (rare, childhood), Lewy body dementia, multisystem atrophy (Shy-Drager syndrome), Parkinson disease (PD): 40% of patients with PD have OH. Pure autonomic failure (rare)
  – Peripheral autonomic nervous system diseases: Acute autonomic neuropathy and Guillain-Barré syndrome (acute onset, frequently preceded by viral syndrome); alcoholic polyneuropathy; amyloidosis; autoimmune autonomic ganglionopathy (rare); chronic renal failure: Uremic or β-2 microglobulin neuropathy (dialysis). Diabetes: Diabetic autonomic neuropathy (very common). Exposure to neurotoxins. Hereditary sensory and autonomic neuropathies: Dopamine-β-hydroxylase deficiency (rare). HIV neuropathy. Paraneoplastic autonomic neuropathy: SCLC, NSCLC, GI neoplasias, prostate, breast, bladder, kidney, testicle, and ovary. Spinal cord pathologies: Trauma, myelitis, tumors, tabes dorsalis, multiple sclerosis, syringomyelia, infarction, vitamin B_{12} deficiency
- Nonneurogenic causes:
  – Cardiac disorders: Heart failure, arrhythmias, pericardial disease, severe aortic stenosis, idiopathic hypertrophic subaortic stenosis (IHSS), hypertrophic obstructive cardiomyopathy (HOCM), acute aortic regurgitation, acute myocardial infarction
  – Deconditioning
  – Intravascular volume depletion: Bleeding, diarrhea, diabetes insipidus, diuretics, poor oral intake, vomiting
  – Metabolic: Adrenal insufficiency, hypoaldosteronism, pheochromocytoma, carcinoid syndrome, hypokalemia (severe), hypothyroidism
  – Sepsis
  – Systemic mastocytosis
  – Venous pooling: Heat or vigorous exercise, postprandial splanchnic dilation, prolonged recumbency or standing

RISK FACTORS
- Elderly, particularly in long-term care facilities
- Multiple comorbidities, including HTN, diabetes, neurodegenerative disorders, and neuropathy
- Polypharmacy (See "Epidemiology" section).

GENERAL PREVENTION
Avoid polypharmacy and monitor drug interactions, maintain adequate fluid balance

COMMONLY ASSOCIATED CONDITIONS
Diabetes mellitus with neuropathy, uncontrolled HTN and antihypertensive treatment, PD

 DIAGNOSIS

Initial approach: Detailed history and physical examination with a focus on neurodegenerative disorders and neuropathy; thorough medication review; screening for reversible causes: 12-lead ECG, CBC, and BMP

HISTORY
- Postural symptoms: Dizziness, lightheadedness, palpitations, syncope or presyncope. Elderly patients may have vague complaints even before frank syncope: Generalized weakness, fatigue, nausea, difficulty with concentration or cognition, leg buckling, pure vertigo, visual blurring, headache or "coat-hanger" pattern neck-shoulder pain, orthostatic dyspnea, or angina
- Aggravating factors: Warm environments, exertion, prolonged standing, ingestions of large/carbohydrate-rich meals, alcohol intake (vasodilation)
- Volume depletion: Vomiting, diarrhea, poor oral intake, polyuria
- Cardiac pump failure: Orthopnea, edema, paroxysmal nocturnal dyspnea, angina
- Peripheral neuropathy: Numbness, pain, paresthesia, imbalance, or falls
- Associated diseases: Diabetes, PD, dementia
- Autonomic symptoms: Altered sweating (hyper- or hypohidrosis), GI dysfunction (bloating, nausea, vomiting, constipation), impotence, bladder dysfunction, sicca symptoms

PHYSICAL EXAM
- Measure BP while supine and standing: Patient should be supine for 5 minutes, then after standing, check the BP at 3 minutes. Use sitting measurements only if the patient is too dizzy or weak to stand. Use fall precautions: Do not check for OH in patients with supine SBP <90 mm Hg (shock) as it adds no useful information. Tachycardic response to standing may be a sign of hypovolemia or cardiac pump failure, whereas minimal or no change in heart rate may suggest a neurogenic cause. Orthostatic tachycardia without a significant drop in BP does not meet criteria for OH and may suggest postural orthostatic tachycardia syndrome (POTS).
- Cardiac exam: Jugular venous distention, pulse irregularity, edema, murmurs, S_3
- Neurologic exam: Hypomimia, gait, tremor, cogwheel rigidity, motor strength, fine-touch, pain sensation, proprioception, Romberg maneuver, cerebellar signs, and myoclonus

DIFFERENTIAL DIAGNOSIS
Neurally mediated (reflex) syncope: Vasovagal syncope, situational syncope (cough, micturition, defecation, swallowing), carotid sinus hypersensitivity. Falls related to a neurologic disorder. Postprandial hypotension. POTS. Shock (must have a normal lying BP before testing)

DIAGNOSTIC TESTS & INTERPRETATION
Initial Tests (lab, imaging)
- CBC, BMP (hypokalemia, alkalosis, and renal insufficiency suggesting volume depletion), thyroid-stimulating hormone (TSH)
- ECG and/or Holter monitor/event monitor: To rule out arrhythmias and detect structural heart disease. Echocardiogram: For abnormal ECG, new murmurs, or suspected heart failure. MRI: For suspected neurodegenerative disorders or spinal disease

Follow-Up Tests & Special Considerations
- If neuropathy is found on exam consider, vitamin B$_{12}$ levels and serum and urine protein electrophoresis (amyloidosis). Nerve conduction studies and electromyography: For suspected neuropathy
- Adrenal insufficiency and pheochromocytoma evaluation is warranted in OH of uncertain cause: 8 a.m. cortisol level: If <18 μg/dL, consider cosyntropin testing. 24-hour urinary or plasma fractionated metanephrines: Consider further testing, depending on results.
- Antibodies to the neuronal nicotinic receptor (nAChR) in cases of suspected autoimmune autonomic ganglionopathy

Diagnostic Procedures/Other
- Tilt table testing: Indicated if orthostatic symptoms are persistent, significant, and characteristic despite a nondiagnostic clinical examination. Provocation with nitroglycerin or IV isoproterenol is not recommended, as it may cause false-positive results (3).
- Autonomic testing: Useful in cases where neurally mediated syncope vs. orthostatic syncope is unclear, and to diagnose subclinical cases. Includes heart rate (HR) and BP variability with deep inspiration and Valsalva maneuver, sudomotor evaluation, orthostatic vascular resistance, plasma norepinephrine response to orthostasis, and pharmacologic challenges (4,5).

TREATMENT

- Abdominal binder or compression stockings (not TED hose), preferably waist high with 20 mm Hg of pressure (worn before rising) (3,4,6)[B]
- Perform gradual staged movements with postural changes: Arise slowly from supine to seated and rest before standing (3,4,6)[C]. Also, physical counter maneuvers (to increase vascular resistance and preload): Isometric contraction of leg muscles for 30 seconds at a time, repeated feet dorsiflexion, leg crossing and contraction, squatting, bending at the waist, leg elevation, and respiratory maneuvers, such as inspiration through pursed lips and inspiratory sniffing (3,4,6)[B]
- Moderate exercise (supine or sitting isotonic exercise if symptoms are severe): Improves orthostatic tolerance and reduces venous pooling (3,4,6)[B]
- Increase water and sodium intake: 2–2.5 L of fluid a day, and up to 10 g/d of sodium (if needed, salt tablets starting at 500 mg PO t.i.d. may be used). Encourage drinking water with meals and before exercise. Rapid ingestion of two 8-oz glasses of water (500 mL) over 3–4 minutes elicits a marked pressor response lasting for up to 1 hour (3,4,6)[B].
- Elevate the head of the bed 20 degrees (4–6 inches) to reduce supine HTN and nocturnal diuresis (3,4,6)[B].

- Avoid: Prolonged recumbency, increased intrathoracic pressure (straining, coughing), large meals, especially if high in carbohydrates, and alcohol (3,4,6)[C]

MEDICATION
1st identify and discontinue all potentially aggravating medications. Medication is indicated only when nonpharmacologic measures are insufficient to control symptoms. Goal of therapy is to improve functional capacity and quality of life without causing excessive supine HTN, rather than to eliminate orthostatic drops in BP.

First Line
- Fludrocortisone: Synthetic mineralocorticoid that increases sodium and fluid retention and increases peripheral vascular resistance. Starting at 0.1 mg/d, titrate for symptoms every week up to 0.5 mg/d. Contraindicated in patients with heart failure (HF) and chronic renal insufficiency due to volume expansion (3,4,6)[B].
- Midodrine: Selective peripheral α-agonist that increases vascular resistance. Only drug currently FDA approved to treat OH. Start at 2.5 mg PO t.i.d. and titrate for symptoms up to 10 mg t.i.d. Avoid within 4 hours of bedtime to prevent worsening supine HTN, and use with caution in patients with coronary artery disease (3,4,6)[A].

Second Line
- Pyridostigmine: Acetylcholinesterase inhibitor, increases sympathetic ganglionic neurotransmission, 30–60 mg PO t.i.d. (4,6)[B]
- Caffeine: Methylxanthine with pressor effect due to blockade of adenosine receptors, 100–250 mg PO t.i.d., as tablets or caffeinated beverages
- Erythropoietin: Increases RBC mass. Consider only when significant anemia coexists, 25–75 U/kg SQ 3×/wk (maintenance dose may be lower). Iron studies and supplementation usually are required (3,4)[B].
- Ephedrine: Mixed α- and β-agonist, 25–50 mg PO t.i.d. (avoid within 4 hours before bedtime to prevent worsening supine HTN) (3,4)[C]
- Pseudoephedrine: Mixed α- and β-agonist, 30–60 mg PO t.i.d. (avoid within 4 hours before bedtime) (4)[C]
- Desmopressin: Vasopressin analogue, 5–40 μg/d nasal spray, or 100–800 μg/d PO (3,4)[C]
- L-dihydroxyphenylserine (Droxidopa): Prodrug that is converted to noradrenaline by dopa decarboxylase enzyme, 200–400 mg/d PO (3,5)[A]
- Non-steroidal antiinflammatory drugs: May supplement treatment with fludrocortisone or a sympathomimetic agent. They are believed to act by limiting the vasodilating effects of circulating prostaglandins.

ADDITIONAL THERAPIES
Consider bedtime nitrates or nifedipine to treat severe, sustained supine HTN; may increase the risk of syncope and falls (4)[C]

ISSUES FOR REFERRAL
Consider cardiology referral if there is significant heart disease or tilt table testing will be required. Consider neurology referral for confirmed or suspected primary neurologic pathologies.

ONGOING CARE
FOLLOW-UP RECOMMENDATIONS
Monitor for significant supine HTN, fluid overload, electrolyte abnormalities, and HF in patients under medical treatment. In patients without an apparent cause of OH, follow-up is essential because OH alone may be the initial presentation of neurologic disorders.

PATIENT EDUCATION
Recognize symptoms and avoid aggravating factors. Educate on nonpharmacologic measures.

COMPLICATIONS
Syncope, falls (hip fracture, head trauma)

REFERENCES
1. Freeman R. Consensus statement on the definition of orthostatic hypotension, neurally mediated syncope and the postural tachycardia syndrome. *Auton Neurosci.* 2011;161:46–48.
2. Benvenuto LJ, Krakoff LR. Morbidity and mortality of orthostatic hypotension: Implications for management of cardiovascular disease. *Am J Hypertens.* 2011;24:135–144.
3. Lahrmann H, Cortelli P, Hilz M, et al. EFNS guidelines on the diagnosis and management of orthostatic hypotension. *Eur J Neurol.* 2006; 13:930–936.
4. Freeman R. Clinical practice. Neurogenic orthostatic hypotension. *N Engl J Med.* 2008;358:615–624.
5. Goldstein DS, Sharabi Y. Neurogenic orthostatic hypotension: A pathophysiological approach. *Circulation.* 2009;119:139–146.
6. Figueroa JJ, Basford JR, Low PA, et al. Preventing and treating orthostatic hypotension: As easy as A, B, C. *Cleve Clin J Med.* 2010;77:298–306.

CODES

ICD10
I95.1 Orthostatic hypotension

CLINICAL PEARLS
- OH is a clinical finding, not a disease. Treatment should be guided by symptoms rather than by absolute BP drop.
- Always check the medication list and volume status. Drug-related OH may be a sign of underlying autonomic dysfunction.
- Pharmacologic treatment is indicated only when nonpharmacologic measures are insufficient to control symptoms.

H

HYPOTHERMIA
Scott T. Henderson, MD

 BASICS

DESCRIPTION
- A core temperature of <35°C (95°F)
- May take several hours to days to develop
- Patients with cold-water immersion can appear to be dead but can still be resuscitated (1)[C].
- System(s) affected: All body systems
- Synonym(s): Accidental hypothermia

EPIDEMIOLOGY
- Predominant age: Very young and the elderly
- Predominant sex: Male > Female

Geriatric Considerations
More common due to lower metabolic rate, impaired ability to maintain normal body temperature, and impaired ability to detect temperature changes.

Prevalence
Estimates vary widely due to lack of pathologic evidence, and it is typically a secondary cause when diagnosing disorders.

ETIOLOGY AND PATHOPHYSIOLOGY
- Overwhelming environmental cold stress
- Decreased heat production
- Increased heat loss
- Impaired thermoregulation

RISK FACTORS
- Alcohol consumption
- Bronchopneumonia
- Cardiovascular disease
- Cold-water immersion
- Dermal dysfunction (burns, erythrodermas)
- Drug intoxication
- Endocrinopathies (myxedema, severe hypoglycemia)
- Excessive fluid loss
- Hepatic failure
- Hypothalamic and CNS dysfunction
- Malnutrition
- Mental illness; Alzheimer disease
- Prolonged cardiac arrest
- Prolonged environmental exposure
- Renal failure
- Sepsis
- Trauma (especially head)
- Uremia

GENERAL PREVENTION
- Appropriate clothing, with particular attention to head, feet, and hands
- For outdoor activities, carry survival bags with rescue foil blanket for use if stranded or injured.
- Avoid alcohol.
- Alertness to early symptoms and initiating preventive steps (e.g., drinking warm fluids)
- Identify medications that may predispose to hypothermia (e.g., neuroleptics, sedatives, hypnotics, tranquilizers).

COMMONLY ASSOCIATED CONDITIONS
- Addison disease
- CNS dysfunction
- Congestive heart failure
- Diabetes
- Hypopituitarism
- Hypothyroidism
- Ketoacidosis
- Pulmonary infection
- Sepsis
- Uremia

 DIAGNOSIS

HISTORY
Presentation varies with the temperature of the patient at the time of presentation.

ALERT
History of prolonged exposure to cold may make the diagnosis obvious, but hypothermia may be overlooked in other situations, especially in comatose patients.

PHYSICAL EXAM
Exam findings vary with the temperature of the patient at the time of presentation:
- Mild (32–35°C):
  - Lethargy and mild confusion
  - Shivering
  - Tachypnea
  - Tachycardia
  - Loss of fine motor coordination
  - Increased BP
  - Peripheral vasoconstriction
- Moderate (28–32°C):
  - Delirium
  - Bradycardia
  - Hypotension
  - Hypoventilation
  - Cyanosis
  - Arrhythmias (prolonged PR interval, AV junctional rhythm, idioventricular rhythm, prolonged QT interval, altered T waves)
  - Semicoma and coma
  - Muscular rigidity
  - Generalized edema
  - Slowed reflexes
- Severe (<28°C):
  - Very cold skin
  - Rigidity
  - Apnea
  - Bradycardia
  - No pulse: Ventricular fibrillation or asystole
  - Areflexia
  - Unresponsive
  - Fixed pupils

ALERT
Use specially designed thermometers that can record low temperatures and measure core temperatures.

Pediatric Considerations
- Infants may present with bright red, cold skin and very low energy.
- A child's body temperature drops faster than an adult's does when immersed in cold water.

DIFFERENTIAL DIAGNOSIS
- Cerebrovascular accidents
- Intoxication
- Drug overdose
- Complications of diabetes, hypothyroidism, hypopituitarism

DIAGNOSTIC TESTS & INTERPRETATION
Initial Tests (lab, imaging)
- Arterial blood gases (corrected for temperature)
- CBC and platelet counts
- Serum electrolytes
- Urinalysis
- Coagulation studies
- Fibrinogen levels
- Blood culture
- BUN/creatinine
- Glucose
- Amylase
- Liver function studies
- Cardiac enzymes
- Calcium
- Magnesium
- Alcohol level
- Drug screen
- Cervical spine, chest, and abdomen x-rays, if appropriate

Follow-Up Tests & Special Considerations
Serum cortisol and TSH if underlying endocrine dysfunction (hypothalamus stimulates release of hormones in response to hypothermia)

Diagnostic Procedures/Other
EKG

Test Interpretation
Serum potassium >12 mmol/ L associated with nonsurvival

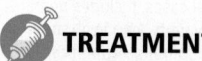 **TREATMENT**

GENERAL MEASURES
- Prehospital (2)[C]:
  - ABCs of basic life support
  - Remove wet garments.
  - Protect against heat loss and wind chill.
  - If far from definitive care, begin active rewarming but do not delay transport:
    - Mild hypothermic patients with shivering ability will have improved comfort and might have a reduced cold-stress response with active rewarming (3)[B].
  - Give warm humidified oxygen if available.
- See "Initial Stabilization."

MEDICATION
- For sepsis or bacterial infections: Antibiotics based on site and etiology
- For hypoglycemia, D50W at a dose of 1 mg/kg
- Thiamine: 100 mg, if alcoholic or cachectic
- Naloxone: 2 mg
- Levothyroxine: 150–500 μg for myxedema
- For severe acidosis: Sodium bicarbonate
- Precautions:
  - Medications including epinephrine, lidocaine, and procainamide, can accumulate to toxic levels if used repeatedly. Should be avoided until core temperature is >30°C:
    - When temperature reaches >30°C, IV medications are indicated, but at longer than the standard intervals.
  - It may be reasonable to consider vasopressors during cardiac arrest according to standard ACLS algorithm with concurrent rewarming (2)[C].

- *Significant possible interactions:*
  – Use all drugs cautiously due to impaired metabolism and renal elimination.
- Once rewarming has occurred, there is mobilization of depot stores.
- Routine use of steroids or antibiotics does not increase survival or decrease postresuscitative damage.

IN-PATIENT CONSIDERATIONS
Admission Criteria/Initial Stabilization
- Rewarming depends on severity of hypothermia and presence of cardiac arrest.
- If no cardiac arrest, consider active external rewarming (4)[B].
- If cardiac arrest present, consider active internal rewarming (4)[B].
- Warm center of body 1st (5)[C].
- The rate of rewarming is determined by whether a perfusing cardiac output is present:
  – If a perfusing cardiac output is present, 1–2°C/hr is appropriate.
  – If not, then a faster rate of >2°C/hr should be used.
- Monitor core temperature; use a consistent method.
- Monitor BP and cardiac rhythm.
- Correct metabolic acidosis.
- Evaluate for frostbite and other trauma.
- Mild hypothermia:
  – Passive rewarming
  – Administration of heated IV solutions (D5NS)
  – Provide warm fluids by mouth if fully alert.
- Moderate hypothermia:
  – Active external rewarming with forced warm air systems (6)[B]
- Severe hypothermia (active internal [core] rewarming):
  – Minimally invasive
  – Heated IV fluids
  – Heated humidified oxygen
  – Body cavity lavage:
    ○ Thoracic cavity lavage (43°C)
    ○ GI, colonic, or bladder lavage with warm fluids (43°C)
    ○ Peritoneal dialysis
  – Extracorporeal blood rewarming (6)[B]:
    ○ Cardiopulmonary bypass
    ○ Extracorporeal membrane oxygenation
    ○ Continuous arteriovenous rewarming
    ○ Hemodialysis and hemofiltration
- Cardiac arrhythmias:
  – Atrial fibrillation and sinus bradycardia are common, but patients usually convert to normal sinus rhythm with rewarming.
  – If ventricular fibrillation is present, it should be treated with 1 shock. If patient does not respond, consider deferring further attempts until rewarm has occurred.
  – Do not treat transient ventricular arrhythmias.
  – If cardiac pacing required, preferable to use external noninvasive pacemaker
- Admit patients, preferably to the ICU, with underlying disease, physiologic abnormalities, or core temperature <32°C.

IV Fluids
Heat IVs to 40–42°C when possible, but should be no colder than the patient's core temperature.

ALERT
- Avoid fluid overload.
- Avoid lactated Ringer's solution because of decreased lactate metabolism.

Nursing
Because of the cold, heart is irritable and susceptible to arrhythmias; take special care in moving and transporting.

Discharge Criteria
Discharge from emergency department once normothermic, if mild hypothermia and no predisposing conditions or complications, and has suitable place to go.

ONGOING CARE

FOLLOW-UP RECOMMENDATIONS
Patient Monitoring
- During acute episode:
  – Monitor cardiac rhythm.
  – Monitor electrolytes and glucose frequently.
  – Monitor urinary output.
  – Follow blood gases.
- Following acute episode:
  – Continued therapy for any underlying disorder

DIET
Warm fluids only, if alert and able to swallow

PATIENT EDUCATION
- Alcohol intake increases risk of becoming hypothermic in cold conditions.
- Encourage persons with cardiovascular disease to avoid outdoor exercise in cold weather.
- Refer to social service agency for help with adequate housing, heat, and/or clothing, if appropriate.

PROGNOSIS
- Mortality rates are decreasing due to increased recognition and advanced therapy.
- Mortality usually depends on the severity of underlying cause of hypothermia.
- In previously healthy individuals, recovery is usually complete:
  – Mortality rate in healthy patients is <5%.
- Mortality rate in patients with coexisting illness is >50%.

Geriatric Considerations
Mortality rates increase with increasing age.

COMPLICATIONS
- Cardiac arrhythmias
- Hypotension
- Hyperkalemia
- Hypoglycemia
- Rhabdomyolysis
- Sepsis
- Pneumonia (aspiration and broncho)
- Pulmonary edema
- Acute respiratory distress syndrome
- Pancreatitis
- Peritonitis
- GI bleeding
- Acute tubular necrosis
- Bladder atony
- Intravascular thromboses/disseminated intravascular coagulation

- Metabolic acidosis
- Gangrene of extremities
- Compartment syndromes
- Seizures
- Cerebral ischemia
- Delirium

REFERENCES
1. Schweitzer KS. Cold but not dead. *Air Med J.* 2008;27:94–98.
2. Part 12: cardiac arrest in special situations: 2010 American Heart Association Guidelines for Cardiopulmonary Resuscitation and Emergency Cardiovascular Care. *Circulation.* 2010; 122(18Suppl 3):S829–61.
3. Lundgren P, Henriksson O, Naredi P, et al. The effect of active warming in prehospital trauma care during road and air ambulance transportation—a clinical randomized trial. *Scand J Trauma Resusc Emerg Med.* 2011;19:59. Epub 2011 Oct 21.
4. Kempainen RR, Brunette DD. The evaluation and management of accidental hypothermia. *Respir Care.* 2004;49:192–205.
5. van der Ploeg GJ, Goslings JC, Walpoth BH, et al. Accidental hypothermia: Rewarming treatments, complications and outcomes from one university medical centre. *Resuscitation.* 2010;81(11): 1550–1555.
6. McCullough L, Arora S. Diagnosis and treatment of hypothermia. *Am Fam Physician.* 2004;70: 2325–2332.

ADDITIONAL READING
- Brown DJA, Brugger H, Boyd J, et al. Accidental hypothermia. *N Engl J Med.* 2012;367:1930–1938.
- Headdon WG, Wilson PM, Dalton HR, et al. The management of accidental hypothermia. *BMJ.* 2009;338:b2085.

SEE ALSO

- Frostbite; Near Drowning
- Algorithm: Hypothermia

CODES

ICD10
- T68.XXXA Hypothermia, initial encounter
- T68.XXXD Hypothermia, subsequent encounter
- T68.XXXS Hypothermia, sequela

CLINICAL PEARLS
- Most common cause of hypothermia in the US is cold exposure due to alcohol intoxication.
- With a severely decreased core temperature, one should assume resuscitation is possible unless there are obvious lethal injuries. Continue resuscitation and rewarm to 33–35°C ("not dead until warm and dead").
- ECG changes are associated with hypothermia: Slowing of sinus rate with T-wave inversion; QT, QRS, and PR interval prolongation; atrial and ventricular arrhythmias; hypothermic J waves (Osborn waves) characterized by a notching of the QRS complex and ST segment

HYPOTHYROIDISM, ADULT

Gisela M. Lopez-Payares, MD • Fozia Ali, MD

 BASICS

DESCRIPTION
- Clinical and metabolic state resulting from decreased circulating levels of free thyroid hormone or from resistance to hormone action
- Can be primary (intrinsic thyroid disease) >95% of cases, or secondary (hypothalamic-pituitary disease)
- Subclinical hypothyroidism: Elevated thyroid-stimulating hormone (TSH) (>4.5) with normal free T4
- System(s) affected: Endocrine/Metabolic
- Synonym(s): Myxedema (Severe Hypothyroidism)

EPIDEMIOLOGY
Incidence
- Predominant age: middle-aged. Female > male 5–8:1
- and more common in woman with small body size at birth and during childhood.

Prevalence
- Prevalence varies from 0.1–2% in general population
- Prevalence of subclinical hypothyroidism is higher, ranging from 4–10% of adults, with higher frequency in elderly woman.
- Common in elderly:
  – >65 years of age, (6–10% women, 2–3% men)
  – Mean serum TSH concentrations higher in white or Mexican-Americans than in African Americans
  – Up to 20% of patients with major depressive disorder

ETIOLOGY AND PATHOPHYSIOLOGY
- Primary: >95% of cases: the commonest cause is autoimmune thyroid disease: Hashimoto thyroiditis or Ord disease.
  – Hashimoto thyroidits (goitrous hypothyroidism)
  – Ord disease (atrophic hypothyroidism)
- Secondary:
  – Postablative: Follows radioactive iodine therapy or thyroid surgery; delayed hypothyroidism may develop in patients treated with thioamide drugs (e.g., propylthiouracil or methimazole) 4–25 years later.
  – Surgical thyroidectomy
  – Radiotherapy for neck malignancies.
  – Transient hypothyroidism during the course of subacute or painless thyroiditis (silent thyroditis, most common during postpartum period) and subacute granulomatous thyroiditis
  – Infiltrative disease (fibrous thyroiditis, hemochromatosis, sarcoidosis)
  – Genetics or deficiency of thyrotropin-releasing hormone (TRH) from hypothalamus or TSH from pituitary
- Other causes: Heritable biosynthetic defects, iodine deficiency (rare in the US), or drugs (iodides, lithium, phenylbutazone, acetylsalicylic acid (ASA), amiodarone, aminoglutethimide, and IFN-α)
- No known genetic pattern for idiopathic primary hypothyroidism
- May be associated with type 2 autoimmune polyglandular syndrome, which is associated with HLA-DR3 and -DR4
- Secondary hypothyroidism frequently results from treatment for Graves disease, which may be familial.

RISK FACTORS
- Personal or family history of autoimmune diseases, including type 1 diabetes mellitus, Addison disease, Hashimoto thyroiditis
- Previous postpartum thyroiditis
- Previous head or neck irradiation
- History of Graves disease
- Treatment with lithium, immune modulators, such as IFN-α, or the iodine-containing amiodarone
- More common in persons of Japanese descent

COMMONLY ASSOCIATED CONDITIONS
- Hyponatremia
- Macrocitic anemia
- Idiopathic adrenocorticoid deficiency
- Diabetes mellitus/metabolic syndrome
- Hypoparathyroidism
- Myasthenia gravis
- Vitiligo
- Hypercholesterolemia
- Mitral valve prolapse
- Depression
- Rapid-cycling bipolar disorder
- Ischemic heart disease
- Down syndrome
- Celiac disease
- Elevated creatine kinase

 DIAGNOSIS

HISTORY
- Onset may be insidious, subtle
- Weakness, fatigue, lethargy
- Cold intolerance
- Decreased memory, concentration
- Hearing impairment
- Constipation
- Muscle cramps, arthralgias, paresthesias
- Modest weight gain (10 lb [4.5 kg])
- Decreased sweating
- Menorrhagia
- Depression
- Hoarseness
- Carpal tunnel syndrome

PHYSICAL EXAM
- Dry, coarse skin, reduced body and scalp hair
- Dull facial expression
- Coarsening or huskiness of voice
- Periorbital puffiness
- Swelling of hands and feet (nonpitting)
- Bradycardia
- Hypothermia
- Reduced systolic BP; increased diastolic BP
- Delayed relaxation of deep-tendon reflexes
- Macroglossia
- Weight gain
- Goiter (particularly in patient with Hashimoto thyroiditis)
- Impalpable thyroid gland (often in Ord disease or atrophic hypothyroidism)

Geriatric Considerations
- Characteristic signs and symptoms frequently changed or absent or sometimes unspecific symptoms
- Diagnosis based on laboratory criteria

DIFFERENTIAL DIAGNOSIS
- Nephrotic syndrome/chronic nephritis
- Neurasthenia
- Depression
- Euthyroid sick syndrome
- Congestive heart failure
- Primary amyloidosis
- Dementia from other causes
- Primary adrenal insufficiency
- Recovery from nonthyroidal illness
- Thyrotropin-secreting pituitary adenoma

DIAGNOSTIC TESTS & INTERPRETATION
Initial Tests (lab, imaging)
No imaging necessary, unless signs of cardiac involvement. Chest radiograph may show enlarged heart (often due to pericardial effusion).
- Primary hypothyroidism:
  – TSH elevated
  – Serum free T4 decreased
- Central hypothyroidism:
  – TSH low
  – Serum-free T4 decreased
  – Impaired TSH response to TRH
  – MRI of brain should be performed.
- Severe hypothyroidism:
  – Macrocitic anemia
  – Elevated cholesterol
  – Elevated creatine phosphokinase, lactate dehydrogenase, aspartate aminotransferase
  – Hyponatremia
- Subclinical hypothyroidism:
  – TSH elevated (>4.5 mIU/L)
  – Serum-free T4 normal

Follow-Up Tests & Special Considerations
- Antithyroid antibodies may define the cause of primary hypothyroidism, but are not necessary in all settings.
- Drugs that may alter lab results:
  – Drugs that decrease TSH:
    ○ Thyroid supplement, cortisone, dopamine, octreotide
  – Drugs that increase TSH:
    ○ phenytoin, amiodarone, dopamine antagonist (metoclopramide/domperidone, salicylates, oral colecystographic dyes (sodium ipodate), or estrogen or androgen in excess of replacement.
- Disorders that may alter lab results:
  – Any severe illness, pregnancy, chronic protein malnutrition, hepatic failure, or nephrotic syndrome

Test Interpretation
- Thyroid may be small, atrophic, or enlarged.
- SCREENING
  – Patient with risks factors:
    ○ H/o autoimmune disease, DM type 1.
    ○ H/o previous radioactive iodine therapy
    ○ H/o neck or head radiation
    ○ Family history of thyroid disease
    ○ Use of medications that may impair thyroid function
    ○ Clinical evidence of goiter
  – Patient with laboratory or imaging abnormalities:
    ○ Substantial hyperlipidemia or change in lipid pattern
    ○ Hyponatremia, often resulting from inappropriate production of antidiuretic hormone
    ○ High serum muscle enzyme concentrations

- o Macrocitic anemia
  - o Pericardial or pleural effusion
  - o Pituitary or hypothalamic disorder
- – Pregnant woman:
  - o If they from an area of moderate to severe iodine insufficiency
  - o Symptomatic hypothyroidism
  - o Personal or family history of thyroid disease
  - o DM type 1
  - o Personal history of thyroid peroxidase antibodies
  - o H/o Recurrent miscarriage, morbid obesity, or infertility
- Recommendations by expert groups:
  - – AAFP recommends periodic assessment in older woman >50 years.
  - – ACP recommends screening of older woman >50 years
  - – ATA and AACE recommend screening of any patient with risk factors and >60 years.
  - – United States Preventive Services Task Force does not recommend routine screening for children or adults.

TREATMENT

MEDICATION
First Line

- Levothyroxine (Synthroid, Levothroid) (1)[B]:
  - – 1.6 mcg/kg/d; increase by 12–25 mcg/d every 4–6 weeks until TSH in normal range (2)[B]
  - – Dosage requirements may vary with age, gender, residual secretory capacity of thyroid gland, other drugs being taken by patient, and intestinal function.
  - – Elderly patients may require 2/3 of dose used in young adults because clearance is decreased.
  - – Levothyroxine should be taken on an empty stomach, ideally an hour before breakfast. Administering at bedtime may result in higher levels than administering in the morning (3)[B].
  - – Medications that interfere with its absorption should be taken 4 hours after the T4 dose: ferrous sulfate, proton pump inhibitors, calcium carbonate, bile acid resins.
- Contraindications:
  - – Thyrotoxic heart disease
  - – Uncorrected adrenocorticoid insufficiency
  - – MI, acute
  - – TSH suppression, pre-existing
- Precautions:
  - – Start with lower doses, such as 25 mcg, in elderly and in patients with heart disease.
  - – Diabetic patients may need readjustment of hypoglycemic agents with institution of thyroxine.
  - – Dosage of oral anticoagulants may need adjustment; monitor prothrombin time while initiating treatment.
- Significant possible interactions:
  - – Oral anticoagulants, insulin, oral hypoglycemic, estrogen, oral contraceptives, cholestyramine, proton pump inhibitors,
  - – Ferrous sulfate, calcium carbonate, antacids, laxatives, colestipol, sucralfate, ciprofloxacin, and cholestyramine may decrease absorption.
  - – Malabsorption of levothyroxine in celiac disease

- Controversy exists whether subclinical hypothyroidism should be treated if asymptomatic (4)[C]. Cochrane Review found no improvement in survival, cardiovascular morbidity, or health-related quality of life. Some evidence indicates improvement in lipid profiles and left ventricular function (5)[B]. Subclinical hypothyroidism should be treated in patients with iron deficiency anemia, and in patients with TSH >10. Treatment may be indicated for patients with TSH between 4.5 and 10 if they are symptomatic.

Pregnancy Considerations
- Replacement therapy may need adjustment, average dose increase from 25–50%.
- TSH levels should be monitored monthly during 1st trimester (6)[C].
- Postpartum: Check TSH levels at 6 weeks.
- Painless subacute thyroiditis may occur in postpartum period, leading to transient hypothyroidism lasting 3 months. Treatment with replacement therapy may be warranted. Up to 30% of these individuals develop permanent hypothyroidism.

Second Line
No benefit to adding triiodothyronine (T3) to thyroxine

ISSUES FOR REFERRAL
- Central hypothyroidism, with low TSH and low free T4, would benefit from an endocrinology referral.
- Hypothyroidism unresponsive to treatment
- Serum TSH remains elevated despite full-dose treatment with levothyroxine

IN-PATIENT CONSIDERATIONS
Admission Criteria/Initial Stabilization
Myxedema coma, hypothermia

ONGOING CARE

FOLLOW-UP RECOMMENDATIONS
Patient Monitoring
- Monitor TSH every 6–12 weeks until stabilized, then annually.
- Follow cardiac status closely in older patients.
- Check TSH more frequently in pregnancy, initiation of estrogen supplementation, or after large changes in body weight.
- In central hypothyroidism, TSH unreliable; must monitor free T4, T3

PATIENT EDUCATION
- Stress importance of compliance with thyroid replacement therapy.
- Explain need for lifelong treatment.
- Instruct to report to physician any signs of infection or heart problems.
- Describe signs of thyrotoxicity.
- High-bulk diet may help avoid constipation.

PROGNOSIS
- Return to normal state is the rule.
- Relapses will occur if treatment is interrupted.
- If untreated, may progress to myxedema coma.

COMPLICATIONS
- Hypothyroid patients (mild to moderate) tolerate surgery, with mortality and complications similar to euthyroid patients.
- If surgery is elective, render patient euthyroid prior to procedure.

- If surgery is urgent, proceed with procedure with individualized replacement therapy preoperatively and postoperatively.
- Treatment-induced congestive heart failure in people with coronary artery disease
- Myxedema coma: Mortality 30–60%
- Increased susceptibility to infection
- Megacolon
- Sexual dysfunction
- Organic psychosis with paranoia
- Adrenal crisis with vigorous treatment of hypothyroidism, especially in patients with undiagnosed polyendocrine syndromes
- Infertility
- Hypersensitivity to opiates
- Treatment over long periods can lead to bone demineralization.
- Subclinical hypothyroidism is associated with increased ischemic heart disease and increased all-cause mortality in men, but not in women.

REFERENCES
1. Khandelwal D, Tandon N. Overt and subclinical hypothyroidism: Who to treat and how. *Drugs*. 2012:17–33.
2. Åsvold BO, Vatten LJ, Midthjell K, et al. Serum TSH within the reference range as a predictor of future hypothyroidism and hyperthyroidism: 11-year follow-up of the HUNT Study in Norway. *J Clin Endocrinol Metab*. 2012;97(1):93–99. Epub 2011 Nov 2.
3. Nienke B, Visser TJ, Nijman J, et al. Effects of evening vs morning levothyroxine intake, a randomized, double blind crossover trial. *Arch Int Med*. 2010;170(22):1996–2003.
4. Cooper DS, Biondi B. Subclinical thyroid disease. *Lancet*. 2012;379(9821):1142–1154. Epub 2012 Jan 23.
5. Villar HC, Saconato H, Valente O, et al. Thyroid hormone replacement for subclinical hypothyroidism. *Cochrane Database Syst Rev*. 2007;(3):CD003419. Epub 2007 Jul 18.
6. Alexander EK, Marqusee E, Lawrence J, et al. Timing and magnitude of increases in levothyroxine requirements during pregnancy in women with hypothyroidism. *N Engl J Med*. 2004;351:241–249.

CODES

ICD10
- E03.8 Other specified hypothyroidism
- E03.9 Hypothyroidism, unspecified
- E89.0 Postprocedural hypothyroidism

CLINICAL PEARLS
- Start low and go slow when initiating thyroxine in an elderly patient or if known cardiovascular disease.
- Once a patient has attained the euthyroid state, maintain on the same brand of thyroxine. There can be up to 12.5% difference in brands considered bioequivalent.
- Monitor TSH every 8–12 weeks until stabilized, then annually.
- The symptoms of hypothyroidism may be vague and diffuse. Maintain a high index of suspicion, especially in women age >50 years.

H

ID REACTION
Michael Terzella, DO • Muhammad Durrani

 BASICS

DESCRIPTION
A generalized skin reaction associated with various infectious (fungal, bacterial, viral, or parasitic) and inflammatory cutaneous conditions distant from the main rash of the disease.

- Id is a word termination often combined with a root reflecting the causative factor (i.e., bacterid, syphilid, and tuberculid). The dermatophytid is the most frequently referenced id reaction in dermatology. A dermatophytid is an autosensitization reaction in which a secondary cutaneous reaction occurs at a site distant to a primary fungal infection. The eruption begins typically within 1–2 weeks of the onset of the main lesion or following exacerbation of the main lesion (1).
- Degrees of Illness: Most commonly localized vesicular lesions, erythema nodosum, and erythema multiforme (1)
- System(s) affected: Skin/Exocrine
- Synonym(s): Dermatophytid, Trichophytid, Autoeczematization

EPIDEMIOLOGY
- Predominant age: All ages
- Predominant sex: Male = Female
- Predominant race: All races

Incidence
Unknown; no good data source

Prevalence
Common

ETIOLOGY AND PATHOPHYSIOLOGY
Precise pathophysiology is uncertain. Circulating antigens may react with antibodies at sensitized areas of the skin, or abnormal immune recognition of autologous skin antigens may occur. It has also been postulated that inflammatory processes may lower irritation threshold of the skin and that hematogenous spread of cytokines from the introductory source may additionally play a role.

- Etiology:
  - Infectious:
    - Fungal Infections: Commonly *T. mentagrophytes, T. rubrum, E. floccosum,* and *Candida* spp. (1,2)
    - Bacterial Infections: Commonly *S. pyogenes, S. aureus,* and *M. tuberculosis* (1)
    - Viral Infections: Commonly HSV, *M. contagiosum,* orf, and milker's nodules (1)
    - Parasitic Infections: Commonly *S. scabiei* and *Leishmania* spp. (1)

  - Allergic:
    - Id reactions have been known to occur in patients with nickel and aluminum allergy
  - Miscellaneous:
    - Rarely, id reaction can develop due to retained sutures postoperatively
    - Rarely, id reaction has been documented in a patient receiving intravesical BCG live therapy for transitional cell carcinoma

RISK FACTORS
- Fungal infection of the skin, especially tinea pedis (1,3)
- Stasis dermatitis

GENERAL PREVENTION
- Minimize factors for developing fungal infections.
- Promptly treat any developing fungal infection.

COMMONLY ASSOCIATED CONDITIONS
- Primary fungal infection
- Stasis dermatitis

 DIAGNOSIS

HISTORY
Itchy rash: Assess for the primary fungal or infectious lesions that would have preceded the onset of the id reaction by days to weeks.

PHYSICAL EXAM
- Common:
  - Symmetric, pruritic vesicles on the palms of hands and, most commonly, on lateral aspects of fingers (2,4)
  - Tinea infection on the feet; contact or other eczematous dermatosis; or bacterial, fungal, or viral infection of the skin
  - Generalized reactions can occur.
- Less common:
  - Papules
  - Lichenoid eruption
- Eczematoid eruption

DIFFERENTIAL DIAGNOSIS
- Pompholyx (dyshidrotic eczema)
- Contact dermatitis
- Drug eruptions
- Pustular psoriasis
- Folliculitis
- Scabies

DIAGNOSTIC TESTS & INTERPRETATION
- Fungal infection at the primary site proven by potassium hydroxide (KOH) or fungal culture
- No fungal elements demonstrable at the site of the presumed id reaction (1)
- Special tests: Skin shows a positive trichophyton reaction (1). A wheal >10 mm at 20 minutes and induration >5 mm at 72 hours is a positive response

Follow-Up Tests & Special Considerations
- The id reaction resolves with successful eradication of the primary skin condition.

- It is important to distinguish dermatophytids from drug-induced allergic reactions, as continued treatment is essential to clear the underlying infection (1)[B].

Test Interpretation
- Histology:
  - Vesicles in the upper dermis
  - Superficial perivascular lymphohistiocytic infiltrate (1)
  - Small numbers of eosinophils (1)
  - Increased granular cell layer (1)
  - No infectious agents present in biopsy specimen (1)

 TREATMENT

GENERAL MEASURES
- Appropriate healthcare: Outpatient

- Treatment of the underlying infection or eczematous dermatitis (1)[B]
- Symptomatic treatment of pruritus with antihistamines and/or topical steroids if needed (may require class 1 or 2 steroid) (1)[B]
- Treatment for secondary bacterial infection (1)[B]

MEDICATION
First Line

- PO antihistamines for pruritus (1,5,6)[A]:
  - Chlorpheniramine: 4 mg (pediatric: 6–12 years 2 mg PO q4-6h PRN; max 12 mg/24 hr; >12 years 4 mg PO q4-6h PRN; max 24 mg/24 hr) PO q4–6h PRN; max 24 mg/24 hr
  - Diphenhydramine: 25–50 mg (pediatric: 5 mg/kg/24 hr divided q6h PRN; 2–5 years max 37.5 mg/24 hr; 6–11 years max 150 mg/24 hr; >12 years max 400 mg/24 hr) PO q4–6h PRN; max 400 mg/24 hr
  - Hydroxyzine: 25–100 mg (pediatric: 2 mg/kg/24 hr divided q6h PRN) PO q6–8h PRN; max 600 mg/24 hr

- Topical treatments for pruritus(5,6,7)[B]:
  - Triamcinolone 0.1% ointment t.i.d.
  - Hydrocortisone 0.5%, 1%, 2.5%: Up to q.i.d.
  - Capsaicin 0.025%, 0.075% cream: Apply t.i.d.–q.i.d.
  - Doxepin 5% cream: Apply q.i.d. for up to 8 days (to max of 10% of the body)
  - EMLA (2.5% lidocaine + 2.5% prilocaine): Apply prior to capsaicin
  - Permethrin 5% cream (for scabies):
    - Apply from neck down after bath.
    - Wash off thoroughly with water in 8–12 hours.
    - May repeat in 7 days
  - Permethrin 1% cream rinse (for lice):
    - Shampoo, rinse, towel dry, saturate hair and scalp (or other affected area), leave on 10 minutes, then rinse.
    - May repeat in 7 days
  - White petrolum emollients: Apply after short bath/shower in warm (not hot) water (5)[A],(6).
- Systemic steroids only if reaction is severe or generalized (e.g., prednisone 20 mg) (1)[C]

Second Line
- Topical and/or systemic antifungals for identified associated fungal infection (common):
  - Tinea cruris/corporis:
    - Topical azole antifungal compounds Econazole (Spectazole), ketoconazole (Nizoral): Usually applied b.i.d. × 2–4 weeks
    - Terbinafine (Lamisil): Over-the-counter (OTC) compound; can be applied once or b.i.d. × 1–2 weeks
    - Butenafine (Mentax): Applied once daily × 2 weeks; also very effective
  - Tinea capitis:
    - PO griseofulvin for *Trichophyton* and *Microsporum* sp.; microsized preparation available; dosage 125 mg/d in patients weighing 10–20 kg; 250 mg/d if weight is 20–40 kg; 500 mg/d if weight is >40 kg; taken b.i.d. or as a single dose daily × 6–12 weeks
    - PO terbinafine can be used for *Trichophyton* sp. at 62.5 mg/d in patients weighing 10–20 kg; 125 mg/d if weight 20–40 kg; 250 mg/d if weight >40 kg; use for 4–6 weeks.
- Topical or systemic antibiotics for any secondary bacterial infection (1)
- Treatment with antiviral agents for erythema multiforme associated with HSV is required (1).

 ONGOING CARE

PATIENT EDUCATION
Avoid hot, humid conditions that promote fungal growth. Aerate susceptible body areas (e.g., wear sandals or open footwear). If possible, wear boxer shorts or loose-fitting clothing, dry off wet skin after bathing, and use powders and antiperspirants to make the environment less conducive to fungal growth. Treat primary dermatitis promptly.

PROGNOSIS
After appropriate treatment, complete resolution in a few days to 2 weeks

COMPLICATIONS
- Secondary bacterial infection (cellulitis)
- After resolution of dermatophytid, post-inflammatory hyperpigmentation is common and disappears without treatment in 1 month (1)

REFERENCES
1. Ilkit M, Durdu M, Karaka M. Cutaneous id reactions: A comprehensive review of clinical manifestations, epidemiology, etiology, and management. *Crit Rev Microbiol*. 2012;38(3): 191–202. Epub 2012 Feb 3.
2. Veien NK. Acute and recurrent vesicular hand dermatitis. *Dermatol Clin*. 2009;27(3):337–353.
3. Stachler RJ, Al-khudari S. Differential diagnosis in allergy. *Otolaryngol Clin North Am*. 2011;44(3): 561–590.
4. Paulsen LL, Geller DD, Guggenbiller M. Symmetrical vesicular eruption on the palms. *Am Fam Physician*. 2012;85(8):811–812.
5. Cotes MES, Swerlick RA. Practical guidelines for the use of steroid-sparing agents in the treatment of chronic pruritus. *Dermatol Ther*. 2013;26(2): 120–134.
6. Yosipovitch G, Bernhard JD. Chronic pruritus. *N Engl J Med*. 2013;368(17):1625–1634.
7. Elmariah SB, Lerner EA. Topical therapies for pruritus. *Semin Cutan Med Surg*. 2011;30(2): 118–126.

ADDITIONAL READING
Greaves MW. Recent advances in pathophysiology and current management of itch. *Ann Acad Med Singap*. 2007;36(9):788–792.

 CODES

ICD10
- B35.9 Dermatophytosis, unspecified
- L30.2 Cutaneous autosensitization

CLINICAL PEARLS
- When assessing an itchy rash, assess for the primary fungal or bacterial lesions that preceded the onset of the id reaction by days to weeks.
- This is a diagnosis in the category of "If you don't think of it, you won't find it," so when you see 1 skin lesion follow another, think of the id reaction.

IDIOPATHIC THROMBOCYTOPENIC PURPURA (ITP)

Kyu K. Jana, MD

 BASICS

DESCRIPTION
- Idiopathic thrombocytopenic purpura (ITP) is an acquired, isolated thrombocytopenia with platelet counts of $<100 \times 10^9$/L caused by accelerated destruction and/or impaired thrombopoiesis by antiplatelet antibodies.
- ITP is classified by:
  - Age: Adult or pediatric
  - Duration: Newly diagnosed (<3 months), persistent, or chronic (>12 months)
  - Whether it occurs in isolation or in association with another disorder: Primary (idiopathic) or secondary
- ITP is a relatively common disease of childhood that often follows viral infection or vaccination. Onset is within 1 week, and spontaneous resolution occurs within 2 months in 83% of patients.
- In adults, ITP is usually a chronic disease and spontaneous remission is rare (9% in 1 series) (1).
- System(s) affected: Heme, Lymphatic, Immunologic
- Synonym(s): Immune thrombocytopenia; Immune thrombocytopenic purpura; and Werlhof disease

EPIDEMIOLOGY
- Peak age:
  - Pediatric ITP: 2–4 years
  - Chronic ITP: >50 years
  - Uncommon in geriatric population
- Predominant gender:
  - Pediatric ITP: Male = Female
  - Chronic ITP: Female > Male (1.2–1.7:1)

Incidence
Meta-analysis of 3 studies from Europe estimated incidence at:
- 1.9–6.4/100,000 children/year
- 3.3/100,000 adults/year (2)

Prevalence
- Based on insurance data, overall prevalence of 9.5/100,000 persons
- Based on survey of hematologists in 2004:
  - Overall prevalence of 11.2/100,000 persons
  - In children (<16 years), 8.1/100,000 with average age of 6 years
  - In adults (>16), 12.1/100,000 persons with average age of 55 (3)

ETIOLOGY AND PATHOPHYSIOLOGY
- Accelerated platelet uptake and destruction by reticuloendothelial phagocytes results from action of IgG autoantibodies against platelet membrane glycoproteins IIb/IIIa. There is also cell-mediated platelet destruction by CD8+ T cells.
- Autoantibodies interfere with megakaryocyte maturation, resulting in decreased production.

RISK FACTORS
- Autoimmune thrombocytopenia (e.g., Evan syndrome)
- Common variable immune deficiency
- Drug side effect (e.g., quinidine, gold, penicillin, procainamide, methyldopa, sulfamethoxazole)
- Infections: *H. pylori*, hepatitis C, HIV, varicella zoster
- Vaccination side effect
- Bone marrow transplantation side effect
- Connective tissue disease, such as systemic lupus erythematosus, antiphospholipid antibody syndrome
- Lymphoproliferative disorders

COMMONLY ASSOCIATED CONDITIONS
- Viral infections, such as measles, rubella, varicella, influenza, and EBV
- Live virus vaccinations carry a lower risk than natural viral infection: 2.6/100,000 cases MMR vaccine doses vs. 6–1,200/100,000 cases of natural rubella or measles infections

 DIAGNOSIS

A careful history, physical exam, and review of CBC and peripheral blood smear remain the key components of the diagnosis of ITP.

HISTORY
- Can be asymptomatic; often found incidentally on routine CBC
- Posttraumatic bleeding occurs at counts of 40–60×10^9/L.
- With counts $<30 \times 10^9$/L, bruising tendency, epistaxis, menorrhagia, and gingival bleeding are common.
- GI bleeding, hematuria, and hemoptysis are less common.
- Spontaneous bleeding may occur with platelet count $<20 \times 10^9$/L.
- Intracerebral bleeding is rare and may occur with counts $<20 \times 10^9$/L and associated trauma or vascular lesions, resulting in neurologic symptoms.
- Constitutional symptoms are absent except for fatigue unrelated to treatment.

PHYSICAL EXAM
- Purpura, which are nonpalpable and nonblanching ecchymosis and petechiae, may be present in extremities and areas exposed to pressure.
- Mucocutaneous hemorrhages may be present.
- Hemorrhagic bullae on buccal mucosa reflect acute, severe thrombocytopenia.
- Absence of splenomegaly is an essential diagnostic criterion. Also absent: Hepatomegaly, lymphadenopathy, stigmata of congenital disease

DIFFERENTIAL DIAGNOSIS
- Acute leukemia
- Thrombotic thrombocytopenia purpura
- Hemolytic uremic syndrome
- Factitious: Platelet clumping on peripheral smear
- Thrombocytopenia secondary to sepsis
- Myelodysplastic syndrome, particularly in older patients
- Decreased marrow production: Malignancy, drugs, viruses, megaloblastic anemia
- Posttransfusion
- Gestational thrombocytopenia
- Isoimmune neonatal purpura
- Congenital thrombocytopenias
- Disseminated intravascular coagulation
- Alcohol-induced thrombocytopenic purpura

DIAGNOSTIC TESTS & INTERPRETATION
Initial Tests (lab, imaging)
- CBC with differential and peripheral smear:
  - Isolated decreased platelet count $<100 \times 10^9$/L
  - Giant platelets are usually present.
- For patients with history, exam, CBC, and peripheral smear typical of ITP, only the following tests may be needed:
  - PT/PTT is normal.

- In adult ITP, serologies to exclude hepatitis B and C and HIV infections are recommended.
- In pediatric ITP, immunoglobulins levels to exclude common variable immunodeficiency are commonly obtained.
- Other tests are not necessary for patients with typical ITP presentation: Antiplatelet, antinuclear, antiphospholipid antibodies; *H. pylori* testing; thrombopoietin; platelet parameters; direct antiglobulin test; reticulocyte count; urinalysis; and thyroid function tests

Diagnostic Procedures/Other
- Imaging is not necessary.
- Bone marrow aspiration/biopsy:
  - Not part of routine workup, and not necessary for diagnosis irrespective of age of patients presenting with typical ITP
  - Can be considered for a patient with atypical symptoms, such as fever and weight loss and multiple abnormalities in blood count

Test Interpretation
- Peripheral smear: Normal red and white cells with large or giant platelets, but diminished in number
- Marrow reveals abundant megakaryocytes with normal erythroid and myeloid precursors.

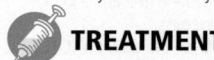 **TREATMENT**

GENERAL MEASURES
- Outpatient management unless patient has platelet count $<20 \times 10^9$/L and is at risk for bleeding.
- Admit patients with active bleeding.

MEDICATION
First Line
- Pediatric ITP:
  - For children with no or mild bleeding (bruising and petechiae only and no mucosal bleeding), observation alone regardless of platelet count (4)[A].
  - For children with significant bleeding:
    - Single-dose γ-globulin (IVIg) 0.8–1 g/kg (4)[A], especially when a more rapid increase in platelet count is desired. Do not administer in patients with IgA deficiencies because of anaphylaxis risk.
    - A short course of corticosteroids (4)[C] (e.g., PO prednisone 2 mg/kg/d for 2 weeks with 3 weeks taper)
    - For nonsplenectomized children who are Rh-positive, single dose of anti-Rho(D) immunoglobulin (anti-D), 50–75 μg/kg (4)[C]. Do not use in children with low hemoglobin or evidence of hemolysis (4)[A].
- Adult ITP (4):
  - Treatment is recommended for newly diagnosed patients with platelet count $<30 \times 10^9$/L (4)[C].
  - Longer course of corticosteroids preferred (e.g., PO prednisone 1 mg/kg/d for 21 days then tapered (5)[B] with addition of IVIg to corticosteroids when a more rapid increase in platelet count is required (4)[C])
  - If corticosteroids are contraindicated:
    - IVIg, 1–2 g/kg once, repeating as necessary
    - OR anti-D, 50–75 μg/kg once, repeating as necessary for Rh+, nonsplenectomized patients (4)[C]. Do not use anti-D in patients with low hemoglobin or evidence of hemolysis.

- ITP in pregnancy:
  - Preeclampsia or gestational thrombocytopenia may cause thrombocytopenia unrelated to ITP.
  - Corticosteroids or IVIg are considered safe and are considered first line.
  - ITP management at time of delivery is based on maternal bleeding risks, and mode of delivery should be based on obstetric indications. Platelet autoantibodies can cross the placenta and cause neonatal thrombocytopenia.
  - Caesarean section can be considered if platelet count >50 × 10^9/L.
  - Prednisone and/or IVIg may be considered 2–3 weeks prior to delivery.
- ITP secondary to HIV:
  - Antivirals should be considered before other treatment.
  - If treatment is required, corticosteroids, IVIg, anti-D, or splenectomies are initial options.
- ITP secondary to HCV:
  - Antivirals should be considered before other treatment.
  - If treatment required, IVIg is initial treatment.
- Emergency treatment of patients with intracranial or GI bleeding, massive hematuria, internal hematoma, or who need emergent surgery include (6):
  - IV corticosteroids (e.g., IV methylprednisolone, 1 g/d for 3 days); caution in patients with GI bleeding.
  - IVIg 1 g/kg, repeat following day for count <50 × 10^9/L
  - Platelet transfusions may also be considered for significant bleeding.
  - Other agents that may be considered: Recombinant factor VIIa promotes hemostasis but also increases risk of thrombosis. Efficacy of antifibrinolytic agents, aminocaproic acids, and tranexamic acid, is unproved; they may be used as adjunctive treatments only.

Second Line
- Pediatric and adolescent ITP:
  - Splenectomy if ITP persistent (4)[C]
  - Rituximab (Rituxan) 375 mg/m² weekly for 4 weeks (7)[C]
  - High-dose dexamethasone 0.6 mg/kg/d for 4 days every 4 weeks (8)[C]
  - Others without adequate data: azathioprine, cyclosporin A, danazol, mycophenolate mofetil, anti-CD52 monoclonal antibody, and interferon
- Adult ITP:
  - Splenectomy for patients who failed corticosteroid therapy (4)[A]
  - Rituximab, 375 mg/m² weekly for 4 weeks, for patients at high risk of bleeding who have failed one line of therapy or post-splenectomy (4)[A]
  - Consider combination therapy with dexamethasone and rituximab (9)[B]
  - For patients for whom splenectomy is contraindicated, thrombopoietin receptor agonists: eltrombopag (Nplate), 50 mg/d PO *OR* romiplostim (Promacta), 1 mcg/kg SC weekly; may be used for patients at high risk of bleeding (5,9)[A].
  - Thrombopoietin receptor agonists can be considered for patients at risk of bleeding who failed 1 line of therapy (4)[A].

  - Others to consider: azathioprine, cyclosporine A, cyclophosphamide, danazol, dapsone, mycophenolate mofetil, and vincristine.

ISSUES FOR REFERRAL
Hematology consultation recommended for acute bleeding or for those who fail to respond to first-line therapies.

ADDITIONAL THERAPIES
Traditional Chinese medicine which has shown benefit in small, nonrandomized controlled trials: Dihuang Zhixue, Kami-kihi-to, Minor Decoction of Bupleurum, Replenishing Qi and Tonifying Kidney, Roasted Licorice Decoction, Sairei-to, Shengxueling, and Zhinu-I and Zhinu-II. Unclear or conflicting evidence for active hexose correlated compound, berberine, dong quai, ginseng, licorice, melatonin and periwinkle (10).

SURGERY/OTHER PROCEDURES
Splenectomy:
- Mortality rate is very low (<1%) even in patients with severe thrombocytopenia.
- Necessary vaccinations prior to splenectomy: Polyvalent pneumococcal vaccine and quadrivalent meningococcal vaccine every 3–5 years; and 1-time *H. influenza b* (Hib).
- Consider lifelong prophylactic antibiotics with penicillin or erythromycin.
- Should raise the platelet count to at least 20 × 10^9/L prior to surgery.
- Reported 5–10-year efficacy is ~65% for all patients (5).
- Open and laparoscopic splenectomy have similar efficacies (4)[A].

 ONGOING CARE

FOLLOW-UP RECOMMENDATIONS
Patient Monitoring
Platelet counts weekly for patients on prednisone and monthly for stable patients are reasonable.

DIET
- Evidence demonstrating benefit of an anti-inflammatory diet in ITP is lacking.
- The following foods and supplements can cause significant bleeding: Garlic, ginger, *Gingko biloba*, and saw palmetto (10).
- Some foods and supplements that may inhibit platelets: evening primrose oil, fish oil, feverfew, ginseng, liquorice, soy, vitamin C, vitamin E, and wintergreen (10).
- Partial list of foods and supplements with coumarin or salicylate components: alfalfa, angelica, anise, asafetida, aspen bark, birch, black cohosh, celery, chamomile, cinnamon, dandelion, fenugreek, heartsease, horse chestnut, meadowsweet, poplar, prickly ash, quassia, sarsaparilla, sweet birch, sweet clover, and willow bark (10).

PATIENT EDUCATION
- Modified activity to prevent injury or bruising; avoid contact sports.
- Avoid anticoagulants; aspirin and other platelet-inhibiting drugs; and NSAIDs.

PROGNOSIS
- Acute ITP:
  - ~80–85% of patients completely recover within 2 months.
  - 15% proceed to chronic ITP.
- Chronic ITP:
  - ~10–20% of the patients recover spontaneously.
  - Remainder with diminished platelets for months to years
  - May see spontaneous remissions (5%) and relapses

- ~10% are refractory (fail medical therapy and splenectomy)

COMPLICATIONS
- Related to thrombocytopenia: 1% mortality due to intracranial hemorrhage and severe blood loss
- Related to treatment: e.g., corticosteroid adverse effects; anaphylaxis and renal failure with IVIg; hepatotoxicity with eltrombopag; reports of progressive multifocal leukoencephalopathy with rituximab; hemolysis with anti-D; and septicemia for splenectomized patients

REFERENCES
1. Fogarty PF. Chronic immune thrombocytopenia in adults: Epidemiology and clinical presentation. *Hematol Oncol Clin North Am.* 2009;23: 1213–1221.
2. Terrell DR, Beebe LA, Vesely SK, et al. The incidence of immune thrombocytopenic purpura in children and adults: A critical review of published reports. *Am J Hematol.* 2010;85:174–180.
3. Terrell D, Beebe LA, George JN, et al. Prevalence of immune thrombocytopenic purpura. 50th ASH Annual Meeting and Exposition Oral and Poster Abtracts, December 6, 2008, updated October 26, 2010.
4. Neunert C, Lim W, Crowtha M, et al. The American Society of Hematology 2011 evidence-based practice guideline for immune thrombocytopenia. *Blood.* 2011;117(16): 4190–4207.
5. Bussel JB. Traditional and new approaches to the management of immune thrombocytopenia: Issues of when and who to treat. *Hematol Oncol Clin North Am.* 2009;23:1329–1341.
6. Stasi R, Evangelista ML, Stipa E, et al. Idiopathic thrombocytopenic purpura: Current concepts in pathophysiology and management. *Thromb Haemost.* 2008;99(1):4–13.
7. Parodi E, Rivetti E, Amendola G, et al. Long-term follow-up analysis after rituximab therapy in children with refractory symptomatic ITP: Identification of factors predictive of a sustained response. *Br J Haematol.* 2009;144(4):552–558. Epub 2008 Nov 22.
8. Gudbrandsodttir S, Birgens HS, Frederiksen H, et al. Rituximab and dexamethasone vs dexamethasone monotherapy in newly diagnosed patients with primary immune thrombocytopenia. *Blood* 2013:121(11):1976–1981.
9. Tarantino MD. The treatment of immune thrombocytopenic purpura in children. *Curr Hematol Rep.* 2006;5:89–94.
10. Naturalstandard.com accessed Jun 3 2013.

 CODES

ICD10
D69.3 Immune thrombocytopenic purpura

CLINICAL PEARLS
- ITP: Platelet counts of <100 × 10^9/L caused by accelerated destruction and/or impaired thrombopoiesis by antiplatelet antibodies
- Pediatric ITP: Relatively common, with spontaneous remission in 2 months.
- Adult ITP: Usually persistent; requires treatment, with rare spontaneous remission.

IGA NEPHROPATHY

Mony Fraer MD, FACP, FASN • Tomoki Tsukahara, MD

 BASICS

DESCRIPTION

- Most common form of glomerulonephritis in the world (particularly high incidence in Asia) resulting from deposition of large amounts of a modified IgA molecule in the glomerular mesangium.
- A heterogeneous condition ranging from asymptomatic to end-stage renal disease (ESRD)

EPIDEMIOLOGY

Incidence

30–40% in Asia, 15–20% in Europe, and 5–10% in North America of all renal biopsies performed

Prevalence

- More common in Asians (particularly in Japan and Korea), Caucasians, and American Indians
- Less common in blacks in the US and Africa
- Most common in 2nd and 3rd decades of life
- Male > Female

ETIOLOGY AND PATHOPHYSIOLOGY

- Polymeric, abnormally glycosylated IgA1 deposition within the mesangium leads to an inflammatory reaction and IgG autoantibodies production.
- The cytokines, chemokines, and local complement activation leads to podocyte injury.

Genetics

Rare familial forms of IgA nephropathy (IgAN) exist.

COMMONLY ASSOCIATED CONDITIONS

Diseases associated with glomerular IgA deposition and secondary forms of IgA nephropathy (1):

- Henoch-Schönlein purpura
- Diseases of the liver (alcoholic, primary biliary, or cryptogenic cirrhosis, etc.)
- Diseases of the intestine (celiac disease, inflammatory bowel disease)
- Diseases of the skin (dermatitis herpetiformis, psoriasis)
- Diseases of the lung (sarcoidosis, idiopathic pulmonary hemosiderosis, cystic fibrosis, etc.)
- Malignancy
- Infection (HIV)
- Other systemic or immunologic disorders (systemic lupus erythematosus, rheumatoid arthritis, cryoglobulinemia, etc.)

 DIAGNOSIS

HISTORY

- Classically presents with painless recurrent episodes of macroscopic hematuria concurrent to or immediately after viral URIs.
- Wide spectrum from asymptomatic microscopic hematuria to acute renal failure

PHYSICAL EXAM

- Hypertension (HTN)
- Edema

DIFFERENTIAL DIAGNOSIS

Other conditions associated/presenting with microscopic hematuria:

- Thin basement membrane disease
- Alport syndrome
- Lupus nephritis
- Postinfectious glomerulonephritis
- Nephrolithiasis
- Urinary tract malignancy
- Henoch-Schönlein purpura (also presenting with IgA deposition)

DIAGNOSTIC TESTS & INTERPRETATION

Initial Tests (lab, imaging)

- Serum BUN and creatinine to evaluate for renal insufficiency
- Complement levels should be normal.
- Urinalysis with microscopy to evaluate for proteinuria, hematuria, dysmorphic RBCs and RBC casts
- Spot urine protein to creatinine ratio or 24-hour urine protein
- Imaging may be indicated to rule out other urologic causes of hematuria

Diagnostic Procedures/Other

Renal biopsy is the gold standard and the only definitive method for the diagnosis IgAN.

Test Interpretation

- Light microscopy: Variable findings ranging from mesangial cell proliferation and expansion to crescentic or chronic sclerosing glomerulonephritis
- Immunofluorescence staining: Pathognomonic finding of IgA deposits in a diffuse pattern within the mesangium
- Electron microscopy: Electron-dense deposits in the mesangium

 TREATMENT

GENERAL MEASURES

KDIGO guidelines:

- Monitor low-risk patients with no HTN, normal GFR, and proteinuria <0.5 g/d
- Supportive treatment with ACE inhibitor (ACEI) or angiotensin receptor blocker (ARB) is the cornerstone of the treatment.
- Good, randomized clinical trials to determine optimal treatments are still lacking.

MEDICATION

First Line

- Antiproteinuric and antihypertensive ACEI or ARB to achieve BP target of 130/80 mm Hg (125/75 mm Hg if proteinuria is >1 g/d) and decrease proteinuria to <0.5 g/d (2)[A]
- 6-month trial of pulse or oral corticosteroids in addition to RAS blockade in patients with persistent (>3–6 months) proteinuria (>1 g/d) (3,4)[B]
- Cyclophosphamide in combination with steroids has been shown to improve renal survival in patients with crescentic forms of IgAN if eGFR >30 mL/min (5)[B]

Second Line

Omega-3 fatty acids in large doses (12 g/d) may be beneficial in preserving renal function for persistent proteinuria despite ACEI/ARB use (6)[B].

ISSUES FOR REFERRAL

Any patients with significant hematuria, proteinuria, or abnormal renal function should be referred to a nephrologist early.

ADDITIONAL THERAPIES

Prevention of CKD progression and its consequence:
- Lipid-lowering therapies with a statin ($\pm$ ezetimibe)
- Low-salt diet ($\pm$ diuretics)
- Antihypertensives
- Smoking cessation, etc.

SURGERY/OTHER PROCEDURES

Consider referring for kidney transplant evaluation when the patient is reaching CKD stage 5.

IN-PATIENT CONSIDERATIONS

Admission Criteria/Initial Stabilization
Acute kidney injury or complications related to CKD

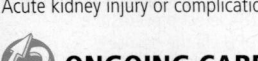

ONGOING CARE

FOLLOW-UP RECOMMENDATIONS
- Patients with mild proteinuria (<500 mg/d), normal renal function, and normal BP may be treated conservatively with regular follow-up at 6-month intervals.
- Patients with more aggressive disease characterized by persistent hematuria, higher grade proteinuria, difficult-to-control HTN, or decreased GFR will require closer monitoring.

Patient Monitoring
- Blood pressure
- Serum electrolytes
- Serum creatinine
- Urine microscopy to evaluate disease activity
- Quantification of urine protein

DIET
Low-sodium diet

PATIENT EDUCATION
- Avoid NSAIDs
- Avoid IV contrast exposure
- In patients approaching ESRD, educate regarding options for RRT

PROGNOSIS
- HTN, proteinuria (>1 g/d), and decreased GFR are risk factors for progressiong of CKD (7).
- Specific histologic findings also have some prognostic significance.

COMPLICATIONS
- 25–30% of patients will require renal replacement therapy (RRT) (e.g., dialysis, transplant) within 20–25 years of presentation (8).
- 1.5% of patients reach ESRD each year (8).
- 5% risk of kidney graft failure secondary to a reccurrent IgAN 5 years after renal transplant (8).

REFERENCES

1. Donavio JV and Grande JP. IgA Nephropathy. *N Engl J Med*. 2002;347:738–748.
2. Cheng J. ACEI/ARB therapy for IgA nephropathy: A meta analysis of randomized controlled trials. *Int J Clin Pract*. 2009;63(6):880–888.
3. Cheng J. Efficacy and safety of glucocorticoids therapy for IgA nephropathy: A meta-analysis of randomized controlled trials. *Am J Nephrol*. 2009;30:315–322.
4. Manno C. Randomized controlled clinical trial of corticosteroids plus ACE-inhibitors with long-term follow-up in proteinuric IgA nephropathy. *Nephrol Dial Transplant*. 2009;24:3694–3701.
5. Tumlin J. Crescentic, proliferative IgA nephropathy: Clinical and histological response to methylprednisolone and intravenous cyclophosphamide. *Nephrol Dial Transplant*. 2003;18:1321–1329.
6. Donadio J. A controlled trial of fish oil in IgA nephropathy. *NEJM*. 1994;331:1194–1199.
7. Barbour SJ, Reich HN. Risk stratification of patients with IgA nephropathy. *AJKD*. 2012;59:865–873.
8. Barratt J, Feehally J. IgA nephropathy. *J Am Soc Nephrol*. 2005;16:2088–2097.

ADDITIONAL READING
- Floege J and Eitner F. Current therapy for IgA nephropathy. *J Am Soc Nephrol* 2011;22: 1785–1794.
- Kidney Disease: Improving Global Outcomes (KDIGO) glomerulonephritis work group. KDIGO Clinical Practice Guideline for Glomerulonephritis. *Kidney Int*. 2012;(Suppl 2):139–274.

 CODES

ICD10
N02.8 Recurrent and persistent hematuria w oth morphologic changes

CLINICAL PEARLS
- IgAN is the most common cause of glomerulonephritis in the world.
- It has a wide clinical spectrum from asymptomatic microscopic hematuria to ESRD.
- Clinical risk factors for progressive disease are an abnormal GFR, HTN, and moderate to severe proteinuria.
- Control of proteinuria and hypertension via RAAS blockade with ACE inhibitors and/or ARBs is the mainstay of therapy.

IMMUNODEFICIENCY DISEASES

Brian P. Peppers, DO, PhD • Robert W. Hostoffer, DO, FACOP, FAAP

BASICS

DESCRIPTION

- Diseases of the immune system can be either primary or secondary (acquired). There are numerous causes; each may lead to increased risk of infections, autoimmune diseases, and cancers.
- Primary immunodeficiency disease (PID): An intrinsic defect in the immune system affecting receptor function, cytoplasmic enzymes, and gene regulatory proteins. These defects affect the maturation and function of B-cells, T-cells, phagocytes, the complement system, and NK-cells. Depending on the defect, effects may be seen directly or indirectly in ≥1 systems.
- B-cells: Humoral immunodeficiencies: Defects in antibody production that typically present clinically as recurrent sinopulmonary infections > gastrointestinal. Most common form of PID (~2/3). Aliments are not normally seen before 6 months of age due to maternal antibodies:
  - IgA deficiency: Most common primary immunodeficiency: Clinical symptoms range from asymptomatic/mild to severe. Sporadic more common than inherited. Spanish and Arabian populations more so than European (~1:150 to 1:400+, respectively). Asian population least at risk (~1:2,600–1:18,000). At risk for autoimmune diseases such as rheumatoid arthritis (RA) (at any age), systemic lupus erythematosus (SLE). Children <5 presenting with IgA deficiency may out grow it.
  - Common variable immunodeficiency: A heterogeneous form of severe antibody deficiency. Low immunoglobulins (IgG, IgA, and/or IgM) leaves the individual susceptible to pyogenic infections. Moderate to severe clinical systems are more common than mild/asymptomatic. Adult onset (mid-20s) more so than childhood. Sporadic (~90%) more common than inherited. Incidence for CVID 1:25,000–1:66,000. Northern European descent more so than African, Asian, and Hispanic. Men/women equal risk. Similar risks and family history as with IgA deficiency. Treatment is important to prevent bronchiectasis, malabsorption, vitamin deficiencies.
  - X-linked agammaglobulinemia (XLA): Xq22; Bruton tyrosine kinase. Recurrent infections with encapsulated bacteria a few months after birth are common. Growth and development are usually normal. All serum immunoglobulins are extremely low. T and NK cells function are preserved. On physical exam the tonsils, adenoids, and peripheral lymph nodes are greatly diminished in size.
  - Hyper-IgM syndrome (HIMG): Similar infections as XLA. Pneumocystis jiroveci pneumonia on initial presentation is possible along with neutropenia. Defect of either B-cell's isotype switching from IgM-secreting to IgG, A, or E (HIMG1-4: autosomal recessive [AR], NEMO) or help T-cell's inability to signal/activate B cells (X-linked: Xq26 and formerly a T-cell PID). Serum IgM concentration is normal to elevated and polyclonal.
  - Other examples: Defects in Ig heavy chain gene, hypogammaglobulinemia.
- T-cells (cellular-mediated immunodeficiencies): Defects in maturation or function of T-lymphocytes. Predisposed to infections such as Candida, parasite and P. jiroveci:

- 22q11.2 deletion syndrome/DiGeorge syndrome: Defect of embryogenesis. Structures involved include thymus, parathyroid, aortic arch. De novo or autosomal dominant (AD). Prevalence is ~1:4000. Normally diagnosed in infancy. Characteristics (CATCH 22): Cardiac abnormalities, hypognathus, long philtrum, low set ears, hypertelorism, downward slanted eyes, "carp shaped" mouth, thymic abnormalities (absent thymic shadow), cleft palate, hypoparathyroidism
- Chronic mucocutaneous candidiasis: A heterogenous group of disorders involving recurrent Candida infections. May occur anywhere on the body and at any point in life. Disease can be familial (STAT 1: AD). Although Candida is the defining infection, it may expand to incorporate other organisms. Endocrine abnormalities are normally involved.
- Combined immunodeficiencies: Defects in the cellular effector and humoral mechanisms directly involving a combination of B-, T-lymphocytes, and NK cells. Typically present as failure to thrive, often with diarrhea and severe eczema.
  - Severe combined immunodeficiency (SCID): Depending on genetic mutation, patients may have absent T cells with/without impairment to B cells and/or NK-cells. Presents in infancy with failure to thrive, recurrent or persistent thrush, gastrointestinal illnesses. Prevalence 1/50,000–100,000. If treatment is unsuccessful or delayed, death normally occurs before 1–2 years of age. X-linked, AR, and mutations in adenosine deaminase deficiency gene, purine nucleoside phosphorylase deficiency gene, interleukin-γ chain, JAK3, CD45, ZAP70, RAG1, and RAG2 genes are known.
  - Major histocompatibility complex (MHC) class II deficiency: Absence of human leukocyte antigen (HLA) class II expression. Primarily found in infants born in Saudi Arabia. AR mutations affect 1–4 regulatory factors: CIITA, RFXANK, RFX5, and RFXAP. Illness patterns are similar to SCID.
  - Other examples: Wiskott-Aldrich syndrome (X-linked) and ataxia telangiectasia (AR)
- Phagocytic immunodeficiencies: Defects in the function and/or quantity of phagocyte cells. Recurrent pyogenic infections such as staphylococcal and Aspergillus, Klebsiella, Pseudomonas. Granulomatous formations and poor wound healing are common.
  - Chronic granulomatous disease: 90% inherited disorder (X-linked and AR) of phagocytic cells; results from an inability of phagocytes to undergo respiratory burst (key enzyme: NADPH oxidase). Recurrent life-threatening bacterial and fungal infections, often involving lymph nodes, liver, spleen, and skin. Normally occurs early in life. X-linked: Mutation of cytochrome gp91 or b558 genes, called CYBB. AR: Chromosome 7, gene called NCF1 (p47phox).
  - Myeloperoxidase deficiency: Myeloperoxidase is an enzyme that facilitates the use of hydrogen peroxide to oxidize chloride and iodide to make perchloric and periodic acid, respectively. Deficiency results in the attenuation of killing bacteria by PMNs. Other mechanisms seem to compensate; there is only a slight increase in the infection rate and rarely life-threatening. Most individuals are asymptomatic, but some may have recurrent candidal infections. AR: 17q21.3-q23.

- Leukocyte adhesion deficiency: An AR disorder resulting in a dysfunction of cell surface adhesion. The defect is in CD18; common to several members of the integrin family. They are important in stabilizing macrophage interaction with T cells and opsonize most pathogenic Staphylococci species for removal by macrophages. Delayed separation of the umbilical cord may be seen in the neonatal period. Later in life, recurrent pyogenic infections without pus formation are common.
- Glucose-6-phosphate dehydrogenase deficiency: This X-linked (Xq28) defect prevents the generation of NADPH via the hexose monophosphate shunt. The resultant lack of NADPH oxidase produces a clinical picture very similar to CGD. Differs by a later age of onset (>10 years). Also associated with hemolytic anemia and commonly presents as such.
- Other examples: Chediak-Higashi syndrome and lazy leukocyte syndrome.
- Complement deficiencies: Deficiencies of the complement components have been reported for most of the constituents. These deficiencies can be inherited or acquired and complete or partial:
  - Classical (C1, C4, C2): Immune complex diseases (e.g., discoid or systemic lupus erythematosus, pneumococcal infections)
  - Alternative (properdin, factor B, factor D): Severe fulminant pyogenic neisserial infections with a high mortality rate
  - Mannose-binding lectin: Recurrent infections, accelerated course of SLE and rheumatoid arthritis.
  - Other examples: C3, factor H, and factor I (pyogenic bacterial infections). Terminal pathway C5–C9 (neisserial and bacterial infections).
- Gene regulatory protein defects MISC
- Immune dysregulation polyendocrinopathy Enteropathy X- linked (IPEX): Classically seen as a syndrome of diarrhea, polyendocrinopathy, and fatal infection in infancy. Involves neonatal onset diabetes mellitus, hypothyroidism, enteritis (diarrhea/villous atrophy), hemolytic anemia and thrombocytopenia, dermatitis: Erythema, eczema, psoriasiform. Death normally occurs by 1–2 years of age. Missense mutations in FOXP3 result in a rheostat of the immune response, impaired development and function of CD4+CD25 and regulatory T cells, and may function as a transcriptional repressor of cytokine promoters.
- Hyper-IgE syndrome: Recurrent severe staphylococcal abscesses (skin, lungs, and viscera). Characteristic facial features include prominent forehead, deep-set eyes, a broad nasal bridge, a wide fleshy nasal tip, mild prognathism, facial asymmetry, hemihypertrophy. Extremely high serum IgE, elevated serum IgD, and normal concentrations of IgG, IgA, and IgM. STAT3 gene mutation (AD form of inheritance with incomplete penetrance).

- Secondary immunodeficiency disease: Either acquired as a result of age, malnutrition, pregnancy, illness, treatment(s), or injury. May be transient (newborn) or permanent (HIV) (1)[A]. Also more common than PID and tend to be occur later in life:
- Age: Premature, newborn infants and the elderly
- Illnesses: HIV/AIDS, cancers, leukemias, lymphomas, myeloma, aplastic anemia, autoimmune diseases, cirrhosis, depression/stress
- Medications/treatments: Corticosteroids, radiation, chemotherapy, immunosuppressants (tacrolimus, cyclosporine, rituximab), splenectomy

– Injury: Burns, trauma (accidental, intentional, surgical).

GENERAL PREVENTION

- Early identification is key to prevent infection and possible comorbid conditions. For newborns: Those with known family history may use genetic counseling and prenatal diagnostic tests to help diagnose prior to birth.
- Proper hygiene and nutrition for all ages regardless of type of immunodeficiency.
- For certain secondary immunodeficiencies such as HIV, Hepatitis B and C, safe needle practices and safe sexual practices are helpful for prevention.

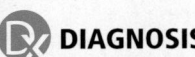 DIAGNOSIS

HISTORY

- Both a complete personal and family history is key to direct diagnosis; limit blood work, radiation exposure, and time invested for both patient and physician. Recurrent respiratory infections are the most common clinical manifestations of PID.
- 10 signs of possible primary immunodeficiency:
  - ≥4 new ear infections in 1 year
  - ≥2 serious sinus infections in 1 year
  - ≥2 months on antibiotics with little effect
  - ≥2 pneumonias within 1 year
  - Failure of an infant to gain weight or grow
  - Recurrent deep skin or organ abscesses
  - Persistent thrush or fungal infections on skin
  - Need for IV antibiotics to clear an infection
  - ≥2 deep-seated infections (e.g., sepsis)
  - Family history of primary immunodeficiency
- Infection history and possible clues:
  - Pneumococcus, *Haemophilus* influenza, etc.: Think B-cell defect
  - PCP, *Candida*, parasites: Think T-cell defect
  - *Aspergillus, Klebsiella, Pseudomonas*: Think PMN defect
  - Meningococcus: Think complement defect
- Family history: Similar symptoms, known PID, autoimmune diseases, early infant deaths, cancers, or hemolytic diseases
- Newborn screening: SCID testing is currently included in WI, MA, NY, CA, CT, MI, CO, MS, DE, FL, TX, MN, IA, PA, UT, OH, and Ontario, Canada (2).

PHYSICAL EXAM

Highly dependent on ailment: such as DiGeorge, dysmorphology listed above, and CVID: Sinus tenderness, PNA

DIAGNOSTIC TESTS & INTERPRETATION
Initial Tests (lab, imaging)

- Complete blood count with differential
- Serum protein electrophoresis for immunoglobulin levels, including IgG, IgA, IgM, and IgE
- X-rays or CT scans if indicated (concern for SCID or DiGeorge, absent thymic shadow, PNA, abscesses)
- Analogous to differences in radiographs among infants, children, and adults, it is equally important to keep in mind differences in lab values as well.

Follow-Up Tests & Special Considerations

It is generally considered appropriate to consult an immunologist before ordering any additional test. Based on clinical and preliminary lab results, here are some additional tests that can be ordered (3,4)[A]:

- Flow cytometry to examine lymphocyte subsets (CD4, CD8, CD3, CD19, CD20): Helps to detect deficiency in T, B, NKT, and NK cells.

- B-cells: Antibody responses to vaccines (e.g., *Pneumococcus*, tetanus): Helps to test the function of the humoral systems response to antigens
- T-cells: T-cell enumeration, mitogen/antigen stimulation, FISH.
- Combined immunodeficiencies: T-cell enumeration, mitogen/antigen stimulation, ADA/PNP activity, ZAP 70, and IL2-γ chain evaluation
- Phagocyte immunodeficiencies: Nitroblue tetrazolium test, dihydrorhodamine reductase test, chemiluminescence, biopsy of granules, chemotaxis assay
- Complement deficiencies: CH50, AH 50, individual complement components
- NK cell deficiency: NK-cell function test

 TREATMENT

GENERAL MEASURES

- All live attenuated viral vaccines should be avoided in patients with severe cellular or antibody immunodeficiencies. These include intranasal influenza, varicella, zoster, measles, mumps, rubella, oral polio, smallpox, Bacille Calmette-Guérin. Please consult the CDC's Advisory Committee on Immunization Practices (ACIP) regarding vaccine safety for up-to-date recommendations.
- Those receiving or who have received immunoglobulin replacement therapy (IgG) in the past 6 months are considered passively immune and do not require vaccination.
- Blood transfusions must use irradiated and CMV-negative blood products for those with cellular or combined defects.
- Bone marrow, stem cell, or thymic transplants for certain immunodeficiencies such as SCID, MHC II, etc.

MEDICATION

- Highly variable depending on form and severity of PID or acquired immunodeficiency.
- Antibiotics: Specific to organism if known, broad coverage until known. May need prophylactic or chronic medications
- Antifungal agents if fungal infection is suspected or known
- Immunoglobulin replacement therapy for the humoral deficiencies (e.g., CVID, XLA, HIMG)

ISSUES FOR REFERRAL

All individuals suspected of a primary immunodeficiency, especially with clinical manifestations, should be referred to a physician specializing in clinical immunology.

 ONGOING CARE

FOLLOW-UP RECOMMENDATIONS
Patient Monitoring

- Highly variable, depending on deficiency
- Recurrence of infections or failure to fully treat current infection
- Those on IgG should have levels checked regularly (<600 at risk for infections).

PATIENT EDUCATION

- Immune Deficiency Foundation, 40 West Chesapeake Ave. Suite 308, Towson, MD 21204. Tel: (800) 296-4433. www.primaryimmune.org.
- Local Library and Allergy and Immunologist

PROGNOSIS

Highly variable; depends on specific deficiency and compliance with preventative and active treatments. Timing of diagnosis and initiation of treatments is also very important (e.g., SCID).

COMPLICATIONS

- Immunoglobulin replacement therapy: Allergic reactions, increased risk of blood clots
- Transplants: Graft-versus-host disease, infection
- Frequent/prophylactic antibiotic use: Development of resistant stains

REFERENCES

1. Chinen J, Shearer WT. Secondary immunodeficiencies, including HIV infection. *J Allergy Clin Immunol*. 2010;125:S195–S203.
2. Severe combined immunodeficiency: www.scid.net. Accessed August 23, 2013.
3. Orange JS, Ballow M, Stiehm ER, et al. Use and interpretation of diagnostic vaccination in primary immunodeficiency: A working group report of the Basic and Clinical Immunology Interest Section of the American Academy of Allergy, Asthma & Immunology. *J Allergy Clin Immunol*. 2012;130: S1–S24.
4. Oliveira JB, Fleisher TA. Laboratory evaluation of primary immunodeficiencies. *J Allergy Clin Immunol*. 2010;125:S297–S305.

ADDITIONAL READING

- Bousfiha AA, Jeddane L, Ailal, et al. Primary immunodeficiency diseases worldwide: More common than generally thought. *J Clin Immunol* 2013;13:1–7.
- Notarangelo LD. Primary immunodeficiency. *J Allergy Clin Immunol*. 2010;125:S182–194.

 CODES

ICD10

- D80.2 Selective deficiency of immunoglobulin A [IgA]
- D80.9 Immunodeficiency with predominantly antibody defects, unspecified
- D84.9 Immunodeficiency, unspecified

CLINICAL PEARLS

- Patients with immunodeficiencies may appear healthier than they are. This is due to attenuated inflammatory response (e.g., mild to no fever).
- Those with humoral deficiencies may have comorbid autoimmune illnesses yet have in-range/negative antibody test (e.g., ANA).
- Those with T-cell deficiencies may not react to purified protein derivative testing for TB.
- High potential for interactions with chronic and acute medications or therapies.

IMPETIGO

Elisabeth Backer, MD

BASICS

DESCRIPTION
- A contagious, superficial, intraepidermal infection occurring prominently on exposed areas of the face and extremities
- Infected patients usually have multiple lesions.
- Cultures are positive in >80% cases for *Staphylococcus aureus* either alone or combined with group A *β*-hemolytic streptococci; *S. aureus* is more common pathogen since 1990s.
- Nonbullous impetigo: Most common form of impetigo. Formation of vesiculopustules that rupture, leading to crusting with a characteristic golden appearance; local lymphadenopathy may occur.
- Bullous impetigo: Staphylococcal impetigo that progresses rapidly to small to large flaccid bullae (newborns/young children) caused by epidermolytic toxin release; less lymphadenopathy; trunk more often affected; <30% of patients
- Folliculitis: Considered by some to be *S. aureus* impetigo of hair follicles
- Ecthyma: A deeper, ulcerated impetigo infection often with lymphadenitis
- System(s) affected: Skin/Exocrine
- Synonym(s): Pyoderma; Impetigo contagiosa; Impetigo vulgaris; Fox impetigo

EPIDEMIOLOGY
Incidence
- Predominant sex: Male = Female
- Predominant age: Children ages 2–5 years

Prevalence
In the US: Not reported, but common

Pediatric Considerations
- Poststreptococcal glomerulonephritis may follow impetigo (in young children).
- Impetigo neonatorum may occur due to nursery contamination.

ETIOLOGY AND PATHOPHYSIOLOGY
- Coagulase-positive staphylococci: Pure culture ~50–90%; more contagious via contact
- *β*-hemolytic streptococci: Pure culture only ~10% of the time (primarily group A)
- Mixed infections of streptococci and staphylococci common; data suggest increasing importance of staphylococci over past 20 years (1)
- Direct contact or insect vector
- Can result from contamination at trauma site
- Regional lymphadenopathy

RISK FACTORS
- Warm, humid environment
- Tropical or subtropical climate
- Summer or fall season
- Minor trauma, insect bites
- Poor hygiene, poverty, crowding, epidemics, wartime
- Familial spread
- Poor health with anemia and malnutrition
- Complication of pediculosis, scabies, chickenpox, eczema/atopic dermatitis
- Contact dermatitis (*Rhus* spp.)
- Burns
- Contact sports
- Children in daycare
- Possibly tobacco exposure
- Carriage of group A streptococcus and *S. aureus*

GENERAL PREVENTION
- Close attention to family hygiene, particularly hand washing among children
- Covering of wounds
- Avoidance of crowding and sharing of personal items
- Treatment of atopic dermatitis

COMMONLY ASSOCIATED CONDITIONS
- Malnutrition and anemia
- Crowded living conditions
- Poor hygiene
- Neglected minor trauma
- Any chronic/underlying dermatitis

DIAGNOSIS

HISTORY
- Lesions are often described as painful.
- May be slow and indolent or rapidly spreading
- Most frequent on face around mouth and nose or at site of trauma

PHYSICAL EXAM
- Tender red macules or papules as early lesions (contact dermatitis presents with pruritic lesions)
- Thin-roofed vesicles to bullae: Usually nontender
- Pustules
- Weeping, shallow, red ulcers
- Honey-colored crusts
- Satellite lesions
- Often multiple sites
- Bullae on buttocks, trunk, face

DIFFERENTIAL DIAGNOSIS
- Nonbullous:
  - Chickenpox
  - Herpes
  - Folliculitis
  - Erysipelas
  - Insect bites
  - Severe eczematous dermatitis
  - Scabies
  - Tinea corporis
- Bullous:
  - Burns
  - Pemphigus vulgaris
  - Bullous pemphigoid
- Stevens-Johnson syndrome

DIAGNOSTIC TESTS & INTERPRETATION
Initial Tests (lab, imaging)
- None usually done; cultures of pus/bullae fluid may be helpful if no response to empiric therapy:
  - Culture: Taken from the base of lesion after removal of crust will grow both staphylococci and group A streptococci
  - Antistreptolysin-O (ASO) titer: Can be weak positive for streptococci
  - Antideoxyribonuclease B (anti-Dnase B) and antihyaluronidase (AHT) response more reliable than ASO response
  - Streptozyme: Positive for streptococci
- Disorders that may alter lab results: Streptococcal pharyngitis will alter streptococcal enzyme tests.

Follow-Up Tests & Special Considerations
Monitor for spread of disease and systemic manifestations

Test Interpretation
Acute purulent infection of the skin due to *S. aureus*, group A *β*-hemolytic streptococci, or mixed bacteria

TREATMENT

GENERAL MEASURES
- Treatment important for healing and avoidance of spread of disease.
- Prevent with mupirocin or triple antibiotic ointment t.i.d. to sites of minor skin trauma.
- Remove crusts, clean with gentle washing 2–3 × daily; clean with antibacterial soap, chlorhexidine, or Betadine.
- Washing of entire body may prevent recurrence at distant sites.

MEDICATION

- In 2005, the Infectious Disease Society of America (IDSA) recommended topical treatment for limited lesions and oral medication when the disease is more severe/extensive (2)[C].
- Optimal treatment is unclear due to limited quality of evidence (3,4)[A]. Treatment reduces spread of infection and enhances resolution.
- Penicillin and macrolide therapy is no longer recommended. Fluoroquinolones are not indicated due to resistance patterns.
- Consult the local hospital or health department for microbial resistance information.
- Nonbullous (minor spread, treat 7 days; widespread, treat 10 days); bullous (treat 10 days):
  – Retapamulin 1% ointment to be applied b.i.d. × 5 days (5)[B]
  – Mupirocin (Bactroban) topical ointment applied t.i.d. × 7–10 days (nonbullous only); not as effective on scalp as around mouth
  – Dicloxacillin: Adult 250 mg PO q.i.d.; pediatric 12–25 mg/kg/d divided q6h
- Dicloxacillin, cephalexin, clindamycin, topical mupirocin, and fusidic acid are effective unless local staphylococcal strains are resistant. (For methicillin-resistant *S. aureus* [MRSA] infections, treatment options include clindamycin and linezolid.) Oral doses given for 7 days are usually sufficient.
- 1st-generation cephalosporins:
  – Children:
    ○ Cephalexin 25–50 mg/kg/d divided, q6h–q12h
    ○ Cefaclor 20–40 mg/kg/d divided q8h
    ○ Cephradine 25–50 mg/kg/d divided q6h–q12h
    ○ Cefadroxil 30 mg/kg/d divided b.i.d.
  – Adults:
    ○ Cephalexin 250 mg up to q.i.d.
    ○ Cefaclor 250 mg t.i.d.
    ○ Cephradine 500 mg b.i.d.
    ○ Cefadroxil 1 g/d in divided doses
- Clindamycin
- Severe bullous disease may require IV therapy such as nafcillin or cefazolin.

ISSUES FOR REFERRAL
If resistant or extensive infections occur, especially in immunocompromised patients

ADDITIONAL THERAPIES
Monitor for microbial resistance patterns.

ONGOING CARE

FOLLOW-UP RECOMMENDATIONS
- Athletes restricted from contact sports
- School and day care contagious restrictions

Patient Monitoring
If not clear within 7–10 days, culture the lesions

PATIENT EDUCATION
Avoidance of infection spread is key; hand washing is vital, especially for reducing spread in children.

PROGNOSIS
- Complete resolution in 7–10 days with treatment
- Antibiotic treatment will not prevent or halt glomerulonephritis, as it will rheumatic fever.
- If not clear within 7–10 days, culture is necessary to find resistant organism.
- Recurrent impetigo: Evaluate for carriage of *S. aureus* in nares (also perineum, axillae, toe web). Apply mupirocin ointment to nares b.i.d. × 5 days for clearance/decolonization.

COMPLICATIONS
- Ecthyma
- Erysipelas
- Poststreptococcal acute glomerulonephritis
- Cellulitis
- Bacteremia
- Osteomyelitis
- Septic arthritis
- Pneumonia
- Lymphadenitis

REFERENCES

1. Britton JW, Fajardo JE, Krafte-Jacobs B. Comparison of mupirocin and erythromycin in the treatment of impetigo. *J Pediatr*. 1990;117:827–829.
2. Stevens DL, Bisno AL, Chambers HF, et al. Practice guidelines for the diagnosis and management of skin and soft-tissue infections. *Clin Infect Dis*. 2005;41:1373–1406.
3. Koning S, van der Sande R, Verhagen AP, et al. Interventions for impetigo. *Cochrane Database Syst Rev*. 2012;1:CD003261.
4. George A, Rubin G. A systematic review and meta-analysis of treatments for impetigo. *Br J Gen Pract*. 2003;53:480–487.
5. Parish LC, Jorizzo JL, Breton JJ, et al. Topical retapamulin ointment (1%, wt/wt) twice daily for 5 days versus oral cephalexin twice daily for 10 days in the treatment of secondarily infected dermatitis: Results of a randomized controlled trial. *J Am Acad Dermatol*. 2006;55:1003–1013.

ADDITIONAL READING

- Del Giudice P, Hubiche P. Community-associated methicillin-resistant *Staphylococcus aureus* and impetigo. *Br J Dermatol*. 2010;162:905.
- Hirschmann JV. Impetigo: etiology and therapy. *Curr Clin Top Infect Dis*. 2002;22:42.
- Stanley JR, Amagai M. Pemphigus, bullous impetigo, and the staphylococcal scalded-skin syndrome. *N Engl J Med*. 2006;355:1800.

SEE ALSO

Algorithm: Rash, Focal

CODES

ICD10
- L01.00 Impetigo, unspecified
- L01.01 Non-bullous impetigo
- L01.03 Bullous impetigo

CLINICAL PEARLS

- Superficial, intraepidermal infection.
- Predominantly staphylococcal in origin.
- Microbial resistance patterns need to be monitored.
- Topical treatment recommended for limited lesions and oral medication only when the disease is more severe/extensive.

INCONTINENCE, FECAL

Auguste Turnier, M.D. • *Frank J. Domino, MD*

BASICS

Continuous/Recurrent uncontrolled passage of fecal material (>10 mL) for >1 month

DESCRIPTION
- Involuntary passage of fecal material through the anal canal for >1 month in an individual >3 years of age
- Major incontinence is the involuntary excretion of feces. Minor incontinence includes incontinence to flatus and occasional seepage of liquid stool.
- Fecal incontinence was the 2nd-leading cause of nursing home placement:
  - Recurrent, involuntary loss of solid/liquid stools
  - Careful rectal exam to assess for rectal tone, voluntary squeeze, and overflow incontinence from fecal impaction
  - Endorectal ultrasound (EUS) is the simplest, most reliable, and least invasive test to find anatomic defects in the anal sphincters.
  - The goal of treatment should be to restore continence and improve quality of life.

Geriatric Considerations
- The prevalence of fecal incontinence increases with age.
- Idiopathic fecal incontinence: No identified cause; more common in middle-aged or elderly women.

EPIDEMIOLOGY
Incidence
Patients underreport fecal incontinence unless prompted. Studies may underestimate the number of patients affected.
Prevalence
- In younger persons: Women > Men
- 8% of adults overall
- 15% of adults age >70 years
- 56–66% of hospitalized older patients and >50% in nursing home residents
- 50–70% of patients who have urinary incontinence also suffer from fecal incontinence.

Pregnancy Considerations
Obstetrical injury to the pelvic floor, during pregnancy/delivery, may result in initial temporary incontinence, which usually improves, but many years later can result in subsequent incontinence.

Geriatric Considerations
- Fecal impaction and overflow diarrhea leading to fecal incontinence is a common scenario in older patients.
- Surgical history:
  - Anal surgery, including hemorrhoidectomy, anal fissure repair (sphincterotomy), and anal dilatation, may predispose to fecal incontinence as a short-term or long-term complication.

ETIOLOGY AND PATHOPHYSIOLOGY
- Continence depends on the complex relationships involving temporal coordination of a variety of muscles, nerves, and reflex arcs.
- Important factors in maintaining continence include stool consistency, stool volume, colonic transit time, anorectal sensation, rectal compliance, anorectal reflexes, external and internal muscle sphincter tone, puborectalis muscle function, and the mental capacity.

- Disease processes/structural defects that alter any of these aspects can contribute to fecal incontinence.
- Diabetes is the most common metabolic disorder that may lead to fecal incontinence secondary to neuropathy of pudendal nerve.
- Congenital: Spina bifida and myelomeningocele with spinal cord damage
- Trauma: Anal sphincter damage from vaginal delivery and surgical procedures
- Medical: Diabetes, stroke, spinal cord trauma, degenerative disorders of the nervous system, inflammatory conditions, rectal neoplasia

RISK FACTORS
- Physical status:
  - Older age, female sex, obesity, limited physical activity
- Neuropsychiatric conditions:
  - Multiple sclerosis, spinal cord injury, dementia, depression, stroke, diabetic neuropathy
- Trauma:
  - Prostatectomy, radiation
  - Risk factors at the time of delivery include the use of forceps and the need for an episiotomy.
  - Forceps delivery, occipitoposterior position, and prolonged 2nd stage of labor
- Other:
  - Diarrhea, inflammatory bowel disease (IBD), irritable bowel syndrome (IBS), menopause, smoking, constipation
  - Potential association with child abuse and sexual abuse
  - Congenital abnormalities, such as imperforate anus/rectal prolapse
  - Fecal impaction is a common cause of fecal incontinence in the elderly.
  - See "Etiology" for other specific causes

GENERAL PREVENTION
- Behavioral and lifestyle changes: Obesity, limited physical activity/exercise, poor diet, and smoking are modifiable risk factors.
- Postmeal bowel regimen
- Pelvic floor muscle training during pregnancy

COMMONLY ASSOCIATED CONDITIONS
- Age >70 years
- Urinary incontinence/pelvic organ prolapse
- Chronic medical conditions, such as diabetes, dementia, cerebrovascular accidents, cord compression, dementia, depression, immobility, chronic obstructive pulmonary disease, IBS, urinary incontinence, or colectomy
- Obstetric injury at young age
- Surgeries in the anorectal area
- Stroke
- History of pelvic/rectal irradiation

DIAGNOSIS

Diagnosis of fecal incontinence is primarily based on clinical history and physical findings.

HISTORY
- Patients seldom volunteer information about fecal incontinence, so direct questioning is important.
- Determine by history:
  - Severity (soiling by liquid stools only/gross incontinence of solid stools)
  - Onset and duration (recent onset vs. chronic)
  - Frequency, presence of constipation/diarrhea
  - Review of medications
  - Assess diet, medical and obstetrical history, lifestyle, and mobility.
- Evaluate cognition with Mini-Mental Status Exam.
- Possible overlapping history of social withdrawal and depression

PHYSICAL EXAM
- Inspect the perianal area.
- Inspect the perineum for chemical dermatitis, hemorrhoids, fistula, surgical scars, skin tags, rectal prolapse, soiling, and ballooning of the perineum (sarcopenia of pelvic musculature).
- A gaping anal orifice may indicate myopathy/neurologic disorder.
- Evaluate the external sphincter in response to perineal skin stimulation (anal wink). Absence is suggestive of a neuropathic component.
- Ask the patient to bear down, preferably in standing position, to look for subclinical rectal prolapse.
- Digital rectal exam to estimate anal canal pressure while resting and during voluntary squeeze, rectal bleeding, hemorrhoids, neoplasm, fecal consistency, and clues to diarrhea/distal fecal impaction.
- Neurologic examination, including perianal sensation

DIFFERENTIAL DIAGNOSIS
- Anorectal disorders:
  - Inflammatory/infectious disorders
  - Neoplasms, radiation, ischemia, fistulas
  - Prolapsing internal hemorrhoids/rectal prolapse
  - Trauma: Obstetric, surgical, radiation, accidental
- Neurologic disorders:
  - Stroke, dementia, neoplasms, spinal cord injury, and/or diseases of altered level of consciousness
  - Pudendal neuropathy, neurosyphilis, multiple sclerosis, diabetes mellitus
- Miscellaneous causes:
  - Infectious diarrhea, fecal impaction and overflow, IBS, laxative abuse, IBD, short bowel syndrome, muscle diseases, senescence and frailty, collagen vascular disease, psychological and behavioral problems, radiotherapy

DIAGNOSTIC TESTS & INTERPRETATION
History and physical exam will usually be enough for diagnosis. In selected patients, consider:
- EUS: Currently the simplest, most reliable, and least invasive test for defining anatomic defects in the external and internal anal sphincters, rectal wall, and the puborectalis muscle. Can be used to predict the therapeutic response to sphincteroplasty.
- Plain abdominal x-ray (impaction, constipation)
- Sigmoidoscopy/Anoscopy/Colonoscopy

- Defecography can measure the anorectal angle, evaluate pelvic descent, and detect occult/overt rectal prolapse.
- MRI defecography (dynamic MRI imaging) to further define pelvic floor anatomy
- Anorectal manometry: Measure parameters, such as maximal resting anal pressure, amplitude and duration of squeeze pressure, the rectoanal inhibitory reflex, threshold of conscious rectal sensation, rectal compliance, and rectal and anal pressure during straining.
- Pudendal nerve terminal motor latency (PNTML): This technique is operator-dependent and has poor correlation with clinical symptoms and histologic findings.
- Electromyography: Sometimes is helpful in evaluating neurogenic/myopathic damage in patients with fecal incontinence.

Initial Tests (lab, imaging)
- If history of travel, antibiotics, tube feedings, or have signs and symptoms of sepsis, the following stool studies may be indicated:
  – Culture and sensitivity
  – Ova and parasites
  – *Clostridium difficile* toxin assay
- Measure thyroid-stimulating hormone (TSH), electrolytes, and BUN in elderly patients with impaction.
- EUS may demonstrate anal sphincters, rectal wall, and the puborectalis muscle structural abnormalities (1).
- EUS can detect a sphincter injury in up to 35% of women who delivered vaginally.
- The approach to the problem of fecal incontinence in older patients should be individualized, minimally invasive, convenient, and practically feasible.

Follow-Up Tests & Special Considerations
Anorectal physiology laboratory

TREATMENT

GENERAL MEASURES
- If ambulatory, prompted and scheduled defecation (effective particularly in patients who have overflow incontinence)
- If bed-bound, schedule osmotic laxatives, or stimulant laxatives if constipated.
- Enemas, laxatives, and suppositories may help to promote more complete bowel emptying in appropriate patients and minimize further postdefecation leakage.
- Scheduled toileting and use of stool deodorants (Periwash, Derfil, Devrom).

MEDICATION
No specific medication has been proven to be of benefit for fecal incontinence (2)[A].

First Line
Specific treatment of underlying cause of diarrhea (e.g., infectious diarrhea/IBD) may improve fecal continence.

Second Line
- Increase dietary fiber in milder forms of fecal incontinence is recommended to reduce symptoms. Stool-bulking agents include high-fiber diet, psyllium products, or methylcellulose (3)[B].
- Antidiarrheal agents, such as adsorbents or opium derivatives, may reduce fecal incontinence (3)[C].

- Patients with a fecal impaction and overflow incontinence should be disimpacted and treated with a bowel regimen to prevent recurrence.

ADDITIONAL THERAPIES
- Biofeedback: Training involves teaching patient to recognize small volumes of rectal distension and to contract the external anal sphincter while keeping intra-abdominal pressure low (4)[A]. Diabetics, in particular, may benefit.
- Biofeedback plus electrical stimulation is more effective than either alone (5)[A].

- Patients with systemic neurologic disease, anal deformity, or frequent episodes of incontinence respond poorly.

SURGERY/OTHER PROCEDURES
- Surgery should be considered only when the nonsurgical approaches have failed.

- Sphincter repair should be offered for highly symptomatic patients with a defined defect of external anal sphincter (3)[B].
- Injectable therapy (tissue-bulking agent injected proximal to anus) seems to be safe and effective for patients with internal anal sphincter dysfunction (3)[B].
- Artificial anal sphincter implantation/dynamic graciloplasty (where gracilis muscle transposed into anus as modified sphincter) may be considered in patients with severe fecal incontinence with irreparable sphincter damage (3)[B].
- Stoma (colostomy/ileostomy) creation may be appropriate in patients with disabling fecal incontinence when other available therapeutic options have failed or when preferred by patient (3)[B].
- Sacral nerve stimulation (neuromodulation) via the implantation of SC electrodes that deliver low-amplitude electrical stimulation to sphincter muscles to improve overall rectal tone (6)[B]

IN-PATIENT CONSIDERATIONS
Admission Criteria/Initial Stabilization
If secondary to fecal impaction, manual fragmentation and extraction of fecal mass (after lubrication with lidocaine jelly)

Nursing
- Avoid catharsis.
- No hot water, soap, or hydrogen peroxide enemas.

Discharge Criteria
Outpatient care

ONGOING CARE

FOLLOW-UP RECOMMENDATIONS
Periodic rectal exam

Patient Monitoring
Fewer than 1 bowel movement every other day with fecal incontinence might suggest impaction.

DIET
- High fiber (25 g/d) and at least 1.5 L fluid daily
- Avoid foods known to worsen symptoms (caffeine).

PATIENT EDUCATION
Kegel/Sphincter training exercises alone do not work for fecal incontinence, but may supplement.

PROGNOSIS
- Reimpaction likely if bowel program not followed.
- 50% failure rate over 5 years following overlapping sphincteroplasty

COMPLICATIONS
- Depression and social isolation
- Skin ulcerations
- Artificial bowel sphincter: 30% infection rate

REFERENCES
1. Woodfield CA, Krishnamoorthy S, Hampton BS, et al. Imaging pelvic floor disorders: Trend toward comprehensive MRI. *AJR Am J Roentgenol*. 2010;194:1640–1649.
2. Cheetham MJ, Brazzelli M, Norton C, et al. Drug treatment for faecal incontinence in adults. *Cochrane Database Syst Rev*. 2008;16(3): CD002116.
3. Tjandra JJ, Dykes SL, Kumar RR, et al. Practice parameters for the treatment of fecal incontinence. *Dis Colon Rectum*. 2007;50:1497–1507.
4. Norton C, Cody J. Biofeedback and or sphincter exercises for the treatment of faecal incontinence in adults. *Cochrane Library*. 2006;3:CD002111.
5. Vonthein R, Heimerl T, Schwandner T, et al. Electrical stimulation and biofeedback for the treatment of fecal incontinence: A systematic review. *Int J Colorectal Dis*. 2013;28(11): 1567–1577. Epub 2013 Jul 31.
6. Wexner SD. Sacral nerve stimulation: Time for critical appraisal. *Ann Surg*. 2011;254:175–176.

ADDITIONAL READING
Maeda Y, Laurberg S, Norton C, et al. Perianal injectable bulking agents as treatment for faecal incontinence in adults. *Cochrane Database Syst Rev*. 2010;5:CD007959.

 ## CODES

ICD10
- F98.1 Encopresis not due to a substance or known physiol condition
- R15.1 Fecal smearing
- R15.9 Full incontinence of feces

CLINICAL PEARLS
- New onset of fecal incontinence may indicate spinal cord compression when observed with other neurologic symptoms.
- True incontinence must be differentiated from frequency and urgency without loss of bowel contents.

INCONTINENCE, URINARY ADULT FEMALE

Cara Marshall, MD

BASICS

DESCRIPTION
- Urinary incontinence: Involuntary loss of urine that is objectively demonstrable and is of medical, financial, social, or hygienic concern
- Stress incontinence: Associated with increased intra-abdominal pressure, such as coughing, laughing, sneezing, or exertion
- Urge incontinence: Sudden uncontrollable loss of urine (also known as overactive bladder or detrusor overactivity)
- Mixed incontinence: Loss of urine from a combination of stress and urge incontinence
- Overflow incontinence: High residual or chronic urinary retention leading to urinary spillage from an overdistended bladder
- Functional incontinence: Loss of urine due to deficits of cognition and/or mobility
- Total incontinence: Continuous leakage of urine; leakage without awareness

EPIDEMIOLOGY
- Affects 25% of premenopausal and 45% of postmenopausal women (1)
- Affects 60–78% of women in nursing homes (2)
- Women 19–64 years of age have predominantly stress incontinence (20–25%), followed by mixed (15–20%), and urge (4–9%) incontinence.
- In women 65–80 years of age, mixed is the most common (18%), followed by stress (16%), and urge (13%) incontinence.
- In women >80 years of age, mixed is the most common (28%), followed by urge (11%), and stress (8%) incontinence (3).

ETIOLOGY AND PATHOPHYSIOLOGY
- Stress incontinence: Occurs with increased intra-abdominal pressure. 2 types:
  - Anatomic: Due to urethral hypermobility from lack of pelvic support
  - Intrinsic sphincter deficiency (ISD): Impaired closure of urethra. Urethral mucosal seal and inherent closure from collagen, fibroelastic tissue, smooth and striated muscles, etc., may be lost secondary to surgical scarring, radiation, or hormonal and senile changes.
- Urge incontinence: May be due to detrusor overactivity (however, association on urodynamic testing is weak), or may be idiopathic (4)
- Overflow incontinence: Urinary retention (usually from lower motor paralytic neurogenic bladder)
- Total incontinence: Constant loss of urine in epispadias–exstrophy complex due to absence of bladder neck and urethra. Ectopic ureters in females usually open in the urethra distal to the sphincter or in the vagina, causing continuous leakage. Also may occur with fistulous connections between bladder, ureters, or urethra and vagina or uterus.

RISK FACTORS
Advanced age, impaired functional status, obesity (BMI >30), menopause, pregnancy, vaginal childbirth, pelvic surgery or radiation, urethral diverticula, genital prolapse, smoking, chronic obstructive pulmonary disease (COPD), cognitive impairment, constipation, and pelvic floor dysfunction

GENERAL PREVENTION
Obesity avoidance, smoking cessation, high-fiber diet to reduce constipation

COMMONLY ASSOCIATED CONDITIONS
Pelvic organ prolapse, UTI, COPD, diabetes mellitus, neurological disease, obesity, chronic constipation, depression, low libido, dyspareunia, and any disease that results in chronic cough

DIAGNOSIS

HISTORY
- Age: Stress incontinence is more common in women aged 19–64, whereas mixed incontinence is more common in women >65 years. Incontinence dating from childhood indicates congenital causes (e.g., ectopic ureter, epispadias).
- Amount and frequency of leakage
- Stress incontinence: Occurs in small spurts; patients typically remain dry at night in bed
- Urge incontinence: Sudden urge followed by leakage of large amounts, usually associated with frequency and nocturia. Sensory stimuli may trigger (e.g., cold)
- Continuous slow leakage in between regular voiding indicates ectopic ureter, urinary fistula, etc.
- Pain: Suprapubic pain with dysuria implies urinary infection, dyspareunia, interstitial cystitis, etc.
- Medical history:
  - Neurologic conditions or suggestive symptomatology: Cerebrovascular accident, parkinsonism, multiple sclerosis, myelodysplasia, diabetes, spinal cord injury
  - Radiation to pelvic and vaginal areas: Causes ISD, overactive bladder, fibrotic changes of pelvic floor musculature, and low bladder compliance
  - Obstetrical history: Weakness of the pelvic floor is more likely in multiparous women.
  - History of smoking and COPD with a chronic cough can aggravate incontinence.
  - Constipation can aggravate incontinence.
- Medications:
  - Sympatholytic α-blockers (terazosin, prazosin, doxazosin, tamsulosin, alfuzosin, silodosin) can cause or worsen incontinence.
  - Sympathomimetic agents, tricyclic antidepressants, anticholinergics and narcotics (e.g., ephedrine, imipramine, amitriptyline, duloxetine, opiates) can cause retention with overflow incontinence.
- Surgical history: Previous pelvic surgery, including gynecologic and bowel surgery, can injure the pelvic floor support and musculature, and affect neurologic function.

PHYSICAL EXAM
- General status:
  - Obesity (BMI)
- General neurologic examination:
  - Mental status, speech, intellectual performance
  - Motor status: Gait, generalized or focal weakness, rigidity, tremor
  - Sensory status: Impairment of perineal-sacral area sensation helps localize the level of neurologic deficit.
- Urologic examination:
  - Abdomen: Masses, visible exstrophy–epispadias, incisional scars of previous surgeries
  - Suprapubic tenderness: May indicate cystitis
  - Palpable, distended bladder: Chronic urinary retention

- Pelvic examination:
  - Examination of the perineum and external genitalia, including tissue quality and sensation
  - Vaginal (half-speculum) examination for prolapse
  - Bimanual pelvic and anorectal examination for pelvic masses, fecal impaction, pelvic floor function, etc.:
    ○ Urethral hypermobility: Gauged by palpation of the descent of the proximal urethra on straining
    ○ Assessment of pelvic floor resting tone and function (ability to isolate and contract pelvic floor musculature)
  - Stress test for urinary incontinence: Patient is asked to cough or strain to reproduce stress incontinence
  - Cystocele: If evident, stage (grade 0–4)
  - Rectocele: If evident, stage (stage 0–IV)

DIFFERENTIAL DIAGNOSIS
- Nocturnal enuresis: Idiopathic, detrusor overactivity, neurogenic, cardiogenic, or sleep apnea
- Continuous leakage: Ectopic ureter, urinary fistulas, exstrophy–epispadias complex
- Postvoid dribbling: Urethral diverticulum, idiopathic, iatrogenic, surgical
- Interstitial cystitis: Bladder and/or pelvic pain (5)

DIAGNOSTIC TESTS & INTERPRETATION
- Urinalysis and urine culture
- Atypical urinary infections including *Ureaplasma* and *Mycoplasma*
- Renal function assessment: Recommended if renal impairment is suspected

Initial Tests (lab, imaging)
- Unnecessary in uncomplicated patients (5)
- Bladder scan to evaluate postvoid residual if overflow suspected (<50–100 mL expected) (4)
- Upper tract imaging if upper tract involvement is suspected: CT scan or renal US
- ICIQ (International Consultation of Incontinence Modulator Questionnaire) is highly recommended for assessment of patient's perspective of symptoms of incontinence and their impact on quality of life.
- 3IQ Questionnaire helps differentiate between stress and urge incontinence (www.overactivebladder.com/3IQ.aspx) (1)[A].
- Voiding diary to evaluate fluid intake, caffeine intake, timing of leakage, and patient habits

Follow-Up Tests & Special Considerations
Asymptomatic bacteriuria is common. With a positive urine culture, initial treatment is indicated; however, if this is ineffective, repeat treatment is not indicated (4).

Diagnostic Procedures/Other
Urodynamic studies (may consider when initial treatment fails or surgery is planned):
- Cystometric study of detrusor function
- Uroflow with electromyography
- Valsalva leak point pressure
- Videourodynamic studies
- Results on urodynamic testing are not predictive of treatment or surgery success (4)[C].

💉 TREATMENT

GENERAL MEASURES
- Treat correctable causes (e.g., UTI).
- Encourage weight loss in obese patients.
- Aggressively correct constipation.

MEDICATION
First Line
Lifestyle changes and behavioral modification are 1st-line interventions and, when properly trained, as effective as medications at reducing incontinence episode frequency. Should be maintained for 8–12 weeks prior to reassessment:
- Lifestyle changes:
  - Weight loss of 8% can reduce frequency of incontinence episodes by 47% (5)[A].
  - Caffeine avoidance
- Behavioral modification:
  - Kegel exercises/pelvic floor muscle training
    - 3 sets of 15 contractions for 10 seconds each (4)[A]
    - Proper technique should be confirmed on exam; training by physical therapists
    - 40% improvement (6)(A)
  - Supervised bladder training/scheduled voiding

Second Line
After behavioral therapies
- Urge incontinence: Anticholinergic agents (4)[A]:
  - Tolterodine (Detrol LA): 2–8 mg/d PO
  - Oxybutynin (Ditropan XL): 5–15 mg/d PO
  - Solifenacin (Vesicare): 5–10 mg/d PO
  - Darifenacin (Enablex): 7.5–15 mg/d PO
  - Trospium chloride (Sanctura XR): 60 mg/d PO
  - Transdermal oxybutynin (Gelnique): 10% applied daily
  - Transdermal oxybutynin patch (Oxytrol): Twice weekly
  - Fesoterodine (Toviaz): 4–8 mg/d PO
  - Imipramine (Tofranil): 10–60 mg PO at bedtime
  - Amitriptyline (Elavil): 10–100 mg PO at bedtime
  - Research is ongoing on β-3 agonists such as mirabegron (5).
  - Dry mouth, dry eyes, constipation, impaired cognitive function, and other anticholinergic side effects can limit use.
  - Avoid with narrow-angle glaucoma, urinary retention, impaired gastric emptying and frail elders.
  - No 1 agent has been shown to be superior, with overall 20% continence rates (6)[A].
  - Extended-release medications cause fewer side effects (5)[B].
- Stress incontinence:
  - Pelvic floor rehabilitation (1)[A]
  - Anticholinergics may be successful in mixed incontinence.
  - Duloxetine (Cymbalta) may be beneficial, but has not been approved for this indication.
  - Estrogen may be beneficial in topical form, but transdermal estrogen may worsen symptoms (6)[B].

Third Line
Nonsurgical management: Helps about 50–65% of patients with milder symptoms:
- Biofeedback and electrostimulation of pelvic floor muscles
- Occlusive and supportive devices (e.g., cones, pessaries, and super tampons) (1)[A]
- Acupuncture (in selected cases)

SURGERY/OTHER PROCEDURES
- Surgical management for stress incontinence:
  - Periurethral injection of bulking agents: Collagen, carbon beads, hyaluronic acid, calcium hydroxylapatite, Macroplastique (polydimethylsiloxane) (6)[B]
  - Slings (minimally invasive, results similar to abdominal approaches) (1)[A]:
    - Tension-free vaginal tape procedures
    - Transobturator tape procedures
    - Single-incision sling (Mini-arc, Solyx)
  - Vaginal needle suspension: Raz, Stamey (not used commonly today)
  - Abdominal approaches: Marshall-Marchetti-Krantz cystourethropexy, Burch colposuspension, laparoscopic colposuspension (1)[A]
  - Artificial urinary sphincter placement (not approved by FDA in women)
- Of note: Up to 1/3 of women who have surgery undergo a 2nd procedure during their lifetime. Quality of life improves, but it is rare to have complete resolution of symptoms after surgery.
- Surgical management for urge incontinence:
  - Sacral nerve stimulation: 50% reduction in episodes in 2/3 of patients who have failed other treatments. Invasive with frequent complications (4)[A]
  - Percutaneous tibial nerve stimulation: Office-based therapy, requires frequent visits
  - Intradetrusor Onabotulinum toxin A has a role with some patients (not FDA approved, urinary retention common, self-catheterization may be needed) (5)[C].
  - Bladder augmentation (4)[C]

ONGOING CARE

FOLLOW-UP RECOMMENDATIONS
Patient Monitoring
- Postoperative assessment: Rule out UTI, check postvoid residual, check suture lines
- Periodic long-term follow-up with outcome-based questionnaire surveys

PROGNOSIS
Significant improvements are usually obtained with most patients.

COMPLICATIONS
- Prolonged exposure to urine causes skin breakdown and dermatitis, which may lead to ulceration and secondary infection.
- Inability for self-care is the precipitating factor for many nursing home admissions.
- Social isolation/depression
- Weight gain (due to self-limiting exercise from fear of leakage)
- Impaired sexual function
- Impaired quality of life

REFERENCES

1. Rogers RG. Clinical practice. Urinary stress incontinence in women. *N Engl J Med*. 2008;358(10):1029–1036.
2. Landefeld CS, Bowers BJ, Feld AD, et al. National Institutes of Health State-of-the-Science Conference Statement: Prevention of fecal and urinary incontinence in adults. *Ann Intern Med*. 2008;148(6):449–458.
3. Shamliyan T, Wyman J, Bliss DZ, et al. Prevention of urinary and fecal incontinence in adults. *Evid Rep Technol Assess (Full Rep)*. 2007;(161):1–379.
4. Nygaard I. Clinical practice. Idiopathic urgency urinary incontinence. *N Engl J Med*. 2010; 363(12):1156–1162.
5. Gormley E, Lightner D, Burgio K, et al. Diagnosis and treatment of overactive bladder (non-neurogenic) in adults: AUA/SUFU Guideline. *J Urol*. 2012;188(6Suppl):2455–2563.
6. Seehusen D. Treatments for urinary incontinence in women. *Am Fam Physician*. 2013;87(10):726–8.

ADDITIONAL READING

- Abrams P, Andersson KE, Birder L, et al. Fourth International Consultation on Incontinence Recommendations of the International Scientific Committee: Evaluation and treatment of urinary incontinence, pelvic organ prolapse, and fecal incontinence. *Neurourol Urodyn*. 2010;29:213–240.
- Atiemo HO, Vasavada AS. Evaluation and management of refractory overactive bladder. *Curr Urol Rep*. 2006;7:370–375.

🔢 CODES

ICD10
- N39.3 Stress incontinence (female) (male)
- N39.41 Urge incontinence
- R32 Unspecified urinary incontinence

CLINICAL PEARLS
- Urinary incontinence is the involuntary loss of urine that is objectively demonstrable, markedly detrimental to quality of life, and is of medical, financial, social, or hygienic concern.
- Stress incontinence: Associated with increased intra-abdominal pressure, such as coughing, laughing, sneezing, or exertion
- Urge incontinence: Sudden uncontrollable urgency, leading to leakage of urine (also known as overactive bladder or detrusor overactivity)
- Rule out UTI or STI by culture.
- Assume that a great percentage of women can be significantly helped by treatment.
- Physical therapy/pelvic floor rehabilitation by select physical therapists can be highly effective.
- Aggressively treat constipation.

I

INCONTINENCE, URINARY ADULT MALE

Abhijeet Patil, MD

 BASICS

DESCRIPTION

- Urinary incontinence (UI) refers to the involuntary loss of urine that presents a medical, financial, social, or hygienic problem. The 2 main types of incontinence: Stress incontinence and urge incontinence
- Stress incontinence: Involuntary urine leaks secondary to increased intra-abdominal pressure being greater than the sphincter can control; may be precipitated by sneezing, laughing, coughing, exertion
- Urge incontinence: Involuntary leakage of urine associated with urgency; is believed to be secondary to uncontrolled contraction of the urinary bladder. It is also called detrusor overactivity.
- Mixed incontinence: Involuntary leakage of urine with urgency and with sneezing, laughing, coughing, exertion

EPIDEMIOLOGY

- Stress incontinence in men is rare, unless it is attributable to prostate surgery, neurologic disease, or trauma.
- Reported rates of incontinence range from 1% after transurethral resection to 2–60% after radical prostatectomy, although rates decline with time (1).

Prevalence

- Systematic reviews have shown prevalence of daily UI in men ranged from 2–11% (1).
- Prevalence of UI in men increases sharply with age: Up to 2.4% of men age <39 years have UI, whereas up to 22% of those age ≥80 years experience symptoms (1).
- No difference in prevalence between racial/ethnic groups (2).
- Prevalence of moderate/severe UI is 4.5% (2).
- Urge UI is most common (40–80%) followed by mixed UI (10–30%) and stress UI (<10%) (1).
- Incontinence in men of all ages is approximately half as prevalent as it is in women (1).

ETIOLOGY AND PATHOPHYSIOLOGY

- Incontinence secondary to bladder abnormalities:
  - Detrusor overactivity results in urge incontinence.
  - Detrusor overactivity commonly is associated with bladder outlet obstruction from benign prostatic hyperplasia (BPH).
- Incontinence secondary to outlet abnormalities:
  - Sphincteric damage secondary to pelvic surgery or radiation
  - Sphincteric dysfunction secondary to neurologic disease
- Mixed incontinence is caused by abnormalities of both the bladder and the outlet overflow or by enlarged prostate/bladder neck contracture from prostate surgery.

RISK FACTORS

- Age
- Hypertension
- Neurologic disease
- Prostate surgery
- Pelvic trauma
- History of urinary tract infections
- Major depression
- Diabetes

GENERAL PREVENTION

Proper management of conditions, such as symptomatic bladder outlet obstruction caused by BPH, early in the course may prevent continence problems later in life. No evidence for screening in men.

COMMONLY ASSOCIATED CONDITIONS

- Neurologic disease (cerebrovascular accident, parkinsonism, multiple sclerosis, myelodysplasia, spinal cord injury)
- Pelvic radiation
- Pelvic trauma
- BPH
- Prostate surgery

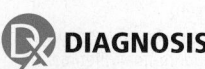 DIAGNOSIS

HISTORY

- Voiding symptoms:
  - Duration and characteristics of incontinence
  - Stress, urge, total
  - Precipitants and associated symptoms
  - Use of pads, briefs, diapers
  - Fluid intake
  - Alteration in bowel habits
  - Previous treatments and effect on incontinence
  - BPH symptoms
- Diabetes mellitus
- Associated conditions, such as neurologic disease
- Medication use: Diuretics, drugs for BPH
- Alcohol and drug use, including caffeine
- Radical pelvic surgery/radiation:
  - Abdominoperineal resection
  - Prostatectomy: Radical for cancer, open/transurethral for benign disease

PHYSICAL EXAM

- Abdominal examination:
  - Suprapubic mass suggests retention
  - Suprapubic tenderness suggests UTI.
  - Surgical scars suggesting pelvic surgery
  - Skin lesions associated with neurologic disease (e.g., neurofibromatosis and café au lait spots)
- External genitalia
- Prostate
- Spine/Back
- Skeletal deformities
- Scars from previous spinal surgery

- Sacral abnormalities may be associated with neurogenic bladder dysfunction:
  - Cutaneous signs of spinal dysraphism:
    - SC lipoma
    - Vascular malformation, tuft of hair, or skin dimple on lower back
  - Cutaneous signs of sacral agenesis:
    - Low, short gluteal cleft
    - Flattened buttocks
    - Coccyx is not palpable
- Focal neurologic exam:
  - Motor function:
    - Inspect muscle bulk for atrophy.
    - Tibialis anterior (L4-S1): Dorsiflexion of foot
    - Gastrocnemius (L5-S2): Plantarflexion of foot
    - Toe extensors (L5-S2): Toe extension
- Sensory function
- Reflexes:
  - Anal reflex (S2-S5):
    - Gently stroke mucocutaneous junction of circumanal skin.
    - Absent visible contraction (wink) suggests peripheral nerve/sacral (conus medullaris) abnormality.
  - Bulbocavernosus reflex (BCR) (S2–S4):
    - Elicited by squeezing glans to cause reflex contraction of anal sphincter
    - Absence of BCR suggests sacral nerve damage

DIFFERENTIAL DIAGNOSIS

- Urge incontinence
- Stress incontinence
- Mixed incontinence
- Overflow incontinence
- Intrinsic sphincter deficiency

DIAGNOSTIC TESTS & INTERPRETATION

- Creatinine if significant retention suspected
- Urinalysis and urine culture to check for glucosuria, infection
- Prostate-specific antigen (PSA)
- Postvoid residual volume
- IV pyelogram, renal ultrasound, or CT of abdomen to confirm normality of upper tracts
- Voiding cystogram in select cases

Diagnostic Procedures/Other

- Urodynamics is useful for confirming bladder outlet obstruction as a possible cause of detrusor overactivity.
- Prostate ultrasound and biopsy if indicated by physical exam or PSA
- Consider referral to a urologist for complicated UI, which includes: Pelvic pain, prior pelvic surgery/radiation, elevated PSA.

TREATMENT

- Best managed by combining lifestyle modification and medication
- Lifestyle changes: Weight loss (especially if overweight), limit fluids (especially at night), toilet on a scheduled basis, eliminate certain foods that may make symptoms worse (e.g., caffeine, acidic foods, alcohol)
- Bladder relaxation techniques (when trained by expert); unclear if pelvic floor exercises (Kegel) are effective for men; biofeedback
- Following radical prostatectomy, it is best to try conservative management and watchful waiting for 6–12 months to allow for spontaneous resolution (3).

GENERAL MEASURES
- Bladder diaries are invaluable in helping patients understand patterns of incontinence.
- Time voiding to avoid significant bladder distention.

MEDICATION
First Line
- Urge incontinence (all equally efficacious; selection based on side effect tolerance):
  - Oxybutynin (Ditropan XL) 5–15 mg PO every day
  - Tolterodine (Detrol LA) 2–4 mg PO every day
  - Darifenacin (Enablex) 7.5–15 mg PO every day
  - Solifenacin (Vesicare) 5–10 mg PO every day
  - Trospium chloride (Sanctura XR) 60 mg PO every day
  - Transdermal oxybutynin (Gelnique) 10% apply daily
  - Fesoterodine (Toviaz) 4–8 mg PO every day
- Stress incontinence:
  - No generally accepted drug therapy
  - Tricyclics sometimes used: Imipramine 10–25 mg PO b.i.d./t.i.d.
  - Duloxetine 40 mg PO b.i.d. is approved in the European Union

Second Line
- Urge incontinence
- Tricyclic antidepressants:
  - Imipramine 10–25 mg PO b.i.d./t.i.d.
- Desmopressin (DDAVP) for nocturnal symptoms:
  - 0.1–0.5 mg PO or intranasal at bedtime
- Intradetrusor botulinum toxin injections (not FDA approved)
- Mirabegron (Myrbetriq) New β-3 agonist (FDA approved) 25–50 mg PO daily. *Caution*: HTN (4)[A]

Geriatric Considerations
- Anticholinergics and tricyclics may result in significant cognitive impairment in elderly patients.
- DDAVP should be avoided in patients with known/potential cardiac disease.

ADDITIONAL THERAPIES
- Pelvic floor rehabilitation (Kegel exercises) may significantly reduce both stress and urge incontinence in male patients and should be considered a part of initial management for stress UI.

- Timed voiding is a useful therapy for patients with urge incontinence.
- Overflow incontinence is usually caused by poor bladder contractility with urinary retention:
  - Indwelling catheter
  - Intermittent catheterization
  - Evaluate for outlet obstruction.

SURGERY/OTHER PROCEDURES
- Urge incontinence:
  - Sacral neuromodulation
  - Augmentation cystoplasty
  - Botulinum toxin injection via cystoscopy
- Stress incontinence:
  - Urethral bulking agents: Modest success rates with low cure rates (5)[C]
  - Male sling procedures: Promising short-term and intermediate results, but no long-term studies (5)[C]
  - Artificial urinary sphincter implant has excellent long-term continence rates and is considered gold standard (5)[A].

COMPLEMENTARY AND ALTERNATIVE MEDICINE
- Acupuncture in selected cases
- Physical therapy in selected cases

ONGOING CARE

FOLLOW-UP RECOMMENDATIONS
Patient Monitoring
Must monitor residual volume after voiding in patients taking anticholinergic medications

PROGNOSIS
Continence can be improved in almost all patients.

COMPLICATIONS
- Dermatitis
- Candidiasis
- Skin breakdown
- Social isolation
- Avoidance of sex
- Weight gain

REFERENCES

1. Buckley BS, Lapitan MC, Epidemiology Committee of the Fourth International Consultation on Incontinence, Paris, 2008. Prevalence of urinary incontinence in men, women, and children—current evidence: Findings of the Fourth International Consultation on Incontinence. *Urology*. 2010;76:265–270.
2. Markland AD, Goode PS, Redden DT, et al. Prevalence of urinary incontinence in men: Results from the national health and nutrition examination survey. *J Urol*. 2010;184:1022–1027.

3. Bauer RM, Bastian PJ, Gozzi C, et al. Postprostatectomy incontinence: All about diagnosis and management. *Eur Urol*. 2009;55:322–333.
4. Khullar V, Amarenco G, Angulo JC, et al. Efficacy and tolerability of mirabegron, a β(3)-adrenoceptor agonist, in patients with overactive bladder: Results from a randomised European-Australian phase 3 trial. *Eur Urol*. 2013;63:283–295.
5. Herschorn S, Bruschini H, Comiter C, et al. Surgical treatment of stress incontinence in men. *Neurourol Urodyn*. 2010;29:179–190.

ADDITIONAL READING
- Landefeld CS, Bowers BJ, Feld AD, et al. National Institutes of Health State-of-the-Science Conference Statement: Prevention of fecal and urinary incontinence in adults. *Ann Intern Med*. 2008;148:449–458.
- Stewart WF, Van Rooyen JB, Cundiff GW, et al. Prevalence and burden of overactive bladder in the United States. *World J Urol*. 2003;20:327–336.

CODES

ICD10
- N39.3 Stress incontinence (female) (male)
- N39.41 Urge incontinence
- R32 Unspecified urinary incontinence

CLINICAL PEARLS
- Think "outside" the lower urinary tract: Comorbid medical illness and impairments are independently associated with UI, treat contributing comorbidities and medicines.
- Always check postvoid residual to rule out overflow incontinence.
- Have patient complete the International Prostate Symptom Score and do uroflow.
- Check PSA.
- Urodynamics can be very helpful.
- Pelvic floor rehabilitation may have a significant effect for male patients.

INFILITY

Sharon L. Koehler, DO, FACS • David Tegay, DO, FACMG, FACOI • Sara H. Soshnick

BASICS

DESCRIPTION

- Definition: Failure to conceive after ≥12 months of regular unprotected intercourse, or after ≥6 months if the woman is over 35 (1). Primary infertility: Couple has NEVER been pregnant. Secondary infertility: Couple HAS been pregnant.

- Evaluation: Thorough evaluation is warranted if couple fails to conceive after 12 months of unprotected intercourse if patient is ≤35 years of age and after 6 months if patient is ≥35 years. Evaluation may commence earlier in women over 40 years. Evaluation of both partners should be simultaneous when applicable (1)[A],(2).

EPIDEMIOLOGY
Incidence
Defined as the probability of achieving a pregnancy within 1 year. ~85% of couples will conceive within 12 months of unprotected intercourse (2).

Prevalence
- In the US, 5–15%% of all women currently trying to conceive are infertile.
- ~11.5% of all married couples between the ages 15 and 34 years and 42% between ages 35 and 44 years meet the criteria for being infertile.
- May increase as more women delay childbearing; 20% of women in the US have their 1st child >35.

ETIOLOGY AND PATHOPHYSIOLOGY
- Most cases multifactorial: Approximately 50% of cases due to female factors (of which 20% are due to ovulatory dysfunction and 30% due to tubal and pelvic pathology), 30% due to male factors, and 20% of all cases are of unknown etiology (3).
- Acquired etiologies: The most common cause of infertility in the US is pelvic inflammatory disease secondary to chlamydia infection (causes tubal scaring and Fitz-Hugh-Curtis syndrome), endometriosis, polycystic ovary syndrome (PCOS), premature ovarian failure, and increased maternal age.
- Diminished ovarian reserve (DOR)—low fertility due to low quantity or functional quality of oocytes (2).
- Congenital etiologies: anatomic anomalies, genetic abnormalities (Turner syndrome (45X), Kleinfelter syndrome (XXY), fragile X syndrome, cystic fibrosis (CF) causing congenital bilateral absence of vas deferens (CBAVD) (3).

Genetics
- Higher incidence of genetic abnormalities among infertile population, including Klinefelter syndrome (47XXY), Turner syndrome (45X or mosaic), and fragile X syndrome.
- Y chromosomal microdeletions are associated with isolated defects of spermatogenesis → found in 16% of men with azo/severe oligospermia (4).
- Cystic Fibrosis Transmembrane Conductance Regulator (CFTR) gene mutation → CBAVD (4).

RISK FACTORS
- Female:
  - Gynecologic history: Irregular/abnormal menses, sexually transmitted infection (STI), dysmenorrhea, fibroids, prior pregnancy.
  - Medical history: Endocrinopathy (i.e., diabetes, hypo/hyperthyroidism, pituitary), autoimmune disease, thrombophilia, obesity, cancer.

- Surgical history: Appendicitis, pelvic surgery, intrauterine surgery (i.e., dilation and curettage, myomectomy), tubal ligation.
  - Social history: Smoking, alcohol/other substance abuse, eating disorders, excessive exercise, advanced maternal age.
- Male:
  - Medical history: STI, prostatitis, medication use (i.e., β-blockers, calcium channel blocker, antiulcer medication), endocrinopathy, cancer.
  - Surgical history: Orchiopexy, hernia repair, vasectomy with/without reversal.
  - Social: Smoking, alcohol, anabolic steroids or other substance abuse, environmental exposures (e.g., lead), occupations leading to increased scrotal temperature.

GENERAL PREVENTION
Normal diet and exercise, avoid smoking and other substance abuse, decrease risk of STIs.

COMMONLY ASSOCIATED CONDITIONS
- Sexual behavior increasing risk for STIs.
- Pelvic pathology: Endometriosis, ovarian cysts, endometrial polyps, and uterine fibroids.
- Endocrine dysfunction (thyroid, glucose metabolism, menstrual cycle abnormalities, prolactin).
- Anovulation is commonly associated with hyperandrogenism and PCOS (5).

DIAGNOSIS

HISTORY
- Complete reproductive history:
  - Age at menarche, regularity of cycles, physical development, previous methods of contraception, history of abnormal Pap smears and any treatment (2).
  - History of induced abortion, bilateral tubal ligation, vasectomy, or other pelvic or abdominal surgery (2).
- Frequency of intercourse and sexual dysfunction.
- Abdominal pain or other abdominal symptoms.
- STIs, especially those that were diagnosed without symptoms and those requiring hospitalization.
- History of endocrine abnormalities (e.g., thyroid).
- History of malignancy or chronic illness? If so, what kind of illness (cancer, diabetes, HIV/AIDS, CF)? How was it treated?
- Family history: Close relatives with congenital abnormalities or mental retardation; infertility/early menopause in close relatives of female partner.
- Medications (including alternative medicine), drug abuse (tobacco, alcohol, other), allergies, occupation and exposure to known environmental hazards.

PHYSICAL EXAM
- BMI and distribution of body fat.
- Female:
  - Pubertal development with Tanner staging.
  - Signs of PCOS: androgen excess (such as acne or hirsutism), obesity, signs of insulin resistance (acanthosis nigricans).
  - Breast exam: Galactorrhea.
  - Vaginal exam: Describe rugation (indicator of estrogen status), discharge, anatomic variation (i.e., blind vagina).
  - Uterine size/shape (fibroids), mobility (scar tissue), and tenderness (endometritis, endometriosis).
  - Adnexal tenderness (Chandelier sign), (infection) or mass.

- Male:
  - Abnormalities of the penis or urethral meatus.
  - Testes: Volume, symmetry, masses (varicocele, hydrocele), presence vs. absence of vas deferens (4).

DIAGNOSTIC TESTS & INTERPRETATION
Initial Tests (lab, imaging)
Evaluation is directed by history:
- Assessment of ovulation:
  - Irregular or infrequent menses, not accompanied by consistent premenstrual or moliminal characteristics, that are inconsistent in flow and duration are indicative of ovulatory dysfunction and no diagnostic tests are necessary for diagnosis (3)[A]. Additional tests should then focus on determining the underlying cause of ovulatory disturbance (6)[A].
  - Luteal-phase progesterone ≥3 ng/mL confirms ovulation has recently occurred but does not indicate when it occurred (3)[A].
  - Luteinizing hormone (LH) testing kit: Identifies mid-cycle LH surge, which occurs approximately 14–26 hours prior to ovulation. Greatest fertility on day of LH surge and 2 days after. Only test that predicts time of ovulation in advance so couples can time intercourse (3).
  - Basal body temperature (BBT): ~1° increase in BBT taken upon wakening indicates ovulation has occurred: Greatest fertility spans 7 days PRIOR to rise in BBT. Not preferred due to unreliability and subjectivity of test (3).
- Assessment of ovarian reserve:
  - Follicle-stimulating hormone (FSH)/estradiol (E2): FSH and E2 levels on cycle days (CD) 2–5 are used to predict response to ovulation induction and pregnancy. High FSH levels >10 mIU/mL and high estradiol (>80 pg/mL) indicate a low chance of pregnancy with in vitro fertilization (IVF).
  - Anti-Müllerian hormone (AMH) and antral follicle counts (AFC): The number of antral follicles measured by transvaginal ultrasound at any one time in the ovary is termed the "antral follicle count." AMH is secreted by the granulosa cells of the antral follicles and decreases as a woman approaches menopause. AMH <0.7 mcg/dL and total AFC <10 between both ovaries during the follicular phase indicate DOR (6).
  - Clomiphene citrate challenge test: Measure FSH on CD 3, administer 100 mg clomiphene CDs 5–9, and recheck FSH on CD 10. FSH >≥10 mIU/mL on CDs 3 or 10 indicates DOR (6). May increase the sensitivity of the standard day 3 FSH test.
- Semen analysis:
  - Warranted in all infertile couples. Semen analysis alone not used to predict male fertility potential: Normal results in 6–27% of infertile males, abnormal results in fertile males (4).
  - Semen collection: Collected after 2–5 days of abstinence (submitted to lab within 1 hour of collection). Repeat test 2–3× due to inherent variability within same individual (4).
  - Parameters for male subfertility: sperm concentration <13.5 mill/mL, sperm motility <32%, sperm morphology <9% normal (4).
- Additional labs:
  - Prolactin, thyroid-stimulating hormone, 17-hydroxyprogesterone, androgen levels.
  - HIV, HSV 1&2, chlamydia gonorrhea antibody, RPR, Hepatitis B&C, CMV (3).
  - Genetic testing based on family history (3).

- Transvaginal ultrasound for anatomic abnormality (fibroid, polycystic ovaries, Müllerian anomalies).
- Hysterosalpingogram (HSG) will evaluate patency of tubes and contour of the cavity; may be both diagnostic and therapeutic (5)[A].
- Sonohysterography (SHG) may provide a more detailed evaluation of the uterine cavity, if indicated.

Follow-Up Tests & Special Considerations
- Any abnormal lab value warrants re-evaluation or possible referral.
- Abnormal imaging may require surgical evaluation.

Diagnostic Procedures/Other
- Hysteroscopy: Gold standard, used to directly visualize the endometrial cavity. May be indicated to evaluate filling defects on HSG or SHG.
- Laparoscopy: Utilized to directly visualize the peritoneal cavity and may be indicated to evaluate abnormal findings on HSG. It is the only way to definitively diagnose endometriosis.

TREATMENT

GENERAL MEASURES
- Be aware of insurance coverage for each patient.
- Infertility and its treatment involve emotional issues. Many patients may benefit from counseling and support measures.
- All female fertility patients should be taking folate supplementation of at least 400 μg/d.
- IVF is the most effective infertility treatment available:
  - Eggs are removed from the female and fertilized outside the body. The embryo is monitored for 3–5 days and then implanted into the uterus on day 3 or day 5 (5).
  - Is an option for all causes of infertility.
  - Anatomic causes (i.e., tubal blockage) should be referred immediately for IVF, although surgical consult may be required.
- Male factor:
  - Consider lifestyle changes. Note: Because it takes ~70–90 days to make sperm, lifestyle modifications will not be immediately apparent.
  - Intrauterine insemination (IUI): Sperm are placed via a catheter directly in the uterus. IUI effectively increases the sperm count.
  - Intracytoplasmic sperm injection (ICSI) is performed in conjunction with IVF. This procedure is performed for males with severe abnormalities (i.e., <5 million sperm) or those that have failed to conceive with IUI. With this procedure, a single sperm is injected directly into the cytoplasm of the egg. Fertilization occurs ~70% of the time.
  - Frozen donor sperm can be obtained from banks for severe male factor or for women lacking a male partner.

MEDICATION
First Line
- Treatment of infertility depends on the etiology.
- Anovulation: Must determine if HYPOgonadotrophic or NORMOgonadotrophic:
  - Hypogonadotrophic anovulation patients: Standard treatment to induce ovulation consists of daily injections of both FSH and LH. These injections need to be carefully monitored to avoid overstimulation, resulting in ovarian hyperstimulation syndrome (OHSS).

  - Normogonadotrophic anovulation patients: Most commonly due to PCOS. Ovulation induction with clomiphene citrate (Clomid). Regimen: 50 mg/d for 5 days beginning on CD 2, 3, 4, or 5 after spontaneous or progestin-induced withdrawal bleed. If no ovulation, then increase dose by 50 mg/d in subsequent cycles; maximum, 250 mg/d. Some will increase dose with ovulation, but no pregnancy. Most effective with ~10% body weight loss if obese (5)[A].
- Unexplained infertility: IVF most effective, IUI, clomiphene, or LH/FSH yield minor improvements, better outcomes when used in combination.
- Coital or cervical problems: IUI.
- Endometriosis: Either IVF or surgery; medical therapy for endometriosis does not increase pregnancy rates.

Second Line
- If clomiphene fails to induce ovulation: metformin (given initially as a low dose, but treatment dosing ultimately is ~1,500 mg/d; test renal function first). Metformin may take up to 3 months to be effective. Consider also oral contraceptive pills (OCPs) for ≥2 cycles, and then retry the clomiphene immediately after stopping the OCPs.
- Generally in subspecialty care: Gonadotropin therapies (injectable FSH or FSH + LH) are effective, but riskier, treatments for infertility. They are effective for hypothalamic dysfunction for which clomiphene generally is not.

ISSUES FOR REFERRAL
Reproductive endocrinology and/or urology: Specialized lab prep is needed for IUI. FSH + LH therapies and IVF warrant referral in most cases.

ADDITIONAL THERAPIES
- Increased age or with poor ovarian reserve, consideration of donor-egg IVF is warranted.
- Consider using surrogate pregnancy if couple is amenable and female cannot conceive.

SURGERY/OTHER PROCEDURES
Reproductive surgery may be necessary in those with anatomic causes of infertility (e.g., septate uteri, tubal blockage). Polypectomy could be beneficial for large polyps obstructing the lumen of the uterus. Myomectomy has been proven to increase pregnancy success rates for intra-mural fibroids that obstruct or distort the uterine cavity. Salpingectomy is highly recommended and increases fertility in those with hydrosalpinx (6)[A].

COMPLEMENTARY AND ALTERNATIVE MEDICINE
Acupuncture may increase live birth rates with IVF.

IN-PATIENT CONSIDERATIONS
Admission Criteria/Initial Stabilization
Rarely needed; however, may be needed occasionally for problems in early pregnancy and OHSS.

 ONGOING CARE

FOLLOW-UP RECOMMENDATIONS
Patients should be referred to a specialist and consider more aggressive options if not successful after 3–6 cycles of oral ovulation induction.

Patient Monitoring
Cycle monitoring may decrease risks. Ultrasound can show the number of developing follicles per cycle, which may help to predict OHSS and risk of multiple gestations.

DIET
Maintain a healthy diet with sufficient calories to maintain a BMI permissive for ovulation. If obese, then weight loss is recommended.

PATIENT EDUCATION
- American Society for Reproductive Medicine (www.asrm.org)
- Resolve: Patient advocacy group (www.resolve.org)

PROGNOSIS
Excellent; most couples will achieve a pregnancy. Without therapy, ~50% of couples not yet pregnant will conceive during the 2nd and 3rd years of trying.

COMPLICATIONS
Anxiety (stress levels are high during treatment), multiple pregnancy (rates increase with all medical ovulation induction therapies), OHSS (very rare with oral medications, but more common with FSH treatments). Couples with infertility may have a slightly increased risk of congenital abnormalities in offspring

REFERENCES

1. The Practice Committee of the American Society for Reproductive Medicine. Definitions of infertility and recurrent pregnancy loss: a committee opinion. *Fertil Steril.* 2013;1:63.
2. The Practice Committee of the American Society for Reproductive Medicine. Diagnostic evaluation of the infertile female: A committee opinion. *Fertil Steril.* 2012;2:302–307.
3. Fritz MA. The modern infertility evaluation. *Clin Obst Gynecol.* 2012;55:692–705.
4. The Practice Committee of the American Society for Reproductive Medicine. Diagnostic evaluation of the infertile male: A committee opinion. *Fertil Steril.* 2012;98:294–301.
5. Thessaloniki ESHRE/ASRM-Sponsored PCOS Consensus Workshop Group. Consensus on infertility treatment related to polycystic ovary syndrome. *Fertil Steril.* 2008;89:505–522 & 2011;205:223.e1–5.
6. Pavone ME, Hirshfeld-Cytron JE, Kazer RR. The progressive simplification of the infertility evaluation. *Obstet Gynecol Surv.* 2011;66:31–41.

 SEE ALSO

- Endometriosis; Amenorrhea; Infertility; Metabolic Syndrome; Polycystic Ovarian Syndrome
- Algorithm: Infertility

 CODES

ICD10
- N46.9 Male infertility, unspecified
- N97.1 Female infertility of tubal origin
- N97.9 Female infertility, unspecified

CLINICAL PEARLS
- Women <35 years of age should be evaluated for infertility after failing to conceive after 1 year of unprotected intercourse; those ≥35 years should receive evaluation after 6 months, and those ≥40 years should receive assistance immediately.
- Medical therapy for endometriosis does not increase pregnancy rates, but surgical treatment does.

INFLUENZA
Katherine M. Tromp, PharmD • Hershey S. Bell, MD, MS

 BASICS

DESCRIPTION
- Acute, usually self-limited, febrile infection caused by influenza virus types A and B.
- Marked by inflammation of nasal mucosa, pharynx, conjunctiva, and respiratory tract.
- Outbreaks have varying degrees of severity and generally peak in the winter.
- Influenza virus rarely displays antigenic shift (variation). This leads to strains of virus to which little immunologic resistance exists in a population, and it may result in pandemics. Displays minor antigenic variation called *drift*.
- Swine H1N1 also affects the GI system.
- System(s) affected: head/eyes/ears/nose/throat; pulmonary; with complications: Cardiac and CNS.
- Synonym(s): flu; grippe; acute catarrhal fever.

EPIDEMIOLOGY
- Predominant age: Young and school-aged children (3 months–16 years) and young adults:
  - Morbidity: Seasonal morbidity highest in elderly (>75) and those with concurrent medical illnesses, such as lung disease; also higher in young preschool-aged children.
  - Hospitalization rates also higher in infants, elderly, and persons with chronic medical illnesses.
- Predominant sex: Male = Female.
- Pandemic novel H1N1 has increased morbidity and mortality in persons <65 and in those with concurrent medical illnesses and marked obesity.

Incidence
- Seasonal influenza in pre-universal vaccination: 95 million cases per year, typically fall/winter.
- Attack rates in healthy children: 10–40% each year, prior to routine influenza vaccination.

ETIOLOGY AND PATHOPHYSIOLOGY
Orthomyxovirus (influenza types A and B).

RISK FACTORS
- For contracting disease:
  - Semiclosed environments such as nursing homes, schools, and prisons
  - Crowded, close environments during epidemics
- For complications:
  - Neonates, infants, elderly
  - Pregnancy, especially in third trimester
  - Chronic pulmonary diseases
  - Cardiovascular diseases, including valvular problems and congestive heart failure (CHF)
  - Metabolic diseases
  - Hemoglobinopathies
  - Malignancies
  - Immunosuppression
  - Neuromuscular diseases that limit respiratory function and secretion handling

GENERAL PREVENTION
- Incubation is 1–4 days; infected persons are most contagious during peak symptoms.
- Vaccination options include:
  - Inactivated influenza vaccine (IIV) is available with either three (IIV3) or four (IIV4) strains of influenza. IIV also is available in the following formulations: high-dose, intradermal, cell culture-based (ccIV3), and recombinant hemagglutinin influenza vaccine (RIV3).
  - Live attenuated influenza vaccine (LAIV) is an intranasal quadrivalent vaccine.

- IIV recommended annually for:
  - All persons aged ≥6 months
  - Vaccine should be administered annually as soon as the vaccine is available
  - Protection occurs 1–2 weeks after immunization
  - Typically mild side effects include low-grade fever and local reaction at vaccination site
  - Inactivated IM dose: ≤3 years: 0.5 mL; children 6–35 months: 0.25 mL
  - Intradermal formulation for 18–64-year-olds uses a short 30-gauge needle in a single-use prefilled syringe with 0.1 mL vaccine; somewhat higher local reactions given intradermal
  - Single dose every year except for children <9 years, who should receive 2 doses (4 weeks apart) the 1st year they receive influenza vaccine
  - Vaccine contraindication: Severe allergy, such as anaphylaxis to eggs or other IIV components; hives from eggs are no longer considered a contraindication to IIV due to very low ovalbumin dose in current IIV and good safety information; observe egg-allergic patients for 30 minutes after vaccination; no skin testing with influenza vaccine needed in egg-allergic patients. Egg allergy is a contraindication to LAIV. RIV and ccIV3 should be safe in patients with an egg allergy since they do not use eggs in the manufacturing process.
  - Precaution: Guillain-Barré syndrome within 6 weeks after a previous dose of influenza vaccine
- LAIV recommended annually for:
  - Healthy persons 2–49 years old
  - Vaccine contraindications: Anaphylaxis to eggs or other vaccine components, immunocompromising conditions, pregnancy, high-risk conditions including asthma or other chronic cardiopulmonary conditions, history of Guillain-Barré syndrome, chronic aspirin therapy in children
  - Single dose every year except for children <9 years, who should receive 2 doses (4 weeks apart) the 1st year they receive influenza vaccine
- IIV-HD: High-dose trivalent inactivated influenza vaccine:
  - Contains 4× the antigen concentration of IIV
  - Licensed for persons ≥65
  - Results in higher antibody levels but somewhat higher rates of local reactions
  - Effectiveness being studied
  - Advisory Committee on Immunization Practices does not express a preference for or against IIV-HD
- Antiviral prophylaxis depends on current resistance patterns each year; see www.cdc.gov/flu for the current patterns or check with local health department:
  - In high-risk groups that have not been vaccinated or need additional control measures during epidemics. *Not* a substitute for vaccination unless vaccine is contraindicated (1)[B].
  - During influenza season, for those with contraindications to vaccine
  - For staff and residents in nursing home outbreaks
  - For immune-deficient persons who are expected not to respond to vaccination

Pediatric Considerations
- Vaccinate children 6–23 months old with IIV
- Either IIV or LAIV in healthy children 2–18 years

- For prophylaxis, oseltamivir dosage varies by weight and is approved for prophylaxis for children 1 year and older; see package insert; zanamivir is approved for prophylaxis for children ≥5 years at a dosage of 2 inhalations per day. For prophylaxis, the dosage of amantadine and of rimantadine is 5 mg/kg body weight/day up to 150 mg in 2 divided doses. Currently amantadine is not recommended due to resistance.

Pregnancy Considerations
- The CDC recommends vaccinating all women who will be pregnant during influenza season.
- Women at risk for influenza complications should receive inactivated influenza vaccine regardless of trimester.
- Recent evidence of excess morbidity during seasonal influenza supports vaccinating healthy pregnant women in the 2nd or 3rd trimester and those with comorbidities in any trimester (2)[B].
- Recent evidence of excess mortality in 2 previous influenza pandemics supports vaccinating women in any trimester during a pandemic. Oseltamivir, zanamivir, rimantadine, and amantadine are pregnancy Category C.

COMMONLY ASSOCIATED CONDITIONS
Bacterial pneumonia

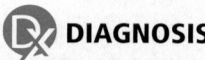 **DIAGNOSIS**

Rule out influenza by the ABSENCE of:
- Systemic symptoms
- Coughing
- Not being able to cope with daily activities
- Being confined to bed.

HISTORY
Sudden onset of:
- Fever (37.7–40.0°C), especially if combined with presenting within 3 days of illness onset
- Anorexia
- Chills, sweats, malaise, myalgia, arthralgia
- Headache
- Sore throat/pharyngitis
- Non-productive cough
- Rhinorrhea, nasal congestion

PHYSICAL EXAM
- Physical exam is not specific for influenza vs. other respiratory pathogens.
- Look for high fever and complications such as otitis media, pneumonia, sinusitis, tracheobronchitis.

DIFFERENTIAL DIAGNOSIS
- Respiratory viral infections including respiratory syncytial virus, parainfluenza, adenovirus, enterovirus
- Infectious mononucleosis
- Coxsackievirus infections
- Viral or streptococcal tonsillitis
- Atypical mycoplasma pneumonia
- Chlamydia pneumoniae
- Q fever
- Less likely possibilities include severe acute respiratory syndrome, primary HIV infection, acute myeloid leukemia, tuberculosis and malaria

DIAGNOSTIC TESTS & INTERPRETATION
Initial Tests (lab, imaging)
- If influenza is prevalent in the community, diagnosis can be based on signs and symptoms:
  – Normal white blood cell count or leukopenia; leukocytosis may indicate bacterial complications
  – Reverse transcription polymerase reaction (RT-PCR) from nasopharyngeal swab or aspirate is the gold stardard; accurate and timely (results in 24 hours)
  – Direct fluorescent antibody or indirect fluorescent antibody staining for influenza antigen; results available within hours but heavily dependent on lab expertise.
  – Commercial rapid enzyme linked immunosorbent assay antigen test. Some rapid tests diagnose influenza A, while others diagnose A and B. Sensitivity and specificity vary by manufacturer, strain of influenza, and age of patient. False negatives are fairly common particularly during periods of peak influenza activity in the population being tested.
  – Viral isolation not particularly useful except in periods of low influenza activity where making the correct diagnosis is critical.
- Imaging:
  – Chest x-ray if secondary bacterial infection is suspected.

Test Interpretation
Inflammation of respiratory tract

TREATMENT
GENERAL MEASURES
- Symptomatic treatment (saline nasal spray, analgesic gargle)
- Cool-mist or ultrasonic humidifier to increase moisture of inspired air
- Droplet precautions: See www.cdc.gov/flu/professionals/infectioncontrol/index.html
- 5 days average shedding in immunocompetent
- Hospitalized patients may require oxygen or ventilatory support
- Avoid smoking

MEDICATION
First Line
- Antiviral treatment depends on current resistance patterns each year; check www.cdc.gov/flu or local health department for current patterns. Antivirals are most effective if administered within first 48 hours and in those with laboratory-confirmed or highly suspected influenza illness.
- Antivirals include amantadine, rimantadine, oseltamivir, zanamivir, and investigational peramivir.
- Antivirals considered for persons not at increased risk of complications from influenza whose onset of symptoms is within the past 48 hours and who wish to shorten the duration of illness and further reduce their relatively low risk of complications.
- Symptomatic treatment for those patients *without risk factors* and *without* signs of lower respiratory tract infection (3).
- Antivirals within 48 hours of symptom onset recommended if at risk of complications (4)[B].
- Antivirals recommended if hospitalized (1)[B].
- Effect is reduction of symptoms by 24 hours and a reduction in complication rates:
  – Zanamivir dose: 2 inhalations b.i.d. for 5 days (age ≥7 years)

- Rimantadine dose: 100 mg b.i.d. for ages 13–64 years; 100 mg/d for >65
- Amantadine dose: 100 mg b.i.d. for ages 13–64 years; 100 mg/d for >65
- Oseltamivir dose: 75 mg PO b.i.d. for 5 days (age ≤13 years)
- If severe renal impairment, 75 mg/d PO
- Oseltamivir for children ≥1 year:
  ○ <15 kg, 30 mg b.i.d.
  ○ >15–23 kg, 45 mg b.i.d.
  ○ >23–40 kg, 60 mg b.i.d.
  ○ >40 kg, 75 mg b.i.d.
- Oseltamivir for children <1 year: 3 mg/kg/dose b.i.d.
- Antipyretics:
  – Acetaminophen: In children
- Precautions:
  – Zanamivir may cause bronchospasm if the patient has COPD or asthma; the patient should have a bronchodilator available.
  – Amantadine: Has anticholinergic properties and should be used with caution in those with psychiatric, addiction, or neurologic disorders, as it may increase risk for suicide attempts or increase neurologic symptoms.
  – Rimantadine may increase the risk of seizures in those with an underlying seizure disorder.
  – Oseltamivir may cause nausea and vomiting; may be less severe if taken with food.
- Decrease dose of certain antivirals if creatinine clearance <30 mL/min.

Second Line
- Ibuprofen or other NSAIDs for symptomatic relief
- Aspirin: Should not be used in children <16 years due to risk of Reye syndrome, a rare and severe complication of aspirin use.

IN-PATIENT CONSIDERATIONS
Admission Criteria/Initial Stabilization
Outpatient except for treatment of severe complications or in high-risk groups

 ONGOING CARE
FOLLOW-UP RECOMMENDATIONS
Patient Monitoring
- Mild cases: Usually no follow-up required
- Moderate or severe cases: Follow until symptoms resolve and any complications are treated effectively.

DIET
Increase fluid intake.

PATIENT EDUCATION
CDC: www.cdc.gov/flu

PROGNOSIS
Favorable

COMPLICATIONS
- Otitis media
- Acute sinusitis
- Croup
- Bronchitis
- Pneumonia (primary viral or secondary bacterial)
- Apnea in neonates
- Reye syndrome
- Rhabdomyolysis/myositis
- Postinfluenza asthenia
- COPD or CHF exacerbation
- Encephalopathy, death

Geriatric Considerations
Complications more likely in elderly

REFERENCES
1. Harper SA, Bradley JS, Englund JA, et al. Seasonal influenza in adults and children–diagnosis, treatment, chemoprophylaxis, and institutional outbreak management: Clinical practice guidelines of the Infectious Diseases Society of America. *Clin Infect Dis*. 2009;48:1003–1032.
2. Mak TK, Mangtani P, Leese J, et al. Influenza vaccination in pregnancy: Current evidence and selected national policies. *Lancet Infect Dis*. 2008;8:44–52.
3. CDC. Seasonal influenza. http://cdc.gov/H1N1flu/flu.
4. Lalezari J, Campion K, Keene O, et al. Zanamivir for the treatment of influenza A and B infection in high-risk patients: A pooled analysis of randomized controlled trials. *Arch Int Med*. 2001;161:212–217.
5. Grayson ML, Melvani S, Druce J, et al. Efficacy of soap and water and alcohol-based hand-rub preparations against live H1N1 influenza virus on the hands of human volunteers. *Clin Infect Dis*. 2009;48:285–291.

ADDITIONAL READING
- American Academy of Pediatrics. Red Book Online Influenza Resource Page: Influenza Information for Health Care Professionals from the American Academy of Pediatrics. http://aapredbook.aappublications.org/flu.
- Centers for Disease Control and Prevention. www.cdc.gov/flu/weekly/fluactivity.htm
- Ebell MH, White LL, Casault T. A systematic review of the history and physical examination to diagnose influenza. *J Am Board Fam Pract*. 2004;17:1–5.
- Osterholm MT, Kelley NS, Sommer A, et al. Efficacy and effectiveness of influenza vaccines: A systematic review and meta-analysis. *Lancet Infect Dis*. 2012; 12(1):36–44.
- Tricco AC, Chit A, Soobiah C, et al. Comparing influenza vaccine efficacy against mismatched and matched strains: A systematic review and meta-analysis. *BMC Med*. 2013;11:153.

 CODES
ICD10
- J09.X2 Flu due to ident novel influenza A virus w oth resp manifest
- J10.1 Flu due to oth ident influenza virus w oth resp manifest
- J11.1 Influenza due to unidentified influenza virus with other respiratory manifestations

CLINICAL PEARLS
- Influenza is an acute, usually self-limited, febrile infection caused by influenza virus types A and B.
- Preventative measures are key, including vaccinations.
- Infection can cause significant morbidity and even mortality in the very young, very old, and those with pre-existing comorbidities.
- Hand hygiene either with soap and water (slightly superior) or with alcohol-based hand rubs are proven to reduce human influenza virus A on human hands (5)[C].

I

INGROWN TOENAIL

Steven E. Roskos, MD

 BASICS

DESCRIPTION
- In ingrown toenail, the distal margin of the nail plate grows into the lateral nail fold, causing irritation, inflammation, and sometimes bacterial or fungal infection:
  - Stage 1 (inflammation): Erythema, slight edema, tenderness of lateral nail fold
  - Stage 2 (abscess): Increased pain, erythema, and edema, as well as drainage (purulent or serous)
  - Stage 3 (granulation): Further increased erythema, edema, and pain, with granulation tissue growing over the nail plate
- Can be recurrent
- Synonym(s): Onychocryptosis

EPIDEMIOLOGY
- Great toenail is almost exclusively affected.
- Lateral edge of nail is more commonly affected than the medial edge.
- Most common in males aged 16–25 years.
- More common in elderly females than in elderly males.
- More common in those with lower incomes.

Prevalence
- 24.5/1,000 overall
- 50/1,000 ≥65 years

ETIOLOGY AND PATHOPHYSIOLOGY
- Nail plate penetrates the nail fold.
- This causes a foreign body reaction (inflammation).
- Bacteria or fungi may enter through the opening in the nail fold, causing infection and abscess formation.
- The inflamed and infected tissue hypertrophies, further covering the nail plate.

RISK FACTORS
- Genetic factors:
  - Increased nail fold width
  - Decreased nail thickness
  - Medial rotation of the toe
- Many others proposed; none proven, including:
  - Distorted, thickened nail (onychogryphosis)
  - Fungal infection (onychomycosis)
  - Hyperhidrosis
  - Improper trimming of the lateral nail plate
  - Poorly fitting shoes
  - Trauma to nail or nail fold

GENERAL PREVENTION
- Properly fitting shoes
- Proper nail trimming

 DIAGNOSIS

HISTORY
- Pain
- Redness
- Swelling
- Drainage

PHYSICAL EXAM
- Tenderness of lateral nail fold
- Erythema
- Edema
- Drainage (serous or purulent)
- Granulation tissue
- Hypertrophy of lateral nail fold

DIFFERENTIAL DIAGNOSIS
- Cellulitis
- Felon (deep abscess on plantar aspect of toe)
- Onychogryphosis (gross thickening and hardening of the nail)
- Onycholysis (separation of nail from nail bed)
- Onychomycosis (fungal infection of the nail)
- Osteomyelitis
- Paronychia
- Subungual exostosis (osteochondroma beneath the nail)

DIAGNOSTIC TESTS & INTERPRETATION
Initial Tests (lab, imaging)
None needed unless patient appears septic: Then consider CBC and blood cultures
- Consider MRI, x-ray, or bone scan if osteomyelitis is suspected.
- Consider x-ray if subungual exostosis is suspected.

TREATMENT

- Surgical Interventions are more effective than non-surgical interventions in preventing recurrence(1)[A].
- The use of phenol for nail bed ablation is probably more effective than nail avulsion alone in preventing recurrence (1,2)[A].
- Surgical interventions include two general types: nail avulsion (described below) and nail fold debulking (not described in this article). Although nail avulsion is more commonly performed, it is not clear which surgical procedure is best.
- Non-surgical interventions, such as a flexible gutter splint, are another option for treatment of stage 2 or 3 ingrown nails (3,4)[B].

GENERAL MEASURES
For stage 1:
- Warm water soaks twice a day
- Proper nail trimming
- Properly fitted shoes

MEDICATION
- Some experts recommend oral or topical antibiotics for conservative management.
- Neither oral nor topical antibiotics are useful as an adjunct to surgical treatment (2,5)[B].
- NSAIDs are usually adequate for analgesia.
- Some experts use topical corticosteroids on the hypertrophic lateral nail fold, but this is not commonly practiced.

ADDITIONAL THERAPIES
- For stage 1 ingrown nails, several treatments are available:
  - Cotton wool:
    - Bluntly insert a wisp of cotton under the ingrown portion of the nail.
    - Instruct the patient to reinsert new cotton if the other comes out until the nail grows beyond the nail fold.
    - Consider adding silver nitrate cautery to the nail fold, which the patient then repeats at home.
  - Dental floss:
    - Bluntly insert some dental floss to lift the nail away from the lateral nail fold.
    - Instruct the patient to replace the floss as necessary if it comes out or gets dirty.
    - Keep floss in place until the nail grows beyond the nail fold.
  - Taping:
    - Apply surgical tape to both sides of toe.
    - Use another piece of tape from 1 side to the other to pull the lateral nail fold away from the nail plate.
    - Instruct the patient to keep taping until the nail grows beyond the fold.
  - Cryotherapy of the lateral nail fold
- For stage 2 ingrown nails, consider attempting conservative treatment, as above, especially cotton wool or cryotherapy.

SURGERY/OTHER PROCEDURES

- For stage 2 ingrown nails where conservative treatment has failed, stage 3 ingrown nails, or recurrent ingrown nails, consider either:
  - Partial avulsion of the nail with phenol nail matrix ablation (1,2)[A]:
    - Achieve local anesthesia as described below.
    - Place a tourniquet around the base of the toe.
    - Incise the nail longitudinally with scissors or a nail splitter a few millimeters from the ingrown border, starting at the distal edge and proceeding to the matrix.
    - Elevate the ingrown part of the nail from the nail bed with a periosteal (Freer) elevator or hemostat.
    - Pull this portion gently out with a hemostat.
    - Dip a urethral swab in 80–88% phenol solution.
    - Apply the phenol for 1 minute to the nail matrix under the proximal nail fold. Use multiple swabs if necessary.
    - Wash the area with isopropyl (rubbing) alcohol to neutralize phenol.
  - Flexible gutter splint (3,4)[B]:
    - Cut a 1–2-cm-long piece of sterilized plastic tube, such as IV tubing, 2–3 mm in diameter (alternatively, you may use a cap from a 29-gauge needle).
    - Make a slit in the tubing lengthwise, and cut the end off at an angle.
    - Apply local anesthesia.
    - Release the ingrown edge of the nail from the nail fold with a hemostat.
    - Slide the tube, angled end first, along the ingrown edge of the nail.
    - Consider fixing the tube in place with self-curing formable acrylic resin (used for dentures and sculptured nails), tape, or a single suture though the nail plate.
    - Leave the tube in place until nail has grown beyond the nail fold.
- Other options for nail matrix ablation include:
  - Electrocautery with a special flattened tip coated with Teflon on 1 side to protect the proximal nail fold
  - Curettage
  - Surgical excision
- Local anesthesia can be achieved with either:
  - Distal wing block: Infuse 1% lidocaine without epinephrine near the junction of the proximal and lateral nail folds. Continue infusing until the nail folds and the tip of the digit under the distal nail are white from the pressure of the anesthetic.
  - Digital ring block: Infuse 1% lidocaine without epinephrine on the medial and lateral surfaces of the involved digit to anesthetize the plantar and dorsal digital nerves. Lidocaine with epinephrine may be used in selected patients (no peripheral vascular disease, diabetes, cardiac problems, or any evidence of digital infection, gangrene, or bone fracture) (6).

ONGOING CARE

FOLLOW-UP RECOMMENDATIONS

- Dress with antibiotic ointment or sterile petroleum jelly; cover with sterile gauze and tube gauze.
- Postop instructions should include:
  - Rest and elevate the foot for 12–24 hours.
  - Take NSAIDs for discomfort.
  - Change dressing and wash with soap and water daily.
  - Expect a sterile exudate for 2–6 weeks.
  - Avulsed nails may take 6–12 months to grow completely out (if no matrix ablation).
  - Call for increasing pain, redness, or swelling.
  - Average time to return to normal activities is 2 weeks.
- Patients treated conservatively should be followed-up in the office every 7–10 days until marked improvement is noted.

PATIENT EDUCATION

- Trim nails straight across (do not round corners) and not too short.
- Wear properly fitting, comfortable shoes.

COMPLICATIONS

- Cellulitis after surgical procedure (uncommon)
- Damage to fascia or periosteum from overly aggressive matrix ablation
- Damage to nail bed
- Distal toe ischemia due to prolonged use of a tourniquet during surgery (rare)
- Nail plate deformity (due to damage to nail matrix)
- Osteomyelitis (rare)
- Permanent narrowing of nail (if matrix ablation is performed)
- Postop wound drainage
- Recurrence (40–80% with avulsion alone, 0.6–14% with matrix ablation, 6–13% with gutter splint)

REFERENCES

1. Eekhof JA, Van Wijk B, Knuistingh Neven A, et al. Interventions for ingrowing toenails. *Cochrane Database Syst Rev.* 2012;4:CD001541.
2. Bos AM, van Tilburg MW, van Sorge AA, et al. Randomized clinical trial of surgical technique and local antibiotics for ingrowing toenail. *Br J Surg.* 2007;94:292–296.
3. Arai H, Arai T, Nakajima H, et al. Formable acrylic treatment for ingrowing nail with gutter splint and sculptured nail. *Int J Dermatol.* 2004;43:759–765.
4. Nazari S. A simple and practical method in treatment of ingrown nails: Splinting by flexible tube. *J Eur Acad Dermatol Venereol.* 2006;20: 1302–1306.
5. Reyzelman AM, Trombello KA, Vayser DJ, et al. Are antibiotics necessary in the treatment of locally infected ingrown toenails? *Arch Fam Med.* 2000;9:930–932.
6. Altinyazar HC, Demirel CB, Koca R, et al. Digital block with and without epinephrine during chemical matricectomy with phenol. *Dermatol Surg.* 2010;36:1568–1571.

ADDITIONAL READING

- Chapeskie H. Ingrown toenail or overgrown toe skin?: Alternative treatment for onychocryptosis. *Can Fam Physician.* 2008;54:1561–1562.
- Richert B. Basic nail surgery. *Dermatol Clin.* 2006;24:313–322.
- Woo SH, Kim IH. Surgical pearl: Nail edge separation with dental floss for ingrown toenails. *J Am Acad Dermatol.* 2004;50:939–940.

SEE ALSO

For a video of this procedure, go to: http://5minuteconsult.com/procedure/1508006 or http://emedicine.medscape.com/article/149627-overview#a01

CODES

ICD10
L60.0 Ingrowing nail

CLINICAL PEARLS

- The best treatment for a stage 1 ingrown toenail is to insert a wisp of cotton or dental floss between the nail plate and lateral nail fold.
- The best treatment for a stage 3 ingrown toenail is probably partial nail avulsion with phenol matrix ablation.
- A patient can prevent ingrown toenails by trimming nails properly and wearing properly fitting shoes.
- Antibiotics are not useful in the treatment of ingrown nails in conjunction with surgical treatment; they may be useful for conservative treatment.

INJURY AND VIOLENCE
Monica Elizabeth Kaitz, MD • Edward Feller, MD

BASICS

DESCRIPTION
- Injury, intentional or not, is both predictable and preventable, with elderly and children most susceptible. Yearly, 1 in 3 adults >65 have falls. In women from 2004–2007, 54% of injuries occurred at home compared to 41% in men. Men acquired injuries more frequently than women in recreational (17%) and occupational settings (13%) (1).]
- Injuries are the 5th leading cause of death overall, the leading cause in persons 1–44, and the primary source of years of productive life lost in the US for individuals <44 (2).

EPIDEMIOLOGY
Injuries are common in the US, accounting for 37.3% of all ED visits.

Incidence
- Per CDC data, most common nonfatal injuries by surveillance data, fatal injuries by death reports:

Age	Most Common Fatal	Most Common Nonfatal
<1	Congenital anomalies	Unintentional fall
1–44	Unintentional injury	Unintentional fall
15–24	Unintentional injury	Unintentional struck by/against
45–64	Malignant neoplasm	Unintentional fall
65+	heart disease	Unintentional fall
All ages	Heart disease (injury 5th)	Unintentional fall

- Children mostly die of unintentional injuries: (In order) motor vehicle accidents (MVAs), fire/burn, drowning, and suffocation (3)
- MVAs are the most common type of injury in adolescents, followed by firearm-associated injuries, including both homicide and suicide. MVAs, homicide and suicide are most common in adults. Suicide by suffocation is also pervasive in both adolescence (4th) and adulthood (5th) (4)
- Poisoning is particularly deadly in adults, with both unintentional (2nd) and suicidal (6th) combined causing more deaths than MVAs.
- Homicide from firearm is 4th in children, 2nd in adolescents, and 4th in adults, whereas suicide by firearm is 3rd in adolescents and adults, and 4th in the elderly.
- *Watch for homicide in infants (3rd) and intentional poisoning in the elderly.*
- Most firearm deaths are homicides in children and adolescents, suicides in adults and the elderly. In 2001, 35% of adults reported living in a home with at least 1 firearm

ETIOLOGY AND PATHOPHYSIOLOGY
Multifactorial

RISK FACTORS
- MVAs:
  - 3 in 10 people are involved in an alcohol-related MVA in their lifetime. 1 in 4 teens killed in a MVA (2008) had a blood alcohol level (BAL) >0.08 g/dL.
  - MVAs and children: Only 37% of children are restrained in age-appropriate devices. 18% of high school students do not wear seat belts. 86% of youth <14 wear seat belts, yet 65% of these wear restraints that are inappropriate for their age or weight. Of children killed in MVAs, 68% are killed while riding with a driver under the influence of alcohol. 16–19-year-olds are at highest risk for MVAs; boys have twice the risk of girls.
  - Mortality rate for male MVAs is >3× females. 50% of road traffic injuries are cyclists, pedestrians, and motorcycle riders.
  - Risk of death by an MVA increases with male driver, inexperience, nighttime driving, speeding, tailgating, driving with other teenagers, cell phones, unrestrained occupants, alcohol and drug use. In elderly, poor vision, medical condition, and comorbidities increases risk of death by an MVA.
  - Pedestrian injury: At risk >65 (18% of pedestrian deaths), children (1:5 5–9-year-olds killed in an MVA were pedestrians), alcohol (reported in 48% of fatal pedestrian injuries; 36% of pedestrians also had BAL over the legal limit) per CDC.
- Bicycle: Collision with motor vehicle, self-reported speed >15 mph, age <6 or >39 years; less likely to wear helmet based on race, ethnicity, child age, household income, household education, helmet law. Cycling on streets rather than cycle tracks (RR 0.72, (95% CI 0.6–0.85)
- Suffocation (children <1 year): Loose bedding, wedging, co-sleeping, entrapment, hanging, sleeping in environments not intended for infants (couches, adult bed)
- Drowning: Males, inadequate supervision, residential swimming pools. 86% of boating accident fatalities were not wearing personal flotation devices
- Falls: Walkers, open windows, open stairways, inadequate supervision, hazardous playground equipment
- Homicide:
  - 2nd leading cause of death for children 1–19
  - Leading cause of death among African Americans 15–24
  - Lack of access to social capital, community organization, and economic resources; familial instability; community and family violence; access to firearms
  - Homicide and suicide: Access to firearms, mental health, alcohol and drug use, exposure to suicidal behavior, history of aggressive behavior, cognitive deficits, poor supervision, exposure to violence, parental drug and alcohol use, poor peer-to-peer interaction, academic failure, poverty, lower socioeconomic class

- Adolescent violence (5):
  - 33% of students are involved in fights annually; 13% of students participated in ≥1 fights at school in the last year.
  - 17% of students have carried a weapon in the last 30 days; 6.1% of students have carried a weapon to school. 9% of students have been injured by a weapon at school.
- Injury (sports-related):
  - Youth are affected disproportionately, accounting for ~30% of potential life years lost before age 65 (more than cancer and heart disease combined)
  - 37.3% of all ED visits are injury-related.
  - In addition, individuals from low-income and racial and ethnic minority groups are at a greater risk for injury.
- Bullying (6):
  - Prevalence is 30% for children either bullying and/or being bullied in 6th–10th-graders
  - Bullying associated with low self-esteem, social isolation, and depression
  - 1:9 middle school students report being cyberbullied (via the Internet or cell phones). ~50% of victims don't know perpetrator's identity.
- Interpersonal violence (IPV):
- Nearly 31% of women and 26% of men report having some form of IPV in their lifetime (7).
  - 40–70% of female homicides killed by boyfriends or husbands.
  - Dating violence: Prevalence has been reported to range from 9–46%.
  - Female, young (33% of rapes occur prior to 12 years of age; 50% by 18 years), history of IPV or sexual assault or child abuse, drugs, marital difficulties, unemployment, depression, minority status, income or educational disparity, poverty, weak legal sanctions
- Falls: Poor vision, medications, weakness, gait imbalance, environmental risk factors (loose rugs, poor lighting, lack of stair railings)
- Poisonings:
  - 2nd leading cause of injury death overall, 1st for ages 35–54, with incidence tripling from 4,000 in 1999 to 13,800 in 2006, 90% involving drugs, 40% involving opioid analgesics, in particular methadone. Risk varies with gender (males account for 75% of 2006 deaths), age, non-Hispanic white ethnicity, and state.
  - Prescription drug overdose is a leading cause of accidental death in adults.

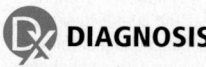 DIAGNOSIS

HISTORY
- Mechanism, timing, and location of injury:
  - Blunt vs. penetrating; intentional vs. unintentional; others injured vs. isolated injury; circumstances (weather, substance use, restrained vs. unrestrained)
  - Does history correlate with level of injury (i.e., level of suspicion for abuse [elderly, child, or partner])?
- IPV: Neurologic deficits, seizures, chronic pain, GI, STI, pregnancy, psychiatric. Recent evidence per USPTF recommends routine screening of women for IPV, but there is insufficient evidence to screen the elderly (7)[B].

TREATMENT

- Prevention: Experts agree that most injuries are preventable. Prevention efforts have been framed as "the 5 E's": Enhanced education, engineering strategies, economic incentives, and enforcement/enactment of laws (8,9)[C].
- Prevention by level of intervention: Primary (i.e., prevent crash), secondary (i.e., prevent injury upon crash), and tertiary (i.e., prevent poor outcomes upon injury)
- Motor vehicle injuries:
  - Infants, toddlers, and children: Age-appropriate child safety seats and passenger restraints with distribution programs, education programs for parents and caregivers, safety seat checkpoints, harsh penalties for drivers transporting children under the influence of drugs and/or alcohol, legislation regarding restraint of motor vehicle occupants
  - Adolescents and adults: Graduated driver licensing programs, blood alcohol concentration laws, minimum drinking age laws, sobriety checkpoints, programs for alcohol servers, zero alcohol tolerance laws for young drivers, school-based education programs on drinking and driving. Emergency medical services (EMS) response times, engineering cars for rapid extraction, organized trauma systems; collapsible automobile steering columns have been shown to decrease injury mortality and morbidity. Avoid alcohol: Effects on motorcycle riding skills observed at blood level as low as 0.05 g/dL. Motorcycle helmets decrease risk of death by 42%, head injury by 69%.
  - Older adults: Alternative transportation programs, screening for high-risk drivers, gradual curtailment of driving privileges, more frequent license renewal process
  - Bicycle helmets can reduce risk of head injury by 63–88%. Canadian helmet legislation decreased mortality by 52%.
  - Pedestrian injury: Reflective clothing, crosswalks.
- Falls:
  - Infants/Toddlers: Home safety assessments, window guards, elimination of walker use. Educational interventions targeting high-risk families decreased injuries by RR 0.82 (CI 0.71–0.95).
  - Older adults: Home safety assessments, installation of handrails and grab bars, removal of tripping hazards, nonslip mats, exercise programs (improve strength and balance), night lights
  - Reduces rate of falls: Exercise 17%, vitamin D dosed 700–1,000 IU/d 19%, expedited 1st-eye cataract surgery 34%, gradual withdrawal from psychotropic medications
- Drowning:
  - Improved supervision of young children (especially children with seizure disorders and in bathtubs); current recommendations: Swimming lessons in those >4 years; trained lifeguard supervision; fencing (1.2 m high, inclining toward climbers), locked gates, and pool alarms; personal flotation devices and boating safety awareness; parental and caregiver certification in CPR

- Fire and burns:
  - Reducing temperature of hot water heaters to <54.4°C (130.1°F)
  - Smoke and carbon monoxide detectors; fire exit planning
  - Educational campaigns for those at highest risk for home fires (homes with children <4, adults >65, lower socioeconomic class, rural communities)
- Violence (homicide, suicide, assaults):
  - Most effective strategies focus on younger age groups' positive sense of self, emotional and behavioral regulation, decision-making skills, moral system of belief, and a positive connection with family and community.
  - Limited access to firearms and/or firearm safety training
  - Suicide: Access to mental health services, improved family and community support, development of healthy coping and problem-solving skills
  - IPV: Proved to be reduced by alcoholism treatment, intense interventions of >12 hours. Refer women who screen positive for intervention.
  - Dating violence: 1 randomized trial of a school program was shown to be effective in decreasing self-reported dating violence 4 years out from the intervention.
- Sports-related injuries:
  - Proper equipment. Helmets can prevent 85% of bicyclist head injuries. States without helmet laws have double the fatality rate from head injuries.
  - Plan of action for dealing with injuries such as concussion in young athletes, with guidelines regarding if or when it is safe to return to play.
- Musculoskeletal workplace injuries:
  - Caffeine was found to decrease errors, improve cognitive performance in shift workers (unclear effect on injury)
  - Back injuries: NIOSH review of literature shows insufficient evidence to substantiate backbelts as effective. Recommends employer implement comprehensive ergonomics program. Due to mechanical patient lifting devices, Bureau of Labor Statistics reported 35% decline in low back injuries in nurses 2003–2009.
  - Follow guidelines: Annual cost of farm-associated injuries among youth has been estimated at $1 billion annually. Guidelines established for parents match chores with their child's development, with follow-up unpublished data showing a 56% decline in youth farm injury rates from 1998–2009. CDC prevention guidelines are available at: http://wonder.cdc.gov/wonder/prevguid/topics.html.
- Poisoning: High rates in children: Call poison center hotline immediately after ingestion of toxin (90% occur at home).

ONGOING CARE

COMPLICATIONS
- Injury-related medical expenditures are ~10% of US health care spending; $224–406 billion annually.
- Social burden of injury: Loss of productivity, emotional loss, nonmedical expenditures, reduced quality of life, litigation, rehabilitation, mental health costs, altered family and peer relationships, chronic pain, substance use and abuse, changes in lifestyle

REFERENCES

1. Chen LH, Warner M, Fingerhut L, et al. Injury episode and circumstances: National Health Interview Survey, 1997–2007. *Vital Health Stat.* 2009;10(241). Available at www.cdc.gov/nchs/data/series/sr_10/sr10_241.pdf.
2. Centers for Disease Control and Prevention. National Center for Injury Prevention and Control. Web-based Injury Statistics Query and Reporting System (WISQARS). Available at: www.cdc.gov/ncipc/wisqars.
3. Mack KA. Fatal unintentional injuries in the home in the U.S., 2000–2008. *Am J Prev Med.* 2013;44: 239–246.
4. Centers for Disease Control and Prevention. National Suicide Statistics at a Glance. Available at: http://www.cdc.gov/ViolencePrevention/suicide/statistics/index.html.
5. Committee on Injury, Violence, and Poison Prevention. Policy statement–Role of the pediatrician in youth violence prevention. *Pediatrics.* 2009;124(1):393–402. Epub 2009 Jun 11.
6. Donnerstein E. Internet bullying. *Pediatr Clin N Am.* 2012;59:623–633.
7. Moyer VA. Screening for intimate partner violence and abuse of elderly and vulnerable adults. *USPSTF. Ann Intern Med.* 2013;158:478–486.
8. Sleet DA. Injury prevention, violence prevention, and trauma care: building the scientific base. *MMWR Surveill Summ.* 2011;60(Suppl 4):78–85.
9. Curry P, Ramaiah R, Vavilala MS. Current trends and update on injury prevention. *Int J Crit Illn Inj Sci.* 2011;1:57–65.

CODES

ICD10
- R29.6 Repeated falls
- T14.8 Other injury of unspecified body region
- T14.90 Injury, unspecified

CLINICAL PEARLS

- Injury is the primary source of lost years of productive life for individuals younger than age 44.
- MVAs cause most deaths in children and adolescents.
- Children die of unintentional injuries (in order): MVA, drowning, fire/burn, and suffocation.
- Homicide from firearm is 4th cause of death in children, 2nd in adolescents, 4th in adults, whereas suicide by firearm is 3rd in adolescents and adults, 4th in the elderly.
- Nearly 31% of women and 26% of men report having some form of IPV in their lifetime.

I

INSOMNIA
Susanne Wild, MD

 BASICS

DESCRIPTION
- Difficulty initiating or maintaining sleep, or nonrestorative sleep despite adequate opportunity and circumstances for sleep
- Causes at least 1 of the following forms of daytime impairment related to nighttime sleep difficulty:
  – Fatigue or malaise
  – Attention, concentration, or memory impairment
  – Social or vocational dysfunction or poor school performance
  – Mood disturbance or irritability
  – Daytime sleepiness
  – Motivation, energy, or initiative reduction
  – Proneness for errors or accidents at work or while driving
  – Tension, headaches, or GI symptoms in response to sleep loss
  – Concerns or worries about sleep

Geriatric Considerations
Caution (risk of falls and confusion) when prescribing benzodiazepines or other sedative hypnotics; if absolutely necessary, use short-acting nonbenzodiazepine benzodiazepine agonists at half the dosage or melatonin agonists for short-term treatment

Pregnancy Considerations
Transient insomnia occurs secondary to change of sleep position, nocturia, gastritis, back pain, anxiety.

EPIDEMIOLOGY
- Predominant age: Increases with age
- Predominant sex: Female > Male (5:1)

Prevalence
- Insomnia (transient and chronic): 5–35% of the population
- Chronic insomnia: 10% middle-aged adults; 1/3 of people >65 years

ETIOLOGY AND PATHOPHYSIOLOGY
- Transient/Intermittent (<30 days):
  – Stress/Excitement/Bereavement
  – Shift work
  – Medical illness
  – High altitude
- Chronic (>30 days):
  – Medical: Gastroesophageal reflux disease, sleep apnea, chronic pain, congestive heart failure, Alzheimer disease, Parkinson disease, chronic fatigue syndrome, irritable bowel syndrome
  – Psychiatric: Mood, anxiety, psychotic disorders
  – Primary sleep disorder: Idiopathic, psychophysiologic (heightened arousal and learned sleep-preventing associations), paradoxical (sleep state misperception)
  – Circadian rhythm disorder: Irregular pattern, jet lag, delayed/advanced sleep phase, shift work
  – Environmental: Light (liquid crystal display [LCD] clocks), noise (snoring, household, traffic), movements (partner/young children/pets)
  – Behavioral: Poor sleep hygiene, adjustment sleep disorder
  – Substance-induced
  – Medications: Antihypertensives, antidepressants, corticosteroids, levodopa-carbidopa, phenytoin, quinidine, theophylline, thyroid hormones

RISK FACTORS
- Age
- Female gender
- Medical comorbidities
- Unemployment
- Psychiatric illness
- Impaired social relationships
- Lower socioeconomic status
- Shift work
- Separation from spouse or partner
- Drug and substance abuse

GENERAL PREVENTION
- Practice consistent sleep hygiene:
  – Fixed wake-up times and bedtimes regardless of amount of sleep obtained (weekdays and weekends)
  – Go to bed only when sleepy
  – Avoid naps
  – Sleep in cool, dark, quiet environment
  – No activities or stimuli in bedroom associated with anything but sleep or sex
  – 30-minute wind-down time before sleep
  – If unable to sleep within 20 minutes, move to another environment and engage in quiet activity until sleepy
- Limit caffeine intake to mornings
- No alcohol after 4 PM
- Fixed eating times
- Avoid medications that interfere with sleep
- Regular moderate exercise

COMMONLY ASSOCIATED CONDITIONS
- Psychiatric disorders
- Painful musculoskeletal conditions
- Obstructive sleep apnea
- Restless leg syndrome
- Drug or alcohol addiction/dependence

DIAGNOSIS

HISTORY
- Daytime sleepiness and napping
- Unintended sleep episodes (driving, working)
- Insomnia history:
  – Duration, time of problem
  – Sleep latency, difficulty in maintaining sleep (repeated awakening), early morning awakening, nonrestorative sleep, or patterns (weekday vs. weekend, with or without bed partner, home vs. away)
- Sleep hygiene:
  – Bedtime/Wakening time
  – Physical environment of sleep area: LED clocks, TV, room lighting, ambient noise
  – Activity: Nighttime eating, exercise, sexual activity
  – Intake: Caffeine, alcohol, herbal supplements, diet pills, illicit drugs, prescriptions, over-the-counter (OTC) sleep aids

- Symptoms or history of depression, anxiety, obsessive-compulsive disorder, or other major psychological symptomatology
- Symptoms of restless leg syndrome and periodic limb movement disorder
- Symptoms of heightened arousal
- Snoring and other symptoms of sleep apnea
- Symptoms or history of drug or alcohol abuse
- Current medication use
- Chronic medical conditions
- Acute change or stressors such as travel or shift work
- Sleep diary: Sleep log for 7 consecutive days

DIFFERENTIAL DIAGNOSIS
- Sleep-disordered breathing, such as obstructive sleep apnea
- CNS hypersomnias (e.g., narcolepsy)
- Circadian rhythm sleep disturbances
- Sleep-related movement disorders (e.g., restless leg syndrome)
- Substance abuse
- Insomnia due to medical or neurologic disorder
- Mood and anxiety disorders, such as depression or anxiety

DIAGNOSTIC TESTS & INTERPRETATION
- Diagnostic testing usually not required; consider polysomnography if sleep apnea or periodic limb movement disorder is suspected (1)[C].
- Primary insomnia:
  – Symptoms for at least 1 month: Difficulty in initiating/maintaining sleep or nonrestorative sleep
  – Impairment in social, occupational, or other important areas of functioning
  – Does not occur exclusively during narcolepsy, breathing-related sleep disorder, circadian rhythm sleep disorder, or parasomnia
  – Does not occur exclusively during major depressive disorder, generalized anxiety disorder, delirium
  – Is not secondary to physiologic effects of substance or general medical condition
  – Sleep disturbance (or resultant daytime fatigue) causes clinically significant distress.
- Secondary insomnia:
  – Due to substance abuse, medication-induced (diuretics, stimulants, etc.), primary depressive disorder, generalized anxiety disorder or phobias, acute situational stress, posttraumatic stress disorder, pain

Initial Tests (lab, imaging)
Testing to consider based on history and physical exam:
- Thyroid-stimulating hormone
- Urine toxicology

Diagnostic Procedures/Other
Polysomnography or multiple sleep latency test not routinely indicated but may be considered if:
- Initial diagnosis is uncertain.
- Treatment interventions have proven unsuccessful.

TREATMENT

- Transient insomnia:
  - May use medications for short-term use only; benzodiazepines favored
  - Self-medicating with alcohol can increase awakenings and sleep-stage changes
- Chronic insomnia:
  - Treatment of underlying condition (major depressive disorder, generalized anxiety disorder, medications, pain, substance abuse)
  - Advise good sleep hygiene
  - Cognitive-behavioral therapy is first-line treatment for chronic insomnia, especially in >60 population, especially when sedatives are not advantageous (2)[A].
  - Behavioral therapy effective treatment for insomnia and a potentially more effective long-term treatment than pharmacotherapy (3)[B].
  - Ramelteon is the only agent without abuse potential (4)[B].

MEDICATION

- Reserved for transient insomnia, such as with jet lag, stress reactions, transient medical condition
- Nonbenzodiazepine hypnotics:
  - Act on benzodiazepine receptor so have abuse potential:
    ○ Zaleplon (Sonata) 5–20 mg; half-life 1 hour
    ○ Zolpidem (Ambien) 5–10 mg; half-life 2.5 hours
    ○ Zolpidem (Ambien CR) 6.25–12.5 mg; half-life 2.8 hours
    ○ Eszopiclone (Lunesta) 1–3 mg; half-life 6 hours
- Benzodiazepine hypnotics:
  - Intermediate-acting:
    ○ Temazepam 7.5–30 mg; half-life 8.8 hours
    ○ Oxazepam 10–30 mg; half-life 8.2 hours
  - Long-acting:
    ○ Alprazolam 0.25–1 mg; half-life 12–20 hours
    ○ Lorazepam 1–4 mg; half-life 14 hours
    ○ Clonazepam 0.5mg; half-life 20–50 hours
    ○ Diazepam 5–10 mg; half-life 30–60 hours
  - Contraindications/Precautions:
    - Not indicated for long-term treatment due to risks of tolerance, dependency, daytime attention and concentration compromise, incoordination, rebound insomnia
    - Avoid in elderly, pregnant, breastfeeding, substance abusers, patients with suicidal or parasuicidal behaviors.
    - Avoid in patients with untreated obstructive apnea and chronic pulmonary disease.
    - No good evidence for benzodiazepines for patients undergoing palliative care (5)[A]
    - Nonbenzodiazepine benzodiazepine receptor agonists may occasionally induce parasomnias (sleepwalking, sleep eating)
    - Clonazepam and oxazepam are not FDA approved for treatment of insomnia
- Melatonin receptor agonist:
  - Ramelteon 8 mg; half-life 1–2.6 hours:
    ○ Effective to reduce sleep time onset for short- and long-term use in adults, without abuse potential; no comparative studies with older agents have been completed (4)[B].

- Serotonergic antidepressants:
  - Trazodone 25–200 mg; half-life 3–9 hours
  - Doxepin 10–50 mg; half-life 15.3 hours
  - Amitriptyline 25–150 mg; half-life 10–26 hours
  - Mirtazapine 15–45 mg; half-life 20–40 hours
- Sedating antihistamines are not recommended and should be used conservatively for insomnia due to insufficient evidence of efficacy and significant concerns about risks of these medications.

ADDITIONAL THERAPIES

Associated with hypertension, congestive heart failure, anxiety and depression, and obesity; management of these chronic conditions will help with incidence and symptoms of insomnia.

COMPLEMENTARY AND ALTERNATIVE MEDICINE

- Melatonin: Decreases sleep latency when taken 30–120 minutes prior to bedtime, but there is no good evidence for efficacy in insomnia, and long-term effects are unknown (6)[B].
- Valerian: Inconsistent evidence supporting efficacy, and its slow onset of action (2–3 weeks) makes it unsuitable for the acute treatment of insomnia.
- Acupuncture: Insufficient evidence on effect of needle acupuncture and its variants (7).
- Cognitive-behavioral therapy (including relaxation therapy): Effective and considered more useful than medications; recommended initial treatment for patients with chronic insomnia.

 ONGOING CARE

FOLLOW-UP RECOMMENDATIONS

- Daily exercise improves quality of sleep and may be more effective than medication.
- Avoid exercise within 4 hours of bedtime.

Patient Monitoring

- Reassess need for medications periodically; avoid standing prescriptions.
- Caution patients that nonbenzodiazepine benzodiazepine agonists (zolpidem, zaleplon, eszopiclone), as well as benzodiazepines, can be habit forming.
- Studies suggest an association between receiving a hypnotic prescription and a >3-fold increase in hazards of death, even when prescribed <18 pills per year (8)[B].

DIET

- Avoid caffeine or reserve for morning only
- Avoid heavy late-night snacks (light snack at bedtime may help)
- Avoid alcohol within 6 hours of bedtime

PROGNOSIS

- Situational insomnia should resolve with time
- Treatment of underlying etiology and consistent sleep hygiene are the mainstays of treatment.

COMPLICATIONS

- Transient insomnia can become chronic.
- Daytime sleepiness, cognitive dysfunction
- Pulmonary hypertension if chronic sleep apnea left untreated
- Sleep apnea may lead to hypertension, stroke, or cardiac ischemia.

REFERENCES

1. Kushida CA, Littner MR, Morgenthaler T, et al. Practice parameters for the indications for polysomnography and related procedures: An update for 2005. *Sleep.* 2005;28:499–521.
2. Montgomery P, Dennis J. Cognitive behavioural interventions for sleep problems in adults aged 60+. *Cochrane Database Syst Rev.* 2003;2: CD003161.
3. Ebben MR, Spielman AJ. Non-pharmacological treatments for insomnia. *J Behav Med.* 2009;32: 244–245.
4. Reynoldson JN, Elliott ES, Nelson LA. Ramelteon: A novel approach in the treatment of insomnia (CE) (September). *Ann Pharmacother.* 2008;42: 1262–1271.
5. Hirst A, Sloan R. Benzodiazepines and related drugs for insomnia in palliative care. *Cochrane Database Syst Rev.* 2002;4:CD003346.
6. Verster GC. Melatonin and its agonists, circadian rhythms, and psychiatry. *Afr J Psychiatry (Johannesbg).* 2009;12:42–46.
7. Cheuk DK, Yeung WF, Chung K et al. Acupuncture for insomnia. *Cochrane Database Syst Rev.* 2012;9: CD005472
8. Kripke DF, Langer RD, Kline LE. Hypnotics' association with mortality or cancer: A matched cohort study. *BMJ Open.* 2012;2:e000850.

ADDITIONAL READING

Glass J, Lanctôt KL, Herrmann N, et al. Sedative hypnotics in older people with insomnia: Meta-analysis of risks and benefits. *BMJ.* 2005;331:1169.

 SEE ALSO

- Anxiety; Depression; Fibromyalgia; Sleep Apnea, Obstructive
- Algorithms: Anxiety; Insomnia, Chronic; Restless Leg Syndrome (RLS)

 CODES

ICD10

- F51.01 Primary insomnia
- F51.02 Adjustment insomnia
- G47.00 Insomnia, unspecified

CLINICAL PEARLS

- Treatment of underlying etiology of the insomnia and consistent sleep hygiene are key.
- Most medications are indicated for short-term use only.
- Sedative hypnotics are not recommended in the elderly because risks may outweigh benefits.
- Patients with chronic insomnia may benefit from cognitive-behavioral therapy.

INTELLECTUAL DISABILITY (INTELLECTUAL DEVELOPMENTAL DISORDER)

Jennifer L. Ayres, PhD

BASICS

- Intellectual disability (ID) is a global deficit in cognitive functioning evidenced by a significant difference between one's mental and chronological ages (also known as *intelligence quotient* [IQ]) and significantly impaired adaptive functioning (1).
- Although these cognitive issues typically have a pervasive impact, patients with ID will display highly variable levels of functioning and subsequent service needs.
- Patients must be evaluated individually. Treatment plans must be tailored to specific needs.
- The term *mental retardation* was deleted from the *Diagnostic statistical manual of mental disorders, 5th edition (DSM-5)* and replaced with "intellectual disability" or "intellectual developmental disorder." The rationale was that the term *mental retardation* is considered pejorative and culturally insensitive.

DESCRIPTION

- ID is defined as an IQ $\leq 70 + 5$ and a significant impairment in intellectual functioning, including verbal and nonverbal reasoning, planning, academic learning, problem solving and experiential learning. The intellectual functioning is confirmed by both IQ testing and clinical assessment (1).
- A diagnosis of ID also requires deficits in adaptive functioning, such as communication, socialization, and independent living (1).
- By definition, ID is a neurodevelopmental disorder that typically is present from birth or determined during early childhood (1).
- Currently, ID is subgrouped according to the patient's level of adaptive functioning and level of support needed. Severity levels: Mild (typical development in some domains, mild impairment in others), Moderate (skills are markedly behind same-age peers), Severe (skills are quite limited, compared to peers), Profound (very limited awareness of concepts, language, dependent on others for all aspects of adaptive functioning) (1).
- The 3 most common causes of ID are Down syndrome, fragile X syndrome, and fetal alcohol syndrome (FAS).
- If the ID reflects a loss of previously acquired intellectual skills, comorbid diagnoses of ID and neurocognitive disorder may be appropriate.

ALERT
For some causes of ID, prenatal testing is available.

EPIDEMIOLOGY
Incidence
- 1 of 6 children (2)
- Predominant sex: Male > Female: 1.6:1 for mild ID, 1.2:1 for severe ID (1)

Prevalence
In the US, 1% of the general population. The prevalence for severe ID is 6/1,000.

ETIOLOGY AND PATHOPHYSIOLOGY
- Causes:
  - Maternal substance abuse (e.g., alcohol); fetal alcohol syndrome (FAS) is a leading environmental cause of ID.
  - Maternal infections: TORCH viruses (Toxoplasma, Other infections, Rubella, Cytomegalovirus, and Herpes simplex)

- Down syndrome
- Sex chromosome abnormalities: Fragile X, Turner syndrome, Klinefelter syndrome
- Autosomal–dominant conditions: Neurocutaneous syndromes (e.g., neurofibromatosis, tuberous sclerosis)
- Autosomal–recessive conditions:
  - Amino acid metabolism (e.g., phenylketonuria, maple-syrup urine disease)
  - Carbohydrate metabolism (e.g., galactosemia, fructosuria)
  - Lipid metabolism
  - Tay-Sachs disease
  - Gaucher disease
  - Niemann-Pick disease (e.g., mucopolysaccharidosis)
  - Purine metabolism (e.g., Lesch-Nyhan disease)
  - Other (e.g., Wilson disease)
- Maternal use of prescription medications (e.g., Accutane, dilantin)
- Perinatal factors:
  - Prematurity
  - Birth injuries
  - Perinatal anoxia
- Postnatal factors:
  - Childhood diseases (e.g., meningitis, encephalitis, hypothyroidism, seizure disorders)
  - Trauma (e.g., accidents, physical abuse, hypoxia)
  - Severe deprivation
  - Poisoning (e.g., lead, carbon monoxide, household products)

Genetics
A number of genetic and epigenetic causes are known, and more are under investigation (3).

RISK FACTORS
- Maternal substance abuse during pregnancy
- Maternal infection during pregnancy
- For some causes, family history

GENERAL PREVENTION
- Public health efforts to reduce alcohol and drug use by pregnant women
- Prenatal folic acid supplementation

COMMONLY ASSOCIATED CONDITIONS
- Seizures
- Mood disorders
- Behavioral disorders
- Constipation

DIAGNOSIS

A diagnosis of ID should be made only through a psychodiagnostic assessment conducted by a mental health provider who is trained and licensed to conduct formal psychological testing.

HISTORY
- Children with profound/severe ID typically are diagnosed at birth or during the newborn period and are may have dysmorphic features.
- Children with ID often are identified because they fail to meet motor/language milestones.

PHYSICAL EXAM
Careful examination by a physician trained in the assessment of morphologic features suggestive of a specific etiology for ID (e.g., microcephaly) (4)

DIFFERENTIAL DIAGNOSIS
- Brain tumors
- Auditory, visual, and/or speech/language impairment
- Autistic disorder (language and social skills are more affected than other cognitive abilities); however, 75% of individuals with an autistic disorder may meet criteria for a comorbid diagnosis of ID.
- Expressive/Receptive language disorders
- Cerebral palsy
- Emotional/Behavioral disturbance
- Learning disorders (reading, math, written expression)
- Auditory/Sensory processing difficulties
- Lack of environmental opportunities for appropriate development

DIAGNOSTIC TESTS & INTERPRETATION
- Visual and hearing tests to rule out these etiologies as a cause of impairment and provide an assessment of visual and auditory functioning, which often are impaired in children and adults with ID
- Formal testing of intellectual and adaptive functioning:
  - A child's communication skills must be considered in test selection. For example, a patient with auditory processing issues/limited expressive/receptive language skills may need to be assessed using a nonverbal IQ test, such as the Leiter-R, Test of Nonverbal Intelligence, or other nonverbal measures.
  - Commonly used intelligence tests (e.g., Bayley Scales of Infant Development, Stanford-Binet Intelligence Scale, Wechsler Intelligence Scales) are determined by age/developmental level of the child.
  - Common tests of adaptive functioning include the Vineland Adaptive Behavior Scales, 2nd ed., and Adaptive Behavior Assessment System, 2nd ed. These tests assess areas of functioning, such as age-appropriate communication, social skills, activities of daily living, and motor skills.

- Metabolic screening is not routine unless evidence in history and physical or no newborn screening records (5)[B].
- Lead as per current targeted guidelines (5)[B]
- Thyroid-stimulating hormone if systemic features present/no newborn screening (5)[B]
- Routine cytogenetic testing (karyotype) (5)[B]:
  - Fragile X screening (*FMR1* gene), particularly with a family history of intellectual disability (5)[B]
  - Rett syndrome (*MECP2* gene) in women with unexplained moderate-to-severe intellectual disability (5)[B]
- Molecular screening, such as array comparative genomic hybridization, is used increasingly and may yield a diagnosis in 10% of undiagnosed cases (4)[B].
- Neuroimaging (MRI more sensitive than CT) is routinely recommended. The presence of physical findings (microcephaly, focal motor deficit) will increase the yield of a specific diagnosis (5)[B].
- MRI may show mild cerebral abnormalities, but is unlikely to establish etiology of ID (4).

Follow-Up Tests & Special Considerations
- Electroencephalogram is not routine unless epilepsy or a specific epileptiform syndrome is present (5)[C].
- Assessment of quality of life provides salient information about a patient's general sense of well-being and life satisfaction; however, quality of life may be difficult to assess when significant behavioral issues confound an individual's self-report and socialization.

TREATMENT

- Early intervention services tailored to the individual's specific needs
- Caregiver support, including:
  - Training caregiver(s) to address behavioral issues and support socialization development
  - Encouraging caregivers to create a structured home environment that is based on the child's developmental level and specific needs rather than age-appropriate expectations
  - Providing caregiver(s) with an opportunity to address their reactions to the diagnosis and their child's special needs
  - Informing caregivers about advocacy groups and available community, state, and national resources (6,7,8)
  - Encouraging caregiver(s) to seek social support to increase overall sense of well-being
- Individualized education plans and, depending on the level of impairment, social skills and behavioral plans/training
- Refer to job training programs and independent living opportunities, if appropriate.
- Notice all changes in behavior, which may be indicative of pain/illness, particularly in individuals with limited communication skills.
- Assess for abuse and neglect

MEDICATION
Medication may be appropriate for comorbid conditions (e.g., anxiety, ADHD, depression).

ONGOING CARE

The physician should match his/her communication of exam procedures, test results, and treatment recommendations to the patient's level of cognitive functioning and receptive language skills:
- Most patients with ID will fall within the mild range and are fully capable of understanding information if it is provided at the appropriate level.
- Provide oral and written explanations directly to the patient instead of solely to his/her caregivers. The dignity of the patient must be respected at all times. This includes providing honest information, responding to patient's questions with respect, and not infantilizing the patient due to his/her intellectual disability.

FOLLOW-UP RECOMMENDATIONS
- Many adults and children with ID exhibit poor physical fitness. Preliminary studies suggest structured exercise programs are effective to engage this population in healthy activities (9)[A].
- Linkage to community-based resources for job training, independent living, caregiver support, school-based services

Patient Monitoring
- Primary care with attention to associated medical conditions
- Vision testing at least once before age 40 (age 30 in Down syndrome) and every 2 years thereafter (10)[B]
- Hearing evaluations every 5 years after age 45 (every 3 years throughout life in Down syndrome) (10)[B]
- Screen for sexual activity and offer contraception and testing for STIs (10)[B].
- Abuse and neglect of people with ID are common. Screen at least annually and if behavior change is noted. Report abuse/neglect to appropriate protective agencies (10)[B].
- Dysphagia and aspiration are common; consider speech pathology evaluation and swallowing study (11)[B].
- Monitor for and treat constipation (11)[B]
- Osteoporosis: Common; low threshold to order imaging studies after traumatic injury (11)[B]

DIET
No restrictions, except in cases of metabolic and storage disorders (e.g., phenylketonuria)

PATIENT EDUCATION
- Association for Retarded Citizens: www.thearc.org
- American Association of Intellectual and Developmental Disabilities: www.aaidd.org
- Family support groups (Parent to Parent, local Down Syndrome or Autism Association)
- Special Olympics: www.specialolympics.org

PROGNOSIS
Although ID is a lifelong diagnosis, individuals with ID are capable of living a fulfilling, purposeful life that includes having a career, living independently, marrying/participating in a committed relationship, and becoming a parent. Also, the level of severity and support needed may vary over the course of the individual's life.

COMPLICATIONS
- Constipation is a commonly overlooked problem and can lead to significant morbidity.
- Polypharmacy, often associated with psychotropic medication use to control behaviors, should be addressed to minimize adverse side effects.

REFERENCES

1. American Psychiatric Association. *Diagnostic and statistical manual of mental disorders*, 5th ed. (DSM-5). Arlington, VA: American Psychiatric Association; 2013.
2. Centers for Disease Control and Prevention. Developmental disabilities. Available at: www.cdc.gov/ncbddd/dd/
3. Grant ME. The epigenetic origins of mental retardation. *Clin Genet*. 2008;73:528–530.
4. van Karnebeek CDM, Jansweijer MCE, Offringa M. Diagnostic investigations in individuals with mental retardation: A systematic literature review of their usefulness. *Eur J Human Genet*. 2005;13:6–25.
5. Shevell M, Ashwal S, Donley D, et al. Practice parameter: Evaluation of the child with global developmental delay: Report of the Quality Standards Subcommittee of the American Academy of Neurology and the Practice Committee of the Child Neurology Society. *Neurology*. 2003;60:367–380.
6. Shogren KA, Bradley VJ, Gomez SC, et al. Public policy and the enhancement of desired outcomes for persons with intellectual disability. *Intellect Dev Disabil*. 2009;47:307–319.
7. Rizzolo MC, Hemp R, Braddock D, et al. Family support services for persons with intellectual and developmental disabilities: Recent national trends. *Intellect Dev Disabil*. 2009;47:152–155.
8. Samuel PS, Hobden KL, LeRoy BW, et al. Analysing family service needs of typically underserved families in the USA. *J Intellect Disabil Res*. 2012;56:111–128.
9. Heller T, Hsieh K, Rimmer JH. Attitudinal and psychosocial outcomes of a fitness and health education program on adults with down syndrome. *Am J Ment Retard*. 2004;109: 175–185.
10. Sullivan WF, Heng J, Cameron D, et al. Consensus guidelines for primary health care of adults with developmental disabilities. *Can Fam Physician*. 2006;52:1410–1418.
11. Prater CD, Zylstra RG. Medical care of adults with mental retardation. *Am Fam Physician*. 2006;73: 2175–2183.

 # CODES

ICD10
- F70 Mild intellectual disabilities
- F71 Moderate intellectual disabilities
- F79 Unspecified intellectual disabilities

CLINICAL PEARLS

- The term *mental retardation* may be interpreted as culturally insensitive and disrespectful to patients and their caregivers. Intellectual disability is the correct diagnosis.
- Overall functioning with ID is highly variable and influenced by multiple factors, including appropriateness of school placement/special education services, exposure to early intervention, behavioral therapy, parent training, self-esteem, and social skills.
- Previous stereotypes of people with ID (e.g., always happy, poor prognosis, unable to function independently) have been refuted. People with ID are showing a level of functioning variability that parallels what is found in the non-ID population.
- Be aware of the unique parenting needs that caregivers may face. Link families to community resources that can provide practical and emotional support when appropriate.
- Because children with developmental disabilities are at higher risk of being abused than their peers without developmental disabilities, discuss with caregivers how to educate children about safety precautions in a developmentally appropriate manner.

INTERSTITIAL CYSTITIS
Montiel Teresa Rosenthal, MD

 BASICS

DESCRIPTION
- A disease of unknown cause, probably representing a final common pathway from several etiologies.
- Likely pathogenesis is disruption of urothelium, impaired lower urinary tract defenses, and loss of bladder muscular wall elasticity. The symptoms in many patients are insidious, and the disease progresses for years before diagnosis is established.
- Mild: Normal bladder capacity under anesthesia. Ulceration, cracking, or glomerulation of mucosa (or not) with bladder distention under anesthesia. No incontinence. Symptoms wax and wane and may not progress. Interstitial cystitis is a bladder sensory problem.
- Severe: Progressive bladder fibrosis. Small true bladder capacity under anesthesia. Poor bladder wall compliance. Often, ulcers present at cystoscopy. May have overflow incontinence and/or chronic bacteriuria unresponsive to antibiotics.
- System(s) affected: Renal/Urologic
- Synonym(s): Urgency frequency syndrome; painful bladder syndrome

Pregnancy Considerations
Unpredictable symptom improvement or exacerbation during pregnancy. No known fetal effects from interstitial cystitis. Usual problems of unknown effect on fetus with medications taken during pregnancy.

EPIDEMIOLOGY
- Occurs predominantly among whites
- Predominant sex: Female > Male (10:1)
- Patients <30 have predominant symptoms: Dysuria, frequency, urinary urgency, pain in external genitals and dyspareunia; and those >60 more commonly have nocturia, urinary incontinence, or Hunner's ulcer disease (1)
- Predominant age:
  – Mild: 20–40 years
  – Severe: 20–70 years
- Pediatric considerations:
  – <10 years old and again at 13–17 years
  – Daytime enuresis, dysuria without infection

Prevalence
In the US:
- Up to 1 million affected, but many cases likely are unreported
- 0.052%, but may be higher, up to 10%

ETIOLOGY AND PATHOPHYSIOLOGY
- Unknown, but is not primarily psychosomatic
- Possible causes:
  – Subclinical urinary infection
  – Damage to glycosaminoglycan mucus layer increasing bladder wall permeability to irritants such as urea
  – Autoimmune
  – Mast cell histamine release
- Neurologic upregulation/stimulation

RISK FACTORS
Unknown

COMMONLY ASSOCIATED CONDITIONS
- Fibromyalgia
- Allergies
- Chronic fatigue syndrome
- Depression
- Vulvodynia
- Sleep disturbance
- Migraines
- Syncope
- Dyspepsia
- Chronic prostatitis
- Chronic pelvic pain
- Irritable bowel syndrome
- Anal/rectal disease

 DIAGNOSIS

- Frequent, urgent, relentless urination day and night; >8 voids in 24 hours
- Pain with full bladder that resolves with bladder emptying (except if bacteriuria is present)
- Urge urinary incontinence if bladder capacity is small
- Sleep disturbance
- Dyspareunia, especially with full bladder
- Secondary symptoms from chronic pain and sleeplessness, especially depression

HISTORY
- Pelvic Pain and Urgency/Frequency Symptom Scale (2)[B]: Self-reporting questionnaire for screening potential interstitial cystitis patients (www.wgcaobgyn.com/files/urgency_frequency_pt_symptom_scale.pdf)
- Frequent UTIs, vaginitis, or symptoms during the week before menses
- O'Leary/Sant Voiding and Pain Indices (www.ichelp.org.document.doc?id=306)

PHYSICAL EXAM
- Perineal/prostatic pain in men
- Anterior vaginal wall pain in women

DIFFERENTIAL DIAGNOSIS
- Uninhibited bladder (urgency, frequency, urge incontinence, less pain, symptoms usually decrease when asleep)
- Urinary infection: Cystitis, prostatitis
- Bladder neoplasm
- Bladder stone
- Neurologic bladder disease
- Nonurinary pelvic disease (STIs, endometriosis, pelvic relaxation)

DIAGNOSTIC TESTS & INTERPRETATION
Initial Tests (lab, imaging)
- Urinalysis: Normal except with chronic bacteriuria (rare)
- Urine culture from catheterized specimen: Normal except with chronic bacteriuria (rare) or partial antibiotic treatment
- Urine cytology:
  – Normal: Reserve for men >40 years old and women with hematuria

Diagnostic Procedures/Other
- Cystoscopy (especially in men >40 years old or women with hematuria):
  – Bladder wall visualization
  – Hydraulic distention: No improved diagnostic certainty over history and physical alone
- No role for urodynamic testing

- K^+ sensitivity test (2)[B]:
  – Insert catheter, empty bladder, instill 40 mL H_2O over 2–3 minutes, rank urgency on scale of 0–5 in intensity, rank pain on scale of 0–5 in intensity, drain bladder, instill 40 mL Potassium chloride (KCl) 0.4 mol/L solution:
    ∘ If immediate pain, flush bladder with 60 mL H_2O and treat with bladder instillations
    ∘ If no immediate pain, wait 5 minutes and rate urgency and pain
  – If urgency or pain >2, treat as above
- Pain or urgency >2 is considered a positive test and strongly correlates with interstitial cystitis if no radiation cystitis or acute bacterial cystitis is present.

Test Interpretation
- Nonspecific chronic inflammation on bladder biopsies
- Urine cytology negative for dysplasia and neoplasia
- Possible mast cell proliferation in mucosa

 TREATMENT

GENERAL MEASURES
- Appropriate health care: Outpatient
- Eliminate foods and liquids that exacerbate symptoms on individual basis
- Biofeedback bladder retraining

MEDICATION
- Randomized controlled trials of most medications for interstitial cystitis demonstrate limited benefit over placebo; there are no clear predictors of what will benefit an individual. Prepare the patient that treatment may involve trial and error.
- Intravesical injections of botulinum toxin are not effective in the treatment of ulcer type interstitial cystitis.

First Line
- Pentosan polysulfate (Elmiron) 100 mg t.i.d. May take several months to become effective; rated as modestly beneficial in systematic drug review (only FDA-approved treatment for interstitial cystitis).
- Tolterodine 1–2 mg b.i.d.
- Triple drug therapy: 6 months of pentosan, hydroxyzine, doxepin
- Behavioral therapy combined with oral agents found improved outcomes compared to medications alone.
- Antibacterials for bacteriuria
- Hydroxyzine
- Amitriptyline $\geq$50 mg/d (3)[C]
- Oxybutynin, hyoscyamine, and other anticholinergic medications decrease frequency.
- Prednisone (only for ulcerative lesions)
- Montelukast
- Doxepin decreases frequency.
- NSAIDs for pain and any inflammatory component
- Bladder instillations:
  – Lidocaine, sodium bicarbonate, and heparin or pentosan polysulfate sodium
  – Dimethyl sulfoxide (DMSO) every 1–2 weeks for 3–6 weeks, then PRN
  – Heparin sometimes added to DMSO
  – Intravesical liposomes (4)
  – Other agents: Steroids, silver nitrate, oxychlorosene (Clorpactin)
- Contraindications:
  – No anticholinergics for patients with closed-angle glaucoma
- Significant possible interactions:
  – Refer to manufacturer's profile of each drug.

Second Line
Phenazopyridine, a local bladder mucosal anesthetic, usually is not very effective.

ISSUES FOR REFERRAL
- Need for clarity with respect to diagnosis
- Surgical intervention

ADDITIONAL THERAPIES
Myofascial physical therapy (targeted pelvic, hip girdle, abdominal trigger point massage) (5)[C]

SURGERY/OTHER PROCEDURES
- Hydraulic distention of bladder under anesthesia: Symptomatic but transient relief
- Cauterization of bladder ulcer
- Augmentation cystoplasty to increase bladder capacity and decrease pressure, with or without partial cystectomy. Expected results in severe cases: Much improved, 75%; with residual discomfort, 20%; unchanged, 5%
- Urinary diversion with total cystectomy only if disease is completely refractory to medical therapy
- Sacral neuromodulation

COMPLEMENTARY AND ALTERNATIVE MEDICINE
Guided imagery

 ## ONGOING CARE

FOLLOW-UP RECOMMENDATIONS
Patient Monitoring
Not specifically needed unless symptoms are unresponsive to treatment

DIET
- Variable effects from person to person
- Common irritants include caffeine, chocolate, citrus, tomatoes, carbonated beverages, K^+-rich foods, spicy foods, acidic foods, and alcohol.

PATIENT EDUCATION
Interstitial Cystitis Association, 110 Washington St. Suite 340, Rockville, MD 20850; 1-800-HELPICA; www.ichelp.org

PROGNOSIS
- Mild: Exacerbations and remissions of symptoms; may not be progressive; does not predispose to other diseases
- Severe: Progressive problems that usually require surgery to control symptoms

COMPLICATIONS
Severe, with long-term, continuous high bladder pressure could be associated with renal damage.

REFERENCES

1. Rais-Bahrami S, Friedlander JI, Herati AS, et al. Symptom profile variability of interstitial cystitis/painful bladder syndrome by age. *BJU Int*. 2012; 109:1356–1359.
2. Parsons CL, Dell J. Increased prevalence of interstitial cystitis; previously unrecognized urologic and gynecological cases identified using a new symptom questionnaire and intravesical potassium sensitivity. *Urology*. 2002;60:573–578.
3. Foster HE, Hanno PM, Nickel JC, et al. Effect of amitriptyline on symptoms in treatment naive patients with interstitial cystitis/painful bladder syndrome. *J Urol*. 2010;183:1853–1858.
4. Lee WC, Chuang YC, et al. Safety and dose flexibility clinical evaluation of intravesical liposome in patients with interstitial cystitis or painful bladder syndrome. *Kaohsiung J Med Sci*. 2011;27:437–440.
5. Fitzgerald MP, Payne CK, Lukacz ES, et al. Randomized multicenter clinical trial of myofascial physical therapy and women with interstitial cystitis/painful bladder syndrome and pelvic floor tenderness. *J Urol*. 2012;187:2113–2118.

 ## SEE ALSO

- Urinary Tract Infection (UTI) in Females
- Algorithm: Pelvic Girdle Pain (Pregnancy or Postpartum Anterior Pelvic Pain)

 ## CODES

ICD10
- N30.1 Interstitial cystitis (chronic)
- N30.10 Interstitial cystitis (chronic) without hematuria
- N30.11 Interstitial cystitis (chronic) with hematuria

CLINICAL PEARLS
- The potassium sensitivity test has been the most useful in confirming an initial diagnosis of interstitial cystitis.
- K^+ sensitivity test (2):
  – Insert catheter, empty bladder, instill 40 mL H_2O over 2–3 minutes, rank urgency on scale of 0–5 in intensity, rank pain on scale of 0–5 in intensity, drain bladder, instill 40 mL KCl 0.4 mol/L solution.
- Submucosal petechial hemorrhages and/or ulceration at the time of bladder distention and cystoscopy further support the diagnosis.
- At present, there is no definitive treatment for interstitial cystitis.
- Most patients with severe disease receive multiple treatment approaches. Regular multidisciplinary follow up, pharmacologic therapy, avoidance of symptom triggers, and psychological and supportive therapy are all important because this disease tends to wax and wane. Monitor patients for comorbid depression.
- Empowering patients to manage their symptoms, communicate regularly with their physicians, and learn as much as they can about this disease can help them to optimize their outcome.

I

INTERSTITIAL NEPHRITIS

Neil Patel, DO • Christi Woods, DO

BASICS

DESCRIPTION
- Acute interstitial nephritis (AIN) is an inflammatory response of the kidney involving interstitial edema and, at times, tubular cell damage. It may be an acute reaction or a result of long-term damage.
- System(s) affected: Renal/Urologic, Endocrine/Metabolic, Immunologic
- Synonym(s): Tubulointerstitial nephritis (TIN), Acute interstitial allergic nephritis

EPIDEMIOLOGY
Pediatric Considerations
Children exposed to lead poisoning are more likely to develop nephritis as a young adult:
- TIN with uveitis presents in adolescent females.
- Atherosclerotic or ischemic nephritis is more common in the elderly.

Incidence
- Interstitial nephritis accounts for 10–15% of kidney disease in the US.
- Analgesic-induced nephritis is 5–6× more common in women.
- Peak incidence in women 60–70 years of age

Geriatric Considerations
The elderly have more severe disease and increased risk of permanent damage.

ETIOLOGY AND PATHOPHYSIOLOGY
- AIN:
  - Delayed drug hypersensitivity reactions
  - May cause acute renal insufficiency
  - Regardless of the severity of the damage to the tubular epithelium, the renal dysfunction generally is reversible, possibly reflecting the regenerative capacity of tubules with a preserved basement membrane.
- Chronic interstitial nephritis (CIN):
  - Follows long-term exposure to offending agents
  - Often found on routine labs or evaluation for hypertension (HTN)
  - Characterized by interstitial scarring, fibrosis, and tubular atrophy, resulting in progressive chronic renal insufficiency
- TIN is sometimes associated with uveitis.
- AIN:
  - Hypersensitivity to drugs (70%):
    ○ Antibiotics: Penicillin, cephalosporins, sulfonamides, rifampin
    ○ NSAIDs/Analgesics/Cox-2 inhibitors
    ○ Sulfa-containing diuretics
    ○ Phenytoin
    ○ Allopurinol
    ○ Cimetidine
    ○ Proton pump inhibitors (omeprazole and lansoprazole)
    ○ Indinavir
  - Infectious sources include *Legionella*, *Leptospira*, streptococcal organisms, cytomegalovirus, *Mycoplasma tuberculosis*
  - AIN is associated with primary renal infections, such as acute bacterial pyelonephritis, renal tuberculosis, and fungal nephritis.
  - Acute transplant rejection
  - Immunologic: Systemic lupus erythematosus (SLE), Sjögren syndrome, sarcoidosis, Wegener granulomatosis, cryoglobulinemia
  - Idiopathic (isolated or with uveitis)

- CIN:
  - Drugs: Analgesics, lithium, antineoplastics, antibiotics, anticonvulsants, antihypertensives, immunosuppressants, diuretics, Chinese herbal medicines
  - Heavy metals: Lead, cadmium
  - Obstructive: Stones, neoplasm, prostatic hypertrophy
  - Metabolic: Hypercalcemia, hyperoxaluria, chronic hypokalemia, cystinosis
  - Vascular changes: Cholesterol emboli, HTN, sickle hemoglobinopathy, radiation
  - Toxins: Snakebite venom (hemotoxic or myotoxic)
  - Other: Balkan-endemic nephropathy, Epstein-Barr virus

GENERAL PREVENTION
- Early recognition and prompt discontinuation of offending agents
- Removal of all sources of heavy metals, including ceramics
- Avoid further nephrotoxic substances.

COMMONLY ASSOCIATED CONDITIONS
- Alport syndrome
- Medullary cystic disease
- Inflammatory bowel disease
- Multiple myeloma
- Primary biliary cirrhosis

DIAGNOSIS

- AIN:
  - Fever: 80%
  - Transient maculopapular rash: 25–50%
  - Acute renal insufficiency:
    ○ Decreased urine output: 50%
    ○ Signs of fluid overload or depletion
    ○ Altered mental status
    ○ Nausea, vomiting
- CIN:
  - HTN
  - Decreased urine output or polyuria
  - Inability to concentrate urine
  - Polydipsia
  - Acidosis
  - Anemia
  - Fanconi syndrome

HISTORY
- Medications
- Alcohol and illicit drug use
- Exposure to heavy metals
- Tobacco use
- Dyslipidemia/Atherosclerosis
- Cancer
- HTN

PHYSICAL EXAM
- Increased BP
- Altered mental status
- Rash accompanying renal findings in acute AIN
- Pericardial rub if uremic pericarditis
- Lung crackles if fluid overloaded
- Fluid retention/extremity swelling/weight gain

DIFFERENTIAL DIAGNOSIS
- Acute renal failure
- Urinary tract obstruction

DIAGNOSTIC TESTS & INTERPRETATION
- CBC:
  - Eosinophilia (80%): NSAID-induced AIN is only associated with eosinophilia in ~15% of cases
  - Anemia
- Chemistry:
  - Acidosis
  - Hypokalemia/Hyperkalemia
  - Elevated BUN and creatinine
- Urinalysis with urine electrolytes:
  - Hematuria (95%)
  - Mild proteinuria (present to variable degrees, usually <1 g/24 h, except in AIN associated with NSAIDs)
  - Specific gravity
  - Pyuria, WBC casts
  - Eosinophiluria
- Serologic testing for immunologic disease: Sarcoidosis, Sjögren syndrome, Wegener granulomatosis, Behçet syndrome
- Lead level:
  - Not useful in chronic lead exposure
  - >90% of lead resides in bone
  - If chronic lead exposure is suspected, consider EDTA lead mobilization test.
- Liver function tests: Elevated serum transaminase levels (in patients with associated drug-induced liver injury)
- Kidneys, ureters, and bladder (KUB)
- Gallium scan (a negative gallium scan does not preclude the diagnosis because false–negative results can be seen)
- Renal US may demonstrate kidneys that are normal to enlarged in size with increased cortical echogenicity, but no US findings will reliably confirm or exclude AIN vs. other causes of acute renal failure.
- The role of IV pyelography (IVP) remains in question (in many instances, similar information can be obtained by US without exposing the patient to potentially nephrotoxic contrast dye).

Follow-Up Tests & Special Considerations
Patients who do not recover renal function and those with chronic TIN should receive long-term follow-up care to protect kidneys from further potentially nephrotoxic therapies.

Diagnostic Procedures/Other
- Renal biopsy is the gold standard and definitive method of establishing the diagnosis of AIN. However, it is not needed in all patients.
- Indications for renal biopsy: Patients who do not improve following withdrawal of likely precipitating medications and who are being considered for steroid therapy are good candidates for renal biopsy.
- Contraindications: Renal biopsy is contraindicated in bleeding diathesis, solitary kidney, end-stage renal disease (ESRD) with small kidneys, severe uncontrolled HTN and sepsis, or renal parenchymal infection.

Test Interpretation
- Acute:
  - Cellular infiltration with eosinophilia
  - In cholesterol microembolism of the kidney, the finding of a characteristic needle-shaped cleft in medium- or small-sized renal arterioles is diagnostic.
- Chronic: Chronic TIN is characterized by tubular atrophy, fibrosis, and cellular infiltration with mononuclear cells.

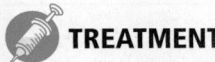
TREATMENT

For AIN, data on corticosteroids' efficacy have been limited (1)[B].

GENERAL MEASURES
- Discontinue offending agent.
- Reduce exposure to other nephrotoxic agents.
- Supportive measures
- Maintain adequate hydration.
- Symptomatic relief for fever, rash, and systemic symptoms
- Control of BP and anemia.
- Correct electrolyte imbalances.
- Possible short-term dialysis until recovery of renal function

MEDICATION
- Mainstay of treatment is supportive therapy.
- Offending drugs should be discontinued.
- If patient is taking multiple offending drugs, a reasonable clinical approach should include whether any suspected drug can be substituted easily with another medication.
- If renal failure persists after removing the agent, attempt medication therapy.

First Line
- Prednisone 1 mg/kg/d PO or equivalent IV dose to a max of 40–60 mg/d × 1–2 weeks, followed by a gradual taper over 3–4 weeks
- In patients who do not respond to corticosteroids within 2–3 weeks, consider treatment with cyclophosphamide (Cytoxan).
- Studies support steroid use in chronic, not acute, interstitial nephritis (1)[B],(2,3)[C],(4)[A].
- Continue corticosteroids for 6 months in patients with sarcoidosis (2)[C].

Second Line
- Lead toxicity: Repeated chelation therapy may improve renal function (5)[A]:
  – Succimer 10 mg/kg PO q8h × 5 days, then q12h × 14 days, or
  – EDTA 2 g IV/IM; if IM, use with 2% lidocaine.
- SLE nephritis: Steroids +cyclophosphamide or azathioprine (4)[A]
- Urate nephropathy:
  – Allopurinol to decrease urate level (2)[C]
  – Use with caution because allopurinol is nephrotoxic.
- Lithium-induced nephritis: Use amiloride as adjunct (2)[C].
- Cidofovir-induced nephritis: Use probenecid as adjunct (2)[C].

ISSUES FOR REFERRAL
Most patients presenting with renal insufficiency, proteinuria, and/or acid–base electrolyte disorders require consultation with a nephrologist.

IN-PATIENT CONSIDERATIONS
Patients with acute renal failure or with serious electrolyte or acid–base disorders may require inpatient care until stabilization or resolution.

Admission Criteria/Initial Stabilization
- Persistent oliguria or anuria
- Severe electrolyte abnormalities
- ECG changes
- Arterial blood gases
- ECG

Discharge Criteria
- Stable vitals, correction of all electrolyte imbalances, including magnesium, and resolution of acute ECG changes
- Normal urine production

ONGOING CARE

FOLLOW-UP RECOMMENDATIONS
Patient Monitoring
If patients must remain on nephrotoxic medications, measure renal function, electrolytes, and phosphorus frequently.

DIET
- Low fat/low cholesterol
- Low protein (6)[A]
- Low sodium
- Low potassium

PATIENT EDUCATION
Printed materials for patients are available at the National Kidney Disease Education Program, (866) 4-KIDNEY, www.nkdep.nih.gov.

PROGNOSIS
- If the associated AIN is detected early (within 1 week of the rise in serum creatinine) and the drug is discontinued promptly, the long-term outcome is favorable for a return to baseline serum creatinine.
- Renal biopsy reveals extent of damage.
- AIN:
  – Recovery within weeks to months
  – Acute dialysis is needed for 1/3 of patients before resolution.
  – Rarely progresses to ESRD
- CIN: Can progress to ESRD
- TIN with uveitis:
  – Renal disease remits in 1 year if untreated.
  – Uveitis has relapsing course, requiring systemic corticosteroids.
- Untreated acute renal failure has 45–70% mortality.

COMPLICATIONS
- Papillary necrosis
- Chronic tubulointerstitial disease may progress to ESRD requiring dialysis or transplantation.
- Analgesics increase the risk of transitional cell cancers of the uroepithelium.

REFERENCES

1. Clarkson MR. Acute interstitial nephritis: Clinical features and response to corticosteroid therapy. *Nephrol Dialysis Transplant*. 2004;19:2778–2783.
2. Braden GL, O'Shea MH, Mulhern JG. Tubulointerstitial diseases. *Am J Kidney Dis*. 2005;46:560–572.
3. Markowitz GS, Perazella MA. Drug-induced renal failure: A focus on tubulointerstitial disease. *Clinica Chimica Acta*. 2005;351:31–47.
4. Flanc RS. Treatment for lupus nephritis. *Cochrane Database Sys Rev*. 2004;1:CD002922.
5. Lin JL, Lin-Tan DT, Hsu KH, et al. Environmental lead exposure and progression of chronic renal diseases in patients without diabetes. *N Engl J Med*. 2003;348:277–286.
6. Fougue D, Laville M. Low-protein diets for chronic kidney disease in nondiabetic adults. *Cochrane Database Sys Rev*. 2009;(3):CD001892.

ADDITIONAL READING
- Muriithi AK, Nasr SH, Leung N. Utility of urine eosinophils in the diagnosis of acute interstitial nephritis. *Clin J Am Soc Nephrol*. 2013 Sep 19. [Epub ahead of print]
- www.aafp.org/afp/20030615/2527.htm
- www.jasn.asnjournals.org/cgi/reprint/9/3/506
- www.nature.com/ki/journal/v77/n11/abs/ki201089a.html

SEE ALSO

Algorithm: Hematuria

CODES

ICD10
- N10 Acute tubulo-interstitial nephritis
- N11.9 Chronic tubulo-interstitial nephritis, unspecified
- N12 Tubulo-interstitial nephritis, not spcf as acute or chronic

CLINICAL PEARLS
- Symptoms of AIN are more dramatic and sudden (days to weeks) than those of CIN, which is slower and progressive.
- The best treatment is to first remove the offending agent.
- Hypercalcemia is both a cause and an effect of CIN. Treating hypercalcemia slows the progression of CIN.
- Eosinophilia on the CBC occurs only in ~15% of NSAID-induced AIN cases.
- The gold standard in diagnosing interstitial nephritis is a renal biopsy.

I

INTESTINAL PARASITES

Douglas W. MacPherson, MD, MSc(CTM), FRCPC

 BASICS

DESCRIPTION
- Parasites are divided into 2 groups:
  - Protozoa: Single-cell organisms; typically multiply within the host. Intestinal protozoa: Transmission by direct fecal–oral route; do not cause eosinophilia.
  - Helminths (worms): Multicellular organisms; rarely multiply within the host (exceptions: *Strongyloides stercoralis, Hymenolepis nana*); infection may cause a degree of eosinophilia. Level of eosinophilia is associated with the degree of tissue invasiveness. Worms have a limited life span and, without reinfection, most eventually die on their own.
- Some are invasive, and some do not release their infective forms into the bowel. This latter group (e.g., *Toxoplasma gondii, Echinococcus* sp., *Trichinella spiralis*) is not reviewed here.
- Most worms require incubation outside the host before being infectious or need a vector for transmission. *Enterobius vermicularis (*pinworm) eggs are infectious shortly after being passed; autoinfection occurs readily.
- Person-to-person transmission of worms is uncommon, except for pinworm.
- System(s) affected: Gastrointestinal (GI)

Pediatric Considerations
Most common age group affected

Pregnancy Considerations
Many of the treatments are contraindicated.

EPIDEMIOLOGY
Acquisition involves personal, food, and/or water sanitation and migration from higher-prevalence areas.

Incidence
- Predominant sex: Male = Female
- Predominant age: Pediatric

Prevalence
- US laboratory statistics: 5–30% of general population. Random testing finds at least 1 GI parasite in 5–10% of all people.
- From day care surveys: Asymptomatic 20–30%; symptomatic 50–80%
- Intestinal protozoa account for most parasite findings in North America. Helminths account for <10% of GI parasites.
- *Blastocystis hominis* is a commensal enteric fungus of no clinical significance found in 20–30% of stools.

ETIOLOGY AND PATHOPHYSIOLOGY
- The pathophysiology of GI parasitic infections is host–parasite-specific.
- Most intestinal parasitic infections are eventually self-limiting. Most worms have a defined life expectancy in the host. Autoreinfection does occur in some worm infections (e.g., strongyloidiasis, pinworm).
- Protozoan pathogens:
  - *Giardia lamblia*: Common
  - *Entamoeba histolytica, Cryptosporidium* sp., *Isospora belli, Balantidium coli, Cyclospora cayetanensis, Microsporida*
- Possible protozoan pathogens: *Dientamoeba fragilis*

- Probable nonpathogenic protozoa:
  - Amoebas: All other *Entamoeba* sp., *Endolimax nana*
  - All other intestinal flagellates
- Helminthic pathogens:
  - Nematodes (roundworms): *Enterobius vermicularis, Trichuris trichiura, Ascaris lumbricoides*, hookworm (*Necator americanus, Ancylostoma duodenale*), *Strongyloides stercoralis, Capillaria philippinensis, Trichostrongylus* sp.
  - Trematodes (flukes): *Fasciolopsis buski, Clonorchis sinensis, Opisthorchis viverrini, Heterophyes, Fasciola hepatica, Paragonimus westermani, Schistosoma mansoni, S. japonicum, S. haematobium, S. mekongi*
  - Cestodes (tapeworms): *Taenia saginata, T. solium, Diphyllobothrium latum, Hymenolepis nana, H. diminuta, Dipylidium caninum*

RISK FACTORS
- Age (children)
- Low socioeconomic status and poor sanitation: Personal, food, water; crowding: Day care centers, institutional care
- International travel or migration
- Multiple medical conditions, pregnancy, gastric hypoacidity, immunosuppression (AIDS)

GENERAL PREVENTION
- Intestinal parasites are usually acquired by direct fecal–oral contact via ingested contaminated food or water. Rarely, infected arthropod vectors are involved in transmission. Person-to-person transmission may occur through this mechanism.
- Safe food and water precautions ("Wash it, cook it, peel it, or forget it"); enteric and hand hygiene is the means of preventing infections. Infrastructure systems for safe food and water processing contribute to the low prevalence of intestinal parasites.

COMMONLY ASSOCIATED CONDITIONS
- GI parasitic infections and diseases may be associated with HIV infection or AIDS, steroid use, immune deficiencies, and blood type.
- Intestinal parasite infection appears to protect against allergic sensitization (1)[A].

 DIAGNOSIS

HISTORY
Historical or physical features alone cannot separate intestinal parasites from other GI infections or the noninfectious enteric diseases except the actual finding of a typical worm: i.e., a tapeworm segment or roundworm: Ascarid, whipworm, or pinworm)
- Acute bacterial or viral GI syndromes tend to be sudden onset and short duration.
- Fever is uncommon with GI parasites unless there is tissue invasion (e.g., amoebiasis, strongyloidiasis).
- Chronic bloating, excessive gas, and intermittent/unpredictable diarrhea without blood is typical of giardiasis.
- Extraintestinal symptoms and signs are uncommon with GI parasites, except invasive strongyloidiasis.
- A water, food, or fecal contamination exposure history (e.g., international travel, migration, high-risk environments [day care centers, camping]) may suggest a particular parasitic agent.

- A family or personal history of inflammatory or irritable bowel syndromes does not exclude GI parasites.

PHYSICAL EXAM
- Will generally appear well even if distressed with GI complaints; usually afebrile
- Diffuse, migratory rash (cutaneous larva currens) with invasive strongyloidiasis; this is a medical emergency.
- Weight loss and anorexia may be present (e.g., chronic giardiasis, invasive amoebiasis, chronic helminths).
- Anemia may be present with heavy hookworm infections.
- Excessive gas: Bloating, eructation, flatulence, borborygmi
- Nausea or vomiting: Intermittent, recurrent
- Abdominal pain/tenderness
- May have bowel tenderness, but liver and spleen are usually normal
- Diarrhea: Persistent and recurrent, chronic but dysentery (i.e., frank GI bleeding) is rare, except with *E. histolytica, B. coli.*
- Pruritus ani: *E. vermicularis, T. trichiura, S. stercoralis*, tapeworms. Perirectal or vulvar rash
- Passing a roundworm or tapeworm or a worm segment

DIFFERENTIAL DIAGNOSIS
- Other nonparasitic intestinal infections
- Food poisoning
- Malabsorption: Commonly lactose, gluten enteropathy; rarely celiac disease, tropical or nontropical sprue
- Inflammatory and irritable bowel diseases
- Hemorrhoid or rectal fissures

DIAGNOSTIC TESTS & INTERPRETATION
- Stool specimens that are properly collected, preserved, and transported for examination in a qualified and proficient laboratory by a dedicated parasitology technologist team have the highest diagnostic yield for GI parasites.
- Special diagnostics for *Cryptosporidium, I. belli, Cyclospora, Microsporidia*, and *Strongyloides*: Give specific laboratory notice.
- Pinworm paddles provide a greater diagnostic yield for *E. vermicularis*. Multiple tests (2) may be needed to exclude pinworms.
- Parasite culture is possible for *G. lamblia, E. histolytica*, and *S. stercoralis* but is rarely indicated; only done in reference laboratories.
- Rarely, a biopsy and histology will demonstrate the presence of an invasive helminth on tissue section.
- Tissue biopsies of intestine, liver, or bladder may show granulomatous reactions of schistosome eggs.
- A single stool specimen collected into a preservative (i.e., sodium acetate formalin [SAF]), well mixed to fix and preserve all elements, yields an accurate diagnosis of 90%. Additional specimens improve diagnostic accuracy (3)[A].
- Newer lab techniques for stool specimens currently provide little diagnostic advantage. Exception: *Giardia* antigen—fluorescent antibody (FA) and ELISA tests: A single FA or ELISA may be at least as sensitive as 3 stools for ova and parasites.

- Serology: Useful if parasite is not found in stool samples normally or if low numbers of parasites; available only through reference centers, that is, *Strongyloides*, amebiasis, schistosomiasis
- Drugs that may alter lab results: Use of antibiotics; oil-based laxatives, and barium in the stool interfere with microscopy.

Initial Tests (lab, imaging)
Screening blood eosinophilia is not recommended.
- Diagnostic radiology is rarely needed. Exception: Invasive disease due to amebiasis for colitis, amebomas, and liver abscesses

Follow-Up Tests & Special Considerations
- A single negative stool examination does not rule out intestinal parasitic infection, but when performed under best conditions, it is highly accurate. Repeat testing may be indicated for primary diagnosis.
- Population-based intestinal parasite screening in North America (e.g., day care attendees, personal-care providers, food handlers, immigrants) has low diagnostic utility and is not recommended.

Diagnostic Procedures/Other
- Invasive diagnostic procedures are rarely needed or indicated.
- Egg granulomata of schistosomiasis may be demonstrated in affected tissues.
- With hemorrhagic colitis due to invasive amebiasis, sigmoidoscopy is diagnostic.
- Upper intestinal endoscopy can yield fluid to be examined for *G. lamblia* trophozoites and *S. stercoralis* larvae.

Test Interpretation
- Most intestinal parasites are not invasive and produce nonspecific or no changes in bowel histology.
- Invasive amebiasis produces a classic endoscopic and histologic picture of ulceration and inflammation in the colon.
- Protozoa or helminths may be seen in bowel biopsy histology.

TREATMENT

Specific antiparasitic treatment should be selected on patient needs, parasite biology, and epidemiology.

GENERAL MEASURES
- Not all patients need to be treated with drugs.
- Symptomatic treatment is indicated for patient comfort once specific therapy has been initiated.
- Drugs inhibiting intestinal motility are relatively contraindicated in patients with diarrhea caused by invasive organisms.

MEDICATION
- Protozoa (4)[A]:
  – *E. histolytica*: Asymptomatic infection needs individual assessment.
  – *E. histolytica* symptomatic intestinal: Iodoquinol or diloxanide furoate
  – *E. histolytica* invasive disease: Iodoquinol or diloxanide furoate plus metronidazole alone or metronidazole alone or emetine + chloroquine phosphate
  – *G. lamblia*: Metronidazole or tinidazole or furazolidone or quinacrine. *Note:* Albendazole, available in the US only from manufacturer, may have activity against *G. lamblia*.
- *Cryptosporidium*: None proven effective

- *I. belli* protozoa: Trimethoprim–sulfamethoxazole
- *B. coli*: Tetracycline or iodoquinol or metronidazole
- *Cyclospora*: Sulfamethoxazole-trimethoprim
- *Microsporidia*: Albendazole (some species)
- Helminths:
  – Nematodes (except *Strongyloides* and *Trichostrongylus*): Mebendazole or pyrantel pamoate or piperazine citrate or albendazole (available in US only from manufacturer)
  – *Strongyloides* and *Trichostrongylus*: Thiabendazole or albendazole (available in the US only from manufacturer)
  – Cestodes: Praziquantel or niclosamide
  – Trematodes: Niclosamide or praziquantel

Pediatric Considerations
Nitazoxanide 7.5 mg/kg PO b.i.d. × 3 days or single-dose tinidazole 50 mg/kg (not available in the US) may be used.

ISSUES FOR REFERRAL
Treatment failures, complex patients (including drug intolerances or allergies), multiple parasitic infections, and complicated medical (e.g., HIV/AIDS, diabetes, chronic steroid use) or surgical conditions: Specialist in tropical medicine or infectious diseases

SURGERY/OTHER PROCEDURES
- Surgical procedures play little role, except for amebic liver abscesses, which may need to be drained, especially left lobe abscesses.
- Surgery possible for bowel or organ obstruction, *A. lumbricoides* migration, or for complicated amebic colitis

COMPLEMENTARY AND ALTERNATIVE MEDICINE
- Many complementary and alternative therapies exist, but none are effective for primary treatment.
- Consequences of intestinal parasitic infections include lactose intolerance, irritable bowel syndrome, or nutritional calorie–protein deficiencies, dehydration, vitamin B_{12} deficiency.

IN-PATIENT CONSIDERATIONS
Nosocomial intestinal parasitic infections are rare, as are hospital-based parasitic GI outbreaks. Invasive strongyloidiasis may occur in hospitals for other reasons (e.g., surgery, use of high-dose steroids, etc.).

Admission Criteria/Initial Stabilization
Admission is rarely required except for intestinal obstruction, dysentery, or systemic invasion.

ONGOING CARE

FOLLOW-UP RECOMMENDATIONS
Patient Monitoring
For most intestinal parasitic infections, testing for clearance is not indicated. Repeat stool examination for clearance should be timed, taking into account the life cycle of the parasite and the risk of reinfection.

DIET
Many patients experience symptoms of irritable bowel syndrome and/or lactose intolerance during and following bowel infections, especially when infected with *G. lamblia*.

PATIENT EDUCATION
Important to reduce the risk of reinfection or transmission

COMPLICATIONS
Complications are rare; they include chronic persistent diarrhea, irritable bowel syndrome, and chronic malabsorption.

REFERENCES

1. Feary J, Britton J, Leonardi-Bee J. Atopy and current intestinal parasite infection: A systematic review and meta-analysis. *Allergy*. 2011;66:569–578.
2. Strand EA, Robertson LJ, Hanevik K, et al. Sensitivity of a *Giardia* antigen test in persistent giardiasis following an extensive outbreak. *Clin Microbiol Infect*. 2008;14:1069–1071.
3. Senay H, MacPherson DW. Parasitology: Diagnostic yield of stool examination. *Can Med Assoc J*. 1989;140:1329–1331.
4. Abramowicz M, ed. Drugs for parasitic infections. In: *The medical letter*. New York: The Medical Letter; 2007:1–15.

ADDITIONAL READING

- Barry MA, Weatherhead JE, Hotez PJ, et al. Childhood parasitic infections endemic to the United States. *Pediatr Clin North Am*. 2013;60:471–485.
- Centers for Disease Control and Prevention. Parasites and health. Parasites of the intestinal tract. Available at: www.dpd.cdc.gov/dpdx/html/para_health.htm
- Granados CE, Reveiz L, Uribe LG, et al. Drugs for treating giardiasis. *Cochrane Database Syst Rev*. 2012;12:CD007787.
- Lal A, Baker MG, Hales S, et al. Potential effects of global environmental changes on cryptosporidiosis and giardiasis transmission. *Trends Parasitol*. 2013;29:83–90.
- Leonardi-Bee J, Pritchard D, Britton J. Asthma and current intestinal parasite infection: Systematic review and meta-analysis. *Am J Respir Crit Care Med*. 2006;174:514–523.
- van Lieshout L, Verweij JJ. Newer diagnostic approaches to intestinal protozoa. *Curr Opin Infect Dis*. 2010;23:488–493.

 SEE ALSO

Algorithm: Hematemesis (Bleeding, Upper GI)

 CODES

ICD10
- A07.9 Protozoal intestinal disease, unspecified
- B82.0 Intestinal helminthiasis, unspecified
- B82.9 Intestinal parasitism, unspecified

CLINICAL PEARLS
- Consider GI parasites when dealing with a history of travel, recent immigration, children, or other vulnerable populations; a story of chronic or persistent diarrhea; or seeing worms in the stool.
- Stools correctly collected in the proper preservative will detect most intestinal parasites. Exceptions: *S. stercoralis*, *E. vermicularis*, *Cryptosporidium*, *Cyclospora*, and *Microspora* sp.
- Checking for eosinophilia is not a reliable screening method.

IRRITABLE BOWEL SYNDROME

Patricia Lacsina, MD, • Fozia Ali, MD

 BASICS

DESCRIPTION
- A condition characterized by:
  - Chronic abdominal pain associated with:
    - Alteration in bowel habits *AND*
    - Absence of organic pathology.
- May be characterized as diarrhea predominant or constipation predominant; or may alternate between diarrhea and constipation
- Synonym(s): Spastic colon; Irritable colon

EPIDEMIOLOGY
Irritable bowel syndrome (IBS) accounts for up to 50% of GI visits in some practices:
- Second to upper respiratory infection as cause for lost workdays

Prevalence
- 5–10% of the population of North America:
  - However, only 15% of these patients actually seek medical attention.
- Predominant age: 20–39 years
- If age >50 years, consider other diagnoses.
- Predominant sex: In the US, Female > Male (2:1)
- Common in low socioeconomic community

ETIOLOGY AND PATHOPHYSIOLOGY
- The etiology is unknown, but patients demonstrate intestinal motility abnormalities with enhanced sensitivity to visceral stimuli.
- The trigger may be luminal or environmental.

Genetics
Unknown, but more common in families of IBS patients

RISK FACTORS
- Other family members with similar GI disorder
- History of childhood sexual abuse
- Sexual/Domestic abuse in women
- Depression
- Can occur after an infectious colitis (1)

Pregnancy Considerations
No risk to mother or fetus

GENERAL PREVENTION
See "Diet."

COMMONLY ASSOCIATED CONDITIONS
- Migraine
- Urinary frequency and urgency
- Fibromyalgia
- Dyspareunia
- Depression
- Anxiety
- Posttraumatic stress disorder

DIAGNOSIS

HISTORY
- Abdominal pain/discomfort described as cramping worsened by emotional stress and eating
- Rome II criteria: ≥12 weeks in past 12 months of abdominal pain or discomfort that has 2 of 3 features:
  - Relieved by defecation
  - Onset associated with change in frequency of stool
  - Onset associated with change in form of stool
- Symptoms can also include:
  - Mucus in stools
  - Constipation
  - Bloating
  - Diarrhea
  - Abdominal distention
  - Upper abdominal discomfort after eating
  - Straining for normal consistency stools
  - Urgency of defecation
  - Feelings of incomplete evacuation
  - Abnormal stool form
  - Nausea, vomiting (rarely)
- May have history of abuse or depression
- Patient may note worsening of symptoms with stress or around menses.
- IBS is unlikely in patients with a history of:
  - Weight loss
  - Bleeding
  - Nocturnal diarrhea
  - Fever
  - Anemia

PHYSICAL EXAM
Generally normal, but may have abdominal tenderness to palpation

DIFFERENTIAL DIAGNOSIS
- Inflammatory bowel disease
- Lactose intolerance
- Infections (*Giardia lamblia, Entamoeba histolytica, Salmonella, Campylobacter, Yersinia, Clostridium difficile*)
- Celiac sprue
- Microscopic colitis
- Cathartic use
- Magnesium-containing antacids
- Hypo-/Hyperthyroidism
- Pancreatic insufficiency
- Depression
- Small bowel bacterial overgrowth
- Somatization
- Villous adenoma
- Endocrine tumors
- Diabetes mellitus
- Radiation damage to colon or small bowel

DIAGNOSTIC TESTS & INTERPRETATION
- In the setting of a typical history and in the absence of danger signs, such as anemia or weight loss, it is reasonable to obtain baseline labs and begin treatment.
- In those who do not respond to treatment, further evaluation with imaging studies and endoscopy is warranted to exclude organic pathology.

Initial Tests (lab, imaging)
As needed to rule out other pathology specific to the patient's symptoms:
- Diarrhea-predominant: ESR, CBC, tissue transglutaminase, thyroid-stimulating hormone (TSH), and stool for ova and parasites
- Constipation-predominant: CBC, TSH, electrolytes, calcium
- Abdominal pain: LFTs and amylase
- Abdominal CT scan or abdominal ultrasound to evaluate pain is generally normal
- Small-bowel series or video capsule endoscopy to rule out Crohn disease of small intestine may be considered and will also be normal.
- Sitz Marker study may be used to evaluate colon transit in patients with constipation

Follow-Up Tests & Special Considerations
- Consider lactulose breath test to assess for small bowel bacterial overgrowth associated with IBS (2)[C].
- Given high rates of false-positive and negative test results, some clinicians opt for an empiric trial of antibiotics.

Diagnostic Procedures/Other
Sigmoidoscopy/colonoscopy may be used to rule out inflammatory bowel disease or microscopic colitis.

> **ALERT**
> Colonoscopy should be performed in all persons >50 years of age for colorectal cancer screening

Test Interpretation
None

 TREATMENT

- Goals: Symptomatic relief and improvement of quality of life
  - Work with primary care physician to determine appropriate measure
  - Determine if diarrhea predominant, constipation predominant, or mixed type
- Lifestyle modification:
  - Vigorous exercise 3–5 times per week decreases IBS severity
  - Make a food diary to determine triggers that worsen symptoms
- Medications:
  - Fiber supplements such as Metamucil can help increase stool bulk but does not relieve abdominal pain; may be used for all types.

- Medications that can improve abdominal pain, global symptoms, and symptom severity in all types:
  – Antispasmodics such as hyoscyamine (Levsin) and dicyclomine can be used for all types but have adverse effects such as dry mouth, dizziness, and blurred vision.
  – Probiotics such as lactobacillus, bifidobacterium, and streptococcus
  – Serotonin antagonists 5-HT3 and 5-4T agonists (alosetron, cilansetron, and tegaserod) have been shown to improve IBS symptoms (vs. placebo)
- Diarrhea predominant:
  – Anti-diarrheal such as loperamide decreases stool frequency and increases stool consistency but does not help with abdominal pain. May also use Lomotil.
  – Antibiotics such as 2 week course of rifaximin improve bloating, pain, and stool consistency
  – Alosetron (Lotronex) used for women with severe symptoms but associated with ischemic colitis, constipation, and death in a small number of patients
- Constipation predominant:
  – Laxatives such as MiraLAX (polyethylene glycol) may improve stool frequency but not pain
  – Antibiotics such as neomycin and selective chloride channel activators such as lubiprostone (Amitiza) can improve global symptoms and severity.
  – Linaclotide (guanylate cyclase-C agonist) has been shown to improve bowel function and reduces abdominal pain and overall severity in adults only (3)[A]
- Mixed picture:
  – May use medications as above for either picture
- Treat underlying psychologic issues:
  – Use SSRIs such as Prozac, sertraline, Paxil, and tricyclic antidepressants such as imipramine can improve abdominal pain and symptom score.
  – Cognitive behavior therapy, interpersonal psychotherapy and relaxation, and stress management

ISSUES FOR REFERRAL
Possible psychiatric referral for those with uncontrolled depression

ADDITIONAL THERAPIES
Evidence for the role of small intestine bacterial overgrowth (SIBO) in IBS and subsequent antibiotic therapy is conflicting; older age and female gender are predictors of SIBO within IBS (4)[C].

 ## ONGOING CARE

FOLLOW-UP RECOMMENDATIONS
Patient Monitoring
May use the IBS severity score to assess severity of symptoms and monitor treatment.

DIET
- Increase fiber slowly to avoid increased intestinal gas production.
- During initial evaluation, may wish to try 2 weeks of lactose-free diet to rule out lactose intolerance as etiology of symptoms.
- Avoid large meals, fatty foods, and caffeine, which can often exacerbate symptoms.
- Some patients note reduction in all symptoms with a low-carbohydrate diet.
- A subgroup of patients (especially diarrhea predominant IBS) will feel relief of symptoms on a gluten-free diet despite negative testing for celiac sprue (5)[C]

PATIENT EDUCATION
Patients should not be given the impression that this is a psychiatric illness.

PROGNOSIS
- No increased risk of death or development of other GI disease such as chronic pancreatitis, GI cancers, small bowel obstruction or gastric ulcers
- Expect recurrences, especially when under stress.

REFERENCES
1. Wilkins T. Diagnosis and management of IBS in adults. *Am Fam Physician*. 2012;86:419–426.
2. Shah ED, Basseri RJ, Chong K, et al. Abnormal breath testing in IBS: A meta-analysis. *Dig Dis Sci*. 2010;55:2441–2449.
3. Videlock EJ, Cheng V, Cremonini F. Effects of linaclotide in patients with irritable bowel syndrome with constipation or chronic constipation: A meta-analysis. *Clin Gastroenterol Hepatol*. 2013;11:1084–1092.e3.
4. Schey R, Rao SS. The role of rifaximin therapy in patients with irritable bowel syndrome without constipation. *Expert Rev Gastroenterol Hepatol*. 2011;5:461–464.
5. Vazquez-Roque MI, Camilleri M, Smyrk T, et al. A controlled trial of gluten-free diet in patients with irritable bowel syndrome-diarrhea: effects on bowel frequency and intestinal function. *Gastroenterology*. 2013;144:903–911.e3.
6. Carroccio A, Mansueto P, Iacono G, et al. Non-celiac wheat sensitivity diagnosed by double-blind placebo-controlled challenge: Exploring a new clinical entity. *Am J Gastroenterol*. 2012;107:1898–1906.

ADDITIONAL READING
- Ciorba MA. A gastroenterologist's guide to probiotics. *Clin Gastroenterol Hepatol*. 2012;10: 960–968.
- Drossman DA, Chey WD, Johanson JF, et al. Clinical trial: Lubiprostone in patients with constipation-associated irritable bowel syndrome—results of two randomized, placebo-controlled studies. *Aliment Pharmacol Ther*. 2009;29:329–341.

- Ford AC, Brandt LJ, Young C, et al. Efficacy of 5-HT3 antagonists and 5-HT4 agonists in irritable bowel syndrome: Systematic review and meta-analysis. *Am J Gastroenterol*. 2009;104:1831–1844.
- Hong KS, Kang HW, Im JP, et al. Effect of probiotics on symptoms in Korean adults with irritable bowel syndrome. *Gut Liver*. 2009;3:101–107.
- Hungin AP, Mulligan C, Pot B, et al. Systematic review: Probiotics in the management of lower gastrointestinal symptoms in clinical practice—an evidence-based international guide. *Aliment Pharmacol Ther*. 2013;38:864–886.
- Jackson JL, O'Malley PG, Tomkins G, et al. Treatment of functional gastrointestinal disorders with antidepressant medications: A meta-analysis. *Am J Med*. 2000;108:65–72.
- Poynard T, Regimbeau C, Benhamou Y. Meta-analysis of smooth muscle relaxants in the treatment of irritable bowel syndrome. *Aliment Pharmacol Ther*. 2001;15:355–361.
- Rahimi R, Nikfar S, Abdollahi M. Efficacy and tolerability of alosetron for the treatment of irritable bowel syndrome in women and men: A meta-analysis of eight randomized, placebo-controlled, 12-week trials. *Clin Ther*. 2008;30:884–901.
- Rahimi R, Nikfar S, Rezaie A, et al. Efficacy of tricyclic antidepressants in irritable bowel syndrome: A meta-analysis. *World J Gastroenterol*. 2009;15:1548–1553.
- Reddymasu SC, Sostarich S, McCallum RW, et al. Small intestinal bacterial overgrowth in irritable bowel syndrome: Are there any predictors? *BMC Gastroenterol*. 2010;10:23.
- Ruepert L, Quartero AO, de Wit NJ, et al. Bulking agents, antispasmodics and antidepressants for the treatment of irritable bowel syndrome. *Cochrane Database Syst Rev*. 2011;8:CD003460.

 ## SEE ALSO

Algorithm: Diarrhea, Chronic

 ## CODES

ICD10
- K58 Irritable bowel syndrome
- K58.0 Irritable bowel syndrome with diarrhea
- K58.9 Irritable bowel syndrome without diarrhea

CLINICAL PEARLS

- Aim treatment at predominant symptom (6)[A].
- Bulking agents or fiber generally useful, but must be added slowly to avoid aggravating symptoms.

KAWASAKI SYNDROME
Manjula Cherukuri, MD, FAAFP

BASICS

DESCRIPTION
- Kawasaki syndrome (KS) is an acute, self-limited, systemic inflammatory process that causes a febrile, exanthematous, vasculitic disease in young children, and is notable for its cardiac sequelae:
  - Vasculitis of coronary arteries resulting in aneurysms/ectasia, further leading to myocardial infarction (MI)/ischemia or sudden death.
- System(s) affected: Cardiovascular; gastrointestinal; hematologic/lymphatic/immunologic; musculoskeletal; nervous; pulmonary; renal/urologic; skin/exocrine
- Synonym(s): Mucocutaneous lymph node syndrome (MCLS); Infantile polyarteritis, Kawasaki syndrome

ALERT
KS should be considered in any child with extended high fever unresponsive to antibiotics or antipyretics, rash, and nonexudative conjunctivitis.

EPIDEMIOLOGY
Incidence
- Worldwide: Affects all races, but most prevalent in Asia; Japan annual incidence rate ~200/100,000 in children <5 years of age
- In the US, the annual incidence in children <5 years is 33/100,000 for Americans of Asian and Pacific Islander descent, 17/100,000 for non-Hispanic blacks, 11/100,00 for Hispanics, and 9/100,000 for whites. Highest incidence in Hawaii.
- Leading cause of acquired heart disease in children in developed countries:
  - Predominant age: 1–5 years
  - 85% of cases are children <5 years of age and 50% <2 years of age

Prevalence
- Highest to lowest prevalence: Asians > African Americans > Hispanics > Caucasians
- Seasonal variation: Increased in winter and early spring in temperate places, summer in Asia, and outbreaks at 2–3-year intervals

ETIOLOGY AND PATHOPHYSIOLOGY
- Acute KS causes inflammation in the smooth muscle layer of medium arteries, especially the coronary arteries.
- Inflammatory cells in the media secrete cytokines, interleukins, and matrix metalloproteases that cause fragmentation of the internal elastic lamina.
- Necrosis may develop and result in aneurysm.
- A prominence of IgA plasma cells and IgA deposits are characteristic features of KS. Similar IgA plasma cells are found in the respiratory tract of patients with KS (1).
- During greatest vascular damage, platelet count increases.
- As the process resolves, active inflammatory cells are replaced by fibroblasts and monocytes; tissue repair/remodeling may cause vascular fibrosis and stenosis.
- Unknown; believed to be infectious due to the acute, self-limited nature, community-wide outbreaks, age distribution, seasonality, and laboratory features indicating respiratory route of entry (1).
- Possible links to New Haven human corona virus, human bocavirus, cytomegalovirus

Genetics
- The risk of occurrence in twins is ~13%; possible genetic predisposition.
- Siblings of patients in Japan have a 10-fold relative risk and >50% develop KS within 10 days of first case. Increased occurrence of KS in children whose parents also had illness in childhood (2).

GENERAL PREVENTION
No preventive measures available

DIAGNOSIS

≥5 days of fever and ≥4 of the following 5 principal clinical features; or <4 features and presence of coronary artery disease on 2D echocardiography:
- Nonpurulent conjunctival injection with limbic sparing
- Erythematous mouth and pharynx, tongue, and lips
- A polymorphous, generalized, erythematous rash
- Changes in the skin of the peripheral extremities
- Cervical lymphadenopathy

Pediatric Considerations
- Prolonged fever without rash and treated with antibiotics may cause clinicians to believe that later rash development is due to a drug reaction.
- Can be diagnosed on day 4 of illness if ≥4 principal features present.
- Incomplete Kawasaki syndrome:
  - ≥5 days of fever, ≥2 principal clinical features, labs indicating systemic inflammation, and exclusion of other diseases
  - Incomplete cases that exhibit <4 clinical criteria often occur in infants ≤6 months of age or older children/adolescents. The frequency of coronary artery aneurysms (CAAs) is often higher in patients with missed diagnosis/delayed treatment. For this reason, in infants with prolonged fever and few or no clinical features, consider echocardiography and labs for inflammation.

HISTORY
- Fever is the 1st sign during the acute phase.
- Symptoms may not occur all at once, but usually occur in close proximity.

PHYSICAL EXAM
- High-spiking and remittent fever for ≥5 days:
  - Fever is high (103–105°F [39.4–40.5°C]) and unresponsive to antibiotics.
  - May be prolonged (3–4 weeks, with mean duration of 11 days)
  - Extreme irritability is a very common feature.
- Bilateral painless nonpurulent conjunctival injection without corneal ulceration, or edema. Limbic sparing usually seen.
- Changes in lips and oral cavity:
  - Redness and swelling of lips in the acute stage; cracking, fissuring, bleeding in subacute phase
  - Strawberry/erythematous tongue
- Extensive erythematous polymorphous rash: Within 5 days of fever:
  - Morbilliform is most common. May be maculopapular, scarlatiniform; can resemble erythema multiforme, erythroderma, urticarial exanthem; rarely micropustular
  - Perineal desquamation, especially in skin folds

- Extremity changes:
  - Reddened palms and soles on days 3–5
  - Edema of hands and feet on days 4–7; painful induration
  - Desquamation of fingers and toes that begins in periungual area at 2–3 weeks
- Acute, unilateral cervical lymphadenopathy (least common symptom):
  - ≥1 lymph nodes >1.5 cm, firm and nonfluctuant. Usually no to slight tenderness
  - Generalized lymphadenopathy usually absent
- Cardiac exam: Tachycardia, gallop rhythms, hyperdynamic precordium, innocent flow murmurs, depressed contractility
- Other organ system involvement:
  - Cardiovascular: Myocarditis; pericarditis (often subclinical), CAA, and other medium-sized arterial aneurysms
  - GI: Anorexia, abdominal pain, vomiting/diarrhea, acute gallbladder hydrops, hepatic enlargement, jaundice
  - Renal: Nephritis, urethritis
  - Respiratory: Pneumonitis, atelectasis/pleural effusion, cough
  - Joints: Polyarthritis of small joints in acute phase; weight-bearing joints affected after 10th day from onset of fever
  - Neurologic: Irritability, aseptic meningitis, peripheral neuropathy (unilateral facial palsy), transient high-frequency hearing loss

DIFFERENTIAL DIAGNOSIS
- Bacterial: Staphylococcal scalded-skin syndrome, toxic shock syndrome, scarlet fever, bacterial cervical lymphadenitis, *Mycoplasma* infection, leptospirosis, Lyme disease, Rocky Mountain spotted fever
- Viral: Measles, adenovirus, Epstein-Barr virus infections
- Toxoplasmosis
- Reiter syndrome
- Hypersensitivity drug reactions (erythema multiforme minor, Stevens-Johnson syndrome)
- Juvenile rheumatoid arthritis
- Acrodynia (mercury poisoning)
- Other vasculitides

DIAGNOSTIC TESTS & INTERPRETATION
- Initial workup: CBC with differential, urinalysis (UA)/culture, blood culture; lumbar puncture if <4 months of age or if signs of meningitis:
  - Leukocytosis (12K–40K cells/mm³) with immature and mature granulocytes
  - Anemia: Normochromic, normocytic
  - Thrombocytosis (500,000 to >1,000,000/mm³) in 2nd and 3rd weeks. Thrombopenia during acute phase is associated with CAA and MI.
- Elevated CRP (>35 mg/L in 80% cases), ESR (>60 mm/hr in 60% cases), and α_1-antitrypsin

ALERT
ESR can be artificially high after IVIG therapy. CRP is a better test.
- Hyponatremia
- Moderately elevated AST, ALT, GGT, and bilirubin
- Decreased albumin and protein
- Abnormal plasma lipids: Low cholesterol, high-density lipoprotein (HDL), and apolipoprotein A-I (apo-AI)
- CSF pleocytosis may be seen (lymphocytic with normal protein and glucose)
- *N*-terminal brain natriuretic peptide might be elevated in acute phase
- Sterile pyuria, but not seen in suprapubic collection
- Nasal swab to rule out adenovirus

Initial Tests (lab, imaging)
- If KS is suspected, obtain ECG and echocardiogram:
  - ECG may show arrhythmias, prolonged PR interval, and ST/T wave changes.
  - Echocardiography has a high sensitivity and specificity for detection of abnormalities of proximal left main coronary artery and right coronary artery may show perivascular brightening, ectasia, decreased left ventricular contractility, pericardial effusion, or aneurysms.
  - Cardiac stress test if CAA seen on echocardiogram
- Baseline chest x-ray (CXR): May show pleural effusion, atelectasis, and congestive heart failure (CHF)
- Hydrops of the gallbladder may be associated with abdominal pain or may be asymptomatic

Diagnostic Procedures/Other
- No laboratory study is diagnostic; diagnosis rests on constellation of clinical features and exclusion of other illnesses.
- Patients with complex coronary artery lesions may benefit from coronary angiography after the acute inflammatory process has resolved; generally recommended in 6–12 months

Test Interpretation
Severe lymphadenitis with necrosis and thrombotic arteriolitis on lymph nodes biopsy

TREATMENT

Inpatient care

GENERAL MEASURES
Use antibiotics until bacterial etiologies are excluded (e.g., sepsis or meningitis).

MEDICATION
- Optimal therapy is IVIG 2 g/kg IV over 10 hours with high-dose aspirin preferably within 7–10 days of fever, followed by low-dose aspirin until follow-up echocardiograms indicate a lack of coronary abnormalities (3)[A].
  - IVIG lowers the risk of CAA and may shorten fever duration.
  - The extreme irritability often resolves very quickly after IVIG is given.
- Retreatment with IVIG if clinical response is incomplete or fever persists/returns >36 hours after start of IVIG treatment:
  - ≥10% of patients do not respond to initial IVIG treatment. 2/3 of nonresponders respond to the 2nd dose of IVIG.

- Nonresponders tend to have ↑ bands, ↓ albumin, and an abnormal echo.
- Aspirin, 80–100 mg/kg/d in 4 doses beginning with IVIG administration. Switch to low-dose aspirin (3–5 mg/kg/d) when afebrile for 48–72 hours or continue until day 14 of illness. Maintain low dose for 6–8 weeks until follow-up echocardiogram is normal. Continue salicylate regimen in children with coronary abnormalities long term or until documented regression of aneurysm.
- Contraindications:
  - IVIG: Documented hypersensitivity, IgA deficiency, anti-IgE/IgG antibodies, severe thrombocytopenia, coagulation disorders
  - Aspirin: Vitamin K deficiency, bleeding disorders, liver damage, documented hypersensitivity, hypoprothrombinemia
- Precautions:
  - No statistically significant difference noted between different preparations of IVIG (3)[A]
  - High-dose aspirin therapy can result in tinnitus, decrease of renal function, and increased transaminases
  - Do not use ibuprofen in children with coronary artery aneurysms who are taking aspirin for antiplatelet effects
  - Significant possible interactions: Aspirin therapy has been associated with Reye syndrome in children who develop viral infections, especially influenza B and varicella. Yearly influenza vaccination thus is recommended for children requiring long-term treatment with aspirin. Delay any live vaccines, especially varicella and measles, for 11 months after IVIG treatment.

Second Line
- Corticosteroids should be used only if ≥2 IVIG treatments have failed. The addition of corticosteroids to IVIG and aspirin during initial treatment might improve CA outcomes in severe KS in Japanese children but role in primary management remains controversial.
- In patients refractory to IVIG and steroids, consider infliximab.

ISSUES FOR REFERRAL
Pediatric cardiologist if abnormalities on echo or if extensive stenosis

ADDITIONAL THERAPIES
- Treatment and prevention of thrombosis are crucial.
- Antiplatelet agents (clopidogrel, dipyridamole), heparin, low-molecular-weight heparin, or warfarin are sometimes added to the low-dose aspirin regimen, depending on severity of coronary involvement.

SURGERY/OTHER PROCEDURES
- Rarely needed; coronary artery bypass grafting for severe obstruction/recurrent MI. Younger patients have a higher mortality rate.
- Coronary revascularization via percutaneous coronary intervention for patients with evidence of ischemia on stress testing.

IN-PATIENT CONSIDERATIONS
IV Fluids
Normal saline (NS) for rehydration and 1/2 NS for maintenance

Discharge Criteria
Discharge if afebrile after IVIG treatment × 24 hours.

ONGOING CARE

FOLLOW-UP RECOMMENDATIONS
With aneurysms, contact and high-risk sports should be avoided.

Patient Monitoring
- Repeat ECG and echocardiogram at 6–8 weeks. If abnormal, repeat at 6–12 months.
- Patients with complex coronary artery lesions may benefit from coronary angiography at 6–12 months.

PROGNOSIS
- Usually self-limited
- Moderate-sized aneurysms usually regress in 1–2 years, resolving in 50–66% of cases.
- Recurrence (3% in Japan, <1% in the US)
- Sudden death in early adulthood (rare)

COMPLICATIONS
- 15–25% of untreated patients develop CAAs in convalescent phase.
- 2–7% of treated patients develop aneurysms. 1% develop giant aneurysms.
- Risk factors for aneurysm:
  - Male, <1 year of age, ↑ ESR >4 weeks, fever >2 weeks, fever >48 hours after IVIG treatment
- Mortality of 0.08–0.17% is due to cardiac disease.

REFERENCES

1. Rowley AH, Shulman ST. Pathogenesis and management of Kawasaki disease. *Expert Rev Anti Infect Ther*. 2010;8:197–203.
2. Takahashi K, Oharaseki T, Yokouchi Y, et al. Pathogenesis of Kawasaki disease. *Clin Exp Immunol*. 2011;164(Suppl 1):20–22.
3. Oates-Whitehead RM, Baumer JH, Haines L, et al. Intravenous immunoglobulin for the treatment of Kawasaki disease in children. *Cochrane Database Syst Rev*. 2003;4:CD004000.

ADDITIONAL READING

Kobayashi T, Saji T, Otani T, et al. Efficacy of immunoglobulin plus prednisolone for prevention of coronary artery abnormalities in severe Kawasaki disease (RAISE study): A randomised, open-label, blinded-endpoints trial. *Lancet*. 2012;84:1613–1620.

CODES

ICD10
M30.3 Mucocutaneous lymph node syndrome [Kawasaki]

CLINICAL PEARLS

- The diagnosis of KS rests on a constellation of clinical features.
- Once KS is suspected, all patients need an inpatient cardiac evaluation, including ECG and echocardiogram.
- Optimal therapy is IVIG 2 g/kg IV over 10 hours with high-dose aspirin 80–100 mg/kg/d in 4 doses.

K

KELOIDS

Mary Lauren Worthen, MD • David Worthen • Adrian Worthen

BASICS

DESCRIPTION
- Keloids are benign hyperproliferative growths of dermal fibroblasts characterized by the excessive deposition of extracellular matrix components, especially collagen, fibronectin, elastin, proteoglycans, and growth factors such as transforming growth factor-β (TGF-β) (1)[B].
- Keloids present as abnormal scar tissue proliferations at a site of injury.
- System(s) affected: Skin/Exocrine

EPIDEMIOLOGY
Incidence
- Predominant age: 10–30 years
- Higher incidence during puberty and pregnancy
- Predominant sex: Female > Male

Prevalence
- 4–16% of the black and Hispanic populations
- Higher incidence in the Asian population
- Data from the UK demonstrated that <1% of Caucasians had keloids

ETIOLOGY AND PATHOPHYSIOLOGY
- The mechanisms of keloid formation include alterations in growth factors, collagen turnover, and skin tension alignment, as well as genetic and immunological contributions.
- Trauma, foreign-body reactions, infections, and endocrine dysfunctions have all been proposed as risk factors for the development of keloids after surgery in genetically susceptible people.
- Rarely occur in places on body lacking sebaceous glands; thus, sebaceous glands, and the body's reaction to this sebum, are hypothesized to be an etiologic factor in keloid development. Moreover, humans are the only mammals with sebaceous glands and the only mammals affected by keloids.
- Wounds: Traumatic, surgical, body piercing (foreign-body reaction)
- Wound infection
- Burn injury
- Other injuries:
  – Insect bite
  – Folliculitis barbae and nuchae
  – Acne
  – Chickenpox
- Vaccination (especially bacille Calmette-Guérin [BCG])
- Increased ratio of type I to type III collagen
- Increased density and proliferation rate of fibroblasts

Genetics
- More common in blacks and Asians (5–15×) than in whites; in all races, more darkly pigmented individuals are at higher risk.
- Both autosomal-dominant and autosomal-recessive familial inheritance have been reported.
- Several genes have been implicated in the etiology of keloid disease, but no single gene mutation has thus far been found to be responsible.
- High frequency of identical twins both developing keloids strongly supports a role for genetics in keloid etiology.

RISK FACTORS
- Family history of keloids
- Race
- Darker skin pigmentation
- Location on the body (e.g., deltoids, chest, neck, earlobes)
- Pregnancy
- Adolescence
- Repeated abnormal wound healing (e.g., earring sites)

GENERAL PREVENTION
- Primary prevention: Avoid elective surgery, body piercing, and tattooing in high-risk patients.
- Wounds should be kept clean to prevent infection.
- When feasible, laparoscopic approaches are preferred in keloid formers.
- Compressive pressure dressings may be useful in high-risk (e.g., burn) patients. Local steroid injection postoperatively in high-risk patients is also effective.
- Physicians should be alert to delays in wound healing, persistent erythema, or pruritus as impending symptoms of possible keloid formation. Attempts to reduce inflammation and tension on the skin with appropriate methods is vital for prevention.

DIAGNOSIS

HISTORY
- Pain
- Tenderness
- Hyperesthesia
- Pruritus and burning (occasional)
- Abnormal growth beyond the border of the original wound
- May be asymptomatic

PHYSICAL EXAM
- Firm, smooth, elevated scar with sharply demarcated borders
- Initially may be pale or mildly erythematous
- Older lesion hypo- or hyperpigmented
- Scar extends beyond margins of the initial wound
- Over period of years, keloids may continue to grow and may develop claw-like projections
- Keloids occur more frequently on the chest, shoulders, upper back, back of the neck, and earlobes

DIFFERENTIAL DIAGNOSIS
- Hypertrophic scar (usually regresses spontaneously, does not cross wound margins, and rarely >1 cm in thickness and width)
- Dermatofibroma
- Infiltrating basal cell carcinoma
- Sclerosing metastatic malignancies
- Desmoplastic melanoma
- Sarcoidosis
- Leprosy (nodular LL type)
- Other fibronodular skin diseases (e.g., neurofibromatosis, post–kala-azar dermal leishmaniasis)

DIAGNOSTIC TESTS & INTERPRETATION
Biopsy only if unable to differentiate from carcinoma or infectious disease, as biopsy may increase the keloid's size. Use a 2-mm punch biopsy to minimize trauma.

Test Interpretation
Histology shows whorl-like arrangements of hyalinized collagen bundles, with pressure thinning of papillary dermis and minimal elastic tissue. Cellular fibrous bands are also noted.

TREATMENT

- Given the high recurrence rates and significant expense associated with treatment, prevention of keloids should take priority. Avoidance of known risk factors such as piercings, tattoos, and elective surgery is highly recommended in people with either a family or personal history of keloids.
- A recent meta-analysis of 70 studies has shown that all currently accepted treatment options have fairly comparable efficacy, with a mean improvement of 60% (2).
- Treatment options should be based on the type of keloid. Characteristics to take into consideration: (i) presence or absence of scar contractures; (ii) size; and (iii) number of keloids:
  – Small, single keloids can be treated more aggressively.
  – Large or multiple keloids are typically more complicated to treat and should be evaluated on an individual basis (3).
- Anti-mitotic drugs described in the literature, such as steroid injection, 5-FU, mitomycin C, and bleomycin, mainly target the fibroblasts in scar tissue (4)[B].

GENERAL MEASURES
- Appropriate health care: Outpatient
- Intralesional corticosteroid injection causes atrophy, telangiectasia, and pigment changes in 1/2 of patients but is a very successful therapy (5)[A].
- Pressure bandages must maintain 24 mm Hg and should be worn for 6–12 months (5)[C]. Bandages should not be removed for >30 min/d.
- Pressure clips (Zimmer splints) are useful for earlobes. Designer splints look like fashion earrings.
- Cryotherapy may be useful for small keloids (e.g., acne scars) (5)[C].
- Use 10–30-second freeze–thaw cycles every month; may cause permanent hypopigmentation.
- Topical agents: No evidence to support efficacy of retinoic acid, vitamin E, allantoin, or onion extract (5); some evidence for imiquimod. Generally, retinoids are tolerated in patients with pigmented skin; however, the treating physician must be cognizant of the development of retinoid dermatitis, which can induce hyperpigmentation.

MEDICATION
First Line
- 5-FU (5-fluorouracil):
  – 5-FU tattooing was more effective than intralesional triamcinolone for the treatment of keloids (6)[A].
  – In 1 study with keloids treated with intralesional 5-FU weekly with a total of 16 injections, ~1/2 of the patients showed >50% flattening. The older keloids (>5 years) were more difficult to treat (4)[B].
  – Side effects are local erythema, swelling, pain, molting, pigmentation, and occasional ulcers.
  – Effectiveness rate of 5-FU injection alone is 62.5%, whereas the efficacy of 5-FU in combination with glucocorticoids is significantly better at 92% (4).

- Triamcinolone (Kenalog) suspension 10 mg/mL (5)[A]:
  – Most commonly used treatment option. Likely more effective if combined with cryotherapy, pulsed dye laser, or 5-FU. No difference when combined with excision vs. monotherapy (3).
  – 72% showed symptomatic improvement in 1 trial (5).
  – Use 27–30-gauge needle and a TB syringe (total dose 20–30 mg triamcinolone); may inject 3 lesions at a time using 10 mg/lesion.
  – Advance the needle while injecting to distribute medication evenly.
  – Early keloids are more responsive to this therapy than are older lesions.
  – Reinject every 4 weeks until keloid shrinks to near skin surface.
  – If no response to 10 mg/mL triamcinolone suspension, may try 40 mg/mL suspension.
  – May mix dilute triamcinolone (5–10 mg/mL) with local anesthetic for excision of keloids; postoperative steroid injections at 2–4 weeks and then monthly for 6 months help to prevent recurrences.
  – Contraindications: Active skin infection at injection site.
  – Precautions:
    ○ Systemic absorption with reversible adrenal suppression, hyperglycemia
    ○ Local effects: Skin atrophy, ulceration, depigmentation, telangiectasias
    ○ Both types of side effects are more common with 40 mg/mL triamcinolone suspension.
  – Significant possible interactions: Rare interactions (only with very large doses of corticosteroids and systemic absorption)
- Silica gel sheeting: 1st-line prophylaxis after surgical procedure or keloid excision (5)[A],(7)[C]:
  – Patient compliance limits effectiveness.
  – Sheets are cut to fit and must be worn for at least 12 hours and, optimally, 24 hours a day.
  – Unclear whether benefit is from silicone or occlusive effect.
  – Adverse effects are generally from irritation: pruritus, rash, erosion, and maceration. There is complete resolution within a few days of removal.

Second Line
- Cryotherapy is likely to be more useful in early, smaller lesions. It is not recommended for larger areas because of pain and decreased skin pigmentation (3).
- Verapamil locally may be helpful as an adjuvant following excision and topical silicone (5)[C].
- Interferon-α2b may be helpful after excision (5)[C].
- Topical imiquimod (Aldara) may be helpful after excision.
- Intralesional bleomycin (5)[C], retinoic acid, mitomycin C, colchicine (4)[B].
- Radiation therapy has greater success rates when used in combination with surgical excision. There are some concerns about precipitating malignant lesions with radiation; however, a direct correlation has not been made (3)[C].

Pregnancy Considerations
Radiation therapy, 5-fluorouracil, and bleomycin are unsafe in pregnancy. Triamcinolone should be used with caution.

ISSUES FOR REFERRAL
When intralesional steroids fail, referral to dermatologist or plastic surgeon may be indicated.

ADDITIONAL THERAPIES
- Local radiotherapy may be effective after excision but carries a small risk of carcinogenesis.
- Physical therapy is useful in associated contractures.

SURGERY/OTHER PROCEDURES
- Surgery: High recurrence rate (45–100%) if used alone; therefore, is used only for the debulking of large keloids or if a lesion is unresponsive to steroid injections or other therapy; combine with preoperative steroid injection and possibly other modalities (5). Debulking just enough for symptomatic improvement is recommended (3).
- Pulsed-dye laser surgery: No definitive evidence of efficacy or advantage over other methods; therefore, use only if other methods fail, and then use in conjunction with them (5)[C]; some promise is seen in combination with triamcinolone and 5-FU (7)[C].

 ## ONGOING CARE

FOLLOW-UP RECOMMENDATIONS
Patient Monitoring
Monthly visits for up to 1 year for evaluation and possible steroid reinjections.

PATIENT EDUCATION
- Stress the possibility of recurrence despite appropriate treatment.
- May require many months of treatment with combined modalities.
- Prevention: In those with risk factors or previous keloids, caution against activities or procedures that may entail dermal disruption, and suggest early treatment of any such events.

PROGNOSIS
When treatment is successful, lesions gradually diminish over 6–18 months with therapy, leaving a flat, shiny scar. Although keloids can improve with treatment, cure is unlikely.

COMPLICATIONS
Skin atrophy, ulceration, depigmentation, and telangiectasias can occur as a result of local steroid injections.

REFERENCES
1. Halim AS, Emami A, Salahshourifar I, et al. Keloid scarring: Understanding the genetic basis, advances, and prospects. *Arch Plast Surg*. 2012;39: 184–189.
2. Leventhal D, Furr M, Reiter D. Treatment of keloids and hypertrophic scars: A meta-analysis and review of the literature. *Arch Facial Plast Surg*. 2006;8: 362–368.
3. Ogawa R. The most current algorithms for the treatment and prevention of hypertrophic scars and keloids. *Plast Reconstr Surg*. 2010;125:557–568.
4. Wang XQ, Liu YK, Qing C, et al. A review of the effectiveness of antimitotic drug injections for hypertrophic scars and keloids. *Ann Plast Surg*. 2009;63:688–692.

5. Mustoe TA, Cooter RD, Gold MH, et al. International clinical recommendations on scar management. *Plast Reconstr Surg*. 2002;110: 560–571.
6. Sadeghinia A, Sadeghinia S. Comparison of the efficacy of intralesional triamcinolone acetonide and 5-fluorouracil tattooing for the treatment of keloids. *Dermatol Surg*. 2012;38:104–109.
7. Asilian A, Darougheh A, Shariati F. New combination of triamcinolone, 5-fluorouracil, and pulsed-dye laser for treatment of keloid and hypertrophic scars. *Dermatol Surg*. 2006;32: 907–915.

ADDITIONAL READING
- Davison SP, Dayan JH, Clemens MW, et al. Efficacy of intralesional 5-fluorouracil and triamcinolone in the treatment of keloids. *Aesthet Surg J*. 2009;29: 40–46.
- Geria AN, Lawson CN, Halder RM. Topical retinoids for pigmented skin. *J Drugs Dermatol*. 2011;10: 483–489.
- Seifert O, Mrowietz U. Keloid scarring: Bench and bedside. *Arch Dermatol Res*. 2009;301:259–272.
- Viera MH, Caperton CV, Berman B. Advances in the treatment of keloids. *J Drugs Dermatol*. 2011;10: 468–480.

 ## SEE ALSO

Bites; Burns; Leprosy; Warts

 ## CODES

ICD10
L91.0 Hypertrophic scar

CLINICAL PEARLS
- The most successful treatment of hypertrophic scar or keloid is achieved while the scar is still immature but the overlying epithelium is intact, although this is not as yet confirmed in the literature.
- Differentiation of keloids from hypertrophic scars is vital. Keloids extend beyond the margins of the original wound and do not regress with time but hypertrophic scars do. Treatment is similar, but keloids are much more likely to recur.
- Closing wounds with a minimum of suture tension, avoiding midsternal incisions and crossing joint lines, and injecting steroids into the incision postoperatively reduce the chance of keloids forming following unavoidable surgery.

K

KERATOACANTHOMA

Shannon N. Sharpe, DO • Jenifer Lloyd, DO

 BASICS

DESCRIPTION

- Rapidly proliferating, solitary dome-shaped, erythematous or flesh-colored papule or nodule with a central keratinous plug, typically reaching 1–2 cm in diameter
- Classified as a variant of a well-differentiated squamous cell carcinoma (SCC); histologic differentiation of a keratoacanthoma (KA) from an SCC may be difficult and unreliable
- Majority are benign and resolve spontaneously, but lesions do have the potential for invasion and metastasis; therefore require treatment
- Three clinical stages of KAs:
  - Proliferative: Rapid growth of the lesion over weeks to several months
  - Maturation/Stabilization: Lesion stabilizes and growth subsides
  - Involution: Spontaneous resolution of the lesion, leaving a hypopigmented, depressed scar; most, but not all lesions will enter this stage
- System(s) affected: Integumentary

EPIDEMIOLOGY

- Greatest incidence over the age of 50; but may occur at any age
- Presentation increased during summer and early fall seasons
- Most frequently on sun-exposed, hair-bearing skin; but may occur anywhere
- Predominant sex: Male > Females (2:1)
- Most commonly in fair-skinned individuals; highest rates in Fitzpatrick I–III
- 104 cases per 100,000 individuals

ETIOLOGY AND PATHOPHYSIOLOGY

- Derived from an abnormality causing hyperkeratosis within the follicular infundibulum
- Squamous epithelial cells proliferate to extend upward around the keratin plug and proceed downward into the dermis; followed by invasion of elastic and collagen fibers (1)
- Cellular mechanism responsible for the hyperkeratosis is currently unknown
- Regression may be due to immune cytotoxicity or terminal differentiation of keratinocytes
- Multiple etiologies have been suggested:
  - UV radiation
  - Trauma: Accidental or iatrogenic, including surgery, cryotherapy, laser therapy
  - Viral infections: Human papillomavirus (HPV) or Merkel cell polyomavirus
  - Genetic predisposition: Muir-Torre syndrome, xeroderma pigmentosum, Ferguson-Smith syndrome
  - Immunosuppression
  - Chemical carcinogen exposure

Genetics

- Mutation of p53 or H-Ras
- Ferguson-Smith (AD)
- Witten-Zak (AD)
- Muir-Torre (AD)
- Xeroderma pigmentosum (AR)
- Gzybowski (sporadic)
- Incontinentia pigmenti (XLD)

RISK FACTORS

- UV exposure/damage: Outdoor and/or indoor tanning
- Fitzpatrick skin type I–III
- Trauma (typically appears within 1 month of injury): Accidental, surgery, cryotherapy, tattoos
- Chemical carcinogens: Tar, pitch, and smoking
- Immunocompromised state
- Discoid lupus erythematosus

GENERAL PREVENTION

Sun protection

COMMONLY ASSOCIATED CONDITIONS

- Frequently, the patient has concurrent sun-damaged skin: Solar elastosis, solar lentigines, actinic keratosis, nonmelanoma skin cancers (basal cell carcinoma, squamous cell carcinoma [SCC])
- In Muir-Torre syndrome, KAs are found with coexisting sebaceous neoplasms and malignancy of the GI and GU tracts

 DIAGNOSIS

HISTORY

- Lesion begins as a small, solitary pink macule that undergoes a rapid growth phase; classically reaching a diameter of 1–2 cm; size may vary
- Once the proliferative stage has subsided, lesion size remains stable
- May decrease in size, indicating regression
- Asymptomatic, occasionally tender
- If multiple lesions present, important to elicit a family history
- If sebaceous neoplasms present, must review history for signs/symptoms of GI or GU malignancies

PHYSICAL EXAM

- Firm, solitary, erythematous or flesh-colored, dome-shaped papule or nodule with a central keratin plug, giving a crateriform appearance
- Surrounding skin and borders of lesion may show telangiectasia, atrophy, or dyspigmentation
- Solitary; although multiple lesions can occur
- Most commonly seen on sun-exposed areas: Face, neck, scalp, dorsum of upper extremities, and posterior legs
- May also be seen on areas without sun exposure: Buttocks, anus, subungual, mucosal surfaces
- Subungual KAs are very painful and seen on the 1st 3 digits of the hands
- Lesion may enlarge up to 30 cm as a KA centrifugum marginatum
- Examine for regional lymphadenopathy due to chance of lesion invasion and metastasis
- Dermoscopy:
  - Central keratin
  - White circles, blood spots (2)

DIFFERENTIAL DIAGNOSIS

- SCC
- Nodular or ulcerative basal cell carcinoma
- Cutaneous horn
- Merkel cell carcinoma
- Metastasis to the skin
- Molluscum contagiosum
- Prurigo nodularis
- Verruca vulgaris
- Verrucous carcinoma
- Hypertrophic actinic keratosis
- Sebaceous adenoma
- Hypertrophic lichen planus
- Hypertrophic lupus erythematosus
- Deep fungal infection
- Atypical mycobacterial infection
- Nodular Kaposi sarcoma

DIAGNOSTIC TESTS & INTERPRETATION

- Excisional biopsy is the diagnostic test of choice
  - Important to include the center of the lesion as well as the margin
- A shave biopsy may be insufficiently deep to distinguish KA from an SCC
  - Questionable as to whether a KA can be reliably differentiated from an SCC
- If unable to perform an excisional biopsy, a deep shave (saucerization) of the entire lesion, extending into the subcutaneous fat, can be done
- Punch biopsies should be avoided because they give an insufficient amount of tissue to represent the entire lesion

Initial Tests (lab, imaging)

- Subungual KA: Radiograph of the digit to monitor for osteolysis (cup-shaped radiolucent defect)
- Aggressive tumors may need CT with contrast for evaluation of lymph nodes and MRI if there is concern of perineural invasion.
- Most lesions do not need any form of imaging

Test Interpretation

- Pathology of biopsy: A well-demarcated central core of keratin surrounded by well-differentiated, mildly pleomorphic, atypical squamous epithelial cells with a characteristic glassy eosinophilic cytoplasm (1)
- May see elastic and collagen fibers invading into the squamous epithelium
- KAs have a greater tendency than SCC to display fibrosis and intraepidermal abscesses of neutrophils and eosinophils
- Regressing KA shows flattening and fibrosis at base of lesion.

TREATMENT

- Treatment of choice is surgical excision with 3–5 mm surgical margins (3)
- Aggressive tumors (>2 cm) or lesions in cosmetically sensitive areas (face, digits, genitalia) that require tissue sparing, consider mohs micrographic surgery
  - Mohs is the treatment of choice in cases with perineural or perivascular invasion
- Small lesions (<2 cm) of the extremities may undergo electrodessication and curettage (1)
- Immunocompromised patients should receive immediate surgical treatment
- If opting for medical treatment, therapy course should be limited to 4 weeks and discontinued if no regression seen on follow-up examination

MEDICATION

- Indicated for lesions not amenable to surgery due to lesion number, size, or location; also for patients with multiple comorbidities who are unwilling or unable to withstand surgery
- Limited data available for the best initial medical treatment, listed below in no particular order:
  - Intralesional methotrexate 12.5–25 mg in 0.5 mL normal saline over 2–4 injections (3)
    - Monitor for pancytopenia with complete blood count
  - 5% Imiquimod cream every 2 days (4)
  - Topical 5% 5-fluorouracil cream daily
  - Intralesional 5-fluorouracil 0.2–0.5 of 50 mg/mL 2–5 doses weekly
  - IFNα2b for actinic or HPV-related lesions
  - Isotretinoin 1.5 mg/kg/d

ISSUES FOR REFERRAL

Dermatology referral if lesions are >2 cm, numerous, mucosal, or subungual.

ADDITIONAL THERAPIES

- Photodynamic therapy with methyl aminolevulinic acid and red light
- Cryotherapy
- Argon or YAG lasers
- Radiotherapy, primary or adjuvant: KAs may regress with low doses of radiation, but may require doses up to 40–50 Gy in 10–20 fractions for possible SCC.

SURGERY/OTHER PROCEDURES

- KA has been highly debated as to whether it is a benign or malignant variant of SCC
- Despite spontaneous regression in many cases, KA requires treatment as an SCC.

ONGOING CARE

FOLLOW-UP RECOMMENDATIONS

After the surgical site has healed or lesion has resolved, patient should be seen every 6 months due to increased risk of developing new lesions or skin cancers.

Patient Monitoring

Skin self-exams should be routinely performed with detailed instructions by:

- The Skin Cancer Foundation: www.skincancer.org/
- The American Academy of Dermatology: www.aad.org/skin-conditions/skin-cancer-detection/about-skin-self-exams

PATIENT EDUCATION

- Sun protection measures: Sun block with SPF >30, wide-brimmed hats, long sleeves, dark clothing, avoiding indoor tanning
- Tar, pitch, and smoking should be avoided

PROGNOSIS

- Atrophic scarring and hypopigmentation will occur with self-resolution but may be significantly reduced by intervention
- Very few cases of invasion and metastasis
- 4–8% recurrence
- Mucosal and subungual lesions do not regress, must undergo treatment
- If multiple KAs are present in patient or family members, evaluate for Muir-Torre syndrome and obtain a colonoscopy beginning at age 25, as well as testing for genitourinary cancer.

REFERENCES

1. Sarabi K, Selim A, Khachemoune A. Sporadic and syndromic keratoacanthomas: Diagnosis and management. *Dermatol Nurs.* 2007;19:166–170.
2. Rosendahl C, Cameron A, Argenziano G, et al. Dermoscopy of squamous cell carcinoma and keratoacanthoma. *Arch Dermatol.* 2012;148:1386–1392.
3. Patel NP, Cervino AL. Treatment of keratoacanthoma: Is intralesional methotrexate an option? *Can J Plast Surg.* 2011;19:15–18.
4. Jeon HC, Choi M, Paik SH, et al. Treatment of keratoacanthoma with 5% imiquimod cream and review of the previous report. *Ann Dermatol.* 2011;23:357–361.

ADDITIONAL READING

Zalaudek I, Bonifazi E, Ferrara G, et al. Keratoacanthomas and spitz tumors: Are they both "self-limiting" variants of malignant cutaneous neoplasms? *Dermatology.* 2009;219:3–6.

 SEE ALSO

Cutaneous Squamous Cell Carcinoma

 CODES

ICD10

L85.8 Other specified epidermal thickening

CLINICAL PEARLS

- Suspect KA with a solitary, dome-shaped, erythematous, or flesh-colored papule or nodule with a central keratinous plug.
- If KA is in the differential diagnosis, elicit time frame of onset during patient encounter; rapid onset supports diagnosis.
- Due to the unreliable histologic differentiation of a KA and an SCC, as well as the ability of KAs to metastasize, a KA should be treated as an SCC with surgical excision as 1st-line therapy.
- Excisional biopsy is the test of choice to diagnose KA.
- Consider KA in subungual lesions if it is painful and does not regress.
- Medical therapy is available for patients who are not surgical candidates or for lesions that are undesirable for surgery.

K

KERATOSIS PILARIS

Zoltan Trizna, MD, PhD

BASICS

- Keratosis pilaris (KP) is a benign skin disorder resulting in hyperkeratinization of the hair follicles (1).
- Generally asymptomatic, often improving with age

DESCRIPTION
Small (1–2 mm) keratotic papules are localized to hair follicles, most frequently on the lateral aspects of the arms and thighs. Often described as chicken skin or goose bumps.

EPIDEMIOLOGY
There is a slight female predominance.

Prevalence
KP affects up to 80% of adolescents, often worsening during puberty, and up to 40% of adults.

ETIOLOGY AND PATHOPHYSIOLOGY
- The abrasive ("sandpaper-like," "chicken-skin," or "goose bump-like") texture of the skin is caused by excess buildup of keratin. An underlying hair may be found in some of the papules. In the inflammatory variant, mild perifollicular erythema is present.
- Autosomal-dominant inheritance, with incomplete penetrance. Keratosis pilaris is more frequent in obese patients (2).

Genetics
Autosomal-dominant inheritance, with incomplete penetrance and variable expressivity, has been described, and many (30–50%) will report a positive family history of the disorder.

GENERAL PREVENTION
Moisturize to prevent excessive drying of the skin. Use only mild soaps (cleansers). Avoid hot showers.

COMMONLY ASSOCIATED CONDITIONS
Ichthyosis, xerosis, atopic dermatitis

DIAGNOSIS

HISTORY
- Patients often complain about a "rough" skin, sometimes with pruritus (which indicates inflammation).
- Most patients are asymptomatic, but some are concerned about their cosmetic appearance.
- Family history is positive in up to 50% of cases.

PHYSICAL EXAM
- Firm, minimally rough, 1–2-mm, follicle-based papules, some with perilesional erythema. Distribution is frequently symmetric.
- Most common on the lateral-proximal aspects of the arms and thighs; less common on the cheeks and gluteal areas.

DIFFERENTIAL DIAGNOSIS
- Acne
- Folliculitis
- Rare dermatologic conditions (e.g., keratosis follicularis, lichen spinulosus, lichen nitidus, perforating folliculitis)

DIAGNOSTIC TESTS & INTERPRETATION
Diagnosis is visual.

Diagnostic Procedures/Other
Skin biopsy if diagnosis in doubt.

Test Interpretation
Hyperkeratosis, hypergranulosis, and follicular plugging are typical. A mild superficial perivascular inflammatory infiltrate may be noted.

TREATMENT

Daily measures to prevent dry skin, such as using mild cleansers, along with moisturizers, are the mainstay of treatment.

GENERAL MEASURES
Moisturize. Use emollients.

MEDICATION
First Line
- Lactic acid 12% creams/lotions (e.g., ammonium lactate: AmLactin, Lac-Hydrin)
- Urea (in 40–50% topical preparations)

Second Line
Emollient-based topical steroids (e.g., Cloderm, Locoid Lipocream)

ADDITIONAL THERAPIES
- Topical retinoids: Tretinoin (Retin-A), adapalene (Differin), tazarotene (Tazorac)
- Tacrolimus (Protopic) ointment

SURGERY/OTHER PROCEDURES
Microdermabrasion, laser (Nd:YAG, pulsed dye)

 ONGOING CARE

PROGNOSIS
Most cases improve with age.

COMPLICATIONS
Hair loss is rare. If the lateral eyebrows are involved, consider the diagnosis of KP atrophicans faciei (ulerythema ophryogenes).

REFERENCES

1. Hwang S, Schwartz RA. Keratosis pilaris: A common follicular hyperkeratosis. *Cutis*. 2008;82:177–180.
2. Boza JC, Trindade EN, Peruzzo J, et al. Skin manifestations of obesity: A comparative study. *J Eur Acad Dermatol Venereol*. 2012;26:1220–1223.

 CODES

ICD10
L85.8 Other specified epidermal thickening

CLINICAL PEARLS

- KP is frequently mistaken for acne.
- Patients often self-manage with over-the-counter acne treatment products/medications originally prescribed for their facial acne.
- Daily measures to prevent dry skin, such as using mild cleansers, along with moisturizers, are the mainstay of treatment.

K

KERATOSIS, ACTINIC
Zoltan Trizna, MD, PhD

BASICS

DESCRIPTION
- Common, usually multiple, premalignant lesions of sun-exposed areas of the skin
- Common consequence of excessive cumulative ultraviolet (UV) light exposure
- A small percentage of lesions progress to squamous cell carcinoma (SCC) of the skin
- Synonym(s): Solar keratosis

Geriatric Considerations
Frequent problem

Pediatric Considerations
Rare (if child, look for freckling and other stigmata of xeroderma pigmentosum)

EPIDEMIOLOGY
Incidence
- Rates vary with age group and exposure to sun
- Predominant age: ≥40 years; progressively increases with age
- Predominant sex: Male > Female
- Common in those with blonde and red hair; rare in darker skin types

Prevalence
- Age-adjusted prevalence rate for actinic keratoses (AKs) in US Caucasians is 6.5%
- For 65–74-year-old males with high sun exposure: ~55%; low sun exposure, ~18%

ETIOLOGY AND PATHOPHYSIOLOGY
- The epidermal lesions are characterized by atypical keratinocytes at the basal layer with occasional extension upward. Mitoses are present. The histopathologic features resemble those of SCC in situ or SCC, and the distinction depends on the extent of epidermal involvement. Most AKs do not progress to SCC, although most SCCs arise from pre-existing AKs.
- Cumulative UV exposure is etiologic.

Genetics
The *p53* chromosomal mutation has been shown consistently in both AKs and SCCs. Many new genes have been shown recently to have similar expression profiles in AKs and SCCs.

RISK FACTORS
- Exposure to UV light (especially long-term and/or repeated exposure due to outdoor occupation or recreational activities, indoor or outdoor tanning)
- Skin type: Burns easily, does not tan
- Immunosuppression, especially organ transplantation

GENERAL PREVENTION
Sun avoidance and protective techniques are helpful.

COMMONLY ASSOCIATED CONDITIONS
- SCC
- Other features of chronic solar damage: Lentigines, elastosis, and telangiectasias

DIAGNOSIS

HISTORY
- The lesions are frequently asymptomatic; symptoms may include pruritus, burning, and mild hyperesthesia.
- Lesions may enlarge, thicken, or become more scaly. They also may regress or remain unchanged.
- Most lesions occur on the sun-exposed areas (head and neck, hands, forearms).

PHYSICAL EXAM
- Usually small (<1 cm), often multiple red, pink, or brown macules, papules, or plaques that are rough to palpation
- Yellow or brown adherent scale is often present on top of the lesion.
- Several clinical variants exist:
  – Atrophic: Dry, scaly macules with indistinct borders and an erythematous base
  – Hypertrophic: Overlying hyperkeratosis (in an extreme form, cutaneous horn) may be impossible to differentiate from SCC clinically.
  – Pigmented: Smooth tan/brown plaque, spreading centrifugally
  – Bowenoid: Red scaly plaques with distinct borders
  – Actinic cheilitis: Inflammatory lesion involving usually the lower lip

DIFFERENTIAL DIAGNOSIS
- SCC (hypertrophic type)
- Keratoacanthoma
- Bowen disease
- Basal cell carcinoma
- Verruca vulgaris
- Less likely: Verrucous nevi, warty dyskeratoma, lichenoid keratoses, seborrheic keratoses, porokeratoses, seborrheic dermatitis or psoriasis (near hairline), lentigo maligna, solar lentigo, discoid lupus erythematosus

DIAGNOSTIC TESTS & INTERPRETATION
Diagnostic Procedures/Other
- The diagnosis is usually made clinically, except where there is a suspicion of carcinoma.
- Skin biopsy is especially recommended if large, ulcerated, indurated, or bleeding or if the lesions are nonresponsive to treatment.

Test Interpretation
- Dysplastic keratinocytes in lower levels of epidermis with a dermal lymphocytic infiltrate
- Neoplastic cells, mostly found in the lower epidermal layers, are cytologically identical to those of SCCs.
- If neoplastic cells extend throughout entire epidermis or into the dermis, the lesions will qualify as an SCC in situ or invasive SCC, respectively.
- Malignant cells are sparse except for the bowenoid variety.
- Hypertrophic, atrophic, bowenoid, acantholytic, and pigmented varieties show the corresponding epidermal findings.

TREATMENT

Although only few AKs progress to SCC, it is impossible to predict which will. Therefore, most authorities recommend treatment. First-line treatment for individual or small numbers of AKs (based on ease of treatment, efficacy, cost, and tolerability) is usually cryotherapy (technically, this is considered surgery, especially by insurance companies) (1,2). Comparative efficacy of treatment is difficult to establish. A recent Cochrane review ranked fluorouracil most efficacious, followed by photodynamic therapy (which was similar in efficacy to imiquimod and ingenol mebutate). Cryotherapy was ranked next, followed by topical diclofenac (3)[A].

GENERAL MEASURES
- Sun-protective techniques
- Sunscreens and physical sun protection recommended

MEDICATION
Cost of pharmaceuticals reflects lowest cash costs of medications collected from a pricing website and from Medicare's allowables for the southern US (2013). Actual costs, insurance coverage, and out-of-pocket costs of patients are subject to change and significant regional variations. Always evaluate current data.

First Line
- Topical treatments target both visible and subclinical lesions and may be most useful for large numbers of lesions and at-risk skin.
- Topical fluorouracil (Efudex, Carac, Fluoroplex cream, Fluoroplex solution):
  – Every day–b.i.d. for 3–6 weeks, depending on the brand, concentration, and formulation
  – Can be very irritating
  – Fluorouracil (generic) 5% 40 g: $97; various brands (0.5–5%, 30-40 g): $271–438.
- Topical imiquimod 5% (Aldara) cream:
  – Apply every day, 2 days per week, for up to 4 months to an area not larger than the forehead or 1 cheek.
  – Can be irritating
  – Imiquimod 5% 12 packets, generic: $105, brand: $439.
- Topical imiquimod 3.75% (Zyclara) cream:
  – Apply once a day for 2 weeks, followed by no treatment for the next 2 weeks; then apply once a day for another 2 weeks.
  – Can be irritating

- Topical ingenol mebutate 0.015% (Picato) and ingenol mebutate 0.05% gel:
  – Apply to the face and scalp once a day for 3 consecutive days.
  – Apply to the trunk and extremities once a day for 2 consecutive days.
  – Picato 0.015% (ingenol mebutate) 3 tubes: $454; 2 tubes of ingenol mebutate 0.05%: $1,016
- 3% diclofenac (Solaraze) gel:
  – Apply b.i.d. for up to 3 months.
  – Solaraze (diclofenac 3%): 100 g: $825

Second Line
- Topical tretinoin (Retin-A) or tazarotene (Tazorac): May be used to enhance the efficacy of topical fluorouracil
- Systemic retinoids: Used infrequently

ADDITIONAL THERAPIES
Close monitoring with no treatment is an appropriate option for mild lesions.

SURGERY/OTHER PROCEDURES
- Cryosurgery ("freezing," liquid nitrogen):
  – Most common method
  – Cure rate: 75–98.8%
  – May leave scars
  – May be superior to photodynamic therapy for thicker lesions
- Photodynamic therapy with a photosensitizer (e.g., aminolevulinic acid) and illumination with blue light 14–18 hours later:
  – May clear >90% of AKs
  – Less scarring than cryotherapy
  – May be superior to cryotherapy, especially in the case of more extensive skin involvement
  – 2 office visits are needed
  – Photodynamic therapy: $145 per visit
- Curettage and electrocautery (scraping and burning)
- Medium-depth peels, especially for the treatment of extensive areas
- CO_2 laser therapy
- Dermabrasion
- Surgical excision (excisional biopsy)

 ## ONGOING CARE

FOLLOW-UP RECOMMENDATIONS
Patient Monitoring
Depends on associated malignancy and frequency with which new AKs appear

PATIENT EDUCATION
- Teach sun-protective techniques:
  – Limit outdoor activities between 10 AM and 4 PM
  – Wear protective clothing and wide-brimmed hat
  – Proper use (including reapplication) of sunscreens with SPF >30, preferably a preparation with broad-spectrum (UV-A and UV-B) protection
- Teach self-examination of skin (melanoma, squamous cell, basal cell).
- Patient education materials:
  – http://dermnetnz.org/lesions/solar-keratoses.html
  – www.skincarephysicians.com/actinickeratosesnet/index.html
  – www.skincancer.org/Actinic-Keratosis-and-Other-Precancers.htm

PROGNOSIS
Very good. A significant proportion of the lesions may resolve spontaneously (4).

COMPLICATIONS
- AKs are premalignant lesions that may progress to SCCs. The rate of malignant transformation is unclear; reported percentages vary (estimates ~1–20%).
- Patients with AKs are at increased risk for other cutaneous malignancies.

REFERENCES
1. Helfand M, Gorman AK, Mahon S, et al. AHRQ evidence report from OHSU Evidence-Based Practice Center. 2001.
2. de Berker D, McGregor JM, Hughes BR, et al. Guidelines for the management of actinic keratoses. *Br J Dermatol*. 2007;156:222–230.
3. Gupta AK, Paquet M. Network meta-analysis of the outcome 'participant complete clearance' in nonimmunosuppressed participants of eight interventions for actinic keratosis: A follow-up on a Cochrane review. *Br J Dermatol*. 2013;169: 250–259.
4. Criscione VD, Weinstock MA, Naylor MF, et al. Actinic keratoses: Natural history and risk of malignant transformation in the Veterans Affairs Topical Tretinoin Chemoprevention Trial. *Cancer*. 2009;115:2523–2530.

ADDITIONAL READING
- Kanellou P, Zaravinos A, Zioga M, et al. Genomic instability, mutations and expression analysis of the tumour suppressor genes p14(ARF), p15(INK4b), p16(INK4a) and p53 in actinic keratosis. *Cancer Lett*. 2008;264:145–161.
- Rossi R, Mori M, Lotti T. Actinic keratosis. *Int J Dermatol*. 2007;46:895–904.

 ## CODES

ICD10
L57.0 Actinic keratosis

CLINICAL PEARLS
- AKs are premalignant lesions, although most do not progress.
- Often more easily felt than seen.
- Therapy-resistant lesions should be biopsied, especially on the face.

K

KERATOSIS, SEBORRHEIC

Christina N. Alavian, MD • Melissa McEnery-Stonelake, MD

 BASICS

DESCRIPTION
- One of the most common benign tumors of the epidermis
- Formed from keratinocytes
- Frequently appears in multiples on the head, neck and trunk of older individuals, but may occur on any hair-bearing area of the body
- Typically are brown, sharply demarcated, round or elongated lesions with a velvety, verrucous-like, "stuck-on" appearance; lesions may also appear waxy yellow or pink.
- Clinical variants include (1):
  – Common seborrheic keratosis
  – Dermatosis papulosa nigra
  – Stucco keratosis
  – Flat seborrheic keratosis
  – Pedunculated seborrheic keratosis
- System(s) affected: Integumentary
- Synonym(s): Verruca seborrhoica; Seborrheic wart; Senile wart; Basal cell papilloma; Verruca senilis; Basal cell acanthoma; Benign acanthokeratoma (2)

EPIDEMIOLOGY
Incidence
- Predominant age:
  – Usually appear after the 3rd decade (3)
  – Most commonly seen during middle and older age (1,2,3)
  – Can occasionally arise as early as adolescence (1,2,3)
- Predominant sex: Male = Female
- Most common among Caucasians, except for the dermatosis papulosa nigra variant, which usually presents in darker skinned individuals

Prevalence
- 80–100% in patients >50 (3)
- The prevalence rate increases with advancing age (1,2,3).

ETIOLOGY AND PATHOPHYSIOLOGY
- Seborrheic keratoses are monoclonal tumors (2).
- The exact pathogenesis is not well understood; the following mechanisms are thought to be involved (2,3):
  – Activating somatic mutations of fibroblast growth factor receptor 3 (FGFR3), a membrane-bound tyrosine kinase
  – Oncogenic phosphoinositide-3-kinase (PIK3CA) pathway mutations
  – Elevated p16 levels, suggesting senescence of epidermal cells in the G1 phase of the cell cycle
  – Apoptosis inhibition
- Etiology still is largely unclear.
- Ultraviolet (UV) light and genetics are thought to be involved.
- The role of human papillomavirus is uncertain (2,3).

Genetics
An autosomal dominant inheritance pattern is suggested (2).

RISK FACTORS
- Advanced age
- Exposure to UV light and genetic predisposition are possible factors (2,3).

GENERAL PREVENTION
Sun protection methods may help prevent seborrheic keratoses from developing.

COMMONLY ASSOCIATED CONDITIONS
- Sign of Leser-Trélat: A paraneoplastic syndrome characterized by a sudden eruption of multiple seborrheic keratoses in association with an internal malignancy, most commonly stomach or colon adenocarcinoma. Usually represents a poor prognosis. The validity of this syndrome as a marker for internal malignancy is controversial (rare) (2,3).
- Documentation of other cutaneous lesions, such as basal cell carcinoma, malignant melanoma, Bowen disease, or squamous cell carcinoma, growing adjacent to or within a seborrheic keratosis, has been reported. The exact relationship between lesions is unclear (rare) (2,3).

 DIAGNOSIS

HISTORY
- Usually asymptomatic
- Trauma or irritation of the lesion may result in pruritus, erythema, bleeding, pain, and/or crusting.
- Rarely, vision or hearing may be hindered by a seborrheic keratosis located near the eyelid or external auditory canal.

PHYSICAL EXAM
- Typically begin as oval- or round-shaped, flat, dull, sharply demarcated patches.
- As they mature, may develop into thicker, elevated, uneven, verrucous-like papules, plaques, or peduncles with a waxy or velvety surface, and appear "stuck on" to the skin.
- Commonly appear on sun-exposed areas of the body, predominately the head, neck, or trunk, but may appear on any hair-bearing skin.
- Vary in color from black, brown, tan, gray to white, or skin-colored, and range in size, from 1 mm to 4 cm.
- Usually occur as multiples, with patients having >100 not uncommon.
- May grow along folds on truncal skin, forming a "Christmas tree" pattern.
- If irritated, may be bleeding, inflamed, painful, pruritic, or crusted.
- Common clinical variants include (1)[C]:
  – Common seborrheic keratoses: On hair-bearing skin, usually on the face, neck, and trunk; verrucous-like, waxy, or velvety lesions that appear "stuck on" to the skin
  – Dermatosis papulosa nigra: Small black papules that usually appear on the face, neck, chest, and upper back; most common in darker skinned individuals, more common in females; most have a positive family history
  – Stucco keratoses: Small gray-white, rough, verrucous papules; usually occur in large numbers on the lower extremities or forearms; more common in men
  – Flat seborrheic keratoses: Oval-shaped, brown patches or macules on face, chest, and upper extremities; increases with age
  – Pedunculated seborrheic keratoses: Hyperpigmented peduncles appear on areas of friction (neck, axilla)

DIFFERENTIAL DIAGNOSIS
Consider the following diagnoses if the seborrheic keratosis is:
- Pigmented:
  – Malignant melanoma
  – Melanocytic nevus
  – Angiokeratoma
  – Pigmented basal cell carcinoma
- Lightly pigmented:
  – Basal cell carcinoma
  – Bowen disease
  – Condyloma acuminatum
  – Fibroma
  – Verruca vulgaris
  – Eccrine poroma
  – Invasive squamous cell carcinoma
  – Acrochordon
  – Acrokeratosis verruciformis of Hopf
  – Follicular infundibulum tumor
- Flat:
  – Solar lentigo
  – Verrucae planae juveniles
- Hyperkeratotic:
  – Actinic keratosis

DIAGNOSTIC TESTS & INTERPRETATION
Initial Tests (lab, imaging)
Not needed unless internal malignancy is suspected.

Diagnostic Procedures/Other
- The diagnosis can usually be made based on clinical appearance.
- Dermoscopy (1)[C],(2)[C]:
  – Can aid in diagnosis
  – Common findings are comedo-like openings, fissures, ridges, sharply demarcated borders, milia-like cysts (1), pseudofollicular openings, and horn pseudocysts (2)[C].
- Biopsy and histologic exam should be performed if the seborrheic keratosis (2)[C],(3)[C]:
  – Is atypical
  – Has inflammation
  – Recently changed in appearance
  – Diagnosis remains unclear

Test Interpretation
- Histologic findings include:
  – Acanthosis and papillomatosis due to basaloid cell proliferation
  – "Squamous eddies" or squamous epithelial cell clusters
  – Hyperpigmentation
  – Hyperkeratosis
  – Horn cysts
  – Pseudocysts
- Several histologic variants exist

TREATMENT

- Treatment is not usually necessary, due to the benign nature of the lesions (2)[C],(3)[C].
- Removal of seborrheic keratoses may be indicated if:
  - Symptomatic
  - Aesthetically displeasing or undesirable (common)
  - There is a question of malignancy

MEDICATION

Current topical treatments of seborrheic keratoses are less effective than a surgical approach (2)[C],(3)[C],(4)[C].

ISSUES FOR REFERRAL

- New seborrheic keratoses appear abruptly
- A seborrheic keratosis becomes inflamed or changes in appearance.

SURGERY/OTHER PROCEDURES

- A surgical approach to treatment is preferred.
- Choice depends on physician preference and availability of the treatment.
- The following procedures are used:
  - Cryotherapy (liquid nitrogen) (5)[B]:
    - Spray flat lesions for 5–10 seconds; may require more time or additional treatments if the seborrheic keratosis is thicker.
    - Possible complications include scarring, hypopigmentation, recurrence.
  - Curettage (5)[B]
  - Electrodessication
  - Shave excision
  - Excisional biopsy
  - Chemical peel
- Use of following laser treatments has been reported (4)[C]:
  - Ablative CO_2
  - Ablative erbium-YAG
  - Argon
  - 492 nm
  - 510 nm
  - Alexandrite lasers
- A recent study indicated that the majority of patients preferred cryotherapy over curettage, over both the short and long term. This was mainly due to decreased postoperative wound care, despite the increased discomfort experienced and increased frequency of seborrheic keratosis remaining after cryotherapy when compared to curettage (5)[B].
  - No statistically significant differences were found in patient's ratings of cosmetic appearance between cryotherapy and curettage.
- Both petrolatum-based skin protectant ointment and combination antibiotic first-aid ointment provide equivalent efficacy for wound healing (6)[B].
  - Antibiotic ointment may not be necessary for satisfactory wound healing and may promote allergic contact dermatitis.

ONGOING CARE

FOLLOW-UP RECOMMENDATIONS
Patient Monitoring
After initial diagnosis, follow-up is not usually required unless:
- Inflammation or irritation develops
- There is a change in appearance
- New seborrheic keratoses suddenly appear

PATIENT EDUCATION
- Sun-protective methods may help reduce seborrheic keratosis development.
- Patient education materials:
  - www.aad.org/skin-conditions/dermatology-a-to-z/seborrheic-keratoses
  - www.cdc.gov/cancer/skin/basic_info/prevention.htm

PROGNOSIS
- Seborrheic keratoses generally do not become malignant (2,3).
- Sign of Leser-Trélat usually represents a poor prognosis.

COMPLICATIONS
- Irritation and inflammation due to mechanical irritation (i.e., from clothing, jewelry)
- Possible complications of surgical treatment include hypopigmentation, hyperpigmentation, scarring, incomplete removal, and recurrence.
- Misdiagnosis (rare)

REFERENCES

1. Rajesh G, Thappa DM, Jaisankar TJ, et al. Spectrum of seborrheic keratoses in South Indians: A clinical and dermoscopic study. *Indian J Dermatol Venereol Leprol*. 2011;77:483–488.
2. Hafner C, Vogt T. Seborrheic keratosis. *J Dtsch Dermatol Ges*. 2008;6:664–677.
3. Noiles K, Vender R. Are all seborrheic keratoses benign? Review of the typical lesion and its variants. *J Cutan Med Surg*. 2008;12:203–210.
4. Herron MD, Bowen AR, Krueger GG, et al. Seborrheic keratoses: A study comparing the standard cryosurgery with topical calcipotriene, topical tazarotene, and topical imiquimod. *Int J Dermatol*. 2004;43:300–302.
5. Wood LD, Stucki JK, Hollenbeak CS, et al. Effectiveness of cryosurgery vs curettage in the treatment of seborrheic keratoses. *JAMA Dermatol*. 2013;149:108–109.
6. Draelos ZD, Rizer RL, Trookman NS. A comparison of postprocedural wound care treatments: do antibiotic-based ointments improve outcomes? *J Am Acad Dermatol*. 2011;64:S23–S29.

ADDITIONAL READING

- Culbertson GR. 532-nm diode laser treatment of seborrheic keratoses with color enhancement. *Dermatol Surg*. 2008;34:525–528; discussion 528.
- Garcia MS, Azari R, Eisen DB. Treatment of dermatosis papulosa nigra in 10 patients: A comparison trial of electrodesiccation, pulsed dye laser, and curettage. *Dermatol Surg*. 2010;36:1968–1972.
- Krupashankar DS, IADVL Dermatosurgery Task Force. Standard guidelines of care: CO2 laser for removal of benign skin lesions and resurfacing. *Indian J Dermatol Venereol Leprol*. 2008;74:S61–S67.
- Luba MC, Bangs SA, Mohler AM, et al. Common benign skin tumors. *Am Fam Physician*. 2003;67:729–738.
- Taylor SC, Averyhart AN, Heath CR, et al. Postprocedural wound-healing efficacy following removal of dermatosis papulosa nigra lesions in an African American population: A comparison of a skin protectant ointment and a topical antibiotic. *J Am Acad Dermatol*. 2011;64:S30–S35.

CODES

ICD10
- L82.0 Inflamed seborrheic keratosis
- L82.1 Other seborrheic keratosis

CLINICAL PEARLS

- Seborrheic keratoses are one of the most common benign tumors of the epidermis.
- Prevalence increases with age.
- Underlying internal malignancy should be considered if large numbers of seborrheic keratoses appear suddenly.

K

KLINEFELTER SYNDROME

Nisha Nathan, MD

BASICS

DESCRIPTION
- Abnormal body regional proportion, decreased trunk-to-leg ratio, eunuchoid body habitus.
- Clinical features of hypergonadotropic hypogonadism: Gynecomastia, small firm testicles, decreased facial and pubic hair.
- Most common karyotype is 47,XXY.
- Virtually all men are infertile.
- Diagnosis is made during adolescence and adulthood; may remain undiagnosed because symptoms are usually subtle.
- Klinefelter syndrome (KS) has been associated with both increased morbidity and mortality believed to be related to genetic, hormonal, behavioral, and socioeconomic factors (1).

EPIDEMIOLOGY
Prevalence
~1 in 600 males.

ETIOLOGY AND PATHOPHYSIOLOGY
- Primary hypergonadotropic hypogonadism.
- Unclear whether many aspects of syndrome are caused by hormonal abnormalities or extra X chromosome.
- Mutations are spontaneous and patients have no family history.
- Recurrence risk is that of the general population.

Genetics
- The most common sex chromosome abnormality.
- The classic form of KS (47,XXY) occurs following meiotic nondisjunction of the sex chromosomes during gametogenesis:
  - 40% during spermatogenesis, 60% during oogenesis.
- Mosaic forms of KS (46,XY/47,XXY) are thought to result from chromosomal mitotic nondisjunction within the zygote and occur in ~10% of individuals with KS.
- Other chromosome variants of KS (48,XXYY, 48,XXXY) have been identified, but are much less common.
- Severity of phenotype is directly correlated with extra number of X-chromosomes, suggesting an effect related to gene dosage:
  - Each extra X is associated with a decrease in IQ of ~15–16 points.

RISK FACTORS
Weakly associated with advanced maternal age; X-chromosome nondisjunction increases with age.

Pregnancy Considerations
- Prenatal diagnosis is possible by karyotyping cells obtained from amniocentesis.
- Diagnosis made via amniocentesis is usually incidental.

COMMONLY ASSOCIATED CONDITIONS
- Clinical manifestations of hypogonadism:
  - Infertility (>99%)
  - Azoospermia (>95%)
  - Osteopenia/Osteoporosis (50%)
  - Erectile dysfunction

- Neurodevelopmental sequelae:
  - Low IQ
  - Gross motor delay or dysfunction
  - Learning disabilities: Speech, language, and reading difficulties
  - Autism spectrum behavior
  - ADHD, attention deficits
  - Emotional and behavior problem
- Cardiovascular and metabolic disorders:
  - Thromboembolic disease
  - Mitral valve prolapse and aortic valve disease
  - Metabolic syndrome (46%) and diabetes (10–39%)
- Autoimmune diseases (uncommon):
  - Rheumatoid arthritis
  - Chronic thyroiditis
- Malignancies (rare):
  - Breast cancer (>50× risk than the general population)
  - Extragonadal germ cell tumors, mainly mediastinal (>65× risk than the general population)

DIAGNOSIS

HISTORY
- Adolescence: Delayed or absent puberty or persistent gynecomastia
- Middle age: Erectile dysfunction, infertility, decreased libido
- Older age: Metabolic syndrome, osteoporosis
- Learning disabilities, psychosocial problems, psychiatric illness

PHYSICAL EXAM
- Small, firm testes (4–6 mL) (95%)
- Eunuchoid body habitus (long legs, short torso, narrow shoulders, broad hips)
- Decreased facial hair (60–80%)
- Gynecomastia (38–75%)
- Decreased muscle strength (70%)
- Decreased pubic hair (30–60%)
- Varicose veins (40%)
- Sparse facial and body hair (88%); female pubic hair distribution (53%)
- Increased fat-to-muscle ratio; abdominal adiposity
- Mitral valve prolapse
- Specific mild dysmorphic features (2)[C]:
  - Clinodactyly (74%)
  - Hypertelorism (69%)
  - Mild elbow dysplasia (36%)
  - High arched palate (37%)

Pediatric Considerations
<10% diagnosed before puberty.

DIFFERENTIAL DIAGNOSIS
- Primary hypogonadism (high follicle-stimulating hormone [FSH]/luteinizing hormone [LH]):
  - Congenital:
    - Pure gonadal dysgenesis
    - Congenital anorchia
    - Hemochromatosis
  - Acquired:
    - Mumps orchitis
    - Injury to the testicles
    - Chemotherapy or radiation therapy

- Secondary hypogonadism (low FSH/LH):
  - Kallmann syndrome
  - Pituitary tumor
  - Inflammatory disorders: Sarcoidosis, TB, histiocytosis
  - HIV/AIDS
  - Medications: Steroids, opiate pain medication
  - Obesity
  - Old age

DIAGNOSTIC TESTS & INTERPRETATION
Initial Tests (lab, imaging)
- Confirm diagnosis of primary hypogonadism:
  - Testosterone levels are low.
  - Elevated gonadotropins: FSH, LH
- Karyotype analysis to confirm genetic abnormality:
  - Cytogenetic analysis (karyotype)
  - Polymerase chain reaction (PCR) looking at the copy number of the androgen receptor (AR) gene (located on Xq11.2–q12) has been described as a screen for KS and other X-chromosome aneuploidies, not commonly used (3)[C].

Follow-Up Tests & Special Considerations
- Fertility:
  - Semen analysis
  - Most men are infertile; although rare, fertility is possible in mosaics
- Screening for associated conditions:
  - Look for metabolic abnormalities; fasting glucose, lipids, thyroid function
  - Vitamin D levels
- Adequacy of androgen replacement:
  - Testosterone levels
- Chest x-ray to rule out mediastinal tumor
- Bone density screening
- Echocardiogram to evaluate for valve disease
- Testes and breast ultrasound

Test Interpretation
Testicular biopsy in an adult demonstrates hyalinization of the seminiferous tubules and hyperplasia of Leydig cells.

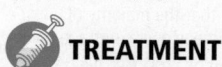

TREATMENT

GENERAL MEASURES
- Preventive dental care
- Calcium and vitamin D supplementation

MEDICATION
First Line
Testosterone therapy:
- Benefits:
  - Develops secondary male sex characteristics:
    - Increases body hair and penis length and improves libido
    - May reduce gynecomastia and abdominal adiposity and increase muscle mass (4)[C] (not replicated in all studies)
  - Improves libido/decrease erectile dysfunction
  - Metabolic:
    - Improves bone density (4)[C]
    - May lower serum total cholesterol (4) and improve metabolic syndrome (5)[C]

– Other:
  ○ May improve mood, energy level, cognition, and social functioning and decrease aggression (4)[B]
  ○ May possibly reduce hypercoagulability (6), improve autoimmune disease (7)[C]
- Risks and side effects:
  – Erythrocytosis
  – Acne
  – Lowering of HDL
  – Worsening of aggression
  – Peliosis hepatitis, hepatic adenomas, and hepatocellular carcinoma
  – Worsening of subclinical prostate cancer
  – May accelerate infertility in adolescents and young men
- Contraindications:
  – Prostate cancer
  – Liver disease
- Dosage:
  – IM injection
  – Transdermal gel

Pediatric Considerations
- Testosterone therapy, beginning at age 11–13, is recommended by experts (8)[C]
- Monitor bone age
- Micropenis in infants and children has been treated with topical or IM testosterone (8)[C]

ISSUES FOR REFERRAL
- Most men have azoospermia at time of diagnosis. Adolescents and young men wishing to preserve fertility should be referred for cryopreservation of existing sperm if sperm are present on semen analysis.
- If viable sperm are noted on semen analysis, fertility treatment may be offered using testicular fine-needle aspiration (TEFNA) or testicular sperm extraction (TESE) followed by in vitro fertilization. Embryos are at a modestly increased risk of cytogenetic abnormalities, but most of the resulting pregnancies are healthy.

ADDITIONAL THERAPIES
Individual or family counseling, if indicated

SURGERY/OTHER PROCEDURES
Mastectomy can be performed to correct gynecomastia and reduce the risk of breast cancer, which can be a cause of psychological strain.

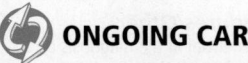 ## ONGOING CARE

FOLLOW-UP RECOMMENDATIONS
Men who are treated with testosterone will require frequent follow up.

Patient Monitoring
- Annual lipid and diabetes screening
- Annual clinical breast exam ± breast imaging
- Periodic bone density testing

PATIENT EDUCATION
- Presentation is variable, with most patients appearing physically normal.
- Patients are likely infertile, but there may be options for reproductive therapy.
- There should be careful thought and discussion between the patient and the provider about the risks and benefits of androgen replacement. Patients should know that testosterone can induce puberty and increase libido.
- There is a high incidence of learning disabilities and psychiatric illness. Appropriate therapy should be utilized.
- Risk of diabetes and importance of regular screening and maintaining a healthy weight.
- Risk of osteoporosis and importance of calcium, vitamin D, and weight-bearing exercise.
- Regular dental care.
- American Association for Klinefelter Syndrome Information and Support: www.aaksis.org
- Klinefelter Syndrome Support Group: http://klinefeltersyndrome.org

PROGNOSIS
- Hypogonadism is permanent.
- There is an increased risk for comorbidities associated with KS.
- On average, adults have modestly reduced intelligence, verbal reasoning, language skills, and motor dexterity.
- Increased number of X chromosomes is correlated with increased phenotypic severity.

REFERENCES
1. Bojesen A, Gravholt CH. Morbidity and mortality in Klinefelter syndrome (47,XXY). *Acta Paediatr.* 2011;100:807–813.
2. Zeger MP, Zinn AR, Lahlou N, et al. Effect of ascertainment and genetic features on the phenotype of Klinefelter syndrome. *J Pediatr.* 2008;152:716–722.
3. Ottesen AM, Garn ID, Aksglaede L, et al. A simple screening method for detection of Klinefelter syndrome and other X-chromosome aneuploidies based on copy number of the androgen receptor gene. *Mol Hum Reprod.* 2007;13:745–750.
4. Wang C. Long-term testosterone gel (AndroGel) treatment maintains beneficial effects on sexual function and mood, lean and fat mass, and bone mineral density in hypogonadal men. *J Clin Endo Metab.* 2004;85:2085–2098.
5. Spark RF. Testosterone, diabetes mellitus, and the metabolic syndrome. *Curr Urol Rep.* 2007;8:467–471.
6. Zitzmann M, Junker R, Kamischke A, et al. Contraceptive steroids influence the hemostatic activation state in healthy men. *J Androl.* 2002;23:503–511.
7. Koçar IH, Yesilova Z, Ozata M, et al. The effect of testosterone replacement treatment on immunological features of patients with Klinefelter's syndrome. *Clin Exp Immunol.* 2000;121:448–452.
8. Bojesen A. Klinefelter syndrome in clinical practice. *Nat Clin Prac.* 2007;4:192–201.

ADDITIONAL READING
- Radicioni AF, Ferlin A, Balercia G, et al. Consensus statement on diagnosis and clinical management of Klinefelter syndrome. *J Endocrinol Invest.* 2010;33:839–850.
- Wattendorf DJ, Muenke M. Klinefelter syndrome. *Am Fam Physician.* 2005;72:2259–2262.

 ## CODES

ICD10
- Q98.0 Klinefelter syndrome karyotype 47, XXY
- Q98.1 Klinefelter syndrome, male with more than two X chromosomes
- Q98.4 Klinefelter syndrome, unspecified

CLINICAL PEARLS
- Klinefelter syndrome males have ≥1 additional X chromosome (XXY karyotype) with associated features of hypergonadotropic hypogonadism.
- Accounts for 3% of male infertility.
- Most men do not have "textbook features" and, therefore, frequently remain undiagnosed until adulthood.
- Testosterone therapy, beginning in adolescence, has many benefits.

K

KNEE PAIN

Gregory Murphy, MD • J. Herbert Stevenson, MD

 ## BASICS

DESCRIPTION
Knee pain is a common complaint in the outpatient setting with a broad differential:
- Knee pain may be acute, chronic, or an acute exacerbation of a chronic condition.
- Trauma, overuse, and degenerative conditions are frequent causes.
- Obtaining a detailed history, including patient age, pain onset and location, mechanism of injury, and associated symptoms, can help narrow the differential diagnosis.
- A thorough but focused exam, including examination of the hips, is key to making a correct diagnosis and determining appropriate treatment.

EPIDEMIOLOGY
Incidence
- Knee pain accounts for 1.9 million primary care visits annually.
- The incidence of knee osteoarthritis is 240 cases/100,000 person-years (1).

Prevalence
- The knee is a common site of lower extremity injury among runners (2):
  - Patellar tendonopathy and patellofemoral syndrome are the most common causes of knee pain in runners.
- Osteoarthritis (OA) is one of the leading causes of disability in the US.

ETIOLOGY AND PATHOPHYSIOLOGY
- Trauma (ligament or meniscal injury, fracture, dislocation)
- Overuse (tendinopathy, patellofemoral syndrome, bursitis, apophysitis)
- Age related (arthritis, degenerative conditions, apophysitis [young])
- Rheumatologic (rheumatoid arthritis [RA], gout, pseudogout)
- Infectious (bacterial, postviral, Lyme disease)
- Referred pain (hip, back)
- Vascular: (popliteal artery aneurysm, deep vein thrombosis)
- Other (tumor, cyst)

RISK FACTORS
- Obesity
- Malalignment
- Poor flexibility, muscle imbalance or weakness
- Rapid increases in training frequency and intensity
- Improper footwear, training surfaces, technique
- Activities involving cutting, jumping, deceleration, kneeling
- Previous injuries

GENERAL PREVENTION
- Maintain normal body mass index; lose weight if obese.
- Use appropriate exercise training principles.
- Correct strength and flexibility imbalances.
- Proper activity-specific techniques, equipment (i.e., jumping and landing, knee pads).

COMMONLY ASSOCIATED CONDITIONS
- Fracture, contusion
- Effusion, hemarthrosis
- Patellar dislocation/subluxation
- Meniscal injury
- Ligamentous injury
- Tendinopathy
- Bursitis
- Osteochondral injury
- Arthritis
- Septic joint
- Muscle strain

DIAGNOSIS

HISTORY
- Pain:
  - Diffuse pain: Osteoarthritis, patellofemoral pain syndrome/chondromalacia
  - Pain ascending/descending stairs: Meniscal injury, patellofemoral pain syndrome/chondromalacia
  - Pain with prolonged sitting, standing from sitting: Patellofemoral pain syndrome/chondromalacia
- Mechanism of injury:
  - Hyperextension, deceleration, cutting: Anterior cruciate ligament (ACL) injury
  - Hyperflexion, fall on flexed knee, "dashboard injury": Posterior cruciate ligament (PCL) injury
  - Lateral force (valgus load): Medial collateral injury
  - Twisting on planted foot: Meniscal injury
- Effusion:
  - Rapid onset (2 hours): ACL tear, patellar subluxation, tibial plateau fracture. Hemarthrosis is common.
  - Slower onset (24–36 hours), smaller: Meniscal injury, ligament sprain
  - Swelling behind the knee: Popliteal cyst. Prepatellar: Bursitis

PHYSICAL EXAM
- Observe for antalgic gait, patellar tracking abnormalities.
- Inspect for malalignment, atrophy, swelling, ecchymosis, or erythema.
- Palpate for effusion, warmth, and tenderness.
- Evaluate active/passive range of motion (ROM) and flexibility.
- Evaluate strength, muscle tone.
- Pay attention to joint instability, locking, catching.
- Evaluate hip ROM, strength, stability.
- Special tests:
  - Patellar apprehension test: Patellar instability. Patellar grind test: Patellar dysfunction
  - Lachman, anterior drawer test: ACL integrity. Lachman is more sensitive and specific.
  - Posterior drawer, posterior sag sign: PCL integrity
  - Valgus/Varus stress test: Medial/Lateral collateral ligament (MCL/LCL) integrity
  - McMurray test: Meniscal injury
  - Ober test: Iliotibial band (ITB) tightness
  - Pivot shift test: Positive with ACL rupture, may have false positive in patients with greater knee laxity
  - Dial test: Positive with posterolateral corner laxity
  - Patellar tilt test and squatting may help suggest patellofemoral pain syndrome, but there is not yet one definitive test (3)[A]

DIFFERENTIAL DIAGNOSIS
- Acute onset: Fracture, contusion, cruciate or collateral ligament tear, meniscal tear, patellar dislocation/subluxation. If systemic symptoms: Osteomyelitis, septic arthritis, gout, pseudogout, Lyme disease
- Insidious onset: Patellofemoral pain syndrome/chondromalacia, iliotibial band syndrome, osteoarthritis, RA, bursitis, tumor, tendinopathy, loose body, bipartite patella, degenerative meniscal tear
- Anterior pain: Patellofemoral pain syndrome, chondromalacia, patellar injury, patellar tendinopathy, pre- or suprapatellar bursitis, tibial apophysitis, fat pad impingement, quadriceps tendinopathy, OA
- Posterior pain: PCL injury, posterior horn meniscal injury, popliteal cyst/aneurysm, hamstring or gastrocnemius injury, deep venous thrombosis (DVT)
- Medial pain: MCL injury, medial meniscal injury, pes anserine bursitis, medial plica syndrome, OA
- Lateral pain: LCL injury, lateral meniscal injury, ITB syndrome, OA

DIAGNOSTIC TESTS & INTERPRETATION
Initial Tests (lab, imaging)
- Suspected septic joint, gout, pseudogout:
  - Arthrocentesis with cell count, Gram stain, culture, protein/glucose, synovial fluid analysis
- Suspected RA:
  - CBC, ESR, rheumatoid factor
- Consider Lyme titer
- Radiographs may be needed to rule out fracture in patients with acute knee trauma per the Ottawa rules:
  - Age >55 years *or*
  - Tenderness at the patella or fibular head *or*
  - Inability to bear weight 4 steps *or*
  - Inability to flex knee to 90°
- Radiographs may help in diagnosing OA, osteochondral lesions, patellofemoral pain syndrome:
  - Weightbearing, upright anteroposterior, lateral, merchant/sunrise, notch/tunnel views

Follow-Up Tests & Special Considerations
- CT to evaluate fracture suspected on x-ray (4[C]
- MRI is "gold standard" for imaging muscle, ligamentous, and intra-articular structures (4)[C].

Diagnostic Procedures/Other
Arthroscopy may be beneficial in the diagnosis of certain conditions, including meniscus and ligament injuries.

Geriatric Considerations
OA, degenerative meniscal tears, and gout are more common.

Pediatric Considerations
- 3 million pediatric sports injuries occur annually.
- Must be concerned about physeal/apophyseal and joint surface injuries in skeletally immature:
  - Acute: Patellar subluxation, avulsion fractures, ACL tear
  - Overuse: Patellofemoral pain syndrome, apophysitis, osteochondritis dissecans, patellar tendonitis, stress fracture
  - Other: Neoplasm, juvenile RA, infection, referred pain from slipped capital femoral epiphysis.

TREATMENT

GENERAL MEASURES
Acute injury: PRICEMM therapy (**p**rotection, **r**elative rest, **i**ce, **c**ompression, **e**levation, **m**edications, **m**odalities)

MEDICATION
First Line
- Oral medications:
  - Acetaminophen: Up to 3–4 g/d. Safe and effective in OA (1)[A].
  - NSAIDs:
    ○ Ibuprofen: 200–800 mg t.i.d.
    ○ Naproxen: 250–500 mg b.i.d.:
      ▪ Useful for acute ligament sprains, muscle strains (5)[C]
      ▪ Useful for short-term pain reduction in OA. Long-term use not recommended due to side effects (1)[A].
      ▪ Not recommended for fracture, stress fracture, chronic muscle injury: May be associated with delayed healing; low dose and brief course only if necessary (5)[C].
  - Tramadol/Narcotics: Not recommended as first-line treatment (1). Can be used with acute injuries.
- Topical medications:
  - Topical NSAIDs may provide pain relief in OA and are more tolerable than oral medications (6)[C].
  - Topical capsaicin may be an adjuvant for pain management in OA (6)[A].
- Injections:
  - Intra-articular corticosteroid injection may provide short-term benefit in knee OA (1,7)[A].
  - Viscosupplementation may reduce pain and improve function in patients with OA after other methods have been exhausted (1,8)[A].

ISSUES FOR REFERRAL
- Acute trauma, young athletic patient
- Joint instability
- Lack of improvement with conservative measures
- Salter-Harris physeal fractures (pediatrics)

ADDITIONAL THERAPIES
- Physical therapy is recommended as initial treatment for patellofemoral pain syndrome (9)[A].
- Exercise, muscle strengthening improves outcome in OA (1)[A].
- Foot orthoses, acupuncture (10)[C]
- May need bracing for stability

SURGERY/OTHER PROCEDURES
- Surgery may be required for ligamentous and cartilaginous injuries.
- Chronic conditions refractory to conservative therapy may require surgical intervention.

COMPLEMENTARY AND ALTERNATIVE MEDICINE
May reduce pain and improve function in OA:
- Glucosamine sulfate (500 mg t.i.d.) (1),(11)[B]
- Chondroitin (400 mg t.i.d.) (11)[B]
- S-adenosylmethionine (SAMe), ginger extract, methylsulfonylmethane: Less reliable improvement and evidence
- Acupuncture (10)[C]

 ONGOING CARE

FOLLOW-UP RECOMMENDATIONS
- Activity modification in overuse conditions
- Rehabilitative exercise in OA:
  - Low-impact exercise: Walking, swimming, cycling
  - Strength, ROM, and proprioception training

Patient Monitoring
- After initial treatment in acute injury, consider rehabilitation.
- In chronic and overuse conditions, assess functional status, rehabilitation exercise compliance, and pain control at follow-up visit.

DIET
Weight reduction for overweight patient with OA

PATIENT EDUCATION
- Review activity modifications.
- Encourage the patient to play an active role in the rehabilitation process.
- Review risks and benefits of pharmaceutical interventions.

PROGNOSIS
Varies with diagnosis, injury severity, chronicity of condition, patient motivation to participate in rehabilitative exercises, and whether surgical intervention is required

COMPLICATIONS
- Disability
- Arthritis
- Chronic joint instability
- Deconditioning

REFERENCES
1. Bijlsma JW, Berenbaum F, Lafeber FP. Osteoarthritis: An update with relevance to clinical practice. *Lancet*. 2011;377:2115–2126.
2. Lopes AD, Hespanhol LC, Yeung SS, et al. What are the main running-related musculoskeletal injuries?: A systematic review. *Sports Med*. 2012;42:891–905.
3. Nunes GS, Stapait EL, Kirsten MH, et al. Clinical test for diagnosis of patellofemoral pain syndrome: Systematic review with meta-analysis. *Phys Ther Sport*. 2013;14:54–59.
4. Teh J, Kambouraglou G, Newton J. Investigation of acute knee injury. *BMJ*. 2012;344:e3167.
5. Ziltener JL, Leal S, Fournier PE. Non-steroidal anti-inflammatory drugs for athletes: An update. *Ann Phys Rehabil Med*. 2010;53:278–282.
6. Derry S, Moore RA, Rabbie R. Topical NSAIDs for chronic musculoskeletal pain in adults. *Cochrane Database of Syst Rev*. 2012;9:CD007400.
7. Bellamy N, Campbell J, Welch V, et al. Intraarticular corticosteroids for treatment of osteoarthritis of the knee. *Cochrane Database Syst Rev*. 2006;2:CD005328.
8. Bellamy N, Campbell J, Welch V, et al. Viscosupplementation for the treatment of osteoarthritis of the knee. *Cochrane Database Sys Rev*. 2006;2;CD005321.
9. Bolgla LA, Boling MC. An update for the conservative management of patellofemoral pain syndrome: A systematic review. *Int J Sports Phys Ther*. 2011;6:112–125.
10. Collins NJ, Bissett LM, Crossley KM, et al. Efficacy of nonsurgical interventions for anterior knee pain: Systematic review and meta-analysis of randomized trials. *Sports Med*. 2012;42:31–49.
11. Vangsness CT, Spiker W, Erickson J. A review of evidence based medicine for glucosamine and chondroitin sulfate use in knee osteoarthritis. *Arthroscopy*. 2009;25:86–94.

ADDITIONAL READING
- Debbi EM, Agar G, Fichman G, et al. Efficacy of a methylsulfonylmethane supplement on osteoarthritis of the knee- a randomized control trial. *BMC Complement Altern Med*. 2011;11:50.
- Ringdahl E, Pandit S. Treatment of knee osteoarthritis. *Am Fam Physician*. 2011;83: 1287–1292.

 SEE ALSO

Algorithms: Knee Pain; Popliteal Mass

CODES

ICD10
- M17.9 Osteoarthritis of knee, unspecified
- M25.569 Pain in unspecified knee
- M76.50 Patellar tendinitis, unspecified knee

CLINICAL PEARLS
- Knee pain is a common presentation for both acute and chronic injuries.
- Presence of an effusion in a patient <30 years of age signifies a significant knee injury needing accurate/prompt diagnosis.
- Acute mechanism: Consider ligamentous injury, meniscal tear, fracture.
- Overuse mechanism: Consider osteoarthritis, patellofemoral pain syndrome, tendinopathy, bursitis, and stress fracture.
- Pediatric patient with knee pain: Consider possible physeal, apophyseal, or articular cartilage injuries.
- Do not forget referred pain from the hip/back (slipped capital femoral epiphysis, Legg-Calve-Perthes disease)!!

K

LABYRINTHITIS
Anne Marie C. Zeller, DO • Emily Drummond, DO

 BASICS

DESCRIPTION
- Acute inflammation of the labyrinth (the organs of hearing and balance that comprise the bony inner ear). Infection (viral/bacterial) with subsequent inflammation of the inner ear is felt to be the most common etiology. Labyrinthitis is a clinical diagnosis in absence of neurologic deficits.
- Typically presents with false sense of motion (i.e., vertigo) or room spinning vertigo lasting for hours or days and often sudden hearing loss in 1 ear.
- System(s) affected: Nervous; Special sensory (auditory and vestibular)
- Synonym(s): Acute peripheral vestibulopathy; Vestibular neuronitis (vertigo/dizziness only); Vestibular neuritis (vertigo/dizziness only)

ALERT
- "Vertigo" and "dizziness" are commonly used terms. Clarify symptoms by giving options of alternative descriptions, such as light-headedness, dysequilibrium, room-spinning vertigo, or imbalance.
- Benign paroxysmal positional vertigo (BPPV) is the most common cause of room-spinning vertigo. Unlike labyrinthitis, BPPV is episodic and is diagnosed using the Dix-Hallpike maneuver. The associated vertigo is often severe, but lasts <1 minute each time. Rarely, some may report a sense of dysequilibrium lasting for hours after the initial event.

Geriatric Considerations
- Acute infectious labyrinthitis is often associated with vestibular hypofunction of the involved ear. Peripheral vertigo improves over time with central compensation.
- Elderly less likely to compensate fully and may report symptoms of dysequilibrium lasting weeks after resolution of the acute vertigo.
- Avoid excessive use of scopolamine, meclizine, and other vestibular suppressants following the initial event, especially in the elderly, as this will delay central compensation.

Pediatric Considerations
Unusual in this age group, except meningogenic suppurative labyrinthitis, which more commonly affects children <2 years of age.

EPIDEMIOLOGY
- Rare in children; most common in middle age (30–60 years)
- Predominant sex: Female = Male

Incidence
- Viral labyrinthitis is the most common etiology.
- Suppurative or serous labyrinthitis secondary to otitis media is increasingly rare in the postantibiotic era. Estimated 0.5–3% of intratemporal complications of otitis media in recent studies. Higher rates in cases with cholesteatoma

Prevalence
In the US, 2nd most common cause of dizziness due to persistent peripheral vestibular hypofunction (9%); benign positional vertigo (16%) is most common. These numbers are believed to be underestimated.

ETIOLOGY AND PATHOPHYSIOLOGY
Acute inflammation/damage to the inner ear, involving the peripheral special sensory organs of hearing and balance:
- Viruses may pass hematogenously into the labyrinth or directly from the middle ear to labyrinth via the round/oval window.
- Bacterial toxins and host inflammatory mediators (e.g., cytokines) from a middle ear infection may reach the inner ear. In serous labyrinthitis, bacteria are not present in the inner ear.
- In suppurative labyrinthitis, the infecting organism obtains direct access into the inner ear:
  – Otogenic: Usually unilateral. Enters via round/oval window to the labyrinth. May also enter via dehiscent horizontal semicircular canal if there is associated cholesteatoma.
  – Meningogenic: Can be bilateral. Enters by way of CSF via internal auditory canal or cochlear aqueduct.
- Ischemia: Ischemic or thromboembolic events involving the labyrinthine artery can cause symptoms that mimic acute labyrinthitis. May have other associated neurologic symptoms
- Autoimmune: Local or systemic inflammatory processes may affect the inner ear directly via autoantibodies or indirectly via a vasculitis of the labyrinthine artery.
- Infections:
  – Common viral: Cytomegalovirus, mumps, varicella zoster, rubeola, influenza, parainfluenza, herpes simplex, adenovirus, coxsackievirus, respiratory syncytial virus, HIV
  – Common bacterial: *Streptococcus pneumoniae, Haemophilus influenzae, Moraxella catarrhalis, Neisseria meningitidis, Streptococcus* spp., *Staphylococcus* spp., *Borrelia burgdorferi*
  – Treponemal: *Treponema pallidum*
- Autoimmune:
  – Wegener granulomatosis
  – Cogan syndrome
  – Systemic lupus erythematous
  – Polyarteritis nodosa
  – Behçet disease
- Ischemia/Infarction
- Ototoxic drugs (e.g., aspirin, aminoglycosides, cisplatin)

Genetics
No known genetic link.

RISK FACTORS
- Viral upper respiratory infection
- Otitis media
- Cholesteatoma
- History of allergies
- Smoking
- Excessive alcohol consumption
- Herpes zoster infection
- Head trauma
- Meningitis
- Vestibulotoxic/Ototoxic medications
- Otosyphilis (congenital or acquired)
- Tuberculosis
- Cerebrovascular disease
- Autoimmune disease

GENERAL PREVENTION
- Scheduled immunizations (to prevent common viral pathogens)
- Prevent maternal transmission of pathogens, including syphilis, HIV

COMMONLY ASSOCIATED CONDITIONS
- Viral upper respiratory infection
- Allergies
- Otitis media
- Cholesteatoma
- Head injury

 DIAGNOSIS

HISTORY
- Vertigo *AND* (often) hearing loss in 1 ear
- Vertigo is acute in onset and lasts days to weeks.
- Nausea and vomiting are common.
- Fullness of affected ear
- Tinnitus of affected ear (roaring, ringing)
- Upper respiratory tract infection symptoms (preceding/concurrent)
- Otorrhea (not common with viral causes)
- Otalgia (not common with viral causes)
- Severe headache, fever, and nuchal rigidity in the setting of meningitis.
- Recurrent/Progressive symptoms should raise suspicion for autoimmune causes.
- Profound imbalance or associated focal neurologic signs (motor/sensory weakness) are not typical and should prompt imaging.

PHYSICAL EXAM
- Nystagmus:
  – Fast-beating nystagmus toward affected ear (acutely)
  – Fast-beating nystagmus away from affected ear (chronically)
- Symptoms abate in supine position and with eyes closed
- Otologic exam may be unremarkable in the setting of viral labyrinthitis.
- Serous/Purulent effusion may be present in the middle ear.
- Retraction of the tympanic membrane and keratinaceous debris may be present in the setting of cholesteatoma.

DIFFERENTIAL DIAGNOSIS
- Vestibular neuritis/neuronitis
- BPPV: Episodic, vertigo lasting seconds/minutes, worse when lying down or looking up
- Ménière disease: Episodic vertigo lasting minutes to hours, associated with ear fullness, tinnitus, and hearing loss
- Idiopathic sudden single-sided deafness
- Autoimmune inner ear disease
- Postconcussive syndrome
- Acute otitis media
- Ototoxicity
- Cardiovascular accident (CVA)/brainstem infarct

- Cerebellopontine-angle tumors (e.g., vestibular schwannoma)
- Vestibular migraine
- Multiple sclerosis
- Parainfectious encephalomyelitis
- Parainfectious cranial polyneuritis
- Ramsay Hunt syndrome
- Cerebral/Systemic vasculitis
- Temporal lobe epilepsy
- HIV infection
- Perilymphatic fistula
- Superior canal dehiscence
- Syphilis

DIAGNOSTIC TESTS & INTERPRETATION

- Routine lab studies not helpful in making the diagnosis unless an autoimmune cause is highly suspected. There is no confirmatory investigation of sufficient sensitivity and specificity for this condition (1,2)[A]
- Consider culture of otorrhea or middle ear fluid to direct antibiotic choice.
- Consider lumbar puncture if associated meningitis is suspected.
- Rapid plasmin reagin (RPR) or Venereal Disease Research Laboratory (VDRL) test to screen for syphilis when clinically indicated by risk factors/history.
- Imaging is not required for the diagnosis of acute labyrinthitis; however, if associated neurologic symptoms are present, an MRI and MR angiography of brain and brainstem would be indicated.
- Vertigo usually spontaneously resolves, and there is a low risk of developing Ménière disease or migraines (3)[C].

Follow-Up Tests & Special Considerations
Labyrinthitis ossificans is fibrosis of the internal auditory canal following bacterial meningitis and is thought to occur due to a suppurative labyrinthitis. This can occur rapidly, especially after *S. pneumoniae* meningitis.

Diagnostic Procedures/Other
- Audiogram should be obtained.
- Vestibular tests are not typically indicated in the acute setting. However, if vertigo and dizziness persist after expected resolution of symptoms, electronystagmography should be utilized.

Test Interpretation
- Audiogram may show varying degrees of both hearing loss and discrimination.
- Caloric testing may show relative weakness of the horizontal semicircular canal of the affected side. Sensitivity and specificity of this test are variable within literature.

TREATMENT

- Symptom management and reassurance.
- Vestibular suppressants as needed (see "Medication"). Optimally used for severe acute attacks of vertigo only. Patients should be advised *NOT* to use these medications as a scheduled medication or for prophylaxis without symptoms.
- Persistent dizziness following acute labyrinthitis should be managed with vestibular physical therapy through a licensed physical therapist. Geriatric patients with labyrinthitis should follow up with physical therapy for balance assessments.

- Sudden single-sided hearing loss (onset within 2 weeks) should be managed with high-dose oral steroids ASAP.
- For suppurative labyrinthitis, appropriate antibiotics to eradicate infection, supportive care, prevention of spread of infection

GENERAL MEASURES
Visual–vestibular exercises for prolonged symptoms and unilateral vestibular loss

MEDICATION
Use of the following drugs should be on a PRN basis. No patient should take vestibular suppressants as chronic medication.
- Vestibular suppressants:
  – Lorazepam (Ativan): 0.5–2 mg SL/PO b.i.d. PRN or diazepam (Valium) 2–5 mg q.i.d. PO PRN
  – Meclizine (Antivert, Bonine, Zentrip [dissolvable]) 12.5–25 mg PO b.i.d.–t.i.d. PRN
  – Dimenhydrinate (Dramamine) 25–50 mg PO q4h PRN
- Antiemetics:
  – Ondansetron (Zofran) 4–8 mg PO t.i.d. PRN or granisetron (Kytril) 1 mg PO t.i.d. PRN
  – Meclizine (Antivert, Bonine) 12.5–25 mg PO q4h PRN
  – Promethazine (Phenergan) 12.5–25 mg PO/PR q.i.d. PRN or prochlorperazine (Compazine) 25 mg PR q.i.d. PRN
  – Metoclopramide (Reglan) 10 mg PO t.i.d. PRN
  – Scopolamine (Transderm Scop Patch) 1 transdermal q3d PRN (avoid in the elderly)
- Antivirals:
  – Acyclovir 800 mg PO 5 × per day for 7 days is used in labyrinthitis associated with herpes zoster. Not indicated otherwise
- Steroids:
  – Adults: Methylprednisolone initially 100 mg PO daily, then tapered to 10 mg PO daily over 3 weeks (2).
  – Pediatrics: Prednisone 1 mg/kg PO daily × 1 week, then taper over 3 weeks.
  – Given early in the setting of bacterial meningitis, may decrease the otologic sequelae, specifically labyrinthitis ossificans
  – Used in treatment of labyrinthitis for associated sudden sensorineural hearing loss

Pregnancy Considerations
Of the vestibular suppressants and antiemetics listed above, dimenhydrinate, diphenhydramine, ondansetron, granisetron, and metoclopramide are pregnancy Class B.

First Line
- Benzodiazepines, which are better vestibular suppressants, are preferred over antihistamine/anticholinergics, such as meclizine. Sublingual benzodiazepines are very effective for vertigo and should be considered first-line therapy.
- Urgent steroid treatment in acute setting

ISSUES FOR REFERRAL
- Consider neuro-otology referral for other peripheral causes of vertigo or unremitting vertigo
- Consider neurology referral for suspected central causes of vertigo or dizziness
- Consider otolaryngology referral for progressive bilateral hearing loss and vertigo after preliminary laboratory workup excluding rheumatologic causes

IN-PATIENT CONSIDERATIONS
Admission Criteria/Initial Stabilization
- Systemic infection, young age, intractable vertigo with nausea and vomiting (e.g., unable to tolerate oral diet or function independently)
- Usually outpatient management

ONGOING CARE
FOLLOW-UP RECOMMENDATIONS
Patient Monitoring
Follow hearing loss weekly with audiograms until hearing stabilizes

DIET
Avoid alcohol as this may exacerbate symptoms

PATIENT EDUCATION
Lie still with eyes closed in a darkened room during acute attacks. Otherwise, encourage activity as tolerated. Minimize rapid head movement until symptoms resolve.

PROGNOSIS
Pathology needs to be determined, prognosis depends on cause of labyrinthitis

COMPLICATIONS
Permanent hearing loss and chronic impairment of balance

REFERENCES
1. Hanley K, O'Dowd T, Considine N. A systematic review of vertigo in primary care. *Br J Gen Pract.* 2001;51:666–671.
2. Post RE, Dickerson LM. Dizziness: A diagnostic approach. *Am Fam Physician.* 2010;82:361–368.
3. Lee HK, Ahn SK, Jeon SY, et al. Clinical characteristics and natural course of recurrent vestibulopathy: A long-term follow-up study. *Laryngoscope.* 2012;122:883–886.

ADDITIONAL READING
Neuhauser HK. Epidemiology of vertigo. *Curr Opin Neurol.* 2007;20:40–46.

SEE ALSO
Ménière Disease; Postconcussive Syndrome; Tinnitus

CODES
ICD10
- H83.01 Labyrinthitis, right ear
- H83.02 Labyrinthitis, left ear
- H83.09 Labyrinthitis, unspecified ear

CLINICAL PEARLS
- "Vertigo" and "dizziness" are commonly used terms. Clarify symptoms by giving options of alternative descriptions, such as lightheadedness, dysequilibrium, room-spinning vertigo, or imbalance.
- Benzodiazepines, which are better vestibular suppressants, are preferred over antihistamine/anticholinergics, such as meclizine.

LACRIMAL DISORDERS
Robert A. Baldor, MD

 BASICS

DESCRIPTION
- Diseases and abnormalities of tear production and maintenance of tear film
- The most common lacrimal disorder is dry eye syndrome, which is often referred to as dysfunctional tear syndrome.
- Lacrimal duct disorders usually result in overflow tearing.
- System(s) affected: Skin/Exocrine

EPIDEMIOLOGY
Prevalence
Very common throughout the US; more often seen in arid climates:
- Predominant gender: Female > Male
- Predominant age: Dry eye symptoms increase with age and are most often seen in the elderly.

ETIOLOGY AND PATHOPHYSIOLOGY
- Tear film is composed of 3 layers:
  - Mucin layer: Allows spread of aqueous tears
  - Thick aqueous layer: Produced by lacrimal gland
  - Lipid layer: Controls tear evaporation
- Results from poor tear production, rapid tear evaporation, and/or an abnormal concentration of mucin or lipid in tear film
- Most common cause of dry eye symptoms is aqueous tear deficiency
- Decreased androgens are thought to contribute to a decrease in tear production.

RISK FACTORS
- Exposure to dry environments (e.g., high altitudes)
- History of collagen vascular disease, such as rheumatoid arthritis, Sjögren syndrome, thyroid disease, rosacea, Bell palsy, eyelid abnormalities
- Medications, including oral contraceptives, diuretics, β-blockers, antihistamines, and antidepressants
- Posttraumatic stress disorder
- Smoking
- Vitamin A deficiency
- Eye surgery: Blepharoplasty, cataract, laser vision correction

GENERAL PREVENTION
- Prevent exposure to eye irritants from pollution, cigarette smoke, and sun exposure
- Ensure adequate vitamin A intake through diet or as a supplement
- Patients with prior laser vision correction should wait at least 6 months before undergoing blepharoplasty because of the effects on corneal sensation, tear production, and tear film alteration (1)[C].
- Increasing awareness of this condition among people residing in dry environments

COMMONLY ASSOCIATED CONDITIONS
- Sjögren syndrome
- Rheumatoid arthritis
- Thyroid disease
- Rosacea
- Pregnancy
- Menopause
- Malnutrition

 DIAGNOSIS

HISTORY
- Dry sensation in eyes
- Foreign-body sensation
- Blurry vision
- Itching
- Ocular pain
- Photophobia
- Burning
- Occasional tearing due to excessive reflex tearing:
  - Patient's symptoms usually worsen in dry, smoky environments, while reading, driving, or using a computer for extended periods.

Pediatric Considerations
Lacrimal duct obstruction should be suspected in an infant presenting with excessive tearing (epiphora).

PHYSICAL EXAM
Slit-lamp exam reveals decreased tear film and may reveal punctate epithelial defects on cornea.

DIFFERENTIAL DIAGNOSIS
- Ocular: Allergy, conjunctivitis, contact lens complication, exposure keratopathy
- Other: Ocular rosacea, thyroid ophthalmopathy, ocular manifestation of HIV, Bell palsy, vitamin A deficiency

DIAGNOSTIC TESTS & INTERPRETATION
Initial Tests (lab, imaging)
Tear production can be measured using a Schirmer filter strip after instillation of topical anesthetic. Wetting of <10 mm of the slip after 5 minutes is indicative of insufficient tear production.

Diagnostic Procedures/Other
- Staining of the ocular surface with fluorescein will show areas of abnormal uptake and patches of drying. It allows the tear break-up time (TBUT) to be calculated. A TBUT of <10 seconds is abnormal.
- Rose bengal will be taken up by dead or dying epithelial cells, and it may be a more sensitive test.

Test Interpretation
In Sjögren syndrome, infiltration of the lacrimal gland with inflammatory cells may be evident.

 TREATMENT

GENERAL MEASURES
- Those with systemic illnesses predisposed to dry eye should be informed and instructed in the appropriate use of artificial tear supplements.
- Symptoms of dry eye may decrease with an increase in home humidification and hydration.

MEDICATION
First Line
- Preservative-free artificial tears: 1 drop in each eye several times a day to prevent discomfort (2)[A],(3)[C]
- Ophthalmic lubricating ointment may be used in each eye at bedtime (4)[B].

Second Line
- Dry eye has been identified as having an inflammatory component that responds in refractory cases to topical immunosuppressives, such as cyclosporine 0.05% (Restasis), 1 drop to each eye b.i.d. (5,6)[A].
- Emerging therapies include topical androgens, secretagogues (e.g., oral pilocarpine), cytokine-blocking agents, and a P2Y2 receptor agonist (Diquafosol).

ISSUES FOR REFERRAL
Rheumatology referral if systemic collagen vascular disease is suspected

ADDITIONAL THERAPIES
Lid massage and warm compresses several times a day

Pediatric Considerations
For most babies born with nasolacrimal duct obstructions, the obstructions will clear spontaneously during the 1st year of life. On occasion, surgical probing is necessary.

SURGERY/OTHER PROCEDURES
Punctal occlusion, with either punctal plugs or laser, is used in moderate to severe dry eye if medical therapy fails.

COMPLEMENTARY AND ALTERNATIVE MEDICINE
Fatty acid (omega-3), linoleic acid, and γ-linoleic acid supplements (7)[B]

ONGOING CARE

FOLLOW-UP RECOMMENDATIONS
Patient Monitoring
- Monitor early to assess efficacy of treatment
- The viscosity of artificial tears and frequency of use can be increased for symptom relief.

DIET
- Diet rich in omega-3 fatty acids and/or linoleic acids may benefit some patients
- Adequate vitamin A intake

PATIENT EDUCATION
All individuals with systemic illnesses predisposed to dry eye, postmenopausal women, residing in arid climates, or those >60 years of age should be instructed in the use of artificial tear supplements to combat dry eye symptoms.

PROGNOSIS
- Lacrimal disorders can be adequately managed with artificial tear supplements.
- Blocked tear ducts can be managed with probing and punctal dilation and/or dacryocystorhinostomy procedures in more severe cases.

COMPLICATIONS
Severe dry eye may lead to the following:
- Corneal breakdown
- Secondary invasion by bacteria
- Eye infections

REFERENCES

1. Lee WB, McCord CD, Somia N, et al. Optimizing blepharoplasty outcomes in patients with previous laser vision correction. *Plast Reconstr Surg.* 2008;122:587–594.
2. Ousler GW, Michaelson C, Christensen MT. An evaluation of tear film breakup time extension and ocular protection index scores among three marketed lubricant eye drops. *Cornea.* 2007;26: 949–952.
3. Karadayi K, Ciftci F, Akin T. Increase in central corneal thickness in dry and normal eyes with application of artificial tears: A new diagnostic and follow-up criterion for dry eye. *Ophthalmic Physiol Opt.* 2005;25:485–491.
4. Tauber J. Efficacy, tolerability and comfort of a 0.3% hypromellose gel ophthalmic lubricant in the treatment of patients with moderate to severe dry eye syndrome. *Curr Med Res Opin.* 2007;23: 2629–2636.
5. Hardten DR, Brown MJ, Pham-Vang S. Evaluation of an isotonic tear in combination with topical cyclosporine for the treatment of ocular surface disease. *Curr Med Res Opin.* 2007;23:2083–2091.
6. Roberts CW, Carniglia PE, Brazzo BG. Comparison of topical cyclosporine, punctal occlusion, and a combination for the treatment of dry eye. *Cornea.* 2007;26:805–809.
7. Barabino S, Rolando M, Camicione P. Systemic linoleic and gamma-linoleic acid therapy in dry eye syndrome with an inflammatory component. *Cornea.* 2003;22:97–101.

ADDITIONAL READING

- Behrens A, Doyle JJ, Stern L, et al. Dysfunctional tear syndrome: A Delphi approach to treatment recommendations. *Cornea.* 2006;25:900–907.
- Galor A, Feuer W, Lee DJ, et al. Prevalence and risk factors of dry eye syndrome in a United States veterans affairs population. *Am J Ophthalmol.* 2011;152:377–384.

 SEE ALSO

Sjögren Syndrome

 CODES

ICD10
- H04.121 Dry eye syndrome of right lacrimal gland
- H04.122 Dry eye syndrome of left lacrimal gland
- H04.129 Dry eye syndrome of unspecified lacrimal gland

CLINICAL PEARLS
- Dry eye syndrome is common in the US, affecting postmenopausal women more than any other population.
- Symptoms are usually adequately managed with preservative-free artificial tears and humidified environments.
- Dry eye symptoms that are refractory to medical treatment and/or punctal plugs should raise suspicion of an underlying systemic condition, and a rheumatology consult should be considered.

L

LACTOSE INTOLERANCE

Nihal Patel, MD • Jill A. Grimes, MD, FAAFP

 BASICS

DESCRIPTION

- Inability to digest lactose into its constituents (glucose and galactose) secondary to low levels of lactase in the brush border of the small intestinal mucosa causes bloating, borborygmi (audible stomach "rumblings"), abdominal pain, and diarrhea
  - Congenital lactose intolerance: Very rare
  - Primary lactose intolerance: Common in adults in whom a low level of lactase has developed after childhood
  - Secondary lactose intolerance: Inability to digest lactose caused by any condition injuring the intestinal mucosa (e.g., infectious enteritis, celiac disease, eosinophilic gastroenteritis, or inflammatory bowel disease) or a reduction of available mucosal surface (e.g., resection)
- Lactase activity peaks at birth, then starts to decrease after the 1st few months of life and continuously during lifetime. *However, only 50% of lactase activity is needed to digest lactose without causing symptoms of lactose intolerance.*
- Lactose malabsorption results from reduction of lactase activity, but it is an asymptomatic condition, fairly common in patients with functional bowel disorders, but no more common than in healthy individuals (1).
- System(s) affected: Endocrine/Metabolic; Gastrointestinal

Pediatric Considerations

- Primary lactose intolerance usually begins in late childhood.
- No consensus exists on whether young children (<5 years of age) should avoid lactose following diarrheal illness.
- Lactose-free formulas are available.
- Exclude a milk protein allergy

EPIDEMIOLOGY

Incidence

- ≥50% of infants with acute or chronic diarrheal disease have lactose intolerance, especially with rotavirus disease.
- Lactose intolerance also is fairly common with giardiasis and ascariasis, irritable bowel syndrome (IBS), tropical and nontropical sprue, and the AIDS malabsorptive syndrome.

Prevalence

- In South America, Africa, and Asia, rates of lactose intolerance are >50%.
- In the US, the prevalence is 15% among whites, 53% among Hispanic Americans, and 80% among African Americans.
- In Europe, it varies from 15% in Scandinavian countries to 70% in Italy.
- Predominant age:
  - Primary: Teenage and adult
  - Secondary: Depends on underlying condition
- Predominant sex: Male = Female

ETIOLOGY AND PATHOPHYSIOLOGY

- Primary lactose intolerance: Normal decline in the lactase activity in the intestinal mucosa is genetically controlled and permanent after weaning.
- Secondary lactose intolerance: Associated with gastroenteritis in children
- Secondary lactose intolerance is also associated with nontropical and tropical sprue, regional enteritis, abetalipoproteinemia, cystic fibrosis, inflammatory bowel disease, celiac disease, and immunoglobulin deficiencies in both adults and children.

Genetics

- In the white population, lactase deficiency has been associated with a single nucleotide polymorphism (SNP) consisting of a nucleotive switch of T for C 13,910 bp above the initiation codon of the gene coding for lactase enzyme on chromosome 2. This results in variants CC-13910 (lactase nonpersistence) *OR* CT-13910/TT-13910 (lactase persistence) (2).
- SNP (C/T-13910) is associated with lactase persistence predominantly in northern Europeans.
- Other SNPs (G/C-14010, T/G-13915, and C/G-13907) have been linked to lactase persistence in Africans.

RISK FACTORS

- Race: Adult-onset lactase deficiency varies widely among countries.
- Age:
  - Signs and symptoms usually do not become apparent until after age 6–7 years; recent studies actually have shown that hypolactasia may begin even after age 20.
  - Symptoms may not be apparent until adulthood, depending on dietary lactose intake and rate of decline of intestinal lactase activity.
  - Lactase enzyme activity is highly correlated with age, regardless of symptoms.

GENERAL PREVENTION

Avoidance of lactose in large quantities will relieve symptoms. Patients can learn what level of lactose is tolerable in their diet.

COMMONLY ASSOCIATED CONDITIONS

- Tropical or nontropical sprue
- Giardiasis
- Inflammatory bowel disease
- Immunoglobulin deficiencies
- Celiac disease
- Cystic fibrosis

 DIAGNOSIS

- Evaluation of lactose intolerance includes a careful medical history, review of symptoms, and physical examination. Lactose intolerance is defined as a combination of a positive lactose hydrogen breath test result plus accompanying clinical symptoms.
- Lactose intolerance can mimic symptoms of functional gastrointestinal disorders, but can also coexist with them (one does not rule out the other) (3).

HISTORY

- Assess patient's daily lactose consumption, since a single dose of lactose (up to 12 g, equivalent to 1 cup of milk) consumed alone produces no or minor symptoms in persons with lactose intolerance or maldigestion.
- Lactose doses of 15–18 g are well tolerated with other nutrients. Doses >18 g causes more symptoms progressively and quantities >50 g elicit symptoms in most individuals (4)[A].
- Symptoms may arise 30 minutes to 2 hours after consumption of products containing lactose.
- Symptoms include bloating, cramping, abdominal discomfort, diarrhea or loose stools, and flatulence.
- Abdominal pain may be crampy in nature and often is localized to the periumbilical area or lower quadrant.
- Stools usually are bulky, frothy, and watery.
- Only 1/3–1/5 of the people with lactose malabsorption will develop symptoms.

PHYSICAL EXAM

Borborygmi may be audible on physical examination and to the patient.

DIFFERENTIAL DIAGNOSIS

- Sucrase deficiency
- Cow's milk protein allergy
- IBS
- Bacterial overgrowth
- Celiac disease
- Inflammatory bowel disease

DIAGNOSTIC TESTS & INTERPRETATION

Initial Tests (lab, imaging)

- The lactose breath hydrogen test (LBT) is considered the best tool to diagnose lactose intolerance because it is noninvasive, easy to perform, and cost-effective. Its main limitation is nonoptimal sensitivity. LBT relies on the ability of intestinal bacteria to digest carbohydrates, producing hydrogen and methane and leading to the release of measurable levels of these gases in air exhaled from the lungs (2):
  - The test is begun by giving oral lactose in the fasting state, at a usual dose of 2 g/kg (max dose 25 g). Breath hydrogen is sampled at baseline and at 30-minute intervals after the ingestion of lactose for 3 hours. The postlactose and baseline values are compared. A breath hydrogen value of 10 ppm is normal. Values between 10 and 20 ppm may be indeterminate unless accompanied by symptoms, whereas values >20 ppm are considered diagnostic of lactose malabsorption.
- The biochemical assay of lactase activity on duodenal sample is as sensitive as LBT in detecting lactase deficiency; it seems to be more accurate than LBT in predicting the clinical response to a lactose-free diet; but cost and invasiveness limit its clinical use as a first-line test. However, for patients who report symptoms of lactose intolerance and are referred to upper endoscopy for other reasons, a biochemical assay on duodenal biopsies could be the best test to rule out lactose malabsorption (3).

- Of note, a positive LBT confirms that lactose malabsorption may explain the patient's symptoms. However, it does not indicate the etiology of the lactose intolerance.
- Low fecal pH and reducing substances are only valid when stools are collected fresh and assayed immediately. Test is fairly insensitive.

Diagnostic Procedures/Other
Lactose absorption test: Alternative to lactose breath hydrogen test in adults (more invasive and equivalent in sensitivity and specificity to breath test). Following oral administration of a 50-g test dose in adults (2 g/kg in children), blood glucose levels are monitored at 0, 60, and 120 minutes. An increase in blood glucose by <20 mg/dL (1.1 mmol/L) plus the development of symptoms is diagnostic. False-negative results may occur in patients with diabetes or bacterial overgrowth.

Test Interpretation
Lactase deficiency in intestinal mucosa may be patchy or focal.

 # TREATMENT

Overall, there is insufficient evidence on therapeutic effectivity of most lactose intolerance treatments including probiotics, colonic adaptation, and other supplements (4)[A].

- Treatment of lactose malabsorption in the absence of a correctable underlying disease includes 4 general principles:
  – Initially patients should avoid milk and dairy products in order to improve symptoms.
  – Up to 12–15 g of lactose can be tolerated in patients with lactose intolerance without significant symptoms (1 cup of milk) (4)[A].
  – Lactose should be gradually reintroduced along with other nutrients until the patient's threshold for symptoms is reached. Spreading lactose servings throughout the day instead of a single dose has been shown to improve tolerance (4)[A].
  – If symptoms persist, patients can be encouraged to substitute lactose for fermented and matured milk products (2)[C].
- Certain strains, concentrations, and preparations of probiotics may alleviate symptoms of lactose intolerance (5)[A].
- Some studies have looked at treating the symptoms of lactose intolerance with incremental doses of lactose to induce colonic adaptation with limited success (4)[A].
- To date, insufficient scientific evidence exists to strongly recommend lactose-reduced or hydrolyzed milk, lactase supplements taken with milk, probiotics, or colonic adaptation to treat lactose intolerance, mainly because most studies are small, heterogeneous, and poor in quality (4)[A]. However, use of these supplements should be assessed in a case-by-case fashion.
- It is very important to maintain calcium and vitamin D intake.

MEDICATION
First Line
Lactase (Lactaid, Lactrase):
- Commercially available "lactase" preparations are actually bacterial or yeast β-galactosidases.
- Take 1–2 capsules or tablets prior to ingesting milk products.
- These vary in effectiveness at preventing symptoms.
- Can add tablets or contents of capsules to milk before drinking; also available in milk in some areas.
- Not effective for all people with lactose intolerance
- High-quality, large, randomized controlled trials showing efficacy and safety are lacking.

COMPLEMENTARY AND ALTERNATIVE MEDICINE
Certain probiotic formulations taken with meals may alleviate some of the symptoms of lactose intolerance.

 # ONGOING CARE

DIET
- Reduce or restrict dietary lactose to control symptoms.
- Yogurt and fermented products, such as hard cheese, are better tolerated than milk.
- Supplement calcium in the form of calcium carbonate.
- Prehydrolyzed milk (Lactaid) is available.

PATIENT EDUCATION
- Patients must read labels on commercial products because milk sugar is used in many products and may cause symptoms.
- Lactose-intolerant patients may tolerate whole milk or chocolate milk better than skim milk due to slower rate of gastric emptying.
- Lactose consumed with other food products is better tolerated than when it is consumed alone.
- Primary lactase deficiency is permanent; secondary lactose intolerance usually is temporary, although it may persist for several months after the inciting disease has been cured.
- 20% of prescription drugs and 6% of over-the-counter (OTC) medicines use lactose as a base.
- Most patients still can tolerate 12–15 g of lactose, despite their lactose intolerance or malabsorption (2).

PROGNOSIS
- Normal life expectancy
- Symptoms can be controlled through diet alone if lactase tablets are ineffective.

COMPLICATIONS
Calcium deficiency: Avoidance of milk and other dairy products can lead to reduced calcium intake, which may increase the risk for osteoporosis and fracture.

REFERENCES
1. Fernández-Bañares F. Reliability of symptom analysis during carbohydrate hydrogen-breath tests. Curr Opin Clin Nutr Metab Care. 2012;15:494–498.
2. Mattar R, de Campos Mazo DF, Carrilho FJ. Lactose intolerance: Diagnosis, genetic, and clinical factors. Clin Exp Gastroenterol. 2012;5:113–121.
3. Furnari M, Bonfanti D, Parodi A, et al. A comparison between lactose breath test and quick test on duodenal biopsies for diagnosing lactase deficiency in patients with self-reported lactose intolerance. J Clin Gastroenterol. 2013;47:148–152.
4. Shaukat A, Levitt MD, Taylor BC, et al. Systematic review: Effective management strategies for lactose intolerance. Ann Intern Med. 2010;152:797–803.
5. Levri KM, Ketvertis K, Deramo M, et al. Do probiotics reduce adult lactose intolerance? A systematic review. J Fam Pract. 2005;54:613–620.

ADDITIONAL READING
- Almeida CC, Lorena SL, Pavan CR, et al. Beneficial effects of long-term consumption of a probiotic combination of Lactobacillus casei Shirota and Bifidobacterium breve Yakult may persist after suspension of therapy in lactose-intolerant patients. Nutr Clin Pract. 2012;27:247–251.
- Boettcher E, Crowe SE. Dietary proteins and functional gastrointestinal disorders. Am J Gastroenterol. 2013;108:728–736.
- Law D, Conklin J, Pimentel M. Lactose intolerance and the role of the lactose breath test. Am J Gastroenterol. 2010;105:1726–1728.
- Tan-Dy CR, Ohlsson A. Lactase treated feeds to promote growth and feeding tolerance in preterm infants. Cochrane Database Syst Rev. 2013;3:CD004591.

 # CODES

ICD10
- E73.0 Congenital lactase deficiency
- E73.8 Other lactose intolerance
- E73.9 Lactose intolerance, unspecified

CLINICAL PEARLS
- Most patients still can tolerate 12–15 g of lactose, despite their lactose intolerance or malabsorption.
- Lactose-intolerant patients may better tolerate yogurt and fermented products.
- Keeping a food diary with symptomatic episodes documented can help to identify food sources that may be problematic.
- Patients should read ingredient labels to look for milk or lactose, but also for ingredients such as whey and curd, which indicate the presence of lactose.
- Interestingly, lactose-intolerant patients may tolerate whole milk or chocolate milk better than skim milk due to a slower rate of gastric emptying.
- Many patients with lactose intolerance avoid dairy products to an unnecessary degree, causing inadequate intake of calcium and vitamin D, which may predispose them to osteoporosis.

LARYNGEAL CANCER

Hugh J. Silk, MD, MPH • Sheila O'Grady Stille, DMD, MAGD

BASICS

DESCRIPTION
- A friable, granular tumor of the larynx that leads to hoarseness, hemoptysis, and cough
- Of all malignant lesions, <1%; squamous cell carcinomas constitute 95–98% of all malignant neoplasms of the larynx.
- Laryngeal cancer accounts for <2% of all carcinomas.
- At the time of diagnosis, 62% will have local disease, 26% regional disease, and 8% distant disease in the lungs, liver, and/or bone.
- System(s) affected: Pulmonary; Ear, Nose, Throat (ENT)
- Synonym(s): Cancer of the larynx; Throat cancer; Cancer of the voice box

EPIDEMIOLOGY
Incidence
- Per year, 3.4/100,000 (12,250 new cases per year in the US; prevalence: 89,000 in 2010). These are usually squamous cell carcinomas (1)[A].
- Predominant age:
  – Median age of occurrence in 6th and 7th decades
  – <1% of laryngeal cancers arise in patients <30.
- Predominant sex: Male > Female (4:1); blacks > whites; increasing incidence in women who smoke; synergistic with alcohol abuse (1)[A]

Prevalence
- About 3,700 deaths from disease in the US yearly
- 2nd most common site for head and neck cancer (26% of all cases)
- 11th most common cancer in males

ETIOLOGY AND PATHOPHYSIOLOGY
- Smoking (dose dependent) (2)[C]
- Heavy alcohol use (2)[C]
- Smoking plus moderate alcohol use (2)[C]
- Possibly chronic laryngopharyngeal reflux (small studies)
- Occupational hazards (asbestos, pesticides, polycyclic aromatic hydrocarbons, woodworkers)
- HPV (less than oropharyngeal; 35% vs. 24%) (3,4)[A]

Genetics
Unknown

RISK FACTORS
See "Etiology and Pathophysiology."

GENERAL PREVENTION
- Avoid or cease smoking and/or alcohol abuse (85% attributed to smoking or alcohol abuse)
- Wear proper respiratory masks/respirators if chronic exposure to certain chemicals, gases, and wood dust
- Treat chronic laryngopharyngeal reflux
- Indirect laryngoscopy for at-risk patients with persistent hoarseness lasting beyond 2–3 weeks

COMMONLY ASSOCIATED CONDITIONS
Up to 10% of patients may have a synchronous squamous cell carcinoma in the lower or upper aerodigestive tract, most notably in the esophagus or lungs.

DIAGNOSIS

- Early laryngeal cancer generally has a good prognosis, with a 5-year disease-specific survival rate of >90% for T1 tumors.
- 57% are diagnosed at this local stage (1)[A].

HISTORY
- Persistent hoarseness in an elderly or middle-aged cigarette smoker (5)[C]
- Dyspnea and/or stridor
- Ipsilateral otalgia
- Dysphagia
- Odynophagia
- Chronic cough
- Hemoptysis
- Weight loss due to poor nutrition
- Halitosis due to tumor necrosis
- Chronic exposure to known risk factors (see "Etiology and Pathophysiology")

PHYSICAL EXAM
- Visualization of larynx initially by mirror and then a full nasolaryngoscopic exam
- Physical observation of vocal cord mobility, airway patency, and any regional spread
- Cervical lymph node exam and cranial nerve exam
- Mass in the neck from metastatic lymph node
- Laryngeal tenderness secondary to tumor necrosis or suppuration
- Broadening of the larynx on palpation with loss of crepitation
- Fullness of the cricothyroid membrane

DIFFERENTIAL DIAGNOSIS
- Acute or chronic laryngitis secondary to allergies, voice overuse, chemical exposures
- Benign vocal cord lesions such as polyps, nodules, and papillomas
- Tuberculosis or fungal infection (candidiasis) of the larynx (6)[B]

DIAGNOSTIC TESTS & INTERPRETATION
Initial Tests (lab, imaging)
- CT scan or MRI to rule out suspected chest, liver, or brain metastasis
- Bone scan if bone metastasis suspected

Diagnostic Procedures/Other
Indirect and/or direct laryngoscopy and biopsy to determine stage of disease, as well as histologic confirmation

Test Interpretation
- Laryngoscopy: Fungating, friable tumor with heaped-up edges and granular appearance, with multiple areas of central necrosis and exudate surrounding areas of hyperemia
- Squamous cell carcinoma in 95% of cases

TREATMENT

- Radiotherapy tends to be the treatment of choice in northern Europe, Australasia, and Canada, whereas surgery tends to be the treatment of choice in southern Europe and many centers in the US (7)[B].
- Increased use of transoral endoscopic laser microsurgery, improved delivery of radiotherapy, and concomitant chemoradiotherapy have been used over the past 10+ years with promising results (8,9)[A].

GENERAL MEASURES
- Tracheotomy care, when applicable
- If patient is diagnosed during pregnancy: Natural history of disease and treatment side effects have to be weighed against the possibilities of continuing on to delivery.

MEDICATION
- Narcotics may be necessary for pain control during treatment for mucositis (of the mouth) secondary to radiation therapy. Swishing with viscous lidocaine can be helpful as well.
- Nystatin mouth rinses for oral thrush

ISSUES FOR REFERRAL
- ENT for direct visualization of larynx; biopsy and surgery
- Depending on patient's management plan, nutritional and dental consults needed.
- Treatment may result in need for voice rehabilitation and be the cause of social isolation, job loss, and depression; therefore, refer to speech therapist, psychology, social work, and/or support groups as indicated (8)[A].

ADDITIONAL THERAPIES
Radiotherapy:
- There is increased focus on radiation therapy (RT), combined chemotherapy and RT, and function-preserving laryngectomy surgery due to patient fear of voice loss (8)[A].
- Early disease may be treatable by either RT or laser cordectomy on an outpatient basis. No randomized controlled trial has proven superiority of either when last reviewed by Cochrane in 2007. 90% cure rates are the rule.
- BCCIP protein (BRCA2 and CDKN1A [p21(Waf1/Cip1)] interacting protein) can be a prognostic marker for RT, with loss of the protein indicating a worse prognosis (10)[C].

SURGERY/OTHER PROCEDURES

- Tracheotomy may be necessary if a tumor is large enough to cause upper airway obstruction.
- More advanced disease needs inpatient care, necessitating partial or total laryngectomy and postoperative RT 4–5 weeks after surgery depending on the stage of disease (11)[A].

IN-PATIENT CONSIDERATIONS

Admission Criteria/Initial Stabilization
- More advanced disease, surgical intervention, and complication management
- Nutritional or airway issues/complications
- Primarily outpatient care

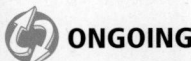 # ONGOING CARE

FOLLOW-UP RECOMMENDATIONS
Patient may remain fully active unless debilitated from more advanced disease and/or greater degree of surgery.

Patient Monitoring
- Repeat indirect laryngoscopy and complete head and neck exams periodically for at least 5 years after treatment to detect early recurrence or 2nd primary
- Yearly chest x-rays (and liver function test monitoring) for metastatic disease
- Patients with dysphagia should undergo barium swallow and/or esophageal endoscopy to rule out 2nd synchronous tumor in the esophagus.
- Patients with unexplained pain should have appropriate radiologic or nuclear medicine bone scans.
- Mental status change warrants CT scan of the brain to rule out brain metastases.

DIET
- Nasogastric or gastrostomy feeding may be necessary if tumor involves esophageal inlet.
- No special diet otherwise

PATIENT EDUCATION
- Material is available from local Cancer Society branch.
- Secondary prevention to address all risk factors especially smoking cessation

PROGNOSIS
- Early disease is expected to have >90% cure rate, with laryngeal and voice preservation.
- If lesion enlarges or metastasizes to regional cervical lymph nodes, the cure rate usually drops by 50%.
- Most recurrences occur within the 2 years of initial treatment.

COMPLICATIONS
- Temporary odynophagia or dysphagia secondary to mucositis and/or thrush during RT
- Persistent hoarseness despite adequate treatment, necessitating further adjunctive procedures and/or speech therapy
- Tracheostoma stenosis requiring stenting with laryngectomy tubes or further surgery
- Dysphagia secondary to upper esophageal stricture after total laryngectomy, necessitating dilation
- Aspiration after partial laryngectomy, necessitating complete laryngectomy or tracheotomy
- Inability to decannulate after partial laryngectomy because of laryngeal stenosis and/or aspiration
- Radiation-induced chondronecrosis, which mimics tumor recurrence
- Radiation edema, necessitating emergent tracheotomy
- Hypothyroidism secondary to laryngectomy and RT (12)[C]

REFERENCES

1. Howlader N, Noone AM, Krapcho M, et al. eds. *SEER cancer statistics review, 1975–2010*. Bethesda, MD: National Cancer Institute, 2013. Available at: http://seer.cancer.gov/csr/1975_2010/
2. La Vecchia C, Zhang ZF, Altieri A. Alcohol and laryngeal cancer: An update. *Eur J Cancer Prev*. 2008;17:116–124.
3. Centers for Disease Control. Human papillomavirus associated cancers—United States 2004–2008. *MMWR*. 2012;61:258–261.
4. Bisht M, Bist SS. Human papilloma virus: A new risk factor in a subset of head and neck cancers. *J Cancer Res Ther*. 2011;7:251–255.
5. Chu EA, Kim YJ. Laryngeal cancer: Diagnosis and preoperative work-up. *Otolaryngol Clin North Am*. 2008;41:673–695.
6. Nunes FP, Bishop T, Prasad ML. Laryngeal candidiasis mimicking malignancy. *Laryngoscope*. 2008;118:1957–1959.
7. Silver CE, Beitler JJ, Shaha AR, et al. Current trends in initial management of laryngeal cancer: The declining use of open surgery. *Eur Arch Otorhinolaryngol*. 2009;266:1333–1352.
8. American Society of Clinical Oncology, Pfister DG, Laurie SA. American Society of Clinical Oncology clinical practice guideline for the use of larynx-preservation strategies in the treatment of laryngeal cancer. *J Clin Oncol*. 2006;24:3693–3704.
9. Samson DJ, Ratko TA, Rothenberg BM, et al. Comparative effectiveness and safety of radiotherapy treatments for head and neck cancer. AHRQ Comparative Effectiveness Reviews, No. 20, May 2010.
10. Rewari A, Lu H, Parikh R. BCCIP as a prognostic marker for radiotherapy of laryngeal cancer. *Radiother Oncol*. 2009;90:183–188.
11. D'Cruz AK, Sharma S, Pai PS. Current status of near-total laryngectomy: Review. *J Laryngol Otol*. 2012;126:556–562.
12. Alkan S, Baylancicek S, Ciftçic M. Thyroid dysfunction after combined therapy for laryngeal cancer: A prospective study. *Otolaryngol Head Neck Surg*. 2008;139:787–791.

ADDITIONAL READING

- Ferlito A, Bradley PJ, Rinaldo A. What is the treatment of choice for TI squamous cell carcinoma of the larynx? *J Laryngol Otol*. 2004;118:747–749.
- Huang SH, Lockwood G, Irish J, et al. Truths and myths about radiotherapy for verrucous carcinoma of larynx. *Int J Radiat Oncol Biol Phys*. 2009;73:1110–1115.
- Hutcheson KA, Lewin JS. Functional outcomes after chemoradiotherapy of laryngeal and pharyngeal cancers. *Curr Oncol Rep*. 2012;14:158–165.
- Sherman EJ, Fisher SG, Kraus DH, et al. TALK score: Development and validation of a prognostic model for predicting larynx preservation outcome. *Laryngoscope*. 2012;122:1043–1050.

 ## CODES

ICD10
- C32.3 Malignant neoplasm of laryngeal cartilage
- C32.8 Malignant neoplasm of overlapping sites of larynx
- C32.9 Malignant neoplasm of larynx, unspecified

CLINICAL PEARLS

- Persistent hoarseness in an at-risk older person should prompt investigation with indirect and/or direct laryngoscopy.
- RT and multimodal therapies have reduced the need for laryngectomy except in advanced cases. ENT and radiation oncology consultations are recommended.
- Counsel all patients about primary prevention (no smoking, limit alcohol use), and counsel patients with cancer on secondary prevention.

L

LARYNGITIS

Hugh J. Silk, MD, MPH • Sheila O'Grady Stille, DMD, MAGD

BASICS

DESCRIPTION
- Laryngitis is inflammation, erythema, and edema of the mucosa of the larynx and/or vocal cords. Characterized by hoarseness, loss of voice, throat pain, or coughing
- There is a range of severity, but most cases are acute and are associated with viral upper respiratory infection, irritation, or acute vocal strain.
- System(s) affected: Pulmonary; Ears, Nose, Throat (ENT)
- Synonym(s): Laryngotracheitis; Acute laryngitis; Chronic laryngitis; Croup (in children)

EPIDEMIOLOGY
- Predominant age: Affects all ages
- Children more susceptible than adults due to increased risk of symptomatic inflammation from smaller airways.
- Predominant sex: Male = Female

Incidence
Common

Prevalence
Common

ETIOLOGY AND PATHOPHYSIOLOGY
- Misuse or abuse of voice
- Virus infections: Influenza A, B; parainfluenza; adenovirus; coronavirus; rhinovirus; human papillomavirus; cytomegalovirus; varicella-zoster virus; herpes simplex virus; respiratory syncytial virus; coxsackievirus
- Bacterial infections (uncommon): β-hemolytic streptococcus, *Streptococcus pneumoniae*, *Haemophilus influenzae*, tuberculosis (TB), leprosy, *Moraxella catarrhalis*, *Mycoplasma pneumoniae*, *Chlamydophila pneumoniae*
- Fungal infections (rare): Histoplasmosis, blastomycosis, coccidioides, cryptococcus, and candida
- Secondary syphilis left untreated
- Leprosy (in 30–55% of those with leprosy, larynx is affected; tropical and warm countries)
- Laryngeal TB
- Inhaling irritating substances (e.g., air pollution, cigarette smoke)
- Aspiration of caustic chemicals
- Aging changes: Muscle atrophy, loss of moisture in larynx, and bowing of vocal cords
- Gastroesophageal reflux disease (GERD)/laryngopharyngeal reflux disease (LPRD)
- Excessively dry environment
- Allergic
- Idiopathic
- Iatrogenic: Inhaled steroids, such as those used to treat asthma, surgical injury, or compression of recurrent laryngeal nerve
- Vocal cord nodules/polyps ("singer's nodes")
- Bowing of vocal cords with age
- Local cancer
- Neuromuscular disorder (e.g., myasthenia gravis); stroke
- Rheumatoid arthritis
- Trauma (e.g., endotracheal intubation, blunt or penetrating trauma to neck)

RISK FACTORS
- Acute:
  – Upper respiratory tract infection
  – Voice overuse-excess talking, singing, or shouting
  – Pneumonia
  – Influenza
  – Lack of immunization for pertussis or diphtheria
  – Immunocompromised
- Chronic:
  – Allergy
  – Chronic rhinitis/sinusitis
  – Voice abuse
  – GERD/LPRD (rare) (1)[A]
  – Smoking: Primary or secondhand
  – Excessive alcohol use
  – Stroke
  – Constant exposure to dust or other irritants; environmental pollution
  – Previous endotracheal intubation
  – Medications: Inhaled steroids, anticholinergics, and antihistamines

Geriatric Considerations
May be more ill, slower to heal

Pediatric Considerations
- Common in this age group
- Consider congenital causes.

GENERAL PREVENTION
- Avoid overuse of voice (voice training helpful for vocal musicians/public speakers)
- Influenza virus vaccine is suggested for high-risk individuals
- Quit smoking and avoid secondhand smoke
- Limit or avoid alcohol/caffeine/acidic foods
- Control GERD
- Maintain proper hydration status
- Avoid allergens
- Good hand washing (infection prevention)

COMMONLY ASSOCIATED CONDITIONS
- Viral pharyngitis
- Diphtheria (rare): Membrane can descend into larynx
- Pertussis: Larynx involved as part of the respiratory system
- Bronchitis
- Pneumonitis

DIAGNOSIS

HISTORY
- Hoarseness, throat tickling, dry cough, and rawness
- Abnormal-sounding voice
- Constant urge to clear the throat
- Possible fever
- Malaise
- Dysphagia/Odynophagia
- Regional cervical lymphadenopathy
- Stridor or possible airway obstruction in children (2)[C]
- Cough may be worse at night in children
- Hemoptysis
- Laryngospasm or sense of choking
- Allergic rhinitis/rhinorrhea/postnasal drip (PND)
- Occupation or other reasons for voice overuse
- Smoking history
- Blunt or penetrating trauma to neck
- GERD/LPRD

PHYSICAL EXAM
- Head and neck exam, including cervical nodes; cranial nerve exam
- ENT referral for persistent symptoms (>2–3 weeks) or concern for foreign body

DIFFERENTIAL DIAGNOSIS
- Diphtheria
- Vocal nodules or polyps
- Laryngeal malignancy
- Thyroid malignancy
- Upper airway malignancy
- Epiglottitis
- Pertussis
- Laryngeal nerve trauma/injury

DIAGNOSTIC TESTS & INTERPRETATION
- Rarely needed
- WBCs elevated in bacterial laryngitis
- Viral culture (seldom necessary)

Follow-Up Tests & Special Considerations
- Barium swallow, only if needed for differential diagnosis
- CT scan if foreign body suspected

Diagnostic Procedures/Other
- Fiber-optic or indirect laryngoscopy: Looking for red, inflamed, and occasionally hemorrhagic vocal cords; rounded edges and exudate (Reinke edema)
- Consider otolaryngologic evaluation and biopsy: Laryngitis lasting >2 weeks in adults with history of smoking or alcohol abuse to rule out malignancy.
- pH probe (24-hour): No difference in incidence of pharyngeal reflux as measured by pH probe between patients with chronic reflux laryngitis and healthy adults (3)[C]
- Strobovideo laryngoscopy for diagnosis of subtle lesions (e.g., vocal cord nodules or polyps)

TREATMENT

- Evidence is limited, but good, that treatment beyond supportive care is ineffective.
- Antibiotics appear to have no benefit because it is viral (4)[A]. The bacterial form is rare.
- Corticosteroids in severe cases of laryngitis to reduce inflammation, such as croup
- May need voice training, if voice overuse
- Racemic epinephrine reduces symptoms at 30 minutes, but effect lasts only 2 hours (5)[A].

GENERAL MEASURES
- Acute:
  - Usually a self-limited illness lasting <3 weeks and not severe
  - Antibiotics of no value (4)[A]
  - Avoid excessive voice use, including whispering
  - Steam inhalations or cool-mist humidifier
  - Increase fluid intake, especially in cases associated with excessive dryness
  - Avoid smoking (or secondhand exposure)
  - Saltwater gargles
- Chronic:
  - Symptomatic treatment, as above
  - Voice therapy (for patients with intermittent dysphagia and vocal abuse)
  - Stop smoking
  - Reduce or stop alcohol intake
  - Occupational change or modification, if exposure
  - Consider discontinuing inhaled corticosteroids
- Reflux laryngitis: Elevate head of bed, diet changes, other antireflux lifestyle change management; proton pump inhibitors

MEDICATION
Usually none

First Line
- Analgesics
- Antipyretics (rare)
- Cough suppressants
- Throat lozenges
- Plenty of fluids

Second Line
- Inhaled corticosteroids (consider if allergy induced)
- Oral corticosteroids: Only if urgent need in adults (presenter, singer, actor)
- Oral corticosteroids: Evidence of benefit has been studied with single-dose dexamethasone in children ages 6 months to 5 years for moderate severity croup; reduces symptoms within 6 hours, reduces hospitalizations, hospital length of stay, and revisits to office (6)[A]
- Standard of care is to prescribe proton pump inhibitors for chronic laryngitis if GERD or LPRD is suspected; however, evidence suggests only a modest benefit, if any (7,8)[C].
- Treat nonviral infectious underlying causes
- Candidal laryngitis:
  - Mild cases: Oral antifungal (fluconazole)
  - Amphotericin B or an echinocandin can be given in life-threatening cases.

ISSUES FOR REFERRAL
- Consider otolaryngologic evaluation and biopsy for laryngitis lasting >2 weeks in adults with history of smoking or alcohol abuse to rule out malignancy.
- Consider GI consult to rule out GERD/LPRD.

SURGERY/OTHER PROCEDURES
- Vocal cord biopsy of hyperplastic mucosa and areas of leukoplakia if cancer or TB is suspected
- Removal of nodules or polyps if voice therapy fails

COMPLEMENTARY AND ALTERNATIVE MEDICINE
The following, although not well studied, have been recommended by some experts:
- Barberry, blackcurrant, echinacea, eucalyptus, German chamomile, goldenrod, goldenseal, hot lemon and honey, licorice, marshmallow, peppermint, saw palmetto, slippery elm, vitamin C, zinc

 ONGOING CARE

PATIENT EDUCATION
- Educate on the importance of voice rest, including whispering
- Provide assistance with smoking cessation
- Help the patient with modification of other predisposing habits or occupational hazards

PROGNOSIS
Complete clearing of the inflammation without sequelae

COMPLICATIONS
Chronic hoarseness

REFERENCES
1. Joniau S. Reflux and laryngitis: A systemic review. *Otolarygol Head Neck Surg.* 2007;136:686–692.
2. Gallivan GJ, Gallivan KH, Gallivan HK. Inhaled corticosteroids: Hazardous effects on voice—an update. *J Voice.* 2007;21:101–111.
3. Johnson DA. Medical therapy of reflux pharyngitis. *J Clin Gastroenterol.* 2008;42:589–593.
4. Reveiz L, Cardona AF. Antibiotics for acute laryngitis in adults. *Cochrane Database Syst Rev.* 2013;3:CD004783.
5. Bjornson C, Russell KF, Vandermeer B, et al. Nebulized epinephrine for croup in children. *Cochrane Database Syst Rev.* 2011;2:CD006619.
6. Russell KF, Liang Y, O'Gorman K, et al. Glucocorticoids for croup. *Cochrane Database Syst Rev.* 2011;1:CD001955.
7. Tulunay OE. Laryngitis—Diagnosis and management. *Otolaryngol Clin North Am.* 2008;41:437–452.
8. Moore JM, Vaezi MF. Extraesophageal manifestations of gastroesophageal reflux disease: Real or imagined? *Curr Opin Gastroenterol.* 2010;26:389–394.

CODES

ICD10
- J04.0 Acute laryngitis
- J04.2 Acute laryngotracheitis
- J37.0 Chronic laryngitis

CLINICAL PEARLS
- Laryngitis is usually self-limited and needs only comfort care. Standard treatment is voice rest.
- Refer to ENT for direct visualization of vocal cords for prolonged laryngitis.
- Corticosteroids have some benefits for children with moderately severe croup.

L

LAXATIVE ABUSE
Lauren Michal de Leon, MD • Edward Feller, MD

 BASICS

DESCRIPTION
- Laxative abuse may be intentional or unintentional and manifests commonly as watery diarrhea caused by self-medication or as apparent diarrhea caused by adding various fluids to stool:
  - Common cause of chronic diarrhea are diverse, reflecting demographics of individual or population studied.
- System(s) affected: Gastrointestinal; Nervous; Psychiatric; Skin
- Synonym(s): Factitious diarrhea; Cathartic colon; Münchausen syndrome (self or by proxy)—most dramatic form

EPIDEMIOLOGY
- Predominant age: 18–40 years with bulimia or anorexia nervosa; 40–60 years without eating disorders
- Common in the elderly as a result of treatment for constipation, either by MD or self-directed (*unintentional*)
- Predominant sex (*intentional abuse*): Female (90%) > Male
- Children may be given excess laxation by caregivers (especially mothers), an example of Münchausen syndrome by proxy.
- May coexist with diverse manifestations of factitious illness (endocrine, skin, neurologic)

Prevalence
Laxative abuse in different groups (1):
- As many as 15% undergoing evaluation for chronic diarrhea
- Unexplained chronic diarrhea after routine investigations: 3.5–7%
- Patients with binging/purging anorexia and bulimia nervosa: As high as 70%
- Referrals to tertiary-care centers for evaluation of chronic diarrhea: As high as 15%
- Chronic use of constipating medications such as opioids

Geriatric Considerations
Elderly in nursing homes at increased risk for laxative overuse (usually inadvertent)

ETIOLOGY AND PATHOPHYSIOLOGY
- Chronic ingestion of any laxative agent:
  - Osmotic diarrhea: Magnesium sulfate, nonabsorbable sugars, sodium phosphate
  - Secretory diarrhea: Dihydroxy bile salts, castor oil, docusate sodium
- Psychologic factors:
  - Bulimia or anorexia nervosa
  - Secondary gain of attention: Disability claims or need for concern, caring from others
  - Hysterical behavior
  - Inappropriate perceptions of "normal" bowel habits
  - Chronic constipation, especially in the elderly

RISK FACTORS
In patients with eating disorders (2):
- Longer duration of illness
- Comorbid psychiatric diagnoses (e.g., major depression, obsessive–compulsive disorder, posttraumatic stress disorder, anxiety, borderline personality disorder)
- Early age of appearance of eating disorder symptoms

GENERAL PREVENTION
- Educate patients about proper nutrition, normal bowel function, potential adverse effects of excessive laxation, and use of additional medications (e.g., magnesium-containing antacids) that can cause diarrhea.
- Ask patients specifically about laxative use. Inadvertent overuse is common.

COMMONLY ASSOCIATED CONDITIONS
- Anorexia nervosa, bulimia nervosa
- Use of constipating medications (opioids, iron supplements)
- Any chronic disorder associated with constipation
- Depression and anxiety
- Borderline personality
- Self-injurious behaviors/suicidal ideation
- Impulsive behavior
- Münchausen syndrome/Münchausen syndrome by proxy (children); may have associated factitious symptoms involving diverse organ systems

 DIAGNOSIS

Chronic diarrhea can be characterized into 4 types: Secretory, osmotic, inflammatory, and fatty. Be certain to rule out other causes of chronic diarrhea, even if laxative abuse is a high probability on the differential diagnosis list.

HISTORY
- Suspicion in patients with undiagnosed chronic diarrhea, especially when refractory; some patients may not be aware of the association of some over-the-counter medications with chronic diarrhea (3).
- Signs and symptoms: Increasing frequency of bowel movements; large volume, watery diarrhea; nocturnal bowel movements that are typically absent in osmotic diarrhea or in irritable bowel syndrome.
- Additional symptoms: Abdominal pain, rectal pain, nausea, vomiting, weight loss, malaise, muscle weakness; be wary of chronic constipation with long-term laxative abuse.
- Absence of nocturnal bowel movements, night sweats, or fever argue against inflammatory process.
- Additional signs: Hypokalemia, hyperphosphatemia, hypernatremia, skin pigmentation, finger clubbing, cyclic edema, kidney stones, melanosis coli, cardiac arrhythmias with severe hypokalemia.
- Monitor "doctor hopping" and potential for associated factitious symptoms.

PHYSICAL EXAM
- No specific findings, but may include cachexia, evidence of dehydration, abdominal pain or distension, and edema; fever may be due to self-infected wounds or thermometer manipulation
- Bulimics or anorexics who purge may have Reynold sign (excoriation of fingers from repeated self-induced retching).
- Rarely, severe cases may be associated with renal failure, cardiac arrhythmias, skeletal muscle paralysis, signs of anemia from blood-letting or self-induced skin wounds.

DIFFERENTIAL DIAGNOSIS
Any etiology of chronic diarrhea, especially in high-risk groups

DIAGNOSTIC TESTS & INTERPRETATION
If patient has not had an initial workup for chronic diarrhea, infectious, inflammatory, and malignant causes must be ruled out as appropriate based on patient demographics and risk factors.

Initial Tests (lab, imaging)
- Serum electrolytes will show hypokalemia secondary to increased intestinal fluid loss:
  - Acute diarrhea: Metabolic acidosis due to hypovolemia
  - Chronic diarrhea: Metabolic alkalosis secondary to hypokalemia-induced inhibition of chloride uptake in the intestine, thereby inhibiting bicarbonate secretion
- CBC, stool cultures, *Clostridium difficile* polymerase chain reaction (PCR): Rule out infectious cause if history is suspicious.
- Not usually necessary for diagnosis of laxative abuse; colonoscopy, small-bowel endoscopy, or imaging studies may be needed to evaluate other causes of chronic diarrhea.
- *Melanosis coli* on sigmoidoscopy may document overuse of anthracene laxatives.

Follow-Up Tests & Special Considerations
If history and initial lab tests are suspicious for laxative abuse, the following algorithm can be used to confirm diagnosis and determine what type of laxative is being used (4):
- Collect 24-hour stool: If solid, workup is over.
- Obtain stool osmolality, stool electrolytes, and calculate osmolal gap ($= 290 - 2(Na^+ + K^+)$, where Na^+ and K^+ are the concentrations from the stool sample):
  - If osmolality >400 mOsm/kg, rule out urine contamination of stool. Measure urea and creatinine of sample.
  - If osmolality <250–400 mOsm/kg, rule out water added to stool (colon cannot dilute stool to osmolality of plasma).
  - If osmolality = 250–400 mOsm/kg, measure osmolal gap:
    - Gap >50: Unmeasured solute; check fecal fat and stool magnesium levels.
    - Gap <50: Rule out use of secretory laxative; urinalysis and stool analysis for laxative titers. Do not obtain serum laxative titers as they peak 1–2 hours after ingestion. Urine titers can be 10× as high as plasma titers.
- Confirm diagnosis with multiple stool analyses before confronting patient with intentional use.

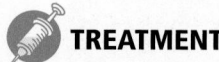 **TREATMENT**

GENERAL MEASURES
- Psychological support is essential in intentional use.
- Determine motive behind excessive laxative abuse without being confrontational.
- Wean patient off laxatives, substitute high-fiber diet and bulk preparations or short-term saline enemas.
- Treat constipation.
- Treat metabolic abnormalities with potassium supplements, etc. (oral preferred).

MEDICATION

Replace needed fluid, vitamins, electrolytes, and minerals (5).

First Line

- Nonstimulant laxatives if needed to treat constipation:
  - Senna best during pregnancy and lactation
  - Lactulose
  - High-fiber diet
- Avoid danthron due to hepatotoxicity.
- Precautions: Patients may be manipulative in attempts to deny problem; may hide laxatives in hospital rooms.
- Significant possible interactions:
  - Increased rate of intestinal motility may affect rate of absorption of medications (e.g., antibiotics, hormones).
  - Docusate sodium may potentiate hepatotoxicity of other drugs.

ISSUES FOR REFERRAL

In cases of Münchausen syndrome by proxy, legal proceedings must be considered, especially because most victims are children.

SURGERY/OTHER PROCEDURES

Avoid exploratory surgery and repetitive evaluations with invasive procedures.

IN-PATIENT CONSIDERATIONS

Admission Criteria/Initial Stabilization

- Persistent diarrhea with evidence of hemodynamic instability
- Electrolyte/Metabolic complications, including lactic acidosis
- Cardiac arrhythmias
- Inability to contract for safety

IV Fluids

Resuscitate based on clinical presentation. If patient is hemodynamically stable and without significant abnormalities in serum sodium, give normal saline boluses or oral replacement to correct metabolic alkalosis (chronic) or acidosis (acute) as needed. If patient is hemodynamically unstable, treat volume status as in hypovolemic shock, while monitoring serum electrolytes closely (especially sodium, potassium, and bicarbonate).

Nursing

- If stable, patient does not need continuous telemetry. Depending on psychiatric history, patient may need constant observation. Special care must be taken to ensure adequate nutrition, discard laxatives. If patient is unstable, telemetry and appropriate vital-signs monitoring may be necessary.
- If surreptitious laxative ingestion is suspected, do not perform unauthorized room searches due to legal constraints.

Discharge Criteria

- Psychological support
- Diet and bowel programs

 ## ONGOING CARE

FOLLOW-UP RECOMMENDATIONS

Patient Monitoring

- Careful psychological counseling
- Careful medical support; show concern by frequent visits as needed.
- Assess serum electrolytes.

DIET

Ensure good nutritional habits:

- Increase fiber intake.
- Avoid constipating substances.
- Adequate calories, especially with bulimia.

PROGNOSIS

- Natural history is unclear and varied, depending on underlying cause.
- Prognosis is related to psychological response in intentional abuse or underlying etiology when organic disease is present.
- Prognosis is poor with anorexia nervosa; very poor in Münchausen syndrome.
- Cathartic colon is commonly refractory to treatment.

COMPLICATIONS

- Risk of multiple tests, procedures, and surgeries (intentional use)
- Malnutrition
- Electrolyte imbalances (hypokalemia)
- Renal failure
- Fatalities, especially in children given laxatives by parents; eating disorders
- Renal calculi
- Cathartic colon with constipation as a consequence of prolonged irritant laxative use; no diarrhea, fever, or blood loss
- Fecal impaction in elderly
- Recurrences are common for factitious abuse, even after confrontation.

REFERENCES

1. Roerig JL, Steffen KJ, Mitchell JE, et al. Laxative abuse: Epidemiology, diagnosis and management. *Drugs*. 2010;70:1487–1503.
2. Sim LA, McAlpine DE, Grothe KB, et al. Identification and management of eating disorders in the primary care setting. *Mayo Clin Proc*. 2010;85:746–751.
3. Abraham BP, Sellin JH. Drug-induced, factitious, and idiopathic diarrhea. *Best Pract Res Clin Gastroenterol*. 2012;26:633–648.
4. Shelton JH, Santa Ana CA, Thompson DR, et al. Factitious diarrhea induced by stimulant laxatives: Accuracy of diagnosis by a clinical reference laboratory using thin layer chromatography. *Clin Chem*. 2007;53:85–90.
5. Kent AJ, Banks MR. Pharmacologic management of diarrhea. *Gastroenterol Clin North Am*. 2010;39: 495–507.

ADDITIONAL READING

- Mascolo M, Trent S, Colwell C, et al. What the emergency department needs to know when caring for patients with eating disorders. *Int J Eat Disord*. 2012;45:977–981.
- Pomeranz JL, Taylor LM, Austin SB. Over-the-counter and out-of-control: Legal strategies to protect youths from abusing products for weight control. *Am J Public Health*. 2013;103:220–225.
- Schiller LR. Definitions, pathophysiology, and evaluation of chronic diarrhea. *Best Pract Res Clin Gastroenterol*. 2012;26:551–562.
- Sweetser S. Evaluating the patient with diarrhea: A case-based approach. *Mayo Clin Proc*. 2012;87: 596–602.

 ## SEE ALSO

Algorithm: Diarrhea, Chronic

 ## CODES

ICD10

F55.2 Abuse of laxatives

CLINICAL PEARLS

- Laxative abuse may be intentional or unintentional; it is a common feature of eating disorders and has a female predilection.
- As many as 15% of patients referred to tertiary-care centers for unexplained chronic diarrhea abuse laxatives.
- Presentation is diverse and nonspecific, including weight loss, weakness, and hypotension without acknowledgment of diarrhea, when intentional.
- Consider the diagnosis in patients with watery diarrhea, especially when unexplained or refractory.

L

LEAD POISONING

Jason Chao, MD, MS

 BASICS

DESCRIPTION
- Consequence of a high body burden of lead (Pb), an element with no known physiologic value
- Synonym(s): Lead poisoning, Inorganic

EPIDEMIOLOGY
- Predominant age: 1–5 years; adult workers
- Predominant sex: Male > Female (1:1 in childhood)

Prevalence
- 2007–2010: Centers for Disease Control (CDC) estimated that 2.6% of US children aged 1–5 years had blood Pb levels >5 μg/dL, but levels are variable among communities and populations
- Sporadic cases in adults

ETIOLOGY AND PATHOPHYSIOLOGY
- Pb replaces calcium in bones. Pb interferes with heme synthesis, causes interstitial nephritis, and interferes with neurotransmitters, especially glutamine; high levels affect blood–brain barrier and lead to encephalopathy, seizures, and coma.
- Inhalation of Pb dust or fumes or ingestion of Pb

RISK FACTORS
- Children with pica or with iron-deficiency anemia
- Residence in or frequent visitor to deteriorating pre-1960 housing with lead-painted surfaces, or recent renovation
- Soil/Dust exposure near older homes, Pb industries, or urban roads
- Sibling or playmate with current or past Pb poisoning
- Dust from clothing of Pb worker or hobbyist
- Pb dissolved in water from Pb or Pb-soldered plumbing
- Pb-glazed ceramics, especially with acidic food or drink
- Recent refugee
- Folk remedies and cosmetics:
  - Mexico: Azarcon, greta
  - Dominican Republic: Litargirio, a topical agent
  - Asia and Middle East: Chuifong tokuwan, pay-loo-ah, ghasard, bali goli, kandu, ayurvedic herbal medicine from South Asia, kohl (alkohl, ceruse), surma, saoott, cebagin
- Hobbies: Glazed pottery making, target shooting, Pb soldering, preparing Pb shot or fishing sinkers, stained-glass making, car or boat repair, home remodeling
- Occupational exposure: Plumbers, pipe fitters, Pb miners, auto repairers, glass manufacturers, shipbuilders, printers, plastics manufacturers, Pb smelters and refiners, steel welders or cutters, construction workers, rubber product manufacturers, battery manufacturers, bridge reconstruction workers
- Dietary: Zinc or calcium deficiency
- Imported toys with Pb

Pediatric Considerations
- Children are at increased risk because of incomplete development of the blood–brain barrier at <3 years of age, allowing more Pb into the CNS; ingested Pb has 40% bioavailability in children compared with 10% in adults.
- Common childhood behaviors such as frequent hand-to-mouth activity and pica (repeated ingestion of nonfood products), greatly increase the risk of ingesting Pb.

GENERAL PREVENTION
- Family should receive counseling on potential sources of Pb and methods to decrease Pb exposure. Children at high risk should receive blood Pb screening (1)[C].
- Warn parents about the dangers posed by unsafe renovation methods.
- Wet mopping and dusting with a high-phosphate solution (e.g., powdered automatic dishwasher detergent with 1/4 cup/gal of water) will help to control Pb-bearing dust. But high-phosphate detergent is no longer available in some states.
- Pregnant women with community-specific or any individual risk factor for Pb poisoning should be screened for Pb toxicity (2)[C].

COMMONLY ASSOCIATED CONDITIONS
Iron-deficiency anemia

 DIAGNOSIS

HISTORY
- Often asymptomatic
- Mild-to-moderate toxicity:
  - May cause myalgia or paresthesia, fatigue, irritability, lethargy
  - Abdominal discomfort, arthralgia, difficulty concentrating, headache, tremor, vomiting, weight loss, muscular exhaustibility
- Severe toxicity: 3 major clinical syndromes:
  - Alimentary type: Anorexia, metallic taste, constipation, severe abdominal cramps due to intestinal spasm and sometimes associated with abdominal wall rigidity
  - Neuromuscular type (characteristic of adult plumbism): Peripheral neuritis, usually painless and limited to extensor muscles
  - Cerebral type or Pb encephalopathy (more common in children): Seizures; coma; and long-term sequelae, including neurologic defects, retarded mental development, and chronic hyperactivity
- Chronic exposure may cause renal failure.

PHYSICAL EXAM
Often normal; abdominal tenderness may be severe. Neurologic exam may reveal neuropathy or encephalopathy.

DIFFERENTIAL DIAGNOSIS
- Alimentary type may be confused with acute abdomen.
- Neuromuscular type may be confused with other polyneuropathies.
- Cerebral type may be confused with ADD, mental retardation, autism, dementia, and other causes of seizures.
- Elevated erythrocyte protoporphyrin may be caused by iron-deficiency anemia or, less commonly, hemolytic anemia.
- Erythropoietic protoporphyria produces a very high erythrocyte protoporphyrin level.

DIAGNOSTIC TESTS & INTERPRETATION
- Blood Pb >5 μg/dL (0.24 μmol/L), collected with Pb-free container
- Use a laboratory that can achieve routine performance within 2 μg/dL
- In 2012, CDC recommended using a reference value as the basis for management, currently >5 μg/dL

- Screening capillary Pb levels >5 μg/dL (0.24 μmol/L) should be confirmed with a venous sample
- Hemoglobin and hematocrit slightly low; eosinophilia or basophilic stippling on peripheral smear may be seen but is not diagnostic of Pb toxicity
- Renal function is decreased in late stages
- Abdominal radiograph for Pb particles in gut if recent ingestion is suspected
- Radiograph of long bones may show lines of increased density in the metaphyseal plate resulting from growth arrest, but does not usually alter management and is not routinely recommended.
- X-ray fluorescence for the total body burden of Pb is experimental.

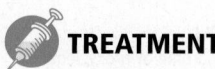 TREATMENT

Blood level (μg/dL)	Time to confirmation testing
≥Ref value–9	1–3 months
10–44	1 week–1 month
45–59	48 hours
60–69	24 hours
≥70	Urgently as emergency test

ALERT
- For any blood lead levels persistently >15 μg/dL, contact local public health department for home inspection.
- If Pb level is between 5–45 μg/dL, the higher the Pb level, the more urgent the need for confirmation testing.
- For all elevated levels: Educate family on sources of Pb (3)[C]
- Pb level > Ref level to <45: Complete history and physical exam; follow-up Pb monitoring; complete inspection of home or workplace to determine source of Pb and Pb hazard reduction; neurodevelopmental monitoring: iron status, Hgb or Hct (4)[C]
- Pb level 45–69: Actions for lower level plus: Free erythrocyte protoporphyrin; oral chelation therapy or hospitalization if lead–safe environment cannot be ensured (4)[C]
- Pb >70: Hospitalize for chelation therapy (5)[C].

MEDICATION
- Consider oral chelation for asymptomatic and Pb >45 and <70; chelation (preferably parenteral) for Pb >70 or symptomatic Pb <70 (5)[C].
- Do not begin chelation until Pb particles present in gut are cleared (5)[C].

First Line
- Oral chelation: Succimer (Chemet), dimercaptosuccinic acid (DMSA) 10 mg/kg q8h × 5 days; then 10 mg/kg q12h × 2 weeks. This may be repeated after 2 weeks off if Pb levels are not stabilized at <15 μg/dL (<0.72 μmol/L) (5)[C].

- Parenteral chelation (begin after establishment of adequate urine output):
  - Dimercaprol (British anti-Lewisite [BAL]) 75 mg/m^2 given deep IM; then BAL 450 mg/m^2/d divided q4h × 5 days plus Ca edetate calcium disodium (EDTA) 1,500 mg/m^2/d continuous IV infusion × 5 days. If rebound Pb level ≥45 μg/dL (≥2.17 μmol/L), chelation may be repeated after 2-day interval if symptomatic, or after 5-day interval if asymptomatic.
  - Ca EDTA 1,000 mg/m^2/d × 5 days; may be repeated after 5–7 days
- Diazepam for initial control of seizures; further control maintained with paraldehyde
- Contraindications: BAL should not be given to patients allergic to peanuts (the drug solution contains peanut oil).
- Precautions:
  - Succimer: GI upset, rash, nasal congestion, muscle pains, elevated liver function tests
  - Ca EDTA: Renal failure, increased excretion of zinc, copper, and iron
  - BAL: Nausea, vomiting, fever, headache, transient hypertension, hepatocellular damage
- Significant possible interactions:
  - Vitamins should not be given concurrently with oral chelation.
  - BAL may precipitate hemolytic crisis in a patient with glucose-6-phosphate dehydrogenase deficiency.

Second Line
Oral chelation with penicillamine (d-penicillamine, Depen, Cuprimine) (5)[C]:
- Penicillin-allergic patient should not receive penicillamine (cross-sensitivity is common).
- 10–15 mg/kg/d given b.i.d. mixed in apple juice/sauce on empty stomach (*not* approved by the FDA)
- Penicillamine may cause GI upset, renal failure, granulocytopenia, liver dysfunction, iron deficiency, and drug-induced lupus-like syndrome.

ISSUES FOR REFERRAL
Consider consultation if parenteral chelation is required.

ADDITIONAL THERAPIES
Remove patient from potential source of Pb for Pb level >45 until complete home inspection is performed.

IN-PATIENT CONSIDERATIONS
Admission Criteria/Initial Stabilization
- Blood Pb level >70 μg/dL
- If symptomatic, blood Pb level >35 μg/dL
- Outpatient care unless parenteral chelation is required or immediate removal from contaminated environment

Discharge Criteria
If Pb source is in the home, the patient must reside elsewhere until the abatement process is completed.

ONGOING CARE

FOLLOW-UP RECOMMENDATIONS
Avoid visit to any site of potential contamination.

Patient Monitoring
- After chelation, check for rebound Pb level in 7–10 days. Follow with regular monitoring, initially biweekly or monthly.
- Correct iron deficiency or any other nutritional deficiencies present.

- Once Pb <35 μg/dL, repeat testing every 1-3 months until level <25 μg/dL is achieved. Then monitor every 3–6 months until level <10 μg/dL. Once <9 μg/dL, test every 6–9 months (4)[C].

DIET
- If symptomatic, avoidance of excessive fluids
- Avoidance of pica
- Adequate calcium, iron, zinc, and vitamin C to reduce absorption and retention of Pb (6)[B]

PATIENT EDUCATION
- Needleman HL, Landrigan PJ. *Raising children toxic free: How to keep your child safe from lead, asbestos, pesticides, and other environmental hazards.* New York: Avon Books; 1995.
- National Lead Information Center, 422 South Clinton Avenue, Rochester, NY 14620; 800-424-5323; www.epa.gov/lead/
- National Safety Council, 1121 Spring Lake Drive, Itasca, IL 60143-3201; 800-621-7615; www.nsc.org/safety'home/HomeandRecreationalSafety/Poisoning/Pages/LeadPoisoning.aspx

PROGNOSIS
- Symptomatic Pb poisoning without encephalopathy generally improves with chelation, but subtle CNS toxicity may be long lasting or permanent.
- If encephalopathy occurs, permanent sequelae (e.g., mental retardation, seizure disorder, blindness, and hemiparesis) occurs in 25–50%.

COMPLICATIONS
- CNS toxicity may be long lasting or permanent.
- Long-term Pb exposure may cause chronic renal failure (Fanconi-like syndrome), gout, or Pb line (blue–black) on gingival tissue.
- Pb exposure in pregnancy is associated with reduced birth weight and premature birth.
- Pb is an animal teratogen.

REFERENCES

1. Centers for Disease Control and Prevention. Recommendations for blood lead screening of Medicaid-eligible children aged 1–5 years: An updated approach to targeting a group at high risk. *MMWR.* 2009;58(RR-9):1–11.
2. Centers for Disease Control and Prevention. *Guidelines for the identification and management of lead exposure in pregnant and lactating women.* U.S. Department of Health and Human Services. Atlanta, GA; November 2010.
3. Binns HJ, Campbell C, Brown MJ, et al. Interpreting and managing blood lead levels of less than 10 microg/dL in children and reducing childhood exposure to lead: Recommendations of the Centers for Disease Control and Prevention Advisory Committee on Childhood Lead Poisoning Prevention. *Pediatrics.* 2007;120:e1285–e1298.
4. Advisory Committee on Childhood Lead Poisoning Prevention, Centers for Disease Control and Prevention. *Low level lead harms children: A renewed call for primary prevention.* Atlanta, GA: Centers for Disease Control and Prevention; 2012.
5. American Academy of Pediatrics Committee on Drugs. Treatment guidelines for lead exposure in children. *Pediatrics.* 1995;96:155–160.
6. Woolf AD, Goldman R, Bellinger DC. Update on the clinical management of childhood lead poisoning. *Pediatr Clin North Am.* 2007;54:271–294, viii.

ADDITIONAL READING
- American Academy of Pediatrics Committee on Environmental Health. Lead exposure in children: Prevention, detection, and management. *Pediatrics.* 2005;116:1036–1046.
- Chandramouli K, Steer CD, Ellis M, et al. Effects of early childhood lead exposure on academic performance and behaviour of school age children. *Arch Dis Child.* 2009;94:844–848.

SEE ALSO

Anemia, Iron Deficiency

CODES

ICD10
- T56.0X1A Toxic effect of lead and its compounds, accidental, init
- T56.0X4A Toxic effect of lead and its compounds, undetermined, init

CLINICAL PEARLS
- The following children should have Pb screening:
  - 6–11 months of age with ≥1 risk factors:
    - Live in or visit a house built before 1960 with peeling paint or recent renovation
    - Sibling/Playmate with elevated Pb
    - Live with adult with job or hobby involving Pb
    - Live near industry likely to release Pb
  - Children living in high-risk communities (>12% elevated Pb) should be tested yearly from ages 1–5.
  - Newly arrived refugees
  - Children in low-risk areas should be screened by a questionnaire containing the above risk factors.
- There is no clear safe Pb level. A level <10 μg/dL is used to define "normal," but there is increasing evidence that levels <10 μg/dL are detrimental to neural development in young children. Many experts are treating Pb levels >4 μg/dL as elevated.
- There are no studies that show benefit of chelation at asymptomatic class III. Removal of sources of Pb is paramount.

L

LEGIONNAIRES' DISEASE

Mary Lindholm, MD

 BASICS

DESCRIPTION
- The term *Legionnaires' disease* was coined for an epidemic of lower respiratory tract disease occurring among people attending an American Legion convention in Philadelphia in 1976. Until this outbreak, the causative bacterium was unknown. It was isolated, identified, and named *Legionella pneumophila*, due to its ability to cause pneumonia and flulike illnesses. The bacteria inhabit man-made water system in hotels, hospitals, and air conditioning cooling towers.
  - Ranks among the 3 most common pneumonias in the clinical setting
  - Most common atypical pneumonia
- System(s) affected: Gastrointestinal; Pulmonary
- Synonym(s): Legionella pneumonia; Legionellosis

EPIDEMIOLOGY
- Predominant age: 15 months–84 years; increased >50 years
- Predominant gender: Male > Female

Incidence
- Reported cases increased from 1,310 in 2002, to 2,223 in 2003, with >2,000 cases/year from 2003–2005.
- Outbreaks occur most often at the end of the summer and early fall.

ETIOLOGY AND PATHOPHYSIOLOGY
- *Legionella pneumophila*, a weak gram-negative aerobic organism, is a saprophytic freshwater bacterium, widely distributed in soil and water. Bacteria are motile by bipolar flagella. Optimum temperature for growth is 40–45°C.
- Exists as an intracellular parasite of protozoa, colonizes surfaces and grows in biofilms, which persist in nematodes
- Serogroups 1–6 account for cases of disease.
- In the lung, *Legionella* infects alveolar macrophages.
- Mode of transmission:
  - Aspiration
  - Direct transmission into the lungs by equipment, such as respiratory equipment
  - Most important mode: Aerosolization and airborne dissemination of contaminated water, such as inhaling organisms while showering
- Recently, community outbreaks have been associated with whirlpools, spas, and fountains.
- Not spread among humans

RISK FACTORS
- Impaired cellular immunity (*Legionella* are intracellular pathogens)
- Smoking
- Alcohol abuse
- Immunosuppression/HIV
- Chronic cardiopulmonary disease
- Surgery
- Advanced age
- Transplant recipients
- Diabetes mellitus
- Use of antimicrobials within the past 3 months

GENERAL PREVENTION
- *Not transmitted person to person* (isolation is unnecessary)

- Superheat and flush water systems: Water is heated to 70°C, and distal outlets are flushed with hot water for 30 minutes.
- Ultraviolet light or copper-silver ionization are bactericidal.
- Monochloramine disinfection of municipal water supplies is associated with decreased risk for *Legionella* infection.

COMMONLY ASSOCIATED CONDITIONS
Pontiac fever: Self-limited flulike illness without pneumonia caused by *Legionella* species

 DIAGNOSIS

- Range of illness is from asymptomatic seroconversion, mild febrile illness, to severe pneumonia.
- Wound infections with *Legionella* have been reported.
- Incubation period of 2–14 days

HISTORY
- Signs and symptoms (percentage that can be affected):
  - Dry cough: 92%, which may become productive
  - Fever/Chills: 90%
  - Dyspnea: 62%
  - Pleuritic chest pain: 35%
  - Headache: 48%
  - Myalgia/Arthralgia: 40%
  - Watery diarrhea: 50%
  - Nausea and vomiting: 49%
  - Neuropsychiatric symptoms of encephalopathy, confusion, disorientation, obtundation, depression, hallucinations, insomnia, seizure: 53%
- History:
  - Identify immunosuppression risk factors.

PHYSICAL EXAM
- Fever
- Relative bradycardia (key sign):
  - Defined as a temperature ≥102°F with an inappropriately low pulse pressure <100 beats/minute (normal compensatory reaction to fever is tachycardia >110 beats/minute)
- Rales on lung auscultation with signs of consolidation

DIFFERENTIAL DIAGNOSIS
- Other bacterial pneumonias, especially atypical pneumonias such as *Mycoplasma pneumonia*, Q fever (*Coxiella burnetii*), *Chlamydophila pneumoniae*, *C. psittaci*, *Francisella tularensis*
- Viral pneumonias, especially adenovirus, influenza (human, avian, swine) (1), cytomegalovirus (CMV), H5N1

DIAGNOSTIC TESTS & INTERPRETATION
Initial Tests (lab, imaging)
- Diagnosis:
  - Gold standard is sputum culture for *Legionella*. Alert lab about possible diagnosis (sample needs buffered charcoal yeast extract agar) (2)[C]. This method has variable sensitivity (10–80%) (3), and is time consuming (up to 7 days for results). Another difficulty is that <50% of patients produce sputum.

- Urinary antigen test (UAT) detects serogroup 1, which causes most human disease (2,3)[A]. Urinary antigen tests are highly specific (99%), but variably sensitive (3,4,5)[A]. *Legionella* antigenuria can be detected within 1–2 days after onset of disease and persists for days to weeks. It is limited by that it only detects serogroup 1, and it is estimated that it may miss up to 40% of cases.
  - Indications for UAT: ICU admission, failure of outpatient antibiotic treatment, active alcohol abuse, recent travel (within past 2 weeks), pleural effusion
- The combination of respiratory specimen cultures and urine *Legionella* antigen testing are optimal for diagnosis.
- Serology via monoclonal direct fluorescence assay (DFA) on respiratory secretions is diagnostic:
  - Sensitivity is 41–94% (3).
  - Primary limitation is that seroconversion usually takes 4–6 weeks.
- Silver and Gimenez stains are used for lung tissue/specimens.
- Disorders that may alter lab results: Direct immunofluorescence can cross-react with *Pseudomonas* and *Bacteroides* sp., *Escherichia coli*, and *Haemophilus sp.*
- Other lab abnormalities, notable because these are not seen with other forms of pneumonia:
  - Hyponatremia
  - Hypophosphatemia (transient)
  - Lymphopenia
  - Mildly elevated serum transaminases
  - Elevated creatinine kinase
  - Microscopic hematuria
  - Highly elevated C-reactive protein (CRP) (>30)
  - Highly elevated ferritin (≥2× normal)
- Chest radiograph (6)[B]:
  - Not specific for *Legionella*
  - Commonly shows lower lobe patchy alveolar infiltrate with consolidation, usually unilateral
  - Cavitation/Abscess formation, more common in immunocompromised
  - Pleural effusion in up to 50%
  - May take from 1–4 months for the radiograph to return to normal. Progression of infiltrate on x-ray can be seen despite antibiotic therapy.

Diagnostic Procedures/Other
Transtracheal aspiration/bronchoscopy may be needed for sputum/lung samples.

Test Interpretation
- Multifocal pneumonia with alveolitis and bronchiolitis, with fibrinous pleuritis; may have serous/serosanguineous pleural effusion
- Abscess formation occurs in up to 20% of patients.
- Progression of infiltrates, despite appropriate therapy, may be suggestive of Legionnaires' disease. Also, improvement on radiograph may not correlate with clinical findings (longer lag times on radiographic findings).

 TREATMENT

GENERAL MEASURES
- Illness severity and the support available in the outpatient setting will dictate the appropriate site for care.

- Supportive care:
  – Oxygenation, hydration, and electrolyte balance with antibiotic therapy
- Extrapulmonary complications and higher mortality rate occur in patients with AIDS.

MEDICATION
First Line

- Antibiotics that achieve high intracellular concentrations (e.g., macrolides, tetracyclines, fluoroquinolones) are most effective. First-line treatment is levofloxacin (7,8,9)[B]; however, no prospective randomized controlled trials have compared fluoroquinolones to macrolides for the treatment of *Legionella*. In retrospective and observational studies, levofloxacin has been shown to result in more rapid defervescence, in fewer complications, and in decreased hospital stay compared with macrolide antibiotics. Antibiotics should be initiated via the parenteral route due to the GI symptoms associated with *Legionella*:
  – Levofloxacin is the preferred agent (7,8,9)[B]:
    ○ Levofloxacin 750 mg/d IV (switch to PO when patient is afebrile/tolerating PO) for 10–14 days
  – Azithromycin may also be used first line (7,8)[B]. It requires a shorter duration of treatment than levofloxacin due to a longer half-life:
    ○ Azithromycin 500 mg/d IV (switch to PO when afebrile/tolerating PO) for 7–10 days
- Contraindications: Hypersensitivity reactions
- Precautions: Liver disease
- Significant possible interactions:
  – Can increase theophylline, carbamazepine, and digoxin levels; can increase activity of oral anticoagulants
  – May decrease the effectiveness of oral anticoagulants, steroids, digoxin, quinidine, oral contraceptives, and hypoglycemic agents
- Longer courses of treatment (up to 21 days) may be needed in immunocompromised patients.

Second Line

- Doxycycline 200 mg IV/PO q12h for 72 hours; then 100 mg IV/PO q12h for total 14 days
- Doxycycline cannot be used in pregnant patients and is not approved for children <8 years of age.

IN-PATIENT CONSIDERATIONS
Admission Criteria/Initial Stabilization

- Inability to tolerate oral antibiotics
- Hypoxemia
- Criteria for direct admission to the ICU (10):
  – Any of the major criteria for severe CAP:
    ○ Septic shock that requires vasopressors
    ○ Acute respiratory failure that requires intubation and/or mechanical ventilation
  – At least 3 of the minor criteria for severe CAP:
    ○ RR ≥30 breaths/min; PaO_2:FiO_2 ratio ≤250; multilobular infiltrates; confusion/disorientation; uremia (BUN ≥20 mg/dL); leukopenia (WBC <4,000 cells/mm³); thrombocytopenia (PLT <100 K cells/mm³); hypothermia (temperature <36°C); hypotension requiring aggressive fluid resuscitation

Discharge Criteria

- Afebrile
- Able to tolerate oral antibiotics
- Normal oxygen saturation

 ## ONGOING CARE

FOLLOW-UP RECOMMENDATIONS
Patient Monitoring

- Respiratory status, hydration, and electrolyte status should be monitored closely.
- A chest radiograph is not useful to monitor the clinical response.

PATIENT EDUCATION

- Educate patients regarding prevention/avoidance measures, risk reduction, the expected disease progression, and the lack of person-to-person transmission.
- Disease prevention: Elimination of the pathogens from water supplies, focusing on low-emission cleaning procedures of cooling towers combined with control measurements of water and air samples (11)[A]

PROGNOSIS

- Recovery is variable:
  – During the 1st 2–3 days of recovery with anti-Legionella therapy, patients may clinically worsen despite treatment.
  – Usually rapid improvement with defervescence in 3–5 days and complete recovery in 6–10 days, whereas others may have a much more protracted course despite treatment.
- Mortality rate can approach 50% with nosocomial infections.

COMPLICATIONS

- Dehydration
- Hyponatremia
- Respiratory insufficiency requiring ventilator support
- Bacteremia/Abscess formation in immunocompromised patients
- Extrapulmonary disease can occur in the form of:
  – Encephalitis
  – Cellulitis
  – Sinusitis
  – Pancreatitis
  – Pyelonephritis
  – Endocarditis (most common extrapulmonary site)
  – Pericarditis
  – Perirectal abscess
- Renal failure
- Disseminated intravascular coagulation
- Multiple organ dysfunction syndrome (MODS)
- Coma
- Death occurs in 10% of treated immunocompetent patients, and in up to 80% of untreated immunocompromised patients.

REFERENCES

1. Cunha BA, Klein NC, Strollo S, et al. Legionnaires' disease mimicking swine influenza (H1N1) pneumonia during the "herald wave" of the pandemic. *Heart Lung*. 2010;39(3):242–248.
2. Yzerman EP, den Boer JW, Lettinga KD, et al. Sensitivity of three urinary antigen tests associated with clinical severity in a large outbreak of Legionnaires' disease in The Netherlands. *J Clin Microbiol*. 2002;40:3232–3236.
3. Tronel H, Hartemann P. Overview of diagnostic and detection methods for legionellosis and *Legionella* spp. *Lett Appl Microbiol*. 2009;48(6): 653–656.
4. Shimada T, Noguchi Y, Jackson JL, et al. Systemic review and metaanalysis: Urinary antigen tests for legionellosis. *Chest*. 2009;136(6):1576–1585.
5. Bartlett JG. Diagnostic tests for agents of community-acquired pneumonia. *Clin Infect Dis*. 2011;52(Suppl 4):S296–S304.
6. Tan MJ, Tan JS, Hamor RH, et al. The radiologic manifestations of Legionnaire's disease. The Ohio Community-Based Pneumonia Incidence Study Group. *Chest*. 2000;117:398–403.
7. Blázquez Garrido RM, Espinosa Parra FJ. Antimicrobial chemotherapy for Legionnaires' disease: Levofloxacin versus macrolides. *Clin Infect Dis*. 2005;40:800–806.
8. Mykietiuk A, Carratalà J, Fernández-Sabé N, et al. Clinical outcomes for hospitalized patients with Legionella pneumonia in the antigenuria era: The influence of levofloxacin therapy. *Clin Infect Dis*. 2005;84(6):794–799. Epub 2005 Feb 17.
9. Sabria M, Pedro-Botet ML, Gomez J, et al. Fluoroquinolones vs macrolides in the treatment of Legionnaires disease. *Chest*. 2005;(128): 1401–1405.
10. Mandell LA, Wunderink RG, Anzueto A, et al. Infectious Diseases Society of America/American Thoracic Society Consensus Guidelines on the Management of Community-Acquired Pneumonia in Adults. *Clin Infect Dis*. 2007;44:S27–S72.
11. Walser SM, Gerstner DG, Brenner B, et al. Assessing the environmental health relevance of cooling towers: A systematic review of legionellosis outbreaks. *Int J Hyg Environ Health*. 2013 Sep 9. pii: S1438-4639(13)00114-4. [Epub ahead of print]

 ## SEE ALSO

Pneumonia, Bacterial

 ## CODES

ICD10
- A48.1 Legionnaires' disease
- A48.2 Nonpneumonic Legionnaires' disease [Pontiac fever]

CLINICAL PEARLS

- Consider Legionnaires' disease in patients with pneumonia, extrapulmonary findings (atypical CAP) and relative bradycardia, accompanied by any 3 of the following: Otherwise unexplained relative lymphopenia, early/mildly elevated serum transaminases (aspartate aminotransferase/alanine aminotransferase), highly increased ferritin levels, or hypophosphatemia.
- *Legionella* is an intracellular organism and must be grown on buffered charcoal yeast extract agar; Gram stain of respiratory secretions with many neutrophils, but few organisms
- Consider Legionnaires' disease in nosocomial pneumonia.
- Because an increase in *Legionella* antibody titers cannot be detected >3–4 weeks, serology is not useful in early stages of the disease.
- The combination of respiratory specimen cultures and urine *Legionella* antigen testing are optimal for diagnosis.

L

LEUKEMIA, ACUTE LYMPHOBLASTIC IN ADULTS (ALL)

Richard A. Larson, MD

BASICS

DESCRIPTION
- ALL in adults is a malignant proliferation and accumulation of immature lymphocytes.
- ALL is the most common malignancy in children (see "Acute Lymphoblastic Leukemia, Pediatric")
- System(s) affected: Hemic/Lymphatic/Immunologic
- Synonym(s): Acute lymphocytic leukemia

Pregnancy Considerations
Many chemotherapy drugs are teratogenic.

EPIDEMIOLOGY
- Predominant age: Median age, 35–40 years; incidence increases with age
- Predominant sex: Male > Female (slightly)

Incidence
In the US: 1,000 adult cases per year

ETIOLOGY AND PATHOPHYSIOLOGY
- Unknown
- Epstein-Barr virus is implicated in Burkitt leukemia/lymphoma

Genetics
- Increased incidence in children with Down syndrome or in rare familial diseases such as ataxia-telangiectasia, Bloom syndrome, Fanconi anemia, Klinefelter syndrome, and neurofibromatosis
- Can rarely occur in adult identical twins

RISK FACTORS
- Age >60 years
- Incidence seems to increase after exposure to chemical agents, such as benzene, or to radiation, but acute myeloid leukemia (AML) is more common.
- May follow aplastic anemia

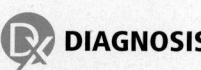

DIAGNOSIS

HISTORY
- Anemia: Fatigue, shortness of breath, lightheadedness, angina, headache
- Thrombocytopenia: Easy bruising
- Neutrocytopenia: Fever, infection
- Lymphocytosis: Bone pain
- CNS: Confusion

PHYSICAL EXAM
- Thrombocytopenia: Petechiae, ecchymoses, epistaxis, retinal hemorrhages
- Anemia: Pallor
- Neutrocytopenia: Fever, infection
- Lymphocytosis: Lymphadenopathy, splenomegaly; less often, hepatomegaly
- CNS: Cranial nerve palsies, confusion

DIFFERENTIAL DIAGNOSIS
- Malignant disorders: Other leukemias, especially AML; chronic myeloid leukemia in lymphoid blast phase; prolymphocytic leukemia; malignant lymphomas; multiple myeloma; bone marrow metastases from solid tumors (breast, prostate, lung, renal); myelodysplastic syndromes (1)[A]
- Nonmalignant disorders: Aplastic anemia, myelofibrosis, autoimmune diseases (Felty syndrome, lupus), infectious mononucleosis, pertussis, autoimmune thrombocytopenic purpura, leukemoid reaction to infection

DIAGNOSTIC TESTS & INTERPRETATION
Initial Tests (lab, imaging)
CBC with differential, liver function tests, uric acid, Anemia: Normochromic, normocytic
- Thrombocytopenia
- Peripheral blood lymphoblasts
- Elevated lactate dehydrogenase
- Elevated uric acid

Follow-Up Tests & Special Considerations
Special tests:
- Immunophenotyping of marrow/blood lymphoblasts: B lineage (CD19, CD20, CD22, CD24); T lineage (CD2, CD5, CD7); common ALL antigen (CD10); human leukocyte antigen (HLA)-DR; terminal deoxynucleotidyl transferase (TdT); aberrant myeloid antigens (CD13, CD33); stem cell antigen (CD34)
- Cytochemical stains: Myeloperoxidase, negative; Sudan black B, usually negative; TdT, positive; periodic acid Schiff ± is variable, depending on subtype
- Cytogenetics: Specific recurring chromosomal abnormalities have independent diagnostic and prognostic significance (hyperdiploidy >50 chromosomes or t(14q11q13) are favorable; the Philadelphia chromosome, t[9;22], t[4;11], −7 and +8 are unfavorable). A translocation t(8;14) or t(2;8) or t(8;22) identifies Burkitt-type leukemia that requires specific therapy.
- Reverse transcription polymerase chain reaction for rapid diagnosis of BCR/ABL + ALL
- HLA typing of patient and siblings for hematopoietic cell transplantation
- Chest CT scan and/or chest radiograph to evaluate for mediastinal mass or hilar adenopathy and for pulmonary infiltrates suggestive of infection
- US exam to assess splenomegaly or renal enlargement suggestive of leukemic infiltration

Diagnostic Procedures/Other
- Bone marrow examination with aspiration, biopsy, immunophenotyping, cytochemistry, cytogenetics, and molecular diagnostics
- Lymph node biopsy is rarely necessary but can be diagnostic.
- Lumbar puncture is typically done both for diagnosis of CNS involvement and for intrathecal treatment. It should be done immediately if neurological symptoms or signs are present. Repeat lumbar puncture after bone marrow remission is achieved to evaluate occult CNS involvement and continue prophylactic CNS treatment.

Test Interpretation
Diffuse replacement of marrow and lymph node architecture by sheets of malignant lymphoblasts

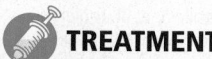

TREATMENT

GENERAL MEASURES
- Appropriate health care:
  - Inpatient care during remission induction chemotherapy
  - Postremission therapy is usually outpatient.
- Protective isolation from infection
- Adequate calcium and vitamin D supplementation may reduce bone injury from corticosteroids and avascular necrosis of large joints.

MEDICATION
First Line
Optimal therapy is not yet known (1,2)[A]. ALL should be treated at a comprehensive oncology center. All treatment regimens are still investigational, but clearly effective for some fraction of patients. Younger adults (<40 years old) may benefit from pediatric regimens (3,4)[A]. Cancer and Leukemia Group B protocol 9111 is an example of therapy (5)[A]:
- Remission induction:
  - Cyclophosphamide: 1,200 mg/m^2 IV on day 1 (800 mg/m^2 if >60)
  - Daunorubicin: 45 mg/m^2 IV on days 1, 2, and 3 (30 mg/m^2 if >60)
  - Vincristine: 2 mg IV on days 1, 8, 15, and 22
  - Asparaginase (L-asparaginase): 6,000 units/m^2 SC or IM on days 5, 8, 11, 15, 18, and 22 (or pegylated asparaginase 2000 U/m^2 (maximum 3,750 U) given on day 5)
  - Prednisone: 60 mg/m^2 on days 1–21 (days 1–7 if >60) (or dexamethasone 10 mg/m^2 on days 1–14)
  - Filgrastim, G-CSF: 5 μg/kg/d SC starting on day 4 has been shown to shorten the duration of neutropenia and improve the complete remission rate, especially in older patients.
  - Imatinib mesylate: 600–800 mg/d (or dasatinib 70 mg b.i.d.) are effective alone and in combination with chemotherapy for Philadelphia chromosome–positive ALL (6)[B].
- Consolidation (repeat twice in 8 weeks):
  - Cyclophosphamide: 1,000 mg/m^2 IV on day 1
  - Intrathecal (IT) methotrexate: 15 mg with hydrocortisone 50 mg on day 1
  - Mercaptopurine (6-mercaptopurine): 60 mg/m^2 on days 1–14
  - Cytarabine: 75 mg/m^2 SC on days 1–4 and 8–11
  - Vincristine: 2 mg IV on days 15 and 22
  - Asparaginase: 6,000 U/m^2 SC or IM on days 15, 18, 22, and 25 (or pegylated asparaginase 2,000 U/m^2 (maximum 3,750 U) on day 15.
- CNS prophylaxis and interim maintenance: 24 Gy cranial irradiation:
  - IT-methotrexate: 15 mg with hydrocortisone 50 mg on days 1, 8, 15, 22, and 29
  - Mercaptopurine (6-mercaptopurine): 60 mg/m^2 on days 1–70, taken in the evening
  - Oral methotrexate: 20 mg/m^2 on days 36, 43, 50, 57, and 64
- Late intensification:
  - Doxorubicin: 30 mg/m^2 IV on days 1, 8, and 15
  - Vincristine: 2 mg IV on days 1, 8, and 15
  - Dexamethasone: 10 mg/m^2 on days 1–14
  - Cyclophosphamide: 1,000 mg/m^2 IV on day 29
  - Thioguanine (6-thioguanine): 60 mg/m^2 on days 29–42
  - Cytarabine: 75 mg/m^2 SC on days 29–32 and 36–39
- Prolonged maintenance:
  - Vincristine: 2 mg/mo IV for 16 months
  - Prednisone: 60 mg/m^2 for 5 days with the vincristine
  - Mercaptopurine (6-mercaptopurine): 60 mg/m^2/d for 16 months, taken in the evening
  - Oral methotrexate: 20 mg/m^2/wk for 16 months
  - Special: Philadelphia chromosome–positive ALL:
    - Imatinib mesylate (400–800 mg/d) is effective alone and in combination with chemotherapy (6)[B].

- Dasatinib (140 mg/d) is effective in combination with dexamethasone or with chemotherapy.
- Contraindications: Doses and schedule may need to be altered for older patients and for concurrent infection and organ toxicity (2)[B].
- Precautions:
  - Tumor lysis syndrome (elevated uric acid, potassium, and phosphate with decreased calcium, leading to renal failure, disseminated intravascular coagulation, and cardiac arrhythmias) may be prevented by administering allopurinol 300 mg/d. Begin 2 days before chemotherapy begins. Reduce doses if used with mercaptopurine or azathioprine. Give increased fluids; IV urate oxidase (rasburicase) can be used to treat hyperuricemia rapidly.
  - Oral sulfamethoxazole-trimethoprim or aerosolized pentamidine is given for *Pneumocystis carinii* prophylaxis.
  - Profound immunosuppression: Take appropriate precautions when patient is neutropenic.
  - High-dose cyclophosphamide causes severe nausea and vomiting. Use appropriate antiemetic regimen to prevent.
  - Neurotoxicity, ileus with vincristine
  - Asparaginase may cause severe allergic reactions as well as impaired pancreatic and liver function. Monitor serum glucose concentrations frequently and carefully. Pancreatitis or thrombosis may occur. Peg-asparaginase has been approved and can be used IV or IM in place of native *Escherichia coli* asparaginase.
  - Avascular (osteo)necrosis (AVN) of bone may occur in adolescents and young adults after alkylating agents and corticosteroids
  - Rituximab (anti-CD20 monoclonal antibody) appears to improve the outcome of patients with ALL if CD20 is expressed on more than 20% of their blast cells.
  - Also note: Burkitt leukemia/lymphoma (ALL-L3):
    - The outcome is clearly better if high-dose methotrexate and alkylating agents are used as part of initial therapy.
    - Only 18 weeks of treatment are required.
    - Rituximab (anti-CD20 monoclonal antibody) improves the outcome of patients with Burkitt leukemia when added to chemotherapy.

Second Line
- Clofarabine has been approved for relapsed childhood ALL. Pegylated asparaginase (IV or IM) has been used in place of *E. coli*–derived L-asparaginase. Liposomal vincristine has been recently approved for single-agent use for the treatment of relapsed ALL in adults.
- Other anthracyclines, investigational chemotherapy agents, and monoclonal antibodies (e.g., rituximab; alemtuzumab). Immunoconjugates such as inotuzumab ozogamicin and bifunctional antibodies such as blinatumomab are under investigation.
- Allogeneic hematopoietic stem cell transplantation is recommended for any patient with relapsed ALL (7,8)[A].

ISSUES FOR REFERRAL

ALERT
ALL can become a fatal disorder quickly. As soon as the diagnosis is suspected, patients should be referred immediately to an appropriate oncology center.

SURGERY/OTHER PROCEDURES
Surgical placement of a percutaneous, silastic, double-lumen central venous catheter

COMPLEMENTARY AND ALTERNATIVE MEDICINE
Unproven; may result in drug interactions with chemotherapy

 ## ONGOING CARE

FOLLOW-UP RECOMMENDATIONS
Ambulatory as tolerated

Patient Monitoring
- Daily during induction chemotherapy for metabolic and infectious complications
- Weekly during remission consolidation chemotherapy
- Monthly during maintenance therapy
- Every 3 months thereafter

DIET
- Nutritional support; if needed IV hyperalimentation
- Avoid alcohol.
- Calcium and vitamin D

PATIENT EDUCATION
- Risks of infection, transfusion, chemotherapy
- Stop smoking.

PROGNOSIS
- ~80–95% of patients <60 will achieve a complete remission, and 35–60% will remain free of disease at 5 years (3,4,5,8,9)[A].
- Older patients (>60 years) do less well, but 80% may achieve a complete remission (2)[B].
- Patients with unfavorable cytogenetic subtypes [especially t(9;22) and t(4;11)] should undergo allogeneic stem cell transplantation in 1st remission if an HLA-identical donor is available (1,6,7,8)[A]. Autologous stem cell transplantation should be considered for Ph+ ALL patients who become reverse transcription–polymerase chain reaction negative for BCR/ABL and lack an allogeneic donor.

COMPLICATIONS
- Infections (*P. carinii* pneumonia, bacterial pneumonia or sepsis, fungal pneumonia)
- Bleeding
- Coagulopathy (deep vein thrombosis) from asparaginase therapy
- Need for transfusions
- Sterility from treatment
- Arachnoiditis and CNS effects from intrathecal chemotherapy and irradiation
- Pancreatitis and liver dysfunction from chemotherapy
- Osteonecrosis of joints (avascular necrosis) related to corticosteroids
- Relapse of ALL in marrow or extramedullary sites (CNS, testis)

REFERENCES

1. Faderl S, O'Brien S, Pui CH, et al. Adult acute lymphoblastic leukemia: Concepts and strategies. *Cancer*. 2010;116:1165–1176.
2. Gokbuget N. How I treat older patients with ALL. *Blood*. 2013;122:1366–1375.
3. McNeer JL, Raetz EA. Acute lymphoblastic leukemia in young adults: which treatment? *Curr Opin Oncol*. 2012;24:487–494.
4. Stock W, La M, Sanford B, et al. What determines the outcomes for adolescents and young adults with acute lymphoblastic leukemia treated on cooperative group protocols? A comparison of Children's Cancer Group and Cancer and Leukemia Group B studies. *Blood*. 2008;112:1646–1654.
5. Larson RA, Dodge RK, Linker CA, et al. A randomized controlled trial of filgrastim during remission induction and consolidation chemotherapy for adults with acute lymphoblastic leukemia: CALGB study 9111. *Blood*. 1998;92:1556–1564.
6. Stock W. Current treatment options for adult patients with Philadelphia chromosome-positive acute lymphoblastic leukemia. *Leuk Lymphoma*. 2010;51:188–198.
7. Oliansky DM, Larson RA, Weisdorf D, et al. The role of cytotoxic therapy with hematopoietic stem cell transplantation in the treatment of adult acute lymphoblastic leukemia: Update of the 2006 evidence-based review. *Biol Blood Marrow Transplant*. 2012;18:16–17.
8. Mattison RJ, Larson RA. Role of allogeneic hematopoietic cell transplantation in adults with acute lymphoblastic leukemia. *Curr Opin Oncol*. 2009;21:601–608.
9. Mulligan C. The molecular genetic makeup of acute lymphoblastic leukemia. *Hematology*. 2012;2012:389–396.

 ## CODES

ICD10
- C91.00 Acute lymphoblastic leukemia not having achieved remission
- C91.01 Acute lymphoblastic leukemia, in remission
- C91.02 Acute lymphoblastic leukemia, in relapse

CLINICAL PEARLS
- ALL can become fatal quickly; as soon as diagnosis is suspected, refer the patient to an oncology center.
- Optimal therapy is not yet known (1,2)[A]. ALL should be treated at a comprehensive oncology center. All treatment regimens are still investigational, but clearly are effective for some fraction of patients.

L

LEUKEMIA, ACUTE MYELOID

Jan Cerny, MD, PhD

BASICS

DESCRIPTION

- Acute myeloid leukemia (AML) is characterized by proliferation and accumulation of abnormal immature myeloid progenitors (blasts) with reduced capacity to differentiate into more mature cellular elements. This leads to bone marrow failure and results in a variety of systemic symptoms.
- Previously the French–American–British (FAB) classification system divided AML based on the cell morphology with the addition of cytogenetics (subtypes M0–M7).
- The World Health Organization (WHO) classification attempts to provide more meaningful prognostic information (1)[C]:
  – AML with characteristic genetic abnormalities: Translocation t(8;21), t(15;17), and inversion in chromosome 16 inv(16)
  – AML with multilineage dysplasia: Presence of a prior myelodysplastic syndrome (MDS) or myeloproliferative neoplasm (MPN) that transformed into AML
  – AML and MDS, therapy related
  – AML not otherwise categorized
  – Acute leukemias of ambiguous lineage (biphenotypic acute leukemia)

EPIDEMIOLOGY

- ~13,500 cases diagnosed in 2007; 2nd most common type of leukemia in adults
- Predominant sex: Male ≥ Female

Incidence

The incidence of AML increases with age and median age is >70 years.

ETIOLOGY AND PATHOPHYSIOLOGY

Precise causes unknown, but some risk factors have been identified (see "Risk Factors")

Genetics

- Unknown; some are familial
- Cytogenetics and genetics play an important role in diagnosis and prognosis of AML and have implications for therapy.
- 3 risk groups:
  – Good risk: inv(16), t(8;21), t(15;17)
  – Standard risk: Normal karyotype
  – Poor risk: Monosomy 5 and 7 (typically secondary AML), deletion 5q, abnormalities of 11q23 or complex karyotype
- FLT3 gene mutations, especially internal transmembrane duplications (FLT3-ITD), have been associated with poor survival in AML. These and growing list of (onco)gene (e.g., NPM1, DNMT3A, and P53) mutations have been studied to further risk-stratify patients (2).

RISK FACTORS

- Genetic predisposition (e.g., Down syndrome); other familial disorders are Bloom syndrome (~25% develop AML), Fanconi anemia (52%), neurofibromatosis, Li-Fraumeni syndrome, Wiskott-Aldrich syndrome, Kostmann syndrome, and Diamond-Blackfan anemia
- Radiation exposure
- Immunodeficiency states
- Chemical and drug exposure (nitrogen mustard and alkylating agents; benzene)
- Myelodysplastic syndrome
- Cigarette smoking

GENERAL PREVENTION

None currently identified, but treatment of high-risk myelodysplastic syndrome with demethylating agents (Vidaza, 5-azacytidine) has been shown to prolong time to transformation from MDS into AML (3).

COMMONLY ASSOCIATED CONDITIONS

The following are oncologic emergencies:

- Disseminated intravascular coagulopathy (DIC) especially in acute promyelocytic leukemia (APL), but may be seen in any AML
- Leukostasis (high blast number and increased adhesive ability of blasts)
- Tumor lysis syndrome (TLS): Spontaneous or in response to chemotherapy

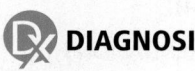

DIAGNOSIS

HISTORY

Fatigue (anemia or tumor burden); bleeding (low platelets or DIC); difficulty clearing infections (neutropenia or immune dysregulation)

PHYSICAL EXAM

- Mostly nonspecific and related to marrow or tissue infiltration:
  – Fever
  – Bleeding
  – Pallor
  – Splenomegaly
  – Hepatosplenomegaly
  – Lymphadenopathy (usually reactive)
- If CNS is involved, symptoms of increased intracranial pressure can be present.
- Occasionally patients will present with prominent extramedullary sites of leukemia (e.g., skin infiltration or ultimately as a myeloid sarcoma).

DIFFERENTIAL DIAGNOSIS

- Virus-induced cytopenia, lymphadenopathy, and organomegaly
- Immune cytopenias (including systemic lupus erythematosus [SLE])
- Drug-induced cytopenias
- Other marrow failure and infiltrative diseases (e.g., aplastic anemia, paroxysmal nocturnal hemoglobinuria, myelodysplastic syndromes, Gaucher disease)

DIAGNOSTIC TESTS & INTERPRETATION

- CBC shows subnormal RBCs, neutrophils, and platelets
- Bone marrow for histology, flow cytometry, and cytogenetics to establish diagnosis and prognosis
- ESR
- Lactate dehydrogenase (LDH) and uric acid can be elevated (e.g., TLS).
- Coagulation profile can be normal or prolonged (e.g., DIC).
- Drugs that may alter lab results: Chemotherapy agents, corticosteroids
- Other special tests: Spinal tap may reveal fluid with leukemic cells.
- Ultrasonography or CT scan of the abdomen may discover organomegaly.

Diagnostic Procedures/Other

Bone-marrow studies are usually necessary to make the diagnosis:

- Aspirates: For cell morphology, cytochemistries, immunophenotyping (can confirm differentiation stage of AML); cytogenetics: Chromosomal aberration (prognostic value; see "Genetics")
- Biopsies provide valuable information for cellularity, architecture, and so forth.

Test Interpretation

- Marrow is usually hypercellular and the normal architecture effaced; leukemic blast count is 20% or more.
- Liver and spleen may be infiltrated with leukemic cells.

TREATMENT

- Chemotherapy is the backbone of AML therapy; it consists of induction and consolidation phase ± maintenance (APL).
- Bone marrow transplantation (BMT) for high-risk AML
- Only modest improvements have been made in AML induction chemotherapy. Supportive care has improved significantly.

GENERAL MEASURES

- Ongoing assessment of bone marrow, liver, heart, and kidney functions during therapy
- Close monitoring of coagulation parameters (risk for DIC)
- Supportive therapy with:
  – Good hydration
  – Transfusions of packed RBCs and platelets based on patient's needs (threshold as for platelets as low as 5,000); use leuko-reduced, irradiated blood products as all patients can be considered for BMT.
  – Avoid antiplatelet agents (e.g., aspirin products).
  – Follow febrile neutropenic guidelines in neutropenic patient who becomes febrile (even low-grade fever).

Geriatric Considerations

- Older patients (>60–65 years) remain a therapeutic challenge. These patients are offered so-called reduced-intensity or nonmyeloablative BMT.
- Adding growth factors (granulocyte-colony stimulating factor [G-CSF]) may reduce toxicity in older patients (but is not broadly accepted).
- Hypomethylating agent, such as 5-azacitidine, significantly prolongs survival in older adults with low marrow blast count (<30%) (4).

Pediatric Considerations

Tolerate intense treatments better

Pregnancy Considerations

Chemotherapy is a viable option in the 2nd and 3rd trimesters.

MEDICATION

First Line

- Acute promyelocytic leukemia [APL, AML with t(15;17)]:
  – All-trans retinoic acid (ATRA) and arsenic trioxide both promote maturation to granulocytes.
  – Idarubicin is often added to induction therapy.

- Treatment of AML in younger adults: AML (other than APL)
  - Induction (daunorubicin or idarubicin [anthracycline and cytarabine]): The generally accepted combination is 3 + 7 (anthracycline is given for 3 and cytarabine for 7 days) or more intensive regimens with high dose of cytarabine (HiDAC) or high dose of anthracycline.
- Remission is typically consolidated in younger patients by:
  - In good-risk AML, 3–4 cycles of HiDAC and BMT is reserved for time of recurrence.
  - In poor-risk patients, 1–2 cycles of HiDAC (until donor is identified) are followed by allogeneic BMT.
  - Intermediate-risk AML should be treated based on individual patient's features, donor availability, and access to clinical trials. A meta-analysis showed that even intermediate-risk patients benefit from allogeneic BMT (5).
- Treatment of AML in older adults (>65 years) remains a challenge. These patients have poor performance status, more likely secondary AML, higher incidence of unfavorable cytogenetics, comorbidities, shorter remissions, and shorter overall survival:
  - Intensive chemotherapy may be feasible for patients with good performance status; alternative regimens with mitoxantrone, fludarabine, and clofarabine. New drugs (hypomethylating agents as above (4), FLT3 inhibitors, monoclonal antibodies, etc.) are being studied in clinical trials.
- Contraindications: Comorbidities; therapy has to be individualized
- Precautions:
  - If organ failure, some drugs may be avoided or dose-reduced (e.g., no anthracyclines in patients with pre-existing cardiac problems).
  - Patients will be immunosuppressed during treatment. Avoid live vaccines. Administer varicella-zoster or measles immunoglobulin as soon as exposure of patient occurs.
- Significant possible interactions: Allopurinol accentuates the toxicity of 6-mercaptopurine.

Second Line
Healthy, younger patients usually are offered reinduction chemotherapy and allogeneic BMT.

ISSUES FOR REFERRAL
- AML should be managed by specialized team led by a hematologist/oncologist.
- Refer patient to a transplant center early because a search for a donor may be necessary.

SURGERY/OTHER PROCEDURES
- BMT: Decision between myeloablative and nonmyeloablative approach should be based on patient's performance status, comorbidities, and AML risk factors:
  - Allogeneic BMT is acceptable in 1st remission in intermediate- or high-risk AML or in 2nd remission in all other AML patients. Matched related donor used to be preferred over matched unrelated donor (lower risk of graft-versus-host disease); recent data suggest equal outcomes as allogeneic transplant regimens and posttransplant care have improved significantly.
- Haploidentical transplants and cord blood may be used as alternative sources of hematopoietic stem cells for adults.
- Autologous BMT may be acceptable in specific situations (e.g., no donor is available).

IN-PATIENT CONSIDERATIONS
Admission Criteria/Initial Stabilization
Induction treatment for AML requires inpatient care, usually on a specialized ward. Episodes of febrile neutropenia typically require admission and IV antibiotics.

IV Fluids
Appropriate hydration to prevent TLS

Nursing
IV may lead to chemical burns in the event of extravasation.

ONGOING CARE

FOLLOW-UP RECOMMENDATIONS
Ambulatory, as tolerated; no intense or contact sports; no aspirin due to risk of bleeding

Patient Monitoring
- Repeat bone-marrow studies to document remission and also if a relapse is suspected.
- Follow CBC with differential, coagulation studies, uric acid level, and other chemistries related to TLS (creatinine, potassium, phosphate, calcium); monitor urinary function at least daily during induction phase and less frequently later.
- Physical evaluation, including weight and BP, should be done frequently during treatment.

DIET
Ensure adequately balanced calorie/vitamin intake. Total parenteral nutrition (TPN) in case of severe mucositis

PATIENT EDUCATION
- Leukemia Society of America, 600 Third Avenue, New York, NY 10016, 212-573-8484
- National Cancer Institute, Bethesda, MD, has pamphlets and telephone education.
- Baker LS. *You and leukemia: A day at a time.* Saunders.

PROGNOSIS
AML remission rate is 60–80%, with only 20–40% long-term survival. The wide variable prognosis is due to prognostic group (age, cytogenetics, and genetics).

COMPLICATIONS
- Acute side effects of chemotherapy, including febrile neutropenia
- TLS
- DIC
- Late-onset cardiomyopathy in patients treated with anthracyclines
- Chronic side effects of chemotherapy (secondary malignancies)
- Graft-versus-host disease in patients who have received allogeneic BMT

REFERENCES
1. Patel JP, Gönen M, Figueroa ME, et al. Prognostic relevance of integrated genetic profiling in acute myeloid leukemia. *N Engl J Med*. 2012;366: 1079–1089.
2. Döhner H, Estey EH, Amadori S, et al. Diagnosis and management of acute myeloid leukemia in adults: Recommendations from an international expert panel, on behalf of the European Leukemia. *Net Blood*. 2010;115:453–474.
3. Fenaux P, Mufti GJ, Hellstrom-Lindberg E, et al. Efficacy of azacitidine compared with that of conventional care regimens in the treatment of higher-risk myelodysplastic syndromes: A randomised, open-label, phase III study. *Lancet Oncol*. 2009;10:223–232.
4. Fenaux P, Mufti GJ, Hellström-Lindberg E, et al. Azacitidine prolongs overall survival compared with conventional care regimens in elderly patients with low bone marrow blast count acute myeloid leukemia. *J Clin Oncol*. 2010;28:562–569.
5. Koreth J, Schlenk R, Kopecky KJ, et al. Allogeneic stem cell transplantation for acute myeloid leukemia in first complete remission: Systematic review and meta-analysis of prospective clinical trials. *JAMA*. 2009;301:2349–2361.

ADDITIONAL READING
O'Donnell MR, Appelbaum FR, Coutre SE, et al. Acute myeloid leukemia. *J Natl Compr Canc Netw*. 2008;6:962–993.

 SEE ALSO

Disseminated Intravascular Coagulopathy (DIC); Leukemia Acute Lymphoblastic in Adults (ALL); Leukemia, Chronic Myelogenous (CML); Myelodysplastic Syndromes (MDS); Myeloproliferative Neoplasms

 CODES

ICD10
- C92.00 Acute myeloblastic leukemia, not having achieved remission
- C92.01 Acute myeloblastic leukemia, in remission
- C92.02 Acute myeloblastic leukemia, in relapse

CLINICAL PEARLS
- Prognosis of leukemia depends on the cytogenetic and molecular profile of the disease.
- Allogeneic transplant remains the only therapy with curative potential for patients with intermediate- and high-risk AML.

LEUKEMIA, CHRONIC LYMPHOCYTIC
Jan Cerny, MD, PhD • Horace Tang, MD

BASICS

DESCRIPTION
- Chronic lymphocytic leukemia (CLL) is a monoclonal disorder characterized by a progressive accumulation of mature but functionally incompetent lymphocytes.
- CLL should be distinguished from prolymphocytic leukemia (PLL); based on percentage of prolymphocytes, the disease may be regarded as CLL (<10% prolymphocytes), PLL (>55% prolymphocytes), or CLL/PLL (>10% and <55% prolymphocytes).
- Small lymphocytic lymphoma is a lymphoma variant of CLL.
- System(s) affected: Hematologic; Lymphatic; Immunologic

EPIDEMIOLOGY
Incidence
- With 15,000–17,000 new cases reported every year, CLL *represents the most common form of leukemia in adults in the US*.
- In 2013, an estimated 4580 adults in US will die from CLL, which makes it the second-leading cause of death among adults with leukemia US after acute myeloid leukemia (1).
- Predominant age: CLL primarily affects elderly individuals, median age of diagnosis being 70 years. The incidence continues to rise in those age >55 years.
- Predominant sex: Male > Female (1.7:1)
- The incidence is higher among whites than among African Americans

ETIOLOGY AND PATHOPHYSIOLOGY
- The cell of origin in CLL is a clonal B cell arrested in the B-cell differentiation pathway, intermediate between pre-B cells and mature B cells. In the peripheral blood, these cells resemble mature lymphocytes and typically show B-cell surface antigens: CD19, CD20, CD21, and CD23. In addition, they express CD5 (usually found on T cells).
- The bcl2 proto-oncogene is overexpressed in B-CLL. Bcl2 is a known suppressor of apoptosis (programmed cell death), resulting in extremely long life of the affected lymphocytes.
- Unknown, but genetic mutations leading to disrupted function and prolonged survival of affected lymphocytes are suspected.

Genetics
CLL is an acquired disorder, and reports of truly familial cases are exceedingly rare. CLL has been shown, however, to occur at higher frequency among 1st-degree relatives of patients with the disease, and several somatic gene mutations have been identified at significantly higher rates among CLL patients (2)[C].

RISK FACTORS
- As in the case of most malignancies, the exact cause of CLL is uncertain.
- Possible chronic immune stimulation is suspected but is still being elucidated.
- Monoclonal B-cell lymphocytosis: 1% risk progression to CLL.

GENERAL PREVENTION
Unknown

COMMONLY ASSOCIATED CONDITIONS
- Immune system dysregulation is common.
- Autoimmune hemolytic anemia (AIHA) may accompany CLL.
- Immune thrombocytopenic purpura (ITP) may accompany CLL.
- Pure red cell aplasia (PRCA) may accompany CLL.

DIAGNOSIS

HISTORY
- Insidious onset; it is not unusual for CLL to be discovered incidentally. Up to 40% of patients are asymptomatic at the time of diagnosis.
- Others may have:
  - Repetitive infections (e.g., pneumonia, but also mucocutaneous herpetic infections)
  - Enlarged lymph nodes
  - Early satiety and/or abdominal discomfort related to an enlarged spleen
  - Mucocutaneous bleeding and/or petechiae due to thrombocytopenia
  - Fatigue-related and/or other symptoms of anemia
  - Fevers, night sweats, >10% weight loss (B symptoms)

PHYSICAL EXAM
- Localized or generalized lymphadenopathy
- Splenomegaly (30–40%)
- Hepatomegaly (20%)
- Mucocutaneous bleeding (thrombocytopenia)
- Skin petechiae (thrombocytopenia)
- Pallor

DIFFERENTIAL DIAGNOSIS
- Infectious causes:
  - Bacterial (tuberculosis)
  - Viral (mononucleosis)
- Malignant causes:
  - Leukemic phase of non-Hodgkin lymphomas
  - Hairy cell leukemia
  - Waldenstrom macroglobulinemia
  - Large granular lymphocytic leukemia

DIAGNOSTIC TESTS & INTERPRETATION
Initial Tests (lab, imaging)
- CBC with differential shows B cell absolute lymphocytosis with >5000 B lymphocytes/μL. The blood smear also shows ruptured lymphocytes ("smudge" cells) and morphologically mature-appearing small lymphocytes.
- Exam of the blood smear is important in diagnosis of CLL.
- Diagnosis can be confirmed by immunophenotyping: CLL cells are positive for CD19, CD20, and CD24, as well as CD5. They have low levels of surface membrane immunoglobulin (Ig) M or IgD. The monoclonality is proven by the presence of a single immunoglobulin light chain (κ or λ). FMC7 is absent.
- CBC shows anemia and/or thrombocytopenia.
- Plasma β_2 microglobulin may be elevated.
- Serum protein electrophoresis (some patients may have monoclonal gammopathy)
- Lactate dehydrogenase (LDH) may be elevated (due to disease activity or to AIHA).

- Hypogammaglobulinemia
- In cases associated with AIHA, labs consistent with hemolysis may be present (elevated LDH, total bilirubin; reticulocyte count does not have to be elevated due to bone marrow infiltration).
- Liver/spleen ultrasound may demonstrate organomegaly and may also detect enlarged abdominal lymph nodes.
- CT scan of chest/abdomen/pelvis typically is not necessary for staging. However, it may help to identify compression of organs or internal structures from enlarged lymph nodes.
- Positron emission tomography (PET) scan might be helpful to guide biopsy if Richter transformation is suspected (see below).

Follow-Up Tests & Special Considerations
Frequency and type of follow up depend on severity of symptoms as well as risk factors (see "Prognosis").

Diagnostic Procedures/Other
- Although bone marrow biopsy has its prognostic value (diffuse infiltration is a risk factor), it is not done routinely.
- Consider a lymph node biopsy if lymph node(s) begins to enlarge rapidly in a patient with known CLL to assess the possibility of transformation to a high-grade lymphoma (Richter syndrome), especially when accompanied by fever, weight loss, and pain.

Test Interpretation
- A bone marrow aspirate usually shows >30% lymphocytes.
- Cytogenetic (fluorescence in situ hybridization) may show chromosomal changes, which are prognostic (i.e., del(13q), del(11q), del(17p), trisomy 12, and del(6q)).
- *SF3B1* mutation is associated with rapid disease progression and shorter survival in CLL (3).

TREATMENT

GENERAL MEASURES
Patients with frequent infections associated with hypogammaglobulinemia are likely to benefit from monthly infusions of intravenous immunoglobulin (IVIG).

MEDICATION
First Line
- Most patients are asymptomatic and do not need active treatment unless they have generalized (so-called B) symptoms, progressive marrow failure, AIHA or thrombocytopenia, progressive splenomegaly, massive lymphadenopathy, or progressive lymphocytosis (increase >50% in 2 months or a doubling time of <6 months) (4)[C].
- Low-risk disease, Rai stage 0, and Binet stage A require only periodic follow up.
- Intermediate-risk group, Rai stages I and II, and Binet stage B could be observed until evidence of disease progression or development of symptoms.
- Treatment should be initiated in high-risk patients, Rai stage III and IV, and Binet stage C.
- Early treatment in low-risk group is not recommended.

- 3 main groups of drugs used are alkylating agents (chlorambucil and, recently, bendamustine), purine analogues (fludarabine and pentostatin), and monoclonal antibodies (rituximab and alemtuzumab)
- Single-agent (fludarabine, bendamustine, or chlorambucil) or combination regimens commonly used
- Fludarabine-based regimens are FC (in combination with cyclophosphamide), FR (fludarabine + rituximab), and FCR (fludarabine + cyclophosphamide + rituximab).
- FCR is the widely used regimen of choice if patient can tolerate it.
- Steroids (prednisone) are useful in patients with autoimmune manifestations of CLL (e.g., AIHA, ITP).

Second Line
- Combinations of chemotherapeutic agents that patient did not fail yet. Occasionally, some patients can be retreated with a drug used previously.
- Alemtuzumab (anti-CD52) has shown activity in relapsed and refractory disease.
- Newer agents, like ofatumumab (novel anti-CD20), lenalidomide, and others, have shown promising activity.
- Consider splenectomy (surgery/radiation) if massive splenomegaly causes significant anemia and thrombocytopenia.
- Allogenic and autologous stem cell transplant can be considered in high-risk and younger patients (limited data available).
- Ibrutinib, is a Bruton tyrosine kinase inhibitor from a novel class of agents, which has a high level of activity in refractory CLL (5).

ISSUES FOR REFERRAL
- Surgical consultation for splenectomy in selected patients
- Bone marrow transplant in young patients with refractory disease (however, still considered experimental therapy):
  – Allogeneic hematopoietic stem cell transplant (HSCT) with nonmyeloablative conditioning offers lower treatment-related mortality and may be appropriate for certain patients.

ADDITIONAL THERAPIES
Patients requiring therapy who are high risk for tumor lysis syndrome should be given allopurinol to prevent uric acid nephropathy.

SURGERY/OTHER PROCEDURES
- Splenectomy in selected patients with splenomegaly and refractory cytopenia
- Radiation (if compression symptoms from bulky lymphadenopathy)

IN-PATIENT CONSIDERATIONS
Admission Criteria/Initial Stabilization
No specific criteria, but due to complications of disease (e.g., AIHA) or of therapy (e.g., febrile neutropenia) or significant tumor lysis syndrome after initiation of chemotherapy

 ONGOING CARE

FOLLOW-UP RECOMMENDATIONS
Patient Monitoring
Patients with low-risk CLL and/or patients in remission:
- CBC with differential (lymphocytosis) every 3–6 months, LDH, β_2 microglobulin, IgG level
- Physical exam (lymphadenopathy, splenomegaly)

DIET
- Ensure adequately balanced calorie/vitamin intake
- Follow weight

PATIENT EDUCATION
Leukemia and Lymphoma Society has educational pamphlets: www.webmd.com/cancer/tc/leukemia-topic-overview

PROGNOSIS
There are 2 staging systems used: The Rai in the US and the Binet in Europe. Neither is completely satisfactory.
- Rai staging system:
  – Stage 0: Lymphocytosis only; median survival of 120 months
  – Stage I: Lymphocytosis and adenopathy; median survival of 95 months
  – Stage II: Lymphocytosis and splenomegaly and/or hepatomegaly; median survival of 72 months
  – Stage III: Lymphocytosis and anemia (hemoglobin <10 g/dL); median survival of 30 months
  – Stage IV: Lymphocytosis and thrombocytopenia (platelets $<100 \times 10^9$/L); median survival of 30 months
- Binet staging system:
  – Stage A: Hemoglobin ≥10 g/dL, platelets $\geq 100 \times 10^9$, and <3 lymph node areas involved (Rai stages 0, I, and II); survival >120 months
  – Stage B: Hemoglobin and platelet levels as in stage A and 3 or more lymph node areas involved (Rai stages I and II); survival is 61 months
  – Stage C: Hemoglobin <100 g/L, platelets $<100 \times 10^9$, or both (Rai stages III and IV); survival is 32 months
- Adverse risk factors:
  – Advanced Rai or Binet stage
  – Peripheral lymphocyte doubling time <12 months
  – Diffuse marrow infiltration
  – Increased number of prolymphocytes or cleaved cells
  – Poor response to chemotherapy
  – High β_2 microglobulin and thymidine kinase levels and low micro RNAs (miRNAs)
  – Abnormal karyotyping: Deletion 17p (del(17p) *P53* mutation or deletion) and del(11q)
  – New IgVH unmutated status (expression of ZAP-70 >20% or CD38 >30% evaluated by immunophenotyping are surrogate markers)
  – NOTCH1 mutation (also associated with unmutated IgVH)

COMPLICATIONS
- Acute or long-term effects of chemotherapy
- Richter syndrome (above)
- AIHA (in some cases may be related to the use of fludarabine)
- Slightly increased risk of solid tumors (especially Kaposi sarcoma, malignant melanoma, laryngeal cancers, lung cancers)
- Infection (especially gram negative and encapsulated organisms)
- Membranoproliferative glomerulonephritis (MPGN) or other glomerular pathology

REFERENCES
1. Siegel R, Naishadham D, Jemal A. Cancer statistics, 2013. *CA Cancer J Clin*. 2013;63:11–30.
2. Chiorazzi N, Rai KR, Ferrarini M. Chronic lymphocytic leukemia. *N Engl J Med*. 2005;352:804–815.
3. Wan Y, Wu CJ. SF3B1 mutations in chronic lymphocytic leukemia. *Blood*. 2013;121:4627–4634.
4. Shanafelt TD, Kay NE. Comprehensive management of the CLL patient: A holistic approach. *Hematology Am Soc Hematol Educ Program*. 2007:324–331.
5. Advani RH, Buggy JJ, Sharman JP, et al. Bruton tyrosine kinase ibrutinib (PCI-32765) has significant activity in patients with relapsed/refractory B-cell malignancies. *J Clin Oncol*. 2013;31:88–94.

ADDITIONAL READING
National Comprehensive Cancer Network guidelines at www.nccn.org

 CODES

ICD10
- C91.10 Chronic lymphocytic leuk of B-cell type not achieve remis
- C91.11 Chronic lymphocytic leukemia of B-cell type in remission
- C91.12 Chronic lymphocytic leukemia of B-cell type in relapse

CLINICAL PEARLS
- CLL represents the most common form of leukemia in adults in the US.
- Predominant age: CLL primarily affects elderly individuals, median age of diagnosis being 70 years. The incidence continues to rise in those age >55 years.
- Clinical monitoring of asymptomatic and low-risk patients is a reasonable approach ("watch and wait").
- High-risk patients, bulky disease, or patients who fail fludarabine- and rituximab-based therapies have typically poor prognosis and may require intensive therapies, including allogeneic transplantation.
- Median survival is 3–10 years, depending on stage.

LEUKEMIA, CHRONIC MYELOGENOUS

Jan Cerny, MD, PhD

BASICS

DESCRIPTION
- Chronic myelogenous leukemia (CML) is a myeloproliferative neoplasm characterized by clonal proliferation of myeloid precursors in the bone marrow with continuing differentiation into mature granulocytes.
- Hallmark of CML is Philadelphia chromosome [translocation t(9;22)]
- Natural history of the disease evolves in 3 clinical phases: A chronic phase, an accelerated phase, and blast phase or crisis (transformation to acute leukemia)

EPIDEMIOLOGY
Incidence
- Per year, 1.6 cases/100,000 persons
- Predominant age: 50–60 years
- Predominant sex: Male > Female (1.3:1)

Prevalence
Accounts for 15–20% of adult leukemias

ETIOLOGY AND PATHOPHYSIOLOGY
Philadelphia chromosome is a balanced translocation between *BCR* (on chromosome 22) and *ABL* (on chromosome 9) genes t(9;22)(q34;q11). This fusion gene, *BCR-ABL*, codes for an abnormal constitutively active tyrosine kinase that affects numerous signal transduction pathways, resulting in uncontrolled cell proliferation and reduced apoptosis.

Genetics
Acquired genomic changes

RISK FACTORS
Ionizing radiation exposure (uncommon)

GENERAL PREVENTION
None currently identified

DIAGNOSIS

85–90% of patients present in the chronic phase and the disease can be found accidentally during routine screening.

HISTORY
- Chronic phase: Fatigue, weight loss, night sweats, abdominal fullness owing to enlarged spleen, early satiety, dyspnea, bleeding. Rare: Bruising, left upper quadrant abdominal pain, sternal pain (owing to expanding bone marrow), and gouty arthritis; up to 30% of patients are asymptomatic.
- Accelerated phase: Progressive splenomegaly and left upper quadrant abdominal pain occasionally referred to the left shoulder (owing to splenic infarction or rupture), progressive weight loss and sweats, unexplained fever or bone pain, chloromas (extramedullary tumors)
- Blast phase: Bleeding, bruising, infections, prominent constitutional symptoms

PHYSICAL EXAM
- Splenomegaly (50–90%), hepatomegaly (up to 50%)
- Less common: Splenic friction rub, lymphadenopathy

DIFFERENTIAL DIAGNOSIS
- Chronic myelomonocytic leukemia, chronic neutrophilic leukemia, chronic eosinophilic leukemia, juvenile myelomonocytic leukemia, infectious mononucleosis, leukemoid reaction, polycythemia vera, and treatment with granulocyte-stimulating factors
- Acute myelogenous leukemia resembles blast crisis with myeloid blasts, and acute lymphoblastic leukemia resembles blast crisis with lymphoid blasts.
- Atypical CML is a chronic myeloproliferative disorder with a clinical hematologic picture similar to CML, but it lacks Philadelphia chromosome and *BCR-ABL* rearrangement.

DIAGNOSTIC TESTS & INTERPRETATION
- CBC:
  - Hematocrit: May be normal, slightly increased, or decreased
  - WBC count: Markedly increased (50,000–100,000/μL), with granulocytes in all stages of development, including occasional blasts <10% in chronic phase, basophilia, eosinophilia
  - Platelets: Normal, elevated (34%), or occasionally low
  - In accelerated phase: Anemia, 10–19% blood or marrow blasts, basophils plus eosinophils >20%, thrombocytopenia
  - Blast phase: Blood or marrow blasts >20%
- Genetics:
  - Demonstration of the Philadelphia chromosome, t(9,22), by cytogenetic techniques, fluorescence in situ hybridization (FISH), or reverse-transcription-polymerase chain reaction (RT-PCR)
  - Additional cytogenetic abnormalities occur in the accelerated and blast phases [monosomy 7, t(3,21), trisomy 8 and 19, Philadelphia chromosome duplication, abnormalities of chromosome 17, such as monosomy, trisomy, and isochromosome mutations]. These may contribute to resistance to tyrosine kinase inhibitors (TKIs; e.g., imatinib). Further molecular testing (mutations within *BCR-ABL*) is suggested in case of loss of response to therapy.
- Others:
  - Low or absent leukocyte alkaline phosphatase in neutrophils
  - High lactate dehydrogenase (LDH)
  - Elevated uric acid

Initial Tests (lab, imaging)
- CBC, LDH, uric acid, bone marrow biopsy and aspirate, cytogenetics on bone marrow, and FISH for *BCR-ABL*, RT-PCR, LFTs
- Abdominal ultrasound or CT scan shows splenomegaly; not mandatory

Follow-Up Tests & Special Considerations
- Mutation analysis of tyrosine kinase domain of *ABL* kinase, as they may cause resistance to therapy with TKIs.
- HLA-A*02 positive is associated with CML and a protective effect is seen with the HLA-B*35 allele (pooled odds ratio 0.64, 95% confidence interval 0.48–0.86 (1)[A].

Diagnostic Procedures/Other
Bone marrow aspiration and biopsy

Test Interpretation
Myeloid hyperplasia with elevated myeloid: Erythroid ratio, normal maturation, marrow basophilia, and increased reticulin fibrosis

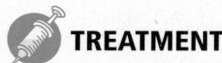

TREATMENT

MEDICATION
- TKIs (e.g., imatinib) provide durable, long-term control of disease.
- The response to TKIs is assessed at specific time points from the beginning of treatment and is categorized as follows:
  - Complete hematologic response (CHR): Normalization of peripheral counts, no disease symptoms, no immature cells
  - Minor/Partial/Complete cytogenetic response (CCR): 1–34%, 35–90%, no Philadelphia-positive metaphases
  - Major molecular response (MMR): Decreased level of *BCR-ABL* transcript by PCR 3-log
  - Complete molecular response (CMR): *BCR-ABL* transcript is undetectable by PCR.

First Line
- Imatinib mesylate (Gleevec), an oral TKI, 400 mg/d
- Side effects: Thrombocytopenia, anemia, elevated liver enzymes, edema, GI disturbances, rash
- International Randomized Study of Interferon versus STI571 (IRIS) established imatinib as first-line therapy (2).
- Imatinib dose can be increased to 600 and 800 mg/d if only suboptimal response is achieved with standard dose.
- 2nd-generation TKIs have shown higher efficacy and fewer side effects and are approved for first-line therapy of chronic phase CML: Nilotinib (Tasigna) and dasatinib (Sprycel) (3,4,5).

Second Line
- Dasatinib, 2nd-generation TKI, active against most of *BRC-ABL* mutants, not active in *T315I* mutation:
  - 100 mg/d in patients resistant or intolerant to imatinib and 70 mg b.i.d. for patients in accelerated or blastic phase
  - Side effects: Pleural effusions, cytopenias
- Nilotinib, also 2nd-generation TKI, highly selective and more potent *BCR-ABL* TKI, active against most *BRC-ABL* mutants, not active in *T315I* mutation:
  - 400 mg PO b.i.d. in patients resistant or intolerant to imatinib in chronic or accelerated phase
  - Side effects: Cytopenias, QTc prolongation, pancreatitis
- Ponatinib, bosutinib, and omacetaxine are now approved for patient who failed or did not tolerate 2 TKIs previously. Ponatinib and omacetaxine are the only effective agents in patients with *T315I* mutation. Agents targeting leukemic stem cells are being developed for clinical use.

ISSUES FOR REFERRAL
All patients with CML should be referred to a hematologist. Patients with inadequate response to TKIs or with *T315I* mutation should consult with a bone marrow transplant physician.

SURGERY/OTHER PROCEDURES
Allogenic bone marrow transplant (BMT):

- It is the only known cure; however, 71% of patients who achieve complete cytogenetic response with imatinib maintain that response for 7 years, and no patient progressed on the trial between years 5 and 6 of treatment (2).
- Most effective in patients <50 years of age who are in the chronic phase
- Initial mortality is higher (related to the use of myeloablative regimens) than medical management, but provided higher rates of survival in pre-imatinib era.
- Significant improvement in transplant techniques leading to better outcomes, such as alternative sources of stem cells; nonmyeloablative regimens have shown improvements in transplant-related mortality.
- Transplant option should be thoroughly discussed with young patients in chronic phase and considered an alternative to imatinib, dasatinib, or nilotinib, especially if the patient does not tolerate TKIs or disease is not responding.
- Can be considered in patients who fail to achieve complete hematologic response by 3 months, have no cytogenetic response or cytogenetic relapse, or have *T315I* mutation.

IN-PATIENT CONSIDERATIONS
Admission Criteria/Initial Stabilization
Acute abdominal symptoms (infarcted or ruptured spleen); tumor lysis syndrome owing to initial therapy; complications of BMT:

- Hydroxyurea might be given, with the goal of reduction of the WBC count, but it has minimal impact on patient response to TKIs.
- Induction chemotherapy (for acute leukemia) in setting of blastic phase
- Allopurinol to prevent tumor lysis syndrome in patients with very high counts; however, probably not necessary when TKIs are used

Discharge Criteria
Abatement of acute symptoms

 ## ONGOING CARE

FOLLOW-UP RECOMMENDATIONS
- Frequency depends on stage at presentation and response to first-line therapy.
- While splenomegaly persists, avoid contact sports or trauma to abdomen.

Patient Monitoring
- CBC with differential: Weekly until blood counts stable, then every 2–4 weeks during complete hematologic response; once in CCR and stable, patient can be followed less frequently (3-month intervals)
- Bone marrow cytogenetics (evaluation for clonal evolution) every 6 months while in CHR, every 12–18 months while in complete cytogenic response, MMR, CMR
- Quantitative RT-PCR every 3 months (peripheral blood)
- ECGs (concern for QT prolongation), liver function tests while on TKIs. Nilotinib, bosutinib, and ponatinib can cause pancreatitis.

PROGNOSIS
- With treatment and good response, the survival is similar to the normal population.
- Without treatment: CML invariably will progress to accelerated phase within 2–5 years and blast phase within several months of the accelerated phase.
- Poor prognosis: Patients presenting in accelerated or blastic phase or presenting with very large spleen size, platelets >700,000/μL, and patients resistant to TKIs (*T315I* mutation)

COMPLICATIONS
- Splenic infarct or rupture
- Progression to accelerated or blastic phase
- Thrombotic events owing to elevated platelets
- Bleeding owing to low or dysfunctional platelets
- Sequelae of anemia

REFERENCES
1. Naugler C, Liwski R. Human leukocyte antigen class I alleles and the risk of chronic myelogenous leukemia: A meta-analysis. *Leuk Lymphoma.* 2010;51:1288–1292.
2. O'Brien SG, Guilhot F, Goldman JM, et al. International randomized study of interferon versus STI571 (IRIS) 7-year follow-up: Sustained survival, low rate of transformation and increased rate of major molecular response (MMR) in patients (pts) with newly diagnosed chronic myeloid leukemia in chronic phase (CMLCP) treated with imatinib (IM). *ASH Ann Meeting Abstracts.* 2008;112:186.
3. Kantarjian HM, Baccarani M, Jabbour E, et al. Second-generation tyrosine kinase inhibitors: The future of frontline CML therapy. *Clin Cancer Res.* 2011;17:1674–1683.
4. Kantarjian H, Shah NP, Hochhaus A, et al. Dasatinib versus imatinib in newly diagnosed chronic-phase chronic myeloid leukemia. *N Engl J Med.* 2010;362:2260–2270.
5. Saglio G, Kim DW, Issaragrisil S, et al. Nilotinib versus imatinib for newly diagnosed chronic myeloid leukemia. *N Engl J Med.* 2010;362:2251–2259.

ADDITIONAL READING
- Goldman JM, Marin D. Management decisions in chronic myeloid leukemia. *Semin Hematol.* 2003;40:97–103.
- Kantarjian H, Pasquini R, Hamerschlak N. Dasatinib or high-dose imatinib for chronic-phase chronic myeloid leukemia after failure of first-line imatinib: A randomized phase 2 trial. *Blood.* 2007;109:5143–5150.

 ## CODES

ICD10
- C92.10 Chronic myeloid leukemia, BCR/ABL-positive, not having achieved remission
- C92.11 Chronic myeloid leukemia, BCR/ABL-positive, in remission
- C92.12 Chronic myeloid leukemia, BCR/ABL-positive, in relapse

CLINICAL PEARLS
- CML belongs to the myeloproliferative disorders group.
- The gold standard for diagnosis of CML is detection of the Philadelphia chromosome or its products, *BCR-ABL* mRNA, and fusion protein.
- TKIs provide durable, long-term control of the disease and have dramatically altered treatment.
- Atypical CML is a form of clinically typical CML, but without the presence of the typical *BCR-ABL* translocation.
- Blast crisis is a form of acute leukemia that is a possible complication of CML.

L

LEUKOPLAKIA, ORAL

Christine K. Jacobs, MD

 BASICS

DESCRIPTION
- Oral leukoplakia is a nonspecific clinical term used to describe a white patch on the oral mucosa that remains despite attempts to rub or scrape it off:
  - It has no pathologic or microscopic correlation with any specific disease and may be related to a variety of lesions, from benign hyperkeratosis to squamous cell carcinoma.
- System(s) affected: Gastrointestinal

EPIDEMIOLOGY
- Develops in middle age, increases with age
- Most common in India, where more people smoke and chew tobacco and areca nuts.

Prevalence
- 1–3% of the adult population is affected.
- Mean age of onset is 40 years.

Geriatric Considerations
Malignant transformation to carcinoma is more common in older patients.

ETIOLOGY AND PATHOPHYSIOLOGY
Hyperkeratosis or dyskeratosis of the oral squamous epithelium
- Tobacco use in any form
- Alcohol consumption/alcoholism
- Oral infections
- *Candida albicans* infection (1)
- Human papillomavirus, types 11 and 15
- Sunlight
- Vitamin deficiency
- Syphilis
- Dental restorations/Prosthetic appliances
- Estrogen therapy
- Chronic trauma or irritation
- Epstein-Barr virus (oral hairy leukoplakia)
- Areca nut/Betel (Asian populations)
- Mouthwash preparations and toothpaste containing the herbal root extract sanguinaria

Genetics
P53 overexpression correlates with leukoplakia and particularly squamous cell carcinoma (2).

RISK FACTORS
- 70–90% of oral leukoplakia is related to tobacco, particularly smokeless tobacco or areca/betel nut use.
- Repeated or chronic mechanical trauma from dental appliances or cheek biting
- Chemical irritation to oral regions
- Diabetes
- Age
- Socioeconomic status
- Risk factors for malignant transformation of leukoplakia (3):
  - Female
  - Long duration of leukoplakia
  - Nonsmoker (idiopathic leukoplakia)
  - Located on tongue or floor of mouth
  - Size >200 mm^2
  - Nonhomogenous type
  - Presence of *C. albicans*
  - Presence of epithelial dysplasia

GENERAL PREVENTION
- Avoid tobacco of any kind, alcohol, habitual cheek biting, tongue chewing
- Use well-fitting dental prosthesis
- Regular dental check-ups to avoid bad restorations
- Diet rich in fresh fruits and vegetables may help to prevent cancer

COMMONLY ASSOCIATED CONDITIONS
- Leukokeratosis nicotina palati is rarely malignant.
- Oral frictional hyperkeratosis is generally benign (4).
- HIV infection is closely associated with hairy leukoplakia.
- Erythroplakia in association with leukoplakia, "speckled leukoplakia," or erythroleukoplakia is a marker for underlying dysplasia.
- Proliferative verrucous leukoplakia may develop into either squamous cell carcinoma or verrucous hyperplasia.

 DIAGNOSIS

Leukoplakia is an asymptomatic white patch on the oral mucosa.

HISTORY
- Usually asymptomatic
- History of tobacco or alcohol use or oral exposure to irritants

PHYSICAL EXAM
- Location:
  - 50% on tongue, mandibular alveolar ridge, and buccal mucosa
  - Also seen on maxillary alveolar ridge, palate, and lower lip
  - Infrequently seen on floor of the mouth and retromolar areas
  - Floor of mouth, ventrolateral tongue, and soft palate complex are more likely to have dysplastic lesions.
- Appearance:
  - Varies from homogeneous, nonpalpable, faintly translucent white areas to thick, fissured, papillomatous, indurated plaques
  - May feel rough or leathery
  - Lesions can become exophytic or verruciform.
  - Color may be white, gray, yellowish white, or brownish gray.
  - Cannot be wiped or scraped off.
- World Health Organization classification (5)[C]:
  - Homogeneous refers to color:
    - Flat, corrugated, wrinkled or pumice
  - Nonhomogeneous refers to color and texture (more likely to be dysplastic or malignant):
    - Erythroleukoplakia (mixture of red and white)
    - Exophytic: Papillary or verrucous texture

DIFFERENTIAL DIAGNOSIS
- White oral lesions that can be wiped away: Acute pseudomembranous candidiasis
- White oral lesions that cannot be rubbed off:
  - Chronic hyperplastic candidiasis
  - Traumatic or frictional keratosis (e.g., linea alba)
  - Leukoedema (benign milky opaque lesions that disappear with stretching)
  - Aspirin burn (from holding aspirin in cheek)
  - Lichen planus (bilateral fairly symmetric lesions, reticular pattern of slightly raised gray-white lines)
  - Verrucous carcinoma
  - Lupus
  - Squamous cell carcinoma
  - Oral hairy leukoplakia, commonly on the lateral border of the tongue with a bilateral distribution (in HIV patients with Epstein-Barr virus infection)
  - Smoker's palate (leukokeratosis nicotina palati)
  - White sponge nevus (congenital benign spongy lesions)
  - Syphilitic oral lesion
  - Dyskeratosis congenita (a rare inherited multisystem disorder)

DIAGNOSTIC TESTS & INTERPRETATION
Biopsy to rule out carcinoma if lesion is persistent, changing, or unexplained.

Initial Tests (lab, imaging)
- Laboratory tests generally are not indicated:
  - Consider saliva culture if *C. albicans* infection is suspected.
- No imaging is indicated.

Follow-Up Tests & Special Considerations
If no clear diagnosis, consider CBC, rapid plasma reagin, and biopsy.

Diagnostic Procedures/Other
- Biopsy is necessary to rule out carcinoma if lesion is persistent, changing, or unexplained.
- Noninvasive brush biopsy and analysis of cells with DNA–image cytometry constitute a sensitive and specific screening method.
- Patients with dysplastic or malignant cells on brush biopsy should undergo more formal excisional biopsy.

Test Interpretation
- Biopsy specimens range from hyperkeratosis to invasive carcinoma.
- At initial biopsy, 6% are invasive carcinoma.
- 0.13–6% subsequently undergo malignant transformation.
- Location is important: 60% on floor of mouth or lateral border of tongue are cancerous; buccal mucosal lesions are generally not malignant but require biopsy if not resolving.

TREATMENT

- All oral leukoplakias should be treated.
- Treatment may include:
  - For 2–3 circumscribed lesions, surgical excision
  - For multiple or large lesions where surgery would cause unacceptable deformity, cryosurgery, laser surgery, or topical bleomycin (6)[C].
  - Removal of predisposing habits (alcohol and tobacco)
- Complete excision is standard treatment for dysplasia or malignancy.
- After treatment, up to 30% of leukoplakia recurs, and some leukoplakia still transforms to squamous cell carcinoma (6)[C].

GENERAL MEASURES
- Eliminate habitual lip biting.
- Correct ill-fitting dental appliances, bad restorations, or sharp teeth.
- Stop smoking and using alcohol.
- Some small lesions may respond to cryosurgery.
- Beta-carotene, lycopene, retinoids, and cyclooxygenase 2 (COX-2) inhibitors may cause partial regression (7)[B].
- For hairy tongue: Tongue brushing

MEDICATION
- Leukoplakia:
  - Isotretinoin (Accutane), 1–2 mg/kg/d PO may lead to temporary remission, but side effects are poorly tolerated.
  - Systemic administration of lycopene may have some efficacy in patients, similar to a subcontinental Indian population, for the short-term resolution of oral epithelial dysplasia (7)[B].
  - Bleomycin may be used for extensive leukoplakia.
- Hairy leukoplakia:
  - Acyclovir, 2–4 g/d PO systemically is effective, but the lesions recur when the treatment is stopped.
  - Topical retinoids
  - Topical podophyllin 25% resin applied twice, 1 week between applications; however, the bad taste is poorly tolerated.

ISSUES FOR REFERRAL
Consider otolaryngologist or oral surgery referral for extensive disease.

SURGERY/OTHER PROCEDURES
- Scalpel excision, laser ablation, electrocautery, or cryoablation
- Cryotherapy slightly less effective than photodynamic therapy response (73% vs. 90%) and recurrence (27% vs. 24%) (8)[A].
- CO_2 laser had 20% recurrence and 10% malignant transformation within 5 years (9)[B].

IN-PATIENT CONSIDERATIONS
Admission Criteria/Initial Stabilization
- Eliminate etiologic factors.
- Re-evaluate in 7–14 days.
- Biopsy if lesion is persistent.

 # ONGOING CARE

FOLLOW-UP RECOMMENDATIONS
Patient Monitoring
- Regular, close follow-up, even after successful treatment
- Biopsy as needed.

DIET
Regular

PATIENT EDUCATION
- If biopsy is negative, stress importance of periodic and careful follow up.
- Initiate a dental referral to eliminate dental factors.
- Stress importance of stopping tobacco and alcohol use.
- Encourage participation in smoking-cessation program.

PROGNOSIS
- Most leukoplakia is benign.
- Leukoplakia may regress, remain stable, or progress.
- 0.13–6% of initially benign lesions subsequently develop into cancer.
- More likely to be cancerous if on floor of mouth or lateral border of tongue.

COMPLICATIONS
- New lesions may develop after treatment.
- Without surgical intervention, 4% develop carcinoma after 6.6 years (10)[B].
- Larger lesions and nonhomogeneous leukoplakia are associated with higher rates of malignant transformation.

REFERENCES
1. Cao J, Liu HW, Jin JQ, et al. The effect of oral candida to development of oral leukoplakia into cancer. *Zhonghua Yu Fang Yi Xue Za Zhi*. 2007; 41(Suppl):90–93.
2. Duarte EC, Ribeiro DC, Gomez MV, et al. Genetic polymorphisms of carcinogen metabolizing enzymes are associated with oral leukoplakia development and p53 overexpression. *Anticancer Res*. 2008;28:1101–1106.
3. Dietrich T, Reichart PA, Scheifele C, et al. Clinical risk factors of oral leukoplakia in a representative sample of the US population. *Oral Oncol*. 2004; 40:158–163.
4. Cam K, Santoro A, Lee JB, et al. Oral frictional hyperkeratosis (morsicatio buccarum): An entity to be considered in the differential diagnosis of white oral mucosal lesions. *Skinmed*. 2012;10: 114–115.
5. Axéll T, Pindborg JJ, Smith CJ, et al. Oral white lesions with special reference to precancerous and tobacco-related lesions: Conclusions of an international symposium held in Uppsala, Sweden, May 18–21 1994. International Collaborative Group on Oral White Lesions. *J Oral Pathol Med*. 1996;25:49–54.
6. Feller L, Lemmer J. Oral Leukoplakia as it relates to HPV infection: A Review. *Int J Dent*. 2012;2012: 540561.
7. Lodi G, Sardella A, Bez C, et al. Interventions for treating oral leukoplakia. *Cochrane Database Syst Rev*. 2006;4:CD001829.
8. Kawczyk-Krupka A, Waśkowska J, Raczkowska-Siostrzonek A, et al. *Photodiagnosis Photodyn Ther*. 2012;2:148–155.
9. Jerjes W, Upile T, Hamdoon Z, et al. CO2 laser of oral dysplasia: Clinicopathological features of recurrence and malignant transformation. *Lasers Med Sci*. 2012;27:169–179.
10. Holmstrup P, Vedtofte P, Reibel J, et al. Long-term treatment outcome of oral premalignant lesions. *Oral Oncol*. 2006;42:461–474.

ADDITIONAL READING
- Reamy BV, Derby R, Bunt CW. Common tongue conditions in primary care. *Am Fam Physician*. 2010;81:627–634.
- Warnakulasuriya S, Dietrich T, Bornstein MM, et al. Oral health risks of tobacco use and effects of cessation. *Int Dent J*. 2010;60:7–30.

 ## SEE ALSO

Epstein-Barr Virus Infections; HIV Infection and AIDS

 ## CODES

ICD10
- K13.3 Hairy leukoplakia
- K13.21 Leukoplakia of oral mucosa, including tongue

CLINICAL PEARLS
- Linea alba: A white line on the buccal mucosa along the occlusal plane.
- After treatment, up to 30% of leukoplakia recurs, and some leukoplakia still transforms to squamous cell carcinoma; thus, long-term surveillance is essential.
- To lessen risk of malignant transformation, encourage tobacco and alcohol cessation, and consider *C. albicans* eradication.
- Oral leukoplakia is a nonspecific clinical term used to describe a white patch on the oral mucosa that remains despite attempts to rub or scrape it off:

LICHEN PLANUS

Mercedes E. Gonzalez, MD • Herbert P. Goodheart, MD

 BASICS

Lichen planus (LP) is an idiopathic eruption with characteristic shiny, flat-topped (Latin: *planus*, "flat") purple (violaceous) papules and plaques on the skin, often accompanied by characteristic mucous membrane lesions. Itching may be severe.

DESCRIPTION

- Classic (typical) LP is a relatively uncommon inflammatory disorder of the skin and mucous membranes; hair and nails may also be affected:
  - Skin lesions are small, flat, angular, red-to-violaceous, shiny, pruritic papules and/or plaques with overlying fine, white lines (called Wickham striae) or gray-white puncta. Most commonly seen on the flexor surfaces of the upper extremities, extensor surfaces of the lower extremities, the genitalia, and on the mucous membranes.
  - On the oral mucosa, lesions typically appear as raised white lines in a lace-like pattern seen most often on the buccal mucosa.
  - Onset is abrupt or gradual. Course is unpredictable; may resolve spontaneously, recur intermittently, or persist for many years.
- Drug-induced LP:
  - Clinical and histopathologic findings may mimic those of classic LP. Lesions usually lack Wickham striae (see below), and oral involvement is rare.
  - There is generally a latent period of months from drug introduction until lesions appear.
  - Lesions resolve when the inciting agent is discontinued, often after a prolonged period.
- LP variants:
  - Follicular: Also called lichen planopilaris; typically seen on the scalp, can lead to scarring alopecia
  - Annular: Papules spread centrifugally as central area resolves, occur on glans penis, axillae, and oral mucosa
  - Linear: May be an isolated finding
  - Hypertrophic: itchy, hyperkeratotic, thick plaques on dorsal legs and feet
  - Atrophic: Rare, most often the result of resolved lesions
  - Bullous LP: Intense inflammation in the dermis leads to blistering of epidermis
  - LP pemphigoides: A combination of LP and bullous pemphigoid (immunoglobulin G autoantibodies to collagen 17)
  - Nail LP: Affects the nail matrix, lateral thinning, longitudinal ridging, and fissuring
- System(s) affected: Skin/Exocrine
- Synonym(s): Lichenoid eruptions

EPIDEMIOLOGY

- Predominant age: 30–60 years old; rare in children and the geriatric population
- Predominant sex: Female > Male

Prevalence

In the US, 450/100,000

ETIOLOGY AND PATHOPHYSIOLOGY

LP is considered to be a T-cell–mediated autoimmune response to self-antigens on damaged keratinocytes.

RISK FACTORS

Exposure to certain drugs or chemicals:

- Thiazides, furosemide, β blockers, sulfonylureas, antimalarials, penicillamine, gold salts, and angiotensin-converting enzyme inhibitors
- Rarely: Photo-developing chemicals, dental materials, tattoo pigments

COMMONLY ASSOCIATED CONDITIONS

- An association has been noted between LP and hepatitis C virus infection, particularly in certain geographic regions (Asia, South America, the Middle East, Europe) (1). Hepatitis should be considered in patients with widespread presentations of LP and those with primarily oral disease.
- In addition, chronic active hepatitis, lichen nitidus, and primary biliary cirrhosis have been noted to coexist with LP.
- Association with dyslipidemia has been reported (2).
- LP has also been reported in association with other diseases of altered immunity, more often than would be expected by chance:
  - Bullous pemphigoid
  - Alopecia areata
  - Myasthenia gravis
  - Vitiligo
  - Ulcerative colitis
  - Graft vs. host reaction
  - Lupus erythematosus (lupus erythematosus–LP overlap syndrome)
  - Morphea and lichen sclerosis et atrophicus

 DIAGNOSIS

LP is most commonly diagnosed by its appearance, despite its range of clinical presentations. A skin biopsy should be performed if the diagnosis is in doubt.

HISTORY

A minority of patients have a family history of LP. Affected families have an increased frequency of human leukocyte antigen B7 (HLA-B7). A thorough drug history should be performed.

PHYSICAL EXAM

- Skin (often severe pruritus):
  - Papules: 1–10 mm, shiny, flat-topped (planar) lesions that occur in crops; lesions may have a fine scale.
  - Evidence of scratching (i.e., crusts and excoriations) is usually absent.
  - Color: Violaceous, with white lacelike pattern (Wickham striae) on surface of papules. Wickham striae are best seen after topical application of mineral oil, and, if present, are virtually pathognomonic for LP.
  - Shape: Polygonal or oval. Annular lesions may appear on trunk and mucous membranes. Various shapes and sizes may be noted (polymorphic).
  - Arrangement: May be grouped, linear, or scattered individual lesions
  - Koebner phenomenon (isomorphic response): New lesions may be noted at sites of minor injuries, such as scratches or burns.

- Distribution: Ventral surface of wrists and forearms, dorsa hands, glans penis, dorsa feet, groin, sacrum, shins, and scalp. Hypertrophic (verrucous) lesions may occur on lower legs and may be generalized.
- Postinflammatory hyperpigmentation: Lesions typically heal, leaving darkly pigmented macules in their wake.
- Mucous membranes (40–60% of patients with skin lesions; 20% have mucous membrane lesions without skin involvement):
  - Most commonly asymptomatic, nonerosive, milky-white lines with an elegant, lacy, netlike streaked pattern
  - Usually seen on buccal mucosa, but may appear on tongue, gingiva, palate, or lips
  - Less commonly, LP may be erosive; rarely bullous
  - Painful, especially if ulcers present
  - Lesions may develop into squamous cell carcinoma (1–3%).
  - Glans penis, labia minora, vaginal vault, and perianal areas may be involved.
- Hair/Scalp:
  - Lichen planus of the hair follicle (lichen planopilaris) presents with keratotic plugs at the follicle orifice with a violaceous rim, may result in atrophy and permanent destruction of hair follicles (scarring alopecia)
- Nails (10%):
  - Involvement of nail matrix may cause proximal-to-distal linear grooves and partial or complete destruction of nail bed with pterygium formation.

DIFFERENTIAL DIAGNOSIS

- Skin:
  - Lichen simplex chronicus
  - Eczematous dermatitis
  - Psoriasis
  - Discoid lupus erythematosus
  - Other lichenoid eruptions (those that resemble lichen planus)
  - Pityriasis rosea
  - Lichen nitidus
- Oral mucous membranes:
  - Leukoplakia
  - Oral hairy leukoplakia
  - Candidiasis
  - Squamous cell carcinoma (particularly in ulcerative lesions)
  - Aphthous ulcers
  - Herpetic stomatitis
  - Secondary syphilis
- Genital mucous membranes:
  - Psoriasis (penis and labia)
  - Nonspecific balanitis, Zoon balanitis
  - Fixed drug eruption (penis)
  - Candidiasis (penis and labia)
  - Pemphigus vulgaris, bullous pemphigoid, and Behçet disease (all rare)
- Hair and scalp:
  - Scarring alopecia (central centrifugal cicatricial alopecia)

DIAGNOSTIC TESTS & INTERPRETATION

If suggested by history:
- Serology for hepatitis
- Liver function tests

Diagnostic Procedures/Other
- Skin biopsy
- Direct immunofluorescence helps to distinguish LP from discoid lupus erythematosus.

Test Interpretation
- Dense, bandlike (lichenoid) lymphocytic infiltrate of the upper dermis
- Vacuolar degeneration of the basal layer
- Hyperkeratosis and irregular acanthosis, increased granular layer
- Basement membrane thinning with "saw-toothing"
- Degenerative keratinocytes, known as colloid or Civatte bodies, are found in the lower epidermis
- Melanin pigment in macrophages

 TREATMENT

Although LP can resolve spontaneously, treatment is usually requested by patients who may be severely symptomatic or troubled by its cosmetic appearance.

GENERAL MEASURES
- Goal is to relieve itching and resolve lesions
- Asymptomatic oral lesions require no treatment.

MEDICATION

First Line
- Skin:
- Superpotent topical steroids (e.g., 0.05% clobetasol propionate) b.i.d. for 2 weeks
  - Potent topical steroids such as triamcinolone acetonide 0.1% or fluocinonide 0.05% under occlusion
  - Intralesional corticosteroids (e.g., triamcinolone [Kenalog] 5–10 mg/mL) for recalcitrant and hypertrophic lesions
  - Antihistamines (e.g., hydroxyzine, 25 mg PO q6h) have limited benefit for itching, but may be helpful for sedation at bedtime.
  - "Soak and smear" technique: Can lead to a rapid improvement of symptoms in even 1–2 days and may obviate the need for systemic steroids. Soaking allows water to hydrate the stratum corneum and allows the anti-inflammatory steroid in the ointment to penetrate more deeply into the skin. Smearing of the ointment traps the water in the skin because water cannot move out through greasy materials:
    - Soaking is done in a bathtub using lukewarm plain water for 20 minutes, then, without drying the skin, the affected area is immediately smeared with a thin film of the steroid ointment containing clobetasol or another superpotent topical steroid.
    - Soak and smear may be done for 4–5 days or longer, if necessary. The treatments are best done at night because the greasy ointment applied to the skin gets on pajamas (instead of on daytime clothes) and the ointment is on the skin during sleep. A topical steroid cream is applied thereafter during the daytime hours, if necessary.

- Mucous membranes:
  - For oral, erosive, painful lichen planus, a Cochrane review found at best weak evidence for the effectiveness of any intervention (3)[A]:
    - Topical corticosteroids (0.1% triamcinolone [Kenalog] in Orabase) or 0.05% clobetasol propionate ointment b.i.d.
    - Intralesional corticosteroids
    - Topical 0.1% tacrolimus (Protopic ointment) b.i.d. or 1% pimecrolimus (Elidel) cream b.i.d. A Cochrane review found no evidence that calcineurin inhibitors are better than placebo (4)[A].
    - Topical retinoids (e.g., 0.05% tretinoin [retinoic acid] in Orabase)

Pediatric Considerations
Children may absorb a proportionally larger amount of topical steroid because of larger skin surface-to-weight ratio.

Second Line
Skin and mucous membranes:
- Intralesional corticosteroids
- Topical 0.1% tacrolimus (Protopic ointment) b.i.d. (4,5) or topical 1% pimecrolimus (Elidel) cream b.i.d. (4)
- Oral prednisone: Used only for a short course (e.g., 30–60 mg/d for 2–4 weeks) or IM triamcinolone (Kenalog) 40–80 mg every 6–8 weeks:
  - Precautions with systemic steroids:
    - Systemic absorption of steroids may result in hypothalamic-pituitary-adrenal axis suppression, Cushing syndrome, hyperglycemia, or glucosuria.
    - Increased risk with high-potency topical steroids (i.e., use over large surface area, prolonged use, occlusive dressings)
    - In pregnancy: Usually safe, but benefits must outweigh the risks
- Oral retinoids: Isotretinoin in doses of 10 mg PO for 2 months and acitretin 30 mg have resulted in improvement in some refractory cases. Observe carefully for resultant dyslipidemia.
- Oral metronidazole 500 mg b.i.d. for 20–60 days can be given as a safer alternative to systemic corticosteroids.
- Cyclosporine may be used in severe cases, but cost and potential toxicity limit its use. Topical use for severe oral involvement refractory to other treatments.
- Thalidomide
- Psoralen ultraviolet-A (PUVA), broad- or narrow-band ultraviolet-B (UVB) (5)
- Griseofulvin
- Azathioprine
- Mycophenolate mofetil

ALERT
Avoid oral and topical retinoids during pregnancy.

IN-PATIENT CONSIDERATIONS
Admission Criteria/Initial Stabilization
Outpatient care

 ONGOING CARE

FOLLOW-UP RECOMMENDATIONS
Patient Monitoring
Serial oral examinations for erosive/ulcerative lesions

PATIENT EDUCATION
- Oral, erosive, or ulcerative LP: Annual follow-up to screen for malignancy (6).
- Avoid spicy foods, cigarettes, and excessive alcohol.
- Avoid crispy foods such as corn chips, pretzels, and toast.

PROGNOSIS
- Spontaneous resolution in weeks is possible, but disease may persist for years, especially oral lesions and hypertrophic lesions on the shins.
- There is a tendency toward relapse.
- Recurrence in 12–20%, especially in those with generalized involvement.

COMPLICATIONS
- Alopecia
- Nail destruction
- Squamous cell carcinoma of the mouth or genitals

REFERENCES

1. Shengyuan L, Songpo Y, Wen W, et al. Hepatitis C virus and lichen planus. A reciprocal association determined by a meta-analysis. *Arch Dermatol*. 2009;145:1040–1047.
2. Arias-Santiago S, Buendía-Eisman A, Aneiros-Fernández J, et al. Cardiovascular risk factors in patients with lichen planus. *Am J Med*. 2011;124:543–548.
3. Cheng S, Kirtschig G, Cooper S, et al. Interventions for erosive lichen planus affecting mucosal sites. *Cochrane Database Syst Rev*. 2012;2:CD008092.
4. Thongprasom K, Carrozzo M, Furness S, et al. Interventions for treating oral lichen planus. *Cochrane Database Syst Rev*. 2011;7:CD001168.
5. Pavlotsky F, Nathansohn N, Kriger G, et al. Ultraviolet-B treatment for cutaneous lichen planus: Our experience with 50 patients. *Photodermatol Photoimmunol Photomed*. 2008;24:83–86.
6. Gonzalez-Moles MA, Scully C, Gil-Montoya JA. Oral lichen planus: Controversies surrounding malignant transformation. *Oral Dis*. 2008;14:229–243.

 CODES

ICD10
- L43.0 Hypertrophic lichen planus
- L43.1 Bullous lichen planus
- L43.9 Lichen planus, unspecified

CLINICAL PEARLS

- Remember the 7 Ps of LP: **P**urple, **p**lanar, **p**olygonal, **p**olymorphic, **p**ruritic (not always), **p**apules that heal with **p**ostinflammatory hyperpigmentation.
- Serial oral or genital exams are indicated for erosive/ulcerative LP lesions to monitor for the development of squamous cell carcinoma.
- An association has been noted between LP and hepatitis C virus infection, chronic active hepatitis, and primary biliary cirrhosis.
- The "soak and smear" technique can lead to a rapid improvement of symptoms in 1–2 days and may obviate the need for systemic steroids.

L

LICHEN SIMPLEX CHRONICUS
Vibin Roy, MD • Manjula Julka, MD, FAAFP

BASICS

DESCRIPTION
- Lichen simplex chronicus (LSC) is a chronic dermatitis resulting from chronic, repeated rubbing or scratching of the skin. Skin becomes thickened with accentuated lines ("lichenification").
- System(s) affected: Skin
- Synonym(s): LSC; lichen simplex; localized neurodermatitis; neurodermatitis circumscripta

EPIDEMIOLOGY
Geriatric Considerations
Most common in middle aged and elderly

Pediatric Considerations
Rare in preadolescents

Incidence
- Common
- Peak incidence 35–50 years
- Predominant sex: Females > Males (2:1)

Prevalence
Common

ETIOLOGY AND PATHOPHYSIOLOGY
- Common triggers are excess dryness of skin, heat, sweat, and psychological stress.
- Scratching may be secondary to habit or a conditioned response to anxiety.
- The formation of a itch–scratch cycle leads to a chronic dermatosis. Repeated scratching or rubbing causes inflammation and pruritus → continued scratching.
- Secondary forms begin as a pruritic skin disease that evolves into neurodermatitis after resolution of the primary dermatitis. Precursor dermatoses include atopic dermatitis, contact dermatitis, lichen planus, stasis dermatitis, psoriasis, fungal infections, and insect bites.
- There is a possible relation between disease development and underlying neuropathy, particularly radiculopathy or nerve root compression.
- Pruritus-specific C neurons are temperature sensitive, which may explain itching that occurs in warm environments.

RISK FACTORS
- Anxiety disorders
- Dry skin
- Insect bites

GENERAL PREVENTION
Avoid common triggers such as psychological distress, environmental factors such as heat and excessive dryness, skin irritation, and the development of pruritic dermatoses.

COMMONLY ASSOCIATED CONDITIONS
- Prurigo nodularis is a nodular variety of the same disease process.
- Atopic dermatitis
- Anxiety, depression, and obsessive–compulsive disorders

DIAGNOSIS

HISTORY
- Gradual onset
- Begins as a localized area of pruritus
- Most patients acknowledge that they respond with vigorous rubbing, itching, or scratching, which brings temporary satisfaction.
- Pruritus is typically paroxysmal, worse at night, and may lead to scratching during sleep.

PHYSICAL EXAM
- Well-defined plaques of thickened skin with varying amounts of overlying excoriation or scaling
- Accentuation of normal skin lines (lichenification)
- In cases of long-standing duration, hyperpigmentation or hypopigmentation can be seen.
- Scarring may result following ulcer formation or secondary infection.
- Most commonly involves easily accessible areas:
  – Lateral portions of lower legs/ankles
  – Nape of neck
  – Vulva/Scrotum/Anus
  – Extensor surfaces of forearms
  – Scalp

DIFFERENTIAL DIAGNOSIS
- Psoriasis
- Atopic dermatitis
- Contact, irritant, or stasis dermatitis
- Extramammary Paget disease
- Lichen planus
- Mycosis fungoides
- Lichen amyloidosis
- Fungal infection
- Nummular eczema

DIAGNOSTIC TESTS & INTERPRETATION
Initial Tests (lab, imaging)
- None is diagnostic
- Microscopy and culture preparation may be helpful in identifying a superimposed bacterial or fungal infection.

Diagnostic Procedures/Other
- Skin biopsy to identify characteristic changes on pathology can be beneficial if the diagnosis is in question.
- Patch testing may be used to rule out a contact dermatitis.

Test Interpretation
- Hyperkeratosis
- Acanthosis
- Lengthening of rete ridges
- Hyperplasia of all components of epidermis
- Mild to moderate lymphohistocytic inflammatory infiltrate with prominent lichenification

TREATMENT

GENERAL MEASURES
- Patient education
- Treat pruritus to interrupt the scratch–itch cycle:

  – Itching may occur at night while the patient is asleep; occlusion may be helpful in these cases.
- Treat underlying pruritic skin conditions.

MEDICATION
First Line
- Reducing inflammation:
  – Topical steroids are first-line agents.
  – High-potency steroids alone, such as 0.05% betamethasone dipropionate cream or 0.05% clobetasol propionate cream, can be used initially but not on the face, anogenital region, or intertriginous areas. They should be used on small areas only, for no longer than 2 weeks except under the close supervision of a physician.
  – Switch to intermediate- or low-potency steroids as response allows.
  – An intermediate-potency steroid, such as 0.1% triamcinolone cream, may be used for initial, brief treatment of the face and intertriginous areas, and for maintenance treatment of other areas.
  – A low-potency steroid, such as 1% hydrocortisone cream, should be used for maintenance treatment of the face and intertriginous areas.
  – Steroid tape, flurandrenolide, has optimized penetration and provides a barrier to continued scratching. Change tape once daily.
  – Intralesional steroids, such as triamcinolone acetate, are also safe and effective (1)[C].
  – Contraindications: High-potency topical steroids should not be used on the face or intertriginous areas.
  – Precautions: Topical steroid therapy can cause epidermal and dermal atrophy, as well as hypopigmentation.
- Preventing the itch–scratch cycle:
  – Antipruritic agents, such as 1% menthol preparations and pramoxine
  – 1st-generation oral antihistamines such as diphenhydramine and hydroxyzine for antipruritic and sedative effects
  – Sedating tricyclics, such as doxepin and amitriptyline, for nighttime itching

Second Line
All recommendations:
- Topical aspirin has been shown to be helpful in treating neurodermatitis.
- Topical 5% doxepin cream has significant antipruritic activity.
- Topical capsaicin cream can be helpful for treatment of early disease manifestations.
- A case report showed that topical 0.1% tacrolimus was effective in treating lichen simplex chronicus of the face.

- Topical pimecrolimus may decrease the symptoms of vulvar lichen simplex chronicus.
- Gabapentin was found to decrease symptoms in patients who are nonresponsive to steroids.
- Botulinum toxin injected intradermally has been reported to improve symptoms in patients with recalcitrant pruritus.
- Transcutaneous electrical nerve stimulation may relieve pruritus in patients for whom topical steroids were not effective.
- SSRIs may be effective in controlling compulsive scratching.

ISSUES FOR REFERRAL
- No response to treatment
- Presence of signs and symptoms suggestive of a systemic cause of pruritus
- Consultation with a psychiatrist for patients with severe stress, anxiety, or compulsive scratching
- Consultation with an allergist for patients with multisystemic atopic symptoms

ADDITIONAL THERAPIES
- Cooling of the skin with ice or cold compresses
- Soaks and lubricants to improve barrier layer function
- Provide barrier protection with bandages or Unna boots
- Nail trimming

COMPLEMENTARY AND ALTERNATIVE MEDICINE
- Cognitive-behavioral therapy may improve awareness and help to identify coping strategies (2)[C].
- Hypnosis may be beneficial in decreasing pruritus and preventing scratching (2)[C].
- Homeopathic remedies (i.e., thuja and graphites) have been utilized.

 ONGOING CARE

FOLLOW-UP RECOMMENDATIONS
Patient Monitoring
Patients should be followed closely and regularly for response to therapy, complications from therapy, and secondary infections.

DIET
Regular balanced diet

PATIENT EDUCATION
- Patients should understand the cause of this disease and their role in its resolution:
  - Emphasize that scratching and rubbing must stop for lesions to heal.
- Stress reduction techniques can be useful for patients for whom stress plays a role.
- Avoid exposure to known triggers.

PROGNOSIS
- Often chronic and recurrent
- Good prognosis if the itch–scratch cycle can be broken
- After healing, the skin should return to normal appearance but may also retain accentuated skin markings or postinflammatory hyperpigmentation.
- Postinflammatory pigmentary changes may be slow to resolve.

COMPLICATIONS
- Secondary infection
- Scarring is rare.
- Complications related to therapy, as mentioned in medication precautions
- Squamous cell carcinoma within affected regions is rare.

REFERENCES
1. Richards RN. Update on intralesional steroid: Focus of dermatoses. *J Cutan Med Surg.* 2010;14:19–23.
2. Shenefelt PD. Biofeedback, cognitive-behavioral methods, and hypnosis in dermatology: Is it all in your mind? *Dermatol Ther.* 2003;16:114–122.

ADDITIONAL READING
- Aschoff R, Wozel G. Topical tacrolimus for the treatment of lichen simplex chronicus. *J Dermatolog Treat.* 2007;18:115–117.
- Datz B, Yawalkar S. A double-blind, multicenter trial of 0.05% halobetasol propionate ointment and 0.05% clobetasol 17-propionate ointment in the treatment of patients with chronic, localized atopic dermatitis or lichen simplex chronicus. *J Am Acad Dermatol.* 1991;25(6 Pt 2):1157–1160.
- Drake LA, Millikan LE. The antipruritic effect of 5% doxepin cream in patients with eczematous dermatitis. Doxepin Study Group. *Arch Dermatol.* 1995;131:1403–1408.
- Engin B, Tufekci O, Yazici A, et al. The effect of transcutaneous electrical nerve stimulation in the treatment of lichen simplex: A prospective study. *Clin Exp Dermatol.* 2009;34:324–328.
- Gencoglan G, Inanir I, Gunduz K. Therapeutic hotline: Treatment of prurigo nodularis and lichen simplex chronicus with gabapentin. *Dermatol Ther.* 2010;23:194–198.
- Goldstein AT, Parneix-Spake A, McCormick CL, et al. Pimecrolimus cream 1% for treatment of vulvar lichen simplex chronicus: An open-label, preliminary trial. *Gynecol Obstet Invest.* 2007;64:180–186.
- Heckmann M, Heyer G, Brunner B, et al. Botulinum toxin type A injection in the treatment of lichen simplex: An open pilot study. *J Am Acad Dermatol.* 2002;46:617–619.
- Hercogová J. Topical anti-itch therapy. *Dermatol Ther.* 2005;18:341–343.
- Kantor GR, Resnik KS. Treatment of lichen simplex chronicus with topical capsaicin cream. *Acta Derm Venereol.* 1996;76:161.
- Kirtak N, Inaloz HS, Akçali C, et al. Association of serotonin transporter gene-linked polymorphic region and variable number of tandem repeat polymorphism of the serotonin transporter gene in lichen simplex chronicus patients with psychiatric status. *Int J Dermatol.* 2008;47:1069–1072.
- Konuk N, Koca R, Atik L, et al. Psychopathology, depression and dissociative experiences in patients with lichen simplex chronicus. *Gen Hosp Psychiatry.* 2007;29:232–235.
- Lotti T, Buggiani G, Prignano F. Prurigo nodularis and lichen simplex chronicus. *Dermatol Ther.* 2008;21:42–46.
- Lynch PJ. Lichen simplex chronicus (atopic/neurodermatitis) of the anogenital region. *Dermatol Ther.* 2004;17:8–19.
- Rajalakshmi R, Thappa DM, Jaisankar TJ, et al. Lichen simplex chronicus of anogenital region: A clinico-etiological study. *Indian J Dermatol Venereol Leprol.* 2011;77:28–36.
- Solak O, Kulac M, Yaman M, et al. Lichen simplex chronicus as a symptom of neuropathy. *Clin Exp Dermatol.* 2009;34:476–480.
- Wu M, Wang Y, Bu W, et al. Squamous cell carcinoma arising in lichen simplex chronicus. *Eur J Dermatol.* 2010;20:858–859.
- Yosipovitch G, Sugeng MW, Chan YH, et al. The effect of topically applied aspirin on localized circumscribed neurodermatitis. *J Am Acad Dermatol.* 2001;45:910–913.
- Yüksek J, Sezer E, Aksu M, et al. Transcutaneous electrical nerve stimulation for reduction of pruritus in macular amyloidosis and lichen simplex. *J Dermatol.* 2011;38:546–552.

 CODES

ICD10
L28.0 Lichen simplex chronicus

CLINICAL PEARLS
- Primary lichen simplex chronicus originates de novo, whereas secondary lichen simplex chronicus occurs in the setting of a pruritic dermatologic condition.
- This is a chronic inflammatory condition that results from repeated scratching and rubbing.
- The diagnosis is made clinically, based on history and skin examination.
- If the diagnosis is unclear, consider empiric treatment with close monitoring or skin biopsy.
- Stopping the itch–scratch cycle through patient education, skin lubrication, and topical antipruritic medications is key.

LIPOMA

Manjula Cherukuri, MD, FAAFP

BASICS

DESCRIPTION
- Lipomas are the most common benign SC tumors.
- They are composed of mature fat cells, enveloped by a thin, fibrous capsule.
- Slow growing, often asymptomatic, and usually have a soft doughy feel on palpation
- Some lipomas are believed to have developed following blunt trauma.
- Lipomas rarely, if ever, become malignant, but must be differentiated from liposarcomas and other tumors.

EPIDEMIOLOGY
- They can occur at any age, but are most common in middle-aged adults, peaking in the 40–60-year group.
- They are rare in children.

Incidence
The incidence of lipomas is 1/1,000 individuals annually.

Prevalence
Occur in ~1% of population

ETIOLOGY AND PATHOPHYSIOLOGY
- The pathogenetic link between soft-tissue trauma and the formation of posttraumatic lipomas is still controversial.
- There are 2 potential explanations to correlate soft-tissue trauma and adipose tissue tumor growth:
  – Formation of so-called posttraumatic pseudolipomas by prolapsing adipose tissue through fascia resulting from direct impact
  – Lipoma formation as a result of preadipocyte differentiation and proliferation mediated by cytokine release following soft-tissue trauma and hematoma formation.
- They are reported to occur after trauma, but most are idiopathic.

Genetics
- May appear as a hereditary syndrome in patients with hereditary multiple lipomatosis, an autosomal dominant condition. This is found most frequently in men, characterized by extensive, symmetric, sometimes giant lipomas, mostly on extremities and trunk.
- Congenital lipomas have been observed in children.

RISK FACTORS
- Soft-tissue trauma frequently has been cited as a cause, especially if the patient develops a posttraumatic hematoma.
- Alcohol consumption may be a predisposing factor for Madelung disease or benign symmetric lipomatosis, with lipomas on the head, neck, shoulders, and proximal upper extremities. This may present with the characteristic "horse collar" cervical appearance, resulting in swallowing or respiratory problems and sudden death.

COMMONLY ASSOCIATED CONDITIONS
- Admixture of other tissue types leads to fibrolipomas, angiolipomas, and myolipomas.
- Unusual presentations of lipoma can occur, like giant lipomas in hereditary multiple lipomatosis, adiposis dolorosa (multiple tender, diffuse lesions), Gardner syndrome with intestinal polyposis, and Madelung disease (numerous symmetrically distributed lipomas of the upper trunk).
- Liposarcomas rarely develop from benign lipomas. They can occur anywhere in the body, mostly in deep structures.

DIAGNOSIS

HISTORY
- Useful questions on history gathering are duration, associated symptoms, tenderness, recurrence, progression, similar lesions, and weight loss.
- Generally slow growing; may take years to be noticed
- If fast growing, may indicate a liposarcoma
- Individuals can have single lesions or a few. In ~5% of cases, patients have multiple lesions.
- Lipomas are usually SC and often found in the upper trunk, especially the shoulders, back, neck, and head, but can be anywhere in or on the body.
- Lipomas have been reported in anatomic locations as varied as cardiac, intrathoracic, endobronchial, retroperitoneal, breast, intermuscular, calf, thigh, scapular, intraosseous, fingers, palmar, toe, epidural, spinal, intra-articular (knee), parapharyngeal, nasopharyngeal, adrenal, inguinal, bladder, scrotal, ovarian, intracranial, intraneural, and GI tract (most often in the ileum).
- Usually asymptomatic
- Infrequently may cause pain; seen with angiolipoma, a highly vascular lipoma
- Depending on location, lipomas can cause respiratory distress due to bronchial obstruction if in major airways or can cause cord compression if in dural/medullary components of the spinal cord.
- Neuropathic symptoms from compression may develop (mass effect from lipoma) in locations such as the forearm or ankle.
- In the GI tract, lipomas can present as submucosal fatty tumors. The most common locations include the esophagus, stomach, and small intestine. Symptoms may occur from luminal obstruction or bleeding.
- Most often, patients show lipomas to physicians for explanation and reassurance.
- They may be 1st noted by physicians on a physical exam.

PHYSICAL EXAM
- Lipomas are usually soft, homogeneous, oval, and nontender, and the overlying skin is mobile over them.
- They are commonly from 1–5 cm in diameter. If larger, this raises suspicion for liposarcoma.
- Rubbery or doughy consistency; if harder, suspect liposarcoma, sebaceous (epidermoid) cyst, or abscess.
- Overlying skin is normal; if erythematous, might indicate an abscess.
- The tumor will be felt to slip out from under your fingers ("slippage sign") as opposed to a sebaceous cyst or an abscess, which is tethered by surrounding induration.

DIFFERENTIAL DIAGNOSIS
- Differential diagnosis includes epidermoid cyst (sebaceous cyst), hematoma, vasculitis, panniculitis, rheumatic nodules, metastatic disease, or infections.
- Sebaceous (epidermoid) cysts are also rounded and SC. They can be differentiated from lipomas by their characteristic central punctum and surrounding induration.
- Abscess typically has pain, along with overlying induration and erythema.
- Benign lipomas must be differentiated from liposarcomas. Rapid growth and hard consistency should prompt consideration of malignancy.

DIAGNOSTIC TESTS & INTERPRETATION
Most SC lipomas can be diagnosed based on history and physical, and no imaging studies are required.

Initial Tests (lab, imaging)
- MRI and CT scan are used mostly for atypical locations and as a preoperative measure.
- Because of differences in treatment, prognosis, and long-term follow up, it is important to preoperatively distinguish simple lipomas from well-differentiated liposarcomas.
- MRI is extremely sensitive in the detection of well-differentiated liposarcomas and very specific in the diagnosis of simple lipomas. When an extremity or body wall lesion is considered suspicious for well-differentiated liposarcoma, it is more likely (64%) to represent 1 of many benign lipoma variants (1).
- Reported MRI findings suggestive of liposarcoma include a partially ill-defined margin, neurovascular involvement, enhancing thick/nodular septum, and a partially bright signal intensity on T_1-weighted images. A thick/nodular septum was identified as the most statistically significant predictor of liposarcoma (2).
- If liposarcoma is suspected, fine- and core-needle aspirations have been proposed along with imaging. A core-needle biopsy has been proposed as the preferred biopsy method; it can provide accurate diagnosis and assessment of malignant potential and grade if examined by an experienced pathologist (3).

Diagnostic Procedures/Other
If diagnosis is uncertain, excisional biopsy is a preferred assessment tool.

Test Interpretation
- Lipomas are composed of adipose tissue, with varying amounts of a network of connective tissue.
- Lipomas are surrounded by a fibrous, well-defined capsule that is separate from the surrounding tissue.
- Lipomas differ from normal fat, with increased levels of lipoprotein lipase and a larger number of precursor cells.

TREATMENT

- Most lipomas can be observed without treatment (4)[C].
- Treat if diagnostic uncertainty, hard consistency on palpation, rapid growth, associated pain, compression of nerves/vital organs, or cosmetic concern.
- Treatment of lipoma varies from nonsurgical treatments like steroid injection or liposuction, which can be cosmetically useful in certain locations (such as facial), or surgical treatments like excision or enucleation by "squeeze technique" (4)[C].
- A successful trial of lipomas treated with SC deoxycholate injections has been reported, suggesting that low-concentration deoxycholate may be a relatively safe and effective treatment for small collections of fat. However, controlled clinical trials will be necessary to substantiate these observations (5)[C].
- Spinal lipomas should be operated on as soon as possible on a prophylactic basis, and careful and constant follow up should be carried out to permit prompt reintervention in cases with deterioration (6)[C].

SURGERY/OTHER PROCEDURES
- Plan the incision to follow skin lines, if possible, to minimize scarring. Use a surgical marker to draw out the palpable margins of the lipoma and the planned incision. The incision should be ~60% of the lipoma width. Be prepared to extend the incision if needed.
- After anesthetizing the skin with a local anesthetic, a linear incision is carried out down to the level of the capsule using a number 11 or 15 blade.
- Blunt dissection (curved hemostat) and sharp dissection (iris scissor) are used to separate the fibrous capsule from the surrounding soft tissue. Care must be taken not to invade the capsule to maintain proper aesthetics.
- As the lobule is lifted, the dissection is continued to free up the entire tumor.
- Apply pressure to the outside of the lipoma to express it through the skin opening (7)[C]. In many cases, the lipoma will simply pop out. If not, more dissection may be needed or the incision may be lengthened.
- After the lipoma is out, pressure with gauze is usually all that is needed to obtain good hemostasis. If bleeding persists, use electrocoagulation before closing the incision.
- The dead space may be closed with deep absorbable sutures, but often this is not necessary.
- The skin may be closed with nonabsorbable simple interrupted sutures. For small lipomas, closure may be performed with wound-closure strips or the linear incision left open.
- If excessive skin remains, the linear incision can be turned into an ellipse to avoid redundant skin.

ONGOING CARE

FOLLOW-UP RECOMMENDATIONS
Usual surgical follow up is needed to monitor for any complications, such as hematoma formation or infection.

PATIENT EDUCATION
Handout: "What are lipomas?" *Am Fam Physician*. 2002;65:905. Available at: www.aafp.org/afp/20020301/905ph.html

PROGNOSIS
Most lipomas grow very slowly and are benign, asymptomatic, and remain stable. Recurrence after excision is rare unless excision was incomplete.

COMPLICATIONS
- Hematoma and seroma formation or infection is rare but possible.
- Occasionally, a bilobar lipoma may be missed, resulting in "recurrence." The local recurrence rate of simple lipomas involving SC tissues is ~1–2%.
- Lipomas that grow rapidly or become painful or nodular must be evaluated for liposarcoma.

REFERENCES

1. Gaskin CM, Helms CA. Lipomas, lipoma variants, and well-differentiated liposarcomas (atypical lipomas): Results of MRI evaluations of 126 consecutive fatty masses. *AJR Am J Roentgenol*. 2004;182:733–739.
2. Jaovisidha S, Suvikapakornkul Y, Woratanarat P, et al. MR imaging of fat-containing tumours: The distinction between lipoma and liposarcoma. *Singapore Med J*. 2010;51:418–423.
3. Strauss DC, Qureshi YA, Hayes AJ, et al. The role of core needle biopsy in the diagnosis of suspected soft tissue tumours. *J Surg Oncol*. 2010;102: 523–529.
4. Bancroft LW, Kransdorf MJ, Peterson JJ, et al. Benign fatty tumors: Classification, clinical course, imaging appearance, and treatment. *Skeletal Radiol*. 2006;35:719–733.
5. Rotunda AM, Ablon G, Kolodney MS. Lipomas treated with subcutaneous deoxycholate injections. *J Am Acad Dermatol*. 2005;53:973–978.
6. Jindal A, Mahapatra AK. Spinal lipomatous malformations. *Indian J Pediatr*. 2000;67:342–346.
7. Salam GA. Lipoma excision. *Am Fam Physician*. 2002;65:901–904.

ADDITIONAL READING

- Aust MC, Spies M, Kall S, et al. Posttraumatic lipoma: Fact or fiction? *Skinmed*. 2007;6:266–270.
- Blount JP, Elton S. Spinal lipomas. *Neurosurg Foc*. 2001;10:e3.
- Pandya KA, Radke F. Benign skin lesions: Lipomas, epidermal inclusion cysts, muscle and nerve biopsies. *Surg Clin North Am*. 2009;89:677–687.

CODES

ICD10
- D17.0 Ben lipomatous neoplm of skin, subcu of head, face and neck
- D17.9 Benign lipomatous neoplasm, unspecified
- D17.79 Benign lipomatous neoplasm of other sites

CLINICAL PEARLS
- Lipomas are slow growing, often asymptomatic, and usually diagnosed by palpation.
- Asymptomatic SC lipomas can be followed clinically and only need treatment if they cause pain, are growing rapidly, or causing compression of vital organs/nerves.
- Most symptomatic lipomas are removed surgically, but for small ones, liposuction or steroid injection is reported successful.
- In the SC location, the primary differential diagnosis is a sebaceous (epidermoid) cyst or an abscess.
- Consider referral to subspecialty if a lipoma in a delicate anatomic location needs removal or if there is concern that the lesion might be malignant.

L

LONG QT INTERVAL

Balakumar Pandian, MD

 BASICS

DESCRIPTION

- QT interval: Electrocardiogram (ECG) measurement that measures the duration of repolarization of myocardial cells. Measured from the onset of the QRS complex to the end of the T wave.
- Corrected QT interval (QTc): QT interval corrected for heart rate (duration of repolarization depends on heart rate). See formulas.
- Prolonged QTc is any prolongation from baseline.
  - Normal QTc interval in men <440 msec
  - Normal QTc interval in women <460 msec
  - Normal QTc in children 1–15 years <450 msec
- Most cases of prolonged QT are acquired, but genetic mutations can also cause hereditary long QT syndromes (LQTS).
- Prolonged QTc from any cause can precipitate polymorphic ventricular tachycardia called torsade de pointes (TdP), leading to dizziness, syncope, and sudden cardiac death from ventricular fibrillation.

EPIDEMIOLOGY

Incidence
Incidence of medication-induced QTc prolongation and torsade de pointes varies with medication and a host of other factors. Exact incidences are difficult to estimate.

Prevalence
- Hereditary LQTS is estimated to occur in 1/2500–1/7000 births (1)
- Five thousand people across the US may die yearly due to LQTS related cardiac arrhythmia (2)

ETIOLOGY AND PATHOPHYSIOLOGY
- Acquired
  - Antiarrhythmic medications (class Ia such as quinidine and procainamide, and class III meds, such as sotalol, and others, such as amiodarone)
  - Electrolyte abnormalities, such as hypokalemia, hypomagnesemia
  - Hypothyroidism
  - Underlying heart disease
  - Antipsychotic medications (haloperidol and, to a lesser extent, the atypical antipsychotics)
  - Tricyclic antidepressants
  - Antibiotics (macrolides and quinolones)
  - Methadone
- Congenital
  - Defective membrane proteins that work as channels for sodium and potassium in myocytes

- Pathophysiology (3)
  - Depolarization of the myocardium results from the rapid influx of sodium through sodium channels and causes myocyte contraction, with resulting cardiac muscle contraction and systole (seen on ECG as the QRS complex).
  - During repolarization, there is an efflux of potassium from the cell through both rapid (I_{Kr}) and slow (I_{Ks}) potassium channels. The T wave on an ECG represents myocyte repolarization.
  - Normally, as the heart rate increases, repolarization speeds up (and QT interval is shortened accordingly). Calculating the QTc accounts for the heart rate to measure the QT interval more accurately.
  - Medications, medical conditions, electrolyte disturbances, and genetic mutations that affect functioning of these membrane channels can cause delayed repolarization.
  - Delayed repolarization can lead to a propensity for re-entry and initiate torsades de pointes.
  - Torsades de pointes type rhythm may be self-limited, but symptomatic (syncope or near syncope). It can also degrade into ventricular fibrillation.

Genetics
- 12 different genes have been linked to LQTS (2).
- Incomplete penetrance makes both diagnosis and management of asymptomatic disease challenging.
- LQTS 1 (42–54%) is the most common. Mutation causes a defect in the I_{Ks} transport protein. Arrhythmias can be triggered by tachycardia due to exercise (swimming seems to be especially problematic) and other high catecholamine states.
- LQTS 2 (35–45%) is a defect in the I_{Kr} transport protein that is sensitive to catecholamine surges. Sudden loud noises or emotional arousal can provoke arrhythmias.
- LQTS 3 (8%) is a defect in the sodium channel that allows an excess of sodium into the cell, increasing repolarization time. Arrhythmias tend to manifest more during rest or sleep (3).
- Jervell and Lange-Nielsen syndrome: Autosomal recessive form of LQTS that features homozygous mutations that affect the I_{Ks} channel and presents with severe form of LQTS1. Features also include deafness.
- Romano-Ward syndrome: Autosomal dominant form of LQTS with variable penetrance. Hearing is normal.

RISK FACTORS
- Female
- QTc >500 msec
- History of syncope or presyncope
- History of torsades de pointes
- Bradycardia in acquired QTc prolongation
- Medications that cause QTc prolongation
  - High doses
  - Fast infusions
  - Combination of medications
- Electrolyte abnormalities
  - Hypokalemia
  - Hypomagnesemia
  - Hypocalcemia
- For hereditary LQTS
  - Catecholamine surges from exercise (especially swimming), emotional stress, loud noises

GENERAL PREVENTION
- Avoid (or use with caution) causative medications.
- Avoid combinations of medications that can have additive effects on the QTc.
- Replete electrolytes
- Treat underlying medical disease (hypothyroidism, cardiac disease).
- Avoid strenuous sports in LQTS.
- Avoid sudden loud noises in LQTS (alarm clocks, doorbells, telephones).

 DIAGNOSIS

HISTORY
- Evaluate for syncope, near syncope, and associated precipitating events.
- Evaluate for history of seizures in patient or in family (tonic–clonic movement may due to cerebral hypoperfusion during episodes of ventricular arrhythmia or due to seizure-like activity during a syncopal episode).
- Detailed medication history
- Evaluate for family history of sudden death, syncope.
- Congenital deafness

PHYSICAL EXAM
- Usually normal physical exam
- If underlying cardiac disease present, may have findings specific to cardiac condition
- Evaluate for signs of hypothyroidism.
- Congenital deafness may be present in some forms of LQTS.

DIAGNOSTIC TESTS & INTERPRETATION
Initial Tests (lab, imaging)
- Electrocardiogram
- Metabolic panel
- Calcium level
- Magnesium level
- TSH

Follow-Up Tests & Special Considerations
- Echocardiogram to evaluate for cardiomyopathy
- Outpatient cardiac rhythm monitoring
- Consider cardiac stress testing to evaluate for QTc interval changes and/or to evaluate for coronary artery disease.
  – Genetic testing for LQTS mutations

Test Interpretation
- QTc calculation using ECG is best done by measuring the QT interval in lead II and measuring the RR interval immediately preceding this QT interval. The easiest and most commonly used formula to calculate QTc is the Bazett formula, although it has its limitations (It overcorrects for tachycardia and under corrects with bradycardia).
- Bazett formula: $QTc = QT / RR$ (all measurements in seconds) (4)
- U wave is not included in the calculation unless it is merged in with the T wave and is 50% of the T wave amplitude (2).

TREATMENT

GENERAL MEASURES
- Ventricular tachycardia (VT), torsades de pointes(TdP) and ventricular fibrillation (VF) should be treated emergently as per ACLS guidelines.
- Cardiac pacing may be needed emergently for drug-induced torsade de pointes to prevent bradycardia.

MEDICATION
First Line
- For torsades de pointes: Magnesium sulfate 2 g infused over 1–2 minutes. May repeat twice every 5–15 minutes. May start a magnesium sulfate drip at 3–10 mg/min if needed. Monitor for magnesium toxicity in those with renal insufficiency.
- Propranolol 40 mg PO twice daily (max: 640 mg/day) has been shown to be more efficacious than other beta blockers for management of LQTS 1 and LQTS 2. Beta blockers are effective in decreasing (but not eliminating) the risk of fatal arrhythmias. Minimal effect of beta blockers is seen in those with LQTS3 (5)

Second Line
Nadolol 40 mg PO once daily (max: 320 mg/day) may also be used (5).

ISSUES FOR REFERRAL
- Refer to cardiologist for establishing diagnosis, especially for hereditary LQTS.
- Symptomatic prolonged QT

SURGERY/OTHER PROCEDURES
- Implanted cardioverter-defibrillator for those with a history of major cardiac events
- Left cervical-thoracic sympathetic denervation was used for symptomatic LQTS prior to the advent of beta blockers. It is still an option for those patients with LQTS who are refractory to beta blocker therapy.

IN-PATIENT CONSIDERATIONS
Admission Criteria/Initial Stabilization
- Patients with TdP, VT, and VF should be promptly treated as per ACLS guidelines. Correct electrolytes on an emergent basis. Evaluate for acquired QT prolongation. If no cause is found, consider hereditary LQTS.
- Patients with prolonged QTc and syncope, near syncope should be monitored on telemetry during evaluation.
- Monitor ECG if initiating medications or combining medications that may prolong QT.
- Monitor electrolytes and urgently treat hypokalemia, hypomagnesemia, and hypokalemia in those with significantly prolonged QT.

Nursing
For those who have LQTS type 2, avoid sudden loud noises.

 ONGOING CARE

FOLLOW-UP RECOMMENDATIONS
On routine visits, ask about syncope, pre-syncope and palpitations in those who have QTc prolongation.
- Patient monitoring: Consider ECG and/or outpatient cardiac rhythm monitoring with any medication additions or dosage changes that may cause further prolongation of the QTc.
- For those who may have symptomatic QTc prolongation of any cause, prompt evaluation is warranted.
- Check labs for electrolyte imbalances as needed.

PATIENT EDUCATION
- Educate patients with QTc prolongation about medications side effects and possibility of medication interactions.
- Patients with congenital forms of LQTS should be aware of, and avoid situations that may trigger, torsades (depending on their specific gene mutation).

REFERENCES
1. Levine E, Rosero S, Budzikowski AS, et al. Congenital long QT syndrome: Considerations for primary care physicians. *Clev Clin J Med.* 2008;8:591–600.
2. Webster G, Berul C. Congenital long-QT syndromes: A clinical and genetic update from infancy through adulthood. *TCM.* 2008;6:216–224.
3. Morita H, Wu J. The QT syndromes: Long and short. *The Lancet.* 2008;372:750–763.
4. Yap Y, Camm A. Drug induced QT prolongation and torsades de pointes. *Heart.* 2003;89:1363–1372.
5. Chockalingam P, Crotti L, Girardengo G, et al. Not all beta-blockers are equal in the management of long QT syndrome types 1 and 2. Higher recurrence of events under metoprolol. *J Am Coll Cardiol.* 2012;20:2092–2099.

 SEE ALSO

www.qtdrugs.org (for lists of drugs that can affect the QT interval)

 CODES

ICD10
I45.81 Long QT syndrome

CLINICAL PEARLS
- Evaluate the corrected QT interval (QTc)/
- For accurate diagnosis, calculate QTc manually.
- Magnesium sulfate is the treatment of choice during ACLS for torsades de pointes.
- Beta blockers are initial treatment of choice for hereditary LQTS.

L

LUMBAR (INTERVERTEBRAL) DISC DISORDERS

Sheldon C. Yao, DO • John P. Flaherty, DO

 BASICS

DESCRIPTION

- Lumbar disc degeneration is a common age-related process that can lead to chronic debilitating pain with significant negative effects on quality of life.
- Degeneration may be histologically evident as early as 15 years of age and, once initiated, is a progressive and irreversible process modified by a variety of intrinsic and extrinsic factors (1)[B].
- This process eventually leads to radiologically evident degeneration of disc structures: Herniation, collapse, nerve impingement, intervertebral narrowing, and osteophyte formation.
- Low back pain may be categorized into four groups: Mechanical (80–90%), neurologic involvement (5–15%), specific spinal pathology (1–2%), nonspinal origin (1–3%) (2)[A].
- Chronic low back pain is defined by low back pain that persists of over a 3-month period (2)[A].
- Initial management should be handled in the primary care setting and based on the extent of symptoms, disability, and goals of the patient.
- Pain should be considered in a biopsychosocial context, modified by the patient's beliefs, coping strategies, distress, and social interactions (2)[A].
- Diagnosis should integrate a focused history, physical exam, psychosocial factors, and correlated radiologic findings.
- Predictors of persistent disabling low back pain include maladaptive pain coping skills, nonorganic signs, functional impairment, general health status, and psychiatric comorbidities.
- System(s) affected: Musculoskeletal; Nervous; Psychiatric
- Synonym(s): Degenerative disc disease; Intervertebral disc dislocation; Herniated disc; Herniated nucleus pulposus

EPIDEMIOLOGY

Incidence
- Low back pain is the 5th most common reason for physician visits in the US, with direct and indirect costs estimated at $118 per year.
- Accounts for 2.3% of all physician visits, with an annual incidence rate of 5–8%.
- Among patients with acute back pain, only 4% have nerve root symptoms due to a herniated disc.

Prevalence
- An estimated 33% of individuals age <40 years and nearly all individuals 60–80 years will have identifiable disc degeneration on MRI. *Most lesions will be asymptomatic.*
- Lifetime prevalence of low back pain is 70–80%, with disc degeneration as a potential cause.

Pediatric Considerations
May emerge rapidly after adolescence, leading to significant and chronic low back pain. No evidence-based standard of care. Usually involves NSAIDs, physical therapy, and potential lumbosacral brace.

Pregnancy Considerations
Increased incidence of low back pain, sacroiliac dysfunction, and/or sciatica. Conservative management.

Geriatric Considerations
Usually multifactorial, disc degeneration, lesions of spine, spondylolisthesis, spinal stenosis, and osteoporotic fractures

ETIOLOGY AND PATHOPHYSIOLOGY

- Age-dependent reduction of cellular maintenance of disc structural matrix. Progressive degeneration of disc plate, nucleus, and annulus. This process is modified by intrinsic and extrinsic factors; genetics, metabolic, mechanical, toxic, and nutritional (1)[B].
- Degenerative changes have a significant influence on biomechanic and kinematic lumbar functions.
- Symptomatic degenerative disc disease results from inflammatory irritation of adjacent tissues (ligament, nerve root, and vertebrae) or compression of structures (bulging disc, herniated nucleus pulposus, degenerative changes of the spine). No studies demonstrate correlation of disc height and symptomatology.

RISK FACTORS

- Normal aging process following adolescence
- Smoking
- Genetics
- Elevated BMI
- Osteoporosis
- Occupational: Prolonged standing, heavy lifting, vibrating tools
- Low mood or somatization
- Trauma: Major or minor

GENERAL PREVENTION

- Most episodes of low back pain are not preventable.
- Modification of occupational risk factors
- Management of bone mineral density, diabetes mellitus, and BMI
- Smoking cessation or reduced exposure
- Routine exercise

COMMONLY ASSOCIATED CONDITIONS

- Obesity
- Diabetes mellitus
- Osteoarthritis
- Osteoporosis
- Depression

DIAGNOSIS

HISTORY

- Assess location, onset, aggravating/relieving factors, and associated symptoms. Establish baseline pain and functional deficits (3)[A].
- Red flags: May indicate a more serious etiology:
  – Cauda equina syndrome: Saddle anesthesia, bladder dysfunction, neurologic deficits in lower extremities
  – Fracture: Major/minor trauma, strenuous lifting, steroid use, osteoporosis
  – Cancer: Age >50 or <20, weight loss, severe nighttime pain
  – Infection: IV drug use, skin infection, UTI, immunosuppression
- Yellow flags: Indicate risk for development of prolonged pain
  – Depression, impaired global function, job dissatisfaction, disputed compensation claims

PHYSICAL EXAM

- Assess gait, posture, range of motion, reflexes, dermatomal sensation, and strength (toe walk, heal walk).
- Palpate and assess bony landmarks.
- For radiculopathy:
  – Straight leg raise (SLR) test: (sensitivity = 0.91; specificity = 0.26)
  – Crossed SLR test: (sensitivity = 0.29; specificity = 0.88)
  – Positive results of femoral stretch test, crossed femoral stretch test, medial ankle pin prick, patellar reflex support midlumbar (L2-4) impingement, especially when used in combination (4)[B].
  – Loss of Achilles reflex supports lower lumbar (L5-S1) impingement (4)[B].
  – Combined femoral stretch test, patellar reflex, medial ankle sensation, crossed femoral stretch test support L4 impingement (4)[B].

DIFFERENTIAL DIAGNOSIS

- Acute or chronic lumbosacral strain
- Facet joint disease
- Piriformis syndrome
- Spondylosis
- Spondylolisthesis
- Spinal arthritis
- Sciatica
- Fibromyalgia
- Compression fracture
- Metastatic and primary tumors
- Vertebral infection
- Pain referred from hip, retroperitoneum, aneurysms, or pelvis; neurogenic claudication
- Cauda equina syndrome

DIAGNOSTIC TESTS & INTERPRETATION

Initial Tests (lab, imaging)
- Labs indicated if red flags are present or organic causes are suspected. CBC, ESR, or C-reactive protein (elevation may signify infection, autoimmune arthropathy, or cancer).
- Urinalysis if suspecting urinary system etiology.
- *Initial imaging and routine imaging are rarely indicated.* MRI preferred over CT.
  – Indicated in patients presenting with red flags, severe progressive neurologic deficits, or failed conservative care at 6 weeks.

Follow-Up Tests & Special Considerations
- Lumbosacral plain films: Rarely indicated; may identify tumor, vertebral compression fracture, osteoarthritis, spondylolisthesis
- Lumbar MRIs on asymptomatic individuals regularly find disc herniation (33%) and disc bulging (>50%).
- Degenerative findings in asymptomatic patients on MRI is not reliably predictive of development or duration of future symptomatology.
- Negative MRI is the only significant indicator to decrease diagnostic likelihood of discogenic pain.

Diagnostic Procedures/Other
- Myelograms are not common (used for surgical candidate evaluation or to help rule out more serious etiology).
- Electromyography may be useful to distinguish peripheral neuropathy from cord or nerve root impairment and may confirm level of lesion.

LUMBAR (INTERVERTEBRAL) DISC DISORDERS

Test Interpretation

Difficult to distinguish the normal aging process of disc degeneration from specific lesions causing low back pain and sciatica. Must correlate history, physical exam, and radiologic findings.

 TREATMENT

GENERAL MEASURES

- Initial conservative therapy is recommended for 6 weeks. Self-care: Daily activities as tolerated, local heat, exercise, avoid bed rest beyond a few days. Consider also: Analgesics as needed, physical therapy, spinal manipulation (3)[A].
- Failed conservative management past 6 weeks, consider re-evaluation and imaging studies.
- Patients with significant radicular symptoms that fail to resolve after 6 weeks conservative care may be considered for epidural steroid injections (5)[A].
- Surgery should be considered in patients with chronic low back pain that has failed prolonged conservative care (2)[A].
- Discussion is recommended at each stage of patient care to address expectations, risks, and short- and long-term benefits (3)[A].

MEDICATION

First Line

Analgesia with acetaminophen or NSAIDs (with consideration of side effect profile), muscle relaxants for acute pain only (2)[A].

Second Line

- May consider short- or long-term use of mild opiates or tramadol (2)[A].
- Epidural steroid injection indicated only for patients with persistent radicular pain (2)[A].
- Antidepressants: Escitalopram or duloxetine (2)[A].
- Gabapentin or pregabalin effective when combined with NSAID or opiate (2)[A].

ISSUES FOR REFERRAL

- Emergent surgical referral for cauda equina syndrome: Urinary incontinence (90% sensitivity)
- Underlying organic disease (fracture, cancer, infection)
- Progressive, persistent, severe neurologic deficit or pain

SURGERY/OTHER PROCEDURES

- Absolute indications: Cauda equina syndrome, multiple episodes of radiculopathy, progressive severe neurologic deficit, and persistent dysfunctional pain
- Decompressive surgery (open discectomy, microdiscectomy, laminectomy): For patients with neurologic impingement such as spinal stenosis or disc herniation. Most evidence supports minimally invasive approach (2)[A].
- Disc arthroplasty (disc prosthesis): Appropriate for patients with degenerative changes confined to one localized lesion (2)[A]. Contraindications include vertebral abnormalities, nerve root compression, and spinal stenosis (1)[B].
- Spinal fusion: Indicated for unstable vertebral segment caused by severe degenerative changes.
- Chemonucleolysis: Limited evidence. Enzymatic injection to decrease bulge/herniation.
- Spinal cord stimulation: Limited evidence. Indicated for pain refractory to operative management (2)[A].

COMPLEMENTARY AND ALTERNATIVE MEDICINE

- Manipulation, physical therapy, exercise, acupuncture, and yoga have been shown to be beneficial (3)[A].
- Psychosocial constructs are important mediators for long-term improvement. Consider referral to a psychiatrist.

IN-PATIENT CONSIDERATIONS

Admission Criteria/Initial Stabilization

Inpatient admission uncommon; evaluate for more serious causes, consider pain management consult.

 ONGOING CARE

FOLLOW-UP RECOMMENDATIONS

- Follow up if pain or neurologic deficit is increasing.
- Return visit 10 days to 2 weeks following initial visit.
- Thereafter, monitor every 2–4 weeks until fully functional.

Patient Monitoring

Follow pain level, neurologic status, and preventative care measures.

PATIENT EDUCATION

Encourage exercise, proper posture and body mechanics, avoidance of risk factors.

PROGNOSIS

- Acute low back pain (90%) or radiculopathy (75–90%) can be expected to recover spontaneously within 6 weeks of conservative care.
- 25% of patients treated nonsurgically who had at least 1 month of herniation-induced radicular symptoms will report recurrence within 1 year (6)[B].
- Chronic radicular and nonradicular discogenic low back pain: Most patients respond to conservative management; however, careful selection of surgical candidates leads to satisfactory results (90%). Improved outcomes are associated with the male gender, younger, active individuals, and exercise program initiated weeks 4–6 postop (7)[A].
- A number of studies indicate long-term success rates are poorer (64%). Risk factors for long-term regression include return to work before full postop recovery, occupation requiring manual labor, and low education level.
- Most helpful predictors of persistent disabling low back pain are maladaptive pain coping skills, nonorganic signs, functional impairment, general health status, and psychiatric comorbidities.

COMPLICATIONS

- Foot drop with weakness of anterior tibial, posterior tibial, and peroneal muscles
- Bladder and rectal sphincter weakness, with retention or incontinence
- Limitation of movement, restricted activity, long-term disability, decreased quality of life

REFERENCES

1. Siepe CJ, Heider F, Haas E, et al. Influence of lumbar intervertebral disc degeneration on the outcome of total lumbar disc replacement: A prospective clinical, histological, X-ray and MRI investigation. *Eur Spine J*. 2012;21:2287–2299.
2. Morlion B. Chronic low back pain: Pharmacological interventional and surgical strategies. *Nat Rev Neurol*. 2013;9:462–473.
3. Chou R, Qaseem A, Snow V, et al. Diagnosis and treatment of low back pain: A joint clinical practice guideline from the American College of Physicians and the American Pain Society. *Ann Intern Med*. 2007;147:478–491.
4. Suri P, Rainville J, Katz JN, et al. The accuracy of the physical examination for the diagnosis of midlumbar and low lumbar nerve root impingement. *Spine*. 2011;36:63–73.
5. Chou R, Loeser JD, Owens DK, et al. Interventional therapies, surgery, and interdisciplinary rehabilitation for low back pain: An evidence-based clinical practice guideline from the American Pain Society. *Spine*. 2009;34:1066–1077.
6. Suri P, Rainville J, Hunter DJ, et al. Recurrence of radicular pain or back pain after nonsurgical treatment of symptomatic lumbar disk herniation. *Arch Phys Med Rehabil*. 2012;93:690–695.
7. Schoenfeld AJ, Weiner BK. Treatment of lumbar disc herniation: Evidence-based practice. *Int J Gen Med*. 2010;3:209–214.

 SEE ALSO

- Low Back Pain
- Algorithm: Low Back Pain, Acute

 CODES

ICD10

- M51.06 Intervertebral disc disorders with myelopathy, lumbar region
- M51.26 Other intervertebral disc displacement, lumbar region
- M51.36 Other intervertebral disc degeneration, lumbar region

CLINICAL PEARLS

- In the absence of red flags, the first 6 weeks of care should:
  - Focus on conservative pain management
  - Self-care, such as minimal rest, local heat, and return to daily activities as tolerated
- Initial imaging and routine imaging are rarely indicated.
- Indications for imaging include patients with:
  - Signs/symptoms suggesting red flags
  - Severe, progressive neurologic deficits
  - Failed conservative care at 6 weeks
- Patients with persistent and disabling pain that fails to resolve after prolonged conservative care should be considered for surgical consult.
- Adverse psychosocial factors to resolving back pain: Pending litigation or compensation; depressed or hostile patient; prolonged use of narcotics or alcohol.
- Acute low back pain (90%) or radiculopathy (75–90%) can be expected to recover spontaneously within 6 weeks of conservative care.

713

LUNG, PRIMARY MALIGNANCIES
Maryann R. Cooper, PharmD, BCOP • Gerald Gehr, MD

 BASICS

DESCRIPTION
- Lung cancers (primary) are the leading cause of cancer-related death in the US (estimated 159,480 deaths in 2013, 27% of all cancer-related deaths) (1).
- Divided into 2 broad categories:
  - Non–small-cell lung cancer (NSCLC) (>85% of all lung cancers):
    - Adenocarcinoma (~40% of NSCLC): Most common type in the US, most common type in nonsmokers, metastasizes earlier than squamous cell, poor prognosis; bronchoalveolar, a subtype of adenocarcinoma has better prognosis
    - Squamous cell carcinoma (<25% of NSCLC): Dose-related effect with smoking; slower growing than adenocarcinoma
    - Large cell (~10% of NSCLC): Prognosis similar to adenocarcinoma
  - Small-cell lung cancer (SCLC) (16% of all lung cancers): Centrally located, early metastases, aggressive
- Other: Mesothelioma, carcinoid tumor, and sarcoma
- Staging:
  - NSCLC: Staged from 0–IV based on: Primary tumor (T), lymph node status (N), and presence of metastasis (M)
  - SCLC: Staged based on disease location: Limited to ipsilateral hemithorax (stages I–IIIB); extensive if metastatic beyond hemithorax (stages IIIB and IV)
- Tumor locations: Upper: 60%; lower: 30%; middle: 5%; overlapping and main stem: 5%
- May spread by local extension to involve chest wall, diaphragm, pulmonary vessels, vena cava, phrenic nerve, esophagus, or pericardium
- Most commonly metastasize to lymph nodes (pulmonary, mediastinal), then liver, adrenal, bone (osteolytic), kidney, brain

EPIDEMIOLOGY
Incidence
- Estimated 228,190 new cases in the US in 2013 (1)
- Predominant age: >40 years; peak at 70 years
- Predominant sex: Male > Female

Prevalence
- Most common cancer worldwide
- Lifetime probability (1):
  - Men: 1 in 13
  - Women: 1 in 16

ETIOLOGY AND PATHOPHYSIOLOGY
Multifactorial; see "Risk Factors."

Genetics
NSCLC:
- Oncogenes: Ras family (H-ras, K-ras, N-ras)
- Tumor suppressor genes: Retinoblastoma, *p53*

RISK FACTORS
- Smoking (relative risk [RR] 10–30)
- Secondhand smoke exposure
- Radon
- Environmental and occupational exposures:
  - Asbestos exposure (synergistic increase in risk for smokers)
  - Air pollution
  - Ionizing radiation

- Mutagenic gases (halogen ethers, mustard gas, aromatic hydrocarbons)
- Metals (inorganic arsenic, chromium, nickel)
- Lung scarring from tuberculosis
- Radiation therapy to the breast or chest

GENERAL PREVENTION
- Smoking cessation and prevention programs
- Screening controversial; the risks of screening (e.g., radiation, biopsy) may offset the benefit.
- Consider for high-risk patients, but best approach remains unclear:
  - High-risk patients: Age 55–74 years with a ≥30-pack year history of smoking tobacco, or if a former smoker, quit within 15 years
  - Annual low-dose CT until age 74 years:
    - Decreased lung cancer mortality (but not life expectancy) compared with chest x-ray alone (2)
- Prevention via aggressive smoking-cessation counseling and therapy; a 20–30% risk reduction occurs within 5 years of cessation
- Avoid supplemental β-carotene and vitamin E in smokers
- Avoid hormone replacement therapy in postmenopausal smokers or former smokers (increased risk of death from NSCLC)

COMMONLY ASSOCIATED CONDITIONS
- Paraneoplastic syndromes: Hypertrophic pulmonary osteoarthropathy, Lambert-Eaton syndrome, Cushing syndrome, hypercalcemia from ectopic parathyroid releasing hormone, syndrome of inappropriate antidiuretic hormone (SIADH)
- Hypercoagulable state
- Pancoast syndrome
- Superior vena cava syndrome
- Pleural effusion
- Chronic obstructive pulmonary disease (COPD), other sequelae of cigarette smoking

 DIAGNOSIS

HISTORY
- May be asymptomatic for most of course
- Pulmonary:
  - Cough (new or change in chronic cough)
  - Wheezing and stridor
  - Dyspnea
  - Hemoptysis
  - Pneumonitis (fever and productive cough)
- Constitutional:
  - Malaise
  - Bone pain (metastatic disease)
  - Fatigue
  - Weight loss, anorexia
  - Fever
  - Anemia
  - Clubbing of digits
- Other presentations:
  - Chest pain (dull, pleuritic)
  - Shoulder/arm pain (Pancoast tumors)
  - Dysphagia
  - Plethora (redness of face or neck)
  - Hoarseness (involvement of recurrent laryngeal nerve)
  - Horner syndrome
  - Neurologic abnormalities (e.g., headaches, syncope, weakness, cognitive impairment)
  - Pericardial tamponade (pericardial invasion)

PHYSICAL EXAM
- General: Pain, performance status, weight loss
- Head, eye, ear, nose, throat (HEENT): Horner syndrome, dysphonia, stridor, scleral icterus
- Neck: Supraclavicular/cervical lymph nodes, mass
- Lungs: Effusion, wheezing, airway obstruction, pleural effusion
- Abdomen/Groin: Hepatomegaly or lymphadenopathy
- Extremities: Signs of hypertrophic pulmonary osteoarthropathy, deep venous thrombosis (DVT)
- Neurologic: Rule out cognitive and focal motor defects

DIFFERENTIAL DIAGNOSIS
- COPD (may coexist)
- Granulomatous (tuberculosis, sarcoidosis)
- Cardiomyopathy
- Congestive heart failure (CHF)

DIAGNOSTIC TESTS & INTERPRETATION
Initial Tests (lab, imaging)
- CBC
- BUN, serum creatinine
- Liver function tests (LFTs), LDH
- Electrolytes:
  - Hypercalcemia (Paraneoplastic syndrome)
  - Hyponatremia (SIADH)
- Sputum cytology
- Chest x-ray (CXR) (compare with old films):
  - Nodule or mass, especially if calcified
  - Persistent infiltrate
  - Atelectasis
  - Mediastinal widening
  - Hilar enlargement
  - Pleural effusion
- CT scan of chest (with IV contrast material):
  - Nodule or mass (central or peripheral)
  - Lymphadenopathy
- Evaluation for metastatic disease:
  - Brain MRI: Lesions may be necrotic, bleeding.
  - CT abdomen: Hepatic, adrenal, renal masses
- PET scan: To evaluate metastasis
- Bone scan: Advanced disease or bone pain

Follow-Up Tests & Special Considerations
CBC, BUN, serum creatinine, LFTs prior to each cycle of chemotherapy

Diagnostic Procedures/Other
- Biopsy with pathology review to determine NSCLC vs. SCLC
- In patients with metastatic NSCLC, determination of epidermal growth factor receptor (EGFR)-activating mutations, *KRAS* mutations and *ALK* gene rearrangements
- Pulmonary function tests
- Enlarged mediastinal lymph nodes necessitate staging by mediastinoscopy, video-assisted thoracoscopy, or fine-needle aspiration
- Transbronchial biopsy (Wang needle)
- Bronchoscopy for surgical planning
- Bone marrow aspirate (small cell)
- Cervical mediastinoscopy (the upper, middle peritracheal, and subcarinal lymph nodes)
- Anterior mediastinotomy (the posterior mediastinum and peritracheal, subazygous, hilar, and aortopulmonary window nodal regions)
- Video-assisted thoracoscopy (associated pleural disease and suspected mediastinal nodal spread)

Test Interpretation

Pathologic changes from smoking are progressive: Basal cell proliferation, development of atypical nuclei, stratification, metaplasia of squamous cells, carcinoma in situ, and then invasive disease.

TREATMENT

GENERAL MEASURES
- NSCLC (3)[C]:
  - Stage I, stage II, and selected stage III tumors are surgically resectable. Neoadjuvant or adjuvant therapy is recommended for many patients with stages II and III NSCLC. Patients with resectable disease who have medical contraindications to surgery are candidates for curative radiation therapy.
  - Patients with unresectable or N2, N3 disease are treated with radiation therapy in combination with chemotherapy. Selected patients with T3 or N2 disease can be treated effectively with surgical resection and either preoperative or postoperative chemotherapy or chemoradiation therapy.
  - Patients with distant metastases (M1) can be treated with radiation therapy or chemotherapy for palliation or best supportive care alone.
- SCLC (4)[C]:
  - Limited stage: Concurrent chemotherapy and radiation
  - Extensive stage: Combination chemotherapy
  - Consider prophylactic cranial irradiation (PCI) in patients achieving a complete response (5)[B].
- Quality-of-life assessments: Karnofsky performance scale (KPS), Eastern Cooperative Oncology Group (ECOG)
- Discussions with patient and family about end-of-life care

MEDICATION
- Chemotherapy is the mainstay of treatment for SCLC and advanced NSCLC.
- Adjuvant chemotherapy following surgery improves survival in patients with fully resected stage II–III NSCLC (6)[A].
- Palliative measures: Analgesics
- Dyspnea: Oxygen, morphine

First Line
- NSCLC:
  - Stages II–III: adjuvant chemotherapy:
    - Cisplatin-based doublets (combination with paclitaxel, etoposide, vinorelbine, docetaxel)
    - Carboplatin is an alternative to cisplatin-based regimens in patients who are unlikely to tolerate cisplatin
    - Cisplatin plus pemetrexed (nonsquamous cell)
  - Unresectable stage IIA, IIIB:
    - Concurrent chemoradiation
      - Cisplatin plus etoposide, vinblastine, or pemetrexed (nonsquamous cell) plus concurrent radiation
      - Carboplatin plus pemetrexed (nonsquamous cell) plus concurrent radiation
  - Stage IV:
    - Cisplatin-based doublets with or without bevacizumab (nonsquamous cell) or cetuximab
    - Erlotinib for patients with tumors with EGFR mutations

- Crizotinib for patients with tumors with EML4-ALK translocations
- Maintenance therapy after 4–6 cycles of original regimen in patients achieving a complete response, partial response, or stable disease:
  - Continue original regimen, continue a single agent from original regimen, bevacizumab, cetuximab, pemetrexed, erlotinib, or observation
- SCLC:
  - Cisplatin or carboplatin + etoposide

Second Line
- NSCLC:
  - Cisplatin-based doublets with or without bevacizumab (nonsquamous cell) or cetuximab
  - Docetaxel or pemetrexed (nonsquamous cell only) or erlotinib (EGFR-positive tumors)
- SCLC:
  - Topotecan or CAV (cyclophosphamide, doxorubicin, vincristine), gemcitabine, docetaxel, paclitaxel

ADDITIONAL THERAPIES
- Smoking cessation counseling
- Consider bisphosphonates or denosumab in patients with bone metastases to reduce skeletal related events.

SURGERY/OTHER PROCEDURES
- Resection for NSCLC, for stages I, II, and IIIa, if medically fit to undergo surgery.
- Resection of isolated, distant metastases has been achieved and may improve survival.
- Resection involves lobectomy in 71%, wedge in 16%, and complete pneumonectomy in 18%.
- Resection should be accompanied by lymph node dissection for pathologic staging.

ONGOING CARE

FOLLOW-UP RECOMMENDATIONS
Patient Monitoring
- Depends on clinical history; in general, postoperative visits every 3–6 months in the year after surgery with physical exam and CXR
- Follow-up CT scans, as indicated

PATIENT EDUCATION
- www.cancer.gov/cancertopics
- www.smokefree.gov/

PROGNOSIS
- For combined, all types and stages, 5-year survival rate is 16% (NSCLC: 17%; SCLC 6%) (1)
- NSCLC (3):
  - Localized disease (stages I and II): 49%
  - Regional disease: 16%
  - Distant metastatic disease: 2%
- SCLC (4):
  - Without treatment: Median survival from diagnosis of only 2–4 months
  - Limited-stage disease: Median survival of 16–24 months; 5-year survival rate: 14%
  - Extensive-stage disease: Median survival of 6–12 months; long-term disease-free survival is rare.

COMPLICATIONS
- Development of metastatic disease, especially to brain, bones, adrenals, and liver
- Local recurrence of disease
- Postoperative complications
- Side effects of chemotherapy or radiation

REFERENCES

1. American Cancer Society. *Cancer Facts and Figures 2013*. Atlanta, GA: American Cancer Society; 2013.
2. National Lung Screening Trial Research Team, Aberle DR, Adams AM, et al. Reduced lung-cancer mortality with low-dose computed tomographic screening. *N Engl J Med*. 2011;365:395–409.
3. National Cancer Institute. www.cancer.gov/cancertopics/pdq/treatment/non-small-cell-lung/healthprofessional.
4. National Cancer Institute. www.cancer.gov/cancertopics/pdq/treatment/small-cell-lung/healthprofessional.
5. Slotman B, Faivre-Finn C, Kramer G, et al. Prophylactic cranial irradiation in extensive small cell lung cancer. *N Engl J Med*. 2007;357:664–672.
6. Pignon JP, Tribodet H, Scagliotti GV, et al. Lung adjuvant cisplatin evaluation: A pooled analysis by the LACE Collaborative Group. *J Clin Oncol*. 2008;26:3552–3559.

ADDITIONAL READING

- Collins LG, Haines C, Perkel R, et al. Lung cancer: Diagnosis and management. *Am Fam Physician*. 2007;75:56–63.
- Shepherd FA, Rodrigues Pereira J, Ciuleanu T, et al. Erlotinib in previously treated non-small-cell lung cancer. *N Engl J Med*. 2005;353:123–132.

CODES

ICD10
- C34.90 Malignant neoplasm of unsp part of unsp bronchus or lung
- C34.91 Malignant neoplasm of unsp part of right bronchus or lung
- C34.92 Malignant neoplasm of unsp part of left bronchus or lung

CLINICAL PEARLS
- Prognosis and treatment of lung cancer differs greatly between small-cell and non–small-cell histologies.
- Adjuvant cisplatin-based chemotherapy improves survival in patients with completely resected stage II-III NSCLC.
- Chemotherapy, with or without radiation, can be offered to patients with advanced NSCLC or SCLC.
- There is little role for surgery in the treatment of SCLC.

L

LUPUS ERYTHEMATOSUS, SYSTEMIC

Katherine M. Tromp, PharmD • Hershey S. Bell, MD, MS

BASICS

DESCRIPTION
- Systemic lupus erythematosus (SLE) is a multisystem autoimmune inflammatory disease characterized by a chronic relapsing/remitting course; can be mild to severe and may be life threatening (CNS and renal forms)
- System(s) affected: Mucocutaneous; Musculoskeletal; Renal; Nervous; Pulmonary; Cardiac; Hematologic; Vascular; Gastrointestinal
- Synonym(s): SLE; Lupus

ALERT
Women with SLE have a 7–50-fold increased risk of coronary artery disease and may present with atypical/nonspecific symptoms.

EPIDEMIOLOGY
Predominant age: 15–45 years

Incidence
- Per year, 1.6–7.6/100,000
- Most common: African American women (8.1–11.4/100,000/year)
- Least common: Caucasian men (0.3–0.9/100,000/year)

Prevalence
Occurs in 30–50/100,000

ETIOLOGY AND PATHOPHYSIOLOGY
- Skin: Photosensitivity; scaly erythematous, plaques with follicular plugging, dermal atrophy, and scarring; nonscarring erythematous psoriasiform/annular rash; alopecia; mucosal ulcers
- Musculoskeletal: Nonerosive arthritis; ligament and tendon laxity, ulnar deviation, and swan neck deformities; avascular necrosis
- Renal: Glomerulonephritis
- Pulmonary: Pleuritis, pleural effusion, alveolar hemorrhage, pneumonitis, interstitial fibrosis, shrinking lung, pulmonary hypertension, pulmonary embolism (PE)
- Cardiac: Nonbacterial verrucous endocarditis, pericarditis, myocarditis, atherosclerosis
- CNS: Thrombosis of small intracranial vessels ± perivascular inflammation resulting in micro- or macroinfarcts ± hemorrhage
- Peripheral nervous system: Mononeuritis multiplex, peripheral neuropathy
- GI: Pancreatitis, peritonitis, colitis
- Hematologic: Hemolytic anemia, thrombocytopenia, leukopenia, lymphopenia
- Vascular: Vasculitis, thromboembolism
- Most cases are idiopathic.
- Genetic and environmental factors
- Drug-induced lupus: Hydralazine, quinidine, procainamide, minocycline, isoniazid, tumor necrosis factor alpha (TNF-α) inhibitors, etc.

Genetics
- Identical twins: 24–58% concordance
- Fraternal twins and siblings: 2–5% concordance
- 8-fold risk if 1st-degree relative with SLE
- Major histocompatability complex associations: HLA-DR2, HLA-DR3
- Deficiency of early complement components, especially C1q, C2, and C4

- Immunoglobulin receptor polymorphisms: *FCγR2A* and *FCγR3A*
- Polymorphism in genes associated with regulation of programmed cell death, protein tyrosine kinases, and interferon production

RISK FACTORS
- Race: African Americans, Hispanics, Asians, and Native Americans
- Predominant sex: Females > Males (8:1)
- Environmental: UV light, infectious agents, stress, diet, drugs, hormones, and tobacco

COMMONLY ASSOCIATED CONDITIONS
- Overlap syndromes: Rheumatoid arthritis (RA), Sjögren syndrome, scleroderma
- Antiphospholipid syndrome; coronary artery disease; nephritis; depression

DIAGNOSIS

Consider SLE in multisystem disease including fever, fatigue, and signs of inflammation.

HISTORY
- Fever, fatigue, malaise, weight loss, headache
- Rash (butterfly/*hyperpigmented ears or scalp*), photosensitivity, alopecia
- Oral/nasal ulcers (usually painless)
- Arthritis, arthralgia, myalgia, weakness
- Pleuritic chest pain, cough, dyspnea, hemoptysis
- Early stroke (age <50 years), seizure, psychosis, cognitive deficits
- Proteinuria, cellular casts
- Hemolytic anemia, leukopenia, lymphopenia, thrombocytopenia
- Abdominal pain, anorexia, nausea, vomiting
- Raynaud phenomenon

PHYSICAL EXAM
- Vital signs: Fever, hypertension
- Malar, discoid, psoriasiform, or annular rash, alopecia
- Oral/nasal ulcers (*often minimally symptomatic*)
- Lymphadenopathy, splenomegaly
- Acrocyanosis
- Inflammatory arthritis, tenosynovitis
- Pleural/Pericardial rub, heart murmur
- Bibasilar rales
- Cranial/Peripheral neuropathies

DIFFERENTIAL DIAGNOSIS
Undifferentiated connective tissue disease, Sjögren syndrome, fibromyalgia, RA, vasculitis, idiopathic thrombocytopenia purpura, antiphospholipid antibody syndrome, drug-induced lupus

DIAGNOSTIC TESTS & INTERPRETATION
Initial Tests (lab, imaging)
- Antinuclear antibody (ANA):
  – High sensitivity (98%), low specificity
  – False-positive rate of 5–30%: Elderly, autoimmune thyroid/liver disease, chronic infection, etc.
  – Low titers <1:160 of limited clinical utility
- Anti–double-stranded DNA (dsDNA) and anti-Smith antibodies: High specificity for SLE:
  – Correlates with disease activity
- RNA protein antibodies (anti-RNP, anti-Ro, anti-La): Less specific for SLE

- False-positive Venereal Disease Research Laboratory (VDRL) test: High sensitivity, low specificity. Surrogate marker of cardiolipin antibody presence
- Low serum complement levels: C3, C4
- Erythrocyte sediment rate (ESR): Nonspecific, often high in active disease
- CBC: Hemolytic anemia, thrombocytopenia, leukopenia, or lymphopenia
- Serum creatinine: Elevated in lupus nephritis
- Urinalysis (UA): Proteinuria, hematuria, cellular cast
- Phospholipid antibodies: Cardiolipin immunoglobulin (Ig) G/IgM, lupus anticoagulant, β_2-glycoprotein IgG/IgM
- Anti-P (ribosomal autoantibodies) are associated with SLE arthritis and disease activity.
- Initial imaging is highly dependent on presenting symptoms.
- Radiograph of involved joints
- Chest x-ray: Infiltrates, pleural effusion, low lung volumes
- Chest CT scan, V-Q scan, duplex ultrasound for PE or deep vein thrombosis
- Head CT scan: Ischemia, infarct, hemorrhage
- Brain MRI: Focal areas of increased signal intensity
- Echocardiogram: Pericardial effusion, valvular vegetations, pulmonary hypertension
- Contrast angiography for medium-size artery vasculitis: Mesenteric/Limb ischemia, CNS symptom

Follow-Up Tests & Special Considerations
- Hemolytic anemia: Elevated reticulocyte count and indirect bilirubin, low haptoglobin, positive direct Coombs test
- Confirm positive phospholipid antibodies results in 12 weeks.
- If phospholipid antibodies are initially negative, but symptoms arise, repeat as they may become positive over time.
- 24-hour urine collection/spot protein/creatinine to quantify proteinuria
- Histone antibodies present in >95% of drug-induced lupus (vs. 80% of idiopathic SLE)
- Fasting lipid panel and glucose
- Follow vitamin D[25(O)H] levels and replenish PRN

Diagnostic Procedures/Other
- Renal biopsy to diagnose lupus nephritis (if UA abnormal)
- Skin biopsy with immunofluorescence on involved and uninvolved non–sun-exposed skin (*lupus band test*) may help differentiate SLE rash from others.
- Lumbar puncture in patients with fever and CNS/meningeal symptoms
- EEG for seizures/global CNS dysfunction
- Neuropsychiatric testing for cognitive impairment
- EMG/NCS for peripheral neuropathy and myositis
- Nerve and/or muscle biopsy
- ECG, cardiac enzymes, stress tests
- American College of Rheumatology classification (not diagnostic) criteria: Any 4 of the 11 listed (95% specificity and 85% sensitivity):
  – Malar (butterfly) rash
  – Discoid rash
  – Photosensitivity: By patient history/physician observation
  – Oral/nasopharyngeal ulcers
  – Nonerosive arthritis: Involving ≥2 peripheral joints
  – Pleuritis *OR* pericarditis

- Renal disorder: Proteinuria (>0.5 g/d or >3+) *OR* cellular casts (red cell, hemoglobin, granular, tubular, or mixed)
- Neurologic disorder: Psychosis/seizures
- Hematologic disorder: Hemolytic anemia, leukopenia (<4,000/mm^3 on ≥2 tests), lymphopenia (<1,500/mm^3 on ≥2 tests), thrombocytopenia (<100,000/mm^3)
- Immunologic disorder: Anti-DNA, anti-Sm, anticardiolipin IgG/IgM, lupus anticoagulant, or false–positive VDRL findings
- Positive ANA in absence of drugs known to cause positive ANA

Test Interpretation
- Skin: Vascular/Perivascular inflammation, immune-complex deposition at dermal–epidermal junction, mucinosis, basal layer vacuolar changes:
  - Similar findings seen in other connective tissue disorders such as dermatomyositis
- Renal: Mesangial hypercellularity/matrix expansion, subendothelial/subepithelial immune deposits, glomerular sclerosis, fibrous crescents:
  - Vary depending on degree of involvement
- Vascular: Immune-complex deposition in vessel walls with fibrinoid necrosis and perivascular mononuclear cell infiltrates, intraluminal fibrin thrombi

 TREATMENT

GENERAL MEASURES
- Education, counseling, and support
- Influenza/pneumococcus vaccines are safe; avoid live vaccines in immunocompromised patients.
- Low-estrogen oral contraceptives safe in mild SLE (1)[A]

MEDICATION
First Line
- *Antimalarial agents and NSAIDs are first-line therapy for patients with mild SLE* (2)[A]:
  - Hydroxychloroquine for constitutional and musculoskeletal symptoms, rash, mild serositis; may reduce flares and increase long-term survival (1,3)[A]. Chloroquine also is effective; however, it is associated with more side effects (3)[A].
  - NSAIDs for musculoskeletal manifestations, mild serositis, headache, and fever (1)[C]
- Systemic glucocorticoids (prednisone or equivalent):
  - Low dose (<0.5 mg/kg) for minor disease activity not responsive to NSAIDs or when NSAIDs are contraindicated (1)[A]
  - High-dose (1–2 mg/kg/d) or IV pulse methylprednisolone for organ-threatening disease, particularly CNS and renal; often combined with immunosuppressive agent (1)[A]
- Topical/Intralesional glucocorticosteroids for skin manifestations

Second Line
- Belimumab as adjunct for preventing flares in patients with active lupus despite first-line therapy (4)[A]:
  - 10 mg/kg IV every 2 weeks × 3 doses, then monthly
- Methotrexate (1)[A], azathioprine (1)[B], mycophenolate mofetil (1)[C], or leflunomide as steroid-sparing agent for persistent active disease or to maintain remission:
  - Requires periodic laboratory monitoring for toxicity

- Treatments under investigation: Rituximab, epratuzumab, abatacept, interferon-α inhibitors, abetimus sodium (LJP 394), prasterone, N-acetylcysteine
- Immunosuppressive agents for severe disease:
  - Cyclophosphamide (1)[A]: Ensure adequate hydration to reduce risk of hemorrhagic cystitis
  - Mycophenolate mofetil (1)[A]: More efficacious for lupus nephritis (2)[A]

SURGERY/OTHER PROCEDURES
Renal transplant for end-stage renal disease (1)[B]

COMPLEMENTARY AND ALTERNATIVE MEDICINE
Biofeedback, visual imagery, cognitive therapy

IN-PATIENT CONSIDERATIONS
Admission Criteria/Initial Stabilization
- Difficult to differentiate SLE flare from infection; may need to treat both pending full evaluation
- IV pulse Solu-Medrol 1 g/d × 3–5 days for life- or organ-threatening disease (1)[A]

 ONGOING CARE

FOLLOW-UP RECOMMENDATIONS
Patient Monitoring
- Clinical evaluation for signs and symptoms:
  - Weekly to monthly for active disease
  - Every 3–6 months for mild/inactive disease
- Measures of disease activity and damage: Systemic Lupus Erythematosus Disease Activity Index, British Isles Lupus Assessment Group Index, European Consensus Lupus Activity Measure
- Laboratory studies:
  - CBC with differential
  - Serum creatinine, UA
  - Declining C3/C4 and rising DS-DNA and ESR may correlate with disease activity (1)[B].
- Monitor for adverse effects of treatment:
  - NSAIDs: GI bleeding and/or ulceration
  - Glucocorticoids: Glucose, lipids, bone density
  - Hydroxychloroquine: Ophthalmologic exam every 6–12 months
  - Methotrexate: CBC, creatinine, albumin, AST, ALT every 2 months
  - Azathioprine and mycophenolate mofetil: CBC every 1–3 months
  - Cyclophosphamide:
    - CBC, creatinine, UA every 2 weeks and liver function tests monthly during treatment
    - UA every 6–12 months for life

DIET
- No special diet unless for complications, such as renal failure, diabetes, hyperlipidemia (1)[C]
- Adequate calcium/vitamin D intake in patients on corticosteroids (1)[A]
- Low glycemic index or calorie-restricted diet in patients on corticosteroids (5)[B]

PATIENT EDUCATION
- Avoid UV light exposure: Sunscreens (SPF ≥30), protective clothing (1)[B]
- Weight control, smoking cessation, exercise (1)[C]
- Stress avoidance/management

PROGNOSIS
- Permanent treatment-free remission is uncommon.
- 5-year survival after diagnosis is 95%.
- Poor prognostic factor: Major organ involvement

- Drug-induced lupus resolves within weeks to months after discontinuation of the offending drug.

COMPLICATIONS
Infections, neoplasms, cardiac disease, nephritis, neuropsychiatric lupus

Pregnancy Considerations
- Exacerbations during pregnancy are less common when in remission for 6 months prior to conception.
- Fetal loss is increased, especially in those with active lupus/antiphospholipid antibodies.
- A 2% risk of congenital heart block if anti-SS-A (Ro) or anti-SS-B (La) antibodies are present.
- See "Antiphospholipid Antibody Syndrome" for recommendations regarding use of aspirin and heparin to prevent pregnancy complications.

REFERENCES
1. Bertsias G, Ioannidis JP, Boletis J. EULAR recommendations for the management of systemic lupus erythematosus. Report of a Task Force of the EULAR Standing Committee for International Clinical Studies Including Therapeutics. *Ann Rheum Dis*. 2008;67:195–205.
2. Yildirim-Toruner C, Diamond B. Current and novel therapeutics in the treatment of systemic lupus erythematosus. *J Allergy Clin Immunol*. 2011; 127:303–312.
3. Ruiz-Irastorza G, Ramos-Casals M, Brito-Zeron P. Clinical efficacy and side effects of antimalarials in systemic lupus erythematosus: A systematic review. *Ann Rheum Dis*. 2010;84:20–28.
4. Sandra V, Navarra SV, Guzman RM, et al. Efficacy and safety of belimumab in patients with active systemic lupus erythematosus: A randomised, placebo-controlled, phase 3 trial. *Lancet*. 2011; 377:721–731.
5. Davies RJ, Lomer MC, Yeo SI, et al. Weight loss and improvements in fatigue in systemic lupus erythematosus: a controlled trial of low glycaemic index diet versus a calorie restricted diet in patients treated with corticosteroids. *Lupus*. 2012;21: 649–655.

 SEE ALSO

Antiphospholipid Antibody Syndrome

 CODES

ICD10
- M32.9 Systemic lupus erythematosus, unspecified
- M32.10 Systemic lupus erythematosus, organ or system involv unsp
- M32.14 Glomerular disease in systemic lupus erythematosus

CLINICAL PEARLS
- *Aggressiveness of therapy should reflect intensity of disease.*
- Most important diagnostic test is the urinalysis: If abnormal, order kidney biopsy; *serum and urine lab values often do not reveal extent of kidney disease.*
- Atherosclerotic and atheroembolic complications are the major cause of death.
- ANA has 5–30% false-positive rate; low titers <1:160 of limited clinical utility.

L

LUPUS NEPHRITIS

Weizhen Tan, MD • Neena R. Gupta, MD

BASICS

DESCRIPTION
- Lupus nephritis (LN) is the renal manifestation of systemic lupus erythematosus (SLE).
- Per American College of Rheumatology (ACR) criteria: Renal involvement defined as persistent proteinuria >500 mg/d or ≥3 on dipstick and/or presence of cellular casts. Alternatively, spot urine protein-to-creatinine ratio >0.5 and "active urinary sediment" (>5 RBC/hpf, >5 WBC/hpf in absence of infection, or cellular casts—RBC or WBC casts) (1).
- Clinical manifestations primarily due to immune complex–mediated glomerular disease, but tubulointerstitial and vascular involvement are often seen. Diagnosis by clinical, urinary abnormalities, autoantibodies; requires renal biopsy.
- Treatment and prognosis depend on International Society of Nephrology/Renal Pathology Society (ISN/RPS) 2003 histologic class—risk of end-stage renal disease (ESRD) highest in class IV.
- Delay in diagnosis/treatment increases risk of ESRD.
- For proliferative LN (class III, IV, V + III/IV features): Induction of remission by steroids + IV cyclophosphamide or mycophenolate mofetil (MMF) and maintenance of remission by low-dose steroids and azathioprine (AZA) or MMF.

EPIDEMIOLOGY
- Peak incidence of SLE is 15–45 years,
- Predominant sex: Female > Male (10:1)
- Once SLE develops, LN affects both genders equally; it is more severe in children and men, and less so in older adults.

Incidence
- SLE: 1.4–21.9/100,000 (2)
- Up to 60% of SLE patients develop LN over time, and 25–50% present initially with nephritis.

Pediatric Considerations
LN is more common and severe in children: 60–80% have LN at or soon after SLE onset.

Prevalence
SLE: 7.4–159.4/100,000 (2)

ETIOLOGY AND PATHOPHYSIOLOGY
- Immune complex–mediated inflammatory response injures glomeruli, tubules, interstitium, and vasculature.
- Glomeruli: Varying degrees of mesangial proliferation, crescent formation, fibrinoid necrosis causing reduced glomerular filtration rate (GFR)
- Persistence of inflammation (chronicity) leads to sclerosis and loss of glomeruli.
- Tubulointerstitial injury (seen as edema, inflammatory cell infiltrate acutely, and tubular atrophy in chronic phase) with or without tubular basement membrane immune complex deposition contributes to reduced renal function.
- Vascular lesions: Immune complex deposition and noninflammatory necrosis in arterioles
- SLE is a multifactorial disease, with a multigenic inheritance, but exact etiology is still elusive.
- Defective T-cell autoregulation and polyclonal hyperactivity of B cells
- Dysregulated apoptosis and impaired clearance of apoptotic cells causes breakdown of self-tolerance to nuclear antigens.

- Development of anti-DNA, anti-C1q, anti-α-actin, and other nuclear component autoantibodies
- Deposition of circulating immune complexes or formation of complexes by these antibodies attaching to local nuclear antigens leads to complement activation; plays a key role in tissue injury and inflammation.
- Interaction of genetic, hormonal, and environmental factors leads to great variability in LN severity.

Genetics
No clear pattern, but multigenic inheritance supported by racial differences, clustering in families, ~25% concordance in identical twins

RISK FACTORS
Risk factors for LN include younger age, African American or Hispanic race, more ACR criteria met for diagnosis of SLE, longer disease duration, hypertension, lower socioeconomic status, family history of SLE, anti-dsDNA antibodies.

COMMONLY ASSOCIATED CONDITIONS
Other organ systems, such as skin, hematologic, cerebral, pulmonary, GI, and cardiac, are often involved as part of SLE.

DIAGNOSIS

HISTORY
- LN can present with proteinuria, hematuria, active urine sediment, edema, hypertension, or increased creatinine. Other symptoms related to acute kidney injury or reduced renal function.
- Symptoms related to other organ involvement
- Renal involvement is relatively uncommon in drug-induced lupus.

PHYSICAL EXAM
- Detailed exam for signs of active SLE
- High BP, peripheral edema

DIFFERENTIAL DIAGNOSIS
- LN has to be differentiated from other primary glomerular disease, secondary renal involvement in other systemic disorders, such as antineutrophil cytoplasmic autoantibody (ANCA) associated vasculitis, Henoch-Schönlein purpura (HSP), antiglomerular basement membrane disease, and viral infections.
- Mixed connective tissue disorder may have glomerulonephritis indistinguishable from LN.
- Clinical data have to be combined with serologic and renal biopsy patterns to differentiate LN from other processes.

DIAGNOSTIC TESTS & INTERPRETATION
- Active urine sediment suggests nephritis.
- Autoantibodies, low C3, C4, CH50 complement levels
- Renal biopsy is gold standard for diagnosis, treatment, and prognostication.

Initial Tests (lab, imaging)
- Urinalysis may show hematuria, proteinuria, and active urine sediment (3)[C].
- Serum electrolytes, BUN, creatinine, albumin, routine serological markers of SLE like antinuclear antibody (ANA), anti-dsDNA, anti-Ro, anti-La, anti-RNP, anti-Sm, antiphospholipid antibody, C3,C4, CH50, CBC with differential and C-reactive protein (CRP) (3)[C]
- Renal ultrasound (3)[C]

Follow-Up Tests & Special Considerations
- Monitor every 3 months for disease activity (3)[C]: Urinalysis for hematuria, proteinuria; blood for C3, C4, anti-dsDNA, serum albumin, and creatinine
- Patients with epidermal growth factor receptor (EGFR) <60 mL: Follow National Kidney Foundation guidelines for chronic kidney disease.
- Drug level monitoring if on immunosuppressants

Pregnancy Considerations
- Pregnancy leads to worsening of renal function in LN. Risk factors include renal impairment at baseline, active disease, hypertension, and proteinuria.
- Risk factors for fetal loss include elevated serum creatinine, heavy proteinuria, hypertension, and anticardiolipin antibodies.

Diagnostic Procedures/Other
Renal biopsy is the gold standard for diagnosing and classifying LN.

Test Interpretation
- Adequate renal biopsy (at least 10 glomeruli for light microscopy or total 20–25 glomeruli) is essential. Light, immunofluorescence, and electron microscopy needed for accurate classification.
- On immunofluorescence microscopy: Immune complex deposits consisting of immunoglobulin (Ig) G, A, M, C1q, and C3 (full house) highly suggestive of LN.
- Revised ISN/RPS 2003 histologic classification guides therapeutic decisions.
- LN is classified as purely mesangial (class I, II), focal proliferative: <50% glomeruli (class III), diffuse proliferative: ≥50% (class IV), membranous (class V), and advanced sclerosis (class VI). Subdivisions for activity (A) and chronicity (C) in class III/IV and for segmental (S) or global (G) glomerular involvement in class IV [Class III A, C, A/C and class IV S(A), G(A), S(A/C), S(C), G(C)].
- Lesions may change to another class over time or with therapy.
- Focal and diffuse proliferative LN (classes III and IV) are common forms of LN and are the ones most likely to progress to ESRD.

TREATMENT

GENERAL MEASURES
- Monitor bone density, optimize vitamin D and calcium intake in patients on glucocorticoids.
- Low-salt diet for hypertension, edema. For EGFR <60 mL: Follow National Kidney Foundation guidelines for chronic kidney disease.
- Avoid sun or ultraviolet light exposure.

MEDICATION
First Line
- Class I + II LN: No specific therapy needed, as long-term renal prognosis is good. Renin–angiotensin system blockade for BP and proteinuria
- Proliferative LN (Class III, IV, V + III/IV): Treatment involves induction and maintenance phase (1).
- Principles of treatment:
  – Avoid delay in treatment.
  – Inducing response/remission in a short time period (3–6 months)
  – Maintaining response and avoiding iatrogenic morbidity (5–10 years)

- Induction: Steroids + immunosuppressive agent (for mild class III, high-dose steroids alone may be enough):
  - Glucocorticoids: Methylprednisolone pulse 0.5–1 g/d for 3 days followed by oral prednisone 0.5–1 mg/kg/d PO (max 60 mg/d, taper after 4–8 weeks) (4,5)[A] *AND*
  - Cyclophosphamide: IV cyclophosphamide (high dose = 0.75–1 g/m^2 monthly × 6 doses— National Institutes of Health (NIH) regimen; low dose = 0.5 g q2wk × 6 doses—EuroLupus regimen) or daily oral cyclophosphamide (1.5 mg/kg/d) for no longer than 6 months (to prevent premature ovarian failure) (6)[A] *OR*
  - MMF (Mycophenolate mofetil): 1–3 g/d PO divided b.i.d. (target 3 g/d as tolerated) for 6 months (7)[A]
- Maintenance:
  - Glucocorticoids: Oral prednisone tapered to low doses (generally <10 mg/d by 6 months) *AND*
  - MMF *OR* AZA (azathioprine): MMF 1–2 g/d divided b.i.d. PO or AZA 1–2.5 mg/kg/d (4,5)[A]
  - In the ALMS (Aspreva Lupus Management Study) MMF was shown to be superior to AZA for maintenance therapy (8)[A].
  - Cyclophosphamide IV quarterly for 1–2 years after renal remission; not used now due availability of less toxic regimen.
- Class V LN: Good prognosis in general, treatment not standardized:
  - For subnephrotic patients, no specific treatment except renin–angiotensin system blockade.
  - Options for nephrotic patients include steroids with either calcineurin inhibitors, IV cyclophosphamide, AZA, or MMF (5)[B].
  - Class V LN with presence of class III or class IV biopsy findings needs aggressive combination regimen as for class III/IV.

Second Line
Other treatments used in selected patients: Rituximab, plasma exchange, IVIG, calcineurin inhibitors. Many biologics are in trials. Belimumab was approved by FDA in 2011, but trials excluded patients with severe active LN (9)[C].

ISSUES FOR REFERRAL
Refer to a nephrologist for initial management and relapses.

ADDITIONAL THERAPIES
- KDIGO 2012 guidelines for LN state that all patients with LN of any class be treated with hydroxychloroquine (maximum daily dose of 6–6.5 mg/kg ideal body weight), unless they have a specific contraindication to this drug (10)[C].
- BP control; treat dyslipidemia and other modifiable cardiovascular risk factors.
- Anticoagulation for symptomatic antiphospholipid antibody syndrome.

SURGERY/OTHER PROCEDURES
- Renal transplant for ESRD when clinical and serologic inactivity for a year
- Patient and graft survival rates are similar to non-SLE patients (2)[C].
- Risk of recurrent LN in renal transplant recipients usually low, but ranges between 0% and 30% in different studies; graft loss due to recurrence is rare.

IN-PATIENT CONSIDERATIONS
Admission Criteria/Initial Stabilization
- Uncontrolled hypertension, acute kidney injury
- Severe extrarenal manifestation
- Control hypertension and proteinuria, if present.
- Labs to help confirm SLE/LN, renal ultrasound
- Consult nephrologist for further management and renal biopsy.

IV Fluids
Patients who have nephrotic syndrome or acute kidney injury should be fluid restricted.

Discharge Criteria
Once the patient is stabilized and renal biopsy is performed, management may be as an outpatient.

 ## ONGOING CARE

FOLLOW-UP RECOMMENDATIONS
Patient Monitoring
- Monitor urine protein-to-creatinine ratio, urine microscopy, serum albumin and creatinine, antibody titers (especially anti-dsDNA), C3, C4, BP at least every 3 months for first 2–3 years (3)[C].
- Once stable on maintenance therapy with no active disease, follow up can be spaced every 6–12 months (3)[C].

DIET
Low-salt diet. For EGFR <60 mL: Follow National Kidney Foundation guidelines for chronic kidney disease.

PATIENT EDUCATION
Teach the patient the importance of medication adherence to control disease and self-monitoring for relapse of symptoms.

PROGNOSIS
- LN has negative impact on survival in SLE patients: 10-year survival 88% and 94% in patients with and without renal involvement (1).
- Relapse rate of about 35%. 10–20% of patients progress to ESRD within 10 years (6) depending on population studied, histologic class, activity and chronicity index, response to treatment, and many other factors.
- 5-year renal survival of class IV LN was <30% before 1970 and is >80% in past 2 decades (2).
- Early and complete remission with treatment is the best prognostic factor. Predictors of remission include low baseline proteinuria, normal creatinine, Caucasian race, and treatment initiation within 3 months of clinical diagnosis.
- Indicators of poorer prognosis: Diffuse proliferative LN, especially crescentic, higher activity/chronicity index, African American race, lower socioeconomic status, poor response to treatment, high creatinine at baseline, uncontrolled hypertension, and relapse

COMPLICATIONS
- Risks from immunosuppression: Infections, malignancy
- Treatment side effects: Cyclophosphamide causes primary amenorrhea.
- MMF may cause GI upset and nausea and is a teratogen. (Azathioprine recommended for women who desire pregnancy.)
- Risk of vascular thromboses (hypercoagulable state from antiphospholipid antibodies)
- About 10–20% of patients will eventually develop ESRD from progressive disease refractory to treatment and require dialysis/kidney transplantation.

REFERENCES

1. Hahn BH, McMahon MA, Wilkinson A, et al. American College of Rheumatology guidelines for screening, treatment, and management of lupus nephritis. *Arthritis Care Res (Hoboken).* 2012;64: 797–808.
2. Ortega LM, Schultz DR, Lenz O, et al. Review: Lupus nephritis: Pathologic features, epidemiology and a guide to therapeutic decisions. *Lupus.* 2010;19:557–574.
3. Mosca M. EULAR recommendations for monitoring patients with SLE in clinical practice and in observational studies. *Ann Rheum Dis.* 2010;69:1269–1274.
4. Ponticelli C, Glassock RJ, Moroni G, et al. Induction and maintenance therapy in proliferative lupus nephritis. *J Nephrol.* 2010;23:9–16.
5. Bomback AS, Appel GB. Updates on the treatment of lupus nephritis. *J Am Soc Nephrol.* 2010;21:2028–2035.
6. Houssiau FA, Ginzler EM. Current treatment of lupus nephritis. *Lupus.* 2008;17:426–430.
7. Appel GB, Contreras G, Dooley MA, et al. Mycophenolate mofetil versus cyclophosphamide for induction treatment of lupus nephritis. *J Am Soc Nephrol.* 2009;20:1103–1112.
8. Dooley MA, Jayne D, Ginzler EM, et al. Mycophenolate versus azathioprine as maintenance therapy for lupus nephritis. *N Engl J Med.* 2011;365:1886–1895.
9. Lo MS, Tsokos GC. Treatment of systemic lupus erythematosus: New advances in targeted therapy. *Ann N Y Acad Sci.* 2012;1247:138–152.
10. Kidney Disease: Improving Global Outcomes (KDIGO) Glomerulonephritis Work Group (2012) KDIGO Clinical Practice Guideline for Glomerulonephritis. *Kidney Int Suppl.* 2012;2: 139–274.

ADDITIONAL READING

- Henderson L, Masson P, Craig JC, et al. Treatment for lupus nephritis. *Cochrane Database Syst Rev.* 2012;12:CD002922.
- Weening JJ, D'Agati VD, Schwartz MM, et al. The classification of glomerulonephritis in systemic lupus erythematosus revisited. *J Am Soc Nephrol.* 2004; 15:241–250.

 ## CODES

ICD10
M32.14 Glomerular disease in systemic lupus erythematosus

CLINICAL PEARLS

- Early diagnosis, classification via biopsy, and treatment are imperative for improved renal survival in patients with LN.
- Treatment of proliferative/progressive LN is based on the principle of short induction course followed by longer maintenance course with glucocorticoids and immunosuppressants.
- KDIGO 2012 guidelines for LN state that all patients with LN of any class be treated with hydroxychloroquine (maximum daily dose of 6–6.5 mg/kg ideal body weight), unless they have a specific contraindication to this drug.

L

LYME DISEASE
Jennifer N. Smith, MD • Felix Chang, MD

 BASICS

DESCRIPTION
- A multisystem infection caused by the spirochetes of *Borrelia* strains, which is transmitted primarily by ixodid ticks:
  - *Ixodes scapularis* (deer ticks) in the New England and Great Lakes areas
  - *I. pacificus* in the West, also known as black-legged ticks and Western black-legged ticks
  - *I. ricinus* in Europe
  - *I. persuladas* in Asia and Russia
- Early localized Lyme disease includes a characteristic expanding skin rash (erythema migrans) (70%) and constitutional flulike symptoms.
- Disseminated Lyme disease may present with involvement of ≥1 organ systems. Neurologic, cardiac, and pauciarticular arthritis are most common.
- Post-Lyme disease syndrome involves arthritis (50%) and chronic neurologic syndromes.
- System(s) affected: Hemic/Lymphatic/Immunologic; Musculoskeletal; Skin/Exocrine; Cardiac; Neurologic
- Synonym(s): Lyme arthritis; Lyme borreliosis

EPIDEMIOLOGY
Incidence
- 96% of US cases in 2011 were reported from 13 states: New England, NY, NJ, DE, PA, MD, MN, and WI (1).
- In states where Lyme disease is endemic, the incidence is 0.5 per 1,000, but can be substantially higher in local areas.
- Cases have been reported from all 50 states.

Prevalence
- The most reported vector-borne illness in the US
- Annually Europe: 65,500; North America: 30,158 in 2011 or average over 8 years was 26,947; Asia: 3,500; North Africa: 10 (2)
- Predominant age: Can occur in all ages, but most common in children ages 5–14 and in the 55–70 age group
- Predominant sex: Male > Female in the US

ETIOLOGY AND PATHOPHYSIOLOGY
- Infection with spirochete *Borrelia burgdorferi* in the US, or *B. afzelii* or *B. garinii* in Europe, transmitted by the bite of ixodid ticks
- Approximately 90% of contracted cases are transmitted during the nymph stage of the tick life cycle
- If a tick is infected, the chance of transmission increases with time attached: 12% at 48 hours, 79% at 72 hours, and 94% at 96 hours of attachment (3)
- Primary animal reservoir is the white-footed mouse

Genetics
Human leukocyte antigen: Haplotype DR4 or DR2 may be more susceptible to prolonged arthritis.

RISK FACTORS
- Exposure in tick-infested area; most common April–November
- Those who reside or are employed in areas where ticks are found are at increased risk.
- Ixodid ticks are commonly found on deer. Hunters may be at an increased risk.

GENERAL PREVENTION
- Prevention of infection is possible by careful exam of skin for ticks after outdoor activities.
- Removal of ticks within 36 hours is most effective in limiting transmission.
- Clothing that covers the ankles should be worn in endemic areas, and the use of insect repellants containing DEET is recommended.
- Permethrin may be applied to clothes, shoes, tents.
- No vaccine is currently available.
- Antibiotic prophylaxis is recommended for the prevention of Lyme disease in endemic areas following an *Ixodes* tick bite.
- Prophylactic treatment with 1 dose of 200 mg of doxycycline within 72 hours of a tick bite in highly endemic areas is 87% effective. (This is contraindicated in pregnancy and children; no prophylactic agent is approved for these groups.)

COMMONLY ASSOCIATED CONDITIONS
Southern tick–associated rash illness may be mistaken for Lyme disease. It is seen in the southeastern and south central US and is associated with the bite of the Lone Star tick, *Amblyomma americanum*.

 DIAGNOSIS

HISTORY
- History of a tick bite followed by illness with erythema migrans is the key to diagnosis.
- Early Lyme disease: Incubation period 3–30 days:
  - Some patients may be asymptomatic.
  - Fever
  - Headache
  - Myalgias
  - Arthralgias
- Disseminated Lyme disease:
  - Carditis with A-V block
  - Facial palsies or other cranial neuropathies
  - Joint pain (early disease: polyarthritis/algias; late disease: monoarthritis-like knee)
  - Iritis, conjunctivitis
  - Migratory musculoskeletal pain
- Late untreated Lyme disease:
  - Recurrent synovitis
  - Recurrent tendonitis and bursitis
  - Encephalopathic symptoms:
    - Headaches
    - *Cognitive slowing*
    - Confusion
    - Profound fatigue
  - Symptoms mimicking other CNS diseases:
    - Multiple sclerosis-like symptoms
    - Stroke-like symptoms
    - Transverse myelitis
  - Peripheral neuropathic symptoms; motor, sensory, or autonomic neuropathies
  - Meningitis

PHYSICAL EXAM
- Early Lyme disease:
  - Erythema migrans
- Disseminated Lyme disease:
  - Multiple erythema migrans
  - Facial palsies or other cranial neuropathies
  - Heart block
  - Pericarditis
  - Arthritis
  - Other neurologic signs

DIFFERENTIAL DIAGNOSIS
- Juvenile rheumatoid arthritis
- Viral syndromes
- Later stages may mimic many other diseases.
- Coinfection with babesiosis has been reported. Suggested by high fever.

DIAGNOSTIC TESTS & INTERPRETATION
Initial Tests (lab, imaging)
- Testing and treatment not indicated if tick attachment is <48 hours
- Diagnosis is based mainly on clinical findings in endemic areas.
- Serology: Enzyme-linked immunosorbent assay (ELISA) for immunoglobulin (Ig) M and IgG *B. burgdorferi* antibodies, followed by a Western blot test if positive or equivocal, or an indirect immunofluorescence assay.
- Culture of CSF for *B. burgdorferi*
- Use of plasma polymerase chain reaction (PCR) is of little value, but PCR of synovial fluid may be helpful.
- No imaging indicated

Follow-Up Tests & Special Considerations
- Disorders that may alter lab results: False-positive response has been seen with Rocky Mountain spotted fever (RMSP), syphilis, systemic lupus erythematosus, and rheumatoid arthritis.
- Arthritis: Serology + PCR for Lyme disease in synovial fluid, which is both sensitive and specific
- Neuroborreliosis: Serology + CSF pleocytosis (PCR of CSF has a very low sensitivity for Lyme meningitis)
- Late-stage disease with negative serology may be seen in patients who received early antibiotic treatment.
- After an infection, antibodies may persist for months to years. *Serologic tests do not distinguish active from past infection.*
- Antibodies are not protective.
- CDC warns against using nonvalidated testing methods, including urine antigen test, immunofluorescent staining for cell wall-deficient forms of *B. burgdorferi*, and lymphocyte transformation tests to aid in the diagnosis of Lyme disease

Diagnostic Procedures/Other
Lumbar puncture when neurologic findings are present, with ELISA of CSF for *B. burgdorferi* antibodies

Test Interpretation
Culture of *B. burgdorferi* from blood or skin biopsy has a very low yield.

TREATMENT

GENERAL MEASURES

Early and disseminated Lyme disease can usually be treated as an outpatient except in the case of complications, such as carditis or meningitis, requiring parenteral antibiotics.

MEDICATION

First Line

- Erythema migrans:
  – Doxycycline (Vibramycin) 100 mg PO b.i.d. for 10 days (10–21) (do not use in children <8 or in pregnancy); *or*
  – Amoxicillin 500 mg PO t.i.d. for 14 days (14–21) (pediatric dose 50 mg/kg/d); *or*
  – Cefuroxime axetil 500 mg PO b.i.d. for 14 days (14–21) (4)[A]:
    ○ Advantage to using doxycycline is treatment of other tick-borne infections such as Ehrlichiosis, Anaplasmosis, RMSF.
    ○ Alternative: Azithromycin 500 mg qd for 7 days (7–10) or clarithromycin 500 mg b.i.d. for 14 days (14–21).
- Neurologic disease:
  – Normal CSF, treat for 14–21 days: Doxycycline 100 mg PO b.i.d. or amoxicillin 500 mg PO t.i.d.
  – Abnormal CSF, treat for 4 weeks: Ceftriaxone 2 g qd IV, cefotaxime 2 g q8h, *or* penicillin G 5 millU q6h
  – Cardiac disease:
    ○ Mild (1st-degree AV block, PR <300 ms): Doxycycline 100 mg PO b.i.d. or amoxicillin 500 mg PO t.i.d. for 14 days (14–21)
    ○ More serious: Ceftriaxone 2 g qd IV for 30 days
- Arthritis without neurologic disease:
  – Oral treatment for 28 days with doxycycline 100 mg b.i.d. or amoxicillin 500 mg t.i.d.
  – If oral treatment fails, may repeat oral regimen for 28 days or begin an IV treatment with ceftriaxone 2 g qd for 2–4 weeks (5)(6)[A].
- Contraindications:
  – Allergy to agent
  – Doxycycline is contraindicated in children and in women who are pregnant or breastfeeding.
- Precautions: Refer to the manufacturer's profile of each drug:
  – In ~15% of patients treated with IV therapy, a Jarisch-Herxheimer–type reaction develops within 24 hours of initiation of therapy.
- Significant possible interactions:
  – If the patient is taking oral anticoagulants, it may be necessary to reduce the dose.
  – Oral contraceptives may be less effective.

Pediatric Considerations
- The drug of choice in pediatrics is amoxicillin.
- Tetracyclines are contraindicated.

Pregnancy Considerations
- Because *B. burgdorferi* can cross the placenta, pregnant patients with active disease should receive parenteral antibiotics.
- Doxycycline should not be used in pregnancy.

Second Line
- Azithromycin, 500 mg PO daily for 7 days, can be used for those allergic to β lactams and unable to take tetracyclines, but is less effective.
- Evidence is lacking for any meaningful clinical benefit from prolonged treatment or re-treatment of patients with persistent unexplained symptoms despite previous antibiotic treatment of Lyme disease (7)[A].

IN-PATIENT CONSIDERATIONS
Admission Criteria/Initial Stabilization
- Admission and monitoring are recommended for patients with Lyme carditis and symptoms of chest pain, syncope, or dyspnea, and for those with 2nd- or 3rd-degree heart block or 1st-degree heart block of ≥300 ms.
- Also for symptoms of meningitis

 ONGOING CARE

FOLLOW-UP RECOMMENDATIONS
Patient Monitoring
Based on the severity of symptoms, patients with Lyme carditis, neurologic syndromes, or arthritis may require monitoring for months to years.

DIET
No restrictions

PATIENT EDUCATION
In endemic areas, patients should be advised to protect themselves against tick exposure.

PROGNOSIS
- Early treatment with antibiotics can shorten the duration of symptoms and prevent later disease.
- Response of late-stage disease is variable and may take several weeks to resolve after beginning treatment.

COMPLICATIONS
- Recurrent synovitis, tendonitis, bursitis
- Chronic neurologic symptoms
- Peripheral neuropathies

REFERENCES

1. Centers for Disease Control and Prevention. Statistics on Lyme disease. Available at: www.cdc.gov/lyme/stats/index.html
2. Stanek G, Wormser G, Gray J, et al. Lyme borreliosis. *Lancet*. 2012;379:461–473.
3. Overstreet M. Tick bites and Lyme disease: The need for timely treatment. *Crit Care Nurs Clin North Am*. 2013;25:165–172.
4. Bartlett J. Lyme disease. In Johns Hopkins antibiotic guide, 3rd ed. Burlington, MA: Jones and Bartlett Learning; 2012.
5. Nadelman R, Hanincová K, Mukherjee P, et al. Differentiation of reinfection from relapse in recurrent Lyme disease. *N Engl J Med*. 2012;367: 1883–1890.
6. Delong A, Blossom B, Maloney EL, et al. Antibiotic retreatment of Lyme disease in patients with persistent symptoms: A biostatistical review of randomized, placebo-controlled, clinical trials. *Contemp Clin Trials*. 2012;33:1132–1142.
7. Klempner MS, Baker PJ, Shapiro ED, et al. Source treatment trials for post-Lyme disease symptoms revisited. *Am J Med*. 2013;126:665–669.

ADDITIONAL READING

Massachusetts Department of Public Health, Division of Epidemiology and Immunization. *Tickborne diseases in Massachusetts: A physician's reference manual*. 2nd edition. Available at: www.mass.gov/eohhs/docs/dph/cdc/lyme/tickborne-diseases-physician-manual.pdf

 CODES

ICD10
- A69.20 Lyme disease, unspecified
- A69.21 Meningitis due to Lyme disease
- A69.23 Arthritis due to Lyme disease

CLINICAL PEARLS
- The presence of erythema migrans following a tick bite in an area endemic for Lyme disease warrants empiric treatment.
- Doxycycline is the drug of choice; avoid in pregnant women and children <8 years.
- Repeat episodes of erythema migrans in appropriately treated patients are due to reinfection and not relapse.
- Antibodies are not protective against recurrent disease.

L

LYMPHANGITIS
Jennifer S. Daly, MD • Lorena Ceci

 ## BASICS

DESCRIPTION
Local inflammation of lymphatic vessels due to a distal skin breach or local trauma that classically presents as red, tender streaks extending proximally with involvement of regional lymph nodes:
- May be acute or chronic
- May result from compromised lymphatic drainage due to surgical procedures leading to inflammation and infection.

ETIOLOGY AND PATHOPHYSIOLOGY
- Acute or chronic infection of the skin causing inflammation of lymphatic channels
- Acute infection:
  - Usually caused by group A β-hemolytic *Streptococcus* (1)
  - Less commonly caused by:
    - *Staphylococcus aureus*
    - *Pasteurella multocida*
    - *Spirillum minus* (rat-bite disease)
    - *Pseudomonas*
    - Other *Streptococcus* sp.
    - Immunocompromised patients can be infected with gram-negative rods, gram-negative bacilli, or fungi.
    - In fresh water, think *Aeromonas hydrophila*
- Nodular lymphangitis:
  - Also known as sporotrichoid lymphangitis
  - Presents as painful or painless nodular subcutaneous swellings along the course of the lymphatic vessels
  - Lesions may ulcerate with accompanying regional lymphadenopathy (2)
  - Typical of infections from: *Sporothrix schenckii*, *Nocardia brasiliensis*, *Mycobacterium marinum*, leishmanisis, tularemia, and systemic mycoses.
  - Pathology may show granulomas (3)
- Noninfectious granulomatous lymphangitis:
  - Rare acquired lymphedema of the genitalia in children (3)
  - May be due to atypical Crohn disease or sarcoidosis
- Filarial lymphangitis:
  - Parasites in the lymphatic vessels cause inflammation and dilatation. Can predispose to secondary bacterial infection.
  - Usually caused by *Wuchereria bancrofti*, *Wuchereria bancrofti*. Others are *Brugia malayai*, *Brugia timori* (4)
- Lymphangitis due to surgery:
  - May occur after surgical procedures and lymph node dissection (5)

RISK FACTORS
- Impaired lymphatic drainage due to surgery, nodal dissection or irradiation.
- Diabetes mellitus
- Chronic steroid use
- Peripheral venous catheter (5)
- Varicella infection
- Immunocompromising condition
- Human, animal, or insect bites
- Fungal skin infections
- Mycobacterium skin infections
- Any trauma to the skin
- IV drug abuse
- Residence in endemic areas of filariasis

GENERAL PREVENTION
- Avoid skin trauma
- Reduce chronic lymphedema via usage of compression devices or treatment of underlying process
- Insect repellant
- Proper wound care (6)

COMMONLY ASSOCIATED CONDITIONS
- Lymphedema
- Lymph node dissection
- Athlete's foot
- Sporotrichosis
- Cellulitis (may coexist)
- Erysipelas (often coexists)
- Filarial infection (*Wuchereria bancrofti*)

 ## DIAGNOSIS

HISTORY
- History of trauma to skin, cut, abrasion, or fungal infection (e.g., athlete's foot)
- Systemic symptoms:
  - Malaise
  - Fever and chills
  - Loss of appetite
  - Headache
  - Muscle aches
- Travel to a tropical region

PHYSICAL EXAM
Local signs:
- Red, macular linear streaks from site of infection toward the regional draining lymph node
- Tenderness and warmth over affected skin or lymph nodes (1)
- May have blistering of affected skin
- Look for fluctuance, swelling, or pus
- Nodular lymphangitis can present with subcutaneous swellings along the lymphatic channels.
- Sporotrichosis may present with papulonodular lesions that may ulcerate.

DIFFERENTIAL DIAGNOSIS
- Superficial thrombophlebitis. Feel for induration over the vein:
  - May be due to noninfected thrombus or infection within the thrombosis (septic thrombophlebitis)
- Contact dermatitis (7)
- Allergic reaction : Less likely to be allergic if >24 hours after exposure (e.g., insect bite)
- Lymphangitis carcinomatosa:
- Malignant cell causing inflammation in the lymphatic vessels (8)

DIAGNOSTIC TESTS & INTERPRETATION
- CBC may show leukocytosis or blood smear may show filarial infection (9)
- Blood cultures for bacteria
- Biopsy cultures

Initial Tests (lab, imaging)
Plain radiology unnecessary

Diagnostic Procedures/Other
- Aspirate and culture any pus.
- Routine blood cultures
- Swab, aspirate, and/or biopsy primary site, nodule or distal ulcer for histology and microscopy.
- Serology (e.g., *Francisella tularensis*, histoplasma)
- Blood film/smear (e.g., Filaria)
- Aspirate and culture any pus for routine bacteria or in nodular type send for cultures acid fast bacilli and fungi
- Imaging for anatomic abnormalities
- Lymphangiography to determine lymphedema or lymphatic obstruction (5)

 ## TREATMENT

GENERAL MEASURES
- Hot, moist compresses to affected area
- If lymphedema is involved, compression garments and weight loss may help.

MEDICATION
- Empirically treat common organisms than use culture and susceptibility to guide antibiotic treatment
- If mild systemic signs and limited local signs treat as an outpatient with oral antibiotics.
- If no improvement after 48 hours of oral antibiotics reassess and consider IV antibiotics.
- If systemic involvement, start IV antibiotics
- If necrotizing fasciitis due to group A hemolytic *Streptococcus* is suspected, treat aggressively with antibiotics and surgical consults.

First Line
- Antibiotics for suspicion of group A streptococcal infection:
  - Amoxicillin (if patient known to have only group A *Streptococcus*):
    - Dosing:
      - Adults:
        - Mild to moderate: 500 mg PO q12h
        - Severe: 875 mg PO q12h or 500 mg PO q8h
      - Children <3 months: 30 mg/kg/d PO divided q12h
      - Children ≥3 months, ≤40 kg:
        - Mild to moderate: 25 mg/kg/d PO divided q12h or 20 mg/kg/d divided q8h
        - Severe: 45 mg/kg/d PO divided q12h or 40 mg/kg/d divided q8h
      - Children ≥40 kg:
        - Refer to adult dosing
    - Common adverse effects:
      - Allergic reaction
      - Diarrhea
    - Serious adverse effects:
      - Anaphylaxis, Stevens-Johnson syndrome (SJS), toxic epidermal necrolysis (TENS)
    - Drug interactions:
      - Methotrexate, venlafaxine, warfarin, hormonal contraceptives
    - Contraindications:
      - Hypersensitivity to penicillins
- Ampicillin/Sulbactam:
  - Dosing:
    - Adults and children ≥40 kg: 1.5–3 g (ampicillin + sulbactam component) IV/IM q6h; maximum 4 g sulbactam/d
    - Children <40 kg: 300 mg/kg/d IV infusion, in divided doses q6h; maximum 4 g sulbactam per day
  - Common adverse effects:
    - Diarrhea, rash, and injection site reactions

- Serious adverse effects:
  - *Clostridium difficile* diarrhea, pseudomembranous enterocolitis, dysuria
- Drug interactions:
  - Hormonal contraceptives
- Contraindications:
  - Hypersensitivity reactions
- Ceftriaxone:
  - Dosing:
    - Adults: 1–2 g IV/IM q24h
    - Children: 50–75 mg/kg/d IV/IM once daily or in divided doses q12h; maximum 2 g/d
  - Common adverse effects:
    - Injection site reactions, diarrhea, thrombocytosis, eosinophilia
  - Serious adverse effects: Same as amoxicillin or ampicillin
  - Drug interactions:
    - Do not administer calcium-containing IV solutions in the same IV line
  - Contraindications:
    - Hypersensitivity to cephalosporins
    - Concurrent use of calcium-containing IV fluids
    - Use in neonates; increased risk of kernicterus, salt precipitation in lungs and kidneys in neonates <28 days (use cefotaxime)
- Cephalexin:
  - Dosing:
    - Adults: 500 mg PO q.i.d.
    - Children: 25–50 mg/kg/d divided q12h
  - Common adverse effects:
    - Diarrhea
  - Serious adverse effects:
    - SJS, TENS, interstitial nephritis, renal failure, pseudomembranous enterocolitis, anaphylaxis
  - Drug interactions:
    - Cholestyramine, metformin
  - Contraindications:
    - Hypersensitivity to cephalosporins
- Azithromycin (if penicillin or cephalosporin allergy):
  - Dosing:
    - Adults: 500 mg PO on day 1 followed by 250 mg/d PO on days 2–5
    - Children ≥2 years: 12 mg/kg/d PO (maximum dose: 500 mg/d) once daily for 5 days (FDA off-label use for skin infections in children)
  - Common adverse effects:
    - Abdominal pain, nausea, vomiting, diarrhea, increased liver enzymes, headache
  - Serious adverse effects:
    - Prolonged QT interval, torsades de pointes, liver failure, Lambert-Eaton syndrome, myasthenia gravis, corneal erosion, anaphylaxis
  - Drug interactions:
    - Contraindicated with the use of ergot derivatives and drugs metabolized by CYP450 isoforms including: disopyramide, class III antiarrhythmics, ziprasidone, warfarin, digoxin, fentanyl, simvastatin, azole class antifungals, tacrolimus
  - Contraindications:
    - Hepatic dysfunction or cholestatic jaundice with prior treatment
    - Hypersensitivity to macrolide (azithromycin, erythromycin, clarithromycin)
- Diethylcarbamazine, ivermectin, albendazole, and doxycycline are used to treat filarial infection.
- Acetaminophen or ibuprofen (NSAIDs) for pain and fever

SURGERY/OTHER PROCEDURES
- Incision and drainage of abscess if present
- Necrotizing fasciitis may need debridement

IN-PATIENT CONSIDERATIONS
Admission Criteria/Initial Stabilization
- Fluids if in hypotensive shock
- Antibiotics
- ICU or surgery as indicated
- If patient requires IV antibiotic therapy beyond 1 dose and this cannot be given as outpatient
- If symptoms are severe :
  - High fever
  - Rigor
  - Systemic toxicity
  - Shock
- Altered mental status

Discharge Criteria
Patient can be discharged on oral antibiotics after systemic symptoms resolve or send home on IV antibiotics if feasible.

 ONGOING CARE

FOLLOW-UP RECOMMENDATIONS
- Elevate affected area when at rest, if possible
- 48-hour follow up to ensure continued improvement if outpatient

Patient Monitoring
Close follow up to ensure decreasing inflammation

PATIENT EDUCATION
Instruct patients on proper wound care (and foot care, if applicable).

PROGNOSIS
- Good prognosis for uncomplicated lymphangitis
- Antimicrobial therapy is effective in 90% of patients.
- Untreated, can spread rapidly, especially group A *Streptococcus*

COMPLICATIONS
- Sepsis
- Bacteremia
- Cellulitis
- Necrotizing fasciitis
- Myositis

REFERENCES
1. Falagas ME, Bliziotis IA, Kapaskelis AM. Red streaks on the leg. *Am Fam Physician*. 2006;73:1061–1062.
2. Schubach A, Barros MB, Wanke B. Epidemic sporotrichosis. *Curr Opin Infect Dis*. 2008;21:129–133.
3. Kostman JR, DiNubile MJ. Nodular lymphangitis: A distinctive but often unrecognized syndrome. *Ann Intern Med*. 1993;118:883–888.
4. Taylor MJ, Hoerauf A, Bockarie M, et al. Lymphatic filariasis and onchocerciasis. *Lancet*. 2010;376:1175–1185.
5. Edlich RF, Winters KL, Britt LD. Bacterial diseases of the skin. *Long-Term Effects Med Implants*. 2005;15:499–510.
6. Smego RA Jr, Castiglia M, Asperilla MO. Lymphocutaneous syndrome. A review of non-sporothrix causes. *Medicine (Baltimore)*. 1999;78:38–63.
7. Bonnetblanc JM, Bédane C. Erysipelas: Recognition and management. *Am J Clin Dermatol*. 2003;4:57–163.
8. Raja A, Seshadri RA, Sundersingh S. Lymphangitis carcinomatosa: Report of a case and review of literature. *Indian J Surg Oncol*. 2010;1:274–276.
9. Smith JA, Ridell J 4th, Kauffman CA. Cutaneous manifestations of endemic mycoses. *Curr Infect Dis Rep*. 2013;15:440–449.

ADDITIONAL READING
- Badger C, Seers K, Preston N, et al. Antibiotics/anti-inflammatories for reducing acute inflammatory episodes in lymphoedema of the limbs. *Cochrane Database Syst Rev*. 2004;1:CD003143.
- Del Giudice P. Cutaneous complications of intravenous drug abuse. *Br J Dermatol*. 2004;150:1–10.
- Haddad FG, Waked CH, Zein EF. Peripheral venous catheter-related inflammation. A randomized prospective trial. *J Med Liban*. 2006;54:139–145.

 CODES

ICD10
- I89.1 Lymphangitis
- L03.91 Acute lymphangitis, unspecified

CLINICAL PEARLS
- The classic presentation of lymphangitis is red, linear streaks along the skin from an infected site (e.g., bite, cut, abrasion) to the draining lymph node for that region.
- Patients who have lymph node dissection as part of their breast cancer treatment may have difficulty draining lymphatic fluid properly, leading to lymphedema and an increased predisposition to infection and lymphangitis.
- A patient with severe systemic symptoms (e.g., high fever, rigors, shock, septic, altered mental status) should be admitted and treated with IV antibiotics. A patient with moderate systemic symptoms (e.g., fever, chills, muscle aches) should be monitored closely for worsening, but could be treated as an outpatient.
- Patients can take ibuprofen or acetaminophen for the pain and/or fever associated with lymphangitis. Ibuprofen also helps with inflammation at high doses.
- Parasitic or fungal infections can cause chronic lymphangitis.
- Treatment of underlying skin infection such as tinea pedis may prevent recurrence.

LYMPHEDEMA

Jon S. Parham, DO, MPH • Sandra N. Berryman, DrNP

 BASICS

DESCRIPTION
- Accumulation of lymphatic fluid in the interstitial tissue causing swelling
- Lymphedema can develop when lymphatic vessels are missing or impaired (primary), or when lymph vessels are damaged or lymph nodes removed (secondary).
- Most common in the lower limb (80%), but also can occur in the arms, face, trunk, and external genitalia

EPIDEMIOLOGY
Incidence
- Predominant sex: Female > Male
- Predominant age: Any age
- 13% of patients with breast cancer treated with surgery; 42% of those treated with surgery and radiation therapy; 25% after GYN cancer surgery
- Milroy disease presents at birth. Estimated to be between 1/6,000 and 1/300 live births
- Meige disease develops during puberty.

Prevalence
- 120 million people worldwide are affected with lymphatic filariasis in 73 countries, but no primary infections in US.
- 10 million people are affected by non-filarial secondary lymphedema in the US.

ETIOLOGY AND PATHOPHYSIOLOGY
Secondary lymphedema:
- Postoperative: Gradual failure of distal lymphatics, which have to "pump" lymph at a greater pressure through damaged proximal ducts
- Risk is higher with postoperative radiation because radiation reduces regrowth of ducts due to fibrous scarring.
- Trauma; recurrent infection; malignancy, including metastatic disease
- Developing countries: Most common cause is filariasis (*Wucheria bancrofti*)

Genetics
- Milroy disease: Autosomal-dominant; diagnosed either at birth or the 1st year of life
- Lymphedema praecox has onset between the ages of 1 and 35 years.
- Lymphedema tarda occurs in those >35 years of age.

RISK FACTORS
- Filariasis: Most common cause worldwide
- Mastectomy
- Prior trauma; Infection of affected limb
- History of prior surgical (particularly, if lymph nodes were removed) or radiation therapy for malignancy (radiation can damage lymph nodes and cause skin dermatitis)
- Long history of venous insufficiency
- Obesity; DVT

GENERAL PREVENTION
Healthy body weight maintenance. Treatment of congestive heart failure (CHF) and venous insufficiency

COMMONLY ASSOCIATED CONDITIONS
Venous disease

 DIAGNOSIS

HISTORY
Recent surgery: Vein stripping can significantly exacerbate mild lymphedema (1)[B]:
- 1st symptom: Painless swelling
- Feeling of heaviness in the limb, especially at the end of the day and in hot weather

PHYSICAL EXAM
- Initial: Pitting edema, can spread proximally
- Later: Non-pitting; after 1st year, does not spread proximally/distally, but spreads radially
- Hyperkeratosis (thicker skin)
- Papillomatosis (rough skin)
- Increase in skin turgor
- Positive Stemmer sign (inability to pinch the skin of the dorsum of the 2nd toe between the thumb and forefinger): Exclude heart failure.

DIFFERENTIAL DIAGNOSIS
- CHF; Renal failure; Lipidemia
- Hypoalbuminemia; Protein-losing nephropathy
- DVT; Chronic venous disease
- Postoperative complications following ipsilateral surgery
- Cellulitis; Baker cyst; Idiopathic edema

DIAGNOSTIC TESTS & INTERPRETATION
- Lack of response to elevation or diuretic therapy may indicate a lymphatic insufficiency
- Diuretics increase excretion of salt and water, thereby decreasing plasma volume, venous capillary pressure, and filtration. Diuretics improve filtration edema, but do not improve lymph drainage over the long term.
- Some relevant protein biomarkers for lymphedema have been identified and show promise for early and latent stage diagnosis (2)[B]

Initial Tests (lab, imaging)
- Comprehensive chemistry panel: Evaluate for hepatic or renal impairment.
- Urinalysis: Protein-losing nephropathy
- Ultrasound: Evaluate for acute/chronic DVT. Gives information about soft tissue changes, but does not tell about truncal anatomy of the lymphatics (1)[B].
- Duplex ultrasound: Lymphedema causes gradual impedance of venous return that aggravates the edema; 82% of patients with unexplained limb edema were diagnosed using a combination of duplex ultrasound and lymphoscintigram (3)[A].

Follow-Up Tests & Special Considerations
- Lymphangiogram: Direct cannulation of lymphatics through the skin; risk for infection, local inflammation; not used commonly (3)[C]
- Lymphoscintigram: Radiolabeled protein technetium-99m–labeled colloid:
  - Measures lymphatic function, lymph movement, lymph drainage, and response to treatment
  - Sensitivity, 73–97%; specificity, 100%
  - Best to use 1-hour and delayed images together (3)[A].
- Indocyanine green lymphography: reported accurately screens post surgically for subclinical lymphedema (4)[B]
- CT scan: Calf skin thickening, thickening of the SC compartment, increased fat density, thickened perimuscular aponeurosis; typical honeycomb appearance (3)[B]
- MRI: Circumferential edema, increased volume of SC tissue, honeycomb pattern above the fascia between the muscle and subcutis; cannot differentiate primary from secondary lymphedema (3)[B]

 TREATMENT

GENERAL MEASURES
- Seek optimal weight, early treatment of cellulitis, avoid trauma to affected area (direct injury, venipunctures, inept nail care, extreme heat/cold).
- Achieve mechanical reduction and maintenance of limb size: compression garments via professionals.
- Elevate affected limb/area, but avoid stasis.
- Avoid BP cuffs in affected limbs.
- Prevent skin infection with daily cleansing, inspection and skin care (with emollients).
- Treatment of varicose veins may benefit some.

MEDICATION
Benzopyrenes (flavonoids and coumarin) (not available for prescription use in the US):
- Micronized purified flavonoid fraction (Daflon 500 mg) is effective in decreasing venous stasis and idiopathic cyclic edema, chronic venous insufficiency, and postmastectomy lymphedema. It also reduces capillary permeability and the inflammatory component (5)[C].
- Coumarin reduces edema fluid by increasing the number of macrophages and enhancing proteolysis, resulting in the removal of protein, increasing softness in the limbs, and decreasing elevated skin temperature with subsequent symptom improvement and decreased secondary infection. Some reports of hepatotoxicity (5)[C]

ISSUES FOR REFERRAL

- Refer to physical therapist with lymphedema training for manual decongestive therapy.
  - In patients with recurrent or metastatic disease, discuss with oncologist prior to initiation of complete decongestive therapy in order not to promote the spread of cancer.
- Provide education for patient/family for self-administration of therapy in future.
- Education for family about bandaging
- Fitting for compression garments

ADDITIONAL THERAPIES

- Exercise: Lymph flow occurs as a result of inspiratory reduction in the intrathoracic pressure associated with inspiration. Best results are achieved with combination of flexibility, strength, and aerobic training (3)[B].
- Compression with custom-made elastic stocking (minimum pressure is 40 mm Hg):
  - Protection against external incidental trauma
  - Decreases the intrinsic trauma on the skin due to chronically increased interstitial pressures, which cause stretch of the skin and SC tissues
  - No data on preference of custom-made vs. prefabricated
  - Replace every 3–6 months or when starting to lose elasticity (1)[B].
- Multilayer bandaging: Inner layer of tubular stockinette followed by foam and padding to protect the joint flexures and to even out the contours of the limb so that pressure is distributed evenly; outer layer of at least 2 short-stretch extensible bandages; more effective than hosiery alone (1)[B]
- Pneumatic pumps: Development of high pressure up to 150 mm Hg; can reduce limb girth by 37–68.6%; wear a compression stocking when not using pump; high risk of genital edema; no metastasis in limb due to risk of spread (1)[B]

SURGERY/OTHER PROCEDURES

- Bypass procedures: Creation of lymphatic–venous anastomosis: Reserved for highly refractory cases only
- Debulking procedures (Charles procedure): Radical excision of SC tissue with primary or staged skin grafting:
  - Men had less improvement than women.
  - Main risk is infection and necrosis of the skin graft.
  - Liposuction is cosmetically preferred to debulking.

COMPLEMENTARY AND ALTERNATIVE MEDICINE

Heat therapy: Hot water immersion, microwave, and electromagnetic irradiation may be helpful (1)[C].

IN-PATIENT CONSIDERATIONS

Admission Criteria/Initial Stabilization

Systemic signs of infection:

- May admit to specialized rehabilitation unit for combination treatment in patients with heart failure or severe pulmonary disease
- IV antibiotics for infection

Nursing

- Leg elevation
- Encourage patient mobilization/exercise.
- Patient education for bandaging/wound care

Discharge Criteria

- Resolution of signs/symptoms of infection (e.g., elevated WBC count, fever, abnormal vital signs)
- Clinical improvement in wound appearance

 ## ONGOING CARE

FOLLOW-UP RECOMMENDATIONS

Lymphedema will return in several days if patient stops wearing compression garments during the day and bandaging at night.

Patient Monitoring

- Daily visit to therapist for acute treatment
- Monthly visits for maintenance care

DIET

Low sodium; weight loss oriented if needed

PATIENT EDUCATION

- Use compression garments, especially when exercising.
- Avoid affected limb(s) being dependant for long period of time: Patient should perform daily skin examination.
- http://www.nlm.nih.gov/medlineplus/lymphedema.html

PROGNOSIS

No cure, but treatment can produce good results with daily care

COMPLICATIONS

- Infection (local vs. systemic): Common
- Risk of wound formation (venous wounds/abrasions) that are difficult to heal: Common
- Lymphangiosarcoma: Found in lymphedematous arms of patients following radical mastectomy; also in patients with Milroy disease. Treatment is radiotherapy with surgery, reserved for patients with discrete nonmetastatic disease

REFERENCES

1. Warren A. Lymphedema: A comprehensive review. *Ann Plastic Surg*. 2007;59(4):464–472.
2. Akita S, Mitsukawa N, Rikihisa N, et al. *Plast Reconstr Surg*. 2013;131(2):283–290. Doi:10.1097/PRS.0b013e318277870f.
3. Brennan MJ, Miller LT. Overview of treatment options and review of the current role and use of compression garments, intermittent pumps, and exercise in the management of lymphedema. *Cancer*. 1998;83:2821–2827.
4. Tiwari A, Cheng KS, Button M, et al. Differential diagnosis, investigation, and current treatment of lower limb lymphedema. *Arch Surg*. 2003;138: 152–161.
5. Lin S, Kim J, Lee M-J, Roche L, et al. Prospective Transcriptomic Pathway Analysis of Human Lymphatic Vascular Insufficiency: Identification and Validation of a Circulating Biomarker Panel. *PLoS ONE*. 2012;7(12):e52021. doi:10.1371/journal.pone.0052021

ADDITIONAL READING

Rockson SG. Causes and consequences of lymphatic disease. *Ann NY Acad Sci*. 2010;1207:e2–e6. Doi: 10.1111/j.1749-6632.2010.05804.X

 ## CODES

ICD10

- I89.0 Lymphedema, not elsewhere classified
- I97.2 Postmastectomy lymphedema syndrome
- I97.89 Oth postproc comp and disorders of the circ sys, NEC

CLINICAL PEARLS

- Use short-stretch bandages for wrapping (not ACE wraps).
- Avoid heat/whirlpool: Typically worsens condition.
- Much higher risk for cutaneous-sourced infections than patients with only venous insufficiency.

Jennifer Greene Welch, MD

BASICS

DESCRIPTION
- Burkitt lymphoma is a mature B-cell neoplasm arising in lymph node germinal centers.
- Highly aggressive, rapidly growing malignancy
- Can present as lymphoma or leukemia
- 3 distinct forms, differing in epidemiology, clinical presentation, and genetics:
  - Endemic, or African
  - Sporadic
  - Immunodeficiency-related:
    - HIV/AIDS-related
    - Post-solid organ transplant
    - Congenital immunodeficiency
- Associated with Epstein-Barr virus (EBV):
  - Almost 100% of endemic cases
  - Up to 30% of sporadic cases
- Specific chromosome translocation [t(8;14)]
- Similar disease characteristics to diffuse large B-cell lymphoma (DLBCL)
- System(s) affected: Hematologic, Lymphatic
- Synonym(s): Mature B-cell high-grade lymphoma; Mature B-cell acute lymphoblastic leukemia; L3 type (FAB classification); Burkitt cell leukemia

Pediatric Considerations
Common age group (30% of cases in the US)

Geriatric Considerations
Unusual in this age group. Toxicity with chemotherapy may be increased in the elderly.

Pregnancy Considerations
With aggressive treatment, good maternal and fetal outcome

EPIDEMIOLOGY
- Varies by disease form
- Endemic:
  - One of most common tumors of childhood in Africa, most frequently occurring in children age 4–7 years
  - Rare in adults
- Sporadic:
  - In the US, trimodal peaks of age incidence around ages 10, 40, and 75
  - More common in Caucasians
  - Predominant sex: Male > Female (3:1 or 4:1)

Incidence
Rare in the US, incidence 0.27 per 100,000 person-years; 50 times more common in endemic regions of Africa

Prevalence
Comprises <1% of adult non-Hodgkin lymphoma (NHL); accounts for 30–40% of NHL in children in the US and Western Europe

ETIOLOGY AND PATHOPHYSIOLOGY
- Activation and overexpression of *c-myc* oncogene
- Monoclonal proliferation of B lymphocytes resulting from dysregulation of *c-myc*:
  - Translocation of *c-myc* to immunoglobulin coding regions results in constitutive expression of gene product.
  - EBV-infected cells in germinal-center reactions may increase the risk of translocation.
- Poorly regulated proliferation of genetically unstable B cells increases chance of translocations:
  - Immunodeficient patients with persistent generalized lymphadenopathy and polyclonal B-cell activation

RISK FACTORS
Pediatric Considerations
Endemic: Children with early acquisition of EBV infection are at increased risk. Coinfection with malaria and EBV increases incidence 100-fold.

GENERAL PREVENTION
No known methods to prevent Burkitt lymphoma

COMMONLY ASSOCIATED CONDITIONS
- EBV infection
- Immunodeficiency, especially AIDS

DIAGNOSIS

HISTORY
- Rapidly progressive bulky adenopathy or extranodal mass
- Symptoms of bone marrow involvement:
  - Fatigue, exercise intolerance, bruising, epistaxis, other bleeding, fever
- Abdominal presentation:
  - Abdominal pain, nausea, vomiting, bowel obstruction, GI bleeding, symptoms mimicking acute appendicitis or intussusception
- Endemic (African): Jaw or facial bone tumor, with mouth pain, loose teeth, or jaw mass
- Nonendemic: Extranodal disease, abdominal presentation typical
- Can present as acute leukemia (L3-ALL) with predominant bone marrow involvement and no mass lesions
- Renal function impairment and significant metabolic derangement may quickly manifest due to the rapid progression and spread of the tumor.

PHYSICAL EXAM
- Endemic: Mass on jaw or facial bone, pallor, petechiae, hepatosplenomegaly
- Sporadic: Lymphadenopathy, any mass lesion, abdominal tenderness, pallor, petechiae, hepatosplenomegaly

DIFFERENTIAL DIAGNOSIS
- Other non-Hodgkin lymphomas:
  - Burkitt-like lymphoma: Intermediate immunophenotype and molecular characteristics between classic Burkitt lymphoma and DLBCL
  - DLBCL: Large, irregular cells, often with BCL rearrangement
  - Precursor B-lymphoblastic lymphoma
  - Precursor T-lymphoblastic lymphoma
  - Mantle cell lymphoma, blastoid variant
- Hodgkin lymphoma
- Acute lymphoblastic leukemia
- Other causes of lymphadenopathy:
  - Infection (e.g., bacterial lymphadenitis, mononucleosis, tuberculosis, atypical mycobacterium, cat-scratch disease)
  - Reactive lymphoid hyperplasia
  - Histiocytosis
- Other primary malignancies of childhood (e.g., Wilms tumor, neuroblastoma, peripheral neuroectodermal tumor)
- Other metastatic malignancies

DIAGNOSTIC TESTS & INTERPRETATION
Initial Tests (lab, imaging)
- Biopsy of mass lesion: Diagnosis by cellular morphology on histologic examination
- CBC with differential: Anemia, neutropenia, or thrombocytopenia
- Tumor lysis syndrome: Hyperkalemia, hyperphosphatemia, hyperuricemia, renal failure. Order electrolytes, BUN, creatinine, calcium, magnesium, phosphorus, serum lactate dehydrogenase (LDH), uric acid
- Consider hepatitis B virus serologies prior to rituximab
- Chest x-ray
- CT scan of chest, abdomen, pelvis
- Consider whole body PET to identify active disease
- Dedicated imaging of any site suspected to be involved by tumor

Follow-Up Tests & Special Considerations
- Diagnosis requires immunophenotypic and cytogenetic data
- Immunophenotype studies:
  - Cells express surface immunoglobulin (Ig) M- and B-associated antigens (CD19, CD20, CD22, CD79a), as well as CD10, HLA-DR, and CD43
  - Cells also show nuclear staining for BCL-6 protein
- Cytogenic studies to visualize chromosomal translocation:
  - Reciprocal chromosome translocation involving *c-myc* and immunoglobulin heavy chain (IgH) gene [t(8;14)] (80% of cases) or immunoglobulin light chain (IgL) genes [t(2;8) or t(8;22)]
  - Fluorescence in situ hybridization (FISH) or long-segment polymerase chain reaction (PCR) may be necessary to identify translocation.
- EBV testing in lesional cells
- Gene expression profiling can help distinguish Burkitt lymphoma from DLBCL.

Diagnostic Procedures/Other
- Bone marrow aspiration and biopsy for morphology and flow cytometry
- Lumbar puncture for CSF cell count, differential, and cytology
- Lymph node biopsy: Most lymph nodes suggestive of disease should be selected for excisional biopsy:
  - Frozen sections and needle biopsies discouraged as lymph node architecture helpful for diagnosis
- Diagnostic laparotomy with resection of localized disease

Test Interpretation
- Monotonous diffuse infiltrate of medium-size round cells, with round or oval nuclei, several nucleoli, and coarse chromatin. Cytoplasm is intensely basophilic and moderately abundant.
- Mitotic rate is high; close to 100% of viable cells will be actively engaged in cell cycle.
- Classic starry-sky histologic appearance:
  - Results from the presence of scattered macrophages with phagocytic cell debris
  - Characteristic of, although not pathognomonic, for Burkitt's lymphoma

TREATMENT

If available, all patients should be offered participation in an appropriate clinical trial.

MEDICATION
First Line
- Intensive, short-term, multiagent chemotherapy administered in cycles (1,2,3)[A]:
  – Chemotherapeutic agents include cyclophosphamide, methotrexate, vincristine, prednisone, high-dose methotrexate, high-dose cytarabine, etoposide, isophosphamide, and doxorubicin.
  – Type and extent of therapy depend on stage of disease.
- Rituximab in combination with chemotherapy may improve outcome (2)[B].
- Nonintensive chemotherapy protocols utilized in developing countries can be effective (4)[B]:
  – Cyclophosphamide, methotrexate
  – Areas with limited financial and medical resources
- CNS prophylaxis for most patients:
  – Not necessary for limited disease far from CNS
  – Intrathecal methotrexate, with or without IV methotrexate and cytarabine, may be used for CNS prophylaxis.
  – Prophylactic irradiation does not improve outcome.
- Chemotherapy cycles should be initiated as soon as hematologic recovery permits:
  – Delay of chemotherapy may result in regrowth of resistant tumor between cycles.
- Management of tumor lysis syndrome with initial cycle of chemotherapy

Second Line
- Rituximab may be effective if not used previously
- Hematopoietic stem cell transplantation in combination with high-dose chemotherapy (3)[B]

ISSUES FOR REFERRAL
All patients should be treated by a pediatric or adult hematologist/oncologist.

SURGERY/OTHER PROCEDURES
- Biopsy and staging:
  – All patients require a biopsy to establish the diagnosis pathologically.
- Surgical resection:
  – Treatment for small, completely resectable abdominal tumors (in addition to chemotherapy)
  – For patients with intestinal obstruction who cannot begin chemotherapy immediately
  – Aggressive upfront resection of disease is not indicated
  – Patients require placement of a central venous line for administration of chemotherapy.

COMPLEMENTARY AND ALTERNATIVE MEDICINE
Many complementary therapies exist to assist in management of side effects of chemotherapy.

IN-PATIENT CONSIDERATIONS
Admission Criteria/Initial Stabilization
- Almost all patients should be admitted to the hospital for initial care.
- Burkitt lymphoma has high-growth fraction and short doubling time:
  – Rapid initiation of definitive chemotherapy is essential.
- Management of tumor lysis syndrome with initial cycle of chemotherapy:
  – Aggressive hydration without potassium
  – Close monitoring of electrolytes, renal function, and uric acid initially q6–8h
  – Rasburicase (0.2 mg/kg IV once daily for up to 5 days, depending on response to therapy) to break down uric acid
  – Allopurinol (10 mg/kg PO divided 2–3/d) if rasburicase not available:
    ○ Consider alkalization of urine with bicarbonate-containing IV fluids (goal urine pH 7–8) when using allopurinol
  – Phosphate binder if serum phosphorus becomes elevated
  – Avoid supplemental calcium unless symptomatic hypocalcium develops
  – Medical management of hyperkalemia

IV Fluids
Aggressive IV hydration with first cycle of chemotherapy:
- Typically D5/0.5 NS at 125 cc/m^2/h (twice the maintenance rate)
- No potassium in IV fluids

 ONGOING CARE

FOLLOW-UP RECOMMENDATIONS
Patient Monitoring
- Close monitoring of serum chemistries is critical due to high risk of tumor lysis syndrome and uric acid nephropathy.
- CBC, liver function, and renal function should also be closely monitored throughout chemotherapy.
- Surveillance physical exam and imaging for detection of recurrence
- All patients, particularly children, should be followed indefinitely for long-term effects of chemotherapy.

PATIENT EDUCATION
Educational materials are available online from:
- Leukemia and Lymphoma Society (www.leukemia-lymphoma.org)
- CureSearch (www.curesearch.org)

PROGNOSIS
- Low stage localized disease, 5-year event-free survival >95%
- Aggressive treatment of advanced disease yields >80% 5-year event-free survival.
- Recurrent disease more resistant to therapy.
- Mortality for endemic form remains high where access to health care is limited.

COMPLICATIONS
- Complications of extensive abdominal disease include obstructive jaundice and pancreatitis, bowel obstruction, and intestinal perforation.
- Tumor lysis syndrome with renal failure (uric acid nephropathy) may occur prior to, and especially following, the start of chemotherapy.
- Rituximab has been associated with reactivation of hepatitis B virus resulting in fulminant liver failure.
- Other effects of chemotherapy include alopecia, myelosuppression, life-threatening infection, nausea, mucositis, infusion reactions, peripheral neuropathy, seizures, infertility, congestive heart failure, and secondary malignancy.

REFERENCES
1. Okebe JU, Skoetz N, Meremikwu MM, et al. Therapeutic interventions for Burkitt lymphoma in children. *Cochrane Database Syst Rev.* 2011;7: CD005198.
2. Molyneux EM, Rochford R, Griffin B, et al. Burkitt's lymphoma. *Lancet.* 2012;379:1234–1244.
3. Todeschini G, Bonifacio M, Tecchio C, et al. Intensive short-term chemotherapy regimen induces high remission rate (over 90%) and event-free survival both in children and adult patients with advanced sporadic Burkitt lymphoma/leukemia. *Am J Hematol.* 2012;87:22–25.
4. Beogo R, Nacro B, Ouedraogo D, et al. Endemic Burkitt lymphoma of maxillofacial region: Results of induction treatment with cyclophosphamide plus methotrexate in West Africa. *Pediatr Blood Cancer.* 2011;56:1068–1070.

ADDITIONAL READING
Gross TG, Hale GA, He W, et al. Hematopoietic stem cell transplantation for refractory or recurrent non-Hodgkin lymphoma in children and adolescents. *Biol Blood Marrow Transplant.* 2010;16:223–230.

 CODES

ICD10
- C83.70 Burkitt lymphoma, unspecified site
- C83.71 Burkitt lymphoma, lymph nodes of head, face, and neck
- C83.73 Burkitt lymphoma, intra-abdominal lymph nodes

CLINICAL PEARLS
- Burkitt lymphoma is an aggressive, mature B-cell malignancy most commonly diagnosed in childhood.
- Burkitt lymphoma is strongly associated with t(8;14) and with EBV and malaria infections.
- Burkitt lymphoma is highly treatable with intense multiagent systemic and intrathecal chemotherapy.

L

MACULAR DEGENERATION, AGE-RELATED

Richard W. Allinson, MD

BASICS

DESCRIPTION
- Age-related macular degeneration (ARMD) results in pigmentary changes in the macula or typical drusen associated with visual loss to the 20/30 level or worse, not caused by cataract or other eye disease, in individuals >50 years of age, although some definitions exclude age or visual acuity criteria.
- Leading cause of irreversible, severe visual loss in persons age >65 years
- Stages:
  - Atrophic/nonexudative
  - Neovascular/exudative
- System(s) affected: Nervous
- Synonym(s): Senile macular degeneration; Subretinal neovascularization; Age-related macular degeneration

EPIDEMIOLOGY
- Neovascular/exudative form is rare in blacks and more common in whites
- Predominant sex: Female

Incidence
- In the Framingham Eye Study (FES), drusen were noted in 25% of all participants who were ≥52 years of age. ARMD-associated visual loss was noted in 5.7%.
- Atrophic/nonexudative stage accounts for 20% of cases of severe visual loss
- Neovascular/exudative stage accounts for 80% of cases of severe visual loss

Prevalence
Per FES study:
- People 65–74 years old: 11%
- People ≥75 years old: 27.9%

ETIOLOGY AND PATHOPHYSIOLOGY
- Breaks in the Bruch membrane allow choroidal neovascular membranes (CNVMs) to invade the retinal pigment epithelium (RPE) and grow into the subretinal space.
- Atrophic/nonexudative: Drusen and/or pigmentary changes in the macula
- Neovascular/exudative: Growth of blood vessels underneath the retina
- Visible light can result in the formation and accumulation of metabolic by-products in the RPE, a pigment layer underneath the retina that normally helps remove metabolic byproducts from the retina. Excess accumulation of these metabolic by-products interferes with the normal metabolic activity of the RPE and can lead to the formation of drusen.
- Neovascular stage generally arises from the atrophic stage
- Most do not progress beyond the atrophic/nonexudative stage; however, those who do are at a greater risk of severe visual loss.

Genetics
- Genetic susceptibility may be a factor in ARMD: ~25% genetically determined.
- Complement factor H is an important susceptibility gene for ARMD.
- While the development of ARMD may be predicted by specific alleles, the clinical response to anti-vascular growth factor is not (1)[A].

RISK FACTORS
- Obesity
- Ethnicity: Non-Hispanic whites
- Cigarette smoking
- *Chlamydia pneumoniae* infection
- Family history
- Excess sunlight exposure
- Blue or light iris color
- Hyperopia
- History of cardiovascular disease
- Short stature
- Aspirin use (2)[A]

GENERAL PREVENTION
- Ultraviolet (UV) protection for eyes
- Routine ophthalmologic visits:
  - Every 2–4 years for patients age 40–64 years
  - Every 1–2 years after age 65
- Patients who take statins, which modify lipid profiles, may have a reduced risk.

COMMONLY ASSOCIATED CONDITIONS
- Presumed ocular histoplasmosis syndrome
- Exudative retinal detachment
- Vitreous hemorrhage
- Other causes of CNVMs

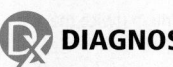

DIAGNOSIS

HISTORY
- Patients frequently notice distortion of central vision.
- Patients may notice straight lines appear crooked (e.g., telephone poles).

PHYSICAL EXAM
- Atrophic/nonexudative stage retinal exam:
  - Drusen (small yellowish white lesions):
    ○ Subtypes: Hard drusen and soft drusen
  - Atrophy of the RPE
- Neovascular/exudative stage retinal exam:
  - Blood vessels growing underneath the retina from the choroid are called CNVMs or subretinal neovascularization (SRN). The choroid is the vascular layer underneath the RPE.
  - Subretinal fluid or hemorrhage
  - Exudates
  - On Amsler grid testing, the horizontal or vertical lines may become broken, distorted, or missing.
- Disciform scar: An advanced stage resulting in a fibrovascular scar

DIFFERENTIAL DIAGNOSIS
- Idiopathic SRN
- Presumed ocular histoplasmosis syndrome
- Diabetic retinopathy
- Hypertensive retinopathy

DIAGNOSTIC TESTS & INTERPRETATION
Diagnostic Procedures/Other
- Amsler grid testing
- Fluorescein angiography:
  - Detection of CNVMs
  - Differentiate between atrophic and neovascular ARMD.
- Indocyanine green video angiography: May identify occult or hidden CNVMs

- Optical coherence tomography (OCT) may be useful in identifying CNVMs, subretinal fluid, and retinal thickening:
  - Fluorescein angiography is better than time-domain OCT in detecting new-onset CNVMs (3)[C].

Test Interpretation
Drusen: Deposits of hyaline material between the RPE and Bruch membrane (the limiting membrane between the RPE and the choroid)

TREATMENT

MEDICATION
First Line
- Ranibizumab (Lucentis):
  - Antibody fragment that inhibits all active forms of vascular endothelial growth factor (VEGF)
  - Approved for neovascular (wet) age-related macular degeneration
  - Injected intravitreally, at a dose of 0.5 mg, every 4 weeks
  - 1 year after treatment, up to 40% of patients treated with ranibizumab gained at least 3 lines of vision, and ~95% maintained vision.
  - Ranibizumab is superior to verteporfin in the treatment of predominately classic CNVMs.
  - The PrONTO study demonstrated optical coherence tomography (OCT)-guided, variable-dosing regimen with ranibizumab resulted in similar results to the MARINA and ANCHOR studies with monthly injections.
  - When comparing ranibizumab and bevacizumab in a multicenter study, both treatments were effective in stabilizing visual loss, and no difference was found in the visual outcome between the 2 treatment groups. A slightly higher rate of serious systemic adverse events was noted in the bevacizumab group (4)[A].
- VEGF Trap-Eye/Aflibercept (Eylea):
  - A decoy VEGF receptor that inhibits all isoforms of VEGF-A and placental growth factor (PlGF), the members of the VEGF family in mammals primarily involved in ocular neovascularization.
  - Approved for neovascular (wet) age-related macular degeneration
  - Injected intravitreally, at a dose of 2 mg, every 4 weeks for 12 weeks, then every 8 weeks
  - Dosed as need after the 12-week fixed dosing schedule resulted in a 5.3-letter gain in best corrected visual acuity at 52 weeks (5)[B].
  - Routine use of prophylactic antibiotics after intravitreal injections may be unnecessary (6)[B].

Second Line
- Pegaptanib sodium (Macugen) is a compound that binds to and neutralizes VEGF. The usual dose is 0.3 mg injected intravitreally every 6 weeks as needed for the treatment of neovascular ARMD. Pegaptanib preserves vision rather than improving it. 70% of treated patients lost fewer than 15 letters of visual acuity at 1 year.
- Bevacizumab (Avastin) is a full-length antibody to VEGF, administered intravitreally at a dose of 1.25 mg; it is being evaluated in the treatment of neovascular ARMD. Widely used off-label because of its lower cost.
- Agents that block platelet-derived growth factor (PDGF) are being investigated.

GENERAL MEASURES
Low-vision aids may be helpful.

SURGERY/OTHER PROCEDURES
- Neovascular/exudative macular degeneration:
  - The Macular Photocoagulation Study (MPS) demonstrated a treatment benefit for laser treatment of CNVMs that were ≥200 microns (200 microns = 0.2 mm) from the center of the macula.
- Treatment of CNVMs 1–199 microns from the center of the macula has been studied by the Age-Related Macular Degeneration Study-Krypton Laser (ARMDS-K). The benefit of laser treatment was greatest among patients without evidence of hypertension (HTN). No benefit was observed among patients who had highly elevated BP or used antihypertensive medication.
- Vitrectomy has been used to remove CNVMs, but this is generally not recommended.
- CNVMs can bleed spontaneously, leaving blood underneath the retina. Vitrectomy to remove subretinal blood may be of benefit and should be performed within 7 days of the bleed. Tissue plasminogen activator (tPA) instilled into the eye may help remove a subretinal hemorrhage. In some cases, intravitreal gas with or without tPA may displace submacular blood:
  - Intravitreal bevacizumab may be helpful in the treatment of neovascular ARMD associated with a large submacular hemorrhage.
- Macular translocation involves intentionally creating a retinal detachment and attempting to shift the macula away from the CNVM. Laser is then applied to the CNVM after the retina is translocated. This procedure is associated with potentially serious surgical risks.
- Photodynamic therapy (PDT) with verteporfin reduces vision loss in patients with >50% "classic" subfoveal CNVMs. Verteporfin is administered IV, and a diode laser at 689 nm is applied to the CNVM:
  - After 24 months of follow up in patients who underwent PDT to treat predominately classic subfoveal CNVM, 59% of the verteporfin-treated eyes vs. 31% of the placebo-treated eyes lost fewer than 15 letters from baseline.
  - Patients should be informed of a ~4% risk of acute, severe vision loss after PDT.
  - Ranibizumab has greater clinical efficacy than PDT.
  - Intravitreal triamcinolone combined with PDT may result in improved visual acuity for patients with CNVMs.
- Combination therapy combining intravitreal ranibizumab with PDT and/or intravitreal triamcinolone is being evaluated:
  - Combination treatment with intravitreal ranibizumab and PDT appears to offer similar gain in visual acuity when compared with ranibizumab monotherapy (7)[B].
  - Combination treatment with ranibizumab and PDT may reduce the number of ranibizumab retreatments.
- Stereotactic radiotherapy is being investigated in the treatment of neovascular ARMD.
- Laser photocoagulation to treat drusen is not recommended.

COMPLEMENTARY AND ALTERNATIVE MEDICINE
Free radical formation in the retina, induced by visible light, may play a role in cellular damage that results in atrophic/nonexudative macular degeneration. The Age-Related Eye Disease Study (AREDS) found that a high-dose regimen of antioxidant vitamins and mineral supplements reduced progression of ARMD in some cases.
- Recommended daily doses: Vitamin C 500 mg, vitamin E 400 IU, β-carotene 15 mg, zinc oxide 80 mg, and cupric oxide 2 mg
- Exercise caution with β-carotene use in smokers due to potential link to lung cancer.
- The Age-Related Eye Disease Study 2 (AREDS2) found the addition of lutein with zeaxanthin alone or in combination with omega-3 fatty acids had no overall effect in further reducing the risk of progression to advanced ARMD (8)[A].

 ONGOING CARE

FOLLOW-UP RECOMMENDATIONS
Patient Monitoring
- Laser-treated patients should be re-examined promptly if new visual symptoms occur.
- Amsler grid can aid in discovering visual disturbances.
- Patients with soft drusen or pigmentary changes in the macula are at an increased risk of visual loss. They should monitor their vision, such as by daily Amsler grid testing, and subjective measures of visual acuity, such as reading ability. If no new symptoms, follow-up examination in 6–12 months.

DIET
- Eating dark green, leafy vegetables (spinach/collard greens), which are rich in carotenoids, may decrease the risk of developing the neovascular/exudative stage.
- Fish consumption with omega-3 fatty acid intake reduces the risk of ARMD.

PATIENT EDUCATION
Instruct visually impaired patients to check with the local low-vision center for aids.

PROGNOSIS
- Patients with bilateral soft drusen and pigmentary changes in the macula, but no evidence of exudation, have an increased likelihood of developing CNVMs and subsequent visual loss.
- Patients with bilateral drusen carry a cumulative risk of 14.7% over 5 years of suffering significant visual loss in 1 eye from the neovascular stage of ARMD.
- Patients with neovascular stage in 1 eye and drusen in the opposite eye are at an annual risk of 5–14% of developing the neovascular stage in the opposite eye with drusen.
- High incidence of recurrence after thermal laser treatment for CNVMs.
- After 2 years of monthly ranibizumab injections, visual loss is commonly associated with impaired function of the photoreceptors and RPE and not from active leakage from CNVMs (9)[A].

COMPLICATIONS
Blindness

REFERENCES
1. Hagstrom SA, Ying GS, Pauer GJ, et al. Parmacogenetics for genes associated with age-related macular degeneration in the Comparison of AMD Treatment Trials (CATT). Ophthalmology. 2013;120:593–599.
2. Klein BE, Howard KP, Gangnon RE, et al. Long-term use of aspirin and age-related macular degeneration. JAMA. 2012;308:2469–2478.
3. Do DV, Gower EW, Cassard SD, et al. Detection of new-onset choroidal neovascularization using optical coherence tomography: The AMD DOC Study. Ophthalmology. 2012;119:771–778.
4. Comparison of Age-related Macular Degeneration Treatments Trials (CATT) Research Group, Martin DF, Maguire MG, et al. Ranibizumab and bevacizumab for treatment of neovascular age-related macular degeneration: Two-year results. Ophthalmology. 2012;119:1388–1398.
5. Heier JS, Boyer D, Nguyen QD, et al. The 1-year results of CLEAR-IT 2, a phase 2 study of vascular endothelial growth factor trap-eye dosed as-needed after 12-week fixed dosing. Ophthalmology. 2011;118:1098–1106.
6. Yin VT, Weisbrod DJ, Eng KT, et al. Antibiotic resistance of ocular surface flora with repeated use of a topical antibiotic after intravitreal injection. JAMA Ophthalmol. 2013;131:456–461.
7. Larsen M, Schmidt-Erfurth U, Lanzetta P, et al. Verteporfin plus ranibizumab for choroidal neovascularization in age-related macular degeneration: Twelve-month MONT BLANC study results. Ophthalmology. 2012;119:992–1000.
8. The Age-Related Eye Disease Study 2 (AREDS2) Research Group. Lutein+zeaxanthin and omega-3 fatty acids for age-related macular degeneration: The Age-Related Eye Disease Study 2 (AREDS2) randomized clinical trial. JAMA. 2013;309:2005–2015.
9. Rosenfeld PJ, Shapiro H, Tuomi L, et al. Characteristics of patients losing vision after 2 years of monthly dosing in the phase III ranibizumab clinical trials. Ophthalmology. 2011;118:523–530.

 ## CODES

ICD10
- H35.30 Unspecified macular degeneration
- H35.31 Nonexudative age-related macular degeneration
- H35.32 Exudative age-related macular degeneration

CLINICAL PEARLS
- Patients frequently notice distortion of central vision.
- Patients may notice straight lines appear crooked (e.g., telephone poles).
- Hyperopia is a risk factor for ARMD.
- The AREDS study found that a high-dose regimen of antioxidant vitamins and mineral supplements reduces progression of ARMD in some cases.

M

MALARIA
Paul M. Arguin, MD

BASICS

DESCRIPTION
- Acute or chronic infection transmitted to humans by *Anopheles* spp. mosquitoes
- Most morbidity and mortality is caused by *Plasmodium falciparum*; it is responsible for 216 million cases annually, including 655,000 deaths, the majority of which occur in children <5 years in sub-Saharan Africa.
- Nonimmune individuals are most susceptible to rapid progression to severe disease.
- System(s) affected: Lymphatic; Immunologic; Vascular; Hematologic; Renal; Cerebral

EPIDEMIOLOGY
Incidence
- Most US cases (>99%) are imported. Very rare cases reported from local transmission after introduction, transfusion transmission, and congenital transmission.
- ~1,500 cases and 5 deaths per year in the US
- Cases imported to the US: 58% *P. falciparum*; 19% *P. vivax*; 2% *P. malariae*; 2% *P. ovale*; 1% mixed; 18% unknown

Prevalence
- Predominant age: All ages
- Predominant sex: Male = Female

ETIOLOGY AND PATHOPHYSIOLOGY
- Malarial parasites digest red cell proteins and make the RBC membrane less deformable, causing hemolysis, increased splenic clearance, and anemia.
- Red cell lysis stimulates release of cytokines and tumor necrosis factor-α (TNF-α).
- *P. falciparum* induces human RBCs to secrete a protein that makes RBCs stick to the intravascular surface of small blood vessels, causing obstruction and end-organ ischemia.
- *P. falciparum*, *P. malariae*, *P. vivax*, *P. ovale*, and *P. knowlesi* in parts of Southeast Asia

Genetics
Unknown genetic predilection, but inherited conditions may affect disease severity and susceptibility (glucose-6-phosphate deficiency, sickle cell disease or trait, and hereditary elliptocytosis)

RISK FACTORS
- Traveling and/or migration from an area where malaria is endemic (most from sub-Saharan Africa)
- Rarely, blood transfusion, mother-to-fetus transmission, and autochthonous transmission

GENERAL PREVENTION
- Mosquito avoidance measures: Insect repellent, clothing that covers most of the body, mosquito nets treated with permethrin, air conditioning, and avoiding outdoor activity dusk to dawn (1)[A]
- *Malarial chemoprophylaxis when in endemic area:*
  - Mefloquine: Begin at least 2 weeks before arrival and continue for 4 weeks after leaving area. Adults, 250 mg (1 tablet) weekly; children ≤9 kg, 5 mg/kg; children >9–19 kg, 1/4 tablet weekly; children >19–30 kg, 1/2 tablet weekly; children >30–45 kg, 3/4 tablet weekly; children >45 kg as adult:
    ○ Caution: Mefloquine-resistant areas

- Atovaquone/Proguanil: Begin 1–2 days before arrival and continue for 1 week after leaving area. Adults, 1 adult tablet daily; children 5–8 kg, 1/2 pediatric tablet daily; children >8–10 kg, 3/4 pediatric tablet daily; children >10–20 kg, 1 pediatric tablet daily; children >20–30 kg, 2 pediatric tablets daily; children >30–40 kg, 3 pediatric tablets daily; children >40 kg, 1 adult tablet daily
- Doxycycline: Begin 1–2 days before arrival and continue for 4 weeks after leaving area. Adults, 100 mg daily; children, 2 mg/kg up to 100 mg daily (not for children <8 years old)
- Chloroquine: Begin 1–2 weeks before arrival and continue for 4 weeks after leaving area. Adults, 300 mg base (500 mg salt) weekly; children, 5 mg base/kg weekly up to 300 mg:
  ○ Caution: Chloroquine-resistant areas
- Primaquine: Begin 1–2 days before arrival and continue for 1 week after leaving area; adults 30 mg/d; children, 0.5 mg/kg/d up to adult dose:
  ○ For use only in areas predominantly endemic for *P. vivax*
  ○ Caution: Glucose-6-phosphate dehydrogenase deficiency must be excluded prior to first use.

COMMONLY ASSOCIATED CONDITIONS
Bacterial co-infections are not common but can sometimes occur.

DIAGNOSIS

HISTORY
- 1st symptoms of malaria are nonspecific; suspect in anyone ill returning from endemic area:
  - Fever, malaise, myalgias, chills, headache, nausea, splenomegaly (with chronic infection), hypotension, anemia (with chronic or severe disease), thrombocytopenia, jaundice, vomiting and diarrhea resembling gastroenteritis
- *P. falciparum:*
  - Incubation usually 12–14 days, symptoms within 1 month of infection in most individuals (partially immune individuals such as immigrants may become ill up to 1 year after last exposure)
  - Severe disease and complications: Vascular collapse, CNS impairment, renal failure, and acute respiratory distress syndrome
- *P. vivax* and *P. ovale:*
  - Incubation period 12–18 days for primary infection and up to 12 months (and longer) for relapses; generally presents with fevers
  - Dormant parasites may remain in liver and reactivate years after initial infection.
  - Can be severe
- *P. malariae* (benign quartan malaria):
  - Incubation period ~35 days
  - May become chronic; untreated can persist asymptomatically in human host for years
- *P. knowlesi:*
  - Incubation period ~12 days
  - Possibly severe

PHYSICAL EXAM
- Often not specific
- General: Elevated temperature, fatigue, tachycardia, tachypnea
- Chronic: Pallor, splenomegaly (hyperactive malarial splenomegaly syndrome)

DIFFERENTIAL DIAGNOSIS
- Infections (disseminated or localized): Abscess, viral, gastroenteritis, typhoid/paratyphoid, other bacteremias, rickettsial disease, mycobacteria
- Collagen vascular disease (SLE, vasculitides)
- Neoplasms (lymphoma, leukemia, other blood dyscrasias, other tropical causes of splenomegaly)
- Severe malaria infection may mimic hepatitis, pneumonia, stroke, or sepsis.

DIAGNOSTIC TESTS & INTERPRETATION
- Malarial smear thick and thin preparations:
  - Microscopy to evaluate for presence of parasite forms, determine species, and quantify the percentage of RBCs that are infected
  - Test should be performed on site, immediately, with results available within hours.
  - Rapid antigen capture enzyme: Can detect the presence of malaria parasites within minutes. Cannot determine species or quantify parasitemia. Positive and negative results must always be confirmed by microscopy.
  - Other tests: Species-specific PCR; species confirmation by PCR is encouraged)
- General laboratory findings (nonspecific):
  - In uncomplicated infection:
    ○ Elevated liver function tests and lactate dehydrogenase
    ○ Thrombocytopenia, anemia, and leukopenia
- Note: A low to low-normal platelet count or a slightly high bilirubin is typical and should alert the clinician to the diagnosis after exposure in an endemic setting.
- Note: Antimalarial agents may reduce parasitemia.

Initial Tests (lab, imaging)
- CBC with differential and platelets
- Basic chemistry panel including bilirubin
- Malaria thick and thin blood films (if negative, repeat q12–24h for at least 3 sets)
- Use only for respiratory disease (chest x-ray) or cerebral malaria (scan prior to spinal tap)

Follow-Up Tests & Special Considerations
Nonimmune individuals with suspected or confirmed *P. falciparum* should be hospitalized.

Test Interpretation
Malaria causes hemolysis

TREATMENT

MEDICATION
First Line

- For uncomplicated chloroquine-resistant *P. falciparum* (most *P. falciparum*), chloroquine-resistant *P. vivax*, or when species is unknown, the following regimens are recommended (2)[A]:
  - Atovaquone-proguanil (Malarone): Adult tablet: 250 mg atovaquone and 100 mg proguanil. Pediatric tablet: 62.5 mg atovaquone and 25 mg proguanil. Adults: 4 adult tablets once per day for 3 days. Children 5–8 kg: 2 pediatric tablets once per day for 3 days; children 9–10 kg: 3 pediatric tablets once per day for 3 days; children 1–20 kg: 1 adult tablet once per day for 3 days; children 21–30 kg: 2 adult tablets once per day for 3 days; children 31–40 kg: 3 adult tablets once per day for 3 days; children >40 kg: 4 adult tablets once per day for 3 days (1,2)[A]

– Artemether-lumefantrine (Coartem): Tablet contains 20 mg artemether and 120 mg lumefantrine. Persons 5–<15 kg: 1 tablet b.i.d. for 3 days; persons 15–<25 kg: 2 tablets b.i.d. for 3 days; persons 25–<35 kg: 3 tablets b.i.d. for 3 days; persons ≥35 kg: 4 tablets b.i.d. for 3 days (1)[A]

– Quinine sulfate plus doxycycline or clindamycin: Adults: Quinine sulfate 650 mg (salt) t.i.d. for 3 days (should be extended to 7 days for infections acquired in southeast Asia). Doxycycline 100 mg b.i.d. for 7 days. Clindamycin 20 mg (base)/kg/d divided t.i.d. for 7 days. Children: Quinine sulfate 10 mg (salt)/kg t.i.d. for 3 days (should be extended to 7 days for infections acquires in Southeast Asia) plus clindamycin dosed as above.

– Mefloquine: Adults: 750 mg followed by 500 mg 8 hours later. Children: 15 mg/kg followed by 10 mg/kg 8 hours later (not to exceed adult dose)

- PO therapy for *P. ovale, P. malariae,* chloroquine-sensitive *P. falciparum* (rare), and chloroquine-sensitive *P. vivax* (New Guinea has highest rates of chloroquine-resistant *P. vivax*):

– Chloroquine: Adults: 600-mg base followed by 300 mg at 6, 24, and 48 hours. Children: 10 mg base/kg (max 600 mg), then 5 mg/kg at 6, 24, and 48 hours

– Primaquine (should be added to chloroquine therapy for cure of dormant forms of *P. vivax* and *P. ovale*): Adults: 30-mg base (52.6 mg) daily for 2 weeks or 45-mg base (79 mg) weekly for 8 weeks. Children: 0.6-mg base/kg/d for 2 weeks (2)[A].

- Therapy for severe *P. falciparum:*
  – Clinical features defining severe malaria:
    ○ Impaired level of consciousness (LOC)
    ○ Respiratory distress, jaundice
    ○ Repeated convulsions, shock
    ○ Renal failure
  – Laboratory features:
    ○ Hypoglycemia
    ○ Acidosis (usually lactic acidosis)
- Parenteral therapy:
  – Quinidine gluconate 10 mg/kg in normal saline over 1–2 hours followed by 0.02 mg/kg/min continuous infusion.
  – Intensive care monitoring is necessary, especially when initiating quinidine therapy.
- In severe malaria, CDC should be contacted for assistance; CDC Malaria Branch: 770-488-7100; www.cdc.gov/Malaria/
- In 2007, CDC made artesunate available in the US for severe malaria and in special circumstances under an investigational protocol. Contact the CDC for assistance, as noted above.

ISSUES FOR REFERRAL
Infectious disease or tropical medicine expert for most cases

ADDITIONAL THERAPIES
None

Pediatric Considerations
- Children are particularly susceptible to severe disease.
- All children, even infants, should receive chemoprophylaxis if traveling to an endemic area.

- Malaria commonly resembles acute gastroenteritis in children.
- Children with severe disease are particularly prone to hypoglycemia. IV fluids with glucose should be used for maintenance and frequent blood glucose measurements taken.

Pregnancy Considerations
- Chloroquine is safe in the doses recommended for prevention and treatment of malaria; FDA pregnancy Category C.
- Mefloquine is safe in the doses recommended for prevention and treatment of malaria; FDA pregnancy Category B.
- Atovaquone-proguanil (Malarone) has not been studied in pregnant women; it has not been shown to cause birth defects or other problems in animal studies; FDA pregnancy Category C.
- No primaquine (FDA class undetermined) or tetracyclines (FDA pregnancy class D) in pregnancy.
- Quinine/Quinidine (FDA pregnancy class X/C, respectively) should be used during pregnancy because benefit outweighs risk.

COMPLEMENTARY AND ALTERNATIVE MEDICINE
None. Many deaths have resulted from using unapproved alternatives to medications.

SURGERY/OTHER PROCEDURES
Rarely, splenectomy must be performed in patients with hepatosplenic schistosomiasis mansoni (HSM) and medically unresponsive hematologic disorders.

IN-PATIENT CONSIDERATIONS
Initial Stabilization
- Inpatient care for all cases of *P. falciparum* malaria in nonimmune patients or any patient, despite the species, with signs of severe illness; outpatient care for others (1)[C]
- Nonimmune with *P. falciparum* may progress from mild symptoms to death within 12 hours. All patients treated on outpatient basis should have follow up within 24 hours.

Admission Criteria/Initial Stabilization
- All nonimmune patients with confirmed or suspected *P. falciparum*
- All patients with signs of severe disease (see "Treatment")

IV Fluids
Maintenance IV fluids with glucose, because of risk of hypoglycemia, is recommended if unable to tolerate fluids by mouth. Excess fluids may result in iatrogenically induced pulmonary edema.

Nursing
Observe for fluid excess, renal insufficiency (urine output), and hypoglycemia.

Discharge Criteria
Clinical improvement, ability to tolerate oral medications and fluids, with documented decreasing parasitemia levels

ONGOING CARE

PATIENT EDUCATION
- Malarial chemoprophylaxis prior to travel
- Travel information may be obtained at the CDC travel Web site: www.cdc.gov/travel

PROGNOSIS
Malaria infection carries a poor prognosis, with high mortality if untreated. However, if diagnosed early and treated appropriately, the prognosis is excellent.

COMPLICATIONS
- If not treated early, may cause cerebral malaria, acute renal failure, acute gastroenteritis, respiratory distress syndrome, and massive hemolysis
- Other complications: Seizures, anuria, delirium, coma, dysentery, algid malaria, blackwater fever, hyperpyrexia
- *P. malariae*: Nephrotic syndrome may develop in patients with chronic infection

REFERENCES
1. Centers for Disease Control and Prevention. Treatment of Malaria (Guidelines for clinicians). Updated July 1, 2013. Available at: www.cdc.gov/malaria/resources/pdf/treatmenttable.pdf
2. Griffith KS, Lewis LS, Mali S, et al. Treatment of malaria in the United States: A systematic review. *JAMA.* 2007;297:2264–2277.

ADDITIONAL READING
- Hill J, Hoyt J, van Eijk AM, et al. Factors affecting the delivery, access, and use of interventions to prevent malaria in pregnancy in sub-saharan Africa: A systematic review and meta-analysis. *PLoS Med.* 2013;10:e1001488.
- Mali S, Kachur SP, Arguin PM, et al. Malaria surveillance—United States, 2010. *MMWR Surveil Summ.* 2012;61:1–17.
- Manyando C, Njunju EM, D'Alessandro U, et al. Safety and efficacy of co-trimoxazole for treatment and prevention of Plasmodium falciparum malaria: A systematic review. *PLoS One.* 2013;8:e56916.
- Steinhardt LC, Magill AJ, Arguin PM. Review: Malaria chemoprophylaxis for travelers to Latin America. *Am J Trop Med Hyg.* 2011;85:1015–1024.

CODES

ICD10
- B50.9 Plasmodium falciparum malaria, unspecified
- B51.9 Plasmodium vivax malaria without complication
- B54 Unspecified malaria

CLINICAL PEARLS
- Rapid malaria tests are useful in the acute setting for determining if a patient has *P. falciparum* malaria (high negative predictive value). However, blood smears should also be performed on all suspected cases.
- Children with malaria frequently clinically appear to have gastroenteritis or nonspecific viral infections.
- Nonimmune persons with suspected or confirmed *P. falciparum* malaria are at high risk and must be managed aggressively (i.e., hospitalized).

M

MARFAN SYNDROME

Michele Roberts, MD, PhD • Helio Pedro, MD

BASICS

DESCRIPTION
- Marfan syndrome (MFS) is an inherited disorder of connective tissue.
- Because many features of MFS appear in the general population, specific diagnostic criteria (Ghent nosology) were established recognizing a constellation of features with major and minor criteria for establishing the diagnosis (1).
- The nosology was revised (2,3) because the previous criteria were not sufficiently validated, were not consistently applicable in children, or necessitated expensive and specialized tests.
- System(s) affected: Musculoskeletal; Cardiovascular; Ocular; Pulmonary; Skin/Integument; Connective tissue (dura)

Pediatric Considerations
Early surgical intervention may reduce the degree of scoliosis.

Pregnancy Considerations
- Manage pregnancy in MFS as high risk, preferably with a cardiologist. Prepregnancy evaluation should include a screening transthoracic echocardiogram for aortic root dilation.
- β-blockers should be considered in all pregnancies to minimize the risk of aortic dilation throughout the pregnancy.
- 1% complication rate if aortic root diameter <40 mm; 10% if >40 mm. Consider elective surgery before pregnancy if >47 mm.

EPIDEMIOLOGY
- Congenital; although clinical manifestations may be apparent in infancy, affected individuals may not present until adolescence or young adulthood.
- No gender, ethnic, or racial predilection; with advanced paternal age, a slightly increased risk of de novo mutation resulting in MFS in offspring.

Prevalence
1/3,000–1/5,000

ETIOLOGY AND PATHOPHYSIOLOGY
Genetic abnormality; mutations of the *FBN1* (fibrillin) gene. Fibrillin is an extracellular matrix protein widely distributed in elastic and nonelastic connective tissue.

Genetics
- Mutations of the fibrillin-1 *(FBN1)* gene on chromosome 15q21.1 are responsible for MFS, OMIM 154700.
- MFS is an autosomal-dominant condition with complete penetrance and variable expressivity. Apparent nonpenetrance may be due to lack of recognition of MFS in a mildly affected individual.
- Each child of an affected parent has a 50% chance of inheriting the disorder and may be more or less severely affected. 25% of cases result from de novo mutation.

GENERAL PREVENTION
- Prenatal diagnosis is possible in families with a known mutation.
- Antibiotic prophylaxis against endocarditis for dental and other procedures is no longer routinely recommended by the American Heart Association (AHA)/American Dental Association (ADA).
- Athletes who are especially tall should be screened for aortic root dilation.

COMMONLY ASSOCIATED CONDITIONS
- High prevalence of obstructive sleep apnea in MFS; may be a risk factor for aortic root dilatation (4)
- Increased prevalence of migraine in MFS

DIAGNOSIS

- In the revised Ghent nosology:
  - Cardiovascular manifestations (aortic root aneurysm/dissection) and ectopia lentis have more weight.
  - Molecular genetic testing for *FBN1* plays a more prominent diagnostic role, but is not required.
  - Less specific manifestations were removed or made less influential, thus avoiding obligate thresholds that were not evidence based. Careful follow up diminishes risk of missed diagnosis.
  - New criteria explicitly allow for alternative diagnoses, when additional features warrant: Shprintzen-Goldberg syndrome (SGS), Loeys-Dietz syndrome (LDS), or vascular-type Ehlers-Danlos syndrome (vEDS).
  - Z-score calculator for aortic root enlargement: www.marfan.org
- In the absence of a family history of MFS:
  - Aortic root dilatation or dissection (Z ≥2) (Ao) *and* ectopia lentis (EL): Unequivocal diagnosis of MFS, irrespective of systemic features, except when they are diagnostic of SGS, LDS, or vEDS
  - Ao *and* a bona fide *FBN1* mutation: Diagnostic of MFS, even in the absence of EL
  - Where Ao is present but EL is absent and the *FBN1* status is negative (or unknown), diagnosis of MFS requires systemic findings score of ≥7 points using new scoring system (see below) and exclusion of SGS, LDS, and vEDS.
  - With EL but without Ao, *FBN1* mutation previously associated with Ao is required for diagnosis of MFS.
- Systemic features, scoring system (see "Physical Exam"):
  - Wrist *and* thumb sign +3; wrist *or* thumb sign +1
  - Pectus carinatum deformity +2; pectus excavatum or chest asymmetry +1
  - Hindfoot deformity +2; pes planus +1
  - Pneumothorax +2
  - Dural ectasia +2
  - Protrusio acetabuli +2 by x-ray, CT, or MRI
  - Reduced upper-to-lower segment ratio (US/LS) *and* increased arm/height *and* no severe scoliosis +1
  - Scoliosis or thoracolumbar kyphosis +1
  - Reduced elbow extension +1
  - Facial features (3/5) +1
  - Skin striae +1
  - Myopia >3 diopters +1
  - Mitral valve prolapse (all types) +1
- Maximum: 20 points; score ≥7 indicates systemic involvement
- Positive family history requires a family member independently diagnosed using above criteria.
- With a positive family history, MFS can be diagnosed with ectopia lentis, *or* systemic score ≥7, *or* aortic root dilatation with Z ≥2 in persons >20 years old, *or* Z ≥3 in persons <20.
- In persons <20 who have negative family history and suggestive findings but who do not meet Ghent criteria, "nonspecific connective tissue disorder" is diagnosed and close clinical follow up is recommended.

- In the presence of a relevant *FBN1* mutation, "potential MFS" is diagnosed and close follow up is recommended.
- In adults who have suggestive findings but who do not meet Ghent criteria, consider alternative diagnoses: Ectopia lentis syndrome (ELS), mitral valve prolapse syndrome (MVPS), MASS (**M**itral valve prolapse, **A**ortic dilation, **S**kin, and **S**keletal) phenotype.

PHYSICAL EXAM
- Facial features: Dolichocephaly (head length longer than expected compared with width), enophthalmos, down-slanting palpebral fissures, malar hypoplasia, retrognathia
- Thumb sign: Distal phalanx of thumb protrudes from clenched fist. Wrist sign: Thumb and 5th digit overlap when circling wrist.
- Pectus carinatum deformity: Pectus excavatum or chest asymmetry beyond normal variation
- Hindfoot valgus with forefoot abduction and lowering of the midfoot; should be distinguished from pes planus
- Reduced upper segment-to-lower segment (US/LS) ratio: 0.93 in unaffected individuals vs. ≤0.85 in affected white adults, ≤0.78 in affected black adults. US is measured from the top of the head to the top of the mid-pubic bone; LS is measured from the top of the pubic bone to the sole of the foot. In children, abnormal US/LS: US/LS <1, age 0–5 years; US/LS <0.95, 6–7 years; US/LS <0.9, 8–9 years; <0.85, age ≥10 years.
- Increased arm span to height ratio >1.05
- Scoliosis or thoracolumbar kyphosis is diagnosed if, on bending forward, there is a vertical difference ≥1.5 cm between the ribs of the left and right hemithorax.
- Reduced elbow extension if angle between upper and lower arm measures ≤170 degrees on full extension
- Skin: Striae atrophicae are significant if not associated with significant weight changes (or pregnancy) and if located on midback, lumbar region, upper arm, axilla, or thigh.
- Because of lack of specificity, the following criteria were removed from the current nosology: Joint hypermobility, high arched palate, and recurrent or incisional herniae (2).

DIFFERENTIAL DIAGNOSIS
Several conditions present clinical manifestations overlapping with MFS in cardiovascular, ocular, and skeletal systems:

- Ectopia lentis syndrome: No aortic root dilatation
- Mitral valve prolapse syndrome: MVP, limited systemic features may include pectus excavatum, scoliosis, mild arachnodactyly; aortic enlargement and ectopia lentis preclude this diagnosis.
- MASS phenotype: *M*itral valve prolapse; myopia; borderline, nonprogressive *a*ortic enlargement (Z <2); and nonspecific *s*keletal and *s*kin involvement. Aortic involvement in MASS is usually nonprogressive; some risk for more severe vascular involvement.
- Shprintzen-Goldberg; Loeys-Dietz; Ehlers-Danlos syndromes
- Homocystinuria: Marfanoid habitus, thrombosis, mental retardation; urine amino acid analysis is diagnostic; lens dislocates downward.
- Familial thoracic aortic aneurysm

- Stickler syndrome, congenital contractural arachnodactyly; Weill-Marchesani syndrome, multiple endocrine neoplasia, type 2B

DIAGNOSTIC TESTS & INTERPRETATION

- Initial testing: Order serum for FBN1 genetic testing and urine for homocystine.
- FBN1 is the only gene mutation thought to be causative of MFS.
- In patients whose physical exam is suggestive of MFS, urinary homocystine should be measured to rule out homocystinuria, an inborn error of methionine metabolism. Sequencing of FBN1 is the preferred method for molecular diagnosis.
- Specific criteria have been established (2) for FBN1 mutations causative of MFS, including those found in families with MFS. FBN1 mutation is a valuable marker for risk or aortic dissection (5). In a small subset of patients with unequivocal MFS, no known FBN1 mutation was found.
- Anteroposterior (AP) radiograph: Diagnosis of protrusio acetabuli; results from deepening of hip sockets during growth; does not cause problems during childhood
- Scoliosis: Cobb angle ≥20 degrees on radiographs; imaging for MFS diagnosis, or as per clinical exam.
- Hindfoot valgus with forefoot abduction and lowering of the midfoot: Anterior and posterior views if clinically indicated
- Echocardiography: Measure aortic root at the level of sinuses of Valsalva; check for mitral valve prolapse.
- MRI or CT to evaluate for dural ectasia for diagnosis and if symptomatic, symptoms highly variable, nonspecific, and include lower back pain

Diagnostic Procedures/Other

- Ectopia lentis is diagnosed on slit-lamp examination after maximal dilatation of the pupil; lens dislocation is most often upward and temporal.
- Myopia: Common in the general population; myopia >3 diopters contributes to MFS systemic score.

Test Interpretation

- Cystic medial necrosis of the aorta
- Myxomatous degeneration of cardiac valves

 ## TREATMENT

MEDICATION

- Prevention of aortic complications: Labetalol or other β-adrenergic blockers. Dosage adjusted to target heart rate (resting rate 60 bpm, increase to ≤110 bpm after moderate exertion; or <100 bpm after submaximal exercise) (2)[C]
- Other agents used if β-blockers contraindicated: Calcium channel blockers, angiotensin-converting enzyme inhibitors, and angiotensin receptor blockers also retard aortic dilation in children and adolescents (6)[B].

ISSUES FOR REFERRAL

Genetics, Cardiology, Orthopedics, Ophthalmology

SURGERY/OTHER PROCEDURES

- When cardiac symptoms develop or aortic root diameter is ≥5 cm, consider surgical intervention (7). Many MFS patients will ultimately require reconstructive cardiovascular surgery:
  – Dissection of ascending aorta (type A) is a surgical emergency. Consider prophylactic surgery when diameter of sinus of Valsalva approaches 5 cm (2). Other considerations: Family history, rate of change, other cardiac pathology, pregnancy

– Dissection of descending thoracic aorta (type B): Surgical indications include intractable pain, limb or organ ischemia, aortic diameter >5.5 cm (or rapidly increasing) (2).
- Mitral valve repair: For severe mitral valve regurgitation or progressive LV dilatation or dysfunction, or in patients undergoing valve-sparing root replacement (2).
- Lens subluxation: Incidence of glaucoma is high, so surgery is performed only if the condition cannot be treated with corrective lenses. Surgical removal of lens in lens opacity, impending complete luxation, lens-induced glaucoma or uveitis, or anisometropia or refractive error not amenable to optical correction (2).
- Severe pectus excavatum may require surgery.
- Scoliosis: Bracing for curves 20–40 degrees until growth is complete or surgery if >40 degrees
- Surgery only for most severe cases of dural ectasia
- Hip replacement in middle age or later if protrusio acetabula has led to severe arthritic change

 ## ONGOING CARE

FOLLOW-UP RECOMMENDATIONS

- Avoid sports that can increase aortic root enlargement or pneumothorax, including weightlifting and acceleration/deceleration sports. Low-risk sports include bowling, golf, skating (but not ice hockey), snorkeling, brisk walking, treadmill walking or stationary biking, modest hiking (8)[C].
- Exercise restrictions based on individual circumstances (8): Follow recommendation from the National Marfan Foundation (www.marfan.org) and guidelines from the American Heart Association/ American College of Cardiology task forces; in general, avoid contact sports, Valsalva, and exhaustion.

Patient Monitoring

Frequent exams (at least 2× per year) while patient is still growing, with particular attention to cardiovascular system and to scoliosis:

- Yearly echocardiograms (initially), more frequent if aortic diameter is increasing rapidly (≥5 cm/yr) or is approaching the surgical threshold (≥4.5 cm in adults)
- Aortic root dilatation in MFS is usually progressive, warrants vigilance even when not seen on initial examination; age <20, yearly echocardiogram; adults with repeatedly normal aortic root measurements, echocardiogram every 2–3 years (2).
- Regular imaging after surgical repair of aorta
- Scoliosis or pectus deformity: Standard orthopedic management; clinical evaluation for scoliosis earlier than in general population; plain radiographs of spine during growth years to detect and measure scoliosis
- Annual ophthalmologic evaluation for detection of ectopia lentis, myopia, cataract, glaucoma, and retinal detachment; myopia is very common in MFS and may have early onset, rapid progression, and high degree of severity; early monitoring, aggressive refraction to prevent amblyopia (2).

PATIENT EDUCATION

- National Marfan Foundation, 382 Main St., Port Washington, NY 11959; 800-8MARFAN, www.marfan.org
- American Heart Association at www.americanheart.org

PROGNOSIS

Life-threatening complications involve cardiovascular dysfunction. In 1972, lifespan was 32 years. Currently, lifespan is nearly normal.

COMPLICATIONS

Bacterial endocarditis, aortic dissection, aortic or mitral valve insufficiency, dilated cardiomyopathy, retinal detachment, glaucoma, pneumothorax

REFERENCES

1. De Paepe A, Devereux RB, Dietz HC, et al. Revised diagnostic criteria for the Marfan syndrome. Am J Med Genet. 1996;62:417–426.
2. Loeys BL, Dietz HC, Braverman AC, et al. The revised Ghent nosology for the Marfan syndrome. J Med Genet. 2010;47:476–485.
3. Faivre L, Collod-Beroud G, Callewaert B, et al. Pathogenic FBN1 mutations in 146 adults not meeting clinical diagnostic criteria for Marfan syndrome: Further delineation of type 1 fibrillinopathies and focus on patients with an isolated major criterion. Am J Med Genet A. 2009;149A:854–860.
4. Kohler M, Blair E, Risby P, et al. The prevalence of obstructive sleep apnoea and its association with aortic dilatation in Marfan's syndrome. Thorax. 2009;64:162–166.
5. Faivre L, Collod-Beroud G, Child A, et al. Contribution of molecular analyses in diagnosing Marfan syndrome and type I fibrillinopathies: An international study of 1009 probands. J Med Genet. 2008;45:384–390.
6. Williams A, Davies S, Stuart AG, et al. Medical treatment of Marfan syndrome: A time for change. Heart. 2008;94:414–421.
7. Benedetto U, Melina G, Takkenberg JJ, et al. Surgical management of aortic root disease in Marfan syndrome: A systematic review and meta-analysis. Heart. 2011;97:955–958.
8. Maron BJ, Chaitman BR, Ackerman MJ, et al. Recommendations for physical activity and recreational sports participation for young patients with genetic cardiovascular diseases. Circulation. 2004;109:2807–2816.

 ## CODES

ICD10

- Q87.40 Marfan's syndrome, unspecified
- Q87.43 Marfan's syndrome with skeletal manifestation
- Q87.418 Marfan's syndrome with other cardiovascular manifestations

CLINICAL PEARLS

- Because many features of MFS appear in the general population, diagnostic criteria have been established. Molecular diagnostic testing for FBN1 mutations will play an increasing role.
- Early diagnosis of homocystinuria is important because clinical complications can be minimized with appropriate diet and medication.

M

MARIJUANA USE DISORDER

Adriana C. Linares, MD, MPH, DrPH

 BASICS

DESCRIPTION

Marijuana or cannabis use disorder is classified in *DSM-5* in different categories (mild, moderate or severe) depending on the presence of criteria for abuse and dependence. The criteria are:

- Failure to fulfill major obligations
- Use of substances in hazardous situations
- Use of substances even though person is having recurrent social or interpersonal problems
- Tolerance, defined by using increased amounts of cannabis to achieve the desired effect or intoxication or diminished effect with continued use of the same amount of cannabis
- Withdrawal
- Use of substances in greater amounts
- Desire to cut down substances
- Time spent in activities necessary to obtain the substance
- Important activities are given up due to use of substance
- Continued use of substance even though having problems associated with the use of it
- Presence of craving for the substance

EPIDEMIOLOGY

- The US is ranked 1st among 17 European and North American countries by the World Health Organization for prevalence of marijuana use.
- ~42% of teens will have tried marijuana by the time they graduate from high school (1).
- An estimated 2.2 million Americans used marijuana for the 1st time in 2008; >50% were under age 18 (1).
- In the US, 10% of those who ever use marijuana become daily users, and 20–30% become weekly users.
- In the United States, some states have approved medical marijuana use and 2 states (Washington and Colorado) have approved recreational use of marijuana
- There have been some concerns about the legalization of marijuana and increased in use and abuse of it

ETIOLOGY AND PATHOPHYSIOLOGY

- Main active ingredient in marijuana: Delta-9-tetrahydrocannabinol (THC)
- When marijuana is smoked, THC rapidly passes from the lungs into the blood and to the brain, where it binds to cannabinoid receptors (CBRs).
- CBRs are responsible for memory, thinking, concentration, sensory and time perception, pleasure, movement, and coordination.
- THC artificially stimulates the CBRs, disrupting the function of endogenous cannabinoids. A marijuana "high" results from overstimulation of these receptors.
- Over time, overstimulation alters the function of CBRs, which can lead to addiction and to withdrawal symptoms when drug use stops.
- Effects of smoked marijuana can last 1–3 hours.
- Effects from marijuana consumed in foods or beverages appear later, usually in 30 minutes to 1 hour, but can last up to 4 hours.
- Smoking marijuana delivers significantly more THC into the bloodstream than eating or drinking the drug.

RISK FACTORS

- Age (highest use among those 18–25 years)
- Male sex
- Comorbid psychiatric disorders (i.e., bipolar disorder, posttraumatic stress disorder [PTSD])
- Other substance use (i.e., alcohol, cocaine)
- Lower educational achievement (rates of dependence lowest among college graduates)

 DIAGNOSIS

- Screen for marijuana use along with other lifestyle questions, such as tobacco and alcohol use
- Ask for frequency and amount used (e.g., "How long does a nickel bag last you?").
- Unexplained deterioration in school or work performance may be a red flag for abuse (2)[C].
- Problems with, or changes in, social relationships (e.g., spending more time alone or with persons suspected of using drugs) and recreational activities (e.g., giving up activities that were once pleasurable) may indicate abuse.
- If available, information from concerned parents or spouses should be obtained (2)[C].
- *DSM-5* criteria for cannabis use dependence has been changed from *DSM-IV*. The legal issues associated with use of cannabis were dropped and the presence of cravings was added.

HISTORY

- Clinical presentation of acute intoxication:
  - Euphoria, elation, laughter, heightened sensory perception, altered perception of time, increased appetite
  - Poor short-term memory, concentration
  - Fatigue, depression
  - Occasionally, distrust, fear, anxiety, panic
  - With large doses, acute psychosis: Delusions, hallucinations, loss of sense of personal identity
- Withdrawal symptoms include:
  - Nausea
  - Weight loss
  - Decreased appetite
  - Insomnia
  - Depressed mood

PHYSICAL EXAM

- Evaluate for:
  - Conjunctival injection
  - Xerostomia
  - Nystagmus
  - Increased heart rate
  - Altered pulmonary status
  - Altered body temperature
  - Reduced muscle strength
  - Decreased coordination
- Withdrawal findings include:
  - Restlessness/Agitation
  - Irritability
  - Tremor
  - Diaphoresis
  - Increased body temperature

DIAGNOSTIC TESTS & INTERPRETATION

Positive urine drug screen. Cannabinoids can be detected in urine weeks to months after marijuana use.

 TREATMENT

- 4 methods of behavioral-based interventions:
  - Cognitive-behavioral therapy
  - Motivational interviewing
  - Motivational enhancement therapy
  - Contingency management
- No intervention to date has proved consistently effective for marijuana abuse (3)[C].
- Despite this, trials on cognitive-behavioral therapy and contingency management have shown better outcomes in reduction in marijuana use and maintaining abstinence (4)[A].
- For younger persons, family-based interventions may be more effective (3)[C].

- With marijuana abuse, most prevalent among patients suffering from other psychiatric disorders, studies indicate that treating the mental health disorder may help reduce marijuana use, particularly among heavy users and those with more chronic mental disorders (1)[C].
- Advice to give to patients for management of withdrawal (3)[C]:
  – Gradually reduce amount of marijuana used before cessation.
  – Delay 1st use of marijuana until later in the day
  – Consider use of nicotine replacement therapy if planning to stop separate tobacco use at the same time
  – Relaxation, distraction
  – Avoid cues and triggers associated with cannabis use
- Prescribe short-term analgesia and sedation for withdrawal symptoms, if required (3)[C].
- If irritability and restlessness are marked, consider prescribing very low-dose diazepam for 3–4 days (3)[C].
- Provide user and family members with information regarding marijuana abuse and withdrawal to increase understanding of the abuse and reduce likelihood of relapse.
- Withdrawal symptoms peak on day 2 or 3, and most are over by day 7. Sleep and vivid dreams can continue for 2–3 weeks.

MEDICATION
- No effective medication for the treatment of marijuana abuse
- 1 study suggested oral THC could be used to abate marijuana withdrawal in individuals who are trying to quit (5)[C].
- Another study concluded medications used to treat other drug use disorders, such as buspirone, lithium, and fluoxetine, may have therapeutic benefit (6)[C].

 ## ONGOING CARE

FOLLOW-UP RECOMMENDATIONS
- Monitor cessation of marijuana use with urine tests over several weeks for the inactive metabolite of cannabis (carboxy-tetrahydrocannabinol).
- Heavy smokers may continue to be positive for marijuana for up to 6 weeks.

PATIENT EDUCATION
To learn more about marijuana abuse, visit the National Institute on Drug Abuse (NIDA) Web site at www.drugabuse.gov. Other NIDA Web sites include:
- http://backtoschool.drugabuse.gov
- http://marijuana-info.org
- http://teens.drugabuse.gov

COMPLICATIONS
- Acute adverse effects:
  – Anxiety and panic, especially in naive users
  – Psychotic symptoms at high doses
  – Motor vehicle accidents if a person drives while intoxicated
- Chronic adverse effects:
  – Subtle cognitive impairment
  – Poor educational outcomes, lower income, greater welfare dependence, and unemployment
  – Chronic bronchitis and impaired respiratory function in regular smokers
  – Psychotic symptoms and disorders in heavy users, especially those with a history of psychotic symptoms or a family history of these disorders

REFERENCES
1. National Institute on Drug Abuse. *Research report series: Marijuana Abuse*, 2010.
2. Hubbard J, Franco S, Onaivi E. Marijuana: Medical implications. *Am Fam Physician*. 1999;60: 2583–2593.
3. Winstock A, Ford C, Witton J. Assessment and management of cannabis use disorders in primary care. *BMJ*. 2010;340:800–804.
4. Denis C, Lavie E, Fatseas M, et al. Psychotherapeutic interventions for cannabis abuse and/or dependence in outpatient settings. *Cochrane Database Syst Rev*. 2008;3:CD005336.
5. Budney A, Vandrey R, Hughes J, et al. Oral delta-9-tetrahydrocannabinol suppresses cannabis withdrawal symptoms. *Drug Alcohol Depend*. 2007;86:22–29.
6. Vandrey R, Haney M. Pharmacotherapy for cannabis dependence: How close are we? *CNS Drugs*. 2009;23:543–553.

ADDITIONAL READING
- American Psychiatric Association. *Diagnostic and statistical manual of mental disorders*, 5th ed. Washington, DC: APA; 2013.
- Fergusson D, Boden J. Cannabis use and later life outcomes. *Addiction*. 2008;103:969–976.
- Hall W, Degenhardt L. Adverse health effects of non-medical cannabis use. *Lancet*. 2009;374: 1383–1391.

 ## CODES

ICD10
- F12.10 Cannabis abuse, uncomplicated
- F12.19 Cannabis abuse with unspecified cannabis-induced disorder
- F12.90 Cannabis use, unspecified, uncomplicated

CLINICAL PEARLS
- Marijuana abuse may result in poor performance in school or work, legal problems, and arguments with family.
- Patients should be screened for marijuana use. Asked about frequency and amount used.
- Effects of smoked marijuana can last 1–3 hours. Effects from foods or beverages containing marijuana appear later, usually in 30 minutes to 1 hour, but can last up to 4 hours.
- Smoking marijuana delivers significantly more THC into the bloodstream than eating or drinking the drug.
- Acute marijuana intoxication is manifested by conjunctival injection, increased heart rate, euphoria, heightened sensory perception, altered perception of time, increased appetite, poor short-term memory and concentration, and fatigue. Large doses may result in acute psychosis, delusions, or hallucinations.
- Withdrawal symptoms include nausea, weight loss, decreased appetite, insomnia, and depressed mood. Peaks on day 2 or 3, and most are over by day 7.
- Cognitive-behavioral therapy, motivational interviewing, motivational enhancement therapy, and contingency management are 4 methods of behavioral-based interventions used in the treatment of marijuana abuse.

MASTALGIA

Eduardo Lara-Torre, MD, FACOG • Amanda Murchison, MD • Patrice M. Weiss, MD, FACOG

 BASICS

DESCRIPTION
- Painful breast tissue, often bilateral, that can be cyclic or noncyclic:
  – 2/3 of breast pain is cyclic and is usually associated with hormonal changes related to menses, external hormones, pregnancy, or menopause.
  – 1/3 is noncyclic and often is related to a breast or chest wall lesion.
- Synonym(s): Mastodynia; Breast pain

EPIDEMIOLOGY
Incidence
- Predominant sex: Most common in women, but occurs occasionally in men
- Predominant age: Generally seen from adolescence through menopause
- Frequency of breast cancer with those reporting breast pain ranges from 1.2–6.7% (1).
- Up to 70% of women report some degree of breast pain at some point in their lives (2).
- Most describe mild pain, but 11% describe pain as moderate to severe.

ETIOLOGY AND PATHOPHYSIOLOGY
- Causative pathophysiology remains unclear, but is thought to be related to hormonal or nutritional factors.
- When fibrocystic disease is the source, growth and distension of the cyst with hormonal fluctuation can cause pain.
- Hormonal factors (e.g., hormone-replacement therapy, oral contraceptives, pregnancy, menses, puberty, and menopause) may influence the diverse conditions that cause mastalgia or may themselves cause breast tenderness and pain.
- Benign breast disorders (e.g., fibrocystic changes)
- Trauma (including sexual abuse/assault)
- Diet and lifestyle (e.g., poor fitting exercise breast support)
- Lactation problems (e.g., engorgement, mastitis, breast abscess)
- Breast masses, including breast cancer
- Hidradenitis suppurativa
- Costochondritis (Tietze syndrome)
- Postthoracotomy syndrome
- Spinal and paraspinal disorders
- Potential side effects of medications
- Postradiation effects
- Referred pain (e.g., pulmonary, cardiac, or gallbladder disease)
- Ductal ectasia

Genetics
Familial tendency

RISK FACTORS
- Diet high in saturated fats
- Cigarette smoking
- Recent weight gain
- Pregnancy
- Large, pendulous breasts (caused by stretching of Cooper ligaments)
- Exogenous hormones
- Caffeine has *not* been shown to be a risk factor (3).

GENERAL PREVENTION
- Avoid exposure to risk factors
- Properly fitted bra support

 DIAGNOSIS

HISTORY
- Location, duration, frequency, severity, associated symptoms, related activities (e.g., trauma), and aggravating and ameliorating factors
- Complete medical history with focus on gynecologic/obstetric history
- Complete systematic review of systems
- Diet/smoking history
- Detailed family history for risk assessment for breast cancer
- There may be an association with other pain syndromes such as fibromyalgia (4)[B].

PHYSICAL EXAM
- Examine breasts systematically in both standing and sitting positions.
- Assess for skin changes, breast symmetry and contour, dimpling, localized tenderness, bruising, masses, nipple discharge, and lymphadenopathy. Look for signs that are suggestive of breast malignancy.

DIFFERENTIAL DIAGNOSIS
- The most important disease to rule out is breast cancer (although uncommon), particularly if pain is localized.
- Manipulation or trauma also can worsen symptoms.
- Chest wall pain or referred pain resulting from splenomegaly also must be differentiated from mastalgia.
- Sometimes cyclic pain is concurrent with premenstrual syndrome.
- Ductal ectasia of the breast

DIAGNOSTIC TESTS & INTERPRETATION
Initial Tests (lab, imaging)
- If galactorrhea is found, check a fasting prolactin level
- Consider thyroid-stimulating hormone (TSH)
- Consider an ultrasound in women with focal, persistent breast pain
- Mammogram ± ultrasound in women aged ≥30–35 years

Pediatric Considerations
Ultrasound is the imaging test of choice for children and adolescents. A mammogram is not useful.

Diagnostic Procedures/Other
- Cysts may need to be aspirated to relieve symptoms or verify diagnosis.
- Biopsies may be indicated based on the results of examination, ultrasound, or mammography.

Pediatric Considerations
In children and adolescents, do not perform biopsies unless there is suspicion for cancer. Refer to a specialist in pediatric breast disease.

Test Interpretation
- Normal breast tissue
- Benign: Fibrocystic changes, duct ectasia, solitary papillomas, simple fibroadenomas
- Small increased risk of breast cancer: Ductal hyperplasia without atypia, sclerosing adenosis, diffuse papillomatosis, complex fibroadenomas
- Moderate increased risk: Atypical ductal hyperplasia, atypical lobular hyperplasia
- Breast cancer

 TREATMENT

GENERAL MEASURES
- Stop or modify the current hormonal therapy
- A repeat examination may help to establish any cyclic nodularity pattern.
- Wear a properly fitted support bra (may be fitted by a professional)
- Reassurance (sufficient for most patients)
- Weight loss for obese patients
- Smoking cessation
- Relaxation training

MEDICATION

First Line

Acetaminophen, NSAIDs either oral or topical (e.g., diclofenac sodium or piroxicam) (5)[A]

Second Line

- Oral contraceptives may help some patients prevent fibrocystic disease, but may worsen pain in some sensitive patients.
- If the patient is on an oral contraceptive, switch to one that has a lower estrogen component.
- In some patients with mastalgia only during their menses, menstrual suppression with continuous oral contraceptives may be of benefit.
- Oral progesterone: 10 mg PO daily
- Other possibilities for patients with refractory symptoms, used infrequently because of potential side effects, include:
  - Danazol: 100 mg b.i.d. (possibly lower doses) may be the most effective; major adverse effects include menstrual irregularities, weight gain, acne, hirsutism, and voice change; *may be used during luteal phase only;* approved by the FDA for this indication
  - Toremifene: 30 mg PO daily (6)[B]
  - Bromocriptine: 5 mg PO daily and cabergoline 0.5 mg PO weekly, both during the 2nd half of the menstrual cycle are equally effective, but cabergoline has fewer side effects (7)[B].

ADDITIONAL THERAPIES

If the patient is breastfeeding, correct any breastfeeding difficulties; treat underlying mastitis or breast abscess.

Pediatric Considerations

Children and adolescents may require referrals to a specialist.

SURGERY/OTHER PROCEDURES

Some patients may need surgical breast reduction.

COMPLEMENTARY AND ALTERNATIVE MEDICINE

- Vitamin E and evening primrose oil have not been found to be of benefit for chronic mastalgia (3)[A].
- Flaxseed oil is not effective for the treatment of mastalgia (3)[C].

 ONGOING CARE

FOLLOW-UP RECOMMENDATIONS

As needed

Patient Monitoring

- As needed for patients not receiving pharmacotherapy
- Time of follow up will vary by type of pharmacotherapy and patient's particular problems

DIET

- Decrease fat intake to 20% of total calories
- No evidence suggests that reduction in caffeine intake may help to decrease the severity or incidence of the disease (3)[A]

PATIENT EDUCATION

Avoid or adjust risk factors

PROGNOSIS

- Premenstrual mastalgia increases with age and then generally stops at menopause unless the patient is receiving hormone therapy (HT).
- Most patients can control symptoms without receiving HT.
- Several months of HT may provide several more months of relief, but mastalgia may recur.
- Cyclic mastalgia responds better than noncyclic mastalgia to treatment.
- Effects of long-term HT are unknown.

REFERENCES

1. Smith RL. Evaluation and management of breast pain. *Mayo Clinic Proc.* 2004;79:353.
2. Ader DN, Shriver CD. Cyclical mastalgia: Prevalence and impact in an outpatient breast clinic sample. *J Am Coll Surg.* 1997;185:466–470.
3. Chase C, Wells J, Eley S, et al. Caffeine and breast pain: Revisiting the connection. *Nurs Womens Health.* 2011;15:286–294.
4. Genc V, Genc A, Ustuner E, et al. Is there an association between mastalgia and fibromyalgia? Comparing prevalence and symptom severity. *Breast.* 2011;20:314–318.
5. Ahmadinejad M, Delfan B, Haghdani S, et al. Comparing the effect of diclofenac gel and piroxicam gel on mastalgia. *Breast J.* 2010;16:213–214.
6. Gong C, Song E, Jia W. A double-blind randomized controlled trial of toremifene therapy for mastalgia. *Arch Surg.* 2006;141:43–47.
7. Aydin Y, Atis A, Kaleli S, et al. Cabergoline versus bromocriptine for symptomatic treatment of premenstrual mastalgia: A randomised, open-label study. *Eur J Obstet Gynecol Reprod Biol.* 2010;150: 203–206.

ADDITIONAL READING

- Blommers J, de Lange-De Klerk ES, Kuik DJ. Evening primrose oil and fish oil for severe chronic mastalgia: A randomized, double-blind, controlled trial. *Am J Obstet Gynecol.* 2002;187:1389–1394.
- Brennan M, Houssami N, French J. Management of benign breast conditions. Part 1—Painful breasts. *Aust Fam Physician.* 2005;34:143–144.
- Colak T, Ipek T, Kanik A. Efficacy of topical nonsteroidal antiinflammatory drugs in mastalgia treatment. *J Am Coll Surg.* 2003;196:525–530.
- Miltenburg DM, Speights VO. Benign breast disease. *Obstet Gynecol Clin North Am.* 2008;35:285–300, ix.
- Olawaiye A, Withiam-Leitch M, Danakas G, et al. Mastalgia: A review of management. *J Reprod Med.* 2005;50:933–939.
- Rosolowich V, Saettler E, Szuck B. Mastalgia. SOGC clinical guideline. Ottawa, Canada: Society of Obstetricians and Gynaecologists of Canada. 2006. Retrieved from www.sogc.org/guidelines/public/170E-CPG-January2006.pdf

 SEE ALSO

- Premenstrual Syndrome (PMS) and Premenstrual Dysphoric Disorder
- Algorithms: Breast Discharge; Breast Pain

 CODES

ICD10

N64.4 Mastodynia

CLINICAL PEARLS

- When evaluating a patient with breast pain, always rule out cancer first.
- In the adolescent population, do not biopsy; instead, refer to a pediatric specialist.
- Premenstrual mastalgia increases with age and then generally stops at menopause unless the patient is receiving HT.

M

MASTITIS

Montiel Teresa Rosenthal, MD

BASICS

DESCRIPTION
- Mastitis is an inflammation of the breast parenchyma, and possibly associated tissues (areola, nipple, subcutaneous [SC] fat).
- Usually associated with bacterial infection (and milk stasis in the postpartum mother)
- Usually an acute condition, but can become chronic cystic mastitis

EPIDEMIOLOGY
- Predominantly affects females
- Mostly in the puerperium; epidemic form rare in the age of reduced hospital stays for mothers and newborns
- Neonatal form
- Posttraumatic: Ornamental nipple piercing increases risk of transmission of bacteria to deeper breast structures: *Staphylococcus aureus* is the predominant organism.

Incidence
- 2.5% of breastfeeding mothers develop nonepidemic mastitis.
- Greatest incidence among breastfeeding mothers 2–3 weeks postpartum
- Neonatal form occurs at 1–5 weeks of age, with equal gender risk and unilateral presentation
- Pediatric form:
  – Around or after puberty
  – 82% of cases in girls

ETIOLOGY AND PATHOPHYSIOLOGY
- Microabscesses along milk ducts and surrounding tissues
- Inflammatory cell infiltration of breast parenchyma and surrounding tissues
- Nonpuerperal (infectious):
  – *S. aureus*, *Bacteroides* sp., *Peptostreptococcus*, *Staphylococcus* (coagulase neg.), *Enterococcus faecalis*
  – *Histoplasma capsulatum*
  – *Salmonella enterica*
  – Rare case of *Actinomyces europaeus*
- Puerperal (infectious):
  – *S. aureus*, *Streptococcus pyogenes* (group A or B), *Corynebacterium* sp., *Bacteroides* sp., *Staphylococcus* (coagulase neg.), *Escherichia coli*, *Salmonella* sp.
  – Methicillin-resistant *S. aureus* (MRSA) (1)
- Rare secondary site for tuberculosis in endemic areas (1% of mastitis cases in these areas): Single breast nodule with mastalgia
- *Corynebacterium* sp. associated with greater risk for development of chronic cystic mastitis

- Granulomatous mastitis:
  – Idiopathic:
    ○ Predilection for Asian and Hispanic women
    ○ Association with α-1-antitrypsin deficiency, hyperprolactinemia with galactorrhea, oral contraceptive use, *Corynebacterium* sp. infection, and breast trauma
    ○ Most women have a history of lactation in previous 5 years.
  – Lupus; autoimmune
- Puerperal:
  – Retrograde migration of surface bacteria up milk ducts
  – Bacterial migration from nipple fissures up breast lymphatics
  – Secondary monilial infection in the face of recurrent mastitis or diabetes
  – Seeding from mother to neonate in cyclical fashion
- Nonpuerperal:
  – Ductal ectasia
  – Breast carcinoma
  – Inflammatory cysts
  – Chronic recurring SC or subareolar infections
  – Parasitic infections: *Echinococcus*; filariasis; Guinea worm in endemic areas
  – Herpes simplex
  – Cat-scratch disease
- Lupus

RISK FACTORS
- Breastfeeding
- Milk stasis:
  – Inadequate emptying of breast:
    ○ Scarring of breast due to prior mastitis
    ○ Scarring due to previous breast surgery (breast reduction, biopsy or partial mastectomy)
  – Breast engorgement: Interruption of breastfeeding
- Ornamental nipple piercing increases risk of transmission of bacteria to deeper breast structures: *S. aureus* predominant organism
- Neonatal colonization with epidemic *Staphylococcus*
- Neonatal:
  – Bottle-fed babies
  – Manual expression of "witch's milk"
  – Can predispose to lethal necrotizing fasciitis
- Maternal diabetes
- Maternal HIV
- Maternal vitamin A deficiency (in animal models)

GENERAL PREVENTION
Regular emptying of both breasts and nipple care to prevent fissures when breastfeeding (2)

COMMONLY ASSOCIATED CONDITIONS
Breast abscess

DIAGNOSIS

- Fever and malaise
- Nausea ± vomiting
- Localized breast tenderness, heat, and redness
- Possible breast mass

HISTORY
- Breast pain
- "Hot cords burning in chest wall"

PHYSICAL EXAM
- Breast tenderness
- Localized breast induration, redness, and warmth
- Peau d'orange appearance to overlying skin

DIFFERENTIAL DIAGNOSIS
- Abscess (bacterial, idiopathic granulomatous mastitis, fungal, tuberculosis)
- Tumor:
  – Idiopathic granulomatous mastitis
  – Inflammatory breast cancer
  – Wegener granulomatosis
  – Sarcoidosis
  – Foreign-body granuloma
- Ductal cyst (ductal ectasia)
- Consider monilial infection in lactating mother, especially if mastitis is recurrent.

DIAGNOSTIC TESTS & INTERPRETATION
Initial Tests (lab, imaging)
Mastitis is typically a clinical diagnosis. Labs rarely needed. In those ill enough to need hospitalization, consider:
- CBC
- Blood culture
- In epidemic puerperal mastitis:
  – Milk leukocyte count
  – Milk culture
  – Neonatal nasal culture
- No imaging required for postpartum mastitis in a breastfeeding mother that responds to antibiotic therapy
- Mammography for women with nonpuerperal mastitis
- Breast ultrasound to rule out abscess formation in women:
  – Special consideration for this in women with breast implants who have mastitis

Follow-Up Tests & Special Considerations
Lactating mothers produce salty milk from affected side (higher Na and Cl concentrations) as compared with unaffected side.

Diagnostic Procedures/Other
Options if further progression to abscess formation:
- Needle aspiration
- Incision and drainage
- Excisional biopsy

TREATMENT

A recent Cochrane review found that insufficient evidence exists to confirm or refute the effectiveness of antibiotic therapy for the treatment of lactational mastitis (3)[A].

MEDICATION

- Prioritized on the basis of likelihood of MRSA as etiologic factor and clinical severity of condition
- Treat for 10–14 days
- For idiopathic granulomatous mastitis, prednisone in 1 mg/kg prolonged taper (± methotrexate or azathioprine)

First Line

- Outpatient:
  – Dicloxacillin 500 mg q.i.d.
  – Cephalexin 500 mg q.i.d.
  – Trimethoprim/Sulfamethoxazole (TMP/SMX); DS b.i.d. (MRSA possible)
- Inpatient:
  – Nafcillin 2 g q4h
  – Oxacillin g q4h
  – Vancomycin 1 g q12h (MRSA possible)
- Breastfeeding beyond 1 month:
  – Penicillin, ampicillin, or erythromycin (4)[A]

Pediatric Considerations

- TMP/SMX given to breastfeeding mothers with mastitis can potentiate jaundice for neonates.
- Clindamycin IM, IV, or PO with dosing based on age and weight

Second Line

- If mastitis is odoriferous and localized under areola, add metronidazole 500 mg t.i.d. IV or PO.
- If yeast is suspected in recurrent mastitis, add topical and oral nystatin.

ISSUES FOR REFERRAL

- Abscess formation
- Need for breast biopsy

ADDITIONAL THERAPIES

- Warm packs (or ice packs) to affected breast for comfort
- The use of a breast pump may aid in breast emptying, especially if the infant is unable to assist in doing this.
- Wear supporting bra that is not too tight

SURGERY/OTHER PROCEDURES

In cases of biopsy-proven idiopathic granulomatous mastitis, surgical removal can result in a 5–50% chance of recurrence, fistula formation, and poor wound healing.

IN-PATIENT CONSIDERATIONS

If a new mother is admitted to the hospital for treatment of her mastitis, rooming-in of the infant with the mother is mandatory so that breastfeeding can continue. In some hospitals, rooming-in may require hospital admission of the infant (4).

Admission Criteria/Initial Stabilization

- Failure of outpatient/oral therapy:
  – Patient unable to tolerate oral therapy
  – Patient noncompliant with oral therapy
  – Severe illness without adequate supportive care at home
- Neonatal mastitis
- Oral antibiotics
- Frequent emptying of breasts, if breastfeeding
- Analgesics for pain:
  – Acetaminophen
  – Ibuprofen

Nursing

- Breastfeeding/Pumping of breasts encouraged
- Start infant with feedings on affected side
- Abscess drainage is not a contraindication for breastfeeding.

Discharge Criteria

- Afebrile
- Tolerating oral antibiotics well

ONGOING CARE

FOLLOW-UP RECOMMENDATIONS

Rest for lactating mothers, up to bathroom

DIET

- Encourage oral fluids
- Multivitamin, including vitamin A

PATIENT EDUCATION

- Encourage oral fluids
- Rest essential
- Regular emptying of both breasts with breastfeeding
- Nipple care to prevent fissures

PROGNOSIS

- Puerperal:
  – Good with prompt (within 24 hours of symptom onset) antibiotic treatment and breast emptying; 96% success rate
  – 11% risk of abscess if left untreated with antibiotics
  – Antibodies develop in breast glands within first few days of infection, which may provide protection against infection or reinfection.
- Rare risk of abscess formation beyond 6 weeks postpartum if no recurrent mastitis

COMPLICATIONS

- Breast abscess
- Recurrent mastitis with resumption of breastfeeding or with breastfeeding after next pregnancy
- Bacteremia
- Sepsis

REFERENCES

1. Gastelum DT, Dassey D, Mascola L, et al. Transmission of community-associated methicillin-resistant *Staphylococcus aureus* from breast milk in the neonatal intensive care unit. *Pediatr Infect Dis J.* 2005;24:1122–1124.
2. Crepinsek MA, Crowe L, Michener K, et al. Interventions for preventing mastitis after childbirth. *Cochrane Database Syst Rev.* 2012;3:CD007239.
3. Jahanfar S, Ng CJ, Teng CL, et al. Antibiotics for mastitis in breastfeeding women. *Cochrane Database Syst Rev.* 2013;3:CD005458.
4. Academy of Breastfeeding Medicine Protocol Committee. ABM clinical protocol #4: Mastitis. Revision, May 2008. *Breastfeed Med.* 2008;3: 177–180.

ADDITIONAL READING

Spencer JP. Management of mastitis in breastfeeding women. *Am Fam Physician.* 2008;78:727–731.

 SEE ALSO

Algorithms: Breast Discharge; Breast Pain

CODES

ICD10

- N61 Inflammatory disorders of breast
- O91.22 Nonpurulent mastitis associated with the puerperium
- O91.23 Nonpurulent mastitis associated with lactation

CLINICAL PEARLS

- Complete emptying of the breasts on a regular schedule, avoiding constrictive clothing or bras that might obstruct breast ducts, meticulous attention to nipple care, "adequate rest," and a liberal intake of oral fluids for the mother can all reduce the risk of a breastfeeding mother's developing mastitis.
- First-line treatment for puerperal mastitis is dicloxacillin 500 mg PO q.i.d. × 10–14 days. Most mastitis can be treated with oral therapy.
- Among breastfeeding mothers, if the symptoms of mastitis fail to resolve within several days of appropriate management, including antibiotics, further investigations may be required to confirm resistant bacteria, abscess formation, an underlying mass, or inflammatory or ductal carcinoma.
- More than 2 recurrences of mastitis in the same location or with associated axillary lymphadenopathy warrant evaluation with ultrasound or mammography to rule out an underlying mass.

M

MASTOIDITIS
Roger Wu, MD, MBA • Patrick Axtmayer, MD • Francesca L. Beaudoin, MD, MS

BASICS

Mastoiditis is a suppurative complication of acute otitis media (AOM) affecting the mastoid air cells or posterior process of the temporal bone.

DESCRIPTION
- Inflammatory process of the mastoid bone
- Acute mastoiditis is a suppurative infection that typically presents after acute otitis media. Symptoms are present for <1 month. Subdivided into 2 stages:
  – Acute mastoiditis with periosteitis: Involvement of the periosteum of the mastoid bone, purulence within the mastoid air cells
  – Acute mastoid osteitis (coalescent mastoiditis): Destruction of the bony septae that separate air cells; leads to an empyema and involvement of more serious head and neck complications
- Subacute mastoiditis (masked mastoiditis): Indolent process, may occur with recurrent AOM that was not sufficiently treated
- Chronic mastoiditis: Due to chronic suppurative otitis media that has failed treatment; usually associated with cholesteatoma; symptoms lasting months to years

EPIDEMIOLOGY
- Children > Adults
- Most common in children <2 years of age
- In pediatrics: Males > Females
- Incidence down since introduction of antibiotics; controversial whether incidence is now rising due to antibiotic-resistant *Staphylococcus pneumoniae*

Incidence
1–4 cases/100,000/yr (1)

ETIOLOGY AND PATHOPHYSIOLOGY
- Subclinical stage begins with acute otitis media causing inflammation of mastoid air cells (likely present in all cases of AOM).
- Obstruction of the aditus ad antrum (the connection between the tympanic cavity and the mastoid) during severe cases of AOM:
  – Blocks outflow tract of mastoid air cells
  – Accumulation of edema and purulent material with penetration of mucosa and periosteum (acute mastoiditis with periosteitis)
- Increased pressure from fluid within the air cells leads to destruction of bony septae (acute mastoid osteitis/acute coalescent mastoiditis)
- Acute mastoid osteitis can then lead to pus dissecting to adjacent areas in head and neck and subsequent abscess formation:
  – Subperiosteal abscess (most common complication), Bezold abscess, suppurative labyrinthitis, suppurative CNS complications
- AOM: *Haemophilus influenzae*, *Streptococcus pneumoniae*
- Acute mastoiditis: *S. pneumoniae* (most common organism), *Streptococcus pyogenes*, *H. influenzae*, *Staphylococcus aureus* (including methicillin-resistant *S. aureus* [MRSA]):
  – Introduction of the 7-valent pneumococcal conjugate vaccine in 2000 has led to increase in multidrug-resistant *S. pneumoniae* serotype 19A
- Chronic mastoiditis: *Pseudomonas aeruginosa*, *S. aureus*, Enterobacteriaceae, anaerobic bacteria, polymicrobials (2)

Genetics
No known genetic pattern

RISK FACTORS
- Cholesteatoma
- Recurrent acute otitis media or chronic suppurative otitis media
- Immunocompromised patient

GENERAL PREVENTION
- Pneumococcal conjugate vaccine
- Early referral to ENT for chronic otitis media
- Adequate antibiotic treatment for acute otitis media when indicated
- Prevention of recurrent acute otitis media
- Treatment of chronic eustachian tube dysfunction (i.e., pressure equalization tubes)
- Early identification of cholesteatoma

DIAGNOSIS

HISTORY
- At time of admission (1)[A]:
  – 42% of children had previous history of otologic disease.
  – 54% were on antibiotic therapy
  – Average duration of symptoms 9.8 days
- Most common symptoms in infancy (1)[A]:
  – Lethargy/malaise/irritability
  – Fever
  – Poor feeding/decreased appetite
- Otalgia/possible otorrhea
- Hearing loss
- Headache
- Pain/redness/swelling noted over mastoid

PHYSICAL EXAM
- Postauricular changes: Erythema, tenderness, edema, and/or fluctuance (81–85%) (1)[A]
- Bulging, erythematous, or dull tympanic membrane (60–71%)
- Protrusion of auricle (79%)
- Fever (76%)
- Possible otorrhea, if tympanic membrane is perforated
- Narrowing of external auditory canal
- Subperiosteal abscess
- Tympanic membrane (TM) can be normal in 10% of patients: Suspicious for mastoiditis when symptoms of acute otitis media persist >2 weeks

DIFFERENTIAL DIAGNOSIS
- Postauricular inflammatory adenopathy
- Severe external otitis
- Postauricular cellulitis
- Benign neoplasm: Aneurysmal bone cyst, fibrous dysplasia
- Malignant neoplasm: Rhabdomyosarcoma, neuroblastoma
- Deep neck space infections
- Furuncle of ear meatus
- Parotitis
- Local trauma to auricula

DIAGNOSTIC TESTS & INTERPRETATION
Initial Tests (lab, imaging)
- CBC with differential: Increased leukocyte count (3)[C]
- Elevated erythrocyte sedimentation rate (ESR) and C-reactive protein (CRP) (2,3)
- Blood cultures
- Myringotomy/tympanocentesis: Send for cultures, Gram stain, acid-fast stain (1)[B]
- Mastoiditis is often a clinical diagnosis, but CT imaging is often pursued to confirm the diagnosis and look for complications.
- If obvious physical exam and/or historical findings are absent, temporal bone imaging is recommended for patients with cervical or postauricular findings (4).
- Plain radiographs of mastoid area (low diagnostic yield):
  – Distortion of mastoid outline or clouding of mastoid air cells (not diagnostic, also seen in AOM)
  – Coalescence of air cells; diagnostic but rare
- CT scan findings (97% sensitivity; 94% predictive value) (5):
  – Clouding/opacification of air cells (a finding also present in AOM)
  – Mastoid air cell coalescence
  – Cortical bone erosion
  – Rim-enhancing fluid collections
- CT of temporal bone with contrast (4)[C]:
  – Useful for identifying suppurative extension or asymptomatic complications
- Technetium-99m bone scan: More sensitive to osteolytic changes than CT
- Indications for CT scan in pediatrics (5)[C]:
  – Neurologic signs
  – Vomiting/lethargy
  – Suspected cholesteatoma
  – Fever after 48–72 hours of therapy
  – Local disease progression
- MRI is being used with increasing frequency; may see increased fluid signal of mastoid air cells on T_2-weighted MRI:
  – Not an effective screening tool, often an incidental finding in the absence of clinical signs

Follow-Up Tests & Special Considerations
Interpret normal WBC with caution in immunocompromised patient with symptoms.

Diagnostic Procedures/Other
- Tympanocentesis should be performed to obtain middle ear fluid for culture and sensitivity (1)[B].
- Myringotomy with culture (also therapeutic)
- Audiography if suspected hearing loss
- Obtain CSF if suspect intracranial extension
- Biopsy if tissue protruding through TM or tympanostomy tube

Test Interpretation
- Inflammatory tissue in air cell system
- Granulation tissue
- Osteitis

TREATMENT

- IV antibiotics and myringotomy (± tympanostomy tubes) is now the mainstay of therapy for uncomplicated acute mastoiditis, reflecting a shift away from surgical treatment.
- Simple mastoidectomy is recommended for nonresponders after 3–5 days to avoid intracranial complications (6)[C].

GENERAL MEASURES
- Inpatient care during acute phase for IV antibiotics
- Keep affected ear dry

MEDICATION
First Line
- Empiric antibiotics directed against most common organisms: *S. pneumoniae* (including multiple resistant strains), *S. pyogenes*, *S. aureus* (including MRSA), *P. aeruginosa*
- Use 3rd-generation cephalosporin with additional coverage for resistant strain (4)[C].
- Ceftriaxone 1–2 g IV q24h:
  – Pediatric dosing: 50–75 mg/kg/d IV divided q12–24h
  – Precaution: Adjust dose with renal impairment
- New recommendation of adding clindamycin to ceftriaxone for coverage of ceftriaxone-resistant *S. pneumoniae* in pediatric patients (4)[C]:
  – Clindamycin pediatric dosing: 20–40 mg/kg/d IV divided q6–8h
- Cefotaxime 1–2 g IV q4–8h, depending on severity:
  – Pediatric dosing: 100–200 mg/kg/d divided q6–8 hours
- Add vancomycin 30–60 mg/kg/d divided q8–12 hours if concerned for MRSA:
  – Pediatric dosing: 15 mg/kg/dose q6–8h
  – Precaution: Adjust dose with renal impairment.
- For patients with a history of recurrent AOM or recent antibiotic administration, treat with piperacillin/tazobactam 3.375 g IV q6h:
  – Pediatric dosing: 300 mg/kg/d based on piperacillin component divided q6–8h
- For other significant contraindications, precautions, or interactions, please refer to the manufacturer's literature.

Second Line
- Oral antibiotics are given after 7–10 days of IV antibiotics and once myringotomy/blood cultures narrow pathogen and sensitivities, typically:
  – Amoxicillin-clavulanate (Augmentin) or clindamycin + 3rd-generation cephalosporin for 3 weeks or total treatment duration of 4 weeks
- For chronic mastoiditis: Use topical drops, ofloxacin otic solution (0.3%), neomycin, polymyxin B, and hydrocortisone 3 drops, 3–4×/d.

ISSUES FOR REFERRAL
All cases of mastoiditis, both adult and pediatric patients, should be referred to ENT specialists.

SURGERY/OTHER PROCEDURES
- Tympanocentesis should be performed to obtain cultures and guide antibiotic choice (1)[B].
- Myringotomy to allow drainage of the middle ear is performed in most patients, with tympanostomy tubes to allow for prolonged drainage (6)[C].
- Mastoidectomy is definitive treatment either initially, for those patients whose condition fails to improve or progress within 24–48 hours despite IV antibiotics and myringotomy, or those with meningeal or intracranial complications (5,6)[C].

- For management of subperiosteal abscesses, if a trial of conservative therapy with drainage, myringotomy and IV antibiotics fails, simple mastoidectomy remains the most effective procedure (7)[C].
- Frequent cleaning of ear canal under microscope to ensure pressure-equalization tube patency and adequate drainage of middle ear
- Topical antibiotic drops are also usually used after insertion of pressure-equalization tubes.

IN-PATIENT CONSIDERATIONS
Admission Criteria/Initial Stabilization
- Clinical or imaging evidence of acute mastoiditis
- Hospitalize any patient with acute mastoiditis; start IV antibiotics

Nursing
Caution patient about getting affected ear wet

Discharge Criteria
- Afebrile for 48 hours before IV antibiotics are discontinued
- Clinical improvement
- Able to take oral antibiotics

 ONGOING CARE

FOLLOW-UP RECOMMENDATIONS
- Oral antibiotics for 3 weeks following satisfactory course of IV antibiotics (total duration of antibiotics is 4 weeks)
- For chronic mastoiditis, consider antimicrobial prophylaxis with amoxicillin for several months

Patient Monitoring
- Postoperative: Audiogram after acute flare-up has subsided to assess for hearing loss
- Follow up with ENT as outpatient, with closer follow up for patients who had intracranial complications or hearing loss

PATIENT EDUCATION
- Precaution about getting affected ear wet
- Follow up with ENT as outpatient

PROGNOSIS
- Depends on severity and stage of disease
- Conductive hearing loss may require reconstructive surgery
- Most cases of mastoiditis recover fully when early treatment is initiated.

COMPLICATIONS
Total estimated complication rate 17.9% (3)
Extracranial:
- Subperiosteal abscess (most common complication)
- Bezold abscess (abscess of sternocleidomastoid muscle, insidious, risk of mediastinitis)
- Citelli abscess (osteomyelitis of the calvaria)
- Osteomyelitis of the temporal bone
- Suppurative labyrinthitis (resulting in deafness)
- Facial nerve paralysis
Intracranial:
- Intracranial abscess: epidural/ subdural/ cerebral
- Meningitis/ Cerebritis/ Periosteitis
- Gradenigo syndrome (palsy of the sixth cranial nerve, draining ear, and retro-orbital pain)
- Sigmoid sinus thrombosis
- Central venous sinus thrombosis

REFERENCES
1. van den Aardweg MT, Rovers MM, de Ru JA, et al. A systematic review of diagnostic criteria for acute mastoiditis in children. *Otol Neurotol.* 2008;29: 751–757.
2. Chien JH, Chen YS, Hung IF, et al. Mastoiditis diagnosed by clinical symptoms and imaging studies in children: Disease spectrum and evolving diagnostic challenges. *J Microbiol Immunol Infect.* 2012;45:377–381.
3. Bilavsky E, Yarden-Bilavsky H, Samra Z, et al. Clinical, laboratory, and microbiological differences between children with simple or complicated mastoiditis. *Int J Pediatr Otorhinolaryngol.* 2009;73:1270–1273.
4. Lin HW, Shargorodsky J, Gopen Q, et al. Clinical strategies for the management of acute mastoiditis in the pediatric population. *Clin Pediatr (Phila).* 2010;49:110–115.
5. Bakhos D, Trijolet JP, Morinière S, et al. Conservative management of acute mastoiditis in children. *Arch Otolaryngol Head Neck Surg.* 2011;137:346–350.
6. Psarommatis IM, Voudouris C, Douros K, et al. Algorithmic management of pediatric acute mastoiditis. *Int J Pediatr Otorhinolaryngol.* 2012;76:791–796.
7. Psarommatis I, Giannakopoulos P, Theodorou E, et al. Mastoid subperiosteal abscess in children: drainage or mastoidectomy? *J Laryngol Otol.* 2012;126:1204–1208.

ADDITIONAL READING
- Minks DP, Porte M, Jenkins N. Acute mastoiditis—The role of radiology. *Clin Radiol.* 2013;68:397–405.
- Pritchett CV, Thorne MC. Incidence of pediatric acute mastoiditis: 1997–2006. *Arch Otolaryngol Head Neck Surg.* 2012;138:451–455.
- Tamir S, Shwartz Y, Peleg U, et al. Shifting trends: Mastoiditis from a surgical to a medical disease. *Am J Otolaryngol.* 2009;31:467–471.

CODES
ICD10
- H70.009 Acute mastoiditis without complications, unspecified ear
- H70.099 Acute mastoiditis with other complications, unspecified ear
- H70.90 Unspecified mastoiditis, unspecified ear

CLINICAL PEARLS
- TM can be normal in 10% of patients: Suspect mastoiditis when symptoms of acute otitis media persist >2 weeks with a normal TM.
- Hospitalize all patients with acute mastoiditis and involve ENT consultation early.
- Start with broad-spectrum IV antibiotics and collect middle ear fluid cultures to further guide treatment.
- If conservative treatment fails after 3–5 days, simple mastoidectomy should be performed to avoid intracranial complications.

M

MEASLES (RUBEOLA)

Herbert L. Muncie, Jr., MD

BASICS

DESCRIPTION
- A highly communicable, acute viral illness characterized by a maculopapular rash; begins at the head, spreads inferiorly to trunk and extremities
- Rash is preceded by fever and the classic triad: Cough, coryza, and conjunctivitis, and pathognomonic Koplik spots.
- Public health problem in the developing world, with significant morbidity and mortality
- System(s) affected: Hematologic; Lymphatic; Immunologic; Pulmonary; Skin
- Synonym(s): Rubeola

EPIDEMIOLOGY
- Transmission: Direct contact with infectious droplets over short distances or airborne spread (less common):
  - Droplets can remain in the air for hours.
  - In 2000, ongoing transmission declared eliminated in the US due to high rates of vaccination.
- Infectivity: Highly infectious; 75–90% of susceptible contacts will develop the disease:
  - Infectivity: Greatest during the prodromal phase
  - Patients are considered contagious from 5 days before symptoms until 4 days after rash appears.
  - Immunocompromised patients are considered contagious for entire duration of disease.
- Incubation period: Averages 12.5 days from exposure to onset of prodromal symptoms (1)
- Predominant age: Varies based on local vaccine practices and disease incidence. In developing countries, most cases occur in children <2 years of age.

Incidence
- In the US: No longer considered an endemic disease by the CDC; isolated outbreaks still occur.
- In 2011, more cases of measles (220) were reported in the US than during any period since 1996:
  - Of these, 89% were imported
  - Many were vaccine-eligible but declined owing to philosophic or religious beliefs
  - Children aged 6–23 months traveling abroad are at increased risk if unvaccinated.
- Worldwide: An estimated 20 million measles cases occur each year, with 164,000 measles deaths in 2008. Of great concern are the recent measles outbreaks in southern and eastern Africa. In 2009, 36,000 cases were reported from 46 African countries; however, in 2010 the number had increased to 172,824. Over 95% of measles deaths occur in countries with per capita gross national income of <US$1,000 and limited health infrastructure (2).

ETIOLOGY AND PATHOPHYSIOLOGY
Measles virus enters respiratory mucosa and replicates locally, then spreads to regional lymphatic tissues, then on to other reticuloendothelial sites via the bloodstream.
- Measles virus, a spherical, enveloped, nonsegmented, single-stranded, negative-sense RNA virus of genus *Morbillivirus*, family *Paramyxoviridae*
- Because humans are the only natural host, measles virus can only be maintained by an unbroken chain of human infections.

RISK FACTORS
- For developing measles:
  - Not being immunized or failure to receive 2 doses of vaccine
  - Travel to countries where measles is endemic
  - Contact with exposed individuals, travelers, or immigrants
- For severe measles or measles complications:
  - Immunodeficiency
  - Malnutrition
  - Pregnancy
  - Vitamin A deficiency
  - Age <5 years or >20 years

GENERAL PREVENTION
- Totally preventable disease with vaccination and positive externalities due to herd immunity (3)
- Measles vaccine (active immunization):
  - Vaccine is usually given in combination with mumps and rubella (MMR); another combination is with varicella (ProQuad)
  - Primary vaccination of general population requires 2 doses (0.05 mL SC):
    - 1st dose given at 12–15 months; 95% develop immunity.
    - 2nd dose given at time of school entry (or any time >4 weeks after 1st measles vaccine); initial nonresponders almost always develop immunity.
    - HIV-infected children should be vaccinated while asymptomatic or before CD4+ cell count drops <500/mm^3.
    - Health care workers should have immunity verified and if not immune receive the vaccine if not contraindicated.
  - Common adverse reactions:
    - Fever and, rarely, febrile seizures 6–12 days after vaccination (5%)
    - Transient, mild, measles like rash 7–10 days after vaccination (2%, with decreasing incidence during 2nd vaccination)
    - Mild allergic reaction
    - If hypersensitivity reaction occurs, test for immunity; if immune, 2nd dose not needed
    - Epidemiologic evidence has not substantiated any link between MMR vaccine and autism (4)[A].
  - Contraindications:
    - Pregnancy: Live vaccine is contraindicated (theoretical risk of fetal infection).
    - Anaphylactic reaction to gelatin or neomycin; consult allergist before vaccination
    - Egg anaphylaxis is not considered a contraindication.

COMMONLY ASSOCIATED CONDITIONS
- Immunosuppression
- Malnutrition

DIAGNOSIS

HISTORY
- Prodromal period: Usually 2–3 days before rash, but may be up to 8 days:
  - Fever:
    - Begins 8–12 days after exposure; persists until 2–3 days after onset of rash
    - High temperatures seen >102°F (39–40.5°C); can precipitate febrile seizures
    - Fever onset >3 days after rash suggests a complication

- Classic triad of "croupy" cough, coryza, and conjunctivitis
  - Cough may persist for 2 weeks.
  - Prodromal symptoms typically intensify over 2–4 days and peak on 1st day of rash before subsiding.
- Loose stools, malaise, irritability, photophobia (from iridocyclitis), sore throat, headache, and abdominal pain

PHYSICAL EXAM
- Koplik spots:
  - Pathognomonic of prodromal measles
  - 2–3-mm, gray–white, raised lesions on erythematous base that appear on buccal mucosa
  - Occur ~48 hours before measles exanthem
- Rash (not pathognomonic):
  - Maculopapular, blanches
  - Begins at ears and hairline and spreads head to toe, reaching hips by day 2
  - Discrete erythematous patches become confluent over time, with greater confluence on upper body than lower body.
  - Clinical improvement usually occurs within 48 hours of appearance of rash.
  - 3–4 days after rash appears, it fades and changes to brown color, followed by fine desquamation.
- Lymphadenopathy and pharyngitis may be seen during exanthem period.

DIFFERENTIAL DIAGNOSIS
- Drug eruptions
- Rubella
- *Mycoplasma pneumoniae* infection
- Infectious mononucleosis
- Parvovirus B19 infection
- Roseola
- Enteroviruses
- Rocky Mountain spotted fever
- Dengue
- Toxic shock syndrome
- Meningococcemia
- Kawasaki disease

DIAGNOSTIC TESTS & INTERPRETATION
Initial Tests (lab, imaging)
- Measles virus specific IgM assay from serum and saliva (or respiratory) is gold standard for the WHO:
  - IgM may be undetectable on 1st day of exanthem; usually detectable 3 days after exanthem:
    - False positive may occur with other infections; therefore, using molecular testing of serum and respiratory specimens is the best opportunity to confirm diagnosis.
    - Sensitivity: 77% within 72 hours of rash onset; 100% 4–11 days after rash onset; if negative but rash lasts >72 hours, repeat.
    - IgM falls to undetectable levels 4–8 weeks after rash onset.
- Measles virus–specific IgG is undetectable up to 7 days after exanthem; peaks about 14 days after exanthem:
  - An IgG concentration with a 4-fold increase from at least 7 days after rash onset vs. 14 days later by standard serologic assay is confirmatory.

- Culturing measles virus is difficult; not commonly performed.
- Mild neutropenia is common.
- Liver transaminases and pancreatic amylase may be elevated, particularly in adults.

ALERT
- Suspected measles cases in the US must be reported to the local or state health department.
- Chest x-ray (CXR) is appropriate when suspicion exists of secondary pneumonia.

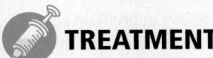 TREATMENT

GENERAL MEASURES
- Supportive therapy (i.e., antipyretics, antitussives, humidification, increased consumption of oral fluids)
- Control:
  - All patients with measles should be placed in respiratory isolation until 4 days after onset of rash; immunocompromised patients should be isolated for duration of illness.
  - Notify public health officials of suspected cases.

MEDICATION
- No approved antiviral therapy is available. Immunosuppressed children with severe measles have been treated with IV or aerosolized ribavirin, but no controlled data exist, and this use is not FDA approved.
- Vitamin A: WHO recommends:
  - Children <6 months of age receive 50,000 IU as 1 daily dose for 2 consecutive days.
  - Children 6–12 months of age receive 100,000 IU as 1 daily dose for 2 consecutive days (4).
  - Children >12 months of age receive 200,000 IU as 1 daily dose for 2 consecutive days (2).
- Antibiotics:
  - Reserved for patients with clinical signs of bacterial superinfection.
  - A 2013 Cochrane review suggests a "beneficial effect of antibiotics in preventing complications such as pneumonia, purulent otitis media and tonsillitis in children with measles," but does not define guidelines for choice or duration of antibiotics (5)[A].
  - A small 2006 randomized, double-blinded trial resulted in an 80% (number needed to treat [NNT] = 7) decrease in measles-associated pneumonia with use of prophylactic antibiotics; authors suggest the use of prophylactic antibiotics in patients with a high risk of complications (6)[B].
- Outbreak control:
  - The CDC defines an outbreak of measles as a single case.
  - Prompt immunization (within 72 hours) of people at risk of exposure or already exposed who cannot provide documentation of measles immunity:
    - Monovalent vaccine may be given to infants 6 months–1 year of age, but 2 further doses of vaccine after 12 months must be given for appropriate immunization.
    - Monovalent or combination vaccine may be given to all measles-exposed susceptible individuals where not contraindicated.
    - Individuals who have not been immunized within 72 hours of exposure should be excluded from school, child care, and health care settings until 2 weeks after onset of rash in last case of measles.

- Immunoglobulin (passive immunity) may be necessary for these high-risk individuals exposed to measles where vaccine is inappropriate:
  - Children age <1 year
  - Pregnant women
  - Individuals with severe immunosuppression
  - IM immunoglobulin should be given within 6 days of exposure to measles; CDC recommends 0.25 mL/kg to maximum of 15 mL; immunocompromised individuals receive 0.5 mL/kg to a maximum of 15 mL.

IN-PATIENT CONSIDERATIONS
Outpatient care is appropriate, except where complications develop (e.g., encephalitis, pneumonia).

 ONGOING CARE

FOLLOW-UP RECOMMENDATIONS
Patients are advised to call their doctor if they develop:
- Difficulty breathing or noisy breathing
- Changes in vision
- Changes in behavior, confusion
- Chest or abdominal pain

PATIENT EDUCATION
- Avoid exposure to other individuals, particularly unimmunized children and adults, pregnant women, and immunocompromised persons, until 4 days after rash onset.
- Avoid contact with potential sources of secondary bacterial pathogens until respiratory symptoms resolve.
- Centers for Disease Control and Prevention. Measles. Available at: www.cdc.gov/measles/about/index.html

PROGNOSIS
- Typically self-limited; prognosis good
- High fatality rates may be seen among malnourished or immunocompromised children, particularly in developing countries.
- Girls may have a higher mortality rate.

COMPLICATIONS
- Otitis media (occurs in 5–15%)
- The immune response to measles infection paradoxically depresses response to non-measles-virus antigens, which renders individuals more susceptible to pneumonia and diarrhea.
- Respiratory complications:
  - Bronchopneumonia (occurs in 5–10%):
    - Accounts for most measles-related deaths
    - May be viral or bacterial
  - Interstitial pneumonitis: In immunocompromised patients
  - Laryngotracheobronchitis ("measles croup"): Occurs in younger age group (<2 years)
- GI complications: Diarrhea (may lead to dehydration)
- Neurologic complications:
  - Febrile seizures
  - Acute disseminated encephalomyelitis with seizures and variety of neurologic abnormalities (occurs in 1/1,000 cases): Presents within 2 weeks of rash, probably an autoimmune response
  - Inclusion body encephalitis is a rare but fatal complication in persons with defective cellular immunity

- Subacute sclerosing panencephalitis:
  - Rare degenerative CNS disease resulting from persistent measles infection following natural disease, usually fatal
  - Presents 5–15 years after infection
  - Most often in persons infected before age 2
- Ocular complications:
  - Keratitis:
    - Can lead to permanent scarring, blindness
    - Vitamin A deficiency predisposes to more severe keratitis and its complications
- Other secondary bacterial infections
- Death: Results from complications, mainly pneumonia, rather than the virus itself. CDC statistics show that for every 1,000 children who get measles, 1 or 2 will die.

REFERENCES
1. Lessler J, Reich NG, Brookmeyer R, et al. Incubation periods of acute respiratory viral infections: A systematic review. *Lancet Infect Dis*. 2009;9: 291–300.
2. Moss W, Griffin D. Measles. *Lancet*. 2012;379: 153–164.
3. Althouse BM, Bergstrom TC, Bergstrom CT, et al. Evolution in health and medicine Sackler colloquium: A public choice framework for controlling transmissible and evolving diseases. *Proc Natl Acad Sci U S A*. 2010;107(Suppl 1): 1696–1701.
4. Demicheli V, Jefferson T, Rivetti A, et al. Vaccines for measles, mumps and rubella in children. *Cochrane Database Syst Rev*. 2005;4:CD004407.
5. Kabra SK, Lodha R. Antibiotics for preventing complications in children with measles. *Cochrane Database Syst Rev*. 2013;8:CD001477.
6. Garly ML, Balé C, Martins CL, et al. Prophylactic antibiotics to prevent pneumonia and other complications after measles: Community based randomised double blind placebo controlled trial in Guinea-Bissau. *BMJ*. 2006;333:1245.

 CODES

ICD10
- B05.2 Measles complicated by pneumonia
- B05.9 Measles without complication
- B05.89 Other measles complications

CLINICAL PEARLS
- Measles is a highly communicable viral disease whose natural transmission has been halted in the US by mass immunization.
- Immunization requires 2 doses: 1 at 12–15 months of age and 1 at school age (4–6 years of age).
- Presentation includes a prodrome of fever, cough, coryza, and conjunctivitis, followed by a descending maculopapular rash that begins on the face and progresses to the chest and lower body centrifugally.
- Health care providers should consider measles in the differential diagnosis of a febrile rash illness especially in unvaccinated individuals with recent international travel.
- Suspected measles cases must be reported to state or local health departments and measures taken to contain outbreak.
- Measles-associated pneumonia is the most common cause of mortality.

M

MEASLES, GERMAN (RUBELLA)

Ekaterina Brodski-Quigley, MD, EdM

BASICS

DESCRIPTION
- Rubella is a mild viral exanthematous infection of children and adults, generally self-limiting, with rare complications. Nonimmune women who become infected with rubella while pregnant may have devastating fetal effects. Up to 50% of infections may be asymptomatic (1,2).
- System(s) affected: Hematologic; Nervous; Pulmonary; Exocrine; Ophthalmologic; Skeletal.
- Synonym(s): German measles; 3-day measles

Pregnancy Considerations
- Pregnancy-associated rubella infection may lead to congenital rubella syndrome (CRS) with potentially devastating fetal outcomes.
- CRS is present in 90% of fetuses exposed during the 1st 11 weeks' gestation and 20% of fetuses exposed by 20 weeks' gestation (2).
- Most effective prevention of CRS is screening pregnant women for rubella immunity and immunizing nonimmune women (2)[B].
- Women vaccinated against rubella are advised not to become pregnant for 28 days: The vaccine-type virus can cross the placenta. No case of CRS has occurred after inadvertent vaccination, but a risk of 0.5–1.3% cannot be ruled out (2)[C].
- Polymerase chain reaction (PCR)–based method (87–100% sensitive) of detecting viral RNA in amniotic fluid allows rapid diagnosis of fetal infection if performed after 15 weeks' gestation; however, recent studies have indicated that fetal blood sampling at the same gestation yielded rubella-specific RNA where amniotic fluid failed (3)[B].

EPIDEMIOLOGY
- A 50–70 nm RNA togavirus of the genus *Rubivirus* (1).
- 13 genotypes have been identified (4).
- Live attenuated vaccine first available in the US in 1969
- Since 2004, not endemic in the US. All cases are of imported origin: Travelers with inadequate immunity (1).
- Average incubation: 14 days; range 12–23 days
- Infectious period between 7 days before and 5–7 days after rash onset
- Transmitted by respiratory droplets
- Temporal association: Late winter and early spring
- Only natural host is the human (1).

Incidence
- US incidence <10/100,000 since 2001
- 5 cases were reported in the US in 2010.
- Still occurs worldwide in developing countries: 100,000 cases of CRS reported annually.

ETIOLOGY AND PATHOPHYSIOLOGY
- Virus invades the respiratory epithelium, replicates in nasopharynx and regional lymph nodes, then spreads hematogenously throughout the body. An infected patient starts shedding the virus from the nasopharynx 3–8 days after inoculation, lasting 7 or more days after the rash starts.
- Progression from prodromal stage (1–5 days), to lymphadenopathy (5–10 days), and finally to a light pink, pruritic, maculopapular rash. Rash starts on the face and spreads to the trunk and extremities, sparing the palms and soles (14–17 days after onset of initial symptoms).
- 90% of fetuses exposed to rubella in the first 11 weeks' gestation (organogenesis) will develop CRS. 20% chance of developing CRS if exposed 12–20 weeks' gestation, and after 20 weeks' gestation the risk drops to 2% (2).
- German measles 1st described by German authors in the mid-18th century; thought to be a variant form of either measles or scarlet fever.
- In 1815, described in the English literature by Manton; felt to be a separate entity from measles or scarlet fever.
- Given the name rubella in 1866 by Veale.
- 1962–1965: Global pandemic resulting in an estimated 12.5 million cases in the US, with a devastating 2,000 cases of encephalitis, 11,250 cases of therapeutic or spontaneous abortions, 2,100 neonatal deaths, and 20,000 infants born with CRS (1).
- Live attenuated vaccine (LAV) licensed in the US in 1969 for the purpose of preventing CRS

Genetics
Children with CRS and children with type 1 diabetes mellitus (DM) share a high frequency of HLA-DR3 histocompatibility Ag and a high prevalence of islet cell Ab.

RISK FACTORS
Inadequate immunization or immunity after prior vaccination, immunodeficiency states, immunosuppressive therapy, crowded living/working conditions, international travel (1).

GENERAL PREVENTION
- Vaccination is the most effective preventive strategy.
- Available combined with measles and mumps (MMR) or combined MMR and varicella (MMRV). Single rubella vaccine is not available in the US.
- Rubella vaccine (strain RA 27/3):
  - A 2-dose schedule combined MMR vaccine recommended for those born after 1957. The 1st dose recommended at ages 12–15 months; 2nd dose recommended either at 4–6 or at 11–12 years of age. Children with HIV should receive MMR vaccine at 12 months of age if no contraindications exist. If an outbreak occurs, immediate vaccination for infants 6–11 months old is recommended (2).
  - Recommended for nonimmune people in the following groups: Prepubertal boys and girls, all women of reproductive age, college students, day care personnel, health care workers, and military personnel
- Contraindicated: Pregnancy, immunodeficiency (except HIV infection), within 3 months of IVIG or blood administration, severe febrile illness, or hypersensitivity to vaccine components. Patients who receive rubella vaccine do not transmit rubella to others, although the virus can be isolated from the pharynx. Breastfeeding is not a counter-indication (1).
- During outbreaks, serologic screening before vaccination is *NOT* recommended because rapid mass vaccination is necessary to stop the spread of the disease (2)[A].
- Debate about safety of MMR vaccine: Continued studies conducted prove the dissociation of the MMR vaccine with autism (5). Cochrane systematic review stated that it is unlikely to be associated with Crohn disease or ulcerative colitis. It is likely to be associated with benign thrombocytopenic purpura, parotitis, joint and limb complaints, febrile seizures, and aseptic meningitis (mumps).
- Children who receive the MMRV vaccine experience a 2-fold increase in incidence of febrile seizures than those who receive MMR and varicella vaccines separately (5).
- Because the US has adequate vaccination capabilities, antibody screening in prenatal care is recommended by the CDC and the ACOG, and should be reinforced (6)[B].

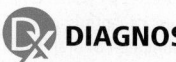

DIAGNOSIS

Counsel of State and Territorial Epidemiologists (CSTE) Case Definition Classifications of Rubella (1):
- Clinical case definition:
  - Acute onset of pink, coalescent macules on the face that spreads to the trunk and extremities, becoming discrete macules; fading in previously affected areas,
  - Temperature >99°F (37.2°C), if measured,
  - Arthralgia or arthritis, lymphadenopathy, or conjunctivitis
- Laboratory criteria for diagnosis:
  - Isolation of virus from: Throat or nasal swabs, serum, CSF, urine, or cataracts if removed from infected infant
  - 4-fold rise in acute- and convalescent-phase titers of serum IgG Ab
  - Positive serologic test for IgM Ab
  - PCR positive for virus

HISTORY
- Most cases of postnatal rubella are due to inadequately immunized travelers returning from endemic areas.
- Rubella can spread quickly among persons residing in close quarters.
- Postnatal rubella: Low-grade fever, sore throat, nausea, anorexia, arthritis, arthralgia, malaise. 50% may be asymptomatic.
- CRS: Parental concerns about hearing or vision impairment, jaundice, or developmental delay
- Deafness could be the only manifestation and not be noticed until 2nd year of life (2).

PHYSICAL EXAM
- Postnatal rubella: Low-grade fever, lymphadenopathy (postauricular, occipital, posterior cervical), exanthem (mild, pink, discrete 1–4 mm maculopapular), soft palate petechiae (Forchheimer sign) (20%)
- CRS: Microcephaly, large anterior fontanelle, sensorineural hearing loss (58%), cataracts, glaucoma, microphthalmia, pigmentary retinopathy, purpuric ("blueberry muffin") skin lesions, murmur (50%) consistent with patent ductus arteriosus (PDA), hepatosplenomegaly with jaundice, cryptorchidism, inguinal hernia, radiolucent bone disease

DIFFERENTIAL DIAGNOSIS
- Postnatal rubella:
  - Measles virus (rubeola)
  - Scarlet fever (strep A)
  - Infectious mononucleosis
  - Erythema infectiosum (parvovirus B19/Fifth disease)

- Roseola infantum (i.e., exanthem subitum)
- Toxoplasmosis
- Drug eruptions
- Other exanthematous enteroviral infections
- Congenital rubella:
  - Measles
  - Parvovirus B19
  - Human herpesvirus 6
  - Other exanthematous entero- or arboviruses

DIAGNOSTIC TESTS & INTERPRETATION

- Because 50% of cases are subclinical, laboratory testing is the only way to confirm the diagnosis (1,2).
- Detection of wild-type virus is considered the gold standard (1).
- Enzyme immunoassay (EIA): Preferred testing for IgM antibodies, which may not be detectable before 5 days after the onset of rash (1).
- Hemagglutination inhibition (HAI) test: Was once the standard. A 4-fold increase of IgG Ab levels from acute to convalescent phase is diagnostic for recent infection (1).
- Latex agglutination (LA) test: Appears to be sensitive and specific, but dependent on experienced lab personnel (1).
- Immunofluorescent antibody (IFA) assay: Used for detection of IgG and IgM Ab to the virus (1).
- Avidity test: Not routine and should be performed in reference labs. Purpose: Distinguish between recent and past infections (1).
- Serum collection should be performed within 7–10 days after the onset of the illness. When testing for IgM, repeat collection may be necessary if the sample was taken before day 5. When testing for seroconversion, a 2nd sample for IgG testing should be collected 2–3 weeks after the first specimen (acute to convalescent phase). In most cases, IgG is detectable 8 days after rash onset (1).
- The virus may be isolated from 1 week prior to 2 weeks after the onset of rash. Maximal viral shedding occurs up to day 4 after rash onset. Best results yielded from throat swabs (1).
- Viral genotyping by reverse transcription (RT)-PCR is performed to help determine the country of origin for epidemiology. For typing, throat swabs should be collected 4 days after the rash onset and sent directly to the CDC (1).
- Viral cultures of CSF are only reserved for suspected cases of CRS or rubella encephalitis (1).
- If a pregnant female is exposed, amniotic fluid for PCR or fetal blood may be obtained at 15 weeks' gestation for viral detection. Placental biopsy may be done at 12 weeks' gestation, but is performed less often. If positive, the parents should be offered genetic counseling (1).
- As the incidence of rubella decreases, the positive predictive value (PPV) of IgM results decreases. False-positive findings can occur in patients with parvovirus B19, mononucleosis, and positive rheumatoid factor (1).
- After re-exposure, a person with a low level of Ab from past infection or vaccination may experience an acute, small rise in Ab levels. This is not associated with a high incidence of contagion to others or of fetal risk (1).

Follow-Up Tests & Special Considerations

- Reporting: State dependent. Samples should be sent to the CDC for genotyping. Cases of CRS are reported to the National Congenital Rubella Syndrome Registry (1,2).

- Infants with CRS may shed virus up to 1 year. Place on contact isolation during all admissions until child's 1st birthday, unless child has 2 negative throat cultures and urine specimens a month apart once the child is 3 months old (2).

TREATMENT

- Supportive for mild cases
- Isolate patients for 5–7 days after the rash onset
- Postnatal rubella: Mild and self-limited; treat for symptomatic relief. Hospitalize for complications: Idiopathic thrombocytopenic purpura (ITP) or encephalitis, which may be associated with the vaccine.
- CRS: Supportive care unless neurologic or hemorrhagic complications develop; phototherapy may be indicated for jaundice; multidisciplinary management of long-term complications.

MEDICATION

No specific therapy available for mild cases.

First Line

- Age- and dose-appropriate antipyretics
- NSAIDs can be used for arthritis and arthralgias in adults and infants age >6 months.
- IVIG can be given in severe thrombocytopenia, but most cases are self-limited.

ONGOING CARE

FOLLOW-UP RECOMMENDATIONS

Patient Monitoring

- People immune to rubella via natural infection or vaccine may be reinfected when re-exposed; such infection is usually asymptomatic and detectable only by serology. Those who have received the vaccine have lower measurable IgG levels than those who had the natural disease.
- In CRS, it is extremely important to detect auditory and visual impairment early so that adequate education and counseling can begin (2).
- 2/3 of internationally adopted children have no written record of immunizations (4).

PATIENT EDUCATION

- JAMA patient page on rubella: Available at: www.jama.com; go to Patient Page Index; click on "Previous Topics, Rubella (1/23–30/2002)."
- www.cdc.gov/rubella/
- www.nlm.nih.gov/medlineplus/ency/article/001574.htm

PROGNOSIS

- Postnatal rubella: Complete and full recovery without sequelae is the rule.
- CRS:
  - Varied and unpredictable spectrum, ranging from stillbirth to completely normal infancy and childhood (1,2).
  - Detectable levels of IgG persist for years and then may decline (does not drop at the expected 2-fold dilution/month). By age 5, 20% have no detectable antibody (2).
  - IgM may not be detectable until 1 month after birth and may persist for 6–12 months (2).
  - Overall mortality 10%, greatest during first 6 months
  - 70% of encephalitis cases develop residual neurological defects, including autistic syndrome.
  - Prognosis is excellent when only minor congenital defects are present.

COMPLICATIONS

- Postinfectious encephalitis (1/5,000 cases)
- Thrombocytopenic purpura (1/3,000 cases)
- CRS: Incidence dependent on trimester exposed
- Rubella vaccine may rarely cause encephalitis or ITP:
  - ITP is self-limited and is not a contraindication to the vaccine.

REFERENCES

1. Centers for Disease Control and Prevention. *Manual for the surveillance of vaccine-preventable diseases*, 5th ed; Chapter 14-Rubella. 2012. Available at: www.cdc.gov/vaccines/pubs/surv-manual/chpt14-rubella.html
2. Centers for Disease Control and Prevention. Manual for surveillance of vaccine-preventable diseases 5th ed; Chapter 15-Congenital rubella syndrome. 2012. Available at: www.cdc.gov/vaccines/pubs/surv-manual/chpt15-crs.html
3. Tang J, Aarons E, Hesketh L, et al. Prenatal diagnosis of congenital rubella infection in the second trimester of pregnancy. *Prenat Diagn*. 2003;23:509–512.
4. Abernathy E, Hubschen J, Muller C, et al. Status of global virologic surveillance for rubella viruses. *JID*. 2011;204:524–532.
5. Lai J, Fay K, Bocchini J. Update on childhood and adolescent immunizations: Selected review of US recommendations and literature: Part 2. *Curr Opin Pediatr*. 2011;23:470–481.
6. Centers for Disease Control and Prevention. Recommendations of the Advisory Committee on Immunization Practices. *MMWR*. 2011;60(RR02):1–60.

ADDITIONAL READING

- Centers for Disease Control and Prevention. Epidemiology and prevention of vaccine-preventable diseases, 12th ed. Chapter 19, 2012. Available at www.cdc.gov/vaccines/pubs/pinkbook/rubella.html
- Mongua-Rodriguez N, Díaz-Ortega JL, García-García L, et al. A systematic review of rubella vaccination strategies implemented in the Americas: Impact on the incidence and seroprevalence rates of rubella and congenital rubella syndrome. *Vaccine*. 2013;31:2145–2151.
- Walling A. Measles, mumps, and rubella in pregnant women. *Am Fam Physician*. 2006;73:907–908.

CODES

ICD10

- P35.0 Congenital rubella syndrome
- B06.00 Rubella with neurological complication, unspecified
- B06.9 Rubella without complication

CLINICAL PEARLS

- Rubella is a mild viral exanthematous infection of children and adults, generally self-limiting, with rare complications.
- Nonimmune women who become infected with rubella while pregnant may have devastating fetal effects.

M

MELANOMA

Mona Mislankar, MD • Adam Anthony Ingraffea, MD

 BASICS

DESCRIPTION

- Melanoma is a tumor arising from malignant transformation of cells from the melanocytic system:
  - Most arise in the skin, but may also present as a primary lesion in any tissue: Ocular, GI, GU, lymph node, and leptomeninges
  - Metastatic spread to any site in body
- 4 main types of cutaneous melanoma:
  - Superficial spreading melanoma: 50–80% cases, occurs in sun-exposed areas (trunk, back, and extremities), most ~6 mm diameter at diagnosis, when seen in younger patients, presents as a flat, slow growing, irregularly bordered lesion (1)
  - Nodular: 20–30%, present in older patients, often ulcerate and hemorrhage, most commonly thick and pigmented
  - Acral lentiginous: <5% of all melanomas; however, most common melanoma in African Americans, found in palmar, plantar, and subungual areas:
    ○ Subungual melanoma: Dark longitudinal band in nail bed, Hutchinson sign when proximal nail fold involved
  - Lentigo maligna: Slowest growing, least likely to metastasize, older population, occurs in sun-exposed areas (head, neck, forearms) (1)
  - Desmoplastic melanoma: sarcoma-like tendencies with increased hematogenous spread (1)
- System(s) affected: Skin/Exocrine

Geriatric Considerations
Lentigo maligna, slowly enlarging pigmented lesion, is most common in elderly patients. This type usually found on face, beginning as a circumscribed macular patch of mottled pigmentation showing shades of dark brown, tan, or black.

Pediatric Considerations
Large congenital nevi (>5 cm) are risk factors and have a >2% lifetime risk of malignant conversion. Blistering sunburns in childhood significantly increase risk.

Pregnancy Considerations
No increased risk of melanoma in pregnancy. However, it is suggested waiting 1–2 years if further pregnancy desired in case of recent melanoma. Melanomas can spread to the placenta (2).

EPIDEMIOLOGY

Incidence
- In 2012, an estimated 76,250 Americans were diagnosed with melanoma with 9,180 expected deaths (1)
- 5th most common cancer in men, 7th most common cancer in women (1)
- Predominant age: Median age: 62 and 54 for men and women respectively, >50% of all individuals with melanoma are between 20 and 40 years of age.
- Predominant sex: Male > Female (1.5×)
- Incidence among whites greater than that among minority groups including, blacks or Hispanics
- Minority groups demonstrate increased rates of metastasis, advanced stages at diagnosis, thicker initial lesions, earlier age at diagnosis, and overall poorer outcomes (1).
- Low socioeconomic status associated with higher incidence of melanoma

Prevalence
- Lifetime risk: Men: 1/37; Female: 1/56
- 2% of all cancer deaths

ETIOLOGY AND PATHOPHYSIOLOGY
- DNA damage by UV-A/UV-B exposure
- Tumor progression: Initially may be confined to epidermis with lateral growth, may then grow into dermis with vertical growth

Genetics
- Dysplastic nevus syndrome is a risk factor for development of melanoma. Close surveillance warranted.
- 8–12% of patients with melanoma have a family history of disease.
- Mutation in *CDKN2A* found in 1/3 of patients with family incidence of melanoma (3).
- Mutations in *BRAF (V600E)* implicated in 50–60% of cutaneous melanomas (1)
- Additional susceptibility genes include *NRAS, CKIT, GNAQ/GNA11, BRCA2, MCR1, and OCA1* (1)

RISK FACTORS
- Genetic predisposition
- UVA-A and UV-B exposure
- History of >5 sunburns during lifetime
- History of intense intermittent sun exposure
- Previous pigmented lesions (especially dysplastic melanocytic nevi)
- Fair complexion, freckling, blue eyes, and blond/red hair
- Highest predictor of risk is increased number of nevi (>100).
- Family/personal history of melanoma
- Tanning bed use: 75% increased risk if 1st exposure before age 35
- Changing nevus
- Large (>5 cm) congenital nevi
- Other skin cancers
- Chronic immunosuppression (chronic lymphocytic leukemia, non-Hodgkin's lymphoma, AIDS, or posttransplant)
- Blistering sunburns in childhood
- Living at high altitude (>700 m or 2,300 ft above sea level)
- Occupational exposure to ionizing radiation
- The HARMM acronym identifies the five most important independent factors for increased likelihood of melanoma. A score of 5 represents high-risk patients versus 0-1 confer a low risk of melanoma (4).
  - **H**istory of prior melanoma
  - **A**ge greater than 50 years
  - Absence of a **R**egular dermatologist
  - A changing **M**ole
  - **M**ale gender

GENERAL PREVENTION
- Avoidance of sunburns, especially in childhood
- Use of sunscreen with at least SPF 30 to all skin exposed to sunlight
- Avoid tanning beds; class 1 carcinogen by World Health Organization (WHO) (3)
- Screening of high-risk individuals, especially males over the age of 50
- Education for proper diagnosis plays a large factor in prevention

- Any suspicious lesions should be biopsied with a narrow excision encompassing the entire breadth plus sufficient depth of the lesion. Options include elliptical excisions, punch, or shave biopsies (1).

COMMONLY ASSOCIATED CONDITIONS
- Dysplastic nevus syndrome
- >50 nevi. These individuals have higher lifetime risk of melanoma than the general population as 50% of all melanoma arise in pre-existing nevi.
- Giant congenital nevus: 6% lifetime incidence of melanoma
- Xeroderma pigmentosum rare condition associated with an extremely high risk of skin cancers, including melanoma
- Psoriasis after psoralen-UV-A (PUVA) therapy

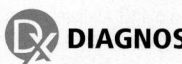 DIAGNOSIS

HISTORY
- Change in a pigmented lesions: either hypo- or hyperpigmentation, bleeding, scaling, ulceration, or changes in size or texture.
- Obtain family and personal history of melanoma or nonmelanoma skin cancer.
- Obtain social history on sunbathing, tanning, and other sun exposure.

PHYSICAL EXAM
- ABCDE: **A**symmetry, **B**order irregularity, **C**olor variegation (especially red, white, black, blue), **D**iameter >6 mm, **E**levation above skin surface
- Any new and/or changing nevus, bleeding/ulcerated.
- Location on Caucasians is primarily back and lower leg, on African Americans is the hands, feet, and nails
- Individuals at high risk for melanoma should have careful ocular exam to assess for presence of melanoma in the iris and retina.

DIFFERENTIAL DIAGNOSIS
- Dysplastic and blue nevi
- Vascular skin tumor
- Pigmented actinic keratosis
- Traumatic hematoma
- Pigmented squamous cell and basal cell carcinomas, seborrheic keratoses, other changing nevi

DIAGNOSTIC TESTS & INTERPRETATION
- Lactate dehydrogenase (LDH) may be helpful in monitoring progression in metastatic disease
- Imaging studies only helpful in detecting, and evaluating for progression of metastatic disease

Diagnostic Procedures/Other
- Dermoscopy allows for magnification of lesions, allowing for a decreased number of biopsies of benign skin lesions in addition to providing increased diagnostic accuracy
- Surgical biopsy remains the standard of care. Any suspicious nevus should be excised, either by scalpel incision or a scoop shave technique.
- Sentinel lymph node biopsies often recommended for patients with T2, T3, T4 staging
- Melafind is a new computer vision system designed to aid dermatologists in detecting early pigmented cutaneous melanoma.

Test Interpretation
- Nodular melanoma is primarily vertical growth, whereas the other 3 types are horizontal.
- Estimated that 1/10,000 dysplastic nevi become melanoma annually.
- Immunohistochemical testing increases sensitivity of lymph node biopsies (2)
- Staging based on the tumor-node-metastasis (TNM) criteria

 TREATMENT

GENERAL MEASURES
Full surgical excision of melanoma is the standard of care. See below for recommended surgical margins.

MEDICATION
- Stages I–III, surgical excision is curative in most cases; patients with stage IV disease, systemic treatment with chemotherapy is recommended (e.g., dacarbazine [DTIC], temozolomide, paclitaxel, carmustine [BCNU], cisplatin, carboplatin, vinblastine).
- Treatment with the cytokine interleukin-2 (IL-2) has demonstrated efficacy in treatment trials, especially with combination treatment with interferon and other chemotherapeutic agents (1)[A]:
  – Approved for metastatic melanoma and may induce remission in some patient, however, due to its toxicity, not all patients will be able to tolerate or be candidates for treatment (4).
- Interferon-α is FDA approved to treat advanced melanoma; shown to slightly increase survival rate (5)[C]
  – Pegylated interferon offers an increased patient friendly dosing regimen in addition to a decreased side effect profile (5)
  – Additional cytokines with some benefit include IL-21
- Biochemotherapy is advocated by some (i.e., chemo- + immunotherapy combination)
- Ipilimumab (YERVOY), monoclonal antibody against CTLA-4, is FDA approved for treatment of advanced melanoma, increased patient survival by 10 months in stage III and IV trials (1)[A]
- Vemurafenib (Zelboraf) is a new BRAF inhibitor approved for metastatic, unresectable melanoma expressing BRAFV600E (1)[A]

ISSUES FOR REFERRAL
- Consultation with oncologist recommended for consideration of chemotherapeutic options.
- Plastic surgery sometimes needed after final excision

ADDITIONAL THERAPIES
New studies have demonstrated that vaccinations targeting gp100, tyrosinase, and MART-1 may open new doors for melanoma treatment in the future (1).

SURGERY/OTHER PROCEDURES
- Standard of care for melanoma includes early surgical excision (4)[A]:
  – Excision margins for invasive melanoma should include a minimum of 1-cm margins
  – In situ tumors should have excisions with 0.5–1.0-cm margins
  – Lesions less than 2 mm in thickness can be safely excised with 1-cm margins
  – Any lesion more than 2 mm in thickness should be excised with 2-cm margins
- Sentinel lymph node biopsy should be strongly considered in patients with T2, T3, and T4 staged melanomas (1)[A]:
  – Selected patients with stage T1a and T1b melanoma should also be considered for sentinel lymph node biopsy
- Mohs surgery often used for lesions with ill-defined borders, or lesions of head and neck (6)
- Radiotherapy can be used to treat lentigo maligna in addition to certain head and neck lesions.

COMPLEMENTARY AND ALTERNATIVE MEDICINE
Many have been tried with no proven benefits

IN-PATIENT CONSIDERATIONS
Admission Criteria/Initial Stabilization
Most surgeries are done as outpatients with no stabilization needed.

 ONGOING CARE

FOLLOW-UP RECOMMENDATIONS
Once diagnosed, close follow up and skin protection (i.e., sunblock, UV protective clothing) are highly advised.

Patient Monitoring
- Skin exams every 3–6 months in patients with a history of melanoma, which can then be increased to every 6–12 months
- Physician skin exams annually for all persons over the age of 40 is controversial and without proven benefit.
- Total body photography and dermoscopy should be used for surveillance of skin lesions, most commonly used for patients with >5 atypical nevi
- Screening blood work is an ineffective tool to detect metastases and is not recommended (1)[C]

DIET
No data suggesting the benefit/risk of dietary manipulations

PATIENT EDUCATION
- Teach patients who are at risk, or have had melanoma, the principles of ABCDE examinations.
- High risk patients should perform monthly skin self-examinations and be taught to examine inaccessible areas.
- Patients with a history of melanoma or dysplastic nevus syndrome must have frequent total-body examinations.

PROGNOSIS
- Median age at death 68 years
- Highest survival seen in women <45 years of age at diagnosis

- Metastatic melanoma has an average survival of 6–9 months
- Palliative radiation therapy used with metastatic melanoma

COMPLICATIONS
- Metastatic spread
- Unsatisfactory cosmetic results following the primary surgery

REFERENCES
1. Ingraffea A. Facial skin: Contemporary topics for the surgeon, melanoma. *Facial Plas Surg Clin North Am.* 2013;21:33–42.
2. Markovic SN, Erickson LA, Rao RD, et al. Malignant melanoma in the 21st century, part 1: Epidemiology, risk factors, screening, prevention and diagnosis. *Mayo Clin Proc.* 2007;82:364–380.
3. Riker AI, Zea N, Trinh T. The epidemiology, prevention and detection of melanoma. *Ochsner.* 2010;10:56–65.
4. Tuong W, Cheng LS, Armstrong AW, et al. Melanoma: Epidemiology, diagnosis, treatment, and outcomes. *Dermatol Clin.* 2012;30:113–124, ix.
5. Coit D, Olszanski A. Progress in the management of melanoma. *J Natl Compr Canc Netw.* 2013; 11:645–648.
6. Erickson C, Miller SJ. Treatment options in melanoma in situ: Topical and radiation therapy, excision and Mohs surgery. *Int J Dermatol.* 2010;49:482–491.

ADDITIONAL READING
- Balch CM, Gershenwald JE, Soong SJ, et al. Final version of 2009 AJCC melanoma staging and classification. *J Clin Oncol.* 2009;27:6199–6206.
- MelaFind. Available at: INTER REF www.melasciences.com

 CODES

ICD10
- C43.4 Malignant melanoma of scalp and neck
- C43.9 Malignant melanoma of skin, unspecified
- C43.30 Malignant melanoma of unspecified part of face

CLINICAL PEARLS
- Always consider melanoma if a regional lymph node is enlarged and nontender.
- Do not forget that amelanotic melanomas exist; the physician should biopsy new sites of no pigment/loss of pigment.
- 80% of cutaneous melanomas arise in existing nevi. Any changing nevi should be considered for full-thickness biopsy.

M

MÉNIÈRE DISEASE

Robert A. Baldor, MD

 BASICS

DESCRIPTION

- An inner ear (labyrinthine) disorder characterized by recurrent attacks of hearing loss, tinnitus, vertigo, and sensations of aural fullness. Generally believed to be caused by, or related to, an increase in the volume and pressure of the inner ear endolymph fluid (endolymphatic hydrops)
- Often unilateral initially, but it is estimated that nearly half become bilateral over time.
- Severity and frequency of vertigo may diminish over time, but hearing loss is often progressive and/or fluctuating.
- Usually idiopathic (Ménière disease), but may be secondary to another condition causing endolymphatic hydrops (Ménière syndrome)
- System(s) affected: Nervous
- Synonym(s): Ménière syndrome; Endolymphatic hydrops

EPIDEMIOLOGY

- Predominant age of onset: 40–60 years
- Predominant gender: Female > Male (1.3:1)
- Race/Ethnicity: White, northern European > blacks

Incidence
Estimates 1–150/100,000 per year

Prevalence
Varies from 7.5 to >200/100,000

ETIOLOGY AND PATHOPHYSIOLOGY

- Not fully understood; theories include increased pressure of the endolymph fluid due to increased fluid production or decreased resorption. This may be caused by endolymphatic sac pathology, abnormal development of the vestibular aqueduct, or inflammation caused by circulating immune complexes. Increased endolymph pressure may cause rupture of membranes and changes in endolymphatic ionic gradient.
- Idiopathic (Ménière *disease*); but Ménière *syndrome* may be secondary to injury or other disorders (e.g., reduced middle ear pressure, allergy, endocrine disease, lipid disorders, vascular, viral, syphilis, autoimmune). Any disorder that could cause endolymph hydrops could be implicated in Ménière *syndrome*.

Genetics
Some families show increased incidence, but genetic vs. environmental influences are not well understood.

RISK FACTORS
Not well understood, but *may* include:
- Stress
- Allergy
- Increased salt intake
- Caffeine, alcohol, or nicotine intake
- Chronic exposure to loud noise
- Family history of Ménière
- Certain vascular abnormalities (patients may also have history of migraines)
- Certain viral exposures (especially herpes simplex virus [HSV])

GENERAL PREVENTION
Reduce risk factors: Stress; salt, alcohol, and caffeine intake; smoking; noise exposure; ototoxic drugs (e.g., aspirin, quinine, aminoglycosides).

COMMONLY ASSOCIATED CONDITIONS
- Anxiety (secondary to the disabling symptoms)
- Migraines
- Hyperprolactinemia

 DIAGNOSIS

Diagnosis is clinical (1)[C]

HISTORY
Attacks are typically spontaneous but may be preceded by an aura of increasing fullness in the ear and tinnitus. These may occur in clusters, with long intervening symptom-free remissions. Signs and symptoms to look for include:
- Formal criteria for diagnosis from American Academy of Otolaryngology–Head and Neck Surgery:
  - At least 2 episodes of rotational-horizontal vertigo >20 minutes in duration
  - Tinnitus or aural fullness
  - Hearing loss: Low frequency (sensorineural) confirmed by audiometric testing
  - Other causes (e.g., acoustic neuroma) excluded
  - During severe attacks: Pallor, sweating, nausea, vomiting, falling, prostration
  - Symptoms are exacerbated by motion.
- Between attacks, affected patients may experience motion-related imbalance without vertigo.
- *Caution*: Many conditions may produce auditory and vestibular findings identical to those associated with Ménière disease.

PHYSICAL EXAM
- Physical exam rules out other conditions; no finding is unique to Ménière disease
- Horizontal nystagmus may be seen during attacks.
- Otoscopy is typically normal.
- Triggering of attacks in the office with Dix-Hallpike maneuver suggests diagnosis of benign paroxysmal positional vertigo, not Ménière.

DIFFERENTIAL DIAGNOSIS
- Acoustic neuroma or other CNS tumor
- Syphilis
- Perilymphatic fistula
- Viral labyrinthitis
- Transient ischemic attack (TIA), migraine
- Vertebrobasilar disease
- Other labyrinthine disorders that produce similar symptoms (e.g., Cogan syndrome, benign positional vertigo, temporal bone trauma)
- Diabetes or thyroid dysfunction
- Vestibular neuronitis
- Medication side effects
- Otitis media

DIAGNOSTIC TESTS & INTERPRETATION
Testing is done to rule out other conditions but does not necessarily confirm or exclude Ménière disease.

Initial Tests (lab, imaging)
- Consider serologic tests specific for *Treponema pallidum* in at-risk populations (1)[C]
- Thyroid, fasting blood sugar, and lipid studies
- Consider MRI to rule out acoustic neuroma or other CNS pathology, including tumor, aneurysm, and multiple sclerosis (MS).

Diagnostic Procedures/Other
- Auditory:
  - Audiometry using pure tone and speech to show low-frequency sensorineural (nerve) loss and impaired speech discrimination. Usually shows low-frequency sensorineural hearing loss.
  - Tuning fork tests (i.e., Weber and Rinne) will confirm validity of audiometry.
  - Auditory brainstem response audiometry to rule out acoustic neuroma
  - Electrocochleography may be useful to confirm etiology (1)[C].
- Vestibular:
  - Caloric testing: Electronystagmography may show reduced caloric response. Can obtain reasonably comparable information with use of 0.8 mL of ice water caloric testing. Reduced activity on either side is consistent with Ménière diagnosis, but is not itself diagnostic.
  - Drugs that may alter lab results: Any sedating medication may affect and invalidate vestibular testing.

Test Interpretation
Histologic temporal bone analysis (at autopsy). Dilation of inner ear fluid system may be seen.

 TREATMENT

- Can usually be managed in outpatient setting
- A paucity of evidence-based guidelines exists regarding treatment for Ménière disease; therefore, there is no gold standard treatment.
- Medications are given primarily for symptomatic relief of vertigo and nausea, not to change disease progression.
- During attacks, bed rest with eyes closed and protection from falling. Attacks rarely last >4 hours.

MEDICATION
First Line
- Acute attack: Initial goal is immediate stabilization and symptom relief. For severe episodes, choose 1 (2)[C]:
  - Benzodiazepines (such as diazepam): Decrease vertigo and anxiety
  - Antihistamines (meclizine/dimenhydrinate): Decrease vertigo and nausea
  - Anticholinergics (transdermal scopolamine): Prevent nausea and emesis associated with motion sickness
  - Antidopaminergic (metoclopramide, promethazine): Decreases nausea, anxiety
  - Rehydration therapy and electrolyte replacement
  - Steroid taper for acute hearing loss
- Maintenance (goal is to prevent/reduce attacks)
- Lifestyle changes (e.g., low-salt diet) are needed.

- Diuretics are frequently used and may help reduce attacks by decreasing the pressure and volume of endolymphatic fluid; however, there is insufficient evidence at this time (2)[C],(3)[A]:
  - Hydrochlorothiazide/triamterene (Dyazide, Maxzide)
  - Acetazolamide (Diamox)

- Contraindications:
  - Atropine: Cardiac disease, especially supraventricular tachycardia and other arrhythmias, prostatic enlargement
  - Scopolamine: Children and elderly, prostatic enlargement
  - Diuretics: Electrolyte abnormalities, renal disease
- Precautions:
  - Sedating drugs should be used with caution, particularly in the elderly. Patients cautioned not to operate motor vehicles or machinery. Atropine and scopolamine should be used with particular caution.
  - Diuretics: Monitor electrolytes.
- Significant possible interactions: Transdermal scopolamine: Anticholinergics, antihistamines, tricyclic antidepressants, other

Second Line
- Steroids have been used, both intratympanic and systemically (PO or IV) for longer treatment of hearing loss:
  - Intratympanic administration results in higher steroid levels in the inner ear and may be more effective and safer than systemic (2)[C].
  - Addition of prednisone 30 mg/d to diuretic treatment reduced severity and frequency of tinnitus and vertigo in 1 pilot study.
- In Europe, 1 of the preferred drugs is betahistine, a histamine agonist (unavailable in the US). Insufficient evidence to state effectiveness. Other vasodilators, such as isosorbide dinitrate, niacin, and histamine, have also been used, but evidence of their effectiveness is sparse (2)[C].
- Famvir evidence is lacking, but indicates more improvement in hearing than balance.
- Inner ear perfusion with gentamicin and steroids have helped control and stabilize vertigo and hearing loss in Ménière disease (4)[A].

ISSUES FOR REFERRAL
- Consider ear, nose, throat/neurology referral for confirmation, further testing
- All patients need formal audiometry to confirm hearing loss.

ADDITIONAL THERAPIES
- Application of intermittent pressures via a myringotomy using a Meniett device has been found in some studies to relieve dizziness:
  - Safe; requires a long-term tympanostomy tube
- Vestibular rehabilitation may be beneficial for patients with persistent vestibular symptoms (5)[A]:
  - Safe and effective treatment for unilateral vestibular dysfunction
  - When attacks are disabling, the patient should be encouraged to resume activity slowly as soon as able.

SURGERY/OTHER PROCEDURES
- Interventions that preserve hearing (6)[B]:
  - Endolymphatic sac surgery, either decompression or drainage of endolymph into mastoid or subarachnoid space:
    ○ Less invasive; may decrease vertigo, may influence hearing/tinnitus
    ○ Insufficient evidence of the beneficial effect of endolymphatic sac surgery in Ménière disease (7)[A]
  - Vestibular nerve section (intracranial procedure):
    ○ More invasive due to intracranial location
    ○ Decreases vertigo and preserves hearing
  - Tympanostomy tube: May decrease symptoms by decreasing the middle ear pressure
- Interventions for patients with no serviceable hearing (6)[B]:
  - Labyrinthectomy: Very effective at controlling vertigo, but causes deafness
  - Vestibular neurectomy
  - Many patients may be candidates for cochlear implantation if they have lost serviceable hearing.

COMPLEMENTARY AND ALTERNATIVE MEDICINE
Insufficient evidence to support effectiveness, but many integrative techniques have been tried, including (2)[C]:

- Acupuncture (8)[A], acupressure, tai chi
- Niacin, bioflavonoids, lipoflavonoids, ginger, ginkgo biloba, and other herbal supplements

 ## ONGOING CARE

FOLLOW-UP RECOMMENDATIONS
Patient Monitoring
Due to the possibility of progressive hearing loss despite eventual decrease in vertiginous attacks, it is important to have close follow up to monitor changes in hearing and to continue surveillance for more serious underlying causes (e.g., acoustic neuroma).

DIET
- Diet is usually not a factor, unless attacks are brought on by certain foods.
- Some physicians restrict salt, but this is not supported by randomized controlled trials (1)[B].

PATIENT EDUCATION
- Limit activity during attacks
- Between attacks, patient may be fully active, but is often limited due to fear or lingering symptoms. This can be severely disabling.
- Patient information, including support group contacts, is available from the Vestibular Disorders Association (www.vestibular.org) and the American Academy of Otolaryngology-Head and Neck Surgery (www.entnet.org/HealthInformation/menieresDisease.cfm).

PROGNOSIS
- Alternating attacks and remission
- Of cases, 50% resolve spontaneously within 2–3 years, but can last >20 years. Severity and frequency of attacks diminish, but hearing loss is often progressive.
- Of patients, 90% can be treated successfully with medication; 5–10% of patients require surgery for incapacitating vertigo.
- Clinicians must not overlook possibility of acoustic tumor, which produces an identical clinical picture.

COMPLICATIONS
Loss of hearing; injury during attack; inability to work

REFERENCES

1. Sajjadi H, Paparella MM. Meniere's disease. *Lancet*. 2008;372:406–414.
2. Coelho DH, Lalwani AK. Medical management of Ménière's disease. *Laryngoscope*. 2008;118:1099–1108.
3. Thirlwall AS, Kundu S. Diuretics for Ménière's disease or syndrome. *Cochrane Database Syst Rev*. 2006;3:CD003599.
4. Hamid M. Medical management of common peripheral vestibular diseases. *Curr Opin Otolaryngol Head Neck Surg*. 2010;18:407–412.
5. Hillier SL, Hollohan V. Vestibular rehabilitation for unilateral peripheral vestibular dysfunction. *Cochrane Database Syst Rev*. 2007;2:CD005397.
6. van Benthem PP, Giard JL, Verschuur HP. Surgery for Ménière's disease (Protocol). *Cochrane Database Syst Rev*. 2005;3:CD005395.
7. Pullens B, Giard JL, Verschuur HP, et al. Surgery for Ménière's disease. *Cochrane Database Syst Rev*. 2010;1:CD005395.
8. Long AF, Xing M, Morgan K, et al. Exploring the evidence base for acupuncture in the treatment of Ménière's syndrome—a systematic review. *Evid Based Complement Alternat Med*. 2011;2011:429102.

 ## SEE ALSO

- Hearing Loss; Labyrinthitis; Tinnitus
- Algorithm: Vertigo

 ## CODES

ICD10
- H81.01 Meniere's disease, right ear
- H81.02 Meniere's disease, left ear
- H81.09 Meniere's disease, unspecified ear

CLINICAL PEARLS

- Diagnosis of Ménière disease is clinical, based on repeated episodes of vertigo, hearing loss, and tinnitus/aural fullness.
- Multiple medical, surgical, and rehabilitative treatments are available to decrease the severity and frequency of attacks. Some of these may preserve hearing, whereas some destroy it.
- A patient is likely to have progressive hearing loss despite a natural progression toward fewer vertigo attacks.
- When considering Ménière disease in a patient with vertigo and hearing loss, also consider acoustic neuromas.
- Take symptoms seriously, as they may be disabling.

M

MENINGITIS, BACTERIAL

Jennifer N. Smith, MD • Felix B. Chang, MD

BASICS

DESCRIPTION
- Bacterial meningitis is an inflammation of the pia-arachnoid, its fluid, and fluid of the ventricles:
  - Always cerebrospinal
- System affected: Nervous

EPIDEMIOLOGY
- Predominant age: Neonates, infants, and elderly
- Predominant sex: Male = Female

Incidence
Varies with age:
- <2 months: 80/100,000
- 2–23 months: 7/100,000
- 2–10 years: 0.5/100,000
- 11–17 years: 0.4/100,000
- 18–34 years: 0.66/100,000
- 35–49 years: 0.95/100,000
- ≥65 years: 1.92/100,000 (1)

Varies with pathogen:
- *Streptococcus pneumoniae*: 0.81/100,000
- Group B *streptococcus*: 0.25/100,000
- *Neisseria meningitidis*: 0.19/100,000
- *Haemophilus influenzae*: 0.08/100,000
- *Listeria monocytogenes*: 0.05/100,000

ETIOLOGY AND PATHOPHYSIOLOGY
Bacterial infection causes inflammation of the pia-arachnoid and its fluid and the fluid of the ventricles. Bacteria are divided into age groups to guide empiric therapy. Guide therapy by culture whenever possible:
- Newborns (<2 months):
  - Group B *Streptococcus*
  - *Escherichia coli*
  - *Listeria monocytogenes*
- Infants and children:
  - Streptococcus pneumoniae
  - Neisseria meningitidis
  - Haemophilus influenzae
- Adolescents and young adults:
  - Neisseria meningitidis
  - Streptococcus pneumoniae
- Older adults:
  - Streptococcus pneumoniae
  - Neisseria meningitidis
  - Listeria monocytogenes

Genetics
Individuals of Navajo Indian or American Eskimo descent may have genetic or acquired vulnerability to invasive disease.

RISK FACTORS
- Immunocompromising condition
- Alcoholism, diabetes, chronic conditions
- Neurosurgical procedure/head injury
- Abdominal surgery
- Neonates: Prematurity, low birth weight, premature rupture of membranes, maternal peripartum infection, and urinary tract abnormalities

GENERAL PREVENTION
- Prompt medical treatment for infections.
- Strict aseptic techniques when treating patients with head wounds or skull fractures.

- Look for CSF fistula with recurrent meningitis.
- Meningitis caused by *Haemophilus influenzae* type B has decreased in incidence by 55% due to routine vaccinations in infants (1).
- Conjugate vaccines against *S. pneumoniae* may reduce the burden of disease in childhood and may produce herd immunity among adults.
- Persons with close contact to patients with meningococcal meningitis must receive chemoprophylaxis to eradicate carriage.

COMMONLY ASSOCIATED CONDITIONS
Conditions associated with a worse prognosis:
- Alcoholism
- Old age
- Infancy
- Diabetes mellitus
- Multiple myeloma
- Head trauma
- Seizures
- Coma

DIAGNOSIS

HISTORY
- Antecedent upper respiratory infection
- Fever
- Headache
- Vomiting
- Photophobia
- Seizures
- Confusion
- Nausea
- Rigors
- Profuse sweats
- Weakness
- Elderly: Subtle findings including confusion
- Infants: Irritability, lethargy, poor feeding

PHYSICAL EXAM
The triad of fever, neck stiffness, and altered mental status has low sensitivity (44%). However, almost all patients present with at least 2 of 4 symptoms: Headache, fever, neck stiffness, and altered mental status.
- Meningismus
- Signs of cerebral dysfunction
- Focal neurologic deficits
- Meningococcal rash: Macular and erythematous at first, then petechial or purpuric

DIFFERENTIAL DIAGNOSIS
- Bacteremia
- Sepsis
- Brain abscess
- Seizures
- Other nonbacterial meningitides

DIAGNOSTIC TESTS & INTERPRETATION
Initial Tests (lab, imaging)
- Prompt lumbar puncture
  - Head CT first if focal neuro findings, papilledema, or depressed mentation

- Typical CSF analysis: Turbid
  - Adults:
    - >500 cells/mL WBCs
    - Glucose <40 mg/dL
    - <2/3 blood to glucose ratio
    - CSF protein >200 mg/dL
    - CSF opening pressure >30 cm
    - Suspect ruptured brain abscess when WBC count is unusually high (>100,000)
- CSF Gram stain and cultures
- Bacterial CSF testing using polymerase chain reaction (PCR) particularly in those with negative cultures for suspected viral meningitis
- Bacterial antigen tests should be reserved for cases in which the initial CSF Gram stain is negative and CSF culture is negative at 48 hours of incubation.
- Serum blood cultures
- Serum electrolytes
- Evaluation of clotting function if petechiae or purpuric lesions are noted
- CT scan of head if concern for increased intracranial pressure or warning signs of space-occupying lesion (new-onset seizure, papilledema, or brain herniation)
- Chest radiograph may reveal pneumonitis or abscess
- Sinus/skull radiographs may reveal cranial osteomyelitis, paranasal sinusitis, or skull fracture, but rarely indicated
- Later in course: Head CT if hydrocephalus, brain abscess, subdural effusions, and subdural empyema are suspected or if no clinical response after 48 hours of appropriate antibiotics

Diagnostic Procedures/Other
Lumbar puncture

TREATMENT

GENERAL MEASURES
- Initiate empiric antibiotic therapy immediately after lumbar puncture (LP > Abx); or if head CT scan is needed, then immediately after blood cultures (Abx > CT > LP)
- Vigorous supportive care with constant nursing to ensure prompt recognition of seizures and prevention of aspiration
- Therapy for coexisting conditions
- Measures to prevent hypothermia and dehydration

MEDICATION
Empiric IV therapy, with adjunctive dexamethasone when indicated, until culture results available:
- Consider local patterns of bacterial sensitivity.

First Line
- Neonates:
  - Ampicillin: 100–400 mg/kg/d divided q6–12h AND
  - Tobramycin: 7.5 mg/kg/d q6–8h (premature or <1 week of age, 2.5 mg/kg q12h)
- Infants >4 weeks of age:
  - Ampicillin: 300–400 mg/kg/d divided q4–6h (max, 2 g q3–4h) AND
  - Chloramphenicol: 75–100 mg/kg/d divided q6h OR
  - Ceftriaxone: 100 mg/kg/d divided q12–24h (max, 2 g q12h) or cefotaxime 200 mg/kg/d divided q4–6h AND
  - Vancomycin: 10–15 mg/kg q12h (max, 1,500 mg q12h)

- Adults:
  - Vancomycin: loading dose 25–30 mg/kg IV then 22.5 mg/kg q12h with goal trough of 20 AND
  - Ceftriaxone: 2 g IV q12 OR
  - Cefotaxime: 2 g IV q4–6h
  - Over age of 50, add Ampicillin: 2 g IV q4h for Listeria
  - Immunocompromised use vancomycin, ampicillin, ceftazidime, AND acyclovir
- Precaution: Ototoxicity from aminoglycoside
- Penicillin-allergic patients:
  - Chloramphenicol: 1 g IV q6h AND
  - Vancomycin: loading dose 25–30 mg/kg IV then 22.5 mg/kg q12h with goal trough of 20
- Treatment duration:
  - S. pneumoniae: 10–14 days
  - N. meningitidis, H. influenzae: 7–10 days
  - Group B Streptococcus organisms, E. coli, L. monocytogenes: 14–21 days
  - Neonates: 12–21 days or at least 14 days after a repeated culture is sterile
- Corticosteroids:
  - Pediatrics:
    - Early treatment with dexamethasone (0.15 mg/kg IV q6h × 4 days) decreases mortality and morbidity for patients >1 month of age with acute bacterial meningitis with no increased risk of GI bleeding.
    - Corticosteroids are associated with lower rates of severe hearing loss, any hearing loss, and neurologic sequelae (2)[A].
  - Adults:
    - Initiate in adults, then only continue if CSF Gram stain is gram-positive diplococcus or if blood or CSF positive for S. pneumoniae
  - Dexamethasone: 10 mg IV q6h started 15–20 minutes before or with antibiotic for 4 days.
- Osmotic diuretics:
  - Glycerol may reduce brain edema and reduce deafness but have not been demonstrated to decrease mortality (3)[A].

Second Line
- Anti pseudomonal penicillins
- Aztreonam
- Quinolones (e.g., ciprofloxacin)
- Meropenem

ISSUES FOR REFERRAL
Consultation from ICU specialist

IN-PATIENT CONSIDERATIONS
Admission Criteria/Initial Stabilization
Bacterial meningitis requires hospitalization.

Nursing
- ICU monitoring may be needed to recognize changes in the patient's consciousness and the development of new neurologic signs, subtle seizures, and to treat severe agitation effectively.
- Patients with suspected meningococcal infection require respiratory isolation for 24 hours.

Discharge Criteria
May consider home therapy for completion of IV antibiotics once clinically stable and culture and sensitivity results are known.

 ONGOING CARE

FOLLOW-UP RECOMMENDATIONS
Patient Monitoring
- Brainstem auditory-evoked response test should be performed on infants before hospital discharge. Further follow up will depend on its results and course of meningitis while in hospital.
- Vaccinations:
  - H. influenzae Hib conjugate vaccine is recommended during infancy for 4 doses.
  - Meningococcal conjugate vaccine quadrivalent (MCV4) is given to children aged 11–12 with a booster at 16 years.
  - Immunizing infants <3 months old does not reduce morbidity or mortality; and vaccinating pregnant women has not been proven to reduce infant infections (4)[A].
  - Administer 2 doses MCV4 at least 2 months apart to adults with:
    - HIV
    - Functional asplenia
    - Persistent complement deficiencies
  - Administer 1 dose of meningococcal vaccine to:
    - Military recruits
    - Microbiologists routinely exposed to isolates of Neisseria meningitidis
    - Those who travel to or live in countries where meningitis is hyperendemic or epidemic
    - First-year college students up through age 21 years who live in residence halls if they have not received a dose on or after their 16th birthday
  - MCV4 is preferred for adults with any of the preceding indications who are ≤55 years; meningococcal polysaccharide vaccine (MPSV4) is preferred for adults aged ≥56 years.
  - Revaccination with MCV4 every 5 years is recommended for adults previously vaccinated with MCV4 or MPSV4 who remain at increased risk.
- Prophylaxis:
  - Only for close contacts of patients
  - Rifampin is effective in eradicating N. meningitidis up to 4 weeks after treatment but may lead to resistance (5)[A].
    - Rifampin: 600 mg PO bid × 2 days
  - Ciprofloxacin and ceftriaxone are effective up to 2 weeks after treatment without leading to resistance (5)[A].
    - Ciprofloxacin: 500 mg PO × 1 dose
    - Ceftriaxone: 250 mg IM × 1 dose

DIET
Regular, as tolerated, except with syndrome of inappropriate secretion of antidiuretic hormone.

PROGNOSIS
Overall case fatality: 14%
- Pediatrics: 7%
- Adults: 16%
  - Fatality rate increases linearly with increasing age (1).

COMPLICATIONS
- Seizures: 20–30%
- Focal neurologic deficit
- Cranial nerve palsies (III, VI, VII, VIII):
  - Comprises 10–20% of the cases
  - Usually disappear within a few weeks
- Sensorineural hearing loss: 10% in children
- Neurodevelopmental sequelae: 30% subtle learning deficits
- Obstructive hydrocephalus
- Subdural effusions
- Decline in consciousness that may be due to meningoencephalitis

REFERENCES
1. Thigpen M, Whitney C, Messonnier NE, et al. Bacterial meningitis in the United States, 1998-2007. N Engl J Med. 2011;364:2016–2025.
2. Brouwer MC, McIntyre P, Prasad K, et al. Corticosteroids for acute bacterial meningitis. Cochrane Database Syst Rev. 2013;6:CD004405.
3. Wall E, Ajdukiewicz K, Heyderman RS, et al. Osmotic therapies added to antibiotics for acute bacterial meningitis. Cochrane Database Syst Rev. 2013;3:CD008806.
4. Chaithongwongwatthana S, Yamamasmit W, Limpongsanurak S, et al. Pneumococcal vaccination during pregnancy for preventing infant infection. Cochrane Database Syst Rev. 2012;7:CD004903.
5. Trestioreanu A, Fraser A, Gafter-Gvili A, et al. Antibiotics for preventing meningococcal infections. Cochrane Database Syst Rev. 2011;8:CD004785.

ADDITIONAL READING
- Centers for Disease Control and Prevention. Meningitis. Available at: www.cdc.gov/meningitis/bacterial.html
- Kulik DM, Uleryk EM, Maguire Jl. Does this child have bacterial meningitis? A systematic review of clinical prediction rules for children with suspected bacterial meningitis. J Emerg Med. 201345:508–519.

 SEE ALSO

- Meningitis, Viral; Meningococcemia
- Algorithm: Delirium

 CODES

ICD10
- G00.2 Streptococcal meningitis
- G00.8 Other bacterial meningitis
- G00.9 Bacterial meningitis, unspecified

CLINICAL PEARLS
- Suspected bacterial meningitis is a medical emergency requiring immediate diagnostics.
- Antibiotic therapy should be initiated immediately after the lumbar puncture if the clinical suspicion for meningitis is high.
- Corticosteroids significantly reduced hearing loss and neurological sequelae, but did not reduce overall mortality.
- Most beneficial to treat bacterial meningitis with corticosteroids only in high-income countries (2)[A].

M

MENINGITIS, VIRAL

Luis K. Abrishamian, MD • Gabriela F. Abrishamian-Garcia

BASICS

DESCRIPTION
- Viral meningitis (VM) is a clinical syndrome characterized by acute meningeal inflammation without an identifiable bacterial pathogen in the CSF.
- System(s) affected: Nervous
- Synonym(s): Abacterial meningitis, Aseptic meningitis

EPIDEMIOLOGY
Incidence
- Estimated 10,000–75,000 cases of VM occur annually in the US
- Estimated 26,000–42,000 hospitalizations each year in the US for VM
- In 2006, there were 72,000 meningitis-related hospitalizations, with 58% of those having meningitis as the primary reason for hospitalization. Of all 72,000 hospitalizations, 56.4% were determined to be viral cases.
- More common than bacterial meningitis:
  – Annual incidence of VM is higher than total number cases of meningitis caused by all other etiologies combined.
- Peaks June 1 through October 31:
  – Enteroviruses and arthropod-borne viruses predominate in warm months
  – Mumps usually occurs in the winter and spring, often in epidemics
- Occurs in both outbreak and sporadic forms

ETIOLOGY AND PATHOPHYSIOLOGY
- First described by Wallgren in 1925
- In immunocompetent hosts, VM is generally caused by a systemic viral infection with predilection to neurologic involvement.
- Less commonly, direct neural transmission occurs from a self-limited infection such as HSV already present in the immunocompetent host.
- >90% of cases caused by enterovirus family, which includes coxsackievirus A and B, echovirus, poliovirus, and E variants: E9 and E30 strains specifically implicated in eastern and western hemispheres, respectively.
- Less common causes include HSV-1 and HSV-2, varicella-zoster virus (VZV), adenovirus, lymphocytic choriomeningitis virus (LCMV), cytomegalovirus (CMV), Epstein-Barr virus (EBV), HIV, and mumps
- Increasing frequency of neonatal morbidity and mortality associated with human parechovirus strains
- Recurrent (Mollaret's) meningitis shows 80% association with herpes simplex virus-2 (HSV-2).
- Arthropod-borne viruses: West Nile virus, St. Louis encephalitis virus, and California encephalitis virus
- Parvovirus B19 is found in the CSF of 4.3% of undiagnosed meningoencephalitis patients (1)[B].

Genetics
None

RISK FACTORS
- Close contact with known cases of VM
- Immunocompromised hosts may be more susceptible to CMV, HSV, and adenovirus.

- LCMV is commonly transmitted via exposure to rodent feces, bodily fluids, or nesting materials:
  – Rodent bites and vertical transmission as mechanisms of infection are possible, but unconfirmed

Geriatric Considerations
Cases of VM in the elderly are rare but are documented. Consider alternative diagnoses (e.g., carcinomatous meningitis, NSAID- or medication-induced meningitis) in the elderly population.

GENERAL PREVENTION
Limit exposure to known hosts; handwashing, and general hygiene.

COMMONLY ASSOCIATED CONDITIONS
Encephalitis; neurologic deficits; myopericarditis; neonatal enteroviral sepsis

DIAGNOSIS

Predominant symptoms include:
- Fever
- Headache
- Photophobia
- Myalgias
- Nausea
- Vomiting
- Malaise

HISTORY
- Travel and exposure history
- Sexual activity (e.g., HSV, HIV)
- Outdoor exposure (Lyme disease)
- Rodent feces and/or urine exposure (LCMV)
- Solid-organ transplant (LCMV, CMV)

PHYSICAL EXAM
- Nuchal rigidity
- Altered mental status
- Fever (>100.4°F/38°C)
- Meningeal signs (should not be used exclusively to diagnose or rule out meningitis) (2)[C]:
  – Nuchal rigidity
  – Brudzinski sign: Neck flexion elicits involuntary knee flexion in supine patient.
  – Kernig sign: Resistance to knee extension following flexion of hips and knees by physician
- In the presence of erythema chronicum migrans or cranial neuropathy, consider Lyme meningitis given correlation with exposure and endemic area.
- Patients do not manifest neurologic abnormalities since inflammation in VM is limited to the meninges and does not involve brain parenchyma (3)
- Mucocutaneous findings include dermatologic manifestations (e.g., vesicular rash in hand, foot, and mouth disease), herpangina, and generalized maculopapular rash:
  – Zoster rash usually occurs after meningeal infection with VZV meningitis.

DIFFERENTIAL DIAGNOSIS
- Bacterial meningitis
- Encephalitis
- Epidural abscess
- Other infectious agents:
  – Tuberculosis; syphilis; leptospirosis; Lyme disease
- Parameningeal infections (e.g., subdural empyema)
- Postinfectious encephalomyelitis
- Viral syndrome (e.g., influenza)

- Leukemia and carcinomatous meningitis
- Migraine headache
- Acute metabolic encephalopathy
- Chemical meningitis
- Brain abscess

DIAGNOSTIC TESTS & INTERPRETATION
Initial Tests (lab, imaging)
- Lumbar puncture (LP) is standard of care in patients with high clinical suspicion:
  – Indications for LP include fever, sudden abrupt mental status change, headache, and/or lethargy.
  – In patients with high suspicion of bacterial meningitis, antibiotic treatment should be started immediately.
- CSF analysis: Glucose, protein, WBC count with differential, RBC count, Gram stain, culture
- Typical CSF findings in viral meningitis:
  – Elevated WBC count: 10–1,000/mm³, classically with a lymphocyte predominance
  – Initial phase of illness (first 24–48 hours) may show neutrophil predominance
  – Protein normal to slightly elevated (<150 mg/dL):
    ○ One 3-year retrospective study found elevated CSF protein levels in patients with meningitis secondary to HSV-2 or VZV infection compared with those with enteroviruses.
  – Negative Gram stain and bacterial culture
  – Rule out bacterial meningitis (BM): Bacterial Meningitis Score (BMS) was first validated model to distinguish VM from BM based on Gram stain, CSF neutrophil count and seizure activity (4). BM unlikely with score of zero.
  – Elevated opening pressure:
    ○ Culture CSF for enteroviruses, HSV, and mumps. However, viral culture may yield no additional benefit when nucleic acid amplification has been employed (5)[C].
    ○ In diagnosing EBV infections, nucleic acid tests are more sensitive than cultures.
    ○ Polymerase chain reaction (PCR) has a sensitivity of 95–100% for HSV-1 and -2, EBV, and enterovirus, allowing for earlier hospital discharge and less intervention.
    ○ Reverse-transcriptase PCR test is approved by the FDA for enteroviral meningitis. Results are available within 2.5 hours.
- Peripheral polymorphonuclear (PMN) count of >16 × 10⁹/L, serum C-reactive protein of >100 mg/L, and hemorrhagic rash are shown to correlate strongly and independently with the diagnosis of bacterial meningitis and meningococcal septicemia.
- EEG in some cases, especially if encephalitis is a consideration
- CBC: Normal or mildly elevated WBCs
- Serum procalcitonin and CSF lactate concentrations appear to be highly discriminative parameters for the differential diagnosis of BM and VM, respectively.
- Viral cultures and/or antibody titers
- Serum procalcitonin (>0.5 ng/mL) and CSF protein (>0.5 g/L) have high correlation with pediatric bacterial vs. aseptic meningitis.
- *Some authors contend that if meningeal symptoms have been present >48 hours with a normal neurologic exam in an immunocompetent patient with confirmed normal level of alertness, BM is extremely unlikely and lumbar puncture is not warranted. Others contend that BM cannot be excluded clinically and to exercise caution*

discharging meningitic patients without lumbar puncture (3,6).
- Indication for imaging rests with consideration of alternative diagnoses; may be performed prior to LP in the presence of papilledema, spinal cord trauma, altered mental status, or focal neurologic findings. Prior to performing LP, CT scan may not be clinically necessary in the absence of risk factors.
- Standard techniques include noncontrast brain CT scan or MRI.

Follow-Up Tests & Special Considerations
- Exercise clinical judgment regarding contraindications to LP. They include:
  – Increased intracranial pressure owing to mass lesion
  – Ventricular obstruction
  – Local infection at potential LP site or suspected epidural abscess
  – Anticoagulation or coagulopathy:
    ○ Level of coagulopathy that increases risk is unclear
  – Possibility of cardiorespiratory compromise secondary to patient positioning during procedure
- Disorders that may alter lab results:
  – Diabetes: Consider blood sugar level to correlate with CSF glucose level
  – Pre-existing neurologic diseases (e.g., intracranial neoplasm, demyelinating disease)

 TREATMENT

GENERAL MEASURES
- Management is largely supportive care
- IV fluids if oral intake is poor or vomiting is present
- Pain management

MEDICATION
First Line
- Analgesics (adult doses):
  – Morphine: 0.05–0.1 mg/kg IV, titrated to pain relief
  – Hydromorphone (Dilaudid): 1–2 mg IV, titrated to pain relief
  – Hydrocodone (Norco): 5/325 mg 1–2 tablets PO q6h *OR* oxycodone (Percocet) 5/325 mg 1–2 tablets PO q4–6h
- Antiemetics:
  – Ondansetron (Zofran): 4–8 mg IV q8h
  – Metoclopramide (Reglan): 10–20 mg IV/IM q4–6h
- Antipyretics: Acetaminophen (Tylenol): 650 mg PO or rectal suppository q4h

- Antiviral agents: Initiate empiric acyclovir at 10 mg/kg IV q8h for patients with CSF pleocytosis, negative Gram stain, and suspicion for HSV while awaiting results of definitive (e.g., HSV PCR) testing (7)[A].
  – Study found that young infants (<60 days old) most likely to receive acyclovir compared with older children (>60 days old) (8)
- Antibiotics:
  – Not indicated for treatment of VM
  – If unclear etiology, treat symptomatically, and follow the patient closely in the hospital setting.
  – If in doubt, initiate an IV or IM broad-spectrum antibiotic with good CSF penetration.
- Precautions: Aspirin should be avoided in children and adolescents owing to a possible association with Reye syndrome.
- Minority of patients receive corticosteroids (8)

IN-PATIENT CONSIDERATIONS
Admission Criteria/Initial Stabilization
Generally, VM is treated on an outpatient basis, in contrast to BM; those with VM plus complicating factors may be hospitalized.
- Study of ED visits found that most children diagnosed with VM were hospitalized (91%) (8)

IV Fluids
May use normal saline bolus or continuous infusion, based on clinical judgment

Nursing
- Neurologic monitoring for changes in mental status, fever, and so forth to assess disease progression or alternate diagnosis
- Contact precautions until bacterial meningitis is ruled out
- Private room indicated with sterile precautions
- Encourage handwashing

Discharge Criteria
Likelihood of BM, CFS WBC count and clinical parameters, such as dehydration, functional level, social circumstances and degree of discomfort (4)

 ONGOING CARE

FOLLOW-UP RECOMMENDATIONS
Follow up with primary care physician
Patient Monitoring
- Monitor for relapse or exacerbation of symptoms after treatment course.
- Observe for potential neurologic and neuroendocrine complications:
  – Seizures
  – Cerebral edema
  – Syndrome of inappropriate antidiuretic hormone (SIADH) secretion
  – Assess ability to have companion monitor change in mental/neurologic status (3)

DIET
- Determined by symptoms
- May need to order NPO owing to nausea or vomiting, with advancement to clear fluids and regular diet, as tolerated

PATIENT EDUCATION
- Discuss possibility, but low probability, of transmission to contacts
- Expected duration of illness (5–10 days)
- For patient education materials, refer patients to the online EBSCO Health Library article Viral Meningitis (http://healthlibrary.epnet.com/GetContent.aspx?token=38405ca3-6cab-4817-9cba-dc64dc5c69f1&chunkiid=11469).

PROGNOSIS
- Complete recovery generally within 7–10 days
- Headaches and other uncomfortable symptoms may persist intermittently for 1–2 weeks
- Only 0.6% of hospitalizations for VM resulted in death in a recent study.
- European studies have shown some residual postmeningeal cognitive impairment.

COMPLICATIONS
- Post-LP headache:
  – 36.5% of patients within 48 hours
- Fatigue
- Irritability
- Muscle weakness
- Seizures (rare)

REFERENCES
1. Barah F. Association of human parvovirus B19 infection with acute meningoencephalitis. *Lancet*. 2001;358(9299):2168.
2. Thomas KE. The diagnostic accuracy of Kernig's sign, Brudzinski's sign, and nuchal rigidity in adults with suspected meningitis. *Clin Infect Dis*. 2002;35:46–52.
3. Ciovacco WA, Baraff LJ. Lumbar puncture is not needed for all patients suspected to have viral meningitis. *Ann Emerg Med*. 2012;59:228–229.
4. Mohseni MM, Wilde JA. Viral meningitis: Which patients can be discharged from the emergency department? *J Emerg Med*. 2012;43:1181–1187.
5. Polage CR, Petti CA. Assessment of the utility of viral culture of cerebrospinal fluid. *Clin Infect Dis*. 2006;43:1578–1579.
6. Talan DA. Bacterial cause of suspected meningitis cannot be safely excluded without cerebrospinal fluid analysis. *Ann Emerg Med*. 2012;59:227–228.
7. Swadron SP. Pitfalls in the management of headache in the emergency department. *Emerg Med Clin North Am*. 2010;28:127–147.
8. Nigrovic LE, et. al Trends in the viral management of viral meningitis at US children's hospitals. *Pediatrics*. 2013;131:670–675.

ADDITIONAL READING
Studahl M, Lindquist L, Eriksson BM, et al. Acute viral infections of the central nervous system in immunocompetent adults: Diagnosis and management. *Drugs*. 2013;73:131–158.

 SEE ALSO

Algorithm: Delirium

CODES

ICD10
- A87.0 Enteroviral meningitis
- A87.1 Adenoviral meningitis
- A87.9 Viral meningitis, unspecified

CLINICAL PEARLS
- Viral vs. bacterial meningitis cannot be distinguished clinically; refer all suspected meningitis cases to hospital for diagnosis and management.
- Viral meningitis is more common than bacterial meningitis in the pediatric population. As age increases, the likelihood of a bacterial cause also increases.
- Antibiotic administration hours or days prior to CSF analysis may result in "partially treated" BM that mimics VM.
- IV acyclovir should be administered with a high clinical suspicion for herpetic VM/encephalitis.
- If BM is in the differential diagnosis, broad-spectrum antibiotics with effective CSF penetration should be given:
- Antibiotics should be continued until the diagnosis of BM is ruled out.
- Morbidity with VM is low, but increases with associated encephalitis.
- No evidence supports meningitis prophylaxis in basilar skull fracture with or without CSF leakage.

M

BASICS

DESCRIPTION
- Meningococcemia is caused by *Neisseria meningitidis* in the blood, which results in a broad spectrum of clinical manifestations.
- Bacteremia without sepsis: Meningococcal bacteremia rarely occurs without sepsis
- Bacteremia without meningitis: Patient is acutely ill and may have skin manifestations (rashes, petechiae, and ecchymosis) and hypotension
- Bacteremia with meningitis:
  – Predominant clinical picture of meningitis: Sudden onset of fever, nausea, vomiting, headache, decreased ability to concentrate, and myalgias
  – Disease progression is usually rapid with a transition from healthy to severe disease in a matter of hours.
  – Skin manifestations and hypotension may also be present:
    ○ A petechial rash appears as discrete lesions 1–2 mm in diameter, most frequently on the trunk and lower portions of the body and will be seen in >50% of patients on presentation.
    ○ Purpura fulminans is a severe complication of meningococcal disease and occurs in up to 25% of cases. It is characterized by acute onset of cutaneous hemorrhage and necrosis due to vascular thrombosis and disseminated intravascular coagulopathy.

EPIDEMIOLOGY
Incidence
- The US mortality rate is 0.5–1.1/100,000, or ~13%:
  – 11–19% of survivors suffer serious sequelae, including deafness, neurologic deficit, or limb loss.
- Disease is seasonal, with cases peaking in December and January.
- Annually, ~1,000 cases of invasive meningococcal disease occur in the US (1):
  – Among adolescents and young adults, 14–24, occurrence is 20%.
  – Among infants <1 year, occurrence is 16%.

ETIOLOGY AND PATHOPHYSIOLOGY
- *Neisseria meningitidis*, a gram-negative diplococcus with at least 13 serotypes
- Major serogroups in the US: B, C, Y, and W-135:
  – Serogroup B is the predominant cause of meningococcemia in children <1 year.
  – Serogroup C is the most common cause of cases in the US.
  – Serogroup Y is the predominant cause of meningococcemia in the elderly (2).
- Major serogroups worldwide are A, B, C, Y, and W-135:
  – W-135 is the major cause of disease in the "meningitis belt" of sub-Saharan Africa.

Genetics
Late complement component deficiency has an autosomal-recessive inheritance.

RISK FACTORS
- Age: 3 months–1 year
- Late complement component deficiency (C5, C6, C7, C8, or C9)
- Asplenia (1)
- Close contacts (e.g., household, nurseries, day care, dormitories, military barracks)
- Exposure to active and passive tobacco smoke (1)

GENERAL PREVENTION
- 2 vaccines are currently licensed for use in the US. Each contains antigens to serogroups A, C, Y, and W-135. Neither provides immunity against serotype B, which is responsible for 1/3 of US cases (2):
  – Meningococcal polysaccharide vaccine (MPSV4): Recommended for patients ≥55 with elevated risk (1):
    ○ Duration of protection is short: 1–3 years for patients <5 years; 3–5 years for adolescents and adults (2)
    ○ Reasonable for patients requiring short protection such as those traveling to endemic areas, college freshmen, those experiencing community outbreaks (2)
  – Meningococcal conjugate vaccine (MCV4): Recommended for patients 2–55 (1)
- Protective levels of antibody are achieved in ~7–10 days after primary immunization (2).
- Vaccine is recommended for all persons 11–18 and persons 19–55 at increased risk for the disease:
  – Guillain-Barré syndrome has been associated with the MCV4 vaccine, so a personal history of Guillain-Barré is a relative contraindication for receiving this vaccine.
- CDC International Travel Advisory:
  – Vaccine is required by the Government of Saudi Arabia for Hajj pilgrims >2.
  – The vaccine should be given to travelers to sub-Saharan Africa ("meningitis belt") during dry season.

DIAGNOSIS

HISTORY
- Symptoms:
  – Sudden onset of fever, nausea, vomiting, headache, myalgias, chills, rigor, and/or sore throat (nonsuppurative):
    ○ Pharyngitis may be mistaken for streptococcal pharyngitis.
    ○ Myalgia may be mistaken for severe "flu," with a peak incidence coinciding in winter months.
  – Changes in mental status, decreased ability to concentrate, stiff neck, convulsions
  – Atypical presentations may include acute arthritis or neuritis (3).
- Be sure to ask about possible exposures.

PHYSICAL EXAM
- Neurological: Nuchal rigidity, focal neurologic findings, coma, seizure:
  – Focal neurologic findings and seizures are more commonly seen with *Haemophilus influenzae* or *Streptococcus pneumoniae*.
- Cardiovascular: Hypotension, tachycardia, shock, heart failure with pulmonary edema
- Dermatologic: Maculopapular rash, petechiae, ecchymosis, purpura
- Median time of onset of specific meningitis symptoms (e.g., neck stiffness, photophobia, bulging fontanelle) was ~12–15 hours after onset of illness (4).
- Late signs of meningitis (e.g., unconsciousness, delirium, or seizures) occurred at a median of 15 hours in infants <1 year and at a median of 24 hours in older children (4).

DIFFERENTIAL DIAGNOSIS
- Septicemia due to other microorganisms
- Meningitis due to other pyogenic bacteria
- Gonococcemia
- Acute bacterial endocarditis
- Rocky Mountain spotted fever
- Hemolytic uremic syndrome
- Gonococcal arthritis dermatitis syndrome
- Influenza

DIAGNOSTIC TESTS & INTERPRETATION

ALERT
- The gold standard for the diagnosis of systemic meningococcal infection is the isolation of *N. meningitidis* from a usually sterile body fluid, such as blood or CSF.
- Antibiotic administration may render blood and/or CSF culture negative within 2 hours, so begin treatment and then test.

Initial Tests (lab, imaging)
- CBC with differential:
  – Leukocytosis or leukopenia
  – Left shift of leukocytes, toxic granulation
  – Thrombocytopenia
- Lactic acid:
  – Lactic acidosis
- Coagulation studies:
  – Prolonged prothrombin time/partial thromboplastin time
  – Low fibrinogen
  – Elevated fibrin degradation products
- Blood culture:
  – Blood culture growing *N. meningitis*
  – Positive in 50–60% of cases
- CSF:
  – Cloudy
  – Increased WBCs with polymorphonuclear cells predominant
  – Gram stain showing gram-negative diplococci
  – Glucose-to-blood glucose ratio <0.4
  – Protein >45 mg/dL
  – Positive for *N. meningitidis* antigen (MAT or PCR)
  – Culture positive for *N. meningitidis*: Positive in 80–90% of cases
- CT scan of head if there is concern for space-occupying lesions

Diagnostic Procedures/Other
- Blood culture
- Lumbar puncture:
  – If brief history and physical suggest meningitis, initiate antibiotics within 30 minutes, then proceed with a lumbar puncture.

Test Interpretation
- Disseminated intravascular coagulation (DIC)
- Exudates on meninges
- Polymorphonuclear infiltration of meninges
- Hemorrhage of adrenal glands

TREATMENT

MEDICATION

First Line

- Dexamethasone:
  - Indications:
    - Known or suspected pneumococcal meningitis in selected adults
    - Children with *H. influenzae* type B meningitis
  - Dexamethasone is often given initially in adults and children with bacterial meningitis while awaiting microbiologic data.
  - Dexamethasone has not been shown to be of benefit in meningococcal meningitis and should be discontinued once this diagnosis is established.
  - Dosage:
    - Infants and children >6 weeks: IV 0.15 mg/kg/dose q6h for the first 2–4 days of antibiotic treatment
    - Start 10–20 minutes before or with the first dose of antibiotic.
- Antibiotics:
  - Treatment for suspected meningococcal meningitis must begin as soon as possible; coverage for other possible causes of meningitis must be given until a definitive diagnosis is made.
  - Age influences the etiologic organism:
    - Preterm to <1 month: Ampicillin plus cefotaxime or ampicillin plus gentamicin:
      - Cefotaxime:
        - 0–7 days: 50 mg/kg q12h
        - 8–28 days: 50 mg/kg q8h
      - Ampicillin:
        - >2,000 g:
          - 0–7 days: 50 mg/kg q8h
          - 8–28 days: 50 mg/kg q6h
        - <2,000 g:
          - 0–7 days: 50 mg/kg q12h
          - 8–28 days: 50 mg/kg q8h
    - 1 month–50 years: Cefotaxime or ceftriaxone plus vancomycin:
      - If severe penicillin allergy: Chloramphenicol plus trimethoprim-sulfamethoxazole (TMP-SMX) plus vancomycin
    - >50 years of age or patients with alcoholism, debilitating disease, or impaired immunity: Ampicillin plus ceftriaxone plus vancomycin:
      - Ampicillin: 2 g IV q4h
      - Ceftriaxone: 2 g IV q12h
      - Vancomycin: 500–750 mg IV q6h
      - If severe penicillin allergy: TMP-SMX plus vancomycin
  - Penicillin G:
    - Meningococcal meningitis is well treated with penicillin G if the isolate is proven to be penicillin susceptible.
    - Penicillin can be used if the isolate has a penicillin minimum inhibitory concentration (MIC) of <0.1 mcg/mL.
    - For isolates with a penicillin MIC of 0.1–1 mcg/mL, treatment with high-dose penicillin is effective, but a 3rd-generation cephalosporin is preferred (5).
    - Penicillin G: 4 million units IV q4h (pediatric dose: 0.25 mU/kg IV q4–6h) *OR* ampicillin: 2 g IV q4h (pediatric dose: 200–300 mg/kg IV q6h)
- Duration of treatment: 7 days (5)
- Chemoprophylaxis:
  - Indications:
    - Close contacts: Those who have had prolonged (>8 hours) contact while in close proximity (<3 feet) to the patient or who have been

directly exposed to the patient's oral secretions between 1 week before the onset of the patient's symptoms until 24 hours after initiation of appropriate antibiotic therapy (2):
    - Examples: Household members and personnel in nurseries, day care centers, nursing homes, dormitories, and other closed institutions
    - No chemoprophylaxis is indicated for casual contacts, including most health care workers, unless there is exposure to respiratory secretion.
  - Timing:
    - Ideally <24 hours after identification of the index patient
    - Chemoprophylaxis administered >14 days is not recommended by the CDC
  - Regimens:
    - Rifampin, ciprofloxacin, and ceftriaxone:
      - Ceftriaxone:
        - Recommended for pregnant women
        - Adults: 250 mg IM as a single dose
      - Rifampin (meningococcal meningitis prophylaxis):
        - Adult: 600 mg IV or PO q12h for 2 days
        - Pediatric:
          - <1 month: 10 mg/kg/d in divided doses q12h for 2 days
          - Infants and children: 20 mg/kg/d in divided doses q12h for 2 days (max: 600 mg/dose)
      - Ciprofloxacin:
        - Adults: 750 mg PO as a single dose (6)[B]
      - Vaccination:
        - For household contacts (if the case is from a vaccine-preventable serogroup)
- Precautions:
  - Adjust the dosage of both medications in patients with severe renal dysfunction.

Second Line

- For meningitis:
  - Chloramphenicol: 1 g IV q6h (pediatric dose: 75–100 mg/kg q6h) or ceftriaxone 2 g IV q12h (pediatric dose: 80–100 mg/kg q12–24h)
  - In large outbreaks, a single dose of long-acting chloramphenicol has been used. Single-dose ceftriaxone shows equal efficacy in one randomized controlled trial.
- Precautions:
  - Ceftriaxone should not be used in patients with a history of anaphylactic reactions to penicillin (e.g., hypotension, laryngeal edema, wheezing, hives).
  - Chloramphenicol may cause aplastic anemia.

ISSUES FOR REFERRAL

Potential complications:

- Seizure activity
- DIC
- Acute respiratory distress syndrome
- Renal failure
- Adrenal failure

IN-PATIENT CONSIDERATIONS

Admission Criteria/Initial Stabilization

- If meningitis is suspected, initiate antibiotics, then proceed to an immediate lumbar puncture.
- Droplet isolation for 24 hours from the beginning of antibiotic therapy

IV Fluids

Replace volume as needed; with septic shock, large volumes of crystalloid needed

ONGOING CARE

PATIENT EDUCATION

- Educate family and close contacts regarding the risk of contracting meningococcal infections.
- Educate health care personnel who are not at risk of contracting meningococcal infections.

PROGNOSIS

Overall mortality is 13%.

COMPLICATIONS

- DIC
- Acute tubular necrosis
- Neurologic: Sensorineural hearing loss, cranial nerve palsy, seizures
- Obstructive hydrocephalus
- Subdural effusions
- Acute adrenal hemorrhage
- Waterhouse-Friderichsen syndrome

REFERENCES

1. Centers for Disease Control and Prevention. Factsheet: Meningococcal disease and meningococcal vaccine. Available at: www.cdc.gov/vaccines/vpd-vac/mening/vac-mening-fs.htm
2. Gardner P. Prevention of meningococcal disease. *N Engl J Med.* 2006;355:1466–1473.
3. Rodríguez CL, Octavio JG, Isea C, et al. Acute polyarthritis as sole manifestation of meningococcal disease. *J Clin Rheumatol.* 2012;18:42–43.
4. Thompson MJ, Ninis N. Clinical recognition of meningococcal disease in children and adolescents. *Lancet.* 2006;367:397.
5. Tunkel AR. Practice guidelines for the management of bacterial meningitis. *Clin Infect Dis.* 2004;39: 1267.
6. Fraser A, Gafter-Gvili A, Paul M. Antibiotics for preventing meningococcal infections. *Cochrane Database Syst Rev.* 2005;4:CD004785.

ADDITIONAL READING

- Visintin C, Mugglestone MA, Fields EJ, et al. National Institute for Health and Clinical Excellence Management of bacterial meningitis and meningococcal septicaemia in children and young people: Summary of NICE guidance. *BMJ.* 2010;340:c3209.
- Wright C, Wordsworth R, Glennie L. Counting the cost of meningococcal disease: Scenarios of severe meningitis and septicemia. *Paediatr Drugs.* 2013;15:49–58.

CODES

ICD10

- A39.0 Meningococcal meningitis
- A39.2 Acute meningococcemia
- A39.4 Meningococcemia, unspecified

CLINICAL PEARLS

- Chemoprophylaxis is needed for close contacts.
- Prevention with vaccinations is key.
- Treatment should never be delayed for diagnostic tests.

M

MENISCAL INJURY
Jennifer Schwartz, MD

 BASICS

DESCRIPTION
- There are 2 menisci: Medial and lateral C-shaped fibrocartilaginous structures located intra-articularly between the femoral condyles and tibial plateaus.
- Each meniscus has a body, anterior horn, and posterior horn.
- The menisci help in load distribution, stabilizing the knee, and in joint lubrication.
- After the age of 10, the menisci begin to devascularize:
  – In adults, the outer 1/3 remains vascularized.
  – The inner 2/3 is avascular and heals poorly
- The medial meniscus is attached to the joint capsule and medial collateral ligament (MCL).
- Concurrent MCL and anterior cruciate ligament (ACL) injuries common.

Geriatric Considerations
Meniscal tears in older patients are more likely due to chronic degeneration of the meniscus.

Pediatric Considerations
- Meniscal injuries are rare in children <10 years old or prior to physial fusion.
- Meniscal tears in young children are often due to a *discoid meniscus*:
  – Anatomic variant (thicker and wider) primarily involving the lateral meniscus (incidence of 3.5–5%).
- MRI is less sensitive and specific in diagnosing meniscal tears in children <12 (1)[B]:
  – Normal still-vascularized meniscal tissue can be misinterpreted as a tear

EPIDEMIOLOGY
- More common in the 3rd–5th decades of life
- More common in males:
  – Male > Female (2.5:1–4:1)

Incidence
- Medial meniscus more commonly injured because of its reduced mobility and role as the primary weight-bearing surface.
- Injuries can be *acute* or *degenerative*:
  – Degenerative tears more likely >40
  – Acute traumatic tears more likely <40; 80–90% occur during athletics

Prevalence
One of the most common musculoskeletal injuries; frequency of 23.8 per 100,000 per year (2)[B]

ETIOLOGY AND PATHOPHYSIOLOGY
- Acute tears typically occur due to a twisting motion of the knee while the foot is planted. Also can occur due to a hyperflexion event.
- Degenerative tears occur due to minimal trauma.

Genetics
A congenital abnormality leading to discoid meniscus increases the risk of meniscal tear among children. No specific gene locus has been identified.

RISK FACTORS
- Increased age (>60), male, work-related kneeling/squatting (3)[B]
- Obesity
- High degree of physical activity (especially pivot/cutting sports like soccer and rugby)
- ACL, posterior cruciate ligament (PCL) insufficiency
  – Waiting >12 months between ACL injury and surgery is a risk factor for medial meniscal tear (3)[B].

GENERAL PREVENTION
- Treatment and rehabilitation of previous knee injuries, particularly ACL injuries
- Strengthening and increased flexibility of quadriceps and hamstring muscles

COMMONLY ASSOCIATED CONDITIONS
- ACL is concomitantly torn in 1/3 of cases
- MCL and lateral collateral ligament (LCL) tears
- Tibial plateau fractures
- Femoral shaft fractures
- Tibiofemoral joint dislocation (seen occasionally)

 DIAGNOSIS

HISTORY
- Noncontact twisting or hyperflexion mechanism
- Delayed swelling, typically >24 hours after the injury
- Knee pain (on the side of the knee where the meniscal tears is present):
  – Increased with flexion of the knee (i.e., climbing stairs or squatting)
- Locking, catching, popping
- Buckling, giving out

PHYSICAL EXAM
- Clinical exam by an experienced provider can be valuable and sufficient in diagnosing meniscal injury, especially medial meniscus (4,5)[B]
- Pertinent findings on physical exam:
  – Effusion (mild–moderate)
  – Joint line tenderness
  – Positive McMurray test
    ○ Pain, clicking of meniscus being stressed
  – The Apley grind test for meniscal tear is neither sensitive nor specific.
  – Decreased range of motion, locking
  – Pain with full flexion (posterior horn tear) or extension (anterior horn tear)
- May need further imaging if not improving or if planning arthroscopy

DIFFERENTIAL DIAGNOSIS
- ACL or collateral ligament tear
- Contusion
- Pathologic plica
- Osteochondritis dissecans
- Loose body or fracture
- Osteoarthritis (OA)
- Patellofemoral syndrome
- Gout, pseudogout
- Rheumatoid arthritis

DIAGNOSTIC TESTS & INTERPRETATION
- Laboratory evaluation generally not indicated unless signs of septic joint
- Plain radiographs can detect fractures, loose bodies, or arthritic changes

Follow-Up Tests & Special Considerations
- MRI is the primary imaging study for diagnosing meniscal tears:
  – Increased signal within a meniscus corresponds to degenerative changes; signal contacting the articular surface indicates an acute tear.
- Meniscal tears are often found incidentally on MRI and may not be the cause of patient's symptoms:
  – 36–76% of meniscal tears found on MRI were asymptomatic. Asymptomatic tears increase with age and in the setting of OA (2)[B].

Diagnostic Procedures/Other
Arthroscopy may be needed for diagnostic purposes if the MRI is indeterminate.

 TREATMENT

GENERAL MEASURES
- Treatment depends on the type, location, and extent of the tear, as well as the age and activity level of the patient.
- Conservative treatment (RICE [Rest, Ice, Compression, Elevation], activity modification, physical therapy, intra-articular corticosteroid injections) should be offered 1st to most patients, especially those with degenerative tears:
  – No increased benefit found to surgery vs. physical therapy in treating symptomatic meniscal tears in patients with mild–moderate OA (6,7)[B].
  – Meniscal preservation should be the goal of treatment, to decrease future complications of OA.
  – Small, partial thickness, or peripheral tears may heal on their own or remain asymptomatic.
- Consider surgical intervention if:
  – Mechanical symptoms, locking
  – Concurrent injuries (i.e., ACL tear)
  – Persistent symptoms following 3–6 months of conservative treatment, symptoms interfering with activities of daily living/sport
  – Young patients (<30) or very active patients with an acute tear

MEDICATION
First Line
- NSAIDs
- Narcotic analgesics if needed for severe pain

ISSUES FOR REFERRAL
Surgical consult for above situations that may require intervention

ADDITIONAL THERAPIES
- Rehabilitation is required for both surgical and nonsurgical patients.
- Weight control–weight gain associated with increased cartilage loss and pain in adults with medial meniscal tears (8)[C]

SURGERY/OTHER PROCEDURES

- Most surgeries can be performed arthroscopically
- Meniscectomy (partial or total) removes the injured portion of the meniscus:
  - Can lead to articular cartilage degeneration and OA
- Meniscal repairs reapproximate the meniscus with sutures or other fixation techniques:
  - Better functional outcome and decreased risk of OA compared with meniscectomy for isolated, traumatic tears (9)[B]
- Meniscal allograft transplantation improves function in patients with prior meniscectomy

ONGOING CARE

FOLLOW-UP RECOMMENDATIONS

- Return to play requires a patient to be pain free, have full range of motion, and full strength.
- Following meniscal repair, patients can generally return to all activities in 3–6 months.
- Combined ACL and meniscal repair requires 6 months of postoperative rehabilitation before the patient can return to sports.

PATIENT EDUCATION

Teach the patient about the risks and benefits of surgical vs. conservative treatment.

PROGNOSIS

- Prognosis is more favorable if surgery is done within 8 weeks, patient is <30, or tear is peripheral/lateral <2.5 cm.
- Young athletes generally recover faster than older patients.

COMPLICATIONS

- Meniscectomies may eventually lead to OA. Consequently, meniscal repair should be performed over meniscectomy when appropriate.
- Risk of developing OA increases 6-fold 20 years after a meniscectomy (10)[B].

REFERENCES

1. Carter CW, Kocher MS. Meniscus repair in children. *Clin Sports Med*. 2012;31:135–154.
2. Maak TG, Fabricant PD, Wickiewicz TL. Indications for meniscus repair. *Clin Sports Med*. 2012;31:1–14.
3. Snoeker BA, Bakker EW, Kegel CA, et al. Risk factors for meniscal tears: A systematic review including meta-analysis. *J Orthop Sports Phys Ther*. 2013;43:352–367.
4. Ercin E, Kaya I, Sungur I, et al. History, clinical findings, magnetic resonance imaging, and arthroscopic correlation in meniscal lesions. *Knee Surg Sports Traumatol Arthrosc*. 2012;20:851–856.
5. Siddiqui MA, Ahmad I, bin Sabir A, et al. Clinical examination vs MRI: Evaluation of diagnostic accuracy in detecting ACL and meniscal injuries in comparison to arthroscopy. *Polish Orthop Traumatol*. 2013;78:59–63.
6. Rathleff CR, Cavallius C, Jensen HP, et al. Successful conservative treatment of patients with MRI-verified meniscal lesions. *Knee Surg Sports Traumatol Arthrosc* 2013; in press.
7. Katz JN, Brophy RH, Chaisson CE, et al. Surgery versus physical therapy for a meniscal tear and osteoarthritis. *N Engl J Med*. 2013;368:1675–1684.
8. Teichtahl AJ, Wluka AE, Wang Y, et al. The longitudinal relationship between changes in body weight and changes in medial tibial cartilage, and pain among community-based adults with and without meniscal tears. *Ann Rheum Dis*. 2013; in press.
9. Paxton ES, Stock MV, Brophy RH. Meniscal repair versus partial meniscectomy: A systematic review comparing reoperation rates and clinical outcomes. *Arthroscopy*. 2011;27:1275–1288.
10. Englund M, Roemer FW, Hayashi D, et al. Meniscus pathology, osteoarthritis and the treatment controversy. *Nat Rev Rheumatol*. 2012;8:412–419.

ADDITIONAL READING

- Englund M, Guermazi A, Gale D. Incidental meniscal findings on knee MRI in middle-aged and elderly persons. *N Engl J Med*. 2008;359:1108–1115.
- Herrlin SV, Wange PO, Lapidus G, et al. Is arthroscopic surgery beneficial in treating non-traumatic, degenerative medial meniscal tears? A five year follow-up. *Knee Surg Sports Traumatol Arthrosc*. 2013;21:358–364.
- Konan S, Rayan F, Haddad FS. Do physical diagnostic tests accurately detect meniscal tears? *Knee Surg Sports Traumatol Arthrosc*. 2009;17:806–811.
- LaPrade RF, Wills NJ, Spiridonov SI, et al. A prospective outcomes study of meniscal allograft transplantation. *Am J Sports Med*. 2010;38:1804–1812.
- Rosas HG, De Smet AA. Magnetic resonance imaging of the meniscus. *Top Magn Reson Imaging*. 2009;20:151–173.
- Stein T, Mehling AP, Welsch F, et al. Long-term outcome after arthroscopic meniscal repair versus arthroscopic partial meniscectomy for traumatic meniscal tears. *Am J Sports Med*. 2010;38:1542–1548.
- Strouse PJ. MRI of the knee: Key points in the pediatric population. *Pediatr Radiol*. 2010;40:447–452.
- Subhas N, Sakamoto FA, Mariscalco MW, et al. Accuracy of MRI in the diagnosis of meniscal tears in older patients. *AJR Am J Roentgenol*. 2012;198:W575–580.
- Surgery or physiotherapy for meniscal tears? *BMJ*. 2013;346:f1921.

SEE ALSO

Algorithm: Knee Pain

CODES

ICD10

- S83.209A Unsp tear of unsp meniscus, current injury, unsp knee, init
- S83.249A Oth tear of medial meniscus, current injury, unsp knee, init
- S83.289A Oth tear of lat mensc, current injury, unsp knee, init

CLINICAL PEARLS

- Increasing core proprioception and quadricep/hamstring flexibility may prevent knee injuries, especially in female athletes.
- MRI is the preferred imaging modality to identify meniscal pathology.
- 36–76% of meniscal tears found on MRI are asymptomatic.
- Nonsurgical and surgical candidates require rehabilitation.
- Meniscal preservation should be the goal of treatment to prevent OA.
- Meniscal repairs have a better functional outcome and decrease the risk of OA compared with meniscectomy.
- Don't forget the posterior horns of the menisci in patients with posterior knee/posterolateral corner pain.

MENOPAUSE
Jeremy Golding, MD

BASICS

DESCRIPTION
- Natural menopause: Permanent cessation of menstrual periods for at least 12 consecutive months in a nonpregnant woman ≥40 years of age:
  - Resulting from ovarian follicular depletion
  - Not associated with a pathologic etiology
- Perimenopause: From the onset of menstrual changes through the 1st year of menopause (average length of perimenopause is 4–5 years)
- Postmenopause: Usually accounts for >1/3 of a woman's life
- Premature menopause: Menopause occurring before age 40; may be associated with sex chromosome abnormalities

EPIDEMIOLOGY
- Average age of perimenopause onset is 51 years.
- Mean age of menopause onset is 51–52 years.
- Earlier menopause occurs in Hispanic women as compared with Caucasian women.

Incidence
In the US, 1.3 million women reach menopause annually.

ETIOLOGY AND PATHOPHYSIOLOGY
Normal physiologic process:
- As women age, the number of ovarian follicles decreases: Ovarian production of estrogen and inhibin decreases, and luteinizing (LH) and follicle-stimulating (FSH) hormone production increases:
  - Without estrogen, failure of endometrial development occurs and menstrual cycles become irregular, then cease.
  - Symptoms directly or indirectly due to decrease in estrogen
- Surgical: Removal of functioning ovaries due to disease or incidental to total hysterectomy
- Other:
  - Treatment of endometriosis
  - Treatment of breast cancer with antiestrogens (which is reversible)
  - May occur after cancer chemotherapy (permanent or reversible)

RISK FACTORS
- Aging
- Oophorectomy
- Sex chromosome abnormalities (e.g., Turner syndrome)
- Age of maternal menopause
- Reproductive history: Nulliparous, short cycles during adolescence
- Smoking (reduces age of onset by 2 years)

GENERAL PREVENTION
Goal is not to prevent menopause, but to retard development of osteoporosis related to menopause:
- Weight-bearing exercise
- Avoid smoking.
- Avoid excessive alcohol and caffeine intake.
- Maintain healthy weight.
- Calcium intake 1,200 mg/d beginning in adolescence, best from diet and not from supplements
- Adequate vitamin D (800–1,200 IU daily)

DIAGNOSIS

HISTORY
- Cessation of menses:
  - Generally preceded by a period of irregular cycles as well as heavy or diminished bleeding
- Vasomotor symptoms: Hot flashes and sweating, often at night (80%):
  - First and most common manifestation of menopause
  - Prevalence of symptoms varies across cultures
  - Last ~3–4 minutes, occur at unpredictable intervals
  - Frequency usually declines with time
- Mood changes (8–38%), anxiety, depression: More common in women with less education attainment and/or personal history of depression
- Sleep disorders (35–60%):
  - Lengthening of latent phase
  - Less time spent asleep
- Urogenital atrophy:
  - Atrophic vaginitis causes vaginal dryness (17–30%), itch, dyspareunia, and possibly sexual dysfunction.
  - Urethral atrophy causes urgency, frequency, dysuria, and stress incontinence.
  - Atrophy of paravaginal tissues that support bladder and rectum can lead to urocele, rectocele, and uterine prolapse.
  - Increased pH and atrophy increase risk of vaginal infections and UTIs.
- Osteopenia and osteoporosis
- Change in intensity and severity of migraines
- Skin thinning, hair loss, hirsutism, brittle nails
- Breast pain

Geriatric Considerations
Vaginal bleeding in postmenopausal women is abnormal; endometrial cancer must be ruled out.

PHYSICAL EXAM
- Decrease in breast size and change in breast texture
- External, speculum, and bimanual pelvic exams: Atrophic vaginal mucosa (urogenital atrophy)

DIFFERENTIAL DIAGNOSIS
Pregnancy, polycystic ovarian syndrome, pituitary adenoma, anorexia nervosa causing amenorrhea, hypothalamic dysfunction, Asherman syndrome, obstruction of uterine outflow tract, Sheehan syndrome, thyroid disease

DIAGNOSTIC TESTS & INTERPRETATION
Initial Tests (lab, imaging)
- Generally none required; the patient's age and symptoms establish the diagnosis.
- If laboratory confirmation is desired:
  - Elevated serum FSH level >30 mIU/mL indicates ovarian failure.
  - Symptoms may precede changes in lab parameters.
- Drugs that may alter lab results: Estrogens, androgens, oral contraceptive pills (OCPs)
- LH has no role in diagnosing menopause.
- In the US, mammography is recommended for menopausal women (upper age limit for discontinuation remains uncertain) with recommendations varying from yearly to every 3 years. In the UK, mammography is recommended every 3 years.

Follow-Up Tests & Special Considerations
- Brain MRI if pituitary tumor suspected
- Abnormal vaginal bleeding in a postmenopausal patient should be evaluated by transvaginal ultrasound (TVUS) and/or endometrial biopsy. If endometrial stripe is <5 mm on TVUS, endometrial carcinoma is unlikely.
- Bone mineral density (BMD) testing with dual energy x-ray absorptiometry (DEXA) scan in postmenopausal women <65 years with additional risk factors may be indicated if the risk for fracture is equivalent to that of a 65 year old woman (using the FRAX tool to assess, http://www.shef.ac.uk/FRAX/). Risk factors for fracture include a previous history of fractures, low body weight, cigarette smoking, and family history of osteoporotic fracture.

Test Interpretation
- Abnormal BMD and DEXA scan results:
  - T-score on DEXA of −1 to −2.5 = Osteopenia
  - T-score <−2.5 = Osteoporosis
  - Defer to femoral neck T-score value over spine T-score
- Z-score measures age-matched mean bone density (not clinically useful)

TREATMENT

Treatment choice depends on the severity of symptoms.

MEDICATION
First Line
Hormone therapy (HT) (1,2): Developing an individual risk-benefit profile is essential for every woman considering any HT regimen. The major influence to use HT for most women is effect on menopausal sx and their effect on quality of life. The absolute risks for use of HT in healthy women ages 50–59 years are low. In contrast, long-term HT or HT initiation in older women is associated with greater risks.

- The primary indication for HT is the treatment of moderate to severe vasomotor symptoms. Combination estrogen–progestin therapy is effective treatment for these symptoms, and other menopausal symptoms (e.g., sleep disorders, urogenital atrophy). It is also useful for preventing osteoporotic fractures and colorectal cancer and may help with mood symptoms (3,4)[A].

- Current recommendations for HT suggest use for a limited duration (i.e., 2–3 years, no more than 5 years) in treating menopausal symptoms in women who do not have a history of, and are not at high risk for, coronary artery disease (CAD), stroke, breast cancer, or thromboembolism. If these risk factors are present, or if the woman is asymptomatic, consider alternative treatments to prevent bone loss. For women in whom progestin is not necessary, unopposed estrogen therapy may be continued for longer than 3–5 years (2).

- If HT is selected, estrogen should be given in combination with progestin for women with an intact uterus. Depending on duration of use, unopposed estrogen carries a 2–6.7-fold higher risk of endometrial cancer. Most data available are for continuous treatment (as opposed to cyclical) with combined conjugated equine estrogen (CEE) 0.625 mg and medroxyprogesterone acetate 2.5 mg. However, considerable evidence supports the use of low-dose HT, which is associated with 50% lower

rates of irregular bleeding. Low dose = 0.3 mg conjugated estrogen and 0.5 mg estradiol.
- Precautions:
  - The Women's Health Initiative (WHI) study, in 2002, done in women without established coronary heart disease (CHD), found those treated with combination estrogen–progestin therapy had an increased relative risk of invasive breast cancer, CHD, stroke, and pulmonary embolism at 5 years of use (4)[A]. This risk of breast cancer was found to be independent of mammography screening frequency (1)[B]. For every 100 women treated with HT for 5 years, 1 woman will have a serious adverse event.
  - The Heart and Estrogen/Progestin Replacement Study (HERS), done in women with established CHD, demonstrated improvements in the lipid profiles of women on HT, but the overall risk of vascular mortality did not decline.
  - An increased risk of ovarian cancer is seen in women who take HT. Of every 8,300 women who take hormone replacement therapy, each year 1 woman has been shown to suffer from ovarian cancer (5)[B].
  - Higher doses of estrogen can cause hypercoagulability, breast tenderness, gallbladder disease, and hypertension (HTN).
  - Contraindications to HT:
    - Estrogen-dependent malignancies
    - Unexplained uterine bleeding
    - History of thromboembolism or stroke
    - CAD
    - Active liver disease
- For osteoporosis:
  - Women with a history of hip or vertebral fracture or personal history of osteoporosis should be treated per below, in addition to taking vitamin D and possibly calcium supplementation (not to exceed 1,200 mg daily), engaging in weight-bearing exercise, and not smoking.
  - Bisphosphonates inhibit osteoclast action and resorption of bone:
    - Alendronate (Fosamax): 70 mg/wk or 10 mg/d.
    - Risedronate (Actonel): 35 mg once a week or 5 mg/d.
    - Zoledronic acid (Reclast or Zometa): 5 mg IV annually.
    - Ibandronate (Boniva): 150 mg/mo PO or 3 mg IV q3mo:
      - The BONE trial demonstrated that ibandronate decreased the risk of vertebral fracture, but failed to demonstrate a decrease in the risk of extravertebral fractures.
  - Selective estrogen receptor modulators (SERMs) selectively inhibit or stimulate estrogen-like action in various tissues. The SERM used for the treatment of osteoporosis is the following:
    - Raloxifene (Evista): 60 mg/d for prevention and treatment; because raloxifene is less effective than alendronate, risedronate, or estrogen, it is best suited for the prevention or treatment of mild osteoporosis (6)[A].
    - Raloxifene should be used in postmenopausal women who cannot tolerate bisphosphonates and/or those who are at risk for invasive breast cancer. Of note, it increases the risk of thromboembolism and hot flashes.
    - Raloxifene should be used primarily in postmenopausal women with predominantly spinal osteoporosis (6,7)[A].

- The EFFECT trial demonstrated that raloxifene decreased the risk of vertebral fracture, but failed to demonstrate a decrease in the risk of extravertebral fractures.
- For atrophic vaginitis: Topical estrogen therapy (ET): Conjugated estrogens (Premarin cream); best for local therapy of atrophic vaginitis. ET applied to vaginal mucosa as needed reverses vaginal atrophy, enhances blood flow, reduces pH and UTIs. Data are insufficient to recommend annual endometrial surveillance in women using ET with no vaginal bleeding. ET should be continued as long as distressing symptoms remain. Treatment is initiated with daily or alternate day vaginal cream, and tapered to maintenance of 1–3 times weekly as desired improvement attained. Women with a history of hormone-dependent cancer should consult with an oncologist before using.

Second Line
Nonhormonal treatments may be helpful to treat vasomotor symptoms in women who wish to or need to avoid HT (e.g., breast cancer):
- Antidepressants venlafaxine (37.5–75 mg/d), paroxetine (10–20 mg/d), or fluoxetine (20 mg/d) are options that have been shown to result in 1 fewer hot flashes per day.
- Gabapentin (300–900 mg/d) has been shown to have some effect in reducing vasomotor symptoms by up to 2 hot flashes per day (8)[A].
- Clonidine may be used to treat mild hot flashes, although it is less effective than antidepressants or gabapentin. Initial oral dose is 0.05 mg b.i.d.; some women may require 0.1 mg b.i.d.
- All trials of second-line therapies have been brief (i.e., a few months) (7,8)[A].

COMPLEMENTARY AND ALTERNATIVE MEDICINE
Trials of nonprescribed therapies are difficult to interpret due to variability of components and doses:
- Soy isoflavone in placebo-controlled trials showed a mixed effect in reducing hot flashes.
- Red clover, black cohosh, reflexology, aerobics, and magnet therapy showed no impact on hot flashes when compared with placebo.
- Small clinical trials of evening primrose, dong quai, ginseng, and wild yam do not support their use for relief of hot flashes.

 ONGOING CARE

FOLLOW-UP RECOMMENDATIONS
Patient Monitoring
A DEXA scan is indicated at age 65 for all women for younger women with risk equivalent to age 65.

DIET
Calcium-rich diet and vitamin D supplements as above. Calcium supplements may have adverse effects including increased risk of kidney stone and coronay calcification.

PATIENT EDUCATION
Encourage lifestyle modifications:
- Smoking cessation
- Weight-bearing exercise at least 30 minutes 3× weekly
- Avoid excess alcohol and caffeine.
- Address cardiovascular risk factor modification.

PROGNOSIS
If untreated:
- Ultimate disappearance of vasomotor symptoms usually takes several years.
- Osteoporosis: Possible fractures of the hip, vertebrae, and wrists

COMPLICATIONS
- Osteoporosis: At menopause, women have accelerated bone loss up to 3–5%/yr for 5–7 years.
- Increased risk of CAD

REFERENCES

1. Chlebowski RT, Kuller LH, Prentice RL, et al. Breast cancer after use of estrogen plus progestin in postmenopausal women. *N Engl J Med*. 2009;360: 573–587.
2. The 2012 hormone therapy position statement of the North American Menopause Society. *Menopause*. 2012;19(3):257–271.
3. Nelson HD. Commonly used types of postmenopausal estrogen for treatment of hot flashes: Scientific review. *JAMA*. 2004;291: 1610–1620.
4. Rossouw JE, Anderson GL, Prentice RL, et al. Risks and benefits of estrogen plus progestin in healthy postmenopausal women: Principal results from the Women's Health Initiative randomized controlled trial. *JAMA*. 2002;288:321–333.
5. Mørch LS, Løkkegaard E, Andreasen AH, et al. Hormone therapy and ovarian cancer. *JAMA*. 2009;302:298–305.
6. Riggs BL, Hartmann LC. Selective estrogen-receptor modulators—mechanisms of action and application to clinical practice. *N Engl J Med*. 2003;348:618–629.
7. North American Menopause Society. The role of local vaginal estrogen for treatment of vaginal atrophy in postmenopausal women: 2007 position statement of The North American Menopause Society. *Menopause*. 2007;14(3 Pt 1):355–369; quiz 370–371.
8. USPSTF. www.ahrq.gov/clinic/epcsums/ osteoporosis.pdf.

ADDITIONAL READING
National Guideline Clearinghouse. Menopause. www.guideline.gov

CODES

ICD10
- E28.310 Symptomatic premature menopause
- N95.1 Menopausal and female climacteric states
- Z78.0 Asymptomatic menopausal state

CLINICAL PEARLS
- Menopause is usually diagnosed by history alone.
- HT can be used short term for relief of moderate to severe vasomotor symptoms, but should not be used long term for prevention of cardiovascular disease.

M

MENORRHAGIA

Donald Nelson, MD

 BASICS

DESCRIPTION
- Menorrhagia is an excessive amount or duration of menstrual flow, at more or less regular intervals. Flow ≥80 mL/cycle, compared with normal average 30–40 mL (1,2).
- Distinguishable from, but may overlap with, the following:
  - Metrorrhagia: Irregular or frequent flow, noncyclic
  - Menometrorrhagia: Frequent, excessive, irregular flow (menorrhagia plus metrorrhagia)
  - Polymenorrhea: Frequent flow, cycles of ≤21 days
  - Intermenstrual bleeding: Bleeding between regular menses
  - Dysfunctional uterine bleeding (DUB): Abnormal endometrial bleeding of hormonal cause and related to anovulation
- System affected: Reproductive

EPIDEMIOLOGY
Prevalence
- The prevalence of abnormal uterine bleeding (AUB) is estimated at 11–13% in the general population and increases with age, reaching 24% in those aged 36–40 years (3).
- ~30% of women complain of excessive bleeding at some point (1).
- Predominant sex: Female only
- Predominant age:
  - Menarche to menopause; ~50% of cases occur in patients age >40 years
  - Dysfunctional bleeding is fairly common in adolescence and near menopause.
  - In adolescence, irregular bleeding due to anovulation and immaturity of the hypothalamic-pituitary-ovarian axis is common.
  - In adolescence, severe menorrhagia may be associated with a bleeding disorder more than 40% of the time, with platelet function defects and von Willebrand disease being the most common (4).

Pediatric Considerations
Genital bleeding before puberty can result from trauma, foreign bodies, vaginal infection, or exogenous hormone administration.

Pregnancy Considerations
Bleeding in pregnancy is not menorrhagia. Complications of pregnancy or cervical/vaginal lesions should be considered.

Geriatric Considerations
True menorrhagia cannot occur after menopause. However, genital atrophy as well as uterine and ovarian cancers may be associated with vaginal bleeding in the elderly.

ETIOLOGY AND PATHOPHYSIOLOGY
- Hypothyroidism
- Endometrial proliferation/excess/hyperplasia:
  - Anovulation, oligo-ovulation
  - Ovarian tumor or other estrogen-producing tumor
  - Prolonged estrogen, progestin, or oral contraceptive administration
  - Polycystic ovarian syndrome
- Local factors:
  - Endometrial atrophy, postmenopause
  - Abnormal endometrial prostaglandin levels
  - Endometrial polyps
  - Endometrial neoplasia

  - Adenomyosis/endometriosis
  - Uterine myomata (fibroids)
  - Intrauterine device (IUD)
  - Uterine sarcoma
- Coagulation disorders:
  - Thrombocytopenia, platelet disorders
  - von Willebrand disease, factor deficiencies
  - Leukemia
  - Ingestion of aspirin/acetylsalicylic acid or anticoagulants
  - Renal failure/dialysis

RISK FACTORS
- Obesity
- Anovulation
- Estrogen administration (± progestin)
- Prior treatment with progestational agents or oral contraceptives increases risk of endometrial atrophy, but it decreases the risk of endometrial hyperplasia or neoplasia.

GENERAL PREVENTION
Periodic Pap smears and pelvic examinations at appropriate intervals based on age and risk factors

COMMONLY ASSOCIATED CONDITIONS
Metrorrhagia, menometrorrhagia, androgenic disorders

 DIAGNOSIS

HISTORY
- Excessive menstrual flow is defined subjectively and varies greatly from woman to woman.
- Useful features:
  - Bleeding substantially heavier than usual flow (or >80 mL/cycle, if quantified)
  - Bleeding lasting >7 days
  - Flow associated with significant clots
  - Anemia
- Symptoms that suggest cycles are ovulatory:
  - Regular menstrual interval
  - Midcycle pain (mittelschmerz)
  - Dysmenorrhea
  - Premenstrual symptoms: Breast soreness/tenderness, mood changes
- Abdominal pain or cramps at other times of the cycle may be associated with structural causes:
  - Myomas
  - Polyps
  - Ovarian tumors
- Symptoms that may indicate a more general bleeding disorder (4):
  - Epistaxis, bleeding gums
  - Easy bruising, increased bleeding with minor trauma
  - Family history of bleeding disorder

PHYSICAL EXAM
- Hirsutism, acne, or obesity may accompany chronic anovulation.
- Signs of nongenital or general bleeding, bruising, petechiae
- Pelvic/rectal examination to detect/exclude other causes of bleeding:
  - Cervical or vaginal bleeding
  - Pelvic or adnexal masses
  - Signs of pelvic infection

DIFFERENTIAL DIAGNOSIS
- Pregnancy complications:
  - Threatened abortion
  - Incomplete abortion
  - Ectopic pregnancy
- Nonuterine bleeding:
  - Cervical ectropion/erosion
  - Cervical neoplasia/polyp
  - Cervical or vaginal trauma/foreign body
  - Condylomata
  - Atrophic vaginitis
- Pelvic inflammatory disease:
  - Endometritis
  - Tuberculosis

DIAGNOSTIC TESTS & INTERPRETATION
Initial Tests (lab, imaging)
- Pregnancy test: Exclude pregnancy first.
- CBC to assess severity of blood loss and to rule out thrombocytopenia and leukemia (2)
- In selected cases:
  - Thyroid stimulating hormone test
  - Coagulation screen, with follow-up testing and platelet function testing if screen is abnormal (4)
  - Creatinine, BUN
  - Serum progesterone: 5–20 ng/mL (15.9–63.6 nmol/L) in luteal phase, <1 ng/mL (<3.18 nmol/L) in follicular phase or anovulatory cycle
- Transvaginal ultrasonography can help distinguish bleeding due to atrophy from bleeding caused by hyperplasia, polyps, or myomas.
- Ultrasonography to evaluate adnexal masses or myomas suspected from pelvic exam.
- A CT is used to investigate potentially malignant pelvic masses.
- An MRI is not recommended as a first-line procedure (3).

Diagnostic Procedures/Other
- Endometrial biopsy detects hyperplasia, dysplasia, or atrophy. If done before expected menses, it may also help confirm the diagnosis of anovulation or luteal phase defect.
- After age 35–40, endometrial carcinoma is a significant cause of bleeding. Obtain endometrial sampling before attempting hormonal treatment (5)[C].

Test Interpretation
- Vary with etiology. In ~50% of cases, no uterine pathology is found (1).
- Progestins used before endometrial biopsy may cause decidualization and obscure correct diagnosis.

 TREATMENT

MEDICATION
First Line
- For acute control of severe bleeding:
  - Estrogen, conjugated (Premarin): 25 mg IV q4h up to 6 doses or 10–20 mg/d PO in 4 divided doses until bleeding abates (5)[C]
- For less severe bleeding (usual case) or after control of acute bleeding has been achieved:
  - Medroxyprogesterone acetate (Provera): 10–30 mg/d for 5–10 days
  - Any combination oral contraceptive (i.e., usually a high-dose oral contraceptive) 1 tablet q.i.d. for 5–7 days

- To prevent heavy bleeding in subsequent cycles:
  – Medroxyprogesterone acetate: 5–30 mg/d for 10 d/mo
  – Usual cyclic dose of a combination oral contraceptive (5)[C]
  – Vaginal hormonal contraceptive ring (NuvaRing) is an alternative to an oral contraceptive (6)[B].

Second Line
- Nonsteroidal prostaglandin-synthetase inhibitors (e.g., naproxen, mefenamic acid, ibuprofen) can reduce blood loss ~25% with ovulatory cycles and reduce dysmenorrhea (7)[B].
- Tranexamic acid (Cyklokapron), a plasminogen activation inhibitor, 2 g/d PO is equally or more effective than medroxyprogesterone 10 mg b.i.d. (8)[B], but is much more expensive.
- Norethindrone acetate (Aygestin): 2.5–10 mg/d for 10–21 d/mo
- Levonorgestrel intrauterine system (Mirena IUD) can reduce blood loss >90% (7)[B].
- Danazol and gonadotropin-releasing hormone agonists are also effective therapies but are more likely to have adverse side effects. Mifepristone (RU-486) has been used experimentally (1).

ADDITIONAL THERAPIES
Nausea and vomiting are common from IV estrogen; antiemetics are helpful.

SURGERY/OTHER PROCEDURES
- Endometrial ablation by laser or electrosurgical, microwave, or thermal means is a conservative alternative to hysterectomy and usually successful, although some patients require additional therapy in the long term (1)[A].
- Hysterectomy when indicated to treat coexisting conditions (myomas, endometrial dysplasia) or for bleeding unresponsive to other measures (1)

IN-PATIENT CONSIDERATIONS
Admission Criteria/Initial Stabilization
- Bleeding leading to orthostatic hypotension
- Hematocrit <25%
- Most cases can be managed as outpatient in an office or emergency department.
- Rule out pregnancy complications and nonuterine bleeding
- Treat severe or life-threatening bleeding acutely:
  – Circulatory support; transfusion, if necessary
  – IV estrogen
  – Curettage, if necessary
  – Hysterectomy in extreme cases

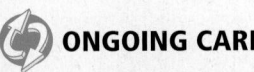
ONGOING CARE

FOLLOW-UP RECOMMENDATIONS
Proceed to identify the underlying cause of bleeding and treat to prevent recurrence:
- Hormonal therapy
- Dilatation and curettage for cases that fail to respond to hormone therapy

- Consider endometrial ablation or hysterectomy in persistent cases in which fertility is not a concern
- Specific treatment for neoplasia, polyps, systemic disease
- Patients in whom fertility is a consideration may also need appropriate treatment for anovulation, endometriosis, and myomas.

Patient Monitoring
- Varies with cause of bleeding
- Medical treatment of hyperplastic/dysplastic endometrium should be followed by a repeat biopsy to confirm that histologic structure has returned to normal.

DIET
Iron supplementation may help correct for increased blood loss.

PATIENT EDUCATION
Information about side effects of medications should be provided.

PROGNOSIS
- Varies with cause of bleeding
- Most patients whose condition results from hormonal causes will respond to hormonal manipulation.

COMPLICATIONS
- Anemia
- Estrogen may precipitate acute, intermittent porphyria or cholestatic jaundice in susceptible patients.

REFERENCES

1. Oehler MK, Rees MC. Menorrhagia: An update. *Acta Obstet Gynecol Scand*. 2003;82:405–422.
2. Siegel JE. Abnormalities of hemostasis and abnormal uterine bleeding. *Clin Obstet Gynecol*. 2005;48:284–294.
3. Marret H, Fauconnier A, Chabbert-Buffet N, et al. Clinical practice guidelines on menorrhagia: Management of abnormal uterine bleeding before menopause. *Eur J Obstet Gynecol Reprod Biol*. 2010;152:133–137.
4. Sokkary NA, Venkateswaran L, Dietrich JE. Platelet function disorders and menorrhagia in adolescents: A review. *J Pediatr Adolesc Gynecol*. 2012;25:233–237.
5. Management of anovulatory bleeding. *ACOG Practice Bulletin* 14, March 2000, reaffirmed *2009*.
6. Abu Hashim H, Alsherbini W, Bazeed M. Contraceptive vaginal ring treatment of heavy menstrual bleeding: A randomized controlled trial with norethisterone. *Contraception*. 2012;85:246–252.
7. Reid PC, Virtanen-Kari S. Randomised comparative trial of levonorgestrel intrauterine system and mefenamic acid for the treatment of idiopathic menorrhagia. *BJOG*. 2005;112:1121–1125.
8. Kriplani A, Kulshrestha V, Agarwal N. Role of tranexamic acid in management of dysfunctional uterine bleeding in comparison with medroxyprogesterone acetate. *J Obstet Gynaecol*. 2006;26:673–678.

ADDITIONAL READING
- Practice Committee of American Society for Reproductive Medicine. Indications and options for endometrial ablation. *Fertil Steril*. 2008;90(5 Suppl): S236–S240.
- Showstack J, Lin F, Learman LA, et al. Randomized trial of medical treatment versus hysterectomy for abnormal uterine bleeding: Resource use in the Medicine or Surgery (Ms) trial. *Am J Obstet Gynecol*. 2006;194:332–338.

SEE ALSO

- Abnormal Pap and Cervical Dysplasia; Amenorrhea; Cervical Malignancy; Cervical Polyps; Cervicitis, Ectropion, and True Erosion; Dysfunctional Uterine Bleeding; Dysmenorrhea; Menopause; Polycystic Ovarian Syndrome (PCOS); Uterine Myomas
- Algorithm: Menorrhagia (Excessive Bleeding)

CODES

ICD10
- N92.0 Excessive and frequent menstruation with regular cycle
- N92.1 Excessive and frequent menstruation with irregular cycle
- N93.8 Other specified abnormal uterine and vaginal bleeding

CLINICAL PEARLS
- Menorrhagia is defined as an excessive amount or duration of menstrual flow at more or less regular intervals and has a wide variety of potential causes.
- Pregnancy should be ruled out as part of the initial evaluation.
- Because endometrial carcinoma is a significant cause of bleeding in women age >35 years, an endometrial biopsy to rule out endometrial carcinoma is recommended before using any hormonal treatments.
- Iron supplementation will help correct for increased blood loss while the underlying etiology is being identified and treated.

M

MERKEL CELL CARCINOMA

Frank J. Domino, MD

 BASICS

- Rare, aggressive, cutaneous neuroendocrine carcinoma most commonly found in the elderly on sun-exposed skin
- System(s) affected: Skin
- Synonym(s): Neuroendocrine carcinoma of the skin; Trabecular carcinoma; Anaplastic carcinoma of the skin; Primary undifferentiated carcinoma of the skin

EPIDEMIOLOGY

Incidence
- Age-adjusted incidence is estimated to be 0.24/100,000 person-years in the US.
- Incidence has tripled since 1986, with an average annual increase of 8%.
- Highest in the elderly: Median age at diagnosis is 74; 5% of cases diagnosed <50

Prevalence
- Rare, <1% of all skin cancers in the US.
- 1,500 cases diagnosed in 2007.
- 0.24/100,000 person-years

ETIOLOGY AND PATHOPHYSIOLOGY
- May arise from Merkel cells, a slowly adapting fine-touch mechanoreceptor, in the basal epidermis.
- Some suggest derivation from immature pluripotential cells in dermis.
- Merkel cell polyomavirus (MCPyV) may contribute to development and has been detected in 80% of tumors tested.

RISK FACTORS
- UV exposure (natural or artificial)
- History of prior skin cancer
- Fair skin
- Age >65
- Chronic immune suppression (HIV, leukemia, organ transplantation)
- Possible association with arsenic exposure

GENERAL PREVENTION
Avoid sun exposure; early referral for symptoms listed below

COMMONLY ASSOCIATED CONDITIONS
Increased risk for developing other malignancies, including lymphomas and other skin cancers

 DIAGNOSIS

Complete examination of skin and regional lymph nodes, followed by biopsy (1)[C]. Sentinel lymph node biopsy should be considered for all patients as even small tumors have been shown to have a ≥15% risk of lymph node disease (2).

HISTORY
Rapidly growing, painless nodule

PHYSICAL EXAM
- Distribution:
  - Usually develops on chronically sun-exposed skin such as head, neck, arms.
- Morphology:
  - Nonspecific appearance; may be mistaken for more common skin lesions
  - Solitary nodule or firm plaque
  - Flesh, bluish-red, or violaceous color
  - Shiny, may have telangiectasias
- Associated signs:
  - Grows rapidly, ulcerates rarely

DIFFERENTIAL DIAGNOSIS
- Cyst
- Basal cell carcinoma
- Squamous cell carcinoma
- Amelanotic melanoma
- Lymphoma cutis
- Kaposi sarcoma
- Pyogenic granuloma
- Adnexal tumor
- Dermatofibrosarcoma protuberans

DIAGNOSTIC TESTS & INTERPRETATION
- Biopsy with histological stains (see below)
- In cases of confirmed Merkel cell carcinoma (MCC), evaluate for metastatic disease. This includes clinical lymph node examination evaluating for gross lymph node disease and sentinel lymph node biopsy to evaluate for microscopic lymph node disease. Radiologic imaging can be used to evaluate for distant metastases if indicated.
- CT/MRI/PET scans are most valuable in cases of confirmed lymph node disease to evaluate for visceral or bone metastases. Imaging may also be utilized to evaluate patients with primary lesions >2 cm who are known to have a higher risk of metastasis and/or to monitor for disease progression (2).

Follow-Up Tests & Special Considerations
MRI may help plan target volume for radiation therapy.

Diagnostic Procedures/Other
Skin biopsy

Test Interpretation
- Morphology:
  - Small, round, blue cells; basophilic nuclei; minimal cytoplasm; frequent mitoses; high apoptotic index
  - Dermal tumor nodule frequently extending into subcutaneous fat, usually sparing papillary dermis and adnexa
  - Similar histological appearance as small cell lung cancer, small cell melanoma, lymphoma
- Immunohistochemistry:
  - Stains positive for epithelial and neuroendocrine markers, negative for lymphoid and melanoma markers
  - Positive for low-molecular-weight intermediate filament CK20 in perinuclear dot pattern, a highly sensitive marker
  - Negative for thyroid transcription factor-1, S100, or leukocyte common antigen
  - The histological differential diagnosis for MCC includes small cell lung cancer and melanoma. Small cell lung cancer is generally negative for CK 20 and positive for TTF-1. Melanoma stains positive for S100 and negative for CK20.

TREATMENT

Wide local excision and radiation therapy are mainstays of therapy. Merkel cell carcinoma is a highly radiosensitive tumor, and radiation therapy of affected lymph node basins should also be performed.

GENERAL MEASURES
- Wide local excision (2–2.5 cm) with pathologically clear margins and sentinel lymph node biopsy (3,4)[A]
- Adjuvant radiation to primary site ± draining regional nodes decreases locoregional recurrence and improves survival (3,4)[A].
- Radiation may be used as monotherapy in inoperable disease and has been used alone to control local disease (3,4)[A].

ISSUES FOR REFERRAL
Early referral to dermatologist if MCC is suspected. Recommend multidisciplinary tumor board with surgeon and radiation oncologist (1)[C].

ADDITIONAL THERAPIES
Chemotherapy reserved for palliative care for patients with stage IV disease; can shrink advanced metastatic disease, but may not increase survival (3,4)[A]

SURGERY/OTHER PROCEDURES
Mohs surgery may be indicated for MCC on the head, where it may not be possible to obtain a margin of at least 2 cm.

 ## ONGOING CARE

FOLLOW-UP RECOMMENDATIONS
- Regular follow-up appointments with dermatologist every 1–3 months for the 1st year, every 3–6 months in 2nd year, and annually thereafter.
- CT scans every 6 months after a high-risk diagnosis.

Patient Monitoring
Patients should perform routine skin checks for any new nodules or pigmentation changes.

PATIENT EDUCATION
- http://www.merkelcell.org
- http://www.cancer.gov/cancertopics/pdq/treatment/merkelcell/Patient/page1

PROGNOSIS
- 70–80% of patients with MCC present with localized disease.
- Locoregional recurrence usually develops within 8 months of diagnosis and is associated with distant metastasis in the future.
- 2-year mortality rate is 30–50%.
- Distant metastasis found at mean of 18 months: Mean survival <6 months

COMPLICATIONS
Metastasizes via lymphatics, commonly to skin, liver, lung, bone, and brain.

REFERENCES
1. Miller SJ, Alam M, Andersen J, et al. Merkel cell carcinoma. *J Natl Compr Canc Netw*. 2009;7(3): 322–332.
2. Schwartz JL, Griffith KA, Lowe L, et al. Features predicting sentinel lymph node positivity in Merkel cell carcinoma. *J Clin Oncol*. 2011;29(8): 1036–1041. Epub 2011 Feb 7.
3. Nicolaidou E, Mikrova A, Antoniou C, et al. Advances in Merkel cell carcinoma pathogenesis and management: A recently discovered virus, a new international consensus staging system and new diagnostic codes. *Br J Dermatol*. 2012;166(1):16–21. Epub 2011 Nov 17.
4. Schrama D, Ugurel S, Becker JC. Merkel cell carcinoma: Recent insights and new treatment options. *Curr Opin Oncol*. 2012;24(2):141–149.

 ## CODES

ICD10
- C4A.4 Merkel cell carcinoma of scalp and neck
- C4A.9 Merkel cell carcinoma, unspecified
- C4A.30 Merkel cell carcinoma of unspecified part of face

CLINICAL PEARLS
- MCC is a rare, aggressive cutaneous neuroendocrine carcinoma with a rising incidence and high mortality rate.
- It usually presents in elderly individuals with fair skin on chronically sun-exposed areas.
- It has a nonspecific appearance but grows rapidly.

M

MESENTERIC ADENITIS
Jill A. Grimes, MD, FAAFP

BASICS

Mesenteric adenitis is inflammation of the mesenteric lymph nodes, typically a self-limited disease.

DESCRIPTION
- Characterized by benign inflammation of the mesenteric lymph nodes.
- The condition is generally self-limited, and both acute and chronic episodes of mesenteric adenitis have been described:
  – May clinically mimic acute appendicitis

EPIDEMIOLOGY
- Commonly misdiagnosed condition, making definite incidence unknown.
- Estimated at ~20% in patients presenting for appendectomy (1).

Prevalence
- Mesenteric adenitis generally affects males and females equally:
  – However, adenitis secondary to *Yersinia* infection is more prevalent in boys than girls (2).
- The prevalence of etiologic agent *Y. enterocolitica* is most common in North America, Eastern Europe, and Australia (2).

ETIOLOGY AND PATHOPHYSIOLOGY
- On gross inspection, lymph nodes are enlarged and soft.
- Adjoining mesentery may be edematous and may or may not present with fluid collections (3).
- In instances of infectious etiologies, pathogens are ingested, translocate through the intestinal epithelium, and gain access to lymph nodes via intestinal lymphatics via Peyer's patches (3).
- Underlying infectious process or intra-abdominal inflammatory process:
  – Infectious agents include (3,4):
    ○ *Y. enterocolitica*
    ○ *β*-hemolytic *Streptococcus* spp.
    ○ *Staphylococcus* spp.
    ○ *Streptococcus viridans*
    ○ *Escherichia coli*
    ○ *Mycobacterium tuberculosis*
    ○ *Giardia lamblia*
    ○ Epstein–Barr virus (EBV)
    ○ Acute HIV infection
    ○ Coxsackie viruses
    ○ Rubeola virus
    ○ Cat-scratch disease
    ○ Adenovirus species

Genetics
- Mesenteric adenitis can occur in adults but is more common in children and adolescents <15.
- This condition during childhood or adolescence is linked to a significantly reduced risk of ulcerative colitis in adulthood (3).

RISK FACTORS
- Typically preceded by upper respiratory infection or pharyngitis
- History of ingesting undercooked pork (2)

GENERAL PREVENTION
Minimize risk by eating fully cooked foods, especially meat (2).

COMMONLY ASSOCIATED CONDITIONS
- Appendicitis (4,5)
- Crohn disease (1,5)
- Enteritis

DIAGNOSIS

HISTORY
The onset of symptoms is variable; nausea or abdominal pain usually are the 1st presenting symptoms. Generally, symptoms are nonspecific:
- Nausea and vomiting (which may precede abdominal pain)
- Abdominal pain: Nonspecific and diffuse tenderness
- Malaise or fatigue
- Diarrhea
- Fevers
- Anorexia
- Recent history of upper respiratory tract infection

PHYSICAL EXAM
- Fevers
- Right lower quadrant tenderness, may or may not exhibit rebound tenderness
- Peripheral/Generalized lymphadenopathy
- Toxic appearance
- Rectal tenderness
- Rhinorrhea
- Hyperemic pharynx

DIFFERENTIAL DIAGNOSIS
- Appendicitis, intussusception, intestinal duplication, regional enteritis
- Epiploic appendagitis, chronic mesenteric ischemia, inflammatory bowel disease
- UTI, pyelonephritis
- Salpingitis, pelvic inflammatory disease, ectopic pregnancy

DIAGNOSTIC TESTS & INTERPRETATION
Initial Tests (lab, imaging)
- CBC: Leukocytosis
- Basic metabolic panel: May show contraction alkalosis and azotemia
- Stool cultures for diarrhea
- Serologic testing of etiologic agents
- Blood cultures: Patients with septicemia
- CT scan: Enlarged mesenteric lymph nodes that tend to be increased in size, number, and distribution compared with that seen in appendicitis:
  – A specific CT appearance is described as ≥3 clustered lymph nodes measuring at least 5 mm in the short axis (6,7)[B]. This cluster of lymph nodes is most commonly located to the right of the psoas muscle.
  – May or may not have evidence of ileal or ileocecal wall thickening
  – Appendix appears normal
- US: Used for exclusion of other potential differential diagnoses:
  – Preferred imaging modality in children (8)[C]
  – May elicit focal tenderness with transducer pressure (7)[B]
  – May be used to also evaluate appendix for signs of appendicitis

Diagnostic Procedures/Other
- Lymph node biopsy: Applicable only for those patients already subjected to laparotomy to isolate the causative organism.
- Surgery is usually indicated in cases of suppuration and/or abscess formation, with signs of peritonitis, or if acute appendicitis cannot be excluded with certainty.

Test Interpretation
- Microscopically, lymph nodes display nonspecific hyperplasia. If a suppurative infection is present, lymph nodes may contain necrotic material with pus formation (1)[B],(4)[C].
- Lymphatic sinuses may be enlarged
- Immune cell infiltration may be observed
- In cases of *Y. enterocolitica* infection, lymph node capsules may be thickened, with surrounding edema present. There may be lymph node hyperplasia, with infiltration from immune-mediated cells and plasma cells (4)[C].

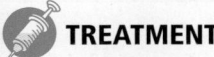 **TREATMENT**

MEDICATION

First Line
- Supportive and symptomatic treatment for uncomplicated cases
- IV fluid resuscitation for patients with clinical evidence of hypovolemia
- Correction of any underlying electrolyte aberrations

Second Line
- Empiric broad-spectrum antibiotic administration for moderately to severely ill patients with adjustment for subsequently isolated pathogens
- Treatment duration is variable based on cause and severity of illness. For uncomplicated cases, antibiotic treatment is not necessary.

SURGERY/OTHER PROCEDURES
- Surgery is usually indicated in cases of suppuration and/or abscess formation, with signs of peritonitis, or if acute appendicitis cannot be excluded with certainty.
- At laparotomy, the diagnosis is generally clear. An appendectomy should be performed in light of the difficulty in differentiating adenitis from appendicitis.

IN-PATIENT CONSIDERATIONS

Admission Criteria/Initial Stabilization
- Indicated for patients with complications and hemodynamic instability
- Volume resuscitation as needed and correction of any underlying electrolyte abnormalities

IV Fluids
- IV fluid hydration may be indicated for patients who cannot tolerate PO intake secondary to nausea or vomiting.
- Aggressive fluid hydration is indicated for patients who show evidence of sepsis.

Discharge Criteria
Hemodynamic stability, able to tolerate a PO diet.

 ONGOING CARE

FOLLOW-UP RECOMMENDATIONS

Patient Monitoring
Close outpatient monitoring is needed to ensure total resolution of symptoms.

DIET
There are no specific dietary recommendations. Oral intake can be temporarily held until nausea and vomiting resolve.

PATIENT EDUCATION
In cases of *Yersinia* infection, patients should avoid unpasteurized milk, raw pork, and contaminated water.

PROGNOSIS
- Generally self-limiting and benign condition
- Increased morbidity/mortality for patients presenting with concomitant sepsis

COMPLICATIONS
- Increased GI losses leading to hypovolemia and electrolyte imbalance
- Abscess formation
- Peritonitis
- Sepsis
- Latent extraintestinal manifestations, including arthralgias, truncal and extremity rashes, and erythema nodosum in instances of *Y. enterocolitica* infection
- Postinfectious chronic complications of *Yersinia* infection including reactive arthritis, conjunctivitis, and urethritis

REFERENCES

1. Frisch M, Pedersen BV, Andersson RE. Appendicitis, mesenteric lymphadenitis, and subsequent risk of ulcerative colitis: Cohort studies in Sweden and Denmark. *BMJ.* 2009;338:b716.
2. Currie B. *Yersinia enterocolitica. Pediatr Rev.* 1998;19:250–251.
3. Blattner RJ. Acute mesenteric lymphadenitis. *J Pediatr.* 1969;74:479–481.
4. Kelly CS, Kelly RE. Lymphadenopathy in children. *Pediatr Clin North Am.* 1998;45:875–888.
5. Zganjer M, Roic G, Cizmic A. Infectious ileocecitis—appendicitis mimicking syndrome. *Bratisl Lek Listy.* 2005;106:201–202.
6. Rao PM, Rhea JT, Novelline RA. CT diagnosis of mesenteric adenitis. *Radiology.* 1997;202:145–149.
7. Sivit CJ. Imaging children with acute right lower quadrant pain. *Pediatr Clin North Am.* 1997;44:575–589.
8. Toorenvliet B, Vellekoop A, Bakker R, et al. Clinical differentiation between acute appendicitis and acute mesenteric lymphadenitis in children. *Eur J Pediatr Surg.* 2011;21:120–123.

ADDITIONAL READING

- Bhandarkar DS, Shah RS, Katara AN, et al. Laparoscopic biopsy in patients with abdominal lymphadenopathy. *J Minim Access Surg.* 2007;3:14–18.
- Ikeda Y, Ikeda Y, Nakai T, et al. A case of mesenteric lymphadenitis with long-acting symptom, showing marked response to corticosteroid. *Nihon Shokakibyo Gakkai Zasshi.* 2007;104:1371–1376.
- Millet I, Alili C, Pages E, et al. Infection of the right iliac fossa. *Diagn Interv Imaging.* 2012;93:441–452.

 CODES

ICD10
I88.0 Nonspecific mesenteric lymphadenitis

CLINICAL PEARLS
- This is a self-limited inflammatory process involving the mesenteric lymph nodes, and it may mimic appendicitis.
- Mesenteric adenitis is more common in children than adults and may follow an upper respiratory tract infection.
- Treatment is mainly supportive.

M

METABOLIC SYNDROME

Deepali Nivas Tukaye, MD, PhD

BASICS

DESCRIPTION
- A cluster of metabolic abnormalities that confer an increased risk factor for type 2 diabetes mellitus (DM), cardiovascular disease, stroke, fatty liver and certain cancers
- Involves the following metabolic abnormalities:
  - Intra-abdominal obesity
  - Dyslipidemia
  - Hypertension
  - Insulin resistance with or without impaired glucose tolerance
  - Proinflammatory state
  - Prothrombotic state

EPIDEMIOLOGY
- Predominant age: >60 years old (~50% of cases)
- Predominant sex: Male = Female
- Ethnicity: Mexican Americans (highest risk)

Prevalence
- Affects 34% of US adults age >20 years; increasing with the aging population and the prevalence of obesity
- Data vary among populations, depending on the criteria used, but available literature suggests that metabolic syndrome is a rapidly growing epidemic worldwide.

Pediatric Considerations
- Obese children and adolescents are at high risk for the metabolic syndrome (prevalence of 6.4% in the US). Risk factors of metabolic syndrome in children and adolescents include heredity, low birth weight, childhood weight gain and obesity, endocrine abnormalities, hostility, maternal gestational diabetes, and poor health habits.
- International Diabetes Federation consensus report (1) defined criteria in 3 age groups (6 ≤10 years; 10 ≤16 years; 16+ years, adult criteria applicable). Obesity defined by waist circumference ≥90th percentile; rest of the diagnostic criteria (triglycerides [TGs], high-density lipoprotein-cholesterol [HDL-C], hypertension [HTN], and fasting blood sugar/type 2 DM) are largely the same as in adults for children ≥10 years, with some exceptions, and warrant treatment. Clinical significance of metabolic syndrome in pediatric population is not well established. Focus on established risk factors rather than diagnosis.

ETIOLOGY AND PATHOPHYSIOLOGY
- Adipose tissue dysfunction and insulin resistance
- Decreased levels of adiponectin, an adipocytokine, known to protect against type 2 DM, HTN, atherosclerosis, and inflammation
- Increase in intra-abdominal and visceral adipose tissue
- Abnormal fatty acid metabolism, endothelial dysfunction, systemic inflammation, oxidative stress, elevated renin-angiotensin system activation, and a prothrombotic state (increased tissue plasminogen activator inhibitor-1) are also associated.
- The main etiological factors are:
  - Obesity (particularly abdominal)/excess adipose tissue
  - Insulin resistance

- Other contributing factors:
  - Advancing age
  - Proinflammatory state
  - Genetics
  - Endocrine (e.g., postmenopausal state)

Genetics
Genetic factors contribute significantly to causation. Most identified genes are transcription factors or regulators of transcription and translation. It is a multifactorial disease with evidence of complex interactions between genetics and environment.

RISK FACTORS
- Obesity/Intra-abdominal obesity
- Insulin resistance
- Older age
- Ethnicity
- Family history
- Physical inactivity
- High-carbohydrate diet
- Smoking
- Postmenopausal status
- Low socioeconomic status
- Alteration of gut flora

GENERAL PREVENTION
- Effective weight loss and maintenance of normal body weight long term
- Regular and sustained physical activity
- Diet low in saturated fats and simple sugars

COMMONLY ASSOCIATED CONDITIONS
- Polycystic ovary syndrome
- Fatty liver disease (nonalcoholic steatohepatitis)
- Chronic renal disease
- Obstructive sleep apnea
- Gallstones (cholesterol)
- Erectile dysfunction (in men)
- Hyperuricemia and gout

DIAGNOSIS

HISTORY
- Family history of metabolic syndrome, type 2 DM, and cardiovascular disease
- Symptoms indicating cardiovascular disease or diabetes
- Comprehensive lifestyle history:
  - Diet, including intake of carbohydrates and fats
  - Weight history, including onset of obesity and previous weight loss attempts
  - Exercise regimen
  - Alcohol intake
- Cigarette smoking
- Assess cardiovascular risk with Framingham risk assessment tool.

PHYSICAL EXAM
Various criteria-based definitions have been proposed, including those by the World Health Organization, the International Diabetes Federation, and the National Cholesterol Education Program's Adult Treatment Panel III (ATP III). According to ATP III, a diagnosis of metabolic syndrome can be made when ≥3 of the following 5 characteristics are present (2)[C]:
- Abdominal obesity: Men >102 cm, women >88 cm (ATP III recommends lowering threshold in population susceptible to insulin resistance, especially Asian Americans)

- BP ≥130/85 mm Hg
- TGs ≥150 mg/dL
- HDL: Men <40 mg/dL, women <50 mg/dL
- Fasting glucose ≥100 mg/dL

DIFFERENTIAL DIAGNOSIS
Individual components of the syndrome may be present without fulfilling all the ATP III diagnostic criteria.

DIAGNOSTIC TESTS & INTERPRETATION
Initial Tests (lab, imaging)
- Fasting lipids (particularly TGs and HDL)
- Fasting glucose

Follow-Up Tests & Special Considerations
- Formal 75-mg oral glucose tolerance test for diagnosis of impaired fasting glucose/impaired glucose tolerance (IGT)
- Serum-free testosterone, sex hormone-binding globulin
- LFTs
- Measurement of insulin levels is controversial.
- None necessary to diagnose metabolic syndrome

Diagnostic Procedures/Other
- May require 24-hour BP monitoring (rules out white coat hypertension)
- ECG, stress test, coronary angiography may be used for diagnosis of cardiovascular disease arising as a complication of the syndrome.

Test Interpretation
- Microalbuminuria
- Increased WBC count
- Increased C-reactive protein
- Increased fibrinogen
- Increased proinflammatory cytokines (e.g., tumor necrosis factor-α)
- Increased uric acid
- Increased homocysteine
- Type 2 DM
- Fatty liver (complicated by end-stage liver disease and hepatocellular carcinoma)
- Hypertensive and/or diabetic eye disease
- Renal impairment/failure
- Peripheral vascular disease
- Coronary artery disease
- Cerebrovascular disease

TREATMENT

Primary therapeutic goal is to prevent or reduce obesity. Aggressive lifestyle modification (diet and exercise) is considered first-line therapy.

GENERAL MEASURES
- Aggressive treatment of individual risk factors
- Avoid or stop smoking.
- Avoid excess alcohol intake.

MEDICATION
- Daily treatment with aspirin is recommended for patients with cardiovascular disease or those at high risk.
- Consult clinical guidelines for treatment of dyslipidemia, hypertension, IGT, and diabetes.
- Multiple medications usually are required to achieve adequate BP control.
- Diagnosis and treatment of insulin resistance is controversial.

First Line
Lifestyle modification alone as initial strategy is applicable to individuals with low 10-year Framingham risk for coronary artery disease (CAD). In individuals with higher 10-year risk, more aggressive risk factor-based approach is recommended in addition to lifestyle modifications (3)[B]:

- Obesity: Lifestyle changes are the cornerstone of treatment. Aim for a gradual ~5–10% weight reduction. Any amount of weight loss is associated with significant benefits.
  - Combination of phentermine and delayed-release topiramate has recently been approved by the FDA for management of obesity with promising outcomes on weight, BP, dylipidemia and other metabolic/glycemic parameters. Long-term safety data is awaited (4).
- Physical activity: 30–60 minutes of moderate-intensity aerobic activities such as brisk walking 5–7 d/wk; increase in daily lifestyle activities and resistance training 1–2 d/wk. In patients with established CAD, assess detailed history of physical activity and exercise tolerance to guide activity prescription. Advise medically supervised programs for high-risk population (recent acute coronary syndrome [ACS], congestive heart failure, recent revascularization). Cumulative exercise time over the day contributes to health benefit.
- Dyslipidemia: Drug therapy can be commenced after 6 weeks of lifestyle modification. Target of therapy depends of patient's level of cardiovascular risk:
  - Statin if predominantly high low-density lipoprotein (LDL)
  - Fibrate with fish oils if predominantly high TGs and/or low HDL
  - Target LDL-cholesterol based on Framingham risk: High risk, <100 mg/dL; moderate risk, <130 mg/dL; low risk, <160 mg/dL.
  - If TGs are >200 mg/dL after achieving goal LDL-cholesterol, consider additional therapies for non–HDL-C (the goal is 30 mg/dL higher than LDL-cholesterol goal for each risk group).
  - If HDL-C remains low after non–HDL-C goal is achieved, intensify lifestyle modification or add drug therapy, depending on patients risk category.
- HTN: Aim for similar targets to patients with diabetes (<130/80 mm Hg).
  - ACE inhibitor or angiotensin receptor blocker (e.g., losartan 50 mg/d if ACE inhibitor intolerance) is usually prescribed for patients with diabetes.
- Impaired glucose tolerance:
  - Current guidelines emphasize that treatment should be with diet and exercise. The role of oral hypoglycemic agents to prevent diabetes in patients with the metabolic syndrome is unclear. Metformin, 500 mg to 1 g, 1–3× daily, may be considered (5)[B].
- Prothrombotic state: Low-dose aspirin for patients with 10-year risk for CAD ≥10% or known atherosclerotic CAD or type 2 DM or others in high-risk category. Use clopidogrel if aspirin is contraindicated in these groups.
- If CAD or type 2 DM is already evident, treat as per guidelines.

ISSUES FOR REFERRAL
- Nutrition
- Exercise program
- Smoking cessation

SURGERY/OTHER PROCEDURES
- Surgery to treat obesity in severely obese patients who have failed trials of lifestyle modification and pharmacotherapy (5)[C]; surgery recommended if body mass index (BMI) >40 or BMI >35 with obesity-related comorbidities.
- Liposuction of abdominal adipose tissue does not reduce insulin resistance or cardiovascular risk factors.

COMPLEMENTARY AND ALTERNATIVE MEDICINE
Fish oils and plant sterol esters for cardioprotective effects

IN-PATIENT CONSIDERATIONS
Management usually does not require admission.

Admission Criteria/Initial Stabilization
Serious complications (e.g., ACS, hypertensive crisis, diabetic coma)

 ## ONGOING CARE

FOLLOW-UP RECOMMENDATIONS
- Regular 30-minute exercise will improve all components of the metabolic syndrome. Cumulative small periods of exercise over the day provide significant health benefits.
- Encourage changing sedentary activity choices (e.g., driving car, taking elevator, and the like) to more active ones (e.g., walking, cycling).
- Regular monitoring of weight, abdominal circumference measurements, BP, fasting lipids, and sugar levels

Patient Monitoring
- Regular monitoring of weight, abdominal circumference measurements, BP, fasting lipids, and sugar levels
- Fasting lipids, fasting sugar, and/or oral glucose tolerance test should be checked annually.

DIET
- Weight reduction to correct abdominal obesity is a primary goal achieved by reduction of energy intake and increased physical activity (6)[A]. Reduction by 500 calories/d will usually achieve a weight loss of 0.5 kg/wk.
- Current recommendations include: Saturated fats <7% total calories; reduction in transfats; dietary cholesterol <200 mg/d; total fat 25–35% of total calories. Diet composed of unsaturated fat with limitation of simple sugars. Encourage salt restriction, increased consumption of fresh fruits and vegetables, alcohol moderation, and increased fiber and whole grains.

PROGNOSIS
Increased risk of type 2 DM (~5-fold), CAD (~1.5–3-fold), acute myocardial infarction (~2.5-fold), and all-cause mortality (~1.5-fold) (7)

COMPLICATIONS
Long-term complications are primarily CAD and type 2 DM. Recent evidence demonstrates an increased risk of nonalcoholic fatty liver disease, stroke, and an increased risk of developing certain cancers, especially breast cancer in postmenopausal women.

REFERENCES
1. Zimmet P, Alberti KG, Kaufman F, et al. The metabolic syndrome in children and adolescents—an IDF consensus report. Pediatr Diabetes. 2007;8:299–306.
2. National Cholesterol Education Program (NCEP) Expert Panel on Detection, Evaluation, and Treatment of High Blood Cholesterol in Adults (Adult Treatment Panel III). Third Report of the National Cholesterol Education Program (NCEP) Expert Panel on Detection, Evaluation, and Treatment of High Blood Cholesterol in Adults (Adult Treatment Panel III) final report. Circulation. 2002;106(25):3143–3421.
3. Grundy SM, Cleeman JI, Daniels SR, et al. Diagnosis and management of the metabolic syndrome: An American Heart Association/National Heart, Lung, and Blood Institute scientific statement: Executive Summary. Crit Pathw Cardiol. 2005;4:198–203.
4. Shin JH, Gadde KM. Clinical utility of phentermine/topiramate (Qsymia™) combination for the treatment of obesity. Diabetes Metab Syndr Obes. 2013;6:131–139
5. National Institutes of Health. Clinical Guidelines on the Identification, Evaluation, and Treatment of Overweight and Obesity in Adults: The Evidence Report. Obes Res. 1998;6(Suppl 2):51S–209S.
6. Slentz CA, Duscha BD, Johnson JL, et al. Effects of the amount of exercise on body weight, body composition, and measures of central obesity: STRRIDE—a randomized controlled study. Arch Intern Med. 2004;164:31–39.
7. Kassi E, Pervanidou P, Kaltsas G, et al. Metabolic syndrome: Definitions and controversies. BMC Med. 2011;9:48.

 ## CODES

ICD10
E88.81 Metabolic syndrome

CLINICAL PEARLS
- Abdominal circumference should be measured as part of a cardiovascular risk assessment.
- Prevention or reduction of obesity is the cornerstone of management of metabolic syndrome. Cumulative physical activity over the day significantly adds to the benefit of regular 30–60-minute exercise regimen.
- Aggressive lifestyle modification is first-line lifelong treatment for all patients.

M

METATARSALGIA
Kenneth M. Bielak, MD, FACSM, FAAFP

 BASICS

DESCRIPTION
- Metatarsalgia is defined as pain in the metatarsal region of the foot, but more commonly refers to pain of the plantar surface of the forefoot in the metatarsal head region.
- System affected: Musculoskeletal

EPIDEMIOLOGY
Incidence
Especially common in athletes in high-impact sports involving the lower extremities (running, jumping, dancing) and in rock climbers (12.5%) (1)[B]

Prevalence
Common

ETIOLOGY AND PATHOPHYSIOLOGY
- General:
  - Excessive or repetitive stress: Wearers of high heels, ballet dancers, competitive athletes
  - Soft-tissue dysfunction: Intrinsic muscle weakness, laxity in the Lisfranc ligament
  - Abnormal foot posture: Forefoot varus or valgus, cavus or equinus deformities, loss of the metatarsal arch, splay foot, pronated foot
  - Dermatologic: Warts, calluses
- Great toe:
  - Hallux valgus (bunion), either varus or rigidus
- Lesser metatarsals:
  - Freiberg infraction (i.e., aseptic necrosis of the metatarsal head usually due to trauma in adolescents who jump or sprint)
  - Hammer toe or claw toe
  - Morton syndrome (i.e., long 2nd metatarsal)
- Abnormal pressure distribution plantar to the metatarsal heads

RISK FACTORS
- Obesity
- High heels, narrow shoes, or overly tight fitting shoes (rock climbers wear shoes sized 2 or 3 sizes smaller) (1)[B]
- Competitive athletes in weight-bearing sports (e.g., ballet, basketball, running, soccer, baseball, football)
- Foot deformities (e.g., pes planus, pes cavus, tight Achilles tendon, tarsal tunnel syndrome, hallux valgus, prominent metatarsal heads, excessive pronation, hammer toe deformity, tight toe extensors)

Geriatric Considerations
- Arthritis should be ruled out early
- More frequent in older athletes
- Symptoms are more pronounced in older people
- Age-related atrophy of the metatarsal fat pad may increase the risk for metatarsalgia

Pediatric Considerations
- Muscle imbalance disorders (e.g., Duchenne muscular dystrophy) are a cause of foot deformities in children.
- In adolescent girls, consider Freiberg infraction (i.e., aseptic necrosis of the metatarsal head usually due to trauma in adolescents who jump or sprint).
- Salter I injuries may affect subsequent growth and healing of the epiphysis.

Pregnancy Considerations
- Forefoot pain during pregnancy usually results from change in gait, increased weight, and joint laxity.
- Properly fitted, low-heeled shoes are especially important in this group of patients.

GENERAL PREVENTION
- Wear properly fitted shoes with good padding.
- Start weight-bearing exercise programs gradually.

COMMONLY ASSOCIATED CONDITIONS
See "Etiology and Pathophysiology."

 DIAGNOSIS

HISTORY
- Gradual chronic onset is more common than acute presentation.
- Predisposition with pes cavus deformity and hyperpronation
- Acute, chronic, or recurrent symptoms located in the region of the metatarsal heads usually on the plantar surface
- Pain: Often described as seeming like walking with a pebble in the shoe; aggravated during midstance or propulsion phases of walking or running

PHYSICAL EXAM
- Point tenderness over plantar metatarsal heads
- Pain in the interdigital space or a positive metatarsal squeeze test suggests Morton neuroma.
- Plantar keratosis (callus formation) often noted
- Swelling
- Tenderness of the metatarsal head(s) with pressure applied by the examiner's finger and thumb
- Erythema (occasionally)

DIFFERENTIAL DIAGNOSIS
- Stress fracture (most commonly 2nd metatarsal)
- Morton neuroma (i.e., interdigital neuroma)
- Sesamoiditis or sesamoid fracture
- Salter I fracture in pediatric population
- Arthritis (e.g., gouty, rheumatoid, inflammatory, osteoarthritis, septic, calcium pyrophosphate dihydrate crystal deposit disease [CPPD])
- Lisfranc injury
- Avascular necrosis of the metatarsal head
- Plantar plate tear
- Infection (e.g., cellulitis, diabetic foot, Lyme disease, leprosy)
- Bone tumors (rare)
- Ganglion cyst
- Foreign body
- Vasculitis (diabetes)
- Cavovarus foot

DIAGNOSTIC TESTS & INTERPRETATION
Initial Tests (lab, imaging)
- Only if diagnosis is in question:
  - Erythrocyte sedimentation rate
  - Rheumatoid factor
  - Human leukocyte antigen (HLA)
  - Rapid plasma reagin (RPR)
  - Uric acid
  - Glucose
  - CBC with differential

- Disorders that may alter lab results: Acute infections
- Weight-bearing radiographs: Anteroposterior, lateral, and oblique views:
  - Occasionally metatarsal or sesamoid axial films (to rule out sesamoid fracture) or skyline view of the metatarsal heads to assess the plantar declination of the metatarsal heads: Obtained with the metatarsophalangeal joints in dorsiflexion (to evaluate alignment)
- Increasing use of ultrasound and MRI, but still no benefit over clinical assessment
- MR arthrography of the metatarsophalangeal (MTP) joint can delineate capsular tears, typically of the distal lateral border of the plantar plate, an often underrecognized cause of metatarsalgia (2)[C].
- Bone scan if high index of suspicion of stress fracture exists

Diagnostic Procedures/Other
Plantar pressure distribution analysis: Although still early in its development, this modality may be helpful to distinguish patterns of pressure distribution due to malalignment.

Test Interpretation
- Because of its 2 sesamoid bones, the 1st metatarsal head usually carries ~30% of the weight when walking.
- A normal metatarsal arch also ensures this balance.
- The 1st metatarsal head has adequate padding to accommodate it.
- A pronated splayfoot disturbs this balance, causing equal weight-bearing on all metatarsal heads.
- Any foot deformity also changes distribution of weight to areas of the foot that do not have sufficient padding.
- Reactive tissue can build up a callus around the metatarsal head, which compounds the pain.

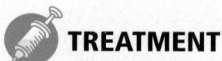 TREATMENT

MEDICATION
- NSAIDs (ibuprofen 800 mg t.i.d. 7–14 days or naproxen 500 mg b.i.d. 7–14 days)
- Contraindications: GI bleeding or ulcer
- Precautions in patients with:
  - Renal disease
  - Hepatic disease
  - Coagulation disorders
- Significant possible interactions:
  - Anticoagulants
  - Digoxin
  - Lithium
  - Methotrexate
  - Cyclosporin

ISSUES FOR REFERRAL
Athletes may warrant early podiatric or orthopedic evaluation.

ADDITIONAL THERAPIES
- Low-heeled (<2 cm height) wide-toe-box shoes
- Metatarsal bars, pads, and arch supports. Metatarsal bars may be more effective than pads (3).

- Orthotics/Rocker bar (prescriptive orthotics have been shown to be effective treatment)
- Thick-soled shoes
- Shaving the callus may provide temporary relief, but should not be excised.
- Improve flexibility and strength of the muscles of the foot with:
  – Exercises (e.g., towel grasps, pencil curls)
  – Physical therapy to maintain range of motion and restore normal biomechanics

SURGERY/OTHER PROCEDURES
- If no improvement with conservative therapy for 3 months, referral to foot/ankle orthopedic or surgical podiatrist may be necessary.
- If a correctable anatomic abnormality exists: Bunionectomy, partial osteotomy, or surgical fusion (4)[C]. Success rates vary depending on procedure.
- Direct plantar plate repair (Grade II type tear) combined with Weil osteotomy can restore normal alignment of the MTP joint, leading to diminished pain with improved functional scores (5)[B].
- The Weil osteotomy (distal metatarsal oblique osteotomy) is a safe and effective treatment for metatarsalgia (6)[C]. The most commonly reported complication was floating toe with an overall occurrence of 36%. Recurrence was reported in 15% of the cases. Transfer metatarsalgia was reported in 7% of the cases, whereas delayed union, nonunion, and malunion were collectively reported in 3% of the cases (7)[C].
- Morton neurectomy for the treatment of metatarsalgia reported 82% excellent or good results (8)[C]. Partial or total treatment response was found in 66% of patients undergoing ultrasound-guided alcohol ablation of Morton's neuroma (9)[B].
- Surgery only as a last resort if no anatomic abnormality is present (10)[C]

COMPLEMENTARY AND ALTERNATIVE MEDICINE
Magnetic insoles not effective for chronic nonspecific foot pain

IN-PATIENT CONSIDERATIONS
Admission Criteria/Initial Stabilization
- Relieve pain
- Ice initially
- Rest: Temporary alteration of weight-bearing activity; use of cane or crutch. For more physically active patients, suggest an alternative exercise or cross-training:
  – Moist heat later
  – Taping or gel cast
  – Stiff-soled shoes will act as a splint
- Relieve the pressure beneath the area of maximal pain by redistributing the pressure load of the foot, which can be achieved by weight loss.

 ONGOING CARE

FOLLOW-UP RECOMMENDATIONS
Patient Monitoring
If stress fracture has been ruled out and patient's condition has not improved >3 months of conservative treatment, consider surgical evaluation.

PATIENT EDUCATION
- Instruct about wearing proper shoes and gradual return to activity
- Cross-training until symptoms subside
- Patient teaching: Prevention
- Biomechanical evaluation by appropriately skilled clinician is advised

PROGNOSIS
Outcome depends on the severity of the problem and whether surgery is required to correct it.

COMPLICATIONS
- Back, knee, and hip pain due to change in gait
- Transfer metatarsalgia following surgical intervention, which subsequently transfers stress to other areas

REFERENCES
1. Buda R, Caprio F, Bedetti L, et al. Foot overuse diseases in rock climbing; an epidemiologic study. *J Am Podiatr Med Assoc.* 2013;103:113–120.
2. Kier R, Abrahamian H, Caminear D, et al. MR arthrography of the second and third metatarsophalangeal joints for the detection of tears of the plantar plate and joint capsule. *AJR Am J Roentgenol.* 2010;194:1079–1081.
3. Deshaies A, Roy P, Symeonidis PD, et al. Metatarsal bars more effective than metatarsal pads in reducing impulse on the second metatarsal head. *Foot (Edinb).* 2011;21:172–175.
4. Thomson CE, Gibson JN, Martin D. Interventions for the treatment of Morton's neuroma. *Cochrane Database Syst Rev.* 2004;3:CD003118.
5. Nery C, Coughlin MJ, et al. Lesser metatarsophalangeal joint instability: Prospective evaluation and repair of plantar plate and capsular insufficiency. *Foot Ankle Int.* 2012;33:301–311.
6. Khurana A, Kadamabande S, James S, et al. Weil osteotomy: Assessment of medium term results and predictive factors in recurrent metatarsalgia. *Foot Ankle Surg.* 2011;17:150–157.
7. Highlander P, Vonherbulis E, Gonzalez A, et al. Complications of the Weil osteotomy. *Foot Ankle Spec.* 2011;4:165–170.
8. Pace A, Scammell B, Dhar S, et al. The outcome of Morton's neurectomy in the treatment of metatarsalgia. *Int Orthop.* 2010;34:511–515.
9. Musson RE, Sawhney JS, Lamb L, et al. Ultrasound guided alcohol ablation of Morton's neuroma. *Foot Ankle Int.* 2012;33:196–201.
10. Espinosa N, Brodsky JW, Maceira E, et al. Metatarsalgia. *J Am Acad Orthop Surg.* 2010;18:474–485.

ADDITIONAL READING
- Adams WR. Morton's neuroma. *Clin Podiatr Med Surg.* 2010;27:535–545.
- Birbilis T, Theodoropoulou E, Koulalis D. Forefoot complaints–the Morton's metatarsalgia. The role of MR imaging. *Acta Medica (Hradec Kralove).* 2007;50:221–222.
- Burns J, Landorf KB, Ryan MM, et al. Interventions for the prevention and treatment of pes cavus. *Cochrane Database Syst Rev.* 2007;4:CD006154.
- Clinical Practice Guideline Forefoot Disorders Panel, Thomas JL, Blitch EL, et al. Diagnosis and treatment of forefoot disorders. Section 2. Central metatarsalgia. *J Foot Ankle Surg.* 2009;48:239–250.
- Gregg JM, Schneider T, Marks P. MR imaging and ultrasound of metatarsalgia—the lesser metatarsals. *Radiol Clin North Am.* 2008;46:1061–1078, vi–vii.
- Janisse DJ, Janisse E. Shoe modification and the use of orthoses in the treatment of foot and ankle pathology. *J Am Acad Orthop Surg.* 2008;16:152–158.
- Kanatli U, Yetkin H, Simek A, et al. [Pressure distribution patterns under the metatarsal heads in healthy individuals]. *Acta Orthop Traumatol Turc.* 2008;42:26–30.
- Ko PH, Hsiao TY, Kang JH, et al. Relationship between plantar pressure and soft tissue strain under metatarsal heads with different heel heights. *Foot Ankle Int.* 2009;30:1111–1116.

 SEE ALSO

Morton Neuroma (Interdigital Neuroma)

 CODES

ICD10
- M77.40 Metatarsalgia, unspecified foot
- M77.41 Metatarsalgia, right foot
- M77.42 Metatarsalgia, left foot

CLINICAL PEARLS
- Pain of the plantar surface of the forefoot in the metatarsal head region.
- Common especially in athletes with high-impact sports involving the lower extremities (running, jumping, dancing, etc.).
- Point tenderness over plantar metatarsal heads.
- Athletes may warrant early podiatric or orthopedic evaluation.
- Remind pregnant patients of the importance of properly fitted, low-heeled shoes.
- Pain is often described as seeming like walking with a pebble in the shoe; aggravated during midstance or propulsion phases of walking or running.

M

METHANOL POISONING

Cynthia M. Waickus, MD, PhD

 BASICS

DESCRIPTION

- Methanol (wood alcohol) is a clear, colorless liquid with an odor similar to ethanol (drinking alcohol), but with a slightly sweeter taste. It is commonly used as an antifreeze, solvent, fuel, and as a denaturant for ethanol (1).
- Ingestion of methanol may occur by patients seeking ethanol substitutes, as a suicide attempt, by accidental ingestion, or by ingestion of denatured alcohol or from methanol contamination in products from illicit distillation ("moonshine").
- Methanol ingestion leads to CNS depression and inebriation. The metabolism of methanol leads to the formation of formic acid, which leads to the symptoms of cellular hypoxia and metabolic acidosis, among other metabolic disturbances (2).
- Nonetheless, even with large ingestions, a favorable prognosis is possible if the patient arrives at the hospital early enough and the poisoning is identified and treated in a timely manner (3,4).

EPIDEMIOLOGY

Incidence

Most prominent in males >18 years of age, or by accidental ingestion by children

Prevalence

In 2010, 9,000 cases of methanol ingestion were reported to the US Poison Control Centers (4).

ETIOLOGY AND PATHOPHYSIOLOGY

- Methanol itself is rapidly absorbed, but is relatively nontoxic, causing mainly CNS sedation.
- Toxic effects of methanol ingestion occur over several hours as it is slowly converted by liver alcohol dehydrogenase to formaldehyde, which is then rapidly oxidized via aldehyde dehydrogenase to formic acid (formate anion).
- Formate anion can lead to retinal injury, with optic disc hyperemia, and can lead to permanent blindness.
- Secondary symptoms of methanol poisoning generally arise ≥10 hours after the initial exposure. These include blurring or loss of vision and metabolic acidosis. Death by respiratory failure may occur (4,5).

RISK FACTORS

- Chronic alcoholism
- Access to illicitly distilled alcohol products
- Accidental ingestion of solvents or cleaning supplies by children

GENERAL PREVENTION

- Education of at-risk populations
- Proper storage of methanol-containing products and the use of embittering agents

COMMONLY ASSOCIATED CONDITIONS

Chronic alcoholism

 DIAGNOSIS

Initial presentation will typically include symptoms of alcohol inebriation (CNS depression, nausea, and vomiting). Several hours after ingestion, symptoms will include visual disturbances and metabolic acidosis.

HISTORY

- Establish the source and nature of the methanol exposure.
- It is important to establish the timing of the ingestion and whether ethanol was ingested subsequently or concurrently.
- Establish the intent of the exposure (accidental or intentional).

PHYSICAL EXAM

- Key physical findings (6)[A]:
  – Initially, the patient will present with inebriation and gastric disturbances.
  – Hyperpnea and hypotension suggest that toxic metabolites have begun to accumulate.
  – An afferent papillary defect suggests advanced methanol poisoning. Eye exam may also reveal mydriasis, retinal edema, and hyperemia of the optic disk.

DIFFERENTIAL DIAGNOSIS

- Ingestion of other alcohols, including ethyl alcohol, ethylene glycol, and isopropyl alcohol
- Possible exposure to formaldehyde, ethylene glycol, or metabolic acidosis due to renal failure

DIAGNOSTIC TESTS & INTERPRETATION

- Serum methanol and/or ethanol may be elevated.
- Electrolytes, osmolarity, and anion gap determinations, including lactate determination
- Serum formate may be elevated.
- Pregnancy test in women of childbearing age
- After a latent period, serum formate is a better measure of toxicity.
- A CT scan of the brain, if indicated by neurologic exam, may reveal optic pathway damage.

 TREATMENT

GENERAL MEASURES

- Prioritize management on timing and amount of exposure; if patient is intoxicated, history may be unreliable.
- A low or nondetectable methanol level does not rule out ingestion.
- Initial stabilization: IV access and isotonic fluids to maintain adequate urine output and prevent renal failure
- Initial management: Focused on preventing metabolic acidosis and ophthalmic complications

MEDICATION

- Administration of sodium bicarbonate to correct systemic acidosis
- Inhibition of alcohol dehydrogenase with either fomepizole (this is the preferred treatment) or ethanol. Do not administer ethanol in women in the 1st trimester of pregnancy.
- If serum methanol levels are elevated, hemodialysis may minimize general organ toxicity.
- Cofactor treatment (folic acid, thiamine, pyridoxine) may promote elimination of the alcohol or its metabolites (3,7)[B].

First Line

- Fomepizole (8)[A]:
  – Load 15 mg/kg IV infusion over 30 minutes
  – Maintain 10 mg/kg IV q12h for 4 doses, then increase to 15 mg/kg q12h
  – Maintain serum level of 8.6–24.6 mg/L
  – Treat until methanol levels are <20 mg/dL
  – Dialysis may also be required.

Second Line

- Folinic acid (Leucovorin): May enhance formic acid metabolism (8)[A]:
  – 50–75 mg IV q4h × 24 h
  – Folic acid can be given q6h at the same dose until metabolic acidosis resolves
- Ethanol:
  – Loading dose:
    ○ 600 mg/kg IV (i.e., 7.6 mL/kg of 10% EtOH solution)
    ○ 600–700 mg/kg PO/NG using a 95% solution diluted to ≤20% with water or juice
  – Maintenance dose:
    ○ 65–155 mg/kg/h, depending on alcohol consumption status (lower for nondrinker)
  – Oral maintenance = 0.15 mL/kg/h (IV = 1.4 mL/kg/h) 10% ethanol
  – Chronic alcoholics and hemodialysis patients need increased dose; increased maintenance by 50%; nonusers may need less (7)[B]
  – Avoid ethanol therapy as a treatment for methanol poisoning during the 1st trimester of pregnancy; may substitute fomepizole, which is a pregnancy Category C drug.

ISSUES FOR REFERRAL

- For patients with substance abuse, referral to detox, rehabilitation, and/or AA/NA
- Ophthalmology follow up for patients with visual disturbances

IN-PATIENT CONSIDERATIONS

Consider urgent hemodialysis with the following (7,9):

- Significant acidosis (pH <7.2) unresponsive to therapy
- Deteriorating vital signs despite intensive support
- Renal failure
- Severe electrolyte imbalance
- Visual or funduscopic abnormalities
- Serum methanol concentration >50 mg/dL or >30 g ingested

IV Fluids

Isotonic IV fluid to maintain urine output

ONGOING CARE

FOLLOW-UP RECOMMENDATIONS

- Restricted activity if patient is inebriated, has altered level of consciousness, or has visual impairments
- Referral to psychiatry for suicidal patients

DIET

Thiamine supplementation for patients with long-term alcoholism

PATIENT EDUCATION

- Anticipatory guidance for parents regarding storage of hazardous chemicals
- Motivational interviewing for those with substance dependence and referral for additional treatment

PROGNOSIS

- Outcome varies, depending on time to presentation and the quantity of methanol ingested (4)
- Outcome is related to the degree of acidosis, coma, or seizures at time of presentation
- Diagnostic and treatment delays are correlated with a poor outcome

COMPLICATIONS

- Blindness and other visual disturbances
- Myoglobinuric renal failure
- Pancreatitis
- Parkinson syndrome

REFERENCES

1. National Institute for Occupational Safety and Health. The Emergency Response Safety and Health Database: Methanol. Available at: http://www.cdc.gov/niosh/ershdb/EmergencyResponseCard_29750029.html
2. Liesivuori J, Savolainen H. Methanol and formic acid toxicity: Biochemical mechanisms. *Pharmacol Toxicol*. 1991;69:157–163.
3. Kruse JA. Methanol and ethylene glycol intoxication. *Crit Care Clin*. 2012;28:661–711.
4. Coulter CV, Farquhar SE, McSherry CM, et al. Methanol and ethylene glycol acute poisonings—predictors of mortality. *Clin Toxicol (Phila)*. 2011;49:900–906.
5. Schep LJ, Slaughter RJ, Vale JA, et al. A seaman with blindness and confusion. *BMJ*. 2009;339: b3929.
6. Jammalamadaka D, Raissi S. Ethylene glycol, methanol and isopropyl alcohol intoxication. *Am J Med Sci*. 2010;339:276–281.
7. Barceloux DG. American Academy of Clinical Toxicology practice guidelines on the treatment of methanol poisoning. *Clin Toxicol*. 2002;40: 415–446.
8. Brent J. Fomepizole for ethylene glycol and methanol poisoning. *N Engl J Med*. 2009;360: 2216–2223.
9. Mégarbane B, Borron SW, Baud FJ. Current recommendations for treatment of severe toxic alcohol poisonings. *Intensive Care Med*. 2005;31: 189–195.

ADDITIONAL READING

- Hovda KE. Methanol outbreak in Norway 2002–2004. *J Int Med*. 2005;258:181–190.
- Kraut JA, Kurtz I. Toxic alcohol ingestions: Clinical features, diagnosis, and management. *Clin J Am Soc Nephrol*. 2008;3:208–225.

 CODES

ICD10

- T51.1X1A Toxic effect of methanol, accidental (unintentional), initial encounter
- T51.1X2A Toxic effect of methanol, intentional self-harm, initial encounter
- T51.1X4A Toxic effect of methanol, undetermined, initial encounter

CLINICAL PEARLS

- Formic acid, the toxic agent in methanol poisoning, causes anion-gap metabolic acidosis, optic disc edema, and myelin breakdown by direct toxic effects (3,7)[B].

- Ethanol has the longest history of use: It is inexpensive and is widely available. Fomepizole is preferred because dosing is simpler; it does not require hourly blood draws, and it is not a CNS depressant. No direct comparison of the 2 treatments is available.

- Common indications for hemodialysis in a methanol overdose include severe acidosis, visual symptoms, unstable vital signs, refractory electrolyte disturbances, and methanol level >50 mg/dL (7)[B].
- Recent literature has suggested that, in the absence of neurologic impairment, ocular symptoms, and severe metabolic acidosis, fomepizole may obviate the need for hemodialysis (8,9)[A].

M

MILD COGNITIVE IMPAIRMENT

Birju B. Patel, MD, FACP, AGSF • N. Wilson Holland, MD, FACP

 BASICS

DESCRIPTION
- Mild cognitive impairment (MCI) is defined as significant cognitive impairment in the absence of dementia, as measured by standard memory tests:
  - Concern regarding change in cognition
  - Preservation of independence in functional activities (activities of daily living (ADLs)
  - Impairment in ≥1 cognitive domains (attention, executive dysfunction, memory, visuospatial, language) (1)[B]
  - Other terms used in the literature relating to MCI: Isolated memory impairment; cognitive impairment not dementia (CIND); predementia; mild cognitive disorder; age-associated memory impairment; age-related cognitive decline; benign senescent forgetfulness. Some of these conditions do not progress to dementia (i.e., benign senescent forgetfulness, age-associated memory impairment, age-related cognitive decline).
- Annual rates of conversion of MCI to dementia are 2–15% in the elderly.

EPIDEMIOLOGY
Incidence
- Predominant sex: Male > Female
- Predominant age:
  - Higher in older persons and in those with less education
  - 12–15/1,000 person-years in those age ≥65 years
  - 54/1,000 person-years in those age ≥75 years

Prevalence
- MCI is more prevalent than dementia in the US.
- 3–5% for those age ≥60 years
- 15% for those age ≥75 years

ETIOLOGY AND PATHOPHYSIOLOGY
- Subtypes of MCI:
  - Single-domain amnestic
  - Multiple-domain amnestic
  - Nonamnestic single-domain
  - Nonamnestic multiple-domain
- The amnestic subtype is higher risk for progression to Alzheimer disease (2)[A].
- Vascular, degenerative, traumatic, metabolic, psychiatric, or a combination

Genetics
Apolipoprotein (APO) E4 genotype: Various pathways exist leading to amyloid accumulation and deposition thought to be associated with dementia.

RISK FACTORS
- Age
- Diabetes
- Hypertension
- Hyperlipidemia
- Cerebrovascular disease
- Smoking
- Sleep apnea
- APO E4 genotype

COMMONLY ASSOCIATED CONDITIONS
See "Risk Factors."

 DIAGNOSIS

HISTORY
- Focus on cognitive deficits and impairment
- Review all medications that may affect cognition; give particular emphasis to anticholinergic medications (patients on these may mistakenly be classified as having MCI)
- Rule out depression
- Assess function (ADLs, instrumental ADLs) and subtle changes in daily function (e.g., in the workplace).
- Impact on interpersonal relationships and caregiver stress
- Assess vascular risk factors (hypertension, diabetes, hyperlipidemia, and cerebrovascular disease)
- Assess behavioral changes.

PHYSICAL EXAM
- A general exam focusing on clinical clues to identifying vascular disease (e.g., bruits, abnormal BP)
- Neurologic exam to rule out reversible CNS causes of cognitive impairment or other causes of cognitive impairment (e.g., Parkinson disease)
- Office measures of cognitive function, depression, and functional status.

DIFFERENTIAL DIAGNOSIS
- Delirium
- Dementia
- Depression
- "Reversible" cognitive impairment:
  - Medications (anticholinergics and medications with anticholinergic properties)
  - Hypothyroidism
  - Vitamin B₁₂ deficiency
- Reversible CNS conditions
- Give consideration to sleep conditions, especially sleep apnea, that can contribute to cognitive deficits

DIAGNOSTIC TESTS & INTERPRETATION
Initial Tests (lab, imaging)
- CBC
- Comprehensive metabolic profile
- Thyroid-stimulating hormone
- Vitamin B₁₂
- Lipids
- Consider HIV testing in the appropriate risk setting
- Imaging tests are helpful when there are focal neurologic deficits or rapid or atypical presentations:
  - CT scan can detect structural CNS conditions leading to cognitive impairment:
    ○ Subdural hematoma
    ○ Normal-pressure hydrocephalus
    ○ Metastatic disease
  - MRI further evaluates vascular, infectious, neoplastic, and inflammatory conditions
- Rule out reversible causes of cognitive impairment
- Cognitive testing is important (e.g., Montreal Cognitive Assessment [MOCA] and Saint Louis University Mental Status [SLUMS]); MOCA may be more sensitive for detecting MCI.

- Neuropsychological testing for complex and atypical presentations
- Vascular risk factor reduction and treatment (3)[C].

Follow-Up Tests & Special Considerations
- Document progression of functional impairment, cognitive decline, concurrent depression, and comorbid conditions.
- Advanced planning while patient is competent
- Early education of caregivers on safety, maintaining structure, managing stress, and future planning

Test Interpretation
- Little is known about MCI pathology due to a lack of longitudinal studies.
- Alzheimer dementia pathophysiology:
  - Neurofibrillary tangles in hippocampus
  - Senile plaques (amyloid deposition)
  - Neuronal degeneration
- Those with MCI have intermediate amounts of pathologic findings of Alzheimer disease with amyloid deposition and neurofibrillary tangles in the mesial temporal lobes compared with those with dementia.
- Amnestic MCI is associated with white-matter hyperintensity volume on MRI, whereas nonamnestic MCI is associated with infarcts.

TREATMENT

GENERAL MEASURES
Atherosclerotic risk factors should be treated aggressively.

MEDICATION
The use of cholinesterase inhibitors (ChEIs) in MCI is not associated with any delay in the onset of Alzheimer disease or dementia. Moreover, the safety profile showed that the risks associated with ChEIs are significant (4)[A]. Therefore, ChEIs are not recommended routinely (5)[A].

ISSUES FOR REFERRAL
Consider referral to a memory specialist (i.e., geriatrician, neurologist, geropsychiatrist, neuropsychologist) to evaluate and differentiate subtypes of MCI and specific cognitive deficits.

COMPLEMENTARY AND ALTERNATIVE MEDICINE
- No evidence suggests the efficacy of vitamin E in the prevention or treatment of people with MCI. More research is needed to identify the role of vitamin E, if any, in the management of cognitive impairment.
- Long-term use of ginkgo biloba extract has shown to have no benefit in the treatment of MCI and in terms of progression to dementia. In addition, ginkgo biloba can be associated with increase in bleeding risk including CNS bleeds (6)[C].

IN-PATIENT CONSIDERATIONS

- Delirium is more common in patients hospitalized with all forms of cognitive impairment.
- Avoid medications that may worsen or precipitate cognitive decline (e.g., anticholinergics, antihistamines).
- Patients may be extremely sensitive to the hospital environment:
  - Moderate level of stimulation is best.
  - Avoid sensory deprivation. Make sure that patients have access to hearing aids and eyeglasses.
  - Use frequent cueing and have caregivers or family in the room whenever possible with patient.
  - Frequently orient patients to date and time.

 ONGOING CARE

FOLLOW-UP RECOMMENDATIONS

Patients should be re-evaluated every 6–12 months to determine if symptoms are progressing.

Patient Monitoring

Appropriate cognitive and functional testing should be used to evaluate progression, along with clinical history and exam. If a medication is started, patients need to be followed more frequently to evaluate for efficacy, side effects, dose titration, and so forth. Declining executive function may be an early marker to progression of MCI to dementia, and clinicians should monitor and advise patients and families proactively to look for this (7)[C]. Impairments in ADL function is a good clue to progression to dementia from MCI.

DIET

Diets that are promoted by the American Heart Association to minimize atherosclerotic risk factors should be emphasized.

PATIENT EDUCATION

- Encourage lifestyle changes:
  - Physical activity, such as walking 30 minutes daily on most days of the week
  - Mental activity that stimulates language skills and psychomotor coordination should be encouraged. Computer activities, reading books, crafts, crossword puzzles, and games may be linked to decreased risk of development of MCI.

- Cognitive rehabilitation strategies may be beneficial in helping with daily activities relating to memory tasks in MCI.
- Participation in exercise programs modestly improved some measures of cognition in some studies (8)[B].
- Treatment of vascular risk factors (hypertension, diabetes, cerebrovascular disease, and hyperlipidemia) is important in lowering risk of progression to dementia (3)[C].

PROGNOSIS

- Conversion rates from MCI to dementia range from 5–15% annually.
- Amnestic subtypes of MCI are most likely to progress to dementia.

REFERENCES

1. Albert MS, DeKosky ST, Dickson D, et al. The diagnosis of mild cognitive impairment due to Alzheimer's disease: Recommendations from the National Institute on Aging-Alzheimer's Association workgroups on diagnostic guidelines for Alzheimer's disease. *Alzheimers Dement*. 2011;7:270–279.
2. Peterson RC. Mild cognitive impairment. *N Engl J Med*. 2011;364:2227–2234.
3. Li J, Wang YJ, Zhang M, et al. Vascular risk factors promote conversion from mild cognitive impairment to Alzheimer disease. *Neurology*. 2011;76:1485–1491.
4. Patel BP, Holland NW. Adverse effects of acetylcholinesterase inhibitors clinical geriatrics. *Clin Geriatr*. 2011;19:27–30.
5. Russ TC, Morling JR. Cholinesterase inhibitors for mild cognitive impairment. *Cochrane Database Syst Rev*. 2012;9:CD009132.
6. Vellas B, Coley N, Ousset PJ, et al. Long-term use of standardised ginkgo biloba extract for the prevention of Alzheimer's disease (GuidAge): a randomised placebo-controlled trial. *Lancet Neurol*. 2012;11:851.
7. Marshall GA, Rentz DM, Frey MT, et al. Executive function and instrumental activities of daily living in mild cognitive impairment and Alzheimer's disease. *Alzheimers Dement*. 2011;7:300–308.
8. Nagamatsu LS, Handy TC, Hsu CL, et al. Resistance training promotes cognitive and functional brain plasticity in seniors with probable mild cognitive impairment. *Arch Intern Med*. 2012;172:666–668.

ADDITIONAL READING

Petersen RC, Roberts RO, Knopman DS, et al. Prevalence of mild cognitive impairment is higher in men. The Mayo Clinic Study of Aging. *Neurology*. 2010;75:889–897.

 CODES

ICD10

G31.84 Mild cognitive impairment, so stated

CLINICAL PEARLS

- Amnestic MCI affects primarily memory and is more likely to progress to Alzheimer dementia.
- Screen for reversible factors, particularly anticholinergic medications, depression, and sleep disorders.
- Look closely at vascular risk factors and modify them as best as possible.
- ChEIs should not be used routinely unless memory complaints are affecting quality of life in patients. Potential side effects of these medications should be thoroughly discussed with patients and their families. A baseline EKG should be done prior to initiation of ChEIs due to risk of bradycardia and syncope.
- Encourage both physical and mental exercises.

MITRAL REGURGITATION

Yongkasem Vorasettakarnkij, MD, MSc

 BASICS

DESCRIPTION

- Disorder of mitral valve (MV) closure, either organic or functional, resulting in a backflow of the left ventricular (LV) stroke volume into the left atrium (LA); uncompensated, this leads to LV and LA enlargement, elevated pulmonary pressures, atrial fibrillation, heart failure, and sudden cardiac death.
- Types of mitral regurgitation (MR):
  - Acute vs. chronic
  - Organic vs. functional:
    - Functional: No valvular abnormalities are found, and the disease results from valve deformation, caused by LV remodeling or dilatation.
    - MV structures include not only the mitral annulus, MV leaflets, chordae tendineae, and papillary muscles, but also posterior LA wall and LV wall.
- System(s) affected: Cardiac; Pulmonary

EPIDEMIOLOGY

Moderate to severe MR affects 2.5 million people in the US (2000 data). It is the most common valvular disease, and its prevalence is expected to double by 2030 (1).

Prevalence

- By severity on echocardiography:
  - Mild MR: 19% (up to 40% if trivial jets included)
  - Moderate MR: 1.9%
  - Severe MR: 0.2%
- By category (1):
  - Degenerative (myxomatous disease, annular calcification): 60–70%
  - Ischemic: 20%
  - Endocarditis: 2–5%
  - Rheumatic: 2–5%

ETIOLOGY AND PATHOPHYSIOLOGY

- Acute MR: Acute damage to MV leads to sudden LA and LV volume overload. Sudden rise in LV volume load without compensatory LV remodeling results in impaired forward cardiac output and possible cardiogenic shock.
- Chronic MR: LV eccentric hypertrophy compensates for increased regurgitant volume to maintain forward cardiac output and alleviate pulmonary congestion. However, ongoing LV remodeling can result in LV dysfunction. Simultaneously, LA compensatory dilatation for the larger regurgitant volume predisposes patients to develop atrial fibrillation (AF).
- Ischemic MR: Papillary muscle rupture, ischemia during acute MI, and incomplete coaptation of valve leaflets or restricted valve movement resulting from ischemia
- Acute MR:
  - Flail leaflet: Myxomatous disease, infective endocarditis, or trauma
  - Ruptured chordae tendineae: Trauma, spontaneous rupture, infective endocarditis, or rheumatic fever
  - Ruptured or displaced papillary muscle: Acute myocardial infarction (MI), severe myocardial ischemia, or trauma
- Chronic MR:
  - Structural:
    - Degenerative: Mitral annular calcification, mitral valve prolapse (MVP)
    - Infective endocarditis

- Rheumatic heart disease (RHD)
- Inflammatory diseases: Lupus, eosinophilic endocardial disease
- Anorectic drugs
- Congenital (cleft leaflet)
  - Functional:
    - Ischemic: Coronary artery disease (CAD)/MI
    - Nonischemic: Cardiomyopathy, LV dysfunction from any cause, hypertrophic cardiomyopathy

RISK FACTORS

Age, hypertension, RHD, endocarditis, anorectic drugs

GENERAL PREVENTION

- Risk factor modification for CAD
- Antibiotic prophylaxis for poststreptococcal RHD
- Endocarditis prophylaxis for MR is no longer recommended

COMMONLY ASSOCIATED CONDITIONS

MVP with MR common in Marfan syndrome

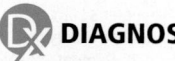 **DIAGNOSIS**

HISTORY

- Associated conditions: RHD, prior MI, connective tissue disorder
- Acute MR:
  - Sudden onset of dyspnea
  - Orthopnea, paroxysmal nocturnal dyspnea
  - Chronic MR:
    - Exertional dyspnea
    - Fatigue
    - Palpitation: Paroxysmal/persistent AF

PHYSICAL EXAM

- Acute MR:
  - Rapid and thready pulses
  - Sign of poor tissue perfusion with peripheral vasoconstriction
  - Hyperdynamic precordium without apical displacement
  - S_3 and S_4 (if in sinus rhythm)
  - Systolic murmur at left sternal border and base:
    - Early, middle, or holosystolic murmur
    - Often soft, low-pitched, decrescendo murmur
  - Rales
- Chronic MR:
  - Brisk upstroke of arterial pulse
  - Leftward displaced LV apical impulse
  - Systolic thrill at the apex (suggests severe MR)
  - Soft S_1 and widely split S_2, S_3 gallop
  - Loud P_2 (if pulmonary hypertension)
  - Holosystolic murmur at apex that radiates to axilla
  - Ankle edema, jugular venous distension, and ascites, if development of right-sided heart failure

DIFFERENTIAL DIAGNOSIS

- Aortic stenosis (AS): Usually midsystolic, but can be long; difficult to distinguish from holosystolic, at apical area, and radiating to the carotid arteries (unlike MR)
- Tricuspid regurgitation: Holosystolic, but at left lower sternal border; does not radiate to axilla or increase in intensity with inspiration (unlike MR)
- Ventricular septal defect (VSD): Harsh holosystolic murmur at lower left sternal border, but radiates to right sternal border (not axilla)

DIAGNOSTIC TESTS & INTERPRETATION

- Chest x-ray (CXR):
  - Acute MR: Pulmonary edema, normal heart size
  - Chronic MR: LA and LV enlargement
- ECG:
  - Acute MR:
    - Varies depending on etiologies (e.g., acute MI)
  - Chronic MR:
    - P mitrale from LA enlargement, AF
    - LV hypertrophy
    - Q waves from prior MI

Initial Tests (lab, imaging)

- Cardiac enzymes and brain natriuretic peptide (BNP), if appropriate
- See workup for MI, CAD, and congestive heart failure (CHF)

Transthoracic echocardiogram (TTE):

- Indications for TTE (2):
  - Baseline evaluation of LV function, right ventricular and LA size, pulmonary artery pressure, and severity of MR
  - Delineation of mechanism of MR
  - Surveillance of asymptomatic moderate to severe LV function (ejection fraction [EF] and end-systolic dimension [ESD])
  - Evaluate MV apparatus and LV size and function after a change in signs/symptoms in a patient with MR
  - Evaluate after MV repair or replacement
- Findings in acute MR:
  - Evidence of etiology: Flail leaflet or infective vegetations
  - Normal LA and LV size
- Findings in chronic MR:
  - Evidence of degenerative, rheumatic, ischemic, congenital, and other causes
  - Enlarged LA and LV

Follow-Up Tests & Special Considerations

- Intervals for follow up TTE: See "Follow-Up Recommendations"
- Transesophageal echocardiogram (TEE):
  - Intraoperatively to define severity/cause of MR and/or LV function
  - Nondiagnostic TTE
  - Evaluation of prosthetic heart valves
- Exercise Doppler echo:
  - Assess exercise tolerance and the effects of exercise on pulmonary artery pressure in asymptomatic patients with severe MR (2)[C].
- Cardiovascular magnetic resonance: When regurgitant severity is indeterminant on echocardiography, especially in patients with LV dysfunction

Diagnostic Procedures/Other

Cardiac catheterization (2):

- Hemodynamic measurements: Pulmonary pressure is discordant to the severity of MR as assessed by noninvasive testing.
- Left ventriculography and hemodynamic measurement:
  - Noninvasive tests are inconclusive regarding severity of MR
  - Regurgitant severity is discordant between clinical and noninvasive findings
- Coronary angiography: Prior to MV surgery in patients at risk for CAD

774

Test Interpretation

Quantification of severe MR requires integration of:

- Structural parameters:
  - LA size: Dilated, unless acute
  - LV size: Dilated, unless acute
  - Leaflets: Abnormal
- Doppler parameters
- Quantitative parameter

 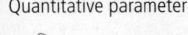

TREATMENT

MEDICATION

- Acute, severe MR (2):
  - Medical therapy has a limited role and is aimed primarily to stabilize hemodynamics preoperatively.
- Chronic MR:
  - Structural:
    - Asymptomatic: No proven long-term medical therapy
    - Symptomatic: Diuretics and vasodilators
  - Functional: LV dysfunction or symptomatic: angiotensin-converting enzyme inhibitors, angiotensin receptor blockers, β-blockers (particularly carvedilol and long-acting metoprolol)

SURGERY/OTHER PROCEDURES

- Isolated MV surgery is not indicated for patients with mild to moderate MR (2)[C].
- Acute, severe MR secondary to acute MI:
  - Acute rupture of papillary muscle: Emergency MV repair/replacement
  - Papillary muscle displacement:
    - Aggressive medical stabilization and intra-aortic balloon pump
    - Valve surgery usually required in addition to revascularization
- Chronic severe MR:
  - MV repair in an experienced center is recommended over MV replacement in most circumstances (3):
    - Survival rate: Early and overall mortality were lower after MV repair than after MV replacement.
    - 10-year rate of stroke: 10% (repair) vs. 12% (bioprosthetic-valve replacement) vs. 23% (mechanical-valve replacement)
    - Risk of endocarditis: 1.5% at 15 years vs. 0.3–1.2% per year
    - Overall rates of reoperation are similar.
  - Indications for MV surgery in chronic severe degenerative MR (2):
    - Symptomatic (NYHA functional class II–IV):
      - Absence of severe LV dysfunction (EF ≥30% and ESD ≤55 mm)
      - Severe LV dysfunction (EF <30% and/or ESD >55 mm). Only if repair is highly likely to be successful.
    - Asymptomatic:
      - Mild to moderate LV dysfunction (EF 30–60% and/or ESD ≥40 mm)
      - Preserved LV function (EF >60% and ESD <40 mm): MV repair in experienced surgical centers is reasonable if chance of successful repair without residual MR is >90%
      - Preserved LV function with new onset AF or with pulmonary hypertension (pulmonary artery systolic pressure [PASP] >50 mm Hg at rest or PASP >60 mm Hg with exercise)

- Indications for surgery in chronic ischemic MR (4)[C]:
  - Severe MR: left ventricular ejection fraction (LVEF) >30% undergoing coronary artery bypass graft (CABG)
  - Moderate MR: Undergoing CABG if repair is feasible
  - Symptomatic, severe MR: LVEF <30%, and option for CABG
  - Severe MR, LVEF >30%: No option for revascularization, refractory to medical therapy, and low comorbidity
- Percutaneous edge-to-edge procedure may be considered in symptomatic patients who fulfill the echo criteria of eligibility, inoperable, or at high surgical risk, and have a life expectancy >1 year (4)[C]:
  - Severe primary MR
  - Severe secondary MR: refractory to optimal medical therapy including cardiac resynchronization therapy if indicated
- Nonischemic functional, severe MR: In selected patients, consider the following:
  - Cardiac resynchronization therapy
  - Percutaneous mitral annuloplasty
  - Percutaneous repair with mitral valve clip

Geriatric Considerations

- Medical therapy alone for patients >75 years of age with MR is preferred owing to increased operative mortality and decreased survival (compared with those with AS), especially with pre-existing CAD or need for MV replacement.
- MV repair is preferable to MV replacement.

IN-PATIENT CONSIDERATIONS

Admission Criteria/Initial Stabilization

Acute MR: Stabilize ABCs (airway, breathing, circulation). Initiate IV, O_2, and monitoring. Nitroprusside (+ dobutamine and/or aortic balloon counterpulsation if hypotensive) (3)[C]. Treat underlying causes (e.g., MI). Treat acute pulmonary edema with furosemide, morphine. Obtain urgent surgical consultation.

 ONGOING CARE

FOLLOW-UP RECOMMENDATIONS

Chronic MR: Asymptomatic:

- Mild MR with normal LV size and function and no pulmonary hypertension: Annual clinical evaluation to assess symptom progression
- Moderate MR: Annual clinical evaluation and echocardiography to assess LV function
- Severe MR: Clinical evaluation and echocardiography every 6–12 months
- Consider serial CXRs and ECGs, and consider stress test if exercise capacity is doubtful.

PATIENT EDUCATION

- Exercise after MV repair: Avoid sports with risk for bodily contact or trauma. Low-intensity competitive sports are allowed.
- Competitive athletes with MR:
  - Asymptomatic with normal LV size and function, normal pulmonary artery pressures, and sinus rhythm: No restrictions
  - Mildly symptomatic and those with LV dilatation: Activities with low to moderate dynamic and static cardiac demand allowed
- AF and anticoagulation: No contact sports

PROGNOSIS

- Acute, severe MR: Mortality risk with surgery is 50%; mortality risk with medical therapy alone, 75% in first 24 hours; 95% at 2 weeks
- Chronic MR: Asymptomatic severe MR with normal LVEF: 10% yearly rate of progression to symptoms and subnormal resting LVEF. Symptomatic severe MR: 8-year survival rate, 33% without surgery; mortality rate, 5% yearly

Pregnancy Considerations

MR with NYHA functional class III–IV at high risk for maternal and/or fetal risk

COMPLICATIONS

Acute pulmonary edema, CHF, AF, bleeding risk with anticoagulation, endocarditis, sudden cardiac death

REFERENCES

1. Enriquez-Sarano M, Akins CW, Vahanian A. Mitral regurgitation. *Lancet*. 2009;373:1382–1394.
2. Bonow RO, Chatterjee K, Faxon DP, et al. 2008 Focused update incorporated into the ACC/AHA 2006 guidelines for the management of patients with valvular heart disease. *Circulation*. 2008;118: e523–661.
3. Foster E. Clinical practice. Mitral regurgitation due to degenerative mitral-valve disease. *N Engl J Med*. 2010;363:156–165.
4. Vahanian A, Alfieri O, Andreotti F, et al. Guidelines on the management of valvular heart disease: The Joint Task Force on the Management of Valvular Heart Disease of the ESC and the EACTS. *Eur Heart J*. 2012;33:2451–2496.

ADDITIONAL READING

- Feldman T, Foster E, Glower DG, et al. Percutaneous repair or surgery for mitral regurgitation. *N Engl J Med*. 2011;364:1395–1406.
- Whitlow PL, Feldman T, Pedersen WR, et al. Acute and 12-month results with catheter-based mitral valve leaflet repair: The EVEREST II (Endovascular Valve Edge-to-Edge Repair) High Risk Study. *J Am Coll Cardiol*. 2012;59:130–139.

 CODES

ICD10

- I05.1 Rheumatic mitral insufficiency
- I34.0 Nonrheumatic mitral (valve) insufficiency
- Q23.3 Congenital mitral insufficiency

CLINICAL PEARLS

- Follow up for mild to moderate MR: Serial exam and/or echo unless LV structural changes.
- Severe MR is usually managed with MV repair.
- Endocarditis prophylaxis is not recommended.

M

MITRAL STENOSIS

Wasiq Faraz Rawasia, MD • Nirmanmoh Bhatia, MD • Marcus F. Stoddard, MD

BASICS

DESCRIPTION

- Mitral stenosis (MS) presents as resistance to diastolic filling of the left ventricle (LV) due to narrowing of mitral valve orifice
- Normal valve orifice 4–6 cm^2; symptoms typically seen when orifice is <2.5 cm^2
- Hemodynamic consequences are due to passive transmission of left atrial (LA) pressure to the pulmonary circulation.

EPIDEMIOLOGY

- Most common acquired valvular disease secondary to rheumatic heart disease (60% of cases)
- Predominant age: Symptoms primarily occur in 4th–7th decades
- Predominant sex: Female > Male (2:1)

Incidence

Decreased incidence of MS seen in the US because of decreased incidence of rheumatic fever (primarily shift in prevalence away from rheumatogenic strains of group A strep [GAS] and also treatment of GAS infection). However, global burden remains significant (1).

ETIOLOGY AND PATHOPHYSIOLOGY

- Obstruction between LA and LV impairs LV filling during diastole and leads to increased LA pressure.
- Increased LA pressure is transmitted passively ("back pressure") to the pulmonary circulation; over time, pulmonary hypertension (HTN) results.
- Over time, LA pressure overload can dilate the chamber and interrupt the cardiac conduction system, resulting in atrial fibrillation.
- Pulmonary HTN can also cause increased collateralization between pulmonary and bronchial circulation, resulting in intraparenchymal hemorrhage with hemoptysis.
- Rheumatic fever: Most common (see "Risk Factors")
- Aging (extension of mitral annular calcification)
- Rare causes:
  - Congenital (associated with mucopolysaccharidoses)
  - Autoimmune: systemic lupus erythematosus (SLE), rheumatoid arthritis
  - Malignant carcinoid
  - Other acquired: LA myxoma, LA thrombus

RISK FACTORS

- Rheumatic fever is the greatest risk factor:
  - 30–40% of rheumatic fever patients eventually develop MS, presenting an average of 20 years after diagnosis of rheumatic fever.
  - Acute rheumatic fever occurs 2–3 weeks after episode of untreated GAS pharyngitis caused by rheumatogenic organism in a genetically susceptible host.
  - Low socioeconomic status (i.e., crowded conditions) favors the spread of streptococcal infection.
- Aging (increasing valvular calcification)
- Chest irradiation (increasing tissue fibrosis)

GENERAL PREVENTION

- Prompt recognition and treatment of GAS infection; recognition of cardinal signs and symptoms of acute rheumatic fever via Jones criteria

- Modified Jones criteria: Diagnosis requires evidence of streptococcal infection plus 2 major criteria or 1 major plus 2 minor criteria (2)[B].

Evidence of strep infection	Antistreptolysin O titer or positive throat culture
Major criteria	Carditis, polyarthritis, Sydenham chorea, erythema marginatum, subcutaneous nodules
Minor criteria	Migratory arthralgias, fever, acute phase reactants (elevated erthrocyte sedimentation rate [ESR], leukocytosis), prolonged PR interval on ECG

COMMONLY ASSOCIATED CONDITIONS

- Atrial fibrillation (30–40% of symptomatic patients) and thromboembolic complications
- Associated valve lesions due to chronic inflammation (aortic stenosis, aortic insufficiency)
- Pulmonary congestion and pulmonary hypertension
- Pulmonary embolism (10%)
- Systemic congestion
- Systemic embolism
- Infection (1–5%)

DIAGNOSIS

HISTORY

- History of rheumatic fever
- Severity of presentation depends on valve area; most early cases will be asymptomatic
- Presenting features usually due to pulmonary vascular congestion: Palpitations, dyspnea on exertion, fatigue, pulmonary edema, paroxysmal nocturnal dyspnea
- Atrial fibrillation, embolic event
- In advanced disease, symptoms of pulmonary hypertension and right-heart failure predominate: Jugular venous distention, hepatomegaly, ascites, and peripheral edema
- Rare presentations: Hemoptysis, hoarseness (compression of recurrent laryngeal nerve by enlarged pulmonary artery or LA), dysphagia (compression)

PHYSICAL EXAM

- Auscultation:
  - Classic murmur: Accentuated S$_1$, opening snap, apical early decrescendo diastolic rumble with presystolic accentuation
  - Murmur variability seen in severe stenosis:
    - With mobile, noncalcified valve, murmur persists throughout diastole and S$_1$, and the opening snap remains loud
    - With a heavily calcified valve, murmur often is difficult to hear. S$_1$ and the opening snap may be soft to absent.
    - In contrast to tricuspid stenosis, the intensity of the murmur from MS increases with inspiration and a prominent *a*-wave in jugular venous pulse
- If pulmonary hypertension is present: Right ventricle (RV) lift, increased P$_2$, high-pitched decrescendo diastolic murmur of pulmonic insufficiency (Graham Steell murmur)
- May also find associated aortic or, less commonly, tricuspid murmurs due to aortic or tricuspid valve involvement from rheumatic heart disease

DIAGNOSTIC TESTS & INTERPRETATION

Initial Tests (lab, imaging)

- ECG:
  - LA enlargement (manifested by broad, notched P waves in lead II [P mitrale] with a negative terminal deflection of the P wave in lead V$_1$)
  - Atrial fibrillation common
  - Right ventricular hypertrophy (RVH), right axis deviation and a large R wave in V$_1$ possible
- Chest radiograph:
  - LA enlargement, straightening of the left heart border, a "double density" and elevation of the left main stem bronchus
  - Prominent pulmonary arteries at the hilum with rapid tapering
  - RVH
  - Pulmonary edema pattern with Kerley B lines (late presentation)
- Echocardiogram indications:
  - Class I:
    - Diagnosis of mitral stenosis
    - Assess severity
    - Reassess after change in symptoms
    - Exercise Doppler for discrepancies between symptoms and echo findings
    - Transesophageal echocardiogram (TEE) to evaluate possible LA thrombus
    - TEE when transthoracic echo nondiagnostic
  - Class II:
    - Reassess asymptomatic patients
    - Severe MS: Yearly
    - Moderate MS: Every 1–2 years
    - Mild MS: Every 3–5 years
  - Class III:
    - Satisfactory result of transthoracic echo
- Echocardiogram findings (3):
  - MV anterior leaflet doming, immobility of the posterior leaflet
  - Echo can demonstrate alternative causes of MS if not rheumatic.
  - Mitral valve area defined:
    - Normal: 4–6 cm^2
    - Mild MS: <2 cm^2
    - Moderate MS: 1–1.5 cm^2
    - Severe MS: <1 cm^2
- Cardiac catheterization indications:
  - Class I recommendations:
    - When echo is inconclusive
    - Discrepancy between echo and symptoms
    - Discrepancy between echo and valve area
  - Class II recommendations:
    - To assess response of LA and pulmonary artery pressures to exercise when symptoms and echo findings do not match
    - Assess cause of severe pulmonary hypertension out of proportion to echo results
  - Class III recommendations: Satisfactory result of echo

Follow-Up Tests & Special Considerations

- If valve area >1.5 cm^2 and mean pressure gradient <5 mm Hg, then no further initial workup is needed
- If valve area is <1.5 cm^2, then do further workup prior to surgical correction

Diagnostic Procedures/Other

Exercise or dobutamine stress test:

- When symptoms are severe but echo findings are mild
- To determine if surgery is needed

Test Interpretation

Rheumatic fever–induced pathologic changes: Leaflet thickening, leaflet calcification, commissural fusion, chordal shortening

 TREATMENT

GENERAL MEASURES
- Exercise:
  – Patients with mild MS are usually asymptomatic even with strenuous exercise.
  – Usually recommend low-level aerobic exercise, limited by symptoms of dyspnea
- Counsel patients that MS usually is slowly progressive but can have sudden onset of atrial fibrillation, which could become rapidly fatal. Call 911 for marked worsening of symptoms.
- Atrial fibrillation accompanying MS impairs LV filling, especially with a rapid ventricular response:
  – Rate control with β- or calcium channel blockers or amiodarone
  – Cardioversion for medical failure or if patient is unstable
  – If the atrial fibrillation has been present for >24–48 hours, then: Anticoagulate for 3 weeks then cardiovert, or alternatively, heparinize, perform TEE, and, if no atrial thrombus, then cardiovert
  – After cardioversion, patient needs long-term anticoagulation
  – These patients can critically decompensate due to loss of atrial contractility, causing an inability to fill the LV.

MEDICATION

First Line
- Since MS is a mechanical anomaly, medical management is always considered adjunctive to interventional management when the latter is indicated.
- Antibiotic prophylaxis against rheumatic fever and/or carditis is recommended for patients with history of rheumatic fever:
  – Penicillin V PO or penicillin G IM: IM is more effective than PO (4)[A]
  – Sulfadiazine
  – Erythromycin
  – Take antibiotic continuously to prevent recurrence of rheumatic fever or carditis
  – Duration of rheumatic fever prophylaxis:
    ○ Rheumatic fever without carditis: Take for 5 years or until age 21, whichever is longer
    ○ Rheumatic fever with carditis but no residual heart disease: Take for 10 years or well into adulthood, whichever is longer.
    ○ Rheumatic fever with carditis plus residual heart disease: Take for 10 years or until 40 years old, whichever is longer.
- Antibiotic prophylaxis against infective endocarditis is not routinely recommended (5)[C].
- β-blockers for tachycardia or exertional symptoms
- Calcium channel blockers for tachycardia or exertional symptoms
- Diuretics for symptoms of pulmonary congestion
- Digitalis for atrial fibrillation if LV or RV dysfunction
- Anticoagulation:
  – Class I recommendations:
    ○ MS and atrial fibrillation or history of atrial fibrillation
    ○ MS and prior embolic event
    ○ MS and left atrial thrombus

  – Class IIb recommendations:
    ○ Asymptomatic MS but with severe MS and LA dimension >54 mm by echo
    ○ Severe MS, enlarged LA and spontaneous contrast on echo
- Warfarin (international normalized ratio) range 2–3
- Heparin in the acute atrial fibrillation setting.
- The new oral anticoagulants (factor Xa inhibitor and direct thrombin inhibitor) are not approved for use in atrial fibrillation that is secondary to mitral stenosis.

Second Line
Amiodarone for rate control if β-blockers or calcium channel blockers cannot be used

SURGERY/OTHER PROCEDURES
- Balloon valvotomy: Symptomatic patients with NYHA class II, III, or IV symptoms with valves that look favorable and with favorable comorbidities
- Mitral valve surgery (6): When MS is severe and balloon valvotomy is contraindicated due to unfavorable anatomy

Pregnancy Considerations
Volume expansion during pregnancy can exacerbate heart failure symptoms. For this reason, MS often presents during the intrapartum period. For patients with known severe MS, intervention should be pursued prior to pregnancy. Pregnancy in a patient with severe MS has a high rate of both maternal and fetal complications, including death. Percutaneous balloon valvotomy can be performed in symptomatic pregnant patients.

 ONGOING CARE

FOLLOW-UP RECOMMENDATIONS
- Ascertain the valve gradient and pulmonary arterial pressure with echocardiogram.
- Follow up will depend on the severity of the MS and the patient's symptoms:
  – Asymptomatic patients: Annual history and examination; follow-up serial echocardiography based on the severity of MS
  – Symptomatic patients are reviewed according to individual therapy, symptoms, and signs; echocardiogram to evaluate for changes

DIET
Salt restriction for pulmonary congestion

PROGNOSIS
Natural history:
- Asymptomatic latent period after rheumatic fever for 10–30 years. 10-year survival for asymptomatic or minimally symptomatic patients is 80%. 10-year survival after onset of symptoms is 50–60%.
- Symptoms typically become debilitating 10 years after onset.
- 10-year survival after onset of debilitating symptoms is only 0–15%.
- Mean survival with significant pulmonary hypertension is <3 years.
- The severity of MS progresses over time in almost all patients. There are no known definitive medical therapies, apart from prevention of recurrent rheumatic fever, that alter its natural history. When symptoms develop, balloon valvotomy, open mitral commissurotomy, or closed mitral commissurotomy provides effective means of reducing stenosis but is not curative. Restenosis sometimes occurs and can be early (<5 years) or late (>20 years).

- Appropriate medical treatment can delay necessity for surgery, and surgical treatment substantially prolongs survival in patients with severe MS.

COMPLICATIONS
Left- and right-heart failure, atrial fibrillation and systemic embolization, pulmonary HTN, bacterial endocarditis

REFERENCES

1. Ray S. Changing epidemiology and natural history of valvular heart disease. *Clin Med*. 2010;10: 168–171.
2. Chandrasekhar Y. Mitral stenosis. *Lancet*. 2009; 374:1271–1283.
3. Maganti K. Valvular heart disease: Diagnosis and management. *Mayo Clin Proc*. 2010;85:483–500.
4. Manyemba J, Mayosi BM. Penicillin for secondary prevention of rheumatic fever. *Cochrane Database Syst Rev*. 2002;3:CD002227.
5. Nishimura RA. ACC/AHA 2008 guideline update on valvular heart disease: Focused update on infective endocarditis: A report of the American College of Cardiology/American Heart Association Task Force on Practice Guidelines endorsed by the Society of Cardiovascular Anesthesiologists, Society for Cardiovascular Angiography and Interventions, and Society of Thoracic Surgeons. *Catheter Cardiovasc Interv*. 2008;72:E1–E12.
6. Zakkar M. Rheumatic mitral valve disease: Current surgical status. *Prog Cardiovasc Dis*. 2009;51: 478–481.

 CODES

ICD10
- I05.0 Rheumatic mitral stenosis
- I05.8 Other rheumatic mitral valve diseases
- I34.2 Nonrheumatic mitral (valve) stenosis

CLINICAL PEARLS
- Asymptomatic patients may be followed clinically with yearly exams for development of symptoms, with periodic echo to evaluate valve area.
- Once symptoms of MS develop, initiate appropriate medical therapy but advise patient that, for most, surgical therapy will be needed to prolong survival. Almost all cases of mitral valve stenosis progress in severity over time.
- MS often presents during the intrapartum period. For patients with known severe MS, intervention should be pursued prior to pregnancy. Pregnancy in a patient with severe MS has a high rate of both maternal and fetal complications, including death.

M

MITRAL VALVE PROLAPSE

Wasiq Faraz Rawasia, MD • Nirmanmoh Bhatia, MD • Marcus F. Stoddard, MD

 BASICS

DESCRIPTION
- Mitral valve prolapse (MVP) is a systolic billowing of 1 or both mitral leaflets into the left atrium during systole ± mitral regurgitation (MR).
- More specifically, MVP is a single or bileaflet prolapse of at least 2 mm superior displacement into the left atrium during systole on the parasternal long-axis annular plane of the valve on echocardiogram ± leaflet thickening:
  - Classic: Prolapse with >5 mm of leaflet thickening
  - Nonclassic: Prolapse with <5 mm of leaflet thickening (1)
- Synonym(s): Systolic click-murmur syndrome; Billowing mitral cusp syndrome; Myxomatous mitral valve; Floppy valve syndrome; Redundant cusp syndrome; Barlow syndrome

EPIDEMIOLOGY
Incidence
- Predominant age: MVP has been described in all age groups.
- Initial descriptions based on clinical examinations suggested a 2:1 female predominance. Using modern echocardiogram criteria, men and women are affected equally (2).
- The most serious consequences of hemodynamically significant MR occur in men age >50 years.

Prevalence
MVP is the most common valvular abnormality, affecting 1–2.5% of the general population (2,3), depending on the precise definition.

ETIOLOGY AND PATHOPHYSIOLOGY
- The pathology causing MVP is multifactorial and includes the following:
  - Abnormal valve tissue:
    - Myxomatous degeneration: Redundant layers of leaflet "hooding" the cords, chordal elongation, and annular dilatation
    - Myxoid leaflets are more elastic and less stiff than normal valves.
    - Chordal rupture is more common.
  - Disparity in size between the mitral valve and the left ventricle
  - Connective tissue disorders (1)
- MVP is often associated with variable degrees of MR.
- Frequently there is enlargement of the left atrium (LA) and left ventricle (LV).
- Mitral annulus is often dilated.
- Involvement of other valves may occur (tricuspid valve prolapse 40%, pulmonic prolapse and aortic prolapse 2–10%)
- Possible increased vagal tone
- Possible increased urine epinephrine and norepinephrine
- MVP patients often have orthostatic hypotension and tachycardia.
- Genetics causes proliferation of the spongiosa layer of the leaflets (3).
- Fibrosis on surface of leaflets (3)
- Thinning and elongation of chordae tendineae
- The mitral valve differentiates during days 35–42 of fetal development, the same time as differentiation of the vertebrae and ribs.

Genetics
- Familial MVP is inherited as an autosomal-dominant trait, but with variable expressivity and incomplete penetrance.
- 2 genetic loci identified:
  - MMVP1 on chromosome 16p11.2-p12.1
  - MMVP2 on chromosome 11p15.4 (1)

RISK FACTORS
- MVP is a primary cardiovascular disorder.
- MVP is more likely to occur in patients with connective tissue disorders (see "Commonly Associated Conditions").
- Physical characteristics associated with MVP:
  - Straight thoracic spine
  - Pectus excavatum
  - Asthenic body hiatus
  - Low body mass index (BMI)
  - Scoliosis or kyphosis
  - Hypermobility of the joints
  - Arm span > height
  - Narrow anteroposterior (AP) diameter of the chest

COMMONLY ASSOCIATED CONDITIONS
- Marfan syndrome (91% of Marfan syndrome patients have mitral valve prolapse) (1)
- Ehlers-Danlos syndrome
- Hypertrophic cardiomyopathy
- Pseudoxanthoma elasticum
- Osteogenesis imperfecta
- von Willebrand disease (3)
- Primary hypomastia

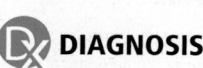 **DIAGNOSIS**

Physical exam and echocardiography

HISTORY
- Most patients are asymptomatic.
- The most frequent symptom is palpitations.
- Symptoms related to autonomic dysfunction:
  - Anxiety and panic attacks
  - Arrhythmias
  - Exercise intolerance
  - Palpitations and chest pains that are atypical for coronary artery disease (CAD)
  - Fatigue
  - Orthostasis, syncope, or presyncope
  - Neuropsychiatric symptoms
- Symptoms related to progression of mitral regurgitation:
  - Fatigue
  - Dyspnea
  - Exercise intolerance
  - Orthopnea
  - Paroxysmal nocturnal dyspnea
  - Congestive heart failure (CHF)
- Symptoms occur as a result of an associated complication (stroke, arrhythmia).

PHYSICAL EXAM
- Auscultatory examination:
  - Mid- to late systolic click:
    - May vary in timing and intensity based on ventricular beat-to-beat volume variations
    - At low ventricular volumes, the valve may prolapse earlier during systole and further into the left atrium (LA) than during volume overload.

  - It may or may not be followed by a high-pitched, mid- to late systolic murmur at the cardiac apex.
  - Murmur: A mid- to late crescendo systolic murmur best heard at apex, middle- to high-pitched, occasionally musical or honking in quality
  - Occasionally, only the ejection click is present.
  - The duration of the murmur corresponds with the severity of MR.
- Dynamic auscultation:
  - Maneuvers that move the click and murmur toward S_1:
    - Arterial vasodilation
    - Amyl nitrite
    - Valsalva
    - Augmented contractility
    - Decreased venous return (which can be induced by standing up)
  - Maneuvers that move the click and murmur toward S_2:
    - Squatting
    - Leg raise
    - Isometric exercise
  - Valsalva maneuver may help differentiate hypertrophic obstructive cardiomyopathy (HOCM) from MVP because it increases the intensity of the murmur in HOCM while it makes it longer but not louder in MVP.

DIFFERENTIAL DIAGNOSIS
- Mitral regurgitation
- Tricuspid regurgitation
- Tricuspid valve prolapse
- Papillary muscle dysfunction
- Hypertrophic cardiomyopathy
- Ejection clicks (do not change timing with systole)

DIAGNOSTIC TESTS & INTERPRETATION
Initial Tests (lab, imaging)
- Echocardiogram:
  - Indicated for the diagnosis of MVP and assessment of MR, leaflet morphology, and left ventricular systolic function in asymptomatic patients with physical signs of MVP
  - Routine repetition of echocardiography is not indicated for the asymptomatic patient who has MVP and no MR, or MVP and mild MR with no changes in clinical signs and symptoms.
  - Most useful and definitive imaging study
  - Parasternal long-axis view most specific for diagnosis
  - Valve prolapse of ≥2 mm above the mitral annulus is most highly associated with MVP ± leaflet thickening.
  - Other findings may include the following:
    - Anterior leaflet billowing
    - Leaflet thickening of ≥5 mm
    - Leaflet redundancy
    - Mitral regurgitation
    - Posterior leaflet displacement
  - Nondiagnostic transthoracic echocardiogram: ≤10%
  - Transesophageal echocardiography particularly with 3D imaging is helpful to visualize the leaflet anatomy, especially if a valve repair operation is being considered or if there is a flail leaflet.
- Angiography indicated in patients with severe and symptomatic MR for whom cardiac surgical referral is being contemplated:
  - Impaired LV systolic function to evaluate for mitral valve surgery
  - Rarely used for diagnostic purposes

- ECG is usually normal:
  - May be nonspecific ST-T wave changes
  - T-wave inversions
  - Prominent Q waves
  - QT prolongation
- A chest x-ray (CXR) is not necessary for diagnosis:
  - Typically, the CXR is normal.
  - Other findings:
    - Possible pulmonary edema: Pulmonary edema may be asymmetric with acute chordal rupture and flail leaflet.
    - Possible calcification of the mitral annulus
- Holter monitoring is optional if patient has palpitations. Order Holter monitoring as usual for syncope or dizziness.
- Tilt table testing may be of value in patients with MVP who presents with syncope of unknown etiology.

Follow-Up Tests & Special Considerations
Patients with a 1st-degree relative who has myxomatous MVP should be screened with echocardiography (1)[A].

Test Interpretation
- Myxomatous proliferation of the middle layer (spongiosa) of the valve, resulting in increased mucopolysaccharide deposition and myxomatous degeneration
- By electron microscopy, the collagen fibers in the valve leaflets are disorganized and fragmented.
- With increased stroma deposition, the valve leaflets enlarge and become redundant.
- The endothelium is usually noncontiguous and a frequent site for thrombus or infective vegetation.

 TREATMENT

GENERAL MEASURES
Treat MVP with orthostatic symptoms by liberalizing fluid and salt intake. If severe, mineralocorticoids or clonidine may rarely be used. Support stockings may also be beneficial.

MEDICATION
- Asymptomatic MVP is treated with reassurance; normal lifestyle and regular exercise is encouraged (3)[A].
- MVP and transient ischemic attacks (TIA) are treated with aspirin 75–325 mg daily (Class I recommendation) (3)[C].
- MVP with history of cryptogenic stroke, or atrial fibrillation with CHADS$_2$ (acronym for **C**ongestive heart failure, **H**ypertension, **A**ge >75, **D**iabetes mellitus, and prior **S**troke or transient ischemic attack) score <2, is generally treated with aspirin 75–325 mg daily (3)[C].
- MVP with atrial fibrillation with CHADS$_2$ score ≥2 is treated with warfarin (3)[C].
- MVP with history of stroke plus atrial fibrillation or left atrial appendage thrombus is treated with warfarin (3)[C].
- MVP with palpitations is treated with β-blockers and/or recommendation to discontinue alcohol, cigarettes, and caffeine. Continuous ambulatory ECG monitoring may be useful to detect significant arrhythmias (3)[C].

ADDITIONAL THERAPIES
- Endocarditis prophylaxis is no longer recommended for MVP (3)[B].
- Patients with prior endocarditis undergoing dental, respiratory tract, infected skin, or musculoskeletal procedures should receive prophylaxis for endocarditis with amoxicillin 30–60 minutes prior to procedure (3)[B]. Ampicillin, cefazolin, or ceftriaxone IM or IV may be used if unable to tolerate oral medications.

SURGERY/OTHER PROCEDURES
- Referral for surgery is recommended for patients with severe MR with impaired LV systolic function or flail leaflet owing to ruptured chordae tendineae (3)[A].
- Minimally invasive mitral valve repair patients have shorter postoperative hospital stay compared with conventional median sternotomy open repair for patients with bileaflet prolapse and severe mitral regurgitation (4)[B].
- Surgical repair of mitral regurgitation due to isolated posterior leaflet prolapse is associated with a low reoperation rate (5)[A].

 ONGOING CARE

FOLLOW-UP RECOMMENDATIONS
- Asymptomatic MVP patients with no significant MR can be followed clinically every 3–5 years.
- Patients who are symptomatic or have high-risk features on initial echocardiogram, including moderate to severe MR, may need serial echocardiograms and should be followed clinically once per year.
- Patients with MVP and severe MR may require coronary angiography and transesophageal echocardiography if cardiac surgical referral is planned.

PATIENT EDUCATION
Patient education on avoidance of alcohol, caffeine, stimulants, and nicotine may be sufficient to control symptoms in some instances:
- No contraindication to pregnancy
- Restriction from competitive sports if patient has MVP with one of the following features (6):
  - A history of syncope associated with document arrhythmia
  - A family history of MVP-related sudden cardiac death
  - Sustained or repetitive and nonsustained supraventricular tachycardia or frequent and/or complex ventricular tachyarrhythmias on ambulatory Holter monitoring
  - Severe MR
  - A prior embolic event
  - LV systolic dysfunction
- Explain the hereditary nature of familial MVP.

PROGNOSIS
- Excellent prognosis for asymptomatic patients
- For patients with severe MR or reduced ejection fraction, the prognosis is similar to that for nonischemic MR.

COMPLICATIONS
- Sudden cardiac death (yearly rate of 1.9/10,000 per year) is twice the rate in the general population; risk is 50–100 times greater (0.9–1.9% per year) if significant MR is present.

- Chordae rupture with acute mitral insufficiency (higher risk of cardiac death; up to 2% per year)
- Endocarditis
- Cerebrovascular ischemic event
- Fibrin emboli
- Heart failure with progressive MR
- Arrhythmia:
  - Atrial premature beats, 35–90%
  - Supraventricular tachycardia, 3–32%
  - Ventricular premature beats, 58–89%
  - Complex ventricular ectopy, 30–56%
- Pulmonary hypertension

REFERENCES

1. Hayek E, Gring CN, Griffin BP. Mitral valve prolapse. *Lancet*. 2005;365:507–518.
2. Freed LA, Levy D, Levine RA, et al. Prevalence and clinical outcome of mitral-valve prolapse. *N Engl J Med*. 1999;341:1–7.
3. Bonow RO, Carabello BA, Chatterjee K. 2008 focused update incorporated into the ACC/AHA 2006 guidelines for the management of patients with valvular heart disease: A report of the American College of Cardiology/American Heart Association Task Force on Practice Guidelines (Writing Committee to revise the 1998 guidelines for the management of patients with valvular heart disease). Endorsed by the Society of Cardiovascular Anesthesiologists, Society for Cardiovascular Angiography and Interventions, and Society of Thoracic Surgeons. *J Am Coll Cardiol*. 2008;52: e1–142.
4. Speziale G, Nasso G, Esposito G, et al. Results of mitral valve repair for Barlow disease (bileaflet prolapse) via right minithoracotomy versus conventional median sternotomy: A randomized trial. *J Thorac Cardiovasc Surg*. 2011;142:77–83.
5. Johnston DR, Gillinov AM, Blackstone EH, et al. Surgical repair of posterior mitral valve prolapse: Implications for guidelines and percutaneous repair. *Ann Thorac Surg*. 2010;89:1385–1394.
6. Maron BJ, Ackerman MJ, Nishimura RA. Task Force 4: HCM and other cardiomyopathies, mitral valve prolapse, myocarditis, and Marfan syndrome. *J Am Coll Cardiol*. 2005;45:1340–1345.

 CODES

ICD10
I34.1 Nonrheumatic mitral (valve) prolapse

CLINICAL PEARLS
- MVP patients may have orthostatic hypotension and tachycardia.
- Asymptomatic MVP patients with no significant MR can be followed clinically every 3–5 years. Patients who are symptomatic or have high-risk features on initial echocardiogram, including moderate to severe MR, may need serial echocardiograms and should be followed clinically once per year.
- Endocarditis prophylaxis is no longer recommended for MVP.

M

MOLLUSCUM CONTAGIOSUM

Gillian S. Stephens, MD, MSc • Erica F. Pearce, PharmD, BCPS

 BASICS

DESCRIPTION
- Molluscum contagiosum is a common, benign, viral (Poxviridae) skin infection.
- 1–5 mm, "pearly" white or flesh-colored dome-shaped papules; central umbilication (difficult to see in young children)
- Highly contagious; autoinoculation, skin-to-skin contact, sexual contact, shared clothing, towels, bathing water
- Self-limited in immunocompetent
- Difficult to treat/disfiguring in immunocompromised

EPIDEMIOLOGY
Incidence
- Up to 20% children in tropics
- 30% in AIDS patients

Prevalence
- Children 2–15 years
- Sexually active young adults
- 5–18% HIV population

ETIOLOGY AND PATHOPHYSIOLOGY
- Virions invade and replicate in cytoplasm of epithelial cells
- Cause abnormal cell proliferation
- Genome encodes proteins to evade host immune system
- Incubation period: 2–6 weeks
- Not associated with malignancy
- DNA virus; Poxviridae family
- 4 major types, clinically indistinguishable
- No cross-hybridization or reactivation by other poxviruses

RISK FACTORS
- Skin-to-skin contact with infected person
- Contact sports
- Sexual activity with infected partner
- Immunocompromised: HIV, chemotherapy, corticosteroid therapy, transplant patients

GENERAL PREVENTION
- Avoid skin-to-skin contact with host (e.g., contact sports, sexual activity).
- Avoid sharing clothing, towels, bathing water.

COMMONLY ASSOCIATED CONDITIONS
- Atopic dermatitis
- HIV/AIDS
- Immunosuppression: Corticosteroids, chemotherapy

 DIAGNOSIS

HISTORY
- Contact with known infected person
- Participation in contact sports
- Sexual activity

PHYSICAL EXAM
- Discrete, firm papules with a central umbilication
- Umbilication not obvious in small children
- White curdlike core under umbilicated center
- Lesions are flesh, pearl, or red in color
- May have surrounding erythema or dermatitis
- Immunocompetent hosts: Average of 11–20 lesions, 2–5 mm diameter (range: 1–10 mm)
- Hosts with HIV/AIDS: Hundreds of widespread lesions
- Children: Trunk, extremities, face, anogenital region
- Sexually active: Inner thighs, anogenital area
- Perform thorough skin exam including conjunctiva and anogenital area.

Pediatric Considerations
- Infants <3 months, consider vertical transmission
- Children: Fever, >50 lesions, limited response to therapy, consider immunodeficiency (1)
- Children: Anogenital lesions, consider autoinoculation/possible sexual abuse (1)

DIFFERENTIAL DIAGNOSIS
- AIDS patients: Cryptococcus, penicilliosis, histoplasmosis, coccidiomycosis
- Basal cell carcinoma
- Benign appendageal tumors: Syringomas, hydrocystomas, ectopic sebaceous glands
- Condyloma acuminatum
- Dermatofibroma
- Eyelid: Abscess, chalazion, foreign-body granuloma
- Folliculitis/furunculosis
- Keratoacanthoma
- Oral squamous cell carcinoma
- Trichoepithelioma
- Verruca vulgaris
- Warty dyskeratoma

DIAGNOSTIC TESTS & INTERPRETATION
Initial Tests (lab, imaging)
- Virus cannot be cultured.
- Scrape lesion; Tzanck preparation; molluscum cytoplasmic inclusion bodies (1)
- Culture lesion if concern is secondary infection
- Sexual transmission: Test for other sexually transmitted infections, including HIV
- Microscopy

Diagnostic Procedures/Other
Clinical; using magnifying lens

Test Interpretation
Molluscum cytoplasmic inclusion bodies within keratinocytes

 TREATMENT

GENERAL MEASURES
- Natural resolution
- No single intervention is shown to be convincingly more effective than any other in treating molluscum contagiosum (2).

MEDICATION
First Line
- Cantharidin solution 0.7–0.9%: Apply sparingly to lesions, cover with occlusion dressing, wash off in 2–6 hours or sooner if blistering. Repeat treatment every 2–4 weeks until lesions resolve (in-office treatment) (1,3)[C]:
  - Adverse effects: Blistering, erythema, pain, pruritus
  - Precautions: Do not use on face or on genital mucosa
- Cimetidine 40 mg/kg/d divided t.i.d. for 2 months. Maximum dose 800 mg t.i.d. (1,4)[C]:
  - Adverse effects: Headache, diarrhea, gynecomastia
  - Precautions: Pregnancy Category B; not recommended for use while nursing
- Imiquimod cream 5%: Optimal dosing regimen unknown. Genital area: Apply to lesions once daily 3 times per week until lesions resolve, up to 16 weeks (1,3)[C]:
  - Adverse effects: Erythema, edema, pruritus, postinflammatory pigment changes
  - Contraindications: Pregnancy

Second Line
- Limit treatment to small areas 4–10 cm^2:
  - Podofilox cream 0.5%: Apply to lesions b.i.d. for 3 days, none for 4 days; may repeat this cycle 4–6 times (3)[C]:
    - Adverse effects: Erythema, edema, pain, pruritus
    - Contraindications: Pregnancy
  - Podophyllin 10–25% solution: Apply sparingly to lesions 1 time weekly for 4–6 weeks (in-office treatment) (3)[C]:
    - Adverse effects: Erythema, edema, pain
    - Contraindications: Pregnancy, infants, children, oral mucosa
- For HIV/AIDS patients with refractory lesions, consider:
  - Starting or maximizing HAART therapy (1)[C]
  - IV or topical cidofovir (1,3)

SURGERY/OTHER PROCEDURES
- Cryotherapy: 5–10 seconds with 1–2 mm margins; repeat every 3–4 weeks as needed until lesions disappear (1,3)[C]:
  - Adverse effects: Erythema, edema, pain, blistering
  - Contraindications: Cryoglobulinemia, Raynaud disease
- Curettage (± electrodessication) under local or topical anesthesia (1,3)[C]:
  - Adverse effects: Pain, scarring
- Incision and expression of central particle (1):
  - Adverse effects: High rate of scarring
- CO_2 (3) or pulsed dye (1,3)[C] lasers (for recalcitrant lesions, usually in HIV/AIDS patients):
  - Adverse effects: Pain, edema, scarring, postinflammatory pigment changes
- Photodynamic therapy (ALA/MAL-PDT) (5)[C]

COMPLEMENTARY AND ALTERNATIVE MEDICINE
- Australian lemon myrtle oil: Apply 10% solution once daily for 21 days (6)[C]
- Tea tree oil and iodine: Apply twice daily for up to 30 days (7)[C]
- KOH 0.5%: Apply nightly for 4 weeks (8)[C]

Pediatric Considerations
- Surgical interventions: 2nd line in small children; pain associated
- Pain control: Pretreat with topical lidocaine or EMLA before surgical treatment.
- Note: Adverse effect:
  - Lidocaine or EMLA over large body surface area: Methemoglobinemia and CNS toxicity. Refer to manufacturer's recommendations on dosing and use in children.

Pregnancy Considerations
- Safe in pregnancy: Curettage, cryotherapy, incision, and expression
- Contraindicated: Podophyllin, podofilox, or imiquimod; teratogenic

 ONGOING CARE

FOLLOW-UP RECOMMENDATIONS
Patient Monitoring
Depends on type of treatment

PATIENT EDUCATION
- Cover lesions to prevent spread
- Avoid scratching
- Avoid contact sports
- Avoid sharing towels, baths
- Avoid sexual activity when lesions present
- Avoid swimming pools

PROGNOSIS
- Immunocompetent: Self-limited, resolves in 3–12 months (range: 2 months–4 years)
- Immunocompromised: Lesions difficult to treat, may persist for years

COMPLICATIONS
- Secondary infection
- Scarring, hyper-/hypopigmentation

REFERENCES
1. Brown J, Janniger CK, Schwartz RA, et al. Childhood molluscum contagiosum. *Int J Dermatol.* 2006;45:93–99.
2. van der Wouden JC, Menke J, Gajadin S, et al. Interventions for cutaneous molluscum contagiosum. *Cochrane Database Syst Rev.* 2009;4:CD004767.
3. Ting PT, Dytoc MT. Therapy of external anogenital warts and molluscum contagiosum: A literature review. *Dermatol Ther.* 2004;17:68–101.
4. Jones S, Kress D. Treatment of molluscum contagiosum and herpes simplex virus cutaneous infections. *Cutis.* 2007;79(Suppl 4):11–17.
5. Rossi R, Bruscino N, Ricceri F, et al. Photodynamic treatment for viral infections of the skin. *G Ital Dermatol Venereol.* 2009;144:79–83.
6. Burke BE, Baillie JE, Olson RD. Essential oil of Australian lemon myrtle (*Backhousia citriodora*) in the treatment of molluscum contagiosum in children. *Biomed Pharmacother.* 2004;58:245–247.
7. Markum E, Baillie, J. Combination of essential oil of *Melaleuca alternifolia* and iodine in the treatment of molluscum contagiosum in children. *J Drugs Derm.* 2012;11:349–354.
8. Rajouria EA, Amatya A, Karn D. Comparative study of 5% potassium hydroxide solution versus 0.05% tretinoin cream for Molluscum Contagiosum in children. *Katmandu Univ Med J.* 2011;9:291–294.

ADDITIONAL READING
- Connell CO, Oranje A, Van Gysel D, et al. Congenital molluscum contagiosum: Report of four cases and review of the literature. *Pediatr Dermatol.* 2008;25:553–556.
- Dohil MA, Lin P, Lee J, et al. The epidemiology of molluscum contagiosum in children. *J Am Acad Dermatol.* 2006;54:47–54.

 CODES

ICD10
B08.1 Molluscum contagiosum

CLINICAL PEARLS
- Natural resolution is preferred treatment in healthy patients (2)[A].
- Reassure parents that lesions will heal naturally and generally resolve without scarring (2)[A].
- No 1 specific treatment has been identified as superior to any other (2)[A].
- Consider topical corticosteroids or antihistamines for pruritus or associated dermatitis (1)[C].

M

MONONUCLEOSIS

Neil Nixdorff, MD, MA, MS, MPH • Katherine L. Margo, MD

BASICS

DESCRIPTION
Formerly known as *glandular fever*, infectious mononucleosis (IM) is an acute illness resulting most commonly from a primary infection of Epstein-Barr virus (EBV).

EPIDEMIOLOGY
Incidence
Not a reportable disease: Incidence is estimated to be ~500 cases per 100,000 person years in the US.

Prevalence
- Viral shedding is highest 1st year postinfection, but can continue for life in asymptomatic hosts.
- By age 5 years, 50% of all Americans demonstrate immunologic exposure to EBV:
  – 90% by age 25 years

ETIOLOGY AND PATHOPHYSIOLOGY
- EBV replicates primarily in B lymphocytes but also replicates in the epithelial cells of the pharynx and parotid duct.
- Symptoms arise from cytokines released from activated T-cells:
  – Response is thought to be proportional to initial viral load.
- EBV is spread by saliva, but has also been isolated in cervical epithelial cells and seminal fluid.
- The incubation period is 4–8 weeks.
- EBV is a double-stranded DNA herpesvirus.
- ~10% of acute mono syndromes are caused by other infectious agents, primarily cytomegalovirus (CMV) (1):
  – Consider other etiologies if EBV and CMV negative (see "Differential Diagnosis").

Genetics
Unknown

RISK FACTORS
Populations that include many young adults in close proximity:
- Active-duty military personnel
- High schools
- College dormitories

GENERAL PREVENTION
- Avoid saliva of infected person.
- Vaccine is under development.

COMMONLY ASSOCIATED CONDITIONS
- Streptococcal pharyngitis may be associated in 30% of patients.
- There is considerable evidence that EBV infection is a strong risk factor for the development of multiple sclerosis (2)[A].

DIAGNOSIS

HISTORY
- Although primary infection is frequently asymptomatic especially in children, adolescents and adults frequently develop a spectrum of symptoms.
- The syndrome is often heralded by malaise, headache, and low-grade fever.
- Prodrome typically evolves into the classic triad:
  – Fever
  – Tonsillar pharyngitis
  – Lymphadenopathy

PHYSICAL EXAM
- Lymphadenopathy:
  – Typically symmetric
  – More commonly involves the posterior cervical chain, but it also may become more generalized.
  – Peaks in the 1st week and then subsides gradually over 2–3 weeks
- Fever
- Pharyngitis
- Splenomegaly
- A generalized maculopapular, urticarial, or petechial rash is seen occasionally. Rash is common following the administration of ampicillin or amoxicillin.

DIFFERENTIAL DIAGNOSIS
- Cytomegalovirus
- Primary HIV infection
- Toxoplasmosis
- Rubella
- Adenovirus
- Herpesviruses
- Streptococcal pharyngitis
- Viral tonsillitis
- Diphtheria
- Viral hepatitis
- Lymphoma or leukemia
- Human herpesvirus 6
- Roseola
- Mumps
- Drug-induced atypical lymphocytosis with mononucleosislike symptoms (dilantin, carbamazepine, isoniazid, minocycline)

DIAGNOSTIC TESTS & INTERPRETATION
Initial Tests (lab, imaging)
- CBC: An increase in total lymphocyte >35% and atypical lymphocytes of at least 10%. Monocytosis is not associated with IM.
- Elevated aminotransferases: Seen in the majority of patients, but typically self-limited
- Autoantibodies: Acute EBV infection can be associated with production of rheumatoid factor and antinuclear antibodies
- Heterophile antibodies (monospot test):
  – In 40% of patients, positive in 1st week
  – 90% of patients in 3rd week
  – May remain positive for 2 years for up to 20% of infected individuals
- EBV-specific antibodies:
  – Viral capsid antigen (VCA):
    ○ IgG and IgM peak at 3–4 weeks.
    ○ IgG then declines but persists for life.
    ○ IgM declines rapidly and is undetectable by 3 months.
  – EB nuclear antigen (EBNA):
    ○ Develops after 2 months and persists indefinitely
    ○ Presence early in the course of illness excludes acute EBV infection.
  – Early antigen (EA):
    ○ IgG to EA is present at the onset of clinical illness and persists for 2–3 months.
    ○ With viral capsid antigen (VCA) IgG, VCA IgM and EBV nuclear antigen (EBNA)-1 IgG], it is normally possible to distinguish acute from past infection: the presence of VCA IgM and VCA IgG without EBNA-1 IgG indicates acute infection, whereas the presence of VCA IgG and EBNA-1 IgG without VCA IgM is typical of past infection (3)[A].
- Imaging usually not indicated.

Follow-Up Tests & Special Considerations
- With high clinical suspicion in a patient with a negative heterophile antibody, the monospot test should be repeated because this test can be negative during the 1st week of clinical illness.
- EBV-specific antibodies should be tested if the patient has a repeatedly negative monospot test.
- US if clinically important to diagnose or follow splenomegaly
- CT scan of abdomen is the preferred methodology to rule out splenic rupture.

Pregnancy Considerations
Differentiating between IM caused by EBV and a similar syndrome owing to CMV or HIV infection often is not possible clinically, but it is particularly important if the patient is pregnant because CMV, HIV, and *Toxoplasma* infections can have significant adverse effects on pregnancy outcomes.

Pediatric Considerations
EBV acquired during childhood years is often subclinical:
- Sensitivity of Monospot in children <4 years is poor, and EBV-specific antibodies should be checked.

TREATMENT

GENERAL MEASURES
Symptomatic treatment, the mainstay of care, includes:
- Adequate hydration
- Analgesics
- Antipyretics
- Adequate rest: *Complete bed rest is unnecessary.*

MEDICATION
First Line
- Acetaminophen
- NSAIDs
- Lozenges

Second Line
- Acyclovir (Zovirax):
  – No clinical benefit in moderate presentations.
  – Weak evidence that antivirals may confer benefit in severe cases in immunocompetent hosts (4)[B]
  – There is a Cochrane review pending on this treatment.
- Corticosteroids:
  – Recommended in patients with significant pharyngeal edema that threatens respiratory compromise
  – There is insufficient evidence to recommend routine treatment (5)[A], but may improve pharyngitis in the short-term and may shorten course of illness.
  – A 2012 Cochrane review found that corticosteroids increased the likelihood of complete resolution of pain (in children over the age of 3 years with a sore throat) at 24 hours by more than three times (6)[A]

ADDITIONAL THERAPIES
The preferred treatment for splenic rupture is nonoperative with intensive supportive care and splenic preservation, but some require splenectomy.

SURGERY/OTHER PROCEDURES
Splenectomy and tonsillectomy are rarely required to manage complications.

IN-PATIENT CONSIDERATIONS
Admission Criteria/Initial Stabilization
- Suspicion of splenic rupture or airway obstruction
- Outpatient usually; 95% of patients recover without persistent morbidity.

ONGOING CARE

DIET
Soft diet followed by gradually advanced diet if severe sore throat

PATIENT EDUCATION
- For athletes planning to resume noncontact sports, training can be restarted gradually 3 weeks from symptom onset:
  – For strenuous contact sports or activities associated with increased intra-abdominal pressure, patient should wait a minimum of 4 weeks after illness onset.
  – Imaging of the spleen is not required prior to return to contact sport participation (7)[B].
- There is no set time to go back to school or work:
  – Individuals with IM tend to be most contagious during the incubation period, the 4–6 weeks before they develop symptoms, and during the acute phases of their illness.
  – Some people may shed EBV when they are no longer symptomatic.
- Because the EBV resides in the body for life, it can reactivate, but in most cases it will not cause symptoms unless the immune system becomes severely compromised.

PROGNOSIS
- IM is typically self-limiting, but occasionally can be associated with complications causing significant morbidity.
- Fatigue, myalgias, and need for sleep may persist for several months after the acute infection has resolved.

COMPLICATIONS
- Chronic EBV infections (i.e., chronic fatigue syndrome, the diagnosis of which remains highly controversial)
- Splenic rupture (rare, 0.1–0.5% of patients with proven IM)
- Hemolytic anemia (mild)
- Thrombocytopenia
- Hemolytic-uremic syndrome
- Seizures and other neurologic abnormalities
- Nerve palsies
- Meningoencephalitis
- Reye syndrome
- Myocarditis/ECG changes
- Airway obstruction
- Acute interstitial nephritis

REFERENCES
1. Bravender T. Epstein-Barr virus, cytomegalovirus, and infectious mononucleosis. *Adolesc Med State Art Rev.* 2010;84(2):251–264, ix.
2. Handel AE, Williamson AJ, Disanto G, et al. An updated meta-analysis of risk of multiple sclerosis following infectious mononucleosis. *PLoS ONE.* 2010;84(9). Epub 2010 Sep 1.
3. De Paschale M, Clerici P. Serological diagnosis of Epstein-Barr virus infection: Problems and solutions. *World J Virol.* 2012;1(1):31–43.
4. Vouloumanou EK, Rafailidis PI, Falagas ME. Current diagnosis and management of infectious mononucleosis. *Curr Opin Hematol.* 2012;84(1):14–20.
5. Candy B, Hotopf M. Steroids for symptom control in infectious mononucleosis. *Cochrane Database Syst Rev.* 2006;(3):CD004402. Epub 2006 Jul 19.
6. Hayward G, Thompson MJ, Perera R, et al. Corticosteroids as stand alone or add-on treatment for sore throat. *Cochrane Database Syst Rev.* 2012;10:CD008268.
7. Putukian M, O'Connor FG, Stricker P, et al. Mononucleosis and athletic participation: An evidence-based subject review. *Clin J Sport Med.* 2008;84(4):309–315.

ADDITIONAL READING
- Permpalung N, Ungprasert P, Chongnarungsin D, et al. A diagnostic blind spot: Acute infectious mononucleosis or acute retroviral syndrome. *Am J Med.* 2013;126(9):e5–6.
- Singer-Leshinsky S. Pathogenesis, diagnostic testing, and management of mononucleosis. *JAAPA.* 2012;84(5):58–62.

 # CODES

ICD10
- B27.10 Cytomegaloviral mononucleosis without complications
- B27.90 Infectious mononucleosis, unspecified without complication
- B27.99 Infectious mononucleosis, unsp with other complication

CLINICAL PEARLS
- IM should be suspected in patients 10–30 years who present with sore throat and significant fatigue, palatal petechiae, posterior cervical or auricular adenopathy, marked axillary adenopathy, or inguinal adenopathy.
- Patients with suspected IM, based on history and physical exam, should have a CBC with differential and a heterophile antibody test. In addition, patients should have a diagnostic evaluation for streptococcal infection by culture or antigen test, as well as an HIV test.
- In a patient with a compatible syndrome and a negative heterophile antibody test, the monospot test can be repeated because this test can be negative during the 1st week of clinical illness. EBV-specific antibodies (e.g., VCA IgM and IgG and EBNA) should be determined if the patient has repeatedly negative monospot tests.
- The presence of IgG EBNA or the absence of IgG and IgM VCA excludes primary EBV infection and should prompt consideration of alternative etiologies of a mononucleosislike illness.
- An increase in monocytes does not suggest mononucleosis; an increase in total lymphocytes >35% and atypical lymphocytes >10% does suggest mononucleosis.

M

MORTON NEUROMA (INTERDIGITAL NEUROMA)

Anila Khaliq, MD • Mahpara Khaliq, MD • Komel Safdar, MBBS

BASICS

DESCRIPTION
- Perineural fibrosis of the common digital nerve as it passes between metatarsals
  - The most common site is the interspace between the 3rd and 4th metatarsals.
  - The interspace between the 3rd and 2nd metatarsals is the next most common site.
- System(s) affected: Musculoskeletal; Nervous
- Synonym(s): Plantar digital neuritis

EPIDEMIOLOGY
Prevalence
- Unknown
- Mean age: 45–50 years
- Predominant sex: Female > Male (8:1)

ETIOLOGY AND PATHOPHYSIOLOGY
- Lateral plantar nerve combines with part of medial plantar nerve, creating a nerve with a larger diameter than nerves going to other digits.
- Nerve lies in SC tissue, deep to the fat pad of foot, just superficial to the digital artery and vein.
- Overlying the nerve is the strong, deep transverse metatarsal ligament that holds the metatarsal bones together.
- With each step the patient takes, the inflamed nerve becomes compressed between the ground and the deep transverse metatarsal ligament.
- Excessive stress of the forefoot
- Repetitive trauma
- Congenitally enlarged plantar digital nerve

RISK FACTORS
- High-heeled shoes:
  - Cause more weight to be transferred to the front of the foot
- Tight-toed shoes (tight toe boxes):
  - Cause lateral compression
- Pes planus (flat feet):
  - Causes nerve to be pulled more medially, which increases irritation
- Obesity
- Ballet dancing, basketball, aerobics, tennis, running, and similar activities

GENERAL PREVENTION
- Wear properly fitting shoes.
- Avoid high heels and shoes with narrow toe boxes.

DIAGNOSIS

HISTORY
- Most common complaint is pain localized to interspace between 3rd and 4th toes.
- Pain is less severe when not bearing weight.
- Pain, cramping, or numbness of the forefoot during weight bearing or immediately after strenuous foot exertion
- Radiation of pain to the toes
- Pain is relieved by removing the shoe and massaging the foot.
- Patients often state: "It feels like I am walking on a marble."
- A burning pain in the ball of the foot that may radiate into the toes
- Tingling or numbness in the toes
- Aggravated by wearing tight or narrow shoes

PHYSICAL EXAM
- A palpable nodule in the metatarsal interspace is an occasional finding.
- Positive Mulder sign: See "Diagnostic Procedures/Other."
- Intense pain on pressure between metatarsal heads
- Assess midfoot motion and digital motion to determine if arthritis or synovitis.
- Palpate along metatarsal shafts to assess for metatarsalgia or stress fractures.

DIFFERENTIAL DIAGNOSIS
- Stress fracture
- Hammer toe
- Metatarsophalangeal synovitis
- Metatarsalgia
- Arthritis
- Bursitis
- Foreign body

DIAGNOSTIC TESTS & INTERPRETATION
Initial Tests (lab, imaging)
- Radiographs may help to rule out osseous pathology if diagnosis is in question, but films usually are normal in patients with a Morton neuroma.
- US may show a hypoechoic nodule between the metatarsal interspace.
- US had a 65% specificity and a 98% sensitivity for Morton neuromas but is poor at assessing the size of the lesion (1)[C].
- MRI is used to ensure that compression is not caused by a malignant tumor in the foot. MRI is helpful in determining how much of the nerve to resect surgically; it has a sensitivity of 83% and a specificity of 99% (1)[C].

Diagnostic Procedures/Other
- Mulder sign: A "click" and pain produced by squeezing the metatarsal heads together and simultaneously compressing the neuroma between the thumb and index finger of the other hand
- Corticosteroid injection can significantly reduce symptoms:
  - Inject 1–2 mL lidocaine and 0.5–1 mL dexamethasone just proximal to the metatarsal heads.
  - >1 injection is often needed, usually once a week for 3 weeks (2,3).

Test Interpretation
Chronic fibrosis and thickening of the digital nerve

TREATMENT

GENERAL MEASURES
- Wear flat shoes with a roomy toe box (4)[A].
- Metatarsal pads placed immediately proximal to the 2 involved metatarsal heads (4)[A]
- Corticosteroid injection into the dorsal part of the foot with medium- or long-acting steroid (e.g., betamethasone, methylprednisolone) mixed with local anesthetic (e.g., lidocaine) (4)[A]
- If patient has pes planus, use an arch support (4)[A].
- Literature suggests wide variability in success rate (50–98%) (4)[A].

MEDICATION

First Line
Injectable steroids (e.g., betamethasone phosphate/acetate or methylprednisolone): Use if general measures fail (2,3)[C]

Second Line
NSAIDs for temporary symptom relief (1,2)[C]

ISSUES FOR REFERRAL
Continued pain despite conservative treatments and injections

ADDITIONAL THERAPIES
- US-guided alcohol ablation therapy to sclerose the nerve has been successful (5,6)[C].
- A pilot study has demonstrated that injection with onabotulinumtoxinA is of possible usefulness to relieve the pain and improve function in Morton neuroma (7)[C].

SURGERY/OTHER PROCEDURES
Surgical removal of the neuroma, release of the transverse metatarsal ligament, or both in refractory cases

ONGOING CARE

FOLLOW-UP RECOMMENDATIONS
If no improvement after 3 months of conservative treatment, consider corticosteroid injection:
- Repeat injection if no improvement after 2–4 weeks.

PATIENT EDUCATION
Wear properly fitted, comfortable shoes

PROGNOSIS
- 40–50% improve after 3 months of conservative treatment.
- 45–50% improve after steroid injection.
- 96% improve after surgery.

COMPLICATIONS
Hip and knee pain related to gait changes

REFERENCES

1. Sharp RJ. The role of MRI and ultrasound imaging in Morton's neuroma and the effect of size of lesion on symptoms. *Br J Bone Joint Surg.* 2003;85: 999–1005.
2. Tallia AF, Cardone DA. Diagnostic and therapeutic injection of the ankle and foot. *Am Fam Physician.* 2003;68:1356–1362.
3. Schreiber K, Khodaee M, Poddar S, et al. Clinical inquiry. What is the best way to treat Morton's neuroma? *J Fam Pract.* 2011;60:157–158, 168.
4. Thomson CE, Gibson JN, Martin D, et al. Interventions for the treatment of Morton's neuroma. *Cochrane Database Syst Rev.* 2004;3: CD003118.
5. Hughes RJ, Ali K, Jones H, et al. Treatment of Morton's neuroma with alcohol injection under sonographic guidance: Follow-up of 101 cases. *Am J Roentgenol.* 2007;188:1535–1539.
6. Musson RE, Sawhney JS, Lamb L, et al. Ultrasound guided alcohol ablation of Morton's neuroma. *Foot Ankle Int.* 2012;33:196–201.
7. Climent JM, Mondéjar-Gómez F, Rodríguez-Ruiz C, et al. Treatment of Morton neuroma with botulinum toxin A: A pilot study. *Clin Drug Investig.* 2013;33:497–503.

ADDITIONAL READING
- Clinical Practice Guideline Forefoot Disorders Panel, Thomas JL, Blitch EL, et al. Diagnosis and treatment of forefoot disorders. Section 3. Morton's intermetatarsal neuroma. *J Foot Ankle Surg.* 2009;48:251–256.
- Smith RW. Steroid injection for Morton neuroma— Data-based justification. *J Bone Joint Surg Am.* 2013;95:e641–e642.

CODES

ICD10
- G57.60 Lesion of plantar nerve, unspecified lower limb
- G57.61 Lesion of plantar nerve, right lower limb
- G57.62 Lesion of plantar nerve, left lower limb

CLINICAL PEARLS
- Diagnosis of Morton neuroma usually is made clinically.
- Footwear modification, metatarsal pads, and shoe inserts are the mainstays of treatment.
- Corticosteroid injection into the neuroma may be helpful.
- US-guided alcohol ablation therapy to sclerose the nerve has been successful.

M

MOTION SICKNESS

Courtney I. Jarvis, PharmD • Allison Hargreaves, MD

 BASICS

DESCRIPTION
- Motions sickness is not a true sickness, but a normal response to a situation in which sensory conflict about body motion exists among visual receptors, vestibular receptors, and body proprioceptors.
- Also can be induced when patterns of motion differ from those previously experienced
- System affected: Nervous
- Synonym(s): Car sickness; Sea sickness; Air sickness; Space sickness; Physiologic vertigo

EPIDEMIOLOGY
Incidence
Predominant sex: Female > Male

Prevalence
Estimation is complex; syndrome occurs in ~25% due to travel by air, ~29% by sea, and ~41% by road. Estimates for vomiting are 0.5% by air, 7% by sea, and 2% by road.

ETIOLOGY AND PATHOPHYSIOLOGY
- Precise etiology unknown; thought to be due to a mismatch of vestibular and visual sensations
- Nausea and vomiting occur as a result of increased levels of dopamine and acetylcholine, which stimulate chemoreceptor trigger zone and vomiting center in CNS.

Genetics
Heritability estimates range from 55–75%.

RISK FACTORS
- Motion (auto, plane, boat, amusement rides)
- Travel
- Visual stimuli (e.g., moving horizon)
- Poor ventilation (fumes, smoke, carbon monoxide)
- Emotions (fear, anxiety)
- Zero gravity
- Pregnancy, menstruation, oral contraceptive use
- History of migraine headaches, especially vestibular migraine
- Other illness or poor health

GENERAL PREVENTION
See "General Measures."

Pediatric Considerations
- Rare in children <2 years of age
- Incidence peaks between 3 and 12 years
- Antihistamines may cause excitation in children

Geriatric Considerations
- Age confers some resistance to motion sickness
- Elderly are at increased risk of anticholinergic side effects from treatment

Pregnancy Considerations
- Pregnant patients are more likely to experience motion sickness.
- Treat with medications thought to be safe during morning sickness (e.g., meclizine, dimenhydrate) (1)[C].

COMMONLY ASSOCIATED CONDITIONS
Migraine headache

 DIAGNOSIS

HISTORY
Presence of the following signs and symptoms in the context of a typical stimulus (2)[C]:
- Nausea
- Vomiting
- Diaphoresis
- Pallor
- Hypersalivation
- Yawning
- Hyperventilation
- Anxiety
- Panic
- Malaise
- Fatigue
- Weakness
- Confusion
- Dizziness

PHYSICAL EXAM
No specific findings

DIFFERENTIAL DIAGNOSIS
- Mountain sickness
- Vestibular disease, central and peripheral
- Gastroenteritis
- Metabolic disorders
- Toxin exposure

DIAGNOSTIC TESTS & INTERPRETATION
None indicated

TREATMENT

- Follow guidelines under "General Measures" section to prevent motion sickness (2)[C].

- Premedicate before travel with antidopaminergic, anticholinergic, or antihistamine agents (2)[A]:
  - For extended travel, consider treatment with scopolamine transdermal patch (3)[A].
  - 2nd-generation (nonsedating) antihistamines are not effective at preventing motion sickness (4)[B].
  - Serotonin (5-HT3) antagonists (e.g., ondansetron) do not appear effective in preventing motion sickness (5)[B].
- Conflicting data exist on the efficacy of acupressure for nausea and vomiting associated with motion sickness (6)[B].

- Benzodiazepines suppress vestibular nuclei but would not be considered first line due to sedation and addiction potential (7)[C].

GENERAL MEASURES
- Minimize exposure (sit in middle of plane or boat, front of car)
- Improve ventilation; avoid noxious stimuli
- Use semirecumbent seating or laying supine
- Fix vision on horizon, avoid fixation on moving objects, keep eyes fixed on still, distant objects
- Avoid reading while actively traveling
- Frequent and graded exposure to stimulus that triggers nausea (habituation)
- Minimize food intake before travel; avoid alcohol
- Increase airflow around face

- Acupressure on point PC6 has been shown to reduce feelings of nausea but not the incidence of vomiting during pregnancy, after surgery, and in cancer chemotherapy. However, conflicting evidence of efficacy has been found for motion sickness. Point PC6 (Neiguan on pericardium meridian): 2 cm proximal of transverse crease of palmar side of wrist between tendons of the palmaris longus and the flexor carpi radialis (6)[B].

MEDICATION
First Line
- Scopolamine transdermal patch: Apply 2.5 cm² (4-mg) patch behind ear at least 4 hours (preferably 6–12 hours) before travel, and replace every 3 days (3)[A]:
  - Scopolamine may also be given in tablets, capsules, or oral solution; all are more effective than placebo (3)[A].

- Dimenhydrinate (Dramamine): Take 30–60 minutes before travel:
  - Adults and adolescents: 50–100 mg q4–6h, maximum 400 mg/d
  - Children 6–12 years of age: 25–50 mg q6–8h, maximum 150 mg/d
  - Children 2–6 years of age: 12.5–25 mg q6–8h, maximum 75 mg/d
- Meclizine (Antivert): Take 30–60 minutes before travel. Adults and adolescents >12 years of age: 12.5–25 mg q12–24h
- Cyclizine (Marezine): Take 30–60 minutes before travel:
  - Adults and adolescents: 50 mg q4–6h, maximum 200 mg/d
  - Children 6–12 years of age: 25 mg up to t.i.d.
- Promethazine (Phenergan): Take 30–60 minutes before travel:
  - Adults and adolescents: 25 mg q12h; 25–50 mg IM if already developed severe motion sickness
  - Children 2–12 years of age: 0.5 mg/kg q12h, maximum 25 mg b.i.d. *Caution:* Increased risk of dystonic reaction in this age group

- Contraindications: Patients at risk for acute-angle closure glaucoma
- Precautions:
  – Young children
  – Elderly
  – Pregnancy
  – Urinary obstruction
  – Pyloric-duodenal obstruction
- Adverse reactions:
  – Drowsiness
  – Dry mouth
  – Blurred vision
  – Confusion
  – Headache
  – Urinary retention
- Significant possible interactions:
  – Sedatives (antihistamines, alcohol, antidepressants)
  – Anticholinergics (belladonna alkaloids)

Second Line
- Benzodiazepines: Take 1–2 hours before travel:
  – Diazepam 2–10 mg PO q6–12h
  – Lorazepam 1–2 mg PO q8h
- Contraindications:
  – Severe respiratory dysfunction
  – Severe liver dysfunction
- Precautions:
  – Alcohol/drug abuse
  – Elderly
  – Sedation
  – Addiction is possible

COMPLEMENTARY AND ALTERNATIVE MEDICINE
Ginger: 940 mg or 1 g; take 4 hours before travel (evidence controversial) (8)[B]

 ## ONGOING CARE

FOLLOW-UP RECOMMENDATIONS
- Semirecumbent seating
- Avoid reading while actively traveling

DIET
- Decrease oral intake or take frequent small feedings
- Avoid alcohol

PROGNOSIS
- Symptoms should resolve when motion exposure ends.
- Resistance to motion sickness seems to increase with age.

COMPLICATIONS
- Hypotension
- Dehydration
- Depression
- Panic
- Syncope

REFERENCES

1. Carroll ID, Williams DC. Pre-travel vaccination and medical prophylaxis in the pregnant traveler. *Travel Med Infect Dis*. 2008;6:259–275.
2. Committee to Advise on Tropical Medicine and Travel. Statement on motion sickness. *CCDR*. 2003;29:1–12.
3. Spinks A, Wasiak J, Bernath V. Scopolamine (hyoscine) for preventing and treating motion sickness. *Cochrane Database Syst Rev*. 2011;6:CD002851.
4. Cheung BS, Heskin R, Hofer KD. Failure of cetirizine and fexofenadine to prevent motion sickness. *Ann Pharmacother*. 2003;37:173–177.
5. Hershkovitz D, Asna N, Shupak A, et al. Ondansetron for the prevention of seasickness in susceptible sailors: An evaluation at sea. *Aviat Space Environ Med*. 2009;80:643–646.
6. Streitberger K, Ezzo J, Schneider A. Acupuncture for nausea and vomiting: An update of clinical and experimental studies. *Auton Neuro*. 2006;129:107–117.
7. Zajonc TP, Roland PS. Vertigo and motion sickness. Part II: Pharmacologic treatment. *Ear Nose Throat J*. 2006;85:25–35.
8. White B. Ginger: An overview. *Am Fam Physician*. 2007;75:1689–1691.

ADDITIONAL READING

Murdin L, Golding J, Bronstein A. Managing motion sickness. *BMJ*. 2011;343:d7430.

 ## SEE ALSO

Algorithm: Vertigo

 ## CODES

ICD10
- T75.3XXA Motion sickness, initial encounter
- T75.3XXD Motion sickness, subsequent encounter
- T75.3XXS Motion sickness, sequela

CLINICAL PEARLS

- The scopolamine patch should be applied at least 4 hours before travel, although it may be more effective if placed 6–12 hours before departure.
- Oral medications should be administered 30–60 minutes before departure.
- Although acupressure wristbands have been found to be effective by systematic reviews in postoperative and chemotherapy-induced nausea and vomiting, conflicting data exist for motion sickness.

M

MRSA SKIN INFECTIONS

Stephen A. Martin, MD, EdM • Paul P. Belliveau, PharmD, RPh

BASICS

DESCRIPTION
- Community-acquired methicillin-resistant *Staphylococcus aureus* (CA-MRSA) has properties that allow it to create skin and soft tissue infections (SSTIs) in otherwise healthy hosts:
  - CA-MRSA has a different virulence and disease pattern than hospital-acquired MRSA (HA-MRSA).
- MRSA infections acquired by persons who have not been recently (<1 year) hospitalized or had a medical procedure (e.g., dialysis, surgery, catheters) are known as CA-MRSA infections:
  - This definition is evolving, given the increasing intersection of HA- and CA-MRSA.
- *The prevalence of CA-MRSA is rapidly increasing in the US.*
- CA-MRSA typically causes mild to moderate SSTIs, particularly abscesses, furuncles, and carbuncles:
  - Severe disease from CA-MRSA is less frequent, but can include:
    - Necrotizing pneumonia with abscesses
    - Necrotizing fasciitis
    - Septic thrombophlebitis
    - Sepsis
  - In 1 review, 77% of CA-MRSA infections were SSTIs; only 6% of infections were invasive (e.g., bacteremia, osteomyelitis).
- Although less frequent, HA-MRSA can still cause SSTIs in the community, and clinicians should be alert to this possibility. 1 study showed no significant difference in hospitalization rates among CA-MRSA, HA-MRSA, and methicillin-sensitive *S. aureus* (MSSA) infections.
- System(s) affected: Skin; Soft tissue

EPIDEMIOLOGY
- Predominant age: All ages, generally younger
- Predominant sex: Female > Male

Incidence
- 316/100,000/year (2004–2005)
- 25/100,000/year pediatric MRSA SSTI hospitalizations (2006)

Prevalence
- Still significantly affected by local epidemiology
- 25–30% of US population are colonized with *S. aureus*; up to 7% are colonized with MRSA.
- CA-MRSA was isolated in 59% of skin and soft tissue infections presenting to 11 emergency departments (range 15–74%). In 1993, 1.5 million SSTIs were seen in US emergency rooms. In 2005, this had increased to 3.4 million. Hospital admission data indicate a 29% increase in SSTIs from 2000–2004.
- CA-MRSA accounts for up to 75% of all community staphylococcal infections in children.

ETIOLOGY AND PATHOPHYSIOLOGY
- First noted in 1980, CA-MRSA's current US epidemic began in 1999. The USA 300 clone is predominant.
- CA-MRSA is currently distinguished from HA-MRSA by:
  - Lack of a multidrug-resistant phenotype
  - Presence of exotoxin virulence factors
  - Type IV staphylococcus cassette cartridge (contains the methicillin-resistance gene *mecA*)

RISK FACTORS
- Although several factors are associated with CA-MRSA, their presence or absence cannot reliably predict CA-MRSA itself; in 1 study, almost 1/2 of the patients with CA-MRSA had no established risk factor. Physician suspicion for MRSA has been found to be a poor predictor.
- Any antibiotic use in the past month
- Presence of an abscess
- Reported "spider bite"
- History of MRSA infection
- Close contact with a similar infection
- Children, particularly in day care centers
- Competitive athletes
- Incarceration
- High prevalence in the community
- Hospitalization in the past 12 months (although *S. aureus* can colonize for years)

GENERAL PREVENTION
- Prior research has established colonization (particularly of the anterior nares) as a risk factor for subsequent *S. aureus* infection. It is not yet clear whether this is also the case for CA-MRSA. Oropharyngeal and inguinal colonization appear to be equally prevalent.
- CA-MRSA may be transmitted much more through the environment, including households, than via nares colonization.
- Health care workers have been found to be a major vector of MRSA for hospitalized patients, reinforcing the need for aggressive cleaning of hands and common equipment.
- Research for a vaccine is under way.

COMMONLY ASSOCIATED CONDITIONS
Many patients are otherwise healthy

DIAGNOSIS

HISTORY
- Potential risk factors
- Complaint of "spider bite"
- Prior MRSA skin infection

- Risk factors alone cannot rule in or rule out a CA-MRSA infection (1)[B].

PHYSICAL EXAM
- Exam consistent with a furuncle/carbuncle (boils) or abscess, sometimes with a surrounding cellulitis. A nonsuppurative cellulitis is also possible, although it is a less common presentation of CA-MRSA.
- Erythema
- Increased warmth
- Tenderness
- Swelling
- Fluctuance
- Infected wound
- Folliculitis, pustular lesions
- Appearance like an insect or spider bite
- Tissue necrosis

DIFFERENTIAL DIAGNOSIS
SSTIs due to another cause

DIAGNOSTIC TESTS & INTERPRETATION
Initial Tests (lab, imaging)
- Wound cultures are essential for diagnosis.
- Susceptibility testing; many labs use oxacillin instead of methicillin.
- A "D-zone disk-diffusion test" evaluates for inducible clindamycin resistance in CA-MRSA resistant to erythromycin (2)[C].

- In unclear cases, ultrasound may help delineate an abscess.
- Although CT or MRI may show fascial plane edema in necrotizing fasciitis, it should not delay intervention.

Diagnostic Procedures/Other
Purulent lesions should be incised and drained (I&D), cultured, and tested for susceptibilities.

TREATMENT

- Evidence for the treatment of CA-MRSA SSTIs, including oral antibiotics, is generally based on results of small case series, anecdotal reports, and anticipated susceptibility profiles. Randomized controlled trials are beginning to accumulate and generally show no additional benefit to antibiotic treatment over I&D alone.
- A recent guideline recommends antibiotics with certain conditions, such as severe, systemic infection; immunosuppression; extremes of age; location difficult to drain; drainage failure (3)[C].
- Systematic review does not recommend routine use of agents to eliminate MRSA colonization for patients with infection or their close contacts (4)[C].
- Most CA-MRSA infections are localized SSTIs and do not require hospitalization or vancomycin therapy (4)[C].
- Initial empirical antibiotic coverage should be based on local CA-MRSA prevalence and individual patient risk factors. In 1 pediatric model, cephalexin was the optimal antibiotic for an SSTI only when CA-MRSA prevalence was <10%.

GENERAL MEASURES
- Modify therapy, as necessary, based on culture and susceptibility testing
- Determine if household or other close contacts have SSTI or other infections and facilitate evaluation
- Treat underlying condition (e.g., tinea pedis)
- Restrict contact if wound cannot be covered
- Elevate affected area

MEDICATION
ALERT
- For purulent infections, basic principles include surgical drainage and debulking, wound culture, and narrow-spectrum antimicrobials:
  - *Successful I&D may have more of an effect than antibiotics in mild cases for both adults and children* and is important in general.
  - Moist heat may work for small furuncles.
  - Patients with an abscess are frequently cured by drainage alone.
- CA-MRSA is resistant to β-lactams (including oral cephalosporins and antistaphylococcal penicillins) and often macrolides, azalides, and quinolones.
- Although most CA-MRSA isolates are susceptible to rifampin, this drug should *never* be used as a single agent because of concerns for rapid emergence of resistance. The role of combination therapy with rifampin in CA-MRSA SSTIs is still not clearly defined.
- There has been increasing resistance to clindamycin, both initial (~33%) and induced. However, 1 recent retrospective study found clindamycin to be associated with fewer treatment

failures or recurrences in areas of low clindamycin resistance.
- Although CA-MRSA isolates are susceptible to vancomycin, oral vancomycin cannot be used for CA-MRSA SSTIs due to limited GI absorption.

First Line
CA-MRSA SSTIs: Treat with a 7–14-day course of one of the following agents (duration of therapy depends on severity and clinical response):
- Trimethoprim/sulfamethoxazole (TMP-SMX): DS (160 mg TMP and 800 mg of SMX) 1–2 tablet(s) PO b.i.d. daily (8–12 mg/kg/d of trimethoprim component in 2 divided doses for children)
- Doxycycline or minocycline: 100 mg PO b.i.d. (children >8 years and <45 kg; 2–5 mg/kg/d PO in 1–2 divided doses, not to exceed 200 mg/d; children >8 years and >45 kg, use adult dosing), taken with a full glass of water
- Clindamycin: 300–600 mg PO t.i.d. (10–20 mg/kg/d PO in 3 divided doses for children), taken with full glass of water. Check D-zone test in erythromycin-resistant, clindamycin-susceptible *S. aureus* isolates (if the test is positive, this shows induced resistance and a new antibiotic should be chosen)

Second Line
The above medication options are not sufficient for treatment of severe CA-MRSA SSTIs requiring hospitalization or for HA-MRSA SSTIs. For such infections, consider 1 of the following (3)[A]:
- Vancomycin: Generally 1 g IV q12h (30 mg/kg/d IV in 2 divided doses; in children: 40 mg/kg/d IV in 4 divided doses)
- Linezolid: 600 mg IV/PO b.i.d. (Uncomplicated: Children <5 years of age, 30 mg/kg/d in 3 divided doses; 20 mg/kg/d IV/PO in 2 divided doses for children 5–11 years of age; children >11 years, use adult dosing. Complicated: Birth–11 years, 30 mg/kg/d IV/PO in 3 divided doses; older, use adult dosing).
  – Linezolid seems to be more effective than vancomycin for treating people with SSTIs, but current studies have high risk of bias (5)[A]
- Clindamycin: 600 mg IV t.i.d.; in children, 10–13 mg/kg/dose q6–8h up to 40 mg/kg/d
- Daptomycin: 4 mg/kg/d IV (safety/efficacy not established in patients <18 years of age) if no pulmonary involvement
- Tigecycline: 100 mg IV once, then 50 mg IV q12h (safety/efficacy not established in patients <18 years of age). An increase in all-cause mortality was observed in early studies involving tigecycline-treated patients.
- Telavancin: 10 mg/kg/d IV once a day (for adults)

Pediatric Considerations
- Tetracyclines (including tigecycline) not recommended <8 years
- TMP-SMX not recommended <2 months

Pregnancy Considerations
- Tetracyclines are contraindicated. Tigecycline may cause fetal harm when administered to a pregnant woman.
- TMP-SMX not recommended in 1st or 3rd trimester

Geriatric Considerations
A recent review notes no prospective trials in this age group and recommends use of general adult guidelines.

ISSUES FOR REFERRAL
In addition to inpatient concerns, consider consultation with an infectious disease specialist in cases of:
- Refractory CA-MRSA infection
- Plan to attempt decolonization

SURGERY/OTHER PROCEDURES
Progression to serious SSTIs, including necrotizing fasciitis, is possible and mandates prompt surgical evaluation.

IN-PATIENT CONSIDERATIONS
Admission Criteria/Initial Stabilization
Consider admission in patients either:
- Systemically ill (e.g., febrile) with stable comorbidities, or
- Systemically well with comorbidities that may delay or complicate resolution of their SSTI
- Depends on severity of SSTI, presence of SSTI complications (sepsis, necrotizing fasciitis), and comorbidities

Nursing
Contact precautions

Discharge Criteria
If admitted for IV therapy:
- Afebrile for 24 hours
- Clinically improved
- Able to take oral medication
- Has adequate social support and available for outpatient follow up

 ONGOING CARE

FOLLOW-UP RECOMMENDATIONS
Patient Monitoring
For outpatients:
- Return promptly if patient develops systemic symptoms, worsening local symptoms, or does not improve within 48 hours.
- Consider a follow up within 48 hours of initial visit to assess response and review culture.

PATIENT EDUCATION
- Keep wounds that are draining covered with clean, dry bandages.
- Clean hands regularly with soap and water or alcohol-based gel. Hot shower daily with soap.
- Do not share items that may be contaminated (including razors or towels).
- Clean clothes, towels, and bed linens.
- The CDC has gathered information for health care professionals, including clinical guides, via the National MRSA Education Initiative available at: www.cdc.gov/mrsa/.
- Clinical Infectious Diseases Advance Access. Clinical Practice Guidelines by the Infectious Diseases Society of America for the Treatment of Methicillin-Resistant *Staphylococcus Aureus* Infections in Adults and Children. Available at: www.idsociety.org/uploadedFiles/IDSA/Guidelines-Patient_Care/PDF_Library/MRSA.pdf

PROGNOSIS
- In outpatients, improvement should occur within 48 hours.
- Data are limited as to risk of recurrence.

COMPLICATIONS
- Necrotizing pneumonia or empyema (after an influenza-like illness)
- Necrotizing fasciitis
- Sepsis syndrome
- Pyomyositis and osteomyelitis
- Purpura fulminans
- Disseminated septic emboli
- Endocarditis

REFERENCES
1. Daum RS. Clinical practice. Skin and soft-tissue infections caused by methicillin-resistant *Staphylococcus aureus*. *N Engl J Med*. 2007;357: 380–390.
2. Moellering RC. A 39-year-old man with a skin infection. *JAMA*. 2008;299:79–87.
3. Liu C, Bayer A, Cosgrove SE, et al. Clinical practice guidelines by the Infectious Diseases Society of America for the treatment of methicillin-resistant *Staphylococcus aureus* infections in adults and children. *Clin Infect Dis*. 2011;52:e18–e55.
4. Stryjewski ME, Chambers HF. Skin and soft-tissue infections caused by community-acquired methicillin-resistant *Staphylococcus aureus*. *Clin Infect Dis*. 2008;46(Suppl 5):S368–S377.
5. Yue J, Dong BR, Yang M, et al. Linezolid versus vancomycin for skin and soft tissue infections. *Cochrane Database Syst Rev*. 2013;7:CD008056.
6. Chuck EA, Frazee BW, Lambert L, et al. The benefit of empiric treatment for methicillin-resistant *Staphylococcus aureus*. *J Emerg Med*. 2010;38: 567–571.

ADDITIONAL READING
- Breen JO. Skin and soft tissue infections in immunocompetent patients. *Am Fam Physician*. 2010;81:893–899.
- Chen LF, Chastain C, Anderson DJ. Community-acquired methicillin-resistant *Staphylococcus aureus* skin and soft tissue infections: Management and prevention. *Curr Infect Dis Rep*. 2011;13:442–450.
- Dryden MS. Complicated skin and soft tissue infection. *J Antimicrob Chemother*. 2010; 65(Suppl 3):iii35–iii44.
- Gurusamy KS, Koti R, Toon CD, et al. Antibiotic therapy for the treatment of methicillin-resistant *Staphylococcus aureus* (MRSA) infections in surgical wounds. *Cochrane Database Syst Rev*. 2013;8: CD009726.

 CODES

ICD10
- A49.02 Methicillin resis staph infection, unsp site
- L08.9 Local infection of the skin and subcutaneous tissue, unspecified
- Z22.322 Carrier or suspected carrier of methicillin resis staph

CLINICAL PEARLS
- Incise and drain purulent lesions and send for wound culture.
- Know the prevalence and susceptibilities of CA-MRSA in your location. Consider use of an algorithm to help guide clinical decisions (6)[B].
- Use 1/4-cup household bleach diluted in 1 gallon of water to clean surfaces; no evidence that widespread cleaning (with sprays/foggers) works any better than focused cleaning of frequently touched areas.

M

MULTIPLE MYELOMA

Jasmine S. Beria, DO, MPH • Maria Plummer, MD

 BASICS

DESCRIPTION
- Multiple myeloma (MM) is a clonal proliferation of malignant plasma cells.
- This clonal proliferation in the bone marrow can cause extensive skeletal destruction with osteolytic lesions and pathologic fractures.
- The malignant plasma cells produce monoclonal protein in the blood and urine.
- MM is also characterized by hypercalcemia, increased susceptibility to infections, renal impairment, and end organ damage (1).
- Monoclonal gammopathy of undetermined significance (MGUS) is a common disorder with limited monoclonal plasma cell proliferation that progresses to MM at rate of ~1% per year.
- MGUS progresses to smouldering or asymptomatic MM and eventually to symptomatic MM.
- Synonym(s): Plasma cell myeloma; Plasma cell leukemia

EPIDEMIOLOGY
- Accounts for ~1% of all cancers and slightly >10% of hematologic malignancies in the US.
- Median age of diagnosis is 69 years; 62.2% diagnosed at age ≥65 years
- Slight male predominance. Blacks about 2–3× more commonly affected than whites. Less common in Asians.

Incidence
4–5 new cases/100,000 annually

Prevalence
In 2010, there were 77,617 cases in the US (2).

ETIOLOGY AND PATHOPHYSIOLOGY
- Clonal proliferation of plasma cells derived from postgerminal center B cells (3)
- Plasma cells undergo multiple chromosomal mutations to progress to MM
- Genetic damage in developing B lymphocytes at time of isotype switching, transforming normal plasma cells into malignant cells, arising from single clone
- Earliest chromosomal translocations involve immunoglobulin heavy chains on chromosome 14q32 and partner genes c-MAF (16q23), FGFR3/MMSET (4p16.3), cyclin D1 (11q13), and cyclin D3 (6p21).
- Activation of K-RAS and N-RAS, mutations in TP53, and changes in c-myc are associated with disease progression (4).
- Malignant cells multiply in bone marrow, suppressing normal bone marrow cells and producing large quantities of monoclonal immunoglobulin (M) protein.
- There is suppression of humoral and cell-mediated immunity and increased cell-mediated immunity with increased interleukin -6 (IL-6) (1).
- Malignant cells stimulate osteoclasts that cause bone resorption and inhibit osteoblasts that form new bone, causing lytic bone lesions.

Genetics
Rare family clusters

RISK FACTORS
- Most cases have no known risks associated.
- Older age, immunosuppression and chemicals like dioxin, herbicides, insecticides, petroleum, heavy

metals, plastics, and ionizing radiation increase the risk of MM.
- MGUS stage consistently precedes MM.

COMMONLY ASSOCIATED CONDITIONS
Secondary amyloidosis commonly due to MM

 DIAGNOSIS

HISTORY
- 34% of patients are asymptomatic at the time of presentation.
- Hypercalcemia (28%): Anorexia, nausea, somnolence, and polydipsia
- Renal failure (20–50%)
- Anemia (73%)
- Bony lesions (80%): Lytic lesions causing bone pain (58%) (3), osteoporosis or pathologic fracture (26–34%)
- Other symptoms: Fatigue (32%), peripheral neuropathy, weight loss (24%), recurrent infections, hyperviscosity syndrome, and cord compression

PHYSICAL EXAM
- Dehydration
- Skin findings of amyloidosis: Waxy papules, nodules, or plaques that may be evident in the eyelids, retroauricular region, neck, or inguinal and anogenital regions; petechiae and ecchymosis; "pinch purpura"
- Extramedullary plasmacytomas can present as large, purplish, subcutaneous masses
- Hyperviscosity syndrome in 7%: Retinal hemorrhages, prolonged bleeding, neurologic changes
- Tender bones and masses

DIFFERENTIAL DIAGNOSIS
- MGUS
- Smouldering MM
- Metastatic carcinoma (kidney, breast, non-small cell lung cancer)
- Waldenström macroglobulinemia
- AL amyloidosis
- Solitary plasmacytoma
- POEMS (Polyneuropathy, Organomegaly, Endocrinopathy, M protein, Skin changes) syndrome

DIAGNOSTIC TESTS & INTERPRETATION
Criteria for diagnosis: The diagnosis of MM requires all of the following (3)[A]:
- Bone marrow (BM) involvement with ≥10% of plasma cells (PC) or the presence of a plasmacytoma
- Monoclonal protein (M-spike) in the blood and/or urine
- Presence of one or more of the following: calcium elevation (>11.5 g/dL), renal insufficiency (creatinine >2 mg/dL), anemia (hemoglobin <10 g/dL or 2 g/dL < normal), bone disease (lytic or osteopenic)

Initial Tests (lab, imaging)
- CBC with differential to evaluate anemia and other cytopenias with evaluation of peripheral blood smear
- BUN, creatinine (elevated creatinine due to myeloma cast nephropathy)

- Serum electrolytes, serum albumin, serum calcium
- Serum lactate dehydrogenase (LDH), β_2-microglobulin
- Serum protein electrophoresis (SPEP), serum immunofixation electrophoresis (SIFE): M protein level elevated
- Quantitative serum immunoglobulin levels: Immunoglobulin (Ig) G, IgA, and IgM
- Quantitative serum free light chain (FLC) levels: κ and λ chains
- Elevated ESR, C-reactive protein
- Urine analysis: 24-hour urine for protein, urine protein electrophoresis (UPEP), urine immuno-fixation electrophoresis (UIFE); 20% positive urine protein (3)[A]:
  – Urinalysis dip is often negative for protein, as this test identifies albumin and the protein in MM is Bence Jones (BJ) monoclonal protein.
- Bone marrow aspirate and biopsy for histology, immunohistochemistry, flow cytometry, cytogenetics, and fluorescence in situ hybridization (FISH)
- Skeletal survey: For lytic bone lesions, osteopenia, osteoporosis, or compression fractures
- MRI for any back pain or earliest signs/symptoms of spinal cord compression

Follow-Up Tests & Special Considerations
- CT scan: If high suspicion for bone lesions despite normal skeletal survey; can differentiate malignant from benign vertebral compression fractures in patients who are not MRI candidates
- PET scans: Used if bone involvement is suspected despite a normal skeletal survey, MRI, and CT
- Baseline bone densitometry may be indicated (3)[A]
- Bone marrow aspirate and biopsy to monitor response to treatment
- SPEP with SIFE: M protein helps to track progression of myeloma and response to treatment
- Serum immunoglobulins and free light chains can be used to monitor response or relapse
- Plasma cell labeling index may be helpful to identify the fraction of the myeloma cell population that is proliferating (3)[A].

Diagnostic Procedures/Other
Staging:
- Durie Salmon stage:
  – Stage I: Low cell mass: $<0.6 \times 10^{12}$ cells/m^2 plus all of the following: Hemoglobin >10 g/dL, serum IgG <5 g/dL, serum IgA <3 g/dL, normal serum calcium, urine BJ protein >12 g/24 h, no generalized lytic bone lesions
  – Stage II: Neither stage I nor stage III
  – Stage III: High cell mass: $>1.2 \times 10^{12}$ cells/m^2 plus one or more of the following: Hemoglobin <8.5 g/L, serum calcium >12 mg/dL, bone lesions, IgG >7 g/dL, IgA >5 g/dL, urine BJ protein >12 g/24 h, advanced lytic bone lesions
- International staging system (ISS):
  – Stage I: Albumin ≥3.5 g/dL and β_2-microglobulin <3.5 μg/mL
  – Stage II: Neither stage I nor stage III
  – Stage III: β_2-microglobulin ≥5.5 μg/mL
- Mayo Clinic risk stratification (mSMART):
  – Standard risk: t(11;14), t(6;14), and hyperdiploidy
  – Intermediate risk: t(4;14), del 13q by cytogenetics, hypodiploidy
  – High risk: t(14;16), t(14;20), del 17 p, and plasma cell labeling index >3%

Test Interpretation

Bone marrow involvement with plasma cells ≥10%; Russell bodies

TREATMENT

- Treatment varies depending on level of disease activity and stage of MM.
- Treatment for smoldering MM is close monitoring at 3-month intervals. Clinical trials are ongoing to determine whether newer agents delay progression.
- Key determinant factor in choosing chemotherapy regimen is to establish if the patient is an autologous stem cell transplant (ASCT) candidate or not.
- Treatment protocols vary by institution and patient.
- ASCT following induction chemotherapy is standard of care for patients with symptomatic disease.

GENERAL MEASURES

Maintain adequate hydration to prevent renal insufficiency. All patients receiving primary melanoma therapy should be given bisphosphonates initially (3)[A].

MEDICATION

- Induction chemotherapy for ASCT eligible patients (5)[C]:
  - Standard risk: Rd (lenalidomide/low-dose dexamethasone)
  - Intermediate risk: VCD (bortezomib/ cyclophosphamide/dexamethasone)
  - High risk: VRD (bortezomib]/lenalidomide/ dexamethasone)

  - After ASCT, maintenance can include a bortezomib compound for the high or intermediate risk group; lenalidomide can be considered for the standard group. Maintenance lenalidomide after ASCT has shown to improve progression free survival (PFS) 41 vs. 23 months with placebo (6)[A].

- Induction chemotherapy for ASCT-ineligible patients:
  - Same regimens as ASCT eligible patients; however, the number of treatment cycles are increased (5)[C].

First Line

- Bortezomib:
  - A proteasome inhibitor, it blocks the ubiquitin-proteasome catalytic pathway in cells by binding to the 20S proteasome complex.
  - Toxicity: Peripheral neuropathy, cytopenia, nausea
  - Consider herpes simplex virus (HSV) prophylaxis.
- Cyclophosphamide:
  - Nitrogen mustard–derivative alkylating agent
  - Often used in combination with prednisone or thalidomide in cases of relapsed disease
  - Toxicity: Cytopenia, anaphylaxis, interstitial pulmonary fibrosis, secondary malignancy, impaired fertility
- Immunomodulators:
  - Thalidomide and lenalidomide:
    o Works by antiangiogenesis inhibition, immunomodulation, and inhibition of tumor necrosis factor
    o Toxicity: Birth defects, deep vein thrombosis (DVT), neuropathy, rash, nausea, bradycardia
    o DVT prophylaxis, usually with aspirin

- Dexamethasone:
  - Low doses (40 mg/wk) superior to higher doses
  - Increases risk of DVT
- Bisphosphonates (7)[A]:
  - No effect on mortality but decrease pain, pathological vertebral fractures, and fractures of other bones
  - IV pamidronate or zoledronic acid can be used; evidence that zoledronic acid may be superior in preventing skeletal-related events
  - Dose-adjust/monitor renal function
  - Monitor for osteonecrosis of jaw
- Alternative options:
  - As first-line treatment for patients with newly diagnosed MM, bortezomib/melphalan/ prednisone was associated with significantly increased PFS (31 months) compared with melphalan/prednisone followed by placebo (14 months) or melphalan – prednisone (13 months) (8)[A].

Second Line

- May be treated with any of the agents not already utilized
- The following agents can be used as salvage therapy to treat relapsed or refractory MM:
  - bortezomib/lenalidomide
  - liposomal doxorubicin
  - carfilzomib: Second-generation selective proteasome inhibitor
- Emerging options: pomalidomide, thalidomide analog
- Interferon-α may be appropriate in selected patients, but because of its toxicity and availability of better alternatives, it has a limited role in treating MM.

ISSUES FOR REFERRAL

For spinal or other bone pathology, refer to orthopedics for support.

ADDITIONAL THERAPIES

- Local radiation therapy for bone pain
- ASCT (investigational)
- Effective pain management: Avoid NSAIDs due to nephrotoxicity
- Kyphoplasty/vertebroplasty: Consider for symptomatic vertebral compressions
- Plasmapheresis: For hyperviscosity syndrome (a rare complication)
- Erythropoietin: For selected patients with anemia
- Patients should receive vaccines for pneumococcus and influenza.
- Do not administer zoster vaccine and other live-virus vaccines.

IN-PATIENT CONSIDERATIONS

Admission Criteria/Initial Stabilization

Indications: Pain, infections, cytopenia, renal failure, bone complications, spinal cord compression

- Avoid IV radiographic contrast materials due to risk for contrast-induced nephropathy
- Adequate hydration
- Manage hypercalcemia and control hyperuricemia

ONGOING CARE

PATIENT EDUCATION

www.myeloma.org
www.nccn.org/patients/patient_guidelines/myeloma/index.html

PROGNOSIS

- Median survival overall is 3 years. The 5-year survival rate is around 35%.
- Median survival by ISS stage:
  - Stage I: 62 months
  - Stage II: 44 months
  - Stage III: 29 months
- Median survival in patients with high-risk multiple myeloma (see "Staging" for definition) is <2–3 years, even after ASCT; standard risk have median overall survival of 6–7 years (5)[C].

COMPLICATIONS

Many, including infection, pain, lytic bone lesions, hypercalcemia, hyperuricemia, spinal cord compression, anemia, hyperviscosity syndrome, amyloidosis, renal insufficiency

REFERENCES

1. Singhal S, Mehta J. Multiple myeloma. *Clin J Am Soc Nephrol*. 2006;1:1322–1330.
2. Howlader N, Noone AM, Krapcho M, et al. SEER cancer statistics review, 1975–2010. National Cancer Institute. Bethesda, MD. Available at: http://seer.cancer.gov/csr/1975_2010/ (based on November 2012 SEER data submission, posted to the SEER website, 2013).
3. NCCN multiple myeloma clinical practice guidelines in oncology (Version 2.2013). 2013 National Comprehensive Cancer Network, Inc. Available at: www.nccn.org
4. Palumbo A, Anderson K. Multiple myeloma. *N Engl J Med*. 2011;364:1046–1060.
5. Rajkumar SV. Multiple myeloma: 2013 update on diagnosis, risk-stratification, and management. *Am J Hematol*. 2013;88:226–235.
6. Attal M, Lauwers-Cances V, Marit G, et al. Lenalidomide maintenance after stem-cell transplantation for multiple myeloma. *N Engl J Med*. 2012;366:1782–1791.
7. Mhaskar R, Redzepovic J, Wheatley K, et al. Bisphosphonates in multiple myeloma. *Cochrane Database Syst Rev*. 2010;3:CD003188.
8. Palumbo A, Hajek R, Delforge M, et al. Continuous lenalidomide treatment for newly diagnosed multiple myeloma. *N Engl J Med*. 2012;366:1759–1769.

 CODES

ICD10

- C90.00 Multiple myeloma not having achieved remission
- C90.01 Multiple myeloma in remission
- C90.02 Multiple myeloma in relapse

M

CLINICAL PEARLS

- MM is a plasma cell malignancy that causes end-organ damage.
- Look for presence of "CRAB" (hypercalcemia, renal insufficiency, anemia, and bone lesions).
- Suspect MM if high total protein-to-albumin ratio is present.
- Maintain high index of suspicion for spinal cord compression.
- Avoid nephrotoxins (radiographic contrast material, NSAIDs, dehydration).
- Patients with MM are immunocompromised.

MULTIPLE SCLEROSIS

Rasai L. Ernst, MD • Carmen Tran, MD • Matthew Goldman, MD

 BASICS

DESCRIPTION

- Multiple sclerosis (MS) is an autoinflammatory disease causing demyelination, neuronal loss, and scarring within the white matter of the brain and spinal cord (1,2)
- 4 recognized forms of MS (1,2,3):
  – Relapsing/Remitting MS (RRMS) (85%): Episodic flare ups occurring over days to weeks between periods of neurologic stability. During attacks, new symptoms may present while previous symptoms may worsen. Complete recovery or residual deficits may ensue following each bout.
  – Secondary progressive MS (SPMS): Beginning as RRMS, progressive deterioration in neurologic function, unassociated with attacks, eventually ensues (progression may continue or halt). ~2% risk per year of RRMS becoming SPMS.
  – Primary progressive MS (PPMS) (~15%): Steady decline of neurologic function from onset of disease without episodic flares.
  – Progressive/Relapsing MS (PRMS) (~5%): Steady decline of neurologic function from onset of disease with episodic flare ups.

Pregnancy Considerations
- Most patients experience lower exacerbation rates during pregnancy. Following delivery, the immune system reverts and MS flares become more likely (4).
- Breastfeeding does not affect the risk of MS relapse (4).
- Relapse during postpartum can be safely treated by IVIG and corticosteroids (4).

EPIDEMIOLOGY
- Age: Peak incidence occurs between 20–40 years (slightly earlier in women than men) (2)
- Gender: Women are ~3 × more likely to develop MS than men (5)
- Latitude: Prevalence tends to rise with increasing distance from the equator, though newer data reveals this latitude gradient may be declining (6,7)

Incidence
- Women (worldwide): 3.6 cases/100,000 person-years (7)
- Men (worldwide): 2.0 cases/100,000 person-years (7)

Prevalence
- US: ~350,000 MS patients
- Worldwide: ~2.5 million MS patients

ETIOLOGY AND PATHOPHYSIOLOGY
- MS lesions: Inflammatory cells, mainly T lymphocytes and macrophages, surround vasculature within the CNS, creating sites of inflammation. These cells then disrupt the blood–brain barrier and infiltrate the surrounding white matter, meanwhile preserving the vessel wall. B lymphocytes as well as myelin-specific autoantibodies also infiltrate the CNS and cause degeneration of the myelin sheaths (2).
- Following demyelination, faster salutatory nerve conduction velocities (impulses jumping between nodes of Ranvier) are replaced with considerably slower continuous nerve velocities (2).
- Astrocytes begin to proliferate and cause gliosis (2).
- Oligodendrocytes, which have survived, or those formed from precursor cells, are able to partially remyelinate stripped axons, producing irreversible scars (2).

- In each MS lesion, axonal damage may occur, but it is the cumulative axonal loss over time that is responsible for the progressive and irreversible neurologic disability seen in MS patients (1,2).
- Most axons are typically lost from the lateral coticospinal (motor) tracts of the spinal cord (2).

Genetics
- Strong predisposition: HLA *DRB1* (2)
- Proposed predisposition: *IL2RA* and *IL7RA* (2)
- Race: Whites > Africans or Asians (2)

RISK FACTORS
- Genetic: *DRB1* locus on chromosome 6 has strongest MS risk association; *DRB1*15* and *16* produce major histocompatibility complexes (MHC) with high binding affinity to myelin basic proteins (MPBs) (2,6)
- Geographic: Sun exposure to the skin provides the ultraviolet-B (UVB) radiation necessary for endogenous vitamin D production. Insufficient UVB radiation exposure, especially in higher latitudes during winter months, is more common in temperate zones (6).
- Infectious: Epstein-Barr virus, human herpes viruses (2,6)
- Race: White > African or Asian (2)
- Others: Tobacco smoking (5)

GENERAL PREVENTION
Further research is required to determine prevention from environmental risk factors. A goal of therapy is to prevent new attacks and disability (1,5,6).

COMMONLY ASSOCIATED CONDITIONS
- Internuclear ophthalmoplegia (INO): Injury to the medial longitudinal fasciculus (MLF) causes impaired adduction to the affected eye
- Optic neuritis: Inflammation of optic nerve resulting in loss of vision
- Uhthoff's phenomenon: Symptoms worsen with exposure to higher than usual temperature.
- L'hermitte's sign: Electric-like shocks extending down spine caused by neck movement, especially flexion.

 DIAGNOSIS

- A person with MS can have almost any neurologic symptom or sign depending on the location of the lesions within the CNS (2).
- Clinical diagnosis: ≥2 attacks; objective clinical evidence of ≥2 lesions or objective clinical evidence of 1 lesion with history of a previous episode. Flare up duration must be at least >24 hours. Relapses must be separated by ≥1 month. ≥1 of 2 neurologic signs must be present. The 2nd clinical sign may be obtained through an abnormal paraclinical exam such as MRI or evoked potentials (EPs) or may be supported by an abnormal paraclinical exam (2,8,9).
- For patients with steady decline of neurologic function for ≥6 months without flares, intrathecal immunoglobulin (Ig) G may be used to support the diagnosis (2,9).

HISTORY
Symptoms may include fatigue, depression, emotional instability, epilepsy, memory loss, diplopia, sudden vision loss, facial palsy, dysarthria, dysphagia, muscle weakness or spasms, ataxia, vertigo, falls, hypesthesia or paraesthesia, pain, bowel or bladder incontinence, urinary frequency or retention or impotence (2,8).

PHYSICAL EXAM
- Optic disc swelling or pallor
- Internuclear ophthalmoplegia
- Nystagmus in abducting eye
- Ataxia
- Intention tremor
- Hypesthesia or paresthesia
- Cerebellar dysarthria (scanning speech)
- Spasticity (especially in lower extremities)

DIFFERENTIAL DIAGNOSIS
- Lyme disease
- Systemic lupus erythematosus (SLE)
- Antiphospholipid antibody syndrome
- Epilepsy
- Progressive multifocal leukoencephalopathy (PML)
- CNS neoplasms
- Guillain-Barré syndrome
- Metachromatic leukodystrophy
- Sarcoidosis
- Stroke
- Vascular malformation
- HIV, neurosyphilis
- Cobalamin (B₁₂) deficiency
- Acute disseminated encephalomyelitis (ADEM)
- Behçet disease

DIAGNOSTIC TESTS & INTERPRETATION
- CSF: Increased monocyte cell count and intrathecally formed IgG levels. Total protein within CSF may be normal or increased. The presence of oligoclonal bands (OCB) is used to determine amount of IgG intrathecally synthesized. ≥2 OCBs is diagnostic (2,9)[B].

- Tests used for exclusion of alternative diagnoses: Antinuclear antibodies (ANAs), serum cobalamin level, erythrocyte sedimentation rate (ESR), and testing for syphilis

- MRI of head/spine (more sensitive than CT) (2)[B]:
  – T₂ (spin-echo) image: Hyperintense lesions
  – T₁ image: Hypointense lesions
  – Gadolinium (Gd): Given IV, leakage of Gd into the parenchyma represents an increase in blood–brain barrier permeability due to vascular breakdown.

- McDonald criteria (2,9)[C]:
  – Dissemination in space: ≥1 T₂ lesion on MRI in at least 2 of 4 CNS regions typically affected by MS: Periventricular, juxacortical, infratentorial, or spinal cord or by waiting for another clinical attack implying a different CNS location
  – Dissemination in time: Simultaneous presentation of asymptomatic Gd-enhanced and nonenhancing lesions at any moment or a new T₂ and/or Gd-enhanced lesion on an MRI when compared with baseline scans

Diagnostic Procedures/Other
Evoked potentials (EP): Assesses function in visual, auditory, and somatosensory or motor CNS pathways by measuring CNS electric potentials evoked by stimulation of either the brain or selected peripheral nerves; a marked delay in a provoked CNS EP, without a clinical manifestation, is suggestive of a dymyelinating disorder (2,9)[B].

TREATMENT

Currently, there is no treatment for promoting remyelination or neuronal repair.

GENERAL MEASURES
- 3 main categories currently exist for MS treatment: Treatment for acute relapses, treatment for reducing MS related activity using disease-modifying agents, and symptomatic therapy (2,4).
- For apparent acute relapse, rule out infectious etiology prior to treatment.

MEDICATION
- Acute relapses (4):
  – Methylprednisolone 1 g/d IV for 3–5 days; without subsequent oral tapering; a 2nd course may be given.
    ○ Adverse effects: Fluid retention, potassium loss, weight gain, GI disturbances, acne, and emotional lability

- Reduction of MS biological activity (1,2,10)[B]:
  – Interferon-β (IFN-β):
    ○ Avonex (IFN-β_{1a}) 30 mcg IM weekly
    ○ Rebif (IFN-β_{1a}) 22 or 44 mcg SC 3 × per week
      ■ Betaseron (IFN-β_{1b}) 0.25 mg SC every other day
      ■ Extavia (IFN-β_{1b}) 0.25 mg SC every other day
        □ CBC w/ diff., platelet count, liver function test at 1, 3, 6 months after starting treatment
        □ Thyroid function tests every 6 months if history of thyroid dysfunction
  – Glatiramer acetate:
    ○ Copaxone 20 mg SC daily
      ■ Common adverse reactions: Injection site reaction, nausea, chest pain, hypertonia, diaphoresis
      ■ No routine monitoring tests recommended
  – Natalizumab (Tysabri): 300 mg IV every 4 weeks
    ○ Restricted distribution in the US; Call 1-800-456-2255 for more information.
    ○ MRI at baseline
  – Fingolimod (Gilenya): 0.5 mg PO daily
    ○ ECG at baseline
    ○ Serious adverse reactions: QT prolongation, AV block; 6-hour observation following 1st dose
  – Teriflunomide (Aubagio): 7–14 mg PO daily
    ○ Avoid pregnancy, teratogenic; pregnancy test at baseline
    ○ Use reliable contraception during treatment

- Symptomatic therapies (2)[C]:
  – Ataxia: Clonazepam, Propanolol, Ondansetron
  – Spasticity: Baclofen, diazepam, tizanidine, dantrolene, cyclobenzaprine hydrochloride
  – Pain: NSAIDs, carbamazepine, gabapentin, phenytoin, amitriptyline, mexiletine
  – Bladder dysfunction: (Urgency) propantheline bromide, oxybutynin, tolterodine tartrate; (Retention) Phenoxybenzamine, terazosin hydrochloride, bethanechol
  – Constipation: High-fiber diets, fluids, natural or other laxatives, stool softeners, bulk-producing agents, suppositories
  – Sexual dysfunction: Tadalafil, sildenafil, vardenafil
  – Weakness/fatigue: Dalfampridine, amantadine, methylphenidate
  – Tremors: Clonazepam, β-blockers, primidone
  – Depression: Fluoxetine other selective serotonin reuptake inhibitors (SSRIs), tricyclic antidepressants, nontricyclic antidepressants

ADDITIONAL THERAPIES
- Cognitive behavioral therapy
- Physical and occupational therapy
- Water therapy: Swimming, in cool water, is typically well tolerated

COMPLEMENTARY AND ALTERNATIVE MEDICINE
- Omega-3: immunomodulary properties
- Vitamin D supplementation, sunlight exposure

 ONGOING CARE

FOLLOW-UP RECOMMENDATIONS
Treat relapses with corticosteroids to minimize disease progression and duration of relapse. Maintain regular activity, but avoid overwork and fatigue. Rest during periods of acute relapse (4).

Patient Monitoring
Assessing the severity of neurologic impairment from MS can be done using the Kurtzke Expanded Disability Status Score (EDSS): 0 indicates a normal neurologic exam and 10 indicate death due to MS. The EDDS uses a functional status (FS) score, covering the following: Pyramidal symptoms, cerebellar, brainstem, sensory, bowel and bladder, visual/optic and cerebral/mental functions (11):
- 0.0: Normal neurological examination
- 1.0: No disability, minimal signs in 1 FS
- 2.0: Minimal disability in 1 FS
- 3.0: Moderate disability in 1 FS or mild disability in 3–4 FS, but fully ambulatory
- 4.0: Ambulatory without aid or rest for ~500 m
- 5.0: Ambulatory without aid or rest for ~200 m
- 6.0: Intermittent or constant unilateral assistance (cane, crutch, or brace) required to walk 100 m with or without rest
- 7.0: Unable to walk beyond 5 m even with aid, essentially restricted to wheelchair, wheels self and transfers alone; active in wheelchair for ~12 h/day
- 8.0: Essentially restricted to bed, chair, or wheelchair, but may be out of bed most of the day; retains self-care functions, generally effective use of arms
- 9.0: Helpless, bed-bound, but can communicate, eat
- 9.5: Unable to effectively communicate, eat/swallow

DIET
High-fiber diet with bulk laxatives and plenty of fluids to prevent constipation (2)[B]

PATIENT EDUCATION
National Multiple Sclerosis Society: 1-800-344-4867 or www.nationalmssociety.org/

PROGNOSIS
- Differs in each individual; depends on the form of MS, the individual's sex and age, the initial presentation of the disease, and the amount of disability the patient has (2).
- Average life expectancy is 5–10 years less than unaffected people (3).
- Specific clinical features suggest a more favorable course: Early onset, RRMS form, female sex, <2 relapses within 1st year of diagnosis, and minimal functional decline after 5 years (2)
- Mortality secondary to an MS relapse is very rare; death is more commonly associated with a complication of MS such as an infection in a person who is more disabled (3).

COMPLICATIONS
Depression or emotional instability, paraplegia, chronic pain, sexual dysfunction, delirium, impaired vision (11)

REFERENCES
1. Compston A, Coles A. Multiple sclerosis. *Lancet*. 2008;372:1502–1517.
2. Rejdak K, Jackson S, Giovannoni G. Multiple sclerosis: a practical overview for clinicians. *Br Med Bull*. 2010;95:79–104.
3. Weinshenker BG. Natural history of multiple sclerosis. *Ann Neurol*. 1994;36(Suppl):S6–S11.
4. Thrower BW. Relapse management in multiple sclerosis. *Neurologist*. 2009;15:1–5.
5. Ascherio A, Munger KL. Environmental risk factors for multiple sclerosis. Part II: Noninfectious factors. *Ann Neurol*. 2007;61:504–513.
6. Ascherio A, Munger KL. Environmental risk factors for multiple sclerosis. Part I: The role of infection. *Ann Neurol*. 2007;61:288–299.
7. Alonso A, Hernán MA. Temporal trends in the incidence of multiple sclerosis: A systematic review. *Neurology*. 2008;71:129–135.
8. Polman CH, Reingold SC, Banwell B, et al. Diagnostic criteria for multiple sclerosis: 2010 revisions to the McDonald criteria. *Ann Neurol*. 2011;69:292–302.
9. Mcdonald WI, Compston A, Edan G, et al. Recommended diagnostic criteria for multiple sclerosis: Guidelines from the International Panel on the diagnosis of multiple sclerosis. *Ann Neurol*. 2001;50:121–127.
10. Zintzaras E, Doxani C, Mprotsis T, et al. Network analysis of randomized controlled trials in multiple sclerosis. *Clin Ther*. 2012;34:857–869.e9.
11. Kurtzke JF. Rating neurologic impairment in multiple sclerosis: An expanded disability status scale (EDSS). *Neurology*. 1983;33:1444–1452.

CODES

ICD10
G35 Multiple sclerosis

CLINICAL PEARLS
- Immune mediated inflammatory disease causing demyelination, neuronal loss, and scarring within the white matter of the CNS.
- Charcot's classical MS triad: Nystagmus, intention tremor, and dysarthria.
- Acute relapses are treated with steroids.
- Disease modifying medications are used for chronic treatment; currently, there is no treatment for promoting remyelination or neuronal repair.

M

MUMPS

Frances Yung-tao Wu, MD

 BASICS

Mumps is an acute, generalized paramyxovirus infection usually presenting with unilateral or bilateral parotitis.

DESCRIPTION
- Painful parotitis occurs in 95% of symptomatic mumps, but 1/3 of mumps cases may be asymptomatic.
- Epidemics in late winter and spring, with transmission by respiratory secretions
- Incubation ~14–24 days
- System(s) affected: Hematologic/Lymphatic/Immunologic; Reproductive; Skin/Exocrine
- Synonym(s): Epidemic parotitis; Infectious parotitis

EPIDEMIOLOGY
- Predominant age: 85% occur before age 15:
  – Adult cases typically more severe
- Predominant sex: Male = Female
- Geriatric population: Most are immune
- Acute epidemic mumps:
  – Most cases occur in children aged 5–15 years.
  – Recent (2006) US epidemic in vaccinated college students aged 18–24 years with 5,700 US cases:
    ○ Another US epidemic 2009–2010 in NY/NJ, >1,500 cases (1)
  – Unusual in children <2 years of age
  – Most infants <1 year are immune.
  – Urban epidemics among nonvaccinated populations
  – Communicable period 24 hours before to 72 hours after parotitis onset
  – Incubation period 18 days

Incidence
- 404 cases in the US in 2011
- Occasional epidemic outbreaks in a given region

Prevalence
- 0.0064/100,000 persons
- 90% of adults are seropositive even without history.

ETIOLOGY AND PATHOPHYSIOLOGY
Mumps virus replicates in glandular epithelium of parotids, pancreas, and testes:
- Leads to interstitial edema and inflammation
- Interstitial glandular hemorrhage may occur.
- Pressure caused by edema of the testes against the tunica albuginea can lead to necrosis.
- Mumps paramyxovirus
- Other viruses, such as coxsackievirus (rare)

RISK FACTORS
- Foreign travel/exposure: 38% of other nations do *not* vaccinate for mumps, including most of Africa and South Asia.
- Crowded environments such as dormitories
- Waning immunity after single-dose vaccination:
  – After 2 doses, immunity drops from 95% to 86% in 9 years (2)[C].

GENERAL PREVENTION
- Vaccination:
  – 2 doses of live mumps vaccine or measles-mumps-rubella (MMR) vaccine recommended, 1st at 12–15 months and 2nd at 4–6 years of age

  – 95% effective in studies, but field trials show 75–95% efficacy, which may be below level needed for herd immunity to prevent epidemic spread (3)[C].
  – Successful prevention (Finland) may require 95% 1st-dose plus >80% 2nd-dose compliance (4).
  – Adverse effects: Most common proven effect is idiopathic thrombocytopenic purpura (ITP), with incidence of 3.3/100,000 doses.
  – *No relationship between MMR vaccine and autism* (5)[A]
- Immunoglobulin (Ig) is not effective in prevention.
- Postexposure vaccination does not protect from recent exposure.
- Isolate hospitalized patients until 5 days past onset (6)[C].
- Exclude nonimmune individuals for 26 days after last case onset.

Pregnancy Considerations
- There are no proven complications of vaccine, but theoretically one should not vaccinate in pregnancy.
- Immunization of family may protect against later exposures but not the present one.

 DIAGNOSIS

HISTORY
- Initial parotid swelling just behind jaw
- Swelling peaks in 1–3 days, lasts 3–7 days
- Sour foods cause pain in parotid gland region
- Moderate fever, usually not >104°F (40°C):
  – High fever frequently is associated with complications.

PHYSICAL EXAM
- Parotid pain and swelling in one or both glands
- Rare prodrome of fever, neck muscle ache, and malaise
- Meningeal signs in 15%, encephalitis in 0.5%
- Rarely arthritis, orchitis, thyroiditis, mastitis, pancreatitis, oophoritis, myocarditis
- Rare maculopapular, erythematous rash
- Up to 50% of cases may be very mild
- Obscures angle of mandible
- Elevates earlobe
- Redness at opening of Stensen duct but no pus
- Swelling in sternal area; rare, but pathognomonic of mumps

DIFFERENTIAL DIAGNOSIS
- If not epidemic, other viruses are more common: Parainfluenza parotitis, Epstein-Barr virus, coxsackievirus, adenovirus, parvovirus B19
- Suppurative parotitis: Often associated with *Staphylococcus aureus* (presence of Wharton duct pus on massaging parotid gland nearly excludes diagnosis of mumps)
- Recurrent allergic parotitis
- Salivary calculus with intermittent swelling
- Lymphadenitis from any cause, even HIV infection
- Cytomegalovirus parotitis in immunocompromised patients

- Mikulicz syndrome: Chronic, painless parotid and lacrimal gland swelling of unknown cause that occurs in tuberculosis, sarcoidosis, lupus, leukemia, lymphosarcoma, and malignant or benign salivary gland tumors
- Sjögren syndrome, diabetes mellitus, uremia, malnutrition
- Drug-related parotid enlargement (iodides, guanethidine, phenothiazine)
- Other causes of the complications of mumps (meningoencephalitis, orchitis, oophoritis, pancreatitis, polyarthritis, nephritis, myocarditis, prostatitis)
- Mumps orchitis must be differentiated from testicular torsion and from chlamydial or bacterial orchitis. (Testicular sonogram can be useful.)

DIAGNOSTIC TESTS & INTERPRETATION
- The following 3 special tests to confirm an outbreak should be ordered and reported to health department:
  – IgM titer (positive by day 5 in 100% of nonimmunized patients)
  – Swab of parotid duct or other affected salivary ducts for viral isolation
  – Rise in IgG titer samples; test should be ordered if patient previously immunized, 1st sample within 5 days of onset, 2nd, 2 weeks later.
- Other potential findings: Serum amylase may be elevated; CSF leukocytosis and leukopenia may be present.
- Testicular ultrasound may be useful to differentiate mumps orchitis from testicular torsion.
- Clinical diagnosis (swelling of one or both parotid glands):
  – Lasting ≥2 days
  – No other apparent cause
  – Rare presentation of meningitis without parotitis (1–10%)

Diagnostic Procedures/Other
If meningitis is present, lumbar puncture may be required to prove aseptic meningitis.

Test Interpretation
Periductal edema and lymphocytic infiltration in affected glands

 TREATMENT

- No specific antiviral therapy
- Analgesics to relieve pain
- Avoid corticosteroids for mumps orchitis because they can reduce testosterone concentrations and increase testicular atrophy.
- IVIG only successful for certain autoimmune-based sequelae:
  – Postinfectious encephalitis
  – Guillain-Barré syndrome
  – ITP
- Interferon-α2b improved severe bilateral orchitis and decreased testicular atrophy in small studies.

GENERAL MEASURES
- High fever and testicular pain: May hospitalize for steroids or interferon
- Orchitis:
  - Ice packs to scrotum can help to relieve pain.
  - Scrotal support with adhesive bridge while recumbent and/or athletic supporter while ambulatory

MEDICATION
First Line
- Corticosteroids or NSAIDs may diminish pain and swelling in acute orchitis and arthritis mumps, but usually not necessary.
- May use acetaminophen for fever and/or pain.
- Contraindications: Refer to manufacturer's profile for each drug.
- Precautions: Avoid aspirin for pain in children. Aspirin use in children with viral infections has been associated with Reye syndrome.
- Significant possible interactions: Refer to manufacturer's profile for each drug.

Second Line
- Mumps arthritis may improve with corticosteroids or an NSAID.
- Interferon-α2b × 7 days has been used experimentally in small studies (2)[C] for severe bilateral orchitis to prevent infertility.

IN-PATIENT CONSIDERATIONS
Admission Criteria/Initial Stabilization
- Hospitalize only if CNS symptoms occur.
- Outpatient supportive care if no complications

IV Fluids
If severe nausea or vomiting accompanies pancreatitis

 ONGOING CARE

FOLLOW-UP RECOMMENDATIONS
Mumps orchitis:
- Bed rest and local supportive clothing (e.g., 2 pairs of briefs) or adhesive-tape bridge
- Must be out of school until no longer contagious: About 9 days after onset of pain

Patient Monitoring
Most cases will be mild. Monitor hydration status.

DIET
Liquid diet if cannot chew

PATIENT EDUCATION
Orchitis is common in older children but rarely results in sterility, even after bilateral orchitis.

PROGNOSIS
- Complete recovery is usual; immunity is lifelong.
- Transient sensorineural hearing loss occurs in 4% of adults.
- Rare recurrence after 2 weeks may be recurrent nonepidemic parotitis.

COMPLICATIONS
- May precede, accompany, or follow salivary gland involvement and may occur (rarely) without primary involvement of the parotid gland
- Orchitis is common (30%) in postpubertal boys:
  - It starts within 8 days after parotitis.
  - Fever, swollen testis of 4 days' duration
  - Impaired fertility in 13%, but absolute sterility is rare.
- Meningitis (1–10%) or encephalitis (0.1%) may present 5–10 days after 1st symptoms of illness. Aseptic meningitis typically is mild, but meningoencephalitis may lead to seizures, paralysis, hydrocephalus, or, in 2% of encephalitis patients, death.
- Acute cerebellar ataxia has been reported after mumps infections; self-resolving in 2–3 weeks.
- CSF pleocytosis, usually lymphocytes, found in 65% of patients with parotitis
- Oophoritis in 7% of postpubertal females; no decreased fertility
- Pancreatitis, usually mild
- Nephritis, thyroiditis, and arthralgias are rare.
- Myocarditis: Usually mild, but may depress ST segment; may be linked to endocardial fibroelastosis
- Deafness: 1/15,000 unilateral nerve deafness; may not be permanent
- Inflammation about the eye (keratouveitis) rarely
- Dacryoadenitis, optic neuritis

Pediatric Considerations
- Orchitis is more common in adolescents.
- Young children are less likely to develop complications.
- Most complications occur in postpubertal group.
- Avoid aspirin use in children with viral symptoms.

Pregnancy Considerations
Disease may increase the rate of spontaneous abortion in first trimester; however, perinatal mumps has been reported to take a benign course.

REFERENCES

1. Centers for Disease Control and Prevention (CDC). Update: Mumps outbreak—New York and New Jersey, June 2008–Jan 2010. *Morb Mortal Wkly Rep.* 2010;59:125–129.
2. Hviid A, Rubin S, Mühlemann K. Mumps. *Lancet.* 2008;371:932–944.
3. Hindiyeh MY, Aboudy Y, Wohoush M, et al. Characterization of large mumps outbreak among vaccinated Palestinian refugees. *J Clin Microbiol.* 2009;47:560–565.
4. MacDonald N, Hatchette T, Elkout L, et al. Mumps is back: Why is mumps eradication not working? *Adv Exp Med Biol.* 2011;697:197–220.
5. Flaherty DK. The vaccine-autism connection: A public health crisis caused by unethical medical practices and fraudulent science. *Ann Pharmacother.* 2011;45:1302–1304.
6. Centers for Disease Control and Prevention (CDC). Updated recommendations for isolation of persons with mumps. *Morb Mortal Wkly Rep.* 2008;57:1103–1105.

ADDITIONAL READING
- Myung NS, Kim YJ, Kim YJ, et al. Complicated mumps viral infection: An unusual presentation affecting only submandibular gland. *Am J Otolaryngol.* 2013;34:600–602.
- Shirts BH, Welch RJ, Couturier MR. Seropositivity rates for measles, mumps and rubella IgG and costs associated with testing and revaccination. *Clin Vaccine Immunol.* 2013;20:443–445.

 CODES

ICD10
- B26.1 Mumps meningitis
- B26.2 Mumps encephalitis
- B26.9 Mumps without complication

CLINICAL PEARLS
- Mumps is a clinical diagnosis, including swelling of ≥1 parotid glands for ≥2 days without other obvious cause, but confirmatory tests must be done for epidemics.
- Ultrasound is useful to distinguish testicular torsion from testicular pain related to mumps orchitis.
- MMR vaccine is only 75–95% effective in field trials; therefore, expect some cases of mumps despite completed vaccinations.

M

MUSCULAR DYSTROPHY

Austin Larson, MD

BASICS

- Primary inherited myopathies caused by dysfunctional proteins of muscle fibers and extracellular matrix
- Distribution of weakness, other associated symptoms, and disease prognosis depend on the specific gene affected and severity of the mutation

DESCRIPTION

- Duchenne muscular dystrophy (DMD):
  - Highest-incidence muscular dystrophy, X-linked inheritance, early onset, progressive
  - Patients are wheelchair dependent prior to age 13
- Becker muscular dystrophy (BMD):
  - Less-severe phenotype than Duchenne, also caused by mutation in *DMD* gene
  - Distinction from DMD is clinical: Patients are wheelchair dependent after age 16
  - Collectively referred to as dystrophinopathies
- Myotonic muscular dystrophy (MMD):
  - Myotonia (slow relaxation after muscle contraction), distal and facial weakness
  - 2nd most common inherited muscle disease
- Fascioscapulohumeral muscular dystrophy (FSHMD):
  - Facial and shoulder muscles most affected
  - 3rd most common inherited muscle disease
- Limb-girdle muscular dystrophy (LGMD):
  - Proximal weakness and atrophy, variable prognosis with many different identified mutations
- Oculopharyngeal muscular dystrophy (OPMD):
  - Usually adult onset, affects extraocular and pharyngeal muscles
- Emery-Dreifuss muscular dystrophy (EDMD):
  - Early development of joint contractures, often cardiomyopathy
- Congenital muscular dystrophies (CMD):
  - Heterogeneous group of myopathic diseases presenting in infancy with generally poor prognosis
  - Includes Fukuyama CMD, Ullrich CMD, Walker Warburg syndrome, Muscle-eye-brain disease, other conditions

EPIDEMIOLOGY

Incidence
- Duchenne: 1/3,500 male births
- Myotonic dystrophy: 1/10,000 births
- Other muscular dystrophies vary widely by population, but are generally rare

ETIOLOGY AND PATHOPHYSIOLOGY

Mutations affect proteins connecting cytoskeleton to cell membrane and extracellular matrix causing muscle fibers to become fragile and easily damaged; muscle weakness and atrophy result:

- DMD/BMD:
  - Defective protein is dystrophin, product of the largest human gene, *DMD;* Duchenne phenotype results from mutations that cause profound loss of dystrophin function
  - Becker phenotype results from less severe mutations in *DMD* gene; patients have low but detectable levels of functional dystrophin
- MMD: Trinucleotide repeat expansion in the untranslated region of the gene *DMPK* on chromosome 19; encodes myotonin-protein kinase
- LGMD: Mutations in genes encoding proteins associated with dystrophin: calpain-, dysferlin-, and fukutin-related proteins are affected most commonly

- EDMD: Dysfunctional proteins are associated with the nuclear membrane in muscle fibers; emerin in X-linked form, lamin A/C in autosomal forms
- OPMD: Trinucleotide repeat expansion in *PABPN1* results in nuclear inclusions in muscle cells
- FSHMD: Deletion in untranslated region of chromosome 4 that likely affects expression of multiple genes by epigenetic effects

Genetics

- X-linked:
  - Duchenne and Becker muscular dystrophy:
    - 30% of affected males have a de novo mutation (mother is not a carrier).
    - 20% of female carriers have some manifestation of the mutation (usually mild muscle weakness or cardiomyopathy)
- Autosomal dominant:
  - Generally later onset and less severe than diseases with recessive or X-linked inheritance
  - FSHMD, OPMD, some forms of LGMD and EDMD
  - Myotonic dystrophy:
    - Trinucleotide repeat expansion with more severe phenotype in subsequent generations due to accumulation of repeats
- Autosomal recessive:
  - Most types of CMD

GENERAL PREVENTION

Genetic counseling for known carriers

COMMONLY ASSOCIATED CONDITIONS

- Decreased IQ: On average, 1 SD below the mean in DMD
- Dilated cardiomyopathy and conduction abnormalities:
  - Can be severe in EDMD
  - Can affect otherwise asymptomatic female carriers of DMD

DIAGNOSIS

HISTORY

- DMD: Normal attainment of early motor milestones with subsequent abnormal gait and slowing gross motor development; clumsiness, weakness in toddlers and young children
- BMD: Progressive difficulty with ambulation and frequent falls in later childhood
- MMD: Slurred speech, muscle wasting, difficulty with ambulation; often with family history
- LGMD: Back pain, lordosis/inability to rise from a chair, climb stairs, and use arms overhead
- FSHMD: Facial weakness, inability to close eyes completely
- EDMD: Contractures of elbows and ankles, difficulty with ambulation in teens
- OPMD: Ptosis and dysphagia; often with family history

PHYSICAL EXAM

- DMD/BMD:
  - Proximal muscle weakness; Gower sign: Use of arms to push upper body into standing posture from lying prone
  - Trendelenburg gait (hip waddling)
  - Winged scapulae and lordosis
  - Pseudohypertrophy of the calf (caused by proliferation of fat and connective tissue)
  - Contractures of lower extremity joints and elbows

- MMD:
  - Characteristic facial appearance: Narrow face, open triangular mouth, high arched palate, concave temples, drooping eyelids, frontal balding in males
  - Myotonia: Inability to relax muscles after contraction
  - Distal muscle weakness and wasting
- CMD:
  - Arthrogryposis (multiple joint contractures); diffuse hypotonia and muscle wasting in an infant

DIFFERENTIAL DIAGNOSIS

- Glycogen storage diseases and other metabolic myopathies
- Mitochondrial myopathies: MELAS (**M**itochondrial **E**ncephalopathy, **L**actic **A**cidosis, and **S**troke-like episodes), MERRF (**M**yoclonus with **E**pilepsy and **R**agged-**R**ed **F**ibers)
- Inflammatory myopathies: Polymyositis, dermatomyositis, inclusion-body myositis
- Neuromuscular junction diseases: Myasthenia gravis, Lambert-Eaton syndrome
- Motor neuron diseases: Amyotrophic lateral sclerosis, spinal muscular atrophy
- Charcot-Marie-Tooth disease
- Friedreich ataxia

DIAGNOSTIC TESTS & INTERPRETATION

Initial Tests (lab, imaging)
- Creatine kinase (CK): Initial screening test if MD is suspected (1)
- Elevated in DMD (10–100×); elevated at birth, peaks at time of presentation and falls through course of illness
- Initial detected lab abnormality may be elevated aspartate transaminase/alanine transaminase (AST/ALT) (originating from muscle)
- Genetic testing:
  - For definitive diagnosis in patient with characteristic presentation and elevated creatine kinase (CK)
  - Deletion and duplication analysis will identify most patients; can sequence *DMD* gene for point mutations
  - Genetic testing is available clinically for most other muscular dystrophies

Diagnostic Procedures/Other
- Muscle biopsy: rarely performed in DMD, may be helpful in other cases
- Electromyography and nerve conduction studies are not necessary unless considering alternative diagnoses
- ECG: Abnormalities found in >90% of males and up to 10% of female carriers of DMD; Q waves in anterolateral leads, tall R waves in V_1, shortened PR interval, arrhythmias (2)

Test Interpretation
- Heterogeneic muscle fibers: Atrophy and hypertrophy of fibers with proliferation of connective tissue in muscle
- Immunohistochemical staining for dystrophin protein:
  - DMD: No detectable dystrophin in most fibers; occasional revertant fibers with normal dystrophin
  - BMD: Highly variable staining for dystrophin throughout muscle

TREATMENT

Trials of agents that affect gene expression, such as antisense oligonucleotides, and small molecules that cause skipping of premature stop codons are ongoing (3); however, steroid treatment is the only clinically available therapy that affects disease progression.

GENERAL MEASURES
- Ambulation prolonged by use of knee-ankle-foot orthoses
- Serial casting to treat contractures
- Diagnose sleep apnea with polysomnography; treat with noninvasive ventilation
- Adaptive devices to improve function
- Avoid overexertion and strenuous exercise (4)

MEDICATION
- Prednisone 0.75 mg/kg/d (1,5,6)[A]:
  - Alternative dosing regimens, such as weekend-only treatment or 10 days on/off, are under investigation and appear to have slightly different profiles of benefits and adverse effects
  - Slows the decline in muscle function, progression to scoliosis and degradation of pulmonary function; prolongs functional ambulation; prolongs lifespan; improved cardiac outcomes (7)
  - Initiate therapy when motor function ceases to improve, prior to decline in function
  - Monitor adverse effects and intervene to mitigate harm:
    - Consider bisphosphonates for preventing loss of bone density; annual exam for cataracts; monitor hypertension; avoid NSAID use due to risk of ulcers; stress-dose steroids during surgeries and illnesses due to adrenal suppression
    - Patients should be aware of immune suppression and notify emergency providers
  - Deflazacort is an alternative oral steroid that is also considered first-line therapy in DMD (1)
- ACE inhibitors:
  - Treatment of cardiomyopathy; may be used in conjunction with β-blockers (8)[A]

ISSUES FOR REFERRAL
- Refer to neuromuscular diseases center for definitive diagnosis and coordinated multidisciplinary care (9)
- Cardiology for management of cardiomyopathy
- Pulmonology for monitoring of pulmonary function and clearance regimen
- Physical medicine and rehabilitation for management of adaptive devices

SURGERY/OTHER PROCEDURES
- Spinal surgery for scoliosis—conflicting evidence of efficacy (10)[B]
- Scapular fixation for scapular winging may be beneficial, also lacking clinical trials (11)[B]
- May consider surgical treatment of ankle/knee contractures
- Surgical procedures should be performed at a center experienced in DMD; total IV anesthesia should be used

ONGOING CARE

- Individualized education plan and developmental evaluation for school accommodations (9)
- Maintenance of current influenza and pneumococcal vaccination status

FOLLOW-UP RECOMMENDATIONS
Patient Monitoring
- ECG, echocardiogram, and consultation with a cardiologist at diagnosis and annually after age 10 (12):
  - Female carriers of *DMD* mutation should be monitored every 5 years.
- Annual spinal radiography for scoliosis
- Dual-energy x-ray absorptiometry (DEXA) scanning and serum marker testing for osteoporosis
- Pulmonary function testing twice yearly if no longer ambulatory

DIET
- Obesity is common due to steroid treatment and wheelchair confinement: weight control can improve quality of life
- Diet may be limited by dysphagia; swallow evaluation can determine appropriate foods
- Calcium and vitamin D supplementation is indicated for patients on steroids; vitamin D levels should be monitored

PATIENT EDUCATION
Muscular Dystrophy Association: www.mda.org

PROGNOSIS
- DMD/BMD:
  - Progressive weakness, contractures, inability to walk
  - Kyphoscoliosis and progressive decline in respiratory vital capacity with recurrent pulmonary infections
  - Significantly shortened lifespan (DMD: 16 ± 4 years; BMD: 42 ± 16 years)
- Other types: Slow progression and near-normal life span with functional limitations

COMPLICATIONS
- Cardiac arrhythmia, cardiomyopathy
- Dysphagia, gastroesophageal reflux disease (GERD), constipation
- Scoliosis, joint contractures
- Obstructive sleep apnea
- Malignant hyperthermia-like reaction to anesthesia
- Respiratory failure and early death

REFERENCES

1. Bushby K, Finkel R, Birnkrant DJ, et al. Diagnosis and management of Duchenne muscular dystrophy, part 1: Diagnosis, and pharmacological and psychosocial management. *Lancet Neurol*. 2010;9:77–93.
2. Takami Y, Takeshima Y, Awano H, et al. High incidence of electrocardiogram abnormalities in young patients with Duchenne muscular dystrophy. *Pediatr Neurol*. 2008;39:399–403.
3. Fairclough RJ, Bareja A, Davies KE. Progress in therapy for Duchenne muscular dystrophy. *Exp Physiol*. 2011;84:1101–1113.
4. van der Kooi EL, Lindeman E, Riphagen I. Strength training and aerobic exercise training for muscle disease. *Cochrane Database Syst Rev*. 2005;1: CD003907.
5. Manzur AY, Kuntzer T, Pike M, et al. Glucocorticoid corticosteroids for Duchenne muscular dystrophy. *Cochrane Database Syst Rev*. 2008;1:CD003725.
6. Cossu G, Sampaolesi M. New therapies for Duchenne muscular dystrophy: Challenges, prospects and clinical trials. *Trends Mol Med*. 2007;13:520–526.
7. Schram G, Fournier A, Leduc H, et al. All-cause mortality and cardiovascular outcomes with prophylactic steroid therapy in duchenne muscular dystrophy. *J Am Coll Cardiol*. 2013;61:948–954.
8. Ishikawa Y, Bach JR, Minami R. Cardioprotection for Duchenne's muscular dystrophy. *Am Heart J*. 1999;137:895–902.
9. Bushby K, Finkel R, Birnkrant DJ, et al. Diagnosis and management of Duchenne muscular dystrophy, part 2: Implementation of multidisciplinary care. *Lancet Neurol*. 2010;9: 177–189.
10. Cheuk DKL, Wong V, Wraige E, et al. Surgery for scoliosis in duchenne muscular dystrophy. *Cochrane Database Syst Rev*. 2013;2:CD005375.
11. Orrell RW, Copeland S, Rose MR. Scapular fixation in muscular dystrophy. *Cochrane Database Syst Rev*. 2010;1:CD003278.
12. American Academy of Pediatrics Section on Cardiology and Cardiac Surgery. Cardiovascular health supervision for individuals affected by Duchenne or Becker muscular dystrophy. *Pediatrics*. 2005;116:1569–1573.

CODES

ICD10
- G71.0 Muscular dystrophy
- G71.2 Congenital myopathies
- G71.11 Myotonic muscular dystrophy

CLINICAL PEARLS

- Pediatricians should have a low threshold to obtain serum CK as a screening test in the face of gross motor delay/muscular weakness, especially in boys.
- Steroids should be initiated in patients with DMD when gross motor function ceases to progress.
- High-quality care of patients with MD requires a medical home; a multidisciplinary team of physicians, therapists, and other providers; and extensive patient and family support.

M

MYASTHENIA GRAVIS

Robert A. Baldor, MD

BASICS

DESCRIPTION
Primary disorder of neuromuscular transmission characterized by fluctuating muscle weakness:
- Ocular myasthenia gravis (MG) (15%): Weakness limited to eyelids and extraocular muscles
- Generalized MG (85%): Commonly affects ocular as well as a variable combination of bulbar, proximal limb, and respiratory muscles
- 50% of patients who present with ocular symptoms develop generalized MG within 2 years.
- Onset may be sudden and severe, but it is typically mild and intermittent over many years.
- System(s) affected: Neurologic; Hematologic; Lymphatic; Immunologic; Musculoskeletal

EPIDEMIOLOGY
Occurs at any age, but a bimodal distribution to the age of onset:
- Female predominance: 20–40 years
- Male predominance: 60–80 years

Incidence
Estimated annual incidence 2–4/1 million

Prevalence
In the US, 100–200/1 million; increasing over the past 5 decades

Pediatric Considerations
A transient form of neonatal MG seen in 10–20% of infants born to mothers with MG. It occurs as a result of the transplacental passage of maternal antibodies that interfere with function of the neuromuscular junction. Resolves in weeks to months.

ETIOLOGY AND PATHOPHYSIOLOGY
- Reduction in the acetylcholine receptors (AChR) at muscle endplates, resulting in insufficient neuromuscular transmission
- Seropositive MG: 80–85% of all MG patients:
  – Antiacetylcholine receptor (anti-AChR): A humoral, antibody-mediated, T-cell–dependent attack of the AChRs or receptor-associated proteins at the postsynaptic membrane of the neuromuscular junction.
  – Patients without anti-AChR antibodies may have antibodies against muscle-specific kinase (MuSK) (1). Females tend to be anti-MuSK positive, and respiratory and bulbar muscles are frequently involved.
  – Seronegative MG (SNMG): 6–12% (2).
- Antibody-mediated autoimmune disorder
- Also documented immediately after viral infections (measles, Epstein-Barr [EBV], HIV, and human T-lymphotropic virus [HTLV])

Genetics
- Congenital MG syndrome describes a collection of rare hereditary disorders. This condition is not immune-mediated, but instead results from the mutation of a component of the neuromuscular junction (autosomal-recessive).
- Familial predisposition seen in 5% of cases.

RISK FACTORS
- Familial MG
- D-Penicillamine (drug-induced MG)
- Other autoimmune diseases

COMMONLY ASSOCIATED CONDITIONS
- Thymic hyperplasia (60–70%)
- Thymoma (10–15%)
- Autoimmune thyroid disease (3–8%)

DIAGNOSIS

Myasthenia Gravis Foundation of America Clinical Classification (3)[C]:
- Class I: Any eye muscle weakness, possible ptosis, no other evidence of muscle weakness elsewhere
- Class II: Eye muscle weakness of any severity; mild weakness of other muscles:
  – Class IIa: Predominantly limb or axial muscles
  – Class IIb: Predominantly bulbar and/or respiratory muscles
- Class III: Eye muscle weakness of any severity; moderate weakness of other muscles:
  – Class IIIa: Predominantly limb or axial muscles
  – Class IIIb: Predominantly bulbar and/or respiratory muscles
- Class IV: Eye muscle weakness of any severity; severe weakness of other muscles:
  – Class IVa: Predominantly limb/axial muscles
  – Class IVb: Predominantly bulbar and/or respiratory muscles (can also include feeding tube without intubation)
- Class V: Intubation needed to maintain airway

HISTORY
The hallmark of MG is fatigability:
- Fluctuating weakness, often subtle, that worsens during the day and after prolonged use of affected muscles, may improve with rest
- Early symptoms are transient with asymptomatic periods lasting days or weeks.
- With progression, asymptomatic periods shorten and symptoms fluctuate from mild to severe.
- >50% of patients present with ocular symptoms (ptosis and/or diplopia). Eventually, 90% of patients with MG develop ocular symptoms.
- Ptosis might be unilateral, bilateral, or shifting from eye to eye.
- 15% present with bulbar symptoms.
- <5% present with proximal limb weakness alone.

ALERT
Myasthenic crisis: Respiratory muscle weakness producing respiratory insufficiency and pending respiratory failure

PHYSICAL EXAM
- Ptosis may worsen with propping of opposite eyelid (curtain sign) or sustained upward gaze.
- "Myasthenic sneer," in which the midlip rises, but corners of mouth do not move.
- Muscle weakness is usually proximal and symmetric.
- Test for muscle fatigability by repetitive or prolonged use of individual muscles.
- Important to test and monitor respiratory function.

DIFFERENTIAL DIAGNOSIS
- Thyroid ophthalmopathy
- Oculopharyngeal muscular dystrophy
- Myotonic dystrophy
- Kearns-Sayre syndrome
- Chronic progressive external ophthalmoplegia
- Brainstem and motor cranial nerve lesions
- Botulism
- Motor neuron disease (e.g., amyotrophic lateral sclerosis [ALS])
- Lambert-Eaton myasthenic syndrome
- Drug-induced myasthenia
- Congenital myasthenic syndrome
- Dermatomyositis/Polymyositis
- Neurosarcoidosis
- Tolosa-Hunt syndrome

DIAGNOSTIC TESTS & INTERPRETATION
Initial Tests (lab, imaging)
- Anti-AChR antibody (74–85% are seropositive):
  – Generalized myasthenia: 75–85%
  – Ocular myasthenia: 50%
  – MG and thymoma: 98–100%
  – Poor correlation between antibody titer and disease severity (4)[C]
  – False–positive results in thymoma without MG, Lambert-Eaton myasthenic syndrome, small cell lung cancer, and rheumatoid arthritis treated with penicillamine
- Anti-MuSK antibody:
  – Used if MG suspected, patient seronegative
  – Present in 40–50% of seronegative patients with generalized MG; absent in ocular MG (1,4)[C]
  – These patients are less likely to respond to acetylcholine esterase inhibitors, which may actually worsen symptoms, but they are more likely to respond to plasmapheresis and selected immunotherapy (4)[C].
- Antistriated muscle (anti-SM) antibody:
  – Present in 84% of patients with thymoma who are <40 years of age
  – Anti-SM antibody can be present without thymoma in patients >40 years of age.
- Chest radiographs or CT scans may identify a thymoma.
- MRI of brain and orbits to rule out other causes of cranial nerve deficit

Diagnostic Procedures/Other
- Tensilon (Edrophonium) test:
  – Initial 2-mg IV dose, followed by another 2 mg every 60 seconds up to a maximum dose of 10 mg
  – A positive test shows improvement of strength within 30 seconds of administration.
  – Sensitivity 80–90% (4)[C]
  – Cardiac disease and bronchial asthma are relative contraindications, especially in elderly.
  – Atropine: 0.4–0.6 mg IV may rarely be required as antidote; must be available.
- Ice pack test:
  – For patients with ptosis in whom tensilon test is contraindicated
  – Ice pack applied to closed eyelid for 60 seconds, then removed; extent of ptosis immediately assessed
  – Ice will decrease the ptosis induced by MG.
  – Sensitivity 80% in patients with prominent ptosis

- Electrophysiology testing:
  - Repetitive nerve stimulation (RNS):
    - Widely available, most frequently used
    - Moderately sensitive for both generalized MG (75%) and ocular MG (50%) (4)[C]
  - Single-fiber electromyogram (SFEMG):
    - Assesses temporal variability between 2 muscle fibers within same motor unit (jitter).
    - Sensitive (90–95%), but less specific (4)[C]
    - Technically difficult to perform; limited availability

Test Interpretation
- Lymphofollicular hyperplasia of thymic medulla occurs in 65% of patients with MG, thymoma in 15%
- Immunofluorescence: IgG antibodies and complement on receptor membranes

TREATMENT

GENERAL MEASURES
- Treatment based on age, gender, and disease severity and progression.
- 3 basic approaches: Symptomatic, immunosuppressive, and supportive. Few should receive a single therapeutic modality.

MEDICATION
First Line
Symptomatic treatments (anticholinesterase agents):
- Pyridostigmine bromide (Mestinon):
  - Most commonly prescribed since available in oral tablet
  - Starting dose of 30 mg PO t.i.d.
  - Maximum dose: 120 mg q3–4h
- Neostigmine methylsulfate (Prostigmin):
  - Starting dose of 0.5 mg SC or IM q3h
  - Titrate dosage to clinical need.
- Ambenonium (Mytelase):
  - Longer duration of action than neostigmine, which leads to longer effect at night and on waking (5)[C]
  - Use with caution in patients with asthma and Parkinson disease
  - Starting dose of 5 mg PO t.i.d. or q.i.d.
  - Maintenance dose of 15–100 mg/d, usual 40 mg/d
  - Maximum dose: 50–75 mg PO t.i.d. or q.i.d.

Second Line
- Immunosuppressants (6)[B]: Oral corticosteroids are 1st choice of drugs when immunosuppression is necessary:
  - Prednisone: Start as inpatient with a 60 mg/d PO; taper the dosage every 3 days; switch to alternate-day regimen within 2 weeks. Taper very slowly to establish the minimum dosage necessary to maintain remission.
  - Cyclophosphamide: Adults: 1–5 mg/kg/d PO; Children: 2–8 mg/kg/d PO
  - Cyclosporine: Adults: 5 mg/kg/d PO (nephrotoxicity and drug interactions)
  - Mycophenolate: 1 g PO or IV b.i.d.
  - Azathioprine: 100–200 mg/d PO:
    - Most frequently used for long-term immunomodulation
    - Benefit may not be apparent for up to 18 months after initiation of therapy
    - Prednisolone + azathioprine may be effective when used as a corticosteroid-sparing agent.

- Acute immunomodulating treatments:
  - Plasmapheresis: Bulk removal of 2–3 L of plasma 3 × per week, repeated until rate of improvement plateaus (5)[B]:
    - Improves weakness in nearly all and can last up to 3 months
  - Immunoglobulin: 2 g/kg IV over 2–5 days (6)[B]
  - Plasmapheresis and immunoglobulin have comparable efficacy in treating moderate to severe MG (7)[C].
  - Rapid onset of effect, but short duration of action
  - Used for acute worsening of MG to improve strength prior to surgery, prevent acute exacerbations induced by corticosteroids, and as a chronic intermittent treatment to provide relief in refractory MG
- Other immunosuppressant therapies:
  - Tacrolimus
  - Rituximab
    - Seronegative MuSK-antibody positive MG patients may have better response to rituximab than conventional therapies.

ALERT
Use caution with drugs that can precipitate weakness: Aminoglycosides, fluoroquinolones, β-blockers, calcium channel blockers, neuromuscular blockers, statins, diuretics, oral contraceptives, gabapentin, phenytoin, lithium, among others.

SURGERY/OTHER PROCEDURES
- Thymectomy recommended for most patients
- No clear clinical benefit if onset at ≥60 years unless thymoma present

Pediatric Considerations
- Infants with severe weakness from transient neonatal myasthenia may be treated with oral pyridostigmine; general support is necessary until the condition clears.
- Corticosteroids limited only to severe disease

IN-PATIENT CONSIDERATIONS
Admission Criteria/Initial Stabilization
- Management of pulmonary infections
- Myasthenic/Cholinergic crises
- Plasmapheresis
- IV γ-globulin

ONGOING CARE

PATIENT EDUCATION
MG Foundation of America (MGFA): www.myasthenia.org

PROGNOSIS
- Overall good, but highly variable
- Myasthenic crisis associated with substantial morbidity and 4% mortality
- Seronegative patients are more likely to have purely ocular disease, and those with generalized SNMG have a better outcome after treatment (8)[C].

COMPLICATIONS
Acute respiratory arrest; chronic respiratory insufficiency

REFERENCES

1. McConville J, Farrugia ME, Beeson D. Detection and characterization of MuSK antibodies in seronegative myasthenia gravis. *Ann Neurol*. 2004;55:580–584.
2. Chan KH, Lachance DH, Harper CM. Frequency of seronegativity in adult-acquired generalized myasthenia gravis. *Muscle Nerve*. 2007;36: 651–658.
3. Jaretzki A, Barohn RJ, Ernstoff RM. Myasthenia gravis: Recommendations for clinical research standards. Task Force of the Medical Scientific Advisory Board of the Myasthenia Gravis Foundation of America. *Neurology*. 2000;55: 16–23.
4. Meriggioli MN, Sanders DB. Myasthenia gravis: Diagnosis. *Semin Neurol*. 2004;24:31–39.
5. Angelini C. Diagnosis and management of autoimmune myasthenia gravis. *Clin Drug Investig*. 2011;31:1.
6. Hart IK, Sathasivam S, Sarshar T. Immunosuppressive agents for myasthenia gravis. *Cochrane Database Syst Rev*. 2007;17:CD005224.
7. Barth D, Nabavi Nouri M, Ng E, et al. Comparison of IVIg and PLEX in patients with myasthenia gravis. *Neurology*. 2011;76:2017–2023.
8. Deymeer F, Gungor-Tuncer O, Yilmaz V. Clinical comparison of anti-MuSK- vs anti-AChR-positive and seronegative myasthenia gravis. *Neurology*. 2007;68:609–611.

ADDITIONAL READING

Merrigioli, Matthew N. Myasthenia gravis: Immunopathogenesis, diagnosis, and management. *Continuum Lifelong Learning Neurol*. 2009;15:35–62.

CODES

ICD10
- G70.00 Myasthenia gravis without (acute) exacerbation
- G70.01 Myasthenia gravis with (acute) exacerbation
- P94.0 Transient neonatal myasthenia gravis

CLINICAL PEARLS

- An autoimmune disease, marked by abnormal fatigability and weakness of selected muscles, which is relieved by rest.
- Anticholinesterase medication and a thymectomy lessen symptom severity.
- Steroid therapy, plasma exchange, or immunoglobulin can be used in severely affected patients.

M

MYELODYSPLASTIC SYNDROMES

Richard A. Larson, MD

 BASICS

DESCRIPTION

Myelodysplastic syndromes (MDSs) constitute a heterogeneous group of acquired hematopoietic stem cell disorders characterized by cytologic dysplasia in the bone marrow and blood and by various combinations of anemia, neutropenia, and thrombocytopenia.

- The natural progression of disease evolves as cellular maturation becomes more arrested and blast cells accumulate. There is an overlap between arbitrary diagnostic subgroups.
- World Health Organization (WHO) classification (1):
  - Refractory cytopenia with unilineage dysplasia:
    - Refractory anemia (RA); refractory neutropenia; refractory thrombocytopenia
    - <5% blasts and <15% ring sideroblasts in marrow; <1% blasts in blood
  - Refractory anemia with ring sideroblasts (RARS):
    - <5% blasts in marrow; ≥15% of erythroid precursors are ring sideroblasts; no blasts in blood
    - Also known as acquired idiopathic sideroblastic anemia
  - Refractory anemia with ring sideroblasts and marked thrombocytosis
  - Refractory cytopenia with multilineage dysplasia:
    - Marked trilineage dysplasia, but without excess blasts in marrow; no Auer rods; <1% blasts in blood
  - Refractory cytopenia with multilineage dysplasia and ring sideroblasts
  - Refractory anemia with excess blasts-1 (RAEB-1):
    - 5–9% blasts in marrow; no Auer rods; <5% blasts in blood; <1,000 monocytes/mm^3
  - RAEB-2:
    - 10–19% blasts in marrow; 5–19% blasts in blood; ± Auer rods; <1,000 monocytes/mm^3
  - MDS associated with isolated del(5q) (2):
    - RA with erythroid hyperplasia, increased megakaryocytes with hypolobated nuclei, and normal or increased platelets; <5% blasts in marrow; <1% blasts in blood
  - Acute MDS with sclerosis:
    - RAEB with marked myelosclerosis
  - Chronic myelomonocytic leukemia (CMMoL) is now grouped with myelodysplastic/myeloproliferative disorders:
    - <20% blasts and promonocytes in marrow and blood with >1,000 monocytes/mm^3
  - RAEB in transformation is now considered acute myeloid leukemia (AML):
    - 20–30% blasts in marrow; >20% blasts in blood
    - Incidence: 2:1 (Female > Male)
  - Therapy-related MDS (t-MDS) (3,4):
    - Seen 3–7 years after treatment with alkylating agents and/or radiotherapy
    - Evolves to AML over ~6 months
    - Classified by the WHO as therapy-related myeloid neoplasm
- System(s) affected: Hematologic; Lymphatic; Immunologic
- Synonym(s): Dysmyelopoietic syndrome; Hemopoietic dysplasia; Preleukemia; Smoldering or subacute myeloid leukemia

Pediatric Considerations
Pediatric presentations of MDS:
- Monosomy 7 syndrome
- Juvenile chronic myelogenous leukemia

EPIDEMIOLOGY
- Predominant age: Median age, >65 years; uncommon in children and young adults
- Predominant sex: Male = Female

Incidence
Apparent increased incidence (1–2/100,000 per year) in recent years may be due to improved diagnosis; incidence increases markedly with older age.

Genetics
- Most are clonal neoplasms by cytogenetics, G6PD isoenzyme analysis, or restriction fragment length polymorphism analysis
- Mutations in *RAS* oncogene
- Mutations in *RPS14* gene on chromosome 5q
- *TET2* mutations

RISK FACTORS
- Primary MDS is associated with older age, occupational exposure to petroleum solvents (benzene, gasoline), and smoking.
- Secondary (therapy-related) MDS is associated with prior treatment with alkylating agents or radiotherapy.

COMMONLY ASSOCIATED CONDITIONS
- Anemia
- Neutropenia
- Thrombocytopenia
- Pancytopenia
- Opportunistic infections
- Bleeding, bruising
- Sweet syndrome (neutrophilic dermatosis)

 DIAGNOSIS

HISTORY
- Fatigue
- Fever
- Easy bruising

PHYSICAL EXAM
- Anemia:
  - Fatigue
  - Shortness of breath
  - Lightheadedness
  - Angina
- Leukopenia:
  - Fever
  - Infection
- Thrombocytopenia:
  - Ecchymoses
  - Petechiae
  - Epistaxis
  - Purpura
- Splenomegaly (uncommon):
  - Mild to moderate enlargement may be encountered, particularly in CMMoL.
- Skin infiltrates:
  - Sweet syndrome

DIFFERENTIAL DIAGNOSIS
- Other malignant disorders:
  - Evolving AML or erythroleukemia
  - Chronic myeloproliferative disorders
  - Polycythemia vera
  - Myeloid metaplasia with myelofibrosis
  - Malignant lymphoma
  - Metastatic carcinoma
- Nonmalignant disorders:
  - Aplastic anemia
  - Autoimmune disorders (Felty syndrome, lupus, hemolytic anemia)
  - Nutritional deficiencies (vitamin B$_{12}$, pyridoxine, copper, protein malnutrition)
  - Heavy metal intoxication
  - Alcoholism
  - Chronic liver disease
  - Hypersplenism
  - Chronic inflammation
  - Recent cytotoxic therapy or irradiation
  - HIV infection
  - Paroxysmal nocturnal hemoglobinuria

DIAGNOSTIC TESTS & INTERPRETATION
Initial Tests (lab, imaging)
- CBC
- Reticulocyte count and serum erythropoietin level if anemia were present.
- Review of the peripheral blood smear for the presence of dysplasia
- Liver/Spleen scan or CT, although rarely necessary, may disclose occult splenomegaly or lymphadenopathy.
- Cytogenetics (5,6)[A]:
  - At least 50% of patients with primary MDS and nearly all with t-MDS have clonal chromosomal abnormalities: +8, −7, del(5q), del(7q), del(20q), iso(17), and complex karyotypes
  - Detection of clonal abnormality establishes a diagnosis of neoplasm and rules out a nutritional, toxic, or autoimmune disorder.
  - Cytogenetic analysis of metaphase cells from a bone marrow aspirate provides more information than fluorescence in situ hybridization analysis on blood cells.
- Granulocyte function tests: Abnormal in 50% (decreased myeloperoxidase activity, phagocytosis, chemotaxis, and adhesion)
- Platelet function tests: Impaired aggregation
- Marrow colony assays in vitro:
  - Results are variable and correlate poorly with clinical course.
  - Poor clonal growth may suggest more rapid evolution to AML.
- Immunophenotyping:
  - Nonspecific myeloid markers are present.
  - Occasionally, evidence can be found for concomitant lymphoproliferative disorder.
  - Loss of CD59 expression suggests paroxysmal nocturnal hemoglobinuria (PNH).

Follow-Up Tests & Special Considerations
- Anemia: Often macrocytic; occasional poikilocytosis, anisocytosis; variable reticulocytosis
- Granulocytopenia: Hypogranular or agranular neutrophils with poorly condensed chromatin; Pelger-Huet anomaly with hyposegmented nuclei
- Thrombocytopenia: Occasionally giant platelets or hypogranular platelets
- Fetal hemoglobin may be elevated.
- Flow cytometry to detect loss of CD59 on RBCs, CD16 on granulocytes, and CD14 on monocytes; typical of PNH
- Direct antiglobulin (Coombs) test
- Paraprotein: Present in some

- Erythropoietin: Usually normally elevated for the degree of anemia unless renal failure is present
- Increased serum and tissue iron (ferritin), especially if anemia has been long-standing
- Serum copper level

Diagnostic Procedures/Other
- Review peripheral blood smear
- Bone marrow aspiration, biopsy, and cytogenetics

Test Interpretation
- Ineffective hematopoiesis with dysplasia in 1 or more cell lineages dominates the bone marrow picture in MDS (1,7)[A].
- Marrow cellularity usually is normal or increased for the patient's age, but may be hypoplastic in ~10%.
- Reticulin fibrosis usually is minimal except in t-MDS and acute MDS with sclerosis.
- Myeloblasts may be clustered in the intertrabecular spaces with abnormal localization of immature precursors.

 ## TREATMENT

GENERAL MEASURES
- Immunize for pneumococcal pneumonia, pertussis, influenza, and hepatitis B
- RBC transfusions to alleviate symptoms
- Platelet transfusions only for bleeding or before surgery to avoid alloimmunization
- Early use of antibiotics for fever, even while culture results are pending, due to quantitative and qualitative granulocyte disorder
- Iron chelation therapy to avoid iron overload from chronic transfusions

MEDICATION
First Line
- Epoetin alfa or darbepoetin can increase hemoglobin levels in MDS patients who have low serum erythropoietin levels at baseline.
- Only azacitidine, decitabine, and lenalidomide have been approved by the FDA for MDS (7,8)[B].
- Azacitidine and decitabine have been proven in randomized controlled trials to be more effective for these heterogeneous disorders than only supportive care, with antibiotics and transfusions, as needed (9,10)[A].
- Vitamins, iron, corticosteroids, androgens, or thyroid hormone are rarely helpful, unless evidence of a specific deficiency exists.
- Clinical trials show azacitidine, 75 mg/m^2 SC for 7 days and repeated every 28 days, decreases RBC transfusion requirements, yields longer times to AML or death, and improves quality of life (9,10)[A].
- Decitabine was approved with a continuous IV schedule that usually requires hospitalization (9,10)[A]. More commonly, it is given at 20 mg/m^2/d IV over 1 hour as an outpatient, repeated every 4 weeks.
- Lenalidomide, 10 mg PO daily for 21 days every 4 weeks has yielded complete remission in patients with MDS and del(5q) (2)[A]. It is less effective in patients with MDS without del(5q).
- Intensive chemotherapy:
  – Younger patients with MDS may benefit from AML chemotherapy, especially if Auer rods are present, but toxicity may be severe for older patients.
  – Remission durations are variable (median, ~1 year).

- Allogeneic hematopoietic stem cell transplantation:
  – Recommended for younger patients with HLA antigen–matched donors to eradicate the malignant clone and resupply normal hematopoietic stem cells (11)[A]
- Aminocaproic acid (epsilon-aminocaproic acid) or tranexamic acid may benefit patients with chronic, severe thrombocytopenia and bleeding.
- Contraindications: Cytotoxicity of chemotherapy may increase the risk of bleeding and infection and the need for transfusion support.
- Precautions: Aspirin, salicylates, and NSAIDs should be avoided

Second Line
- Danazol or prednisone may be of benefit for concomitant autoimmune thrombocytopenia.
- Investigational agents:
  – Low doses of cytarabine, tretinoin (all-trans retinoic acid), homoharringtonine, 13-cis retinoic acid, arsenic trioxide, histone/protein deacetylase inhibitors, interferon, cyclosporine, antithymocyte globulin, granulocyte macrophage colony-stimulating factor or granulocyte colony-stimulating factor, and interleukin-3
  – Agents, such as thalidomide, that inhibit the production of tumor necrosis factor in the marrow
- Amifostine may stimulate the proliferation of normal hematopoiesis.

ISSUES FOR REFERRAL
- Refer younger adults for allogeneic hematopoietic cell transplantation.
- Refer patients with symptoms or transfusion requirements for clinical trials.

 ## ONGOING CARE

FOLLOW-UP RECOMMENDATIONS
Usually outpatient, except when necessary to hospitalize for the treatment of infection, blood transfusions, or intensive chemotherapy

Patient Monitoring
- At least monthly during supportive care
- More frequently if receiving treatment

DIET
Reduce alcohol use and iron intake (unless patient is iron deficient)

PATIENT EDUCATION
- Stop smoking
- Seek early medical attention for fever, bleeding, or symptoms of anemia
- Advise about the risks of chronic transfusion therapy

PROGNOSIS
- Median survival for RA and RARS is 5 years, but it may extend much longer.
- RA with del(5q) syndrome is favorable (2).
- Median survival for RAEB, RCMD, and CMMoL is ~1 year; 50% of patients evolve to AML and the other 50% die of infection or bleeding.

COMPLICATIONS
- Infection
- Bleeding
- Complications of anemia and transfusions

REFERENCES
1. Swerdlow SH, Campo E, Harris NL, et al., eds. WHO classification of tumours of haematopoietic and lymphoid tissues. Lyon, France: IARC Press; 2008.
2. List A, Dewald G, Bennett J, et al. Lenalidomide in the myelodysplastic syndrome with chromosome 5q deletion. *N Engl J Med*. 2006;355:1456–1465.
3. Singh ZN, Huo D, Anastasi J, et al. Therapy-related myelodysplastic syndrome: Morphologic subclassification may not be clinically relevant. *Am J Clin Pathol*. 2007;127:197–205.
4. Larson RA, Le Beau MM. Therapy-related myeloid leukaemia: A model for leukemogenesis in humans. *Chem Biol Interact*. 2005;153–154: 187–195.
5. Voso MT, Fenu S, Latagliata R, et al. Revised International Prognostic Scoring System (IPSS) predicts survival and leukemic evolution of myelodysplastic syndromes significantly better than IPSS and WHO Prognostic Scoring System: Validation by the Gruppo Romano Mielodisplasie Italian Regional Database. *J Clin Oncol*. 2013;31: 2671–2677
6. Cheson BD, Greenberg PL, Bennett JM, et al. Clinical application and proposal for modification of the International Working Group (IWG) response criteria in myelodysplasia. *Blood*. 2006; 108:419–425.
7. Greenberg PL. The multifaceted nature of myelodysplastic syndromes: clinical, molecular, and biological prognostic features. *J Natl Compr Canc Netw*. 2013;11:877–885.
8. Larson RA. Myelodysplasia: When to treat and how. *Best Pract Res Clin Haematol*. 2006;19: 293–300.
9. Malcovati L, Hellström-Lindberg E, Bowen D, et al. Diagnosis and treatment of primary myelodysplastic syndromes in adults: Recommendations from the European Leukemia Net. *Blood*. 2013;122:2943–2964.
10. Fenaux P, Adès L. How we treat lower-risk myelodysplastic syndromes. *Blood*. 2013;121: 4280–4286.
11. Koreth J, Pidala J, Perez WS, et al. Role of reduced-intensity conditioning allogeneic hematopoietic stem-cell transplantation in older patients with de novo myelodysplastic syndromes: An international collaborative decision analysis. *J Clin Oncol*. 2013;31:2662–2670.

 ## CODES

ICD10
- D46.B Refract cytopenia w multilin dysplasia and ring sideroblasts
- D46.4 Refractory anemia, unspecified
- D46.9 Myelodysplastic syndrome, unspecified

CLINICAL PEARLS
- MDS constitutes a heterogeneous group of acquired, hematopoietic stem cell disorders characterized by cytologic dysplasia in the bone marrow and blood and by various combinations of anemia, neutropenia, and thrombocytopenia.
- The natural progression of disease evolves as cellular maturation becomes more arrested and blast cells accumulate.
- Initial lab: CBC with WBC differential and review of peripheral smear for dysplasia.

M

MYELOPROLIFERATIVE NEOPLASMS

Shannon Nicole Sharpe, DO • Jamil A. Alarafi, DO

BASICS

DESCRIPTION
- Myeloproliferative neoplasms (MPNs) are defined as disorders of the pluripotent hematopoietic stem cells of bone marrow.
- MPNs are characterized by proliferation of a specific stem cell lineage such as myeloid, erythroid, or megakaryocyte; resulting in granulocytosis, erythrocytosis, or thrombocytosis, respectively.
- The "classic" MPNs include chronic myelogenous leukemia (CML), polycythemia vera (PV), essential thrombocythemia (ET), and primary myelofibrosis (PMF). The classification now includes the "nonclassic" conditions of chronic neutrophilic leukemia (CNL), chronic eosinophilic leukemia not otherwise specified (CEL-NOS), systemic mastocytosis (SM), and myeloproliferative neoplasm unclassifiable (MPN-u). This topic focuses on the classic MPNs.
- CML is classified as a Philadelphia-positive MPN; whereas ET, PMF, and PV are classified as Philadelphia-negative MPNs.
- CML: Characterized by uninhibited growth and production of granulocytes at varying stages, primarily neutrophils, leading to granulocytosis
- PMF: Progressive fibrosis of the bone marrow due to clonal stem cell proliferation that has become hypersensitive to the effects of cytokines, leading to extramedullary hematopoiesis
- ET: Characterized by a clonal proliferation of megakaryocytes, leading to thrombocytosis
- PV: Trilineage growth of hematopoietic stem cells with erythroid precursors predominating, leading to erythrocytosis

EPIDEMIOLOGY
Incidence
- CML: 0.6–2.0/100,000/year; median age at diagnosis 66 years; Male > Female (1.6:1)
- PMF: 0.5–1.5/100,000/year; median age at diagnosis 65 years; Male = Female
- ET: 0.6–2.5/100,000/year; median age at diagnosis 60 years, 2nd peak in younger patients at ~30 years; Female > Male (2:1)
- PV: 1–2/100,000/year; Male > Female (1.3:1)

ETIOLOGY AND PATHOPHYSIOLOGY
- CML: *BCR-ABL1* gene leads to increased and unrestrained activity of tyrosine kinase resulting in activity of downstream signaling pathways, unchecked proliferation, incomplete differentiation, inhibition of apoptosis and extended survival of hematopoietic cells, as well as mobilization of progenitor cells, leading to the neutrophilic changes seen in CML.
- PMF: Hematopoietic stem cells become hyperreactive to the effects of circulating cytokines, causing clonal proliferation of the stem cells leading to bone marrow fibrosis and resultant extramedullary hematopoiesis, accounting for most of the signs/symptoms of PMF.
- ET: Thrombopoietin binds to a pluripotent stem cell receptor to induce proliferation of a megakaryocyte and eventually a platelet; this process is normally regulated by a negative feedback loop, which is nonfunctioning in ET, leading to unrestrained growth and development of platelets.

- PV: Gain-of-function mutation (*JAK2*) leads to increased erythrocyte production regardless of an intact negative feedback mechanism (normal expression of cell surface receptors and decreased renal production of erythropoietin).
- Unknown; familial component described in PV, ET, and PMF

Genetics
- Philadelphia chromosome (*BCR-ABL1* gene): Translocation and fusion of the *BCR* gene on chromosome 22 and the *ABL* gene on chromosome 9; seen in all patients with CML
- *JAK2* mutations: Point mutations in the tyrosine kinase domain of *JAK2*, causing a substitution of valine for phenylalanine at position 617 (*JAK2V617F*); leading to unrestrained *JAK2* activation with a deactivation of typical feedback mechanism:
  – Seen in >95% of PV cases; 50% of ET and PMF cases
- Myeloproliferative leukemia virus (*MPL*) gene: Mutation found in 5–10% of patients with PMF and in 3–5% of those with ET

RISK FACTORS
- Rare familial cases have been reported.
- CML: Exposure to ionizing radiation

COMMONLY ASSOCIATED CONDITIONS
- Progression to acute myeloid leukemia; most common with CML
- Thrombosis/Hemorrhage

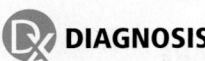

DIAGNOSIS

HISTORY
- Many MPN cases are found incidentally on routine blood work.
- CML: Most patients are asymptomatic at time of diagnosis:
  – Fatigue, malaise, weight loss, excessive perspiration, abdominal fullness, early satiety, bleeding episodes
- PMF: Symptoms depend on the degree of anemia and splenomegaly:
  – Fatigue, shortness of breath, early satiety, constitutional symptoms, cachexia, Budd-Chiari syndrome, splenic infarcts, osteosclerosis
- ET: Characterized by thrombotic and hemorrhagic events:
  – Thrombotic events (deep vein thrombosis, pulmonary embolism, Budd-Chiari syndrome), microvascular occlusive events (digital ischemia, erythromelalgia), major/minor hemorrhagic events; headaches, dizziness, syncope, tingling, visual changes, transient ischemic attacks
- PV: Symptoms are due to level of erythrocytosis and the resultant increased blood viscosity:
  – Erythromelalgia, pruritus after hot baths, headaches, tinnitus, paresthesias, gout attacks

PHYSICAL EXAM
- CML: Splenomegaly, hepatomegaly
- PMF: Splenomegaly seen in nearly all patients, hepatomegaly, paleness
- ET: Possible petechiae, purpura, ecchymosis
- PV: Cyanotic blush (lips, nose, ears, distal extremities), increased blood pressure, splenomegaly, epistaxis, ecchymosis

DIFFERENTIAL DIAGNOSIS
- CML: Leukemoid reaction (elevated LAP), juvenile myelomonocytic leukemia, chronic myelomonocytic leukemia (CMML), chronic eosinophilic leukemia, chronic neutrophilic leukemia
- PMF: Other MPNs, lymphoma, hairy cell leukemia, multiple myeloma, metastatic cancer, connective tissue disease, rickets, renal osteodystrophy
- ET: Reactive thrombocytosis, CML, PV, PMF, and myelodysplastic syndromes
- PV: Hypoxic states (e.g., chronic obstructive pulmonary disease [COPD], anemia), renal cell carcinoma, Wilms tumor, hepatoma, polycystic kidney disease, exogenous androgens

DIAGNOSTIC TESTS & INTERPRETATION
- CML: White blood cell count $>100,000 \times 10^9$/L with differential showing increased neutrophils at varying stages of development and an increased percentage of myelocytes; neutrophils have decreased leukocyte alkaline phosphatase; platelet count $>600,000 \times 10^9$/L and a normochromic, normocytic anemia.

- PMF (1)[A] (World Health Organization [WHO] criteria): Diagnosis requires meeting all 3 major criteria and >2 minor criteria:
  – *Major criteria*: (i) Megakaryocyte proliferation and atypia accompanied by either reticulin or collagen fibrosis. (ii) Not meeting WHO criteria for CML, PV, MDS, or other myeloid neoplasm. (iii) Demonstration of *JAK2V617F* or other clonal marker or absence of marker with no evidence of secondary marrow fibrosis
  – *Minor criteria*: (i) Leukoerythroblastosis. (ii) Increased serum lactate dehydrogenase (LDH) level. (iii) Anemia. (iv) Palpable splenomegaly
- ET (1)[A] (WHO criteria): Diagnosis requires meeting all 4 major criteria:
  – *Major criteria*: (i) Thrombocytosis with persistent platelet level $\geq 450 \times 10^9$/L. (ii) Megakaryocyte proliferation with large and mature morphology. (iii) Not meeting WHO criteria for CML, PV, PMF, MDS, or other myeloid neoplasm. (iv) Demonstration of *JAK2V617F* or other clonal marker or absence of clonal marker with no evidence of reactive thrombocytosis
- PV (1)[A] (WHO criteria): Diagnosis requires either both major criteria and 1 minor criterion or the first major criterion and 2 of the minor criteria:
  – *Major criteria*: (i) Hemoglobin >18.5 g/dL in men, >16.5 g/dL in women or other evidence of increased red cell volume. (ii) Presence of *JAK2V617F* or other functionally similar mutation (e.g., *JAK2* exon 12 mutation)
  – *Minor criteria*: (i) Bone marrow biopsy showing hypercellularity for age with trilineage myeloproliferation. (ii) Low serum erythropoietin level. (iii) Endogenous erythroid colony formation in vitro

Initial Tests (lab, imaging)
If clinical suspicion of MPN, obtain a CBC and peripheral blood smear; if positive, obtain bone marrow biopsy.
- PMF: Radiographic osteosclerosis in 25–66%
- ET: Ultrasonic imaging if venous thrombosis suspected

Diagnostic Procedures/Other

- CML: Diagnosis with identification of Philadelphia chromosome: Karyotyping of metaphase chromosomes is the gold standard for diagnosis; fluorescence in situ hybridization (FISH) used when karyotypic analysis is negative/inconclusive; polymerase chain reaction (PCR) for monitoring response to tyrosine kinase inhibitors (2)[A]:
  - Bone marrow biopsy: Granulocytic hyperplasia with dwarf megakaryocytes
- PMF, ET and PV: Genotypic analysis and bone marrow biopsy as described in above WHO criteria; "dry tap" for bone marrow aspiration in PMF
- Risk stratification
  - CML: 3 phases of CML:
    - (i) Chronic phase (85% patients at diagnosis; <5% blast counts). (ii) Accelerated phase (poorly controlled regardless of treatment, 10–19% blast counts). (iii) Blast crisis (resembles acute leukemia, >20% blast counts)
  - PMF (3)[A]: International Prognostic Scoring System (IPSS) at diagnosis and Dynamic IPSS (DIPSS-plus) throughout disease
    - IPSS: Age >65 years, constitutional symptoms, hemoglobin <10 g/dL, leukocyte count >25 × 10^9, circulating blasts >1%:
      - Low risk = 0 of above; intermediate-1 risk = 1 of above; intermediate-2 risk = 2 of above; high risk = ≥3 of above
    - DIPSS-plus: Same 5 risk factors in the IPSS + the need for red cell transfusion, platelets <100 × 10^9/L and unfavorable karyotype:
      - Low risk = 0 of above; intermediate-1 risk = 1 of above; intermediate-2 risk = 2–3 of above; high risk = ≥4 of above
  - ET (4)[A]: Low risk = age <40 years, no prior thromboembolic events, no cardiovascular risk factors, platelet count <1,500 × 10^9/L; intermediate risk = age 40–59, presence of cardiovascular risk factors, platelet count <1,500 × 10^9/L; high risk = age ≥60 and/or prior thromboembolic or hemorrhagic episode and/or platelet count >1,500 × 10^9/L
  - PV (1)[A]: Low risk = age <60, no history of thrombosis/cardiovascular risk factors; intermediate risk = platelets >1,000 × 10^9/L and cardiovascular risk factors; high risk = age >60 or a history of thrombosis

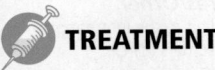

TREATMENT

GENERAL MEASURES
Splenectomy has no impact on mortality, but is occasionally carried out for symptomatic relief.

MEDICATION
First Line

- CML (5)[A]:
  - Chronic phase: Imatinib mesylate (Gleevec): 400 mg/d, a potent tyrosine kinase inhibitor (TKI)
  - Accelerated or blast phase: Increase imatinib to 800 mg/d and consider allogeneic stem cell transplant (aSCT).
  - While awaiting confirmation of diagnosis, hydroxyurea can be used to lower the WBC count.
- PMF (1,3)[A]: Main goal is symptomatic relief:
  - Low and intermediate-1 risk: No drug therapy indicated, palliative measures if necessary
  - Intermediate-2 and high risk: Hydroxyurea or consider aSCT

- Palliative treatment:
  - Anemia (keep hemoglobin >10 g/dL): Transfusions, low-dose prednisone; erythropoiesis-stimulating agents, androgens, danazol, or thalidomide 50 mg/d
  - Splenomegaly: Hydroxyurea, splenectomy or IV cladribine monthly for refractory cases
  - Thrombosis: Hydroxyurea and low-dose aspirin
- ET (1,4)[A] low and intermediate risk: "Watch and wait" + low-dose aspirin if microvascular disturbances present and no contraindications; high risk: hydroxyurea 15 mg/kg/d to reduce platelet count to <450 × 10^9/L
- PV (1)[A]:
  - Low and intermediate risk: Phlebotomy and low-dose aspirin
  - High risk (or those who do not tolerate phlebotomy): Hydroxyurea 500–1,000 mg/d

Second Line
- CML: Only curable treatment is aSCT; reserved for accelerated/blast phase due to high rates of morbidity and mortality with aSCT:
  - 2nd-generation TKIs: Dasatinib, nilotinib, and bosutinib; increasing evidence for improved, deeper responses with these medications; ongoing studies assessing role of 2nd-generation TKIs for first-line therapy (5)[A]
- ET (4)[A]: If resistant/intolerant to hydroxyurea, use anagrelide:
  - If resistant/intolerant to hydroxyurea or anagrelide, pregnant or age <40: Use interferon-α.
- PMF (1,3)[A]: Only curable treatment is aSCT; reserved for intermediate-2 or high-risk patients age <50
  - If unresponsive to hydroxyurea, use pegylated interferon-α.
- Ongoing investigations for *JAK2* inhibitors in the treatment of PV, PMF, and ET
  - Ruxolitinib, a JAK2 Inhibitor, has completed phase III trials for the treatment of PMF (6)[A]

ISSUES FOR REFERRAL
Patients with MPNs are usually referred to hematology/oncology. May consult palliative care or surgical/radiation oncology if necessary.

SURGERY/OTHER PROCEDURES
May require splenectomy/palliative radiation for foci of extramedullary hematopoiesis.

IN-PATIENT CONSIDERATIONS
Admission Criteria/Initial Stabilization
- Severe cachexia; renal failure and hepatomegaly secondary to extramedullary hematopoiesis; massive splenomegaly requiring treatment; severe thrombotic/hemorrhagic episodes; anemia; tumor lysis syndrome
  - Treatment aimed at symptom relief and pain control

IV Fluids
Optimal hydration to prevent tumor lysis syndrome

 ONGOING CARE

PROGNOSIS
- CML: 10-year survival rate ~80% from time of diagnosis; 85% will die in blast crisis; 12- to 18-month median survival for accelerated phase; 3–6-month median survival for blast phase
- PMF: Worst prognosis of the MPNs; drug therapy does not modify disease course, but treats the

symptoms; median survival for low risk = 135 months, intermediate-1 risk = 95 months; intermediate-2 risk = 48 months; high risk = 27 months
- ET and PV: Near-normal life expectancy

COMPLICATIONS
- CML: Blast crisis, transformation to acute leukemia, gout, or nephropathy due to hyperuricemia
- PMF: 10% develop acute myeloid leukemia; anemia, massive hepatosplenomegaly, thrombohemorrhagic events, osteosclerosis, secondary gout, splenic infarcts, paraspinal/epidural extramedullary hematopoiesis
- ET: <10% develop post-ET myelofibrosis, 2% develop acute myeloid leukemia; thrombohemorrhagic events
- PV: Erythromelalgia, pruritus, secondary gout, headaches, vascular occlusive events

REFERENCES

1. Bittencourt RI, Vassallo J, Chauffaille Mde L, et al. Philadelphia-negative chronic myeloproliferative neoplasms. *Rev Bras Hematol Hemoter*. 2012;34:140–149.
2. Tohami T, Nagler A, Amariglio N. Laboratory tools for diagnosis and monitoring response in patients with chronic myeloid leukemia. *Isr Med Assoc J*. 2012;14:501–507.
3. Vannucchi AM. Management of myelofibrosis. *Hematology Am Soc Hematol Educ Program*. 2011;2011:222–230.
4. Cervantes F. Management of essential thrombocythemia. *Hematology Am Soc Hematol Educ Program*. 2011;2011:215–221.
5. Ferdinand R, Mitchell SA, Batson S, et al. Treatments for chronic myeloid leukemia: A qualitative systematic review. *J Blood Med*. 2012;3:51–76
6. Sonbol MB, Firwana B, Zarzour A, et al. Comprehensive review of JAK inhibitors in myeloproliferative neoplasms. *Ther Adv Hematol*. 2013;4:15–35.

ADDITIONAL READING

Koopmans SM, van Marion AM, Schouten HC. Myeloproliferative neoplasia: A review of clinical criteria and treatment. *Neth J Med*. 2012;70:159–167.

 SEE ALSO

Leukemia, Chronic Myelogenous; Polycythemia Vera

 CODES

ICD10
- D47.1 Chronic myeloproliferative disease
- C92.10 Chronic myeloid leukemia, BCR/ABL-positive, not having achieved remission
- D45 Polycythemia vera

CLINICAL PEARLS

Myeloproliferative neoplasms (MPNs) are defined as disorders of the pluripotent hematopoietic stem cells of bone marrow.

M

NARCOLEPSY
Jeffrey F. Minteer, MD

 BASICS

DESCRIPTION
- Disorder of unknown etiology characterized by excessive daytime sleepiness typically associated with cataplexy (sudden bilateral weakness of skeletal muscles) and other rapid eye movement (REM) sleep phenomena, such as sleep paralysis and hypnagogic hallucinations (e.g., vivid auditory or visual perceptions without an external stimulus that occur as one is falling asleep).
- Frequently overlooked disorder, with an average of 15 years of symptoms prior to diagnosis
- System affected: Nervous

EPIDEMIOLOGY
Incidence
- Onset usually in teenage years
- Bimodal distribution peak at 15 and 36 years of age
- Predominant sex: Male > Female (1.6:1)
- Occurrence: 0.74/100,000 persons

Pediatric Considerations
Uncommon in childhood

Prevalence
25–50 cases/100,000 people.

ETIOLOGY AND PATHOPHYSIOLOGY
- Unknown
- Neurodegenerative disorder resulting from selective loss of neurons containing hypocretin (orexin) in the hypothalamus; may be autoimmune (associated with influenza A or *Streptococcus pyogenes*)
- Orexin neurons also regulate metabolism, feeding, reward and autonomic tone; weight gain especially in children from reduction of metabolism
- 85% of patients with narcolepsy and cataplexy have low hypocretin in CSF.
- Possible involvement of immune system and environmental influences

Genetics
- Increased incidence in families with positive history: 1–2% in 1st-degree relative of index case (10–40× the general population)
- Twin concordance is 25–31% (suggests environmental contribution)
- Most are sporadic
- 85–95% of patients with narcolepsy and cataplexy have biologic human leukocyte antigen (HLA) DQB1*0602; 40% of patients with narcolepsy without cataplexy express this antigen. (HLA) DQB1*0602 is present in 24% of the general population.
- Autosomal-recessive inheritance pattern
- 12% of Asians, 25% of whites, and 38% of African Americans are gene carriers.

RISK FACTORS
- Head trauma
- CNS infectious disease
- Anesthesia
- Psychological stress
- Pregnancy
- Family history
- High BMI

COMMONLY ASSOCIATED CONDITIONS
Obstructive sleep apnea (up to 25%), obesity, anxiety

 DIAGNOSIS

HISTORY
- Classic tetrad of excessive daytime sleepiness, cataplexy, sleep paralysis, and hypnagogic hallucinations (4 most common symptoms): Only 10–20% of patients have all 4 symptoms.
- 3 general forms:
  – Narcolepsy without cataplexy: 40%
  – Narcolepsy with cataplexy: 60%
  – Narcolepsy due to a medical condition: Unknown (e.g., Parkinson disease with sleep disturbance)
- Excessive daytime sleepiness and sleep attacks (cardinal symptom):
  – Primary symptom and required for diagnosis
  – Instantaneous, irresistible REM sleep
  – First and most disabling symptom
  – Tendency to take naps lasting 5–10 minutes
  – Episodes last minutes to hours
  – 1–8 naps/day, but normal 24-hour sleep duration
  – Associated with dreaming
  – Nap restores wakefulness for several hours
  – More likely in a monotonous, warm environment, after a large meal, or with strong emotions
- Cataplexy: Auxiliary symptom (60%; cardinal symptom):
  – Pathognomonic if present
  – Sudden bilateral weakness of skeletal muscles
  – Provocation by sudden strong wave of emotion
  – Consciousness and memory are not impaired.
  – Short duration (less than a few minutes)
  – Can be limited to a particular muscle group (e.g., jaw droop with inability to speak; arm, neck, or leg weakness, eye muscles not affected)
  – Status catapleticus: In children or on withdrawal of drugs
- Sleep paralysis: Auxiliary symptom (50%):
  – When falling asleep or on awakening, the patient wants to but cannot move; this can end abruptly when the patient is touched or spoken to.
  – Brain wakes from sleep while body remains paralyzed in REM sleep.
  – Lasts seconds to minutes
  – Patients are aware of events around them but cannot open eyes or move.
  – Can be preceded by hallucinatory phenomena
  – 50% of the normal population have ≥1 episodes (thus, this symptom is nonspecific).
- Hypnagogic hallucinations: Auxiliary symptom (60%):
  – Vivid, frightening visual or auditory illusions or hallucinations at onset of sleep
  – Dreamlike experiences that occur during wakefulness or suddenly at sleep onset
  – Characteristic hallucinations include seeing human or animal faces or feeling that someone else is in the room.
  – Hallucinations also can be auditory.
- Disturbed nocturnal sleep (66%):
  – Normal total sleep with decreased sleep efficiency
  – More frequent transitions from wakefulness to sleep
  – Retrograde amnesic and automatic behavior lasting minutes to hours
  – Increased periodic leg movements (50%)
  – Depression (18–37%)
  – Automatic behavior: Activity without memory of the event

PHYSICAL EXAM
- A complete exam is useful to rule out other causes of hypersomnia.
- If cataplexy is witnessed, examiner will be unable to elicit deep tendon reflexes.

DIFFERENTIAL DIAGNOSIS
Excessive daytime sleepiness is present in 4% of the general population, although most individuals are not narcoleptic. Possible etiologies include:
- Sleep apnea syndromes (40–50% of those with excessive somnolence); increased incidence in narcolepsy, up to 26% prevalence
- Epileptic seizures and syncope
- Idiopathic CNS hypersomnolence (5–10% of those with excessive somnolence)
- Nocturnal myoclonus
- Psychomotor seizures
- Recurrent hypersomnia that lasts days to weeks and recurs months later
- Hypersomnia related to a medical condition, such as Parkinson disease

DIAGNOSTIC TESTS & INTERPRETATION
Initial Tests (lab, imaging)
- Nighttime polysomnography (PSG): Monitoring of patients in a sleep laboratory will usually document fragmented sleep with a normal amount of REM sleep but a pattern of sleep-onset REM. The PSG is useful to rule out other causes of excessive daytime sleepiness, including sleep apnea syndromes and nocturnal myoclonus.
- Multiple sleep latency test (MSLT): Begins ≥90 minutes after nighttime test:
  – The patient is monitored during 4–5 naps taken at 2-hour intervals; rapidity of sleep onset and type of sleep pattern are documented. The supportive test includes mean sleep latency (time to fall asleep) of ≤8 minutes and ≥1 sleep-onset REM periods.
  – Sensitivity 77%; specificity 97%; positive predictive value 73%

Follow-Up Tests & Special Considerations
- HLA typing for DQB1 in ambiguous cases
- Low CSF hypocretin-1 level: 99% specificity, 87% sensitivity in patients with cataplexy; useful in children unable to do an MSLT (described below)

Diagnostic Procedures/Other
- Diagnostic criteria according to the International Classification of Sleep Disorders (1)[C]
- Minimal criteria are B + C or A + D + E + G or B + E + H:
  – A. Excessive sleepiness—required
  – B. Recurrent lapses into sleep daily for ≥3 months (daytime latency average <8 min)
  – C. Cataplexy
  – D. Associated features: Sleep paralysis, hypnagogic hallucinations, disrupted sleep
  – E. MSLT abnormalities (as described above)
  – F. Biologic markers (see "Genetics")
  – G. Absence of medical or psychiatric disorder
  – H. Low CSF hypocretin-1 level <110 pg/mL; use if unable to do MSLT, especially in children

TREATMENT

GENERAL MEASURES

- None of the currently available medications enables people with narcolepsy to consistently maintain a fully normal state of alertness.
- Drug therapy should be supplemented by various behavioral strategies.
- Well-timed 20-minute naps may be helpful.
- Avoid sedative drugs.
- Use safety precautions, particularly when driving. People with untreated narcoleptic symptoms are involved in automobile accidents roughly 10× more frequently than the general population. However, accident rates are at normal levels among patients who have received appropriate medication therapy.

MEDICATION

First Line

- Excessive daytime sleepiness:
  - Modafinil (Provigil):
    - Structurally distinct from amphetamines
    - 200–400 mg/d; start with 100 mg/d and increase over 3–4 days (2)[A].
    - First-line treatment: 60% effective and 20% partially effective
    - Half-life of 14 hours, can dose daily
    - No decrease in cataplexy
  - Armodafinil (Nuvigil):
    - Enantiomeric form of modafinil with slightly longer half-life of 15 hours
    - 150–250 mg every morning
  - Sodium oxybate (Xyrem):
    - 2.5–9 mg; may take 3 months to achieve full response
    - Preferred treatment for narcolepsy with cataplexy and disturbed nocturnal sleep
    - Give 1/2 dose at bedtime and 1/2 dose 4 hours later; date rape drug with abuse potential (2)[A]
    - Can use with modafinil in severe cases
    - May worsen sleep-disordered breathing in patients with obstructive sleep apnea
- Cataplexy:
  - Sodium oxybate: See above
  - Serotonin-norepinephrine reuptake inhibitors:
    - Venlafaxine: 75–375 mg/d
  - Tricyclic antidepressants:
    - High side-effect profile
    - Abrupt withdrawal causes rebound cataplexy
    - Protriptyline: 2.5–10 mg/d
  - Amphetamines:
    - Methylphenidate (Ritalin): Initial dose 30 mg/d divided b.i.d. or t.i.d.; maximum dose 100 mg/d (2)[B], short-acting
    - Dextroamphetamine: Initial dose 15 mg/d divided b.i.d. or t.i.d.; maximum dose 100 mg/d (2)[B]
    - Combination regimen of long- and short-acting medicines: Pemoline plus single or multiple doses of methylphenidate
- Auxiliary symptoms (e.g., cataplexy [3][C], hypnagogic hallucination, sleep paralysis [3][C]):
  - Antidepressants suppress REM sleep:
    - Imipramine: 75–150 mg/d
    - Protriptyline: 10–40 mg/d
    - Clomipramine: 150–250 mg/d
    - Fluoxetine: 20–60 mg/d
    - Venlafaxine: 75–150 mg b.i.d.
  - Although often used, quality evidence is lacking to demonstrate improvement in cataplexy symptoms from antidepressants (3)[A].
- Contraindications: Stimulants in hypertensive patients
- Precautions:
  - Amphetamines:
    - If the patient develops a tolerance to stimulants, switch drugs rather than increase dose; there is little cross-tolerance.
    - Headaches, irritability, hypertension (HTN), psychosis, anorexia, habituation, rebound hypersomnia
    - Pemoline: Fewer cardiovascular side effects, longer acting, liver toxicity, little abuse potential
  - Other:
    - Imipramine: Dry mouth, sedation, urinary retention, impotence
    - Modafinil: Less rebound hypersomnia; may become drug of choice; does not affect BP; tolerance limited; best if initial treatment; does not treat cataplexy; main side effect is headache; increased metabolism of oral contraceptives (use 50-μg pill)
    - The patient may develop a tolerance to the anticataplectic effect of tricyclic antidepressants (TCAs) and can have rebound cataplexy when a drug is withdrawn.
- Significant possible interactions: Combination of TCAs and stimulants can lead to significant HTN.

Second Line

- Excessive daytime sleepiness:
  - Amphetamines:
    - Methylphenidate (Ritalin): Initial dose 30 mg/d divided b.i.d. or t.i.d.; maximum dose 100 mg/d (2)[B], short acting, most potent amphetamine available
    - Dextroamphetamine: Initial dose 15 mg/d divided b.i.d. or t.i.d.; maximum dose 100 mg/d (2)[B]
  - Selegiline: Selective MAO-B inhibitor; anticataplectic effective for excessive daytime sleepiness; 20–40 mg/d divided morning and noon (2)[B]
- Contraindications: Stimulants in hypertensive patients
- Precautions:
  - Amphetamines:
    - If the patient develops a tolerance to stimulants, switch drugs rather than increase dose; there is little cross-tolerance.
    - Headaches, irritability, HTN, psychosis, anorexia, habituation, rebound hypersomnia
  - Other: Selegiline: Doses >20 mg require a low-tyramine diet because the drug begins to lose selectivity.
  - The patient may develop a tolerance to the anticataplectic effect of antidepressants and can have rebound cataplexy when a drug is withdrawn.

ISSUES FOR REFERRAL

- Unresponsive to primary medications
- Patient support groups can be very beneficial.

 ONGOING CARE

FOLLOW-UP RECOMMENDATIONS

Patient Monitoring

Frequent BP checks and regular follow ups (approximately every 6 months) are recommended.

DIET

Selegiline: Doses >20 mg require a low-tyramine diet because the drug begins to lose selectivity.

PATIENT EDUCATION

- Narcolepsy information from the National Institute of Neurological Disorders and Stroke at www.ninds.nih.gov/disorders/narcolepsy/narcolepsy.htm
- Narcolepsy Network, Inc., North Kingstown, RI 02852; www.narcolepsynetwork.org

PROGNOSIS

Narcolepsy is a lifelong disease. Symptoms can worsen with aging. In women, symptoms can improve after menopause.

REFERENCES

1. American Academy of Sleep Medicine. *International classification of sleep disorders*, 2nd ed: *Diagnostic and coding manual*. Westchester, IL: American Academy of Sleep Medicine; 2005.
2. Mohsenin V. Narcolepsy—master of disguise: Evidence-based recommendations for management. *Postgrad Med*. 2009;121:99–104.
3. Vignatelli L, D'Alessandro R, Candelise L. Antidepressant drugs for narcolepsy. *Cochrane Database Syst Rev*. 2008;1:CD003724.

ADDITIONAL READING

- Dauvilliers Y, Arnulf I, Mignot E. Narcolepsy with cataplexy. *Lancet*. 2007;369:499–511.
- Zaharna M, Dimitriu A, Guilleminault C. Expert opinion on pharmacotherapy of narcolepsy. *Expert Opin Pharmacother*. 2010;11:1633–1645.

 CODES

ICD10

- G47.411 Narcolepsy with cataplexy
- G47.419 Narcolepsy without cataplexy
- G47.429 Narcolepsy in conditions classified elsewhere w/o cataplexy

CLINICAL PEARLS

- Narcolepsy is a frequently missed disorder, with an average of 15 years of symptoms before a definitive diagnosis is made.
- The classic tetrad of symptoms includes excessive daytime sleepiness, cataplexy, sleep paralysis, and hypnagogic hallucinations.
- The International Classification of Sleep Disorders has specific diagnostic criteria for narcolepsy.
- Medications are helpful but not curative.

N

NASAL POLYPS

Erika L. LeBaron, DO, MSN • Diana Ponsky, MD

 BASICS

DESCRIPTION
- Chronic inflammatory lesion of nasal mucosa
- Appearance of edematous pedunculated mass in the nasal cavity or within the paranasal sinus
- Often causes symptoms of blockage, discharge, or loss of smell
- Most commonly bilateral; suspect tumor, such as inverted papilloma, if unilateral

EPIDEMIOLOGY
Incidence
- Estimated to be ~2–4% in adults
- Much rarer in children: ~0.1%
- Increases with age

Prevalence
- Estimated to be 2–4% in general population
- Predominant sex: Female > Male (2:1)

ETIOLOGY AND PATHOPHYSIOLOGY
- No clearly delineated pathway; research has demonstrated separate TH1, TH2, and TH17 driven pathways.
- Remains unclear; multiple inflammatory and infectious pathways resulting from chronic rhinosinusitis is most common.

RISK FACTORS
- Chronic sinusitis
- Allergic fungal sinusitis
- Aspirin sensitivity
- Cystic fibrosis
- Primary ciliary dyskinesia (Kartagener syndrome)

GENERAL PREVENTION
Use of intranasal corticosteroids after polyp removal surgery has shown effectiveness against recurrence.

COMMONLY ASSOCIATED CONDITIONS
- Bronchial asthma
- Aspirin hypersensitivity
- Allergy

 DIAGNOSIS

HISTORY
- Nasal obstruction/restricted nasal airflow: Persistent mouth breathing
- Nasal discharge:
  - Rhinorrhea
  - Postnasal drip
- Reduction/loss of smell
- Dull headaches
- Facial pain/discomfort
- Symptoms of acute, recurrent, or chronic rhinosinusitis

PHYSICAL EXAM
- Anterior rhinoscopy looking for a pale translucent mass of tissue:
  - Most commonly from lateral wall of middle meatus
  - Otoscope with nasal speculum or even otologic speculum is typically used.
- Flexible/rigid endoscopy is required to assess the nasal cavity fully:
  - Endoscopy is the gold standard for diagnosis.
  - Topical anesthesia nasal spray should be used prior to the endoscopy if patient is awake.
- Tympanic membrane examination for eustachian tube dysfunction secondary to large posterior nasal polyps
- Examine the posterior pharynx via oral cavity for large posterior polyps.

DIFFERENTIAL DIAGNOSIS
- Antrochoanal polyp
- Benign or malignant tumor:
  - Papilloma
  - Intranasal glioma
  - Encephalocele
  - Rhabdomyosarcoma
  - Mycetoma

DIAGNOSTIC TESTS & INTERPRETATION
Initial Tests (lab, imaging)
- Allergy testing:
  - Skin prick test
  - Immunocap testing
  - Radioallergosorbent test (RAST)
- Testing for cystic fibrosis in children with multiple benign polyps: Sweat test: Often requires repeat tests
- CT scanning:
  - May be helpful to corroborate history and endoscopic findings
  - Unable to differentiate polyp from other soft tissue masses
- MRI:
  - May aid in unilateral polyposis if concern for neoplasia, mycetoma, or encephalocele

Follow-Up Tests & Special Considerations
Histologic exam to exclude malignancy if unilateral polyp

Diagnostic Procedures/Other
- Diagnosis is made by the combination of rhinoscopy, endoscopy, and CT scanning.
- CT reveals extent of disease and is necessary to formulate a plan for surgical intervention.

Test Interpretation
- Ciliated pseudostratified columnar epithelium: With areas of transitional or squamous epithelium
- Chronic infiltration of inflammatory cells
- Eosinophils are the predominant cells in most patients.

TREATMENT

MEDICATION

First Line

Intranasal corticosteroids: Treat for a minimum of 12 weeks; minimal systemic absorption, side effects rare—minor nose bleeding is most common (1,2)[A]:

- Budesonide 280 mcg/d (3)[A]
- Beclomethasone dipropionate 320 mcg/d (2)[B]
- Fluticasone dipropionate 400 mcg/d (4)[B]
- Mometasone furoate 200 mcg b.i.d. (5)[A]

Second Line

Oral systemic corticosteroids: Less definitive benefit; more systemic adverse effects; use with caution in patients with diabetes mellitus, hypertension, or peptic ulcer disease:

- Prednisolone (6)[B]:
  - Weight-based dosing burst with taper

ISSUES FOR REFERRAL

Patients with severe obstruction symptoms should be referred for surgery.

ADDITIONAL THERAPIES

Antileukotrienes: Clinical improvement without aspirin hypersensitivity (7)[B]

- Aspirin desensitization may have a role in reducing recurrence of nasal polyposis (8)[C].
- Anti-interleukin-5 immunomodulators: May benefit those with T_H2 eosinophilic disease process (7)

SURGERY/OTHER PROCEDURES

- Most surgeries are approached endonasally.
  - Endoscopic sinus surgery has become the mainstay of treatment.
  - The external (Caldwell-Luc) approach is used for more difficult cases, but carries higher risk of complications.
- Functional endonasal sinus surgery has slightly lower revision rate than intranasal polypectomy. Both modalities provide effective symptom relief (9)[B].
- Postoperative use of nasal corticosteroids delay the recurrence of nasal polyps and hence the timing of revision surgery (10)[B].

- Postoperative use of steroid releasing stents to prevent polyp recurrence by decreasing mucosal inflammation
- Intrapolyp steroid injection may be considered in cases refractory to other interventions, but has risk of visual loss (11)

ONGOING CARE

COMPLICATIONS

- Acute/chronic sinus infection
- Heterotropic bone formation within the sinus cavity
- Recurrence:
  - Of patients, 5–10% with severe disease
  - Twice as likely in those with asthma

REFERENCES

1. Rudmik L, Schlosser RJ, Smith TL, et al. Impact of topical nasal steroid therapy on symptoms of nasal polyposis: A meta-analysis. *Laryngoscope.* 2012;122:1431–1437.
2. Bachert C. Evidence-based management of nasal polyposis by intranasal corticosteroids: From the cause to the clinic. *Int Arch Allergy Immunol.* 2011;155:309–321.
3. Filiaci F, Passali D, Puxeddu R, et al. A randomized controlled trial showing efficacy of once daily intranasal budesonide in nasal polyposis. *Rhinology.* 2000;38:185–190.
4. Aukema AA, Mulder PG, Fokkens WJ. Treatment of nasal polyposis and chronic rhinosinusitis with fluticasone propionate nasal drops reduces need for sinus surgery. *J Allergy Clin Immunol.* 2005;115:1017–1023.
5. Small CB, Stryszak P, Danzig M, et al. Onset of symptomatic effect of mometasone furoate nasal spray in the treatment of nasal polyposis. *J Allergy Clin Immunol.* 2008;121:928–932.
6. Hissaria P, Smith W, Wormald PJ, et al. Short course of systemic corticosteroids in sinonasal polyposis: A double-blind, randomized, placebo-controlled trial with evaluation of outcome measures. *J Allergy Clin Immunol.* 2006;118:128–133.
7. DeMarcantonio MA, Han JK. Nasal polyps: Pathogenesis and treatment implications. *Otolaryngol Clin North Am.* 2011;44:685–695, ix.
8. Aouad RK, Chiu AG. State of the art treatment of nasal polyposis. *Am J Rhinol Allergy.* 2011;25:291–298.
9. Hopkins C, Slack R, Lund V, et al. Long-term outcomes from the English national comparative audit of surgery for nasal polyposis and chronic rhinosinusitis. *Laryngoscope.* 2009;119:2459–2465.
10. Stjärne P, Olsson P, Alenius M. Use of mometasone furoate to prevent polyp relapse after endoscopic sinus surgery. *Arch Otolaryngol Head Neck Surg.* 2009;135:296–302.
11. Becker SS, Duncavage JA. The role of steroid injection in the management of sinonasal polyps. *Curr Opin Otolaryngol Head Neck Surg.* 2008;16:38–43.

ADDITIONAL READING

Fokkens WJ, Lund VJ, Mullol J, et al. EPOS 2012: European position paper on rhinosinusitis and nasal polyps 2012. A summary for otorhinolaryngologists. *Rhinology.* 2012;50:1–12.

CODES

ICD10

- J33.0 Polyp of nasal cavity
- J33.8 Other polyp of sinus
- J33.9 Nasal polyp, unspecified

CLINICAL PEARLS

- Allergy testing is very important.
- Sampter's triad consists of asthma, aspirin hypersensitivity, and nasal polyps.
- Never biopsy a nasal polyp in the office.
- Patients with severe obstruction should be referred for surgery.
- Unilateral nasal polyp needs malignancy workup (MRI).

NEAR DROWNING
Kevin M. Curtis, MD, MS

 BASICS

DESCRIPTION
- Survival, at least temporarily, after suffocation in liquid
- System(s) affected: Cardiovascular; Nervous; Pulmonary; Renal
- Synonym(s): Submersion injury

EPIDEMIOLOGY
Incidence
- From 2005–2009, an average of 3,533 deaths/year occurred from drowning in the US (1).
- 54 infants accidentally drowned in the US in 2007 (1).
- Three age-related peaks: Toddlers and young children (1–5 years), adolescents and young adults (15–25 years), and the elderly
- Predominant sex: Male > Female

Prevalence
- Drowning was the 5th most common cause of accidental death in the US in 2007 and the 2nd most common for children aged 1–14 years.
- For every child age <15 years who dies from drowning, 5 more children are seen in the emergency room for nonfatal submersion injuries.

ALERT
Proper water safety techniques may help to avoid this problem.

ETIOLOGY AND PATHOPHYSIOLOGY
Hypoxemia via aspiration and/or reflex laryngospasm causing cerebral hypoxia and multisystem organ involvement
- Bathtub and bucket drowning in children <1 year of age
- Pool drowning in children 1–4 years of age
- Drug or alcohol overdose
- Boating mishaps, water sports, scuba diving
- Motor vehicle accidents (e.g., automobile submerged in water)
- Head trauma while swimming or diving
- Hyperventilation before underwater swimming
- Suicide
- "Dry lungs": ~10–20% of victims drown without aspiration; may be due to prolonged laryngospasm, but some controversy exists
- "Wet drowning": 80–90% of victims show aspiration of water, sand, and/or mud into the lungs.
- Pulmonary: Dilution of surfactant with decreased gas transfer across alveoli, atelectasis, development of intrapulmonary right-to-left shunting; acute respiratory distress syndrome (ARDS); bronchospasm
- Cardiac: Arrhythmia (primary or secondary)
- Renal: Acute tubular necrosis from hypoxemia, shock, hemoglobinuria, myoglobinuria
- Neurologic: Hypoxic-ischemic brain injury with damage especially to the hippocampus, insular cortex, and basal ganglia; cerebral edema
- Coagulation: Hemolysis and coagulopathy

RISK FACTORS
- Alcohol ingestion
- Use of illicit drugs
- Seizure disorder
- Inability to swim
- Hyperventilation prior to underwater swimming
- Risk-taking behavior
- Improper pool fencing
- Trauma, including boating accidents
- Inadequate adult supervision of children
- Concomitant stroke, or myocardial infarction (MI)
- Hypothermia
- Cardiac arrhythmias: Familial long QT and familial polymorphic ventricular tachycardia (VT)
- Residence within sunbelt states
- African Americans
- Low socioeconomic status

GENERAL PREVENTION
- Proper adult supervision of children
- Knowledge of water safety guidelines
- Mandatory pool fencing and pool alarms
- Fences higher than 54 inches (137 cm) for home pools
- Avoidance of alcohol or recreational drugs around water
- Swimming instruction at an early age
- Cardiopulmonary resuscitation (CPR) instruction for pool owners, parents
- Boating safety knowledge
- Personal flotation device (e.g., preserver, if necessary)

Pediatric Considerations
Children should never be left alone near water. Young children can drown in very small amounts of water, such as in bathtubs, buckets, and toilets.

COMMONLY ASSOCIATED CONDITIONS
- Trauma
- Seizure disorder
- Alcohol or illicit drug use
- Hypothermia
- Concomitant stroke, or MI
- Cardiac arrhythmias: Familial long QT and familial polymorphic VT
- Hyperventilation

 DIAGNOSIS

HISTORY
- Victim found in or near water
- Duration of submersion
- Loss of consciousness
- Period of apnea
- Artificial ventilation/CPR performed
- History of associated trauma
- Approximate water temperature
- Recent use of alcohol or drugs
- Known seizure disorder
- Known cardiac disease, including arrhythmia or prolonged QT
- Preceding syncope

PHYSICAL EXAM
- Airway status and degree of respiratory effort and/or distress
- Pulse: Absent, weak, or normal
- Vital signs, including pulse oximetry
- Glasgow Coma Scale (GCS)
- Wheezing
- Evidence of trauma

DIFFERENTIAL DIAGNOSIS
Head trauma, arrhythmia, seizure, alcohol or other substance overdose, nonaccidental trauma

DIAGNOSTIC TESTS & INTERPRETATION
Initial Tests (lab, imaging)
May be unnecessary if initial GCS and pulse oximetry are normal and remain that way for 6–8 hours (2):
- CBC with differential
- Arterial blood gases (ABGs): Hypoxia, hypercarbia, acidosis
- Electrolytes: Hypokalemia, hyponatremia, hypernatremia
- Blood glucose: May be low as cause of near drowning; increased levels may impair neurologic recovery after ischemic brain injury.
- BUN, creatinine: Acute tubular necrosis
- Troponin
- Creatine kinase (CK) and urine myoglobin: Rhabdomyolysis
- Coagulation studies
- Urinalysis/urine drug screen
- A chest x-ray (CXR) may be unnecessary for patients with all of the following (2):
  – Normal initial GCS and pulse oximetry
  – No evidence of respiratory distress
  – No change after 6–8 hours of observation
- For others, a CXR may show evidence of aspiration, atelectasis, pneumothorax, or ARDS.
- Head CT and/or C-spine imaging as needed for associated trauma

Follow-Up Tests & Special Considerations
- Patients with an initial GCS of 15 and pulse oximetry >95% should be observed for 6–8 hours in the emergency department (ED) (2).
- CXR findings may be minimal or absent on early imaging.

Diagnostic Procedures/Other
- Continuous cardiac monitoring
- Continuous pulse oximetry
- Continuous core temperature monitoring if hypothermic
- ECG
- Central venous pressure (CVP) monitoring for critically ill
- Electroencephalogram (EEG) if question of seizure as cause

TREATMENT

Early resuscitation and reversal of hypoxemia optimizes outcome.

GENERAL MEASURES
- Prehospital:
  – Never approach a struggling victim alone.
  – Start with the basics: Airway, breathing, circulation (ABCs).
  – For severely hypothermic patients, the pulse check should be performed for at least 1 minute
  – CPR as soon as possible and prior to removal from water if able
  – Two initial rescue breaths should precede chest compressions
  – Remove from water quickly and place in a normal CPR position (3).
  – Avoid abdominal thrusting or Heimlich maneuvers (3).

– Routine cervical collar use and spinal precautions are not needed unless a high suspicion for trauma exists (4).

– Supplemental oxygen and early intubation, as needed (4)[A]

– If patient is breathing on his or her own and does not need spinal precautions, place in the right lateral decubitus position to prevent aspiration of vomit or gastric contents (3).

- Emergency Department:
  – Oxygen, as needed, to maintain saturation >94%
  – Continuous positive airway pressure (PAP), BiPAP or intubation if O_2 alone unsuccessful
  – Indications for intubation:
    ○ Neurologic deterioration
    ○ Inability to protect the airway
    ○ Inability to maintain oxygen saturation >90% or PaO_2 >60 mm Hg on high-flow supplemental oxygen
    ○ $PaCO_2$ >50 mm Hg
  – Routine cervical collar use and spinal precautions are not needed unless a high suspicion for trauma exists (4).
  – Remove wet clothing and initiate rewarming
  – Core temperature reading for possible hypothermia
  – Core warming with pleural and peritoneal lavage with warm saline; warm, humidified oxygen; warm IV fluids; warmed, humidified oxygen; or cardiopulmonary bypass as needed for severe hypothermia (4)[C]

MEDICATION
First Line
- High flow oxygen, as needed (3)[A]
- For bronchospasm: Aerosolized bronchodilator (3)[C]: Albuterol (Proventil, Ventolin), 3 mL of 0.083% solution or 0.5 mL of 0.5% solution diluted in 3 mL of saline
- Pressors, as needed, for hypotension refractory to IV fluid resuscitation
- Prophylactic antibiotics and steroids are not helpful (4)[B].

Second Line
With pneumonia: Antibiotics based on sputum or endotracheal lavage culture (4)[A]

IN-PATIENT CONSIDERATIONS
Admission Criteria/Initial Stabilization
- All symptomatic patients
- Patients with abnormalities in vital signs, mental status, oxygenation, CXR, or laboratory analysis

IV Fluids
To maintain adequate intravascular volume (3)[C]

Nursing
- Continuous cardiac monitoring
- Continuous pulse oximetry monitoring
- Frequent monitoring of vital signs and clinical reassessment
- Careful monitoring of neurologic status

Discharge Criteria
Patients can be discharged from the ED after 6–8 hours of observation if the following criteria are met (2):
- GCS = 15
- Normal CXR, if indicated
- Lack of clinical evidence of respiratory difficulty
- Normal lung exam
- Normal vital signs
- Oxygen saturation ≥95% on room air (4)

ONGOING CARE

FOLLOW-UP RECOMMENDATIONS
Appropriate follow up with orthopedic, neurologic, cardiac, pulmonary, and so forth specialists as warranted

Patient Monitoring
- Continuous cardiac monitoring
- Continuous pulse oximetry monitoring
- Frequent monitoring of vital signs and clinical reassessment
- Careful monitoring of neurologic status
- ABG monitoring, as indicated (4)
- A pulmonary artery catheter may be needed for hemodynamic monitoring in unstable patients (3)[C].
- Intracranial pressure monitoring in selected patients (3)[C]
- Serum electrolyte determinations (4)

DIET
NPO until mental status normalizes

PATIENT EDUCATION
Re-emphasize preventive measures on discharge from hospital. Educate parents and recommend pool safety, and so on.

PROGNOSIS
- 75% of drowning victims survive; 6% of these with residual neurologic deficits
- Patients with an initial GCS ≥13 and an oxygen saturation ≥95% have a low risk of complications and an excellent chance for a full recovery.
- Patients who are comatose or receiving CPR at the time of presentation or who have dilated and fixed pupils and no spontaneous respiratory activity have a more guarded and often poor prognosis.
- Secondary drowning from neurogenic pulmonary edema may occur within 48 hours of initial presentation.

COMPLICATIONS
- Early:
  – Bronchospasm
  – Vomiting/Aspiration
  – Hypoglycemia
  – Hypothermia
  – Seizure
  – Hypovolemia
  – Electrolyte abnormalities
  – Arrhythmia from hypoxia or hypothermia (rarely from electrolyte imbalance)
  – Hypotension
- Late:
  – ARDS
  – Anoxic encephalopathy
  – Pneumonia
  – Lung abscess/Empyema
  – Renal failure
  – Coagulopathy
  – Sepsis
  – Barotrauma
  – Seizure

REFERENCES
1. Centers for Disease Control and Prevention. CDC 24/7: Saving lives. protecting people. unintentional drowning: Get the facts. Available at: www.cdc.gov/HomeandRecreationalSafety/Water-Safety/waterinjuries-factsheet.html/
2. Causey AL, Tilelli JA, Swanson ME. Predicting discharge in uncomplicated near-drowning. *Am J Emerg Med*. 2000;18:9–11.
3. Orlowski JP, Szpilman D. Drowning. Rescue, resuscitation, and reanimation. *Pediatr Clin North Am*. 2001;48:627–646.
4. Salomez F, Vincent JL. Drowning: A review of epidemiology, pathophysiology, treatment and prevention. *Resuscitation*. 2004;63:261–268.

ADDITIONAL READING
- American Academy of Pediatrics Committee on Injury, Violence, and Poison Prevention. Prevention of drowning. *Pediatrics*. 2010;126:178–185.
- American Heart Association guidelines for cardiopulmonary resuscitation and emergency cardiovascular care. Part 10.3: Drowning. *Circulation*. 2005;112(24S):133–135.
- Giesbrecht GG, Hayward JS. Problems and complications with cold-water rescue. *Wilderness Environ Med*. 2006;17:26–30.
- Guenther U, Varelmann D, Putensen C, et al. Extended therapeutic hypothermia for several days during extracorporeal membrane-oxygenation after drowning and cardiac arrest: Two cases of survival with no neurological sequelae. *Resuscitation*. 2009;80:379–381.
- Kochanek PM, Fink EL, Bell MJ, et al. Therapeutic hypothermia: Applications in pediatric cardiac arrest. *J Neurotrauma*. 2009;26:421–427.

 ## CODES

ICD10
- T75.1XXA Unsp effects of drowning and nonfatal submersion, init
- T75.1XXD Unsp effects of drowning and nonfatal submersion, subs
- T75.1XXS Unsp effects of drowning and nonfatal submersion, sequela

CLINICAL PEARLS
- The single most important treatment for near-drowning victims is prompt reversal of the hypoxic state. This should form the cornerstone for all other treatment modalities. Without oxygenation, other treatment is futile.
- Family physicians and pediatricians should review water safety tips and guidelines with parents and children at yearly visits. Encourage pool owners and parents with young children to become CPR certified. Prevention of drowning can save many lives each year.
- Despite successful resuscitation, patients are at risk for ARDS due to delayed pulmonary edema that may start hours after their submersion incident. For this reason, careful monitoring of every resuscitated patient is essential.
- Patients with an initial GCS ≥13 and an oxygen saturation ≥95% have a low risk of complications and an excellent chance for a full recovery.

N

NEPHROTIC SYNDROME

Carla M. Nester, MD, MSA

 BASICS

DESCRIPTION
- A clinical syndrome of heavy proteinuria (>3.5 g/1.73 m^2/24 hours), hypoalbuminemia, hyperlipidemia, and edema
- Includes both primary and secondary forms
- Associated with many types of kidney disease

EPIDEMIOLOGY
Based on definitive diagnosis:
- Diabetic nephropathy: Most common cause of secondary nephrotic syndrome (1)
- Minimal change disease (MCD):
  - Most common nephrotic syndrome in children, peaks at 2–8 years
  - Associated with drugs or lymphoma in adults
- Amyloidosis: Rare
- Lupus nephropathy (LN): Adult women are affected about 10 × more often than men.
- Focal segmental glomerulosclerosis (FSGS):
  - 25% of nephrotic syndrome in adults
  - Most common primary nephrotic syndrome in African Americans
  - Has both primary and secondary forms
- Membranous nephropathy:
  - Most common primary nephrotic syndrome in Caucasians
  - Associated with malignancy and infection
- Membranoproliferative glomerulonephritis (MGN):
  - May be primary or secondary
  - May present in the setting of a systemic viral or rheumatic illness

ETIOLOGY AND PATHOPHYSIOLOGY
- Increased glomerular permeability to protein molecules, especially albumin
- Edema results primarily from renal salt retention, with arterial underfilling from decreased plasma oncotic pressure playing an additional role.
- Hyperlipidemia is thought to be a consequence of increased hepatic synthesis resulting from low oncotic pressure and urinary loss of regulatory proteins.
- The hypercoagulable state that can occur in some nephrotic states is likely due to loss of antithrombin III in urine.
- Primary renal disease:
  - MCD
  - FSGS
  - MGN
  - IgA nephropathy
  - Membranoproliferative glomerulonephritis
- Secondary renal disease (associated primary renal disease shown in parentheses):
  - Diabetic nephropathy
  - Amyloidosis
  - LN
  - FSGS
  - Infections (MGN)
  - Cancer (MCD or MGN)
  - Drugs (MCD or MGN)

Genetics
Genetic factors are likely to play a role in susceptibility to the various nephrotic syndromes, although these have not been sufficiently defined to be useful clinically.

RISK FACTORS
- Drug addiction (e.g., heroin [FSGS])
- Hepatitis B and C, HIV, other infections
- Immunosuppression
- Nephrotoxic drugs
- Vesicoureteral reflux (FSGS)
- Cancer (usually MGN, may be MCD)
- Chronic analgesic use/abuse
- Preeclampsia
- Diabetes mellitus

GENERAL PREVENTION
In general, there are few preventive measures, except avoidance of known causative medications.

DIAGNOSIS

HISTORY
- Inquire about signs or symptoms of systemic disease: Joint complaint, rash, edema, infectious complaint, fevers, anorexia, oliguria, foamy urine, acute flank pain, hematuria
- Obtain a recent drug history for medications that may be causative, especially NSAIDs
- Assess for risk factors

PHYSICAL EXAM
A complete physical exam may discover clues to systemic disease as a potential cause and/or may suggest the severity of disease:
- Fluid retention: Abdominal distention, abdominal fluid shift, extremity edema, puffy eyelids, scrotal swelling, weight gain, shortness of breath. Pericardial rub and decreased breath sounds with pleural effusions may develop.
- Hypertension
- Orthostatic hypotension

ALERT
The potential for thromboembolic disease leading to pulmonary embolism is one of the most life-threatening aspects of a patient who is actively nephrotic.

DIFFERENTIAL DIAGNOSIS
- Edema and proteinuria: See "Etiology and Pathophysiology."
- Edema alone: Other diseases to rule out in patients who have edema without proteinuria include congestive heart failure, cirrhosis, hypothyroidism, nutritional hypoalbuminemia, protein-losing enteropathy.

DIAGNOSTIC TESTS & INTERPRETATION
Initial Tests (lab, imaging)
- Confirm proteinuria is present: By urine dipstick initially, and then quantitate by 24-hour urine or urine protein-to-creatinine ratio
- Rule out urine infection with urine culture
- Full blood count and coagulation screen
- Renal function tests: BUN, creatinine with estimated glomerular filtration rate (GFR)
- Glucose to rule out overt diabetes
- Consider blood cultures to rule out a postinfectious process
- Lipid panel
- Liver function tests to exclude liver disease or infection
- Look for autoimmune disease:
  - Antinuclear antibody and/or antidouble-stranded DNA positivity suggest lupus.
  - Complement levels: A low C3 may suggest a postinfectious or membranoproliferative process, whereas both low C3 and C4 point to lupus.
- Serum protein electrophoresis/urine immune electrophoresis to rule in a paraproteinemia
- Hepatitis B and C screen
- HIV and syphilis testing
- Urinalysis to evaluate for the presence of cellular casts
- Renal US to verify the presence of 2 kidneys of normal shape and size
- Chest x-ray to detect presence of pleural effusion or infection
- If thrombosis suspected:
  - Doppler US of the legs
  - MRI or venography for renal vein thrombosis
  - Ventilation/Perfusion nuclear medicine lung scan and/or CT may be required to rule out pulmonary embolism.

Diagnostic Procedures/Other
Renal biopsy:
- Rarely done in children with 1st episode of nephrotic syndrome, as MCD is common and empiric steroid therapy is the standard of care
- Required to confirm the clinical diagnosis in adults and assist with making a treatment plan

Test Interpretation
- Light microscopy:
  - May see nothing (e.g., MCD)
  - Sclerosis (e.g., FSGS or diabetic nodules in diabetes)
  - Diffuse hypercellularity suggests a proliferative disease such as IgA nephropathy, LN, or postinfectious GN.
- Immunofluorescence: Mesangial IgA suggests IgA nephropathy, Henoch-Schönlein; other staining patterns are specific for other disease processes.
- Electron microscopy: The location of immunoglobulin deposits is useful in pointing to a particular diagnosis.

TREATMENT

MEDICATION

First Line

- Edema: Salt restriction and salt-wasting diuretics (loop and thiazide diuretics):
  - Salt restriction to <6 g of sodium chloride (<2.4 g sodium/d)
  - Restrict fluid intake to <1.5 L/d if hyponatremic
  - Target weight loss of 0.5–1 kg/d (1–2 lb/d)
- Statins have been shown to improve endothelial function (2) and may decrease proteinuria (3), but effect (if any) on GFR and preservation of renal function is small. The major role for statin use is in cardiovascular risk reduction.
- ACE inhibitors or angiotensin II receptor blockers thought to reduce proteinuria, hyperlipidemia, thrombotic tendencies, progression of renal failure (2,4)[A], and to control hypertension if present.
- For steroid-responsive disease (MCD and FGS), steroids dosed in consultation with nephrologist

Second Line

- Many of the nephrotic diseases will require escalation in therapy above steroids. These include rapidly relapsing forms, as well as MGN, LN, and IgA nephropathy. Bolus steroids and other immunosuppressives are required in this circumstance (cyclophosphamide, mycophenolate mofetil, chlorambucil, cyclosporine) (5)[A].
- Randomized controlled data have been insufficient to determine which patients require prophylactic anticoagulation (6)[A]. 1 practice is to anticoagulate with heparin and then warfarin in patients who have persistent nephrotic-range proteinuria. This decision is made based on the patient's history of edema, hypoalbuminemia, thromboembolism, or immobility.
- Hypocalcemia from vitamin D loss should be treated with oral vitamin D (dihydrotachysterol) 0.2 mg/d.

ISSUES FOR REFERRAL

Consultation with a nephrologist is often required to assist with renal biopsy to confirm diagnosis and to assist with management of edema. Cytotoxic medications may be called for, depending on the disease process, and this may best be handled by a nephrologist.

ADDITIONAL THERAPIES

Ambulation or range-of-motion exercises to lower risk of deep vein thrombosis (DVT)

IN-PATIENT CONSIDERATIONS

Admission Criteria/Initial Stabilization

Respiratory distress, sepsis/severe infection, thromboses, renal failure, hypertension, or other complications

Discharge Criteria

Hemodynamically stable patients without complications may be managed as outpatients.

 ONGOING CARE

FOLLOW-UP RECOMMENDATIONS

Patient Monitoring

- Frequent monitoring is required for relapse, disease progression, and for detecting signs of toxicity of medical management.
- Re-evaluate for azotemia, urine protein, hypertension, edema, loss of renal function, cholesterol, and weight.

DIET

- Normal protein (1 g/kg/d)
- Low fat (cholesterol)
- Reduced sodium
- Supplemental multivitamins and minerals, especially vitamin D and iron
- Fluid restriction if hyponatremic

PATIENT EDUCATION

- Printed material for patients: National Kidney Foundation, 30 E. 33rd Street, Suite 1100, New York, NY 10016; 800-622-9010:
  - Childhood nephrotic syndrome
  - Diabetes and kidney disease
  - Focal glomerulosclerosis
- Website: National Institutes of Health: Nephrotic syndrome

PROGNOSIS

Nephrotic syndrome in children (MCD) is typically self-limited and carries a good prognosis. In the adult, the prognosis is variable. Complete remission is expected if the basic disease is treatable (infection, malignancy, drug-induced); otherwise, a relapsing and remitting course is possible, with progression to dialysis seen in more aggressive forms (diabetic glomerulosclerosis).

COMPLICATIONS

- Thromboembolism:
  - DVT and/or renal vein thrombosis may occur.
  - The risk appears to be greater the lower the serum albumin.
  - Pulmonary embolism is a known complication.
- Pleural effusion
- Ascites
- Hyperlipidemia, cardiovascular disease
- Acute renal failure, progressive renal failure
- Protein malnutrition/muscle wasting
- Infection secondary to low serum IgG concentrations, reduced complement activity, and depressed T-cell function: Peritonitis, pneumonia, or cellulitis
- Loss of vitamin D (vitamin D–binding protein loss in urine) leading to bone disease

REFERENCES

1. Kodner C. Nephrotic syndrome in adults: Diagnosis and management. *Am Fam Physician*. 2009;80: 1129–1134.
2. Randomised placebo-controlled trial of effect of ramipril on decline in glomerular filtration rate and risk of terminal renal failure in proteinuric, non-diabetic nephropathy. The GISEN Group (Gruppo Italiano di Studi Epidemiologici in Nefrologia) *Lancet*. 1997;349:1857–1863.
3. Fried LF, Orchard TJ, Kasiske BL. Effect of lipid reduction on the progression of renal disease: A meta-analysis. *Kidney Int*. 2001;59:260–269.
4. Kunz R, Friedrich C, Wolbers M, et al. Meta-analysis: Effect of monotherapy and combination therapy with inhibitors of the renin angiotensin system on proteinuria in renal disease. *Ann Intern Med*. 2008;148:30–48.
5. Hodson EM, Willis NS, Craig JC, Interventions for idiopathic steroid-resistant nephrotic syndrome in children. *Cochrane Database Syst Rev*. 2010;11: CD003594.
6. Kulshrestha S, Grieff M, Navananeethan SD. Interventions for preventing thrombosis in adults and children with nephrotic syndrome (protocol). *Cochrane Database Syst Rev*. 2006;2:CD006024.

ADDITIONAL READING

- Madaio MP, Harrington JT. The diagnosis of glomerular diseases: Acute glomerulonephritis and the nephrotic syndrome. *Arch Intern Med*. 2001;161:25–34.
- Meyrier A. An update on the treatment options for focal segmental glomerulosclerosis. *Expert Opin Pharmacother*. 2009;10:615–628.

 SEE ALSO

Amyloidosis; Diabetes Mellitus, Type 1; Diabetes Mellitus, Type 2; Glomerulonephritis, Acute; HIV Infection and AIDS; Lupus Erythematosus, Discoid; Multiple Myeloma; Renal Failure, Acute

CODES

ICD10

- N04.1 Nephrotic syndrome w focal and segmental glomerular lesions
- N04.2 Nephrotic syndrome w diffuse membranous glomerulonephritis
- N04.9 Nephrotic syndrome with unspecified morphologic changes

CLINICAL PEARLS

- Nephrotic syndrome is a clinical syndrome of >3.5 g/d proteinuria, hypoalbuminemia, hyperlipidemia, and edema often associated with diabetes and NSAIDs use.
- Pediatric nephrotic syndrome typically carries a good prognosis and is easily treated with steroids. Recurrences are common.
- Nondiabetic adults with nephrotic syndrome will require a renal biopsy to determine cause.
- Have a high index of suspicion for symptoms that may represent an embolic event.

N

NEUROFIBROMATOSIS TYPE 1

Rayna Goldstein, MD • Michele Roberts, MD, PhD

 BASICS

DESCRIPTION

- Neurofibromatosis types 1 (NF1) and 2 (NF2) are neurocutaneous syndromes (phakomatoses). Although they share a name, they are distinct and unrelated conditions with genes on different chromosomes.
  - NF2 is a rare condition that causes bilateral vestibular schwannomas.
  - NF1 is a multisystem disorder that may affect any organ. It is the most common of the phakomatoses.
- System(s) affected: Musculoskeletal; Nervous; Skin/Exocrine; Cardiovascular; Neuroophthalmologic
- Synonym(s): Von Recklinghausen disease, formerly peripheral NF

EPIDEMIOLOGY

Incidence
- Predominant sex for NF1: Male = Female
- Birth incidence NF1: 1:2,500–3,000

Prevalence
1:3,000–1:4,000

ETIOLOGY AND PATHOPHYSIOLOGY
- Neurofibromin is a guanosine triphosphatase–activating protein that acts as a tumor suppressor by downregulating a cellular proto-oncogene, *p21-ras*, that enhances cell growth and proliferation.
- Neurofibromata are benign tumors composed of Schwann cells, fibroblasts, mast cells, and vascular components that develop along nerves.
- The 2-hit hypothesis has been invoked to explain malignant transformation in *NF1*.

Genetics
- Online Mendelian Inheritance in Man 162200
- Caused by a mutation in the *NF1* gene on chromosome 17q11.2; autosomal-dominant inheritance; protein product is called *neurofibromin*
- 50% of cases are due to new mutations. Prenatal diagnosis possible if family history is positive.
- Penetrance is nearly 100%; expressivity is highly variable.
- Gene is large, with a variety of mutations causing NF1. Molecular technology can detect 95% of clinically important *NF1* mutations, but it is usually not indicated because clinical diagnosis frequently can be made in childhood.
- ~5% of individuals with NF1 have a large deletion of the entire *NF1* gene (or nearly so); they usually have a more severe phenotype.
- *Segmental NF* (an NF1 variant) is limited to a single body region and is caused by mosaicism for the *NF1* mutation.

RISK FACTORS
- Having an affected 1st-degree relative is a diagnostic criterion for NF1, although relatives may be unaware of their condition.
- Affected individuals with a positive family history, as well as those with a new mutation, have a 50% risk of transmitting NF1 to each of their offspring; 1 in 12 will be severely affected.
- Individuals with segmental NF1 may have gonadal mosaicism and may be at risk for transmission of the mutated gene.

COMMONLY ASSOCIATED CONDITIONS
Congenital heart disease, pulmonary stenosis, hypertension, renal artery stenosis

 DIAGNOSIS

- NF1 can be diagnosed by routine exam by age 4 years, with attention to skin stigmata; diagnostic criteria for include ≥2 of the following (1):
  - ≥6 café-au-lait (light brown) macules, ≥5 mm in prepubertal individuals or ≥15 mm in adults
  - ≥2 neurofibromata of any type or 1 plexiform (noncircumscribed) neurofibroma
  - Axillary or inguinal freckling
  - ≥2 Lisch nodules (benign iris hamartomas, asymptomatic)
  - Optic glioma by MRI
  - Characteristic osseous lesions: Sphenoid dysplasia, long-bone cortical thinning, ribbon ribs, angular scoliosis
  - 1st-degree relative with NF1 by above criteria
- Prenatal diagnosis is possible with known mutation or by linkage testing (with positive family history), although not predictive of clinical course.

HISTORY
- Family history of a 1st-degree relative with NF1
- Manifestations generally are not visible at birth, although plexiform neurofibromata usually are congenital and tibial bowing is congenital.
- In addition to cutaneous lesions, NF1 may present with painful neurofibromata, pathologic fractures, or headaches secondary to hypertension caused by pheochromocytomas.
- Optic gliomata may present as involuntary eye movement, squinting, loss of vision, or as diencephalic syndrome.

PHYSICAL EXAM
- Skin:
  - Café-au-lait macules develop during the first 3 years of childhood and are usually the presenting feature of NF1. Evenly pigmented, irregularly shaped (coast-of-California), light brown macules present in 97% of patients with NF1; many unaffected individuals have 1–3 such macules.
  - Neurofibromata: Can be cutaneous, SC, or plexiform and may be soft or firm; buttonhole invagination is pathognomonic. Cutaneous neurofibromata usually begin to appear during late childhood or adolescence.
  - Plexiform neurofibromata are present in up to 50% of individuals with NF1:
    ○ Usually congenital; may be subtle in infancy
    ○ Freckling or hypertrichosis may be present over plexiform neurofibromata; may affect underlying structures or cause focal hyperplasia.
    ○ Many are internal, not obvious on exam.
    ○ Most grow slowly over may years, but can have rapid growth, especially in early childhood.
  - Evaluate for new lesions and progression of pre-existing ones. Rapidly growing cutaneous lesions should be evaluated thoroughly.
  - Axillary freckling (Crowe sign) or inguinal freckling (91%)
- Ophthalmologic:
  - Lisch nodules (benign iris hamartomas) in 30%: well-defined, dome-shaped, gelatinous hamartomatous lesions projecting from the iris, varying from clear yellow to brown.

  - Essentially unique to NF, Lisch nodules are asymptomatic and are significant only for diagnosis
  - Pallor or atrophy of optic disc, bulging of orbit, loss of vision may be signs of optic glioma.
- Skeletal:
  - Scoliosis and vertebral angulation
  - Localized bone hypertrophy, especially of the face
  - Limb abnormalities:
    ○ Pseudoarthrosis of the tibia
    ○ Tibial dysplasia (anterolateral bowing of the tibia) is congenital, if present.
    ○ Nonossifying fibromas of the long bones in adolescents and adults are uncommon but can increase risk of fracture.
- Pay particular attention to neurologic examination or new focal pain.
- Measure BP yearly. Hypertension is more common in patients with NF1 and could be secondary to renal artery stenosis, aortic stenosis, or pheochromocytoma.
- Evaluate neurodevelopmental progress in children. Learning disabilities occur in 50–75%.

DIFFERENTIAL DIAGNOSIS
Familial café-au-lait spots (autosomal dominant, no other NF1 features), Watson syndrome, LEOPARD syndrome, McCune-Albright syndrome, neurocutaneous melanosis, proteus syndrome, lipomatosis

Geriatric Considerations
In NF1, cutaneous lesions and tumors increase in size and number with age.

Pediatric Considerations
- Children who have inherited the *NF1* gene of an affected parent usually are identified by age 1, but external stigmata may be subtle. If there are no stigmata by age 2, NF is unlikely but the child should be re-examined within the next few years. Definite diagnosis can be made by age 4 using National Institute of Health (NIH) criteria (1).
- Young children with multiple café-au-lait spots, but no other stigmata after careful physical and ophthalmologic evaluation, should be followed clinically as if they have NF1 (2).
- Molecular confirmation may be appropriate, especially with atypical presentation (3).

DIAGNOSTIC TESTS & INTERPRETATION
- DNA sequence and deletion/duplication analysis of the *NF1* gene can identify mutations in ~96% of those with a clinical diagnosis.
- Molecular genetic testing is available, although often not necessary for diagnosis. Diagnostic laboratory information: www.genetests.org
- Confirmatory genetic testing is appropriate in those who are suspected of having NF1 but do not fulfill diagnostic criteria or for prenatal diagnosis or preimplantation genetic diagnosis (PGD) (4).

Initial Tests (lab, imaging)
- Characteristic radiographic findings: Sphenoid dysplasia, long-bone cortical thinning, ribbon ribs, and angular scoliosis. Screening radiographs of the knees in adolescents is controversial. CT can demonstrate bony changes.

- MRI findings of the orbits, brain, or spine (86%). Routine head MRI scanning in asymptomatic individuals with NF1 is controversial. Optic gliomata (seen on MRI, 11–15%) may lead to blindness. Although areas of increased T_2 signal intensity (unidentified bright objects) are common on brain MRI, they are not diagnostic of NF1 and are of no clinical significance.
- The NIH Consensus Development Conference does not recommend routine neuroimaging as a means of establishing a diagnosis (1,5).

Diagnostic Procedures/Other
- Ophthalmologic evaluation, including slit-lamp exam of the irides; visual field testing to evaluate optic gliomata
- Neuropsychological testing: Intelligence usually normal, but may have significant deficits in language, visuospatial skills, and neuromotor skills

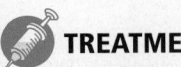

TREATMENT

MEDICATION
First Line
Anticonvulsants for seizures, medications for ADHD.

Second Line
Multiple clinical trials for NF1 are recruiting patients (see www.clinicaltrials.gov).

ISSUES FOR REFERRAL
- Patients with more than minimal manifestations of NF1: Refer to a multidisciplinary NF clinic
- Referral for psychosocial issues of family and affected individuals
- Educational intervention for children with learning disabilities or ADHD (40%)
- Early referral to orthopedics for congenital tibial bowing

ADDITIONAL THERAPIES
- Occupational therapy for children with NF1 who present with fine motor difficulties
- There is no evidence supporting laser therapy for café-au-lait spots.
- The Children's Tumor Foundation (CTF) has established the NF Clinical Trials Consortium and the CTF NF Clinic Network to facilitate future clinical trials and help identify best practices (6).

SURGERY/OTHER PROCEDURES
Surgical treatment for severe scoliosis, plexiform neurofibromata, or malignancy

ONGOING CARE

FOLLOW-UP RECOMMENDATIONS
NF1 health supervision 2008 guidelines (7):
- Infancy to 1 year:
  - Growth and development: Mild short stature, macrocephaly (increased brain volume); aqueductal stenosis/obstructive hydrocephalus, hydrocephalus
  - Check for focal neurologic signs or asymmetric neurologic exam
  - Skeletal abnormalities, especially spine and legs
  - Neurodevelopmental progress
- 1–5 years:
  - Café-au-lait spots and axillary freckling have no clinical significance.
  - Annual ophthalmologic exam
  - Brain MRI for visual changes, persistent headaches, seizures, marked increase in head size, plexiform neurofibroma of the head

- Assess speech and language: Hypernasal speech due to velopharyngeal insufficiency and delayed expressive language development
- Developmental evaluation of learning and motor abilities; may benefit from speech/language and/or motor therapy, and special education
- Monitor BP annually
- 5–13 years:
  - Evaluate for skin tumors causing disfigurement and obtain consultation if surgery is desired to improve appearance or function.
  - Evaluate for premature or delayed puberty. If sexual precocity is noted, evaluate for an optic glioma or hypothalamic lesion. Review the effects of puberty on NF.
  - Evaluate for learning disabilities and ADHD
  - Evaluate social adjustment, development, and school placement
  - Monitor ophthalmologic status yearly until age 8; complete eye exam every 2 years
  - Monitor BP annually.
  - Refer patient to a clinical psychologist or child psychiatrist for problems with self-esteem
  - Discuss growth of neurofibromata during adolescence and pregnancy
  - Counsel parents about discussing diagnosis with child
- 13–21 years:
  - Examine the adolescent for abnormal pubertal development
  - Perform a thorough skin examination for plexiform neurofibromata and a complete neurologic exam for findings suggestive of deep plexiform neurofibromata; seek surgical consultation for signs of pressure on deep structures.
  - Continue to monitor BP yearly
  - Continue ophthalmologic examination every 2 years until age 18
  - Discuss genetics of NF1 or refer for genetic counseling
  - Discuss sexuality, contraception, and reproductive options
  - Discuss effects of pregnancy on NF1, if appropriate. Neurofibromata may enlarge and new tumors may develop during pregnancy.
  - Review prenatal diagnosis or refer the patient to a geneticist

PATIENT EDUCATION
- Genetic counseling and patient education regarding future complications about family planning
- The CTF: www.CTF.org. Support groups are important.

PROGNOSIS
Variable; most patients have a mild expression of NF1 and lead normal lives.

COMPLICATIONS
- Disfigurement: Skin neurofibromata develop primarily on exposed areas. The number tends to increase with puberty or pregnancy.
- Scoliosis: 10–30% (most cases mild); bowing of long bones, 2%; osteopenia and osteoporosis
- A large head is common but rarely associated with hydrocephalus.
- Increased risk of malignancy: Malignant peripheral nerve sheath tumor (MPNST) (5–10%) usually in adults (1), especially within the field of previous radiotherapy (typically arises from a plexiform neurofibroma); slightly increased risk for pheochromocytoma, rhabdomyosarcoma, leukemia, Wilms tumor; CNS tumors (5–15%), especially optic pathway glioma (most common CNS tumor), most

often asymptomatic, but if symptomatic, usually presents before age 6. Symptomatic lesions are usually stable or only slowly progressive.
- Learning disability: ~50%; may be associated with ADHD; mental retardation in 4–8%
- GI neurofibromata may cause GI disturbances
- Seizures 6–7%
- Hypertension is a frequent finding in adults and may occur during childhood.
- Disorders of puberty

Pregnancy Considerations
Increased risk of perinatal complications, stillbirth, intrauterine growth constriction; risk of cord compression and outlet obstruction by pelvic neurofibromata

REFERENCES

1. DeBella K, Szudek J, Friedman JM. Use of the National Institutes of Health Criteria for diagnosis of neurofibromatosis 1 in children. *Pediatrics.* 2000;105:608–614.
2. Nunley KS, Gao F, Albers AC, et al. Predictive value of café au lait macules at initial consultation in the diagnosis of neurofibromatosis type 1. *Arch Dermatol.* 2009;145:883–887.
3. Burkitt Wright EM, Sach E, Sharif S, et al. Can the diagnosis of NF1 be excluded clinically? A lack of pigmentary findings in families with spinal neurofibromatosis demonstrates a limitation of clinical diagnosis. *J Med Genet.* 2013;50:606–613.
4. Neurofibromatosis 1. GeneReviews at GeneTests Medical Genetics Information Resource (database online). Copyright, University of Washington, Seattle. 1997–2012. Available at: www.genetests.org
5. National Institutes of Health Consensus Development Conference Statement: Neurofibromatosis. Bethesda, MD; July 13–15, 1987. *Neurofibromatosis.* 1988;1:172–178.
6. Williams VC, Lucas J, Babcock MA, et al. Neurofibromatosis type 1 revisited. *Pediatrics.* 2009;123:124–133.
7. Hersh JH, American Academy of Pediatrics Committee on Genetics. Health supervision for children with neurofibromatosis. *Pediatrics.* 2008;84:633–642.

 SEE ALSO

Tuberous Sclerosis Complex; von Hippel–Lindau Disease

 CODES

ICD10
Q85.01 Neurofibromatosis, type 1

CLINICAL PEARLS
- NF1 and NF2 are 2 distinct genetic disorders.
- NF1 has marked clinical variability. External stigmata may be subtle or absent in young children. Minimally affected children may become severely affected adults.
- A single café-au-lait spot is of no concern in a child, but having ≥6 is a diagnostic criterion for NF1.

N

NEUROLEPTIC MALIGNANT SYNDROME

Anubhav Kaul, MD, MPH • Sakshi Jasra, MD • Rekha Bhandari, MD

 BASICS

DESCRIPTION
- Neuroleptic malignant syndrome (NMS) is a life-threatening condition that may develop anytime during therapy with neuroleptics; most cases develop within the 1st 2 weeks of starting 1 of these medications.
- Non-neuroleptic medications that have antidopaminergic activity have also been implicated.
- Characterized by muscular rigidity due to dopamine antagonism in the nigrostriatal pathway
- Hyperthermia from the blockage of hypothalamic thermoregulation (more likely in the setting of benzodiazepine withdrawal)
- Autonomic dysfunction
- Altered mental status
- May be indistinguishable from other causes of drug-induced hyperthermia (e.g., malignant hyperthermia, serotonin syndrome, lethal catatonia, anticholinergic toxins, or sympathomimetic poisoning); detailed history can help differentiate between these causes

EPIDEMIOLOGY
Incidence
- Variably reported from prospective studies as 0.01–3%
- 2,000 new cases annually in the US
- Predominant sex: Male > Female
- Predominant age: <40 years

Prevalence
0.15% ± 0.05% among patients receiving neuroleptics

ETIOLOGY AND PATHOPHYSIOLOGY
- Exact mechanism unknown
- Most likely due to central dopaminergic blockade of nigrostriatal, hypothalamic, mesocortical/limbic pathways
- Certain theories suggest a role of sympathoadrenal hyperactivity; defects in neuronal calcium regulatory proteins may also contribute to the pathogenesis.
- Most commonly seen in treatment with typical neuroleptics: Phenothiazines (e.g., fluphenazine), butyrophenones (e.g., haloperidol), and thiothixene
- May also be seen with atypical antipsychotics (e.g., clozapine, risperidone, olanzapine) (1,2)
- Nonneuroleptic agents with anti–dopaminergic activity (e.g., metoclopramide, promethazine and droperidol) have also been implicated.
- Rare cases have occurred with usage of medications not known to have any central anti-dopaminergic activity (e.g., lithium, phenelzine and desipramine).
- Also associated with withdrawal from dopamine agonists in Parkinson disease, CNS shunt failure, and functional hemispherectomy (3)

Genetics
- Some studies show a genetic predisposition to NMS.
- Polymorphisms: Loss of del allele in 141C Ins/Del of the dopamine D_2 receptor gene and Ser9Gly in the dopamine D_3 receptor gene

RISK FACTORS
- Newly administered medication/rapid increase in the dose of an existing agent
- Intramuscular or depot administration of medications
- Concurrent use of multiple neuroleptic agents
- Administration of neuroleptics with other drugs known to cause NMS, such as lithium
- Previous episodes of NMS
- Exposure to heat
- Dehydration/malnutrition
- Use of psychoactive agents
- Presence of an underlying structural/functional brain disorder (tumor, encephalitis, delirium/dementia)
- Postpartum women may be at an increased risk of developing NMS.

 DIAGNOSIS

HISTORY
- Neuroleptic use or an increase in dose
- Discontinuation of antiparkinsonian drug

PHYSICAL EXAM
- Extrapyramidal symptoms: Dysphagia, short shuffling gait, resting tremor, and significant skeletal muscle rigidity—lead-pipe rigidity (these symptoms are less likely with clozapine-induced NMS) (1)
- Hyperthermia (temperature may be as high as 106–107°F [41°C])
- Altered level of consciousness (ranging from mild drowsiness, agitation, or confusion to a severe delirium/coma)
- Autonomic instability (e.g., diaphoresis, flushing, skin pallor, tachycardia, tachypnea, labile BP, urinary incontinence)

DIFFERENTIAL DIAGNOSIS
- Infectious: Meningitis, encephalitis, brain abscess, pneumonia/sepsis
- Metabolic: Acute renal failure, thyrotoxicosis, pheochromocytoma
- Malignant hyperthermia, severe dystonic reaction
- Lethal catatonia
- Serotonin syndrome
- Anticholinergic poisoning, salicylate poisoning
- Sympathomimetic poisoning
- Acute hydrocephalus or spinal cord injury
- Tetanus
- Rabies
- Heat stroke
- Strychnine poisoning
- Vascular CNS event
- Acute intermittent porphyria
- Nonconvulsive status epilepticus
- Drug withdrawal: From alcohol, benzodiazepines, baclofen, sedatives, and hypnotics

DIAGNOSTIC TESTS & INTERPRETATION
- CBC (evaluate for leukocytosis)
- Elevated creatine phosphokinase (CPK)
- Serum electrolyte abnormalities (hypocalcemia, hypomagnesemia, hypo-/hypernatremia, hyperkalemia, metabolic acidosis)
- Consider: Lactate dehydrogenase levels, liver function tests, urine myoglobin, BUN and creatinine, uric acid, serum iron, and coagulation studies

Initial Tests (lab, imaging)
- Chest x-ray (if aspiration pneumonia is suspected)
- Head CT scan (before lumber puncture and to rule out underlying brain etiology)
- MRI to detect restricted diffusion in cerebellar hemispheres, basal ganglia, and cerebellum (4)[C]

Diagnostic Procedures/Other
- Lumbar puncture (rule out other causes of fever/altered mental status)
- Urinalysis (rule out UTI)
- Blood culture (as part of sepsis workup)
- Urinary drug screen
- Electroencephalography (rule out nonconvulsive status epilepticus)

 TREATMENT

- Discontinue offending agent immediately (5)[C]; if symptoms are due to CNS insult and do not subside on alleviation of insult, consider use of intrathecal baclofen (3)[C]
- Provide supportive care (6)[C]:
  – Hydration
  – Maintain renal function
  – Regulate temperature

GENERAL MEASURES
- Volume repletion
- Correct electrolyte abnormalities.
- Relief of muscle rigidity
- Recognize complications (e.g., rhabdomyolysis, respiratory failure, acute renal failure); mortality can be as high as 50%.

MEDICATION
- Dopamine agonists can be used, but their role in NMS is still uncertain:
  – Bromocriptine: May play a role in longer-term management: 5–10 mg PO b.i.d.; max 40 mg/d
  – Amantadine: 100 mg PO b.i.d.; increase, as needed, to a max 400 mg/d
- Skeletal muscle relaxant: Dantrolene (may play a role in longer-term management: 100–200 mg/d PO; max 400 mg/d or 0.8–2.5 mg/kg q6h; max 10 mg/kg/d)
- Benzodiazepines are the drugs of choice:
  – Diazepam: 5 mg IV q5min
  – Lorazepam: 1 mg IV q5min
- Electroconvulsive therapy may be used for refractory symptoms not responding to medical treatment (5).
- Neither bromocriptine nor dantrolene has a rapid onset, and neither has been demonstrated to alter outcome.

ISSUES FOR REFERRAL
- The patient's psychiatric disease should be evaluated by a psychiatrist during withdrawal of neuroleptic medications.
- All patients should be transferred to an acute-care facility where intensive monitoring is available.
- Nephrologist should be consulted in the setting of renal failure.

IN-PATIENT CONSIDERATIONS

Admission Criteria/Initial Stabilization

- All patients with the diagnosis of NMS should be admitted.
- Patients often will require intensive care.
- Airway intervention and circulatory support, as needed; ventilation may be difficult because of chest wall rigidity.
- IV fluids, supplemental O$_2$, cardiac monitor
- Immediate IV benzodiazepines (e.g., diazepam, lorazepam); may require repeated large doses to control agitation.
- If symptoms are not controlled within a few minutes, rapid-sequence intubation and neuromuscular blockade are necessary; nondepolarizing neuromuscular blockers (e.g., vecuronium, rocuronium, pancuronium) are preferable to succinylcholine.
- Cool the patient (ice packs, cooling blankets, ice water gastric lavage); fast cooling therapy is strongly recommended to reduce residual impairment.
- Treat arising symptoms, such as seizures and high blood pressure, appropriately.
- Aggressive IV fluid therapy with lactated Ringer solution or normal saline (NS), and alkalinization of urine to prevent renal failure from rhabdomyolysis (high CPK levels)
- Check fingerstick glucose to monitor for hyperosmolar hyperglycemic state (HHS)
- Administer heparin/low molecular weight heparin to prevent deep venous thrombosis

IV Fluids

Hydration with IV NS (6)[C]

ONGOING CARE

FOLLOW-UP RECOMMENDATIONS

- Allow 2 weeks after recovery to rechallenge neuroleptic; rechallenge should not be with the medication implicated in the original NMS episode; consider lower potency neuroleptic agent (6)[C].
- For pregnant women, untreated psychosis by discontinuing neuroleptics in the setting of NMS can lead to adverse effect such as miscarriage, stillbirth, prematurity, and small size for gestational age; consider risk and benefit before restarting neuroleptic therapy.
- Start at low dose and titrate gradually
- Carefully monitor for signs and symptoms of recurrent NMS (5)[C].

PATIENT EDUCATION

- Discuss risk-to-benefit ratio of restarting therapy vs. a recurrence of NMS.
- NMS information service: www.nmsis.org

PROGNOSIS

- Mortality rate is estimated at 5–11.6% (dropped from 25% in 1984).
- Signs that may warn of a poor prognosis include temperature >104°F, renal failure, and cardiopulmonary complications.
- In the absence of complications, the prognosis for recovery is good; most patients recover in 15 days.
- Prognosis is better when NMS is detected early.
- NMS complicated by HHS is rare but carries a poor prognosis (7).

COMPLICATIONS

- Dehydration
- Electrolyte imbalance
- Rhabdomyolysis (causing acute renal failure and, possibly, disseminated intravascular coagulation)
- Cardiac arrest (cardiac arrhythmia, myocardial infraction)
- Respiratory failure (aspiration pneumonia, pulmonary embolism, chest wall rigidity)
- Deep venous thrombophlebitis/thrombosis (due to immobilization)
- Seizure
- Hepatic failure
- Sepsis
- Uncontrolled psychosis; persistent neuropsychiatric complications (6)
- Death (6)

REFERENCES

1. Trollor JN, Chen X, Sachdev PS. Neuroleptic malignant syndrome associated with atypical antipsychotic drugs. *CNS Drugs*. 2009;23: 477–492.
2. Neuhut R, Lindenmayer JP, Silva R, et al. Neuroleptic malignant syndrome in children and adolescents on atypical antipsychotic medication: A review. *J Child Adolesc Psychopharmacol*. 2009;19:415–422.
3. Wait SD, Ponce FA, Killory BD, et al. Neuroleptic malignant syndrome from central nervous system insult: 4 cases and a novel treatment strategy. Clinical article. *J Neurosurg Pediatr*. 2009;4: 217–221.
4. Lyons JL, Cohen AB. Selective cerebellar and basal ganglia injury in neuroleptic malignant syndrome. *J Neuroimaging*. 2013;23:240–241.
5. Strawn JR, Keck PE, Caroff SN. Neuroleptic malignant syndrome. *Am J Psychiatry*. 2007;164: 870–876.
6. Seitz DP, Gill SS. Neuroleptic malignant syndrome complicating antipsychotic treatment of delirium or agitation in medical and surgical patients: Case reports and a review of the literature. *Psychosomatics*. 2009;50:8–15.
7. Rock W, Elias M, Lev A, et al. Haloperidol-induced neuroleptic malignant syndrome complicated by hyperosmolar hyperglycemic state. *Am J Emerg Med*. 2009;27:1018.e1–e3.

ADDITIONAL READING

- Berman BD. Neuroleptic malignant syndrome: A review for neurohospitalists. *Neurohospitalist*. 2011;1:41–47.
- Halloran LL, Bernard DW. Management of drug-induced hyperthermia. *Curr Opin Pediatr*. 2004;16:211–215.
- Perry PJ, Wilborn CA. Serotonin syndrome vs neuroleptic malignant syndrome: A contrast of causes, diagnoses, and management. *Ann Clin Psychiatry*. 2012;24:155–162.
- Tural U, Onder E. Clinical and pharmacologic risk factors for neuroleptic malignant syndrome and their association with death. *Psychiatry Clin Neurosci*. 2010;64:79–87.

 SEE ALSO

Algorithms: Coma; Delirium

 CODES

ICD10

G21.0 Malignant neuroleptic syndrome

CLINICAL PEARLS

- Of cases, 2/3 occur within the 1st week of starting a neuroleptic, but NMS may occur years later.
- NMS may be triggered by discontinuation of Parkinson medications.
- Elevated serum creatinine kinase is the most consistent lab abnormality in patients with NMS.

NEUROPATHIC PAIN
Cassandra Dorvil, MBS, DO • Felix Chang, MD

BASICS

DESCRIPTION
- Neuropathic pain is a complex pain state that arises as a direct consequence of injured, damaged or dysfunctional nerve fibers of the somatosensory system.
- Can arise from damage to the nerve pathways at any point from the terminals of the peripheral nociceptors to the cortical neurons in the brain
- Distinct from nociceptive pain in the way that the latter is induced by activation of peripheral nociceptor nerve fibers
- May be triggered by direct nerve injury, infection, metabolic dysfunction, autoimmune disease, neoplasm, drugs, radiation, and neurovascular disorders
- May reflect the pathologic operation of a dysfunctional nervous system rather than a manifestation of any underlying pathology itself (i.e., phantom limb pain, complex regional pain syndrome [CRPS]):
  - Patients may paradoxically experience pain and hypersensitivity in an area of denervation

EPIDEMIOLOGY
Incidence
Epidemiologic data are limited. Depending on the inclusion criteria: Radiculopathies, peripheral neuropathy, >3 million Americans suffer from painful diabetic neuropathy (PDN).
- 1 million Americans suffer from postherpetic neuralgia (PHN).

Prevalence
Estimated at 1.5% of the population

ETIOLOGY AND PATHOPHYSIOLOGY
- Positive symptoms due to changes in peripheral nerves, loss of inhibitory mechanisms in CNS, and central sensitization
- Negative symptoms likely due to axonal or neuronal loss
- Associated with a predisposing factor
- Risk factors:
  - Demyelinating disorders (multiple sclerosis [MS], Guillain-Barré)
  - Neoplasm (primary/metastatic)
  - Neurovascular (central poststroke syndrome, trigeminal neuralgia)
  - Autoimmune disease (Sjögren syndrome, polyarteritis nodosa)
  - Structural disease (herniated disc disease)

RISK FACTORS
- Radiculopathy
- Polyneuropathy (diabetes mellitus, alcohol-induced, postchemotherapy, heritable neuropathies)
- Trauma (nerve entrapment, postsurgical, nerve injury)
- Infection (HIV, herpes zoster)
- Central mechanisms (stroke, MS, spinal cord injury, limb amputation)
- Nutritional deficiencies (B_{12}, folate)
- Medications (AIDS medications DDC and DDI, antibiotics metronidazole and isoniazid, some chemotherapeutics, amiodarone, hydralazine, phenytoin, nitrofurantoin)

COMMONLY ASSOCIATED CONDITIONS
- Depression/anxiety
- Sleep disturbance
- Fibromyalgia

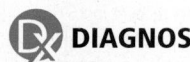

DIAGNOSIS

HISTORY
- May have history of nerve trauma; however, absence does not exclude the diagnosis of neuropathic pain
- Clinical manifestation can include both negative and positive sensory symptoms and signs. Motor dysfunction is rare.
- Pain is often described as burning, shocklike, tingling, numbing, or intensely hot or cold.

PHYSICAL EXAM
- Positive signs/symptoms:
  - Hyperalgesia: An exaggerated pain response to a noxious stimulus
  - Allodynia: Perception of pain due to a nonnoxious stimuli; for instance, gentle mechanical pressure, light pinprick, hot or cold stimuli, and vibration cause pain.
- Negative signs/symptoms: Reduced sensation to touch, pinprick, temperature, or vibration
- Motor signs and symptoms: Signs may include hypotonia, tremor, dystonia, ataxia, hypo-/hyperreflexia, or motor neglect. Motor symptoms include weakness, fatigability, decreased range of motion, joint stiffness, and spontaneous muscle spasm.

DIAGNOSTIC TESTS & INTERPRETATION
Initial Tests (lab, imaging)
None specifically for neuropathic pain, but tests to rule out other causes should be considered:
- Serum B_{12}
- 25 hydroxy vitamin D
- Thyroid-stimulating hormone (TSH)
- Rapid plasma reagin (RPR) or venereal disease reaction level (VDRL)
- Fasting glucose, creatinine
- Lyme serology
- Used to rule out other causes for pain
- Consider imaging based on affected area: MRI shows greatest anatomic detail for spine.
- PET and SPECT scans, and standard and functional MRI all have been used to map synaptic activity in the thalamus and somatosensory cortex. Initial studies using these imaging techniques have suggested maladaptive reorganization of the thalamus and somatosensory cortex.

Follow-Up Tests & Special Considerations
Studies may include nerve conduction, electromyography, evoked potentials, quantitative sensory testing, thermography, radiologic imaging.

Diagnostic Procedures/Other
- Sympathetic nerve blocks
- Epidural steroids
- Peripheral nerve blocks
- Dorsal column stimulator and peripheral nerve stimulator

TREATMENT

GENERAL MEASURES
- Use heat or cold packs on painful area
- Stay active
- Learn ways to relax body and mind

MEDICATION
First Line
- Calcium channel alpha-2-delta ligands:
  - Gabapentin (1)[A]
    - Primarily been studied and found effective for the treatment of postherpetic neuralgia (PHN) and painful diabetic neuropathy (PDN).
    - Dosing: Start 300 mg PO daily × 1 day, then 300 mg PO b.i.d. × 1 day, then 300 mg PO t.i.d.; max: 3,600 mg/d
    - Taper over >7 days to discontinue
    - An adequate trial can require ≥2 months before considering failure.
    - Contraindication (C/I): Hypersensitivity to drug/class/components, avoid abrupt withdrawal
    - Precaution: If renal impairment, history of depression, CNS depressant use, ethanol (EtOH) use or drug abuse history.
    - Interactions: Propoxyphene, buprenorphine, levomethadyl acetate, sodium oxybate
    - Adverse effects: Dizziness, somnolence, ataxia, fatigue, fever, tremor, blurred vision, asthenia, GI symptoms, peripheral edema, URI, headache, weight gain, xerostomia
  - Pregabalin (2)[A]
    - Used for the treatment of PDN, spinal cord injury, PHN, fibromyalgia
    - Dosing: Diagnosis dependent; max 600 mg/d
    - C/I: same as gabapentin
    - Precaution: In elderly patients, renal impairment, CHF Class III or IV NYHA, angioedema history or risk, depression or history, CNS depressant use or EtOH use
    - Interactions: Same as gabapentin
    - Adverse effects: Dizziness, Somnolence, thrombocytopenia, GI symptoms, peripheral edema
- Tricyclic antidepressants (3)[A]:
  - Amitriptyline (4)[A]
  - Dosing: Start at 10–25 mg at bedtime, then titrate up to antidepressant drug levels
  - Adequate trial: 6–8 weeks, including 2 weeks at the highest dose tolerated; onset of analgesia may be after 1 week
  - C/I: Hypersensitivity to drug/class/components, recovery from acute myocardial infarction, avoid abrupt withdrawal. Absolute contraindication with monamine oxidase inhibitors (MAOIs).
  - Precaution: In elderly or patients <25 years old, cardiovascular disease, urinary retention, prostatic hypertrophy, close-angle glaucoma, seizure disorder, thyroid disease, diabetes mellitus, Parkinson disease, hepatic impairment, schizophrenia, bipolar disorder, EtOH abuse, suicide risk, GI/GU obstruction
  - Interactions: Numerous possible drug–drug interactions (type 1C antiarrhythmics, SSRIs, anticholinergics, sympathomimetics, CNS depressants)

- Adverse effects: QT interval abnormalities, arrhythmias, sedation, dry mouth, constipation, sexual dysfunction, weight gain, postural hypotension, urinary retention
- Secondary amines (nortriptyline, desipramine) are safer than amitriptyline and imipramine.
- Obtain a pretreatment ECG for documentation/ monitoring any arrhythmias.
- Serotonin norepinephrine reuptake inhibitors (SNRIs) (5)[A]:
  - Duloxetine (6)[A]
  - Effective in the treatment of PDN, fibromyalgia, and more recently chronic low back pain
  - Dosing: 60 mg PO daily max dose: 120 mg/d
  - C/I: Hypersensitivity, hepatic impairment, uncontrolled close-angle glaucoma, EtOH abuse
  - Precaution: Patients <25 years old, elderly, pregnancy 3rd trimester, creatinine clearance (CrCl) <30, hypertension (HTN), seizure history, GI motility disorder, suicidal, hypomania or mania history
  - Interactions: Co-administered with any CNS stimulant (i.e., phentermine, amphetamine, methylphenidate, methamphetamine, cocaine) leading to increased risk for serotonin syndrome
  - Adverse effects: GI symptoms, dizziness, somnolence, insomnia, fatigue, anorexia, blurred vision, headache, erectile dysfunction, tremor, weight changes, elevated BP, elevated liver function tests, postural hypotension
  - Venlafaxine (Effexor XR)
  - Efficacy in PDN and painful polyneuropathies of different origins, but not in PHN
  - Dosages evaluated varied considerably based on etiology of chronic pain conditions in the range of 75–225 mg/d; onset of relief may occur in 1–2 weeks, or take up to 6 weeks for full benefit
  - C/I: hypersensitivity, concurrently with MAOIs (or discontinue MAOIs within 14 days)
  - Precaution: Suicidal thinking/behavior
  - Interactions: Linezolid
  - Adverse effects: Anxiety, insomnia, bleeding risk, HTN, hypercholesteremia, sexual dysfunction
- Local anesthetics such as lidocaine, mexiletine, tocainide, and flecainide have been shown to give an analgesic effect when administered orally or parenterally. Adjuvant therapy to first line medications (7)[A].

Second Line

- Anticonvulsants: Topiramate, zonisamide (Zonegran), carbamazepine, lamotrigine (8)[I]

  - Oxcarbazepine (9)[A]: shown to be better tolerated and more efficacious than carbamazepine

  - Oxcarbazepine is primarily used for diabetic neuropathy and radiculopathy.
  - Lamotrigine does not have a significant place in therapy based on available evidence

- Opioids (10)[A]:
  - World Health Organization suggested adding to nonopioid agents if they are insufficient. However, this is usually for palliative cancer patients. Chronic opioid therapy can be detrimental to psychosocial environment of the patient.
  - Increased efficacy when used in conjunction with gabapentin
  - Controlled-release opioids recommended (controlled-release oxycodone, morphine, transdermal fentanyl, methadone)

- Dosage: Start with short-acting analgesic equivalent to oral morphine sulfate 5–15 mg q4h; after 1–2 weeks of treatment, calculate equivalent dose of long-acting agent and use short-acting opioids for breakthrough.
- No clear maximum dosage, but trials do not show benefits at doses >180 mg/d of morphine.
- Precaution: Avoid in those with history of substance abuse, use with caution in the elderly, may cause respiratory depression.
- Interactions: Additive effects with CNS depressants, increased risk of serotonin syndrome with serotonergic agents
- Adverse effects: Constipation, sedation, nausea, lightheadedness
- Adjuvant therapies with opioids should be used to treat nausea/vomiting, constipation, sedation, pruritus, and so forth.
- Tramadol (11)[A]:
  - Norepinephrine and serotonin inhibitor with a major metabolite that acts as an opioid (μ-receptor) agonist
  - Dosage: 250 mg/d divided doses, max 400 mg/d
  - Precautions: Avoid in those with seizure history.
  - Interactions: Increased seizure risk in those taking SSRIs, tricyclic antidepressants, MAOIs, neuroleptics concomitantly; increased risk of serotonergic symptoms if used with SSRIs, MAOIs; adjust dose for renal insufficiency, hepatic disease.
  - Adverse effects: Dizziness, nausea, constipation, somnolence, orthostatic hypotension

Third Line

- NMDA receptor antagonists: Ketamine, dextromethorphan (5)[B]
- Other agents: Baclofen, clonidine, capsaicin (12)[A]

ISSUES FOR REFERRAL
Referral to pain clinic or neurosurgery is appropriate if refractory to initial treatment.

ADDITIONAL THERAPIES

- Transcutaneous electrical nerve stimulation (TENS) may be helpful; optimal dosing is yet to be established (13)[B].
- Spinal cord stimulation may be effective for chronic pain, especially if back surgery failed (10)[B].

SURGERY/OTHER PROCEDURES
Nerve destructive procedures:

- Caution, as a refractory to treatment to different pain can ensue.
- Sympathectomy: More studies needed
- Dorsal root entry zone lesion (dorsal rhizotomy)
- Lateral cordotomy
- Trigeminal nerve ganglion ablation

ONGOING CARE

FOLLOW-UP RECOMMENDATIONS
- Multidisciplinary team
- Opioid contracts to prevent abuses

Patient Monitoring
Random urinalysis for specific prescribed drug and all drugs of abuse for patients receiving opioid therapy

PROGNOSIS
Chronic course of pain symptoms often requires management with numerous medications and adjunctive therapies.

COMPLICATIONS
Long-term disability and drug addiction are possible.

REFERENCES

1. Moore RA, Wiffen PJ, Derry S, et al. Gabapentin for chronic neuropathic pain and fibromyalgia in adults. *Cochrane Database Syst Rev.* 2011;3: CD007938.
2. Moore RA, Straube S, Wiffen PJ, et al. Pregabalin for acute and chronic pain in adults. *Cochrane Database Syst Rev.* 2009;3:CD007076.
3. Saarto T, Wiffen PJ. Antidepressants for neuropathic pain: A Cochrane Review. *J Neurol Neurosurg Psychiatry.* 2010;81:1372.
4. Moore RA, Derry S, Aldington D, et al. Amitriptyline for neuropathic pain and fibromyalgia in adults. *Cochrane Database Syst Rev.* 2012;12;CD008242.
5. Galluzzi KE. Managing neuropathic pain. *J Am Osteopath Assoc.* 2007;107:ES39–ES48.
6. Lunn MPT, Hughes RAC, Wiffen PJ. Duloxetine for treating painful neuropathy or chronic pain. *Cochrane Database Syst Rev.* 2010;2:CD007115.
7. Challapalli V, Tremont-Lukats IW, McNicol ED, et al. Systemic administration of local anesthetic agents to relieve neuropathic pain. *Cochrane Database Syst Rev.* 2009;2:CD003345.
8. Wiffen PJ, Derry S, Moore RA. Lamotrigine for acute and chronic pain. *Cochrane Database Syst Rev.* 2011;3:CD006044.
9. Zhou M, Chen N, He L, et al. Oxcarbazepine for neuropathic pain. *Cochrane Database Syst Rev.* 2013;2:CD007963.
10. Finnerup NB, Sindrup SH, Jensen TS. The evidence for pharmacological treatment of neuropathic pain. *J Pain.* 2010:150:573.
11. Hollingshead J. Tramadol for neuropathic pain. *Cochrane Database Syst Rev.* 2007;2:CD003726.
12. Derry S, Rice ASC, Cole P, et al. Topical capsaicin (high concentration) for chronic neuropathic pain in adults. *Cochrane Database Syst Rev.* 2013;3: CD007393.
13. Nnoaham KE, Kumbang J. Transcutaneous electrical nerve stimulation (TENS) for chronic pain. *Cochrane Database Syst Rev.* 2008;3: CD003222.

ADDITIONAL READING

Attal N, Cruccu G, Baron R, et al. EFNS guidelines on the pharmacological treatment of neuropathic pain: 2010 revision. *Eur J Neurol.* 2010;17:1113.

CODES

ICD10
- E10.40 Type 1 diabetes mellitus with diabetic neuropathy, unsp
- E11.40 Type 2 diabetes mellitus with diabetic neuropathy, unsp
- M79.2 Neuralgia and neuritis, unspecified

CLINICAL PEARLS

- Opioids should be reserved for selected patients with moderate to severe pain that adversely impacts function or quality of life.
- Lamotrigine does not have a significant place in therapy based on available evidence

NEUROPATHY, PERIPHERAL

Amy Chen, MD, PhD • David N. Herrmann, MBBCh

BASICS

DESCRIPTION
- Peripheral neuropathy (PN) is a functional or structural disorder of the peripheral nervous system (PNS).
- PN affects any combination of motor, sensory, or autonomic nerves.
- The motor PNS comprises spinal cord motor neurons, their nerve roots that combine to form plexus, and branches that form individual nerves innervating skeletal muscles. Peripheral motor involvement causes muscle atrophy, weakness, cramps, and fasciculations.
- The sensory PNS consists of sensory organs, which transmit touch, vibration, and position sensation in larger-diameter myelinated fibers and pain and temperature in small-diameter lightly myelinated and unmyelinated C fibers to the dorsal root ganglia. Sensory signals are relayed to the central nervous system (CNS) for integration. Disorders of sensory nerves produce negative phenomena (loss of sensibility, lack of balance) or heightened phenomena (tingling or pain). Large sensory fiber dysfunction impairs touch and vibration sensation, while small fiber sensory neuropathy (SFN) affects pin and thermal sensation and causes neuropathic pain.
- The autonomic nervous system (ANS) includes the sympathetic and parasympathetic systems. ANS dysfunction causes cardiovascular, gastrointestinal, and sudomotor symptoms.
- The PNS can be affected from the cell body (sensory ganglionopathy or motor neuronopathy), root (radiculopathy), or plexus (plexopathy) to the nerve (demyelinating or axonal neuropathy).

EPIDEMIOLOGY
Prevalence
Approximately 2.4% of general population, or 8% of people over age 55, are affected by distal symmetric PN, the most common form of PN.

ETIOLOGY AND PATHOPHYSIOLOGY
- PN can be acquired or hereditary
- The most common cause of acquired PN is diabetes
- Other categories of acquired PN with illustrative examples:
  - Vascular: Ischemia, vasculitis
  - Infectious: HIV, hepatitis C, cryoglobulinemia, Lyme disease
  - Traumatic
  - Autoimmune: Rheumatoid arthritis, Sjögren's, postinfectious Guillain-Barré syndrome (GBS), chronic inflammatory demyelinating polyneuropathy (CIDP)
  - Metabolic: Diabetes, renal failure, hypothyroidism, vitamin B_{12} deficiency, celiac disease
  - Iatrogenic/toxic: Chemotherapy, platinum, taxanes, metronidazole, colchicine, infliximab, alcoholism
  - Idiopathic: 30% of PN
  - Neoplastic/paraneoplastic: paraproteinemia, Waldenstrom macroglobulinemia, multiple myeloma, amyloidosis, neurofibromatosis
- PN occurs due to demyelination or axonal degeneration

- Demyelination results from Schwann cell dysfunction, mutations in myelin protein genes, or direct damage to myelin sheaths
- Axonal degeneration occurs when injury/dysfunction occurs at the cell body or axon

Genetics
- Approximately 50% of undiagnosed PN is hereditary
- Currently over 50 known genetic causes of hereditary PN
- Charcot-Marie-Tooth (CMT) neuropathies: Most common hereditary PN
  - CMT1A (duplication of the *PMP22* gene) is the most common CMT
  - A *PMP22* deletion causes PN with liability to pressure palsy (HNPP)

RISK FACTORS
Systemic disorders predispose to PN

GENERAL PREVENTION
- Healthy nutrition and avoidance of alcoholism and of pressure at nerve entrapment sites
- Surveillance for glucose dysmetabolism and tight glycemic control may prevent diabetic PN

DIAGNOSIS

HISTORY
- A detailed inquiry for symptoms of sensory, motor, or autonomic dysfunction:
  - Numbness, tingling, prickling, burning pain, a "tightly wrapped" sensation, and an "unsteady gait"
  - Distal weakness manifests as foot drop (tripping, foot slapping) or difficulty with grip; proximal weakness (e.g., difficulty arising from a chair) is less common
  - Orthostatic dizziness, abnormal sweating, constipation, or voiding difficulties
- Symptom onset:
  - Acute: Consider infection (e.g., Lyme disease), postinfectious dysimmune process (e.g., GBS), ischemia (e.g., vasculitis), toxin, or trauma
  - Subacute: Consider metabolic, neoplastic, paraneoplastic, or dysimmune processes
  - Chronic: Consider dysimmune process (CIDP), idiopathic, or hereditary
- Progression: Stable or indolent; slowly or rapidly progressive; monophasic or relapsing or remitting
- Anatomic pattern: Focal, multifocal, diffuse

ALERT
Hemi body symptoms suggest CNS rather than PNS pathology

PHYSICAL EXAM
- Based on exam, a functional (*sensory*: small-fiber vs. large-fiber vs. mixed, *sensorimotor*, *motor*, *autonomic*) and anatomic pattern of PN (*distal symmetric*, *multifocal*, or *focal*) should be established.
- Cognition preserved in isolated PN
- Cranial nerves may be involved with focal or multifocal PN (e.g., bifacial weakness may occur with GBS, Lyme disease, sarcoidosis, among other causes)
- Stocking/glove sensory loss is typical of distal symmetric sensory PN (e.g., diabetes)

- Isolated reduced pin or thermal sensation or allodynia suggests a pure small-fiber neuropathy (SFN)
- Reduced vibration and joint position sense suggests large-fiber sensory neuropathy; when severe, a Romberg sign is present and gait is wide-based or ataxic
- Distal muscle atrophy and weaknesses of toe extension and finger abduction are often present with distal symmetric axonal PN
- In acquired demyelinating PN (e.g., GBS or CIDP), weakness is commonly both proximal and distal
- Deep tendon reflexes may be reduced or absent, distally at the ankles in large-fiber axonal PN, or diffusely in demyelinating PN
- High arched or flat feet or hammer toes suggest hereditary PN

ALERT
Hemi body sensory loss or loss of sensation below a spinal cord level suggest a CNS process.

ALERT
Hyperreflexia and spasticity are upper motor neuron signs not seen with isolated PN.

DIFFERENTIAL DIAGNOSIS
The following categories of PN can be identified (differential diagnosis [DDx] listed when applicable):
- Pure sensory neuropathy:
  - DDx: SFN, sensory ganglionopathy, polyradiculopathy
- Distal symmetric sensorimotor axonal PN:
  - Most common type of PN
  - DDx: Distal acquired demyelinating symmetric PN (DADS)
- Motor predominant PN:
  - DDx: Motor neuron disease, polyradiculopathy, immune-mediated multifocal motor neuropathy (MMN)
- Mononeuropathy:
  - Most likely due to compression, entrapment, or trauma
  - DDx: Monoradiculopathy
- Mononeuropathy multiplex:
  - DDx: Plexopathy, polyradiculopathy

DIAGNOSTIC TESTS & INTERPRETATION
Initial Tests (lab, imaging)
- Nerve conduction studies and electromyography (NCS/EMG):
  - Best performed by physicians with specialty training in electrodiagnostic medicine
  - Delineate axonal vs. demyelinating, anatomic pattern, chronicity and severity of PN
- Specialized skin biopsy:
  - In clinically suspected SFN if NCS/EMG normal
  - Analysis of lower limb epidermal nerve fiber density (ENFD)
- Blood tests (1)[C]:
  - CBC, BUN, creatinine, fasting glucose, HgA1C, vitamin B_{12}, serum protein electrophoresis and immunofixation
- Autonomic tests:
  - Not routinely done but useful to characterize autonomic PN

- Neuroimaging:
  - Generally not indicated in evaluation of PN, but useful in evaluation of brachial plexopathies, radiculopathies, or where findings are attributable to the CNS

Follow-Up Tests & Special Considerations
- Additional blood tests are tailored to the medical history, the PN type, and NCS/EMG findings
- Genetic testing for diagnosis of hereditary PN should be ordered by neurologists expert in PN.

ALERT
Ordering of laboratory batteries (e.g., peripheral nerve antibody panels) without careful consideration of the clinical and NCS/EMG features should be avoided.

Diagnostic Procedures/Other
Nerve biopsy (sural or superficial peroneal nerve): Useful if vasculitic PN, amyloidosis, granulomatous disorders, or neoplastic infiltration is suspected.

ALERT
Nerve biopsies are rarely helpful in late-onset chronic, slowly progressive distal symmetric PN.
- Lumbar puncture:
  - Cytoalbuminemic dissociation in GBS or CIDP
  - Infection, inflammation, or neoplasia in polyradiculopathies

Test Interpretation
- Demyelinating PN: Disproportionate slowing of conduction velocities on NCS
- Axonal PN: Reduced amplitude in sensory or motor responses, with relatively preserved conduction velocities on NCS
- Reduced ENFD on distal leg skin biopsies is supportive of SFN

 TREATMENT

GENERAL MEASURES
Manage associated medical conditions; disease modifying therapy for specific forms of PN (e.g., CIDP); symptomatic relief of pain and dysautonomia; rehabilitation to optimize function

MEDICATION
First Line
- Targeted treatment for underlying systemic conditions:
  - Glycemic control, thyroid hormone supplementation, vitamin supplementation, antimicrobial therapy (e.g., Lyme disease, HIV), glucocorticoids for sarcoidosis, cytotoxic therapy for vasculitis
- Immunotherapy for dysimmune PN:
  - Intravenous immunoglobulin (IVIG): Within the first 2 weeks of GBS to hasten recovery (2)(A); as a 1st-line alternative for CIDP (3)(A); and for prevention of secondary axonal loss in multifocal motor neuropathy (MMN) (4)(A)
    - Loading dose 2 g/kg body weight divided into 2–5 days; maintenance regimen variable for CIDP and MMN
    - Adverse effects (AE): Headache, fever, hypertension, and rarely pulmonary embolism
  - Plasma exchange: 1st agent shown to improve functional outcome for patients with GBS (5)(A); short-term benefit in CIDP (6)(A)
    - AE: Catheter complication, hypotension and others
  - Corticosteroids: 1st agent used in treatment of CIDP (7)(C)

- Treatment of autonomic symptoms:
  - Compression stockings, hydration, midodrine, fludrocortisone for orthostatic hypotension
  - Pyridostigmine for immune-mediated dysautonomia (off-label)
- Treatment of neuropathic pain: Evidence of efficacy derived from clinical trials in diabetic painful neuropathy (DPN) and postherpetic neuralgia (PHN):
  - Pregabalin: For DPN and PHN
  - Duloxetine: For DPN
  - Lidocaine patch: For PHN
  - Gabapentin (off-label)
  - Tricyclic antidepressants (TCA) (off-label)
  - Venlafaxine (off-label)
  - Tramadol (off-label)

ISSUES FOR REFERRAL
- Rapidly progressive symptoms or suspected demyelinating or hereditary PN should be referred to a neurologist with expertise in neuromuscular disorders.
- Rheumatology referral for vasculitic PN
- Patients with paraproteinemia should have a skeletal bone survey and be referred to hematology
- Physical therapy for gait and balance training

ADDITIONAL THERAPIES
- Combination therapy (e.g., gabapentin with TCA or venlafaxine or tramadol) can be more effective than monotherapy for neuropathic pain
- Long-acting opiates for refractory neuropathic pain
- Additional immunosuppressant agents (e.g., cyclophosphamide) may be used in refractory chronic dysimmune PN

ALERT
Opiates have significant side effects and may cause rebound headaches, tolerance, and dependence.

SURGERY/OTHER PROCEDURES
- Decompressive surgery for entrapment neuropathy (e.g., carpal tunnel syndrome)
- Foot and ankle surgery to improve symptoms or function in hereditary PN
- Radiation, surgery, or bone marrow transplantation for plasmacytoma or osteosclerotic myeloma or POEMS syndrome
- Liver transplantation for amyloidotic PN

COMPLEMENTARY AND ALTERNATIVE MEDICINE
Low-intensity transcutaneous electrical nerve stimulation (TENS), acupuncture, mediation

ALERT
Vitamin B_6 supplementation may cause peripheral neurotoxicity and should be avoided except for a deficiency state.

IN-PATIENT CONSIDERATIONS
Admission Criteria/Initial Stabilization
- Patients with suspected GBS should be admitted for diagnosis, monitoring (30–60% may develop cardiovascular or respiratory failure), and for acute treatment
- Elective intubation may be required in GBS when forced vital capacity is <15 mL/kg body weight
- Other rapidly progressive undiagnosed PNs that impair independent ambulation may require admission

 ONGOING CARE

FOLLOW-UP RECOMMENDATIONS
- Physical therapy
- Gait assistive devices as needed
- Flu vaccination should be avoided in the 1st year following GBS

PROGNOSIS
- Late onset idiopathic distal symmetric axonal PN are indolent
- 80% of GBS have a near complete or good recovery; 80% of CIDP have moderate or good response with treatment but can be relapsing

REFERENCES

1. England JD, Gronseth GS, Franklin G, et al. Practice parameter: Evaluation of distal symmetric polyneuropathy: Role of laboratory and genetic testing (an evidence-based review): Report of the American Academy of Neurology, American Association of Neuromuscular and Electrodiagnostic Medicine, and American Academy of Physical Medicine and Rehabilitation. *Neurology*. 2009;72:185–192.
2. Hughes RA, Swan AV, van Doorn PA. Intravenous immunoglobulin for Guillain-Barré syndrome. *Cochrane Database Syst Rev*. 2012;7:CD002063.
3. Hughes RA, Donofrio P, Bril V, et al. ICE study group. Intravenous immune globulin (10% caprylate–chromatography purified) for the treatment of chronic inflammatory demyelinating polyradiculoneuropathy (ICE study): A randomized placebo-controlled trial. *Lancet Neurol*. 2008;7: 136–144.
4. Cats EA, Van der Pol WL, Piepers S, et al. Correlates of outcome and response to IVIg in 88 patients with multifocal motor neuropathy. *Neurology*. 2010;75:818–825.
5. The Guillain-Barré syndrome study group. Plasmapheresis and acute Guillain-Barré syndrome. *Neurology* 1985;35:1096–1104.
6. Dyck PJ, Daube J, O'Brien P, et al. Plasma exchange in chronic inflammatory demyelinating polyradiculoneuropathy. *N Engl J Med*. 1986;314: 461–465.
7. Dyck PJ, O'Brien PC, Oviatt KF, et al. Prednisone improves chronic inflammatory polyradiculoneuropathy more than no treatment. *Ann Neurol*. 1982;11:136–141.

 CODES

ICD10
- G62.9 Polyneuropathy, unspecified
- G62.89 Other specified polyneuropathies

CLINICAL PEARLS
- There are many causes of PN. Diagnosis is made by history and physical exam, targeted laboratory testing, NCS/EMG, skin biopsy, or ANS testing.
- Consider hereditary neuropathy if patient has an early age of PN symptom onset, family history of PN, or foot deformity.
- GBS is monophasic and progresses for up to 4 weeks; CIDP progresses beyond 8 weeks, and untreated usually has a progressive course.

N

NICOTINE ADDICTION
Brett White, MD • Benjamin N. Schneider, MD

BASICS

DESCRIPTION
Nicotine addiction is characterized by signs of dependence and compulsive use despite knowledge of its adverse effects.

EPIDEMIOLOGY
Incidence
20–25% of the US population smoke

Prevalence
70 million in US $\geq$12 years of age reported current use of tobacco (58.7 million were cigarette smokers, 13.3 million smoked cigars, 8.6 million used smokeless tobacco, 2.1 million smoked pipes) (1)[B].

Pediatric Considerations
Nicotine use is common and often underrecognized in this population. The following are the percentages from 1 study of those who reported using cigarettes or smokeless tobacco in the past 30 days: 8th graders: 4.9% and 2.8%, 10th graders: 10.8% and 6.4%, 12th graders: 17.1% and 7.9% (2).

ETIOLOGY AND PATHOPHYSIOLOGY
- Nicotine causes changes in brain nicotinic acetylcholine receptors (nAChRs) during smoking that initiate addiction, including nicotine-induced upregulation in nAChR binding sites.
- Nicotine has both stimulating and depressing effects within the CNS; relaxing and euphoric effects may contribute to psychological dependence. It is likely that endogenous opioid peptides and their receptors play an important role in the psychoactive properties of nicotine.
- Polymorphisms in neuronal nAChR genes could be associated with increased susceptibility to tobacco dependence.

Genetics
- Mutation in the α_4 subunit of nAChRs expressed by neurons was found to lower the threshold for the induction of nicotine dependence.
- Specific genes have been isolated that are associated with nicotine dependence, including *CHRNB3*, the β_3 nicotine receptor subunit gene.
- T-variant gene associated with decreased activity of CYP2B6 (enzyme that breaks down nicotine in the brain); may lead to increased craving during smoking cessation. These patients are also 1.5 × more likely to resume smoking during treatment.

RISK FACTORS
- Mental illness (depression, posttraumatic stress disorder, bipolar disorder, and schizophrenia)
- Low socioeconomic status
- Low educational status
- Early 1st-hand nicotine experience increases risk for chronic abuse
- Environmental factors are critical for smoking initiation; genetic factors contribute to smoking persistence and difficulty quitting.

GENERAL PREVENTION
- The US Preventive Services Task Force (USPSTF) strongly recommends clinicians screen all (A Rating):
  - Adults for tobacco use and provide tobacco cessation interventions for those who use tobacco products.
  - Pregnant women for tobacco use and provide augmented pregnancy-tailored counseling to those who smoke.
- The USPSTF concludes the evidence is insufficient to recommend for or against routine screening for tobacco use or interventions to prevent and treat tobacco use and dependence among children or adolescents.
- School-based smoking-prevention education

Pregnancy Considerations
- Carbon monoxide and nicotine may interfere with oxygen supply to the fetus, resulting in fetal growth restriction and decreased birth weight.
- Smoking may increase the incidence of spontaneous abortion and sudden infant death syndrome (SIDS), as well as learning or behavioral problems and an increased risk of obesity in children (1).

COMMONLY ASSOCIATED CONDITIONS
- Chronic obstructive pulmonary disease (COPD) (emphysema and chronic bronchitis)
- Cancers (lung, oral/pharyngeal, kidney, bladder, cervical, anal)
- Coronary artery disease
- Periodontal disease

DIAGNOSIS

HISTORY
- Amount and duration of smoking
- Previous attempts to quit

PHYSICAL EXAM
Cardiovascular exam

DIFFERENTIAL DIAGNOSIS
- Depression
- COPD
- α_1-antitrypsin deficiency
- Asthma
- Congestive heart failure (CHF)
- Respiratory infections
- Lung cancer
- Cystic fibrosis

DIAGNOSTIC TESTS & INTERPRETATION
Spirometry: Decreased FEV$_1$ (forced expiratory volume in 1 second; if COPD suspected)

Diagnostic Procedures/Other
- Using spirometry to determine "lung age" (approximation of age of patient's lungs based on the faster decline in FEV$_1$ than is expected with normal aging)
- American College of Chest Physicians Lung Cancer Screening Recommendations 2013:
  - Low-dose CT screening for individuals aged 55–75 with a history of 30 or more pack-years who are still smoking or have quit within the past 15 years in settings that can deliver the comprehensive care provided to National Lung Screening Trial participants.
  - Screening is not recommended (Grade 2C) for individuals with a smoking history of fewer than 30 pack-years, those who fall outside the age guidelines, or those with comorbidities that might limit their life expectancy.

TREATMENT

Counseling:
- Advice from medical providers helps improve quit rates (number needed to treat [NNT] 75) (3).
- Providing brief, simple advice about quitting smoking increases the likelihood that someone who smokes will successfully quit and remain a nonsmoker 12 months later. More intensive advice (i.e., motivational interviewing) may result in higher rates of quitting. Providing follow-up support after offering the advice may increase the quit rates slightly (3)[A].
- The USPSTF strongly recommends screening all adults for tobacco use and providing cessation interventions for those using tobacco products (Level A recommendation).

GENERAL MEASURES
- Brief strategies to help the patient willing to quit tobacco use—the "5 As":
  - Ask the patient if he or she uses tobacco.
  - Advise him or her to quit.
  - Assess willingness to make a quit attempt.
  - Assist those who are willing to make a quit attempt.
  - Arrange for follow-up contact to prevent relapse (4).
- Enhancing motivation to quit tobacco—the "5 Rs":
  - Relevance: Encourage the patient to indicate why quitting is personally relevant.
  - Risks: Ask the patient to identify potential negative consequences of tobacco use.
  - Rewards: Ask the patient to identify potential benefits of stopping tobacco use.
  - Roadblocks: Ask the patient to identify barriers or impediments to quitting, and provide treatment (e.g., problem-solving counseling or medication) that could address barriers.
  - Repetition: The motivational intervention should be repeated every time an unmotivated patient visits the clinic setting (5)[A].

MEDICATION
- There are 7 FDA-approved medications for tobacco use and all are efficacious: Bupropion SR, nicotine gum, nicotine inhaler, nicotine lozenge, nicotine nasal spray, nicotine patch, and varenicline.
- Varenicline and combination nicotine replacement therapy (long acting patch + PRN short acting agent) should be considered first line as they have been shown to be more effective than nicotine patch alone.
- All medications for cessation have side effects and some have FDA warnings, providers should be familiar with these.

First Line
- Varenicline (Chantix) is a nicotinic acetylcholine partial agonist for the treatment of nicotine addiction. Trials have suggested this agent may be more efficacious than bupropion (6)[A]. Longer-term therapy (up to 24 weeks) may delay or prevent relapse:
  - Starter package includes 0.5 mg/d for 3 days, then 0.5 mg b.i.d. for 4 days, then 1 mg/d starting on day 7.
  - Maintenance package includes 1 mg b.i.d. (continue for 12 weeks total).
- Combination nicotine replacement therapy (NRT): All forms of NRT increase the chance of stopping smoking by 50–70%. No overall difference in effectiveness of different forms of NRT (6) and combining long- with short-acting NRTs has been shown to be more effective than using the patch alone (e.g., patch + inhaler, patch + gum). Heavier smokers may need higher doses. Starting NRT before planned a quit date may increase the chances of success (7)[A]:

– Nicotine gum (Nicorette): For >25 cigarettes/d habit, 4-mg gum q1–2h for 6 weeks; for <25 cigarettes/d habit, 2-mg gum q1–2h for 6 weeks; decrease dosing by q1–2h for 3 weeks; chew, then tuck between cheek and gingiva

– Nicotine transdermal (NicoDerm CQ): For >10 cigarettes/d habit, 21-mg patch/d for 6 weeks, then 14-mg patch/d for 2 weeks, then 7-mg patch/d for 2 weeks; for <10 cigarettes/d habit, 14-mg patch/d for 6 weeks, then 7-mg patch/d for 2 weeks

– Nicotine lozenge (Commit): For patients who have 1st cigarette within 30 minutes of waking, 4-mg lozenge PO q1–2h for 6 weeks; 1st cigarette >30 minutes after waking, 2-mg lozenge PO q1–2h for 6 weeks; decrease dosing by q1–2h for 3 weeks.

– Nicotine nasal (Nicotrol NS): 1–2 sprays (0.5 mg/spray) each nostril q1h for 8 weeks, then taper; max 10 sprays/h and 80 sprays/d

– Nicotine inhaler (Nicotrol inhaler): 6–16 cartridges inhaled (4 mg/cartridge) per day for 6–12 weeks, then taper

ALERT
Varenicline (Chantix) carries a boxed warning for risks of serious neuropsychiatric events, including changes in behavior, hostility, agitation, depressed mood, and suicidal thoughts or actions. It should be used with extreme caution in patients with serious psychiatric disorders (bipolar disorder, depression, or schizophrenia); use may exacerbate these conditions. Chantix may also increase the risk of certain cardiovascular adverse events in patients with cardiovascular disease.

Second Line
- Single-agent NRT: See above for prescribing information
- Bupropion SR (Zyban): An antidepressant; start 150 mg/d PO for 3 days, then 150 mg PO b.i.d.; stop smoking 5–7 days after starting treatment; continue 7–12 weeks
  – 1:1,000 risk of seizure
- Nortriptyline: Tricyclic antidepressant; start 25 mg/d, gradually increase to target dose of 75–100 mg/d; stop smoking 2–4 weeks after starting treatment; continue for 12 weeks:
  – Contraindications: Narrow-angle glaucoma or heart disease (acute myocardial infarction, atrioventricular or bundle-branch block, QT prolongation)
  – Caution: Pregnancy Category D

Third Line
- Clonidine: 0.1-mg patch/week, increase dose as needed; continue for 3–10 weeks:
  – Caution: Must monitor blood pressure closely and taper when discontinuing.
- Benzodiazepines: Although this class of drug has not improved rates of abstinence from smoking, patients with a high level of anxiety possibly could benefit from anxiolytics as a smoking-cessation intervention.

ADDITIONAL THERAPIES
Some Internet-based interventions can assist smoking cessation, especially if the information is appropriately tailored to the users and frequent automated contacts with the users are ensured (8).
- Other interventions:
  – Smokers who get support from partners and other people are more likely to quit.

– Group programs double cessation rates more than being given self-help materials without face-to-face instruction and group support. It is unclear whether groups are better than individual counseling or other advice, but they are more effective than no treatment. Not all smokers making a quit attempt want to attend group meetings, but for those who do, they are likely to be helpful.
- Smokers should be given a choice of quitting methods, either reducing smoking before quitting or abruptly quitting, as neither has demonstrated superior quit rates.
- E-Cigarettes: Currently there are questions from the FDA and others around safety, consistency of nicotine dose, and possible benefits from these devices. There are clinical trials set to report results in late 2013 or early 2014 looking at their efficacy and safety.

Pregnancy Considerations
- Interventions were effective in helping women to stop smoking during pregnancy (overall by ~6%). The most effective intervention appeared to be providing incentives, which helped ~24% of women to quit smoking during pregnancy. The smoking cessation interventions reduced the number of babies with low birth weight and preterm births.
- NRT is metabolized faster in pregnant women, so higher doses may be required. A 2012 Cochrane review found insufficient evidence for efficacy or change in adverse birth outcomes.

COMPLEMENTARY AND ALTERNATIVE MEDICINE
- Acupuncture: No consistent evidence acupuncture is effective for smoking cessation
- Hypnotherapy: No good evidence to show whether or not hypnotherapy can help people trying to quit smoking

IN-PATIENT CONSIDERATIONS
- Programs to stop smoking that begin during a hospital stay and include follow-up support for at least 1 month after discharge are effective. Programs are effective when administered to all hospitalized smokers, regardless of admitting diagnosis.
- Consider NRT to all inpatients who smoke to decrease withdrawal symptoms (9).

 ## ONGOING CARE

FOLLOW-UP RECOMMENDATIONS
- Patients motivated to quit smoking and who have initiated therapy should follow up routinely with the physician to monitor response and observe for any medication side effects.
- Encourage routine exercise as a component of smoking-cessation treatment.

DIET
Weight gain (4–5 kg over 10 years) possible after smoking cessation

PATIENT EDUCATION
- www.smokefree.gov
- www.nicotine-anonymous.org
- http://quitnet.com

PROGNOSIS
>85% of those who try to quit on their own relapse, most within a week (1).

REFERENCES

1. National Institute on Drug Abuse. *Tobacco addiction*. NIH Publication Number 09-4342. Bethesda, MD: National Institute of Health; 2009.
2. Johnston LD, O'Malley PM, Bachman JG, et al. (2012). *Monitoring the future national results on adolescent drug use: Overview of key findings, 2011*. Ann Arbor: Institute for Social Research, University of Michigan, 2012.
3. Stead LF, Bergson G, Lancaster T. Physician advice for smoking cessation. *Cochrane Database Syst Rev*. 2008;2:CD000165.
4. Dixon LB, Medoff D, Goldberg R, et al. Is implementation of the 5 A's of smoking cessation at community mental health centers effective for reduction of smoking by patients with serious mental illness? *Am J Addict*. 2009;18:386–392.
5. The Clinical Practice Guideline Treating Tobacco Use and Dependence 2008 Update Panel, Liaisons, and Staff. A clinical practice guideline for treating tobacco use and dependence: 2008 update. A U.S. Public Health Service Report. *Am J Prev Med*. 2008;35:158–176.
6. Cahill K, Stead LF, Lancaster T. Nicotine receptor partial agonists for smoking cessation. *Cochrane Database Syst Rev*. 2008;3:CD006103.
7. Stead LF, Perera R, Bullen C, et al. Nicotine replacement therapy for smoking cessation. *Cochrane Database Syst Rev*. 2008;1:CD000146.
8. Civljak M, Sheikh A, Stead LF, et al. Internet-based interventions for smoking cessation. *Cochrane Database Syst Rev*. 2010:CD007078.
9. Rigotti NA, Clair C, Munafo MR, et al. Interventions for smoking cessation in hospitalised patients. *Cochrane Database Syst Rev*. 2012;3:CD001837.

ADDITIONAL READING

National Guideline Clearinghouse (NGC). Guideline synthesis: Tobacco use cessation. In: National Guideline Clearinghouse (NGC). Rockville, MD: Agency for Healthcare Research and Quality (AHRQ); 2001 July (revised 2012 Feb). Available at: www.guideline.gov.

CODES

ICD10
- F17.200 Nicotine dependence, unspecified, uncomplicated
- F17.201 Nicotine dependence, unspecified, in remission
- F17.203 Nicotine dependence unspecified, with withdrawal

CLINICAL PEARLS

- Smoking cessation should be encouraged for all patients who smoke.
- No 1 type of NRT is best; they are equally effective. Choice, therefore, should be based on patient preference and risk factors for side effects.
- Consider NRT for all hospitalized patients who smoke to decrease withdrawal symptoms.

N

NOSOCOMIAL INFECTIONS

Cheryl Durand, PharmD • Edward L. Yourtee, MD, FACP

 BASICS

DESCRIPTION

- Also known as health care–associated infections (HAIs)
- Infection must not have been present or incubating on admission to a health care facility
- CDC categories:
  - Catheter-associated urinary tract infection (CAUTI)
  - Surgical site infection (SSI)
  - Ventilator-associated pneumonia (VAP)
  - Central line–associated bloodstream infection (CLABSI)
  - *Clostridium difficile* infection (*C. diff, C. difficile,* CDAD, CDI)
- The National Healthcare Safety Network (NHSN) at www.cdc.gov/nhsn monitors the epidemiology of emerging HAI pathogens and their mechanisms of resistance and evaluates alternative surveillance and prevention strategies.
- *Medicare and Medicaid will not provide payment for the treatment of certain hospital-acquired conditions (HAC), including catheter-associated UTIs, central line–associated bloodstream infections, and some surgical site infections.*

EPIDEMIOLOGY

- General:
  - 13/1,000 patient-days in the ICU (1)
  - 6.9/1,000 patient-days in high-risk nurseries
  - 2.6/1,000 patient-days in nurseries (1)
  - Estimated cost of HAIs is $20 billion per year (2)
- Infection-specific:
  - CAUTI:
    ○ Hospital stay increased by 1–3 days
    ○ Cost up to $600/infection
  - VAP:
    ○ Hospital stay increased by 6 days
    ○ Cost up to $5,000/infection
  - CLABSI:
    ○ Hospital stay increased by 7–20 days
    ○ Cost up to $56,000/infection
  - SSI:
    ○ Hospital stay increased by 7.3 days
    ○ Cost >$3,000/infection
    ○ May not be apparent until 1 month after surgery
  - *C. difficile* infection (see topic "*Clostridium Difficile* Infection")

Incidence

- 1.7 million HAIs in 2002 (1)
- 5–10% of hospital stays are complicated by HAIs (2)
- Most patients affected have a single-site infection
- UTI: 36% of HAIs (1):
  - 424,060 cases in 2002 in the US (1)
  - 2.39/100 admissions
- Pneumonia: 11% of HAIs (1):
  - 129,519 cases in 2002 in the US (1)
  - 0.60/100 admissions
- Bloodstream infection: 11% of HAIs (1):
  - 133,368 cases in 2002 in the US (1)
  - 0.27/100 admissions
- SSI: 20% of HAIs (1):
  - 244,385 cases in 2002 in the US (1)
  - 3% of all surgeries
  - 20% of emergency abdominal surgeries
- Others: 22% of HAIs (1): 263,810 cases in 2002 in the US (1)
- There is increasing prevalence of nosocomial infections caused by gram-negative rods resistant to almost all antibiotics, including ESBL (extended spectrum beta-lactamase) producing organisms and CPE (carbapenemase-producing Enterobacteriaceae).

- In 2008, 70% of nosocomial infections were resistant to at least 1 antimicrobial drug that was effective previously.
- 50% of sepsis cases originate in inpatients

ETIOLOGY AND PATHOPHYSIOLOGY

- Endogenous spread: Patient's own normal flora causes invasive disease (most cases).
- Exogenous route: Flora acquired from within health care facility causes invasive disease
- UTI: *Escherichia coli, Klebsiella* spp., *Serratia* spp., *Enterobacter, Pseudomonas aeruginosa, Enterococcus* spp., *Candida albicans*
- Pneumonia: Aerobic gram-negative bacilli, *S. aureus, P. aeruginosa*
- Bloodstream infection: *Staphylococcus* spp.
- SSI: *S. aureus,* gram-negative bacilli

RISK FACTORS

- Extremes of age
- Chronic disease (including diabetes, renal failure, and malignancy)
- Immunodeficiency
- Malnutrition
- Medications (e.g., recent antibiotics, proton pump inhibitors, and sedatives)
- Colonization with pathogenic strains of flora
- Breakdown of mucosal/cutaneous barriers, including trauma and battle wounds
- Anesthesia

GENERAL PREVENTION

- Prevention efforts should address both patient-specific and facility-related risk factors.
- Hand hygiene (3)[C]:
  - Upon entering and leaving a patient room (3)
  - After contact with blood, excretions, body fluids, wound dressings, nonintact skin, mucous membranes (3)
  - After contact with intact skin (3)
  - Wash hands before using and after removing gloves (gloves are permeable to bacteria)
  - When hands will be moving from contaminated to clean body site (3)
  - Alcohol-based product: When hands are not visibly soiled (3)
  - Soap and water:
    ○ When visibly soiled (3)
    ○ When in contact with spores (3)
- Antibiotic stewardship:
  - Judicious use of antibiotics reduces the emergence of multidrug resistant organisms and the occurrence of *C. difficile* infection (2).
  - Use narrow spectrum early-generation antibiotics when possible
  - Take an antibiotic "time out" at 72 hours to review clinical status and culture results
  - "Streamline" antibiotics at 72 hours by eliminating redundant/unnecessary antibiotics
  - Shorter courses of antibiotics may be as effective as and less toxic than traditional longer courses.
- Hospital-based surveillance programs
- Infection control programs with specially trained employees (3)[C]
- Employee education on HAIs (3)[C]
- Disinfection of hospital rooms with hydrogen peroxide vapor in addition to standard cleaning reduces environmental contamination and the risk of infection with multidrug-resistant organisms (4)[C]
- Minimize invasive procedures.
- Caregiver stethoscope cleaning:
  - Stethoscope bacterial contamination is common, and regular cleaning with alcohol-based preparations reduces bacterial load; however, evidence is lacking to confirm whether stethoscope contamination causes nosocomial infections (5)[A].
- Isolation of known pathogen carriers (3)[A]:
  - Contact precautions:
    ○ Pathogens spread by direct contact.
    ○ Gloves when entering room (3)[B]
    ○ Gown if clothing will touch patient or environment (3)[B]
    ○ Includes methicillin-resistant *Staphylococcus aureus* (MRSA), vancomycin-resistant *Enterococcus, C. difficile,* extended-spectrum β-lactamase–producing gram-negative rods, and carbapenemase-producing gram-negative rods
  - Droplet precautions:
    ○ Infectious particles measure >5 μm
    ○ Mask when entering room (3)[B]
    ○ Shed via talking, coughing, sneezing, mucosal shedding, airway suctioning, bronchoscopy
    ○ Includes *Neisseria meningitis,* influenza, *Haemophilus influenzae,* diphtheria, *Bordetella pertussis*
  - Airborne precautions:
    ○ Infectious particles measure <5 μm
    ○ Fit-tested National Institute of Occupational Safety and Health (NIOSH)–approved ≥N-95 respirator on entering room (3)[B]
    ○ Shed via coughing
    ○ Includes tuberculosis, varicella-zoster virus, measles
- Infection-specific measures:
  - CAUTI:
    ○ Employee education on urinary catheters (e.g., indications, placement, maintenance) (6)[C]
    ○ Sterile catheter placement technique (6)[C]
    ○ Closed urine collection system (6)[C]
    ○ Use of catheter only as necessary (6)[B]
    ○ Removal of catheter as early as possible (6)[B]
    ○ Consider nurse-driven protocols for guideline-driven catheter removal
    ○ Do not confuse catheter-associated asymptomatic bacteriuria with CAUTI (6).
    ○ Do not screen for bacteriuria by routinely performing a urine culture when the catheter is withdrawn.
  - VAP:
    ○ Intubation only as necessary (7)[C]
    ○ Perform oral decontamination with an antiseptic agent (8)[A]
    ○ Avoidance of nasotracheal intubation (7)[B]
    ○ Inline suctioning (7)[C]
    ○ Head elevation of 30–45 degrees (7)[C]
  - CLABSI:
    ○ Employee education on IV catheters (e.g., indications, placement, maintenance) (9)[A]
    ○ Sterile catheter placement technique (including chlorhexidine prep, maximal barrier precautions) (9)[A]
    ○ Use order "bundles" to improve adherence to catheter insertion guidelines

- ○ Prompt removal of catheter (9)[A]
- ○ Hand hygiene in addition to glove use (9)[A]
- ○ Regular monitoring of catheter site (9)[B]
- – SSI:
  - ○ Proper surgical hand hygiene (2)[B]
  - ○ Prophylactic antibiotic therapy when indicated (2)[A]
  - ○ Elimination of underlying infections before surgery (2)[A]
  - ○ Hair removal with electric clippers/depilatory agent (2)[B]
  - ○ Postoperative blood sugar control
- – *C. difficile* infection:
  - ○ Hand hygiene with soap and water (spores are resistant to alcohol-based products) (2)
  - ○ Restrict use of fluoroquinolones, cephalosporins, and clindamycin when possible (2)
  - ○ *C. difficile* is strongly associated with the use of proton pump inhibitors: Use H2 blockers for acid suppression whenever feasible (10)[A]
  - ○ Accumulating evidence suggests that probiotics may reduce nonspecific antibiotic-associated diarrhea; but the effectiveness of probiotics and selection of probiotic for prevention of *C. difficile* remains unclear (10).
- – Bloodstream infections
  - ○ Daily bathing of ICU patients with chlorhexidine-impregnated washcloths can reduce bloodstream infections by 28% (11)[B]
  - ○ Screen inpatients routinely for systemic inflammatory response (SIRS) by established criteria for early detection of sepsis

DIAGNOSIS

Consistent with nature of infection

HISTORY
- Exposure to health care facility
- Recent surgery/open wounds
- History of invasive procedure:
  - – Urinary catheter placement
  - – Indwelling vascular catheter
- Recent intubation/mechanical ventilation
- Past infections (e.g., MRSA)

PHYSICAL EXAM
Consistent with nature of infection

DIFFERENTIAL DIAGNOSIS
- Community-acquired infection
- Noninfectious process

DIAGNOSTIC TESTS & INTERPRETATION
As appropriate for suspected infection

Test Interpretation
Consistent with underlying infection

TREATMENT

GENERAL MEASURES
- Treat the underlying infection as indicated.
- The use of an sepsis protocol order bundle may improve adherence to sepsis guidelines and has been shown to improve survival.
- Specific measures as appropriate for type of infection:
  - – UTI: Remove urinary catheters
  - – CLABSI: Remove IV catheter
  - – *C. difficile*: Stop all antibiotics not being used to treat *C. difficile* infection

MEDICATION
First Line
- As appropriate for specific nature of infection
- Several agents have been approved recently for the treatment of antibiotic-resistant gram-positive infections:
  - – Linezolid
  - – Daptomycin
  - – Telavancin
  - – Tigecycline
  - – Ceftaroline
- *Some emerging resistant gram-negative infections have been found to be resistant to nearly all antibiotics and require expert consultation for management.*

ISSUES FOR REFERRAL
As appropriate

SURGERY/OTHER PROCEDURES
- As appropriate for specific nature of infection
- Screening for nasal carriage of MRSA and isolation have been shown to reduce the nosocomial spread of MRSA.
- Treating proven nasal carriers of *Staphylococcus* or MRSA with mupirocin prevents *S. aureus* nosocomial infections after surgery. This screen-and-treat approach is cost-saving as long as the prevalence of mupirocin resistance is low (12)[B].

IN-PATIENT CONSIDERATIONS
IV Fluids
As needed

Nursing
- Handwashing should be performed on entering and exiting the patient room even with no direct contact with the patient.
- Isolation precautions as indicated

Discharge Criteria
When infection has resolved or patient is stable

ONGOING CARE

FOLLOW-UP RECOMMENDATIONS
Patient Monitoring
As appropriate for specific type of infection

PROGNOSIS
- 99,000 deaths in 2002 in the US (1)
- Bloodstream infection mortality: 27%
- Pneumonia mortality: 33–50%
- SSI mortality: 11% (1)

COMPLICATIONS
Related to specific nature of infection

REFERENCES

1. Klevens RM, Edwards JR, Richards CL, et al. Estimating health care-associated infections and deaths in U.S. hospitals, 2002. *Public Health Rep.* 2007;122:160–166.
2. Yokoe DS, Mermel LA, Anderson DJ, et al. A compendium of strategies to prevent healthcare-associated infections in acute care hospitals. *Infect Control Hosp Epidemiol.* 2008;29(Suppl 1):S12–S21.
3. Siegel JD, Rhinehart E, Jackson M, et al. 2007 guideline for isolation precautions: Preventing transmission of infectious agents in health care settings. *Am J Infect Control.* 2007;35:S65–S164.
4. Passaretti CL, Otter JA, Reich NG, et al. An evaluation of environmental decontamination with hydrogen peroxide vapor for reducing the risk of patient acquisition of multidrug-resistant organisms. *Clin Infect Dis.* 2013;56:27–35.
5. Bandi S, Conway A. Question 2. Does regular cleaning of stethoscopes result in a reduction in nosocomial infections? *Arch Dis Child.* 2012;97:175–177.
6. Hooton TM, Bradley SF, Cardenas DD, et al. Diagnosis, prevention, and treatment of catheter-associated urinary tract infection in adults: 2009 International Clinical Practice Guidelines from the Infectious Disease Society of America. *Clin Infect Dis.* 2010;50:625–663.
7. Tablan OC. Guidelines for preventing health-care associated pneumonia, 2003: Recommendations of CDC and the Healthcare Infection Control Practices Advisory Committee. *MMWR.* 2004;53:1–40.
8. Chan EY, Ruest A, Meade MO, et al. Oral decontamination for prevention of pneumonia in mechanically ventilated adults: Systematic review and meta-analysis. *BMJ.* 2007;334:889.
9. O'Grady NP, Alexander M, Burns LA, et al. Guidelines for the prevention of intravascular catheter-related infections, 2011. Available at: www.cdc.gov/hicpac/BSI/01-BSI-guidelines-2011.html
10. Surawicz CM, Brandt LJ, Binion DG, et al. Guidelines for diagnosis, treatment, and prevention of *Clostridium difficile* infections. *Am J Gastroenterol.* 2013;108:478–498.
11. Climo MW, Yokoe DS, Warren DK, et al. Effect of daily chlorhexidine bathing on hospital-acquired infection. *N Engl J Med.* 2013;368:533–542.
12. Van Rijen M, Bonten M, Wenzel R, et al. Mupirocin ointment for preventing *Staphylococcus aureus* infections in nasal carriers. *Cochrane Database Syst Rev.* 2009;1:CD006216.

CODES

ICD10
- T81.4XXA Infection following a procedure, initial encounter
- T82.7XXA Infect/inflm react d/t oth cardi/vasc dev/implnt/grft, init
- T83.51XA Infect/inflm reaction due to indwell urinary catheter, init

CLINICAL PEARLS
- Nosocomial infections are associated with increased mortality, length of hospital stay, and admission cost.
- Prevention efforts should address both patient-specific and facility-related risk factors.
- Proper use of an alcohol-based hand product should be carried out before and after each patient encounter, even when gloves are used. Alcohol-based hand rubs are not effective for killing spores formed by *C. difficile*. Handwashing with soap and water after exposure to spores is the appropriate alternative.
- Contact, droplet, or airborne precautions should be used when appropriate to reduce the spread of infection.
- The risk of developing a resistant nosocomial infection can be reduced by antibiotic streamlining, emphasizing the use of narrow-spectrum antibiotics and frequent evaluation of the necessity of continuing antibiotics in the health care setting.

N

NOVEL INFLUENZA A (2009 H1N1)
Sumanth Gandra, MD, MPH

 BASICS

DESCRIPTION
Novel influenza (2009 H1N1):
- 2009 H1N1 virus, a novel influenza A virus originated from a reassortment of influenza viruses that circulated in North American and Eurasian pig herds.
- The 2009 H1N1 pandemic started in March 2009 in Mexico and then spread to many countries, including the US.
- The pandemic was declared in August 2010 by the World Health Organization (WHO) (1).
- Although pandemic is over, 2009 H1N1 virus still exists and continues to cause disease.
- Generally self-limited and uncomplicated disease course
- Typically presents with influenza-like symptoms, but patients may be symptomatic with diarrhea and vomiting (2)
- Susceptible to neuraminidase inhibitors, but resistant to adamantine antiviral agents (3)

EPIDEMIOLOGY
- The CDC estimates that between 43 million and 89 million cases of 2009 H1N1 occurred between April 2009 and April 2010 in the US, including ~274,000 hospitalizations and 12,470 deaths (4).
- 90% of the reported cases were accounted for by patients <64 (4).

Incidence
- Predominant sex: Male = Female
- Affects mostly young people
- Older people are protected because they have pre-existing antibodies that cross-react with 2009 H1N1.

ETIOLOGY AND PATHOPHYSIOLOGY
- 2009 H1N1 influenza was a quadruple-reassortant strain with the individual gene segments of the virus originating from humans, birds, North American pigs, and Eurasian pigs.
- Reservoirs included infected human and pig populations.

RISK FACTORS
- Similar to regular influenza transmission, with exposure to respiratory secretions accounting for the main avenue of infection
- Close contact (<6 feet) with confirmed case increases the possibility for large-droplet transmission (2)
- Risk factors for complications of or severe illness with 2009 H1N1 virus infection (5):
  - Age <5 or >65 years
  - Pregnancy
  - Morbid obesity
  - Chronic medical conditions (diabetes, chronic cardiovascular conditions, cirrhosis, end-stage renal disease [ESRD] on hemodialysis [HD])

- Chronic lung disorders (chronic obstructive pulmonary disease [COPD], asthma, cystic fibrosis)
- Immunosuppression (associated with HIV infection, organ transplantation, receipt of chemotherapy or corticosteroids, or malnutrition)
- Immunoglobulin (Ig) G2 subclass deficiency
- Sickle cell disease
- Native Americans/Alaska Natives
- Persons aged <19 years who are receiving long-term aspirin therapy
- Residents of nursing homes and other chronic-care facilities

GENERAL PREVENTION
- 2009 H1N1 vaccination, monovalent or trivalent. The 2011–2012 and 2012–2013 seasonal influenza vaccines had 2009 H1N1 virus included.
- CDC recommends 2009 H1N1 vaccine for all persons ≥6 months.
- No safety concerns were identified with 2009 H1N1 vaccine among pregnant women, infants, and children.
- Observe hand hygiene and appropriate cough etiquette
- Health care personnel must observe droplet precautions (surgical mask or N95 mask and protective goggles) in addition to contact precautions for patients presenting with symptoms of an influenza-like illness (fever with cough or sore throat).
- When leaving their rooms, patients should be outfitted with a surgical mask to contain their respiratory secretions.

 DIAGNOSIS

HISTORY
- Incubation period: 1.5–3 days but may be as long as 7 days
- Close contact with a suspected or confirmed case
- Clinical spectrum ranges from afebrile upper respiratory illness to fulminant viral pneumonia
- Symptoms similar to regular seasonal influenza; most patients present with (5):
  - Fever
  - Sore throat
  - Cough
  - Myalgias
  - Nasal congestion
  - Rhinorrhea
- GI symptoms (more common than with seasonal influenza):
  - Nausea
  - Vomiting
  - Diarrhea

- Extrapulmonary complications include:
  - Hepatitis
  - Myocarditis
  - Rhabdomyolysis
  - Renal failure
  - Systemic or pulmonary vascular thrombosis
  - Reactive hemophagocytosis
  - In children, acute necrotizing encephalopathy or encephalopathy

DIFFERENTIAL DIAGNOSIS
- Seasonal influenza
- Respiratory viral infections from such agents as coronavirus, rhinovirus, and adenovirus
- Croup
- Pneumonia (typical and atypical)
- Infectious mononucleosis
- Pharyngitis (viral or streptococcal)
- HIV syndrome

DIAGNOSTIC TESTS & INTERPRETATION
- Rapid flu tests (6):
  - The rapid antigen test and direct fluorescent antibody (DFA) have low sensitivities to detect 2009 H1N1 (17.8% and 46.7%, respectively)
- Viral culture and polymerase chain reaction (PCR) test are highly sensitive (88.9% vs. 97.8%) (6)
- Reverse transcription-polymerase chain reaction (RT-PCR; respiratory viral panel) is the test of choice (5).

Initial Tests (lab, imaging)
- CBC with differential
- Basic metabolic panel
- Blood cultures
- Liver function tests (LFTs)
- Chest x-ray (CXR): Among those hospitalized for 2009 H1N1 infection, 50% had infiltrates on CXR (2).

Test Interpretation
Most consistent histopathologic findings are varying degrees of diffuse alveolar damage with hyaline membranes and septal edema, tracheitis, and necrotizing bronchiolitis.

 TREATMENT

- Most infections are self-limited and uncomplicated.
- Treatment for seasonal influenza with neuraminidase inhibitors is most effective when administered within 48 hours of symptom onset (7)[A].
- Patients with 2009 H1N1 who were treated with oseltamivir had faster resolution of symptoms and a more rapid clearance of viral shedding in hospitalized patients of all ages, organ transplant recipients, and pregnant women (5)[B].

- Poor outcomes were seen in patients with delayed oseltamivir therapy for severe cases of 2009 H1N1.
- Antiviral treatment is recommended as soon as possible (even if patient presents >48 hours after illness onset) for all persons with suspected or confirmed 2009 H1N1 infection requiring hospitalization or who have progressive, complicated illness regardless of previous health or vaccination status (7)[B].
- High-risk patients (mentioned in "Risk Factors") with confirmed or suspected 2009 H1N1 should be treated with antiviral agents, when treatment can begin within 48 hours after symptom onset (7)[A].
- Consider antiviral treatment for high-risk patients with illness that is not improving and who have a positive 2009 H1N1 test result from a specimen obtained >48 hours after onset of symptoms (7)[C].

MEDICATION
- 2009 H1N1 is susceptible to the neuraminidase inhibitors oseltamivir (Tamiflu) and zanamivir (Relenza) (3).
- Oseltamivir resistance is reported in <2% of strains tested globally, due to H275Y mutation, but remained susceptible to zanamivir.
- Genetic sequencing indicated resistance to the adamantine antivirals (e.g., amantadine).

First Line
- Oseltamivir:
  - Adult dosage: 75 mg PO b.i.d. × 5 days
  - Pediatric dosage (safety and efficacy not established for children <1 year):
    - ≤15 kg: 30 mg PO b.i.d. × 5 days; 16–23 kg: 45 mg PO b.i.d. × 5 days; 24–40 kg: 60 mg PO b.i.d. × 5 days; >40 kg: 75 mg PO b.i.d. × 5 days
  - Pediatric dosage <1 year old: <3 months: 3 mg/kg PO b.i.d. × 5 days; 3–11 months: 3 mg/kg PO b.i.d. × 5 days
  - Longer treatment courses can be considered for patients who are hospitalized and remain severely ill after 5 days of treatment.
  - Adverse effects:
    - Most common symptoms include nausea and vomiting, occurring in 9–10% of patients.
    - Neuropsychiatric events (e.g., hallucinations, delirium, and abnormal behavior) are rare symptoms.
    - Other rare symptoms include anaphylaxis and severe skin reactions, such as Stevens-Johnson syndrome and toxic epidermal necrolysis.
  - Other considerations: Metabolized by liver
  - Pregnancy Class C medication

- Zanamivir (not recommended for patients with respiratory conditions such as COPD or asthma):
  - Adult dosage: 2 puffs of 5 mg inhaled b.i.d. × 5 days
  - Pediatric dosage: >7 years old: 2 puffs of 5 mg inhaled b.i.d. × 5 days
  - Limited quantities of IV zanamivir were made available.
  - Adverse effects:
    - Most notably may cause bronchospasm, especially in patients with pre-existing respiratory illnesses
    - Common adverse symptoms include headache, nausea, dizziness, and cough.
    - Rare symptoms are similar to those of oseltamivir, including neuropsychiatric symptoms, anaphylaxis, and severe skin reactions.
  - Other considerations: Metabolized by liver
  - Pregnancy Class C medication
- Peramivir:
  - FDA issued emergency use authorization (EUA) for peramivir, an investigational neuraminidase inhibitor for treatment of severely ill cases of confirmed or suspected cases of 2009 H1N1.
  - Administered IV
  - EUA for peramivir expired in June 2010

ADDITIONAL THERAPIES
- Broad-spectrum antibiotics as needed for treatment of bacterial co-infections
- In patients with 2009 H1N1 who had acute respiratory distress syndrome (ARDS), extracorporeal membrane oxygenation was utilized.

COMPLICATIONS
- ARDS
- Rapidly progressive pneumonia
- Respiratory failure
- Bacterial superinfection of lungs
- Encephalitis/encephalopathy
- Seizures

REFERENCES
1. World Health Organization. In focus: H1N1 now in the post-pandemic period. August 10, 2010. Available at: www.who.int/csr/disease/swineflu/en/index.html
2. Novel Swine-Origin Influenza A (H1N1) Virus Investigation Team, Dawood FS, Jain S, et al. Emergence of a novel swine-origin influenza A (H1N1) virus in humans. N Engl J Med. 2009;360:2605–2615.
3. Centers for Disease Control and Prevention (CDC). Update: Drug susceptibility of swine-origin influenza A (H1N1) viruses, April 2009. MMWR. 2009;58:433–435.
4. Updated CDC Estimates of 2009 H1N1 Influenza Cases, Hospitalizations and Deaths in the United States, April 2009–April 10, 2010. Available at: www.cdc.gov/h1n1flu/estimates_2009_h1n1.htm
5. Cheng VC, To KK, Tse H, et al. Two years after pandemic influenza A/2009/H1N1: What have we learned? Clin Microbiol Rev. 2012;25:223–263.
6. Ginocchio CC, Zhang F, Manji R, et al. Evaluation of multiple test methods for the detection of the novel 2009 influenza A (H1N1) during the New York City outbreak. J Clin Virol. 2009;45:191–195.
7. Fiore AE, Fry A, Shay D, et al. Antiviral agents for the treatment and chemoprophylaxis of influenza—recommendations of the Advisory Committee on Immunization Practices (ACIP). MMWR Recomm Rep. 2011;60:1–24.

ADDITIONAL READING
- Marshall HS, Collins J, Sullivan T, et al. Parental and societal support for adolescent immunization through school based immunization programs. Vaccine. 2013;31:3059–3064.
- Tooher R, Collins JE, Street JM, et al. Community knowledge, behaviours and attitudes about the 2009 H1N1 influenza pandemic: A systematic review. Influenza Other Respi Viruses. 2013; in press.

 ### CODES

ICD10
- J10.00 Flu due to oth ident flu virus w unsp type of pneumonia
- J10.01 Flu due to oth ident flu virus w same oth ident flu virus pn
- J10.1 Flu due to oth ident influenza virus w oth resp manifest

CLINICAL PEARLS
- 2009 H1N1 pandemic started in March 2009 and was declared over in August 2010.
- Affected mostly young people because older people had pre-existing antibodies that cross-reacted with 2009 H1N1.
- Most cases are self-limited and uncomplicated.
- Up to 25% of patients reported vomiting and diarrhea in addition to fever, headache, sore throat, and cough.
- RT-PCR (respiratory viral panel) was the test of choice.
- Susceptible to neuraminidase inhibitors (oseltamivir and zanamivir), but resistant to adamantine antiviral agents.

N

OBESITY

Maya Leventer-Roberts, MD, MPH

BASICS

DESCRIPTION
- Obesity refers to excess adipose tissue. Weight status is characterized by calculating the body mass index [BMI = body weight (kg)/(body height (m))^2] and classified as underweight, normal weight, overweight, or obese:
  - For adults, a BMI $\geq$30 kg/m^2 is consistent with obesity.
- Obesity is associated with negative health outcomes:
  - The increased risk of morbidity and mortality is most closely related to abdominal obesity.
- System(s) affected: Endocrine/Metabolic; Cardiac; Respiratory; Gastrointestinal; Musculoskeletal; Dermatologic; Mental Health
- Synonym(s): Overweight; Adiposity

Geriatric Considerations
BMI associated with the lowest risk of mortality increases as age increases.

EPIDEMIOLOGY
- Predominant age: Incidence rises in the early 20s
- Predominant sex: Female > Male

Prevalence
- Mean prevalence of obesity among adults is 32.2% in the US.
- Overweight: 40% of men and 25% of women
- Obese: 20% of men and 25% of women

Pediatric Considerations
- Pediatric obesity is categorized as $\geq$95th percentile, as established by CDC growth curves, by age and sex.
- The incidence of obesity among the pediatric population has risen.
- Obesity during adolescence and young adulthood is strongly associated with obesity in adulthood.
- Risk factors include insufficient physical activity, consumption of sweetened beverages, and excess television viewing.

ETIOLOGY AND PATHOPHYSIOLOGY
- Obesity is caused by an imbalance among food intake, absorption, and energy expenditure.
- Underlying organic causes may be psychiatric disturbances, hypothyroidism, hypothalamic disorders, insulinoma, and Cushing syndrome.
- Medications: Corticosteroids, neuroleptics (particularly the "atypical" antipsychotics), and antidepressants

Genetics
- Genetic syndromes such as Prader-Willi and Bardet-Biedl are responsible for a minor percentage of people with obesity.
- Studies are insufficiently powered to isolate genes as predictors of obesity.

RISK FACTORS
- Parental obesity
- Sedentary lifestyle
- Calorie dense food
- Low socioeconomic status
- >2 hours/d of television viewing

GENERAL PREVENTION
- Encourage 1 hour of daily exercise, limited television viewing, and moderation in portion size.
- Avoid calorie-dense and nutrient-poor foods such as sweetened beverages and processed foods.
- Most patients underestimate daily calorie consumption.

DIAGNOSIS

HISTORY
- Prior attempts at weight loss
- Reported readiness to change lifestyle
- Social support and resources
- Diet and exercise habits
- Associated risk factors: Diabetes mellitus type 2, hypertension, hyperlipidemia, sleep apnea
- Psychiatric history
- Symptoms suggesting hypothyroidism, Cushing syndrome, genetic syndromes

PHYSICAL EXAM
Elevated BMI and excess adipose tissue:
- BMI = body weight (kg)/body height (m^2):
  - Overweight: BMI = 25–29.9 kg/m^2
  - Obese: BMI $\geq$30 kg/m^2
- BMI obesity threshold by height

Height	BMI = 25 Weight (lb/kg)	BMI = 27 Weight (lb/kg)	BMI = 30 Weight (lb/kg)
5'0	128/58	138/63	153/70
5'2	136/61	147/67	164/74
5'4	145/66	157/71	174/79
5'6	155/70	167/76	186/84
5'8	164/74	177/81	197/89
5'10	174/79	188/85	209/95
6'0	184/83	199/90	221/100
6'2	194/88	210/95	233/106
6'4	205/92	221/101	246/112

- Fat distribution pattern:
  - Waist circumference is measured around the abdomen at the level of the umbilicus:
    - >40 inches (102 cm) for men and >35 inches (88 cm) for women is associated with increased risk for most obesity-related medical conditions (1)[C].

DIAGNOSTIC TESTS & INTERPRETATION
- Consider screening as well as routine laboratory assessment.
- Used to monitor underlying physiologic causes as well as associated comorbid conditions.
- Labs should be done while fasting, although nonfasting labs within normal limits do not need to be repeated.
- Preserved glucose, total insulin, hemoglobin A1C
- Serum lipid panel
- Thyroid function tests
- LFTs
- Imaging interpretation:
  - Hypertrophy and/or hyperplasia of adipocytes
  - Cardiomegaly
  - Hepatomegaly

TREATMENT

GENERAL MEASURES
- Begin with the following assessment:
  - Degree of health risk from BMI and waist circumference (1)[C] (see "Diagnosis")
  - Motivation to lose weight (1)[C]
  - Patient-specific goals of therapy
  - Referral for intensive counseling for diet, exercise, and behavior modification (1)[B]
  - Long-term follow-up (1)[C]
- Goal for therapy is to achieve and sustain weight loss up of at least 10% of body weight for overweight and obese patients (1)[A].
- Tracking of PO intake and exercise on a daily basis using index cards or software (www.myfitnesspal.com, www.loseit.com, others)
- Goal is to limit carbohydrates to less than 40% of total calories (typically by limiting all sweetened drinks, including fruit juices and encouraging 5–10 servings of fruits and vegetables per day)
- Behavior therapy and cognitive-behavioral methods can result in modest weight loss, but are most effective when combined with dietary and exercise treatments (2)[A].
- Use of commercial weight loss programs (e.g., Weight Watchers) can be more effective than "standard of care" counseling (3)[B].

MEDICATION
- National Institute of Health guidelines suggest nonpharmacologic treatment for at least 6 months.
- Medication treatment may be initiated for unsatisfactory weight loss in those with a BMI >30 or with a BMI >27 combined with associated risk factors (e.g., coronary artery disease, diabetes, sleep apnea, hypertension, hyperlipidemia).
- Diet, exercise, and behavior therapy *must* be included with pharmacologic treatment for those without comorbid conditions (1)[B].

First Line

- Medications may produce modest weight loss (4)[A].
- The lipase inhibitor orlistat decreases the absorption of dietary fat. Dose: 120 mg PO t.i.d. with meals. Patients must avoid taking fat-soluble vitamin supplements within 2 hours of taking orlistat. The FDA has approved orlistat to be sold over the counter as a weight-loss aid.
- Contraindications:
  – Orlistat: Chronic malabsorption syndromes, cholestasis
- Precautions: Relapse after discontinuation of drug
- Significant possible interactions:
  – Pulse and BP elevations possible with sibutramine.
  – Concurrent use with general anesthetics may cause arrhythmias.
  – Serotonergic agents may cause "serotonin syndrome" in combination with sibutramine.

Second Line

- Appetite suppressants recommended for short-term treatment (≤6 months)
- Only beneficial in patients who exercise and eat reduced calorie diet:
  – Lorcaserin (Belviq) 10 mg PO bid (D/C if weight loss is <5% after 12 weeks)
  – Topiramate 200 mg PO bid (initiate by 25 bid and increase by 50 mg/week); not FDA approved for the treatment of obesity, but effective (5)[A]
- Schedule IV drugs:
  – Diethylpropion: 25 mg before meals t.i.d.; discontinue if no response after 4 weeks.
  – Phentermine: 15, 30, 37.5 mg PO every morning; discontinue if tolerance or no response after 4 weeks.
  – Phentermine/Topiramate (37.5/23 ER, 7.5/46 ER, 11.25/69 ER, 15/92 ER); initiate at 7.5/46 or 15/92 once PO every morning

Pregnancy Considerations

- Weight loss is not appropriate for most pregnant women (1)[C].
- During pregnancy, obese women should gain fewer pounds than recommended for nonobese women.

SURGERY/OTHER PROCEDURES

Patients meeting criteria should be evaluated for gastric bypass or lap band procedures:

- Requires complex presurgical evaluation, surgery, and follow-up in a skilled treatment center (1)[C]
- Surgical treatment is the most effective long-term weight-loss treatment available for morbidly obese patients (6)[B].

ONGOING CARE

FOLLOW-UP RECOMMENDATIONS

- Exercise is an integral part of any weight-loss program, yet exercise alone rarely results in significant weight loss (1)[A].
- Combination of weight training and aerobic activity is preferred over aerobic activity alone.

Patient Monitoring

Long-term routine follow-up is crucial to prevent relapse after weight loss or further weight gain.

DIET

- Long-term studies suggest net calorie reduction of 500–1,000 kcal/d and ease of use are more important than diet composition for long-term results:
  – A reduction of 500 kcal/d intake can result in ~1 lb (0.45 kg) weight loss per week (1)[A].
  – Portion-controlled servings are recommended.
- Low glycemic index diet: Foods that result in slowed absorption of carbohydrates
- Very-low-calorie diet (400–800 kcal/d):
  – Can result in more rapid weight loss than higher-calorie diets, but are less effective in the long term
  – Complications can include dehydration, orthostatic hypotension, fatigue, muscle cramps, constipation, headache, cold intolerance, and relapse after discontinuation.
  – Contraindications: Recent myocardial infarction or cerebrovascular accident, renal disease, cancer, pregnancy, insulin-dependent diabetes mellitus, and some psychiatric disturbances

PATIENT EDUCATION

- Emphasize the value of a healthy BMI.
- Recommended Web sites:
  – www.nal.usda.gov/fnic/foodcomp/search for the FDA nutritional content in common foods

PROGNOSIS

- Lowest mortality associated with a BMI of 22
- Long-term maintenance of weight loss is extremely difficult.
- A motivated patient is most likely to achieve successful weight loss.

COMPLICATIONS

- Cardiovascular disease
- Stroke (in men)
- Thromboembolism
- Heart failure
- Hypertension
- Hypoventilation and sleep apnea syndromes
- Higher death rates from cancer: Colon, breast, prostate, endometrial, gallbladder, liver, kidney
- Diabetes mellitus
- Skin changes
- Hyperlipidemia
- Gallbladder disease
- Osteoarthritis
- Gout
- Poor self-esteem
- Discrimination
- Increased sick leave

REFERENCES

1. National Institutes of Health Clinical guidelines on the identification, evaluation, and treatment of overweight and obesity in adults: The evidence report. NIH Publication No. 98-4083, 1998.
2. Shaw K, O'Rourke P, Del Mar C, et al. Psychological interventions for overweight or obesity. *Cochrane Database Syst Rev.* 2005;(2):CD003818. Epub 2005 Apr 18.
3. Jebb SA, Ahern AL, Olson AD, et al. Primary care referral to a commercial provider for weight loss treatment versus standard care: A randomised controlled trial. *Lancet.* 2011;378:1485–1492.
4. Padwal R, Li SK, Lau DCW. Long-term pharmacotherapy for obesity and overweight (Cochrane Review). *Cochrane Library.* Issue 4. Chichester, UK: Wiley & Sons; 2005.
5. Kramer CK, Leitão CB, Pinto LC, et al. Efficacy and safety of topiramate on weight loss: A meta-analysis of randomized controlled trials. *Obes Rev.* 2011;12(5):e338–e347.
6. Colquitt J, Clegg A, Loveman E, et al. Surgery for morbid obesity. *Cochrane Database Syst Rev.* 2005;(4):CD003641. Epub 2005 Oct 19.

ADDITIONAL READING

- Flegal K, Graubard B, Williamson D, et al. Excess deaths associated with underweight, overweight, and obesity. *JAMA.* 2005;293(15):1861–1867.
- Thomas DE, Elliott EJ, Baur L. Low glycaemic index or low glycaemic load diets for overweight and obesity. *Cochrane Database Syst Rev.* 2007;(3):CD005105. Epub 2007 Jul 18.

CODES

ICD10

- E66.01 Morbid (severe) obesity due to excess calories
- E66.8 Other obesity
- E66.9 Obesity, unspecified

CLINICAL PEARLS

- Drug treatment with a 1st-line medication may be indicated when nonpharmacologic treatment for 6 months has been ineffective and the patient has a BMI >30 or a BMI >27 with associated risk factors. Medications produce (at most) a modest long-term weight loss.
- Surgical treatment may be indicated in patients with a BMI >40 who have failed more conservative treatment, particularly when there are associated risk factors, such as diabetes mellitus.
- No convincing evidence indicates that any specific diet is more effective than any other diet of equivalent caloric content.

OBSESSIVE-COMPULSIVE DISORDER

Anila Khaliq, MD • Mahpara Khaliq, MD • Komel Khaliq, MBBS

BASICS

DESCRIPTION
- A psychiatric condition classified as an anxiety disorder characterized by obsessions (recurrent intrusive thoughts, ideas, or images) and compulsions (repetitive, ritualistic behaviors, or mental acts) causing significant patient distress
- Not to be confused with obsessive-compulsive personality disorder

EPIDEMIOLOGY
Incidence
- Predominant age: Mean age of onset 22–36 years:
  - Male = Female (males present at younger age)
  - Child/Adolescent onset in 33% of cases
  - 1/3 of cases present by age 15 years
  - 85% of cases present at <35 years of age
  - Diagnosis rarely made at >50 years of age
- Predominant gender: Male > Female (3:1)

Pediatric Considerations
Insidious onset; consider brain insult in acute presentation of childhood obsessive-compulsive disorder (OCD).

Geriatric Considerations
Consider neurologic disorders in new-onset OCD in the elderly.

Prevalence
- 2.3% lifetime in adults
- 1–2.3% prevalence in children/adolescents

ETIOLOGY AND PATHOPHYSIOLOGY
- Exact pathophysiology unknown
- Dysregulation of serotonergic pathways
- Dysregulation of corticostriatal–thalamic–cortico (CSTC) pathway
- Exact etiology unknown
- Genetic and environmental factors
- Pediatric autoimmune disorder associated with streptococcal infections

Genetics
- Greater concordance in monozygotic twins
- Positive family history: Prevalence rates of 7–15% in 1st-degree relatives of children/adolescents with OCD

RISK FACTORS
- Exact cause of OCD is not fully elucidated.
- Combination of biologic and environmental factors likely involved:
  - Link between low serotonin levels and development of OCD
  - Link between brain insult and development of OCD (i.e., encephalitis, pediatric streptococcal infection, or head injury)

GENERAL PREVENTION
- OCD cannot be prevented.
- Early diagnosis and treatment can decrease patient's distress and impairment.

COMMONLY ASSOCIATED CONDITIONS
- Major depressive disorder
- Panic disorder
- Phobia/Social phobia
- Tourette syndrome
- Substance abuse
- Eating disorder/body dysmorphic disorder

DIAGNOSIS

HISTORY
- Patient presents with either obsessions or compulsions, which cause marked distress, are time-consuming (>1 h/d), and cause significant occupational/social impairment.
- 4 criteria support diagnosis of obsessions:
  - Patients are aware that they are thinking the obsessive thoughts; thoughts are not imposed from outside (as in thought insertion).
  - Thoughts are not just excessive worrying about real-life problems.
  - Recurrent thoughts are persistent, intrusive, and inappropriate, causing significant anxiety and distress.
  - Attempts to suppress intrusive thoughts are made with some other thought/activity.
- 2 criteria support a diagnosis of compulsions:
  - The response to an obsession is to perform repetitive behaviors (e.g., hand washing) or mental acts (e.g., counting silently) rigidly.
  - Although done to reduce stress, the responses are either not realistically connected with the obsession or they are excessive.
  - In children, check for precedent streptococcal infection.

PHYSICAL EXAM
- Dermatologic problems caused by excessive hand washing may be observed.
- Hair loss caused by compulsive pulling/twisting of the hair (trichotillomania) may be observed.

DIFFERENTIAL DIAGNOSIS
- Obsessive-compulsive personality disorder:
  - In personality disorder, traits are ego-syntonic and include perfectionism and preoccupation with detail, trivia, or procedure and regulation. Patients tend to be rigid, moralistic, and stingy. These traits are often rewarded in the patient's job as desirable.
- Impulse-control disorders: Compulsive gambling, sex, or substance abuse: The compulsive behavior is not in response to obsessive thoughts, and the patient derives pleasure from the activity.
- Major depressive disorder
- Eating disorder
- Tics (in tic disorder) and stereotyped movements
- Schizophrenia: Patient perceives thought to be true and coming from an external source
- Generalized anxiety disorder, phobic disorders, separation anxiety: Similar response on heightened anxiety, but presence of obsessions and rituals signifies OCD diagnosis.
- Anxiety disorder due to a general medical condition: Obsessions/Compulsions are assessed to be a direct physiologic consequence of a general medical condition.

DIAGNOSTIC TESTS & INTERPRETATION
According to *DSM5*, diagnostic criteria for OCD are:
- Presence of obsessions, compulsions, or both
  - Recurrent or persistent thoughts, urges, or images that are experienced at sometime during the disturbance, as intrusive and unwanted, and that in most individuals cause marked anxiety or distress

- The individual attempts to ignore or suppress such thoughts, urges, or images or to neutralize them with some other thought or actions (i.e., by performing compulsion)

Compulsions are defined by:
- Repetitive behavior (e.g., hand washing, ordering, checking) or mental acts (e.g., praying, counting, repeating words silently) that the individual feels driven to perform in response to an obsession or according to rules that must be applied rigidly.
- The behavior or mental acts are aimed at preventing or reducing anxiety or distress or preventing some dreaded event or situation. However, these behavior or mental acts are not connected in a realistic way with what they are designed to neutralize or prevent or are clearly excessive.
- The obsessions or compulsions are time-consuming (e.g., take more than 1 hour per day) or cause clinically significant distress or impairment in social, occupational, or other important areas of functioning.
- The obsessive-compulsive symptoms are not attributable to the physiological effects of a substance (e.g., a drug of abuse, a medication or other medical condition.
- The disturbance is not better explained by the symptoms of another mental disorder (e.g., excessive worries, as in generalized anxiety disorder, preoccupation with appearance, as in body dysmorphic disorder etc.)
- Specify if:
  - With good or fair insight: The individual recognizes the OCD beliefs are definitely or probably not true or that they may or may not be true.
  - With poor insight: The individual thinks that OCD beliefs are probably true.
  - With absent insight/delusional beliefs: The individual is completely convinced that OCD beliefs are true.
- Specify if:
  - Tic related: The individual has a current or past history of tic disorder.

Diagnostic Procedures/Other
- Yale-Brown Obsessive-Compulsive Scale (Y-BOCS) or CY-BOCS for children
- Maudsley Obsessive-Compulsive Inventory (MOCI)

Test Interpretation
- Compulsions are designed to relieve the anxiety of obsessions; they are not inherently enjoyable (ego-dynastic) and do not result in completion of a task.
- Common obsessive themes:
  - Harm (i.e., being responsible for an accident)
  - Doubt (i.e., whether doors/windows are locked or the iron is turned off)
  - Blasphemous thoughts (i.e., in a devoutly religious person)
  - Contamination, dirt, or disease
  - Symmetry/Orderliness
- Common rituals or compulsions:
  - Hand washing, cleaning
  - Checking
  - Counting
  - Hoarding
  - Ordering, arranging
  - Repeating

- Neither obsessions nor compulsions are related to another mental disorder (i.e., thoughts of food and presence of eating disorder).
- 80–90% of patients with OCD have obsessions and compulsions.
- 10–19% of patients with OCD are pure obsessional.

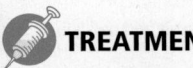

TREATMENT

GENERAL MEASURES
- Combined medications and cognitive–behavioral therapy (CBT) is most effective (1,2)[A].
- Family psychoeducation
- Parent behavior management training if patient is a child/adolescent

MEDICATION
First Line
- Adequate trial at least 10–12 weeks
- Doses may exceed typical doses for depression.

- SSRIs recommended first-line agents (1,2)[A]:
  – Fluoxetine (Prozac):
    ○ Adults: 20 mg/d; increase by 10–20 mg every 4–6 weeks until response; range: 20–80 mg/d
    ○ Children (7–17 years of age): 10 mg/d; increase 4–6 weeks until response; range: 20–60 mg/d
  – Sertraline (Zoloft):
    ○ Adults: 50 mg/d; increase by 50 mg every 4–7 days until response; range: 50–200 mg/d; may divide if above 100 mg/d
    ○ Children (6–17 years of age): 25 mg/d; increase by 25 mg every 7 days until response; range: 50–200 mg/d
  – Paroxetine (Paxil):
    ○ Adults: 20 mg/d; increase by 10 mg every 4–7 days until response; range: 40–60 mg/d
    ○ Children: Safety and effectiveness in patients <18 years have not been established.
  – Fluvoxamine (Luvox):
    ○ Adult: 100 mg/d; increase by 50 mg every 4–7 days until response; range: 200–300 mg/d
    ○ Children (8–17 years of age): 25 mg/d; increase by 25 mg every 4–7 days until response; range: 50–200 mg/d
  – Absolute SSRI contraindications:
    ○ Hypersensitivity to SSRIs
    ○ Within 14 days of monoamine oxidase inhibitor (MAOI)
  – Relative SSRI contraindications:
    ○ Severe liver impairment
    ○ Seizure disorders (lower seizure threshold)
  – Precautions:
    ○ Watch for suicidal behavior/worsening depression during 1st few months of therapy/after dosage changes with antidepressants, particularly in children, adolescents, and young adults.
    ○ Long half-life of fluoxetine (>7 days) may be troublesome if patient has an adverse reaction.
    ○ May cause drowsiness and dizziness when therapy initiated; warn patients about driving and heavy-equipment hazards.

Pregnancy Considerations
All SSRIs are pregnancy Category C, except paroxetine, which is Category D.

Second Line
- Try switching to another SSRI.
- Tricyclic acid (TCA), clomipramine (Anafranil):
  – Adults: 25 mg/d; increase gradually over 2 weeks to 100 mg/d, then to 250 mg/d (max dose) over next several weeks, as tolerated.
  – Children (10–17 years of age): 25 mg/d; titrate as needed and tolerated up to 3 mg/kg or 200 mg/d (whichever is less).
  – Absolute clomipramine contraindications:
    ○ Within 6 months of a myocardial infarction (MI)
    ○ Hypersensitivity to clomipramine or other TCA
    ○ Within 14 days of an MAOI
    ○ 3rd-degree atrioventricular (AV) block
  – Relative clomipramine contraindications:
    ○ Narrow-angle glaucoma (increased intraocular pressure)
    ○ Prostatic hypertrophy (urinary retention)
    ○ 1st- or 2nd-degree AV block, bundle-branch block, and congestive heart failure (proarrhythmic effect)
    ○ Pregnancy Category C
  – Precautions:
    ○ Dangerous in overdose
    ○ Pretreatment ECG for patients >40 years of age
    ○ Watch for suicidal behavior/worsening depression during 1st few months of therapy or after dosage changes with antidepressants, particularly in children, adolescents, and young adults.
    ○ May cause drowsiness and dizziness when therapy is initiated; warn patients about driving and heavy-equipment hazards.

ISSUES FOR REFERRAL
- Psychiatric referral for CBT (in vivo exposure and prevention of compulsions)
- Psychiatric evaluation if obsessions and compulsions significantly interfere with patient's functioning in social, occupational, or educational situations

ADDITIONAL THERAPIES
Dopamine receptor antagonists (antipsychotic agents) alone are not effective in treatment of OCD. They can be used as augmentation to SSRI therapy for treatment-resistant OCD; they also can worsen OCD symptoms (2). Some evidence that addition of quetiapine or risperidone to antidepressants will increase efficacy; data with olanzapine too limited to draw conclusions (3):
- Pimozide (Orap): Initial dose: 0.5 mg/d; target dose: 1–6 mg/d
- Haloperidol (Haldol): Initial dose: 0.5 mg/d; target dose: 0.5–6 mg/d
- Risperidone (Risperdal): Initial dose: 0.5 mg/d; target dose: 0.5–2 mg/d
- Olanzapine (Zyprexa): Initial dose: 1.25 mg/d; target dose: 1.25–30 mg/d
- Quetiapine (Seroquel): Initial dose: 25 mg/d; target dose: 600 mg/d

ONGOING CARE

FOLLOW-UP RECOMMENDATIONS
Y-BCOS or MOCI surveys to track progress

Patient Monitoring
Monitor for decrease in obsessions and time spent performing compulsions.

DIET
No dietary modifications/restrictions recommended

PATIENT EDUCATION
- Importance of medication adherence
- Importance of psychotherapy (CBT)
- International OCD Foundation, Boston, MA 617-973-5801; www.ocfoundation.org
- Obsessive Compulsive Anonymous, New Hyde Park, NY http://obsessivecompulsiveanonymous.org

PROGNOSIS
- Chronic waxing and waning course in most patients:
  – 24–33% fluctuating course
  – 11–14% phasic periods of remission
  – 54–61% chronic progressive course
- Early onset a poor predictor

COMPLICATIONS
- Depression in 1/3 patients with OCD
- Avoidant behavior (phobic avoidance):
  – Children may drop out of education.
  – Adults may become homebound.
- Anxiety and panic-like episodes associated with obsessions

REFERENCES
1. Gava I. Psychological treatments versus treatment as usual for obsessive compulsive disorder (OCD). Cochrane Database Sys Rev. 2007;2:CD005333.
2. Stein DJ. Obsessive-compulsive disorder: Diagnostic and treatment issues. Psychiatr Clin North Am. 2009;32:665–685.
3. Komossa K, Depping AM, Meyer M, et al. Second-generation antipsychotics for obsessive compulsive disorder. Cochrane Database Sys Rev. 2010;12:CD008141.

ADDITIONAL READING
- Koran LM. Practice guideline for the treatment of patients with obsessive-compulsive disorder. Am J Psychiatry. 2007;164:5–53.
- Kurlan R, Kaplan EL. The pediatric autoimmune neuropsychiatric disorders associated with streptococcal infection (PANDAS) etiology for tics and obsessive-compulsive symptoms: Hypothesis or entity? Practical considerations for the clinician. Pediatrics. 2004;113:883–886.
- McGuire JF, Lewin AB, Horng B, et al. The nature, assessment, and treatment of obsessive-compulsive disorder. Postgrad Med. 2012;124:152–165.
- Nestadt G. Genetics of obsessive compulsive disorder. Psychiatr Clin North Am. 2010;33:141–158.

 CODES

ICD10
- F42 Obsessive-compulsive disorder
- F63.9 Impulse disorder, unspecified
- F63.89 Other impulse disorders

CLINICAL PEARLS
- CBT is the initial treatment of choice for mild OCD.
- CBT plus an SSRI or an SSRI alone is the treatment choice for more severe OCD.
- >65–70% of patients with OCD respond to 1st SSRI treatment.
- Improvement in symptoms is often incomplete, ranging from 25–60%.

OCULAR CHEMICAL BURNS
Robert J. Hyde, MD, MA • Ariel M. Hubert, GSM

BASICS

DESCRIPTION
- Chemical exposure to the eye can result in rapid, devastating, and permanent damage, and is one of the true emergencies in ophthalmology.
- Separate alkaline from acid chemical exposure:
  - Alkali burns: More severe. Alkaline compounds are lipophilic, penetrating rapidly into eye tissue; saponification of cells leads to necrosis and may produce injury to lids, conjunctiva, cornea, sclera, iris, and lens (cataracts).
  - Acid burns: Acid usually does not damage internal structures because its associated anion causes protein denaturation, creating a barrier to further acid penetration. (Hydrofluoric acid is an exception to this rule; see below.) Injury is often limited to lids, conjunctiva, and cornea.
- System(s) affected: Nervous; Skin/Exocrine
- Synonym(s): Chemical ocular injuries

EPIDEMIOLOGY
- Predominant age: Can occur at any age, peak from 16–25 years of age
- Predominant sex: Male > Female

Incidence
- Estimated 300/100,000 per year
- Alkali burns twice as common as acid burns

ETIOLOGY AND PATHOPHYSIOLOGY
- Acidic compounds:
  - Anion leads to protein denaturing and protective barrier formation by coagulation necrosis forming an eschar. This more superficial mechanism of injury tends to have prominent scarring that may lead to vision loss:
    - Hydrofluoric acid is an exception. In its nonionized form, it behaves like an alkaline substance, capable of penetrating the corneal stroma and leading to extensive anterior segment lesions. When ionized, it may combine with intracellular calcium and magnesium to form insoluble complexes, leading to potassium ion movements and cell death. Once systemically absorbed, severe hypocalcemia can occur.
- Alkaline compounds:
  - Lipophilic compounds that penetrate into deep structures on disassociation into cations and OH−
  - OH− causes saponification of fatty acids in cell membranes, leading to cell death.
  - Cation causes hydration of glycosaminoglycans, leading to corneal opacification and hydration of collagen, resulting in rapid shortening and thickening of collagen fibrils that leads to elevated intraocular pressure secondary to distortion of trabecular meshwork.
  - Penetration into deep structures may also affect perfusing vessels, leading to ischemia of affected area.

Sources of alkaline and acidic compounds

Alkaline compounds	Typical sources
Calcium hydroxide (Lime)	Cement, whitewash
Sodium hydroxide (Lye)	Drain cleaner, airbags
Potassium hydroxide (Lye)	Drain cleaner
Ammonia	Cleaning agents
Ammonium hydroxide	Fertilizers
Acidic compounds	**Typical sources**
Sulfuric acid	Car batteries
Sulfurous acid	Bleach
Hydrochloric acid	Chem labs, swimming pools
Acetic acid	Vinegar
Hydrofluoric acid	Glass polish

RISK FACTORS
- Construction work (plaster, cement, whitewash)
- Use of cleaning agents (drain cleaners, ammonia)
- Automobile battery explosions (sulfuric acid)
- Industrial work (many possible agents)
- Alcoholism
- Any risk factor for assault (~10% of injuries due to deliberate assault)

GENERAL PREVENTION
Safety glasses to safeguard eyes

COMMONLY ASSOCIATED CONDITIONS
Facial (including eyelids) cutaneous chemical or thermal burns

DIAGNOSIS

HISTORY
- Most often complaints of pain, photophobia, blurred vision and a foreign body sensation
- In alkali burns, can have initial pain that later diminishes
- Mild burns: Pain and blurred vision
- Moderate-to-severe burns: Severe pain and markedly reduced vision

PHYSICAL EXAM
- Acidic compound may present with a ground-glass appearance secondary to superficial scar formation.
- Alkaline compounds may present with corneal opacification secondary to glycosaminoglycan hydration; however, severe acid burns may also present with this finding.
- Mild burns:
  - Blurry vision
  - Eyelid skin erythema and edema
  - Corneal epithelial defects or superficial punctate keratitis
  - Conjunctival chemosis, hyperemia, and hemorrhages without perilimbal ischemia
  - Mild anterior chamber reaction

- Moderate-to-severe burns:
  - Reduced vision
  - 2nd- and 3rd-degree burns of eyelid skin
  - Corneal edema and opacification
  - Corneal epithelial defects
  - Marked conjunctival chemosis and perilimbal blanching
  - Moderate anterior chamber reaction
  - Increased intraocular pressure
  - Local necrotic retinopathy

DIFFERENTIAL DIAGNOSIS
- Thermal burns
- Ocular cicatricial pemphigoid
- Other causes of corneal opacification
- Ultraviolet radiation keratitis

DIAGNOSTIC TESTS & INTERPRETATION
Not necessary unless suspicion of intraocular or orbital foreign body is present. In this case, CT should be used and MRI is contraindicated.

Diagnostic Procedures/Other
- Measure pH of tear film with litmus paper or electronic probe:
  - Irrigating fluid with nonneutral pH (e.g., normal saline has pH of 4.5) may alter results.
- Careful slit-lamp exam, fundus ophthalmoscopy, tonometry, and measurement of visual acuity
- Full extent of damage from alkali burns may not be apparent until 48–72 hours after exposure.

Test Interpretation
- Corneal epithelial defects or superficial punctate keratitis, edema, opacification
- Conjunctival chemosis, hyperemia, and hemorrhages
- Perilimbal ischemia
- Anterior chamber reaction
- Increased intraocular pressure

TREATMENT

Copious irrigation and removal of corneal or conjunctival foreign bodies are always the initial treatment (1,2,3)[A]:

- Passively open patient's eyelid and have patient look in all directions while irrigating.
- Be sure to remove all reservoirs of chemical from the eyes.
- Continue irrigation until the tear film and superior/inferior cul-de-sac is of neutral pH (7+/−0.1) and pH is stable (2)[C]:
  - Severe burns should be irrigated for at least 15 minutes to as much as 2–4 hours; this irrigation should not be interrupted during transportation to hospital (2)[C].
  - Irrigation via Morgan lens (polymethylmethacrylate scleral lens) is a good way to achieve continuous irrigation over a prolonged period of time.
  - It is impossible to overirrigate.
- Initial pH testing should be done on both eyes even if the patient claims to only have unilateral ocular pain/irritation so that a contralateral injury is not neglected.

- Use whatever nontoxic fluid is available for irrigation on scene. In hospital, sterile water, normal saline, normal saline with bicarbonate, balanced salt solution (BSS), or lactated Ringer's solution may be used:
  – No therapeutic difference in effectiveness has been noted between types of solutions (1)[C].
- A topical anesthetic can be used to provide patient comfort (e.g., proparacaine, tetracaine).
- Sweep the conjunctival fornices every 12–24 hours to prevent adhesions (2)[C].
- Eye patching may relieve pain but has not been shown to improve outcomes (4)[C].

MEDICATION

First Line

- Further treatment (depending on severity and associated conditions):
  – Topical prophylactic antibiotics: Any broad-spectrum agent (e.g., bacitracin–polymyxin B [Polysporin] ointment q2–4h, ciprofloxacin [Ciloxan] drops q2–4h, chloramphenicol [Chloroptic] ointment q2–4h) (1)[C]:
    ○ Some experts suggest that systemic tetracycline 250 mg PO q6h and especially derivatives such as doxycycline 100 mg PO b.i.d. may be beneficial to encourage healing of persistent corneal epithelial defects by inhibiting metalloproteinases (5)[C].
  – Tear substitutes: Hydroxypropyl methylcellulose (HypoTears PF, Refresh Plus) drops q4h, carboxymethylcellulose (Refresh PM) ointment at bedtime (1)[C]:
    ○ Most beneficial in those with impaired tear production (elderly patients)
  – Cycloplegics for photophobia and/or uveitis: Cyclopentolate 1% t.i.d., or scopolamine 1/4% b.i.d. (1)[C]
  – Antiglaucoma for elevated intraocular pressure (IOP): Latanoprost (Xalatan) 0.005% q24h, or timolol (Timoptic) 0.5% b.i.d., or levobunolol (Betagan) 0.5% b.i.d., and/or acetazolamide (Diamox) 125–250 mg PO q6h, or methazolamide (Neptazane) 25–50 mg PO b.i.d., and/or IV mannitol 20% 1–2 g/kg as needed (1)[C]
  – Corticosteroids for intraocular inflammation: Prednisolone (Pred-Forte) 1% or equivalent q1–4h for 7–10 days; if severe, prednisone 20–60 mg PO daily for 5–7 days. Taper rapidly if epithelium is intact by this time (1)[C]:
    ○ Use of corticosteroids > 10 days may do harm by inhibiting repair and cause corneoscleral melt (1,6)[C].
  – Consider vitamin C (ascorbic acid) 500 mg PO q.i.d. and/or acetylcysteine (Mucomyst) 10–20% topically q4h if corneal melting occurs (1)[C].
- Precautions:
  – Timolol and levobunolol: History of congestive heart failure (CHF) or chronic obstructive pulmonary disease (COPD)
  – Acetazolamide and methazolamide: History of nephrolithiasis or metabolic acidosis
  – Mannitol: History of CHF or renal failure
  – Scopolamine: History of urinary retention
  – Topical corticosteroids must be used with caution in the presence of damaged corneal epithelium because iatrogenic infection can occur. Daily follow-up or consultation with an ophthalmologist is recommended.

SURGERY/OTHER PROCEDURES

- Goal of subacute treatment is restoration of the normal ocular surface anatomy, control of glaucoma, and restoration of corneal clarity.
- Surgical options include:
  – Débridement of necrotic tissue (1)[C]
  – Conjunctival/Tenon advancement (tenoplasty) to restore vascularity in severe burns (1)[C]
  – Tissue adhesive (e.g., isobutyl cyanoacrylate) for impending or actual corneal perforation of <1 mm (1)[C]:
    ○ Tectonic keratoplasty for acute perforation >1 mm (1)[C]
  – Limbal autograft transplantation for epithelial stem cell restoration (1)[C]
  – Amniotic membrane transplantation to promote epithelial regeneration (6)[C]
  – Conjunctival or mucosal membrane transplant to restore ocular surface in severe injury (1)[C]
  – Lamellar or penetrating keratoplasty for tectonic stabilization or visual rehabilitation (1)[C]

IN-PATIENT CONSIDERATIONS

Admission Criteria/Initial Stabilization

Based on ophthalmologic consultation and concomitant burn injuries

 ONGOING CARE

FOLLOW-UP RECOMMENDATIONS

Patient Monitoring

- Depending on severity of ocular injury:
  – From daily to weekly visits initially
- May be inpatient
- If on mannitol or prednisone, consider frequent serum electrolytes.

PATIENT EDUCATION

- Safety glasses
- Need for immediate ocular irrigation with any available water following chemical exposure to the eyes

PROGNOSIS

- Depends on severity of initial injury: increased Limbal involvement in clock hours and greater percentage of conjunctival involvement correlate with poorer prognosis (Dua classification system).
- For mildly injured eyes, complete recovery is the norm.
- For severely injured eyes, permanent loss of vision is not uncommon.

COMPLICATIONS

- Orbital compartment syndrome
- Persistent epitheliopathy
- Fibrovascular pannus
- Corneal ulcer/perforation
- Corneal scarring
- Progressive symblepharon and entropion
- Neurotrophic keratitis
- Lid malposition secondary to cicatricial changes
- Glaucoma
- Cataract
- Hypotony
- Phthisis bulbi
- Blindness

REFERENCES

1. Wagoner MD. Chemical injuries of the eye: Current concepts in pathophysiology and therapy. *Survey Ophthalmol.* 1997;41:275–313.
2. Kuckelkorn R, Schrage N, Keller G, et al. Emergency treatment of chemical and thermal eye burns. *Acta Ophthalmol Scand.* 2002;80:4–10.
3. Chau JP, Lee DT, Lo SH. A systematic review of methods of eye irrigation for adults and children with ocular chemical burns. *Worldviews Evid Based Nurs.* 2012;9(3):129–138. Epub 2011 Jun 7.
4. Spector J, Fernandez WG. Chemical, thermal, and biological ocular exposures. *Emerg Med Clin North Am.* 2008;26:125–136, vii.
5. Ralph RA. Tetracyclines and the treatment of corneal stromal ulceration: A review. *Cornea.* 2000;19:274–277.
6. Fish R, Davidson RS. Management of ocular thermal and chemical injuries, including amniotic membrane therapy. *Curr Opin Ophthalmol.* 2010;21:317–321.

ADDITIONAL READING

- Gicquel JJ. Management of ocular surface chemical burns. *Br J Ophthalmol.* 2011;95(2):159–161.
- Lin A, Patel N, Yoo D, et al. Management of ocular conditions in the burn unit: Thermal and chemical burns and Stevens-Johnson syndrome/toxic epidermal necrolysis. *J Burn Care Res.* 2011;32:547–560.
- Roblin I, Urban M, Flicoteau D, et al. Topical treatment of experimental hydrofluoric acid skin burns by 2.5% calcium gluconate. *J Burn Care Res.* 2006;27:889.

 SEE ALSO

Burns

 CODES

ICD10

- T26.50XA Corrosion of unsp eyelid and periocular area, init encntr
- T26.60XA Corrosion of cornea and conjunctival sac, unsp eye, init
- S05.00XA Inj conjunctiva and corneal abrasion w/o fb, unsp eye, init

CLINICAL PEARLS

- Prompt irrigation of all chemical burns, even prior to arrival to the emergency department, is essential to ensure best outcomes. It is impossible to overirrigate.
- All patients with chemical injuries to their eyes should have urgent ophthalmology consultation and/or referral.

O

ONYCHOMYCOSIS

Tabasum Nazir, MD • Nora Gimpel, MD

 BASICS

DESCRIPTION
- Chronic fungal infection of fingernails/toenails
- Caused mostly by dermatophytes, but also yeasts, molds
- Toenails more commonly affected than fingernails
- System(s) affected: Skin; Exocrine
- Synonym(s): Tinea unguium; Ringworm of the nail

EPIDEMIOLOGY
Prevalence
- Occurs in 2–8% in general population
- Predominant age: 14–28% in adults >60 years of age
- Rare before puberty

ETIOLOGY AND PATHOPHYSIOLOGY
- Dermatophytes: *Trichophyton* (*T. rubrum* most common), *Epidermophyton*, *Microsporum*
- Yeasts: *Candida albicans* (most common), *C. parapsilosis, C. tropicalis, C. krusei*
- Molds: *Scopulariopsis brevicaulis, Hendersonula toruloidea, Aspergillus* sp., *Alternaria tenuis, Cephalosporium, Scytalidium hyalinum*
- Dermatophytes cause 90% of toenail and most of fingernail onychomycoses.
- Fingernail onychomycosis is more often caused by yeasts than is the case for toenail onychomycosis.
- Dermatophytes can invade normal keratin, whereas molds invade altered keratin (dystrophic/injured nails).

RISK FACTORS
- Older age
- Tinea pedis
- Cancer
- Diabetes
- Peripheral vascular disease
- Psoriasis
- Cohabitation with others with onychomycosis
- Immunodeficiency
- Swimming
- Smoking
- Peripheral vascular disease
- Children with Down syndrome

COMMONLY ASSOCIATED CONDITIONS
- Immunodeficiency/chronic metabolic disease
- Tinea pedis/manuum

 DIAGNOSIS

PHYSICAL EXAM
- Dermatophytes: Commonly preceded by dermatophyte infection at another site; 80% involve toenails, especially hallux; simultaneous infection of fingernails and toenails is rare. 5 clinical forms occur:
  - Distal/Lateral subungual onychomycosis (most common): Spreads from distal/lateral margins to nail bed to nail plate; subungual hyperkeratosis; onycholysis; nail dystrophy; discoloration— yellow–brown; yellow streaking laterally; bois vermoulu ("worm-eaten wood"); onychomadesis
  - Proximal subungual onychomycosis (rare): Hands/feet; leukonychia—begins at proximal part of nail plate, appearing to occur from the proximal underside of the nail (or direct invasion of the nail

plate from above); spreads to nail plate and lunula; seen with immunodeficiency
  - Superficial white onychomycosis (rare): Hallux preferentially affected; infection of outer surface of nail plate; opaque white spots on nail plate eventually merge to involve entire surface of the nail
  - Endonyx onychomycosis involves interior of nail plate sparing nail bed. Subungual hyperkeratosis is absent (1).
  - Totally dystrophic onychomycosis causes complete destruction of nail plate by fungus resulting in thickened and ridged nail bed covered with keratotic debris (1).
- Candidal:
  - Hands, 70%, especially for the dominant hand
  - Middle finger most common
  - Pain mild, unless secondarily infected
  - Increases on prolonged contact with water
  - Primarily affects tissue surrounding nail
  - Begins with cuticle detachment
  - White or whitish-yellow nail discoloration
  - Secondary ungual changes: Convex, irregular, striated nail plate with dull, rough surface
  - Onycholysis, especially on hands
  - Distal subungual onychomycosis may occur
  - Primary involvement of the nail plate is uncommon (thin, crumbly, opaque, brownish nail plate deformed by transverse grooves)
  - Periungual edema/erythema may occur (club-shaped, bulbous fingertips).
- Molds:
  - More common in those >60 years of age
  - More common in nails of hallux
  - Resembles distal and lateral onychomycosis

Pediatric Considerations
Candidal infection presents more commonly as superficial white onychomycosis

DIFFERENTIAL DIAGNOSIS
- Psoriasis (most common alternate diagnosis)
- Traumatic dystrophy
- Lichen planus
- Onychogryphosis ("ram's horn nails")
- Eczematous conditions
- Hypothyroidism
- Drugs and chemicals
- Yellow nail syndrome
- Neoplasms (0.7–3.5%) of all melanoma cases are subungual.
- Only 50% of dystrophic nails are due to onychomycosis.

DIAGNOSTIC TESTS & INTERPRETATION
- Accurate diagnosis requires both laboratory and clinical evidence.
- If onychomycosis is suspected clinically and initial diagnostic laboratory tests are negative, the tests should be repeated.

Initial Tests (lab, imaging)
- Direct microscopy with potassium hydroxide (KOH) preparation:
  - Clip away diseased, discolored nail plate.
  - Collect debris from stratum corneum of most proximal area (beneath nail or crumbling nail itself) with 1-mm curette/scalpel
  - Larger sample improves sensitivity
  - KOH (5%) + gentle heat
  - High sensitivity if >2 preparations examined

- Cultures: False-negative finding in 30% (secondary to loss of dermatophyte viability; improved by immediate culture on Sabouraud cell culture medium)
- Histologic examination of nail clippings/nail plate punch biopsy: Proximal lesions; stain both with periodic acid–Schiff (PAS) stain
- KOH treated nail clipping stained with PAS: Significantly higher rates of detection of onychomycosis as compared with standard methods of KOH preparation and fungal culture (2)
- Polymerase chain reaction (PCR) increases sensitivity of detection of dermatophytes in nail specimen, can be used as complementary to direct microscope exam and fungal culture (3)
- Fluorescence microscopy can be used as a rapid screening tool for identification of fungi in nail specimens (3)
- Discontinue all topical medication for at least 1 week before obtaining a sample.

Test Interpretation
Pathogens within the nail keratin

TREATMENT

GENERAL MEASURES
- Avoid factors that promote fungal growth (i.e., heat, moisture, and occlusion)
- Treat underlying disease risk factors
- Treat secondary infections

MEDICATION
Pregnancy Considerations
Oral antifungals and ciclopirox are pregnancy Category B (terbinafine, ciclopirox) or C (itraconazole, fluconazole, and griseofulvin). Because treatment of onychomycosis usually can be postponed until after pregnancy, treatment should be avoided during pregnancy.

First Line
- Oral antifungals are preferred due to higher rates of cure, but they have systemic adverse effects and drug–drug interactions.
- Terbinafine: 250 mg/d PO × 6 weeks for fingernails and 3 months for toenails, most effective in cure and prevention of relapse (4)[A], most cost-effective with higher patient satisfaction compared with other antifungals and with itraconazole pulse, although evidence quality is not excellent. It has similar tolerance to terbinafine pulse (500 mg/d × 1 week/month for 3 months), and fewer drug–drug interactions, but efficacy of pulse dosed terbinafine is 13% less than continued dose (3).
- Itraconazole pulse: 400 mg/d PO or 200 mg PO b.i.d. × 1 week, then 3 weeks off, repeat for 2 cycles for fingernails and 3–4 cycles for toenails (lower cost and lower pill burden than itraconazole continuous, more effective than terbinafine for *Candida* and molds, do not need to monitor liver function tests (LFTs).
- Itraconazole continuous: 200 mg/d PO × 6 weeks for fingernails and 3 months for toenails (may be more effective than itraconazole pulse, more effective than terbinafine for *Candida* and molds)

Second Line
- Fluconazole pulse: 150–300 mg PO weekly × 6 months (less frequent dosing, but lower cure rate)
- Griseofulvin: 500–1,000 mg/d PO for up to 18 months (lower cure rate, needs to be continued until the diseased nail is completely replaced)
- Posaconazole: 100, 200, or 400 mg once daily for 24 weeks; 400 mg once daily for 12 weeks is comparable to terbinafine (250 mg/d for 12 weeks). However, due to its higher cost limits, its use is second-line treatment (5)[B].
- Ciclopirox: 8% nail lacquer: Apply once daily to affected nails (if without lunula involvement) for up to 48 weeks, and every 7 days; remove lacquer with alcohol, then file away loose nail material and trim nails (low cure rate, avoids systemic adverse effects, less cost-effective). Application after PO treatment may reduce recurrences (3).
- Amorolfine: 8% nail lacquer. Once a week until cure is achieved. Not available in US (3)[A].
- Contraindications for oral antifungals:
  – Hepatic disease
  – Pregnancy (see "Pregnancy Considerations")
  – Current or history of congestive heart failure (CHF) (itraconazole)
  – Porphyria (griseofulvin)
- Other treatments:
  – Vicks VapoRub application to nails daily for 48 weeks has been found safe and cost effective alternative for toenail onychomycosis (6)[C].
  – Not available in US: Albaconazole: 100 to 400 mg once a week for 24 or 36 weeks and Efinaconazole topical 10% solution
- Precautions/Adverse effects:
  – Oral antifungals:
    ○ Hepatotoxicity
    ○ Neutropenia
    ○ Hypersensitivity
    ○ Photosensitivity, lupus-like symptoms, proteinuria (griseofulvin)
    ○ Chronic kidney disease (avoid terbinafine for patients with creatine clearance (CrCl) <50 mL/min, decrease fluconazole dose)
    ○ CHF, peripheral edema, pulmonary edema (itraconazole)
  – Ciclopirox: Rash, nail disorders; avoid contact with skin other than skin immediately surrounding nail; use with caution on broken skin or in vascular compromise.
- Significant drug–drug interactions:
  – Terbinafine (inhibits CYP2D6): β-blockers, cimetidine, cyclosporine, dextromethorphan, monoamine oxidase inhibitors (MAOIs), rifampin, SSRIs, tricyclic antidepressants (TCAs), warfarin
  – Itraconazole, fluconazole (inhibit CYP3A4): Antiarrhythmics, benzodiazepines, cisapride, ergot alkaloids, HMG CoA reductase inhibitors, alfentanil, buspirone, calcium channel blockers, carbamazepine, cimetidine, corticosteroids, cyclosporine, haloperidol, hydrochlorothiazide, hypoglycemics, losartan, oral contraceptives, phenytoin, pimozide, protease inhibitors, rifamycins, sirolimus, tacrolimus, tricyclic antidepressants, theophylline, tolterodine, vinca alkaloids, warfarin, zidovudine, zolpidem
  – Griseofulvin: Barbiturates, cyclosporine, oral contraceptives, salicylates, warfarin

SURGERY/OTHER PROCEDURES
- Nail debridement to remove infected keratin (efficacy not well studied): May be best suited for those with few nails involved or those who are not candidates for systemic therapy:
  – Mechanical: Soften with occlusive dressing with 40% urea gel; detach from nail bed with tweezers, file with abrasive stone or curette.
  – Chemical: Protect peripheral tissue with adhesive strips; apply ointment of 30% salicylic acid, 40% urea, or 50% potassium iodide under occlusive dressing
  – Debridement may be combined with topical antifungal therapy.
  – Surgical avulsion: For involvement of a few nails; used by some for pain control
- Laser treatment has shown positive results to treat onychonycosis. Patients are treated 2–3 × with minimum 3-week interval between sessions (3).
- Phototherapy is appropriate for superficial nail infections and lacks side effects concerning kidney, liver functions, lacks risk to patient with systemic diseases and has absence of drug interactions (3).

COMPLEMENTARY AND ALTERNATIVE MEDICINE
Melaleuca alternifolia (tea tree oil) has a 10% mycologic cure.

 ## ONGOING CARE
FOLLOW-UP RECOMMENDATIONS
- Formation of a new fingernail takes 4–6 months and a new toenail takes 12–18 months.
- Cure defined as :
  – 100% absence of clinical signs and/or
  – Negative mycology with ≥1 of the following clinical signs:
    ○ Distal subungual hyperkeratosis/onycholysis leaving <10% of the nail plate affected
    ○ Nail plate thickening that does not improve with treatment because of comorbid condition

Patient Monitoring
- Topical agents: Slow response expected; visits every 6–12 weeks
- Terbinafine, griseofulvin: Baseline and, as needed, LFTs and CBC
- Itraconazole continuous: Baseline and, as needed, LFTs.

PATIENT EDUCATION
- Advise patient to:
  – Keep affected area clean and dry
  – Avoid rubber/other occlusive footwear
  – Avoid tight/ill-fitting footwear
  – Wear absorbent cotton socks; avoid synthetic fibers
  – Change clothing and towels frequently, and launder them in hot water
  – Avoid sharing nail implements. Avoid use of same nail implements on normal and abnormal nails.
- Cure of all toenails may not be attainable.
- Nails may not appear normal after cure.

PROGNOSIS
- Complete clinical cure in 25–50% (higher mycologic cure rates)
- Recurrence is 10–50% (relapse/reinfection)
- Poor prognostic factors:
  – Areas of nail involvement >50%
  – Significant proximal/lateral disease
  – Subungual hyperkeratosis >2 mm
  – White/Yellow or orange/brown streaks in the nail (includes dermatophytoma)
  – Total dystrophic onychomycosis (with matrix involvement)
  – Nonresponsive organisms (e.g., *Scytalidium* mold)
  – Patients with immunosuppression
  – Diminished peripheral circulation

COMPLICATIONS
- Secondary infections with progression to soft tissue infection/osteomyelitis
- Toenail discomfort/pain that can limit physical mobility or activity
- Anxiety, negative self-image

REFERENCES
1. Hay RJ, Baran R. Onychomycosis: A proposed revision of the clinical classification. *J Am Acad Dermatol.* 2011;65:1219.
2. Haghani I, Shokohi T, Hajheidari Z, et al. Comparison of diagnostic methods in the evaluation of onychomycosis. *Mycopathologia.* 2013;175:315–321.
3. Tchernev G, Kolev Penev P, Nenoff P, et al. Onychomycosis: Modern diagnostic and treatment approaches. *Wien Med Wochenschr.* 2013;163:1–12.
4. Crawford F, Young P, Godfrey C, et al. Oral treatments for toenail onychomycosis: A systematic review. *Arch Dermatol.* 2002;138:811–816.
5. Elewski B, Pollak R, Ashton S, et al. A randomized, placebo- and active-controlled, parallel-group, multicentre, investigator-blinded study of four treatment regimens of posaconazole in adults with toenail onychomycosis. *Br J Dermatol.* 2012;166:389–398.
6. Derby R, Rohal P, Jackson C, et al. Novel treatment of onychomycosis using over-the-counter mentholated ointment: A clinical case series. *J Am Board Fam Med.* 2011;24:69–74.

ADDITIONAL READING
Gupta A, Simpson F. Device-based therapies for onychomycosis treatment. *Skin The Lett.* 2012;17:4–9.

 ## CODES
ICD10
- B35.1 Tinea unguium
- B37.2 Candidiasis of skin and nail

CLINICAL PEARLS
- Psoriasis and chronic nail trauma are commonly mistaken for fungal infection.
- Diagnosis should be based on both clinical and mycologic laboratory evidence.
- Oral antifungals generally are well tolerated and more effective than topical antifungals, with terbinafine being the most effective. Take care in those on multiple medications as drug–drug interactions are common with antifungals.
- LFT monitoring is necessary for most oral antifungal regimens.
- Patient should understand that treatment is long term, recurrence is common, and nails may not appear normal even after treatment.

OPTIC NEURITIS

Olga M. Ceron, MD • Pablo I. Hernandez-Itriago, MD

 BASICS

DESCRIPTION
- Inflammation of the optic nerve (cranial nerve II)
- Most common form is acute demyelinating optic neuritis (ON), but other causes include infectious disease and systemic autoimmune disorders.
- Optic disc may be normal in appearance at onset (retrobulbar ON, 67%) or swollen (papillitis, 33%).
- Key features:
  - Abrupt visual loss (typically monocular)
  - Periorbital pain with eye movement (90%)
  - Pain in the distribution of the 1st division of the trigeminal nerve
  - Dyschromatopsia: Color vision deficits
  - Relative afferent pupillary defect (RAPD)
- Usually unilateral in adults; bilateral disease more common in children
- Presenting complaint in 25% of patients with multiple sclerosis (MS)
- In children, headaches are common.
- System(s) affected: Nervous
- Synonym(s): Papillitis; Demyelinating optic neuropathy; Retrobulbar optic neuritis

EPIDEMIOLOGY
Incidence
- 1–5/100,000 cases per year
- More common in northern latitudes
- More common in whites than in other races
- Predominant age:18–45 years; mean age 30
- Predominant sex: Female > Male (3:1)

ETIOLOGY AND PATHOPHYSIOLOGY
- In both MS-associated and isolated monosymptomatic ON, the cause is presumed to be a demyelinating autoimmune reaction.
- Possible mechanisms of inflammation in immune-mediated ON are the cross-reaction of viral epitopes and host epitopes, and the persistence of a virus in CNS glial cells.
- Neuromyelitis optica (NMO) IgG autoantibody, which targets the water channel aquaporin-4
- Primarily idiopathic
- MS
- Viral infections: Measles, mumps, varicella-zoster, coxsackievirus, adenovirus, hepatitis A and B, HIV, herpes simplex virus, cytomegalovirus
- Nonviral infections: Syphilis, tuberculosis, meningococcus, cryptococcosis, cysticercosis, bacterial sinusitis, streptococcus B, *Bartonella*, typhoid fever, Lyme disease, fungus
- Systemic inflammatory disease: Sarcoidosis, systemic lupus erythematosus, vasculitis
- Local inflammatory disease: Intraocular or contiguous with the orbit, sinus, or meninges
- Toxic: Lead, methanol, arsenic, radiation
- Vascular lesions affecting the optic nerve
- Posterior uveitis (i.e., birdshot retinochoroidopathy, toxoplasmosis, toxocariasis)
- Tumors
- Medications: Ethambutol, chloroquine, isoniazid, chronic high-dose chloramphenicol, tumor necrosis factor α-antagonist, infliximab (Remicade), adalimumab (Humira), etanercept (Enbrel)

COMMONLY ASSOCIATED CONDITIONS
- MS (common): ON is associated with an increased risk of MS.
- Other demyelinating diseases: Guillain-Barré syndrome, Devic neuromyelitis optica, multifocal demyelinating neuropathy, acute disseminated encephalomyelitis

 DIAGNOSIS

HISTORY
- Decreased visual acuity, deteriorating in hours to days, usually reaching lowest level after 1 week
- Usually unilateral but can also be bilateral
- Brow ache, globe tenderness, deep orbital pain exacerbated by eye movement (92%)
- Retro-orbital pain may precede visual loss.
- Desaturation of color vision (dull or faded colors), especially red tones
- Apparent dimness of light intensities
- Impairment of depth perception (80%); worse with moving objects (Pulfrich phenomenon)
- Transient increase in visual symptoms with increased body temperature and exercise (Uthoff phenomenon)
- May present with a recent flulike viral syndrome
- Detailed history and review of systems, looking for a history of demyelinating, infectious, or systemic inflammatory disease

PHYSICAL EXAM
Complete general exam, full neurologic exam, and ophthalmologic exam looking for the following:
- Decreased visual acuity and color perception
- Central, cecocentral, arcuate, or altitudinal visual field deficits
- Papillitis: Swollen disc ± peripapillary flame-shape hemorrhage or often normal disc exam
- Temporal disc pallor seen later at 4–6 weeks (1)[A]
- Relative afferent pupillary defect (Marcus-Gunn pupil): The pupil of the affected eye dilates with a swinging light test unless disease is bilateral.

DIFFERENTIAL DIAGNOSIS
- Demyelinating disease, especially MS
- Infectious/systemic inflammatory disease
- Neuroretinitis: Virus, toxoplasmosis, *Bartonella*
- Toxic or nutritional optic neuropathy
- Acute papilledema (bilateral disc edema)
- Compression:
  - Orbital tumor/abscess compressing the optic nerve
  - Intracranial tumor/abscess compressing the afferent visual pathway
  - Orbital pseudotumor
  - Carotid–ophthalmic artery aneurysm
- Temporal arteritis or other vasculitides
- Trauma or radiation
- Neuromyelitis optica (Devic disease)
- Anterior ischemic optic neuropathy
- Leber hereditary optic neuropathy
- Kjer-type autosomal-dominant optic atrophy
- Severe systemic hypertension
- Diabetic papillopathy

DIAGNOSTIC TESTS & INTERPRETATION
Initial Tests (lab, imaging)
- In typical presentations, ESR is standard, but other labs are unnecessary. Antinuclear antibodies (ANAs), angiotensin-converting enzyme level, fluorescent treponemal antibody absorption (FTA-ABS), and chest radiograph have been shown to have no value in typical cases (1)[A].
- In atypical presentations, including absence of pain, a very swollen optic nerve, >30 days without recovery, or retinal exudates, labs may be indicated to rule out underlying disorders:
  - CBC
  - ANA test
  - Rapid plasma reagin test
  - FTA-ABS test
- MRI of brain and orbits: Thin cuts (2–3 mm) gadolinium-enhanced and fat-suppression images to look for Dawson fingers of MS (periventricular white matter lesions oriented perpendicular to the ventricles) and also to look for enhancement of the optic nerve
- CT scan of chest to rule out sarcoidosis if clinical suspicion is high
- OCT (ocular coherence tomography) of the retinal nerve fiber layer (RNFL); a noninvasive imaging technique of the optic nerve. May serve as a diagnostic tool to quantify thickness of the nerve fiber layer objectively and, thus, monitor structural change (axonal loss) of the optic nerve in the course of the disease.

Follow-Up Tests & Special Considerations
- Visual field test (Humphrey 30–2) to evaluate for visual field loss: Diffuse and central visual loss more predominant in the affected eye at baseline (2)[A].
- Low-contrast visual acuity (as a measure of disease progression)
- A novel blood test called an NMO-IgG checks for antibodies for neuromyelitis optica.

Diagnostic Procedures/Other
- In atypical cases, including bilateral deficits, young age, or suspicion of infectious etiology, lumbar puncture (LP) with neurology consultation is indicated.
- LP for suspected MS is a physician-dependent decision. Some studies indicate that it may not add value to MRI for MS detection (1)[A], but no consensus on the subject exists.

TREATMENT

Most persons with optic neuritis recover spontaneously.

MEDICATION
First Line
- IV methylprednisolone has been shown to speed up the rate of visual recovery, but without significant long-term benefit; consider for patients who require fast recovery (i.e., monocular patients or those whose occupation requires high-level visual acuity). For significant vision loss, parenteral corticosteroids may be considered on an individualized basis: ONTT (Optic Neuritis Treatment Trial):
  - Observation and corticosteroid treatment are both acceptable courses of action (3)[A].
  - High-dose IV methylprednisolone (250 mg q6h × 3 days) followed by oral corticosteroids (1 mg/kg/d PO × 11 days, taper over 1–2 weeks) (3)[A]
- Others use IV Solu-Medrol infusion (1 g in 250 mL D₅ 1/2 normal saline infused over 1 hour daily for 3–5 days):
  - No evidence of long-term benefit (1)[A],(4)[B]
  - May decrease recovery time (3)[A],(4)[B]
  - May decrease risk of MS at 2 but not 5 years (3)[A]
- Give antiulcer medications with steroids.

Second Line
- Disease-modifying agents, such as interferon-β1a (IFN-β1a; Avonex, Rebif) and IFN-β1b (Betaseron), are used to prevent or delay the development of MS in people with ON who have ≥2 brain lesions evident on MRI (5).
  - These medications have been proposed for use in patients with 1 episode of ON (clinically isolated syndrome) at high risk of developing MS (1+ lesion on brain MRI).
- The Controlled High Risk Avonex Multiple Sclerosis (CHAMPS) trial study has shown that IFN-β1a reduces the conversion to clinically definite MS in high-risk patients by ~50%.
- Decisions should be made individually with neurology consultation.

ALERT
Never use oral prednisone alone as the primary treatment because this may increase the risk for recurrent ON (3)[A].

Pediatric Considerations
- No systematic study defining high-dose corticosteroids in children with ON have been conducted.
  - Consensus recommends: 3 to 5 days of intravenous methylprednisolone (4–30 mg/kg per day), followed by a 2–4 week taper of oral steroids.
- Optic disc swelling and bilateral disease are more common in children, as is severe loss of visual acuity (20/200 or worse).
- Consider infectious and postinfectious causes of optic nerve impairment.

ISSUES FOR REFERRAL
Referral to a neurologist and/or ophthalmologist

ONGOING CARE

FOLLOW-UP RECOMMENDATIONS
Patient Monitoring
Monthly follow up to monitor visual changes and steroid side effects (6)

PATIENT EDUCATION
- Provide reassurance about recovery of vision.
- If the disease is believed to be secondary to demyelinating disease, patient should be informed of the risk of developing MS.
- For patient education materials favorably reviewed on this topic, contact:
  - National Eye Institute, Information Officer, Department of Health and Human Services, 9000 Rockville Pike, Bethesda, MD 20892, 301-496-5248
  - North American Neuro-Ophthalmology Society (NANOS), 5841 Cedar Lake Road, Suite 204, Minneapolis, MN 55416, 952-646-2037, fax: 952-545-6073, www.nanosweb.org

PROGNOSIS
- Orbital pain usually resolves within 1 week.
- Visual acuity:
  - Rapid spontaneous improvement at 2–3 weeks and continues for several months (may be faster with IV corticosteroids)
  - Often returns to normal or near-normal levels (20/40 or better) within 1 year (90–95%), even after near blindness
- Other visual disturbances (e.g., contrast sensitivity, stereopsis) often persist after acuity returns to normal.
- Recurrence risk of 35% within 10 years: 14% affected eye, 12% contralateral, 9% bilateral; recurrence is higher in MS patients (48%).
- ON is associated with an increased risk of developing MS; 35% risk at 7 years, 58% at 15 years:
  - Brain MRI helps to predict risk:
    - 0 lesions: 16%
    - 1–2 lesions: 37%
    - 3+ lesions: 51% (7)
- Poor prognostic factors:
  - Absence of pain
  - Low initial visual acuity
  - Involvement of intracanalicular optic nerve
- Children with bilateral visual loss have a better prognosis than adults.

COMPLICATIONS
Permanent loss of vision

REFERENCES

1. Vedula SS. Corticosteroids for treating optic neuritis. Cochrane Database Syst Rev. 2007;1:CD001430.
2. Keltner JL, Johnson CA, Cello KE, et al. Visual field profile of optic neuritis: A final follow-up report from the optic neuritis treatment trial from baseline through 15 years. Arch Ophthalmol. 2010;128: 330–337.
3. Simsek I, Erdem H, Pay S. Optic neuritis occurring with anti-tumour necrosis factor alpha therapy. Ann Rheum Dis. 2007;66:1255–1258.
4. Gleicher N. Principles and practice of medical therapy in pregnancy, 3rd ed. Norwalk, CT: Appleton and Lange; 1998:1396–1399.
5. Galetta SL. The controlled high risk Avonex multiple sclerosis trial (CHAMPS Study). J Neuroophthalmol. 2001;21:292–295.
6. Bonhomme GR, Mitchell EB. Treatment of pediatric optic neuritis. Curr Treat Options Neurol. 2012; 14(1):93–102.
7. Kaufman DI, Trobe JD, Eggenberger ER. Practice parameter: The role of corticosteroids in the management of acute monosymptomatic optic neuritis. Report of the Quality Standards Subcommittee of the American Academy of Neurology. Neurology. 2000;54:2039–2044.

ADDITIONAL READING
- Arnold AC. Evolving management of optic neuritis and multiple sclerosis. Am J Ophthalmol. 2005;139:1101–1108.
- Balcer LJ. Clinical practice. Optic neuritis. N Engl J Med. 2006;354:1273–1280.
- Optic Neuritis Study Group. Visual function 15 years after optic neuritis: A final follow-up report from the Optic Neuritis Treatment Trial. Ophthalmology. 2008;115:1079–1082.e5.

SEE ALSO

Multiple Sclerosis

CODES

ICD10
- H46.00 Optic papillitis, unspecified eye
- H46.9 Unspecified optic neuritis
- H46.10 Retrobulbar neuritis, unspecified eye

CLINICAL PEARLS
- MRI is the procedure of choice for determining relative risk and possible therapy for MS prevention.
- The ONTT showed that high-dose IV methylprednisolone followed by oral prednisone accelerated visual recovery, but did not improve the 6-month or 1-year visual outcome compared with placebo, whereas treatment with oral prednisone alone did not improve the outcome and was associated with an increased rate of recurrence of ON.

ALERT
Results of 15-year Optic Neuritis Study Group:
- After the initial period of recovery following an acute episode of ON, visual acuity remained stable in most patients.
- Overall, 72% of affected eyes had visual acuity of 20/20 or better, with 2/3 of patients having 20/20 or better vision in both eyes.
- In most patients, there was little change in vision between the 10- and 15-year follow-up examinations: 6 patients (2%) had visual acuity of 20/40 or worse in both eyes. Visual function was slightly better in patients without MS compared with those with MS.

O

ORAL REHYDRATION

Kevin M. Curtis, MD, MS

 BASICS

DESCRIPTION

- Oral rehydration therapy (ORT) is a clinically useful, cost-effective, and safe technique to treat mild and moderate dehydration from diarrheal illness (1),(2,3)[B],(4)[A].
- ORT is as effective as IV hydration, and the treatment of choice, for children with mild to moderate dehydration caused by diarrhea.
- ORT should be divided into rehydration and maintenance phases.
- ORT should have an osmolality of ~245 mosom/kg, a sodium (Na) content of ~75 mEq/L, and a glucose concentration of ~75 mmol/L (13.5 g/L).
- Fruit juices, soda, popsicles, sports drinks, and broth have inappropriate sodium and/or electrolyte concentrations for ORT.
- Although ORT can be prepared at home, commercially prepared solutions eliminate the potential major errors that can occur from homemade solutions.
- System(s) affected: Endocrine/Metabolic; Gastrointestinal

EPIDEMIOLOGY
Incidence
- Diarrheal disease is a leading cause of childhood morbidity and mortality in the world, causing ~2 million deaths per year (5).
- Diarrhea and the resulting dehydration is the source of >200,000 hospitalizations annually in the US and >1.5 million outpatient visits (6).
- Predominant age: Primarily infants and children, but ORT is effective for all ages.

ETIOLOGY AND PATHOPHYSIOLOGY
This therapy takes advantage of the preserved coupled transport of Na and glucose in the small intestine during infectious gastroenteritis. Water follows osmotically after Na entry. Potassium is passively absorbed via solvent drag. An equimolar concentration of glucose and sodium is most effective for ORT (7).

 DIAGNOSIS

HISTORY
- Vomiting: Duration and amount
- Diarrhea: Duration and amount
- Fever
- Weight loss: Amount
- Frequency and volume of urination
- Exposure to others with gastroenteritis
- Travel
- Recent antibiotic use
- Past medical history of short gut, or carbohydrate malabsorption

PHYSICAL EXAM
- Assessment of the degree of dehydration (Table 1).
- The 3 most useful of these signs to predict ≥5% dehydration may be prolonged capillary refill (LR 4.1), abnormal skin turgor (LR 2.5), and abnormal respiratory pattern (LR 2.0) (8)

Table 1 Signs and symptoms of dehydration in children with rehydration requirements

Sign or symptom	Mild (3–5%)	Moderate (6–10%)	Severe (>10%)
General	Increased thirst	Listlessness, irritability	Grunting, lethargy, coma
Pulse	Normal/mildly increased	Increased	Rapid and/or weak
Blood pressure	Normal	Normal	Low
Respirations	Normal	Normal	Increased
Mucous membranes	Normal/mildly dry	Dry	Very dry
Urine output	Normal/slightly decreased	Decreased	Absent
Skin turgor	Normal	Reduced	Tenting
Skin	Normal	Cool	Mottled
Eyes	Normal	Sunken	Sunken
Rehydration requirements	30–50 mL/kg	60–100 mL/kg	>100 mL/kg

DIAGNOSTIC TESTS & INTERPRETATION
Initial Tests (lab, imaging)
- Most with mild dehydration from diarrheal illness do not need lab tests.
- For some with moderate dehydration and all with severe dehydration, obtain Na, potassium, bicarbonate, chloride, glucose, BUN, creatinine.

 TREATMENT

GENERAL MEASURES
- The composition of oral rehydration solution (ORS) according to the WHO and UNICEF is (9):
  - Total osmolality: 200–310 mmol/L
  - Equimolar concentrations of glucose and sodium
- Glucose ≤20 g/L (111 mmol/L)
  - Sodium concentration 60–90 mEq/L
  - Potassium concentration 15–25 mEq/L
  - Citrate concentration 8–12 mmol/L
  - Chloride concentration 50–80 mEq/L
- See Table 2
- ORS is not to be diluted.
- Effective at all ages:
  - If child refuses because of taste, flavor with a commercial flavoring, such as sugar-free grape-flavored drink mix, and use ~1/4 tsp to 4 oz ORS.
  - Prepackaged ORS-flavored freeze pops are often well accepted
- Begin feeding as soon as rehydration is achieved.
- Contraindications:
  - Conditions predisposing to risk of aspiration:
    ◦ Significantly depressed level of consciousness, seizure activity
    ◦ Severe dehydration
    ◦ Underlying disorders of intestinal absorption
- For those in whom ORT is unsuccessful or contraindicated, IV rehydration should be performed

- Precautions:
  - The ingredients should be provided in premixed packets to avoid iatrogenic errors in mixing. In the US, Pedialyte premixed powder packets are to be diluted in 8 oz (240 mL) of water.
  - If water contamination is a concern, it should be boiled/treated for purification.
  - Discard the solution after 12 hours if held at room temperature or 24 hours if refrigerated.
  - After rehydration is complete, ORT should not continue as the only fluid intake because the high Na content may lead to hypernatremia.

MEDICATION
First Line
- The overall approach is to perform initial rehydration over 3–4 hours, followed by maintenance hydration.
- In the rehydration phase, ORT should be given as frequent, small amounts by spoon or syringe.
- 5 mL every 1–2 minutes is often well tolerated and supplies 150–300 mL/h (11).
- For the child who will not take adequate oral fluids, ORT via nasogastric tube, and/or the addition of ondansetron, are alternatives to IV fluid.
- For rehydration fluid goals, see Table 1.
- During the maintenance hydration stage, the fluid goals are as follows:
  - 1st 0–10 kg body weight: 4 mL/kg/h
  - Next 10–20 kg: Additional 2 mL/kg/h
  - Additional body weight >20 kg: Additional 1 mL/kg/h
- Example: An 18-kg child who has moderate dehydration would require:
  - Rehydration phase: 100 mL/kg = 1,800 mL over 3–4 hours = 450–600 mL/h = ~15–20 mL every 2 minutes
  - Maintenance phase: 56 mL/h [(10 kg × 4 mL/h) + (8 kg × 2 mL/h)] = ~15 mL every 15 minutes

Table 2 Comparison of effective oral rehydration products (10)

Solution	Osmolality (mosm/kg H₂O)	Na⁺ (mEq/L)	K⁺ (mEq/L)	HCO₃ (mEq/L)	Carbohydrate (g/L)
WHO	245	75	20	10	13.5
Pedialyte	250	45	20	25	25
Enfalyte	200	50	25	34	30
Rehydralyte	310	75	20	30	25

– The child should receive additional ORT for any ongoing losses.

- In addition to the standard volumes of hydration provided, in both rehydration and maintenance phases, ongoing losses should be additionally replaced according to:
  – 10 mL/kg body weight of ORT for each watery/loose stool
  – 2 mL/kg body weight for each episode of emesis
- ORT can be used for both rehydration and maintenance hydration.
- Many comparable generic formulations are available.

Second Line

- In developing countries and areas where malnutrition is prevalent, supplementation with 20 mg oral zinc daily shortens the course of diarrhea and lessens costs (12)[B].
- For children with vomiting, ondansetron (0.1–0.15 mg/kg) decreases vomiting, allows easier administration of ORT, and decreases the need for IV fluids. Ondansetron ODT can be particularly effective based on its ease of administration and tolerance in the vomiting child (13)[A].

IN-PATIENT CONSIDERATIONS
Admission Criteria/Initial Stabilization
Failure of oral therapy: Estimated failure rate is 4% (4)[A].

IV Fluids
To be used for initial resuscitation in severe cases or for ORS failure.

Nursing
If vomiting occurs, small amounts of ORS given frequently are usually effective.

 ## ONGOING CARE

FOLLOW-UP RECOMMENDATIONS
- Primarily outpatient
- Designed to be administered by family members

DIET
- For breastfeeding infants, the mother should continue nursing.
- For bottle-fed babies, there should be an early institution of formulas. Lactose-free formulas rarely are required.
- Age appropriate:
  – Complex carbohydrate-rich (e.g., rice, bread, potato, cereal), low-fat foods should be offered as soon as the dehydration deficit is replaced.
- Cow's milk can be added to diet after several days.

PATIENT EDUCATION
- Awareness and availability of ORT markedly diminishes morbidity from gastroenteritis.
- Early use of ORT at home for children with diarrhea reduces outpatient visits, hospitalizations, and costs (7).
- Travelers concerned with severe diarrhea should carry ORT packets on trips.

PROGNOSIS
- Rapid clinical improvement despite continuing diarrhea is the usual course.
- The overall complication rate for oral rehydration is similar to that for parenteral rehydration in cases of mild and moderate dehydration (2)[B],(4)[A].

COMPLICATIONS
Change to IV hydration if the patient has increasing weight loss (fluid deficit), clinical deterioration, or intractable vomiting.

REFERENCES

1. Victora CG, Bryce J, Fontaine O, et al. Reducing deaths from diarrhoea through oral rehydration therapy. *Bull World Health Organ*. 2000;78: 1246–1255.
2. Spandorfer PR, Alessandrini EA, Joffe MD, et al. Oral versus intravenous rehydration of moderately dehydrated children: A randomized, controlled trial. *Pediatrics*. 2005;115:295–301.
3. Hahn S, Kim S, Garner P. Reduced osmolarity oral rehydration solution for treating dehydration caused by acute diarrhoea in children. *Cochrane Database Syst Rev*. 2002;1:CD002847.
4. Hartling L, Bellemare S, Wiebe N. Oral versus intravenous rehydration for treating dehydration due to gastroenteritis in children. *Cochrane Database Syst Rev*. 2006;3:CD004390.
5. Bryce J, Boschi-Pinto C, Shibuya K, et al. WHO estimates of the causes of death in children. *Lancet*. 2005;365:1147–1152.
6. Santosham M, Keenan EM, Tulloch J, et al. Oral rehydration therapy for diarrhea: An example of reverse transfer of technology. *Pediatrics*. 1997;100:E10.
7. Duggan C, Fontaine O, Pierce NF. Scientific rationale for a change in the composition of oral rehydration solution. *JAMA*. 2004;291: 2628–2631.
8. Steiner MJ, DeWalt DA, Byerley JS. Is this child dehydrated? *JAMA*. 2004;291:2746–2754.
9. World Health Organization. Reduced osmolarity oral rehydration salts (ORS) formulation. UNICEF House, New York, NY 2001. Available at: www.who.int/child-adolescent-health/New_Publications/NEWS/Expert_consultation.thm
10. Murphy CK, Hahn S, Volmink J. Reduced osmolarity oral rehydration solution for treating cholera. *Cochrane Database Syst Rev*. 2004;4:CD003754.
11. Practice parameter: The management of acute gastroenteritis in young children. American Academy of Pediatrics, Provisional Committee on Quality Improvement, Subcommittee on Acute Gastroenteritis. *Pediatrics*. 1996;97:424–435.
12. Lazzerini M, Ronfani L. Oral zinc for treating diarrhoea in children. *Cochrane Database Syst Rev*. 2008;3:CD005436.
13. Alhashimi D, Al-Hashimi H, Fedorowicz Z. Antiemetics for reducing vomiting related to acute gastroenteritis in children and adolescents. *Cochrane Database Syst Rev*. 2009;2:CD005506.

ADDITIONAL READING

- Canani RB, Cirillo P, Terrin G. Probiotics for treatment of acute diarrhoea in children: Randomised clinical trial of five different preparations. *BMJ*. 2007;335:340.
- Fonseca BK, Holdgate A, Craig JC. Enteral vs intravenous rehydration therapy for children with gastroenteritis: A meta-analysis of randomized controlled trials. *Arch Pediatr Adolesc Med*. 2004;158:483–490.

 ## CODES

ICD10
- A09 Infectious gastroenteritis and colitis, unspecified
- E86.0 Dehydration
- K52.9 Noninfective gastroenteritis and colitis, unspecified

CLINICAL PEARLS

- ORT is as effective and less costly than IV hydration for mild and moderate dehydration, yet is under utilized in the developed world.
- ORT should not be diluted.
- The addition of ondansetron can augment the effectiveness of ORT.

OSGOOD-SCHLATTER DISEASE

David Sealy, MD

 BASICS

DESCRIPTION
- A syndrome associated with traction apophysitis and patellar tendinosis:
  - Adolescent boys and girls
  - Pain and swelling in the tibial tubercle
- System(s) affected: Musculoskeletal

EPIDEMIOLOGY
Incidence
Incidence in girls increasing

Prevalence
Not known, but common (13% of athletes in a Finnish study)

ETIOLOGY AND PATHOPHYSIOLOGY
Traction apophysitis of the tibial tubercle due to repetitive strain on the secondary ossification center of the tibial tuberosity, concurrent patellar tendinosis, and proximal tibial apophysis disruption (1)
- Basic etiology unknown, but clearly exacerbated by exercise:
  - Jumping and pivoting sports are the worst—repetitive trauma the most likely source
- Possible association with tight hip flexors, quadriceps, and hamstring muscle groups

RISK FACTORS
- Ages 11–18 years:
  - Girls 8–12
  - Boys 10–16
- Male sex slightly more common
- Rapid skeletal growth
- Involvement in repetitive-jumping sports such as:
  - Football
  - Volleyball
  - Basketball
  - Hockey
  - Soccer
  - Skating
  - Gymnastics
  - Ballet (2-fold risk compared with nonathletes)
- Sports involving heavy quadriceps activity

GENERAL PREVENTION
- Avoidance of sports involving heavy quadriceps loading, especially deceleration mechanisms
- Patients may compete if pain is minimal.
- Increase hamstring and quadriceps flexibility

COMMONLY ASSOCIATED CONDITIONS
Shortened (tight) rectus femoris found in 75% with Osgood-Schlatter disease (OSD) (2)[C]

 DIAGNOSIS

HISTORY
- Unilateral or bilateral (30%) tibial tuberosity pain
- Pain exacerbated by exercise, especially jumping and landing after jumping
- Pain upon kneeling on the affected side(s)
- Antalgic or straight-legged gait

PHYSICAL EXAM
- Knee pain with squatting or crouching
- Absence of effusion or condyle tenderness
- Tibial tuberosity swelling and tenderness
- Pain increased with knee extension against resistance or kneeling
- Erythema over tibial tuberosity

DIFFERENTIAL DIAGNOSIS
- Stress fracture of the proximal tibia
- Pes anserinus bursitis
- Quadriceps tendon avulsion
- Patellofemoral stress syndrome
- Chondromalacia patellae
- Proximal tibial neoplasm
- Osteomyelitis of the proximal tibia
- Tibial plateau fracture
- Sinding-Larsen-Johansson syndrome (patellar apophysitis)—pain over inferior patellar tendon
- Patellar fracture
- Infrapatellar bursitis
- Patellar tendinitis—pain over inferior patellar tendon and inferior pole of patella

DIAGNOSTIC TESTS & INTERPRETATION
Initial Tests (lab, imaging)
- No blood tests are indicated unless other diagnostic considerations are entertained.
- Radiographic imaging of the proximal tibia and knee may show heterotopic calcification in the patellar tendon:
  - X-rays are rarely diagnostic, but appearance of a separate fragment at the tibial tuberosity increases potential for surgical intervention (3)[C].
  - Calcified thickening of the tibial tuberosity with irregular ossification at insertion of tendon to tibial tubercle

Diagnostic Procedures/Other
- Bone scan may show increased uptake in the area of the tibial tuberosity:
  - Increased uptake in apophysis exists in any child, but with OSD *may be more than the opposite side.*
- Ultrasound is becoming an excellent alternative, with characteristic findings and marked thickening of the distal patellar tendon (4)[C].
- MRI has characteristic findings of fragmentation of the tibial tubercle and bone edema.

Test Interpretation
Biopsy is not necessary, but would show osteolysis and fragmentation of the tibial tubercle.

TREATMENT

GENERAL MEASURES

- Frequent ice applications after exercise
- Rest
- Knee immobilization in extension (severe cases)
- In more severe cases, avoidance of activities that increase pain or swelling
- Consider physical therapy referral for quadriceps isometric strengthening, hip extensions, adductor strengthening, and hamstring and quadriceps stretching exercises.
- Open- and closed-chain eccentric quadriceps strengthening
- If tibial tuberosity fracture or complete avulsion is likely, surgery is likely to be needed.
- Electrical stimulation is not proven but may be beneficial in isolated cases (5).
- Patients with marked pronation may benefit from orthotics.
- Hypertonic glucose and/or xylocaine injections have recently been shown of benefit (1)[C].

MEDICATION

First Line

- None in particular, but all analgesics may be considered.
- NSAIDs are of minimal benefit.
- Narcotics are not recommended.

Second Line

- More potent analgesics, such as narcotics, may be considered for short-term use or in extreme situations.
- Injectable corticosteroids universally not recommended.

ISSUES FOR REFERRAL

When conservative therapy is unsuccessful, consideration of surgery warrants referral.

SURGERY/OTHER PROCEDURES

- Debridement of a thickened, cosmetically unsatisfactory tibial tubercle (rare) or removal of mobile heterotopic bone (3)[C]
- Surgical excision of a painful tibial tubercle is rarely needed (<5%).
- 75% return to normal sport activity and 89% are not restricted from competition due to recurrent pain (6)[B].

 ONGOING CARE

FOLLOW-UP RECOMMENDATIONS

- Athletes may return to play if able to tolerate pain
- Presence of pain does not preclude competition.

Patient Monitoring

With worsening of symptoms only

PATIENT EDUCATION

- Consider avoidance of jumping sports
- Assure family that symptoms and findings will diminish with time and rest
- Can play sports with mild pain
- Quad stretching and strengthening important

PROGNOSIS

- Except in rare complicated cases, this is a self-limiting illness that resolves within 2 years of full skeletal maturation.
- However, up to 60% of adults with prior OSD still report occasional symptoms and have pain with kneeling.
- Strength and endurance of quads in adults with prior OSD improves with growth maturity but does not reach normal (4)[C].
- Most persons with OSD will have residual "knobby" tibial tubercles that never completely resolve:
  – The tubercles may decline in size, but will remain throughout life to some extent.

COMPLICATIONS

Rarely, the heavily fragmented and inflamed tibial ossicle will avulse and require surgery.

REFERENCES

1. Topol GA, Podesta LA, Reeves KD, et al. Hyperosmolar dextrose injection for recalcitrant Osgood-Schlatter disease. *Pediatrics*. 2011;128: e1121–e1128.
2. de Lucena GL, dos Santos GC, Guerro RO. Prevalence and associated factors of Osgood Schlatter syndrome in a population based sample of Brazilian adolescents. *Am J Sports Med*. 2011;39:414–420.
3. Nierenberg G, Falah M, Keren Y, et al. Surgical treatment of residual Osgood-Schlatter disease in young adults: Role of the mobile osseous fragment. *Orthopedics*. 2011;34:176.
4. Kayce DO, Toprak U, Baltaci G, et al. Long-term functional and sonographic outcomes in OSD. *Knee Surg Sports Traumatol Arthros*. 2013;21: 1131–1139.
5. Weller R, Ingram M, Wolman R. 10 minute consultation: OSD. *BMJ*. 2011;343.
6. Pihlamajaki HK, Visuri TI. Long-term outcome after surgical treatment of unresolved Osgood Schlatter disease in young men: Surgical technique. *J Bone Joint Surg Am*. 2010;92(Suppl 1, Pt 2):258–264.

 CODES

ICD10

- M92.50 Juvenile osteochondrosis of tibia and fibula, unsp leg
- M92.51 Juvenile osteochondrosis of tibia and fibula, right leg
- M92.52 Juvenile osteochondrosis of tibia and fibula, left leg

CLINICAL PEARLS

- Pain starting below the patella in an athlete during rapid growth spurt is OSD, patellar tendinosis, or Sinding-Larsen-Johansson syndrome.
- Always consider lumbar disc disease, osteogenic sarcoma, or hip etiologies in the differential diagnosis of OSD.
- Though most return to normal activity, over 50% of OSD patients will have residual weakness or knee pain.

O

OSTEOCHONDRITIS DISSECANS

Luke R. Miller, MD • Jack Spittler, MD, MS

 BASICS

DESCRIPTION
- Osteochondritis dissecans (OCD) is a lesion of the subchondral bone that may cause separation and instability of the overlying articular cartilage.
- The loose piece of bone and cartilage may migrate into the joint causing instability, pain, or a locking sensation.
- OCD is the most common cause of an intra-articular loose body in adolescents.
- Knee is the most commonly affected joint (usually posterolateral aspect of the medial femoral condyle).
- OCD can also occur in any other diarthrodial joint, including, in decreasing order of frequency:
  - Elbow (capitellum)
  - Ankle (talar dome or tibial plafond)
  - Tarsal navicular
  - Hip (femoral capital epiphysis)
  - Shoulder (humeral head or glenoid)
  - Wrist (scaphoid)
- System(s) affected: Musculoskeletal

EPIDEMIOLOGY
Incidence
- Unknown: Estimated 2–5:10,000 persons
- Predominant age: 10–40 years
- Juvenile type (JOCD) in children and adolescents prior to physeal closure
- Predominant sex: Male > Female (5:3)

ETIOLOGY AND PATHOPHYSIOLOGY
- Primary change happens in the bone and necrosis occurs in a focal area.
- Overlying cartilage changes are secondary to these bony changes.
- Loss of subchondral bone support leads to degenerative cartilage changes: Softening and fibromatous fissuring.
- A fragment may detach and become a loose body within the affected joint.
- Cartilage itself is without a vascular supply and healing occurs by vascular supply to underlying bone, which stimulates inflammation, repair, and remodeling.
- Difficult to predict which lesions will go on to heal and remodel
- Controversial and unclear; histologic studies have been inconsistent (1)[B]
- Theories include:
  - Trauma or repetitive microtrauma
  - Ischemia
  - Familial predisposition
  - Fragile blood supply of the physeal line
  - Epiphyseal abnormalities
  - Endocrine imbalance

- Currently, the most credited theory is repetitive microtrauma with possible vascular insufficiency (2).
- Most commonly affected joints are:
  - Knee: Overuse, and with patellar dislocation and injury to the anterior cruciate ligament; bilateral involvement noted in up to 30% of patients
  - Elbow: Overuse injury in overhead throwers and racket sports, as well as gymnasts
  - Ankle: Frequently associated with history of previous ankle sprain
- Relationship between adult and juvenile forms of OCD remains unclear.

Genetics
No genetic pattern known but bilateral lesions have been noted in up to 30% of patients. Case reports of bilateral involvement in twins exist but this is rare.

RISK FACTORS
- Trauma
- High physical activity level (children and adults)
- Participating in multiple sports, especially gymnastics and overhead sports
- Abnormal mechanical axis of the leg (3)[C]:
  - Varus axis and medial condyle OCD
  - Valgus axis and lateral condyle OCD

Pediatric Considerations
Although still idiopathic, the mean age in JOCD is decreasing, and the prevalence in girls is increasing with changes in athletic participation by children (4)[C].

GENERAL PREVENTION
There is no clear way to avoid the development of OCD.

 DIAGNOSIS

HISTORY
- Insidious (most common) or posttraumatic onset of pain, which improves with rest
- Pain usually is described as a deep and vague ache.
- Pain may be associated with clicking, swelling, locking (usually with a loose body), and stiffness.

PHYSICAL EXAM
- May be associated with secondary muscle atrophy, mild effusion, decreased range of motion (ROM), joint-line tenderness, or tenderness over the lesion
- The Wilson test may be positive (i.e., pain with knee extension and tibial internal rotation) in some patients with knee involvement. Pain may be relieved by external rotation of the tibia.

DIFFERENTIAL DIAGNOSIS
- In the knee:
  - Meniscal tear
  - Patellofemoral pain syndrome
  - Gout
- Osteoarthritis
- Stress fracture
- Tendinopathy
- Avascular necrosis
- Acute fracture
- Neoplasm

DIAGNOSTIC TESTS & INTERPRETATION
Initial Tests (lab, imaging)
No specific laboratory tests are helpful in the diagnosis of OCD.
- The diagnosis is usually made by standard radiographs.
- Typical findings include small articular surface radiolucency or irregularity and bony fragmentation with partial or complete separation of the articular cartilage:
  - Knee: Anteroposterior (AP), lateral, sunrise, and tunnel views (most likely location for abnormality in the posterolateral portion of the medial femoral condyle)
  - Elbow: Routine AP and lateral elbow series (common involvement of the humeral capitellum)
  - Ankle: AP, lateral, and mortise views (lesions most commonly involve the posteromedial or anterolateral talar dome)
- MRI can delineate the bony lesion, involvement of cartilage, and any fluid behind the fragment and is useful to detect the stability or instability of the lesion (5)[A]. It also allows for staging of the lesion (Anderson MRI classification):
  - Stage I: Bone marrow edema (subchondral trabecular compression; radiograph results are negative with positive bone scan findings)
  - Stage IIa: Subchondral cyst
  - Stage IIb: Incomplete separation of the osteochondral fragment
  - Stage III: Fluid around an undetached, undisplaced osteochondral fragment
  - Stage IV: Displaced osteochondral fragment
- CT scan provides architectural description of the bony lesion; however, it provides less information than MRI.
- Bone scan may be useful in evaluation of healing potential, but this is controversial at present.

 TREATMENT

GENERAL MEASURES
- Goals of treatment:
  - Maintain a smooth, congruous joint surface
  - Alleviate pain
  - Prevent degenerative joint disease
  - Promote revascularization of necrotic fragment and regeneration of affected cartilage
- There are no randomized, controlled trials, but in JOCD, initial nonsurgical treatment is the standard of care.
- Treatment options include periods of immobilization, activity modification, and non–weight-bearing. Type and duration of immobilization remain controversial.
- Casting is sometimes used for 6-week intervals, especially with JOCD, due to issues of compliance in this age group.
- If non–weight-bearing immobilization is used, add intermittent maintenance of ROM.
- Physical therapy can often be helpful to establish an exercise plan.
- Follow closely for at least 12 weeks to ensure healing

MEDICATION

First Line

Acetaminophen (650–1,000 mg q.i.d. PRN), NSAIDs (ibuprofen 600–800 mg t.i.d. PRN), or other pain medications for symptomatic relief

ISSUES FOR REFERRAL

- Patients in whom surgery may be considered as an early treatment option (loose fragments, adults, or lesions >1 cm)
- Unstable lesions on MRI, including presence of an intra-articular loose body
- Failure of conservative, symptomatic treatment

SURGERY/OTHER PROCEDURES

- Surgical treatment is used when:
  - Conservative measures have failed
  - Physeal closure has occurred, which carries a worse prognosis for healing (adult form)
  - Unstable lesions are visualized on MRI, including presence of an intra-articular loose body
  - Lesion are large (>1 cm)
- Arthroscopic surgery is the preferred method. In addition, arthroscopy is a valuable tool to evaluate the stability of the lesion and visualize the overlying cartilage.
- Surgical treatment includes fragment excision, microfracture technique (drilling) to increase blood supply, screw fixation of the loose fragment, allograft insertion, and autologous chondrocyte implantation.
- Both transarticular drilling for stable lesions and bioabsorbable pin fixation for unstable lesions show similar favorable results (6)[A].
- Fragment excision has fallen out of favor due to poor long-term results (2)[B].

 ## ONGOING CARE

FOLLOW-UP RECOMMENDATIONS

- Outpatient care usually utilized
- Inpatient treatment usually not indicated, unless postoperative

Patient Monitoring

- Initially should be followed every 6 weeks with serial radiographs to evaluate healing and monitor for possible displacement
- Healing is expected within 4–6 months
- In JOCD, radiographs at 1 year may show no residual abnormality
- If postoperative patient remains symptomatic, may be followed with MRI or SPECT/CT to evaluate healing (7)[C].

DIET

Vitamin D supplementation

PATIENT EDUCATION

The critical importance of compliance with the treatment plan should be stressed.

PROGNOSIS

- Factors associated with good prognosis:
  - Younger age
  - Open growth plate
  - Smaller lesions (<160 mm^2)
  - Stable lesions
  - Non–weight-bearing location of the lesion
- The absence of a sclerotic rim on x-rays at the time diagnosis can be an indication for conservative treatment for OCD of the knee, due to the resultant high probability for spontaneous recovery (8)[C].
- An incongruous joint surface may lead to degenerative changes in the future.
- Clinical improvement may proceed radiologic healing.

COMPLICATIONS

- Failure to revascularize and heal
- Displacement of a fragment becoming a loose body within a joint
- Predisposition for early osteoarthritis in the affected joint

REFERENCES

1. Edmonds EW, Polousky J. A review of knowledge in osteochondritis dissecans: 123 years of minimal evolution from König to the ROCK study group. *Clin Orthop Relat Res*. 2013;471:1118–1126.
2. Pape D, Filardo G, Kon E, et al. Disease-specific clinical problems associated with the subchondral bone. *Knee Surg Sports Traumatol Arthrosc*. 2010;18:448–462.
3. Jacobi M, Wahl P, Bouaicha S, et al. Association between mechanical axis of the leg and osteochondritis dissecans of the knee: Radiographic study on 103 knees. *Am J Sports Med*. 2010;38:1425–1428.
4. Kocher MS, Tucker R, Ganley TJ, et al. Management of osteochondritis dissecans of the knee: Current concepts review. *Am J Sports Med*. 2006;34:1181–1191.
5. Quatman CE, Quatman-Yates CC, Schmitt LC, et al. The clinical utility and diagnostic performance of MRI for identification and classification of knee osteochondritis dissecans. *J Bone Joint Surg Am*. 2012;94:1036–1044.
6. Abouassaly M, Peterson D, Salci L, et al. Surgical management of osteochondritis dissecans of the knee in the paediatric population: A systematic review addressing surgical techniques. *Knee Surg Sports Traumatol Arthrosc*. 2013; in press.
7. Hirschmann MT, Davda K, Rasch H, et al. Clinical value of combined single photon emission computerized tomography and conventional computer tomography (SPECT/CT) in sports medicine. *Sports Med Arthrosc Rev*. 2011;19:174–181.
8. Ramirez A, Abril JC, Chaparro M, et al. Juvenile osteochondritis dissecans of the knee: Perifocal sclerotic rim as a prognostic factor of healing. *J Pediatr Orthop*. 2010;30:180–185.

ADDITIONAL READING

- Chambers HG, Shea KG, Anderson AF, et al. American Academy of Orthopaedic Surgeons clinical practice guideline on: the diagnosis and treatment of osteochondritis dissecans. *J Bone Joint Surg Am*. 2012;94:1322–1324.
- Parikh SN, Allen M, Wall EJ, et al. The reliability to determine "healing" in osteochondritis dissecans from radiographic assessment. *J Pediatr Orthop*. 2012;32:e35–e39.
- Vasiliadis HS, Danielson B, Ljungberg M, et al. Autologous chondrocyte implantation in cartilage lesions of the knee: Long-term evaluation with magnetic resonance imaging and delayed gadolinium-enhanced magnetic resonance imaging technique. *Am J Sports Med*. 2010;38:943–949.

 ## CODES

ICD10

- M93.20 Osteochondritis dissecans of unspecified site
- M93.229 Osteochondritis dissecans, unspecified elbow
- M93.269 Osteochondritis dissecans, unspecified knee

CLINICAL PEARLS

- OCD is an acquired lesion of the subchondral bone, causing separation and instability of the overlying articular cartilage; it may sometimes become loose in the joint, causing it to "lock up"; the knee is most commonly affected.
- With adherence to a conservative management plan, many lesions may heal without surgical intervention.
- Compliance with immobilization and possibility of further trauma should be emphasized, especially with younger athletes.
- Frequent follow up every 6 weeks is important to ensure healing.
- In certain patients, surgery may be considered as an early treatment option (loose fragments, adults, or lesions >1 cm).

O

OSTEOMALACIA AND RICKETS

Elizabeth Nelson, MD

 BASICS

DESCRIPTION
- A metabolic bone disorder due to decreased bone mineralization (calcification) and increased organic bone matrix that results in decreased bone density
- Referred to as *renal osteodystrophy* when secondary to renal disease
- System(s) affected: Musculoskeletal

EPIDEMIOLOGY
- Children: Median age of presentation is 15 months.
- Adults: Elderly

Incidence
In the US, occurs almost exclusively in breast-fed infants without vitamin D supplementation or sun exposure.

ETIOLOGY AND PATHOPHYSIOLOGY
- Children: Defective mineralization of cartilage in the epiphyseal growth plates:
  - Failure of growing bone to mineralize due to inadequate substrate (low calcium or phosphate) or interference with mineralization (e.g., vitamin D deficiency or toxic exposure)
  - Lack of calcified osteoid and accumulation of unossified cartilage
- Adults: Disorder of mineralization of newly formed bone matrix
- Hypophosphatemia from secondary hyperparathyroidism, due to vitamin D deficiency is the primary cause in adults.
- Vitamin D metabolism abnormalities, including hepatic or renal disease
- Resistance to vitamin D
- Inadequate dietary calcium
- Impaired intestinal absorption of calcium/phosphorus due to celiac disease, cystic fibrosis, or postgastrectomy
- Inadequate dietary phosphorus
- Impaired renal phosphate absorption associated with proximal or distal renal tubular defects
- Causes that inhibit mineralization of the growth plate and osteoid:
  - Alkaline phosphatase deficiency
  - Aluminum toxicity
  - Fluoride toxicity
  - Primary hyperparathyroidism
- Drugs that may affect absorption or metabolism of calcium, phosphorus, or vitamin D:
  - Antacids
  - Antiepileptic drugs
  - Corticosteroids
  - Loop diuretics
- Drugs that inhibit mineralization: Bisphosphonates
- Oncogenic osteomalacia

Genetics
Rare causes of rickets in children include:
- Vitamin D–dependent rickets: An autosomal-recessive disorder caused by deficiency of renal 25-hydroxyvitamin D_3 1-α-hydroxylase or altered calcitriol receptors
- Vitamin D–resistant rickets: An X-linked dominant or autosomal disorder caused by decreased proximal renal tubular reabsorption of phosphorus

RISK FACTORS
- Children:
  - Nutritional rickets:
    ○ Breastfeeding as a sole source of nutrition without vitamin D supplementation
    ○ Dark skin
    ○ Limited exposure to sunlight
    ○ Vegetarian diet without vitamin supplementation
    ○ Malabsorption syndromes
  - Prematurity
  - Maternal vitamin D deficiency
- Adults:
  - Poor diet
  - Poverty
  - Primary biliary cirrhosis
  - Anorexia nervosa
  - Renal failure
  - Gastrectomy

GENERAL PREVENTION
- Adequate vitamin D intake: Encourage foods, such as fatty fish, cod liver oil, egg yolks, and fortified foods:
  - Adults: Vitamin D, 400–800 IU/d
- American Academy of Pediatrics recommends a minimum vitamin D intake of 400 IU/d starting within the 1st few days of life (1)[C]:
  - Infants who consume >1 L/d of vitamin D–fortified formula or whole milk will receive the recommended vitamin D intake.
  - Supplementation is recommended for breast-fed infants and children consuming <1 L/d of vitamin D–fortified formula or milk.
- Sunlight exposure: 10–15 minutes on face, hands, and arms 2–3 d/wk
- Adequate calcium intake: Encourage high-calcium foods or supplements.

COMMONLY ASSOCIATED CONDITIONS
- Children with vitamin D–deficiency rickets:
  - Secondary hyperparathyroidism
  - Dilated cardiomyopathy
  - Marrow fibrosis with pancytopenia or microcytic hypochromic anemia
  - Dysregulation of immune function and cellular differentiation and proliferation
- Adults with osteomalacia:
  - Chronic renal disease
  - Gastrectomy
  - Epilepsy
  - Malnutrition

Rx **DIAGNOSIS**

HISTORY
- Common presentations in children:
  - Muscle weakness: May not be able to stand until age 3
  - Bowed legs
  - Diffuse limb pain
  - Hypocalcemic seizures
  - Carpopedal spasms

- Signs and symptoms of hypocalcemia:
  ○ Muscle cramps
  ○ Numbness
  ○ Paresthesia
  ○ Tetany
  ○ Seizures
  ○ Diarrhea
- Common presentations in adults:
  - Dull bony pain and tenderness typically in lower spine and pelvis that is aggravated by activity and weight bearing
  - Muscle weakness, especially the proximal lower extremity
  - Fractures may occur with little or no trauma.

PHYSICAL EXAM
Perform a complete physical and dental examination in children:
- General:
  - Palpate entire skeletal system to search for tenderness and bony abnormalities.
  - Evaluate for growth abnormalities, such as decreased height and spinal deformity.
- Head, ears, eyes, nose, and throat (HEENT):
  - Craniotabes (thinning and softening of occipital and parietal bones)
  - Late closing of fontanelles
  - Fontal bossing of skull
  - Tooth abnormalities
- Chest:
  - Rachitic rosary (enlarged costochondral joints felt lateral to nipple line)
  - Harrison groove (flaring of ribs at diaphragm level)
  - Pigeon breast (protrusion of the sternum)
- Back:
  - Lordosis/Kyphosis
  - Scoliosis
- Extremities:
  - Bowing or widening of the physis
  - Genu valgum (leg bowing)
  - Flaring of the wrists
  - Fraying and cupping of metaphysis
  - Genu varum (knock knees)
- Neurologic:
  - Gait disturbances in an ambulatory child
  - Signs of hypocalcemia:
    ○ Hyperreflexia
    ○ Neuromuscular instability: Chvostek sign (tap cranial nerve VII), Trousseau sign (carpopedal spasm 2–3 minutes after BP cuff is inflated proximally)
    ○ Tetany, myopathy, seizures, spasm, muscle weakness
- In adults:
  - Proximal muscle weakness, possible muscle wasting, hypotonia, and discomfort with movement
  - Waddling gait
  - Bone pain and tenderness to palpation: Most pronounced in the lower spine, pelvis, and lower extremities

DIFFERENTIAL DIAGNOSIS

- Children:
  - Liver disease
  - Anticonvulsant drugs
  - Failure to thrive
  - Developmental delay
  - Orthopedic abnormalities
  - Congenital syphilis
  - Osteogenesis imperfecta
  - Child abuse
  - Alkaline phosphatase deficiency
  - Aluminum toxicity
  - Fluoride toxicity
  - Primary hyperparathyroidism (rare)
- Adults:
  - Osteoporosis
  - Hyperparathyroidism
  - Metastatic bone disease
  - Lymphoma/myeloma
  - Fibromyalgia

DIAGNOSTIC TESTS & INTERPRETATION

- In children with vitamin D–deficiency rickets (2)[C]:
  - Serum phosphorus: Decreased
  - Serum calcidiol (25-hydroxy vitamin D_3): Decreased:
    - Indicative of overall vitamin D status
  - Urinary calcium: Decreased
- In adults with vitamin D–deficiency osteomalacia (2)[C]:
  - Serum phosphorus: Decreased
  - Plasma calcium: Decreased/Normal
  - Serum calcidiol: Decreased
  - Alkaline phosphatase: Increased
- In adults with phosphate-wasting osteomalacia (2)[C]:
  - Serum phosphorous: Decreased
  - Phosphate clearance: Increased
  - Serum calcium: Normal
  - Alkaline phosphatase: Normal

Initial Tests (lab, imaging)

- Blood tests:
  - Serum calcium (total and ionized), phosphate, BUN, creatinine, electrolytes
  - Serum calcidiol (25-hydroxy vitamin D_3)
  - Alkaline phosphatase
  - Parathyroid hormone
- Urinalysis:
  - Calcium, phosphate, creatinine in spot urine sample
  - pH, protein, and glucose
- Anteroposterior radiograph of rapidly growing skeletal areas, include knees, wrists, and anterior rib ends may show Looser's transformation zones.
- Children: Radiographic changes in rapidly growing skeletal areas (knee, wrist), including widening of the distal epiphysis, fraying and widening of the metaphysis, and angular deformities of the arm and leg bones (1)[C]

Diagnostic Procedures/Other

The most accurate diagnosis is made by bone biopsy using double tetracycline labeling. Tetracyclines are deposited as a band at the mineralization front and, because they are fluorescent, they are easily visualized under a fluorescence microscope. After 2 courses of the antibiotic, separated by a period of days, the growth rate of the skeleton can be estimated in iliac crest biopsies by measuring the distance between the bands of deposited tetracycline. In normal adults, this distance is ~1 micron/d:

- 2 changes occur in osteomalacia:
  - Distance between tetracycline bands is reduced
  - Unmineralized matrix appears as a widened osteoid seam (>15 microns), and the osteoid volume is >10%.
- Both features are necessary for the diagnosis because other disorders may show one of these findings (2)[C].
- Bone biopsy is not usually done in adults because the diagnosis can be made from the history, physical exam, and a combination of laboratory and radiologic studies.

Test Interpretation

- Children (1)[C]:
  - Widening of distal physis
  - Fraying and widening of the metaphysis
  - Angular deformities of arm and leg bones
- Adults:
  - Most common: Reduced bone density with thinning of the cortex
  - Changes in vertebral bodies: Loss of radiologic distinctness and concavity of the vertebral body
  - Characteristic finding: Looser's zones:
    - Pseudofractures, fissures, or narrow radiolucent lines, 2–5 mm in width with sclerotic borders
    - Usually located at the femoral neck, on the medial part of the femoral shaft, immediately under the lesser trochanter, or a few centimeters beneath the pubic and ischial rami

 TREATMENT

A combination of calcium and vitamin D is recommended:

- A study in Nigerian children with nutritional rickets showed that treatment with calcium and vitamin D combined compared with treatment with vitamin D alone is more likely to produce radiographic evidence of nearly complete healing of rickets (58% vs. 19%) (3)[B].

MEDICATION

First Line

- Children with vitamin D–deficiency rickets:
  - Ergocalciferol (calciferol) 150,000/300,000 IU single dose:
    - Can be administered IM or PO in liquid or capsule form
    - Capsules can be softened in water and mixed with food
  - Calcium 1,000 mg/d PO
- Adults with vitamin D–deficiency osteomalacia:
  - Ergocalciferol (calciferol) 50,000 IU once or twice per week for 6–12 months
  - Followed by ergocalciferol 400 IU/d
  - If the deficiency is due to malabsorption:
    - Ergocalciferol: 10,000–50,000 IU/d
    - Calcidiol: 0.05–0.125 mg/d
  - Calcium 1,000 mg/d PO:
    - If the patient has malabsorption, 4 g/d of calcium

ADDITIONAL THERAPIES

Calcium and phosphorus supplementation if serum levels are low

SURGERY/OTHER PROCEDURES

Surgery may be necessary to repair severe bone abnormalities.

 ONGOING CARE

FOLLOW-UP RECOMMENDATIONS

- For children, monitor:
  - Serum calcium, phosphorus, alkaline phosphatase, calcidiol:
    - Serum phosphorus should increase during the 1st week of treatment, followed by an increase in serum calcium
  - Urinary calcium and phosphorus levels, spot urine calcium
- For adults taking calcium supplements, monitor:
  - Plasma concentration and urinary levels of calcium

PROGNOSIS

- Varies depending on the etiology
- Vitamin D deficiency causes of rickets:
  - Radiographic findings will normalize within 1 week of treatment.
  - Reversible physical findings will normalize within 6 months of treatment.

COMPLICATIONS

- Fractures: Typically involve the ribs, vertebrae, and long bones
- Osteomyelitis
- Renal failure
- Renal tubular acidosis
- Hypocalcemic seizures/muscle spasms
- Growth deformity and bowing of the long bones in children

REFERENCES

1. Wagner CL, Greer FR, American Academy of Pediatrics Section on Breastfeeding, et al. Prevention of rickets and vitamin D deficiency in infants, children, and adolescents. *Pediatrics*. 2008;122(5):1142–1152.
2. Bingham CT, Fitzpatrick LA. Noninvasive testing in the diagnosis of osteomalacia. *Am J Med*. 1993; 95:519.
3. Thacher TD, Fischer PR, Pettifor JM, et al. A comparison of calcium, vitamin D or both for nutritional rickets in Nigerian children. *N Engl J Med*. 1999;341(8):563.

 CODES

ICD10

- E55.0 Rickets, active
- M83.9 Adult osteomalacia, unspecified
- N25.0 Renal osteodystrophy

CLINICAL PEARLS

In the US, occurs almost exclusively in breast-fed infants without vitamin D supplementation or sun exposure. Ensure adequate vitamin D supplementation.

O

OSTEOMYELITIS

Colleen M. Prinzivalli, PharmD, BCPS • Michael C. Barros, PharmD, BCPS, BCACP • J. Michael O'Connell, Jr., MD

BASICS

DESCRIPTION

- An acute or chronic inflammation of the bone. Osteomyelitis can occur as a result of hematogenous seeding, contiguous spread of infection, or direct inoculation into intact bone (trauma or surgery).
- 2 major classification systems (1):
  - Waldvogel classification:
    ○ Classified according to the duration of the disease (acute or chronic), the mechanism of infection (hematogenous or contiguous), and the presence of vascular insufficiency
  - Cierny-Mader classification:
    ○ Based on the portion of bone affected, the physiologic status of the host, and other risk factors
- Special situations:
  - Vertebral osteomyelitis (2,3):
    ○ Acute, subacute, or chronic
    ○ May result from hematogenous seeding, direct inoculation, or contiguous spread
    ○ Back pain is most common initial symptom.
    ○ Lumbar spine is most commonly involved, followed by thoracic spine.
  - Infections of prosthetic joints:
    ○ Obtaining specific diagnosis and targeted therapy quicker (easy access)
    ○ X-ray of joint initially done, then 3-phase bone scan, since MRI/CT scans of limited use in this circumstance
    ○ Treat with combination of antibiotics, including rifampin, especially in prosthetic joint infections.
  - Posttraumatic infections:
    ○ Depends on type of fracture, level of contamination, and severity of tissue injury
    ○ Tibia most commonly involved
- System(s) affected: Musculoskeletal

EPIDEMIOLOGY

- Predominant age: Commonly seen in older adults
- Predominant sex: Male > Female
- Hematogenous osteomyelitis:
  - Adults (most patients >50): Vertebral
  - Children: Long bones
- Contiguous osteomyelitis: Predominantly found in patients with diabetes mellitus or vascular insufficiency

Incidence

- Incidence is low due to high resistance of normal bone to infection; occurs in patients with risk factor.
- 25% lifetime risk of diabetics of developing foot complication

Prevalence

Up to 66% of diabetics with foot ulcers (1)

ETIOLOGY AND PATHOPHYSIOLOGY

- Infection is caused by biofilm bacteria, which protects bacteria from antimicrobial agents and host immune responses (3).
- Acute: Suppurative infection of bone with edema and vascular compromise leading to sequestra
- Chronic: Presence of necrotic bone or sequestra or recurrence of previous infection
- Hematogenous osteomyelitis (commonly a monomicrobial infection) (1):
  - *S. aureus* (most common) with high percentage of MRSA (50%) (3)

- Coagulase-negative staphylococci and aerobic gram-negative bacteria
  - *Salmonella* sp. (sickle-cell patients)
  - *M. tuberculosis* and fungi (rare) in endemic areas or in immunocompromised hosts
- Contiguous focus osteomyelitis (commonly a polymicrobial infection):
  - Diabetes or vascular insufficiency:
    ○ Coagulase-positive and -negative staphylococci
    ○ Streptococci, gram-negative bacilli, anaerobes (*Peptostreptococcus* sp.)
  - Prosthetic device:
    ○ Coagulase-negative staphylococci and *S. aureus*

RISK FACTORS

- Diabetes mellitus
- Recent trauma/surgery
- Foreign body (e.g., prosthetic implant)
- Neuropathy and vascular insufficiency
- Immunosuppression
- Sickle cell disease
- Injection drug use
- Previous osteomyelitis

GENERAL PREVENTION

- Antibiotic prophylaxis:
  - Clean bone surgery:
    ○ Antibiotics should be administered IV from 30 minutes before skin incision to no longer than 24 hours after the operation.
  - Closed fractures:
    ○ Antistaphylococcal penicillins or 1st- or 2nd-generation cephalosporins
  - Open fractures:
    ○ In patients who can receive antibiotics within 6 hours of injury and who receive prompt operative treatment, give antistaphylococcal penicillins or 1st- or 2nd-generation cephalosporins for 24 hours.
- All patients with diabetes mellitus should have a complete annual foot examination by a health care professional (1).

COMMONLY ASSOCIATED CONDITIONS

See "Risk Factors."

DIAGNOSIS

HISTORY

- Hematogenous osteomyelitis:
  - Conditions predisposing to bacteremia (diabetes, renal insufficiency, invasive procedures, IV drug use) (3)
  - Other sites of infection
- Contiguous osteomyelitis and vascular insufficiency–associated infection:
  - Recent trauma/surgery within 1–2 months
  - Presence of prosthetic device
  - History of diabetes
- Chronic osteomyelitis:
  - History of acute osteomyelitis

PHYSICAL EXAM

- Restriction of movement of the involved extremity or refusal to bear weight
- Pain or tenderness in the infected area
- Signs of localized inflammation
- Fever and/or chills
- Motor and sensory deficits (vertebral infection)

- Visible or palpable bone with a metal probe ("positive probe-to-bone test")
- Ulcer >2 cm wide and >3 mm deep increases likelihood in diabetic foot ulcers (1)[B].
- In patients with diabetes, classic signs and symptoms of infection may be masked due to vascular disease and neuropathy.
- In diabetics, otherwise unexplained deviations in glycemic control may be evident, such as hyperglycemia.

DIFFERENTIAL DIAGNOSIS

- Systemic infection from other source
- Aseptic bone infarction
- Localized inflammation or infection of overlying skin and soft tissues (e.g., gout)
- Brodie abscess
- Neuropathic joint disease (Charcot foot)
- Fractures/Trauma
- Tumor

DIAGNOSTIC TESTS & INTERPRETATION

Initial Tests (lab, imaging)

Labs (1)[C]:
- WBC is not a reliable indicator and can be normal even when infection is present (3).
- CRP is usually elevated but nonspecific.
- ESR is high in most cases:
  - ESR >70 mm/h increases likelihood in diabetic lower extremity ulcer (4)[B].
- Drugs that may alter lab results: Antimicrobial agents given prior to culture
- Disorders that may alter lab results: Immunosuppression, chronic inflammatory disease, other/adjacent sites of infection
- Routine radiography standard first-line imaging (5)[C]: Classic triad for osteomyelitis is demineralization, periosteal reaction, and bone destruction:
  - Bone destruction is not apparent on plain films until after 10–21 days of infection.
  - Bone must undergo 30–50% destruction before damage is evident on films.
- MRI:
  - For visualization of septic arthritis, spinal infection, and diabetic foot infections (5)[C]
  - T_1-weighted image: Low signal intensity
  - T_2-weighted image: High signal intensity
  - MRI with gadolinium sensitivity and specificity range from 60–100% and 50–90%, respectively (3)[C].
- CT:
  - Better than standard radiography in fragments and sequestration, but inferior to MRI in soft-tissue and bone marrow assessment
  - Useful to define surrounding soft tissues and identify sequestra
  - Bone scan is typically 1st test after plain x-ray in setting of joint prosthesis.

Follow-Up Tests & Special Considerations

- A persistently elevated CRP but not ESR at 4–6 weeks can be associated with persistent osteomyelitis (1)[C].
- Patients receiving prolonged antimicrobial therapy should have the following tests to monitor for adverse reactions (1)[C]:
  - Weekly CBC
  - Liver and kidney function tests

844

- Radionuclide scanning (e.g., technetium, indium, or gallium) is useful when diagnosis is ambiguous or extent of disease is in question, but is limited by reports of low sensitivity and specificity.
- MRI is not helpful in assessing the response to therapy due to persistence of bony edema (1)[C].

Diagnostic Procedures/Other
- Cultures:
  - Definitive diagnosis is made by blood culture (hematogenous) and by needle aspiration/bone biopsy, with subsequent demonstration of the micro-organism by culture and sensitivity or histology.
  - Appropriate pathogen isolated in blood culture combined with radiographic evidence may obviate need for bone culture.
  - Wound swabs and sinus tract cultures have utility for infection control and correlate well with the presence of *S. aureus* in deep cultures.
- Image-guided bone biopsy for vertebral osteomyelitis unless positive blood culture and positive radiographic evidence

Test Interpretation
Inflammatory process of bone with pyogenic bacteria, necrosis

 ## TREATMENT

GENERAL MEASURES
- Adequate nutrition
- Smoking-cessation counseling
- Control of diabetes

MEDICATION
- Empiric therapy should be directed toward most probable organism and tailored once culture results are available.
- Optimal antimicrobial concentration at infection site is essential, hence vascular perfusion to site should be considered.
- Antibiotic dosing depends on creatinine clearance (utilizing Cockroft-Gault equation).
- Duration of therapy 4–6 weeks for acute osteomyelitis and generally >8 weeks for chronic osteomyelitis or MRSA infection
- In children, evidence suggests that early transition from intravenous to oral therapy, after 3–4 days in patients responding well, followed by oral therapy to a total of 3 weeks, may be as effective as longer courses for uncomplicated acute osteomyelitis (6)[A].
- Resistance to fluoroquinolones develops quickly; however, they may be considered as oral options for chronic suppression.

First Line
- *S. aureus* or coagulase-negative staphylococci (1)[C]:
  - MSSA: β-lactam at high dose (nafcillin or oxacillin 2 g IV q6h) *or* cefazolin 2 g IV q8h (2,7)
  - MRSA: Vancomycin 15 mg/kg IV q8–12h (use q8h interval if CrCl >70 mL/min) with target trough of 15–20 mcg/mL
  - Vancomycin and clindamycin often used together (8)[A]
- *Streptococcus* sp. (2):
  - Penicillin G 4 million U q4–6h

- *Enterobacter* sp. (2,6):
  - Fluoroquinolone (levofloxacin 750 mg IV/PO q24h or moxifloxacin 400 mg IV/PO q24h) *or* ceftriaxone 2 g IV q24h
- *Pseudomonas aeruginosa* (2):
  - Cefepime or ceftazidime 2 g IV q8–12h (consider adding aminoglycoside)
- Anaerobes (2,6):
  - Clindamycin 600 mg IV q8h (300–450 mg PO q6–8h)

Second Line
- *S. aureus* (1)[C],(2):
  - MSSA: Fluoroquinolone plus rifampin (levofloxacin 750 mg IV/PO q24h plus rifampin 300 mg PO q12h *or* 600 mg PO q24h)
  - MRSA: Linezolid 600 mg PO/IV q12h *or* daptomycin 6 mg/kg IV q24h
- *Streptococcus* sp. (2):
  - Ceftriaxone 2 g IV q24h *or* cefazolin 2 g IV q8h
- *Enterobacter* sp. (quinolone-resistant, including extended-spectrum β-lactamase–producing *E. coli*) (2):
  - Carbapenem (imipenem/cilastatin) 500 mg IV q6h
- *Pseudomonas aeruginosa* (2):
  - Piperacillin/Tazobactam 4.5 g IV q6h
- Anaerobes (2):
  - Metronidazole 500 mg IV/PO q6–8h

ADDITIONAL THERAPIES
- Hyperbaric oxygen therapy may be useful as an adjunctive treatment, but data are limited.
- Negative pressure wound therapy is also a possible adjunctive treatment.

SURGERY/OTHER PROCEDURES
Surgical drainage, dead-space management, adequate soft tissue coverage, restoration of blood supply, and removal of necrotic tissues are of utmost importance to effect cure.

Pediatric Considerations
Medullary osteomyelitis (stage 1) in children may be treated without surgical intervention.

IN-PATIENT CONSIDERATIONS
Admission Criteria/Initial Stabilization
Correct electrolyte imbalances, hyperglycemia, azotemia, and acidosis; control pain.

Nursing
Bed rest and immobilization of the involved bone and/or joint

Discharge Criteria
Clinical and laboratory evidence of resolving infection and appropriate outpatient therapy

 ## ONGOING CARE

FOLLOW-UP RECOMMENDATIONS
Patient Monitoring
Blood levels of antimicrobial agents, ESR, CRP, and repeat plain radiography

PATIENT EDUCATION
Diabetic glycemic control and foot care

PROGNOSIS
- Superficial and medullary osteomyelitis treated with antimicrobial and surgical therapy have a response rate of 90–100%.
- Up to 36% recurrence in diabetics
- Increased mortality after amputation

COMPLICATIONS
- Abscess formation
- Bacteremia
- Fracture/nonunion
- Loosening of prosthetic implant
- Postoperative infection
- Sinus tract formation can be associated with neoplasms, especially in presence of long-standing infection.

REFERENCES

1. Sia IG, Berbari EF. Osteomyelitis. *Best Prac Res Clin Rheum*. 2006;20:1065–1081.
2. Zimmerli W. Clinical practice. Vertebral osteomyelitis. *N Engl J Med*. 2010;362: 1022–1029.
3. Bhavan KP, Marschall J, Olsen MA, et al. The epidemiology of hematogenous vertebral osteomyelitis: A cohort study in a tertiary care hospital. *BMC Infect Dis*. 2010;10:158.
4. Dinh MT. Diagnostic accuracy of the physical examination and imaging tests for osteomyelitis underlying diabetic foot ulcers: Meta analysis. *Clin Inf Dis*. 2008;47:519–527.
5. Stumpe KD, Strobel K. Osteomyelitis and arthritis. *Semin Nucl Med*. 2009;39:27–35.
6. Howard-Jones AR, Isaacs D. Systematic review of duration and choice of systemic antibiotic therapy for acute haematogenous bacterial osteomyelitis in children. *J Paediatr Child Health*. 2013;48: 760–768.
7. Fraimow HS. Systemic antimicrobial therapy in osteomyelitis. *Semin Plast Surg*. 2009;23:90–99.
8. Vardakas KZ, Kontopidis I, Gkegkes ID. Incidence, characteristics, and outcomes of patients with bone and joint infections due to community-associated methicillin-resistant Staphylococcus aureus: A systematic review. *Eur J Clin Microbiol Infect Dis*. 2013;32:711–721.

 ## CODES

ICD10
- M86.00 Acute hematogenous osteomyelitis, unspecified site
- M86.9 Osteomyelitis, unspecified
- M86.10 Other acute osteomyelitis, unspecified site

CLINICAL PEARLS
- Hematogenous osteomyelitis is usually monomicrobial, whereas osteomyelitis due to contiguous spread or direct inoculation is usually polymicrobial.
- Acute osteomyelitis typically presents with gradual onset of pain.
- Treatment of osteomyelitis often requires both surgical debridement and at least 6 weeks of antimicrobial therapy.

O

OSTEOPOROSIS

Nora E. Gimpel, MD

 BASICS

DESCRIPTION
A skeletal disease characterized by compromised bone strength that predisposes an individual to an increased risk of fracture

EPIDEMIOLOGY
- Predominant age: Elderly >60 years of age
- Predominant sex: Female > Male (80%/20%)

Incidence
Of persons age >50 years, 9% had osteoporosis at either the femoral neck or lumbar spine.

Prevalence
- 12 million Americans older than 50 years have osteoporosis.
- Women >50 years of age: 24%
- Men >50 years of age: 7.5%
- 50% of postmenopausal women will have an osteoporotic fracture during their lifetime and 15% will experience a hip fracture

ETIOLOGY AND PATHOPHYSIOLOGY
- Imbalance between bone resorption and bone formation
- Trabecular bone (vertebral) more active than cortical (hip) bone
- Aging
- Hypoestrogenemia

Genetics
- Familial predisposition
- More common in Caucasians and Asians than in African Americans and Hispanics

RISK FACTORS
- Nonmodifiable:
  - Advanced age (>65 years)
  - Female gender
  - Caucasian or Asian
  - Family history of osteoporosis
  - History of atraumatic fracture
- Modifiable:
  - Low body weight (58 kg or body mass index [BMI] <21)
  - Calcium/Vitamin D deficiency
  - Inadequate physical activity
  - Cigarette smoking
  - Excessive alcohol intake (>3 drinks/d)
  - Medications: Chronic corticosteroids, excessive thyroid hormone replacement, medroxyprogesterone acetate, heparin, proton pump inhibitors

GENERAL PREVENTION
The aim in the prevention and treatment of osteoporosis is to prevent fracture:
- Depending on the severity of the osteoporosis, between 9–60 patients need to be treated for 3 years to prevent 1 vertebral fracture (1).
- Regularly perform weight-bearing exercise
- Current evidence is insufficient to assess the balance of the benefits and harms of combined vitamin D and calcium supplementation for primary prevention of fractures in premenopausal women and men [I statement] (2).
- There is good evidence that daily supplementation with 400 IU of vitamin D and 1,000 mg of calcium has no effect on the incidence of fractures in postmenopausal women.

- The benefits and harms of higher doses taken to prevent fractures in noninstitutionalized postmenopausal women are not well defined.
- Avoid smoking
- Limit alcohol consumption (<3 drinks/d).
- Take measures to avoid falls
- Screen:
  - All women ≥65 years of age
  - Screen women <60 years of age with ≥10-year fracture risk (utilizing the WHO's Fracture Risk Assessment Tool [FRAX]) >9.3%
  - The National Osteoporosis Foundation recommends screening men age >70 years.

COMMONLY ASSOCIATED CONDITIONS
- Malabsorption syndromes: Gastrectomy, inflammatory bowel disease, celiac disease
- Hypoestrogenism: Menopause, hypogonadism, eating disorders, elite athletes
- Chronic liver disease, hemochromatosis
- Endocrinopathies: Hyperparathyroidism, hyperthyroidism, hypercortisolism
- Multiple myeloma, multiple sclerosis, osteomalacia, rheumatoid arthritis, chronic obstructive pulmonary disease (COPD), HIV/AIDS
- Medications: Antiepileptics, aromatase inhibitors (raloxifene), SSRI, warfarin, thyroid hormone (in supraphysiologic doses)

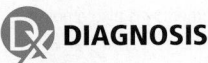 **DIAGNOSIS**

HISTORY
- Review risk factors
- Online risk factor assessment tools are available:
  - FRAX (www.sheffield.ac.uk/FRAX/index.htm)
  - Garvan (http://garvan.org.au/promotions/bone-fracture-risk/calculator/)
- Often no clinical findings until fracture occurs

PHYSICAL EXAM
- Thoracic kyphosis
- Height loss >1.5 cm

DIFFERENTIAL DIAGNOSIS
- Multiple myeloma/other neoplasms
- Osteomalacia
- Type I collagen mutations
- Osteogenesis imperfecta

DIAGNOSTIC TESTS & INTERPRETATION
Dual-energy x-ray absorptiometry (DEXA) of the lumbar spine/hip is considered the gold standard for osteoporosis diagnosis.

Initial Tests (lab, imaging)
Consider in screening for secondary osteoporosis:
- Serum 25-hydroxyvitamin D
- CBC
- Serum chemistry, including serum calcium, phosphorus, total protein, albumin, liver enzymes, creatinine, alkaline phosphatase, electrolytes
- Urinalysis (24-hour collection) for calcium, sodium, and creatinine (to identify calcium malabsorption of hypercalciuria)
- DEXA of the lumbar spine/hip is the gold standard for measuring bone mineral density (BMD) and making a diagnosis of osteoporosis.
- A minimum of 2 years may be needed to reliably measure a change in BMD

- BMD is expressed in terms of T-scores and Z-scores:
  - T-score is the number of standard deviations (SDs) a patient's BMD deviates from the mean for young, normal (age 25–40 years) control individuals of the same sex.
  - WHO defines normal BMD as a T-score ≥−1, osteopenia as a T-score between −1 and −2.5, and osteoporosis as a T-score ≤−2.5.
  - WHO thresholds can be used for postmenopausal women and men >50 years of age.
  - The Z-score is a comparison of the patient's BMD with an age-matched population.
  - A Z-score <−2 should prompt evaluation for causes of secondary osteoporosis.
- Ultrasound densitometry is not as accurate as DEXA, and no studies support its use in determining therapy.
- Plain radiographs lack sensitivity to diagnose osteoporosis, but an abnormality (e.g., widened intervertebral spaces, rib fractures, vertebral compression fractures) should prompt evaluation.

Follow-Up Tests & Special Considerations
Further labs depending on initial evaluation, Z-score −2.5 or lower or young age:
- Parathyroid hormone (PTH) and ionized calcium
- Thyroid-stimulating hormone (TSH)
- Testosterone levels (hypogonadism in men)
- Serum protein electrophoresis and free κ and λ light chains (multiple myeloma)
- Urinary-free cortisol (Cushing disease)
- Tissue transglutaminase antibodies (celiac disease)
- Markers of bone resorption (urine N-telopeptides of type 1 collagen, serum C-telopeptides of type 1 collagen, serum N-terminal propeptide of type 1 procollagen): No prospective studies supporting use in osteoporosis diagnosis and management; potential role for identifying patients at high risk for fracture and monitoring response to therapy

Diagnostic Procedures/Other
Bone biopsy recommended for patients with bone disease and renal failure to establish the correct diagnosis.

Test Interpretation
- Reduced skeletal mass, trabecular bone thinned or lost more than cortical bone
- Osteoclast and osteoblast number variable
- No evidence of other metabolic bone diseases and no increase in unmineralized osteoid
- Bone marrow normal/atrophic

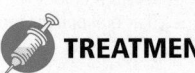 **TREATMENT**

- Patients with a T-score ≤−2.5 with no risk factors
- All postmenopausal women who have had an osteoporotic vertebral/hip fracture
- All postmenopausal women who have BMD values consistent with osteoporosis (T-score ≤2.5) at the lumbar spine, femoral neck, or total hip region.
- Postmenopausal women with T-scores from −1.0 to −2.5 and a 10-year risk, based on the FRAX calculator, of a major osteoporotic fracture (spine, hip, shoulder, and wrist) of at least 20% or hip of at least 3% (3)[B]

- Treat men >50 years who present with a hip or vertebral fracture or a T-score <−2.5 after appropriate evaluation; however, evidence for the effectiveness of treatment of osteoporosis in men is limited.

MEDICATION
Vitamin D 800 IU/d

First Line
- Bisphosphonates:
  - Alendronate 10 mg PO daily or 70 mg PO weekly
  - Risedronate 5 mg PO daily, 35 mg PO weekly, 75 mg PO twice monthly, or 150 mg PO monthly
  - Zoledronic acid 5 mg IV yearly
- These drugs become incorporated into skeletal tissue, where they inhibit the resorption of bone by osteoclasts.
- The evidence on the risk for atrial fibrillation with bisphosphonates is conflicting (4).
- Osteonecrosis of the jaw has been associated with bisphosphonates in case reports, particularly in patients with cancer who receive high doses.
- Possible risk of midfemur fractures in patients receiving bisphosphonates for more than 5 years (4)
- Avoid oral bisphosphonates in patients with (5):
  - Delayed esophageal emptying owing to esophageal abnormalities such as achalasia/stricture
  - Inability to stand/sit upright for at least 30–60 minutes after taking the bisphosphonates
  - Hypocalcemia (correct prior to initiating therapy)
  - Severe renal impairment (creatine clearance [CrCl] ≤30 mL/min for risedronate and ibandronate and ≤35 mL/min for alendronate and zoledronic acid)
  - Ibandronate increases bone density but does not appear to decrease fractures.

Second Line
- Raloxifene 60 mg PO daily:
  - Selective estrogen receptor modulator with positive effects on BMD and fracture risk, but no stimulatory action on breasts/uterus
  - Nonvertebral of hip fracture efficacy has not been demonstrated (6); increases risk of thromboembolism
  - Additional side effects include menopausal symptoms (hot flashes and night sweats)
- Teriparatide 20 mg SC daily:
  - Recombinant formulation of PTH
  - Works anabolically to stimulate the growth of bone through osteoblastic activation
  - Primarily indicated for those with severe osteoporosis that necessitates aggressive therapy
  - Studies have shown a reduction in the incidence of vertebral fractures by 65% and nonvertebral fractures by 54% (3).
  - No data exist on its safety and efficacy after >2 years of use.
- Estrogen 0.625 mg PO daily (with progesterone if patient has a uterus): Effective in prevention and treatment of osteoporosis (35% reduction in hip and vertebral fractures after 5 years of use), but the risks (e.g., increased rates of myocardial infarction, stroke, breast cancer, pulmonary embolus, and deep vein thrombosis) must be weighed against the benefits and have decreased interest in this regimen.
- Strontium 2 g PO daily (5)[C]:
  - Appears to inhibit bone resorption and increase bone formation
  - Available for use in Europe

- Denosumab (6)[C]:
  - Human monoclonal antibody receptor activator of nuclear factor kappa-B ligand (RANKL) receptor
  - Inhibits osteoclast formation
- Calcitonin:
  - PTH antagonist that reduces osteoclastic activity, therefore decreasing bone turnover
  - Has been shown to increase BMD, but no studies have shown conclusively a reduction in the occurrence of fractures
  - May decrease acute vertebral compression-fracture pain (analgesic)

ISSUES FOR REFERRAL
Endocrinology for recurrent bone loss/fracture

ADDITIONAL THERAPIES
- Weight-bearing exercise 30 min 3/week
- Smoking cessation
- Physical therapy to help with muscle strengthening

SURGERY/OTHER PROCEDURES
Options for patients with painful vertebral compression fractures failing medical treatment:
- Vertebroplasty: Orthopedic cement is injected into the compressed vertebral body.
- Kyphoplasty: A balloon is expanded within the compressed vertebral body to reconstruct volume of vertebrae. Cement is injected into the space.

COMPLEMENTARY AND ALTERNATIVE MEDICINE
Isoflavones not better than placebo for fracture risk

IN-PATIENT CONSIDERATIONS
Admission Criteria/Initial Stabilization
Inpatient care for pain control of acute back pain secondary to new vertebral fractures and for acute treatment of femoral and pelvic fractures

Discharge Criteria
Rehabilitation, nursing home, or home care may be needed following peripheral fractures

 ## ONGOING CARE

FOLLOW-UP RECOMMENDATIONS
Patient Monitoring
- Weight-bearing exercises, such as walking, jogging, stair climbing, and tai chi, have been shown to decrease falls.
- All successful studies on the treatment of osteoporosis involve weight-bearing exercise.
- BMD should be tested no earlier than 2 years after starting bisphosphonate. It is uncertain whether repeat DEXA scanning is of value.
- For many women, 5 years of treatment with a bisphosphonate is as good as 10 years of treatment. Those at high risk for vertebral fracture or with very low BMD may benefit by continuing treatment beyond 5 years.
- Physicians prescribing bisphosphonates should advise patients of the small risk of osteonecrosis and encourage dental examinations (7)
- Limited data to guide decision-making about "drug holiday." Drug holiday may not be justified for patients at high risk but could be done for patients at low risk (1).

DIET
- Diet to maintain normal body weight
- Vitamin D (see "General Prevention")

PATIENT EDUCATION
- National Osteoporosis Foundation: www.nof.org

PROGNOSIS
- With treatment, 80% of patients stabilize skeletal manifestations, increase bone mass and mobility, and have reduced pain.
- 15% of vertebral and 20–40% of hip fractures may lead to chronic care and/or premature death.

COMPLICATIONS
- Severe, disabling pain

REFERENCES
1. McClung M, Harris S, Miller P, et al. Bisphosphonates therapy for osteoporosis: Benefits, risk, and drug holiday. *Am J Med*. 2013;126: 13–20.
2. U.S. Preventive Services Task Force recommendation statement. *Ann Intern Med*. 2013;158:I–36.
3. Christenson ES, Jiang X, Kagan R, et al. Osteoporosis management in post-menopausal women. *Minerva Ginecol*. 2012;64:181–194.
4. Nordin C. Screening for osteoporosis: U.S. Preventive Services Task Force recommendation statement. *Ann Intern Med*. 2011;155:276.
5. Poole KE, Compston JE. Bisphosphonates in the treatment of osteoporosis. *BMJ*. 2012;344:e3211.
6. Watts NB, Bilezikian JP, Camacho PM, et al. American Association of Clinical Endocrinologists medical guidelines for clinical practice for the diagnosis and treatment of postmenopausal osteoporosis. *Endocr Pract*. 2010;16(Suppl 3): 1–37.
7. Heng C, Badner VM, Johson R, et al. Bisphosphonates-related osteonecrosis of the jaw in patients with osteoporosis. *Am Fam Physician*. 2012;85:1135–1137.

ADDITIONAL READING
Rao SS, Budhwar N, Ashfaque A, et al. Osteoporosis in men. *Am Fam Physician*. 2010;82:503–508.

 ## CODES

ICD10
- M80.00XA Age-rel osteopor w current path fracture, unsp site, init
- M81.0 Age-related osteoporosis w/o current pathological fracture
- M80.08XA Age-rel osteopor w current path fracture, vertebra(e), init

CLINICAL PEARLS
- Screen all women ≥65 years of age with DEXA scans.
- Screen both men and women ≥60 years of age at increased risk for osteoporosis with DEXA scans.
- Premenopausal women with osteoporosis should be screened for secondary causes, such as malabsorption syndromes, hyperparathyroidism, hyperthyroidism, and medication sensitivity.
- Evaluate and treat all patients presenting with fractures from minimal trauma.
- If the patient is not responding to treatment, consider screening for a secondary, treatable cause of osteoporosis.

0

OTITIS EXTERNA
Douglas S. Parks, MD

 BASICS

DESCRIPTION
Inflammation of the external auditory canal:
- Acute diffuse otitis externa: The most common form; an infectious process, usually bacterial, occasionally fungal (10%)
- Acute circumscribed otitis externa: Synonymous with furuncle; associated with infection of the hair follicle, a superficial cellulitic form of otitis externa
- Chronic otitis externa: Same as acute diffuse but of longer duration (>6 weeks)
- Eczematous otitis externa: May accompany typical atopic eczema or other primary skin conditions
- Necrotizing malignant otitis externa: An infection that extends into the deeper tissues adjacent to the canal; may include osteomyelitis and cellulitis; rare in children
- System(s) affected: Skin/Exocrine
- Synonym(s): Swimmer's ear

EPIDEMIOLOGY
Incidence
- Unknown; higher in the summer months and in warm, wet climates
- Predominant age: All ages
- Predominant sex: Male = Female

Prevalence
- Acute, chronic, and eczematous: Common
- Necrotizing: Uncommon

ETIOLOGY AND PATHOPHYSIOLOGY
- Acute diffuse otitis externa:
  - Traumatized external canal (e.g., from use of cotton swab)
  - Bacterial infection (90%): *Pseudomonas* (67%), *Staphylococcus, Streptococcus,* gram-negative rods
  - Fungal infection (10%): *Aspergillus* (90%), *Candida, Phycomycetes, Rhizopus, Actinomyces, Penicillium*
- Chronic otitis externa: Bacterial infection: *Pseudomonas*
- Eczematous otitis externa (associated with primary skin disorder):
  - Eczema
  - Seborrhea
  - Psoriasis
  - Neurodermatitis
  - Contact dermatitis
  - Purulent otitis media
  - Sensitivity to topical medications
- Necrotizing otitis externa:
  - Invasive bacterial infection: *Pseudomonas,* increasing incidence of MRSA
  - Associated with immunosuppression

RISK FACTORS
- Acute and chronic otitis externa:
  - Traumatization of external canal
  - Swimming
  - Hot, humid weather
  - Hearing aid use

- Eczematous: Primary skin disorder
- Necrotizing otitis externa in adults:
  - Advanced age
  - Diabetes mellitus (DM)
  - Debilitating disease
  - AIDS
  - Immunosuppression
- Necrotizing otitis externa in children (rare):
  - Leukopenia
  - Malnutrition
  - DM
  - Diabetes insipidus

GENERAL PREVENTION
- Avoid prolonged exposure to moisture.
- Use preventive antiseptics (acidifying solutions with 2% acetic acid [white vinegar] diluted 50/50 with water or isopropyl alcohol, or 2% acetic acid with aluminum acetate [less irritating]) after swimming and bathing.
- Treat predisposing skin conditions.
- Eliminate self-inflicted trauma to canal with cotton swabs and other foreign objects.
- Diagnose and treat underlying systemic conditions.
- Use ear plugs when swimming.

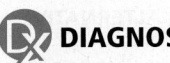 **DIAGNOSIS**

HISTORY
Variable-length history of itching, plugging of ear, ear pain, and discharge from ear

PHYSICAL EXAM
- Ear canal red, containing purulent discharge and debris
- Pain on manipulation of the pinnae
- Possible periauricular adenitis
- Possible eczema of pinna
- Cranial nerve (VII, IX–XII) involvement (extremely rare)

DIFFERENTIAL DIAGNOSIS
- Idiopathic ear pain
- Otitis media with perforation
- Hearing loss
- Cranial nerve (VII, IX–XII) palsy with necrotizing otitis externa
- Wisdom tooth eruption
- Basal cell or squamous cell carcinoma

DIAGNOSTIC TESTS & INTERPRETATION
- Gram stain and culture of canal discharge (occasionally helpful)
- Antibiotic pretreatment may affect results.
- Radiologic evaluation of deep tissues in necrotizing otitis externa with high-resolution CT scan, MRI, gallium scan, and bone scan

Test Interpretation
- Acute and chronic otitis externa: Desquamation of superficial epithelium of external canal with infection
- Eczematous otitis externa: Pathologic findings consistent with primary skin disorder; secondary infection on occasion
- Necrotizing otitis externa: Vasculitis, thrombosis, and necrosis of involved tissues; osteomyelitis

 TREATMENT

Outpatient treatment, except for resistant cases and necrotizing otitis externa

GENERAL MEASURES
- Cleaning the external canal may facilitate recovery.
- Analgesics as appropriate for pain
- Antipruritic and antihistamines (eczematous form)
- Ear wick (Pope) for nearly occluded ear canal

MEDICATION
- Resistance is an increasing problem. *Pseudomonas* is the most common bacteria, and it is more susceptible to fluoroquinolones such as ciprofloxacin or ofloxacin, whereas *Staphylococcus* is equally susceptible to both fluoroquinolones and polymyxin B combinations (1)[B]. If a patient has recurring episodes or is not improved in 2 weeks, change the class of antibacterial and consider cultures and sensitivities.
- Oral antibiotics are indicated only if there is associated otitis media or cellulitis of the outer ear (red canal without discharge). Oral antibiotics alone are not effective and markedly increase the risk of progressing to chronic otitis externa.
- Analgesics as needed; narcotics may be necessary. Recurrent otitis externa may be prevented by applying equal parts white vinegar and isopropyl alcohol (OTC rubbing alcohol) to external auditory canals after bathing and swimming.

First Line
- Acute bacterial and chronic otitis externa:
  - Ciprofloxacin 0.3% and dexamethasone 0.1% suspension (Cipro Dex): 3–4 drops b.i.d. × 7 days or ofloxacin (Floxin Otic): 0.3% solution 10 drops once a day × 7 days (2)[A]. Less ototoxicity and reported antibiotic resistance (3)[A], but branded drugs are far more expensive.
  - Neomycin/Polymyxin B/Hydrocortisone (Cortisporin): 5 drops q.i.d. If the tympanic membrane is ruptured, use the suspension; otherwise, the solution may be used; may be ototoxic and resistance-developing in *Staphylococcus* and *Streptococcus* sp. (4)[B]; least expensive
  - Acetic acid 2% with hydrocortisone 1%: 3–5 drops q4–8h × 7 days; may cause minor local stinging. This is as effective as neomycin–polymyxin B (5)[B] but is expensive. It may take up to 2 days longer to achieve resolution of symptoms (2)[A]. A wick may be helpful in severe cases by keeping the canal open and keeping antibiotic solution in contact with infected skin (6)[C].
- Fungal otitis externa:
  - Topical therapy, antiyeast for *Candida* or yeast: 2% acetic acid 3–4 drops q.i.d.; clotrimazole 1% solution; itraconazole oral
  - Parenteral antifungal therapy: Amphotericin B
  - Patients with Ramsay-Hunt syndrome: Acyclovir IV

- Eczematous otitis externa: Topical therapy:
  - Acetic acid 2% in aluminum acetate
  - Aluminum acetate (5%; Burow solution)
  - Steroid cream, lotion, ointment (e.g., triamcinolone 0.1% solution)
  - Antibacterial, if superinfected
- Necrotizing otitis externa:
  - Parenteral antibiotics: Antistaphylococcal and antipseudomonal
  - 4–6 weeks of therapy
  - Quinolones PO × 2–4 weeks

Second Line
- Acute bacterial and chronic otitis externa:
  - Betamethasone 0.05% solution may be as effective as a polymyxin B combination without the risk of ototoxicity or antibiotic resistance. However, the data are not very robust and more study is needed (2)[A].
- Azole antifungals for fungal otitis externa

ISSUES FOR REFERRAL
Resistant cases or those requiring surgical intervention

SURGERY/OTHER PROCEDURES
For necrotizing otitis externa or furuncle

COMPLEMENTARY AND ALTERNATIVE MEDICINE
- OTC white vinegar; 3 drops in affected ear for minor case
- Tea tree oil in various concentrations has been used as an antiseptic (7)[B]. Ototoxicity has been reported in animal studies at very high doses.
- Grapefruit seed extract in various concentrations has been described as useful in the lay literature.

IN-PATIENT CONSIDERATIONS
Admission Criteria/Initial Stabilization
Necrotizing otitis media requiring parenteral antipseudomonal antibiotics

Discharge Criteria
Resolution of infection

ONGOING CARE

FOLLOW-UP RECOMMENDATIONS
No restrictions

Patient Monitoring
- Acute otitis externa:
  - 48 hours after therapy instituted to assess improvement
  - At the end of treatment

- Chronic otitis externa:
  - Every 2–3 weeks for repeated cleansing of canal
  - May require alterations in topical medication, including antibiotics and steroids
- Necrotizing otitis externa:
  - Daily monitoring in hospital for extension of infection
  - Baseline auditory and vestibular testing at beginning and end of therapy

DIET
No restrictions

PROGNOSIS
- Acute otitis externa: Rapid response to therapy with total resolution
- Chronic otitis externa: With repeated cleansing and antibiotic therapy, most cases will resolve. Occasionally, surgical intervention is required for resistant cases.
- Eczematous otitis externa: Resolution will occur with control of the primary skin condition.
- Necrotizing otitis externa: Usually can be managed with débridement and antipseudomonal antibiotics; recurrence rate is 100% when treatment is inadequate. Surgical intervention may be necessary in resistant cases or if there is cranial nerve involvement. Mortality rate is significant, probably secondary to the underlying disease.

COMPLICATIONS
- Mainly a problem with necrotizing otitis externa; may spread to infect contiguous bone and CNS structures
- Acute otitis externa may spread to pinna, causing chondritis.

REFERENCES
1. Dohar JE, Roland P, Wall GM, et al. Differences in bacteriologic treatment failures in acute otitis externa between ciprofloxacin/dexamethasone and neomycin/polymyxin B/hydrocortisone: Results of a combined analysis. *Curr Med Res Opin*. 2009;25: 287–291.
2. Kaushik V, Malik T, Saeed SR, et al. Interventions for acute otitis externa. *Cochrane Database Syst Rev*. 2010;(1):CD004740.
3. Mösges R, Nematian-Samani M, Hellmich M, et al. A meta-analysis of the efficacy of quinolone containing otics in comparison to antibiotic-steroid combination drugs in the local treatment of otitis externa. *Curr Med Res Opin*. 2011;27:2053–2060.
4. Cantrell HF, Lombardy EE, Duncanson FP. Declining susceptibility to neomycin and polymyxin B of pathogens recovered in otitis externa clinical trials. *South Med J*. 2004;97:465–471.
5. van Balen FA, Smit WM, Zuithoff NP. Clinical efficacy of three common treatments in acute otitis externa in primary care: Randomised controlled trial. *BMJ*. 2003;327:1201–1205.
6. Block SL. Otitis externa: Providing relief while avoiding complications. *J Fam Pract*. 2005;54: 669–676.
7. Farnan TB, McCallum J, Awa A. Tea tree oil: In vitro efficacy in otitis externa. *J Laryngol Otol*. 2005;119: 198–201.

SEE ALSO
Algorithm: Ear Pain

CODES
ICD10
- H60.90 Unspecified otitis externa, unspecified ear
- H60.319 Diffuse otitis externa, unspecified ear
- H60.339 Swimmer's ear, unspecified ear

CLINICAL PEARLS
- Acute diffuse otitis externa is the most common form: Bacterial (90%), occasionally fungal (10%).
- Acute circumscribed otitis externa is associated with infection of a hair follicle.
- Chronic otitis externa is the same as acute diffuse but of longer duration (>6 weeks).
- Eczematous otitis externa may accompany typical atopic eczema or other primary skin conditions.
- Necrotizing malignant otitis externa is an infection that extends into the deeper tissues adjacent to the canal. It may include osteomyelitis and cellulitis; it is rare in children.

OTITIS MEDIA
Serena Hon, MD • David B. Gilchrist, MD

 BASICS

DESCRIPTION
- Inflammation of the middle ear; usually accompanied by fluid collection
- Acute otitis media (AOM): Inflammation of the middle ear. Rapid onset; cause may be infectious, either viral (AOM-v) or bacterial (AOM-b), but there is also a sterile etiology (AOM-s)
- Recurrent AOM: ≥3 episodes in 6 months or ≥4 episodes in 1 year
- Otitis media with effusion (OME): Persistent middle ear fluid that is associated with AOM but can arise without prior AOM
- Chronic otitis media with or without cholesteatoma
- System(s) affected: Nervous; ENT
- Synonym(s): Secretory or serous otitis media

EPIDEMIOLOGY
Incidence
- AOM:
  - Predominant age: 6–24 months; declines >7 years; rare in adults
  - Predominant sex: Male > Female
  - By age 7 years, 93% of children have had ≥1 episodes of AOM; 39% have had ≥6.
  - Placement of tympanostomy tubes is 2nd only to circumcision as the most frequent surgical procedure in infants.
  - Increased incidence in the fall and winter
- OME:
  - By age 4, 90% of children have had at least 1 episode

Prevalence
- Most common infection for which antibacterial agents are prescribed in the US
- Diagnosed 5 million times per year in the US

ETIOLOGY AND PATHOPHYSIOLOGY
- AOM-b (bacterial): Usually, a preceding viral upper respiratory infection (URI) produces eustachian tube dysfunction:
  - *Streptococcus pneumoniae*: 20–35%, *Haemophilus influenzae*: 20–30%, *Moraxella (B.) catarrhalis*: 15%, group A streptococci: 3%, *Staphylococcus aureus*: 12% produce β-lactamases that hydrolyze amoxicillin and some cephalosporins.
- AOM-v (viral): 15–44% of AOM infections are caused primarily by viruses (e.g., respiratory syncytial virus, parainfluenza, influenza, enteroviruses, adenovirus, human metapneumovirus, and parechovirus).
- AOM-s (sterile/nonpathogens): 25–30%
- OME: Eustachian tube dysfunction; allergic causes are rarely substantiated.

Genetics
- Strong genetic component in twin studies for recurrent and prolonged AOM
- May be influenced by skull configuration or immunologic defects

RISK FACTORS
- Premature birth
- Bottle-feeding while supine
- Routine daycare attendance
- Frequent pacifier use after 6 months of age
- Smoking in household; environmental smoke exposure
- Male gender
- Native American/Inuit ethnicity
- Low socioeconomic status
- Family history of recurrent otitis
- AOM before age 1 is a risk for recurrent AOM
- Presence of siblings in the household
- Underlying ear, nose, or throat (ENT) disease (e.g., cleft palate, Down syndrome, allergic rhinitis)

GENERAL PREVENTION
- Pneumococcal vaccine (PCV)-7 immunization reduces the number of cases of AOM by about 6–28% (however, evidence shows that this is offset by an increase in AOM caused by other bacteria) (1)[C]. The effect of the introduction of the PCV-13 vaccine on the incidence of AOM has yet to be studied.
- Influenza vaccine reduces AOM by ~30% in children age >2 (by preventing influenza).
- Breast-feeding for ≥6 months is protective.
- Avoiding supine bottle-feeding, passive smoke, and pacifiers >6 months may be helpful.
- Secondary prevention: Adenoidectomy and adenotonsillectomy for recurrent AOM has limited short-term efficacy for children >3 years of age and is associated with its own adverse risks.
- Vitamin D supplementation (1,000 U/d to maintain vitamin D levels >30) may be helpful in reducing cases in children with recurrent AOM (2)[B].

COMMONLY ASSOCIATED CONDITIONS
URI

 DIAGNOSIS

HISTORY
- AOM: Acute history, signs, and symptoms of middle ear inflammation and effusion:
  - Earache
  - Preceding or accompanying URI symptoms
  - Decreased hearing
- AOM in infants and toddlers:
  - May cause few symptoms in the 1st few months of life
  - Irritability may be the only symptom
- OME: Usually asymptomatic
  - Decreased hearing

PHYSICAL EXAM
- Infectious AOM:
  - Fever (although it is debatable whether OM itself causes fever or fever is due to accompanying viral illness)
  - Decreased eardrum mobility (with pneumatic otoscopy)
  - Eardrum bulging, cloudy, distinctly red; presence of air–fluid level behind the tympanic membrane
  - Redness alone is not a reliable sign.
  - Otorrhea if eardrum is perforated
- OME:
  - Eardrum often dull, but not bulging
  - Decreased eardrum mobility (pneumatic otoscopy)
  - Presence of air–fluid level
  - Weber test is positive to affected ear for an ear with effusion.

DIFFERENTIAL DIAGNOSIS
- Tympanosclerosis
- Tympanic membrane erythema secondary to crying, fever, or manipulation of the ear canal
- Trauma
- Referred pain from the jaw, teeth, or throat
- Otitis externa
- Otitis-conjunctivitis syndrome

DIAGNOSTIC TESTS & INTERPRETATION
Initial Tests (lab, imaging)
WBC count may be higher in bacterial AOM than in sterile AOM, but this is almost never useful.

Diagnostic Procedures/Other
- To document the presence of middle ear fluid, pneumatic otoscopy can be supplemented with tympanometry and acoustic reflex measurement.
- Hearing testing is recommended when hearing loss persists for ≥3 months or at any time suspecting language delay, significant hearing loss, or learning problems.
- Language testing should be performed for children with hearing loss.
- Tympanocentesis for microbiologic diagnosis is recommended for treatment failures; may be followed by myringotomy.

 TREATMENT

- Significant disagreement exists about the usefulness of antibiotic treatment for this often self-resolving condition. Studies suggest that ~15 children need to be treated with antibiotics to prevent 1 case of persisting AOM pain at 1–2 weeks; the number needed to treat to cause harm (primarily diarrhea) is 8–10.
- If antibiotics are not used, 81% of patients >2 years of age are better in 1 week vs. 94% if antibiotics are used.
- Delay of antibiotics found a modest increase in mastoiditis from 2/100,000 to 4/100,000.
- American Academy of Pediatrics/American Academy of Family Physicians (AAP/AAFP) guidelines recommend the following for observation vs. antibacterial therapy, although these guidelines are not rigorously evidence based:
  - <6 months of age: Antibacterial therapy should be administered to any child, regardless of the degree of diagnostic certainty.
  - Children >6 months: Antibacterial therapy is recommended when the diagnosis of AOM is certain and the illness is severe (i.e., moderate to severe otalgia or fever ≥39°C in the previous 24 hours).
  - Observation is an option when the diagnosis is certain, but illness is not severe, and in patients with an uncertain diagnosis.
- OME: Watchful waiting for 3 months per AAP/AFPP guidelines for those not at risk (see "Complications"). Of these cases, 25–90% will recover spontaneously over this period. No benefit of antihistamines or decongestants (3)[A] or antibiotics or systemic steroids. Autoinflation may be beneficial (4)[B].

GENERAL MEASURES
- Assess pain
- Acetaminophen, ibuprofen, benzocaine drops (additional but brief benefit over acetaminophen)

MEDICATION
First Line

- AOM: AAP/AAFP Consensus Guideline recommends amoxicillin, 80–90 mg/kg/d; children >2 years with no complications, 5–7-day course; 10-day course for children <2 years. Unclear if daily or b.i.d. dosing is as effective as t.i.d. or q.i.d. dosing (5)[A].
- If penicillin allergic:
  – Non–type 1 hypersensitivity reaction: Cefdinir, 14 mg/kg/d; cefpodoxime, 10 mg/kg/d; or cefuroxime 30 mg/kg b.i.d.
  – Type 1 hypersensitivity to penicillin: Azithromycin (10 mg/kg/d [max dose 500 mg/d] as a single dose on day 1 and 5 mg/kg/d [max dose 250 mg/d] for days 2–5)
  – Other alternatives: Clarithromycin, 15 mg/kg/d (b.i.d. dose); erythromycin-sulfisoxazole, 50 mg/kg/d; or sulfamethoxazole–trimethoprim, 6–10 mg/kg/d based on trimethoprim
- A single dose of parenteral ceftriaxone (50 mg/kg) is as effective as a full course of antibiotics in uncomplicated AOM.
- A single dose of azithromycin has been approved by the FDA, but studies did not include otitis-prone children or have criteria for AOM diagnosis.
- Consider treatment of children between ages 6 months and 2 years with antibiotics to reduce duration of symptoms (6)[A].
- OME: See "General Measures"; no benefit to treatment. Medications promote transitory resolution in 10–15%, but the effect is short-lived.

Second Line
- Alternative antibiotics are indicated for the following AOM patients:
  – Persistent symptoms after 48–72 hours of amoxicillin
  – AOM within 1 month of amoxicillin therapy
  – Severe earache
  – Age <6 months with high fever
  – Immunocompromised:
    ○ Amoxicillin-clavulanate, 90 mg/kg–6.4 mg/kg/d, divided b.i.d.
    ○ Ceftriaxone, 50 mg/kg IM or IV q24h for 3 consecutive days can be reserved for those who are too sick to take oral medications or who unsuccessfully took amoxicillin-clavulanate. Neither erythromycin-sulfisoxazole nor trimethoprim-sulfamethoxazole should be used as a second-line agent in treatment failures.
- Recurrent AOM: Antibiotic prophylaxis for recurrent AOM (>3 distinct, well-documented episodes in 6 months) with amoxicillin, 20 mg/kg/d for 3 months, resulted in a benefit of ~1 fewer episode per child per year. The possibility of increased resistance and side effects are not thought to be worth risking.

SURGERY/OTHER PROCEDURES
- Recurrent AOM: Consider referral for surgery if ≥3 episodes of well-documented AOM within 6 months, ≥4 episodes within 12 months, or AOM episodes occur while on chemoprophylaxis.
- Tympanostomy tubes may be effective in selective patients, particularly children age <2 years with recurrent AOM (7)[A].
- Adenoidectomy has limited or no effect.
- Adenotonsillectomy reduced the rate of AOM by 0.7 episode per child only in the 1st year after surgery and had a 15% complications rate.

- OME: Referral for surgery for tympanostomy should be individualized. It can be considered if >4–6 months of bilateral OME and/or >6 months of unilateral OME and/or hearing loss >25 dB or for high-risk individuals at any time.
- Tympanostomy tubes may reduce recurrence of AOM minimally, but it does not lower the risk of hearing loss (8)[A].
- Adenoidectomy is indicated in specific cases; tonsillectomy or myringotomy is never indicated.

COMPLEMENTARY AND ALTERNATIVE MEDICINE
- It is unclear whether alternative and homeopathic therapies are effective for AOM, including mixed evidence about the effectiveness of zinc supplementation of reducing AOM.
- Xylitol, probiotics, herbal ear drops, and homeopathic interventions may be beneficial in reducing pain duration, antibiotic use, and bacterial resistance.

IN-PATIENT CONSIDERATIONS
Admission Criteria/Initial Stabilization
Outpatient, except if surgery is indicated, or for AOM in febrile infants age <2 months or children requiring ceftriaxone who also require monitoring for 24 hours

 ## ONGOING CARE

FOLLOW-UP RECOMMENDATIONS
Patients with otitis media who do not respond within 48–72 hours should be re-evaluated:
- If therapy was delayed and diagnosis is confirmed, start therapy with high-dose amoxicillin.
- If therapy was initiated, consider changing the antibiotic; options are limited because macrolides have limited benefit against H. influenza over amoxicillin, and most oral cephalosporins have no improved outcomes.

Patient Monitoring
- AOM: Up to 40% may have persistent middle ear effusion at 1 month, with 10–25% at 3 months.
- OME: Repeat otoscopic or tympanometric exams at 3 months, as indicated, as long as OME persists or sooner if there are red flags (see above).

PROGNOSIS
- See "General Measures."
- Recurrent AOM and OME: Usually subsides in school-aged children; few have complications.

COMPLICATIONS
- AOM: Serious complications are rare: Tympanic membrane perforation/otorrhea, acute mastoiditis, facial nerve paralysis, otitic hydrocephalus, meningitis, hearing impairment
- OME: Speech and language disabilities may occur. Hearing loss is not caused by OME, but in children who are at risk for speech, language, or learning problems (e.g., autism spectrum, syndromes, craniofacial disorders, developmental delay, and children already with speech/language delay), it could lead to further problems because they are less tolerant of a hearing impairment.
- Recurrent AOM and OME: Atrophy and scarring of eardrum, chronic perforation and otorrhea, cholesteatoma, permanent hearing loss, chronic mastoiditis, other intracranial suppurative complications

REFERENCES

1. Eskola J, Kilpi T, Palmu A. Efficacy of a pneumococcal conjugate vaccine against acute otitis media. N Engl J Med. 2001;344:403–409.
2. Marchioso P, Consonni D, Baggi E, et al. Vitamin D supplementation reduces the risk of acute otitis media in otitis-prone children. Pediatr Infect Dis J. 2013;32:1055–1060.
3. Coleman C, Moore M. Decongestants and antihistamines for acute otitis media in children. Cochrane Database Syst Rev. 2008;3:CD001727.
4. Perera R, Glasziou PP, Heneghan CJ, et al. Autoinflation for hearing loss associated with otitis media with effusion. Cochrane Database Syst Rev. 2013;5:CD006285.
5. Thanaviratananich S, Laopaiboon M, Vatanasapt P. Once or twice daily versus three times daily amoxicillin with or without clavulanate for the treatment of acute otitis media. Cochrane Database Syst Rev. 2008;4:CD004975.
6. Hoberman A, Paradise JL, Rockette HE, et al. Treatment of acute otitis media in children under 2 years of age. N Engl J Med. 2011;364:105–115.
7. Kujala T, Alho OP, Luotonen J, et al. Tympanostomy with and without adenoidectomy for the prevention of recurrences of acute otitis media: A randomized controlled trial. Pediatr Infect Dis J. 2012;31:565–569.
8. Lous J, Burton MJ, Felding JU. Grommets (ventilation tubes) for hearing loss associated with otitis media with effusion in children. Cochrane Database Syst Rev. 2005;1:CD001801.

ADDITIONAL READING
- Gould JM, Matz PS. Otitis media. Pediatr Rev. 2010;31:102–116.
- Shaikh N, Hoberman A, Kaleida PH, et al. Videos in clinical medicine. Diagnosing otitis media—otoscopy and cerumen removal. N Engl J Med. 2010;362:e62.

 ## SEE ALSO

Algorithm: Ear Pain

 ## CODES

ICD10
- H65.90 Unspecified nonsuppurative otitis media, unspecified ear
- H66.90 Otitis media, unspecified, unspecified ear
- H65.00 Acute serous otitis media, unspecified ear

CLINICAL PEARLS
- Pneumatic otoscopy is the single most specific and clinically useful test for diagnosis.
- Consider a delay of antibiotics for 24–48 hours in uncomplicated children age >2 years who do not have severe illness.
- First-line treatment is amoxicillin, 80–90 mg/kg/d for 10 days for children age <2 years; consider a 5–7-day course in children age >2 years.
- Erythema and effusion can persist for weeks.
- Antibiotics, antihistamines, and steroids are not indicated for OME.

OTITIS MEDIA WITH EFFUSION

Leanne Zakrzewski, MD • Daniel T. Lee, MD, MA

 BASICS

DESCRIPTION
- Also called serous otitis media, secretory otitis media, or "glue ear"
- Otitis media with effusion (OME) is defined as the presence of a middle-ear effusion (MEE) in the absence of acute signs of infection.
- In children, OME most often arises following acute otitis media (AOM). In adults, it often occurs in association with eustachian tube dysfunction.

EPIDEMIOLOGY
Incidence
- It is difficult to determine the incidence of OME because it is asymptomatic. In addition, many cases self-resolve quickly, making it challenging to diagnose OME.
- Studies have shown an MEE incidence of 31–61% over a 1–2-year examination period, depending on the child's age.
- Nearly all children have experienced 1 episode of OME by the age of 3 years.
- Predominant sex: Male = Female

Prevalence
The prevalence of OME varies with age and the time of year. It is more prevalent in the winter months than in the summer months.

ETIOLOGY AND PATHOPHYSIOLOGY
- In children, it was thought that OME resulted from chronic inflammation after AOM, and that the effusions frequently were sterile; however, some recent studies have demonstrated that a biofilm forms by bacterial otopathogens. A bacterial pathogen is identified in ~1/3 of effusions from OME in children who undergo myringotomy and tube placement. The common pathogens include nontypeable *Haemophilus influenzae*, *Streptococcus pneumoniae*, and *Moraxella catarrhalis*.
- The contribution of allergies to OME in children is still controversial. One study of 209 children with OME in a UK allergy clinic found a history of allergic rhinitis, asthma, and eczema in 89%, 36%, and 24%, respectively (1).
- Gastroesophageal reflux has been hypothesized to be a cause of OME in children as well. However, studies measuring the concentration of pepsin and pepsinogen in middle-ear fluid have reported conflicting results.
- In adults, OME often occurs in association with eustachian tube dysfunction, but can also result from barotrauma or allergy.

RISK FACTORS
- Risk factors for children include a family history of OME, bottle-feeding, attending daycare, and exposure to tobacco smoke.
- In adults, eustachian tube dysfunction may be a predisposing factor.

GENERAL PREVENTION
OME is generally not preventable, although lowering smoke exposure may reduce risk.

 DIAGNOSIS

HISTORY
- OME is often asymptomatic. It can be characterized by hearing loss or a sense of aural fullness. Older children and adults usually recognize the hearing impairment. An infant will not be able to express the hearing loss, but it may be apparent to the parent when observing and interacting with the child. Sleep disturbances are often reported by the affected child's parents.
- OME is transient in most children and may not be diagnosed.
- Vertigo may occur, although it is not a common complaint. In the young child, vertigo can be recognized by imbalance, falling, stumbling, or clumsiness. The older child or adult with vertigo may describe a feeling of spinning.
- In adults, there may be a history of recurrent episodes of AOM or a recent upper respiratory tract infection. There may also be an exacerbation in seasonal allergy symptoms or recent airplane travel.

PHYSICAL EXAM
- Clinical signs of acute illness or AOM are, by definition, absent in patients with OME, including bulging or erythema of the tympanic membrane (TM).
- Otoscopic findings of OME are fluid (often yellowish, but sometimes clear) visible behind a retracted TM.

DIFFERENTIAL DIAGNOSIS
- Acute otitis media
- Bullous myringitis
- Tympanosclerosis (may cause decreased/absent motion of the TM)
- Sensorineural hearing loss

DIAGNOSTIC TESTS & INTERPRETATION
Diagnostic Procedures/Other
- A subcommittee composed of members from the American Academy of Pediatrics, the American Academy of Family Physicians, and the American Academy of Otolaryngology-Head and Neck Surgery (AAP/AAFP/AAOHNS) developed a clinical practice guideline that delineates current diagnosis and management of children between 2 months and 12 years of age with OME (2)[A].
- The primary standard to make the diagnosis is pneumatic otoscopy, which demonstrates reduced/absent mobility of the TM secondary to fluid in the middle ear (2)[A].
- Tympanometry and acoustic reflectometry may also be used to support the diagnosis, especially when the presence of MEE is difficult to determine based on routine physical exam and pneumatic otoscopy.

 TREATMENT

- OME resolves without medical intervention in most patients.
- Management goals are to eliminate the effusion, restore normal hearing, and prevent future episodes, if possible.
- Management options include watchful waiting, medications in limited situations, and surgery. Which strategy is chosen depends on many factors, including the risk/presence of any associated speech, language, or learning delays and on the severity of any associated hearing loss.
- Many studies support the strategy of watchful waiting:
  - A 2010 Cochrane review was done on the use of tympanostomy tubes for hearing loss associated with OME in children. While children who received tympanostomy tubes spent less time with effusion during the initial postoperative period, the gains seen in hearing disappeared by 12–18 months. In addition, no significant effects were seen on language development or cognition in otherwise healthy children (3)[A].
  - Another longitudinal study evaluated children <3 years of age with persistent MEE and timing of tympanostomy tubes. Children were randomly assigned to prompt (<3 months) or delayed insertion of tubes, and development outcomes were assessed at periodic intervals from 3–11 years of age. No difference was noted between the 2 groups in literacy, attention, social skills, and academic achievement (4)[B].

MEDICATION
- The AAP/AAFP/AAOHNS guideline recommends against routine use of antibiotics in treatment of OME (2)[A]:
  - Antibiotics have been found in a meta-analysis to improve clearance of the effusion within the 1st month after treatment, but relapses of an effusion were common, and no benefit was noted past the 1st month.
  - Amoxicillin is preferred for treatment of OME when antibiotics are used. Other antibiotics, including amoxicillin-clavulanate and ceftibuten, have been tested in clinical trials, but none has been clearly shown to have significant advantage over the others.
- Antihistamines and decongestants have little effect on OME in children and are not recommended (2)[A]. A 2011 Cochrane review found children receiving antihistamines and decongestants were unlikely to have significant improvements in their symptoms (5).
- The AAP/AAFP/AAOHNS guideline recommends against administering oral or intranasal corticosteroids (2)[A]. While these may help to clear an MEE faster, no effect has been noted on hearing loss or other patient-centered outcomes.

- In adults, eustachian tube dysfunction secondary to allergic rhinitis or recent upper respiratory infection (URI) can be the cause of OME. As a result, most patients are treated with decongestants, antihistamines, and/or nasal steroids, despite a lack of data demonstrating a clear benefit. Most effusions will self-resolve over the course of 12 weeks, and most adult patients can be observed during this time.

ISSUES FOR REFERRAL

- The following are indications for referral to a surgeon for evaluation of tympanostomy tube placement:
  - Children with hearing loss ≥40 dB
  - Children who have structural damage to the TM/middle ear (prompt referral is recommended)
  - Children who have OME of ≥4 months' duration with persistent hearing loss (≥21 dB) or other signs/symptoms related to the effusion (2)[B]
- It is also recommended that children with recurrent/persistent OME who are at risk of speech, language, or learning problems have early referral to a specialist, regardless of hearing status.

ADDITIONAL THERAPIES

- Autoinflation, which refers to the process of opening the eustachian tube by raising intranasal pressure (e.g., by forced exhalation with closed mouth and nose) has been evaluated, and it may be beneficial in the short term. A 2006 Cochrane review of 6 studies comparing any form of autoinflation to no autoinflation in children with OME found improvement in patients' tympanogram or audiometry results beyond 1 month (6)[A].
- Studies of autoinflation in adults have not been published to date, but the maneuver is free, without significant adverse effects, and may be helpful for some patients.

SURGERY/OTHER PROCEDURES

- Adenoidectomy should not be performed in children with persistent OME alone unless there is a distinct indication for the procedure for another problem (e.g., chronic sinusitis/nasal obstruction) (2)[B]. Adenoidectomy (and concurrent tube placement) may be considered when repeat surgery for OME is necessary (e.g., when effusion recurs after tubes have fallen out or are removed) (2)[B]. In these cases, adenoidectomy has been shown to decrease the need for future procedures for OME.
- Tonsillectomy does not appear to improve the outcome for OME and is generally not advised (2)[B].
- In adults, myringotomy may be effective with few adverse effects; however, no randomized trials have been published to date evaluating myringotomy and tube placement in adults.

ONGOING CARE

FOLLOW-UP RECOMMENDATIONS
Patient Monitoring
- Children who are at risk for speech, language, or learning problems and whose OME persists for ≥3 months should undergo hearing evaluation. The results of the hearing test can help determine the management strategy:
  - Children with hearing loss ≤20 dB and without speech, language, or developmental problems can be managed with watchful waiting.
  - Children with hearing loss 21–39 dB can be managed with watchful waiting or referred for surgery.
  - Children with hearing loss ≥40 dB should be referred for surgical evaluation (2)[B].
- Re-evaluation and repeat hearing tests should be performed every 3–6 months until the effusion has resolved or the child develops an indication for surgical referral. It is also reasonable to refer a patient for surgical evaluation if the child has had bilateral OME for ≥3 months, unilateral OME ≥6 months, or cumulative duration of OME ≥12 months.
- For children with mild conductive hearing loss (21–39 dB) whose parents prefer the watchful waiting strategy, interventions in the home can help. These include speaking in close proximity to the child, facing the child and speaking clearly, and providing preferential seating in the classroom.

PROGNOSIS
Regular follow up and evaluation are important to detect any hearing loss or speech, language, or learning delay. Surgical referral is important when indicated to prevent long-term sequelae. The prognosis for OME is otherwise good in low-risk children and adults.

COMPLICATIONS
- The most significant complication of OME is permanent conductive hearing loss, but pain, balance disturbance, and tinnitus may also occur.
- If the TM becomes severely retracted, a cholesteatoma can occur. Another potential complication is tympanosclerosis, which is characterized by whitish plaques in the TM.

REFERENCES

1. Alles R, Parikh A, Hawk L, et al. The prevalence of atopic disorders in children with chronic otitis media with effusion. *Pediatr Allergy Immunol.* 2001;12:102–106.
2. American Academy of Family Physicians, American Academy of Otolaryngology-Head and Neck Surgery, American Academy of Pediatrics Subcommittee on Otitis Media with Effusion, et al. Otitis media with effusion. *Pediatrics.* 2004;113: 1412–1429.
3. Browning GG, Rovers MM, Williamson I, et al. Grommets (ventilation tubes) for hearing loss associated with otitis media with effusion in children. *Cochrane Database Syst Rev.* 2010;10: CD001801.
4. Paradise JL, Feldman HM, Campbell TF, et al. Effect of early or delayed insertion of tympanostomy tubes for persistent otitis media on developmental outcomes at the age of three years. *N Engl J Med.* 2001;344:1179.
5. Griffin G, Flynn CA. Antihistamines and/or decongestants for otitis media with effusion (OME) in children. *Cochrane Database Syst Rev.* 2011;9: CD003423.
6. Perera R, Haynes J, Glasziou P, et al. Autoinflation for hearing loss associated with otitis media with effusion. *Cochrane Database Syst Rev.* 2006;4: CD006285.

ADDITIONAL READING

- Hall-Stoodley L, Hu FZ, Gieseke A, et al. Direct detection of bacterial biofilms on the middle-ear mucosa of children with chronic otitis media. *JAMA.* 2006;296:202.
- Lieu JE, Muthappan PG, Uppaluri R. Association of reflux with otitis media in children. *Otolaryngol Head Neck Surg.* 2005;133:357.
- Lous J, Burton MJ, Felding JU, et al. Grommets (ventilation tubes) for hearing loss associated with otitis media with effusion in children. *Cochrane Database Syst Rev.* 2005;1:CD001801.
- O'Reilly RC, He Z, Bloedon E, et al. The role of extraesophageal reflux in otitis media in infants and children. *Laryngoscope.* 2008;118:1.
- Paradise JL, Feldman HM, Campbell TF, et al. Tympanostomy tubes and developmental outcomes at 9 to 11 years of age. *N Engl J Med.* 2007;356: 248.
- Simpson SA, Lewis R, van der Voort J, et al. Oral or topical nasal steroids for hearing loss associated with otitis media with effusion in children. *Cochrane Database Syst Rev.* 2011;5:CD001935.

CODES

ICD10
- H65.00 Acute serous otitis media, unspecified ear
- H65.20 Chronic serous otitis media, unspecified ear
- H65.90 Unspecified nonsuppurative otitis media, unspecified ear

CLINICAL PEARLS

- OME is defined as the presence of an MEE in the absence of acute signs of infection.
- In children, OME most often arises following an AOM. In adults, it often occurs in association with eustachian tube dysfunction.
- The primary standard for diagnosis is pneumatic otoscopy.
- Avoid the use of antihistamines, decongestants, or corticosteroids (oral/intranasal) routinely for the treatment of OME in children, as they have not been shown to offer significant benefit.
- Management options include watchful waiting, medications in limited situations, and surgery (when indicated). Which strategy is chosen depends on many factors, including the risk/presence of any associated speech, language, or learning delays and on the severity of any associated hearing loss.

OVARIAN CANCER

Susan L. Zweizig, MD

 BASICS

There are >22,000 new cases of ovarian cancer annually, and >15,000 women will die of their disease, making this the most lethal of gynecologic cancers.

DESCRIPTION

Malignancy that arises from the epithelium (90%), stroma, or germ cells of the ovary; also, tumors metastatic to the ovary; histologic types include:

- Epithelial:
  - Serous (tubal epithelium)
  - Mucinous (cervical and GI mucinous epithelium)
  - Endometrioid (endometrial epithelium)
  - Clear cell (mesonephroid)
  - Brenner (transitional cell epithelium)
  - Carcinosarcoma
- Stromal:
  - Granulosa cell tumor
  - Theca cell tumor
  - Sertoli–Leydig cell tumors
  - Gynandroblastoma
  - Lipid cell tumor
- Germ cell:
  - Teratoma (immature)
  - Dysgerminoma
  - Embryonal carcinoma
  - Gonadoblastoma
  - Endodermal sinus tumor
  - Embryonal carcinoma
  - Choriocarcinoma
- Metastatic disease from:
  - Breast
  - Endometrium
  - Lymphoma
  - GI tract (Krukenberg tumor)
  - Primary peritoneal
- System(s) affected: Gastrointestinal; Reproductive; Endocrine; Metabolic

EPIDEMIOLOGY

Incidence

- 21,990 new cases/yr in the US; 15,460 deaths/yr
- Leading cause of gynecologic cancer death in women; mortality from ovarian cancer has decreased only slightly during the past 4 decades.
- 75% diagnosed at advanced stage
- Predominant age:
  - Epithelial: Mid-50s
  - Germ cell malignancies: Usually observed in patients <20 years of age

Prevalence

Lifetime risk for general population: 1 in 70 women develops ovarian cancer.

ETIOLOGY AND PATHOPHYSIOLOGY

- Malignant transformation of the ovarian epithelium from repeated trauma during ovulation may lead to this change. Many of these cancers originate in the distal fallopian tube.
- Most ovarian cancer (75%) presents as advanced disease. Metastatic disease may develop at the same time as the primary tumor.

Genetics

- Hereditary Breast/Ovarian cancer syndrome: Early-onset breast or ovarian cancer, autosomal dominant transmission, usually associated with *BRCA-1* or *BRCA-2* mutation
- Lynch II syndrome: Autosomal-dominant inheritance; increased risk for colorectal, endometrial, stomach, small bowel, breast, pancreas, and ovarian cancers; defect in mismatch repair genes

RISK FACTORS

- 90% of ovarian cancer is sporadic and not inherited, but family history is the most significant risk factor. One 1st-degree relative increases risk to 5%; 2 relatives to 7%; individuals in families with familial cancer syndromes have 20–60% risk of developing ovarian cancer.
- Nulligravidity (or infertility), early menarche, late menopause, endometriosis
- Environmental (talc, smoking, obesity)

GENERAL PREVENTION

For epithelial cancer, frequency of ovulation appears to be important. The following factors are *protective*:

- Use of oral contraceptives: 5 years of use decreases risk by 20%; 15 years by 50%:
  - The progestin component of oral contraceptive preparations (OCPs) may protect against ovarian cancer by regulating apoptosis of the ovarian epithelium.
- Multiparity
- Breastfeeding
- Tubal ligation or hysterectomy
- Recent studies have shown no clear association exists between ovarian cancer and use of ovulation-induction agents such as clomiphene, but more long-term studies are necessary.

- NSAIDs and acetaminophen use have been shown to reduce risk of ovarian cancer (1)[B].
- Recommendations for high-risk (family history of a hereditary ovarian cancer syndrome) population:
  - Women should undergo pelvic examinations, CA-125 level measurement, and transvaginal US every 6–12 months beginning at age 25–35.
  - Women with family histories of ovarian cancer or premenopausal breast cancer should be referred for genetic counseling.
  - Prophylactic oophorectomy is advised for mutation carriers after child-bearing is completed or by age 35:
    - Risk of primary peritoneal carcinoma is 1% after prophylactic oophorectomy.
- Screening: No effective screening exists for ovarian cancer:
  - Routine use of CA-125 and transvaginal US for screening in women of average risk is discouraged. Annual pelvic examinations are recommended, particularly in postmenopausal women. An adnexal mass in a premenarchal female or a palpable adnexa in a postmenopausal female warrants further evaluation.

COMMONLY ASSOCIATED CONDITIONS

- Ascites
- Pleural effusion
- Decrease of serum albumin
- Breast carcinoma
- Bowel obstruction
- Carcinomatosis

 DIAGNOSIS

HISTORY

- Bloating
- Early satiety, anorexia, dyspepsia
- Sense of abdominal fullness, increased abdominal size
- Abdominopelvic pain or cramping
- Urinary frequency or urgency in absence of infection
- Fatigue
- Dyspareunia
- Weight loss
- Severe pain secondary to ovarian rupture or torsion; most frequent in germ cell tumors
- Precocious puberty (choriocarcinoma, embryonal carcinoma)

PHYSICAL EXAM

- Ascites
- Cul-de-sac and/or pelvic nodularity
- Pelvic mass
- Pleural effusion
- Omental mass
- Cachexia
- Adenopathy
- Hirsutism in androgen-secreting germ cell tumors

DIFFERENTIAL DIAGNOSIS

- GI, fallopian, or endometrial malignancies
- Irritable bowel syndrome
- Colitis
- Hepatic failure with ascites
- Diverticulitis
- Pelvic kidney
- Tubo-ovarian abscess or hydrosalpinx
- Uterine fibroids
- Endometriomas
- Physiologic cysts
- Benign or borderline neoplasms

DIAGNOSTIC TESTS & INTERPRETATION

Initial Tests (lab, imaging)

- Obtain with confirmed or suspected disease:
- CA-125 (not specific for ovarian cancer)
- Liver function tests (LFTs) to rule out hepatic disease
- CBC
- Urinalysis
- Serum albumin
- Carcinoembryonic antigen (CEA) if GI primary suspected
- If nonepithelial tumor suspected: Chorionic gonadotropin (β-hCG [dysgerminoma, choriocarcinoma, embryonal carcinoma]), α-fetoprotein (endodermal sinus tumor, embryonal carcinoma), lactate dehydrogenase (LDH [dysgerminoma]), or inhibin (granulosa cell tumor)

- Pelvic US
- CXR
- Abdominopelvic CT scan with contrast material

Follow-Up Tests & Special Considerations
Disorders that may alter lab results: CA-125 may be elevated from gynecologic causes (e.g., menses, pregnancy, endometriosis, peritonitis, myomas, pelvic inflammatory disease) and with ascites, pleural effusion, congestive heart failure (CHF), pancreatitis, systemic lupus erythematosus (SLE), or liver disease.
- Patients with ovarian cancer need current mammography.
- Barium enema or colonoscopy if a colon primary is suspected

Diagnostic Procedures/Other
- Endometrial biopsy if abnormal bleeding present
- Surgery is necessary for definitive diagnosis.
- Paracentesis if patient with symptomatic ascites and not an operative candidate

Test Interpretation
Epithelial ovarian cancer commonly involves the peritoneal surfaces of the abdomen and pelvis, especially the cul-de-sac, paracolic gutters, and diaphragmatic surfaces.

 TREATMENT

MEDICATION
First Line
- After surgery, most patients will require chemotherapy. Stage 1a, grade 1 and most stage 1b, grade 1 tumors do not require adjuvant therapy. Patients with clear cell carcinomas, grade 3 tumors, or tumors staged 1c or worse require adjuvant therapy. Patients should be encouraged to participate in clinical trials whenever possible.
- Paclitaxel (Taxol) is recommended in combination with platinum-based therapy as the 1st-line treatment of epithelial ovarian cancer.
- Intraperitoneal (IP) chemotherapy in combination with IV chemotherapy improves survival in advanced ovarian cancer (2)[A]. IP chemotherapy is associated with more toxicity.
- Germ cell cancers: Bleomycin, etoposide, platinum agent (3)[A]
- Contraindications: Poor functional status, excessive toxicity, hypersensitivity
- Precautions: All regimens cause bone marrow suppression. Cisplatin is associated with ototoxicity, renal toxicity, and peripheral neuropathy. Taxol can cause neutropenia and neuropathy.
- Antiemetic: Ondansetron (Zofran), dronabinol (Marinol), metoclopramide (Reglan), prochlorperazine (Compazine), promethazine (Phenergan)

Second Line
- Liposomal doxorubicin
- Carboplatin/Gemcitabine
- Topotecan
- Taxotere
- Etoposide
- Bevacizumab
- Cyclophosphamide
- Tamoxifen may be used in recurrent disease when chemotherapy is not appropriate (4)[B].

ADDITIONAL THERAPIES
Some patients with advanced disease and poor functional status and/or extreme tumor burden are managed with preoperative chemotherapy (neoadjuvant treatment) followed by interval cytoreductive surgery. These patients receive more chemotherapy after tumor debulking.

SURGERY/OTHER PROCEDURES
- Surgical exploration with staging and debulking is critical. Maximal cytoreduction of tumor burden enhances effectiveness of adjuvant therapy and is associated with longer survival.
- For epithelial malignancies, careful staging, tumor excision/debulking includes:
  – Cytologic evaluation of peritoneal fluid (or washings from peritoneal lavage)
  – Bilateral salpingo-oophorectomy with hysterectomy and tumor reductive surgery
  – Excision of omentum
  – Inspection and palpation of peritoneal surfaces
  – Cytologic smear of right hemidiaphragmatic surface
  – Biopsy of adhesions or any suspicious areas
  – Biopsy of paracolic recesses, pelvic sidewalls, posterior cul-de-sac, and bladder peritoneum
  – Pelvic and para-aortic lymph node biopsies
- Germ cell cancers (less likely to be bilateral): Salpingo-oophorectomy (unilateral if only 1 ovary involved) in young patient

 ONGOING CARE

FOLLOW-UP RECOMMENDATIONS
Patient Monitoring
- Physical exam every 3 months for the first 2 years after diagnosis; every 6 months until 5 years and then yearly thereafter (5)[C]
- If CA-125 elevated at diagnosis, follow levels after treatment to detect recurrence (is often elevated 2–5 months before clinical detection of relapse) (5,6)[C].
- Germ cell/sex-cord stromal cancer: Physical exam and tumor markers every 3 months for the first 2 years after diagnosis:
  – Tumor markers for sex-cord stromal cancers should be checked every 6 months for 10 years, as recurrences can occur remote from initial diagnosis (5)[C].
- CT scan of chest, abdomen, and pelvis and/or PET scan when recurrence suspected
- Screening with CXR, MRI, CT, or PET not recommended; insufficient data to support

PROGNOSIS
- Recurrence rates:
  – Early-stage disease: 25%
  – Advanced disease: >80%
- 5-year survival rates for ovarian cancer based on FIGO data:

Stage I	a 90%	b 86%	c 83%
Stage II	a 71%	b 66%	c 71%
Stage III	a 47%	b 42%	c 33%
Stage IV	19%		

COMPLICATIONS
- Pleural effusion
- Pseudomyxoma peritonei
- Ascites
- Toxicity of chemotherapy
- Bowel obstruction
- Malnutrition
- Electrolyte disturbances
- Fistula formation

REFERENCES

1. Collaborative Group on Epidemiological Studies of Ovarian Cancer, Beral V, Doll R, et al. Ovarian cancer and oral contraceptives: Collaborative reanalysis of data from 45 epidemiological studies including 23,257 women with ovarian cancer and 87,303 controls. *Lancet*. 2008;371(9609): 303–314.
2. Armstrong DK, Bundy B, Wenzel L, et al. Intraperitoneal cisplatin and paclitaxel in ovarian cancer. *N Engl J Med*. 2006;354:34–43.
3. Schumer ST, Cannistra SA. Granulosa cell tumor of the ovary. *J Clin Oncol*. 2003;21:1180–1189.
4. Orlando M, Costanzo MV, Chacon RD. Randomized trial of combination chemotherapy versus monotherapy in relapsed ovarian carcinoma: A meta-analysis of published data. *J Clin Oncol*. 2007;25:280s.
5. Salani R, Backes F, Fung M, et al. Posttreatment surveillance and diagnosis of recurrence in women with gynecologic malignancies: Society of Gynecologic Oncologists recommendations. *Am J Obstet Gynecol*. 2011;204:466–476.
6. Gadducci A, Cosio S, Zola P, et al. Surveillance procedures for patients treated for epithelial ovarian cancer: A review of the literature. *Int J Gynecol Cancer*. 2007;17:21–31.

CODES

ICD10
- C56.1 Malignant neoplasm of right ovary
- C56.2 Malignant neoplasm of left ovary
- C56.9 Malignant neoplasm of unspecified ovary

CLINICAL PEARLS
- Family history of ovarian cancer or early-onset breast cancer is the most significant risk factor for the development of ovarian cancer, yet the vast majority of cases remain sporadic.
- The diagnosis of ovarian cancer should be suspected in women with persistent bloating, upper abdominal discomfort, or GI symptoms of unknown etiology.
- Surgery is the mainstay of diagnosis and treatment for ovarian cancer, and many patients benefit from adjuvant chemotherapy.
- The prognosis of advanced ovarian cancer is poor and requires close follow-up by physical exam, tumor markers, and imaging when indicated.

O

OVARIAN CYST, RUPTURED

Leah C. Wilson, MD • Mark J. Manning, DO, MsMEL

BASICS

- Ovarian cysts are very common. Women of reproductive age develop ovarian cysts with each ovulatory cycle.
- Ovarian cyst rupture and hemorrhage (of follicle or corpus luteum) are essentially physiologic events.
- A ruptured ovarian cyst is usually asymptomatic but sometimes causes pain ranging from mild to severe due to peritoneal irritation (blood and sebaceous material most irritating).
- Symptomatic ruptured ovarian cysts can usually be managed as an outpatient but occasionally require surgical intervention.

DESCRIPTION

Types of ovarian cysts that may rupture fall into 2 groups: Physiologic and pathologic (1,2):

- Physiologic or functional cysts form as a result of hormonal stimulation of the ovary. Most are asymptomatic and spontaneously resolve in 60–90 days:
  - Follicular cysts form when a growing follicle fails to rupture and release an egg:
    - Most common type of functional cyst
    - Unilateral and filled with serous fluid
  - Corpus luteum cysts occur when an egg is released and pregnancy does not occur. The residual structure does not regress and may hemorrhage internally (hemorrhagic cysts).
  - Theca-lutein cysts result from excessive stimulation of β-human chorionic gonadotropin such as in infertility patients, molar pregnancies, or choriocarcinoma. These cysts are also susceptible to internal hemorrhage.
- Pathologic cysts are caused by a process other than normal hormonal stimulation. When followed, these cysts remain stable in size or may grow:
  - Endometriomas are cysts or collections of blood clots that form as a result of cycling endometrial tissue on the ovary. Also called "chocolate cysts" due to their appearance.
  - Mature cystic teratoma (dermoid) develop from totipotent germ cells:
    - Most commonly, they contain mucinous material and hair.
    - Up to 14% are bilateral and can grow very large.
    - <1% rupture spontaneously but if they do, may lead to shock, hemorrhage, and acute peritonitis.
  - Cystadenomas may have solid or mucinous areas. They are typically benign but may have borderline malignant areas. They rarely rupture.
  - Other cystic-appearing adnexal structures include paratubal cysts, tubo-ovarian abscess, hydrosalpinx, ectopic pregnancy.

EPIDEMIOLOGY

- The exact incidence is difficult to determine due to the asymptomatic nature of most cysts and cyst rupture.
- Annual incidence of acute pelvic pain attributed to ovarian cysts in the US has been estimated at 65,000.
- 4% of women have been admitted to a hospital with an ovarian cyst by age 65.

RISK FACTORS

Increased risk of developing physiologic cysts associated with:

- Smoking
- Levonorgestrel IUD
- Tamoxifen

GENERAL PREVENTION

For patients with painful, recurrent ovarian cysts, oral contraceptive pills can be prescribed to suppress ovulation: This may help prevent the formation of new cysts but will not impact cysts that have already formed (3)[A].

DIAGNOSIS

- A ruptured ovarian cyst may be asymptomatic or present as acute abdominal pain, varying from mild to severe.
- The broad range of presentations can prove to be a diagnostic dilemma for many physicians.

HISTORY

- A general past medical and surgical history should be reviewed.
- Risk factors for gynecologic pain should be elicited:
  - Possibility of pregnancy
  - Menstrual history, with attention to symptoms suggestive of endometriosis or history of cysts
  - STD history
  - Levonorgestrel-containing intrauterine device (up to 12% of users experience ovarian cysts) (4)[B]
  - Infertility treatment
- Typical features of pain due to ruptured ovarian cyst include:
  - Pain often begins during strenuous activity (exercise or intercourse)
  - Sudden-onset, unilateral pelvic pain that becomes more dull and generalized over time
  - Pain is worse with movement
- Other causes of acute abdominal pain should also be considered, including GI and urologic etiologies.

ALERT

Patients with bleeding diathesis or undergoing anticoagulation therapy may experience significant bleeding from hemorrhagic cysts.

PHYSICAL EXAM

- Vital signs are typically normal.
- Low-grade fever may be present.
- If significant blood loss has occurred, may have signs of hypovolemic shock (uncommon)
- Tenderness in unilateral lower quadrant (right side more common)
- Peritoneal signs may be present depending on degree of peritoneal irritation.
- On bimanual exam, unilateral adnexal mass may be palpable.
- May have cervical motion tenderness

DIFFERENTIAL DIAGNOSIS

Should include all causes of acute abdominal pain, both gynecologic and nongynecologic

ALERT

The first objective should be to exclude ectopic pregnancy. It has a similar presentation and can be life threatening. Then:

- Ovarian torsion
- Pelvic inflammatory disease tubo-ovarian abscess
- Ovarian hyperstimulation syndrome (OHSS)
- Ovarian cancer with ascites
- Appendicitis
- Diverticulitis
- Nephrolithiasis
- Bowel obstruction or perforation

DIAGNOSTIC TESTS & INTERPRETATION

- Pregnancy test is an important 1st step for ruling out ectopic pregnancy as a cause of the pain.
- CBC is useful:
  - Hematocrit is best compared to a baseline hematocrit.
  - Elevated WBC count or left shift may indicate infectious etiology
  - Low platelets can worsen bleeding.
- Cervical cultures and/or testing for gonorrhea and chlamydia if pelvic inflammatory disease is suspected
- Urinalysis to evaluate possibility of infection or stones
- Blood type and cross-matching if the patient is hemodynamically unstable and surgery is planned
- Tumor markers (i.e., CA-125): Not recommended for initial evaluation. May be elevated in a number of benign conditions including hemoperitoneum. Not likely to help in diagnosis or management
- Transvaginal US is first-line imaging modality (1,2)[C]
- Findings may include:
  - Adnexal mass: Features may suggest type of cyst/tumor
  - Free fluid in pelvis: Usually small amount but large amount may indicate ongoing hemorrhage
- CT scan is second-line and not typically helpful. Most useful for excluding nongynecologic pathology (2).
- MRI can be useful in distinguishing a ruptured ovarian cyst from other gynecologic etiologies, such as tubo-ovarian abscess, but is expensive and rarely necessary (5)[C].

TREATMENT

MEDICATION

- For uncomplicated cyst ruptures (absence of hemodynamic instability, acute abdomen, enlarging hemoperitoneum, or US evidence of malignancy), goal should be conservative therapy if possible.
- Pain due to an uncomplicated cyst rupture is usually self-limiting and can be managed on an outpatient basis with pain medication and rest (6)[B].

First Line
NSAIDs are the most effective at relieving pain due to peritoneal irritation.

Second Line
Narcotic pain medications may also be necessary acutely.

ISSUES FOR REFERRAL

- The vast majority of ruptured ovarian cysts in reproductive-age women are a result of functional cysts, and the risk of malignancy is very low.
- Referral to a gynecologic oncologist should be made in any postmenopausal woman with an adnexal mass that has concerning US findings, an elevated CA-125, ascites, a nodular, fixed pelvic mass, and a family history of breast or ovarian cancer (1)[C],(5)[B].

SURGERY/OTHER PROCEDURES

For complicated ovarian cyst rupture (hemodynamic instability, significant hemoperitoneum, concern for ovarian torsion) or if patient is deteriorating, surgical evaluation is recommended (6):

- Laparoscopy is typically preferred but approach should be based on surgeon's comfort and expertise, and patient factors (clinical condition, body habitus, previous abdominal surgeries, etc.) (1)[C],(5)[B].
- Surgery includes suction-evacuation of any fluid or blood found in the pelvis, as well as achieving hemostasis, if needed, at the site of the cyst: If a cyst wall is present, it should be removed.
- In the vast majority of cases, oophorectomy is not necessary.
- Laparoscopic excision of the cyst and capsule of endometriomas substantially decreases risk of recurrence (7)[A].

IN-PATIENT CONSIDERATIONS

Inpatient management may include IV hydration, monitoring of vital signs, serial hematocrits, and pain control.

 ONGOING CARE

FOLLOW-UP RECOMMENDATIONS

- Patient should have follow-up US in 6 weeks.
- Most functional cysts resolve spontaneously without treatment, and watchful waiting with serial transvaginal US for 2–3 cycles is appropriate.
- If cysts fail to resolve or develop concerning US findings (increasing size or complexity, nodules, septations, excrescences), they may be pathologic and surgical evaluation is recommended (3)[A].
- With an uncomplicated cyst rupture, fluid typically resorbs in 24 hours and symptoms resolve within 2–3 days.

Pregnancy Considerations
Ovarian cysts in pregnancy:

- With the widespread use of US during pregnancy, up to 4% of pregnant women are found to have adnexal masses, most of which are follicular cysts that spontaneously resolve by 16 weeks' gestation.
- <2% will spontaneously rupture or torse during pregnancy; however, this can lead to preterm labor and delivery, which may cause poor obstetric outcomes.
- If they are painful, large (>8 cm), or have US characteristics that are concerning for malignancy, elective surgical evaluation may be considered (1)[C],(5)[B].

PATIENT EDUCATION
Patient handout on pelvic pain at aafp.org

REFERENCES

1. Stany MP, Hamilton CA. Benign disorders of the ovary. *Obstet Gynecol Clin North Am*. 2008;35: 271–284, ix.
2. Roch O, et al. Radiologic appearances of gynaecologic emergencies. *Insights Imaging*. 2012;3:265–275.
3. Grimes DA, Jones LB. Oral contraceptives for functional ovarian cysts. *Cochrane Database Syst Rev*. 2009;2:CD006134.
4. Mirena [package insert]. Wayne, NJ: Bayer HealthCare Pharmaceuticals Inc.; 2009.
5. American College of Obstetricians and Gynecologists. ACOG Practice Bulletin. Management of adnexal masses. *Obstet Gynecol*. 2007;110:201–214.
6. Bottomley C, Bourne T. Diagnosis and management of ovarian cyst accidents. *Best Pract Res Clin Obstet Gynaecol*. 2009;23:711–724.
7. Hart RJ, Hickey M, Maouris P, et al. Excisional surgery versus ablative surgery for ovarian endometriomata. *Cochrane Database Syst Rev*. 2008;2:CD004992.

ADDITIONAL READING

- Falcone T. Risk of complications from gynecological surgery is lower with laparoscopy than with laparotomy. *Evidence Based Obstet Gynecol*. 2004;4:185–186A.
- Hoo WL, Yazbek J, Holland T, et al. Expectant management of ultrasonically diagnosed ovarian dermoid cysts: Is it possible to predict outcome? *Ultrasound Obstet Gynecol*. 2010;36:235–240.
- Huchon C, Staraci S, Fauconnier A, et al. Adnexal torsion: A predictive score for pre-operative diagnosis. *Hum Reprod*. 2010;25:2276–2280.
- Kruszka PS, Kruszka SJ. Evaluation of acute pelvic pain in women. *Am Fam Physician*. 2010;82: 141–147.
- Møller LM. [Complications of gynaecological operations. A one-year analysis of a hospital database]. *Ugeskr Laeg*. 2005;167:4654–4659.
- Raziel A, Ron-El R, Pansky M, et al. Current management of ruptured corpus luteum. *Eur J Obstet Gynecol Reprod Biol*. 1993;50:77–81.
- Saunders BA, Podzielinski I, Ware RA, et al. Risk of malignancy in sonographically confirmed septated cystic ovarian tumors. *Gynecol Oncol*. 2010;118: 278–282.
- Suzuki S, Yasumoto M, Matsumoto R, et al. MR findings of ruptured endometrial cyst: Comparison with tubo-ovarian abscess. *Eur J Radiol*. 2012;81: 3631–3637.

 CODES

ICD10
- N83.0 Follicular cyst of ovary
- N83.1 Corpus luteum cyst
- N83.20 Unspecified ovarian cysts

CLINICAL PEARLS

- Functional ovarian cysts are very common in reproductive-age women and usually resolve spontaneously in 60–90 days.
- First objective should be to exclude ectopic pregnancy.
- If a cyst does rupture, the pain is usually self-limited and can be treated with oral pain medications on an outpatient basis.
- Surgery may be necessary if pain is extreme or if the patient is unstable. This usually involves laparoscopically evacuating irritating fluid and blood from the abdominal cavity, achieving hemostasis, and removing the cyst wall if possible.

O

OVARIAN TUMOR, BENIGN

Kristin D'Orsi, DO • Mark J. Manning, DO, MsMEL

BASICS

DESCRIPTION
- The ovaries are a source of many tumor types (benign and malignant) because of the histologic variety of their constituent cells.
- Benign ovarian tumors create difficulties in differential diagnosis because of the need to identify malignancy and discriminate tumor from cysts, infectious lesions, ectopic pregnancy, and endometriomas.
- Tumors are often clinically silent until well developed; may be solid, cystic, or mixed; and they may be functional (producing sex steroids, as with arrhenoblastomas and gynandroblastomas) or nonfunctional.
- System(s) affected: Endocrine/Metabolic; Reproductive

Geriatric Considerations
Because incidence of malignancy increases with age, postmenopausal patients warrant comprehensive evaluation and follow up.

Pediatric Considerations
Malignancy must be ruled out in premenarchal patients. Early neonatal cysts are rare.

EPIDEMIOLOGY
Incidence
- 30% of regularly cycling females
- 50% of women without regular cycles
- Predominant age: Premenarchal girls have a 6–11% risk of cancer in an ovarian tumor, and postmenopausal women have a 29–35% risk. A high percentage of ovarian tumors are malignant in girls <15 years of age.

ETIOLOGY AND PATHOPHYSIOLOGY
- Endometriosis with localized, repeated ovarian hemorrhage
- Physiologic cysts
- Tumorigenesis, with genetics as yet poorly defined

RISK FACTORS
- As yet poorly characterized for benign tumors; cigarette smoking doubles the relative risk for developing functional ovarian cysts.
- Possible contributory factors are early menarche, obesity, infertility, and hypothyroidism.
- Tamoxifen increases risk of ovarian cyst formation (15–30%).
- Risks for ovarian cancer include age >60 years; early menarche; late menopause; nulligravidity; infertility; endometriosis; polycystic ovarian syndrome; family history of ovarian, breast, or colon cancer; a personal history of breast/colon cancer; or *BRCA* mutation.
- Risk for ovarian cancer is decreased in women who have used oral contraceptive pills (OCPs), are multiparous, have a history of a tubal ligation, or who have breast fed.

GENERAL PREVENTION
- Although OCPs do not appear to increase rates of cyst resolution, they do decrease the risk for forming new ovarian cysts.
- Resection of benign cysts has no impact on future risk for ovarian cancer.
- A case-control study of 299 women found no evidence that ovulation-induction treatment predisposes women to the development of borderline ovarian growths (1).

DIAGNOSIS
- A careful history is important.
- Usually asymptomatic
- Pain related to torsion, endometriosis, or rupture

HISTORY
- Early satiety
- Dyspepsia/bloating
- Increased abdominal girth
- Bowel pressure or bladder pressure sensations
- Menstrual irregularities
- Dyspareunia
- Deepening of the voice
- Hormonal status (OCPs, hormone replacement therapy [HRT] or fertility drugs)

PHYSICAL EXAM
- Severe acne
- Examine lymph nodes for enlargement.
- Chest auscultation can reveal a pleural effusion.
- Abdominal exam may identify ascites, masses, or increased abdominal girth.
- Hirsutism/sexual precocity
- Pelvic exam
- Virilization

DIFFERENTIAL DIAGNOSIS
- Ovarian malignancies
- Endometrioma
- Uterine leiomyoma
- Appendicular cysts
- Diverticulitis/bowel abscess
- Pelvic inflammatory disease (PID) with tubo-ovarian abscess
- Distended urinary bladder
- Ectopic pregnancy
- Hydrosalpinx
- Paraovarian cyst
- Peritoneal inclusion cysts
- Functional cysts (follicular and corpus luteum cysts)
- Polycystic ovaries
- Ovarian lipoma

DIAGNOSTIC TESTS & INTERPRETATION
Initial Tests (lab, imaging)
- CBC for WBCs helpful if PID or ovarian torsion suspected
- Serum β-human chorionic gonadotropin (β-hCG)
- Urinalysis
- Serum estrogens and androgens if signs of androgen excess (although only as part of polycystic ovarian [PCO] workup)
- Serum tumor markers may be considered, but often confuse rather than help to resolve diagnosis; choose carefully (2):
  - CA-125 should not be ordered in a premenopausal patient for screening purposes. If an ovarian tumor in a premenopausal patient is highly suspicious for cancer by ultrasound, a CA-125 level >200 U is concerning. In a postmenopausal patient, cancer must be ruled out and a CA-125 >35 U is concerning (value is lab dependent).
  - α-Fetoprotein and hCG can be ordered for suspected germ cell tumor.
- Disorders that may alter lab results:
  - CA-125: Endometriosis, peritonitis, PID, Meigs syndrome, uterine fibroids, hepatitis, pancreatitis, systemic lupus erythematosus (SLE), diverticulitis
  - β-hCG: Pregnancy, hydatidiform mole
  - α-Fetoprotein: Hepatocellular carcinoma, hepatic cirrhosis, acute/chronic hepatitis
  - Human epididymis protein 4 (HE4) may offer superior specificity compared to CA-125 for the differentiation of benign and malignant adnexal masses in premenopausal women (3).
- Transvaginal ultrasound is the best means to determine the architecture of an ovarian cyst or mass (4).
- Transvaginal ultrasonography may differentiate tumors from other pelvic lesions and identify features that place the patient at greater risk for malignancy (e.g., solid component, papillations, multiple septations, ascites, bilaterality, fixed and irregular, rapidly enlarging, accompanied by cul-de-sac nodules).
- Transabdominal ultrasonography can help identify ascites.
- Color-flow Doppler evaluation also may be helpful. Color flow to the solid component of the tumor is concerning for cancer. Gray scale may be an important method of differential diagnosis of ovarian growths.
- MRI with apparent diffusion coefficient mapping may be useful in the differential diagnosis of cystic masses. MRI can be helpful in better defining masses in women with low risk of ovarian cancer but who have an "indeterminant" mass on ultrasound. Usually not necessary as decision for surgery can proceed without MRI if indicated. Can add greatly to cost of care.
- Cystoscopy if hematuria is present in the absence of infection or if IV pyelogram reveals intravesical surface irregularity
- Abdominopelvic CT scan with contrast material, if MRI unavailable, although ultrasound still far superior (5)
- Barium enema, colonoscopy, or IV pyelogram, as indicated

Diagnostic Procedures/Other
Exploratory laparoscopy/laparotomy

Test Interpretation
- Follicular (fluid distension of atretic follicle) and corpus luteum cysts (corpus luteum hematoma). Follicular cysts are the most common ovarian cysts in the premenopausal nonpregnant female.
- Endometrioma (extrauterine endometrial tissue)
- Pregnancy luteoma (composed of hyperplastic stromal theca–lutein cells)
- Serous and mucinous cystadenomas and mixed serous/mucinous cystadenomas
- Granulosa cell tumors
- Benign connective tissue tumors (thecomas, fibromas, Brenner tumors)
- Cystic teratoma (dermoid cyst); teratomas are the most common benign neoplasms.
- Germinal inclusion cyst (regarded by some as the precursor for epithelial ovarian cancer)

Pregnancy Considerations
- Most cysts discovered during pregnancy are corpus luteum/follicular cysts.
- The 2 most commonly encountered tumors during pregnancy are cystadenomas (serous/mucinous) and dermoid cysts.

TREATMENT

GENERAL MEASURES
- In premenopausal patients with cystic lesions <10 cm in diameter, simple observation for 4–6 weeks is acceptable. Simple and hemorrhagic cysts <3 cm, are not suspicious and do not likely need follow up.
- Premenopausal women should have a repeat ultrasound ideally during their follicular phase (day 3-10 of cycle) (6).
- If a large cyst remains unchanged after 4–6 weeks of observation, then surgical exploration is indicated.
- In postmenopausal patients cysts <1 cm are likely benign.

MEDICATION
Oral contraceptives decrease the risk for forming new ovarian cysts. They do not aid in resorption of current ovarian cysts.

First Line
NSAIDs or narcotics may be helpful for discomfort.

SURGERY/OTHER PROCEDURES
- Cystectomy/wedge resection for cyst with benign features (7)
- Surgical removal of tumor to establish diagnosis when:
  – Premenopausal cysts >5 cm that persist >12 weeks
  – Mass is solid.
  – Mass is >10 cm.
  – Mass in a premenarchal/postmenopausal female
  – Suspicion of torsion/rupture
  – Postmenopausal cysts
  – Cysts with worrisome features on ultrasound (e.g., papillations)
  – For masses that are worrisome for cancer, consider referral to a gynecologist/oncologist for initial surgery.

ONGOING CARE

FOLLOW-UP RECOMMENDATIONS
Patient Monitoring
- Most require only yearly exams
- Varies by diagnosis

PATIENT EDUCATION
A variety of excellent patient education materials (e.g., "Ovarian Cyst") can be downloaded from the American Association of Family Physicians and American College of Obstetricians and Gynecologists Internet sites: www.aafp.org/afp and www.acog.com

PROGNOSIS
Complete cure

COMPLICATIONS
Complications of untreated dermoid and mucinous cysts may include rupture and pseudomyxoma peritonei.

REFERENCES

1. Cusidó M, Fábregas R, Pere BS, et al. Ovulation induction treatment and risk of borderline ovarian tumors. *Gynecol Endocrinol*. 2007;23:373–376.
2. Clarke-Pearson D. Screening for ovarian cancer. *N Engl J Med*. 2009;361:170–177.
3. Holcomb K, Vucetic Z, Miller MC, et al. Human epididymis protein 4 offers superior specificity in the differentiation of benign and malignant adnexal masses in premenopausal women. *Am J Obstet Gynecol*. 2011;205:358.e1–358.e6.
4. Givens V, Mitchell G. Diagnosis and management of adnexal masses. *Am Fam Physician*. 2009;80: 815–822.
5. Iyer VR, Lee SI. MRI, CT, and PET/CT for ovarian cancer detection and adnexal lesion characterization. *AJR Am J Roentgenol*. 2010;194:311–321.
6. Levine D, Brown D, Andreotti RF, et al. Management of asymptomatic ovarian and other adnexal cysts imaged at US: Society of Radiologists in Ultrasound Consensus Conference Statement. *Radiology*. 2010;256:943–954.
7. Labarge PY. Short-term morbidity and long-term recurrence rate of ovarian dermoid cysts treated by laparoscopy vs. laparotomy. *J Obstet Gynecol Can*. 2006;28:789–793.

ADDITIONAL READING

- Crayford TJ, Campbell S, Bourne TH, et al. Benign ovarian cysts and ovarian cancer: A cohort study with implications for screening. *Lancet*. 2000;355: 1060–1063.
- Holt VL, Cushing-Haugen KL, Daling JR. Oral contraceptives, tubal sterilization, and functional ovarian cyst risk. *Obstet Gynecol*. 2003;102: 252–258.
- Kirilovas D, Schedvins K, Naessén T, et al. Conversion of circulating estrone sulfate to 17beta-estradiol by ovarian tumor tissue: A possible mechanism behind elevated circulating concentrations of 17beta-estradiol in postmenopausal women with ovarian tumors. *Gynecol Endocrinol*. 2007;23:25–28.
- Marchesini AC, Magrio FA, Berezowski AT, et al. A critical analysis of Doppler velocimetry in the differential diagnosis of malignant and benign ovarian masses. *J Womens Health (Larchmt)*. 2008;17:97–102.

CODES

ICD10
- D27.0 Benign neoplasm of right ovary
- D27.1 Benign neoplasm of left ovary
- D27.9 Benign neoplasm of unspecified ovary

CLINICAL PEARLS
- In perimenopausal patients follicles and simple cysts <3 cm are normal physiologic findings.
- Transvaginal pelvic ultrasound is the imaging test of choice to initially determine the architecture of an ovarian cyst or mass.
- Malignancy must be ruled out in both premenarchal and postmenopausal patients.
- Do not order CA-125 on premenopausal patients with an ovarian mass unless it is highly suspicious for cancer.

O

PAGET DISEASE OF THE BREAST
Dawnielle C. Endly, DO • Tracy O. Middleton, DO

 BASICS

DESCRIPTION
- Rare disease of the nipple–areolar complex associated with underlying in situ or invasive carcinoma
- Characterized by eczematous changes, erythema, ulceration, crusting, bleeding, and/or itching (1,2)
- System(s) affected: Skin/Exocrine

EPIDEMIOLOGY
Incidence
- 1–3% of breast cancers in females (1)
- Incidence of Paget disease of the breast has been decreasing since 1988, despite an increased incidence of breast cancer (3).
- Median age at diagnosis = 64 (3)
- Extremely uncommon in males

Prevalence
<1% of population

ETIOLOGY AND PATHOPHYSIOLOGY
Cause is unknown, but risk factors for Paget disease are similar to those for developing breast cancer in general (see below):
- Epidermotropic theory:
  – Ductal carcinoma cells migrate from underlying mammary ducts to epidermis of the nipple to become Paget cells (3,4)
- Transformation theory (not favored):
  – Epidermal cells of nipple/areola transform into Paget cells that can invade the basement membrane into the dermis (3,5,6).

Genetics
No known genetic pattern, although studies suggest up to 88% display *Her2/Neu* overexpression (1,7)

RISK FACTORS
Same risk factors apply as for noninherited breast cancers:
- Female gender
- Age >40
- Previous breast cancer
- Benign breast disease (atypical ductal/lobular hyperplasia, fibroadenoma, sclerosing adenosis, intraductal papilloma)
- 1st-degree relative with history of breast cancer
- Jewish/Caucasian
- Menarche <12 years of age
- Menopause >50 years of age
- Nulliparity or 1st child after age 34
- History of ionizing radiation exposure
- History of alcohol abuse

COMMONLY ASSOCIATED CONDITIONS
- Underlying in situ or invasive breast cancer in 82–94% of patients, although there is often no associated breast mass or mammographic abnormality (1,3,8)
- The underlying carcinomas are multifocal/multicentric in 32–41% of patients (1,2).

 DIAGNOSIS

HISTORY
- Scaly, raw, vesicular, or ulcerated lesion that begins on the nipple and then spreads to the areola (1,2)
- Pain, burning, pruritus may be present even before clinically evident disease
- Nipple/areolar skin changes that have not responded to conservative topical treatment
- Median duration of symptoms is 9 months prior to histologic diagnosis (9)

PHYSICAL EXAM
- Eczematous nipple changes
- Nipple erythema and scaling
- Nipple erosion or ulceration
- Bloody or serous nipple discharge
- Nipple retraction
- Nipple fissures with crusting
- Palpable breast mass, when present, is often >2 cm from nipple–areolar complex
- Thickening in breast tissue without nipple change (2)

DIFFERENTIAL DIAGNOSIS
- Eczema/atopic dermatitis
- Contact dermatitis
- Psoriasis
- Bowen's disease
- Squamous cell carcinoma
- Basal cell carcinoma
- Superficially spreading malignant melanoma
- Lichen simplex chronicus
- Erosive adenomatosis of the nipple

DIAGNOSTIC TESTS & INTERPRETATION
Mammography and breast ultrasound:
- Bilateral mammography should be performed in all cases to evaluate for synchronous invasive cancer or ductal carcinoma in situ (DCIS) (10).
- Mammographic appearance can be normal in 22%–50% of cases (10).
- Breast US is also helpful in initial diagnosis, especially if mammogram is negative (1,8,10)
- Both US *and* mammogram were negative in 13% of Paget cases in one study (10).

Follow-Up Tests & Special Considerations
Breast MRI:
- More sensitive than mammography or breast ultrasound in detecting multifocal or multicentric breast cancer (1,8)[B]
- Recommended if negative mammography and ultrasound to detect occult disease (8,10,11)[B]
- Recommended in those patients with abnormalities limited to the central breast tissue on mammogram or US (8,10,11)[B].
- Recommended if considering breast-conserving surgery (12,13)[C]
- Some recommend breast MRI for all patients with a new Paget disease diagnosis (12)[C]
- Higher false-positive rate—patients should be followed up by confirmatory biopsy

Diagnostic Procedures/Other
- Full-thickness skin biopsy and cone biopsy of any associated breast lesion provides definitive diagnosis and should be performed if there are:
  – Positive findings on clinical exam or imaging
  – Chronic or nonhealing nipple lesions (6)[B]

Test Interpretation
- Histologic evidence of Paget cells with abundant pale cytoplasm and hyperchromatic nuclei (2,7)
- Immunohistochemistry positive for cytokeratin 7, carcinoembryonic antigen (CEA), and epithelial membrane antigen (EMA), and about 50% positive for hormone receptor expression (6)

TREATMENT

MEDICATION
Systemic adjuvant chemotherapy and/or endocrine therapy is based on the stage and hormone receptor status of the associated cancer.
- In Paget's disease without an associated cancer, or in estrogen-receptor positive DCIS, consider tamoxifen (13)[C]
- In Paget's disease with associated invasive breast cancer, treat per oncology study protocols. See www.nccn.org for the most recent guidelines (13)[C].
- Possible agents include:
  – Tamoxifen
  – Anastrozole, letrozole, or exemestane
  – Doxorubicin
  – Cyclophosphamide
  – Paclitaxel
  – Docetaxel
  – Carboplatin
  – Trastuzumab

ISSUES FOR REFERRAL
- Surgery
- Medical oncology
- Radiation oncology

ADDITIONAL THERAPIES
Possible breast reconstructive surgery with plastic surgery

SURGERY/OTHER PROCEDURES
- Mastectomy with axillary dissection or breast conservation therapy followed by radiation therapy, depending on extent and location of malignancy (1,10)[C]
- Multicentric lesions or diffuse calcifications require mastectomy (1)[C]
- Studies show no difference in long-term survival with mastectomy vs. central lumpectomy (1,3)[A]
- Axillary lymph node dissection and sentinel node biopsy:
  – Recommended in patients diagnosed with invasive cancer (1)[C]
  – Recommended in patients undergoing mastectomy (8,11)[B]
  – Considered for patients with underlying DCIS (13)[C]

IN-PATIENT CONSIDERATIONS
Admission Criteria/Initial Stabilization
Dependent on cancer histology, size, and stage (see topic on "Breast Cancer"):
- Surgery
- Radiotherapy
- Chemotherapy
- Hormone therapy

 ONGOING CARE

FOLLOW-UP RECOMMENDATIONS
Oncology consultation

Patient Monitoring
- After successful treatment for Paget disease of the breast, patients should start an individualized cancer surveillance program to include regular history, physical examination, and mammograms.
- Routine screening for average risk women who have never been diagnosed with breast cancer or Paget disease is per USPSTF guidelines:
  – Biennial screening mammography for women ages 50–74.

PATIENT EDUCATION
- National Cancer Institute, Department of Health and Human Services, Public Inquiries Section, Office of Cancer Communications, Building 31, Room 101-18, 9000 Rockville Pike, Bethesda, MD 20892; 301-496-5583
- www.cancer.gov/cancertopics/factsheet/Sites-Types/paget-breast

PROGNOSIS
- Factors of unfavorable prognosis (1,4,14):
  – Palpable breast mass
  – Multifocal disease
  – Lymph node enlargement
  – Vascular Invasion/Invasive disease
  – Higher stage of disease
  – Her2/Neu overexpression
  – Age <60
- Prognosis by presence/absence of palpable mass:
  – 22% 10-year survival if palpable mass present prior to excision
  – 82% 10-year survival if no palpable mass prior to excision
- Prognosis by lymph node status:
  – 47% 10-year survival if positive nodes
  – 93% 10-year survival if negative nodes (14)
- Prognosis by stage of underlying breast carcinoma (15):
  – (See (16) for Breast Cancer staging descriptions)

Stage	5-yr relative survival
I	96%
II	78%
III	46%
IV	14%

COMPLICATIONS
Risk factors for recurrence (17):
- Axillary lymph node metastases
- Underlying invasive cancer
- Negative hormone receptor expression
- Her2/Neu overexpression

REFERENCES
1. Caliskan M, Gatti G, Sosnovskikh I, et al. Paget's disease of the breast: The experience of the European Institute of Oncology and review of the literature. Breast Cancer Res Treat. 2008;112: 513–521.
2. Kim HS, Seok JH, Cha ES, et al. Significance of nipple enhancement of Paget's disease in contrast enhanced breast MRI. Arch Gynecol Obstet. 2010;282:157–162.
3. Chen CY, Sun LM, Anderson BO. Paget disease of the breast: Changing patterns of incidence, clinical presentation, and treatment in the U.S. Cancer. 2006;107:1448–1458.
4. Kanitakis J. Mammary and extramammary Paget's disease. J Eur Acad Dermatol Venereol. 2007;21: 581–590.
5. Sanders MA, Dominici L, Denison C, et al. Paget disease of the breast with invasion from nipple skin into the dermis: an unusual type of skin invasion not associated with an adverse outcome. Arch Pathol Lab Med. 2013;137:72–76.
6. Karakas C. Paget's disease of the breast. J Carcinog. 2011;10:31.
7. Sek P, Zawrocki A, Biernat W, et al. HER2 molecular subtype is a dominant subtype of mammary Paget's cells. An immunohistochemical study. Histopathology. 2010;57:564–571.
8. Siponen E, Hukkinen K, Heikkilä P, et al. Surgical treatment in Paget's disease of the breast. Am J Surg. 2010;200:241–246.
9. Marshall JK, Griffith KA, Haffty BG, et al. Conservative management of Paget disease of the breast with radiotherapy: 10- and 15-year results. Cancer. 2003;97:2142.
10. Lim HS, Jeong SJ, Lee JS, et al. Paget disease of the breast: Mammographic, US, and MR imaging findings with pathologic correlation. Radiographics. 2011;31:1973–1987.
11. Morrogh M, Morris EA, Liberman L, et al. MRI identifies otherwise occult disease in select patients with Paget disease of the nipple. J Am Coll Surg. 2008;206:316–321.
12. Zakhireh J, Gomez R, Esserman L, et al. Converting evidence to practice: A guide for the clinical application of MRI for the screening and management of breast cancer. Eur J Cancer. 2008;44:2742–2752.
13. NCCN Clinical Practice Guidelines in Oncology and Breast Cancer (version 3.2013) 2013. Breast Cancer National Comprehensive Cancer Network, Inc. Available at: www.nccn.org
14. Kawase K, Dimaio DJ, Tucker SL, et al. Paget's disease of the breast: There is a role for breast conservative therapy. Ann Surg Oncol. 2005;12: 391–397.
15. National Cancer Institute. Paget disease of the breast. Available at: www.cancer.gov/cancertopics/factsheet/Sites-Types/paget-breast
16. American Cancer Society. How is breast cancer staged? Available at: www.cancer.org/Cancer/BreastCancer/DetailedGuide/breast-cancer-staging
17. Lohsiriwat V, Martella S, Rietjens M, et al. Paget's disease as a local recurrence after nipple-sparing mastectomy: clinical presentation, treatment, outcome, and risk factor analysis. Ann Surg Oncol. 2012;19:1850–1855.

ADDITIONAL READING
Ceccherini AF, Evans AJ, Pinder SE, et al. Is ipsilateral mammography worthwhile in Paget's disease of the breast? Clin Radiol. 1996;51:35.

 CODES

ICD10
- C50.011 Malignant neoplasm of nipple and areola, right female breast
- C50.012 Malignant neoplasm of nipple and areola, left female breast
- C50.019 Malignant neoplasm of nipple and areola, unsp female breast

CLINICAL PEARLS
- Any chronic or nonhealing nipple or breast lesions should be biopsied to rule out malignancy.
- Paget disease is an uncommon presentation of breast malignancy involving the nipple–areolar complex and characterized by eczematous changes, erythema, ulceration, bleeding, and/or itching.

PALLIATIVE CARE

Felix B. Chang, MD • Rocio I. Nordfeldt, MD

 BASICS

Care of patients whose disease is not responsive to curative treatment

DESCRIPTION
- Focuses on relieving and preventing suffering
- Goals are patient centered, which arise following an informed discussion of the current disease(s), prognosis, and treatment options
- Hospice eligibility: Terminal illness with an estimated prognosis of ≤6 months.
- Skills: Communication, decision making, management of complications, psychosocial care of the patient and family, symptom control, care of the dying, coordination

EPIDEMIOLOGY
- Estimate palliative care covers >500,000 patients
- By 2008, 31% had cancer and 69% died from chronic diseases.
- More than 80% of hospice beneficiaries are >65 years and 1/3 are >85 years.

Incidence
- Difficult to measure. The most common reason to enter palliative care is advanced cancer.

GENERAL PREVENTION
- State-by-state laws: www.aarp.org/relationships/caregiving/info-01-2011/caregiver_map.html

COMMONLY ASSOCIATED CONDITIONS
- Headache, bone pain, ascites, chest pain.
- Shortness of breath (60%) commonly due to lung cancer and advanced congestive heart failure (CHF)
- 62% have anorexia, nausea and vomiting, constipation, dysphagia, anxiety, depression, and hopelessness.
- Delirium (40–85%)
- Pruritus causes considerable discomfort and affects the quality of life (1).

 DIAGNOSIS

The PEACE tool evaluates:
- Physical symptoms
- Emotive and cognitive symptoms
- Autonomy and related issues
- Communication: Contribution to others, and closure of life affairs–related issues
- Economic burden and other practical issues, also transcendent and existential issues

HISTORY
- Assessment: Pain/symptom, social, spiritual, understanding illness/prognosis treatment options, identification of patient-centered goals of care, and transition of care postdischarge
- Personhood issues (spiritual/faith, cultural, family/community resource support)
- Evaluate possible barriers to timely consideration of a palliative approach to care:
  - The impression that palliation means "there is nothing else to do," "giving up"
  - Difficulty in recognizing when "aggressive" interventions have lost ability to prolong life

- Assessment (2):
  - Emotive and cognitive symptoms: Sadness (grief), anxiety, depression, and delirium
  - Autonomy:
    ○ Do you feel in control of your care? Are we doing all and only the things you desire? Do you know the nature of your illness and what to expect of it?
    ○ Do you feel heard/listened to? Are we following your directions to your satisfaction? Are your treatment preferences in writing?
  - Closure of life affairs: Is there anyone you have not seen or with whom you need to talk? Do you have regrets? What do you still want to accomplish in your life?
  - Economic burden: Are you worried about financial burden? Do you worry that you may become a burden to your family? Do you need help with insurance agencies?
- Transcendental and existential issues: Evaluate sense of peace, meaning, and hopes vs. torment or agony. Are you suffering? Would you like a chaplain/counselor to visit?

PHYSICAL EXAM
- Pain, genitourinary (incontinence); respiratory (dyspnea, cough); GI (nausea, constipation, vomiting, diarrhea); ulcerations and other skin complaints; level of functioning; fatigue or asthenia; and side effects
- Vitals: Weight, midarm circumference
- General: Orientation, cognition
- ENT, adequate vision and hearing for communication purposes
- Oral: tongue (moist/dry, thrush). Check for presence of ketone breath, gag reflex, dentures, gingivitis, tooth decay, and abscess; assess risk for aspiration
- Neck: Assess lymphadenopathy, thyromegaly, hepatojugular reflux, stiff/supple neck, paracervical pain triggers (common cause of headaches in elderly), and kyphosis
- Cardiovascular: Murmurs/splits/gallops, point of maximal impulse (PMI)
- Lungs: Inspection, palpation, percussion, auscultation; blood pressure (sitting and standing); pulse and respiration
- Abdomen/Genitourinary: Distention, presence of artificial feeding device. Digital rectal exam for constipation/impaction and Hemoccult.
- Musculoskeletal/Neurologic: Pain sites, weakness, paresthesia, pathologic reflexes (Hoffman, Babinski), contractures, posture, range of motion
- Skin: Presence of rash, bed sores, wounds

DIAGNOSTIC TESTS & INTERPRETATION
Initial Tests (lab, imaging)
Urinalysis, comprehensive metabolic panel, CBC.
Should be reserved for the identification of conditions that will change treatment when present.

Follow-Up Tests & Special Considerations
Teamwork: Physician, nurse, social worker, home health aide, pastor, administrator, pharmacist, medical supplier (beds, nebulizers, oxygen, commodes, wheelchairs), respite and home health agencies, community resources (Meals on Wheels, volunteers), allied health practitioners (e.g., aromatherapy, massage, osteopathic manipulative medicine, acupuncture, meditation, ethicist)

 TREATMENT

GENERAL MEASURES
- Symptoms management
- Polypharmacy is common

MEDICATION
- Consider trimming medications that offer little improvement in the quality of life
- Assure compliance by addressing patient/caregiver understanding and written consensus.
- Pain: Immediate-release opioids PO/IV treat dyspnea effectively and typically at doses lower than would be necessary for the relief of moderate pain (3)
  - Once pain is controlled, convert to a long-acting opioids with short-acting agents made available as tolerance develops and/or patient develops breakthrough pain.
- Vomiting associated with a particular opioid may be relieved by substitution with an equianalgesic dose of another opioid or a sustained-release formulation. Dopamine-receptor antagonists (metoclopramide, prochlorperazine, promethazine) are commonly used.
- Droperidol: Insufficient evidence to advise on the use for the management of nausea and vomiting (4)[A]
- Constipation: Prophylactic stool softeners (docusate) and stimulants (bisacodyl or senna). Polyethylene glycol should be started when opioid treatment is begun to avoid constipation (5)[A].
- Subcutaneous methylnaltrexone is effective in inducing bowel movements without inducing withdrawal with opioid-induced constipation (5)[A].
- Dyspnea: Oxygen, narcotics, and, if CHF, diuretics and/or long-acting nitrates, benzodiazepines (3)
- Delirium: Lowest doses necessary of benzodiazepines or antipsychotics (Haldol, others)
- Patient safety and nonpharmacologic strategies to assist orientation (clocks, calendars, environment, and redirection). When cause of delirium cannot be identified/corrected rapidly, consider neuroleptics (haloperidol or risperidone)
- Pruritus: No optimal therapy recommended (1)
- Anxiety: Insufficient data for recommendations (6)
- Megestrol acetate improves appetite and slight weight gain (7)

ALERT
Bone pain: NSAIDs added to narcotics are more effective than narcotics alone.

ISSUES FOR REFERRAL
- Eligibility for hospice care:
  - I. The patient's condition is life limiting, and the patient and/or family have been informed of this condition.
  - II. The patient and/or family have elected treatment goals directed toward the relief of symptoms, rather than a cure of the underlying disease.

– III. The patient has either of the following:
A. Documented disease clinical progression:
1. Progression of the primary disease process documented by serial assessments, laboratory, radiologic, or other studies. 2. Multiple emergency department visits or inpatient hospitalizations over the prior 6 months. 3. For homebound patients receiving home health services, nursing assessment may be documented. For patients who do not qualify for 1, 2, or 3, a recent decline in functional status may be documented.
B. Documented recent impaired nutritional status related to the terminal process. 1. Unintentional, progressive weight loss of >10% over the prior 6 months. 2. Serum albumin <2.5 g/dL may be a helpful prognostic indicator, but should not be used in isolation from other factors in I–III

- Eligibility: Eligibility for Medicare part A (hospital insurance), Medicare approved hospice. The patient signs a statement choosing hospice care instead of regular Medicare. The patient's physician and the hospice medical director both certify that the patient has a terminal illness and <6 months to live. (There is no penalty to certifier if patient lives >6 months.)

 ONGOING CARE

PATIENT EDUCATION
www.getpalliativecare.org

PROGNOSIS
- For seriously ill patients with advanced COPD, HF, or end-stage liver disease, clinical prediction criteria are not effective in identifying a population with a survival prognosis of ≤6 months.
- Determining prognosis in noncancer diseases:
  – Heart disease: For CHF symptoms at rest; uncontrollable arrhythmias, history of cardiac arrest/resuscitation; cardiogenic brain embolism
  – Pulmonary disease:
    ○ Dyspnea at rest from decreased functional activity, exacerbated by fatigue, cough
    ○ Presence of cor pulmonale or right-sided heart failure
    ○ Hypoxemia at rest on supplemental oxygen; hypercapnia; unintentional weight loss of >10% of body weight over 6 months; resting tachycardia (>100/min) in COPD
  – Dementia:
    ○ Functional assessment ≥ stage 7: Unable to ambulate, dress or bathe; urinary/fecal incontinence; unable to communicate meaningfully
    ○ Comorbid conditions: Aspiration pneumonia, pyelonephritis, or urinary infections; septicemia; decubitus ulcer; recurrent fever; difficulty swallowing or refusal to eat

– HIV:
  ○ CD4+ count <25 cells/mm^3
  ○ Viral load >100,000 copies/mL
  ○ Life-threatening concomitant conditions
  ○ Chronic persistent diarrhea for 1 year; persistent serum albumin <2.5 gm/dL; substance abuse; age >50; decision to forgo retroviral, chemotherapeutic prophylaxis drug therapy related specifically to HIV disease, CHF
– Liver disease:
  ○ Laboratory indicators of severely impaired liver function: Prothrombin time prolonged >5 sec over control; serum albumin <2.5 g/dL
  ○ Clinical indicators of end-stage liver disease: Patient noncompliant, refractory ascites, spontaneous bacterial peritonitis, hepatorenal syndrome, refractory hepatic encephalopathy, recurrent variceal bleeding
  ○ Worsening prognosis: Progressive malnutrition, muscle wasting with reduced strength and endurance; continued active alcoholism, >80 g/d ethanol, hepatocellular carcinoma, hepatitis B surface antigen positivity
– Renal diseases:
  ○ Renal failure: Creatinine clearance of <10 mL/min (<15 mL/min for diabetes) and serum creatinine of <8 mg/dL (>6 mg/dL in diabetics)
  ○ ESRD discontinuing dialysis, or dialysis eligible and refusing, with renal failure: Uremia; oliguria; intractable hyperkalemia; uremic pericarditis; hepatorenal syndrome; intractable fluid overload
  ○ Early mortality: Mechanical ventilation; malignancy; chronic lung disease; advanced cardiac disease; sepsis; immunosuppression/AIDS; albumin <3.5 g/dL; cachexia; platelet count <25,000; age >75; disseminated intravascular congestion; GI bleeding
– Stroke and coma: I. During the acute phase immediately following a hemorrhagic or ischemic stroke: A. Coma or persistent vegetative state >3 days. B. In postanoxic stroke, coma or severe obtundation, accompanied by severe myoclonus, persisting >3 days past the anoxic event. C. Comatose patients with any 4 of the following on day 3 of coma: Abnormal brainstem response; absent verbal response; absent withdrawal response to pain; serum creatinine >1.5 mg/dL, age >70. D. Dysphagia severe enough to prevent the patient from receiving food and fluids necessary to sustain life. E. CT or MRI findings indicating decreased likelihood of survival. II. Once the patient has entered the chronic phase: A. Age >70. B. Poor functional status, as evidenced by Karnofsky score of <50%. C. Poststroke dementia, as evidenced by a FAST (Functional Assessment Staging) score >7. D. Poor nutritional status, whether on artificial or not: Aspiration pneumonia; upper urinary track infection, sepsis; refractory stage 3–4 decubitus ulcer; fever recurrent after antibiotics.

REFERENCES

1. Xander C, Meerpohl J, Galandi D, et al. Pharmacological intervention for pruritus in adult palliative care patients. *Cochrane Database Syst Rev.* 2013;6:CD008320.
2. Chan EY, Wu HY, Chan YH. Revisiting the Palliative Performance Scale: Change in scores during disease trajectory predicts survival. *Palliat Med.* 2013;27:367–374.
3. Ben-Aharon I, Gaffer-Gvili A, Paul M, et al. Interventions for alleviating cancer-related dyspnea: A systematic review. *J Clin Oncol.* 2008;26:2396–2404.
4. Dorman S, Perkins P. Droperidol for treatment of nausea and vomiting in palliative care patients. *Cochrane Database Syst Rev.* 2010;10:CD006938.
5. Candy B, Jones L, Goodman ML, et al. Laxatives or methylnaltrexone for the management of constipation in palliative care patients. *Cochrane Database Syst Rev.* 2011;1:CD003448.
6. Bridget C, Jackson K, Jones L, et al. Drug therapy for symptoms associated with anxiety in adult palliative care patients. *Cochrane Database Syst Rev.* 2012;10:4596.
7. Ruiz Garcia V, Lopez Briz E, Carbonell Sanchis R, et al. Megestrol acetate for treatment of anorexia-cachexia syndrome. *Cochrane Database Syst Rev.* 2013;3:CD004310.

ADDITIONAL READING

Gomes B, Calanzani N, Curiale V, et al. Effectiveness and cost effectiveness of home palliative care services for adults with advanced illness and their caregivers. *Cochrane Database Syst Rev.* 2013;6:CD007760.

 CODES

ICD10
Z51.5 Encounter for palliative care

CLINICAL PEARLS

Workforce shortages, late referrals, and palliative care program resources constrain present significant barriers to meeting the needs of hospitalized patients facing serious illness.

PANCREATIC CANCER

Edward Feller, MD

 BASICS

DESCRIPTION
- Carcinoma of the exocrine pancreas is the 4th most common cause of cancer death in the US.
- Rarely curable: Overall 1-year and 5-year relative survival rates of 25% and 5%, respectively.
- 60–70% occur in the head, 15% in the body, 5% in the tail, 20% diffusely involve the gland
- <20% are localized at diagnosis. For localized, small cancers (<2 cm) with no lymph node metastases and no extension beyond the capsule, surgical resection has 5-year survival of 18–24%.
- In apparently resectable disease, 20–40% have unresectable lesions at surgery.
- Ampullary, duodenal, or distal bile duct tumors may mimic pancreatic carcinoma and are more likely to be resectable and curable.
- For advanced or unresectable cancers, survival is <1% at 5 years; most patients die within 1 year.

EPIDEMIOLOGY
During 2003–2007, median age at diagnosis = 72 years; rare younger than age 45; after 45, occurrence rises.

Incidence
- An estimated 42,470 people diagnosed in 2009 (21,040 men and 21,420 women); 35,240 deaths
- More common in black and white races, 16.7 and 10.3 in 100,000 men and 14.4 and 10.3 in 100,000 women, respectively. Among Hispanic and Asian/Pacific Islanders there is an incidence of 10.9 and 8.3 in 100,000 men and 10.1 and 8.3 in 100,000 women, respectively (1).

Prevalence
In 2008, in the US, ~34,600 men and women (16,811 men and 17,846 women) were alive who had a history of pancreatic cancer.

RISK FACTORS
- Smoking: Relative risk (RR) = 1.5; correlates with amount smoked
- Diabetes: RR = 2.1 (95% confidence interval, 1.6–2.8); as many as 1 in 6 become diabetic within 6 months before diagnosis.
- Prior partial gastrectomy or cholecystectomy: 2–5-fold increased risk 15–20 years after gastrectomy
- Familial aggregation/genetic factors: 5–10% of patients have a 1st-degree relative with the disease, which confers a 9-fold increase in risk vs. the general population; subgroup may carry germline mutations of DNA repair genes (*BRCA2*) (2).
- Hereditary chronic pancreatitis: Cumulative risk by ages 50 and 75 is 10% and 54%, respectively
- Chronic pancreatitis: Tropical and nontropical
- Non-O blood type
- High intake of dietary fat and obesity
- Alcohol: Recent data indicate a modest increase in risk confined to heavy alcohol consumers (3).
- Coffee intake, aspirin, and NSAID use *NOT* regarded as risk factors.

GENERAL PREVENTION
Routine screening is not recommended. Even with a strong family history or predisposition syndromes, utility and cost-effectiveness of screening are unclear.

COMMONLY ASSOCIATED CONDITIONS
Chronic pancreatitis; diabetes mellitus; inherited cancer syndromes

 DIAGNOSIS

HISTORY
- Dependent on tumor location; majority become symptomatic late in disease. Majority develop in the pancreatic head and may block the periampullary bile duct, causing obstructive jaundice.
- Weight loss 90%; pain 75% (progressive midepigastric dull ache that often radiates to the back); malnutrition 75%; jaundice 70%; anorexia 60%; pruritus 40%; diabetes mellitus 15%; weakness, fatigue, malaise 30–40%; alcoholic stools, dark urine, steatorrhea; depression is common
- Pancreatic cancer is a consideration in acute pancreatitis in the elderly and with new-onset diabetes, but most new-onset diabetes is not associated with cancer; thus, evaluation for cancer is warranted only in selected cases.
- Uncommon: Unexplained thrombophlebitis; acute pancreatitis from tumor obstruction of the pancreatic duct; duodenal obstruction or GI bleeding (4)

PHYSICAL EXAM
- Muscle wasting and malnutrition are common; skin lesions are indicative of pruritus.
- Palpable abdominal mass or ascites in 20%
- Jaundice: 70% if tumor obstructs bile duct; 10% with body or tail carcinoma
- Courvoisier sign (painless jaundice with a palpable gallbladder): Uncommon; usually associated with pancreatic head tumors, periampullary or primary bile duct tumors; hepatomegaly in advanced disease
- Virchow node (left supraclavicular) and Sister Mary Joseph node (umbilical) in metastatic disease; palpable rectal shelf (nonspecific sign of carcinomatosis)
- Migratory thrombophlebitis (uncommon); due to hypercoagulability in mucin-producing pancreatic cancer
- GI bleeding from tumor erosion into adjacent viscera (colon); portal hypertension-related bleeding (uncommon)
- Pancreatic panniculitis: Subcutaneous areas of nodular fat necrosis

DIFFERENTIAL DIAGNOSIS
- Duodenal cancer, cholangiocarcinoma, lymphoma, islet cell tumor, sarcoma, cystic neoplasms, tumor metastatic to pancreas (rare)
- Nonmalignant conditions: Choledocholithiasis, acute or chronic pancreatitis, biliary tract stricture, adenoma; chronic mesenteric ischemia
- Tuberculosis or fungal abscess in AIDS
- Patients may present with back pain mimicking musculoskeletal disease.

DIAGNOSTIC TESTS & INTERPRETATION
- Cross-sectional imaging, usually CT scan, is used to evaluate symptoms or abnormal lab results.
- Endoscopic ultrasound-guided biopsy: Best modality for tissue diagnosis; sensitivity 75–90%; specificity ~100% for diagnosis of a mass
- Routine laboratory tests may reveal elevated serum bilirubin and alkaline phosphatase (cholestasis), anemia, or decreased serum albumin (malnutrition).

Initial Tests (lab, imaging)
- Most patients do not require measurement of serum tumor markers (CA19-9) for diagnosis or management. Some evidence suggests utility in predicting outcome and response to adjuvant chemotherapy (5,6).
- Elevated CA19.9 antigen: 80% sensitivity; 90% specificity; individuals with Lewis-negative blood group antigen phenotype (5–10%) are unable to synthesize CA19-9. Elevations can occur in benign pancreatic or biliary diseases and in nonpancreatic malignancy. Not recommended as a screening test.

Follow-Up Tests & Special Considerations
- During therapy, increase in CA19-9 may identify progressive tumor growth. Normal CA19-9 does not exclude recurrence.
- CT scan using thin section, multiphase multidetector helical CT with a pancreatic protocol is the choice for diagnosis and staging: 85–90% sensitivity; 90–95% specificity; useful for evaluation of distant metastasis and prediction of resectability (7).
- Abdominal ultrasound: Common initial test to assess jaundice and duct dilatation; less sensitive than CT for pancreatic masses.
- Endoscopic ultrasound (EUS) is accurate for tissue biopsy, local tumor and node staging, predicting vascular invasion (90% specificity; 73% sensitivity), and when no mass is identified on CT.
- Endoscopic retrograde cholangiopancreatography (ERCP): Invasive procedure with 90% sensitivity; 95% specificity for ductal cancer; useful if endoscopic stent is indicated for biliary obstruction; generally confined to high probability for therapeutic intervention on biliary or pancreatic ductal systems
- MRI: No advantage over contrast-enhanced CT
- MR cholangiopancreatography: Noninvasive: 90% sensitivity; 95% specificity. Preferred in specific settings: Gastric outlet or duodenal stenosis or after surgical rearrangement (Billroth II) or ductal disruption; to detect bile duct obstruction, after attempted ERCP is unsuccessful or provides incomplete information
- Cystic pancreatic lesions may be benign or malignant; must be differentiated from pancreatic pseudocysts (8)

Diagnostic Procedures/Other
- Percutaneous fine-needle biopsy with US or CT guidance: 80–90% sensitivity; 98–100% specificity
- EUS-guided biopsy: 85–90% sensitivity; virtually 100% specificity for pancreatic mass
- Staging laparoscopy and US: 92% sensitivity; 88% specificity; 89% accuracy

- Positive peritoneal cytology has a positive predictive value of 94%; specificity of 98%; sensitivity of 25% for determining unresectability (5).
- PET scan: 90% sensitivity, but 70% specificity; limited anatomic information
- Tumor staging:
  - Stage I: Tumors limited to the pancreas
  - Stage II: Regionally invasive; may involve lymph nodes, but without celiac or mesenteric artery involvement
  - Stage III: Direct involvement of celiac or superior mesenteric artery involvement
  - Stage IV: Distant metastases

Test Interpretation
- Duct cell carcinoma: 90%
- Others: Acinar, papillary mucinous, signet ring, adenosquamous, mucinous, giant or small cell, cystadenocarcinoma, undifferentiated, unclassified carcinoma

ALERT
Chronic pancreatitis can present with similar pain, weight loss, jaundice, and an inflammatory mass on imaging.

TREATMENT

- Surgical resection: Only chance of cure; no role for resection in metastatic disease. As few as 15–20% are candidates for resection.
- Criteria for unresectability: Extrapancreatic spread, encasement or occlusion of major vessels, distant metastases
- New combination chemotherapy regimens may offer advantages over gemcitabine-based therapies.

MEDICATION
- Analgesics
- Stages I and II:
  - Radical pancreatic resection + chemotherapy
  - ESPAC-3 trial after resection: Compared with 5-fluorouracil (5-FU) and folinic acid, gemcitabine did not improve overall survival (9)[A].
  - Currently, postoperative gemcitabine alone or in combination with 5-FU–based chemoradiation is the current standard of care; preoperative neoadjuvant treatment trials are in progress (4).
- Stage III:
  - Standard: Chemotherapy with gemcitabine-based regimens (10)[A]; added chemoradiation is controversial, but recent data suggest efficacy in advanced disease.
  - Palliation of biliary obstruction by endoscopic, surgical, or radiologic methods
  - Intraoperative radiation therapy and/or implantation of radioactive substances
- Stage IV:
  - Chemotherapy: Gemcitabine with erlotinib, a platinum agent, or a fluoropyrimidine may modestly prolong survival compared with gemcitabine alone (10)[A].
  - Pain-relieving procedures (celiac or intrapleural block); supportive care; palliative decompression

ADDITIONAL THERAPIES
- For resected tumors: Postoperative radiation therapy with other chemotherapeutic agents
- Intraoperative radiation therapy and/or implantation of radioactive substances (ongoing trials)
- Biliary decompression with endoprosthesis or transhepatic drainage
- Celiac axis and intrapleural nerve blocks can provide effective pain relief for some patients.
- Opiates may be needed for pain control.

SURGERY/OTHER PROCEDURES
- Standard treatment options:
  - Pancreaticoduodenectomy, Whipple procedure, en bloc resection of the head of the pancreas, distal common bile duct, duodenum, jejunum, and gastric antrum
  - Total pancreatectomy
  - Distal pancreatectomy for body and tail tumors
- Nonstandard surgeries:
  - Pylorus-preserving pancreaticoduodenectomy, regional pancreatectomy
  - Palliative bypass:
    - Biliary decompression; gastrojejunostomy for gastric outlet obstruction; duodenal endoprosthesis for obstruction

ONGOING CARE

DIET
- Anorexia, asthenia, pain, and depression may contribute to cachexia.
- Fat malabsorption due to exocrine pancreatic insufficiency may contribute to malnutrition; pancreatic enzyme replacement may help to alleviate symptoms.
- Fat-soluble vitamin deficiency may require replacement therapy.

PROGNOSIS
- Median survival: 10–20 months
- 5-year survival: ~30% if node-negative; 10% if node-positive
- Metastatic cancer: 1–2% 5-year survival
- For localized disease and small cancers (<2 cm) with no lymph node involvement and no extension beyond the capsule, complete surgical resection can yield a 5-year survival of 18–24%.

COMPLICATIONS
- Diabetes mellitus, malabsorption, thrombophlebitis
- Surgical complications: Intra-abdominal abscess, postgastrectomy syndromes, pancreaticojejunostomy, gastric and biliary anastomotic leaks; operative mortality varies

REFERENCES

1. Yadav D, Lowenfels AB. The epidemiology of pancreatitis and pancreatic cancer. *Gastroenterology*. 2013;144:1252–1261.
2. Vincent A, Herman J, Hruban RH, et al. Pancreatic cancer. *Lancet*. 2011;378:607–620.
3. Luncenforte E, Vecchia, Silverman D, et al. Alcohol consumption and pancreatic cancer: A pooled analysis in the International Pancreatic Cancer Case-Control Consortium. *Ann Oncol*. 2012;23: 374–382.
4. Hidalgo M. Pancreatic cancer. *N Engl J Med*. 2010;362:1605–1617.
5. Callery MP, Chang KJ, Fishman EK, et al. pretreatment assessment of resectable and borderline resectable pancreatic cancer; expert consensus statement. *Ann Surg Oncol*. 2009;16: 1727–1733.
6. Winter JM, Yeo CJ, Brody JR. Diagnostic, prognostic, and predictive biomarkers in pancreatic cancer. *J Surg Oncol*. 2013;107:15–22.
7. Kinney T. Evidence-based imaging of pancreatic malignancies. *Surg Clin North Am*. 2010;90: 411–425.
8. Verbesey JE, Munson JL. Cystic pancreatic neoplasms. *Surg Clin North Am*. 2010;90: 411–425.
9. Neoptolemos JP, Stocken DD, Ghaneh P, et al. Adjuvant chemotherapy with fluorouracil plus folinic acid vs gemcitabine following pancreatic cancer resection. *JAMA*. 2010;304:1073–1081.
10. Oberstein PE, Olive KP. Pancreatic cancer: Why is it so hard to treat ? *Ther Adv Gastroenterol*. 2013;6:321–337.

 CODES

ICD10
- C25.0 Malignant neoplasm of head of pancreas
- C25.1 Malignant neoplasm of body of pancreas
- C25.9 Malignant neoplasm of pancreas, unspecified

CLINICAL PEARLS
- Sudden onset of diabetes mellitus in nonobese adults aged >40 years may warrant consideration of pancreatic cancer in selected cases.
- Cancer of the exocrine pancreas is rarely curable; overall 5-year survival rate of <4%. Fewer than 20% of cases are localized at diagnosis.
- Be wary of chronic pancreatitis, which can present with similar pain pattern, weight loss, jaundice, and an inflammatory mass on imaging.

PANCREATITIS, ACUTE
Robert L. Frachtman, MD

BASICS

DESCRIPTION
Acute inflammatory process of the pancreas with variable involvement of regional tissue or remote organ systems:
- Inflammatory episode with symptoms related to intrapancreatic activation of enzymes with pain, nausea, and vomiting and associated intestinal ileus
- Varies widely in severity, complications, and prognosis, accounting for 280,000 hospital admissions per year in the US
- Complete structural and functional recovery, provided no necrosis or pancreatic ductal disruption

EPIDEMIOLOGY
Incidence
- 1–5/10,000
- Predominant age: None
- Predominant sex: Male = Female

Prevalence
Acute: 19/10,000

ETIOLOGY AND PATHOPHYSIOLOGY
- Alcohol
- Gallstones (including microlithiasis)
- Trauma/surgery
- Acute discontinuation of medications for diabetes or hyperlipidemia
- Following endoscopic retrograde cholangiopancreatography (ERCP)
- Medications (most common, but not exhaustive list):
  – ACE inhibitors
  – Angiotensin receptor blockers (ARBs)
  – Thiazide diuretics and furosemide
  – Antimetabolites (Purinethol and azathioprine) (1)[A]
  – Corticosteroids
  – Exenatide (Byetta) (2)[A]
  – Pentamidine
  – Statins, especially simvastatin (1)[A]
  – Pancreatitis may occur only after several months' administration of some of the implicated medications.
  – When a patient presents with pancreatitis, all medications should be reviewed in the *Physicians' Desk Reference* and accessible literature and should be continued only if the benefit justifies the risk of continuing a potential cause of pancreatitis, especially if no other causes are identified.
- Metabolic causes:
  – Hypertriglyceridemia (>1,000 mg/dL)
  – Hypercalcemia
  – Acute renal failure
  – Hereditary causes (uncommon)
  – Systemic lupus erythematosus/polyarteritis
  – Infections (list not exhaustive):
    ○ Mumps, coxsackie, cryptosporidiosis
- Penetrating peptic ulcer (rare)
- Cystic fibrosis and *CFTR* gene mutations
- Tumors (e.g., ampullary)
- Pancreas divisum
- Sphincter of Oddi dysfunction
- Scorpion venom
- Vascular disease
- Acute fatty liver of pregnancy

- Idiopathic/autoimmune
- Autodigestion of the pancreas, interstitial edema with severe 3rd spacing, hemorrhage, necrosis, release of vasoactive peptides, acute fluid collection (within 6 weeks), pseudocyst or acute necrotic collection (>6 weeks), pancreatic ductal disruption, injury to surrounding vascular structures such as the splenic vein (thrombosis) and splenic artery (pseudoaneurysm)

Genetics
Hereditary pancreatitis is a rare condition with an autosomal-dominant inheritance pattern.

GENERAL PREVENTION
- Avoidance of alcohol excess, especially over a prolonged period
- Avoidance of cigarette smoking
- Correction of underlying causes (hypertriglyceridemia or hypercalcemia)
- Discontinuation of medications associated with pancreatitis as soon as it is diagnosed
- Cholecystectomy if symptomatic cholelithiasis

COMMONLY ASSOCIATED CONDITIONS
- Consider coexistent alcohol withdrawal, alcoholic hepatitis, diabetic ketoacidosis, and ascending cholangitis
- Obesity increases severity, local complications, and mortality (3)[A].

DIAGNOSIS

Symptoms and objective evidence (imaging, amylase/lipase) do not always correlate

HISTORY
- Fairly rapid onset of epigastric pain, which may radiate posteriorly, often with emesis
- Alcohol use
- History or family history of gallstones
- Medication use
- Abdominal trauma
- Recent significant rapid weight loss (via induction of cholelithiasis)

PHYSICAL EXAM
- Abdominal findings: Epigastric tenderness, loss of bowel sounds
- Other findings: Fever, tachycardia, hypotension/shock, jaundice, rales/percussive dullness
- Rare (with hemorrhagic pancreatitis):
  – Flank discoloration (Grey–Turner sign) or umbilical discoloration (Cullen sign)

DIAGNOSTIC TESTS & INTERPRETATION
The laboratory/radiographic assessment of both acute and chronic pancreatitis must be used together, as there can be many false-positive and false-negative findings.
- Elevated serum amylase >3 × upper limit of normal (ULN) (severity is not related to degree of elevation)
- Elevated serum lipase >3 × ULN (may stay elevated longer than amylase in mild cases)
- Elevated total bilirubin to 3 mg/dL is not uncommon with pancreatitis per se, but more elevated levels create consideration of common bile duct obstruction.

- Transaminases can quickly rise to near 1,000 U/L with acute bile duct obstruction, but should rapidly fall as the alkaline phosphatase rises; a 3-fold elevation in the alanine aminotransferase (ALT) in the setting of acute pancreatitis has a 95% positive predictive value for gallstone pancreatitis. Triglyceride levels >1,000 mg/dL suggest hypertriglyceridemia as the cause.
- Glucose is increased in severe disease.
- Calcium is decreased in severe disease.
- WBCs can be 10,000–25,000/μL without active infection.
- Rising hemoglobin is a poor prognostic sign (severe 3rd spacing). Rising BUN and creatinine imply volume depletion or acute renal failure.

DIFFERENTIAL DIAGNOSIS
- Penetrating peptic ulcer
- Acute cholecystitis or cholangitis
- Macroamylasemia, macrolipasemia
- Mesenteric vascular occlusion and/or infarction
- Perforation of a viscus
- Intestinal obstruction
- Aortic aneurysm (dissecting or rupturing)
- Inferior wall myocardial infarction
- Lymphoma
- Disorders that may alter results for amylase or lipase:
  – Biliary tract disease, penetrating peptic ulcer, intestinal obstruction, intestinal ischemia/infarction, ruptured ectopic pregnancy, renal insufficiency, burns, macroamylasemia, or macrolipasemia

Initial Tests (lab, imaging)
- Admit labs should be supplemented by early and frequent follow-up labs to assess renal function, hydration, sepsis, biliary obstruction, and O_2 saturation.
- Plain film of abdomen is useful to rule out mechanical small bowel obstruction, but ileus secondary to pancreatitis is common.
- Chest x-ray (CXR) is useful to evaluate for early acute respiratory distress syndrome (ARDS) and pleural effusion; if upright, can rule out free subdiaphragmatic air.
- Ultrasound is useful to rule out cholelithiasis; choledocholithiasis can occasionally be seen.
- CT scan:
  – Will confirm the diagnosis, assess the severity, establish a baseline, and rule out other possibilities, but will not rule out noncalcified cholelithiasis. Acute fluid collections often resolve spontaneously.
  – IV contrast, regarding evaluation for necrosis, is not essential on the initial CT scan and should be avoided in volume-depleted patients.
  – If not contraindicated, a CT scan with IV contrast at day 3 can assess the degree of necrosis when necrotizing pancreatitis is suspected because of O_2 saturation <90%, systolic BP <90 mm Hg, etc.
- MRCP is useful to assess the likelihood of choledocholithiasis; as a bonus, pancreas divisum, a dilated pancreatic duct, or chronic ductal changes could be found.
- Esophagogastroduodenoscopy (EGD) may occasionally be necessary to rule out a penetrating duodenal ulcer or an obstructing ampullary neoplasm if suggested by laboratory or imaging studies.

- ERCP may be necessary for emergency common bile duct decompression due to an impacted stone.
- Endoscopic ultrasonography (EUS) when a patient with "idiopathic pancreatitis" has 2nd episode.

Follow-Up Tests & Special Considerations

If renal function is stable, a contrast-enhanced CT scan at day 3 to assess for necrosis, a major prognostic indicator. Later in the course, if there is a sudden worsening in the temperature curve, material can be aspirated via CT scan to assess for secondary infection.

 TREATMENT

MEDICATION

First Line

- Analgesia: No consensus; guidelines vary widely on types and dosing for analgesia (4):
  - Hydromorphone (Dilaudid) 0.5–1 mg IV q1–2h PRN (morphine sulfate can increase sphincter of Oddi pressure, worsening the pancreatitis)
  - AVOID Demerol due to the potential of accumulation of a toxic metabolite.
- Antibiotics:
  - Carbapenems can be considered for initial treatment, before cultures (especially of aspirated collections) return, if there is a strong suspicion of active infection, particularly in patients with necrotizing pancreatitis
  - β-lactam blockers with semisynthetic penicillin (e.g., Zosyn) or fluoroquinolones if cholangitis
  - Be vigilant for monilial superinfections when giving prophylactic antibiotics.
  - The use of prophylactic antibiotics is no longer recommended, even with necrotizing pancreatitis.

GENERAL MEASURES

- Confirm diagnosis and rule out other possibilities, if needed (see above).
- Unless extremely mild, most cases require hospitalization; ICU if multiorgan dysfunction or hypotension/respiratory failure that fails to respond to initial resuscitation. There is a progression from mild to severe pancreatitis, which may include persistent organ failure in 15–20% of cases.
- Fluid resuscitation (4):
  - If moderate or severe pancreatitis, there could easily be a 3-L deficit due to 3rd spacing.
  - Infusion of a bolus of 1,000–2,000 mL (lactated Ringers may be better than normal saline, unless hypercalcemic) in the ER, followed by a rate of 250–300 mL/h, adjusted on the basis of age, weight, PE findings, and comorbid conditions. (Caution regarding elderly patients and those with cardiac or renal disease.)
  - Urine output goal should be 0.5–1 mL/kg/h. Lower infusion rate when this goal is achieved or once BUN decreases, 4 L should be the maximum fluid on day 1.
- Eliminate all unnecessary medications, especially those that could potentially cause pancreatitis.
- Nasogastric (NG) tube is needed if there is intractable emesis, which could be secondary to a generalized ileus or a gastric outlet obstruction secondary to extrinsic duodenal compression.
- Follow status regarding renal function, volume, calcium, and oxygenation. Organ failure is more important than pancreatic necrosis.
- Intermittent pneumatic compression device
- Enteral nutrition at level of ligament of Treitz if oral feeding will not be possible within 5–7 days (preferable to total parenteral nutrition [TPN] due to

decreased infection rate and decreased mortality), to be discontinued with increases in pain, amylase/lipase levels, or fluid collection volume
- TPN (without lipids if triglycerides are elevated) if oral or nasoenteric feedings are not tolerated

ISSUES FOR REFERRAL

Refer to a tertiary center if pancreatitis is either already severe or actively evolving and when advanced imaging or endoscopic therapy is being considered.

SURGERY/OTHER PROCEDURES

- Consider cholecystectomy before discharge in patients with cholelithiasis because of risk of near term post-discharge recurrent acute pancreatitis
- Necrosectomy for infected necrosis, after 2–4 weeks of antibiotics. If not infected, walled off necrosis should be observed, unless symptomatic.
- ERCP early if evidence of acute cholangitis or at 72 hours if evidence of ongoing biliary obstruction. ERCP/stent late if ongoing disrupted pancreatic duct.
- Resection or embolization for bleeding pseudoaneurysms
- Plasma exchange with insulin if necrotizing pancreatitis secondary to hypertriglyceridemia

IN-PATIENT CONSIDERATIONS

Discharge Criteria

- Pain control
- Diet tolerance
- Alcohol rehab and smoking cessation, if needed
- Low-grade fever and mild leukocytosis do not necessarily indicate infection and may take weeks to resolve. Infections may occur even after 10 days (33% of patients with necrotizing pancreatitis) due to secondary infection of necrotic material, which will require surgical debridement.

 ONGOING CARE

FOLLOW-UP RECOMMENDATIONS

- Follow-up imaging studies may be required in several weeks, especially if the original CT scan showed a fluid collection or necrosis or if the amylase/lipase continues to be elevated:
  - Pseudocyst (may occur in 10%) or abscess (sudden onset of fever): Conservative management is reasonable for asymptomatic pseudocysts, even if 6 cm in diameter.
  - Splenic vein thrombosis (gastric variceal hemorrhage can occur rarely)
  - Pseudoaneurysm (splenic, gastroduodenal, intrapancreatic) hemorrhages (life threatening)
- Mild exocrine and endocrine dysfunction occur but are usually subclinical. However, patients with necrotizing pancreatitis, steatorrhea, or ductal obstruction should receive enzyme supplementation.

DIET

- Begin diet after pain, tenderness, and ileus have resolved; small amounts of high-carbohydrate, low-fat, and low-protein foods; advance as tolerated; NPO or NG tube if patient is vomiting.
- Enteral nutrition at level of ligament of Treitz is preferable to TPN if tolerated.
- TPN if oral or enteral route is not tolerated (no lipids if triglycerides are increased) (5)[A]

PROGNOSIS

- 85–90% resolve spontaneously; 3–5% mortality (17% in necrotizing pancreatitis). BMI >30 is another risk factor; APACHE II scoring is most accurate, but difficult to apply (6)[A]; BISAP, SIRS

(temp, pulse, resp, and WBC), and HAPS are newer, more rapidly applicable calculations. Ranson criteria (see below) have a sensitivity of ~40%:

- On admission: Age >55 years, WBCs >16,000/mm, blood glucose >200 mg/dL (11.1 mmol/L), serum lactate dehydrogenase (LDH) >350 IU/L, aspartate aminotransferase (AST) >250 IU/L
- Within 48 hours: Hematocrit decreases >10%, serum calcium <8 mg/dL, BUN increase >8 mg/dL, arterial PO_2 <60 mm Hg, base deficit >4 mEq/L, fluid retention >6 L
- Ranson scoring:
  - Ranson score of 0–2: Minimal mortality
  - Ranson score of 3–5: 10–20% mortality
  - Ranson score of >5: >50% mortality

REFERENCES

1. Nitsche CJ, Jamieson N, Lerch MM, et al. Drug induced pancreatitis. *Best Pract Res Clin Gastroenterol*. 2010;24:143–155.
2. Wang SQ, Li SJ, Feng QX, et al. Overweight is an additional prognostic factor in acute pancreatitis: A meta-analysis. *Pancreatology*. 2011;11:92–98.
3. Wu BU, Conwell DL. Acute pancreatitis part I: Approach to early management. *Clin Gastroenterol Hepatol*. 2010;8:410–416.
4. Oláh A, Romics L. Evidence-based use of enteral nutrition in acute pancreatitis. *Langenbecks Arch Surg*. 2010;395:309–316.
5. Gravante G, Garcea G, Ong SL, et al. Prediction of mortality in acute pancreatitis: A systematic review of the published evidence. *Pancreatology*. 2009;9:601–614.
6. Lu X, Aoun E. Complications of Acute Pancreatitis. *Practical Gastroenterology*. 2012;36:11–26.

ADDITIONAL READING

- Fisher J, Gardner T. The "golden hours" of management in acute pancreatitis. *Am J Gastroenterol*. 2012;107:1146–1150.
- Wu B, Banks P. Clinical management of patients with acute pancreatitis. *Gastroenterology*. 2013;144:1272–1281.

 CODES

ICD10

- K85.2 Alcohol induced acute pancreatitis
- K85.8 Other acute pancreatitis
- K85.9 Acute pancreatitis, unspecified

CLINICAL PEARLS

- Review all medications upon admission and discontinue any that have been implicated as causing pancreatitis, especially ACE inhibitors.
- Many patients identified as having mild pancreatitis progress to severe pancreatitis over the initial 48 hours, often due to inadequate fluid replacement.
- Referral to tertiary center is needed if acute pancreatitis is severe or evolving/worsening.
- Outpatient follow up, particularly re-imaging, is important.

PANCREATITIS, CHRONIC

Robert L. Frachtman, MD

BASICS

DESCRIPTION
Irreversible:
- Progressive destruction of the pancreas
- May result in either or both exocrine and endocrine insufficiency
- Major features:
  - Pain
  - Malabsorption
  - Diabetes mellitus
  - Increased risk of pancreatic cancer

EPIDEMIOLOGY
Incidence
Predominant age:
- 35–45 years (usually related to alcohol)
- Predominant sex: Male = Female

Prevalence
8.3/10,000

Genetics
Hereditary pancreatitis is a rare condition with an autosomal-dominant inheritance pattern.

GENERAL PREVENTION
- Avoid smoking
- Avoid excess alcohol

DIAGNOSIS

Symptoms and objective evidence (imaging, amylase/lipase) do not always correlate.

HISTORY
- Fairly rapid onset of epigastric pain, which may radiate posteriorly
- Often presents with emesis, with acute superimposed on chronic pancreatitis
- Chronic vague abdominal pain occurs with classical chronic pancreatitis
- Alcohol use
- Steatorrhea
- Weight loss
- Symptoms may not be present
- Children:
  - Recurrent postprandial epigastric pain
  - Family history of chronic pancreatitis
  - Growth failure
  - Diabetes

PHYSICAL EXAM
- Acute superimposed on chronic pancreatitis:
  - See "Pancreatitis, Acute"
  - Epigastric tenderness
  - Loss of bowel sounds
  - Fever
  - Tachycardia
  - Hypotension/shock
  - Jaundice
  - Rales/percussive dullness
- Chronic pancreatitis:
  - Mild, diffuse tenderness
  - Ascites

DIAGNOSTIC TESTS & INTERPRETATION
The laboratory and radiographic assessment of both acute and chronic pancreatitis must be used together, as there can be many false positives and negatives.

Initial Tests (lab, imaging)
Features and considerations:
- Amylase and lipase usually normal or near normal
- Hyperglycemia
- Steatorrhea (fecal fat >7 g/d on 100 g of fat per day diet), with other malabsorptive consequences such as low B_{12} level
- Flare-ups may mimic acute pancreatitis
- Elevated alkaline phosphatase and bilirubin imply obstruction of the intrapancreatic common bile duct by extrinsic fibrosis or cancer.
- Hereditary pancreatitis: Mutations in *PRSSI* gene and *SPINKI* gene
- Autoimmune pancreatitis: Elevated serum IgG4, autoantibodies to lactoferrin and carbonic anhydrase
- Pancreatic insufficiency: Fecal elastase-1 <200 mcg/g in moderate to severe pancreatic insufficiency
- Plain film of abdomen: Might show pancreatic calcification if severe
- US: Not very helpful for pancreas, but will assess the common bile duct diameter
- CT scan of abdomen: Pseudocysts, pancreatic duct dilation, and calcifications
- Magnetic resonance cholangiopancreatography (MRCP): Pancreatic ductal deformities/strictures (with or without pancreatic ductal stones), retained common bile duct stones
- Endoscopic US (EUS): Might help diagnose pancreatic cancer arising out of chronic pancreatitis

Follow-Up Tests & Special Considerations
Disorders that may alter results for amylase or lipase:
- Biliary tract disease
- Penetrating peptic ulcer
- Intestinal obstruction
- Intestinal ischemia/infarction
- Ruptured ectopic pregnancy
- Renal insufficiency
- Burns
- Macroamylasemia
- Macrolipasemia

DIFFERENTIAL DIAGNOSIS
- Pancreatic cancer
- Lymphoma
- Other malabsorptive processes, such as bacterial overgrowth, celiac disease, etc.

TREATMENT

MEDICATION
First Line
- Analgesics (no consensus on specific medications or doses):
  - Transdermal fentanyl might be useful when tablet ingestion is difficult, but higher doses are needed and more skin side effects noted (1)[C].
- Traditional pancreatic enzyme supplements are microencapsulated and do not require acid inhibition for protection. Dosage is 25–40,000 IU at the beginning of the meal.
- Some experts believe that uncoated enzymes (Viokase) are much more efficacious for pain control (when given with proton pump inhibitors [PPIs] to protect their integrity) than are coated enzymes (2)[C],(3)[B].
- Octreotide (Sandostatin) can be supplemental therapy for pancreatic ductal fistulae

GENERAL MEASURES
- Discontinue cigarette smoking, which can exacerbate chronic pancreatitis (4)[B]
- Analgesia: Consider pain management consultation regarding narcotic requirements
- Exocrine and endocrine replacement therapy (enzymes and insulin, respectively) (5)[C]
- Consider more advanced therapy for pain: Celiac ganglion block, endoscopic or surgical decompression of partially obstructed pancreatic duct

SURGERY/OTHER PROCEDURES

- Pseudocyst drainage:
  - Conservative approach recommended if asymptomatic
  - Endoscopic (via endoscopic ultrasound) or surgical approach if mature wall
  - Percutaneous approach if rapidly enlarging or if thin wall
- Pancreatic ascites with disruption of the main pancreatic duct:
  - Endoscopic placement of pancreatic ductal stent is preferred, if possible (6)[B].
  - Lateral pancreaticojejunostomy if endoscopic therapy is not possible
- Biliary obstruction (secondary to chronic pancreatitis, not choledocholithiasis):
  - Placement of retrievable metal stent or multiple plastic stents, if possible
  - Choledochojejunostomy if endoscopic therapy is not possible
- Pancreatic ductal obstruction by stone:
  - Endoscopic pancreatic sphincterotomy with stone extraction
- Total pancreatectomy and islet autotransplantation (7)[A]:
  - Favorable outcomes with pain reduction
  - Indication for timing of procedure uncertain

IN-PATIENT CONSIDERATIONS

Discharge Criteria
- Pain control
- Resolution of problems secondary to ductal disruption, if present
- Alcohol rehab and smoking cessation, if needed

 ONGOING CARE

FOLLOW-UP RECOMMENDATIONS
Depends on the source of the pain and whether a ductal disruption exists

DIET
- Small meals high in protein, ~20 g/d of fat; adjust if diabetes mellitus is present
- Pancreatic enzyme replacement therapy (coated/microencapsulated if treating pancreatic insufficiency, but noncoated with PPI if treating pancreatic pain)

PROGNOSIS
- Patient may have recurrent episodes of acute pancreatitis, which is a strong predictor for chronic pancreatitis.
- Slow progression
- May "burn out" with resolution of symptoms
- Narcotic addiction occurs frequently.
- Pancreatic exocrine and/or endocrine insufficiency may occur years later.

REFERENCES

1. Niemann T, Madsen LG, Larsen S, et al. Opioid treatment of painful chronic pancreatitis. *Int J Pancreatol*. 2000;27:235–240.
2. Slaff J. Protease-specific suppression of pancreatic exocrine secretion. *Gastroenterology*. 1984;87: 44–52.
3. Puylaert M, Kapural L, Van Zundert J, et al. Pain in chronic pancreatitis. *Pain Pract*. 2011;11:492–505.
4. Yadav D. Alcohol consumption, cigarette smoking, and the risk of recurrent acute and chronic pancreatitis. *Arch Intern Med*. 2009;169:1035.
5. Giuliano CA, Dehoorne-Smith ML, Kale-Pradhan PB. Pancreatic enzyme products: Digesting the changes. *Ann Pharmacother*. 2011;45:658–666.
6. Kozarek R, Ball T, Patterson D, et al. Endoscopic transpapillary therapy for disrupted pancreatic duct and peripancreatic fluid collections. *Gastro-enterology*. 1991;100(5 Pt 1):1362.
7. Bornman PC, Botha JF, Ramos JM, et al. Guideline for the diagnosis and treatment of chronic pancreatitis. *S Afr Med J*. 2010;100(12 Pt 2): 845–860.

ADDITIONAL READING

- Bramis K, Gordon-Weeks AN, Friend PJ, et al. Systematic review of total pancreatectomy and islet autotransplantation for chronic pancreatitis. *Br J Surg*. 2012;99:761–766.
- Yadav D, O'Connell M, Papachristou GI. Natural history following the first attack of acute pancreatitis. *Am J Gastroenterol*. 2012;107: 1096–1103.

 SEE ALSO

Choledocholithiasis; Peptic Ulcer Disease; Substance Use Disorders; Systemic Lupus Erythematosus

 CODES

ICD10
- K86.0 Alcohol-induced chronic pancreatitis
- K86.1 Other chronic pancreatitis

CLINICAL PEARLS

- Pancreatic enzyme replacement therapy and avoidance of cigarettes and alcohol are always the cornerstone of therapy.
- Pancreatic ductal injury must be considered and addressed.
- All patients with chronic pancreatitis do not yet necessarily have clinically significant pancreatic insufficiency.
- Fat malabsorption precedes carbohydrate and protein malabsorption.
- It may be very difficult to differentiate between chronic pancreatitis and pancreatic cancer arising from chronic pancreatitis.

PANIC DISORDER

Michael Golding, MD

 BASICS

DESCRIPTION
- The key feature of a panic attack is a brief period of sympathetic nervous system hyperarousal accompanied by psychological terror.
- In panic disorder, multiple panic attacks occur, some unexpected, over the course of at least 1 month, with worry about them.

EPIDEMIOLOGY
Incidence
- Predominant age: All ages; in school-aged children, panic disorder can be confused with conduct disorder and school avoidance.
- Peak age of onset is early to mid-20s
- Predominant sex: Female > Male (2:1)

Prevalence
- Lifetime prevalence: 1–3%
- ~8% of patients in a primary care practice population have panic disorder.
- Of patients presenting with chest pain in the emergency room, 25% have panic disorder.
- Chest pain is more likely due to panic if atypical, younger age, female, known problems with anxiety

ETIOLOGY AND PATHOPHYSIOLOGY
Unknown:
- Biologic theories focus on limbic system malfunction in dealing with anxiety-evoking stimuli.
- Psychological theories speak of deficits in managing strong affects, such as fear and anger.
- Agoraphobia may be a learned response to panic attacks or a learned response to a cluster of subclinical panic symptoms; e.g., if a person has a panic attack in the grocery store, he may learn to fear the grocery store and other situations in which subclinical or clinical panic attacks occur.
- Noradrenergic neurotransmission from the locus coeruleus causes increased sympathetic stimulation throughout the body.
- Current neurobiologic research focuses on abnormal responses to anxiety-producing stimuli in the hippocampus, amygdala, and prefrontal cortex; e.g., there appears to be limbic kindling in which an original frightening experience dominates future responses even when subsequent exposures are not objectively threatening.
- Brain pH disturbances (e.g., excess lactic acid) from normal mentation in genetically vulnerable patients may activate the amygdala and generate unexpected fear responses.

Genetics
Twin and family studies support a genetic predisposition.

RISK FACTORS
- Life stressors of any kind can precipitate attacks.
- History of sexual abuse and physical abuse, anxious and overprotective parents
- Substance abuse, bipolar disorder, major depression, obsessive–compulsive disorder (OCD), simple phobia

COMMONLY ASSOCIATED CONDITIONS
- Of patients with panic disorder, >70% also have ≥1 other psychiatric diagnoses: PTSD (recalled trauma precedes panic attack), social phobia (fear of scrutiny precedes panic attack), simple phobia (fear of something specific precedes panic), major depression, bipolar disorder, substance abuse, OCD, separation anxiety disorder
- Panic disorder is more common in patients with hypertension, mitral valve prolapse, reflux esophagitis, interstitial cystitis, irritable bowel syndrome, fibromyalgia, nicotine dependence.
- Suicidality

DIAGNOSIS

- Panic attack: A discrete period of intense fear, reaching a peak within 10 minutes in which ≥4 of the following symptoms develop abruptly: (a) palpitations, pounding heart, or accelerated heart rate; (b) sweating; (c) trembling or shaking; (d) sensations of shortness of breath or feeling smothered; (e) a choking sensation; (f) chest pain or discomfort; (g) nausea or abdominal distress; (h) feeling dizzy, unsteady, lightheaded, or faint; (i) derealization (feelings of unreality) or depersonalization (feeling detached from oneself); (j) fear of losing control or going crazy; (k) fear of dying; (l) paresthesias; (m) chills or hot flushes.
- Panic disorder: Recurrent unexpected panic attacks not better accounted for by another psychiatric condition (e.g., PTSD, OCD, separation anxiety disorder) *and* not induced by drugs of abuse, medical conditions, or prescribed drugs *and* with >1 month of at least 1 of the following: (a) worry about additional attacks; (b) worry about the implications of the attack (e.g., losing control, having a heart attack, "going crazy"); and/or (c) a significant change in behavior related to the attacks.
- Specify "panic with agoraphobia" if anxiety about being in places or situations from which escape might be difficult (or embarrassing).

HISTORY
- Panic attacks are not subtle, but obtaining a clear history, especially with a new patient, is difficult for 2 reasons:
  – In the throes of a panic attack, many patients are convinced that the disorder is physically dangerous because of the frightening physical symptoms they are experiencing.
  – Patients are often deeply embarrassed by their problem, which they see as a personal failure.
- The best way to get a good history is through tactful, nonjudgmental questioning after the worst of the attack is over.
- A thorough medication and substance abuse history is important.
- Patients must have a month of fear of out-of-the-blue panic attacks to diagnose panic disorder.

PHYSICAL EXAM
- During an attack, there will be tachycardia, hyperventilation, and sweating.
- Check the thyroid for fullness or nodules.
- Cardiac exam to check for a murmur or arrhythmias
- Lung exam to rule out asthma (limited airflow, wheezing)

DIFFERENTIAL DIAGNOSIS
- Medication use may mimic panic disorder and create anxiety: Antidepressants to treat panic may paradoxically initially cause panic; antidepressants in bipolar patients can cause anxiety/mania/panic; short-acting benzodiazepines (alprazolam), β-blockers (propranolol), and narcotics can cause interdose rebound anxiety; benzodiazepine treatment causes panic when patients take too much and run out of these medicines early; bupropion, levodopa, amphetamines, steroids, albuterol, sympathomimetics, fluoroquinolones, and interferon can cause panic.
- Substances of abuse: Alcohol withdrawal, benzodiazepine withdrawal, narcotic withdrawal, caffeine, marijuana (panic with paranoia), amphetamine abuse, MDMA, hallucinogens (PCP, LSD), dextromethorphan abuse, synthetic cathinones (bath salts) abuse.
- Medical conditions: Hypo-/Hyperthyroidism, mitral valve prolapse, asthma/chronic obstructive pulmonary disease (COPD), reflux esophagitis with hyperventilation, tachyarrhythmias, premenstrual dysphoric disorder, menopause, pregnancy, hypoglycemia (in diabetes), hypoxia, inner ear disturbances (labyrinthitis), myocardial infarction, pulmonary embolus, TIAs, carcinoid syndrome, pre- and postictal states (e.g., in TLE), autoimmune disease, pheochromocytoma, Cushing syndrome, hyperaldosteronism, Wilson disease
- Psychiatric conditions that have overlapping symptomatology include mood, anxiety, and personality disorders such as major depression, bipolar disorder, PTSD, borderline personality disorder, social phobia, OCD, and generalized anxiety disorder. In PTSD, there is always a recollection or visual image that precedes the panic attack. In social phobia, fear of scrutiny precedes the panic attack. In bipolar disorder, major depression, borderline personality disorder, and particularly substance abuse, the patient often complains 1st of panic symptoms and anxiety and minimizes other potentially relevant symptoms and behaviors.
- Somatization disorder is also an illness of multiple unexplained medical symptoms, but the presenting picture is usually one of chronic symptoms rather than the acute, dramatic onset of a panic attack. Somatization disorder and panic can be (and often are) diagnosed together.

DIAGNOSTIC TESTS & INTERPRETATION

Consider ECG and pulse oximetry to rule out certain serious causes of panic; consider Holter monitoring. No specific lab tests are indicated except to rule out conditions in the differential diagnosis. Consider these tests:

- Finger-stick blood sugar in acute setting in a diabetic patient
- Thyroid-stimulating hormone (TSH), electrolytes, CBC
- Consider ordering echocardiogram if you suspect mitral valve prolapse.

Diagnostic Procedures/Other

If a medical cause of anxiety is strongly suspected, do the workup appropriate for that condition.

 TREATMENT

Combined antidepressant therapy and psychotherapy is superior to either alone during active treatment. Cognitive-behavioral therapy (CBT) provides long-lasting treatment, often without subsequent need for medications (1)[A].

GENERAL MEASURES

CBT, tailored for panic disorder, consists of several steps: Education, changing cognitions about the attack and the illness, relaxation and controlled breathing techniques, and, if appropriate, exposure to anxiety-provoking conditions coupled with in vivo relaxation exercises.

MEDICATION

- Medication management is indicated if psychotherapy is not successful or may be initiated together with psychotherapy.
- Patient preference plays a big part in this decision.
- Because patients typically are anxious about their treatment, the therapeutic alliance is critical for the chronic care of this disorder.
- If medications are started, they should be maintained for at least 6 months after symptom control.

First Line

- In nonbipolar patients, start a low-dose antidepressant (e.g., 5 mg escitalopram, 25 mg sertraline, 10 mg paroxetine) and consider doubling the dose after 2 or 3 weeks; while waiting for the antidepressant to work, schedule frequent visits, give the patient reassurance, teach a relaxation technique, encourage the patient to do vigorous aerobic exercise as soon as a panic attack begins (if medically appropriate and in an appropriate situation) (2)[B]; refer the patient to a competent therapist for CBT.
- In bipolar patients, treat the underlying bipolar disorder with a mood stabilizer rather than an antidepressant, and panic symptoms often resolve.
- FDA-approved choices for the treatment of panic disorder include sertraline, paroxetine, fluoxetine, alprazolam, and clonazepam, but avoid giving benzodiazepines to those with a history of substance abuse or those who are currently abusing alcohol or benzodiazepines, unless utilizing a detoxification protocol.
- All antidepressants except bupropion can treat panic disorder, but fluoxetine and selegiline patch can cause more initial nervousness than other antidepressants.

Second Line

- Tricyclic antidepressants, particularly imipramine (start 25 mg/d in the evening and increase up to 25 mg every 3 days to a maximum of 200 mg/d); slower titration and lower doses are often as effective. Imipramine is as efficacious as SSRIs in the treatment of panic. Tricyclic antidepressants are considered 2nd-line because of difficulty in dosing, more side effects, and greater risk associated with overdose compared with SSRIs.
- Alprazolam (0.5–1 mg) and lorazepam (0.5–1 mg) can be given as a single dose to help with panic symptoms. If antidepressants are only partially effective, consider adding a longer-acting benzodiazepine like clonazepam (0.5–1.5 mg b.i.d.).
- Benzodiazepines, particularly longer-acting benzodiazepines like clonazepam, can be considered as single agents to treat panic in patients with bipolar disorder and those with no mood symptoms or anxiety symptoms other than panic.

ISSUES FOR REFERRAL

Consider referral to a psychiatrist for panic disorder that is comorbid with bipolar disorder, borderline personality disorder, schizophrenia, suicidality, alcohol or substance abuse.

ADDITIONAL THERAPIES

Aerobic exercise reduces symptoms better than placebo (3)[B].

IN-PATIENT CONSIDERATIONS

Admission Criteria/Initial Stabilization

- In an outpatient clinic or emergency room, if certain life-threatening mimics of panic disorder have not been ruled out, such as a myocardial infarction (MI) or pulmonary embolus (PE), inpatient hospitalization is needed to complete the evaluation.
- If a panic disorder patient is suicidal with intention to act on the idea, a psychiatric admission is indicated.

 ONGOING CARE

PATIENT EDUCATION

- www.nlm.nih.gov/medlineplus/panicdisorder.html
- Patient information handouts in *American Family Physician* 2005;71:740 and 2006;74:1393.
- www.nimh.nih.gov/health/publications/when-fear-overwhelms-panic-disorder/index.shtml

PROGNOSIS

- Most patients recover with treatment.
- Although it can recur, panic can be successfully treated again.

COMPLICATIONS

- Iatrogenic benzodiazepine dependence.
- Iatrogenic mania in bipolar patients treated for panic with unopposed antidepressants
- Misdiagnosis of more difficult to treat psychiatric conditions as panic and vice-versa

REFERENCES

1. Furukawa TA, Watanabe N, Churchill R. Combined psychotherapy plus antidepressants for panic disorder with or without agoraphobia. *Cochrane Database Syst Rev*. 2007(1);CD004364.
2. Esquivel G, Díaz-Galvis J, Schruers K, et al. Acute exercise reduces the effects of a 35% CO_2 challenge in patients with panic disorder. *J Affect Disord*. 2008;107(1–3):217–220.
3. Broocks A, Bandelow B, Pekrun G, et al. Comparison of aerobic exercise, clomipramine, and placebo in the treatment of panic disorder. *Am J Psychiatry*. 1998;155:603–609.

ADDITIONAL READING

- McIntosh A. Clinical Guidelines for the Management of Anxiety. *Management of anxiety (panic disorder, with or without agoraphobia, and generalized anxiety disorder) in adults in primary, secondary and community care*. National Institute for Clinical Evidence NICE, 2004.
- Yaseen ZS, Chartrand H, Mojtabai R, et al. Fear of dying in panic attacks predicts suicide attempt in comorbid depressive illness: Prospective evidence from the National Epidemiological Survey on Alcohol and Related Conditions. *Depress Anxiety*. 2013; 30(101):930–939.

 SEE ALSO

Algorithm: Anxiety

CODE ICD-9 301. CODES

ICD10

- F40.01 Agoraphobia with panic disorder
- F41.0 Panic disorder without agoraphobia

CLINICAL PEARLS

- Encouraging patients (who are medically able) to do 10 minutes of vigorous aerobic exercise the moment a panic attack seems to be starting is often a very effective way to help patients feel safe during panic attacks. They often notice, and you can point out, that through exercise they can raise their heart rate beyond that which occurs in a panic attack. If a normal, healthy activity like exercise can do that, they conclude, panic attacks probably are not endangering their hearts after all. In addition, such exercise often makes patients feel better in itself and can treat panic.
- Always check that a patient with panic is not suicidal: Patients with panic disorder are at increased risk, particularly if depressed and fear dying.
- Once the panic attacks are eliminated, agoraphobia often needs to be separately treated by gentle exposure to the feared environment, even though the physiological effects of panic are no longer present.

PARKINSON DISEASE

Sheldon Yao, DO • Christopher J. Husko

BASICS

DESCRIPTION
- Parkinson disease (PD) is a progressive neurodegenerative disorder caused by degeneration of dopaminergic neurons in the substantia nigra pars compacta.
- Cardinal symptoms include resting tremor, rigidity, bradykinesia, and postural instability.
- Diagnosis is based primarily on history and examination.

EPIDEMIOLOGY
Incidence
- Average age of onset: ~60 years
- Slightly more common in men than women

Prevalence
- Second most common neurodegenerative disease after Alzheimer disease
- 0.3% of general population and 1–2% of those ≥60 years of age and up to 4% of those ≥80 years of age
- Affects approximately 1 million people in the US and 5 million worldwide (1)

ETIOLOGY AND PATHOPHYSIOLOGY
Dopamine depletion in the substantia nigra and the nigrostriatal pathways results in the major motor complications of PD.
- Pathologic hallmark: Selective loss of dopamine-containing neurons in the pars compacta of the substantia nigra
- Loss of neurons accompanied by presence of Lewy bodies, pale bodies (predecessor of the Lewy body), and Lewy neuritis

Genetics
Mutations in multiple autosomal-dominant and autosomal-recessive genes have been linked to PD/parkinsonian syndrome particularly when the age at symptom onset is younger than 50 years old. Genes investigated in PD include *MAPT, SNCA, HLA-DRB5, BST1, GAK,* and *LRRK2* (2)

RISK FACTORS
- Age and family history of PD or tremor are the greatest risk factors.
- History of smoking as well as coffee and caffeine intake may reduce risk
- Weak association with exposure to toxins (herbicides and insecticides); however, relationship is not clear

COMMONLY ASSOCIATED CONDITIONS
Non–motor-associated symptoms include cognitive abnormalities, autonomic dysfunction (e.g., constipation, urinary urgency), sleep disturbances, mental status changes (depression, psychosis, hallucinations, dementia), orthostatic hypotension, and pain.

DIAGNOSIS

- Diagnosis is based on clinical impression.
- Gold standard for diagnosis is neuropathologic exam.
- Generally, bradykinesia plus either tremor or rigidity must be present in order to make the diagnosis of idiopathic PD.
- Clinical features supportive of the diagnosis include: unilateral onset, resting tremor, persistent asymmetry with the side of onset most affected, and significant response to dopaminergic therapy

HISTORY
Symptoms often subtle or attributed to aging:
- Decreased emotion displayed in facial features
- General motor slowing and stiffness (1 or both arms do not swing with walk)
- Resting tremor (often initially 1 hand)
- Speech soft/mumbling
- Falls/difficulty with balance (tends to occur with disease progression)

PHYSICAL EXAM
- Tremor:
  – Resting tremor (4–6 Hz) that is often asymmetric
  – Disappears with voluntary movement
  – Frequently emerges in a hand while walking and may present as pill rolling
  – May also present in jaw, chin, lips, tongue
- Bradykinesia
- Rigidity: Cogwheel (catching and releasing) or lead pipe (continuously rigid)
- Postural instability

DIFFERENTIAL DIAGNOSIS
- Essential tremor: Bradykinesia is not present; often symmetric, and occurs mostly during action or when holding hands outstretched
- SWEDD: Scans Without Evidence of Dopaminergic Deficit; isolated upper extremity resting and postural tremor resembling PD but failing to progress to generalized PD
- Dementia with Lewy bodies: characterized clinically by visual hallucinations, fluctuating cognition, and parkinsonism
- Multiple system atrophy: Presets with parkinsonism but with varying degrees of dysautonomia, cerebellar involvement, and pyramidal signs
- Progressive supranuclear palsy: Impairment in vertical eye movements (particularly down gaze), hyperextension of neck, and early falling
- Idiopathic basal ganglia calcification
- Associated neurodegenerative disorders: Late stages of Alzheimer disease, Huntington disease, Frontotemporal dementia, Spinocerebellar ataxias
- Secondary parkinsonism
  – Drug-induced: Reversible, may take weeks/months after offending medication is stopped
    ○ Neuroleptics (most common cause)
    ○ Antiemetics (e.g., prochlorperazine and promethazine), metoclopramide
    ○ SSRIs
    ○ Calcium channel blockers (e.g., flunarizine and cinnarizine)
    ○ Amiodarone
    ○ Lithium
    ○ Cholinergics
    ○ Chemotherapeutics
    ○ Amphotericin B
    ○ Estrogens
    ○ Valproic acid

DIAGNOSTIC TESTS & INTERPRETATION
Initial Tests (lab, imaging)
- Diagnosis is mainly clinical and there are no physiologic or blood tests to confirm the diagnosis
- Excellent response to an acute dopaminergic challenge test supports the diagnosis
- MRI of brain is nondiagnostic but can be used to rule out structural abnormalities
- DaT scan: Striatal dopamine transporter imaging can distinguish PD and other parkinsonian syndromes but cannot differentiate between them
- PET and single-photon emission CT may be helpful with diagnosis, but are not required

TREATMENT

GENERAL MEASURES
- Multidisciplinary rehabilitation with standard physical and occupational therapy components to improve functional outcomes
- Physiotherapy to help with gait re-education, enhancement of aerobic capacity, improvement in movement initiation, improvement in functional independence, and help with home safety

MEDICATION
- PD goal: Improve motor and nonmotor deficits
- Agents are chosen based on patient age and symptoms present

First Line
- First-line agents in early PD: Levodopa, dopamine agonists, monoamine oxidase (MAO)-B inhibitors (1)[A]:
  – Levodopa vs. dopamine agonist is controversial (2)[B]:
    ○ Most patients eventually will develop motor fluctuations with levodopa. Younger patients are more likely to develop motor fluctuations. Some recommend delaying initiation of levodopa to decrease drug-induced motor fluctuations early in the disease.
    ○ Older patients often are unable to tolerate the adverse events of dopamine agonists.
    ○ All patients eventually will require levodopa.
  – MAO-B inhibitors (rasagiline) should be considered as initial monotherapy (2)[B]; investigated for potential neuroprotective effects
- Carbidopa + levodopa (carbidopa inhibits peripheral conversion of levodopa):
  – Immediate release (Sinemet):
    ○ Tablets (mg): 10/100, 25/100, 25/250
    ○ Usual initial maintenance dose: 25/100 mg PO t.i.d. Most patients require 25 mg of carbidopa to inhibit peripheral conversion of levodopa.
    ○ Watch for nausea, orthostatic hypotension, sedation, vivid dreams, and vomiting
  – Orally disintegrating (Parcopa):
    ○ Tablets (mg): 10/100, 25/100, 25/25
  – Sustained release (Sinemet CR):
    ○ Tablets (mg): 25/100, 50/200
    ○ Dose agents initially b.i.d.

- Carbidopa + levodopa + entacapone (Stalevo):
  – Tablets (mg): 12.5/50/200, 18.75/75/200, 25/100/200, 31.25/125/200, 37.5/150/200, 50/200/200
  – Addition of entacapone as a single agent should be initiated prior to use of this combination:
    ○ Once daily dose of carbidopa/levodopa has been identified, may convert to Stalevo
    ○ Dose of levodopa may need to be decreased with the addition of entacapone
  – Side effects are the same, plus diarrhea and brownish orange urine
- Dopamine agonists (Nonergot): Side effects nausea, vomiting, hypotension, sedation, edema, vivid dreaming, compulsive behavior, confusion, lightheadedness, and hallucinations:
  – Pramipexole (Mirapex): Tablets (mg): 0.125, 0.25, 0.5, 1, 1.5:
    ○ Start with 0.125 mg t.i.d., gradually increase every 5–7 days to 0.5–1.5 mg t.i.d.
    ○ CrCl 35–59 mL/min 0.125 mg PO b.i.d.
    ○ CrCl 15–34 mL/min 0.125 mg PO daily
  – Pramipexole ER (Mirapex ER): Tablets (mg): 0.375, 0.75, 1.5, 3, 4.5; start with 0.375 PO daily
  – Ropinirole (Requip): Tablets (mg): 0.25, 0.5, 1, 2, 3, 4, 5; start with 0.25 mg t.i.d., increase gradually to 3–8 mg t.i.d.
  – Requip XL: Tablets (mg): 2, 4, 6, 8, 12; start at a 2-mg dose once daily, increase in 1–2 weeks
- Dopamine agonists (ergot): Increased adverse event profile makes these agents nonpreferred to nonergot dopamine agonists
- Bromocriptine (Parlodel):
  – Tablets: 2.5 mg
  – Capsules: 5 mg
  – Start with 1.25 mg b.i.d., increase by 2.5 mg every 2–4 weeks up to effective dose (30–90 mg/d in 3 divided doses).
  – Same as nonergot and increases risk for pulmonary fibrosis (decreased efficacy compared with other agents)
- Selective MAO-B inhibitors: Side effects insomnia, jitteriness, hallucinations; mostly found with selegiline; rasagiline similar adverse events as placebo in clinical trials. Rasagiline is metabolized via *CYP1A2*; caution with other medications utilizing this enzyme system (e.g., ciprofloxacin):
  – Both agents contraindicated with meperidine band numerous other agents metabolized via *CYP1A2*
  – At therapeutic doses, unlikely to induce a "cheese reaction" (tyramine storm)
- Selegiline (Eldepryl):
  – Tablets: 5 mg; initiate 5 mg PO b.i.d.
  – Orally disintegrating tablet (Zelapar): 1.25 mg; 1.25 mg PO daily for 6 weeks; increase as needed to max of 2.5 mg daily
  – Transdermal patch (Emsam): 6 mg/24 h, 9 mg/24 h, 12 mg/24 h; start with 6 mg/24 h and titrate up every 2 weeks as needed to a maximum of 12 mg/24 h
- Rasagiline (Azilect): Tablets: 0.5 mg, 1.0 mg; initiate 0.5–1 mg daily

Second Line

- Second-line agents in early PD: β-adrenergic antagonists (postural tremor), amantadine, anticholinergics (young patients with tremor) (1)[A]; there is lack of good evidence for symptom control

- Treatment of levodopa-induced motor complications:
  – End of dose wearing off:
    ○ Entacapone (with each levodopa dose) or rasagiline preferred (3)[A]
    ○ May also consider dopamine agonist, apomorphine, selegiline (4)[B]
  – Dyskinesias:
    ○ Typically occur at peak dopamine level
    ○ Amantadine may be considered; however, its efficacy is questionable (1)[B].
- Anticholinergic agents: Usually avoided due to lack of efficacy (only useful for tremor) and increased adverse event profile, including blurred vision, confusion, constipation, dry mouth, memory difficulty, sedation, and urinary retention:
  – Trihexyphenidyl:
    ○ Tablets: 2 mg, 5 mg
    ○ Start with 1–2 mg daily, increase by 2 mg every 3–5 days until usual dose is 5–15 mg in 3–4 divided doses
  – Benztropine (Cogentin):
    ○ Tablets: 0.5 mg, 1 mg, 2 mg
    ○ Start with 0.5–6 mg in 1–2 divided doses; increase by 0.5 mg every 5–6 days
- *N*-methyl-D-aspartic acid antagonist: Exact mechanism is unknown and efficacy is questionable; however, it may be useful for dyskinesias. Side effects include confusion, dizziness, dry mouth, livedo reticularis, and hallucinations:
  – Amantadine (Symmetrel):
    ○ Tablets: 100 mg
    ○ Start with 100 mg b.i.d.; may increase to 300 mg daily in divided doses; renally adjusted
- Catechol-O-methyl transferase (COMT) inhibitors: Entacapone preferred due to hepatotoxicity associated with tolcapone. Adverse events include nausea and orthostatic hypotension:
  – Tolcapone (Tasmar):
    ○ Tablets: 100 mg, 200 mg
    ○ Start 100 mg t.i.d.; max dose 600 mg/d; must be taken with carbidopa/levodopa
  – Entacapone (Comtan):
    ○ Tablets: 200 mg
    ○ 200 mg with each dose of carbidopa/levodopa; max dose, 1,600 mg/d
- Apomorphine (Apokyn): Nonergot-derived dopamine agonist given SC for off episodes. Adverse events nausea, vomiting, dizziness, hallucinations, orthostatic hypotension, somnolence:
  – Effective dose ranges from 2–6 mg/injection; most patients require 0.06 mg/kg
  – Monitor for orthostatic hypotension after initial dose; this is a potent emetic, so initiate an antiemetic (e.g., trimethobenzamide) 3 days prior to start and continue for 2 months. Avoid ondansetron (combination causes severe hypotension and syncope) and dopamine antagonists, such as prochlorperazine and metoclopramide.
  – Only for "off" episodes with levodopa therapy

ISSUES FOR REFERRAL
Early specialty referral for patients with suspected PD for an accurate diagnosis and management

ADDITIONAL THERAPIES
- Emotional psychological support of patient family
- Physical therapy and manual medicine has been shown to improve balance, muscle strength, and walking speed
- Speech therapy: May be helpful in improving speech volume and maintaining voice quality

SURGERY/OTHER PROCEDURES
Deep brain stimulation (bilateral subthalamic nucleus/globus pallidus interna) is an effective therapeutic option for patients with motor complications refractory to best medical treatment who are healthy, have no significant comorbidities, are responsive to levodopa, and do not have depression or dementia.

 ONGOING CARE

DIET
- Increase dietary fluids and fiber, and increase activity for constipation
- For dysphagia, consider soft food, swallowing evaluation, and increased time for meals
- Avoid large, high-fat meals that slow digestion and interfere with medication absorption

PATIENT EDUCATION
- www.apdaparkinson.org
- www.parkinson.org
- www.michaeljfox.org

PROGNOSIS
PD is a chronic progressive disease; prognosis varies based on patient-specific symptoms.

COMPLICATIONS
Most commonly the result of adverse effects of medications used to treat

REFERENCES

1. Gazewood JD, Richards DR, Clebak K. Parkinsons disease: An update. *Am Fam Physician*. 2013;87:267–273.
2. International Parkinson Disease Genomics Consortium, Nalls MA, Plagnol V, et al. Imputation of sequence variants for identification of genetic risks for Parkinson's disease: A meta-analysis of genome-wide association studies. *Lancet*. 2011;377:641–649.
3. Pahwa R, Factor SA, Lyons KE, et al. Practice parameter: Treatment of Parkinson disease with motor fluctuations and dyskinesia (an evidence based review): Report of the Quality Standards Subcommittee of the American Academy of Neurology. *Neurology*. 2006;66:983–995.
4. Diaz NL, Waters CH. Current strategies in the treatment of Parkinson's disease and a personalized approach to management. *Expert Rev. Neurother*. 2009;9:1781–1789.

 CODES

ICD10
- G20 Parkinson's disease
- G21.9 Secondary parkinsonism, unspecified
- G31.83 Dementia with Lewy bodies

CLINICAL PEARLS

- Emphasize the importance of exercise and movement to help preserve function.
- Pharmacotherapeutic regimens need to be individualized based on patient-specific symptoms and age.

PARONYCHIA
Robert S. Freelove, MD

 BASICS

DESCRIPTION
- Inflammation of the lateral and posterior folds of skin surrounding the fingernail or toenail:
  - Acute: Characterized by pain, erythema, and swelling; usually a bacterial infection, often appearing 2–5 days after trauma (1)
  - Chronic: Characterized by swelling, tenderness, cuticle loss/separation, and nail dystrophy (1)
  - May be considered work-related among bartenders, waitresses, nurses, and others who often wet their hands (1)
- System(s) affected: Skin/Exocrine
- Synonym(s): Eponychia; Perionychia

Pediatric Considerations
Thumb/Finger-sucking is a risk factor (anaerobes and *Escherichia coli* may be present)

EPIDEMIOLOGY
Incidence
- Common in the US
- Predominant age: All ages
- Predominant sex: Female > Male (3:1)

ETIOLOGY AND PATHOPHYSIOLOGY
- Acute: *Staphylococcus aureus* and *Streptococcus pyogenes*; less frequently, *Pseudomonas pyocyanea* and *Proteus vulgaris*. In digits exposed to oral flora, also consider *Eikenella corrodens, Fusobacterium,* and *Peptostreptococcus*.
- Chronic: Eczematous reaction with secondary *Candida albicans* (~95%); less frequently, dermatophytes, and, occasionally, molds (*Scytalidium, Fusarium*)
- A paronychial infection usually starts in the lateral nail fold.
- Occasionally, the infection includes the complete margin of skin around the nail plate, which results from mechanical separation of the nail plate from the perionychium.
- Early in the course of this disease process (<24 hours), cellulitis alone may be present. An abscess can form if the infection does not resolve quickly.
- Chronic infections most likely represent eczematous reaction with secondary infection and multifocal etiology.

RISK FACTORS
- Acute: Trauma to skin surrounding nail, ingrown nails, manicured/sculptured nails, diabetes mellitus (DM), nail biting, and thumbsucking
- Chronic: Frequent immersion of hands in water (e.g., cooks, chefs, bartenders, housekeepers, swimmers), DM, immunosuppression (reported association with antiretroviral therapy for HIV and with use of epidermal growth factor inhibitors)

GENERAL PREVENTION
- Acute: Avoid nail biting; prevent thumbsucking.
- Chronic: Avoid allergens; keep fingers/hands dry; wear rubber gloves with a cotton liner.
- Good diabetic control

COMMONLY ASSOCIATED CONDITIONS
- DM
- Eczema or atopic dermatitis
- Certain medications: Cetuximab, paclitaxel, antiretroviral therapy (especially protease inhibitors and lamivudine, with toes more commonly involved)
- Immunosuppression
- If multiple, consider pemphigus vulgaris (rare)

 DIAGNOSIS

HISTORY
- Localized pain or tenderness, swelling, and erythema:
  - Acute: Fairly rapid onset
  - Chronic: 6 weeks duration
- Previous trauma (bitten nails, ingrown nails, manicured nails)
- Contact with herpes infections
- Contact with allergens or irritants (frequent water immersion, latex)

PHYSICAL EXAM
- Acute: Red, hot, tender, tense nail fold ± abscess
- Chronic: Swollen, tender, boggy nail fold ± abscess
- Occasional elevation of nail bed
- Separation of nail fold from nail plate
- Red, painful swelling of skin around nail plate
- Fluctuance, purulence at the nail margin, or purulent drainage
- Secondary changes of nail plate
- Green changes in nail (*Pseudomonas*)
- Positive digital pressure test (light pressure over the area causes digital blanching and demarcation of the abscess) (1)
- Chronic: Retraction of nail fold and absence of adjacent cuticle, thickening of nail plate with prominent transverse ridges known as Beau lines (1)

DIFFERENTIAL DIAGNOSIS
- Herpetic whitlow (similar in appearance, very painful, often associated with vesicles)
- Felon (abscess of fingertip pulp; urgent diagnosis required)
- Allergic contact dermatitis (latex, acrylic)
- Reiter disease
- Pustular psoriasis
- Proximal/Lateral onychomycosis
- Malignancy: Squamous cell carcinoma, malignant melanoma, metastatic disease

DIAGNOSTIC TESTS & INTERPRETATION
None required unless condition is severe; resistant to treatment, or methicillin-resistant *S. aureus* (MRSA) is suspected, then:
- Gram stain
- Culture and sensitivity
- Potassium hydroxide wet mount plus fungal culture
- Drugs that may alter lab results: Use of over-the-counter antimicrobials or antifungals

Diagnostic Procedures/Other
- Scraping for wet mount and culture in chronic cases
- Incision and drainage for suppurative or cases not responding to conservative management
- Tzanck testing or viral culture in suspected viral cases
- Biopsy in cases not responding to conservative management or when malignancy suspected

TREATMENT

GENERAL MEASURES
- Acute: Warm water soaks (t.i.d.–q.i.d.), warm compresses, elevation, splint protection if pain severe
- Chronic: Keep fingers dry; apply moisturizing lotion after hand washing; avoid exposure to irritants; improved diabetic control

MEDICATION
First Line
- Tetanus booster when appropriate
- Acute (mild cases):
  - Antibiotic cream alone or in combination with a topical steroid
  - Antibiotic cream applied t.i.d.–q.i.d. after warm soak (e.g., mupirocin or gentamicin/neomycin/polymyxin B) for 5–10 days
  - If eczematous: Topical steroid applied b.i.d. (e.g., betamethasone 0.05% cream) for 7–14 days
- Acute (exposure to oral flora):
  - Clindamycin (Cleocin) 300–450 mg t.i.d.–q.i.d. for 7 days; pediatric, 10 mg/kg q8h
  - Amoxicillin–clavulanate potassium (Augmentin): 875 mg/125 mg q12h or 500 mg/125 mg t.i.d. for 7 days; pediatric, 45 mg/kg q12h (for <40 kg)
- Acute (no exposure to oral flora):
  - Dicloxacillin 250 mg t.i.d. for 7 days
  - Cephalexin (Keflex) 500 mg b.i.d.–t.i.d. for 7 days
- Acute (suspected MRSA):
  - Trimethoprim/Sulfamethoxazole 160 mg/800 mg b.i.d. for 7 days
  - Doxycycline 100 mg b.i.d. for 7 days
- Chronic:
  - Topical steroids: Betamethasone 0.05%; applied b.i.d. for 7–14 days with or without antifungal (2)[A]
  - Topical antifungal: Econazole, clotrimazole, or nystatin; applied topically t.i.d. for up to 30 days
  - Other topical: Tacrolimus (Protopic) 0.1% ointment b.i.d. for up to 21 days has been shown to be effective but is more expensive (3)[B].
- Contraindications: Allergy to antibiotic; may consider erythromycin as alternative
- Precautions: Erythromycin may cause significant GI upset.

Second Line
- Systemic antifungals (rarely needed):
  - Itraconazole (Sporanox) 200 mg/d for 90 days (may have longer action because it is incorporated into nail plate); pulse therapy may be useful (200 mg b.i.d. for 7 days, repeated monthly for 2 months)
  - Terbinafine (Lamisil) 250 mg/d for 6 weeks (fingernails) or 12 weeks (toenails)
  - Fluconazole (Diflucan) 150 mg/wk for 4–6 months
- Antipseudomonal drugs (e.g., 3rd-generation cephalosporins, aminoglycosides)

ISSUES FOR REFERRAL
Chronic; in treatment failure, consider biopsy and/or in cases of recalcitrant chronic paronychia referral for possible en bloc excision of the nail fold or eponychial marsupialization with or without nail removal.

SURGERY/OTHER PROCEDURES
- Incision and drainage of abscess, if present (4)[A]
- A subungual abscess or ingrown nail requires partial or complete removal of nail.

 ONGOING CARE

FOLLOW-UP RECOMMENDATIONS
Chronic: Avoid frequent immersion, triggers, allergens, or nail biting and finger sucking.

DIET
If patient is diabetic, institute appropriate dietary changes for better control.

PATIENT EDUCATION
Avoid trimming cuticles; avoid nail trauma; stress importance of good diabetic control; avoid contact irritants; use rubber gloves with cotton liners to avoid exposure to moisture; use moisturizing lotion after washing hands; do not bite nails/suck on fingers.

PROGNOSIS
- With adequate treatment and prevention, healing can be expected.
- If no response in chronic lesions, rarely benign or malignant neoplasm may be present and referral should be considered (5)[C].

COMPLICATIONS
- Acute: Subungual abscess
- Chronic: Secondary ridging, thickening, and discoloration of nail, nail loss

REFERENCES
1. Rigopoulos D, Alevizos A. Acute and chronic paronychia. *Am Fam Physician*. 2008;177: 339–346.
2. Tosti A, Piraccini BM, Ghetti E, et al. Topical steroids versus systemic antifungals in the treatment of chronic paronychia: An open, randomized double-blind and double dummy study. *J Am Acad Dermatol*. 2002;47:73–76.
3. Rigopoulos D, Gregoriou S, Belyayeva E, et al. Efficacy and safety of tacrolimus ointment 0.1% vs. betamethasone 17-valerate 0.1% in the treatment of chronic paronychia: An unblinded randomized study. *Br J Dermatol*. 2009;160:858–860.
4. Shaw J, Body R. Best evidence topic report. Incision and drainage preferable to oral antibiotics in acute paronychial nail infection? *Emerg Med J*. 2005;22: 813–814.
5. Rockwell PG. Acute and chronic paronychia. *Am Fam Physician*. 2001;63:1113–1116.

 SEE ALSO

Onychomycosis

 CODES

ICD10
- L03.011 Cellulitis of right finger
- L03.019 Cellulitis of unspecified finger
- L03.039 Cellulitis of unspecified toe

CLINICAL PEARLS
- Administer tetanus booster when appropriate.
- Incision and drainage is recommended for an obvious abscess.
- For chronic paronychia, topical steroid is first-line treatment.
- Antibiotic selection for acute paronychia is influenced by presence or absence of exposure to oral flora.

PAROTITIS, ACUTE AND CHRONIC

Kathleen Ferrer, MD, FAAP, AAHIVS • Julia Emanuel, MD, MSc

 BASICS

DESCRIPTION
- Parotitis is inflammation of the parotid gland caused by infection (viral or bacterial), noninfectious systemic illnesses, mechanical obstruction, or medications.
- Parotitis can be unilateral or bilateral, acute or chronic. Unilateral parotitis is usually associated with duct obstruction, whereas bilateral parotitis more commonly indicates a systemic cause.
- The parotid gland is the largest of the salivary glands, located lateral to the masseter muscle anteriorly and extending posteriorly over the sternocleidomastoid muscle behind the angle of the mandible. It produces exclusively serous secretions, which lack the bacteriostatic properties of mucinous secretions, making the parotid gland more susceptible to infection than other salivary glands.
- The parotid duct, also called Stensen's duct, pierces the buccinator muscle to enter the buccal mucosa just opposite the 2nd maxillary molar.
- The branches of the 7th cranial nerve or "facial nerve" divide the gland into lobes.
- The parotid gland contains lymph nodes.

EPIDEMIOLOGY
- Prior to widespread vaccination, parotitis was primarily caused by mumps virus, with 150,000 cases of parotitis per year; in 2011, 370 cases occurred.
- Acute bacterial parotitis occurs more frequently in elderly patients, neonates (especially preterm infants), and postoperative patients.
- Neonatal parotitis and juvenile recurrent parotitis are more common in males than females.
- Juvenile recurrent parotitis is the 2nd most common inflammatory cause of parotitis in the US after viral parotitis; 1st episode usually occurs between the ages of 3 and 6.
- Chronic parotitis mainly affects adults, more often females. The average age of presentation is between 40 and 60 years.
- Chronic bilateral parotid enlargement is a common manifestation of HIV infection; for perinatally HIV-infected children, the average age of onset for parotid enlargement is 5 years.

RISK FACTORS
- Acute viral parotitis: Lack of mumps, measles, rubella (MMR) vaccination.
- Acute bacterial parotitis:
  - Conditions that predispose to salivary stasis, such as dehydration, debilitation, poor oral hygiene, Sjögren syndrome, cystic fibrosis, bulimia/anorexia, sialolithiasis (stones), ductal stenosis, trauma
  - Immunosuppression, HIV, chemotherapy, radiation, malnutrition, alcoholism
- Neonatal parotitis: Prematurity, low birth weight, ductal obstruction, oral trauma, structural abnormalities, immunosuppression
- Juvenile recurrent parotitis: Dental malocclusion, congenital duct malformation, genetic factors, immunological anomalies
- Drug-induced parotitis: Medications such as anticholinergics, antihistamines, diuretics, tricyclic antidepressants, antipsychotics, antineoplastic agents, and iodine
- Chronic parotitis: Ductal stenosis, HIV, tuberculosis, Sjögren syndrome, and sarcoidosis

GENERAL PREVENTION
- MMR vaccination with the 1st dose between 12 and 15 months and 2nd dose between 4 and 6 years of age; of note, mumps vaccination does not guarantee prevention, possibly due to waning immunity in adolescence.
- Maintain adequate hydration and good dental hygiene
- Suck on hard or sour candy and use hot compresses with parotid massages to stimulate salivary flow and prevent salivary stasis
- Smoking cessation, abstinence from alcohol, and avoidance of chronic purging

ETIOLOGY AND PATHOPHYSIOLOGY
- Acute viral parotitis begins as a systemic infection that localizes to the parotid gland, resulting in inflammation and swelling of the gland:
  - Mumps, or paramyxovirus, has a predilection for the parotid gland and classically has been linked to parotitis.
- Acute bacterial parotitis results from stasis of salivary flow that allows retrograde introduction of bacterial pathogens into the parotid gland, resulting in localized infection.
- Acute parotitis pathogens:
  - Viral:
    ○ Paramyxovirus (mumps), parainfluenza virus types 1 and 3, influenza A, coxsackie viruses, Epstein-Barr virus (EBV)
    ○ Cytomegalovirus (CMV) and adenovirus have been seen in patients with HIV.
  - Bacterial:
    ○ *Staphylococcus aureus* and anaerobes (oral flora) are most commonly seen.
    ○ *Streptococcus pneumoniae*, viridans streptococci, *Escherichia coli*, and *Haemophilus influenza* (less common)
    ○ Gram-negative rods such as *E. coli*, *Klebsiella*, *Enterobacter*, and *Pseudomonas* can be seen in chronically ill or hospitalized patients.
  - Fungal:
    ○ *Candida* has been isolated in chronically ill or hospitalized patients.
    ○ *Actinomyces* can be found in patients with a history of trauma or dental caries.
- Acute, recurrent parotitis:
  - Juvenile recurrent parotitis may be secondary to chronic inflammation; etiology is unknown, but a genetic predisposition may exist.
  - Mechanical: Sialolithiasis, ductal stenosis; repeated sialolith formation can lead to ductal wall damage, fibrosis, and stricture formation which further decreases salivary flow and perpetuates obstruction.
  - Pneumoparotitis may occur when air is trapped in the ducts of the parotid gland; may be seen in wind instrument players, glass blowers, scuba divers, and with dental cleaning.
  - Medications: Anticholinergics, antihistamines, tricyclic antidepressants, antipsychotics (especially phenylbutazone, thioridazine, clozapine), iodine (especially contrast media), and L-asparaginase (1)[C].
  - Other: Diabetes, alcoholism, bulimia, "anesthesia mumps" (possible mechanisms include transient mechanical compression of Stensen's duct by airway devices, loss of muscle tone around the Stensen orifice after neuromuscular relaxants, increased salivary secretion, and increased flexion or rotation of the head during general anesthesia)

- Chronic parotitis may occur due to chronic ductal stenosis but is often due to a chronic infectious or inflammatory condition:
  - HIV
  - Tuberculosis, syphilis (rare)
  - Autoimmune: Sjögren syndrome (parotid enlargement, xerostomia, and keratoconjunctivitis)
  - Inflammatory: Sarcoidosis:
    ○ Heerfordt syndrome (parotid enlargement, facial palsy, and uveitis) is a rare manifestation of sarcoidosis.
- Chronic parotitis in HIV-infected patients can be due to the presence of benign lymphoepithelial cysts, follicular hyperplasia of parotid lymph nodes, or diffuse infiltrative lymphocytosis syndrome (DILS), causing infiltration of the parotid gland by CD8 cells:
  - Parotitis may also be secondary to immune reconstitution after initiation of combination antiretroviral therapy in HIV-infected patients.

COMMONLY ASSOCIATED CONDITIONS
HIV, Sjögren syndrome, sarcoidosis, sialolithiasis

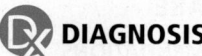 DIAGNOSIS

HISTORY
- Acute parotitis presents with sudden-onset pain and swelling of the cheek usually extending to and obscuring the angle of the mandible:
  - Viral parotitis is usually bilateral and accompanied by a prodrome of malaise, anorexia, headaches, myalgias, arthralgias, and fever; typically, overlying skin is not warm or erythematous and no pus is reported at the opening of Stensen's duct.
  - Bacterial parotitis is typically unilateral with induration, warmth, and erythema over the affected cheek; fever is often present.
  - Juvenile recurrent parotitis is usually unilateral; pain and swelling usually resolve within 2 weeks and exacerbations occur until puberty; purulent exudate is not typical, but superinfection may occur.
  - Sialolithiasis is characterized by recurrent acute swelling and pain, exacerbated by eating; sialolithiasis affects the submandibular gland more frequently.
  - Other frequently reported symptoms include trismus (inability to open mouth), pain exacerbated by chewing or worsened by foods that stimulate production of saliva (i.e., sour candies), dry mouth with abnormal taste, difficulty with drinking/eating, anorexia, or dehydration.
- Chronic parotitis presents with recurrent or chronic nontender swelling of one or both parotid glands; can have periods of remission lasting weeks to years:
  - Sjögren syndrome, sarcoidosis, HIV, tuberculosis
  - Chronic parotitis may predispose to superinfection, which would present similarly to an acute parotitis.

PHYSICAL EXAM
- Parotitis is characterized by swelling or enlargement of the parotid gland(s) overlying the masseter muscle; may obscure the angle of the mandible or cause the ear to protrude upward and outward.
- Palpation of the parotid gland is best done by using 1 hand to start at the attachment of the earlobe and palpating anteriorly and inferiorly along the mandibular ramus while the other hand simultaneously palpates the Stensen duct orifice:

– Tender and bilateral suggests viral etiology, whereas tender, erythematous, warm, and unilateral suggests bacterial etiology.
– Nontender in HIV, tuberculosis, Sjögren, sarcoidosis
- Trismus may be noted.
- Pus from Stensen's duct is suggestive of bacterial parotitis or superinfection; opening of duct may appear edematous and erythematous in both bacterial and viral parotitis.
- In juvenile recurrent parotitis, Stensen's duct is often enlarged, dilated, erythematous, and swollen.
- Halitosis and dental decay are often associated with acute exacerbations.
- Facial nerve palsy can be seen in severe cases.

DIFFERENTIAL DIAGNOSIS
- Lymphoma, neoplasm, lymphangitis, cervical adenitis, otitis externa, dental abscess, odontogenic infections, Ludwig angina, and cellulitis should be considered in the differential.
- Parotid swelling or enlargement typically obscures the angle of the mandible (unlike cervical adenitis).
- Involvement of Stensen's duct is unique to parotitis.

DIAGNOSTIC TESTS & INTERPRETATION
- History and physical exam are usually sufficient for diagnosis of parotitis.
- Performing aerobic culture and Gram stain of purulent drainage from Stensen's duct or aerobic and anaerobic culture from needle aspiration of gland or abscess can be helpful to identify causative organism:
– Anaerobic culture from Stensen's duct will likely contain oropharyngeal contamination; hence, it is recommended to perform anaerobic cultures only from needle aspirate fluid.
- Aerobic and anaerobic blood culture may also identify causative organism.
- Acute bacterial parotitis often demonstrates an elevated white blood cell count and amylase.
- For suspected mumps, obtain mumps IgM antibody or mumps reverse transcription-polymerase chain reaction (RT-PCR). A 4-fold increase of mumps IgG antibody indicates infection.
- Consider sending EBV titers and respiratory virus PCR panel if viral parotitis suspected; CMV titers should be sent in immunocompromised patients.
- For chronic, recurrent, or nontender parotitis, obtain HIV test, PPD, SS-A SS-B antibodies, rheumatoid factor, and antinuclear antibodies to evaluate for underlying etiology.
- Consider obtaining ultrasound or CT scan of parotid area to assess for abscess, cystic masses, parotid tumors, ductal stenosis, or sialolithiasis if no response to initial treatment.
- Consider sialography with chronic parotitis to assess the anatomy and functional integrity of the gland; can be diagnostic and therapeutic.

Diagnostic Procedures/Other
Consider performing a biopsy or fine-needle aspiration of gland if there is suspicion for tuberculosis, Sjögren syndrome, or sarcoidosis.

Test Interpretation
- Findings characteristic of HIV are described in the "Etiology and Pathophysiology" section.
- Noncaseating granulomas may be seen in sarcoidosis, and caseating granulomas may be found in tuberculosis.

 TREATMENT

- Usually a self-limiting course that requires primarily supportive treatment with rest, adequate hydration, analgesia, and antipyretics:
– Can stimulate glands to produce saliva by sucking on hard candies or glycerin swabs.
– Local heat and gentle massage of gland can provide symptomatic relief.
– For chronic presentations, encourage good dental hygiene and treat underlying etiology of parotitis (HIV, Sjögren, etc.).
- For suspected bacterial component, can empirically initiate antibiotics to cover *S. aureus,* anaerobes (oral flora), and *S. pneumoniae*
- Patients diagnosed with mumps should be isolated with standard and droplet precautions for 5 days after onset of parotid swelling.

MEDICATION
- Acute bacterial parotitis:
– Outpatient management: amoxicillin/clavulanate, 1st-generation cephalosporin, clindamycin
– Chronically ill or hospitalized: ampicillin/sulbactam or clindamycin and nafcillin; if methicillin resistance is probable, consider vancomycin or linezolid
- Pilocarpine and cevimeline can stimulate saliva production and inhibit ascending infection as well as provide symptomatic relief for patients with underlying Sjögren syndrome.

SURGERY/OTHER PROCEDURES
- Consider needle aspiration for bacterial parotitis with abscess formation or clinical deterioration with increasing pain, erythema, and swelling not responding to medication.
- May perform serial drainage for symptomatic cysts.
- Consider superficial parotidectomy for severe recurrent parotid infections in patients with underlying predisposing etiology (such as Sjögren syndrome).
- For sialolithiasis, ductal stenosis, or for patients with > 1 recurrence per year, consult otolaryngology for possible duct ligation, ductoplasty, or parotidectomy; sialendoscopy has been shown to be a therapeutic tool for many pediatric salivary disorders while allowing for gland preservation (2)[C].
- Sclerotherapy with methyl violet or tetracycline has been shown to be effective in the treatment of cysts in HIV parotitis (3)[C] and is also considered definitive treatment for chronic parotitis.

 ONGOING CARE

FOLLOW-UP RECOMMENDATIONS
Antibiotic therapy initiated at diagnosis combined with adequate hydration should result in improvement within 48 hours. If not, patient should be re-evaluated.

DIET
- Ensure adequate fluid intake
- Hard or sour candies to promote salivary flow

PROGNOSIS
- Viral infection in immunocompetent individuals often resolves with excellent prognosis.
- Parotid cysts found in HIV-infected patients are usually benign lymphoepithelial lesions with infrequent malignant transformation.

- Increased incidence of malignant lymphoma or lymphoepithelial carcinoma may be seen in patients with Sjögren syndrome.

COMPLICATIONS
- For mumps, potential complications include orchitis, oophoritis, mastitis, meningitis, pancreatitis, sensorineural hearing loss, and nephritis.
- Untreated bacterial parotitis can lead to local extension, abscess formation, and facial paralysis.

REFERENCES
1. Brooks KG, Thompson DF. A review and assessment of drug-induced parotitis. *Ann Pharmacother.* 2012;46:1688–1699.
2. Hackett A, Baranano C, Reed M, et al. Sialoendoscopy for the treatment of pediatric salivary gland disorders. *Arch Otolaryngol Head Neck Surg.* 2012;128:912–915.
3. Berg EE, Moore CE. Office-based sclerotherapy for benign parotid lymphoepithelial cysts in the HIV-positive patient. *Laryngoscope.* 2009;119: 868–870.

ADDITIONAL READING
- Armstrong MA, Turturro MA. Salivary gland emergencies. *Emerg Med Clin North Am* 2013;31:485–494.
- Brook I. The bacteriology of salivary gland infections. *Oral Maxillofac Surg Clin North Am.* 2009;21:269–274.
- Capaccio P, Sigismund PE, Luca N, et al. Modern management of juvenile recurrent parotitis. *J Laryngol Otol.* 2012;126:1254–1260.
- Harbison JM, Liess BD, Templer JW, et al. Chronic parotitis: A challenging disease entity. *Ear Nose Throat J.* 2011;90:E13–E16.
- Ortega KL, Ceballos-Salobreña A, Gaitán-Cepeda LA, et al. Oral manifestations after immune reconstitution in HIV patients on HAART. *Int J STD AIDS.* 2008;19:305–308.
- Patel R, Karlis V. Diagnosis and management of pediatric salivary gland infections. *Oral Maxillofac Surg Clin North Am.* 2009;21:345–352.

 CODES

ICD10
- K11.20 Sialoadenitis, unspecified
- K11.21 Acute sialoadenitis
- K11.23 Chronic sialoadenitis

CLINICAL PEARLS
- History and physical exam are usually sufficient for diagnosis (parotid swelling and tenderness with or without purulent drainage from Stensen's duct).
- In recurrent or chronic cases, consider other underlying etiologies, such as HIV.
- *S. aureus* and anaerobes (oral flora) are the most common organisms isolated in acute bacterial parotitis.
- Encouraging good oral hygiene and adequate hydration in chronically ill, debilitated, and hospitalized patients can reduce the occurrence of parotitis.

PARVOVIRUS B19 INFECTION

David Krulak, MD, MPH, MBA, FAAFP

 BASICS

DESCRIPTION

- Human parvovirus B19 is the primary cause of erythema infectiosum (EI, or fifth disease).
- Complications in susceptible individuals include transient aplastic crisis (TAC) in patients with increased RBC turnover (e.g., sickle cell anemia), pure red cell aplasia (PRAC) and chronic anemia in immunocompromised individuals, and arthritis and arthralgias in normal hosts:
  – Pregnant women who are not immune are at risk of intrauterine infection, with potentially significant consequences to the fetus.
- System(s) affected: Hemic/Lymphatic/Immunologic; Musculoskeletal; Skin/Exocrine; possibly Central Nervous System; Cardiac; Renal

Pregnancy Considerations
Acute infection during pregnancy should prompt referral to a maternal–fetal medicine specialist. Maternal B19 infection between 9 and 20 weeks' gestation may carry a significant risk for developing fetal anemia.

EPIDEMIOLOGY
- Infection is common in childhood.
- Extremely low mortality rate
- Predominant age: Peak age for EI is 4–12 years.
- Predominant sex: Male = Female
- Adult females are more likely to develop postinfectious arthritis
- No racial predilection is known.
- In temperate climates, infections often occur from late winter to early summer.
- Local outbreaks occur every 2–4 years.

Prevalence
- Extremely common in the US.
- Antibody immunoglobulin (Ig) G prevalence:
  – 1–5 years: 2–15%
  – 6–15 years: 20–40%
  – 16–40 years: 50–60%
  – >40 years: 70–85%

ETIOLOGY AND PATHOPHYSIOLOGY
- Small (20–25 mm), nonenveloped, single-stranded DNA virus belongs to the family *Parvoviridae*:
  – Only known parvovirus to infect humans; it does not cross-infect dogs or cats.
- Natural host of B19 is human erythroid progenitor.
- Respiratory, hematogenous, and vertical transmission are sources of human spread of virus.
- 4–14 day incubation. Rash and joint symptoms occur 2–3 weeks after initial infection.
- Contagiousness greatest 5–10 days after exposure
- In EI, the rash is thought to be autoimmune due to IgM complexes; signals the clearance of viremia.
- Cytotoxic infection of proerythroblasts causes cessation of RBC production.

Genetics
Erythrocyte P antigen-negative individuals are resistant to infection.

RISK FACTORS
- School-related epidemic and nonimmune household contacts have a secondary attack rate of 20–50%.
- Highest secondary attack rates are for daycare providers and school personnel in contact with affected children.

- Those with increased cell turnover (e.g., hemoglobinopathy, sickle cell [SS] anemia, thalassemia) are at risk for transient aplastic crisis.
- Immunodeficiency (e.g., HIV, congenital) may increase risk of PRAC and chronic anemia.
- Of pregnant women, as many as 40% are not immune, with 1.5% seroconversion per year.

GENERAL PREVENTION
- Standard hygienic practices include frequent hand washing and wearing barrier protection, such as surgical masks, when treating patients with possible respiratory viral infections.
- Because EI is so common, it is impossible to avoid exposure completely, particularly because the period of contagion is before clinical illness (rash) appears.
- Pregnant health care workers should avoid caring for patients with transient aplastic crises.
- No significant risk of infection based on occupational exposure. Exclusion from the workplace is not recommended.
- No vaccine is available to prevent the disease.
- Droplet precautions recommended around patients with TAC, chronic infection, or anemia.

COMMONLY ASSOCIATED CONDITIONS
- Nondegenerative arthritis:
  – *In adults, 80% of patients may manifest polyarthritis and/or arthralgia (female > male).*
  – In children, joint symptoms are less common.
  – Knees, hands, wrists, and ankles (frequently symmetric) are most commonly involved.
  – Joint symptoms usually subside within 3 weeks, but may persist for months. No joint erosions on x-ray.
- Transient aplastic crisis:
  – Seen in patients with increased RBC turnover, such as sickle cell anemia, spherocytosis, thalassemia, or decreased RBC production (iron deficiency anemia).
  – Patients often present with weakness, lethargy, and pallor due to anemia.
  – Aplastic event may be life threatening but is self-limited, with reticulocytes reappearing in 7–10 days and full recovery in 2–3 weeks.
  – In children with sickle cell hemoglobinopathies and heredity spherocytosis, fever is the most common symptom (73%), and rash is unlikely.
- Chronic anemia:
  – Seen in immunocompromised individuals (HIV, cancer, transplant) with no IgM response
  – Usually no manifestations of fever, rash, or joint symptoms
- Fetal/Neonatal infection:
  – Risk of transplacental spread of virus ~33% in infected mothers
  – A pregnant woman with a new rash or arthralgia should be tested for the virus.
  – Clinical manifestations range from asymptomatic seroconversion and normal pregnancy (most commonly), to variable degrees of fetal hydrops, to 2nd- and 3rd-trimester intrauterine fetal demise without hydrops.
  – B19 infection always should be suspected in cases of nonimmune hydrops.
  – The principal organ involved in the fetus is the bone marrow. RBC survival is shortened, and profound anemia can result, leading to high output heart failure.

- >95% of fetal complications (fetal hydrops and death) occur within 12 weeks of acute parvovirus B19 infection in pregnancy.
- Risk of fetal loss in pregnancy is highest with B19 infections in the 1st trimester but is only between 2% and 5%.
- Parvovirus B19 infection may be associated with long-term neurodevelopmental impairment in infants requiring intrauterine transfusions (1).
- Papular purpuric gloves and socks syndrome (PPGSS): Severe petechial and ecchymotic rash in hand–foot distribution with associated febrile tonsillopharyngitis and oral ulcerations (2).

 DIAGNOSIS

HISTORY
- Rash
- Headache
- Pharyngitis
- Coryza and rhinorrhea
- Arthralgias and arthritis
- Nausea and GI disturbances are more frequent and severe in adults (nonspecific flulike illness)
- Pruritus (especially soles of feet).
- Fever, myalgia, and malaise

PHYSICAL EXAM
- Onset of rash is first noted on the face, sparing the nasolabial folds ("slapped-cheek" appearance).
- A lacy, reticular rash on the trunk, buttocks, and limbs can follow 1–4 days later and lasts 1–6 weeks.
- The rash may be pruritic and characterized by recrudescence, sometimes associated with bathing, exercise, sun exposure, or heat or emotional stress.
- Alternatively, B19 may manifest as painful pruritic papules and purpura on the hands and feet.

DIFFERENTIAL DIAGNOSIS
- Rubella
- Enteroviral disease
- Systemic lupus erythematosus
- Drug reaction
- Lyme disease
- Rheumatoid arthritis

DIAGNOSTIC TESTS & INTERPRETATION
Initial Tests (lab, imaging)
- Usually no need for lab studies because diagnosis is made clinically and illness is mild and self-limiting.
- If testing immunocompetent individuals, IgG and IgM serology is preferred.
- B19-specific DNA detection by polymerase chain reaction (PCR) analysis for fetus (via cord blood or amniotic fluid) and patients with chronic infection and immunocompromise
- PCR increases diagnostic sensitivity and specificity to confirm/exclude suspected infections in those who are IgM antibody negative.
- For patients with TAC, CBC with reticulocyte count shows anemia and reticulocytopenia. IgM antibodies are present by day 3, and IgG antibodies are detectable at time of recovery. PCR will show high levels of viremia.
- Pregnant women exposed to B19 require IgG and IgM serology to assess fetal risk.

Follow-Up Tests & Special Considerations
- Fetal/Neonatal infection:
  - To exclude congenital B19 in infants with negative B19 IgM, an infant's B19 IgG serology must be followed in the 1st year of life.
  - Maternal serum α-fetoprotein may be increased in fetuses with hydrops fetalis.
  - Documented acute maternal infection in the 1st trimester warrants weekly fetal ultrasound for 8–12 weeks to assess for hydrops development: ascites, pericardial effusion, oligohydramnios, cardiomegaly, and thickened placenta (3)[C].
  - Weekly peak systolic velocity measurements of the middle cerebral artery by Doppler US is also recommended to evaluate for heart failure and fetal anemia and need for intrauterine transfusion (>1.5 MoM) (4)[C].
  - Cerebral MRI studies to assess for CNS damage in infected neonates with prolonged hydrops fetalis or hematocrit <15%.

Diagnostic Procedures/Other
- Skin biopsy usually normal, but may show mild inflammation consisting of perivascular infiltrations of mononuclear cells
- In stillbirths related to maternal B19 infection, virus can be detected in all tissues.
- In hydrops fetalis, may see intranuclear inclusions in nucleated RBCs

TREATMENT

GENERAL MEASURES
- No therapy is usually needed.
- Cessation of immunosuppressive therapy has allowed some patients to clear chronic infections. B19-associated anemia in HIV-positive patients may resolve with highly active antiretroviral therapy.

MEDICATION
First Line
- Anti-inflammatory agents may alleviate arthritic symptoms.
- Antipyretics may be used for fever. Avoid aspirin in children.

Second Line
- RBC transfusions often required for aplastic crisis.
- Intravenous immunoglobulin (IVIG) for B19-related refractory anemia or PRAC, especially if patient is immunodeficient (5)[C]
- Intrauterine RBC transfusions have been shown to reduce mortality significantly in hydrops/anemia diagnosed by US or cordocentesis (6)[A].

ISSUES FOR REFERRAL
- Acute infection during pregnancy should prompt referral to a maternal–fetal medicine specialist.
- TAC patients require treatment by a hematologist.
- Patients with chronic or abnormal B19 infections may benefit from consultation to immunology or infectious disease specialists.

IN-PATIENT CONSIDERATIONS
Admission Criteria/Initial Stabilization
- Outpatient management for EI
- Inpatient management for aplastic crisis, which may require RBC transfusions

ONGOING CARE

FOLLOW-UP RECOMMENDATIONS
Patient Monitoring
Periodic blood counts for anemic patients

PATIENT EDUCATION
- Parvovirus B19 (fifth disease): www.cdc.gov/parvovirusB19/fifth-disease.html
- Parvovirus B19: What you should know: www.aafp.org/afp/2007/0201/p377.html
- Parvovirus B19 infection and pregnancy: www.cdc.gov/parvovirusB19/pregnancy.html
- March of Dimes fifth disease in pregnancy: www.marchofdimes.com/pregnancy/complications_fifthdisease.html
- Physicians should counsel pregnant women with respect to prevention and management of maternal B19 infection.
- Pregnant women should avoid exposure to patients with active/chronic infections. However, exclusion of pregnant women from the workplace where EI is occurring is not recommended.
- Children with symptoms such as rash are no longer infectious and may attend childcare or school.

PROGNOSIS
- Usually self-limited
- Joint symptoms subside in weeks (often by 2 weeks, but may last months).
- ~20% of infections result in delayed virus elimination and viremia persisting for several months to years.
- Full recovery from aplastic crisis in 2–3 weeks

COMPLICATIONS
Conditions associated with B19, but not proven causal:
- Chronic fatigue syndrome
- Glomerulonephritis, nephrotic syndrome, and other renal diseases
- Hepatitis
- Neurologic manifestations/stroke/meningoencephalitis
- Henoch-Schönlein purpura, idiopathic thrombocytopenic purpura, and vasculitis
- Myocarditis and pericarditis
- Hemophagocytic syndrome

REFERENCES

1. De Jong EP, Lindenburg IT, van Klink JM, et al. Intrauterine transfusion for parvovirus B19 infection: Long-term neurodevelopmental outcome. *Am J Obstet Gynecol*. 2012;206:204.e1–e5.
2. Santonja C, Nieto-González G, Santos-Briz A, et al. Immunohistochemical detection of parvovirus B19 in "gloves and socks" papular purpuric syndrome: Direct evidence for viral endothelial involvement. *Am J Dermatopathol*. 2011;33:790–795.
3. Enders M, Weidner A, Rosenthal T, et al. Improved diagnosis of gestational parvovirus B19 infection at the time of nonimmune fetal hydrops. *J Infect Dis*. 2008;197:58.
4. Lamont RF, Sobel JD, Vaisbuch E, et al. Parvovirus B19 infection in human pregnancy. *BJOG-Int J Obstet Gy*. 2011;118:175–186.
5. Orange JS, Hossny EM, Weiler CR, et al. Use of intravenous immunoglobulin in human disease: A review of evidence by members of the Primary Immunodeficiency Committee of the American Academy of Allergy, Asthma and Immunology. *J Allergy Clin Immunol*. 2006;117:S525–S553.
6. de Jong EP, de Haan TR, Kroes AC, et al. Parvovirus B19 infection in pregnancy. *J Clin Virol*. 2006;36: 1–7.

ADDITIONAL READING

- Azevedo KM, Setbal S, Camacho LA, et al. Parvovirus B19 seroconversion in a cohort of human immunodeficiency virus-infected patients. *Mem Inst Oswaldo Cruz*. 2012;107:356–361.
- Beigi RH, Wiesenfeld HC, Landers DV, et al. High rate of severe fetal outcomes associated with maternal parvovirus b19 infection in pregnancy. *Infect Dis Obstet Gynecol*. 2008;2008:524601.
- De Jong EP, Walther FJ, Kroes AC, et al. Parvovirus B19 infection in pregnancy: New insights and management. *Prenat Diagn*. 2011;31:419–425.
- Snyder M, Wallace R. Clinical inquiry: What should you tell pregnant women about exposure to parvovirus? *J Fam Pract*. 2011;60:765–766.

CODES

ICD10
- B08.3 Erythema infectiosum [fifth disease]
- B34.3 Parvovirus infection, unspecified

CLINICAL PEARLS
- Parvovirus B19 infection is usually a benign, self-limited illness with no long-term effects.
- The rash of EI, initially presenting with a "slapped cheeks appearance," signifies that the patient is no longer infectious.
- Patients with increased RBC turnover (SS, thalassemia) are at risk for transient aplastic crisis.
- Immunocompromised patients may be at risk for chronic anemia.
- Documentation of acute infection <20 weeks gestation warrants maternal–fetal consultation for serial monitoring of fetal well-being for 3 months via ultrasound.

PATELLOFEMORAL PAIN SYNDROME

Howsen Kwan, MD, MRCS • Robert Dimeff, MD

BASICS

DESCRIPTION
- Peri- or retropatellar pain resulting from repetitive motion and abnormal tracking of the patella over the knee joint, leading to pathologic changes in the articular cartilage.
- System(s) affected: Musculoskeletal

EPIDEMIOLOGY
Prevalence
- May affect 25% of athletes (1)
- Common among adolescents
- Difference between sexes is negligible (a 3% higher prevalence has been reported among female vs. male athletes).
- Higher incidence during the 2nd and 3rd decades of life: Incidence decreases with age in both men and women.

ETIOLOGY AND PATHOPHYSIOLOGY
- Precise cause unknown, likely multifactorial; can be categorized into 3 subsets:
  - Anatomic (malalignment, abnormal patellar height, shallow trochlear groove, muscular dysfunction)
  - Dynamic (muscle imbalance, overload, or overuse)
  - Specific (chondral, plica, or neuroma)
- Repetitive contact of the undersurface of the patella against the trochlea of the femur with or without maltracking of the patella

Genetics
Unknown

RISK FACTORS
- Increased Q angle (>20°); normal range: 13–15° (2,3)[B]
  - Q angle: angle between the line of tension of the quadriceps and the line of the patellar tendon
- Weakness of the quadriceps, gastrocnemius, or hamstring (2,3)[B]
- Iliotibial (IT) band tightness (2)[B]
- Inflexibility of the hamstrings, quadriceps, or hip flexors (2)[B]
- Generalized ligamentous laxity (2)[B]
- Lateral retinacular tightness (2)[B]

GENERAL PREVENTION
Limited evidence exists regarding interventions that prevent patellofemoral pain syndrome:
- In runners, wearing properly fitting footwear: There is mixed evidence for and against the use of custom/shock-absorbing insoles.
- Training programs with appropriate slow increases in mileage and dynamic stretching
- Mixed evidence exists for the use of knee braces in distance runners.

COMMONLY ASSOCIATED CONDITIONS
- Overuse
- Obesity
- Knee ligament injury/surgery
- Patellar tendinopathy
- Prolonged synovitis
- IT band friction syndrome
- Immobilization

DIAGNOSIS

HISTORY
- An accurate history should differentiate pain from instability (e.g., pain quality, swelling, giving way, mechanical symptoms, and grinding, inciting events, overuse, and history of trauma)
- Most common symptom: Anteromedial knee pain exacerbated by physical activity or an increase in physical activity
- Pain often exacerbated when squatting
- Anterior knee pain when descending/ascending stairs, ambulating over uneven surfaces, or running
- Theater sign or movie-goer sign: Anterior knee pain upon arising after prolonged sitting
- Crepitus with knee range of motion
- Often can have pain after activity as well as during activity

PHYSICAL EXAM
- In some athletes, physical findings may be subtle or absent. Observe patellar position in the knee at 90° and track for a J sign (3).
- Pain and/or crepitus at the area of the patellofemoral articulation (e.g., patella facets, trochlea, and peripatellar area) (3).
- Apprehension sign: Compress the patella against the femur and ask the patient to contract quadriceps muscles; pain upon contraction is consistent with patellofemoral pain syndrome (3), although pain may be present in normal individuals as well.
- Reproduction of pain with compression of patella against the trochlea (3)
- Q angle is assessed by taking the angle of the intersection of 2 lines: 1 drawn from the anterior superior iliac spine to the midpatella and the other line drawn from the midpatella to the tibial tubercle. An angle of >20° is a potential risk factor.
- Assessing strength of hip adductors with bilateral/single squat test

DIFFERENTIAL DIAGNOSIS
- Patellofemoral joint osteoarthritis (2)
- Chondromalacia patella
- Patellar tendinopathy
- Articular cartilage injury
- Hoffa disease
- IT band syndrome
- Loose bodies
- Neuromas
- Osgood-Schlatter disease
- Osteochondritis dissecans
- Patellar instability/subluxation
- Patellar fracture
- Patellar stress fracture
- Pes anserine bursitis
- Plica synovialis
- Bone tumors
- Prepatellar bursitis
- Previous surgery
- Quadriceps tendinopathy

- Referred pain from lumbar spine or hip joint pathology
- Saphenous neuritis
- Sinding-Larsen-Johansson syndrome
- Symptomatic bipartite patella

DIAGNOSTIC TESTS & INTERPRETATION
- None indicated. *In general, imaging is unnecessary and not helpful in diagnosing this condition.* If imaging is indicated because of severity, atypical symptoms, or persistence of symptoms despite treatment, 4 views of the knee are recommended to view patellar tilt and to rule out other potential etiologies of anterior knee pain:
  - Lateral
  - Merchant (also called sunrise)
  - Standing anteroposterior
  - Posteroanterior tunnel views
- Radiographic findings may not correlate with symptoms.

Follow-Up Tests & Special Considerations
Radiographic images may be normal until late stages, when the posterior patellar surface becomes irregular and cartilage erosion becomes radiographically detectable.

Test Interpretation
Should be absent, and any presence of pathology indicates other diagnosis

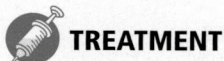

TREATMENT

Most important is abstaining from activity thought to induce the problem, relative rest with low-impact training, and analgesia as needed.

GENERAL MEASURES
- Physical therapy referral for exercises (McConnell regimen) to reduce pain and increase strength over 6 weeks (1,4)[A].
- Specific home exercises may be employed, but guidance from a physical therapist is preferred (1,4)[A], particularly for athletes.
- Knee braces and taping can be helpful at the initiation of physical therapy, but do not replace a well-designed exercise program (1,4,5)[A].
- Orthotic arch support may be helpful, but has not been well studied (4)[C].
- Rest from painful activity and substitute aggravating activities with cross-training exercises (e.g., swimming) (4)[C].
- Applying ice for 10–15 minutes at a time may be helpful (4)[C].
- Physical therapy for hip adductor strengthening

MEDICATION

- There is limited evidence for the effectiveness of NSAIDs for short-term pain relief (6)[C].
- The evidence for glycosaminoglycan polysulfate is conflicting and merits further investigation (6).
- Nandrolone may be effective, but it is too controversial to recommend for treatment (6).

ISSUES FOR REFERRAL

Referral for surgery is a last resort after all conservative measures fail. Surgery is rarely needed if appropriately managed.

ADDITIONAL THERAPIES

Ice packs after activity have been found to improve clinical symptoms.

SURGERY/OTHER PROCEDURES

- Attempts to correct maltracking of the patellofemoral joint with a lateral retinacular release or tibial tubercle transposition have shown variable results.
- Rarely indicated

 ONGOING CARE

PATIENT EDUCATION

Patient education and exercises: http://familydoctor.org/online/famdocen/home/healthy/physical/injuries/479.html

PROGNOSIS

- Often improves spontaneously with rest and physical therapy
- Conversely, established chondromalacia patella (see "Differential Diagnosis") has poor prognosis.

REFERENCES

1. Collado H, Fredericson M. Patellofemoral pain syndrome. *Clin Sports Med*. 2010;29:379–398.
2. Waryasz GR. Patellofemoral pain syndrome (PFPS): A systematic review of anatomy and potential risk factors. *Dynam Med*. 2008;7:1476–1459.
3. Fredericson M, Yoon K. Physical examination and patellofemoral pain syndrome. *Am J Phys Med Rehabil*. 2006;85:234–243.
4. Dixit S, DiFiori JP, Burton M, et al. Management of patellofemoral pain syndrome. *Am Fam Physician*. 2007;75:194–202.
5. Callaghan MJ, Selfe J. Patellar taping for patellofemoral pain syndrome in adults. *Cochrane Database Syst Rev*. 2012;4:CD006717.
6. Heintjes E, Berger MY, Bierma-Zeinstra SM, et al. Pharmacotherapy for patellofemoral pain syndrome. *Cochrane Database Syst Rev*. 2004;3:CD003470.

ADDITIONAL READING

- Barton CJ, Lack S, Malliaras P, et al. Gluteal muscle activity and patellofemoral pain syndrome: A systematic review. *Br J Sports Med*. 2013;47:207.
- Lankhorst NE, Bierma-Zeinstra SM, van Middelkoop M. Factors associated with patellofemoral pain syndrome: A systematic review. *Br J Sports Med*. 2013;47:193.
- Lankhorst NE, Bierma-Zeinstra SM, van Middelkoop M. Risk factors for patellofemoral pain syndrome: A systematic review. *J Orthop Sports Phys Ther*. 2012;42:81–94.

 SEE ALSO

Algorithm: Knee Pain

 CODES

ICD10

- M25.561 Pain in right knee
- M25.562 Pain in left knee
- M25.569 Pain in unspecified knee

CLINICAL PEARLS

- Patellofemoral pain syndrome is the most common cause of anterior knee pain in active adults (age 20–39), affecting men and women almost equally.
- The clinical diagnosis is made by taking a history and the use of the apprehension sign (compress the patella against the femur and ask the patient to contract quadriceps muscles; pain with contraction is consistent with patellofemoral pain syndrome).
- Well-designed exercises geared at quadriceps strengthening, hamstring, and IT band flexibility and hip stabilizers are the most effective evidence-based treatment.

PEDICULOSIS (LICE)

Kaelen C. Dunican, PharmD • Cynthia Jeremiah, MD

BASICS

DESCRIPTION
- A contagious parasitic infection caused by lice (blood-sucking insects, obligate parasites)
- 2 species of lice infest humans:
  - *Pediculus humanus* has 2 subspecies: The head louse (var. *capitis*) and the body louse (var. *corporis*). Both species are 1–3 mm long, flat, and wingless and have 3 pairs of legs that attach closely behind the head.
  - *Phthirus pubis* (pubic or crab louse): Resembles a sea crab and has widespread claws on the 2nd and 3rd legs
- System(s) affected: Skin/Exocrine
- Synonym(s): Lice; Crabs

EPIDEMIOLOGY
Incidence
- In the US: 6–12 million new cases per year
- Predominant age:
  - Head lice: Most common in children 3–12 years of age; more common in girls than boys
  - Pubic lice: Most common in adults

Prevalence
Head lice: 1–3% in industrialized countries

ETIOLOGY AND PATHOPHYSIOLOGY
Itching is a hypersensitivity reaction to the saliva of the feeding louse.
- Infestation by lice: *P. humanus* (var. *capitis*), *P. humanus* (var. *corporis*), or *P. pubis*
- Characteristics of lice:
  - Adult louse is dark grayish and moves quickly, but does not jump or fly.
  - Eggs (sometimes referred to as nits) camouflage with the individuals' hair color and are cemented to the base of the hair shaft (within 4 mm of the scalp).
  - Nits (empty egg casings) appear white (opalescent) and remain cemented to the hair shaft.
  - Lice feed solely on human blood by piercing the skin, injecting saliva, and then sucking blood.
- Transmission: Direct human-to-human contact:
  - Head lice: Direct head-to-head contact or contact with infested fomite (less common)
  - Body lice: Contact with contaminated clothing or bedding
  - Pubic lice: Typically transmitted sexually (fomite transmission is unlikely)

RISK FACTORS
- General: Overcrowding and close personal contact
- Head lice:
  - School-aged children, gender (girls)
  - Sharing combs, hats (including helmets), clothing, and bed linens
  - African Americans rarely have head lice; theories include twisted hair shaft and increased use of thick hair products
- Body lice: Poor hygiene, homelessness
- Pubic lice: Promiscuity (very high transmission rate)

GENERAL PREVENTION
- Environmental measures: Wash, dry-clean, or vacuum all items that may have come in contact with infected individuals.
- Screen and treat affected household contacts

- Head lice: Follow up by school nurses may help to prevent recurrence and spread.
- Pubic lice: Limit the number of sexual partners (Note: Condoms do not prevent transmission nor does shaving pubic hair).
- Body lice: Proper hygiene

COMMONLY ASSOCIATED CONDITIONS
Up to 1/3 of patients with pubic lice have at least one concomitant STI.

DIAGNOSIS

HISTORY
- Pruritus is common, mostly at night
- Investigate contacts of infected individuals

PHYSICAL EXAM
- Diagnosis is confirmed clinically by visualization of live lice.
- *P. capitis* (head lice):
  - Found most often on the back of the head and neck and behind the ears (warmer areas)
  - Eyelashes may be involved
  - Eggs, found cemented on the base of a hair shaft, are difficult to remove.
  - Pruritus may be accompanied by local erythema and small papules.
  - May see excoriations around hairline
  - Scratching can cause inflammation and secondary bacterial infection
  - Pyoderma and lymphadenopathy in severe infestation
- *P. corporis* (body lice):
  - Poor hygiene
  - Adult lice and nits in the seams of clothing
  - Intense pruritus involving area covered by clothing (trunk, axillae, and groin)
  - Uninfected bites present as erythematous macules, papules, and wheals.
  - Pyoderma and excoriation may be seen.
- *P. pubis* (pubic louse):
  - Pubic hair is the most common site, but lice may spread to hair around anus, abdomen, axillae, chest, beard, eyebrows, and eyelashes.
  - Eggs are present at the base of hair shafts.
  - Anogenital pruritus
  - Blue macules may be seen in surrounding skin.
  - Delay in treatment may lead to development of groin infection and regional adenopathy.

DIFFERENTIAL DIAGNOSIS
- Scabies and other mite species that can cause cutaneous reactions in humans
- Dandruff and other hair debris can sometimes look like head lice but do not stick to hair shafts as do eggs and nits.

DIAGNOSTIC TESTS & INTERPRETATION
- Head lice: Comb hair thoroughly with a fine-toothed louse comb (0.2–0.3 mm between teeth) to identify live lice (1,2)[C]. Simple visual inspection is of similar sensitivity to wet combing, but ~25% as effective as dry combing with a metal comb (3).
- Body lice: Examine the seams of clothing to locate lice and their eggs (2)[C].
- Carefully examine hair shafts under the microscope; lice and eggs can be seen easily under a microscope.
- In contrast to dandruff, eggs and nits cannot be removed easily from a hair shaft.

Follow-Up Tests & Special Considerations
- Empty nits will remain on hair shafts for months after eradication of the live infestation. On Wood's lamp exam, live nits fluoresce white and empty nits fluoresce gray.
- Pubic lice: Patients should be evaluated for other STIs.

TREATMENT

Since the early 1990s, lice have acquired some degree of resistance to insecticides (3).

MEDICATION
Permethrin (over the counter [OTC]), synergized pyrethrin (OTC), spinosad (Rx), benzyl alcohol (Rx), malathion (Rx), and topical ivermectin (Rx) are effective for head lice (1,4,5)[A]. Permethrin, synergized pyrethrin, and malathion are effective for pubic lice (4)[A].
- Permethrin may be preferred because it has residual activity for up to 3 weeks (2)[C]. However, newer shampoos and conditioners may reduce the residual effect (1)[C].
- Malathion and spinosad are considered second line for head lice, but may be more effective due to ovicidal activity (1,5)[B].
- Ivermectin 0.5% lotion is also effective for head lice and does not require a second treatment (6)[B].

First Line
- Head and pubic lice:
- Pyrethrum insecticides: Permethrin 1% cream rinse (Nix) or pyrethrins 0.33% with piperonyl butoxide 4% (synergized pyrethrin, Rid, Pronto): Apply for 10 minutes, then wash:
  - Reapplication in 7–10 days (day 9 is optimal) is always required with use of synergized pyrethrin and may be necessary with use of permethrin, if live lice are observed.
  - Side effects: Application-site erythema, ocular erythema, and application-site irritation
- Body lice: Best treated with synergized pyrethrin lotion applied once and left on for several hours.
- Eyelash infestation: Apply petroleum jelly b.i.d. × 10 days.
- Precautions:
  - Pyrethrin: Avoid in patients with ragweed allergy (may cause respiratory symptoms).
  - Pediculicides should never be used to treat eyelash infections.

Second Line
- Head lice and pubic lice:
  - Malathion 0.5% lotion (Ovide):
    ○ Apply for 8–12 hours, then wash off
    ○ Excipients isopropyl alcohol (78%) and terpineol (12%) may contribute to its efficacy
    ○ Flammable and has a bad odor
    ○ Despite ovicidal activity, a 2nd application may be necessary after 7–10 days (day 9 is optimal) if live lice are observed.
  - Lindane 1% shampoo: Apply for 4 minutes, then wash (should *not* be repeated):
    ○ Side effects: Neurotoxicity (seizures, muscle spasms), aplastic anemia
    ○ Contraindications: Uncontrolled seizure disorder, premature infants

○ Precautions: Do not use on excoriated skin, in immunocompromised patients, conditions that increase seizure risk, or with medications that decrease seizure threshold.
○ Possible interactions: Concomitant use with medications that lower the seizure threshold
- Head lice:
  – Spinosad 0.9% lotion (Natroba):
    ○ Apply to dry hair and scalp for 10 minutes, then rinse with warm water. Repeat in 7 days if live lice are observed.
    ○ Side effects: Application-site erythema, ocular erythema, and application-site irritation
  – Benzyl alcohol 5% lotion (Ulesfia):
    ○ Apply to dry hair using a sufficient amount to saturate scalp and hair (amount depends on hair length), rinse after 10 minutes, and repeat in 7 days.
    ○ Side effects: Pruritus, erythema, pyoderma, ocular irritation, application-site irritation
  – Ivermectin 0.5% lotion (Sklice):
    ○ Apply to dry hair by using a sufficient amount to saturate the scalp and hair (max. 4 oz) then rinse after 10 minutes
    ○ Mechanical removal of lice and nits by wetting hair and then systematically combing with a fine-toothed comb every 3–4 days × 2 weeks to remove all lice as they hatch

ALERT
Lindane: FDA black box warning of severe neurologic toxicity (use only when first-line agents have failed). The National Pediculosis Association strongly advises against using lindane at all.

GENERAL MEASURES
- Head lice: Wash all bedding, towels, clothes, headgear, combs, brushes, and hair accessories in hot water (60°C).
- Vacuum furniture and carpets
- Any personal articles that cannot be washed in hot water, dry cleaned, or vacuumed should be sealed in a plastic bag and stored for at least 2 weeks.
- All household members and close contacts should be examined and treated concurrently if infested.
- Insecticide sprays are not necessary.
- Pubic lice: Avoid sexual activity until both partners are successfully treated.
- Nit and egg removal:
  – It is important to remove eggs that are within 1 cm of the scalp to prevent reinfestation.
  – After treatment with shampoo or lotion, eggs and nits remain in the scalp or pubic hair until mechanically removed.
  – Eggs and nits are best removed with a very fine nit comb.

Pediatric Considerations
- Avoid synergized pyrethrin and permethrin in infants <2 months of age; benzyl alcohol, topical ivermectin, and spinosad in children <6 months of age; and malathion in children <2 years of age
- Lindane: Not recommended in patients who weigh <50 kg, including infants

Pregnancy Considerations
Permethrin, synergized pyrethrin, malathion, spinosad, and benzyl alcohol are pregnancy Category B. Lindane and topical ivermectin are Category C.

ADDITIONAL THERAPIES
- For "difficult to treat" cases of head lice, oral ivermectin 400 μg/kg (not approved by the FDA for lice), given twice at a 7-day interval, had superior efficacy when compared with topical 0.5% malathion lotion (7)[A].
- Dual therapy with 1% permethrin and oral trimethoprim/sulfamethoxazole (TMP/SMX) only for cases of multiple treatment failures or suspected cases of lice-related resistance to therapy (TMP/SMX is not approved by the FDA for lice)

COMPLEMENTARY AND ALTERNATIVE MEDICINE
- Ivermectin: 200 μg/kg PO repeated in 7–10 days:
  – Should not be used in children weighing <15 kg; pregnancy Category C
  – Not approved by the FDA for lice
- Head lice:
  – Dry-on, suffocation-based pediculicide: Nuvo or Cetaphil lotion:
    ○ Apply thoroughly to hair, comb, dry with hairdryer, shampoo after 8 hours
    ○ Repeat once a week until cured, up to a maximum of 3 applications
    ○ Not approved by the FDA for lice
  – Dimethicone 4% lotion: Apply to hair for 8 hours; repeat in 1 week (not approved by the FDA for lice)
  – No home remedies (e.g., vinegar, isopropyl alcohol, olive oil, mayonnaise, melted butter, and petroleum jelly) have been proven effective to treat head lice infestations.
  – Herbal shampoos and pomades have not been evaluated in clinical trials and are not approved by the FDA for lice.
  – Lavender oil and tea tree oil have been implicated in triggering prepubertal gynecomastia in boys, so they should not be used against lice (3).

ONGOING CARE

FOLLOW-UP RECOMMENDATIONS
Children may return to school after completing topical treatment, even if nits remain in place. No-nit policies are not necessary (1).

Patient Monitoring
Drug resistance should be suspected if live lice are still present 24 hours after treatment.

PATIENT EDUCATION
- National Pediculosis Association at www.headlice.org
- CDC at www.cdc.gov/parasites/lice/

PROGNOSIS
- With appropriate treatment, >90% cure rate
- Recurrence common, mainly from reinfection or failure to comply with treatment, although resistance to synthetic pyrethroids is increasing (8)

COMPLICATIONS
- Poor sleep due to pruritus
- Persistent itching may be caused by too frequent use of the pediculicide
- Missed school; social stigma
- Secondary bacterial infections
- Body lice can transmit typhus and trench fever.

REFERENCES
1. Frankowski BL, Bocchini JA. The Council on School Health and Committee on Infectious Disease. Head lice. Pediatrics. 2010;126:392–403.
2. Orion E, Marcos B, Davidovici B. Itch and scratch: Scabies and pediculosis. Clin Dermatol. 2006;24:168–175.
3. Burgess IF. Current treatments for pediculosis capitis. Curr Opin Infect Dis. 2009;22:131–136.
4. Flinders DC, De Schweinitz P. Pediculosis and scabies. Am Fam Physician. 2004;69:341–348.
5. Cole SW, Lundquist LM. Spinosad for treatment of head lice infestation. Ann Pharmacother. 2011;45:954–959.
6. Pariser DM, Meinking TL, Bell M, et al. Topical 0.5% ivermectin lotion for treatment of head lice. N Engl J Med. 2012;367:1687–1693.
7. Chosidow O, Giraudeau B, Cottrell J, et al. Oral ivermectin versus malathion lotion for difficult-to-treat head lice. N Engl J Med. 2010;362:896–905.
8. Durand R, Bouvresse S, Berdjane Z, et al. Insecticide resistance in head lice: Clinical, parasitological and genetic aspects. Clin Microbiol Infect. 2012;18:338–344.

 SEE ALSO

Arthropod Bites and Stings; Scabies

CODES

ICD10
- B85.0 Pediculosis due to Pediculus humanus capitis
- B85.1 Pediculosis due to Pediculus humanus corporis
- B85.3 Phthiriasis

CLINICAL PEARLS
- Proper product application is essential; improper product application should be considered when assessing treatment failure.
- Prevalence of resistant infestations is increasing, so if live lice are present 24 hours after proper treatment, resistance should be suspected and an alternative agent from another class should be used.
- Routine re-treatment on day 9 is commonly recommended for nonovicidal products (permethrin and synergized pyrethrin).
- With all treatment options, patients' hair should be reinspected after 7–9 days and, if live lice are detected, treatment should be repeated on day 9.
- No-nit policies are not necessary because empty nits may remain on hair shafts for months after eradication.

PELVIC INFLAMMATORY DISEASE

Fozia Akhtar Ali, MD

BASICS

DESCRIPTION
- Pelvic Inflammatory disease (PID) is an infectious and inflammatory disorder of the upper female genital tract, including the uterus, fallopian tubes, and adjacent pelvic structures.
- Salpingitis is the most important component due to its impact on future fertility (1).
- Diagnosis may be challenging and incorrect in up to 1/3 of cases. No set of criteria is both sensitive and specific for the disease.
- System(s) affected: Reproductive

EPIDEMIOLOGY
- Predominant age: 15–25 years; this number has remained constant since early 1900s (2).
- Predominant sex: Female only

Incidence
770,000 cases of acute PID diagnosed annually in the US. Incidence decreased from 1885–2001. The CDC has estimated that more than 1 million women experience an episode of PID every year. The disease leads to approximately 2.5 million office visits and 125,000–150,000 hospitalizations yearly. The cost of PID is approximately $2,000 per patient, which equals about $1.5 billion annually.

ETIOLOGY AND PATHOPHYSIOLOGY
Multiple organisms may be etiologic agents in PID. Most cases are polymicrobial:
- *Chlamydia trachomatis, Neisseria gonorrhoeae,* genital tract mycoplasmas (particularly *Mycoplasma genitalium*), aerobic and anaerobic (*Bacteroides fragilis*), and vaginal flora (e.g., *Prevotella, Peptostreptococci, Gardnerella vaginalis, Escherichia coli, Haemophilus influenza*) are recognized as etiologic agents.
- Many nongonococcal, nonchlamydial micro-organisms recovered from upper genital tract in acute PID are associated with bacterial vaginosis (especially *Prevotella bivius, P. disiens,* and *P. capillosus)* (3)
- The precise mechanism by which micro-organisms ascend from the lower genital tract is unclear. Possible mechanisms include: (i) Travel from cervix to endometrium to salpinx to peritoneal cavity; (ii) lymphatic spread via infection of the parametrium (from an IUD); and (iii) hematogenous route, although this is rare (2).
- Of cases, 75% occur within 7 days of menses, when cervical mucus favors ascent of organisms.

RISK FACTORS
- Sexually active and age <25 years
- First sexual activity at young age (<15 years)
- New/multiple sexual partners
- Nonbarrier contraceptive methods (i.e., oral contraceptive pills)
- Previous history of PID; 20–25% will have a recurrence.
- History of *C. trachomatis*; 10–40% will develop PID.
- History of gonococcal cervicitis; 10–20% will develop PID (2).
- Gynecologic procedures such as endometrial biopsy, curettage, and hysteroscopy break the cervical barrier, predisposing women to ascending infections.

GENERAL PREVENTION
- Educational programs about safer sex practices such as barrier contraceptives, especially condoms and spermicidal creams or sponges, provide some protection.
- The U.S. Preventive Services Task Force recommends screening for chlamydia in all sexually active women younger than 25 years and in those 25 years and older at increased risk (new sex partner/multiple sex partners)
- Routine STI screening in pregnancy
- Early medical care with occurrence of genital lesions or abnormal discharge

COMMONLY ASSOCIATED CONDITIONS
- If PID is suspected in a patient with an IUD and a pelvic abscess is present, an *Actinomyces* infection requiring penicillin treatment may be present.
- Rupture of an adnexal abscess is rare but life threatening. Early surgical exploration is mandatory.
- Chlamydial or gonococcal perihepatitis may occur with PID. This combination is called Fitz-Hugh-Curtis (FHC) syndrome and is characterized by severe pleuritic right upper quadrant pain. FHC syndrome complicates 10% of PID cases.

DIAGNOSIS

- The diagnosis of PID is based primarily on clinical evaluation. Clinical diagnosis alone is 87% sensitive and 50% specific.
- Physicians must consider PID in the differential diagnosis in women 15–44 years of age who present with lower abdominal or pelvic pain and cervical motion or pelvic tenderness, even if these symptoms are mild.
- The CDC recommends empiric treatment for PID if ≥1 of the following minimum criteria are present on pelvic exam in an at-risk patient: Cervical motion tenderness, uterine tenderness, and adnexal tenderness in the presence of lower abdominal or pelvic pain.
- Additional criteria used to enhance specificity: Fever >101°F, new/abnormal vaginal discharge, presence of abundant numbers of WBCs on wet prep, elevated ESR, and laboratory documentation of cervical infection with *N. gonorrhoeae* or *C. trachomatis* (2)
- Most specific criteria for diagnosing PID: Endometrial biopsy reveals endometritis/plasma cells; transvaginal ultrasound showing thickened, fluid-filled salpinges; and laparoscopic abnormalities consistent with PID (1)

HISTORY
- Lower abdominal or pelvic pain: Typically described as dull, aching or crampy, bilateral, and constant; accentuated by motion, exercise, or coitus
- New/abnormal vaginal discharge (~75% of cases)
- Fever, chills, cramping, dyspareunia
- Low back pain (2)
- Urinary discomfort
- Unanticipated vaginal bleeding, often postcoital, is reported in about 40% of cases
- Recent hysterosalpingogram (HSG)
- IUD insertion within the past 21 days (2)

PHYSICAL EXAM
- Fever
- Lower abdominal and particularly cervical motion tenderness
- Findings of cervicitis with/without vaginal discharge

DIFFERENTIAL DIAGNOSIS
- Appendicitis
- Ectopic pregnancy
- Ovarian tumor/torsion
- Hemorrhagic/ruptured ovarian cyst
- Endometriosis/dysmenorrhea
- Functional pelvic pain
- Inflammatory bowel disease
- Diverticulitis
- UTI/pyelonephritis
- Nephrolithiasis (2)

DIAGNOSTIC TESTS & INTERPRETATION
Initial Tests (lab, imaging)
- Pregnancy test: Must be performed to rule out ectopic pregnancy and complications of an intrauterine pregnancy
- Specific testing for chlamydia and gonorrhea (usually nucleic acid amplification test (NAAT) and/or ligase chain reaction)
- Urinalysis
- Saline microscopy of vaginal fluid (for WBC)
- Consider CBC: WBC count $\geq 10,500/mm^3$, although $\leq 50\%$ of PID cases present with leukocytosis
- Consider transvaginal ultrasound: Not necessary for diagnosis. May show thickened, fluid-filled tubes (hydrosalpinges) ± free fluid or tubo-ovarian abscess (TOA)

Follow-Up Tests & Special Considerations
- ESR >15 mm/h or elevated C-reactive protein used in some diagnostic criteria
- Consider HIV testing in patients with PID
- Follow-up ultrasound as outpatient for resolution of adnexal abscess (4).

Diagnostic Procedures/Other
- Culdocentesis with culture is rarely necessary
- Laparoscopy is best used for confirming, as opposed to making, the diagnosis of PID and should be reserved for the following situations:
  – Ill patient with competing diagnosis (e.g., appendicitis)
  – Ill patient who has failed outpatient treatment
  – Any patient not improving after 72 hours of inpatient treatment
- Endometrial biopsy (rarely indicated): Reveals endometritis/plasma cells

TREATMENT

- Outpatient treatment, if appropriate
- Criteria for hospitalization and parenteral treatment are described below.

GENERAL MEASURES
Avoid intercourse until treatment is completed.

MEDICATION
First Line
- Several antibiotic regimens are highly effective, with no single regimen of choice.
- Outpatient treatment regimen A:
  – Ceftriaxone 250 mg IM or cefoxitin 2 g IM in a single dose *plus*
  – Doxycycline 100 mg PO b.i.d. × 14 days ±
  – Metronidazole 500 mg PO b.i.d. × 14 days
- On the basis of the recent emergence of fluoroquinolone-resistant gonococci, the CDC no longer recommends the use of these agents for the treatment of gonococcal infections and associated conditions such as PID (1).
- Metronidazole should be considered in cases where risk of infection with anaerobic organisms is considered high (1).

Second Line
- Many other antibiotic regimens have been proposed and used with success. Examples:
  – Tobramycin in place of gentamicin
  – Tetracycline in place of doxycycline
- In persons with documented severe allergic reactions to penicillin or cephalosporins, azithromycin or spectinomycin might be an option for therapy of uncomplicated gonococcal infections (1).
- Special consideration:
  – Refer sex partners for appropriate evaluation and treatment if they had sexual contact with patient during preceding 60 days or most recent sexual contact (1). Partners should be treated, irrespective of evaluation, with regimens effective against *chlamydia* and gonorrhea.

SURGERY/OTHER PROCEDURES
Reserved for failures of medical treatment and for suspected ruptured adnexal abscess with resulting acute surgical abdomen

IN-PATIENT CONSIDERATIONS
Admission Criteria/Initial Stabilization
- Hospitalization recommended in the following:
  – Surgical emergencies (e.g., appendicitis)
  – Suspected pelvic abscess
  – Pregnancy
  – Severe illness, nausea, vomiting, or high fever
  – Intolerance/inability to adhere to outpatient regimen
  – Failure to respond to outpatient therapy (1)
- For inpatient treatment of PID, the CDC also lists 2 currently accepted treatment regimens:

– Parenteral regimen A:
  ○ Cefotetan 2 g IV q12h or cefoxitin 2 g IV q6h + doxycycline 100 mg PO or IV q12h
  ○ Parenteral therapy × 24 hours after clinical improvement; continue doxycycline for a total of 14 days
– Parenteral regimen B:
  ○ Clindamycin 900 mg IV q8h + gentamicin loading dose IV or IM (2 mg/kg of body weight) followed by a maintenance dose (1.5 mg/kg) q8h
  ○ Parenteral therapy for 24 hours after clinical improvement; continue doxycycline as above or clindamycin 450 mg PO q.i.d. for a total of 14 days

ONGOING CARE

FOLLOW-UP RECOMMENDATIONS
Patient Monitoring
- Close observation of clinical status, particularly for fever, symptoms, degree of peritonitis, serum WBC
- Retest for gonorrhea and chlamydia in 3–6 months. The likelihood of reinfection is high.
- Follow adnexal abscess size and position with serial ultrasound.

PATIENT EDUCATION
- Abstinence from any type of sexual contact until treatment of patient/partner (if necessary) is complete
- Consistent and correct condom use should be enforced
- Hepatitis B and human papilloma virus (HPV) vaccines should be given to patients who meet criteria
- Advise comprehensive STI screening

PROGNOSIS
- Wide variation with good prognosis if early, effective therapy is instituted and further infection is avoided
- Poor prognosis related to late therapy and continued high-risk sexual behavior
- Nongonococcal nonchlamydial PID is more often associated with severe PID and with worse prognosis for future fertility

COMPLICATIONS
- Tubo-ovarian abscess will develop in ∼7–16% of patients with PID.
- Recurrent infection occurs in 20–25% of patients.
- Risk of ectopic pregnancy is increased 7–10-fold among women with a history of PID.
- Tubal infertility occurs in 8%, 19.5%, and 40% of women after 1, 2, and 3 episodes of PID, respectively (1).
- Chronic pelvic pain occurs in 20% of cases and is related to adhesion formation, chronic salpingitis, or recurrent infection.

REFERENCES

1. Workowski KA, Berman S, Centers for Disease Control and Prevention (CDC). Sexually transmitted diseases treatment guidelines, 2010. *MMWR Recomm Rep.* 2010;59(RR-12):1–110.
2. Gradison M. Pelvic inflammatory disease. *Am Fam Physician.* 2012;85:791–796.
3. Sweet RL. Treatment of acute pelvic inflammatory disease. *Infect Dis Obstet Gynecol.* 2011;2011: 561909.
4. Lareau SM, Beigi RH. Pelvic inflammatory disease and tubo-ovarian abscess. *Infect Dis Clin North Am.* 2008;22:693–708, vii.

ADDITIONAL READING
- Judlin P. Current concepts in managing pelvic inflammatory disease. *Curr Opin Infect Dis.* 2010;23:83–87.
- Jung SI, Kim YJ, Park HS, et al. Acute pelvic inflammatory disease: Diagnostic performance of CT. *J Obstet Gynaecol Res.* 2011;37:228–235.
- Weinstein SA, Stiles BG. A review of the epidemiology, diagnosis and evidence-based management of *Mycoplasma genitalium*. *Sex Health.* 2011;8:143–158.

CODES

ICD10
- N73.0 Acute parametritis and pelvic cellulitis
- N73.2 Unspecified parametritis and pelvic cellulitis
- N73.9 Female pelvic inflammatory disease, unspecified

CLINICAL PEARLS
- Most often PID starts with gonorrhea or *chlamydia*, but it can be polymicrobial.
- Physicians should treat on the basis of clinical judgment without waiting for confirmation from laboratory or imaging tests. PID is a common cause of infertility.
- Complications include hydrosalpinx, adhesions, pelvic pain, and 10-fold increased risk of ectopic pregnancy.
- 3 major predictors of preserved post-PID fertility: (i) Short duration of symptoms (<72 hours) prior to initiation of treatment, (ii) first episode of PID, and (iii) nongonococcal PID.

PEMPHIGOID, BULLOUS

Cinthya Peña Orbea, MD • Felix B. Chang, MD

BASICS

DESCRIPTION
- Bullous pemphigoid (BP) is an acquired autoimmune subepidermal blistering skin disorder caused by deposition of linear autoantibodies against the epithelial basal membrane zone.
- Pruritic, tense, symmetric, localized, widespread blisters or urticarial plaques
- Flexural surface (80%), axillary, inguinal folds and abdomen (20%)
- Oral lesions develop in 10–20% of cases, rarely affecting mucosae of eyes, nose, pharynx and anogenital zones.

EPIDEMIOLOGY
- Most common autoimmune blistering disease
- Typical between 60 and 80 years old, but juvenile bullous pemphigoid can occur.
- Affects both females and males, possibly with higher incidence in females.
- No association with race or geographic location

Incidence
- BP is probably the only autoimmune disease that increases in likelihood with age
- In France and Germany, the reported incidence is 6.6 cases per million people per year.
- 4.8 new cases/100 elder-years.

ETIOLOGY AND PATHOPHYSIOLOGY
- Autoantibodies react against hemidesmosomal proteins: The 230-kDa BP antigen within basal keratinocytes and 180-kDa type XVII collagen in the basement membrane zone (BMZ).
- IgG is usually the predominant autoantibody leading to C3 complement activation, recruitment of inflammatory cells, and liberation of proteolytic enzymes that break down the dermoepidermal junction.
- The noncollagenous 16A domain (NC16A) located at the membrane proximal region of BP180 is considered the major target epitope and is recognized in 80–90% of BP patients.
- It has recently been shown that IgE antibodies correlate with a severe form of BP, and those who test positive for IgE anti-BP180 antibodies required longer duration for remission and therapy.

Genetics
- Certain class II antigens of the major histocompatibility complex (MHC) alleles DQB1*0301 predominate.
- Expression of this allele on antigen-presenting cells is thought to be involved in the presentation to autoreactive T cells in patients with BP.
- Molecular mimicry has been proposed as a mechanism by which exogenous agents may trigger the immune response.

RISK FACTORS
- Advanced age.
- No clear precipitating factors but can be related to infections such as hepatitis B, hepatitis C, *Helicobacter pylori*, *Toxoplasma gondii*, cytomegalovirus (CMV).
- Associated with autoimmune disorders and inflammatory dermatoses like lichen planus, psoriasis, and other forms of bullous disease

- Increased risk in patients with neurologic disorders, such as multiple sclerosis, dementia, stroke, Parkinson disease, and psychiatric disorders
- Although drug-induced BP is rare, chronic intake of neuroleptics, aldosterone antagonists, furosemide, dopaminergic drugs, opioids, salicylates, NSAIDs, and phenacetin have been associated.
- Less frequent: Trauma, burns, surgical scars, UV radiation, and x-ray therapy.

COMMONLY ASSOCIATED CONDITIONS
- Underlying malignancy can be found in patients with BP <60 years old
- Several autoimmune disorders such as rheumatoid arthritis, Hashimoto thyroiditis, dermatomyositis, lupus erythematosus inflammatory dermatoses-like psoriasis, and lichen planus have been reported.

DIAGNOSIS

HISTORY
- BP occurs sporadically without any obvious trigger factor.
- Prodromal nonbullous phase: Mild to severe pruritus, associated with excoriated, eczematous, papular and/or urticarial skin lesions
- Mucosal lesions can be mild, transient, and are often seen with extensive cutaneous disease.
- Bullous stage: Single or numerous tense bullae on erythematous, noninflammatory, urticarial skin
- Unusual clinical presentations:
  – Localized form: 30% of cases (e.g., disease limited to lower leg, anogenital region, site of trauma)
  – Urticarial variant: Presents initially with mild to intractable pruritus and urticarial lesions; no blisters
  – Vegetative form: Uncommon, vegetating plaques in intertriginous areas
  – Lichen planus pemphigoides: Rare variant, bullae on site of previously normal skin or mucosa, after the onset of lichen planus

PHYSICAL EXAM
- Lesions usually are 1–3 cm round or oval, tense blisters localized on either normal or inflamed skin
- 80–90% appear in the lower trunk, axilla, and groin and 10–20% oral and intertriginous spaces
- Blister rupture leads to painful erosions that may become crusted and occasionally invaded by organisms
- Fluid is clear but sometimes presents with hemorrhagic exudates
- Negative active acantholysis (Nikolsky sign) and no extension of bullae into the surrounding, unblistered skin when vertical pressure is applied to the top of the bulla (Asboe-Hansen sign) support the diagnosis.

DIFFERENTIAL DIAGNOSIS
- Blistering diseases with antibodies: Pemphigus, cicatricial pemphigoid, pemphigoid gestationis, epidermolysis bullosa acquisita, linear IgA dermatosis, dermatitis herpetiformis, bullous erythema multiforme
- Blistering diseases without antibodies: Erythema multiforme, toxic epidermal necrolysis, porphyria, epidermolysis bullosa, allergic contact dermatitis, bullous impetigo, staphylococcal scaled-skin syndrome, friction blisters

DIAGNOSTIC TESTS & INTERPRETATION
Initial Tests (lab, imaging)
- Diagnosis of BP is based on a combination of clinical features and immunopathologic findings.
- Half of patients will have elevated total serum IgE.
- ~ 50% of patients have peripheral blood eosinophilia that does not correlate with serum IgE levels.
- Diagnosis of atypical and nonbullous variants relies on findings of immunofluorescence microscopy with specific circulating antibodies.
- Considerations:
  – BP has a waxing and waning course with spontaneous remission in the absence of treatment.
  – ELISA for the NC16A domain of BP180 is available at some centers, reported sensitivity 82–94%; specificity 93–99.9%.
  – Old age and poor general health along with presence of anti-BP180 have been related to poor prognosis.

Diagnostic Procedures/Other
- Diagnosis is made by biopsy and direct immunofluorescence exam.
- Histopathology: 4-mm punch biopsy from the edge of an intact bulla. Staining shows subepidermal blister and multiple eosinophils.
- Immunohistochemistry: Studies have suggested that the detection of C3d deposits at the dermoepidermal junction in formalin-fixed tissue is helpful for the diagnosis (1).
- Direct immunofluorescence (DIF): Second 4-mm perilesional punch biopsy will show linear deposition of IgG and/or C3 along BMZ.
- Serological studies: Indirect immunofluorescence (IIF) and ELISA are done when DIF is negative, there is a strong suspicion of BP, and when the skin biopsy cannot be performed. Both detect circulating IgG antibodies against 230BP (specificity 96%) and 180BP (specificity 90%) (1).

TREATMENT

GENERAL MEASURES
- Discontinue trigger factors
- In oral lesions: Avoid hard consistency, spicy and hot food. Soft and liquid meals should be given instead.
- Strict control of wounds to avoid complications.

MEDICATION
First Line
- Treatment of BP depends on the extent of the disease.
- Potent topical corticosteroids should be considered in the management of localized and moderate disease (2)[A].
  – Topical clobetasol propionate 0.05% cream: 10–30 mg/d, apply 2 × per day. Low doses compared to larger amount (40 g/d) has been found to be just as effective as larger amounts (40 g) and mortality appears to be decreased 43% in 1 year in patients with moderate disease treated with this regimen (2)[A].
  – Side effects: Skin atrophy, striae, hypertrichosis, acne, and ecchymosis

- Systemic therapy:
  - Oral prednisolone: 0.5 mg/kg/d for disease control. Goal is to achieve the lowest maintenance dosage that will prevent new lesion formation and reduce adverse reactions (2)[A]
  - Clinical response is usually obtained within 1–2 weeks and is indicated by healing of existing lesions and cessation of new blister formation (3).
  - Evidence shows that higher doses >0.75 mg/kg/d do not improve healing rate but do increase mortality (2)[A].
  - Taper the dose gradually within 1–2 years to avoid relapse
  - Side effects: Cutaneous atrophy, osteoporosis, GI ulcers, Cushing syndrome, diabetes mellitus, hypertension
- Immunosuppressive agents like azathioprine, mycophenolate mofetil, and methotrexate are used in severe cases; they may be beneficial especially in patients taking systemic corticosteroids.
  - Addition of azathioprine to prednisone regimen reduces the total maintenance dose of prednisone by 45% without increasing serious side effects or mortality (2)[A].
  - Azathioprine: 0.5–2.5 mg/kg/d, most common side effect: myelosuppression.
  - Mycophenolate mofetil: 1.5–2 g/d, most common side effect: GI disturbance
  - Methotrexate: 5–20 mg/wk, low dose usually initiated (5 mg/wk) plus folic acid replacement. Adverse effects: myelosuppression, hepatotoxicity. Higher rate of remission with the use of prednisone (4)[B]
- Tetracycline and nicotinamide may be beneficial in disease control and longer remission period (5)[C].

Second Line
- Plasmapheresis: Reduce the amount of prednisolone required to achieve disease control (5)[C]
- Omalizumab: Used in patients who have high levels of IgE antibodies (5)[C]
- IVIG: For patients who did not respond to first-line therapy or at risk of potentially fatal side effects from conventional therapy. The recommended dose is 1–2 g/kg divided over a 3- or 5-day cycle every 3–4 weeks (6)[B].

ISSUES FOR REFERRAL
- Gastroenterology, otorhinolaryngology referral in patients who have esophageal, pharyngeal, laryngeal involvement.
- Ophthalmologic consult when patient complains of: burning sensation, itching, visual changes and in those patients who require high doses of steroids

IN-PATIENT CONSIDERATIONS
Admission Criteria/Initial Stabilization
Extensive denuding of skin, dehydration, and electrolyte imbalance requiring IV fluid reposition

 ONGOING CARE

FOLLOW-UP RECOMMENDATIONS
Patient Monitoring
- Taper medication when disease is stable and control side effects.
- Perform periodic skin examination for new lesions.
- Frequent bacterial cultures of cutaneous erosions are essential to identify early infections.

DIET
- Liquid or soft diet with active oral lesions
- After lesions are resolved, advance diet. Avoid hard or crunchy foods, as they may cause flare ups.
- Supplement with calcium and vitamin D for patients on systemic corticosteroids

PATIENT EDUCATION
- Symptoms of infection, worsening lesions
- Education in good skin hygiene and wound care
- Wash clothing and linens if they come in contact with oozing, crusting, or infected skin.
- Protect from sun exposure and physical trauma to the skin.

PROGNOSIS
- Disease length can persist from weeks to years even under treatment.
- Around 47% of patients experience relapse within 1 year of therapy and ~50% of patients can achieve remission within 2.5–6 years.
- Yearly mortality varies from 6–40%
- Poor prognosis and high mortality: Old age, poor general condition, and the presence of antibodies in serum
- Other factors that may be included are: Age >80 years, prednisolone dose >37 mg/d after hospitalization, serum albumin levels of <3.6 g/dL, ESR >100 mm/h.

COMPLICATIONS
- Most often secondary to medication: Osteoporosis, cataracts, adrenal insufficiency, bone marrow suppression
- Skin infections
- Dehydration and electrolytes imbalance

REFERENCES

1. Ujiie H, Nishie W, Shimizu H. Pathogenesis of bullous pemphigoid. *Dermatol Clin*. 2011;29:439–446.
2. Garcia-Romero M, Werth VP. Randomized controlled trials needed for bullous pemphigoid intervention. *Arch Dermatol*. 2012;148:244–246.
3. Mutasim DF. Autoimmune bullous dermatoses in the elderly: An update on pathophysiology, diagnosis and management. *Drugs Aging*. 2010;27:1–19.
4. Gürcan HM, Ahmed AR. Analysis of current data on the use of methotrexate in the treatment of pemphigus and pemphigoid. *Br J Dermatol*. 2009;161:723–731.
5. Venning VA, Taghipor K, Mohd MF, et al. British Association of Dermatologists' guidelines for the management of bullous pemphigoid 2012. *Br J Dermatol*. 2012;167:1200–1214.
6. Kirtschig G, Middleton P, Bennett C, et al. Interventions for bullous pemphigoid. *Cochrane Database Syst Rev*. 2010;10:CD002292.

ADDITIONAL READING

- Marzano AV, Tedeschi A, Berti E, et al. Activation of coagulation in bullous pemphigoid and other eosinophil-related inflammatory skin diseases. *Clin Exp Immunol*. 2011;165:45–50.
- Schmidt E, della Torre R, Borradori L. Clinical features and practical diagnosis of bullous pemphigoid. *Dermatol Clin*. 2011;29:427–438.

 CODES

ICD10
L12.0 Bullous pemphigoid

CLINICAL PEARLS
- Tense bullae differentiates the lesions of bullous pemphigoid from the flaccid bullae of pemphigus vulgaris.
- Low doses of potent topical steroid have been shown to be just as effective as larger amounts in the initial therapy of BP.

PEMPHIGOID, CICATRICIAL

Miesha Merati, DO • Jenifer Lloyd, DO

BASICS

DESCRIPTION
- An acquired autoimmune subepithelial blistering disorder, mainly affecting mucous membranes
- In descending order of involvement, affects the oral cavity (85% of patients), conjunctivae (65%), skin (25–30%), nasal cavity (20–40%), anogenital region (20%), pharynx (20%), larynx (5–10%), and esophagus (5–15%) (1)
- Clinical hallmark is scarring (cicatrix), however, it may not be apparent, especially in the oral mucosa
- Synonym(s): Mucous membrane pemphigoid, oral pemphigoid, desquamative gingivitis, ocular cicatricial pemphigoid (CP), ocular pemphigus (incorrect nomenclature) (2)

EPIDEMIOLOGY
- Mean onset at age 60–80 years
- Prevalent sex: Female > Male (1.5–2:1)
- No racial or geographic predilection (3)

Incidence
1/1 million annually (3)

ETIOLOGY AND PATHOPHYSIOLOGY
- Autoantibodies binding to specific epithelial basement membrane components:
  - Type XVII collagen (bullous pemphigoid antigen 2), type VII collagen, laminin-5, laminin-6, α-6 and β-4 integrin subunits, 120 kDa undefined epithelial antigen:
    - Exclusive ocular mucosal involvement: autoantibodies to β-4 subunit of integrin
    - Exclusive oral mucosal involvement: autoantibodies to α-6 subunit of integrin
    - Association with internal malignancy: autoantibodies to antilaminin-5
- "Epitope spreading": Previous inflammatory event may predispose epithelial basement membrane components to autoreactive T cells
  - Several patients with Stevens-Johnson syndrome developed CP
  - Association with Sjögren syndrome and ocular CP
- Mechanism linking the binding of the antibodies to the epithelial basement membrane zone and subsequent scarring process yet to be defined (4)

Genetics
Association with HLA *DQB1*0301* (1)

GENERAL PREVENTION
None identified

COMMONLY ASSOCIATED CONDITIONS
Antilaminin-5 autoantibody–positive patients have a higher risk of internal malignancy (4)

DIAGNOSIS

Diagnosis is based on direct immunofluorescence and clinical presentation

HISTORY
- Oral: Pain, sensitivity, bleeding, mucosal lesions
- Ocular: Burning, dryness/tearing, itching, foreign body sensation, vision changes, photosensitivity (1,3)
- Nasal: Discharge, pain, congestion, epistaxis
- Larynx: Hoarseness, sore throat, frequent throat clearing, loss of voice
- Esophagus: Dysphagia, odynophagia, unintentional weight loss
- Anogenital: Blisters, erosions, scarring, dyspareunia, hematuria (3)
- Skin: Tense vesicles and bullae, hair loss, pruritus (1)

PHYSICAL EXAM
- Oral (especially on gingival and palatal mucosa, and less commonly on labial, buccal, and tongue mucosa): Erythematous patches, blisters, erosions, reticulate scarring, and/or pseudomembrane-covered erosions, adhesions (2,3,4)
  - Patients with restricted oral involvement have mild to moderate disease process with less chance of scarring (4)
- Ocular: Unilateral/bilateral involvement, conjunctival inflammation and erosions, malalignment of eyelashes, or tarsal conjunctivitis may proceed to scar formation, causing symblepharon, trichiasis, neovascularization, and eventually blindness (1,3):
  - All patients should be seen by an ophthalmologist. Early disease detection requires slit-lamp examination and eversion of eyelids (1,3)
- Nasal: Scarring, tissue loss, epistaxis, discharge; may resemble upper respiratory infections
- Larynx: Erosions and edema leading to life-threatening airway obstruction requiring tracheostomy (3)
- Esophagus: Life-threatening stenosis
- Anogenital: Blisters, erosions, scarring, urethral strictures, vaginal/anal stenosis, fusion of labial tissues
- Skin: Tense vesicles/bullae, erosions generally on head, neck, and upper trunk; lesions heal with atrophic scars and milia (2,3)

DIFFERENTIAL DIAGNOSIS
- Bullous pemphigoid
- Pemphigus vulgaris
- Linear IgA bullous dermatosis
- Paraneoplastic pemphigus
- Epidermolysis bullosa acquisita
- Stevens-Johnson syndrome
- Erythema multiforme major
- Drug-induced conjunctival cicatrization
- Ocular chemical/radiation trauma
- Lupus erythematosus
- Lichen planus
- Lichenoid drug eruptions

DIAGNOSTIC TESTS & INTERPRETATION
- Direct immunofluorescence (DIF):
  - Linear deposition of IgG, IgA, and/or C3 along the epithelial basement membrane zone:
    - Biopsy for DIF:
      - Single mucous membrane involvement: Take biopsy from adjacent inflamed tissue
      - Multiple mucous membrane involvement: Take biopsy from adjacent nonocular inflamed tissue
      - Both mucous membrane and skin involvement: Take biopsy from adjacent inflamed skin lesion
- Indirect Immunofluorescence (low sensitivity)
  - Serum samples tested with chemically separated normal human epithelial substrate split by 1.0 mol/L NaCl
  - At low titres (1:10–1:40), contain anti-dermal-epidermal junction antibodies
  - Combined IgA and IgG reactivity is associated with more severe disease (1,2,4)
- Enzyme-linked immunosorbent assay (ELISA):
  - More sensitive test for target antigen, but limited access to the test (4)

Test Interpretation
Histopathologic (hematoxylin-eosin [H+E]):
- Early lesions: Subepidermal blisters with lymphohistiocytic infiltrates, granulocytes, and plasma cells
- Late lesions: Subepidermal blisters with scant infiltrates, fibroblast proliferations, upper dermis lamellar fibrosis (2,3,4)
- H+E is not a required criterion secondary to difficulty in biopsying a blister, especially in difficult areas such as ocular mucosae
  - Ocular biopsy may worsen inflammation (4)

TREATMENT

- Low-risk patients (oral mucosa +/− skin involvement):
  - Topical corticosteroids (moderate to high potency): Can use an oral insertable prosthetic device (2)[A]
  - Tetracycline hydrochloride (1–2 g/d) (2)[B]
  - Nicotinamide (2–2.5 g/d) (2)[B]
  - Non-responsive disease:
    - Prednisone (0.5 mg/kg/d) + dapsone (2,4,5)[A]:
      - Serious adverse effects of dapsone are rare
      - Starting dose: 24 mg/d for 4 weeks
      - Increase to 50 mg/d for another 4 weeks
      - Increase to 100 mg/d for last 4 weeks
    - If no response with prednisone + dapsone, add azathioprine (100–150 mg/d) or mycophenolate mofetil (1 g/d) (4)[A]
- High-risk patients (involvement of any of the following mucosae: Ocular, genital, nasopharyngeal, esophageal, laryngeal):
  - Slow-moderate progression of disease: Dapsone + corticosteroids (1 mg/kg/d) + azathioprine (100–150 mg/d) or mycophenolate mofetil (1–1.5 g/d) (2,4)[A]
  - Patients with rapid progression of disease (especially ocular, esophageal, or laryngeal involvement): Prednisone (1–1.5 mg/kg/d) + cyclophosphamide (1–2 mg/kg/d) (2)[A]
  - After control of disease, taper prednisone and continue cyclophosphamide
  - Preliminary reports show rituximab ± IV immunoglobulin is effective for treatment-resistant ocular disease (2,4)[C]
  - Ocular involvement requires lubricant without preservative:
    - Blepharitis may be treated with tetracycline and lid hygiene (4)
      - Patients should see the appropriate specialists for systems involved
- Extensive side-effect profiles, condensed to most important ones—appropriate monitoring required (4):
  - Azathioprine and mycophenolate mofetil: Severe liver toxicity, bone marrow suppression
  - Cyclophosphamide: Hemorrhagic cystitis, bone marrow suppression

ADDITIONAL THERAPIES
For patients receiving long-term prednisone and immunosuppressive treatment, add anti-Candida medication to prevent osteoporosis (5).

SURGERY/OTHER PROCEDURES
Surgery for patients with ocular involvement: Entropion surgery, tarsorrhaphy, mucous membrane grafting, amniotic membrane transplantation, tectonic keratoplasty, keratoprosthesis (4)

 ONGOING CARE

FOLLOW-UP RECOMMENDATIONS
- Cancer screening for patients with antilaminin-5 autoantibodies
- All patients should be seen by an ophthalmologist: Early detection of disease is key (4)
- Long-term follow up with appropriate specialists

PROGNOSIS
- IgG and IgA anti-basement membrane autoantibodies are associated with more severe disease (3)
- Prognosis mostly depends on site involved:
  - Better prognosis and better response to treatment: Oral +/− skin involvement
  - Poorer prognosis, high likelihood for loss of function and scarring: Ocular, genital, nasopharyngeal, esophageal, laryngeal
    - Ocular scarring and blindness
    - Genital and urinary scarring
    - Scarring can only be prevented, not reversed (2,3)
    - Airway obstruction
    - Esophageal strictures

REFERENCES
1. Schmidt E, Zillikens D. Pemphigoid diseases. *Lancet.* 2013;381:320–332.
2. Chan LS, Ahmed AR, Anhalt GJ, et al. The first international consensus on mucous membrane pemphigoid: Definition, diagnostic criteria, pathogenic factors, medical treatment, and prognostic indicators. *Arch Dermatol.* 2002; 138:370–379.
3. Kirtschig G, Murrell D, Wojnarowska F, et al. Interventions for mucous membrane pemphigoid and epidermolysis bullosa acquisita. *Cochrane Database Syst Rev.* 2009;1:CD004056.
4. Chan LS. Ocular and oral mucous membrane pemphigoid (cicatricial pemphigoid). *Clin Dermatol.* 2012;30:34–37.
5. Kourosh, AS, Yancey KB. Pathogenesis of mucous membrane pemphigoid. *Dermatol Clin.* 2011;29: 479–484.

ADDITIONAL READING
- Culton DA, Diaz LA. Treatment of subepidermal immunobullous diseases. *Clin Dermatol.* 2012;30: 95–102.
- Kirtschig G, Murrell D, Wojnarowska F, et al. Interventions for mucous membrane pemphigoid/ cicatricial pemphigoid and epidermolysis bullosa acquisita. *Arch Dermatol.* 2002;138:380–384.
- Schiavo AL, Puca RV, Ruocco V, et al. Adjuvant drugs in autoimmune bullous diseases, efficacy vs safety: Facts and controversies. *Clin Dermatol.* 2010;28:337–343.

CODES

ICD10
L12.1 Cicatricial pemphigoid

CLINICAL PEARLS
- Patients diagnosed with cicatricial pemphigoid require thorough mucous membrane and skin examinations.
- Scarring is the clinical hallmark of disease, although not always evident.
- Prognosis depends on site involved; oral and/or skin involvement has a better prognosis and better response to treatment. Ocular, genital, nasopharyngeal, esophageal, and laryngeal mucosal involvement are more likely to scar and can lead to life-threatening emergencies such as blindness and airway obstruction.

PEMPHIGUS VULGARIS

Michelle A. Tinitigan, MD

BASICS

Pemphigus is derived from the Greek word *pemphix* meaning "bubble" or "blister."

DESCRIPTION
- Rare, potentially fatal autoimmune mucocutaneous blistering disease that involves the skin and the mucous membranes (1).
- Flaccid, painful, nonhealing bullae or ulcerations that appear spontaneously on the skin and mucosal surfaces, typically begin in the oropharynx, and then may spread to the skin, having a predilection for the scalp, face, chest, axillae, groin, and pressure points.
- Patient often presents with erosions and no intact bullae.
- System(s) affected: Skin; Gastrointestinal; Genitourinary

EPIDEMIOLOGY
Incidence
- Disease of the middle-aged population, typically occurring after the age of 50 years, although some cases have been reported in younger adults and children (1).
- Affects both sexes equally
- 0.1–3.2 cases per 100,000 individuals annually worldwide (1).

Prevalence
- Uncommon, affects <200,000 people in the US
- Seen more frequently in people of Mediterranean decent and Ashkenazi Jew (1)

ETIOLOGY AND PATHOPHYSIOLOGY
- Autoantibodies (IgG) are directed against desmoglein (Dsg) 1 and 3 adhesion molecules. Desmogleins interact with desmosomes, which hold epidermal cells together. The antibodies against Dsg molecules cause intraepidermal blister formation and acantholysis.
- Dsg 3 is predominantly expressed in oral epithelium, while both Dsg 1 and Dsg 3 are expressed in the skin.
- Dsg 1 is expressed more intensely in the superficial layer, while Dsg 3 is found more abundantly in basal and suprabasal layers.
- Autoimmune; stimulus is unknown
- Inducing factors include physical trauma, such as thermal burns, UV light, and ionizing radiation; neoplasm, emotional stress, drugs, and infections. Most patients lack a recognized inducing factor.

Genetics
Strong association with certain human leukocyte antigens (HLA), especially HLA DR4, DR14, DQ1, and DQ3, although the susceptibility gene differs depending on ethnic origin.

COMMONLY ASSOCIATED CONDITIONS
- Thymoma
- Myasthenia gravis
- Paraneoplastic pemphigus is a type of pemphigus defined by the fact that the patient has a malignancy at the time the pemphigus is diagnosed.
- Gastric adenocarcinoma

DIAGNOSIS

HISTORY
- Hoarseness, sore mouth
- Mucosal lesions (in 50–70% of patients) may be the sole sign for an average of 5 months before skin lesions or may be the sole manifestation of the disease.
- Cutaneous lesions: Primary lesion is a flaccid blister developed by most patients; affected skin is often painful but rarely pruritic.
- Drug-induced: Penicillamine, ACE inhibitors, thiol-containing compounds, rifampin

PHYSICAL EXAM
- Mucosal lesions: Intact bullae rare; commonly are ill-defined, irregularly shaped gingival, buccal, or palatine erosions that are painful and slow healing; most often affected area is the oral cavity; may involve conjunctiva, oropharynx esophagus, labia, vagina, cervix, penis, urethra, and anus
- Cutaneous lesions: Painful, flaccid blisters with clear fluid found on normal skin or on erythematous base; fragile bullae rupture easily, leading to painful, open, denuded areas that can become secondarily infected.
- Nails: Acute or chronic paronychia, onychomadesis, subungual hematomas, and nail dystrophies may be present.
- Nikolsky sign: Involves application of pressure to skin causing intraepidermal cleavage that allows the superficial skin to slip free from the deeper layers, producing an erosion; can be elicited on normal skin or at the margin of a blister
- Asboe-Hansen sign: Lateral pressure on the edge of a blister may spread the blister into clinically unaffected skin.

DIFFERENTIAL DIAGNOSIS
- Predominance of oral mucous lesions: Herpes simplex virus (HSV), aphthous ulcers, lichen planus, erythema multiforme
- Predominance of widespread cutaneous lesions: Bullous pemphigoid, cicatricial pemphigoid, bullous drug eruptions, pemphigus erythematosus, pemphigus foliaceus, paraneoplastic pemphigus, impetigo, contact dermatitis, dermatitis herpetiformis, erythema multiforme, Stevens-Johnson syndrome, toxic epidermal necrolysis, pemphigoid gestationis, and linear IgA dermatosis

DIAGNOSTIC TESTS & INTERPRETATION
Diagnosis is achieved via 3 different parameters: Perilesional tissue biopsy, histologic, and immunologic examinations

Initial Tests (lab, imaging)
- Shave or 4-mm punch biopsy of edge of fresh bullous lesion
- A second 4-mm punch biopsy of the perilesional skin is sent for direct immunofluorescence (DIF).
- Serum for indirect immunofluorescence (IDIF) is positive for circulating autoantibodies against desmogleins in 80–90% if DIF is positive.

Follow-Up Tests & Special Considerations
IDIF corresponds loosely to disease activity and may be useful to gauge disease activity.

Test Interpretation
- Light microscopy: Intradermal blister; loss of cohesion between epidermal cells (acantholysis) with an intact basement membrane; "row of tombstones appearance"
- DIF looking for deposits of IgG between epidermal cells

TREATMENT

Reduce inflammatory response and autoantibody production by suppression of the immune system to decrease blister formation and promote healing of blisters and erosions.

MEDICATION
First Line
- High-dose systemic glucocorticoids (e.g., prednisone 1–1.5 mg/kg/d) are the mainstay of treatment (2). If clinical response is insufficient, can increase dose to 2 mg/kg/d.
- Glucocorticoids can be used alone or in combination with other steroid-sparing immunosuppressive drugs (azathioprine [starting at 1 mg/kg/d and increasing by 0.5 mg/kg/d every 2–3 weeks to reach a maintenance dose of 2.5 mg/kg/d], cyclophosphamide [2–3 mg/kg/d], dapsone [50–200 mg/d], mycophenolate mofetil [MMF] [2–3 g/d]) (3)[A] and appear to be the most effective treatment.
- Combination therapy is particularly useful within the first 6 months and indicated if uncontrolled on relatively low doses of prednisone (5–10 mg/d to every other day) within a year of starting therapy.
- Dexamethasone-cyclophosphamide pulse therapy is a beneficial treatment, sparing the adverse effects of conventional regimens, and has been claimed to induce remission in many patients (4)[A]. Methylprednisolone and azathioprine regimen is similar in efficacy (3)[A].
- For mild-to-moderate disease: Combination therapy of MMF and prednisone is an effective treatment regimen to achieve rapid and complete control of pemphigus vulgaris (PV). For those patients who fail treatment with MMF and prednisone, rituximab is an efficacious alternative therapy (5).
- Rapidly progressive lesions necessitate high prednisone dose (1.5–2.5 mg/kg/d) for early and adequate control of the disease. Patients with impaired physical status, especially those with relatively stable lesions at baseline, might safely and effectively be treated with low-dose oral prednisone on alternate days plus azathioprine every day (Lever's minitreatment [LMT]) for oral pemphigus (2)[B].
- For oropharyngeal disease: Perilesional/Intralesional triamcinolone acetonide injections combined with conventional immunosuppressive therapy shortened the time of complete clinical remission and reduced the total amount of corticosteroids used.
- Oral analgesics: Use before eating for painful oral lesions (viscous lidocaine, Benadryl).

Second Line

For refractory disease:

- Rituximab (anti-CD20 monoclonal antibody): Alone or in combination with intravenous immunoglobulin (IVIG) is an effective therapy for patients with refractory PV (1).
- Other options: Methotrexate (10–20 mg/wk), hydroxychloroquine, gold
- Cyclosporine (2.5–5 mg/kg/d) may be ineffective as a steroid-sparing agent (3)
- Tumor necrosis factor (TNF)-α antagonist, etanercept, may be an effective therapeutic agent and may reduce healing time of skin lesions in PV (3) and for patients presenting with recalcitrant disease.
- Plasmapheresis in aggressive disease if combined with systemic steroids and immunosuppressant drugs
- IVIG may have a moderate effect as an adjuvant or alone on treatment-resistant pemphigus or in patients who have contraindications (3)[A]. Experience with IVIG in patients with autoimmune skin blistering disease is limited (2).

GENERAL MEASURES

- Minimize activities that may cause trauma to skin and precipitate blisters
- Avoid use of dental plates, dental bridges, or contact lenses that may precipitate or exacerbate mucosal disease
- Wound care: Daily gentle cleaning, topical agents to promote wound healing, and use of nonadhesive dressings
- Clobetasol propionate 0.05% ointment 2 × daily in conjunction with systemic steroids for hard to treat lesions
- For persistent lesions: Intralesional triamcinolone acetonide (20 mg/mL)

ISSUES FOR REFERRAL

- Ophthalmologist referral in suspected ocular involvement and prolonged use of high-dose steroids
- Referral to a dentist and/or otolaryngologist for patients with extensive oral disease

IN-PATIENT CONSIDERATIONS

Admission Criteria/Initial Stabilization

- Secondary infections requiring IV antibiotics
- Severe oral lesions leading to dehydration requiring fluid resuscitation

 ONGOING CARE

A minority (10%) achieve complete remission after initial treatment and do not need continued drug therapy; most require maintenance therapy to stay in remission.

FOLLOW-UP RECOMMENDATIONS

- Patients taking steroids long term should be screened for osteopenia/osteoporosis, avascular necrosis, HPA-axis suppression, cataract, cushingoid features, hyperlipoproteinemia, myopathy, mood changes, and immunosuppression. Patients on systemic steroids should maintain adequate vitamin D and calcium intake through diet and supplements.
- Patients taking azathioprine should have CBC, Cr, LFT checked at baseline and every 2 weeks the 1st 3 months then every 3 months after.

Patient Monitoring

Seek medical care for any unexplained blisters and if treated for PV and develop any of the following symptoms:

- Fever, chills
- General ill feeling
- Myalgias, joint pain
- New blisters or ulcers

DIET

- Patients with active oral lesions may benefit from liquid or soft diet and then advance as tolerated.
- Avoid spicy and acidic food when oral ulcers are present.
- Hard food that may cause mechanical trauma to epithelium, such as nuts, chips, and hard vegetables and fruits, may be best avoided in cases of active oral disease.

PATIENT EDUCATION

- Minimize activities that may cause trauma to skin and precipitate blisters, such as contact sports. Nontraumatic exercises, such as swimming, may be helpful.
- Explain wound care of erosions: Daily gentle cleaning, covering open areas with clean petrolatum and nonadhesive dressings
- Educate patients about the chronicity of the disease and the need for long-term follow up
- For oral pemphigus:
  - Soft diets and soft toothbrushes help to minimize local trauma
  - Explain the need for meticulous oral hygiene to prevent dental decay. Encourage gentle tooth brushing, dental flossing, and visits to the dentist/dental hygienist at least every 6 months.
  - Discuss how dental plates, dental bridges, or contact lenses may precipitate or exacerbate mucosal disease
  - Topical analgesics or anesthetics (e.g., benzydamine hydrochloride 0.15% or viscous lidocaine) may be useful in alleviating oral pain, particularly prior to eating or tooth brushing.

PROGNOSIS

- Mortality rate with combination therapy is ~5%, with most deaths due to drug-induced complications, including sepsis.
- 10% of patients achieve complete remission after initial treatment; most require maintenance therapy to stay in remission.
- Morbidity and mortality are related to the extent of disease, the maximum dose of oral steroids required to induce remission, and the presence of other diseases. Prognosis is worse in older persons and patients with extensive disease.
- Most deaths occur during the 1st few years of the disease; if a patient survives 5 years, prognosis is good.

COMPLICATIONS

- Secondary infection, localized to skin or systemic, may occur because of impaired immune response due to use of immunosuppressive drugs. Most frequent cause of death is *Staphylococcus aureus* septicemia.
- Osteoporosis in patients requiring long-term systemic steroids

- Adrenal insufficiency has been reported following prolonged use of glucocorticoids
- Bone marrow suppression and malignancies have been reported in patients receiving immunosuppressants, with an increased incidence of leukemia and lymphoma.
- Growth retardation has been reported in children taking systemic corticosteroids and immunosuppressants.

REFERENCES

1. Zakka LR, Shetty SS, Ahmed AR. Rituximab in the treatment of pemphigus vulgaris. *Dermatol Ther (Heidelb)*. 2012;2:17.
2. Chaidemenos G, Apalla Z, Koussidou T, et al. High dose oral prednisone vs. prednisone plus azathioprine for the treatment of oral pemphigus: A retrospective, bi-centre, comparative study. *J Eur Acad Dermatol Venereol*. 2011;25:206–210.
3. Singh S. Evidence-based treatments for pemphigus vulgaris, pemphigus foliaceus, and bullous pemphigoid: A systematic review. *Indian J Dermatol Venereol Leprol*. 2011;77:456–469.
4. Zivanovic D, Medenica L, Tanasilovic S, et al. Dexamethasone-cyclophosphamide pulse therapy in pemphigus: A review of 72 cases. *Am J Clin Dermatol*. 2010;11:123–129.
5. Strowd LC, Taylor SL, Jorizzo JL, et al. Therapeutic ladder for pemphigus vulgaris: Emphasis on achieving complete remission. *J Am Acad Dermatol*. 2011;64:490–494.

ADDITIONAL READING

- Ishii N, Hashimoto T, Zillikens D, et al. High-dose intravenous immunoglobulin (IVIG) therapy in autoimmune skin blistering diseases. *Clin Rev Allergy Immunol*. 2010;38:186–195.
- Schmidt E, Goebeler M, Zillikens D, et al. Rituximab in severe pemphigus. *Ann N Y Acad Sci*. 2009;1173:683–691.

 CODES

ICD10

L10.0 Pemphigus vulgaris

CLINICAL PEARLS

- Pemphigus vulgaris is a rare, chronic, potentially fatal autoimmune vesiculobullous disease of the mucous membranes and skin.
- Biopsy immediately with rush processing.
- When clinical suspicion is high, initiate therapy without delay using systemic corticosteroids.
- Minimize activities that may cause trauma to skin and precipitate blisters, such as contact sports.

PEPTIC ULCER DISEASE
Fozia Akhtar Ali, MD

 BASICS

DESCRIPTION
- Duodenal ulcer:
  - Most common form of peptic ulcer
  - Usually located in the proximal duodenum
  - Multiple ulcers or ulcers distal to the second portion of duodenum raise possibility of gastrinoma (Zollinger-Ellison syndrome).
- Gastric ulcer:
  - Less common than duodenal ulcer in absence of NSAID use
  - Commonly located along lesser curvature of the antrum
- Esophageal ulcers:
  - Located in the distal esophagus; usually secondary to gastroesophageal reflux disease (GERD); also seen with gastrinoma
- Ectopic gastric mucosal ulceration:
  - May develop in patients with Meckel's diverticulum

GENERAL PREVENTION
- NSAID ulcers: Avoid salicylates and NSAIDs:
  - Alternatives include acetaminophen and tramadol. COX-2 inhibitor use (e.g., celecoxib) is controversial due to potential cardiac safety risks.
  - If NSAIDs are needed, adjust the ibuprofen dose to <1,200 mg/d to decrease risk of ulcerogenesis, and add a proton pump inhibitor (PPI) or H_2 blocker.
  - To reduce ulcer risk, consider testing for and eradicating *Helicobacter pylori* before starting therapy with NSAIDs.
- Maintenance therapy with PPIs or H_2 blockers is indicated for patients with a history of ulcer complications, recurrences, refractory ulcers, or persistent *H. pylori* infection.
- Should also consider maintenance PPI treatment in patients with *H. pylori*-negative, non–NSAID-induced ulcer.
- Imbalance between aggressive factors (e.g., gastric acid, pepsin, bile salts, pancreatic enzymes) and defensive factors maintaining mucosal integrity (e.g., mucus, bicarbonate, blood flow, prostaglandins, growth factors, cell turnover)
- May be multifactorial
- *H. pylori* infection: 90% of duodenal ulcers and 70–90% of gastric ulcers:
  - Lifetime risk for peptic ulcer disease (PUD) in *H. pylori*–infected people: 10–20%
  - Annual risk of developing duodenal ulcer in *H. pylori*–infected people: ≤1%
- Ulcerogenic drugs (e.g., NSAIDs)
- Hypersecretory syndromes (e.g., gastrinoma)
- Retained gastric antrum
- Less common: Crohn disease, vascular insufficiency, radiation therapy, cancer chemotherapy, smoking

EPIDEMIOLOGY
Incidence
- Predominant sex: Male = Female
- Predominant age:
  - 70% of ulcers occur in patients ages 25—64
  - Ulcer incidence increases with age
- Peptic ulcer: 500,000 new cases/yr
- Recurrence: 4 million/yr
- Global incidence rate: 0.1–0.19%

Prevalence
- Peptic ulcer: 1.8% in the US
- Lifetime prevalence is 5–10% for patients not infected with *H. pylori;* 10–20% if infected.

Genetics
Increased incidence of PUD in families is likely due to familial clustering of *H. pylori* infection and inherited genetic factors reflecting response to the organism.

RISK FACTORS
- *H. pylori* infection
- NSAID use (5–20%)
- Smoking cigarettes
- Family history of ulcers
- Stress (after acute illness, ventilator support, extensive burns, head injury)
- Gastrinoma
- Medications: Corticosteroids (high-dose and/or prolonged therapy), bisphosphonates, potassium chloride, chemotherapeutic agents (e.g., IV fluorouracil)

COMMONLY ASSOCIATED CONDITIONS
- Gastrinoma (Zollinger-Ellison syndrome)
- Multiple endocrine neoplasia type 1
- Carcinoid syndrome
- Chronic illness: Crohn disease, chronic obstructive pulmonary disease (COPD), chronic renal failure, hepatic cirrhosis, cystic fibrosis
- Hematopoietic disorders (rare): Systemic mastocytosis, myeloproliferative disease, hyperparathyroidism, polycythemia rubra vera

 DIAGNOSIS

HISTORY
- Signs and symptoms:
  - Episodic gnawing or burning epigastric pain
  - Pain occurring after meals or on an empty stomach
  - Nocturnal pain
  - Pain relieved by food intake, antacids, or antisecretory agents
  - Nonspecific dyspeptic complaints: Indigestion, nausea, vomiting, loss of appetite, and heartburn
- Alarm symptoms:
  - Anemia, hematemesis, melena, or heme-positive stool suggest bleeding
  - Vomiting and early satiety suggest obstruction
  - Anorexia/weight loss
  - Persisting upper abdominal pain radiating to the back suggests penetration
  - Severe, spreading upper abdominal pain suggests perforation
- NSAID-induced ulcers are often silent; perforation/bleeding may be the initial presentation.

PHYSICAL EXAM
Physical exam for uncomplicated peptic ulcer may be unreliable and nonspecific: Epigastric tenderness (absent in at least 30% of older patients); guaiac-positive stool from occult blood loss

DIFFERENTIAL DIAGNOSIS
Functional dyspepsia, gastritis, GERD, biliary colic, pancreatitis, cholecystitis, Crohn disease, intestinal ischemia, cardiac ischemia, GI malignancy

DIAGNOSTIC TESTS & INTERPRETATION
Initial Tests (lab, imaging)
- Routine lab tests to consider when evaluating PUD:
  - CBC: Rule out anemia
  - Fecal occult blood test
  - If multiple/refractory ulcers: Consider fasting serum gastrin to rule out gastrinoma
- Indications for *H. pylori* testing: New-onset PUD, history of PUD, persistent symptoms after empirical antisecretory therapy, gastric mucosa–associated lymphoid tissue (MALT) lymphoma, noninvestigated dyspepsia in patients <50 years of age without alarm symptoms
- *H. pylori* diagnostic tests: False-negative results may occur if patient was recently treated with antibiotics, bismuth, or PPIs; or in patients with active bleeding. Diagnostic yield improved by checking 2 different tests in a patient with an ulcer to be sure *H. pylori* is not present:
  - Noninvasive tests:
    - Serology antibody: Most commonly used for testing in primary care, but slow to normalize after treatment, so it cannot be used to document successful eradication (sensitivity, 85%; specificity, 79%) (1)[A]
    - Urea breath test: Identifies active *H. pylori* infection; also used for posttreatment testing (sensitivity, >95%; specificity, >90%) (1)[A]
    - Stool antigen: Can be used for screening and posttreatment testing (sensitivity, 91%; specificity, 94%) (1)[A]
  - Invasive tests:
    - Upper endoscopy with gastric biopsy, which can be evaluated with Steiner stain for direct visualization of organism (sensitivity, >95%; specificity, >95%) (1)[A]
    - Rapid urease test: Conducted on gastric biopsies (sensitivity, 93–97%; specificity, 95%) (1)[A]
- Barium or Gastrografin contrast radiography (double-contrast hypotonic duodenography): Indicated when endoscopy is unsuitable or not feasible

Diagnostic Procedures/Other
Indications for upper endoscopy: Patients with suspected peptic ulcers who are >55 years of age, those who have alarm symptoms, and those with ulcers that do not respond to treatment (2)[A]

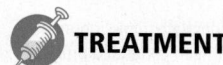 **TREATMENT**

MEDICATION
First Line
- Acid suppression: PPIs:
  - Omeprazole 20 mg/d PO; lansoprazole 30 mg/d PO; rabeprazole 20 mg/d PO; esomeprazole 40 mg/d PO; *or* pantoprazole 40 mg/d PO
  - Administer PPIs before breakfast.
  - Insufficient evidence for concluding superiority, inferiority or equivalence of high-dose PPI treatment over lower doses in peptic ulcer bleeding (3)[A]

Pregnancy Considerations
PPIs are *not* associated with an increased risk for major congenital birth defects, spontaneous abortions, or preterm delivery (4)[A]:

- H$_2$ blockers: Ranitidine or nizatidine 150 mg PO b.i.d. or 300 mg PO at bedtime; cimetidine 400 mg PO b.i.d. or 800 mg PO at bedtime; famotidine 150 mg PO b.i.d. or 300 mg PO at bedtime
- Treat ulcers for 8 weeks or until healing is confirmed in patients with complicated ulcers.
- PPIs heal peptic ulcers more rapidly and should not be taken with H$_2$ blockers.
- Optimal *H. pylori* eradication regimens (1)[A]: Triple therapy: 2 antibiotics + a PPI × 14 days: Omeprazole 20 mg PO b.i.d. or lansoprazole 30 mg PO b.i.d., or pantoprazole 40 mg PO b.i.d. or rabeprazole 20 mg PO b.i.d. or esomeprazole + clarithromycin 500 mg PO b.i.d. + amoxicillin 1 g PO b.i.d. or metronidazole 500 mg PO b.i.d. in patients with allergy to amoxicillin:
  - Triple and quadruple therapy have similar eradication rates for primary infection (5)[A].
- Bacterial resistance: Clarithromycin 10%; amoxicillin 1.4%; metronidazole 37%: Culture-guided choice of triple therapy is more clinically and cost-effective.
- Treatment of *H. pylori*–negative ulcers (usually due to NSAIDs):
  - Discontinue NSAID use
  - Treat acutely with PPIs for 8 weeks; may use longer as maintenance for patients with recurrent, complicated, or idiopathic ulcers; or in patients who require long-term aspirin or NSAID use.
- Precautions:
  - Renal insufficiency: Decrease H$_2$ blocker dosage by 50%.
  - Cimetidine: Avoid with theophylline, warfarin, phenytoin, and lidocaine.
  - PPIs may decrease bone density. Obtain interval bone densitometry with long-term PPI use
  - PPIs may cause hypomagnesemia. Consider baseline and interval levels in patients, especially for long-term use and in patients taking diuretics.
  - PPIs may be associated with increased risk of *Clostridium difficile* infection.
  - Despite earlier concerns, PPIs do not appear to decrease the efficacy of clopidogrel.

Second Line

- For *H. pylori* eradication: Use 2nd-line therapy if 1st line fails (1)[A]:
  - Bismuth quadruple therapy × 14 days:
    - Bismuth subsalicylate 525 mg PO q.i.d. +
    - Metronidazole 500 mg PO q.i.d. +
    - Tetracycline 500 mg PO q.i.d. +
    - PPI × 14 days
  - Alternative 2nd-line therapy:
    - Levofloxacin 250 mg PO b.i.d. +
    - Amoxicillin 1,000 mg PO b.i.d. +
    - PPI PO b.i.d.
  - Another alternative salvage therapy:
    - Rifabutin 300 mg PO daily +
    - Amoxicillin 1,000 mg PO b.i.d. +
    - PPI PO b.i.d.
- Alternative ulcer-healing drugs: Sucralfate 1 g PO q.i.d. or 2 g PO b.i.d. × 4–8 weeks
- Precautions: Renal insufficiency:
  - Reduce H$_2$ blocker dosage by 50%
  - Avoid magnesium-containing antacids
- Significant possible interactions:
  - Cimetidine inhibits cytochrome P450 isozymes (avoid with theophylline, warfarin, phenytoin, and lidocaine).

- Omeprazole may prolong elimination of diazepam, warfarin, and phenytoin.
- Sucralfate reduces absorption of tetracycline, norfloxacin, ciprofloxacin, and theophylline; it leads to subtherapeutic levels.

SURGERY/OTHER PROCEDURES

- Endoscopy indicated for patients age >50 years with new onset of dyspeptic symptoms, those who do not respond to treatment, and those of any age with alarm symptoms, such as bleeding and weight loss.
- At endoscopy:
  - Biopsy of stomach for *H. pylori* testing
  - Biopsy of margin of gastric ulcer to confirm benign etiology
  - Interventions to stop active bleeding or prevent rebleeding in those with certain stigmata, include injection with epinephrine, heater probe treatment, or placement of endoscopic clips.
- Indications for surgery: Ulcers that are refractory to treatment and patients at high risk for complications (e.g., transplant recipients, patients dependent on steroids/NSAIDs); surgery also may be needed acutely for treatment of perforation and bleeding that is refractory to endoscopic therapy.
- Surgical options:
  - Duodenal ulcers: Truncal vagotomy and drainage (pyloroplasty/gastrojejunostomy), selective vagotomy (preserving the hepatic and/or celiac branches of the vagus) and drainage, or highly selective vagotomy
  - Gastric ulcers: Partial gastrectomy, Billroth I or II
  - Perforated ulcers: Laparoscopy/open patching (6)

IN-PATIENT CONSIDERATIONS
Admission Criteria/Initial Stabilization

- Discontinue ulcerogenic agents (e.g., NSAIDs)
- Bleeding peptic ulcers:
  - Stable: Give PPI to reduce transfusion requirements, need for surgery, and duration of hospitalization (2)[A]
  - Unstable: Fluid/packed RBC resuscitation followed by emergent esophagogastroduodenoscopy (EGD); use IV PPI
- After endoscopic therapy, oral PPIs are as effective as IV (7).
- Perforated peptic ulcers: Free peritoneal perforation with bacterial peritonitis is a surgical emergency.

 ## ONGOING CARE

FOLLOW-UP RECOMMENDATIONS
Patient Monitoring

- *H. pylori* eradication: Expected in >90% (with double antibiotic regimen): Confirm eradication by urea breath test.
- Acute duodenal ulcer: Monitor clinically.
- Acute gastric ulcer: Confirm healing via endoscopy after 12 weeks if biopsy is not done initially to confirm that the lesion is benign.

PROGNOSIS

After *H. pylori* eradication:
- Low ulcer relapse rate; if relapse, consider surreptitious use of NSAIDs
- Reinfection rates <1% per year
- Low risk of rebleeding
- Decreased NSAID ulcer recurrence

COMPLICATIONS

- Hemorrhage: Up to 25% of patients (initial presentation in 10%)

- Perforation: <5% of patients
- Gastric outlet obstruction: Up to 5% of duodenal or pyloric channel ulcers; male predilection found
- Risk of gastric adenocarcinoma increased in *H. pylori*–infected patients

REFERENCES

1. Saad R, Chey WD. A clinician's guide to managing Helicobacter pylori infection. *Cleve Clin J Med*. 2005;72:109–110, 112–113, 117–118.
2. Ramakrishnan K, Salinas RC. Peptic ulcer disease. *Am Fam Physician*. 2007;76:1005–1012.
3. Neumann I, Letelier LM, Rada G, et al. Comparison of different regimens of proton pump inhibitors for acute peptic ulcer bleeding. *Cochrane Database Syst Rev*. 2013;6:CD007999.
4. Gill SK, O'Brien L, Einarson TR. The safety of proton pump inhibitors (PPIs) in pregnancy: A meta-analysis. *Am J Gastroenterol*. 2009;104: 1541–1545.
5. Luther J, Higgins PD, Schoenfeld PS, et al. Empiric quadruple vs. triple therapy for primary treatment of Helicobacter pylori infection: Systematic review and meta-analysis of efficacy and tolerability. *Am J Gastroenterol*. 2010;105:65–73.
6. Bertleff MJ, Lange JF. Perforated peptic ulcer disease: A review of history and treatment. *Dig Surg*. 2010;27:161–169.
7. Yen HH, Yang CW, Su WW, et al. Oral versus intravenous proton pump inhibitors in preventing re-bleeding for patients with peptic ulcer bleeding after successful endoscopic therapy. *BMC gastroenterology*. 2012;12:66.

ADDITIONAL READING

- Gisbert JP, Calvet X, Cosme A, et al. Long-term follow-up of 1,000 patients cured of *Helicobacter pylori* infection following an episode of peptic ulcer bleeding. *Am J Gastroenterol*. 2012;107: 1197–1204.
- Laine L, Jensen DM. Management of patients with ulcer bleeding. *Am J Gastroenterol*. 2012;107: 345–360; quiz 361.

CODES

ICD-9-CM 301

ICD10

- K25.9 Gastric ulcer, unspecified as acute or chronic, without hemorrhage or perforation
- K26.9 Duodenal ulcer, unspecified as acute or chronic, without hemorrhage or perforation
- K27.9 Peptic ulc, site unsp, unsp as ac or chr, w/o hemor or perf

CLINICAL PEARLS

- In patients with PUD, *H. pylori* should be eradicated to assist in healing and to reduce the risk of gastric and duodenal ulcer recurrence (2)[A].
- Upper endoscopy is indicated in patients with suspected peptic ulcers who are >55 years of age, those who have alarm symptoms, and those who do not respond to treatment (2)[A].

PERFORATED TYMPANIC MEMBRANE
Sarah Mowry MD • Brian Ho, MD

BASICS

DESCRIPTION

- The ear drum, or tympanic membrane (TM), is a thin barrier that separates the external auditory canal (EAC) from the middle ear and vibrates in response to sound waves, creating amplification as well as providing protection.
- Rupture of the TM can disrupt hearing while also allowing pathogens to access the middle ear space from the EAC.
- Perforations are classified by location:
  – Central: Not involving the annulus (the tendon-like structure that attaches the TM to the ear canal) can occur after a case of acute otitis media that leads to perforation.
  – Marginal: Involves the annulus and may be associated with cholesteatoma and are thus less likely to heal spontaneously.
  – Subtotal: A large defect surrounded with an intact annulus; requires surgery to close.
- Classification of perforations by etiology:
  – Infectious: Acute/chronic suppurative otitis media
  – Traumatic: barotrauma (e.g., diving), acoustic trauma (e.g., explosion), self-inflicted/penetrating (e.g., cotton swab)
  – Middle ear mass: Cholesteatoma or neoplasm
  – Iatrogenic: Persistent perforation after myringotomy tube placement
- The TM possesses the ability for spontaneous closure, resulting in formation of a dimeric membrane (outer squamous and inner mucosal). However, if this does not occur, a persistent perforation will result.

EPIDEMIOLOGY

Incidence in the general population is unknown, since many perforations heal spontaneously.

Genetics

Genetic susceptibility has been reported for recurrent acute otitis media (AOM) and chronic otitis media with effusion (COME), 2 of the etiologies of perforations (1).

GENERAL PREVENTION

- Avoid ear trauma or self-inserted foreign objects in the EAC
- Treat otitis media in a timely fashion prior to resultant TM perforation

ETIOLOGY AND PATHOPHYSIOLOGY

- Chronic eustachian tube dysfunction or chronic negative middle-ear pressure can lead to OM.
- Insertion of foreign objects into ear (cotton swab)
- Otitis media: A purulent, serous, or mucoid fluid builds up behind the TM leading to perforation
- A ruptured TM that chronically drains painlessly may be due to cholesteatoma.
- Iatrogenic: For the treatment of chronic eustachian tube dysfunction, a myringotomy is performed and tympanostomy tubes are placed; after tubes are extruded, a chronic perforation may result.

COMMONLY ASSOCIATED CONDITIONS

- Chronic eustachian tube dysfunction (e.g., cleft palate)
- OME
- Cholesteatoma
- Tympanosclerosis
- Ossicular chain damage (if traumatic perforation)

DIAGNOSIS

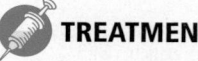

HISTORY

- Otorrhea or drainage from the ear (pus, blood, or clear fluid)
- Otalgia or earache consistent with AOM, followed by sudden relief of symptoms (because of TM rupture)
- Tinnitus or buzzing
- Self-audible whistling from the ear with valsalva maneuver or nose blowing
- Hearing loss (can be due to loss of amplification from large TM perforation or from concomitant ossicular chain discontinuity due to trauma)
- Vertigo
- Nausea and vomiting
- History of ear infections as a child or difficulty equalizing pressure during flights (chronic eustachian tube dysfunction)
- Ear surgery (prior placement of pressure equalizing [PE] tubes)
- Recurrent ear infections

PHYSICAL EXAM

- Otoscopic exam: Pay attention to location, purulent drainage, or involvement of annulus or the malleus. Also inspect ear canal to look for concomitant otitis externa.
- Pneumatic-otoscopy will reveal no motion because air passes freely into the middle ear space
- Note foreign bodies (cotton swabs, PE tubes); Batteries are an emergency and ENT should be consulted for immediate removal
- Retraction pocket (chronic eustachian tube dysfunction and resultant cholesteatoma)
- Thinned TM (prior perforations or severe chronic retraction)
- Keratin debris consistent with cholesteatoma (pearl white mass or chronically draining ear)
- Mass in the middle ear space behind the TM (cholesteatoma, paragangliomas, CN7 schwannomas, etc.)
- Ulcerations in the EAC that carry on to the annular surface causing perforations should lead to suspicion of squamous cell carcinoma (ENT consult)
- If history of hearing loss on that side: Weber (512 kHz tuning fork to center of forehead; if conductive hearing loss, sound should lateralize to the perforated side) and Rinne tests (place tuning fork to mastoid, when vibration no longer heard, transfer tuning fork next to outside ear canal; air conduction should be greater than bone conduction)
- Facial nerve palsy is uncommon with an isolated TM perforation. This is likely due to more occult pathology and ENT consult should be placed.
- Inspection of oropharynx noting tonsillar asymmetry or neoplasms that can cause eustachian tube obstruction leading to unilateral AOM and TM perforation

DIAGNOSTIC TESTS & INTERPRETATION

- Audiogram can reveal normal hearing or a mild conductive hearing loss:
  – A simple perforation will typically result in a low-frequency conductive hearing loss.
  – An audiogram that demonstrates a worse-than-expected conductive hearing loss or sensorineural hearing loss is more suspicious for ossicular chain damage or middle ear pathology.

- Tympanometry demonstrates an increased volume in the ear, decreased pressure (can demonstrate perforation even if not present on otoscopic exam); acoustic emittance demonstrates a volume >2 mL.
- MRI and CT imaging are not indicated for routine TM perforations.
- If there is suspicion for cholesteatoma or a CN VII palsy, then obtain noncontrast CT of the temporal bone as initial imaging study.
- Follow up should be established with an otolaryngologist for proper management, possible debridement, identification of cholesteatoma, and possible surgery for chronic perforations.

DIFFERENTIAL DIAGNOSIS

- Tympanosclerosis
- Dimeric membrane from prior perforation (thin membrane may be hard to discern)
- Otitis externa can obscure a perforation
- Cholesteatoma causing chronic drainage
- Iatrogenic: Previous ear surgery
- Trauma (baro or foreign body)
- Infectious: AOM/OME (rare pathogens such as TB)

TREATMENT

- Most TM perforations are nonurgent and do not require immediate evaluation by an otolaryngologist. Often these can be managed as an outpatient with drops and pain control to decrease inflammation. ENT follow up in few days to a week.
- A significant portion of TM perforations heal spontaneously without intervention because of the TM's regenerative abilities.
- Most are uncomplicated with minimal hearing loss (<40 dB) and lack vestibular complaints
- Observation of >3 months is a feasible option in select patients with uncomplicated, small perforations
- Debate exists over dry-ear precautions. But conservatively, patient should avoid getting water into the external auditory canal and into middle ear space.
- Treatment of purulence with topical antibiotics will reduce otorrhea
- If significant bleeding, topical Afrin can also be instilled in the ear canal
- Perforations with hearing loss >40 dB, any degree of ipsilateral facial weakness, those associated with vestibular symptoms, or those associated with cholesteatoma require referral to ENT; for traumatic perforation, obtain evaluation within 48 hours.

MEDICATION

- Some topical antibiotics (gentamicin, neomycin sulfate, or tobramycin) may rarely cause ototoxicity with TM perforations because they absorb through the round window
- Nonototoxic drops are preferred, but cost and availability may be relevant considerations given the rarity of oto- and vestibulotoxicity (2)[C].
- Oral antibiotics can be used if perforation is suspectedly due to AOM. But oral antibiotics are rarely indicated for the isolated TM perforation.
- Topical drops can be used for 5–7 days. Topical antibiotic drops should be continued if persistent otorrhea. May need evaluation by an otolaryngologist if drainage does not resolve with ototopical medication

First Line
- Ciprofloxacin ear drops ± dexamethasone
- Ofloxacin ear drops

ADDITIONAL THERAPIES
- Some advocate dry-ear precautions (cotton ball with petroleum jelly while showering and use of hairdryer to dry out ear if water enters the EAC).
- Most agree that dry-ear precautions should be used if patients will be swimming in lakes/rivers.

GENERAL MEASURES
- For some patients with chronic eustachian tube dysfunction, having a perforated TM is a favorable situation since it allows for the equalization of pressure in the middle ear that would otherwise be more difficult because of the decreased eustachian tube function, thus obviating the need for tympanostomy tube placement later. For these patients, dry-ear precautions are recommended.
- For patients who participate in water sports as a part of daily life, such as swimmers and divers, repair is recommended to provide the patient a "safe ear."
- Because there is a connection from the outer ear to the middle ear, dry-ear precautions are needed to prevent a nidus of infection, such as using a cotton ball in the ear during showers and gentle hairdryer use over ear if water enters the ear canal.
- A case-by-case risk–benefit analysis must be performed in cases of conductive hearing loss, since surgery entails the risk of hearing loss.
- Prevent infection primarily with eardrops or oral antibiotics as a secondary measure.

SURGERY/OTHER PROCEDURES
- Myringoplasty can be performed if the perforation is small and appears to be favorable. This is often performed with gel or paper patch which provides a scaffold across which the TM can heal.
- Tympanoplasty is performed for larger perforations, persistent perforations, or anteriorly based perforations. Perichondrium, fat, cartilage, pericranium, and temporalis fascia are often used in reconstructing the TM.
- A combined tympanoplasty/mastoidectomy surgery might be required for large perforations, chronic draining ears, presence of cholesteatoma, damage to the ossicular chain, or with evidence of mastoid disease.
- Surgery is often outpatient procedure and may be done under sedation and local anesthesia. General anesthesia can also be used.
- Patients often receive mastoid compressive dressings and instructions for postoperative antibiotics.
- Potential major complications of surgery include: Worsening of hearing, facial nerve damage, CSF leak, bleeding, and repair failure
- Ossiculoplasty might also be performed if pathology involves the ossicular chain; full repair of the ossicular chain can be performed at primary procedure or as a second look.
  - If ossicular chain discontinuity is repaired, patients will require postoperative audiogram to evaluate airborne gap

IN-PATIENT CONSIDERATIONS
Inpatient care is generally not required for TM perforation. The presence of comorbid disease like mastoiditis or meningitis would require inpatient stabilization with IV antibiotics and appropriate care for those disorders.

ONGOING CARE

FOLLOW-UP RECOMMENDATIONS
Patient Monitoring
- Follow up should be established with an otolaryngologist to confirm TM healing and to obtain an audiogram.
- It is vital to re-examine the ear, especially after an episode of infection associated with a perforation, to rule out underlying cholesteatoma or chronic eustachian tube dysfunction which may be contributing to the perforation.
- Follow up after surgery is necessary

DIET
No dietary restrictions

PATIENT EDUCATION
- Dry-ear precautions
- Avoid cotton swabs in the ear
- Call physician for worsening hearing loss, vertigo, facial nerve palsy, fever, or persistent drainage

PROGNOSIS
- Most perforations will heal spontaneously; however, large perforations and those associated with a chronic draining ear often require surgery.
- Mortality associated with this condition is low, but there is a potential for infection to spread to the mastoid, leading to meningitis, if proper aural care is not maintained.

COMPLICATIONS
- Nonhealing perforation
- Infection (otitis media, mastoiditis, meningitis)
- Conductive hearing loss
- Facial paralysis (rare and likely due to additional pathology)
- Ossicular chain disruption (traumatic induced)

REFERENCES
1. Rye MS, Blackwell JM, Jamieson SE. Genetic susceptibility to otitis media in childhood. *Laryngoscope.* 2012;122:665–675.
2. Haynes DS, Rutka J, Hawke M, et al. Ototoxicity of ototopical drops—an update. *Otolaryngol Clin North Am.* 2007;40:669–683, xi.

ADDITIONAL READING
- Jensen RG, Koch A, Homøe P, et al. Long-term tympanic membrane pathology dynamics and spontaneous healing in chronic suppurative otitis media. *Pediatr Infect Dis J.* 2011;31:139–144.
- Lou ZC, Lou ZH, Zhang QP. Traumatic tympanic membrane perforations: A study of etiology and factors affecting outcome. *Am J Otolaryngol.* 2012;33:549–555.
- Morris PS, Leach AJ. Acute and chronic otitis media. *Pediatr Clin North Am.* 2009;56:1383–1399.

 CODES

ICD10
- H72.00 Central perforation of tympanic membrane, unspecified ear
- H72.2X9 Other marginal perforations of tympanic membrane, unsp ear
- H72.90 Unsp perforation of tympanic membrane, unspecified ear

CLINICAL PEARLS
- To evaluate a patient with a suspected TM perforation, history and physical exam will usually suffice and does not require imaging.
- Nonhealing perforations associated with malodorous or recurrent infections are often associated with cholesteatoma and require otolaryngology consultation.
- Retraction pockets and history of AOM are suspicious for chronic eustachian tube dysfunction.
- Tympanoplasty surgery might be required for a perforation that does not spontaneously heal.
- If the presentation is a sudden sensorineural hearing loss, this should warrant referral and initiation of steroid therapy the same day.
- If presentation is also with sudden facial paralysis, this should warrant urgent referral and initiation of steroid therapy +/– antiviral treatment.

PERICARDITIS
Jeremy Golding, MD

BASICS

DESCRIPTION
Inflammation of the pericardium, with or without associated pericardial effusion. Myopericarditis or perimyocarditis refers to cases that have myocardial involvement in addition to the pericardial sac.

EPIDEMIOLOGY
Incidence
Epidemiologic studies lacking. Exact incidence unknown, but occurs in up to 5% of patients evaluated in the emergency room for chest pain without myocardial infarction (MI) (1)

ETIOLOGY AND PATHOPHYSIOLOGY
- Inflammation of the pericardial sac can be *acute* or *chronic* (recurrent). Chronic/recurrent inflammation may result in constrictive pericarditis.
- Can produce serous/purulent fluid/dense fibrinous material (depending on etiology), which may or may not lead to hemodynamic compromise (cardiac tamponade).

Genetics
No known genetic factors:
- Idiopathic: 85–90% of cases. Likely related to viral infection (2)[B]
- Infectious:
  – Viral: Coxsackievirus, echovirus, adenovirus, Epstein-Barr virus, cytomegalovirus, hepatitis viruses, influenza virus, HIV, measles, mumps, varicella
  – Bacterial: Gram-positive and gram-negative organisms
  – Fungal (more common in immunocompromised populations): *Blastomyces dermatitidis*, *Candida* sp., *Histoplasma capsulatum*
  – Mycobacterial: *Mycobacterium tuberculosis*
  – Parasites: *Echinococcus*
- Noninfectious causes:
  – Acute MI (2–4 days after MI), Dressler syndrome (weeks to months after MI)
  – Aortic dissection
  – Renal failure, uremia
  – Malignancy (e.g., breast cancer, lung cancer, Hodgkin disease, leukemia, lymphoma)
  – Radiation therapy
  – Trauma
  – Postpericardiotomy
  – After cardiac procedures (e.g., catheterization, pacemaker placement, ablation) (3)
  – Autoimmune disorders: Connective tissue disorders, systemic lupus erythematosus (SLE), rheumatoid arthritis, scleroderma, hypothyroidism, inflammatory bowel disease, spondyloarthropathies, Wegener granulomatosis
  – Sarcoidosis
- Medication induced: Dantrolene, doxorubicin, hydralazine, isoniazid, mesalamine, methysergide, penicillin, phenytoin, procainamide, rifampin (1)

COMMONLY ASSOCIATED CONDITIONS
Depends on etiology

DIAGNOSIS

HISTORY
- Prodrome of fever, malaise, myalgias
- Acute, sharp, stabbing chest pain
- Duration typically hours to days
- Pleuritic pain
- Pain reduced by leaning forward, worsened by lying supine

PHYSICAL EXAM
- Heart rate is usually rapid and regular.
- Pericardial friction rub: Coarse, high-pitched sound best heard during end expiration at left lower sternal border with patient leaning forward. Highly specific for diagnosis (but not sensitive). May be transient and mono-, bi-, or triphasic (1)
- New S$_3$ may suggest myopericarditis.
- Cardiac tamponade suggested by the presence of:
  – Systemic arterial hypotension
  – Elevated jugular venous pressure
  – Pulsus paradoxus (inspiratory fall in arterial pressure of at least 10 mm Hg)
- Diagnostic clinical criteria (4):
  – Acute pericarditis (at least 2 of 4 criteria):
    ○ Typical (pleuritic) chest pain
    ○ Pericardial friction rub
    ○ ECG changes with widespread ST elevation
    ○ New/Increasing pericardial effusion
  – Myopericarditis:
    ○ Definite pericarditis *plus*
    ○ Symptoms (dyspnea, chest pain, or palpitations) *and* ECG changes not previously documented (ST/T wave abnormalities, supraventricular/ventricular tachycardia) *or* focal/diffuse depressed left ventricular (LV) function documented on imaging study
    ○ Absence of evidence of other cause
    ○ 1 of the following: Elevated cardiac enzymes (creatine kinase [CK]-MB, troponin I or T), *or* new focal/diffuse depressed LV function *or* abnormal imaging consistent with myocarditis (MRI with gadolinium, gallium-67 scanning, anti-myosin antibody scanning)
  – Case definitions:
    ○ *Suspected myopericarditis*: Criteria 1, 2, and 3
    ○ *Probable myopericarditis*: Criteria 1, 2, 3, and 4
    ○ *Confirmed myopericarditis*: Histopathologic evidence of myocarditis by endomyocardial biopsy (EMB) or autopsy. (Note: In the clinical setting, for self-limited cases with predominantly pericarditis, EMB is rarely indicated.)

DIAGNOSTIC TESTS & INTERPRETATION
Initial Tests (lab, imaging)
- It is not necessary to order tests for uncomplicated cases or when the diagnosis is clear. Following labs may be helpful:
  – CBC: Typically shows leukocytosis
  – Inflammatory markers: Elevated erythrocyte sedimentation rate (ESR), C-reactive protein (CRP)
  – Cardiac biomarkers: Typically elevated creatine kinase, troponins:
    ○ Elevated troponins associated with younger age, male sex, pericardial effusion at presentation, and ST-segment elevation on ECG
    ○ Adverse outcomes not predicted by elevated troponin (5)
- ECG: Findings include widespread upward concave ST-segment elevation and PR-segment depression that may evolve through 4 stages (but ECG may be normal/show nonspecific abnormalities) (1):
  – Stage 1: Diffuse ST-segment elevation and PR-segment depression
  – Stage 2: Normalization of the ST and PR segments
  – Stage 3: Widespread T-wave inversions
  – Stage 4: Normalization of T waves; may have persistent inversions if chronic pericarditis

- ECG may demonstrate low voltage and electrical alternans with tamponade.
- Additional testing (if clinically appropriate based on history or atypical presentation or course) may include tuberculin skin test, sputum cultures, rheumatoid factor, antinuclear antibody, and HIV serology.
- Viral cultures and antibody titers rarely clinically useful
- Chest x-ray (CXR) is performed to rule out pulmonary/mediastinal pathology. Enlarged cardiac silhouette suggests large pericardial effusion (at least 200 mL).
- Transthoracic echocardiogram recommended to evaluate for the presence of pericardial effusion, tamponade, or myocardial disease (presence of effusion helps to confirm diagnosis of pericarditis) (6)[B].
- CT and MRI allow visualization of pericardium to assess for complications or if initial workup is inconclusive.

Diagnostic Procedures/Other
- Pericardiocentesis indicated for cardiac tamponade and for suspected purulent, tuberculous, or neoplastic pericarditis
- Surgical drainage with pericardial biopsy recommended if recurrent tamponade/ineffective pericardiocentesis

Test Interpretation
- Microscopic examination may reveal hyperemia, leukocyte accumulation, or fibrin deposition.
- Purulent fluid with neutrophilic predominance if bacterial etiology
- Lymphocytic predominance in viral, tuberculous, and neoplastic pericarditis

TREATMENT

- Goal of treatment is to relieve pain and reduce complications (e.g., recurrence, tamponade, chronic restrictive pericarditis).
- Outpatient therapy is reported to be successful in 85% patients with low-risk features (3)[B].

GENERAL MEASURES
Specific therapy directed toward underlying disorder for patients with identified cause other than viral/idiopathic disease

MEDICATION
First Line
- NSAIDs are considered the mainstay of therapy for acute pericarditis; dosage is tapered every 1–2 weeks to reduce recurrence rate:
  – Ibuprofen 600 mg t.i.d. Wean to 600 mg b.i.d. or 400 mg t.i.d., then 600 mg/d.
  – Aspirin 750–1,000 mg t.i.d. Wean to 750–1,000 mg b.i.d., then 750–1,000 mg/d. Preferable for patients with recent MI because other NSAIDs impair scar formation in animal studies.
  – Indomethacin 50 mg t.i.d. Wean by decreasing total daily dose by 25 mg every 1–2 weeks.
  – GI protection should be provided.

- Colchicine 0.5–0.6 mg b.i.d. (≥70 kg patient) or once daily for those who weight less, × 3 months (6–12 months for recurrences) (7)[B], Taper over 2–4 weeks. A higher initial loading dose is associated with adverse GI events (3)[B]. More effective as an adjunct to NSAIDs or steroids than monotherapy for initial attack and prevention of recurrences.
- Tapering should be done only if the patient is asymptomatic and CRP/ESR are normal and are done every 1–2 weeks.
- Treatment duration using NSAIDs for initial attacks is 1–2 weeks, but for recurrences, consider 2–4 weeks of therapy.
- Monitoring: NSAIDs: CBC and CRP at baseline and weekly until CRP normalizes; Colchicine: Consider CBC, CRP, transaminases, creatine kinase, and creatinine at baseline and at least after 1 month (3)[B].
- Contraindications: Hypersensitivity to aspirin or NSAIDs, active peptic ulcer/GI bleeding
- Precautions: Use with caution in patients with asthma, 3rd-trimester pregnancy, coagulopathy, and renal/hepatic dysfunction.
- Pregnant: <20 weeks' gestation: Aspirin is 1st choice, but NSAIDs and prednisone are also allowed; >20 weeks' gestation: Prednisone is allowed with avoidance of NSAIDs, aspirin, and colchicine (6)[B].

Second Line
- Colchicine is significantly effective in primary prevention and in secondary prevention of recurrent pericarditis (8)[A].
- Corticosteroid treatment is indicated in connective tissue disease, uremic/tuberculous pericarditis, or severe recurrent symptoms unresponsive to NSAIDs or colchicine (5)[B]; should be avoided in uncomplicated acute pericarditis. *Corticosteroid use alone has been found to be an independent risk factor for recurrence.*
- If steroids are used, consider low dose (0.2–0.5mg/kg/d × 2 weeks for 1st attack, 0.2–0.5 mg/kg/d × 2–4 weeks for recurrence) with slow taper (>50 mg: 10 mg/d every 1–2 weeks; 50–25 mg: 5–10 mg/d every 1–2 weeks; 25–15 mg: 2.5 mg/d every 2–4 weeks; <15 mg/d: 1–2.5 mg/d every 2–6 weeks) following remission with symptom resolution and normalization of CRP. Remember to use adequate prophylaxis treatment for osteoporosis prevention (3)[B].
- Intrapericardial administration of steroids may be effective and limits systemic side effects (5)[B].

ISSUES FOR REFERRAL
- Refractory cases include those on unacceptably high long-term steroid doses (>25 mg/d).
- Consider trial of aspirin and/or NSAIDs + steroid and colchicine (3)[C].

SURGERY/OTHER PROCEDURES
- Pericardiocentesis is indicated in cases of cardiac tamponade, high likelihood of tuberculous/purulent/neoplastic pericarditis, and large symptomatic effusions refractory to medical therapy (3)[B].
- Pericardial biopsy may be considered for diagnosis in those with persistent worsening pericarditis without a definite diagnosis (3)[B].

- Pericardioscopy for targeted diagnostic imaging may be performed at experienced tertiary referral centers in refractory and difficult cases (3)[B].
- Pericardial window may be performed in cases of recurrent cardiac tamponade with large pericardial effusion despite medical therapy and severe symptoms (3)[B].
- Pericardiectomy can be considered for frequent and highly symptomatic recurrences with cardiac tamponade and constrictive pericarditis (3)[B]. The 2004 European Society of Cardiology guidelines recommend pericardiectomy (Class IIa) for frequent and highly symptomatic recurrences of pericarditis refractory to medical therapy (5)[B]. However, this is rarely performed in the US.

IN-PATIENT CONSIDERATIONS
Admission Criteria/Initial Stabilization
Inpatient therapy recommended for pericarditis associated with clinical predictors of poor prognosis (3)[B]:
- Major predictors: Fever >38°C, subacute onset, large pericardial effusion, cardiac tamponade, lack of response to NSAID/aspirin therapy after at least 1 week
- Minor predictors: Immunosuppressed state, trauma, oral anticoagulation therapy, myopericarditis

IV Fluids
IV fluids considered for hypotension in the setting of pericardial tamponade

Discharge Criteria
- Response to therapy with symptom improvement
- Hemodynamic stability

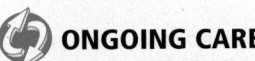 ONGOING CARE

FOLLOW-UP RECOMMENDATIONS
- 7–10 days to assess response to treatment
- 1 month to check CBC and CRP and thereafter if symptoms continue to be present
- Those with clinical predictors of poor prognosis may require closer follow-up based on lab data and echocardiographic findings.

Patient Monitoring
Myopericarditis (3)[B]:
- Use lower doses of anti-inflammatory drugs to control symptoms for 1–2 weeks while minimizing deleterious effects on myocarditic process.
- Exercise restrictions for 4–6 weeks
- Echocardiographic monitoring at 1, 6, and 12 months (especially in those with left ventricular dysfunction)

DIET
No restrictions

PROGNOSIS
Overall good prognosis; disease usually benign and self-limiting

COMPLICATIONS
- Recurrent pericarditis (1): Occurs in ~24% of patients, with most instances resulting from idiopathic, viral, or autoimmune pericarditis; inadequate treatment of the initial attack; and, less commonly, neoplastic etiologies. Recurrence usually within 1st weeks following initial episode, but may occur months to years later. Rarely associated with tamponade/constriction

- Cardiac tamponade: Rare complication with increased incidence in neoplastic, purulent, and tuberculous pericarditis
- Effusive-constrictive pericarditis (6): Reported in 24% of patients undergoing surgery for constrictive pericarditis and in 8% of patients undergoing pericardiocentesis and cardiac catheterization for cardiac tamponade. Failure of right atrial pressure to fall by 50% or to a level below 10 mm Hg after pericardiocentesis is diagnostic.
- Constrictive pericarditis: Rare complication in which rigid pericardium produces abnormal diastolic filling with elevated filling pressures. Pericardiectomy remains definitive therapy.

REFERENCES
1. Tingle LE, Molina D, Calvert CW. Acute pericarditis. *Am Fam Physician.* 2007;76:1509–1514.
2. Khandaker MH, Espinosa RE, Nishimura RA, et al. Pericardial disease: Diagnosis and management. *Mayo Clin Proc.* 2010;85:572–593.
3. Imazio M, Spodick DH, Brucato A, et al. Controversial issues in the management of pericardial diseases. *Circulation.* 2010;121:916–928.
4. Imazio M, Trinchero R. Triage and management of acute pericarditis. *Int J Cardiol.* 2007;118:286–294.
5. Maisch B, Seferovi PM, Risti AD, et al. Guidelines on the diagnosis and management of pericardial diseases executive summary: The task force on the diagnosis and management of pericardial diseases of the European Society of Cardiology. *Eur Heart J.* 2004;25:587–610.
6. Imazio M, Brucato A, Trinchero R, et al. Diagnosis and management of pericardial diseases. *Nat Rev Cardiol.* 2009;6:743–751.
7. Imazio M, Brucato A, Cemin R, et al. A randomized trial of colchicine for acute pericarditis. *N Engl J Med.* 2013;369:1522–1528.
8. Imazio M, Brucato A, Forno D, et al. Efficacy and safety of colchicine for pericarditis prevention. Systematic review and meta-analysis. *Heart.* 2012;98:1078–1082.

 CODES

ICD10
- I30.1 Infective pericarditis
- I30.9 Acute pericarditis, unspecified
- I31.9 Disease of pericardium, unspecified

CLINICAL PEARLS
- Consider *major* predictors and *minor* predictors in deciding which patients should be admitted.
- Therapy aimed at symptomatic relief and NSAIDs are first-line treatment. Colchicine is recommended as an adjunct to NSAIDs.
- Pericardiocentesis is recommended in the setting of cardiac tamponade or possible purulent pericarditis.

PERIODIC LIMB MOVEMENT DISORDER

Donald E. Watenpaugh, PhD • John R. Burk, MD

BASICS

DESCRIPTION
- Sleep-related movement disorder with these features (1,2):
  - Episodes of periodic limb movements (PLMs) during sleep
  - Movements consist of bilateral ankle dorsiflexion, sometimes with knee and hip flexion.
  - Arm or more generalized movements occur less commonly.
  - Movements may cause brief microarousals from sleep unbeknownst to the patient.
  - Complaints include insomnia, unrestorative sleep, daytime fatigue, and/or somnolence.
  - Bed partner may complain of movements.
  - Another sleep disorder (e.g., obstructive sleep apnea) does not cause the PLMs.
- System(s) affected: Musculoskeletal; Nervous
- Synonym(s): Nocturnal myoclonus; Sleep myoclonus; Periodic leg movements of sleep

EPIDEMIOLOGY
Incidence
- Increases with age: 1/3 of patients >60 exhibit PLMs, but not necessarily periodic limb movement disorder (PLMD) (1).
- Predominant sex: Male = Female
- PLMs in 15% of insomnia patients

Prevalence
- PLMs in sleep: Common and often of no clinical consequence
- PLMs constituting PLMD (causing sleep complaints and/or daytime consequences) much less common: <5% of adults (but underdiagnosed)

ETIOLOGY AND PATHOPHYSIOLOGY
- Unstudied
- Primary: Probable CNS dopaminergic impairment
- Secondary:
  - Iron deficiency
  - Peripheral neuropathy
  - Arthritis
  - Renal failure
  - Synucleinopathies (multiple-system atrophy)
  - Spinal cord injury
  - Pregnancy
  - Medications:
    ○ Most antidepressants (not bupropion or desipramine).
    ○ Some antipsychotic and antidementia medications
    ○ Antiemetics (metoclopramide)
    ○ Antihistamines

Genetics
Unstudied, but see Restless Legs Syndrome (RLS)

RISK FACTORS
- Family history of RLS (3)
- Iron deficiency and associated conditions (e.g., pregnancy, gastric surgery, renal disease)
- Attention-deficit hyperactivity disorder (ADHD) (4)
- Aging
- Peripheral neuropathy
- Arthritis, orthopedic problems
- Chronic limb pain or discomfort

GENERAL PREVENTION
- Regular physical activity
- Adequate nightly sleep
- Avoid causes of secondary PLMD.
- Avoid causes of RLS.

COMMONLY ASSOCIATED CONDITIONS
- RLS
- Rapid eye movement (REM) sleep behavior disorder
- Narcolepsy
- Iron deficiency
- Renal failure
- Cardiovascular disease; stroke
- Gastric surgery
- Pregnancy
- Arthritis
- Synucleinopathies (multiple-system atrophy)
- Lumbar spine disease; spinal cord injury
- Peripheral neuropathy
- Insomnia, insufficient sleep
- ADHD
- Depression

Pediatric Considerations
- PLMD may precede overt RLS by years.
- Association with RLS is more common than in adults
- Symptoms may be more consequential than in adults
- Associated with ADHD (4)[B]

Pregnancy Considerations
- May be secondary to iron or folate deficiency
- Most severe in 3rd trimester
- Usually subsides after delivery

Geriatric Considerations
- May become a significant source of sleep disturbance
- May cause or exacerbate circadian disruption and "sundowning"
- Many medications given to the elderly cause or exacerbate PLMs, which can lead to PLMD or RLS.

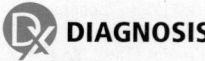

DIAGNOSIS

HISTORY
- Episodes of PLMs during sleep (often reported by bed partner)
- Insomnia: Difficulty maintaining sleep
- Unrestorative sleep
- Daytime fatigue, tiredness, and/or somnolence
- Oppositional behaviors
- Memory impairment
- Depression
- ADHD, particularly in children (4)

PHYSICAL EXAM
No specific findings

DIFFERENTIAL DIAGNOSIS
- When PLMs occur along with RLS, REM sleep behavior disorder, or narcolepsy, those disorders are diagnosed as "with PLMs," and PLMD is not diagnosed separately.
- Obstructive sleep apnea: LMs occur during microarousals from apneas; treatment of sleep apnea eliminates these LMs (1).
- Sleep starts: Nonperiodic, generalized, occur only at wake–sleep transition, <0.2 seconds duration
- Sleep-related leg cramps: Isolated and painful
- Fragmentary myoclonus: 75–150 ms of EMG activity, minimal movement, no periodicity
- Nocturnal seizures: Epileptiform EEG, motor pattern incongruent with PLMs
- Fasciculations, tremor: No sleep association
- Sleep-related rhythmic movement disorder: Voluntary movement during wake–sleep transition; higher frequency than PLMs

DIAGNOSTIC TESTS & INTERPRETATION
- Polysomnography with finding of repetitive, stereotyped limb movements (2):
  - Tibialis anterior electromyographic (EMG) activity lasting 0.5–10 seconds
  - EMG amplitude increases >8 μV from baseline.
  - Movements occur in a sequence of $\geq$4 at intervals of 5–90 seconds
  - Children: $\geq$5 movements/hr; adults, 15
  - Movement may also involve arms
  - Associated with heart rate variability from autonomic-level arousals
  - Most PLM episodes occur in the 1st hours of non-REM sleep.
  - Significant night-to-night PLM variability
- Serum ferritin to assess for iron deficiency

Diagnostic Procedures/Other
- Ankle actigraphy for in-home use
- EMG or nerve conduction studies for peripheral neuropathy/radiculopathy

Test Interpretation
Serum ferritin <75 ng/mL

TREATMENT

- Daily exercise
- Adequate nightly sleep
- Treatment paradigm similar to that for RLS (5,6)[A], except that all medications are off-label for PLMD

GENERAL MEASURES

- Daily exercise
- Adequate nightly sleep
- Warm the legs (long socks, leg warmers, electric blanket, etc.).
- Hot bath before bedtime
- Avoid nicotine and evening caffeine and alcohol.

MEDICATION

- Use minimum effective dose.
- Consider risks, side effects, and interactions individually (e.g., benzodiazepines in elderly).
- Daytime sleepiness is unusual with the doses and timing employed for PLMD.

First Line

- Dopamine agonists: Take 1 hour before bed; titrate weekly to optimal dose (5,6)[A]:
  - Pramipexole (Mirapex): 0.125–1.5 mg; titrate by 0.125 mg
  - Ropinirole (Requip): 0.25–4 mg; titrate by 0.25 mg
  - Transdermal rotigotine (Neupro): 1–3 mg patch; titrate by 1 mg weekly to effectiveness
- Avoid dopamine agonists in psychotic patients, especially if taking dopamine antagonists.

Second Line

- Anticonvulsants: Useful for associated neuropathy:
  - Gabapentin enacarbil (Horizant): 300–600 mg/d
  - Pregabalin (Lyrica): 50–300 mg/d
- Opioids: Low risk for tolerance with bedtime dose:
  - Hydrocodone: 5–20 mg/d
  - Oxycodone: 2.5–20 mg/d
- Benzodiazepines and agonists:
  - Clonazepam (Klonopin): 0.5–3 mg/d
  - Zaleplon, zolpidem, temazepam, triazolam, alprazolam, diazepam

Pediatric Considerations

- First-line treatment is nonpharmacologic (4)[B].
- Consider low-dose clonidine or clonazepam.

Pregnancy Considerations

- Initial approach: Fe supplementation, nonpharmacologic therapies
- Most medications are Class C or D
- In 3rd trimester, low-dose opioids or clonazepam may be considered.

Geriatric Considerations

In weak or frail patients, avoid medications that may cause dizziness or unsteadiness.

ADDITIONAL THERAPIES

- If iron-deficient, iron supplementation:
  - 325 mg ferrous sulfate with 200 mg vitamin C between meals t.i.d.
  - Repletion may require months.
  - Symptoms continue without other treatment.
- Vitamin/Mineral supplements, including calcium, magnesium, B_{12}, folate
- Clonidine: 0.1–0.7 mg/d

SURGERY/OTHER PROCEDURES

Correction of orthopedic, neuropathic, or peripheral vascular problems

IN-PATIENT CONSIDERATIONS

- Control during recovery from orthopedic procedures
- Addition or withdrawal of medications that affect PLMD
- Changes in medical status may require medication changes (e.g., Mirapex contraindicated in renal failure and Requip contraindicated in liver disease).

IV Fluids

- Consider iron infusion when oral supplementation is ineffective, not tolerated, or contraindicated.
- When NPO, consider IV opiates.

Nursing

- Evening walks, hot baths, leg warming
- Sleep interruption risks prolonged wakefulness.

ONGOING CARE

FOLLOW-UP RECOMMENDATIONS

Patient Monitoring

- At monthly intervals until stable
- Annual and PRN follow-up thereafter
- If Fe-deficient, remeasure ferritin to assess repletion.

DIET

Avoid caffeine and alcohol late in the day.

PATIENT EDUCATION

- National Sleep Foundation: www.sleepfoundation.org; e-mail: nsf@sleepfoundation.org; (703) 243-1697

PROGNOSIS

- Primary PLMD: Lifelong condition with no current cure
- Secondary PLMD: May subside with resolution of cause(s)
- Current therapies usually control symptoms.
- PLMD often precedes emergence of RLS.

COMPLICATIONS

- Tolerance to medications requiring increased dose or alternatives
- Augmentation (increased PLMs and sleep disturbance, emergence of RLS) from prolonged use of dopamine agonists:
  - Higher doses increase risk.
  - Fe deficiency increases risk.
  - Add alternative medication, then detitrate dopaminergic agent (5)[A].
- Iatrogenic PLMD (from antidepressants, etc.)

REFERENCES

1. Natarajan R. Review of periodic limb movement and restless leg syndrome. *J Postgrad Med*. 2010;56:157–162.
2. Sateia MJ. Periodic limb movement disorder. In: *International classification of sleep disorders diagnostic & coding manual*, 2nd ed. Westchester, IL: American Academy of Sleep Medicine, 2005;182–186.
3. Picchietti DL, Rajendran RR, Wilson MP, et al. Pediatric restless legs syndrome and periodic limb movement disorder: Parent-child pairs. *Sleep Med*. 2009;10(8):925–931.
4. Picchietti MA, Picchietti DL. Restless legs syndrome and periodic limb movement disorder in children and adolescents. *Semin Pediatr Neurol*. 2008; 15:91–99.
5. Aurora RN, Kristo DA, Bista SR, et al. The treatment of restless legs syndrome and periodic limb movement disorder in adults-an update for 2012: Practice parameters with an evidence-based systematic review and meta-analyses: An American Academy of Sleep Medicine Clinical Practice Guideline. *Sleep*. 2012;35(8):1039–1062.
6. Garcia-Borreguero D, Stillman P, Benes H, et al. Algorithms for the diagnosis and treatment of restless legs syndrome in primary care. *BMC Neurol*. 2011;11:28. Epub 2011 Feb 27.

SEE ALSO

Restless Legs Syndrome

CODES

ICD10

G47.61 Periodic limb movement disorder

CLINICAL PEARLS

- Many patients with PLMs may not require treatment; however, when sleep disturbance from PLMs causes insomnia and/or daytime consequences, PLMD exists and should be treated.
- Many antidepressants and some antihistamines cause or exacerbate PLMs.
- Accumulating data indicate that sleep disturbance, including that from PLMs, may cause or exacerbate ADHD (4)[B].

PERIORAL DERMATITIS

Heather Summe, MD • Nikki A. Levin, MD, PhD

 BASICS

DESCRIPTION
- A common facial eruption of women and children
- Presents as tiny, flesh-colored, or erythematous monomorphic papules or pustules around the mouth with characteristic sparing of the area immediately adjacent to the vermilion border
- May also involve the periocular, perinasal, and glabellar regions of the face
- Etiology is unknown, but a relation to topical steroid use has been suggested
- Without treatment, the course is usually fluctuating and chronic
- Variants in children include granulomatous periorificial dermatitis (GPD) and facial Afro-Caribbean childhood eruption (FACE).
- Synonym(s): Periorificial dermatitis (POD); Chronic papulopustular facial dermatitis; Granulomatous perioral dermatitis; Light-sensitive seborrhea; Lupus-like perioral dermatitis; Papulopustular facial dermatitis; Rosacea-like dermatitis; Stewardess disease

EPIDEMIOLOGY
- Occurs worldwide, especially in fair-skinned populations
- Predominantly affects children between 6 months and 16 years and women aged 17–45
- ~90% of adult cases are in women (1)
- Childhood cases may be more common in boys.
- All races are affected, but the granulomatous form is more common in African American and dark-skinned children.
- Some believe the number of cases peaked in the 1960s–1970s and decreased in the 1980s–1990s when the side effects of topical steroids were recognized. Others believe that cases are still increasing.

Incidence
- Peak incidence is in the 2nd and 3rd decades of life.
- In children, peak incidence is in the prepubertal period.

Prevalence
- Represents ~2% of patients presenting to dermatology clinics (2)
- ~3% of children using inhalational steroids develop some form of POD (3)

ETIOLOGY AND PATHOPHYSIOLOGY
- Exposure to an irritant results in breakdown of the epidermal barrier and subsequent water loss and sensation of dryness; this encourages use of facial products and corticosteroids, which may worsen the condition.
- This inflammatory cycle eventually leads to clinical features of the disease.
- The exact cause is unknown, and there may be more than 1 contributing factor.
- The most widely cited factor implicated in POD is use of potent topical corticosteroids on the face.
- Inhaled corticosteroids, especially when used with a spacer and nebulizer or mask, have also been reported to cause POD.
- Intranasal steroids have been associated with POD beginning in the nasolabial folds.
- Two cases associated with systemic steroid use have been reported in children (4).

- Use of foundation, moisturizer, and night cream was associated with a 13-fold increased risk of POD in 1 study (5).
- Other factors implicated but not proven:
  – Drugs: Oral contraceptives
  – Toothpastes: Fluoridated, tartar control, whitening
  – Physical factors: UV light, heat, wind, salivary leakage
  – Infectious factors: Fusiform bacteria, *Candida* species, *Demodex folliculorum*
  – Miscellaneous factors: Atopy, GI disturbances, stress, contact allergy, lip-licking, immunosuppression, bubble gum, formaldehyde, varicella vaccination

Genetics
55% of pediatric patients with POD have a family history of atopy (5)

RISK FACTORS
See "Etiology and Pathophysiology."

GENERAL PREVENTION
- Avoid using potent topical corticosteroids on the face.
- Avoid using excessive foundation, moisturizer, and night cream.
- Avoidance of tartar-control and whitening toothpastes may also be helpful.

COMMONLY ASSOCIATED CONDITIONS
Atopic dermatitis

 DIAGNOSIS

HISTORY
- Patient reports a history of facial rash, which may improve with use of topical corticosteroids and flare with discontinuation
- Affected skin may be pruritic or have a burning sensation
- Course may be chronic and fluctuating
- Recent topical, inhaled, or systemic steroid use in 72% of patients (6)
- May worsen with sun exposure

PHYSICAL EXAM
- Monomorphic, minute, flesh-colored to erythematous papules or pustules, sometimes surmounted with scale, in a perioral distribution, often asymmetrical, with sparing of the vermilion border 3–5 mm around the lips
- Granulomatous form can usually be distinguished clinically by the absence of pustules and the presence of yellow-brown papules
- Common locations are alar creases, nasolabial folds, chin, periocular skin, eyelids, and glabella.
- Diameter of lesions is usually 1–2 mm
- Distribution (2):
  – Perioral area (39%)
  – Perinasal (13%)
  – Periocular (1%)
  – Perioral and perinasal (14%)
  – Perioral and periocular (6%)
  – Perinasal and periocular (6%)
  – Perioral, perinasal, and periocular (10%)
- Lupus-like variant diagnosed by yellowish discoloration of lesions on diascopy

DIFFERENTIAL DIAGNOSIS
- Acne vulgaris
- Contact dermatitis
- Rosacea
- Seborrheic dermatitis
- Lip-licker's dermatitis
- Papular sarcoidosis
- *Demodex* infestation
- Acrodermatitis enteropathica
- Biotin deficiency
- Glucagonoma syndrome
- Xanthomas
- Eruptive syringomas
- Polymorphous light eruption
- Acne agminata
- Lupus miliaris disseminatus faciei
- Haber syndrome (familial rosacea-like dermatosis)

DIAGNOSTIC TESTS & INTERPRETATION
Diagnosis is usually clinical:
- No laboratory abnormalities expected
- Prick tests and IgE testing may show evidence of atopy, but are not routinely done
- Patch testing may be used to rule out contact dermatitis
- Scrapings for *Demodex* mites

Diagnostic Procedures/Other
Skin biopsy is not routinely performed, but can be helpful in atypical cases

Test Interpretation
Histopathology of skin biopsy:
- Mild, nonspecific inflammation with variable perifollicular or perivascular lymphohistiocytic infiltrate
- Eczematous changes, acanthosis, parakeratosis, and spongiosis
- Occasionally, follicular abscesses are seen.
- Older lesions may contain diffuse hypertrophy of connective tissue and hyperplasia of sebaceous follicles with occasional noncaseating granulomas in the dermis (1).
- Caseating granulomas are seen with granulomatous variant.

 TREATMENT

GENERAL MEASURES

"Zero therapy" can be an effective treatment in adherent patients (2)[B]:
- Reduce use of facial soaps, makeup, and moisturizers and wash with only water
- Discontinue use of potent topical corticosteroids on the face:
  – This may result in a flare.
  – Flares may be decreased with use of less-potent topical steroids, calcineurin inhibitors, or IM steroid injection.
- Discontinue use of fluoridated, whitening, and tartar-control toothpaste

MEDICATION
Based on disease severity and patient's tolerance for adverse effects

First Line
- Severe disease:
  - Oral antibiotics:
    - Tetracycline has been proven as an effective treatment (2)[A]:
    - 250–500 mg b.i.d. for 8–10 weeks
    - Dose may be halved after 3–4 weeks if improvement noted
    - Contraindicated in children and pregnant women
    - Common side effects: Photosensitivity, GI upset, rash, candidiasis, headache, dizziness, tinnitus
  - Doxycycline or minocycline (5)[C]:
    - 100 mg b.i.d. for 6–8 weeks
    - Dose may be halved after 3–4 weeks if improvement noted
    - Contraindicated in children and pregnant women
    - Common side effects of doxycycline: GI upset, esophagitis, joint pain, upper respiratory infection (URI) symptoms, rash, dysmenorrhea, candidiasis, headache, dizziness, photosensitivity, elevated BUN
    - Common side effects of minocycline: GI upset, lightheadedness, vertigo, ataxia, headache, fatigue, tinnitus, rash, urticaria, candidiasis, hyperpigmentation
  - Alternatively, doxycycline 40 mg/d modified-release capsule may achieve the anti-inflammatory effect without the microbial activity that promotes emergence of resistant bacterial strains (7)[C].
  - Erythromycin (5)[C] may be used when tetracyclines are contraindicated or not tolerated:
    - 250 mg b.i.d.–t.i.d. for 6–8 weeks
    - Dose may be halved after 3–4 weeks if improvement noted
    - May be used in children or pregnant women
    - Common side effects: GI upset, diarrhea, rash, urticaria
    - Rarer serious side effects: Erythema multiforme, pancreatitis, convulsions, QT prolongation, and ventricular arrhythmias
- Moderate disease:
  - Topical antibiotics:
    - May be slower than systemic antibiotics in clearing lesions
    - Metronidazole cream 0.75% b.i.d. (2)[B]
    - Erythromycin 2% gel, solution, or ointment b.i.d. (2)[B]
    - Clindamycin 1% gel, lotion, or cream b.i.d.
- Mild disease:
  - "Zero therapy" (see "General Measures") (2)[B]

Second Line
- Severe disease:
  - Clarithromycin (250 mg/d) may be used when tetracyclines and erythromycin are contraindicated or not tolerated (2)[C]:
    - Common side effects: GI upset, headache, rash, abnormal taste sensation, urticaria
  - Oral isotretinoin may be useful in granulomatous cases that are not responsive to a full dose of tetracyclines (1)[C]:
    - 0.2 mg/kg initially followed by 0.1 mg/kg after notable improvement

- Isotretinoin is a pregnancy Category X drug and may cause severe birth defects. Use with caution with in women of reproductive age. Physician and patient must register with iPLEDGE program.
  - Common side effects: Dry skin, cheilitis, arthralgias/myalgias, hypertriglyceridemia, elevated liver function tests (LFTs), hair loss, visual disturbances, depression, tinnitus
  - Pimecrolimus 1% cream may accelerate healing (2)[A] and tacrolimus 0.1% ointment use has been reported with success (2):
    - Rare cases of lymphoma and skin malignancies have been reported. Avoid long-term use.
- Moderate disease:
  - Topical therapies:
    - Antiacne drugs, such as azelaic acid and adapalene, may be helpful (2).
    - Ichthyol (ammonium bituminosulfonate) (2)

ADDITIONAL THERAPIES
A number of other therapies have been reported in the literature, including photodynamic therapy with 5-aminolevulinic acid (2)[B], radiotherapy, and liquid nitrogen. There has also been a case reported of oral metronidazole (250 mg b.i.d.) resulting in complete clearance of GPD without scarring after 1 month of use (8).

COMPLEMENTARY AND ALTERNATIVE MEDICINE
Compress with chamomile tea or physiologic solution may be used if the patient struggles with "zero therapy" (1)[C]

 ## ONGOING CARE

DIET
No restrictions

PATIENT EDUCATION
- Lesions may take many weeks to resolve.
- Symptoms may temporarily worsen, especially with discontinuance of steroids.
- Recurrence is rare.
- Topical corticosteroid use on the face should be avoided in the future.

PROGNOSIS
- Most cases resolve without recurrence.
- Oral or topical antibiotics usually lead to remission within 6–10 weeks.
- Untreated disease may persist for months to years and be characterized by unpredictable flares.
- Disease is not associated with significant morbidity.

COMPLICATIONS
- Most cases resolve without complications.
- Emotional stress can result from bothersome appearance of lesions and chronic course of disease.
- Scarring may be problematic with lupus-like variant.

REFERENCES

1. Lipozencic J, Ljubojevic S. Perioral dermatitis. *Clin Dermatol*. 2011;29:157–161.
2. Wollenberg A, Bieber T, Dirschka T, et al. Perioral dermatitis. *J Dtsch Dermatol Ges*. 2011;9: 422–427.
3. Henningsen E, Bygum A. Budesonide-induced periorificial dermatitis presenting as chalazion and blepharitis. *Pediatr Dermatol*. 2011;28:596–597.
4. Clementson B, Smidt A. Periorificial dermatitis due to systemic corticosteroids in children: Report of two cases. *Pediatr Dermatol*. 2012:29:331–332.
5. Vanderweil SG, Levin NA. Perioral dermatitis: It's not every rash that occurs around the mouth. *Dermatol Nurs*. 2009;21:317–320, 353; quiz 321.
6. Nguyen V, Eichenfield LF. Periorificial dermatitis in children and adolescents. *J Am Acad Dermatol*. 2006;55:781–785.
7. Rosso JQ. Management of papulopustular rosacea and perioral dermatitis with emphasis on Iatrogenic causation or exacerbation of inflammatory facial dermatoses: Use of doxycycline-modified release 40 mg capsule once daily in combination with properly selected skin care as an effective therapeutic approach. *J Clin Aesthet Dermatol*. 2011;4:20–30.
8. Rodriguez-Caruncho C, Bielsa I, Fernandez-Figueras MT, et al. Childhood granulomatous periorificial dermatitis with a good response to oral metronidazole. *Pediatr Dermatol*. Epub 2013;30:e98–99.

ADDITIONAL READING

- Hafeez ZH. Perioral dermatitis: An update. *Int J Dermatol*. 2003;42:514–517.
- Kim YJ, Shin JW, Lee JS, et al. Childhood granulomatous periorificial dermatitis. *Ann Dermatol*. 2011;23:386–388.
- Peralta L, Morais P. Perioral dermatitis—the role of nasal steroids. *Cutan Ocul Toxicol*. 2012;31: 160–163.
- Weber K, Thurmayr R. Critical appraisal of reports on the treatment of perioral dermatitis. *Dermatology (Basel)*. 2005;210:300–307.

 ## CODES

ICD10
L71.0 Perioral dermatitis

CLINICAL PEARLS
- Suspect POD when an acneiform eruption involves the perioral, perinasal, or periocular areas with characteristic sparing of the skin immediately adjacent to the vermilion border.
- Ask patients about a history of recent corticosteroid use, facial product use, and use of fluoridated, whitening, or tartar-control toothpastes.
- Substitution of low-potency steroids may allow patients to discontinue higher-potency steroids while avoiding a rebound flare.

PERIPHERAL ARTERIAL DISEASE

Zhen Lu, MD

 BASICS

DESCRIPTION
Peripheral arterial disease (PAD) is a manifestation of systemic atherosclerosis in which there is partial or total blockage in the arteries, exclusive of the coronary and cerebral vessels. Objectively, PAD is defined as a resting ankle-brachial index (ABI) of <0.90.

EPIDEMIOLOGY
- Predominant age: >40 years
- Predominant sex: Male > Female (2:1), based on the Framingham study
- Patients with symptomatic PAD have a 5-year mortality rate of 30%.
- Highly prevalent syndrome that affects 8–12 million individuals in the US

Incidence
Incidence overall: 1–2.7/1,000/year

Prevalence
- US prevalence: 2.7–4.1%
- Age-adjusted prevalence of PAD is close to 12%.
- Up to 29% among patients in primary care practices

ETIOLOGY AND PATHOPHYSIOLOGY
- In patients with PAD, arterial stenoses cause inadequate blood flow in distal limbs, which fails to meet the metabolic demand during exertion:
  - The degree of ischemia is proportional to the size and proximity of the occlusion to the end organ.
  - Acidic products of anaerobic metabolism build up within the muscle and result in claudication clinically.
  - Arterial occlusion also causes significantly diminished distal pressure in patients with PAD due to atherosclerotic lesions.
- Most common cause of arterial stenoses is atherosclerosis.

Genetics
Current NIH–funded research focuses on single-nucleotide polymorphisms in candidate genes that are regulated in the vasculature in an attempt to explore genetic factors responsible for PAD.

RISK FACTORS
- Age >40 years
- Cigarette smoking
- Diabetes mellitus
- Obesity
- Hypertension
- Hyperlipidemia
- Hyperhomocysteinemia

GENERAL PREVENTION
Control risk factors

COMMONLY ASSOCIATED CONDITIONS
- See "Risk Factors."
- Associated with other common complications of atherosclerosis, including myocardial infarction (MI), transient ischemic attack, stroke, and limb amputation
- Occurs in ~40% of patients with cardiovascular disease

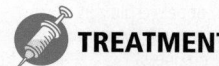 **DIAGNOSIS**

HISTORY
- Intermittent claudication, with symptoms typically resolving within 2–5 minutes of rest (although it is regarded as the classic symptom for PAD, intermittent claudication is present in only 10% of patients with PAD)
- Rest leg pain (especially in a supine position)
- Skin ulceration (in advanced PAD)
- Gangrene (in advanced PAD)
- Impotence

PHYSICAL EXAM
- Skin pallor when leg is elevated above the level of the heart (in mild PAD)
- Dependent rubor
- Dry and scaly skin
- Poor nail growth
- Hair loss
- Reduced/Absent extremity pulses (in advanced PAD)

DIFFERENTIAL DIAGNOSIS
- Arterial embolism
- Deep venous thrombosis
- Thromboangiitis obliterans (Buerger disease)
- Osteoarthritis
- Restless legs syndrome
- Peripheral neuropathy
- Spinal stenoses (pseudoclaudication)
- Intervertebral disc prolapse

DIAGNOSTIC TESTS & INTERPRETATION
Serum glucose is recommended screening for diabetes mellitus in suspected or confirmed PAD.

Initial Tests (lab, imaging)
- Fasting lipid profile is indicated for risk assessment of hyperlipidemia.
- Duplex ultrasonography and Doppler color-flow imaging, which are useful in detecting stenosed segments and assessing lesion severity, are initial imaging tests of choice.
- Magnetic resonance angiography, coupled with 3D reconstruction, is highly sensitive and specific for the localization of occluded lesions.
- CT scanning has a limited role in the evaluation of PAD.
- Angiography remains the gold standard in the diagnosis of PAD.

Diagnostic Procedures/Other
- Doppler ankle brachial index (ABI) measures the ratio of the higher systolic BPs between the dorsalis pedis and the posterior tibial artery vs. the higher of the systolic BPs in the 2 brachial arteries: Values for the ABI should be reported as "incompressible" if >1.40; "normal" if 1.00–1.40; "borderline" if 0.91–0.99; and "abnormal" if ≤0.90 (1). ABI <0.4: Severe ischemia
- Segmental limb pressures: Usually obtained if abnormal ABI measurement is identified; a ≥20-mm Hg reduction in pressure is considered significant for PAD.
- Treadmill exercise test assesses the severity of claudication and the response to treatment.
- Segmental volume plethysmography: Often used in conjunction with segmental limb pressures to measure the volume change in an organ or limb; the study is indicated for calcified vessel when the ABI cannot be applied diagnostically.

 TREATMENT

GENERAL MEASURES
- Claudication exercise rehabilitation program: Patient to walk until symptoms develop, then rest and start again, for a total of 30 minutes initially; walking then is increased by 5 minutes until 50 minutes of intermittent walking is achieved.
- Modification of risk factors, including smoking, diabetes mellitus, hypertension, and hyperlipidemia:
  - Weight loss is associated with a decrease in the risk of cardiovascular disease, but has not been shown to improve PAD (2)[C].
  - Antiplatelet therapy (aspirin) is recommended for patients with PAD when there is no other contraindication; however, neither the addition of an anticoagulant nor anticoagulant therapy alone has demonstrated superior outcome in PAD patients (3)[A].
  - Simvastatin (20–40 mg/d) has been shown to reduce the incidence of new intermittent claudication from 3.6–2.3% in patients with coronary artery disease (CAD) (4)[A].
  - No statistical significance for overall improvement of exercise performance or reduction in claudication symptoms for patients on niacin ER–lovastatin combined therapy.
  - β-adrenergic antagonists should be used with caution in individuals with severe PAD (2)[B].
  - Smoking cessation is likely to reduce the severity of claudication (2)[C].

MEDICATION

First Line

Antiplatelet therapy has been the mainstay treatment to prevent ischemic events in patients with PAD. However:

- The effect of aspirin on the risk reduction of overall ischemic events is inconclusive. Some suggest that aspirin delays disease progression and reduces the need for surgical intervention. AHA/ACCF guidelines (1) note that the use of antiplatelet therapy to reduce cardiovascular risks in asymptomatic patients with borderline ABIs is characterized as "not well established." Aspirin is recommended to reduce the risk of MI, stroke, and vascular death in symptomatic patients with PAD (1)[A]
- Low-dose aspirin (75–150 mg/d) is as effective as higher doses of aspirin (2).
- Ticlopidine (250 mg b.i.d.) reduces the risk of MI, stroke, and death in patients with PAD, but it has a complication of thrombocytopenia in 2–3% of patients (2)[A].

Second Line

- Clopidogrel (75 mg/d) is approved by the FDA for the secondary prevention of thrombotic events in patients with symptomatic lower-extremity PAD (4)[A] and is recommended as an alternative to aspirin (1)[A].
- Neither vasodilators nor anticoagulant therapy (e.g., heparin, low-molecular-weight heparin, or oral anticoagulant) has shown any clinically proven efficacy for the treatment of claudication (2)[B] and may be harmful.
- Other medications that may reduce claudication include pentoxifylline (1.2 g/d), cilostazol (100 mg b.i.d.), naftidrofuryl (600 mg/d), and prostaglandins (120 μg/d).

ADDITIONAL THERAPIES

- Weight reduction, smoking cessation, and BP control are essential in treating claudication.
- A walking program should include walking at least 3 × per week for 30–60 minutes each time and has been shown to improve quality of life as much as or more so than medication (see below).
- A healthy diet high in complex carbohydrates (e.g., whole grains and pastas), fruits, and vegetables, and low in salt and animal fats

SURGERY/OTHER PROCEDURES

Surgical interventions, such as revascularization, are warranted for individuals who have debilitating intermittent claudication, ischemic rest pain, or tissue loss:

- Transluminal balloon angioplasty is a percutaneous method of dilating arterial stenoses or recanalizing occluded vessels with or without stents (reserved for short, isolated, and hemodynamically significant lesions of the iliac or proximal superficial femoral artery).
- Bypass surgery is the standard operative treatment for lower extremity peripheral occlusive disease.

COMPLEMENTARY AND ALTERNATIVE MEDICINE

- Acupuncture, biofeedback, chelation therapy, and supplements such as *Ginkgo biloba,* omega-3 fatty acids, and vitamin E have been studied.
- *G. biloba* modestly reduces the symptoms of intermittent claudication (120 mg/d for up to 6 months) and can be considered as an adjunct to exercise therapy. Inconclusive evidence exists for the use of vitamin E.

 ONGOING CARE

FOLLOW-UP RECOMMENDATIONS

- An exercise training program composed of walking/bicycle riding improves maximal treadmill walking distance and, therefore, enhances functional capacity (4)[A].
- However, little added benefit exists from *G. biloba* treatment when added to supervised exercise training in patients with PAD as compared with patients in exercise training program alone (5)[C].

DIET

A low-fat cardiac diet is recommended.

PROGNOSIS

- Among patients with intermittent claudication, 15–20% will experience worsening claudication; 5–10% will undergo lower extremity bypass surgery; and 2–5% will need primary amputation (rates for smokers and diabetics are much higher).
- 30,000–50,000 people in the US undergo amputations annually because of PAD.

REFERENCES

1. Rooke TW, Hirsch AT, Misra S, et al. 2011 ACCF/AHA focused update of the guideline for the management of patients with peripheral artery disease (updating the 2005 guideline). *J Am Coll Cardiol.* 2011;58:2020–2045.
2. Hankey GJ, Norman PE, Eikelboom JW. Medical treatment of peripheral arterial disease. *JAMA.* 2006;295:547–553.
3. Duprez DA. Pharmacological interventions for peripheral artery disease. *Expert Opin Pharmacother.* 2007;8:1465–1477.
4. Gey DC, Lesho EP, Manngold J. Management of peripheral arterial disease. *Am Fam Physician.* 2004;69:525–532.
5. Wang J, Zhou S, Bronks R, et al. Supervised exercise training combined with ginkgo biloba treatment for patients with peripheral arterial disease. *Clin Rehabil.* 2007;21:579–586.

ADDITIONAL READING

Hiatt WR, Hirsch AT, Creager MA, et al. Effect of niacin ER/lovastatin on claudication symptoms in patients with peripheral artery disease. *Vasc Med.* 2010;15:171–179.

 CODES

ICD10

- I70.209 Unsp athscl native arteries of extremities, unsp extremity
- I70.219 Athscl native arteries of extrm w intrmt claud, unsp extrm
- I73.9 Peripheral vascular disease, unspecified

CLINICAL PEARLS

- Screening of a general medical population for PAD is not recommended. Studies have indicated that screening for PAD among asymptomatic adults in the general population could lead to false-positive results and unnecessary workups. The prevalence among the general public who are asymptomatic is low.
- A patient already receiving medical treatment should be referred for further surgical evaluation for any of the following scenarios:
  - Unsatisfactory results despite medical therapy
  - No definitive diagnosis can be made
  - Critical limb ischemia is present, such as rest pain, gangrene, or ulceration.
- The clopidogrel (75 mg/d) vs. aspirin (325 mg/d) study in the Patients at Risk of Ischemic Events (CAPRIE) trial found a 23.8% relative risk ratio for MI, stroke, or cardiovascular death in PAD patients treated with clopidogrel compared with aspirin, but no statistically significant difference in overall mortality reduction. Clopidogrel is much more expensive than aspirin.

PERITONITIS, ACUTE

Bradley Anderson, MD • Justin Ertle • Marie L. Borum, MD, EdD, MPH

 BASICS

DESCRIPTION

- Acute inflammation of the peritoneum. Peritonitis can be a localized or diffuse reaction that is either bacterial or aseptic. Aseptic peritonitis can be caused by chemical irritants or systemic inflammatory conditions and can progress to bacterial peritonitis. Bacterial peritonitis is categorized based on etiology that determines treatment and prognosis.
- Bacterial peritonitis types:
  – Primary/Spontaneous bacterial peritonitis (SBP): Spontaneous infection of ascitic fluid without detectable surgically treatable intra-abdominal infectious source; defined by an ascites absolute polymorphonuclear (PMN) count >250 cells/mm^3 (1). Most frequent, life-threatening infection in liver cirrhosis (2,3). Typically monomicrobial.
  – Secondary bacterial peritonitis: Infection of peritoneal fluid from a detectable, intra-abdominal source. Most commonly occurs secondary to perforated viscus and typically polymicrobial. Ascitic fluid PMN >250 cells/mm^3.
  – Tertiary bacterial peritonitis: Persistent or recurrent infection after adequate initial therapy.

EPIDEMIOLOGY

Incidence
- SBP: In patients with ascites, the incidence of SBP in a 1-year period is 10–25% (4).
- Secondary bacterial peritonitis: Correlated to the incidence of the underlying pathology (e.g., colitis, appendicitis, diverticulitis, or peptic ulcer disease).
- Tertiary bacterial peritonitis: 57% with secondary bacterial peritonitis progress to tertiary (5).

Prevalence
- SBP: In outpatients with cirrhosis without symptoms, the prevalence is <3.5% and 8–36% in the nosocomial setting (2).
- In patients with cirrhosis and concomitant ascites, 5% of peritonitis is secondary rather than SBP (6).

ETIOLOGY AND PATHOPHYSIOLOGY
- SBP: Ascites are caused mainly by cirrhosis, but may be cardiac, renal, or malignant:
  – Major mechanism is bacterial translocation via lymphatic spread through mesenteric lymph nodes into ascitic fluid.
  – Cirrhosis leads to small intestinal bacterial overgrowth (SIBO) and increased intestinal mucosal permeability to bacteria, increasing bacterial translocation. SBP rarely occurs in the absence of SIBO (2).
  – Decreased cellular and humoral immunity secondary to cirrhosis increases susceptibility to bacterial translocation.
  – SBP major organisms: *Escherichia coli* (46%), *Streptococcus* spp. (30%), *Klebsiella* (9%), *and Staphylococcus* (6%) (4). Increasing rate of gram-positive and resistant organisms (e.g., extended-spectrum β-lactamase-producing [ESBL] *E. coli*, MRSA, enterococcus) in the nosocomial setting (2).
- Secondary bacterial peritonitis: Inflamed, traumatically injured, necrotic, or perforated intraperitoneal organs lead to spillage or translocation, irritating the peritoneum and introducing bacteria and leading to infection.
  – Bowel perforation: Appendicitis, diverticulitis, PUD, ischemic bowel, colitis, iatrogenic causes (endoscopy, anastomotic dehiscence, mechanical/thermal bowel injury), or blunt/penetrating abdominal trauma
  – Organ perforation/fluid translocation: Cholecystitis, pancreatitis, bladder rupture, PID, ruptured ectopic pregnancy
  – Peritoneal cavity damage: Peritoneal dialysis, intraperitoneal chemotherapy
  – Secondary bacterial peritonitis organisms: *E. coli*, *Klebsiella*, *Proteus*, *Streptococcus*, *Enterococcus*, *Bacteroides*, *Clostridium* (4)
- Tertiary bacterial peritonitis: Most commonly following secondary peritonitis, with inadequacy of source control or patient immune response.

RISK FACTORS
- SBP: Advanced cirrhosis with large volume ascites, prior SBP, ascitic fluid protein <1.0 g/dL, elevated serum bilirubin >2.5 mg/dL, malnutrition, upper GI bleed, bacterascites, and proton pump inhibitor (PPI) usage:
  – Acid suppression with PPIs has been shown to promote SIBO, increasing SBP (2).
  – 70% of cases of SBP are seen in patients with Child-Pugh class C cirrhosis (4).
  – Nonselective β-blockers may decrease SBP long term (2).
- Secondary bacterial peritonitis: Underlying disease factors associated with perforation (e.g., *H. pylori* causing PUD, diet/constipation causing diverticulitis, vascular disease predisposing to intestinal ischemia).

GENERAL PREVENTION
- SBP prophylaxis:
  – Prior SBP: Long-term norfloxacin PO daily (or trimethoprim/sulfamethoxazole [TMP/SMX]) (1)[A].
  – Cirrhosis and GI bleed: ceftriaxone 2 g IV daily or norfloxacin PO b.i.d. for a total of 7 days, IV during bleeding and PO if oral intake is tolerated (1)[A].
  – Cirrhosis and ascites with ascitic fluid protein <1.5 g/dL and either renal impairment (creatinine ≥1.2, BUN ≥25, or serum Na ≤130) or liver failure (Child score ≥9, bilirubin ≥3): Long-term norfloxacin PO daily (1,2)[A].
  – Avoid intermittent antibiotic use to avoid bacterial resistance (1,2)[C]

DIAGNOSIS

HISTORY
- SBP: History of liver disease. Fever, chills, nausea/vomiting, abdominal pain, altered mental status, GI bleed. 30% of patients asymptomatic (4)[C].
- Secondary bacterial peritonitis: History of perforation or abscess. Acute abdominal pain, nausea/vomiting, anorexia, altered mental status.
- Tertiary: History of recurrent peritonitis despite adequate treatment.

PHYSICAL EXAM
- Abdominal distention, ascites, abdominal wall guarding and rigidity, rebound tenderness, hypoactive/absent bowel sounds
- Fever, tachycardia, tachypnea

- Signs and symptoms are frequently absent, particularly in children and elderly patients (2)[B].

DIFFERENTIAL DIAGNOSIS
- Alcoholic hepatitis: Fever, leukocytosis, and abdominal pain can mimic SBP. Ascitic fluid will be sterile with normal PMN count.
- Abscess formation, ileus, volvulus, intussusception, mesenteric adenitis, pancreatitis, cholecystitis, malignancy, peritoneal carcinomatosis
- Ruptured ectopic pregnancy, tubo-ovarian abscess, PID, severe UTI and/or pyelonephritis
- Tuberculosis, pneumonia, MI, porphyria, SLE.

DIAGNOSTIC TESTS & INTERPRETATION
Initial Tests (lab, imaging)
Initial studies:
- Early diagnosis is essential to reducing mortality.
- Paracentesis should be performed in any patient with ascites, including suspected SBP. SBP is not a clinical diagnosis and requires paracentesis (1)[B].
- Perform paracentesis, blood, and urine cultures before administration of antibiotics. Ascitic fluid culture should be performed with aerobic and anaerobic blood culture bottles (1,4)[B].
- Ascitic fluid should be analyzed with culture, gram stain, cell count with differential, total protein, LDH, glucose, amylase, and albumin (1)[B].

Lab interpretation:
- Nonneutrocytic bacterascites: Positive ascites culture, ascitic fluid PMN <250 cells/mm^3.
- SBP: Bacterascites with ascitic fluid PMN >250 cells/mm^3. Typically monomicrobial. However, ascitic fluid culture is negative in up to 50% of patients with SBP (3,4)[A].
- Culture-negative neutrocytic ascites: Negative ascites culture, ascitic fluid PMN >250 cells/mm^3. Retain high suspicion of SBP due to high culture failure rate.
- Secondary peritonitis: PMN >250 cells/mm^3 on ascitic fluid analysis, with any of the following criteria:
  – Polymicrobial culture or 2 of the following: ascitic fluid total protein >1 g/dL, glucose <50 mg/dL, or lactate dehydrogenase (LDH) >225 mU/mL. Sensitivity for perforation 96%, sensitivity for nonperforation secondary peritonitis 50% (1,3)[B].
  – Secondary peritonitis with perforation is likely with alkaline phosphatase >240 U/l or carcinoembryonic antigen (CEA) >5 ng/mL, sensitivity 92% (1)[B].

Imaging:
- Criteria or clinical suspicion for secondary peritonitis necessitates emergent CT scan. CT diagnostic for secondary peritonitis in 85% (1)[B].
- Ultrasound/CT scan with enteral and IV contrast: Intra-abdominal mass, ascites, abscess, extravasation of contrast
- Abdominal or chest x-ray: Free air in peritoneal cavity, large/small bowel dilatation, intestinal wall edema

Follow-Up Tests & Special Considerations
- If asymptomatic bacterascites, recent antibiotic exposure, nosocomial atypical organism, or no clinical improvement, repeat paracentesis in 48 hours to resolution, defined as decrease in PMNs of 25% or negative cultures (4)[C].

- PMN count can be manual or automated (2)[B].

In hemorrhagic ascites, PMN count can be corrected by subtracting 1 PMN per 250 RBCs (2)[A].

- SBP caused by gram-positive cocci can result in ascitic PMN <250 cells/mm^3 (2)[A].
- Leukocyte esterase reagent strips (LERS) are not yet recommended for diagnosis of peritonitis, as are not yet confirmed in large trials (2)[C].
- Bacterial DNA, procalcitonin, lactoferrin, and C-reactive protein are not yet recommended diagnostics tests in peritonitis (2,3)[C].

TREATMENT

GENERAL MEASURES
- For SBP, control the effects of cirrhosis/ascites with salt restriction, spironolactone ± furosemide, albumin infusion after large volume paracentesis, and/or lactulose for encephalopathy (1)[A].
- Nonselective β-blockers may reduce long-term risk of SBP but can acutely cause systemic hypotension (1)[B].
- Limit use of PPIs to data-proven indications (1)[B].
- Avoid nephrotoxic medications (e.g., NSAIDs) or other renal insults (1)[C].

MEDICATION
- SBP empiric treatment:
  - Community-acquired SBP without recent β-lactam antibiotic use: Third generation cephalosporins, preferably cefotaxime, 2 g IV q8h × 5 days. Cefotaxime has excellent penetration into ascites (1)[A].
  - SBP in absence of previous quinolone use/prophylaxis, vomiting, shock, grade II or higher hepatic encephalopathy or serum creatinine >3 mg/dL: Ofloxacin 400 mg PO can be substituted for cefotaxime (1)[B].
    - Nosocomial SBP or recent β-lactam antibiotic use: Empiric therapy based on local susceptibility of patients with cirrhosis for resistant bacteria (e.g., ESBL Enterobacteriaceae, MRSA, etc.) (1)[B].
    - Bacterascites with PMN count <250 cells/mm^3 and symptoms: cefotaxime 2 g IV q8h while awaiting culture results (1)[B].
    - SBP with renal or hepatic impairment (serum creatinine >1 mg/dL, BUN >30 mg/dL or total bilirubin >4 mg/dL): Albumin 1.5 g/kg within 6 hours and 1 g/kg on day 3 (1)[B].
  - Alternative antibiotic regimens include fluoroquinolones (levofloxacin), piperacillin/tazobactam, or vancomycin (1,3)[C].
- Secondary bacterial peritonitis:
  - Empiric broad spectrum antibiotic coverage
- Tertiary treatment
  - If no unrepaired perforations or leaks, treatment of choice is conservative management. This includes antibiotics and early enteral nutrition to prevent atrophy and maintain immunocompetence (5)[B].

SURGERY/OTHER PROCEDURES
- SBP: Surgery is rarely indicated.
- Secondary bacterial peritonitis: Emergent surgical management is first-line treatment (2)[A]. Open laparotomy to repair the perforated viscus and eradicate infected material (6)[B]:
  - Peptic ulcer perforation—omental patch; perforated small intestine resection with primary anastomosis; perforated appendix-appendectomy; perforated colon-colectomy with ostomy formation
- Tertiary treatment
  - Reoperation for abdominal infection correlated with significant mortality (5).

IN-PATIENT CONSIDERATIONS
Admission Criteria/Initial Stabilization
- Initial stabilization: Patients who present with peritonitis can be severely hypovolemic. IV fluid resuscitation is critical to reduce the risk of secondary organ dysfunction. Obtain large-bore IV access. Nasogastric tube placement will prevent aspiration in patients with vomiting or GI bleeding.
- In patients with cardiogenic or septic shock, invasive monitoring required with goal-directed fluid therapy.
- SBP: Albumin administration to prevent renal failure and aid volume resuscitation (1)[B].
- Secondary bacterial peritonitis: Volume resuscitation titrated to improve tachycardia, hypotension, and urine output as needed
- Failure to respond to volume resuscitation necessitates consideration of vasoactive agents (e.g., norepinephrine and vasopressin).

ONGOING CARE

FOLLOW-UP RECOMMENDATIONS
Patient Monitoring
- Patients can be admitted to a close observation unit, for potential intensive monitoring. Hourly monitoring of vital signs and urinary output will aid in evaluating response to treatment.
- Normalization of vital signs with resolution of leukocytosis indicates improvement:
  - SBP: If follow-up paracentesis is performed after 48 hours to evaluate resolution, PMN decrease ≥25% is expected.
  - Development of leukopenia indicates immune exhaustion and poor prognosis.

DIET
- NPO, total parental nutrition as necessary
- Enteral feeding after return of bowel function
- Sodium restriction can reduce future ascites (2)[A]

PROGNOSIS
SBP:
- For inpatients with first episode of SBP, mortality ranges from 10–50% (2).
- Patients with prior SBP have 1-year recurrence rate of 40–70% and 1-year mortality of 31–93% (2,4).
- Strongest prognostic indicator is renal insufficiency. Other poor prognostic factors include nosocomial acquisition, elderly, poor liver function (high Child-Pugh-Turcotte or MELD scores), malnutrition, malignancy, peripheral leukopenia, and antibiotic resistance (2).
- Prognosis is improved if antibiotics are started early, prior to onset of shock or renal failure.
- Mortality rate approaches 80% if a patient with SBP receives unnecessary exploratory laparotomy (4).

Secondary bacterial peritonitis:
- Mortality approaches 100% if not treated surgically, especially if secondary to perforation (2,4).
- In-hospital mortality of treated patients is 67% (6).
- Prognosis is worse in perforated etiologies

COMPLICATIONS
- Renal failure, liver failure, encephalopathy, coagulopathy
- Secondary infection, iatrogenic infection, abscess, fistula formation, abdominal compartment syndrome
- Sepsis/septic shock, cardiovascular collapse, adrenal insufficiency, respiratory failure, ARDS

REFERENCES
1. Runyon, B. AASLD practice guideline—Management of adult patients with ascites due to cirrhosis: Update 2012. *Hepatology.* 2013;57:1651–1653.
2. Wiest R, Krag A, Gerbes A. Spontaneous bacterial peritonitis: Recent guidelines and beyond. *Gut* 2012;61:297–310.
3. Bajaj J, O'Leary J, Wong F, et al. Bacterial infections in end-stage liver disease: current challenges and future directions. *Gut.* 2012;61:1219–1225.
4. Alaniz C, Regal RE. Spontaneous bacterial peritonitis: A review of treatment options. *Pharm Therapeut.* 2009;34:204–210.
5. Panhofer P, Izay B, Riedl M, et al. Age, microbiology and prognostic scores help to differentiate between secondary and tertiary peritonitis. *Langenbecks Arch Surg.* 2009;394:265–271.
6. Soriano G, Castellote J, Alvarez C, et al. Secondary bacterial peritonitis in cirrhosis: A retrospective study of clinical and analytical characteristics, diagnosis and management. *J Hepatol.* 2010;52:7–9.

SEE ALSO

Appendicitis, Acute; Cirrhosis of the Liver; Diverticular Disease; Peptic Ulcer Disease

CODES

ICD10
- K65.0 Generalized (acute) peritonitis
- K65.2 Spontaneous bacterial peritonitis
- K65.8 Other peritonitis

CLINICAL PEARLS
- Maintain a high index of suspicion for SBP in cirrhotic patients with ascites. SBP occurs in pre-existing ascites and carries a high mortality, especially if presenting with GI bleed.
- Paracentesis is necessary to establish the diagnosis of SBP. Clinical suspicion is not adequate.
- Distinguishing SBP from secondary bacterial peritonitis is essential, as SBP treatment consists of antibiotic therapy, secondary bacterial peritonitis necessitates surgical intervention.
- Renal function is the most important prognostic indicator for SBP. Albumin administration decreases the incidence of renal failure and mortality after large-volume paracentesis and decreases mortality in SBP with renal or hepatic impairment.

PERSONALITY DISORDERS

Moshe S. Torem, MD, DLFAPA

 BASICS

DESCRIPTION

- Personality disorders (PDs) are a group of conditions, with onset at or before adolescence, characterized by enduring patterns of maladaptive and dysfunctional behavior that deviates markedly from one's culture and social environment, leading to functional impairment and distress to the individual, coworkers, and family.
  - These behaviors are perceived by patients to be "normal" and "right," and they have little insight as to their ownership, responsibility, and abnormal nature of these behaviors.
  - These conditions are classified based on the predominant symptoms and their severity.
- System(s) affected: Nervous/Psychiatric
- Synonym(s): Character disorder; Character pathology (1)

Geriatric Considerations
Coping with the stresses of aging is challenging.

Pediatric Considerations
A history of childhood neglect, abuse, and trauma is not uncommon.

Pregnancy Considerations
Pregnancy adds pressure in coping with the activities of daily living (ADLs).

EPIDEMIOLOGY
Prevalence
- General population: 15% (1)
- Cluster A: 5.7% (1)
- Cluster B: 6.0% (1)
- Cluster C: 9.1% (1)
- Outpatient psychiatric clinic: 3–30% (2)
- In male prisoners, the prevalence of antisocial personality disorder is ~60%.
- Predominant age: Starts in adolescence and early 20s and persists throughout patient's life
- Predominant sex: Male = Female; some personality disorders are more common in females, and others are more common in males.

ETIOLOGY AND PATHOPHYSIOLOGY
- Environmental and genetic factors (3)
- Criteria for a PD includes an enduring pattern of:
  - Inner experience and behavior that deviates markedly from the expectations of one's culture in ≥2 of the following areas: Cognition, affectivity, interpersonal functioning, or impulse control
  - Inflexibility and pervasiveness across a broad range of personal and social situations
  - Significant distress or impairment in social or occupational functioning
  - The pattern is stable and of long duration
  - The enduring pattern is not better explained as a manifestation of another psychiatric disorder
  - The enduring pattern is not attributable to the effects of a drug or a medical condition
- PDs are classified into 3 major clusters (1):
  - Cluster A: Eccentricism and oddness:
    - *Paranoid PD:* Unwarranted suspiciousness and distrust of others
    - *Schizoid PD:* Emotional, cold, or detached; socially isolated
    - *Schizotypal PD:* Eccentric behavior, odd belief system/perceptions, social isolation, and general suspiciousness

  - Cluster B: Dramatic, emotional, or erratic behavioral patterns:
    - *Antisocial PD:* Aggressive, impulsive, irritable, irresponsible, dishonest, deceitful
    - *Borderline PD:* Unstable interpersonal relationships, high impulsivity from early adulthood, intense fear of abandonment, mood swings, poor self-esteem, chronic boredom, and feelings of inner emptiness
    - *Histrionic PD:* Needs to be the center of attention, with self-dramatizing behaviors and attention seeking in a variety of contexts
    - *Narcissistic PD:* Grandiose sense of self-importance and preoccupation with fantasies of success, power, brilliance, beauty, or ideal love; lack of empathy for other people's pain or discomfort
  - Cluster C: Anxiety, excessive worry, fear, and unhealthy patterns of coping with emotions:
    - *Avoidant PD:* Social inhibition, feelings of inadequacy, hypersensitivity to negative evaluation, avoidance of occupational and interpersonal activities that involve the risk of criticism by others, views self as socially inept and personally unappealing or inferior to others
    - *Dependent PD:* Excessive need to be taken care of, leading to submissive and clinging behavior with fears of separation, avoids expressing disagreements with others due to fear of losing support and approval, usually seeks out strong and confident people as friends or spouses and feels more secure in such relationships
    - *Obsessive–compulsive PD:* Preoccupation with cleanliness, orderliness, perfectionism; preoccupation with excessive details, rules, lists, order, organization, and schedules to the extent that the major point of the activity is lost
  - Personality change due to another medical condition: It is a persistent personality disturbance that is caused by the physiological effects of a medical condition such as frontal lobe lesion, epilepsy, MS, Parkinson disease, lupus, etc.
  - Other specified *PD and unspecified PD:* A category provided for 2 situations: (i) the individual's personality pattern meets the general criteria for PD and traits of several PDs are present but the criteria for any specific PD are not met; (ii) the individual's personality pattern meets the general criteria for PD but the individual is considered to have a PD that is not included in *DSM-V* classification such as: passive-aggressive PD, depressive PD, masochistic PD, and dangerous and severe PD (1)

Genetics
Major character traits are inherited; others result from a combination of genetics and environment.

RISK FACTORS
- Positive family history
- Pregnancy risk factors:
  - Nutritional deprivation
  - Use of alcohol or drugs
  - Viral and bacterial infections
- Dysfunctional family with child abuse/neglect

COMMONLY ASSOCIATED CONDITIONS
Depression, other psychiatric disorders in patient and family members

 DIAGNOSIS

HISTORY
- Comprehensive interview and mental status examination
- Screen to rule out alcohol and drug abuse
- Interview of relatives and friends helpful in establishing an enduring pattern of behavior

DIAGNOSTIC TESTS & INTERPRETATION
Psychological testing (e.g., MMPI-II)
Initial Tests (lab, imaging)
- CBC
- Comprehensive metabolic panel
- Thyroid-stimulating hormone
- HIV
- Toxicology screen for substance abuse
Follow-Up Tests & Special Considerations
- EEG to rule out a chronic seizure disorder
- CT and MRI of the brain may be necessary in newly developed symptoms to rule out organic brain disease (e.g., frontal lobe tumor).

DIFFERENTIAL DIAGNOSIS
- Medical disorders with behavioral changes
- Other psychiatric disorders with similar symptoms:
  - In obsessive–compulsive disorder (OCD), symptoms are ego-dystonic (i.e., perceived as foreign and unwanted). In addition, OCD has a pattern of relapse and partial remission.
  - In obsessive–compulsive personality disorder (OCPD), symptoms are perceived as desirable behaviors (ego-syntonic) that the patient feels proud of and wants others to emulate. In addition, OCPD has a lifelong pattern (i.e., without significant relapse or remission).

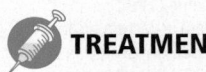 **TREATMENT**

Psychotherapy with family involvement is the foundation of treatment. No specific drugs are indicated to treat PDs; some medications can reduce the intensity, frequency, and dysfunctional nature of certain behaviors (4)[B].

GENERAL MEASURES
- Long-term psychotherapy and cognitive-behavioral therapy (5)
- Group therapy is helpful in the use of therapeutic confrontation and increasing one's awareness of and insight regarding the damaging effects of dysfunctional behavior patterns (6)[B].

MEDICATION
Medications are effective in the treatment of comorbid conditions such as anxiety and depression.

First Line

- Symptom management (7)[B]:
  - Minipsychosis (associated with paranoid, schizoid, borderline, and schizotypal PDs): Atypical antipsychotics: Risperidone (Risperdal), quetiapine (Seroquel), olanzapine (Zyprexa), ziprasidone (Geodon), aripiprazole (Abilify), asenapine (Saphris), lurasidone (Latuda); start with a low dose, gradually adjusting to the patient's needs
  - Anxiety: Anxiolytics (benzodiazepines, buspirone [BuSpar], and serotonin reuptake inhibitors)
  - Depressed mood: Antidepressants
  - Many patients with borderline PD respond well to small doses of atypical neuroleptics and mood stabilizers (8)[B].
- Precautions: Some atypical neuroleptic drugs may be associated with hyperglycemia and insulin-resistant metabolic syndrome.

Second Line

Mood stabilizers: Lithium carbonate, lamotrigine (Lamictal), carbamazepine (Tegretol, Equetro), and valproate (Depacon, Depakene, Depakote) (9)[B]

ISSUES FOR REFERRAL

- When psychiatric comorbidity of Axis I disorders is present (e.g., mood disorders, anxiety disorders, substance abuse, etc.)
- Suicidal ideation or attempts

ADDITIONAL THERAPIES

- Dialectical behavior therapy
- Psychoanalytic therapy
- Interactive psychotherapy
- Group therapy

IN-PATIENT CONSIDERATIONS

Admission Criteria/Initial Stabilization
Disorders with complications of suicide attempts

 ONGOING CARE

FOLLOW-UP RECOMMENDATIONS

Continue outpatient treatment, potentially long term

Patient Monitoring

- Regular physical exercise (e.g., 30–45 min/d, helps with stress and the ADLs)
- If substance abuse is suspected, check drug screens.
- Infrequent sessions with relatives or friends are helpful in monitoring behavioral progress.

DIET

Emphasize variety of healthy foods; avoid obesity

PATIENT EDUCATION

- Bibliotherapy and writing therapy, specific assignments, and watching certain movies to better understand the nature and origin of one's specific condition are helpful:
  - Kreger R. *The essential family guide to borderline personality disorder.* Center City, MN: Hazelden; 2008.
  - Mason PT, Kreger R. *Stop walking on eggshells.* Oakland, CA: New Harbinger Publishers; 2010.
- The movie *As Good as It Gets* illustrates someone with obsessive–compulsive behaviors and their impact on ADLs and relationships with family and friends.

- The movie series *The Godfather* includes several characters with antisocial PD and shows how this affects their interpersonal relationships and their own physical and mental health.
- The movie *What About Bob?* illustrates the challenges involved in treating certain patients with a borderline PD, especially in the management of boundaries in the doctor–patient relationship.
- The movie *A Streetcar Named Desire* illustrates an example of a woman with a histrionic PD.
- The movie *Wall Street* illustrates an example of a person with a narcissistic PD.
- The movie *The Caine Mutiny* illustrates an example of a person with a paranoid PD.
- The movie *Four Weddings and a Funeral* illustrates an example of a person with an avoidant PD.

PROGNOSIS

PDs are enduring patterns of behavior throughout one's lifetime and are not readily responsive to treatment.

COMPLICATIONS

- Disruptive family life with frequent divorces and separations, alcoholism, substance abuse, and drug addiction
- Disruptive behaviors in the workplace may cause absenteeism and loss of productivity.
- Violation of the law and disregard for the concerns and rights of others

REFERENCES

1. American Psychiatric Association (APA). *Diagnostic and statistical manual*, 5th ed. Arlington, VA: American Psychiatric Association Press; 2013:645–684.
2. Angstman K, Rasmussen NH. Personality disorders: Review and clinical application in daily practice. *Am Fam Physician.* 2011;84;1253–1260.
3. Reichborn-Kjennerud T. Genetics of personality disorders. *Clin Lab Med.* 2010;30:893–910.
4. Hadjipavlou G. Promising psychotherapies for personality disorders. *Can J Psychiatry.* 2010;55:202–210.
5. Clarkin JE. An integrated approach to psychotherapy techniques for patients with personality disorder. *J Pers Disord.* 2012;26:43–62.
6. Livesley WJ. Integrated treatment: A conceptual framework for an evidence-based approach to the treatment of personality disorder. *J Pers Disord.* 2012;26:17–42.
7. Ripoll LH, Triebwasser J, Siever LJ. Evidence-based pharmacotherapy for personality disorders. *Focus.* 2013;11:225–248.
8. Ripoll LH. Clinical psychopharmacology of borderline personality disorder: An update on the available evidence in light of the Diagnostic and Statistical Manual of Mental Disorders—5. *Curr Opin Psychiatry.* 2012;25:52–58.
9. Lieb K. Pharmacotherapy for borderline personality disorder: Cochrane systematic review of randomised trials. *Br J Psychiatry.* 2010;196:4–12.

ADDITIONAL READING

- Borschmann R, Henderson C, Hogg J, et al. Crisis interventions for people with borderline personality disorder. *Cochrane Database Syst Rev.* 2012;6:CD009353.
- Cosci F. Assessment of personality in psychosomatic medicine: Current concepts. *Adv Psychosom Med.* 2012;32:133–159.
- Feurino L, Silk KR. State of the art in the pharmacologic treatment of borderline personality disorder. *Curr Psychiatry Rep.* 2011;13:69–75.
- Kealy D, Ogrodniczuk JS. Narcissistic interpersonal problems in clinical practice. *Harv Rev Psychiatry.* 2011;19:290–301.
- Leichsenring F, Leibing E, Kruse J, et al. Borderline personality disorder. *Lancet.* 2011;377:74–84.
- Mauchnik J, Schmahl C. The latest neuroimaging findings in borderline personality disorder. *Curr Psychiatry Rep.* 2010;12:46–55.
- Molina JD, López-Muñoz F, Stein DJ, et al. Borderline personality disorder: A review and reformulation from evolutionary theory. *Med Hypotheses.* 2009;73:382–386.
- Ronningstam E. Narcissistic personality disorder: A current review. *Curr Psychiatry Rep.* 2010;12:68–75.
- Stoffers J, Völlm BA, Rücker G, et al. Pharmacological interventions for borderline personality disorder. *Cochrane Database Syst Rev.* 2010;6:CD005653.

 SEE ALSO

Obsessive–Compulsive Disorder

 CODES

ICD10

- F60.0 Paranoid personality disorder
- F60.1 Schizoid personality disorder
- F60.9 Personality disorder, unspecified

CLINICAL PEARLS

- PDs are enduring patterns of behavior throughout one's lifetime and are not readily responsive to treatment.
- No specific drugs treat PDs; however, specific medications can reduce the intensity, frequency, and dysfunctional nature of certain behaviors, thoughts, and feelings.
- Most patients with a PD require a well-trained and experienced mental health professional.
- A stable, trustful alliance with the patient is the foundation for any therapeutic progress.

PERTUSSIS

Mary Cataletto, MD • Margaret McCormick, MS, RN

 BASICS

Highly contagious disease

DESCRIPTION
- Human host: Adults most common reservoir
- Can affect all ages
- Worldwide distribution
- May be endemic or epidemic with outbreaks every 3–5 years
- Seasonality: Can occur year round; peaks late summer–autumn
- Transmission: Person to person via aerosolizes respiratory droplets
- Effective vaccine available but neither vaccine nor infection confer lifelong or 100% immunity
- System(s) Affected: Respiratory
- Synonym(s): Whooping cough

EPIDEMIOLOGY
Incidence
- Worldwide: Estimated 48.5 million cases and nearly 295,000 deaths/year (1,2)
- US: 27,550 cases in 2010; 18,719 in 2011(1)

ETIOLOGY AND PATHOPHYSIOLOGY
- Toxin mediated
- Infectious process with predilection for ciliated respiratory epithelium
- *Bordetella pertussis* (responsible for ~95% of cases)
- *B. parapertussis*

RISK FACTORS
- Exposure to a confirmed case
- Non- or underimmunized infants and children
- Pregnancy
- Premature birth
- Chronic lung disease
- Immunodeficiency (e.g., AIDS)

GENERAL PREVENTION
- Public health measures:
  - Surveillance activities
  - Prevention programs
  - Outbreak management
- Care of exposed persons:
  - Household and close contacts
  - Childcare workers
  - Health care workers
- Immunization:
  - Vaccine products
  - Boosters
- In 2011, the CDC 2011 CDC and Prevention's Advisory Committee on Immunization Practices recommends 1 Tdap (tetanus toxoid, reduced diphtheria toxoid and acellular pertussis) vaccination for all adults age 19 years and to provide increased herd immunity.

Pediatric Considerations
- Primary immunization series against pertussis followed by boosters (1)
- Adult immunization and cocooning (3) are alternative strategies to protect unimmunized infants

Pregnancy Considerations

ALERT
2011 CDC and Prevention's Advisory Committee on Immunization Practices approved new recommendations permitting Tdap (tetanus toxoid, reduced diphtheria toxoid and acellular pertussis) vaccine during pregnancy, preferably during late second (>20 weeks) or 3rd trimester in women who previously have not received Tdap (4)

Geriatric Considerations
The incidence of pertussis in individuals age 50 and older has increased between 2006 and 2010 (5)

COMMONLY ASSOCIATED CONDITIONS
- Apnea
- Secondary bacterial pneumonia
- Sinusitis
- Seizures
- Encephalopathy
- Urinary incontinence

 DIAGNOSIS

HISTORY
- Exposure to pertussis
- Incubation period 7–10 days (range 5–21 days)
- Classic symptoms are more common in adults and adolescents and include paroxysmal cough, posttussive whoop and/or vomiting
- Infants with pertussis may present with apnea or sudden death (6,7)

PHYSICAL EXAM
- Classic pertussis has 3 phases, which occur over 6–10 weeks:
  - Catarrhal phase: Rhinorrhea, mild cough, low grade fever
  - Paroxysmal phase: Cough occurs in bursts, with increased intensity and frequency, often followed by an inspiratory whoop and/or posttussive vomiting
  - Convalescent phase: Coughing paroxysms decrease in frequency and intensity
- In the absence of paroxysms or complications, the physical exam may be normal.

ALERT
Infants <6 months of age may have atypical presentations.

DIFFERENTIAL DIAGNOSIS
- *Bordetella parapertussis*
- *Mycoplasma pneumonia*
- *Chlamydia trachomatis*
- *Chlamydophilia pneumonia*
- *Bordetella bronchiseptica*
- Respiratory syncytial virus
- Adenovirus

DIAGNOSTIC TESTS & INTERPRETATION
Initial Tests (lab, imaging)
- Nasopharyngeal Culture (gold standard): 100% specific and permits strain identification and antimicrobial resistance testing. Collect secretions from the back of the throat through the nose, using a Dacron or calcium alginate swab or syringe filled with saline. For best results collect specimen during the first 2 weeks of cough—sensitivity decreases after 2 weeks.
- Polymerase chain reaction (PCR) Assays: Frequently used because they are quick and sensitive. Specificity may vary between assays and must be interpreted within clinical context and local pertussis epidemiology. CDC "Best Practice" guidelines exist for PCR assays although they have not yet received FDA approval. 6 accurate results can be obtained during the first 3 weeks from onset of cough. Dacron swabs should be used as calcium alginate swabs are inhibitory to PCR.
- Serology: Available commercially; however there is no FDA-approved test or standardization (7).
  - The Centers for Disease Control (CDC) uses single point serology obtained between 2 and 8 weeks following cough onset when titers are expected to be at their peak.

Follow-Up Tests & Special Considerations
- Evaluation and follow-up for associated conditions and complications
- Chest radiograph (2 views) to evaluate for the presence of pneumonia.
- EEG/Neuroimaging may be considered in infant with seizures or acute life-threatening events (ALTEs).
- Infants <1 month of age who are treated with macrolides should be monitored for the possible development of hypertrophic pyloric stenosis.

TREATMENT

GENERAL MEASURES
Waiting rooms, during transport and procedures: Patients with suspected pertussis should wear masks (7).

MEDICATION
Pertussis illness may be less severe if antibiotics are started early, i.e. before the onset of paroxysms or during the catarrhal phase (1,2). Antibiotics can also help to prevent the spread of pertussis to close contacts and is necessary for stopping the spread of pertussis.

First Line
- For children > 1 year of age through adulthood, TREAT WITHIN 3 WEEKS OF COUGH ONSET
- For infants <1 year of age, pregnant women, especially those near term, TREAT WITHIN 6 WEEKS OF COUGH ONSET
  - AZITHROMYCIN
  - CLARITHROMYCIN
  - ERYTHROMYCIN

ALERT
Risk of infantile hypertrophic pyloric stenosis has been associated with the use of macrolides in infants <1 month of age. Consultation and monitoring are recommended (8).

ALERT
Due to reports of fatal cardiac dysrhythmias with azithromycin, consider alternate drugs in the elderly and in those with cardiovascular disease.

Second Line
TRIMETHOPRIM SULFAMETHOXAZOLE (for persons >2 months of age) if:
- They cannot tolerate macrolides OR
- They are infected with a macrolide resistant strain

ALERT
- TMP-SMX is contraindicated in infants <2 months of age.
- Clarithromycin is not recommended in infants <1 month of age

ISSUES FOR REFERRAL
Evaluation and treatment of infants <6 months of age, especially those born prematurely, who are unimmunized and those who require hospitalization.

ADDITIONAL THERAPIES
Symptomatic treatment of the cough in pertussis (e.g., corticosteroids, B2 adrenergic agonists, pertussis-specific immunoglobulin, antihistamine and leukotriene receptor antagonist) have not shown consistent benefit (2).

IN-PATIENT CONSIDERATIONS
Admission Criteria/Initial Stabilization
- Small, frequent meals may be necessary to ensure adequate nutrition
- Correct fluid and electrolyte abnormalities
- Infants may require IV fluids

IV Fluids
Indicated for dehydration and when oral fluids are either contraindicated or poorly tolerated.

Nursing
- In addition to standard precautions, hospitalized patients should be isolated with respiratory precautions for 5 days after the initiation of effective antibiotic treatment; for 3 weeks after onset of paroxysms in older patients if antibiotics are not used.
- Gentle suctioning of nasal secretions
- Avoid stimuli that trigger paroxysms.
- Respiratory monitoring including pulse oximetry
- Educate each family about the importance of immunizations.
- Discuss chemoprophylaxis with each family

Discharge Criteria
- Clinically stable
- Able to tolerate oral feedings

ONGOING CARE

Supportive
FOLLOW-UP RECOMMENDATIONS
- Monitor infants who received EES or azithromycin for pyloric stenosis
- Neurologic and/or pulmonary follow-up as necessary

Patient Monitoring
ICU care may be necessary for severely ill or compromised patients

DIET
IV fluids/nutrition may be required to treat dehydration or supplement poor oral intake

PATIENT EDUCATION
- American Academy of Pediatrics http://www.aap.org
- Centers for Disease Control http://www.cdc.gov

PROGNOSIS
- Complete recovery in most cases
- Most severe morbidity and highest mortality in infants <6 months of age

COMPLICATIONS
- Highest and most severe in infants. May include: Apnea, cyanosis, and sudden death.
- In children: May include conjunctival hemorrhage, inguinal hernia, pneumonia and seizures.
- More frequent in adults than adolescents: May include sinusitis, otitis media, pneumonia, weight loss, fainting, rib fracture, urinary incontinence, seizures, encephalopathy, and death

REFERENCES
1. CDC. Pertussis (Whooping Cough). Available at: http://www.cdc.gov/pertussis.
2. Bettiol, S, Wang, K, Thompson, MJ, et al, Symptomatic treatment of the cough in whooping cough, *Cochrane Database Syst Rev.* 2012;5: CD003257.
3. Wiley, KE, Zuo, Y, Macartney, KK, McIntyre, PB, Sources of pertussis infection in young infants: A review of key evidence informing targeting of the cocoon strategy, *Vaccine.* 2013;31: 618–625.
4. American College of Obstetrics and Gynecology. Committee Opinion No 521, Update on Immunizations and Pregnancy. *Obstet Gynecol.* 2012;19:690–691.
5. Balderston-McGuiness C, Hill J, Fonseca E, et al. The disease burden of pertussis in adults 50 years old and older in the United States: A retrospective study. *BMC Infect Dis.* 2013;13:32.
6. CDC. Best Practices for Healthcare Professionals on the use of Polymerase Chain Reaction (PCR) for diagnosing pertussis 2011. Atlanta, GA: CDC; 2011.
7. Snyder J, Fisher D. Pertussis in childhood. *Pediatr Rev.* 2012;33(9):412–421.
8. *American Academy of Pediatrics, Red Book Committee: 2012 Report of the Committee on Infectious Diseases*, Pickering, LK, Ed. 29th edition Elk Grove Village, Il: American Academy of Pediatrics; 2012.

CODES

ICD10
- A37.10 Whooping cough due to Bordetella parapertussis w/o pneumonia
- A37.80 Whooping cough due to other Bordetella species w/o pneumonia
- A37.90 Whooping cough, unspecified species without pneumonia

CLINICAL PEARLS
- Pertussis is a highly contagious infection.
- A high index of suspicion is needed. During the primary or catarrhal phase, the presentation may be non specific.
- Immunization (Primary series & boosters), isolation and early treatment of affected cases as well as chemoprophylaxis are key components to controlling the spread of pertussis.

PHARYNGITIS

Jimmy J. Brown, MD • Brian Ho, MD

 BASICS

DESCRIPTION
- Acute or chronic Inflammation of the pharynx
- Most commonly caused by acute viral infection
- Group A *streptococcus* pharyngitis is a common clinical focus due to its potential for preventable rheumatic sequelae
- Synonym(s): Sore throat; Tonsillitis; Strep throat
- Generally infection mediated, but can be due to caustic injury, allergies, GERD, smoking, endotracheal intubation, vocal abuse

EPIDEMIOLOGY
- Estimated 30 million cases diagnosed yearly
- 12–25% of all sore throats are thought to prompt visits to physicians or the care provider.
- All age groups, but some etiologies may predilect specific age groups
- No gender predilection

Incidence
- Respiratory infections account for 38% of the 129 million physician visits per year in the US. This accounts for ~200 visits to a physician per 1,000 population in the US annually (1)
- Most commonly viral (40–60%)
- Group A *streptococcus* is the most common bacterial cause of acute pharyngitis, accounting for ~15–30% and 5–10% of bacterial pharyngitis cases in children/adults, respectively.
- Rheumatic fever is rare in the US; 112 cases reported to the CDC in 1994 (the last year this was a reportable disease) due to the preponderance of early antibiotic intervention.

Pediatric Considerations
Rheumatic fever has its greatest incidence in children aged 5–18 years, but is currently a rare sequel of streptococcal pharyngitis in the US.

ETIOLOGY AND PATHOPHYSIOLOGY
- Acute, viral: (lower grade fever)
  - Rhinovirus
  - Adenovirus (associated with conjunctivitis)
  - Parainfluenza virus
  - Coxsackievirus (hand-foot-mouth disease)
  - Coronavirus
  - Echovirus
  - *Herpes simplex* virus (vesicular lesions)
  - Epstein-Barr virus (EBV/mononucleosis)
  - Cytomegalovirus
  - HIV
- Acute, bacterial (higher fevers):
  - Group A β-hemolytic streptococci <10% of adult pharyngitis
  - *Neisseria gonorrhoeae*
  - *Corynebacterium diphtheriae* (diphtheria)
  - *Haemophilus influenzae*
  - *Moraxella (Branhamella) catarrhalis*
  - Groups C and G *streptococcus*, rarely
- Chronic:
  - More likely noninfectious
  - Chemical irritation (GERD)
  - Smoking
  - Neoplasms
  - Vasculitis
  - Radiation changes

Genetics
Patients with a positive family history of rheumatic fever have a higher risk of rheumatic sequelae following an untreated group A β-hemolytic streptococcal infection.

RISK FACTORS
- Epidemics of group A β-hemolytic streptococcal disease occurrence.
- Age (i.e., younger patients are more susceptible)
- Family history
- Living at close quarters, such as in military recruits
- Immunosuppression
- Fatigue
- Smoking
- Oral sex
- Diabetes mellitus
- Recent illness (secondary postviral bacterial infection)
- Chronic colonization of bacteria in tonsils/adenoids bed

GENERAL PREVENTION
Avoid contact with infectious patients (viral and bacterial)

 DIAGNOSIS

- Group A (β-hemolytic) streptococcus is almost always not associated with cough
- Modified Centor clinical prediction rule for group A streptococcal infection (2)[A]:
  - +1 point: Tonsillar exudates
  - +1 point: Tender anterior chain cervical adenopathy
  - +1 point: Fever by history
  - +1 point: Age <15 years
  - 0 point: Age 15–45 years
  - –1 point: Age >45 years
  - –1 point: Cough
- Scoring:
  - If 3–4 points, positive predictive value (PPV) of ~80%; treat empirically
  - If 2 points, PPV of ~50%, rapid strep antigen + culture; treat if either positive
  - If 1 point, PPV <50%, positive rapid strep. antigen or culture likely false-positive finding
  - If 0 or –1 point, PPV <20%; do not test; close follow up as needed
- Coryza (nasal congestion), hoarseness, cough, diarrhea, conjunctivitis, or rash highly suggestive of viral cause.

HISTORY
- Sore throat (odynophagia)
- Cough
- Hoarseness
- Fever
- Anorexia
- Chills
- Malaise
- Contacts with similar symptoms or diagnosed infection

PHYSICAL EXAM
- Enlarged tonsils (tonsillar exudate or possible peritonsillar abscess)
- Pharyngeal erythema
- Tonsillar/soft palate petechiae (suggest EBV)
- Cervical adenopathy
- Fever
- Pharyngeal ulcers (CMV, HIV, Crohn's, Other autoimmune vasculitides)
- Scarlet fever rash: Punctate erythematous macules with reddened flexor creases and circumoral pallor (suggestive of streptococcal pharyngitis)
- Gray oral pseudomembrane found in diphtheria and, occasionally, infectious mononucleosis
- Characteristic erythematous-based clear vesicles are found in herpes simplex virus infection.
- Conjunctivitis is found more commonly with adenovirus infections.

DIFFERENTIAL DIAGNOSIS
- Viral syndrome
- Streptococcal Infection
- Allergic rhinitis
- GERD
- Malignancy (lymphoma or squamous cell carcinoma)
- Irritants/chemicals
- Atypical bacterial (e.g., gonococcal, syphilis, pertussis, diphtheria)
- Oral candidiasis (patients typically complain mostly of dysphagia)

DIAGNOSTIC TESTS & INTERPRETATION
- Testing, if performed, is usually for the presence of group A β-hemolytic streptococci (GAS). Options include:
  - Rapid screening for streptococci can be done from throat swab with antigen agglutination kits; 5–10% false-negative results
  - Blood agar throat culture from swab. Bacitracin disk sensitivity of hemolytic colonies suggests group A streptococci
  - Antistreptolysin-O (carrier state suspected if positive culture, and unchanged antistreptolysin-O [ASO] titers).
- Special tests usually are done only if history is suggestive of a different diagnosis.
- Screening for gonococcal infection requires warm Thayer-Martin plate or antigen testing
- Viruses can be cultured in special media(e.g., herpes simplex), but rarely indicated
- Mono spot test for EBV
- Recent American Heart Association scientific statement is "some form of microbiological confirmation, with either a throat culture or a rapid antigen detection test, is required for the diagnosis of GAS pharyngitis" (3).

Test Interpretation
Culture of pathogens may help to identify which is causative, but are not cost-effective or influence outcome. Cultures should be considered when patients fail primary treatment.

TREATMENT

- Clinicians should remember that acute pharyngitis is caused considerably more often by viruses rather than by bacteria. 1st-line therapy is conservative management.
- Empirical therapy leads to overuse of antibiotics in adults, by some reports (4).
- Streptococcal infections should be treated to prevent rheumatic fever. Each episode should be documented to support need for patient to undergo tonsillectomy/adenoidectomy.
- Ulcers related to autoimmune diseases usually require steroids systemically or steroid injections into ulcers.
- HIV-related ulcers are due to decreasing counts of CD4 and respond when patient's CD4 titers increase.
- Guidelines in 2000, updated by American Academy of Otolaryngology, state tonsillectomy is indicated for 3 or more strep positive infections per year or if a patient misses >2 weeks of school/work per year.
- Conservative measures:
  – Salt water gargles
  – Viscous lidocaine 2% 5–10 mL PO q4h swish/spit
  – Acetaminophen 15–20 mg/kg (pediatric) q4h for analgesia. In adults they should not exceed >4 g of acetaminophen in 24 hours
  – Anesthetic lozenges
  – Cool-mist humidifier
  – PO or IV fluid resuscitation

MEDICATION
First Line
For streptococcal pharyngitis, penicillin is the standard therapy. Only penicillin has been proven to prevent rheumatic fever. Penicillin courses <10 days are not as effective (5)[A]. Other antibiotics use streptococcal eradication as a proxy of effectiveness due to the low incidence of rheumatic fever and the ethics of further controlled studies (6)[A]:

- Penicillin V 250 mg PO t.i.d. or 500 mg b.i.d. (25–50 mg/kg/d) (5)[A] or
- Amoxicillin 20 mg/kg up to 750 mg divided t.i.d. Use with caution if diagnosis is unclear because amoxicillin and *EBV infection may induce rash*.
- For patients allergic to penicillin, erythromycin ethylsuccinate 300–400 mg PO t.i.d. (30 mg/kg/d) (5)[B] or
- Cephalexin 250 mg PO t.i.d. (30 mg/kg/d) (5)[C]
- Clindamycin 300 mg PO q6h

Second Line
- Penicillin is the most documented treatment to prevent rheumatic sequelae, but cephalosporins have a lower rate of antimicrobial failure.
- Other cephalosporins are generally effective for streptococcal pharyngitis, but more expensive than cephalexin.
- May also consider the newer macrolides, azithromycin and clarithromycin; while effective against streptococcal pharyngitis, they are more expensive.
- Macrolide-resistant strains of GAS are currently <10% in the US, but more prevalent worldwide.
- If tonsillar hypertrophy, may consider short steroid burst in addition to antibiotic therapy.

 ONGOING CARE

FOLLOW-UP RECOMMENDATIONS
- Patient must complete antibiotic course for strep, regardless of symptom response.
- Patients may consider themselves noninfectious after 24 hours of antibiotic therapy.
- Follow-up culture is not recommended.

DIET
As tolerated. Encourage the consumption of fluids.

PROGNOSIS
- Streptococcal pharyngeal infection runs a 5–7-day course with peak fever at 2–3 days.
- Symptoms will resolve spontaneously without treatment, but rheumatic complications are still possible.

COMPLICATIONS
- Rheumatic fever (e.g., carditis, valve disease, arthritis)
- Poststreptococcal glomerulonephritis
- Peritonsillar abscess: also called Quinsy tonsillitis; considered a clinical diagnosis and does not require imaging. Will generally require percutaneous or more commonly transoral drainage. Surgery may also involve a so-called Quinsy tonsillectomy.
- Acute airway compromise (rare) can typically be bypassed with nasal trumpets (requires consult to anesthesia/otolaryngology).

REFERENCES

1. Armstrong GL, Pinner RW. Outpatient visits for infectious diseases in the United States, 1980 through 1996. *Arch Intern Med*. 1999;159: 2531–2536.
2. McIsaac WJ, Kellner JD, Aufricht P, et al. Empirical validation of guidelines for the management of pharyngitis in children and adults. *JAMA*. 2004; 291:1587–1595.
3. Gerber MA, Baltimore RS, Eaton CB, et al. Prevention of rheumatic fever and diagnosis and treatment of acute streptococcal pharyngitis. A scientific statement from the American Heart Association Rheumatic Fever, Endocarditis, and Kawasaki Disease Committee of the Council on Cardiovascular Disease in the Young, the Interdisciplinary Council on Functional Genomics and Translational Biology, and the Interdisciplinary Council on Quality of Care and Outcomes Research. *Circulation*. 2009;119:1541–1551.
4. Humair JP, Revaz SA, Bovier P, et al. Management of acute pharyngitis in adults: Reliability of rapid streptococcal tests and clinical findings. *Arch Intern Med*. 2006;166:640–644.
5. Denny FW. Prevention of rheumatic fever. Treatment of the preceding streptococcic infection. *JAMA*. 1950;143:151–153.
6. Spinks A, Glasziou PP, Del Mar CB. Antibiotics for sore throat. *Cochrane Database Syst Rev*. 2011;9: CD00023.

ADDITIONAL READING

Pichichero ME, Cohen R. Shortened course of antibiotic therapy for acute otitis media, sinusitis and tonsillopharyngitis. *Pediatr Infect Dis*. 1997;16: 680–695.

 SEE ALSO

- Herpes simplex; Mononucleosis; Rheumatic fever
- Algorithm: Pharyngitis

 CODES

ICD10
- J02.0 Streptococcal pharyngitis
- J02.9 Acute pharyngitis, unspecified
- J03.00 Acute streptococcal tonsillitis, unspecified

CLINICAL PEARLS

- Most cases of pharyngitis are viral.
- Risk of missed case of group A β-hemolytic strep is rheumatic fever, a very rare complication (112 cases reported to CDC in 1994; last year it was reported)
- Use Modified Centor Score to guide testing and treatment.
- Presence of coryza (nasal congestion), hoarseness, cough, diarrhea, conjunctivitis, or viral rash highly suggests viral cause.

PHEOCHROMOCYTOMA

Maya Campara, PharmD, BCPS • Anna Porter, MD

 BASICS

DESCRIPTION
- A pheochromocytoma is a rare neuroendocrine tumor arising from the adrenal or extra-adrenal chromaffin tissue and, less commonly, the sympathetic ganglia.
- These tumors are catecholamine-producing: Norepinephrine (NE) > epinephrine (EPI) >>> dopamine (DA).
- System(s) affected: Endocrine; Nervous; Cardiovascular
- Synonym(s): Chromaffin tumors; Paragangliomas

EPIDEMIOLOGY
Incidence
- 500–1,000 cases per year diagnosed in the US
- <0.2% of people with severe hypertension (HTN)

Prevalence
- 1:6,500–1:2,500 in Western countries
- Affects all genders and ages; usually diagnosed in 4th–5th decades of life, familial cases diagnosed 1 decade earlier

ETIOLOGY AND PATHOPHYSIOLOGY
Pheochromocytoma is a tumor that releases catecholamines into the circulation. Catecholamines bind to adrenergic receptors to produce various effects that could induce severe or lethal cardiovascular and cerebrovascular complications:
- Stimulation of α_1 receptors (NE > EPI) causes smooth muscle constriction resulting in high BP (arteriolar vasoconstriction).
- Stimulation of α_2 receptors (EPI > NE) causes smooth muscle contraction, cardiac muscle relaxation, and inhibition of hormones, such as insulin, resulting in elevated blood glucose levels.
- Stimulation of β_1 receptors (EPI = NE) causes heart muscle contraction resulting in increased heart rate.
- Stimulation of β_2 receptors (EPI >> NE) causes smooth muscle relaxation.
- In 80% of cases, it is a sporadic disease of unknown etiology.
- In 20% of cases, it has familial origin and is a component of 1 of the following 4 autosomal-dominant diseases:
  – Multiple endocrine neoplasia type 2 (MEN-2)
  – Von Hippel-Lindau syndrome (VHL)
  – Hereditary paraganglioma syndrome (PGL)
  – Neurofibromatosis type 1 (NF-1)
- Tumor location:
  – 80% are solitary and unilateral.
  – 20% are divided between bilateral lesions and extra-adrenal masses (organ of Zuckerkandl, neck, mediastinum, abdomen, pelvis)

Genetics
Genetic testing is recommended; genes identified in the pathogenesis:
- Rearranged during transfection (*RET*) proto-oncogene
- Von Hippel-Lindau disease tumor suppressor gene (*VHL*)
- Neurofibromatosis type 1 tumor suppressor gene (*NH-1*)
- Genes encoding 4 succinate dehydrogenase complex (*SDH*) subunits
- Gene encoding the enzyme responsible for flavination of the SDHA subunit
- Tumor suppressor *TMEM127* gene

RISK FACTORS
- Familial pheochromocytoma
- Familial paraganglioma
- MEN-2
- VHL disease
- von Recklinghausen NF-1

COMMONLY ASSOCIATED CONDITIONS
- Multiple endocrine neoplasia type IIA (medullary thyroid carcinoma and primary hyperparathyroidism)
- Multiple endocrine neoplasia type IIB (medullary thyroid carcinoma and mucosal neuromas)
- VHL disease (retinal angiomas, cerebellar hemangioblastomas, renal cysts, carcinomas, pancreatic cysts, epididymal cystadenomas)
- NF-1
- Sturge-Weber syndrome
- Tuberous sclerosis
- Carney syndrome (gastric epithelioid leiomyosarcoma, pulmonary chondroma, extra-adrenal paraganglioma)
- Familial paraganglioma
- Ataxia-telangiectasia
- Renal artery stenosis

Dx DIAGNOSIS

HISTORY
- Classic "triad" of symptoms includes headache, palpitations, and diaphoresis.
- 5 P's mnemonic:
  – Paroxysmal spells
  – Pressure: Sudden increase in BP
  – Pain: Headache, chest, abdominal pain
  – Perspiration (profuse sweating common in children)
  – Palpitations and pallor
- Additional symptoms: Constipation, tremor, weight loss, anxiety, paresthesias, flushing, shortness of breath, nausea/vomiting
- Sudden death may occur in patients with an undiagnosed tumor who undergo surgery or biopsy due to lethal hypertensive crises and multiorgan failure.
- Dopamine-secreting pheochromocytomas lack the classic presentation of catecholamine excess.

PHYSICAL EXAM
- HTN: Paroxysmal in 50% of affected patients; most common clinical sign
- Tachyarrhythmias
- Orthostatic hypotension
- Café au lait spots and Lisch nodules of the eye (*in neurofibromatosis*)
- Grades II–IV retinopathy
- Transient ischemic attacks/stroke
- Cardiomyopathy
- GI crisis
- Diabetes mellitus/insipidus
- Fever
- Hypercalcemia
- Erythrocytosis

DIFFERENTIAL DIAGNOSIS
- Labile essential HTN
- Anxiety and panic attacks
- Paroxysmal cardiac arrhythmia
- Thyrotoxicosis
- Menopausal syndrome
- Hypoglycemia
- Withdrawal of adrenergic-inhibiting medications
- Angina
- Hyperventilation
- Migraine headache
- Amphetamine or cocaine use
- Sympathomimetic ingestion/overdose

DIAGNOSTIC TESTS & INTERPRETATION
Initial Tests (lab, imaging)
Diagnosis is typically confirmed by measurements of urine catecholamines and their metabolites (NE/EPI → [nor]metanephrine, NE/EPI → vanillylmandelic acid (VMA), dopamine → homovanillic acid). Their amount in the urine correlates with tumor size.
- Elevated metanephrine and catecholamines in 24-hour urine collection (sensitivity, 90%; specificity, 98%):
  – A positive test is considered to be a 2-fold elevation above the upper limit of normal in urine.
- Elevated plasma fractionated metanephrine (sensitivity, 97%; specificity, 85%): (1)[A]:
  – Measured while patient is at rest
  – Pheochromocytoma cannot be excluded if normal catecholamine values are obtained when the patient is normotensive and asymptomatic (record BP at time of blood draw) (1)[A].
- Elevated VMA in 24-hour urine collection (sensitivity, 64%; specificity, 95%)
- Dopamine-secreting pheochromocytomas are often missed if urine or plasma dopamine is not included as part of the catecholamine screening. Urine and plasma dopamine are the most widely used methods in the diagnosis of dopamine-secreting tumors.
- Proceed with imaging after positive laboratory evaluation:
  – Abdominal imaging with MRI/CT have similar specificity and sensitivity.
  – If CT/MRI is negative, but clinical suspicion is high, imaging can be done with 123-I-metaiodobenzylguanidine (MIBG) scan/pentetreotide scan.

Follow-Up Tests & Special Considerations
- Drugs that may increase measured levels of catecholamines and metabolites should be discontinued at least 2 weeks before assessment:
  - Tricyclic antidepressants
  - Monoamine oxidase inhibitors (MAOIs)
  - Levodopa, methyldopa
  - Drugs containing adrenergic receptor agonists (e.g., decongestants)
  - Amphetamines
  - Cocaine
  - Buspirone and most psychoactive agents (but not SSRIs)
  - Prochlorperazine
  - Reserpine
  - Withdrawal from clonidine and other drugs
  - Ethanol
  - Acetaminophen (may increase measured levels of fractionated plasma metanephrine in some assays)
- Drugs that may decrease measured levels of catecholamines and metabolites:
  - Reserpine
  - Centrally acting α_2 receptor agonists (dexmedetomidine, clonidine, tizanidine, guanfacine)
- Conditions that may alter lab results include major physical stress due to surgery, stroke, myocardial infarction, congestive heart failure, and so forth.

Diagnostic Procedures/Other
Clonidine-suppression test distinguishes between pheochromocytoma and essential HTN when urine and plasma tests are equivocal. In essential HTN, plasma and urine catecholamines decrease 3 hours after oral clonidine; in pheochromocytoma, they do not.

Test Interpretation
Pathology shows a tumor that demonstrates staining for chromogranin-A (catecholamine secretory granules).

 TREATMENT

MEDICATION
First Line
Surgical resection of the tumor is the treatment of choice (2)[C]. Medical management of BP is essential prior to surgery (3)[C]:
- Preoperative control of BP (target <120/80 mm Hg) achieved first with α-adrenergic blockade followed by β-adrenergic blockade starting 1 week before surgical removal of pheochromocytoma (longer for patients with recent history of cardiovascular complication). Never initiate β-adrenergic blockade before α-adrenergic blockade, as unopposed α-stimulation will result in worsened HTN:
  - α-adrenergic blockade is achieved with the nonselective α-blocker phenoxybenzamine starting at a dose of 10 mg PO b.i.d. and increasing by 10–20 mg every 2 days as needed and tolerated for BP control (normal dose 100 mg/d, but up to 240 mg/d has been reported). Warn patient of postural hypotension.
  - After adequate α-adrenergic blockade, β-blockade is initiated at low doses using short-acting agent propranolol 10 mg PO q6h that can be titrated up until resting heart rate of 60–80 beats/min is achieved (max dose 120 mg/d). Avoid β-blockers in acute decompensated heart failure, bradycardia, and patients with uncontrolled asthma.

Second Line
- Treat hypertensive crisis with nitroprusside, nicardipine, or phentolamine.
- For inoperable tumors requiring long-term medical management, specific α_1 blocking agents can be used due to a more favorable side effect profile: Prazosin, terazosin, doxazosin
- Selective β_1 blockers (no β_2 activity): Atenolol, metoprolol, nadolol
- Combined β- and α-blockers: Labetalol and carvedilol
- Catecholamine synthesis inhibitor: Metyrosine only if intolerant to first-line treatment (Mayo Clinic protocol). Avoid long-term use due to adverse reactions (sedation, depression, diarrhea, crystalluria or urolithiasis, and extrapyramidal signs).

SURGERY/OTHER PROCEDURES
- Removal of pheochromocytoma is treatment of choice.
- It is a high-risk surgical procedure requiring experienced surgical and anesthesia teams.
- Laparoscopic approach for tumors in the adrenal gland may result in shorter hospitalization.
- Cortical-sparing subtotal adrenalectomy may preserve adrenocortical function in those with bilateral disease.

IN-PATIENT CONSIDERATIONS
Admission Criteria/Initial Stabilization
- Severe/Refractory HTN
- Control of HTN and replacement of volume with IV normal saline

Nursing
Monitor BP closely

Discharge Criteria
When hemodynamically stable

 ONGOING CARE

FOLLOW-UP RECOMMENDATIONS
Patient Monitoring
- Monitor BP daily before surgery.
- Invasive hemodynamic monitoring intraoperatively
- Monitor urine metanephrine and catecholamine 2 weeks postoperatively and, if normal, recheck annually
- Ensure resolution of HTN and normalization of blood glucose

DIET
- Preoperatively, after initiation of α-blocker, encourage high-sodium diet (>5,000 mg/d) to increase blood volume and prevent orthostasis. May be contraindicated in setting of renal or heart failure.
- Postoperatively, resume general diet.

PATIENT EDUCATION
National Adrenal Disease Foundation (NADF), 505 Northern Blvd., Great Neck, NY 11021; 516-487-4992; e-mail: nadfmail@aol.com

PROGNOSIS
- Survival after surgical removal of a benign tumor is similar to age-matched controls.
- Recurrence rate is 8–15%.
- 5-year survival for malignant disease is <50%.

COMPLICATIONS
- The most common lethal complications are myocardial infarction and cerebrovascular accident.
- Postural hypotension due to α-blockade can be ameliorated with saline volume expansion/high-sodium diet.
- Intraoperative hypertensive crisis can be managed with IV nitroprusside, nicardipine, and phentolamine.

REFERENCES
1. Karagiannis A, Mikhailidis DP, Athyros VG, et al. Pheochromocytoma: An update on genetics and management. *Endocr Relat Cancer.* 2007;14: 935–956.
2. Scholz T, Eisenhofer G, Pacak K, et al. Clinical review: Current treatment of malignant pheochromocytoma. *J Clin Endocrinol Metab.* 2007;92:1217–1225.
3. Bruynzeel H, Feelders RA, Groenland TH, et al. Risk factors for hemodynamic instability during surgery for pheochromocytoma. *J Clin Endocrinol Metab.* 2010;95:678–685.

 SEE ALSO

Hypertension, Essential; Multiple Endocrine Neoplasia

 CODES

ICD10
- D35.00 Benign neoplasm of unspecified adrenal gland
- D35.01 Benign neoplasm of right adrenal gland
- D35.02 Benign neoplasm of left adrenal gland

CLINICAL PEARLS
- Rare catecholamine-secreting tumor with serious and potentially lethal cardiovascular complications.
- Clinical presentation is variable, but classic triad consists of episodic headaches, diaphoresis, and tachycardia/palpitations in association with HTN.
- Diagnosis by urine screen for catecholamines and their metabolites followed by imaging studies (CT, MRI).
- Surgical removal of tumor is standard therapy that must be preceded by a period of BP stabilization with nonselective α-adrenergic blockade followed by β-adrenergic blockade several days later.
- High-salt diet is initiated after α-blockade to minimize orthostasis and ensure volume expansion.
- Never initiate a β-blocker before adequate α-blockade is achieved.

PHOTODERMATITIS

Aamir Siddiqi, MD

 BASICS

DESCRIPTION
- Light-induced eruptions seen in a pattern of photodistribution:
  - Phototoxic reactions: Result of an acute toxic effect on skin of ultraviolet (UV) light alone (sunburn) or together with a photosensitizing substance (nonallergic) (1)
  - Photoallergic eruptions: A form of allergic dermatitis resulting from combined effects of a photosensitizing substance (drugs or chemical) plus UV light (immunologic/delayed hypersensitivity)
  - Polymorphous light eruption (PLE): Chronic, intermittent, light-induced eruption with erythematous papules, urticaria, or vesicles on areas exposed to sunlight
- System(s) affected: Skin/Exocrine
- Synonym(s): Sun poisoning; Sun allergy

EPIDEMIOLOGY
Incidence
- PLE usually occurs after the 1st intense exposure to the sun in the spring or summer
- Predominant age: All ages
- Predominant sex: Male = Female

Prevalence
May be as high as 20% in some areas

ETIOLOGY AND PATHOPHYSIOLOGY
- Sunlight
- Phenothiazines
- Diuretics
- Tetracyclines, sulfonamides
- Oral contraceptives
- Topicals: Psoralens, coal tars, photoactive dyes (eosin, acridine orange)
- 5-fluorouracil
- Quinine
- Sunscreens containing *para*-aminobenzoic acid (PABA)
- In the US, ~115 chemical agents used topically are known to cause photodermatitis.

Genetics
Predisposition occurs in inbred populations (e.g., Pima Indians)

RISK FACTORS
- Job-related exposure to sunlight
- Light and fair-colored skin

GENERAL PREVENTION
- Sunlight avoidance/protective clothing
- Identification and avoidance of causative drugs (see "Etiology and Pathophysiology")
- Sunscreens: Apply before exposure:
  - Zinc oxide: Opaque, cosmetically less acceptable
  - Chemical: Use sun-protective factor (SPF) >30 for maximum protection; substantively resistant to sweat and swimming; cosmetically more acceptable (2)
- Avoid direct sun exposure
- Wear appropriate gear to avoid sunlight exposure

COMMONLY ASSOCIATED CONDITIONS
- Sunlight aggravation of systemic lupus erythematosus (SLE)
- Persistent light reactivity
- Actinic reticuloid

 DIAGNOSIS

HISTORY
Pruritic and often painful rash developing in sun-exposed areas

PHYSICAL EXAM
- Phototoxic (3):
  - Erythema
  - With increasing severity: Vesicles and bullae
  - Classic example: Sunburn
  - Nails may exhibit onycholysis
  - Chronic: Epidermal thickening, elastosis, telangiectasia, and pigmentary changes
  - Sharp lines of demarcation between involved and uninvolved skin (sunlight exposure)
  - Phototoxic eruption due to topicals: Area of application
  - Usually develops shortly after sun exposure
  - Hyperpigmentation may follow resolution
  - Pain

- Photoallergic (3):
  - Papules with erythema and occasionally vesicles
  - Area exposed to light with less distinct borders
  - Usually delayed ≥24 hours after exposure
  - May spread to unexposed areas
  - Pruritus
- PLE:
  - Erythematous papules
  - Occasionally urticaria or vesicles
  - Scattered over sun-exposed areas with normal skin in between
  - Can spread to nonexposed areas
  - Often flares in spring or early summer
  - Desensitization effect (lessens over the course of the summer)
  - Burning or pruritus may precede lesions.

DIFFERENTIAL DIAGNOSIS
SLE

DIAGNOSTIC TESTS & INTERPRETATION
Follow-Up Tests & Special Considerations
Antinuclear antibody to rule out SLE if suspected

Diagnostic Procedures/Other
- Phototesting: Exposing patient to UV light
- Photopatch testing: Applying suspected agents and chemicals to patient's skin
- Skin biopsy: To rule out other disorders if necessary

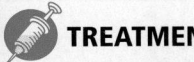

TREATMENT

GENERAL MEASURES
- Appropriate health care: Outpatient
- Avoid sunlight/limit exposure
- Protective clothing/sunscreens
- Ice packs/cold water compresses

MEDICATION
- Topical corticosteroids (triamcinolone 0.25%, 0.1%, 0.5%; betamethasone valerate 0.1% cream, others)

ALERT
Limit use of fluorinated steroids on face; use hydrocortisone ointments.
- NSAIDs (ibuprofen 600 mg q.i.d., indomethacin 25 mg PO t.i.d., aspirin, others)
- Prednisone for severe reactions (0.5–1 mg/kg/d PO) × 3–10 days
- Antihistamines for pruritus (hydroxyzine 25–50 mg PO q.i.d.)
- Sunscreens (>30 SPF) for prevention: Use broad-spectrum sunscreen to block both UVA and UVB. PABA may aggravate photodermatitis in sensitized patients (due to the sulfa moiety) (2).
- Aspirin and ibuprofen taken orally or applied topically (diclofenac) before sun exposure may modestly reduce erythema and pain of sunburn.

Geriatric Considerations
More likely to experience adverse reactions to causative drugs

COMPLEMENTARY AND ALTERNATIVE MEDICINE
- PO β-carotene seems to modestly reduce the risk of sunburn in individuals who are sensitive to sun exposure (4).
- Omega-3 fatty acid intake may decrease the sensitivity of skin to UV exposure (5).
- Compresses made from tea bags steeped in a small amount of water may reduce itching and burning of sunburn.

ONGOING CARE

FOLLOW-UP RECOMMENDATIONS
Avoid direct sunlight

PATIENT EDUCATION
- Avoidance of direct sunlight exposure
- Avoidance of photosensitizing drugs
- Protective clothing (e.g., hats, long sleeves)
- Sunscreens >30 SPF

PROGNOSIS
Good with avoidance/protection measures

COMPLICATIONS
Rare (secondary bacterial infection)

REFERENCES

1. Smith E, Kiss F, Porter RM, et al. A review of UVA-mediated photosensitivity disorders. *Photochem Photobiol Sci.* 2012;11:199–206.
2. Kalia S, Laurentiu Haiducu M. Sunscreen and sun protection: Shedding light on recent advances. *J Cutan Med Surg.* 2011;15(Suppl 1):S382–S386.
3. Glatz M, Hofbauer GF. Phototoxic and photoallergic cutaneous drug reactions. *Chem Immunol Allergy.* 2012;97:167–179.
4. Stahl W, Sies H. β-Carotene and other carotenoids in protection from sunlight. *Am J Clin Nutr.* 2012; 96:1179S–1184S.
5. Pilkington SM, Watson RE, Nicolaou A, et al. Omega-3 polyunsaturated fatty acids: Photoprotective macronutrients. *Exp Dermatol.* 2011;20:537–543.

CODES

ICD10
- L56.4 Polymorphous light eruption
- L56.8 Oth acute skin changes due to ultraviolet radiation
- L57.8 Oth skin changes due to chr expsr to nonionizing radiation

CLINICAL PEARLS
- Choose a sunscreen with an SPF of at least 30 with full-spectrum protection (UVA and UVB) for the best efficacy.
- The most common medications that predispose to photosensitivity include tetracyclines and sulfonamide. However, many other medications may cause photosensitivity.

PILONIDAL DISEASE

Jeremy Golding, MD

 BASICS

DESCRIPTION
- Pilonidal disease results from an abscess, or sinus tract, in the upper part of the natal (gluteal) cleft.
- Synonym(s): Jeep disease

EPIDEMIOLOGY
Incidence
- 26/100,000 per year
- Predominant sex: Male > Female (3–4:1)
- Predominant age: 2nd–3rd decade, rare >45 years
- Ethnic consideration: Whites > Blacks > Asians

Prevalence
Surgical procedures show male:female ratio of 4:1, yet incidence data are 10:1.

ETIOLOGY AND PATHOPHYSIOLOGY
Pilonidal means "nest of hair"; hair in the natal cleft allows hair to be drawn into the deeper tissues via negative pressure caused by movement of the buttocks (50%); follicular occlusion from stretching, and blocking of pores with debris (50%)
- Inflammation of SC gluteal tissues with secondary infection and sinus tract formation
- Polymicrobial, likely from enteric pathogens given proximity to anorectal contamination

Genetics
- Congenital dimple in the natal cleft/spina bifida occulta
- Follicular-occluding tetrad: Acne conglobata, dissecting cellulitis, hidradenitis suppurativa, pilonidal

RISK FACTORS
- Sedentary/Prolonged sitting
- Excessive body hair
- Obesity/Increased sacrococcygeal fold thickness
- Congenital natal dimple
- Trauma to coccyx

GENERAL PREVENTION
- Weight loss
- Trim hair in/around gluteal cleft weekly
- Hygiene
- Ingrown hair prevention/follicle unblocking

 DIAGNOSIS

HISTORY
3 distinct clinical presentations:
- Asymptomatic: Painless cyst or sinus at the top of the gluteal cleft
- Acute abscess: Severe pain, swelling, discharge from the top of the gluteal cleft that may or may not have drained spontaneously
- Chronic abscess: Persistent drainage from a sinus tract at the top of the gluteal cleft

PHYSICAL EXAM
- Common: Inflamed cystic mass at the top of the gluteal cleft with limited surrounding erythema ± drainage or a sinus tract
- Less common: Significant cellulitis of the surrounding tissues near the gluteal cleft

DIFFERENTIAL DIAGNOSIS
- Furunculosis
- Hidradenitis suppurativa
- Anal fistula
- Perirectal abscess
- Crohn disease

DIAGNOSTIC TESTS & INTERPRETATION
Initial Tests (lab, imaging)
- Consider CBC and wound culture, but generally not necessary for less-severe infections
- MRI might be considered to differentiate between perirectal abscess and pilonidal disease.

 TREATMENT

GENERAL MEASURES
Shave area; remove hair from crypts weekly.

MEDICATION
- Antibiotics not indicated unless there is significant cellulitis
- If antibiotics are needed, a culture to direct therapy might be useful.
- Cefazolin and metronidazole or amoxicillin-clavulanate are often used empirically

ISSUES FOR REFERRAL
- Patients who cannot comply with frequent dressing changes required after incision and drainage (I&D)
- Patients who have recurrence after I&D
- Patients who have complex disease with multiple sinus tracts

ADDITIONAL THERAPIES
- I&D with only enough packing to allow the cyst to drain; overpacking not indicated
- Antibiotics only if significant cellulitis; temporizing, not curative

SURGERY/OTHER PROCEDURES
6 levels of care based on severity or recurrence of disease; recent innovations in technique are aimed at expediting healing and minimizing recurrence (1,2)[C]:
- I&D, remove hair, curette granulation tissue
- Excision of midline "pits" allows drainage of lateral sinus tracts (pit picking) (3)[C].
- Pilonidal cystotomy: Insert probe into sinus tract, excise overlying skin, and close wound (4)[B].

- Marsupialization: Excise overlying skin and roof of cyst, and suture skin edges to cyst floor.
- Excision: Use of flap closure (5)[B]. No clear benefit for open healing over surgical closure (6)[A].
- Off-midline surgical excision (cleft lift or modified Karydakis procedure): A systematic review showed a clear benefit in favor of off-midline rather than midline wound closure. When closure of pilonidal sinuses is the desired surgical option, off-midline closure should be the standard management (6)[A].

IN-PATIENT CONSIDERATIONS
Admission Criteria/Initial Stabilization
- Severe cellulitis
- Large area excision

 ## ONGOING CARE

FOLLOW-UP RECOMMENDATIONS
- Frequent dressing changes required after I&D
- Follow-up wound checks to assess for recurrence

Patient Monitoring
Monitor for fever, more extensive cellulitis

PATIENT EDUCATION
- Wash area briskly with washcloth daily
- Shave the area weekly
- Remove any embedded hair from the crypt
- Avoid prolonged sitting

PROGNOSIS
- Simple I&D has a 55% failure rate; median time to healing is 5 weeks.
- More extensive surgical excisions involve hospital stays and longer time to heal.

COMPLICATIONS
Malignant degeneration is a rare complication of untreated chronic pilonidal disease.

REFERENCES

1. Kement M, Oncel M, Kurt N, et al. Sinus excision for the treatment of limited chronic pilonidal disease: Results after a medium-term follow-up. *Dis Colon Rectum*. 2006;49:1758–1762.
2. Theodropoulos GE. Modified Bascom's asymmetric midgluteal cleft closure technique for recurrent pilonidal disease: Early experience in a military hospital. *Dis Colon Rectum*. 2003;49:1755–1757.
3. Iesalnieks I, Deimel S, Kienle K, et al. [Pit-picking surgery for pilonidal disease.] *Chirurg*. 2011;82:927–931.
4. Rao MM, Zawislak W, Kennedy R, et al. A prospective randomised study comparing two treatment modalities for chronic pilonidal sinus with a 5-year follow-up. *Int J Colorectal Dis*. 2010;25:395–400.
5. Washer JD, Smith DE, Carman ME, et al. Gluteal fascial advancement: An innovative, effective method for treating pilonidal disease. *Am Surg*. 2010;76:154–156.
6. Al-Khamis A, McCallum I, King PM, et al. Healing by primary versus secondary intention after surgical treatment for pilonidal sinus. *Cochrane Database Syst Rev*. 2010;1:CD006213.

ADDITIONAL READING
- Ates M, Dirican A, Sarac M, et al. Short and long-term results of the Karydakis flap versus the Limberg flap for treating pilonidal sinus disease: A prospective randomized study. *Am J Surg*. 2011;202:568–573.
- Aygen E, Arslan K, Dogru O, et al. Crystallized phenol in nonoperative treatment of previously operated, recurrent pilonidal disease. *Dis Colon Rectum*. 2010;53:932–935.
- Bradley L. Pilonidal sinus disease: A review. Part one. *J Wound Care*. 2010;19:504–508.
- Harlak A, Mentes O, Kilic S, et al. Sacrococcygeal pilonidal disease: Analysis of previously proposed risk factors. *Clinics (Sao Paulo)*. 2010;65:125–131.
- Humphries AE, Duncan JE. Evaluation and management of pilonidal disease. *Surg Clin North Am*. 2010;90:113–124.
- Oram Y, Kahraman F, Karincaolu Y, et al. Evaluation of 60 patients with pilonidal sinus treated with laser epilation after surgery. *Dermatol Surg*. 2010;36:88–91.

 ## CODES

ICD10
- L05.01 Pilonidal cyst with abscess
- L05.91 Pilonidal cyst without abscess
- L05.92 Pilonidal sinus without abscess

CLINICAL PEARLS
- Avoid prolonged sitting.
- Lose weight.
- Trim hair in gluteal cleft weekly.
- Refer recurring infections for more definitive surgical management.

PINWORMS

Jonathan MacClements, MD, FAAFP

 BASICS

DESCRIPTION
- Intestinal infection with *Enterobius vermicularis*:
  - Characterized by perineal and perianal itching
  - Usually worse at night
- System(s) affected: Gastrointestinal; Skin/Exocrine
- Synonym(s): Enterobiasis

EPIDEMIOLOGY
Predominant age: 5–14 years

Prevalence
- Most common helminthic infection in the US:
  - 20–42 million people harboring the parasite
- ~30% of children are infected throughout the world.

Pediatric Considerations
More common in children, who are more likely to become reinfected

ETIOLOGY AND PATHOPHYSIOLOGY
- Small white worms (2–13 mm) inhabit the cecum, appendix, and adjacent portions of the ascending colon following ingestion.
- Female worms migrate to the perianal and perineal areas at night, depositing ~11,000 eggs, resulting in irritation and itching of the perianal area.
- Scratching of the perianal and perineal areas followed by touching of the mouth can lead to ingestion of the eggs and continuation of pinworm's life cycle in the host.
- Infestation by the intestinal nematode *E. (Oxyuris) vermicularis*

RISK FACTORS
- Institutionalization
- Crowded living conditions
- Poor hygiene
- Warm climate
- Handling of infected children's clothing or bedding

GENERAL PREVENTION
- Careful hand washing, especially after bowel movements
- Clip and maintain short fingernails
- Wash anus and genitals at least once a day, preferably during a shower
- Do not scratch anus or put fingers near nose or mouth.

COMMONLY ASSOCIATED CONDITIONS
Pruritus ani (1)

 DIAGNOSIS

HISTORY
Many patients are asymptomatic, but symptoms can include:
- Perianal itching
- Perineal itching
- Vulvovaginitis
- Dysuria
- Abdominal pain (rare)
- Insomnia
- Restless sleep

PHYSICAL EXAM
Perineal and perianal exam

DIFFERENTIAL DIAGNOSIS
- Idiopathic pruritus ani
- Atopic dermatitis
- Contact dermatitis
- Psoriasis
- Lichen planus
- Infection with human papillomavirus
- Herpes simplex
- Fungal infections
- Erythrasma
- Scabies
- Vaginitis
- Hemorrhoids

DIAGNOSTIC TESTS & INTERPRETATION
Diagnostic Procedures/Other
- Adhesive tape test:
  - A piece of transparent cellophane tape is stuck to the perianal skin in the early morning before bathing and then affixed to a microscope slide after removal.
  - This procedure must be performed at least 3 times to achieve 90% sensitivity.
  - Alternatively, anal swabs or a pinworm paddle coated with adhesive material also can be useful (2,3,4)[C].
- Digital rectal exam with saline slide preparation of stool on gloved finger (2)[C]
- *Routine stool examination for ova and parasites is positive in only 10–15% of infected patients.*

Test Interpretation
Identification of ova on low-power microscopy or direct visualization of the female worm (10 mm long); ova are asymmetric, flattened on 1 side, and measure $56 \times 27 \ \mu m$.

 TREATMENT

MEDICATION
First Line
- Treatment options include any of the following (2,5)[A]:
  - Mebendazole (Vermox): Chewable 100-mg tablet as a single dose in adults and children >2 years of age; use with caution in children <2 years of age
  - Albendazole (Albenza): 400 mg PO as a single dose in adults and children >2 years of age; 100 mg PO as a single dose repeated in 7 days in children ≤2 years of age
  - Pyrantel pamoate (Pin-X, Reese's Pinworm Medicine): Oral liquid or tablet 11 mg/kg as a single dose in adults and children >2 years of age; maximum dose 1 g. Use with caution in children <2 years of age.
- Many clinicians recommend repeat treatment after 2 weeks due to the high frequency of reinfection and autoinfection. Occasionally, refractory cases may require retreatment every 2 weeks for 4–6 cycles.
- All symptomatic family members should be treated.

Pregnancy Considerations
Drug therapy should be avoided in pregnancy. Treatment should be delayed until after delivery (6)[C].

ONGOING CARE

FOLLOW-UP RECOMMENDATIONS
Unnecessary unless symptoms do not abate following drug therapy

PATIENT EDUCATION
- Take medicine with food
- Practice good hygiene
- Encourage frequent and careful hand washing
- Clip fingernails short
- All clothing and bedding should be washed to prevent reinfection.
- Do not share washcloths.
- Do not shake linen and clothing before laundering because this may spread the eggs.
- Do not allow children to co-bathe during treatment and for 2 weeks after the final treatment; showering is preferred.

PROGNOSIS
- Asymptomatic carriers are common.
- Symptomatic infections are cured >90% of the time by pharmacotherapy.
- Reinfection is common, especially among children.

COMPLICATIONS
- Perianal scratching may lead to bacterial superinfection.
- Females: Vulvovaginitis, urethritis, endometritis, salpingitis
- UTIs
- Rarely, ectopic disease involving granulomas of the pelvis, urinary tract, female genitourinary tract, and appendix

REFERENCES

1. Stermer E, Sukhotnic I, Shaoul R. Pruritus ani: An approach to an itching condition. *J Pediatr Gastroenterol Nutr*. 2009;48:513–516.
2. Jones JE. Pinworms. *Am Fam Physician*. 1988;38: 159–164.
3. Cram EB. Studies on oxyuriasis, 28. Summary and conclusions. *Am J Dis Child*. 1943;65:46–59.
4. Kucik CJ. Common intestinal parasites. *Am Fam Physician*. 2004;69:1161–1168.
5. *Enterobius vermicularis*. In: *Drugs for parasitic infections. Treatment guidelines from The Medical Letter*, Vol. 8 (Suppl), 2010.
6. Hamblin J. Pinworms in pregnancy. *J Am Board Fam Practice*. 1995;8:321–324.

ADDITIONAL READING

- CDC Resources for Health Professionals. Parasites—Enterobiasis (also known as Pinworm Infection). Available at: www.cdc.gov/parasites/pinworm/health_professionals/index.html
- Johansson J, Ignatova S. Pinworm infestation mimicking Crohns' disease. *Case Rep Gastrointest Med*. 2013;2013:706197.
- Lamps LW. Infectious causes of appendicitis. *Infect Dis Clin North Am*. 2010;24:995–1018.
- Xiao SH, Utzinger J, Tanner M, et al. Advances with the Chinese anthelminthic drug tribendimidine in clinical trials and laboratory investigations. *Acta Trop*. 2013;126:115–126.

SEE ALSO

Pruritus Ani

CODES

ICD10
B80 Enterobiasis

CLINICAL PEARLS

- Treatment for pinworms includes use of mebendazole, albendazole, or pyrantel pamoate (2,5)[A].
- Close contacts should be treated as well.
- Retreatment after 2 weeks is recommended by many experts due to difficulty eradicating this parasite (2)[C].

PITUITARY ADENOMA

Anup Sabharwal, MD, MBA, FACE, CCD • Lewis S. Blevins, Jr, MD

 BASICS

DESCRIPTION
Typically benign, slow-growing tumors that arise from cells in the pituitary gland:
- Pituitary adenomas have been identified as the 3rd most frequent intracranial tumor; accounts for 10–25%.
- Subtypes (hormonal): Prolactinoma (PRL) 50%, nonfunctioning pituitary adenomas 30%, somatotroph adenoma (growth hormone [GH]) 15–20%, corticotroph adenoma (adrenocorticotrophic hormone [ACTH]) 5–10%, thyrotroph adenoma (thyroid-stimulating hormone [TSH]) <1%, gonadotropinoma (luteinizing hormone/follicle-stimulating hormone [LH/FSH]), mixed
- Defined as microadenoma <10 mm and macroadenoma ≥10 mm
- May secrete hormones and/or cause mass effects

EPIDEMIOLOGY
- Predominant age: Age increases incidence
- Predominant sex: Female > Male (3:2) for microadenomas (often delayed diagnosis in men)

Incidence
- Autopsy studies have found microadenomas in 3–27% and macroadenomas in <0.5% of people without any pituitary disorders.
- MRI scans illustrate abnormalities consistent with pituitary adenoma in 1/10 persons.
- Clinically apparent pituitary tumors are seen in 18/100,000 persons.

ETIOLOGY AND PATHOPHYSIOLOGY
- Monoclonal adenohypophysial cell growth
- Hormonal effects of functional microadenomas often prompt diagnosis before mass effect.
- Prolactin increased by functional prolactinomas or inhibited dopaminergic suppression by stalk effect

Genetics
- Carney complex
- Familial isolated pituitary adenomas: ~15% have mutations in the aryl hydrocarbon receptor-interacting protein gene (*AIP*). Present at a younger age and are larger in size.
- McCune-Albright syndrome
- Multiple endocrine neoplasia type 1 (MEN-1)-like phenotype (MEN-4): Germline mutation in the cyclin-dependent kinase inhibitor 1B (CDKN1B)

RISK FACTORS
Multiple endocrine neoplasias

 DIAGNOSIS

HISTORY
- Common:
  - Hyperprolactinemia: Infertility, amenorrhea, galactorrhea, gynecomastia, impotence
  - Headache (sellar expansion)
  - Visual disturbances: Bitemporal hemianopsia
- Less common:
  - Hypersomatotropinemia: Acromegaly (coarse facial features, hand/foot swelling, carpal tunnel syndrome, hyperhidrosis, left ventricular hypertrophy)
  - Hyposomatotropinemia: Failure to thrive (FTT) (children), asymptomatic (adults)

- Intracranial pressure (ICP) elevation: Headache, nausea, seizures
- Hypercorticotropinemia: Cushing disease (supraclavicular/dorsocervical fat pad thickening, moon face, hirsutism, acne, plethora, abdominal striae, centripetal obesity with thin limbs, easy bruising and bleeding, hyperglycemia)
- Rare:
  - Apoplexy: Headache, sudden collapse
  - Secondary hyperthyroidism: Palpitations, diaphoresis, heat intolerance, diarrhea
  - Secondary adrenal insufficiency: Weakness, irritability, anorexia, nausea/vomiting
- Hypothalamic compression: Temperature, thirst/appetite disorders

PHYSICAL EXAM
- Common:
  - Visual disturbances: Bitemporal hemianopsia
  - Hyperprolactinemia: Hypogonadism, galactorrhea, gynecomastia
  - Hypersomatotropinemia: Acromegaly (coarse features, hand/foot swelling, diaphoresis)
  - Hyposomatotropinemia: FTT (children)
- Less common:
  - ICP elevation: Papilledema, dementia
  - Cushing disease: Centripetal obesity, supraclavicular fat pad thickening, moon face, hirsutism, acne
- Rare:
  - Apoplexy: Hypotension, hypoglycemia, tachycardia, oliguria
  - Secondary hyperthyroidism: Tachycardia, tachypnea, diaphoresis, warm/moist skin, tremor
  - Adrenal crisis: Orthostatic hypotension
- Hypothalamic compression: Temperature dysregulation, obesity, increased urination

DIFFERENTIAL DIAGNOSIS
Pituitary hyperplasia (e.g., pregnancy, primary hypothyroidism, menopause), Rathke cleft cyst, granulomatous disease (e.g., tuberculosis), lymphocytic hypophysitis, metastatic tumor, germinoma, craniopharyngioma

DIAGNOSTIC TESTS & INTERPRETATION
Select based on dysfunction(s) suspected:
- Somatotrophic (GH secreting): 40–130/million):
  - Acromegaly/hypersomatotropinemia: Serum IGF-1 elevated; oral glucose tolerance test with GH given at 0, 30, and 60 minutes (normally suppresses GH to <1 g/L)
  - Hyposomatotropinemia: Low growth hormone-releasing hormone response
- Corticotrophic:
  - Cushing disease/hypercorticotropinemia
  - 24-hour urinary-free cortisol >50 mcg
  - Overnight low-dose dexamethasone suppression test (DMST): Normal plasma cortisol (FPC) >1.8 μg/dL at 8 A.M. (after 1 mg given at 11 P.M. on night prior)
  - ACTH level assay (if DMST results abnormal): <20 pg/mL = adrenal tumor; ≥20 pg/mL = ectopic/pituitary source
  - Hypocorticotropinemia/secondary glucocorticoid deficiency: High-dose corticotropin stimulation test: FPC <10 g/dL at baseline, with an increase of <25% 1 hour after 250 mcg; metyrapone test: 11-deoxycortisol <150 ng/L after 2 g given (prepare to give steroids because test may worsen insufficiency)

- Gonadotrophic/hypogonadotropinism: Gonadotropin-releasing hormone stimulation of LH/FSH blunted in pituitary hypergonadism, but increased in primary hypogonadism
- Lactotrophic (prolactin secreting): Hyperprolactinemia: Serum PRL >20 ng/mL
- Thyrotrophic (TSH secreting): Hyper-/hypothyroidism: TSH and free T$_4$ both increased for pituitary hyperthyroidism and both decreased for pituitary hypothyroidism

Initial Tests (lab, imaging)
- A typical panel for asymptomatic tumors: Prolactin, GH, IGF-1, ACTH, 24-hour urinary-free cortisol or overnight DMST, βHCG, FSH, LH, TSH, free T$_4$
- Screening for *AIP* mutations may be offered to families of patients with pituitary adenoma, where available (1)[B].
- MRI preferred (>90% sensitivity and specificity) after biochemically confirmed
- Octreotide scintigraphy is useful in identifying tumors with somatostatin receptors.

Diagnostic Procedures/Other
Inferior petrosal sinus sampling: ACTH sampled from inferior petrosal sinuses to distinguish Cushing disease (pituitary source) from ectopic ACTH

Test Interpretation
- Cell types identified by immunohistochemistry
- Light microscope: Eosinophilic (GH, PRL), basophilic (FSH/LH, TSH, ACTH), chromophobic

 TREATMENT

Medical therapy is primary therapy for prolactinomas and adjunct for other tumors (2)[A].

MEDICATION
First Line
- Hyperprolactinemia: Dopamine agonists increase dopaminergic suppression of PRL:
  - Cabergoline (Dostinex): D$_2$ receptor-specific:
    ○ Initial dose: 0.25 mg PO once or twice weekly
    ○ Maintenance dose: Increase q4wk by 0.25 mg 2 ×/week per PRL (max 2 mg/week)
    ○ Contraindications: Hypersensitivity (ergots), hypertension (HTN), pregnancy
    ○ Precautions: Caution with liver impairment
    ○ Interactions: May be inhibited by tricyclic antidepressants, phenothiazines, opiates
    ○ Adverse reactions: Orthostatic hypotension, vertigo, dyspepsia, hot flashes
  - Bromocriptine (Parlodel): D$_2$ receptor-specific:
    ○ Initial dose: 1.25–2.5 mg PO daily (give with food)
    ○ Maintenance dose: Increase by 2.5 mg/d q2–7d (max 100 mg/d)
    ○ Contraindications: Hypersensitivity (ergots), HTN, pregnancy; preferred over cabergoline if required
    ○ Precautions: Caution with liver impairment
    ○ Interactions: May be inhibited by tricyclic antidepressants, phenothiazines, opiates
    ○ Adverse reactions: Orthostatic hypotension, seizures, hallucinations, stroke, myocardial infarction

---

- Somatotropinoma:
  - Long-acting analogues of somatostatin (Sandostatin LAR and Lanreotide Autogel):
    - Sandostatin LAR: 20 mg q28d; Lanreotide Autogel 90 mg q28d; titrate per package insert.
    - Contraindication: Hypersensitivity
    - Precautions: Caution with biliary, thyroid, cardiac, liver, or kidney disease
    - Interactions: Pimozide increases risk of QT prolongation; variable effects with β-blockers, diuretics, oral glycemic agents
    - Adverse reactions: Ascending cholangitis, arrhythmias, congestive heart failure, glycemic instability
    - More effective as adjuvant than as primary treatment for somatotropinomas (2)[A]
  - Pegvisomant (Somavert): Growth hormone receptor antagonist:
    - Initial dose: 40 mg SC × 1, then 20 mg daily and titrate by 5 mg every 4–6 weeks based on IGF-1 levels (maximum 30 mg/d maintenance dose)
    - Contraindication: Hypersensitivity
    - Precautions: Caution if GH-secreting tumors, diabetes mellitus, impaired liver function
    - Interactions: NSAIDs, opiates, insulins, oral glycemic agents
    - Adverse reactions: Hepatitis, tumor growth, GH-secretion
- Corticotropinemia: Peripheral inhibitors:
  - Mitotane (Lysodren):
    - Initial dose: 2–6 g PO t.i.d. (max 19 g/d)
    - Maintenance dose: 2–16 g t.i.d.
    - Contraindication: Hypersensitivity
    - Precautions: Caution with liver dysfunction and brain damage
    - Interactions: Contraindicated with rotavirus vaccine; caution with other vaccines
    - Adverse reactions: HTN, orthostatic hypotension, hemorrhagic cystitis, rash
  - Ketoconazole:
    - Dosing: 200 mg PO t.i.d. (max 1,200 mg/d)
    - Contraindications: Hypersensitivity, achlorhydria, fungal meningitis, impaired liver function
    - Precautions: Caution with liver dysfunction
    - Interactions: Contraindicated with cisapride, niacin, statins, pimozide, sirolimus; caution with other antifungals
    - Adverse reactions: Adrenal insufficiency, thrombocytopenia, hepatic failure, hepatotoxicity, anaphylaxis, leukopenia, hemolytic anemia
  - Signifor (Pasireotide):
    - Dosing: Initially, 0.6–0.9 mg twice daily, then 0.3–0.9 mg twice daily
    - Contraindication: None
    - Precautions: Hypocortisolism, hyperglycemia, bradycardia or QT prolongation, liver test elevations, cholelithiasis, other pituitary hormone deficiencies
  - Korlym (Mifepristone):
    - Dosing: Administer PO once daily with a meal. The recommended starting dose is 300 mg once daily. Not to exceed 600 mg daily in renal impairment.
    - Contraindication: Pregnancy, use of simvastatin or lovastatin and CYP3A substrates with narrow therapeutic range, concurrent long-term corticosteroid use, women with history of unexplained vaginal bleeding, women with endometrial hyperplasia with atypia or endometrial carcinoma
    - Precautions: Adrenal insufficiency, hypokalemia, vaginal bleeding and endometrial changes, QT

interval prolongation, use of strong CYP3A inhibitors
    - Interactions: Potential interactions with drugs metabolized by CYP3A, CYP2C8/9, CYP2B6, and hormonal contraceptives. Nursing mothers should discontinue drug or discontinue nursing.
    - Adverse reactions: Most common adverse reactions in Cushing's syndrome (≥20%): Nausea, fatigue, headache, decreased blood potassium, arthralgia, vomiting, peripheral edema, HTN, dizziness, decreased appetite, endometrial hypertrophy
- Gonadotropinemia:
  - Bromocriptine: See above
- Thyrotropinemia:
  - Somatostatin analogues: See above.

Second Line
- Corticotropinemia: Peripheral inhibitors:
  - Metyrapone:
    - Dose: 250–600 mg/d PO
    - Contraindication: Porphyria
    - Precautions: Caution in liver/thyroid disease
    - Interactions: Dilantin increases metabolism.
    - Adverse reactions: Nausea, hypotension
- Gonadotropinemia:
  - Octreotide: See above.

ISSUES FOR REFERRAL
- Neurosurgery consultation for symptomatic tumors (except for prolactinoma)
- Ophthalmologist evaluation prior to surgery

ADDITIONAL THERAPIES
- Fractionated radiotherapy: Often effective as adjunctive when surgery is inadequate (3)[A]
- Stereotactic radiosurgery: Alternative to surgery in high-risk patients or as adjunct (3)[B]

SURGERY/OTHER PROCEDURES
- Most are now done endoscopically via translabial/transsphenoidal approach
- Indications: Symptoms or treatment-resistant
- Follow-up: Serial neurologic/hormonal evaluations to evaluate complications (e.g., diabetes insipidus, CNS damage) and need for more treatment (4)
- Remission rates: 72–87% for microadenoma, but only 50–56% for macroadenomas (4)

IN-PATIENT CONSIDERATIONS
Admission Criteria/Initial Stabilization
Outpatient management unless apoplexy or adrenal crisis
- Treat pituitary apoplexy immediately to prevent death (see "Complications").
- Consider stress-dose steroids in frail or hemodynamically unstable patients.
- Maintain BP with fluids and/or pressor agents.
- Check serum sodium, serum osmolality, and urine specific gravity if polyuric or electrolytes are imbalanced.
- Contact neurosurgery.

IV Fluids
- Diabetes insipidus: Hyposmolar IV fluids
- Adrenal crisis: Normal saline

Nursing
- Pituitary apoplexy: Monitor inputs/outputs (I/Os), central venous pressure, and ICP; and do frequent neurologic checks.
- Adrenal crisis: Monitor BP and I/Os.

Discharge Criteria
Keep as inpatient postoperatively until diabetes insipidus and/or adrenal insufficiency is managed.

ONGOING CARE
FOLLOW-UP RECOMMENDATIONS
Patient Monitoring
- Follow-up MRIs at 6 and 12 months after discharge
- Involved hormone(s) are followed postoperatively, especially after radiation, because hypopituitarism may develop 10–15 years after treatment (2).

PROGNOSIS
- Depends on type, size, symptoms, therapy

COMPLICATIONS
- Postoperative diabetes insipidus and/or hypogonadism (usually transient/common)
- Pituitary apoplexy (acute/uncommon): Acute hemorrhagic pituitary infarction; adrenal crisis with severe headache; surgical decompression required to prevent shock, coma, and death
- Nelson syndrome (subacute/uncommon): Rapid adenoma growth postadrenalectomy
- Pituitary hormone insufficiency (chronic/uncommon): Often years after treatment
- Optic nerve neuropathy and brain necrosis after >60 Gy radiotherapy (chronic/rare)

REFERENCES
1. Georgitsi M, Raitila A, Karhu A. Molecular diagnosis of pituitary adenoma predisposition caused by aryl hydrocarbon receptor-interacting protein gene mutations. *Proc Natl Acad Sci U S A.* 2007;104:4101–4105.
2. Tichomirowa MA, Daly AF, Beckers A. Treatment of pituitary tumors: Somatostatin. *Endocrine.* 2005; 28:93–100.
3. Mondok A, Szeifert GT, Mayer A. Treatment of pituitary tumors: Radiation. *Endocrine.* 2005;28: 77–85.
4. Buchfelder M. Treatment of pituitary tumors: Surgery. *Endocrine.* 2005;28:67–75.

SEE ALSO

Cushing Disease and Cushing Syndrome; Galactorrhea

CODES

ICD10
D35.2 Benign neoplasm of pituitary gland

CLINICAL PEARLS

- An incidentaloma is an asymptomatic microadenoma found on imaging. General labs include PRL, GH, IGF-1, ACTH, 24-hour urinary-free cortisol/overnight DMST, β-subunit FSH, LH, TSH, and free T_4. Obtain follow-up MRIs at 6 and 12 months if normal, but consult endocrinology if not.
- Initial treatment selected for symptomatic pituitary adenoma includes a dopamine agonist for prolactinomas and surgical resection for all others.
- Pituitary apoplexy is a rapid hemorrhagic pituitary infarction due to compression of the blood supply. It is fatal within hours unless surgically decompressed.

PITYRIASIS ALBA

Courtney R. Schadt, MD • W. Brooke Veith, MD • Mark Haeberle, MD

BASICS

DESCRIPTION
- A chronic skin disorder characterized by ≥1 groups of poorly marginated, pale pink, or tan/white patches and plaques that most commonly appear on the cheeks, neck, and lateral arms of children and young adults
- Subtypes: (i) Endemic; (ii) Atopic-dermatitis-related
- System(s) affected: Skin/Exocrine
- Synonym(s): Pityriasis streptogenes; Pityriasis simplex; Pityriasis sicca faciei; Erythema streptogenes

Geriatric Considerations
Rare in this age group

Pediatric Considerations
More common in children aged 3–16 years

EPIDEMIOLOGY
Incidence
- Common; exact incidence unknown, but seen frequently in people with dark skin in sunnier climates
- Predominant age: 90% of affected patients are aged 6–12 years; rare >25 years
- Predominant sex: Male = Female

ETIOLOGY AND PATHOPHYSIOLOGY
- Unknown
- Atopic-dermatitis-related type likely due to eczema exacerbation and postinflammatory hypopigmentation
- Other implicated causes: Infectious, nutritional deficiencies, excessive sun exposure, or a skin barrier defect

Genetics
- Associated with carriers of a loss-of-function mutation in the gene for filaggrin, important for structural integrity and hydration of the epidermis.
- Mutations in this gene are also associated with atopic dermatitis.

RISK FACTORS
Children with a genetic predisposition to atopic disease

GENERAL PREVENTION
No known preventive measures (sun protection may minimize visibility of lesions)

COMMONLY ASSOCIATED CONDITIONS
Atopic dermatitis

DIAGNOSIS

HISTORY
- Usually asymptomatic
- Pruritus (rare)
- More apparent in summertime in light-skinned people
- Lesions do not tan in summer
- Even a small amount of sunlight exposure causes lesions to redden

PHYSICAL EXAM
- Description: Small, ill-defined, pale pink or tan/white patches 0.5–5 cm
- Rash evolves from pink patch to white macule with fine scale to smooth hypopigmented macule
- Location: Most commonly cheeks, forehead, and lateral arms
- Number: ≥1–12 patches
- Palpation: Smooth or slightly rough, but dry
- Appearance: Pinpoint white papules (representing accentuation and keratinization of follicular orifices)
- Scale is either invisible or fine and light.

DIFFERENTIAL DIAGNOSIS
- Tinea versicolor
- Vitiligo
- Postinflammatory hypomelanosis
- Chemical leukoderma
- Indeterminate or uncharacteristic leprosy
- T-cell lymphoma
- Sarcoidosis

DIAGNOSTIC TESTS & INTERPRETATION
- Wood's lamp exam
- Microscopy of skin scraping with KOH preparation
- Biopsy for histology (rarely needed) to rule out other skin diseases if clinically appropriate

Test Interpretation
- Negative skin scraping and absence of fluorescence under Wood's lamp help to rule out fungal etiology (tinea versicolor)
- Early histology: Follicular dilatation, plugging, spongiosis, superficial perivascular infiltrate, and dermal edema
- Late histology: Nonspecific; hyperkeratosis, focal parakeratosis, and spongiosis with variable reduction in basal melanocytes

TREATMENT

GENERAL MEASURES
Sun protection, including protective apparel and sunscreen, is essential.

MEDICATION
First Line
- Treatment is primarily symptomatic, as lesions tend to resolve spontaneously.
- Topical emollients and lubricants can be used to relieve dryness and/or roughness.
- Topical steroids (e.g., hydrocortisone acetate 1%) if needed to reduce redness and/or pruritus due to sunburn or spontaneous inflammation

Second Line
- Limited evidence to support the use of topical corticosteroids for resolution or treatment of extensive disease. Corticosteroids are not FDA approved for use in this condition (1)[C]. Long-term use has the potential to cause further depigmentation.
- Calcineurin inhibitors, pimecrolimus 1% cream applied topically b.i.d. (2)[C] and tacrolimus 0.1% ointment applied topically b.i.d. (3)[C] have been used with good effect for pityriasis alba associated with atopic dermatitis or more extensive involvement. Neither are currently FDA approved.
- 0.0003% calcitriol ointment has been shown to be as effective as 0.1% tacrolimus ointment for resolution of lesions without risk of carcinoma or skin atrophy (4)[B].
- Coal tar preparations (e.g., Alphosyl, Estar, Balnetar) applied topically once daily or b.i.d. for symptomatic relief

ALERT
- Extended duration or potent topical corticosteroid use on the face should be avoided.
- Black box warning for topical tacrolimus: Questionable increased risk of lymphoma and skin malignancies. Avoid long-term use.
- Use precaution in pediatric populations
- Precautions: Refer to the manufacturer's literature for each drug.

ADDITIONAL THERAPIES
- Psoralen plus UVA (PUVA) considered for extensive involvement only (4)[C]
- 308-nm UVB excimer laser therapy effective for treatment of facial pityriasis alba lesions (5)[C]

IN-PATIENT CONSIDERATIONS
Admission Criteria/Initial Stabilization
Outpatient

 ONGOING CARE

FOLLOW-UP RECOMMENDATIONS
Patient Monitoring
As needed, only if lesions become symptomatic

DIET
No special diet

PATIENT EDUCATION
- Stress long-term chronicity and likely permanent resolution of condition in 2nd or 3rd decade of life
- Sun protection

PROGNOSIS
- Permanent resolution during 2nd or 3rd decade of life in almost all cases
- Worse prognosis in patients with higher Fitzpatrick skin types (darker skin)

COMPLICATIONS
None expected

REFERENCES
1. Lin RL, Janniger CK. Pityriasis alba. *Cutis*. 2005;76:21–24.
2. Fujita WH, McCormick CL, Parneix-Spake A, et al. An exploratory study to evaluate the efficacy of pimecrolimus cream 1% for the treatment of pityriasis alba. *Int J Dermatol*. 2007;46:700–705.
3. Rigopoulos D, Gregoriou S, Charissi C, et al. Tacrolimus ointment 0.1% in pityriasis alba: An open-label, randomized, placebo-controlled study. *Br J Dermatol*. 2006;155:152–155.
4. Landeck L, Visser M, Kezic S, et al. Genotype-phenotype associations in filaggrin loss-of-function mutation carriers. *Contact Dermatitis*. 2013;68:149–155.
5. Di Lernia V, Ricci C. Progressive and extensive hypomelanosis and extensive pityriasis alba: Same disease, different names? *J Eur Acad Dermatol Venereol*. 2005;19:370–372.

ADDITIONAL READING
- Al-Mutairi N, Hadad AA. Efficacy of 308-nmm xenon chloride excimer laser in pityriasis alba. *Dermatol Surg*. 2012;38:604–609.
- Halder RM, Nandedkar MA, Neal KW. Pigmentary disorders in ethnic skin. *Dermatol Clin*. 2003;21:617–628, vii.
- In SI, Yi SW, Kang HY, et al. Clinical and histopathological characteristics of pityriasis alba. *Clin Exp Dermatol*. 2009;34:591–597.
- Jadotte YT, Janniger CK. Pityriasis alba revisited: Perspectives on an enigmatic disorder of childhood. *Cutis*. 2011;87:66–72.

- Miller DC. Pigmentation disorders in adults. *Clin Fam Pract*. 2003;5:691.
- Moreno-Cruz B, Torres-Alvarez B, Hernandez-Blanco D, et al. Double-blind, placebo-controlled, randomized study comparing 0.0003% calcitriol with 0.1% tacrolimus ointments for the treatment of endemic pityriasis alba. *Dermatol Res Pract*. 2012;303275:1–6.
- Patel AB, Kubba R, Kubba A. Clinicopathological correlation of acquired hypopigmentary disorders. *Indian J Dermatol*. 2013;79:376–382.
- Plensdorf S, Martinez J. Common pigmentation disorders. *Am Fam Physician*. 2009;79:109–116.

 SEE ALSO

Keratosis, Actinic; Tinea Versicolor; Vitiligo

 CODES

ICD10
L30.5 Pityriasis alba

CLINICAL PEARLS
- More common in patients with atopic dermatitis.
- Use of KOH preparation and Wood's lamp is a quick way to differentiate this from a fungal infection.
- Treatment is largely symptomatic, and sun protection is essential.
- Topical calcineurin inhibitor therapy may become primary treatment for extensive pityriasis alba or when associated with atopic dermatitis.

PLACENTA PREVIA

Dawn S. Tasillo, MD • Laura Ferraro

 BASICS

DESCRIPTION
- Placental implantation in the lower uterine segment in advance of presenting fetal part and in proximity to/covering the internal os
- Complete/Total previa: Placenta covers entire internal cervical os.
- Partial previa: Placenta covers part of internal cervical os.
- Marginal previa: Placental edge is adjacent to cervical os by US, but not overlapping, usually within 2 cm of os.
- Low-lying placenta: Placental edge located in the lower uterine segment, but does not encroach on/cover the os; has been defined as within 2–3 cm of cervical os by US
- System(s) affected: Cardiovascular; Reproductive

EPIDEMIOLOGY
- Average gestational age of 1st bleed, 27–36 weeks
- Most common cause of minimally painful bleeding after 20 weeks' gestational age
- 10% of low-lying placentas at 10–20 weeks persist to term (1).

Incidence
- 0.4% of primiparous pregnancies, with increasing incidence with cesarean deliveries/other uterine scarring
- Up to 5% incidence in grand multiparous (>5 deliveries) women

Prevalence
- Prevalence decreases from early pregnancy to mid pregnancy.
- Placenta previa complicates 0.3–0.5% of deliveries (1).

ETIOLOGY AND PATHOPHYSIOLOGY
- Not well understood
- Uterine scaring may predispose to placental implantation in the lower uterine segment.
- As lower uterine segment expands and the trophoblastic tissue expands toward the fundus, many marginal or low-lying placentas will resolve to a safe distance from the cervix to allow vaginal delivery (2).

Genetics
No genetic links have been identified.

RISK FACTORS
- History of placenta previa (relative risk [RR] = 8)
- Advanced maternal age (RR = 9 if >40 years of age)
- Multiparity (5% if >5 deliveries) (RR = 1.1–1.7)
- Assisted reproductive technology (RR = 2)
- Multiple gestation
- Smoking (RR = 1.4–3)
- Cocaine use
- Male fetus (RR = 1.4)
- Asian (RR = 1.9)
- Previous cesarean deliveries:
  – 1 previous C-section: RR = 4.5 (95% CI 3.6–5.5) (1)
  – 4 previous C-sections: RR = 44.9 (95% CI 13.5–15) (1)
- Induced/Spontaneous abortion/Curettage (Asherman syndrome) (RR = 1.6)
- Leiomyoma/History of lower uterine segment surgery

GENERAL PREVENTION
Once pregnancy is diagnosed, risk factors are not modifiable. If patient has any risk factors for previa and anatomic survey is suggestive of previa, serial US should be performed for monitoring purposes. Patient should be counseled regarding potential bleeding and should be triaged with all bleeding episodes.

COMMONLY ASSOCIATED CONDITIONS
- Abnormal presentations (e.g., oblique and/or transverse fetal lie)
- Antepartum/Intrapartum/Postpartum hemorrhage (RR = 9.81 for antepartum bleeding) (1)
- Small for gestational age/intrauterine growth restriction (up to 16% in some reports after controlling for confounders)
- Vasa previa/velamentous insertion of the cord (particularly after resolution of early placenta previa)
- Premature rupture of membranes
- Evidence that shortened cervical length in the 3rd trimester is an independent risk factor for bleeding episodes (3)
- Placenta previa is an independent risk factor for placenta accreta (OR = 54; 95% CI = 18–166) (4):
  – Placenta accreta encompasses various types of abnormal placentations in which chorionic villi attach directly to/invade the myometrium.
  – Placenta previa in cases of prior cesarean delivery increases risk of accreta.
  – Elective delivery may be planned earlier (34–36 weeks) if accreta is suspected (5).

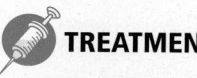 **DIAGNOSIS**

HISTORY
- Painless, bright-red vaginal bleeding in 2nd/3rd trimester (classic presentation)
- Painful bleeding if contractions are also present
- Decreased fetal movement/nonreassuring fetal heart tracing

PHYSICAL EXAM

ALERT
- Do not perform digital cervical exam in any woman with a complaint of bleeding until placental position has been verified.
- Careful sterile speculum exam can be performed to evaluate for vaginal/cervical source of bleeding.
- Evaluate for rupture of membranes as cause for bleeding.

DIFFERENTIAL DIAGNOSIS
- Abruptio placentae
- Vasa previa
- Labor
- Vaginal and cervical pathology, including polyps, erosion, cancer, trauma, or infections

DIAGNOSTIC TESTS & INTERPRETATION
- Transvaginal/Translabial US is gold standard to identify placental position accurately (1).
- Transabdominal US may be performed bedside if skilled sonographer is not available.
- Contraction and fetal heart rate monitoring should be performed during evaluation.

Initial Tests (lab, imaging)
- Maternal blood type and antibody screen
- CBC: Normocytic, normochromic anemia may be present with acute bleeding.
- Prothrombin time (PT)/International normalization ratio (INR), and partial thromboplastin time (PTT): Coagulopathy is rare, but may occur with significant blood loss.
- Fibrinogen is optional, and disseminated intravascular coagulation (DIC) panel is often inconclusive.
- Kleihauer-Betke test: Positive test indicates fetal–maternal transfusion may be present and can determine Rho (D) immunoglobulin dosing in Rh-negative patients (1).
- Cross-match at least 4 units of packed RBCs if clinically significant bleeding.
  – Development of US, especially the transvaginal scan, has helped in the definitive diagnosis and management of placenta previa.
  – External abdominal US with full, then empty bladder: Full bladder can cause compression of lower uterine segment causing a false appearance of previa.
  – Careful assessment may still miss some posterior previas if fetal vertex is low.
  – Vaginal probe sonography using 8.4 MHz transducer to define placental position further. Translabial US may also be utilized, but may not be able to discern specifically the characteristics of previas.
  – 3D US may help define placenta to cervical os distance for management of delivery (6)[C]
- Given increased risk of accreta, the placental–uterine interface should be closely examined for evidence of lakes/other abnormal vasculature.
- MRI if concerned for placenta accreta without definitive US diagnosis; important also for surgical planning

Follow-Up Tests & Special Considerations
- Repeat hemoglobin/hematocrit determinations as needed to assess blood loss.
- Previas found on US before 35 weeks should have a repeat US prior to delivery:
  – 10% of previas at 10–20 weeks persist until term (1).
  – 62% of previas at 28–31 weeks persist until term.
  – 75% of previas at 32–35 weeks persist until term.

Test Interpretation
Placental pathology often shows giant trophoblasts at placental interface, evidence of abruption.

TREATMENT

GENERAL MEASURES
- Many patients with placenta previa will have no antepartum bleeding, and delivery may be electively planned between 36 and 38 weeks (1,5).
- Avoid vaginal exams, sexual intercourse, douching, or other vaginal manipulation.
- Amniocentesis can determine fetal lung maturity for elective delivery before 38 weeks but not recommended to guide the timing of delivery (5).
- A trial of labor may be considered in a tertiary care institution with placenta position >2 cm away from the cervix (7)[B].

- Blood volume is increased in pregnancy; patient can lose >30% maternal blood volume before shock develops.
- Rh-negative women should receive 300 μg Rho(D) immunoglobulin (RhoGAM).

MEDICATION
First Line
- Oxygen supplementation if needed
- Adequate IV access via large bore catheters
- Aggressive IV fluids/blood products as needed: Fresh-frozen plasma, platelets, and packed RBCs
- Tocolytics for uterine contractions may be used with caution, especially to allow for steroids for fetal lung maturity if possible (8)[A]. Calcium channel blockers such as nifedipine, loading dose of 10 mg PO q20min × 3, then q4–6h:
  – Watch for placental hypoperfusion (late decelerations on the fetal heart tracing).
  – Contraindications: Term fetus/unstable maternal/fetal cardiovascular status

Second Line
Alternative tocolytics:
- Magnesium sulfate: 4–6 g IV load over 20 minutes, then 2–3 g/hr continuous infusion (9)[A]; watch for toxicity: Loss of reflexes, pulmonary edema, cardiac arrest

ISSUES FOR REFERRAL
- Maternal–fetal medicine consult for delivery decisions regarding stable patients
- Neonatal ICU team should be alerted for high-risk delivery and consulted for preterm delivery.
- Appropriate interdisciplinary planning with blood bank, anesthesia, nursing staff in anticipation of placenta previa delivery
- Hospitals with obstetric units should consider massive transfusion protocols and staff training.

ADDITIONAL THERAPIES
Recombinant factor VII is an alternative blood product for DIC when fresh-frozen plasma and cryoprecipitate fail (10)[C].

SURGERY/OTHER PROCEDURES
- Cesarean delivery is indicated for partial/complete previa.
- Timing of delivery depends on maternal stability and fetal lung maturity.
- Threshold for delivery is lower after 34 completed weeks gestation and is planned by 38 weeks.

IN-PATIENT CONSIDERATIONS
Admission Criteria/Initial Stabilization
- Heavy vaginal bleeding warrants inpatient observation at least until 48 hours resolved.
- 1st bleed usually is self-limited. Patients should be observed and steroids for fetal lung maturity administered at gestational age 24–34 weeks. Once stable, preterm patients may be observed on an outpatient basis without difference in outcome (1)[B],(11).
- Patients managed outpatient should have reliable, rapid (within 20 minutes) transportation available to a tertiary care OB center.
- Multiple large bleeds may necessitate admission until scheduled delivery between 34 and 36 weeks, depending on institutional guidelines.

- May consider transfer to high-risk perinatology service based on patient condition, local services, and concern for accreta.
- Bed rest and NPO until delivery decision made
- 2 large-bore IV sites and IV fluids as needed for resuscitation
- Continuous fetal heart and contraction monitoring

Nursing
- Continuous fetal heart and contraction monitoring
- Frequent vital signs, including fluid intake and output
- Monitor pad count, amount of vaginal bleeding

Discharge Criteria
- Demonstration of fetal well-being by fetal heart tracing/biophysical profile
- Demonstration of maternal hemodynamic stability: No active bleeding for >48 hours
- Proximity of patient to health care facility and patient reliability
- Final determination made based on number of bleeding episodes, gestational age, and other mitigating factors

ONGOING CARE

FOLLOW-UP RECOMMENDATIONS
- Repeat US of placenta location if last US was done at <37 weeks gestational age.
- Placentas should be sent for pathologic evaluation.

DIET
No restrictions once stable; NPO if delivery possible

PATIENT EDUCATION
www.nlm.nih.gov/medlineplus/ency/article/000900.htm

PROGNOSIS
- Maternal mortality 0.03% with placenta previa (1)
- Greatest fetal risk is preterm delivery and consequences of hypoxemia if delay in delivery with fetal tracing abnormalities.

COMPLICATIONS
- Peripartum hysterectomy (RR = 33) (1):
  – Increased risk with prior C-section
- Blood transfusion (RR = 10) (1)
- DIC risk is low unless massive bleeding is present.
- Fetal anemia and Rh isoimmunization
- Intra- and postpartum hemorrhage due to placental insertion into noncontractile lower uterine segment (1)

REFERENCES
1. Oyelese Y, Smulian JC. Placenta previa, placenta accreta, and vasa previa. *Obstet Gynecol*. 2006;107:927–941.
2. Predanci M. A sonographic assessment of different patterns of placenta previa "migration" in the third trimester of pregnancy. *J Ultrasound Med*. 2005;24:773.
3. Stafford IA, Dashe JS, Shivvers SA, et al. Ultrasonographic cervical length and risk of hemorrhage in pregnancies with placenta previa. *Obstet Gynecol*. 2010;116:595–600.
4. Publications Committee, Society for Maternal-Fetal Medicine, Belfort MA. Placenta accreta. *Am J Obstet Gynecol*. 2010;84(5):430–439.
5. Committee opinion no. 560: medically indicated late-preterm and early-term deliveries. *Obstet Gynecol*. 2013;121:908.
6. Simon EG, Fouche CJ, Perrotin F. Three-dimensional transvaginal sonography in third-trimester evaluation of placenta previa. *Ultrasound Obstet Gynecol*. 2013;41:465.
7. Bhide A, Prefumo F, Moore J, et al. Placental edge to internal os distance in the late third trimester and mode of delivery in placenta praevia. *BJOG*. 2003;110:860–864.
8. Sharma A, Suri V, Gupta I. Tocolytic therapy in conservative management of symptomatic placenta previa. *Int J Gynaecol Obstet*. 2004;84:109–113.
9. Briggs GG, Wan SR. Drug therapy during labor and delivery, part 2 [Review]. *Am J of Health-System Pharm*. 2006;63(12):1131–1139.
10. Alfirevic Z, Elbourne D, Pavord S, et al. Use of recombinant activated factor VII in primary postpartum hemorrhage: The Northern European registry 2000–2004. *Obstet Gynecol*. 2007;110:1270–1278.
11. Neilson JP. Interventions for suspected placenta praevia. *Cochrane Database Syst Rev*. 2003;(2):CD001998.

 SEE ALSO

Abruptio Placentae

 CODES

ICD10
- O44.10 Placenta previa with hemorrhage, unspecified trimester
- O44.11 Placenta previa with hemorrhage, first trimester
- O44.12 Placenta previa with hemorrhage, second trimester

CLINICAL PEARLS
- Placenta previa is a major cause of antepartum bleeding in the 2nd and 3rd trimesters.
- Do *not* perform digital cervical exam, only careful speculum exam.
- US, both transvaginal and transabdominal, is used to verify placenta location and diagnosis.
- Delivery is by cesarean section with rare exceptions.

PLANTAR FASCIITIS
Katie M. Crowder, MD • Alan J. Williamson, MD

 BASICS

DESCRIPTION
- Degenerative change of plantar fascia at origin from medial tuberosity of calcaneus
- Pain on plantar surface, usually at calcaneal insertion of plantar fascia upon weightbearing, especially in morning or on initiation of walking after prolonged rest

EPIDEMIOLOGY
Prevalence
- Lifetime: 10–15% of population
- Data suggest persistence with BMI >30.
- Condition is self-limiting; typically resolves within 10 months.

ETIOLOGY AND PATHOPHYSIOLOGY
- Repetitive partial tearing of plantar fascia
- Chronic degenerative change (-osis/-opathy rather than -itis) of plantar fascia generally at insertion on medial tuberosity of calcaneus

RISK FACTORS
- Dancers, runners, court sport athletes
- Obesity (BMI >30)
- Pes planus (flat feet), pes cavus (high arch), overpronation, leg length discrepancy
- Occupations with prolonged standing, especially on hard surfaces (nurses, letter carriers, warehouse/factory workers)
- Female, pregnancy
- Age (>40–60 years)
- Tightness of calf and hamstring tendons
- Decreased ankle range of motion in dorsiflexion (tight heel chord; <10 degrees of dorsiflexion)
- Systemic connective tissue disorders

GENERAL PREVENTION
- Maintain normal body weight
- Avoid prolonged standing on bare feet, sandals, or slippers
- Avoid training errors (increasing intensity, distance, duration, and frequency of high-impact activities too rapidly)
- Proper foot gear (appropriate cushioning and arch support)
- Runners should replace footwear after every 250–500 miles
- Avoid excessive use

COMMONLY ASSOCIATED CONDITIONS
- Usually isolated
- Heel spurs common, but not marker of severity
- Posterior tibial neuropathy

 DIAGNOSIS

HISTORY
- Pain on plantar surface of foot, usually at fascial insertion at calcaneus (medial calcaneal tubercle), but can have pain anywhere along length of plantar fascia.
- Pain is typically worse with first few steps in the morning or after prolonged rest (poststatic dyskinesia).
- Pain typically improves after those first few steps only to recur toward the end of the day
- Pain can be dull and constant in chronic plantar fasciitis
- Pain with prolonged ambulation or standing
- Limp with excessive toe walking
- Numbness and burning of medial hindfoot when associated with posterior tibial nerve compression

PHYSICAL EXAM
- Point tenderness on medial tuberosity of calcaneus at insertion of plantar fascia
- Pain along plantar fascia with foot dorsiflexion
- Windlass test: Pain with passive dorsiflexion of the toes.
- High specificity, low sensitivity. Sensitivity improves (13.5–31.8%) if performed while standing
- Decreased passive range of motion with dorsiflexion of ankle
- Evaluate for pes planus, pes cavus, overpronation
- Loss of heel fat pad suggests heel fat pad syndrome
- Point tenderness on posteriosuperior aspect of heel suggests Achilles' tendinopathy

DIFFERENTIAL DIAGNOSIS
- Calcaneal stress fracture
- Heel fat pad syndrome (painful or atrophic heel pad)
- Longitudinal arch strain
- Nerve entrapment (posterior tibial nerve–tarsal tunnel syndrome, medial calcaneal branch of posterior tibial nerve, abductor digit quinti)
- Achilles' tendinopathy
- Calcaneal contusion
- Plantar calcaneal bursitis
- Tendonitis of posterior tibialis
- Plantar fascia tear
- Calcaneal apophysitis (Sever disease)—adolescents
- Pain from neoplasm or infection
- Spondyloarthropathy (Reiter syndrome)
- In association with connective tissue disorder:
  - Rheumatoid arthritis
  - Polymyositis

DIAGNOSTIC TESTS & INTERPRETATION
- None necessary for the diagnosis
- Consider further imaging only if diagnosis is in question
- 2 radiographic views of foot can rule out fracture, tumor, cyst, periostitis, bony erosions; weightbearing preferred
- Ultrasound: Demonstrates signs of inflammation at insertion (hypoechoic), including thickened plantar fascia (≥4 mm)
- MRI can evaluate for other soft tissue etiologies
- CT or technetium-99 bone scan can rule out calcaneal stress fracture and evaluate for infection
- Nerve conduction studies can rule out nerve entrapment

TREATMENT
Nonoperative management is mainstay of treatment

GENERAL MEASURES
- Supportive footwear with stable midfoot; avoid wearing sandals or walking barefoot
- Relative rest/activity modification
- Stretching: Plantar fascial stretches more effective than Achilles' tendon stretches (1)[B]
- Weight reduction if BMI >25
- Orthotics:
  - Custom orthotics show no benefit over prefabricated orthotics and are more costly
  - Improved effectiveness of night splints when used in association with orthotics
- Strengthening of calf and next interosseous muscles, utilizing the towel drag/pick-up exercise
- Night splints: Can be uncomfortable for the 1st few nights, but generally become less bothersome with time. Especially effective with calf and Achilles' tightness
- Ice (frozen water bottle roll)
- Massage (golf ball roll)

MEDICATION
First Line
- Use only as an adjunct to general measures to control pain and increase compliance
- NSAIDs (1): Naproxen 500 mg PO b.i.d. *or* ibuprofen 600–800 mg PO t.i.d. PRN for pain (2)[A]
- Acetaminophen 1,000 mg PO t.i.d. PRN for pain

Second Line
None

ISSUES FOR REFERRAL
- Podiatry, surgery: Consider referral for more invasive treatments if conservative measures fail after 3–6 months
- Consider physical therapy referral for patient instruction on proper stretching and strengthening techniques

ADDITIONAL THERAPIES
- Low-dye taping (3)[B]:
  - Limited evidence
  - Less effective in severe cases
- Corticosteroid injections (4)[A]:
  - Short-term pain relief
  - Recommend ultrasound guidance
  - Risk for plantar fascial rupture and calcaneal fat pad atrophy with resultant permanent heel pain
  - Can cause injection pain and postinjection pain for up to 5–7 days
- Extracorporeal shock wave therapy (ESWT) (5)[A]:
  - Growing body of evidence showing benefit
  - Meta-analysis comparing effectiveness of focused shock wave therapy of different intensity levels vs. radial shock wave therapy shows consistent benefit; radial shock wave therapy likely more beneficial
  - Uncomfortable to patients but less risk than injection or surgery
  - May be more effective in patients with an obvious spur on x-ray

- Some orthopedic surgeons prefer casting in severe cases.
- Promising therapies:
  – Botulinum toxin (BT) A injection:
    ◦ RCT comparing steroid injection to BT injection showed similar results in pain reduction and other measures of foot function at 1 month; improvements in these areas persisted at 6 months more so with BT than with steroid injection (6)[B]
    ◦ Randomized, multicenter, double-blind, placebo-controlled study comparing BT injection to placebo showed no statistical difference in pain and global assessment
  – Platelet-rich plasma injections: Limited evidence
  – Myofascial trigger point manual therapy
  – Intralesional autologous blood injection
  – Intracorporeal pneumatic shock application
  – Low-level laser therapy (LLLT)
  – Pulsed radiofrequency electromagnetic field therapy
  – Percutaneous bipolar radiofrequency microdebridement

SURGERY/OTHER PROCEDURES

- Only necessary in a small percentage of patients (10%)
- Recommended after resistance to conservative treatment of 6–12 months and pain is unrelenting
- Open/endoscopic plantar fasciotomy (less risk and complications with endoscopic technique but requires specialized equipment and skills and is not widely used)
- Calcaneal spur resection
- Other: Cryosurgery (leads to long-term heel numbness), radiofrequency nerve ablation (uses heat), Coblation therapy (uses Topaz wand)
- More likely beneficial in severely obese

COMPLEMENTARY AND ALTERNATIVE MEDICINE

- Heel cup with magnet has proven ineffective
- Acupuncture shows limited benefit in a few studies

 ## ONGOING CARE

FOLLOW-UP RECOMMENDATIONS

- Ensure patient is adhering to proper stretching exercises
- Following 3–6 months of unsuccessful conservative treatment, consider additional therapies or referrals

PATIENT EDUCATION

- Weight reduction if BMI >25
- Proper footwear (adequate cushion and arch support)
- Stretch plantar fascia: Pull toes into dorsiflexion prior to walking after prolonged sitting or sleep
- Ice the foot using a frozen water bottle: Roll foot over bottle for 10 minutes in morning and after work
- Massage plantar fascia: Roll foot over a golf ball
- Strengthen foot muscles: Grab cloth or carpet by plantar flexing the toes
- Decrease repetitive stress
- Video overview for patients: www.youtube.com/watch?v=Pnithn4EYQk

PROGNOSIS

- Good
- Self-limited condition (resolves within 2 years) in up to 85–90% of patients

COMPLICATIONS

- Rupture of plantar fascia (more common with repeated corticosteroid injections)
- Chronic pain
- Gait abnormality

REFERENCES

1. Digiovanni BF, Nawoczenski DA, Malay DP, et al. Plantar fascia-specific stretching exercise improves outcomes in patients with chronic plantar fasciitis. A prospective clinical trial with two-year follow-up. *J Bone Joint Surg Am.* 2006;88:1775–1781.
2. Donley BG, Moore T, Sferra J, et al. The efficacy of oral nonsteroidal anti-inflammatory medication (NSAID) in the treatment of plantar fasciitis: A randomized, prospective, placebo-controlled study. *Foot Ankle Int.* 2007;28:20–23.
3. Speksnijder C, van de Water A. Efficacy of taping for the treatment of plantar fasciosis. A systematic review of controlled trials. *J Am Podiatr Med Assoc.* 2010;100:41–51.
4. McMillan AM, Landorf KB, Gilheany MF. Ultrasound guided corticosteroid injection for plantar fasciitis: Randomized controlled trial. *BMJ.* 2012;344:1–12.
5. Chang K, Chen S, Chen WS, et al. Comparative effectiveness of focused shock wave therapy of different intensity levels and radial shock wave therapy for treating plantar fasciitis: A systematic review and network meta-analysis. *Arch Phys Med Rahabil.* 2012;93:1259–1268.
6. Jabbari B, Machado D. Treatment of refractory pain with botulinum toxins—An evidence-based review. *Pain Med.* 2011;12:1594–1606.

ADDITIONAL READING

- Aksahin E, Dogruyol D, Yuksel HY, et al. The comparison of the effect of corticosteroids and protein rich plasma (PRP) for the treatment of plantar fasciitis. *Arch Orthop Trauma Surg.* 2012;132:781–785.
- Burns J, du Toit V, Hawke F, et al. Custom-made foot orthoses for the treatment of foot pain. *Cochrane Database Sys Rev.* 2008;3:CD006801.
- Crawford F. Interventions for treating plantar heel pain. *Cochrane Database Sys Rev.* 2006;1:CD000416.
- Diaz-Llopis IV, Rodriguez-Ruiz CM, et al. Randomized controlled study of the efficacy of the injection of botulinum toxin type A versus corticosteroids in chronic plantar fasciitis: Results at one and six months. *Clin Rehab.* 2011;26:594–606.
- Dogramaci Y, Kalaci A, Emir A, et al. Intracorporeal pneumatic shock application for the treatment of chronic plantar fasciitis: A randomized, double blind prospective clinical trial. *Arch Orthop Trauma Surg.* 2010;130:541–546.
- Goff JD, Crawford R. Diagnosis and treatment of plantar fasciitis. *Am Fam Physician.* 2011;84:676–682.
- Healey K, Chen K. Plantar fasciitis: Current diagnostic modalities and treatments. *Clin Podiatr Med Surg.* 2010;27:369–380.
- Huang YC, Wei SH, Wang HK, et al. Ultrasonographic guided botulinum toxin type A treatment for plantar fasciitis: An outcome-based investigation for treating pain and gait changes. *J Rehabil Med.* 2010;42:136–140.

- Ibrahim MI, Donatelli RA, Schmitz C, et al. Chronic plantar fasciitis treated with two sessions of radial extracorporeal shock wave therapy. *Foot Ankle Int.* 2010;31:391–397.
- Kiritsi O, Tsitas K, Malliaropoulos N, et al. Ultrasonographic evaluation of plantar fasciitis after low-level laser therapy: Results of a double-blind, randomized, placebo-controlled trial. *Lasers Med Sci.* 2010;25:275–281.
- Lee TG, Ahmad TS. Intralesional autologous blood injection compared to corticosteroid injection for treatment of chronic plantar fasciitis. A prospective, randomized, controlled trial. *Foot Ankle Int.* 2007;28:984–990.
- Peterlein CD, Funk JF, Holscher A, et al. Is botulinum toxin A effective for the treatment of plantar fasciitis? *Clin J Pain.* 2012;28:527–533.
- Ragab EM, Othman AM. Platelets rich plasma for treatment of chronic plantar fasciitis. *Arch Orthop Trauma Surg.* 2012;132:1065–1070.
- Renan-Ordine R, Alburquerqe-Sendin F, et al. Effectiveness of myofascial trigger point manual therapy combined with a self-stretching protocol for the management of plantar heel pain: A randomized controlled trial. *J Ortho Sports Phys Ther.* 2011;41:43–50.
- Thomas J, Christensen J, Kravitz S, et al. The diagnosis and treatment of heel pain: A clinical practice guideline—Revision 2010. *J Foot Ankl Surg.* 2010;49:S1–S19.
- Uden H, Boesch E, Kumar S. Plantar fasciitis—To jab or to support? A systematic review of the current best evidence. *J Multidiscip Healthc.* 2011;4:155–164.
- Young C. In the clinic. Plantar fasciitis. *Ann Intern Med.* 2012;156(1 Pt 1):ITC1-1–ITC1-15; quiz ITC1-16.

 ## SEE ALSO

Algorithm: Heel Pain

 ## CODES

ICD10

M72.2 Plantar fascial fibromatosis

CLINICAL PEARLS

- Degeneration of plantar fascia at origin from plantar tuberosity of calcaneum.
- Pain on plantar surface on weightbearing, especially first few steps in the morning or after prolonged rest.
- Conservative treatment is the mainstay of therapy:
  – Wear supportive footwear to help avoid excess pronation, provide adequate cushion, and provide arch support
  – Arch supports are beneficial
  – Activity modification
  – Weight reduction if BMI >25
  – Stretch plantar fascia after prolonged rest
  – NSAIDs and acetaminophen treat pain only
  – Ice (frozen water bottle roll)
  – Massage (golf ball roll)

PLEURAL EFFUSION

Felix B. Chang, MD • Jose F. Vargas, MD

BASICS

Abnormal accumulation of fluid in the pleural space

DESCRIPTION
Types:
- Congestive heart failure 40%
- Pneumonia 25%, malignancy 15%, and pulmonary embolism PE 10% account for exudative effusions.
- Malignant: Lung cancer and metastases of breast, ovary, and lymphoma

EPIDEMIOLOGY
Incidence

Estimated 1.3 million cases/year in the US; CHF: 500,000; pneumonia 300,000; malignancy 150,000; PE 150,000; cirrhosis 150,000; tuberculosis 2,500; pancreatitis 20,000; collagen-vascular disease 6,000.

Prevalence
- Estimated 320 cases/100,000 people in industrialized countries. In hospitalized patients with AIDS prevalence is 7–27%
- No gender predilection: ~2/3 of malignant pleural effusions occur in women.

ETIOLOGY AND PATHOPHYSIOLOGY
- Pleural fluid formation exceeds pleural fluid absorption.
- Transudates result from imbalances in hydrostatic and oncotic forces:
  - Increase in hydrostatic and/or low oncotic pressures; increase in pleural capillary permeability; lymphatic obstruction or impaired drainage; movement of fluid from the peritoneal or retroperitoneal space
- Transudates:
  - CHF: 40% of transudative effusions; 80% bilateral. Constrictive pericarditis, atelectasis; superior vena cava syndrome
  - Cirrhosis (hepatic hydrothorax); nephrotic syndrome, hypoalbuminemia; mixedema
  - Urinothorax, central line misplacement; peritoneal dialysis
- Exudates:
  - Lung parenchyma infection, bacterial (parapneumonic, tuberculous pleurisy) fungal, viral, parasitic (amebiasis, *Echinococcus*)
  - Cancer: Lung cancer, metastases (breast, lymphoma, ovaries), mesothelioma
  - Pulmonary embolism 25% of PEs are transudate
  - Collagen-vascular disease: Rheumatoid arthritis, systemic lupus erythematosus, Wegener granulomatosis, sarcoidosis
  - GI: Pancreatitis, esophageal rupture, abdominal abscess, after liver transplant. Chylothorax: Thoracic duct tear, malignancy
  - Hemothorax: Trauma, PE, malignancy, coagulopathy, aortic aneurysm
  - Others: After coronary artery bypass graft; Dressler syndrome; uremia, asbestos exposure, radiation; drug-induced: Nitrofurantoin, bromocriptine, amiodarone, procarbazine, methysergide, hydralazine, procainamide, quinidine, methotrexate, methysergide;
  - Meigs syndrome; yellow-nail syndrome; ovarian stimulation syndrome; lymphangiomatosis; acute respiratory distress syndrome (ARDS)
  - Chylothorax: Thoracic duct tear, malignancy

RISK FACTORS
- Occupational exposures/drugs
- PE; TB; bacterial pneumonias
- Opportunistic infections (in HIV patients when CD4 count is <150 cells/μL)

COMMONLY ASSOCIATED CONDITIONS
Hypoproteinemia, heart failure, cirrhosis

DIAGNOSIS

Presumptive diagnosis in 50%. Small pleural effusions, radiographic area <2 intercostal spaces (<300 mL) are asymptomatic.

HISTORY
Dyspnea, fever, malaise, and weight loss; chest pain, cough, hemoptysis

PHYSICAL EXAM
- Pleural effusion >300 mL: Tachypnea, asymmetric expansion of the thoracic cage; decrease/absent tactile fremitus; dullness to percussion; decreased/inaudible breath sounds, egophony, pleural friction rub

DIFFERENTIAL DIAGNOSIS
- Empyema, Malignancy, Inflammatory, Fungal, Tubercular, others

DIAGNOSTIC TESTS & INTERPRETATION
Initial Tests (lab, imaging)
- Pleural fluid: Appearance, pH, WBC differential, total protein, lactate dehydrogenase (LDH), glucose, Gram stain and culture, acid-fast bacilli staining. Consider polymerase chain reaction (PCR) for *Mycobacterium tuberculosis* and *Streptococcus pneumoniae*.
- By scenario: Amylase, triglycerides, cholesterol, LE cells, cytology, antinuclear antibodies (ANAs), adenosine deaminase, tumor markers, rheumatoid factor, cytology, creatinine
- Light's criteria, transudate vs. exudate (98% sensitivity; 80% specificity) fluid is considered an exudate if any of the following (1)[B]:
  - Ratio of pleural fluid/serum protein levels >0.5; Ratio of pleural fluid-to-serum LDH levels >0.6; pleural fluid LDH level >2/3 the upper limit for serum LDH level
- Other exudate criteria:
  - Serum-effusion albumin gradient ≤1.2 (sensitivity 87%; specificity 92%); cholesterol effusion >45 mg/dL and LDH effusion >200 mg/dL (sensitivity 90%; specificity 98%)
- Empyema: Pus, putrid odor; culture; a putrid odor suggests an anaerobic empyema: LDH levels >1,000 IU/L (normal serum = 200 IU/L); glucose, <60 mg/dL; low pH
- Malignancy: Cytology, red, bloody; glucose normal to low, depending on the tumor burden; RBCs, >100,000/mm^3
- Lupus pleuritis: LE cells present; pleural fluid serum ANAs >1; glucose <60 mg/dL; pleural fluid/serum glucose ratio <0.5
- Fungal: Positive KOH, culture; peritoneal dialysis: Protein, <1 g/dL; glucose, 300–400 mg/dL
- Urinothorax: Creatinine pleural/blood >0.5; high LDH pleural fluid, with low protein levels

- Hemothorax: Hematocrit pleural/blood >0.5; benign asbestos effusion: Unilateral, exudative; have elevated eosinophil count.
- TB pleuritis: Lymphocytes >80% predominance effusion; elevated levels of adenosine deaminase >50 U/L and interferon-γ >140 pg/mL; positive acid fast bacillus (AFB) stain, culture; total protein >4 g/dL (2)[B]
- Chylothorax: Milky; triglycerides >110 mg/dL; lipoprotein electrophoresis (chylomicrons)
- Amebic liver abscess: Anchovy paste effusion; Waldenström macroglobulinemia and multiple myeloma: Protein >7 g/dL
- Esophageal rupture: High salivary amylase; pleural fluid acidosis, pH <6; amylase-rich: Acute pancreatitis, chronic pancreatic pleural effusion, malignancy, esophageal rupture; rheumatoid pleurisy: Glucose <60 mg/dL; pleural fluid/serum glucose <0.5
- Lymphocytosis: Tuberculous pleurisy, lymphoma, sarcoidosis, chronic rheumatoid pleurisy, yellow-nail syndrome, or chylothorax (80–95% of the nucleated cells). Carcinomatosis in half of cases (50–70% are lymphocytes)
- Pleural fluid eosinophilia (>10% of total nucleated cells): Pneumothorax, hemothorax, malignancy, drugs, pulmonary infarction, fungal (coccidiomycosis, cryptococcosis, histoplasmosis), benign asbestos pleural effusion
- Low glucose (<60 mg/dL): TB, malignancy, rheumatoid pleurisy, parapneumonic, empyema, hemothorax, paragonimiasis, Churg-Strauss syndrome
- RBC count >100,000/mm^3: Trauma, malignancy, PE, injury after cardiac surgery, asbestos pleurisy, pancreatitis, TB
- Pleural fluid LDH >1,000 IU/L: Suggests empyema, malignant effusion, rheumatoid effusion, or pleural paragonimiasis
- pH >7.3: Rheumatoid pleurisy, empyema, malignant effusion, TB, esophageal rupture, or lupus nephritis
- Mesothelial cells in exudates: TB is unlikely if there are >5% of mesothelial cells.
- *S. pneumoniae* accounts for 50% of cases of parapneumonic effusions in AIDS patients, followed by *Staphylococcus aureus*, *Haemophilus influenzae*, *Mycoplasma pneumoniae*, *Legionella*, *Nocardia*, and *Bordetella bronchiseptica*. Exudate with low count of nucleated cells.
- *Pneumocystis jiroveci* is an uncommon cause in HIV. Usually it is a small effusion, unilateral or bilateral, serous to bloody in appearance. Demonstration of the trophozoite or cyst is mandatory.
- Cancer-related HIV pleural effusion: Kaposi sarcoma, Castleman disease, and primary effusion lymphoma. Kaposi sarcoma: Mononuclear predominance, exudate, pH >7.4; LDH, 111–330 IU/L; glucose >60 mg/dL.

- Chest x-ray (CXR): Posteroanterior–anteroposterior views:
  - Upright x-rays show a concave meniscus in the costophrenic angle that suggests >250 mL of pleural fluid; homogeneous opacity, with visibility of pulmonary vessels through diffuse haziness and absence of air bronchogram; 75 mL of fluid will obliterate the posterior costophrenic sulcus.
  - Lateral x-rays show blunting of the posterior costophrenic angle and the posterior gutter. Decubitus x-rays to exclude a loculated effusion and underlying pulmonary lesion or pulmonary thickening
  - Supine x-rays show costophrenic blunting, haziness, obliteration of the diaphragmatic silhouette, decreased visibility of the lower lobe vasculature, and widened minor fissure.
- Ultrasonography (US): Detects as 5–50 mL of pleural fluid; identifies loculated effusions; site for thoracocentesis, pleural biopsy, or pleural drainage
- Chest CT scan with contrast for patients with undiagnosed pleural effusion. CT pulmonary angiography if pulmonary embolism is suspected

Follow-Up Tests & Special Considerations
- 75% of patients with exudative effusions have a non-CHF cause:
  - NT-ProBNP: Biomarker of CHF-associated effusion. >1,500 pg/mL. Sensitivity and specificity 94% (3)[A]
- Observation in uncomplicated asymptomatic patients (i.e., CHF, cirrhosis),viral pleurisy, thoracic or abdominal surgery

Diagnostic Procedures/Other
Diagnostic thoracentesis indicated for:
- Clinically significant pleural effusion (>10 mm thick on US or lateral decubitus x-ray with no known cause)
- CHF: Asymmetric effusion, fever, chest pain, or failure to resolve after diuretics
- Parapneumonic effusions

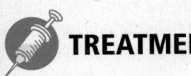

TREATMENT

Oxygen support

GENERAL MEASURES
- Therapeutic thoracentesis, if symptomatic
- Chest tube thoracostomy drainage: >1/2 hemithorax; complicated parapneumonic effusion (positive Gram stain or culture, pH <7.2, or glucose <60 mg/dL); empyema; hemothorax. Recommended limit is 1,000–1,500 mL in a single thoracentesis procedure.

MEDICATION
First Line
CHF: Diuretics (75% clearing in 48 hours); Parapneumonic effusion: Antibiotics; heumatologic conditions/inflammation: Steroids and NSAIDs

Second Line
Symptomatic nonmalignant effusions that are refractory to treatment may be managed with repeated therapeutic thoracentesis or pleurodesis.

ISSUES FOR REFERRAL
- Uncertain etiology; malignant effusion; high-risk diagnostic thoracentesis; decortication
- Video-assisted thoracoscopy for sclerosis. Peritoneal shunts for symptomatic recurrence

ADDITIONAL THERAPIES
- Pleurodesis for symptomatic patients whose pleural effusion reaccumulates too quickly for repeat therapeutic thoracentesis
- Tunneled pleural catheter is the preferred treatment for patients with malignant plerural effusion and limited survival (4)[B]
- Sclerosing agents for malignant effusions: Doxycycline, bleomycin, talc, and minocycline; talc is more efficacious. The relative risk of nonrecurrent effusion was 1.34 (95% confidence interval 1.16–1.55) in favor of talc compared with bleomycin, tetracycline, or mustine (5)[A].

SURGERY/OTHER PROCEDURES
- Percutaneous pleural biopsy if a cause is not clear after thoracentesis:
  - Close pleural biopsy: Pleura is diffusely involved (TB pleuritis, noncaseating granuloma in rheumatoid pleuritis)
  - CT-guided needle biopsy: Pleural mass; video-assisted thoracoscopic pleural biopsy: Negative percutaneous biopsy, patchy disease, or CT scan does not show obvious mass.
- Parapneumonic effusion should be sampled if free-flowing but layer is >10 mm on a lateral decubitus film. Loculated, thickened pleura on a contrast-enhanced CT scan, clearly delineated by ultrasound. Open pleural biopsy by thoracotomy.
- Contraindications for thoracocentesis: Anticoagulation, bleeding diathesis, thrombocytopenia <20,000/mm^3, mechanical ventilation
- Bronchoscopy: When malignancy is suspected (pulmonary infiltrate or mass on CXR or CT scan, hemoptysis, massive pleural effusion, or shift of the mediastinum toward the side of effusion)
- Thoracoscopy

IN-PATIENT CONSIDERATIONS
Admission Criteria/Initial Stabilization
Treat any underlying medical disorder.

 # ONGOING CARE

FOLLOW-UP RECOMMENDATIONS
Patient Monitoring
- Check for the amount and quality of fluid drained, air leak (bubbling), oscillation.
- Repeat a CXR when drainage decreases to <100 mL/d to evaluate complete clearing.
- For a large effusion,re-evaluate catheter position;if positioned appropriately, consider fibrinolytics.

DIET
Cardiac diet in patients with heart failure. Correct hypoproteinemia.

PROGNOSIS
- Malignant effusion: Poor
- Low-pH malignant effusions have shorter survival and poorer response to chemical pleurodesis than those with pH >7.3.
- Low pleural fluid pH (≤7.15): High likelihood of pleural space drainage

COMPLICATIONS
- Pleural effusion: Constrictive fibrosis, pleurocutaneous fistula
- Thoracentesis: Pneumothorax (5–10%); hemothorax (~1%); empyema; spleen/liver laceration; re-expansion pulmonary edema (if >1.5 L is removed)

REFERENCES
1. Bielsa S, Porcel JM, Castellote J, et al. Solving the Light's criteria misclassification rate of cardiac and hepatic transudates. *Respirology.* 2012;17: 721–726.
2. Garcia-Zamalloa A, Taboada-Gomez J. Diagnostic accuracy of adenosine deaminase and lymphocyte proportion in pleural fluid for tuberculous pleurisy in different prevalence scenarios. *PLoS ONE.* 2012;7(6):e38729.
3. Porcel JM. Utilization of B-type natriuretic peptide and NT-proBNP in the diagnosis of pleural effusions due to heart failure. *Curr Opin Pulm Med.* 2011; 17:215–219.
4. Puri V. Treatment of malignant pleural effusion: a cost effective analysis. *Ann Thorac Surg.* 2012; 94(2):379–380.
5. Davies HE, Mishra EK, Kahan BC, et al. Effect of an indwelling pleural catheter vs chest tube and talc pleurodesis for relieving dyspnea in patients with malignant pleural effusion: The TIME2 randomized controlled trial. *JAMA.* 2012;307:2383–2389.

ADDITIONAL READING
- Clive A, Bhatnagar R, Preston NJ, et al. Interventions for the management of malignant pleural effusions (protocol). *Cochrane Database Syst Rev.* 2013;5:CD010529.
- Light RW. Pleural effusions. *Med Clin North Am.* 2011;95(6):1055–1070.
- Shaw P, Agarwal R. Pleurodesis for malignant pleural effusions. *Cochrane Database Syst Rev.* 2004;(1):CD002916.

CODES

ICD10
- J90 Pleural effusion, not elsewhere classified
- J91.0 Malignant pleural effusion
- J94.0 Chylous effusion

CLINICAL PEARLS
- All patients with pleural effusion >1 cm of unknown origin should have thoracentesis.
- Urgent thoracentesis is mandatory if suspected hemothorax or empyema.

PNEUMONIA, BACTERIAL

Archana Govindan, MD, MS • Rahele Lameh, MD

BASICS

Bacterial pneumonia is an infection of the pulmonary parenchyma by a bacterial organism.

DESCRIPTION
Bacterial pneumonia can be classified as:
- Community-acquired pneumonia (CAP): Lower-respiratory tract infection not acquired in a hospital, long-term care facility, or during other recent contact with the health care system
- Hospital-acquired pneumonia (HAP): Pneumonia that occurs ≥48 hours after admission and did not appear to be incubating at the time of admission
- Ventilator-associated pneumonia (VAP): Pneumonia that develops >48–72 hours after endotracheal intubation
- Health care–associated pneumonia (HCAP): Pneumonia that occurs in a nonhospitalized patient with extensive health care contact, such as:
  - IV therapy/wound care within the past 30 days
  - Residing in a nursing home/long-term care facility
  - Hospitalization in an acute care hospital for ≥2 days within the past 90 days
  - Visited a hospital/hemodialysis clinic within the past 30 days

EPIDEMIOLOGY
- Influenza and pneumonia are the 8th leading cause of death in the US, with about 53,692 deaths in 2010.
- HAP is the leading cause of death among hospital-acquired infections and is the primary cause of death in the ICU.

Incidence
- CAP: 5–11 cases/1,000 persons with increased incidence occurring in the winter months
- HAP: 5–10 cases/1,000 admissions; incidence increase 6–20 fold in ventilated patients (1)

ETIOLOGY AND PATHOPHYSIOLOGY
- Adults, CAP:
  - Typical: *Streptococcal pneumoniae, Haemophilus influenzae, Staphylococcus aureus*, group A *Streptococcus, Moraxella catarrhalis*
  - Atypical: *Legionella* sp., *Mycoplasma pneumoniae, Chlamydophila pneumoniae*
- Adults, HCAP/HAP/VAP:
  - Aerobic gram-negative bacilli: *Pseudomonas aeruginosa, Escherichia coli, Klebsiella pneumoniae*, and *Acinetobacter* sp.
  - Gram-positive cocci: *Streptococcus* sp. and *S. aureus* (including MRSA)
- Children (2)[B]:
  - Birth to 20 days: *E. coli*, group B streptococci, *Listeria monocytogenes*
  - 3 weeks to 3 months: *Chlamydia trachomatis, S. pneumoniae*
  - 4 months to 18 years:
    - Typical: *S. pneumoniae*
    - Atypical: *C. pneumoniae, M. pneumoniae*

RISK FACTORS
- CAP:
  - Age >65 years
  - HIV/Immunocompromised
  - Recent antibiotic therapy/resistance to antibiotics
  - Asthma, CAD, COPD, chronic renal failure, CHF, diabetes, liver disease, neoplasm's VAP, HAP, HCAP
  - Hospitalization for ≥2 days during past 90 days
  - Severe illness
  - Antibiotic therapy in the past 6 months
  - Poor functional status as defined by activities-of-daily living score
  - Immunosuppression

GENERAL PREVENTION
- All children 2–59 months of age should be routinely vaccinated with PCV-13; given at 2, 4, and 6 months of age; a 4th at 12–15 months of age. PCV-13 is now currently FDA approved for those >50 years age (3).
- 23-valent pneumococcal polysaccharide vaccine is recommended for (3):
  - Age ≥65: 2nd dose recommended if patient received vaccine 5 years prior and was <65 years at the time of the 1st vaccination
  - Age 19–64 with chronic cardiovascular disease, chronic pulmonary disease (including asthma), diabetes mellitus, chronic liver disease, CSF leaks, cochlear implants, alcoholism, or who smoke cigarettes/live in chronic care facilities. Revaccination not recommended <65 years of age.
  - Age 19–64 who are immunocompromised: 2nd dose recommended if ≥5 years have elapsed since 1st dose
- Annual influenza vaccine is recommended according to current guidelines.

DIAGNOSIS

HISTORY
- Fever, chills, rigors, malaise, fatigue
- Dyspnea
- Cough, with/without sputum
- Pleuritic chest pain
- Myalgias
- GI symptoms

ALERT
High fever (>104°F [40°C]), male sex, multilobar involvement, and GI and neurologic abnormalities have been associated with CAP caused by *Legionella* infection.

Geriatric Considerations
Older adults with pneumonia often present with weakness and mental status change.

PHYSICAL EXAM
- Fever >100.4°F (38°C), tachypnea, tachycardia
- Rales, rhonchi, egophony, increased fremitus, bronchial breath sounds, dullness to percussion, asymmetric breath sounds, abdominal tenderness (4)

DIFFERENTIAL DIAGNOSIS
Bronchitis, asthma exacerbation, pulmonary edema, lung cancer, pulmonary tuberculosis, pneumonitis

DIAGNOSTIC TESTS & INTERPRETATION
Initial Tests (lab, imaging)
- Routine laboratory testing to establish an etiology in outpatients with CAP is usually unnecessary.
- For hospitalized patients with CAP, a CBC, sputum Gram stain, and 2 sets of blood cultures
- More extensive diagnostic testing in patients with CAP is recommended if:
  - Blood cultures: ICU admission, cavitary infiltrates, leukopenia, alcohol abuse, chronic severe liver disease, asplenia, positive pneumococcal urine antigen test (UAT), pleural effusion
  - Sputum Gram stain and cultures: ICU admission, failure of outpatient treatment, cavitary infiltrates, alcohol abuse, severe COPD/structural lung disease, positive *Legionella* UAT, positive pneumococcal UAT, pleural effusion
  - *Legionella* UAT: ICU admission, failure of outpatient treatment, alcohol abuse, travel in past 2 weeks, pleural effusion
  - Pneumococcal UAT: ICU admission, failure of outpatient treatment, leukopenia, alcohol abuse, chronic severe liver disease, asplenia, pleural effusion
- A chest x-ray (CXR) is indicated when pneumonia is suspected or with an acute respiratory infection and:
  - Vital signs: Temperature >100°F (37.8°C); heart rate (HR) >100 beats/min; respiratory rate (RR) >20 breaths/min
  - At least 2 of the following clinical findings: Decreased breath sounds, rales, absence of asthma
- Early in the course of the disease, a CXR may be negative.
- Evidence of necrotizing/cavitary pneumonia should raise suspicion for MRSA pneumonia, especially with history of prior MRSA skin lesions.

Diagnostic Procedures/Other
- For VAP/HAP: By bronchoscopic or nonbronchoscopic means, obtain a lower respiratory tract sample for culture prior to initiation/change of therapy. Serial evaluations may be needed (1)[A].
- Safe cessation of antibiotics can be done from a good quality negative sputum culture.

TREATMENT

MEDICATION
First Line
- Adults:
  - CAP, outpatient:
    - No significant differences in efficacy between antibiotic option in adults (4)[A]:
      - Previously healthy, no antibiotics in past 3 months:
        □ Azithromycin 500 mg PO 1 time, then 250 mg PO daily for 4 days; clarithromycin 500 mg PO b.i.d. for 10 days; erythromycin 500 mg PO b.i.d. for 10 days, or
        □ Doxycycline 100 mg PO b.i.d. for 10 days
      - Comorbid conditions, immunosuppressed, antibiotic use in past 3 months:
        □ Levofloxacin 750 mg PO daily for 5 days; moxifloxacin 400 mg PO daily for 10 days; gatifloxacin 400 mg PO daily for 10 days, osr
      - Amoxicillin 1 g PO t.i.d.; Amoxicillin-clavulanate 2 g PO b.i.d.) + macrolide

- CAP, inpatient (non-ICU):
  - IV antibiotics initially, then switch to oral after clinical improvement.
  - Cefotaxime; ceftriaxone; ampicillin-sulbactam + macrolide (clarithromycin; erythromycin) for 14 days, or
  - Gatifloxacin; levofloxacin for 14 days
  - If *pseudomonas* is a consideration:
    - Piperacillin-tazobactam; cefepime; imipenem; meropenem + levofloxacin, or
    - Piperacillin-tazobactam; cefepime; imipenem; meropenem + azithromycin or
    - Piperacillin-tazobactam; cefepime; imipenem; meropenem + aminoglycoside + levofloxacin
  - If MRSA is a consideration:
    - Add vancomycin or linezolid
- HCAP/HAP/VAP:
  - Use IV antibiotics.
  - Early onset (<5 days), and no risk factors for multidrug-resistant pathogens:
    - Ceftriaxone; ampicillin-sulbactam; ertapenem, or
    - Levofloxacin; moxifloxacin
  - Late onset (≥5 days) or risk factors for multidrug-resistant pathogens (antibiotic therapy in preceding 90 days; high frequency of antibiotic resistance in community/hospital; immunosuppressive disease/therapy; risk factors for HCAP):
    - MRSA coverage: linezolid or vancomycin + β-Lactam cefepime; ceftazidime; imipenem; meropenem; piperacillin-tazobactam + either fluoroquinolone (levofloxacin) or aminoglycoside (amikacin; gentamicin; tobramycin) [B]
    - Short-course vs. prolonged-course antibiotic therapy for HAP in critically ill adults is just as effective and reduced recurrence of VAP associated multi-drug resistance (5).
    - Drug-resistant *S. pneumonia* should be treated with high-dose amoxicillin, amoxicillin/clavulanate, cefpodoxime with a macrolide, or a respiratory fluoroquinolone (4).
- Adult IV antibiotic doses:
  - β-Lactams (ampicillin-sulbactam 3 g q6h; aztreonam 2 g q6h; cefepime 1–2 g q8–12h; cefotaxime 1 g q6–8h; ceftazidime 2 g q8h; ceftriaxone 1 g daily; imipenem 500 mg q6h; meropenem 1 g IV q8h)
  - Aminoglycosides (amikacin 20 mg/kg daily; gentamicin 7 mg/kg daily; tobramycin 7 mg/kg daily)
  - Fluoroquinolones (levofloxacin 750 mg daily; gatifloxacin 500 mg daily)
  - Macrolides (azithromycin 500 mg daily; clarithromycin 500 mg daily; erythromycin 500–1,000 mg q6h)
  - Vancomycin 15 mg/kg q12h
  - Linezolid 600 mg q12h

- Pediatric, outpatient (≥3 months):
  - Antibiotic treatment in preschool-aged children is not routinely required because viral pathogens are more common (6)[A].
  - Oral antibiotics are as efficacious as IV antibiotics in CAP (length of stay and oxygen requirement were reduced in those given oral antibiotics).
  - Typical bacterial pneumonia:
    - Amoxicillin 90 mg/kg/d PO b.i.d. (max 4 g/d) (6)[A]
    - Amoxicillin-clavulanate 90 mg/kg/d PO b.i.d. (max 4 g/d) (6)[A]
    - Alternative: Levofloxacin 16–20 mg/kg/d PO b.i.d. for children 6 months to 5 years, 8–10 mg/kg/d daily for children ≥5 years (max 750 mg/d) (6)[C]
  - Atypical bacterial pneumonia:
    - Azithromycin 10 mg/kg PO on day 1, then 5 mg/kg/d on days 2–5 (max 500 mg day 1, 250 mg days 2–5) (6)[C]
    - Clarithromycin 15 mg/kg PO b.i.d. (max 1 g/d) (6)[C]
    - Erythromycin 40 mg/kg/d PO daily (6)[C]

IN-PATIENT CONSIDERATIONS
Admission Criteria/Initial Stabilization
Clinical judgment and use of a validated severity-of-illness score are recommended to determine if inpatient management is indicated:

- The Pneumonia Severity Index (PSI) is a clinical prediction rule used to calculate the probability of morbidity and mortality among patients with CAP. PSI is risk stratified from I–V. PSI risk class from I–III can be treated as outpatients and IV–V should be hospitalized. PSI can be calculated at: http://pda.ahrq.gov/clinic/psi/psicalc.asp
- The CURB-65 or CRB 65 (Confusion, Urea nitrogen, Respiratory rate, Blood pressure, age >65) (www.mdcalc.com/curb-65-severity-score-community-acquired-pneumonia/) is a severity-of-illness score for stratifying adults with CAP into different management groups (4).
- The SMART-COP (systolic BP, multilobar chest radiography, albumin, respiratory rate, tachycardia, confusion, oxygen level, arterial pH) is a new method to predict which patients will require intensive respiratory/vasopressor support. A score of ≥3 has sensitivity of 92% to identify those patients who will receive intensive treatment (4).
- Patients with COPD or CHF are more likely to require ICU admission when suffering from CAP.
- Clinical prediction tools do not replace a physician's clinical judgment.

Pediatric Considerations
In-patient treatment of children is recommended in the following settings: Infants ≤3–6 months (6)[C]; presence of respiratory distress (tachypnea, dyspnea, retractions, grunting, nasal flaring, apnea, altered mental status, O₂ sat <90%) (6)[A]; or if known to have CAP as result of a virulent pathogen such as community-associated MRSA should be hospitalized (7).

Discharge Criteria
Clinical stability: Temperature ≤100°F (37.8°C); HR ≤100 beats/min; RR ≤24 beats/min; systolic BP ≥90 mm Hg; O₂ sat ≥90% or pO₂ ≥60 mm Hg on room air; ability to maintain oral intake; normal mental status

ONGOING CARE
FOLLOW-UP RECOMMENDATIONS
Patient Monitoring
Consider chest CT if patient is failing to improve on current management.

PATIENT EDUCATION
Smoking cessation, vaccinations

COMPLICATIONS
Necrotizing pneumonia, respiratory failure, empyema, abscesses, cavitation, bronchopleural fistula, sepsis

REFERENCES
1. File TM. Recommendations for treatment of hospital-acquired and ventilator-associated pneumonia: Review of recent international guidelines. *Clin Infect Dis.* 2010;51(Suppl 1): S42–S47.
2. Schrock-Stuckey K, Hayes LB, George MC. Community-acquired pneumonia in children. *Am Fam Physician.* 2012;86:661–667.
3. Vila-Corcoles A, Ochoa-Gondar O, Guzmán JA, et al. Effectiveness of the 23-valent polysaccharide pneumococcal vaccine against invasive pneumococcal disease in people 60 years or older. *BMC Infect Dis.* 2010;10:73.
4. Watkins RR, Lemonovich LT. Diagnosis and management of community-acquired pneumonia in adults. *Am Fam Physician.* 2011;83:1299–1306.
5. Pugh R, Grant C, Cooke RP, et al. Short-course versus prolonged-course antibiotic therapy for hospital-acquired pneumonia in critically ill adults. *Cochrane Database Syst Rev.* 2011;10:CD007577.
6. Bradley JS, Byington CL, Shah SS, et al. The management of community-acquired pneumonia in infants and children older than 3 months of age: Clinical practice guidelines by the Pediatric Infectious Diseases Society and the Infectious Diseases Society of America. *Clin Infect Dis.* 2011;53:e25–e76.
7. Delvitt M. PIDS and IDSA issue management guidelines for community-acquired pneumonia in infants and young children. *Am Fam Physician.* 2012;86:196–202.

 ## CODES

ICD10
- J14 Pneumonia due to Hemophilus influenzae
- J15.4 Pneumonia due to other streptococci
- J15.9 Unspecified bacterial pneumonia

CLINICAL PEARLS
- Bacterial pneumonia can usually be treated empirically based on its classification as CAP or HCAP/HAP/VAP.
- A severity-of-illness score is helpful in determining the need for hospitalization of adult patients, but does not replace a physician's clinical judgment.

PNEUMONIA, MYCOPLASMA

Rebecca M. Wight, MD • Aaron Winnick, MD

BASICS

DESCRIPTION
- Bronchopulmonary infection caused by the mycoplasma species, *Mycoplasma pneumoniae*
- Smallest free-living organism; fastidious and slow-growing; first isolated in cattle in 1898
- Most common cause of community-acquired pneumonia
- Most frequently affects children/young adults, but can also occur in the elderly; often causes epidemics in close communities
- Infection may be asymptomatic, most often confined to the upper respiratory tract, however may progress to pneumonia (5–10%)
- Course is usually acute with an incubation period of 2–3 weeks
- Synonym(s): Primary atypical pneumonia (PAP); Eaton agent pneumonia; Cold agglutinin-positive pneumonia; Walking pneumonia

Geriatric Considerations
Uncommonly isolated as a single agent in elderly patients

Pediatric Considerations
- Unusual in infants and children <5 years; (pneumonia <5 years is more commonly viral)
- Increased incidence of asthma exacerbation in older children
- All infants 3–6 months with suspected bacterial pneumonia should be hospitalized (1)

EPIDEMIOLOGY
Incidence
- Estimated 1 million cases per year in the US (1).
- Responsible for 20% of community-acquired pneumonia (CAP) requiring hospitalizations annually
- Seasonal variation is low, however, infection is more common in late summer/fall months, accounting for up to 50% of pneumonia cases in summer.

Prevalence
- Predominant sex: Male = Female
- Predominant age group affected: 5–20 years:
  – May occur at any age
  – Rare in children <5 years of age
- Responsible for 15–20% of all cases of CAP yearly:
  – Most common cause of pneumonia in school children and young adults who do not have a chronic underlying condition

ETIOLOGY AND PATHOPHYSIOLOGY
- *M. pneumoniae* is a short rod mucosal pathogen which lacks a cell wall thus not visible on Gram stain
- Can grow under both aerobic and anaerobic conditions
- Highly contagious, *M. pneumoniae* is transmitted by contact and aerosols
- Pathogenicity linked to its filamentous tips, which adhere selectively to respiratory epithelial cell membrane proteins with production of H_2O_2 and superoxide radicals, damaging cilia (1)

- Toll-like receptor-2 binding involved in activating cytokine pathways causing inflammation
- Decreased ciliary movement produces prolonged paroxysmal, hacking cough

ALERT
- Macrolide-resistant *M. pneumoniae* has emerged in cases of adult CAP and pediatric pneumonias.
- Infection by *M. pneumoniae* has come to be recognized as a worldwide cause of CAP.

RISK FACTORS
- Immunocompromised state (e.g., HIV, transplant recipients, chemotherapy)
- Smoking
- Close community living (e.g., military bases, prisons, hospitals, fraternity houses, schools, household contacts)

GENERAL PREVENTION
Consider droplet isolation of active cases

COMMONLY ASSOCIATED CONDITIONS
- Asthma exacerbations as a result of proinflammatory cytokine release
- Chronic obstructive pulmonary disease

DIAGNOSIS

HISTORY
- Infection may be asymptomatic
- Gradual onset of headache, malaise, low-grade fevers, chills
- Symptoms of upper respiratory infection then occur including incessant, nonproductive, worsening cough (which may become mildly productive late in the disease); rhinorrhea, pharyngitis, and sinusitis
- Pneumonia may occur with associated pleural effusion, however, dyspnea and pleuritic chest pain are rare.
- Extrapulmonary findings may develop in 5–10% of patients, including arthralgias, skin rashes, cervical adenopathy, hemolysis, CHF, and cardiac conduction abnormalities.
- Neurologic symptoms develop more commonly in children and may include encephalitis, aseptic meningitis, cranial nerve palsies, cerebellar ataxia, ascending paralysis, and coma.
- Persistent cough is common during convalescence; other sequelae are rare.

PHYSICAL EXAM
- Patients generally appear nontoxic
- Hacking/pertussis-like cough may be present along with fever and lassitude
- Normal lung findings with early infection but rhonchi, rales, and/or wheezes may develop several days later
- Mild pharyngeal injection without exudates
- Minimal/no cervical adenopathy
- Erythematous tympanic membranes or bullous myringitis in patients >2 years of age is an uncommon, but unique, sign.
- Some patients may develop a pleural friction rub.
- Various exanthems, including erythema multiforme and Stevens-Johnson syndrome

DIFFERENTIAL DIAGNOSIS
- Viral/bacterial/fungal pneumonia
- Tuberculosis
- Other atypical pneumonias, including *Chlamydia pneumoniae*, *C. psittaci*, *Coxiella burnetii* (Q fever), *Francisella tularensis* (tularemia), *Pneumocystis jiroveci*, *Legionella pneumophila*

DIAGNOSTIC TESTS & INTERPRETATION
- Labs are typically not necessary to make a diagnosis, but they may be indicated depending on the clinical presentation.
- Serology (ELISA) is the mainstay of laboratory diagnosis (2).

Initial Tests (lab, imaging)
- WBC count may be normal or elevated
- Hemolytic anemia has been described, but is rare.
- Elevated erythrocyte sedimentation rate (ESR) may be present, but is nonspecific.
- Positive Coombs test with cold agglutinin titers are elevated in >50% of patients, however, also nonspecific.
- When available, polymerase chain reaction (PCR) for *M. pneumoniae* DNA in respiratory secretions, CSF, and tissue samples may be the most sensitive and specific (2).
- CXR shows reticulonodular pattern with patchy areas of lower lobe consolidation, may be bilateral. Small pleural effusion may be present in 10–15% cases.

Follow-Up Tests & Special Considerations
- Sputum Gram stains are not helpful because *M. pneumoniae* lacks a cell wall and cannot be stained.
- *M. pneumoniae* is difficult to culture and requires 7–21 days to grow; culturing is successful in 40–90% of cases but does not provide information to guide treatment, thus infrequently performed.
- Complement fixation serologic assay shows 4-fold rise in IgM antibody titer at 2–4 weeks after symptom onset; this is an older technique.
- Positive cold agglutinins (titer of ≥1:128 or rising 4-fold) in 50% of infections, but can take 1–2 weeks to develop; not sensitive/specific; not routinely recommended
- CT of chest may show a combination of patchy tree-in-bud opacities with segmental ground-glass opacities

TREATMENT

GENERAL MEASURES
- Avoid sick contacts
- Treatment is usually empiric and must be comprehensive to cover all likely pathogens in the context of the clinical setting.
- Calculation of pneumonia severity score (CAP score: www.mdcalc.com/psi-port-score-pneumonia-severity-index-adult-cap) may be helpful in determining inpatient vs. outpatient treatment (3).

ALERT
Pediatric patients should receive a macrolide and amoxicillin to cover *M. pneumoniae* and other likely agents causing CAP (4).

Pregnancy Considerations
- Azithromycin: Pregnancy Class B (preferred treatment)
- Clarithromycin and levofloxacin: Pregnancy Class C
- Doxycycline: Pregnancy Class D (contraindicated)

MEDICATION
First Line
- Azithromycin:
  - <6 months of age: not established
  - >6 months of age: day 1, 10 mg/kg PO × 1 (not to exceed 500 mg); days 2–5: 5 mg/kg PO daily (not to exceed 250 mg/d).
  - Adults: 500 mg PO × 1 followed by 250 mg PO daily × 4 days (5)[A]
- Erythromycin:
  - Children: 20–50 mg/kg/d PO divided q6–8h × 10–14 days
  - Adults: 400 mg PO q6h × 10–14 days (5)[A]
- Clarithromycin:
  - Children <6 months of age: Not established
  - Patients >6 months of age: 15 mg/kg/d PO divided q12h × 10–14 days
  - Adults: 250–500 mg PO b.i.d. × 10–14 days (5)[A]
- Doxycycline:
  - Children <8 years of age: Not recommended
  - Patients >8 years of age: 2–4 mg/kg/d up to 200 mg/d PO divided b.i.d. × 10–14 days
  - Adults: 100 mg PO b.i.d. × 7–14 days (5)[C]

Second Line
- Levofloxacin:
  - Children <18 years of age: Not recommended
  - Adults: 500 mg PO daily × 7–10 days
- Telithromycin:
  - Children <18 years of age: Not recommended
  - Adults: 800 mg/d PO × 7–10 days
- Levofloxacin and moxifloxacin show good activity against *M. pneumoniae*. Consider use with comorbid conditions and other pneumonia pathogens (5)[A].

ADDITIONAL THERAPIES
- Albuterol inhaler: 2 puffs q4–6h (with spacer for pediatric patients) as needed for wheezing
- Dexamethasone may downregulate cytokine release (6)[B]
- Acetaminophen/Ibuprofen as needed for fever
- Up to 10.9% of hospitalized patients may require mechanical ventilation

IN-PATIENT CONSIDERATIONS
Admission Criteria/Initial Stabilization
- CAP score risk class IV/V
- Advanced age with comorbidities
- Complicating neoplastic disease
- Significant cerebrovascular, cardiac, renal, liver, or GI symptoms
- Altered mental status
- Inability to maintain oxygen saturation
- Tachycardia/tachypnea
- Hypotension
- Neurologic symptoms
- Signs of Stevens-Johnson syndrome
- Significant hemolysis (autoimmune hemolytic anemia, cold agglutinin disease)

Discharge Criteria
- Change from IV to PO antibiotic may be made when:
  - Respiratory distress and hypoxia have resolved
  - Patients are tolerating oral hydration
  - No significant complications present
- Generally no need for 24-hour observation on PO antibiotics prior to discharge

 ONGOING CARE

FOLLOW-UP RECOMMENDATIONS
- Clearing of condition on CXR should be documented in patients >50 years of age
- In smokers document a clear CXR in 6–8 weeks
- Worsening symptoms/development of rash or meningeal/neurologic signs should prompt immediate presentation to medical attention
- Antibiotic prophylaxis for exposed contacts is not routinely recommended
- For household contacts who may be predisposed to severe mycoplasmal infection, macrolide or doxycycline prophylaxis should be used.

DIET
- No special diet considerations
- Ensure adequate hydration

PATIENT EDUCATION
- Smoking cessation
- Contact and droplet precautions
- Adequate hand-washing techniques

PROGNOSIS
- Symptoms usually resolve in 2 weeks
- Some constitutional symptoms may persist for several weeks
- With correct therapy, even most severe cases can expect complete recovery

COMPLICATIONS
- All complications are rare, except reactive airway disease, hemolytic anemia, and erythema multiforme (1).
- Reactive airway disease may persist indefinitely and can cause acute chest syndrome in patients with sickle cell anemia.
- Meningoencephalitis
- Aseptic meningitis
- Peripheral neuropathy
- Transverse myelitis/acute transverse myelitis
- Cerebellar ataxia
- Acute disseminated encephalomyelitis
- Guillain-Barré syndrome
- Encephalitis (especially in children)
- Polyneuritis/Polyarthritis
- Stevens-Johnson syndrome
- Pericarditis/myocarditis
- Respiratory distress syndrome
- Cerebral ataxia
- Thromboembolic phenomena
- Pleural effusion
- Nephritis
- Occasional deaths occur primarily among the elderly and persons with sickle cell disease.

REFERENCES
1. Atkinson TP, Balish MF, Waites KB. Epidemiology, clinical manifestations, pathogenesis and laboratory detection of *Mycoplasma pneumoniae* infections. *FEMS Microbiol Rev.* 2008;32:956–973.
2. Wang K, Gill P, Perera R, et al. Clinical symptoms and signs for the diagnosis of *Mycoplasma pneumoniae* in children and adolescents with community acquired pneumonia. *Cochrane Database Syst Rev.* 2012;10:CD009175.
3. Fine MJ, Auble TE, Yealy DM, et al. A prediction rule to identify low-risk patients with community-acquired pneumonia. *N Engl J Med.* 1997;23:243–250.
4. Bradley JS, Byington CL, Shah SS, et al. The management of community-acquired pneumonia in infants and children older than 3 months of age: Clinical practice guidelines by the Pediatric Infectious Diseases Society and the Infectious Diseases Society of America. *Clin Infect Dis.* 2011;53:e25–e76.
5. Mandell LA, Wunderink RG, Anzueto A. Infectious Diseases Society of America/American Thoracic Society consensus guidelines on the management of community-acquired pneumonia in adults. *Clin Infect Dis.* 2007;44:S27–S72.
6. Remmelts HHE, Meijvis SCA, Biesma DH, et al. Dexamethasone downregulates the systemic cytokine response in patients with community-acquired pneumonia. *Clin Vaccine Immunol.* 2012;19:1532–1538.

ADDITIONAL READING
- Carbonara S, Monno L, Longo B. Community-acquired pneumonia. *Curr Opin Pulm Med.* 2009;15:261–273.
- Eliakim-Raz N, Robenshtok E, Shefet D, et al. Empiric antibiotic coverage of atypical pathogens for community-acquired pneumonia in hospitalized adults. *Cochrane Database Syst Rev.* 2012;9:CD004418.
- Mulholland S, Gavranich JB, Gillies MB, et al. Antibiotics for community-acquired lower respiratory tract infections secondary to *Mycoplasma pneumoniae* in children. *Cochrane Database Syst Rev.* 2012;9:CD004875.

 CODES

ICD10
J15.7 Pneumonia due to Mycoplasma pneumoniae

CLINICAL PEARLS
- Most common atypical respiratory pathogens include *M. pneumoniae*, *C. pneumoniae*, and *L. pneumophila*.
- Atypical pneumonia is typically a clinical diagnosis; if labs are indicated, serology is the mainstay of diagnosis.
- Watch closely for complicating symptoms that could indicate worsening disease.

PNEUMONIA, PNEUMOCYSTIS JIROVECI
Thomas J. Hansen, MD • Tejesh Srinivasa Reddy, MD

 BASICS

DESCRIPTION
- The fungus that causes this pneumonia in humans was previously called *Pneumocystis carinii*.
- The name was formally changed to *Pneumocystis jiroveci* in 2001 following the discovery that the fungus that infects humans is unique and distinctive from the fungus that infects animals (1).
- *P. jiroveci* causes pneumonia primarily in immunocompromised patients.
- *P. jiroveci* is extremely resistant to traditional antifungal agents, including both amphotericin and azole agents (2).
- To prevent confusion, the term PCP, which is used to represent *P. carinii* pneumonia, now represents *Pneumocystis* pneumonia (3).

ALERT
No combination of symptoms, signs, blood chemistries, or radiographic findings is diagnostic of *P. jiroveci* pneumonia (4).

EPIDEMIOLOGY
- *P. jiroveci* has a worldwide distribution, and most children have been exposed to the fungus by 2–4 years (5).
- The reservoir and mode of transmission for *P. jiroveci* is still unclear:
  - Human studies favor an airborne transmission model with person-to-person spread being the most likely mode of infection acquisition (4).

Incidence
- Infants with HIV infection have a peak incidence of PCP between 2 and 6 months (5).
- HIV-infected infants have a high mortality rate, with a median survival of only 1 month.

Prevalence
- The prevalence of *P. jiroveci* colonization among healthy adults is 0–20% (2).
- Recent studies have demonstrated the transient nature of *P. jiroveci* colonization in asymptomatic, immunocompetent patients (4).
- 50% of patients with PCP are coinfected with ≥2 strains of *P. jiroveci* (5).
- There is evidence that distinct strains are responsible for each episode in patients who develop multiple episodes of PCP (5).

ETIOLOGY AND PATHOPHYSIOLOGY
Mode of transmission is unknown; respiratory likely important

RISK FACTORS
Individuals at risk (4):
- Patients with HIV/AIDS infection, especially if not receiving prophylactic treatment for PCP
- Patients who are receiving high doses of glucocorticoids
- Patients who have an altered immune system not due to HIV
- Patients who are receiving chronic immunosuppressive medications
- Patients who have hematologic or solid malignancies resulting in malignancy-related immune depression

GENERAL PREVENTION
- Medication:
  - Trimethoprim-sulfamethoxazole (TMP-SMX):
    - Adults: 1 double-strength tablet daily or 1 double-strength tablet 3 × week
    - Children >2 months: 150 mg TMP/m^2/d in divided doses q12h for 3 × week
  - Atovaquone suspension:
    - Adults: 1,500 mg PO once daily
    - Children: Not to exceed 1,500 mg/d:
      - 1–3 months: 30 mg/kg/d PO once daily
      - 4–24 months: 45 mg/kg/d PO once daily
      - >24 months: 30 mg/kg/d PO once daily
  - Dapsone:
    - Adults only: 50 mg b.i.d. or 100 mg once daily
  - Pentamidine:
    - Adults only: 300 mg aerosolized every 4 weeks
- Indications for prophylaxis:
  - HIV-infected adults (5):
    - Should start when CD4 count is <200 cells/μL or if the patient develops oropharyngeal candidiasis
  - HIV-infected children (5):
    - Prophylaxis should be provided for children ≥6 years based on adult guidelines
    - For children aged 1–5, start when CD4 count is <500 cells/μL
    - For infants <12 months, start when the CD4 is <15%
  - Non-HIV-infected adults receiving immunosuppressive medications or with underlying immune system deficits should receive PCP prophylaxis, but currently there are no specific guidelines on when to start this.
- Discontinuation of prophylaxis:
  - When CD4+ cell counts are >200 cells/μL for a period of 3 months in the adult population (2)[C]
  - There are no clear guidelines for discontinuation of prophylaxis in children

COMMONLY ASSOCIATED CONDITIONS
- HIV/AIDS
- Chronic obstructive lung disease (COPD)
- Interstitial lung disease
- Connective tissue diseases treated with corticosteroids
- Cancer and organ-transplant patients on immunosuppressive medication

 DIAGNOSIS

HISTORY
- HIV-infected patients:
  - Subacute onset over several weeks:
    - Progressively worsening dyspnea
    - Tachypnea
    - Cough: Nonproductive or productive of clear sputum
    - Low-grade fever, chills
    - Weakness, fatigue, malaise
- Non–HIV-infected immunocompromised patients:
  - More acute onset with fulminant respiratory failure:
    - Abrupt tachypnea, dyspnea
    - Fever
    - Dry cough

PHYSICAL EXAM
- Fever
- Tachypnea
- Tachycardia
- Lung exam is normal or near normal

DIFFERENTIAL DIAGNOSIS
- Tuberculosis
- Bacterial pneumonia
- Fungal pneumonia
- Viral pneumonia

DIAGNOSTIC TESTS & INTERPRETATION
P. jiroveci cannot be cultured. Therefore, a diagnosis relies on detection of the organism by colorimetric or immunofluorescent stains or by polymerase chain reaction (PCR) (5)[C].
- ABG: Reveals hypoxemia and increased alveolar–arterial (A-a) gradient that varies with severity of disease
- LDH: Serum lactate dehydrogenase is frequently increased (nonspecific; likely due to underlying lung inflammation and injury)
- CD4 cell count is generally <200 in HIV-infected patients with PCP.
- S-adenosylmethionine levels are significantly lower in a patient with PCP. The levels increase with successful treatment (6)[B].
- Comprehensive metabolic profile
- Chest x-ray (CXR) (4)[C]:
  - Bilateral, symmetric, fine, reticular interstitial infiltrates involving perihilar areas. Becomes more homogeneous and diffuse as severity of infection progresses
  - Less common patterns include upper lobe involvement in patients receiving aerosolized pentamidine, solitary or multiple nodular opacities, lobar infiltrates, pneumatoceles, and pneumothoraces
  - May be normal in up to 30% of patients with PCP (3)[C]
- High-resolution CT is more sensitive than CXR

Diagnostic Procedures/Other
- Fiber-optic bronchoscopy with bronchoalveolar lavage (BAL) is the preferred diagnostic procedure to obtain samples for direct fluorescent antibody staining:
  – Sensitivities range from 89% to >98%.
- *Pneumocystis* trophic forms or cysts obtained from induced sputum, BAL fluid, or lung tissue, which can be visualized using conventional stains
- PCR can detect *Pneumocystis* from respiratory sources, but the potential remains for false positives (4)[C].

TREATMENT

The recommended duration of therapy differs in patients with or without AIDS:
- In patients with PCP who do not have AIDS, the typical duration of therapy is 14 days.
- Treatment of PCP in patients who have AIDS was increased to 21 days due to the risk for relapse after only 14 days of treatment (4)[C].

MEDICATION
Pediatric Considerations
Only medications that are FDA approved are listed for pediatric dosing.
- Trimethoprim-sulfamethoxazole (TMP-SMX) (2,4)[C]
- Adult dosing:
  – TMP: 15–20 mg/kg/d, PO or IV, divided into 4 doses
  – SMX: 75–100 mg/kg/d, PO or IV, divided into 4 doses
- Pediatric dosing (>2 months) (4)[C]:
  – TMP: 15–20 mg/kg/d in divided doses q6–8h
- Reduce doses of TMP-SMX in patients with renal failure
- Treatment response to *Pneumocystis* therapy often requires at least 7–10 days before clinical improvement is documented (2)[C]
- Pregnancy risk factor: Class C (4)[C]
- Precautions:
  – History of sulfa allergy
  – There is an emergence of drug-resistant PCP, especially against TMP-SMX.

Second Line
- Pentamidine (for moderate to severe cases):
  – Adults and children: 4 mg/kg IV or IM once daily
- Dapsone ± trimethoprim (adults only):
  – Dapsone 100 mg PO once daily, *plus*
  – Trimethoprim 5 mg/kg PO t.i.d.
    ○ Check the glucose-6-phosphate dehydrogenase level before beginning dapsone, as hemolysis may result.
- Clindamycin ± primaquine (adults only):
  – Clindamycin 600 mg IV q8h or 300–450 mg PO q.i.d., *plus*
  – Primaquine 30 mg PO once daily
- Atovaquone:
  – Adults: 750 mg PO b.i.d. (>13 years of age)
  – Children: 40 mg/kg/d PO divided b.i.d. (max 1,500 mg)
- Note: Pentamidine has greater toxicity than TMP-SMX: Hypotension, hypoglycemia, pancreatitis (4)[C]

ADDITIONAL THERAPIES
Adjunctive corticosteroid (prednisone or methylprednisolone) (4)[C],(7)[A]:
- Adjunctive corticosteroids are shown to provide benefits in patients who have AIDS and symptoms of moderate to severe PCP.
- Corticosteroids provide the greatest benefit to HIV patients who have hypoxemia manifested as a partial pressure of arterial oxygen <70 mm Hg or an alveolar-arteriolar gradient >35 on room air.
- Adults and children >13 years of age: Prednisone, 40 mg PO b.i.d. on days 1–5; 40 mg daily on days 6–11; 20 mg daily on days 12–21

IN-PATIENT CONSIDERATIONS
- No set criteria for hospital admission
- 5 predictors of mortality in HIV-associated *Pneumocystis* pneumonia (8):
  – Increased age of the patient
  – Recent IV drug use
  – Total bilirubin >0.6 mg/dL
  – Serum albumin <3 g/dL
  – Alveolar-arterial oxygen gradient ≥50 mm Hg (8)[C]

ONGOING CARE

FOLLOW-UP RECOMMENDATIONS
In patients with HIV/AIDS: Patients with previous episodes of PCP should receive lifelong secondary prophylaxis unless they respond well to highly active antiretroviral therapy (HAART) and have a CD4 count >200 cells/μL for at least 3 months.

Patient Monitoring
Serum lactate dehydrogenase levels, pulmonary function test results, and ABG measurements generally normalize with treatment.

DIET
No special diet needed

PATIENT EDUCATION
- Centers for Disease Control and Prevention at www.cdc.gov/ncidod/dpd/parasites/pneumocystis/default.htm
- Family Doctor.org at http://familydoctor.org/online/famdocen/home/common/sexinfections/hiv/475.html

REFERENCES

1. Catherinot E, Lanterneier F, Bougnoux ME. *Pneumocystis jirovecci* pneumonia. *Infect Dis Clin North Am*. 2010;24:107–138.
2. Limper AH, Knox KS, Sarosi GA, et al. An official American Thoracic Society statement: Treatment of fungal infections in adult pulmonary and critical care patients. *Am J Respir Crit Care Med*. 2011;183:96.
3. D'Avignon LC, Schofield CM, Hospenthal DR. *Pneumocystis* pneumonia. *Semin Repir Crit Care Med*. 2008;29:132–140.
4. Krajicek BJ, Thomas CF, Limper AH. Pneumocystis pneumonia: Current concepts in pathogenesis, diagnosis, and treatment. *Clin Chest Med*. 2009;30:265–278, vi.
5. Kovacs JA, Masur H. Evolving health effects of Pneumocystis: One hundred years of progress in diagnosis and treatment. *JAMA*. 2009;301:2578–2585.
6. Skelly MJ, Holzman RS. S-adenosylmethionine levels in the diagnosis of *Pneumocystis carinii* pneumonia in patients with HIV infection. *Clin Infect Dis*. 2008;46:467.
7. Briel M, Bucher H, Boscacci R, et al. Adjunctive corticosteroids for *Pneumocystis jiroveci* pneumonia in patients with HIV-infection. *Cochrane Database Syst Rev*. 2006;3:CD006150.
8. Fei WM, Kim EJ, Sant CA, et al. Predicting mortality from HIV-associated *Pneumocystis* pneumonia at illness presentation: An observational cohort study. *Thorax*. 2009;64:1007–1076.

ADDITIONAL READING
- Centers for Disease Control. Guidelines for preventing opportunistic infections among HIV-infected persons—2002 recommendations of the US Public Health Service and the Infectious Disease Society of America. *MMWR*. 2002;51(RR-8):1–46.
- Centers for Disease Control. Treating opportunistic infections among HIV-infected adults and adolescents: Recommendations from CDC, the National Institutes of Health, and the HIV Medicine Association/Infectious Disease Society of America. *MMWR*. 2004;53(RR-15):1–112.
- Green H, Paul M, Vidal L, et al. Prophylaxis for *Pneumocystis pneumonia* (PCP) in non-HIV immunocompromised patients. *Cochrane Database Syst Rev*. 2007;3:CD005590.
- Shankar SM, Nania JJ. Management of *Pneumocystis jiroveci* pneumonia in children receiving chemotherapy. *Paediatr Drugs*. 2007;9:301–309.
- Stringer JR, Beard CB, Miller RF. A new name (*Pneumocystis jiroveci*) for *Pneumocystis* from humans. *Emerg Infect Dis*. 2002;8:891–896.

 SEE ALSO

HIV Infection and AIDS

 CODES

ICD10
B59 Pneumocystosis

CLINICAL PEARLS
- Colonization with *P. jiroveci* is common in the pediatric population.
- PCP only occurs in immunocompromised patients.
- Patients with HIV are at risk once their CD4 count is <200. At that time, trimethoprim-sulfamethoxazole should be initiated as prophylaxis. Prophylaxis may end after HAART has been initiated and the CD4 count is >200 for 3 months.
- Patients who are immunocompromised are also at risk. Currently, no clear clinical guidelines are available as to when to initiate or end prophylaxis.
- The first-line treatment is trimethoprim-sulfamethoxazole. The typical duration of therapy is 14 days in non-AIDS-infected patients and 21 days in AIDS-infected patients.

PNEUMONIA, VIRAL
Aaron Lambert, MD

BASICS

DESCRIPTION
- Inflammatory disease of the lungs due to a viral infection
- Most viral pneumonia results from exposure infection in the form of aerosolized secretions.
- Hematogenous and direct spread also possible

Geriatric Considerations
High rates of morbidity and mortality in the elderly

Pediatric Considerations
- Adenoviral infections in children are serious.
- More serious respiratory viral infections are almost always seen in infants and in immunocompromised patients.

Pregnancy Considerations
- Pregnant patients should avoid contact with anyone who has a viral infection.
- Influenza vaccination is recommended for all pregnant women during the influenza season.

EPIDEMIOLOGY
Incidence
- Predominant age: Children <5 years
- Predominant sex: Male = Female

Prevalence
- Prevalence is unknown and varies with seasonal outbreaks, but the disease is more common during winter months.
- ~90% of all cases of childhood pneumonias have a viral cause.
- Between 4–39% of pneumonia diagnosed in adults has been attributed to viral causes.

ETIOLOGY AND PATHOPHYSIOLOGY
Overall: Influenza A and respiratory syncytial virus (RSV) are leading causes followed by adenovirus and the parainfluenza viruses (1):
- Adults:
  – Influenza A, B, and C
  – Influenza H1N1
  – Adenovirus
  – Parainfluenza
  – Coronavirus/SARS
- Children:
  – Influenza A, B, and C
  – Influenza H1N1
  – Rhinovirus
  – Adenovirus
  – Parainfluenza
  – Rubeola (measles)
  – RSV (particularly for those born prematurely)
- Miscellaneous:
  – Cytomegalovirus (CMV) (particularly in immunocompromised patients)
  – Varicella
  – Herpes simplex virus (HSV)
  – Enterovirus
  – Rubeola
  – Epstein-Barr virus
  – Hantavirus
  – Human metapneumovirus
  – Viruses often isolated but not the cause of symptoms

Genetics
No known genetic pattern has been recognized.

RISK FACTORS
- Immunocompromised (HIV, transplant recipient, medication-induced)
- Living in close quarters
- Seasonal: Epidemic upper respiratory illness
- Age >65 years or < 5 years
- Altered mental status (due to dysphagia)
- Cardiac disease
- Chronic pulmonary disease (e.g., COPD, emphysema)
- Cystic fibrosis
- Recent upper respiratory infection
- Travel to endemic area
- Nonvaccinated person
- Kartagener syndrome

GENERAL PREVENTION
- General hand-hygiene techniques are the first-line prevention in transmission of infectious particles.
- Influenza vaccination: Routine vaccination is now recommended for ALL persons aged ≥6 months.
  – Children who are 6 months to 8 years of age and receiving seasonal vaccination for the *first* time should receive 2 doses 4 weeks apart.
  – Children who are 6 months to 8 years of age who received 2 doses of the influenza vaccine should receive 1 dose of the seasonal influenza vaccine the following year (2).
  – See the CDC guidelines regarding the use of live, attenuated vaccine vs. inactivated vaccine
- For those patients who are unable to receive influenza vaccine (e.g., with an egg allergy or other) and are at very high risk because of age, comorbid illness, or another risk factor, oseltamivir or zanamivir may be used for the duration of the season, with special recognition for potential viral resistance (3).
- For those who did not receive the vaccine and have been exposed to influenza, use of oseltamivir or zanamivir is recommended for 7 days following exposure (3).

COMMONLY ASSOCIATED CONDITIONS
- Rate of mixed viral–bacterial coinfection is ~20% and can lead to more severe illness or hospitalization
- Fungal infection and *Pneumocystis jiroveci* pneumonia in immunocompromised patients

DIAGNOSIS

HISTORY
- Gradual onset
- May have preceding URI symptoms
- Fever/chills
- Headache
- Myalgias
- Malaise
- Anorexia/decreased feeding in adults/infants
- Cough (with or without purulent sputum production)
- Dyspnea
- Rhinorrhea
- Pharyngitis
- Pleurisy
- Upper abdominal pain in children

PHYSICAL EXAM
- Fever
- Tachypnea
- Tachycardia
- Hypoxemia with severe disease
- Altered breath sounds (bronchophony, tactile fremitus, whispered pectoriloquy)
- Pulmonary rales and rhonchi
- Friction rub
- Possible associated rash (i.e., measles, HSV)

DIFFERENTIAL DIAGNOSIS
- Bacterial pneumonia (especially atypical etiologies: *Chlamydophila pneumoniae* and *C. psittaci*, *Mycoplasma pneumoniae*, *Legionella pneumophila*)
- Pulmonary edema
- *Pneumocystis pneumonia/P. jiroveci* pneumonia
- Aspiration pneumonia
- Hypersensitivity pneumonitis
- Bronchiolitis obliterans, with organizing pneumonia
- Pulmonary embolus/infarction
- Cystic fibrosis (in infants)
- Severe acute respiratory syndrome or severe acute respiratory syndrome–associated coronavirus

DIAGNOSTIC TESTS & INTERPRETATION
- No standard labs to diagnose viral pneumonia
- Specific lab investigations should be based on the clinical scenario.

Initial Tests (lab, imaging)
- CBC:
  – Normal or near normal granulocyte count, occasionally leukopenic with increased lymphocyte percentage
  – Hemoconcentration (hantavirus)
- Chest x-ray (CXR): Interstitial or alveolar infiltrates, peribronchial thickening, pleural effusion
- ESR/CRP may be helpful in children

Follow-Up Tests & Special Considerations

Clinicians can also consider additional testing, as clinically indicated:

- Appropriate direct fluorescent antibody or enzyme immunoassay from throat nasopharyngeal washings (children) or swab (adults), tracheal aspirate, or bronchoalveolar lavage specimens (HSV, varicella-zoster virus, influenza viruses A and B, RSV, adenovirus)
- Viral culture (1,4):
  - Limitations: Results take 3–14 days. False-negative results occur with lower viral titers.
  - Rapid antigen detection: Nasopharyngeal swab for rapid influenza testing
  - Cytopathology (cytoplasmic inclusion bodies [CMV], HSV, measles virus)
  - Serology (4-fold rise in acute compared with convalescent titers): Confirm diagnosis retrospectively, but not clinically useful
  - Serologic testing for hantavirus: Enzyme immunoassay if available from health departments
  - Polymerase chain reaction (PCR) detection if modality available (1):
    - Highly sensitive and specific, but a positive result does not imply causality
- Sputum Gram stain and culture to identify bacterial copathogens, if present
- Chest CT may show consolidations surrounded by ground glass opacities.

Diagnostic Procedures/Other
Bronchoscopy with bronchoalveolar lavage

TREATMENT

- Outpatient treatment for most patients
- Inpatient treatment for infants <4 months of age, elderly, or for any patient with diffuse, severe infection (e.g., hypoxemia, hypercarbia, hypotension or shock, acute respiratory distress syndrome [ARDS]) or significant comorbidity (e.g., congestive heart failure [CHF], coronary artery disease, COPD)
- The Pneumonia Severity Index Calculator (http://pda.ahrq.gov/clinic/psi/psicalc.asp) from the Agency for Healthcare Research and Quality may be used to assess the need for hospitalization as well as mortality risk (5)[A].
- Consider concomitant treatment for bacterial coinfection if severely ill or not responding to treatment

MEDICATION
First Line
- Influenza viruses A and B:
  - Oseltamivir (Tamiflu): Patients >18, 75 mg PO q12h for 5 days; dosage adjusted to 75 mg PO q24h in cases where creatinine clearance rate is <30 mL/min. Effectiveness is maximal when started within 48 hours of symptom onset (3)[A].
  - Zanamivir (Relenza): Patients >18, 2 inhalations (10 mg) q12h for 5 days

- Varicella-zoster virus:
  - Acyclovir:
    - Adults: For immunocompetent patients, 800 mg PO q6h for 5–7 days; use ideal body weight for dosing (1)[B]
    - Children >2 years: For immunocompetent patients, 80 mg/kg/d PO divided q6h for 5 days. Start within 24 hours of symptom onset; immunocompromised patients 30 mg/kg/d PO divided q6h for 5 days. Start within 24 hours of symptom onset; immunocompromised patients 30 mg/kg/d IV divided q8h for 7–10 days (1)[B]
- CMV or HSV:
  - Acyclovir:
    - Immunocompromised adults: 5 mg/kg IV q8h for 7 days (1)[B]
    - Children: Contact an infectious disease specialist or an experienced pharmacist regarding dosing
  - Ganciclovir: Use should be in conjunction with infectious disease consultation (4)[B].
- RSV:
  - Ribavirin: Indicated in few, select cases (20 mg/mL via continuous aerosol administration for 12–18 h/d for 3–7 days). Ribavirin is teratogenic and should not be administered by pregnant health care personnel: Its cost is high and benefits are marginal (1)[C].

Second Line
- Influenza: Amantadine and rimantadine are no longer recommended due to high levels of resistance among circulating influenza A viruses (3)[A].
- CMV, HSV, varicella virus infections:
  - Foscarnet (Foscavir): 60 mg/kg IV q8h in conjunction with infectious disease consultation (1,4)[C]

GENERAL MEASURES
- Most healthy individuals will only require symptomatic treatment.
- Encourage coughing and deep breathing exercises to clear secretions.
- Careful disposal of secretions/universal precautions
- Hydration
- Respiratory isolation with negative pressure room for varicella virus, which is highly contagious

ONGOING CARE

FOLLOW-UP RECOMMENDATIONS
Patient Monitoring
- Physical exams
- Repeat a CXR only if warranted by clinical presentation. A CXR may take weeks to resolve after clinical illness has resolved.
- Oxygenation if illness severe enough for hospitalization

PATIENT EDUCATION
- For patient education materials on this topic, contact American Lung Association, 1301 Pennsylvania Avenue, NW, Suite 800, Washington, DC 20004; 800-LUNG-USA
- Centers for Disease Control and Prevention. Seasonal influenza (flu). Available at: www.cdc.gov/flu.

PROGNOSIS

- Usually favorable prognosis, with illness lasting several days to a week
- Postviral fatigue is common.
- Death can occur, especially in pediatric or bone marrow transplant recipients with adenovirus infections or in older people with influenza.
- The 2009 H1N1 influenza pandemic resulted in higher-than-usual mortality rates among the pediatric, young adult, and pregnant populations.

COMPLICATIONS

- Superimposed bacterial infections, such as *Streptococcus pneumoniae*, *Staphylococcus aureus*, *Haemophilus influenzae*, and others
- Respiratory failure requiring mechanical ventilation
- ARDS
- Reye syndrome after influenza in children (avoid aspirin)

REFERENCES

1. Marcos MA. Viral pneumonia. *Curr Opin Infect Dis.* 2009;22:143–147.
2. Prevention & Control of Influenza with Vaccines—Recommendations of the Advisory Committee on Immunization Practices (ACIP) 2011. *MMWR.* 2011;60:1128–1132.
3. Prevention & Control of Influenza with Vaccines—Recommendations of the Advisory Committee on Immunization Practices (ACIP) 2010. *MMWR.* 2010;59(RR08):1–62.
4. Ruuskanen O, Lahti E, Jennings LC, et al. Viral pneumonia. *Lancet.* 2011;377:1264–1275.
5. Pneumonia Severity Index Calculator: About. December 2003. Agency for Healthcare Research and Quality. Rockville, MD. Available at: http://pda.ahrq.gov/psiabout.htm

ADDITIONAL READING

Centers for Disease Control and Prevention. Seasonal influenza (flu). Available at: www.cdc.gov/flu

 SEE ALSO

Bronchiolitis Obliterans and Organizing Pneumonia; Respiratory Distress Syndrome, Acute

CODE
ICD-9
301 CODES

ICD10
- J12.0 Adenoviral pneumonia
- J12.1 Respiratory syncytial virus pneumonia
- J12.9 Viral pneumonia, unspecified

CLINICAL PEARLS

- Laboratory testing may confirm the diagnosis of viral pneumonia, but this may not change therapy and must not replace clinical judgment.
- Influenza vaccination is recommended for all persons age ≥6 months.
- Amantadine and rimantadine are no longer recommended for use against influenza.

PNEUMOTHORAX
Muhammad Imran Khan, MD • Najm Hasan Siddiqui, MD

BASICS

DESCRIPTION
- Gas within the pleural space
- Primary spontaneous pneumothorax (PSP): This does not have a precipitating event in a person who does not have known lung disease.
- Secondary spontaneous pneumothorax (SSP): Associated with underlying lung disease. The most common: Chronic obstructive pulmonary disease (COPD), cystic fibrosis, *Pneumocystis jiroveci* infection, and tuberculosis (TB).

EPIDEMIOLOGY
Incidence
- PSP: 7.4 and 1.2/100,000/year in men and women in the US, respectively
- SSP: 6.3 and 2/100,000/year in men and women in the US, respectively

Prevalence
- 70% of cases of SSP occur with COPD
- Rupture of apical blebs
- 30% of patients with pneumocystis pneumonia develop SSP
- 6% of all patients with cystic fibrosis will have an episode of SSP
- 1–3% of patients hospitalized with TB

ETIOLOGY AND PATHOPHYSIOLOGY
- Loss of negative intrapleural pressure, lung collapse
- Simple pneumothorax: Pleural pressure in the affected hemithorax remains subatmospheric and is only more positive than the pleural pressure in the contralateral hemithorax.
- Tension pneumothorax (TP): Pleural pressure in the affected hemithorax exceeds atmospheric pressure, particularly during expiration.
- Open pneumothorax: Traumatic chest wall defect persists, and ambient air enters the pleural space during inspiration. Mediastinum shifts to the normal hemithorax, and the lung within the injured hemithorax remains collapsed. During expiration, the air exits the pleural space through the chest wall defect, and the mediastinum swings back toward the injured hemithorax.
- Pneumothorax ex vacuo: This is the result of rapid atelectasis, producing an abrupt decrease in the intrapleural pressure with the subsequent release of nitrogen from pleural capillaries.
- Perforation of the visceral pleura and entry of gas from the lung; penetration of the chest wall, diaphragm, mediastinum, or esophagus
- Blunt thoracic trauma: Gas generated by microorganisms in an empyema
- Spontaneous rupture of pulmonary/subpleural bleb into pleural space
- Rupture of large subpleural cysts caused by subpleural necrosis is the cause of most SSP in patients with *Pneumocystis jiroveci*
- Cystic fibrosis: Rupture of apical subpleural cysts, coinfection with *Pseudomonas aeruginosa*, *Burkholderia cepacia* complex, or *Aspergillus* spp. or a prior episode of massive hemoptysis
- TB: Rupture of a tuberculous cavity into the pleural space
- Pulmonary barotrauma: 10% on mechanical ventilation

Genetics
- PSP: A family history of autosomal-dominant, autosomal-recessive, polygenic, and X-linked recessive inheritance has been proposed.
- Birt-Hogg-Dubé syndrome: Autosomal-dominant, associated with lung cysts, benign skin tumor, renal cancer; the *FLCN* mutation has been mapped to chromosome 17p11.2
- Marfan syndrome: Some patients develop lung bullae, which predispose them to PSP. Genes implicated: Mutations in fibrillin-1 (*FBN1*), transforming growth factor-β receptor (*TGFBR*)

RISK FACTORS
- PSP: Smoking, family history, Marfan syndrome, homocystinuria, and thoracic endometriosis
- SSP:
  – Airway disease: COPD, asthma, cystic fibrosis, α_1-antitrypsin deficiency
  – Infection: *Pneumocystis* pneumonia, TB, necrotizing pneumonia
  – Malignancy: Lung cancer, synovial sarcoma
  – Connective tissue disorder: Marfan or Ehlers-Danlos syndrome, scleroderma, rheumatoid arthritis, ankylosing spondylitis, polymyositis/dermatomyositis
  – Interstitial lung disease: Sarcoidosis, idiopathic pulmonary fibrosis, histiocytosis X, lymphangioleiomyomatosis, esophageal rupture, bronchial obstruction/foreign body (also complications from scuba diving or a loss of airplane cabin pressure)
  – Traumatic pneumothorax:
    ○ Trauma (penetrating injury, broken rib, ruptured bronchus, perforated esophagus)
    ○ Iatrogenic/Postprocedure: Intubation, central line placement, liver biopsy, mechanical ventilation, thoracentesis, cardiopulmonary resuscitation
    ○ IV drug abusers (who attempt to access the internal jugular vein)

GENERAL PREVENTION
Patients should cease smoking and wear seatbelts while driving.

COMMONLY ASSOCIATED CONDITIONS
See "Risk Factors."

DIFFERENTIAL DIAGNOSIS
- Acute coronary syndrome
- Acute respiratory distress syndrome
- Pericarditis
- Congestive heart failure
- Pulmonary edema
- Aortic dissection
- Pneumonia
- Pulmonary embolism
- Pleural effusion
- Flail chest
- Myocardial infarction
- Hemothorax
- Asthma/COPD
- Airway obstruction/foreign body
- Esophageal perforation
- Diaphragmatic hernia
- Should be differentiated from bullae, skin folds, and stomach herniation into chest following rupture of the left hemidiaphragm

DIAGNOSIS

HISTORY
- Chest pain (sudden onset, maximum intensity, sharp, usually lateral and pleuritic), dyspnea; cough, palpitations, and Horner syndrome are less common
- Moderate to severe: Profound respiratory distress, shock, circulatory collapse; referred pain to shoulder/back; history of chest trauma, lung disease, family history, previous hemothorax

PHYSICAL EXAM
- Asymmetry of respirations: Diminished/absent breath sounds on the affected side
- Decreased fremitus: Absent egophony and bronchophony on the affected side
- Hyperresonance to percussion: Crepitus over the chest wall and neck (SC emphysema), tachycardia, respiratory distress, cyanosis
- Tension pneumothorax: Hypotension, cyanosis, tachycardia. The tracheal deviation is away from the affected side. The patient usually has a weak, rapid pulse; pallor; neck vein distention; anxiety; and an altered mental status.
- Consider TP with the sudden onset of tachycardia and hypotension in patients on a ventilator.

DIAGNOSTIC TESTS & INTERPRETATION
Initial Tests (lab, imaging)
- Arterial blood gases (ABGs): Elevated A–a gradient and acute respiratory alkalosis, hypoxemia
- ECG: May show axis deviation, nonspecific ST-segment changes, T-wave inversion
- Chest x-ray (CXR):
  – White visceral pleural line outlines the edge of lung, separated by a space with no lung/vascular markings adjacent to chest wall
  – Upright: ~50 mL of pleural gas; mostly apicolateral location
  – Supine: ~500 mL of pleural gas; most pleural gas accumulates in subpulmonic location; anterior pleural reflexion
  – Deep sulcus sign: Low lateral costophrenic angle on the affected side
  – Lateral decubitus: ~5 mL of pleural gas; gas in nondependent lateral location
- CT scan: This is the most sensitive technique and is valuable for locating small collections of gas, loculated pneumothoraces, atypical collections, and pleural pathology:
  – Occult pneumothorax (OP) is not suspected on the basis of a clinical exam or plain radiography, but is detected with thoracoabdominal CT scanning.
- Ultrasound: Sliding lung sign: Visceral and parietal pleura move relative to one another during the respiratory cycle. Comet-tail artifacts are echogenic lines that originate at the visceral-parietal-pleural interface and extend to the bottom of the sonographic image (1).
- Simple pneumothorax: No mediastinal shift
- Tension pneumothorax: Radiograph shows the shift of the mediastinum to the contralateral side and flattening/inversion of the ipsilateral hemidiaphragm.
- Open pneumothorax: Radiograph shows a visible chest wall defect and massive expiratory mediastinal shift toward the injured side.
- Pneumothorax ex vacuo: Forms adjacent to an atelectasis lobe

TREATMENT

MEDICATION

First Line

- Providing 100% O_2 accelerates the rate of pleural air absorption.

ALERT

TP: Within the 2nd or 3rd intercostal space of the midclavicular line, use needle decompression with a 14-gauge needle.

SURGERY/OTHER PROCEDURES

- For 1st-time PSP:
  - If small (<2–3 cm, <20%) and few symptoms: Patient may be observed in the emergency department for 3–6 hours and discharged if repeat x-ray shows no progression (2).
  - If larger and/or patient is symptomatic:

    - Aspiration technique: (i) Position patient semisupine at 45°, (ii) prep and anesthetize the skin, (iii) insert a 16-gauge over-the-needle catheter into the 2nd anterior intercostal space and aspirate air, (iv) extract the needle and connect a 3-way stopcock and 60-mL syringe, and (v) aspirate until no more air can be removed. Disagreement exists to whether a failed aspiration should be reattempted (3)[A].

    - Radiologists can place small-bore catheters/small-caliber chest tubes over a guide wire and connect to a Heimlich valve/water seal. However, no trials have compared their effectiveness.
    - One trial has shown no difference in outcomes between aspiration and a chest tube, and fewer hospitalizations with aspiration, but this should be accepted with caution owing to the small sample size in the study.
  - Surgical therapy can be considered in cases with pneumothorax size ≥50% after the 1st episode (4)
- If the pneumothorax is large, the patient is unstable, or prior treatment has failed:
  - Insert a thoracostomy tube (16–22F) into the 4th, 5th, or 6th intercostal space at the midaxillary line and connect to a water seal device. Clamp the tube after 12 hours of no further air leakage.
- Video-assisted thoracoscopic surgery (VATS) can be used for persistent air leakage and when the lung is <90% expanded. VATS has the advantage of reducing hospitalization time, the use of analgesic drugs, and disease recurrence.
- For recurrent PSP:
  - Options: Pleurodesis via VATS, chemical pleurodesis via tube thoracostomy, and thoracotomy
  - VATS pleurodesis: The rate of recurrent pneumothorax is <5% after VATS with bleb/bullae resection and pleurodesis.
  - Pleurodesis with sclerosing agent via chest tube or thoracostomy: Superior to simple drainage in reducing recurrence rate; by symphysis between parietal and visceral pleura:
    - Intrapleural talc: 5 g in 250 mL of isotonic saline; more effective than tetracycline derivatives, but safety concerns still exist (5).
    - Intrapleural doxycycline: 5 mg/kg or 500 mg in total of 50 mL

- Sclerosing agents are contraindicated if the patient is a possible candidate for a future lung transplant because the agents increase the risk of bleeding during surgery. Side effects are fever, pain, and acute lung injury.
  - VATS with pleurodesis is recommended for:
    - Recurrent PSP, initial SSP, with persistent air leakage after 3 days
    - Persistent bronchopleural fistula
    - Patient preference or patient with a high-risk occupation (e.g., pilot, diver)
    - Open thoracotomy if failed or unavailable VAT
- For traumatic/OP:
  - Usually both overt and occult pneumothorax patients get chest tubes.
  - Small to moderate OP can be treated conservatively.
- Aspiration is done with an 18-gauge needle with an 8–9F catheter inserted into the pleural space; the catheter is threaded deeper into the pleural space, and then the needle is withdrawn.
- A 16–24F chest tube is generally used for spontaneous/iatrogenic pneumothorax.
- For traumatic pneumothoraces, 28–40F tubes are used to drain blood as well as add air if necessary.

IN-PATIENT CONSIDERATIONS

Admission Criteria/Initial Stabilization

Admit all patients with large PSPs that do not resolve completely with simple aspiration; recurrent pneumothorax; SSP; or traumatic pneumothorax.

ONGOING CARE

FOLLOW-UP RECOMMENDATIONS

- A follow-up CXR showing a stable or smaller pneumothorax in 24 hours suggests adequate treatment.
- No air travel should be taken until radiographs are normal.
- Athletes with pneumothorax may return to sports after 2–3 weeks of rest as symptoms permit; athletes who require inpatient care should have a normal CXR before resuming sports activity.
- Deep-sea diving is contraindicated in patients with PSP until bilateral surgical pleurodectomy is performed.

Patient Monitoring

- Aspiration: A closed stopcock can be attached and the in-dwelling catheter is secured to the chest wall. Obtain a CXR 4 hours later. If adequate lung expansion had occurred, the catheter can be removed. Following 2 hours of observation, another chest radiograph should be performed. The patient can be discharged if the lung remains expanded on this chest radiograph. If not, the catheter can be left in place and attached to a Heimlich valve. The patient can then be discharged with follow up within 2 days.
- Bed rest while chest tube is in place
- The chest tube might be clamped 12 hours after the last evidence of an air leak and a chest radiograph should be performed 24 hours after the last evidence of an air leak. The tube can be removed if the pneumothorax has not reaccumulated.
- If the lung has not fully re-expanded after 7 days, consider persistent bronchopleural fistula.
- Outpatient management should include a follow-up CXR to document the resolution of the pneumothorax, typically within several days after discharge.

PROGNOSIS

- Air is reabsorbed in days to weeks. Chest pain typically resolves in 24 hours in PSP.
- Prognosis is worse depending on comorbidities. It is more severe with SSP.
- Occurrence of SSP due to PCP has a poor prognosis.
- The 5-year recurrence rate for PSP is 28–31% and for SSP it is 43%.

COMPLICATIONS

- Recurrent PSP: 25–50%, with most recurrences occurring within the 1st year
- Failure of lung re-expansion; persistent air leak

REFERENCES

1. Havelock T, Teoh R. Pleural procedures and thoracic ultrasound: British Thoracic Society Pleural Disease Guideline 2010. *Thorax*. 2010;65(Suppl 2): ii61–ii76.
2. Management of spontaneous pneumothorax: An American College of Chest Physicians Delphi consensus statement. *Chest*. 2001;119:590.
3. Wakai A, O'Sullivan RG, McCabe G. Simple aspiration versus intercostal tube drainage for primary spontaneous pneumothorax in adults. *Cochrane Database Syst Rev*. 2007;1:CD004479.
4. Sayar A, Kök A, Citak N, et al. Size of pneumothorax can be a new indication for surgical treatment in primary spontaneous pneumothorax. *Ann Thorac Cardiovasc Surg*. 2013; in press.
5. MacDuff A, Arnold A, Harvey J, et al. Management of spontaneous pneumothorax. British Thoracic Society Pleural Disease Guideline 2010. *Thorax*. 2010;65(Suppl 2):ii18–ii31.

ADDITIONAL READING

Abdala OA, Levy RR, Bibiloni RH, et al. [Advantages of video assisted thoracic surgery in the treatment of spontaneous pneumothorax]. *Medicina (B Aires)*. 2001;61:157–160.

CODES

ICD10

- J93.9 Pneumothorax, unspecified
- J93.11 Primary spontaneous pneumothorax
- J93.12 Secondary spontaneous pneumothorax

CLINICAL PEARLS

- PSP is rare in patients age >40 years; consider more aggressive workup if this occurs.
- Do not wait for a chest x-ray if there is a respiratory/hemodynamic compromise.
- With tension pneumothorax, use needle decompression. Insert a ≥19F needle (14–16-gauge, 5-cm needle) into the 2nd intercostal space at the midclavicular line over the superior aspect of the rib to avoid vessels and attach a 3-way stopcock. Use a large syringe to withdraw air. Follow with a chest tube.

POLYARTERITIS NODOSA
Katherine S. Upchurch, MD • Nida Chaudhary, MD

BASICS

DESCRIPTION
- Polyarteritis nodosa (PAN) is a necrotizing arteritis of medium or small arteries without glomerulonephritis or vasculitis in arterioles, capillaries, or venules, and not associated with antineutrophil cytoplasmic antibodies (ANCAs).
- Systemic symptoms are prominent at presentation.
- Most common organ involvement: GI tract, peripheral nervous system (sensory and motor), kidney, skin, testes/epididymis, cardiac, CNS
- Most common features of PAN include mesenteric ischemia-related symptoms, renal involvement, mononeuritis multiplex, and purpuric skin lesions.
- Renal disease in PAN usually manifests as hypertension (HTN) and mild proteinuria with/without azotemia.
- PAN formerly encompassed several distinct entities (classic PAN, microscopic PAN, cutaneous PAN). With the advent of antineutrophil cytoplasmic antibody (ANCA) testing, it is now apparent that microscopic PAN may not be related to the other 2 entities pathophysiologically (1):
  - Patients with classic PAN (now commonly referred to as PAN) are *typically ANCA negative*.
  - In contrast, patients with microscopic PAN have ANCAs directed against myeloperoxidase (MPO) and generally involvement of small arterioles (as opposed to medium-sized arteries). This disease is also known as microscopic polyangiitis and is now classified as 1 of the ANCA-associated vasculitides.
  - Cutaneous (or limited) PAN is a chronic disease with cutaneous lesions with characteristic histopathologic features of PAN. There are no systemic manifestations, although myalgias and peripheral neuropathy may be present in the area of skin involvement ANCA positivity is variable.
- Synonym(s): Periarteritis; Panarteritis; Necrotizing arteritis

EPIDEMIOLOGY
Incidence
- Predominant age: Peak onset is in the 5th–6th decade, but all ages can be affected.
- Predominant sex: Male > Female (2.5:1)
Prevalence
Rare: 31 cases/1 million adults in 1 study

ETIOLOGY AND PATHOPHYSIOLOGY
- Segmental, transmural, necrotizing inflammation of medium and small muscular arteries, with subsequent intimal proliferation at the sites of inflammation, thrombosis, and ischemia of the organ/tissue supplied by the affected arteries. Aneurysm formation is prominent.
- Most frequent sites for inflammatory lesions: Bifurcations of vessels
- Disease mechanism in hepatitis B-related PAN: Direct injury to the vessel due to viral replication or secondary to deposition of immune complexes, with consequent activation of the complement cascade leading to an inflammatory response
- Most cases are idiopathic; 20% are related to hepatitis B or C infection
- The cause is unknown but immune-complex mediation has been postulated.
- In patients with PAN and hepatitis B, studies have shown immune complexes containing the hepatitis B antigen in involved vessel walls.

Genetics
Unknown

RISK FACTORS
Hepatitis B infection >> hepatitis C infection (cutaneous PAN)

COMMONLY ASSOCIATED CONDITIONS
- Hepatitis B (strong association with classic PAN)
- Hepatitis C (less strongly linked to cutaneous PAN)
- Hairy cell leukemia
- 27 case reports of systemic PAN following hepatitis B vaccination (2)
- Case reports of various drugs, such as amphetamines, minocycline, and interferon

DIAGNOSIS

Suspect PAN in patients with:
- Acute, sometimes fulminant multisystem disease with a relatively short prodrome (i.e., weeks to months); (single organ involvement can occur)
- Vasculitic skin rash (see "Physical Exam") with sensorimotor symptoms/findings
- Recent onset HTN with systemic symptoms
- Unexplained sensory and/or motor neuropathy with systemic symptoms
- Hepatitis B infection with multisystem disease

HISTORY
General: Systemic symptoms with multiorgan involvement (3):
- Constitutional symptoms (e.g., fever, weight loss, malaise)
- Symptoms highly dependent on specific organ system involved:
  - Focal muscular weakness/extremity numbness
  - Myalgia and arthralgia
  - Rash
  - Recurrent postprandial pain, intestinal angina, nausea, vomiting, and bleeding
  - Altered mental status, headaches, mononeuritis multiplex
  - Testicular/Epididymal pain, neurogenic bladder (rare)

PHYSICAL EXAM
Related to organ system involved by vasculitic process (may dominate clinical picture and course):
- Peripheral nervous system: Mononeuritis multiplex, peripheral neuropathy
- Renal: HTN
- Skin: Purpura, urticaria, polymorphic rashes, subcutaneous nodules (uncommon, but characteristic), livedo reticularis; deep skin ulcers, especially in lower extremities; Raynaud phenomenon (rare)
- GI: Acute abdomen due to bowel infarction and perforation, cholecystitis, and gallbladder infarctions (4)
- CNS: Seizures, altered mental status, thrombotic stroke (with cerebral artery involvement), papillitis
- Lung: Pleural effusion, rarely bronchial arteritis:
  - Capillaritis/Other lung parenchymal involvement by vasculitis strongly suggests another process (microscopic PAN, Wegener granulomatosis, Churg-Strauss syndrome, or antiglomerular basement membrane disease).
- Cardiac: Congestive heart failure (CHF) and/or myocardial infarction associated with HTN; pericarditis (rare)

- Genitourinary: Testicular/Epididymal tenderness
- Musculoskeletal: Arthritis (usually large joint in lower extremities)

DIFFERENTIAL DIAGNOSIS
- Other forms of vasculitis (ANCA-associated, such as Wegener granulomatosis, Churg-Strauss syndrome, and microscopic polyangiitis; Henoch-Schönlein purpura, drug-induced vasculitis, cryoglobulinemia)
- Buerger disease
- Systemic lupus erythematosus (SLE)
- Embolic disease, such as atrial myxoma, cholesterol emboli
- Thrombotic disease, such as catastrophic antiphospholipid antibody syndrome
- Dissecting aneurysm
- Goodpasture syndrome
- Ehlers-Danlos syndrome (may cause aneurysmal formation)
- Multiple sclerosis, systemic amyloidosis
- Infection (subacute endocarditis, HIV infection, trichinosis, some rickettsial diseases)
- Spider bites

DIAGNOSTIC TESTS & INTERPRETATION
- Diagnosis should be confirmed by biopsy if possible.
- Angiography may be helpful to reveal microaneurysms and/or beading of blood vessels.
- CT angiography and MR angiography may be substituted for conventional angiography.
- Avoid contrast in the setting of renal disease.
- Specific: No specific laboratory abnormalities
- Nonspecific:
  - Erythrocyte sedimentation rate (ESR) and C-reactive protein (CRP) elevation
  - Mild proteinuria, elevated creatinine
  - Hepatitis B surface antigen positive in 10–50% of patients (strong circumstantial evidence)
  - Hepatitis C antibody/hepatitis C virus RNA may be positive.
  - ANCA, anti-proteinase 3 (PR3), anti-MPO typically negative
  - Rheumatoid factor may be positive
  - Anemia of chronic disease
  - Hypergammaglobulinemia

Initial Tests (lab, imaging)
Lab tests performed to look for evidence of systemic disease and address broad differential:
- CBC (anemia of chronic disease), ESR, CRP (elevated)
- Chemistries: Elevated creatinine/BUN
- Hepatitis B serology: Often positive; hepatitis C serology less commonly positive
- LFTs: Abnormal in unusual cases, such as PAN involving the liver/biliary tract
- Urinalysis: Proteinuria/Hematuria, but generally no cellular casts/active urinary sediment
- Antinuclear antibody, cryoglobulins
- ANCA testing as well as specific tests for anti-MPO and anti-PR3
- Angiographic demonstration of aneurysmal changes/beading of small and medium-sized arteries: Mesenteric, renal, hepatic

Diagnostic Procedures/Other
- Electromyography and nerve conduction studies in patients with suspected mononeuritis multiplex. If abnormal, may support a sural nerve biopsy.
- Arterial/Tissue biopsy wherever involvement suspected, biopsy feasible

- Skin biopsy from edges of ulcers; include deep dermis and subcutaneous (SC) fat to look for small muscular artery involvement (excisional *not* punch biopsy)

Test Interpretation
- Necrotizing inflammation with fibrinoid necrosis of small and medium-sized muscular arteries; segmental, often at bifurcations and branchings. Involvement of venules is not seen in classic PAN.
- Acute lesions with infiltration of polymorphonuclear cells through vessel walls into perivascular area with subsequent proliferation, degeneration, appearance of monocytes, necrosis with thrombosis, and infarction of involved tissue
- Aneurysmal dilatations characteristic, including aortic aneurysm with dissection
- Peripheral nerves: 50–70% (vasa nervorum with necrotizing vasculitis)
- GI vessels: 50% (at autopsy) with bowel necrosis; gallbladder and appendix vasculature: 10%
- Muscle vessels: 50%
- Testicular vasculature often involved when males are symptomatic.
- *The key differences from other necrotizing vasculitides are lack of granuloma formation and sparing of veins and pulmonary arteries.*

 TREATMENT

GENERAL MEASURES
Aggressive treatment of HTN to prevent associated complications (stroke, myocardial infarction, acute heart failure)

MEDICATION
First Line
- Severe (life-threatening) disease: Corticosteroids (CS) (high-dose prednisone or parenteral Solu-Medrol ± pulse for stabilization):
  – Only 50% of patients achieved and maintained remission with CS, and 40% of patients required additional immunosuppressive therapy (5).
  – Cyclophosphamide (CTX) in combination with CS: Improved survival and steroid-sparing in moderate/severe PAN (5):
    ○ CTX can have long-term sequelae of infertility and malignancy
  – Plasma exchange for refractory disease (efficacy not established)
- Less severe disease: CS alone ± other immunosuppressive agents: Azathioprine (5), methotrexate
- HBV associated PAN: Antiviral agents, short-term CS, plasma exchange (no large evidence-based trials (1,6)

Second Line
- Tumor necrosis factor inhibitors (anecdotal evidence)
- PAN disease activity correlates with serum IL-6 levels; tocilizumab, an inhibitor of IL-6 approved for use in rheumatoid arthritis, may be a treatment option, although no evidence-based studies support this approach (7).

ADDITIONAL THERAPIES
- For patients receiving IV CTX, suggest concurrent administration of mercaptoethane sulfonate (Mesna) to reduce bladder exposure to carcinogenic metabolites.
- For patients on CTX, recommendation is prophylactic treatment against *Pneumocystis jiroveci* (*carinii*) pneumonia with trimethoprim sulfamethoxazole (or atovaquone in patients who are intolerant/allergic).

IN-PATIENT CONSIDERATIONS
Admission Criteria/Initial Stabilization
Depends on extent and involvement of specific organs

 ONGOING CARE

FOLLOW-UP RECOMMENDATIONS
Patient Monitoring
- CBC, urinalysis, renal and hepatic profiles, as indicated
- Acute-phase reactants (e.g., ESR, CRP) may be helpful in monitoring activity level during treatment and follow-up.
- Careful monitoring for:
  – Infection during treatment
  – Delayed appearance of neoplasms after treatment, especially bladder malignancy in patients treated with CTX (check annual U/A, urinary cytology with urologic evaluation if microscopic hematuria)

DIET
Low salt if patient has attendant HTN

PATIENT EDUCATION
Advise patient that materials are available from Arthritis Foundation, 1314 Spring St, N.W., Atlanta, GA 30309; 800-283-7800.

PROGNOSIS
- Expected course of untreated PAN is poor, with an estimated 5-year survival of 13%.
- Steroid and cytotoxic therapy treatment may increase survival rate significantly (8), with a 5-year survival rate of 75–80% (9).
- Survival is greater for hepatitis B–related PAN as a result of the introduction of antiviral treatments (1,6).
- Patients presenting with proteinuria, renal insufficiency, GI tract involvement, cardiomyopathy, or CNS involvement have a poor prognosis.
- Rate of mortality from PAN remains high for elderly patients (3).

COMPLICATIONS
- End organ damage from ischemia (including renal failure, tissue organ necrosis, stroke, myocardial infarction, mononeuritis, perforated bowel)
- Complications of treatment with immunosuppressive agents (10)

REFERENCES

1. Jennette JC, Falk RJ, Bacon PA, et al. 2012 Revised International Chapel Hill Consensus Conference nomenclature of vasculitides. *Arthritis Rheum*. 2013;65:1–11.
2. Carvalho JF, Pereira RM, Shoenfeld Y. Systemic polyarteritis nodosa following hepatitis B vaccination. *Eur J Intern Med*. 2008;19:575–578.
3. Pagnoux C, Seror R, Henegar C, et al. Clinical features and outcomes in 348 patients with polyarteritis nodosa: A systematic retrospective study of patients diagnosed between 1963 and 2005 and entered into the French Vasculitis Study Group Database. *Arthritis Rheum*. 2010;62:616–626.
4. Ebert EC, Hagspiel KD, Nagar M, et al. Gastrointestinal Involvement in polyarteritis nodosa. *Clin Gastroenterol Hepatol*. 2008;6:960–966.
5. Ribi C, Cohen P, Pagnoux C, et al. Treatment of polyarteritis nodosa and microscopic polyangiitis without poor-prognosis factors: A prospective randomized study of one hundred twenty-four patients. *Arthritis Rheum*. 2010;62:1186–1197.
6. Guillevin L, Mahr A, Callard P, et al. Hepatitis B virus-associated polyarteritis nodosa: Clinical characteristics, outcome, and impact of treatment in 115 Patients. *Medicine (Baltimore)*. 2005;84:313–322.
7. Murakami M, Nishimoto N. The value of blocking IL-6 outside of rheumatoid arthritis: Current perspective. *Curr Opin Rheumatol*. 2011;23:273–277.
8. Bourgarit A, Le Toumelin P, Pagnoux C, et al. Deaths occurring during the first year after treatment onset for polyarteritis nodosa, microscopic polyangiitis, and Churg-Strauss syndrome: A retrospective analysis of causes and factors predictive of mortality based on 595 patients. *Medicine (Baltimore)*. 2005;84:323–330.
9. Phillip R, Luqmani R. Mortality in systemic vasculitis: A systematic review. *Clin Exp Rheumatol*. 2008;26:94–104.
10. Chan M, Lugmani R. Pharmacotherapy of vasaculitis. *Expert Opin Pharmacother*. 2009;10:1273–1289.

ADDITIONAL READING

- de Menthon M, Mahr A. Treating polyarteritis nodosa: Current state of the art. *Clin Exp Rheumatol* 2011;29:S110–S116.
- Nakamura T, Kanazawa N, Ikeda T, et al. Cutaneous polyarteritis nodosa: Revisiting its definition and diagnostic criteria. *Arch Dermatol Res*. 2009;301:117–121.
- Villa-Forte A, European League Against Rheumatism, European Vasculitis Study Group. European League Against Rheumatism/European Vasculitis Study Group recommendations for the management of vasculitis. *Curr Opin Rheumatol*. 2010;22:49–53.

 SEE ALSO

Hepatitis B; Hepatitis C

 CODES

ICD10
- M30.0 Polyarteritis nodosa
- M30.1 Polyarteritis with lung involvement [Churg-Strauss]

CLINICAL PEARLS

- PAN is a necrotizing vasculitis of small to medium-sized muscular arteries with lack of granuloma formation and sparing of veins and pulmonary arteries. Clinical features depend on tissue supply of involved vessels.
- Skin biopsy should be collected at the edges of ulcers and include deep dermis and SC fat for high yield of diagnosis.
- Check hepatitis B and C serologies.
- ANCA negative.

POLYCYSTIC KIDNEY DISEASE
Maricarmen Malagon-Rogers, MD

 BASICS

DESCRIPTION
- A group of monogenic disorders that results in renal cyst development
- The most frequent are 2 genetically distinct conditions: Autosomal-dominant polycystic kidney disease (ADPKD) and autosomal-recessive polycystic kidney disease (ARPKD).
- ADPKD is one of the most common human genetic disorders.

EPIDEMIOLOGY
- ADPKD is generally late onset:
  - Mean age of end-stage kidney disease (ESKD) 57–69 years
  - More progressive disease in men than in women
  - Up to 90% of adults have cysts in the liver.
- ARPKD usually presents in infants:
  - A minority in older children and young adults may manifest as liver disease.
  - Nonobstructive intrahepatic bile dilatation is sometimes seen.
  - Found on all continents and in all races

Incidence
As ESKD:
- ADPKD: 8.7/1 million in the US; 7/1 million in Europe
- Mean age of ESRD: *PKD1*, 54.3 years vs. *PKD2*, 74 years

Prevalence
- ADPKD affects 1/400–1,000 live births.
- ARPKD affects 1/20,000 live births; carrier level is 1/70.

ETIOLOGY AND PATHOPHYSIOLOGY
- ADPKD:
  - Protein product of *PKD1*: Polycystin-1 mechanosensor in cilia; detects changes in flow, interacts with surrounding matrix and cell membrane proteins, and influences Ca^{2+} influx through *PKD2* product, polycystin-2 channel
  - Intracellular Ca^{2+} is reduced in cyst-derived cells, decreasing the Ca^{2+} inhibition of adenyl cyclase and increasing the concentration of cyclic adenosine monophosphate (cAMP).
  - cAMP stimulates cell proliferation and fluid secretion with cyst expansion.
  - Abnormal extracellular matrix and cell–cell interactions cause cells to detach and form cysts.
- ARPKD:
  - *PKHD1* product fibrocystin is also located in cilia; might be a cell surface receptor implicated in protein–protein interactions and is capable of enhancing the channel function of polycystin-2.
  - An alteration also occurs in intracellular calcium homeostasis.
- ADPKD: Cysts arise from only 5% of nephrons:
  - Autosomal-dominant pattern of inheritance, but a molecularly recessive disease with the 2-hit hypothesis
  - Requires genetic and environmental factors
- ARPKD: Mutations are scattered throughout the gene with genotype–phenotype correlation.

Genetics
- ADPKD:
  - Autosomal-dominant inheritance
  - 50% of children of an affected adult are affected.
  - 100% penetrance; genetic imprinting and genetic anticipation are seen as well.
  - 2 genes isolated:
    - *PKD1* on chromosome 16p13.3 (85% of patients)
    - *PKD2* on chromosome 4q21 (15% of patients)
    - Presumed *PKD3* not yet identified
- ARPKD:
  - Autosomal-recessive inheritance
  - Siblings have a 1:4 chance of being affected; gene *PKHD1* on chromosome 6p21.1–p12

RISK FACTORS
- Large inter- and intrafamilial variability
- A more rapidly progressive clinical course is predicted by onset of hypertension (HTN) <35 years, male gender in *PKD2*, diagnosis <30 years, hyperlipidemia, kidney size (1), increased glomerular filtration (2)

GENERAL PREVENTION
Genetic counseling

COMMONLY ASSOCIATED CONDITIONS
- ADPKD:
  - Cysts in other organs:
    - Polycystic liver disease in 58% of young age group to 94% of 45-year-olds
    - Pancreatic cysts: 5%
    - Seminal cysts: 40%
    - Arachnoid cysts: 8%
  - Vascular manifestations:
    - Intracerebral aneurysms in 6% of patients without family history and in 16% with family history
    - Aortic dissections
  - Cardiac manifestations: Mitral valve prolapse: 25%
  - Diverticular disease
- ARPKD: Liver involvement: Affected in inverse proportion to renal disease; congenital hepatic fibrosis with portal HTN

 DIAGNOSIS

HISTORY
- ADPKD:
  - Positive family history
  - Flank pain: 60%
  - Hematuria
  - UTI
  - HTN: 50% aged 20–34 years; 100% with ESKD
  - Renal failure
- ARPKD:
  - 30% of affected neonates die:
    - Enlarged echogenic kidneys and oligohydramnios are diagnosed in utero.
    - Later in childhood: HTN
  - Adolescents and adults present with complications of portal HTN: Esophageal varices
  - Hypersplenism

PHYSICAL EXAM
- HTN
- Flank masses

DIFFERENTIAL DIAGNOSIS
- ADPKD and ARPKD
- Tuberous sclerosis: Prevalence 1/6,000
- Von Hippel–Lindau syndrome: Prevalence 1/36,000
- Nephronophthisis: Accounts for 10–20% of cases of renal failure in children; medullary cystic kidney disease
- Renal cystic dysplasias: Multicystic dysplastic kidneys: Grossly deformed kidneys; most common type of bilateral cystic diseases in newborns (prevalence: 1/4,000)
- Simple cysts: Most common cystic abnormality:
  - Localized or unilateral renal cystic disease
  - Medullary sponge kidney
  - Acquired renal cystic disease
- Renal cystic neoplasms: Benign multilocular cyst (cystic nephroma)

DIAGNOSTIC TESTS & INTERPRETATION
Electrolytes, BUN/creatinine, urine analysis plus urinary citrate

Initial Tests (lab, imaging)
- ADPKD:
  - Renal dysfunction:
    - Impaired renal concentration (3), hypocitraturia aciduria
    - Hyperfiltration (2)
    - Elevated creatinine
  - Urinalysis: Hematuria and mild proteinuria
- ARPKD:
  - Electrolyte abnormalities and renal insufficiency
  - Anemia, thrombocytopenia, leukopenia
- ADPKD:
  - US: Diagnostic method of choice:
    - Renal enlargement is universal.
    - In at-risk patients: By age 30, 2 renal cysts (bilateral or unilateral) are 100% diagnostic. In children, it sometimes appears similar to ARPKD; may be diagnosed in utero.
    - Presence of hepatic cysts in young adults is pathognomonic for ADPKD.
    - In the absence of family history, bilateral renal enlargement and cysts make the diagnosis.
  - CT scan/MRI:
    - Kidney volume assessed by CT or MRI is a main predictor of progression (1).
    - Helpful in identifying cysts in other organs
- ARPKD:
  - US: Kidneys are enlarged, homogeneously hyperechogenic (cortex and medulla)
  - CT scan is more sensitive if diagnosis is in doubt.
  - Presence of hepatic fibrosis helps the diagnosis.

Follow-Up Tests & Special Considerations
- Diagnosis and prevention of secondary problems because of renal and liver abnormalities
- Follow up of combined renal volume to assess disease severity
- Beyond age 2, renal size decreases in ARPKD but continues to grow in ADPKD at an average rate of 5.27% per year.
- Diagnosis of ADPKD in at-risk asymptomatic children may not need to be done because of psychological and insurance issues.
- Counseling should be done before testing.

Diagnostic Procedures/Other
- Genetic testing is available for *PKD1* and *PKD2* in ADPKD when imaging results are equivocal and for potential living related donors (4).
- For *PKHD1* in ARPKD, a prenatal diagnosis is feasible in about 72% of patients.

Test Interpretation
- ADPKD:
  - Kidneys are diffusely cystic and, although enlarged, retain their general shape.
  - Cysts range from a few millimeters to several centimeters and are distributed evenly throughout the cortex and medulla.
  - They arise in all segments of the nephron, although they are initially from the collecting ducts.
  - 1 kidney may be larger than the other.
- ARPKD:
  - Disease is a spectrum, ranging from severe renal disease with mild liver damage to mild renal disease with severe liver damage.
  - Renal enlargement is due to fusiform dilatation of the collecting ducts in the cortex and medulla in the newborn period.
  - Liver lesion is diffuse but limited to fibrotic portal areas.

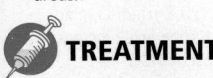 TREATMENT

GENERAL MEASURES
- HTN: Moderate sodium restriction, weight control, and regular exercise
- Medications: ACE inhibitors; angiotensin receptor blockers (ARBs)
- Pain: Narcotics and other analgesics; bed rest; limit NSAIDs (they worsen renal function)
- Urolithiasis: Treated with alkalinization of urine and hydration therapy; surgery as needed
- UTIs/Infections of cysts: Lipid-soluble antibiotics more effective (e.g., trimethoprim-sulfamethoxazole and chloramphenicol); fluoroquinolones also useful
- Dialysis for ESKD patients
- Hematuria: Reduce physical activity

MEDICATION
- No specific drug therapy is yet available for PKD.
- HTN: Should be very well controlled to prevent complications. ACE inhibitors may have an advantage.
- The use of antihypertensive medications has been found to decrease mortality (5).

ISSUES FOR REFERRAL
- Nephrologist primary management
- Urologic consultation for management of symptomatic/infected cysts
- Genetic counseling is critical.

SURGERY/OTHER PROCEDURES
- Indications for surgical intervention:
  - Uncontrollable HTN
  - Severe back and loin pain, abdominal fullness
  - Renal deterioration due to enlarging cysts
  - Hematuria/Hemorrhage or recurrent UTI
- Open and laparoscopic cyst unroofing: May decrease pain and narcotics requirements; has not been proven to prevent renal failure or to prolong current renal function
- Percutaneous cyst aspiration ± injection of sclerosing agent; not usually performed secondary to recurrent fluid accumulation
- Renal transplant for ESKD
- Vasopressin V2 receptor inhibitors: Decrease cAMP: Slowed decline in kidney function (6)

IN-PATIENT CONSIDERATIONS
Admission Criteria/Initial Stabilization
Severe pain, gross hematuria with clots

 ONGOING CARE

FOLLOW-UP RECOMMENDATIONS
None in early stages of the disease; avoid vigorous activity if disease advances. Recurrent gross hematuria is secondary to trauma, associated with faster decline of renal function.

Patient Monitoring
- Monitor BP and renal function. Encourage hydration. Treat UTI and stone disease aggressively.
- Avoid nephrotoxic drugs
- Creatinine and BP monitoring at least twice a year; more often as needed
- Screening for intracranial aneurysms (7)

DIET
- Low-protein diet may retard renal insufficiency.
- Limit caffeine, because this might increase cyst's growth.

PROGNOSIS
- Renal failure in 2% by age 40 years; 23% by age 50; 48% by age 73
- ADPKD accounts for 10–15% of dialysis patients.
- No increased incidence of renal cell cancer

COMPLICATIONS
- Cyst rupture, infection, or hemorrhage
- Progression to renal failure
- Renal calculi

REFERENCES

1. Chapman AB, Bost JE, Torres VE, et al. Kidney volume and functional outcomes in autosomal dominant polycystic kidney disease. *Clin J Am Soc Nephrol.* 2012;7:479–486.
2. Helal I, Fick-Brosnahan GM, Reed-Gitomer B, et al. Glomerular hyperfiltration: Definitions, mechanisms and clinical implications. *Nat Rev Nephrol.* 2012; 8:293–300.
3. Zittema D, Boertien WE, van Beek AP, et al. Vasopressin, copeptin, and renal concentrating capacity in patients with autosomal dominant polycystic kidney disease without renal impairment. *Clin J Am Soc Nephrol.* 2012;7:906–913.
4. Harris PC, Rossetti S. Molecular diagnostics for autosomal dominant polycystic kidney disease. *Nat Rev Nephrol.* 2010;6:197–206.
5. Patch C, Charlton J, Roderick PJ, et al. Use of antihypertensive medications and mortality of patients with autosomal dominant polycystic kidney disease: A population-based study. *Am J Kidney Dis.* 2011;57:856–862.
6. Torres VE, Chapman AB, Devuyst O, et al. Tolvaptan in patients with autosomal dominant polycystic kidney disease. *N Engl J Med.* 2012; 367:2407–2418.
7. Rozenfeld MN, Ansari SA, Shaibani A, et al. Should patients with autosomal dominant polycystic kidney disease be screened for cerebral aneurysms? *AJNR Am J Neuroradiol.* 2013, in press.

ADDITIONAL READING
- Harris PC, Torres VE. Polycystic kidney disease. *Annu Rev Med.* 2009;60:321–337.
- Mochizuki T, Tsuchiya K, Nitta K. Autosomal dominant polycystic kidney disease: Recent advances in pathogenesis and potential therapies. *Clin Exp Nephrol.* 2013;17:317–326.
- Torres VE, Harris PC. Polycystic kidney disease in 2011: Connecting the dots toward a polycystic kidney disease therapy. *Nat Rev Nephrol.* 2012; 8:66–68.
- Torres VE, Harris PC, Pirson Y. Autosomal dominant polycystic kidney disease. *Lancet.* 2007;369: 1287–1301.
- Wilson PD. Polycystic kidney disease. *N Engl J Med.* 2004;350:151–164.

 SEE ALSO

Kidney Failure, Chronic; Nephrolithiasis

 CODES

ICD10
- Q61.2 Polycystic kidney, adult type
- Q61.3 Polycystic kidney, unspecified
- Q61.19 Other polycystic kidney, infantile type

CLINICAL PEARLS
- Although many PKD patients eventually develop ESKD, many do not.
- No specific treatment has been proven to prevent ESRD, but hydration and control of BP are reasonable goals.
- Patients may benefit from a nephrology consultation after the initial diagnosis to counsel regarding disease progression prevention. They then can be followed by primary care if the disease was an incidental finding or no significant kidney dysfunction is present.

POLYCYSTIC OVARIAN SYNDROME

Maria de La Luz Nieto, MD

 BASICS

DESCRIPTION

- Polycystic ovarian syndrome (PCOS) is a common endocrine disorder with heterogeneous manifestations that affect up to 7% of the US population.
- Hyperandrogenism leading to anovulation, typically presenting as amenorrhea or oligomenorrhea
- Diagnosis is based on clinical assessment and ultrasound findings.
- Diagnostic clinical characteristics include menstrual dysfunction, infertility, hirsutism, acne, obesity, and metabolic syndrome. The ovaries are often polycystic on imaging.
- The etiology of PCOS is unknown but can be modified by lifestyle factors.
- System(s) affected: Reproductive; Endocrine/Metabolic; Skin/Exocrine
- Synonym(s): Stein-Leventhal syndrome; Polycystic ovary disease

ALERT
- Condition may begin at puberty.
- Pregnancy does not resolve the syndrome.
- Predisposes to and is associated with obesity, hypertension, diabetes, metabolic syndrome, hyperlipidemia, infertility, insulin-resistance syndrome

EPIDEMIOLOGY
Prevalence
- Incidence and prevalence are still highly debated due to a wide spectrum of diagnostic features: The National Institutes of Health (NIH) criteria require chronic anovulation in addition to clinical or biochemical signs of hyperandrogenism. The prevalence based on NIH criteria is 6.5–8%.
- Predominant age: Reproductive age
- Predominant sex: Females only

ETIOLOGY AND PATHOPHYSIOLOGY
- PCOS is a multifactorial functional disorder of unclear etiology.
- Recent evidence points to a primary role for insulin resistance with hyperinsulinemia (1).
- Androgenism: Ovaries are the main source of excess androgens. Polycystic ovaries have thickened thecal layers, which secrete excess androgens in response to luteinizing hormone (LH). LH receptors are overexpressed in thecal and granulosa cells of polycystic ovaries.
- Ovarian follicles: Abnormal androgen signaling may account for abnormal folliculogenesis causing polycystic ovaries. The mechanism that determines abnormal number of follicles is unknown but may be due to abnormal androgen signaling on the ovarian stroma.
- Insulin resistance: Women with PCOS have insulin resistance similar to that in type 2 diabetes. Elevated levels of insulin decrease sex hormone binding protein (SHBG), increasing bioavailability of testosterone. Insulin may also act directly on adrenal, ovary, and hypothalamus to regulate androgen and gonadotropin release. Insulin resistance causes elevated insulin levels.
- Insulin resistance may cause the frequently associated metabolic syndrome and frank diabetes mellitus (DM).

Genetics
Ultimate expression is likely a combination of polygenic and environmental factors.

RISK FACTORS
See "Commonly Associated Conditions"; cause and effect are difficult to disentangle in this disorder.

GENERAL PREVENTION
None known; focus on early diagnosis and treatment to prevent long-term complications.

COMMONLY ASSOCIATED CONDITIONS
- Infertility
- Obesity
- Obstructive sleep apnea
- Hypertension
- Diabetes mellitus
- Endometrial hyperplasia/carcinoma
- Fatty liver disease
- Mood disturbances and depression

 DIAGNOSIS

HISTORY
- A comprehensive history, including a family history of diabetes and premature onset of cardiovascular disease, is important in the differential diagnosis.
- Focus on the onset and duration of the various signs of androgen excess, menstrual history, and concomitant medications, including the use of exogenous androgens.

PHYSICAL EXAM
- Vital signs: Body mass index (BMI), high BP
- General appearance: Central obesity, deepened voice, hirsutism, acne
- Skin: Hair pattern and growth, acne, seborrhea, acanthosis nigricans
- Genitalia: Clitoromegaly and ovarian enlargement

ALERT
Look specifically for signs of virilization, such as hair pattern, deepened voice, and clitoromegaly.

DIFFERENTIAL DIAGNOSIS
- Cushing syndrome
- HAIR-AN syndrome
- Testosterone-producing ovarian or adrenal tumor
- Prolactin-producing pituitary adenoma
- Hyperthecosis
- Adult-onset adrenal hyperplasia
- Partial congenital adrenal hyperplasia (21-hydroxylase deficiency)
- 11β-hydroxylase deficiency
- 17β-hydroxysteroid dehydrogenase deficiency
- Acromegaly
- Drug-induced hirsutism, oligo-ovulation (e.g., danazol, steroids, valproic acid)
- Thyroid disease

DIAGNOSTIC TESTS & INTERPRETATION
- The measurement of circulating androgens to document PCOS is uncertain, but should include measuring free testosterone concentration directly by equilibrium dialysis.
- Most commonly diagnostic criteria used is Rotterdam criteria (need 2 of 3):
  – Oligo- or anovulation
  – Clinical and/or biochemical signs of hyperandrogenism
  – Transvaginal ultrasonographic polycystic ovaries and exclusion of other etiologies; therefore, consider exclusion of Cushing disease, congenital adrenal hyperplasia, and androgen-secreting tumors.
- More recent criteria also focus on similar criteria while acknowledging that there may be forms of PCOS without overt evidence of hyperandrogenism (2).

Initial Tests (lab, imaging)
- Screening workup should include human chorionic gonadotropin (hCG), TSH, prolactin, FSH (exclude premature ovarian failure), DHEAS, 17-OH progesterone, and testosterone level.
- LH determination may be ordered, but is not usually necessary:
  – Hirsute women should have a testosterone or free testosterone determination and a DHEAS determination.
  – Consider 17-OH progesterone if congenital adrenal hyperplasia is a possibility.
- LH/FSH level ≥2.5–3/L in ~50% of women with PCOS, but LH testing is not generally necessary.
- Testosterone increased, but <200 ng/dL (6.94 nmol/L)
- Typical findings in PCOS include mild elevation in DHEAS, but <800 μg/dL (20.8 μmol/L), mild increase in 17-OH progesterone level, increased estrogen level, and decreased SHBG.
- Drugs that may alter lab results:
  – Oral contraceptives (OCs)
  – Steroids
  – Antidepressants
- Transvaginal ultrasound: Findings: 1 or both ovaries with ≥12 follicles measuring 2–9 mm or increased ovarian volume to 10 cm^3

Follow-Up Tests & Special Considerations
- Consider fasting serum glucose, insulin level, and plasminogen activator inhibitor-1 determinations to establish presence of insulin resistance and glucose intolerance, especially if diagnosis is in doubt.
- Overnight dexamethasone suppression test (Decadron 1 mg PO at 11:00 PM and fasting serum cortisol at 8:00 AM the next morning) to rule out Cushing syndrome in the appropriate setting
- Endometrial biopsy to rule out hyperplasia and/or carcinoma, if indicated
- If the syndrome is diagnosed, determination of fasting glucose and fasting lipid levels should be performed and formal glucose tolerance test considered.

Test Interpretation
- Ovary usually enlarged with a smooth white glistening capsule
- Ovarian cortex lined with follicles in all stages of development, but most atretic
- Thecal cell proliferation with an increase in the stromal compartment

TREATMENT

GENERAL MEASURES
- No ideal treatment exists.
- Therapy must be individualized according to the needs and desires of each patient.

MEDICATION
Drug costs related to this condition are high.

First Line
- The goal of treatment in PCOS depends on symptoms and patient's goals for fertility.
- Treatment can be divided into 5 main categories: Lifestyle changes; appropriate nutrition and exercise to decrease body weight can restore ovulation and increase insulin sensitivity.
- Menstrual irregularity when pregnancy not desired:
  – Low-dose OCs (30–35 μg); newer formulations containing progestins with lower androgenicity (e.g., norethindrone, desogestrel, norgestimate, drospirenone) may be particularly beneficial, but all OCs increase SHBG and decrease excess androgen and estrogen. If unable to tolerate OCs, then intermittent medroxyprogesterone (Provera) 10 mg PO × 10 days given every 1–2 months.
  – Metformin may help to correct metabolic abnormalities in women who are shown to be insulin resistant. Initial dose is 500 mg at dinner time × 1 week, increasing by 500 mg/wk to a total of 1,500–2,000 mg/d divided b.i.d.; take with food:
    ○ Overall, data support the usefulness of metformin on both cardiometabolic risk and reproduction assistance in PCOS women (3)[B].
    ○ Thiazolidinediones may increase likelihood of ovulation and treat insulin resistance.
- If pregnancy desired:
  – Ovulation induction with clomiphene (Clomid, Serophene) and/or exogenous gonadotropins. Birth rate with Clomid is 22.5%, 7.2% with metformin, and 26.8% in women who use both medications (4)[B].
  – Metformin: 500–2,000 mg PO divided b.i.d. has been shown to improve hyperandrogenism and restore ovulation. Many times the drug is continued throughout the 1st trimester or the entire pregnancy if there is a history of spontaneous abortion or glucose intolerance. It does improve clinical pregnancy rates, but does not improve live birth rates alone or in combination with clomiphene when used for ovulation induction (5)[B].
  – Has been demonstrated that metformin reduces the incidence of gestational diabetes

Second Line
- Spironolactone for androgen-excess hirsutism not addressed by OC therapy
- Cosmetic issues due to hyperandrogenism: Acne may respond best with OCs with low doses of cyproterone or drospirenone.
- Eflornithine hydrochloride 13% cream to inhibit hair growth

ADDITIONAL THERAPIES
- Weight loss in overweight women results in biochemical and symptomatic improvement in most.

ISSUES FOR REFERRAL
- To reproductive endocrinologist for all women who cannot achieve pregnancy with Clomid
- High-risk pregnancies
- To endocrinologist if Cushing syndrome, congenital adrenal hyperplasia, or adrenal or ovarian tumors are found during the workup

SURGERY/OTHER PROCEDURES
- Ovarian wedge resection and laparoscopic laser drilling are controversial and rarely used today.
- Mechanical means of hair removal, including electrolysis, waxing, and depilatory, may improve cosmesis.

COMPLEMENTARY AND ALTERNATIVE MEDICINE
Acupuncture assists with cycle normalization and weight loss (6)[B].

 ONGOING CARE

FOLLOW-UP RECOMMENDATIONS
Follow up at 6-month intervals to evaluate response to therapy and to monitor weight as well as medication side effects.

Patient Monitoring
- Counsel patient about the risk of endometrial and breast carcinoma, insulin resistance, and diabetes, as well as obesity and its role in infertility.
- See patient frequently throughout the menstrual cycle, depending on which drug combination is used to induce ovulation.

DIET
In overweight patients, weight loss is the most successful therapy because it improves cardiovascular risk, insulin sensitivity, and menstrual patterns: Counsel on lifestyle dietary changes; consider referral to nutritionist and weight center.

PATIENT EDUCATION
- Provide patient with information about PCOS, such as from www.acog.org.
- Discuss the chronic nature of this condition and the risks and benefits and side effects of potential treatments
- Review the importance of weight loss, if applicable. Modest weight loss of 5–10% of initial body weight has been demonstrated to improve many of the features of PCOS.

PROGNOSIS
- Fertility prognosis is good but may need assisted reproductive technologies.
- Proper follow up and screening can prevent endometrial carcinoma.
- Early detection of diabetes may decrease morbidity and mortality associated with cardiovascular risk factor.

COMPLICATIONS
- Reproductive: Infertility
- Metabolic: Insulin resistance, diabetes mellitus, cardiovascular disease
- Psychosocial: Increased anxiety, mood disorder, eating disorder, depression

REFERENCES

1. Moran LJ, Misso ML, Wild RA, et al. Impaired glucose tolerance, type 2 diabetes and metabolic syndrome in polycystic ovary syndrome: A systematic review and meta-analysis. *Hum Reprod Update*. 2010;16:347–363.
2. Azziz R, Carmina E, Dewailly D, et al. The Androgen Excess and PCOS Society criteria for the polycystic ovary syndrome: The complete task force report. *Fertil Steril*. 2009;91:456–488.
3. Diamanti-Kandarakis E, Economou F, Palimeri S, et al. Metformin in polycystic ovary syndrome. *Ann N Y Acad Sci*. 2010;1205:192–198.
4. Legro RS, Barnhart HX, Schlaff WD, et al. Clomiphene, metformin, or both for infertility in the polycystic ovary syndrome. *N Engl J Med*. 2007;356:551–566.
5. Tang T, Lord JM, Norman RJ, et al. Insulin-sensitising drugs (metformin, rosiglitazone, pioglitazone, D-chiro-inositol) for women with polycystic ovary syndrome, oligo amenorrhoea and subfertility. *Cochrane Database Syst Rev*. 2010;1: CD003053.
6. Lim CE, Wong WS. Current evidence of acupuncture on polycystic ovarian syndrome. *Gynecol Endocrinol*. 2010;26:473–478.

ADDITIONAL READING

- Carmina E, Oberfield SE, Lobo RA, et al. The diagnosis of polycystic ovary syndrome in adolescents. *Am J Obstet Gynecol*. 2010;203: 201.e1–e5.
- Chang RJ. A practical approach to the diagnosis of polycystic ovary syndrome. *Am J Obstet Gynecol*. 2004;191:713–717.
- Hirschberg AL. Polycystic ovary syndrome, obesity and reproductive implications. *Womens Health (Lond Engl)*. 2009;5:529–540; quiz 541–542.
- Rotterdam ESHRE/ASRM Sponsored PCOS Consensus Workshop Group. Revised 2003 Consensus on diagnostic criteria and long-term health risks related to polycystic ovary syndrome. *Fertil Steril*. 2004;81:19–25.

 SEE ALSO

Algorithm: Amenorrhea

CODES

ICD10
E28.2 Polycystic ovarian syndrome

CLINICAL PEARLS
- In the US, 40% of women with PCOS are not obese.
- Chronic anovulation should be treated because chronic estrogen stimulation in absence of progesterone may lead to endometrial hyperplasia.
- Specific therapies must be individualized according to the needs and desires of each patient.

POLYCYTHEMIA VERA

Jennifer C. Colvin, MD

 BASICS

DESCRIPTION
- Polycythemia vera (PV) is a myeloproliferative clonal disorder marked by increased production of red blood cells (erythrocytosis) with excessive erythroid, myeloid, and megakaryocytic elements in the bone marrow.
- Morbidity and mortality are primarily related to complications from blood hyperviscosity as well as malignant transformation. Myelofibrosis can develop in the "spent" phase of the disease.
- Synonym(s): Primary polycythemia; Vaquez disease; Polycythemia, splenomegalic; Vaquez-Osler disease

EPIDEMIOLOGY
Incidence
- Predominant age: Middle to late years; mean is 60 years (range 15–90 years)
- Predominant sex: Male > Female (slightly)
Prevalence
Incidence in the US: 1.9/100,000 person-years

ETIOLOGY AND PATHOPHYSIOLOGY
Clonal proliferative disorder commonly associated with *JAK2 V617F* mutation.
Genetics
JAK2 V617F (tyrosine kinase) mutation: Prevalence 95–99%; is helpful in differentiating from secondary polycythemia. Homozygote carriers will have higher incidence of symptoms such as pruritus but will not have higher incidence of disease than heterozygotes (1)[A].

RISK FACTORS
- Ashkenazi Jewish ancestry (may have increased frequency)
- Familial history (rare)

COMMONLY ASSOCIATED CONDITIONS
- Budd-Chiari syndrome
- Mesenteric artery thrombosis
- Myocardial infarction
- Cerebrovascular accident or transient ischemic attack
- Venous thromboembolism and pulmonary embolism

 DIAGNOSIS

HISTORY
- Patients may be asymptomatic or present with nonspecific complaints, such as fatigue, malaise, and subjective weakness, in early stages.
- Erythromelalgia (burning pain of feet/hands, occasionally with erythema, pallor, cyanosis, or paresthesias)
- Arterial and venous occlusive events
- Headaches
- Blurred vision
- Pruritus
- Spontaneous bruising/bleeding
- Peptic ulcer disease (due to alterations in gastric mucosal blood flow)
- Bone pain (ribs and sternum)

PHYSICAL EXAM
- Bone tenderness (ribs and sternum)
- Splenomegaly
- Hepatomegaly
- Facial plethora
- Skin excoriations if significant pruritus
- Gouty tophi or arthritis
- Hypertension

DIFFERENTIAL DIAGNOSIS
- Secondary polycythemias
- Hemoglobinopathy
- Ectopic erythropoietin production
- Spurious polycythemia

DIAGNOSTIC TESTS & INTERPRETATION
CBC; if suspicion is high, obtain erythropoietin level and gene testing for *JAK2 V617F*.

Initial Tests (lab, imaging)
- Polycythemia Vera Study Group (PVSG) (1960s) major (A) and minor criteria (B):
  - A_1: Increased red cell mass (RCM): Female ≥ 32 mL/kg; male ≥ 36 mL/kg
  - A_2: Normal arterial oxygen saturation ($\geq 92\%$)
  - A_3: Splenomegaly
  - B_1: Thrombocytosis (platelet count >400,000/L)
  - B_2: Leukocytosis >12,000/L
  - B_3: Leukocyte alkaline phosphatase increased
  - B_4: Increased serum vitamin B_{12} or increased unsaturated vitamin B_{12} binding capacity
- PVSG diagnosis acceptable with following combinations:
  - $A_1 + A_2 + A_3$
  - $A_1 + A_2 +$ any 2 from B category (splenomegaly absent in ~25% of patients)
- Recent advances have prompted development of other diagnostic models, namely, the discovery of *JAK2 V617F* and improved assays for erythropoietin (EPO) measurement. Although the RCM was traditionally included in diagnostic criteria, it is difficult to perform and has been shown no longer to be a necessary component of diagnosis, given that additional laboratory tests and clinical evaluation are easily attainable.
- 2008 World Health Organization diagnostic criteria: Requires both major criteria or 1 major criterion and 2 minor criteria (1):
  - Major criteria:
    - Hemoglobin (Hgb) >18.5 g/dL (men); Hgb >16.5 g/dL (women); Hgb >17 g/dL (men) or Hgb >15 g/dL (women) if there is a sustained increase of ≥ 2 g/dL above baseline that cannot be attributed to iron-deficiency correction
    - Presence of *JAK2 V617F* or similar mutation
  - Minor criteria:
    - Bone marrow trilineage myeloproliferation
    - Subnormal serum EPO level
    - Endogenous erythroid colony growth
- Some authors feel diagnosis can be made reliably based on clinical symptoms, presence of *JAK2 V617* mutation, and low EPO (2).
- Other lab findings:
  - Hyperuricemia
  - Hypercholesterolemia
  - Elevated blood histamine level

- Conditions can be confused with polycythemia vera (actual false-positive rate is <1%):
  - Cirrhosis
  - Tobacco use
  - Diuretic use
  - Other myeloproliferative disorders
- Conditions in which patients with PV may not be recognized:
  - GI bleeding (dilution of hemoglobin)
  - Early in disease course
  - Obesity (leads to low RCM)
- CT to assess for splenomegaly (if not palpable), although not necessary for diagnosis

Diagnostic Procedures/Other
- Bone marrow aspiration shows increased cellularity and low storage iron.
- Cytogenetic testing (*JAK2 V617F*)

Test Interpretation
- Plethoric congestion in all organs and tissues
- Major vessels contain thick, viscous blood.
- Splenic sinuses engorged with RBCs

 TREATMENT

GENERAL MEASURES
- Individualized management considering the patient's risk factors and comorbidities (3)
- Risk factors: Age, disease duration, disease phenotype, complications, disease activity
- Currently, phlebotomy is the mainstay of therapy. Beyond this, differences exist among authorities about use and effectiveness of myelosuppressives.
- Phlebotomy:
  - To reduce hematocrit to ~45%
  - Performed as often as every 2–3 days until normal hematocrit reached; phlebotomies of 250–500 mL. Reduce to 250–350 mL in elderly patients or patients with cerebrovascular disease.
  - May require concurrent myelosuppressive agent if at high risk for thrombosis
- Other therapy:
  - Maintain hydration
  - Pruritus therapy
  - Manage thrombotic/hemorrhagic complications the same as with nonpolycythemic patient
  - Uric acid reduction therapy

MEDICATION
First Line
- Primary therapies (4)[C]:
  - Low-dose aspirin 81 mg PO has been demonstrated in 1 study to reduce the risk of thrombotic events without increasing bleeding complications when used in conjunction with phlebotomy. A follow-up meta-analysis, however, did not show a statistically significant benefit to aspirin therapy nor increase in major bleeding (5,6)[A].
  - Hydroxyurea if unable to maintain on phlebotomy alone or if at high risk for thrombosis (age >60 or history of thrombotic event). Common starting dose 15–20 mg/kg/d. Be aware that hydroxyurea can lead to higher risk of leukemic transformation (3).
  - Radioactive phosphorous in selected patients when life expectancy is <10 years given mutagenic potential
  - Use of the novel tyrosine kinase inhibitor imatinib has been explored. This has been reported to reduce the amount of phlebotomy needed, but ultimately has little effect on the course of the disease.
  - Studies have shown pegylated interferon α2a is effective in controlling erythrocytosis, although dosing is generally limited secondary to intolerable side effects (7).
  - Refer to hematologist/oncologist for further dosing and instructions.
- Symptomatic/Adjunctive:
  - Allopurinol 300 mg/d PO for uric acid reduction
  - Cyproheptadine 4–16 mg PO as needed for pruritus
  - H_2-receptor blockers or antacids for GI hyperacidity; cimetidine is also used for pruritus (8)[A].
  - SSRIs have shown some efficacy in controlling pruritus in setting of PV.
  - Aspirin 81 mg daily has been effective in managing erythromelalgia as well.

Second Line
Myelosuppression: Chlorambucil; controversial as some believe this is contraindicated

ISSUES FOR REFERRAL
Referral to hematologist to assist in management

ONGOING CARE

FOLLOW-UP RECOMMENDATIONS
Patient Monitoring
- Frequent monitoring during early treatment until target hematocrit is reached
- Monitor hematocrit often and phlebotomize, as needed, to maintain target goal

DIET
Avoid iron supplements

PATIENT EDUCATION
- Stress the importance of lifelong maintenance
- Continuous education regarding possible complications and importance of seeking treatment early should complications appear

PROGNOSIS
- Currently, survival is >15 years with treatment (1).
- Patients are at risk for developing postpolycythemic myelofibrosis (PPMF). One study showed that the risk of developing PPMF was 16% at 10 years and 34% at 15 years (9).
- Patients are also at increased risk of malignant transformation.

COMPLICATIONS
- Uric acid stones
- Secondary gout
- Vascular thromboses (major cause of death)
- Transformation to leukemia
- Transformation to myelofibrosis
- Hemorrhage
- Peptic ulcer
- Increased risk for complications and mortality from surgery procedures. Assess risk/benefits and ensure optimal control of disorder before any elective surgery.

REFERENCES
1. Tefferi A. Essential thrombocythemia, polycythemia vera, and myelofibrosis: Current management and the prospect of targeted therapy. *Am J Hematol.* 2008;83:491–497.
2. Tefferi A. The diagnosis of polycythemia vera: New tests and old dictums. *Best Prac Res Clin Haematol.* 2006;19:455.
3. Finazzi G, Barbui T. Evidence and expertise in the management of polycythemia vera and essential thrombocythemia. *Leukemia.* 2008;22:1494–1502.
4. Koopmans SM, van Marion AM, Schouten HC, et al. Myeloproliferative neoplasia: A review of clinical criteria and treatment. *Neth J Med.* 2012;70: 159–167.
5. Squizzato A, Romualdi E, Middeldorp S, et al. Antiplatelet drugs for polycythaemia vera and essential thrombocythaemia. *Cochrane Database Syst Rev.* 2008;2:CD006503.
6. Landolfi R, Marchioli R, Kutti J, et al. Efficacy and safety of low-dose aspirin in polycythemia vera. *N Engl J Med.* 2004;350:114–124.
7. Quintás-Cardama A, Kantarjian H, Manshouri T, et al. Pegylated interferon alfa-2a yields high rates of hematologic and molecular response in patients with advanced essential thrombocythemia and polycythemia vera. *J Clin Oncol.* 2009;27: 5418–5424.
8. Tefferi A, Fonseca R. Selective serotonin reuptake inhibitors are effective in the treatment of polycythemia vera-associated pruritus. *Blood.* 2002;99:2627.
9. Alvarez-Larrán A, Bellosillo B, Martínez-Avilés L, et al. Postpolycythaemic myelofibrosis: Frequency and risk factors for this complication in 116 patients. *Br J Haematol.* 2009;146:504–509.

ADDITIONAL READING
- Kiladjian JJ, Cassinat B, Chevret S, et al. Pegylated Interferon-alfa-2a induces complete hematological and molecular responses with low toxicity in polycythemia vera. *Blood.* 2008;112:3065–3072.
- Landolfi R, Di Gennaro L. Thrombosis in myeloproliferative and myelodysplastic syndromes. *Hematology.* 2012;17(Suppl 1):S174–S176.
- Levine RL, Gilliland DG. Myeloproliferative disorders. *Blood.* 2008;112:2190–2198.
- Nussenzveig RH, Cortes J, Sever M, et al. Imatinib mesylate therapy for polycythemia vera: Final result of a phase II study initiated in 2001. *Int J Hematol.* 2009;90:58–63.
- Passamonti F. How I treat polycythemia vera. *Blood.* 2012;120:275–284.

SEE ALSO
Myeloproliferative Neoplasms

CODES
ICD10
- D45 Polycythemia vera
- D75.1 Secondary polycythemia

CLINICAL PEARLS
- *JAK2* mutations are an important component of myeloproliferative disorders.
- Common complications include thrombosis, malignant transformation, and myelofibrosis.
- Phlebotomy is 1st-line treatment, although multiple therapies exist and consultation with an experienced hematologist is recommended.

POLYMYALGIA RHEUMATICA

Amrutha Pavle, MD • Amimi Osayande, MD

BASICS

DESCRIPTION
- Polymyalgia rheumatica (PMR) is a clinical syndrome characterized by pain and stiffness of the shoulder, hip girdles, and neck:
  – Disease of the elderly, associated with morning stiffness and elevated markers of inflammation
- System(s) affected: Musculoskeletal; Hematologic/Lymphatic/Immunologic
- Synonym(s): Senile rheumatic disease; Polymyalgia rheumatica syndrome; Pseudo-polyarthrite rhizomélique

Geriatric Considerations
- Incidence increases with age
- Average age of onset ~70 years

Pediatric Considerations
Does not occur in patients <50 years

EPIDEMIOLOGY
Incidence
- Predominant age: Peak incidence between 70 and 80
- Incidence increases after age 50. Incidence of PMR and giant cell arteritis (GCA) in the US population is 50 and 18 per 100,000 people
- Predominant sex: Female > Male (2:1)
- Most common in Caucasians, especially those of northern European ancestry

Prevalence
Prevalence in population >50 years old: 700/100,000 people

ETIOLOGY AND PATHOPHYSIOLOGY
- Unknown
- Pathogenesis:
  – Polygenic where multiple environmental and genetic factors play a role.
  – Significant association found between histologic evidence of GCA and parvovirus B19 DNA in temporal-artery specimen

Genetics
Associated with human leukocyte antigen determinants (HLA-DRB1*04 and DRB1*01 alleles)

RISK FACTORS
- Age >50 years
- Presence of GCA

COMMONLY ASSOCIATED CONDITIONS
GCA (temporal arteritis) may occur in 15–30% of patients, more commonly in females than males with PMR.

DIAGNOSIS

- Suspect PMR in an elderly patient with new onset of proximal limb pain and stiffness.
- Nighttime pain
- Difficulty arising from a chair or raising the arms
- Systemic symptoms in ~25% (fatigue, weight loss, low-grade fever)

PHYSICAL EXAM
- Decreased range of motion (ROM) of shoulders, neck, and hips may be seen.
- Muscle strength is usually normal, although it may be limited by pain.
- Muscle tenderness may be seen.
- Disuse atrophy of muscles may be seen.
- Synovitis of the small joints and tenosynovitis may be seen.
- Coexisting carpal tunnel syndrome

DIFFERENTIAL DIAGNOSIS
- RA
- Palindromic rheumatism
- Late-onset seronegative spondyloarthropathies (e.g., psoriatic arthritis, ankylosing spondylitis)
- Systemic lupus erythematosus
- Sjögren syndrome
- Fibromyalgia
- Depression
- Polymyositis-dermatomyositis (check creatine phosphokinase, aldolase)
- Thyroid disease
- Hyperparathyroidism, hypoparathyroidism
- Hypovitaminosis D
- Viral myalgia
- Osteoarthritis
- Rotator cuff syndrome
- Adhesive capsulitis
- RS3PE syndrome (remitting seronegative symmetrical synovitis with pitting edema)
- Occult infection
- Occult malignancy (e.g., lymphoma, leukemia, myeloma, solid tumor)
- Myopathy (e.g., steroid, alcohol, electrolyte depletion)

DIAGNOSTIC TESTS & INTERPRETATION
- Temporal artery biopsy if symptoms of GCA are present
- ESR (Westergren) elevation >40 mm/hr:
  – ESR is elevated in most patients, sometimes >100 mm/hr.
  – ESR may be normal (<40 mm/hr) in 7–22% of patients.
- Elevated C-reactive protein
- Normochromic/normocytic anemia common
- Anti-CCP antibodies usually negative (in contrast to elderly onset rheumatoid arthritis [RA])

- Rheumatoid factor: Negative (5–10% of patients >60 will have positive rheumatoid factor without RA)
- Mild elevations in liver function tests, especially alkaline phosphatase
- Antibodies to ferritin peptide may be a useful marker (1).
- Drugs that may alter lab results: Prednisone
- Disorders that may alter lab results: Other disorders causing elevation of the sedimentation rate (e.g., infection, neoplasm, renal failure)
- Normal EMG
- Normal muscle histology

Initial Tests (lab, imaging)
- ESR
- C-reactive protein
- CBC
- MRI of the joints may show periarticular inflammation, tenosynovitis, and bursitis. However, MRI typically is not necessary for diagnosis.
- US of the shoulder or hip may show bursitis, tendinitis, and synovitis.
- MRI, PET, and temporal artery US may all play a role in diagnosis of PMR.

Diagnostic Procedures/Other
If patients have symptoms suggestive of GCA, a temporal artery biopsy is indicated.

Test Interpretation
- A scoring algorithm was devised consisting of morning stiffness >45 minutes (2 points), hip pain/limited range of motion (1 point), absence of RF and ACPA (2 points), and absence of peripheral joint pain (1 point). A score of >4 has been associated with 68% sensitivity and 78% specificity. Sensitivity and specificity increase with positive temporal artery US (2).
- Consider PMR in a patient >50 with proximal pain and stiffness. Obtain laboratory work recommended above. Consider a diagnostic and therapeutic trial of low-dose steroids.

TREATMENT

GENERAL MEASURES
- A crucial step in management is to make a well-documented, firm diagnosis since once glucocorticoids are started they can mask symptoms of many other diseases.
- Address risk of steroid-induced osteoporosis: Obtain dual energy x-ray absorptiometry, check 25-OH vitamin D levels, and consider antiresorptive therapies (bisphosphonates) based on recommendations for treatment of corticosteroid-induced osteoporosis.
- Advise patient on adequate calcium (1,500 mg/d) and vitamin D (800–1,000 U/d) supplementation.
- Physical therapy for ROM exercises, if needed

MEDICATION

First Line

- Prednisone: 10–20 mg/d PO initially; typically, expect a dramatic (diagnostic) response within days. 15 mg/d is effective in almost all patients (3)[A]:
  - May increase to 20 mg/d if no immediate response
  - If no response to 10–20 mg/d within a week, reconsider diagnosis.
- Divided-dose steroids (b.i.d. or t.i.d.) may be useful initially (especially if symptoms recur in the afternoon).
- Consider using delayed-release prednisone taken at bedtime, which may be more efficient in treating morning stiffness compared to conventional immediate-release prednisone (4).
- Begin slow taper by 2.5 mg decrements every 2–4 weeks to a dose of 7.5–10 mg/d. Below this dose, taper by 1 mg/mo to prevent relapse.
- Increase prednisone for recurrence of symptoms (relapse common).
- Corticosteroid treatment often lasts at least 1–2 years (5)[A].
- May be stopped at 6–12 months without any symptoms, normal ESR on maintenance dose.
- Contraindications:
  - Use steroids with caution in patients with chronic heart failure, diabetes mellitus, and systemic fungal or bacterial infection.
  - Must treat infections concurrently if steroids are absolutely necessary.
- Precautions:
  - Long-term steroid use mostly after 2 years is associated with several significant adverse effects, including sodium and water retention, exacerbation of chronic heart failure, hypokalemia, increased susceptibility to infection, osteoporosis, fractures, hypertension, cataract, glaucoma, avascular necrosis, depression, and weight gain.
  - Patients may develop temporal arteritis while on low-dose corticosteroid treatment for polymyalgia. This requires an immediate increase in dose to 40–60 mg.
  - Alternate-day steroids are not effective.

Second Line

- NSAIDs usually are not adequate for pain relief (6)[B].
- Methotrexate has a modest effect in reducing relapse rate and lowering the cumulative dose of steroid therapy (3,7)[A].
- There is conflicting evidence for antitumor necrosis factor agents (anti-TNF) (infliximab, etanercept) regarding whether they have been shown to add any steroid-sparing effects (8)[B],(9)[A],(10)[A].
- Shoulder corticosteroid injection may help reduce pain and duration of morning stiffness (11).

 ONGOING CARE

FOLLOW-UP RECOMMENDATIONS

Patient Monitoring

- Follow monthly initially and during taper of medication; every 3 months otherwise.
- Follow ESR as steroids are tapered; both ESR and CRP should decline as symptoms improve.

- Follow-up with patient for symptoms of GCA. Educate patient to report such symptoms immediately (e.g., headache, visual loss, and diplopia).
- Monitor side effects of corticosteroid such as osteoporosis, hypertension, and hyperglycemia.
- If patient is asymptomatic, do not treat the ESR (i.e., do not increase the steroid dose in an attempt to normalize the ESR).

DIET

- Regular diet
- Aim for adequate calcium and vitamin D.

PATIENT EDUCATION

- Review adverse effects of corticosteroids.
- Discuss the symptoms of GCA; instruct the patient to contact the physician immediately if any occur.
- Instruct patient to contact physician if symptoms recur during the steroid taper.
- Instruct the patient to never abruptly stop taking steroids without a taper.
- Counsel patients on calcium and vitamin D requirements.
- Resources for patients:
  - Arthritis Foundation: www.arthritis.org/
  - American College of Rheumatology: http://www.rheumatology.org/Practice/Clinical/Patients/Diseases_And_Conditions/Polymyalgia_Rheumatica/

PROGNOSIS

- Most patients require at least 2 years of corticosteroid treatment.
- Exacerbation if steroids are tapered too fast (12)
- Prognosis is very good if treated.
- Relapse is common (in 25–50% of patients).
- Higher age at diagnosis, female sex, high baseline ESR, increased plasma viscosity, increased levels of soluble IL-6 receptor or high initial prednisolone dose have been associated with a prolonged disease course and greater number of disease flares.

COMPLICATIONS

- Medication: Complications related to steroid use
- Disease: Exacerbation of disease with taper of steroids; development of GCA (may occur when PMR is being treated adequately)

REFERENCES

1. Régent A, Ly KH, Blet A, et al. Contribution of antiferritin antibodies to diagnosis of giant cell arteritis. *Ann Rheum Dis.* 2013;72(7):1269–1270.
2. Dasgupta B, Cimmino MA, Maradit-Kremers H, et al. 2012 provisional classification criteria for polymyalgia rheumatica: a European League Against Rheumatism/American College of Rheumatology collaborative initiative. *Ann Rheum Dis.* 2012;71(4):484–492.
3. Hernández-Rodríguez J, Cid MC, López-Soto A, et al. Treatment of polymyalgia rheumatica: A systematic review. *Arch Intern Med.* 2009; 169(20):1839–1850.
4. Buttgereit F, Gibofsky A. Delayed-release prednisone: A new approach to an old therapy. *Expert Opin Pharmacother.* 2013;14(8): 1097–1106.
5. Dasgupta B, Borg FA, Hassan N, et al. BSR and BHPR guidelines for the management of polymyalgia rheumatica. *Rheumatology (Oxford).* 2010;49:186–190.
6. Michet CJ, Matteson EL. Polymyalgia rheumatica. *BMJ.* 2008;336:765–769.
7. Spies CM, Burmester GR, Buttgereit F. Methotrexate treatment in large vessel vasculitis and polymyalgia rheumatica. *Clin Exp Rheumatol.* 2010;28(5 Suppl 61):S172–S177.
8. Salvarani C, Macchioni P, Manzini C, et al. Infliximab plus prednisone or placebo plus prednisone for the initial treatment of polymyalgia rheumatica: A randomized trial. *Ann Intern Med.* 2007;146:631–639.
9. Kreiner F, Galbo H. Effect of etanercept in polymyalgia rheumatica: A randomized controlled trial. *Arthritis Res Ther.* 2010;12(5):R176.
10. Aikawa NE, Pereira RM, Lage L, et al. Anti-TNF therapy for polymyalgia rheumatica: Report of 99 cases and review of the literature. *Clin Rheumatol.* 2012;31(3):575–579.
11. Salvarani C, Cantini F, Olivieri I, et al. Corticosteroid injections in polymyalgia rheumatica: A double-blind, prospective, randomized, placebo controlled study. *J Rheumatol.* 2000;27(6):1470–1476.
12. Kremers HM, Reinalda MS, Crowson CS, et al. Relapse in a population based cohort of patients with polymyalgia rheumatica. *J Rheumatol.* 2005;32:65–73.

ADDITIONAL READING

Camellino D, Cimmino MA. Imaging of polymyalgia rheumatica: Indications on its pathogenesis, diagnosis and prognosis. *Rheumatology (Oxford).* 2012;51(1): 77–86. Epub 2011 May 12.

 SEE ALSO

Arteritis, Temporal; Arthritis, Osteo; Arthritis, Rheumatoid; Depression; Fibromyalgia; Polymyositis/Dermatomyositis

 CODES

ICD10

- M31.5 Giant cell arteritis with polymyalgia rheumatica
- M35.3 Polymyalgia rheumatica

CLINICAL PEARLS

- Consider PMR in an elderly patient with proximal limb girdle pain and stiffness.
- Markers of inflammation are usually elevated, but a normal ESR does not exclude the diagnosis.
- If the patient does not report a dramatic and rapid response to low-dose steroids, reconsider the diagnosis.
- Adjust steroids according to patient's symptoms, not based on the ESR.

POLYMYOSITIS/DERMATOMYOSITIS

Christopher Wise, MD

 BASICS

DESCRIPTION
- Systemic connective tissue disease characterized by inflammatory and degenerative changes in proximal muscles, sometimes accompanied by characteristic skin rash:
  - If skin manifestations (Gottron sign [symmetric, scaly, violaceous, erythematous eruption over the extensor surfaces of the metacarpophalangeal and interphalangeal joints of the fingers]; heliotrope [reddish violaceous eruption on the upper eyelids]) are present, it is designated as dermatomyositis (1).
  - Different types of myositis include:
    ○ Idiopathic polymyositis
    ○ Idiopathic dermatomyositis
    ○ Polymyositis/dermatomyositis as an overlap (usually with lupus or systemic sclerosis or as part of mixed connective-tissue disease)
    ○ Myositis associated with malignancy
    ○ HIV-associated myopathy
- Inclusion-body myositis (IBM), a variant with atypical patterns of weakness and biopsy findings (2)
- System(s) affected: Cardiovascular; Musculoskeletal; Pulmonary; Skin/Exocrine
- Synonym(s): Myositis; Inflammatory myopathy; Antisynthetase syndrome (subset with certain antibodies)

EPIDEMIOLOGY
Incidence
- Estimated at 0.5–0.8/100,000 population/year
- Predominant age: 5–15 years, 40–60 years, peak incidence in mid-40s
- Predominant sex: Female > Male (2:1)

Prevalence
1–2 patients/100,000 population

Geriatric Considerations
Elderly patients with myositis or dermatomyositis are at increased risk of neoplasm.

Pediatric Considerations
Childhood dermatomyositis is likely a separate entity associated with cutaneous vasculitis and muscle calcifications.

ETIOLOGY AND PATHOPHYSIOLOGY
- Inflammatory process, mediated by T cells and cytokine release, leading to damage to muscle cells (predominantly skeletal muscles)
- In patients with IBM, degenerative mechanisms may be important.
- Unknown; potential viral, genetic factors

Genetics
Mild association with human leukocyte antigen (HLA)–DR3, HLA-DRw52

RISK FACTORS
Family history of autoimmune disease (e.g., systemic lupus, myositis) or vasculitis

COMMONLY ASSOCIATED CONDITIONS
- Malignancy (in 15–25%)
- Progressive systemic sclerosis
- Vasculitis
- Systemic lupus erythematosus (SLE)
- Mixed connective-tissue disease

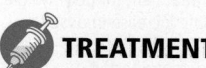 **DIAGNOSIS**

HISTORY
- Symmetric proximal muscle weakness causing difficulty when:
  - Arising from sitting or lying positions
  - Climbing stairs
  - Raising arms
- Joint pain/swelling
- Dysphagia
- Dyspnea
- Rash on face, eyelids, hands, arms

PHYSICAL EXAM
Proximal muscle weakness:
- Shoulder muscles
- Hip girdle muscles (trouble standing from seated or squatting position, weak hip flexors in supine position)
- Muscle swelling, stiffness, induration
- Distal muscle weakness is seen only in patients with IBM.
- Rash over face (eyelids, nasolabial folds), upper chest, dorsal hands (especially knuckle pads), fingers ("mechanic's hands")
- Periorbital edema
- Calcinosis cutis (childhood cases)
- Mesenteric arterial insufficiency/infarction (childhood cases)
- Cardiac impairment; arrhythmia, failure

DIFFERENTIAL DIAGNOSIS
- Vasculitis
- Progressive systemic sclerosis
- SLE
- Rheumatoid arthritis
- Muscular dystrophy
- Eaton-Lambert syndrome
- Sarcoidosis
- Amyotrophic lateral sclerosis
- Endocrine disorders:
  - Thyroid disease
  - Cushing syndrome
- Infectious myositis (viral, bacterial, parasitic)
- Drug-induced myopathies:
  - Cholesterol-lowering agents
  - Colchicine
  - Corticosteroids
  - Ethanol
  - Chloroquine
  - Zidovudine
- Electrolyte disorders (magnesium, calcium, potassium)
- Heritable metabolic myopathies
- Sleep-apnea syndrome

DIAGNOSTIC TESTS & INTERPRETATION
- Diagnosis of muscle component (myositis) usually relies on 4 findings:
  - Weakness
  - Creatine kinase and/or aldolase elevation
  - Abnormal electromyogram
  - Findings on muscle biopsy
- Presence of compatible skin rash of dermatomyositis

Initial Tests (lab, imaging)
- Increased creatine kinase (CK), aldolase
- Increased serum AST (aspartate aminotransferase)
- Increased LDH (lactate dehydrogenase)

- Myoglobinuria
- Increased ESR
- Positive rheumatoid factor (<50% of patients)
- Positive ANA (antinuclear antibody) (>50% of patients)
- Leukocytosis (<50% of patients)
- Anemia (<50% of patients)
- Hyperglobulinemia (<50% of patients)
- Myositis-specific antibodies (antisynthetase antibodies) described in a minority of patients:
  - Anti-Jo-1 is the most common, but has been found in <20% of patients
  - Associated with an increased incidence of interstitial lung disease
- Chest radiograph as part of initial evaluation to assess for associated pulmonary involvement or malignancy

Follow-Up Tests & Special Considerations
- Changes in muscle enzymes (CK or aldolase) correlate with improvement and worsening.
- MRI to assess muscle edema and inflammation may be used in some patients to determine best biopsy site or response to therapy.

Diagnostic Procedures/Other
- EMG: Muscle irritability, low-amplitude potentials, polyphasic action potentials, fibrillations
- Muscle biopsy (deltoid or quadriceps femoris)

Test Interpretation
- Microscopic findings:
  - Muscle fiber degeneration
  - Phagocytosis of muscle debris
  - Perifascicular muscle fiber atrophy
  - Inflammatory cell infiltrates in adult form
  - Via electron microscopy: Inclusion bodies (IBM only)
  - Sarcoplasmic basophilia
- Muscle fiber increased in size
- Vasculopathy (childhood polymyositis/dermatomyositis)

💉 TREATMENT

GENERAL MEASURES
General evaluation for malignancy in all adults, particularly with dermatomyositis, at initial evaluation and during follow up

First Line
- Prednisone (3)[B],(4):
  - 40–80 mg/d PO in divided doses
  - Consolidate doses and reduce prednisone slowly when enzyme levels are normal.
  - Probably need to continue 5–10 mg/d for maintenance in most patients
- For steroid-refractory or -dependent patients (3)[B],(5)[B]:
  - Azathioprine 1 mg/kg PO (arthritis dose) once daily or b.i.d.
  - Methotrexate 10–25 mg PO weekly, useful in most steroid-resistant patients

- Rash of dermatomyositis may require topical steroids or oral hydroxychloroquine.
- Patients with IBM have very poor response to steroids and other first- and second-line drugs in general.

Second Line
- Other immunosuppressant drugs (e.g., cyclophosphamide, chlorambucil, cyclosporine, mycophenolate, tacrolimus) can be added to steroids.
- Combination methotrexate and azathioprine also may be useful in refractory cases (3)[B].
- IVIG (6)(B) and rituximab (7)[A] have been reported to be helpful in a small series of patients with refractory disease.
- Contraindications: Methotrexate is contraindicated with previous liver disease, alcohol use, pregnancy, and underlying renal disease (use with extreme caution in patients with serum creatinine >1.5 mg/dL in general).
- Precautions:
  - Prednisone: Adverse effects associated with long-term steroid use include adrenal suppression, sodium and water retention, hypokalemia, osteoporosis, cataracts, and increased susceptibility to infection
  - Azathioprine: Adverse effects include bone marrow suppression, increased liver function tests, and increased risk of infection
  - Methotrexate: Adverse effects include stomatitis, bone marrow suppression, pneumonitis, and risk of liver fibrosis and cirrhosis with prolonged use

ISSUES FOR REFERRAL
- Diagnostic uncertainty, usually related to elevated muscle enzymes without typical symptoms of findings of muscle weakness
- Poor response to initial steroid therapy
- Excessive steroid requirement (unable to taper prednisone to <20 mg/d after 4–6 months)

SURGERY/OTHER PROCEDURES
None indicated, other than initial biopsy

IN-PATIENT CONSIDERATIONS
Admission Criteria/Initial Stabilization
- Inability to stand, ambulate
- Respiratory difficulty
- Fever or other signs of infection
- Inpatient evaluation seldom needed

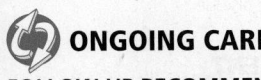

ONGOING CARE

FOLLOW-UP RECOMMENDATIONS
Patient Monitoring
- Follow muscle enzymes along with muscle strength and functional capacity
- Monitor for steroid-induced complications (e.g., hypokalemia, hypertension, and hyperglycemia)
- Bone densitometry and consideration of calcium, vitamin D, and bisphosphonate therapy
- If azathioprine, methotrexate, or other immunosuppressant is used, appropriate laboratory monitoring should be done periodically (e.g., hematology, liver enzymes, and creatinine).
- Attempt to decrease and/or discontinue steroid dose as patient responds to therapy.
- Maintain immunosuppression until patient's muscle strength stabilizes for prolonged period depending on individual patient parameters, risks of medication, risk of relapse; time period undefined (months, years).

DIET
Moderation of caloric and sodium intake to avoid weight gain from corticosteroid therapy

PATIENT EDUCATION
- Curtail excess physical activity in early phases when muscles enzymes are markedly elevated
- Emphasize range-of-motion exercises
- Gradually introduce muscle strengthening when muscle enzymes are normal or improved and stable

PROGNOSIS
- Residual weakness: 30%
- Persistent active disease: 20%
- 5-year survival 65–75%, but mortality is 3-fold higher than general population (5,8)
- Survival is worse for women and African Americans and those with dermatomyositis, IBM, or cancer.
- Most patients improve with therapy.
- Patients with IBM respond poorly to most therapies.
- 20–50% have full recovery (8)

COMPLICATIONS
- Pneumonia
- Infection
- Myocardial infarction
- Carcinoma (especially breast, lung)
- Severe dysphagia
- Respiratory impairment due to muscle weakness, interstitial lung disease
- Aspiration pneumonitis
- Steroid myopathy
- Steroid-induced diabetes, hypertension, hypokalemia, osteoporosis

REFERENCES
1. Khan S, Christopher-Stine L. Polymyositis, dermatomyositis, and autoimmune necrotizing myopathy: Clinical features. *Rheum Dis Clin North Am*. 2011;37:143–158, v.
2. Solorzano GE, Phillips LH. Inclusion body myositis: Diagnosis, pathogenesis, and treatment options. *Rheum Dis Clin North Am*. 2011;37:173–183, v.
3. Choy EH, Hoogendijk JE, Lecky B, et al. Immunosuppressant and immunomodulatory treatment for dermatomyositis and polymyositis. *Cochrane Database Syst Rev*. 2005;3:CD003643.
4. Aggarwal R, Oddis CV. Therapeutic approaches in myositis. *Curr Rheumatol Rep*. 2011;13:182–191.
5. Schiopu E, Phillips K, MacDonald PM, et al. Predictors of survival in a cohort of patients with polymyositis and dermatomyositis: Effect of corticosteroids, methotrexate and azathioprine. *Arthritis Res Ther*. 2012;14:R22.
6. Wang DX, Shu XM, Tian XL, et al. Intravenous immunoglobulin therapy in adult patients with polymyositis/dermatomyositis: A systematic literature review. *Clin Rheumatol*. 2012;31:801–806.
7. Oddis CV, Reed AM, Aggarwal R, et al. Rituximab in the treatment of refractory adult and juvenile dermatomyositis and adult polymyositis: A randomized, placebo-phase trial. *Arthritis Rheum*. 2013;65:314–324.
8. Marie I. Morbidity and mortality in adult polymyositis and dermatomyositis. *Curr Rheumatol Rep*. 2012;14:275–285.

ADDITIONAL READING
- Airio A, Kautiainen H, Hakala M. Prognosis and mortality of polymyositis and dermatomyositis patients. *Clin Rheumatol*. 2006;25:234–239.
- Ponyi A, Borgulya G, Constantin T, et al. Functional outcome and quality of life in adult patients with idiopathic inflammatory myositis. *Rheumatology (Oxford)*. 2005;44:83–88.

 CODES

ICD10
- M33.20 Polymyositis, organ involvement unspecified
- M33.90 Dermatopolymyositis, unspecified, organ involvement unspecified
- M33.92 Dermatopolymyositis, unspecified with myopathy

CLINICAL PEARLS
- Corticosteroids alone may be sufficient in patients who have rapid improvement in weakness and muscle enzymes. However, most patients require azathioprine, methotrexate, or other immunosuppressive medications.
- The risk of associated malignancy is higher in patients >50 and in those with cutaneous manifestations.
- Elevated muscle enzymes (e.g., CK and aldolase) are seen frequently as transient phenomena in patients with febrile illness and injuries; may return to normal on repeat.
- In patients with persistently elevated muscle enzymes and symptoms and findings of muscle weakness, EMG followed by muscle biopsy should be the initial studies considered.
- Suspect IBM in older patients with very slow onset and progression of symptoms, poor response to steroids and immunosuppressive therapy, and atypical patterns (asymmetric, sometimes distal) of muscle weakness.

PORTAL HYPERTENSION

Walter M. Kim, MD, PhD • Jyoti Ramakrishna, MD

BASICS

DESCRIPTION
- Increased portal venous pressure >5 mm Hg that occurs in association with splanchnic vasodilatation, portosystemic collateral formation, and hyperdynamic circulation
- Most commonly secondary to elevated hepatic venous pressure gradient (HVPG; the gradient between portal and central venous pressures)
- Course is generally progressive, with risk of complications including acute variceal bleeding, ascites, encephalopathy, and hepatorenal syndrome

EPIDEMIOLOGY
Incidence
- Prevalence: <200,000 persons in the US
- Predominant age: Adult
- Predominant sex: Male > Female

ETIOLOGY AND PATHOPHYSIOLOGY
- Causes generally classified as:
  - Prehepatic (portal vein thrombosis or obstruction)
  - Intrahepatic (most commonly cirrhosis)
  - Posthepatic (hepatic vein thrombosis, Budd-Chiari syndrome, right-sided heart failure)
- Cirrhosis accounts for 90% of intrahepatic cases; may be due to:
  - Virus (hepatitis B, hepatitis C, hepatitis D)
  - Alcoholism
  - Schistosomiasis
  - Wilson disease
  - Hemochromatosis
  - Primary biliary cirrhosis (PBC)
  - Sarcoidosis
- Increased HVPG results in venous collateral formation in the distal esophagus, proximal stomach, rectum, and umbilicus
- Intrahepatic portal hypertension is specifically associated with gastroesophageal variceal formation.

Genetics
No known genetic patterns except those associated with specific hepatic diseases that cause portal hypertension

RISK FACTORS
See "Etiology"

Pediatric Considerations
In children, portal vein thrombosis is the most common extrahepatic cause; intrahepatic causes are more likely to be biliary atresia, viral hepatitis, and metabolic liver disease.

DIAGNOSIS

HISTORY
- Weakness/Fatigue
- Jaundice
- Symptoms of heart failure including chest pain, shortness of breath, and/or edema
- Hematemesis
- Melena
- Oliguria
- History of chronic liver disease
- Alcoholic hepatitis
- Alcohol abuse

PHYSICAL EXAM
- Exam findings may be general or related to specific complications
- General:
  - Pallor
  - Icterus
  - Digital clubbing
  - Palmar erythema
  - Splenomegaly
  - Caput medusa
  - Spider angiomata
  - Umbilical bruit
  - Hemorrhoids
  - Gynecomastia
  - Testicular atrophy
- Gastroesophageal varices:
  - Hypotension
  - Tachycardia
- Ascites:
  - Distended abdomen
  - Fluid wave
  - Shifting dullness with percussion
- Hepatic encephalopathy:
  - Confusion/Coma
  - Asterixis
  - Hyperreflexia

DIFFERENTIAL DIAGNOSIS
Usually related to specific presentations:
- Gastroesophageal varices with hemorrhage:
  - Portal hypertensive gastropathy
  - Hemorrhagic gastritis
  - Peptic ulcer disease
  - Mallory-Weiss tear
- Ascites:
  - Spontaneous bacterial peritonitis (SBP)
  - Pancreatic ascites
  - Peritoneal carcinomatosis
  - Tuberculous peritonitis
  - Nephrotic syndrome
  - Fluid overload from heart failure
- Hepatic encephalopathy:
  - Delirium tremens
  - Intracranial hemorrhage
  - Sedative abuse
  - Uremia
- Hepatorenal syndrome:
  - Drug nephrotoxicity
  - Renal tubular necrosis

DIAGNOSTIC TESTS & INTERPRETATION
Initial Tests (lab, imaging)
Nonspecific changes associated with underlying disease:
- Hypersplenism: Anemia (also may be due to malnutrition or bleeding), leukopenia, thrombocytopenia
- Hepatic dysfunction:
  - Hypoalbuminemia
  - Hyperbilirubinemia
  - Elevated alkaline phosphatase
  - Elevated liver enzymes (AST, ALT)
  - Abnormal clotting (prothrombin time, international normalized ratio, partial thromboplastin time)
- GI bleeding:
  - Iron-deficiency anemia
  - Elevated serum ammonia
  - Fecal occult blood
- Hepatorenal syndrome:
  - Elevated serum creatinine (Cr), blood urea nitrogen (BUN)
  - Urine Na <5 mEq/L (<20 mmol/L)
- US and CT scan/MRI may detect cirrhosis, splenomegaly, ascites, and varices.
- US/Duplex Doppler:
  - Can determine presence and direction of flow in portal and hepatic veins
  - Useful in diagnosing portal vein thrombosis, shunt thrombosis, or the presence of ascites
- CT scan/MRI: Angiographic measurement of hepatic venous wedge pressure via jugular or femoral vein:
  - Correlates with portal pressure
  - Risk of variceal bleeding is increased if hepatic venous pressure gradient >12 mm Hg
- Upper GI series may outline varices in esophagus and stomach.

Diagnostic Procedures/Other
Endoscopy can diagnose esophageal and gastric varices and portal hypertensive gastropathy.

Test Interpretation
Specific for underlying disease

TREATMENT

GENERAL MEASURES
- Avoid sedatives that may precipitate encephalopathy.
- Limit sodium intake because cirrhotic patients avidly retain sodium.
- Restrict protein only if encephalopathic.

MEDICATION
Therapy for encephalopathy: See "Hepatic Encephalopathy."

First Line
- Prophylaxis against variceal bleeding (1)[B]:
  - Nonselective β-blockade (2)[B]:
    ○ Propranolol: Start with 10–20 mg/d PO b.i.d.–t.i.d.; pediatric dose: 0.5–1 mg/kg/d divided q6–8h
    ○ Nadolol: 40–80 mg/d PO once-daily dosing
  - Doses may be titrated up as tolerated to maximum recommended doses.

- Therapy for acute variceal hemorrhage (3)[B]:
  – Vasopressin: Start with 0.2–0.4 U/min IV; increase to maximum dose 0.9 U/min as needed; pediatric dose: 0.002–0.005 U/kg/min; do not exceed 0.01 U/kg/min. After bleeding stops, continue at same dose for 12 hours and then taper off over 24–48 hours.
  – Somatostatin: 250 μg IV bolus, followed by 250 μg/hr continuous infusion; continue for 2–5 days if successful
  – Octreotide: 25–50 μg/hr continuous infusion; pediatric dose: 1 μg/kg bolus followed by 1 μg/kg/hr is used traditionally; treat for up to 5 days
- For prevention of recurrence and for overall reduction in mortality:
  – Propranolol: 10–60 mg/d PO b.i.d.–q.i.d.; pediatric dose: 0.5–1 mg/kg/d PO divided q6–8h
  – Nadolol: 40–80 mg/d PO reduces portal venous blood inflow by blocking the adrenergic dilatation of the mesenteric arterioles.
  – Tetrandrine, a calcium-channel blocker, also has been found to reduce the rate of rebleeding with fewer side effects.
- Treatment for ascites (along with salt and fluid restriction):
  – Furosemide: 20–40 mg/d PO; pediatric dose: 1–2 mg/kg/dose PO $\pm$ IV albumin infusion
  – Spironolactone: 50–100 mg/d PO; pediatric dose: 1–3 mg/kg/d PO

Second Line
- Terlipressin (1–2 mg IV q4–6h for up to 48 hours) is a more selective splanchnic vasoconstrictor and may be associated with fewer complications (2)[B]. It is currently used when standard therapy with somatostatin or octreotide fails.
- Addition of nitrates, such as nitroglycerin or isosorbide mononitrate, reduces portal pressures and bleeding rates and has been shown to reduce mortality. Since the risk–benefit ratio is not clear, nitrates are not considered 1st-line treatment.

ISSUES FOR REFERRAL
Patients with portal hypertension should be managed longitudinally by both a primary care physician and a gastroenterologist.

SURGERY/OTHER PROCEDURES
- Treatments available for specific complications of portal hypertension (in addition to or if refractory to medications) (4)[B]:
  – Gastroesophageal varices with hemorrhage:
    ○ Endoscopic variceal sclerosis or banding (the first-line treatment in many cases for acute hemorrhage)
    ○ Balloon tamponade (not used commonly when endoscopic treatment is available)
    ○ Transjugular intrahepatic portosystemic shunt (TIPS)
    ○ Portocaval shunting
  – Ascites refractory to medical management:
    ○ Large-volume paracentesis
    ○ Peritoneovenous shunt
    ○ TIPS
- Liver transplantation should be considered for patients with advanced disease (2)[B].

IN-PATIENT CONSIDERATIONS
- Acute GI bleeding should be managed in the inpatient setting, either on the regular medical floor if the patient is hemodynamically stable or occasionally in the ICU if the patient is unstable.
- Patients with mental status changes from encephalopathy need to be evaluated in the inpatient setting.

Admission Criteria/Initial Stabilization
- Acute bleeding from the intestinal tract, either vomiting or per rectum
- Acute confusional state/mental status changes
- If acute variceal bleeding (5)[B]:
  – Type and cross patient's blood.
  – Initial resuscitation with isotonic fluid until packed RBCs are available
  – Correct coagulopathy with vitamin K and fresh-frozen plasma (FFP).
  – Endoscopy as soon as the patient is stabilized (for diagnosis and treatment)
- Avoid sedatives that may precipitate encephalopathy.
- Limit sodium administration because cirrhotic patients avidly retain sodium.
- Restrict protein only if encephalopathic.

ALERT
If the patient is an active alcohol drinker, watch for signs and symptoms of withdrawal. Follow inpatient protocols for alcohol withdrawal management.

IV Fluids
Use isotonic fluid for hydration.

Discharge Criteria
- For GI bleeding:
  – No active bleeding in 24 hours
  – Stable hemoglobin and hematocrit
  – Hemodynamically stable (especially heart rate)
- For encephalopathy: Improvement in or resolution of mental status changes to baseline

ONGOING CARE

DIET
- In patients with cirrhosis, sodium restriction is important because cirrhotic patients avidly retain sodium.
- Restrict protein only in patients who are encephalopathic.

PATIENT EDUCATION
Refrain from drinking alcohol. Resources for patients who have difficulty with not drinking alcohol can be obtained from Alcoholics Anonymous at www.aa.org.

PROGNOSIS
- Hepatic reserve defined by Child-Pugh classification: Rating based on encephalopathy, ascites, bilirubin, albumin, prothrombin
- Variceal bleeding:
  – 1/3 of patients with known varices will bleed eventually.
  – 50% rebleed, usually within 2 years, unless portal pressure is reduced by surgical or transjugular intrahepatic portosystemic shunt procedure.
  – 15–20% mortality rate
- Ascites and encephalopathy often recur.
- Prognosis of patients with ascites is poor: 50% 1-year survival without liver transplant (compared with 90% for patients with cirrhosis and no ascites)

REFERENCES
1. Bosch J. The management of portal hypertension: Rational basis, available treatments and future options. *J Hepatology.* 2008;48:S68–S92.
2. Abraldes JG, Angermayr B, Bosch J. The management of portal hypertension. *Clin Liver Dis.* 2005;9:685–713, vii.
3. Garcia-Tsao G, Sanyal AJ, Grace ND, et al. Prevention and management of gastroesophageal varices and variceal hemorrhage in cirrhosis. *Hepatology.* 2007;46(3):922–938.
4. Sanyal AJ, Bosch J, Blei A, et al. Portal hypertension and its complications. *Gastroenterology.* 2008; 134:1715–1728.
5. Sass DA, Chopra KB. Portal hypertension and variceal hemorrhage. *Med Clin North Am.* 2009; 93(4):837–853.

 CODES

ICD10
K76.6 Portal hypertension

CLINICAL PEARLS
- Endoscopic treatment is successful for acute variceal hemorrhage 85% of the time.
- Prognosis of patients with ascites is poor: 50% 1-year survival without liver transplant (compared with 90% for patients with cirrhosis and no ascites).
- Advantages and disadvantages of balloon tamponade for acute variceal bleed:
  – Advantages include rapid and often effective control of bleeding and common availability of device.
  – Disadvantages include recurrence of bleeding when balloon is deflated, patient discomfort, and risk of esophageal perforation.

POSTCONCUSSION SYNDROME (MILD TRAUMATIC BRAIN INJURY)

Tyler H. Wheeler, MD • Jeanne M. Cawse-Lucas, MD

 BASICS

DESCRIPTION

- Postconcussion syndrome (PCS) is an evolving clinical diagnosis involving physical, cognitive, and/or behavioral symptoms that develop 2–12 weeks after a concussion and persist for weeks to months.
- Symptoms of PCS (1)[C]:
  - Cognitive:
    - Poor focus
    - Poor organization
    - Diminished academic/intellectual performance
    - Slowed response time
  - Physical:
    - Headache
    - Nausea
    - Visual changes
    - Light and nose sensitivity
    - Tinnitus
    - Dizziness and balance problems
    - Fatigue and sleep disturbance
  - Behavioral:
    - Depression
    - Irritability/Emotional lability
    - "Clinginess"
    - Apathy
    - Increased sensitivity to alcohol
- Diagnosis is a clinical one based on history, and clinical symptoms and signs.

EPIDEMIOLOGY

Incidence

The reported range of mild traumatic brain injury (MTBI) in patients who develop PCS varies widely between 5% and 80%.

- The variation is due to difficulty in differentiating normal postconcussion *symptoms* from postconcussion *syndrome*.
- Consensus from the 3rd International Conference on concussion in sport (2008) is that 80–90% of concussion victims recover from postconcussion *symptoms* within 7–10 days, or maybe slightly longer in children/adolescents (2,3).

Prevalence

- MTBI accounts for most head trauma seen in emergency departments.
- Predominant sex: Female > Male, although female gender is not universally considered a risk factor.

ETIOLOGY AND PATHOPHYSIOLOGY

- Controversial; exact mechanism(s) unknown
- It is postulated that microscopic axonal injury from shearing forces leads to inflammation that causes the secondary brain injury.
- Conflicting data on structural brain damage and the correlation of imaging findings with physical symptoms (1,3,4,5,6)
- Strong correlation between existing psychiatric disease and development of PCS:
  - PCS symptoms develop in patients with non-brain injury trauma at similar rates to those with MTBI. These findings suggest a psychiatric component to the pathophysiology of PCS (5,6)[B].
- Concussion: A difficult-to-define pathophysiologic process affecting the brain. It is characterized by rapid development of impaired neurologic function following direct head injury/transmitted force to the head (2):
  - Symptoms are similar to those of PCS, but generally resolve within 7–10 days (2)[C].
  - Loss of consciousness is not required to sustain a concussion.
- Most commonly related to:
  - Motor vehicle accidents
  - Falls
  - Occupational accidents
  - Recreational accidents
  - Assaults
- Because the pathophysiology of PCS is still not well understood, and because of significant symptom overlap (notably among depression, anxiety, and PTSD), PCS remains a difficult condition to diagnose and to manage:
  - Only some people with MTBI develop PCS; it is unclear what causes PCS symptoms to occur and to persist (5,6)[B].
  - As above, psychiatric factors are commonly associated with, and likely play a role in, the development of PCS (5,6)[B].

RISK FACTORS

- Amnesia, migraine, self-reported cognitive decline, noise and light sensitivity, depression/anxiety developing or worsening in the 1st days to weeks after MTBI are thought to be the major risk factors (1,3,4)[A].
- Preexisting psychiatric disease including depression, anxiety, personality disorder, and posttraumatic stress disorder (PTSD)
- Preexisting expectation of poor outcomes in patients following concussion/MTBI (1,3,4)[B]
- Unclear if previous history of concussion(s) is likely a risk factor for PCS (1)[C]
- Poor coping strategies, namely premature return to play following MTBI ("all-or-nothing behavior") (1,4)[B]
- Low socioeconomic status

GENERAL PREVENTION

- Education of players, coaches, parents, and athletic trainers about concussion, PCS, and following game safety rules designed to protect players
- Head injury precautions with activities (e.g., helmets, mouth guards, and standard safety practices) advised, but no good evidence that these decrease incidence of MTBI or PCS
- Early screening and intervention(s) for anxiety and depression

COMMONLY ASSOCIATED CONDITIONS

- PTSD
- Depression
- Anxiety
- Fibromyalgia
- Personality disorders (namely, compulsive, histrionic, and narcissistic)

DIAGNOSIS

HISTORY

- Detailed history of recent impact/closed head injury, including:
  - Mechanism
  - Amount and type of force
  - Timing of injury related to symptoms
  - Previous head injuries, including concussion, and timing of those injuries
  - Previous medical, psychiatric, and social (e.g., drug/alcohol use) history
- Report of neurologic, cognitive, or behavioral symptoms by patient/family

PHYSICAL EXAM

Complete neurologic exam, including:

- Glasgow Coma Scale (GCS)
- Depression/Anxiety screening:
  - PHQ-9
  - GAD-7
- Sport Concussion Assessment Tool (SCAT2: http://www.scribd.com/doc/35128754/SCAT2-form, NFL Sideline Concussion Assessment tool, or computerized neuropsychological testing (CNP) both pre- and post-MTBI is common practice, although data are limited on validity (2)[C]. More info regarding CNP below.

DIFFERENTIAL DIAGNOSIS

- PTSD
- Anxiety
- Depression
- Personality disorder
- Migraine headaches
- Chronic fatigue syndrome, fibromyalgia
- Evolving intracranial hemorrhage
- Exposure to toxins, including prescription and recreational drugs
- Endocrine/Metabolic abnormality (e.g., hypothyroidism, hyponatremia).

DIAGNOSTIC TESTS & INTERPRETATION

Initial Tests (lab, imaging)

If clinically warranted, consider evaluation for infection, intoxication, and endocrine/metabolic abnormality.

- Brain imaging both on initial evaluation of MTBI and PCS is generally neither fruitful nor indicated.
- Consider the use of cervical imaging when concomitant cervical spine injury is suspected.

Follow-Up Tests & Special Considerations

- Several computerized neuropsychologic testing programs can be used to guide decisions regarding return to play. Consensus is that baseline testing should be done and scores used as controls against scores achieved after MTBI. However, few data support this approach. Formal neuropsychiatric evaluations are likely superior when available. None of these tests should be used alone in decision-making, especially if a patient is still having symptoms despite improving or "baseline" scores (2).
- Common neuropsychologic testing programs for PCS:
  - Immediate Post-Concussion Assessment and Cognitive Testing (ImPACT)
  - Axon Sports Computerized Cognitive Assessment Tool (CCAT)
  - Post Concussion Symptom Scale (PCSS)
  - Balance Error Scoring System (BESS)
  - Automated Neuropsychological Assessment Metrics (ANAM)

 TREATMENT

GENERAL MEASURES

Return to play guidelines (2,3)[C]:

- Stage 1. No activity: Complete physical and cognitive rest, until symptom free.
  – Consider school/work accommodations to allow earlier return to school/work in an attempt to prevent patients from getting too far behind (3)[C].
- Stage 2. Light aerobic exercise: Walking, swimming, or stationary cycling keeping intensity <70% max predicted heart rate. No resistance training
- Stage 3. Sport-specific exercise: Drills (e.g., skating in ice hockey, running in soccer). No head impact activities
- Stage 4. Noncontact training drills: Progression to more complex training drills (e.g., passing drills in football and ice hockey). May start progressive resistance training
- Stage 5. Full contact practice: Following medical clearance, participate in normal training activities
- Stage 6. Return to play: Normal game play
- Each step should take 24 hours. If PCS symptoms occur at any step, the patient should drop back to the previous asymptomatic level and try to progress again after 24 hours of rest (2)[C].
- Persons with concussion or PCS should be restricted from sport activity until they are off all medications used to treat PCS symptoms and the clinical symptoms of PCS have resolved (1,2)[C].

MEDICATION
First Line
Headache/Neck pain:
- Nonnarcotic pain control if possible (e.g., NSAIDs, Tramadol):
  – Sedation may obscure cognitive evaluation.
  – Possible association with use of opiates and increased risk of depression and anxiety in PCS patients (5)[B].
  – Occipital nerve block may be considered for persistent pain.

ALERT
Avoid opiates and benzodiazepines for patients with MTBI (5)[B].
- Depression/Sleep disorders:
  – Depression/Anxiety screening starting in the 1st week post MTBI:
    ○ SSRIs
    ○ Tricyclic antidepressants, specifically trazodone if there is concomitant sleep disturbance, may be beneficial
  – Consider referral to mental health specialist(s).
- Cognitive disorders (6):
  – Evaluation by neuropsychiatrist
  – Some evidence suggests computerized neuropsychologic (CNP) testing and rehab programs are beneficial.
  – Methylphenidate may be considered.
  – SSRIs may be considered, especially if concomitant depression/anxiety.

Second Line
- Dopaminergic agents, such as amantadine, levodopa, and bromocriptine (1)[B]
- Dehydroepiandrosterone sulfate (DHEAS) (7).

ISSUES FOR REFERRAL
- Psychiatric treatment, including behavioral therapy for anxiety and depression symptoms. Specifically neuropsychiatric therapy can be of benefit.
- Occupational therapy for vocational rehabilitation, if needed

- Neurology referral if primary care interventions for seizures, headache, vertigo, or cognition are unsuccessful
- Comprehensive cognitive evaluation for potential TBI rehabilitation
- Cognitive–behavioral therapy
- Substance abuse counseling, if needed

COMPLEMENTARY AND ALTERNATIVE MEDICINE
Massage therapy/osteopathic manipulative treatment for headache and neck pain

 ONGOING CARE

FOLLOW-UP RECOMMENDATIONS
Schedule regular follow-up to evaluate for persistent symptoms, efficacy of/need for neuropsychiatric evaluation, and the efficacy of/need for pharmacologic therapy.

Patient Monitoring
- Consider serial neuropsychologic testing.
- Follow return-to-play guidelines.

PATIENT EDUCATION
- NCAA Concussion Program: http://www.ncaa.org/wps/wcm/connect/public/NCAA/Health+and+Safety/Concussion+homepage/Concussion+Landing+Page
- Centers for Disease Control and Prevention: http://www.cdc.gov/concussion/sports
- Mayo Clinic Health Information: http://www.mayoclinic.com/health/post-concussion-syndrome/DS01020
- Brain Injury Association of America: www.biausa.org; (800) 444-6443

PROGNOSIS
- Prognosis generally is good (8).
- Young children may recover more slowly than young adults.

COMPLICATIONS
- Repeat head injury/return to play before resolution of PCS symptoms can worsen/prolong symptoms.
- Case studies of 2nd-impact syndrome, a rare but fatal condition owing to a 2nd head injury soon after the 1st, have been reported.

REFERENCES
1. Jotwani V, Harmon KG. Postconcussion syndrome in athletes. *Curr Sports Med Rep.* 2010;9:21–26.
2. McCrory P, Meeuwisse W, Johnston K, et al. Consensus statement on Concussion in Sport 3rd International Conference on Concussion in Sport held in Zurich, November 2008. *Clin J Sport Med.* 2009;19:185–200.
3. Harmon KG, Drezner JA, Gammons M, et al. American Medical Society for Sports Medicine position statement: Concussion in sport. *Br J Sports Med.* 2013;47:15–26.
4. Hou R, Moss-Morris R, Peveler R, et al. When a minor head injury results in enduring symptoms: A prospective investigation of risk factors for postconcussional syndrome after mild traumatic brain injury. *J Neurol Neurosurg Psychiatr.* 2012;83: 217–223.
5. Silverberg ND, Iverson GL. Etiology of the post-concussion syndrome: Physiogenesis and Psychogenesis revisited. *NeuroRehabilitation.* 2011;29:317–329.

6. Meares S, Shores EA, Batchelor J, et al. The relationship of psychological and cognitive factors and opioids in the development of the postconcussion syndrome in general trauma patients with mild traumatic brain injury. *J Int Neuropsychol Soc.* 2006;12:792–801.
7. Lee H, Kim S, Kim J, et al. Comparing effects of methylphenidate, sertraline and placebo on neuropsychiatric sequelae in patients with traumatic brain injury. *Hum Psychopharmacol Clin Exp.* 2005;20:97–104.
8. Milman A, Zohar O, Maayan R, et al. DHEAS repeated treatment improves cognitive and behavioral deficits after mild traumatic brain injury. *Eur Neuropsychopharmacol.* 2008;84(3):181–187. Epub 2007 Jul 31.

ADDITIONAL READING
- Barlow M, Schlabach D, Peiffer J, et al. Differences in change scores and the predictive validity of three commonly used measures following concussion in the middle school and high school aged population. *Int J Sports Phys Ther.* 2011;84(3):150–157.
- Broglio SP, Ferrara MS, Macciocchi SN, et al. Test-retest reliability of computerized concussion assessment programs. *J Athl Train.* 2007;42(4): 509–514.
- Leddy JJ, Kozlowski K, Donnelly JP, et al. A preliminary study of subsymptom threshold exercise training for refractory post-concussion syndrome. *Clin J Sport Med.* 2010;20(1):21–27.
- Leddy JJ, Snadhu H, Sodhi V, et al. Rehabilitation of concussion and post-concussion syndrome. *Sports Health.* 2012;4(2):147–154.
- Nampiaparampil DE. Prevalence of chronic pain after traumatic brain injury: A systematic review. *JAMA.* 2008;300(6):711–719.
- Stulemeijer M, van der Werf S, Borm GF, et al. Early prediction of favourable recovery 6 months after mild traumatic brain injury. *J Neurol Neurosurg.* 2008;79:936–942.

 SEE ALSO

Concussion

 CODES

ICD10
- F07.81 Postconcussional syndrome
- S06.9X0A Unsp intracranial injury w/o loss of consciousness, init
- S06.9X9A Unsp intracranial injury w LOC of unsp duration, init

CLINICAL PEARLS
- Head CT scan is the test of choice for acute injury in which it is necessary to exclude intracranial bleeding.
- Coordinate multidisciplinary treatment plans for patients with persistent symptoms, namely mental health professionals.
- Return to play/activity should not occur until symptom free and off all medications started to treat PCS symptoms. Any return to activity with persistent symptoms should be discussed in detail with the patient and the patient's family (1)[B].

POSTTRAUMATIC STRESS DISORDER

Rachel Bramson, MD • Michael L. Brown, MD • Robert E. Rogers

 BASICS

DESCRIPTION

- Posttraumatic stress disorder (PTSD) is an anxiety disorder defined as a reaction that can occur after exposure to an extreme traumatic event involving death, threat of death, serious physical injury, or a threat to physical integrity.
- This reaction has 3 cardinal characteristics:
  – Re-experiencing the trauma
  – Avoidance of anything related to the traumatic event and/or numbing of general responsiveness
  – Increased arousal
- Traumatic events that may trigger PTSD include natural/human disasters, serious accidents, war, sexual abuse, rape, torture, terrorism, hostage-taking, or being diagnosed with life-threatening disease.
- PTSD can be:
  – Acute: Symptoms lasting <3 months
  – Chronic: Symptoms lasting ≥3 months
  – Delayed onset: 6 months (from event to symptom onset) in 25% of diagnosed cases

EPIDEMIOLOGY

- ~30% of men and women who have spent time in a war zone experience PTSD
- Current estimates of PTSD in military personnel who served in Iraq range from 12–20%.

Incidence
~7.7 million American adults aged ≥18 years (3.5% of this age group) are diagnosed with PTSD each year

Prevalence
Lifetime prevalence for PTSD is 8–9%.

ETIOLOGY AND PATHOPHYSIOLOGY

- During trauma, the locus coeruleus mediates sympathetic outflows to the amygdala (rapid effect) and adrenal medulla (sustained effect). The adrenal medulla then releases catecholamines, which stimulate peripheral afferent vagal β-receptors. Vagal afferents innervate the nucleus tractus solitarius (NTS) in the brainstem medulla. NTS fibers innervate the amygdala with norepinephrine (NE).
- With an increase in NE, the amygdala mediates coupling of emotional valence to declarative memories via long-term potentiation, forming deeply engraved trauma memories and leading to intrusive memories and emotions, potentially leading to PTSD.
- The orbitoprefrontal cortex (which usually exerts an inhibiting effect on this activation) appears less capable of inhibiting this activation due to stress-induced atrophy of specific nuclei in this region.

Genetics
- Monozygotic twins exposed to combat in Vietnam were at increased risk of the co-twin having PTSD compared with twins who were dizygotic.
- Some data suggest an association between dopamine transporter gene (DAT) *SLC6A3 3′* (VNTR) polymorphism, and PTSD.

RISK FACTORS
- Pretrauma environment:
  – Female sex
  – Younger age
  – Psychiatric history
  – Sexual abuse
- Peritrauma environment:
  – Severity of the trauma
  – Peritrauma emotionality

- – Perception of threat to life
  – Perpetration of the trauma
- Posttrauma environment:
  – Perceived injury severity
  – Medical complications
  – Perceived social support
  – Persistent dissociation from traumatic event
- Subsequent exposure to trauma-related stimuli

GENERAL PREVENTION

- Although some evidence of benefit of pharmacologic interventions, including propranolol and corticosteroids, no standard intervention prevents the onset of PTSD (1)[A].
- Compulsory psychological debriefing immediately after a trauma (critical incident stress management) does not prevent PTSD and may be harmful (2)[A].

COMMONLY ASSOCIATED CONDITIONS
- Major depressive disorder
- Alcohol/Substance abuse
- Panic disorder
- Obsessive compulsive disorder
- Agoraphobia and/or social phobia
- Traumatic brain injury
- Smoking (especially with assaultive trauma)
- Major neurocognitive disorders, dementia or amnesia

Pediatric Considerations
- Oppositional defiant disorder and separation anxiety are common comorbid conditions

 DIAGNOSIS

HISTORY
Diagnosis is based on *DSM-V* criteria:
- Criterion A: Exposure to trauma (≥1 of the following):
  – Direct experience of a traumatic event
  – In-person witnessing of a traumatic event
  – Learning of a traumatic event involving a close friend or family member
  – Repeated exposure to details of a traumatic event
- Criterion B: Intrusive symptoms associated with the traumatic event (≥1 of the following):
  – Recurrent, involuntary, and intrusive distressing memories of the event
  – Recurrent distressing dreams related to the event
  – Dissociative reactions that simulate a recurrence of the event
  – Intense or prolonged distress to stimuli that resemble an aspect of the event
- Criterion C: Avoidance of stimuli associated with the trauma (≥1 of the following):
  – Avoidance of memories, thoughts, or feelings about the event
  – Avoidance of external reminders that trigger memories, thoughts, or feelings about the event
- Criterion D: Negative cognitive and mood changes associated with the trauma (≥2 of the following):
  – Inability to remember aspects of event
  – Persistent and exaggerated negative opinion of self, others, or the world
  – Distorted beliefs about the cause or consequences of the event
  – Negative emotional state
  – Diminished interest in significant activities
  – Feeling detached from others
  – Inability to experience positive emotions
- Criterion E: Hyperarousal (≥2 of the following):

- – Difficulty sleeping/falling asleep
  – Decreased concentration
  – Hypervigilance
  – Outbursts of anger/irritable mood
  – Exaggerated startle response
  – Self-destructive behavior
- Criterion F: Duration of the relevant criteria symptoms should be >1 month.
- Criterion G: Clinically significant distress/impairment in functioning
- Criterion H: Relevant criteria not attributed to substance effects or other medical conditions

Pediatric Considerations
- Memories of the traumatic event may not appear distressing and may be seen as play reenactment.
- Frightening dreams of children may not have content attributable to the traumatic event.
- Reactions can include a fear of being separated from a parent, crying, whimpering, screaming, immobility and/or aimless motion, trembling, frightened facial expressions, excessive clinging, and regressive behavior.
- Older children may show extreme withdrawal, disruptive behavior, and/or an inability to pay attention. Regressive behaviors, nightmares, sleep problems, irrational fears, irritability, refusal to attend school, outbursts of anger, fighting, somatic complaints with no medical basis, and decline in schoolwork performance are often seen. Furthermore, depression, anxiety, feelings of guilt, and emotional numbing are often present.

- Parental posttraumatic stress has been shown to be a robust predictor of pediatric PTSD (3)[A].

PHYSICAL EXAM
- Patients may present with physical injuries from the traumatic event.
- Mental status examination:
  – Thoughts and perceptions (e.g., hallucinations, delusions, suicidal ideation, phobias)
  – General appearance: Disheveled, poor hygiene
  – Behavior: Agitation; startle reaction extreme
  – Psychological numbness
  – Orientation may be affected
  – Memory: Forgetfulness, especially concerning the details of the traumatic event
  – Poor concentration
  – Poor impulse control
  – Altered speech rate and flow
  – Mood and affect may be changed: Depression, anxiety, guilt, and/or fear

Pediatric Considerations
Elevated heart rate immediately following trauma is associated with development of PTSD (3)[A].

DIFFERENTIAL DIAGNOSIS
- Acute stress disorder (symptoms <4 weeks)
- Generalized anxiety disorder
- Adjustment disorder
- Obsessive-compulsive disorder
- Schizophrenia
- Major depressive disorder
- Mood disorder with psychotic features
- Substance abuse
- Personality disorders
- Dissociative disorders
- Conversion disorder

TREATMENT

- Better prognosis if treated with a combination of psychotherapy and pharmacotherapy, initiated soon after the trauma.

MEDICATION
First Line

- SSRIs: Depression, panic attacks, startle response, sleep disruption (4,5)[A]. All commonly used SSRIs have been shown to be effective in the treatment of PTSD and are the first-line treatment:
  - Sertraline: 50–200 mg every day (FDA approved)
  - Paroxetine: Starting dose: 10 mg every day; may be increased in 10-mg increments at intervals ≥1 week (FDA approved)
  - Fluoxetine: 20 mg every day/b.i.d. not to exceed 80 mg/d (demonstrates some efficacy for all 3 symptom clusters) (5)[A]
- Sleep disruption: Sleep disruption due to hyperarousal is ubiquitous in PTSD. Standard sedatives, such as trazodone 50–300 mg at bedtime, mirtazapine 7.5–30 mg qhs, or amitriptyline 25–100 mg qhs
- Nightmares/Nighttime hyperarousal: Prazosin 2–15 mg qhs (6)[A], clonidine 0.1–0.2 mg qhs, amitriptyline 25–100 mg qhs

Second Line

Refractory/Residual symptoms: Consider augmentation with (6)[A]:

- Depression: Mirtazapine 15–45 mg/d; consider switch to a serotonin-norepinephrine reuptake inhibitor (SNRI), such as venlafaxine XR 37.5–300 mg/d, duloxetine 60–120 mg/d or desvenlafaxine 50–100 mg/d. Nefazodone 300–600 mg/d in divided doses can be very effective, but requires quarterly LFTs.
- Re-experiencing/intrusive thoughts: 1st-/2nd-generation antipsychotic medications: Aripiprazole 5–15 mg/d, risperidone 0.5–2 mg/d, olanzapine 2.5–10 mg/d, quetiapine 50–400 mg/d. 2nd-generation Rx less prone to extrapyramidal symptoms (EPS), cognitive dulling.
- Hyperarousal: Clonidine, start 0.05 mg b.i.d./t.i.d.; slowly titrate to as much as 0.45 mg/d divided doses; guanfacine 1–3 mg/d in divided doses (long-acting forms of both clonidine and guanfacine now available). Also consider 2nd-generation antipsychotics quetiapine, risperidone, and olanzapine as above. Divided doses often more helpful.
- Impulsivity/Explosiveness: Anticonvulsants: Valproic acid 500–2,000 mg/d, carbamazepine 200–600 mg/d, topiramate 50–200 mg/d
- Anxiety: Benzodiazepines (see "ALERT"), including clonazepam, 1–4 mg/d in divided doses for a limited duration. Consider also hydroxyzine 25–50 mg t.i.d./q.i.d. PRN, or risperidone 0.25–0.5 mg t.i.d. PRN

ALERT

Given risk of substance abuse and questionable benefit in PTSD, recommended benzodiazepines be avoided (7)[A]. Short-acting benzodiazepines, present the greatest risk.

ADDITIONAL THERAPIES

- Psychotherapeutic interventions:

  - Exposure therapies have shown the highest effectiveness for treatment of PTSD (8)[A]:
    - Behavioral and cognitive-behavioral therapy (CBT): Early CBT has been shown to speed recovery. CBT is currently considered the standard of care for PTSD by the U.S. Department of Defense.
    - Internet-based CBT has shown benefit in reduction of PTSD symptoms.
    - Prolonged exposure therapy: Re-experience distressing trauma-related memories and reminders to facilitate habituation and successful emotional processing of memory.
    - EMDR (eye movement desensitization and reprocessing) has been shown to benefit patients with PTSD (9)[A].
    - Emotional Freedom Technique has been shown to benefit veterans with PTSD (10)[A].

  - Stress-reduction techniques:
    - Immediate symptom reduction (e.g., rebreathing in a bag for hyperventilation)
    - Early recognition and removal from a stress
    - Relaxation, meditation, and exercise techniques are also helpful in reducing the reaction to stressful events.
- Interpersonal psychotherapy:
  - Supportive psychotherapy with an emphasis on the here and now
- Social:
  - Establish the social framework of the problem. Clarifying this allows the patient to begin viewing it within the proper context (e.g., change of job/relocation of adult-dependent offspring)

IN-PATIENT CONSIDERATIONS

Inpatient care is necessary only if the patient becomes suicidal/homicidal or for treatment of comorbid conditions (e.g., depression, substance abuse).

ONGOING CARE

PATIENT EDUCATION

National Center for PTSD: www.ptsd.va.gov

PROGNOSIS

- Varies significantly from patient to patient
- In 50% of cases, the symptoms spontaneously remit after 3 months; however, in other cases, symptoms may persist, often for many years, and cause long-term impairment in life functioning.
- Factors associated with a good prognosis include:
  - Rapid engagement of treatment
  - Early and ongoing social support
  - Avoidance of retraumatization
  - Positive premorbid function
  - Absence of other psychiatric disorders/substance abuse

COMPLICATIONS

- Increased risk for panic disorder, agoraphobia, obsessive–compulsive disorder, social phobia, specific phobia, major depressive disorder, somatization disorder; impulsive behavior, suicide, and homicide. Victims of sexual assault are at especially high risk for developing mental health problems and committing suicide.
- Benzodiazepines lead to abuse and dependence.
- Avoidance of stimuli associated with the trauma can generalize to wide-ranging avoidance. This leads to a far greater negative impact on the patient's life.

REFERENCES

1. Searcy CP, Bobadilla L, Gordon WA, et al. Pharmacological prevention of combat-related PTSD: A literature review. *Mil Med*. 2012;177: 649–654.
2. Rose S, Bisson J, Churchill R, et al. Psychological debriefing for preventing post traumatic stress disorder (PTSD). *Cochrane Database Syst Rev*. 2002;2:CD000560.
3. Brosbe MS, Hoefling K, Faust J. Predicting posttraumatic stress following pediatric injury: A systematic review. *J Pediatr Psychol*. 2011;36: 718–729.
4. Stein DJ, Ipser JC, Seedat S, et al. Pharmacotherapy for post traumatic stress disorder (PTSD). *Cochrane Database Syst Rev*. 2006;1:CD002795.
5. Xu JJ, Chan MJ, Yang YC. Fluoxetine as a treatment for post-traumatic stress disorder. *Neurosciences (Riyadh)*. 2011;16:257–262.
6. Bajor LA, Ticlea AN, Osser DN, et al. The psychopharmacology algorithm project at the Harvard South shore program: An update on posttraumatic stress disorder. *Harv Rev Psychiatry*. 2011;19:240–258.
7. Jeffreys M, Capehart B, Friedman MJ. Pharmacotherapy for posttraumatic stress disorder: Review with clinical applications. *J Rehabil Res Dev*. 2012;49:703–715.
8. Kornør H, Winje D, Ekeberg Ø, et al. Early trauma-focused cognitive-behavioural therapy to prevent chronic post-traumatic stress disorder and related symptoms: A systematic review and meta-analysis. *BMC Psychiatry*. 2008;8:81.
9. Goodson J, Helstrom A, Halpern JM, et al. Treatment of posttraumatic stress disorder in U.S. combat veterans: A meta-analytic review. *Psychol Rep*. 2011;109:573–599.
10. Church D, Hawk C, Brooks AJ, et al. Psychological trauma symptom improvement in veterans using emotional freedom techniques: A randomized control trial. *J Nerv Ment Dis*. 2013;201:153–160.

ADDITIONAL READING

American Psychiatric Association. *Diagnostic and Statistical Manual of Mental Disorders DSM-V*. 5th ed. Washington, DC: American Psychiatric Publishing; 2013.

CODES

ICD10

- F43.10 Post-traumatic stress disorder, unspecified
- F43.11 Post-traumatic stress disorder, acute
- F43.12 Post-traumatic stress disorder, chronic

CLINICAL PEARLS

- Treatment is often best accomplished with a combination of psychotherapy and pharmacotherapy.
- The sooner therapy is initiated after the trauma, the better the prognosis.

PREECLAMPSIA AND ECLAMPSIA (TOXEMIA OF PREGNANCY)
Konstantinos E. Deligiannidis, MD, MPH

 BASICS

DESCRIPTION
- Preeclampsia is a disorder of pregnancy developing at the 20th week (or beyond), with hypertension (HTN), proteinuria, and/or edema and poor perfusion of vital organs:
  - May progress from mild to life threatening in hours to days
  - The disease may include rapid weight gain and edema on the face and hands. The disorder is reversible by delivery if at term or, if maternal/fetal health are in danger, by preterm delivery.
  - Eclampsia is defined as seizure activity or coma in a patient with preeclampsia without underlying neurologic disease.
  - Most postpartum cases occur within 48 hours of delivery, but can occur up to 4 weeks postpartum.
- System(s) affected: Cardiovascular; Renal; Reproductive; Feto-placental; Central Nervous System (CNS); Hepatic
- Synonym(s): Toxemia of pregnancy

EPIDEMIOLOGY
Incidence
- Predominant age:
  - Most cases occur in younger women because of the higher incidence of preeclampsia in younger (nulliparous) women.
  - However, older (>40 years) patients with preeclamsia have 4× the incidence of seizures compared with patients in their 20s.
- Pregnancy-induced HTN: 6% of pregnancies
- Preeclampsia: 5–7%
- Eclampsia develops in 1/2,000 deliveries in developed countries. In developing countries, estimates range from 1/100–1/1,700.
- 40% of eclamptic seizures occur before delivery; 16% occur >48 hours after delivery.

ETIOLOGY AND PATHOPHYSIOLOGY
Systemic derangements in eclampsia include:
- Cardiovascular: Generalized vasospasm
- Hematologic: Decreased plasma volume, increased blood viscosity, hemoconcentration, coagulopathy
- Renal: Decreased glomerular filtration rate
- Hepatic: Periportal necrosis, hepatocellular damage, subcapsular hematoma
- CNS: Cerebral vasospasm and ischemia, cerebral edema, cerebral hemorrhage

Genetics
Increased incidence in pregnant women whose mothers/sisters had the disease

RISK FACTORS
- Nulliparity: 3:1 (relative risk [RR])
- Age >40 years: 2:1 (RR)
- High body mass index: 2:1 (RR)
- Antiphospholipid syndrome: 10:1 (RR)
- Diabetes: 3.5:1 (RR)
- Twin pregnancy: 3:1 (RR)
- Preeclampsia during a previous pregnancy
- Family history of preeclampsia: 3:1 (RR)
- Father of fetus previously experienced a preeclamptic pregnancy with another woman.

GENERAL PREVENTION
- Adequate prenatal care: Women who do not receive prenatal care are 7× more likely to die from complications.
- Good control of pre-existing HTN
- Recent systematic reviews and meta-analyses show that low-dose aspirin started early in pregnancy lowers the risk of developing preeclampsia in moderate- to high-risk patients, lowers the rate of preterm delivery and neonatal death, and has no significant effect on the rate of placental abruption/neonatal bleeding complications, with number needed to treat (NNT) to prevent 1 case of preeclampsia ~100 (1)[A].
- Calcium supplementation has been shown to reduce the risk of preeclampsia by 30%. The risk reduction seems to be greatest in women with a high risk of preeclampsia (RR = 0.22) (2)[A].
- Some evidence suggests vitamin C (1,000 mg/d) and vitamin E (400 U/d) reduce the risk for preeclampsia (3)[B], although some guidelines recommend against their use (4).

COMMONLY ASSOCIATED CONDITIONS
- Abruptio placenta
- Placental insufficiency
- Fetal growth restriction
- Preterm delivery
- Fetal demise
- Maternal seizures (eclampsia)
- Maternal pulmonary edema
- Maternal liver/kidney failure
- Maternal death

 DIAGNOSIS

Diagnosis is dependent on new onset of elevated BP and proteinuria after 20 weeks of gestation.

HISTORY
May be asymptomatic. In some cases, rapid excessive weight gain (>5 lb/wk; >2.3 kg/wk); more severe cases are associated with epigastric pain, headache, altered mental status, and visual disturbance.

PHYSICAL EXAM
- Preeclampsia:
  - Mild: Elevated BP ≥140 mm Hg systolic or 90 mm Hg diastolic on 2 BP readings 6 hours apart; proteinuria (>300 mg/24 hr or >1 g/L)
  - Severe: Elevated BP ≥160 systolic mm Hg or 110 mm Hg diastolic on 2 BP readings 6 hours apart:
    ○ Proteinuria (>5 g/24 hr)
    ○ Facial/Hand edema
    ○ Hyperreflexia
    ○ Retinal arteriolar spasm, papilledema
    ○ Epigastric/Right upper quadrant (RUQ) pain
    ○ Oliguria or anuria

- Eclampsia:
  - Headache, visual disturbance, and epigastric or RUQ pain often precede seizure.
  - Tonic–clonic seizure activity (focal/generalized)
  - Seizures may occur once/repeatedly.
  - Postictal coma, cyanosis (variable)
  - Temperatures >39°C, consistent with CNS hemorrhage
  - Normal BP, even in response to treatment, does not rule out potential for seizures. Up to 30% may not have edema; 20% may not have proteinuria.

DIFFERENTIAL DIAGNOSIS
- Chronic HTN: HTN before pregnancy; high BP before the 20th week; diagnosis during pregnancy, but persisting beyond postpartum day 84
- Gestational HTN: Increased BP first discovered during pregnancy, with no proteinuria; normal BP by 12 weeks postpartum
- Seizures in pregnancy: Epilepsy, cerebral tumors, meningitis/encephalitis, ruptured cerebral aneurysm. Until other causes are proven, however, all pregnant women with convulsions should be considered to have eclampsia.

DIAGNOSTIC TESTS & INTERPRETATION
Initial Tests (lab, imaging)
- Routine spot urine testing for protein should be done at each prenatal visit.
- CBC, including platelets
- Creatinine
- Serum transaminase levels
- Uric acid
- Coagulation profiles: Abnormalities suggest severe disease.
- 24-hour urine for protein/creatinine clearance: <90 mL/min/1.73 m² is abnormal.
- Daily fetal movement monitoring by mother ("kick counts")
- Nonstress test (NST) at diagnosis and then weekly until delivery
- US is used to monitor growth and cord blood flow; perform, as indicated, based on clinical stability and laboratory findings.
- US imaging for biophysical profile, estimation of fetal age, growth progress, amniotic fluid volume:
  - Weekly for mild preeclampsia
  - Twice weekly in severe preeclampsia
- With seizures, CT scan and MRI should be considered if focal findings persist or uncharacteristic signs/symptoms are present.

Follow-Up Tests & Special Considerations
Disseminated intravascular coagulation, thrombocytopenia, liver dysfunction, and renal failure can complicate preeclampsia associated with HELLP syndrome.

Test Interpretation
CNS: Cerebral edema, hyperemia, focal anemia, thrombosis, and hemorrhage: Cerebral lesions account for 40% of eclamptic deaths.

TREATMENT

- Mild:
  - Outpatient care
  - Maternal: Daily home BP monitoring; daily weights; weekly labs (24-hour protein, platelet count, creatinine, LFTs)
  - Fetal:
    - Patient-measured: Daily "kick counts"
    - Medical provider-measured: NST (see "Imaging" section)
- Severe:
  - Inpatient care if patient condition deteriorates (BP ≥160/110 mm Hg; severe headache; visual changes [scotoma or "flashing lights"]; impaired mentation; pulmonary edema; epigastric/RUQ pain; increasing LFTs; oliguria; thrombocytopenia) or if fetal status is deemed "nonreassuring"
  - Maternal: Daily labs, adding coagulation tests; IV magnesium sulfate as anticonvulsive prophylaxis; IV labetalol and oral nifedipine antihypertensive therapy titrated to keep systolic BP <155 mm Hg and diastolic BP <105 mm Hg. Keep diastolic BP >90 mm Hg to avoid hypoperfusing the uterus.
  - Fetal: Continuous heart monitoring; daily US with BP, amniotic fluid levels, fetal growth assessment as deemed necessary

GENERAL MEASURES
Management by gestational age of severe preeclampsia:
- <23 weeks: Offer to terminate pregnancy.
- At 23–32 weeks: Antihypertensives; evaluate maternal–fetal condition; steroids to enhance fetal lung maturity; plan delivery at 34 weeks with magnesium sulfate prophylaxis or for worsening maternal/fetal jeopardy.
- At 33–34 weeks: Steroids, magnesium sulfate, and delivery
- At >34 weeks: Magnesium sulfate and delivery

ALERT
- Regardless of gestational age, emergent delivery is recommended if there are signs of maternal hypertensive crisis, abruptio placentae, uterine rupture, or fetal distress (5)[B].
- Seizures:
  - Control of convulsions, correction of hypoxia and acidosis, lowering of BP, steps to effect delivery as soon as convulsions are controlled
  - See "Medication" section

MEDICATION
First Line
- For seizure prophylaxis: Magnesium sulfate (MgSO₄): Loading dose 4 g IV in 200 mL normal saline over 20–30 minutes; maintenance dose 1–2 g/hr IV
- For HTN:
  - Nifedipine (PO): 40–120 mg/d (caution with combination of Nifedipine and magnesium sulfate resulting in hypotension and neuromuscular blockade) or
  - Labetalol (IV): 600–2,400 mg/d, both titrated to keep BP <155/105 mm Hg; antihypertensives are inadvisable for mild HTN/preeclampsia.

- For eclampsia/seizures:
  - In recent randomized trials, MgSO₄ was found to be superior to phenytoin in the treatment and prevention of eclampsia and probably more effective and safer than diazepam.
  - Magnesium sulfate for seizures:
    - 2–4 g IV repeated q15min to a maximum of 6 g to achieve resolution of an ongoing convulsion
    - Magnesium then is continued at 1–3 g/hr, with the amount given based on the neurologic examination and patellar reflexes.
  - Levels of 6–8 mEq/mL are considered therapeutic, but clinical status is most important and must ensure that:
    - Patellar reflexes are present.
    - Respirations are not depressed.
    - Urine output is ≥25 mL/hr.
  - May be given safely, even in the presence of renal insufficiency
- Fluid therapy:
  - Ringer lactated solution with 5% dextrose at 60–120 mL/hr, with careful attention to fluid–volume status
- HTN, if present and severe (e.g., >160/110 mm Hg), also should be treated:
  - Hydralazine: 5 mg IV then 5–10-mg boluses as needed q20min or
  - Labetalol: 10–20 mg IV then double dose at 10-minute intervals up to 80 mg; maximum total cumulative dose of 220–230 mg (e.g., 20–40–80–80 or 10–20–40–80–80)
- Precautions: Do not use diuretics. Carefully monitor neurologic status, urine output, respirations, and fetal status.
- Calcium carbonate (1 g, administered slowly IV) may reverse magnesium-induced respiratory depression.

Second Line
- Diazepam 2 mg/min until resolution or 20 mg given or
- Lorazepam 1–2 mg/min up to total of 10 mg or
- Phenytoin 18–20 mg/kg at a rate of 20–40 mg/min or
- Phenobarbital 100 mg/min to a total of 20 mg/kg given

ONGOING CARE

FOLLOW-UP RECOMMENDATIONS
- Mild: Restricted activity
- Severe: Restricted activity, in hospital

DIET
- Salt restriction is inadvisable because the patient often is experiencing intravascular hypovolemia.
- Calcium supplementation is recommended for women who have low calcium intake (<600 mg/d) (4).

PATIENT EDUCATION
American College of Obstetricians and Gynecologists, 409 12th St. SW, Washington, DC 20024-2188; (800) 762-ACOG; www.acog.org

PROGNOSIS
- For nulliparous women with preeclampsia before 30 weeks of gestation, the recurrence rate for the disorder may be as high as 40% in future pregnancies (6).
- Multiparous women have higher rates of recurrence.
- 25% of eclamptic women will have HTN during subsequent pregnancies, but only 5% of these will be severe and only 2% will be eclamptic again.

- Eclamptic, multiparous women may be at higher risk for subsequent essential HTN; they also have higher mortality during subsequent pregnancies than do primiparous women.

COMPLICATIONS
- Most women do not have long-term sequelae from eclampsia, although many may have transient neurologic deficits.
- A history of preeclampsia is equivalent to traditional risk factors for cardiovascular disease. Women with a history of preeclampsia should be strongly advised to avoid obesity and smoking. Other signs of metabolic syndrome should be closely monitored as well (7).
- Maternal and/or fetal death

REFERENCES

1. Gauer R, Atlas M, Hill J. Clinical inquiries. Does low-dose aspirin reduce preeclampsia and other maternal-fetal complications? *J Fam Pract.* 2008;57:54–56.
2. Hofmeyr GJ, Duley L, Atallah A, et al. Dietary calcium supplementation for prevention of pre-eclampsia and related problems: A systematic review and commentary. *Br J Obstet Gynaecol.* 2007;114:933–943.
3. Rumbold A, Duley L, Crowther CA, et al. Antioxidants for preventing pre-eclampsia. *Cochrane Database Syst Rev.* 2008;CD004227.
4. Magee LA, Helewa M, Moutquin J-M, et al. Diagnosis, evaluation, and management of the hypertensive disorders of pregnancy. *JOGC.* 2008;30:3(S1–S48).
5. Sibai BM. Diagnosis and management of gestational hypertension and preeclampsia. *Obstet Gynecol.* 2003;102:181–192.
6. Report of the National High Blood Pressure Education Program Working Group on High Blood Pressure in Pregnancy. *Am J Obstet Gynecol* 2000;183:S1–S22.
7. Carty DM, Delles C, Dominiczak AF, et al. Preeclampsia and future maternal health. *J Hypertens.* 2010;28:1349–1355.

CODES

ICD10
- O14.10 Severe pre-eclampsia, unspecified trimester
- O14.90 Unspecified pre-eclampsia, unspecified trimester
- O15.9 Eclampsia, unspecified as to time period

CLINICAL PEARLS

- Consider prescribing 81 mg aspirin each day to 2 groups of pregnant women: Those who had severe preeclampsia in a prior pregnancy and those who develop signs of preeclampsia/strong risk factors for it before the 3rd trimester in their current pregnancy.
- Management of preeclampsia depends on both the severity of the condition and the gestational age of the fetus.
- The disorder is reversible by delivery if at term or, if maternal or fetal health are in danger, by preterm delivery.

PREMENSTRUAL SYNDROME AND PREMENSTRUAL DYSPHORIC DISORDER

Courtney I. Jarvis, PharmD • Jessica Dalby, MD

 BASICS

DESCRIPTION
- Premenstrual syndrome (PMS), a complex of physical and emotional symptoms sufficiently severe to interfere with everyday life, occurs cyclically during the luteal phase of menses.
- Premenstrual dysphoric disorder (PMDD) is a severe form of PMS characterized by severe recurrent depressive and anxiety symptoms, with premenstrual (luteal phase) onset, that remits a few days after the start of menses.
- PMDD is now included as a full diagnostic category in the fifth edition of the *Diagnostic and Statistical Manual of Mental Disorders* (*DSM-5*).
- System(s) affected: Endocrine/Metabolic; Nervous; Reproductive

EPIDEMIOLOGY
Prevalence
- Many women have some physical and psychic symptoms before menses (this is not premenstrual syndrome).
- 30% of menstruating women suffer from PMS; 3–8% of menstruating women have PMDD.

ETIOLOGY AND PATHOPHYSIOLOGY
Not well understood. Leading theories postulate metabolites of progesterone interact with central neurotransmitter receptors (serotonin and γ-aminobutyric acid [GABA]), provoking downstream effects of decreased GABA-mediated inhibition and decreased serotonin levels. Women with PMS/PMDD have similar levels of progesterone but seem to have an increased sensitivity to its metabolites, compared with women without PMS/PMDD (1).

Genetics
- Role of genetic predisposition is controversial; however, twin studies do suggest a genetic component.
- Involvement of gene coding for the serotonergic *5HT1A* receptor and allelic variants of the estrogen receptor-α gene (*ESR1*) is suggested.

RISK FACTORS
- Age: Usually present in late 20s to mid-30s
- History of mood disorder (major depression, bipolar disorder), anxiety disorder, personality disorder, or substance abuse
- Family history
- Low parity
- Tobacco use
- Psychosocial stressors/history of trauma
- High BMI

 DIAGNOSIS

HISTORY
DSM-5 criteria (2):
- Symptoms occur 1 week before menses, improve in the 1st few days after menses begin, and are minimal/absent in the week following menses (over most menstrual cycles during the past year).

- ≥5 of the following (1 must be among the first 4):
  - Marked depressed mood, feelings of hopelessness, or self-deprecating thoughts
  - Marked anxiety, tension, and/or feelings of being keyed up or on edge
  - Marked affective lability (mood swings)
  - Marked irritability or anger or increased interpersonal conflicts
  - Decreased interest in usual activities and social withdrawal
  - Lethargy, easy fatigability, or lack of energy
  - Appetite change, overeating, food cravings
  - Hypersomnia or insomnia
  - Feeling out of control or overwhelmed
  - Subjective difficulty concentrating
  - Physical symptoms, such as abdominal bloating, breast tenderness, headaches, weight gain, and joint/muscle pain
- For PMDD, emotional symptoms must be sufficiently severe to interfere with work, school, usual social activities, or relationships with others.
- Symptoms may be superimposed on an underlying psychiatric disorder but may not be an exacerbation of another condition, such as panic disorder/major depression.
- Criteria should be confirmed by prospective patient record of symptoms for a minimum of 2 consecutive menstrual cycles (without confirmation, "provisional" should be noted with diagnosis)
  - Use the Daily Record of Severity of Problems (available online at www.aafp.org/afp/2011/1015/p918-fig1.pdf) or similar inventory (3)[A].
- Symptoms should not be attributable to drug abuse, medications, or other medical conditions.

PHYSICAL EXAM
No specific physical exam required; may consider thyroid and pelvic exams if indicated by additional patient symptoms.

DIFFERENTIAL DIAGNOSIS
- Premenstrual exacerbation of underlying psychiatric disorder
- Psychiatric disorders (especially bipolar disorder, major depression, anxiety)
- Thyroid disorders
- Perimenopause
- Premenstrual migraine
- Chronic fatigue syndrome
- Irritable bowel syndrome (painful symptoms)
- Seizures
- Anemia
- Endometriosis (painful symptoms)
- Drug/Alcohol abuse

DIAGNOSTIC TESTS & INTERPRETATION
- The repetitive nature of symptoms precludes need for labs if a classic history is present.
- Consider:
  - Hemoglobin to rule out anemia
  - 25-OH vitamin D level to exclude deficiency, although precise relationship of deficiency with the disorder is unclear
  - Serum thyroid stimulating hormone (TSH) to rule out hypothyroidism
- Imaging with pelvic ultrasound to diagnose causes of pelvic pain and dysmenorrhea may be needed.

 TREATMENT

GENERAL MEASURES
Although evidence is lacking for aerobic exercise in treating PMS/PMDD, it is often recommended as part of an integrated care plan.

MEDICATION
First Line
- SSRIs show a small to moderate effect in the treatment of physical, functional, and behavioral symptoms of PMS and PMDD compared to placebo (4)[A]:
  - Both intermittent luteal phase dosing and continuous full-cycle dosing are effective(4)[A] with no clear evidence of difference between modes of administration.
  - All SSRIs tested appeared effective (4)[A].
  - SSRIs are effective at low doses. Higher doses have increased effect, but are accompanied by increased side effects (4)[A].
- Fluoxetine (Prozac, Sarafem) 20 mg/d every day or 20 mg/d only during luteal phase, or 90 mg once a week × 2 weeks in luteal phase
- Sertraline (Zoloft) 50–150 mg/d every day or 50–150 mg/d only during luteal phase
- Citalopram (Celexa) 10–30 mg/d every day or 10–30 mg/d only during luteal phase
- Adverse effects (number needed to harm [NNH] with moderate dose SSRI): nausea (NNH = 7), asthenia (NNH = 9), somnolence (NNH = 13), fatigue (NNH = 14), decreased libido (NNH = 14), and sweating (NNH = 14) (4)[A]
- Contraindications: Patients taking monoamine oxidase inhibitors (MAOIs)
- Precautions:
  - Increased risk of suicidal thinking and behavior in children and adolescents with depressive disorders; uncertain if this risk applies to those taking SSRIs for PMDD
  - Bipolar disorder
  - Seizure disorder
  - Hepatic dysfunction
  - Renal dysfunction
- Possible interactions:
  - MAOIs
  - Selegiline
  - Pimozide
  - Thioridazine

Second Line
Alternative therapies should be considered if no response to SSRIs:
- Spironolactone (Aldactone) 50–100 mg/d × 7–10 days during luteal phase; helpful for fluid retention. Adverse reactions: Lethargy, headache, irregular menses, hyperkalemia

- Oral contraceptive pills (OCPs):
  - OCPs can cause adverse effects similar to PMDD symptoms.
  - Extended-cycle use of OCPs (e.g., 12 weeks on and 1 week off) or a shorter placebo interval (e.g., 24 active pills with 4 placebo days [24/4] compared with 21/7 preparations) may be beneficial (5)[B].
  - OCPs containing the progestin drospirenone (structurally similar to spironolactone) may improve physical symptoms and mood changes associated with PMDD (6)[A]. Caution: Risk of venous thromboembolism may be modestly higher than with other OCPs.
  - Continuous administration of levonorgestrel/ethinyl estradiol may improve patient symptoms in PMDD (5)[B].
    - Suggested OCP formulations:
      - Ethinyl estradiol/drospirenone (Yasmin/Yaz/Beyaz/Safyral): 1 tablet/d
      - Levonorgestrel 90 μg/ethinyl estradiol 20 μg (Amethyst/Lybrel): 1 tablet/d
- Anxiolytics:
  - Alprazolam (Xanax) 0.25 mg t.i.d.–q.i.d. only during luteal phase; taper at onset of menses (other benzodiazepines not studied for PMDD). Caution: Addictive potential
  - Buspirone (BuSpar) 10–30 mg/d divided b.i.d.–t.i.d. in the luteal phase
- Ovulation inhibitors:
  - Gonadotropin-releasing hormone (GnRH) agonists: Leuprolide (Lupron) depot 3.75 mg/mo IM
    - Precautions: Menopause-like side effects (e.g., osteoporosis, hot flashes, headaches, muscle aches, vaginal dryness, irritability) limit treatment to 6 months; may be 1st step if considering bilateral oophorectomy for severe, refractory PMDD
  - Danazol (Danocrine) 300–400 mg b.i.d.; adverse reactions: Androgenic and antiestrogenic effects (e.g., amenorrhea, weight gain, acne, fluid retention, hirsutism, hot flashes, vaginal dryness, emotional lability)
  - Estrogen, transdermal preferred, 100–200 μg:
    - Precautions: Increased risk of blood clot, stroke, heart attack, and breast cancer
    - Requires concomitant progesterone add-back therapy to protect against uterine hyperplasia and endometrial cancer
- Progesterone: Insufficient evidence to support use (7)[A]

ISSUES FOR REFERRAL
Referral to psychiatrist may be indicated for mood/anxiety disorders if patient has no symptom-free period.

ADDITIONAL THERAPIES
Cognitive–behavioral therapy (CBT) is theoretically helpful for PMS/PMDD given its application for symptom reduction in other mood disorders, but direct evidence is lacking.

SURGERY/OTHER PROCEDURES
Bilateral oophorectomy, usually with concomitant hysterectomy, is an option for rare, refractory cases with severe, disabling symptoms.

COMPLEMENTARY AND ALTERNATIVE MEDICINE
- Acupuncture demonstrated superiority to progestins, anxiolytics, and sham acupuncture with no evidence of harm.

- Some data support the use of the following:
  - Calcium: 600 mg b.i.d.
  - Vitamin B_6: 50–100 mg/d
  - Chasteberry (*Vitex agnus-castus*): 4 mg/d of extract containing 6% of agnuside (or 20–40 mg/d of fruit extract)
  - Omega-3 fatty acids 2 g/d
- Data insufficient regarding the following:
  - Magnesium: 200–400 mg/d
  - Vitamin D: 2,000 IU/d
  - Vitamin E: 400 IU/d
  - Manganese: 1.8 mg/d
  - St. John's wort: 900 mg/d
  - Soy: 68 mg/d isoflavones
  - Ginkgo: 160–320 mg/d
  - Saffron: 30 mg/d
- Evidence supporting efficacy and/or safety of herbal products is lacking; the following products/interventions have *not* been found useful for PMS/PMDD, although not all studies are of high quality and able to eliminate possibility of benefit completely:
  - Evening primrose oil
  - Black current oil
  - Black cohosh
  - Wild yam root
  - Dong quai
  - Kava kava
  - Light-based therapy

 ONGOING CARE

FOLLOW-UP RECOMMENDATIONS
Patient Monitoring
Increased risk of suicidal thinking and behavior in children and adolescents with depressive disorders on initiation of SSRIs; uncertain if this risk applies to those taking SSRIs for PMDD

DIET
- Reduce consumption of salt, sugar, caffeine, dairy products, and alcohol (anecdotal reports)
- Eat small, frequent portions of food high in complex carbohydrates (limited data)

PATIENT EDUCATION
- Counsel patients to eat a balanced diet rich in calcium, vitamin D, and omega-3 fatty acids and low in saturated fat and caffeine.
- Counsel women that they are not "crazy." PMDD is a real disorder with a physiologic basis.
- Although incompletely understood, successful treatment is often possible.

PROGNOSIS
- Many patients can have their symptoms adequately controlled. PMS disappears at menopause.
- PMS can continue after hysterectomy, if ovaries are left in place.

REFERENCES
1. Rapkin AJ, Akopians AL. Pathophysiology of premenstrual syndrome and premenstrual dysphoric disorder. *Menopause Int*. 2012;18:52–59.
2. American Psychiatric Association. *Diagnostic and statistical manual of mental disorders*, 5th ed. Washington, DC: American Psychiatric Association; 2013.
3. Borenstein JE, Dean BB, Yonkers KA, et al. Using the daily record of severity of problems as a screening instrument for premenstrual syndrome. *Obstet Gynecol*. 2007;109:1068–1075.
4. Marjoribanks J, Brown J, O'Brien PMS, et al. Selective serotonin reuptake inhibitors for premenstrual syndrome. *Cochrane Database Syst Rev*. 2013;6:CD001396.
5. Freeman EW, Halbreich U, Grubb GS, et al. An overview of four studies of a continuous oral contraceptive (levonorgestrel 90 mcg/ethinyl estradiol 20 mcg) on premenstrual dysphoric disorder and premenstrual syndrome. *Contraception*. 2012;85:437–445.
6. Lopez LM, Kaptein A, Helmerhorst FM. Oral contraceptives containing drospirenone for premenstrual syndrome. *Cochrane Database Syst Rev*. 2012;2:CD006586.
7. Ford O, Lethaby A, Roberts H, et al. Progesterone for premenstrual syndrome. *Cochrane Database Syst Rev*. 2012;3:CD003415.

ADDITIONAL READING
- Biggs WS, Demuth RH. Premenstrual syndrome and premenstrual dysphoric disorder. *Am Fam Physician*. 2011;84:918–924.
- Cunningham J, Yonkers KA, O'Brien S, et al. Update on research and treatment of premenstrual dysphoric disorder. *Harv Rev Psychiatry*. 2009;17:120–137.
- Freeman EW. Therapeutic management of premenstrual syndrome. *Expert Opin Pharmacother*. 2010;11:2879–2889.
- Kim SY, Park HJ, Lee H, et al. Acupuncture for premenstrual syndrome: A systematic review and meta-analysis of randomised controlled trials. *BJOG*. 2011;118:899–915.
- Whelan AM, Jurgens TM, Naylor H, et al. Herbs, vitamins and minerals in the treatment of premenstrual syndrome: A systematic review. *Can J Clin Pharmacol*. 2009;16:e407–e429.

 CODES

ICD10
N94.3 Premenstrual tension syndrome

CLINICAL PEARLS
- Have the patient keep a daily log of her symptoms and menses. Symptoms beginning in the week before menses and abating before the end of menses, occurring over at least 2 months, and sufficiently severe to interfere with daily functioning are diagnostic of PMS.
- The difference between PMS and PMDD is that PMDD is a severe form of PMS characterized by recurrent depressive and anxiety symptoms with luteal phase onset, sufficiently severe to disrupt social and occupational functioning. These symptoms remit a few days after the onset of menses.
- PMDD is not the same as more generalized depressive/anxiety disorders. PMDD-associated symptoms of depression and anxiety begin to resolve within the 1st few days of menses.
- Luteal phase treatment only is likely as effective as continuous-cycle treatment with SSRIs, but has fewer adverse effects.

PRENATAL CARE AND TESTING
Fozia Ali, MD • Teny Philip, MD

BASICS

- The goal of prenatal care is to ensure the birth of a healthy baby with minimal risk for the mother by:
  - Identifying the patient who is at risk for complications
  - Estimating the gestational age (GA) as accurately as possible
  - Evaluating the health status of mother and fetus
  - Encouraging and empowering the patient to do her part to care for herself and her baby-to-be
  - Intervening when fetal abnormalities are present to prevent morbidity

GENERAL PREVENTION
- A recommended prenatal care schedule consists of:
  - Monthly visits to a health care professional for weeks 4–28 of pregnancy
  - Visits twice monthly from 28–36 weeks
  - Weekly after week 36 (delivery at week 38–40)
- Recommendations for use of dietary supplements in pregnancy:
  - Folic acid supplementation (0.4–0.8 mg) prior to conception; 4 mg for secondary prevention
  - Calcium: 1,000–1,300 mg/d; supplement may be beneficial for women with high risk for gestational hypertension or communities with low dietary calcium intake.
  - Iron: Screen for anemia (Hgb/Hct) and treat if necessary. Recommend 30 mg/d of iron in pregnant women.
  - Vitamin A: Pregnant women in industrialized countries should limit to <5,000 IU/day.
  - Vitamin D: Consider supplementation in women with limited exposure to sunlight.
- Routine thyroid screening and vitamin D deficiency during pregnancy is not recommended.

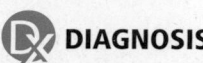

DIAGNOSIS

HISTORY
At the initial visit, a complete medical, obstetrical, family, and psychosocial history should be obtained and updated throughout the pregnancy.

- Assess and counsel as appropriate regarding:
  - Lifestyle, nutrition, safety of medications (teratogenicity, category), tobacco, alcohol, and drug use, toxins, relationship issues/domestic violence, stressors/supports, work environment, risk factors
- Domestic violence:
  - ACOG guidelines recommend that physicians screen *all* pregnant patients for intimate partner domestic violence (1):
    - At the 1st prenatal visit
    - At least once per trimester
    - At the postpartum checkup

PHYSICAL EXAM
- A full physical exam should be performed at the 1st prenatal appointment.
- At each subsequent prenatal visit, the following should be recorded:
  - Weight: Total weight gain range (lbs) should be 25–35 lb, except in obese women, for whom weight gain should be <15 lb.
  - BP:
    - ACOG defines hypertension as BP >140 mm Hg systolic or >90 mm Hg diastolic (2)

- Monitor BP especially closely in patients with chronic hypertension (predating pregnancy), pre-eclampsia/eclampsia, or gestational hypertension
  - UA for glucose and protein; 24-hour protein excretion is the gold standard but not practical
  - Fundal height
  - Fetal heart rate: Usually audible by 12 weeks' GA with a Doppler instrument
  - Routine fetal movement counts *not* recommended
  - Fetal position by abdominal palpation at 36 weeks
  - Pelvic/cervical exam if indicated

DIAGNOSTIC TESTS & INTERPRETATION
Cervical cancer screening:

- A Pap smear should be obtained when indicated by standard Pap screening guidelines, regardless of gestation (ACOG, USPSTF, ASCCP, ACS, and ASCP Guidelines state that women <21 should not be screened regardless of age of sexual initiation or other risk factors).
- Squamous intraepithelial lesions can progress during pregnancy, but often regress postpartum.
- Colposcopy only to exclude the presence of invasive cancer in high-risk women (3)
- Cervical biopsy should be avoided unless a malignancy is suspected. Endocervical sampling is contraindicated (3).
- 1st prenatal visit:
  - Lab tests:
    - Hematocrit or hemoglobin
    - Blood type: A, B, AB, or O
    - Rhesus type and antibody screen: Rh(+) or Rh(−)
    - Hemoglobin electrophoresis for patients at risk for sickle cell disease or thalassemia
    - Urine testing for glucose and protein
    - Urine culture
    - Rubella titer
    - Syphilis test
    - Gonorrhea/*Chlamydia* screening
    - Hepatitis B surface antigen
    - HIV testing (patient may "opt out" if chooses to decline)
    - Routine screening for bacterial vaginosis, toxoplasmosis, CMV, and parvovirus not recommended
    - Cystic fibrosis screening (information should be made available to all couples):
      - Cystic fibrosis carrier screening should be offered before conception or early in pregnancy when 1 partner is of Caucasian, European, or Ashkenazi Jewish descent (4).
      - It is reasonable to offer cystic fibrosis carrier screening to all couples regardless of race or ethnicity as an alternative to selective testing.
- Screening tests (for birth defects), noninvasive (5):
  - U/S nuchal translucency (NT): Measures thickness at the back of the neck of the fetus
  - Blood screens: Human chorionic gonadotropin (hCG), pregnancy-associated plasma protein A (PAPP-A), quad screen: α-Fetoprotein (AFP), unconjugated estriol (UE3), hCG, inhibin-A (INH-A)
  - Currently, cell-free fetal nucleic acids assays are also commercially available for screening purposes. This enables fetal sex determination as early as 7 weeks of gestation, which is especially useful as initial step in X-linked diseases. The assay also allows screening for aneuploidy, rhesus typing in Rh(D) negative women, and single-gene

disorders (limited to detection of paternally inherited mutation). Because of a small but real risk for false-positive results, most experts advise using these assays as screening tests and confirming positive result with invasive prenatal diagnostics.
  - 1st-trimester screening between 11 and 14 weeks GA using both NT and hCG/PAPP-A blood testing is an effective protocol in the general population and is more effective than NT alone, with an 83% detection rate for Down syndrome, with false-positive rate of 5%. Detects trisomy 21 (Down syndrome) and trisomy 18 (Edward syndrome). May be performed either as a single combined stand-alone test (U/S NT + blood [HCG and PAPP-A]) or as part of a sequential "step-by-step" 1st- and 2nd-trimester screening process (see below).
  - 2nd-trimester screening protocols:
    - Obtain "multiple marker"/quad screen between 15 and 21 weeks' GA, optimally between 16 and 18 weeks; ~84% detection rate for trisomy 21, trisomy 18, and neural tube defects (NTDs), with false-positive rate of 5%, *or*
    - 2-step integrated screening protocol: Combines information collected during the 1st and 2nd trimesters of the pregnancy to determine the risk of Down syndrome, trisomy 18, or open NTD:
      - 2 options: Step-wise sequential integrated screen (~91% detection rate with false-positive rate 3.3%):
        - 1st trimester: NT measurement, plus blood (hCG, PAPP-A):
          - If calculated risk for Down syndrome is ≥1:30, then additional steps are recommended (genetic counseling, U/S, and chorionic villi sampling [CVS])
          - If calculated risk for Down syndrome is <1:30 *then*
          - 2nd trimester quad screen (AFP, UE3, hCG, INH-A) is required, *or*
      - Serum integrated screen: 88% detection rate with false-positive rate of 4.5%; requires a 1st-trimester PAPP-A blood test without NT measurement, *and* a 2nd-trimester (16–18 week quad screen)
- Diagnostic tests (for birth defects), invasive:
  - ACOG guidelines: All pregnant women, not just women ≥35, should be offered invasive prenatal diagnostic testing, such as CVS and amniocentesis to detect possible genetic abnormalities in their fetuses (6).
  - Women found to be at increased risk of having a baby with Down syndrome with 1st-trimester screening should be offered genetic counseling and the option of CVS or mid-trimester amniocentesis. If screening tests show increased risk of birth defect, there are 2 possible diagnostic tests:
    - CVS: 1st trimester: Usually done after 10 weeks (10–12 weeks). Small sample of the placenta; chorionic tissue sample obtained either transcervical (TC) or transabdominal (TA). Complication: Pregnancy loss rate of 1.0–1.5%.
    - Amniocentesis:
      - 1st trimester: Usually at 11–13 weeks, but higher rate of pregnancy loss and complication than either CVS or early 2nd-trimester procedures; therefore, not recommended.

- 2nd trimester: Usually done after 15 weeks (15–18 weeks). The prenatal diagnostic technique associated with the lowest risk of pregnancy loss. Small sample of amniotic fluid from the amniotic sac surrounding the developing fetus is obtained by an US-guided TA approach. Complication: Pregnancy loss rate of ≤0.5%.
- 24–28 weeks:
  - Obtain diabetes screen (see below), repeat hematocrit or hemoglobin, and repeat antibody screen in Rh-negative mother prior to receiving prophylactic Rh immunoglobulin:
    - Gestational diabetes mellitus (GDM) screening: Universal recommendation for ideal approach for screening and diagnosis of GDM remains elusive. In 2010, the International Association of Diabetes and Pregnancy Study Group, proposed a new system in which diabetes in pregnancy is classified as overt vs. gestational diabetes. The American Diabetes Association reaffirmed this in 2010 and 2013. Presently, this system is not endorsed by ACOG because there is no evidence that 1-step screening using this criteria leads to clinically significant improvements in maternal and fetal outcomes but would lead to significant increase in health care costs.
    - Overt diabetes (test when women first present for prenatal care): Fasting blood sugar ≥126 mg/dL or A1c ≥6.5%, or random ≥200 mg/dL that is confirmed with subsequent fasting blood sugar or A1c. (These thresholds were chosen due to correlation with adverse vascular events, e.g., retinopathy and CAD).
    - Gestational diabetes: Fasting plasma glucose >92 mg/dL but is <126 mg/dL at any gestational age. At 24–28 weeks of gestation, a 75 g 2-hour oral glucose tolerance test with at least 1 abnormal result: FBG ≥92 mg/dL, but <126 mg/dL, or 1-hour ≥180 mg/dL, or 2-hour ≥153 mg/dL.
    - The prevalence of gestational diabetes in the US can be 2–25%, greater in African Americans, Hispanics, Native Americans, and Asians than in Caucasians. Using the IADPSG criteria for overt vs. gestational diabetes, ~18% of women would be diagnosed with diabetes during pregnancy.
    - The following guidelines for GDM are established by ACOG:
      - Specified cutoffs define GDM:
        - A value of >130 mg/dL will identify 90% of women with GDM, but 20–25% of all women screened will need to continue to the 3-hour oral glucose tolerance test (OGTT) (1,2).
        - Raising the value to >140 mg/dL will identify only 80% of women with GDM but decrease to 14–18% the number of women who will need to continue to the 3-hour OGTT (7).
      - Screening test: 1-hour OGTT (nonfasting):
        - 50 g PO glucose load with blood glucose testing 1 hour later
        - Carpenter and Coustan positive screen: >130 mg/dL
        - National Diabetes Data Group (NDDG) positive screen: >140 mg/dL
      - Diagnostic test: 3-hour OGTT (fasting):
        - If abnormal 1-hour OGTT screening test, may be followed by a 3-hour OGTT
        - 100 g PO glucose load with blood drawn: Fasting, 1, 2, and 3 hours after ingestion of glucose

- Either the plasma or serum glucose level designated by Carpenter and Coustan or by the NDDG are appropriate to use:
  - *A positive diagnosis of GDM requires that ≥2 thresholds be exceeded (8).
    - Carpenter and Coustan standard:
      - *>95 (fasting), >180 (1-hour), >155 (2-hour), >140 (3-hour)
    - National Diabetes Data Group standard:
      - *>105 (fasting), >190 (1-hour), >165 (2-hour), >145 (3-hour)
- 35–37 weeks:
  - Group B streptococcus (GBS) culture: Universal screening for GBS colonization at 35–37 weeks of gestation remains the sole strategy for intrapartum antibiotic prophylaxis (9).
  - High-risk patients: High-risk patients should be screened again for *Gonorrhea, Chlamydia*, HIV, and syphilis.
- Post-term pregnancy:
  - Rate of stillbirth increases with gestational age, 1/3,000 per week at 37 weeks, 3/3,000 per week at 42 weeks, 6/3,000 at 43 weeks. In 1 meta-analysis, routine induction of labor at 41 weeks' gestation reduced rates of perinatal death without increased rates of cesarean delivery (10).
  - For gestational periods beyond 42 weeks, fetal well-being should be assessed with nonstress testing and US assessment of amniotic fluid volume.

 TREATMENT

ISSUES FOR REFERRAL
Abnormal screening labs or imaging may prompt referral to maternal-fetal medicine specialist or other medical specialist, as indicated.

 ONGOING CARE

PATIENT EDUCATION
- Education:
  - Immunizations during pregnancy: The following vaccines are considered safe per CDC: Tdap (recommended for all women in 3rd trimester to increase passive antibody transfer of pertussis antibody to fetus), Hep B, influenza; possibly include meningococcal, rabies. Contraindicated during pregnancy or safety not established: BCG, MMR, varicella.
  - Patients should be made aware of the tests that are performed routinely, as well as other tests that might be elected (e.g., CVS or amniocentesis), as well as the choices that would be available if testing were abnormal (pregnancy termination, preparation for the birth of an infant with congenital anomalies, further testing).
- Prevention:
  - Preconception counseling offers the opportunity to discuss individualized risks.
  - To decrease the risks of NTDs, preconception folate supplementation is indicated.
- Recommendations:
  - Airline travel: Generally safe until up to 4 weeks from EDD. Lengthy trips associated with increased risk of thrombosis.
  - Caffeine: Limit to <200 mg/day. Correlation between IUGR and miscarriage with caffeine is undetermined at this time.

- Exercise: Healthy women with uncomplicated pregnancies should continue to exercise.
- Seat belts/Air bags: ACOG recommends that pregnant women wear lap and shoulder seatbelts and should not turn off air bags.
- Sexual activity: Intercourse is not associated with adverse outcomes.
- Alcohol, cigarettes, and illicit drugs are injurious to fetal and maternal health.
- Pregnancy-safe medications (teratogenicity)

REFERENCES

1. ACOG Screening Tools-Domestic Violence. Accessed August 7, 2012, at www.acog.org/ ACOG_Departments/Violence_Against_Women/ Screening_Tools Domestic Violence.
2. Committee on Obstetric Practice. Committee Opinion No. 514: Emergent therapy for acute-onset, severe hypertension with preeclampsia or eclampsia. *Obstet Gynecol*. 2011;118(6):1465–1468.
3. Fleury AC, Birsner ML, Fader AN, et al. Management of the abnormal Papanicolaou smear and colposcopy in pregnancy: An evidence-based review. *Minerva Ginecol*. 2012;64(2):137–148.
4. American College of Obstetricians and Gynecologists Committee on Genetics. ACOG Committee Opinion No. 486: Update on carrier screening for cystic fibrosis. *Obstet Gynecol*. 2011;117(4):1028–1031.
5. Summers AM, Langlois S, Wyatt P, et al. Prenatal screening for fetal aneuploidy. *J Obstet Gynaecol Can*. 2007;29(2):146–179.
6. American College of Obstetricians and Gynecologists. ACOG Practice Bulletin No. 88, December 2007. Invasive prenatal testing for aneuploidy. *Obstet Gynecol*. 2007;110(6):1459–1467.
7. Berger H, Crane J, Farine D, et al. Screening for gestational diabetes mellitus. *J Obstet Gynaecol Can*. 2002;24(11):894–912.
8. Committee Opinion No. 504: Screening and diagnosis of gestational diabetes mellitus. *Obstet Gynecol*. 2011;118(3):751–753.
9. 2010 Guidelines for the Prevention of Perinatal Group B Streptococcal (GBS) Disease. Accessed July 14, 2012, at www.cdc.gov/groupbstrep/ guidelines/new-differences.html.
10. Crowley P. Interventions for preventing or improving the outcome of delivery at or beyond term. *Cochrane Database Syst Rev*. 2004;(4):CD000170.

 CODES

ICD10
- Z34.00 Encntr for suprvsn of normal first pregnancy, unsp trimester
- Z34.90 Encntr for suprvsn of normal pregnancy, unsp, unsp trimester
- Z36 Encounter for antenatal screening of mother

CLINICAL PEARLS
Prenatal care and screening are best accomplished using standardized flowsheets and checklists to ensure that the complex sequence of evaluations and education is performed consistently and properly.

Drew Grimes, MD • Stacy Jones, MD

BASICS

DESCRIPTION
- Preoperative medical evaluation should determine the presence of established or unrecognized disease or other factors that may increase the risk of perioperative morbidity and mortality in patients undergoing surgery.
- Specific assessment goals include:
  - Conducting a thorough medical history and physical exam to assess the need for further testing and/or consultation
  - Recommending strategies to reduce risk and optimize patient condition prior to surgery
  - Encouraging patients to optimize their health for possible improvement of both perioperative and long-term outcomes
- Synonym(s): Preoperative diagnostic workup; Preoperative preparation; Preoperative general health assessment

EPIDEMIOLOGY
Overall patient morbidity and mortality related to surgery is low. One large study of inpatients looking at 30-day mortality in the US showed a rate of 1.32% (1). This rate varies by type of procedure and varies by country (2). Preoperative patient evaluation and subsequent optimization of perioperative care can reduce both postoperative morbidity and mortality.

RISK FACTORS
- Functional capacity (3): Exercise tolerance is one of the most important determinants of cardiac risk:
  - Self-reported exercise tolerance may be an extremely useful predictive tool when assessing risk. Patients unable to meet a 4 metabolic equivalent (MET) demand (defined in the Diagnosis section) during daily activities have increased perioperative cardiac and long-term risks.
  - Patients who report good exercise tolerance require minimal, if any, additional testing.
- Levels of surgical risk:
  - High: Aortic, major vascular, and peripheral vascular surgery
  - Intermediate: Intraperitoneal, intrathoracic, carotid endarterectomy, head/neck, orthopedic, and prostate surgery
  - Low: Endoscopic, superficial, cataract, breast, and ambulatory surgery
- Clinical risk factors (3): History of ischemic heart disease, the presence of compensated heart failure or a history of prior congestive heart failure (CHF), cerebrovascular disease, diabetes mellitus (DM), and renal insufficiency; these risk factors plus surgical risk can dictate the need for further cardiac testing.
- Age: Patients >70 are at higher risk for perioperative complications and mortality and have a longer length of stay in the hospital postoperatively. (Likely attributed to increasing medical comorbidities with increasing age.) Age alone should not be a deciding factor in the decision to proceed or not proceed with surgery (4).

DIAGNOSIS

HISTORY
- Evaluate pertinent medical records and interview the patient. Many institutions provide standard patient questionnaires that screen for preoperative risk factors:
  - History of present illness and treatments
  - Past medical and surgical history
  - Patient and family anesthetic history and associated complications
  - Current medications (including over-the-counter [OTC] medications, vitamins, supplements, and herbals) as well as reasons for use
  - Allergies (including specific reactions)
  - Social history: Tobacco, alcohol, drug use, and cessation
  - Family history: Prior illnesses and surgeries
- Systems (both history and current status):
  - Cardiovascular: Inquire about exercise capacity:
    - 1 MET: Can take care of self, eat, dress, and use toilet; walk around house indoors; walk a block or 2 on level ground at 2–3 miles/hr
    - 4 METs: Can climb flight of stairs or walk up hill, walk on level ground at 4 miles/hr, run a short distance, do heavy work around house, participate in moderate recreational activities
    - 10 METs: Can participate in strenuous sports such as swimming, singles tennis, football, basketball, or skiing
  - Note presence of CHF, cardiomyopathy, ischemic heart disease (stable vs. unstable), valvular disease, hypertension (HTN), arrhythmias, murmurs, pericarditis, history of pacemaker or implantable cardioverter defibrillator (ICD):
    - Rhythm management devices (pacemakers and automatic ICDs [AICD]) affect the perioperative course. Most importantly, the following information need to be available for proper management: Name of cardiologist who manages the device, type of device, manufacturer, last interrogation, and any problems that have occurred recently. Based on this information and the location and type of surgery, a perioperative plan of management will be made (5).
    - Stents: Patients with coronary stents are maintained on antiplatelet therapy with a thienopyridine, such as clopidogrel, frequently in combination with aspirin. Premature discontinuation of antiplatelet therapy markedly increases the risk of acute stent thrombosis, the results of which can be catastrophic. Elective surgery should be delayed and antiplatelet therapy continued for 4–6 weeks after bare metal stent placement, and for at least 12 months after placement of drug-eluting stents. Even after this time period, any perioperative disruption in the patient's antiplatelet regimen should be discussed with the patient's cardiologist and surgeon. The risk of perioperative bleeding must be weighed against the risks associated with discontinuation of antiplatelet drugs prior to surgery.

- Pulmonary: Chronic and active disease processes should be addressed: Chronic infections, bronchitis, emphysema, asthma, wheezing, shortness of breath, cough (productive or otherwise):
  - Sleep apnea: Patients with obstructive sleep apnea (OSA) are at increased risk for perioperative adverse events. Because of the high incidence of undiagnosed sleep apnea in perioperative patients, many authors are recommending screening questionnaires such as the Berlin or STOP-BANG (6,7). The American Society of Anesthesiologists (ASA) has practice guidelines based on expert review that takes into account the severity of sleep apnea, the invasiveness of surgery, and the projected need for postoperative opioids (8).
  - Patients with OSA frequently are at increased risk for obesity, coronary disease, HTN, atrial fibrillation, CHF, and pulmonary hypertension. Optimizing the management of these comorbidities may be the 1st important step in the preoperative management of patients with OSA. Often, patients with an existing diagnosis of OSA who use continuous positive airway pressure (CPAP) at night are asked to bring their CPAP machine to the hospital or surgery center when they are admitted for surgery.
- GI: Hepatic disease, gastric ulcer, inflammatory bowel disease, hernias (especially hiatal), significant weight loss, nausea, vomiting, history of postoperative nausea and vomiting: Any symptoms consistent with gastroesophageal reflux disease (GERD) should be optimally treated.
- Hematologic: Anemia, serious bleeding, clotting problems, blood transfusions, hereditary disorders
- Renal: Kidney failure, dialysis, infections, stones, changes in bladder function
- Endocrine: Nocturia, parathyroid, pituitary, adrenal disease, thyroid disease
  - Diabetes: Evidence that hyperglycemia in the perioperative period is associated with increased perioperative complications. Although recommendations vary, most experts recommend keeping perioperative blood glucose levels <180.
- Neurologic/Psychiatric: Seizures, stroke, paralysis, tremor, migraine headaches, nerve injury, multiple sclerosis, extremity numbness, psychiatric disorders (e.g., anxiety, depression)
- Musculoskeletal: Arthritis, lower back pain
- Reproductive: Possibility of pregnancy in women of child-bearing potential
- Mouth/Upper airway: Dentures, crowns, partials, bridges, teeth (loose, chipped, cracked, capped)

PHYSICAL EXAM
- Assess vital signs, including arterial BP bilaterally.
- Check carotid pulses; auscultate for bruits.
- Examine lungs by auscultating all lung fields, listening for rales, rhonchi, wheezes, or other sounds indicating disease.
- Examine cardiovascular system by auscultating heart and noting any irregular rhythms or murmurs; precordial palpation.
- Palpate abdomen.
- Examine airway and mouth for ease of intubation, neck mobility, and size of tongue; note any lesions or dental deformities.

- If a regional anesthesia technique is being contemplated, perform a relevant, focused neurologic exam.

DIAGNOSTIC TESTS & INTERPRETATION
Initial Tests (lab, imaging)

- Laboratory testing should not be obtained routinely prior to surgery unless indicated (9)[C]. Specific tests should be requested if the evaluator suspects findings from the clinical evaluation that may influence perioperative patient management.
- Labs performed within the past 4 months prior to evaluation are reliable unless the patient has had an interim change in clinical presentation or is taking medications that require monitoring of plasma level or effect.
- CBC (9)[C]:
  - Hemoglobin: If patient has symptoms of anemia or is undergoing a procedure with major blood loss; extremes of age; liver or kidney disease
  - WBC count: If symptoms suggest infection or myeloproliferative disorder or the patient is at risk for chemotherapy-induced leukopenia
  - Platelet count: If history of bleeding, myeloproliferative disorder, liver or renal disease, or the patient is at risk for chemotherapy-induced thrombocytopenia
- Serum chemistries (electrolytes, glucose, renal and liver function tests): Should be obtained for extremes of age; in known renal insufficiency, CHF, liver dysfunction, or endocrine abnormalities, or the patient is on medications that alter electrolyte levels, such as diuretics
- PT/PTT: If history of a bleeding disorder, chronic liver disease, or malnutrition, or those with recent or chronic antibiotic or anticoagulant use
- Urinalysis (9)[C]: Routine urinalysis is not recommended preoperatively.
- Pregnancy test: Controversial; should be *considered* for all female patients of child-bearing age
- CXR is not generally indicated. It can be considered in patients with recent upper respiratory tract infection and in those with suspected cardiac or pulmonary disease (because there is a likelihood for unanticipated findings), but these indications are not considered unequivocal.

Diagnostic Procedures/Other

- ECG (9)[C]:
  - Evidence indicates that the incidence of ECG abnormalities may be higher in older patients and in patients with multiple cardiac risk factors. In these instances, a preoperative ECG may be warranted. Age alone, however, is not necessarily an indication for a preoperative ECG.
  - ECGs are not indicated for asymptomatic patients undergoing low-risk procedures (3).
- Further cardiac testing should be considered in patients with poor or unknown functional capacity and 3+ clinical risk factors if the surgery is high risk and testing will change management (e.g., dipyridamole-thallium scan).
- PFTs: Definitive data regarding the efficacy of preoperative testing are lacking. The most important factor is preoperative optimization of patients with chronic obstructive pulmonary disease (COPD) or reactive airways disease with indicated use of antibiotics, bronchodilators, and inhaled corticosteroids. Spirometry can help guide therapy. Upper abdominal and thoracic surgery have a higher risk of postoperative pulmonary complications.

TREATMENT
MEDICATION

- Reducing cardiac risk:
  - Elective surgery should be delayed or canceled if the patient has any of the following: Unstable coronary syndromes (unstable or severe angina), recent myocardial infarction (MI) (<30 days), decompensated heart failure, significant arrhythmias, or severe valvular disease.
  - Active CHF should be treated with diuretics, afterload reduction, and β-adrenergic blockers.
  - Perioperative β-blockade has been shown to reduce mortality and the incidence of perioperative MIs in high-risk patients. Studies conflict, however, in which patients need to be treated, the dosage and timing of treatment, and for what surgeries. *Patients chronically on β-blockers should have the medication continued in the perioperative period.* When β-blockers are discontinued in the perioperative period, 30-day mortality increases. β-blockers are reasonable for vascular surgery patients with at least 1 clinical risk factor (3)[C].
  - Perioperative statin use may have a protective effect on reducing cardiac complications. Currently, the American Heart Association (AHA) has a class I indication for perioperative statin therapy for patients already on statins prior to their surgery. There is also evidence that vascular surgery patients benefit from perioperative statins.
- Reducing pulmonary risk:
  - Recommend cigarette cessation for at least 8 weeks prior to elective surgery.
  - Patients with asthma should not be wheezing and should have a peak flow of at least 80% of their predicted or personal-best value.
  - Treatment of COPD and asthma should focus on maximally reducing airflow obstruction and is identical to treatment of nonsurgical patients.
  - Lower respiratory tract infections (bacterial) should be treated with appropriate antibiotic therapy.

REFERENCES

1. Semel ME, Lipsitz SR, Funk LM, et al. Rates and patterns of death after surgery in the United States, 1996 and 2006. *Surgery.* 2012;151(20):171–182.
2. Pearse RM, Moreno RP, Bauer P, et al. Mortality after surgery in Europe: A 7-day cohort study. *Lancet.* 2012;380 (9847):1059–1065.
3. American College of Cardiology Foundation/American Heart Association Task Force on Practice Guidelines, American Society of Echocardiography, American Society of Nuclear Cardiology, et al. 2009 ACCF/AHA focused update on perioperative beta blockade. *J Am Coll Cardiol.* 2009;54:2102–2128.
4. Carrillo PM, González A. Escoboza R, et al. Perioperative risk evaluation. *Internet J Anesthesiol.* 2003;8(2).
5. American Society of Anesthesiologists. Practice advisory for the perioperative management of patients with cardiac implantable electronic devices: Pacemakers and implantable cardioverter-defibrillators: An updated report by the American Society of Anesthesiologists Task Force on Perioperative Management of Patients with Cardiac Implantable Electronic Devices. *Anesthesiology.* 2011;114(2):247–261.
6. Adesanya AO, Lee W, Greilich NB, et al. Perioperative management of obstructive sleep apnea. *Chest.* 2010;138(6):1489–1498.
7. Chung SA, Yuan H, Chung F. A systematic review of obstructive sleep apnea and its implications for anesthesiologists. *Anesth Analg.* 2008;107(5):1543.
8. Gross JB, Bachenberg KL, Benumof JL, et al. Practice guidelines for the perioperative management of patients with obstructive sleep apnea: A report by the American Society of Anesthesiologists Task Force on Perioperative Management of Patients with Obstructive Sleep Apnea. *Anesthesiology.* 2006;104(5):1081–1093; quiz 1117–1118.
9. Committee on Standards and Practice Parameters, Apfelbaum JL, Connis RT, et al. Practice advisory for preanesthesia evaluation: An updated report by the American Society of Anesthesiologists Task Force on Preanesthesia Evaluation. *Anesthesiology.* 2012;116(3):522–538.

ADDITIONAL READING

- Akhtar S, Barash PG, Inzucchi SE, et al. Scientific principles and clinical implications of perioperative glucose regulation and control. *Anesth Analg.* 2010;110:478–497.
- Chung F, Subramanyam R, Liao P, et al. High STOP-Bang score indicates a high probability of obstructive sleep apnoea. *Br J Anaesth.* 2012;108(5):768–775. Epub 2012 Mar 8.
- Lander JS, Coplan NL. Statin therapy in the perioperative period. *Rev Cardiovasc Med.* 2011;12(1):30–37.

SEE ALSO

Algorithm: Preoperative Evaluation of the Noncardiac Surgical Patient

CODES

ICD10
- Z01.811 Encounter for preprocedural respiratory examination
- Z01.812 Encounter for preprocedural laboratory examination
- Z01.818 Encounter for other preprocedural examination

CLINICAL PEARLS

- The preoperative evaluation should include medical record evaluation, patient interview, and physical exam.
- The minimum for the physical exam includes airway, pulmonary, and cardiovascular exams.
- Functional capacity, the level of surgical risk, and clinical risk factors determine if further cardiac testing is needed.
- No preoperative tests are routine.
- Active cardiac conditions should lead to delay or cancellation of nonemergent surgery.

PRESBYCUSIS

Brian Ho, MD • Michael Groves, MD, FACS

BASICS

DESCRIPTION
- Age-related, bilateral sensorineural hearing loss (SNHL)
- Represents a lifetime of insults to the auditory system from toxic noise exposure and natural decline
- Initially presents as high-frequency SNHL
- Impacts the "clarity" of sounds (i.e., ability to detect, identify, and localize sounds)
- Due to mild and progressive nature, presbycusis is often treated with amplification alone
- Can lead to adverse effects on physical, cognitive, emotional, behavioral, and social function in the elderly (e.g., depression, social isolation)

EPIDEMIOLOGY
Incidence
According to recent community-based epidemiological study, the 5-year incidence of HL (1):
- Age 48–59: M (19.1%), F (7%); all (11.6%)
- Age 60–69: M (35%), F (18.1%); all (23.1%)
- Age 70–79: M (59.1%), F (45.2%); all (4%)
- Age 80–92: M (100%), F (94.7%); all (95.5%)

Prevalence
- 10% of the population develops SNHL severe enough to impair communication
- Increases to 40% in the population >65 years of age
- 80% of HL cases occur in elderly patients
- Only 10–20% of older adults with HL have ever used hearing aids (HAs)
- Predominant sex: Male > Female
- Hearing levels are poorer in industrialized societies than in isolated or agrarian societies.

ETIOLOGY AND PATHOPHYSIOLOGY
- The external ear transmits sound energy to the tympanic membrane. The middle ear ossicles amplify and conduct the sound waves into the inner ear (cochlea) via the oval window. The organ of Corti, located in the cochlea, contains hair cells that detect these vibrations and depolarize, producing electrical signals that travel through the auditory nerve to the brain. Toxic noise exposure traumatizes the hair cells and leads to cell death and hearing loss.
  - Sensory presbycusis: Primary loss of the hair cells in the basal end of the cochlea (high frequency loss)
  - Neural presbycusis: Loss of spiral ganglion cells (nerve cells induced by hair cells to produce action potentials to travel to the brainstem)
  - Strial (metabolic) presbycusis: Atrophy of the stria vascularis (the cochlear tissue that generates the endocochlear electrical potential)
  - Cochlear conductive (mechanical) presbycusis: No morphologic findings (presumed stiffening of the basilar membrane)
  - Mixed presbycusis: Combinations of hair cell, ganglion cell, and stria vascularis loss
  - Indeterminate presbycusis: No morphologic findings (presumed impaired cellular function)
- Presbycusis is caused by the accumulated effects of noise exposure, systemic disease, ototoxic drugs, and genetic susceptibility.

Genetics
Presbycusis has a familial aggregation (2):
- Heritability estimates show 35–55% of the variance of sensory presbycusis is from genetic factors; even greater percentage in strial presbycusis.
- Heritability is stronger among women than men.

RISK FACTORS
- Noise exposure
- Ototoxic substances:
  - Organic solvents
  - Heavy metals
  - Carbon monoxide
- Drugs:
  - Aminoglycosides
  - Cisplatin
  - Salicylates
  - Diuretics
- Tobacco smoking
- Alcohol
- Lower socioeconomic status
- Family history of presbycusis
- Head trauma
- Cardiovascular disease (hypertension, atherosclerosis, hyperlipidemia)
- Diabetes mellitus
- Autoimmune disease
- Metabolic bone disease
- Endocrine medical conditions: Levels of aldosterone
- Alzheimer disease
- Otological conditions (e.g., Ménière disease or otosclerosis)

GENERAL PREVENTION
- Avoid hazardous noise exposure
- Use hearing protection
- Maintain healthy diet and exercise
- Screening:
  - In the only published RCT on screening for HL, HA use was significantly higher in 3 screened groups (4.1% in those using a questionnaire, 6.3% using handheld audiometry, and 7.4% using both modalities) vs. unscreened control participants (3.3%) at 1-year follow up (3)[B].
  - Based on a 2011 review, according to the USPSTF, there is insufficient evidence to assess the relative benefits and harms of HL screening in adults ≥50 (4)[A].

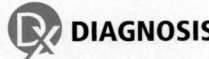

DIAGNOSIS

HISTORY
- Reduced hearing sensitivity and speech understanding in noisy/public environments
- Impaired localization of sound sources
- Increased difficulty understanding conversations, especially with women, due to higher frequency of spoken voice
- Presents bilaterally and symmetrically
- Additional history if HL is suspected or detected (5):
  - Time course of HL
  - Symptoms of tinnitus, otalgia, otorrhea, or vertigo
  - History of noise exposure, ear trauma, or head trauma
  - Presence of any neurologic deficit
- Reports from patient/family/caregiver (5):
  - Confusion in social situations
  - Excessive volume of television/radio/computer
  - Social withdrawal
  - Anxiety in group settings

PHYSICAL EXAM
- Rinne and Weber tests are helpful for determining conductive (CHL) vs. SNHL
- Pneumatic otoscopy to evaluate for simple middle ear effusion as cause of conductive hearing loss

DIFFERENTIAL DIAGNOSIS
- Acute noise-induced traumatic loss (explosion)
- Autoimmune HL
- Perilymph fistula
- Ménière disease
- Acoustic neuroma
- Complete canal occlusion
- Otitis externa
- Chronic otitis media or effusion
- Otosclerosis
- Large middle ear tumors (e.g., facial nerve schwannomas, paragangliomas)
- Vascular anomaly
- Cholesteatoma

DIAGNOSTIC TESTS & INTERPRETATION
- Handheld audiometry; insert probe in ear (sealing canal) and have patient indicate if tones can be heard:
  - Positive likelihood ratio (LR) range, 3.1–5.8; negative LR range, 0.03–0.40 (6)
- Screening audiometry:
  - Symmetric high frequency hearing loss in descending slope pattern.
  - SNHL frequencies > 2 kHz initially
  - Essential to determine if etiology is CHL vs. SNHL, pseudohypacusis, and global clinical hearing status.

TREATMENT

- HA:
  - Types:
    - o Analog HA: Picks up sound waves through a microphone; converts them into electrical signals; amplifies and sends them through the ear canal to the tympanic membrane
    - o Digital HA: Programmable; may reduce acoustic feedback, reduce background noise, detect and automatically accommodate different listening environments, control multiple microphones
  - HAs have an average 16.3 dB gain
  - Associated with hypersensitivity to loud sounds ("loudness recruitment")
- Hearing-assistive technologies (HATs) (7)[B]:
  - Can be used along or in combination with HAs (for difficult listening conditions)
  - Addresses face-to-face communication, broadcast or other electronic media (radio, TV), telephone conversation, sensitivity to alerting signals and environment stimuli (doorbell, baby's cry, alarm clock, etc.)
  - Includes personal FM systems, infrared systems, induction loop systems, hardwired systems, telephone amplifier, telecoil, TDD (telecommunication device for the deaf), situation-specific devices (e.g., television), alerting devices
- Aural rehabilitation (also known as audiological orientation or auditory training) (5)[C]:
  - Adjunct to HA or HATs
  - Involves education regarding proper use of amplification devices, coaching on how to manage the auditory environment, training in speech perception and communication, and counseling for coping strategies to deal with the difficulties of HAs or HATs

ISSUES FOR REFERRAL

Refer to audiologist for formal evaluation and optimal fitting of HAs and/or HATs:

- Individuals receiving post-fitting orientation/education have significantly fewer HA returns.
- Individuals receiving >2 hours of education and counseling report higher levels of satisfaction.

SURGERY/OTHER PROCEDURES

- Cochlear implants (CI) (8)[C]:
  - Indications include hearing no better than identifying ≤50% of key words in test sentences in the best aided condition in the worst ear and 60% in the better ear.
  - Works by bypassing the ear canal, middle ear, and hair cells in the cochlea to provide electric stimulation directly to the auditory nerve.
  - Incoming sounds are received through the microphone in the audio processor component (resembles a small HA), which converts them into electrical impulses and sends them to the magnetic coil (located on the skin). The impulses transmit these across intact skin via radio waves to the implanted component (directly subjacent to the coil). The pulses travel to the electrodes in the cochlea and stimulate the cochlea at high rates.
  - Receiving a unilateral CI is most common; some may receive bilateral CIs (either sequentially or in the same surgery). Others may wear a CI in 1 ear and an HA in the contralateral ear (bimodal fit).
- Active middle ear implants (AMEIs) (8)[C]:
  - Suitable for elderly adults who cannot wear conventional HAs for medical or personal (cosmetic reasons) and whose HL is not severe enough for a CI.
  - Comes in different models and may include components that are implantable under the skin.
- Electric acoustic stimulation: Use of CI and HA together in 1 ear:
  - Addresses the specific needs of patients presenting with good low-frequency hearing (a mild to moderate sensorineural HL in frequencies up to 1,000 Hz) but poorer hearing in the high frequencies (sloping to 60 dB or worse HL above 1,000 Hz) (8)[C]:
    - o Contraindications: Progressive HL, autoimmune disease; HL related to meningitis, otosclerosis, or ossification; malformation of the cochlea; a gap in air conduction and bone conduction thresholds of >15 dB; external ear contraindications, active infection or unwillingness to use amplification devices (8)[C].

ONGOING CARE

FOLLOW-UP RECOMMENDATIONS

Patient Monitoring

- During follow-up visits, check for compliance of HA use:
  - 25–40% of adults will either stop wearing them or use them only occasionally.
- Assess perceived benefit of HA, and, if ineffective, for indications for possible surgical treatments
- Annual audiograms
- Can follow up with audiologists for HA fittings if HA becomes uncomfortable

PATIENT EDUCATION

- Educate the patient that conversations should be face-to-face, spoken clearly and unhurriedly, without competing background noise (e.g., radio, TV), and include a confirmation that the message is received.
- Formal speech reading classes may be beneficial; however, availability may be limited.

REFERENCES

1. Nash SD, Cruickshanks KJ, Klein R, et al. The prevalence of hearing impairment and associated risk factors: The Beaver Dam Offspring Study. *Arch Otolaryngol Head Neck Surg.* 2011;137:432–439.
2. Huang Q, Tang J. Age-related hearing loss or presbycusis. *Eur Arch Otorhinolaryngol.* 2010;267: 1179–1191.
3. Yueh B, Collins MP, Souza PE, et al. Long-term effectiveness of screening for hearing loss. *J Am Geriatr Soc.* 2010;58:427–434.
4. Chou R, Dana T, Bougatsos C, et al. Screening adults aged 50 years or older for hearing loss: A review of the evidence for the U.S. Preventive Services Task Force. *Ann Intern Med.* 2011;154: 347–355.
5. Pacala J, Yueh B. Hearing deficits in the older patient: "I didn't notice anything." *JAMA.* 2012;307:1185–1194.
6. Bagai A, Thavendiranathan P, Detsky AS. Does this patient have hearing impairment? *JAMA.* 2006;295:416–428.
7. Valente M. Summary guidelines: Audiological management of adult hearing impairment. *Audio Today.* 2006;18:32–37.
8. Sprinzl GM, Riechelmann H. Current trends in treating hearing loss in elderly people: A review of the technology and treatment options—a mini-review. *Gerontology.* 2010;56:351–358.

CODES

ICD10

- H91.10 Presbycusis, unspecified ear
- H91.11 Presbycusis, right ear
- H91.13 Presbycusis, bilateral

CLINICAL PEARLS

- Presbycusis is age-related HL, showing increased incidence with age. It is often bilateral and initially begins as high-frequency HL. It presents as difficulty communicating in noisy conditions.
- There are more affected males than females.
- Compliance is only from 25–40% for those who own HAs. A referral to an audiologist is key for optimal evaluation, fitting for HAs, and consideration for HATs or surgical treatment.
- Indication for cochlear implants include hearing no better than identifying ≤50% key words in test sentences in the best-aided condition in the worst ear and 60% in the better ear.

PRESSURE ULCER
Amy M. Zack, MD, FAAFP

BASICS

DESCRIPTION
- A localized area of soft tissue injury resulting from pressure between an external surface and a bony prominence that causes local tissue breakdown classified in stages according to the National Pressure Ulcer Advisory Panel (NPUAP) classification:
  - Stage I: Erythema of localized area, usually nonblanching over bony surface
  - Stage II: Partial loss of dermal layer, resulting in pink ulceration
  - Stage III: Full dermal loss often exposing subcutaneous tissue and fat
  - Stage IV: Full thickness ulceration exposing bone, tendon, muscle. Osteomyelitis may be present
- Synonym(s): Decubitus ulcer; Bed sores

EPIDEMIOLOGY
Incidence
- 2.5 million pressure ulcers treated yearly in US in acute care facilities (1)

Prevalence
- Acute care 0.4–38%; long-term care 2.2–23.9%; home care 0–17%
- Majority occur in patients over 65 years: 36% with hip fracture, 50% in ICU care (2)

ETIOLOGY AND PATHOPHYSIOLOGY
- Pathophysiology of pressure ulcers is changing, differs depending on stage of ulceration
- Stages I–II result largely from prolonged moisture and friction and may not even be related to pressure and hypoxia, as previously believed (3).
- Stages III–IV likely begin with compressive forces, causing muscle damage and tissue hypoxia and leading to reperfusion injury of the deep tissue. The skin ulcer forms after significant deep tissue damage is already under way (3).
- Shearing and friction forces are also components of some ulcer formation, resulting in localized skin damage and early stage ulcers (3).

RISK FACTORS
- Immobility: Greatest risk factor regardless of patient, temporary or permanent immobility (4)
- Urinary and fecal incontinence present in >80% of immobile patients with pressure ulcers
- Poor nutritional status: hypoalbuminemia and low BMI are markers for poor ulcer outcome (4)
- Poor skin perfusion, including vascular disease, diabetes, anemia, and tobacco use, increase risk
- Extended stay in hospital/nursing home, inadequate staffing (5)
- Other risks include history of previous ulcer, age-related skin changes, immunocompromise, impaired skin sensation, impaired awareness
- Assessment scales commonly used for risk evaluation include Braden and Norton scales. The use of these does not decrease incidence, but they are more accurate than clinical judgment alone (6).

GENERAL PREVENTION
- Up to 95% are preventable; identification of at-risk patients is essential, with early multidisciplinary care.
- Pressure relief with proper patient positioning and the use of mattresses, cushions, heel protectors, and other devices to minimize pressure and friction. Regular turning of patients, including the use of angles and rotation of extremities, helps to minimize pressure.
- Minimize duration of immobility, adequate physical, occupational therapies when appropriate
- Aggressive moisture prevention with management of incontinence and maintenance of clean resting area
- Nutrition: Assess nutritional status and form plan for improving/maintaining adequate nutrition, particularly protein intake and albumin levels
- Manage skin health, clean and dry with mild cleansers, skin protection where appropriate

COMMONLY ASSOCIATED CONDITIONS
See "Risk Factors."

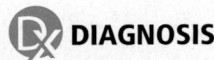

DIAGNOSIS

HISTORY
- Risk factors
- Date of ulcer diagnosis
- Treatment course

PHYSICAL EXAM
- Do full skin examination on admission to hospital or extended-care facility and repeatedly throughout admission, best with bathing/bed changes
- 83% of hospitalized patients with decubitus ulcers develop them in first 5 days of hospitalization.
- Classify ulcer based on NPUAP stages (see "Description")

DIFFERENTIAL DIAGNOSIS
- Venous stasis ulcers
- Arterial ulcers resulting from poor vascular supply
- Diabetic ulcers
- Pyoderma gangrenosum, cancers, vasculitides, and other dermatologic conditions

DIAGNOSTIC TESTS & INTERPRETATION
Initial Tests (lab, imaging)
- Wound culture: Do not culture surface drainage. Do deep tissue culture/bone biopsy.
- If systemic infection or that of bone, muscle is suspected: Add infectious workup, including inflammatory markers, CBC, blood cultures, x-ray. MRI may be necessary to confirm osteomyelitis.
- Nutritional assessment: BMI, protein and calorie intake, albumin, prealbumin, CBC for anemia. No clear evidence in support of specific nutritional supplements including zinc, vitamin C (7)[A],(8)[B].

Follow-Up Tests & Special Considerations
Additional tests may be indicated when additional medical illness complicates assessment. This may include testing for diabetes, vascular disease, and other dermatologic diagnoses.

TREATMENT

GENERAL MEASURES
- Pressure reduction, minimize immobility, manage incontinence, improve nutritional status and skin health (as described in "Prevention")
- Wound management by stage of ulcer:
  - Stage I: Aggressive preventive measures, thin film dressings for protection
  - Stage II: Occlusive dressing to maintain healing, transparent films, hydrocolloids
  - Stages III–IV: Debridement of necrotic tissue. Exudative ulcers will benefit from absorptive dressings like calcium alginates, foams, hydrofibers. Dry ulcers require occlusive dressing to maintain moisture, including hydrocolloids, hydrogels
  - Debridement: Type depends on extent of necrosis, eschar. Incisional with scalpel when extensive, dry. Mechanical with wet-dry dressings; enzymatic debridement is also frequently used.
  - Surgical closure may be necessary in advanced wounds
- Vacuum-assisted closure:
  - Negative pressure reduces wound edema and improves local tissue perfusion.
  - Removes necrotic debris and reduces bacterial load
  - Literature review demonstrates the efficacy of negative pressure wound therapy (9)[A]

MEDICATION
First Line
- See "General Measures" for first-line treatment
- Pain control
- Aggressive management of contributing medical conditions
- Infection: If suspected, treat appropriately for cellulitis, osteomyelitis

Second Line
Nutritional interventions as determined by nutritional assessment

ISSUES FOR REFERRAL
- Vascular surgery is a consideration for improvement of blood flow to wound via vascular bypass.
- Plastic surgery is a consideration for skin graft/flap.

ADDITIONAL THERAPIES
Whirlpool/PulseVac aids in wound debridement

COMPLEMENTARY AND ALTERNATIVE MEDICINE
- Nutritional support as needed
- US and electrical stimulation create new vasculature in affected region (9)[C].

IN-PATIENT CONSIDERATIONS
Admission Criteria/Initial Stabilization
- Refractory cellulitis, osteomyelitis, systemic infection, advanced nutritional decline, suspected patient mistreatment, inability to care for self

Nursing
- Dressing changes 1–3 × daily based on wound assessment and plan of care
- Assess risk factors according to scales
- Assess for new or changing wounds

Discharge Criteria
Clinical improvement in wound and systemic illness; when applicable, safe and appropriate location for discharge

ONGOING CARE

FOLLOW-UP RECOMMENDATIONS
Weekly assessment by nurse with wound experience; biweekly assessment by physician

Patient Monitoring
- Home health nursing
- Change in plan of care if no improvement in 2–3 weeks

DIET
- 1–1.5 kg/d of protein
- Good glycemic control
- Include supply of micronutrients in diet or as supplements

PATIENT EDUCATION
- Check skin regularly
- Signs and symptoms of infection
- Report new or increased pain
- Prevention of new wound where old wound healed
- Skin care, moisture prevention

PROGNOSIS
Variable, depending on:
- Removal of pressure
- Nutrition
- Wound care

COMPLICATIONS
- Infection
- Amputation

REFERENCES

1. Reddy M, Gill S, Rochon P. Preventing pressure ulcers: A systematic review. *JAMA*. 2006;296:974–984.
2. Baumgarten M, Margolis DJ, Orwig DL, et al. Pressure ulcers in elderly patients with hip fracture across the continuum of care. *J Am Geriatr Soc*. 2009;57:863.
3. Sibbald, RG, Krasner, DL, Woo KY. Pressure ulcer staging revisited: Superficial changes and deep pressure framework. *Adv Skin Wound Care*. 2011;24:571–580.
4. Cakmak S, Gul U, Ozer S, et al. Risk factors for pressure ulcers. *Adv Skin Wound Care*. 2009;22:412–415.
5. European Pressure Ulcer Advisory Panel and National Pressure Ulcer Advisory Panel. *Treatment of pressure ulcers: Quick Reference Guide*. Washington, DC: National Pressure Ulcer Advisory Panel; 2009.
6. Pancorbo-Hidalgo PL, Garcia-Fernandez FP, Lopez-Medina IM, et al. Risk assessment scales for pressure ulcer prevention, a systematic review. *J Adv Nurs*. 2006;54:94–110.
7. Langer G, Scholemer G, Knerr A, et al. Nutritional interventions for preventing and treating pressure ulcers. *Cochrane Database Syst Rev*. 2003;4:CD003216.
8. Jamshed N, Schneider E. Is the use of supplemental vitamin C and zinc for the prevention and treatment of pressure ulcers evidence based? *Ann Long-Term Care Med*. 2010;18:28–32.
9. Gregor S, Maegele M, Sauerland S, et al. Negative pressure wound therapy: A vacuum of evidence? *Arch Surg*. 2008;143:189–196.

 CODES

ICD10
- L89.91 Pressure ulcer of unspecified site, stage 1
- L89.92 Pressure ulcer of unspecified site, stage 2
- L89.95 Pressure ulcer of unspecified site, unstageable

CLINICAL PEARLS
- Identify risk, reduce pressure, maximize nutrition, regular skin checks, assess and treat wound appropriately.

PRETERM LABOR

Kara M. Coassolo, MD • John C. Smulian, MD, MPH

 BASICS

DESCRIPTION
Contractions occurring between 20 and 36 weeks' gestation at a rate of 4 in 20 minutes or 8 in 1 hour with at least 1 of the following: Cervical change over time or dilation ≥2 cm

EPIDEMIOLOGY
Preterm birth is the leading cause of perinatal morbidity and mortality in the US.

Incidence
10–15% of pregnancies experience at least 1 episode of preterm labor.

Prevalence
~12% of all births in the US are preterm (9% spontaneous preterm births and 3% indicated preterm births).

ETIOLOGY AND PATHOPHYSIOLOGY
- Premature formation and activation of myometrial gap junctions
- Inflammatory mediator–stimulated contractions
- Weakened cervix (structural defect or extracellular matrix defect)
- Abnormal placental implantation
- Systemic inflammation/infections (e.g., UTI, pyelonephritis, pneumonia, sepsis)
- Local inflammation/infections (intra-amniotic infections from aerobes, anaerobes, *Mycoplasma*, *Ureaplasma*)
- Uterine abnormalities (e.g., cervical insufficiency, leiomyomata, mullerian anomalies, diethylstilbestrol exposure)
- Overdistension (by multiple gestation or polyhydramnios)
- Preterm premature rupture of membranes
- Trauma
- Placental abruption
- Immunopathology (e.g., antiphospholipid antibodies)
- Placental ischemic disease (preeclampsia and fetal growth restriction)

Genetics
Familial predisposition

RISK FACTORS
- Demographic factors, including single parent, poverty, and black race
- Short interpregnancy interval
- No prenatal care
- Prepregnancy weight <45 kg (100 lb), body mass index <20
- Substance abuse (e.g., cocaine, tobacco)
- Prior preterm delivery (common)
- Previous 2nd-trimester dilation and evacuation (D&E)
- Cervical insufficiency or prior cervical surgery (cone biopsy or LEEP)
- Abdominal surgery/trauma during pregnancy
- Uterine structural abnormalities, such as large fibroids or müllerian abnormalities
- Serious maternal infections/diseases
- Bacterial vaginosis
- Bacteriuria

- Vaginal bleeding during pregnancy
- Multiple gestation
- Select fetal abnormalities
- Intrauterine growth restriction
- Placenta previa
- Premature placental separation (abruption)
- Polyhydramnios
- Ehlers-Danlos syndrome

GENERAL PREVENTION
- Patient education at each visit in 2nd and 3rd trimesters for those at risk and periodically in the last 2 trimesters for the general population
- If previous preterm birth, evaluate if etiology is likely to recur and target intervention to specific condition:
  – Weekly injections of 17α-hydroxyprogesterone (250 mg IM every week) from 16–36 weeks if previous spontaneous preterm birth (1,2)[A]
  – Consider cerclage placement before 24 weeks' gestation for those at high risk because of cervical insufficiency or significant or progressive cervical shortening.
- For women with a short cervix in the 2nd trimester (<20 mm on transvaginal US), progesterone 200 mg/d per vagina × 24–34 weeks may decrease the risk of preterm delivery (2)[A].

 DIAGNOSIS

Diagnosis is generally based on a combination of significant cervical changes (such as dilation, effacement) with regular contractions. However, there is no single test that will reliably diagnose or predict true preterm labor. The diagnosis is based on a combination of physical findings and diagnostic tests that are interpreted in the context of the degree of risk to the patient.

HISTORY
- Address risk factors, especially etiologies of previous preterm birth
- Regular uterine contractions or cramping
- Dull, low backache or pain
- Intermittent lower abdominal pain
- Increased low pelvic pressure
- Change in vaginal discharge
- Vaginal bleeding
- Fluid leakage

PHYSICAL EXAM
- Sterile speculum exam for membrane rupture evaluation, cultures, cervical inspection
- Bimanual cervical exam if intact membranes: Dilation of the cervix >1 cm and/or effacement of the cervix >50%

ALERT
Avoid bimanual examination when possible if rupture of the membranes is suspected.

DIFFERENTIAL DIAGNOSIS
- Braxton-Hicks contractions/false labor
- Round ligament pain
- Lumbosacral muscular back pain
- Urinary tract or vaginal infections
- Adnexal torsion

- Degenerating fibroid
- Appendicitis
- Dehydration
- Viral gastroenteritis
- Nephrolithiasis

DIAGNOSTIC TESTS & INTERPRETATION
Initial Tests (lab, imaging)
- In symptomatic women from 22–34 weeks' gestation with intact membranes and no intercourse or bleeding in past 24 hours, obtain a fetal fibronectin (FFN) swab from the posterior vaginal fornix. FFN must be obtained prior to digital cervical exam:
  – If results are positive (≥50 ng/mL), patient is at a modest increased risk of preterm birth (positive predictive value [PPV] 13–30% for delivery within 2 weeks).
  – If results are negative, more than 97% of patients will not deliver in 14 days, so can consider avoiding complicated or high-risk interventions (3)[A]
- Urinalysis and urine culture
- Cultures for gonorrhea and chlamydia
- Wet prep for bacterial vaginosis evaluation (although evidence for improved outcomes with treatment is weak)
- Vaginal introitus and rectal culture for group B *Streptococcus*
- pH and Ferning test of vaginal fluid to evaluate for rupture of membranes
- CBC with differential
- Drug screen when appropriate
- US to identify number of fetuses and fetal position, confirm gestational age, estimate fetal weight, quantify amniotic fluid, and look for conditions making tocolysis contraindicated
- Transvaginal US to evaluate cervical length, funneling, and dynamic changes after obtaining FFN (if clinical assessment of the cervix is uncertain or if the cervix is closed on digital exam).

Follow-Up Tests & Special Considerations
Repeat FFN as indicated by symptoms.
    After successful treatment, progressive changes of the cervix on repeat examination or US (in 1–2 weeks) may indicate need for hospitalization.

Diagnostic Procedures/Other
- Monitor contractions with external tocodynamometer
- Consider amniocentesis at any preterm gestational age to evaluate for intra-amniotic infection (cell count with differential, glucose, Gram stain, aerobic, anaerobic, *Mycoplasma*, *Ureaplasma* cultures)
- Consider amniocentesis if ≥32 weeks' gestation for evaluation of fetal lung maturity (e.g., lecithin/sphingomyelin [L:S] ratio and phosphatidylglycerol [PG]). If L:S ratio >2:1 (nondiabetic) and PG is present, hyaline membrane disease is unlikely, so tocolysis may be withheld.

Test Interpretation
- Placental inflammation:
  – Acute inflammation usually caused by infection
  – Chronic inflammation caused by immunopathology
- Abruption

TREATMENT

GENERAL MEASURES
- Treat underlying risk factors (e.g., antibiotics for infections, hydration for dehydration).
- Liquids only or NPO if delivery imminent
- Hospitalization is necessary if the patient is on IV tocolysis.

MEDICATION
Tocolysis may allow time for interventions such as transfer to tertiary care facility and administration of corticosteroids, but may not prolong pregnancy significantly (1,4)[A].

First Line
- Tocolysis:
  - Nifedipine: 10 mg PO q10min up to 30 mg total; then 10–20 mg q6h × 24 hours; then 10–20 mg PO q8h (do not use sublingual route); check BP often and avoid hypotension. Concurrent use with magnesium sulfate should be avoided to avoid theoretic risk of neuromuscular blockade.
  - Indomethacin: 50–100 mg PO initial dose; then 50 mg q6–8h × 24 hours (or, if available, 100-mg suppository per rectum q12h for 2 doses); then 25 mg q6–8h; use for no longer than 72 hours due to risk of premature closure of ductus arteriosus, oligohydramnios, and possibly neonatal necrotizing enterocolitis. Use with caution in patients with platelet dysfunction, liver dysfunction, or allergy to aspirin.
  - Contraindications to tocolysis: Severe preeclampsia, hemorrhage, chorioamnionitis, advanced labor, intrauterine growth retardation, fetal distress, or lethal fetal abnormalities
- Antibiotics: Antibiotics for group B *Streptococcus* prophylaxis if culture positive or unknown
- Steroids: If mother is at 23–34 weeks' gestation with no evidence of systemic infection, give glucocorticoids to decrease neonatal respiratory distress, intraventricular hemorrhage, necrotizing enterocolitis, and overall perinatal mortality (5)[A]. Betamethasone 12 mg IM × 2 doses 24 hours apart (preferred choice) *or* dexamethasone 6 mg IM q12h for 4 doses.

Second Line
- Magnesium sulfate by IV infusion has not been shown to be superior to placebo in prolonging pregnancy beyond 48 hours. The side effects are generally greater compared with calcium channel blockers or NSAIDs. Therefore, this agent should be used cautiously if at all. (Standard dosages for tocolysis start with a 4–6-g IV bolus over 20 minutes and then 2–3 g/h until contractions stop.):
  - Magnesium may decrease the risk of cerebral palsy when 12-hour course is given prior to an anticipated preterm birth (6)[B].
  - Relative contraindications to magnesium sulfate include myasthenia gravis, hypocalcemia, renal failure, or concurrent use of calcium channel blockers.
- Terbutaline 0.25 mg SC q30min for up to 3 doses until contractions stop, then 0.25 mg SC q6h for 4 doses (optional); if contractions persist or pulse >120 beats/min, change to another tocolytic agent (may be poorly tolerated by mothers)

- Terbutaline PO or by infusion pump has been used in the past for treatment or prevention of preterm labor. Due to reports of serious cardiovascular events and maternal deaths, PO or long-term SC administration of terbutaline should not be given.
- Significant possible interactions include pulmonary edema from crystalloid fluids and tocolytic agents, especially magnesium sulfate.
- PO maintenance therapy with any agent is controversial, and its use is limited.

ISSUES FOR REFERRAL
- If delivery is inevitable but not immediate, consider transport to a tertiary care center or hospital equipped with a neonatal ICU.
- Consider consultation with maternal–fetal medicine specialist.

ADDITIONAL THERAPIES
- Pelvic rest (e.g., no douching or intercourse) and activity restriction are often recommended, however, data to prove the efficacy are lacking. Some reduction in physical activity may be reasonable; this should be individualized.
- Strict bed rest has not been demonstrated to be effective in most situations.

SURGERY/OTHER PROCEDURES
- For malpresentation or fetal compromise, consider cesarean delivery if labor is progressing.
- Cerclage for cervical insufficiency (until 24 weeks' gestation)

IN-PATIENT CONSIDERATIONS
Admission Criteria/Initial Stabilization
Suspected/Threatened preterm labor:
- IV access
- Continuous fetal and contraction monitoring
- Assess cervix for dilatation and effacement

IV Fluids
Hydrate with 500 mL 5% dextrose normal saline solution or 5% dextrose lactated Ringer's solution for 1st half-hour; then at 125 mL/h.

Nursing
Monitor for fluid overload (input/output monitoring, symptoms, lung auscultation, pulse oximetry), especially with tocolysis and multiple gestations.

Discharge Criteria
- Regular contractions and cervical change resolve
- If cervix is dilated ≥3 cm or FFN is positive, individualize decision to discharge by gestational age and patient circumstances

ONGOING CARE

FOLLOW-UP RECOMMENDATIONS
Patient Monitoring
- Weekly office visits with contraction monitoring, cervical checks, or cervical US if at high risk for recurrence
- Routine use of maintenance tocolysis is ineffective in preventing preterm birth

DIET
Regular

PATIENT EDUCATION
Call physician or proceed to hospital whenever regular contractions last >1 hour, bleeding, increased vaginal discharge or fluid, decreased fetal movement

PROGNOSIS
- If membranes are ruptured and no infection is confirmed, delivery often occurs within 3–7 days.
- If membranes are intact, 20–50% deliver preterm.

COMPLICATIONS
Labor resistant to tocolysis, pulmonary edema, infection with preterm rupture of membranes

REFERENCES
1. Simhan HN, Caritis SN. Prevention of preterm delivery. *N Engl J Med*. 2007;357:477–487.
2. Tita AT, Rouse DJ. Progesterone for preterm birth prevention: An evolving intervention. *Am J Obstet Gynecol*. 2009;200:219–224.
3. Goldenberg RL, Goepfert AR, Ramsey PS. Biochemical markers for the prediction of preterm birth. *Am J Obstet Gynecol*. 2005;192(5 Suppl): S36–S46.
4. Haas DM, Caldwell DM, Kirkpatrick P et al. Tocolytic therapy for preterm delivery: Systematic review and network meta-analysis. *Br Med J*. 2012;345:e6226.
5. Roberts D, Dalziel S. Antenatal corticosteroids for accelerating fetal lung maturation for women at risk of preterm birth. *Cochrane Database Syst Rev*. 2006;3:CD004454.
6. American College of Obstetricians and Gynecologists Committee on Obstetric Practice, Society for Maternal-Fetal Medicine. Committee Opinion No. 455: Magnesium sulfate before anticipated preterm birth for neuroprotection. *Obstet Gynecol*. 2010;115:669–671.

ADDITIONAL READING
Berghella V, Rafael TJ, Szychowski JM, et al. Cerclage for short cervix on ultrasonography in women with singleton gestations and previous preterm birth. *Obstet Gynecol*. 2011;117:663–671.

CODES

ICD10
- O60.00 Preterm labor without delivery, unspecified trimester
- O60.02 Preterm labor without delivery, second trimester
- O60.03 Preterm labor without delivery, third trimester

CLINICAL PEARLS
- Treatment of preterm labor may delay delivery to facilitate short-term interventions.
- Steroids improve neonatal outcomes.
- Progesterone therapy can prevent recurrence of preterm birth in next pregnancy.

PRIAPISM

Shenelle N. Wilson, MD • Kelvin A. Moses, MD, PhD

 BASICS

DESCRIPTION
- Penile erection that lasts for >4 hours and is unrelated to sexual stimulation or excitement
- Classified into ischemic and nonischemic types
- Ischemic (low-flow) priapism is painful and requires urgent clinical intervention
- Stuttering priapism is recurrent episodes of short-lived, self-limiting ischemic priapism over an extended period.
- Nonischemic (high-flow) priapism is painless, could be related to prior trauma, and does not require urgent treatment.
- Malignant priapism is a rare condition resulting most commonly from penile metastases from primary bladder, prostatic, rectosigmoid, and renal tumors.
- System(s) affected: Reproductive

Pediatric Considerations
In children, nearly all priapism is caused either by sickle cell anemia or trauma (1).

EPIDEMIOLOGY
Incidence
In the US, 1 study estimates 1,868–2,960 cases of priapism each year. They also noted an increasing incidence from 1998 to 2006, specifically in those from nonhematologic causes (2):
- Mean age: 33.7 years. There has been an age shift in recent years toward men in their 40s.
- Other studies have found the incidence of priapism to double in men aged >40 (2.9 vs. 1.5/100,000 person-years) (3).
- Race: 61.1% black, 30% white, 6.3% Hispanic
- Associations: Sickle cell anemia (41.9%), drug abuse (7.9%), sickle cell trait (2.5%)
- Anatomy and physiology:
  - The penis consists of three longitudinally oriented corpora: Two dorsolaterally paired corpora cavernosa that are responsible for penile erection and a single ventral corpus spongiosum that surrounds the glans penis and extends distally to form the glans penis.
  - In general, the penile artery (which is a branch of the internal pudendal artery that, in turn, is a branch from the internal iliac artery) supplies the penis. It divides into three branches: Dorsal artery, bulbar artery (supplies the corpus spongiosum), and cavernosal artery (the main blood supply to the erectile tissue).
  - During an erection, smooth muscle relaxation of the cavernosal arterioles results in high volume inflow to the sinusoids, resulting in compression of the exiting venules. This leads to significant volume expansion of the corpora cavernosa.
  - During the flaccid resting state, the sympathetic nervous system is predominantly in control. Penile tumescence and erection are driven by the parasympathetic nervous system through the generation of nitric oxide (NO).
  - Smooth muscle relaxation occurs via utilization of the phosphodiesterase type 5 (PDE-5A) pathway, which generates cyclic guanosine monophosphate (cGMP).

ETIOLOGY AND PATHOPHYSIOLOGY
- In ischemic priapism, decreased venous outflow results in increased intracavernosal pressure. This leads to erection, decreased arterial inflow, blood stasis, local hypoxia, and acidosis (a compartment syndrome). Eventually, penile tissue necrosis and fibrosis may occur. The exact mechanism is unknown and may involve trapping of erythrocytes in the veins draining the erectile bodies.
- In nonischemic priapism, there is increased arterial flow without decreased venous outflow. There is increased inflow and outflow, which results in a sustained, nonpainful, partially rigid erection.
- Aberrations in the PDE-5A pathway have been proven in mice to be one mechanism of priapism (4).
- Ischemic priapism:
  - Idiopathic, estimated to about 50% (1)
  - Intracavernosal injections of vasoactive drugs for erectile dysfunction
  - Oral agents for erectile dysfunction
  - Pelvic vascular thrombosis
  - Prolonged sexual activity
  - Sickle cell disease and trait
  - Leukemia from infiltration of the corpora
  - Other blood dyscrasias (G6PD deficiency, thrombophilia)
  - Pelvic hematoma or neoplasia (penis, urethra, bladder, prostate, kidney, rectal)
  - Cerebrospinal tumors
  - Asplenism
  - Fabry disease
  - Tertiary syphilis
  - Total parenteral nutrition, especially 20% lipid infusion (results in hyperviscosity)
  - Bladder calculus
  - Trauma to penis
  - UTIs, especially prostatitis, urethritis, cystitis
  - Several drugs suspected as causing priapism (e.g., chlorpromazine, prazosin, cocaine, trazodone, and some corticosteroids); anticoagulants (heparin and warfarin); phosphodiesterase inhibitors (sildenafil, others); immunosuppressants (tacrolimus); and antihypertensives (hydralazine, propranolol, guanethidine)
  - Intracavernous fat emulsion
  - Hyperosmolar IV contrast
  - Spinal cord injury
  - General or spinal anesthesia
  - Heavy alcohol intake or cocaine use
- Nonischemic priapism:
  - The most common cause is penile or perineal trauma resulting in a fistula between the cavernous artery and the corpora.
  - Acute spinal cord injury
  - Rarely, iatrogenic causes for the management of ischemic priapism can result in nonischemic priapism.
  - Certain urologic surgeries have also resulted in nonischemic priapism.

RISK FACTORS
- Sickle cell anemia, lifetime risk of ischemic priapism 29–42% (1)
- Dehydration

GENERAL PREVENTION
- Avoid dehydration
- Avoid excessive sexual stimulation
- Avoid causative drugs (see "Etiology and Pathophysiology") when possible
- Avoid genital and pelvic trauma

COMMONLY ASSOCIATED CONDITIONS
- Sickle cell anemia or sickle cell trait
- Drug abuse
- G6PD deficiency
- Leukemia
- Neoplasm

 DIAGNOSIS

HISTORY
- Penile erection that is persistent, prolonged, painful, and tender (ischemic)
- Duration of erection, degree of pain
- Perineal or penile trauma
- Prior episodes of priapism
- Urination difficult during erection
- History of any hematological abnormalities
- Cardiovascular disease
- Medications
- Recreational drugs
- Loss of erectile function if treatment is not prompt and effective

PHYSICAL EXAM
- Ischemic priapism:
  - Penis is fully erect, corpora cavernosa are rigid and tender, and corpora spongiosum and glans are flaccid. Usually associated with tenderness and pain
- Nonischemic priapism:
  - Penis is partially erect and the corpora cavernosa are semirigid and nontender, with the glans and corpora spongiosum flaccid. Usually not tender or painful
- Perineum, abdomen, and lymph node exam also valuable to rule out underlying condition
- A complete penile and scrotal exam is necessary. Determine if a penile prosthesis is present.

DIAGNOSTIC TESTS & INTERPRETATION
- CBC with reticulocyte count to detect leukemia or platelet abnormalities
- Sickling hemoglobin (Hgb) solubility test and Hgb electrophoresis
- Coagulation profile
- Platelet count
- Urinalysis
- Urine toxicology if illicit drugs suspected
- Corporal blood gas (CBG) should be used to distinguish ischemic from nonischemic priapism.
- A color duplex ultrasound of the penis and perineum may be necessary to differentiate ischemic from nonischemic priapism. In ischemic priapism, there is no blood flow in the cavernosal arteries, whereas in nonischemic patients there is high blood flow (1); may also see fistulas or pseudoaneurysms suggestive of nonischemic priapism.
- Penile arteriography can be used to identify the presence and site of fistulas in patients with nonischemic priapism.

Diagnostic Procedures/Other
A physical exam is usually able to distinguish ischemic from nonischemic priapism; however, CBG is the most definitive method.

Test Interpretation
- Pelvic vascular thrombosis
- Partial thrombosis of corpora cavernosa of the penis
- Corpus spongiosum, glans penis: No involvement
- Arterial priapism will show arteriocavernous fistula.

TREATMENT

- Ischemic priapism requires immediate treatment to preserve future erectile function (a longer delay in treatment means a higher chance of future impotence):
  - Cavernosal aspiration with a large bore needle with irrigation (success rate ~30%) (1,5)
  - Cavernosal injection of phenylephrine (α-adrenergic sympathomimetic) with monitoring of patient's BP and pulse (success rate ~65%) (5). Inject q5–10min until detumescence
  - Continue aspiration, irrigation, and phenylephrine for several hours. If this fails, shunt procedures are considered (1st a distal shunt).
- Nonischemic priapism:
  - Initial observation
  - If this fails, arteriography and embolization with absorbable materials (5% rate of impotence vs. 39% with permanent materials) or surgical ligation as a last resort (5).
- Treat the underlying condition (i.e., sickle cell disease). Do not delay intracavernous treatment.

GENERAL MEASURES
- Reassure the patient about the outcome, if warranted
- Provide continuous caudal or spinal anesthesia if the etiology is neurogenic
- Treat any underlying cause
- In sickle cell anemia: IV hydration; supplemental oxygen; partial exchange or repeated transfusions to reduce percentage of sickle cells to <50%
- Relieve the patient's pain

MEDICATION
- Narcotics for pain, if needed
- Pseudoephedrine is not recommended by the American Urological Association (5):
  - Efficacy is reported in nonrandomized studies as 28–36% (1).
  - No randomized studies have been conducted to date.
- Terbutaline has been studied and may be effective (uncontrolled trials showed a 65% resolution rate) for priapism caused by self-injection of agents to treat erectile dysfunction (5).
- For stuttering priapism, a trial of gonadotropin-releasing hormone (GnRH) agonists or antiandrogens is effective; self-injection of phenylephrine is also effective.
- PDE-5 inhibitors also have a role in the prevention of priapism in patients suffering from stuttering priapism (6).

ISSUES FOR REFERRAL
A urologist should be consulted in all cases of suspected priapism to ensure the highest likelihood of preserved erectile function.

SURGERY/OTHER PROCEDURES
- Introduction of 18- or 19-gauge needle into corpora cavernosa (best done by urologist if available) at 9 o'clock and 3 o'clock positions with aspiration of 20–30 mL of blood from corpus cavernosum. May follow with intracavernous injection of 100–500 mcg phenylephrine (Mix 0.2 mL [200 mcg]) of 1% phenylephrine in 9.8 cc of normal saline.) If this fails, consider shunts.
- Distal shunts:
  - Percutaneous: Ebbehoj, Winter, or T-shunt (7,8,9)
  - Open: Al-Ghorab or Corporal Snake (10,11)
- Proximal shunts:
  - Open: Quackles or Sacher (12,13)
  - Saphenous vein shunt (14)
  - Deep dorsal vein shunt (15)

ONGOING CARE

FOLLOW-UP RECOMMENDATIONS
Bed rest until priapism resolves

Patient Monitoring
Close follow up with a urologist is required after surgical treatments for priapism.

PATIENT EDUCATION
- Information about long-term outlook, referral for counseling
- Reduction of vasoactive drug therapy if responsible for priapism and elimination of offending drugs if causal

PROGNOSIS
- Even with excellent treatment for a prolonged priapism, detumescence may require several weeks secondary to edema (1).
- Impotence due to irreversible corporal fibrosis is likely in ischemic priapism and is up to 90% if the priapism lasts >24 hours.
- Despite early intervention, ischemic priapism is likely to result in impotence in up to 50% of men.

COMPLICATIONS
Erectile dysfunction (i.e., impotence)

REFERENCES
1. Huang YC, Harraz AM, Shindel AW. Evaluation and management of priapism: 2009 update. Nat Rev Urol. 2009;6:262–271.
2. Chrouser KL, Ajiboye OB, Oyetunji TA, et al. Priapism in the United States: The changing role of sickle cell disease. Am J Surg. 2011;201:468–474.
3. Eland IA, van der Lei J, Stricker BH, et al. Incidence of priapism in the general population. Urology. 2001;57:970–972.
4. Champion HC, Bivalacqua TJ, Takimoto E. Phosphodiesterase-5A dysregulation in penile erectile tissue is a mechanism of priapism. Proc Natl Acad Sci U S A. 2005;102:1661–1666.
5. Montague DK, Jarow J, Broderick GA. American Urological Association guideline on the management of priapism. J Urol. 2003;170:1318–1324.
6. Muneer A, Minhas S, Arya M, et al. Stuttering priapism—a review of the therapeutic options. Int J Clin Pract. 2008;62:1265–1270.
7. Ebbehoj J. A new operation for priapism. Scand J Plast Reconstr Surg. 1974;8:241–242.
8. Winter CC. Cure of idiopathic priapism: New procedure for creating fistula between glans penis and corpora cavernosa. Urology. 1976;8:389–391.
9. Brant WO, Garcia MM, Bella AJ, et al. T-shaped shunt and intracavernous tunneling for prolonged ischemic priapism. J Urol. 2009;181:1699–1705.
10. Borrelli M, Mitre AI, Alfer Jnior W, et al. [Surgical treatment of priapism using Al-Ghorab's technic]. Rev Paul Med. 1983;101:27–28.
11. Burnett AL, Pierorazio PM. Corporal "snake" maneuver: Corporoglanular shunt surgical modification for ischemic priapism. J Sex Med. 2009;6:1171–1176.
12. Quackels R. [Treatment of a case of priapism by cavernospongious anastomosis]. Acta Urol Belg. 1964;32:5–13.
13. Sacher EC, Sayegh E, Frensilli F, et al. Cavernospongiosum shunt in the treatment of priapism. J Urol. 1972;108:97–100.
14. Grayhack JT, Mccullough W, O'Conor VJ, et al. Venous bypass to control priapism. Invest Urol. 1964;1:509–513.
15. Barry JM. Priapism: Treatment with corpus cavernosum to dorsal vein of penis shunts. J Urol. 1976;116:754–756.

ADDITIONAL READING
- Burnett AL. Pathophysiology of priapism: Dysregulatory erection physiology thesis. J Urol. 2003;170:26–34.
- Morrison BF, Reid M, Madden W, et al. Testosterone replacement therapy does not promote priapism in hypogonadal men with sickle cell disease: 12-month safety report. Andrology. 2013;1:576–582.
- Pryor J, Akkus E, Alter G. Priapism. J Sex Med. 2004;1:116–120.

SEE ALSO

Anemia, Sickle Cell; Erectile Dysfunction

CODES

ICD10
- N48.30 Priapism, unspecified
- N48.31 Priapism due to trauma
- N48.39 Other priapism

CLINICAL PEARLS

- Priapism is a prolonged penile erection that lasts >4 hours and is unrelated to sexual stimulation.
- In evaluating priapism, the clinician must distinguish ischemic from nonischemic priapism by history and physical exam, as well as blood gas and possibly ultrasound, if needed.
- Ischemic priapism is an emergent condition that requires immediate urologic evaluation and treatment.
- The most common causes of ischemic priapism are idiopathic, related to treatments for erectile dysfunction, or related to use of substances (medicinal or recreational).
- If an underlying medical condition is identified (sickle cell anemia), proper concomitant treatment is necessary to increase the efficacy of treatment.

PROSTATE CANCER

Sara Valente, MD • Kevan Sternberg, MD

 BASICS

DESCRIPTION

- The prostate gland is often likened in size to a walnut, typically averaging 20–25 g in volume in an adult male; tends to become larger with age.
- 3 distinct zones delineate the functional anatomy of the prostate: Peripheral zone (largest, neighbors rectal wall, palpable on DRE), central zone (contains the ejaculatory ducts), and transition zone (located centrally, adjacent to the urethra)
- Common metastatic locations (most to least common): Pelvic lymph nodes, bone, lung, and liver
- Clinical staging is an objective evaluation of disease extent based upon pretreatment criteria including imaging, digital rectal exam, PSA, biopsy.
- Pathologic stage is determined only once the prostatic tissue and accompanying lymph nodes have been analyzed histologically.
- Staging: Tumor, node, metastasis (TNM) classification: Clinical:
  - Tx: Primary tumor cannot be assessed
  - T0: No evidence of primary tumor
  - T1: Clinically inapparent tumor not palpable or visible by imaging. T1a: Tumor incidental histologic finding in ≤5% of tissue resected (by transurethral resection of prostate [TURP]). T1b: Tumor incidental histologic finding in >5% of tissue resected (by TURP). T1c: Tumor identified by needle biopsy (e.g., because of elevated PSA)
  - T2: Tumor confined within prostate, found in 1 or both lobes. T2a: Tumor involves ≤1/2 of 1 lobe. T2b: Tumor involves >1/2 of 1 lobe. T2c: Both lobes.
  - T3: Tumor extends through the prostatic capsule (invasion into the prostatic apex or into, but not beyond, the prostatic capsule is still T2). T3a: Extracapsular extension (unilateral or bilateral). T3b: Tumor invades seminal vesicle(s).
  - T4: Tumor is fixed or invades adjacent structures other than seminal vesicles (e.g., bladder neck, external sphincter, rectum, levator muscles, and/or pelvic wall).
- Pathologic staging based on histologic findings, pT2–pT4 with analogous groupings. Also includes N (nodes) and M (metastasis). Nodes range from Nx (not assessed) to N0 (no nodes) to N1 (metastasis to regional nodes). Metastasis: Mx (not assessed), M0 (no metastasis), M1 (distant metastasis) including M1a (regional mets), M1b (bones), M1c (other sites w/o bone disease)
- Gleason grade: Tumors are graded from 1 (well differentiated) to 5 (poorly differentiated) based on the degree of glandular differentiation and structural architecture, though only scores 3–5 are reported as cancers. Primary and secondary scores are reported and combined to form the combined Gleason score.
- Gleason score is now recognized by the American Joint Committee on Cancer (AJCC) as the preferred grading system, and this score is an important variable used to risk stratify patients with localized prostate cancer

EPIDEMIOLOGY
Incidence
Mortality from carcinoma of the prostate (CaP) is decreasing. Based on 5 years of mortality data (2006–2010), the overall cancer death rate decreased by 3.1% per year.

Prevalence
- According to the National Cancer Institute, an estimated 238,590 men in the US will be newly diagnosed with CaP in 2013.
- ~29,720 men in the US will die of CaP in 2013.
- Mean age at diagnosis is 66 years.
- Prostate cancer is the most commonly diagnosed non-skin cancer in men in the US (~15.3% lifetime risk) and 2nd leading cause of cancer death in men (only ~3% of all CaP results in CaP-related death).
- Autopsy studies find foci of latent CaP in 50% of men in their 8th decade (1).
- Probability of invasive CaP 12.54% (1 in 8) in men aged ≥70.

ETIOLOGY AND PATHOPHYSIOLOGY
- Adenocarcinoma: >95%; Nonadenocarcinoma: <5% (most common transitional cell carcinoma)
- Cells often stain positive for PSA and prostatic acid phosphatase (PAP)
- Location of CaP: 70% peripheral zone, 20% transitional zone, 5–10% central zone

Genetics
Risk doubled if 1st-degree relative <50 affected.

RISK FACTORS
- Age >50 years, African American race
- Incidence is 152.0 per 100,000 in Caucasians vs. 228.5 per 100,000 in African Americans
- Age is the most important risk factor
- Testosterone therapy does not increase CaP recurrence rates postprostatectomy, even in men with high-risk disease (2)

GENERAL PREVENTION
- Finasteride reduced the risk of prostate cancer by 24.8% *but was associated with an increased risk of high-grade disease* and there were no differences in rates of overall survival with finasteride (3).
- Dutasteride reduces risk *without* increased risk of high-grade tumors
- 5-α-reductase inhibitors are currently not FDA approved for CaP prevention (3).
- No ↓ risk of CaP with selenium or vitamin E supplements; ↑ CaP risk with vitamin E (4)[A].

ALERT
- U.S. Preventive Services Task Force (USPSTF) recommends against PSA-based screen for prostate cancer; concluded harm of screening outweighs benefit (5)
- For men ages 55–69, the AUA panel recommends shared decision making between physician and patient regarding PSA screening (6)[B]

DIAGNOSIS

HISTORY
- Inquire about family history of CaP, symptoms of bladder outlet obstruction, and other voiding symptoms
- Anorexia and weight loss, bone pain (with metastasis), hematuria, hematospermia (rare)

PHYSICAL EXAM
If clinical suspicion (dysuria, hematuria, hematospermia) DRE to assess for prostatic masses/firmness/asymmetry

ALERT
Most patients with CaP are asymptomatic.

DIFFERENTIAL DIAGNOSIS
BPH, benign nodular prostatic growth, subacute prostatitis, prostatic intraepithelial neoplasia (PIN), prostate stones, atypical small acinar proliferation (ASAP)
- The high predictive value of ASAP for subsequent adenocarcinoma warrants repeat biopsy (1)

DIAGNOSTIC TESTS & INTERPRETATION
Initial Tests (lab, imaging)
- PSA is produced by prostatic epithelial cells
- Age/race-adjusted "normal" PSA values (ng/mL):

Age	Asians	Blacks	Whites
40–49	0–2.0	0–2.0	0–2.5
50–59	0–3.0	0–4.0	0–3.5
60–69	0–4.0	0–4.5	0–4.5
70–79	0–5.0	0–5.5	0–6.5

- Total PSA ≥4 ng/mL (sensitivity 21%, specificity 91%); 1st-time PSA >4 ng/mL alone not indication for biopsy:
  - Rectal manipulation will not significantly ↑ PSA
  - Other benign conditions can affect PSA and cause increase (infection, inflammation, normal growth)
- 5-α-reductase inhibitors decrease PSA ~50%
- Other PSA metrics used to aid in CaP diagnosis: PSA velocity, PSA doubling time, PSA density, percentage free PSA
  - Total PSA velocity: ≥0.75 ng/mL/yr increases CaP suspicion if PSA >4.0 ng/mL
  - Free PSA and age/race-adjusted PSA helpful in evaluating risk when total PSA is 4–10 ng/mL
  - Consider CaP if PSAD (PSA density) ≥0.15 or if PSA rises even while on 5-α-reductase inhibitors
- PSA/free PSA and probability of cancer:

PSA (ng/dL)	Cancer rate	% Free PSA	Cancer rate
0–2	1%	0–10%	56%
2–4	15%	10–15%	28%
4–10	25%	15–20%	16%
>10	>50%	20–25%	16%
		>25%	8%

- Abnormal DRE, PSA, PSA kinetics (i.e., velocity), all may trigger transrectal ultrasound (TRUS) guided biopsy of the prostate
- Patient-specific models to predict pathologic stage based on PSA, TRUS biopsy results, and estimated clinical stage have been validated

Test Interpretation
Small, closely packed glandular tissue, loss of basement membrane, perineural invasion, and smaller prostate size are associated with higher-grade disease.

Follow-Up Tests & Special Considerations
- If life expectancy ≤5 years and patient is asymptomatic, no further workup is needed (if high risk may consider ADT or RT in select patients) (7)
- Bone scan: If T1 and PSA >20, if T2 and PSA >10, if Gleason ≥8, T3 or T4, or symptomatic (7)
- Pelvic CT or MRI: If T3, T4, or T1–T2 with >10% nomogram indicated probability of lymph node involvement (7)
- Biopsy if suspicious nodal findings
- Alkaline phosphatase associated with bony mets

- *PCA3* (prostate cancer gene 3) urine testing used in conjunction with PSA may decrease the unnecessary repeat prostate biopsies. Using a *PCA3* cutoff of 10, the number of false-positive CaP diagnoses may be reduced by >35% (6)
- Risk categories:
  - D'Amico et al., classifies men with localized CaP into categories based on risk of biochemical recurrence (BCR) after definitive treatment: Low, intermediate, or high (8,9)
  - Must meet all 3 criteria to be low risk, any 1 criterion moves patient to a higher risk group

Risk category	Clinical stage	Serum PSA	Gleason score
Very low*	T1c	<10 ng/mL	≤6
Low	T1–T2a	<10 ng/mL	≤6
Intermediate	T2b–T2c	>10 and ≤20 ng/mL	7
High	T3a	>20 ng/mL	8–10
Very high	T3b–T4		

*Very low category also includes: PSA density <0.15 ng/mL/g, <3 prostate biopsy cores positive (<50% CaP in any core)

TREATMENT

A treatment decision should be reached after a discussion about options, risks, and benefits. Initial decisions are based on PSA, Gleason score, volume of disease, life expectancy, and patient preference.
- Active surveillance (1)[C]: Close monitoring of PSA, DRE, and repeat biopsy at regular intervals
- Prostatectomy: Retropubic, robotic-assisted laparoscopic ± pelvic lymph node dissection (PLND); nerve-sparing surgery is possible if there is no extracapsular extension
- Radiation therapy: External beam and/or brachytherapy—seed implantation
- Brachytherapy: Radioactive implants placed in prostate; popular option for early clinical stage localized to the prostate
- ADT (see next section)
- Treatment guidelines for clinically localized CaP (7):
  - Very low risk: Active surveillance (if other risk factors, consider moving to low risk)
  - Low risk: Active surveillance, external beam RT, brachytherapy, or radical prostatectomy ± PLND
  - Intermediate risk: If life expectancy <10 years: Active surveillance, RT ± short-term ADT, brachytherapy. If >10 yr radical prostatectomy ± PLND, or RT.
  - High risk: External beam radiotherapy *with* long-term ADT; external beam radiotherapy with brachytherapy ± ADT, or radical prostatectomy with PLND
- Low-volume, high-grade CaP may warrant adjuvant ADT
- Locally advanced:
  - Very high risk: RT with long-term ADT, RT with brachytherapy ± ADT, radical prostatectomy with PLND, or ADT
- Metastatic: ADT or RT with long-term ADT

MEDICATION

Medications are generally indicated for advanced, high-risk, or metastatic disease

First Line
- ADT is for patients at high risk of recurrence or those with metastatic disease who are not candidates for local therapy.

- ADT consists of 2 equally effective options (7):
  - Bilateral orchiectomy (surgical castration)
  - Gonadotropin-releasing hormone (GnRH) agonist or antagonist (medical castration)
- GnRH agonists include leuprolide or goserelin; GnRH antagonist, degarelix
- Side effects of ADT: Osteoporosis, gynecomastia, erectile dysfunction (ED), decreased libido, obesity, lipid alterations, greater risk of diabetes and cardiovascular disease; flare phenomenon (disease flare: hot flashes, fatigue) can occur owing to transient increase in testosterone levels on initiation of GnRH agonist therapy. It can be avoided by giving preceding or concurrent antiandrogen therapy for at least 7 days.

Second Line
- Combined androgen blockade with GnRH agonist and antiandrogen (e.g., bicalutamide, nilutamide, or flutamide)
- Castration-recurrent disease: Most patients develop continued disease after androgen deprivation (either castration or GnRH therapy); continued hormonal treatment may be beneficial
- Chemotherapy with a docetaxel-based regimen has shown survival benefit and is the preferred first-line chemotherapy in metastatic castration-resistant prostate cancer (CRPC). Mitoxantrone-based regimen is another option.
- Abiraterone (Zytiga): 1,000 mg/d PO given with prednisone 5 mg b.i.d. (NNT 25 for additional 4 months of overall survival) for metastatic CRPC patients who have received prior chemotherapy containing docetaxel
- Cabazitaxel is another FDA-approved medication for men with metastatic CRPC previously treated with a docetaxel regimen.
- Sipuleucel-T is an immunotherapeutic agent that can prolong overall survival.
- Bisphosphonate (zoledronic acid) every 4 weeks is recommended together with ADT or systemic chemotherapy for CRPC. This may prevent disease-related skeletal complications.

ADDITIONAL THERAPIES
- Adjuvant RT should be considered for men with ≥2 adverse features (Gleason 8-10, pT3, positive margins) (10)
- Cryoablation: Argon gas–based freezing of tissue

ONGOING CARE

FOLLOW-UP RECOMMENDATIONS
- CT/bone scan if suspected recurrence
- Prostatectomy: PSA/DRE every 6 months for 5 years; yearly thereafter; PSA >0.2 ng/mL after surgery is suggestive of recurrence
- XRT: PSA/DRE every 3 months for 1 year; every 3–6 months for 4 years; yearly thereafter; PSA ≥2 ng/mL from post-XRT nadir is suggestive of recurrence.

PROGNOSIS
- Localized disease should be curable; advanced disease has a favorable prognosis if lesions are hormone-sensitive
- 3-year CaP survival by stage: Local 100%, regional 99.1%, distant 33.1%, unstaged 79.2%
- Recurrence risk increased if extracapsular extension, seminal vesicle invasion, positive surgical margins

COMPLICATIONS
- Urinary incontinence, mild colitis, ED, radiation cystitis, and hematuria are the most common.

- Treatment options for postop ED: PDE5 inhibitors, intracavernosal injections, penile prosthesis
- Skeletal-related events due to bone metastases

REFERENCES

1. Klotz L. Active surveillance for low-risk prostate cancer. *F1000 Med Rep*. 2012;4:16.
2. Pastuszak AW, Pearlman AM, Lai WS, et al. Testosterone replacement therapy in patients with prostate cancer after radical prostatectomy. *J Urol*. 2013;190:639–644.
3. Thompson IM, Goodman PJ, Tangen CM, et al. Long-term survival of participants in the Prostate Cancer Prevention Trial. *N Engl J Med*. 2013; 369:603–610.
4. Klein EA, Thompson IM, Tangen CM, et al. Vitamin E and the risk of prostate cancer: The Selenium and Vitamin E Cancer Prevention Trial (SELECT). *JAMA*. 2011;306:1549–1556.
5. Lin K, Lipsitz R, Miller T, et al. Benefits and harms of prostate-specific antigen screening for prostate cancer: An evidence update for the U.S. Preventive Services Task Force. *Ann Intern Med*. 2008;149(3): 192–199.
6. Crawford ED, Rove KO, Trabulsi EJ, et al. Diagnostic performance of PCA3 to detect prostate cancer in men with increased prostate specific antigen: A prospective study of 1,962 cases. *J Urol*. 2012;188:1726–1731.
7. National Comprehensive Cancer Network. Clinical practice guidelines: Prostate cancer. 2012. Available at: www.nccn.org
8. Lowrance WT, Scardino PT. Predictive models for newly diagnosed prostate cancer patients. *Rev Urol*. 2009;11:117–126.
9. D'Amico AV, Whittington R, Schultz D, et al. Outcome based staging for clinically localized adenocarcinoma of the prostate. *J Urol*. 1997; 158(4):1422–1426.
10. Nomiya T, Tsuji H, Toyama S, et al. Management of high-risk prostate cancer: Radiation therapy and hormonal therapy. *Cancer Treat Rev*. 2013; 39:872–878.

CODES

ICD10
C61 Malignant neoplasm of prostate

CLINICAL PEARLS

- Prostate cancer is clinically diverse, ranging from low-risk/indolent disease to high-risk/aggressive disease.
- Most men with CaP are asymptomatic.
- The incidence of CaP is high, yet the mortality is low and a large percentage are thought to be clinically insignificant.
- The use of PSA for CaP screening is controversial and necessitates an open conversation between medical provider and patient regarding benefits/risks.
- Active surveillance is an important treatment option to consider for low-risk patients.
- The Gleason score is the most commonly used classification system for the histologic grading of CaP.
- In patients taking 5α-reductase inhibitors, must use PSA level times 2 to estimate actual PSA.

PROSTATIC HYPERPLASIA, BENIGN

David Longstroth, MD

BASICS

- Increase in number of cells (both stroma and epithelial cell lines) within prostate, ultimately increasing its size.
- As it grows in volume, the central urethra may become compressed and narrowed, causing symptoms of obstruction, which results in clinical symptoms (difficulty initiating urination, frequency, dysuria).
- May result in increased risk for upper and lower tract infections and may progress to acute renal failure, causing partial, or sometimes virtually complete, obstruction of the urethra, which interferes with the normal flow of urine.

DESCRIPTION

- Benign prostatic hyperplasia (BPH) is one of the most common diseases of older men.
- Diagnosed histologically, characterized by an increase in the total number of stromal and epithelial cells within the prostate gland
- Associated with bothersome lower urinary tract symptoms (LUTS) that affect quality of life
- Disease affects the renal, urologic, and reproductive systems

EPIDEMIOLOGY
In the US, near universal development in men; age dependent

Incidence
- No clear identifying characteristics
- Commonly involves prostate volume >30 mL and high prostate symptom score

Prevalence
From 8% in men aged 31–40; to 40–50% in men 51–60; and >80% in men >80 years

ETIOLOGY AND PATHOPHYSIOLOGY
- Older age and functional Leydig cells in testes are determinant.
- BPH is rare in men with hypogonadism onset before age 40 years not treated with androgens.
- BPH develops in the periurethral or transition zone of the prostate.
- Hyperplastic nodules of stromal and epithelial components increase glandular components.

COMMONLY ASSOCIATED CONDITIONS
- LUTS:
  - LUTS can be divided into 3 groups: Filling/Storage symptoms, voiding symptoms, and postmicturition symptoms.
    - Filling/Storage symptoms include frequency, nocturia, urgency, and urge incontinence
    - Voiding: Irritative: Frequency, urgency, dysuria, nocturia. Obstructive symptoms: Poor stream, hesitancy, terminal dribbling, incomplete voiding, overflow incontinence
    - Postmicturition: Leakage
- BPH symptoms are strong and independent risk factors for sexual dysfunction, including erectile dysfunction and ejaculatory disorders (1)[C].

Genetics
- Males who have a 1st-degree relative with BPH are at increased risk.
- Race has some influence on the risk for BPH severe enough to require surgery.
- Black men <65 years may need treatment more often than white men.
- Asians have a lower risk for nocturia, whereas risks for African American and Caucasian men are similar.

RISK FACTORS
- Increased risk of BPH with higher free prostate-specific antigen (PSA) levels, heart disease, and use of β-blockers
- Decreased risk with higher physical activity
- Conflicting data that tobacco use may lower risk of surgery for BPH symptoms
- Intact testes (BPH rare in eunuchs)
- No evidence of increased or decreased risk with smoking, alcohol, or any dietary factors
- Low androgen levels from cirrhosis/chronic alcoholism can reduce the risk of BPH.

GENERAL PREVENTION
The disease appears to be part of the aging process.

DIAGNOSIS

HISTORY
- International Prostate Symptom Score (IPSS) of LUTS:
  - Questionnaire: Over the past month, how often have you:
    - 1. Had the sensation of not emptying your bladder completely after you finished urinating?
    - 2. Had to urinate again <2 hours after you finished urinating?
    - 3. Found you stopped and started again several times when you urinated?
    - 4. Found it difficult to postpone urination?
    - 5. Had a weak urinary stream?
    - 6. Had to push or strain to begin urination?
    - 7. Been up to urinate from the time you went to bed at night until the time you got up in the morning?
    - 8. How would you feel if you were to spend the rest of your life with your current symptoms?
  - Scoring of the questionnaire:
    - Questions 1–6: No symptoms = 0 points, 1 in 5 times = 1 point, less than half = 2 points, about half = 3 points, more than half = 4 points, most of the time = 5 points
    - Question 7: No occurrence = 0 points, 1 time = 1 point, 2 times = 2 points, 3 times = 3 points, 4 times = 4 points, and 5 times or more = 5 points
    - Question 8: 0 = Delighted, 1 = Pleased, 2 = Mostly satisfied, 3 = Mixed, 4 = Mostly dissatisfied, 5 = Unhappy, 6 = Terrible
    - Symptoms are classified as mild (total score 0–7), moderate (total score 8–19), and severe (total score 20–35)

- Important to include in the history:
  - Gross hematuria
  - History of type 2 diabetes, which can cause nocturia and is a risk factor for BPH; chronically elevated glucose can cause neurogenic bladder
  - Symptoms of neurologic disease
  - Sexual dysfunction, which is correlated with LUTS
  - History of urethral trauma, urethritis, or urethral instrumentation that could lead to urethral stricture
  - Family history of BPH and prostate cancer
  - Treatment with drugs that can impair bladder function (anticholinergic drugs) or increase outflow resistance (sympathomimetic drugs)

PHYSICAL EXAM
- Digital rectal exam finding of enlarged prostate, but *size does not always correlate with symptoms*
- Percussion to detect distended bladder, particularly if postvoid
- Signs of renal failure due to obstructive uropathy (edema, pallor, pruritus, ecchymoses, nutritional deficiencies)

DIFFERENTIAL DIAGNOSIS
- Obstructive:
  - Prostate cancer
  - Urethral stricture or valves
  - Bladder neck contracture (usually secondary to prostate surgery)
  - Prostatitis
  - Inability of bladder neck or external sphincter to relax appropriately during voiding
- Neurologic:
  - Spinal cord injury
  - Stroke
  - Parkinsonism
  - Multiple sclerosis
- Medical:
  - Poorly controlled diabetes mellitus
  - Congestive heart failure (CHF)
- Pharmacologic:
  - Diuretics
  - Sympathomimetics (e.g., cold medications)
  - Anticholinergics
- Other:
  - Bladder carcinoma
  - Overactive bladder
  - Bladder calculi
  - UTI

DIAGNOSTIC TESTS & INTERPRETATION
Initial Tests (lab, imaging)
- PSA may be elevated, but usually <10 ng/mL (10 μg/L). Acute urinary retention, prostatitis, urinary tract instrumentation, or prostatic infarction may elevate PSA.
- Urinalysis: Pyuria if stones or infection present, pH changes due to chronic residual urine
- Urine culture positive (sometimes due to chronic residual urine)
- BUN and creatinine (if concerns for uremia)
- Postvoid residual to detect obstruction/distended bladder

Follow-Up Tests & Special Considerations
- Uroflow: Volume voided per unit time (peak flow <10 mL/s is abnormal)
- Postvoid residual: Either with catheterization or bladder ultrasound (>100 mL demonstrates incomplete emptying)

- Transrectal ultrasound: Assessment of gland size; not necessary in the routine evaluation
- Abdominal ultrasound: Can demonstrate increased postvoid residual or hydronephrosis; not necessary in the routine evaluation

Geriatric Considerations
Drugs to avoid: Anticholinergics, antihistamines, sympathomimetics, tricyclic antidepressants, narcotics, and skeletal muscle relaxants

Diagnostic Procedures/Other
- Pressure-flow studies (urine flow vs. voiding pressures):
  - Best test to determine etiology of voiding symptoms
  - Obstructive pattern shows high voiding pressures with low flow rate
- Cystoscopy:
  - Demonstrates presence, configuration, cause (stricture, stone), and site of obstructive tissue
  - May help determine best minimally invasive therapeutic option
  - Not recommended in initial evaluation unless other factors, such as hematuria, are present

Test Interpretation
Confirmation obtained by biopsy, resection, or surgical removal

TREATMENT

GENERAL MEASURES
- Patients with urinary retention require bladder drainage.
- If catheterization is difficult, consider coude catheter or flexible cystoscopy.
- With postobstructive diuresis, monitor electrolytes.
- Avoid prolonged periods of not voiding.

MEDICATION
The American Urological Association (AUA) recommends watchful waiting for patients without bothersome LUTS who have not developed a serious complication.

First Line
- α-adrenergic antagonists more effective than other methods alone (2)[A]:
  - Nonselective, reduce prostatic smooth muscle tone, improving urinary flow (3):
    - Terazosin (Hytrin): 1–10 mg/d PO (4)[A]
    - Doxazosin (Cardura): 1–8 mg/d PO
  - Selective, may produce fewer side effects; generally more expensive:
    - Tamsulosin (Flomax): 0.4 mg/d PO (5)[A]
    - Alfuzosin (Uroxatral): 10 mg/d PO
- 5-α-reductase inhibitors reduce prostatic volume (useful if prostatic enlargement) (6)[A]:
  - Finasteride (Proscar): 5 mg/d PO
  - Dutasteride (Avodart): 0.5 mg/d PO
  - Also useful in controlling prostatic bleeding
- Combination therapy of α-blocker plus 5-α-reductase inhibitor is superior to monotherapy when used for very large prostates and evaluated over at least 4.5 years (7):
  - Dutasteride and tamsulosin combination known as Jalyn
- Contraindications:
  - α-blockers can cause orthostatic hypotension; less risk with tamsulosin and alfuzosin
  - See specific recommendations for α-blocker use with phosphodiesterase type-5 inhibitors (for erectile dysfunction).

ISSUES FOR REFERRAL
- Recurrent UTIs
- Hematuria
- Failure to respond to medical therapy
- Bladder stones

SURGERY/OTHER PROCEDURES
- Indications for surgery:
  - Urinary retention due to prostatic obstruction, recurrent
  - Intractable symptoms due to prostatic obstruction AUA score >8 and symptoms
  - Obstructive uropathy (renal insufficiency)
  - Recurrent or persistent UTIs due to prostatic obstruction
  - Recurrent gross hematuria due to enlarged prostate
  - Bladder calculi
- Surgical procedures:
  - Transurethral resection of the prostate (TURP): Gold standard
  - Open prostatectomy: Treatment of choice for patients with extremely large prostates (>100 g)
  - Transurethral incision of the prostate: Treatment of choice for men with obstruction and small prostates
  - Transurethral laser ablation: Holmium laser ablation of the tissue; useful in patients on anticoagulant therapy
  - Transurethral needle ablation: Office-based, minimally invasive approach usually used with small prostates
  - Transurethral microwave thermotherapy: Office-based minimally invasive approach usually used with small prostates
  - Transurethral laser resection/enucleation
  - UroLume stent placement: Only for those too ill for other surgical procedures
- Complications of TURP:
  - Bleeding can be significant.
  - TUR syndrome: Hyponatremia secondary to absorption of hypotonic irrigant
  - Retrograde ejaculation
  - Urinary incontinence

COMPLEMENTARY AND ALTERNATIVE MEDICINE
Saw palmetto (Serenoa repens) did not improve LUTS in a Cochrane review (8)[A].

ONGOING CARE

FOLLOW-UP RECOMMENDATIONS
The patient is more likely to void after surgery or illness when able to stand over toilet.

Patient Monitoring
- Symptom index (IPSS) monitored every 3–12 months
- Digital rectal exam yearly
- PSA yearly: Should not be checked while patient is in retention, recently catheterized, or within a week of any surgical procedure to the prostate
- Consider monitoring postvoid residual, if elevated

DIET
Avoid large boluses of oral or IV fluids or alcohol intake

PATIENT EDUCATION
National Kidney and Urologic Diseases Information Clearinghouse, Box NKUDIC, Bethesda, MD 20893; 301-468-6345

PROGNOSIS
- Symptoms improve or stabilize in 70–80% of patients.
- 25% of men with LUTS will have persistent storage symptoms after prostatectomy.
- Of men with BPH, 11–33% have occult prostate cancer.

COMPLICATIONS
- Urinary retention (acute or chronic)
- Bladder stones
- Prostatitis
- Renal failure
- Hematuria

REFERENCES
1. Rosen R, Altwein J, Boyle P. Lower urinary tract symptoms and male sexual dysfunction: The multinational survey of the aging male (MSAM-7). Eur Urol. 2003;44:637–649.
2. Rich KT. FPIN's clinical inquiries. Medical treatment of benign prostatic hyperplasia. Am Fam Physician. 2008;77:665–666.
3. Neal RH, Keister D. What's best for your patient with BPH? J Fam Pract. 2009;58:241–247.
4. Wilt TJ. Terazosin for benign prostatic hyperplasia. Cochrane Database Syst Rev. 2002;4:CD003851.
5. Wilt TJ. Tamsulosin for benign prostatic hyperplasia. Cochrane Database Syst Rev. 2003;1:CD002081.
6. AUA Guidelines: Guideline on the Management of Benign Prostatic Hyperplasia (BPH): Updated 2006. Available at: www.AUAnet.org
7. Hollingsworth JM, Wei JT. Does the combination of an alpha1-adrenergic antagonist with a 5alpha-reductase inhibitor improve urinary symptoms more than either monotherapy? Curr Opin Urol. 2010;20:1–6.
8. Tacklind J, MacDonald R, Rutks I, et al. Serenoa repens for benign prostatic hyperplasia. Cochrane Database Syst Rev. 2009;2:CD001423.

CODES

ICD10
- N40.0 Enlarged prostate without lower urinary tract symptoms
- N40.1 Enlarged prostate with lower urinary tract symptoms

CLINICAL PEARLS
- Although medical therapy has changed the management of BPH, it has only delayed the need for TURP by 10–15 years, not eliminated it.
- Urinary retention, obstructive uropathy, recurrent UTIs, bladder calculi, and recurrent hematuria are indications for surgical management of BPH.
- Indications for referral include recurrent UTIs, elevated PSA, failure of medical therapy, hematuria, retention, and patient desire.

PROSTATITIS

Anne Newbold, DO

 BASICS

DESCRIPTION

- Inflammatory or painful condition affecting the prostate gland; variety of etiologies
- National Institutes of Health's (NIH) prostatitis classification:
  - Class I: Acute bacterial prostatitis: Febrile illness with perineal pain, dysuria, and obstructive symptoms
  - Class II: Chronic bacterial prostatitis: Chronic or recurrent bacterial infection with pain and voiding disturbances
  - Class III: Chronic abacterial prostatitis/chronic pelvic pain syndrome:
    - Inflammatory (subtype IIIa): Chronic symptoms and significant inflammatory cells in prostatic secretions, urine, or semen. No bacterial infection
    - Noninflammatory (subtype IIIb): Chronic symptoms without evidence of inflammation or bacterial infection. Insignificant number of inflammatory cells
  - Class IV: Asymptomatic inflammatory prostatitis (NIH class IV): Incidental finding during prostate biopsy for infertility, cancer workup.
- System(s) affected: Renal/Urologic; Reproductive

EPIDEMIOLOGY

Incidence

- 2 million cases annually in the US
- Predominant age: 30–50 years, sexually active; chronic more common in those >50
- Bacterial prostatitis occurs more frequently in patients with HIV

Prevalence

2.2–9.7% of male population (1)

ETIOLOGY AND PATHOPHYSIOLOGY

- Extension of UTI
- May occur following manipulation/biopsy of prostate or urethra
- Ascending infection through urethra
- Infectious: NIH classes I and II:
  - Aerobic gram-negative bacteria (e.g., *E. coli*, *Klebsiella*, *Proteus*, *Pseudomonas*, *N. gonorrhoeae*, *B. pseudomallei*)
  - Miscellaneous: *C. trachomatis*, Ureaplasma, trichomoniasis
  - Gram-positive bacteria (*S. faecalis*, *S. aureus*)
  - Organisms suspected but unproven (*S. epidermidis*, S. micrococci, non–group D Streptococcus, diphtheroids)
  - Uncommon: *M. tuberculosis*, parasitic, mycoses (blastomycosis, coccidioidomycosis, cryptococcus, histoplasmosis, paracoccidioidomycosis, candidiasis)
- Nonbacterial: Cause unknown: Leading theory suggests nonrelaxation (spasm) of the internal urinary sphincter and pelvic floor striated muscles leading to increased prostatic urethral pressure and intraprostatic urinary reflux.

RISK FACTORS

- Age >50 years
- Prostate biopsy (especially in patients with prior exposure to quinolones) (2)
- Prostatic calculi
- UTI
- Trauma (e.g., bicycle, horseback riding)
- Dehydration
- Sexual abstinence
- Chronic indwelling catheter
- Intermittent catheterization
- HIV infection
- Urethral stricture
- Cystoscopy
- Urethral dilatation
- Transurethral resection of prostate

GENERAL PREVENTION

Antibiotic prophylaxis and enema prior to prostatic biopsy

COMMONLY ASSOCIATED CONDITIONS

- Prostatic hypertrophy
- Cystitis
- Urethritis
- Pyelonephritis
- Sexual dysfunction

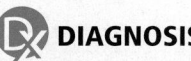 **DIAGNOSIS**

HISTORY

- Acute prostatitis (NIH class I):
  - Fever, chills, malaise
  - Low back pain, myalgias
  - Prostatodynia, perineal pain
  - Obstructive voiding symptoms
  - Frequency, urgency, dysuria, nocturia
- Chronic prostatitis (NIH classes II and III):
  - Prostatodynia, perineal pain
  - Dysuria, irritative voiding
  - Lower abdominal pain
  - Low back, scrotal, and/or penile pain
  - Pain on ejaculation
  - Hematospermia

PHYSICAL EXAM

- Very tender, boggy prostate on rectal exam
- Prostate may be warm, swollen, firm, or irregular

ALERT

Avoid massage of the prostate in acute bacterial prostatitis; may induce iatrogenic bacteremia

DIFFERENTIAL DIAGNOSIS

- Cystitis (bacterial, interstitial)
- Urethritis
- Pyelonephritis
- Malignancy
- Obstructive calculus
- Foreign body
- Acute urinary retention

DIAGNOSTIC TESTS & INTERPRETATION

Initial Tests (lab, imaging)

- Suspected acute prostatitis (NIH class I):
  - Urinalysis (UA), urine and blood cultures, urine Gram stain
  - CBC with differential
- Suspected chronic bacterial prostatitis or abacterial prostatitis (NIH class II or III):
  - Fractional urine exam (4-glass test) (3)[A]:
    - VB1 (voided bladder 1): Initial 10 mL urine from urethra
    - VB2: Next 200 mL discarded; then midstream urine from bladder
    - EPS: Expressed prostate secretion after prostate massage
    - VB3: Urine *after* prostate massage
  - Post-VB3 semen culture increases sensitivity and specificity (3)[A]
  - Many clinicians employ 2-glass test (VB2 and VB3) only
  - Specimen handling:
    - UA, culture, sensitivities, Gram stain on all samples
    - pH of EPS
    - Bacterial antigen-specific IgA and IgG levels in EPS
    - Wet mount of EPS
  - Interpretation:
    - 10–15 WBCs per high-powered field in VB3 suggest bacterial prostatitis
    - Macrophages containing fat (oval bodies) suggest bacterial prostatitis
    - A positive culture in EPS, VB3, or post a VB3 semen sample, but not VB1 or VB2, is diagnostic of bacterial prostatitis
    - In acute bacterial prostatitis, serum and EPS fluid bacterial antigen-specific IgA and IgG can be detected immediately after the onset of the infection. Level declines over 6–12 months after successful antibiotic therapy.
    - Bacteria count is less in chronic prostatitis.
    - In chronic bacterial prostatitis, no serum IgG elevation is seen, whereas EPS fluid IgA and IgG levels are increased. With antibiotic therapy, IgG levels return to normal in several months, but IgA levels remain elevated for 2 years.
    - Prostatic fluid is alkaline in chronic bacterial prostatitis.
    - Inflammatory cells (WBCs) with a negative culture (although false-negative cultures are not uncommon) suggest abacterial prostatitis.
    - No abnormal findings with chronic prostatitis without inflammation (this misnomer refers to patients with symptoms such as perineal pain, ejaculatory pain, and lower abdominal pain but no inflammatory changes on lab studies).
    - Prostate-specific antigen (PSA) level is increased with acute prostatitis (do not order until at least 1 month after prostatitis is treated).
- Drugs that may alter lab results: Antibiotics
- Imaging not required in most cases
- CT or MRI if malignancy or abscess suspected
- Transrectal US if prostatic calculi or abscess suspected

Follow-Up Tests & Special Considerations

- Acute bacterial: Urinalysis and culture 30 days after initiating treatment
- Chronic bacterial: Urinalysis and culture every 30 days (may take several months of treatment to clear)

Diagnostic Procedures/Other
- Needle biopsy or aspiration for culture
- Urodynamic testing (prostatodynia)
- Cystoscopy (in persistent nonbacterial prostatitis to rule out bladder cancer, interstitial cystitis)

 ## TREATMENT
GENERAL MEASURES
- Analgesics/Antipyretics/Stool softeners
- Hydration
- Sitz baths to relieve pain and spasm
- Suprapubic catheter for urinary retention
- Anxiolytics, antidepressants

MEDICATION
First Line
- Acute bacterial (outpatient) (4)[A]:
  – Fluoroquinolone (ciprofloxacin 500 mg PO q12h or levofloxacin 500 mg PO once daily) × 2–4 weeks or
  – Trimethoprim-sulfamethoxazole 1 DS tab PO q12h × 2–4 weeks or
  – If gram-positive cocci are seen in initial urine Gram stain, start with amoxicillin 500 mg PO q8h. Adjust antibiotics once culture and sensitivities report is available.
  – Local sensitivity pattern should guide therapy.
  – Ceftriaxone 250 mg IM or cefixime 400 mg PO × 1 dose plus doxycycline 100 mg PO q12h or azithromycin 500 mg PO once daily for 2 weeks if at risk for sexually transmitted disease (STD) pathogens
- Acute bacterial (inpatient):
  – Ampicillin 1–3 g IV divided q6h or fluoroquinolone (ciprofloxacin 400 mg IV q12h or levofloxacin 750 mg q24h) plus aminoglycoside, gentamicin 2 mg/kg IV loading dose, 1.7 mg/kg IV q8h maintenance; begin oral therapy after afebrile for 24–48 hours
- Chronic bacterial (NIH class II) (5)[B]:
  – Fluoroquinolone: levofloxacin 500 mg PO once daily for 4 weeks (6,7)[A], or ciprofloxacin 500 mg PO q12h for 4–12 weeks
  – Combination therapy with azithromycin may help to eradicate unusual pathogens
  – Anti-inflammatory agents for pain symptoms and α-adrenergic receptor antagonists for urinary symptoms
- Chronic abacterial prostatitis (NIH class III):
  – No universally effective treatment
  – Treatment choice is usually by trial and error (8):
    ○ α-Blockers, antibiotics, and combinations of these therapies achieve greatest improvement in clinical symptom scores (9)[A].
    ○ α-Blockers better than placebo in some trials
    ○ Tamsulosin 0.2 mg PO once daily at bedtime for at least 6 months. Continue if there is a response (10)[A].
- Contraindications: Drug allergies
- Precautions:
  – Renal disease
  – Hepatic disease
  – Glucose-6-phosphate dehydrogenase deficiency may manifest with sulfonamides or NSAIDs
  – Significant possible interactions: Fluoroquinolones, magnesium/aluminum antacids, theophylline, probenecid, NSAIDs, warfarin

Second Line
- Piperacillin or ticarcillin with aminoglycoside, erythromycin, tetracycline, cephalexin, fluoroquinolones, dicloxacillin, nafcillin IV, vancomycin IV
- Finasteride (in patients >45, category IIIa inflammatory chronic prostatitis/chronic pelvic pain syndrome, and enlarged prostate gland)
- Nonbacterial: May benefit from erythromycin, doxycycline, trimethoprim-sulfamethoxazole

ISSUES FOR REFERRAL
Urology referral for surgical drainage if an abscess persists after ≥1 week of therapy, persistent symptoms, hematuria, or elevated PSA

ADDITIONAL THERAPIES
Psychotherapy if sexual dysfunction

SURGERY/OTHER PROCEDURES
Surgical resection for intractable chronic disease or to drain an abscess

COMPLEMENTARY AND ALTERNATIVE MEDICINE
- Neuromodulation, acupuncture, heat therapy; limited data to support
- Myofascial release (11)

IN-PATIENT CONSIDERATIONS
Admission Criteria/Initial Stabilization
- Proven or suspected abscess
- Unstable vital signs (sepsis)
- Immunocompromised

 ## ONGOING CARE
FOLLOW-UP RECOMMENDATIONS
- Most improve in 3–4 weeks
- Consider prostatic abscess in patients who do not respond well to therapy

Patient Monitoring
NIH Chronic Prostatitis Symptom Index (www2.niddk.nih.gov): 13 items tabulated into 3 domain scores:
- Pain
- Urinary symptoms
- Quality of life

PROGNOSIS
- Often prolonged and difficult to cure; 55–97% cure rate depending on population and drug used
- 20% have reinfection or persistent infection

COMPLICATIONS
- Prostatic abscess (common in HIV-infected)
- Gram-negative sepsis, bacteremia
- Urinary retention
- Epididymitis
- Chronic bacterial prostatitis (with acute prostatitis)
- Metastatic infection (spinal, sacroiliac)

REFERENCES
1. Krieger, JN, Lee SW, Jeon J, et al. Epidemiology of prostatitis. Int J Antimicrob Agents. 2008;31 (Suppl 1):S85–S90.
2. Mosharafa AA, Torky MH, Said WM, et al. Rising incidence of acute prostatitis following prostate biopsy: Fluoroquinolone resistance and exposure is a significant risk factor. Urology. 2011;78:511–514.
3. Magri V, Wagenlehner FM, Montanari E, et al. Semen analysis in chronic bacterial prostatitis: Diagnostic and therapeutic implications. Asian J Androl. 2009;11:461–477.
4. Lipsky BA, Byren I, Hoey CT, et al. Treatment of bacterial prostatitis. Clin Infect Dis. 2010;50:1641–1652.
5. Murphy AB, Macejko A, Taylor A, et al. Chronic prostatitis: Management strategies. Drugs. 2009;69:71–84.
6. Paglia M, Peterson J, Fisher AC, et al. Safety and efficacy of levofloxacin 750 mg for 2 weeks or 3 weeks compared with levofloxacin 500 mg for 4 weeks in treating chronic bacterial prostatitis. Curr Med Res Opin. 2010;26:1433–1441.
7. Naber KG, Roscher K, Botto H, et al. Oral levofloxacin 500 mg once daily in the treatment of chronic bacterial prostatitis. Int J Antimicrob Agents. 2008;32:145–153.
8. McNaughton CM, Mac Donald R, Wilt T. Interventions for abacterial prostatitis. Cochrane Database Sys Rev. 2006;4:CD004124.
9. Anothaisintawee T, Attia J, Nickel JC, et al. Management of chronic prostatitis/chronic pelvic pain syndrome: A systematic review and network meta-analysis. JAMA. 2011;305:78–86.
10. Chen Y, Wu X, Liu J, et al. Effects of a 6-month course of tamsulosin for chronic prostatitis/chronic pelvic pain syndrome: A multicenter, randomized trial. World J Urol. 2011;29:381–385.
11. Anderson RU, Wise D, Sawyer T, et al. 6-day intensive treatment protocol for refractory chronic prostatitis/chronic pelvic pain syndrome using myofascial release and paradoxical relaxation training. J Urol. 2011;185:1294–1299.

 ## SEE ALSO
- Prostate Cancer; Prostatic Hyperplasia Benign; Urinary Tract Infection in Males
- Algorithm: Hematuria

CODES
ICD10
- N41.0 Acute prostatitis
- N41.1 Chronic prostatitis
- N41.9 Inflammatory disease of prostate, unspecified

CLINICAL PEARLS
- Prostatic massage is contraindicated in acute prostatitis.
- Antibiotic therapy is not proven to be effective in chronic abacterial prostatitis (NIH class III).
- At least 30 days of antibiotic therapy is required for acute prostatitis.

PROTEIN C DEFICIENCY

Maissaa Janbain, MD • Rebecca Kruse-Jarres, MD, MPH

 BASICS

DESCRIPTION
- Protein C is a vitamin K–dependent factor made by the liver that becomes activated when thrombin binds to the endothelial receptor thrombomodulin.
- Activated protein C, with protein S as a cofactor, inactivates factors Va and VIIIa.
- Patients with protein C deficiency have a thrombotic disorder that primarily affects the venous system, but can also affect the arterial system.
- System(s) affected: Cardiovascular; Hemic/Lymphatic/Immunologic; Pulmonary

EPIDEMIOLOGY
Prevalence
- 0.3% of normal individuals
- 4–5% of persons with venous thrombosis (VT)
- Predominant age: Mean age of 1st thrombosis is 45 years
- Predominant sex: Male = Female

ETIOLOGY AND PATHOPHYSIOLOGY
- Polymorphisms in the promoter region of the protein C gene can affect antigen levels. At least 150 mutations have been described in the protein C gene that can lead to functional deficiency.
- Acquired protein C deficiency can occur with liver disease, acute respiratory distress syndrome (ARDS), disseminated intravascular coagulopathy (DIC), chemotherapy with L-asparaginase, 5-fluorouracil (5-FU), methotrexate, and cyclophosphamide, as well as postoperative state and severe infections, especially meningococcemia. Also, rare patients can develop inhibitors to activated protein C. Neonates have lower levels of protein C than adults.

Genetics
Patients heterozygous for protein C deficiency who start warfarin without concomitant heparin can develop warfarin-induced skin necrosis because the half-life of other vitamin K–dependent clotting factors, prothrombin, factor IX, and factor X is much longer than that of protein C (4–8 hours). These patients develop extremely low levels of protein C and subsequently increased thrombin generation, leading to necrosis of the skin over central areas of the body such as the breast, abdomen, buttocks, and genitalia (1)[A].

GENERAL PREVENTION
Since protein C deficiency is a congenital disease, there are no preventive measures.

COMMONLY ASSOCIATED CONDITIONS
- Deep and superficial venous thrombosis, often spontaneous
- Up to 50% of homozygotes will have thrombosis
- Homozygosity is associated with catastrophic thrombotic complications at birth (e.g., purpura fulminans)
- Sites of thrombosis can be unusual, including the mesentery and cerebral veins, especially when combined with other risk factors like oral contraceptives.
- Arterial thrombosis is rare.
- Skin necrosis can be seen in patients on warfarin.

 DIAGNOSIS

HISTORY
- Venous thrombosis at <40 years without another etiology
- Thrombosis in unusual locations (e.g., mesentery, sagittal sinus, portal vein)
- Family history of thrombosis or spontaneous abortion

PHYSICAL EXAM
Normal

DIFFERENTIAL DIAGNOSIS
- Factor V Leiden (causes resistance to activated protein C, not a deficiency of protein C)
- Protein S deficiency
- Antithrombin deficiency
- Dysfibrinogenemia
- Dysplasminogenemia
- Homocystinemia
- Prothrombin 20210 mutation
- Elevated factor VIII levels

DIAGNOSTIC TESTS & INTERPRETATION
Initial Tests (lab, imaging)
- For evaluation of new clot in patient at risk (see "History"): CBC with peripheral smear, PT/INR, aPTT, thrombin time, lupus anticoagulant, antiphospholipid antibodies, factor VIII, anticardiolipin antibody, anti-β_2-glycoprotein I antibody, activated protein C resistance, protein S antigen and resistance, antithrombin III assay, fibrinogen, factor V Leiden, prothrombin G20210A, homocysteine
- Protein C activity assay using a snake venom protease to activate protein C
- Immunoassay for quantitative assessment of protein C level

- Drugs that may alter lab results:
  - Oral contraceptives can raise protein C levels.
  - Warfarin reduces protein C levels.
  - Patients should be off warfarin for 2–3 weeks before reliable testing (2)[C].
- Disorders that may alter lab results:
  - Liver disease reduces protein C levels.
  - Acute thrombosis can lower protein C levels. Repeat confirmatory test of low protein C level at a separate time is advisable. If a normal level of protein C is obtained at presentation, then deficiency can be excluded.

 TREATMENT

Treat active thrombosis; follow up.

GENERAL MEASURES
- Routine anticoagulation for asymptomatic patients with protein C deficiency is not recommended (1)[A].
- Anticoagulation for 6–12 months is recommended for patients with protein C deficiency and a 1st thrombosis.
- Some argue for lifetime anticoagulation; data are limited.
- Anticoagulation for life is indicated for patients with protein C deficiency and recurrent thromboses.

- The role of family screening for protein C deficiency is unclear because most patients with this mutation do not have thrombosis. Screening should be considered for women considering using oral contraceptives or pregnancy and who have a family history of protein C deficiency (3)[B].
- Treatment with low-molecular-weight heparin (LMWH) is recommended over unfractionated heparin, unless the patient has severe renal failure (4)[B].
- Treat as outpatient, if possible (4)[B].
- Initiate warfarin together with heparin on the first treatment day and discontinue heparin after 5 days and when INR >2 (4)[A].

- For pregnant women with no prior history of venous thromboembolism (VTE), antepartum and postpartum clinical vigilance is suggested. Postpartum prophylaxis for 6 weeks with prophylactic- or intermediate-dose LMWH is reserved only for patients with positive family history of VTE (Grade 2C) (4).

MEDICATION
First Line

- LMWH (1)[A]: Continue until therapeutic on warfarin and for at least 5 additional days:
  - Enoxaparin (Lovenox) 1 mg/kg SC b.i.d.
- Alternatively, enoxaparin 1.5 mg/kg/d SC, which is slightly less effective. Continue until therapeutic on warfarin and for at least 5 additional days:
  - Fondaparinux (Arixtra) 7.5 mg/d SC
  - Tinzaparin (Innohep): 175 anti-Xa IU/kg/d SC
  - Dalteparin (Fragmin) 200 U/kg/d
- Oral anticoagulant: Warfarin (Coumadin), per the most recent guidelines, 10 mg/d PO for 2 doses, then adjusted to an INR of 2–3 for at least 3–6 months (1)[A],(4)
- Contraindications:
  - Active bleeding precludes anticoagulation; risk of bleeding is a relative contraindication to long-term anticoagulation.
  - Warfarin is contraindicated in patients with a prior history of warfarin-induced skin necrosis
- Precautions:
  - Observe patient for signs of embolization, further thrombosis, or bleeding
  - Avoid IM injections
  - Periodically check stool and urine for occult blood; monitor CBC, including platelets
  - Heparin: Thrombocytopenia and/or paradoxical thrombosis with thrombocytopenia
  - Warfarin: Necrotic skin lesions (typically breasts, thighs, and buttocks)
  - LMWH: Adjust dose in renal insufficiency
- Significant possible interactions:
  - Agents that intensify the response to oral anticoagulants: Alcohol, allopurinol, amiodarone, anabolic steroids, androgens, many antimicrobials, cimetidine, chloral hydrate, disulfiram, all NSAIDs, sulfinpyrazone, tamoxifen, thyroid hormone, vitamin E, ranitidine, salicylates, acetaminophen
  - Agents that diminish the response to oral anticoagulants: Aminoglutethimide, antacids, barbiturates, carbamazepine, cholestyramine, diuretics, griseofulvin, rifampin, oral contraceptives

Second Line
- Heparin 80 mg/kg IV bolus followed by 18 mg/kg/h; adjust dose depending on PPT.
- In patients requiring large daily doses of heparin, measure an anti-Xa level for dose guidance
- Alternatively, and for outpatients, unfractionated heparin can be given at 333 U/kg then 250 U/kg SC, without monitoring (4)[C].

ISSUES FOR REFERRAL
Patients with suspected protein C deficiency should be seen by a hematologist.

SURGERY/OTHER PROCEDURES
- Anticoagulation must be held for surgical interventions.
- In patients with acute proximal deep vein thrombosis (DVT) of the leg *and* an absolute contraindication to anticoagulation, IVC filters are recommended; otherwise the use of an inferior vena cava filter in addition to anticoagulants is not recommended in most patients with acute DVT of the leg (Grade 1B) (4).

IN-PATIENT CONSIDERATIONS
Admission Criteria/Initial Stabilization
- Life-threatening VT
- Significant bleeding while on anticoagulant therapy

Nursing
Look for signs of bleeding while on anticoagulation therapy

 ONGOING CARE

FOLLOW-UP RECOMMENDATIONS
Patient Monitoring
- Warfarin requires periodic (monthly after initial stabilization) monitoring of the INR to maintain a range of 2–3.
- LMWH is the treatment of choice in pregnancy. Periodic monitoring with anti-Xa levels is recommended in these patients.

DIET
Unrestricted

PATIENT EDUCATION
- Patients should be educated about use of oral anticoagulant therapy if taking such.
- Avoid NSAIDs while on warfarin

PROGNOSIS
- When compared with normal individuals, persons with protein C deficiency have normal life spans.
- By age 45, 50% of the people heterozygous for protein C deficiency will have VT; half will be spontaneous.

COMPLICATIONS
Recurrent thrombosis (requires indefinite anticoagulation)

REFERENCES

1. Bick RL. Prothrombin G20210A mutation, antithrombin, heparin cofactor II, protein C, and protein S defects. *Hematol Oncol Clin North Am*. 2003;17:9–36.
2. Moll S. Thrombophilias—practical implications and testing caveats. *J Thromb Thrombolysis*. 2006;21:7–15.
3. Langlois NJ, Wells PS. Risk of venous thromboembolism in relatives of symptomatic probands with thrombophilia: A systematic review. *Thromb Haemost*. 2003;90:17–26.
4. Guyatt GH, Akl EA, Crowther M, et al. Executive summary: Antithrombotic therapy and prevention of thrombosis, 9th ed: American College of Chest Physicians Evidence-Based Clinical Practice Guidelines. *Chest*. 2012;141:7S–47S.

 CODES

ICD10
D68.59 Other primary thrombophilia

CLINICAL PEARLS
- Asymptomatic patients with protein C deficiency do not need prophylactic anticoagulation because the risk of thrombosis is low.
- Patients with protein C deficiency who have DVT should be anticoagulated for at least 6 months.

PROTEIN S DEFICIENCY

Maissaa Janbain, MD • Rebecca Kruse-Jarres, MD, MPH

BASICS

DESCRIPTION
- Protein S is a vitamin K–dependent factor made principally by the liver that acts as a cofactor for protein C.
- Protein C becomes activated when thrombin binds to the endothelial receptor, thrombomodulin.
- Activated protein C, with protein S as a cofactor, inactivates clotting factors Va and VIIIa, and it enhances fibrinolysis.
- Protein S is also able to directly inhibit factors Va, VIIa, and Xa independently of activated protein C.
- Patients with protein S deficiency have a thrombotic disorder that primarily affects the venous system.
- System(s) affected: Cardiovascular; Hematologic/Lymphatic/Immunologic; Pulmonary

EPIDEMIOLOGY
Incidence
- Predominant age: Mean age of 1st thrombosis is the 2nd decade.
- Predominant sex: Male = Female

Prevalence
- 0.3% of normal individuals
- Found in 3% of persons with VT

ETIOLOGY AND PATHOPHYSIOLOGY
- More than 131 mutations in the protein S gene leading to an inherited protein S deficiency have been described. Protein S reversibly binds to the C4b-binding protein. Only the free form acts as a cofactor for activated protein C. This leads to conditions in which free protein S is low, but total protein S is normal. These individuals are prone to thrombosis.
- Acquired protein S deficiency from decreased free protein S can occur during pregnancy; in patients taking oral contraceptives or warfarin; and in DIC, liver disease, nephrotic syndrome, inflammation, L-asparaginase chemotherapy, and acute thrombosis.
- Transient autoantibodies can develop to protein S in patients with acute varicella (1)[C].

Genetics
Autosomal dominant. Heterozygotes have an odds ratio of venous thrombosis (VT) of 1.6–11.5. Arterial thrombosis is more frequent in patients with protein S deficiency who smoke. Homozygotes can have a fulminant thrombotic event in infancy, termed neonatal purpura fulminans. Homozygosity or compound heterozygosity, if untreated, is usually incompatible with adult life.

RISK FACTORS
- Oral contraceptives, pregnancy, and the use of hormone replacement therapy (HRT) increase the risk of VT in patients with protein S deficiency (2)[A].
- Patients with protein S deficiency and another prothrombotic state, such as factor V Leiden, have further increased rates of thrombosis (2)[A].
- Patients heterozygous for protein S deficiency who are begun warfarin without concomitant heparin can develop warfarin-induced skin necrosis because the half-life of other vitamin K–dependent clotting factors (e.g., prothrombin, factor IX, and factor X) is much longer than the anticoagulant protein S (4–8 hours), leading to a transient hypercoagulable state when protein S becomes depleted. These patients develop extremely low levels of protein S and develop necrosis of the skin over central areas of the body such as the breast, abdomen, buttocks, and genitalia (2)[A].

Pregnancy Considerations
Increased thrombotic risk in patients with protein C deficiency

GENERAL PREVENTION
Since protein S deficiency is a congenital disease, there are no preventive measures.

COMMONLY ASSOCIATED CONDITIONS
- Deep and superficial VT, often spontaneous
- Up to 50% of homozygotes will have thrombosis.
- Homozygosity is associated with catastrophic thrombotic complications at birth: Neonatal purpura fulminans
- Sites of thrombosis can be unusual, including the mesentery and cerebral and axillary veins.
- Arterial thrombosis is rare, but reported in several case reports.
- Skin necrosis can be seen in patients on warfarin.

DIAGNOSIS

HISTORY
Order testing for patients with VT at age <40 without another etiology; thrombosis in unusual locations (e.g., mesentery, sagittal sinus, portal vein) with a family history of thrombosis or spontaneous abortion.

PHYSICAL EXAM
Normal

DIFFERENTIAL DIAGNOSIS
- Factor V Leiden
- Protein C deficiency
- Antithrombin deficiency
- Dysfibrinogenemia
- Dysplasminogenemia
- Homocystinemia
- Prothrombin 20210 mutation
- Elevated factor VIII levels

DIAGNOSTIC TESTS & INTERPRETATION
Initial Tests (lab, imaging)
- For evaluation of a new clot in patient at risk: CBC with peripheral smear, PT/INR, aPTT, thrombin time, lupus anticoagulant, antiphospholipid antibodies, factor VIII, anticardiolipin antibody, anti-β_2-glycoprotein I antibody, activated protein C resistance, protein S antigen and resistance, antithrombin III assay, fibrinogen, factor V Leiden, prothrombin G20210A, homocysteine
- Protein S activity assay (mainly after obtaining activated protein C [APC] resistance)
- Immunoassay for quantitative assessment of total and free protein S levels
- Disorders that may alter lab results: Liver disease and pregnancy reduce protein S levels.
- Total protein S levels are markedly decreased in newborns and young infants; use age-adjusted norms.

TREATMENT

GENERAL MEASURES
- Routine anticoagulation for asymptomatic patients with protein S deficiency is not recommended (2)[A].
- Anticoagulation for 6–12 months is recommended for patients with protein S deficiency and a 1st thrombosis.
- Some argue for lifetime anticoagulation; data are limited.
- Anticoagulation for life is indicated for patients with protein S deficiency and recurrent thromboses.
- The role of family screening for protein S deficiency is unclear because most patients with this mutation do not have thrombosis. Screening should be considered for women considering using oral contraceptives or pregnancy, and who have a family history of protein S deficiency (3)[B].
- Treatment with low-molecular-weight heparin (LMWH) is recommended over unfractionated heparin, unless the patient has severe renal failure (4)[B]
- Treat as outpatient, if possible (4)[B]
- Initiate warfarin together with heparin on the 1st treatment day and discontinue heparin after a minimum of 5 days and when INR >2 (4)[A].
- For pregnant women with no prior history of venous thromboembolism (VTE), antepartum and postpartum clinical vigilance is suggested. Postpartum prophylaxis is reserved for patients with positive family history only; in that case, prophylactic- or intermediate-dose LMWH for 6 weeks is suggested (Grade 2C) (4).

MEDICATION
First Line

- LMWH (2)[A] initially for at least 5 days and until INR is 2–3, at which time it can be stopped:
  - Enoxaparin (Lovenox) 1 mg/kg SC b.i.d.:
    - Alternatively, 1.5 mg/kg/d SC; initially for at least 5 days and until INR is 2–3, at which time it can be stopped
  - Fondaparinux (Arixtra) 7.5 mg/d SC
  - Tinzaparin (Innohep) 175 anti-Xa IU/kg/d SC
  - Dalteparin (Fragmin) 200 IU/kg/d
- Oral anticoagulant: Warfarin (Coumadin): 10 mg/d PO for the first 2 days then adjusted to an INR of 2–3 for at least 6 months (4)[A]

- Contraindications:
  - Active bleeding precludes anticoagulation; risk of bleeding is a relative contraindication to long-term anticoagulation.
  - Warfarin is contraindicated in patients with a prior history of warfarin-induced skin necrosis.
- Precautions:
  - Observe patient for signs of embolization, further thrombosis, or bleeding
  - Avoid IM injections
  - Periodically check stool and urine for occult blood; monitor CBC, including platelets
  - Heparin: Thrombocytopenia and/or paradoxical thrombosis with thrombocytopenia
  - Warfarin: Necrotic skin lesions (typically breasts, thighs, and buttocks)
  - LMWH: Adjust dose in renal insufficiency
- Significant possible interactions:
  - Agents that intensify the response to oral anticoagulants: Alcohol, allopurinol, amiodarone, anabolic steroids, androgens, many antimicrobials, cimetidine, chloral hydrate, disulfiram, all NSAIDs, sulfinpyrazone, tamoxifen, thyroid hormone, vitamin E, ranitidine, salicylates, acetaminophen
  - Agents that diminish the response to oral anticoagulants: Aminoglutethimide, antacids, barbiturates, carbamazepine, cholestyramine, diuretics, griseofulvin, rifampin, oral contraceptives

Second Line
Heparin 80 mg/kg IV bolus followed by 18 mg/kg/h; adjust dose depending on aPTT:

- In patients requiring large daily doses of heparin, measure an anti-Xa level for dose guidance
- Alternatively, in outpatients, unfractionated heparin can be given at 333 U/kg then 250 U/kg SC, without monitoring (4)[C].
- It does not alter plasma protein S concentration.

ISSUES FOR REFERRAL
Patients with suspected protein S deficiency should be seen by a hematologist.

SURGERY/OTHER PROCEDURES
- Anticoagulation must be held for surgical interventions.
- For most patients with deep vein thrombosis (DVT), recommendations are against routine use of vena cava filter in addition to anticoagulation; inferior vena cava is only recommended in cases of contraindication to anticoagulation (4)[A].

IN-PATIENT CONSIDERATIONS
Admission Criteria/Initial Stabilization
- Life-threatening VT
- Significant bleeding while on anticoagulant therapy

Nursing
Look for signs of bleeding while on anticoagulation therapy.

 ONGOING CARE

FOLLOW-UP RECOMMENDATIONS
Patient Monitoring
- Warfarin requires periodic (monthly after initial stabilization) monitoring of the INR
- Periodic measurement of INR to maintain a range of 2–3
- LMWH is the treatment of choice in pregnancy. Periodic monitoring with anti-Xa levels is recommended in some cases, such as overweight and borderline renal failure.

DIET
Unrestricted

PATIENT EDUCATION
- Patients should be educated about use of oral anticoagulant therapy if taking such.
- Avoid NSAIDs while on warfarin

PROGNOSIS
- Those with protein S deficiency have normal life spans.
- By age 45, 50% of the people heterozygous for protein S deficiency will have VT; half will be spontaneous.

COMPLICATIONS
Recurrent thrombosis (requires indefinite anticoagulation)

REFERENCES
1. Moll S. Thrombophilias—practical implications and testing caveats. *J Thromb Thrombolysis*. 2006;21: 7–15.
2. Bick RL. Prothrombin G20210A mutation, antithrombin, heparin cofactor II, protein C, and protein S defects. *Hematol Oncol Clin North Am*. 2003;17:9–36.
3. Langlois NJ, Wells PS. Risk of venous thromboembolism in relatives of symptomatic probands with thrombophilia: A systematic review. *Thromb Haemost*. 2003;90:17–26.
4. Guyatt GH, Akl EA, Crowther M, et al. Executive summary: Antithrombotic Therapy and Prevention of Thrombosis, 9th Ed: American College of Chest Physicians Evidence-Based Clinical Practice Guidelines. *Chest*. 2012;141:7S–47S.

 CODES

ICD10
D68.59 Other primary thrombophilia

CLINICAL PEARLS
- Asymptomatic patients with protein S deficiency do not require prophylactic anticoagulation because the risk of thrombosis is low; asymptomatic patients do not require anticoagulation.
- Patients with protein S deficiency and DVT should be anticoagulated for at least 6 months, especially if 1st episode.

PROTEIN-ENERGY MALNUTRITION

Robert A. Baldor, MD

 BASICS

DESCRIPTION
- Protein-energy malnutrition (PEM) is present when sufficient energy and/or protein is not available to meet metabolic demands, leading to impairment in normal physiologic processes. It is highly associated with systemic inflammation (1).
- Malnutrition in children is a major underlying factor in ~5 million preventable deaths annually, with 2 distinct phenotypes:
  - Marasmus: A wasting condition due to deficiency of calories and protein
  - Kwashiorkor: Distinguished by generalized edema and ascites, associated with low protein relative to caloric intake
- System(s) affected: Immunologic; Gastrointestinal; Endocrine/Metabolic; Hematologic; Musculoskeletal; Integumentary; Neurologic

EPIDEMIOLOGY
- Children:
  - Most commonly <5 years of age
  - Prevalent sex: Males = Females
  - Globally, malnutrition increases morbidity and mortality from other common childhood diseases.
- Older patients:
  - Highest risk group >age 75, affecting 5–10% of nursing home residents and up to 50% of older patients on hospital discharge (2)
  - Increased mortality and morbidity, including pressure ulcers, infection, and cognitive status changes.
- Malnutrition may be common, but it is difficult to recognize in hospital populations.

Prevalence
- Worldwide, >70 million children suffer from moderate and severe acute malnutrition.
- Prevalence in older patients is between 29% and 61%.

ETIOLOGY AND PATHOPHYSIOLOGY
- Inadequate dietary intake
- Increased metabolic demands
- Increased nutrient losses

RISK FACTORS
- Starvation-related malnutrition:
  - Prolonged and severe reduction of intake
  - Anorexia nervosa (3)
- Mild to moderate inflammatory conditions:
  - Chronic inflammatory states (rheumatoid arthritis, chronic cardiac or lung disease, and cancer)
  - Metabolic disorders (diabetes, hyperthyroidism)
  - Malabsorptive and maldigestive states (celiac disease and pancreatic insufficiency) (2)
  - Protein-losing enteropathy, nephrotic syndrome, enteric fistulas
  - Sarcopenic obesity

- Marked inflammatory conditions: Acute disease, fever, infection, trauma, burns, closed head injury (3)
- Other states in which caloric requirements are increased: Pregnancy and lactation, childhood growth and development

ALERT
- Functional, financial, and social factors may limit access to an adequate diet, particularly in geriatric and pediatric populations.
- Elders with delirium, dementia, or depression or long periods spent NPO or with prolonged hospitalization are at high risk for malnutrition.
- Extreme high or low BMI individuals are also at increased risk (3).

GENERAL PREVENTION
- Observation and recording of patients' nutritional intake and BMI
- In children, routine record of anthropomorphic measurements and developmental milestones
- Early recognition of increased nutritional requirements during stress, infection, and other medical illness
- Frequent interactions among physician, nurse, and dietitian to assess nutritional needs
- Emphasis on food security and nutritional education

COMMONLY ASSOCIATED CONDITIONS
- Infection: Weakened immune system, predisposing to bacterial, viral, and parasitic infections
- Electrolyte disturbances: Loss of cellular integrity, diminished transmembrane pump activity, renal dysfunction
- Hypoglycemia: Decreased glycogen stores, increased glucose utilization (as in infection or trauma)
- Micronutrient deficiencies: Vitamins, including B complex, folic acid, iron, magnesium
- Wounds: Pressure ulcers in older patients (increased incidence if reduced mobility)

DIAGNOSIS

HISTORY
- Diagnostic historical criteria for malnutrition (3)[C]:
  - Inadequate nutrient intake, based on estimated energy needs vs. measured energy consumed (24-hour recall or calorie count).
  - Weight loss
- Presence of ≥2 diagnostic criteria (historical criteria above or exam criteria below) support the diagnosis of malnutrition (3)[C].
- Other historical features:
  - GI tract disorders: Early satiety, constipation, vomiting, diarrhea, dysphagia, dental and oral health problems
  - Decreased urine output (assess for dehydration)
  - Chronic medical illness
  - Impaired work capacity, endurance, and muscle strength
  - Falls and/or reduced physical activity
  - Impaired concentration/cognitive function, delirium, or lethargy
  - Delayed wound healing and recovery
  - In children: Delayed puberty, diminished cognitive and psychosocial development
  - Medications that cause nausea, dry mouth, loss of appetite or taste distortion

PHYSICAL EXAM
- Diagnostic exam criteria for malnutrition (3)[C]:
  - Localized or generalized fluid accumulation
  - Loss of muscle mass or subcutaneous fat
  - Decreased hand grip strength
- Other possible features: Glossitis, cheilosis, loss of vibratory or position sense, sparse hair, nail spooning, night blindness, Bitot spots, loss of taste (4)[C]
- Subnormal heart rate, BP, and core body temperature
- Anthropomorphic measurements:
  - Weight (W) and height (H): In children, measure W:H; in adults, BMI <18.5 kg/m^2 in PEM.
  - Mid–upper arm circumference (MUAC): In adults, MUAC <200 mm is suggestive of PEM.
  - Triceps skin-fold thickness
- Bioelectrical impedance analysis to estimate total body water and fat-free body mass
- Marasmic children: Thin, little subcutaneous fat, wasting at the shoulders, buttocks, arms, and thighs
- Children with Kwashiorkor are irritable, with anasarca, and sparse and brittle hair:
  - They can develop a "flaky paint" dermatosis characterized by blackish discoloration and excoriation.
  - Hepatomegaly from fatty infiltration may be present.

ALERT
- Commonly used markers of dehydration (dry mucous membranes, lack of tears, skin tenting) are not reliable in PEM.
- Poor immune function may make identification of superimposed infection difficult. Fevers, swelling, and redness are often absent.
- Fluid accumulation may mask weight loss (3).

DIFFERENTIAL DIAGNOSIS
- In children, secondary growth failure due to malabsorption, congenital defects, or deprivation
- Pellagra (niacin deficiency = "4 Ds"): Diarrhea, dermatitis, dementia, death
- Nephritis or nephrosis
- Hypo- or hyperthyroidism
- Hyperparathyroidism
- Cardiac failure
- Neoplasm
- Viral or parasitic infection

DIAGNOSTIC TESTS & INTERPRETATION
Initial Tests (lab, imaging)
- Pediatric patients:
  - Serum chemistries: Hypernatremia, hypokalemia, hypocalcemia, hypophosphatemia, hypomagnesemia
  - Hypoglycemia/Hyperglycemia
  - Anemia, decreased lymphocyte count
  - BUN: Decreased
  - Plasma transferrin: Decreased
  - Plasma cortisol, growth hormone: Increased, but insulin is low

- Adult and elderly patients:
  – Serum albumin and prealbumin, inflammatory markers, are affected by acute illness:
    ○ They do not correlate directly with nutritional status or improve with feeding interventions.
    ○ Lower albumin levels do, however, correlate with increased mortality (3).
  – Serum prealbumin measures PEM risk level:
    ○ Normal >15 mg/dL
    ○ Increased risk 5–10 mg/dL:
    ○ Significant risk <5 mg/dL: Poor prognosis, high mortality
  – Elevation of serum alkaline phosphatase and C-reactive protein
  – Chest x-ray (CXR): Evaluate for coexisting pneumonia, neoplasm, or tuberculosis. Cardiomegaly may be present from cardiac failure or marked anemia.

Follow-Up Tests & Special Considerations
In critically ill patients, blood glucose levels >180 mg/dL are associated with increased morbidity and mortality (5)[C].

TREATMENT

GENERAL MEASURES
- Slowly restore and maintain fluid and electrolyte balance.
- Initiate oral iron and folate supplements (begin iron therapy ~2 weeks after initiation of dietary treatment to avoid promotion of bacterial infection).
- Administer blood transfusion in the presence of severe anemia (hemoglobin <4–6 g/dL) or symptomatic moderate anemia.
- Ensure that immunizations are up to date (PEM is not a contraindication to vaccination).

MEDICATION
- Diet prescription in conjunction with a dietician or nutritionist
- Appetite stimulants (e.g., megestrol acetate, mirtazapine, oxandrolone, others) may be appropriate for short-term treatment of anorexia in adults, but may increase thromboembolic risk.
- Medications that have weight gain as a side effect (atypical antipsychotics, carbamazepine, gabapentin, corticosteroids, valproic acid, SSRIs, sulfonylureas, injectable medroxyprogesterone) may be used if otherwise indicated in patients with comorbid conditions.

ISSUES FOR REFERRAL
Consider dentistry referral for oral disorders and speech therapy referral for dysphagia.

IN-PATIENT CONSIDERATIONS
Admission Criteria/Initial Stabilization
- Hemodynamic instability
- Alteration of consciousness (delirium)
- Unsafe living environment (evidence of child/elder mistreatment)
- Profound hypokalemia or hypocalcemia
- Cardiac abnormalities/arrhythmia
- Anemia (hemoglobin <10 g/dL in older patients)
- Reversal of fluid and electrolyte imbalance should occur before IV nutrition, if any, is started.
- Continuous cardiac rhythm monitoring (telemetry) is recommended when electrolyte imbalance or acidosis is present.

IV Fluids
Parenteral (IV) nutrition, which carries a high risk of associated infection, should be reserved for use in patients with severe GI tract dysfunction or anatomic disturbance (4).

Nursing
- Patients should be assessed for risk of pressure ulcer (using a Braden scale or other tool) and a skin care protocol initiated.
- Any patient admitted to the hospital with malnutrition should have a nutritionist consult, if available.
- Physical therapy should be initiated once the patient is stable for assessment.

Geriatric Considerations
Older patients may require assistance with basic activities of daily living (ADLs) and are at high risk of injury due to falls.

Discharge Criteria
- Basic electrolyte abnormalities corrected to tolerance
- Patient demonstrates ability to maintain adequate oral intake of a nutritionally sound diet.
- Social and financial considerations have been identified and addressed.

Geriatric Considerations
Patient may need transfer to alternative level of care (e.g., skilled nursing home, rehabilitation center) temporarily for continued care, depending on level of disability before returning safely home.

ONGOING CARE

FOLLOW-UP RECOMMENDATIONS
Children are discharged from a nutritional rehabilitation program when W:H ratio is >85%, at least 1 week of consistent weight gain has been achieved, and all disease conditions associated with PEM have been addressed.

Patient Monitoring
Frequent assessment until weight stabilized (BMI >18.5 kg/m^2)

DIET
- Slow refeeding of amino acid constituent and calorie-to-BMI-adjusted diet, in consultation with a nutritionist/dietician.
- For children, initiate 100 kcal/kg/d with 3 g/kg/d protein. When tolerated, advance to at least 200 kcal/kg/d with 5 g/kg/d protein:
  – Small, frequent feedings are preferred.
  – Consider low-lactose formulas to decrease diarrhea from disaccharidase deficiency
  – Target growth: 10–15 g/kg/d
  – Supplement with vitamins and micronutrients, especially vitamin A and zinc.

PATIENT EDUCATION
- Emphasis on diet education
- In older patients, caregiver education and supervision may be relevant.

PROGNOSIS
- Excellent when PEM is identified early and managed aggressively
- Mortality varies between 15% and 40%.
- Compromised immune function returns to normal with recovery.
- Behavioral and mental issues may persist following treatment of severe cases.
- Insufficient evidence indicates that enteral tube feeding in patients with advanced dementia improves survival or lowers the prevalence of pressure ulcers (2,5)[A].

COMPLICATIONS
- Fatalities in the early days of treatment usually result from electrolyte imbalance, infection, hypothermia, or circulatory failure. Lethargy, anorexia, stupor, and petechiae are ominous signs.
- Patients who develop PEM have greater risk of hospital-acquired infection (4).

Pregnancy Considerations
Pregnant women with PEM are at risk of delivering a growth-restricted infant.

REFERENCES

1. Soeters PB, Schols AM. Advances in understanding and assessing malnutrition. *Curr Opin Clin Nutr Metab Care*. 2009;12:487–494.
2. Morley JE. Undernutrition in older adults. *Fam Pract*. 2012;29(Suppl 1):i89–i93.
3. White JV, Guenter P, Jensen G, et al. Consensus statement: Academy of Nutrition and Dietetics and American Society for Parenteral and Enteral Nutrition: Characteristics recommended for the identification and documentation of adult malnutrition (undernutrition). *JPEN J Parenter Enteral Nutr*. 2012;36:275–283.
4. Ziegler TR. Parenteral nutrition in the critically ill patient. *N Engl J Med*. 2009;361:1088–1097.
5. Sampson EL, Candy B, Jones L, et al. Enteral tube feeding for older people with advanced dementia. *Cochrane Database Syst Rev*. 2009;2:CD007209.

CODES

ICD10
- E41 Nutritional marasmus
- E46 Unspecified protein-calorie malnutrition
- E61.8 Deficiency of other specified nutrient elements

CLINICAL PEARLS

- Older patients may experience elevated BUN levels from excessive protein supplementation; routine monitoring is suggested.
- Decreased muscle mass in patients with malnutrition may lower creatinine level and lead to overestimation of the glomerular filtration rate.
- Malnourished patients have a higher risk of toxicity from fat-soluble or protein-bound drugs due to weight loss and decrease in albumin (2).

PROTEINURIA
Andrew Allegretti, MD • Douglas Shemin, MD

BASICS

DESCRIPTION
Urinary protein excretion of >150 mg/d:
- Nephrotic-range proteinuria: Urinary protein excretion of >3.5 g/d; also called *heavy proteinuria*
- 3 pathologic types:
  - Glomerular proteinuria: Increased permeability of proteins across glomerular capillary membrane
  - Tubular proteinuria: Decreased proximal tubular reabsorption of proteins
  - Overflow proteinuria: Increased production of low-molecular-weight proteins

Pediatric Considerations
- Proteinuria: Normal is daily excretion of up to 100 mg/m^2 (body surface area)
- Nephrotic-range proteinuria: Daily excretion of >1,000 mg/m^2 (body surface area)

Pregnancy Considerations
- Proteinuria in pregnancy beyond 20 weeks' gestation is a hallmark of preeclampsia/eclampsia and demands further workup.
- Proteinuria in pregnancy before 20 weeks' gestation is suggestive of underlying renal disease.

ETIOLOGY AND PATHOPHYSIOLOGY
- Glomerular proteinuria: Increased filtration/larger proteins (albumin) due to:
  - Increased size of glomerular basement membrane pores and
  - Loss of proteoglycan negative charge barrier
- Tubular proteinuria: Tubulointerstitial disease prevents proximal tubular reabsorption of smaller proteins (β_2-microglobulin, immunoglobulin [Ig] light chains, retinol-binding protein, amino acids).
- Overflow proteinuria: Proximal tubular reabsorption overwhelmed by increased production of smaller proteins
- Glomerular proteinuria:
  - Primary glomerulonephropathy:
    - Minimal-change disease
    - Idiopathic membranous glomerulonephritis
    - Focal segmental glomerulonephritis
    - Membranoproliferative glomerulonephritis
    - IgA nephropathy
  - Secondary glomerulonephropathy:
    - Diabetic nephropathy
    - Autoimmune/collagen-vascular disorders (e.g., lupus nephritis, Goodpasture syndrome)
    - Amyloidosis
    - Preeclampsia
    - Infection (HIV, hepatitis B and C, poststreptococcal, endocarditis, syphilis, malaria)
    - Malignancy (GI, lung, lymphoma)
    - Renal transplant rejection
    - Structural (reflux nephropathy, polycystic kidney disease)
    - Drug-induced (NSAIDs, penicillamine, lithium, heavy metals, gold, heroin)

- Tubular proteinuria:
  - Hypertensive nephrosclerosis
  - Tubulointerstitial disease (uric acid nephropathy, hypersensitivity, interstitial nephritis, Fanconi syndrome, heavy metals, sickle cell disease, NSAIDs, antibiotics)
  - Acute tubular necrosis
- Overflow proteinuria:
  - Multiple myeloma (light chains; also tubulotoxic)
  - Hemoglobinuria
  - Myoglobinuria (in rhabdomyolysis)
  - Lysozyme (in acute monocytic leukemia)
- Benign proteinuria:
  - Functional (fever, exercise, cold exposure, stress, CHF)
  - Idiopathic transient
  - Orthostasis (postural)

RISK FACTORS
- Hypertension
- Diabetes
- Obesity
- Strenuous exercise
- CHF
- UTI
- Fever

Genetics
No known genetic pattern

GENERAL PREVENTION
Control of weight, BP, and blood glucose reduces the risk of proteinuria.

COMMONLY ASSOCIATED CONDITIONS
- Hypertension (common)
- Diabetes mellitus (common)
- Preeclampsia (common)
- Multiple myeloma (rare)

DIAGNOSIS

HISTORY
- Frothy/Foamy urine
- Change in urine output
- Blood- or cola-colored urine
- Recent weight change
- Swelling
- Rule out systemic illness: Diabetes, heart failure, autoimmune, poststreptococcal infection

PHYSICAL EXAM
- BP
- Weight
- Peripheral edema
- Periorbital/Facial edema
- Ascites
- Palpation of kidneys
- Check lungs, heart for signs of CHF

DIFFERENTIAL DIAGNOSIS
Includes all causes listed under "Etiology and Pathophysiology."

DIAGNOSTIC TESTS & INTERPRETATION
Screening for proteinuria is not cost-effective unless directed at groups with hypertension/diabetes, older persons, and so forth.

Initial Tests (lab, imaging)
- Urinalysis (UA) quantitatively estimates proteinuria:
  - Only sensitive to albumin; will not detect smaller proteins of overflow/tubular etiologies
  - False-positive finding if urine pH >7, highly concentrated (specific gravity [SG] >1.015), gross hematuria, mucus, semen, leukocytes, iodinated contrast agents, penicillin analogues, sulfonamide metabolites
  - False-negative finding if urine is dilute (SG 1.005), albumin excretion <20–30 mg/dL, protein is nonalbumin
  - Sensitivity, 32–46%; specificity, 97–100%
  - Also can perform sulfosalicylic acid test to detect nonalbumin protein
- If UA positive, perform urine microscopy. Refer to nephrologist if positive for signs of glomerular disease.
- If UA shows trace to 2+ protein, rule out transient proteinuria with repeat UA at another visit:
  - More common than persistent proteinuria
  - Causes include exercise, fever, CHF, UTI, and cold exposure
  - Reassure patient that transient proteinuria is benign and requires no further workup.

- If initial UA shows 3+ to 4+ protein or repeat UA is positive, measure creatinine clearance and quantify proteinuria with 24-hour urine collection (gold standard) or spot urine protein-to-creatinine (P/C) ratio (acceptable practice) (1)[A]:
  - Numerical P/C ratios correlate with total protein excreted in grams per day (i.e., ratio of 0.2 correlates with 0.2 g during a 24-hour collection).
  - Patients age <30 years with 24-hour urine excretion of <2 g/d and normal creatinine clearance should be tested for orthostatic proteinuria:
    - Benign condition is present in 2–5% of adolescents.
    - Diagnosed with a normal urine P/C ratio in 1st morning void and an elevated urine P/C ratio in a 2nd specimen taken after standing for several hours
- If protein excretion >2 g/d, consider nephrology referral and begin workup for systemic/renal disease.
- Patients with persistent proteinuria not explained by orthostatic changes should undergo renal ultrasound to rule out structural abnormalities (e.g., reflux nephropathy, polycystic kidney).

Follow-Up Tests & Special Considerations
Renal/systemic disease workup can include:

- CBC, ferritin, ESR, serum iron
- Electrolytes, LFTs
- Lipid profile (ideally, fasting)
- Prothrombin time/International normalized ratio
- Antinuclear antibodies: Elevated in lupus
- Antistreptolysin O titer: Elevated after streptococcal glomerulonephritis
- Complement C3/C4: Low in most glomerulonephritis
- HIV, syphilis, and hepatitis serologies: All associated with glomerular proteinuria
- Serum and urine protein electrophoresis: Abnormal in multiple myeloma
- Blood glucose: Elevated in diabetes
- All patients with diabetes should be screened for microalbuminuria.
- Patients with nephrotic-range proteinuria are at increased risk for hypercholesterolemia and thromboembolic events. Optimal duration of prophylactic anticoagulation is unknown, but may extend for the duration of the nephrotic state (2)[C].
- Proteinuric pregnant patients beyond 20 weeks' gestation should be examined for other signs/symptoms of preeclampsia (e.g., hypertension, thrombocytopenia, elevated liver transaminases).

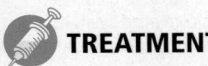 **TREATMENT**

- Systolic BP goal is in the 120 range (3)[A].
- Proteinuria goal is <0.5 g/d (3)[A].

GENERAL MEASURES

- Limit protein intake to 0.7 mg/kg/d. Soy protein may be renoprotective. Monitor protein intake with 24-hour urine urea excretion (3)[A].
- Limit sodium chloride intake to 2–3 g/d to optimize antiproteinuric medications (3)[B]. Effect on BP is further protective (3)[A].
- Limit fluid intake for urine output goal of <2 L/d. Larger urine volumes are associated with increased proteinuria and later glomerular filtration rate (GFR) decline (3)[B].
- Smoking cessation: Smoking is associated with increased proteinuria and faster kidney disease progression (3)[B].
- Encourage supine posture (up to 50% reduction vs. upright) (3)[B].
- Discourage severe exertion (3)[B].
- Encourage weight loss (3)[B].

MEDICATION
First Line

- ACE inhibitors: First choice; use maximally tolerated doses; use even if normotensive (3)[A].
- Angiotensin receptor blockers (ARBs): Proven antiproteinuric and renoprotective; studies ongoing to assess cardioprotection vs. ACE inhibitors; ARBs are 1st choice if ACE inhibitors are not tolerated (3)[A].
- Combination ACE inhibitor and ARB: Shown to reduce proteinuria, but does not reduce poor outcomes and does increase risk of adverse drug reactions (4)[B].
- Statins: In addition to cardioprotection (3)[A], may be antiproteinuric and renoprotective (3)[B]

Second Line

- β-Blockers: Antiproteinuric and cardioprotective (3)[A]
- Dihydropyridine calcium channel blockers (DHCCB): Should be avoided unless needed for BP control; not antiproteinuric (3)[A]
- Non-DHCCB: Antiproteinuric, may be renoprotective (3)[B]
- Aldosterone antagonists: Antiproteinuric independent of BP control (3)[B]
- NSAIDs: Antiproteinuric, but also nephrotoxic; generally should be avoided and reserved for refractory nephrotic syndrome (3)[C]

ISSUES FOR REFERRAL
Consider nephrology referral for possible renal biopsy if:

- Impaired creatinine clearance
- Nephrotic-range proteinuria
- Unclear etiology of nonnephrotic-range proteinuria
- Diabetics with microalbuminuria

COMPLEMENTARY AND ALTERNATIVE MEDICINE

- Corticosteroids: No proven benefit in mortality or need for renal replacement in adults with nephrotic syndrome, although steroids are recommended in some patients who do not respond to conservative treatment. Classically, children with nephrotic syndrome respond better than adults, especially those with minimal-change disease (5)[A].
- Estrogen/Progesterone replacement: May be renoprotective in premenopausal women, but should be avoided in postmenopausal women (3)[B].
- Antioxidant therapy: May be antiproteinuric in diabetic nephropathy (3)[C].
- Sodium bicarbonate: Not antiproteinuric, but may block tubular injury caused by proteinuria; correcting metabolic acidosis may decrease protein catabolism (3)[C].
- Avoid excessive caffeine consumption: Antiproteinuric in diabetic rat models (3)[C]
- Avoid iron overload (3)[C].
- Pentoxifylline: Prevents progression of renal disease by unclear mechanisms (3)[C].
- Mycophenolate mofetil: Antiproteinuric and renoprotective in animal models (3)[C]

 ONGOING CARE

FOLLOW-UP RECOMMENDATIONS
Patient Monitoring
All patients with persistent proteinuria should be followed with serial BP checks, urinalysis, and renal function tests in the outpatient setting. Intervals depend on underlying etiology.

PROGNOSIS

- Transient and orthostatic proteinuria are benign conditions that do not convey a poor prognosis.
- Clinical significance of persistent proteinuria varies greatly and depends on underlying etiology.
- Degree of proteinuria is associated with disease progression in chronic kidney disease.
- Independent of GFR, higher levels of proteinuria likely convey an increased risk of mortality, myocardial infarction, and progression to kidney failure (6).

COMPLICATIONS

- Progression to chronic renal failure and the need for dialysis/renal transplant
- Hypercholesterolemia
- Hypercoagulable state

REFERENCES

1. DOQI: Clinical practice guidelines for chronic kidney disease: Evaluation classification, and stratification: Guideline 5. Assessment of proteinuria. Available at: www.kidney.org/Professionals/Kdoqi/ guidelines_ckd/p5_lab_g5.htm
2. Glassock RJ. Prophylactic anticoagulation in nephrotic syndrome: A clinical conundrum. *J Am Soc Nephrol.* 2007;18:2221–2225.
3. Wilmer WA, Rovin BH, Hebert CJ, et al. Management of glomerular proteinuria: A commentary. *J Am Soc Nephrol.* 2003;14: 3217–3232.
4. ONTARGET Investigators, Yusuf S, Teo KK, et al. Telmisartan, ramipril, or both in patients at high risk for vascular events. *N Engl J Med.* 2008;358: 1547–1559.
5. Kodner C. Nephrotic syndrome in adults: Diagnosis and management. *Am Fam Physician.* 2009;80: 1129–1134.
6. Tonelli M, Muntner P, Lloyd A, et al. Using proteinuria and estimated glomerular filtration rate to classify risk in patients with chronic kidney disease: A cohort study. *Ann Intern Med.* 2011;154:12–21.

 CODES

ICD10

- R80.1 Persistent proteinuria, unspecified
- R80.8 Other proteinuria
- R80.9 Proteinuria, unspecified

CLINICAL PEARLS

- Transient and orthostatic proteinuria are benign conditions that do not convey a poor prognosis.
- Proteinuria >2 g/d likely represents glomerular malfunction and warrants a nephrology consultation.
- Clinical course varies greatly but, in general, the degree of proteinuria correlates with kidney disease progression.
- First-line therapy for persistent proteinuric patients is a high-dose ACE inhibitor.

PROTHROMBIN 20210 (MUTATION)
Maissaa Janbain, MD • Rebecca Kruse-Jarres, MD, MPH

 BASICS

DESCRIPTION
- Prothrombin 20210 mutation is the 2nd most common inherited risk factor for venous thromboembolism after factor V Leiden mutation.
- Polymorphism (replacement of G by A) in the 3′ untranslated end of the prothrombin gene causes increased translation, resulting in elevated synthesis and secretion of prothrombin. This leads to a 2.8-fold increased risk for venous thrombosis.
- System(s) affected: Cardiovascular; Hemic/Lymphatic/Immunologic; Nervous; Pulmonary; Reproductive
- Synonym(s): Prothrombin G20210A mutation; Prothrombin G20210 gene polymorphism; Prothrombin gene mutation; FII A^{20210} mutation

EPIDEMIOLOGY
- Found largely in Caucasian populations. Found in 2–5% of European and Middle Eastern populations, but rarely in nonwhites. Found in 4–8% of persons with venous thromboembolism and in up to 18% of patients with recurrent thrombosis.
- Predominant age: Mean age of 1st thrombosis is in the 2nd decade.
- Predominant gender: Male = Female

Prevalence
3–5% of the population

ETIOLOGY AND PATHOPHYSIOLOGY
- Replacement of G for A in the 3′ untranslated region of the prothrombin gene resulting in relatively higher plasma prothrombin activity, leading to increased risk for venous thrombosis
- Gene mutation

Genetics
Autosomal dominant

RISK FACTORS
- Oral contraceptives, pregnancy, and the use of hormone replacement therapy increase the risk of venous thrombosis in patients with prothrombin 20210 (1).
- Patients with prothrombin 20210 and another prothrombotic state, such as factor V Leiden, have increased rates of thrombosis (1).

Pregnancy Considerations
Increased thrombotic risk in patients with prothrombin 20210

GENERAL PREVENTION
Patients with prothrombin 20210 without thrombosis do not require prophylactic anticoagulation (2)[A].

COMMONLY ASSOCIATED CONDITIONS
Venous thromboembolism

 DIAGNOSIS

HISTORY
- Previous thrombosis
- Family history of thrombosis
- Family history of factor prothrombin 20210 mutation

PHYSICAL EXAM
Arterial thrombosis is rare in adults with prothrombin 20210 gene mutation.

DIFFERENTIAL DIAGNOSIS
- Factor V Leiden mutation
- Protein C deficiency
- Protein S deficiency
- Antithrombin deficiency
- Other causes of activated protein C resistance (e.g., antiphospholipid antibodies)
- Dysfibrinogenemia
- Dysplasminogenemia
- Homocystinemia
- Elevated factor VIII levels

DIAGNOSTIC TESTS & INTERPRETATION
Test patients with thrombosis at age <50, history of recurrent idiopathic thrombosis, those with thrombosis in unusual locations, or those with strong family history.

Initial Tests (lab, imaging)
- For evaluation of a new clot in patients at risk: CBC with peripheral smear, PT/INR, aPTT, thrombin time, lupus anticoagulant, antiphospholipid antibodies, factor VIII, anticardiolipin antibody, anti-B2 glycoprotein I antibody, activated protein C resistance, protein S antigen and resistance, antithrombin III assay, fibrinogen, factor V Leiden, prothrombin G20210A, homocysteine
- DNA analysis for mutation
- Testing is reliable during acute thrombosis and on any kind of anticoagulation (3).
- As appropriate for suspected site of thrombosis: US, CT scan, and V/Q scan

Follow-Up Tests & Special Considerations
Although prothrombin levels are elevated, this is not a sensitive test to make the diagnosis.

Diagnostic Procedures/Other
MR angiography (MRA), venography, or arteriography to detect thrombosis

Test Interpretation
Venous thrombus

 TREATMENT

For acute thrombosis

GENERAL MEASURES
- Patients with prothrombin 20210 mutation and a 1st thrombosis should receive anticoagulation medication initially with heparin or LMWH (1)[A].
- Treatment with LMWH is recommended over unfractionated heparin, unless the patient has severe renal failure (3)[A].
- Treat as outpatient, if possible (3)[B].
- Initiate warfarin together with heparin on the 1st treatment day, and discontinue heparin after 5 days if INR >2 (3)[A].
- Patients should be maintained on warfarin with an INR of 2–3 for at least 6 months (1)[A].
- Recurrent thrombosis requires indefinite anticoagulation (1)[B].

MEDICATION
First Line
- Low-molecular-weight heparin (LMWH) (2)[A]:
  - Enoxaparin (Lovenox): 1 mg/kg SC b.i.d., start warfarin simultaneously, continue Lovenox for at least 5 days and until INR is >2, at which time it can be stopped.
  - Fondaparinux (Arixtra): 7.5 mg/d SC
  - Tinzaparin (Innohep): 175 anti-Xa IU/kg SC daily for 6 days and patient is adequately anticoagulated with warfarin (INR of at least 2 for 2 consecutive days)
  - Dalteparin (Fragmin): 200 IU/kg/d SC
- Oral anticoagulant:
  - Warfarin (Coumadin) 10 mg/d PO for the first 2 days then adjusted to an INR of 2–3 (4)
- Contraindications:
  - Active bleeding precludes anticoagulation (2)[A].
  - Risk of bleeding is a relative contraindication to long-term anticoagulation (2)[A].
  - Warfarin is contraindicated in patients with history of warfarin skin necrosis (2)[A].
- Precautions:
  - Observe patient for signs of embolization, further thrombosis, or bleeding.
  - Avoid IM injections; periodically check stool and urine for occult blood; monitor CBCs, including platelets.
  - Heparins: Thrombocytopenia and/or paradoxic thrombosis with thrombocytopenia
  - Warfarin: Necrotic skin lesions (typically breasts, thighs, or buttocks)
  - LMWH: Adjust dosage in renal insufficiency.

- Significant possible interactions:
  – Agents that intensify the response to oral anticoagulants: Alcohol, allopurinol, amiodarone, anabolic steroids, androgens, many antimicrobials, cimetidine, chloral hydrate, disulfiram, all NSAIDs, sulfinpyrazone, tamoxifen, thyroid hormone, vitamin E, ranitidine, salicylates, acetaminophen
  – Agents that diminish the response to anticoagulants: Aminoglutethimide, antacids, barbiturates, carbamazepine, cholestyramine, diuretics, griseofulvin, rifampin, oral contraceptives

Second Line
- Heparin 80 mg/kg IV bolus followed by 18 g/kg/hr continuous infusion
- Adjust dose, depending on aPTT.
- In patients requiring large daily doses of heparin, measure an anti-Xa level for dose guidance.
- Alternatively, unfractionated heparin can be given for outpatients at 333 U/kg then 250 U/kg SC, without monitoring (4)[A].

ISSUES FOR REFERRAL
- Recurrent thrombosis on anticoagulation
- Difficulty anticoagulating
- Genetic counseling

SURGERY/OTHER PROCEDURES
- Anticoagulation must be held for surgical interventions.
- For most patients with deep venous thrombosis (DVT), recommendations are against routine use of vena cava filter in addition to anticoagulation, except in case with contraindication to anticoagulation (4)[A].
- Thrombectomy may be necessary in some cases.

COMPLEMENTARY AND ALTERNATIVE MEDICINE
Compression stockings for prevention

IN-PATIENT CONSIDERATIONS
Admission Criteria/Initial Stabilization
Complicated thrombosis, such as pulmonary embolus; heparin
Nursing
- Teach LMWH and warfarin use.
- See above for drug interactions.
Discharge Criteria
Stable on anticoagulation

ONGOING CARE
FOLLOW-UP RECOMMENDATIONS
Patient Monitoring
- Warfarin use requires periodic (monthly after initial stabilization) INR measurements, with a goal of 2–3 (2)[A].
- Heterozygous prothrombin 20210 mutations increase the risk for recurrent venous thromboembolism (VTE) only slightly once anticoagulation is stopped and should have the same length of anticoagulation as in someone without the mutation.

DIET
- No restrictions
- Foods rich in vitamin K may interfere with warfarin anticoagulation.

PATIENT EDUCATION
- Patients should be educated about:
  – Use of oral anticoagulant therapy
  – Avoidance of NSAIDs while on warfarin
- The role of family screening is unclear, as most patients with this mutation do not have thrombosis. In a patient with a family history of prothrombin 20210, consider screening during pregnancy or if considering oral contraceptive use.

PROGNOSIS
When compared with normal individuals, persons with prothrombin 20210 have normal lifespans.

COMPLICATIONS
- Recurrent thrombosis
- Bleeding on anticoagulation

REFERENCES
1. Girolami A, Simioni P, Scarano L, et al. Prothrombin and the prothrombin 20210 G to A polymorphism: Their relationship with hypercoagulability and thrombosis. *Blood Rev*. 1999;13:205–210.
2. Girolami A, Scarano L, Tormene D, et al. Homozygous patients with the 20210 G to A prothrombin polymorphism remain often asymptomatic in spite of the presence of associated risk factors. *Clin Appl Thromb Hemost*. 2001; 7:122–125.
3. Moll S. Thrombophilias–practical implications and testing caveats. *J Thromb Thrombolysis*. 2006; 21:7–15.
4. Guyatt GH, Akl EA, Crowther M, et al. Executive summary: Antithrombotic Therapy and Prevention of Thrombosis, 9th Ed: American College of Chest Physicians Evidence-Based Clinical Practice Guidelines. *Chest*. 2012;141(Suppl 2):7S–47S.

ADDITIONAL READING
Seligsohn U, Lubetsky A. Genetic susceptibility to venous thrombosis. *N Engl J Med*. 2001; 344: 1222–1231.

SEE ALSO
Antithrombin Deficiency; Deep Vein Thrombophlebitis (DVT); Factor V Leiden; Protein C Deficiency; Protein S Deficiency

CODES
ICD10
D68.52 Prothrombin gene mutation

CLINICAL PEARLS
- Prothrombin 20210 mutation is the 2nd most common inherited risk factor for VTE after factor V Leiden mutation.
- Asymptomatic patients with prothrombin 20210 mutation do not need anticoagulation.
- Testing for the prothrombin G20210 mutation may be done while the patient is anticoagulated, as it is a genetic assay.
- For pregnant women homozygous for factor V Leiden, or heterozygous for factor V and prothrombin G20210 mutation, but no prior history of VTE, postpartum prophylaxis with prophylactic or intermediate-dose LMWH or vitamin K antagonists with target INR 2–3 for 6 weeks is recommended. Antepartum prophylaxis is added if there is positive family of VTE (4)[B].

PRURITUS ANI

Pia Prakash, MD • Marie L. Borum, MD, EdD, MPH

BASICS

DESCRIPTION
- Intense and often unpleasant anal and perianal itching and/or burning
- Usually acute
- Common complaint seen by many physicians in primary care, dermatology, gastroenterology, and colorectal surgery
- Must be differentiated from other primary dermatologic disorders

EPIDEMIOLOGY
Incidence
- The incidence ranges from 1–5% of the general population
- Predominant age: 40–70
- Predominant sex: Male > Female (4:1)

Prevalence
Difficult to estimate the prevalence as many cases are likely unreported or actually related to hemorrhoids

ETIOLOGY AND PATHOPHYSIOLOGY
- Perianal itching usually due to irritant in stool:
  - Excess alkalinity with antibiotics, tomatoes, wine, caffeine, intermittent stool seepage
- Itch–scratch cycle may be initiated via other mechanical or inflammatory factors and perpetuated by the resulting lichenification caused by scratching.
- 50–90% idiopathic vs. 10–50% associated with colonic or anorectal pathology:
  - Hemorrhoids, anal fissures, skin tags, rectal prolapse, polyps, or cancers of the colon, rectum, or anus in rare cases
- In 50–75% of cases, the associated skin irritation is from feces:
  - Poor hygiene
  - Loose or leaking stool that makes cleansing difficult
  - Laxity of the internal sphincter mechanism
- In the remaining cases, the inciting irritation may be caused by:
  - Dermatologic disorders:
    ○ Allergic contact dermatitis (e.g., to soaps, perfumes or dyes in toilet paper, topical anesthetics, oral antibiotics)
    ○ Excess skin moisture due to hyperhidrosis
    ○ Psoriasis: Lesions tend to be poorly demarcated, pale, and nonscaling
    ○ Erythrasma (*Corynebacterium* infection)
    ○ Atopic dermatitis ± lichen simplex chronicus: Patients likely to have asthma and/or eczema
    ○ Eczema can result from dietary components (citrus, vitamin C supplements, milk products, coffee, tea, cola, chocolate, beer, wine).
    ○ Seborrheic dermatitis
    ○ Lichen planus: May be seen in patients with ulcerative colitis and myasthenia gravis
    ○ Local malignancy: Uncommon, but may be presenting symptom of Bowen or Paget disease
  - Colorectal and anal pathology: Rectal prolapse, internal hemorrhoids, anal fissures, anal fistulas, chronic diarrhea/constipation, papillomas, polyps, and cancer

- Infection with dermatophytes (*Tinea*), bacteria (*Staphylococcus aureus*, β-hemolytic *Streptococcus*, *gonorrhea*, *syphilis*), viruses (herpes simplex virus [HSV], human papillomavirus [HPV]), parasites (pinworms, rarely scabies, or pediculosis)
- Mechanical factors: Vigorous cleaning and rubbing, tight-fitting clothes, or synthetic undergarments
- Associated systemic diseases: Diabetes mellitus (most common), chronic liver disease, renal failure, leukemia or lymphoma, hyperthyroidism, and anemia
- Chemical irritation from chemotherapy or alkaline diarrhea
- Psychogenic: Anxiety–itch–anxiety cycle

RISK FACTORS
- Obesity
- Excess perianal hair growth, excessive perspiration
- Underlying anorectal pathology
- Underlying anxiety disorder

GENERAL PREVENTION
- Practice good perianal hygiene:
  - Absorb excess sweat with talcum powder or cornstarch
- Avoid mechanical irritation of skin (vigorous cleaning or rubbing, harsh soaps or perfumed products, excessive cleansing with dry toilet paper or "baby wipes," scratching with fingernails, or tight or synthetic undergarments).
- May wear cotton gloves at night if difficulty with nocturnal scratching
- Minimize moisture in perianal area (absorbent cotton in anal cleft may help keep area dry)
- Avoid laxative use (loose stool is an irritant)

COMMONLY ASSOCIATED CONDITIONS
See above listing of conditions causing perianal irritation.

DIAGNOSIS

HISTORY
- Patient presents with complaint of anal and/or perianal itching, burning, or excoriations
- Inquire about:
  - Melena or hematochezia
  - Change in bowel habits
  - Recent antibiotic use
  - History of diabetes
  - Skin disorders
  - Rectal or vaginal discharge
  - Poor hygiene or over cleansing
  - Caffeine use and dietary history
  - Family history of colorectal cancer
  - Anal receptive intercourse
  - Change in toiletry products
  - Household members with itching (possible pinworms)
  - Clothing preference (tight, synthetic)

PHYSICAL EXAM
- Perianal inspection for erythema, hemorrhoids, anal fissures, maceration, lichenification, rashes, warts, excoriations, neoplasia
- Digital rectal exam to check for masses and to evaluate internal sphincter tone
- Anoscopy to evaluate for hemorrhoids, fissures, other internal lesions

DIFFERENTIAL DIAGNOSIS
- Dermatologic conditions
- Infections (dermatophytes, bacterial, viral)
- Allergies (topical agents)
- Colorectal pathology: Fistulas, fissures, rectal prolapse, sphincter weakness, hemorrhoids, tumor/malignancy
- Skin cancer: Squamous cell cancer, extramammary Paget disease, Bowen disease, melanoma
- Systemic illness such as diabetes

DIAGNOSTIC TESTS & INTERPRETATION
Initial Tests (lab, imaging)
Depending on patient's history and exam, consider the following:
- Blood glucose and hemoglobin A1C to assess for diabetes
- Test for pinworms via cellophane tape to area; check stool for ova and parasites
- CBC, comprehensive metabolic panel, thyroid studies to identify underlying systemic disease

Pediatric Considerations
Pinworms are more common in children and, therefore, testing is always indicated:
- Skin scraping with potassium hydroxide (KOH) prep for dermatophytes or candidiasis (as etiology or as superinfection) and mineral oil prep for scabies
- Perianal skin culture (bacterial superinfection)
- Hemoccult testing of stool

Follow-Up Tests & Special Considerations
Anal DNA polymerase chain reaction (PCR) probe for gonorrhea and anal Pap smear for HPV (*if receptive anal intercourse*)

Diagnostic Procedures/Other
- Suspicious lesions (e.g., lichenification, ulcerated epithelium, refractory cases) should be biopsied to exclude neoplasia.
- Consider colonoscopy if history, exam, or testing suggests colorectal pathology (family history of colorectal disease, especially if age >40, rectal bleeding).

Geriatric Considerations
- Stool incontinence may be a predisposing factor.
- Consider possible systemic disease
- Higher likelihood of colorectal pathology

TREATMENT

MEDICATION

First Line

- Establish proper anal hygiene by avoiding moisture and keeping the perianal area
- Treat underlying infections: Fungal or dermatophyte infection with topical imidazoles, bacterial infection with topical antibacterials (or oral erythromycin if itch >1 year); cefuroxime has been shown to be more effective than penicillin for perianal strep dermatitis.
- Patients should maintain regular bowel habits by maintaining a high-fiber diet.
- Break itch–scratch cycle with low-potency steroid cream such as hydrocortisone 1% ointment applied sparingly up to 4 × daily. Discontinue when itching subsides. Recommended not to use >12 weeks due to risk of skin atrophy.
- If lichenification or no response with low-potency steroid, use high-potency steroid cream sparingly to area twice daily, totaling <8 weeks of steroid treatment (1).
- Antihistamines may be useful until local measures take effect, particularly sedating antihistamines, which will reduce nighttime itching. Psychotropic medications may be added for additional sedation (2).
- Zinc oxide can be used after completing steroid course; use petroleum jelly as barrier during treatment period (2).
- Topical capsaicin cream also may be used in combination with steroid cream or if refractory itch or hypersensitized skin (3) (although evidence is conflicting)
- Tacrolimus 0.1% ointment has also recently shown effectiveness in patients with resistant idiopathic pruritus ani (4).
- Treat comorbid anxiety or depression
- Recently, methylene blue has shown promise as an effective injectable treatment (5).

Second Line

Radiation may be used to destroy nerve endings (create permanent anesthesia) in intractable cases. This is almost never indicated, but is close to 100% effective for those who require it (1,6).

ISSUES FOR REFERRAL

- Intractable pruritus: Consider referral to gastroenterology (for colonoscopy) or dermatology (for additional treatment, possibly injections). Refractory or persistent symptoms should signal the possibility of underlying neoplasia because pruritus ani of long duration is associated with a greater likelihood of colorectal pathology (7).
- If risks or red flags for colon cancer are present, refer for colonoscopy.

SURGERY/OTHER PROCEDURES

None unless malignancy identified

ONGOING CARE

FOLLOW-UP RECOMMENDATIONS

See patient in 2 weeks if not improving. Check for persistent lichenification. With refractory pruritus or lichenification that does not resolve, underlying malignancy should be considered (7).

DIET

- Trial elimination of foods and beverages known or suspected to exacerbate symptoms: Coffee, tea, chocolate, beer, cola, vitamin C tablets in excessive doses, citrus fruits, tomatoes, or spices (2)
- Eliminate foods or drugs contributing to loose bowel movements. Add fiber supplementation to bulk stools and prevent fecal leakage in patients who have fecal incontinence or partially formed stools.

PATIENT EDUCATION

- Resist overuse of soap and rubbing
- Avoid toiletry products with irritating perfumes and dyes
- Avoid use of ointments to the area
- Wear loose, light clothing
- If moisture is a problem, unmedicated talcum powder or cornstarch may be used to keep the area dry
- Cleanse perianal area after bowel movements with cotton moistened with water or witch hazel
- Following bathing, the area should be dried by patting with a soft towel or with a hair dryer
- Avoid medications that cause diarrhea or constipation
- Use barrier protection if engaging in anal intercourse
- If unable to completely empty rectum with defecation, use small plain-water enema (infant bulb syringe) after each bowel movement to prevent soiling and irritation

PROGNOSIS

- Conservative treatment and reassurance are successful in ~90% of patients.
- Idiopathic form often is chronic, waxing and waning, but regardless of etiology, the condition may be persistent and recurrent.

COMPLICATIONS

- Bacterial superinfection at site of excoriations and potential abscess formation or penetrating infection via self-inoculation with colonic pathogens
- Lichenification

REFERENCES

1. Weichert GE. An approach to the treatment of anogenital pruritus. *Dermatol Ther*. 2004;17: 129–133.
2. Siddiqi S, Vijay V, Ward M, et al. Pruritus ani. *Ann R Coll Surg Engl*. 2008;90:457–463.
3. Lysy J, Sistiery-Ittah M, Israelit Y, et al. Topical capsaicin—a novel and effective treatment for idiopathic intractable pruritus ani: A randomised, placebo controlled, crossover study. *Gut*. 2003;52: 1323–1326.
4. Ucak H, Demir B, Cicek D, et al. Efficacy of topical tacrolimus for the treatment of persistent pruritus ani in patients with atopic dermatitis. *J Dermatolog Treat*. 2013; in press.
5. Markell KW, Billingham RP. Pruritus ani: Etiology and management. *Surg Clin North Am*. 2010;90: 125–135.
6. Mentes BB, Akin M, Leventoglu S, et al. Intradermal methylene blue injection for the treatment of intractable idiopathic pruritus ani: Results of 30 cases. *Tech Coloproctol*. 2004;8:11–14.
7. Handa Y, Watanabe O, Adachi A, et al. Squamous cell carcinoma of the anal margin with pruritus ani of long duration. *Dermatol Surg*. 2003;29: 108–110.

ADDITIONAL READING

- Gooding SM, Canter PH, Coelho HF, et al. Systematic review of topical capsaicin in the treatment of pruritus. *Int J Dermatol*. 2010;49: 858–865.
- Rucklidge JJ, Saunders D. Hypnosis in a case of long-standing idiopathic itch. *Psychosom Med*. 1999;61:355–358.
- Zuccati G, Lotti T, Mastrolorenzo A, et al. Pruritus ani. *Dermatol Ther*. 2005;18:355–362.

SEE ALSO

Pinworms; Pruritus Vulvae

CODES

ICD10
L29.0 Pruritus ani

CLINICAL PEARLS

- Pruritus ani is a condition characterized by intense and often unpleasant anal and perianal itching and/or burning.
- Usually idiopathic or related to skin irritation.
- Conservative treatment and reassurance are successful in 90% of patients.
- Consider trial of dietary elimination of citrus, vitamin C supplements, milk products, coffee, tea, cola, chocolate, beer, and wine as adjuvant measure to proper hygiene.
- Consider infection in immunosuppressed patients.
- Consider underlying malignancy with refractory pruritus.

PRURITUS VULVAE

Laura K. Randolph, DO, MS • Michael P. Hopkins, MD, MEd

 BASICS

DESCRIPTION
- Pruritus vulvae is a symptom as well as a primary diagnosis:
  - The symptom may indicate an underlying pathological process.
  - Only when no underlying disease is identified may this be used as a primary diagnosis.
- Pruritus vulvae as a primary diagnosis may also be more appropriately documented as vulvodynia (see "Vulvodynia" topic) and burning vulva syndrome.

EPIDEMIOLOGY
Symptoms may occur at any given age during a woman's lifetime:
- Young girls most commonly have infectious or hygiene etiology.
- The primary diagnosis is more commonly seen in postmenopausal women.

Incidence
The exact incidence is unknown. However, most women complain of vulvar pruritus at some point in their lifetime.

ETIOLOGY AND PATHOPHYSIOLOGY
Vulvar tissue is more permeable than exposed skin due to differences in structure, occlusion, hydration, and susceptibility to friction. It is particularly vulnerable to irritants (1):
- Perfumes
- Soaps
- Laundry detergent
- Douches
- Toilet paper
- Sanitary napkins

RISK FACTORS
- High-risk sexual behavior
- Immunosuppression
- Obesity

GENERAL PREVENTION
- Attention should be paid to personal hygiene and avoidance of possible environmental factors.
- Tight-fitting clothing should be avoided.
- Only cotton underwear should be worn.

COMMONLY ASSOCIATED CONDITIONS
- Infectious etiology:
  - Vaginal or vulvar candida
  - *Gardnerella vaginalis*
  - *Trichomonas*
  - Human papillomavirus
  - Herpes simplex virus
- Vulvar vestibulitis
- Lichen sclerosis
- Lichen planus
- Lichen simplex chronicus (squamous cell hyperplasia)
- Malignant or premalignant conditions
- Psoriasis
- Fecal or urinary incontinence
- Excessive heat with sweat
- Dietary: Methylxanthines (e.g., coffee, cola), tomatoes, peanuts
- Autoimmune progesterone dermatitis: Perimenstrual eruptions
- Irritant or allergic contact dermatitis
- Atopic dermatitis

 DIAGNOSIS

Pruritus vulvae is a diagnosis of exclusion.

HISTORY
- Persistent itching
- Persistent burning sensation over the vulva or perineum
- Change in vaginal discharge
- Postcoital bleeding
- Dyspareunia

PHYSICAL EXAM
- Visual inspection of the vulva, vagina, perineum, and anus:
  - Superior surfaces of the labia majora—extending from mons to the anal orifice are most involved
  - Vulvar skin is leathery or lichenified in appearance
  - Papillomatosis may be a sign of chronic inflammation
- Light touch identification of affected areas
- Cotton swab–applied pressure to vestibular glands

DIAGNOSTIC TESTS & INTERPRETATION
- Sodium chloride: Gardnerella or Trichomonas
- 10% potassium hydroxide: Candida
- Viral culture and polymerase chain reaction (PCR): Herpes simplex virus
- Directed biopsy: Human papillomavirus, lichen, malignancy
- Colposcopy with acetic acid of Lugol's solution of vagina and vulva

Follow-Up Tests & Special Considerations
- A patch test may be performed by a dermatologist to assist in identifying a causative agent if contact dermatitis is suspected.
- Exam-directed biopsies are essential in the postmenopausal population to rule out malignancy.

Diagnostic Procedures/Other
Biopsies should be collected from any ulceration, discoloration, raised areas, macerated areas, and the area of most intense pruritus.

Test Interpretation
- Only in the absence of pathological findings can the primary diagnosis of pruritus vulvae be made.
- In 1 study, a specific clinicopathologic diagnosis was obtained in 89% of patients by using the most recent 2006 International Society for the Study of Vulvar Diseases (ISSVD) classifications (2).

 TREATMENT

Identify the underlying cause or disease to target treatment:
- Stop all potential irritants (i.e., excessive body hygiene)
- Eliminate bacterial and fungal infection
- Cool the affected area: Use cool gel packs (not ice packs, which may cause further injury)
- Sitz baths and bland emollients to soothe fissured or eroded skin

MEDICATION
First Line
- Antihistamines (3)[C]:
  - Hydroxyzine 10–100 mg before bedtime (slow increase)
  - Doxepin 10–100 mg before bedtime (slow increase)
- SSRIs (3)[C]:
  - Citalopram 20–40 mg in the morning
- Topical steroids (4)[C]:
  - Triamcinolone 0.1% applied daily for 2–4 weeks, then twice weekly
  - Hydrocortisone 1–2.5% cream applied 2–4 times daily (5)
  - Avoid long-term use due to risk of atrophy.
  - One randomized, controlled trial showed no difference between topical triamcinolone and placebo cream (6).

Second Line
Topical pimecrolimus 1% cream applied b.i.d. for 3 weeks (7)[B]:
- May lead to an 80% reduction of pruritus

ISSUES FOR REFERRAL
- Persistent symptoms should prompt additional investigation and referral to a gynecologist or gynecologist oncologist.
- Gynecology oncology referral for proven or suspected malignancy
- Dermatology referral for patch testing to evaluate for contact dermatitis

ADDITIONAL THERAPIES
- SC triamcinolone injections (8)[B]
- Alcohol nerve block (9)[B]
- Laser therapy (10)[B]
- GnRH analogue (11)[C]

ONGOING CARE
- Frequent evaluation, repeat cultures, and biopsies are necessary for cases resistant to treatment.
- Refractory cases may require referral to gynecologist or gynecology oncology for further management.

DIET
Dietary alterations include avoidance of the following:
- Coffee and other caffeine-containing beverages
- Tomatoes
- Peanuts

PATIENT EDUCATION
- American Congress of Obstetricians and Gynecologists: www.acog.org
- National Vulvodynia Foundation: www.nva.org

PROGNOSIS
Conservative measures and short-term topical steroids control most patients' symptoms.

COMPLICATIONS
Malignancy

REFERENCES
1. Farage M, Maibach HI. The vulvar epithelium differs from the skin: Implications for cutaneous testing to address topical vulvar exposures. *Contact Dermatitis*. 2004;51:201–209.
2. Kelecki KH, Adamhasan F, Gencdal S, et al. The impact of the latest classification system of benign vulvar diseases on the management of the women with chronic vulvar pruritus. *Indian J Dermatol Venereol Leprol*. 2011;77:294–299.
3. Margesson LJ. Overview of treatment of vulvovaginal disease. *Skin Therapy Lett*. 2011;16:5–7.
4. Weichert GE. An approach to the treatment of anogenital pruritus. *Dermatol Ther*. 2004;17:129–133.
5. Pincus SH. Vulvar dermatoses and pruritus vulvae. *Dermatol Clin*. 1992;10:297–308.
6. Lagro-Janssen AL, Sluis S. Effectiveness of treating non-specific pruritus vulvae with topical steroids: A randomized controlled trial. *Eur J Gen Pract*. 2009;15:29–33.
7. Sarifakioglu E, Gumus II. Efficacy of topical pimecrolimus in the treatment of chronic vulvar pruritus: A prospective case series—a non-controlled, open-label study. *J Dermatolog Treat*. 2006;17:276–278.
8. Kelly RA, Foster DC, Woodruff JD. Subcutaneous injection of triamcinolone acetonide in the treatment of chronic vulvar pruritus. *Am J Obstet Gynecol*. 1993;169:568–570.
9. Woodruff JD, Babaknia A. Local alcohol injection of the vulva: Discussion of 35 cases. *Obstet Gynecol*. 1979;54:512–514.
10. Ovadia J, Levavi H, Edelstein T. Treatment of pruritus vulvae by means of CO_2 laser. *Acta Obstet Gynecol Scand*. 1984;63:265–267.
11. Banerjee AK, de Chazal R. Chronic vulvovaginal pruritus treated successfully with GnRH analogue. *Postgrad Med J*. 2006;82:e22.

ADDITIONAL READING
- Boardman LA, Botte J, Kennedy CM. Recurrent vulvar itching. *Obstet Gynecol*. 2005;100:1451–1455.
- Bohl TG. Overview of vulvar pruritus through the life cycle. *Clin Obstet Gynecol*. 2005;48:786–807.
- Farage MA, Miller KW, Ledger WJ. Determining the cause of vulvovaginal symptoms. *Obstet Gynecol Surv*. 2008;63:445–464.
- Foster DC. Vulvar disease. *Obstet Gynecol*. 2002;100:145–163.
- Petersen CD, Lundvall L, Kristensen E, et al. Vulvodynia. Definition, diagnosis and treatment. *Acta Obstet Gynecol Scand*. 2008;87:893–901.
- Sener AB, Kuscu E, Seckin NC, et al. Postmenopausal vulvar pruritus–colposcopic diagnosis and treatment. *J Pak Med Assoc*. 1995;45:315–317.

 ## CODES

ICD10
- L29.2 Pruritus vulvae
- N94.819 Vulvodynia, unspecified

CLINICAL PEARLS
- Most women complain of pruritus vulvae at some point in their lifetime.
- Pruritus vulvae is a diagnosis of exclusion once other causes of itching have been ruled out.
- Exam-directed biopsies from any ulceration, discoloration, raised areas, macerated areas, and the area of most intense pruritus are essential to rule out malignancy.
- Initial treatment is conservative.

PSEUDOBULBAR AFFECT

Aaron Hauptman, MD • Sheldon Benjamin, MD

 BASICS

- Pseudobulbar affect (PBA) is a neuropsychiatric disorder consisting of brief emotional outbursts thought to be caused by disruption of corticobulbar or possibly cortico-subcortical-thalamo-cerebellar circuitry (1).
- PBA is frequently undertreated due to misdiagnosis as mood disorder/other psychiatric condition (2).

DESCRIPTION

PBA is marked by emotional outbursts, particularly crying and laughter, that are (1):

- Uncontrollable
- Incongruous with (or exaggerated in comparison to) the patient's subjective, internal emotional state
- Dissociated from external (or internal) emotional stimuli
- Brief in duration (lasting seconds to minutes)
- Disruptive and potentially upsetting to the individual due to incongruity with mood and extremity of outbursts
- Stereotyped in episode semiology within an individual, but differing markedly between individuals (e.g., 1 patient may have only crying episodes, another may have only laughing episodes, whereas a 3rd may have both, although not simultaneously) (1)
- PBA is seen only in patients with underlying neurologic damage (1).
- Terminology surrounding PBA can be confusing
- PBA overlaps with/includes other disorders comorbid with neurologic conditions, particularly:
  - Pathologic laughing and crying (emotional response incongruous to stimulus) (part of PBA)
  - Affective lability (exaggerated affective response to emotional stimulus) (part of PBA)
  - Involuntary emotional expression disorder (synonym for PBA)
  - Pseudobulbar palsy (PBA is one component of this disorder)
- The term pseudobulbar should not give the impression that PBA is not a true neuropsychiatric disorder; rather, it refers to the neurologic and behavioral symptoms of corticobulbar disruption that mimic brainstem dysfunction.

EPIDEMIOLOGY

Incidence

Incidence is unclear

Prevalence

- Seen primarily in multiple sclerosis (MS), amyotrophic lateral sclerosis (ALS), Alzheimer disease, Parkinson disease, stroke, and traumatic brain injury (TBI):
  - Estimated prevalence across patients with these disorders is ~10%, although it may reach as high as 38% (2):
    - Significantly underdiagnosed (2)
- Between 2 and 7 million people in the US are estimated to suffer from PBA (2):
  - Prevalence estimates include ALS 2–49%; stroke 11–52%; MS 7–52%; Alzheimer disease 10–74%; Parkinson disease 7%; and TBI 5% (3)

ETIOLOGY AND PATHOPHYSIOLOGY

- Disruption of emotional motor pathway consisting of cortico-pontine-cerebellar circuitry is hypothesized to be at the root of PBA.
- Summary of pathway (1):
  - Flow from motor and frontotemporal cortices to brainstem drive physical expression of emotion-controlling behaviors such as laughter or crying.
  - These pathways require tuning modification for congruity between stimuli (both the external world and internal emotional states) and behavioral output.
  - This tuning is informed by direct somatosensory cortical inhibition of motor cortex and substantial cortical afferentation that descends to cerebellum.
  - This aggregate information converges at the basis pontis where it is then relayed to the cerebellum for integration.
  - The cerebellum integrates these data and appropriately modifies descending signals, yielding behavioral outputs consistent with emotional states and relevant sensory data.
  - PBA is believed to result from dysfunction anywhere along this circuit from cortex through basis pontis to cerebellum, disrupting coordination of mood and behavioral output and causing disinhibition of emotional motor expression.
- Neurotransmitter dysfunction:
  - Disruption of serotonin and glutamate systems are thought to be central to PBA:
    - This is based on both the known importance of these neurotransmitters to circuitry involved in PBA pathophysiology as well as the fact that effective treatments for this condition are serotonergic or antiglutamatergic (1).

RISK FACTORS

PBA is seen in patients with underlying neurologic dysfunction, including, but not limited to:

- MS, ALS, Parkinson disease, Alzheimer disease, stroke, and TBI (1)

 DIAGNOSIS

No formal set of diagnostic criteria exists in either the *DSM* or the *ICD* system. The following include recently proposed criteria for the diagnosis of PBA (1),(4)[C].

HISTORY

- Careful history is crucial for diagnosis: This disorder should be suspected in neurologic patients presenting with emotional changes since onset of neurologic disease:
  - Incongruence of mood and affect in a patient with emotional changes should raise suspicions of PBA over mood disorder.
  - PBA is frequently misdiagnosed as depression, "just part of underlying condition," posttraumatic stress disorder (PTSD), bipolar disorder, or other psychiatric disorders (2).
- Episodes of emotional expression, particularly laughter or crying, incongruous with emotional stimulus
- The emotional outbursts are typically disturbing to the patient because they do not match the patient's emotional state.
- Events last seconds to minutes
- Outbursts are similar from event to event for a given patient.
- Outbursts are not part of the patient's baseline emotional activity.
- History of underlying brain disorder:
  - If such a history is not present, the diagnosis either is not PBA or a neurologic condition is present that has not been recognized and requires further investigation.
- Proneness to anger may also be noted in the recent history.

PHYSICAL EXAM

- Thorough neurologic examination is crucial, with particular attention to pseudobulbar signs:
  - Increased jaw jerk
  - Exaggerated gag reflex
  - Tongue weakness
  - Dysarthria and dysphagia
- Facial flushing and other autonomic dysfunction may be present

DIFFERENTIAL DIAGNOSIS
- Mood disorder
- Anxiety disorder
- Seizure disorder (particularly dacrystic/gelastic)
- Essential crying
- Witzelsucht (1):
  - Finding significant humor in situations not considered funny by others
  - Seen most frequently in frontal cortical damage
- Pathologic laughing and crying (a subset of PBA):
  - Can be seen in stroke, ALS, Parkinson disease, MS, frontotemporal dementia, TBI, Alzheimer disease, epilepsy, normal pressure hydrocephalus, progressive supranuclear palsy, Wilson disease, or neurosyphilis
- Affective lability (a subset of PBA):
  - Can be seen in similar populations as pathologic laughing and crying, but may also be seen without neurologic disease
- Kluver-Bucy-like syndrome (placidity in situations that normally would evoke emotional responses):
  - Causes include herpes simplex encephalitis, frontotemporal dementia, ischemia/anoxia, temporal lobectomy, progressive subcortical gliosis, adrenoleukodystrophy, systemic lupus erythematosus (SLE), porphyria, or limbic encephalitis (5).

DIAGNOSTIC TESTS & INTERPRETATION
- No diagnostic test for PBA exists. Diagnosis is made by detailed history and observation.
- Brain CT/MR scanning may reveal scattered corticobulbar and subcortical lesions in vascular, traumatic, or demyelinating disease-related cases.

TREATMENT

MEDICATION
The combination of dextromethorphan (N-methyl-D-aspartate blocker)/quinidine (inhibits dextromethorphan metabolism) has not been tested in comparison with antidepressant agents that have been shown to be effective in some studies.

First Line
Dextromethorphan/Quinidine is the only FDA-approved treatment for PBA (6)[A]:
- 20 mg PO daily for the 1st 7 days followed by q12h maintenance dosing
- Side effects:
  - Most significant side effect is QTc prolongation:
    o Recommend baseline ECG before starting medication and follow-up ECG 2–4 hours following 1st dose
  - May be associated with serotonin syndrome when used with SSRIs or tricyclic antidepressants (TCAs).

- Because of dextromethorphan abuse risks, observe patients with substance abuse history when on this medication.
- Dextromethorphan is hepatically metabolized by CYP2D6; quinidine is a CYP2D6 inhibitor, which blocks first-pass metabolism of dextromethorphan, allowing it to be more systemically available.
  - Because of CYP2D6 interactions, attention should be paid when dextromethorphan/quinidine is used in conjunction with other CYP2D6-effecting medications.
  - Coadministration with paroxetine, another CYP2D6 substrate and inhibitor, for example, has been shown to increase plasma concentrations of all 3 medications and increase adverse event risks (7).
  - Clinicians should monitor especially closely for side effects as doses of each medication may need to be reduced.

Second Line
- SSRIs and TCAs have been historically used for PBA treatment and have been shown to be effective for PBA in small controlled trials (8)[B].
- These medications are not FDA approved for this use and have not been tested in large, well-controlled trials. Further testing in large, well-controlled trials is required.
- SSRIs and TCAs are easy to use and much less costly than dextromethorphan/quinidine
- Pharmacotherapies shown in trials to reduce PBA symptoms include (1)[C]:
  - Amitriptyline, nortriptyline, citalopram, fluoxetine, and sertraline.
- Because patients with PBA may be on combined dextromethorphan/quinidine and SSRIs, attention should be paid to increased side effect risk when CYP2D6-modifying medications such as paroxetine are coadministered.
  - As described above, patients should be monitored closely and doses may need to be decreased if side effects present.

REFERENCES
1. Miller A, Pratt H, Schiffer RB, et al. Pseudobulbar affect: The spectrum of clinical presentations, etiologies and treatments. *Expert Rev Neurother*. 2011;11:1077–1088.
2. Work SS, Colamonico JA, Bradley WG, et al. Pseudobulbar affect: An under-recognized and under-treated neurological disorder. *Adv Ther*. 2011;28:586–601.

3. Strowd RE, Cartwright MS, Okun MS, et al. Pseudobulbar affect: Prevalence and quality of life impact in movement disorders. *J Neurol*. 2010;257:1382–1387.
4. Cummings JL, Arciniegas DB, Brooks BR, et al. Defining and diagnosing involuntary emotional expression disorder. *CNS Spectr*. 2006;11:1–7.
5. Arciniegas DB. A clinical overview of pseudobulbar affect. *Am J Geriatr Pharmacother*. 2005;3 (Suppl A):4–8; quiz 16–17.
6. Garnock-Jones KP. Dextromethorphan/quinidine: In pseudobulbar affect. *CNS Drugs*. 2011;25:435–445.
7. Schoedel KA, Pope LE, Sellers EM. Randomized open-label drug-drug interaction trial of dextromethorphan/quinidine and paroxetine in healthy volunteers. *Clin Drug Investig* 2012;32:157–169.
8. Rosen HJ, Cummings J. A real reason for patients with pseudobulbar affect to smile. *Ann Neurol*. 2007;61:92–96.

CODES

ICD10
F48.2 Pseudobulbar affect

CLINICAL PEARLS
- PBA is an underdiagnosed disorder that has an impact on patients already suffering from neurologic disease.
- Available pharmacotherapy can help alleviate symptoms.
- PBA is often misdiagnosed as psychiatric or other illness and thus an opportunity for treatment is missed.

PSEUDOFOLLICULITIS BARBAE

Maurice Duggins, MD

 BASICS

DESCRIPTION
- Foreign-body inflammatory reaction from an ingrown hair resulting in the appearance of papules and pustules. This is found mainly in the bearded area (*barbae*), but may occur in other hairy locations such as the scalp, axilla, or pubic areas where shaving is done.
- A mechanical problem: Extrafollicular and transfollicular hair penetration
- System(s) affected: Skin/Exocrine
- Synonym(s): Chronic sycosis barbae; Pili incarnate; Folliculitis barbae traumatica; Razor bumps; Shaving bumps; Tinea barbae; Pseudofolliculitis barbae (PFB)

EPIDEMIOLOGY
- Predominant age: Postpubertal, middle age (40–75)
- Predominant sex: Male > Female (can be seen in females of all races who wax/shave axillary and pubic areas) (1)

Incidence
- Adult male African Americans: 50,000/100,000
- Adult male whites: 3,000–5,000/100,000

Prevalence
- Widespread in Fitzpatrick skin types 4–6 (darker complexions) who shave
- 45–83% of African American soldiers who shave

ETIOLOGY AND PATHOPHYSIOLOGY
- Transfollicular escape of the low-cut hair shaft as it tries to exit the skin is accompanied by inflammation and often an intraepidermal abscess (2).
- As the hair enters the dermis, more severe inflammation occurs, with down growth of the epidermis in an attempt to sheath the hair.
- A foreign-body reaction forms at the tip of the invading hair, followed by abscess formation.
- Shaving too close
- Plucking/tweezing or wax depilation of hair may cause abnormal hair growth in injured follicles.

Genetics
- People with curly hair have an asymmetric accumulation of acidic keratin hHa8 on hair shaft (3).
- Single-nucleotide polymorphism (disruption Ala12Thr substitution) affects keratin of hair follicle (3).

RISK FACTORS
- Curly hair
- Shaving too close or shaving with multiple razor strokes
- Plucking/Tweezing hairs
- South Mediterranean/American, Middle Eastern, Asia, or African descent (skin types 4–6)

GENERAL PREVENTION
- Prior to shaving, rinse face with warm water to hydrate and soften hairs.
- Use adjustable hair clippers that leave very low hair length above skin.
- Shave with either a manual adjustable razor at coarsest setting (avoids close shaves), a single-edge blade razor (e.g., Bump Fighter), a foil-guarded razor (e.g., PFB razor), or electric triple "O-head" razor.
- Empty razor of hair frequently
- Shave in the direction of hair growth. Do not overstretch skin when shaving.
- Use a generous amount of the correct shaving cream/gel (e.g., Ef-Kay Shaving Gel, Edge Shaving Gel, Aveeno Therapeutic Shave Gel, Easy Shave Medicated Shaving Cream).
- Daily shaving reduces papules/pruritus (4)
- Regular use of depilatories

COMMONLY ASSOCIATED CONDITIONS
- Keloidal folliculitis
- Pseudofolliculitis nuchae

 DIAGNOSIS

HISTORY
Pain on shaving; pruritus of shaved areas, irritated "razor bumps"

PHYSICAL EXAM
- Tender, exudative, erythematous follicular papules or pustules in beard area (less commonly in scalp, axilla, and pubic areas); range from 2–4 mm (5)
- Hyperpigmented "razor or shave bumps"
- Alopecia
- Lusterless, brittle hair

DIFFERENTIAL DIAGNOSIS
- Bacterial folliculitis
- Impetigo
- Acne vulgaris
- Tinea barbae
- Sarcoidal papules

DIAGNOSTIC TESTS & INTERPRETATION
Initial Tests (lab, imaging)
- Clinical diagnosis
- Culture of pustules: Usually sterile; may show coagulase-negative staphylococcal epidermidis (normal skin flora)
- Additional hormonal testing may be indicated in females with hirsutism and/or polycystic ovary syndrome: dehydroepiandrosterone sulfate, luteinizing hormone (LH)/follicle-stimulating hormone (FSH), and free and total testosterone (3).

Test Interpretation
Follicular papules and pustules (2)

 TREATMENT

- Mild cases:
  - Stop shaving or avoid close shaving for 30 days while keeping beard groomed and clean
  - Consider 5% benzoyl peroxide after shaving and application of 1% hydrocortisone cream at bedtime (or LactiCare HC lotion after shaving).
  - Tretinoin 0.025% cream; apply daily
- Moderate cases:
  - Chemical depilatories (barium sulfide; Magic Shave powder); 1st test on forearm for 48 hours (for irritation).
  - Consider eflornithine HCl cream (Vaniqa) to reduce hair growth and stiffness, but it can cause PFB (6).
- Severe cases:
  - Laser therapy (7)[A]: Longer wavelength laser (e.g., neodymium [Nd]:YAG) is safer for dark skin (1)
  - Avoid shaving altogether; grow beard

GENERAL MEASURES
Acute treatment:
- Dislodge embedded hair with sterile needle/tweezers
- Discontinue shaving until red papules have resolved (minimum 3–4 weeks; longer if moderate or severe); can trim to length >0.5 cm during this time
- Massage beard area with washcloth, coarse sponge, or a soft brush several times daily
- Hydrocortisone 1–2.5% cream to relieve inflammation
- Selenium sulfide if seborrhea is present and to help reduce pruritus
- Systemic antibiotics if secondary infection is present

Pregnancy Considerations
Do not use tretinoin (Retin-A), tetracycline, or benzoyl peroxide

MEDICATION
First Line
- Topical or systemic antibiotic for secondary infection:
  - Application of clindamycin (Cleocin T) solution b.i.d. or topical erythromycin
  - Low-dose erythromycin or tetracycline 250–500 mg PO b.i.d. for more severe inflammation
  - Benzoyl peroxide 5%–clindamycin 1% gel b.i.d. (8)[C]: Administer until papule/pustule resolves
- Mild cases: Tretinoin 0.025% cream at bedtime; combination of the above therapies
- Moderate disease/chemical depilatories:
  - Disrupt cross-linking of disulfide bonds of hair to produce blunt (less sharp) hair tip
  - Apply no more frequently than every 3rd day: 2% barium sulfide (Magic Shave) or calcium thioglycollate (Surgex); calcium hydroxide (Nair)

- Contraindications:
  - Clindamycin: Hypersensitivity history; history of regional enteritis or ulcerative colitis; history of antibiotic-associated colitis
  - Erythromycin, tetracycline, tretinoin: Hypersensitivity history
- Precautions:
  - Clindamycin: Colitis, eye burning and irritation, skin dryness; pregnancy Category B
  - Erythromycin: Use cautiously in patients with impaired hepatic function; GI side effects, especially abdominal cramping; pregnancy Category B (erythromycin base formulation).
  - Chemical depilatories: Use cautiously; frequent use and prolonged application may lead to irritant contact dermatitis and chemical burns.
  - Tetracycline: Permanent discoloration of teeth if given during last half of pregnancy
  - Tretinoin: Severe skin irritation; pregnancy Category C
  - Benzoyl peroxide: Skin irritation and dryness, allergic contact dermatitis
  - Hydrocortisone cream: Local skin irritation, skin atrophy with prolonged use, lightening of skin color
- Significant possible interactions:
  - Erythromycin: Increases theophylline and carbamazepine levels; decreases clearance of warfarin; cardiac toxicity with terfenadine and astemizole
  - Tetracycline: Depresses plasma prothrombin activity (therefore, warfarin dosage must be decreased)

Second Line
Chemical peels with either glycolic acid or salicylic acid

ISSUES FOR REFERRAL
- Worsening or poor response to the above therapies after 4–6 weeks should prompt dermatology consultation.
- Occupational demands may also prompt earlier referral to dermatology for more aggressive therapy.

SURGERY/OTHER PROCEDURES
Laser treatment with long-pulsed Nd:YAG is helpful for severe cases (8)

 ## ONGOING CARE

FOLLOW-UP RECOMMENDATIONS
Patient Monitoring
- As needed
- Educate patient on curative and preventive treatment

DIET
- No restrictions
- No dietary studies available

PATIENT EDUCATION
- Dunn JF Jr. Pseudofolliculitis barbae. *Am Fam Physician*. 1988;38:170–172.
- Medlineplus.com

PROGNOSIS
- Good, with preventive methods
- Prognosis is poor in the presence of progressive scarring and foreign-body granuloma formation.

COMPLICATIONS
- Scarring (occasionally keloidal)
- Foreign-body granuloma formation
- Disfiguring postinflammatory hyperpigmentation (use sunscreens; can treat with hydroquinone 4% cream, Retin A, clinical peels) (3)
- Impetiginization of inflamed skin
- Epidermal (erythema, crusting, burns with scarring) and pigmentary changes with laser (1,5)

REFERENCES

1. Bridgeman-Shah S. The medical and surgical treatment of pseudofolliculitis barbae. *Dermatol Ther*. 2004;17:158–163.
2. Kindred C, Oresajo CO, Yatskayer M, et al. Comparative evaluation of men's depilatory composition versus razor in black men. *Cutis*. 2011;88:98–103.
3. Quarles FN, Brody H, Johnson BA, et al. Pseudofolliculitis barbae. *Dermatol Ther*. 2007;20:133–136.
4. Daniel A. Shave frequency and regimen variation effects on the management of pseudofolliculitis barbae. *J Drugs Dermatol*. 2013;12:410–418.
5. Perry PK. Defining pseudofolliculitis barbae in 2001: A review of the literature and current trends. *J Am Acad Dermatol*. 2002;46(Suppl 2):S113–S119.
6. Xia Y, Cho S, Howard RS, et al. Topical eflornithine hydrochloride improves the effectiveness of standard laser hair removal for treating pseudofolliculitis barbae: A randomized, double-blinded, placebo-controlled trial. *J Am Acad Dermatol*. 2012;67:694–699.
7. Weaver SM, Sagaral EC. Treatment of pseudofolliculitis barbae using the long-pulse Nd:YAG laser on skin types V and VI. *Dermatol Surg*. 2003;29:1187–1191.
8. Cook-Bolden FE. Twice daily application of benzoyl peroxide 5% clindamycin 1% gel versus vehicle in treatment of pseudofolliculitis barbae. *Cutis*. 2004;73(6 Suppl):13–24.

ADDITIONAL READING

Shenenberger DW, Utecht LM. Removal of unwanted facial hair. *Am Fam Physician*. 2002;66:1907–1911.

 ## SEE ALSO

Folliculitis; Impetigo

 ## CODES

ICD10
- B35.0 Tinea barbae and tinea capitis
- L73.1 Pseudofolliculitis barbae

CLINICAL PEARLS

- Electrolysis is not recommended as a treatment. It is expensive, painful, and often unsuccessful.
- Combination of laser therapy with eflornithine is more effective than laser alone.
- Use Bump Fighter razor from American Safety Razor Company (www.asrco.com).
- Men may prefer the convenience of the Bump Fighter razor over depilatory products.
- The aversive smell of sulfur could be a problem with some depilatory products.
- Have patient test for skin sensitivity with a small (coin-sized) amount of the depilatory on the bearded area or forearm.

PSEUDOGOUT

Dylan C. Kwait, MD

 BASICS

DESCRIPTION
- Autoinflammatory disease triggered by calcium pyrophosphate dihydrate (CPPD) crystal deposition in the joints.
- 1 of many diseases associated with pathologic mineralization and ossification:
  - Although chondrocalcinosis and pseudogout are characterized by CPPD crystal deposition, ankylosing spondylitis, osteoarthritis, and vascular calcification are characterized by hydroxyapatite deposition (1).
- CPPD crystal deposition may cause a progressive degenerative arthritis in numerous joints:
  - Primarily affects the elderly
  - Usually involves large joints
- Symptom onset is insidious, resulting in symmetric polyarthritis similar to rheumatoid arthritis (RA).
- Definitive diagnosis requires the presence of CPPD crystals in synovial fluid (2).
- System(s) affected: Endocrine/Metabolic; Musculoskeletal

EPIDEMIOLOGY
Prevalence
- Predominant age: 80% of patients >60
- Predominant sex: Male = Female
- Chondrocalcinosis is present in 1:10 adults age 60–75 and 1:3 by >80, however only a small percentage develop arthropathy (3).

ETIOLOGY AND PATHOPHYSIOLOGY
- Arthropathy results from an acute autoinflammatory reaction to CPPD crystals shed into the synovial cavity.
- Neutrophils engulf CPPD crystals, inducing the formation of neutrophil extracellular traps which cause cellular damage and synovitis (4).
- Physical and chemical changes in aging cartilage favor crystal growth.

Genetics
Uncommonly seen in familial pattern with autosomal-dominant inheritance (<1% of patients); most cases are sporadic.

RISK FACTORS
- Advanced age
- Traumatic injury
- Pseudogout often may occur as a complication in patients hospitalized for other medical and surgical illnesses.

GENERAL PREVENTION
Colchicine 0.6 mg b.i.d. may be used prophylactically to reduce frequency of episodes in recurrent CPPD (5)[A].

COMMONLY ASSOCIATED CONDITIONS
- Hyperparathyroidism
- Hemochromatosis
- Gout
- Hypophosphatasia
- Hypothyroidism
- Ochronosis
- Wilson disease
- Amyloidosis
- Hypomagnesemia

 DIAGNOSIS

HISTORY
- Acute pain and swelling of ≥1 or more joints; knee involved in 1/2 of all attacks; ankle, wrist, and shoulder are also commonly involved.
- May present as a chronic progressive arthritis with superimposed acute inflammatory attacks.
- Progressive degenerative arthritis in numerous joints, including wrists, metacarpophalangeal, hips, shoulders, elbows, and ankles.
- Low-grade inflammatory arthritis with multiple symmetric joint involvement (mimicking RA) in <5% of cases.
- Can present in proximal joints (mimicking polymyalgia rheumatica), often accompanied by tibiofemoral and ankle arthritis and tendinous calcifications (6)[C].
- May develop after intra-articular injection of hyaluronic acid (Hyalgan, Synvisc) (7)[C].

PHYSICAL EXAM
- Inflammation, joint effusion, decreased range of motion
- 50% associated with fever
- Any other synovial joint may be involved, including 1st metatarsophalangeal joint

DIFFERENTIAL DIAGNOSIS
- Illnesses that may cause acute inflammatory arthritis in a single or multiple joint(s):
  - Gout
  - Septic arthritis
  - Trauma
- Other illnesses that may present with an acute inflammatory arthritis:
  - Reiter syndrome
  - Lyme disease
  - Acute RA

DIAGNOSTIC TESTS & INTERPRETATION
Initial Tests (lab, imaging)
Synovial fluid analysis consistent with an inflammatory effusion:
- Cell count 2,000–100,000 WBCs/mL
- Differential predominantly neutrophils (80–90%)
- >50,000 WBC count increases likelihood of septic arthritis, 11% prevalence; number needed to treat (NNT) = 9; >100,000 WBCs/mL, 22% prevalence (8)[C]
- Wet prep with polarized microscopy may demonstrate small numbers of weakly *positively birefringent* crystals in the fluid and within neutrophils; false-negative rate is high
- The following metabolic studies should always be obtained in patients <50 and should be considered in the elderly to exclude an underlying etiology:
  - Serum calcium
  - Serum phosphorus
  - Serum alkaline phosphatase
  - Serum parathormone (i-PTH)
  - Serum iron, total iron-binding capacity, and serum ferritin
  - Serum magnesium
  - Serum thyroid-stimulating hormone (TSH) level

- Plain radiographs:
  - Radiographic findings in pseudogout are neither sensitive nor specific (2)[A].
  - Punctate and linear calcifications may be visualized in articular hyaline or fibrocartilage.
  - Knees, hips, symphysis pubis, and wrists are most commonly affected.
  - Patients with chronic CPPD may demonstrate subchondral cysts and loose bodies (i.e., osseous fragmentation with formation of intra-articular radiodense bodies) in joints not typically affected by degenerative joint disease (e.g., osteoarthritis).
- US:
  - US may be more useful than plain radiography for the diagnosis of pseudogout in peripheral joints (2)[A], with a positive predictive value of 92% and negative predictive value of 93% (9)[C].
  - US imaging characteristics of pseudogout include: Joint effusion, synovial thickening, and hyperechoic deposits (9)[C].
- MRI:
  - Chondrocalcinosis may be evident as hypointense lesions on MRI, particularly in association with the menisci of the knee (10).

Diagnostic Procedures/Other
Aspiration of joint fluid with synovial fluid analysis and demonstration of CPPD crystals is required for diagnosis (2)[A]; aspiration may relieve symptoms and speed resolution of the inflammatory process.

Test Interpretation
CPPD crystal deposition in articular cartilage, synovium, ligaments, and tendons.

TREATMENT

GENERAL MEASURES
Current regimens are directed at relieving the symptoms of joint inflammation:
- Rest and elevate affected joint(s)
- Apply ice/cool compresses to affected joints
- Non-weight bearing on affected joint while painful; use crutches or a walker.

MEDICATION
First Line
- A combination of pharmacologic and nonpharmacologic measures is recommended (11)[A].
- Acute attacks should be treated with cool packs, rest, and joint aspiration/steroid injection (11)[A].
- Chronic inflammatory CPPD arthropathy should be managed prophylactically with oral NSAIDs and/or colchicine (11)[A].
- Oral NSAIDs:
  - Ibuprofen (Motrin) 600–800 mg PO t.i.d.–q.i.d. with food; maximum 3.2 g/d
  - Naproxen (Naprosyn) 500 mg PO b.i.d. with food
  - Other NSAIDs at anti-inflammatory doses are effective, although indomethacin has higher complication rates (relative risk [RR] = 2.2) compared with ibuprofen (RR = 1.2) (12)[B].

- Oral colchicine (13)[C]:
  - 0.6 mg q.i.d. or 0.6 mg hourly until symptoms relieved or vomiting/diarrhea develops; maximum dose per attack 4–6 mg; 0.5–1 mg/d may be used (11)[A]; avoid with significant renal insufficiency
- Intra-articular steroid injection:
  - Prednisolone–sodium phosphate 4–20 mg or triamcinolone diacetate 2–40 mg administered with local anesthetic
- Contraindications:
  - History of hypersensitivity to NSAIDs or aspirin
  - Active peptic ulcer disease or history of recurrent upper GI lesions
  - Avoid in renal insufficiency if serum creatinine >1.6 mg/dL
  - Serious GI bleeding can occur without warning; follow the patient carefully for internal bleeding. Administer proton pump inhibitor (PPI) or misoprostol 200 μg PO q.i.d. in patients with peptic ulcer disease history.

ALERT
Significant possible interactions:
- May elevate BP in treated hypertensives
- May blunt antihypertensive effects of ACE inhibitors
- May prolong prothrombin time (PT) in patients taking oral anticoagulants
- Avoid concomitant aspirin use
- May blunt diuretic effect of furosemide and hydrochlorothiazide
- May increase plasma lithium level in patients taking lithium carbonate

Second Line
- Oral prednisone: Begin at 40–60 mg/d and taper over 10 days.
- IM triamcinolone acetonide 60 mg; may repeat in 1–4 days (8)[B].
- Methotrexate may have a role in severe disease resistant to traditional therapy (13,14)[C].

ISSUES FOR REFERRAL
Consider consultation with orthopedist or rheumatologist if septic joint is a serious consideration or patient is not responding.

ADDITIONAL THERAPIES
Physical therapy:
- Isometric exercises to maintain muscle strength during the acute stage (e.g., quadriceps isometric contractions, leg lifts if knee affected)
- Begin joint range-of-motion (ROM) exercises as inflammation and pain subside
- Resume weight bearing when pain subsides

SURGERY/OTHER PROCEDURES
Perform arthrocentesis and joint fluid analysis

IN-PATIENT CONSIDERATIONS
Admission Criteria/Initial Stabilization
Consider admission for septic arthritis if:
- Synovial fluid WBC count >50,000/mL
- Strongly consider if >100,000/mL
- Treat with appropriate antibiotics pending culture results

ONGOING CARE

FOLLOW-UP RECOMMENDATIONS
Patient Monitoring
Re-evaluate patient for response to therapy 48–72 hours after treatment instituted; re-examine 1 week later, then as needed.

DIET
No known relationship to diet

PATIENT EDUCATION
- Rest affected joint
- Symptoms usually resolve in 7–10 days

PROGNOSIS
- Acute attack usually resolves in 10 days; prognosis for resolution of acute attack is excellent.
- Patients may experience progressive joint damage with functional limitation.

COMPLICATIONS
- Recurrent acute attacks
- Erosive destructive arthritis

Geriatric Considerations
Elderly patients treated with NSAIDs require careful monitoring and are at higher risk for GI bleeding and acute renal insufficiency.

REFERENCES

1. Mebarek S, Hamade E, Thouverey C, et al. Ankylosing spondylitis, late osteoarthritis, vascular calcification, chondrocalcinosis and pseudo gout: Toward a possible drug therapy. *Curr Med Chem*. 2011;18:2196–2203.
2. Zhang W, Doherty M, Bardin T, et al. European League Against Rheumatism recommendations for calcium pyrophosphate deposition. Part I: Terminology and diagnosis. *Ann Rheum Dis*. 2011;70:563–570.
3. Richette P, Bardin T, Doherty M. An update on the epidemiology of calcium pyrophosphate dihydrate crystal deposition disease. *Rheumatology (Oxford)*. 2009;84:711–715.
4. Panq L, Hayes CP, Buac K, et al. Pseudogout-associated inflammatory calcium pyrophosphate dihydrate microcrystals induce formation of neutrophil extracellular traps. *J Immunol*. 2013;190:6488–6500.
5. Macmullan P, McCarthy G. Treatment and management of pseudogout: insights for the clinician. *Ther Adv Musculoskelet Dis*. 2012;4:121–131.
6. Pego-Reigosa JM, Rodriguez-Rodriguez M, Hurtado-Hernandez Z, et al. Calcium pyrophosphate deposition disease mimicking polymyalgia rheumatica: A prospective followup study of predictive factors for this condition in patients presenting with polymyalgia symptoms. *Arthritis Rheum*. 2005;53:931–938.
7. Hamburger MI, Lakhanpal S, Mooar PA, et al. Intra-articular hyaluronans: A review of product-specific safety profiles. *Semin Arthritis Rheum*. 2003;32:296–309.
8. Shah K, Spear J, Nathanson LA, et al. Does the presence of crystal arthritis rule out septic arthritis? *J Emerg Med*. 2007;32:23–26.
9. Filippou G, Frediani B, Gallo A, et al. A "new" technique for the diagnosis of chondrocalcinosis of the knee: Sensitivity and specificity of high-frequency ultrasonography. *Ann Rheum Dis*. 2007;66:1126–1128.
10. Demertzis JL, Rubin DA. MR imaging assessment of inflammatory, crystalline-induced, and infectious arthritides. *Magn Reson Imaging Clin North Am*. 2011;19:339–363.
11. Zhang W, Doherty M, Pascual E, et al. EULAR recommendations for calcium pyrophosphate deposition. Part II: Management. *Ann Rheum Dis*. 2011;70:571–575.
12. Richy F, Bruyere O, Ethgen O, et al. Time dependent risk of gastrointestinal complications induced by non-steroidal anti-inflammatory drug use: A consensus statement using a meta-analytic approach. *Ann Rheum Dis*. 2004;63:759–766.
13. Lioté F, Ea HK. Recent developments in crystal-induced inflammation pathogenesis and management. *Curr Rheumatol Rep*. 2007;9:243–250.
14. Chollet-Janin A, Finckh A, Dudler J, et al. Methotrexate as an alternative therapy for chronic calcium pyrophosphate deposition disease: An exploratory analysis. *Arthritis Rheum*. 2007;56:688–692.

ADDITIONAL READING
- Announ N, Guerne PA. Treating difficult crystal pyrophosphate dihydrate deposition disease. *Curr Rheumatol Rep*. 2008;10:228–234.
- Wise CM. Crystal-associated arthritis in the elderly. *Clin Geriatr Med*. 2005;21:491–511, v–vi.

CODES

ICD10
M11.20 Other chondrocalcinosis, unspecified site

CLINICAL PEARLS
- Suspect in arthritis cases with a pattern of joint involvement not usually affected by degenerative joint disease (e.g., metacarpophalangeal joints, wrists).
- Perform joint fluid aspiration and analysis to evaluate acute arthritis.
- If septic arthritis is considered, treat presumptively with antibiotics until culture results are available.
- NSAID therapy is preferred treatment.
- Oral steroids are useful if NSAIDs are contraindicated.
- Intra-articular steroids can be used *if* septic arthritis has been excluded.

PSORIASIS
Alyssa Miceli, DO • Karen Sheflin, DO

 BASICS

DESCRIPTION
- A chronic, multisystem inflammatory disorder most commonly characterized by cutaneous erythematous papules and plaques with silvery scale. A complex genetic and immune-mediated disorder with flares related to systemic, psychological, infectious, and environmental factors. Skin disease with multiple different phenotypic variations and degrees of severity (1).
- Clinical phenotypes:
  - Plaque (vulgaris): Most common variant (>80% of cases); well-demarcated, scaly, pink-to-red plaques of various sizes; symmetrically distributed on scalp, extensor surfaces of extremities, and trunk
  - Guttate: <2% of psoriasis patients, usually in patients <30 years of age; presents abruptly with 1-mm to 10-mm droplet-shaped pink papules and fine scale over trunk and extremities; often preceded by group A beta-hemolytic streptococcal infection 2–3 weeks earlier
  - Inverse: Affects intertriginous areas and flexural surfaces; pink-to-red plaques with minimal scale; absence of satellite pustules distinguishes it from candidiasis
  - Erythrodermic: ~1–2.25% of psoriasis patients; generalized erythema and scaling, affecting >75% of body surface area; associated with desquamation, hair loss, nail dystrophy, and systemic symptoms such as fever, chills, malaise or high-output cardiac failure; may require hospital admission for management of dehydration, electrolyte abnormalities, and high risk of infection
  - Pustular: Sterile pustules; several forms including generalized pustular psoriasis, annular pustular psoriasis, and impetigo herpetiformis; generalized type can result in life-threatening bacterial superinfections, sepsis, and dehydration if left untreated
  - Nail disease: Pitting, oil spots, and thickening; nails involved in up to 50% of patients with psoriasis
  - Psoriatic arthritis: Seronegative inflammatory spondyloarthropathy

EPIDEMIOLOGY
Incidence
- Predominant sex: Male = Female
- Predominant age: Two peaks in incidence between the ages of 20–30 and 50–60

Prevalence
- 2–4.7% (2)
- Similar prevalence in all races
- ~80% of patients have mild to moderate disease; 20% having severe disease (1)

ETIOLOGY AND PATHOPHYSIOLOGY
Antigenic triggers activate dendritic cells and T cells; plasmacytoid dendritic cells produce type I interferon, activating myeloid dendritic cells, which in turn produce interleukin (IL)-20 locally, which speeds keratinocyte proliferation; a subset of myeloid dendritic cells release IL-23 in lymph nodes, recruiting TH1 and TH17 cells to the lesions; T cells produce numerous cytokines, including interferon-γ, IL-17, and IL-22, that stimulate keratinocytes to proliferate and produce proinflammatory antimicrobial peptides and cytokines, which recruit neutrophils to the epidermis and activate dermal fibroblasts (3)

Genetics
- Genetic predisposition (probably polygenic)
- 40% have psoriasis in a 1st-degree relative
- Increased incidence of specific human leukocyte antigens (e.g., HLA-Cw6)
- Multiple susceptibility loci contain genes involved in immune system regulation (e.g., psoriasis-susceptibility [PSORS1] locus on chromosome 6p21; polymorphisms in the IL-12/IL-13 receptor, the p40 subunit of IL-12 and IL-23, and the p19 subunit of IL-12) (2)

RISK FACTORS
- Family history
- Local trauma; local irritation
- Diabetes, obesity, hyperlipidemia, metabolic syndrome
- HIV; Streptococcal infection
- Mental stress
- Withdrawal of steroid therapy
- Medications (lithium, antimalarials, β-blockers, interferon)
- Smoking

GENERAL PREVENTION
Avoid triggers, including trauma, sunburns, smoking, and exposure to certain medications (see above), alcohol and stress; weight loss if obese

COMMONLY ASSOCIATED CONDITIONS
- Psoriatic arthritis
- Obesity, metabolic syndrome, diabetes
- Cardiovascular disease; atherosclerotic disease (2,4)
- Nonalcoholic fatty liver disease (NAFLD)
- Autoimmune: Alopecia areata, celiac disease, Crohn disease, systemic sclerosis
- Psychiatric/Psychologic: Depression, suicide, emotional burden/anxiety
- Malignancy: Lymphoma, nonmelanoma skin cancer with psoralen-UVA (PUVA) therapy

 DIAGNOSIS

HISTORY
- May include sudden onset of clearly demarcated, erythematous plaques with overlying silvery scales exacerbation of chronic plaques; especially on extensor surfaces and scalp; generally no or mild pruritus, although some may have more significant pruritus; dystrophic nails and joint pain may be seen; triggers may include streptococcal/viral infection or trauma
- Family history of similar condition

PHYSICAL EXAM
- Well-demarcated salmon pink to red erythematous papules and plaques; silvery scale
- Distribution favors scalp, auricular conchal bowls and postauricular area; extensor surface of extremities, especially knees and elbows; umbilicus, lower back, intergluteal cleft, and nails
- Nail findings: Pitting, oil spots, onycholysis, subungual hyperkeratosis
- Auspitz sign: Underlying pinpoints of bleeding following scraping of plaques (4)
- Koebner phenomenon: New psoriatic lesions arising at sites of skin injury/trauma (4)
- Sebopsoriasis: Psoriasis can overlap with seborrheic dermatitis as greasy scales on the eyebrows, nasolabial folds, and postauricular and presternal areas

DIFFERENTIAL DIAGNOSIS
- Plaque: Seborrheic dermatitis, nummular eczema, atopic dermatitis, contact dermatitis, lichen planus, lichen simplex chronicus, tinea, pityriasis rubra pilaris, subacute/discoid lupus erythematosus, squamous cell carcinoma in situ
- Guttate: Pityriasis rosea, pityriasis lichenoides chronica, lichen planus, secondary syphilis, small plaque parapsoriasis
- Pustular: Subcorneal pustulosis, acute generalized exanthematous pustulosis, folliculitis, pemphigus foliaceous
- Erythrodermic: Cutaneous T-cell lymphoma, drug-induced erythroderma, Ichthyosiform erythroderma

DIAGNOSTIC TESTS & INTERPRETATION
Initial Tests (lab, imaging)
Clinical diagnosis based on history and physical exam (2). May include negative rheumatoid factor, normal erythrocyte sedimentation rate (ESR), and C-reactive protein (elevated in pustular/erythrodermic variants); uric acid level may be elevated in pustular psoriasis; sterile fluid from pustules with neutrophilic infiltrate; fungal studies in hand and foot psoriasis

Diagnostic Procedures/Other
- Psoriasis Area and Severity Index (PASI) evaluates overall severity and body surface area (BSA) involvement
- Physicians Global Assessment: Target plaque score and the percentage BSA together; 4-mm punch biopsy from affected skin, if necessary

Test Interpretation
Biopsy: Thickening of the stratum corneum (hyperkeratosis) with retention of nuclei (parakeratosis), basal cell hyperplasia, thin/absent granular cell layer; elongation, thickening, and clubbing of rete ridges; dilated tortuous capillary loops in the dermal papillae; perivascular lymphocytic infiltrate, Munro's microabscesses: Neutrophils in stratum corneum

 TREATMENT

GENERAL MEASURES
Adequate topical hydration (emollients), sun exposure (avoid sunburns), stress relief

MEDICATION
First Line
- Mild-to-moderate disease:
  - Emollients b.i.d.: Petrolatum/ointments to maintain skin hydration and minimize pruritus and risk of koebnerization

  - Topical corticosteroids (1,5)[A]:
    ○ Anti-inflammatory, antiproliferative, immunosuppressive and vasoconstrictive effects; tachyphylaxis develops over time, may alternate to prevent
    ○ Local side effects: Skin atrophy, hypopigmentation, striae, acne, folliculitis, and purpura. Systemic side effects: Risk is higher with higher potency formulations used over a large surface for a prolonged period; pregnancy Category C
    ○ Applications are typically twice daily until lesions flatten/resolve, then taper to PRN use for maintenance
    ○ Scalp: Strong potency in solution/foam vehicle; shampoos and sprays also available

- Face, intertriginous areas, infants: Low-potency corticosteroids: 1% hydrocortisone
- Adult initial therapy: Medium-potency corticosteroids daily (e.g., 0.1% mometasone or triamcinolone); strong-potency corticosteroids: 0.05% betamethasone or fluocinonide daily; (4)[A]; superpotency corticosteroids: Clobetasol, halobetasol; limit use to 2–4 weeks; avoid occlusive dressings; reserved for recalcitrant plaques (5,6)[A]
- Vitamin D analogues: Calcipotriene 0.005% ointment b.i.d.; limits keratinocyte hyperproliferation; may be highly effective for short-term control in combination with a superpotent corticosteroid (5,6)[A]; should not be used with products that can alter pH, such as topical lactic acid; local side effects: burning, pruritus, edema, peeling, dryness, and erythema; pregnancy Category C
- Topical retinoids: Tazarotene 0.05% or 0.1% (Tazorac) daily; normalizes abnormal keratinocyte differentiation and diminishes hyperproliferation; may be combined with corticosteroids; side effects: local irritation, photosensitivity; pregnancy Category X (6)[A]
- Topical calcineurin inhibitors: Tacrolimus 0.1% or pimecrolimus 1% may be used as steroid-sparing agents, especially in facial and intertriginous areas (1)[A]
- Comparison of topical therapies: Vitamin D analogues have slower onset of action than topical corticosteroids, but longer disease-free periods
- Severe disease: May need combination therapy
  - Light therapy: Locally immunosuppressive and antiproliferative. Natural sunlight; UVB (broad/narrow band) or PUVA (5)[C]: Broadband UVB up to 20–25 treatments 3 × per week with or without topical tar or anthralin (may increase effectiveness) until remission; UVA administered within 2 hours of receiving psoralen: initially 3 × per week until remission, then 1–2 × per week for maintenance; increased risk of nonmelanoma skin cancers with >350 treatments
  - Systemic therapies:
    - Methotrexate: Blocks DNA synthesis and inhibits proliferation of lymphoid tissue; start 7.5–15 mg/wk IV, PO, IM, or SC, then increase 2.5 mg every 2–3 weeks, up to 25 mg; contraindicated in pregnancy; supplement with folic acid 1–5 mg/d to protect against side effects (5)[C]: Hepatotoxicity, pulmonary toxicity, bone marrow suppression; baseline chest x-ray, monitor LFTs, renal function, CBC, testing for latent tuberculosis (TB); consider liver biopsy when cumulative dose reaches 3.5–4 g; avoid alcohol and medications that interfere with folic acid metabolism, including Bactrim, sulfamethoxazole, or hepatotoxic agents (e.g., retinoids) (5)[C]
    - Cyclosporine: Inhibits T-cell activation; start high dose 3–5 mg/kg/d for 12–16 weeks, and taper to 0.5–1 mg/kg/d for maintenance; pregnancy Class C; side effects: renal toxicity and hypertension, limit long-term use: Monitor renal function, CBC with Mg^{2+} and K^+, and BP
    - Acitretin (Soriatane): Systemic retinoid; onset ranges from 3–6 months; start 25–50 mg/d; effective for pustular psoriasis and as a maintenance therapy after stabilization with other agents; sometimes combined with UV-B/PUVA; teratogenic: Pregnancy test before starting; 2 forms of contraception 1 month before, during, and for at least 3 years after

treatment; avoid alcohol (may convert acitretin to etretinate) (1,5)[C]; side effects: Alopecia, xerosis, cheilitis, hepatotoxicity, hyperlipidemia, cataracts; monitor LFTs, renal function, lipid profile, CBC, regular eye exams (5)[C]

- Biologics: General guidelines: Screen for latent TB at baseline and yearly, hepatitis panel at baseline, avoid live vaccines; monitor CBC with differential, signs/symptoms of infections, heart failure, malignancy, drug-induced lupus, inflammatory bowel disease, demyelinating disorder. Etanercept (Enbrel): Recombinant human TNF-α receptor protein fused with the Fc portion of IgG1; blocks interaction with cell surface receptors; begin at 50 mg SC twice a week × 3 months then maintenance of 50 mg/week (2,5)[B]. Adalimumab (Humira): Human anti-TNF-α monoclonal antibody; specifically binds to soluble membrane-bound TNF-α; dosing starts at 80 mg SC × 1 week, then 40 mg SC every other week (5)[B]. Infliximab (Remicade): Chimeric monoclonal antibody binding TNF-α; 5 mg/kg IV at weeks 0, 2, and 6; maintenance doses of 5 mg/kg every 8 weeks thereafter; adjust interval, as needed (2,4)[B]; anaphylaxis-like infusion reaction occurs in <1% of patients. Ustekinumab (Stelara): Human monoclonal antibody against common p40 subunit of IL-12 and IL-23; Patients <100 kg: 45 mg SC at weeks 0 and 4, then every 12 weeks; >100 kg: 45 or 90 mg can be given

Second Line
Immunosuppressives: Azathioprine, hydroxyurea, 6-thioguanine, fumaric acid esters, and topicals: Salicylic acid; anthralin (6)[C]

ISSUES FOR REFERRAL
Psoriasis >20% of BSA, severe extremity involvement, particularly hands and feet

SURGERY/OTHER PROCEDURES
Psoriasis and psoriatic medications can affect wound healing postoperatively; Methotrexate: Monitor for postoperative infections; hold cyclosporine for 1 week before and after; some surgeons may prefer to hold therapy with biologics for up to 1 month before and after surgery.

IN-PATIENT CONSIDERATIONS
Admission Criteria/Initial Stabilization
Generalized pustular psoriasis/erythrodermic psoriasis: Rule out sepsis; restoration of barrier function of skin with cleaning and bandaging; intensive topical corticosteroid therapy, phototherapy, systemic therapy, particularly medications with a quick onset such as oral cyclosporine; management of electrolytes

ONGOING CARE

FOLLOW-UP RECOMMENDATIONS
Measure BSA involvement to determine if therapy is working; change therapy or add agent if no improvement is seen (2,5).

DIET
Well-balanced diet and exercise to limit cardiovascular risk factors and decrease risk of associated conditions, including obesity, metabolic syndrome, diabetes, and atherosclerosis.

PATIENT EDUCATION
- American Academy of Dermatology: www.aad.org/skin-conditions/dermatology-a-to-z/psoriasis; 866-503-7546
- National Psoriasis Foundation: www.psoriasis.org; 800-723-9166

PROGNOSIS
Guttate form may be self-limited and remit after 4 months; chronic plaque type is lifelong, with intermittent spontaneous remissions and exacerbations; erythrodermic and generalized pustular forms may be severe and persistent

COMPLICATIONS
Psoriatic arthritis, generalized pustular psoriasis, erythrodermic psoriasis

REFERENCES
1. Menter A, Korman NJ, Elmets CA, et al. Guidelines of care for the management of psoriasis and psoriatic arthritis: Section 6. Guidelines of care for the treatment of psoriasis and psoriatic arthritis: Case-based presentations and evidence-based conclusions. J Am Acad Dermatol. 2011;65: 137–174.
2. Villasenor-Park J, Wheeler D, Grandinetti L. Psoriasis: Evolving treatment for a complex disease. Cleve Clin J Med. 2012;79:413–423.
3. Coimbra S, Figueiredo A, Castro E, et al. The roles of cells and cytokines in the pathogenesis of psoriasis. Int J Dermatol. 2012;4:389–395.
4. Kimball AB, Gladman D, Gelfand JM, et al. National Psoriasis Foundation clinical consensus on psoriasis comorbidities and recommendations for screening. J Am Acad Dermatol. 2008;84:1031–1042.
5. Menter A, Gottlieb A, Feldman SR, et al. Guidelines of care for the management of psoriasis and psoriatic arthritis: Section 1. Overview of psoriasis and guidelines of care for the treatment of psoriasis with biologics. J Am Acad Dermatol. 2008;58: 826–850.
6. Mason AR, Mason J, Cork M, et al. Topical treatments for chronic plaque psoriasis. Cochrane Database Syst Rev. 2009;2:CD005028.

 SEE ALSO

Arthritis, Psoriatic

 CODES

ICD10
- L40.0 Psoriasis vulgaris
- L40.4 Guttate psoriasis
- L40.9 Psoriasis, unspecified

CLINICAL PEARLS
Chronic lifelong inflammatory skin condition with remissions and exacerbations; if 1 medication does not work, use/combine with another agent.

PSYCHOSIS

Michael Golding, MD

 BASICS

DESCRIPTION

Syndrome seen with schizophrenia, schizoaffective disorder, mood disorder, substance use, medical problems, delirium, and dementia; symptoms include:

- Positive symptoms: Hallucinations and delusions (fixed false and often paranoid beliefs created as the patient loses the ability to correct errors in thinking)
- Negative symptoms: Apathy, avolition, withdrawal
- Disorganized speech/behavior
- Cognition: Decreased working memory, difficulty with attention, poor and slow information interpretation

EPIDEMIOLOGY

Prevalence

- Schizophrenia: Peak onset 18–25 years in men; women peak onset 25–35 years
  - 1% of the US population; thought to be similar worldwide
- Delusional disorder: 0.03% of population
- Bipolar type I: 1% of population
- Prevalence in major depression not known

ETIOLOGY AND PATHOPHYSIOLOGY

- Neurodevelopmental predisposition + 1st/3rd trimester in utero insult (e.g., 1st trimester infection or 3rd trimester birth hypoxia) leads to exaggerated neuronal apoptosis in late adolescence with subsequent thalamic sensory overload. Increased dopaminergic mesolimbic transmission may contribute to delusions and hallucinations in schizophrenia. Dopamine deficiency in mesocortical pathways may contribute to frontal lobe hypoactivity often associated with apathy and withdrawal in schizophrenia. Glutamate, neurosteroids, and neurodevelopmental abnormalities are active areas of research.
- Postulated stress-diathesis model: Individuals biologically at risk develop psychosis when under stress.

Genetics

Schizophrenia: 50% concordance for monozygotic twins, little or no shared environmental effect; multiple candidate genes involving disruption of neurodevelopment

RISK FACTORS

Substance abuse (particularly marijuana), family history of psychosis, lower socioeconomic status

GENERAL PREVENTION

Community interventions for early detection and treatment of prodromal symptoms show promise.

COMMONLY ASSOCIATED CONDITIONS

- Serious mental illness is associated with metabolic syndrome, autonomic dysfunction, sudden cardiac death.
- Cancer mortality: Particularly breast and lung cancer
- Substance abuse disorders, including nicotine dependence

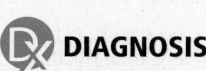 DIAGNOSIS

First rule out delirium: Psychosis should not have fluctuating consciousness/reduced clarity of awareness.

HISTORY

- Delusions (fixed false beliefs): Persecutory (being monitored), bizarre (involving impossible states), somatic (fixed belief in nonexistent serious illness), referential (getting messages from TV, radio, or thoughts inserted/deleted by others), grandiose (belief that one has special powers)
- Hallucinations: Auditory, visual, tactile
- Bipolar illness, depression, and dementia are all associated with psychosis, so screen for symptoms of depression, mania, and memory loss
- Screen for toxidromes of drugs of abuse
- Screen for history of epileptiform activity
- Suicidality: Higher risk with comorbid depression/mania, previous suicide attempts, drug abuse, agitation/akathisia, poor compliance

PHYSICAL EXAM

- Mental Status Exam: Disorganized idea sequencing and/or error correction, not incorrect thought content, is the *condicio sine qua non* of schizophrenia Patients often have negative symptoms (e.g., social withdrawal, lack of initiative, poverty of thought) and disorganized behavior
- Attention to neurologic focalities, antipsychotic-induced parkinsonism, tardive dyskinesia, and akathisia
- May rarely present with catatonia: Extreme excitement/lack of movement; posturing, mutism, grimacing, waxy flexibility

DIFFERENTIAL DIAGNOSIS

- Schizophrenia: Positive symptoms (psychosis) and negative symptoms (flat affect), prodrome of social withdrawal, cognitive impairment; schizophreniform disorder: Psychotic/Prodromal symptoms in <6 months; schizoaffective disorder: Manic/ Depressive mood disorder with hallucinations/ delusions that persist even when euthymic; schizotypal personality disorder: No true psychosis, but distance in relationships and odd beliefs; delusional disorder: Nonbizarre delusion (e.g., erotomanic, grandiose, jealous, persecutory, somatic), no negative/mood symptoms
- Mood disorder with psychotic features: Can occur in mania/depression. Delusions often mood-congruent; psychosis remits when mood improves.
- Substance-induced psychosis: Alcohol and benzodiazepine withdrawal, intoxication with cocaine, bath salts, PCP, cannabis, amphetamines, hallucinogens, and alcohol. May persist beyond acute intoxication.
- Borderline personality disorder: During extreme stress, patients often experience auditory/visual hallucinations (psychosis NOS).
- Posttraumatic stress disorder: Psychosis associated with traumatic recollections. Often visual hallucinations (vs. more auditory in schizophrenia).
- Psychosis due to general medical condition: delirium, stroke, infection, collagen vascular disease, head injury, tumor, interictal, porphyria, syphilis, etc.
- Medication-induced psychosis: Common causes: Steroids, L-dopa, anticholinergic medication, antidepressants in bipolar patients, interferon, digoxin, stimulants

DIAGNOSTIC TESTS & INTERPRETATION

Test for causes of delirium mimicking psychosis, if uncertain.

- Broad screen for medical causes: CBC, metabolic panel, LFTs, thyroid-stimulating hormone (TSH),

rapid plasma reagin (RPR), HIV, vitamin B_{12}, U/A, and screens for subclinical infection in elderly
- Screen for drugs of abuse.
- No imaging necessary for diagnosis. Consider MRI/CT to evaluate for medical cause of symptoms, especially if new onset or in elderly. In research studies, schizophrenia is associated with enlarged lateral ventricles and less frontal activity.

Follow-Up Tests & Special Considerations

Because of elevated risk related to schizophrenia and psychotropic medications, screen for metabolic syndrome.

- Consider: Wilson disease, porphyria, metachromatic leukodystrophy, inflammatory conditions
- Consider ECG: Antipsychotics can prolong corrected QT (QTc) interval, particularly ziprasidone, thioridazine, droperidol, IV haloperidol
- Consider lumbar puncture if unable to distinguish from delirium and/or unexplained rapid-onset psychosis.
- Consider electroencephalogram (EEG) for partial complex seizures and psychosis associated with preictal and postictal events.

 TREATMENT

Before antipsychotic treatment, lipid profile, fasting blood sugar, LFTs, metabolic panel, weight

MEDICATION

- Antipsychotics are the mainstay of treatment. Classified as typical vs. atypical. Dopamine-2 (D_2) antagonists with varied affinity for the receptor. Atypicals also block serotonin 5-HT2A receptors. Help positive symptoms more than negative. Nonspecific effect on agitation begins early; antipsychotic effect takes 1–6 weeks.
- For mania with psychotic features, a mood stabilizer may be used with an antipsychotic.
- For major depression with psychotic features, antidepressant and antipsychotic medications yield better response rate than either medication alone.
- In delirium, must treat underlying cause.
- Risks of antipsychotic medications include:
  - Acute dystonia: Utilize 1–3 mg IM/IV benztropine initially, then 0.5–2 mg b.i.d.–t.i.d. and/or diphenhydramine 50–100 mg IM/IV b.i.d.–t.i.d. max 400 mg/d.
  - Parkinsonism: Lower medication dose; switch to atypical (particularly, quetiapine, olanzapine, or clozapine) or add benztropine 0.5–2 mg PO b.i.d.–t.i.d., diphenhydramine 25–50 mg b.i.d.–t.i.d.
  - Akathisia: Intense restlessness, especially legs. Lower dose; switch or β-blocker, anticholinergic, antihistaminic/benzodiazepine, or utilize quetiapine, olanzapine, iloperidone, or clozapine.
  - Tardive dyskinesia: 20% of those treated long-term with typicals. Switch to clozapine or quetiapine. If cannot, minimize dose.
  - Neuroleptic malignant syndrome: Potentially fatal; rigidity, tremor, fever, autonomic instability, mental status changes; discontinue neuroleptic; ICU; volume resuscitation; cooling blankets; no anticholinergics/antihistaminics; consider dantrolene, amantadine, bromocriptine, electroconvulsive therapy (ECT)
  - Metabolic syndrome, sudden cardiac death (risk higher IM/IV droperidol, IV haloperidol), stroke (elderly), QTc prolonged, pulmonary embolus

First Line

- Benefits of some of the atypical antipsychotics include low risk of extrapyramidal symptoms (quetiapine, olanzapine, iloperidone, or clozapine) and tardive dyskinesia (clozapine, quetiapine); possibly more effective for negative symptoms
- Compared with typicals and some of the atypicals (ziprasidone, aripiprazole), more risk of weight gain, new-onset diabetes, and hyperlipidemia with olanzapine and clozapine.
- Acute psychotic agitation: Olanzapine 5–10 mg IM with up to three 10-mg injections over a 24-hour period, care with subsequent benzodiazepines; ziprasidone 5–20 mg IM q4–6h max 40 mg over a 24-hour period; haloperidol/lorazepam 5 mg/2 mg IM often with 1 mg IM benztropine, max 20 mg haloperidol, and 8 mg lorazepam over a 24-hour period
- Psychosis in schizophrenia:
  - Olanzapine: Start 5–10 mg at bedtime, target dose 5–20 mg/d within 2 days and up to 40 mg/d in treatment-refractory schizophrenia. More likely weight gain, hyperlipidemia, and hyperglycemia than other oral atypicals except clozapine (1)[B]; may have lower rates of discontinuation and rehospitalization than several other atypicals (1)[B], but likely not more efficacy than clozapine (2)[B]. Sedation initially.
  - Quetiapine: Start 25 mg b.i.d. 25–50 mg b.i.d.–t.i.d. on days 2 and 3, up to 300–400 mg in divided doses by day 4. Within 2 weeks, up to 400–800 mg/d divided b.i.d.–t.i.d.; less parkinsonism, useful in Parkinson disease psychosis; more weight gain than aripiprazole, lurasidone. ziprasidone; sedation, restless legs syndrome; more gradual titration tolerated better. Quetiapine XR can start 300 mg/d. Dose increases can be within 1 day and up to 300 mg/d, but slower start and titration may be better; target dose 300–800 mg at bedtime; lower parkinsonism, but more weight gain than aripiprazole, lurasidone, and ziprasidone. Sedation initially.
  - Risperidone: Start 1–2 mg/d; target dose of 1–4 mg/d to be reached over 1–2 weeks; 5–8 mg rarely more effective and higher risk of parkinsonism. Higher risk of prolactinemia/parkinsonism than clozapine, quetiapine, olanzapine.
  - Paliperidone: Start 3 mg/d target dose 3–12 mg/d; titrate over 1–2 weeks. Higher risk of prolactinemia/parkinsonism than clozapine, quetiapine, olanzapine.
  - Ziprasidone: Start 40 mg PO b.i.d., with target dose of 100–200 mg/d in divided doses over 2 weeks; prolongs QTc; less likely to cause weight gain than other atypicals; higher risk of akathisia/parkinsonism than clozapine, quetiapine, olanzapine. Requires meal. Often sedation.
  - Aripiprazole: Start 5–15 mg/d, increase to 10–30 mg/d over a week or 2; less weight gain, but higher rates of akathisia/parkinsonism than clozapine, quetiapine, olanzapine
  - Asenapine: Start 5 mg at bedtime or b.i.d. sublingually, increase to 10 b.i.d. if needed over a week or 2; less weight gain than some, higher rates of akathisia/parkinsonism than clozapine, quetiapine, olanzapine; sedation, numb tongue, nausea, bad taste; black cherry flavor preferred to plain.
  - Lurasidone: Start 20–40 mg at dinner with 350 calories, increase to 80/120 mg at bedtime if needed over 2–4 weeks. Less weight gain than some, but higher rates of akathisia/parkinsonism than clozapine, quetiapine, olanzapine; not antihistaminic, but α-blocking sedation and serotonergic nausea.
  - Iloperidone: Start 1 mg b.i.d., may increase by 2 mg b.i.d. each day, but slower can be better due to significant orthostasis. Increase to max 12 mg b.i.d. Little akathisia/parkinsonism, less weight gain than olanzapine or clozapine, but slower efficacy due to long titration, orthostasis, sedation.

Geriatric Considerations

Increased risk of cerebrovascular accident when antipsychotics are used in the elderly with dementia (3)[B].

Second Line

- Clozapine: More effective for reducing symptoms, preventing relapse, decreasing tardive dyskinesia, and decreasing suicidality than other antipsychotics (2), but 2nd line given risk of fatal agranulocytosis. National registry for all patients on clozapine, weekly CBC and absolute neutrophil count (ANC) for 6 months then every 2 weeks for 6 months, then every 4 weeks. More weight gain, hyperlipidemia, hyperglycemia, seizures, myocarditis, pulmonary embolus, and sedation, but low rate of parkinsonism, tardive dyskinesia. Useful in treatment-refractory psychosis and in Parkinson disease psychosis.
- Despite association with more weight gain than other antipsychotics, clozapine and olanzapine do not appear to increase risk of cardiac and all-cause mortality (4,5).
- Long-acting preparations: Available for 2 typicals (haloperidol and fluphenazine) and 4 atypicals (risperidone, paliperidone, olanzapine, aripiprazole; olanzapine requires registration due to rare delirium syndrome). Test tolerability with oral medication first. Long-acting neuroleptics promote compliance.
- Long-acting haloperidol, paliperidone, olanzapine, aripiprazole administered every 4 weeks; long-acting risperidone and fluphenazine administered every 2 weeks

ISSUES FOR REFERRAL

Encourage contact with advocacy groups for families and patients (National Alliance for the Mentally Ill).

ADDITIONAL THERAPIES

Cognitive-behavioral therapy (CBT) is an effective adjuvant to antipsychotics.

IN-PATIENT CONSIDERATIONS

Admission Criteria/Initial Stabilization

At risk for harm to self or others; extreme functional impairment; unable to care for self; new-onset psychosis

Discharge Criteria

No longer a danger to self or others and adequate outpatient treatment in place

 ONGOING CARE

FOLLOW-UP RECOMMENDATIONS

Close follow-up for inpatient discharge (high risk for suicide), utilize CBT, exercise, teach smoking cessation

PATIENT EDUCATION

National Alliance on Mental Illness: www.nami.org/

PROGNOSIS

Schizophrenia: Fluctuating course, 70% first-episode psychosis patients improve in 3–4 months; 7% will die of suicide; 20–40% will attempt suicide.

REFERENCES

1. Komossa K, Rummel-Kluge C, Hunger H, et al. Olanzapine versus other atypical antipsychotics for schizophrenia. *Cochrane Database Syst Rev.* 2010;(3):CD006654.
2. McEvoy JP, Lieberman JA, Stroup TS, et al. Effectiveness of clozapine versus olanzapine, quetiapine, and risperidone in patients with chronic schizophrenia who did not respond to prior atypical antipsychotic treatment. *Am J Psychiatry.* 2006;163:600–610.
3. van Iersel MB, Zuidema SU, Koopmans RT, et al. Antipsychotics for behavioural and psychological problems in elderly people with dementia: A systematic review of adverse events. *Drugs Aging.* 2005;22:845–858.
4. Tilhonen J, Lonnqvist J, Wahlbeck K, et al. 11-year follow-up mortality in patients with schizophrenia: A population-based cohort study. *Lancet.* 2009;22(9690):620–627.
5. Strom BL, Faich G, Eng SM, et al. Comparative mortality associated with ziprasidone vs. olanzapine in real-world use: The ziprasidone observational study of cardiac outcomes (zodiac). *Eur Psychiatry.* 2008;23:158.
6. Fayek M, Flowers C, Signorelli D, et al. Psychopharmacology: Underuse of evidence-based treatments in psychiatry. *Psychiatr Serv.* 2003;54:1453–1456.

 SEE ALSO

Delirium; Schizophrenia

 CODES

ICD10

- F29 Unsp psychosis not due to a substance or known physiol cond
- F20.9 Schizophrenia, unspecified
- F39 Unspecified mood [affective] disorder

CLINICAL PEARLS

- Antipsychotics are the mainstay of treatment; evidence corroborates decreased all-cause mortality in patients who are adherent to these medications (4).
- Clozapine and long-acting preparations are likely underutilized in schizophrenia in the US and may increase adherence (6), whereas newer atypicals (quetiapine, lurasidone, aripiprazole, olanzapine-fluoxetine combination) may help with depressive symptoms in psychosis.

PULMONARY ARTERIAL HYPERTENSION

Urooj Najm, MBBS • Najm Hasan Siddiqui, MD

 BASICS

DESCRIPTION

- Pulmonary arterial hypertension (PAH) is a category of pulmonary hypertension (PH) characterized by abnormalities in the small pulmonary arteries (precapillary PH) that produce increased pulmonary arterial pressure (PAP) and vascular resistance, eventually resulting in right-sided heart failure. PAH is a progressive disorder associated with increased mortality:
  - Previously, PH was classified as primary PH (without cause: Now idiopathic pulmonary arterial hypertension [IPAH]) or secondary PH (with cause or associated condition); now it is clear that some types of secondary PH closely match primary PH (IPAH) in their histology, natural history, and response to treatment. Therefore, WHO classifies PH into 5 groups based on mechanism, with PAH as group 1 in this classification.
- PAH is diagnosed by right heart catheterization and defined by:
  - Mean PAP $\geq$25 mm Hg at rest
  - Pulmonary capillary wedge pressure $\leq$15 mm Hg (to exclude PH owing to left heart disease i.e., group 2 PH)
  - Mild or absent chronic lung disease or other causes of hypoxemia (excludes PH owing to lung disease or hypoxemia; i.e., group 3 PH)
  - Absent venous thromboembolic disease (excludes chronic thromboembolic PH; i.e., group 4 PH)
  - Absent systemic disorder (like sarcoidosis), hematologic disorders (like myeloproliferative disease), and metabolic disorders (like glycogen storage disease). Purpose is to exclude group 5 PH.
- PAH is divided into 5 main categories:
  - Idiopathic: Sporadic, with no family history or risk factors
  - Heritable: IPAH with mutations or familial cases with or without mutations
  - Drug- or toxin-induced: Mostly associated with anorectics (e.g., fenfluramine), rapeseed oil, L-tryptophan, and illicit drugs such as methamphetamine and cocaine
  - Associated: Connective tissue diseases (e.g., systemic lupus erythematosus, rheumatoid arthritis, scleroderma); HIV infection; portal hypertension; congenital heart disease; schistosomiasis; chronic hemolytic anemia (e.g., sickle cell disease)
  - Persistent PH of the newborn
- System(s) affected: Pulmonary; Cardiovascular

EPIDEMIOLOGY
- Age: Can occur at any age; mean age, 37 years
- Sex (IPAH): Female > Male (~4:1)

Incidence
- Overall PAH: 5–52 cases/million
- IPAH: Low, ~2–6 per million
- Drug-induced PAH: 1/25,000 with >3 months of anorectic use
- HIV associated: 0.5/100
- Portal hypertension associated: 1–6/100
- Scleroderma associated: 6–60%

Prevalence
- PAH: ~15–50 cases per million
- IPAH: ~6 cases per million

ETIOLOGY AND PATHOPHYSIOLOGY
- Pulmonary: Inflammation, vasoconstriction, endothelial dysfunction, and remodeling of pulmonary arteries produced by increased cell proliferation and reduced rates of apoptosis lead to obstruction.
- Cardiovascular: Right ventricular hypertrophy (RVH), eventually leading to right-sided heart failure
- IPAH: By definition, unknown. True IPAH is mostly sporadic or sometimes familial in nature.
- Pulmonary arteriolar hyperactivity and vasoconstriction, occult thromboembolism, or autoimmune (high frequency of antinuclear antibodies)

Genetics
- 75% of heritable pulmonary arterial hypertension (HPAH) cases and 25% of IPAH cases have mutations in BMPR2 (autosomal dominant)
- Mutations in ALK1 and endoglin (autosomal dominant) also are associated with PAH.

RISK FACTORS
- Female sex
- Previous anorectic drug use
- Recent acute pulmonary embolism
- Commonly associated conditions
- 1st-degree relatives of patient with familial PAH

COMMONLY ASSOCIATED CONDITIONS
See Associated PAH, above.

 DIAGNOSIS

Symptoms of PAH are nonspecific, which can lead to missed or delayed diagnosis of this serious disease.

HISTORY
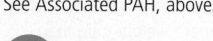
Dyspnea, weakness, syncope, dizziness, chest pain, palpitations, lower extremity edema

PHYSICAL EXAM
- Pulmonary component of S_2 (at apex in >90% of patients)
- Right ventricular (RV) lift
- Early systolic click of pulmonary valve
- Pansystolic murmur of tricuspid regurgitation
- Diastolic murmur of pulmonic insufficiency (Graham-Steell murmur)
- RV S_3 or S_4
- Edema as jugular vein distention, ascites, hepatomegaly, or peripheral edema

DIFFERENTIAL DIAGNOSIS
Other causes of dyspnea:
- Pulmonary parenchymal disease, such as chronic obstructive pulmonary disease
- Pulmonary vascular disease, such as pulmonary thromboembolism
- Cardiac disease, such as cardiomyopathy
- Other disorders of respiratory function, such as sleep apnea

DIAGNOSTIC TESTS & INTERPRETATION
- ECG: RVH and right axis deviation
- Pulmonary function testing and/or arterial blood gas: Arterial hypoxemia, reduced diffusion capacity, hypocapnia
- Ventilation-perfusion ratio (V/Q) scan: Must rule out proximal pulmonary artery emboli and chronic thromboembolic PH (CTEPH)

- Exercise test: Reduced maximal O_2 consumption, high minute ventilation, low anaerobic threshold, increased PO_2 alveolar-arterial gradient; correlation to severity of disease with 6-minute walk test
- Antinuclear antibody positive (up to 40% of patients):
  - LFTs to evaluate for portopulmonary HTN, a complication of chronic liver disease
  - HIV test, thyroid function tests, sickle cell disease screening
- Elevated brain natriuretic peptide (BNP) and N-terminal-proBNP may be useful for early detection of PAH in young, otherwise healthy patients with mild symptoms. It can also be used to assess disease severity and prognosis.
- Chest radiograph:
  - Prominent central pulmonary arteries with peripheral hypovascularity of pulmonary arterial branches
  - RV enlargement is a late finding.
- Echo Doppler:
  - Should be performed with suspicion of PAH; recent studies show some inaccuracy compared with right-sided heart catheterization.
  - Most commonly used screening tool:
    - Estimates mean PAP and assesses cardiac structure and function, excludes congenital anomalies
    - Echo suggests, but does not diagnose, PAH. Invasive hemodynamic evaluation confirms PAH diagnosis.
  - Right atrial and ventricular enlargement; tricuspid regurgitation
  - Important to rule out underlying cardiac disease, such as atrial septal defect with secondary PH or mitral stenosis
- Cardiac magnetic resonance is not commonly used.

Diagnostic Procedures/Other
- Pulmonary angiography:
  - Should be done if V/Q scan suggests CTEPH
  - Use caution; can lead to hemodynamic collapse; use low osmolar agents, subselective angiograms
- Right-sided cardiac catheterization (gold standard for diagnosis of PAH):
  - Essential 1st step to confirm diagnosis and determine severity and prognosis by measuring pulmonary arterial pressures and hemodynamics
  - Rule out underlying cardiac disease (e.g., left-sided heart disease) and response to vasodilator therapy.
- Lung biopsy: Not recommended unless primary pulmonary parenchymal disease exists
- 6-minute walk test: Classifies severity of PAH and estimates prognosis

Test Interpretation
- Distal arterioles show medial hypertrophy, proliferative/fibrotic intima, complex lesions, and thrombosis.
- Pulmonary veins usually are not affected.

 TREATMENT

- PAH remains incurable. Treat underlying diseases/conditions that may cause PAH to relieve symptoms and improve quality of life and survival.
- PAH-specific treatment has been studied mostly in IPAH.

GENERAL MEASURES
Oxygen supplementation to O_2 >90% is indicated for rest, exercise, or nocturnal hypoxemia.

MEDICATION
- Acute vasodilator test (performed during cardiac catheterization) for all IPAH patients who are potential candidates for long-term oral calcium channel blocker (CCB) therapy:
  - Screens for pulmonary vasoreactivity/responsiveness using inhaled nitrous oxide; IV epoprostenol; or IV adenosine: Positive response may be a prognostic indicator.
  - Contraindicated in right-sided heart failure or hemodynamic instability
- Chronic vasodilator therapy:
  - If IPAH with positive response to acute vasodilator test (a fall in mean PAP of $\geq$10 mm Hg and to a value <40 mm Hg, with unchanged/increased cardiac output), use CCBs (1)[C]:
    - ~13% will initially respond. Long-term clinical response to CCB therapy is small (~7%) (1)[C].
    - CCBs include nifedipine (long-acting), diltiazem, amlodipine.
    - Avoid verapamil due to its significant negative inotropic effect.
    - CCBs are contraindicated in patients with a cardiac index of <2 L/min/m^2 or a right atrial pressure >15 mm Hg.
  - PAH with negative response to acute vasodilator test or worsening on therapy; specific vasodilator choice based on risk stratification (1)[C]:
    - Higher risk: Prostanoids: Improve exercise capacity, cardiopulmonary hemodynamics: Epoprostenol (IV) (only drug with demonstrated survival benefit and treatment of choice for most ill; i.e., NYHA functional class IV patients) (1)[B]; treprostinil (IV, SC, or inhaled); iloprost (inhaled)
    - Lower risk:
      - Endothelin receptor antagonists: Improve exercise capacity; reducing mortality has been noted (2)[A]: bosentan (PO); ambrisentan (PO). Monitor LFTs monthly.
      - Phosphodiesterase-5 inhibitors: Suggested improvement in exercise capacity, cardiopulmonary hemodynamics, and symptoms (1)[C]: Sildenafil (PO); tadalafil (PO)
      - It is unclear whether any of the above 3 separate classes of drugs significantly reduces mortality; however, pooling all the vasodilators in a recent systematic review shows 39% reduction in mortality (3)[A]; another recent meta-analysis shows that only prostanoid class has survival benefit, particularly IV prostacyclins (4)[A].
      - If 1 agent fails, vasodilator combination therapy (CT) using 2 vasodilators (e.g., epoprostenol + sildenafil) is currently being studied (5)[C]. A recent meta-analysis found CT did not improve outcomes compared with monotherapy (MT). Only 6-minute walk distance was improved when using CT vs. MT (6)[A].
- Anticoagulation:
  - Improved survival originally suggested in patients with IPAH only. Newer studies show some evidence for favorable effects of anticoagulation on survival in IPAH, HPAH, or PAH associated with anorexigens (1)[B],(7).

- Warfarin with international normalized ratio of 1.5–2.5:
  - Contraindications: Avoid in patients with syncope or significant hemoptysis; consider drug interactions
- Diuretics indicated in patients with RV volume overload (e.g., peripheral edema or ascites) (1)[B].
- Digoxin has little long-term data in PAH: Utilized in RV failure and/or atrial dysrhythmias, increases cardiac output and preserves RV contractility

ISSUES FOR REFERRAL
Refer to a pulmonologist and/or a cardiologist for further evaluation/treatment if PAH is suspected.

SURGERY/OTHER PROCEDURES
- Patients with documented large-vessel thromboembolic disease should be considered for pulmonary thrombectomy.
- Balloon atrial septostomy for severe PAH with right-sided heart failure despite optimized medical therapy to relieve symptoms prior to lung transplant or as a treatment on its own
- Heart-lung or lung transplantation

IN-PATIENT CONSIDERATIONS
Admission Criteria/Initial Stabilization
- Medical therapy, is primarily palliative.
- Hospitalization with invasive monitoring is needed to screen vasodilator responsiveness and initiate vasodilator therapy.
- National registry has been established by the National Heart, Lung, and Blood Institute.

 ONGOING CARE

FOLLOW-UP RECOMMENDATIONS
- Pneumococcal and influenza vaccines
- Exercise: Walking or low-level aerobic activity, as tolerated, once stable; respiratory training

Patient Monitoring
Frequently evaluate disease progression and therapeutic efficacy. Objective tests to measure treatment response include 6-minute walk test and cardiopulmonary exercise test.

DIET
Fluid and salt restrictions, especially with RV failure

PATIENT EDUCATION
Discuss disease, prognosis, lifestyle changes, and all therapeutic options (including transplant)

PROGNOSIS
- Median survival is 2–3 years from diagnosis; 5-year survival rate is 34% for National Institute of Health registry; newer studies show 5-year survival near 70% with new treatment.
- Mode of death: Right-side heart failure (most common), pneumonia, sudden death, cardiac death
- Poor prognostic factors:
  - Rapid symptom progression
  - Clinical evidence of RV failure
  - World Health Organization functional PAH class 4 (or NYHA functional class 3 or 4)
  - 6-minute walk distance <300 m
  - Peak VO$_2$ during cardiopulmonary exercise testing <10.4 mL/kg/min
  - Echocardiography with pericardial effusion, significant RV enlargement/dysfunction, right atrial enlargement
  - Mean right atrial pressure >20 mm Hg
  - Cardiac index <2 L/min/m^2
  - Elevated mean PAP

- Significantly elevated BNP and NT-proBNP; other markers also show promise in predicting survival: RDW, GDF-15, interleukin-6, creatinine
- Scleroderma spectrum of diseases

COMPLICATIONS
- Thromboembolism, heart failure, pleural effusion, and sudden death
- Pregnancy should be avoided due to high maternal mortality (30–50%) and fetal wastage.

REFERENCES
1. Badesch DB, Abman SH, Simonneau G, et al. Medical therapy for pulmonary arterial hypertension: Updated ACCP evidence-based clinical practice guidelines. Chest. 2007;131: 1917–1928.
2. Liu C, Chen J, Gao Y, et al. Endothelin receptor antagonists for pulmonary arterial hypertension. Cochrane Database Syst Rev. 2009;CD004434.
3. Macchia A, Marchioli R, Tognoni G, et al. Systematic review of trials using vasodilators in pulmonary arterial hypertension: Why a new approach is needed. Am Heart J. 2010;159: 245–257.
4. Ryerson CJ, Nayar S, Swiston JR, et al. Pharmacotherapy in pulmonary arterial hypertension: A systematic review and meta-analysis. Respir Res. 2010;11:12.
5. McLaughlin VV, Archer SL, Badesch DB, et al. ACCF/AHA 2009 expert consensus document on pulmonary hypertension a report of the American College of Cardiology Foundation Task Force on Expert Consensus Documents and the American Heart Association developed in collaboration with the American Thoracic Society, Inc.; and the Pulmonary Hypertension Association. J Am Coll Cardiol. 2009;53:1573–1619.
6. Fox BD, Shimony A, Langleben D, et al. Meta-analysis of monotherapy versus combination therapy for pulmonary arterial hypertension. Am J Cardiol. 2011;108:1177–1182.
7. Barst RJ, Gibbs JS, Ghofrani HA, et al. Updated evidence-based treatment algorithm in pulmonary arterial hypertension. J Am Coll Cardiol. 2009; 54:S78.

 SEE ALSO

Cor Pulmonale; Pulmonary Embolism

 CODES

ICD10
- I27.0 Primary pulmonary hypertension
- I27.2 Other secondary pulmonary hypertension

CLINICAL PEARLS
- In patients with PAH, a V/Q scan should be performed to rule out CTEPH; a normal scan effectively excludes a diagnosis of CTEPH.
- CCBs are first-line agents to manage IPAH.

PULMONARY EDEMA

Brandon C. Maughan, MD, MHS

BASICS

DESCRIPTION
- Pulmonary capillaries leak fluid into the lung interstitium and alveoli, leading to hypoxia and respiratory distress.
- Fluid accumulation results from cardiogenic causes (e.g., heart failure), leading to imbalanced hydrostatic and oncotic pressures within pulmonary capillaries or from noncardiogenic causes (e.g., acute lung injury) that increase alveolar membrane permeability.

EPIDEMIOLOGY
Incidence
- Annual heart failure incidence: 650,000 cases (1)
- Heart failure incidence increases with age:
  – Age 35–64: 2 cases per 1,000
  – Age 65–69: 20 cases per 1,000
  – Age >85: >80 cases per 1,000
- Disparities in heart failure incidence by race and sex:
  – Blacks (16.3/1,000) vs. whites (11.9/1,000)
  – Men (15.8/1,000) vs. women (11.7/1,000)
- Acute respiratory distress syndrome (ARDS): 190,000 cases annually in US

Prevalence
Heart failure syndromes: 5.8 million US adults

ETIOLOGY AND PATHOPHYSIOLOGY
- Cardiogenic causes will increase hydrostatic pressure in the pulmonary capillaries, leading to increased transvascular filtration of a protein-poor fluid into lung interstitium.
- Systolic dysfunction is due to decreased contractility of the left ventricle (LV), leading to decreased cardiac output, which in turn stimulates the renin–angiotensin system and increases fluid retention. Diastolic dysfunction is often due to decreased LV compliance secondary to hypertrophy.
- Noncardiogenic causes will increase permeability of the lung vasculature, leading to accumulation of protein-rich fluid in the lung interstitium and air spaces. Many causes of this vascular permeability are associated with ARDS.
- Cardiogenic (left-sided heart failure):
  – Impaired contractility
    ○ Ischemic heart disease
    ○ Dilated cardiomyopathy
    ○ Myocarditis
    ○ Volume overload
    ○ Alcoholic cardiomyopathy
  – Increased LV afterload
    ○ Systemic hypertension (HTN)
    ○ Aortic stenosis
    ○ Cocaine abuse
  – Poor diastolic filling
    ○ LV hypertrophy
    ○ Hypertrophic cardiomyopathy
    ○ Mitral stenosis
    ○ Atrial fibrillation
  – Valvular dysfunction
    ○ Mistral regurgitation
    ○ Acute papillary muscle rupture
  – High cardiac output states
    ○ Thyrotoxicosis
    ○ Systemic arteriovenous fistulas
    ○ Anemia
  – Noncompliance with medications or diet
  – Medications with negative inotropic effects

- Noncardiogenic:
  – Severe systemic inflammatory states:
    ○ Sepsis
    ○ Severe trauma
    ○ Severe burns
    ○ Pancreatitis
    ○ DIC
  – Pneumonia
  – Aspiration or near-drowning
  – Inhalation of smoke or toxic gases
  – Blood product transfusion
  – Preeclampsia
  – Rapid ascent to high altitude (>2,500 m)
  – Drug toxicity (salicylates, opiates)
  – Embolism (thrombus, fat, air, amniotic fluid)
  – Neurogenic (after head trauma/surgery)
  – Re-expansion (after pneumothorax/thoracentesis)

Genetics
Multifactorial

RISK FACTORS
- Cardiogenic: HTN, ischemic heart disease, valvular disease, left ventricular hypertrophy (LVH)
- Noncardiogenic: Sepsis, severe systemic inflammatory states, aspiration, pneumonia, trauma

GENERAL PREVENTION
Early detection and treatment of risk factors

COMMONLY ASSOCIATED CONDITIONS
See "Etiology and Pathophysiology."

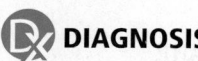

DIAGNOSIS

HISTORY
- Past medical history:
  – Underlying comorbidities, including prior heart failure or prior myocardial infarction (MI)
  – Fever or other symptoms of infection
  – Recent trauma
  – Drug or alcohol abuse
  – Dietary or medication noncompliance
  – Recent weight gain or increasing edema
  – Recent use of negative inotropic agents (calcium channel blockers)
  – Recent use of NSAIDs (increase water retention)
- Symptoms:
  – Progressive dyspnea
  – Orthopnea and paroxysmal nocturnal dyspnea
  – Cough
  – Fatigue and generalized weakness
  – Pink frothy sputum
  – Chest pain

PHYSICAL EXAM
- Vital signs: Tachypnea, tachycardia, and hypoxemia. Patients may be hypotensive or hypertensive.
- General: Respiratory distress, diaphoresis
- HEENT (Head, Eyes, Ears, Nose, Throat): Frothy oral secretions, cyanosis
- Cardiac: S3 or S4, jugular venous distension, murmurs suggestive of valvular disease
- Pulmonary: Crackles or wheezing
- Extremities: Edema, cyanosis, mottled skin

DIFFERENTIAL DIAGNOSIS
- COPD
- Pneumonia
- Pulmonary embolism
- Asthma/reactive airway disease
- Pneumothorax
- Cardiac tamponade

- Asphyxiant or toxic gas exposure
- Inhalational burns

DIAGNOSTIC TESTS & INTERPRETATION
Initial Tests (lab, imaging)
- CBC/differential to screen for anemia or infection
- Chemistry panel to screen for acute kidney injury, hyponatremia (associated with severe heart failure), or electrolyte disturbances leading to dysrhythmias
- Troponin may be elevated from recent infarction causing acute heart failure or from myocardial ischemia secondary to elevated ventricular strain. Elevated cardiac enzymes carry a strongly negative prognosis in heart failure.
- In settings of clinical uncertainty, B-type natriuretic peptide (BNP) can add to clinical judgment in patients with intermediate risk of heart failure. BNP >500 pg/mL suggests heart failure, and BNP <100 pg/mL suggests alternative causes (1,2,3)[A]. BNP may also be elevated due to atrial fibrillation, renal failure, severe valvular disease, or pulmonary HTN, so use the test cautiously.
- Liver function tests (LFTs) to check for elevated transaminases, which can suggest hepatic congestion from heart failure or may indicate heavy alcohol use contributing to cardiomyopathy.
- Drug levels (aspirin, opiates, cocaine, alcohol)
- Arterial blood gas to measure pO_2 and A-a gradient
- Serum lipase if suspicious for pancreatitis
- TSH if suspicious for thyrotoxicosis
- Blood/urine cultures and lactic acid if concerned for severe sepsis or septic shock
- Urinalysis to check for nephrotic syndrome or UTI
- Chest x-ray to evaluate for:
  – Pneumothorax
  – Cardiomegaly
  – Infiltrate suggestive of pneumonia
  – Increased interstitial markings, perihilar alveolar edema, or pleural effusion
- CT pulmonary angiography if concerned for pulmonary emboli
- ECG to evaluate for ischemia or dysrhythmias
- Echocardiography to assess:
  – Systolic function (incl. wall motion abnormalities)
  – Valve function
  – Pericardial effusion

Follow-Up Tests & Special Considerations
Emergent echocardiography if considering cardiogenic shock, tamponade, or papillary muscle rupture

TREATMENT

MEDICATION
First Line
- Guide all treatment based on the suspected cause
- Start with supplemental oxygen
- Preload reduction for acute cardiogenic edema:
  – Loop diuretics: Furosemide 40–80 mg IV, torsemide 10 mg IV, or bumetanide 1 mg IV. If on chronic diuretics, start IV dose at or above home dose and titrate. Onset 15–30 minutes (1,2,3)[B]
  – IV nitrate vasodilators: Rapid onset. Start IV nitroglycerin 20 μg/min, titrate 20–40 μg/min q3–5min until distress resolved or onset of hypotension
  – For severe HTN, consider IV nitroprusside 5–10 μg/min, titrate. Max 400 μg/min. Use <48 hours due to risk of cyanide toxicity (3)[C].

- Afterload reduction for systolic heart failure:
  - Angiotensin-converting enzyme inhibitors (ACEI): Lisinopril 2.5–5 mg/d PO, enalapril 2.5 mg PO b.i.d., or captopril 6.25 mg PO t.i.d. Avoid in acutely ill patients with hypotension, acute renal failure, hyperkalemia, poor diuresis (1)[A].
  - Angiotensin receptor blockers (ARB) for ACEI-intolerant patients: Candesartan 4 mg/d PO, losartan 25 mg/d PO, or valsartan 20 mg PO b.i.d. Use the same precautions as with ACEI.
  - β-Blockers: Carvedilol 3.125 mg PO b.i.d., bisoprolol 1.25 mg/d PO, or metoprolol ER 12.5 mg/d PO. Avoid if patients are hypotensive or recently received inotropic therapy.
- Improve contractility in hypotensive patients with severe systolic heart failure (1,2,3)[C]:
  - Dobutamine: 5–10 μg/kg/min IV, titrate
  - Milrinone: Load 50 μg/kg IV over 10 minutes, then infuse 0.375–0.75 μg/kg/min, titrate
  - Dopamine: 5–10 μg/kg/min IV, titrate
  - Norepinephrine: 2–4 μg/min IV for acute cardiogenic shock following acute MI. Not for use in acute decompensated heart failure.
- High-altitude pulmonary edema:
  - Descent is the only definitive treatment.
  - Adjunctive therapy: Supplemental oxygen. Consider nifedipine ER 30 mg PO q12h or sildenafil 50 mg PO q8h.
- Chronic heart failure: Start daily PO therapy at low dose. Listed values are recommended maximum daily doses (1,2):
  - Loop diuretics: Furosemide 20–80 mg q6–8h, torsemide 20 mg/d, bumetanide 1 mg q12h (1,2)[C]
  - ACEIs: Lisinopril 20–40 mg/d, enalapril 10–20 mg q12h, captopril 50 mg q8h (1,2)[A]
  - ARBs: Candesartan 32 mg/d, valsartan 160 mg q12h, losartan 100 mg/d (1,2)[A]
  - β-Blockers: Carvedilol 25 mg q12h, metoprolol ER 200 mg/d, bisoprolol 10 mg/d (1,2)[A]
  - Nitrates: Isosorbide dinitrate 60 mg q8h (1,2)[B]
- Precautions:
  - Diuretics: Monitor for electrolyte derangement and renal dysfunction. Use very carefully in patients with aortic stenosis.
  - Inotropes increase myocardial oxygen demand and may damage the ischemic myocardium.
  - Monitor the additive hypotensive effects of diuretics, nitrates, and afterload reducers.

Second Line
- Thiazide diuretics: hydrochlorothiazide (HCTZ) 25–50 mg/d PO, metolazone 2.5–10 mg/d PO
- Spironolactone: 25–50 mg/d PO; recheck renal function and electrolytes in 7–10 days
- Digoxin: 125 μg/d PO, titrate to serum concentration of 0.5–0.8 ng/mL

ISSUES FOR REFERRAL
Cardiology referral for underlying cardiac disease

ADDITIONAL THERAPIES
- Noninvasive positive-pressure ventilation (NPPV) should be considered early for emergency department patients with acute respiratory distress from pulmonary edema/congestive heart failure (CHF). NPPV decreases preload and afterload, thereby alleviating symptoms and potentially avoiding intubation by allowing time for medications to work. Use cautiously if patients are hypotensive.
- Nesiritide may help alleviate dyspnea but does not reduce hospitalization, mortality, or renal failure, and it may increase risk of hypotension (4)[B].

SURGERY/OTHER PROCEDURES
- Cardiac catheterization for cardiac ischemia/ACS
- Extracorporeal membrane oxygenation (ECMO) for severe refractory hypoxia/ARDS
- Intra-arterial balloon pump for cardiogenic shock
- Implantable cardioverter defibrillator (ICD) for sudden cardiac death prevention in patients with prior cardiac arrest or ischemic/dilated cardiomyopathy and LVEF <30% (2)[A]
- Cardiac resynchronization therapy (CRT) for severe systolic heart failure and QRS >0.12 ms
- LV assist device (LVAD) for severe systolic dysfunction as bridge to a heart transplant

IN-PATIENT CONSIDERATIONS
Admission Criteria/Initial Stabilization
- Hypotension
- Acute kidney injury
- Altered mental status
- Dyspnea at rest
- O_2 saturation <90%
- Acute coronary syndromes
- Arrhythmias (i.e., new-onset atrial fibrillation)
- Mild distress: Oxygen by nonrebreather mask
- Significant hypoxia: Noninvasive positive pressure ventilation (BiPAP/CPAP) to improve oxygenation and decrease LV afterload (5)[A]
- Intubation for patients with apnea, altered mental status, or hypoxia despite NPPV

IV Fluids
Use crystalloid infusions cautiously. Limit free water.
Nursing
- Daily weights, strict input/output
- Assess for functional improvement
Discharge Criteria
- Underlying condition treated, fluid status optimized
- Started β-blocker and ACEI in patients with CHF
- Patient and family educated about diet/medications

 ONGOING CARE

FOLLOW-UP RECOMMENDATIONS
Patient Monitoring
- Strict input/output measurement, daily weights
- Posthospitalization appointment in 7–10 days
DIET
Low-sodium diet (<2 g/d), fluid restriction (<2 L/d)
PATIENT EDUCATION
- Dietary precautions
- Early signs and symptoms of fluid overload
- Adjust diuretic dose based on recent weight gain
PROGNOSIS
Mortality: 30–60% for noncardiogenic edema/ARDS; up to 80% for cardiogenic causes
COMPLICATIONS
- Acute hypoxic respiratory failure
- CHF increases long-term risk for dysrhythmias and sudden cardiac death.
- ARDS increases short-term risk for pneumonia and pneumothorax. Long-term complications include risks of pulmonary hypertension and fibrosis.

REFERENCES
1. Yancy CW, Jessup M, Bozkurt B, et al. 2013 ACCF/AHA guideline for the management of heart failure: A report of the American College of Cardiology Foundation/American Heart Association Task Force on Practice Guidelines. *J Am Coll Cardiol*. 2013;S0735-1097(13):02114-1.
2. Jessup M. 2009 focused update: ACCF/AHA Guidelines for the Diagnosis and Management of Heart Failure in Adults: A Report of the American College of Cardiology Foundation/American Heart Association Task Force on Practice Guidelines: Developed in collaboration with the International Society for Heart and Lung Transplantation. *Circulation*. 2009;119:1977–2016.
3. Heart Failure Society of America, Lindenfeld J, Albert NM, et al. HFSA 2010 comprehensive heart failure practice guideline. *J Card Fail*. 2010;16: e1–e194.
4. O'Connor CM, Starling RC, Hernandez AF, et al. Effect of nesiritide in patients with acute decompensated heart failure. *N Engl J Med*. 2011;365:32–43.
5. Vital FM, Saconato H, Ladeira MT, et al. Non-invasive positive pressure ventilation (CPAP or bilevel NPPV) for cardiogenic pulmonary edema. *Cochrane Database Syst Rev*. 2008;3:CD005351.

 SEE ALSO

Altitude Illness; Congestive Heart Failure; Respiratory Distress Syndrome, Acute (ARDS)

 CODES

ICD10
- J81.0 Acute pulmonary edema
- J81.1 Chronic pulmonary edema

CLINICAL PEARLS
- Diagnosis of the underlying etiology is essential.
- Initial treatment of acute cardiogenic edema among hypertensive/normotensive patients includes IV diuretics, IV nitrates, and NPPV.
- Hypotensive patients with pulmonary edema due to CHF will require careful use of inotropes and vasopressor to improve hemodynamic stability.
- Pulmonary edema from ARDS has very high mortality and requires ICU-level care.
- Home dietary and medication management are critical for long-term treatment of CHF.

PULMONARY EMBOLISM

Alfonso J. Tafur, MD • Ana I. Casanegra, MD, FSVM, RPVI

 BASICS

DESCRIPTION
- Pulmonary embolism (PE) is the obstruction of the pulmonary arteries, typically due to a thrombus that formed at another site and traveled in the bloodstream until it lodged.
- Venous thromboembolism (VTE) refers to both PE and deep vein thrombosis (DVT).

EPIDEMIOLOGY
The case fatality rate ranges from 1–60% depending on the severity of the clinical presentation.

Incidence
- Incidence increases with age.
- ~23–69 new PE cases per 100,000 per year
- 250,000 hospitalizations per year in the US, 10–60% in hospitalized patients:
  - Highest risk for orthopedic patients
  - 1:1,000 pregnancies (including postpartum)

ETIOLOGY AND PATHOPHYSIOLOGY
- Venous stasis, endothelial damage, and changes in the coagulation properties of the blood trigger the formation of thrombus.
- PE causes increased pulmonary vascular resistance, impaired gas exchange, and decreased pulmonary compliance.
- DVT in the proximal veins is the most common source of PE.
- Upper extremity DVT and pelvic vein thrombi can also cause PE.

Genetics
- Factor V Leiden: The most common thrombophilia. +5.5% in Caucasian, 2.2% in Hispanics, 1.2% in African American, 0.5% in Asian
- Responsible for 20% of all patients with VTE
- Prothrombin G20210A: 3% of Caucasians, rare in African American, Asian, and Native American; 6% in patients with VTE

RISK FACTORS
- Acquired: Age, immobilization, surgery, cancer, oral contraceptives, hormonal replacement therapy, pregnancy/puerperium, previous thrombosis, paroxysmal nocturnal hemoglobinuria, antiphospholipid syndrome, prolonged travel
- Inherited: Antithrombin deficiency, protein C deficiency, protein S deficiency, factor V Leiden, prothrombin gene mutation G20210A, dysfibrinogenemia

GENERAL PREVENTION
- Prevention strategies must be tailored to patient VTE risk and patient bleeding risk (1,2,3).
- Mechanical thromboprophylaxis includes: Early ambulation after surgery, graduated compression stockings, and intermittent pneumatic compression
- Intermediate risk: Medical patients, general surgery, gynecologic or urologic surgery. Pharmacologic prophylaxis is recommended with low-molecular-weight heparin (LMWH), unfractionated heparin (UFH), or fondaparinux (1,2).
- High risk: Hip or knee arthroplasty, pharmacologic prophylaxis with LMWH, fondaparinux, apixaban, dabigatran, rivaroxaban, or low-dose UFH: Hip fracture surgery, LMWH, fondaparinux, UFH, or vitamin K antagonists (VKA); Major trauma, spinal cord injury, LMWH or UFH (3)

- Long-distance travel (>8 hours): Adequate hydration, avoidance of constrictive clothing and frequent calf exercises. If additional risk factors are present, graduated compression stockings below knee (1)
- Patients with factor V Leiden, prothrombin G20210A with no previous thrombosis do not need long-term daily prophylaxis (1)

 DIAGNOSIS

Establish a pretest probability based on clinical criteria such as Wells score or Geneva score (4,5):
- Wells score:
  - Clinical signs and symptoms of DVT +3
  - Alternative diagnosis is less likely than PE +3
  - Heart rate >100 +1.5
  - Immobilization/Surgery in previous 4 weeks +1.5
  - Previous DVT/PE +1.5
  - Hemoptysis +1
  - Malignancy +1:
    - <2 points, low clinical probability; 2–6 points, moderate; >6 points, high

HISTORY
- Provoked or idiopathic
- Presence of risk factors and family history
- Bleeding risk (previous anticoagulation, history of bleeding, recent interventions/surgeries, liver disease)
- Dyspnea (82%), chest pain (49%), cough (20%), syncope (14%), hemoptysis (7%)

PHYSICAL EXAM
- Tachycardia, tachypnea, accentuated pulmonary component in S2
- Pleuritic chest pain, pleural friction rub, rales
- Leg swelling, tenderness along a vein, visible collateral veins
- Signs of right ventricular (RV) failure may be present (rare): Jugular vein distention, 3rd or 4th sound, audible systolic murmur at left sternal edge, hepatomegaly

ALERT
- Massive PE: Acute PE with sustained hypotension, pulselessness, or persistent profound bradycardia (5,6)
- Submassive PE: Acute PE without systemic hypotension but with either RV dysfunction or myocardial necrosis (5,6):
  - RV dysfunction: RV dilation or RV systolic dysfunction on echocardiography, RV dilation (4-chamber RV diameter divided by left ventricle diameter 0.9) on CT, elevation of brain natriuretic peptide (BNP), elevation of N-terminal pro-BNP (500 pg/mL), or consistent ECG changes
- Low-risk PE: Acute PE and the absence of the clinical markers of adverse prognosis that define massive or submassive PE

DIFFERENTIAL DIAGNOSIS
- Pulmonary: Pneumonia, bronchitis, pneumonitis, chronic obstructive pulmonary disease (COPD) exacerbation, pulmonary edema, pneumothorax
- Cardiac: Myocardial infarction (angina pectoris), pericarditis, congestive heart failure (CHF)
- Vascular: Dissection of the aorta

- Musculoskeletal: Rib fracture(s), musculoskeletal chest wall pain

DIAGNOSTIC TESTS & INTERPRETATION
- D-dimer: In patients with low pretest probability; D-dimer can rule out PE if result is negative (high negative predictive value [NPV]). It is not diagnostic if positive (low positive predictive value [PPV]), and it is not helpful if pretest probability is intermediate or high (4).
- CBC, creatinine, aPTT and PT, ABG.
- In young patients with idiopathic VTE, recurrent VTE, or significant family history of VTE, consider testing for hypercoagulable tests:
  - Do not test for protein C, S, factor VIII, and antithrombin in the acute setting or while on treatment, as results may be falsely abnormal.
  - All patients with intermediate or high pretest probability and low probability with elevated D-dimer need further diagnostic testing
- Chest x-ray (CXR): Suggestive findings: Westermark sign (lack of vessels in an area distal to the embolus), Hampton hump (wedge-shaped opacity with base in pleura), Fleischner sign (enlarged pulmonary arteries), atelectasis, pleural effusion, pulmonary infarct, hemidiaphragm elevation
- ECG: Right heart strain, nonspecific rhythm abnormalities, S1Q3T3
- CT pulmonary angiography: Sensitivity 96–100%, specificity 86–89%. NPV 99.8%. Requires IV iodine contrast (1)[B],(7)
- Ventilation/Perfusion scintigraphy (V/Q scan): Use if CT angiography is not available or contraindicated. A high-probability V/Q scan makes the diagnosis of PE; a normal V/Q scan excludes PE (1)[B].
- Pulmonary angiogram: Gold standard but invasive and technically difficult: 2% morbidity and <0.01 mortality risk
- Echocardiogram: Helpful to assess RV function
- Magnetic resonance angiography: Lower sensitivity and specificity than CT angiography
- Compression ultrasound (CUS): Noninvasive. 1/3 of the patients with PE will have a DVT (1)[B]
- CT venography: Can be done at the same time as CT angiography; increases diagnostic yield. Requires IV-iodinated contrast.

ALERT
If your preclinical probability is intermediate or high and the patient has a low bleeding risk, start the treatment while waiting for the diagnostic results (2)[C].

Follow-Up Tests & Special Considerations
Elevated troponin I or T and elevated BNP are markers for higher risk patients.

 TREATMENT

MEDICATION
- If the clinical suspicion is high and there are no contraindications, start treatment as soon as possible (5).
- Start LMWH, fondaparinux, UFH, as initial therapy. VKA can be started the 1st day and must overlap with parenteral treatment for a minimum of 5 days, until the international normalized ratio (INR) is 2–3 for 24 hours (1)[B],(5).

- An oral option for initial and long-term treatment is rivaroxaban (1)[B],(8)
- Patients with massive PE with low bleeding risk: Consider systemic thrombolytics if they have no contraindications (2)[C],(5,6).
- Patients <75 year with submassive PE and low bleeding risk, consider thrombolysis

First Line
- UFH (5):
  – IV bolus of 80 U/kg or 5,000 U followed by continuous infusion (initially at 18 U/kg/h or 1,300 U/h) with dose adjustments to maintain an aPTT that corresponds to antiactivated factor X (anti-Xa) levels of 0.3–0.7
  – SC injection: 2 options:
    ○ Monitored: 17,500 U or 250 U/kg b.i.d. with dose adjustments to maintain an aPTT that corresponds to anti-Xa levels of 0.3–0.7 measured 6 hours after a dose
    ○ Fixed dose: 333 U/kg initial dose, followed by 250 U/kg b.i.d.
- LMWH (5):
  – Enoxaparin (Lovenox) 1 mg/kg/dose SC q12h
  – Dalteparin (Fragmin) 200 U/kg SC q24h
    ○ Fondaparinux (Arixtra) (5): 5 mg (body weight <50 kg), 7.5 mg (body weight 50–100 kg), or 10 mg (body weight >100) SC q24h
- Maintenance therapy: VKA; Warfarin: Start on day 1, if possible; 5 mg/d for 3 days; adjust dose to maintain an INR of 2–3. Needs to overlap with UFH, LMWH or fondaparinux 5–7 days, until 2 consecutive therapeutic INR (1)[B]
- Rivaroxaban: 15 mg twice daily for 3 weeks and then 20 mg once daily to complete treatment (1)[B],(8)

ALERT
Contraindications:
- Active bleeding is a contraindication for any anticoagulation.
- Heparin: Heparin-induced thrombocytopenia (HIT)
- LMWH: HIT, renal failure
- Fondaparinux: Renal failure
- Warfarin: Pregnancy
- Rivaroxaban: renal failure

Pregnancy Considerations
- Warfarin is teratogenic and should not be used in pregnant patients (especially in 1st trimester); safe while breastfeeding
- Dalteparin, enoxaparin, and fondaparinux are Category B for pregnancy; heparin is Category C.
- Rivaroxaban is Category C. No adequate studies.

Second Line
Massive PE: Evaluate the risks and benefits. Consider thrombolytics if the patient has hemodynamic compromise and a low bleeding risk (2)[C],(5,6,9):
- Tissue plasminogen activator (tPA) 100 mg infused through a peripheral vein over 2 hours
- Absolute contraindications: Intracranial hemorrhage, known intracranial cerebrovascular or malignant disease, ischemic stroke within 3 months, suspected aortic dissection, bleeding diathesis, active bleeding, recent neurosurgery, recent major trauma

SURGERY/OTHER PROCEDURES
- Inferior vena cava (IVC) filter placement in patients with contraindication for anticoagulation (1)[B],(5,6)

- Emergency surgical embolectomy can be considered if the patient has massive PE with contraindications for thrombolysis and surgical resources ara available (2)[C],(5,6).
- Consider catheter-based interventions if the patient has massive PE and either contraindications to thrombolytics or if patinet remains unstable despite the use of thrombolytics (2)[C],(5,6).

IN-PATIENT CONSIDERATIONS
Admission Criteria/Initial Stabilization
May require ICU-level care if hemodynamically unstable

 ## ONGOING CARE

Duration of anticoagulation (5):
- Provoked PE (and the trigger is no longer present): 3 months (1)[B]
- Unprovoked (idiopathic) PE: A minimum of 3 months, but consider long-term or prolonged secondary prophylaxis if the bleeding risk is low (1)[B]
- Cancer-related PE: LMWH for the 1st 3–6 months, followed by long-term anticoagulation with LMWH or VKA (2)[B]. LMWH dose can be reduced to 75% after the first 6 months
- Recurrent PE: Long-term anticoagulation (2)[B]
- Low-dose aspirin can be used in patients with unprovoked PE and high bleeding risk after completing anticoagulation (1)[B]

FOLLOW-UP RECOMMENDATIONS
- If concomitant DVT, knee-height compression stockings, 30–40 mm Hg knee height
- Consider retrieval of retrievable IVC filters in anticoagulated patients.

Patient Monitoring
- INR should be checked at regular intervals. Target INR is 2–3 for therapy.
- aPTT needs to be monitored if the patient is on adjustable SC UFH.
- Anti-Xa can be checked in special circumstances in patients treated with LMWH.

DIET
Patients on warfarin need education for a vitamin K consistent diet

PROGNOSIS
- Severity at presentation affects mortality: Massive PE 50% vs. nonmassive PE 8–14%
- Abbreviated Pulmonary Embolism Severity Index score predicts acute mortality (Any one of the following variables defines high risk: age >80 years, history of cancer, chronic cardiopulmonary disease, heart rate ≥110/min, systolic blood pressure <100 mm Hg, O_2 saturation <90%)

COMPLICATIONS
- 1 in 25 PE patients will develop chronic thromboembolic pulmonary hypertension
- Recurrent DVT or PE
- Complications of the treatment, such as anticoagulation-associated bleeding. Incidence of major hemorrhage associated with thrombolytics is 8%; intracerebral bleed is 2% (fatal in 1/2 of cases).

REFERENCES
1. Kahn SR, Lim W, Dunn AS, et al. Prevention of VTE in nonsurgical patients: Antithrombotic therapy and prevention of thrombosis, 9th ed: American College of Chest Physicians Evidence-Based Clinical Practice Guidelines. Chest. 2012;141(2 Suppl): e195S–e226S.
2. Gould MK, Garcia DA, Wren SM, et al. Prevention of VTE in nonorthopedic surgical patients: Antithrombotic therapy and prevention of thrombosis, 9th ed: American College of Chest Physicians Evidence-Based Clinical Practice Guidelines. Chest. 2012;141(2 Suppl): e227S–e277S.
3. Falck-Ytter Y, Francis CW, Johanson NA, et al. Prevention of VTE in orthopedic surgery patients: antithrombotic therapy and prevention of thrombosis, 9th ed: American College of Chest Physicians Evidence-Based Clinical Practice Guidelines. Chest. 2012;141(2 Suppl): e278S–e325S.
4. Douma RA, Mos IC, Erkens PM, et al. Performance of 4 clinical decision rules in the diagnostic management of acute pulmonary embolism: A prospective cohort study. Ann Intern Med. 2011;154:709–718.
5. Kearon C, Akl EA, Comerota AJ, et al. Antithrombotic therapy for VTE disease: Antithrombotic therapy and prevention of thrombosis, 9th ed: American College of Chest Physicians Evidence-Based Clinical Practice Guidelines. Chest. 2012;141:e419S–e494S.
6. Jaff MR, McMurtry MS, Archer SL, et al. Management of massive and submassive pulmonary embolism, iliofemoral deep vein thrombosis, and chronic thromboembolic pulmonary hypertension: A scientific statement from the American Heart Association. Circulation. 2011;123:1788–1830.
7. Sadigh G, Kelly AM, Cronin P, et al. Challenges, controversies, and hot topics in pulmonary embolism imaging. AJR Am J Roentgenol. 2011;196:497–515.
8. EINSTEIN–PE Investigators, Büller HR, Prins MH, et al. Oral rivaroxaban for the treatment of symptomatic pulmonary embolism. N Engl J Med. 2012;366:1287–1297.
9. Dong BR, Hao Q, Yue J, et al. Thrombolytic therapy for pulmonary embolism. Cochrane Database Syst Rev. 2009;3:CD004437.

 ## CODES

ICD10
- I26.99 Other pulmonary embolism without acute cor pulmonale
- I27.82 Chronic pulmonary embolism

CLINICAL PEARLS
- PE can be excluded in patients who have a low pretest probability and negative D-dimer testing.
- Unless contraindicated, CT angiogram can reliably be used to diagnose or rule out PE in the majority of cases (1).
- Perform cancer-oriented review of systems and age- and gender-appropriate cancer screening in patients >40, recurrent VTE, upper extremity DVT (not related to catheter or lines), bilateral lower extremity DVT, intra-abdominal DVT, resistance to treatment.
- In patients with a prolonged baseline aPTT, adjust the heparin dose with anti-Xa levels (therapeutic range 0.3–0.7).

PULMONARY FIBROSIS

Anna G. Rudnicki, MD

 BASICS

DESCRIPTION
- Characterized by fibrosis of the lung parenchyma
- Chest CT shows reticular pattern and honeycombing, with subpleural and lower lobe predominance
- Lung biopsy shows "usual interstitial pneumonia" pattern
- Classified based on etiology:
  – Idiopathic (IPF)
  – Nonidiopathic

EPIDEMIOLOGY
Incidence
- Incidence of IPF is 7–16/100,000 person-years
- IPF is more common in men.
- Most patients with IPF are >60 years.
- Incidence of nonidiopathic pulmonary fibrosis is unknown.

Prevalence
- Prevalence of IPF is 2–39 cases/100,000 people
- Prevalence of nonidiopathic pulmonary fibrosis is unknown

ETIOLOGY AND PATHOPHYSIOLOGY
- Postulated that microinjury to alveolar epithelial cells causes release of cytokines that activates fibroblasts, which in turn leads to excess production of extracellular matrix.
- Causes of the nonidiopathic form include:
  – Occupational exposure
  – Environmental exposure
  – Drugs
  – Systemic connective tissue diseases
  – Granulomatous diseases

Genetics
- <5% of IPF is familial and may involve mutations in surfactant protein A2 and C and/or abnormal telomere shortening.
- Most likely mode of transmission is autosomal-dominant with variable penetrance.

RISK FACTORS
- Family history of pulmonary fibrosis
- Gastroesophageal reflux disease (GERD)
- Smoking
- Exposure to birds, livestock, dust from metals or wood, solvents

GENERAL PREVENTION
Avoid the risk factors mentioned above, such as smoking, certain occupational exposures, or drugs that induce pulmonary fibrosis.

COMMONLY ASSOCIATED CONDITIONS
- Pulmonary hypertension: Occurs in 30–80% of patients with IPF, likely as a result of hypoxemic vasoconstriction
- GERD
- Nonidiopathic pulmonary fibrosis may be associated with connective tissue diseases (e.g., rheumatoid arthritis and scleroderma).

 DIAGNOSIS

HISTORY
- Slowly progressive dyspnea
- Dry cough

PHYSICAL EXAM
- Tachypnea
- Fine inspiratory crackles
- Possible clubbing

DIFFERENTIAL DIAGNOSIS
- Asbestosis
- Berylliosis
- Coal worker's pneumoconiosis
- Chronic hypersensitivity pneumonitis
- Sarcoidosis
- Silicosis

DIAGNOSTIC TESTS & INTERPRETATION
Initial Tests (lab, imaging)
- High-resolution chest CT (HRCT) is required to make diagnosis. Characteristic findings include a reticular pattern, traction bronchiectasis, and honeycombing. There is a subpleural and lower lobe predominance. There is minimal to no evidence of active inflammation (1,2).
- If the patient has characteristic findings of pulmonary fibrosis on chest CT, then lung biopsy may not necessarily be required (1).
- HRCT is needed as part of initial workup (as above).

Follow-Up Tests & Special Considerations
- Surgical lung biopsy should be considered if clinical presentation and HRCT are not entirely characteristic of pulmonary fibrosis (1).
- Blood work to rule out associated collagen vascular disease (1)
- Bronchoscopy with bronchoalveolar lavage may help rule out other types of interstitial lung disease (1).

Diagnostic Procedures/Other
- Pulmonary function testing (PFT): Initially, may see only decrease in diffusing capacity. Later in disease, may develop decrease in lung volumes as well
- Echocardiogram to evaluate for concomitant pulmonary hypertension
- Resting and exercise pulse oximetry to determine need for supplemental oxygen

Test Interpretation
Usual interstitial pneumonitis: Shows interstitial scarring, honeycombing, and fibroblastic foci. There is temporal heterogeneity, meaning there may be areas of normal lung adjacent to fibrosed or inflamed lung.

 TREATMENT

GENERAL MEASURES
- Pulmonary rehabilitation (1)[C]
- Consider treating for GERD, even if asymptomatic (1)[B]
- Consider lung transplant

MEDICATION
First Line
Supplemental oxygen, if needed (1)[C]

ISSUES FOR REFERRAL
- Patients should be evaluated and cared for longitudinally by a pulmonologist.
- If any uncertainty in diagnosis, then consider referral to thoracic surgery for lung biopsy.
- Depending on patient age, comorbidities, and preference, may consider referral for lung transplant.

ADDITIONAL THERAPIES
- A recent study showed an increase in mortality in patients treated with a combination of prednisone, azathioprine, and N-acetylcysteine when compared with those receiving placebo or N-acetylcysteine alone (3).
- Studies have shown a modest benefit with the anti-fibrotic agent pirfenidone in slowing the progression of IPF. This drug is not available for this purpose in the US (4).
- Many other clinical trials are currently under way. Some of the targets being studied include TGF-β, connective tissue growth factor, IL-13, CCL2, CXCR4, and CXCL12, ACE, and angiotensin II (5).

SURGERY/OTHER PROCEDURES
Lung transplant carries a 5-year survival of 50–56% (1).

COMPLEMENTARY AND ALTERNATIVE MEDICINE
None

IN-PATIENT CONSIDERATIONS
Admission Criteria/Initial Stabilization
Worsening shortness of breath and/or increased oxygen requirements:
- Provide adequate supplemental oxygen
- Workup for other possible causes of respiratory decompensation
- If no other cause for respiratory decompensation found, then consider administration of high-dose steroids

Nursing
Supplemental oxygen to keep saturations >90%

ONGOING CARE

FOLLOW-UP RECOMMENDATIONS
Patient should follow up with a pulmonologist

Patient Monitoring
Disease progression can be monitored by periodic PFTs and HRCT

DIET
No specific dietary requirements

PATIENT EDUCATION
- Patients should be counseled extensively regarding the prognosis of this diagnosis and given as much support as possible. Information about support groups in the local community and online may be helpful.
- Patients should be informed about the side effects of corticosteroid and/or cytotoxic therapy to decide whether to initiate pharmacologic treatment.
- American Lung Association: www.lungusa.org/lung-disease/pulmonary-fibrosis/
- Pulmonary Fibrosis Foundation: www.pulmonaryfibrosis.org/, which includes information about active pulmonary fibrosis clinical trials.

PROGNOSIS
- Median survival time was thought to be 2–3 years from time of diagnosis. However, recent data from clinical trials suggest that this may be an underestimate (1).
- Some patients may deteriorate quickly, whereas others can remain stable for an extended period of time. Acute exacerbations carry a high mortality, and ICU treatment (mechanical ventilation) is mostly unsuccessful.
- A higher extent of fibrosis increases the risk of death, whereas a higher percentage-predicted diffusing capacity of lung for carbon monoxide reduced the risk of death.

COMPLICATIONS
- Respiratory failure
- Infection
- Pulmonary hypertension
- Rib fractures secondary to prolonged coughing (especially in elderly patients with decreased bone density)

REFERENCES
1. Raghu G, Collard HR, Egan JJ, et al. An official ATS/ERS/JRS/ALAT statement: Idiopathic pulmonary fibrosis: Evidence-based guidelines for diagnosis and management. *Am J Respir Crit Care Med*. 2011;183:788–824.
2. Lynch DA, Godwin JD, Safrin S, et al. High-resolution computed tomography in idiopathic pulmonary fibrosis: Diagnosis and prognosis. *Am J Respir Crit Care Med*. 2005;172:488–493.
3. Idiopathic Pulmonary Fibrosis Clinical Research Network, Raghu G, Anstrom KJ, et al. Prednisone, azathioprine, and N-acetylcysteine for pulmonary fibrosis. *N Engl J Med*. 2012;366:1968–1977.
4. Spagnolo P, Del Giovane C, Luppi F, et al. Non-steroid agents for idiopathic pulmonary fibrosis. *Cochrane Database Syst Rev*. 2010;9:CD003134.
5. Rafii R, Juarez MM, Albertson TE, et al. A review of current and novel therapies for idiopathic pulmonary fibrosis. *J Thorac Dis*. 2013;5:48–73.

ADDITIONAL READING
- Castriotta RJ, Eldadah BA, Foster WM, et al. Workshop on idiopathic pulmonary fibrosis in older adults. *Chest*. 2010;138:693–703.
- Coward WR, Saini G, Jenkins G. The pathogenesis of idiopathic pulmonary fibrosis. *Ther Adv Respir Dis*. 2010;4:367–388.
- Hoo ZH, Whyte MK. Idiopathic pulmonary fibrosis. *Thorax*. 2012;67:742–746.
- Lee JS, McLaughlin S, Collard HR. Comprehensive care of the patient with idiopathic pulmonary fibrosis. *Curr Opin Pulm Med*. 2011;17:348–354.
- O'Connell OJ, Kennedy MP, Henry MT. Idiopathic pulmonary fibrosis: Treatment update. *Adv Ther*. 2011;28:986–999.

 CODES

ICD10
- J84.10 Pulmonary fibrosis, unspecified
- J84.112 Idiopathic pulmonary fibrosis

CLINICAL PEARLS
- Pulmonary fibrosis can usually be diagnosed based on characteristic chest CT findings, which include a reticular pattern, traction bronchiectasis, and honeycombing with a peripheral and basilar predominance.
- There are idiopathic and nonidiopathic forms of pulmonary fibrosis.
- Treatment options for pulmonary fibrosis are very limited and, at best, serve to slow the progression of disease.

PYELONEPHRITIS

Stephen A. Martin, MD, EdM

BASICS

DESCRIPTION
- Acute pyelonephritis is a syndrome caused by an infection of the renal parenchyma and renal pelvis, often producing localized flank/back pain combined with systemic symptoms, such as fever, chills, and nausea. It has a wide spectrum of presentation, from mild illness to septic shock.
- Chronic pyelonephritis is the result of progressive inflammation of the renal interstitium and tubules, presumed to be caused by recurrent infection, vesicoureteral reflux, or both.
- Uncomplicated vs. complicated: Presentation is considered uncomplicated if the infection is caused by a typical pathogen in an immunocompetent patient who has normal urinary tract anatomy and renal function.
- System(s) affected: Renal; Urologic
- Synonym: Acute upper urinary tract infection (UTI)

Geriatric Considerations
- May present only as confusion; absence of fever is common in this age group.
- Elderly patients with diabetes and pyelonephritis are at higher risk of bacteremia, long hospitalization, and mortality.

Pregnancy Considerations
- Most common medical complication requiring hospitalization
- Affects 1–2% of all pregnancies. Morbidity does not differ between trimesters.
- Urine culture follow-up 1–2 weeks after therapy

Pediatric Considerations
- UTI is present in ~5% of patients age 2 months to 2 years with fever and no source evident from history and physical exam.
- Route for antibiotics and location of care should be based on the clinical situation.

EPIDEMIOLOGY
Incidence
Community-acquired acute pyelonephritis: 28/10,000/year
Prevalence
Adult cases: 250,000/year, with 100,000 hospitalizations

ETIOLOGY AND PATHOPHYSIOLOGY
- Infection with *Escherichia coli* (>80%)
- Other gram-negative pathogens: *Proteus, Klebsiella, Serratia, Clostridium, Pseudomonas,* and *Enterobacter*
- *Enterococcus*
- *Staphylococcus: S. epidermis, S. saprophyticus* (number 2 cause in young women), and *S. aureus*
- *Candida*

RISK FACTORS
- Underlying urinary tract abnormalities
- Indwelling catheter/recent urinary tract instrumentation
- Nephrolithiasis
- Immunocompromise, including diabetes
- Elderly, institutionalized women
- Prostatic enlargement
- Childhood UTI
- Acute pyelonephritis within the prior year

- Frequency of recent sexual intercourse/spermicide use
- Stress incontinence
- Pregnancy
- Hospital-acquired infection
- Symptoms >7 days at presentation

COMMONLY ASSOCIATED CONDITIONS
- Indwelling catheters
- Renal calculi
- Benign prostatic hyperplasia

DIAGNOSIS

HISTORY
- In adults (1)[C]:
  - Flank pain
  - Nausea ± vomiting
  - Malaise, anorexia
  - Myalgia
  - Dysuria, urinary frequency, urgency
  - Suprapubic discomfort
- In infants and children:
  - Irritability
  - GI symptoms

PHYSICAL EXAM
- In adults (1)[C]:
  - Fever: ≥37.8°C (100°F)
  - Costovertebral angle tenderness
  - From no physical findings to septic shock
  - A pelvic exam may be needed in female patients to assess for pelvic inflammatory disease (PID)
- In infants and children:
  - Sepsis
  - Fever
  - Poor skin perfusion
  - Inadequate weight gain/weight loss
  - Jaundice to gray skin color

DIFFERENTIAL DIAGNOSIS
- Obstructive uropathy
- Acute bacterial pneumonia (lower lobe)
- Cholecystitis
- Acute pancreatitis
- Appendicitis
- Perforated viscus
- Aortic dissection
- PID
- Kidney stone
- Ectopic pregnancy
- Diverticulitis

DIAGNOSTIC TESTS & INTERPRETATION
Initial Tests (lab, imaging)
- Urinalysis: Pyuria ± leukocyte casts, hematuria, nitrites, and mild proteinuria
- Urine leukocyte esterase test positive
- Urine Gram stain; urine culture (>10,000 colony-forming units/mL) and sensitivities
- CBC, BUN, and creatinine
- In 1 study of hospitalized patients, C-reactive protein levels were found to correlate with prolonged hospitalization and infection recurrence.
- Imaging generally not indicated in straightforward cases
- Pediatrics: Practice is evolving based on recent studies. A recent guideline recommends renal and bladder US (2)[C], but not voiding cystourethrogram after a 1st UTI (2)[B].

Follow-Up Tests & Special Considerations
- To obtain reliable pediatric urine cultures, catheterization/suprapubic aspirate should be used to obtain samples from non–toilet-trained children.
- In certain geriatric patients, obtaining a clean-catch specimen may be difficult. A new condom catheter, new indwelling catheter (after 2 weeks), or straight catheterization are important considerations.

- Blood culture(s): Indicated in diagnostic uncertainty, immunosuppression, or a suspected hematogenous source (1)[B]
- Drugs that may alter lab results: Antibiotics
- If patient's condition does not respond in >72 hours or if obstruction/anatomic abnormality suspected:
  - CT scan of abdomen and pelvis ± contrast material
  - US, renal with kidneys, ureter, bladder
  - Cystoscopy with ureteral catheterization

Test Interpretation
- Acute: Abscess formation with neutrophils
- Chronic: Fibrosis with reduction in renal tissue

TREATMENT

- Total duration of antibiotic use is guided by the clinical situation:
  - A 2013 systematic review found that 7 days of treatment is equivalent to longer treatment regimens in patients without urogenital abnormalities (3)[A].
  - An RCT of 7 days of ciprofloxacin treatment was found not to be inferior to 14 days for young women in an outpatient setting (4)[A].
- IV antibiotics are indicated for inpatients.

GENERAL MEASURES
- Broad-spectrum antibiotics initially, tailoring therapy to culture and sensitivity results
- Analgesics and antipyretics
- Consider urinary analgesics (e.g., phenazopyridine 200 mg t.i.d.) for severe dysuria.

MEDICATION
- For empirical oral therapy, a fluoroquinolone is recommended. Should fluoroquinolone resistance exceed 10%, a single initial IV dose of a long-acting antibiotic such as ceftriaxone 1 g is recommended (5)[C].
- For parenteral therapy, a fluoroquinolone, aminoglycoside ± ampicillin, or an extended-spectrum cephalosporin ± an aminoglycoside can be used (5)[B].
- Contraindications:
  - Allergies to agents listed
  - Fluoroquinolones are contraindicated in children, adolescents, and pregnant women.
  - Nitrofurantoin does not achieve reliable tissue levels for pyelonephritis treatment.
- Precautions:
  - Most antibiotics require adjustments in dosage in patients with renal insufficiency.
  - Test for aminoglycoside levels and renal function.
  - If *Enterococcus* is suspected based on Gram stain, ampicillin + gentamicin is a reasonable empirical choice, unless patient is penicillin allergic; then use vancomycin. If outpatient, add amoxicillin to

fluoroquinolone pending culture results and sensitivity. Do not use a 3rd-generation cephalosporin for suspected/proven enterococcal infection.

First Line
- Adults:
  - Severe illness: IV therapy until afebrile 24–48 hours and tolerating oral hydration and medications, then oral agents to complete 2 weeks. Adult doses (5)[B].
  - IV agents (assuming normal creatine clearance [CrCl]):
    ○ Ciprofloxacin: 400 mg q12h
    ○ Levofloxacin: 500 mg/d
    ○ Gatifloxacin: 400 mg/d
    ○ Cefotaxime: 1 g q8–12h up to 2 g q4h
    ○ Ceftriaxone: 1–2 g/d
    ○ Cefoxitin: 2 g q4–8h
    ○ Gentamicin: 5–7 mg/kg of body weight daily (± ampicillin 2 g q6h for enterococcus)
  - Oral agents (initial outpatient treatment):
    ○ Ciprofloxacin: 500 mg q12h for 7 days
    ○ Ciprofloxacin XR: 1,000 mg/d for 7 days
    ○ Levofloxacin: 750 mg/d for 5 days
    ○ Trimethoprim/Sulfamethoxazole (TMP-SMX) (160/800 mg): 1 tab PO b.i.d. for 14 days provided uropathogen known to be susceptible and ceftriaxone 1 g initial IV dose given
- Pediatric:
  - IV agents (general indication is for age <2 months or clinical concern in other ages):
    ○ Ceftriaxone: 50–100 mg/kg/d (also can be used IM in outpatient setting)
    ○ Ampicillin: 100 mg/kg/d IV divided in 4 doses + gentamicin 7.5 mg/kg/d divided in 3 doses
  - Oral agents: Cefixime: 16 mg/kg/d PO in 2 divided doses on the 1st day, followed by 8 mg/kg once per day to complete therapy
  - IV agents (general indication is for age <2 months/clinical concern in other ages):
    ○ Ceftriaxone: 50–100 mg/kg/d (also can be used IM in outpatient setting)
    ○ Ampicillin: 100 mg/kg/d IV divided in 4 doses + gentamicin 7.5 mg/kg/d divided in 3 doses
  - Oral agents: Cefixime: 16 mg/kg/d PO in 2 divided doses on the 1st day, followed by 8 mg/kg once per day to complete therapy

Second Line
Adults:
- IV agents:
  - Piperacillin–tazobactam: 3.375 g q6–8h
  - Ticarcillin–clavulanate: 3.1 g q4–6h
- Oral agents:
  - Cefixime: 400 mg PO q12h
  - Cefpodoxime (Proxetil): 200 mg q12h
  - Amoxicillin–clavulanate: 875/125 mg q12h or 500/125 mg t.i.d.
  - TMP-SMX: 60–800 mg q12h (up to 30% E. coli strains are resistant to ampicillin and TMP-SMX in community-acquired infections)

Pediatric Considerations
- Children <2 years of age and children with febrile or recurrent UTI are usually treated for 10 days.
- Empirical coverage should include E. coli. Ampicillin should be added if Enterococcus is suspected:
  - Oral antibiotics (cefixime, ceftibuten, and amoxicillin/clavulanic acid) may be used alone, or
  - IV antibiotics (single daily dosing with aminoglycoside) for 2–4 days, followed by oral antibiotics (6)[A]

- If patient is treated as an outpatient, antibiotic course must be completed successfully.

ISSUES FOR REFERRAL
- Acute pyelonephritis unresponsive to therapy
- Chronic pyelonephritis

SURGERY/OTHER PROCEDURES
Perinephric abscess drainage as indicated

IN-PATIENT CONSIDERATIONS
Admission Criteria/Initial Stabilization
- In-patient therapy for severe illness (e.g., high fevers, severe pain, marked debility, intractable vomiting, possible urosepsis), risk factors for complicated pyelonephritis, or extremes of age
- Outpatient therapy if mild–moderate illness (not pregnant, no nausea/vomiting; fever and pain not severe), uncomplicated, and tolerating oral hydration and medications. Most such patients can be selected for outpatient management (7)[B].

IV Fluids
As indicated for dehydration or renal calculi

Discharge Criteria
Discharge on oral agent (see above) after patient is afebrile 24–48 hours to complete 2 weeks.

ONGOING CARE

FOLLOW-UP RECOMMENDATIONS
- Women: Routine follow-up cultures not recommended unless symptoms resolve, but recur within 2 weeks. If symptoms resolve, but recur after 2 weeks, treat as sporadic episode of pyelonephritis unless ≥2 recurrences; then, urologic evaluation is necessary.
- Men, children, adolescents, patients with recurrent infections, patients with risk factors: Repeat cultures 1–2 weeks after completing therapy; urologic evaluation after 1st episode of pyelonephritis and with recurrences.

Patient Monitoring
- No response within 48 hours (5% of patients): Re-evaluate and review cultures, CT scan, or US, and adjust therapy as needed; may need urologic consult. The 2 most common causes are a resistant organism and nephrolithiasis.
- Mild–moderate illness: Oral therapy for 2 weeks as outpatient
- Close contact should be maintained with children's families to monitor their response.

DIET
Encourage fluid intake.

PROGNOSIS
95% of treated patients respond within 48 hours.

COMPLICATIONS
- Kidney abscess
- Metastatic infection: Skeletal system, endocardium, eye, meningitis with subsequent seizures
- Septic shock and death
- Acute/Chronic renal failure

REFERENCES
1. Colgan R, Williams M, Johnson JR. Diagnosis and treatment of acute pyelonephritis in women. Am Fam Physician. 2011;84(5):519–526.
2. Subcommittee on Urinary Tract Infection, Steering Committee on Quality Improvement and Management, Roberts KB. Urinary tract infection: Clinical practice guideline for the diagnosis and management of the initial UTI in febrile infants and children 2 to 24 months. Pediatrics. 2011;84(3):595–610. Epub 2011 Aug 28.
3. Eliakim-Raz N, Yahav D, Paul M, et al Duration of antibiotic treatment for acute pyelonephritis and septic urinary tract infection: 7 days or less versus longer treatment: Systematic review and meta-analysis of randomized controlled trials. J Antimicrob Chemother. 2013 Oct;68(10):2183–2191.
4. Sandberg T, Skoog G, Hermansson AB, et al. Ciprofloxacin for 7 days versus 14 days in women with acute pyelonephritis: A randomised, open-label and double-blind, placebo-controlled, non-inferiority trial. Lancet. 2012;380(9840):484–490.
5. Gupta K, Hooton TM, Naber KG, et al. International clinical practice guidelines for the treatment of acute uncomplicated cystitis and pyelonephritis in women: A 2010 update by the Infectious Diseases Society of America and the European Society for Microbiology and Infectious Diseases. Clin Infect Dis. 2011;52:e103–e120.
6. Hodson EM, Willis NS, Craig JC, et al. Antibiotics for acute pyelonephritis in children. Cochrane Database Syst Rev. 2007;(4):CD003772.
7. Hooton TM. Clinical practice. Uncomplicated urinary tract infection. N Engl J Med. 2012;84(11):1028–1037.

ADDITIONAL READING
- Beetz R, Westenfelder M. Antimicrobial therapy of urinary tract infections in children. Int J Antimicrob Agents. 2011;38(Suppl):42–50. Epub 2011 Oct 27.
- Hooton TM, Bradley SF, Cardenas DD, et al. Diagnosis, prevention, and treatment of catheter-associated urinary tract infection in adults: 2009 International Clinical Practice Guidelines from the Infectious Diseases Society of America. Clin Infect Dis. 2010;50(5):625–663.
- Matthews SJ, Lancaster JW. Urinary tract infections in the elderly population. Am J Geriatr Pharmacother. 2011;9(5):286–309. Epub 2011 Aug 12.

CODES

ICD10
- N10 Acute tubulo-interstitial nephritis
- N11.9 Chronic tubulo-interstitial nephritis, unspecified
- N12 Tubulo-interstitial nephritis, not spcf as acute or chronic

CLINICAL PEARLS
- Pyelonephritis presentation can be classic or subtle. Early diagnosis can help prevent clinical deterioration.
- Keep pyelonephritis in mind with less common populations (e.g., children and men).
- The most common causes of poor response to antibiotics are antibiotic resistance and kidney stones.

PYLORIC STENOSIS
Ruben Peralta, MD, FACS

 BASICS

DESCRIPTION
- Progressive narrowing of the pyloric canal, occurring in infancy
- Synonym(s): Infantile hypertrophic pyloric stenosis (IHPS)

EPIDEMIOLOGY
- Predominant age: Infancy:
  - Onset usually at 3–6 weeks of age; rarely in the newborn period or as late as 5 months of age
- Considered the most common condition requiring surgical intervention in the 1st year of life
- A recent decline in its incidence has been reported in a number of countries
- Predominant sex: Male > Female (4:1)

Incidence
In Caucasian population, 2–5:1,000 babies; less common in African American and Asian populations

Prevalence
National prevalence level is 1–2:1,000 infants, ranging from 0.5–4.21:1,000 live births.

ETIOLOGY AND PATHOPHYSIOLOGY
- Abnormal relaxation of the pyloric muscles leads to hypertrophy
- Redundant mucosa fills the pyloric canal
- Gastric outflow is obstructed, leading to gastric distension and vomiting.
- The exact cause remains unknown, but multiple genetic and environmental factors have been implicated (1,2,3).
- A recent surveillance study of a population-based birth defects registry identified an association between pyloric stenosis and the use of fluoxetine in the 1st trimester of pregnancy, even after adjustment for maternal age and smoking. The adjusted odds ratio was 9.8 (95% CI: 1.5–62) (4)[B].

Genetics
Recent studies have identified linkage to chromosome 11 and multiple loci and chromosome 16 (1,2,3).

RISK FACTORS
- Incidence higher in firstborn boys
- 5 × increased risk with affected 1st-degree relative
- Strong familial aggregation and heritability (2)

COMMONLY ASSOCIATED CONDITIONS
Associated anomalies present in ~4–7% of infants with pyloric stenosis:
- Hiatal and inguinal hernias (most commonly)
- Other anomalies include:
  - Congenital heart disease
  - Esophageal atresia
  - Tracheoesophageal fistula
  - Renal abnormalities
  - Turner syndrome and trisomy 18
  - Cornelia de Lange syndrome
  - Smith-Lemli-Opitz syndrome
- A common proposed genetic link between breast cancer, endometriosis, and pyloric stenosis has been observed in families.

 DIAGNOSIS

HISTORY
- Nonbilious projectile vomiting after feeding, increasing in frequency and severity
- Emesis may become blood-tinged from vomiting-induced gastric irritation
- Hunger due to inadequate nutrition
- Decrease in bowel movements
- Weight loss

PHYSICAL EXAM
- Firm, mobile ("olive-like") mass palpable in the right upper quadrant (70–90% of the time)
- Epigastric distention
- Visible gastric peristalsis after feeding
- Late signs: Dehydration, weight loss
- Rarely, jaundice when starvation leads to decreased glucuronyl transferase activity resulting in indirect hyperbilirubinemia

DIFFERENTIAL DIAGNOSIS
- Inexperienced or inappropriate feeding
- Gastroesophageal reflux disease (GERD)
- Gastritis
- Congenital adrenal hyperplasia, salt-losing
- Pylorospasm
- Gastric volvulus
- Antral or gastric web

DIAGNOSTIC TESTS & INTERPRETATION
Metabolic disturbances are late findings and are uncommon in present era of early diagnosis and intervention.
- If prolonged vomiting, then check electrolytes for:
  - Hypokalemia
  - Hypochloremia
  - Metabolic alkalosis
- Elevated unconjugated bilirubin level (rare)
- Paradoxical aciduria: The kidney tubules excrete hydrogen to preserve potassium in face of hypokalemic alkalosis.
- Abdominal US is the study of choice:
  - Shows thickened and elongated pyloric muscle and redundant mucosa
- Upper GI series reveals strong gastric contractions; elongated, narrow pyloric canal (string sign); and parallel lines of barium in the narrow channel (double-tract sign or railroad track sign).

Test Interpretation
Concentric hypertrophy of pyloric muscle

 TREATMENT

SURGERY/OTHER PROCEDURES
- Ramstedt pyloromyotomy is curative. The entire length of hypertrophied muscle is divided, with preservation of the underlying mucosa.
- Surgical approaches include open (traditional right upper quadrant transverse) incision; more contemporary circumumbilical incision, and laparoscopic techniques.
- A recent review concluded that the laparoscopic approach results in less postoperative pain and can be performed with no increase in operative time or complications (5,6).
- Conservative approach:
  - Conservative management of infantile hypertrophic pyloric stenosis with atropine can be effective in approximately 6 of 7 cases but has a lower success rate and longer duration of therapy than surgery (7)[B].
  - Atropine therapy may be considered as an alternative to pyloromyotomy for patients unsuitable or at high risk for surgery, and in areas of the world where surgery on small infants is unavailable or unsafe (7)[B].

IN-PATIENT CONSIDERATIONS
Admission Criteria/Initial Stabilization
- Prompt treatment to avoid dehydration and malnutrition
- Correct acid–base and electrolyte disturbances. Surgery should be delayed until alkalosis is corrected.
- Patients need pre- and postoperative apnea monitoring. Patients have a tendency toward apnea to compensate with respiratory acidosis for their metabolic alkalosis.

IV Fluids
To correct dehydration and metabolic abnormalities

 ONGOING CARE

FOLLOW-UP RECOMMENDATIONS
Patient Monitoring
- Routine pediatric health maintenance
- Postoperative monitoring, including monitoring for pain, emesis, apnea

DIET
- No preoperative feeding
- Initiate feeding 12–24 hours after surgery, with goal of advancing to full oral feedings within 36–48 hours of surgery.

PROGNOSIS
Surgery is curative.

COMPLICATIONS
No long-term morbidity. Duodenal perforation is a known, but uncommon, complication of surgery. In a recent systematic review and meta-analysis addressing major complications rates between open vs. laparoscopic pyloromyotomy, no major difference was found in complications, but the laparoscopic group showed faster time to full feed and a shorter hospital stay.

REFERENCES
1. Feenstra B, Geller F, Carstensen L, et al. Plasma lipids, genetic variants near APOA1, and the risk of infantile hypertrophic pyloric stenosis. *JAMA*. 2013;310:714–721.
2. Krogh C, Fischer TK, Skotte L, et al. Familial aggregation and heritability of pyloric stenosis. *JAMA*. 2010;303:2393–2399.
3. Ranells JD, Carver JD, Kirby RS, et al. Infantile hypertrophic pyloric stenosis: Epidemiology, genetics, and clinical update. *Adv Pediatr*. 2011;58:195–206.
4. Bakker MK, De Walle HE, Wilffert B, et al. Fluoxetine and infantile hypertrophic pylorus stenosis: A signal from a birth defects-drug exposure surveillance study. *Pharmacoepidemiol Drug Saf*. 2010;19:808–813.
5. Sola JE, Neville HL. Laparoscopic vs open pyloromyotomy: A systematic review and meta-analysis. *J Pediatr Surg*. 2009;44:1631–1637.
6. Oomen MW, Hoekstra LT, Bakx R, et al. Open versus laparoscopic pyloromyotomy for hypertrophic pyloric stenosis: A systematic review and meta-analysis focusing on major complications. *Surg Endosc*. 2012;26:2104–2110.
7. Mercer AE, Phillips R. Question 2: Can a conservative approach to the treatment of hypertophic pyloric stenosis with atropine be considered a real alternative to surgical pylomyotomy? *Arch Dis Child*. 2013;98:474–477.

ADDITIONAL READING
- Colletti JE. Pyloric stenosis. *CJEM*. 2004;6:444–445.
- Everett KV, Capon F, Georgoula C, et al. Linkage of monogenic infantile hypertrophic pyloric stenosis to chromosome 16q24. *Eur J Hum Genet*. 2008;16:1151–1154.

- Everett KV, Chioza BA, Georgoula C, et al. Genome-wide high-density SNP-based linkage analysis of infantile hypertrophic pyloric stenosis identifies loci on chromosomes 11q14-q22 and Xq23. *Am J Hum Genet*. 2008;82:756–762.
- Georgoula C, Gardiner M. Pyloric stenosis a 100 years after Ramstedt. *Arch Dis Child*. 2012;97:741–745.
- National Birth Defects Prevention Network. Selected birth defects data from population-based birth defects surveillance programs in the United States, 2003–2007. *Birth Defects Res A Clin Mol Teratol*. 2010;88:1062–1174.
- Owen RP, Almond SL, Humphrey GM. Atropine sulphate: Rescue therapy for pyloric stenosis. *BMJ Case Rep*. 2012;2012:pii: bcr2012006489.
- Sommerfield T, Chalmers J, Youngson G, et al. The changing epidemiology of infantile hypertrophic pyloric stenosis in Scotland. *Arch Dis Child*. 2008;93:1007–1011.
- St Peter SD, Holcomb GW, Calkins CM, et al. Open versus laparoscopic pyloromyotomy for pyloric stenosis: A prospective, randomized trial. *Ann Surg*. 2006;244:363–370.

 CODES

ICD10
Q40.0 Congenital hypertrophic pyloric stenosis

CLINICAL PEARLS
- Pyloric stenosis is the most common condition requiring surgical intervention in the 1st year of life.
- The condition classically presents between 1–5 months of life, with projectile vomiting after feeds and a firm, mobile mass in the right upper quadrant.
- Abdominal ultrasound is the study of choice.
- Surgery (laparoscopic Ramstedt pyloromyotomy is the preferred method) is curative.

RABIES

Alan M. Ehrlich, MD

 BASICS

DESCRIPTION
- A rapidly progressive CNS infection caused by a ribonucleic acid (RNA) rhabdovirus affecting mammals, including humans
- The disease is generally considered to be 100% fatal once symptoms develop.
- System(s) affected: Nervous
- Synonym(s): Hydrophobia (due to inability to swallow water)

EPIDEMIOLOGY
Incidence
- Most cases are in developing countries
- Estimated 55,000 deaths worldwide per year
- Only 1 death in the US in 2007
- Only 3 cases in the US in 2006
- Predominant age: Any
- Predominant sex: Male = Female

ETIOLOGY AND PATHOPHYSIOLOGY
Lyssavirus, which is an RNA virus in the family Rhabdoviridae:
- Rabies virus, a neurotropic virus present in saliva of infected animals
- Transmission occurs via bites from infected animals or rarely via saliva coming in contact with open wound or mucous membranes.
- In the US, bats are the most common source of rabies.

RISK FACTORS
- Professions or activities that may expose a person to wild or domestic animals (e.g., animal handlers, lab workers, veterinarians, spelunkers [cave explorers])
- In the US, most cases due to exposure to bats
- Internationally, many countries still have rabies widespread in both domestic and feral dogs.
- Human-to-human transmission has occurred through cornea, solid organs, and other tissue transplants (1).
- International travel to countries where canine rabies is endemic

GENERAL PREVENTION
- Pre-exposure vaccination if at risk of unapparent or unrecognized exposure to rabies, such as traveling to endemic areas
- Pre-exposure vaccination for high-risk groups such as veterinarians, animal handlers, and certain laboratory workers
- Consider pre-exposure vaccination for travelers visiting relatives in areas, such as North Africa, that have increased risk of rabies from domestic animals.
- Immunization of dogs and cats
- People who observe abnormal behavior in any wildlife species should contact animal control and avoid approaching or handling those animals.
- Avoid wild and unknown domestic animals
- Seek treatment promptly if bitten, scratched, or in contact with saliva.
- Infection can be prevented by prompt postexposure treatment of persons bitten by or otherwise exposed to animals known or suspected to be carrying the disease.
- Postexposure prophylaxis should be considered for any person who reports direct contact with bats, unless it is known that an exposure did not occur.

 DIAGNOSIS

HISTORY
- It is important to elicit history of animal exposure, because early diagnosis and treatment are necessary for survival.
- Diagnosis should be considered if there is a bite by an animal capable of transmitting the disease or travel to a rabies-endemic country; however, most patients in the US do not recall exposure.
- 5 stages (may overlap):
  - Incubation period: Time between bite and 1st symptoms of disease: Usually 10 days–1 year, with average of 20–60 days. It is shortest in patients with extensive bites about the head and trunk.
  - Prodrome: Lasts 1–14 days; symptoms include pain or paresthesia at bite site and nonspecific flulike symptoms, including fever and headache.
  - Acute neurologic period: Lasts 2–10 days. CNS symptoms dominate clinical picture; generally takes 1 of 2 forms: (i) Furious rabies: Episodes of hyperactivity last about 5 minutes and include hydrophobia, aerophobia, hyperventilation, hypersalivation, and autonomic instability interspersed with periods of normalcy. (ii) Paralytic rabies: Paralysis dominates clinical picture; may be ascending (as in Guillain-Barré syndrome) or may affect ≥1 limbs differentially.
  - Coma: Lasts hours to days; with intensive care, rarely may last months. May evolve over a few days following acute neurologic period. May be sudden, with respiratory arrest.
  - Death: Usually occurs within 3 weeks of onset as result of complications. Only 6 survivors have been reported in the literature (2)[C].

PHYSICAL EXAM
Findings can range from normal exam up to severe neurologic findings, including paralysis and coma, depending on the stage of rabies at the time of presentation.

DIFFERENTIAL DIAGNOSIS
- Any rapidly progressive encephalitis; important to exclude treatable causes of encephalitis, especially herpes
- Only 2007 rabies case in the US was diagnosed initially as transverse myelitis.

DIAGNOSTIC TESTS & INTERPRETATION
Initial Tests (lab, imaging)
- Spinal tap
- WBC count in CSF examination may be normal or show moderate pleocytosis
- CSF protein may be normal or moderately elevated
- Skin biopsy to detect rabies antigen in hair follicles:
  - Available at state and federal reference labs
- Rabies antibody titer on serum and CSF
- Skin biopsy from nape of neck for direct fluorescent antibody examination
- Viral isolation from saliva or CSF
- Corneal smear stains are positive by immunofluorescence in 50% of patients
- Sodium levels may be low
- Head CT scan: Normal or nonspecific findings consistent with encephalitis
- MRI may allow early diagnosis and can be used to rule out other forms of encephalitis

Follow-Up Tests & Special Considerations
For wild animals, the brain of the biting animal, if available, should be submitted for laboratory testing.
Diagnostic Procedures/Other
Spinal tap

Test Interpretation
Encephalitis may be found on brain biopsy, but abnormal findings may be confined to parts (e.g., brainstem, midbrain, cerebellum) examined only postmortem.

TREATMENT

Thorough wound cleansing with soap and water is the 1st line of treatment. Irrigate wound with virucidal agent, such as povidone-iodine, if available (3).

GENERAL MEASURES
- Physicians should evaluate each possible exposure to rabies and consult local or state public health officials about the need for rabies prophylaxis. In the US, raccoons, skunks, bats, foxes, and coyotes are the animals most likely to be infected, but any carnivore can carry the disease.
- Before specific antirabies treatment is initiated, consider:
  - Type of exposure (bite or nonbite)
  - Epidemiology of rabies in species involved
  - Circumstances of biting incident (provoked vs. unprovoked)
  - Vaccination status of exposing animal

MEDICATION
ALERT
- Immunosuppression, either by medications or disease, can interfere with the development of immunity after vaccination. Immunosuppressive drugs should be avoided during postexposure prophylaxis unless absolutely necessary for the treatment of other conditions. If postexposure prophylaxis is given to an immunosuppressed person, serum samples should be checked for the presence of rabies virus–neutralizing antibody in response to vaccination (4)[B].
- All wounds should be thoroughly cleansed, regardless of whether postexposure prophylaxis was given.
- Assess need for postexposure prophylaxis based on circumstances of possible exposure.
- Increased risk associated with:
  - Bites involving any puncture of the skin constitute a significant risk, whereas saliva is only a risk if it comes in contact with an open wound.
  - Wild or domestic animals that cannot be quarantined
  - Any potential exposure to bats
  - Hybrid animals of wild and domestic species (e.g., wolf-dog)
  - Unprovoked attack (feeding a wild animal is considered a provoked attack)

- Management based on type of animal:
  – Bites from cats, dogs, and ferrets that can be watched for 10 days do not require prophylaxis unless animal shows signs of illness.
  – Skunks, foxes, bats, raccoons, and most carnivores are high risk, and prophylaxis should begin promptly unless animal can be captured and euthanized for pathologic evaluation.
  – For rodents or livestock, consult local public health authorities before initiating prophylaxis.
- Postexposure prophylaxis regimen consists of (2)[B]:
  – Passive vaccination: Rabies immunoglobulin (RIG, Hyperab) administered once: 20 IU/kg of body weight. If anatomically feasible, all the RIG should be thoroughly infiltrated in the area around the wound. Any remaining RIG should be administered IM. RIG never should be administered in the same syringe or into the same anatomic site as vaccine.
  – Active vaccination: Rabies vaccine, human diploid cell (HDCV) or rabies vaccine adsorbed (RVA) or purified chick embryo cell vaccine IM in the deltoid. For children, the anterolateral aspect of the thigh is acceptable. The gluteal area never should be used for vaccine injections. Give the first dose, 1 mL, as soon as possible after exposure. The day of the 1st dose is designated Day 0. Give an additional 1-mL dose on days 3, 7, and 14. If immunocompromised, give 5th dose on day 28.
- For previously vaccinated patients, a 1-mL IM dose of vaccine should be administered immediately and an additional 1-mL dose 3 days later. RIG is not necessary in these patients (2)[B].
- Pre-exposure vaccination: For people in high-risk groups, such as veterinarians, animal handlers, certain laboratory workers, and those spending time in foreign countries where rabies is enzootic (2)[B]:
  – Primary pre-exposure: IM vaccination regimen consists of 3 1-mL injections of HDCV or RVA given in deltoid area, 1 each on days 1, 7, and 28. HDCV also may be given in intradermal doses, administered with a special syringe developed for that purpose (Imovax Rabies ID Vaccine); the 0.1-mL IM dose is administered in the deltoid area; follow the same schedule as for IM doses. Recently, the manufacturer discontinued production of Imovax Rabies ID Vaccine.
  – Pre-exposure boosters: For people at frequent risk of exposure to rabies, serum should be tested every 2 years. A pre-exposure booster (1.0 mL IM) should be administered if this is less than an acceptable level. If titer cannot be obtained, a booster can be administered instead.
- Contraindications: None for postexposure treatment

Pregnancy Considerations
- Pregnancy is not a contraindication to postexposure prophylaxis.
- Rabies vaccination is not associated with a higher incidence of abortion, premature births, or fetal abnormalities.

IN-PATIENT CONSIDERATIONS
Admission Criteria/Initial Stabilization
Clinical rabies

- For diagnosed rabies, comfort care and sedation are indicated for all patients.
- Milwaukee Protocol: Experimental treatment used ketamine, midazolam, and amantadine (originally included ribavirin but no longer recommended) (4,5)[C] (see "Prognosis")
- May also need medication to control cerebral artery vasospasm (such as nimodipine) (5,6)[C]
- Fludrocortisone and hypertonic saline if needed to maintain normal sodium level (6)[C]

 ONGOING CARE

FOLLOW-UP RECOMMENDATIONS
After primary vaccination, serologic testing is necessary only if the patient has a disease or takes a medication that may suppress the immune system.

PATIENT EDUCATION
Homes should be secured from bats by using screens over ventilation areas in the roof.

PROGNOSIS
- No postexposure failures reported in the US since the 1970s
- Rabies has the highest case-fatality rate of any infectious disease.
- The disease is generally considered to be 100% fatal once symptoms develop.
- Survival has been well documented for only 6 patients. In 5 of these, the persons had received rabies vaccination before the onset of disease.
- There have only been a small number of cases of successful recovery from rabies reported, with almost all having received some form of pre- or postexposure immunization. One patient who did not receive pre- or postexposure prophylaxis recovered from clinical rabies in 2004 after being treated with medically induced coma and amantadine in what has become known as the Milwaukee Protocol (4)[C]. 2 years after treatment, there were some persistent neurologic deficits, but overall functioning was normal enough for the patient to finish high school and enroll in college (7)[C]. Another patient similarly treated also recovered (6)[C], but most other patients treated similarly have not survived (5)[C].

COMPLICATIONS
0.6% of people develop mild serum sickness reaction following HDCV boosters. Mild local and systemic reactions are common following vaccination. Mild reactions should not be a cause for interruption of immunization.

REFERENCES

1. Vora NM, Basavaraju SV, Feldman KA, et al. Transplant-Associated Rabies Virus Transmission Investigation Team. Raccoon rabies virus variant transmission through solid organ transplantation. JAMA. 2013;310:398–407.
2. Hankins DG, Rosekrans JA. Overview prevention, and treatment of rabies. Mayo Clin Proc. 2004;79:671–676.
3. Rupprecht CE, Briggs D, Brown CM, et al. Use of a reduced (4-dose) vaccine schedule for postexposure prophylaxis to prevent human rabies: Recommendations of the advisory committee on immunization practices. MMWR Recomm Rep. 2010;59:1–9.
4. Willoughby R. Survival after treatment of rabies with induction of coma. N Engl J Med. 2005;352:2508–2514.
5. Aramburo A, Willoughby RE, Bollen AW, et al. Failure of the Milwaukee protocol in a child with rabies. Clin Infect Dis. 2011;53:572–574.
6. Centers for Disease Control and Prevention (CDC). Recovery of a patient from clinical rabies—California, 2011. MMWR Morb Mortal Wkly Rep. 2012;61:61–65.
7. Hu WT, Willoughby RE, Dhonau H, et al. Long-term follow-up after treatment of rabies by induction of coma. N Engl J Med. 2007;357:945–946.
8. De Serres G, Skowronski DM, Mimault P, et al. Bats in the bedroom, bats in the belfry: Reanalysis of the rationale for rabies postexposure prophylaxis. Clin Infect Dis. 2009;48:1493–1499.

ADDITIONAL READING
- Eckerle I, Rosenberger KD, Zwahlen M, et al. Serologic vaccination response after solid organ transplantation: a systematic review. PLoS One. 2013;8:e56974.
- Manning SE, Rupprecht CE, Fishbein D, et al. Human rabies prevention–United States, 2008: Recommendations of the Advisory Committee on Immunization Practices. MMWR Recomm Rep. 2008;57(RR-3):1–28.

 SEE ALSO

Bites

 CODES

ICD10
- A82.0 Sylvatic rabies
- A82.1 Urban rabies
- A82.9 Rabies, unspecified

CLINICAL PEARLS
- Rare in the US, but quite common in other areas of the world.
- Seek treatment if exposed to scratch, bite, or saliva of potentially infected animal (e.g., feral dog, bat, fox, raccoon, or other wild animals).
- Postexposure prophylaxis consists of 3 steps: Local wound cleansing, passive immunization with rabies immunoglobulin, and active immunization with human diploid cell vaccine.
- Postexposure prophylaxis should be considered for anyone who reports direct contact with bats, unless it is known that an exposure did not occur.
- Exposure to bats in bedrooms while sleeping is not uncommon, but contraction of rabies in this circumstance is rare (8)[B].

RADIATION ENTERITIS
Daniel Jamorabo, MD • Eric J. Mao, MD • Edward Feller, MD

BASICS

- Radiation enteritis (RE) is injury to the colon and small intestine secondary to radiation therapy (RT):
  - RT is used to treat abdominal, pelvic, and retroperitoneal cancers in as many as 200,000 patients yearly in the US.
  - As many as 2/3 of US cancer patients undergo radiation as part of their treatment.
- Toxicity to normal tissues is common and potentially devastating. Limiting radiation dosage to tumors to prevent RT damage is a barrier to curing malignancy.

DESCRIPTION
- Acute RE develops during or shortly after RT, but usually resolves within 2–6 weeks of completion of treatment (1).
- Chronic RE generally develops 6+ months following RT, often 1–6 years later (1,2).
- Chronic RE is usually progressive with potential for significant long-term morbidity and mortality:
  - Therapeutic options other than symptomatic treatment are limited.
  - Surgical resection: Role in selected cases (3)
- Recent introduction of radioembolization of liver tumors using yttrium-90 microspheres has produced gastroduodenal ulceration stemming from ectopic distribution of radioactive microspheres into lining of GI tract (4).
- Incidence of acute RE: 60–80% of patients receiving intra-abdominal/pelvic RT (1)
- Incidence of chronic RE: 20% receiving pelvic RT for gynecologic/urologic tumors (2)

Prevalence
Prevalence of RE in the US: 1.5–2 million people (1)

ETIOLOGY AND PATHOPHYSIOLOGY
- Radiation injury can lead to impaired cell division/immediate cell death from absorption of energy from incident radiation; indirectly, injury may be mediated by release of free radicals, which may damage DNA (2).
- Acute RE: Mucosal atrophy and inflammation, leading to nutrient and fluid loss with possible blood loss
- Chronic RE: Obliterative endarteritis, causing tissue ischemia and necrosis with subsequent transmural fibrosis
- Result: Vascular degeneration, telangiectatic vessel formation, altered intestinal transit, malabsorption, mucosal ulceration, intestinal wall necrosis, serosal adhesion formation, bacterial overgrowth, lactose intolerance, and increased intestinal permeability

RISK FACTORS
- Patient factors:
  - Older age
  - Low body mass index
  - Medical comorbidities: DM, HTN, atherosclerosis, collagen vascular disease, occlusive vascular disease, IBD, HIV, ataxia-telangiectasia
  - Smoking history
  - Prior abdominal/pelvic surgery
  - Prior intra-abdominal infection
- Treatment factors (5):
  - Treatment volume and total dose given
  - Fractionation dose and schedule
  - Concurrent chemotherapy

GENERAL PREVENTION
- Physical measures:
  - Belly board device
  - Surgical placement of intestinal sling
  - Bladder distension during RT
  - Trendelenburg position in pelvic RT
- Treatment measures:
  - Reduce field size
  - Multiple field arrangements
  - Intensity-modulated RT
  - Brachytherapy
- Other: Radiation injury can also occur in settings of terrorist attacks and occupational hazards. Coordination of public health resources is essential to prepare for disasters. Broad-spectrum antibiotics may be useful as these individuals may become immunocompromised (6).

COMMONLY ASSOCIATED CONDITIONS
- Radiation injury to other organs
- Features specific to underlying malignancy

DIAGNOSIS

- All patients with a history of RT should be questioned; many do not seek medical care for chronic morbidity.
- Diagnosis of RE may be difficult and unsuspected because of the complicated, multifactorial causality of these nonspecific symptoms in cancer patients.

HISTORY
Clinical presentation (2):
- Onset:
  - Acute RE within 3 months after RT
  - Chronic RE after 6 months following RT
- Oropharyngeal and Esophageal symptoms:
  - Mucositis
  - Dysphagia/odynophagia
  - Esophageal bleeding or perforation
- Stomach/Small bowel symptoms:
  - Nausea
  - Vomiting
  - Abdominal bloating
  - Dyspepsia and ulceration
  - Obstruction
- Large bowel symptoms:
  - Constipation or diarrhea
  - Abdominal pain
  - Obstruction
  - Intestinal bleeding:
    - Hematochezia, melena, occult blood positivity in stools, or iron deficiency anemia
- Rectal symptoms:
  - Defecation urgency
  - Tenesmus
  - Mucus
  - Incontinence
  - Bleeding
- Malabsorption symptoms:
  - Diarrhea
  - Steatorrhea
  - Weight loss
  - Wasting illness
- Nonspecific symptoms:
  - Weight loss, lethargy, fever, abdominal pain
- Associated conditions: May present as osteoporosis, anemia, bone marrow suppression, dermatitis, or cardiac injury, depending on the nature of RT and the dose distribution

PHYSICAL EXAM
- Nonspecific:
  - May mimic diverse, common abdominal disorders
  - Weight loss and anorexia
  - Nausea, vomiting
  - Fatigue, night sweats
- Adverse RT effect should be considered in patients who have received prior RT and present with:
  - Abdominal tenderness
  - Blood in stool
  - Evidence of malnutrition

DIFFERENTIAL DIAGNOSIS
- Postsurgical adhesions
- Inflammatory bowel disease
- Irritable bowel syndrome
- New/Recurrent neoplasia/metastatic lesions
- Ischemic colitis
- Infectious colitis
- Malabsorption syndromes
- Lymphoma
- Gynecologic disorders
- Medication toxicity

DIAGNOSTIC TESTS & INTERPRETATION
- Acute RE:
  - Diagnostic tests not indicated except to exclude other pathology or if clinical presentation suggests serious disease
- Chronic RE:
  - Diagnostic tests indicated

Initial Tests (lab, imaging)
- Initial labs:
  - CBC
  - Comprehensive metabolic panel
  - Serum albumin and globulin
  - Fecal occult blood test
- First-line investigations:
  - If upper GI or small bowel symptoms:
    - Upper GI endoscopy
    - CT scanning commonly used to visualize small bowel. Upper GI series with small bowel follow through is a second line to visualize distal segments.
    - Video capsule endoscopy, small bowel enteroscopy, and MR enterography are increasingly used because of the relative inaccessibility of small bowel (7).
  - If large bowel symptoms:
    - Colonoscopy with terminal ileal intubation and potential for endoscopic control of bleeding with thermal/laser methodology
  - If nonspecific symptoms (i.e., weight loss or abdominal pain):
    - Abdominopelvic CT/MRI imaging to assess bowel wall thickening, stricture, or alternative diagnosis
- If first-line investigation is negative:
  - Reassess symptoms
  - Stool studies (in selected cases) for pathogens, fecal leukocytes, spot stool for fat and muscle fibers
  - Reconsider other first-line investigations
- If evidence of GI bleeding/iron deficiency with negative first-line tests, investigate small bowel:
  - Small bowel enteroscopy/capsule endoscopy (if strictures excluded)

Follow-Up Tests & Special Considerations
Second-line investigations:

- Diarrhea may be due to: Accelerated bowel transit time; medication effect; malabsorption of bile salts, fat, or carbohydrates; bacterial overgrowth; pancreatic insufficiency; ischemic colitis; mucosal inflammation; short bowel syndrome
  - Vitamin deficiency: Serum vitamin B_{12} and folate, serum carotene, D-xylose test, PT, 25-hydroxy vitamin D; serum iron/iron-binding capacity ratio
  - Carbohydrate: Hydrogen breath test after carbohydrate challenge
  - Pancreatic exocrine/endocrine insufficiency: Spot stool sample for fat and muscle fibers; glucose tolerance test, fasting plasma glucose/hemoglobin A1c

TREATMENT

- Evidence-based treatment of RE is limited.
- Acute RE: Treat symptomatically; spontaneous resolution is common.
- Chronic RE: 1/3 of patients will require surgery for RE complications and must be counseled on likely impaired quality of life (3,8).
- Malnutrition in cancer patients increases hospitalizations and mortality.

MEDICATION
First Line
- Acute RE:
  - First line (antidiarrheal):
    - Loperamide 2–4 mg/d PO (9)[B]
    - Diphenoxylate 5 mg PO t.i.d. (9)[B]
  - First line (antiemetic):
    - Prochlorperazine 5–10 mg PO or by rectal suppository t.i.d.
    - Ondansetron 8 mg PO b.i.d. (1)[B]
  - Second line (antidiarrheal):
    - Octreotide 150 μg SC t.i.d. for diarrhea (1)[B]
- Chronic RE (9)[B]:
  - Treatment options with good evidence:
    - Loperamide 2–4 mg PO b.i.d. for symptomatic treatment of diarrhea (obstruction must be excluded prior to use)
    - Diphenoxylate 5 mg PO q.i.d. for symptomatic treatment of diarrhea (obstruction must be excluded prior to use)
    - Cholestyramine 4 g PO 1–2 × per day for bile salt malabsorption
    - Doxycycline 100 mg/d PO and metronidazole 400 mg PO t.i.d. for 7–10 days for bacterial overgrowth
  - Treatment options with weak evidence:
    - Hyperbaric oxygen, posttreatment failure; expensive, requires special facilities

SURGERY/OTHER PROCEDURES
- Endoscopy:
  - Thermal/Laser coagulation therapy useful for radiation-induced ileitis, hemorrhagic duodenitis, and colonic telangiectasia (7)
  - Endoscopic balloon dilatation of accessible strictures in selected patients
- Surgery:
  - May be more difficult and complicated because of poor nutrition, comorbidity, prior surgery, intra-abdominal adhesions from prior radiotherapy
  - Indications:
    - Obstruction secondary to strictures or adhesions
    - Fistula (colovesical in men, rectovaginal in women)
    - Perforation
  - Wide excision preferable to bypass operations due to higher risk of anastomotic leak, bacterial overgrowth, perforation, fistula formation
  - Strictureplasty for patients with limited intestinal reserve and strictures within long segments of diseased intestine
  - Risk factors for complications: Poor nutritional status, >1 abdominal/pelvic surgery prior to RT, <12 months between RT and surgery; advanced malignancy
  - Postoperative complications (30%); 40–60% will require >1 laparotomy
  - Small bowel transplantation may be indicated in rare, selected, especially challenging cases of chronic RE (8).

ONGOING CARE

FOLLOW-UP RECOMMENDATIONS
Depression is common in chronic, severe illness. Prevalence in the setting of RE is not well documented, but this may contribute to malnutrition, so behavioral support is important (1,2).

DIET
- Malnutrition is common in chronic RE. Many are undernourished before therapy and most suffer significant weight loss during treatment (9).
- Dietary supplementation of selenium and zinc may reduce anorectal sequelae following RT.
- Exclusion diets useful only in selected cases (lactose-free), but high-fiber and fatty foods are associated with worsening symptoms
- Long-term TPN used for patients who cannot manage oral supplementation, but associated with problems maintaining vascular access, infection, ongoing mortality, hepatic dysfunction

REFERENCES

1. Theis VS, Sripadam R, Ramani V, et al. Chronic radiation enteritis. *Clin Oncol (R Coll Radiol).* 2010;22:70–83.
2. Shadad AK, Sullivan FJ, Martin JD, et al. Gastrointestinal radiation injury: symptoms, risk factors, and mechanisms. *World J Gastroenterol.* 2013;19:185–198.
3. Perrakis N, Athanassiou E, Vamakopoulos D, et al. Practical approaches to effective management of radiation injury: Benefit of resectional surgery. *World J Gastroenterol.* 2011;12:4013–4016.
4. Riaz A, Lewandowski RJ, Kulik LM, et al. Complications following radioembolization with yttrium-90 microspheres: A comprehensive literature review. *J Vasc Interv Radiol.* 2009;20: 1121–1130.
5. Samuelian JM, Callister MD, Ashman JB, et al. Reduced acute bowel toxicity in patients treated with intensity-modulated radiotherapy for rectal cancer. *Int J Radiat Oncol Biol Phys.* 2012;84: 1981–1987.
6. Ende N, Kovalenko OA, Azzam EI. The necessity of early antibiotics in treatment of mass casualties from ionizing radiation. *Int J Radiat Biol.* 2012; 88:381.
7. Pasha SF, Leighton JA. Endoscopic techniques for small bowel imaging. *Radiol Clin North Am.* 2013;51:177–187.
8. Zhu W, Sripadam R, Ramani V, Lal S. A retrospective study of surgical treatment for chronic radiation enteritis. *J Surg Oncol.* 2012;105: 632–636.
9. Webb GJ, Brooke R, Niroshan de Silva A. Chronic radiation enteritis and malnutrition. *J Digest Dis.* 2013;14:350–357.

CODES

ICD10
K52.0 Gastroenteritis and colitis due to radiation

CLINICAL PEARLS

- Radiation injury is common, nonspecific, and can occur at any time, even decades after irradiation.
- Index of suspicion is vital, because medications, advanced/ongoing malignancy, or more common GI disorders may mimic radiation injury.
- Acute RE is transient and usually resolves spontaneously.
- Chronic RE is very common, has late onset, and is progressive.
- RE has multifactorial causes; always consider recurrent malignancy.

RAPE CRISIS SYNDROME

Joceyln F. Blackwell, MD, MAJ, MC

 BASICS

DESCRIPTION
- Definitions (legal definitions may vary from state to state):
  - Sexual contact: Intentional touching of a person's intimate parts (including thighs) or the clothing covering such areas, if it is construed as being for the purpose of sexual gratification
  - Sexual conduct: Vaginal intercourse between a male and female, or anal intercourse, fellatio, or cunnilingus between persons, regardless of sex
  - Rape: Any sexual penetration, however slight, using force or coercion against the person's will
  - Sexual imposition: Similar to rape, but without penetration or the use of force (i.e., nonconsensual sexual contact)
  - Gross sexual imposition: Nonconsensual sexual contact with the use of force
  - Corruption of a minor: Sexual conduct by an individual age ≥18 years with an individual <16 years of age
- Most states have expanded rape statutes to include marital rape, date rape, and shield laws.
- System(s) affected: Nervous; Reproductive
- Synonym(s): Sexual assault; Rape trauma

EPIDEMIOLOGY
- Anyone can be sexually assaulted, but some populations are especially vulnerable (1):
  - Adolescents and young women
  - People with disabilities
  - Poor and homeless people
  - Sex workers
  - Those living in institutions/areas of conflict
- Predominant age:
  - The incidence of sexual assault peaks in those 16–19 years of age, with the mean occurring at 20 years of age:
    ○ Adolescent sexual assault has a greater frequency of anogenital injuries.
- Predominant sex: Female > Male:
  - For males:
    ○ 69% of male victims were 1st raped before age 18.
    ○ 41% of male victims were raped before age 12.

Incidence
- 208,830 rapes and sexual assaults reported in 2008 in the US.
- Estimated that only 1:3–1:5 of adult cases are reported:
  - In 2005, only 38% of rape/sexual assaults were reported to the police.
- 20% of American women report being raped during their lifetime (2):
  - Between 20% and 25% of females will experience rape/attempted rape during their college years.
- 1/7 males will be sexually assaulted during a lifetime.
- ~2/1,000 children in the US were confirmed by child protective agencies as having experienced sexual assault in 2003.
- Most rape victims either know or have some acquaintance with their attacker.

RISK FACTORS
- In general, adults are assaulted in their own homes, whereas adolescents are assaulted in their assailant's residence.
- Most perpetrators of sexual violence are males, with all acts against females >90%.
- Most acts against males are >65% male perpetrators.

GENERAL PREVENTION
- Scope of rape prevention is very complex and broad.
- The public health approach should include both prevention and avoidance of vulnerability factors and implementation of protective factors.
- Females may benefit from assertiveness training and self-defense training.
- Universal screening by health care providers for interpersonal violence does assist in identifying victims (2).

 DIAGNOSIS

- In adults:
  - History of sexual penetration
  - Sexual contact/conduct without consent and/or with the use of force
- In children:
  - Actual observation/suspicion of sexual penetration, sexual contact, or sexual conduct
  - Signs include evidence of the use of force and/or evidence of sexual contact (e.g., presence of semen and/or blood).

HISTORY
- Avoid questioning that implies the patient is at fault.
- Record answers in patient's own words insofar as possible. Include date, approximate time, and general location as best as possible. Document physical abuse other than sexual. Describe all types of sexual contact, whether actual/attempted. Take history of alcohol and/or drug use before or after alleged incident.
- Document time of last activity that could possibly alter specimens (e.g., bath, shower, douche).
- Thorough gynecologic history is mandatory, including last menstrual period, last consenting sexual contact, contraceptive practice, and prior gynecologic surgery.

PHYSICAL EXAM
- Use of drawings and/or photographs is encouraged.
- Document all signs of trauma/unusual marks.
- Document mental status/emotional state.
- Use UV light (Wood's lamp) to detect seminal stains on clothing/skin.

ALERT
- A forensic kit or "rape kit" contains swabs that are collected from the vagina and rectum, and instructions are given with the kit as to proper collection.
- Many states and emergency departments across the country are using a Sexual Assault Nurse Examiner (SANE) when available. This has led to more consistent and more accurate collection of evidence in alleged rape cases.
- Complete genital–rectal exam, including evidence of trauma, secretions, or discharge:
  - Use of a nonlubricated, water-moistened speculum is mandatory because commonly used lubricants may destroy evidence.
  - Testing and/or specimen collection, as indicated, and in compliance with state requirements

DIFFERENTIAL DIAGNOSIS
Consenting sex among adults

DIAGNOSTIC TESTS & INTERPRETATION
- In females, obtain a serum or urine pregnancy test.
- Record results of wet mount, screening for vaginitis, but also note the presence/absence of sperm and, if present, whether it is motile/immotile.
- Drug/Alcohol testing as indicated by history and/or physical findings

 TREATMENT

GENERAL MEASURES
- Providing health care to victims of sexual assault/abuse requires special sensitivity and privacy.
- All such cases *must* be reported immediately to the appropriate law enforcement agency.
- With the victim's permission, enlist the help of personnel from local support agencies (e.g., rape crisis center). When available, use of in-house social services is extremely helpful to victim and family.
- SANE programs have been shown to be beneficial, especially in large cities and metropolitan areas with multiple emergency departments of varying capability and staff training/experience.
- Give sedation and tetanus prophylaxis when indicated.
- Discuss possible pregnancy and pregnancy termination with the victim. If hospital policy precludes such a discussion, then information about this option should be offered to the victim via follow-up mechanisms.
- Discuss suspected HIV and hepatitis B exposure and testing with the victim in accordance with hospital, regional, and state policies/protocols. The initial HIV test should be completed within 7 days of the suspected exposure.

MEDICATION
First Line
- Controversy exists regarding empiric antibiotic prophylaxis for victims of sexual assault. However, the Centers for Disease Control (CDC) recommends empiric antibiotic prophylaxis of potential sexually transmitted infections (specifically, gonorrhea, chlamydia, trichomoniasis, and potentially syphilis) as many patients will not return for a follow-up visit and many patients prefer immediate treatment.

- Cultures are *not* required before initiating treatment, but can be considered as part of routine evidence collection.
- Gonorrhea: Ceftriaxone 250 mg IM once or cefixime 400 mg PO once
- Chlamydia: Azithromycin 1 g PO single dose, or doxycycline 100 mg PO b.i.d. × 7 days, *or* erythromycin base 500 mg PO q.i.d. × 7 days, *or* erythromycin ethylsuccinate 800 mg PO q.i.d. × 7 days
- Syphilis: Benzathine penicillin G 2–4 million units IM once, or doxycycline 100 mg PO b.i.d. × 14 days. Some suggest ceftriaxone 1 g/d, either IM/IV, × 8–10 days, or azithromycin 2 g PO single dose, but treatment failures have been reported in several geographic areas.
- Trichomoniasis and bacterial vaginosis, if present (if cultures/wet mount were collected): Metronidazole 2 g PO once, *or* metronidazole 500 mg PO b.i.d. × 7 days (consider single dose to maximize compliance), *or* metronidazole gel 0.75% 1 full applicator (5 g) intravaginally every day × 5 days; *or* clindamycin cream 2% 1 full applicator (5 g) intravaginally at bedtime × 7 days (considered less efficacious than PO metronidazole)
- If pregnancy prophylaxis is indicated, use levonorgestrel 1.5 mg once (Plan B, progestin-only), efficacious for up to 5 days after the incident:
  – Levonorgestrel alone has proved more effective than the Yuzpe regimen, a method of emergency contraception (3)[A].
  – *Alternatively*, ethynil estradiol/levonorgestrel (Yuzpe) 100 mcg/0.5 mg once and repeated in 12 hours can be used.
  – Alternatively, uliprisital acetate (Ella) 30 mcg once can be used.
  – Alternatively, a copper intrauterine device can be inserted up to 5 days after the earliest predicted date of ovulation in that cycle.
- HIV: Currently, there is a low likelihood of HIV transmittance, but the CDC still recommends postexposure prophylaxis for victims of sexual assault. Regimen is lamivudine–zidovudine (Combivir) 1 tablet PO b.i.d. × 28 days *or* zidovudine 300 mg + lamivudine 150 mg PO b.i.d. × 28 days:
  – Most effective if started within 4 hours, and could reduce transmission by as much as 80%; unlikely to be beneficial if started after 72 hours
- Hepatitis B: If prevalent in area or assailant known to be high risk: Hepatitis B immunoglobulin 0.06 mL/kg IM, single dose, and initiate 3-dose hepatitis B virus immunization series. No treatment if the victim has had a complete hepatitis B vaccine series, with documented levels of immunity.

Second Line
Gonorrhea: Cefotaxime 500 mg IM once + probenecid 1 g PO once. Note: Be aware that drug resistance is on the rise in several major cities. Quinolones are no longer recommended for treatment of gonorrhea.

Pregnancy Considerations
Conduct baseline pregnancy test; discuss pregnancy prevention and termination with patient.

Pediatric Considerations
Assure the child that she or he is a good person and was not the cause of the incident.

IN-PATIENT CONSIDERATIONS
Admission Criteria/Initial Stabilization
- Contact appropriate social services agency.

- Most adult victims can be treated as outpatients, unless associated trauma (physical/mental) requires admission.
- Most pediatric sexual assault/abuse victims will require admission/outside placement until appropriate social agency can evaluate home environment.

 ONGOING CARE

FOLLOW-UP RECOMMENDATIONS
Patient Monitoring
- Patient should be seen in 7–10 days for follow-up care, including pregnancy testing and counseling.
- Close exam for vaginitis and treatment if necessary
- Follow-up test for gonorrhea should occur in 1–2 weeks.
- Follow-up testing for syphilis, HIV, and hepatitis B should occur at 6 weeks, 3 months, and 6 months.
- Provide telephone numbers of counseling agency(ies) that can provide counseling/legal services to the patient.
- Strongly consider SANE, if available.

PATIENT EDUCATION
- Local rape crisis support organizations.
- National Sexual Violence Resource Center, 123 Enola Drive, Enola, PA 17025; (877) 739-3895; www.nsvrc.org
- National Domestic Violence Hotline at (800) 799-SAFE(7233) or TTY (800) 787-3224 or www.ndvh.org

PROGNOSIS
- Acute phase (usually 1–3 weeks following rape): Shaking, pain, wound healing, mood swings, appetite loss, crying. Also feelings of grief, shame, anger, fear, revenge, or guilt.
- Late/Chronic phase (also called "reorganization"): Female victim may develop fear of intercourse, fear of men, nightmares, sleep disorders, daytime flashbacks, fear of being alone, loss of self-esteem, anxiety, depression, posttraumatic stress syndrome, and somatic complaints (e.g., nonspecific abdominal pain).
- Recovery may be prolonged. Patients who are able to talk about their feelings seem to have a faster recovery. It is unclear if pharmaco- or psychotherapy results in better outcomes.

COMPLICATIONS
Sequelae include (1):
- Trauma (physical and mental)
- STIs, including HIV
- Unwanted pregnancy (with the possibility of abortion):
  – The rape-related pregnancy rate in the US is 5%/rape among victims of reproductive age, resulting in >32,000 unwanted pregnancies each year (2).
  – Adolescents are at highest risk of pregnancy.
- Depression
- Posttraumatic stress disorder
- Substance abuse

REFERENCES

1. Welch J, Mason F. Rape and sexual assault. *BMJ*. 2007;334:1154–1158.
2. Toohey JS. Domestic violence and rape. *Med Clin North Am*. 2008;92:1239–1252, xii.
3. Cheng L, Gülmezoglu AM, Piaggio G, et al. Interventions for emergency contraception. *Cochrane Database Syst Rev*. 2008;(2):CD001324.

ADDITIONAL READING
- A National Protocol for Sexual Assault Medical Forensic Examinations (Adults/Adolescents). U.S. Department of Justice, Office on Violence Against Women; September 2004.
- Centers for Disease Control and Prevention. *Sexual violence: Facts at a glance*. Atlanta, GA: CDC: 2008.
- Devorett K, Sachs CJ. Sexual assault. *Emerg Med Clin North Am*. 2011;9(3):605–620.
- Linden, JA. Clinical practice. Care of the adult patient after sexual assault. *N Engl J Med*. 2011;365: 384.
- Peterson, ZD et al. Prevalence and consequences of adult male sexual assault: review of empirical findings and state of the literature. *Clin Psychol Rev*. 2011;31:1.

 SEE ALSO

Chlamydial Sexually Transmitted Diseases; Gonococcal Infections; Hepatitis B; Hepatitis C; HIV Infection and AIDS; Posttraumatic Stress Disorder (PTSD); Syphilis

 CODES

ICD10
- T74.21XA Adult sexual abuse; confirmed, initial encounter
- T74.22XA Child sexual abuse, confirmed, initial encounter
- Z04.41 Encounter for exam and obs following alleged adult rape

CLINICAL PEARLS
- *Rape* is a legal term, and the examining physician is encouraged to use terminology such as *alleged rape* or *alleged sexual conduct*.
- Marital rape is a federal offense in all 50 states and the District of Columbia; in some states, also applies to unmarried cohabiting couples.
- Because "consent defense" is common, documentation of evidence supporting the use of force or the administration of drugs/alcohol is imperative.
- Use of a protocol is encouraged to assure every victim a uniform, comprehensive evaluation, regardless of the expertise of the examiner. The protocol must ensure that all evidence is properly collected and labeled, chain of custody is maintained, and the evidence is sent to the most appropriate forensic laboratory.
- All medical records must be well documented and legible.
- All medical personnel must be willing and able to testify on behalf of the patient.

The views expressed in this chapter are those of the author and do not reflect the official policy or position of the Department of the Army, Department of Defense, or the US Government. Opinions, interpretations, conclusions, and recommendations herein are those of the author and are not necessarily endorsed by the US Army.

RAYNAUD PHENOMENON
Herbert L. Muncie, Jr., MD

 BASICS

DESCRIPTION
- Idiopathic intermittent episodes of vasoconstriction of digital arteries, precapillary arterioles, and cutaneous arteriovenous shunts in response to cold temperatures or emotional stress:
  - A triphasic color change of the fingers (occasionally the toes, rarely nipples) is the physical manifestation of the episodes:
    ○ The initial color is white from extreme pallor, then blue from cyanosis, and finally with warming and vasodilatation intense redness develops.
    ○ Thumbs are rarely involved.
  - Swelling, throbbing, and paresthesias are the final symptoms.
  - Primary:
    ○ 80% of patients have primary disease.
    ○ Episodes are bilateral and nonprogressive.
    ○ Diagnosis confirmed only if after 2 years of symptoms, no underlying connective tissue disease develops.
  - Secondary:
    ○ Progressive and asymmetric
    ○ Spasm is more frequent and more severe with time. No gangrene; rarely, ulceration; 13% may progress to atrophy of digital fat pads and ischemic ulcers of fingertips.
    ○ Usually associated with an underlying connective tissue disease
- System(s) affected: Hematologic; Lymphatic; Immunologic; Musculoskeletal; Dermatologic; Exocrine

Pregnancy Considerations
- Raynaud phenomenon can appear as breast pain in lactating women (1).
- Bacterial culture of breast milk can distinguish mastitis from Raynaud phenomenon.

Geriatric Considerations
Initial appearance of Raynaud phenomenon after age 40 frequently indicates an underlying connective tissue disease.

Pediatric Considerations
Associated with systemic lupus erythematosus (SLE) and scleroderma

EPIDEMIOLOGY
Incidence
- Primary:
  - Predominant age: 14 years; ~1/4 begin >40
  - Predominant sex: Female > Male (4:1)
- Secondary:
  - Predominant age: >40
  - Predominant sex: No gender predilection

Prevalence
- Primary: ~3–12.5% of men; 6–20% of women (based on reporting of characteristic skin color changes, intolerance to cold)
- Secondary: only ~1% of population

ETIOLOGY AND PATHOPHYSIOLOGY
Unknown. Functional blood vessel wall abnormalities may cause primary and secondary structural abnormalities. Serotonin receptors (5-HT$_2$ type) may be involved in secondary Raynaud phenomenon. Dysregulation of control mechanisms of vascular motility leads to imbalance between vasodilation and vasoconstriction. Platelet and blood viscosity abnormalities are implicated in secondary.

Genetics
Little information is available, but some studies suggest a dominant inheritance pattern. ~1/4 of primary patients have a 1st-degree relative with Raynaud phenomenon.

RISK FACTORS
- Smoking may reduce digital blood flow but is not associated with increased risk of Raynaud phenomenon.
- Existing autoimmune or connective tissue disorder
- End-stage renal disease with hemodialysis may increase the risk due to a steal phenomenon complicating the arterial-venous shunt.
- An elevated homocysteine level has been associated with primary and secondary disease.

GENERAL PREVENTION
- Avoid exposure to cold.
- Stop smoking.
- Avoid trauma and vibration to hands and fingertips; however, no relationship has been established between etiology of Raynaud phenomenon and occupational vibratory tool use.

COMMONLY ASSOCIATED CONDITIONS
Secondary Raynaud:
- Scleroderma
- SLE
- Polymyositis
- Sjögren syndrome
- Occlusive vascular disease
- Cryoglobulinemia

DIAGNOSIS

HISTORY
- Primary:
  - Symmetric attacks
  - Absence of tissue necrosis, ulceration, or gangrene
  - Absence of secondary cause after history and physical exam
  - If, after ≥2 years of symptoms, no abnormal clinical or laboratory signs have developed, secondary disease is highly unlikely.
- Secondary:
  - Onset typically > age 40
  - Asymmetric episodes more intense and painful
  - Ask about arthritis, myalgias, fever, dry eyes and/or mouth, rash, or cardiopulmonary symptoms.
  - Ask about past or current drug use.
  - Ask about exposure to toxic agents.
  - Ask about repetitive trauma.

PHYSICAL EXAM
Pallor (whiteness) of fingertips with cold exposure, followed by cyanosis, then redness and pain with warming:
- Ischemic attacks evidenced by demarcated or cyanotic skin limited to digits; usually starts on 1 digit and spreads symmetrically to remaining fingers of both hands; however, the thumb is often spared.
- Beau lines: Transverse linear depressions in nail plate of most or all fingernails that can occur after exposure to cold temperature or any disease serious enough to disrupt normal nail growth

- Livedo reticularis: Mottling of the skin of the arms and legs may occur but is completely benign and reversible with warming.
- Primary:
  - Normal physical exam
  - Nail bed capillaries: Place 1 drop of grade B immersion oil on skin at base of fingernail and view capillaries with handheld ophthalmoscope at 10–40 diopters. Normal appearance.
- Secondary:
  - Clinical features suggestive of connective tissue disease (e.g., arthritis, abnormal lung function)
  - Ischemic skin lesions: Ulceration of finger pads, progressing to autoamputation in severe, prolonged cases
  - Nail bed capillaries distorted and anatomically abnormal (2)[C]
  - Videocapillaroscopy is gold standard (200× magnification).

DIFFERENTIAL DIAGNOSIS
- Thromboangiitis obliterans (Buerger disease): Primarily affects men; involves legs and feet; <5% have hand involvement; smoking-related
- Rheumatoid arthritis (RA)
- Progressive systemic sclerosis (scleroderma): Raynaud phenomenon may precede other symptoms by years.
- SLE
- Carpal tunnel syndrome
- Thoracic outlet syndrome
- Hypothyroidism
- CREST syndrome (calcinosis cutis, Raynaud phenomenon, esophageal dysmotility, sclerodactyly, and telangiectasias)
- Cryoglobulinemias
- Waldenström macroglobulinemia
- Acrocyanosis
- Polycythemia
- Occupational (e.g., especially from vibrating tools, masonry work, exposure to polyvinyl chloride)
- Drugs (e.g., clonidine, ergotamine, methysergide, amphetamines, bromocriptine, bleomycin, vinblastine, cisplatin, cyclosporine)

DIAGNOSTIC TESTS & INTERPRETATION
Unnecessary to perform provocative test (e.g., immersion of patient's hand in ice water)
- Primary:
  - Antinuclear antibody: Negative
  - ESR: Normal
- Secondary:
  - Tests for underlying secondary causes (e.g., CBC, ESR)
  - Positive autoantibody has low positive predictive value for an associated connective tissue disease (30%).
  - Antibodies to specific autoantigens more suggestive of secondary disease (e.g., scleroderma with anticentromere or antitopoisomerase antibodies)
  - Rarely necessary; patients may demonstrate osteolysis of distal metaphysial portions of phalanges with tapering and calcification of soft tissue.

Follow-Up Tests & Special Considerations

Periodic assessments could be helpful during the initial years after the diagnosis is made to determine if a connective tissue disease has become manifest.

Diagnostic Procedures/Other

Diagnosis is determined by history and physical exam.

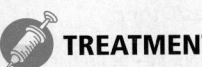

TREATMENT

The effects of treatment can be assessed using a Raynaud Condition Score (3).

GENERAL MEASURES

- Dress warmly, wear gloves, and avoid cold.
- During the attacks, rotating the arms in a windmill pattern or placing the hands under warm water or in a warm body fold may be helpful.
- Stop smoking.
- Avoid β-blockers, amphetamines, ergot alkaloids, and sumatriptan.
- Temperature-related biofeedback may help patients to increase hand temperature, but at the 1-year follow-up no better than control.
- Use finger guards over ulcerated fingertips.

MEDICATION

Calcium-channel blockers (CCBs) have been the primary treatment for many years. Nifedipine has been best studied and is the most frequently used drug in this group.

First Line

- Nifedipine: 30–180 mg/d (sustained-release form); may be needed only during winter; up to 75% experience improvement (4)[A].
- Symptomatic responses do not correlate with objective evidence of improvement.
- Contraindications: Allergy to drug, pregnancy, CHF
- Precautions: May cause headache, dizziness, lightheadedness, edema, or hypotension
- Significant possible interactions:
  – Increases serum level of digoxin; monitor digoxin levels closely after nifedipine is added.
  – May increase PT in patients taking warfarin

Second Line

- Amlodipine (5–20 mg/d) and nicardipine appear to be effective and may have fewer adverse effects.
- No data exist to support use of another CCB if initial one is ineffective.
- Small studies support benefit from losartan, fluoxetine.
- Phosphodiesterase type-5 inhibitors (sildenafil, vardenafil) may reduce symptoms without increasing blood flow.
- Parenteral iloprost, a prostacyclin, even in low doses (0.5 ng/kg/min over 6 hours), has improved ulcerations with severe Raynaud phenomenon when CCBs failed. Oral prostacyclin has not proved useful.
- Nitroglycerin patches may be helpful, but use is limited by the occurrence of severe headache. Nitroglycerin gel has shown promise as a topical therapy (5)[B].
- Prazosin (1–2 mg t.i.d.) is the only well-studied α_1-adrenergic receptor blocker with modest effect, but adverse effects may outweigh any benefit.
- ACE inhibitors are no longer recommended.

ISSUES FOR REFERRAL

If an underlying disease is suspected, consider rheumatology consultation for evaluation and treatment.

ADDITIONAL THERAPIES

- Botulinum toxin has shown some effect in reducing vasospastic episodes (6)[B].
- Aspirin
- Digital or wrist block with lidocaine or bupivacaine (without epinephrine)
- Short-term anticoagulation with heparin if persistent critical ischemia, evidence of large-artery occlusive disease, or both

SURGERY/OTHER PROCEDURES

Effect of cervical sympathectomy is transient; symptoms return in 1–2 years.

COMPLEMENTARY AND ALTERNATIVE MEDICINE

- Although well-designed studies have not been done yet for complementary medicine, some treatments have shown an effect (6).
- *Ginkgo biloba* may reduce the frequency of attacks but did not in 1 randomized trial (7)[B].
- Fish oil supplements may increase digital systolic pressure and time to onset of symptoms after exposure to cold but was not proven in controlled trials.
- Oral arginine is no better than placebo.
- Biofeedback is not helpful (8)[A].

ONGOING CARE

FOLLOW-UP RECOMMENDATIONS

Avoid exposure to cold situations; avoid use of vibrating tools.

Patient Monitoring

Management of fingertip ulcers, including rapid treatment of infection

DIET

No special diet

PATIENT EDUCATION

- Emphasize cessation of smoking.
- Discuss avoiding aggravating factors (e.g., trauma, vibration, cold).
- Dress warmly; wear gloves.
- Warm hands when experiencing vasospasm.

PROGNOSIS

- Attacks may last from several minutes to a few hours.
- 2/3 of attacks are likely to have spontaneous resolution.
- ~13% of Raynaud phenomenon patients develop a secondary disorder, many of which are connective tissue diseases.

COMPLICATIONS

- Primary: Very rare
- Secondary: Gangrene, autoamputation of fingertips

REFERENCES

1. Barrett ME, Heller MM, Stone HF, et al. Raynaud phenomenon of the nipple in breastfeeding mothers: An underdiagnosed cause of nipple pain. *JAMA Dermatol.* 2013 Mar;149(3):300–306.
2. Herrick AL, Cutolo M. Clinical implications from capillaroscopic analysis in patients with Raynaud's phenomenon and systemic sclerosis. *Arthritis Rheum.* 2010;62:2595–2604.
3. Khanna PP, Maranian P, Gregory J, et al. The minimally important difference and patient acceptable symptom state for the Raynaud's condition score in patients with Raynaud's phenomenon in a large randomised controlled clinical trial. *Ann Rheum Dis.* 2010;69:588–591.
4. Goundry B, Bell L, Langree M, et al. Diagnosis and management of Raynaud's phenomenon. *BMJ.* 2012;344:e289.
5. Chung L, Shapiro L, Fiorentino D, et al. MQX-503, a novel formulation of nitroglycerin, improves the severity of Raynaud's phenomenon: A randomized, controlled trial. *Arthritis Rheum.* 2009;60:870–877.
6. Iorio ML, Masden DL, Higgins JP. Botulinum toxin a treatment of Raynaud's phenomenon: A review. *Semin Arthritis Rheum.* 2012;41:599–603.
7. Bredie SJH, Jong MC. No significant effect of ginkgo biloba special extract EGb 761 in the treatment of primary Raynaud phenomenon: A randomized controlled trial. *J Cardiovasc Pharmacol.* 2012;59:215–221.
8. Malenfant D, Catton M, Pope JE, et al. The efficacy of complementary and alternative medicine in the treatment of Raynaud's phenomenon: A literature review and meta-analysis. *Rheumatology (Oxford).* 2009;48:791–795.

ADDITIONAL READING

- Herrick AL. Contemporary management of Raynaud's phenomenon and digital ischaemic complications. *Curr Opin Rheumatol.* 2011;23(6):555–561.
- Huisstede BM, Hoogvliet P, Paulis WD, et al. Effectiveness of interventions for secondary Raynaud's phenomenon: A systematic review. *Arch Phys Med Rehabil.* 2011;92(7):1166–1180.

 SEE ALSO

Algorithm: Raynaud Phenomenon

 CODES

ICD10

- I73.0 Raynaud's syndrome
- I73.00 Raynaud's syndrome without gangrene
- I73.01 Raynaud's syndrome with gangrene

CLINICAL PEARLS

- Initial presentation of Raynaud phenomenon after age 40 suggests underlying disease.
- Remember Raynaud phenomenon in differential diagnosis of a lactating woman with breast pain (vs. mastitis).
- Primary Raynaud phenomenon is symmetric, whereas secondary is asymmetric.
- Digital ulcers are not normal and always reflect secondary Raynaud phenomenon.

REFRACTIVE ERRORS
Robert M. Kershner, MD, MS, FACS

BASICS

DESCRIPTION
- Refraction is the bending of a wave of light as it passes through the optical system of the eye. The degree of bending is dependent on the index of refraction among the air, cornea, and lens and is described quantitatively by Snell's law. A refractive error refers to the inability of the eye to produce a focused image on the fovea or central part of the retina
- Emmetropia: When light rays are in perfect focus, the image being viewed is seen clearly.
- Ametropia: Any refractive error of the eye that prevents normal focusing of the image
- Hyperopia: When the cornea of the eye is too flat or the eye is too short, light rays fall in focus behind the retina, and the individual is "farsighted."
- Myopia: When the cornea is too steep or the length of the eyeball is too long, the focal point for light rays lies short of the retina, and the individual is "nearsighted."
- Presbyopia: The natural tendency of the crystalline lens to harden/become sclerotic with age, limiting the focusing of the eye on near objects (accommodation). By the age of 40, most people do not have enough room within the eye to allow normal excursion of the lens and accommodation; viewing of near objects is blurred, and reading glasses are required.
- Astigmatism: When the cornea is steeper in 1 meridian more than the other or the globe is not round (i.e., is oval or almond-shaped), visual blurriness occurs.
- Anisometropia: An unequal refractive error between the 2 eyes
- System(s) affected: Nervous

Geriatric Considerations
Presbyopia occurs in later life.

Pediatric Considerations
Refractive errors can be detected early in life.

EPIDEMIOLOGY
- Predominant age: Refractive errors may be present at birth and can increase in magnitude with age until the eye is fully developed. Often they are not detected until puberty.
- Predominant gender: Male = Female
- Individuals >40 are more likely to experience presbyopia/the normal loss of accommodation that occurs with age, necessitating the use of reading glasses for close work.

Prevalence
Of the general US population, 70% have some form of ametropia.

ETIOLOGY AND PATHOPHYSIOLOGY
- Developmental (most common)
- Ocular trauma
- Iatrogenic (e.g., postcataract removal)

Genetics
Inherited

GENERAL PREVENTION
No exercises; lenses can prevent/worsen refractive error.

COMMONLY ASSOCIATED CONDITIONS
- Patients with diabetes mellitus have fluctuating myopia as a result of poorly controlled blood glucose and concomitant swelling of the crystalline lens.
- Those who have a pathologic steepening of the cornea due to structural weakness (keratoconus) may have increasing myopia and astigmatism throughout life.

DIAGNOSIS

HISTORY
- Difficulty seeing objects at a distance
- Difficulty focusing on near objects
- Difficulty reading
- Squinting
- Headaches (from squinting)
- In children:
  - Rubbing of the eyes
  - Sitting close to TV/computer screen
  - Problems in sports, particularly declining performance
  - Declining grades
  - Preference for front-row seating
  - Covering of an eye while reading

PHYSICAL EXAM
Snellen Eye Chart (developed by Dr. Hermann Snellen in 1862):
- Test each eye separately.
- The smallest row of letters that the patient can read determines visual acuity in the uncovered eye.
- The standard convention is visual acuity measured at 20 feet with a Snellen Chart. A person with "normal" acuity will see letters clearly at 20 feet as recorded 20/20 (6/6 in meters). A person with 20/200 vision would be considered legally blind and able only to see a letter at 20 feet that a person with normal vision could see clearly at 200 feet.

DIAGNOSTIC TESTS & INTERPRETATION
- Pinhole vision test: To distinguish a refractive error from an organic cause of visual blurring, have the patient look through a pinhole in a card without a corrective lens.
- Patients with a pure refractive error have improved vision because the pinhole blocks nonparallel and unfocused rays of light.
- There are no lab tests for measuring visual acuity.
- A number of digital imaging systems exist for measuring refractive error:
  - The use of US can determine the length of the eye (A-Scan Biometry).
  - Autorefractors can measure myopia, hyperopia, and astigmatism utilizing a projected light into the eye and measuring its return.
  - Corneal topography quantitatively and qualitatively measures the amount of curvature on the surface of the cornea that affects the bending and focusing of light on the retina.
  - Wavefront corneal analysis measures the reflected rays of light as they pass into and out of the entire optical system (cornea, lens, and retina).
- Most corneal and refractive imaging techniques are reserved for individuals who are contemplating refractive surgical correction (intraocular lenses or excimer laser surgery "LASIK").

Follow-Up Tests & Special Considerations
Corneal and refractive imaging are used to monitor changing refractive errors postsurgically and to follow pathologic changes, such as in keratoconus.

Diagnostic Procedures/Other
- Methods:
  - Objective streak retinoscopy may be used to measure the degree of refractive error in spherocylinder correction for the proper spectacle/contact lens.
  - Antimuscarinic agents, such as cyclopentolate (Cyclogyl) or tropicamide (Mydriacyl), applied topically paralyze the ciliary body, preventing accommodation. Cycloplegic refraction can then be performed.
  - α-Adrenergic agents, such as phenylephrine (Neo-Synephrine), can be used concomitantly to stimulate and dilate the pupillary dilator muscle making measurements easier. They have no effect on cycloplegia.
- Age-related testing:
  - Newborns should be examined for general eye health; ophthalmologic evaluation is indicated for any problems discovered.
  - Vision screening should occur at each well-child visit.
  - Visual acuity testing and motility testing should be performed at ~3.5 years of age or at any time that a malposition of the eyes or difficulty following objects is observed.
  - Visual acuity must be performed by age 5 years or prior to the child entering school to screen for and pick up refractive errors early before they lead to amblyopia.
  - Visual acuity should be retested prior to obtaining a driver's license, at age 40 years, and every 2–4 years until age 65, after which age evaluations are recommended every 1–2 years.

DIFFERENTIAL DIAGNOSIS
- Corneal disease
- Cataract
- Retinal abnormalities
- Diseases of the optic nerve
- Neuromuscular disorders
- Neurologic impairment

TREATMENT

GENERAL MEASURES
- Spectacle lenses (glasses)
- Soft/Hard contact lenses

MEDICATION
Precaution: Antimuscarinic agents may induce acute glaucoma via acute-angle closure in susceptible individuals. The elderly and those with high hyperopia or a history of angle closure should not be tested with these agents.

First Line
No medical treatment for refractive error exists.

Second Line
Cycloplegia is sometimes utilized to "fog/blur" the better seeing eye in cases of amblyopia.

ISSUES FOR REFERRAL

Any individual who fails a basic screening visual acuity test should be promptly referred to an eye care professional for evaluation. Children do not outgrow refractive errors. Left untreated, refractive errors can lead to permanent visual loss.

ADDITIONAL THERAPIES

Eye exercises and visual training may improve hand-to-eye coordination and visual awareness, but do not treat refractive error.

SURGERY/OTHER PROCEDURES

- Laser-assisted in-situ keratomileusis (LASIK), approved by the FDA in 1997. A superficial corneal flap is created with a mechanical keratome/femtosecond laser, under which the excimer laser removes a small amount of tissue corresponding to the correction of refractive error, thus reshaping the cornea. LASIK can be used for all refractive errors, but not in all patients. Healing is rapid because re-epithelialization is not required. Surgery is reserved for those with a stable refractive error and a cornea that is thick enough to allow safe removal of tissue. The procedure is permanent.
- Implantable contact lens (ICL): A thin plastic lens is permanently implanted either in the anterior chamber and anchored to the iris (FDA approved in 2005, VERISYES) or in the posterior chamber (Visian Lens, FDA approved 2006) between the iris and the human crystalline lens. All refractive errors can be corrected. Risks include damage to the natural lens during surgery, cataract formation, and intraocular inflammation/infection.
- Excimer laser photorefractive keratectomy: The laser photoablates corneal tissue from the central visual axis, flattening it. Following the procedure, the cornea must re-epithelialize. Healing takes several months, during which there is a mild haze and blurring of vision. FDA approved October 1995.
- Other modifications:
  - LASIK and EPI LASIK involve removing just the superficial epithelium before laser application.
  - IntraLASIK is a femtosecond laser that is used to create the flap as an alternative to a mechanical keratome.
  - Custom ablation: Uses the information from a wavefront map of the cornea and eye to tailor the ablation to remove higher orders of refractive errors.
- Older methods now superseded by LASIK:
  - Radial keratotomy: With topical anesthesia, a surgical keratome is used to incise multiple (4–8) radial incisions into the peripheral cornea to a depth of $\geq$85%. The incisions cause gaping and thus flatten the central, optical zone of the cornea. Radial keratotomy is safe and effective, corrects nearsightedness and astigmatism, but has been replaced by excimer laser surgery for its improved accuracy and stability of correction.
  - Photorefractive keratectomy: Surface corneal tissue is removed with the excimer laser to reshape the cornea, correcting nearsightedness, farsightedness, or astigmatism. Risks and disadvantages include pain, keratitis, and potential scarring. Healing requires 3 months with topical antibiotics and steroids, with associated risks of glaucoma, cataract, chronic inflammation, and scarring.

- Several scleral expansion procedures presently under investigation increase the space within the ciliary body by surgical means to restore lens movement and accommodation. The results have been unsatisfactory.
- Bifocal intraocular lenses (several types have been approved by the FDA: ReSTOR-Alcon, ReZOOM-AMO, Tecnis-AMO) are implanted in the posterior chamber. They increase the depth of field to allow viewing objects both at near and at distance. Side effects include decreased contrast, glare, ghosting of images, and problems with night vision.
- Accommodative intraocular lenses (Crystalens). 1st FDA-approved intraocular lens; several others under clinical investigation. The accommodative intraocular lens moves in response to ciliary body movement to allow focusing at different focal lengths. Side effects are minimal. Present lenses have limited range of focus.

 ONGOING CARE

FOLLOW-UP RECOMMENDATIONS

Patient Monitoring

- Exams recommended when starting school, entering college, with any change in vision quality, and at the age of onset of presbyopia (the need for reading glasses)
- Individuals with any of the known risks of eye disease or conditions that could affect the eyes (e.g., diabetes) need annual ocular examinations.
- Family history of eye diseases/refractive errors necessitates annual re-exam.

DIET

Although refractive error is unaffected by diet, diet has been shown to be important for retinal health. Diets high in fats, cholesterol, along with cigarette smoking or diabetes can lead to an increased risk of age-related macular degeneration (AMD), a potentially blinding disease of the retina. Diets high in vegetables, low in meats, and high in antioxidants (e.g., lutein, β-carotene, vitamins A, C, and E, zinc, and omega-3 fatty acids) have been shown to be protective for retinal degeneration. The AREDS formulation, which has been proven effective in numerous clinical trials, includes a specific daily amount of 500 mg vitamin C, 400 IU of vitamin E, 15 mg of β-carotene (often labeled as the equivalent of 25,000 IU vitamin A), 80 mg of zinc as zinc oxide, and 2 mg of copper as cupric oxide to prevent copper-deficiency anemia, and is taken with meals in 2 equally divided doses in the morning and evening (1)[B].

PATIENT EDUCATION

- All patients should have their eyes examined when starting school and periodically thereafter.
- The options of eyeglasses, contact lenses, and permanent surgical correction of refractive errors can be considered.
- Encourage aggressive control of diabetes mellitus and annual exams by an ophthalmologist. These individuals are at increased risk of blindness from their disease and should not undergo refractive corrective surgery.

PROGNOSIS

- Good, if discovered early and corrected appropriately.
- It is not unusual for refractive errors to be temporarily worsened during pregnancy because of hormonal changes in tear function and corneal swelling.
- It is common that refractive errors worsen as a child ages until complete adult growth has been achieved (this is around age 18–20 for girls and 20–25 for boys). This is a common source of concern for parents. Reassurance that refractive change is often seen with growth spurts, especially at puberty, is advised.
- Any refractive change that is increasing/worsening each year should prompt further investigation by an ophthalmologist.

COMPLICATIONS

- Amblyopia or permanent loss of vision that is not correctable with glasses or contact lenses
- Poor school performance
- Inability to pass a drivers license examination

REFERENCE

1. www.nei.nih.gov/amd/summary.asp

ADDITIONAL READING

- Fax-on-Demand service of American Academy of Ophthalmology for policy statement and patient education materials: (908) 935–2761.
- Frequency of Ocular Exams. *Policy Statement*. San Francisco: American Academy of Ophthalmology; 2009.
- http://www.nei.nih.gov/health/errors/errors.asp
- Kershner RM. *Lessons from the practice: The gift of sight. A guide to understanding your eyes.* Thorofare, NJ: Slack; 1994.
- Vision Screening for Infants and Children. *Policy Statement*. San Francisco: American Academy of Ophthalmology; 2007.

 CODES

ICD10

- H52.00 Hypermetropia, unspecified eye
- H52.7 Unspecified disorder of refraction
- H52.10 Myopia, unspecified eye

CLINICAL PEARLS

- Vision screening should occur at each well-child visit.
- Visual acuity testing should be performed at ~3.5 years of age or at any time that the physician or parent is concerned about the child's eye movements, ability to see, or track objects.
- Children *never* grow out of a refractive error. All suspected refractive errors should be referred to the appropriate eye care professional for evaluation to prevent permanent loss of vision from amblyopia.

REITER SYNDROME

Douglas W. MacPherson, MD, MSc(CTM), FRCPC

BASICS

Reiter syndrome is a seronegative, multisystem, inflammatory disorder classically involving joints, the eye, and the lower genitourinary (GU) tract. Axial joint involvement (e.g., spine, sacroiliac joints) is common. Dermatologic manifestations are also seen frequently.

DESCRIPTION

A classic triad of features, including arthritis, conjunctivitis/iritis, and either urethritis or cervicitis:

- The epidemiology is similar to other reactive arthritis syndromes, characterized by sterile inflammation of joints associated with infections originating at nonarticular sites. A fourth feature of dermatologic manifestations may include buccal ulceration or balanitis or a psoriaform skin eruption. (Having only 2 features present does not rule out the diagnosis.)
- 2 forms:
  – Sexually transmitted: Symptoms generally emerge between 7 and 14 days after exposure to *Chlamydia trachomatis* and other urethral/cervical pathogens acquired during sexual contact
  – Postdysenteric or other bacterial enteric infections (including traveler's diarrhea) (1)[A]
- In a demographic group associated with new or frequent sexual partners, the antecedent triggering infection is more likely to be sexually transmitted than enteric.
- With a preceding history of enteric illness, the antecedent triggering event is more likely to be a bacterial enteric infection than sexually transmitted.
- System(s) affected: Musculoskeletal; Renal/Urologic; Dermatologic/Exocrine
- Synonym(s): Idiopathic blennorrheal arthritis; Arthritis urethritica; Urethro-oculosynovial syndrome; Fiessinger-Leroy-Reiter disease

Pediatric Considerations
Juvenile rheumatoid arthritis has many of the same clinical features of Reiter syndrome.

Pregnancy Considerations
No special considerations, except as related to the usual precautions concerning pharmaceutical therapies

EPIDEMIOLOGY

Incidence
- Predominant age: 20–40 years
- Predominant sex: Male > Female
- 0.24–1.5% incidence after epidemics of bacterial dysentery
- Complicates 1–2% of all cases of nongonococcal urethritis (2,3)

ETIOLOGY AND PATHOPHYSIOLOGY
- The pathophysiology of all the seronegative reactive arthritis syndromes and the immunologic role of infectious diseases as precipitants for clinical illness remain incompletely understood.
- Avoidance of precipitant infections and early management of the multiorgan system inflammatory consequences are important. Scientific evidence does not suggest that antibiotic treatment following onset of syndrome will benefit inflammatory joint, eye, or urinary tract symptoms.
- *C. trachomatis* is the usual causative organism of the postvenereal variety.

- Dysentery-associated form follows enteric bacterial infection owing to *Shigella, Salmonella, Yersinia,* and *Campylobacter* spp. This form is more likely to be seen in women, children, and the elderly than is the postvenereal form.

Genetics
HLA-B27 tissue antigen present in 60–80% of patients

RISK FACTORS
- New or high-risk sexual contacts occurring 7–14 days before the onset of clinical presentation; for sexually acquired precipitants of Reiter syndrome, the primary infection may be subclinical and undiagnosed.
- Food poisoning or bacterial dysentery

GENERAL PREVENTION
- The immune-response characteristics of this syndrome make specific avoidance of infectious precipitants the most important general precaution and potentially the most difficult to achieve.
- Safer sexual exposures and good food and water handling for personal consumption are essential for all persons at all times to maintain health and to avoid infections and the chronic inflammatory consequences associated with infection.
- A family history of seronegative or reactive arthritis syndromes may suggest a genetic predisposition.

COMMONLY ASSOCIATED CONDITIONS
Recent case of:
- Enteric disease from:
  – Shigellosis
  – Salmonellosis
  – Camplyobacteriosis
  – Enteric infection with *Yersinia* spp.
- Urogenital infection from:
  – *Chlamydia* urethritis/cervicitis
  – *Mycoplasma* or *Ureaplasma* spp.
- Infection with HIV

DIAGNOSIS

- Diagnosis of Reiter syndrome is based on the clinical presentation of the classic triad of joint, eye, and GU inflammation and negative serologic testing for rheumatoid factor.
- These 3 symptoms and signs may not all be evident at the same time.
- HLA-B27 testing is not required for diagnosis.
- Treatable STIs should be sought when clinically indicated.
- Screening for enteric infections is rarely useful and generally not indicated diagnostically.

HISTORY
The presence of the clinical syndrome plus:
- Diarrhea, dysentery, urethritis, or genital discharge and risk events for enteric or STIs
- Include a risk history, including travel or migration history and potential exposure to a precipitating infectious agent.

PHYSICAL EXAM
- Musculoskeletal:
  – Asymmetric arthritis (especially knees, ankles, and metatarsophalangeal joints)
  – Enthesopathy (inflammation at tendinous insertion into bone, such as plantar fasciitis, digital periostitis, and Achilles' tendinitis)

- Spondyloarthropathy (spine and sacroiliac joint involvement)
- Urogenital tract:
  – Urethritis
  – Prostatitis
  – Occasionally, cystitis
  – Balanitis
  – Cervicitis: Usually asymptomatic
- Eye:
  – Conjunctivitis of 1 or both eyes
  – Occasionally, scleritis, keratitis, and corneal ulceration
  – Rarely, uveitis and iritis
- Skin:
  – Mucocutaneous lesions (small, painless, superficial ulcers on oral mucosa, tongue, or glans penis)
  – Keratoderma blennorrhagica (hyperkeratotic skin lesions of palms and soles and around nails—can be mistaken for psoriasis)
- Cardiovascular: Occasionally, pericarditis, murmur, conduction defects, and aortic incompetence
- Nervous system: Rarely, peripheral neuropathy, cranial neuropathy, meningoencephalitis, and neuropsychiatric changes
- Constitutional:
  – Fever, malaise, anorexia, and weight loss
  – Patient can appear seriously ill (e.g., fever, rigors, tachycardia, and exquisitely tender joints)

DIFFERENTIAL DIAGNOSIS
- For specific diagnosis, arthritis associated with urethritis for >1 month
- Rheumatoid arthritis (RA)
- Ankylosing spondylitis
- Arthritis associated with inflammatory bowel disease
- Psoriatic arthritis
- Juvenile RA
- Bacterial arthritis, including gonococcal

DIAGNOSTIC TESTS & INTERPRETATION
- Blood:
  – Negative rheumatoid factor
  – Leukocyte count: 10,000–20,000 cells/mm^3
  – Neutrophilic leukocytosis
  – Elevated ESR
  – Moderate normochromic anemia
  – Hypergammaglobulinemia
- Synovial fluid:
  – Leukocyte count: 1,000–8,000 cells/mm^3
  – Bacterial culture negative
- Supportive test results (4):
  – Cultures, antigens, or serology positive for *C. trachomatis* or stool test positive for *Salmonella, Shigella, Yersinia,* or *Campylobacter* spp. supports the diagnosis
  – HIV serology positive (acute retroviral syndrome)
  – HLA-B27-positive status (*not required or recommended for diagnosis*)
  – Drugs that may alter lab results: Antibiotics may affect isolation of the bacterial pathogens.
- X-ray:
  – Periosteal proliferation, thickening
  – Spurs
  – Erosions at articular margins
  – Residual joint destruction
  – Syndesmophytes (spine)
  – Sacroiliitis

Diagnostic Procedures/Other
HLA-B27 histocompatibility antigen: Positive result in 60–80% of cases in non–HIV-related Reiter syndrome; HLA testing is not required or recommended for diagnosis. Rheumatoid factor is negative.

Test Interpretation
- A seronegative spondyloarthropathy (similar to ankylosing spondylitis, enteric arthritis, and psoriatic arthritis)
- Villous formation in joints
- Joint hyperemia
- Joint inflammation
- Prostatitis
- Seminal vesiculitis
- Skin biopsy similar to psoriasis
- Nonspecific conjunctivitis

 TREATMENT

GENERAL MEASURES
Treatment is determined by symptoms:
- Conjunctivitis does not require specific treatment.
- Iritis requires treatment.
- Mucocutaneous lesions do not require treatment.
- Physical therapy (PT) is needed during recovery.
- Arthritis may become prominent and disabling during the acute phase.

MEDICATION
First Line
- Symptomatic management: NSAIDs, including indomethacin, naproxen, and others; intra-articular or systemic corticosteroids for refractory arthritis and enteritis (5)[C]:
  - Contraindications:
    - GI bleeding
    - Patients with peptic ulcer, gastritis, or ulcerative colitis
    - Renal insufficiency
- Specific treatment of pathogenic micro-organism may be attempted if isolated:
  - C. trachomatis: Doxycycline 100 mg PO b.i.d. × 7–14 days (Note: All STIs should be treated whether associated with Reiter syndrome or not.)
  - Salmonella, Shigella, Yersinia, and Campylobacter infections: Ciprofloxacin 500 mg PO b.i.d. × 5–10 days (Note: Emerging antimicrobial resistance may limit this agent's effectiveness in treatment and bacterial clearance. Antibiotic treatment does not reduce GI symptoms or duration of infection or prevent carrier state.)
  - Trials of antibiotic treatment for reactive arthritis have produced mixed results, so the efficacy of antibiotics is uncertain (6)[A].
- GI upset: Antacids
- Iritis: Intraocular steroids
- Keratitis: Topical steroids

Second Line
- Aspirin or other NSAIDs
- Sulfasalazine is promising, but not approved for this indication by the FDA.
- Methotrexate or azathioprine in severe cases (such usage is still experimental and not approved or agreed to be effective); immunosuppressive therapy is relatively contraindicated if patient suffers from HIV-related Reiter syndrome.
- Consultation with specialist is recommended, particularly when considering immunomodulatory agents such as sulfasalazine, methotrexate, or azathioprine.

- Role of antibiotics has been under investigation. They are currently unproven in effectiveness in seronegative arthritis syndromes.
- No published evidence supports the beneficial effect of antibiotics on development of this syndrome or the long-term outcome in patients with Reiter syndrome.

ISSUES FOR REFERRAL
Joint and eye complications; complex management

IN-PATIENT CONSIDERATIONS
Admission Criteria/Initial Stabilization
- Severity, complications, and degree of disability
- Inpatient care may be needed during acute phase.

 ONGOING CARE

FOLLOW-UP RECOMMENDATIONS
Bed rest until joint inflammation subsides

Patient Monitoring
Monitor clinical response to anti-inflammation medications. Observe for complications of therapy, particularly sulfasalazine and immunosuppressive drugs.

PATIENT EDUCATION
- Educate on risk factors for exposure, occurrence, and recurrence
- Teach home PT techniques
- For a listing of sources for patient education materials favorably reviewed on this topic, physicians may contact American Academy of Family Physicians Foundation, P.O. Box 8418, Kansas City, MO 64114, 800-274-2237, ext. 4400.
- Arthritis Foundation, 1314 Spring Street NW, Atlanta, GA 30309, 404-872-7100

PROGNOSIS
- Urethritis occurs 1–15 days after sexual exposure to causative agent.
- Reiter syndrome onset within 10–30 days of either enteric infection or STI
- Mean duration of symptoms is 19 weeks.
- Prognosis is poor in cases involving the heel, eye, or heart.

COMPLICATIONS
- Chronic or recurrent disease in 5–50% of patients (7)[A]
- Ankylosing spondylitis develops in 30–50% of patients who test positive for HLA-B27 antigen.
- Urethral strictures
- Cataracts and blindness
- Aortic root necrosis

REFERENCES
1. Porter CK, Thura N, Riddle MS. Quantifying the incidence and burden of postinfectious enteric sequelae. Mil Med. 2013;178:452–469.
2. Siegel DM. Chronic arthritis in adolescence. Adolesc Med State Art Rev. 2007;18:47–61, viii.
3. Kim PS, Klausmeier TL, Orr DP, et al. Reactive arthritis: A review. J Adolesc Health. 2009;44: 309–315.
4. Contini C, Grilli A, Badia L, et al. Detection of Chlamydophila pneumoniae in patients with arthritis: Significance and diagnostic value. Rheumatol Int. 2011;31:1307–1313.
5. National Guideline Clearinghouse. British Association of Sexual Health and HIV (BASHH) United Kingdom national guideline on management of sexually acquired reactive arthritis. 2009:13596. Available at: www.bashh.org/guidelines
6. Barber CE, Kim J, Inman RD, et al. Antibiotics for treatment of reactive arthritis: A systematic review and metaanalysis. Rheumatology. 2013;40: 916–928.
7. Pope JE. Campylobacter reactive arthritis: A systematic review. Semin Arthritis Rheum. 2007;37: 48–55.

ADDITIONAL READING
- Carter JD, Inman RD. Chlamydia-induced reactive arthritis: Hidden in plain sight? Best Pract Res Clin Rheumatol. 2011;25:359–374.
- Curry JA, Riddle MS, Gormley RP, et al. The epidemiology of infectious gastroenteritis related reactive arthritis in U.S. military personnel: A case-control study. BMC Infect Dis. 2010;10:266.
- Wilson G, Folzenlogen DD. Spondyloarthropathies: New directions in etiopathogenesis, diagnosis and treatment. Mo Med. 2012;109:69–74.

 SEE ALSO

Ankylosing Spondylitis; Arthritis, Psoriatic; Behçet Syndrome

 CODES

ICD10
- M02.30 Reiter's disease, unspecified site
- M02.39 Reiter's disease, multiple sites
- M02.359 Reiter's disease, unspecified hip

CLINICAL PEARLS
- Diagnosis of Reiter syndrome is based on the clinical presentation of the classic triad of joint, eye, and GU inflammation and negative serologic testing for rheumatoid factor (although these signs and symptoms may not all be present at the same time).
- To differentiate Reiter syndrome from other seronegative arthritis syndromes, keep in mind that many of these syndromes may have similar clinical components and overlap in the presenting symptoms. Seek the opinion of a specialist if unsure.
- When the history points toward a sexually acquired infection as a cause, including HIV, associated treatable infectious precipitants of Reiter syndrome must be tested for both personal and public health reasons. Enteric investigations are rarely indicated clinically nor justify a therapeutic response.
- Some patients have a chronic course, experience recurrences, or have clinical complications. If the inflammatory symptoms do not resolve quickly on NSAID agents, consider referral to a specialist.

RENAL CELL CARCINOMA

Jonathon M. Firnhaber, MD

 BASICS

DESCRIPTION
- Renal cell carcinoma (RCC; also called hypernephroma or Grawitz tumor), accounts for 3–4% of all adult cancers and 2.3% of all cancer deaths; 7th most common malignant tumor in men and 9th in women
- Characterized by obscure and varied presentations, including paraneoplastic syndromes, vascular findings, and uncommon metastatic sites
- Early, aggressive surgical management provides the best opportunity for cure.
- System(s) affected: Renal/Urologic

EPIDEMIOLOGY
Incidence
- Predominant age: Patients in 5th–7th decades; median age at diagnosis is 66 years
- Predominant sex: Male > Female (1.6:1)
- Age-adjusted incidence increasing 3% per year, likely due in part to increased detection as an incidental finding on imaging studies
- In males, 10.7 new cases of RCC per 100,000 population per year vs. 6.5 in females
- Between 1975 and 1998, incidence among African Americans increased by 4.5% compared with 2.9% among Caucasians; reasons are unclear

ETIOLOGY AND PATHOPHYSIOLOGY
Unknown

Genetics
- 2–3% of cases are familial, with several autosomal-dominant syndromes described.
- Oncogenes localized to the short arm of chromosome 3 may have etiologic implications. Chromosome 3p12–p26 is specific for clear cell RCC.
- People with HLA types Bw44 and DR8 are prone to develop RCC. These are rare familial RCCs.
- Hereditary papillary RCC is an autosomal-dominant form of disease associated with multifocal papillary renal tumors and a 5:1 male predominance.

RISK FACTORS
- Smoking, active and passive (increases relative risk by 2–3)
- Obesity (linear relationship in women)
- Hypertension (antihypertensive medications are not independently associated with RCC)
- End-stage renal failure
- Acquired renal cystic disease
- Tuberous sclerosis
- HIV infection
- Urban environment
- Heavy metal exposure (cadmium, lead)
- Environmental toxin exposure (asbestos, petroleum by-products, chlorinated solvents)

GENERAL PREVENTION
Smoking may contribute to 1/3 of all cases.

COMMONLY ASSOCIATED CONDITIONS
- Von Hippel–Lindau disease: 30–45% of these patients develop clear cell tumors
- Tuberous sclerosis: Associated primarily with angiomyolipoma and clear cell tumors
- Sickle cell trait: With few exceptions, renal medullary tumor is seen in young African American males with sickle cell trait
- Adult polycystic kidney disease

- Horseshoe kidney
- Acquired renal cystic disease from chronic renal failure

 DIAGNOSIS

HISTORY
>70% of RCC are incidentally discovered in asymptomatic patients due to increased use of ultrasound, CT scanning, and MRI.

PHYSICAL EXAM
- Classic triad of hematuria, abdominal mass, and flank pain in <10%
- Hematuria: 50–60%
- Flank pain: 35–40%
- Palpable mass: 25%
- Hypertension: 22–38%
- Weight loss: 28–36%
- Pyrexia: 7–17%
- Nonmetastatic hepatic dysfunction (Stauffer syndrome): 10–15%
- Neuromyopathy: 3%
- Scrotal varicoceles: 2–11% (most are left-sided)
- Patients with vena cava thrombus present with lower extremity edema, new varicocele, dilated superficial abdominal veins, albuminuria, pulmonary emboli, right atrial mass, or nonfunction of the involved kidney.

DIFFERENTIAL DIAGNOSIS
- Benign renal masses (e.g., renal hamartomas)
- Hydronephrosis
- Pyelonephritis
- Renal abscess
- Polycystic kidneys
- Renal tuberculosis
- Renal calculi
- Renal infarction
- Benign renal cyst
- Transitional cell carcinoma of the renal pelvis
- Wilms tumor
- Metastatic disease, especially melanoma

DIAGNOSTIC TESTS & INTERPRETATION
Initial Tests (lab, imaging)
- Increased ESR: 50–60%
- Anemia: 21–41%
- Hypercalcemia: 3–6%
- Erythrocytosis: 3–4%
- Hematuria
- Urinary neoplastic cells
- Alkaline phosphate may be elevated.
- Increased renin
- Increased plasma fibrinogen
- Ultrasonography: Determine if mass is solid or cystic; simple cystic may be observed or subjected to percutaneous aspiration; solid lesions require further imaging
- Abdominal/Pelvic CT, using 3-phase imaging, with and without IV contrast, is the optimal imaging modality to evaluate the kidneys; it is ~100% sensitive for detecting a renal mass >15 mm in diameter. A solid renal mass with >15–20 Hounsfield units change on multiphase CT has an 80% likelihood of being RCC. A predominantly cystic mass with an irregular, nodular, or enhancing wall, calcifications, and/or septa >2 mm thick has a >70% likelihood of being cystic RCC.

Follow-Up Tests & Special Considerations
- MRI with pre- and postgadolinium phases is superior to ultrasound in evaluating adenopathy, diagnosing intracaval and renal venous thrombus, and demonstrating bony metastases.
- Chest CT scan if initial chest x-ray suggests metastatic disease; brain CT scan if the patient has neurologic symptoms
- Bone scan is indicated if the alkaline phosphatase level is elevated or the patient has bone pain.
- CT or MR angiography for staging evaluation; vascular information helpful in planning resection
- PET is of limited use because of RCC's inconsistent uptake of fluorodeoxyglucose, the most commonly used radiotracer, although this variable uptake may be an asset in predicting response to some targeted agents.

Diagnostic Procedures/Other
- No need to aspirate simple cyst unless symptomatic
- Calcified cysts may contain RCC, requiring open renal biopsy of the cyst wall or partial nephrectomy
- Hemorrhagic cyst: Aspiration cytology may be helpful, but needle biopsy of solid masses is discouraged, particularly if the patient has a normal contralateral kidney.
- Doppler-flow ultrasound of the renal veins or CT scan that shows the renal vein entering the vena cava can be used to rule out tumor thrombus.

Test Interpretation
- RCC tends to bulge out from the cortex, producing a mass effect.
- 48% of RCCs measure <5 cm, are grossly yellow to yellow–orange due to high lipid content in the clear cell variety. Average size has been decreasing due to incidental discovery and is now ~3.6 cm.
- Small tumors are typically homogeneous.
- Large tumors may have areas of necrosis and hemorrhage.
- About 5–10% of RCCs extend into the venous system as tumor thrombi.
- 5 distinct subtypes:
  – Clear cell: 70–80%; proximal tubule, typically solitary
  – Papillary renal cell (previously termed chromophilic): 10–15%; proximal tubule; tumors tend to be bilateral and multifocal; type 1 and more aggressive type 2 variant
  – Chromophobic: 3–5%; intercalated cells; tend to have a less aggressive course
  – Medullary: <1%; typically affect younger patients; most are at an advanced stage with metastases at time of diagnosis; occur almost exclusively in patients with sickle cell trait
  – Collecting duct: <1%

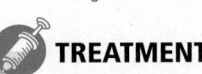 **TREATMENT**

Among small (<4 cm) renal masses, ~20% are benign, 60% represent indolent variants of RCC, and only 20% are potentially aggressive tumors.

MEDICATION
First Line
- Sunitinib represents front-line standard treatment for the good and intermediate prognosis groups of patients with clear cell RCC (1)[C].

- In fit patients with metastatic disease and minimal symptoms, nephrectomy followed by interferon-alfa is the best survival strategy for fully validated therapies (2)[A]. Interferon is the standard comparator for the assessment of new treatments in metastatic RCC.
- Sunitinib and sorafenib are both oral inhibitors of the tyrosine kinase portion of the vascular endothelial growth factor (VEGF) family of receptors. Sunitinib is considered 1st-line treatment in advanced RCC and in patients refractory or intolerant to cytokine therapy. Sunitinib demonstrated improved response (31% vs. 6%; number needed to treat [NNT] = 4) and longer median progression-free survival (11 vs. 5 months) over interferon-alfa in a randomized study of 750 patients (3)[B]. Sorafenib is considered a 2nd-line option.
- Bevacizumab is a monoclonal antibody that binds and neutralizes circulating VEGF protein. Combined with interferon-alfa, bevacizumab offers patients with metastatic RCC a hazard ratio for progression-free survival of 0.63 (95% confidence interval 0.52–0.75; $p = .0001$) compared with interferon alone (4)[B].
- Temsirolimus, an IV mammalian target of rapamycin (mTOR) inhibitor, also approved for advanced RCC, is the 1st-line choice for patients with non–clear-cell histology. It has shown improved response (32% vs. 16%; NNT = 6) and longer median survival (10.9 vs. 7.3 months) over interferon-alfa in a comparative clinical trial of 626 patients.
- A 2008 phase 3 trial of 410 patients comparing everolimus, another mTOR inhibitor, with placebo was stopped early after disease progression was seen in 37% of patients receiving everolimus vs. 65% receiving placebo (hazard ratio = 0.30, 95% confidence interval 0.22–0.40; $p <.0001$) (5)[B].

Second Line
- Response rates with traditional chemotherapeutic agents are typically <15%.
- Despite occasional reports of responses, a review of medroxyprogesterone, the most widely studied progestational agent, concluded that RCCs are neither hormone dependent nor hormone responsive.

ADDITIONAL THERAPIES
- RCC is considered radioresistant, but radiation therapy may be useful to treat a single or limited number of metastases, particularly brain or bone metastases or painful recurrences in the renal bed.
- Targeted agents rarely induce complete responses, and patients eventually develop resistance to therapy, prompting continued interest in immunotherapy for RCC. Phase 1 or 2 trials of vaccination with allogeneic dendritic cell/tumor fusions in patients with RCC have demonstrated immunologic and clinical responses in some patients, and T-cell modulating agents have also shown some efficacy in early clinical trials (6)[B].

SURGERY/OTHER PROCEDURES
- Surgery is curative in most patients with nonmetastatic RCC and is the preferred treatment for all but the most extensive disease.
- There is no current role for adjuvant therapy after nephrectomy for clinically localized disease.
- Assuming a normal contralateral kidney, radical nephrectomy, which can be done laparoscopically and involves node dissection and complete removal of the kidney and Gerota fascia, is the typical preferred approach.

- Partial nephrectomy has shown equal long-term, cancer-specific survival for small to medium (<7 cm) tumors when compared with radical nephrectomy. Partial nephrectomy, however, is a more technically challenging procedure.
- Better cancer-specific quality of life has been reported in patients who underwent radical vs. partial nephrectomy and in those who underwent laparoscopic vs. open surgery (7)[B].
- Surgical intervention in metastatic disease:
  - Metastasectomy in those with limited metastatic disease vs. cytoreductive nephrectomy (debulking) prior to systemic therapy.
  - Transitional cell carcinoma of the renal pelvis or calyces: Nephroureterectomy
  - Wilms tumor in adults: Radical nephrectomy for unilateral disease
  - Cortical adenoma <3 cm (7–22% at autopsy): Wedge resection
- Image-guided radiofrequency or cryoablation has been successful in limited studies for the treatment of small (average 2 cm) peripheral renal tumors; long-term efficacy data are limited.

ONGOING CARE

FOLLOW-UP RECOMMENDATIONS
Patient Monitoring
- CT scan of the abdomen/renal fossa 3–6 months after surgery, to monitor recurrences
- For partial nephrectomy: Renal ultrasound every 6 months for 3 years, then annually
- CXR or CT scan quarterly for 2 years, then periodically.
- Skeletal x-rays and bone scan should be obtained only if patient complains of bone pain or if alkaline phosphatase is elevated.
- Postoperative follow up with plasma transcobalamin II or serum haptoglobin level to detect or monitor recurrences
- Small (<3 cm), incidentally detected tumors may have an indolent behavior; immediate treatment in poor-risk patients may not be of benefit, and active surveillance may be a viable management strategy.

DIET
Red meat intake may increase the risk of RCC. Higher intakes of heterocyclic amines and polycyclic aromatic hydrocarbons generated in the processing and cooking of red meat have been associated with a 2-fold increase in the risk of papillary RCC and a 20–30% increase in the overall risk of RCC (8)[B].

PROGNOSIS
- 5-year survival in the absence of metastases >50%; in the presence of distant metastases, 5-year survival decreases to 10%.
- Median survival for metastatic RCC is in the range of 10–12 months.
- Performance status at diagnosis and histologic grade of tumor also influence prognosis.

COMPLICATIONS
- Paraplegia can result with little warning from spinal vertebral metastasis.
- CNS metastases are not uncommon.
- ~30% of patients with RCC have metastatic disease when the diagnosis is established. Most common sites of metastasis are the lung (50–60%), bone (30–40%), regional nodes (15–30%), brain (10%), and adjacent organs (10%).

REFERENCES
1. Di Lorenzo G, Buonerba C, Biglietto M, et al. The therapy of kidney cancer with biomolecular drugs. *Cancer Treat Rev.* 2010;36(Suppl 3):S16–S20.
2. Coppin C, Porzsolt F, Awa A, et al. Immunotherapy for advanced renal cell cancer. *Cochrane Database Syst Rev.* 2005;2:CD001425.
3. Motzer RJ, Hutson TE, Tomczak P, et al. Sunitinib versus interferon alfa in metastatic renal-cell carcinoma. *N Engl J Med.* 2007;356:115–124.
4. Escudier B, Bellmunt J, Négrier S, et al. Phase III trial of bevacizumab plus interferon alfa-2a in patients with metastatic renal cell carcinoma (AVOREN): Final analysis of overall survival. *J Clin Oncol.* 2010;28:2144–2150.
5. Motzer RJ, Escudier B, Oudard S, et al. Efficacy of everolimus in advanced renal cell carcinoma: A double-blind, randomised, placebo-controlled phase III trial. *Lancet.* 2008;372:449–456.
6. Escudier B. Emerging immunotherapies for renal cell carcinoma. *Ann Oncol.* 2012;23(Suppl 8): viii35–40.
7. Parker PA, Swartz R, Fellman B, et al. Comprehensive assessment of quality of life and psychosocial adjustment in patients with renal tumors undergoing open, laparoscopic and nephron sparing surgery. *J Urol.* 2012;187:822–826.
8. Daniel CR, Cross AJ, Graubard BI, et al. Large prospective investigation of meat intake, related mutagens, and risk of renal cell carcinoma. *Am J Clin Nutr.* 2012;95:155–162.

 CODES

ICD10
- C64.1 Malignant neoplasm of right kidney, except renal pelvis
- C64.2 Malignant neoplasm of left kidney, except renal pelvis
- C64.9 Malignant neoplasm of unsp kidney, except renal pelvis

CLINICAL PEARLS
- RCC represents 3–4% of all cancers and 2% of all cancer deaths; most patients have clear cell histology and do not respond to standard chemotherapy.
- Diverse and obscure presentations are typical; most RCCs are found incidentally during radiologic studies.
- At presentation, up to 30% of patients with RCC have metastatic disease; recurrence develops in ~40% treated for localized disease.
- Only 20% of renal masses <4 cm represent potentially aggressive tumors.
- Surgery is curative in most patients with nonmetastatic RCC and is the preferred treatment for all but the most extensive disease.
- Multiple pharmacologic options are considered first-line for metastatic RCC; sequential treatments are likely to be pursued for most patients.

RENAL TUBULAR ACIDOSIS

Jason M. Kurland, MD

 BASICS

DESCRIPTION
- Renal tubular acidosis (RTA) is composed of a group of disorders characterized by an inability of the kidney to resorb bicarbonate/secrete hydrogen ions, resulting in normal anion gap metabolic acidosis. Renal function (glomerular filtration rate [GFR]) must be normal or near normal.
- Several types have been identified:
  - Type I (distal) RTA: Inability of the distal tubule to acidify the urine; due to impaired hydrogen ion secretion, increased back leak of secreted hydrogen ions, or impaired sodium reabsorption (interfering with the generation of negative luminal charge required for hydrogen/potassium secretion). Urine pH >5.5.
  - Type II (proximal) RTA: Defect of the proximal tubule in bicarbonate (HCO_3) reabsorption. Proximal tubular HCO_3 reabsorption absent; plasma HCO_3 concentration stabilizes at 12–18 mEq/L due to compensatory distal HCO_3 reabsorption. Urine pH <5.5 unless plasma HCO_3 brought above reabsorptive threshold (1).
  - Type III RTA: Extremely rare autosomal–recessive syndrome with features of both type I and type II (may be due to carbonic anhydrase II deficiency).
  - Type IV RTA (hypoaldosteronism): Due to aldosterone resistance/deficiency that results in hyperkalemia. Urine pH usually <5.5.

EPIDEMIOLOGY
Incidence
- Predominant age: All ages
- Predominant sex: Male > Female (with regard to type II RTA with isolated defect in bicarbonate reabsorption)

ETIOLOGY AND PATHOPHYSIOLOGY
- Type I RTA:
  - Genetic: Autosomal dominant, autosomal recessive associated with sensorineural deafness
  - Sporadic
  - Other familial disorders: Ehlers-Danlos syndrome, glycogenosis type III, Fabry disease, Wilson disease
  - Autoimmune diseases: Sjögren syndrome, rheumatoid arthritis (RA), systemic lupus erythematosus (SLE)
  - Hematologic diseases: Sickle cell disease (hyperkalemic), hereditary elliptocytosis
  - Medications: Amphotericin B, lithium, ifosfamide, foscarnet, amiloride, triamterene, trimethoprim, pentamidine
  - Toxins: Toluene, glue
  - Hypercalciuria, diseases causing nephrocalcinosis
  - Vitamin D intoxication
  - Medullary cystic disease
  - Obstructive uropathy (hyperkalemic)
  - Hypergammaglobulinemic syndrome
  - Chronic pyelonephritis
  - Chronic renal transplant rejection
  - Leprosy
  - Hepatic cirrhosis
  - Malnutrition

- Type II RTA:
  - Familial (cystinosis, tyrosinemia, hereditary fructose intolerance, galactosemia, glycogen storage disease type I, Wilson disease, Lowe syndrome, inherited carbonic anhydrase deficiency)
  - Sporadic
  - Multiple myeloma, other dysproteinemic states
  - Amyloidosis
  - Heavy-metal poisoning (e.g., cadmium, lead, mercury, copper)
  - Medications: Acetazolamide, ifosfamide, tenofovir, sulfanilamide, outdated tetracycline, topiramate, aminoglycosides
  - Interstitial renal disease
  - Paroxysmal nocturnal hemoglobinuria
  - Defects in calcium metabolism (hyperparathyroidism)
- Type IV RTA:
  - Medications: NSAIDs, ACE inhibitors, angiotensin receptor blockers, heparin/low molecular weight heparin, ketoconazole, calcineurin inhibitors (tacrolimus, cyclosporine) (2)
  - Diabetic nephropathy
  - Nephrosclerosis due to hypertension
  - Tubulointerstitial nephropathies
  - Primary adrenal insufficiency
  - Pseudohypoaldosteronism (PHA) (end-organ resistance to aldosterone):
    ○ PHA type 1
    ○ PHA type 2 (Gordon's syndrome)

Genetics
- Type I RTA: Hereditary forms due to mutations affecting intercalated cells in collecting tubules (3) May occur in association with other genetic diseases (e.g., Ehlers-Danlos syndrome, hereditary elliptocytosis, or sickle cell nephropathy). The autosomal-recessive form is associated with sensorineural deafness.
- Type II RTA: Autosomal-dominant form is rare. Autosomal-recessive form is associated with ophthalmologic abnormalities and mental retardation. Occurs in Fanconi syndrome, which is associated with several genetic diseases (e.g., cystinosis, Wilson disease, tyrosinemia, hereditary fructose intolerance, Lowe syndrome, galactosemia, glycogen storage disease, and metachromatic leukodystrophy).
- Type IV RTA: Some cases are familial, such as PHA type I (autosomal dominant).

GENERAL PREVENTION
Careful use/avoidance of causative agents

COMMONLY ASSOCIATED CONDITIONS
- Type I RTA in children: Hypercalciuria leading to rickets, nephrocalcinosis
- Type I RTA in adults: Autoimmune diseases (Sjögren syndrome, RA, SLE), hypercalciuria
- Type II RTA: Fanconi syndrome (generalized proximal tubular dysfunction resulting in glycosuria, aminoaciduria, hyperuricosuria, phosphaturia, bicarbonaturia)
- Type II RTA in adults: Multiple myeloma, carbonic anhydrase inhibitors (acetazolamide)
- Type IV RTA: Diabetic nephropathy

 DIAGNOSIS

HISTORY
- Often asymptomatic (particularly type IV)
- In children: Failure to thrive, rickets
- Anorexia, nausea/vomiting, constipation
- Weakness or polyuria (due to hypokalemia)
- Polydipsia
- Osteomalacia in adults

DIFFERENTIAL DIAGNOSIS
- Plasma anion gap should be normal. If not, evaluate for causes of anion-gap metabolic acidosis. (MUDPILES: **M**ethanol, **u**remia, **d**iabetic ketoacidosis, **p**ropylene glycol/paraldehyde, **i**ron/isoniazid ingestion, **l**actic acidosis, **e**thylene glycol, **s**alicylates)
- Extrarenal HCO_3 losses:
  - Diarrhea
  - Small bowel, pancreatic, or biliary fistulas (4)[C]
  - Urinary diversion (e.g., ureterosigmoidostomy, ileal conduit)
- Acidosis of chronic renal failure (develops when GFR ≤20–30 mL/min)
- Excessive administration of acid load via chloride salts ($NaCl$, HCl, NH_4Cl, lysine HCl, $CaCl_2$, $MgCl_2$)

DIAGNOSTIC TESTS & INTERPRETATION
- Electrolytes reveal hyperchloremic metabolic acidosis.
- Plasma anion gap normal (anion gap = Na − [Cl + HCO_3]). Normal values (in mEq/L): Neonates ≤16; infants/children ≤14–16; adolescents/adults 8 ± 4). Must correct calculated anion gap for hypoalbuminemia. Increase calculated anion gap by 2.5 mEq/L for each 1 g/dL decrease in albumin below 4 g/dL.
- Plasma K+: Low in type I (if due to impaired distal H^+ secretion/increased H^+ back leak), type II; high in type IV, type I (if due to impaired distal Na^+ reabsorption)
- Plasma HCO_3 (in untreated RTA): Type I: <10–20 mEq/L; type II: 12–18 mEq/L; type IV: >17 mEq/L
- BUN/Cr normal or near normal (rules out renal failure as cause of acidosis)
- Urinalysis: Urine pH inappropriately alkaline (>5.5) despite metabolic acidosis in type I/II if HCO_3 above reabsorptive threshold (12–18 mEq/L)
- Urine culture: Rule out UTI with urea-splitting organism (may elevate pH) and chronic infection
- Urine anion gap (urine Na^+, K^+, and Cl^- on random urine): Reflects unmeasured urine anions, so inversely related to urine NH_4^+ (or acid) excretion. Positive urine anion gap in an acidemic patient indicates impaired renal acid excretion. Urine Na^+ >25 mEq/L required for accurate interpretation of urine anion gap. Results tend to be:
  - Negative in HCO_3 losses due to diarrhea, UTI caused by urea-splitting organisms, and other extrarenal causes of nonanion gap metabolic acidosis
  - Variable in type II RTA
  - Positive in type I RTA, type IV RTA (4)[C]
  - Positive in impaired acid excretion due to renal failure

- Urine calcium:
  - High in type I
  - Typically normal in type II
- Drugs that may alter lab results:
  - Diuretics
  - Sodium bicarbonate (and other alkali)
  - Cholestyramine

Initial Tests (lab, imaging)
- Serum electrolytes; consider urinalysis, urine culture

Diagnostic Procedures/Other
- Helpful to measure urine pH on fresh sample with pH meter for increased accuracy instead of dipstick. Pour film of oil over urine to avoid loss of CO_2 if pH cannot be measured quickly.
- Urine NH_4^+ excretion (anion gap only provides a qualitative estimate)
- Urinary acidification (impaired in type I RTA) can be assessed by oral administration of furosemide and fludrocortisone; patients with type I RTA unable to reduce urine pH to <5.3 (5).
- Fractional excretion of HCO_3 >15% during HCO_3 infusion (type II RTA) (1)

Test Interpretation
- Nephrocalcinosis
- Nephrolithiasis
- Rickets
- Osteomalacia, osteopenia
- Findings of an underlying disease causing RTA

TREATMENT

MEDICATION
First Line
- Provide oral alkali to raise serum HCO_3 to normal. Start at a low dose and increase until HCO_3 is normal. Give as sodium bicarbonate or citrate mixtures (1 mEq citrate = 1 mEq HCO_3) such as Bicitra (1 mEq Na, 1 mEq citrate/mL, no K) or Polycitra (1 mEq Na, 1 mEq K, 2 mEq citrate/mL) depending on need for potassium. Sodium bicarbonate tablets are available (7.7 mEq $NaHCO_3$/650 mg tab) (6)[C].
- Type I RTA: Typical doses 1–2 mEq/kg/d (in adults), 3–4 mEq/kg/d (in children) PO alkali divided 3–4 × per day (require much higher doses if HCO_3 wasting is present). May require K^+ supplementation.
- Type II RTA: Typical doses 10–15 mEq/kg/d alkali, divided 4–6 × per day. Very difficult to restore plasma HCO_3 to normal, as renal HCO_3 losses increase once plasma HCO_3 is corrected above resorptive threshold. Exogenous HCO_3 increases K^+ losses, requiring supplemental K^+. Often need supplemental PO_4 and vitamin D due to proximal PO_4 wasting. May add thiazide diuretic to induce mild hypovolemia, which increases proximal Na^+/HCO_3^- reabsorption.
- Type IV RTA: Avoid inciting medications; restrict dietary K^+. May augment K^+ excretion with loop diuretic, thiazide diuretic, or Kayexalate. Correcting hyperkalemia increases activity of the urea cycle, augmenting renal ammoniagenesis and adding substrate for renal acid excretion. If necessary, 1–5 mEq/kg/d alkali divided 2–3 × per day. If mineralocorticoid deficiency, fludrocortisone: 0.1–0.3 mg/d.

- Precautions:
  - Sodium-containing compounds will increase urinary calcium excretion, potentially increasing the risk of nephrolithiasis.
  - Sodium-based alkali/mineralocorticoids may lead to hypertension and/or edema.
  - Aluminum-containing medications (antacids, sucralfate) should be avoided if solutions containing citric acid are prescribed, as citric acid increases aluminum absorption.
  - Sodium bicarbonate may cause flatulence because CO_2 is formed, whereas citrate is metabolized to HCO_3 in the liver, avoiding gas production.

Second Line
Thiazide diuretics may be used as adjunctive therapy in type II RTA (after maximal alkali replacement), but are likely to further increase urinary K^+ losses.

SURGERY/OTHER PROCEDURES
If distal RTA is due to obstructive uropathy, surgical intervention may be required.

IN-PATIENT CONSIDERATIONS
Admission Criteria/Initial Stabilization
Generally managed as outpatient; inpatient if acidosis severe, patient unreliable, emesis persistent, or infant with severe failure to thrive

 ONGOING CARE

FOLLOW-UP RECOMMENDATIONS
Patient Monitoring
- Electrolytes 1–2 weeks following initiation of therapy, monthly until serum HCO_3 corrected to desired range, then as clinically indicated
- Monitor underlying disease as indicated
- Poor compliance common due to 3–6 × per day alkali dosing schedule

DIET
Varies based on serum K^+ level and volume status

PATIENT EDUCATION
- National Kidney & Urologic Diseases Information Clearinghouse, Box NKUDIC, Bethesda, MD 20893, 301-468-6345; www.niddk.nih.gov/health/kidney
- National Kidney Foundation: www.kidney.org

PROGNOSIS
- Depends on associated disease; otherwise, good with therapy
- Transient forms of all types of RTA may occur

COMPLICATIONS
- Nephrocalcinosis, nephrolithiasis (type I)
- Hypercalciuria (type I)
- Hypokalemia (type I, type II if given bicarbonate)
- Hyperkalemia (type IV, some causes of type I)
- Osteomalacia (type II due to phosphate wasting), osteopenia (due to buffering of acid in bone) (7)

REFERENCES

1. Reddy P. Clinical approach to renal tubular acidosis in adult patients. *Int J Clin Pract*. 2011;84: 350–360.
2. Heering PJ, Kurschat C, Vo DT, et al. Aldosterone resistance in kidney transplantation is in part induced by a down-regulation of mineralocorticoid receptor expression. *Clin Transplant*. 2004;18: 186–192.
3. Batlle D, Hague SK. Genetic causes and mechanisms of distal renal tubular acidosis. *Nephrol Dial Transplant*. 2012;27:3691–3704.
4. Casaletto J. Differential diagnosis of metabolic acidosis. *Emer Med Clin N Am*. 2005;23:771–787.
5. Walsh SB, Shirley DG, Wrong OM, et al. Urinary acidification assessed by simultaneous furosemide and fludrocortisone treatment: An alternative to ammonium chloride. *Kidney Int*. 2007;71: 1310–1316.
6. Chan JC, Scheinman JI, Roth KS. Consultation with the specialist: Renal tubular acidosis. *Pediatr Rev*. 2001;22:277–287.
7. Domrongkitchaiporn S, Pongskul C, Sirikulchayanonta V, et al. Bone histology and bone mineral density after correction of acidosis in distal renal tubular acidosis. *Kidney Int*. 2002;62: 2160–2166.

ADDITIONAL READING

Liamis G, Milionis HJ, Elisaf M, et al. Pharmacologically-induced metabolic acidosis: A review. *Drug Saf*. 2010;33:371–391.

 CODES

ICD10
N25.89 Oth disorders resulting from impaired renal tubular function

CLINICAL PEARLS

- Consider RTA in cases of normal anion gap metabolic acidosis with normal/near-normal renal function.
- Type I RTA: Urine pH >5.5 in setting of acidemia; positive urine anion gap; acidemia can be severe.
- Type II RTA: Urine pH <5.5 unless HCO_3 raised above reabsorptive threshold (12–18 mEq/L).
- Type IV RTA: Most common subtype; hyperkalemia; urine pH <5.5; acidemia usually mild.
- Treatment includes avoidance of inciting causes, provision of oral alkali (HCO_3 or citrate), and measures to supplement (type II, many type I) or restrict (type IV) potassium.

RESPIRATORY DISTRESS SYNDROME, ACUTE

Muhammad Imran Khan, MD • Najm Hasan Siddiqui, MD

 BASICS

DESCRIPTION
- Acute respiratory distress syndrome (ARDS) is characterized by abrupt onset of diffuse lung injury with severe hypoxemia and bilateral pulmonary infiltrates:
  - Absence of left atrial hypertension (HTN)
  - By consensus, $PaO_2/FiO_2 < 200$
  - Most severe form of acute lung injury
- System(s) affected: Pulmonary; Cardiovascular
- Synonym(s): Shock lung; Wet lung; Noncardiac pulmonary edema

EPIDEMIOLOGY
Incidence
Acute lung injury: 40–75 cases/100,000 annually

ETIOLOGY AND PATHOPHYSIOLOGY
3 phases:
- Acute exudative phase: Characterized by profound hypoxia and associated with inflammation with infiltration of inflammatory and proinflammatory mediators and diffuse alveolar damage
- Fibrosing alveolitis phase: Coincides with recovery or after ~1–2 weeks; patients continue to be hypoxic and have increased dead space and decreased compliance.
- Resolution may require 6–12 months.
- Several mediators are involved in the initiation and perpetuation of ARDS:
  - Cytokines
  - Complement activation
  - Coagulation activation
  - Platelet-activating factor
  - Oxygen free radicals
  - Lipoxygenase pathways
  - Neutrophil proteases
  - Nitric oxide
  - Endotoxin
  - Cyclooxygenase pathway products
- Systemic inflammatory response with activation of the previous mediators can occur with direct or indirect injury to the lung:
  - Direct:
    - Aspiration
    - Pulmonary infections
    - Air, fat, or amniotic fluid emboli
    - Near-drowning
    - Pulmonary contusion
    - Inhalation of toxic gases and dusts
  - Indirect:
    - Sepsis
    - Shock
    - Transfusion
    - Trauma
    - Overdose
    - Pancreatitis, severe
    - Eclampsia

RISK FACTORS
- Severe infection (localized or systemic) most common
- Aspiration of gastric contents
- Shock
- Infection
- Trauma with or without lung contusion
- Pneumonia
- Toxic inhalation
- Pancreatitis
- Fat embolism
- Near-drowning
- Multiple blood transfusions

GENERAL PREVENTION
No effective measures have been identified.

COMMONLY ASSOCIATED CONDITIONS
- Severe sepsis
- Trauma
- Shock

 DIAGNOSIS

HISTORY
- No history of heart disease
- Precipitating event (see "Commonly Associated Conditions"): Abrupt onset of respiratory distress

PHYSICAL EXAM
- Tachypnea and tachycardia during the first 12–24 hours; respiratory distress
- Lethargy, obtundation
- Flat neck veins
- Hyperdynamic pulses
- Physiologic gallop
- Absence of edema
- Moist, cyanotic skin
- Manifestations of underlying disease

DIFFERENTIAL DIAGNOSIS
- Left ventricular failure
- Interstitial and airway diseases
- Hypersensitivity pneumonitis
- Veno-occlusive disease
- Mitral stenosis: Intravascular volume overload
- Toxic shock syndrome

DIAGNOSTIC TESTS & INTERPRETATION
Initial Tests (lab, imaging)
- Arterial blood gases (ABGs) show evidence of severe hypoxemia.
- $PaO_2/FiO_2 < 200$
- ECG: Sinus tachycardia; nonspecific ST-T-wave changes
- Pulmonary artery wedge pressure (PAWP) <15 mm Hg
- Cardiac index >3.5 $L/min/m^2$
- Chest x-ray (CXR): Normal heart size; fluffy, bilateral infiltrates; air bronchograms common
- Chest CT scan: Diffuse interstitial opacities and bullae

Follow-Up Tests & Special Considerations
- Serial blood gases
- Monitor for and treat multisystem organ failure when it occurs.
- Serial CXRs

Diagnostic Procedures/Other
Invasive monitoring of vital signs, cardiac output, and PAWP has been questioned by large clinical trials.

Test Interpretation
- Lungs show exudative, early proliferative, or late proliferative phases.
- Interstitial and alveolar edema is present.
- Inflammatory cells and erythrocytes spill into the interstitium and the alveolus.
- Type 1 cells are destroyed, leaving a denuded basement membrane.
- Protein-rich fluid fills the alveoli.
- Type 2 alveolar cells initially appear unaltered.
- Type 2 cells begin to proliferate within 72 hours of initial insult and cover the denuded basement membrane.
- Aggregates of plasma proteins, cellular debris, fibrin, and surfactant remnants form hyaline membranes.
- Over the next 3–10 days, alveolar septum thickens by proliferating fibroblasts, leukocytes, and plasma cells.
- Capillary injury begins to occur.
- Hyaline membranes begin to reorganize.
- Fibrosis becomes apparent in respiratory ducts and bronchioles.

 TREATMENT

GENERAL MEASURES
- Ensure adequate oxygenation.
- Ventilatory support generally requires endotracheal intubation and use of positive end-expiratory pressure (PEEP) (1).
- Provide appropriate cardiorespiratory monitoring.
- Fluid management

MEDICATION
- No single drug or combination of drugs prevents or treats full-blown ARDS. Treatment is supportive while addressing the underlying cause.
- Supplemental oxygen
- Ventilatory support:
  - Most often requires endotracheal intubation with emphasis on lower tidal volumes per weight and optimization of PEEP.
  - High-frequency oscillation might improve survival and is unlikely to cause harm (2)[A].

ISSUES FOR REFERRAL
- All patients with ARDS should be cared for in an ICU with appropriately trained staff.
- Pregnant patients with ARDS also should be followed by a high-risk perinatologist or obstetrician.

RESPIRATORY DISTRESS SYNDROME, NEONATAL

Mary Cataletto, MD

 BASICS

DESCRIPTION
- Neonatal respiratory distress syndrome (NRDS) is a serious disorder of prematurity with a clinical manifestation of respiratory distress.
- Pulmonary surfactants that are deficient at birth and an overly compliant chest wall cause diffuse lung atelectasis.
- System(s) affected: Pulmonary
- Synonym(s): Hyaline membrane disease; Surfactant deficiency

ALERT
A disorder of the neonatal period

EPIDEMIOLOGY
Incidence
- In 2007, accounted for ~3% of neonatal deaths
- Predominant age: 93% incidence in infants born at or before 28 weeks' gestational age (1)
- Inversely proportional to gestational age and birth weight
- Predominant sex: Slight male predominance

Prevalence
Common disorder in premature infants, especially those born <28 weeks' gestation

ETIOLOGY AND PATHOPHYSIOLOGY
- Structurally immature lungs and surfactant deficiency lead to diffuse atelectasis.
- Exposure to high FiO_2 and barotrauma associated with mechanical ventilation trigger proinflammatory cytokines that further damage alveolar epithelium.
- Decreased lung compliance leads to alveolar hypoventilation and ventilation–perfusion mismatch.
- Impaired surfactant synthesis and secretion

Genetics
No known genetic pattern

RISK FACTORS
- Premature birth
- Infants of diabetic mothers
- Perinatal asphyxia
- History of RDS in a sibling

GENERAL PREVENTION
- Prevention of premature birth with education and regular prenatal care
- Antenatal corticosteroids
- Manage any medical issues appropriately.
- Healthy behaviors including diet, exercise
- Avoid exposure to tobacco smoke, alcohol, and illegal drugs.

 DIAGNOSIS

HISTORY
Preterm neonates with worsening respiratory distress beginning shortly after birth and progressing over 1st few hours of life

PHYSICAL EXAM
- Tachypnea
- Grunting
- Nasal flaring
- Subcostal and intercostal retractions
- Decreased breath sounds
- Cyanosis

DIFFERENTIAL DIAGNOSIS
- Early-onset group B streptococcal pneumonia and/or sepsis
- Transient tachypnea of newborn
- Meconium aspiration pneumonia

DIAGNOSTIC TESTS & INTERPRETATION
- CBC and blood culture to rule out sepsis, pneumonia
- Electrolytes: Monitor for hypoglycemia, hypocalcemia
- Arterial blood gases (ABGs):
  - Hypoxemia (which responds to supplemental oxygen)
  - Features of respiratory and metabolic acidosis
- Chest x-ray (CXR):
  - Diffuse reticulogranular pattern (ground-glass appearance)
  - Air bronchograms
  - Low lung volumes

Diagnostic Procedures/Other
Echocardiogram: Consider if murmur present to evaluate for patent ductus arteriosus (PDA) and contribution to lung disease due to L → R shunting (2)

Test Interpretation
- Macroscopically: Uniformly ruddy, airless appearance of lungs
- Microscopically: Diffuse atelectasis and hyaline membranes (eosinophilic and fibrinous membrane lining air spaces)

 TREATMENT

- Along with antenatal steroids, surfactants improve survival for preterm infants.
- Surfactants are now recommended routinely as early in the course of RDS as possible (3)[A].

GENERAL MEASURES
- Warm, humidified, oxygen-enriched gases if the neonate is ventilating effectively
- Continuous positive airway pressure (CPAP) if infant is active and breathing spontaneously
- Positive-pressure ventilation per ETT via conventional mechanical ventilator (CMV) or high-frequency oscillation ventilator (HFOV) if respiratory failure occurs (i.e., respiratory acidosis, apnea, or hypoxia despite nasal CPAP) (4)
- Transcutaneous monitors to measure CO_2 tension as necessary
- Pulse oximetry
- Umbilical artery catheter placement for continuous BP monitoring and sampling ABGs

MEDICATION
- Pulmonary surfactant (5,6)
- Side effects: Bradycardia, hypotension, airway obstruction/endotracheal tube blockage with administration; rapid changes in tidal volume due to increased compliance can cause a pneumothorax and small risk of pulmonary hemorrhage.
- Precautions: Transient adverse effects seen with the administration of surfactant may require stopping administration and alleviating situation; may proceed with dosing when stable.
- Contraindications: Presence of congenital anomalies incompatible with life beyond neonatal period; infant with laboratory evidence of lung maturity
- Perform frequent clinical and laboratory checks so that oxygen and ventilatory support can be modified to respond to respiratory changes.

ISSUES FOR REFERRAL
Comorbid conditions associated with prematurity may require consultation during the course of the infant's NICU admission, including PDA (cardiology consult), necrotizing enterocolitis (NEC) (gastroenterology), retinopathy of prematurity (ROP) (ophthalmology), etc.

ADDITIONAL THERAPIES
Treat associated problems of prematurity.

IN-PATIENT CONSIDERATIONS
Admission Criteria/Initial Stabilization
All neonates with respiratory distress require evaluation, monitoring, and treatment in a NICU; treatment may be required in the delivery room.

IV Fluids
- To maintain blood pressure and perfusion, when necessary
- To provide optimal fluid balance, provide nutritional support

Nursing
- Supportive care
- Thermoneutral environment
- Respiratory monitoring
- Establish relationship with family to provide education and emotional support.

Discharge Criteria
- Should have stable vital signs and pulse oximetry before discharge.
- Medical home and support services should be in place.

 ONGOING CARE

FOLLOW-UP RECOMMENDATIONS
Following discharge, infants should be followed closely by their physicians to monitor growth and respiratory symptomatology.

DIET
As clinically indicated

PATIENT EDUCATION
- Educate parents regarding the risks in subsequent pregnancies.
- Advise parents regarding potential issues with chronic lung disease.
- For patient education materials favorably reviewed on this topic, go to Boston Children's Hospital Web site (www.childrenshospital.org) and search for respiratory distress syndrome in the "My Child Has" window.

PROGNOSIS
Prognosis and outcome highly dependent on gestational age and birth weight

COMPLICATIONS
- Complications specific to NRDS:
  - Pneumothorax
  - Chronic lung disease, bronchopulmonary dysplasia (BPD)
  - Pulmonary interstitial edema (PIE)
- Additional complications may occur related to therapeutic interventions and comorbid conditions.

REFERENCES
1. Stoll BJ, Hansen NI, Bell EF, et al. Neonatal outcomes of extremely preterm infants from the NICHD Neonatal Research Network. *Pediatrics*. 2010;126:443.
2. Hamrick SE, Hansmann G. Patent ductus arteriosus of the preterm infant. *Pediatrics*. 2010;125: 1020–1030.
3. Sweet DG, Halliday HL. The use of surfactants in 2009. *Arch Dis Child Educ Pract Ed*. 2009;94: 78–83.
4. Sekar KC, Corff KE. To tube or not to tube babies with respiratory distress syndrome. *J Perinatol*. 2009;29(Suppl 2):S68–S72.
5. Engle WA, American Academy of Pediatrics Committee on Fetus and Newborn. Surfactant-replacement therapy for respiratory distress in the preterm and term neonate. *Pediatrics*. 2008;121: 419–432.
6. Moya F. Synthetic surfactants: Where are we? Evidence from randomized, controlled clinical trials. *J Perinatol*. 2009;29(Suppl 2):S23–S28.

ADDITIONAL READING
- Jain NJ, Kruse LK, Demissie K. Impact of mode of delivery on neonatal complications: Trends between 1997 and 2005. *J Matern Fetal Neonatal Med*. 2009:1–10.
- Ramachandrappa A, Jain L. Health issues of the late preterm infant. *Pediatr Clin North Am*. 2009;56: 565–577.
- Soll RF. Multiple versus single dose natural surfactant extract for severe neonatal respiratory distress syndrome. *Cochrane Database Sys Rev*. 1999;2:CD000141.
- Support Study Group of the Eunice Kennedy Shriver NICHD Neonatal Research Network, Finer NN, Carlo WA, et al. Early CPAP vs surfactant in extremely preterm infants. *N Engl J Med*. 2010;362:1970.

 CODES

ICD10
P22.0 Respiratory distress syndrome of newborn

CLINICAL PEARLS
- Surfactants are used routinely as early in the course of RDS as possible.
- If an infant has a murmur, consider an echocardiogram to rule out PDA and shunting.
- Prognosis and outcome are highly dependent on gestational age and birth weight.

RESPIRATORY SYNCYTIAL VIRUS INFECTION

Elizabeth C. McKeen, MD, FAAP

BASICS

Respiratory syncytial virus (RSV) is a medium-sized, membrane-bound ribonucleic acid (RNA) virus that causes acute respiratory tract illness in all ages, with most clinically significant disease in infants and young children.

DESCRIPTION
A major cause of respiratory illness, either of the upper respiratory tract (URT) or of the lower respiratory tract (LRT/bronchiolitis):
- In adults, RSV causes URT infections (URTIs).
- In infants and children, RSV causes URTIs and LRT infections (bronchiolitis).

Pediatric Considerations
- 90–95% of children are infected at least once by the age of 24 months; reinfection is common.
- Leading cause of pediatric bronchiolitis (50–90%)
- Premature infants are at increased risk for severe acute RSV infection.

EPIDEMIOLOGY
- Seasonality: Highest incidence of RSV infection in the US is between December and March.
- Morbidity: RSV infection leads to 75–125,000 hospitalizations annually nationwide.

ETIOLOGY AND PATHOPHYSIOLOGY
- RSV-induced bronchiolitis causes acute inflammation, edema, and necrosis of the epithelial cells lining the small airways, air trapping, bronchospasm, and increased mucus production.
- RSV is a medium-sized, membrane-bound RNA virus. It develops in the cytoplasm of infected cells and matures by budding from the plasma membrane.
- Infection spreads via infected droplets, either airborne or conveyed on hands, that are inoculated in the nose or conjunctivae of a susceptible subject.

Genetics
- A genetic predisposition to severe RSV infections may be associated with polymorphisms in cytokine- and chemokine-related genes, including *CCR5*, *IL4* and its receptor, *IL8*, *IL10*, and *IL13*.
- Infants with transplacentally acquired antibody against RSV are not protected against infection, but may have milder symptoms.

RISK FACTORS
- Risk factors for severe disease:
  - History of prematurity
  - Age <12 weeks
  - Underlying cardiopulmonary disease
  - Immunodeficiency
- Other risk factors:
  - Low socioeconomic status
  - Exposure to environmental air pollutants
  - Childcare attendance
  - Severe neuromuscular disease
  - In adults, occupational exposure: Pediatric hospital staff, teachers, and daycare workers

GENERAL PREVENTION
- Hand decontamination is the most important step in preventing nosocomial spread of RSV:
  - Alcohol-based rubs are preferred; an alternative is hand washing with antimicrobial soap (1)[B].
  - In patients with proven or suspected RSV, infection should be isolated or cohorted.
- Exposure to passive tobacco smoke should be avoided, especially in infants and children (2)[A].
- Palivizumab (Synagis), a monoclonal antibody directed against the F (fusion) protein of RSV, is indicated as prophylaxis for the following groups (as of the 2012–2013 season):
  - Infants and children <24 months of age with:
    ○ Chronic lung disease of prematurity requiring medical therapy within 6 months of the start of RSV season
    ○ Hemodynamically significant cyanotic or acyanotic congenital heart disease
    ○ Congenital abnormalities of the airway or neuromuscular disease
    ○ Prematurity <32 weeks' gestation, even in the absence of chronic lung disease. Those born at ≤28 weeks should receive prophylaxis during their first RSV season whenever that occurs during the first 12 months of life. Those born at 29–32 weeks benefit most from prophylaxis up to 6 months of age.
    ○ Prematurity of <35 weeks' gestation *and* congenital abnormalities of the airway or neuromuscular disease
    ○ Prematurity 32 0/7–34 6/7 weeks' gestation *and* at least 1 of 2 risk factors born within 3 months before the start of RSV season or at any time throughout the RSV season:
      ■ Infant attends childcare, or
      ■ ≥1 more siblings or other children <5 years living permanently in the child's household
  - Dosage: 5 monthly doses beginning in November or December at 15 mg/kg per dose administered IM
  - For most current palivizumab guidelines, see the most current edition of Red Book.

COMMONLY ASSOCIATED CONDITIONS
- Asthma
- Serious bacterial infection (SBI) in infants and children with concurrent RSV infection is rare. When it occurs, the most likely etiology is URTI, followed by acute otitis media.

DIAGNOSIS

ALERT
In most cases, diagnosis should be made by history and physical exam alone. Laboratory and radiologic studies should not be ordered routinely (1)[B].

HISTORY
Patients may present with a variety of symptoms, including but not limited to:
- Upper respiratory congestion
- Respiratory distress
- Cough
- Fever

PHYSICAL EXAM
- Fever
- Rhinorrhea
- Cough
- Wheezing
- Crackles
- Increased work of breathing, manifested as tachypnea, retractions, nasal flaring, and/or grunting
- In infants and children, evidence of poor hydration status, such as feeding difficulty, dry mucous membranes, poor skin turgor
- Repeat examinations over time are most helpful in providing the best overall assessment.

Pediatric Considerations
Young infants with bronchiolitis may develop apnea, which is associated with increased risk of prolonged hospitalization, ICU admission, and mechanical ventilation.

DIFFERENTIAL DIAGNOSIS
- Mild illness/URTI:
  - Other (non-RSV) respiratory viral infections, such as rhinovirus, human metapneumovirus, influenza virus, human bocavirus
  - Allergic rhinitis
  - Sinusitis
- Severe illness/LRTI:
  - Bronchiolitis
  - Asthma
  - Pneumonia
  - Foreign-body aspiration

DIAGNOSTIC TESTS & INTERPRETATION
Initial Tests (lab, imaging)
- Routine laboratory testing is not necessary:
  - If obtained, WBC count may be normal or elevated.
  - Virologic tests for RSV, despite high predictive value, rarely change management decisions or outcomes for patients with clinically diagnosed bronchiolitis.
- Given the low risk of SBI, full septic workups in these patients should not be undertaken routinely.
- Chest x-ray (CXR) has not been proven to affect patient outcomes or predict disease severity.
- A CXR may be most helpful when a patient does not improve as expected, if the severity of the disease requires further investigation, or if another diagnosis is suspected.
- If obtained, typical findings on CXR can include:
  - Hyperinflation and peribronchiolar thickening
  - Atelectasis
  - Interstitial infiltrates
  - Segmental or lobar consolidation
  - Pleural fluid (rare)

TREATMENT

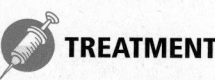

GENERAL MEASURES
- Clinicians must promptly assess hydration status and ability to take fluids orally. Dehydration must be treated adequately with an oral or IV fluid, with special attention to infants.
- Supplemental O_2 is indicated if the saturation of peripheral oxygen (SpO_2) falls persistently <90% in previously healthy patients:
  - An SpO_2 of 90% is an approximate cutoff and should be adjusted in the context of the patient.
  - Continuous O_2 monitoring can be discontinued in a patient whose clinical status is improving.

MEDICATION

First Line
No 1st-line medication for RSV infections; treatment is usually supportive.

Second Line
- Bronchodilators show small, short-term improvements in clinical scores, but this small benefit should be weighed against the costs and adverse effects of these agents:
  - Bronchodilators do not improve oxygen saturation, reduce hospital admission after outpatient treatment, shorten the duration of hospitalization, nor reduce the time to resolution of illness at home.
  - Routine use not recommended
- Epinephrine is superior compared with placebo for short-term outcomes for outpatients, particularly in the first 24 hours of care:
  - Evidence shows the effectiveness and superiority of adrenaline for outcomes of most clinical relevance among outpatients with acute bronchiolitis, and evidence from a single precise trial for combined adrenaline and dexamethasone (3)[A].
- Current evidence does not support a clinically relevant effect of systemic or inhaled glucocorticoids on admissions or length of hospitalization (4)[A]:
  - However, combined dexamethasone and epinephrine may reduce outpatient admissions, but results are exploratory and safety data limited (4)[A].
- A recent study found that montelukast (Singulair) has no effect on the clinical course of acute bronchiolitis (5)[C].
- Ribavirin, a nucleoside analogue and antiviral agent, has not been shown to be efficacious in the treatment of RSV (6)[C], particularly in immunocompromised patients (7)[A].
- There is no current evidence that nebulized rhDNase changes clinical outcomes children <24 months who are hospitalized with acute RSV bronchiolitis (8)[B].
- Use of antibacterial agents should be reserved for patients who have specific signs of a coexisting SBI. When such an infection is present, it should be treated in the same manner as in the absence of RSV infection (9)[B].
- Current evidence suggests nebulized 3% saline may significantly reduce the length of hospital stay and improve the clinical severity score in infants with acute viral bronchiolitis (10)[A].

ADDITIONAL THERAPIES
Bulb suctioning of the nares may provide some comfort to infants and allow for easier feeding.

Pediatric Considerations
Parents must be reminded that the American Academy of Pediatrics strongly recommends against the use of over-the-counter (OTC) cough and cold medications in children <6 years of age due to lack of efficacy and the risk of life-threatening side effects.

COMPLEMENTARY AND ALTERNATIVE MEDICINE
Clinicians should inquire about patients' use of complementary and alternative therapies, such as echinacea and zinc.

IN-PATIENT CONSIDERATIONS

Admission Criteria/Initial Stabilization
- Clinical judgment of the patient's degree of respiratory distress is the most important consideration.
- Significant respiratory distress and/or O_2 requirement to keep SpO_2 >90%
- Inability to hydrate orally
- A full history and physical exam should be completed, including the ABCs. Special attention should be paid to respiratory and hydration status.
- Mechanical ventilation is required in about 5% of infants hospitalized with RSV and 20% of children with underlying congenital heart disease, chronic lung disease, or immunosuppression, and should be instituted in the case of respiratory failure.

IV Fluids
See "Treatment."

Discharge Criteria
No set criteria for discharge exists, but the following guidelines may be helpful:
- Respiratory distress resolving or resolved
- Patient oxygenating well without O_2 therapy
- Adequate oral intake for sustained hydration
- Caretaker able to clear the infant's airway with bulb suctioning
- Home resources adequate to support use of any necessary home therapies
- Education of family complete

 ## ONGOING CARE

FOLLOW-UP RECOMMENDATIONS
Close follow-up with the patient's primary health care provider is essential.

PATIENT EDUCATION
- See "General Prevention."
- *Bronchiolitis and Your Child*, available at http://familydoctor.org/online/famdocen/home/children/parents/common/common/020.html.

PROGNOSIS
Most patients with RSV infection recover fully within 7–10 days, although reinfection is common.

COMPLICATIONS
- Infants hospitalized for RSV may be at increased risk for recurrent wheezing and reduced pulmonary function, particularly during the 1st decade of life.
- Overall mortality for infants and children <24 months of age is <1%.

REFERENCES

1. American Academy of Pediatrics Subcommittee on Diagnosis and Management of Bronchiolitis. *Pediatrics*. 2006;118:1774–1793.
2. Difranza JR, Masaquel A, Barrett AM, et al. Systematic literature review assessing tobacco smoke exposure as a risk factor for serious respiratory syncytial virus disease among infants and young children. *BMC Pediatrics*. 2012;12(1): 81. Epub 2012 Jun 21.
3. Hartling L, Fernandes RM, Bialy L, et al. Steroids and bronchodilators for acute bronchiolitis in the first two years of life: Systematic review and meta-analysis. *BMJ*. 2011;342:d1714.
4. Fernandes RM, Bialy LM, Vandermeer B, et al. Glucocorticoids for acute viral bronchiolitis in infants and young children. *Cochrane Database Syst Rev*. 2010;(10):CD004878.
5. Amirav I, Luder AS, Kruger N, et al. A double-blind, placebo-controlled, randomized trial of montelukast for acute bronchiolitis. *Pediatrics*. 2008;122:e1249–e1255.
6. Ventre K. Ribavirin for respiratory syncytial virus infection of the lower respiratory tract in infants and young children. Cochrane Acute Respiratory Infections Group. *Cochrane Database Sys Rev*. 2009;1:CD000181.
7. Hynicka LM, Ensor CR. Prophylaxis and treatment of respiratory syncytial virus in adult immunocompromised patients. *Ann Pharmacother*. 2012;46(4):558–566. Epub 2012 Mar 6.
8. Enriquez A. Nebulised deoxyribonuclease for viral bronchiolitis in children younger than 24 months. *Cochrane Database Syst Rev*. 2012 Nov 14;11:CD008395.
9. Spurling GKP. Antibiotics for bronchiolitis in children. Cochrane Acute Respiratory Infections Group. *Cochrane Database Sys Rev*. 2007;1:CD005189.
10. Zang L. Nebulized hypertonic saline solution for acute bronchiolitis in infants. *Cochrane Database Syst Rev*. 2008;(4):CD006458.

ADDITIONAL READING

- American Academy of Pediatrics. *Red Book: 2012 Report of the Committee on Infectious Diseases*. Section 3: Respiratory Syncytial Virus. Pickering LK, ed. 29th ed. Elk Grove Village, IL: American Academy of Pediatrics; 2012.
- Gadomski AM, Brower M. Bronchodilators for bronchiolitis. *Cochrane Database Syst Rev*. 2010;CD001266.

 ## CODES

ICD10
- B97.4 Respiratory syncytial virus causing diseases classd elswhr
- J06.9 Acute upper respiratory infection, unspecified
- J21.0 Acute bronchiolitis due to respiratory syncytial virus

CLINICAL PEARLS
- RSV causes 50–90% of pediatric bronchiolitis.
- Hand sanitation is key for prevention in the general population.
- Palivizumab is key for prevention in the high-risk population.
- Diagnosis is clinical in most cases.
- Treatment is usually supportive.
- Routine lab testing is not necessary, including virologic tests for RSV because, despite high predictive value, they rarely change management decisions or outcomes for patients with clinically diagnosed bronchiolitis.

RESTLESS LEGS SYNDROME

Donald E. Watenpaugh, PhD • John R. Burk, MD

BASICS

DESCRIPTION
- Sensorimotor disorder defined by 4 criteria (1):
  – A strong urge to move the legs, usually with paresthesia
  – Symptoms emerge during inactivity.
  – Movement relieves symptoms, but they soon recur with inactivity.
  – Symptoms occur in the evening/night and are not solely accounted for by another disorder.
- Symptoms may involve the arms or be more generalized.
- Patient may also report involuntary leg jerks.
- System(s) affected: Musculoskeletal; Nervous
- Synonym(s): Willis-Ekbom disease

EPIDEMIOLOGY
Incidence
- Onset at any age; increases with age
- Predominant sex: Male = Female (nulliparous); Female (parous) $2\times$ > Male (2)

Prevalence
- 4–15% of Caucasian adults; underdiagnosed (3)
- 1–3% in children and adolescents
- Increases with age
- Lower in non-Caucasians

Pregnancy Considerations
10–30% prevalence; exacerbates existing restless legs syndrome (RLS) (2)

ETIOLOGY AND PATHOPHYSIOLOGY
- Primary RLS: Subcortical dopamine deficiency/dysmetabolism (3)
- Secondary RLS:
  – Iron deficiency and associated conditions
  – Chronic extremity tissue pathology/inflammation
  – Medications:
    ○ Most antidepressants (exceptions: bupropion and desipramine)
    ○ Dopamine-blocking antiemetics (e.g., metoclopramide)
    ○ Some antiepileptic agents (e.g., phenytoin)
    ○ Phenothiazine antipsychotics; donepezil
    ○ Theophylline and other xanthines
    ○ Antihistamines/Over-the-counter (OTC) cold preparations (e.g., pseudoephedrine)
    ○ Adrenergics, stimulants

Genetics
- Primary RLS heritability: ~50%
- Genetically heterogenous (4):
  – Susceptibility loci: 2p14, 2q, 6p21.2, 9p, 12q, 14q, 15q23, and 20p
  – Genes: MEIS1, MAP2K5/LBXCOR1, and BTBD9

RISK FACTORS
- Family history (3,4)
- Aging
- Chronic inactivity
- Inadequate sleep
- Associated conditions (see below)
- Certain medications (see "Etiology")

GENERAL PREVENTION
- Regular physical activity/exercise
- Adequate sleep
- Avoid evening caffeine, alcohol, tobacco.
- Avoid evening use of medications that cause RLS.

COMMONLY ASSOCIATED CONDITIONS
- Periodic limb movements of sleep, insomnia, sleep walking, other parasomnias, delayed sleep phase
- Iron deficiency, renal disease/uremia/dialysis, gastric surgery, liver disease
- Parkinson disease, multiple sclerosis, peripheral neuropathy, migraine
- Orthopedic problems, arthritis, fibromyalgia
- Venous insufficiency/peripheral vascular disease, erectile dysfunction
- Pulmonary hypertension, lung transplantation, chronic obstructive pulmonary disease (COPD)
- ADHD, anxiety/depression, "sundowning"
- Pregnancy (especially if Fe- or folate-deficient)

DIAGNOSIS

- Depends on history, yet often "difficult to describe"
- May go undiagnosed for years by multiple doctors

HISTORY
- Signs/Symptoms (see also "Description") (1,4,5):
  – Limited to evening, night
  – Example descriptions: Burning, achy, itching, antsy, "can't get comfortable"
  – Painful in ~35% of patients
  – Discomfort associated with overwhelming urge to move and relieved by movement
  – Urge to move may be the only "discomfort."
  – Movement frequency every 10–90 seconds (mean ~25 seconds)
  – Some patients must get up and walk.
  – May involve arms or, rarely, whole body
  – Periodic movements in sleep in ~80% of patients
  – Insomnia, fatigue, anxiety
- Severity range: From rare, minor problem to daily severe impact on quality of life
- Primary RLS presents early and progresses slowly.
- Secondary RLS:
  – Precipitated by other conditions/medications
  – Tends to progress rapidly
  – Resolves to extent that cause(es) resolve

Pediatric Considerations
If all 4 diagnostic criteria not met, apply first 3 + 2 of the following (4)[C]:
- Insomnia or sleep disturbance
- RLS in immediate biological relative
- Periodic limb movements during sleep

Geriatric Considerations
For diagnosis in the cognitively impaired (5)[C]:
- Rubbing or kneading the legs in evening
- Evening hyperactivity (foot tapping, pacing, fidgeting, tossing/turning in bed)

PHYSICAL EXAM
Patient may be fidgety, unable to sit still.

DIFFERENTIAL DIAGNOSIS
- Claudication: Movement does not relieve pain and may worsen it.
- Motor neuron disease fasciculation/tremor: No discomfort or circadian pattern
- Peripheral neuropathy: Usually no circadian pattern; unresponsive to dopamine agonists.
- Dermatitis/Pruritus: Movement only to scratch; no circadian pattern
- Sleep-related leg cramps: Isolated and very painful muscle contracture
- Periodic limb movement disorder: No wakeful movements
- Sleep starts: Isolated involuntary events
- Rhythmic movement sleep disorder: Movement periodicity faster than RLS
- Growing pains: No urge to move or relief by movement; circadian pattern opposite RLS
- ADHD: No sleep disorders or complaints in diagnostic criteria.

DIAGNOSTIC TESTS & INTERPRETATION
Serum ferritin to assess for iron deficiency

Diagnostic Procedures/Other
- Sleep study helpful but not required:
  – Frequent, periodic movements during wake
- Suggested immobilization test:
  – Conducted before nocturnal polysomnography
  – Patient attempts to sit still in bed for 1 hour.
  – >40 movements per hour suggests RLS.
- Ankle actigraphy for in-home use
- Electromyography, nerve conduction studies for peripheral neuropathy, radiculopathy

Test Interpretation
- Serum ferritin: <75 ng/mL
- Transferrin saturation: <16%

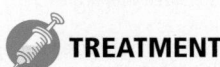

TREATMENT

1st-line treatments (4,6)[B]:
- Prescribed daily exercise; adequate sleep.
- Correct iron deficiency.
- Dopaminergic medications
- For secondary RLS, treat cause(s).
- Multiple possible causes are *not* mutually exclusive.

GENERAL MEASURES
- If iron deficient, supplement:
  – 325 mg $FeSO_4$ with vitamin C between meals t.i.d.
  – Repletion requires months.
- Daily exercise (4,6)[B]
- Unusual activity may exacerbate symptoms.
- Regular and replete sleep
- Hot bath and leg massage
- Warm the legs (long heavy socks, electric blanket)
- Intense mental activity (games, puzzles, etc.)

MEDICATION

- Use minimum effective dose (1,7)[A]
- Daytime sleepiness unusual with doses and timing for RLS.
- Severe/refractory RLS may require combination therapy.

First Line

- Dopamine agonists; titrate every 3 days to minimum necessary dose:
  - Pramipexole (Mirapex): 0.125–1.5 mg 1 hour before symptoms; titrate by 0.125 mg
  - Ropinirole (Requip): 0.25–4 mg 1 hour before symptoms; titrate by 0.25 mg
  - Divide dose for evening and bedtime symptoms.
  - Liver disease: Pramipexole (renal clearance)
  - Renal insufficiency: Ropinirole (hepatic catabolism)
  - Transdermal Rotigotine (Neupro): 1–3 mg patch; titrate by 1 mg weekly
  - Avoid dopamine agonists in psychotic patients, particularly if taking dopamine antagonists.
  - Add a different class of medication before exceeding dopamine agonist recommended dose.
- Gabapentin enacarbil (Horizant): 300–600 mg every day ~5:00 p.m.
- All other medications off-label

Second Line

- Anticonvulsants (for neuropathic RLS):
  - Pregabalin (Lyrica): 50–300 mg/d
  - Carbamazepine: 200–800 mg/d
- Opioids (low risk of tolerance/addiction at bedtime):
  - Hydrocodone: 5–20 mg/d
  - Tramadol: 50 mg/d
  - Oxycodone: 2.5–20 mg/d
- Benzodiazepines and agonists (for associated insomnia or anxiety):
  - Clonazepam (Klonopin): 0.5–3 mg/d
  - Temazepam, triazolam, alprazolam, zaleplon, zolpidem, and diazepam
- Dopamine agonists:
  - Carbidopa-levodopa (Sinemet or Sinemet CR): 25/100–100/400; p.r.n. for sporadic symptoms
  - Cabergoline: 0.25–3 mg (warning: Valvulopathy)

Pregnancy Considerations

- Initial approach: Nonpharmacologic therapies, iron supplements (2)[C]
- Avoid medications Class C or D.
- In 3rd trimester, low-dose opioids or clonazepam may be considered.

Pediatric Considerations

- First-line treatment: Nonpharmacologic (4)[C]
- Low-dose clonidine or clonazepam may be considered.

Geriatric Considerations

- Avoid medications that cause dizziness or unsteadiness.
- Many medications given to elderly cause/exacerbate RLS (5)[C].

ISSUES FOR REFERRAL

- Severe, intractable symptoms
- Augmentation response to dopaminergic therapy
- Peripheral neuropathy; orthopedic problems
- Peripheral vascular disease; intransigent iron deficiency

ADDITIONAL THERAPIES

- Vitamin, mineral supplements: Ca, Mg, B_{12}, folate
- Clonidine: 0.1–0.7 mg/d
- Baclofen: 20–80 mg/d
- Quinine
- Methadone: Up to 30 mg/d
- Prescription or OTC hypnotics

SURGERY/OTHER PROCEDURES

For orthopedic, neuropathic, or leg vascular disease (laser ablation, sclerotherapy, etc.)

COMPLEMENTARY AND ALTERNATIVE MEDICINE

- Sequential pneumatic leg compression
- Enhanced external counterpulsation
- Acupuncture
- MicroVas therapy
- Near-infrared light

IN-PATIENT CONSIDERATIONS

- Control RLS after orthopedic procedures.
- Addition/Withdrawal of medications affecting RLS (e.g., narcotics)
- Changes in medical status may require medication changes.

IV Fluids

- Iron infusion when oral Fe fails or contraindicated.
- When NPO, consider IV opiates.

Nursing

- Evening walks, hot baths, leg massage, and warming
- Sleep interruption risks prolonged wakefulness.

 ONGOING CARE

FOLLOW-UP RECOMMENDATIONS

Patient Monitoring

- At 2-week intervals until stable, then annually
- If taking iron, remeasure ferritin
- If status changes, assess for associated conditions and medications.

DIET

Avoid evening caffeine and alcohol.

PATIENT EDUCATION

- Willis-Ekbom Disease Foundation: www.rls.org
- National Sleep Foundation: www.sleepfoundation.org

PROGNOSIS

- Primary RLS: Lifelong condition with no current cure
- Secondary RLS: May subside with resolution of precipitating factors
- Current therapies usually control symptoms.

COMPLICATIONS

- Augmentation of symptoms from prolonged dopaminergic therapy:
  - Symptoms increase in severity, occur earlier, and/or spread.
  - Higher doses increase risk.
  - Highest risk from daily levodopa or Sinemet
  - Iron deficiency increases risk.
  - Add alternative medication, then slowly down-titrate dopamine agonist.
- Obsessive–compulsive or impulse-control disorders from dopamine agonists
- Vicious cycle between sleep loss from RLS and exacerbation of RLS by sleep loss
- Iatrogenic RLS (from antidepressants, etc.)

REFERENCES

1. Garcia-Borreguero D, Stillman P, Benes H, et al. Algorithms for the diagnosis and treatment of restless legs syndrome in primary care. *BMC Neurol.* 2011;11:28. Epub 2011 Feb 27.
2. Manconi M, Ulfberg J, Berger K, et al. When gender matters: Restless legs syndrome. Report of the "RLS and woman" workshop endorsed by the European RLS Study Group. *Sleep Med Rev.* 2012;16(4):297–307. Epub 2011 Nov 9.
3. Yeh P, Walters AS, Tsuang JW. Restless legs syndrome: A comprehensive overview on its epidemiology, risk factors, and treatment. *Sleep Breath.* 2011. Epub 2011 Oct 26.
4. Picchietti MA, Picchietti DL. Advances in pediatric restless legs syndrome: Iron, genetics, diagnosis and treatment. *Sleep Med.* 2010;11:643–651.
5. Spiegelhalder K, Hornyak M. Restless legs syndrome in older adults. *Clin Geriatr Med.* 2008;24:167–180.
6. Aukerman MM, Aukerman D, Bayard M, et al. Exercise and restless legs syndrome: A randomized controlled trial. *J Am Board Fam Med.* 2006;19:487–493.
7. Aurora RN, Kristo DA, Bista SR, et al. The treatment of restless legs syndrome and periodic limb movement disorder in adults-an update for 2012: practice parameters with an evidence-based systematic review and meta-analyses: An American Academy of Sleep Medicine Clinical Practice Guideline. *Sleep.* 2012;35(8):1039–1062. Epub 2012 Aug 1.

 SEE ALSO

- Periodic Limb Movement Disorder
- Algorithm: Restless Leg Syndrome (RLS)

 CODES

ICD10

G25.81 Restless legs syndrome

CLINICAL PEARLS

- Insomnia with frequent tossing/turning and difficulty "getting comfortable" is often RLS.
- Many antidepressants, antipsychotics, antiemetics, and antihistamines cause or exacerbate RLS.
- RLS may interfere with use of positive airway pressure to treat obstructive sleep apnea.
- RLS and other sleep disorders may cause ADHD.

RETINAL DETACHMENT

Richard W. Allinson, MD

 BASICS

DESCRIPTION
- Separation of the sensory retina from the underlying retinal pigment epithelium
- Rhegmatogenous retinal detachment (RRD): Most common type; occurs when the fluid vitreous gains access to the subretinal space through a break in the retina (Greek *rhegma*, "rent")
- Exudative or serous detachment: Occurs in the absence of a retinal break, usually in association with inflammation or a tumor
- Traction detachment: Vitreoretinal adhesions mechanically pull the retina from the retinal pigment epithelium. The most common cause is proliferative diabetic retinopathy.
- System(s) affected: Nervous

EPIDEMIOLOGY
Incidence
- Predominant age: Incidence increases with age.
- Predominant sex: Male > Female (3:2)
- Per year: 1/10,000 in patients who have not had cataract surgery

Prevalence
After cataract surgery, 1–3% of patients will develop a retinal detachment.

ETIOLOGY AND PATHOPHYSIOLOGY
- Traction from a posterior vitreous detachment (PVD) causes most retinal tears. With aging, vitreous gel liquefies, leading to separation of the vitreous from the retina. The vitreous gel remains attached at the vitreous base, in the retinal periphery, resulting in vitreous traction that produces tears in the retinal periphery. There is an ~15% chance of developing a retinal tear from a PVD.
- PVD associated with vitreous hemorrhage has a high incidence of retinal tears.
- Exudative detachment:
  - Tumors
  - Inflammatory diseases (Harada, posterior scleritis)
  - Miscellaneous (central serous retinopathy, uveal effusion syndrome, malignant hypertension)
- Traction detachment:
  - Proliferative diabetic retinopathy
  - Cicatricial retinopathy of prematurity
  - Proliferative sickle-cell retinopathy
- Penetrating trauma

Genetics
- Most cases are sporadic.
- There is an increased risk of RRD if a sibling has been affected by this condition. The risk increases with higher levels of myopia in the family history (1)[B].

RISK FACTORS
- Myopia (>5 diopters)
- Aphakia or pseudophakia: In patients undergoing small-incision coaxial phacoemulsification with high myopia (axial length ≥26 mm), the incidence of retinal detachment is 2.7%.
- PVD and associated conditions (e.g., aphakia, inflammatory disease, and trauma)

- Trauma
- Retinal detachment in fellow eye
- Lattice degeneration: A vitreoretinal abnormality found in 6–10% of the general population
- Glaucoma: 4–7% of patients with retinal detachment have chronic open-angle glaucoma.
- Vitreoretinal tufts: Peripheral retinal tufts are caused by focal areas of vitreous traction.
- Meridional folds: Redundant retina usually is found in the supranasal quadrant.

GENERAL PREVENTION
Patients at risk for retinal detachment should have regular ophthalmologic exams.

Geriatric Considerations
- Posterior vitreous detachment
- Cataract surgery

Pediatric Considerations
Usually associated with underlying vitreoretinal disorders and/or retinopathy of prematurity

COMMONLY ASSOCIATED CONDITIONS
- Lattice degeneration
- High myopia
- Cataract surgery
- Glaucoma
- History of retinal detachment in the fellow eye
- Trauma

Pregnancy Considerations
Preeclampsia/Eclampsia may be associated with exudative retinal detachment. No intervention is indicated, provided hypertension is controlled. Prognosis is usually good.

 DIAGNOSIS

HISTORY
- Sudden flashes (photopsia)
- Shower of floaters
- Visual field loss: "Curtain coming across vision"
- Central vision will be preserved if the macula is not detached.
- Poor visual acuity (20/200 or worse), with loss of central vision when macula is detached

PHYSICAL EXAM
- Slit-lamp exam
- Dilated fundus exam with binocular indirect ophthalmoscopy

DIFFERENTIAL DIAGNOSIS
Retinoschisis (splitting of the retina):
- Vitreous cells and vitreous hemorrhage are found rarely in the vitreous with retinoschisis, whereas they are seen commonly in RRD.
- Retinoschisis usually has a smooth surface and is dome shaped, whereas RRD often has a corrugated, irregular surface.

DIAGNOSTIC TESTS & INTERPRETATION
Visual field testing: Differentiates RRD from retinoschisis. An absolute scotoma is seen in retinoschisis, whereas RRD causes a relative scotoma.

Initial Tests (lab, imaging)
- US can demonstrate a detached retina and may be helpful when the retina cannot be visualized directly (e.g., with cataracts).
- Fluorescein dye leakage can be seen in exudative retinal detachment; caused by central serous retinopathy and other inflammatory conditions.

Test Interpretation
- Elevation of the neurosensory retina from the underlying retinal pigment epithelium
- Elevation of retina associated with ≥1 retinal tears in RRD or elevation of the retina without tears in exudative detachment
- In 3–10% of patients with presumed RRD, no definite retinal break is found.
- Tenting of the retina without retinal tears in traction detachment
- Pigmented cells within the vitreous ("tobacco dust")

 TREATMENT

GENERAL MEASURES
- Not all retinal tears or breaks need to be treated:
  - Flap or horseshoe tears in symptomatic patients (e.g., patients with flashes or floaters) are treated frequently.
  - Operculated holes in symptomatic patients are treated sometimes.
  - Atrophic holes in symptomatic patients are treated rarely.
- Lattice degeneration with or without holes within the lattice in an asymptomatic patient with prior retinal detachment in the fellow eye may be treated prophylactically.
- Flap retinal tears in asymptomatic patients frequently are treated prophylactically.
- Exudative detachments usually are managed by treating underlying disorder.
- Traction detachments usually are managed by observation. If the fovea is involved, a vitrectomy is needed.

MEDICATION
First Line
- Intraocular gases:
  - Air
  - Perfluoropropane (C_3F_8)
  - Sulfur hexafluoride (SF_6)
- Perfluorocarbon liquids
- Silicone oil
- Contraindications to intraocular gas: Patients with poorly controlled glaucoma
- Precautions with intraocular gas: Expanding intraocular gas bubble increases intraocular pressure; therefore, avoid higher altitudes.
- Significant possible interactions with intraocular gas: Nitrous oxide used in general anesthesia can expand an intraocular gas bubble.

Second Line
Steroids may cause worsening of central serous retinopathy.

SURGERY/OTHER PROCEDURES

- Timing of repairs:
  - Macula attached: Within 24 hours. If the detachment is peripheral and does not have features suggestive of rapid progression (e.g., large and/or superior tears), repair can be performed within a few days.
  - Macula recently detached: Within 10 days of development of a macula-off retinal detachment (2)[B]
  - Old macular detachment: Elective repair within 2 weeks
- If a retinal break has led to the development of a retinal detachment, surgery is needed. Surgical options (and combinations) include:
  - Demarcation laser treatment
  - Pneumatic retinopexy: Head positioning is required postoperatively.
  - Scleral buckle
  - Vitrectomy
  - Perfluorocarbon liquids for giant tears (circumferential tears ≥90°)
  - Silicone oil for complex repairs
- Anesthesia: Local or general
- RRD may have >1 break. If any retinal break is not closed at the time of surgery, the surgery will fail.
- Additional surgery may be required if the retina redetaches secondary to a new retinal break or because of proliferative vitreoretinopathy (PVR).
- Adjuvant combination therapy using 5-fluorouracil (5-FU) and low-molecular-weight heparin (LMWH) may reduce the incidence of PVR in patients undergoing vitrectomy for RRD who are at a greater risk of developing PVR, such as patients with uveitis, but does not seem to be of benefit in cases of established PVR.
- If a vitreous hemorrhage is present, presumably from a retinal tear, and the fundus cannot be well visualized, consideration can be given for early vitrectomy (3)[C].
- There is a trend toward primary vitrectomy in the management of RRD. Eyes undergoing PPV for primary RRD repair may not need the addition of a scleral buckle (4)[B].
- There is a reduced incidence of intraoperative retinal tear formation using a transconjunctival cannulated pars plana vitrectomy system compared to the standard 20-gauge system requiring suture closure (5)[C].

IN-PATIENT CONSIDERATIONS

Admission Criteria/Initial Stabilization

- Recognition of condition is key (see "Diagnosis").
- Refer to an ophthalmologist for exam and treatment, if indicated.

ONGOING CARE

FOLLOW-UP RECOMMENDATIONS

- Bed rest prior to surgery
- Postoperatively, if intraocular gas has been used, the patient may need specific head positioning and should not travel to high altitudes.

Patient Monitoring

- Alert ophthalmologist if there is new onset of floaters or flashes, increase in floaters or flashes, sudden shower of floaters, curtain or shadow in the peripheral visual field, or reduced vision.

- Patients with acute symptomatic PVD should be re-examined by the ophthalmologist in 3–4 weeks. The development of a retinal detachment is unlikely if no retinal tears are present on re-examination in 3–4 weeks.
- If acute symptomatic PVD is associated with gross vitreous hemorrhage that interferes with complete visualization of the retinal periphery by indirect ophthalmoscopy, the patient should be re-examined at short intervals with indirect ophthalmoscopy until the entire retinal periphery can be observed.
- If the examiner is not certain whether the retina is detached in the presence of opaque medium, US should be performed.

DIET
NPO if surgery is imminent

PATIENT EDUCATION
American Academy of Ophthalmology, 655 E. Beach Street, San Francisco, CA 94109-1336

PROGNOSIS

- RRD:
  - 90% of retinal detachments can be reattached successfully after ≥1 surgical procedures. Postoperative visual acuity depends primarily on the status of the macula preoperatively. Also important is the length of time between the detachment and the repair (75% of eyes with macular detachments of <1 week will obtain a final visual acuity of 20/70 or better).
  - 87% of eyes with a retinal detachment not involving the macula attain a visual acuity of 20/50 or better postoperatively. 37% of eyes with a detached macula preoperatively attain 20/50 or better vision postoperatively.
  - In 10–15% of successfully repaired retinal detachments not involving the macula preoperatively, visual acuity does not return to the preoperative level. This decrease is secondary to complications such as macular edema and macular pucker.
- Tractional retinal detachment: When not involving the fovea, the patient usually can be observed because it is uncommon for these to extend into the fovea.
- Exudative retinal detachment:
  - Management is usually nonsurgical.
  - The presence of shifting fluid is highly suggestive of an exudative retinal detachment. Fixed retinal folds, which are indicative of PVR, are seen rarely in exudative retinal detachment. If the underlying condition is treated, the prognosis generally is good.

COMPLICATIONS

- PVR is the most common cause of failed retinal detachment repair; 10–15% of retinas that reattach initially after retinal surgery will redetach subsequently, usually within 6 weeks, as a result of cellular proliferation and contraction on the retinal surface.
- Partial or total loss of vision due to macular detachment and/or PVR
- Moderate-to-severe forms of PVR usually are treated with pars plana vitrectomy and fluid–gas exchange. If a segmental scleral buckle was placed at the initial procedure, it may need to be revised.
- Primary retinectomy can be used in cases of PVR without a scleral buckle (6)[C].
- Scleral buckles may erode the overlying conjunctiva and lead to an infection.
- Optic neuropathy after PPV for macula-sparing primary RRD (7)[C].

REFERENCES

1. Mitry D, Williams L, Charteris DG, et al. Population-based estimate of the sibling recurrence risk ratio for rhegmatogenous retinal detachment. *Invest Ophthalmol Vis Sci.* 2011;52:2551–2555.
2. Hassan TS, Sarrafizadeh R, Ruby AJ, et al. The effect of duration of macular detachment on results after the scleral buckle repair of primary, macula-off retinal detachments. *Ophthalmology.* 2002;109:146–152.
3. Tan HS, Mura M, Bijl HM. Early vitrectomy for vitreous hemorrhage associated with retinal tears. *Am J Ophthalmol.* 2010;150:529–533.
4. Kinori M, Moisseiev E, Shoshany N, et al. Comparison of pars plana vitrectomy with and without scleral buckle for the repair of primary rhegmatogenous retinal detachment. *Am J Ophthalmol.* 2011;152(2):291–297.
5. Covert DJ, Henry CR, Bhatia SK, et al. Intraoperative retinal tear formation and postoperative rhegmatogenous retinal detachment in transconjunctival cannulated vitrectomy systems compared with the standard 20-gauge system. *Arch Ophthalmol.* 2012;130:186–189.
6. Tan HS, Mura M, Oberstein SY. Primary retinectomy in proliferative vitreoretinopathy. *Am J Ophthalmol.* 2010;149:447–452.
7. Bansal AS, Jason H, Sunir JG, et al. Optic neuropathy after vitrectomy for retinal detachment: Clinical features and analysis of risk factors. *Ophthalmol.* 2012;119:2364–2370.

ADDITIONAL READING

Alio JL, Ruiz-Moreno JM, Shabayek MH, et al. The risk of retinal detachment in high myopia after small incision coaxial phacoemulsification. *Am J Ophthalmol.* 2007;144:93–98.

SEE ALSO

Retinopathy, Diabetic

CODES

ICD10

- H33.009 Unsp retinal detachment with retinal break, unspecified eye
- H33.20 Serous retinal detachment, unspecified eye
- H33.40 Traction detachment of retina, unspecified eye

CLINICAL PEARLS

- If a patient complains of the new onset of floaters or flashes of light, the patient should undergo a dilated eye exam to rule out a retinal tear or retinal detachment.
- There is an increased risk of retinal detachment after cataract surgery.
- Proliferative vitreoretinopathy can result in redetachment of the retina after an initially successful repair.

RETINITIS PIGMENTOSA

Richard W. Allinson, MD

 BASICS

DESCRIPTION

- An eye disease in which progressive damage to the retina occurs with gradual loss of peripheral vision that eventually leads to significant visual impairment; signs often seen in childhood, but severe vision problems do not develop until adulthood.
- Characterized by poor night vision, constricted visual fields, bone spiculelike pigmentation of the fundus, and electroretinographic evidence of photoreceptor cell dysfunction
- System(s) affected: Nervous
- Synonym(s): Rod-cone dystrophy; Retinal dystrophy

EPIDEMIOLOGY

Incidence

- Predominant age:
  - X-linked retinitis pigmentosa (RP) has the earliest onset of the major hereditary types; many X-linked patients are legally blind by age 30.
  - Autosomal-dominant RP has a later onset than autosomal-recessive or X-linked–recessive RP.
  - Leber's congenital amaurosis, which is a variant of RP, presents at birth.
  - Late-onset RP typically is asymptomatic and unrecognized until age 40–50 years.
- Predominant sex: Male > Female

Prevalence

Affects ~1/4,000 people in the US

Pediatric Considerations

Leber's congenital amaurosis characterized by reduced vision from birth and impaired electroretinogram responses from both cones and rods.

Geriatric Considerations

Late-onset RP is asymptomatic and generally unrecognized until >40.

ETIOLOGY AND PATHOPHYSIOLOGY

- Mutations in the rhodopsin gene account for ~30% of cases of autosomal-dominant RP.
- Another 4–6% of autosomal-dominant RP is caused by a mutation in the gene for a photoreceptor protein peripherin/rds.

Genetics

- Autosomal dominant: 20%
- Autosomal recessive: 37%
- X-linked recessive: 4.5%
- Sporadic: 38.5%

RISK FACTORS

Family history

GENERAL PREVENTION

- Genetic counseling
- No conclusive evidence demonstrates that the amount of light modifies the course of RP. A study in which 1 eye was covered with an opaque lens did not show any difference in disease progression compared with the fellow eye.
- Ultraviolet (UV)–absorbing sunglasses and brimmed hats are recommended when patients are at the beach or in the snow.

COMMONLY ASSOCIATED CONDITIONS

With systemic disorders:

- Usher syndrome: RP and congenital sensorineural hearing impairment
- Laurence-Moon-Biedl syndrome (also called *Bardet-Biedl syndrome*): Autosomal-recessive disorder associated with retinal dystrophy, mental retardation, obesity, hypogonadism, and postaxial polydactyly
- Cockayne syndrome: Autosomal-recessive disorder in which children at the age of 1–2 years present with retinal dystrophy, sensorineural deafness, cerebellar dysfunction, dementia, and UV light photosensitivity

 DIAGNOSIS

HISTORY

- Headache and light flashes are the most common initial complaints.
- Night blindness (nyctalopia)
- Progressive visual field loss
- Central visual acuity is usually preserved until the end stages.

PHYSICAL EXAM

- Bone spicule pigmentation in the retina
- Retinal arteriolar narrowing
- Optic nerve head pallor, "waxy pallor"
- Most patients are myopic.
- Posterior subcapsular cataracts are common in all forms.
- Cystoid macular edema
- Optic nerve head drusen
- Electroretinogram changes
- Retinal neovascularization
- RP is associated with an exudative retinal vasculopathy; fundus findings include serous retinal detachment, lipid deposition in the retina, and telangiectatic vascular anomalies.
- Variants of RP exist with unusual or regional distribution, including:
  - Sectorial RP
  - Pigmented paravenous atrophy
  - Unilateral RP

DIFFERENTIAL DIAGNOSIS

- Bone spiculelike retinal pigmentation and retinal atrophy are nonspecific findings and may result from conditions other than RP.
- Infections
- Syphilis
- Rubella
- Inflammation (severe uveitis)
- Choroidal vascular occlusion
- Toxicity (chloroquine or thioridazine)
- Choroideremia
- Gyrate atrophy of choroid and retina (10–20-fold elevation of plasma ornithine levels)
- Systemic metabolic disorders such as Refsum disease and abetalipoproteinemia
- Kearns-Sayre syndrome: Usually presents in adolescents; characterized by progressive external ophthalmoplegia—the 1st sign usually being ptosis—pigmentary degeneration of the retina, and a cardiac conduction defect that may cause complete heart block

- Cone-rod dystrophy: Characterized by bilateral and symmetric loss of cone function in the presence of reduced rod function
- Cone dystrophy: Characterized by marked abnormality in cone function with some or no rod involvement
- Congenital stationary night blindness
- Oguchi disease
- Fundus albipunctatus
- Trauma

DIAGNOSTIC TESTS & INTERPRETATION

- Electroretinography: Photoreceptors generate reduced-amplitude A and B waves in RP. Rod and cone responses may be undetectable in advanced RP.
- Visual field testing: A ring scotoma in the midperiphery may be identified. The ring scotoma generally starts as a group of isolated scotomas in the area 20–25 degrees from fixation. Long after the entire peripheral field is gone, a small island of intact central visual field remains.
- Fluorescein angiography can demonstrate cystoid macular edema.
- Fundus photography documents the status of the retina.
- Hearing tests in patients complaining of hearing loss, such as those with Usher syndrome (RP with hearing loss)
- Optical coherence tomography can be used to detect and monitor cystoid macular edema.
- An abnormal hyperautofluorescent ring surrounding the fovea may be present on fundus autofluorescence imaging (FAF). In addition, spectral-domain optical coherence tomography (SD-OCT) has demonstrated a decrease in retinal thickness in the area of the hyperautofluorescent ring in RP patients with loss of the inner segment/ outer segment (IS/OS) junction (1)[B].

Follow-Up Tests & Special Considerations

- Elevated plasma levels of phytanic acid in Refsum disease
- Acanthocytosis of RBCs in peripheral blood smear in abetalipoproteinemia, an autosomal-recessive disorder in which apolipoprotein B is not synthesized, leading to fat malabsorption and deficiencies of fat-soluble vitamins; therapy with vitamins A and E may improve retinal function
- Syphilitic neuroretinitis can be diagnosed by performing a fluorescent treponemal antibody absorption or microhemagglutination *Treponema pallidum* test.
- Elevated plasma ornithine levels in gyrate atrophy of the choroid and retina; usually a 10–20-fold elevation of plasma ornithine levels

Test Interpretation

- Disappearance of the rods, cones, and outer nuclear layers of the retina
- Bone spicule formation in the retina is secondary to the migration of retinal pigment epithelial cells into the overlying retina.

TREATMENT

GENERAL MEASURES
- Supportive care
- Genetic counseling
- Low-vision aids
- Patient education

MEDICATION
- Vitamin A 15,000 IU/d (retinal degeneration slowed, as measured by electroretinogram/visual fields); β-carotene is not a suitable substitute; has not been studied in patients <18 years (2)[A].
- Vitamin E 400 IU/d results in faster retinal degeneration and is not recommended (2)[A].
- Lutein supplementation at a dose of 12 mg/d slowed visual field loss among nonsmoking adults with RP taking vitamin A (3)[B].
- Acetazolamide may be of benefit in the treatment of cystoid macular edema, which may occur in RP; 500 mg/d in a sustained-release capsule was found to be more effective than 250 mg/d.
- Topical dorzolamide may be of benefit in the treatment of cystoid macular edema associated with RP.
- Intravitreal bevacizumab and ranibizumab injection may be of benefit in the treatment of cystoid macular edema associated with RP (4)[C].
- Contraindications: Women who are pregnant or considering pregnancy should not take >8,000 IU/d of vitamin A. There is an increased incidence of birth defects in babies born to women who ingest higher dosages of vitamin A during pregnancy. Women should consult their obstetrician.
- Precautions: Avoid vitamin A supplement dosages >15,000 IU/d because higher dosages may cause liver damage.

Pregnancy Considerations
Risk of teratogenicity with a high intake of vitamin A during pregnancy

SURGERY/OTHER PROCEDURES
- The efficacy of the "Cuban therapy"—electric stimulation, autotransfused ozonized blood, and ocular surgery—has not been proven.
- Macular grid laser photocoagulation may be of benefit in patients with cystoid macular edema secondary to RP.
- Research is being done on photoreceptor and retinal pigment epithelium transplantation, gene therapy, and implantation of a visual prosthesis. The inner retinal neurons may be preserved after death of photoreceptors in RP, which could make some of these experimental procedures feasible:
  – Patients who are blind from RP are able to detect motion with the Argus II retinal prosthesis (5)[B].
- Gene therapy has been successful in treating patients with Leber's congenital amaurosis due to defects in the *RPE65* gene (6)[C].

ONGOING CARE

FOLLOW-UP RECOMMENDATIONS
Caution should be exercised because of reduced peripheral vision and poor night vision.

Patient Monitoring
- Ophthalmic examinations every 1–2 years
- Check for complications (e.g., cataracts).

DIET
A diet rich in omega-3 fatty acids (primarily docosahexaenoic acid), when taken in combination with 15,000 IU/d of vitamin A, may slow the rate of visual acuity loss in patients with RP (7)[B].

PATIENT EDUCATION
- Counsel patients to help them understand RP and its genetics.
- RP is a slowly progressive, chronic disease; patients do not go blind rapidly, and total blindness is not a frequent endpoint of this disease.
- RP Foundation Fighting Blindness, Executive Plaza One, Suite 800, 11350 McCormick Road, Hunt Valley, MD 21031-1014 (800) 683-5555
- The American Academy of Ophthalmology, 655 E. Beach Street, San Francisco, CA 94109-1336 (415) 561-8540

PROGNOSIS
- Reassure about the slow course of RP.
- Most of the deafness in Usher syndrome is congenital. It is unlikely that an RP patient who is not born deaf will become deaf later in life.
- RP severity varies with inheritance pattern.
- Autosomal-recessive form has an early age of onset, and patients may have severely constricted visual fields by age 20. Tends toward more rapid progression compared with autosomal-dominant RP; also increased incidence of cataracts.
- X-linked RP is similar in clinical presentation to autosomal-recessive RP.
- Autosomal-dominant RP generally has less severe findings initially than does autosomal-recessive RP; symptoms may not occur until age 30.
- Good central vision is usually preserved. If the central visual field radius is >30 degrees, >90% of patients will have visual acuities of 20/40 or better. If the central visual field radius is <10 degrees, 30% of patients will have a visual acuity of 20/40 or better.

COMPLICATIONS
- Cataract
- Cystoid macular edema
- Loss of visual field
- Poor night vision
- Blindness

REFERENCES

1. Chen RW, Greenberg JP, Lazow MA, et al. Autofluorescence imaging and spectral-domain optical coherence tomography in incomplete congenital stationary night blindness and comparison with retinitis pigmentosa. *Am J Ophthalmol*. 2012;153:143–154.e2.
2. Berson EL, Rosner B, Sandberg MA, et al. A randomized trial of vitamin A and vitamin E supplementation for retinitis pigmentosa. *Arch Ophthalmol*. 1993;111:761–772.
3. Berson EL, Rosner B, Sandberg MA, et al. Clinical trial of lutein in patients with retinitis pigmentosa receiving vitamin A. *Arch Ophthalmol*. 2010;128:403–411.
4. Artunay O, Yuzbasioglu E, Rasier R, et al. Intravitreal ranibizumab in the treatment of cystoid macular edema associated with retinitis pigmentosa. *J Ocul Pharmacol Ther*. 2009;25:545–550.
5. Dorn JD, Ahuja AK, Caspi A, et al. The detection of motion by blind subjects with the epiretinal 60-electrode (Argus II) retinal prosthesis. *JAM Ophthalmol*. 2013 Feb;131:183–189.
6. Bainbridge JW, Smith AJ, Barker SS, et al. Effect of gene therapy on visual function in Leber's congenital amaurosis. *N Engl J Med*. 2008;358:2231–2239.
7. Berson EL, Rosner B, Sandberg MA, et al. ω-3 intake and visual acuity in patients with retinitis pigmentosa receiving vitamin A. *Arch Ophthalmol*. 2012;130(6):707–711.

CODES

ICD10
H35.52 Pigmentary retinal dystrophy

CLINICAL PEARLS
- Characterized by poor night vision, constricted visual fields, bone spiculelike pigmentation of the fundus, and electroretinographic evidence of photoreceptor cell dysfunction.
- Avoid Vitamin E as it results in faster retinal degeneration and is not recommended.
- RP severity varies with inheritance pattern.

RETINOPATHY, DIABETIC

Richard W. Allinson, MD

BASICS

DESCRIPTION
- Noninflammatory retinal disorder characterized by retinal capillary closure and microaneurysms. Retinal ischemia leads to release of a vasoproliferative factor stimulating neovascularization on retina, optic nerve, or iris.
- Most patients with diabetes mellitus (DM) will develop diabetic retinopathy (DR). It is the leading cause of new cases of legal blindness among residents in the US between the ages of 20 and 64 years.
- Diabetic retinopathy can be divided into 3 stages:
  - Nonproliferative (background)
  - Severe nonproliferative (preproliferative)
  - Proliferative
- System(s) affected: Nervous

Geriatric Considerations
Prevalence will increase as population generally ages and patients with diabetes live longer.

Pregnancy Considerations
- Pregnancy can exacerbate condition.
- Pregnant diabetic women should be examined in 1st trimester, then every 3 months until delivery.

EPIDEMIOLOGY
Incidence
- Peak incidence of type 1, juvenile-onset DM is between the ages of 12 and 15 years.
- Peak incidence of type 2, adult-onset DM is between the ages of 50 and 70 years.
- Incidence of DR is directly related to the duration of diabetes.
- <10 years of age, it is unusual to see DR, regardless of DM duration.

Prevalence
- 6.6% of the US population between ages of 20 and 74 has DM.
- ~25% of the diabetic population has some form of DR.
- Predominant age:
  - Risk increases after puberty.
  - 2/3 of juvenile-onset diabetics who have had DM for at least 35 years will develop proliferative DR, and will develop macular edema. Proportions are reversed for adult-onset diabetes.
- Predominant sex: Male = Female (type 1, juvenile-onset DM); Female > Male (type 2)

ETIOLOGY AND PATHOPHYSIOLOGY
- Related to development of diabetic microaneurysms and microvascular abnormalities
- Reduction in perifoveal capillary blood flow velocity, perifoveal capillary occlusion, and increased retinal thickness at the central fovea in diabetic patients are associated with visual impairment in patients with diabetic macular edema.

RISK FACTORS
- Duration of DM (usually >10 years)
- Poor glycemic control
- Pregnancy
- Renal disease
- Systemic hypertension (HTN)
- Smoking
- Elevated lipid levels associated with increased risk of retinal lipid deposits (hard exudates)
- Myopic eyes (eyes with longer axial length) have a lower risk of DR

GENERAL PREVENTION
- Monitor and control of blood glucose
- Schedule yearly ophthalmologic eye exams.

COMMONLY ASSOCIATED CONDITIONS
- Glaucoma
- Cataracts
- Retinal disease
- Vitreous hemorrhage
- Disc edema (diabetic papillopathy); may occur in type 1/type 2 DM

DIAGNOSIS

HISTORY
Diabetic patients should be encouraged to have an annual ophthalmologic exam because early changes are asymptomatic.

PHYSICAL EXAM
- Eye exam: Measurement of visual acuity and documentation of the status of the iris, lens, vitreous, and fundus
- Nonproliferative (background) DR:
  - Microaneurysms
  - Intraretinal hemorrhage
  - Macular edema causing decrease in central vision
  - Lipid deposits
- Severe nonproliferative (preproliferative) DR:
  - Nerve fiber layer infarctions ("cotton wool spots")
  - Venous beading
  - Venous dilatation
  - Intraretinal microvascular abnormalities
  - Extensive retinal hemorrhage
- Proliferative DR:
  - New blood vessel proliferation (neovascularization) on the retinal surface, optic nerve, and iris
  - Visual loss caused by vitreous hemorrhage, traction retinal detachment

GENERAL MEASURES
- The Diabetes Control and Complications Trial (DCCT) recommended that for most patients with insulin-dependent DM, blood glucose levels should be as close to the nondiabetic range as is safe to reduce the risk and rate of progression of diabetic retinopathy:
  - In the DCCT, insulin-dependent DM patients were randomly assigned into either conventional or intensive insulin treatment. Conventional treatment consisted of 1–2 daily insulin injections, with daily self-monitoring of urine/blood glucose. Intensive treatment consisted of insulin administered ≥3× daily by injection/an external pump, with self-monitored blood glucose levels measured at least 4×/d.
  - The DCCT demonstrated that intensive insulin therapy reduced the risk of macular edema and retinal neovascularization. The benefit of intensive insulin therapy and the reduced risk of DR-associated microvascular complications persist for at least 10 years (1)[A].
  - In the DCCT, intensive insulin therapy was more effective in reducing the risk of progression of DR in the less advanced stages. However, advanced DR also benefited from the intensive insulin therapy.
- The Early Treatment Diabetic Retinopathy Study demonstrated that aspirin therapy did not prevent the development of proliferative DR or reduce the risk of visual loss associated with DR.
- Microvascular complications, including proliferative diabetic retinopathy, are increased when blood sugar levels are ≥200 mg/dL.
- Poor glycemic control is associated with an increased risk both for development and progression of DR, regardless of the type of DM; that hyperglycemia itself is causative is not established, especially for type 2 DM.
- Cataracts are more common among those with DM. Try to delay cataract surgery in DM patients with retinopathy until the symptoms are severe. Cataract surgery can cause retinopathy to worsen and increase the risk for development of diabetic macular edema.
- HTN has a detrimental effect on DR and must be controlled.

DIFFERENTIAL DIAGNOSIS
Other causes of retinopathy (e.g., radiation, retinal venous obstruction, HTN)

DIAGNOSTIC TESTS & INTERPRETATION
Diagnostic Procedures/Other
- Fluorescein angiography demonstrates retinal nonperfusion, retinal leakage, and proliferative DR.
- Optical coherence tomography (OCT) can be used to help detect diabetic macular edema by measuring retinal thickness.

Test Interpretation
- Increased capillary permeability
- Microaneurysms
- Hemorrhages in retina
- Exudates in retina
- Capillary nonperfusion

TREATMENT

MEDICATION

- Treatment with the angiotensin-receptor blocker candesartan has been shown to result in regression of DR in some patients (2)[B].
- Under evaluation: Protein kinase C-β is activated by hyperglycemia and is associated with the development of vascular dysfunction. Inhibition of this enzyme could help to reduce the retinal vascular complications from DM.
- Nutritional antioxidant intake of vitamins C and E and of β-carotene has no protective effect on diabetic retinopathy.
- Atorvastatin may reduce the severity of lipid deposits with clinically significant diabetic macular edema in type 2 DM and dyslipidemia.

SURGERY/OTHER PROCEDURES

- Laser photocoagulation treatment: Recommended for patients with proliferative DR and for those with clinically significant macular edema; destroys leaking blood vessels and areas of neovascularization.
- The Diabetic Retinopathy Study demonstrated that panretinal photocoagulation reduced overall rate of severe visual loss from 15.9% in untreated eyes to 6.4% in treated eyes. In certain subgroups, the incidence of severe visual loss in untreated eyes was as high as 36.9% within 2 years.
- The Early Treatment Diabetic Retinopathy Study demonstrated that eyes with significant diabetic macular edema benefited from focal laser treatment. Clinically significant diabetic macular edema (CSDME) is defined as:
  - Thickening of the retina within 500 μm of the center of the macula
  - Hard exudates within 500 μm of the center of the macula associated with thickening of the adjacent retina
  - Zone of retinal thickening $\geq$1 disc area within 1 disc diameter of the center of the macula
- Patients with CSDME and high-risk proliferative disease can have simultaneous focal and panretinal photocoagulation without adversely affecting the visual outcome.
- Vitrectomy may benefit some with diffuse macular edema. This may apply especially to eyes with vitreomacular traction found on OCT and with persistent CSDME.
- Intravitreal triamcinolone may be used for DM-related macular edema that fails laser treatment. No long-term benefit of intravitreal triamcinolone relative to focal/grid photocoagulation in patients with CSDME. This is an off-label use (3)[C].
- Ranibizumab, an antibody fragment that binds vascular endothelial growth factor (VEGF), can be used to treat CSDME when injected intravitreally. Ranibizumab 0.3 mg given monthly to treat CSDME resulted in improved vision and reduced central foveal thickness (4)[A]:
  - Intravitreal ranibizumab treatment for diabetic macular edema may also improve diabetic retinopathy severity and reduce the risk of diabetic retinopathy progression (5)[A].
- Bevacizumab, a full-length antibody that binds VEGF, can be used to treat CSDME when injected intravitreally. This is an off-label use (6)[B].

- Aflibercept, a soluble decoy receptor for VEGF, is being investigated in the treatment of CSDME when injected intravitreally. This is an off-label use (7)[C].
- Preoperative bevacizumab can be used as an adjuvant to vitrectomy for complications of proliferative DR. This is an off-label use:
  - At ~10 days after intravitreal injection of bevacizumab, the vascular component of proliferation is markedly reduced and the contractile components are not yet very significant. Patients with dense fibrovascular proliferation need to be monitored closely for evidence of traction retinal detachment (8)[C].
- Cryoretinopexy can be used instead of laser treatment in certain patients to decrease the neovascular stimulus and treat proliferative DR.
- Vitrectomy: Recommended for patients with severe proliferative DR, traction retinal detachment involving the macula, and nonclearing vitreous hemorrhage:
  - A transvitreal fibrinoid response can occur after diabetic vitrectomy and present as a pseudoendophthalmitis (9)[C].

ONGOING CARE

FOLLOW-UP RECOMMENDATIONS
Patient Monitoring
Scheduled ophthalmologic eye exams:
- Yearly follow-up if no retinopathy
- Every 6 months with background DR
- At least every 3–4 months with preproliferative DR
- Every 2–3 months with active proliferative DR

DIET
Follow prescribed diet for patients with diabetes.

PATIENT EDUCATION
- Patient education should include regular ophthalmic exams.
- Stress importance of strict blood glucose control through diet, exercise, drugs/insulin, and monitoring of blood glucose.

PROGNOSIS
If the condition is diagnosed and treated early in development, outlook is good. If treatment is delayed, blindness may result.

COMPLICATIONS
Blindness

REFERENCES

1. White NH, Sun W, Cleary PA, et al. Prolonged effect of intensive therapy on the risk of retinopathy complications in patients with type 1 diabetes mellitus: 10 years after the Diabetes Control and Complications Trial. Arch Ophthalmol. 2008;126:1707–1715.
2. Sjølie AK, Klein R, Porta M, et al. Effect of candesartan on progression and regression of retinopathy in type 2 diabetes (DIRECT-Protect 2): A randomised placebo-controlled trial. Lancet. 2008;372:1385–1393.
3. Diabetic Retinopathy Clinical Research Network (DRCR.net), Beck RW, Edwards AR, et al. Three-year follow-up of a randomized trial comparing focal/grid photocoagulation and intravitreal triamcinolone for diabetic macular edema. Arch Ophthalmol. 2009;127:245–251.
4. Brown DM, Nguyen, Marcus DM, et al. Long-term outcomes of ranibizumab therapy for diabetic macular edema: The 36-month results from two phase III trials: Rise and Ride. Ophthalmology. 2013; Epub.
5. Ip MS, Domalpally A, Hopkins JJ, et al. Long-term effects of ranibizumab on diabetic retinopathy severity and progression. Arch Ophthalmol. 2012;130:1145–1152.
6. Rajendram R, Fraser-Bell S, Kaines A, et al. A 2-year prospective randomized controlled trial of intravitreal bevacizumab or laser therapy (BOLT) in the management of diabetic macular edema: 24-month data: report 3. Arch Ophthalmol. 2012;130:972–979.
7. Do DV, Nguyen QD, Boyer D, et al. One-year outcomes of the DA VINCI Study of VEGF Trap-Eye in eyes with diabetic macular edema. Ophthalmology. 2012;119(8):1658–1665.
8. El-Sabagh HA, Abdelghaffar W, Labib AM, et al. Preoperative intravitreal bevacizumab use as an adjuvant to diabetic vitrectomy: Histopathologic findings and clinical implications. Ophthalmology. 2011;118:636–641.
9. Luo C, Ruby A, Neuwelt M, et al. Transvitreal fibrinoid pseudoendophthalmitis after diabetic vitrectomy. Retina. 2013; Epub.

SEE ALSO

Diabetes Mellitus, Type 1; Diabetes Mellitus, Type 2.

CODES

ICD10
- E08.319 Diabetes mellitus due to underlying condition with unspecified diabetic retinopathy without macular edema
- E10.319 Type 1 diabetes mellitus with unspecified diabetic retinopathy without macular edema
- E11.319 Type 2 diabetes mellitus with unspecified diabetic retinopathy without macular edema

CLINICAL PEARLS

- Options for the treatment of diffuse macular edema include focal laser treatment, intravitreal triamcinolone, intravitreal ranibizumab, intravitreal bevacizumab, and vitrectomy.
- High BP should be controlled to reduce the risk of diabetic eye complications.
- Blood glucose levels should be well controlled to help reduce the risk and rate of DR progression.
- Schedule yearly ophthalmologic eye exams.

RH INCOMPATIBILITY
Donald Nelson, MD

 BASICS

DESCRIPTION
- Antibody-mediated destruction of red blood cells (RBCs) that bear Rh surface antigens in individuals who lack the antigens and have become isoimmunized (sensitized) to them
- System(s) affected: Hematologic/Lymphatic/Immunologic
- Synonym(s): Rh isoimmunization; Rh alloimmunization; Rh sensitization

EPIDEMIOLOGY
Incidence
Predominant age and sex: Affects fetuses/neonates of isoimmunized child-bearing females

ETIOLOGY AND PATHOPHYSIOLOGY
- Circulating antibodies to Rh antigens (transplacentally transferred antibodies in the case of a fetus/newborn) attach to Rh antigens on RBCs.
- Immune-mediated destruction of RBCs leads to hemolysis, anemia, and increased bilirubin production.
- Transfusion of Rh-positive blood to Rh-negative recipient
- Maternal exposure to fetal Rh antigens, either antepartum or intrapartum
- Most commonly seen in the Rh-positive fetus or infant of an Rh-negative mother

Genetics
- Complex autosomal inheritance of polypeptide Rh antigens; 3 genetic loci with closely related genes carry an assortment of alleles: Dd, Cc, and Ee (1).
- Individuals who express the D antigen (also called *Rho* or *Rho[D]*) or its weak D (D^u) variant are considered Rh-positive. Individuals lacking the D antigen are Rh-negative. (There is no antigen identified with the d allele.)
- Another variant D antigen, DEL, has been identified in some individuals (predominantly Asians) who are classified as Rh-negative by the usual assays. While testing Rh-negative, these individuals are not likely to be sensitized by exposure to Rh-D antigens through pregnancy or transfusion (2).
- Antibodies may be produced to C, c, D, E, or e in individuals lacking the specific antigen; only D is strongly immunogenic (3).
- Isoimmunization to Rh antigens in susceptible individuals is acquired, not inherited.

RISK FACTORS
- ~15% of the white population and smaller fractions of other races are Rh-negative and susceptible to sensitization (4).
- Any Rh-positive pregnancy in an Rh-negative woman can result in sensitization.
- Native risk of isoimmunization after Rh-positive pregnancy had been estimated at ≤15%, but seems to be decreasing.
- The risk of isoimmunization antepartum is only 1–2%.
- The risk of isoimmunization is 1–2% after spontaneous abortion and 4–5% after induced abortion (5).
- Use of Rho(D) immunoglobulin prophylaxis has reduced incidence of isoimmunization to <1% of susceptible pregnancies.

GENERAL PREVENTION
- Blood typing (ABO and Rh) on all pregnant women and prior to blood transfusions
- Antibody screening early in pregnancy
- Rh immunoglobulin prevents only sensitization to the D antigen.
- For prophylaxis, Rho(D) immunoglobulin (RhIG, RhoGAM, HyperRHO, RHOphylac) given to unsensitized, Rh-negative women after the following (6)[A]:
  - Spontaneous abortion
  - Induced abortion
  - Ectopic pregnancy
  - Antepartum hemorrhage
  - Trauma to abdomen
  - Amniocentesis
  - Chorionic villus sampling
  - Within 72 hours of delivery of an Rh-positive infant
  - Given routinely at 28 weeks' gestation
- Prophylaxis, whether antepartum or postpartum, is to prevent sensitization affecting a subsequent pregnancy and has little effect on the current pregnancy (6).
- Dose for prophylaxis:
  - 50-μg dose for events up to 12 weeks' gestation
  - 300-μg dose for events after 12 weeks' gestation
  - Higher doses may be required in the event of a large fetal–maternal hemorrhage (>30 mL of whole blood).

COMMONLY ASSOCIATED CONDITIONS
- Hemolytic disease of newborn
- Hydrops fetalis
- Neonatal jaundice
- Kernicterus
- See "Erythroblastosis Fetalis" topic.

 DIAGNOSIS

PHYSICAL EXAM
- Jaundice of newborn
- Kernicterus
- Fetal hydrops or fetal death in utero if severe (see "Erythroblastosis Fetalis" topic)

DIFFERENTIAL DIAGNOSIS
- ABO incompatibility
- Other blood group (non-Rh) isoimmunization
- Nonimmune fetal hydrops
- Hereditary spherocytosis
- RBC enzyme defects

DIAGNOSTIC TESTS & INTERPRETATION
Initial Tests (lab, imaging)
- Positive indirect Coombs' test (antibody screen) during pregnancy
- Paternal blood type
- Kleihauer-Betke (fetal hemoglobin acid elution, Hb F slide elution) test to quantify an acute fetal–maternal bleed (7)
- Flow cytometry using antibody to Hemoglobin F is emerging as an alternative to the Kleihauer-Betke test to detect or quantify fetal-maternal bleed (7).
- Congenital or fetal anemia
- Blood type, direct Coombs' test in newborn

Follow-Up Tests & Special Considerations
Prior administration of IgD may lead to weakly (false-) positive indirect Coombs' test in mother and direct Coombs' test in infant.

 TREATMENT

GENERAL MEASURES
- Depending on severity of involvement, treatment of fetus may include:
  - Intrauterine transfusion
  - Early delivery
- Treatment of newborn may include:
  - Exchange transfusion
  - Transfusion after delivery
  - Phototherapy
  - Diuretics and digoxin for hydrops
  - Immunoglobulin infusion has reduced the need for exchange transfusion in a few studies (8)[A].

ISSUES FOR REFERRAL

Because of the specialized, somewhat hazardous treatment measures involved, pregnancies in Rh-sensitized women are usually managed at tertiary-care facilities.

IN-PATIENT CONSIDERATIONS

Admission Criteria/Initial Stabilization

Initial monitoring of the newborn is inpatient or in special care nursery if treatment interventions are needed.

ONGOING CARE

FOLLOW-UP RECOMMENDATIONS

Patient Monitoring

- In most cases, outpatient ambulatory management is appropriate during the antepartum period.
- Antibody titer measured at 20 weeks and every 4 weeks thereafter during pregnancy; a titer of $\geq$1:16 indicates the need for further testing (1).
- If the patient had a previously affected infant, an Rh-positive fetus in the current pregnancy should be considered at risk regardless of antibody titers (9):
  - Fetal heart rate testing/US to assess fetal status
  - Doppler US measurement of cerebral blood flow is now a suitable alternative to invasive tests (amniocentesis, cordocentesis) for diagnosing fetal anemia (9).
  - Umbilical blood sampling (cordocentesis) for fetal blood type, hematocrit, reticulocyte count, and presence of erythroblasts (1)
  - Amniocentesis for amniotic fluid bilirubin levels (1)
  - Amniocentesis for fetal lung maturity if early delivery is a treatment option (1)

PROGNOSIS

- With appropriate monitoring and treatment, infants born of severely affected pregnancies have a survival rate of >80% (1).
- Even with severe disease, the neurologic outcome of survivors is generally good (10)[C].
- Fetuses with hydrops have a higher mortality rate and higher risk of neurologic impairment (10)[C].
- Disease is likely to be more severe in affected subsequent pregnancies.

COMPLICATIONS

- Pregnancy loss from umbilical blood sampling
- Pregnancy loss from intrauterine transfusion
- Fetal distress requiring emergent delivery (1)

REFERENCES

1. Management of alloimmunization during pregnancy. *ACOG Practice Bulletin* 75. Aug 2006, reaffirmed 2008.
2. Shao C, Xu H, Xu Q, et al. Antenatal Rh prophylaxis is unnecessary for "Asia type" DEL women. *Transfus Clin Biol*. 2010;17:260–264.
3. Agre P, Cartron JP. Molecular biology of the Rh antigens. *Blood*. 1991;78:551–563.
4. Bianchi DW, Avent ND, Costa JM, et al. Noninvasive prenatal diagnosis of fetal Rhesus D: Ready for prime(r) time. *Obstet Gynecol*. 2005; 106:841–844.
5. Bowman J. Thirty-five years of Rh prophylaxis. *Transfusion*. 2003;43:1661–1666.
6. Crowther CA, Middleton P, McBain RD. Anti-D administration in pregnancy for preventing Rhesus alloimmunisation (review). *Cochrane Library* 2013;2.
7. Kim YA, Makar RS. Detection of fetomaternal hemorrhage. *Am J Hematology* 2012:417–423.
8. Alcock GS, Liley H. Immunoglobulin infusion for isoimmune haemolytic jaundice in neonates. *Cochrane Database Syst Rev*. 2006;1.
9. Moise KJ. Management of rhesus alloimmunization in pregnancy. *Obstet Gynecol*. 2008;112: 164–176.
10. Lindenberg IT, Smits-Wintjens VE, van Klink JM, et al. Long-term developmental outcome after intrauterine transfusion of the fetus/newborn: The LOTUS study. *Am J Obstet Gynecol*. 2012;206: 141.e1–e8.

ADDITIONAL READING

Prevention of Rh D alloimmunization. *ACOG Practice Bulletin 4*. May 1999, reaffirmed 2009.

SEE ALSO

Anemia, Autoimmune Hemolytic; Erythroblastosis Fetalis; Jaundice

CODES

ICD10

- O36.0990 Maternal care for other rhesus isoimmunization, unspecified trimester, not applicable or unspecified
- P55.0 Rh isoimmunization of newborn
- T80.40XA Rh incompat react due to tranfs of bld/bld prod, unsp, init

CLINICAL PEARLS

- If paternity is certain, determining that the father does not carry the Rh(D) blood group antigen eliminates the need to give RhIG prophylaxis during pregnancy or the need for special fetal surveillance if the mother is already sensitized.
- Attempts have been made to determine the fetal blood type noninvasively by detecting fetal DNA in the maternal blood. Because Rh antigens are polymorphic among racial groups, this technique has both false-positive and false-negative results and should be considered experimental.
- The weak D antigen, formerly called D^u, is a weakly reacting variant of the D antigen. A "weak D–positive" mother or infant should be managed as any other D-positive mother or infant, respectively.
- The dose of RhIG for prophylaxis is affected by gestational age. The fetal blood volume is only a few milliliters at 12 weeks' gestation. Therefore, a 50-μg dose of RhIG may be used for threatened, spontaneous, or induced abortions up to 12 weeks' gestation, instead of the standard 300-μg dose.

RHABDOMYOLYSIS

Caroline Y. Tschibelu, MD • Rajiv Arya, MD, FACEP

 BASICS

DESCRIPTION
- Breakdown of skeletal muscle cells and release of intracellular contents into the circulation
- Rhabdomyolysis typically manifests with muscle aches, pains and weakness, and reddish brown (tea-colored) urine, but up to 50% of patients are asymptomatic.

EPIDEMIOLOGY
Incidence
Annually in the US: 26,000 hospitalized cases

ETIOLOGY AND PATHOPHYSIOLOGY
- Direct muscle trauma (most common cause):
  - Crush injuries
  - Extended periods of muscle pressure (during surgery, unconscious from alcohol ingestion)
  - Burns, electrocution, lightning strike
- Muscle exertion:
  - Intense and/or prolonged physical exercise (marathon runners, athletes, contact sports)
  - Seizures
  - Delirium tremens
- Drugs and toxins:
  - Alcohol
  - Cocaine (most common recreational drug), methamphetamine, phencyclidine
  - Antipsychotics (due to neuroleptic malignant syndrome, malignant hyperthermia, and severe dystonia)
  - Zidovudine
  - Antimalarials
  - Heroin
  - HMG-CoA reductase inhibitors (statins) (risk <0.01%), higher with high dose and in combination with fibrates
  - Fibrates
  - Colchicine
  - Corticosteroids
  - Carbon monoxide
  - Snake envenomation
  - Bath salts: Abuse of these psychogenic substances has been recently shown to be complicated by rhabdomyolysis and acute renal failure (1).
- Muscle ischemia:
  - Thrombosis, embolism, sickle cell disease
  - Compartment syndrome
  - Tourniquets
- Infections:
  - Viral: Influenza A and B, coxsackievirus, HIV, varicella
  - Bacterial: *Streptococcus* or *Staphylococcus* sepsis, gas gangrene, necrotizing fasciitis, *Salmonella*, *Legionella*
  - Malaria
- Hypothermia
- Hyperthermia
- Autoimmune and genetic disorders:
  - Polymyositis, dermatomyositis
  - Muscular dystrophies
  - Disorders of lipid metabolism (e.g., carnitine palmitoyltransferase deficiency)
  - Disorders of carbohydrate metabolism (i.e., phosphofructokinase deficiency, phosphoglycerate mutase, myophosphorylase deficiency, aka McArdle disease/deficiency)
  - Glycogen storage diseases (e.g., phosphorylase B kinase deficiency) and others (e.g., lactate dehydrogenase A deficiency)
  - Metabolic and endocrinologic:
  - Hypothyroidism or thyrotoxicosis
  - Electrolyte imbalances (e.g., hyponatremia, hypernatremia, hypokalemia, hypocalcemia, hypophosphatemia)
  - Diabetic ketoacidosis
  - Hyperosmolar state

Genetics
- Hereditary causes of rhabdomyolysis are rare, but should be suspected for children, patients with recurrent attacks, or patients who have attacks after minimal exertion, mild illness, or starvation.
- The main inherited disorders are described below in "Etiology."

RISK FACTORS
See "Etiology."

GENERAL PREVENTION
- Avoid excessive exertional muscle injury. Preventing hypovolemia is important to prevent renal hypoperfusion, acidemia, and subsequent renal failure.
- Avoid precipitating drugs, metabolic and electrolyte abnormalities.

 DIAGNOSIS

HISTORY
- Crush injury: Direct trauma, prolonged compression/immobility. Causes include motor vehicle accidents (MVA), entrapment in collapsed buildings. The elderly are more susceptible to crush injury due to immobility and falls. Rhabdomyolysis usually occurs after 1 hour of immobilization, but cases reported with compression lasting <20 minutes.
- Possible history of overexertion or use of drug/toxin (e.g., cocaine, amphetamine, statins)
- Patient may complain of muscle aches, cramps, or fatigue.
- Agitation while patients are in restraints

PHYSICAL EXAM
- May have obvious muscle tenderness/injury and swelling on exam, or muscle exam may be completely normal
- Tea-colored urine is indicative of myoglobinuria.
- Decreased urine output may indicate renal failure.

DIFFERENTIAL DIAGNOSIS
- For acute renal failure with rhabdomyolysis: Any disease that causes acute tubular necrosis may be confused with rhabdomyolysis.
- Renal pigment injury from hemoglobin resembles pigment injury from myoglobin.

DIAGNOSTIC TESTS & INTERPRETATION
Initial Tests (lab, imaging)
- Creatine kinase (CK) is the most important diagnostic enzyme: Elevated >5× the upper limit of normal or >1,000 U/L. CK levels >5,000 U/L are causally related to acute renal failure (ARF) (2) and should prompt aggressive fluid resuscitation. Other elevated muscle enzymes are aldolase and lactic dehydrogenase (LDH).

- CK levels peak at ~24 hours and return to normal after 3–5 days, making it a more sensitive marker than myoglobin. CK is also a cheaper and an easier surrogate than myoglobin. Myoglobin, however, is the enzyme responsible for kidney failure (2).
- Serum myoglobin levels peak within a few hours and return to normal after ~24 hours as it is cleared quickly from the circulation. Urine/serum myoglobin levels may be useful markers early on, but normal levels do not rule out rhabdomyolysis because of its rapid clearance.
- Urinalysis: Dipstick test positive for blood without erythrocytes in sediment is suggestive of injury from either hemoglobin or myoglobin. However, rhabdomyolysis often presents with hematuria, which is a limitation to using dipstick due to false-positive results.
- Marked elevations of potassium from the muscle injury sometimes are compounded by ARF.
- Initial hypocalcemia: Calcium enters the injured muscle cells and precipitates as calcium phosphate, leading to calcification of ischemic muscle cells. Only correct initial hypocalcemia if patient is symptomatic/has ECG changes; it will self-resolve during the renal recovery phase.
- Hypercalcemia during renal recovery phase: Unique to rhabdomyolysis-induced ARF for 20–30% of patients (3)[A]. As renal function improves, there is mobilization of the precipitated calcium, increase in calcitriol, and hyperphosphatemia resolves.
- Extreme hyperuricemia may be present and can cause acute uric acid nephropathy in the setting of rhabdomyolysis.
- Elevations in BUN and creatinine are indicative of acute renal failure.
- Reversible hepatic dysfunction can occur. However, elevations in alanine aminotransferase (ALT), aspartate aminotransferase (AST), and LDH may be due to muscle injury and may not indicate any hepatic injury.
- Disseminated intravascular coagulation (DIC) can occur, with increase in coagulation times, fibrin degradation products, and D-dimer; decreases in platelets and fibrinogen.
- Place patient on a 12-lead ECG if rhabdomyolysis is suspected because hyperkalemia can induce fatal arrhythmias.

Follow-Up Tests & Special Considerations
- Delayed renal failure/electrolyte abnormalities despite normal initial levels
- Ongoing muscle injury is manifested by rising creatine phosphokinase (CPK).
- Any renal imaging is similar to other evaluations of acute renal failure.

Diagnostic Procedures/Other
Muscle compartment pressures if compartment syndrome suspected

Test Interpretation
- Muscle necrosis
- Myoglobin-related renal injury may resemble acute tubular necrosis from other causes.

1048

💉 TREATMENT

GENERAL MEASURES

- Aggressive hydration is often necessary. With severe muscle trauma (crush injuries), up to 12 L of fluid may be sequestered in the muscles, leading to intravascular volume depletion and explaining the low urine output despite fluid resuscitation, which increase the risk for renal failure.
- Monitor CK levels to ensure that rhabdomyolysis has ended.
- Monitor renal function and electrolytes.
- Continuous monitoring of potassium levels to prevent hyperkalemic arrhythmias and potential hypokalemia and arrhythmias.
- If DIC/hepatic dysfunction occurs, patients will need treatment and monitoring appropriate to these conditions.

MEDICATION

First Line

- When rhabdomyolysis is identified, appropriate intervention may prevent renal failure.
- Aggressive fluid resuscitation is the most important intervention: Normal saline (NS) and 5% glucose solution with a target urine output of 200 mL/hr. Alternating NS and 5% glucose is recommended to prevent volume overload. Infusion rate should be 500 mL/hr (4).
- Alkalinization of the urine is thought to decrease myoglobin-induced nephrotoxicity in the tubules (sodium bicarbonate to increase urine pH >6.5):
  – Use is controversial without strong evidence of efficacy.
  – Side effects include worsening hypocalcemia.
  – Sodium bicarbonate may be of use in patients with very high CK levels, an acidotic state, or coexisting hyperkalemia.
  – Place 150 mEq, 3 ampules, NaHCO$_3$ in 1 L of D5W and infuse at 200 mL/hr.

- IV mannitol as a bolus, 1–2 g/kg, not to exceed 200 g in 24 hours and cumulative dose up to 800 g. It is used to prevent ARF(3)[A]. Plasma osmolality should be closely monitored and stopped if diuresis is not adequate (>20 mL/hr):
  – Increases prostaglandins production leading to renal vasodilation and diuresis, making the kidneys less susceptible to myoglobin injury. Also an osmotic agent, filtered but not reabsorbed by the tubules, it increases sodium delivery and diuresis. This may remove necrotic cell debris and fluids trapped in damaged muscle cells preventing rise in compartment pressure and compartment syndrome.
  – Use of mannitol is controversial in this setting because no good evidence indicates that it improves outcomes more than aggressive IV hydration. It is a free-radical scavenger and has renal protective effects when used early, before tubular occlusion.
  – Consider adding furosemide to force diuresis if necessary (40–120 mg/d).
  – Diuresis should not be used in anuric renal failure. Customize the regimen for elderly and patients with heart disease.

Second Line

- Hyperkalemia can result from massive release of intracellular potassium stores or ARF. Severe hyperkalemia may be life-threatening. Treatment is warranted when ECG changes are present (tall, thin T waves; P-R prolongation; QRS widening; P-wave flattening).
- Treatments aiming at resolving hyperkalemia:
  – Calcium gluconate: To stabilize the cardiac membrane. IV 1–2 ampules (0.5 mL 10% calcium gluconate = 4 mg elemental calcium; give 4 mg/kg/hr × 4 hours)
  – If acidosis is present: 1–2 ampules (2–3 mL/kg) sodium bicarbonate IV. Remember that bicarbonate administration worsens hypocalcemia.
  – If tolerated: PO sodium polystyrene sulfonate (Kayexalate) as much as 20 g (1 g/kg); also can be given via enema if oral intake is not tolerated or not indicated.
  – Insulin and albuterol will transiently drive potassium into the cells. Administration of glucose can prevent the hypoglycemic effects of insulin.
  – Precautions: See "Etiology," especially drug combinations. Continuous monitoring of potassium levels to prevent overcorrecting with potential hypokalemia and arrhythmias.
  – Indications for dialysis include resistant and symptomatic hyperkalemia (ECG), oliguria (<0.5 mL/kg over 12-hour period), anuria, volume overload, or persistent acidosis (pH <7.1).

ISSUES FOR REFERRAL

- Usually managed as an inpatient
- Diagnosis of muscle entrapment/compartment syndromes may require surgical intervention (fasciotomy) to stop rhabdomyolysis.
- Early escharotomy for compartment syndrome related to burn
- Renal dialysis may be indicated in ARF.

ADDITIONAL THERAPIES

During the oliguric phase, symptomatic hypocalcemia is possible but rare and may benefit from IV calcium gluconate.

SURGERY/OTHER PROCEDURES

For muscle entrapment/compartment syndrome

IN-PATIENT CONSIDERATIONS

Admission Criteria/Initial Stabilization

- Patients with significant elevations of CK should be admitted for IV hydration and serial laboratory monitoring.
- Usually required for symptomatic patients or other complications

IV Fluids

Volume expansion with normal saline to increase urine output to at least 150 mL/hr

Nursing

Monitoring of vital signs and urine output

Discharge Criteria

CK usually peaks 24–36 hours after muscle injury, so monitoring should confirm that the CK is trending down. Renal function should be stable/improving. Electrolytes should be normal. Patients with mild CK elevation, trending down, and normal renal function may be discharged after observation phase.

⟳ ONGOING CARE

FOLLOW-UP RECOMMENDATIONS

Outpatient assessment within a few days to recheck CPK, electrolytes, and renal function

Patient Monitoring

- Contingent on disease: Essential for metabolic myopathies
- Myotoxic drugs should be discontinued/monitored closely.

DIET

- When rhabdomyolysis causes renal failure, restrict protein intake to lower BUN level.
- Potassium intake must be limited.
- With anuria, essential to restrict volume intake; once resolved, no restrictions

PROGNOSIS

Contingent on primary cause of rhabdomyolysis and on recovery from ARF without complications

COMPLICATIONS

- Death, especially from hyperkalemia/renal failure
- With dialysis and supportive care, the prognosis is very good.

REFERENCES

1. Murphy CM, Dulaney AR, Beuhler MC, et al. "Bath salts" and "plant food" products: The experience of one regional US poison center. *J Med Toxicol*. 2012 Jun 26. Epub 2012 Jun 26.
2. Huerta-Alardín AL, Varon J, Marik PE, et al. Bench-to-bedside review: Rhabdomyolysis—an overview for clinicians. *Crit Care*. 2005;9:158–169.
3. Bosch X, Poch E, Grau JM. Rhabdomyolysis and acute kidney injury. *N Engl J Med*. 2009;361: 62–72.
4. Cervellin G, Comelli I, Lippi G. Rhabdomyolysis: Historical background, clinical, diagnostic and therapeutic features. *Clin Chem Lab Med*. 2010;48:749–756.

ADDITIONAL READING

Shawkat H, Westwood MM, Mortimer A. Mannitol: A review of its clinical uses. *Cont Edu Anaesth Crit Care Pain*. 2012;12(2):82–85.

 ## SEE ALSO

Renal Failure, Acute

 ## CODES

ICD10

- M62.82 Rhabdomyolysis
- T79.6XXA Traumatic ischemia of muscle, initial encounter
- T79.6XXD Traumatic ischemia of muscle, subsequent encounter

CLINICAL PEARLS

- Acute CPK elevation into the thousands (often tens of thousands) is necessary before one sees myoglobinuric renal failure.
- The cornerstone of treatment of rhabdomyolysis is aggressive fluid administration.
- Frequent monitoring of potassium, calcium, and creatinine is necessary in the acute period.

RHABDOMYOSARCOMA

Ankur Goel, MD • Olusola Fasusi, MD • Edward Kruse, DO

BASICS

DESCRIPTION
- Rhabdomyosarcoma (RMS) is the most common soft tissue sarcoma in children younger than 20 years of age. (It is exceedingly rare in adults, representing 3% of all soft tissue sarcomas.)
  - 50% occur in the 1st decade of life
- Overall, it is an uncommon malignancy that arises from myoblasts.
- Common anatomic sites:
  - Head and neck (most common primary site in children)
  - Genitourinary
  - Musculoskeletal (extremities are the most common primary sites in adults)
- Subtypes:
  - Alveolar (ARMS): 23% of cases
    ○ More common in the trunk and extremities. Clinically more aggressive.
  - Embryonal (ERMS): Early onset. 57% of cases (most common subtype in children)
    ○ More likely to occur in the head, neck, and genitourinary areas.
      ■ Classic: Comprises 50% of cases
      ■ Botryoid: Sarcoma botryoids is typically seen in girls <4 years of age. 6% of cases
      ■ Spindle cell: 3% of cases Pleomorphic: Usually occurs in adults. 1% of cases
  - Sarcoma (not otherwise specified): Comprises 11% of all cases of RMS (most common subtype in adults, reflects inability for pathologists to characterize tumor)
  - Undifferentiated: Comprises 8% of all cases of RMS
- Associated term(s): Soft tissue sarcoma

EPIDEMIOLOGY

Incidence
- 4.5 cases of RMS per 1 million patients <20 years old per year (1)[A]
  - 50% occur within 1st decade of life (2)
- In adults, RMS represents 3% of all soft tissue sarcomas in adults

Prevalence
- RMS comprises 3% of all childhood cancers.
- Predominant sex: Male > Female (1.37:1)

Genetics
- Alveolar: *PAX3-FOXO1* or *PAX7-FOXO1* fusion genes as a result of t(2;13) and t(1;13), respectively; found in 75% of ARMS (3)[B]
- Embryonal: Loss of alleles on chromosome 11 may be seen.

RISK FACTORS
Smoking, advanced maternal age, in utero x-ray exposure, maternal recreational drug use, and history of still births

COMMONLY ASSOCIATED CONDITIONS
- Neurofibromatosis (NF1) 1: 20-fold increased risk of RMS in patients with NF1
- Li-Fraumeni syndrome: p53 mutations predispose to multiple tumors, including RMS

DIAGNOSIS

HISTORY
- Presents as a progressive painless mass of the head and neck, genitourinary tissue, trunk, or extremities.
- RMS of genitourinary tissue may present as vaginal bleeding in females.

- Other symptoms may be noted due to mass effect of the primary or metastatic lesions.
- Family history of genetic syndromes (i.e., NF1, Li-Fraumeni syndrome)

PHYSICAL EXAM
- Painless, enlarging mass
- Polypoid mass protruding from vagina (botryoid)
- Exophthalmos and chemosis (orbital involvement)
- Abdominal pain
- Compression symptoms, i.e., seizures, visual field defects, nerve palsy, headaches

DIAGNOSTIC TESTS & INTERPRETATION

Initial Tests (lab, imaging)
- Ultrasound: Used for differentiation of cystic vs. solid mass.
- MRI/CT: Used to evaluate tumor.
- Staging tests: Chest X-ray, CT thorax, fluorodeoxyglucose (FDG) PET (4)[B]
  - Most common site of metastasis is lung; evaluated by CT
  - FDG PET scans may be useful to detect lymph node or distant metastases not readily evident on CT or MRI scans

Diagnostic Procedures/Other
- Core needle biopsy, incisional biopsy, or excisional biopsy (based on size of mass):
  - The presence of rhabdomyoblast indicates the diagnosis.
- Immunohistochemical markers (5)[B]:
  - Myogenin: Commonly expressed in ARMS
  - Desmin: Associated with multiple subtypes of RMS
- Pathology
  - Alveolar: Rhabdomyoblasts arranged in what grossly appears to mimic pulmonary alveoli
  - Embryonal:
    ○ Classic: Rhabdomyoblasts configured in sheets without alveolar pattern
    ○ Botryoid: "Grape-like" appearance of rhabdomyoblasts with notable clustering in the subepithelium forming the cambium layer
    ○ Spindle cell: Rhabdomyoblasts with a spindle-like appearance
  - Undifferentiated: Rhabdomyoblast arrangement that cannot be classified as any other subtype
- Staging
  - Based on site, size, regional nodal involvement, and distance spread (6)[A]
  - See table

Stage	Site	T	Tumor diameter	N	M
1	Orbit; head and neck (excluding parameningeal); genitourinary—nonbladder and nonprostate; biliary tract	T1 or T2	a or b	N0 or N1 or NX	M0
2	Bladder or prostate; extremity; cranial parameningeal; other (includes trunk, retroperitoneum, etc.)	T1 or T2	a	N0 or NX	M0
3	Bladder or prostate; extremity; cranial parameningeal; other (includes trunk, retroperitoneum, etc.)	T1 or T2	a	N1	M0
				0 or N1 or NX	M0
4	All sites	T1 or T2	a or b	N0 or N1	M1

Note: a, ≤5 cm in diameter; b, >5 cm in diameter; M0, no distant metastasis present; M1, metastasis present; N0, regional nodes not clinically involved; N1, regional nodes clinically involved by neoplasm; Nx, clinical status of regional nodes unknown; T1, confined to site of origin; T2, extension and/or fixation to surrounding. tissue

TREATMENT

The 3 tenets of treatment for adults and children consist of surgical resection, radiation therapy, and chemotherapy. Patients should be referred to a multidisciplinary treatment team with expertise in oncology for definitive treatment.

SURGERY/OTHER PROCEDURES

- Wide local resection of tumor. If possible resect metastasis as well.
- However, wide resection may not be feasible in cases where grossly impaired functionality results.
  - All children receive chemotherapy:
  - In North America, the 3-drug combination of vincristine, dactinomycin, and cyclophosphamide (VAC) is the standard regimen (7)[B]:
    ○ Vincristine:
      ■ Adverse reactions: Alopecia, constipation, peripheral neuropathy
    ○ Actinomycin-D:
      ■ Adverse reactions: Pancytopenia, hepatotoxicity
    ○ Cyclophosphamide:
      ■ Adverse reactions: Hemorrhagic cystitis(mesna for prophylaxis), sterility, transitional cell carcinoma
- In addition, ifosfamide, topotecan, doxorubicin, etoposide, and irinotecan may also be used.
- Duration of chemotherapy is dependent on risk stratification and ranges from 6 to 12 months.
- Chemotherapy has been less commonly used in adults, who generally undergo treatment with resection and radiation therapy.
- Radiotherapy is currently used for those whose tumor cannot be completely resected.

ONGOING CARE

FOLLOW-UP RECOMMENDATIONS

Patients should follow up with their multidisciplinary treatment team. Long-term follow-up is necessary for detection of recurrence, metastatic disease, and development of secondary malignancies. Follow-up consists of physical exam, chest x-ray, and imaging of the primary tumor site every 3–6 months for the 1st 3 years.

PROGNOSIS

- RMS (all cases): 62% 5-year survival (1)[A]
- ARMS: 48% 5-year survival
- ERMS: 73% 5-year survival
- Prognosis in adults is worse, it is unclear whether this is related to subtype of tumor or lack of clear guidelines for adults; this is a rare presentation in adults.

COMPLICATIONS

- Recurrence
- Secondary neoplasm
- Growth abnormalities
- Treatment side effects

REFERENCES

1. Ognjanovic S, Linabery AM, Charbonneau B, et al. Trends in childhood rhabdomyosarcoma incidence and survival in the United States, 1975–2005. *Cancer*. 2009;115:4218–4226.
2. Kapoor G, Das K. Soft tissue sarcomas in children. *Indian J Pediatr*. 2012;79:936–942.
3. Arndt CA, Rose PS, Folpe AL, et al. Common musculoskeletal tumors of childhood and adolescence. *Mayo Clin Proc*. 2012;87:475-487.
4. Klem ML, Grewal RK, Wexler LH, et al. PET for staging in rhabdomyosarcoma: An evaluation of PET as an adjunct to current staging tools. *J Pediatr Hematol Oncol*. 2007;29:9–14.
5. Parham DM, Ellison DA. Rhabdomyosarcomas in Adults and Children. *Arch Pathol Lab Med*. 2006;130:1454–1465.
6. Malempati S, Hawkins D. Rhabdomyosarcoma: Review of the Children's Oncology Group Soft-Tissue Sarcoma Committee experience and rationale for current COG studies. *Pediatr Blood Cancer*. 2012;59:5–10.
7. Ray A, Huh W. Current state-of-the-art systemic therapy for pediatric soft tissue sarcomas. *Curr Oncol Rep*. 2012;14:311–319.

ADDITIONAL READING

- Hawkins DS, Spunt SL, Skapek SX. Children's Oncology Group's 2013 Blueprint for Research: Soft tissue sarcomas. *Pediatr Blood Cancer*. 2013;60: 1001–1008.
- Sultan I, Qaddoumi I, Yaser S, et al. Comparing adult and pediatric rhabdomyosarcoma in the Surveillance, Epidemiology and End Results Program, 1973 to 2005: An analysis of 2,600 patients. *J Clin Oncol*. 2009;27:3392–3397.

CODES

ICD10

- C49.9 Malignant neoplasm of connective and soft tissue, unsp
- C49.0 Malignant neoplasm of connective and soft tissue of head, face and neck
- C49.5 Malignant neoplasm of connective and soft tissue of pelvis

CLINICAL PEARLS

- RMS is the most common soft tissue sarcoma in children.
- They can arise at any site and in any tissue except bone.
- All persistent soft tissue masses should be evaluated with imaging (ultrasound to rule out cystic vs. solid, then MRI/CT)
- Fine needle aspiration may be helpful but core needle vs. incisional/excisional biopsy for confirmation.

R

RHEUMATIC FEVER
Payal Modi, MD, MPH • Elizabeth Goldberg, MD

BASICS

DESCRIPTION
- Acute rheumatic fever (ARF) is a recurrent inflammatory disease, possibly autoimmune in nature, that affects multiple organ systems.
- Delayed nonsuppurative sequelae of pharyngeal infection with group A streptococci can rarely cause permanent cardiac valvular disease as well as acute cardiac decompensation.
- Recurrences in both adults and children are common if not prevented with prophylactic antibiotic treatment.
- System(s) affected: Cardiovascular, Hematologic/Lymphatic/Immunologic, Musculoskeletal, Nervous, Skin/Exocrine

Pediatric Considerations
- More common in children
- In early studies, ARF developed in 3% of children with untreated group A β-hemolytic streptococcal pharyngitis (1).

EPIDEMIOLOGY
Incidence
- ARF and rheumatic heart disease (RHD) are now largely restricted to developing countries and some poor, mainly indigenous populations of wealthy countries.
- Predominant age: Children ages 5–15 years
- Predominant sex: Male = Female; females are more prone to develop chorea.
- Worldwide, the incidence of rheumatic fever has been declining for decades due to improved living conditions, better access to health care, and the increasing use of antibiotics.
- In the US, ARF had an incidence rate of 10.2/100,000 in the 1970s and currently is <2/100,000. However, since the mid-1980s, a resurgence of cases has occurred, with multiple outbreaks likely due to immigration from high-incidence countries (1)[A].
- Currently, the incidence of ARF is highest in developing countries, exceeding 50/100,000 children in some and accounting for 95% of ARF cases worldwide (1,2)[A].

Prevalence
- Prevalence of RHD in the US is <0.05/1,000 population, with rare regional outbreaks.
- Worldwide, 15.6 million people have RHD. 470,000 new cases of rheumatic fever and 233,000 deaths attributable to rheumatic fever or RHD each year (1).
- The overall prevalence worldwide is rising due to advancements in medical care and longer life expectancies.

ETIOLOGY AND PATHOPHYSIOLOGY
- Presents 1–4 weeks following an untreated group A β-hemolytic streptococcal pharyngitis or tonsillitis
- Molecular mimicry: Antibodies created against the M protein on cells of group A streptococcus also cross-react with various proteins in the heart and vessel walls. They subsequently attack self-cells, initiating an inflammatory cascade and causing the symptoms of rheumatic fever.

Genetics
- Certain human leukocyte antigen (HLA) class II DR and DQ genotypes and haplotypes, particularly DR7 and DR4. Additionally, polymorphisms occur in the promoter region of the TNFα, IL-10, and IL-6 genes (1).
- Increased susceptibility in certain populations, including Australian Aborigines and Pacific Islanders, likely due to genetic predisposition

RISK FACTORS
Possible increased incidence with iron deficiency and low albumin concentrations (3)[C]

GENERAL PREVENTION
- Primary prevention: Antibiotics are effective at reducing the incidence of ARF after known or suspected group A streptococcal (GAS) pharyngitis. To achieve clinical and bacteriologic cures, treat streptococcal pharyngitis with 10 days of penicillin, an oral cephalosporin, or an oral macrolide in patients who are allergic to penicillin. Number needed to treat: 100 (4)[A].
- Secondary prevention: Long-term prophylaxis (with penicillin G or a macrolide) in selected populations

DIAGNOSIS

- Evidence of preceding GAS infection indicated by: Positive throat culture for GAS, positive streptococcal antigen test, or elevated/rising antistreptolysin O antibody titer
- Modified Jones criteria for diagnosis: 2 major manifestations or 1 major and 2 minor manifestations
- Major criteria: Carditis, migratory polyarthritis, Sydenham chorea, erythema marginatum, and SC nodules
- Minor criteria: Fever, arthralgia, leukocytosis, ECG findings (prolonged PR interval, heart block), increased inflammatory markers (elevated ESR or C-reactive protein), and a history of rheumatic fever or heart disease
- Exception to Jones for diagnosis: Only chorea, indolent carditis, recurrent RF (5).

HISTORY
- Pharyngitis usually 1–4 weeks prior
- Acute febrile illness with malaise and muscle weakness
- Migratory large-joint polyarthritis and arthralgia (75%) with dramatic response to small doses of salicylates or NSAIDs:
  – Lower extremity joints are typically involved 1st, and symptoms are usually transient.
  – In patients treated with anti-inflammatory drugs, arthritis may be monoarticular, nonmigratory, or of short duration.
- Chest discomfort, pleuritic chest pain
- Rash
- Choreiform movements: Late manifestation 2–6 months after infection
- Emotional disturbances, outbursts of inappropriate behavior, crying, restlessness

PHYSICAL EXAM
- Pericardial frictional rub
- Pancarditis (50%): Blowing pansystolic murmur, rarely diastolic or new or changing murmurs
- Evidence of heart failure
- SC nodules (<1%): Firm, painless, up to 2 cm; over bony surface, prominences, or near tendons; present for a few weeks
- Erythema marginatum (5–13%): Nonpruritic erythematous rings on trunk that transiently appear and disappear over months; can be accentuated by warming the skin
- Sydenham chorea (10–15%): Nonrhythmic involuntary movements, more marked on 1 side, cease during sleep, may last up to 8 months
- "Milking sign": Diffuse hypotonia with no sensory losses

DIFFERENTIAL DIAGNOSIS
- Systemic lupus erythematosus (SLE)
- Poststreptococcal reactive arthritis
- Juvenile rheumatoid arthritis (JRA)
- Infectious arthritis
- Viral myocarditis
- Innocent cardiac murmurs
- Tourette syndrome
- Kawasaki syndrome
- Pediatric autoimmune neuropsychiatric disorders associated with streptococcal infections (PANDAS)

DIAGNOSTIC TESTS & INTERPRETATION
Initial Tests (lab, imaging)
- Prior treatment with aspirin or steroids may alter lab results.
- CBC with differential: Elevated WBC count and normochromic normocytic anemia
- Increased acute-phase reactants: ESR and CRP
- Throat culture for group A hemolytic streptococci (75% are negative)
- Bacteriologic or serologic evidence of GAS infection:
  – Antistreptolysin O titers (ASO, 80%): Peak at 4–5 weeks
  – If negative, check ASO antideoxyribonuclease (DNase B: detectable for 6–9 months), streptokinase, and antihyaluronidase.
- No change in complement levels
- ECG: All degrees of heart block, including prolonged PR interval, A-V dissociation, evidence of pericarditis
- Joint aspiration of affected joints reveals sterile inflammatory fluid with 10–100,000 WBC/mm³
- Chest x-ray (CXR): Most common radiologic manifestation of carditis is cardiomegaly
- Echocardiogram: Assess for chamber size and function, valvular disease including silent mitral regurgitation, and pericardial effusion; comprehensive echo screening identified ~10× as many children with RHD as were identified by the traditional strategy of clinical screening with echo confirmation (2).
- Antimyosin scintigraphy for detection of carditis (80% sensitive, limited specificity) (6)

Follow-Up Tests & Special Considerations
- Repeat ASO titers every 1–2 weeks until normalized (cannot be used as a measure of rheumatogenic activity)
- CRP and ESR are useful in monitoring rebounds of inflammation.
- Serial CXRs to monitor carditis
- Serial echocardiograms to document the course of valvular lesions

Test Interpretation
- Fibrinous pericardium and Anitschkow cells: Cardiac histiocytes
- Aschoff bodies: Focal inflammation surrounding fibrinoid necrosis
- Aschoff cells: Multinucleated giant cells in mass of fragmented swollen collagen fibers
- SC nodules have a characteristic histologic appearance.

TREATMENT

GENERAL MEASURES
- Mainly anti-inflammatory agents, especially for patients with carditis
- Treat arrhythmias with appropriate agents.
- Pain relief for patients with arthritis
- Heart failure therapy as needed

MEDICATION
First Line
- Symptomatic relief
- Eradication: Treat initially with penicillin as if active streptococcal infection is present; then begin prophylaxis (see "Follow-Up Recommendations"):
  – Penicillin × 10 days IM or IV
  – If the patient is allergic to penicillin, use a narrow-spectrum cephalosporin or a macrolide such as erythromycin.
- If patient has moderate-severe carditis with cardiomegaly/congestive heart failure (CHF), treat with prednisone 2 mg/kg/d (60 mg/d max) × 2 weeks; then taper over 2 weeks. Data on use of steroids are inconclusive (7)[C].
- If no cardiomegaly, start aspirin 80–100 mg/kg/d in children and 4–8 g/d in adults × 4–6 weeks. Start aspirin at beginning of steroid taper, and continue until symptoms are absent and ESR and CRP are normal (~6 weeks).
- For severe cases of chorea, sedation may be required with valproic acid as first line, then haloperidol or carbamazepine. IVIG may be beneficial as well (8).
- Household contacts should be screened with a throat culture and treated with appropriate antibiotics even if asymptomatic.
- Contraindications: Specific drug allergies
- Significant possible interactions: Refer to the manufacturer's profile of each drug.

Second Line
For children, naproxen at 15–20 mg/kg/d divided b.i.d. has been found safe and effective in ARF and has fewer adverse reactions than aspirin (9).

ISSUES FOR REFERRAL
Patients should be managed or comanaged by a cardiologist.

SURGERY/OTHER PROCEDURES
Mitral stenosis is a manifestation of late scarring and calcification of damaged valves that often requires surgical correction (valve repair preferred over replacement), especially in the presence of left atrial enlargement.

IN-PATIENT CONSIDERATIONS
Admission Criteria/Initial Stabilization
- Initial hospitalization may be helpful for diagnosis and to establish patient stability.
- CHF requires prompt hospitalization.

IV Fluids
Only if signs of dehydration present; use cautiously in patients with carditis/CHF

Nursing
- Gradual activity as tolerated
- Bed rest initially for arthralgia and heart failure: Once symptoms are improved, advance activity cautiously.

ONGOING CARE

FOLLOW-UP RECOMMENDATIONS
- ARF patients should be on prophylactic antibiotics throughout childhood and possibly indefinitely in adulthood:
  – The preferred treatment regimen is monthly IM injections of 1.2 million units of benzathine penicillin.
  – PO penicillin V-K 250 mg b.i.d. is an alternative to monthly injections for patients at lower risk for recurrence.
  – Patients should be treated for a minimum of 5 years after an attack or until age 18.
  – In adults with valvular disease, consider treating indefinitely.
  – If the patient is allergic to penicillin, treat with sulfadiazine 500 mg/d for children weighing <27 kg up to a maximum dose of 1 g/d for adults. Fluid intake should be maintained ≥1,500 mL/d to guard against sulfadiazine crystalluria.
- If patients have valvular damage from ARF, they also require bacterial endocarditis prophylaxis for dental and other high-risk procedures.
- Low threshold to test and treat acute episodes of GAS pharyngitis

Patient Monitoring
Initially each week, then every 6 months

Pediatric Considerations
Use aspirin with caution in children, given the potential risk of Reye syndrome.

Pregnancy Considerations
Residual valvular disease may be exacerbated. Refer preconception and pregnant patients to a cardiologist for assistance in management.

DIET
- Regular diet
- Low-sodium diet if the patient has carditis

PATIENT EDUCATION
American Heart Association at www.heart.org

PROGNOSIS
Sequelae are limited to the heart and depend on the severity of carditis during an acute attack.

COMPLICATIONS
- Subsequent attacks of ARF secondary to streptococcal reinfection
- Cardiac sequelae including carditis, RHD (specifically mitral stenosis; more likely in patients with carditis), and CHF

REFERENCES
1. Chang C. Cutting edge issues in rheumatic fever. *Clin Rev Allergy Immunol.* 2012;84(2):213–237.
2. Seckeler MD, Hoke TR. The worldwide epidemiology of acute rheumatic fever and rheumatic heart disease. *Clin Epidemiol.* 2011;3:67–84.
3. Zaman MM, Yoshiike N, Rouf MA, et al. Association of rheumatic fever with serum albumin concentration and body iron stores in Bangladeshi children: Case-control study. *BMJ.* 1998;317: 1287–1288.
4. Del Mar CB, Glasziou PP, Spinks AB, et al. Antibiotics for sore throat. *Cochrane Database Syst Rev.* 2006;(4):CD000023.
5. Ferrieri P, Jones Criteria Working Group. Proceedings of the Jones Criteria workshop. *Circulation.* 2002;106(19):2521.
6. Narula J, Malhotra A, Yasuda T. Usefulness of antimyosin antibody imaging for the detection of active rheumatic myocarditis. *Am J Cardiol.* 1999;84:946–950, A7.
7. Cilliers AM, Manyemba J, Saloojee H. Anti-inflammatory treatment for carditis in acute rheumatic fever. *Cochrane Database Syst Rev.* 2003;(2):CD003176.
8. Weiner SG, Normandin PA. Sydenham chorea: A case report and review of the literature. *Pediatr Emerg Care.* 2007;84(1):20–24.
9. Hashkes PJ, Tauber T, Somekh E, et al. Naproxen as an alternative to aspirin for the treatment of arthritis of rheumatic fever: A randomized trial. *J Pediatr.* 2003;143:399–401.

CODES

ICD10
- I00 Rheumatic fever without mention of heart involvement
- I01.0 Acute rheumatic pericarditis
- I01.9 Acute rheumatic heart disease, unspecified

CLINICAL PEARLS
- ARF is a recurrent inflammatory disease, possibly autoimmune in nature that affects multiple organ systems including the heart.
- The modified Jones criteria for the diagnosis of ARF include 2 major manifestations or 1 major and 2 minor manifestations in the context of a preceding documented GAS infection.
- ARF patients should be on prophylactic antibiotics throughout childhood.

RHINITIS, ALLERGIC
Naureen Rafiq, MD, MBBS

 BASICS

Allergic rhinitis is the collection of symptoms, involving mucous membranes of nose, eyes, ears, and throat after an exposure to allergens like pollen, dust, or dander.

DESCRIPTION
- IgE-mediated inflammation of the nasal mucosa following exposure to an extrinsic protein; an immediate symptomatic response is characterized by sneezing, congestion, and rhinorrhea followed by a persistent late phase dominated by congestion and mucosal hyperreactivity.
- Allergic rhinitis can be classified into seasonal or perennial and can be intermittent or persistent.
- Seasonal responses are usually due to outdoor allergens like tree pollen, flowering shrubs in spring, grasses and flowering plants in summer, and ragweed and mold in fall.
- Perennial responses, or year-round symptoms, are usually associated with indoor allergens like dust mites, mold, and animal dander.
- Occupational allergic rhinitis is caused by allergens at the workplace and can be sporadic or year round.
- Nonallergic rhinitis (e.g., vasomotor, rhinitis of pregnancy, and rhinitis medicamentosa) can occur.

Pediatric Considerations
Chronic nasal obstruction can result in facial deformities, dental malocclusions, and sleep disorders.

Pregnancy Considerations
Physiologic changes during pregnancy may aggravate all types of rhinitis, frequently in the 2nd trimester.

EPIDEMIOLOGY
- Onset usually in first 2 decades, rarely before 6 months of age, with tendency declining with advancing age.
- The mean age of onset is 8–11 years, and about 80% of cases have established allergic rhinitis by age 20.

Prevalence
- ~10–25% of the US adult population and 9–42% of the US pediatric population are affected.
- 44–87% of patients with allergic rhinitis have mixed allergic and nonallergic rhinitis, which is more common than either pure form (1).
- Scandinavian studies have demonstrated cumulative prevalence rate of 14% in men and 15% in women.

ETIOLOGY AND PATHOPHYSIOLOGY
- Aeroallergen-driven mucosal inflammation due to resident and infiltrating inflammatory cells, as well as vasoactive and proinflammatory mediators (e.g., cytokines)
- Inhalant allergens:
  - Perennial: House dust mites, indoor molds, animal dander, cockroach/insect detritus
  - Seasonal: Tree, grass, and weed pollens; outdoor molds
  - Occupational: Latex, plant products (e.g., baking flour), sensitizing chemicals, and certain animals for people working in farms and vet clinics

Genetics
Complex but strong genetic predilection present (80% have family history of allergic disorders)

RISK FACTORS
- Family history of atopy, with a greater risk if both parents have atopy
- Higher socioeconomic status
- Tobacco smoke can exacerbate symptoms and increase risk of developing asthma in patients with allergic rhinitis.
- Having other allergies like asthma
- Unclear evidence regarding risk due to early, repeated exposure to offending allergen and early introduction of solid food.
- Pets in house and houses infested with cockroaches can cause perennial allergic rhinitis.

GENERAL PREVENTION
- Primary prevention of atopic disease has not been proven effective by maternal diet or maternal allergen avoidance (2).
- Symptomatic control or secondary prevention by environmental avoidance by patient is the "first-line treatment."
- Unclear evidence to support use of acaricides with mite-proof mattress and pillow covers, carpet and drape removal, removal of plants in the home, pet control (2,3)[B].
- Air conditioning and limited outside exposure during allergy season (1)[B]
- HEPA air cleaners and vacuum bags are of unclear efficacy.
- Close doors and windows during allergy season.
- Use a dehumidifier to reduce indoor humidity.

COMMONLY ASSOCIATED CONDITIONS
Other IgE-mediated conditions: Asthma, atopic dermatitis, allergic conjunctivitis, food allergy

 DIAGNOSIS

Diagnosis is made primarily by history and physical exam.

HISTORY
- Evaluation of nature, duration, and time course of symptoms
- History of atopic dermatitis and/or food allergies
- History of nasal congestion; rhinorrhea; pruritus of nose, eyes, ears, and/or palate; sneezing; itching; and watering eyes
- Family history of allergic diseases
- History of environmental and occupational exposure and various nasal stimuli can help differentiate between allergic and vasomotor rhinitis.

PHYSICAL EXAM
Many findings are suggestive of but not specific for allergic rhinitis:
- Dark circles under eyes, "allergic shiners" (infraorbital venous congestion)
- Transverse nasal crease from rubbing nose upward; typically seen in children
- Rhinorrhea, usually with clear discharge
- Pale, boggy, blue-gray nasal mucosa
- Postnasal mucus discharge
- Oropharyngeal lymphoid tissue hypertrophy

DIFFERENTIAL DIAGNOSIS
- Infectious rhinitis: Usually viral, commonly with secondary bacterial infection:
  - Usually associated with sinusitis and is known as rhinosinusitis
  - Viral rhinitis averages 6 episodes/yr from ages 2–6 years.
  - IgA deficiency with recurrent sinusitis
  - Rhinitis medicamentosa:
    - Rebound effect associated with continued use of topical decongestant drops and sprays
    - ACE inhibitors, reserpine, β-blockers, oral contraceptive pills (OCPs), guanethidine, methyldopa
    - Aspirin, NSAIDs
  - Vasomotor (idiopathic) rhinitis caused by numerous nasal stimuli like warm or cold air, scents and odors, light or particulate matter
  - Hormonal: Pregnancy, thyroid, OCPs
  - Nonallergic rhinitis with eosinophilia syndrome (NARES)
  - Gustatory: Watery rhinorrhea in response to alcohol or food
  - "Skier's nose": Watery rhinorrhea in response to cold air
- Conditions associated with rhinitis:
  - Nasal polyps, tumor
  - Septal/Anatomic obstruction:
    - Adenoidal hypertrophy, particularly in children
    - Septal abnormality or deflected nasal septum (DNS) in adults

DIAGNOSTIC TESTS & INTERPRETATION
- Lab tests rarely needed
- Skin testing is done to identify the allergen for immunotherapy.

Initial Tests (lab, imaging)
- Testing is rarely indicated.
- If diagnosis implies other causes, consider:
  - CBC with differential may show elevated eosinophils.
  - Increased total serum IgE level
  - Nasal probe smear may show elevated eosinophils.
- Medications that may alter lab results:
  - Corticosteroids may decrease eosinophilia.
  - Antihistamines suppress reactivity to skin tests; stop antihistamines 7 days before testing.
- CT scan of sinuses is not routinely done, but can be used to check for complete opacity, fluid level, and mucosal thickening.

Diagnostic Procedures/Other
- Consider testing in only those cases where allergic symptoms do not respond to treatment and/or considering immunotherapy.
- Specific allergen sensitivity with allergen skin testing or radioallergosorbent testing (RAST); clinical correlation based on history is essential in interpreting results.
- Diagnostic allergen prick tests are used to select agent to determine appropriate environmental control measures, as well as to direct immunotherapy:
  - Prick or puncture: Superficial injury to epidermis with application of test antigen
  - Intradermal

- RAST: More expensive and less sensitive than skin testing; typically used in patients in whom skin testing is not practical or a severe reaction is possible
- Rhinoscopy: Useful to visualize intranasal anatomy and posterior pharyngeal structures, including adenoids, polyps, and larynx

Test Interpretation
- Nasal washing/scraping: Eosinophils predominate but may see basophils, mast cells
- Nasal mucosa: Submucosal edema but without destruction; eosinophilic infiltration; congested mucous glands and goblet cells

 TREATMENT

There are 3 mainstays of treatment of allergic rhinitis:
- Allergen avoidance
- Medication
- Allergy immunotherapy

GENERAL MEASURES
- Establish specific cause(s) by history and appropriate testing.
- Limit exposure to offending allergen.
- Allergen immunotherapy (desensitization):
  – Reserved when symptoms are uncontrollable with medical therapy or have a comorbidity (e.g., asthma)
  – Specific allergen extract is injected SC in increasing doses to induce patient tolerance.

MEDICATION
Oral medication and intranasal sprays are commonly used.

First Line
- Mild symptoms: 2nd-generation nonsedating antihistamines are first-line therapy for mild-to-moderate allergic rhinitis (1,4).
- Adverse effects: Mild sedation, mild anticholinergic effects
- Generic (cetirizine, fexofenadine, loratadine; most to least effective):
  – Levocetirizine is a new 2nd-generation nonsedating antihistamine that is effective, but costly.
- Intranasal corticosteroids are 1st-line therapy for moderate-to-severe allergic rhinitis (1,4)[A]:
  – Most effective drug class for symptoms of allergic rhinitis.
  – Use nasal sprays after showering, and direct spray away from septum to improve deposition on mucosal surface.
  – May be used as needed; however, less effective than regular use (1)
  – Adverse effects: Nosebleed, nasal septal perforation, and systemic corticosteroid effects
- Systemic steroids should be considered only in urgent cases and only for short-term use.
- Generic: Fluticasone

Second Line
1st-generation antihistamines, such as:
- Brompheniramine: 12–24 mg PO b.i.d.
- Chlorpheniramine: 4 mg PO q4–6h PRN
- Clemastine: 1–2 mg PO b.i.d. PRN

- Diphenhydramine: 25–50 mg PO q4–6h PRN:
  – May precipitate urinary retention in men with prostatism and/or hypertrophy
  – Adverse effects: Sedation, prolonged QT interval, performance impairment, and anticholinergic effect
- Nasal antihistamines effective but may be systemically absorbed and thus cause sedation: Azelastine, olopatadine
- Decongestants:
  – Phenylephrine: 10 mg PO q4h PRN
  – Pseudoephedrine: 60 mg PO q4–6h PRN
  – Oxymetazoline nasal spray (Afrin): 2–3 sprays per nostril q10–12h PRN (max 3 days). Intranasal agents should not be used for >3 days due to rebound rhinitis. Discourage use in patients with hypertension (HTN) or cardiac arrhythmia.
- Intranasal anticholinergics such as ipratropium nasal spray 2 sprays per nostril b.i.d.–t.i.d.:
  – Intranasal anticholinergics can increase efficacy in combination with steroid use (1).
- Leukotriene antagonists such as montelukast 10 mg/d PO:
  – Should generally be used as an adjunct, not monotherapy
- Mast cell stabilizers such as Cromolyn nasal spray 1 spray per nostril t.i.d.–q.i.d.:
  – May take 2–4 weeks of therapy for optimal efficacy
  – May be ineffective in patients with nonallergic rhinitis and nasal polyps

ISSUES FOR REFERRAL
Refer to allergist for consideration of immunotherapy.

ADDITIONAL THERAPIES
- Immunotherapy, either by injection (5)[A] or sublingually, which may be better tolerated by children (6)[A]
- Nasal saline use has evidence of efficacy as sole agent or as adjunctive treatment (1,7)[A].

 ONGOING CARE

FOLLOW-UP RECOMMENDATIONS
No specific restrictions on activity; emphasize avoiding activity where exposure to the allergen is likely.

Patient Monitoring
Initiation of patient education is critical.

DIET
- No special diet unless concomitant food reactions are suspected and evaluated
- Some patients with severe sensitivity to seasonal pollens may have oral allergy syndrome, which is associated with itching in the mouth with the ingestion of fresh fruits that may cross-react with the allergens.

PATIENT EDUCATION
- Asthma & Allergy Foundation of America, 1717 Massachusetts Ave., Suite 305, Washington, DC 20036; (800) 7-ASTHMA; www.aafa.org
- Other helpful information available at www.acaai.org and www.aaaai.org

PROGNOSIS
- Acceptable control of symptoms is the goal.
- Treatment is helpful to reduce the risk of comorbidities, such as sinusitis and asthma.

COMPLICATIONS
- Secondary infection such as otitis media or sinusitis
- Epistaxis
- Nasopharyngeal lymphoid hyperplasia
- Airway hyperreactivity with allergen exposure
- Asthma
- Facial changes, especially in children who are mouth breathers
- Sleep disturbance

REFERENCES

1. Wallace DV. The diagnosis and management of rhinitis: An updated practice parameter. *J Allergy Clin Immunol*. 2008;122:S1–S84.
2. Kramer MS, Kakuma R. Maternal dietary antigen avoidance during pregnancy or lactation, or both, for preventing or treating atopic disease in the child. *Cochrane Database Syst Rev*. 2012;9: CD000133. Epub 2012 Sep 12.
3. Sheikh A, Hurwitz B, Nurmatov U, et al. House dust mite avoidance measures for perennial allergic rhinitis. *Cochrane Database Syst Rev*. 2010;(7): CD001563. Epub 2010 Jul 7.
4. Plaut M, Valentine MD. Clinical practice. Allergic rhinitis. *N Engl J Med*. 2005;353:1934–1944.
5. Calderon MA, Alves B, Jacobson M, et al. Allergen injection immunotherapy for seasonal allergic rhinitis. *Cochrane Database Syst Rev*. 2007;(1):CD001936. Epub 2007 Jan 24.
6. Wilson DR, Lima MT, Durham SR. Sublingual immunotherapy for allergic rhinitis: Systematic review and meta-analysis. *Allergy*. 2005;60(1): 4–12.
7. Harvey R, Hannan SA, Badia L, et al. Nasal saline irrigations for the symptoms of chronic rhinosinusitis. *Cochrane Database Syst Rev*. 2007;(3):CD006394. Epub 2007 Jul 18.

 SEE ALSO

Conjunctivitis, Acute

 CODES

ICD10
- J30.1 Allergic rhinitis due to pollen
- J30.2 Other seasonal allergic rhinitis
- J30.9 Allergic rhinitis, unspecified

CLINICAL PEARLS
- Nasal saline irrigation (flushing 6–8 oz) may be very helpful in clearing upper airway of secretions and may precede the use of nasal corticosteroids.
- 2nd-generation antihistamines and intranasal corticosteroids are first-line therapies for allergic rhinitis.
- Referral to allergist is appropriate for identification of offending allergens and consideration of immunotherapy for inadequate symptom control.

ROCKY MOUNTAIN SPOTTED FEVER

Ginny H. Lee, MD • Alison P. Southern, MD

BASICS

DESCRIPTION
- Rocky Mountain spotted fever (RMSF) is a potentially fatal tick-borne systemic small vessel vasculitis caused by the bacterium *Rickettsia rickettsii*.
- RMSF is typically characterized by fever, headache, and myalgias followed by a centripetal (moving from the extremities inward towards the trunk) rash.
- System(s) affected: Cardiovascular, Musculoskeletal, Skin, CNS, Renal, Hepatic, Pulmonary

EPIDEMIOLOGY
Incidence
- In the US, the incidence of RMSF has increased from <2 cases per million persons in 2000 to >8 per million in 2008.
- Although RMSF has been reported in almost all states, most cases occur in the mid-Atlantic and southern states. North Carolina, Oklahoma, Arkansas, Tennessee, and Missouri account for ~60% of cases. RMSF has also been found in areas of Canada and in Central and South America.
- Predominant age: All ages are susceptible, but highest prevalence is in those age 50–64 years.
- Predominant sex: Male > Female, likely a product of outdoor exposure.
- Peak incidence occurs with tick exposure, typically in late spring and summer.

Prevalence
In the US, ~2,000–2,500 cases are reported annually.
- <0.1% of ticks carry virulent Rickettsial species.

ETIOLOGY AND PATHOPHYSIOLOGY
- An adult tick releases *R. rickettsii* from its salivary glands after 6–10 hours of feeding.
- The aerobic obligate intracellular Gram-negative coccobacilli spread hematogenously.
- Infected ticks are primarily the American dog tick, *Dermacentor variabilis*, in the eastern US, the Rocky Mountain wood tick, *Dermacentor andersoni*, in the western US, and the Brown dog tick, *Rhipicephalus sanuineus*, in the southwest.
- Rickettsiae proliferate inside endothelial cells by binary fission and invade contiguous vascular endothelial cells, causing a small-vessel vasculitis and the characteristic rash.
- Subsequent increased vascular permeability can lead to edema, hypovolemia, and hypoalbuminemia, with subsequent end-organ injury.
- Platelets are consumed locally due to vascular injury, but coagulopathy or disseminated intravascular coagulation (DIC) is rare.
- Incubation time: 2–14 d, with a median of 4–7 d.
- Transplacental transmission of infection has not been demonstrated.
- RMSF can rarely be caused by direct inoculation of tick blood into open wounds or conjunctivae.

RISK FACTORS
- Known tick bite, engorged tick, or presence of tick for >20 hours; *likelihood of infection increases with duration of tick attachment*.
- Crushed tick during its removal
- Accumulated outdoor exposure or residence in a wooded area
- Contact with outdoor pets or wild animals

GENERAL PREVENTION
People who will be exposed to the outdoor environment, especially in known tick-prone areas, can take measures to prevent infection (1,2,3)[A]:
- Limit time spent in tall grasses, open areas of low bushy vegetation, and wooded areas.
- Cover exposed skin; wear a hat, long sleeves and pants, closed-toed shoes.
- Use DEET-containing insect repellents on exposed skin. Permethrin can be used in conjunction on clothing.
- Carefully inspect the entire body after possible exposure, especially the scalp, neck, and axillae. Ticks are commonly hidden by hair. Closely inspect legs, groin, external genitalia, and waistlines.
- Remove attached ticks in their entirety with tweezers immediately. Wear gloves if possible.
- Wash hands and site of bite thoroughly after tick removal to avoid potential mucosal inoculation.
- Prophylactic antibiotic treatment is not recommended.

DIAGNOSIS

Delay in presentation and initiation of therapy can increase long-term sequelae and mortality.

HISTORY
Consider RMSF in acute febrile illness, especially with history of potential tick exposure within previous 14 days, travel to an endemic area, and presentation in the late spring or summer. *The painless tick bite often goes unnoticed, so many patients will not report a tick bite.*

PHYSICAL EXAM
- Early disease (days 1–3) presents like a viral illness with headache, fever, malaise, nausea, and vomiting. RMSF is easily mistaken for gastroenteritis, pharyngitis, or mononucleosis.
- On days 3–4, a centripetal rash usually forms (80% of adults), involving the palms and soles, spreading centrally to arms, legs, and trunk. The rash typically starts as an erythematous, macular, or maculopapular exanthem; 50% become petechial or purpuric:
  - ~20% will never develop this "classic" rash, which may delay diagnosis and result in a more severe outcome. Rash may also be difficult to visualize in dark-skinned patients.
  - Rash appearance may be variable. *Do not rely on the presence or absence of the typical rash*.
  - In severe cases, the rash can involve the entire body and mucosal membranes and may progress to necrotic or gangrenous lesions.
  - The rash is not associated with pruritus or urticaria; their presence makes RMSF less likely.

- Signs and symptoms associated with RMSF and their frequency of occurrence:
  - Fever, usually >102°F (99–100%)
  - Rash, macular/maculopapular/petechial (88–90%)
  - Headache (79–91%)
  - "Classic triad" of headache, fever, and rash (50–60%)
  - Myalgias (72–83%)
  - Nausea/Vomiting (56–60%)
  - Abdominal pain, particularly in children (35–52%)
  - Hepatosplenomegaly (12–16%)
  - Lymphadenopathy (27%)
  - Cough, nonproductive (33%)
  - CNS dysfunction, stupor/confusion/coma/focal abnormalities (10–30%)
  - Patients may also have malaise, restlessness, arthralgia, conjunctivitis, peripheral or periorbital edema.

DIFFERENTIAL DIAGNOSIS
- Viral exanthems (e.g., measles, rubella, roseola)
- Meningoencephalitis (viral meningitis or encephalitis, bacterial meningitis)
- Meningococcemia
- Typhus
- Ehrlichiosis
- Lyme disease
- Leptospirosis
- Toxic shock syndrome
- Adenovirus infection
- Drug reaction or serum sickness
- Mononucleosis
- Kawasaki disease

DIAGNOSTIC TESTS & INTERPRETATION
Diagnosis is often clinical in a patient with exposure history in an endemic area. Retrospective confirmation is attained by serology. Treatment should not be delayed awaiting confirmatory serology.

Initial Tests (lab, imaging)
- Specific laboratory diagnosis:
  - Serum indirect fluorescent antibody (IFA): titer of >1:64 is diagnostic. A 4-fold increase of acute and convalescent titers helps confirm an active case of RMSF.
  - Antibodies usually develop 7–10 days after onset of symptoms; optimal time for testing, therefore, is 14–21 days after onset of symptom onset. *Do not delay treatment*.
  - Early treatment may limit antibody formation.
  - Seropositivity is related to increasing age in endemic states. Positive spotted fever group rickettsia antibody does not necessarily signify an acute infection.
- Nonspecific laboratory changes (incidence):
  - WBC count: Variable and frequently normal
  - Thrombocytopenia (32–52%)
  - Anemia, mild (5–24%)
  - Hyponatremia, mild (19–56%)
  - Azotemia (12–14%)
  - Elevated AST (36–62%)
  - Coagulation derangements are not common, despite vascular damage.
  - CSF is usually normal; some patients may have mononuclear pleocytosis, elevated protein and normal glucose.
- Other than occasional nonspecific pneumonic infiltrates on chest radiograph, imaging procedures are rarely helpful.

Diagnostic Procedures/Other

Skin biopsy of a rash lesion can offer definitive diagnosis. A 3-mm punch biopsy is sufficient to perform a rapid direct fluorescent antibody (DFA) test (sensitivity 70%, specificity 100%). Electron microscopy (EM) can also identify rickettsiae within endothelial cells. Western immunoblotting is necessary to confirm the specific spotted fever group species.

Test Interpretation

- Rickettsiae can be demonstrated within endothelial cells by DFA or EM.
- Petechiae due to the vasculitis may be seen on various organ surfaces (e.g., liver, brain, or epicardium).
- Secondary thromboses and tissue necrosis may be seen.

TREATMENT

MEDICATION
First Line

Doxycycline is the treatment of choice in adults and children (1,3,4,5)[A]:

- Untreated rickettsial infections have a high rate of morbidity and mortality. Other antibiotics are considerably less effective.
- The ONLY contraindication to doxycycline is severe allergy.
- For adults: 100 mg PO or IV q12h × 7d, lengthened to 2 days after the patient has become afebrile; 100 mg q24h in renal failure
- For children weighing <45 kg (100 lbs): 2.2 mg/kg/dose q12h
- Fever should subside within 24–72 h with early treatment; may take longer if patient is severely ill.
- If patient has no response to doxycycline, consider an alternate diagnosis. Rickettsial resistance to doxycycline has NOT been documented.
- Side effects of doxycycline:
  – Dyspepsia. Take medication with food and water. Avoid dairy products, iron preparations, or antacids as they may inhibit drug absorption.
  – Photosensitivity may occur. Minimize sun exposure and use sunscreen.
  – Long courses of medication can result in staining teeth in children. This side effect has never been documented in the short courses advocated for rickettsial infections.

Second Line

- Chloramphenicol: 20 mg/kg IV q6h (4 g/d max); same dose in renal failure:
  – Associated with aplastic anemia and an increased case-mortality
- Fluoroquinolones have not been evaluated clinically in RMSF, but they have shown in vitro activity against *R. rickettsii*.
- Sulfa-containing drugs may worsen tick-borne infections.

Pregnancy Considerations

- Doxycycline is appropriate for this life-threatening infection in pregnancy if suspicion is high, despite the potential risk to fetal bones/teeth.
- Chloramphenicol may be considered during the first 2 trimesters, but should be avoided in the 3rd trimester due to potential for gray baby syndrome.

ISSUES FOR REFERRAL
Consider infectious disease consult.

ADDITIONAL THERAPIES
Patients with neurologic injury or loss of limbs caused by gangrene may require prolonged physical and cognitive therapy.

IN-PATIENT CONSIDERATIONS
Admission Criteria/Initial Stabilization
- CNS dysfunction
- Nausea/Vomiting preventing oral antibiotic therapy
- Immunocompromised patients
- Specific acute organ failure
- Failure of oral pain management
- Acutely ill patients with shock should be treated in an ICU.

IV Fluids
Aggressive fluid resuscitation and electrolyte management may be required in critically ill patients.

Discharge Criteria
- Resolution of fever
- Ability to take oral therapy and nutrition

 ONGOING CARE

FOLLOW-UP RECOMMENDATIONS
- Patients with moderate to severe disease typically should be hospitalized.
- Patients with mild disease may be treated as outpatients. Close follow-up is important to identify complications.
- Infection does not confer lifelong immunity.

Patient Monitoring
- Outpatients should be seen every 2–3 days until symptom resolution.
- Consider tracking CBC, electrolytes, and LFTs, when clinically indicated.

DIET
Consider nutritional supplementation if intake is poor.

PROGNOSIS
- Prognosis is closely related to the timeliness of appropriate antibiotics. Treatment before day 5 of illness is essential and can prevent morbidity and mortality.
- When treated promptly, prognosis is usually excellent with resolution of symptoms over several days and no sequelae.
- If complications develop (see "Complications"), course may be more severe and long-term sequelae (especially neurologic sequelae) may be present.
- Death is rare with prompt institution of appropriate therapy.
- Children age 5–9 years and elderly >70 years are at higher risk of significant morbidity and/or mortality.
  – Black males with G6PD deficiency are at highest risk for fulminant RMSF, in which death can occur within 5 days.

COMPLICATIONS
- Encephalopathy (30–40%); most commonly transient impaired level of consciousness or meningismus
- Seizures, focal neurologic deficit (10%)
- Renal injury (10%)
- Hepatitis (10%)
- Congestive heart failure (CHF) (5%)
- Respiratory failure (5%)
- Also proximal muscle weakness, changes in personality, paresthesias, distal necrosis, and deafness.

REFERENCES

1. Lin L, Decker CF. Rocky Mountain spotted fever. *Dis Mon*. 2012;58(6):361–369.
2. Minniear TD, Buckingham SC. Managing Rocky Mountain spotted fever. *Expert Rev Anti Infect Ther*. 2009;7:1131–1137.
3. Elston DM. Tick bites and skin rashes. *Curr Opin Infect Dis*. 2010;23:132–138.
4. Botelho-Nevers E, Raoult D. Host, pathogen and treatment-related prognostic factors in rickettsioses. *Eur J Clin Microbiol Infect Dis*. 2011;30(10):1139–1150.
5. Woods CR. Rocky Mountain spotted fever in children. *Pediatr Clin North Am*. 2013;60(2):455–470. doi: 10.1016/j.pcl.2012.12.001.

ADDITIONAL READING

- Dahlgren FS, Holman RC, Paddock CD, et al. Fatal Rocky Mountain spotted fever in the United States, 1999–2007. *Am J Trop Med Hyg*. 2012;86(4):713–719.
- Salinas LJ, Greenfield RA, Little SE, et al. Tickborne infections in the southern United States. *Am J Med Sci*. 2010;340(3):194–201.
- Stallings SP. Rocky Mountain spotted fever and pregnancy: A case report and review of the literature. *Obstet Gynecol Surv*. 2001;56(1):37–42.

 CODES

ICD10
A77.0 Spotted fever due to Rickettsia rickettsii

CLINICAL PEARLS

- Maintain a high index of clinical suspicion and initiate treatment early: the painless tick bite often goes unnoticed, so many patients will not report a tick bite. Do not delay for serologic confirmation or development of a characteristic rash as some patients may never develop a rash or the classic triad of symptoms.
- The only absolute contraindication to treatment of RMSF with doxycycline is severe allergy.
- Lab testing is nonspecific and frequently normal.
- While prevalence is highest in central and southeastern US, cases have been reported in almost all states.

ROSEOLA

Rebecca Khezri Jacobson, MST, MD • Angela Beeler, MD

 BASICS

DESCRIPTION

- Acute infection of infants or very young children
- Causes a high fever followed by a skin eruption as the fever resolves
- Transmission via contact with salivary secretions from adults shedding human herpesvirus-6 (HHV-6)
- Incubation period of 5–15 days
- System(s) affected: Skin/Exocrine; Metabolic; Gastrointestinal; Respiratory; Neurologic
- Synonym(s): Exanthem subitum; Pseudorubella; sixth disease; 3-day fever

Pediatric Considerations
A disease of infants and very young children

EPIDEMIOLOGY
- Predominant age:
  – Infants and very young children (<2 years old)
  – Peak age HHV-6 infection 7–13 months, rarely congenital or perinatal infection
- Predominant sex: Male = Female

Incidence
- Common

Prevalence
Peak prevalence is between 9 and 21 months (1)[B]

ETIOLOGY AND PATHOPHYSIOLOGY
- HHV-6 and -7 (2)[C]

- Majority of cases (60–74%) due to HHV-6 (3)[A]
  – HHV-6B > HHV-6A (4)[A]
  – HHV-6 binds to CD46 receptors on all nucleated cells (4)[A]
- Latent or persistent asymptomatic infection occurs after primary infection (5)[A]
  – 80–90% population intermittently sheds HHV-6/7 in salivary glands (6)[A]
  – Patients are viremic from 2 days prior to fever until defervescence and onset of rash (2)[C]
  – HHV-6 latency also implicated in CSF (5)[A]

Genetics
No known genetic pattern

RISK FACTORS
- Female gender (1)[B]
- Having older siblings (1)[B]

- At-risk adults: Immunocompromised:
  – Renal, liver, other solid organ and bone marrow transplant (BMT)

  – HHV-6 reactivation can occur in 1st weeks posttransplant accompanied by a cytomegalovirus (CMV) infection (3)[A]
    ○ HHV-6 viremia occurs in 30–45% of BMT within the first several weeks after transplantation (4)[A]
    ○ Usually asymptomatic (4)[A]
    ○ Up to 66% of HHV-6 reactivation/reinfection in solid organ transplant (4)[A]
  – Advanced AIDS (3)[A]

- Nonrisk factors (1)[B]:
  – Child care attendance
  – Method of delivery
  – Breastfeeding
  – Maternal age
  – Season

 DIAGNOSIS

HISTORY
- Irritability (1)[B]
- +/– 3–5 days abrupt fever 102.2–104°F (39–40°C) (3)[A]
  – 50% of cases, afebrile (2)[C]
- Sudden drop of fever:
  – After 3–5 days, fever disappears, skin rash appears (5)[A]
  – +/– Rash on trunk then spreads centrifugally to neck, peripheral extremities, and face (6)[A]
- Diarrhea (1)[B]
- Vomiting (1)[B]
- Mild upper respiratory symptoms (3)[A]
- Rhinorrhea (1)[B]
- Febrile seizure occurs in 10% of cases (2)[C]

PHYSICAL EXAM
- Rash (exanthem subitum):
  – Rose-pink macules and/or papules (2)[C]
  – 1st appears on the neck and trunk then peripherally (2)[C]
  – Fades within 2 days (2)[C]

  – Occurs in as few as 10% of patients (1)[B]
- Inflammation of tympanic membrane (4)[A]

- Erythematous papules on soft palate and uvula (Nagayama spots) (2)[C]
- Uvulo-palatoglossal junctional ulcers (2)[C]

- Cervical lymphadenopathy (3)[A]

DIFFERENTIAL DIAGNOSIS
- Enterovirus infection (7)[A]
- Adenovirus infection (7)[A]
- Epstein-Barr virus (7)[A]
- Fifth disease-parvovirus B19 (7)[A]
- Rubella (7)[A]
- Scarlet fever (7)[A]
- Drug eruption (7)[A]

DIAGNOSTIC TESTS & INTERPRETATION
- A clinical diagnosis

- Tests often cannot differentiate latent or active disease (8)[A]

Initial Tests (lab, imaging)
- HHV-6 and HHV-7 by PCR (5)[A]:
  – Only use noncellular specimen for testing: Serum, CSF, or saliva
  – Becoming more widely available
- HHV-6 IgM immunofluorescence (5)[A]:
  – Diagnostic for acute infection
  – Detected 5–7 days, peak 2–3 weeks
  – Unreliable: High false positive and negative

- HHV-6 IgG immunofluorescence (5)[A]:
  – 4-fold rise in titers needed
  – Suggests primary infection or reactivation
  – Single positive test not diagnostic, need samples 2–3 weeks apart
  – More reliable than single IgM test
  – Not used widely
- Viral culture:
  – Takes 1–3 weeks, rarely done (5)[A]
  – Not widely available (5)[A]
  – Too time consuming (6)[A]

Diagnostic Procedures/Other
- Urine culture: To rule out UTI as source of fever
- Chest x-ray (CXR): If a child has respiratory symptoms

 TREATMENT

No treatment necessary, resolves without sequelae (3)[A]

GENERAL MEASURES
- Symptomatic relief including antipyretics (2)[C],7[A]
- Anticonvulsant if there is a seizure (7)[A]

MEDICATION
First Line
- No specific first-line treatment in immunocompetent hosts (5)[A]
  – Antivirals not suggested in immunocompetent (3)[A]
- No approved antiviral treatment in immunocompromised (8)[A]

Second Line
- IV Ganciclovir, cidofovir, foscarnet tested in vitro studies in stem cell transplant patients (8)[A]:
  – HHV-6B susceptible: Ganciclovir and foscarnet (8)[A]
  – HHV-6A and HHV-7: More resistant to ganciclovir (8)[A]
- Antivirals suggested in individual cases of encephalitis (3)[A]

ONGOING CARE

FOLLOW-UP RECOMMENDATIONS
Patient Monitoring
- None after typical rash appears and fever resolves
- Mean duration of illness is 6 days (4)[A]
- If febrile seizures occur, they will cease after fever subsides and will not cause brain damage

DIET
Encourage fluids

PATIENT EDUCATION
- Parental reassurance that this is usually a benign, self-limited disease
- There is no specific recommended period of exclusion from out-of-home care for affected children
- Patient is viremic a few days prior to fever until time of defervescence and rash onset

PROGNOSIS
- Course: Acute, complete recovery without sequelae
- Reactivation in immunocompromised patients is possible

COMPLICATIONS
- Febrile seizures
- Medication hypersensitivity syndromes
- Reactivation can occur in transplant patients, HIV-1 infection
- Poor association with multiple sclerosis (3,4)[A]
- Poor association with chronic fatigue syndrome (3,4)[A]
- Meningioencephalitis (rare, reported in case reports, conflicting studies) (4,5)[A]

REFERENCES

1. Zerr DM, Meier AS, Selke SS, et al. A population-based study of primary human herpesvirus 6 infection. *N Engl J Med*. 2005; 352:768–776.
2. Dyer JA. Childhood viral exanthems. *Ped Annals*. 2007;36:21–29.
3. Stoeckle MY. The spectrum of human herpesvirus 6 infection: From roseola infantum to adult disease. *Ann Rev Med*. 2000;51:423–430.
4. Caserta MT, Mock DJ, Dewhurst S. Human Herpesvirus 6. *Clin Infect Dis*. 2001;33:829–833.
5. Leach CT. Human herpesvirus-6 and -7 infections in children: Agents of roseola and other syndromes. *Curr Opin Pediatr*. 2000;12:269–274.
6. Wolz MM, Sciallis GF, Pittelkow MR. Human herpesvirus 6, 7, 8 from a dermatologic perspective. *Mayo Clin Proc*. 2012;87:1004–1014.
7. Folster-Holst R, Kreth HW. Viral exanthems in childhood-infectious (direct) exanthems. Part 1: Classic exanthems. *J Dtsch Dermatol Ges*. 2009;7:309–316.
8. Le J, Gantt S, AST Infectious Disease Community of Practice. Human herpesvirus 6, 7 and 8 in solid organ transplantation. *Am J Transpl*. 2013;13: 128–137.

ADDITIONAL READING

- Ablashi DV, Devin CL, Yoshikawa T, et al. Review part 3: Human herpesvirus-6 in multiple non-neurological diseases. *J Med Virol*. 2010;82: 1903–1910.
- Caselli E, Di Luca D. Molecular biology and clinical associations of Roseoloviruses human herpesvirus 6 and human herpesvirus 7. *New Microbiol*. 2007;30:173–187.
- Dockrell DH, Smith TF, Paya CV. Human herpesvirus 6. *Mayo Clin Proc*. 1999;74:163–170.
- Evans CM, Kudesia G, McKendrick M. Management of herpesvirus infections. *Int J Antimicrob Agents*. 2013;42:119–128.
- Huang CT, Lin LH. Differentiating roseola infantum with pyuria from urinary tract infection. *Pediatr Int*. 2013;55:214–218.
- Lowry, M. Roseola infantum. *Pract Nurse*. 2013;43: 40–42.
- Vianna RA, de Oliveira SA, Camacho LA, et al. Role of human herpesvirus 6 infection in young Brazilian children with rash illnesses. *Pediatr Infect Dis J*. 2008;27:533–537.

CODES

ICD10
- B08.20 Exanthema subitum [sixth disease], unspecified
- B08.21 Exanthema subitum [sixth disease] due to human herpesvirus 6
- B08.22 Exanthema subitum [sixth disease] due to human herpesvirus 7

CLINICAL PEARLS

- Roseola infection should be suspected if a young child presents with a high temperature.
- As the fever abates, a macular rash will be seen on the neck and trunk, with eventual spread to the face and extremities.
- Roseola is a clinical diagnosis and laboratory testing is not necessary for most children with classic roseola.
- For atypical presentations, complications, and immunocompromised hosts, several laboratory tools are available, including serologic testing for antibody, viral PCR testing, and viral culture.
- Infection is typically self-limiting and without sequelae.
- Usually only symptomatic treatment is needed.

ROTATOR CUFF IMPINGEMENT SYNDROME

Faren H. Williams, MD, MS

BASICS

DESCRIPTION
- Compression of rotator cuff tendons and subacromial bursa between the humeral head and the structures that make up the coracoacromial arch and humeral tuberosities
- Most common cause of atraumatic shoulder pain in patients age >25 years
- Typical symptom is pain that is most severe with arm abducted between 60° and 120° (the "painful arc").
- Classically divided into 3 stages:
  - Stage I: Acute inflammation, edema, or hemorrhage of the underlying tendons due to overuse (typically in those age <25 years)
  - Stage II: Progressive tendinosis that leads to partial rotator cuff tear along with underlying thickening or fibrosis of surrounding structures (commonly, ages 25–40 years)
  - Stage III: Full-thickness tear (typically in patients age >40 years)

EPIDEMIOLOGY
Incidence
- Shoulder pain accounts for 1.2% of all primary care visits.
- Peak incidence of 25/1,000 patients/year in those aged 42–46.
- Impingement cited as cause in 18–74% of patients with shoulder pain.

Prevalence
Prevalence of shoulder pain in general population thought to range from ~7–30%.

RISK FACTORS
- Repetitive overhead motions, including throwing
- Glenohumeral joint instability or muscle imbalance
- Hooked acromion
- Acromioclavicular (AC) spurs, osteophytes
- Thickened coracoacromial ligament
- Shoulder trauma
- Os acromiale
- Increasing age
- Smoking

GENERAL PREVENTION
- Proper throwing and lifting techniques
- Proper development of rotator cuff and scapula stabilizer muscles

DIAGNOSIS

HISTORY
- Gradual increase in shoulder pain with overhead activities (sudden onset of sharp pain may be suggestive of a tear).
- Pain at night is frequently reported, exacerbated by lying on the involved shoulder or sleeping with the arm above the head.
- Common complaint of anterolateral shoulder pain with overhead activities
- May progress to weakness and decreased range of motion if shoulder is not used through full range of motion.

PHYSICAL EXAM
- Neer Impingement Test: Examiner stabilizes the scapula and asks the patient to forward flex the arm until reporting pain or until full elevation is reached. Sensitivity: 78%. Specificity: 58% (1)[A].
- Hawkins-Kennedy Impingement Test: Examiner places the arm in 90° of forward flexion and then gently internally rotates the arm. Endpoint for internal rotation is when the patient feels pain or when the rotation of the scapula is felt or observed by the examiner. Test is positive when patient experiences pain during the maneuver. Sensitivity: 74%. Specificity: 57% (1)[A].
- Empty Can Test: Examiner asks the patient to elevate and internally rotate the arm with thumbs pointing downward in the scapular plane. Elbow should be fully extended. Examiner applies downward pressure on upper surface of the arm, testing for supraspinatus weakness. Sensitivity: 69%. Specificity: 62% (1)[A].
- Lift-Off Test: Patient internally rotates the shoulder, placing the hand on ipsilateral buttock, then lifts hand off buttock against resistance. A tear in the subscapularis muscle produces weakness of this action. Sensitivity: 42%. Specificity: 97% (1)[A].
- Drop-Arm Test: Patient fully elevates arm and then slowly reverses the motion. If the arm is dropped suddenly or the patient has extreme pain, the test is positive for a possible rotator cuff tear. Sensitivity: 21%. Specificity: 92% (1)[A].
- Resisted External Rotation: Weakness suggestive of infraspinatus and/or teres minor tendon involvement.
- Cervical spine must be evaluated to rule out cervical pathology as source of shoulder pain.

DIFFERENTIAL DIAGNOSIS
- Labral injury (labrum of glenoid is a cartilage cuff that assists in supporting the head of the humerus; tears usually due to trauma)
- Acromioclavicular arthritis (more common as age increases; likely to have pain with cross-arm testing)
- Adhesive capsulitis (rotator cuff tendonitis leads to decreased use and atrophy of rotator cuff muscles, followed by contracture of joint; may be related to prior trauma and has been linked to diabetes).

- Anterior shoulder instability (owing to trauma; more common in those age <25 years)
- Multidirectional instability
- Biceps tendonitis or rupture (perform Speed's and Yergeson's tests and look for visible or palpable defect of biceps)
- Calcific tendonitis
- Cervical radiculopathy (spinal or foraminal stenosis, can test with Spurling's maneuver)
- Glenohumeral arthritis (evaluate with plain films)
- Suprascapular nerve entrapment (look for focal muscle atrophy of supra- or infraspinatus)
- Traumatic rotator cuff tear

DIAGNOSTIC TESTS & INTERPRETATION
Initial Tests (lab, imaging)
- Plain-film radiographs of the shoulder (3 views): Anteroposterior, axillary, scapular Y views.
- Plain film may reveal:
  - Osteoarthritis of the acromioclavicular and glenohumeral joints
  - Superior migration of the humeral head (indicative of a large rotator cuff tear)
  - Cystic change of the humeral head and sclerosis of the inferior acromion (indicative of chronic rotator cuff disease)
  - Calcific tendonitis
- MRI is used to assess rotator cuff tendinopathy, partial tears, and complete tears.
- MR arthrogram is preferred test for detecting suspected labral pathology.
- US is sensitive and specific for rotator cuff tears, but is highly operator dependent.
- CT scan is the preferred imaging study for bony pathology or for those unable to undergo MRI.

Diagnostic Procedures/Other
- Lidocaine injection test:
  - Inject lidocaine into the subacromial space:
    - Repeat impingement tests; if pain is completely relieved and range of motion is improved, likely impingement syndrome
  - Allows for more accurate strength testing on physical examination:
    - If strength is intact, rules out rotator cuff tear.
    - If range of motion does not improve in any plane, more likely adhesive capsulitis
  - Some pain relief and improved range of motion occurs after lidocaine injection with:
    - Glenoid labral tear
    - Capsular strain
    - Glenohumeral osteoarthritis
    - Glenohumeral instability
- A lack of any pain relief suggests other sources or inappropriate placement of injection.

Test Interpretation
May have tendinosis, tendonitis, or muscle/tendon tear

TREATMENT

Anti-inflammatory agents + aggressive rehabilitation can improve and fully resolve rotator cuff tendonitis in most patients.

GENERAL MEASURES
- Rest
- Ice or heat for symptom relief
- Activity modification, with avoidance of aggravating activities, particularly overhead motions
- Range-of-motion exercises
- Rotator-cuff and adjacent muscle strengthening to enhance stability and prevent further injuries

MEDICATION
First Line
NSAIDs or other analgesic, often for 6–12 weeks

ISSUES FOR REFERRAL
Failure of conservative treatment, persistent pain, weakness, or complete tear of rotator cuff

ADDITIONAL THERAPIES
- Supervised- or home-exercise regimens have been shown to provide clinically significant pain reduction and improved function (2)[A].
- Physical therapy has demonstrated evidence of effectiveness for short-term and long-term recovery with respect to function (3)[A]:
  – Initial goal is to restore range of motion.
  – After pain resolves, gradually strengthen rotator cuff muscles in internal rotation, external rotation, and abduction.

SURGERY/OTHER PROCEDURES
- Steroid injections may have a significant benefit on pain and function in the short-term, but do not appear to have a significant long-term effect (5)[A]:
  – No apparent significantly increased risk for rotator cuff tears in those receiving subacromial steroid injections (6)[C]
  – Joint and soft tissue injections appear to be safe in patients receiving warfarin anticoagulation with an INR <3 (7)[A].
- No evidence that surgical treatment is superior to conservative management, or that 1 surgical technique is superior to another to treat impingement syndrome (8)[A]:
  – No apparent effect of platelet-rich plasma injection during arthroscopic rotator cuff repair on overall retear rates or shoulder-specific outcomes (9)[A].

COMPLEMENTARY AND ALTERNATIVE MEDICINE
Possible benefit of acupuncture when used with physical therapy, reducing pain and improving function, with benefit maintained for up to 1 year (4)[A]

 ONGOING CARE

PATIENT EDUCATION
- Patient must understand that physical rehabilitation may be necessary, both in conservative course of treatment (i.e., NSAIDs, physical therapy, home exercises) and with surgical decompression. An aggressive trial of rehabilitation should be encouraged prior to extensive testing or surgical intervention.
- Symptoms often recur if not fully addressed.

PROGNOSIS
- Variable, depends on underlying pathology
- Most patients improve with conservative management, but recovery is often slow.
- Having clinical symptoms for >1 year and increased severity of symptoms are reported to be prognostic factors for a negative outcome on conservative intervention.

COMPLICATIONS
- Progression of injury
- Tendon retraction in complete rotator cuff tear

REFERENCES

1. Alqunaee M, Galvin R, Fahey T, et al. Diagnostic accuracy of clinical tests for subacromial impingement syndrome: A systematic review and meta-analysis. *Arch Phys Med Rehabil*. 2012;93:229–236.
2. Kuhn JE. Exercise in the treatment of rotator cuff impingement: A systematic review and a synthesized evidence-based rehabilitation protocol. *J Shoulder Elbow Surg*. 2009;18(1):138–160.
3. Green S, Buchbinder R, Hetrick S. Physiotherapy interventions for shoulder pain. *Cochrane Database Syst Rev*. 2008;3.
4. Vas J, Ortega C, Olmo V, et al. Single-point acupuncture and physiotherapy for the treatment of painful shoulder: A multicentre randomized controlled trial. *Rheumatology* 2008;47:887–893.
5. Gaujoux-Viala C, Dougados M, Gossec L, et al. Efficacy and safety of steroid injections for shoulder and elbow tendonitis: A meta-analysis of randomised controlled trials. *Ann Rheum Dis*. 2009;68:1843–1849.
6. Bhatia M, Singh B. Correlation between rotator cuff tears and repeated subacromial steroid injections: A case-controlled study. *Ann R Coll Surg Engl*. 2009;91(5):414–416.
7. Conway R, O'Shea FD, Cunnane G, Doran MF. Safety of joint and soft tissue injections in patients on warfarin anticoagulation. *Clin Rheumatol*. 2013 Aug 8. [Epub ahead of print]
8. Gebremariam L, Hay EM, Koes BW, et al. Effectiveness of surgical and postsurgical interventions for the subacromial impingement syndrome: A systematic review. *Arch Phys Med Rehabil*. 2011;92:1900–1913.
9. Chahal J, Van Thiel GS, Mall N, et al. The role of platelet-rich plasma in arthroscopic rotator cuff repair: A systematic review with quantitative synthesis. *Arthroscopy*. 2012;28(11):1718–1727. Epub 2012 Jun 12.

ADDITIONAL READING

- Baumgarten KM, Gerlach D. Cigarette smoking increases the risk for rotator cuff tears. *Clin Orthop Relat Res*. 2010;468(6):1534–1541.
- Burbank KM, Stevenson JH, Czarnecki GR, et al. Chronic shoulder pain: Part I. Evaluation and diagnosis. *Am Fam Physician*. 2008;77:453–460.
- Burbank KM, Stevenson JH, Czarnecki GR, et al. Chronic shoulder pain: Part II. Treatment. *Am Fam Physician*. 2008;77:493–497.
- Cumpston M, Johnston R, Wengier L, et al. Topical glyceryl trinitrate for rotator cuff disease. *Cochrane Database Syst Rev*. 2009;3.
- Hanchard N, Handoll H. Physical tests for shoulder impingements and local lesions of bursa, tendon or labrum that may accompany impingement. *Cochrane Database Syst Rev*. 2008;4.
- Hegedus EJ, Goode A, Campbell S, et al. Physical examination tests of the shoulder: A systematic review with meta-analysis of individual tests. *Br J Sports Med*. 2008;42(2):80–92; discussion 92. Epub 2007 Aug 24.
- Kennedy DJ, Visco CJ, Press J. Current concepts for shoulder training in the overhead athlete. *Curr Sports Med Rep*. 2009;8(3):154–160.
- Speed C. A systematic review of shockwave therapies in soft tissue conditions: focusing on the evidence. *Br J Sports Med*. 2013 Aug 5. doi: 0.1136/bjsports-2012-091961. [Epub ahead of print]

 CODES

ICD10
- M75.40 Impingement syndrome of unspecified shoulder
- M75.41 Impingement syndrome of right shoulder
- M75.42 Impingement syndrome of left shoulder

CLINICAL PEARLS
- Consider impingement syndrome in patients with repetitive overhead arm motion (e.g., swimming, throwing).
- Shoulder pain in middle age without trauma may be secondary to rotator cuff tendonitis.
- Supraspinatus tendon most commonly affected.
- Use Neer and Hawkins tests to check for shoulder impingement.
- Use Empty Can test to test for weakness of supraspinatus muscle.
- Drop-Arm test is highly specific for rotator cuff tear.
- Physical therapy over 6–12 weeks promotes return to function.
- Most patients respond to conservative management; nonresponders should be referred for surgical treatment.

SALICYLATE POISONING
Lars C. Larsen, MD

BASICS

DESCRIPTION
Systemic disorder caused by acute and/or chronic intoxication from salicylate-containing medications:
- Following accidental or intentional exposure, toxic actions of salicylates include:
  - Stimulation of CNS respiratory center
  - Uncoupling of oxidative phosphorylation
  - Inhibition of Krebs cycle dehydrogenases
  - Stimulation of gluconeogenesis
  - Increased lipolysis and lipid metabolism
  - Inhibition of aminotransferases
  - Cyclo-oxygenase inhibition and decreased production of clotting factors
  - Irritation of the gastric mucosa and stimulation of the CNS chemoreceptor trigger zone
- These actions cause sequential and progressively severe physiologic abnormalities with increasing doses of salicylates, time following exposure, duration of chronic exposure, extremes of age, and presence of concurrent medical conditions; abnormalities include:
  - Respiratory alkalosis accompanied by progressive metabolic acidosis
  - Hyperpyrexia
  - GI, renal, pulmonary, and skin losses of body fluids and electrolytes
  - Initial hyperglycemia followed by hypoglycemia, particularly CNS hypoglycemia
  - Abnormal hemostasis and coagulation
- Clinical presentation of patients with salicylate toxicity can range from minor symptoms to a syndrome initially indistinguishable from septic shock with multiple organ failure, including encephalopathy and acute respiratory distress syndrome (ARDS).
- The very young and elderly are particularly prone to develop severe toxicity, as are those with chronic intoxication.
- Conditions causing concurrent acidosis may increase tissue concentrations of salicylate and result in greater morbidity and mortality.
- System(s) affected: Cardiovascular; Endocrine/Metabolic; Gastrointestinal; Hematologic/Lymphatic/Immunologic; Musculoskeletal; Nervous; Pulmonary; Renal/Urologic; Skin/Exocrine

Geriatric Considerations
- Increased risk for chronic toxicity because of decreased renal function
- Increased risk for bleeding or perforated gastric ulcers in patients >70

Pediatric Considerations
Acidosis is often more severe in the very young, particularly in chronic or repeated therapeutic-dose poisonings.

Pregnancy Considerations
- Salicylates may cause premature closure of ductus arteriosus in the fetus.
- Increased risk of ante- and intrapartum hemorrhage

EPIDEMIOLOGY
Incidence/Prevalence in the US:
- >11,100 single-substance ingestions of acetylsalicylic acid (ASA) or ASA combination products reported by poison control centers in 2011.
- 22 deaths in 2011, none in children <6 years of age
- Occurs in children and adults at any age

ETIOLOGY AND PATHOPHYSIOLOGY
- Accidental or intentional ingestion of salicylates or salicylate-containing medications
- Percutaneous absorption of dermatologic medications containing salicylate
- Breastfeeding by mothers ingesting salicylate-containing medications
- Teething gels containing salicylates

RISK FACTORS
- Dehydration
- Conditions causing metabolic or respiratory acidosis
- Extremes of age—very young and elderly
- Psychiatric illness
- History of previous toxic ingestions or suicide attempts
- Concurrent oral poisoning with other substances
- Concurrent use of acetazolamide (Diamox)

GENERAL PREVENTION
- Patient and parent/caregiver education essential; see "Patient Education"
- Emergency telephone numbers (poison control centers): (800) 222–1222

COMMONLY ASSOCIATED CONDITIONS
Reye syndrome with salicylate use and varicella or influenza viral infection

DIAGNOSIS

PHYSICAL EXAM
- Signs and symptoms may differ when the intoxication is acute or chronic.
- Acute intoxication:
  - Symptoms vary with amount ingested, usually begin within 3–8 hours of ingestion, and progress more rapidly in children:
    - <150 mg/kg, minimal symptoms
    - 150–300 mg/kg, moderate symptoms
    - 300–500 mg/kg, severe symptoms
    - >500 mg/kg, potentially fatal
  - Nausea and vomiting
  - Hyperpnea, tachypnea
  - Hyperpyrexia
  - Tinnitus
  - Disorientation, coma, convulsions
  - Cardiac arrhythmias
  - Hypotension
  - Pulmonary edema
- Chronic intoxication:
  - Onset of symptoms is usually gradual.
  - Signs and symptoms similar to acute intoxication may occur and may be advanced at diagnosis and include severe hypotension and ARDS.
  - Neurologic symptoms often predominate, particularly in the elderly; they include agitation, confusion, stupor, hyperactivity, paranoia, bizarre behavior, dysarthria, and restlessness.

DIFFERENTIAL DIAGNOSIS
- All ages:
  - Infection
  - Sepsis
  - Diabetic ketoacidosis
  - Other causes of metabolic acidosis
- In the elderly:
  - Delirium
  - Cerebral vascular accident
  - Myocardial infarction
  - Ethyl alcohol intoxication
  - Congestive heart failure

DIAGNOSTIC TESTS & INTERPRETATION
Initial Tests (lab, imaging)
- Serum salicylate levels initially and ≥6 hours after ingestion; then repeat q2h until the levels are declining and patient's condition has stabilized
- Electrolytes, BUN, creatinine, glucose, LFTs, uric acid
- Arterial blood gases
- PT/INR
- Urinalysis
- Stool guaiac testing may be positive.
- Chest radiograph:
  - Noncardiogenic pulmonary edema
  - Variable severity, from mild to ARDS
- Abdominal plain film: Nonspecific bowel gas pattern with retained contrast material in chronic bismuth subsalicylate ingestion

Diagnostic Procedures/Other
- None, other than correlating serum salicylate concentration with clinical presentation
- Use of the Done nomogram in managing patients is not recommended.

Test Interpretation
- Serum salicylate levels initially on all patients to confirm diagnosis; following acute ingestions, check levels ≥6 hours after ingestion and repeat q2h until the levels are declining and patient's condition has stabilized.
- Acid–base abnormalities common:
  - Usually respiratory alkalosis or mixed respiratory alkalosis and metabolic acidosis
  - Metabolic acidosis often predominates in chronic or severe acute poisonings and in poisonings in young children.
- Increased anion gap, especially in acute poisonings and salicylate-only poisonings
- Initial hyperglycemia may be followed by hypoglycemia.
- Electrolyte abnormalities, such as hypernatremia or hyponatremia and hypokalemia, are common.
- Dehydration findings are common, including an increased BUN:creatinine ratio.
- Prothrombin time (PT)/International normalization ratio (INR) may be increased.
- Liver function abnormalities may be present.
- Proteinuria and renal function abnormalities may be present.
- Stool guaiac testing may be positive.
- Occasional hypouricemia

- Drugs that may alter lab results:
  - Diflunisal (Dolobid) may cross-react with assay of salicylate concentration.
  - Medications affecting similar organ systems, including oral anticoagulants and hypoglycemic agents
- Disorders that may alter lab results: Concurrent medical conditions involving similar organ systems
- Other Findings:
- GI:
  - Antral and prepyloric ulcers
  - Small bowel ulcerations with enteric-coated salicylates
- Renal:
  - Interstitial nephritis
  - Acute tubular necrosis
  - Minimal-change nephrotic syndrome
- Pulmonary:
  - Noncardiogenic pulmonary edema

 TREATMENT

MEDICATION
- Prevent further absorption if the ingestion is felt to be life-threatening:
  - Gastric lavage is rarely indicated.
  - Activated charcoal may be given within 1 hour of toxic ingestion (immediately after gastric lavage if performed) (1,2)[C].
  - Ipecac is no longer recommended for use at home or in health care facilities (3)[C].
- Emergency facility/hospital:
  - Activated charcoal 1 g/kg, single dose, within 1 hour of toxic ingestion
  - Fluid/Electrolyte balance: IV fluids to restore intravascular volume and prevent hypoglycemia
  - With hypotension, give isotonic fluid until orthostatic changes are no longer present.
  - Fluids should contain ≥5% dextrose unless hyperglycemia is a problem.
  - Normal saline or a mixture of 0.45% NaCl with 1 ampule of sodium bicarbonate (43 mEq NaHCO₃) may be administered at 10–15 mL/kg/hr × 1–2 hours, depending on the degree of acidosis.
  - When BP is stable, fluid management is directed toward alkalinizing the urine to enhance salicylate excretion, prevent CNS hypoglycemia, and treat fluid and electrolyte abnormalities.
  - Enhance elimination by alkaline diuresis (4)[C]:
    - Alkaline diuresis (urine pH >7.5) and prevention of hypoglycemia usually can be accomplished by initial bolus of NaHCO₃ 1–2 mEq/kg IV given over 1 hour, followed by infusion of 1,000 mL D₅W plus 2–3 ampules of NaHCO₃ (43 mEq NaHCO₃/ampule) at 1.5–2 times maintenance rate (or, at 2–3 mL/kg/hr). Consider adding 40 mEq of potassium chloride to each liter; monitor potassium levels closely.
    - Goal: Bicarbonate to alkalinize the urine (pH >7.5) and, when appropriate, to correct severe systemic acidosis (for pH <7.1)
    - Potassium should be added for potassium levels <4 mEq/L.
    - Patients with cardiovascular compromise should be monitored closely for fluid overload.
    - Alkalinization can be discontinued when the salicylate level decreases into the therapeutic range.

- Serum electrolytes and glucose should be monitored frequently and urine pH checked hourly until stable at >7.5. Arterial blood gases should be monitored >2–4 hours to ensure blood pH ≤7.5.
- Hemodialysis should be considered in poisonings with markedly elevated salicylate levels (>100 mg/dL in acute poisonings, >40 mg/dL in chronic poisonings), acidosis unresponsive to alkalinization and diuresis, renal and/or hepatic dysfunction with impaired salicylate clearance, endotracheal intubation (excluding for coingestants), noncardiac pulmonary edema, and persistent, severe CNS symptoms.
- Dextrose-containing IV solution to prevent hypoglycemia; CNS hypoglycemia may be present despite a normal serum glucose level.
- Contraindications: Medication allergies
- Precautions:
  - Intravascular overload may result from injudicious use of sodium bicarbonate.
  - Dextrose should not be given to patients with severe hyperglycemia.

ISSUES FOR REFERRAL
Psychiatric and psychological evaluation in emergency department and in close follow-up for intentional overdose

IN-PATIENT CONSIDERATIONS
Admission Criteria/Initial Stabilization
- Evaluate all patients at a health care facility.
- Outpatient for nontoxic accidental ingestions
- Inpatient for toxic and intentional ingestions (3)[C]

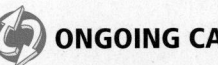 ONGOING CARE

FOLLOW-UP RECOMMENDATIONS
Patient Monitoring
- Fluid, acid–base, blood glucose, and electrolyte status until stable; urine pH (to enhance elimination of salicylate)
- Psychiatric follow-up after intentional ingestions

DIET
No special diet

PATIENT EDUCATION
- Education of parents/caregivers during well-child visits
- Education of patients about chronic salicylate therapy
- Anticipatory guidance for caregivers, family, and cohabitants of potentially suicidal patients
- http://familydoctor.org/familydoctor/en/kids/home-safety/child-safety-keeping-medicines-out-of-reach.html
- Poison control: (800) 222-1222

PROGNOSIS
- Complete recovery with early therapy
- Clinical course and prognosis are worse in the very young and elderly, chronic intoxications, and in patients with concurrent conditions that cause dehydration and/or acidosis.

COMPLICATIONS
- Rare following recovery from poisoning
- Noncardiogenic pulmonary edema
- ARDS

REFERENCES
1. Gaudreault P. Activated charcoal revisited. *Clin Pediatr Emerg Med*. 2005;6:76–80.
2. Heard K. Gastrointestinal decontamination. *Med Clin North Am*. 2005;89:1067–1078.
3. Chyka PA, Erdman AR, Christianson G, et al. Salicylate poisoning: An evidence-based consensus guideline for out-of-hospital management. *Clin Toxicol (Phila)*. 2007;45(2):95–131.
4. Proudfoot AT, Krenzelok EP, Vale JA. Position Paper on urine alkalinization. *J Toxicol Clin Toxicol*. 2004;42:1–26.

ADDITIONAL READING
Bronstein AC, Spyker DA, Cantilena LR, et al. 2011 Annual Report of the American Association of Poison Control Centers' National Poison Data System (NPDS): 29th Annual Report. *Clin Toxicol*. 2012;50:911–1164.

 CODES

ICD10
- T39.012A Poisoning by aspirin, intentional self-harm, init encntr
- T39.014A Poisoning by aspirin, undetermined, initial encounter

CLINICAL PEARLS
- Gastric decontamination should not be done in all poisonings, only in potentially life-threatening ingestions.
- Think of salicylate toxicity with mixed metabolic acidosis and respiratory alkalosis, especially if anion gap.
- Activated charcoal within 1 hour of toxic ingestion (immediately after gastric lavage, if performed) (1,2)[C]
- Ipecac is no longer recommended for use at home or in health care facilities.
- There is a bedside test to evaluate for the presence of salicylates. A few drops of 10% ferric chloride solution added to 1 mL of urine usually will produce a purple color if salicylates are present.

SALIVARY GLAND CALCULI/SIALADENITIS
Mary Lauren Worthen, MD • Adrian Worthen • David Worthen

BASICS

DESCRIPTION
- Inflammation or "stones" involving ≥1 salivary gland
- Sialolithiasis is the cause of ~90% of all obstructive salivary gland diseases.
- Salivary obstruction is clinically characterized by a food-related painful swelling of the affected gland, known as "mealtime syndrome."
- The submandibular gland is more commonly affected by sialolithiasis and infection than is the parotid gland.
- Can be acute or chronic
- Types:
  - Infectious
  - Obstructive (sialolithiasis)
  - Autoimmune
- System(s) affected: Gastrointestinal

EPIDEMIOLOGY
Incidence
- A review of British patients showed an incidence of symptomatic sialolithiasis of 27–59/1 million population per year (1)[B].
- Predominant sex: Male > Female
- Predominant age: Peak incidence is 30–60 years
- Most common in debilitated and dehydrated patients

Prevalence
- Salivary calculi can be found in 1.2% of the adult population.
- Only 3% of all cases occur in the pediatric population.
- In those with sialographic evidence of benign intraductal obstruction, the obstruction is caused by salivary calculi in 73.2% of cases.

ETIOLOGY AND PATHOPHYSIOLOGY
- Decreased salivary outflow from anticholinergics, dehydration, or radiation is thought to allow bacterial infection of salivary glands.
- Salivary calculi are thought to form as the result of deposition of calcium phosphate around an initial organic matrix consisting of altered salivary mucins, bacteria, and desquamated epithelial cells. Predisposing factors include salivary stasis, increased alkalinity of saliva, salivary infection, and physical trauma to salivary duct or gland (2)[B].
- Systemic abnormalities of calcium metabolism do not cause salivary stones. Gout is the only systemic disease known to be associated with salivary stone development. In gout, sialoliths are composed of uric acid.
- Bacterial:
  - *Staphylococcus aureus*
  - *Streptococcus viridans*
  - *Streptococcus pyogenes*
  - *Haemophilus influenza*
  - *Escherichia coli*
  - *Pseudomonas aeruginosa* and group B streptococci (neonates and prepubescent children)

- Viral:
  - Mumps
  - Cytomegalovirus (CMV), Epstein-Barr virus (EBV)
  - HIV
  - Enteroviruses

Genetics
- Sjögren syndrome
- Polygenic cause, with several loci under investigation

RISK FACTORS
- Dehydration
- Anticholinergic use
- Antihistamine use
- Diuretic use
- Poor oral hygiene
- Malnutrition
- Head/Neck radiation
- Tuberculosis (TB)
- HIV
- Failure to immunize (mumps)
- Gout

GENERAL PREVENTION
- Adequate postoperative hydration
- Maintain proper oral care and hygiene
- Avoid antihistamines, anticholinergics, and other causes of xerostomia, especially if predisposed to risk factors

COMMONLY ASSOCIATED CONDITIONS
- Postoperative dehydration
- Radiation-induced xerostomia
- Drug-induced xerostomia
- Sjögren syndrome
- Hypercalcemia

DIAGNOSIS

HISTORY
- Onset, duration of symptoms, previous episodes
- Dental pain, discharge, foul breath (halitosis), pain with chewing
- Fever, unintentional weight loss
- Recent dental work, surgery
- Immunization history
- Radiation, TB, and HIV exposure
- History of alcoholism, bulimia, malnutrition (suggest sialadenosis)

PHYSICAL EXAM
- Palpate all salivary glands, floor of mouth, tongue, and neck to assess symmetry, tenderness, presence of stones, and lymphadenopathy.
- Examine duct openings for purulent discharge.
- Palpate gland gently to express purulent material.
- Examine eyes for interstitial keratitis.
- Note lingual papillary atrophy and loss of tooth enamel.

DIFFERENTIAL DIAGNOSIS
- Acute bacterial parotitis
- Chronic bacterial parotitis
- Dental abscess
- Mumps
- TB
- HIV (in pediatric populations)
- EBV, CMV, enteroviruses
- Tularemia
- Sialolithiasis
- Cystic fibrosis
- Lupus
- Sjögren syndrome
- Alcoholism
- Bulimia
- Hypothyroidism
- Pleomorphic adenoma
- Lymphoma
- Sarcoidosis
- Collagen-vascular disease
- Metal poisoning

DIAGNOSTIC TESTS & INTERPRETATION
Initial Tests (lab, imaging)
- CBC, electrolytes (3)[B]
- Culture and sensitivity of any expressed pus (3)[B]
- CT scan with IV contrast is the preferred imaging modality (4)[B].
- US can localize abscesses, differentiate between solid and cystic disease and extraglandular disease (5)[B].

Follow-Up Tests & Special Considerations
- If autoimmune process is suspected, consider ordering appropriate labs, such as autoantibody titers: Sjögren syndrome A (SS-A) and Sjögren syndrome B (SS-B), rheumatoid factor, and antinuclear antibodies (ANA). Erythrocyte sedimentation rate (ESR) may also be conducted.
- Consider serial CT scans with contrast to evaluate disease resolution.

Diagnostic Procedures/Other
- Sialography to evaluate sialolithiasis and other obstructive lesions
- Sialoscopy to find and remove sialoliths (6)[B]

Test Interpretation
In chronic sialadenitis, loss of acini, fibrosis, and periductal lymphocytosis are evident; degree indicates chronicity.

SALMONELLA INFECTION

Pia Prakash, MD • Neha Jakhete, MD • Marie L. Borum, MD, EdD, MPH

BASICS

DESCRIPTION
- Disease caused by any serotype of the bacterial genus *Salmonella*, a gram-negative bacilli
- *Salmonella enterica*:
  - 2,500 different serotypes
  - Most pathogenic species in humans
- Nontyphoidal *Salmonella* has a number of agricultural animal hosts and is an important cause of foodborne infection.
- Clinical syndromes:
  - Gastroenteritis (75%)
  - Bacteremia (10%)
  - Enteric fever (10%) (see "Typhoid Fever")
  - Localized infection outside GI tract (5%)
  - Chronic carrier state (<1%)
- Pathogenesis: Organisms are ingested, invade the gut mucosa, and produce inflammatory and cytotoxic response. They can then disseminate into systemic circulation via the lymphatic system.
- Chronic carrier state is defined as a positive stool culture >1 year.

Geriatric Considerations
Patients >65 have increased risk of developing invasive disease (1). This population often has comorbidities (atherosclerotic endovascular lesions, prostheses, etc.) that increase risk of seeding and bacteremia.

Pediatric Considerations
Neonates (<3 months) are more susceptible to invasive disease and subsequent complications, including CNS infection.

Pregnancy Considerations
Pregnancy has not been demonstrated to increase the risk or severity of infection.

EPIDEMIOLOGY
Incidence
- Incidence of laboratory-confirmed *Salmonella* infection in 2009 in the US (2):
  - 16.42 cases per 100,000 in 2012 according to the CDC
  - Incidence has been stable over past 6 years
  - 42,000 cases reported to CDC each year; however, actual number of infections is likely greater due to unreported cases
  - Highest incidence in children <4 years
  - Hospitalization rates for infection are higher in patients ≥50
- Peak frequency: July–November
- *Salmonella* is the major cause of bacterial diarrheal illness in the US.
- *Salmonella* is also a common cause of traveler's diarrhea.

ETIOLOGY AND PATHOPHYSIOLOGY
- Ingestion of contaminated food (e.g., poultry, beef, eggs, tomatoes, dairy products, commercially prepared nuts and nut products) or water accounts for 95% of cases (3).
- Person-to-person and/or fecal–oral spread
- Contact with chronic carrier (daycare center)
- Contact with exotic pets with high fecal carriage rates for *Salmonella*, especially reptiles
- Iatrogenic contamination (e.g., blood transfusion, endoscopy)

RISK FACTORS
- Recent travel outside the US
- Chicken and egg consumption
- Contact with reptiles or live poultry:
- Impaired gastric acidity: H_2 receptor blockers, antacids, PPIs, gastrectomy, achlorhydria
- Reticuloendothelial blockade: Sickle cell, malaria, bartonellosis
- Immunosuppression: AIDS, diabetes, corticosteroid use, immunosuppressant use, chemotherapy

GENERAL PREVENTION
- Proper hygiene in production, transport, and storage of food (e.g., refrigerating eggs to minimize multiplication of the bacteria if present, thoroughly cooking eggs prior to consumption)
- Control of animal reservoir, especially by avoiding contact with animal feces and polluted waters
- Hand hygiene
- Updated reports of *Salmonella* outbreaks are available on CDC web site.

COMMONLY ASSOCIATED CONDITIONS
- Gastroenteritis: Typically associated with normal immune function
- Bacteremia: More often seen in immunocompromised patients or those with anatomic disruptions (e.g., cholelithiasis, prostheses)

DIAGNOSIS

HISTORY
- *Salmonella* infections typically result in mild, self-limited gastroenteritis or asymptomatic state.
- Symptoms usually occur 12–72 hours after ingestion of contaminated food and resolve within 4–10 days.
- Acute uncomplicated illness (3)[C]:
  - Sudden onset of nausea, vomiting, diarrhea (rarely bloody)
  - Abdominal cramping
  - Headache
  - Myalgias
  - Fever

PHYSICAL EXAM
- Fever, tachycardia, tachypnea
- Evidence of hypovolemia
- Abdominal tenderness
- Heme-positive stool
- Rash (subtle rash possible if patient is bacteremic)
- Evidence of localized infection: Arthritis, soft-tissue abscesses, osteomyelitis

DIFFERENTIAL DIAGNOSIS
- Viral gastroenteritis
- Other bacterial enteritis
- Other bacterial sources of bacteremia or localized infection
- Pseudomembranous colitis
- Inflammatory bowel disease

DIAGNOSTIC TESTS & INTERPRETATION
Initial Tests (lab, imaging)
- Gastroenteritis:
  - Stool culture should evaluate for *Salmonella*, *E. coli*, *Shigella*, and *Campylobacter*
  - Indications for stool culture include (3):
    ○ Severe diarrhea (≥6 loose stools daily)
    ○ Diarrhea >1 week in duration
    ○ Fever
    ○ Diarrhea containing blood or mucous
    ○ Multiple cases of illness suggestive of an outbreak
  - Fecal leukocytes: Positive
  - CBC: Leukocytosis or normal WBC count
- Bacteremia:
  - Blood cultures: Positive for *Salmonella*
  - Stool cultures: May also be positive because a percentage of patients with gastroenteritis develop bacteremia
- Local infections:
  - CBC: Polymorphonuclear leukocytosis
  - Wound culture: May be positive for *Salmonella*
- Chronic carrier state:
  - Stool culture positive for >1 year
  - Urine culture may be positive as well.
- Endovascular infection is uncommon but possible in nontyphoidal *Salmonella* bacteremia. Consider angiography in patients >50 with bacteremia if aortic or vascular source is suspected.
- Consider CT or MRI for soft-tissue or bone infections.

Follow-Up Tests & Special Considerations
- Asymptomatic excretion of *Salmonella* bacilli may occur for multiple weeks after infection.
- Diarrhea lasting >10 days should lead to consideration of other etiologies.
- Serotyping of isolates can be performed at public health laboratories.
- PCR-based tests can be used in outbreaks to determine the relationship between strains.
- Early, empiric antibiotics may lead to false-negative culture and blunted immunologic response.

Test Interpretation
- Mucosal ulceration, hemorrhage, and necrosis
- Reticuloendothelial hyperplasia and hypertrophy
- Focal organ and soft-tissue abscesses

TREATMENT

- Treatment for nonsevere *Salmonella* gastroenteritis is fluid and electrolyte replacement as the illness is typically self-limited in the immunocompetent patient (4).
- Antibiotics should be considered in an immunocompetent host who has severe diarrhea, high fever, or requires hospitalization.
- Certain populations at increased risk of developing bacteremia benefit from antibiotics for acute gastroenteritis:
  - Infants <3 months
  - Persons >50 years
  - Patients with immunosuppression, hemoglobinopathies, underlying atherosclerotic lesions, and prosthetic valves, grafts, or joints

- Pregnancy: Antibiotic treatment is unnecessary in mild, uncomplicated gastroenteritis early in pregnancy. Antibiotic treatment is indicated in the following clinical settings:
  - Febrile patients with severe disease or bacteremia
  - Infection near term (to limit risk of transmission during childbirth)
- Chronic carriage of nontyphoidal *Salmonella*:
  - 4–6 weeks of antimicrobial therapy
  - Prophylactic therapy in immunocompromised patients

GENERAL MEASURES

Precautions: Avoid antimotility drugs (Lomotil, Imodium). Antimotility drugs may lead to increased contact time of the enteropathogen within the gut mucosa (3)[C].

MEDICATION

First Line

- Gastroenteritis, uncomplicated: None advised (4)[A]
- Gastroenteritis, complicated (risk factors above) (3)[C]:
  - Adults (treat for 14 days if immunocompromised):
    ○ Levofloxacin (or other fluoroquinolone): 500 mg/d PO × 7–10 days; or
    ○ Bactrim: 160/800 mg PO b.i.d. × 7–10 days *or*
    ○ Amoxicillin: 500 mg PO t.i.d. × 7–10 days *or*
    ○ Ceftriaxone: 1–2 g/d IV × 7–10 days *or*
    ○ Azithromycin: 500 mg/d PO × 7 days
  - Children:
    ○ Ceftriaxone: 100 mg/kg/d IV or IM in 2 equally divided doses × 7–10 days; *or*
    ○ Azithromycin: 20 mg/kg/d PO daily × 7 days
- Bacteremia: Due to resistance trends, life-threatening infections in adults should be treated with a fluoroquinolone *and* a 3rd-generation cephalosporin until susceptibilities are determined:
  - Adults:
    ○ Ciprofloxacin (or other fluoroquinolone): 400 mg IV b.i.d. × 7–10 days; *or*
    ○ Ceftriaxone: 1–2 g/d IV × 7–14 days
    ○ Cefotaxime: 2 g IV t.i.d. × 7–14 days
  - Children:
    ○ Ampicillin: 200 mg/kg/d in 4 divided doses × 10–14 days; *or*
    ○ Trimethoprim-sulfamethoxazole: 10–50 mg/kg/d in 2 divided doses × 10–14 days; *or*
    ○ Ceftriaxone: 50–75 mg/kg/d once per day × 10–14 days
- Localized infection (e.g., septic arthritis, osteomyelitis, cholangitis, and pneumonia):
  - Same as for bacteremia
  - In sustained bacteremia, prolonged local infection, or immunocompromised patients, antibiotics can be given PO for 4–6 weeks.
- Chronic carrier state (shedding >1 year duration):
  - Amoxicillin: 1 g/d PO t.i.d. × 12 weeks; *or*
  - Trimethoprim: 160 mg *and* sulfamethoxazole 800 mg PO b.i.d. × 12 weeks; *or*
  - Ciprofloxacin: 500 mg PO b.i.d. × 4 weeks, *or* levofloxacin 500 mg/d × 4 weeks *or* norfloxacin 400 mg PO b.i.d. × 4 weeks if gallstones are present

- Antimicrobial resistance rates:
  - Strains resistant to ampicillin, chloramphenicol, and trimethoprim-sulfamethoxazole have been increasing over the past 15 years. Some strains are rapidly becoming multidrug-resistant (1)[B].
  - Fluoroquinolone resistance has been observed in serotypes common to swine and humans.
  - Extended-spectrum cephalosporin resistance has been reported in the US with increasing frequency. 2.5% of invasive serotypes isolated from 1996–2007 in the US demonstrated resistance to ceftriaxone (1)[B].

Second Line

- Aztreonam is an alternative agent that may be useful in patients with multiple allergies or organisms with unusual resistance patterns.
- Fluoroquinolones are now routinely given to children for 5–7 days in areas of the world where multidrug-resistant *Salmonella typhi* is common.

SURGERY/OTHER PROCEDURES

- Surgical excision and drainage for infected tissue sites, followed by a minimum of 2 weeks antimicrobial therapy
- If biliary tract disease is present, a preoperative 10–14 day course of parenteral antibiotics followed by cholecystectomy is standard.

 ONGOING CARE

FOLLOW-UP RECOMMENDATIONS

Patient Monitoring

- Follow-up fecal cultures are generally not indicated for patients with uncomplicated gastroenteritis. Requirements may differ during a *Salmonella* outbreak.
- Cessation of diarrhea and good hand hygiene are appropriate criteria for return of health care workers to their duties.
- Criteria may vary by state and local regulations. For example, some public health departments require negative stool cultures for health workers and food handlers prior to returning to work. Shedding may last 4–8 weeks.

DIET

As tolerated

PATIENT EDUCATION

- Meticulous hand hygiene to prevent primary and secondary infections; caution when handling raw meat, poultry, and eggs
- Fruits and vegetables should be thoroughly washed prior to consumption.
- Thoroughly cooking meats eliminates *Salmonella*.
- Caution when handling animals (e.g., reptiles) with high fecal carriage rates
- For more details, visit: www.cdc.gov/salmonella/general/prevention.html

PROGNOSIS

- Most cases of *Salmonella* gastroenteritis are self-limited and have an excellent prognosis.
- Increased mortality is seen in the very young (<3 months), the very old (>65), and the immunocompromised.
- Complications of meningitis and endocarditis have a poor prognosis, with fatality approaching 50% of cases.
- Mortality is increased with multidrug-resistant strains.

COMPLICATIONS

Toxic megacolon, hypovolemic shock, metastatic abscess formation, endocarditis, infectious endarteritis, meningitis, septic arthritis, osteomyelitis, pneumonia, appendicitis, cholecystitis

REFERENCES

1. Crump JA, Medalla FM, Joyce KW, et al. Antimicrobial resistance among invasive nontyphoidal Salmonella enterica isolates in the United States: National Antimicrobial Resistance Monitoring System, 1996 to 2007. *Antimicrob. Agents Chemother.* 2011;55:1148–1154.
2. Centers for Disease Control and Prevention (CDC). Preliminary FoodNet data on the incidence of infection with pathogens transmitted commonly through food—10 states, 2009. *MMWR Morb Mortal Wkly Rep.* 2010;84(14):418–422.
3. DuPont HL. Clinical practice. Bacterial diarrhea. *N Engl J Med.* 2009;361:1560–1569.
4. Onwuezobe IA, Oshun PO, Odigwe CC. Antimicrobials for treating symptomatic non-typhoidal Salmonella infection. *Cochrane Database Syst Rev.* 2012;11:CD001167.

ADDITIONAL READING

- Lee MB, Greig JD A review of nosocomial Salmonella outbreaks: Infection control interventions found effective. *Public Health.* 2013; 127(3):199–206. doi: 10.1016/j.puhe.2012.12. 013. Epub 2013 Feb 22.
- Shah N, DuPont HL, Ramsey DJ. Global etiology of travelers' diarrhea: Systematic review from 1973 to the present. *Am J Trop Med Hyg.* 2009;80: 609–614.

 SEE ALSO

Gastroenteritis; Typhoid Fever

 CODES

ICD10

- A02.0 Salmonella enteritis
- A02.1 Salmonella sepsis
- A02.9 Salmonella infection, unspecified

CLINICAL PEARLS

- Nontyphoidal *Salmonella* is a foodborne infection strongly associated with poultry, eggs, and fresh produce.
- Clinical syndromes include gastroenteritis, bacteremia, enteric fever or typhoid fever, localized infection outside the GI tract, or a chronic carrier state. Those at greatest risk of death from *Salmonella* infection include the very young, the elderly, and immunocompromised patients.
- Treatment of uncomplicated gastroenteritis in healthy populations is generally focused on fluid and electrolyte replacement.
- Antibiotics should be used in infants, the elderly, and immunocompromised patients.

SARCOIDOSIS
Donnah Mathews, MD, FACP

 BASICS

DESCRIPTION
- Sarcoidosis is a noninfectious, multisystem granulomatous disease of unknown cause, commonly affecting young and middle-aged adults:
  - Frequently presents with hilar adenopathy, pulmonary infiltrates, ocular and skin lesions
  - In ~50% of cases, it is diagnosed in asymptomatic patients with abnormal chest x-rays (CXRs).
  - Almost any organ may be involved.
- System(s) affected: Primarily Pulmonary, but also Cardiovascular; Gastrointestinal; Hematologic/Lymphatic; Endocrine; Renal; Neurologic; Dermatologic; Ophthalmologic; Musculoskeletal
- Synonym(s): Löfgren syndrome (erythema nodosum, hilar adenopathy, fever, arthralgias); Heerfordt syndrome (uveitis, parotid enlargement, facial palsy, fever); Besnier-Boeck disease; Boeck sarcoid; Schaumann disease (1,2)[C]

EPIDEMIOLOGY
Incidence
Estimated 6/100 person-years
Prevalence
- Estimated 10–20/100,000 persons
- <15% of patients with active disease >60 years of age
- Rare in children (3)

ETIOLOGY AND PATHOPHYSIOLOGY
- Despite extensive research, mostly unknown
- Thought to be due to exaggerated cell-mediated immune response to unknown antigen(s)
- In the lungs, the initial lesion is CD4+ T-cell alveolitis, causing noncaseating granulomata, which may resolve/undergo fibrosis.
- "Immune paradox" with affected organs showing an intense immune response and yet anergy exists elsewhere (4)

Genetics
- Reports of familial clustering
- 3–4× more common in African Americans
- Although worldwide in distribution, increased prevalence in Scandinavians, Japanese, African Americans, and women (3).

RISK FACTORS
Exact etiology and pathogenesis remain unknown (3).

GENERAL PREVENTION
None

COMMONLY ASSOCIATED CONDITIONS
None

DIAGNOSIS

HISTORY
- Patients may be asymptomatic.
- Patients may have nonspecific complaints, such as:
  - Nonproductive cough
  - Shortness of breath
  - Fever
  - Night sweats
  - Weight loss
  - General fatigue
  - Eye pain
  - Chest pain/palpitations
  - Skin lesions
  - Polyarthritis
  - Renal calculi (4)
  - Facial droop due to Bell palsy
  - Encephalopathy, seizures, hydrocephalus (rare)
  - Patients >70 more likely to have systemic symptoms

PHYSICAL EXAM
- Many patients have a normal physical exam.
- Lungs may reveal wheezing/fine interstitial crackles in advanced disease.
- ~30% of patients have extrapulmonary manifestations (1), which may include:
  - Uveitis
  - Other eye findings: Conjunctival nodules, lacrimal gland enlargement, cataracts, glaucoma, papilledema
  - Cranial nerve palsies
  - Salivary gland swelling
  - Lymphadenopathy
  - Arrhythmias
  - Hepatosplenomegaly
  - Polyarthritis
  - Rashes (5):
    ○ Maculopapular of nares, eyelids, forehead, base of neck at hairline, and previous trauma sites
    ○ Waxy nodular of face, trunk, extensor surfaces of extremities
    ○ Plaques (lupus pernio) of nose, cheeks, chin, ears
    ○ Erythema nodosum (component of Löfgren syndrome)
    ○ Atypical lesions

DIFFERENTIAL DIAGNOSIS
- Infectious granulomatous disease, such as tuberculosis and fungal infections
- Hypersensitivity pneumonitis
- Lymphoma
- Other malignancies associated with lymphadenopathy
- Berylliosis

DIAGNOSTIC TESTS & INTERPRETATION
No definitive test for diagnosis, but diagnosis is suggested by:
- Clinical and radiographic manifestations
- Exclusion of other diagnoses
- Histopathologic detection of noncaseating granulomas

Initial Tests (lab, imaging)
- CBC: Anemia/Leukopenia ± eosinophilia can be seen.
- Hypergammaglobulinemia can exist.
- LFTs: Abnormal liver function and increased alkaline phosphatase can be encountered with hepatic involvement.
- Calcium: Hypercalciuria occurs in up to 10% of patients, with hypercalcemia less frequent.
- Serum ACE inhibitors elevated in >75% of patients, but is not diagnostic or exclusionary:
  - Drugs may alter lab results: Prednisone will lower serum ACE and normalize gallium scan. ACE inhibitors will lower serum ACE level.
  - Disorders may alter lab results: Hyperthyroidism and diabetes will increase serum ACE level.
- CXR or CT scan may reveal granulomas/hilar adenopathy. Routine CXRs are staged using Scadding classification (6):
  - Stage 0 = Normal
  - Stage 1 = Bilateral hilar adenopathy alone
  - Stage 2 = Bilateral hilar adenopathy + parenchymal infiltrates
  - Stage 3 = Parenchymal infiltrates alone (primarily upper lobes)
  - Stage 4 = Pulmonary fibrosis
- Chest CT scan may enhance appreciation of lymph nodes.
- High-resolution chest CT scan may reveal peribronchial disease.
- Gallium scan will be positive in areas of acute disease/inflammation, but is not specific.
- Positron emission tomography (PET) scan can indicate areas of disease activity in lungs, lymph nodes, and other areas of the body, but does not differentiate between malignancy and sarcoidosis.
- Cardiac PET scan may detect cardiac sarcoidosis

Diagnostic Procedures/Other
- Pulmonary function tests (PFTs) may reveal restrictive pattern with decreased carbon monoxide diffusing capacity (DLCO).
- Characteristically in active disease, bronchioalveolar lavage fluid has an increased CD4-to-CD8 ratio.
- Ophthalmologic examination may reveal uveitis, retinal vasculitis, or conjunctivitis.
- ECG
- Tuberculin skin test
- Biopsy of lesions should reveal noncaseating granulomas.
- If lungs are affected, bronchoscopy with biopsy of central and peripheral airways is helpful. Endobronchial US (EBUS)-guided transbronchial needle aspiration may potentially have a better diagnostic yield (7)[B].

ALERT
If signs indicate Löfgren syndrome, it is not necessary to perform a biopsy because prognosis is good with observation alone, and biopsy would not change management.

Test Interpretation
Noncaseating epithelioid granulomas without evidence of fungal/mycobacterial infection

TREATMENT

- Many patients undergo spontaneous remission. It is difficult to assess disease activity and severity, however, making it challenging to develop guidelines.
- No treatment may be necessary in asymptomatic individuals, but treatment may be needed for specific indications, such as cardiac, CNS, renal, or ocular involvement.
- No treatment is indicated for asymptomatic patients with stage I–III radiographic changes with normal/mildly abnormal lung function, although close follow-up is recommended.
- Treatment of pulmonary and skin manifestations is done on the basis of impairment. The symptoms that necessitate systemic therapy remain controversial:
  – Worsening pulmonary symptoms
  – Deteriorating lung function
  – Worsening radiographic findings

MEDICATION
Systemic therapy is clearly indicated for hypercalcemia, cardiac disease, neurologic disease, and eye disease not responding to topical therapy.

First Line
- Systemic corticosteroids in the symptomatic individual:
  – The optimal dose of glucocorticoids is not known.
  – Usually prednisone initially, 0.3–0.6 mg/kg ideal body weight (20–40 mg/d) × 4–6 weeks.
  – If stable, taper by 5 mg/wk to 10–20 mg/d over the next 6 weeks.
  – If no relapse, 10–20 mg/d × 8–12 months
  – Relapse is common.
  – Higher doses may be warranted in patients with cardiac, neurologic, or ocular disease.
- In patients with skin disease, topical steroids may be effective.
- Inhaled steroids (budesonide 800–1,600 mcg b.i.d.) may be of some clinical benefit in early disease with mild pulmonary symptoms:
  – Contraindications: Patients with known problems with corticosteroids
  – Precautions: Careful monitoring in patients with diabetes mellitus and/or hypertension
  – Significant possible interactions: Refer to the manufacturer's profile of each drug.

Second Line
- All alternative agents to glucocorticoids carry substantial risk for toxicity, including myelosuppression, hepatotoxicity, and opportunistic infection.
- Methotrexate: initially 7.5 mg/wk, increasing gradually to 10–15 mg/wk
- Azathioprine: 50–100 mg/d
- Leflunomide: 20 mg/d
- Use of immunosuppressants, such as methotrexate or azathioprine, will require regular monitoring of CBC and LFTs.
- Antimalarial agents, such as chloroquine or hydroxychloroquine
- Tumor necrosis factor antagonists, such as Infliximab, have been useful in refractory cases.

ISSUES FOR REFERRAL
May be followed by a pulmonologist, with referrals to other specialists as dictated by involvement of other organ systems

SURGERY/OTHER PROCEDURES
Lung transplantation in severe, refractory cases; long-term outcomes unknown

COMPLEMENTARY AND ALTERNATIVE MEDICINE
None known to be effective

ONGOING CARE

FOLLOW-UP RECOMMENDATIONS
There is limited data on indications for the specific tests and optimal frequency of monitoring of disease activity. Suggestions follow.

Patient Monitoring
- Patients on prednisone for symptoms should be seen q1–2mo while on therapy.
- Patients not requiring therapy should be seen regularly (q3mo) for at least the first 2 years after diagnosis, obtaining a thorough history and physical exam, laboratory testing tailored to sites of disease activity, PFTs, and ambulatory pulse oximetry.
- If active disease:
  – Every 6 months, obtain ophthalmologic exam if on hydroxychloroquine.
  – Annually, CBC, creatinine, calcium, LFTs, ECG, 25-hydroxy vitamin D and 1,25 dihydroxy vitamin D, CXR, and ophthalmologic exam if not on hydroxychloroquine
- Other testing per individual patient's symptoms, including HRCT, echocardiogram, Holter monitoring, urinalysis (UA), thyroid-stimulating hormone (TSH), bone density, MRI of brain
- The serum ACE level is used by some physicians to follow the disease activity. In patients with an initially elevated ACE level, it should fall toward normal while on the therapy or when the disease resolves.
- If inactive disease, follow annually with history and physical exam, PFTs, ambulatory pulse oximetry, CBC, creatinine, calcium, liver enzymes, 1,25 dihydroxy vitamin D, EKG, ophthalmologic exam.

DIET
No special diet

PATIENT EDUCATION
- The American Lung Association at www.lungusa.org/lung-disease/sarcoidosis/?gclid = CPX6zuipm6MCFQxW2godISFepQ
- Sarcoidosis by Medline Plus at www.nlm.nih.gov/medlineplus/sarcoidosis.html

PROGNOSIS
- 50% of patients will have spontaneous resolution within 2 years.
- 25% of patients will have significant fibrosis, but no further worsening of the disease after 2 years.
- 25% of patients (higher in some populations, including African Americans) will have chronic disease.
- Patients on corticosteroids for >6 months have a greater chance of having chronic disease.
- Overall death rate: <5%

COMPLICATIONS
- Patients may develop significant respiratory involvement, including cor pulmonale.
- Pulmonary hemorrhage from infection with aspergillosis in the damaged lung is possible.

- Other organs, especially the heart (congestive heart failure, arrhythmias), eyes (rarely blindness), and CNS can be involved with serious consequences. Cardiac, ocular, and CNS involvement usually manifests early on in patients with these complications of the disease.

REFERENCES
1. Holmes J, Lazarus A. Sarcoidosis: Extrathoracic manifestations. *Dis Mon.* 2009;55:675–692.
2. King CS, Kelly W. Treatment of sarcoidosis. *Dis Mon.* 2009;55:704–718.
3. Rybicki BA, Iannuzzi MC, Frederick MM, et al. Familial aggregation of sarcoidosis. A case-control etiologic study of sarcoidosis (ACCESS). *Am J Respir Crit Care Med.* 2001;164:2085–2091.
4. Dempsey OJ, Paterson EW, Kerr KM, et al. Sarcoidosis. *BMJ.* 2009;339:b3206.
5. Lodha S, Sanchez M, Prystowsky S, et al. Sarcoidosis of the skin: A review for the pulmonologist. *Chest.* 2009;136:583–596.
6. Statement on sarcoidosis. Joint Statement of the American Thoracic Society (ATS), the European Respiratory Society (ERS) and the World Association of Sarcoidosis and Other Granulomatous Disorders (WASOG) adopted by the ATS Board of Directors and by the ERS Executive Committee, February 1999. *Am J Respir Crit Care Med.* 1999;160:736–755.
7. Tremblay A, Stather DR, Maceachern P, et al. A randomized controlled trial of standard vs endobronchial ultrasonography-guided transbronchial needle aspiration in patients with suspected sarcoidosis. *Chest.* 2009;136:340–346.

ADDITIONAL READING
- Hoang DQ, Nguyen ET. Sarcoidosis. *Semin Roentgenol.* 2010;45:36–42.
- Mock B, Richter S, Hein G, et al. [Recurrent panuveitis. First manifestation of Behçet disease in childhood]. *Ophthalmologe.* 1998;95:784–787.
- Polychronopoulos VS, Prakash UB. Airway involvement in sarcoidosis. *Chest.* 2009;136:1371–1380.

CODES

ICD10
- D86.0 Sarcoidosis of lung
- D86.83 Sarcoid iridocyclitis
- D86.9 Sarcoidosis, unspecified

CLINICAL PEARLS
- Sarcoidosis is a noninfectious, multisystem granulomatous disease of unknown cause, typically affecting young and middle-aged adults.
- Any organ can be affected.
- Diagnosis is based on clinical findings, exclusion of other disorders, and pathologic detection of noncaseating granulomas.
- Most patients do not need systemic treatment and the disease resolves spontaneously; a few will have life-threatening progressive organ dysfunction.

SCABIES

Kaelen C. Dunican, PharmD • Brandi Hoag, DO

BASICS

DESCRIPTION
- A contagious parasitic infection of the skin caused by the mite *Sarcoptes scabiei*, var. *hominis*
- System(s) affected: Skin/Exocrine
- Synonym(s): Sarcoptic mange

EPIDEMIOLOGY
Incidence
Predominant age: Children and young adults
Prevalence
- Global prevalence is estimated at 300 million cases.
- May be more prevalent in urban areas and areas of overcrowding

ETIOLOGY AND PATHOPHYSIOLOGY
Itching is a delayed hypersensitivity reaction to the mite saliva, eggs, or excrement.
  S. scabiei, var. *hominis*:
- An obligate human parasite
- Female mite lays eggs in burrows in the stratum corneum and epidermis.
- Primarily transmitted by human-to-human direct skin contact
- Infrequently transmitted via fomites (e.g., bedding, clothing, or furnishings)

RISK FACTORS
- Personal skin-to-skin contact (e.g., sexual promiscuity, crowding, nosocomial infection)
- Poor nutritional status, poverty, and homelessness
- Hot, tropical climates
- Seasonal variation: Incidence may be higher in the winter than in the summer (may be due to overcrowding).
- Immunocompromised patients, including those with HIV/AIDS, are at increased risk of developing severe (crusted/Norwegian) scabies.

GENERAL PREVENTION
Prevent outbreaks by prompt treatment and cleansing of fomites (see "Additional Treatment").

DIAGNOSIS

HISTORY
- Generalized itching is often severe and worse at night.
- Determine any contact with infected individuals.
- Initial infection may be asymptomatic.
- Symptoms may develop after 3–6 weeks.

PHYSICAL EXAM
- Lesions (inflammatory, erythematous, pruritic papules) most commonly located in the finger webs, flexor surfaces of the wrists, elbows, axillae, buttocks, genitalia, feet, and ankles
- Burrows (thin, curvy, elevated lines in the upper epidermis that measure 1–10 mm) may be seen in involved areas—a pathognomic sign of scabies.

- Secondary erosions or excoriations from scratching
- Pustules (if secondarily infected)
- Pruritic nodules in covered areas (buttocks, groin, axillae) resulting from an exaggerated hypersensitivity reaction.
- Crusted scabies (Norwegian scabies) is a psoriasiform dermatosis occurring with hyperinfestation with thousands of mites (more common in immunosuppressed patients).

Geriatric Considerations
The elderly often itch more severely despite fewer cutaneous lesions and are at risk for extensive infestations, perhaps related to a decline in cell-mediated immunity. There may be back involvement in those who are bedridden.

Pediatric Considerations
Infants and very young children often present with vesicles, papules, and pustules and have more widespread involvement, including the hands, palms, feet, soles, body folds, and head (rare for adults).

DIFFERENTIAL DIAGNOSIS
- Atopic dermatitis
- Contact dermatitis
- Folliculitis/impetigo
- Tinea corporis
- Dermatitis herpetiformis
- Eczema
- Insect bites
- Papular urticaria
- Pediculosis corporis
- Pityriasis rosea
- Prurigo
- Psoriasis (crusted scabies)
- Pyoderma
- Seborrheic dermatitis
- Syphilis

DIAGNOSTIC TESTS & INTERPRETATION
- Definitive diagnosis requires microscopic identification of mites, eggs, or feces.
- A failure to find mites does not rule out scabies (1).

Initial Tests (lab, imaging)
CBC is rarely needed but may show eosinophilia.

Diagnostic Procedures/Other
- Examination of skin with magnifying lens:
  – Look for typical burrows in finger webs and on flexor aspect of the wrists, and on the penis.
  – Look for a dark point at the end of the burrow (the mite).
  – Presumptive diagnosis is based on clinical presentation, skin lesions, and identification of burrow (1,2).
  – The mite can be extracted with a 25-gauge needle and examined microscopically.

- Mineral oil mounts (3):
  – Place a drop of mineral oil over a suspected lesion. Nonexcoriated papules or vesicles also may be sampled.
  – Scrape the lesion with a no. 15 surgical blade.
  – Examine under a microscope for mites, eggs, egg casings, or feces.
  – Scraping from under fingernails often may be positive.
- Potassium hydroxide (KOH) wet mount not recommended because it can dissolve mite pellets (1).
- Burrow ink test (3):
  – If burrows are not obvious, apply blue–black ink to an area of rash. Wash off the ink with alcohol. A burrow should remain stained and become more evident.
  – Then apply mineral oil, scrape, and observe microscopically, as noted previously.
- Epiluminescence microscopy and high-resolution video dermatoscopy are expensive and have not been proven to be more sensitive than skin scraping (2).

Test Interpretation
Skin biopsy of a nodule (although performed rarely) will reveal portions of the mite in the corneal layer.

TREATMENT

GENERAL MEASURES
- Treat all intimate contacts and close household and family members.
- Wash all clothing, bed linens, and towels in hot (60°C) water or dry-clean.
- Personal items that cannot be washed or dry-cleaned should be sealed in a plastic bag for 3–5 days.
- Some itching and dermatitis may persist for up to 6 weeks and can be treated with oral antihistamines and/or topical or oral corticosteroids.

MEDICATION
First Line
Permethrin 5% cream (Elimite) is the most effective topical agent for scabies (4,5)[A]:
- After bathing or showering, apply cream from the neck to the soles of the feet paying particular attention to areas that are most involved; then wash off after 8–14 hours. A second application 1 week later is recommended if new lesions develop.
- The adult dose is usually 30 g.
- Side effects include itching and stinging (minimal absorption).
- Crusted scabies may require more frequent application (q2–3d for 1–2 weeks) in combination with PO ivermectin (6)[C].

Pediatric Considerations
Permethrin may be used on infants >2 months of age. In children <5 years of age, the cream should be applied to the head and neck, as well as to the entire body.

Second Line

- Crotamiton (Eurax) 10% cream:
  - Apply from the neck down for 24 hours, rinse off, then reapply for an additional 24 hours, and then thoroughly wash off.
  - Nodular scabies: Apply to nodules for 24 hours, rinse off, reapply for an additional 24 hours, then thoroughly wash off.
- Ivermectin (Stromectol):
  - Not FDA approved for scabies.
  - 200–250 μg/kg PO as single dose; repeated in 1 week
  - Take with food to improve bioavailability and enhance penetration into the epidermis.
  - May need higher doses or may need to use in combination with topical scabicide for HIV-positive patients
- Precipitated sulfur 5–10% in petrolatum:
  - Not FDA approved for scabies.
  - Apply to the entire body from the neck down for 24 hours, rinse by bathing, then repeat for 2 more days (3 days total). It is malodorous and messy but is thought to be safer than lindane, especially in infants <6 months of age, and safer than permethrin in infants <2 months of age.
- Lindane (γ-benzene hexachloride, Kwell) 1% lotion:
  - Apply to all skin surfaces from the neck down and wash off 6–8 hours later.
  - 2 applications 1 week apart are recommended but may increase the risk of toxicity.
  - 2 oz is usually adequate for an adult:
    - Side effects: Neurotoxicity (seizures, muscle spasms), aplastic anemia
    - Contraindications: Uncontrolled seizure disorder, premature infants
    - Precautions: Do not use on excoriated skin, on immunocompromised patients, in conditions that may increase risk of seizures, or with medications that decrease seizure threshold
    - Possible interactions: Concomitant use with medications that lower the seizure threshold

ALERT

Lindane: FDA black box warning of severe neurologic toxicity; use only when first-line agents have failed.

Pediatric Considerations

- The FDA recommends caution when using lindane in patients who weigh <50 kg. It is not recommended for infants and is contraindicated in premature infants.
- PO Ivermectin should be avoided in children <5 years and in those weighing <15 kg.

Pregnancy Considerations

- Permethrin is pregnancy Category B, and lindane, ivermectin, and crotamiton are Category C.
- Permethrin is considered compatible with lactation, but if permethrin is used while breastfeeding, the infant should be bottle-fed until the cream has been thoroughly washed off.

ADDITIONAL THERAPIES

- Crusted scabies may require use of keratolytics to improve penetration of permethrin.
- Benzyl benzoate lotion (not available in the US but used widely in developing countries):
  - Not FDA approved for scabies.
  - Dose for adults is 25–28%; dilute to 12.5% for children and 6.25% for infants
  - After bathing, apply lotion from the neck to soles of feet for 24 hours
- Topical ivermectin 1% lotion (investigational, not available for use in the US)(7):
  - Not FDA approved for scabies.
  - Apply to affected sites and wash off 8 hours later.

COMPLEMENTARY AND ALTERNATIVE MEDICINE

Herbal products such as tea tree oil, eugenol compounds, toto soap, and lippie oil may be effective but require additional evidence to establish efficacy (5).

 ONGOING CARE

FOLLOW-UP RECOMMENDATIONS
Patient Monitoring
Recheck patient at weekly intervals only if rash or itching persists. Scrape new lesions and retreat if mites or products are found.

PATIENT EDUCATION

- Patients should be instructed on proper application and cautioned not to overuse the medication when applying it to the skin.
- A patient fact sheet is available from the CDC: www.cdc.gov/parasites/scabies/

PROGNOSIS

- Lesions begin to regress in 1–2 days, along with the worst itching, but eczema and itching may persist for up to 6 weeks after treatment.
- Nodular lesions may persist for several weeks, perhaps necessitating intralesional or systemic steroids.
- Some instances of lindane-resistant scabies have now been reported. These do respond to permethrin.

COMPLICATIONS

- Poor sleep due to pruritus
- Social stigma
- Secondary bacterial infection (group A streptococci and *Staphylococcus aureus*)
- Sepsis
- Glomerulonephritis
- Eczema
- Pyoderma
- Postscabetic pruritus
- Nodules (nodular scabies) may persist for weeks to months after treatment.

REFERENCES

1. Chosidow O. Scabies. *N Engl J Med.* 2006;354: 1718–1727.
2. Leone PA. Scabies and pediculosis pubis: An update of treatment regimens and general review. *Clin Infect Dis.* 2007;44(Suppl 3):S153–S159.
3. Hengge UR, Currie BJ, Jäger G. Scabies: A ubiquitous neglected skin disease. *Lancet Infect Dis.* 2006;6:769–779.
4. Stong M, Johnstone PW. Interventions for treating scabies. *Cochrane Database Sys Rev.* 2007:3.
5. Hay RJ, Steer AC, Engelman D, et al. Scabies in the developing world—its prevalence, complications, and management. *Clin Microbiol Infect.* 2012; 18(4):313–323.
6. Currie BJ, McCarthy JS. Permethrin and ivermectin for scabies. *N Engl J Med.* 2010;362:717–724.
7. Sunita C, Dave J, Mehta D, Patel V, Shah H. Comparative efficacy and safety of topical permethrin, topical ivermectin, and oral ivermectin in patients of uncomplicated scabies. *Indian J Dermatol Venereol Leprol.* 2012;78:605–610.

ADDITIONAL READING

- Flinders DC, De Schweinitz P. Pediculosis and scabies. *Am Fam Physician.* 2004;69:341–348.
- Heukelbach J, Feldmeier H. Scabies. *Lancet.* 2006;367:1767–1774.
- Orien E, Marcos B, Davidovici B, et al. Itch and scratch: Scabies and pediculosis. *Clin Dermatol.* 2006;24:168–175.

 SEE ALSO

Arthropod Bites and Stings; Pediculosis (Lice)

 CODES

ICD10
B86 Scabies

CLINICAL PEARLS

- Prior to diagnosis, use of a topical steroid to treat pruritic symptoms may mask symptoms and is termed *scabies incognito*.
- Environmental control is recommended. All linens, towels, and clothing used in the previous 4 days should be washed in hot water or dry-cleaned. Personal items that cannot be washed or dry-cleaned should be sealed in a plastic bag for 3–5 days.
- All members of the affected household may require treatment, especially close contacts (those sharing the same bed or who have intimate contact).
- Eczema and itching may persist for up to 6 weeks after treatment, causing many patients to falsely believe that they have failed treatment or are being reinfected.
- In patients with actual reinfection, either the patient has not applied the medication properly or, more likely, the index patient has not been identified and treated.
- Some experts recommend routine reapplication of permethrin between days 8 and 15.

SCARLET FEVER

John C. Huscher, MD

BASICS

DESCRIPTION
- Generally, a childhood disease characterized by fever, pharyngitis, and rash caused by group A β-hemolytic *Streptococcus pyogenes* (GAS) that produces erythrogenic toxin.
- Incubation period: 1–7 days
- Duration of illness: 4–10 days
- Rash usually appears on the 2nd day of illness.
- Rash 1st appears in the upper chest and flexural creases and then spreads rapidly all over the body.
- Rash clears at the end of the 1st week and is followed by several weeks of desquamation.
- System(s) affected: Head; Eyes; Ears; Nose; Throat; Skin/Exocrine
- Synonym(s): Scarlatina

EPIDEMIOLOGY
Incidence
- Fairly common; rare in infancy because of maternal antitoxin antibodies
- Predominant age: 6–12 years
- Peak age: 4–8 years
- Predominant sex: Male = Female
- Rare in the US in those >12 because of high rates (>80%) of lifelong protective antibodies to erythrogenic toxins
- >900 cases of scarlet fever recorded in Hong Kong from January–July, 2011, including 6 cases complicated by toxic shock (with 2 fatalities) (1)[C]

Prevalence
- 5–30% of pediatric sore throats are due to GAS.
- <10% of children with streptococcal pharyngitis develop scarlet fever.

ETIOLOGY AND PATHOPHYSIOLOGY
- Erythrogenic toxin produced by phage is necessary for scarlet fever.
- 3 types: A, B, C
- These toxins damage capillaries (producing rash) and act as superantigens stimulating cytokine release.
- Antibodies to toxins prevent development of rash, but do not protect against underlying infection.
- Site of streptococcal infection usually tonsils; may occur with infection of skin, surgical wounds, or uterus (puerperal scarlet fever)

RISK FACTORS
- Winter/Spring seasons
- Age: School-aged children
- Contact with infected individual(s)
- Crowded living conditions (e.g., lower socioeconomic status, military, child care, schools)

GENERAL PREVENTION
- GAS is spread by contact with airborne respiratory particles.
- Asymptomatic contacts do not require cultures/prophylaxis.
- Symptomatic contacts may be treated ± cultures.
- Children should not return to school/daycare until they have received >24 hours of antibiotic therapy.

COMMONLY ASSOCIATED CONDITIONS
- Pharyngitis
- Impetigo
- Rheumatic fever
- Glomerulonephritis

DIAGNOSIS

HISTORY
Prodrome 1–2 days:
- Sore throat
- Headache
- Myalgias
- Malaise
- Fever (>38°C [100.4°F])
- Vomiting
- Abdominal pain (may mimic acute abdomen)
- Rash
- Cough, conjunctivitis, hoarseness, rhinorrhea more likely viral

PHYSICAL EXAM
- Oral exam:
  - Beefy red tonsils and pharynx with/without exudate
  - Petechiae on palate
  - White coating on tongue: White strawberry tongue appears on days 1–2. This sheds by days 4–5, leaving a red strawberry tongue, which is shiny and red with prominent papillae.
- Exanthem (appears within 1–5 days):
  - Scarlet macules over generalized erythema
  - Orange-red punctate skin eruption with sandpaperlike texture: Sunburn with goose pimples
  - Initially, chest and axillae; then spreads to abdomen and extremities; prominent in skin folds, flexural surfaces (e.g., axillae, groin, buttocks), with sparing of palms and soles
  - Flushed face with circumoral pallor, red lips
  - Pastia lines: Transverse red streaks in skin folds of abdomen, antecubital space, and axillae
  - Desquamation begins on face after 7–10 days and proceeds over trunk to hands and feet; may persist for 6 weeks
  - In severe cases, small vesicular lesions (miliary sudamina) may appear on abdomen, hands, and feet.
  - Rash: Blanches if pressed

DIFFERENTIAL DIAGNOSIS
- Viral exanthem
- Measles
- Rubella
- Infectious mononucleosis
- Roseola
- *Mycoplasma* pneumonia
- Secondary syphilis
- *Arcanobacterium haemolyticum*
- Toxic shock syndrome
- Staphylococcal scalded-skin syndrome
- Kawasaki disease
- Drug hypersensitivity
- Severe sunburn

DIAGNOSTIC TESTS & INTERPRETATION
- Swabbing the pharynx and testing for GAS pharyngitis by rapid antigen detection test (RADT) and/or culture should be performed because the clinical features alone do not reliably discriminate between GAS and viral pharyngitis.
- Testing for GAS pharyngitis is usually *not* recommended for children/adults with clinical and epidemiologic features that strongly suggest a viral etiology (e.g., cough, rhinorrhea, hoarseness, and oral ulcers).

Initial Tests (lab, imaging)
- RADT: Diagnostic if positive, 95% specific; sensitivity approaches that of culture. Negative RADT should be backed up by a throat culture. Positive RADTs do not necessitate a back-up culture because they are highly specific.
- Throat culture: Culture β-hemolytic colonies, catalase negative, sensitive to bacitracin; culture is gold standard for confirming streptococcal infection (99% specific, 90–97% sensitive, but 5–10% of healthy individuals are carriers).
- Serologic tests (includes antistreptolysin O titer and streptozyme tests, antihyaluronidase): Confirm recent GAS infection; not helpful/recommended for diagnosis of acute disease
- Gram stain: Positive cocci in chains
- CBC may show elevated WBC count (12,000–16,000/mm^3); possible eosinophilia later (2nd week)
- Follow-up posttreatment throat cultures or RADT are not recommended routinely, but may be considered in special circumstances.
- Diagnostic testing/empiric treatment of asymptomatic household contacts of patients with acute streptococcal pharyngitis is not routinely recommended.

Follow-Up Tests & Special Considerations
- Drugs that may alter lab results: Prior antibiotic therapy may result in negative throat culture.
- Within 5 days of symptoms, antibiotics can delay/abolish antistreptolysin O response.

Test Interpretation
Skin lesions reveal characteristic inflammatory reaction, specifically hyperemia, edema, and polymorphonuclear cell infiltration.

TREATMENT

GENERAL MEASURES
Supportive care. If warranted, use of an analgesic/antipyretic agent, such as acetaminophen or an NSAID, for treatment of moderate to severe symptoms or control of high fever associated with GAS pharyngitis should be considered as an adjunct to an appropriate antibiotic.

MEDICATION

First Line

- Penicillin (PO; penicillin V and others) for 10 days (2,3)[A]:
  - 250 mg PO b.i.d. or t.i.d. for <27 kg (60 lb); 500 mg b.i.d. or t.i.d. for >27 kg (60 lb) adolescents and adults
  - If compliance is questionable, use penicillin G, benzathine: Single IM dose 600,000 U for <27 kg (60 lb); 1.2 mU for others
- Amoxicillin (PO) 50 mg/kg once daily (4) (use only for definitive GAS because it can induce rash with some viral infections) (2)[A]:
  - Contraindications: Penicillin allergy
- Acetaminophen for fever and pain
- Precautions: Refer to manufacturer's profile of each drug.
- Significant possible interactions: Refer to manufacturer's profile of each drug.

Second Line

- For patients allergic to penicillin:
  - Azithromycin (Zithromax, Z pack): 12 mg/kg/d (max 500 mg) for 5 days (2)[B]
  - Clarithromycin (Biaxin): Children >6 months: 7.5 mg/kg b.i.d. for 10 days; adults: 250 mg b.i.d. for 10 days (2)[B]
- Oral cephalosporins: Many are effective, but 1st-generation cephalosporins are less expensive:
  - Cephalexin 40 mg/kg/d divided t.i.d.; max 250 mg t.i.d. × 10 days (2)[B]
  - Cefadroxil 30 mg/kg/d divided b.i.d.; max 500 mg b.i.d. × 10 days (2)[B]
- Clindamycin 20 mg/kg/d divided t.i.d. × 10 days (2)[B]
- Tetracyclines and sulfonamides should not be used.

ALERT

Avoid aspirin in children due to risk of Reye syndrome

ISSUES FOR REFERRAL

Development of peritonsillar abscess/shock symptoms: Hypotension, disseminated intravascular coagulation (DIC), cardiac, liver, renal dysfunction

SURGERY/OTHER PROCEDURES

- Tonsillectomy may be recommended with recurrent bouts of pharyngitis (≥6 positive strep cultures in 1 year).
- Children still may get strep throat after a tonsillectomy, but for some children with recurring strep throat, tonsillectomy reduces the frequency and severity of strep throat infections.

 ONGOING CARE

FOLLOW-UP RECOMMENDATIONS

Follow-up throat culture is not needed unless the patient is symptomatic.

Patient Monitoring

Because GAS is uniformly susceptible to penicillin, bacteriologic treatment failures are possible due to:

- Poor compliance
- β-Lactamase oral flora hydrolyzing penicillin

- GAS carrier state and concurrent viral rash (requires no treatment)
- Repeat exposure to carriers in family: Strep persists on nonrinsed toothbrushes and orthodontic appliances for up to 15 days.

DIET

No special diet

PATIENT EDUCATION

- Brief delay in initiating treatment while awaiting throat culture results does not increase the risk of rheumatic fever.
- Must take antibiotics for full course
- Children should not return to school/daycare until they have received >24 hours of antibiotic therapy.
- Can spread person to person: Avoid contact, wash hands.
- "Recurring strep throat: When is tonsillectomy useful?" Available at www.mayoclinic.com/health/recurring-strep-throat/AN01626

PROGNOSIS

- Course may be shortened by 12–24 hours with penicillin.
- Recurrent attacks are possible (different erythrogenic toxins).
- Mild disease usually responds well to antibiotics.

COMPLICATIONS

- Suppurative:
  - Sinusitis
  - Otitis media/mastoiditis
  - Cervical adenitis
  - Peritonsillar abscess/Retropharyngeal abscess
  - Pneumonia
  - Bacteremia with metastatic infectious foci: Meningitis, brain abscess, osteomyelitis, septic arthritis, endocarditis, intracranial venous sinus thrombosis, necrotizing fasciitis
- Nonsuppurative:
  - Rheumatic fever: Therapy prevents rheumatic fever when started as long as 10 days after onset of acute GAS infection.
  - Glomerulonephritis: Due to nephritogenic strain of *Streptococcus*; prevention even after adequate treatment of GAS is less certain.
  - Streptococcal toxic shock syndrome: Fever, hypotension, DIC, and cardiac, liver, and/or kidney dysfunction related to other toxin-mediated sequelae
  - Cellulitis
  - Weeks to months later, may develop transverse grooves in nail plates and hair loss (telogen effluvium)

REFERENCES

1. Luk EY, Lo JY, Li AZ. Scarlet fever epidemic, Hong Kong, 2011. *Emerg Infect Dis*. 2012;18(10):1658–1661.
2. Gerber MA. Prevention of rheumatic fever and diagnosis and treatment of acute streptococcal pharyngitis: A statement from the American Heart Association Rheumatic Fever, Endocarditis, and Kawasaki Disease Committee of the Council on Cardiovascular Disease in the Young, the Interdisciplinary Council on Functional Genomics and Translational Biology, and the Interdisciplinary Council on Quality of Care and Outcomes Research: Endorsed by the American Academy of Pediatrics. *Circulation*. 2009;119:1541–1551.
3. Spinks A. Antibiotics for sore throat (Review). *Cochrane Database Syst Rev*. 2010;3.
4. Lennon DR, Farrell E, Martin DR. Once-daily amoxicillin versus twice-daily penicillin V in group A beta-haemolytic streptococcal pharyngitis. *Arch Dis Child*. 2008;93:474–478.

ADDITIONAL READING

- Baltimore RS. Re-evaluation of antibiotic treatment of streptococcal pharyngitis. *Curr Opin Pediatr*. 2010;22:77–82.
- Chen M, Yao W, Wang X, et al. Outbreak of scarlet fever associated with emm12 type group A Streptococcus in 2011 in Shanghai, China. *Pediatr Infect Dis J*. 2012;31(9):e158–162.
- Shulman ST, Bisno AL, Clegg HW, et al. Clinical practice guideline for the diagnosis and management of group A streptococcal pharyngitis: 2012 update by the Infectious Diseases Society of America. *Clin Infect Dis*. 2012;84(10):e86–e102. Epub 2012 Sep 9.

 SEE ALSO

- Pharyngitis
- Algorithm: Tonsillar Exudates

 CODES

ICD10

- A38.0 Scarlet fever with otitis media
- A38.8 Scarlet fever with other complications
- A38.9 Scarlet fever, uncomplicated

CLINICAL PEARLS

- Consider scarlet fever in the differential diagnosis of children with fever and a rash.
- Look for strawberry tongue, circumoral pallor (vs. hyperemic cracked lips as in Kawasaki disease), and a coarse sandpaper rash (especially helpful in dark-skinned individuals). Desquamation may last for several weeks following the illness.
- Perform throat swabs to document streptococcal illness vs. other etiologies. Confirm before treating.

SCHIZOPHRENIA

Jodi J. Weinstein, MD • Jeffrey G. Stovall, MD

BASICS

Schizophrenia is a chronic, severe, and disabling psychiatric disorder.

DESCRIPTION
- Major psychiatric disorder characterized by prodrome, active, and residual psychotic symptoms involving disturbances in appearance, speech, behavior, perception, and thought that last for at least 6 months.
- DSM-V has eliminated subcategories of schizophrenia (1)
- System(s) affected: Nervous

EPIDEMIOLOGY
Incidence
- 7.7–43/100,000 (2)
- Predominant sex: Male > Female (1.4:1)
- Age of onset: Typically <30 years, earlier in males (early to mid-20s) than females (late 20s), with a smaller peak that occurs in women >45 years (3)

Prevalence
- Lifetime (1%): Highest prevalence in lower socioeconomic classes and urban centers (2)
- 1.1% of the population >18 years in all countries

ETIOLOGY AND PATHOPHYSIOLOGY
- Unknown: Not initiated/maintained by a known organic factor
- Probably a complex interaction between inherited and environmental factors

Genetics
Biologic relative with schizophrenia: If 1st-degree relative, risk is 8–10%, a 10-fold increase (4)[B].

GENERAL PREVENTION
- Currently, no known preventive measures decrease the incidence of schizophrenia.
- Interventions to improve the long-term course and outcome and to prevent some of the associated comorbid conditions are employed as approaches to prevention.

COMMONLY ASSOCIATED CONDITIONS
- Substance use disorders and nicotine dependence are common and lead to significant long-term medical and social complications (5).
- Metabolic syndrome, diabetes mellitus, obesity, and certain infectious diseases, including HIV, hepatitis B, and hepatitis C all occur in higher-than-expected rates in individuals with schizophrenia.

DIAGNOSIS

HISTORY
Focus on identifying an insidious social decline associated with the onset of ≥2 of the following characteristic signs and symptoms:
- Delusions
- Hallucinations
- Disorganized thought (derailed or incoherent speech)
- Grossly disorganized/catatonic behavior (hyper- or hypoactive movements)
- Negative symptoms (affective flattening, alogia, avolition) (1)

PHYSICAL EXAM
No characteristic physical findings

DIFFERENTIAL DIAGNOSIS
- Mental disorder due to medical illnesses:
  - Characterized by impaired judgment, orientation, memory, affect, and concentration.
  - Disorientation, in particular, indicates delirium.
  - Illnesses include trauma, infection, tumor metabolic, endocrine, and intoxication and disorders that affect the CNS (i.e., epilepsy, Huntington disease, Wilson disease, lupus cerebritis, metachromatic leukodystrophy)
- Substance-induced psychosis: Cocaine, amphetamines, LSD, phencyclidine, cannabis, alcohol, steroids, anticholinergics and opiates
- Personality disorders (paranoid, schizotypal, borderline personality disorder)
- Mood disorders: Especially bipolar disorder (manic–depressive disorder), schizoaffective disorder, mood disorders with psychotic features
- Delusional disorder
- Cultural belief system

DIAGNOSTIC TESTS & INTERPRETATION
- No tests are available to indicate schizophrenia.
- Imaging and laboratory tests are needed to rule out other causes; these may include:
  - Brain MRI
  - CBC, blood chemistries
  - Thyroid-stimulating hormone (TSH)
  - Rapid plasma reagin (RPR)
  - Urinalysis
  - Vitamin levels (thiamine, vitamin D)
  - Drug/Alcohol screen of blood and urine
  - Heavy-metal exposure: Ceruloplasmin, urine porphobilinogen as indicated

Initial Tests (lab, imaging)
Laboratory tests are needed when starting antipsychotic medications; these may include:
- CBC, blood chemistries
- Blood glucose level, preferably fasting
- Hemoglobin A1C
- Lipid panel
- TSH
- ECG, for baseline QTc

Follow-Up Tests & Special Considerations
Clinical and laboratory tests are needed, at least yearly, for routine monitoring if using antipsychotic medications (6)[A]; these may include:
- Blood pressure, weight, and waist circumference
- CBC, blood chemistries
- Blood glucose level, preferably fasting
- Hemoglobin A1C
- Lipid panel
- TSH
- Pregnancy test and prolactin level, if indicated
- ECG, monitoring for QTc prolongation

Diagnostic Procedures/Other
- Psychological: Not a routine part of assessment
- EEG to rule out seizure disorder
- Lumbar puncture if indicated by clinical presentation

Test Interpretation
No consistent/clinically useful pathologic findings

TREATMENT

MEDICATION
First Line
- Antipsychotics: Risperidone, olanzapine, ziprasidone, aripiprazole, quetiapine:
  - Atypical (2nd-generation): In addition to those listed above, paliperidone, iloperidone, asenapine, lurasidone, clozapine
  - Typical (1st-generation): Chlorpromazine, fluphenazine, trifluoperazine, perphenazine, thioridazine, haloperidol, thiothixene

- Medication choice is based on clinical and subjective response and side effect profile (6)[B]:
  - For sensitivity to extrapyramidal adverse effects: Atypical
  - For tardive dyskinesia: Clozapine
  - For poor compliance/high risk of relapse: Injectable form of long-acting antipsychotic, such as haloperidol, fluphenazine, risperidone, olanzapine, aripiprazole, or paliperidone
  - Special attention needs to be given to motor side effects, metabolic side effects, and cardio-vascular side effects.

- Usual oral daily dose (initial dose may be lower):
  - Aripiprazole: 10–30 mg/d
  - Asenapine: 5 mg b.i.d. (sublingual)
  - Chlorpromazine: 200 mg b.i.d.
  - Clozapine: 200 mg b.i.d.
  - Fluphenazine: 5 mg b.i.d.
  - Haloperidol: 5 mg b.i.d.
  - Iloperidone: 2–12 mg b.i.d.
  - Lurasidone: 40–80 mg/d
  - Olanzapine: 15–30 mg/d
  - Paliperidone: 6–12 mg/d
  - Perphenazine: 24 mg/d divided b.i.d. or t.i.d.
  - Quetiapine: 200–300 mg b.i.d.
  - Risperidone: 3 mg/d
  - Thiothixene: 10 mg b.i.d.
  - Trifluoperazine: 10 mg b.i.d.
  - Ziprasidone: 60–80 mg b.i.d. (with meal)
- Precautions:
  - Risperidone, olanzapine, quetiapine, and clozapine are associated with weight gain and development of metabolic syndrome.
  - For acute side effects of antipsychotics: Dystonic reaction (especially of head and neck): Give diphenhydramine (Benadryl) 25–50 mg IM or benztropine (Cogentin) 1–2 mg IM.
  - For pseudoparkinsonism reaction: trihexyphenidyl (Artane) 2 mg b.i.d. (may be increased to 15 mg/d if needed) or benztropine (Cogentin): 0.5 b.i.d. (range 1–4 mg/d)
  - For neuroleptic malignant syndrome: Hyperthermia, severe extrapyramidal effect, and autonomic dysfunction (e.g., hypertension, tachycardia, diaphoresis, and incontinence): Stop antipsychotic. Acute hyperthermia is treated with dantrolene 1 mg/kg IV push and continued PRN until cumulative total dose is up to 10 mg/kg. Post crisis management is with dantrolene 4–8 mg/kg/d PO in 4 divided doses × 1–3 days to prevent recurrence. Extrapyramidal effects are treated with bromocriptine 2.5 mg t.i.d. to q.i.d. PO/NG.

Second Line
- Clozapine (Clozaril):
  - Effective in treatment of refractory or suicidal patients (6)[B]
  - Serious risk of agranulocytosis mandates weekly CBC with differential and registration with National Clozapine Registry; significant risk of seizure at higher doses.
  - Start at 12.5 mg/d and increase slowly to a dose of 300–400 mg/d given b.i.d.; do not exceed 900 mg/d.
  - Side effects can include constipation, sialorrhea, tachycardia, and weight gain.
- Adjunctive treatments:
  - Benzodiazepines:
    - May be effective adjuncts to antipsychotics during acute phase of illness
    - Useful for the treatment of catatonia
    - Withdrawal reactions can include psychosis or seizures.
    - Individuals with schizophrenia are vulnerable to abuse/addiction.
  - Anticonvulsants: May be effective adjuncts for those with agitated/violent behavior (6,7)[A].
  - Antidepressants: If prominent symptoms of depression are present.

ISSUES FOR REFERRAL
- Patients with schizophrenia should receive multidisciplinary ongoing care from both a primary care physician and a psychiatrist.
- Issues for referral include suicidality, the coexistence of an addiction, difficulty in engagement or self-care
- Additional therapies: Specific psychosocial rehabilitation programs are strongly encouraged.
- Regular supportive therapy and family and patient education are essential.
- Family members often benefit from referral to family advocacy organizations such as the National Alliance for the Mentally Ill (NAMI) (8)[A].

ADDITIONAL THERAPIES
- General measures include family and patient education and engagement in the management of a chronic and severe illness. These include specific treatments to reduce the impact of psychotic symptoms and to enhance the social functioning and rehabilitation of the patient.
- Cognitive–behavioral therapy has been shown to be effective for specific symptoms of schizophrenia (9)[C].

SURGERY/OTHER PROCEDURES
- Electroconvulsive therapy (ECT): For patients presenting with catatonic features, the option of ECT should be considered early, when insufficient response to benzodiazepines is observed (6)[B].
- Surgical interventions are not available.

COMPLEMENTARY AND ALTERNATIVE MEDICINE
No alternative therapies are validated.

IN-PATIENT CONSIDERATIONS
Initial stabilization focuses on maintaining a safe environment and reducing acute psychotic symptoms and agitation through the initiation of pharmacologic treatment.

Admission Criteria/Initial Stabilization
The decision to admit is usually based on the patient's risk of harming him- or herself or someone else and the ability to care for self in the community.

Nursing
Monitor for safety concerns and establish a safe and supportive environment.

Discharge Criteria
The decision to discharge is based on the patient's ability to remain safe in the community and reflects a combination of suicide risk, level of psychotic symptoms, support systems, and the availability of appropriate outpatient services.

 ONGOING CARE

FOLLOW-UP RECOMMENDATIONS
- Long-term symptom management and rehabilitation depend on engagement in ongoing pharmacologic and psychosocial treatment.
- Monitoring is based on evaluation of symptoms (including safety and psychotic symptoms), looking for the emergence of comorbidities and medication side effects, and prevention of complications.

DIET
- Newer atypical antipsychotics confer a higher risk of metabolic side effects, such as diabetes, hypercholesterolemia, and weight gain.
- Although there are no specific dietary requirements, attention should be paid to the high risk of development of obesity, metabolic syndrome, and diabetes mellitus in individuals with schizophrenia.

PATIENT EDUCATION
- National Institute of Mental Health: *Schizophrenia*, at www.nimh.nih.gov/health/topics/schizophrenia/index.shtml
- *Helping a Family Member with Schizophrenia*, at www.aafp.org/afp/20070615/1830ph.html
- National Alliance on Mental Illness (NAMI), at www.NAMI.org

PROGNOSIS
- Chronic course: Remission and exacerbations; complete remission not common.
- Guarded prognosis
- Negative symptoms (consisting of decreased ambition, energy, and emotional responsiveness and social withdrawal) are often most difficult to treat.
- Excessive mortality occurs due to suicide, accidents, coronary artery disease, nicotine dependence, or substance abuse.

COMPLICATIONS
- Side effects from antipsychotic medications, including tardive dyskinesia, orthostatic hypotension, QTc prolongation, and metabolic syndrome
- Self-inflicted trauma and suicide
- Combative behavior toward others
- Comorbid addictions, including nicotine (10)[A]

REFERENCES
1. American Psychiatric Association. *Diagnostic and statistical manual of mental disorders* (5th ed.). Washington, DC, 2013.
2. McGrath JJ. Variations in the incidence of schizophrenia: Data versus dogma. *Schizophr Bull*. 2006;32(1):195–197.
3. Riecher-Rossler A, Hafner H. Gender aspects in schizophrenia: Bridging the border between social and biological psychiatry. *Acta Psychiatr Scand*. 2000;102(suppl 407):58–62.
4. Norman RM, Manchanda R, Malla AK, et al. The significance of family history in first-episode schizophrenia spectrum disorder. *J Nerv Ment Dis*. 2007;195:846–852.
5. Fagerström K, Aubin HJ. Management of smoking cessation in patients with psychiatric disorders. *Curr Med Res Opin*. 2009;25:511–518.
6. Hasan A, Falkai P, Wobrock T, et al. World Federation of Societies of Biological Psychiatry (WFSBP) Guidelines for Biological Treatment of Schizophrenia, Part 1: Update 2012 on the acute treatment of schizophrenia and the management of treatment resistance. *World J Biol Psychiatry*. 2012;13:318–378.
7. Essali A, Al-Haj Haasan N, Li C, et al. Clozapine versus typical neuroleptic medication for schizophrenia. *Cochrane Database Syst Rev*. 2009:CD000059.
8. Mojtabai R, Nicholson RA, Carpenter BN. Role of psychosocial treatments in management of schizophrenia: A meta-analytic review of controlled outcome studies. *Schizophr Bull*. 1998;24:569–587.
9. Grant PM, Huh GA, Periroliotis D, et al. Randomized trial to evaluate the efficacy of cognitive therapy for low-functioning patients with schizophrenia. *Arch Gen Psychiatry*. 2012;69(2):121–127.
10. Saha S, Chant D, McGrath J. A systematic review of mortality in schizophrenia: Is the differential mortality gap worsening over time? *Arch Gen Psychiatry*. 2007;64:1123–1131.

ADDITIONAL READING
Saks E. *The center cannot hold: My journey through madness*. New York: Hyperion, 2007.

 SEE ALSO

Algorithm: Delirium

 CODES

ICD10
- F20.0 Paranoid schizophrenia
- F20.1 Disorganized schizophrenia
- F20.9 Schizophrenia, unspecified

CLINICAL PEARLS
- Schizophrenia is a debilitating chronic mental illness that affects all cultures.
- Schizophrenia is characterized by positive symptoms, including hallucinations, such as voices that converse with/about the patient, delusions that are often paranoid, and negative symptoms, including flattened affect, loss of a sense of pleasure, loss of will/drive, and social withdrawal.
- Multidisciplinary teams are essential to enhance patient and family coping with serious and persistent mental illness, to prevent and treat comorbidities, and to promote recovery.

SCIWORA SYNDROME (SPINAL CORD INJURY WITHOUT RADIOLOGIC ABNORMALITY)

Elizabeth Varadian, DO, MS • Tyler Cymet, DO, FACP, FACOFP

 BASICS

DESCRIPTION
- SCIWORA occurs after trauma; it is an acute spinal cord injury and nerve root trauma resulting in sensory, motor, or combined sensorimotor deficits that can be either transient or permanent.
- These neural injuries occur without a fracture or misalignment visible on radiographic (x-ray, CT) imaging and without radiological explanations for the abnormal examination findings.
- MRI may be able to demonstrate neural and extra-neural injuries occurring primarily in the cervical region (C2–C6) due to fracture through cartilaginous end plates, edema, herniation, interspinous ligamentous injury, or other soft-tissue damage.
- SCIWORA has a broad presentation, from minor positive neurologic symptoms to complete quadriplegia.
- It can occur in all populations, but is primarily observed in pediatric patients.

EPIDEMIOLOGY
Incidence
Variable: In trauma victims, it has been reported to be 19–34%.

ETIOLOGY AND PATHOPHYSIOLOGY
Mechanism:
- The possible mechanisms of traumatic spinal cord injury causing SCIWORA are thought to include:
  – Hyperextension
  – Hyperflexion
  – Longitudinal distraction
  – Ischemic damage
- Neural injury: Edema
- Extraneural injury: Ligamentous injury

Trauma:
- Motor vehicle accident (most common cause of SCIWORA); either unrestrained passengers, pedestrians, or bicyclists struck by motor vehicles
- Sports-related injury
- Significant fall
- Child abuse

- Age: Pediatric patients have a higher incidence of SCIWORA than adults due to several differences that permit increased mobility and flexibility:
  – Anatomy:
    ○ Facet joints are oriented horizontally, which permits increased translational motion in the coronal (AP) plane.
    ○ Superior aspects of vertebral bodies demonstrate anterior wedging.
    ○ Ligaments and joint capsules have increased elasticity, permitting increased intersegmental movement and transient soft disc protrusion.
    ○ In patients age <8 years, head size-to-trunk ratio is disproportionately large.
    ○ Nuchal musculature is immature and lacking in strength.
    ○ Uncovertebral joints are absent.
  – Location: Mostly cervical region; thoracic spine is protected and splinted by the rib cage, preventing forced flexion or extension.

RISK FACTORS
- History of trauma
- Age <8 years
- Location (upper cervical spine)

 DIAGNOSIS

HISTORY
Trauma:
- Motor vehicle accident
- Sports-related injury
- Fall injury
- Child abuse injury

PHYSICAL EXAM
Assess for sensorimotor deficit:
- On neurologic exam abnormal findings are not accounted for by known/visible injuries.
- Abnormalities on musculoskeletal exam increases risk of spinal cord injury causing motor function problems.

DIFFERENTIAL DIAGNOSIS
- Cervical fracture through end-plate (1)[A]
- Central cord syndrome (1)[A]
- Brown-Sequard syndrome (1)[A]
- Anterior spinal artery syndrome (1)[A]
- Partial spinal cord injury (1)[A]
- Complete spinal cord injury (1)[A]

DIAGNOSTIC TESTS & INTERPRETATION
- Depending on the affected area, radiographic images can rule out a fracture:
  – Lateral x-ray C-spine
  – CT scan C-spine
  – If negative and pathology still suspected, flexion/extension views of C-spine on plain films
- No radiographic evidence of a fracture:
  – MRI imaging C-spine
  – Consider bone scan.

Follow-Up Tests & Special Considerations
Adult considerations: Adults are less prone to SCIWORA due to decreased flexibility and mobility in comparison to pediatric patients, although SCIWORA is possible in the setting of acute trauma or cervical spondylosis (1).
- MRI imaging can also rule out reoccurrence of SCIWORA after the initial traumatic event.
- MRI abnormalities correlate closely with neurologic injury.

Diagnostic Procedures/Other
Diagnosis is based on clinical findings of neurologic dysfunction and radiographic or neuroimaging evidence of injury.

 TREATMENT

GENERAL MEASURES
SCIWORA can present with a trauma history and no initial symptoms followed by subsequent neurologic deterioration:
- SCIWORA should be suspected with a history of trauma even if there are no initial neurologic exam findings.
- Unconscious patients should be immobilized until plain x-ray and CT radiographs are obtained or until consciousness improves and a neurologic and pain assessment can be made.
- Transient findings, such as numbness, and a history of trauma should be treated following spinal cord injury protocol with immobilization.
- Immobilization should be implemented for 12 weeks even after the return of normal neurologic function to minimize SCIWORA recurrence.
- If x-ray and CT scan are negative following a history of trauma, an MRI should be obtained as soon as possible to rule out neural injury and formulate a treatment plan.
- Treatment is nonoperative initially. Surgery may be required for spinal cord compression or spine instability secondary to extraneural injury.

MEDICATION
First Line
- Supportive care and observation with serial neurological and musculoskeletal exams (2)[A]
- Corticosteroid use is controversial; if used, start within the first 8 hours after injury

ADDITIONAL THERAPIES
Rigid immobilization for 12 weeks (day and night) if indicated by persistent symptoms

IN-PATIENT CONSIDERATIONS
Admission Criteria/Initial Stabilization
- Unexplained neurologic findings post trauma, MVC (motor vehicle collision)
- Neurologic injury demonstrated through MRI
- Suspected ligamentous lesion
- Trauma and spinal injury protocol
- Immobilization
- Consultation with a neurosurgeon once stable

Discharge Criteria
- Neurologic exam without any deficits
- History of transient cervical neurologic symptoms that have since resolved

ONGOING CARE

FOLLOW-UP RECOMMENDATIONS
Patient Monitoring
- Reassessing neurologic function within 24–48 hours if patient presents with no initial symptoms after a traumatic event considering a possible latency period
- Follow-up MRI before discharge

PROGNOSIS
Initial clinical instability or severity, MRI findings, neurological features, location, age, and persistence of injury have a direct correlation with prognosis:
- Favorable:
  – Initial mild-to-moderate injury is associated with good recovery.
  – Resolution of changes as evidenced by follow-up MRI predicts favorable outcome.
- Unfavorable:
  – Initial severe neural injury is associated with a poor prognosis.
  – MRI findings of spinal cord transection and significant hemorrhage are associated with a poor prognosis.
  – MRI follow-up findings of persistent spinal cord injury result in a less favorable outcome.
  – Higher cervical injuries have greater neurologic trauma and a worse prognosis.
  – Patients age <8 years have greater neurologic trauma and a worse prognosis.

COMPLICATIONS
Recurrent SCIWORA has been reported and should be considered in trauma patients who present themselves to a health care provider.

REFERENCES
1. Kasimatis GB, Panagiotopoulos E. The adult spinal cord injury without radiographic abnormalities syndrome: Magnetic resonance imaging and clinical findings in adults with spinal cord injuries having normal radiographs and computed tomography studies. *J Trauma.* 2008;65:86–93.
2. Launay F, Leet AI, Sponseller PD. Pediatric spinal cord injury without radiographic abnormality: A meta-analysis. *Clin Orthop Relat Res.* 2005;433: 166–170.

ADDITIONAL READING
- Buldini B, Amigoni A. Spinal cord injury without radiographic abnormalities. *Eur J Pediatr.* 2006;165: 108–111.
- Pillai A, Crane E, Chappell A, et al. Traumatic cervical hematomyelia: Report of a rare spinal cord injury without radiographic abnormality. *J Trauma.* 2008;65(4):938–941.

- Trigylidas T, Yuh SJ, Vassilyadi M, et al. Spinal cord injuries without radiographic abnormality at two pediatric trauma centers in Ontario. *Pediatr Neurosurg.* 2010;46(4):283–289. Epub 2010 Dec 15.
- Piatt Jr. JH, Campbell JW Spinal cord injury without radiographic abnormality and the Chiari malformation: Controlled observations. *Pedatr Neurosurg.* 2013 Aug 6 [Epub ahead of print]
- Boese CK, Lechler P. Spinal cord injury without radiographic abnormalities in adults: A systematic review. *J Trauma Acute Care Surg.* 2013;75(2): 320–323.

 # CODES

ICD10
- S14.2XXA Injury of nerve root of cervical spine, initial encounter
- S14.102A Unsp injury at C2 level of cervical spinal cord, init encntr
- S14.109A Unsp injury at unsp level of cervical spinal cord, init

CLINICAL PEARLS
- If a child presents with a history of trauma and neurologic symptoms but has negative x-ray and CT findings, consider SCIWORA.
- There is an association between Chiari malformation type 1 (CM1) and spinal cord injury without radiographic abnormality.

SCLERITIS
Matthew Schear, DO, MS • Michael J. Terzella, DO

BASICS

DESCRIPTION
- Scleritis is a painful, inflammatory process of the sclera, part of the eye's outer coat:
  - Commonly associated with systemic disorders
  - Frequently requires systemic anti-inflammatory therapy
  - Potentially vision-threatening due to the deeper layer of the sclera being involved
- In contrast, episcleritis is a self-limited inflammation of the eye with only mild discomfort.
- System(s) affected: Ocular

EPIDEMIOLOGY
- Predominant age: Most frequently occurs in 4th and 6th decades; mean age for all types of scleritis is ~52 years.
- Predominant sex: Female > Male (1.6:1)

Incidence
- Anterior scleritis (~94% of cases):
  - Diffuse anterior scleritis (most common)
- Remaining 6% have posterior scleritis

Prevalence
Estimated to be 6 cases/100,000 people in the general population

ETIOLOGY AND PATHOPHYSIOLOGY
- Frequently associated with a systemic illness (1):
  - Most commonly associated with rheumatoid arthritis
  - In ~38% of cases, scleritis is the presenting manifestation of an underlying systemic disorder.
  - A recently described T-helper cell population, known as Th-17, has been implicated (2)[A].
- Other etiologies (1):
  - Drug-induced scleritis has been reported in patients on bisphosphonate therapy.
  - Following ocular surgery (surgically induced necrotizing scleritis)
  - Infectious scleritis most commonly after pterygium excision or cataract extraction, and *Pseudomonas aeruginosa* most common causative organism (3)[B]

RISK FACTORS
Individuals with autoimmune disorders are most at risk.

COMMONLY ASSOCIATED CONDITIONS
- Rheumatoid arthritis
- Sjögren syndrome
- Ankylosing spondylitis
- Systemic lupus erythematosus
- Reactive arthritis
- Relapsing polychondritis
- Polyarteritis nodosa
- Wegener granulomatosis
- Sarcoidosis
- Inflammatory bowel disease
- Varicella zoster virus
- Syphilis
- Lyme disease
- Herpes zoster
- Tuberculosis

DIAGNOSIS

HISTORY
- Redness and inflammation of the sclera:
  - Can be bilateral in 1/3 of cases (4)[B]
- Decrease in visual acuity
- Photophobia and tearing
- Pain ranging from mild discomfort to extreme localized tenderness (severe pain not a common feature of most inflammatory eye disease) (1):
  - May be described as constant, deep, boring, or pulsating
  - Pain may be referred to the eyebrow, temple, or jaw (4)[B]
  - Pain may awaken patient from sleep in early hours of morning.

PHYSICAL EXAM
- Examine sclera in all directions of gaze by gross inspection:
  - A bluish hue may suggest thinning of sclera.
  - Inspect for breadth and degree of injection.
- Check visual acuity.
- Slit-lamp exam using red-free light (1):
  - Episcleritis: Conjunctival and superficial vascular plexuses displaced anteriorly
  - Scleritis: Deep episcleral plexus is maximum site of vascular congestion, displaced anteriorly d/t edema of underlying sclera. Characteristic blue or violet color, absent in patients with episcleritis.
- Ocular tenderness
- Dilated fundus exam to rule out posterior involvement
- A complete physical exam, particularly of the skin, joints, heart, and lungs, should be done to evaluate for associated conditions.

DIFFERENTIAL DIAGNOSIS
- Conjunctivitis
- Episcleritis
- Iritis (anterior uveitis)
- Blepharitis
- Trauma
- Ocular rosacea
- Herpes zoster

DIAGNOSTIC TESTS & INTERPRETATION
Consider further tests if warranted by history and physical:
- Routine tests to exclude systemic disease:
  - CBC, serum chemistry, urinalysis, ESR, and/or C-reactive protein
- Specific tests for underlying systemic illness (1),(4)[B]:
  - Rheumatoid factor, anticyclic citrullinated peptide antibodies, antineutrophil cytoplasmic antibody, and antinuclear antibody may aid in the diagnosis.
- Other tests:
  - Fluorescent treponemal antibody absorption (FTA-ABS), rapid plasma reagin, and Lyme titers
- Further imaging studies, such as a chest x-ray and sacroiliac joint films, may be useful if a specific systemic illness is suspected.
- B-scan US to detect posterior scleritis and thickness of sclera
- If indicated, MRI/CT scan to detect orbital disease

Diagnostic Procedures/Other
Biopsy is not routinely required unless diagnosis remains uncertain after above investigations.

Test Interpretation
Different subtypes of scleritis are associated with varying presentations and distinct findings (4)[B]:
- Diffuse anterior scleritis: Widespread inflammation
- Nodular anterior scleritis: Immovable, inflamed nodule
- Necrotizing anterior scleritis:
  - "With inflammation": Sclera becomes transparent.
  - Scleromalacia perforans "without inflammation": Associated with pain fiber necrosis
- Posterior scleritis: Associated with retinal and choroidal complications, adjacent swelling of orbital tissues may occur.

TREATMENT

GENERAL MEASURES
If scleral thinning, glasses/eye shield should be worn to prevent perforation.

MEDICATION
- Diffuse anterior and nodular scleritis initially treated with (1),(2)[A],(5)[B]:
  – Oral NSAID therapy, provided no contraindications exist (36.7% successful)
  – Subconjunctival triamcinolone is highly effective.
  – In severe disease and those with associated systemic disease, start systemic steroids: Prednisone
  – If limited response on systemic steroids, immunosuppressive agents may be indicated, including:
    ○ Cyclophosphamide, cyclosporine, azathioprine, methotrexate, and mycophenolate mofetil
    ○ Infliximab or rituximab has been effective in resistant cases
- Necrotizing anterior scleritis and posterior scleritis (2)[A],(4)[B]:
  – May require immunosuppressive therapy in addition to systemic steroids
  – Treat aggressively due to possible complications if left untreated.
- Infectious (2)[A]:
  – Treat with appropriate antibiotic therapy.

ISSUES FOR REFERRAL
- All patients with scleritis should be managed by an ophthalmologist familiar with this condition.
- Rheumatology referral for coexistent systemic disease is helpful for long-term success.

ADDITIONAL THERAPIES
Immunosuppressants used for autoimmune and collagen vascular disorders may be of help in active scleritis.

SURGERY/OTHER PROCEDURES
- In rare cases, scleral biopsy may be indicated to confirm infection or malignancy.
- Ocular perforation requires scleral grafting.

ONGOING CARE

Follow-Up Tests & Special Considerations
- No restrictions
- Avoid contact lens wear only if there is corneal involvement, which is rare.

Patient Monitoring
- Patient in the active stage of inflammation should be followed very closely by an ophthalmologist to assess the effectiveness of therapy.
- Medication use mandates close surveillance for adverse effects.

DIET
No special diet

PATIENT EDUCATION
Scleritis at PubMed Health: www.ncbi.nlm.nih.gov/pubmedhealth/PMH0001998/

PROGNOSIS
Scleritis is indolent, chronic, and often progressive:
- Diffuse anterior scleritis (best prognosis)
- Necrotizing anterior scleritis (worst prognosis)
- Recurrent bouts of inflammation may occur.
- Scleromalacia perforans has the highest risk of perforation of the globe.

COMPLICATIONS
- Spread to adjacent structures, most commonly cornea and uvea (1)
- Increased intraocular pressure
- Cataract and glaucoma can result from disease or treatment with steroids.
- Visual loss due to posterior extension/adjacent structural involvement
- Ocular perforation can occur in severe stages.

REFERENCES
1. Wakefield D, Girolamo ND, Thurau S, et al. Scleritis: Immunopathogenesis and molecular basis for therapy. *Prog Retin Eye Res*. 2013;35:44–62.
2. Rachitskaya A, Mandelcorn ED, Albini TA, et al. An update on the cause and treatment of scleritis. *Curr Opin Ophthalmol*. 2010;21:463–467.
3. Hodson KL, Galor A, Karp CL, et al. Epidemiology and visual outcomes in patients with infectious scleritis. *Cornea*. 2013;32:466–472.
4. Sainz de la Maza M, Molina N, Gonzalez-Gonzalez LA, et al. Clinical characteristics of a large cohort of patients with scleritis and episcleritis. *Ophthalmology*. 2012;84(1):43–50. Epub 2011 Oct 2.
5. Sainz de la Maza M, Molina N, Gonzalez-Gonzalez LA, et al. Scleritis therapy. *Ophthalmology*. 2012;84(1):51–58. Epub 2011 Oct 19.

ADDITIONAL READING
- Doctor P, Sultan A, Syed S, et al. Infliximab for the treatment of refractory scleritis. *Br J Ophthalmol*. 2010;84(5):579–583. Epub 2009 Dec 2.
- Fraunfelder FW, Fraunfelder FT. Bisphosphonates and ocular inflammation. *N Engl J Med*. 2003;348:1187–1188.
- Iaccheri B, Androudi S, Bocci EB, et al. Rituximab treatment for persistent scleritis associated with rheumatoid arthritis. *Ocul Immunol Inflamm*. 2010;18:223–225.
- Lin P, Bhullar SS, Tessler HH, et al. Immunologic markers as potential predictors of systemic autoimmune disease in patients with idiopathic scleritis. *Am J Ophthalmol*. 2008;84(3):463–471. Epub 2007 Dec 3.
- Smith JR, Mackensen F, Rosenbaum JT. Therapy insight: Scleritis and its relationship to systemic autoimmune disease. *Nat Clin Pract Rheumatol*. 2007;3:219–226.

CODES

ICD10
- H15.009 Unspecified scleritis, unspecified eye
- H15.019 Anterior scleritis, unspecified eye
- H15.039 Posterior scleritis, unspecified eye

CLINICAL PEARLS
- Episcleritis is a self-limited inflammation of the eye with mild discomfort. In contrast, scleritis is a painful, severe, and potentially vision-threatening condition, due to the deeper layer of the sclera being involved, for which active treatment is imperative.
- Uveitis, by definition, involves some combination of the iris, ciliary body, and choroid membrane. Scleritis can spread to involve these structures, but may not always do so. Both conditions can be associated with underlying inflammatory diseases.
- ~35% of all cases of scleritis are associated with a systemic disease, such as rheumatoid arthritis.

SCLERODERMA

Ann M. Lynch, PharmD, RPh, AE-C • Deborah M. DeMarco, MD

BASICS

DESCRIPTION
- Scleroderma (systemic sclerosis [SSc]) is a chronic disease of unknown cause characterized by diffuse fibrosis of skin and visceral organs and vascular abnormalities.
- Most manifestations have vascular features (e.g., Raynaud phenomenon), but frank vasculitis is rarely seen.
- Can range from a mild disease, affecting the skin, to a systemic disease that can cause death in a few months
- The disease is categorized into 2 major clinical variants:
  - Diffuse: Distal and proximal extremity and truncal skin thickening
  - Limited:
    - Restricted to the fingers, hands, and face
    - CREST syndrome (calcinosis, Raynaud phenomenon, esophageal dysmotility, sclerodactyly, telangiectasia)
- System(s) affected: Include, but not limited to Skin; Renal; Cardiovascular; Pulmonary; Musculoskeletal; Gastrointestinal

Geriatric Considerations
Uncommon >75 years of age

Pediatric Considerations
Rare in this age group

Pregnancy Considerations
- Safe and healthy pregnancies are common and possible despite higher frequency of premature births.
- High-risk management must be standard care to avoid complications, specifically renal crisis.
- Diffuse scleroderma causes greater risk for developing serious cardiopulmonary and renal problems. Pregnancy should be delayed until disease stabilizes.

EPIDEMIOLOGY
Incidence
- In the US: 1–2/100,000/yr
- Predominant age:
  - Young adult (16–40 years); middle-aged (40–75 years), peak onset 30–50 years
  - Symptoms usually appear in the 3rd–5th decades
- Predominant sex: Female > Male (4:1)

Prevalence
In the US: 1–25/100,000

ETIOLOGY AND PATHOPHYSIOLOGY
Pathophysiology involves both a vascular component and a fibrotic component. Both occur simultaneously. The inciting event is unknown, but there is an increase in certain cytokines after endothelial cell activation that are pro-fibrotic (TGF-β and PDGF).
- Unknown
- Possible alterations in immune response
- Possibly some association with exposure to quartz mining, quarrying, vinyl chloride, hydrocarbons, toxin exposure
- Treatment with bleomycin has caused a scleroderma-like syndrome, as has exposure to rapeseed oil.

Genetics
Familial clustering is rare but has been seen.

RISK FACTORS
Unknown

DIAGNOSIS

HISTORY
- Raynaud phenomenon is generally the presenting complaint (differentiated from Raynaud disease, generally affecting younger individuals and without digital ulcers).
- Skin thickening, "puffy hands," pruritus, and gastroesophageal reflux disease (GERD) are often noted early in the disease process.

PHYSICAL EXAM
- Skin:
  - Digital ulcerations
  - Digital pitting
  - Tightness, swelling, thickening of digits
  - Hyperpigmentation/Hypopigmentation
  - Narrowed oral aperture
  - Scaling of skin
  - SC calcinosis
- Peripheral vascular system:
  - Telangiectasia
- Joints, tendons, and bones:
  - Flexion contractures
  - Friction rub on tendon movement
  - Hand swelling
  - Joint stiffness
  - Polyarthralgia
  - Sclerodactyly
- Muscle:
  - Proximal muscle weakness
- GI tract:
  - Dysphagia
  - Esophageal reflux due to dysmotility (most common systemic sign in diffuse disease)
  - Malabsorptive diarrhea
  - Nausea and vomiting
  - Weight loss
  - Xerostomia
- Kidney:
  - Hypertension
  - May develop scleroderma renal crisis: Acute renal failure (ARF)
- Pulmonary:
  - Dry crackles at lung bases
  - Dyspnea
- Nervous system:
  - Peripheral neuropathy
  - Trigeminal neuropathy
- Cardiac (progressive disease):
  - Conduction abnormalities
  - Cardiomyopathy
  - Pericarditis
  - Secondary cor pulmonale

DIFFERENTIAL DIAGNOSIS
- Mixed connective tissue disease/Overlap syndromes
- Scleredema
- Nephrogenic systemic fibrosis
- Toxic oil syndrome (Madrid, 1981, affecting 20,000 people)
- Eosinophilia—myalgia syndrome
- Diffuse fasciitis with eosinophilia
- Scleredema of Buschke

DIAGNOSTIC TESTS & INTERPRETATION
Initial Tests (lab, imaging)
- Nail fold capillary microscopy
- CBC
- Creatinine
- Urinalysis (albuminuria, microscopic hematuria)
- Antinuclear antibodies (ANA): Positive in >90% of patients
- Anti–Scl-70 (topoisomerase) antibody is highly specific for systemic disease and confers a higher risk of interstitial lung disease (ILD)
- Anticentromere antibody usually associated with CREST variant
- Chest radiograph:
  - Diffuse reticular pattern
  - Bilateral basilar pulmonary fibrosis
- Hand radiograph:
  - Soft-tissue atrophy and acro-osteolysis
  - Can see overlap syndromes, such as rheumatoid arthritis
  - SC calcinosis

Follow-Up Tests & Special Considerations
- Pulmonary function tests (PFTs):
  - Decreased maximum breathing capacity
  - Increased residual volume
  - Diffusion defect
- Hypergammaglobulinemia
- Antibodies to U3-RNP-higher risk for scleroderma-associated pulmonary hypertension
- Anti-PM-Scl antibodies (for myositis)
- ECG (low voltage): Possible nonspecific abnormalities, arrhythmia, and conduction defects
- Echocardiography: Pulmonary hypertension or cardiomyopathy
- Nail fold capillary loop abnormalities
- Upper GI:
  - Distal esophageal dilatation
  - Atonic esophagus
  - Esophageal dysmotility
  - Duodenal diverticula
- Barium enema:
  - Colonic diverticula
  - Megacolon
- High-resolution CT scan for detecting alveolitis, which has a ground-glass appearance or honeycomb pattern in fibrosis

Diagnostic Procedures/Other
- Skin biopsy:
  - Compact collagen fibers in the reticular dermis and hyalinization and fibrosis of arterioles
  - Thinning of epidermis, with loss of rete pegs and atrophy of dermal appendages
  - Accumulation of mononuclear cells is also seen.
- Right-sided heart catheterization: Pulmonary hypertension is an ominous prognostic feature.

Test Interpretation
- Skin:
  - Edema, fibrosis, or atrophy (late stage)
  - Lymphocytic infiltrate around sweat glands
  - Loss of capillaries
  - Endothelial proliferation
  - Hair follicle atrophy
- Synovium:
  - Pannus formation
  - Fibrin deposits in tendons
- Kidney:
  - Small kidneys
  - Intimal proliferation in interlobular arteries
- Heart:
  - Endocardial thickening
  - Myocardial interstitial fibrosis
  - Ischemic band necrosis
  - Enlarged heart
  - Cardiac hypertrophy
- Lung:
  - Interstitial pneumonitis
  - Cyst formation
  - Interstitial fibrosis
  - Bronchiectasis
- Esophagus:
  - Esophageal atrophy
  - Fibrosis

 TREATMENT

GENERAL MEASURES
- Treatment is symptomatic and supportive.
- Esophageal dilation may be used for strictures.
- Avoid cold; dress appropriately in layers for the weather; be wary of air conditioning.
- Avoid smoking (crucial).
- For chronic digital ulcerations:
  - Débridement after soaking in 1/2-strength hydrogen peroxide solution
  - Digital plaster to immobilize
- Avoid finger sticks (e.g., blood tests).
- Elevate the head of the bed during sleep to help relieve GI symptoms.
- Use softening lotions, ointments, and bath oils to help prevent dryness and cracking of skin.
- Dialysis may be necessary in renal crisis.

MEDICATION
First Line
- ACE inhibitors (ACEIs): For preservation of renal blood flow and for treatment of hypertensive renal crisis (1)[C]
- Corticosteroids: For disabling myositis, pulmonary alveolitis, or mixed connective tissue disease (not recommended in high doses due to increased incidence of renal failure) (1)[C]
- NSAIDs: For joint or tendon symptoms. Caution with long-term concurrent use with ACEIs (potential renal complications)
- Antibiotics: For secondary infections in bowel and active skin infections (1)
- Antacids, proton pump inhibitors: For gastric reflux (1)[B]
- Intestinal dysfunction: Metoclopramide (1)[C]
- Dipyridamole or aspirin: Antiplatelet therapy
- Hydrophilic skin ointments: Skin therapy

- Topical clindamycin, erythromycin, or silver sulfadiazine cream may prevent recurrent infectious cutaneous ulcers.
- Consider immunosuppressives for treatment of life-threatening or potentially crippling scleroderma or interstitial pneumonitis (1)[A].
- Avoidance of caffeine, nicotine, and sympathomimetics may ease Raynaud symptoms.
- Nitrates and dihydropyridine calcium-channel blockers for Raynaud phenomenon (2)[A]
- PDE-5 antagonists (e.g., sildenafil), prostanoids, and endothelin-1 antagonists are changing the management of pulmonary hypertension (1)[B].
- Alveolitis: Immunosuppressants and alkylating agents (e.g., cyclophosphamide) (1)[A]

ADDITIONAL THERAPIES
- Anti-TNF-α therapy: Preliminary suggestion is that these may reduce joint symptoms and disability in inflammatory arthritis, but small sample sizes and observational biases lend to the need for further well-designed, adequately powered, longitudinal clinical trials (3)[A].
- Physical therapy to maintain function and promote strength
- Heat therapy to relieve joint stiffness

SURGERY/OTHER PROCEDURES
- Some success with gastroplasty for correction of GERD
- Limited role for sympathectomy for Raynaud phenomenon

 ONGOING CARE

FOLLOW-UP RECOMMENDATIONS
Patient Monitoring
- Monitor every 3–6 months for end-organ and skin involvement and medications. Provide encouragement.
- Echocardiology and PFTs yearly

DIET
Drink plenty of fluids with meals.

PATIENT EDUCATION
- Stay as active as possible, but avoid fatigue.
- Printed patient information available from the Scleroderma Federation, 1725 York Avenue, No. 29F, New York, NY 10128; (212) 427-7040
- Advise the patient to report any abnormal bruising or nonhealing abrasions.
- Assist the patient about smoking cessation, if needed.

PROGNOSIS
- Possible improvement, but incurable
- Prognosis is poor if cardiac, pulmonary, or renal manifestations present early.

COMPLICATIONS
- Renal failure
- Respiratory failure
- Flexion contractures
- Disability
- Esophageal dysmotility
- Reflux esophagitis
- Arrhythmia
- Megacolon

- Pneumatosis intestinalis
- Obstructive bowel
- Cardiomyopathy
- Pulmonary hypertension
- Possible association with lung and other cancers
- Death

REFERENCES
1. Kowal-Bielecka O, Landewé R, Avouac J, et al. EULAR recommendations for the treatment of systemic sclerosis: A report from the EULAR Scleroderma Trials and Research group (EUSTAR). *Ann Rheum Dis*. 2009;68:620–628.
2. Harding SE, Tingey PC, Pope J, et al. Prazosin for Raynaud's phenomenon in progressive systemic sclerosis. *Cochrane Database Syst Rev*. 1998;2: CD000956.
3. Phumethum V, Jamal S, Johnson SR. Biologic therapy for systemic sclerosis: A systematic review. *J Rheumatol*. 2011;38(2):289–296. Epub 2010 Nov 1.

ADDITIONAL READING
- Herrick AL. Contemporary management of Raynaud's phenomenon and digits ischemic complications. *Curr Opin Rheum*. 2011;23:555.
- Reveille JD, Solomon DH, American College of Rheumatology Ad Hoc Committee of Immunologic Testing Guidelines. Evidence-based guidelines for the use of immunologic tests: Anticentromere, Scl-70, and nucleolar antibodies. *Arthritis Rheum*. 2003;49:399–412.
- Steen VD. Pregnancy in scleroderma. *Rheum Dis Clin North Am*. 2007;33:345–358, vii.
- Valerio CJ, Schreiber BE, Handler C, et al. Borderline mean pulmonary artery pressure in patients with systemic sclerosis. *A&R*. 2013;65:1074–1084.

 SEE ALSO

Morphea

 CODES

ICD10
- M34.0 Progressive systemic sclerosis
- M34.89 Other systemic sclerosis
- M34.9 Systemic sclerosis, unspecified

CLINICAL PEARLS
- Raynaud phenomenon is frequently the initial complaint.
- Skin thickening, "puffy hands," and GERD are often noted early in disease.
- Eosinophilic fasciitis can mimic scleroderma, but differs with the absence of Raynaud symptoms and is responsive to corticosteroid treatment.

SEASONAL AFFECTIVE DISORDER

Christopher C. White, MD, JD • Anna T. Wiley

 BASICS

DESCRIPTION

- Seasonal affective disorder (SAD) is a heterogeneous mood disorder with depressive episodes usually occurring in winter months, with full remissions in the spring and summer.
- Ranges from a milder form (winter blues) to a seriously disabling illness
- Must separate out patients with other mood disorders (such as major depressive disorder and bipolar affective disorder) whose symptoms persist during spring and summer months.

EPIDEMIOLOGY

Incidence
- Affects up to 500,000 people every winter
- Up to 30% of patients visiting a primary care physician (PCP) during winter may report winter depressive symptoms.
- Predominant age: Occurs at any age; peaks in 20s and 30s
- Predominant sex: Female > Male (3:1)

Prevalence
- 1–9% of the general population
- 10–20% of patients identified as having mood symptoms will have a seasonal component.

ETIOLOGY AND PATHOPHYSIOLOGY
The major theories currently involve the interplay of phase-shifted circadian rhythms, genetic vulnerability, and serotonin dysregulation.

- Melatonin produced by the pineal gland at increased levels in the dark has been linked to depressive symptoms; light therapy on the retina acts to inhibit melatonin secretion.
- Serotonin dysregulation, because it is secreted less during winter months, must be present for light therapy to work, and treatment with SSRIs appears to reverse SAD symptoms.
- Decreased levels of vitamin D, often occurring during low-light winter months, may be associated with depressive episodes in some individuals experiencing SAD symptoms.

Genetics
- Some twin studies and a preliminary study on GPR50 melatonin receptor variants have suggested a genetic component.
- Recent studies indicate an association with the melanopsin gene (OPN4).
- Increased incidence of depression, ADHD, and alcoholism in close relatives

RISK FACTORS
- Most common during months of January and February: Patients frequently visit PCP during winter months complaining of recurrent flu, chronic fatigue, and unexplained weight gain.
- Working in a building without windows or other environment without exposure to sunlight

GENERAL PREVENTION
- Consider use of light therapy at start of winter (if prior episodes begin in October), increase time outside during daylight, or move to a more southern location.
- Bupropion (Wellbutrin) is an FDA-approved antidepressant for the prevention of SAD.

COMMONLY ASSOCIATED CONDITIONS
Some individuals with SAD have a weakened immune system and may be more vulnerable to infections.

 DIAGNOSIS

- Carefully document the presence or absence of prior manic episodes.
- Screen for the existence of any suicidal ideation and safety risk factors.
- Remission of symptoms during spring and summer
- Symptoms have occurred for the past 2 years.
- Seasonal episodes associated with winter months substantially outnumber any nonseasonal depressive episodes.

HISTORY
- Symptoms of depression meeting the criteria for major depressive disorder:
  - Sleep disturbance: Either too much or too little
  - Lack of interest in life and absence of pleasure from hobbies/activities
  - Guilt: Feelings of guilt or worthlessness
  - Energy: Fatigue or constantly feeling tired
  - Concentration: Difficulty with concentration and memory
  - Appetite: Changes in appetite and weight
  - Psychomotor retardation: Patients feel slowed down with decreased activity
  - Suicidal thoughts: Patients report thoughts of suicide
- In SAD, hypersomnia, hyperphagia (craving for carbohydrates and sweets), and weight gain usually predominate. Despite sleeping more, patients report daytime sleepiness and fatigue. Cravings may lead to binge eating and weight gains >20 lb.
- Obtain collateral history if patient is unable to provide insight into the seasonal component.

PHYSICAL EXAM
Use exam to exclude other organic causes for symptoms. Focal neurologic deficits, signs of endocrine dysfunction, or stigmata of substance abuse should prompt further testing.

DIFFERENTIAL DIAGNOSIS
- Similar to that of major depression, meaning that organic causes of low energy and fatigue, such as hypothyroidism, anemia, and mononucleosis (or other viral syndromes), need to be considered
- Other mood disorders without a seasonal component, such as major depression, bipolar disorder, adjustment disorder, or dysthymia
- Symptoms should not be better accounted for by seasonal psychosocial stressors, which often accompany the winter holiday seasons.
- Substance abuse

DIAGNOSTIC TESTS & INTERPRETATION
- Thyroid-stimulating hormone to rule out hypothyroidism
- CBC to rule out anemia
- Rule out electrolyte and glucose dysregulation.
- 25-OH vitamin D level
- Pregnancy test for women of child-bearing potential
- Urine tox screen if substance abuse is a concern
- Imaging not useful unless focal neurologic finding or looking to exclude an organic cause.

 TREATMENT

MEDICATION
Lack of evidence to determine whether light therapy or medication should be the first-line agent. Both supported by the literature and in some studies have equal efficacy. Medications have more side effects. Adherence to both remains a critical issue. The ultimate choice depends on the acuity of the patient and the comfort level of the prescribing clinician with each treatment modality (1)[B]:

- SSRIs such as sertraline (Zoloft), paroxetine (Paxil), fluoxetine (Prozac), citalopram (Celexa), and escitalopram (Lexapro) in their traditional antidepressant doses (2)[B]
- Bupropion (Wellbutrin) is the only antidepressant currently approved by the FDA for the prevention of SAD (3)[B].

ISSUES FOR REFERRAL
- Patients with a history of ocular disease should be referred for an ophthalmologic exam before phototherapy and for serial monitoring.
- Patients who fail to respond or who develop manic symptoms or suicidal ideation once treatment is initiated should be considered for psychiatric referral.

ADDITIONAL THERAPIES

Phototherapy using special light sources has been shown to be effective in 60–90% of patients, often providing relief with a few sessions (2,4)[B]:

- Variables that can regulate effect are:
  - Light intensity: Although the minimum light source intensity is under investigation, 2,500 lux is suggested (domestic lights emit, on average, 200–500 lux). There is good evidence for 10,000 lux as the recommended source (2)[B].
  - Treatment duration: Exposure time varies based on intensity of light source, with daily sessions of 30 minutes to a few hours.
  - Time of treatment: Most patients respond better by using the light therapy early in the morning.
  - Color of light source: Emerging data suggest that shorter sessions (20 minutes) of lower-intensity (2,500 lux) light-emitting diodes enriched in the blue spectrum have equal efficacy to the traditional white light treatment (30 minutes; 10,000 lux) (5)[B].
- Light box is placed on table several feet away, and the light is allowed to shine onto the patient's eyes (sunglasses should be avoided). Ensure that the light box has an ultraviolet filter.
- Most common side effects are eye strain and headache. Insomnia can result if the light box is used too late in the day. Light boxes also can precipitate mania in some patients.
- Dawn simulation machines gradually increase illumination while the patient sleeps, simulating sunrise while using a significantly less intense light source.

COMPLEMENTARY AND ALTERNATIVE MEDICINE

- Work to reduce stress levels through meditation, progressive relaxation exercises, and/or lifestyle modification.
- The potential role of vitamin D supplementation is under investigation. Currently, there is a lack of consistent research to satisfactorily demonstrate that treatment improves SAD symptoms. Reported doses vary widely, but typically are between 400 and 800 IU/d (6)[B].

IN-PATIENT CONSIDERATIONS

Admission Criteria/Initial Stabilization

If the patient develops suicidal ideation as part of his or her depression or mania after treatment is initiated

 ONGOING CARE

FOLLOW-UP RECOMMENDATIONS

Regular monitoring by PCP or psychiatrist for response to treatment; patients may become manic when treated with SSRIs or light therapy.

Patient Monitoring

Patients should be seen in the outpatient clinic weekly to biweekly when initiating light or pharmacotherapy to monitor treatment results, side effects, and any increased suicidal thoughts if using SSRIs.

DIET

No specific diet modification needed

PATIENT EDUCATION

- Increase time outdoors during daylight.
- Rearrange home or work environment to get more direct sunlight through windows.

PROGNOSIS

Symptoms, if untreated, generally remit within 5 months with exposure to spring light, only to return in subsequent winters. If treated, patients usually respond within 3–6 weeks.

COMPLICATIONS

Development of suicidal ideation and mania are 2 outcomes the clinician needs to monitor.

REFERENCES

1. Lam RW, Levitt AJ, Levitan RD, et al. The Can-SAD study: A randomized controlled trial of the effectiveness of light therapy and fluoxetine in patients with winter seasonal affective disorder. *Am J Psychiatry*. 2006;163:805–812.
2. Kurlansik SL, Ibay AD. Seasonal affective disorder. *Am Fam Physician*. 2012;86:1037–1041.
3. Niemegeers P, Dumont GJH, Patteet L, et al. Bupropion for the treatment of seasonal affective disorder. *Expert Opin Drug Metab Toxicol*. 2013; 9(9):1229–1240.
4. Terman M, Terman JS. Light therapy for seasonal and nonseasonal depression: Efficacy, protocol, safety, and side effects. *CNS Spectr*. 2005;10: 647–663; quiz 672.
5. Gordijn MC, 't Mannetje D, Meesters Y, et al. The effects of blue-enriched light treatment compared to standard light treatment in seasonal affective disorder. *J Affect Disord*. 2012;136:72–80.
6. Howland RH. Vitamin D and depression. *J Psychosoc Nurs Ment Health Serv*. 2011;49:15–18.

ADDITIONAL READING

- Pail G, Huf W, Pjrek E, et al. Bright-light therapy in the treatment of mood disorders. *Neuropsychobiology*. 2011;64:152–162.
- Thaler K, Delivuk M, Chapman A, et al. Second-generation antidepressants for seasonal affective disorder. *Cochrane Database Syst Rev*. 2011;(12):CD008591.

 SEE ALSO

- Bipolar I Disorder; Bipolar II Disorder; Depression
- Algorithm: Depressive Episode, Major

 CODES

ICD10

- F33.0 Major depressive disorder, recurrent, mild
- F33.1 Major depressive disorder, recurrent, moderate
- F33.9 Major depressive disorder, recurrent, unspecified

CLINICAL PEARLS

- SAD is a subtype of major depressive disorder. Once the patient has a diagnosed mood disorder, such as depression or bipolar, ask whether the symptoms vary in a seasonal pattern to qualify for the diagnosis of SAD. Generally, these patients will report sleeping too much, eating too much (especially carbs and sweets), and gaining weight during winter months.
- As with all psychiatric diagnoses, ensure that the symptoms are not due to an organic process or better explained by substance abuse.
- Lack of good evidence to decide whether light therapy or SSRIs should be the 1st-line agent. Guidelines suggest using SSRIs 1st if the patient is more acute or has contraindications to light therapy or the clinician is not comfortable with light therapy.
- Light therapy boxes are available from numerous online suppliers, but are not extensively regulated; practitioners should take care to ensure that patients are using devices from reputable suppliers.
- If using SSRIs, recent studies indicate that some patients may begin to experience increased suicidal thoughts on therapy; these patients need to be monitored closely as outpatients every 1–2 weeks. Patients on light therapy also should be monitored closely initially in order to adjust treatment. Once stabilized, both groups of patients can be seen every 4–8 weeks during the winter months.
- All patients who demonstrate suicidal ideation or symptoms of mania should be referred for consideration of hospitalization.

SECRETION OF INAPPROPRIATE ANTIDIURETIC HORMONE (SIADH)
Ruben Peralta, MD, FACS

BASICS

DESCRIPTION
- A syndrome of abnormal production of antidiuretic hormone (ADH), despite low serum osmolality, leading to hyponatremia and inappropriately elevated urine osmolality:
  - Resulting abnormal urinary free water retention leads to dilutional hyponatremia (total body sodium levels may be normal or near normal, but the patient's total body water is increased).
  - Often secondary to medications, but may be associated with an underlying disorder, such as neoplasm, pulmonary disorder, or CNS system disease
- Synonym(s): Syndrome of inappropriate secretion of ADH

EPIDEMIOLOGY
Incidence
- Often found in the hospital setting, where incidence can be as high as 35%
- Predominant age: Elderly
- Predominate sex: Females > Males

ETIOLOGY AND PATHOPHYSIOLOGY
- Drugs:
  - Antidepressants (e.g., monoamine oxidase inhibitors [MAOIs], tricyclics, SSRIs)
  - Oral hypoglycemics (e.g., chlorpropamide, metformin)
  - Antineoplastic drugs (e.g., vincristine, vinblastine, cisplatin, cyclophosphamide)
  - Antipsychotic agents (e.g., phenothiazines, thioridazine, haloperidol)
  - Analgesics (e.g., NSAIDs)
  - Antiepileptics (e.g., carbamazepine, valproic acid)
  - Diuretics (thiazides and loop)
  - Others (e.g., vasopressin, DDAVP, ecstasy, oxytocin, α-interferon)
- Neoplasms (ectopic ADH production):
  - Small-cell carcinoma of the lung
  - Oat cell carcinoma of the lung
  - Hodgkin disease
  - Pancreatic carcinoma
  - Thymoma
  - Mesothelioma
  - Bronchogenic carcinoma
- Infectious diseases:
  - Meningitis
  - Encephalitis
  - Pneumonia
  - Pulmonary tuberculosis (TB)
  - Rocky Mountain spotted fever
  - HIV infection
- Miscellaneous cardiopulmonary conditions:
  - Asthma
  - Atelectasis
  - Myocardial infarction
  - Vascular diseases

- Other:
  - CNS injury
  - Mechanical ventilation
  - Multiple sclerosis
  - Guillain-Barré syndrome
  - Lupus erythematosus
  - Porphyria
  - Hypothyroidism, myxedema
- Idiopathic

Genetics
No known genetic pattern

RISK FACTORS
- Use of predisposing drugs
- Advanced age
- Postoperative status
- Institutionalization

GENERAL PREVENTION
- Search for cause, if unknown.
- Administration of 0.9% sodium chloride in adults during the perioperative period is recommended (if hypernatremia is not present) (1)[C].
- Monitor electrolytes in postoperative patients to determine if fluid intake needs restriction.
- Reduce/Change medications, if drug-induced.
- Lifelong restriction of fluid intake

COMMONLY ASSOCIATED CONDITIONS
See "Etiology."

DIAGNOSIS

HISTORY
Early symptoms:
- Fatigue
- Anorexia
- Nausea
- Vomiting
- Diarrhea
- Headaches
- Myalgias
- Increased thirst

PHYSICAL EXAM
Late/Severe hyponatremia (serum Na <100–115 mEq/L):
- Altered mental status
- Confusion
- Lethargy
- Seizures
- Psychosis
- Coma
- Death

DIFFERENTIAL DIAGNOSIS
- Postoperative complications:
  - Usually after major abdominal/thoracic surgery
  - Caused by nonosmotic release of ADH, probably mediated by pain afferents
  - ADH increased by pain and narcotics
- Postprostatectomy syndrome:
  - Irrigating solution must be nonconducting (i.e., electrolyte-free).
  - D_5W absorbed
- Psychogenic polydipsia:
  - Active therapy rarely is needed.
  - Diuresis occurs when intake is stopped.
  - Intake usually >10 L/d
  - Interaction with other psychotropic drugs
- Acute (usually in children):
  - Swallowing water during swimming
  - Diluted formula
  - Tap-water enemas
- Endocrine:
  - Addison disease
  - Hypothyroidism
- Spurious hyponatremia: Caused by increased serum glucose, cholesterol, or proteins
- Appropriate ADH secretion and hyponatremia with decreased effective arterial blood volume (e.g., congestive heart failure [CHF], nephrotic syndrome, cirrhosis)
- Cerebral salt-wasting syndrome (hyponatremia, extracellular fluid depletion, CNS insult)

DIAGNOSTIC TESTS & INTERPRETATION
- Serum Na level: Low
- Serum osmolality: Low
- Urine osmolality: High
- Urinary Na concentration: High (losing sodium, rather than retaining)
- Serum ADH level: High
- Not usually required for diagnosis but to assess for other concerns:
  - Uric acid
  - Serum glucose; BUN; creatinine
  - Thyroid function
  - Morning cortisol

TREATMENT

GENERAL MEASURES
- Fluid restriction (800–1,000 mL/d) is the main form of treatment.
- Mildly symptomatic (serum Na >125 mEq/L [>125 mmol/L]): Restrict fluid to 800–1,000 mL/d.
- Acute (<48 hours duration) or symptomatic (altered mental status, seizure, coma):
  - Hypertonic saline (3% normal saline) bolus
  - Diuresis with loop diuretics
  - Decrease oral free water to maintenance.
  - Increase oral salt.
  - Correct serum Na deficit (mEq Na deficit = [desired Na – actual Na] × 0.5 × body weight [kg]).
  - Increase serum Na slowly with hypertonic saline by 0.5 mEq/L/hr until it reaches 120 mEq/L.

MEDICATION

- Diuretics: Furosemide (Lasix) + hourly NaCl and KCl replacement:
  - Requires frequent monitoring (see "Patient Monitoring")
  - Treatment of choice for acute management
- Hypertonic (3%) saline to increase serum Na cautiously (2),(3)[B]:
  - By 10–12 mEq/L (10–12 mmol/L) q24h (in chronic hyponatremia)
  - 5% over 1st few hours
  - To only 120 mEq/L (120 mmol/L) acutely
  - By 0.5 mEq/h (0.5 mmol/hr)
- Contraindications: Avoid fluids in CHF, nephrotic syndrome, or cirrhosis.
- Precautions: Overly rapid correction (>12 mEq/L/d [>12 mmol/d]) can cause:
  - CHF
  - Subdural and intracerebral hemorrhage
  - Permanent CNS damage, especially with serum Na <120 mEq/L (<120 mmol/L)
  - Demyelination syndrome
- Vasopressin-2 receptor antagonist (the vaptans: Tolvaptan, conivaptan) (4),(5)[C]:
  - Good efficacy and safety profiles in the treatment of mild-to-moderate hyponatremia due to SIADH (1,2,6)[C].
- Demeclocycline (second line):
  - Blocks ADH at renal tubule; produces nephrogenic diabetes insipidus
  - Dosage for long-term management: 600–1,200 mg/d
  - Onset of action within 1 week; therefore, not best for acute management and supplanted by vasopressin-2 receptor antagonist.

ALERT

Increase Na levels slowly, no more than 0.5–1 mEq/L/hr, to prevent complications such as central pontine myelinosis (CPM).

 ## ONGOING CARE

FOLLOW-UP RECOMMENDATIONS
Patient Monitoring
- Careful continuous clinical and laboratory monitoring of hyponatremic state during acute phase:
  - Hourly urine output
  - Urine Na
  - Serum Na and potassium (K)
- Chronic management: Monitor underlying cause, as needed.

DIET
May need increased salt/decreased water intake, depending on cause

PATIENT EDUCATION
Diet and fluid restrictions

PROGNOSIS
- Depends on underlying cause; in general, higher morbidity and mortality in hospitalized patients with hyponatremia
- If symptomatic (seizure, coma): High mortality due to cerebral edema if serum Na <120 mEq/L (<120 mmol/L)

COMPLICATIONS
- Osmotic demyelination: Central pontine and extrapontine irreversible myelinolysis (2,7)
- Chronic hyponatremia: Usually <120 mEq/L (<120 mmol/L)
- Complications of overly rapid correction (see "Treatment, Precautions")
- Chronic hyponatremia is associated with osteoporosis (8).

REFERENCES

1. Ellison DH, Berl T. Clinical practice. The syndrome of inappropriate antidiuresis. *N Engl J Med*. 2007;356:2064–2072.
2. Esposito P, Piotti G, Bianzina S, et al. The syndrome of inappropriate antidiuresis: Pathophysiology, clinical management and new therapeutic options. *Nephron Clinical Pract*. 2011;119:c62–c73.
3. Moritz ML, Ayus JC. 100 cc 3% sodium chloride bolus: A novel treatment for hyponatremic encephalopathy. *Metab Brain Dis*. 2010;25:91–96.
4. Friedman B, Cirulli J. Hyponatremia in critical care patients: Frequency, outcome, characteristics, and treatment with the vasopressin V(2)-receptor antagonist tolvaptan. *J Crit Care*. 2012 Aug 8. Epub 2012 Aug 8.
5. Graziani G, Cucchiari D, Aroldi A, et al. Syndrome of inappropriate secretion of antidiuretic hormone in traumatic brain injury: When tolvaptan becomes a life saving drug. *J Neurol Neurosurg Psychiatr*. 2012;84(5):510–512. Epub 2012 Feb 9.
6. Sherlock M, Thompson CJ. The syndrome of inappropriate antidiuretic hormone: Current and future management options. *Eur J Endocrinol*. 2010;162(Suppl 1):S13–S18.
7. Fleming JD, Babu S. Images in clinical medicine. Central pontine myelinolysis. *N Engl J Med*. 2008;359:e29.
8. Verbalis JG, Barsony J, Sugimura Y, et al. Hyponatremia-induced osteoporosis. *J Bone Miner Res*. 2010;25:554–563.

ADDITIONAL READING

- Adrogué HJ, Madias NE. The challenge of hyponatremia. *J Am Soc Nephrol*. 2012;84(7): 1140–1148. Epub 2012 May 24.
- Babayev R, Terner S, Chandra S, et al. Trimethoprim-associated hyponatremia. *Am J Kidney Dis*. 2013. doi:10.1053/j.ajkd.2013.06.007

 ## SEE ALSO

Hyponatremia

 ## CODES

ICD10
E22.2 Syndrome of inappropriate secretion of antidiuretic hormone

CLINICAL PEARLS

- Fluid restriction to 600–800 mL/d × 2–3 days will result in weight loss and correction of hyponatremia and salt wasting in SIADH. Fluid restriction fails to correct hyponatremia and Na wasting in salt-losing renal disease (1)[C].
- Cerebral salt wasting is a controversial disease entity and is similar to SIADH. However, patients with SIADH are euvolemic, whereas patients with cerebral salt wasting are hypovolemic. The only real way to establish the diagnosis is through fluid restriction. Serum urate and fractional excretion of urate will be corrected with fluid restriction in SIADH, but will not correct in cerebral salt wasting.
- CPM is a cerebral demyelination syndrome that causes quadriplegia, pseudobulbar palsy, seizures, coma, and death. It is caused by an overly rapid rate of Na correction (2,7)[C].
- Safe correction of hyponatremia is important. Online calculators are available: www.medcal.com/sodium.html.

S

SEIZURE DISORDER, ABSENCE

Felicia Chu, MD

BASICS

DESCRIPTION
- An absence seizure is a generalized epileptic seizure characterized by a brief lapse of awareness.
- Absence seizure types:
  - Absence seizure types according to the International League Again Epilepsy (ILAE) 2010 classification include (1):
    - Typical absence:
      - Formerly called *petit mal seizures*
      - Abrupt-onset behavioral arrest, loss of awareness, and blank staring, sometimes with mild upward eye deviation, repetitive blinking
      - May include automatisms, tonic or atonic features, eyelid or facial clonus, autonomic features
      - Lasts 5–30 seconds
      - Immediate return to normal consciousness
      - Associated with genetic generalized epilepsies, namely, childhood absence epilepsy, juvenile absence epilepsy, and juvenile myoclonic epilepsy
    - Atypical absence:
      - Onset and offset less abrupt than typical absence seizures
      - Lasts 10–45 seconds
      - Impairment of consciousness often incomplete with continued purposeful activity
      - Postictal confusion sometimes occurs
      - Associated clinical features more pronounced and frequent than in typical absence; atonia most common
      - Associated with syndromic epilepsies, such as Lennox-Gastaut and nonsyndromic epilepsies in patients with developmental delay
    - Absence with special features:
      - Myoclonic absence:
        - Rhythmic clonic jerking at 2–4 Hz that lasts 5–10 seconds
        - Unlike myoclonic seizures with no impairment of consciousness, brief lapses of awareness are characteristic of myoclonic absence.
      - Eyelid myoclonia:
        - Rhythmic clonic jerking of the eyelids at 5–6 Hz that lasts 3–5 seconds
        - Eyelid myoclonia with absence associated with an impairment of consciousness
- Epilepsy diagnoses:
  - Specific diagnoses according to ILAE (2010):
    - Childhood absence epilepsy (CAE):
      - Also known as *pyknolepsy*
      - Typical absence seizures are the only seizure type in 90% of children.
      - 10% develop additional generalized tonic–clonic seizures.
      - Seizures last ~10 seconds and often occur hundreds of times per day.
      - Normal neurologic state and development
      - Spontaneous remission occurs in 65–70% of patients during adolescence.
    - Juvenile absence epilepsy (JAE):
      - Typical absence seizures are the main seizure type.
      - Seizures last longer than in CAE and occur usually less than once a day.
      - Generalized tonic–clonic seizures occur in most patients, often in the first 1–2 hours after awakening.
      - Seizures often persist into adulthood.

EPIDEMIOLOGY
- Predominant Age:
  - CAE: Onset ages 4–10 years, with peak at ages 5–8 years
  - JAE: Onset ages 9–16 years, with peak at ages 10–12 years
- Predominant gender:
  - Female > Male (3:2–2:1)
  - Absence epilepsy with myoclonus has male predominance.

Incidence
6–8/100,000 per year

Prevalence
5–50/100,000

ETIOLOGY AND PATHOPHYSIOLOGY
- Corticoreticular theory implicates abnormal activity in thalamocortical circuits.
- Thalamic reticular nucleus is responsible for both normal sleep spindles and pathologic slow-wave discharges; contains inhibitory GABAergic neurons.
- These neurons affect low-threshold calcium currents.
- These circuits can fire in oscillatory/rhythmic fashion:
  - Normally, activation of $GABA_A$ receptors causes 10-Hz oscillations in sleep spindle frequency.
  - If $GABA_B$ receptors are strongly activated, oscillation frequency will be 3–4 Hz, similar to spike-and-wave typical absence seizure frequency.

Genetics
- 70–85% concordance occurs in monozygotic twins; 82% share EEG features.
- 33% concordance among 1st-degree relatives
- 15–45% have a family history of epilepsy.
- Complex multifactorial inheritance
- For childhood absence, genes/loci implicated include 6q, 8q24, and 5q14.
- Mutations of $GABA_A$ receptor and voltage-gated Ca^{2+} channel are implicated.

COMMONLY ASSOCIATED CONDITIONS
- 3–8% of CAE cases evolve into juvenile myoclonic epilepsy.
- Associated with difficulties in visual attention and visuospatial skills, verbal learning and memory, and reduced language abilities
- Children with CAE have elevated rates of behavioral and psychiatric comorbidities including attentional deficits, anxiety, depression, isolation, and low self-esteem.
- Large study in 2010 detected overall normal cognition, but 35% of subjects had pretreatment attentional deficits that did not resolve with seizure control.

DIAGNOSIS

Seizures are often so brief that untrained observers are not aware of the occurrence.

HISTORY
- Frequently diagnosed in children being evaluated for poor school performance
- Teachers report that child seems to daydream or zone out frequently.
- Child will forget portions of conversations.
- Child with normal intelligence quotient (IQ) underperforms in school

PHYSICAL EXAM
- Unless a child has another genetic or acquired abnormality, a neurologic exam usually is normal.
- Seizures may be frequent enough to be observed during physical exam:
  - Manifest by behavioral arrest: Child will stop speaking in mid-sentence, stare blankly, etc.
  - Automatisms (repetitive stereotyped behaviors) may be present.
  - Child resumes previous activity
  - Absence seizures can have a variable effect on respiratory rate, but bradypnea is common.
- Seizures may be induced by hyperventilation:
  - Have child blow on pinwheel or similar exercise to provoke seizure.
  - Alternatively, ask the patient to perform hyperventilation with eyes closed and count. Patient will open eyes at onset of seizure and stop counting.
- Patient manifests unresponsiveness but retains postural tone in a typical absence seizure.

DIFFERENTIAL DIAGNOSIS
- Complex partial seizures
- Psychogenic non-epileptic seizures
- Attention deficit hyperactivity disorder (ADHD)
- Confusional states and acute memory disorders
- Migraine variants
- Panic/Anxiety attacks
- Breath holding spells
- Nonepileptic staring spells: Suggestive features include:
  - Events do not interrupt play.
  - Events are 1st noticed by professional such as schoolteacher, speech therapist, occupational therapist, or physician (rather than parent).
  - During a staring spell, child is responsive to touch or other external stimuli.

DIAGNOSTIC TESTS & INTERPRETATION
- No specific hematologic workup
- Follow blood chemistry, hepatic function, and blood counts specific to drug regimen.
- Drug levels are useful in evaluating symptoms of toxicity or for breakthrough seizures.

Initial Tests (lab, imaging)
- EEG is standard for diagnosis:
  - Typical absence features: 3-Hz spike-and-wave activity on normal EEG background
  - Seizures feature bursts of 34-Hz spike-and-wave activity, which may slow to 2.5–3-Hz during seizure.
  - Seizure usually is evident clinically if bursts last >3 seconds; subtle changes of transient cognitive impairment may be evident with briefer seizures.
  - Hyperventilation and occasionally photic stimulation may induce seizure, thus confirming diagnosis of typical absence epilepsy. In contrast, atypical absence seizures are not susceptible to induction by hyperventilation or photic stimulation.
- Imaging is not routinely indicated in children with typical absence and normal neurologic exam and IQ.
  - Brain MRI is indicated in atypical absence and in children with mixed seizure types when combined with abnormal neurologic exam or low IQ.
  - If imaging is performed, MRI is preferable to CT scan due to higher sensitivity for anatomic abnormalities.

– A review of the brain MRIs of 134 patients with idiopathic generalized epilepsy in 2006 showed 24% with structural abnormalities, 88% of which were nonspecific (2)[B].

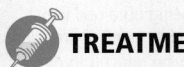 TREATMENT

GENERAL MEASURES
- Review seizure precautions with every patient diagnosed with or suspected of having epilepsy.
- Seizure precautions include bathroom, kitchen, home, driving, outdoors, and sports safety topics, as well as special considerations for parents.

MEDICATION
Concern regarding generic medications allowing more breakthrough seizures has not been supported in evidence-based studies (3)[A].

ALERT
Certain common anticonvulsants may exacerbate absence including carbamazepine, oxcarbazepine, phenytoin, phenobarbital, tiagabine, vigabatrin, pregabalin, and gabapentin.

First Line
- Ethosuximide blocks T-type calcium channels:
  – First-line, except in absence patients with tonic–clonic seizures (lacks efficacy)
  – High efficacy (4)[A], fastest onset of efficacy (5)[B], and fewer adverse attentional effects compared to valproic acid (4)[A]
  – Side effects: Vomiting, diarrhea, abdominal discomfort, hiccups, headache, sedation
  – Adverse effects: Rare blood dyscrasias (monitor CBC)
- Valproic acid has multiple mechanisms:
  – 1st choice in absence patients with tonic–clonic, myoclonic, mixed seizure types
  – Very effective, but has highest rate of adverse events leading to treatment discontinuation, including negative attentional effects (4)[A].
  – Side effects: Tremor, drowsiness, dizziness, weight gain, alopecia, sedation, vomiting
  – Adverse effects: Teratogenicity, pancreatitis, thrombocytopenia, rare fulminant hepatic failure (especially in children <2 years)

Second Line
- Lamotrigine affects sodium channels:
  – Controls seizures, but may be less efficacious than ethosuximide or valproic acid (4)[A]
  – May be equally as efficacious for new-onset CAE (5)[B]
  – Side effects: Rash, diplopia, headache, insomnia, dizziness, nausea, vomiting, diarrhea
  – Adverse effects: Rare Stevens-Johnson rash, more often when coadministered with valproic acid
- Topiramate affects GABA and excitatory neurotransmission:
  – FDA approved for Lennox-Gastaut syndrome
  – Side effects: Psychomotor slowing
  – Adverse effects: Weight loss, renal stones, myopia, glaucoma (rare), anhidrosis
- Levetiracetam is used off-label:
  – Has been used as both monotherapy and adjunct therapy for absence seizures
  – A small multicenter RTC showed modest efficacy, but not statistically significant vs. placebo (6)[C].

- Zonisamide is also used off-label.
- Clonazepam, nitrazepam, and clobazam may be effective in the short-term but are not recommended for long-term management due to development of tolerance (few months to a year) and side effects.

Pregnancy Considerations
Anticonvulsants, especially valproic acid, are associated with an increase in fetal malformations. Use of valproic acid in women who are or are likely to become pregnant generally is contraindicated. Obtain specialty consultation.

ADDITIONAL THERAPIES
- Most absence seizure patients respond to a single medication.
- Male sex and an early age at diagnosis are associated with the need for 2 medications to control the disease (7)[B].
- Vagal nerve stimulator (VNS) may be considered as an option for medically refractory absence epilepsy (8)[C].

IN-PATIENT CONSIDERATIONS
Admission Criteria/Initial Stabilization
- Absence epilepsy rarely requires admission.
- Status epilepticus requires inpatient management.

Discharge Criteria
Resolution of status epilepticus

 ONGOING CARE

FOLLOW-UP RECOMMENDATIONS
- Patients with associated tonic–clonic seizures should avoid high places and swimming alone.
- Absence rarely persists into adulthood, but affected adults may be restricted from driving, working over open flames, etc., as with other generalized and partial epilepsy subtypes.
- Patients should be monitored periodically by a neurologist for evolution of absence epilepsy into tonic–clonic or other seizure types.

PROGNOSIS
- Patient's whose shortest pretreatment EEG seizures are >20 seconds in duration are more likely to achieve seizure freedom, regardless of treatment (9)[A].
- Of those with CAE without tonic–clonic seizures, 90% remit by adulthood.
- 35% of patients with tonic–clonic seizures experience complete remission of absence seizures.
- 15% of patients develop juvenile myoclonic epilepsy.

COMPLICATIONS
Reported frequencies of typical absence status epilepticus range from 5.8–9.4% of patients with CAE.

REFERENCES

1. Berg AT, Berkovic SF, Brodie MJ, et al. Revised terminology and concepts for organization of seizures and epilepsies: Report of the ILAE Commission on Classification and Terminology, 2005–2009. *Epilepsia.* 2010;51(4):676–685.
2. Betting LE, Mory SB, Lopes-Cendes I, et al. MRI reveals structural abnormalities in patients with idiopathic generalized epilepsy. *Neurology.* 2006;67;848–852.
3. Kesselheim AS, Stedman MR, Bubrick EJ, et al. Seizure outcomes following the use of generic versus brand-name antiepileptic drugs: A systematic review and meta-analysis. *Drugs.* 2010;70;605–621.
4. Glauser TA, Cnaan A, Shinnar S, et al. Ethosuximide, valproic acid, and lamotrigine in childhood absence epilepsy: Initial monotherapy outcomes at 12 months. *Epilepsia.* 2013;54; 141–155.
5. Hwang H, Kim H, Kim SH, et al. Long-term effectiveness of ethosuximide, valproic acid, and lamotrigine in childhood absence epilepsy. *Brain Dev.* 2012;34;344–348.
6. Fattore C, Boniver C, Capovilla G, et al. A multicenter, randomized, placebo-controlled trial of levetiracetam in children and adolescents with newly diagnosed absence epilepsy. *Epilepsia.* 2011;52;802–809.
7. Nadler B, Shevell MI. Childhood absence epilepsy requiring more than one medication for seizure control. *Can J Neurol Sci.* 2008;35:297–300.
8. Arya R, Greiner HM, Lewis A, et al. Vagus nerve stimulation for medically refractory absence epilepsy. *Seizure.* 2013;22;267–270.
9. Dlugos D, Shinnar S, Cnaan A, et al. Pretreatment EEG in childhood absence epilepsy: Associations with attention and treatment outcome. *Neurology.* 2013;81;150–156.

ADDITIONAL READING

- Glauser TA, Loddenkemper T. Management of childhood epilepsy. *Continuum.* 2013;19;656–681.
- Tenney, JR. Glauser TA. The current state of absence epilepsy: Can we have your attention? *Epilepsy Curr.* 2013;13;135–140.
- Vrielynck P. Current and emerging treatments for absence seizures in young patients. *Neuropsychiatr Dis Treat.* 2013;9;963–975.

 CODES

ICD10
- G40.401 Oth generalized epilepsy, not intractable, w stat epi
- G40.409 Other generalized epilepsy and epileptic syndromes, not intractable, without status epilepticus
- G40.419 Oth generalized epilepsy, intractable, w/o stat epi

CLINICAL PEARLS
- If parents are unable to determine the cause of a staring spell, try suggesting that parents mention something exciting or unexpected like "ice cream" during a spell to get the child's attention rather than calling their name.
- To help aid with diagnosis during an exam, try having child blow repetitively on pinwheel (causing hyperventilation) to attempt to trigger absence seizure.
- Ethosuximide and valproic acid are first-line agents in treatment of absence seizures. Valproic acid and lamotrigine are recommended for absence patients with tonic-clonic and mixed seizure types.

SEIZURE DISORDER, PARTIAL

Ruben Peralta, MD, FACS • Wynne Morgan, MD

BASICS

DESCRIPTION
- Seizures occur when abnormal synchronous neuronal discharges in the brain cause transient cortical dysfunction.
- Generalized seizures involve bilateral cerebral cortex from the seizure's onset.
- Partial seizures originate from a discrete focus in the cerebral cortex.
- Partial seizures are further divided into simple and complex subtypes:
  – If consciousness is impaired during a partial seizure, it is classified as complex.
  – If consciousness is preserved, it is a simple partial seizure.

EPIDEMIOLOGY
Prevalence
Partial seizures occur in 20/100,000 persons in the US.

ETIOLOGY AND PATHOPHYSIOLOGY
- Partial seizures begin when a localized seizure focus produces an abnormal, synchronized depolarization that spreads to a discrete portion of the surrounding cortex.
- The area of cortex involved in the seizure determines the symptoms; for example, an epileptogenic focus in motor cortex produces contralateral motor symptoms.
- In some cases, etiology is related to structural abnormalities that are susceptible to epileptogenesis. Most common etiologies vary by life stage:
  – Early childhood: Developmental/Congenital malformation, trauma
  – Young adults: Developmental, infection, trauma
  – Adults 40–60 years of age: Cerebrovascular insult, infection, trauma
  – Adults >60 years of age: Cerebrovascular insult, trauma, neoplasm
- Complex partial seizures: A common cause is mesial temporal sclerosis.

Genetics
Benign rolandic epilepsy, a form of partial seizure disorder, has an autosomal-dominant inheritance pattern with penetrance depending on multiple factors.

RISK FACTORS
- History of traumatic brain injury (1)[B]
- Children exposed to a thiamine-deficient formula (2)[C]

COMMONLY ASSOCIATED CONDITIONS
Epilepsy patients have a higher incidence of depression than the general population.

DIAGNOSIS

- Seizure activity usually stereotyped
- Duration: Seconds–minutes, unless status epilepticus develops; status epilepticus may present as focal/generalized convulsions/altered mental status without convulsions.
- Simple partial seizures:
  – Simple partial seizures are characterized by localized symptoms. The patient is conscious. Symptoms may involve motor, sensory, or psychic systems.
  – Motor: Seizure activity in motor strip causes contraction (tonic) or rhythmic jerking (clonic) movements that may involve 1 entire side of body or may be more localized (i.e., hands, feet, or face):
    ○ Jacksonian march: As discharge spreads through motor cortex, tonic–clonic activity spreads in predictable fashion (i.e., beginning in hand and progressing up arm and to the face).
  – Sensory/Psychic:
    ○ Todd paresis: After motor seizure, residual, temporary weakness in the affected area
    ○ Parietal lobe: Sensory loss/paresthesias, dizziness
    ○ Temporal lobe: Déjà vu, rising sensation in epigastrium, auditory hallucinations/forced memories, unpleasant smell/taste
  – Occipital: Visual hallucinations
- Complex partial seizures:
  – Impaired consciousness by definition
  – May have aura; this is start of seizure
- Amnesia for the event, postictal confusion:
  – Most often, focus in complex partial seizures is temporal/frontal.
  – Motor manifestations may include dystonic posturing/automatisms (i.e., simple, repetitive movements of face and hands such as lip smacking, picking, or more complex actions such as purposeless walking).
  – Frontal lobe seizure is characterized by brief, bilateral complex movements, vocalizations, often with onset during sleep.

HISTORY
- A detailed description of the seizure should be obtained from an observer.
- Review medication list for drugs that lower seizure threshold (e.g., tramadol, bupropion, theophylline).
- Drugs of abuse (e.g., cocaine) lower seizure threshold.
- History of traumatic brain injury (1)[B].

PHYSICAL EXAM
Include neurologic exam, with attention to lateralizing signs suggestive of structural lesion.

DIFFERENTIAL DIAGNOSIS
- Nonepileptic seizure
- Syncope/Postanoxic myoclonus
- Hypoglycemia
- For hemiparesis following event:
  – Transient ischemic attack
  – Hemiplegic migraine

DIAGNOSTIC TESTS & INTERPRETATION
EEG: Spikes/Sharp waves over seizure focus:
- Yield of EEG is increased by being obtained in 1st 24 hours following seizure and by sleep deprivation.
- Frontal lobe seizure focus may be difficult to detect by routine EEG.
- If difficulty with diagnosis, continuous video–EEG monitoring may be appropriate.
- Serum electrolytes, including calcium, magnesium, phosphorus; hepatic function panel; CBC; drugs of abuse
- If measured within 10–20 minutes of suspected seizure, an elevated prolactin level may help to differentiate generalized/complex partial seizure from psychogenic seizure (3)[B],(4)[C].
- CSF exam if infection is suspected
- Urinalysis, chest x-ray, levels of antiepileptic drugs for breakthrough seizure
- Technological advances in neuroimaging are usually directed at the diagnosis and prognosis for seizure control (5)[C].
- Emergency evaluation of new seizure: CT scan to screen for hemorrhage, stroke
- After emergency evaluation, MRI with thin cuts through area of interest
- If planning epilepsy surgery, positron emission tomography (PET) scan and/or interictal single-photon emission computed tomography (SPECT) may be of value.
- Magnetoencephalography (MEG) is an evolving technology for localizing seizure focus.

TREATMENT

GENERAL MEASURES
- Ask patient to maintain a seizure diary.
- Note potential triggers, such as stress, sleep deprivation, drug use, discontinuation of alcohol/benzodiazepines, menses.

MEDICATION
- Some physicians do not start medication after a single seizure if EEG and MRI are normal and/or a precipitant is clear and avoidable.
- Antiepileptic drugs (AEDs) act on voltage-gated ion channels, affect neuronal inhibition via enhancement of γ-aminobutyric acid (GABA, an inhibitory neurotransmitter), or decrease neuronal excitation. End result is to decrease the abnormal synchronized firing and to prevent seizure propagation.
- 50% of those with newly diagnosed partial seizures respond to, and tolerate, first AED trial.
- Choose AED based on seizure type, side-effect profile, and patient characteristics. Increase dose until seizure control is obtained/side effects become unacceptable.
- Attempt monotherapy, but many patients will require adjunctive agents.
- *Refractory to medications* is defined as failure of at least 3 anticonvulsants to achieve adequate control.
- Several AEDs induce/inhibit cytochrome P450 enzymes (watch for drug interactions).

First Line
- Carbamazepine: Affects sodium channels; side effects include GI distress, hyponatremia, diplopia, dizziness, rare pancytopenia/marrow suppression, exfoliative rash

- Oxcarbazepine: Affects sodium channels; side effects include dizziness, diplopia, hyponatremia, headache
- Lamotrigine: Affects sodium channels:
  – Side effects include insomnia, dizziness, ataxia
  – Risk of Stevens-Johnson reaction (potentially fatal exfoliative rash) especially when given with valproate; requires slow titration
- Levetiracetam: Multiple mechanisms; side effects include sedation, ataxia, irritability

Second Line
- Phenytoin: Affects sodium channels; side effects include ataxia, dizziness, diplopia, tremor, GI upset, gingival hyperplasia, fever
- Phenobarbital: Multiple mechanisms; side effects include sedation, withdrawal seizures
- Valproate: Multiple mechanisms; side effects include GI upset, weight gain, alopecia, tremor; less common, thrombocytopenia, hepatitis, pancreatitis
- Topiramate: Multiple mechanisms; side effects include anorexia, cognitive slowing, sedation, nephrolithiasis, anhidrosis (6)[C]
- Gabapentin: Multiple mechanisms; side effects include sedation, dizziness, ataxia
- Pregabalin: Affects calcium channels; side effects include sedation, dizziness, weight gain
- Zonisamide: Affects sodium channels:
  – Side effects include sedation, anorexia, nausea, dizziness, ataxia, anhidrosis, nephrolithiasis
  – Cross-reaction with sulfa allergy

Pregnancy Considerations
- Several AEDs induce hepatic metabolism of oral contraceptives, decreasing their efficacy. AED therapy during 1st trimester is associated with doubled risk for major fetal malformations (6% vs. 3%).
- Phenytoin in pregnancy may result in fetal hydantoin syndrome.
- Valproate is associated with neural tube defects.
- Fetal insult from seizures following withdrawal of therapy also may be severe. Risk-to-benefit balance should be evaluated with high-risk pregnancy and epileptology consultations. Most patients remain on anticonvulsants.
- Consider vagal nerve stimulator during pregnancy (7)[B].

ISSUES FOR REFERRAL
For refractory seizures, consider referral to an epilepsy specialist (8)[B].

ADDITIONAL THERAPIES
- Vagal nerve stimulator: Implanted in neck; provides periodic stimulation to vagus nerve; may induce hoarseness, cough, and dysphagia (9)[B].
- New technologies under development include deep brain stimulation.

SURGERY/OTHER PROCEDURES
- For refractory partial complex seizures
- Should have identifiable focus
- Preoperative testing, such as Wada test, should be done to decrease likelihood of inducing aphasia and memory loss.
- Workup also may include MRI, video—EEG monitoring, electrocorticography, MEG, and ictal SPECT.
- 64% will be seizure-free after surgery (with continued medication treatment), 25% will have significant decrease in frequency, and 1/3 continue to have disabling seizures.

- Goal of surgical intervention is to reduce reliance on medications; most patients remain on anticonvulsants postoperatively.

IN-PATIENT CONSIDERATIONS
Admission Criteria/Initial Stabilization
Admit for unremitting seizure (partial/secondary generalized status epilepticus)

 ## ONGOING CARE

FOLLOW-UP RECOMMENDATIONS
- Most states have restrictions on driving for those with seizure disorders.
- Depending on seizure manifestation, may recommend against activities such as swimming, climbing to heights, working over open flames, or operating heavy machinery

Patient Monitoring
AED levels if concern over toxicity, noncompliance, or for breakthrough seizures

DIET
Ketogenic or low-glycemic-index diet may improve seizure control in some patients.

PATIENT EDUCATION
Avoid potential triggers such as alcohol or drug use and sleep deprivation.

PROGNOSIS
- Risk of seizure recurrence: ~30% after 1st seizure; of these, 50% will occur in the 1st 6 months; 90% in the 1st 2 years.
- Depends on seizure type; rolandic epilepsy has a good prognosis; temporal lobe epilepsy is more likely to be persistent.
- ~25–30% of all seizures are refractory to current medications.
- AEDs initiated after an initial seizure have been shown to decrease the risk of seizure over the 1st 2 years, but are not demonstrated to reduce long-term risk of recurrence.
- Long duration of uncontrolled seizure disorder associated with increased cognitive and functional impairments; early pharmacologic intervention is encouraged.
- The potential for AEDs to confer neuroprotection is under investigation.
- The risk of developing seizure after mild traumatic brain injury remains high for a long period (>10 years) (1)[B].
- Patients with history of military brain injury carry a high risk of intractable posttraumatic epilepsy decades after their injury and, thus, require a long-term medical follow-up (10)[B].

COMPLICATIONS
Risk of accidental injury

REFERENCES
1. Christensen J, Pedersen MG, Pedersen CB, et al. Long-term risk of epilepsy after traumatic brain injury in children and young adults: A population-based cohort study. *Lancet*. 2009; 373(9669): 1105–1110.
2. Fattal-Valevski A, Bloch-Mimouni A, Kivity S, et al. Epilepsy in children with infantile thiamine deficiency. *Neurology*. 2009;73:828–833.
3. Chen DK, So YT, Fisher RS, et al. Use of serum prolactin in diagnosing epileptic seizures: Report of the Therapeutics and Technology Assessment Subcommittee of the American Academy of Neurology. *Neurology*. 2005;84(5):668–675.
4. LaFrance WC. Use of serum prolactin in diagnosing epileptic seizures: Report of the Therapeutics and Technology Assessment Subcommittee of the American Academy of Neurology. *Neurology*. 2006;84(8):1287–1288; author reply 1287–1288.
5. Gaillard WD, Cross JH, Duncan JS, et al. Epilepsy imaging study guideline criteria: Commentary on diagnostic testing study guidelines and practice parameters. *Epilepsia*. 2011;52(9):1750–1756.
6. Sankar R, Ramsay E, McKay A, et al. A multicenter, outpatient, open-label study to evaluate the dosing, effectiveness, and safety of topiramate as monotherapy in the treatment of epilepsy in clinical practice. *Epilepsy Behav*. 2009;15(4):506–512.
7. Houser MV, Hennessy MD, Howard BC, et al. Vagal nerve stimulator use during pregnancy for treatment of refractory seizure disorder. *Obstet Gynecol*. 2010;115:417–419.
8. Hemb M, Velasco TR, Parnes MS, et al. Improved outcomes in pediatric epilepsy surgery: The UCLA experience, 1986–2008. *Neurology*. 2010;74: 1768–1775.
9. Siddiqui F, Herial NA, Ali II, et al. Cumulative effect of vagus nerve stimulators on intractable seizures observed over a period of 3 years. *Epilepsy Behav*. 2010;18(3):299–302.
10. Kazemi H, Hashemi-Fesharaki S, Razaghi S, et al. Intractable epilepsy and craniocerebral trauma: Analysis of 163 patients with blunt and penetrating head injuries sustained in war. *Injury*. 2012 Jul 2. Epub 2012 Jul 2.

ADDITIONAL READING
- Adams SM, Knowles PD. Evaluation of a first seizure. *Am Fam Physician*. 2007;75:1342–1347.
- Baker MT. The anticonvulsant effects of propofol and a propofol analog, 2,6-diisopropyl-4-(1-hydroxy-2,2,2-triuoroethyl)phenol, in a 6 Hz partial seizure model. *Anesthesia Analgesia*. 2011;112:340–344.

 ## CODES

ICD10
- G40.109 Local-rel symptc epi w simp prt seiz,not ntrct, w/o stat epi
- G40.119 Local-rel symptc epi w simple part seiz, ntrct, w/o stat epi
- G40.209 Local-rel symptc epi w cmplx prt seiz,not ntrct,w/o stat epi

CLINICAL PEARLS
- It is controversial whether AED treatment is indicated after a 1st seizure. Treatment should be strongly considered when a clear structural cause is identified/risk of injury from seizure is high (e.g., osteoporosis, anticoagulation).
- Consider vagus nerve stimulation in pregnancy and in patients with medically refractory seizures.
- Postictal elevation in prolactin levels can help distinguish physiologic from psychogenic seizures.

SEIZURE DISORDERS

Allison Hargreaves, MD • Ann M. Lynch, PharmD, RPh • Christopher Chang, MD

 BASICS

DESCRIPTION
- Seizure: Sudden change in cortical electrical activity, manifested through motor, sensory, or behavioral changes, and/or an alteration in consciousness
- System(s) affected: Nervous
- Synonym(s): Epilepsy; Convulsion; Attacks; Spells

Geriatric Considerations
Fractures from falls are more common in the osteopenic age range. Differential diagnosis of acute delirium should include status epilepticus.

Pediatric Considerations
Breastfeeding is not contraindicated. Sedation of the infant should be monitored.

Pregnancy Considerations
- Monitor serum levels of antiepileptic drugs (AEDs).
- There is a 2-fold increase in congenital malformations in children born to mothers taking certain anticonvulsants. Some expectant mothers can stop taking anticonvulsants safely for the 1st trimester or initial 6-week period (organogenesis). Avoid valproate and lamotrigine. Epileptic patients should notify their neurologist before conception, if possible.
- Recommend against use of category C or D AEDs during pregnancy/nursing. Levetiracetam and topiramate are alternatives for women of childbearing potential (1)[C].

EPIDEMIOLOGY
Incidence
- 200,000 new cases of epilepsy are diagnosed in the US yearly, with 45,000 new cases in children <15 years of age.
- Pediatric (<2 years) and older adults (>65 years) more commonly present with new-onset seizures.
- Predominant sex: Male = Female

Prevalence
- 2.7 million with seizure disorder
- 4 million people have had ≥1 seizures.
- 326,000 children (≤14 years) and 600,000 adults (>65 years) have a seizure disorder.

ETIOLOGY AND PATHOPHYSIOLOGY
- Synchronous and excessive firing of neurons, resulting in impairment of normal control of CNS
- True seizures may be triggered by the following metabolic/medical conditions, but seizures occurring due to these conditions do not necessarily define the presence of a seizure disorder (see also "Differential Diagnosis"):
  - CNS infection
  - Hyperthyroidism
  - Hypoglycemia or hyperglycemia
  - Hyponatremia
  - Uremia
  - Porphyria
  - Hypoxia
  - Confusional migraine
  - Transient ischemic attack
  - Narcolepsy/Sleep disorder
  - Toxins (e.g., lead, picrotoxin, strychnine)
  - Brain tumor
  - Cerebral hypoxia

- Stroke/Cardiovascular accident (CVA)
- Drug/Alcohol overdose/withdrawal
- Eclampsia
- Head injury
- Heat stroke

Genetics
Family history increases risk 3-fold.

RISK FACTORS
Children delivered breech have a prevalence rate of 3.8% compared with 2.2% in vertex deliveries.

GENERAL PREVENTION
Take measures to prevent head injuries. Reduce exposure to lead-containing products. Avoid excessive alcohol/substance use/abuse.

COMMONLY ASSOCIATED CONDITIONS
Infections, tumors, drug abuse, alcohol and drug withdrawal, trauma, metabolic disorders

 DIAGNOSIS

- Differentiate 1st between epileptiform seizures and nonepileptiform seizures (NESs).
- NESs are psychogenic and usually associated with a history of psychiatric conditions and often with a history of sexual abuse.
- Physiologic seizures are true cortical events and may require acute intervention.
- Conventional classification of seizures (2)[C]:
  - Generalized seizures:
    - Tonic-clonic: Tonic phase: Sudden loss of consciousness; clonic phase: Sustained contraction followed by rhythmic contractions of all 4 extremities; postictal phase: Headache, confusion, fatigue; clinically hypertensive, tachycardic, and otherwise hypersympathetic
    - Absence: Impaired awareness and responsiveness
    - Atonic: Abrupt loss of muscle tone
    - Myoclonic: Repetitive muscle contractions
  - Febrile seizures:
    - Usually ≤6 years
    - Fever without evidence of any other defined cause of seizures
    - Recurrent febrile seizures probably do not increase the risk of epilepsy.
  - Symptomatic focal epilepsies
  - Complex partial seizures
  - Nonconvulsive status epilepticus: Most commonly seen in ICU patients; no tonic–clonic activity seen so must diagnose with bedside EEG
  - Status epilepticus: Repetitive generalized seizures without recovery between seizures; considered a neurologic emergency

HISTORY
- Eyewitness descriptions of event; patient impressions of what occurred before, during, and after the event
- Screen for etiologies, including provoking/ameliorating factors for the event, such as sleep deprivation.
- Ask about bowel/bladder incontinence, tongue biting, other injury, or automatisms.

PHYSICAL EXAM
Thorough neurologic exam

DIFFERENTIAL DIAGNOSIS
Below represents a differential diagnosis for the etiology of actual seizures, not for apparent seizures (see also "Etiology," above):
- Idiopathic
- Hippocampal sclerosis and other neurodevelopmental abnormalities of the brain
- Acute infection (meningitis, abscess, encephalitis)
- Metabolic and endocrine disorders
- Trauma
- Drug and alcohol withdrawal
- Tumor
- Vascular disease, including vasculitis
- Familial/Genetic, infantile and pediatric seizure syndromes (e.g., Lennox-Gastaut, benign familial, myoclonic epilepsy of infancy)
- Other etiologies (by age of onset):
  - Infancy (0–2 years):
    - Hypoxic-ischemic encephalopathy/other injury to cerebral cortex
    - Metabolic: Hypoglycemia, hypocalcemia, hypomagnesemia, vitamin B_6 deficiency, phenylketonuria
  - Childhood (2–10 years): Absence or febrile (usually <6 years) seizure
  - Adolescent (10–18 years): AVM
  - Late adulthood (>60 years):
    - Degenerative disease, including dementia
    - Metabolic: Hypoglycemia, uremia, hepatic failure, electrolyte abnormality

DIAGNOSTIC TESTS & INTERPRETATION
A negative EEG does not rule out a seizure disorder. Interictal EEG sensitivity may be as low as 20%; multiple EEGs may increase sensitivity to 80%. Prognostically, EEG abnormality may predict likelihood of seizure recurrence:
- Sleep deprivation may be helpful prior to EEG, and hyperventilation and photic stimulation during recording may increase sensitivity for spike wave formations.
- Video EEG monitoring is used to differentiate psychomotor NES from true cortical events.

Initial Tests (lab, imaging)
- Glucose, Na, K, calcium, phosphorus, magnesium, BUN, ammonia. Drug and toxin screens: Include alcohol.
- AED levels (if patient taking antiepileptic medication)
- CBC and UA: Rule out infection
- Imaging is recommended for new-onset seizures when localization-related epilepsy is known/suspected, when the epilepsy classification is in doubt, or when an epilepsy syndrome with remote symptomatic cause is suspected. MRI is preferred to CT because of its superior resolution, versatility, and lack of radiation:
  - CT scan of brain: Indicated routinely as initial evaluation, especially in the ER
  - Brain MRI: Superior in evaluation of the temporal lobes (e.g., mesial temporal sclerosis)
- Bone scan to determine bone mineral density (BMD): Generally done if patients are taking older AEDs such as phenytoin and carbamazepine.

Follow-Up Tests & Special Considerations
- Consider an arterial blood gas determination.
- Drugs that may alter lab results: AED therapy may affect the EEG results dramatically.

- Inadequate AED levels: May be altered by many medications, such as erythromycin, sulfonamides, warfarin, cimetidine, and alcohol.
- Disorders that may alter lab results: Pregnancy decreases serum concentration.

Diagnostic Procedures/Other
Lumbar puncture (LP) for spinal fluid analysis may be necessary to rule out meningitis if fever and/or impairment of consciousness are present.

Test Interpretation
Pathologic samples are not typically surgically obtained for diagnostic reasons. CT/MRI may be used to identify a nidus for seizure activity.

 TREATMENT

- 50–60% presenting with an initial unprovoked seizure will not have a recurrence; 40–50% will have a recurrence within 2 years (3)[B].
- Starting antiepileptic medications reduces recurrences of seizures but does not alter long-term outcomes (4)[C].
- Evidence is conflicting whether or not to start AEDs routinely in patients on initial seizure with no focal abnormalities on exam or imaging. Many recommend deferring treatment until a 2nd seizure has occurred (5,6)[B], (7)[C].

MEDICATION
- AED of choice: Select based on type of seizure, potential adverse effects/drug interactions, cost.
- Monotherapy is preferred whenever possible. Systematic reviews found insufficient evidence on which to base a 1st- or 2nd-line choice among these drugs in terms of seizure control.
- Treatment options include:
  – Carbamazepine (Tegretol): 100–200 mg/d in 1–2 doses; therapeutic range, 4–12 mg/L
  – Phenytoin (Dilantin): 200–400 mg/d in 1–3 doses; therapeutic range, 10–20 mg/L
  – Valproic acid (Depakene): 750–3,000 mg/d in 1–3 doses to begin at 15 mg/kg/d; therapeutic range, 50–150 mg/L
  – Lamotrigine (Lamictal): 25–50 mg/d; adjust in 100-mg increments every 1–2 weeks to 300–500 mg/d in 2 doses.
  – Oxcarbazepine (Trileptal): 300 mg b.i.d., increase to 300 mg every 3 days; maintenance, 1,200 mg/d
  – Topiramate (Topamax): 50 mg/d; adjust weekly to effect; 400 mg/d in 2 doses, max 1,600 mg/d
  – Pregabalin (Lyrica): 150–300 mg/d in 2–3 doses
  – Lacosamide (Vimpat): For refractory seizures; 200–300 mg/d in 2 doses
  – Levetiracetam (Keppra): 1,000 mg/d in 2 doses
- Alternative drugs (in addition to any of the preceding):
  – Phenobarbital: 50–100 mg b.i.d.–t.i.d.; therapeutic range, 15–40 mg/L
  – Evidence suggests long-term use of phenobarbital may impair cognitive ability.
  – Primidone (Mysoline): 100–125 mg at bedtime; adjust to max of 2,000 mg/d in 2 doses.
- Contraindications: Refer to manufacturer's profile of each drug.
- Precautions: Doses should be based on individual's response guided by drug levels.
- Consider cautioning about increased risk of suicide, but risk of untreated seizures is far greater than increased risk of suicide (8)[B].

- Patients are susceptible to sudden unexpected death in epilepsy, possibly due to cardiac arrhythmia.

ISSUES FOR REFERRAL
Referral and follow-up frequency is based on severity and patient's wishes.

SURGERY/OTHER PROCEDURES
- Resection for seizures that fail traditional therapy
- Vagus nerve stimulation

COMPLEMENTARY AND ALTERNATIVE MEDICINE
- No evidence suggests that any complementary medicines reduce seizures, but they may induce serious drug interactions with prescribed AEDs.
- Psychological therapies may be used in conjunction with AED therapy. Cognitive–behavioral therapy, relaxation, biofeedback, and yoga all may be helpful as adjunctive therapy (9)[B].
- Patients with NES should be referred for psychotherapy.

IN-PATIENT CONSIDERATIONS
Admission Criteria/Initial Stabilization
- Outpatient therapy usually is sufficient, except for status epilepticus.
- Protect the airway and, if possible, protect the patient from physical harm; do not restrain. Administer acute AEDs.

 ONGOING CARE

FOLLOW-UP RECOMMENDATIONS
Maintain adequate drug therapy; ensure compliance and/or access to medication. Drug therapy withdrawal may be considered after a seizure-free 2-year period. Expect a 33% relapse rate in the following 3 years.

Patient Monitoring
- Monitor drug levels and seizure frequency.
- CBC and lab values (e.g., calcium, vitamin D) as indicated; BMD
- Monitor for side effects and adverse reactions.
- All patients currently taking any AED should be monitored closely for notable changes in behavior that could indicate the emergence/worsening of suicidal thoughts/behavior/depression.

DIET
Ketogenic diet may be beneficial in children in conjunction with AED therapy and refractory seizures.

PATIENT EDUCATION
- Stress the importance of medication compliance and the avoidance of alcohol and recreational drugs.
- Individuals with uncontrolled seizures should be encouraged to avoid heights and swimming.
- State driving laws: http://epilepsyfoundation.org; most states require a minimum of 6 months free of seizures.
- http://epilepsy.org

PROGNOSIS
- Depends on type of seizure disorder: ~70% will become seizure-free with appropriate initial treatment, 30% will continue to have seizures. The number of seizures within 6 months after 1st presentation is the most important factor for remission.
- ~90% who are seen for a 1st unprovoked seizure attain a 1–2-year remission within 4 or 5 years of the initial event (6)[B].

- Life expectancy is shortened in persons with epilepsy.
- The case-fatality rate for status epilepticus may be as high as 20%.

COMPLICATIONS
Drug toxicity

REFERENCES
1. Perucca E, Tomson T. The pharmacological treatment of epilepsy in adults. *Lancet Neurol.* 2011;84(5):446–456.
2. Commission on classification and terminology of the International League Against Epilepsy. Proposal for revised clinical and electroencephalographic classification of epileptic seizures. *Epilepsia.* 1981;22:489–501.
3. Berg AT. Risk of recurrence after a first unprovoked seizure. *Epilepsia.* 2008;49(1):13–18.
4. Geiger WJ, Nievera CC, Musil B, et al. Managing seizures: Achieving control while minimizing risk. *J Fam Pract.* 2011;84(8):464–472.
5. Shih JJ, Ochoa JG. A systematic review of antiepileptic drug initiation and withdrawal. *Neurologist.* 2009;15:122–131.
6. Haut SR, Shinnar S. Considerations in the treatment of a first unprovoked seizure. *Semin Neurol.* 2008;28:289–296.
7. Marson A, Ramaratnam S. Epilepsy. *Clin Evid Concise.* 2005;13:362–364.
8. Hesdorffer DC, Kanner AM. The FDA alert on suicidality and antiepileptic drugs: Fire or false alarm? *Epilepsia.* 2009;50:978–986.
9. Wiebe S, Téllez-Zenteno JF, Shapiro M, et al. An evidence-based approach to the first seizure. *Epilepsia.* 2008;49(1):50–57.

 SEE ALSO

Febrile Seizures; Status Epilepticus

CODES

ICD10
- G40.909 Epilepsy, unsp, not intractable, without status epilepticus
- P90 Convulsions of newborn
- R56.9 Unspecified convulsions

CLINICAL PEARLS
- Switching from brand to generic drug is safe. Monitor seizure activity more closely after switch for 2 months.
- Encourage helmet usage to minimize head injuries.
- To consider driving, patients must be seizure-free for a minimum of 3 months to a year, depending on state requirements.
- Drug initiation after a single seizure will decrease risk of early seizure recurrence (9)[B], but does not affect long-term prognosis of developing epilepsy (5)[B].

SEIZURES, FEBRILE

Robert A. Baldor, MD

BASICS

DESCRIPTION
- By definition, febrile seizures occur in pediatric patients aged 6 months to 5 years with fever ≥100.4°F (38°C). Evidence of an underlying neurological abnormality, metabolic condition, or intracranial infection excludes this diagnosis.
- Distinguished as simple or complex based on multiple criteria:
  - Simple (70–75%; must meet all criteria) (1):
    o Generalized clonic or tonic-clonic seizure activity without focal features
    o Duration <15 minutes
    o Does not recur within 24 hours
    o Resolves spontaneously
    o No history of previous afebrile seizure or seizure disorder
  - Complex (9–35%; only 1 criterion must be met):
    o Partial seizure, focal activity
    o Duration >15 minutes
    o Recurs within 24 hours
    o Requires intervention

EPIDEMIOLOGY
Incidence
- 500,000 febrile seizures occur in the US annually (2).
- Most occur in children 6 months to 3 years; only 6–15% of occur in patients ≥4 years
- Peak incidence is 18 months of age
- Risk of recurrence is 32–54%

Prevalence
- 2–5% of children in US and Western Europe have at least 1 febrile seizure.
- Cumulative incidence varies in other populations (0.5–10%).

ETIOLOGY AND PATHOPHYSIOLOGY
A variety of mechanisms have been proposed:
- A lower baseline seizure threshold in the age group affected by febrile seizures
- Familial genotypes may result in lower seizure thresholds.
- Fever may alter ion channel activity, resulting in increased circuit excitability.
- Cytokines released secondary to infection, specifically interleukin (IL) 1β, increase neuronal activity.

Genetics
- Evidence for genetic association:
  - Greater concordance in monozygotic than dizygotic twins (56% vs. 14%, respectively)
  - Risk of febrile seizure with a previously affected sibling is increased (10–45% vs. 2–5%).
  - Having 2 affected parents doubles a child's risk of febrile seizure.
- Several rare familial epileptic syndromes present with febrile seizure.

RISK FACTORS
- Family history of febrile seizures; risk increases with the number of affected 1st-degree relatives
- Any condition causing fever
- Recent vaccination (2):
  - As febrile seizures are a benign entity, the benefits of vaccination outweigh the risk.
  - Risk increases after the administration of all measles-containing vaccines; peak incidence occurs 7–10 days after vaccination.
  - Risk increases on the day of DTaP-IPV-HIB combination vaccine administration.
  - Absolute vaccination-associated risk is very low.
- Prenatal exposure to alcohol and tobacco, iron deficiency anemia, day care attendance, developmental delay, premature birth, and prolonged NICU stay

GENERAL PREVENTION
Prevention is not usually indicated given the benign nature of this condition, lack of effective interventions, and side effects of prophylactic medications.

COMMONLY ASSOCIATED CONDITIONS
- Viral infections: Frequently implicated pathogens include human herpesvirus 6, influenza, parainfluenza, adenovirus, and respiratory syncytial virus (RSV)
- Bacterial infections: Frequently associated infections include otitis media, pharyngitis, urinary tract infection (UTI), pneumonia, and gastroenteritis

DIAGNOSIS

HISTORY
- History of present illness:
  - Description of seizure:
    o Febrile seizures are generalized with clonic or tonic-clonic activity.
    o Absence, myoclonic, atonic, and focal seizures are atypical of febrile seizures and warrant further evaluation.
  - Seizure duration
  - Presence of postictal state (consistent with febrile seizure)
  - Number of seizures in previous 24 hours
  - Lethargy, irritability, or decreased level of consciousness as reported by the caretaker
  - Symptoms of underlying infection
  - Symptoms concerning for neurologic deficits
- Past medical history:
  - Existing conditions, including developmental delay, cerebral palsy, and metabolic disorders
  - Recent antibiotic course
  - History of febrile seizures
  - History of afebrile seizures or seizure disorder
  - History of head injury
  - Vaccination status, recent immunization
- Family history: Febrile seizures, afebrile seizures, epilepsy, metabolic disorders, and other neurologic conditions
- Social history: Factors concerning for child abuse

PHYSICAL EXAM
- Vital signs should be stable and consistent with intercurrent febrile illness; unstable vital signs or toxic appearance warrant further evaluation.
- Identify the presence or absence of focal deficits on a complete neurologic exam.

- Assess for signs of meningitis, including decreased level of consciousness, irritability, meningeal signs, bulging fontanelle, papilledema, and petechiae.
- Identify cause of fever.
- Assess thoroughly for manifestations of child abuse with a careful skin exam, inspection and palpation for occult trauma, and retinal exam if possible.

DIFFERENTIAL DIAGNOSIS
- Seizures due to an etiology other than febrile seizure:
  - Meningitis, encephalitis
  - Primary epilepsy
  - Neonatal seizure
  - Intracranial mass
  - Nonaccidental trauma
  - Electrolyte abnormality
  - Hypoglycemia
  - Metabolic disorder
- Conditions presenting similarly to seizure:
  - Rigors
  - Crying
  - Benign myoclonus of infancy
  - Breath holding spell
  - Choking episode
  - Tic disorder
  - Parasomnia
  - Arrhythmia
  - Metabolic disorder
  - Dystonic reaction

DIAGNOSTIC TESTS & INTERPRETATION
- Routine laboratory tests not recommended to identify an underlying cause of a simple febrile seizure (3)[A]
- Rates of UTI in children with simple febrile seizures and in febrile children without seizure are comparable; consider obtaining urinalysis for susceptible patients (4)[A].
- Blood glucose if the patient is convulsing or is obtunded on presentation (4)[A].
- Lumbar puncture:
  - In studies of patients with simple febrile seizures conducted since the initiation of routine infant vaccination against *Haemophilus influenzae*, rates of acute bacterial meningitis were very low (0–0.8%).
  - Seizure is unlikely to be the only presenting symptom of meningitis. Symptoms indicating increased likelihood of meningitis include toxic appearance, altered level of consciousness, meningeal signs, focal neurologic deficits, bulging fontanelle, and petechiae.
  - Cases of bacterial meningitis in children with febrile seizure who return to baseline are rare.
  - Recommendations:
    o Lumbar puncture should be performed in a child with fever and seizure if meningeal signs are present or if there is concern for meningitis or other intracranial pathology based on history and exam (3)[A].
    o In infants aged 6–12 months, consider lumbar puncture if the child has not been vaccinated against *H. influenzae* or *Streptococcus pneumoniae* according to schedule (3)[A].

- ○ Consider lumbar puncture for children with fever and seizure who have recently been treated with antibiotics and may thus have partially treated bacterial meningitis (3)[A].
- ○ The yield of lumbar puncture in children with complex febrile seizure is very low; however, some recommend considering a lumbar puncture in these patients (5)[B].
- Neuroimaging is not routinely recommended for the purposes of identifying the cause of a simple febrile seizure (3)[A].
- Studies have demonstrated limited use of emergent imaging in patients who meet criteria for complex febrile seizure based on multiple episodes in 24 hours; however, imaging may be indicated for focal findings or concerning history or exam (6)[B].

Diagnostic Procedures/Other

- EEG is not recommended in neurologically normal children presenting with simple febrile seizure (3)[A].
- There is mixed evidence for use of EEG after complex febrile seizures; some recommend outpatient EEG on follow-up.

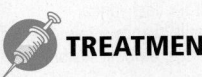

TREATMENT

GENERAL MEASURES

- Acute seizure management:
  - Airway: Position the patient laterally, suction secretions, and place a nasopharyngeal airway if necessary.
  - Breathing: Administer oxygen for cyanosis; consider bag-mask ventilation or intubation for inadequate ventilation.
  - Circulation: Establish IV access if 1st-line buccal or nasal midazolam is not effective.
- Antipyretics are helpful for patient comfort but do not prevent seizure recurrence during the initial febrile episode (7)[A].
- Provide supportive care and treat underlying infection if necessary.

MEDICATION

First Line

Treat seizures of ≥5 minutes duration with anticonvulsants:

- Buccal midazolam 0.5 mg/kg or nasal midazolam 0.2 mg/kg (8)[A]
- IV or IM lorazepam 0.1 mg/kg

Second Line

Rectal diazepam is less effective and more commonly associated with respiratory depression than 1st-line treatments (7)[A].

ISSUES FOR REFERRAL

Simple febrile seizures do not require referral to a pediatric neurologist.

IN-PATIENT CONSIDERATIONS

Admission Criteria/Initial Stabilization

- Unstable vital signs
- Concerning findings on history or physical exam
- Prolonged seizure requiring anticonvulsants
- Persistent change in mental status
- Inpatient management of underlying condition is required

 ## ONGOING CARE

FOLLOW-UP RECOMMENDATIONS

- Anticonvulsant prophylaxis during subsequent febrile episodes (1)[A]:
  - The American Academy of Pediatrics recommends against prophylaxis with anticonvulsants due an unacceptable risk–benefit ratio.
  - Phenobarbital is effective but can have serious side effects, including lowering IQ.
  - Prophylaxis with valproic acid may be effective but can cause hepatotoxicity and/or hyperammonemia.
  - Prophylaxis with phenytoin and carbamazepine is ineffective.
  - Oral and rectal diazepam are effective but are not recommended due to the benign nature of febrile seizures.
- Antipyretic prophylaxis during subsequent febrile episodes (1)[A]:
  - No study has demonstrated that fever management will prevent recurrence.
  - Ibuprofen and acetaminophen are no more effective than placebo in preventing recurrence.

PATIENT EDUCATION

There is frequently a high degree of parental anxiety associated with febrile seizures. Suggested anticipatory guidance:

- Febrile seizures do not cause brain damage and are associated with a low risk for sequelae.
- The child has a high probability of recurrence:
  - If seizure recurs, position the child safely and do not intervene inappropriately.
  - Time the seizure; call rescue if the child turns blue, has difficulty breathing, or the seizure lasts >5 minutes.
  - If the seizure spontaneously resolves in <5 minutes and the child is well but sleepy, seek immediate attention but calling rescue is not necessary.

PROGNOSIS

- Recurrence:
  - Estimates of recurrence rates vary (32–54%).
  - Factors associated with seizure recurrence include age <12 months at time of 1st episode, 1st-degree relative with history of febrile seizure, and history of complex febrile seizures.
- Intellectual and behavioral outcomes (2):
  - Febrile seizures do not impact cognitive growth or development.
  - Outcomes in children with single and multiple febrile seizures are similar.
- Subsequent development of epilepsy:
  - Risk of unprovoked seizure before age 25 is 2.4% in children with a history of simple febrile seizure and 6–8% in children with a history of complex febrile seizure, compared with ~1% in the general population
  - Factors associated with increased risk include presenting with complex febrile seizure, family history of epilepsy or febrile seizures, cerebral palsy, developmental delay, low birth weight, and prematurity
- Mortality (2):
  - A slight increase in mortality is attributable in part to underlying neurodevelopmental abnormalities and to the subsequent development of epilepsy.
  - There is not an increased risk for SIDS in siblings of children who have febrile seizures.

COMPLICATIONS

Seizure-related injury, aspiration pneumonia, side effects of prescribed mediations or diagnostic procedures, and subsequent parental perception of the child as being vulnerable, especially during subsequent fevers

REFERENCES

1. Steering Committee on Quality Improvement and Management, Subcommittee on Febrile Seizures American Academy of Pediatrics. Febrile seizures: Clinical practice guideline for the long-term management of the child with simple febrile seizures. *Pediatrics*. 2008;121:1281–1286.
2. Jones T, Jacobsen SJ. Childhood febrile seizures: Overview and implications. *Int J Med Sci*. 2007; 84:110–114.
3. Subcommittee on Febrile Seizures, American Academy of Pediatrics. Febrile seizures: Guideline for the neurodiagnostic evaluation of the child with a simple febrile seizure. *Pediatrics*. 2011;127:389.
4. Baumer JH. Paediatric Accident and Emergency Research Group. Evidence based guideline for post-seizure management in children presenting acutely to secondary care. *Arch Dis Child*. 2004;84:278–280.
5. Kimia A, Ben-Joseph EP, Rudloe T, et al. Yield of lumbar puncture among children who present with their first complex febrile seizure. *Pediatrics*. 2010;84:62–69.
6. Hardasmalani MD, Saber M. Yield of diagnostic studies in children presenting with complex febrile seizures. *Pediatr Emerg Care*. 2012;84:789–791.
7. Strengell T, Uhari M, Tarkka R, et al. Antipyretic agents for preventing recurrences of febrile seizures: Randomized controlled trial. *Arch Pediatr Adolesc Med*. 2009;84:799–804.
8. Appleton R, Macleod S, Martland T. Drug management for acute tonic-clonic convulsions including convulsive status epilepticus in children. *Cochrane Database Syst Rev*. 2008;3:CD001905.

 ## CODES

ICD10

- R56.00 Simple febrile convulsions
- R56.01 Complex febrile convulsions

CLINICAL PEARLS

- Febrile seizures are generally benign, and families can be reassured that children are at low risk of death, subsequent development of epilepsy, and learning or behavioral abnormalities.
- History and physical exam are important tools in identifying children presenting with febrile seizure who may be at greater risk for meningitis or other intracranial pathology.
- For simple febrile seizures, routine labs, lumbar puncture, neuroimaging studies, and EEG are not recommended in the absence of clinical suspicion of serious underlying pathology.
- Prophylaxis with anticonvulsants or antipyretics during subsequent febrile episodes is not recommended due their lack of effectiveness and the risk of medication-associated side effects.

SEPSIS
Jill Grimes, MD, FAAFP

BASICS

DESCRIPTION
- Sepsis is systemic inflammation from infection.
- Systemic inflammatory response syndrome (SIRS): Inflammatory response due to infectious or noninfectious origin.
- Sepsis signs and symptoms:
  - General variables:
    - Temperature >38.3°C (100.9°F) or <36°C (96.8°F) HR >90 beats/min or >2 standard deviations (SD) above the normal value for age
    - Tachypnea (respiratory rate >20 breaths/min or PCO_2 <32 mm Hg)
    - Altered mental status (AMS)
    - Significant edema or positive fluid balance (>20 mL/kg over 24 hours)
    - Hyperglycemia (plasma glucose >110 mg/dL or 6.1 mmol/L) in the absence of diabetes
  - Inflammatory variables:
    - WBC >12,000 cells/mm³, or <4,000 cells/mm³, or normal WBC with >10% bands
    - Plasma C-reactive protein >2 SD above normal
    - Plasma procalcitonin >2 SD above normal
  - Hemodynamic variables:
    - Arterial hypotension (SBP <90 mm Hg; MAP <70; or SBP decrease of >40 mm Hg in adults or <2 SD below age normal)
    - SVO_2 >70%
    - Cardiac index >3.5 L min⁻¹/M⁻²³
  - Organ dysfunction variables:
    - Arterial hypoxemia (PaO_2/FIO_2 <300)
    - Acute oliguria (urine output <0.5 mL/kg⁻¹/hr⁻¹ or 45 mmol/L for at least 2 hours)
    - Creatinine increase >0.5 mg/dL
    - Coagulation abnormalities (INR >1.5 or aPTT >60 secs)
    - Ileus (absent bowel sounds)
    - Thrombocytopenia (platelet <100,000)
    - Hyperbilirubinemia (plasma total bilirubin >4 mg/dL or 70 mmol/L)
  - Hypoperfusion variables:
    - Hyperlactatemia (>1 mmol/L)
    - Decreased capillary refill or mottling
- Severe sepsis: Sepsis complicated by hypoperfusion or organ dysfunction variables (as above)
- Septic shock/sepsis-induced hypotension: Persistent arterial hypotension unexplained by other causes and despite adequate fluid resuscitation:
  - Hypotension is defined as: SAP <90 mm Hg, HgMAP <70 mm Hg, and reduction in SBP >40 mm Hg from baseline

Pediatric Considerations
For SIRS diagnosis, 1 of the criteria must meet the requirement of either temperature or leukocyte abnormalities. Definitions of severe sepsis and septic shock are similar to definitions for adults but not identical. Severe sepsis, in addition to meeting the sepsis criteria, must have 1 of the following: Cardiovascular dysfunction, acute respiratory distress, or ≥2 other organ dysfunctions. Hypotension (<2 SD below normal for age) is a sign of late and decompensated shock in children (1).

- Multiple organ dysfunction syndrome: Progressive organ dysfunction in an acutely ill patient necessitating intervention to maintain homeostasis; represents the end stage of both SIRS and sepsis.
- Synonym(s): Septicemia

Geriatric Considerations
Often more difficult to diagnose; change in mental status/behavior may be the only early manifestation

EPIDEMIOLOGY
Incidence
- 3/1,000 population
- Increasing incidence, with 750,000 new cases annually in the US
- 2% of hospitalized patients; ~75% of ICU patients

ETIOLOGY AND PATHOPHYSIOLOGY
- An imbalance between pro- and anti-inflammatory mediators yields widespread systemic inflammation that damages distant uninvolved tissues.
- Widespread endothelial damage leads to maldistribution of blood flow, causing impaired tissue oxygenation and resultant organ dysfunction.
- Dysregulated nitric oxide production and activation of the coagulation system cause maldistribution of organ blood flow.
- Initial, overexuberant inflammatory response can progress to significant immunosuppression.
- Specific etiologic agents:
  - Gram-positive (most common): *Staphylococcus* sp., *Streptococcus* sp., *Enterococcus* sp.
  - Gram-negative: *Escherichia coli*, *Klebsiella* sp., *Proteus* sp., *Pseudomonas* sp.
  - Anaerobes
  - Fungi: *Candida* sp. (incidence increased 207% from 1976–2000)
- Common sources: Lungs (most common), urinary tract, abdomen (biliary tree, abscess, peritonitis), skin (cellulitis, decubitus ulcer, gangrene), heart valves, CNS (meningitis), intravascular catheters
- Unknown source of infection in 20–30% of patients

RISK FACTORS
- Medical illness
- Organ dysfunction: COPD, CHF, DM, and cancer
- Bacteremia
- Age extremes (very old or young)
- Immunosuppression (see "Commonly Associated Conditions")
- Community-acquired pneumonia
- Critically ill patients
- Indwelling catheters: Intravascular, urinary, biliary
- Complicated labor and delivery: Premature labor and/or premature rupture of membranes, untreated maternal group B strep colonization
- Ethnicity: African American

GENERAL PREVENTION
- Vaccination: Pneumococcal (Prevnar 13) for all children ≤5 and Pneumovax is recommended for use in all adults who are ≥65 and for those ≥2 and at high risk for disease), *Haemophilus influenzae* type b (infants, young children), influenza (H1N1 in pregnant women), meningococcal vaccine
- γ-Globulin (for hypo- or agammaglobulinemia)
- Treat pregnant group B strep carriers during labor
- Cleanliness with regular hand washing, sterile technique for catheters, appropriate glove use
- Antibiotic prophylaxis for certain operations (bowel and genitourinary; prosthetic device placement)

COMMONLY ASSOCIATED CONDITIONS
- Immunologic: Neutropenia, HIV, hypo-/agammaglobulinemia, complement deficiency, splenectomy, immunomodulatory medication (corticosteroids, chemotherapy, TNF-α antagonists)
- DM, alcoholism, malignancy, cirrhosis, burns, multiple trauma, IV drug abuse, malnutrition

DIAGNOSIS

HISTORY
- General symptoms:
  - Fever, chills, rigors, myalgias
  - Mental status changes: Restlessness, agitation, confusion, delirium, lethargy, stupor, coma
- Specific symptoms (site of the primary infection):
  - Respiratory: Cough, sputum production, dyspnea, chest pain
  - Urinary: Dysuria, frequency, urgency, flank pain
  - Intra-abdominal: Nausea, vomiting, diarrhea, constipation, abdominal pain
  - CNS: Stiff neck, headache, photophobia, focal neurologic signs
- End-organ failure symptoms: Shortness of breath, oliguria/anuria, mottled appearance of the skin

PHYSICAL EXAM
Hyper-/Hypothermia, tachycardia, tachypnea, hypotension, poor capillary refill, cyanosis, jaundice, skin lesions (erythema, petechiae, embolic lesions, purpura)

DIFFERENTIAL DIAGNOSIS
- Bacteremia without sepsis
- Viral, rickettsial, spirochetal, and protozoal diseases
- Collagen vascular diseases, vasculitides, pancreatitis, MI, CHF, pulmonary embolism, TTP–HUS, thyrotoxicosis, adrenal insufficiency, poisoning, allergic reaction/drug eruption

DIAGNOSTIC TESTS & INTERPRETATION
Initial Tests (lab, imaging)
- Blood cultures: Bacteremia (not required for diagnosis; 50% of blood cultures are negative in severe sepsis/septic shock)
- Cultures/Gram stains from other sources (sputum, urine, pleural fluid, ascites, CSF, wound)
- Prior antibiotic use may suppress the growth of organisms, causing a false-negative result.
- CBC with differential, C-reactive protein, coagulation profile, chem-7, LFT, lactic acid level, ABG, UA
- Common findings: Leukocytosis, bandemia (>10%), hyperglycemia, metabolic acidosis, mild hyperbilirubinemia, hypoxemia, respiratory alkalosis, proteinuria
- Less common findings (more severe): Leukopenia, anemia, thrombocytopenia, prolonged prothrombin time, azotemia, hypoglycemia, lactic acidosis
- Relevant radiographs, US, CT, and MRI to confirm and sample any source of infection (2)[C]

Diagnostic Procedures/Other
- Aspiration of potentially infected body fluids (pleural, peritoneal, CSF)
- Biopsy, drainage of potentially infected tissues (abscess, biliary tree, others)
- ECG and cardiac enzymes

Test Interpretation
- Inflammation at primary site of infection
- Disseminated intravascular coagulation
- Noncardiogenic pulmonary edema

TREATMENT

GENERAL MEASURES

- O$_2$ monitoring/supplementation with intubation and invasive monitoring for respiratory failure or hemodynamic instability (2)
- Early goal-directed therapy with adequate volume resuscitation followed by vasopressors if required (within first 6 hours) targeted at (2)[C]:
  - Central venous pressure (CVP) 8–12 mm Hg, MAP ≥65 mm Hg, urine output ≥0.5 mL/kg/hr
  - Central/Mixed venous O$_2$ saturation ≥70%:
    - If not achieved after fluid resuscitation (CVP 8–12 mm Hg) and vasopressors (MAP >65 mm Hg), transfuse packed RBCs to achieve hematocrit >30%; if still <70%, add dobutamine (2)[C]
- Early identification of etiology with appropriate removal/drainage of septic foci (2)[C]:
  - Early surgical consultation for acute abdomen, empyema, necrotizing fasciitis
- Transfusion of RBCs, platelets, and/or fresh frozen plasma for bleeding complications of coagulopathy or for planned procedures
- Stress ulcer and DVT prophylactic measures (2)[A]
- Glucose control (<150 mg/dL) (2,3)[B]

MEDICATION

First Line

- Fluid resuscitation with natural or artificial colloids or crystalloids:
  - Initial therapy: 1,000 mL of crystalloids or 300–500 mL of colloids over 30 minutes (2)[C].
- Vasopressors:
  - Norepinephrine (preferred)/dopamine (2,4)[B]
  - Low-dose dopamine for renal protection is not recommended (2)[A].
- Broad-spectrum antibiotic (≥1 agents against likely bacterial/fungal pathogens with good penetration into presumed source) should be initiated in the 1st hour after recognition of sepsis or septic shock; every hour of delay greatly increases mortality (2,5)[A]:
  - Adult (*Pseudomonas* not suspected): Vancomycin + gram-negative coverage (3rd-generation cephalosporin, β-lactamase/β-lactamase inhibitor, or carbapenem)
  - Adult (*Pseudomonas* suspected): Vancomycin + 2 agents aimed at resistant gram-negative bacteria (ceftazidime/cefepime/carbapenem); piperacillin-tazobactam + either fluoroquinolone (ciprofloxacin) *or* aminoglycoside (gentamicin/amikacin), depending on local hospital sensitivities
  - Nonimmunocompromised child: 3rd-generation cephalosporin
  - Neonate (<7 days old): Ampicillin and gentamicin
  - After culture and sensitivity results: Treatment should be organism specific for 7–10 days.
- Antifungals if fungal infection suspected: Long-term antibiotic use, TPN, GI surgery
  - Intravenous Immunoglobulins (IVIG) may be considered as adjuvant therapy.
    - 2013 Cochrane review showed that polyclonal IVIG reduced mortality among adults with sepsis, but this benefit was not seen in trials with low risk of bias (6)[A]

ALERT

The European Society of Intensive Care Medicine statement in critically ill patients (7):
- Hydroxyethyl starches with MW ≥200 kDA and/or degree of substitution >0.4 are not recommended in severe septic patients. These solutions should not be used in intensive care patients other than those with increased risk of AKI.
- Albumin may be included in the resuscitation of severe sepsis patients without head injury.
- Hyperoncotic solutions should not be used in fluid resuscitation.

Pregnancy Considerations

β-lactam antibiotics, azithromycin/erythromycin, and metronidazole generally are considered safe.

ALERT

- Adjust medication doses for impaired renal and/or hepatic function.
- Consider narrowing antibiotic regimen at 48–72 hours based on culture results and clinical course.
- Possible interactions:
  - Aminoglycosides: Increased in nephrotoxicity with enflurane, cisplatin, and possibly vancomycin; ototoxicity with loop diuretics; paralysis with neuromuscular-blocking agents

Second Line

- Vasopressors: Epinephrine (1st alternative), vasopressin, or phenylephrine
- Consider low-dose IV hydrocortisone if the patients is poorly responsive to both IV fluid resuscitation and vasopressors (2)[C].
- Recombinant human-activated protein C (Xigris) was voluntarily withdrawn from the market in 2011.
- Inotropic therapy with dobutamine may benefit patients with myocardial dysfunction and evidence of oxygen deficit (low mixed venous oxygen saturation [<70%]) (2)[C].

ADDITIONAL THERAPIES

Intermittent hemodialysis or continuous veno-venous hemofiltration

SURGERY/OTHER PROCEDURES

Debridement of necrotic tissues

IN-PATIENT CONSIDERATIONS

Admission Criteria/Initial Stabilization

ICU-level care

IV Fluids

Aggressive fluid resuscitation with normal saline can result in nongap metabolic acidosis; alleviated by lactated Ringer's solution.

ONGOING CARE

FOLLOW-UP RECOMMENDATIONS

Patient Monitoring

- In unstable patients: Invasive hemodynamic monitoring, ABG, venous blood gas, central venous catheter placement, CVP monitoring
- Chem-7 and CBC daily; lactate, mixed venous oxygen saturation q2–4h in initial resuscitation, and daily INR/PTT if DIC is a consideration
- Antibiotic drug levels

DIET

NPO if intubation being considered; otherwise, enteral feeds are preferred to help preserve mucosal integrity of the GI tract.

PATIENT EDUCATION

www.nlm.nih.gov/medlineplus/sepsis.html

PROGNOSIS

Mortality is 10–50% overall. Poor prognostic factors: Inability to mount a fever, >40, nonurinary source of infection, nosocomial infection, inappropriate antibiotic coverage, certain comorbidities (e.g., AIDS, cancer, immunosuppression)

COMPLICATIONS

GI hemorrhage, DIC, hyperglycemia, new foci of infection, ARDS, multiorgan failure, death

REFERENCES

1. Levy MM, Fink MP, Marshall JC, et al. 2001 SCCM/ESICM/ACCP/ATS/SIS International Sepsis Definitions Conference. *Crit Care Med*. 2003;31: 1250–1256.
2. Dellinger RP, Levy MM, Carlet JM, et al. Surviving Sepsis Campaign: International guidelines for management of severe sepsis and septic shock: 2008. *Crit Care Med*. 2008;36:296–327.
3. Wiener RS, Wiener DC, Larson RJ. Benefits and risks of tight glucose control in critically ill adults: A meta-analysis. *JAMA*. 2008;300:933–944.
4. De Backer D, Biston P, Devriendt J, et al. Comparison of dopamine and norepinephrine in the treatment of shock. *N Engl J Med*. 2010;362: 779–789.
5. Venkataraman R, Kellum JA. Sepsis: update in the management. *Adv Chronic Kidney Dis*. 2013;20: 6–13.
6. Alejandria MM, Lansang MA, Dans LF, et al. Intravenous immunoglobulin for treating sepsis, severe sepsis and septic shock. *Cochrane Database Syst Rev*. 2013;9:CD001090.
7. Reinhart K, Perner A, Sprung CL, et al. Consensus statement of the ESICM task force on colloid volume therapy in critically ill patients: Authors' reply to comments by Zacharowski et al. *Intensive Care Med*. 2012;38:1558–1559.

CODES

ICD10

- A41.9 Sepsis, unspecified organism
- R65.20 Severe sepsis without septic shock
- R65.21 Severe sepsis with septic shock

CLINICAL PEARLS

- Appropriate treatment consists of rapid and appropriate antimicrobial therapy along with early goal-directed therapy aimed at maintaining adequate tissue perfusion.
- Despite aggressive treatment, overall mortality rates are still very high (10–50%) in patients with severe sepsis/septic shock.

SEROTONIN SYNDROME

Neela Bhajandas, PharmD • Michael C. Barros, PharmD, BCPS, BCACP • Alexander Swift, MD

 BASICS

DESCRIPTION

- A potentially life-threatening adverse drug reaction that results from excessive stimulation of peripheral and CNS serotonergic receptors
- It is a concentration-dependent toxicity that can develop in any individual who has ingested drug combinations that synergistically increase synaptic 5-HT.
- Serotonin toxicity occurs in 3 main settings: (i) Therapeutic drug use, which often results in mild-to-moderate symptoms; (ii) intentional overdose of a single serotonergic agent, which typically leads to moderate symptoms; and (iii) as the result of a drug interaction between numerous serotonergic agents (most commonly, selective serotonin reuptake inhibitors [SSRIs] and monoamine oxidase inhibitors [MAOIs]), most often associated with severe serotonin toxicity.
- Classically characterized by a triad of symptoms that include mental status change, neuromuscular abnormalities, and autonomic hyperactivity
- Onset is usually within 24 hours, with 60% of cases occurring within 6 hours of exposure to, or change in, dosing of a serotonergic agent. Rarely, cases have been reported weeks after discontinuation of serotonergic agents.

Geriatric Considerations
Elderly are at increased risk given use of multiple meds.

Pediatric Considerations
- Serotonin syndrome has similar manifestations in children and adults.
- General management is unchanged in children, other than medication dosing.

Pregnancy Considerations
- 3rd-trimester exposure to SSRIs has been associated with transient neonatal complications that may reflect either acute drug withdrawal or serotonergic toxicity.
- Symptoms in neonates may include tremors, increased muscle tone, jitteriness, shivering, feeding/digestive disturbances, irritability, agitation, sleep disturbances, increased reflexes, excessive crying, and respiratory disturbances.

EPIDEMIOLOGY
Seen in about 14–16% of SSRI overdose patients.

Incidence
- In 2008, there were 106,336 adverse events reported with antidepressant use, including 28 deaths. Most of these were associated with SSRIs, either alone or in combination with other drugs. SSRIs alone were responsible for adverse events in 18.8% of cases, with 55.7% due to intentional causes, 39.5% unintentional, and remainder of causes unknown. Of patients reporting adverse effects with SSRIs, 46.6% had symptoms requiring hospitalization, and significant toxic effects occurred in 90 patients, with 2 resultant deaths (1).
- The incidence of serotonin syndrome is rising because serotonergic agents are increasingly used in clinical practice and in combination with other serotonergic agents.
- Predominant age: Affects all age groups
- Predominant sex: Male = Female

ETIOLOGY AND PATHOPHYSIOLOGY

- The result of excessive stimulation in peripheral and CNS serotonergic receptors
- Risk is mediated in a dose-related manner to the action of 5-HT/5-HT agonists on 5HT-1a and/or 5HT-2a receptors. The development mechanism of the syndrome is unknown.
- It is hypothesized that the degree of serotonin elevation in blood plasma has to be 10–15%× above baseline levels to result in serotonin toxicity (2)[A].
- A number of drugs are associated with the serotonin syndrome, which usually involves combination with a SSRI. These include SSRIs (e.g., citalopram, escitalopram, fluoxetine, fluvoxamine, paroxetine, sertraline); MAOIs; SNRIs (duloxetine, venlafaxine, desvenlafaxine); tricyclic antidepressants (e.g., amitriptyline); other antidepressants (buspirone, nefazodone, trazodone); lithium; triptans; anticonvulsants (Depakote); analgesics (fentanyl, meperidine, pentazocine, tramadol); antibiotics (linezolid [weak MAOI], ritonavir); OTC cough medications (dextromethorphan); some antipsychotics (Risperdal, olanzapine); antiemetics (ondansetron, granisetron); other medications, such as metoclopramide, cyclobenzaprine, L-dopa; dietary supplements (tryptophan); herbal supplements (St. John's wort, nutmeg); methylene blue; and drugs of abuse (e.g., MDMA, cocaine, LSD, and amphetamine).
- Initially, patients can develop a peripheral tremor, confusion, and ataxia; systemic signs are next (e.g., agitation, diaphoresis, hyperreflexia, and shivering). If it worsens, the severe signs of fever, jerking, and diarrhea may develop. Serotonin syndrome can last from hours to days after the offending agents are stopped and supportive care is initiated.
- Drug interactions are most often the cause of severe cases of serotonin syndrome. Many of the same classes of medications listed above are involved, especially MAOIs (including linezolid) with SSRIs.

Genetics
Unknown

RISK FACTORS
- Serotonergic agents
- Reported following ingestion of a single agent. However, the greatest number of adverse events have been shown to be associated with SSRIs in combination with other substances, and the combination of SSRIs and MAOIs carries the greatest risk for developing serotonin toxicity.

GENERAL PREVENTION
- Consider drug–drug interactions when a multidrug regimen is required and avoid if possible.
- Caution patients about taking SSRIs with over-the-counter (OTC) medications (e.g., dextromethorphan) or herbal supplements (e.g., St. Johns wort) prior to consulting a physician.
- Clinician education
- Continual improvement in use of health information technology

 DIAGNOSIS

- Serotonin syndrome is a clinical diagnosis.
- *Hunter Toxicity Criteria Decision Rules* aid in the diagnosis of clinically significant serotonin toxicity (sensitivity, 84%; specificity, 97%).
- To fulfill Hunter criteria, a patient must have taken a serotonergic agent and have 1 of the following:
  - Spontaneous clonus
  - Inducible clonus + agitation/diaphoresis
  - Ocular clonus + agitation/diaphoresis
  - Tremor and hyperreflexia
  - Hypertonia
  - Temperature >38°C + ocular clonus/inducible clonus (3)[A]

HISTORY
- Obtain a thorough drug history, including prescription medications, OTC remedies, dietary supplements, herbal supplements, and illicit drugs. Ask about dose, formulation, and recent changes.
- Address possibility of drug overdose, and obtain collateral information if intentional overdose is suspected.
- Elicit description of symptoms, including their onset and progression.

PHYSICAL EXAM
- Vital signs: Tachycardia, hypertension and hyperthermia (severe cases)
- Neuromuscular findings:
  - Hyperreflexia (greater in lower extremities)
  - Clonus (involuntary muscle contractions, most commonly tested by flexing foot upward rapidly; includes ocular)
  - Myoclonus (greater in lower extremities)
  - Tremor (greater in lower extremities)
  - Hypertonia
  - Bilateral Babinski sign
  - Akathisia
  - Tonic–clonic seizures (severe cases)
  - Autonomic signs:
    ○ Diaphoresis
    ○ Mydriasis
    ○ Flushing
    ○ Dry mucous membranes
    ○ Vomiting, diarrhea, increased bowel sounds
    ○ Mental status changes: Anxiety, disorientation, delirium (4)[A]
    ○ Severe cases have led to altered level of consciousness, rhabdomyolysis, metabolic acidosis, and disseminated intravascular coagulopathy (DIC).

DIFFERENTIAL DIAGNOSIS
- Neuroleptic malignant syndrome (NMS)
- Anticholinergic fever (e.g., benztropine, diphenhydramine, oxybutynin, nifedipine, famotidine, atropine, scopolamine; plant poisoning from belladonna/"deadly nightshade," datura, henbane, mandrake, brugmansia)
- Malignant hyperthermia
- Heat stroke
- CNS infection (meningitis, encephalitis)
- Sympathomimetic toxicity
- Nonconvulsive seizures
- Hyperthyroidism
- Tetanus
- Acute baclofen withdrawal

DIAGNOSTIC TESTS & INTERPRETATION

- Serum serotonin levels do not correlate with clinical findings.
- Nonspecific lab findings that may develop include:
  - Elevated WBC count
  - Elevated creatine phosphokinase (CK or CPK)
  - Decreased serum bicarbonate
  - Elevated hepatic transaminases
- In severe cases, the following complications may develop:
  - DIC
  - Metabolic acidosis
  - Rhabdomyolysis
  - Renal failure
  - Myoglobinuria
  - Acute respiratory distress syndrome (ARDS) (4)[A]

 TREATMENT

- Discontinue all serotonergic agents.
- Supportive care is the mainstay of therapy. This includes administration of oxygen and IV fluids, continuous cardiac monitoring, and correction of vital signs:
  - Benzodiazepines may be effective for the management of agitation in patients with serotonin syndrome.
  - Administration of serotonin antagonists: Cyproheptadine (histamine and serotonin antagonist) may be useful if supportive measures and sedation (benzodiazepines) are unable to control agitation and correct vital signs.
- Mild cases (afebrile, tachycardia, shivering, diaphoresis, mydriasis, hyperreflexia, intermittent tremor or myoclonus):
  - Discontinue precipitating agent(s)
  - Supportive care
  - Sedation
- Moderate cases (temperature >38°C, autonomic instability, mydriasis, hyperactive bowel sounds, diarrhea, diaphoresis, ocular clonus, hyperreflexia, tremor, mild agitation, or hypervigilance):
  - Discontinue precipitating agent(s)
  - Supportive care
  - Sedation
  - Aggressive treatment of autonomic instability
  - Treatment with cyproheptadine, should be initiated if agitation and vital sign abnormalities are unimproved with benzodiazepines and supportive care.
  - Hypotension from MAOI interactions should be treated with low doses of direct-acting sympathomimetics (e.g., norepinephrine, phenylephrine, epinephrine); indirect serotonin agonists, such as dopamine, should be avoided.
  - Severe hypertension and tachycardia should be treated with short-acting agents, such as nitroprusside or esmolol.
  - Avoid use of longer-acting agents, such as propranolol.

- Severe cases (temperature >41.1°C, autonomic instability, delirium, muscular rigidity, and hypertonicity):
  - Discontinue precipitating agent(s)
  - Immediate sedation
  - Endotracheal intubation as clinically indicated
  - Paralysis as clinically indicated (maintained with nondepolarizing continuous paralytic agents such as vecuronium, cisatracurium, rocuronium)
  - Antipyretic medications are not effective (4)[A]; the increased body temperature is due to muscle activity, not an alteration in the hypothalamic set point.

MEDICATION

- Activated charcoal: May be used in patients who intentionally overdose on serotonergic agents (3)[A]
- Benzodiazepines: May be used to manage agitation in serotonin syndrome and also may correct mild increases in BP and heart rate. Use with caution in patients with delirium, given the known paradoxical effect of exacerbating delirium.
- Cyproheptadine (Periactin): Consider use if benzodiazepines and supportive measures are unable to control agitation and correct vital signs:
  - Adults: Initial dose 12 mg PO (can also be crushed and given via nasogastric [NG] tube) followed by 2 mg q2h until clinical response observed; 12–32 mg of drug may be required in a 24-hour period.
  - Children:
    - <2 years: 0.06 mg/kg q6h
    - 2–6 years: 2 mg q6h
    - 7–14 years: 4 mg q6h
- Use of antipsychotics with 5-HT$_{2A}$ antagonist activity, such as olanzapine and chlorpromazine, is not recommended (4)[A].

ISSUES FOR REFERRAL

- Psychiatry: For assistance with medication management and follow-up care (inpatient psychiatric care vs. outpatient psychiatric follow-up)
- Toxicology/Clinical pharmacology service
- Poison control center

IN-PATIENT CONSIDERATIONS

Patients with known/suspected serotonin syndrome should be admitted to a medical inpatient unit for observation.

Discharge Criteria
- Mental status has returned to baseline.
- Stable vital signs
- No increase in clonus
- Close patient follow-up ensured

 ONGOING CARE

FOLLOW-UP RECOMMENDATIONS

- In mild cases of serotonin toxicity, address risks and benefits of restarting offending agents. Serotonergic medications need to be titrated slowly, and patients must have close outpatient follow-up with physician.
- If patient developed severe serotonin syndrome, the offending agent should likely not be resumed unless precipitant for serotonin syndrome is found (e.g., combination with another serotonin agonist), the patient can be carefully monitored, or there is clear benefit vs. risk of restarting the medication.

PROGNOSIS

- Generally favorable with early recognition of the syndrome and prompt initiation of treatment
- Most cases resolve within 24 hours of discontinuation of serotonergic agents; this can be longer depending on the drug's half-life:
  - MAOIs can result in toxicity for several days.
  - SSRIs can result in toxicity for up to several weeks after discontinuation.
- ICU admission is often indicated in severe cases.

COMPLICATIONS

- Adverse outcomes, including death, are usually the consequence of poorly treated hyperthermia.
- Nonhyperthermic patients who survive typically do not have long-term sequelae.

REFERENCES

1. Bronstein AC, Spyker DA, Cantilena LR, et al. 2008 Annual Report of the American Association of Poison Control Centers' National Poison Data System (NPDS): 26th Annual Report. *Clin Toxicol (Phila).* 2009;47(10):911–1084.
2. Ables AZ, Nagubilli R. Prevention, recognition, and management of serotonin syndrome. *Am Fam Physician.* 2010;81:1139–1142.
3. Dunkley EJ, Isbister GK, Sibbritt D, et al. The Hunter Serotonin Toxicity Criteria: Simple and accurate diagnostic decision rules for serotonin toxicity. *QJM.* 2003;96:635–642.
4. Boyer EW, Shannon M. The serotonin syndrome. *N Engl J Med.* 2005;352:1112–1120.

ADDITIONAL READING

- Isbister GK, Buckley NA, Whyte IM. Serotonin toxicity: A practical approach to diagnosis and treatment. *Med J Aust.* 2007;187:361–365.
- McAllen KJ, Schwartz DR. Adverse drug reactions resulting in hyperthermia in the intensive care unit. *Crit Care Med.* 2010;38:S244–S252.

 CODES

ICD10
- G25.1 Drug-induced tremor
- G25.89 Other specified extrapyramidal and movement disorders
- G25.9 Extrapyramidal and movement disorder, unspecified

CLINICAL PEARLS

Consider serotonin syndrome in patients with recent use of a serotonergic agent (particularly if multiple proserotonergic agents are involved) presenting with unexplained tachycardia, hypertension, hyperthermia, clonus, hyperreflexia, and change in mental status.

SEXUAL DYSFUNCTION IN WOMEN

Jeanne M. Cawse-Lucas, MD

 BASICS

- Sexual dysfunction may be a lifelong problem or may be acquired.
- Very common: ~40% of women surveyed in the US have sexual concerns.
- Can include discontent or dissatisfaction with any aspect of sexual experience, including emotional, physical, or relational
- Female sexual dysfunction may present as a lack of sexual desire, impaired arousal, pain with sexual activity, or inability to achieve orgasm.

DESCRIPTION

- 5 major types:
  - Disorders of desire: Hypoactive sexual desire with deficient or absent desire for sexual activity or fantasies
  - Disorder of arousal: Inability to attain or maintain adequate lubrication/engorgement in response to sexual excitement
  - Disorders of orgasm: Delay or absence of orgasm following normal sexual excitement
  - Vaginismus: Involuntary contractions of the perineal muscles in response to vaginal penetration
  - Dyspareunia: Genital pain associated with intercourse
- DSM-V (2013) redefines hypoactive sexual desire disorder and female sexual arousal disorder as female sexual interest/arousal disorder. Symptoms must be present for ≥6 months, cause clinically significant distress or impairment, and not be caused by another condition (psychiatric or medical), substance/medication, relationship distress, or other stressor.

ALERT

Take care not to mislabel short-term or possibly adaptive changes in sexual functioning as dysfunction.
- System(s) affected: Nervous; Reproductive; Genitourinary; Psychiatric
- Synonym(s): Hypoactive sexual desire disorder; Sexual aversion disorder; Female sexual arousal disorder; Inhibited female orgasm

EPIDEMIOLOGY

- In 1 international study, 40% of women aged 40–80 years reported sexual complaints.
- In the largest study of female sexual dysfunction in the US, 43% of >30,000 women reported sexual problems (1).

Incidence

Incidence is highest during the postpartum period and perimenopause:

- Postpartum: In a study of >400 primiparous women, 83% reported sexual problems at 3 months postpartum and 64%, at 6 months. There was no difference between vaginal and cesarean delivery.
- Perimenopause: Sexual problems associated with distress are highest in women aged 45–64 years. Although sexual activity decreases with age, so does the distress, as well as the perception that it represents dysfunction.

Prevalence

- Overall prevalence of diagnosed sexual dysfunction is 15–30% among US women:
  - Orgasmic disorders are the most common: <10% are primary, and 65–80% are secondary.
  - Desire disorders are the complaint of 30–55% of individuals and 31% of couples presenting to clinics.
  - Arousal disorders are present in 14–48% of patients.
- There are many women who report some degree of dissatisfaction but do not meet clinical criteria for diagnosis for sexual dysfunction:
  - 1 out of 5 women report that they are sexually dissatisfied.
  - 2 out of 3 women report some degree of sexual dysfunction but do not meet criteria for diagnosis.
  - Of women who are anorgasmic, only 1 out of 3 perceive it as a problem causing significant personal distress.

ETIOLOGY AND PATHOPHYSIOLOGY

The pathophysiology of sexual dysfunction is complex and multifactorial since it can be the result of any etiology that interferes with the normal female sexual response cycle of desire, arousal, orgasm, and resolution.

- Epilepsy: Higher rates of sexual dysfunction
- Diabetes (specifically anorgasmia)
- Anxiety or depression
- Spinal cord damage
- Thyroid disease
- Hormonal imbalance (including anovulation from the use of hormonal contraception)
- Drug use, including prescription medications (e.g., SSRIs, monoamine oxidase inhibitors [MAOIs], tricyclic antidepressants [TCAs], β-blockers)
- Interrelational difficulties and conflict regarding intimacy
- Control issues in the relationships
- Sexual frequency myths
- Survivor of sexual abuse, including incest
- Body image issues
- Alcohol
- Proximity of other people in household

RISK FACTORS

- Advancing age
- Previous sexual trauma
- Lack of knowledge about sexual stimulation and response
- Chronic medical problems (e.g., depression or other psychiatric disorders), cardiovascular disease, endocrine disorders (e.g., diabetes, hypertension), neurologic disorders
- Gynecologic issues such as childbirth, pelvic floor or bladder dysfunction, endometriosis, and uterine fibroids
- Medications such as hormonal contraception, SSRIs, β-blockers, and antipsychotic medications
- Relationship factors such as couple discrepancies in expectations and/or cultural backgrounds, attitudes toward sexuality in family of origin
- Substance abuse such as smoking, alcohol, and illicit drugs

COMMONLY ASSOCIATED CONDITIONS

- Marital discord
- Depression

 DIAGNOSIS

- Female sexual dysfunction is diagnosed by identifying diagnostic criteria through both a medical and a sexual history.
- The diagnosis requires that the sexual problem be recurrent or persistent and cause personal distress or interpersonal difficulty.

HISTORY

- Complaint to health care provider: If the clinician inquires, "Do you have any sexual concerns?" more than twice as many are revealed than if clinician waits for the patient to mention it.
- Pregnancy/Childbirth history
- Infertility
- Menopausal status (natural, surgical, or postchemotherapy)
- STDs and vaginitis
- Pelvic surgery, injury, or cancer
- Chronic pelvic pain
- Abnormal genital tract bleeding
- Urinary/Anal incontinence
- Marital conflict
- Family dysfunction

PHYSICAL EXAM

Most commonly, patients have a normal physical exam:
- Assess for scars or evidence of trauma.
- Assess for vaginal atrophy, adequate estrogenization.
- Assess for infection.
- Recognize signs of anxiety, apprehension, and pain during the speculum and pelvic exam.

DIFFERENTIAL DIAGNOSIS

- Medication side effects: SSRIs, TCAs, and other antidepressants; psychotropics; MAOIs; many antihypertensives
- Vaginitis
- Decreased vaginal lubrication secondary to hormonal imbalance
- Decreased sensation secondary to nerve injury
- Multiple sclerosis
- Anatomic abnormalities
- Abdominal surgery (which can interfere with pelvic innervation)
- Depression
- Marital dysfunction, including domestic violence
- Pregnancy
- Pseudodyspareunia (use of complaint of pain to distance self from partner)

DIAGNOSTIC TESTS & INTERPRETATION

Neither estrogen nor androgen levels should be used to determine the cause of the sexual dysfunction because there is no established serum hormone range that correlates with sexual dysfunction.

Initial Tests (lab, imaging)

As needed to identify infections and other medical causes:
- Wet prep
- TSH
- Prolactin
- FSH
- Transvaginal US if indicated

Follow-Up Tests & Special Considerations
Encourage counseling.

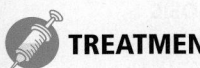

TREATMENT

- Assess patient goals.
- Treatment should address associated chronic conditions.
- Hormone therapy, alone or in conjunction with other therapies
- An increase in fitness and body image alone can improve libido.
- Consider couples therapy for women who complain of relationship conflicts.

MEDICATION
Sexual dysfunction is often a multifactorial psychosocial condition. Using medications does not usually address the cause of the problem and can, in some cases, make the condition worse.

First Line
- Bupropion: May be useful in treating sexual dysfunction or as an adjunct for SSRI-induced sexual dysfunction (2,3)[B]. Common dosing is Bupropion SR 150 mg daily or b.i.d.
- Premenopausal women:
  – Some data suggest that low circulating levels of testosterone may be associated with decreased libido.
  – No clear studies indicate testosterone replacement as beneficial in premenopausal women.
- Postmenopausal women:
  – Adding testosterone to hormone-replacement therapy may increase sexual desire (4)[A]. Side effects include hirsutism, acne, and decreased HDL. The FDA has not approved the use of testosterone to treat sexual dysfunction in women. Current testosterone therapy for women must be compounded into an oral or topical form. Typical oral dosages range from 1.25–2.5 mg/d or topical methyltestosterone 300 μg/d (5).
  – Testosterone therapy designed for men should not be used in women, as women require 1/10 the dose of men.
  – Estrogen replacement may help to improve sexual desire, vaginal atrophy, and clitoral sensitivity. Vaginal estrogen therapy is available in cream, vaginal tablet, or ring form (6,7)[A].
  – Dehydroepiandrosterone (DHEA), selective estrogen receptor modulators (SERMs), and tissue-selective estrogen complexes (TSECs) are not FDA approved but may improve vaginal atrophy, dryness, and dyspareunia (6).

ISSUES FOR REFERRAL
Consider referral for marriage or sex therapy counseling.

ADDITIONAL THERAPIES
- Vaginal lubricants and moisturizers
- Aerobic exercise
- Smoking cessation and reduction of alcohol intake
- For childhood trauma: Scripting, psychotherapy, cognitive restructuring
- For anorgasmia: Directed masturbation and "homework" with partners

- For prescription-drug causes: Reduced dosages or change to different medication
- Other: Family therapy, sensate conditioning; referral to specialized sex therapy

COMPLEMENTARY AND ALTERNATIVE MEDICINE
- Yohimbe: Not recommended, potentially dangerous
- Ginseng and St. John's wort have no evidence to support treatment of sexual dysfunction.

ONGOING CARE

DIET
Weight reduction if needed for either partner

PATIENT EDUCATION
- In the US, sex therapists and counselors can be found through the American Association of Sex Educators, Counselors and Therapists: www.aasect.org.
- National Women's Health Resource Center: www.Healthywomen.org
- North American Menopause Society: www.menopause.org
- National Vulvodynia Association: www.nva.org

PROGNOSIS
Lack of desire is most difficult type to treat, with <50% success.

REFERENCES

1. Shifren JL, Monz BU, Russo PA, et al. Sexual problems and distress in United States women: Prevalence and correlates. *Obstet Gynecol*. 2008;112:970–978.
2. Safarinejad MR, Hosseini SY, Asgari MA, et al. A randomized, double-blind, placebo-controlled study of the efficacy and safety of bupropion for treating hypoactive sexual desire disorder in ovulating women. *BJU Int*. 2010;106:832–839.
3. Safarinejad MR. Reversal of SSRI-induced female sexual dysfunction by adjunctive bupropion in menstruating women: A double-blind, placebo-controlled and randomized study. *J Psychopharmacol (Oxford)*. 2011;25:370–378.
4. Somboonporn W, Davis S, Seif MW, et al. Testosterone for peri- and postmenopausal women. *Cochrane Database Syst Rev*. 2010.CD004509.
5. Woodis CB, McLendon AN, Muzyk AJ, et al. Testosterone supplementation for hypoactive sexual desire disorder in women. *Pharmacotherapy*. 2012;32:38–53.
6. Tan O, Bradshaw K, Carr BR, et al. Management of vulvovaginal atrophy-related sexual dysfunction in postmenopausal women: An up-to-date review. *Menopause*. 2012;19:109–117.
7. Suckling J, Lethaby A, Kennedy R, et al. Local oestrogen for vaginal atrophy in postmenopausal women. *Cochrane Database Syst Rev*. 2006;(4): CD001500.

ADDITIONAL READING
- Barrett G, Pendry E, Peacock J, et al. Women's sexual health after childbirth. *BJOG*. 2000;107:186–195.
- Basaria S, Dobs AS. Safety and adverse effects of androgens: How to counsel patients. *Mayo Clin Proc*. 2004;79:S25–32.
- Basson R, Wierman ME, van Lankveld J, et al. Summary of the recommendations on sexual dysfunctions in women. *J Sex Med*. 2010;7: 314–326.
- Blumel JE, Del Pino M, Aprikian D, et al. Effect of androgens combined with hormone therapy on quality of life in post-menopausal women with sexual dysfunction. *Gynecol Endocrinol*. 2008;24: 691.
- Braunstein GD. Safety of testosterone treatment in postmenopausal women. *Fertil Steril*. 2007;88:1.
- Laumann EO, Nicolosi A, Glasser DB, et al. Sexual problems among women and men aged 40–80 y: Prevalence and correlates identified in the Global Study of Sexual Attitudes and Behaviors. *Int J Impot Res*. 2005;17:39–57.
- Meston CM, Bradford A. Sexual dysfunctions in women. *Annu Rev Clin Psychol*. 2007;3:233–256.
- Modelska K. Female sexual dysfunction in postmenopausal women: Systematic review of placebo-controlled trials. *Am J Obstet Gynecol*. 2003;188:286.
- Rudkin L, Taylor MJ, Hawton K. Strategies for managing sexual dysfunction induced by antidepressant medication. *Cochrane Database Syst Rev*. 2013:CD003382.
- The role of testosterone therapy in postmenopausal women: Position statement of the North American Menopause Society. *Menopause*. 2005;12:497.

CODES

ICD10
- F52.0 Hypoactive sexual desire disorder
- N94.1 Dyspareunia
- R37 Sexual dysfunction, unspecified

CLINICAL PEARLS
- Female sexual dysfunction is a common, complex, multifactorial problem.
- Most commonly, patients with sexual dysfunction have a completely normal physical exam.
- Symptoms of sexual dysfunction peak during perimenopause between the ages of 45 and 64, even though hormone levels of estrogen and testosterone may fall in the normal range; women often benefit from hormone supplementation with estrogen and/or testosterone.
- Encourage follow-up with counseling for marriage, individual, and/or sex therapy.
- Use of hormonal contraception in premenopausal women can be associated with complaints of decreased libido.

SHIN SPLINTS
Kyle Kutsche, MD • Ryan Pearson, MD

BASICS

DESCRIPTION
- American Medical Association defines shin splints as "pain or discomfort in the leg from repetitive running on hard surfaces or forcible excessive use of the foot flexors":
  - Definition excludes stress fracture or pain from ischemic origin
- Periostitis caused by excessive stress on the medial border of the tibia
- Synonym(s): Medial tibial stress syndrome (preferred term); Medial tibial periostalgia; Tibial periostitis; Shin soreness; Tibial stress syndrome; Medial tibial syndrome

EPIDEMIOLOGY
Incidence
Can account for 4–35% of all running injuries (1)

ETIOLOGY AND PATHOPHYSIOLOGY
- Somewhat controversial, with many different theories, including:
  - Bone stress reaction
  - Periostitis
  - Periostalgia
  - Periosteum traction
  - Low bone mineral density
  - Tendinopathy
  - Periosteal remodeling
- Several structures possibly involved or implicated, including:
  - Soleus
  - Deep crural fascia
  - Flexor digitorum longus
  - Flexor hallucis longus
  - Tibialis posterior
- Likely multifactorial, drawing from biomechanical, anatomic, and environmental causes

RISK FACTORS
- Runners (particularly sprinters and hurdlers)
- Dancers (particularly ballet)
- Gymnasts, basketball players
- Military personnel
- Usually categorized into intrinsic (personal) and extrinsic (environmental) factors (1,2):
  - Intrinsic factors:
    - Overpronation/Increased navicular drop
    - Hindfoot valgus
    - Female sex
    - Increased hip internal/external range of motion
    - Higher body mass index
    - Leaner calf girth
  - Extrinsic factors:
    - Previous history of shin splints
    - Inexperienced runner
  - Other factors thought to contribute (but lack study support):
    - Training errors (increased mileage, increased intensity of workout)
    - Low calcium intake in female athletes
    - Running on hard or inclined surfaces
    - Running while wearing worn-out footwear

GENERAL PREVENTION
Suggested recommendations include:
- Screening for overpronation
- Designing appropriate training regimen/identifying training errors
- Regular stretching, strength, and flexibility exercises
- Cross training
- Rehabilitation of previous injuries
- Wearing proper footwear

DIAGNOSIS

HISTORY
- Pain along the junction of the middle and distal thirds of the posteromedial tibia (most common) or anterior tibia, described as "dull ache" or "soreness"
- Pain with exercise (commonly bilateral) that dissipates with rest:
  - Severe shin splints may cause persistent pain at rest or pain with only mild activity, and the character of the pain can become "sharp" or "penetrating."
- Pain subsides or is gone at rest in shin splints, compared with a stress fracture of the tibia (in which pain persists with rest):
  - There can be considerable overlap of signs and symptoms between shin splints and stress fractures.

PHYSICAL EXAM
- Generalized tenderness to palpation along the medial border of the tibia with possible mild swelling
- Pain with resisted plantar flexion or toe raises
- Clinical presentation may closely resemble that of stress fractures and exertional compartment syndrome, which can carry a far worse prognosis:
  - Stress fracture tenderness usually is more localized.
  - Exertional compartment syndrome has characteristic physical findings:
    - Anterolateral leg pain (described as "cramplike, tight, squeezing ache")
    - Most commonly over the anterior compartment
    - Fascial hernias may be present.
    - Tenderness not usually noted on direct palpation.
    - Depending on the compartment affected, characteristic weakness and/or paresthesias also can be present.

DIFFERENTIAL DIAGNOSIS
- Bone:
  - Stress fractures
- Muscle/Tendon:
  - Chronic exertional compartment syndrome
  - Acute tendinitis
  - Muscle strain/muscle tear/fascial defects
- Vascular disease
- Popliteal artery entrapment:
  - Popliteal artery aneurysm
  - Claudication
  - Deep vein thrombosis
- Nerve entrapment:
  - Lumbar radiculopathy
  - Peroneal nerve entrapment
- Infection: Osteomyelitis
- Malignancy: Sarcoma or osteosarcoma (3)

DIAGNOSTIC TESTS & INTERPRETATION
- Serial plain radiographs are often normal but are needed to rule out stress fractures, which usually are positive after 2 weeks of symptoms.
- A bone scan for shin splints reveals diffuse, linear uptake along the posteromedial border of the tibia on the delayed phase, whereas a bone scan for stress fracture reveals localized, more intense, fusiform, or transverse uptake in all phases.
- MRI not necessary but may reveal periosteal edema and can be used to identify a stress fracture earlier (4).
- Compartment pressure measurement with exercise may be needed to diagnose exertional compartment syndrome if pain is anterolateral.

TREATMENT

- Acute-phase treatment includes reducing training activity below symptom level or, if it is a serious case, the patient may need to stop activity altogether; ice the area of injury (5)[C].
- Recovery time is variable.
- Exercises to consider: www.youtube.com/watch?v= kv6ycmOWnq0
- Running in a pool or bicycling can aid in keeping up with conditioning while rehabilitation occurs.
- Options mostly based on expert opinion and clinical experience (5).
- Although exercising and modifying training schedules have been suggested as interventions to reduce injury, there is little to no evidence to support this (6)[A].

MEDICATION
First Line
- NSAIDs
- Analgesics

ADDITIONAL THERAPIES

- Physical therapy (5)[C]:
  - Therapist-determined modalities
  - Strengthening, stretching, and flexibility exercises after acute symptoms disappear
- Whirlpool, phonophoresis, electrical stimulation, US, augmented soft-tissue mobilization, and acupuncture can be considered (5)[C].

SURGERY/OTHER PROCEDURES

- Only after a documented trial of maximal nonoperative treatment (for at least 6 months) has failed should posterior medial fascia release be considered:
  - Consider if there is severe limitation of physical activity or frequent recurrence of pain despite proper rehabilitation (7)[C].
- Extracorporeal shock wave therapy (ESWT) is a possible alternative to surgical treatment and, when combined with a running program, may lead to quicker recovery. More investigation is needed on this mode of therapy (8,9)[B].

COMPLEMENTARY AND ALTERNATIVE MEDICINE

- Orthotic or shoe modification if there is significant foot pronation
- Evidence for shock-absorbing orthotics reducing the incidence of shin splints is limited at best (6)[A].

 # ONGOING CARE

PATIENT EDUCATION

- Identifying training errors and avoiding a rush back to preinjury pace will help to prevent recurrence.
- Emphasize the importance of modified activity followed by stretching and strengthening exercises.
- Resumption of activity should be done gradually, below the level of the symptoms.
- Exercises for stretching: See www.youtube.com/watch?v=7vZVq3ov914

PROGNOSIS

- Most patients respond well to nonoperative treatment.
- Gradual return to activity can be expected.

COMPLICATIONS

- If shin splints are not addressed, the degree of leg pain can interfere with activities of daily living, and stress fractures/true fractures may occur.
- Undiagnosed stress fracture can lead to complete fracture and displacement.
- Undiagnosed chronic compartment syndrome could develop into an acute syndrome with possible tissue necrosis.

REFERENCES

1. Reshef N, Guelich DR. Medial tibial stress syndrome. *Clin Sports Med*. 2012;31(2):273–290.
2. Moen MH, Tol JL, Weir A, et al. Medial tibial stress syndrome: A critical review. *Sports Med*. 2009; 39:523–546.
3. Brewer RB, Gregory AJ. Chronic lower leg pain in athletes: A guide for the differential diagnosis, evaluation, and treatment. *Sports Health*. 2012;4(2):121–127.
4. Spiker AM, Dixit S, Cosgarea AJ. Triathlon: Running injuries. *Sports Med Arthrosc Rev*. 2012;20(4): 206-213.
5. Galbraith RM, Lavallee ME. Medial tibial stress syndrome: Conservative treatment options. *Curr Rev Musculoskelet Med*. 2009;2:127–133.
6. Yeung SS, Yeung EW, Gillespie LD, et al. Interventions for preventing lower limb soft-tissue running injuries. *Cochrane Database Syst Rev*. 2011;CD001256.
7. Yates B, Allen MJ, Barnes MR. Outcome of surgical treatment of medial tibial stress syndrome. *J Bone Joint Surg Am*. 2003;85-A:1974–1980.
8. Moen MH, Rayer S, Schipper M, et al. Shockwave treatment for medial tibial stress syndrome in athletes; a prospective controlled study. *Br J Sports Med*. 2012;46(4):253–257. Epub 2011 Mar 9.
9. Rompe JD, Cacchio A, Furia JP, et al. Low-energy extracorporeal shock wave therapy as a treatment for medial tibial stress syndrome. *Am J Sports Med*. 2010;38:125–132.

ADDITIONAL READING

- Lopes AD, Hespanhol Jnior LC, Yeung SS, Costa LO. What are the main running-related musculoskeletal injuries? A systematic review. *Sports Med*. 2012 Oct 1;42(10):891-905. doi:10.2165/11631170-000000000-00000.
- Aweid O, Gallie R, Morrissey D, et al. Medial tibial pain pressure threshold algometry in runners. *Knee Surg Sports Traumatol Arthrosc*. 2013 Jun 6. Epub ahead of print

 ## CODES

ICD10

- S86.891A Other injury of other muscle(s) and tendon(s) at lower leg level, right leg, initial encounter
- S86.892A Other injury of other muscle(s) and tendon(s) at lower leg level, left leg, initial encounter
- S86.899A Other injury of other muscle(s) and tendon(s) at lower leg level, unspecified leg, initial encounter

CLINICAL PEARLS

- *Medial tibial stress syndrome* is the much more anatomically accurate and preferred term.
- Diagnosis is usually made clinically by pain, most commonly in the middle and distal thirds of the posteromedial border of the tibia that comes on with activity and reduces or resolves with rest; this is contrasted with a stress fracture, in which the pain persists with rest.
- Relative rest, ice, and NSAIDs are the generally agreed-upon mainstays of treatment.

SHOULDER PAIN

Gregory Murphy, MD • J. Herbert Stevenson, MD

 BASICS

DESCRIPTION

Shoulder pain is a common condition, affecting patients of all ages:

- Causes include acute trauma or overuse during sports and activities of everyday living.
- Age plays an important role in determining the etiology of shoulder pain.
- Onset and characteristics of pain, weakness, mechanism of injury, and functional limitation help in accurately diagnosing shoulder pain.

EPIDEMIOLOGY

- Shoulder pain accounts for 16% of all musculoskeletal complaints.
- The lifetime prevalence of shoulder pain is as high as 70% (1).
- Predominant age:
  - <30 years: Shoulder instability
  - >30 years: Rotator cuff (RTC) disorder:
    ○ 30–50 years: Tendinopathy
    ○ 40–60 years: Partial tear
    ○ >60 years: Full-thickness tear
  - >60 years: Osteoarthritis (OA) of the glenohumeral joint

Incidence

The incidence of shoulder pain is 6.6–25 cases/1,000 patients, with a peak incidence in the 4th–6th decades.

ETIOLOGY AND PATHOPHYSIOLOGY

Depends on underlying etiology

- Trauma (fracture, dislocation, ligament/tendon tear, Acromioclavicular (AC) separation)
- Overuse (RTC pathology, biceps tenosynovitis, bursitis, muscle strain):
  - RTC disorders most commonly occur from repetitive overhead activity. This leads to impingement of the RTC that can progress through 3 stages:
    ○ Stage I: Tendinopathy
    ○ Stage II: Partial RTC tear
    ○ Stage III: Full-thickness RTC tear
  - Subacromial bursitis can occur with RTC disorders, but is rarely an isolated diagnosis.
- Age-related (AC and glenohumeral joint OA, adhesive capsulitis, RTC tear; pediatric athletes instability and physial injuries)
- Rheumatologic (rheumatoid arthritis, polymyalgia rheumatica, fibromyalgia)
- Referred pain (neck, gallbladder)

RISK FACTORS

- Repetitive overhead activities
- Overhead and upper extremity weight-bearing sports (baseball, softball, swimming)
- Weight lifting: Acromioclavicular (AC) disorders
- Rapid increases in training frequency, improper technique
- Muscle weakness or imbalance
- Trauma or fall onto the shoulder
- Diabetes, thyroid disorders, female gender, age 40–60 years are risk factors for adhesive capsulitis.

GENERAL PREVENTION

- Maintenance of good shoulder strength and range of motion (ROM)
- Avoidance of repetitive overhead activities
- Proper technique (pitching, weight-lifting)

 DIAGNOSIS

Majority of shoulder pain is diagnosed in the outpatient setting.

HISTORY

- Characteristic of pain:
  - Superior shoulder pain: AC pathology, trapezius strain
  - Lateral/Deltoid pain: RTC pathology (RTC pain typically does not extend past elbow)
  - Diffuse pain: RTC pathology, adhesive capsulitis, glenohumeral OA
  - Nighttime pain: RTC pathology (pain when laying on affected side), adhesive capsulitis, glenohumeral OA
  - Stiff shoulder: Adhesive capsulitis (increased risk in diabetic patients)
  - Pain with cross-body activities: AC pathology
  - Pain with abduction/external rotation (reaching behind): Shoulder instability
  - Pain with overhead activity: RTC pathology, AC pathology, labrum pathology
  - Pain with turning toward neck, pain past elbow: Cervical pathology
- Mechanism of injury:
  - Fall on outstretched hand: Traumatic shoulder instability/dislocation
  - Fall directly onto shoulder: AC joint sprain, clavicle fracture
  - Repetitive overhead activity: RTC pathology
- Age:
  - Shoulder instability (subluxation, dislocation, multidirectional instability) is most common cause of shoulder pain in the young athlete (<30 years old).
  - RTC disorders are the most common cause of shoulder pain in patients >30 years old. Severity of RTC disorder also increases with age:
    ○ Tendinopathy: 30–50 years old
    ○ Partial RTC tear: 40–60 years old
    ○ Full-thickness tear: >60 years old
  - Older patients (>60 years old) more likely to have OA
  - Trauma in a young person <40 more commonly associated with dislocation/subluxation; in a person >40 trauma more commonly associated with RTC tear.

PHYSICAL EXAM

- Observe as patient takes off jacket, moves arm, shakes hand.
- Inspect for malalignment, muscle atrophy, asymmetry, erythema, ecchymosis, or swelling. Scapular winging suggests long thoracic nerve or muscular (trapezius, serratus anterior) dysfunction.
- Palpate for tenderness, warmth, bony step-offs.
- Evaluate active and passive ROM and flexibility:
  - Decreased active AND passive ROM: Adhesive capsulitis:
    ○ Mildly decreased active and/or passive ROM can also indicate glenohumeral OA.
  - Decreased active, full passive ROM: RTC pathology
- Evaluate for muscle strength.
- Special tests:
  - Neer (stabilize the scapula and with the thumb pointing down and passively flex the arm- assess for pain), Hawkins (stabilize the scapula, passively abduct shoulder to 90 degrees, flex shoulder to 30 degrees, flex the elbow to 90 degrees, and internally rotate the shoulder and assess for pain): RTC impingement
  - Pain with strength testing the supraspinatus (empty can test), infraspinatus/teres minor (resisted external rotation), subscapularis (lift-off test, resisted internal rotation): RTC pathology. Weakness could suggest tear.
  - Drop-arm test: RTC tear
  - Cross-arm adduction test: AC joint arthritis
  - Speed test (flex the shoulder to 90 degrees with the arm supinated and provide downward resistance against shoulder flexion) and the Yergason test (flex elbow to 90 degrees, shake hands with patient, and provide resistance against supination and assess for pain): Biceps tendinopathy
  - Apprehension, relocation test: Anterior glenohumeral joint instability
  - Sulcus sign: Inferior glenohumeral joint instability
  - O'Brien, clunk test: Labral pathology
  - Spurling test (with the patient's head extended and rotated toward the painful shoulder, apply an axial load to the cervical spine; assess for pain): Cervical pathology

DIFFERENTIAL DIAGNOSIS

- Fracture (clavicle, humerus, scapula), contusion
- RTC disorder: Impingement, tear, calcific tendonitis
- Subacromial bursitis
- AC joint pathology (AC separation/OA)
- Biceps tenosynovitis or tear
- Glenohumeral joint OA
- Glenohumeral joint instability (acute dislocation or chronic multidirectional instability)
- Adhesive capsulitis
- Labral tear or associated bony pathology
- Muscle strain (trapezius, deltoid, biceps)
- Cervical radiculopathy
- Other: Autoimmune, rheumatologic, referred pain

DIAGNOSTIC TESTS & INTERPRETATION

- Most shoulder pain can be diagnosed by history and physical exam:
  - Adults with nontraumatic shoulder pain of <4 weeks may not require initial imaging.
- When diagnosis remains unclear, surgery is considered.
- History of significant trauma, prolonged symptoms, or red flags (older age, fever, rest pain) suggests that further studies may be indicated.
- Plain radiographs are first-line imaging:
  - Can assess for fracture, degenerative changes, signs of dislocation (Bankart, Hill-Sachs deformity), signs of large RTC tear (sclerosis, humeral head proximal migration), anatomic deformities contributing to impingement, occult tumor
  - Standard views: Anteroposterior, scapular Y, axillary
- EMG study of the upper extremity may help differentiate cervical pain referred to the shoulder from a primary shoulder disorder.
- Obtain ECG if any suspicion for cardiac etiology of left shoulder pain.
- Appropriate rheumatologic tests may be indicated if autoimmune etiology considered.

Follow-Up Tests & Special Considerations

- CT scan may rule out occult fracture.
- MRI is gold standard for noninvasive imaging of soft-tissue structures, including RTC, biceps tendon.
- MR arthrogram may be needed to assess for labral tears or small/partial RTC tears.
- US is gaining recognition in screening for shoulder pathologies, including RTC tears, biceps tendinopathies, and AC joint disorders (1)[B].

Diagnostic Procedures/Other

Diagnostic arthroscopy may be used in the proper setting after noninterventional means have been exhausted and structural injury is suspected.

Test Interpretation

Depends on underlying diagnosis:

- Tendinosis rather than tendonitis is often found with stage I impingement.
- Scarring of the shoulder capsule is the hallmark of adhesive capsulitis.
- Calcifications can be found in rotator cuff tendons with calcific tendonitis.

TREATMENT

Treatment is based on underlying pathology but, in general, conservative therapy includes relative rest, analgesics, and/or anti-inflammatory medicines; there is little evidence to support or refute many common interventions for shoulder pain (2)[A].

MEDICATION

First Line

- Analgesics and anti-inflammatory medications may be required for symptomatic relief of shoulder pain:
  - Ibuprofen: 200–800 mg t.i.d.
  - Naprosyn: 250–500 mg b.i.d.
  - Acetaminophen: Up to 3–4 g/d
- Corticosteroid injections (subacromial, glenohumeral) may acutely relieve pain: RTC pathology, adhesive capsulitis, OA (2,3)[B]. Effect may be enhanced if US-guided (4)[B].

ISSUES FOR REFERRAL

Shoulder pain where etiology remains unclear, nonresponsive to conservative care, complicated or displaced fractures, large RTC tears

ADDITIONAL THERAPIES

- Physical therapy may provide benefit if unimproved with conservative measures—consider for RTC disorders, adhesive capsulitis, shoulder instability (3,5,6)[B].
- Physical therapy/exercise may improve nonspecific shoulder pain, but it does not generally improve ROM or function (7)[B].
- Manual manipulative therapy by chiropractors, osteopathic physicians, or physical therapists can improve pain with adhesive capsulitis, RTC, and soft-tissue disorders (8)[B].

SURGERY/OTHER PROCEDURES

Surgery is necessary for shoulder pain caused by acute displaced fractures, large rotator cuff tears, shoulder dislocation in patients <20 years of age. Surgery may be necessary for shoulder pain unresponsive to conservative measures >3–6 months.

COMPLEMENTARY AND ALTERNATIVE MEDICINE

Acupuncture may help in the acute setting, although there is no conclusive evidence for its effectiveness.

ONGOING CARE

FOLLOW-UP RECOMMENDATIONS

Limiting overhead activity may reduce the symptoms of impingement syndrome.

PATIENT EDUCATION

Refer to specific diagnosis for shoulder pain.

PROGNOSIS

Shoulder pain generally has a favorable outcome with conservative care, but recovery can be slow, with 40–50% with persistent pain or recurrence at 12 months (1).

REFERENCES

1. Cadagon A, Laslett M. A prospective study of shoulder pain in primary care: Prevalence of imaged pathology and response to guided diagnostic blocks. *BMC Musculoskel Disord*. 2011;28(12):119.
2. Gross C, Dhawan A, Harwood D, Gochanour E, Romeo A. Glenohumeral joint injections: A review. *Sports Health*. 2013;(5)2:153–159.
3. Favejee MM, Huisstede BM, Koes BW. Frozen shoulder: The effectiveness of conservative and surgical interventions: A systematic review. *Br J Sports Med*. 2011;45(1):49–56.
4. Soh E, Li W. Image guided versus blind corticosteroid injections in adults with shoulder pain: A systematic review. *BMC Musculoskel Disord*. 2011;12(1):137.
5. Littlewood C, Ashton J, Chance-Larsen K, et al. Exercise for rotator cuff tendinopathy: A systematic review. *Physiotherapy*. 2012;98(2):101–109.
6. Green S, Buchbinder R, Hetrick SE. Physiotherapy interventions for shoulder pain. *Cochrane Database Syst Rev*. 2010:CD004258.
7. van den Dolder PA, Ferriera PH, Refshauge KM. Effectiveness of soft tissue massage and exercise for the treatment of non-specific shoulder pain: A systematic review with meta-analysis. *Br J Sports Med*. 2012.
8. Brantingham JW, Cassa TK. Manipulative therapy for shoulder pain and disorders: An expansion of a systematic review. *J Manipulative Ther*. 2011;34(5):314–316.

ADDITIONAL READING

- Celik D, Sirmen B, Demirhan M. The relationship of muscle strength and pain in subacromial impingement. *Acta Orthop Traumatol Turk*. 2011;45(2):79–84.
- Sipola P, Niemitukia L. Detection and quantification of rotator cuff tears with ultrasonography and MRI—a prospective study in 77 consecutive patients with a surgical reference. *Ultrasound Med Biol*. 2010;36(12):1981–1989.

CODES

ICD10

- M19.019 Primary osteoarthritis, unspecified shoulder
- M25.519 Pain in unspecified shoulder
- S43.429A Sprain of unspecified rotator cuff capsule, init encntr

CLINICAL PEARLS

- Rotator cuff disorders (tendinopathy, tears) are the most common source of shoulder pain in individuals >30 years of age.
- Shoulder instability (acute dislocation/subluxation or chronic instability) is the most common source of shoulder pain in individuals <30 years of age.
- Patients with diabetes are at increased risk for adhesive capsulitis.

SINUSITIS
Adarsh K. Gupta, DO, MS, FACOFP

 BASICS

DESCRIPTION
- Acute sinusitis is a symptomatic inflammation of ≥1 paranasal sinuses of <4 weeks' duration resulting from impaired drainage and retained secretions. Because rhinitis and sinusitis usually coexist, "rhinosinusitis" is the preferred term.
- Disease is subacute when symptomatic for 4–12 weeks and chronic when symptomatic for >12 weeks.
- System(s) affected: Head/Eyes/Ears/Nose/Throat (HEENT); Pulmonary

EPIDEMIOLOGY
- Affects 31 million individuals in the US each year
- Diagnosis of acute bacterial rhinosinusitis remains the 5th leading reason for prescribing antibiotics.
- 2% of viral rhinosinusitis episodes have a bacterial superinfection.

Incidence
Incidence highest in early fall through early spring (related to incidence of viral upper respiratory infection [URI]). Adults have 2–3 viral URIs per year; 90% of these colds are accompanied by viral rhinosinusitis. It is 5th most common diagnosis made during family physician visits.

ETIOLOGY AND PATHOPHYSIOLOGY
- Important features:
  - Inflammation and edema of the sinus mucosa
  - Obstruction of the sinus ostia
  - Impaired mucociliary clearance
- Secretions that are not cleared become hospitable to bacterial growth.
- Inflammatory response (neutrophil influx and release of cytokines) damages mucosal surfaces.
- Viral: Vast majority of cases (rhinovirus, influenza A and B; parainfluenza virus; respiratory syncytial; adeno-, corona-, and enteroviruses)
- Bacterial (complicates 0.2–2% of viral cases):
  - More likely if symptoms worsen after 5–7 days or do not improve >10 days
  - *S. pneumoniae, H. influenzae,* and *M. catarrhalis* are the most common bacterial pathogens.
  - Often overdiagnosed, which leads to overuse of and increasing resistance to antibiotics
  - MRSA present in 0–15.9% of patients (1)
- Fungal: Seen in immunocompromised hosts (uncontrolled diabetes, neutropenia, use of corticosteroids) or as a nosocomial infection

Genetics
No known genetic pattern

RISK FACTORS
- Viral URI
- Allergic rhinitis
- Asthma
- Cigarette smoking
- Dental infections and procedures
- Anatomic variations:
  - Tonsillar and adenoid hypertrophy
  - Turbinate hypertrophy, nasal polyps
  - Cleft palate
- Immunodeficiency (e.g., HIV)
- Cystic fibrosis

GENERAL PREVENTION
Hand washing to prevent transmission of viral infection

 DIAGNOSIS

- History and physical exam suggest and establish the diagnosis, but are rarely helpful in distinguishing bacterial from viral causes.
- Use a constellation of symptoms rather than a particular sign or symptom in diagnosis.

HISTORY
- Symptoms somewhat predictive of bacterial sinusitis:
  - Worsening of symptoms >5–7 days after initial improvement
  - Persistent symptoms for ≥10 days
  - Persistent purulent nasal discharge
  - Unilateral upper tooth or facial pain
  - Unilateral maxillary sinus tenderness
  - Fever
- Associated symptoms:
  - Headache
  - Nasal congestion
  - Retro-orbital pain
  - Otalgia
  - Hyposomia
  - Halitosis
  - Chronic cough
- Symptoms requiring urgent attention:
  - Visual disturbances, especially diplopia
  - Periorbital swelling or erythema
  - Altered mental status

PHYSICAL EXAM
- Fever
- Edema and erythema of nasal mucosa
- Purulent discharge
- Tenderness to palpation over sinus(es)
- Transillumination of the sinuses may confirm fluid in sinuses (helpful if asymmetric; not helpful if symmetric exam).

Pediatric Considerations
- Sinuses are not fully developed until age 20. Maxillary and ethmoid sinuses, although small, are present from birth.
- Since children have an average of 6–8 colds per year, they are at risk for developing sinusitis.
- Diagnosis can be more difficult than in adults because symptoms are often more subtle.

DIFFERENTIAL DIAGNOSIS
- Dental disease
- Cystic fibrosis (CF)
- Wegener granulomatosis
- HIV infection
- Kartagener syndrome
- Neoplasm
- Headache, tension, or migraine

DIAGNOSTIC TESTS & INTERPRETATION
Diagnostic tests are not routinely recommended; no diagnostic tests can adequately differentiate between viral and bacterial rhinosinusitis.
- None indicated in routine evaluation
- Routine use of sinus radiography discouraged because:
  - ≥3 clinical findings have similar diagnostic accuracy as imaging.

- Imaging does not distinguish viral from bacterial etiology.
- Limited coronal CT scan can be useful in recurrent infection or failure to respond to medical therapy.

Diagnostic Procedures/Other
Sinus CT if signs suggest extrasinus involvement or to evaluate chronic rhinosinusitis (2)[C]

Test Interpretation
- Inflammation, edema, thickened mucosa
- Impaired ciliary function
- Metaplasia of ciliated columnar cells
- Relative acidosis and hypoxia within sinuses
- Polyps

 TREATMENT

Most cases resolve with supportive care (treating pain, nasal symptoms). Antibiotics should be reserved for symptoms that persist >10 days or worsen in 5–7 days.

GENERAL MEASURES
- Hydration
- Steam inhalation 20–30 minutes t.i.d.
- Saline irrigation (Neti pot) or nose drops
- Sleep with head of bed elevated.
- Avoid exposure to cigarette smoke or fumes.
- Avoid caffeine and alcohol.
- Antibiotics indicated only when findings suggest bacterial infection
- Analgesics, NSAIDs
- Acute viral sinusitis is self-limiting; antibiotics should not be used.

MEDICATION
First Line
- Decongestants:
  - Pseudoephedrine HCl
  - Phenylephrine nasal spray (limited use)
  - Oxymetazoline nasal spray (e.g., Afrin) (not to be used >3 days)
- Analgesics:
  - Acetaminophen
  - Aspirin
  - NSAIDs
  - Codeine (for severe cases)
- Antibiotics:
  - Antibiotics have a slight advantage over placebo, yet most improve without therapy.
  - Reserve antibiotic use for patients with moderate-to-severe disease (3)[A].
  - Treat for 10–14 days unless otherwise specified.
  - Choice should be based on understanding of antibiotic resistance in the community.
  - Initial therapy (narrow-spectrum antibiotics) (4,5)[A]:
    o Amoxicillin: 500 mg t.i.d. (adults); 80–90 mg/kg/d divided q8h (children)
    o Trimethoprim-sulfamethoxazole (TMP/SMX): 160/800 mg q12h in adults and 8–12 mg/kg/d of trimethoprim component divided q12h for children
    o Doxycycline: 100 mg PO b.i.d. (adults only)
- Since allergies may be a predisposing factor, some patients may benefit from use of the following agents:
  - Oral antihistamines:

- Loratadine (Claritin), fexofenadine (Allegra), cetirizine (Zyrtec), desloratadine (Clarinex), or levocetirizine (Xyzal)
  - Chlorpheniramine (Chlor-Trimeton)
  - Diphenhydramine (Benadryl)
- Leukotriene inhibitors (Singulair, Accolate), especially in patients with asthma
- Nasal steroids (i.e., fluticasone Flonase])

Second Line
- Amoxicillin-clavulanate (Augmentin): 875/125 mg q12h (adults); 30 mg/kg/d of amoxicillin component divided b.i.d. in children
- High-dose amoxicillin-clavulanate (Augmentin XR) b.i.d. in adults and Augmentin ES-600 in children (for both β-lactam and penicillin-binding protein resistance)
- Cefpodoxime (Vantin): 200 mg q12h in adults and 10 mg/kg/d divided b.i.d. in children
- Cefuroxime axetil (Ceftin): 250 mg q12h in adults and 30 mg/kg/d divided q12h in children
- Azithromycin (Zithromax): 500 mg on day 1 and 250 mg on days 2–5 in adults; 10 mg/kg on day 1 and 5 mg/kg on days 2–5 in children
- Clarithromycin (Biaxin): 500 mg b.i.d. (regular) or 1,000 mg/d (extended release) in adults; 15 mg/kg/d divided b.i.d. in children
- Levofloxacin (Levaquin): 750 mg/d for 5 days (adults only)
- If no response to first-line therapy after 72 hours, or if patients have had antibiotics within the past 4–6 weeks, use or change to:
  - High-dose amoxicillin-clavulanate
  - Cephalosporins as above
  - Fluoroquinolones as above
- *Note:* Bacteriologic failure rates of up to 20–25% are possible with use of azithromycin and clarithromycin (4)[C].
- If lack of response to 3 weeks of antibiotics, consider:
  - CT scan of sinuses
  - Ear/Nose/Throat (ENT) referral

ISSUES FOR REFERRAL
Complications or failure of treatment

ADDITIONAL THERAPIES

ALERT
- Meta-analyses have demonstrated no benefit of newer antibiotics over amoxicillin, trimethoprim-sulfamethoxazole, or doxycycline (4)[A].
- Antibiotics recommendations vary with different guidelines. Patients seen by specialists are different from those in a primary care setting. Patients usually do not have complicated sinusitis in primary care setting:
  - American Academy of Otolaryngology-Head and Neck Surgery Foundation (6)[B] recommends:
    - Consider watchful waiting without antibiotics in patients with uncomplicated mild illness (mild pain and temperature <101°F) with assurance of follow-up.
    - If decision is made to treat with antibiotics, use amoxicillin as first-line therapy for most adults.
  - Infectious Disease Society of America (7)[B] recommends:
    - Start antibiotics as soon as clinical diagnosis of acute bacterial sinusitis is made.
    - Use amoxicillin-clavulanate rather than amoxicillin alone.

- Treat for 5–7 days in adults if uncomplicated bacterial rhinosinusitis (IDSA low-moderate-quality evidence). Treat for 10–14 days in children if uncomplicated bacterial rhinosinusitis (IDSA low-moderate-quality evidence).
- American Academy of Pediatrics (8)[B] recommends:
   Amoxicillin: 45–90 mg/kg/d in 2 divided doses if uncomplicated acute bacterial sinusitis in children
  - Amoxicillin-clavulanate: 80–90 mg/6.4 mg/kg/d in 2 divided doses for children with severe illness, recent antibiotics, or attending day care.
- Use of intranasal steroids produces modest improvement in symptoms when used alone or in combination with antibiotics (1)[B].
- Precautions:
  - Decongestants can exacerbate hypertension.
  - Intranasal decongestants should be limited to 3 days to avoid rebound nasal congestion.
  - Significant possible interactions:
    - Warfarin (Coumadin): Increased INR with macrolides or TMP/SMX.
    - Stop statins temporarily with macrolides due to increased risk of myopathy and rhabdomyolysis.

Pregnancy Considerations
- Nasal irrigation with saline, pseudoephedrine, most antihistamines, and some nasal steroids are safe during pregnancy and lactation.
- Antibiotics safe in pregnancy and lactation:
  - Amoxicillin, amoxicillin-clavulanate, cephalosporins, azithromycin
- Antibiotic contraindicated: Clarithromycin
- Antibiotic safe in lactation but not pregnancy: Levofloxacin

SURGERY/OTHER PROCEDURES
- If medical therapy fails, consider sinus irrigation.
- Functional endoscopic sinus surgery is the preferred treatment for medically recalcitrant cases (4)[C].
- Absolute surgical indications:
  - Massive nasal polyposis
  - Acute complications: Subperiosteal or orbital abscess, frontal soft-tissue spread of infection
  - Mucocele or mucopyocele
  - Invasive or allergic fungal sinusitis
  - Suspected obstructing tumor
  - CSF rhinorrhea

IN-PATIENT CONSIDERATIONS
Hospitalization for complications (e.g., meningitis, orbital cellulitis or abscess, brain abscess)

ONGOING CARE

FOLLOW-UP RECOMMENDATIONS
Return if no improvement after 72 hours or no resolution of symptoms after 10 days of antibiotics.

PATIENT EDUCATION
- http://familydoctor.org
- http://medlineplus.gov

PROGNOSIS
Alleviation of symptoms within 72 hours with complete resolution within 10–14 days

COMPLICATIONS
- Serious complications are rare.
- Meningitis, orbital cellulitis, brain abscess
- Cavernous sinus thrombosis
- Osteomyelitis, subdural empyema

REFERENCES

1. Zalmanovici A. Steroids for acute sinusitis. *Cochrane Database Sys Rev.* 2007;2:CD005149.
2. Dykewicz MS, Hamilos DL. Rhinitis and sinusitis. *J Allergy Clin Immunol.* 2010;125:S103–S115.
3. CDC Get Smart. http://www.cdc.gov/getsmart/ (Assessed 5/2/2012)
4. Varonen H, Mäkelä M, Savolainen S, et al. Comparison of ultrasound, radiography, and clinical examination in the diagnosis of acute maxillary sinusitis: A systematic review. *J Clin Epidemiol.* 2000;53:940–948.
5. Williams JW. Antibiotics for acute maxillary sinusitis. *Cochrane Database Sys Rev.* 2003;2: CD000243.
6. Rosenfeld RM, Andes D, Bhattacharyya N, et al. Clinical practice guideline: Adult sinusitis. *Otolaryngol Head Neck Surg.* 2007;137:S1–31.
7. Chow AW, Benninger MS, Brook I, et al. IDSA clinical practice guideline for acute bacterial rhinosinusitis in children and adults. *Clin Infect Dis.* 2012;84(8):e72–e112. Epub 2012 Mar 20.
8. American Academy of Pediatrics. Subcommittee on Management of Sinusitis and Committee on Quality Improvement. Clinical practice guideline: Management of sinusitis. *Pediatrics.* 2001; 108:798–808.

ADDITIONAL READING

McCoul ED, Jourdy DN, Schaberg MR, et al. Methicillin-resistant *Staphylococcus aureus* sinusitis in nonhospitalized patients: A systematic review of prevalence and treatment outcomes. *Laryngoscope.* 2012;122(10):2125–2131.

CODES

ICD10
- J01.00 Acute maxillary sinusitis, unspecified
- J01.20 Acute ethmoidal sinusitis, unspecified
- J01.90 Acute sinusitis, unspecified

CLINICAL PEARLS

- When bacterial infection is present, patients recover somewhat more quickly with antibiotics, but the majority will recover with symptomatic treatment alone, and accurate diagnosis of bacterial sinusitis is very difficult (5)[A].
- Multiple meta-analyses have demonstrated *no* benefit of newer antibiotics over amoxicillin, trimethoprim-sulfamethoxazole, or doxycycline. Overall NNT to prevent 1 persistent case at follow-up = 15; harm due to antibiotic-associated diarrhea is similar.
- Significant patient symptom relief with nasal saline spray or drops or irrigation (Neti pot)

SJÖGREN SYNDROME

Katrina Darlene Zedan, MSPAS, PA-C • Vincent Honrubia, MD

 BASICS

- Chronic inflammatory disorder characterized by lymphocytic infiltrates in exocrine organs
- Typically presents with diminished salivary and lacrimal gland function, manifested as sicca symptoms such as:
  – Dry eyes, dry mouth, and enlargement of the parotid glands
  – Extraglandular symptoms may also be present, such as arthralgia, arthritis, Raynaud phenomenon, myalgia, pulmonary disease, GI disease, leukopenia, anemia, lymphadenopathy, neuropathy, vasculitis, renal tubular acidosis, and lymphoma.
- Primary Sjögren: Not associated with other diseases
- Secondary Sjögren: Complication of other rheumatologic conditions, most commonly rheumatoid arthritis
- The disease is named after Swedish ophthalmologist Henrik Sjögren (1899–1986), who first described it (1).

EPIDEMIOLOGY
Incidence
- Depending on the study, annual incidence is about 4/100,000—4.8% of population. Variability is likely due to the different criteria used in diagnosis.
- People of all races are affected.
- Predominant sex: Female > Male (9:1)
- Predominant age: Can affect patients of any age, but is most common in the elderly; onset typically occurs in the 4th–5th decades of life

Prevalence
Sjögren syndrome (SS) affects 1–4 million people in the US.

ETIOLOGY AND PATHOPHYSIOLOGY
- Systemic autoimmune disease
- Characterized by infiltration of glandular tissue primarily by CD4 T-lymphocytes
- A theory is that glandular epithelial cells present antigen to the T cells. Cytokine production then occurs, and there is also evidence for B-cell activation, resulting in autoantibody production and increased incidence of B-cell malignancies.
- Etiology is unknown. Estrogen may play a role because SS is more common in women.

Genetics
Sjögren syndrome has a familial tendency and seems to be associated with family members with a wide variety of autoimmune diseases.

RISK FACTORS
There are no known modifiable risk factors.

GENERAL PREVENTION
- No known prevention, but complications can be prevented by diagnosing and treating early.
- Dentists can play a key role in early detection of SS, as well as management of oral symptoms that result from salivary dysfunction (2)[A].

COMMONLY ASSOCIATED CONDITIONS
May be primary or secondary (associated with rheumatoid arthritis, scleroderma, systemic lupus erythematosus [SLE], polymyositis, HIV, hepatitis C)

DIAGNOSIS

- There is no single diagnostic test. Diagnosis is made by presence of compatible clinical signs and symptoms, as well as lab tests, and after exclusion of other causes.
- International consensus criteria for SS (3)[C]:
  – Ocular signs and symptoms (at least 1 present):
    ○ Persistent, troublesome dry eyes every day for >3 months
    ○ Recurrent sensation of sand or gravel in the eyes *or*
    ○ Use of tear substitute >3×/d
  – Oral signs and symptoms (at least 1 present):
    ○ Feeling of dry mouth every day for at least 3 months
    ○ Recurrent feeling of swollen salivary glands as an adult *or*
    ○ Need to drink liquids to aid in swallowing dry foods
  – Objective evidence of dry eyes (at least 1 present):
    ○ Schirmer test
    ○ Rose bengal
    ○ Lacrimal gland biopsy sample with focus score >1
  – Objective evidence of salivary gland involvement (at least 1 present):
    ○ Salivary gland scintigraphy
    ○ Parotid sialography
    ○ Unstimulated whole sialometry
  – Laboratory abnormality (at least 1 present):
    ○ Anti-SS-A or anti-SS-B
    ○ Antinuclear antibodies (ANAs)
    ○ IgM rheumatoid factor (anti-IgG Fc)
- Exclusion criteria: Prior head/neck irradiation, infection with hepatitis C, AIDS, lymphoma, sarcoidosis, graft-versus-host disease, recent use of anticholinergic medications (3)[C]
- Patients who fulfill ≥4 of the criteria likely have SS.

HISTORY
- Decreased tear production, burning, scratchy sensation in eyes
- Difficulty speaking/swallowing, dental caries, xerotrachea
- Enlarged parotid glands or intermittent swelling (bilateral)
- Dyspareunia

PHYSICAL EXAM
Common physical exam findings include:

- Eye exam: Dry eyes (keratoconjunctivitis sicca), decreased tear pool in the lower conjunctiva, dilated conjunctival vessels, mucinous threads, and filamentary keratosis can be detected during a slit-lamp examination.
- Mouth exam: Dry mouth (xerostomia), decreased sublingual salivary pool, tongue may stick to the tongue depressor, frequent caries—sometimes in unusual locations such as the incisor surface and the gum line, deep red tongue from prolonged xerostomia
- Ear, nose, and throat exam: Bilateral parotid gland enlargement, submandibular gland enlargement
- Skin exam: Nonpalpable or palpable vasculitic purpura with lesions that are typically 2–3 mm in diameter and located on the lower extremities
- Other manifestations: Chronic arthritis, interstitial nephritis (40%), type I rheumatoid arthritis (20%), vasculitis (25%), vaginal dryness, pleuritis, pancreatitis

DIFFERENTIAL DIAGNOSIS
- Causes of ocular dryness: Hypovitaminosis A, decreased tear production unrelated to autoimmune process, chronic blepharitis or conjunctivitis, impaired blinking (i.e., due to Parkinson disease or Bell palsy), working long hours at a computer, infiltration of lacrimal glands (i.e., amyloidosis, lymphoma, sarcoidosis), low estrogen levels
- Causes of oral dryness: Anticholinergic medications, sialadenitis due to chronic obstruction, chronic viral infections (i.e., hepatitis C or HIV), irradiation of head and neck
- Causes of salivary gland swelling: Unilateral: bacterial infection, neoplasm; bilateral: acute or chronic viral infection (i.e., mumps, Epstein–Barr virus [EBV], coxsackievirus, echovirus, HIV, hepatitis C), granulomatous diseases (i.e., tuberculosis, sarcoidosis), malnutrition, alcoholism, bulimia, acromegaly, diabetes

DIAGNOSTIC TESTS & INTERPRETATION
In addition to history and physical exam, the following tests are recommended when SS is suspected:
- Schirmer test
- Rose bengal test
- Basic labs, special labs (see below)
- MRI with fat suppression, chest x-ray, minor salivary gland biopsy
- Most have autoantibodies: +ANAs (95%), +RF (75%)
- In primary SS: +anti-Ro (anti SS-A, 56%) and +anti-La (anti-SS-B, 30%)

Initial Tests (lab, imaging)
Preliminary lab workup:
- Basic labs: CBC with differential, BUN/creatinine (Cr), AST/ALT, ESR, C-reactive protein (CRP), urinalysis (UA)
- Special labs: ANA, rheumatoid factor (RF), anti-Ro/SS-A, anti-La/SS-B, anti-Sm, anti-RNP, anti-dsDNA, serum C3 and C4, cryoglobulins, SPEP, UPEP, IgM, IgG, IgA
- Other: HIV, hepatitis C, CXR, minor salivary gland biopsy, MRI with fat suppression
- Initial imaging studies may include (4)[C]:
  – Imaging for xerostomia: Salivary gland scintigraphy (insensitive but highly specific)
  – Parotid gland sialography (should not be used in acute parotitis)
  – MRI (correlates well with salivary gland biopsy)
  – MRI with fat suppression (4)[B]

Diagnostic Procedures/Other
- Salivary gland biopsy: Used to confirm suspected diagnosis of SS or exclude other causes of xerostomia and bilateral gland enlargement
- Schirmer test (3)[B]
- Rose bengal test (3)[B]
- Perform a biopsy on the parotid gland if malignancy is suggested.
- Perform a biopsy on an enlarged lymph node to help rule out pseudolymphoma or lymphoma.

Test Interpretation
Salivary gland biopsy: Histology shows focal collections of lymphocytes; immunocytology shows that most of the lymphocytes are CD4+ T cells.

TREATMENT

- Treatment is primarily supportive care and treating symptoms that are problematic to patients.
- Treat dry eyes.
- Use topical therapy for dry mouth.
- Treat systemic manifestations.
- Address fatigue, vague complaints, and pain syndromes.

MEDICATION

- Usually only requires local therapy for sicca symptoms: Secretions and tears
- Immunosuppressive therapy such as hydroxychloroquine can be used for systemic symptoms; however, it has not shown any benefit in relieving refractory sicca symptoms.
- Evoxac (Cevimeline) may be prescribed for Sjögren syndrome associated xerostomia. It works by stimulating muscarinic cholinergic receptors, increasing salivary gland secretion.
- Topical therapy for dry mouth: Can be as simple as liberally drinking sips of water, trying sugar-free lemon drops or artificial saliva preparations such as Salivart, Saliment, Xero-Lube, Mouthkote (5)
- Depends on the severity of eye dryness, which is best determined by an ophthalmologist. Dry eyes are graded according to degree of symptoms, conjunctival injection and staining, corneal damage, tear quality, and lid involvement. Artificial tears may be used; however, artificial tears with hydroxymethylcellulose or dextran are more viscous and can last longer.
- Acetaminophen or NSAIDs can be taken for arthralgias.

First Line

- Xerostomia: Sugar-free lozenges, especially malic acid (4)[B], pilocarpine (4)[A], cevimeline (dose of 30 mg t.i.d. showed significant improvement (4)[A], artificial saliva
- Keratoconjunctivitis sicca: Artificial tears and ocular lubricants for symptomatic relief (4)[C], topical cyclosporine (4)[A]

Second Line

- Xerostomia: Interferon-alfa lozenges may enhance salivary gland flow (4)[B].
- Keratoconjunctivitis sicca: Emerging therapies include diquafosol (pending FDA approval) and topical NSAIDs (use with caution).
- Immunosuppressive therapy: Antimalarials (e.g., hydroxychloroquine) for arthralgias, lymphadeno-pathies, and skin manifestations (4)[B]; may then consider methotrexate or cyclosporine, which showed subjective improvement but no significant objective improvement
- Early studies show improvement in fatigue with rituximab (6)[B].
- For life-threatening extraglandular manifestations, cyclophosphamide (PO or IV), mycophenolate mofetil, and azathioprine are often used.

ISSUES FOR REFERRAL

- Systemic manifestations or resistant symptoms
- Rheumatology, as a rheumatologist is key in the management of patients with Sjögren syndrome
- Dentistry, for routine oral care is necessary
- Ophthalmology, for grading of severity of eye dryness

ADDITIONAL THERAPIES

- Patients should use vaginal lubricants, such as Replens, for vaginal dryness. Vaginal estrogen creams can be considered in postmenopausal women. Watch for and treat vaginal yeast infections (5).
- Xerostomia: Small sips of water, good dental care
- Keratoconjunctivitis sicca: Conservation of tears with side shields or ski/swim goggles, humidifiers, moist washcloths
- DHEA does not offer improvement in fatigue and well-being greater than placebo (7)[B].

SURGERY/OTHER PROCEDURES

Keratoconjunctivitis sicca: If refractory to artificial tears, punctal occlusion is the treatment of choice.

COMPLEMENTARY AND ALTERNATIVE MEDICINE

- Studies show conflicting data on the efficacy of acupuncture on saliva production and dry mouth symptoms.
- There is insufficient evidence to determine the effects of electrostimulation devices on dry mouth symptoms or saliva production in patients with Sjögren' syndrome (8)[A].

IN-PATIENT CONSIDERATIONS

May be required for extraglandular manifestations, such as cardiopulmonary disease, renal involvement, and CNS manifestations (e.g., optic neuritis, transverse myelitis, vasculitis, or ischemic stroke)

ONGOING CARE

FOLLOW-UP RECOMMENDATIONS

Frequency of follow-up depends on severity.

Patient Monitoring

- Monitor for complications, systemic manifestations, and relief of symptoms.
- Medicolegal pitfalls: Failure to monitor and evaluate for parotid tumor or lymphoma

PATIENT EDUCATION

Explanation of SS is essential. In most cases, simple measures are adequate, such as humidifiers, sips of water, chewing gum, or artificial tears.

PROGNOSIS

- Hypocomplementemia is an independent risk factor for premature death.
- Primary Sjögren syndrome is significantly associated with increased risks of overall malignancy, non-Hodgkin lymphoma, and thyroid cancer (9)[A].

COMPLICATIONS

Complications include dental caries, gum disease, dysphagia, salivary gland calculi, keratitis, conjunctivitis, and scarring of the ocular surface.

REFERENCES

1. Ramos-Casals M, Tzioufas AG, Stone JH, et al. Treatment of primary Sjögren syndrome: A systematic review. *JAMA*. 2010;304:452–460.
2. Stewart CM, Berg KM, Cha S, et al. Salivary dysfunction and quality of life in Sjogren syndrome: A critical oral-systemic connection. *J Am Dent Assoc*. 2008;139:291–299.
3. Fox RI. Sjogren's syndrome. *Lancet*. 2005;366: 321.
4. von Bültzingslöwen I, Sollecito TP, Fox PC, et al. Salivary dysfunction associated with systemic diseases: Systematic review and clinical management recommendations. *Oral Surg Oral Med Oral Pathol Oral Radiol Endod*. 2007; 103(Suppl):S57.e1–e15.
5. Miller AV. Sjogren syndrome: Treatment & medications. Available at: http://emedicine.medscape.com/article/332125-treatment. Assessed: 8/21/2010.
6. Dass S, Bowman SJ, Vital EM, et al. Reduction of fatigue in Sjogren's syndrome with rituximab: Results of a randomised, double-blind, placebo controlled pilot study. *Ann Rheum Dis*. 2008; 67(11):1541–1544.
7. Hartkamp A, Geenen R, Godaert GL, et al. Effect of dehydroepiandrosterone administration on fatigue, well-being, and functioning in women with primary Sjögren's syndrome. A randomized controlled trial. *Ann Rheum Dis*. 2008;67(1): 91–97.
8. Furness S, Bryan G, McMillan R, et al. Interventions for the management of dry mouth: Non-pharmacological interventions. *Cochrane Database Syst Rev*. 2013;9:CD009603. [Epub ahead of print]
9. Liang Y, Yang Z, Qin B, et al. Primary Sjogren's syndrome and malignancy risk: A systematic review and meta-analysis. *Ann Rheum Dis*. 2013. [Epub ahead of print]
10. Fischer A, Swigris JJ, du Bois RM, et al. Minor salivary gland biopsy to detect primary Sjogren syndrome in patients with interstitial lung disease. *Chest*. 2009;136(4):1072–1078.

ADDITIONAL READING

- Aragona P, Spinella R, Rania L, et al. Safety and efficacy of 0.1% clobetasone butyrate eyedrops in the treatment of dry eye in Sjögren syndrome. *Eur J Ophthalmol*. 2012;0. Epub 2012 Nov 19.
- Mays JW, Sarmadi M, Moutsopoulos NM. Oral manifestations of systemic autoimmune and inflammatory diseases: Diagnosis and clinical management. *J Evid Based Dent Pract*. 2012; 12(3 Suppl):265–282.
- Pan Q, Angelina A, Zambrano A, et al. Autologous serum eye drops for dry eye. *Cochrane Database Syst Rev*. 2013 Aug 27;8:CD009327.

 CODES

ICD10

- M35.00 Sicca syndrome, unspecified
- M35.03 Sicca syndrome with myopathy
- M35.09 Sicca syndrome with other organ involvement

CLINICAL PEARLS

- Many symptoms can be treated with nonprescription interventions such as artificial tears and sugar-free lozenges.
- Consider lacrimal duct plugs for dry eyes (placed under local anesthetic by an ophthalmologist).
- Consider minor salivary gland biopsy to confirm diagnosis in the setting of interstitial lung disease (10)[B].

SLEEP APNEA, OBSTRUCTIVE

Robert A. Baldor, MD

 BASICS

DESCRIPTION
- Obstructive sleep apnea (OSA) is defined as repetitive episodes of cessation of airflow (apnea) at the nose and mouth during sleep due to obstruction at the level of the pharynx:
  - Apneas often terminate with a snort/gasp
  - Repetitive apneas produce sleep disruption, leading to excessive daytime sleepiness
  - Associated with oxygen desaturation and nocturnal hypoxemia
  - Usual course is chronic
- System(s) affected: Cardiovascular; Nervous; Pulmonary
- Synonym(s): Pickwickian syndrome; Sleep apnea syndrome; Nocturnal upper airway occlusion

EPIDEMIOLOGY
Incidence
- Predominant age: Middle-aged men and women
- Predominant sex: Male > Female (2:1)
Prevalence
- Up to 4% in men, 2% in women
- Prevalence is higher in obese/hypertensive patients

ETIOLOGY AND PATHOPHYSIOLOGY
OSA occurs when the naso- or oropharynx collapses passively during inspiration. Anatomic and neuromuscular factors contribute to pharyngeal collapse:
- Anatomic abnormalities, such as increased soft tissue in the palate, tonsillar hypertrophy, macroglossia, and craniofacial abnormalities, predispose the airway to collapse by decreasing the area of the upper airway or increasing the pressure surrounding the airway.
- During sleep, decreased muscle tone in the naso- or oropharynx contributes to airway obstruction and collapse.
- Upper airway narrowing may be due to:
  - Obesity, redundant tissue in the soft palate
  - Enlarged tonsils/uvula
  - Low soft palate
  - Large/Posteriorly located tongue
  - Craniofacial abnormalities
  - Neuromuscular disorders
  - Alcohol/sedative use before bedtime

RISK FACTORS
- Obesity
- Age >40 years
- Alcohol/Sedative intake before bedtime
- Smoking
- Nasal obstruction (due to polyps, rhinitis, or deviated septum)
- Anatomic narrowing of nasopharynx (e.g., tonsillar hypertrophy, macroglossia, micrognathia, retrognathia, craniofacial abnormalities)
- Acromegaly
- Hypothyroidism
- Neurologic syndromes (e.g., muscular dystrophy, cerebral palsy)

GENERAL PREVENTION
Weight control and avoidance of alcohol and sedatives at night can help to prevent airway collapse.

COMMONLY ASSOCIATED CONDITIONS
- Common:
  - Hypertension
  - Obesity
  - Daytime sleepiness
  - Metabolic syndrome
- Rare:
  - Cardiac arrhythmias
  - Cardiovascular disease
  - Congestive heart failure
  - Pulmonary hypertension
  - Nasal obstructive problems

 DIAGNOSIS

HISTORY
Elicit a complete history of daytime and nighttime symptoms. Symptoms can be insidious and present for years:
- Daytime symptoms:
  - Excessive daytime sleepiness (EDS) or fatigue (cardinal symptom):
    ○ Mild symptoms occur during quiet activities (e.g., reading, watching television)
    ○ Severe symptoms occur during dynamic activities (e.g., work, driving)
  - Tired on morning awakening
  - Sore/Dry throat
  - Poor concentration, memory problems, irritability, mood changes
  - Morning headaches
  - Decreased libido
  - Depression
- Nighttime symptoms:
  - Loud snoring (present in 60% of people with OSA)
  - Snort/Gasp that arouses patient from sleep
  - Disrupted sleep
  - Witnessed apneic episodes at night

PHYSICAL EXAM
- Most patients have a normal physical exam. However, OSA is commonly associated with hypertension, obesity, or sleepiness.
- Focused head and neck exam:
  - Short neck with large circumference
  - Oropharynx:
    ○ Narrowing of the lateral airway wall
    ○ Tonsillar hypertrophy
    ○ Macroglossia
    ○ Micrognathia/retrognathia
    ○ Soft palate edema
    ○ Long/Thick uvula
    ○ High, arched hard palate
  - Nasopharynx:
    ○ Deviated nasal septum
    ○ Poor nasal airflow

DIFFERENTIAL DIAGNOSIS
- Other causes of excessive daytime sleepiness, such as:
  - Narcolepsy
  - Idiopathic daytime hypersomnolence
  - Inadequate sleep time
  - Depressive episodes with excessive daytime sleepiness
  - Periodic limb movements disorder
- Respiratory disorders with nocturnal awakenings, such as:
  - Asthma
  - Chronic obstructive pulmonary disease
  - Congestive heart failure
- Central sleep apnea
- Sleep-related choking/laryngospasm
- Gastroesophageal reflux
- Sleep-associated seizures (temporal lobe epilepsy)

DIAGNOSTIC TESTS & INTERPRETATION
Initial Tests (lab, imaging)
- When clinically indicated:
  - Thyroid-stimulating hormone to evaluate hypothyroidism
  - CBC to evaluate anemia and polycythemia, which can indicate nocturnal hypoxemia
  - Fasting glucose in obesity to evaluate for diabetes
  - Rare: Arterial blood gases to evaluate daytime hypercapnia
- Cephalometric measurements from lateral head and neck radiographs aid in surgical treatment.

Diagnostic Procedures/Other
- The gold standard for OSA is polysomnography (PSG), a nighttime sleep study:
  - Demonstrates severity of hypoxemia, sleep disruption, and cardiac arrhythmias associated with OSA and elevated end-tidal CO_2
  - Shows repetitive episodes of cessation/marked reduction in airflow despite continued respiratory efforts
  - Apneic episodes must last at least 10 seconds and occur 10–15 × per hour to be considered clinically significant.
  - Complete PSG is expensive, and health insurance may not cover the cost.
- Multiple sleep latency testing is a diagnostic tool used to measure the time it takes from the start of a daytime nap period to the 1st signs of sleep (sleep latency). It provides an objective measurement of daytime sleepiness.
- The apnea/hypoapnea index (AHI) is defined as the total number of apneas and hypoapneas divided by the total sleep time:
  - Mild OSA: AHI = 5–15
  - Moderate OSA: AHI = 15–30
  - Severe OSA: AHI >30
- Drugs that may alter the test results include benzodiazepines and other sedatives that can amplify the severity of apnea seen during the sleep study.
- Early data suggest that home-based diagnosis using portable monitoring devices may be an alternative to laboratory-based PSG (1)[B].

TREATMENT

- Lifestyle modification is the most frequently recommended treatment for mild to moderate OSA. This includes weight loss, exercise, and avoidance of alcohol, smoking, and sedatives, especially before bedtime. Weight loss has been shown to decrease the severity of symptoms in obese patients. Lifestyle modifications should be seen as adjunctive rather than curative therapy (2)[A], and a lack of improvement of symptoms with lifestyle modification should not preclude patients from receiving other therapy, such as continuous positive airway pressure (CPAP).
- If OSA is present only when supine, keep the patient off his/her back when sleeping (e.g., tennis ball worn on back of nightshirt).
- The most effective therapy for both mild to moderate (3)[B] and moderate to severe OSA is CPAP. Treatment with CPAP utilizes a mask interface and a flow generator to prevent airway collapse, thus helping to prevent apnea, hypoxia, and sleep disturbance. Compared with inactive controls, CPAP significantly improves both objective (24-hour systolic and diastolic blood pressures) and subjective measures (Epworth Sleepiness Scale) (4)[A] in OSA patients with symptoms of daytime sleepiness. CPAP may also decrease the risk for stroke (5)[C] and atherosclerosis (5)[C] as well as improve insulin resistance in nondiabetic patients (6)[A]. Early data show that these benefits may not be seen in patients who do not have symptoms of daytime sleepiness (7)[B].
- Compliance may be problematic in some OSA patients undergoing CPAP therapy, particularly those with mild disease (8)[A]. Several types of mask interfaces, including nasal masks, oral masks, and nasal pillows exist. Short-term data suggest that nasal pillows are the preferred interface in almost all patients. In patients with compliance difficulty, a different choice of interface may be appropriate (9)[A].
- Oral appliances to treat OSA are available and often subjectively preferred by patients. Although oral appliances have been shown to improve symptoms compared with inactive controls, they are not as effective for reduction of respiratory disturbances as CPAP over short-term data. Treatment with oral appliances may be considered in patients who fail to comply with CPAP therapy (10)[A].

MEDICATION

Medications are yet to be proven effective in treating OSA (11)[A]. Further studies in this area are needed.

First Line

Some short-term data found fluticasone nasal spray, mirtazapine, physostigmine, and nasal lubricant of some benefit; longer-term studies needed (11)[A].

ISSUES FOR REFERRAL

If sleep apnea is suspected, patient should be referred to a sleep specialist/neurologist for a sleep study evaluation.

SURGERY/OTHER PROCEDURES

Surgical corrections of the upper airway include uvulopalatopharyngoplasty (UPPP), tracheostomy, and craniofacial surgery. Currently no evidence supports the use of surgery for the treatment of OSA (12)[A].

IN-PATIENT CONSIDERATIONS

On admission, patients should continue to use CPAP/dental devices if they do so at home. They should bring in their own appliance and know their CPAP settings.

ONGOING CARE

Lifelong compliance with weight loss or CPAP is necessary for successful OSA treatment.

DIET

Overweight and obese patients should be encouraged to lose weight, and all patients must avoid weight gain. Weight loss alone can relieve symptoms of OSA.

PATIENT EDUCATION

- Weight loss and avoidance of alcohol and sedatives can reduce OSA symptoms.
- Significantly sleepy patients should not drive a motor vehicle/operate dangerous equipment.

PROGNOSIS

- EDS is reduced dramatically with appropriate apnea control.
- Lifelong compliance with weight loss or CPAP is necessary for effective treatment of OSA.
- If untreated, OSA is progressive.
- Significant morbidity and mortality with OSA usually are due to motor vehicle accidents or are secondary to cardiac complications, including arrhythmias, cardiac ischemia, and hypertension.

COMPLICATIONS

Untreated OSA may increase the risk for development of hypertension, stroke, myocardial infarction, diabetes, cardiovascular disease, and work-related and driving accidents.

Pediatric Considerations

- The prevalence of pediatric OSA is 1–2% in children 4–5 years of age, and the peak incidence is between 3 and 6 years of age.
- Predominant sex: Male = Female.
- Etiology: The most common cause is tonsillar hypertrophy. Additional causes are obesity and craniofacial abnormalities. OSA is also seen in children with neuromuscular diseases, such as cerebral palsy and spinal muscular atrophy, due to abnormal pharyngeal muscle control.
- Signs and symptoms:
  - Nighttime: Loud snoring, restlessness, and sweating
  - Daytime: Hyperactivity and decreased school performance
  - EDS is not a significant symptom.
- Diagnosis: Gold standard is PSG. Abnormal AHI is different in children: >1–2/hr is abnormal.
- Treatment: Surgery is the first-line treatment in cases due to tonsillar enlargement (reduces symptoms in 70%). Some data suggest improved academic performance if tonsillectomy is performed for OSA. For cases due to obesity/craniofacial abnormalities, patients can use CPAP treatment.

REFERENCES

1. Rosen CL, Auckley D, Benca R, et al. A multisite randomized trial of portable sleep studies and positive airway pressure autotitration versus laboratory-based polysomnography for the diagnosis and treatment of obstructive sleep apnea: The HomePAP study. *Sleep*. 2012;84: 757–767.
2. Anandam A, Akinnusi M, Kufel T, et al. Effects of dietary weight loss on obstructive sleep apnea: A meta-analysis. *Sleep Breath*. 2013;17:227–234.
3. Weaver TE, Mancini C, Maislin G, et al. CPAP treatment of sleepy patients with milder OSA: Results of the CATNAP randomized clinical trial. *Am J Resp Crit Care Med*. 2012;186:677–683.
4. Giles TL, Lasserson TJ, Smith BH, et al. Continuous positive airways pressure for obstructive sleep apnoea in adults. *Cochrane Database Syst Rev*. 2008;4:CD001106.
5. Drager LF, Bortolotto LA, Figueiredo AC, et al. Effects of continuous positive airway pressure on early signs of atherosclerosis in obstructive sleep apnea. *Am J Respir Crit Care Med*. 2007;176: 706–712.
6. Yang D, Liu Z, Yang H, et al. Effects of continuous positive airway pressure on glycemic control and insulin resistance in patients with obstructive sleep apnea: A meta-analysis. *Sleep Breath*. 2013;17:33–38.
7. Barbé F, Durán-Cantolla J, Sánchez-de-la-Torre M, et al. Effect of continuous positive airway pressure on the incidence of hypertension and cardiovascular events in nonsleepy patients with obstructive sleep apnea: A randomized controlled trial. *JAMA*. 2012;84:2161–2168.
8. Madbouly EM, Nadeem R, Nida M, et al. The role of severity of obstructive sleep apnea measured by apnea-hypopnea index in predicting compliance with pressure therapy, a meta-analysis. *Am J Ther*. 2012, in press.
9. Chai CL, Pathinathan A, Smith B. Continuous positive airway pressure delivery interfaces for obstructive sleep apnoea. *Cochrane Database Syst Rev*. 2006;4:CD005308.
10. Lim J, Lasserson TJ, Fleetham J, et al. Oral appliances for obstructive sleep apnoea. *Cochrane Database Syst Rev*. 2009;3:CD004435.
11. Smith I, Lasserson TJ, Wright J. Drug therapy for obstructive sleep apnoea in adults. *Cochrane Database Syst Rev*. 2006;2:CD003002.
12. Sundaram S, Bridgman SA, Lim J, et al. Surgery for obstructive sleep apnoea. *Cochrane Database Syst Rev*. 2005;4:CD001004.

CODES

ICD10

G47.33 Obstructive sleep apnea (adult) (pediatric)

CLINICAL PEARLS

- OSA is characterized by repetitive episodes of apnea at the pharynx often terminating in a snort/gasp.
- Laboratory polysomnography is the key to diagnosis.
- CPAP is the most effective form of treatment for both mild to moderate and moderate to severe OSA.
- Central sleep apnea may mimic OSA.

SLEEP DISORDER, CIRCADIAN RHYTHM—DELAYED PHASE TYPE

Adam J. Sorscher, MD

BASICS

DESCRIPTION

- Circadian rhythm sleep disorders (CRSDs) are a family of conditions that occur when an individual's preferred timing of sleep is not synchronized to commitments to job, school, family, or social engagements. In CRSDs, intrinsic sleep is normal (i.e., no sleep fragmenting condition such as obstructive sleep apnea or periodic limb movement disorder). However, when forced by obligations to attempt sleep at nonpreferred times, individuals with CRSDs complain of both sleep-initiation insomnia and excessive sleepiness in wake time. These symptoms resolve entirely if the individual is allowed to sleep at his or her preferred time.
- Circadian rhythm sleep disorder, delayed-phase type (CRSD-DPT) is marked by a stable but persistent inability to initiate sleep at a desired time. Individuals are typically unable to initiate sleep until 3–6 hours later than societal norms (i.e., after 2 A.M.), and this frequently results in insufficient sleep/sleepiness in the day that follows. This topic addresses circadian rhythm disorder, delayed-phase type.

EPIDEMIOLOGY

CRSD-DPT is the most common circadian rhythm disorder seen by referral in sleep medicine clinics (1).

Prevalence

CRSD-DPT has an estimated prevalence of 0.1–0.2% in the general population. It is most common in adolescents, with a prevalence of 7–16%.

ETIOLOGY AND PATHOPHYSIOLOGY

In all mammals, an oscillating signal from the suprachiasmatic nucleus (SCN) in the anterior hypothalamus establishes circadian rhythms, including the propensity to be awake or asleep. The average period of this signal in humans is 24.2 hours. Certain factors, most significantly light, can shift the timing of the circadian rhythm and thereby synchronize it to the shorter environmental cycle day by day. CRSD-DPT and other circadian rhythm disorders occur when the circadian rhythm is not adequately synchronized to the shorter 24-hour environmental cycle, creating a mismatch between them. Some theories to account for inadequate synchronization are that it occurs in individuals who have an abnormally long circadian period (>25 hours) or whose circadian clock does not properly respond to synchronizing agents such as light.

- Release of melatonin from the pineal gland in the evening initiates a cascade of events that usually triggers sleep behavior several hours later. Studies suggest that the timing of melatonin release within the circadian cycle is delayed by 40–120 minutes in later adolescence compared with prepuberty. This suggests that the tendency for teenagers to delay sleep onset is largely a genetically programmed developmental phenomenon.
- CRSD-DPT is the result of biologic, behavioral, and psychosocial factors. The relative contributions of genetically ordained endogenous factors (the shifting of the circadian phase just described) vs. voluntary behaviors that delay bedtime are not fully delineated.

Genetics

Emerging evidence indicates a genetic component to both CRSD-DPT and morning/evening preference. In 1 familial case report, CRSD-DPT was shown to occur in an autosomal-dominant inheritance pattern. Polymorphisms in circadian rhythm genes such as *hPer3* and *clock* among individuals with CRSD-DPT constitute evidence of a genetic component to the disorder (2).

RISK FACTORS

CRSD-DPT primarily affects adolescents and young adults who have a biologic tendency to delay the onset of sleep yet often need to be up early for school/work responsibilities.

GENERAL PREVENTION

In CRSD-DPT (and all CRSDs), careful attention to sleep hygiene is necessary to establish and maintain a desired sleep schedule. The most important behavioral practices needed to prevent an undesirably late fall-asleep time are:

- Maintain a regular sleep/wake schedule 7 days/week.
- Avoid napping.
- Minimize caffeine and stimulants.
- Avoid stimulating activities in the late evening, such as computer, TV, and social interactions. A 30-minute "wind-down" time prior to bedtime in which homework, socializing, and electronic devices are off-limits is helpful.
- Adolescents who sleep ad lib on the weekends (sometimes into the afternoon) often find that they have especially great difficulty initiating sleep on Sunday night and, thus, get the week off to a bad start; to prevent this, they should be advised to arise at a similar time on weekends as on the school/work mornings.

DIAGNOSIS

HISTORY

- People with CRSD-DPT report both sleep initiation insomnia and excessive sleepiness in the daytime. They struggle to awaken for school/work in the morning.
- Careful questioning should explore for competing/comorbid causes of insomnia (poor sleep hygiene, significant mental health disorders, restless legs syndrome, and medical conditions/medication side effects) and for competing/comorbid causes of hypersomnolence (symptoms of narcolepsy and obstructive sleep apnea, voluntary insufficient sleep, and medication side effects).
- Individuals with psychophysiological insomnia (psychologically conditioned arousal when attempting to initiate sleep) do not usually experience genuine hypersomnolence in the daytime despite short sleep times overnight, but instead complain of fatigue.
- Those who voluntarily stay up late and obtain insufficient sleep do not report insomnia when they do attempt to initiate sleep.
- In contrast to the other disorders in the differential, people with CRSD-DPT will usually assert that they would have no complaint about sleep/wakefulness if they were simply allowed to sleep at their preferred time (e.g., they do not have sleep/wakefulness issues when on summer vacation from school).

PHYSICAL EXAM

Explore for features of sleep apnea: Obesity/Large neck circumference; hypertension, crowded oropharynx.

DIFFERENTIAL DIAGNOSIS

CRSDs are unique in that they are marked by the twin complaints of insomnia when attempting to sleep *and* hypersomnolence in the wake period. Usually, other sleep disorders cause either insomnia or hypersomnolence, but not both. In contrast to other sleep/wakefulness disorders, symptoms of CRSDs resolve entirely if the individual is allowed to sleep at a preferred time.

DIAGNOSTIC TESTS & INTERPRETATION

- Diagnosis of CRSD-DPT is made primarily by thorough history-taking.
- Sleep logs completed over 3 weeks time graphically reveal fall-asleep times that are consistently 3–6 hours later than societal norms and much later wake-up times (not infrequently in the afternoon) on days off from school/work (3)[C].
- Wrist actigraphy (using a wristwatch-like device with an accelerometer), undertaken for 3 weeks, also provides an accurate display of sleep and wake timing, but is currently not reimbursable and is not needed if the individual can complete sleep logs (3)[B].
- Testing in the sleep lab is not indicated unless a suspicion exists of comorbid intrinsic disorders of sleep, such as sleep apnea, narcolepsy, or parasomnias (unusual behaviors arising out of sleep).

TREATMENT

- The goal of treatment in CRSD-DPT is to help the individual consistently initiate sleep at an earlier time. The principal therapies that advance sleep onset are light and melatonin (factors that shift the circadian rhythm are called *zeitgebers*) (4)[A]. Comparatively, light is much more potent than melatonin in its phase-shifting ability. The phase-shifting effects of light and melatonin depend on the timing at which they are provided as depicted in the phase-response curve. Key points: Light will advance sleep onset to an earlier time if provided after the body's temperature nadir that occurs ~2/3 through the habitual sleep phase and up for several hours immediately after arising. Proper timing is critical, since exposure to light in the evening or before the temperature nadir (i.e., in the initial 2/3 of the sleep period) will further delay sleep onset. For melatonin, the most potent phase-advancing occurs if it is provided in the evening, 5–6 hours before an individual's usual sleep onset time.
- Use the following rules to guide prescribing of light in order to advance sleep phase (5)[A]:
  - No single rule exists for intensity, duration, or wavelength for light therapy. Most protocols employ a 2,500–10,000 lux full-spectrum light box, set 2–3 feet from the individual for 30–120 minutes. A common prescription is 10,000 lux box for 30 minutes upon awakening in the morning. Retailers of full-spectrum light boxes abound on the Internet. Sunlight, when present in the morning in warm-weather seasons, is equally effective.

– Prescribe exposure to full-spectrum light immediately upon awakening (Note: Although the phase-advancing effect of light is actually greatest if it is provided immediately after the body temperature nadir that occurs ~2/3 through the sleep period, the strategy of waiting until the habitual waking time is preferred for these reasons: (i) it acknowledges that it is onerous for the individual to wake up artificially early for light therapy and (ii) it minimizes the risk of unintentionally providing light *before* the temperature nadir, which further delays the sleep phase).

– Light exposure in the evening has the effect of delaying sleep phase and worsening CRSD-DPT. Instruct individuals to limit light exposure in the evening (consider using sunglasses or curtailing outdoors activities in warm-weather months).

– Contraindications to phototherapy include retinopathy, photosensitivity, and bipolar disorder.

MEDICATION

• Prescribe melatonin to be taken 5–6 hours before the habitual (usual) fall-asleep time, not at bedtime. Melatonin in minute doses is as effective as higher doses in producing phase-shift; therefore, use the lowest dose available—usually 1 or 3 mg (5)[A].

• Once earlier sleep onset and wake-up occurs, adjust the timing of therapies every 3–5 days—continue to use light directly upon awakening; provide melatonin earlier and earlier in the evening corresponding to 5–6 hours before the newly observed fall-asleep time.

ALERT

Melatonin has a weak sedating effect, and individuals should be counseled not to drive/operate dangerous machines after taking the medication. Other side effects include headache and unusual taste in mouth.

ISSUES FOR REFERRAL

• Referral for evaluation and testing at a sleep clinic is not necessary in most cases of CRSD-DPT. The chief indications for referral are suspicion of the following comorbid disorders:

– Obstructive sleep apnea: Indicated by loud snoring, obesity/large neck, witnessed apneas, and history of hypertension

– Narcolepsy: Indicated by severe levels of daytime sleepiness, despite adequate sleep quantity, and sometimes accompanied by cataplexy (bouts of sudden muscular weakness triggered by strong emotions)

– Parasomnias: Undesirable experiential/behavioral phenomena that arise out of sleep, such as dangerous sleepwalking/dream-enactment

• In addition, many individuals with the complaint of insomnia/sleepiness have comorbid mental health disorders, primarily depression and possibly substance abuse. Referral for mental health disorders/substance abuse treatment is indicated if these are present.

ADDITIONAL THERAPIES

• Chronotherapy is an older strategy in which the individual is instructed to delay sleep and wake times by 2–3 hours every 2–3 days, shifting the sleep cycle across the 24-hour day, until the individual reaches a desired bedtime. Carried out over several weeks, this protocol is extremely disruptive to daytime schedules and also has not been demonstrated to be effective. It is seldom used (3)[C].

• Some early reports suggest that vitamin B_{12} has circadian phase-shifting properties. This finding has not been confirmed in subsequent investigations, and presently no evidence seen of benefit to the use of this supplement in CRSDs (3).

• Use of sedative-hypnotic medications to treat the insomnia component and stimulant medications to treat daytime sleepiness has not been shown to be effective in the context of CRSD-DPT (5).

ONGOING CARE

Remind patients to practice healthy sleep behaviors (see "General Prevention") if they wish to maintain an earlier sleep/wake pattern.

PATIENT EDUCATION

http://www.aafp.org/afp/1999/0401/p1918.html

REFERENCES

1. Dagan Y, Eisenstein M. Circadian rhythm disorders: Toward a more precise definition and diagnosis. *Chronobiol Intern*. 1999;16:213–222.
2. Ebisawa T, Uchiyama M, Kajimura N, et al. Association of structural polymorphisms in the human period3 gene with delayed sleep phase syndrome. *EMBO Rep*. 2001;2:342–346.
3. Morgenthaler TI, Lee-Chiong T, Alessi C, et al. Practice parameters for the clinical evaluation and treatment of circadian rhythm sleep disorders. An American Academy of Sleep Medicine report. *Sleep*. 2007;30:1445–1459.
4. Wilson SJ, Nutt DJ, Alford C, et al. British Association for Psychopharmacology consensus statement on evidence-based treatment of insomnia, parasomnias and circadian rhythm disorders. *J Psychopharmacol (Oxford)*. 2010; 24:1577–1601.
5. Sack RL, Auckley D, Auger RR, et al. Circadian rhythm sleep disorders: Part II, advanced sleep phase disorder, delayed sleep phase disorder, free-running disorder, and irregular sleep-wake rhythm. An American Academy of Sleep Medicine review. *Sleep*. 2007;30:1484–1501.

ADDITIONAL READING

• Barion A, Zee PC. A clinical approach to circadian rhythm sleep disorders. *Sleep Med*. 2007;8: 566–577.

• Kanathur N, Harrington J, Lee-Chiong T, et al. Circadian rhythm sleep disorders. *Clin Chest Med*. 2010;31:319–325.

 ## CODES

ICD10

G47.21 Circadian rhythm sleep disorder, delayed sleep phase type

CLINICAL PEARLS

• The tendency to become night-owlish with adolescence is, to a large extent, a biologically programmed phenomenon, not strictly a behavioral choice. Enlightened public policy would recognize this and allow for later start times for high schools.

• CRSD-DPT can be diagnosed with careful history-taking and sleep logs; referral for formal sleep studies is usually not indicated.

• Use of light and melatonin can shift habitual sleep onset and offset time by their action on the human circadian rhythm.

• To maintain a desirable sleep phase, individuals with CRSD-DPT usually need to maintain meticulous attention to sleep hygiene, including a regular sleep/wake schedule 7 days/week, to avoid lapsing into a delayed phase pattern.

SLEEP DISORDER, SHIFT WORK

Frank J. Domino, MD

BASICS

DESCRIPTION
- The nomenclature of the *International Classifications of Sleep Disorders*, 2nd edition, calls this disorder circadian rhythm sleep disorder, shift work type, but in clinical practice, it is usually called shift work disorder (SWD). As the official name denotes, this is classified among the circadian rhythm sleep disorders.
- A universally accepted definition has not been consistently used in the research, but current best-practice standards require all the general criteria for circadian rhythm disorders be met (see below) and that the complaints are associated with night shifts, early morning shifts, or rotating shifts.
- General criteria for circadian rhythm disorders are the following:
  – A persistent/recurrent sleep disruption due to either an alteration in the circadian (24-hour) timekeeping system or due to a misalignment between endogenous circadian rhythm and exogenous factors that affect sleep
  – A complaint of insomnia/excessive daytime sleepiness or both
  – An impairment in occupational, educational, or social functioning

EPIDEMIOLOGY
Incidence
Both incidence and prevalence depend on the number of shift workers in a given society, which can change over time. Therefore, the literature does not estimate incidence.

Prevalence
- Epidemiologic data are rare, but one study found ~1/3 of night/rotating shift workers met the minimum criteria for SWD (1)[A].
- Often stated in the literature is that ~20% of the population in industrialized countries performs shift work. Therefore, a rough estimate of the prevalence of SWD is 5%.

ETIOLOGY AND PATHOPHYSIOLOGY
- Common understanding is every cell in the human body regulates its physiology according to a 24-hour (i.e., circadian) clock.
- The most powerful *zeitgeber*, or timekeeper, is light. It is not just a social convention that has us sleeping at night and up in the daytime; this is the natural rhythm for most humans and it is difficult to work when both circadian and homeostatic forces are signaling sleep, and it is difficult to sleep when these forces are in alert mode.
- See above.

RISK FACTORS
Shift work, meaning night shifts, early morning shifts, or rotating shifts, is the obvious risk factor. Great individual variability in tolerance for shift work may indicate that certain individuals are at a greater risk for developing SWD as they perform shift work.

Genetics
No genetic predisposition has been described.

GENERAL PREVENTION
As shift work is surely here to stay in industrialized countries, it is best to focus on measures that make it more tolerable. They include the following:
- Limiting rotating shifts
- Using bright light during shifts
- Scheduling brief, 10–20-minute, naps during the shifts, if suitable

COMMONLY ASSOCIATED CONDITIONS
- Some evidence that SWD increases the risk of breast and prostate cancer such that the International Agency for Research on Cancer (IARC) has classified shift work that involves a circadian disruption as a probable carcinogen (2)[A].
- Also, association data link SWD to increased risk of GI disease, specifically peptic ulcer disease, cardiovascular disease (CVD), infertility, and pregnancy complications.

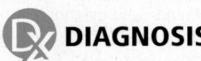

DIAGNOSIS

This is primarily a clinical diagnosis. However, there are some useful diagnostic aids.

HISTORY
- A careful history is critical.
- Special attention should be paid to:
  – Sleep/Wake habits
  – Sleep environment
  – Light exposure before, during, and after the shift
  – Medications as well as over-the-counter (OTC) stimulants such as caffeine and energy drinks
- It is also important to know patients' sleep/wake schedules when they have days off.
- It is essential to ask about other sleep disorders such as:
  – Snoring (obstructive sleep apnea [OSA])
  – Sudden sleep attacks and leg symptoms (restless legs syndrome [RLS])
  – Drop attacks and daytime fatigue (narcolepsy)

PHYSICAL EXAM
Evaluate for signs of OSA, such as obesity, a large neck, and a tight oropharynx.

DIFFERENTIAL DIAGNOSIS
- Another primary sleep disorder, such as OSA, RLS, narcolepsy, and psychophysiological insomnia. Keep in mind shift workers often have another coexisting primary sleep disorder such as OSA in addition to, and separate from, their shift work disorder, which exacerbates symptoms.
- Another circadian rhythm sleep disorder such as delayed sleep phase disorder or jet lag syndrome. Distinguishing among these is challenging even for sleep specialists.

DIAGNOSTIC TESTS & INTERPRETATION
- Although there is no diagnostic test, there are some useful tools.
- Because of a possible increased risk for CVD and cancer among shift workers, consider appropriate screenings.

Initial Tests (lab, imaging)
- Fasting lipid panel, fasting glucose, age-appropriate cancer screenings
- None

Diagnostic Procedures/Other
- The 2 most widely used and recommended tools are sleep diaries and actigraphy (a mechanical device, often worn on the arm/leg, to measure movement) (3)[A].
- Data should be collected for at least 1 week, but 2 weeks is preferable.
- There is no standard, validated sleep diary. Note that the terms "sleep diary" and "sleep log" are used interchangeably by sleep specialists.
- Some sleep specialists use actigraphy, which is a gross measure of time and amount of activity and rest.

Test Interpretation
Both the sleep diary and the actigraph data usually show the following:
- Increased sleep latency
- Decreased total sleep time
- Frequent awakenings
- Also usually show most people revert to nocturnal sleeping on their days off, which means every workweek, they start fresh in their attempts to shift their circadian rhythms to align with work schedules.

TREATMENT

- The American Academy of Sleep Medicine (AASM) published its most recent practice parameters for diagnosis and treatment of circadian rhythm sleep disorders, including SWD, in 2007.
- The only therapeutic modality deemed as "standard" treatment is planned (or prescribed) sleep schedules.
- Regular exercise on a schedule will help with sleep quality and daytime fatigue.
- The 2 most researched and used treatments include bright light therapy and melatonin; research shows such mixed results that neither was ranked as a standard treatment (4)[A].

GENERAL MEASURES

- Bright light therapy with conventional light/light boxes (10,000 lux preferable, but >1,000 lux will help) should be given during the night/early morning shift.
- When night-shift workers are ending their shifts in the morning, bright light should be avoided. We recommend the use of dark sunglasses/special glasses that filter the blue wavelength, as well as a hat.

MEDICATION

- Much research has shown that melatonin may help shift circadian rhythms.
- Although melatonin has little soporific effect when given at night when endogenous levels are high anyway, some research has shown good results in its ability to shorten sleep latency when taken in the daytime, making it useful in treating SWD.
- Melatonin is not considered a medication by the FDA and its use in the treatment of SWD (or anything else) is not approved by the FDA.
- No reports of serious side effects have been reported with melatonin use. A medication, ramelteon (Rozerem), which is a melatonin receptor agonist, is approved as a hypnotic.
- No good research exists on melatonin's use in circadian rhythm disorders.
- For excessive sleepiness, wakefulness-promoting medications (modafinil, armodafinil) may be very beneficial to the patient's quality of life.
- Use of hypnotics such as zolpidem received a "guideline" rating by the AASM.
- While stimulants are an "option" according to the AASM, modafinil, which is a wakefulness-promoting agent, received a guideline rating as a treatment modality.

First Line

Circadian shift/sleep promoting: Melatonin, 3 mg PO or sublingual, 30 minutes before daytime sleep period. It should be taken only when the patient is home and able to go to bed if the hypnotic effects begin.

Second Line

- Wakefulness-promoting:
  - Modafinil (Provigil) 100–200 mg PO 60 minutes before the shift begins
  - Armodafinil (Nuvigil) 150–250 mg is long-acting (12–16 hours, depending on food intake) and should be used judiciously in SWD as not to impede a patient's ability to sleep after the shift.
- Hypnotic: Zolpidem (Ambien) 5–10 mg or eszopiclone (Lunesta) 2–3 mg 30 minutes before desired sleep period

ISSUES FOR REFERRAL

Reasons to refer to a sleep specialist: Suspicion of other primary sleep disorders; dependence on hypnotics, alcohol, or stimulants

ONGOING CARE

PATIENT EDUCATION

- Health care providers should discuss good sleep hygiene and advise on how to optimize the sleep environment.
- Shift workers who need to sleep in the daytime must take serious measures to ensure that their sleep environment is cool, dark, and quiet.
- Remove all telephones, including mobile phones, and disconnect the doorbell.
- Blackout shades are usually necessary in order to achieve the proper darkness. Patients need to understand that the single most powerful wake signal to the brain is light. They need to learn when to seek light and when to avoid it.

PROGNOSIS

- Given the challenge to diagnose SWD appropriately and the limited treatment options, prognosis data are hard to evaluate.
- Shift workers should learn tactics needed to regulate their sleep/wake cycle.

REFERENCES

1. Sack RL, Auckley D, Auger RR, et al. Circadian rhythm sleep disorders: Part I, basic principles, shift work and jet lag disorders. An American Academy of Sleep Medicine review. *Sleep.* 2007;30: 1460–1483.
2. Stevens RG, Hansen J, Costa G, et al. Considerations of circadian impact for defining "shift work" in cancer studies: IARC Working Group Report. *Occup Environ Med.* 2011;68: 154–162.
3. Morgenthaler TI, Lee-Chiong T, Alessi C, et al. Practice parameters for the clinical evaluation and treatment of circadian rhythm sleep disorders. An American Academy of Sleep Medicine report. *Sleep.* 2007;30:1445–1459.
4. Bjorvatn B, Pallesen S. A practical approach to circadian rhythm sleep disorders. *Sleep Med Rev.* 2009;13:47–60.

ADDITIONAL READING

Sleep Diary: http://www.helpguide.org/life/pdfs/sleep_diary.pdf.

CODES

ICD10

G47.26 Circadian rhythm sleep disorder, shift work type

CLINICAL PEARLS

- Shift work is exceedingly and increasingly common in the industrialized world and is negatively impacting both the quality of life and the long-term health of many of those who perform shift work.
- Other primary sleep disorders commonly coexist (OSA, RLS) with, and exacerbate, shift work disorder, as do some OTC agents, like stimulants. Carefully screen for OSA in particular among the shift-work population.
- It is essential to educate the shift worker about the effect that light has on his/her sleep/wake cycle.
- The most important 1st diagnostic step is to obtain a sleep diary.

SMELL AND TASTE DISORDERS
Beth K. Mazyck, MD • Daniel B. Kurtz, PhD

 BASICS

DESCRIPTION
- The senses of smell and taste allow a full appreciation of the flavor and palatability of foods and also serve as a warning system against toxins, polluted air, smoke, and spoiled food.
- Physiologically, the chemical senses aid in normal digestion by triggering GI secretions. Smell/Taste dysfunction may have a significant impact on quality of life.
- Loss of smell occurs more frequently than loss of taste, and patients frequently confuse the concepts of flavor loss (as a result of smell impairment) with taste loss (an impaired ability to sense sweet, sour, salty, or bitter).
- Smell depends on the functioning of CN I (olfactory nerve) and CN V (trigeminal nerve).
- Taste depends on the functioning of CNs VII, IX, and X. Because of these multiple pathways, total loss of taste (ageusia) is rare.
- System(s) affected: Nervous; Upper Respiratory

EPIDEMIOLOGY
Incidence
There are ~200,000 patient visits a year for smell and taste disturbances.

Prevalence
- Predominant sex: Male > Female. Men begin to lose their ability to smell earlier in life than women.
- Predominant age: Chemosensory loss is age-dependent:
  - Age >80 years: 80% have major olfactory impairment; nearly 50% are anosmic.
  - Ages 65–80 years: 60% have major olfactory impairment; nearly 25% are anosmic.
  - Age <65 years: 1–2% have smell impairment.
- Estimated >2 million affected in the US

ETIOLOGY AND PATHOPHYSIOLOGY
- Smell and/or taste disturbances (1,2):
  - Nutritional factors (e.g., malnutrition, vitamin deficiencies, liver disease, anemia)
  - Endocrine disorders (e.g., thyroid disease, diabetes mellitus, renal disease)
  - Head trauma
  - Migraine headache (e.g., gustatory aura, olfactory aura)
  - Sjögren syndrome
  - Toxic chemical exposure
  - Industrial agent exposure
  - Aging
  - Medications (see below)
  - Neurodegenerative diseases (e.g., multiple sclerosis, Alzheimer disease, cerebrovascular accident, Parkinson disease)
  - Infections (e.g., upper respiratory infection [URI], oral and perioral infections, candidiasis, coxsackievirus, AIDS, viral hepatitis, herpes simplex virus)

- Possible causes of smell disturbance:
  - Nasal and sinus disease (e.g., allergies, rhinitis, rhinorrhea)
  - Cigarette smoking
  - Cocaine abuse (intranasal)
  - Hemodialysis
  - Radiation treatment of head and neck
  - Congenital conditions
  - Neoplasm (e.g., brain tumor, nasal polyps, intranasal tumor)
  - Systemic lupus erythematosus (SLE)
  - Bell palsy
  - Oral/Perioral skin lesion
  - Damage to CN I/V
  - Possible association with psychosis and schizophrenia
- Possible causes of taste loss:
  - Oral appliances
  - Dental procedures
  - Intraoral abscess
  - Gingivitis
  - Damage to CN VI, IX, or X
  - Stroke (especially frontal lobe)
- Selected medications that reportedly alter smell and taste:
  - Antibiotics: Amikacin, ampicillin, azithromycin (Zithromax), ciprofloxacin (Cipro), clarithromycin (Biaxin), doxycycline, griseofulvin (Grisactin), metronidazole (Flagyl), ofloxacin (Floxin), tetracycline, terbinafine (Lamisil), β-lactamase inhibitors
  - Anticonvulsants: Carbamazepine (Tegretol), phenytoin (Dilantin)
  - Antidepressants: Amitriptyline (Elavil), clomipramine (Anafranil), desipramine (Norpramin), doxepin (Sinequan), imipramine (Tofranil), nortriptyline (Pamelor)
  - Antihistamines and decongestants: Chlorpheniramine, loratadine (Claritin), pseudoephedrine, zinc-based cold remedies (Zicam)
  - Antihypertensives and cardiac medications: Acetazolamide (Diamox), amiloride (Midamor), betaxolol (Betoptic), captopril (Capoten), diltiazem (Cardizem), enalapril (Vasotec), hydrochlorothiazide (Esidrix) and combinations, nifedipine (Procardia), nitroglycerin, propranolol (Inderal), spironolactone (Aldactone)
  - Anti-inflammatory agents: Auranofin (Ridaura), colchicine, dexamethasone (Decadron), gold (Myochrysine), hydrocortisone, penicillamine (Cuprimine)
  - Antimanic drugs: Lithium
  - Antineoplastics: Cisplatin (Platinol), doxorubicin (Adriamycin), methotrexate (Rheumatrex), vincristine (Oncovin)
  - Antiparkinsonian agents: Levodopa (Larodopa, with carbidopa (Sinemet)
  - Antipsychotics: Clozapine (Clozaril), trifluoperazine (Stelazine)
  - Antithyroid agents: Methimazole (Tapazole), propylthiouracil
  - Lipid-lowering agents: Fluvastatin (Lescol), lovastatin (Mevacor), pravastatin (Pravachol)
  - Muscle relaxants: Baclofen (Lioresal), dantrolene (Dantrium)

Genetics
May be related to underlying genetically associated diseases (Kallmann syndrome, Alzheimer disease, migraine syndromes, rheumatologic conditions, endocrine disorders)

RISK FACTORS
- Age >65 years
- Poor nutritional status
- Smoking tobacco products

GENERAL PREVENTION
- Eat a well-balanced diet, with appropriate vitamins and minerals.
- Maintain good oral and nasal health, with routine visits to the dentist.
- Do not smoke tobacco products.
- Avoid noxious chemical exposures/unnecessary radiation.

Geriatric Considerations
- Elders are at particular risk of eating spoiled food or inadvertently being exposed to natural gas leaks owing to anosmia from aging.
- Anosmia also may be an early sign of degenerative disorders such as Alzheimer disease.

Pediatric Considerations
- Smell and taste disorders are uncommon in children in developed countries.
- In developing countries with poor nutrition (particularly zinc depletion), smell and taste disorders may occur.
- Delayed puberty in association with anosmia (± midline craniofacial abnormalities, deafness, or renal abnormalities) suggests the possibility of Kallmann syndrome (hypogonadotropic hypogonadism).

Pregnancy Considerations
- Pregnancy is an uncommon cause of smell and taste loss or disturbances.
- Many women report increased sensitivity to odors during pregnancy, as well as an increased dislike for bitterness and a preference for salty substances.

COMMONLY ASSOCIATED CONDITIONS
URI, allergic rhinitis, dental abscesses

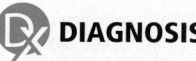 **DIAGNOSIS**

Smell and taste disturbances are symptoms; it is essential to look for possible underlying causes.

HISTORY
- Symptoms of URI, environmental allergies
- Oral pain, other dental problems
- Cognitive/Memory difficulties
- Current medications
- Nutritional status, ovolactovegetarian
- Weight loss or gain
- Frequent infections (impaired immunity)
- Worsening of underlying medical illness
- Increased use of salt and/or sugar to increase taste of food

PHYSICAL EXAM
Thorough HEENT exam

DIFFERENTIAL DIAGNOSIS
- Epilepsy (gustatory aura)
- Epilepsy (olfactory aura)
- Memory impairment
- Psychiatric conditions

DIAGNOSTIC TESTS & INTERPRETATION
Initial Tests (lab, imaging)
Consider (not all patients require all tests):
- Hemoglobin
- WBC count
- BUN
- Blood glucose
- Creatinine
- Bilirubin
- Alkaline phosphatase
- Thyroid-stimulating hormone (TSH)
- Serum IgE
- Plain radiographs have substantial limitations (and are rarely useful).
- CT scanning is the most useful and cost-effective technique for assessing sinonasal disorders and is superior to an MRI in evaluating bony structures and airway patency. Coronal CT scans are particularly valuable in assessing paranasal anatomy.

Follow-Up Tests & Special Considerations
Diagnosis of smell and taste disturbances is usually possible through history (1)[C]; however, the following tests can be used to confirm:
- Olfactory tests:
  - Smell identification test: Evaluates the ability to identify 40 microencapsulated scratch-and-sniff odorants
  - Brief smell identification test
- Taste tests (more difficult because no convenient standardized tests are presently available): Solutions containing sucrose (sweet), sodium chloride (salty), quinine (bitter), and citric acid (sour) are helpful.
- An MRI is useful in defining soft-tissue disease; therefore, a coronal MRI is the technique of choice to image the olfactory bulbs, tracts, and cortical parenchyma. Possible placement of an accessory coil (TMJ) over the nose to assist in imaging.

TREATMENT

GENERAL MEASURES
- Appropriate treatment for underlying cause
- Quit smoking.
- Some drug-related dysgeusias can be reversed with cessation of the agent, but it may take many months.
- Eliminate exposures (e.g., volatile gases, toxins, use of oxygen-liberating mouthwashes).
- Stop repeated oral trauma (e.g., appliances, tongue-biting behaviors).
- Proper nutritional and dietary assessment
- Formal dental evaluation

MEDICATION
- Treat underlying causes as appropriate. Of idiopathic cases, will resolve spontaneously.
- Corticosteroids topically (e.g., aqueous nasal spray) or systemically (e.g., oral prednisone) may be helpful. Prednisone 60 mg/d × 4 days, then taper by 10 mg/d thereafter.
- Artificial saliva (e.g., Xero-Lube) may be helpful in patients with xerostomia.
- Pilocarpine (Salagen) 5–10 mg PO t.i.d. may help with dry mouth/xerostomia; response may take 6–12 weeks.
- Chlorhexidine (Peridex) 0.12% oral rinse may help with gingivitis/dysgeusia.
- Zinc and vitamins (A, B complex) when deficiency is suspected

ISSUES FOR REFERRAL
- Consider referral to an otolaryngologist or neurologist for persistent cases.
- Referral to a subspecialist at a smell and taste center, if needed

SURGERY/OTHER PROCEDURES
If needed for treatment of underlying cause

ONGOING CARE

DIET
- Weight gain/loss is possible because the patient may reject food or may switch to calorie-rich foods that are still palatable.
- Ensure a nutritionally balanced diet with appropriate levels of nutrients, vitamins, and essential minerals.

PATIENT EDUCATION
- Caution patients not to overindulge as compensation for the bland taste of food. For example, patients with diabetes may need help in avoiding excessive sugar intake as an inappropriate way of improving food taste.
- Patients with chemosensory impairments should use measuring devices when cooking and should not cook by taste.
- Optimizing food texture, aroma, temperature, and color may improve the overall food experience when taste is limited.
- Patients with permanent smell dysfunction must develop adaptive strategies for dealing with hygiene, appetite, safety, and health.
- Natural gas and smoke detectors are essential; check for proper function frequently.
- Check food expiration dates frequently; discard old food.

PROGNOSIS
- In general, the olfactory system regenerates poorly after a head injury. Most patients who recover smell function subsequent to head trauma do so within 12 weeks of injury.
- Patients who quit smoking typically recover improved olfactory function and flavor sensation.
- Many taste disorders (dysgeusias) resolve spontaneously within a few years of onset.
- Phantosmias that are flow-dependent may respond to surgical ablation of olfactory mucosa.
- Conditions such as radiation-induced xerostomia and Bell palsy generally improve over time.

COMPLICATIONS
- Permanent loss of ability to smell/taste
- Psychiatric issues with dysgeusias and phantosmia

REFERENCES
1. Bromley SM. Smell and taste disorders: A primary care approach. *Am Fam Physician*. 2000;61:427–436, 438.
2. Nguyen-Khoa B, Goehring EL, Vendiola RM. Epidemiologic study of smell disturbance in 2 medical insurance claims populations. *Arch Otolaryngol Head Neck Surg*. 2007;133(8):748–757.

ADDITIONAL READING
- Cullen MM, Leopold DA. Disorders of smell and taste. *Med Clin North Am*. 1999;83:57–74.
- Lacroix JS, Landis BN. Future perspectives in smell and taste disorders. *B-ENT*. 2009;5(Suppl 13):133–136.

CODES

ICD10
- R43.1 Parosmia
- R43.2 Parageusia
- R43.9 Unspecified disturbances of smell and taste

CLINICAL PEARLS
- Smell disorders are often mistaken as decreased taste by patients.
- Actual taste disorders are often related to dental problems.
- Smell disorders are very common in the elderly; extensive workup in this population may not be indicated if no associated signs/symptoms are present.

SNAKE ENVENOMATIONS, CROTALIDAE

Lee T. Church, MD • Ryan D. Pearson, MD

BASICS

DESCRIPTION
- Symptom complex following envenomation by a snake of the family *Viperidae*, subfamily *Crotalinae* (pit vipers)
- Includes snakes of the genera *Crotalus* (rattlesnakes), *Agkistrodon* (moccasins/cottonmouth/copperhead), and *Sistrurus* (pygmy rattlesnake/massasaugas)
- Occurs most commonly in the southeastern and southwestern US
- North American pit viper characteristics:
  - Triangular-shaped heads, eyes with elliptical pupils, and small heat-sensing facial pits located between the nostril and the eye
  - In contrast, nonpoisonous snakes in the US generally have small, round heads and round pupils, except coral snakes (which are highly venomous and brightly colored).
- System(s) affected: Cardiovascular; Hematologic/Lymphatic/Immunologic; Nervous; Skin/Exocrine
- Synonym(s): Crotalidae envenomation; snakebite; venomous snakebite; pit viper snakebite

EPIDEMIOLOGY
Incidence
- In 2011, per the National Poison Data System 29th Annual Report there were 6,630 reported snakebites in the US with 2 exposures resulting in death (1):
  - ~55% of reported snakebites are identified as crotaline.
  - ~43% are from unidentified snakes.
- The actual incidence of envenomation may be higher due to underreporting or lower due to dry bites.
- Predominant age: >20 years

ETIOLOGY AND PATHOPHYSIOLOGY
Clinical problems related to envenomation include tissue damage, coagulopathy, thrombocytopenia, hypovolemia, and neurotoxicity.
- Pit viper venom is a complex mixture that contains cytotoxins, hemotoxins, neurotoxins, and cardiotoxins.
- Toxin composition varies from bite to bite, even from the same snake.
- Envenomation can affect all major organ systems.
- Mojave rattlesnake venom, which is more neurotoxic than that of other crotalids, can cause respiratory depression.

RISK FACTORS
- Handling, provoking, or pursuing snakes
- Acute ethanol intoxication/other drug intoxication that impairs judgment

GENERAL PREVENTION
- Use preventive measures if handling snakes.
- In snake-infested areas:
  - Wear protective shoes and clothing when walking.
  - Do not insert hands/feet into cracks, crevices, or hollow logs.
  - Carry a flashlight if walking at night.

DIAGNOSIS
- Signs and symptoms vary, from minor local injury to severe systemic illness.
- Snake identification is helpful, but should not place others at risk for being bitten.
- Digital photography may be a safe means to identify the snake.

PHYSICAL EXAM
- Fang mark(s): >90%
- Pain out of proportion to puncture wound, usually within minutes of the bite: >50%
- Edema of site, progressing proximally up extremity: >50%
- Weakness, dizziness: >50%
- Numbness/Tingling in extremity, mouth, tongue: >50%
- Ecchymosis of skin, vesicles around bite, which may take hours to develop: >50%
- Tachycardia: >50%
- Nausea/Vomiting: <50%
- Hypo- or hypertension: <50%
- Muscle fasciculations: <50%
- Mental status changes, including coma: <25%
- Change in taste sensation

DIFFERENTIAL DIAGNOSIS
- Bite of nonvenomous snake
- Bite of venomous species other than those of *Crotalinae* subfamily
- Crotaline bite without envenomation (dry bite)

DIAGNOSTIC TESTS & INTERPRETATION
- CBC: Hemoglobin/Hematocrit and/or platelets decreased in <50%
- Prothrombin time/International normalized ratio, adjusted partial thromboplastin time: Prolonged in >50%
- Fibrinogen (decreased in <50%), fibrin degradation products (increased in <50%)
- Urinalysis: Glycosuria (<50%), proteinuria (<25%), hematuria (<25%)
- Type and crossmatch "to hold" in severe envenomations
- Electrolytes, BUN, creatinine
- LFTs
- Creatine kinase in severe envenomations
- Serum ethanol level if suspicious
- Disorders that may alter lab results:
  - Preexisting anemia/polycythemia
  - Advanced liver disease
  - Kidney disease
  - Platelet disorders
- Drug(s) that may alter lab results: Anticoagulants

TREATMENT
- Patients with true envenomations need emergency department evaluation.
- Rapid transportation should take priority over all but the most basic first aid:
  - Most field snakebite treatments (e.g., cutting the bite, attempting to remove poison with suction, tourniquet, and constriction bandages) are ineffective and potentially harmful.

- Reassure patient; minimize patient movement during transport.
- Splint area of bite, allowing room for swelling.
- Position affected extremity at or below level of heart.
- Support vital signs, place on monitor, O_2 as needed, and obtain IV access.
- Remove rings and constrictive items.

GENERAL MEASURES
- Reassess all prehospital care. Use of tourniquet and pressure dressings is controversial. If tourniquet has been placed in prehospital setting, sudden removal could bolus patient with venom. A tourniquet or constriction band should be removed only after beginning the treatment with antivenom.
- Obtain toxicology consultation by contacting the American Association of Poison Control Centers' regional poison information center (www.AAPCC.org). (800) 222-1222
- Minimal envenomation:
  - If local signs of edema are confined to the bite area, without any other symptom of envenomation, place IV line of crystalloid at maintenance rates and draw baseline laboratory studies.
  - Place reference marks for measuring circumference of extremity at 10 and 20 cm proximal to the site of envenomation. Measure q15min and mark leading edge of swelling.
  - Give tetanus toxoid if needed.
  - Provide pain relief: IV opioids preferred.
  - Repeat laboratory studies in 6 hours. If all remains normal and swelling does not progress, observe 8–12 hours and then follow up as outpatient.
  - If swelling progresses or systemic signs and symptoms appear, patient needs admission and further therapy (progress to moderate–severe envenomation measures).
- Moderate–severe envenomation:
  - If edema, vesicles, erythema progress beyond the immediate bite area, or there are associated systemic signs/symptoms (hypotension, bleeding beyond puncture site, refractory vomiting, diarrhea, angioedema, neurotoxicity) or laboratory abnormalities (elevated ProTime, decreased fibrinogen or platelets), then give IV antivenom + all minimal envenomation management.
  - Intensive care monitoring may be necessary.
  - Repeat laboratory evaluations q6h initially until stable and then less frequently.
  - Blood products are necessary only for coagulopathies with clinical bleeding, not for the treatment of laboratory abnormalities. Antivenom treatment may reverse hematologic abnormalities and should be given 1st.
  - Have equipment and medications readily at hand to treat allergic reactions to antivenom.

MEDICATION
First Line
- Crotalidae polyvalent immune Fab (Ovine) (2,3)[B]:
  - No skin test necessary
  - Initial dose: 4–6 reconstituted vials added to normal saline (total volume 250 mL):
    - 10 mL of sterile water added to each vial; swirl only (do not shake) so as not to denature proteins
    - Infuse IV slowly for the first 10 minutes; then increase the rate to 250 mL/hr to run remainder over 60 minutes

○ For patients in acute shock/with active bleeding, a higher initial dose (8–12 vials) has been recommended (4).

○ After initial infusion is complete, if all signs/symptoms of envenomation have not ceased, give up to ≥2 doses of 4–6 vials until initial control is achieved.

– Maintenance: After initial control of symptoms, administer 3 maintenance doses of 2 vials at 6, 12, and 18 hours following time of initial control.

- Precautions: Papain is used in the manufacturing process of Crotalidae polyvalent immune Fab; patients with papaya allergies may be at risk for an allergic reaction.
- Adverse reactions: Anaphylaxis, serum sickness; 5–19% of patients developed hypersensitivity reaction, but most reactions are mild, easily treated, and do not prevent completion of the antivenom treatment.

Second Line
Pain relief with opiate (e.g., morphine sulfate 0.1–0.2 mg/kg/dose q2–4h, as needed) *or* acetaminophen (10–15 mg/kg/dose q4–6h, as needed; max 4 g/d in adults)

ALERT
Avoid aspirin, NSAIDs, and other anticoagulants.

SURGERY/OTHER PROCEDURES
- Fasciotomy is rarely needed; no current studies show it is beneficial.
- Envenomation may mimic compartment syndrome, making clinical distinction difficult.
- Decision to perform a fasciotomy should be based on measured compartmental pressures.

IN-PATIENT CONSIDERATIONS
Admission Criteria/Initial Stabilization
- Dry bites may be observed for 8–12 hours. The patient can be discharged if there is no evidence of envenomation.
- Anyone receiving antivenom should be admitted, because of frequent evaluation and lab draws; most will require ICU placement.

Patient Monitoring
- Once you have determined if initial control of envenomation has been achieved:
  – Perform serial exams looking for signs/symptoms of worsening envenomation.
  – If worsening envenomation are noted, maintenance antivenom therapy may be given 2 vials of antivenom q6hr ×3 (at 6, 12, and 18 hours after initial control).
  – Repeat labs q6hrs after initial control and prior to discharge.

ONGOING CARE

FOLLOW-UP RECOMMENDATIONS
Patient Monitoring
- Phone follow-up in 12–24 hours for discharged dry bites, then PRN after that.
- If antivenom given, patient should return twice in the 1st week post discharge for repeat labs: First return visit within 48 hours of hospital discharge, then at 1 week and as clinically indicated thereafter.
- Physical therapy referral should be made early for optimal outpatient intervention.

PATIENT EDUCATION
- Return precautions upon discharge:
  – Worsening swelling not relieved by elevation.
  – Abnormal bleeding; melena, gums, or easy bruising
- If patient received antivenom therapy, instruct him to watch for signs serum sickness (rash, fever, polyarthralgias, or polyarthritis).
- Avoid elective surgery, dental work, contact sports, and anticoagulant medications (including aspirin) after discharge for ~2 weeks.

PROGNOSIS
Mortality: 2 of 6,630 total reported snakebites in the U.S. during 2011 resulted in fatality (1).

Geriatric Considerations
- Course may be more severe
- Consider ECG, chest x-ray, and arterial blood gases if underlying conditions may be exacerbated by stress of envenomation.

Pediatric Considerations
- Course may be more severe
- Crotalidae polyvalent immune Fab (Ovine) dosing is the same as for adults and appears to be similarly tolerated (5).
- Fluid overload may be a problem in small children who require multiple vials of antivenom.

Pregnancy Considerations
- Snakebites in pregnant women in North America are rare, but consequences appear to be more severe than in nonpregnant patients. The overall case-fatality rate in pregnant females has been reported as ~4% with a fetal loss rate of ~20% (6).
- Pregnant patients should be counseled about the presence of thiomersal in antivenom. The unknown risks of thiomersal should be weighed against the benefit of antivenom in significant envenomations.
- Treatment that optimizes maternal health is presumed to be the best available treatment for the fetus.
- There are no studies of Crotalidae polyvalent immune Fab (Ovine) in pregnant women.

COMPLICATIONS
- Local wound infection (rare)
- Bleeding after discharge from hospital: Patients should be told to report nosebleeds, excessive bleeding after brushing teeth, blood in stools/vomitus, or excessive menstrual bleeding.

REFERENCES

1. Bronstein AC, Spyker DA, Cantilena LR Jr., et al. 2011 Annual report of the American Association of Poison Control Centers' National Poison Data System (NPDS): 29th Annual Report. *Clin Toxicol (Phila)*. 2012;50(10):911–1164.
2. Dart RC. A randomized multicenter trial of Crotalinae polyvalent immune Fab (ovine) antivenom for the treatment for crotaline snakebite in the United States. *Ann Emerg Med*. 2001;161: 2030–2036.
3. Weant KA, Johnson PN, Bowers RC, et al. Evidence-based, multidisciplinary approach to the development of a Crotalidae polyvalent antivenin (CroFab) protocol at a university hospital. *Ann Pharmacother*. 2010;44:447–455.
4. Lavonas EJ, Ruha AM, Banner W, et al. Unified treatment algorithm for the management of crotaline snakebite in the United States: Results of an evidence-informed consensus workshop. *BMC Emerg Med*. 2011;11:2.
5. Farrar HC, Grayham T, Bolden B, et al. The use and tolerability of Crotalidae Polyvalent Immune FAB (Ovine) in pediatric envenomations. *Clin Pediatr (Phila)*. 2012;84(10):945–949. Epub 2012 Apr 17.
6. Langley RL. Snakebite during pregnancy: A literature review. *Wilderness Environ Med*. 2010; 21(1):54–60.

ADDITIONAL READING

- Cardwell MD. Recognizing dangerous snakes in the United States and Canada: A novel 3-step identification method. *Wilderness Environ Med*. 2011;22:304–308.
- Gold BS, Barish RA, Dart RC. North American snake envenomation: Diagnosis, treatment, and management. *Emerg Med Clin North Am*. 2004;22:423–443, ix.
- World Health Organization venomous snake distribution database http://apps.who.int/bloodproducts/snakeantivenoms/database/default.htm
- Wozniak EJ, Wisser J, Schwartz M. Venomous adversaries: A reference to snake identification, field safety, and bite-victim first aid for disaster-response personnel deploying into the hurricane-prone regions of North America. *Wilderness Environ Med*. 2006;17:246–266.

 ### SEE ALSO

Snake Envenomations, Elapidae (Coral Snake)

 ## CODES

ICD10
- T63.011A Toxic effect of rattlesnake venom, accidental, init
- T63.014A Toxic effect of rattlesnake venom, undetermined, init encntr
- T63.064A Toxic effect of venom of N & S American snake, undet, init

CLINICAL PEARLS
- Poison Control Center: (800) 222-1222
- The best first aid for snakebites is rapidly transporting a calm and still victim. Do *not* cut or attempt to suck out the venom. Cold therapy, electrical shocks, and tourniquets have been shown to be potentially harmful and, at least, unhelpful.
- Skin testing is not necessary before antivenom administration.
- Once moderate–severe envenomation has been diagnosed and antivenom delivered; patient should be admitted to ICU for serial exams, labs, and possible maintenance antivenom therapy if warranted.
- The rate of infection following crotaline snakebite is so low that prophylactic antibiotics are not indicated.

SOMATIZATION DISORDER

Robert A. Baldor, MD

 BASICS

DESCRIPTION
- A pattern of recurring, multiple, clinically significant somatic complaints beginning <30 years of age that occur over a period of several years and result in treatment being sought or significant impairment in social, occupational, or other important areas of functioning
- Each of the following criteria must be met, with individual symptoms occurring at any time during the course of the disturbance:
  - 4 pain symptoms: Different sites or functions
  - 2 GI symptoms: Other than pain
  - 1 sexual symptom
  - 1 pseudoneurologic symptom
- These symptoms are not intentionally produced or feigned.
- Chronic course, fluctuating in severity
- Affected individual rarely goes 1 year without seeking medical attention prompted by unexplained somatic complaints.
- System(s) affected: Multiple
- Synonym: Briquet syndrome

EPIDEMIOLOGY
Incidence
- Usually, 1st symptoms appear in adolescence; full criteria met by 30 years of age.
- Predominant sex: Female > Male (10:1)
- Type and frequency of somatic complaints may differ among cultures, so symptom reviews should be adjusted based on culture.

Prevalence
- Ranges from 0.2–2% among women and <0.2% among men
- 1/500 adults in the US
- Seen in up to 29% of patients presenting to primary care offices (1)
- Prevalence declines after age 65 (2)

ETIOLOGY AND PATHOPHYSIOLOGY
- Unknown
- Adoption studies indicate that both genetic and environmental factors contribute to the risk of somatization disorder (SD).

Genetics
- Observed in 10–20% of female 1st-degree biologic relatives of women with SD
- Male relatives of women with this disorder show an increased risk of antisocial personality disorder and substance-related disorders.

RISK FACTORS
- Child abuse, particularly sexual abuse, has been shown to be a risk factor.
- Symptoms begin or worsen after losses (e.g., job, close relative, or friend).
- Greater intensity of symptoms often occurs with stress.

COMMONLY ASSOCIATED CONDITIONS
Comorbid with other psychiatric conditions, including major depression (55% of patients), anxiety disorders (34%), personality disorders (61%), and panic disorders (26%)

 DIAGNOSIS

HISTORY
- Multiple somatic complaints, usually a grossly positive review of symptoms
- Pain symptoms (≥4) related to different sites, such as head, abdomen, back, joints, extremities, chest, or rectum, or related to body functions, such as menstruation, sexual intercourse, or urination
- GI symptoms (≥2, excluding pain), such as nausea, bloating, vomiting (not during pregnancy), diarrhea, intolerance of several foods
- Sexual symptoms (at least 1, excluding pain), such as indifference to sex, difficulties with erection or ejaculation, irregular menses, excessive menstrual bleeding, or vomiting throughout all 9 months of pregnancy
- Pseudoneurologic symptoms (at least 1), such as impaired balance or coordination, weak or paralyzed muscles, lump in throat or trouble swallowing, loss of voice, retention of urine, hallucinations, numbness (to touch or pain), double vision, blindness, deafness, seizures, amnesia or other dissociative symptoms, loss of consciousness (other than with fainting); none of these is limited to pain

PHYSICAL EXAM
Physical exam remarkable for absence of objective findings to fully explain the many subjective complaints

DIFFERENTIAL DIAGNOSIS
- Other psychiatric illnesses must be ruled out:
  - Depressive disorders
  - Anxiety disorders
  - Schizophrenia
  - Other somatoform disorders: Conversion disorder, factitious disorders, hypochondriasis, pain disorder
- General medical conditions, with vague, multiple, confusing symptoms, must be ruled out:
  - Systemic lupus erythematosus
  - Hyperparathyroidism
  - Hyper- or hypothyroidism
  - Lyme disease
  - Porphyria

DIAGNOSTIC TESTS & INTERPRETATION
Several screening tools are available that help to identify symptoms as somatic:
- Patient Health Questionnaire (PHQ)-15 (screens and monitors symptoms) (3)[C]
- Minnesota Multiphasic Personality Inventory (MMPI) (identifies somatization) (4)[C]
- Perley-Guze Checklist (helps the physician to identify SD)

Initial Tests (lab, imaging)
- Laboratory test results do not support the subjective complaints.
- Imaging studies do not support the subjective complaints.

Test Interpretation
None are identified.

TREATMENT

GENERAL MEASURES

- The goal of treatment is to help the person learn to control the symptoms.
- A supportive relationship with a sympathetic health care provider is the most important aspect of treatment (5)[C]:
  - Regularly scheduled appointments should be maintained to review symptoms and the person's coping mechanisms (at least 15 minutes once a month) (5)[C].
  - Acknowledge and explain test results
- The involvement of a single physician is important because a history of seeking medical attention and "doctor shopping" is common.
- Antidepressant or antianxiety medication and referral to a support group or psychiatrist can help patients who are willing to participate in their treatment.
- Patients usually receive the most benefit from primary care physicians who accept the limitations of treatment, listen to their patient's concerns, and provide reassurance.
- It is not helpful to tell patients that their symptoms are imaginary.

MEDICATION

Antidepressants (e.g., SSRIs) help to treat comorbid depression and anxiety.

ISSUES FOR REFERRAL

- Discourage referrals to specialists for further investigation of somatic complaints
- Referrals to support groups or to a psychiatrist may be helpful.

ADDITIONAL THERAPIES

Treatment typically includes long-term therapy, which has been shown to decrease the severity of symptoms:

- Cognitive–behavioral therapy has been shown to be the most efficacious treatment in SD (6)[B],(7)[A].
- Psychotherapy
- Supportive therapy

ONGOING CARE

FOLLOW-UP RECOMMENDATIONS

Patients should have regularly scheduled follow up with a primary care doctor, psychiatrist, and/or therapist.

PATIENT EDUCATION

Encourage interventions that decrease stressful elements of the patient's life:

- Psychoeducational advice
- Increase in exercise
- Pleasurable private time

PROGNOSIS

- Chronic course, fluctuating in severity
- Full remission is rare.
- Individuals with this disorder do not experience any significant difference in mortality rate or significant physical illness.
- Patients with this diagnosis do experience substantially greater functional disability and role impairment than nonsomatizing patients (8).

COMPLICATIONS

- May result from invasive testing and from multiple evaluations that are performed while looking for the cause of the symptoms
- A dependency on pain relievers or sedatives may develop.

REFERENCES

1. Roca M, Gili M, Garcia-Garcia M, et al. Prevalence and comorbidity of common mental disorders in primary care. *J Affect Disord*. 2009;119:52–58.
2. Hilderink PH, Collard R, Rosmalen JG, et al. Prevalence of somatoform disorders and medically unexplained symptoms in old age populations in comparison with younger age groups: A systematic review. *Ageing Res Rev*. 2012;12:151–156.
3. Kroenke K, Spitzer RL, Williams JB. The PHQ-15: Validity of a new measure for evaluating the severity of somatic symptoms. *Psychosom Med*. 2002;64:258–266.
4. Wetzel RD, Brim J, Guze SB, et al. MMPI screening scales for somatization disorder. *Psychol Rep*. 1999;85:341–348.
5. Servan-Schreiber D, Tabas G, Kolb R. Somatizing patients: Part II. Practical management. *Am Fam Physician*. 2000;61:1423–1428, 1431–1432.
6. Allen LA, Woolfolk RL, Escobar JI, et al. Cognitive-behavioral therapy for somatization disorder: A randomized controlled trial. *Arch Intern Med*. 2006;166:1512–1518.
7. Kroenke K, Swindle R. Cognitive-behavioral therapy for somatization and symptom syndromes: A critical review of controlled clinical trials. *Psychother Psychosom*. 2000;69:205–215.
8. Harris AM, Orav EJ, Bates DW, et al. Somatization increases disability independent of comorbidity. *J Gen Intern Med*. 2009;24:155–161.

ADDITIONAL READING

Mai F. Somatization disorder: A practical review. *Can J Psychiatry*. 2004;49:652–662.

CODES

ICD10

- F45.0 Somatization disorder
- F45.1 Undifferentiated somatoform disorder
- F45.9 Somatoform disorder, unspecified

CLINICAL PEARLS

- Acknowledge the patient's pain, suffering, and disability.
- Do not tell patients the symptoms are "all in their head."
- Emphasize that this is not a rare disorder.
- Discuss the limitations of treatment while providing reassurance that there are interventions that will lessen suffering and reduce symptoms.

SPIDER ANGIOMA

Rebecca Khezri Jacobson, MD • Dori Goldberg, MD

BASICS

DESCRIPTION
Solitary or multiple, blanchable vascular lesions consisting of a central arteriole that is surrounded by thin-walled capillaries that branch outward, which may be benign or indicative of an underlying condition (1):
- System(s) affected: Skin
- Synonym(s): Nevus araneus; Spider nevus; Arterial spider; Vascular spider (1)

EPIDEMIOLOGY
Incidence
Not well studied
Prevalence
- General population: 10–15% of normal adults and children (1)
- No definitive study documents a predominant sex.
- No definitive study documents a predominant race. However, lesions are easier to see in patients with lighter skin.
- Pregnant women and children are most commonly affected:
  - Pregnancy considerations: Occurs in 60–70% of pregnant white women and 10% of pregnant dark-skinned women (2)
  - More common in pregnant woman in their 1st and 2nd trimesters of pregnancy (2)
  - A reported 38% of school-aged children have 1–4 spider angiomas, with increased numbers of lesions with age.

ETIOLOGY AND PATHOPHYSIOLOGY
- Spider angiomas are due to dilation of existing blood vessels rather than the development of new blood vessels (1).
- The pathophysiology remains unclear, however, several hypotheses indicate a role for:
  - Higher levels of plasma estrogen that cause dilation of pre-existing arterioles (1)
  - Increased substance P, which is elevated in patients with spider angiomas and nonalcoholic cirrhosis (1)
  - Increased vascular endothelial growth factor (VEGF)
  - Increased basic fibroblastic growth factor (bFGF)
- The etiology is unclear, but lesions are associated with higher estrogen states including liver disease and pregnancy, but can occur in children without liver problems.

Genetics
No evidence of an inheritance pattern

RISK FACTORS
- An elevated estrogen state, including:
  - Pregnancy
  - An increased estradiol/free testosterone ratio in males with cirrhosis, which is inversely related to liver function (1)
  - Women who are taking oral contraceptives (1)
  - Women taking hormonal therapy
- Liver disease including cirrhosis:
  - Alcoholic cirrhosis > Nonalcoholic cirrhosis
  - Alcohol abuse > Viral hepatitis

GENERAL PREVENTION
No known prevention strategy

COMMONLY ASSOCIATED CONDITIONS
- Thyrotoxicosis
- Oral contraceptive use
- Pregnancy
- Liver disease
- Spider nevi are more common in alcoholic cirrhosis compared with viral or idiopathic cirrhosis.
- Spider nevi are strong predictors of hepatopulmonary syndrome (HPS) (1).
- Spider nevi can help predict the stage and grade of hepatitis C with moderate accuracy (1).
- Spider angiomas were seen in 50% of patients with marked portal and septal fibrosis of the liver and 84% of patients with cirrhosis (3).
- Almost no spider angiomas were seen in patients with minimal portal fibrosis or mild portal fibrosis with some septal fibrosis (3).
- Spider angiomas have a 4.3 (95% CI, 2.4–6.2) likelihood ratio in detecting cirrhosis (4).

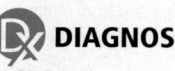

DIAGNOSIS

HISTORY
Obtain a thorough history including:
- A history of alcohol use (type, frequency, duration, pattern of consumption) (1)
- A history of medications including:
  - Estrogen therapy (1)
  - Medications that can cause liver damage (1)
  - Oral contraceptives (1)
- The possibility of pregnancy (1)
- A history of cirrhosis (1)
- The location of the lesion:
  - Located most frequently on the face, neck, arms, and upper part of the chest in adults (1)
  - In children, located on the dorsal portion of hands (1)
  - Infrequently seen in the mucous membranes, including the pharynx, mouth, and nose (1)
  - They can occur as single or multiple lesions (1). A greater number of lesions can be indicative of the extent of hepatic fibrosis.

PHYSICAL EXAM
- Skin: Examine for a lesion with a roughly 1 mm central erythematous papule with or without surrounding, radiating, thin-walled vessels:
  - Diameter may vary from the size of a pinhead to 5 cm (1)
  - Should be blanchable when pressed with a glass slide and rapidly refill at the central arteriole when the pressure is removed (1)
  - Occasionally may pulsate in the center (1)
  - Temperature may be 2–3°C higher than surrounding skin (1).
  - May disappear with improving liver function, hypotension, and discontinuation of medications (1)
  - Appears most commonly in exposed areas of the skin
  - May appear along the path of the superior vena cava in cases of liver disease (4)

- HEENT (Head, Eyes, Ears, Nose, Throat) exam: Examine mucous membranes for lesions:
  - Other signs of liver disease including:
    - Glossy tongue (1)
    - Jaundice
- Abdomen: Exam liver with palpation and percussion for liver span (1):
  - Ascites related to liver disease (1)
- Extremities: Palmar erythema, muscle atrophy, which are stigmata of liver disease:
  - Areas on the arms and buttocks that whiten with cooling of the skin may signify the early stages of a spider nevus (1).
  - Nails: Leukonychia associated with liver disease (1)
- Hair: In males, female distribution of hair secondary to hormonal changes related to liver disease (1).

DIFFERENTIAL DIAGNOSIS
- Cherry hemangioma (1)
- Osler-Weber-Rendu syndrome (1)
- Angioma serpiginosum (1)
- Ataxia telangiectatica
- Angiokeratoma corporis diffusum and circumscriptum as part of Fabry disease (1)
- Disseminated essential telangiectasia (1)
- Senile angioma (1)
- Insect bite (1)
- Acneiform eruptions
- Basal cell carcinoma
- Generalized essential telangiectasia
- Unilateral nevoid telangiectasia
- Hereditary benign telangiectasia
- Rosacea

DIAGNOSTIC TESTS & INTERPRETATION
Initial Tests (lab, imaging)
- Liver function tests: aspartate aminotransferase (AST), alanine aminotransferase (ALT), bilirubin
- Hepatitis panel
- Pregnancy: β-human chorionic gonadotropin (BHcG) test, if appropriate

Follow-Up Tests & Special Considerations
- Free estradiol/testosterone ratio in males with cirrhosis (1)
- Arterial blood gas (ABG) in patients with cirrhosis (1)
- Examine for clubbing in patients with hepatopulmonary syndrome (1)
- Useful sign in diagnosing hepatitis C with moderate accuracy (1)
- Helpful in diagnosing hepatopulmonary syndrome (1)

Diagnostic Procedures/Other
- Confirm the diagnosis by the characteristic morphology of the lesion and by observing refill at the central arteriole with compression (1)[C].
- Skin biopsy if the diagnosis is questionable and lesions such as basal cell carcinoma need to be ruled out
- In vivo reflectance confocal microscopy may be helpful as a noninvasive diagnostic tool to evaluate vascular lesions including spider angiomas (5)[A].

Test Interpretation
- An ascending arteriole that terminates as an ampulla beneath the epidermis with arterial branches in the papillary dermis (1)
- Glomus cells in the wall of the central arteriole (1)
- 5 components of spider nevus:
  - Central arteriole
  - Cutaneous arterial net
  - Subepidermal ampulla
  - Capillaries
  - Star-shaped formation of the radiating vessels (1)

TREATMENT

MEDICATION
First Line
- No treatment may be needed for:
  - Children whose lesions regress spontaneously (1)[C]
  - Young women who discontinue their oral contraception pills
  - Postpartum women since lesions often disappear at the end of pregnancy (2)[C]
  - Patients with liver disease whose disease improves with treatment or transplant
- Electrodesiccation of the central arteriole:
  - For larger telangiectasias; may lead to scarring and bleeding
  - Incomplete electrodesiccation can result in recurrence.
  - Aggressive electrodesiccation can result in a pitted scar.
- Laser treatments include argon, copper vapor, flashlamp-pump dye, pulse dye laser (PDL), and potassium titanul phosphate (KTP)
  - Argon laser:
    - An earlier, more nonselective treatment that led to more scarring and pigmentary changes
    - Treatment is less effective in darker-skinned patients with associated changes in pigmentation (6)[B].
  - Flashlamp-pump dye lasers:
    - In adults, may lead to purpura (6)[B]
    - In 1 retrospective study, 93% clearance after treatment of spider angiomas
    - Most common side effect is posttreatment hyperpigmentation in 10–15% of cases (6)[B]
  - Copper vapor laser:
    - An alternative therapy that does not produce purpura (7)[B]
    - Given its deeper penetrance and shorter interpulse interval (6), it is best used for larger vessels with higher heat tolerance (6).
    - Ross et al. reports 3/20 patients developed either transient postinflammatory hyperpigmentation or specific atrophic areas (7)[B].

- PDL:
  - Effective in treating childhood and adult spider angiomas with less of a risk for pigmentary and textural changes:
    - Spider angiomas cleared within 2 treatments
  - Varying reports of efficacy between 93% and 95% clearance:
    - Rapini et al. reports 585 nm laser produced a 95% initial clearance of the lesion, with a 36% recurrence rate in 73% of patients during an average 37.9 month follow-up period.
    - Tan et al. reports complete clearance of spider angiomas in 93% of patients after 1 treatment.
    - Optimal for smaller vessels
    - Adverse effects include purpura, edema, blistering, and crusting
    - Purpura will resolve in 7–10 days.
    - Unlike other laser treatments, it does not leave a bruise-like pigmentation.
    - Its efficacy is similar to the hyfrecator, but requires fewer treatments without the increased risk of scarring.
  - KTP laser treatments are comparable to PDL treatments.

ADDITIONAL THERAPIES
Often no treatment is needed in pregnant women because lesions disappear within 3 months of delivery. However, if they are disfiguring or do not fade, patients can receive laser treatments or intense pulse light source treatments (2)[C].

ONGOING CARE

PROGNOSIS
- Recurrence of spider angiomas after treatment with PDL, KTP laser, or electrodesiccation is common.
- Resolve in women who discontinue use of oral contraception pills (1)[C]
- Have been known to disappear with improving liver function and hypotension (1)[C]:
  - Reported improvement after liver transplantation

COMPLICATIONS
- Occasionally, bleeding can occur after minor trauma (1)[C].
- Patients may experience cosmetic concerns from spider angiomas (1)[C].

REFERENCES
1. Khasnis A, Gokula RM. Spider nevus. *J Postgrad Med*. 2002;48:307.
2. Henry F, Quatresooz P, Valverde-Lopez JC, et al. Blood vessel changes during pregnancy: A review. *Am J Clin Dermatol*. 2006;7:65–69.
3. Niederau C, Lange S, Fruhauf M, et al. Cutaneous signs of liver disease: Value of prognosis of severe fibrosis and cirrhosis. *Liver Int*. 2008;28:659–666.
4. Udell JA, Wang CS, Tinmouth J, et al. Does this patient with liver disease have cirrhosis? *JAMA*. 2012;307:832–842.
5. Astner S, González S, Cuevas J, et al. Preliminary evaluation of benign vascular lesions using in vivo reflectance confocal microscopy. *Dermatol Surg*. 2010;36:1099–1110.
6. Rothfleisch JE, Kosann MK, Levine VJ, et al. Laser treatment of congenital and acquired vascular lesions. A review. *Dermatol Clin*. 2002;20:1–18.
7. Ross BS, Levine VJ, Ashinoff R, et al. Laser treatment of acquired vascular lesions. *Dermatol Clin*. 1997;15:385–396.

ADDITIONAL READING
Requena L, Sangueza OP. Cutaneous vascular anomalies. Part I. Hamartomas, malformations, and dilation of preexisting vessels. *J Am Acad Dermatol*. 1997;37:523–552.

 # CODES

ICD10
I78.1 Nevus, non-neoplastic

CLINICAL PEARLS
- Spider angiomas are vascular dilations of pre-existing blood vessels that commonly occur in children and adults.
- Pregnant women, patients with liver disease, and patients on hormonal therapy are more at risk for developing spider angiomas.
- Diagnosed by blanching of the lesion with a brisk capillary refill starting at the central arteriole.
- Lesions may resolve spontaneously.
- The best treatment outcomes with the least side effects occur with PDL and KTP laser therapy.

SPINAL STENOSIS

N. Wilson Holland, MD, FACP • Birju B. Patel, MD, FACP, AGSF

 BASICS

DESCRIPTION
Spinal stenosis is a condition in which a narrowing of the spinal canal and foramen occurs:

- Spondylosis or degenerative arthritis is the most common etiology for spinal stenosis and results from compression of the spinal cord by disc degeneration, facet arthropathy, osteophyte formation, and ligamentum flavum hypertrophy.
- The L_4–L_5 level is involved most commonly, but other lumbar levels also can be affected.

EPIDEMIOLOGY
The prevalence of spinal stenosis increases with age because it is essentially an arthritic condition from "wear and tear" on the normal spine.

Incidence
The incidence of symptomatic spinal stenosis is as high as 8% of the general population.

Prevalence
- The prevalence increases with age and can be very high when assessed by imaging studies in elderly patients; however, not all patients with radiographic spinal stenosis are symptomatic.
- Predominant age: Symptoms develop in 5th–6th decades (congenital stenosis becomes symptomatic much earlier).

ETIOLOGY AND PATHOPHYSIOLOGY
- Disc dehydration leads to loss of height with bulging of the disc annulus and ligamentum flavum into the spinal canal, thus increasing joint loading of facets.
- This leads to reactive sclerosis and osteophytic bone growth, resulting in further compression of neural elements in the spinal canal and foramen.
- Spinal stenosis can result from congenital or acquired causes. Degenerative spondylosis is the most common cause. Acquired causes include:
  - Disc degeneration and spondylosis
  - Trauma
  - Neoplasms
  - Neural cysts and lipomas
  - Postoperative changes
  - Rheumatoid arthritis
  - Diffuse idiopathic skeletal hyperostosis
  - Ankylosing spondylitis
  - Metabolic/Endocrine:
    - Osteoporosis
    - Renal osteodystrophy
    - Paget disease

Genetics
No definitive genetic links

RISK FACTORS
Increasing age and degenerative spondylolisthesis

GENERAL PREVENTION
There is no known way to prevent spinal stenosis. Symptoms can be alleviated with flexion at the waist:

- Leaning forward while walking
- Pushing a shopping cart
- Lying in flexed position
- Sitting
- Avoid provocative maneuvers that can cause pain (e.g., back extension, ambulating long distances without resting) (1)[A].

 DIAGNOSIS

HISTORY
- Long-standing back pain that progresses to buttocks and lower extremity pain
- Neurogenic claudication (i.e., pain, tightness, numbness, and subjective weakness of lower extremities) may mimic arterial insufficiency–related claudication
- The history is an extremely important aspect in distinguishing patients with spinal stenosis from those with other causes of back pain and peripheral vascular disease.
- Components of the history that should be considered include:
  - Insidious onset
  - Generally progresses slowly but may rarely have periods of remittance
  - Symptoms worsen with extension of the spine (prolonged standing, walking especially downhill or downstairs)
  - Symptoms improve with flexion (sitting, leaning forward while walking, walking uphill or upstairs, and lying in a flexed position).
  - Intermittent claudication
  - Urinary symptoms
  - Bilateral plantar numbness

PHYSICAL EXAM
Neurologic exam may be normal. There may be very few physical findings even in affected patients:

- Gait alteration (rule out cervical myelopathy or intracranial pathology)
- Loss of lumbar lordosis
- Decreased range of motion of lumbar spine
- Pain with extension of the lumbar spine
- Straight-leg-raise test may be positive if nerve root entrapment is present.
- Muscle weakness is usually mild or subtle and involves the L_4, L_5, and rarely, S_1 nerve roots.
- ~1/2 of patients with symptomatic stenosis have a reduced or absent Achilles reflex, and some have reduced or absent knee-jerk reaction.

DIFFERENTIAL DIAGNOSIS
- Vascular claudication also can cause calf pain with ambulation. Symptoms of vascular claudication do not improve with leaning forward and should not persist with standing.
- Disc herniation
- Cervical myelopathy

DIAGNOSTIC TESTS & INTERPRETATION
Spinal stenosis generally is diagnosed with a combination of history, physical exam, and imaging studies (MRI is best).

Initial Tests (lab, imaging)
- Consider CBC, ESR, C-reactive protein (to look for infection or malignancy).
- New back pain lasting >2 weeks, or accompanied by neurologic findings in those >50 generally warrants neuroimaging.
- MRI is the modality of choice for the diagnosis of spinal stenosis. 3D MR myelography may be more sensitive but is more expensive at diagnosing lumbar spinal stenosis, as shown by a few studies.

- CT myelography is an alternative to MRI but is invasive, with the potential risk of complications.
- Plain radiography may help to support the diagnosis but in general will not reveal the underlying pathology (but may be helpful to help exclude other causes of new back pain).
- Radiological abnormalities in general do not correlate with the clinical diagnosis (2)[B].

Diagnostic Procedures/Other
Surgical decompression is the only definitive treatment in patients who continue to be symptomatic after nonoperative treatment:

- Spinal stenosis generally does not lead to neurologic damage.
- Surgery may be required for pain relief, allowing patients to become more mobile and thus improving overall health.

Test Interpretation
- Decreased disc height
- Facet hypertrophy
- Spinal canal and/or foraminal narrowing

 TREATMENT

- A few studies have shown improvement with decompressive surgery, but the duration of improvement is uncertain.
- In general, nonoperative interventions are tried prior to surgical interventions unless there are progressive or life-threatening neurologic symptoms:
  - Recent review of nonoperative treatment options for lumbar spinal stenosis with claudication suggests that there is not enough evidence in the current literature to guide clinical recommendations for practice; more studies are needed (3)[C].
  - Consider ruling out other forms of neuropathy and peripheral vascular disease.
  - Physical therapy, spinal injections, and medications should be used prior to consideration for surgery.
- If decompressive surgery is performed, it is generally successful in alleviating symptoms of spinal stenosis.
- There is some controversy about whether a fusion should be performed with the decompression because of risk of future spondylolisthesis.

MEDICATION
First Line
- Acetaminophen
- NSAIDs: Consider potential for GI side effects, fluid retention, and renal failure
- Tramadol

Second Line
- There is limited evidence for long-term efficacy of lumbar epidural steroid and/or anesthetic injections. Injections maybe less effective in those with more severe stenosis and those with stenosis involving >3 lumbar levels.
- Consider judicious use of opioids only when other treatments have failed to control severe pain.

Geriatric Considerations
- Anti-inflammatory medications should be used with caution in the elderly due to the risks of GI bleeding, fluid retention, renal failure, and cardiovascular risks.
- Side effects of opioids, including constipation, confusion, urinary retention, drowsiness, nausea, vomiting, and potential for dependence, should be considered.
- >10% of elderly lack Achilles reflexes.

ISSUES FOR REFERRAL
Refer to a spine surgeon when patients are in unremitting pain or have a neurologic deficit.

ADDITIONAL THERAPIES
- General conditioning; these patients are able to ride an exercise bicycle without many problems because they can lean forward and relieve symptoms.
- Aquatic therapy (helpful for muscle and general conditioning)
- Back extensor muscle strengthening
- Abdominal muscle strengthening
- Gait training

SURGERY/OTHER PROCEDURES
- Surgery is indicated when symptoms persist despite conservative measures (4)[B].
- Age alone should not be an exclusion factor for surgical intervention. However, cognitive impairment, multiple comorbidities, and osteoporosis may increase the risk of perioperative complications in the elderly.
- Decompression of neural elements is the mainstay of treatment. The traditional approach is laminectomy and partial facetectomy (5)[B].
- Controversy exists about whether the decompression should be supplemented by a fusion procedure:
  - There is evidence that fusion (simple or complex), as opposed to decompression procedure alone, may be associated with higher risk of major complications, increased mortality, and increased resource use in the elderly (6)[B].
- A less-invasive alternative, known as interspinous distraction (X STOP implant), is also available as a treatment option (7)[C].
- The use of the Aperius Interspinous implant device is inconclusive in terms of evidence for efficacy in lumbar spinal stenosis at this time (8,9)[C].
- A unilateral partial hemilaminectomy combined with transmedial decompression may adequately treat stenosis with less morbidity in the elderly population (10)[C].
- The use of bone morphogenetic proteins (BMP) may improve fusion rates but not clinical outcomes in the elderly (11)[B].
- Transforaminal balloon treatment may be a viable option for resistant spinal stenosis pain and functional impairment (12)[C].

IN-PATIENT CONSIDERATIONS
Admission Criteria/Initial Stabilization
Unremitting pain that prevents the ability to perform the activities of daily living (ADLs) or acute or progressive neurologic deficit
- A brace or corset may help for a short time but is not recommended long term because it leads to paraspinal muscle weakness.

- Patient should be encouraged to continue to be active despite pain to prevent deconditioning.
- Weight loss

Discharge Criteria
Improved pain or after neurologic deficit has been addressed

 ## ONGOING CARE

FOLLOW-UP RECOMMENDATIONS
- Routine follow-up as needed
- No limitations to activity; patients may be as active as tolerated. Exercise should be encouraged.

Patient Monitoring
Patients are monitored for improvement of symptoms and development of any complications.

DIET
If undergoing surgery, optimize nutritional status.

PATIENT EDUCATION
- Activity as tolerated, as long as no other pathology is present (e.g., fractures)
- Patients should be alerted to possibility of progressive motor weakness and bladder/bowel dysfunction.
- Patients should be educated about the natural history of the condition.

PROGNOSIS
- Spinal stenosis generally is benign, but the pain can lead to limitation in ADLs and progressive disability.
- Surgery is usually successful in improving pain and symptoms in patients who fail nonoperative treatment.
- Clinical outcomes in elderly patients after surgery are similar in terms of pain relief and functional improvement compared with younger patients.

COMPLICATIONS
- Severe spinal stenosis can lead to bowel and/or bladder dysfunction.
- Surgical complications include infection, neurologic injury, chronic pain, and disability.

REFERENCES
1. Suri P, Rainville J, Kalichman L, et al. Does this older adult with lower extremity pain have the clinical syndrome of lumbar spinal stenosis? *JAMA*. 2010;204(23):2628–2636.
2. Li AL, Yen D. Effect of increased MRI and CT scan utilization on clinical decision-making in patients referred a surgical clinic for back pain. *Can J Surg*. 2011;54(2):128–132.
3. Ammendolia C, Stuber K, de Bruin LK, et al. Nonoperative treatment of lumbar spinal stenosis with neurogenic claudication: A systematic review. *Spine*. 2012;37:E609–E616.
4. Weinstein JN, Tosteson TD, Lurie JD, et al. Surgical versus nonsurgical therapy for lumbar spinal stenosis. *N Engl J Med*. 2008;358:794–810.
5. Katz JN, Harris MB. Clinical practice. Lumbar spinal stenosis. *N Engl J Med*. 2008;358:818–825.
6. Deyo RA, Mirza SK, Martin BI, et al. Trends, major medical complications, and charges associated with surgery for lumbar spinal stenosis in older adults. *JAMA*. 2010;303:1259–1265.
7. Miller LE, Block JE. Interspinous spacer implant in patients with lumbar spinal stenosis: Preliminary results of a multicenter, randomized, controlled trial. *Pain Res Treat*. 2012;2012:823509. Epub 2012 Feb 7.
8. Surace MF, Fagetti A, Fozzato S, et al. Lumbar spinal stenosis treatment with Aperius perclid interspinous system. *Eur Spine J*. 2012;21(Suppl 1):S69–S74.
9. Postacchini R, Ferrari E, Cinotti G, et al. Aperius interspinous implant versus open surgical decompression in lumbar spinal stenosis. *Spine J*. 2011;11:933–939.
10. Morgalla MH, Noak N, Merkle M, et al. Lumbar spinal stenosis in elderly patients: Is a unilateral microsurgical approach sufficient for decompression? *J Neurosurg Spine*. 2011;14(3):305–312.
11. Deyo RA, Ching A, Matsen L, et al. Use of bone morphogenetic proteins in spinal fusion surgery for older adults with lumbar stenosis: Trends, complications, repeat surgery, and charges. *Spine (Phila Pa 1976)*. 2012;37(3):222–230.
12. Kim SH, Choi WJ, Suh JH, et al. Effects of transforaminal balloon treatment in patients with lumbar foraminal stenosis: A randomized, controlled, double-blind trial. *Pain Physician*. 2013;16(3):213–224.

 ## SEE ALSO

Algorithm: Low Back Pain, Acute

 ## CODES

ICD10
- M48.00 Spinal stenosis, site unspecified
- M48.06 Spinal stenosis, lumbar region
- M48.07 Spinal stenosis, lumbosacral region

CLINICAL PEARLS
- Spinal stenosis may present as neurogenic claudication (pain, tightness, numbness, and subjective weakness of lower extremities) and may mimic arterial insufficiency–related claudication.
- Neurogenic claudication as opposed to vascular claudication is improved by uphill ambulation and lumbar flexion and is not alleviated by standing.
- Positions that cause flexion of the spine such as sitting, bending forward, walking uphill, or walking with a shopping cart generally[*] relieve symptoms and can be helpful in making the diagnosis.
- Positions that cause spinal extension such as prolonged standing, walking downhill, and walking downstairs can worsen symptoms.
- Surgery should be considered urgently in patients who present with rapidly evolving cauda equina/conus medullaris syndrome or newly progressive bladder dysfunction.

SPRAIN, ANKLE

Salwa Khan, MD, MHS, FAAP • Ryan Y. Shields

 BASICS

DESCRIPTION

Ankle sprains, which are the most common cause of ankle injury, make up a significant proportion of sports injuries:

- There are several types of ankle sprains, including lateral, medial, and syndesmotic (or high ankle sprain):
  - Lateral ankle sprains are the most common, accounting for 85% of all ankle sprains:
    - In lateral ankle sprains, the anterior talofibular ligament (ATFL) is the weakest ligament and, therefore, the most likely to be injured.
    - The calcaneofibular ligament (CFL) is the 2nd most likely ligament to be injured.
    - The posterior talofibular ligament (PTFL) is the least likely to be injured.
  - Medial ankle sprains, which make up 5–10% of ankle sprains, result from an injury to the deltoid ligament:
    - The medial deltoid ligament is the strongest ligament.
  - Syndesmotic (or high ankle) sprains are also rare; they account for 5–10% of ankle sprains.
- Ankle sprains can be classified based on degree of injury from grade I–III:
  - Grade I: Mild stretching of a ligament with possible microscopic tears
  - Grade II: Incomplete tear of a ligament
  - Grade III: Complete ligament tear

Geriatric Considerations
Increased risk of fracture in patients who suffer a sprain and have pre-existing bone-weakening conditions (osteoporosis/osteopenia)

Pediatric Considerations
- Increased risk of physial injuries instead of ligament sprain, as ligaments have greater tensile strength than physes.
- Inversion ankle injuries in children may have a concomitant fibular physial injury (Salter Harris type I or higher fracture).

EPIDEMIOLOGY

Incidence
- 2.15/1,000 person-years, with peak age of incidence between 15 and 19 years.
- 1/2 of all ankle sprains are associated with sports; basketball alone is responsible for 41%, football for 9%, and soccer for 8%.
- Most common sports injury.
- Equal incidence in males and females, with males age <30 years more affected and females >30 years more affected.

Prevalence
- 20% of sports injuries in the US
- 75% of all ankle injuries are sprains.

ETIOLOGY AND PATHOPHYSIOLOGY
- Lateral ankle sprains result from an inversion while plantarflexing the ankle.
- Medial ankle sprains are due to forced eversion while in dorsiflexion.
- Syndesmotic sprains result from eversion stress/extreme dorsiflexion along with internal rotation of tibia.

RISK FACTORS
- Previous ankle sprain is the number 1 risk factor: Of people who have had a sprain, 3–34% will sustain another.
- Postural instability, gait change (decreased clearance and more inversion) appear to be risk factors.
- Joint laxity and decreased proprioception were not found to be risk factors.

GENERAL PREVENTION
- Conditioning before participating in sports and throughout the season (1)[A]:
  - Training in agility and flexibility
  - Single-leg balancing
  - Proprioceptive training
- Taping/Wearing ankle braces may help prevent reinjury to a sprained ankle, but has not been found to reduce sprain severity.

COMMONLY ASSOCIATED CONDITIONS
- Contusions
- Fractures:
  - Fibula head fracture/dislocation
  - Base of the 5th metatarsal fracture
  - Distal fibula fracture (including Salter Harris fractures in pediatric patients)

 DIAGNOSIS

HISTORY
- Mechanism of injury (inversion vs. eversion)
- Popping/Snapping sensation during the injury
- Previous history of ankle injuries
- Ability to ambulate immediately after the injury
- Rapid onset of pain and swelling
- Ecchymosis
- Pain on lateral/medial ankle
- Weakness
- Difficulty bearing weight
- Past medical history of systemic/connective tissue disorders

PHYSICAL EXAM
- Compare to uninjured ankle for swelling and laxity.
- Palpate ATFL, CFL, PTFL, and deltoid ligament for tenderness.
- Palpate lateral and medial malleolus, base of 5th metatarsal, and entire fibula.
- Grade I sprain: Mild swelling and pain; no laxity
- Grade II sprain: Moderate swelling and pain; mild laxity with endpoint noted
- Grade III sprain: Severe swelling, pain, and bruising; laxity with no endpoint

- Special tests:
  - Anterior drawer test to check for laxity of ATFL
  - Talar tilt test to check laxity in CFL/deltoid ligament
  - Squeeze test of tibia and fibula midcalf to check for syndesmotic injury. Positive test is causing of pain isolated to the syndesmosis.
  - Dorsiflexion/External rotation test

DIFFERENTIAL DIAGNOSIS
- Tendon injury:
  - Tendinopathy
  - Tendon tear
- Fracture and/or dislocation of the ankle/foot
- Hindfoot/Midfoot injuries
- Nerve injury
- Contusion
- Hematologic

DIAGNOSTIC TESTS & INTERPRETATION
- Use the Ottawa ankle rules to determine whether radiographs are needed to rule out ankle fractures (patient must be 18–55 years; certain patients, e.g., diabetics with diminished sensation, may need radiographs regardless):
  - Pain in malleolar zone AND
  - Inability to bear weight (walk ≥4 steps) immediately and in the ER or office OR
  - Bony tenderness at tip/posterior edge of the lateral/medial malleolus or base of 5th metatarsal.
- Obtain anteroposterior, lateral, and mortise views of the ankle.
- Small avulsion fractures are associated with grade III sprains.
- Consider CT if radiographs are negative but are highly suggestive for occult fracture.
- MRI is gold standard for soft tissue, including ligaments, but is expensive and usually unnecessary.
- US is a good 2nd-line imaging option; it has been shown to have sensitivity comparable to MRI (2)[B].

Follow-Up Tests & Special Considerations
If patient's condition is not improving in 6 weeks, consider CT, MRI, or US.

 TREATMENT

GENERAL MEASURES
- PRICE: Protection, rest, ice, compression, elevation
- Early mobilization and physical therapy may speed recovery (3)[A].
- The majority of grades I, II, and III lateral ankle ligament ruptures can be managed without surgery; grade III should have short-term immobilization followed by a semi-rigid brace (4)[A].
- Wrapping the ankle with an elastic bandage helps decrease swelling, but its use alone leads to a slower return to sports and work and provides less stability than an ankle brace (5)[A].
- Air-filled/Gel-filled ankle brace/an ankle-stabilizing orthoses provides better support than elastic bandage/taping.
- Short-term immobilization (10 days) has been shown to be beneficial for severe ankle sprains (6)[B].

- Do not use heat in an acute injury.
- Activity:
  – Weight-bearing, as tolerated.
  – Crutches may be needed if patient is unable to bear weight.
  – Exercises should be limited to pain-free range of motion and should be started as early as tolerated.
  – Patient can start mobilization by tracing the alphabet with the foot in the air.
  – Elastic resistance exercises to improve balance

MEDICATION
- NSAIDs: Preferably oral, but topical forms may be used if GI side effects are intolerable (7)[A]
- Opioids if severe pain

ISSUES FOR REFERRAL
- Malleolar/Talar dome fracture
- Syndesmotic sprain
- Tendon rupture

ADDITIONAL THERAPIES
Physical therapy:
- After the acute phase of the injury, patients should start physical therapy.
- Physical therapy should include increasing range of motion, strength, flexibility, and proprioceptive balance (wobble board/ankle disk).
- Functional rehabilitation is necessary to prevent chronic instability and can speed healing.
- Athletes should go through a sport-specific rehabilitation before returning to play.

SURGERY/OTHER PROCEDURES
- There is little evidence to show that surgery provides a relatively better result than conservative treatment for ankle sprains. Athletes should go through a sport-specific rehabilitation before returning to play (5).
- Syndesmotic sprains, however, may require surgery.
- Patients with chronic ankle instability who fail functional rehabilitation or with poor tissue quality may need anatomic repair/reconstructive surgery.

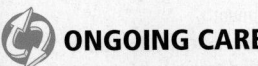 ONGOING CARE

FOLLOW-UP RECOMMENDATIONS
- Ankle-stabilizing orthoses should be worn for high-risk sports after a person has sustained an ankle sprain to prevent future ankle sprains.
- Moderate and severe sprains require ankle orthoses for ≥6 months while participating in sports.
- Return to play for athletes with a grade I lateral ankle sprain is generally 1–2 weeks; grade II sprain is 2–3 weeks; grade III sprain is 4 weeks.
- Return to play with medial/syndesmotic sprains is longer.

Patient Monitoring
If athletes continue to have symptoms when they return to play, consider further rehabilitation.

PATIENT EDUCATION
- Training on how to use crutches
- Training on how to use elastic bandages, brace, and/or orthoses
- Demonstration of mobilization exercises for ankle.

PROGNOSIS
- Earlier physical therapy and mobilization with bracing allows for faster return to daily living and/or sports.
- Grade of ankle sprain does not relate to prognosis.
- Ligamentous strength does not return for months after the injury.

COMPLICATIONS
- Joint instability
- Intermittent swelling and pain if not treated properly
- Accumulation of cartilage damage, leading to degenerative changes
- 5–33% will continue to have pain 1 year post injury.

REFERENCES
1. Abernethy L. Strategies to prevent injury in adolescent sport: A systematic review. Br J Sports Med. 2007;41:627–638.
2. Oae K, Takao M, Uchio Y, et al. Evaluation of anterior talofibular ligament injury with stress radiography, ultrasonography and MR imaging. Skeletal Radiol. 2010;39:41–47.
3. Bleakley CM, O'Connor SR, Tully MA, et al. Effect of accelerated rehabilitation on function after ankle sprain: Randomised controlled trial. BMJ. 2010;340:c1964. Epub 2010 May 10.
4. Petersen W, Rembitzki IV, Koppenburg AG, et al. Treatment of acute ankle ligament injuries: A systematic review. Arch Orthop Trauma Surg. 2013;133(8):1129–1141.
5. Kerkhoffs GM, Handoll HH, de Bie R, et al. Surgical versus conservative treatment for acute injuries of the lateral ligament complex of the ankle in adults. Cochrane Database Syst Rev. 2007;(2):CD000380.
6. Lamb SE, Marsh JL, Hutton JL, et al. Mechanical supports for acute, severe ankle sprain: A pragmatic, multicentre, randomised controlled trial. Lancet. 2009;373:575–581.
7. Massey T, Derry S, Moore RA, et al. Topical NSAIDs for acute pain in adults. Cochrane Database Syst Rev. 2010;(6):CD007402. Epub 2010 Jun 16.

ADDITIONAL READING
- Dizon JM, Reyes JJ. A systematic review on the effectiveness of external ankle supports in the prevention of inversion ankle sprains among elite and recreational players. J Sci Med Sport. 2010;13:309–317.
- Handoll HHG, Rowe BH, Quinn KM, et al. Interventions for preventing ankle ligament injuries. Cochrane Database Syst Rev. 2001;3:CD000018.
- Hiller CE, Nightingale EJ, Lin CW, et al. Characteristics of people with recurrent ankle sprains: A systematic review with meta-analysis. Br J Sports Med. 2011;45:660–672.
- Ivins D. Acute ankle sprain: An update. Am Fam Physician. 2006;74:1714–1720; 1723–1726.

- Jacobs CL, Hincapié CA, Cassidy JD. Musculoskeletal injuries and pain in dancers: A systematic review update. J Dance Med Sci. 2012;84(2):74–84.
- Jones MH. Acute treatment of inversion ankle sprains: Immobilization versus functional treatment. Clin Orthop Relat Res. 2007;455:169–172.
- Kerkhoffs GM, van den Bekerom M, Elders LA, et al. Diagnosis, treatment and prevention of ankle sprains: An evidence-based clinical guideline. Br J Sports Med. 2012;46(12):854–860.
- Mehallo CJ, Drezner JA, Bytomski JR. Practical management: Nonsteroidal antiinflammatory drug (NSAID) use in athletic injuries. Clin J Sport Med. 2006;16:170–174.
- Raymond J, Nicholson LL, Hiller CE, et al. The effect of ankle taping or bracing on proprioception in functional ankle instability: A systematic review and meta-analysis. J Sci Med Sport. 2012;84(5):386–392. Epub 2012 Apr 17.
- Waterman BR, Owens BD, Davey S, et al. The epidemiology of ankle sprains in the United States. J Bone Joint Surg Am. 2010;92:2279–2284.

 CODES

ICD10
- S93.419A Sprain of calcaneofibular ligament of unsp ankle, init
- S93.499A Sprain of other ligament of unspecified ankle, init encntr
- S96.919A Strain of unsp msl/tnd at ank/ft level, unsp foot, init

CLINICAL PEARLS
- Increased risk of physial injuries rather than ligament sprains in pediatric patients because ligaments are stronger than physes
- Conditioning, including proprioceptive training, before participating in sports and throughout the season helps to prevent ankle sprains.
- Taping/Wearing ankle braces may help prevent reinjury to a sprained ankle, but does not help prevent initial ankle sprains/decrease new sprain severity.
- Functional rehabilitation, rather than total immobilization, is recommended for quicker return to sport and work.
- If patient's condition is not improving in 6 weeks, consider CT, MRI, or US.

SPRAINS AND STRAINS

Kylee Eagles, DO • J. Herbert Stevenson, MD

 BASICS

DESCRIPTION
- *Sprains* are complete or partial ligamentous injuries either within the body of the ligament or at the site of attachment to bone:
  - Classified as grade I, II, or III (AMA Ligament Injury Classification):
    - Grade I: Stretch injury without ligamentous laxity
    - Grade II: Partial tear with increased ligamentous laxity but firm endpoint on exam
    - Grade III: Complete tear with increased ligamentous laxity and no firm endpoint on exam
  - Physical exam is the key to diagnosis.
  - Usually secondary to trauma (e.g., falls, twisting injuries, motor vehicle accidents)
- *Strains* are partial or complete disruptions of the muscle, muscle-tendon junction, or tendon:
  - Classified as:
    - 1st degree: Minimal damage to muscle, tendon, or musculotendinous unit
    - 2nd degree: Partial tear to the muscle, tendon, or musculotendinous unit
    - 3rd degree: Complete disruption of the muscle, tendon, or musculotendinous unit
  - Often associated with overuse injuries

Geriatric Considerations
More likely to see associated bony injuries due to decreased joint flexibility and prevalence of osteoporosis and osteopenia

Pediatric Considerations
- Sprains and strains have been found to account for 24% of injuries in pediatric patients.
- 3 million pediatric sports injuries occur annually.
- Must be concerned about physial/apophyseal injuries in the skeletally immature

EPIDEMIOLOGY
Incidence
~80% of all US athletes at some time in their career will experience a sprain or strain.

Prevalence
- Ankle sprains are among the most common injuries seen in the primary care setting and account for up to 30% of sports medicine clinic visits.
- Most ankle sprains are due to inversion injuries (lateral sprains).
- Predominant age:
  - Sprains: Any age when patient is physically active
  - Strains: Usually 15–40 years of age
- Predominant sex: Male > Female; Female > Male for sprain of acromioclavicular ligament

ETIOLOGY AND PATHOPHYSIOLOGY
- Trauma, falls, MVA
- Excessive exercise
- Improper footwear
- Inadequate warm-up and stretching before activity
- Poor conditioning
- Prior sprain or strain

RISK FACTORS
- Prior history of sprain or strain is greatest risk factor for future sprain/strain.
- Change in or improper shoe gear, protective gear, or environment (e.g., surface)
- Sudden increase in training schedule

GENERAL PREVENTION
- Use appropriate warm-up, and cool-down exercises.
- Use proper equipment.
- Balance training programs can improve joint position sense and reduce the risk of ankle sprains (1)[A].
- Semirigid orthoses or air casts may prevent ankle sprains during high-risk sports, especially in athletes with history of sprain (2,3)[A].

COMMONLY ASSOCIATED CONDITIONS
- Effusions, hemarthrosis
- Stress, avulsion, or other fractures
- Syndesmotic injuries
- Contusions
- Wounds
- Dislocations/Subluxations

 DIAGNOSIS

HISTORY
- May describe feeling or hearing pop or snap
- Mechanism (key in diagnosis)

PHYSICAL EXAM
- Gait disturbances present if severe injury
- Inspect for swelling, asymmetry, ecchymosis.
- Palpate for tenderness.
- Evaluate for decreased range of motion (ROM) of joint and joint instability.
- Evaluate for strength.
- Sprains:
  - Grade I: Tenderness without laxity. Minimal pain, swelling. Little ecchymosis. Can bear weight.
  - Grade II: Tenderness with increased laxity on exam but firm endpoint. More pain, swelling. Often ecchymosis. Some difficulty bearing weight.
  - Grade III: Tenderness with increased laxity on exam and no firm endpoint. Severe pain, swelling. Obvious ecchymosis. Difficulty bearing weight.

DIFFERENTIAL DIAGNOSIS
- Tendonitis
- Bursitis
- Contusion
- Hematoma
- Fracture
- Rheumatologic process

DIAGNOSTIC TESTS & INTERPRETATION
- Ankle:
  - Anterior drawer test assesses integrity of anterior talofibular ligament.
  - Talar tilt test assesses integrity of calcaneofibular ligament.
- Knee:
  - Lachman test assesses integrity of anterior cruciate ligament. Posterior drawer assesses integrity of posterior cruciate ligament.
  - Valgus/Varus stress tests assess integrity of collateral ligaments.
- Shoulder:
  - Positive apprehension test may indicate glenohumeral ligament sprain.
- Radiographs may be needed to rule out bony injury; stress views may be helpful. Should obtain bilateral radiographs in children to rule out growth plate injuries.
- Use Ottawa ankles rules (age 18–55) to determine if radiograph is necessary (3,4)[A].
- Ankle films: Required if pain in the malleolar zone *and*:
  - Bone tenderness in posterior aspect distal 6 cm of tibia *or* fibula *or*
  - Inability to bear weight immediately or in emergency department
- Foot films: Required if midfoot zone pain is present *and*:
  - Bone tenderness at base of 5th metatarsal *or*
  - Bone tenderness at navicular *or*
  - Inability to bear weight immediately or in emergency department

Follow-Up Tests & Special Considerations
- CT scan of the affected area may be required if occult fracture is suspected.
- MRI is gold standard for imaging soft-tissue structures, including muscle, ligaments, and intraarticular structures. Using 2 diagnostic criterion on MRI for the diagnosis of anterior talofibular ligament (AITFL) disruption, sensitivity is 100% and specificity is 93%. For the diagnosis of PITFL disruption using 2 criterion on MRI, sensitivity is 100% and specificity is 100% (5).

Diagnostic Procedures/Other
Surgery may be required for some partial and complete sprains. Need for surgery depends on the neurovascular supply to the injured area or the ability to attain full ROM and stability of the affected joint.

TREATMENT

GENERAL MEASURES

- History and physical exam along with treatment of the worst possible suspected injury
- Acutely: PRICEMM therapy (*protection, relative rest, ice, compression, elevation, medications, modalities*)
- Grade I, II ankle sprain: Functional treatment with brace, orthosis, taping, elastic bandage wrap (3)[A]:
  – Ankle braces (lace-up, stirrup-type, air cast) are a more effective functional treatment than elastic bandages or taping (3,6)[B].
- Grade III ankle sprain: Short period of immobilization with cast/crutches may be needed (3)[A].
- Consider aspiration of a joint effusion that lasts >1–2 weeks.
- Early physical therapy
- For high-level athletes with more extensive damage, consider surgery.

MEDICATION

First Line

- Acetaminophen: Up to 3–4 g/d
- NSAIDs:
  – Ibuprofen: 200–800 mg t.i.d.
  – Naproxen: 250–500 mg b.i.d.
  – Diclofenac: 75 mg b.i.d.
- Narcotics for severe pain, acute injury
- Acetaminophen and NSAIDs found to have similar efficacy in reducing pain after ankle sprains
- Topical diclofenac may reduce pain in acute ankle sprains (7)[B].
- Platelet-rich plasma injections may aid recovery in treatment of muscle strains, but more studies are needed (8)[C].
- Refer to manufacturer's profile of each drug for contraindications, precautions, and possible interactions.

ISSUES FOR REFERRAL

- ACL sprain in athletes/physically active
- Salter-Harris physial fractures
- Lack of improvement with conservative measures
- Joint instability
- Tendon disruption (i.e., Achilles, biceps)

ADDITIONAL THERAPIES

Physical therapy is a useful adjunct after a sprain, and early mobilization is crucial (9)[A]:

- Proprioception retraining
- Core strengthening
- Eccentric exercises
- Theraband exercises

SURGERY/OTHER PROCEDURES

Casting and surgery are reserved for select grade III injuries.

ONGOING CARE

FOLLOW-UP RECOMMENDATIONS

If affected joint has full strength and ROM, patient can advance activity as tolerated.

Patient Monitoring

After initial treatment, consider rehabilitation. Direct emphasis toward limiting swelling and providing a pain-free, full ROM.

DIET

Weight loss if obesity is etiologic

PATIENT EDUCATION

- Instructions on how to wrap with elastic bandage
- Prevention of injury
- Give ROM and strengthening exercises with physical therapy prescription since there can be delays in getting an appointment.

PROGNOSIS

With appropriate treatment and rest, 1–8 weeks (or longer) for recovery, depending on the severity of injury

COMPLICATIONS

- Chronic joint instability
- Arthritis
- Muscle contracture

REFERENCES

1. Sefton JM, Yarar C. Six weeks of balance training improved sensorimotor function in individuals with chronic ankle instability. *J Orthop Sports Phys Ther.* 2011;41(2):81–89.
2. Handoll MM, Rowe BH. Interventions for preventing ankle ligament injuries. *Cochrane Database Syst Rev.* 2011:CD000018.
3. Seah R, Mani-Babu S. Managing ankle sprains in primary care: What is the best practice? A systematic review of the last 10 years of evidence. *Br Med Bull.* 2011;97:105–135.
4. Bachmann LH, Kolb E. Accuracy of the Ottawa Ankle Rules to exclude fractures of the ankle and mid-foot: A systematic review. *BMJ.* 2003; 326(7386):417.
5. Oae K, Takao M, Naito K, et al. Injury of the tibiofibular syndesmosis: Value of MR imaging for diagnosis. *Radiology.* 2003;227(1):155–161. Epub 2003 Feb 28.
6. Lardenoye S, Theunissen E, Cleffken B, et al. The effect of taping versus semi-rigid bracing on patient outcome and satisfaction in ankle sprains: A prospective, randomized controlled trial. *BMC Musculoskelet Disord.* 2012;13:81. Epub 2012 May 28.

---

7. Lionberger DR, Joussellin E, Lanzarotti A. Diclofenac epolamine topical patch relieves pain associated with ankle sprain. *J Pain Res.* 2011;4:47–53.
8. Hamilton BH, Best TM. Platelet-rich plasma and muscle strain injuries-challenges imposed by the burden of proof. *Clin J Sports Med.* 2011; 21(1):31–36.
9. Bleakley CM, O'Connor SR. Effect of accelerated rehabilitation on function after ankle sprain: A randomized control trial. *BMJ.* 2010;34:c1964.

ADDITIONAL READING

- Dalton JD, Schweinle JE. Randomized controlled noninferiority trial to compare extended release acetaminophen and ibuprofen for the treatment of ankle sprains. *Ann Emerg Med.* 2006;48:615–623.
- Kerkoffs MMJ, Rowe BH. Immobilisation and functional treatment for acute lateral ankle ligament injuries. *Cochrane Database Syst Rev.* 2010: CD003762.
- McGuine TA, Keene JS. The effect of a balance training program on the risk of ankle sprains in high school athletes. *Am J Sports Med.* 2006;34: 1103–1111.
- Rupp, KA, Saliba SA. Should athletes return to activity after cryotherapy? *J Athl Train.* 2013 May.

SEE ALSO

Tendinitis

CODES

ICD10

- S43.50XA Sprain of unspecified acromioclavicular joint, initial encounter
- S93.409A Sprain of unsp ligament of unspecified ankle, init encntr
- S96.919A Strain of unsp msl/tnd at ank/ft level, unsp foot, init

CLINICAL PEARLS

For acute injury, remember PRICEMM:

- Protection of the joint
- Rest as appropriate
- Apply ice
- Apply compression
- Elevate joint
- Medications for pain
- Other modalities as needed

STEATOHEPATITIS, NONALCOHOLIC

Megan Gillem, DO • Amimi Osayande, MD

BASICS

DESCRIPTION
- The definition of nonalcoholic fatty liver disease (NAFLD) requires evidence of hepatic steatosis, either by imaging or histology and no secondary causes for hepatic fat accumulation (such as alcohol consumption, use of steatogenic medication, or hereditary disorders)
- Most patients with nonalcoholic steatohepatitis (NASH) are asymptomatic.
- Increased aminotransferase activities are the most common abnormality reported in patients with NASH.
- NASH is the most severe form of NAFLD; both are the hepatic manifestations of metabolic syndrome.

EPIDEMIOLOGY
Incidence
- NAFLD and NASH have a worldwide distribution.
- NAFLD is the most common form of chronic liver disease in the Western world.
- Age-adjusted prevalence of NAFLD was highest in Mexican Americans (21.2%), followed by non-Hispanic whites (12.5%), and was lowest in non-Hispanic blacks (11.6%) (1).
- Prevalence of NAFLD and NASH in the US and other Western countries is ~6.3–33%, and 3–5%, respectively.
- 25–35% of NASH patients develop fibrosis, while 9–20% develop cirrhosis.
- 22–33% of cirrhotics die of complications of liver failure or require orthotopic liver transplant. Studies have established that cardiovascular disease is the most common cause of death in patients with NAFLD and NASH (2).

Pediatric Considerations
- Obesity is also increasing in prevalence in children. The overall prevalence of NAFLD in children is estimated at 3–10%, but it may be much higher in obese children.
- First-line treatment for children with NAFLD is weight loss and lifestyle modifications (2)[B].
- Children with fatty liver who are very young or who are not overweight should be tested for other causes of liver disease (i.e., fatty acid oxidation defects, lysosomal storage diseases, peroxisomal disorders, hepatitis, Wilson disease, and autoimmune diseases) (2)[C].
- Reye syndrome: Fatty liver with encephalopathy; characterized by vomiting with dehydration, progressive CNS damage, hypoglycemia, and signs of hepatic injury: Mortality rate is 30–50%.
- Treatment: Mannitol, IV glucose, and fresh frozen plasma

ETIOLOGY AND PATHOPHYSIOLOGY
- NAFLD is closely linked to obesity, insulin resistance, and metabolic syndrome.
- When insulin resistance develops, free fatty acids are inappropriately shifted to nonadipose tissue, including the liver.
- Insulin resistance increases free fatty acid flux to the liver by decreased inhibition of lipolysis and also increased de novo lipogenesis.

- Insulin resistance and visceral obesity also result in decreased levels of adiponectin. Adiponectin inhibits liver gluconeogenesis and suppresses lipogenesis. Thus, decreased adiponectin hinders fatty acid oxidation and increases fat accumulation in the liver.
- Apoptosis and oxidative stress also may contribute to the development and progression of NASH.
- Cause is unknown, but is closely linked to obesity, insulin resistance, and metabolic syndrome.
- Of these, insulin resistance may be the most important trigger of simple fatty liver (steatosis) and NASH.
- Since both these conditions can remain stable for many years, causing little harm, a 2nd hit to the liver may trigger a progression to cirrhosis.
- Triggers may include cytokine-mediated inflammation, lipid peroxidation, and apoptosis.

Genetics
There may be a genetic component; however, screening is not recommended at this time (2)[B].

RISK FACTORS
- NAFLD occurs in individuals who have associated metabolic syndrome/insulin resistance.

- The presence of metabolic syndrome increases the risk of future development of NAFLD by 4–11-fold (1)[A].
- The 3 most important risk factors are closely related to metabolic syndrome and insulin resistance (2)[A]:
  - Obesity: Associated in 57–98% of patients with NAFLD
  - DM: Present in up to 69% of with NAFLD
  - Dyslipidemia: Found in up to 92% of patients with NAFLD

- Insulin resistance is associated strongly with metabolic syndrome and plays a central role in the pathogenesis of NAFLD.
- Other risk factors:
  - Data suggest that hypothyroidism, hypopituitarism, sleep apnea, and polycystic ovary syndrome, independent of obesity, are important risk factors for the presence of NAFLD.
  - Male gender (2)
  - Small bowel resections, gastric bypass, and jejunal bypass operations often lead to rapid weight loss, which may increase risk of NAFLD.
  - Medications: Corticosteroids, synthetic estrogens, amiodarone, tamoxifen, methotrexate
  - Other conditions: Wilson disease, hemochromatosis, abetalipoproteinemia, galactosemia, glycogen storage diseases

GENERAL PREVENTION
- Maintain ideal weight and normal cholesterol and blood sugar levels.
- Avoid alcohol.
- Avoid hepatotoxic substances.

COMMONLY ASSOCIATED CONDITIONS
Preeclampsia

Pregnancy Considerations
- A severe complication of 3rd trimester is acute fatty liver of pregnancy. It presents as an abrupt onset of confusion and restlessness with possible jaundice and right upper quadrant pain.
- Alanine aminotransferase/aspartate aminotransferase (ALT/AST) elevated, usually >1,000 U/L

- Emergency liver biopsy confirms.
- Prompt delivery corrects the liver disease. In most cases, the fetus has an inborn error of lipid metabolism blocking, the same as in the mother.
- Recurrence is rare in subsequent pregnancies.

DIAGNOSIS

HISTORY
- Often asymptomatic
- Fatigue
- Malaise
- A dull ache in the upper right abdomen is a possible sign of an enlarged liver.
- At more advanced stage, such as cirrhosis, NASH may cause lack of appetite, weight loss, nausea, weakness, fatigue, spider nevi, palmar erythema, yellowing of skin and eyes, dark cola-colored urine, light-colored stools, gynecomastia, varices, ascites, pruritus, edema, and encephalopathy.

PHYSICAL EXAM
Hepatomegaly is present in 75% of patients with NASH (3)[A].

DIFFERENTIAL DIAGNOSIS
Viral hepatitis, alcohol hepatitis, autoimmune hepatitis, hemochromatosis, Wilson disease, α_1-antitrypsin deficiency

DIAGNOSTIC TESTS & INTERPRETATION
Initial Tests (lab, imaging)
- Exclude coexisting etiologies for liver disease: Hemochromatosis, autoimmune liver disease, chronic viral hepatitis, and Wilson disease.
- Aminotransferase and alkaline phosphatase levels may be mildly elevated, but serum albumin, prothrombin, and bilirubin levels are usually normal.
- AST:ALT ratio is usually <1 in NASH.
- Mildly elevated serum ferritin is common, and it does not necessarily indicate increased iron stores.
- Right upper quadrant US: Reveals a hyperechoic texture or a bright liver because of diffuse fatty infiltration
- CT scan of abdomen and MRI: Identifies steatosis, but not sufficiently sensitive to detect inflammation or fibrosis

- MR spectroscopy: Better sensitivity, quantitative rather than qualitative (4)[B]

Diagnostic Procedures/Other
- NAFLD fibrosis score is based on 6 readily available variables (age, body mass index [BMI], hyperglycemia, platelet count, albumin, AST:ALT ratio) and is a clinically useful tool for identifying NAFLD patients with higher likelihood of having bridging fibrosis and/or cirrhosis (2)[B].
- Liver biopsy is considered the gold standard for characterizing liver histology in patients with NAFLD Consider biopsy in patients with NAFLD who are at increased risk of steatohepatitis and advanced fibrosis or in whom competing etiologies for hepatic steatosis and coexisting chronic liver disease cannot be excluded (2)[B].

Test Interpretation

- Criteria to establish pathologic diagnosis of NASH have remained controversial.
- Histologic diagnosis of NASH is based on a composite pattern of injury rather than a single defining feature.
- Pathologic scoring system for NAFLD (Nonalcoholic Steatohepatitis Clinical Research Network) (5)[A]:
  – Steatosis (0–3)
  – Lobular inflammation (0–3)
  – Ballooning (0–3)
- NAFLD Activity Score (NAS): 0–2 not NASH; >5 usually NASH

TREATMENT

- Treatment of patients consists of treating liver disease as well as the associated metabolic comorbid conditions, such as obesity, hyperlipidemia, insulin resistance, and type 2 DM (3)[A].
- Preferred treatments include:
  – Weight loss (2)[A]
  – Exercise (2)[B]
  – Avoidance of toxic substances (2)[B]

GENERAL MEASURES
Weight loss and exercise may reduce inflammation, lower elevated levels of liver enzymes, and decrease insulin resistance.

MEDICATION
The decision to start pharmacologic treatment should be restricted to patients at risk for developing advanced liver disease.

First Line
- Despite the large number of agents tested, no established, evidence-based treatment exists for NASH:
  – Weight loss, metformin, thiazolidinediones (especially pioglitazone), and antioxidants have been most extensively evaluated:
    ○ Weight loss is safe and dose-dependently reduced histologic disease activity in NASH, but >50% of patients failed to achieve target weight loss (6).
    ○ Metformin has no significant effect on liver histology and is not recommended for treatment (2)[A].
    ○ Thiazolidinediones reduced steatosis and inflammation, but yielded significant weight gain (7)[B].
    ○ Antioxidants yielded conflicting results and were heterogenous with respect to type and dose of drug, duration, implementation of lifestyle intervention (2):
    ○ Vitamin E administered at daily doses of 800 IU/d improves liver histology in nondiabetic adults with biopsy-proven NASH and should be considered as first-line therapy (2)[B].
- Statins can be used to treat dyslipidemia in patients with NAFLD and NASH, but should not be used specifically to treat NASH (2)[B].
- Fibrates had no significant benefit on histologic, biochemical, or radiologic outcome.
- Ursodeoxycholic acid showed no significant improvement in ALT levels/radiologic steatosis (2)[B].

ISSUES FOR REFERRAL
Referral to a hepatologist, with/without liver biopsy, may help in staging and prognosis.

SURGERY/OTHER PROCEDURES

- Bariatric surgery: Although abdominal weight-loss surgery coupled with rapid weight loss has been implicated as contributing to development of NASH, it is not contraindicated in otherwise eligible obese patients (2)[A].
- Some research suggests that bariatric surgery combined with modest weight loss may reduce the inflammation and scarring associated with NASH (3)[A].
- It is premature to recommend bariatric surgery as a treatment for NASH (2)[B].

COMPLEMENTARY AND ALTERNATIVE MEDICINE
- A number of complementary and alternative therapies claim to improve liver health. Among these are milk thistle, α-lipoic acid, betaine, viusid, vitamin E, N-acetyl cysteine, and Ω-3 fatty acids.
- Antioxidants, such as vitamin E, N-acetyl cysteine, S-adenosylmethionine (SAMe), and betaine, have been investigated in the treatment of NAFLD. The extreme heterogenicity of RCTs prevents any firm conclusion on the effect of antioxidants in NAFLD/NASH.

ONGOING CARE

FOLLOW-UP RECOMMENDATIONS
All patients should be tested for hepatitis A and B and vaccinated if appropriate.

Patient Monitoring
Patients with fatty liver disease should be seen regularly to detect disease progression through:
- Physical exam findings (spider telangiectasia, palmar erythema, splenomegaly)
- Laboratory findings (decreasing platelets, elevated bilirubin, decreasing albumin)
- Patient complaints (encephalopathy, ascites, fatigue)
- Incidental imaging study findings (cirrhotic liver, splenomegaly, varices, ascites)

DIET
Restrictions of total calories, simple carbohydrates, and alcohol are required to control diabetes, weight, and lipids.

PATIENT EDUCATION
Planning for lifelong change in diet, exercise, and alcohol use is required. As such, regular education and motivation sessions are of value.

COMPLICATIONS
- Steatohepatitis may progress to cirrhosis, with complications that include variceal bleeding, ascites, encephalopathy, and liver failure.
- Progression to hepatocellular carcinoma

REFERENCES

1. Schneider AL, Lazo M, et al. Racial differences in nonalcoholic fatty liver disease in the U.S. population. *Obesity (Silver Spring)*. 2013 Mar 20;doi: 10.1002/oby.20426.
2. Chalasani N, Younossi Z, Lavine JE, et al. The diagnosis and management of non-alcoholic fatty liver disease: practice guideline by the American Association for the Study of Liver Diseases, American College of Gastroenterology, and the American Gastroenterological Association. *Hepatology*; 2012;55: 2005–2023.
3. Ramesh S, Sanyal AJ. Evaluation and management of non-alcoholic steatohepatitis. *J Hepatol*. 2005;42(Suppl):S2–S12.
4. Szczepaniak LS, Nurenberg P, Leonard D, et al. Magnetic resonance spectroscopy to measure hepatic triglyceride content: Prevalence of hepatic steatosis in the general population. *Am J Physiol Endocrinol Metabol*. 2005;288:E462–E468.
5. Bondini S, Kleiner DE, Goodman ZD, et al. Pathologic assessment of non-alcoholic fatty liver disease. *Clin Liver Dis*. 2007;11:17–23.
6. Promrat K, Kleiner DE, Niemeier HM, et al. Randomized controlled trial testing the effects of weight loss on nonalcoholic steatohepatitis. *Hepatology*. 2010;51:121–129.
7. Chalasani NP, Sanyal AJ, Kowdley KV, et al. Pioglitazone versus vitamin E versus placebo for the treatment of non-diabetic patients with non-alcoholic steatohepatitis: PIVENS trial design. *Contemp Clin Trials*. 2009;30:88–96.

ADDITIONAL READING

Vernon G, Baranova A, Younossi ZM. Systematic review: The epidemiology and natural history of non-alcoholic fatty liver disease and non-alcoholic steatohepatitis in adults. *Aliment Pharmacol Ther*. 2011;84(3):274–285. Epub 2011 May 30[BluM1].

CODES

ICD10
- K75.81 Nonalcoholic steatohepatitis (NASH)
- K76.0 Fatty (change of) liver, not elsewhere classified

CLINICAL PEARLS

- Prevalence of NAFLD and NASH is much higher in patients who have metabolic syndrome or any one of its components (diabetes, obesity, hypertriglyceridemia).
- Liver biopsy is the gold standard for diagnosis.
- Weight loss and treating components of the metabolic syndrome are central to the treatment of NAFLD.
- Insulin sensitizers, such as metformin and thiazolidinediones are not currently recommended for treatment.
- Vitamin E should be considered as -first line therapy in nondiabetic patients with biopsy-proven NASH, but not in diabetic patients.
- Statins are not contraindicated and should be considered in patients who have NAFLD with dyslipidemia.

STRESS FRACTURE
Omer Jamal, DO • Nitin Budhwar, MD

 BASICS

DESCRIPTION

- Stress fractures are microscopic fractures that occur when bone is subject to repetitive stress. This causes breakdown faster than the formation of new bone.
- Stress fractures can occur in different situations:
  - Fatigue fracture: Abnormal stress applied to normal bone (e.g., young college athletes or new military recruits with inadequate conditioning)
  - Insufficiency fracture: Normal stress applied to abnormal bone (e.g., femoral neck fracture in osteopenic)
  - Combination: Abnormal stress applied to abnormal bone (e.g., female long-distance runners with premature osteoporosis from female athlete triad)
- Weight-bearing bones of the lower extremity are affected the most.
- Commonly affected sites:
  - Tibia
  - Metatarsus
  - Fibula
  - Navicular
  - Femoral neck
  - Pars interarticularis
- Less commonly affected sites:
  - Pelvis
  - Calcaneus
  - Ribs
  - Ulna
- High-risk stress fractures are defined as stress fractures that are more likely to result in fracture displacement and/or nonunion (1)[B]. High-risk sites include:
  - Femoral neck
  - Anterior tibial cortex
  - Sesamoids
  - Pars interarticularis
  - 5th metatarsal metaphyseal
  - Proximal second metatarsal
  - Medial malleolus
  - Tarsal navicular
  - Body of the talus
- Synonym(s): March fracture; Fatigue fracture

EPIDEMIOLOGY
Incidence
- Predominant age: Can occur at any age
- Predominant sex: Female > Male
- Greatest incidence 15–27 years of age
- Affects 8.7–21.1% of track and field athletes annually
- Accounts for as many as 7.8% of visits to sports medicine and orthopedic clinics
- Occurs in <1% of general population
Prevalence
- Affects 5% of military recruits
- Affects 1–2.6% of college athletes

ETIOLOGY AND PATHOPHYSIOLOGY
- Osteoblastic activities lag behind osteoclastic activities during the initial increase in exercise activity.
- Strong and repetitive stress transmits to bone when the surrounding muscles become fatigued.

RISK FACTORS
- Sports involving running and jumping
- Rapid increase in physical training programs
- Female athlete triad (i.e., amenorrhea, eating disorder, premature bone loss)
- History of previous stress fracture
- History of osteoporosis, osteomalacia, rheumatoid arthritis, corticosteroid therapy
- Skeletal malalignment:
  - Pes cavus, pes planus
  - Excessive external rotation of the hip
- Inappropriate footwear
- Increased vertical loading rate (e.g., heel-to-toe running instead of forefoot striking in runners) (2)[A]
- Extremes of body size and composition
- Muscle fatigue and decreased lean muscle mass
- Previous inactivity or low aerobic fitness

GENERAL PREVENTION
- Avoid abrupt increases in physical activity.
- Reduce intensity and duration of activity if new-onset pain.
- Use proper footwear.
- Increasing dynamic physical activity (jumping) has shown to increase bone density and resistance to mechanical stress (3)[A].
- Decrease vertical loading rate either by switching to forefoot strike style running, or, if continuing with heel-to-toe strike, using a heel pad insert (2)[A].
- Shock-absorbing foot inserts may help.
- Increasing calcium, vitamin D, skim milk, and low-fat dairy product intake may reduce the rate of stress fractures in female runners/military recruits (4)[B].

COMMONLY ASSOCIATED CONDITIONS
- Osteoporosis/Osteopenia
- Female athlete triad
- Metabolic bone disorders

 DIAGNOSIS

HISTORY
- Insidious onset of vague, achy pain over period of weeks that occurs at the end or after physical activity
- Rest will relieve the pain initially.
- If untreated, pain will occur earlier during training sessions or even with daily walking and also become more localized.
- Eventual fracture of untreated stress fractures will cause pain at rest.
- More detailed history may reveal recent change in training intensity and/or footwear.
- Attention to diet and possible eating disorders

PHYSICAL EXAM
- Antalgic gait (common in painful weight-bearing)
- Point tenderness or percussion tenderness over injury site
- Placing a vibrating tuning fork over the fracture site may intensify pain.
- Swelling may be present.
- Specific tests may be helpful:
  - Hop test for tibia: Cannot hop on 1 leg 10 times; if able, consider shin splints (i.e., medial tibial stress syndrome)

- Fulcrum test for femur: With patient seated, provoke pain by applying downward force on the distal femur while examiner uses other hand under the midthigh as fulcrum for femoral shaft.
- Single-leg hyperextension (Stork) test for pars interarticularis of lumbar spine: Stand on ipsilateral leg of symptomatic side and extend lumbar spine.
- Anatomic malalignment may be present (e.g., leg-length discrepancy, pes planus/cavus).

DIFFERENTIAL DIAGNOSIS
- Fracture
- Shin splints (i.e., medial tibial stress syndrome) pain resolves with rest, whereas stress fracture pain does not.
- Infection (osteomyelitis)
- Soft-tissue injury (e.g., sprain, tendonitis, and periostitis)
- Compartment syndrome
- Neoplasm (osteoid osteoma)
- Nerve or artery entrapment syndromes
- Intermittent claudication

DIAGNOSTIC TESTS & INTERPRETATION
None unless clinically indicated for suspected disease process (e.g., hyperparathyroidism and vitamin D deficiency)
   Radiography:

- 1st-line management in suspected stress fracture (5)[B]
- Findings typically seen 2–8 weeks after onset of pain
- Sensitivity during early stages (1–2 weeks) may be as low as 10%.
- May see periosteal callus, "gray cortex" sign (cortical region of decreased intensity), osteopenia, endosteal reaction, or ill-defined cortical margin
- Severe cases may show discrete partial or complete fracture.

Follow-Up Tests & Special Considerations
- MRI:
  - Gold standard for imaging stress fractures (5)[B]
  - Very sensitive
  - Better evaluation of surrounding soft tissue
  - Allows for classification of the injury
  - T2 weighting and short time inversion recovery (STIR) methods
- Bone scan:
  - Very sensitive, but lack of specificity may limit clinical utility
  - Should not be used to assess healing process
- CT scan:
  - Less sensitive than MRI for early stress fractures, but has an important role in evaluating occult fractures in certain regions: Foot, tibia, carpal scaphoid, and pars interarticularis (5)[B]
  - Can distinguish diseases such as osteoid osteoma, malignancy, and osteomyelitis that mimic stress fracture on bone scan
  - Useful for evaluating lesions found to be equivocal on other imaging modalities (5)[B]
  - May also be used to determine whether a known stress fracture is complete or incomplete (5)[B]
- US:
  - Not routinely used for the diagnosis of stress fractures

- Able to detect cortical breaks and periosteal reactions
- Of particular use in the evaluation of the foot; may distinguish between metatarsal stress fractures and other causes of metatarsalgia (e.g., Morton's neuroma) (5)[B]
- Classification by radiographic grading:
  - Grade I: Normal x-ray, positive STIR (MRI)
  - Grade II: Normal x-ray, positive STIR + positive T2-weighted MRI
  - Grade III: Discrete line or discrete periosteal reaction on x-ray, positive T1/T2-weighted MRI but with no definite cortical break
  - Grade IV: Fracture or periosteal reaction on x-ray, positive T1/T2-weighted fracture line

 TREATMENT

- Protection, rest, ice, compression, and elevation (PRICE) for acute pain and edema
- Decrease activity below threshold of pain.
- Pain at rest or with range of motion (ROM) may require temporary immobilization.
- Painful ambulation is criterion for crutches with periodic walking trial.
- Gradually increase activity as long as patient remains pain-free.
- Early surgical management of high-risk fractures is indicated in the elite athlete secondary to the high risk of displacement and nonunion, as well as the association with earlier return to sports (1)[C].
- Conservative non–weight-bearing management is the standard of care for initial treatment of both partial and complete stress fractures of the tarsal navicular (6)[A].
- Prophylactic fixation of bisphosphonate associated proximal femoral stress fractures reduces hospital stay and has a lower likelihood of fracture completion compared to nonoperative management (7)[B].

MEDICATION
First Line
- Calcium and vitamin D supplementation should be initiated when deficiencies are found.
- Acetaminophen
- NSAIDs are beneficial for pain and inflammation, but are controversial and discouraged by some authors because of negative impact on bone/tissue healing.
- Bisphosphonates theoretically could treat stress fractures, but their use should be limited because no randomized, controlled trials have been performed that show conclusive evidence (8)[B]. Currently, only case reports have shown benefit.

ISSUES FOR REFERRAL
Orthopedic opinion should be obtained for high-risk fractures, failure to improve with standard treatment, evidence of non union within 3–4 weeks, or inability to tolerate rehabilitation.

ADDITIONAL THERAPIES
- Electrical stimulator may be considered in more severe injuries and/or elite athletes (9)[B].
- Extracorporeal shock wave therapy (ESWT) may be considered and has been shown to be effective in animal models (10).
- Low-intensity pulsed US:
  - No evidence for improved healing in stress fracture
  - May improve healing with subsequent complete fracture

- Physical therapy:
  - Correct training errors predisposing to stress fracture.
  - Correct inappropriate mechanics.
  - Strengthen muscles around the site of stress fracture.
  - Correct anatomic variations.
  - Anti-gravity treadmills

 ONGOING CARE

FOLLOW-UP RECOMMENDATIONS
- After initial treatment, activity should be increased gradually.
- Once the patient is pain-free, low-impact training can be started and advanced as tolerated.
- Once running is resumed, mileage should be increased slowly.

Patient Monitoring
Radiographs every 4–6 weeks to document healing progress

PATIENT EDUCATION
- Gradually increase activity as tolerated as long as patient is pain-free.
- Rest if there is a recurrence of pain.
- Correct mechanical and training errors.
- Strengthen core muscles.

PROGNOSIS
- Stress fractures in young people have a good prognosis.
- Older patients or those with metabolic bone disease typically continue to develop insufficiency fractures in other bones.
- Time to return to full activity:
  - Grade I: 3+ weeks
  - Grade II: 5+ weeks
  - Grade III: 11+ weeks
  - Grade IV: 14+ weeks

COMPLICATIONS
Completion of fracture:
- Delayed union
- Nonunion
- May require surgery with internal fixation

REFERENCES

1. Anderson RB, Hunt KJ, McCormick JJ, et al. Management of common sports-related injuries about the foot and ankle. *J Am Acad Orthop Surg.* 2010;18:546–556.
2. Zadpoor AA, Nikooyan AA. The relationship between lower-extremity stress fractures and the ground reaction force: A systematic review. *Clin Biomech (Bristol, Avon).* 2011;26(1):23–28.
3. Nikander R, Sievanen H, Heinonen A, et al. Targeted exercise against osteoporosis: A systematic review and meta analysis for optimizing bone strength throughout life. *BMC Medicine.* 2010;8:47.
4. Tenforde AS, Sayres LC, Sainani KL, et al. Evaluating the relationship of calcium and vitamin D in the prevention of stress fracture injuries in the young athlete: A review of the literature. *PM R.* 2010;2:945–949.
5. Dixon S, Newton J, Teh J, et al. Stress fractures in the young athlete: A pictorial review. *Curr Probl Diagn Radiol.* 2011;40:29–44.
6. Fowler JR, Gaughan JP, Boden BP, et al. The non-surgical and surgical treatment of tarsal navicular stress fractures. *Sports Med.* 2011; 84(8):613–619.
7. Banffy M, Vrahas M, Ready J, et al. Nonoperative vs. prophylactic treatment of bisphosphonate-associated femoral stress fractures. *Clin Orthop Relat Res.* 2011;469:2028–2034.
8. Shima Y. Use of bisphosphonates for the treatment of stress fractures in athletes. *Knee Surg Sports Traumatol Arthrosc.* 2009;5:542–550.
9. Beck B. Do capacitively coupled electric fields accelerate tibial stress fracture healing?: A randomized controlled trial. *Am J Sports Med.* 2008;3:545–553.
10. Shindle MK, Endo Y, Warren RF, et al. Stress fractures about the tibia, foot, and ankle. *J Am Acad Orthop Surg.* 2012;20:167–176.

ADDITIONAL READING

- Chen YT, Tenforde AS, Fredericson M. Update on stress fractures in female athletes: Epidemiology, treatment, and prevention. *Curr Rev Musculoskelet Med.* 2013;6(2):173–181. doi: 10.1007/s12178-013-9167-x.
- Miller T, Kaeding CC, Flanigan D. The classification systems of stress fractures: A systematic review. *Phys Sportsmed.* 2011;84(1):93–100.
- Torg J, Moyer J, Gaughan J. Management of tarsal navicular stress fractures: Conservative versus surgical treatment: A meta-analysis. *Am J Sports Med.* 2010;38:1048–1053.
- Ward W, Carter C, Wilson S, et al. Femoral stress fractures associated with long-term bisphosphonates treatment. *Clin Orthop Relat Res.* 2012; 470:759–765.

 SEE ALSO

Algorithm: Foot Pain

 CODES

ICD10
- M84.38XA Stress fracture, other site, initial encounter for fracture
- M84.369A Stress fracture, unsp tibia and fibula, init for fx
- M84.376A Stress fracture, unspecified foot, init encntr for fracture

CLINICAL PEARLS
- Diagnosis requires a high index of suspicion because x-rays are often negative initially.
- Emphasis must be placed on rest to allow for proper bone healing.
- Once the patient can walk pain-free, he or she can proceed to low-impact activity, and when low-impact activity can be performed pain-free, proceed to running.
- Gradually increase running mileage.
- Rest if there is a recurrence of pain.
- Recognize high-risk stress fracture for appropriate referral and possible surgery.

STROKE REHABILITATION

Aaron Hauptman, MD • Jordan Eisenstock, MD

BASICS

DESCRIPTION
- Stroke is a compromise in blood supply to an area of the nervous system, secondary to hemorrhage or occlusion, with resultant infarction of nervous tissue.
- Stroke is the 3rd leading cause of death and the leading cause of long-term disability in the US (1).
- Rehabilitation refers to the process of restoring a debilitated person toward baseline level of functionality.
- Specific rehabilitation techniques should be used depending on the individual and based on particular deficits and brain regions impacted.
- Rehabilitation involves cycling through the following (2):
  – Assessment of patient with the goal of identification and quantification of the needs of the individual
  – Setting of objectives that are realistic, concrete, and attainable
  – Repetition of assessment to gauge changes in status, with subsequent alteration of techniques as necessary
- Motor impairment is the most commonly recognized impairment secondary to stroke.
- Speech and language, swallowing, vision, sensation, and cognition are also commonly impaired.

EPIDEMIOLOGY
Incidence
- Each year, about 795,000 people suffer a stroke, ~610,000 of which are 1st attacks and 185,000 are recurrent attacks (3).
- ~14% of survivors of stroke reach full recovery in physical function, but 25–50% require assistance poststroke (1).
- According to the World Health Organization, 15 million people suffer stroke worldwide each year. Of these, 5 million die and another 5 million are permanently disabled.

Prevalence
- ~7 million Americans ≥20 years old have had a stroke (~3%) (3).
- ~50 million stroke survivors worldwide (4)
- >1/2 of strokes in people <65 result in death within 8 years (1).

ETIOLOGY AND PATHOPHYSIOLOGY
Stroke involves a compromise in blood supply to an area, usually by either rupture or blockage of a vessel. Of all strokes, 87% are ischemic, 10% intracerebral hemorrhage, and 3% subarachnoid hemorrhage (3).

RISK FACTORS
Risk factors for stroke are discussed in the topics "Stroke, Acute" and "Atherosclerosis."

GENERAL PREVENTION
See "Stroke, Acute."

DIAGNOSIS

HISTORY
- For acute stroke symptoms, see "Stroke, Acute."
- A wide variety of systems and functions are commonly impacted by stroke, depending on type, severity, location, and other factors. Common functions impacted include (2):
  – Consciousness and psychological functions:

- Orientation, arousal, alertness, attention, intellect, personality, sleep, perception, memory, cognition, perception, behavior, temperament, psychomotor functions, as well as others
  – Perceptual functions, most commonly:
    ○ Vision, proprioception, touch sensation
  – Communication, excretory and sexual functions:
    ○ Vocal control and articulation; intake of food (chewing, swallowing), urinary and bowel functions; sexual function
  – Neuromuscular and activities of daily living (ADLs):
    ○ Muscle strength, stability, endurance, reflexes, tone, gait, voluntary movement

PHYSICAL EXAM
- Neurologic manifestations should be examined based on location of stroke when known but should include investigation of:
  – Sensory or motor deficits, especially unilaterally (i.e., hemiparesis/hemiplegia)
  – Dysarthria or aphasia
  – Visual field deficits (i.e., hemianopsia)
  – Dysphagia
  – Apraxia
  – Unilateral facial palsy
- Neuropsychiatric evaluation should be undertaken to assess cognitive, intellectual, personality, memory, psychomotor, and other system changes that may benefit from treatment during the course of rehabilitation.

DIFFERENTIAL DIAGNOSIS
- Differential diagnosis in stroke rehabilitation should take into account acute changes that are inconsistent with general trend in the individual patient's status.
- New changes in motor function, mental status, etc. could represent new stroke.
- Subacute changes could include a wide range of neuromuscular, neuropsychiatric, or psychiatric diseases that could be related or unrelated to the initial stroke event.

DIAGNOSTIC TESTS & INTERPRETATION
A wide range of standardized, quantifiable scales have been used to track outcomes in stroke rehabilitation. These include (2):
- Neurological scales:
  – Glasgow coma scale, Mini Mental Status Examination, NIH stroke scale among others
- Global ADL scales:
  – Including, but not limited to, Barthel index, Functional Independence Measure, modified Rankin scale, Frenchay activities index, trunk control test, timed up-and-go, stair climbing test, Toronto bedside swallowing screening test, etc.
- Family and caretaker contextual factors are very important to stroke rehabilitation and have been shown to impact outcomes, so thorough assessment should include testing such as:
  – Caregiver Strain Index, Family Assessment Device
- See topic "Stroke, Acute."

Follow-Up Tests & Special Considerations
Monitor the coagulation profile of patients on anticoagulants.

TREATMENT

- Treatments and rehabilitation techniques should be tailored to specific stroke-related sequelae.
- The 3 major stroke rehabilitation goals are (1):
  – Prevention/Treatment of the various complications of prolonged inactivity
  – Prevention of recurrent stroke and cardiovascular events
  – Increase in aerobic fitness

GENERAL MEASURES
Prevention and/or treatment of the complications associated with stroke (4)[C]:
- Aspiration:
  – Immediately after stroke, up to 50% of patients have dysphagia; this improves in many.
  – Patient should be kept NPO until initial bedside swallow assessment
  – Prevention of aspiration involves postural changes, increased sensory input, swallowing maneuvers, active exercise programs, diet modifications, nonoral feeding (if indicated), psychological support, and supportive nursing interventions.
- Pulmonary embolism/seep venous thrombosis:
  – Risk highest during first 3–120 days post stroke
  – Pneumatic compression devices and compression stockings
  – Ambulation as soon as possible
- Skin breakdown:
  – Increased risk due to loss of sensation, impaired circulation, older age, decreased level of consciousness, inability to move due to paralysis, and incontinence of urine or stool
  – Frequent repositioning (at least q2h) with special care to avoid excessive friction
  – Keep skin clean and dry.
- Spasticity:
  – Occurs in ~35% of stroke survivors; treated with a combination of physical and pharmacological modalities:
    ○ Range-of-motion exercises
    ○ Heat, cold, or electric stimulation
    ○ Splinting
    ○ Oral medications for spasticity of cerebral origin (e.g., dantrolene, tizanidine); phenol or botulinum toxin injections for targeting specific muscles or muscle groups
- Malnutrition:
  – Nutritional assessment with a diet history and monitoring by a dietician
- Seizures:
  – More common after hemorrhagic stroke (11%) than after ischemic stroke (9%)
  – Antiepileptic drugs and elimination of disturbances (i.e., toxins, metabolic) that may lower seizure threshold
- Falls:
  – Lifestyle changes:
    ○ Avoid loose rugs; maintain a clear path without obstruction.
    ○ Avoid slippery surfaces (such as wet floors).
    ○ Maintain good lighting.
    ○ Shoes with nonskid soles
    ○ Slow down movements for transfers or walking.
- Severe sleep apnea:
  – Lifestyle changes:
    ○ Stop smoking.
    ○ Lose weight.

○ Sleep on side vs. back.
○ Mouthpieces
○ Breathing devices (i.e., CPAP)
○ Surgery

- Neurocognitive (5):
  – Wide range of deficit patterns that can be focal (e.g., aphasia) or diffuse (general cognitive slowing)
  ○ Most broadly effected are orientation, language, attention, memory
  ○ Common particular deficits include aphasia, neglect, cognitive slowing, memory deficits, executive function deficits,
  ○ Assessment, treatment, and outcomes vary markedly based on stroke type, location, severity, timing, and a variety of additional factors
  ○ Cognitive rehabilitation has shown some success for focal deficits but less for diffuse cognitive changes.
  ○ Pharmacology: There is evidence of efficacy for escitalopram and rivastigmine for cognitive function.
  ○ Additional modalities under investigation: therapies such as rTMS and prism adaptation have sown some benefit in driving plasticity and functional brain changes.
- Depression:
  – May be organic secondary to stroke or reactive to the stroke itself
  – Poststroke depression has been found to cause higher mortality, poorer functional recovery, and less activity socially (1)[B].
  – Treat with a combination of pharmacotherapy and psychotherapy:
  ○ Evidence suggests heterocyclic antidepressants are effective in the setting of poststroke depression but must be closely monitored in older adults due to side effects.
  ○ SSRIs are also effective in treating poststroke depression.
  ○ All stroke patients should be assessed for depression and treated with the appropriate antidepressant for 6 months.

MEDICATION
First Line
- Management of controllable risk factors, including BP reduction, diabetes, and cholesterol (initiate statin therapy, if history of TIA or stroke with evidence of atherosclerosis, LDL $\geq$100, and no CHD)
- Anticoagulation with warfarin for patients mechanical prosthetic heart valves and ischemic stroke or TIA (dosage of warfarin varies depending on optimum INR for patient in setting of comorbidities)
- Antiplatelet drugs (aspirin, aspirin/dipyridamole, clopidogrel, ticlopidine) decrease relative risk of stroke, MI, or death by ~22% (6)[B].

ISSUES FOR REFERRAL
For stroke survivors who require 24-hour care of medical comorbidities, close physician supervision, and specialized nursing care (RN with specialized training or rehabilitation experience) an inpatient rehabilitation facility (IRF) can offer hospital-level care.

ADDITIONAL THERAPIES
Physical, occupational, speech, and recreational therapy

IN-PATIENT CONSIDERATIONS
Admission Criteria/Initial Stabilization
- For stroke survivors who require 24-hour care of medical comorbidities, close physician supervision, and specialized nursing care (RN with specialized training or rehabilitation experience), an IRF can offer hospital-level care.
- Such patients must also require and receive a minimum of 3 hours daily occupational or physical therapy for no less than 5 days each week; this can be combined with other skilled modalities, such as speech-language or prosthetic-orthotic services) to meet the 3-hour requirement.
- Either the aforementioned is required or an IRF is the only reasonable setting in which a low-intensity rehab program may be executed.
- An alternative inpatient setting is a skilled nursing facility that provides nursing care or rehabilitation to residents needing daily rehab or nursing care on an inpatient basis.
- See "Stroke, Acute."

IV Fluids
Avoid D5W in acute setting to avoid hyperglycemia and its secondary effects.

Nursing
An alternative inpatient setting is a skilled nursing facility that provides nursing care or rehabilitation to residents needing daily rehab or nursing care on an inpatient basis.

Discharge Criteria
Chronic care settings support and help make external resources available to manage the patient's level of health; such services must be prescribed by a qualified health care professional, such as a physician.

 ## ONGOING CARE

FOLLOW-UP RECOMMENDATIONS
Patient should follow up regularly with primary care physician for management of risk factors for stroke.

Patient Monitoring
Continue to monitor for risk factors. Lab studies monitored periodically may include hemoglobin A1c (and fingerstick glucose testing in diabetics), lipid panel, CBC including platelets, lipid profile, coagulation studies (PT/INR—of special importance in patients on anticoagulation)

DIET
Low salt, low calorie, low saturated and trans fat, low cholesterol

PATIENT EDUCATION
National Stroke Association: www.stroke.org

PROGNOSIS
- Strong evidence suggests an organized, interdisciplinary stroke care team of physicians, nurses, therapists, family, and patient can reduce mortality rates and the likelihood of institutional care and long-term disability. It can also enhance recovery and increase ADL independence.
- Aggressive rehabilitation beyond the time window of the 1st poststroke months, including treadmill with or without body weight support, can increase aerobic capacity and sensorimotor functionality.

COMPLICATIONS
- Aspiration
- Pulmonary embolism/deep venous thrombosis
- Greater exercise intolerance
- Muscle atrophy

- Osteoporosis
- Skin breakdown
- Spasticity
- Malnutrition
- Seizures
- Falls
- Severe sleep apnea

REFERENCES
1. Gordon NF, Gulanick M, Costa F, et al. Physical activity and exercise recommendations for stroke survivors: An American Heart Association scientific statement from the Council on Clinical Cardiology, Subcommittee on Exercise, Cardiac Rehabilitation, and Prevention; the Council on Cardiovascular Nursing; the Council on Nutrition, Physical Activity, and Metabolism; and the Stroke Council. *Circulation*. 2004;109:2031–2041.
2. Langhorne P, Bernhardt J, Kwakkel G, et al. Stroke rehabilitation. *Lancet*. 2011;377:1693–1702.
3. Roger VL, Go AS, Lloyd-Jones DM, et al. Heart disease and stroke statistics–2011 update: A report from the American Heart Association. *Circulation*. 2011;123:e18–e209.
4. Miller EL, Murray L, Richards L, et al. Comprehensive overview of nursing and interdisciplinary rehabilitation care of the stroke patient: A scientific statement from the American Heart Association. *Stroke*. 2010;41:2402–2448.
5. Cumming TB, Marshall RS, Lazar RM. Stroke, cognitive deficits and rehabilitation: Still an incomplete picture. *Int J Stroke*. 2013;8:38–45.
6. Furie KL, Kasner SE, Adams RJ, et al. Guidelines for the prevention of stroke in patients with stroke or transient ischemic attack: A guideline for healthcare professionals from the American Heart Association/American Stroke Association. *Stroke*. 2011;42:227–276.

 ## SEE ALSO

- Brain Injury—Post Acute Care Issues; Stroke, Acute; Dementia; Delirium
- Algorithm: Stroke

 ## CODES

ICD10
- I63.9 Cerebral infarction, unspecified
- I69.10 Unsp sequelae of nontraumatic intracerebral hemorrhage

CLINICAL PEARLS
- Stroke is the 3rd leading cause of death and the leading cause of long-term disability in the US.
- An essential part of poststroke management is the treatment of controllable risk factors, including BP reduction and cholesterol control (initiate statin therapy, if history of TIA or stroke with evidence of atherosclerosis, LDL $\geq$100).
- Strong evidence suggests an organized, interdisciplinary stroke care team of physicians, nurses, therapists, family, and patient can reduce mortality rates and the likelihood of institutional care and long-term disability. It can also enhance recovery and increase ADL independence.

STROKE, ACUTE
Nihal Patel, MD • Marc Fisher, MD

 BASICS

A cerebrovascular accident (CVA) is an infarction or hemorrhage in the brain.

DESCRIPTION
Stroke is the sudden onset of a focal neurologic deficit(s) resulting from either infarction or hemorrhage within the brain:

- 2 broad categories: Ischemic (thrombotic or embolic; 87%) and hemorrhagic (13%) (1)
- Hemorrhage can be intracerebral or subarachnoid.
- System(s) affected: Neurologic; Vascular
- Synonym(s): Cerebrovascular accident; Cerebral infarct; Brain attack
- Related terms: Transient ischemic attack (TIA), a transient episode of neurologic dysfunction due to focal ischemia without permanent infarction on imaging (see topic "Transient Ischemic Attack [TIA]")

Pediatric Considerations
- Cardiac abnormalities (congenital heart disease, paradoxical embolism, rheumatic fever, bacterial endocarditis)
- Metabolic: Homocystinuria, Fabry disease

EPIDEMIOLOGY
Incidence
Annual incidence in the US is ~795,000.

Prevalence
- Prevalence in the US: 550/100,000
- Predominant age: Risk increases >45 years of age and is highest during the 7th and 8th decades.
- Predominant sex: Male > Female at younger age, but higher incidence in women with age ≥75

ETIOLOGY AND PATHOPHYSIOLOGY
- 87% of stroke is ischemic, 3 main subtypes for etiology: Thrombosis, embolism, and systemic hypoperfusion. Large vessel artherothrombotic strokes are commonly related to the origin of the internal carotid artery. Small vessel lacunar strokes are commonly due to lipohyalinotic occlusion. Embolic strokes are largely from a cardiac source (due to left atrial thrombus, atrial fibrillation, recent MI, valve disease or mechanical valves) or ascending aortic atheromatous disease (>4 mm)
- 13% of stroke is hemorrhagic, most commonly due to HTN. Other causes include intracranial vascular malformations (cavernous angiomas, AVMs), cerebral amyloid angiopathy (lobar hemorrhages in elderly), and anticoagulation.
- Other causes include fibromuscular dysplasia (rare), vasculitis, or drug use (cocaine, amphetamines).

Genetics
Stroke is a polygenic multifactorial disease, with some clustering within families.

RISK FACTORS
- Uncontrollable: Age, gender, race, family history/genetics, prior stroke or TIA
- Controllable/Modifiable/Treatable:
  - Metabolic: Diabetes, dyslipidemia
  - Lifestyle: Smoking, cocaine use, amphetamine use
  - Cardiovascular: Hypertension, atrial fibrillation, valvular heart disease, endocarditis, recent MI, severe carotid artery stenosis, hypercoagulable states, and patent foramen ovale

GENERAL PREVENTION
Smoking cessation, regular exercise, weight control to maintain nonobese BMI and prevent type 2 diabetes, use alcohol in moderation, control BP, and manage hyperlipidemia; use of antiplatelet agent, such as aspirin, in high-risk persons; treatment of nonvalvular atrial fibrillation with dose-adjusted warfarin or dabigatran, apixiban, and rivoroxiban.

COMMONLY ASSOCIATED CONDITIONS
Coronary artery disease is the major cause of death during the first 5 years after a stroke.

 DIAGNOSIS

HISTORY
Acute onset of focal arm/leg weakness, facial weakness, difficulty with speech or swallowing, vertigo, visual disturbances, diminished consciousness; presence of vomiting and severe headache favor diagnosis of hemorrhagic stroke.

PHYSICAL EXAM
- Anterior (carotid) circulation: Hemiparesis/Hemiplegia, neglect, aphasia, visual field defects
- Posterior (vertebrobasilar) circulation: Diplopia, vertigo, gait and limb ataxia, facial paresis, Horner syndrome, dysphagia, dysarthria, alternating sensory loss

DIFFERENTIAL DIAGNOSIS
- Migraine (complicated)
- Postictal state (Todd paralysis)
- Systemic infection, including meningitis or encephalitis (infection also may uncover or enhance previous deficits)
- Toxic or metabolic disturbance (hypoglycemia, acute renal failure, liver failure, drug intoxication)
- Brain tumor, primary or metastases
- Head trauma
- Other types of intracranial hemorrhage (epidural, subdural, subarachnoid)
- Trauma, septic emboli

DIAGNOSTIC TESTS & INTERPRETATION
Primarily used to narrow differential and identify etiology of stroke

Initial Tests (lab, imaging)
- ECG
- Serum glucose level, including finger-stick testing (exclude hypo- and hyperglycemia)
- CBC, including platelets
- Electrolytes, including BUN and creatinine
- Coagulation studies: PT, PTT, INR
- Markers of cardiac ischemia
- Emergent brain imaging with noncontrast CT (or brain MRI with diffusionweighted [DW]-MRI) to exclude hemorrhage can be lifesaving.
- Subsequent multimodal CT (perfusion CT, CTA, unenhanced CT) or MRI to improve diagnosis of acute ischemic stroke (2)

Follow-Up Tests & Special Considerations
Consider LFT, tox screen, blood alcohol, ABG, lumbar puncture if suspected subarachnoid hemorrhage (SAH), EEG if suspect seizures, blood type and cross
- DW-MRI is more sensitive than CT for acute ischemic stroke (3); however, MRI also is better than CT for diagnosis of posterior fossa lesions.

- Emergent treatment (IV thrombolysis) should not be delayed to obtain advanced imaging studies.
- Follow-up imaging of carotid vessels with Doppler ultrasound, CTA, or MRA of head and neck should be completed.

Diagnostic Procedures/Other
Echocardiogram (transthoracic and/or transesophageal) in patients with increased suspicion for cardioembolic source. In cryptogenic stroke patients prolonged ECG monitoring should be performed with a 30-day event monitor.

Test Interpretation
Early CT findings: Hyperdense MCA sign, loss of gray-white differentiation in cortical ribbon, sulcal effacement, loss of insular ribbon

TREATMENT

- BP should be closely monitored in the first 24 hours:
  - Antihypertensives should be withheld unless systolic BP >220 mm Hg or diastolic BP >120 mm Hg, with a goal to lower BP by ~15% during first 24 hours if treatment is indicated (2)[A]. If thrombolytic therapy is to be initiated, BP must be <185/110 prior to thrombolytics.
  - In acute spontaneous intracranial hemorrhagic stroke, goal for BP control is 160/90 or target MAP 110 (see topic, "Subarachnoid Hemorrhage" for details on BP management). With suspicion for elevated ICP, BP should be reduced with goal to keep cerebral perfusion pressure between 61 and 80 mm Hg.
  - Antihypertensive medications should be restarted 24 hours after stroke onset for patients with a history of hypertension who are neurologically stable (2)[A].
- Thrombolysis (2)[A]: IV thrombolysis should be started in patients with measurable neurologic deficits that do not clear spontaneously, presenting within 3–4.5 hours of stroke symptom onset.
- Exclusion criteria for thrombolysis within 3 hours of onset include:
  - Symptoms suggestive of SAH
  - Head trauma or prior stroke within 3 months
  - MI within 3 months
  - GI or gastric ulcer hemorrhage within 21 days
  - Major surgery within 14 days
  - Arterial puncture at noncompressible site within 7 days
  - Any history of intracranial hemorrhage
  - Elevated BP (systolic >185 mm Hg and diastolic >110 mm Hg)
  - Active bleeding or acute trauma on examination
  - Taking anticoagulant and INR ≥1.7
  - Activated PTT not in normal range if heparin received during previous 48 hours; platelet count <100,000 mm³
  - Blood glucose concentration <50 mg/dL
  - Seizure with postictal residual neurologic impairment
  - Multilobar infarction on CT (hypodensity >1/3 cerebral hemisphere)
  - Patient or family members not able to weigh and understand potential risks and benefits of treatment

- Extended exclusion criteria for thrombolysis within 4.5 hours include per AHA/ASA guidelines:
  – Age >80 years
  – All patients taking oral anticoagulants regardless of INR
  – National Institute of Health (NIH) Stoke Scale >25
  – History of stroke and diabetes
- Antiplatelet agents: Oral aspirin (initial dose, 325 mg) should be started within 24–48 hours (2)[A].

MEDICATION
First Line
- BP management: Antihypertensive options include (2)[A]:
  – Labetalol 10–20 mg IV over 1–2 minutes, which may be repeated once
  – Nitropaste 1–2 inches
  – Nicardipine infusion 5 mg/hr, titrate up by 2.5 mg/hr at 5–15-minute intervals to maximum of 15 mg/hr; reduce to 3 mg/hr when target BP is reached
- Thrombolysis, IV administration of rtPA: Infuse 0.9 mg/kg, maximum dose 90 mg over 60 minutes with 10% of dose given as bolus over 1 minute (2)[A]:
  – Admit to ICU or stroke unit, with neurologic exams every 15 minutes during infusion, every 60 minutes for next 6 hours, then hourly until 24 hours after treatment.
  – Discontinue infusion and obtain emergent CT scan if severe headache, angioedema, acute hypertension, or nausea and vomiting develop.
  – Measure BP every 15 minutes for first 2 hours, every 30 minutes for next 6 hours, then every hour until 24 hours after treatment. Maintain BP <185/105. Follow-up CT at 24 hours before starting anticoagulants or antiplatelet agents.
- Antiplatelet: Aspirin 325 mg/d within 48 hours, or 24–48 hours after thrombolytic therapy

Second Line
Carotid endarterectomy (CEA) for carotid artery stenosis rarely is indicated emergently. CEA is indicated for stenosis >70% ipsilateral to TIA or incomplete stroke lesion, and may be indicated for 50–69% stenosis in carefully selected patients, depending on risk factors.

ISSUES FOR REFERRAL
Follow-up with neurologist 1 week after discharge, with subsequent follow-up based on individual circumstances.

ADDITIONAL THERAPIES
- Prophylactic antibiotics are *not* recommended (2)[A].
- Deep vein thrombosis (DVT) prophylaxis should be instituted for immobilized patients.
- Corticosteroids are *not* recommended for cerebral brain edema (2)[A].
- Statin use should be continued without interruption following acute stroke.
- At discharge, patient should be referred for physical therapy, occupational therapy, and speech therapy, as necessary.

SURGERY/OTHER PROCEDURES
- Ventricular drain may be placed for patients with acute hydrocephalus secondary to stroke (most commonly due to cerebellar stroke).
- Decompressive surgery is recommended for major cerebellar infarction; it should be considered for

malignant middle cerebral artery infarction, especially if the patient is <60 years of age.
- Consider mechanical embolus removal with a cerebral infarction device in carefully selected patients with evidence of potentially salvageable tissue on advanced imaging.

COMPLEMENTARY AND ALTERNATIVE MEDICINE
Acupuncture starting within 30 days from stroke onset may improve neurologic functioning.

IN-PATIENT CONSIDERATIONS
Admission Criteria/Initial Stabilization
- Observe closely within first 24 hours for neurologic decline, particularly due to brain swelling.
- Keep head of bed at least 30° when elevated ICP is suspected. Patients with ischemic stroke may benefit from a horizontal bed position during the acute phase.
- Monitor cardiac rhythm for at least first 24 hours to identify any arrhythmias.
- Airway support and ventilatory assistance may be necessary due to diminished consciousness or bulbar involvement; supplemental oxygen should be reserved for hypoxic patients. Consider elective intubation for patients with malignant edema.
- Correct hypovolemia with normal saline.
- All patients should be kept NPO until a formal swallow evaluation has been performed; to reduce risk of aspiration pneumonia, maintain elevated head of bed to 30°.
- Hypoglycemia can cause neurologic dysfunction; rapidly correct during initial evaluation.
- Hyperglycemia within first 24 hours after stroke is associated with poor functional outcomes and AHA/ASA guidelines: Insulin treatment for patients with glucose levels >140–185 mg/dL.
- In patients with ICH secondary to anticoagulant use, correction of an elevated INR is necessary with use of IV vitamin K and fresh frozen plasma or prothrombin concentrate complex. Factor VII infusion should be used in patients needing urgent surgical intervention (i.e. those with cerebellar hemorrhage who are neurologically deteriorating).
- DVT prophylaxis

IV Fluids
IV hydration with maintenance amounts of normal saline until swallowing status is assessed; monitor fluid balance closely.

Nursing
- Regular neurologic exams more frequent in first 24 hours (every 1–2 hours)
- Fall precautions; frequent repositioning to prevent skin breakdown

Discharge Criteria
Medically stable, adequate nutritional support, neurologic status stable or improving

 ## ONGOING CARE

FOLLOW-UP RECOMMENDATIONS
- Secondary prevention of stroke with aggressive management of risk factors
- Platelet inhibition using aspirin, clopidogrel, or aspirin plus extended-release dipyridamole (Aggrenox) based on physician and patient preference.

Patient Monitoring
Follow-up every 3 months for 1st year, then annually.

DIET
Patients with impaired swallowing should receive nasogastric or percutaneous endoscopic gastrostomy feedings to maintain nutrition and hydration.

PATIENT EDUCATION
National Stroke Association (800-STROKES or www.stroke.org)

PROGNOSIS
Variable, depending on subtype and severity of stroke; NIH stroke scale may be used for prognosis.

COMPLICATIONS
- Acute: Brain herniation, hemorrhagic transformation, MI, congestive heart failure, dysphagia, aspiration pneumonia, UTI, DVT, pulmonary embolism, malnutrition, pressure sores
- Chronic: Falls, depression, dementia, orthopedic complications, contractures

REFERENCES
1. Yew KS, Cheng E. Acute stroke diagnosis. *Am Fam Physician*. 2009;80:33–40.
2. Adams HP, del Zoppo G, Alberts MJ, et al. Guidelines for the early management of adults with ischemic stroke: A guideline from the American Heart Association/American Stroke Association Stroke Council, Clinical Cardiology Council, Cardiovascular Radiology and Intervention Council, and the Atherosclerotic Peripheral Vascular Disease and Quality of Care Outcomes in Research Interdisciplinary Working Groups: The American Academy of Neurology affirms the value of this guideline as an educational tool for neurologists. *Stroke*. 2007;38:1655–1711.
3. Chalela JA, Kidwell CS, Nentwich LM, et al. Magnetic resonance imaging and computed tomography in emergency assessment of patients with suspected acute stroke: A prospective comparison. *Lancet*. 2007;369:293–298.

 ## SEE ALSO
- Stroke Rehabilitation; Transient Ischemic Attack (TIA)
- Algorithm: Stroke

CODES
ICD10
- I61.9 Nontraumatic intracerebral hemorrhage, unspecified
- I63.9 Cerebral infarction, unspecified
- I63.50 Cereb infrc due to unsp occls or stenos of unsp cereb artery

CLINICAL PEARLS
- Unless stroke is hemorrhagic or patient is undergoing thrombolysis, BP should not be lowered acutely to maintain perfusion of penumbric region.
- DW-MRI is more sensitive than conventional CT for acute ischemic stroke (3). MRI is also better than CT for diagnosis of posterior fossa lesions.

SUBCONJUNCTIVAL HEMORRHAGE

Cara Marshall, MD

BASICS

DESCRIPTION
- Subconjunctival hemorrhage (SCH) is bleeding from small blood vessels underneath the conjunctiva, the thin clear skin covering the sclera of the eye.
- SCH is diagnosed clinically:
  - Flat, well-demarcated areas of extravasated blood can be seen just under the surface of the conjunctiva of the eye (red patch of blood sign).
  - SCH is more common temporally than nasally.
- Typically, SCH resolves spontaneously within 1–2 weeks.

EPIDEMIOLOGY
Common
- Male = Female, no gender predilection found

Incidence
Incidence increases:
- With increasing age
- In contact lens wearers (5% of cases) (1)
- With systemic diseases, such as diabetes, hypertension (HTN), and coagulation disorders
- During summer months, possibly due to trauma

ETIOLOGY AND PATHOPHYSIOLOGY
- Direct trauma to the blood vessels of the conjunctiva from blunt or penetrating trauma
- Direct trauma to the conjunctiva from improper contact lens placement or improper cleaning
- Increased BP in the vessels of the conjunctiva from hypertension or from the temporary increase in BP from a Valsalva type maneuver (e.g., vomiting)
- Damaged vessels from diabetes and atherosclerotic disease
- Increased bleeding tendencies from either thrombocytopenia or elevated PT/elevated INR (2)
- Trauma to the eye
- Valsalva maneuvers, such as coughing, vomiting, straining, and pushing of a laboring patient
- Hypertension
- Atherosclerotic disease and diabetes

- Bleeding factors, such as thrombocytopenia or elevated PT (from either disease or medication side effects)
- In patients age >60 years, HTN is the most common etiology.
- In patients <40 years, trauma/Valsalva and contact lens use are the most common etiologies.
- In patients >40 years, conjunctivochalasis (redundant conjunctival folds) and presence of pinguecula are strongly associated (1).

RISK FACTORS
- Age
- Contact lens wearer
- Systemic diseases
- Bleeding disorders (3)
- Recent cataract surgery

GENERAL PREVENTION
- Correct cleaning and maintenance of contact lenses
- Protective eyewear in sports and hobbies
- Control of high BP
- Optimizing control of systemic diseases, such as diabetes and atherosclerotic disease
- Control of prothrombin time (PT)/international normalized ratio (INR) in patients on Coumadin therapy (4)

DIAGNOSIS

HISTORY
- Generally asymptomatic; usually the patient noticed the redness in the mirror or another person mentions it to the patient.
- There should be little to no pain involved (4)[C].
- Obtain history of trauma.
- Obtain history of contact lens usage or cataract surgery (3)[C].
- Comprehensive past medical history to evaluate if at risk for systemic diseases or treatments

PHYSICAL EXAM
- Evaluate BP to assess control
- Measure visual acuity; this should be normal in a simple SCH (4)[C].
- Verify that the pupils are equal and reactive to light and accommodation; this should be normal with an SCH (4)[C].
- There should be no discharge or exudate noted (4)[C].
- Look at sclera for a bright red demarcated patch:
  - Demarcated area is most often on inferior aspect of eye due to gravity (1)[C].
- If penetrating trauma is a consideration, do a gentle digital assessment of the integrity of the globe (2)[C].

Geriatric Considerations
In older adults, the area of SCH will be more widespread across the sclera (1). Elastic and connective tissues are more fragile with age, and underlying conditions, such as HTN and diabetes, may contribute.

DIFFERENTIAL DIAGNOSIS
- Conjunctivitis (viral, bacterial, allergic, chemical)
- Foreign body to conjunctiva
- Penetrating trauma
- Acute angle glaucoma
- Iritis

DIAGNOSTIC TESTS & INTERPRETATION

If a foreign body is suspected, perform a fluorescein exam:

- Fluorescein exam of a patient with a SCH should show no uptake of staining (4)[C].
- Typically none; SCH is a clinical diagnosis.
- If an orbital fracture is suspected, may obtain plain facial bone films or CT scan (2)[C]

Follow-Up Tests & Special Considerations

If history and physical exam suggest a bleeding etiology (4)[C]:

- CBC
- PT/INR

ALERT

If a penetrating injury is suspected, may obtain a CT scan of the orbits, but not an MRI (if object may be metal) (2)[C]

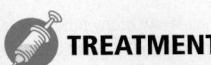

TREATMENT

GENERAL MEASURES

- Control BP
- Control blood glucose
- Control INR
- Wear protective eyewear

MEDICATION

No prescription medications are useful in treatment of SCH.

ISSUES FOR REFERRAL

- If a penetrating eye injury is suspected, send the patient to the emergency room for emergent ophthalmology consultation.
- If the patient complains of any decreased visual acuity or visual disturbances, refer to an ophthalmologist as soon as possible.
- If there is no resolution of SCH within 2 weeks, patient may need referral to an ophthalmologist.

ADDITIONAL THERAPIES

- Warm compresses
- Eye lubricants (4)[C]

ONGOING CARE

FOLLOW-UP RECOMMENDATIONS

- Follow-up only if the area does not resolve within 2 weeks.
- If SCH recurs, then workup patient for systemic sources, such as bleeding disorders (4)[C].

PATIENT EDUCATION

- Reassurance of the self-limited nature of the problem and typical time frame for resolution
- Education to return to clinic if the area does not heal or recurs.
- Correct cleaning and maintenance of contact lenses
- PubMed Health: www.ncbi.nlm.nih.gov/pubmedhealth/PMH0002583/

PROGNOSIS

Excellent

COMPLICATIONS

Rare

REFERENCES

1. Mimura T, Yamagami S, Mori M, et al. Contact lens-induced subconjunctival hemorrhage. *Am J Ophthalmol*. 2010;150(5):656–665.e1. Epub 2010 Aug 14.
2. Wirbelauer C. Management of the red eye for the primary care physician. *Am J Med*. 2006;119: 302–306.
3. Mimura T, Usui T, Yamagami S, et al. Recent causes of subconjunctival hemorrhage. *Ophthalmologica*. 2010;224:133–137.
4. Cronau H, Kankanala RR, Mauger T, et al. Diagnosis and management of red eye in primary care. *Am Fam Physician*. 2010;81:137–144.

ADDITIONAL READING

- Mimura T, Usui T, Yamagami S, et al. Subconjunctival hemorrhage and conjunctivochalasis. *Ophthalmology*. 2009;116(10):1880–1886.
- Mimura T, Yamagami S, Usui T, et al. Location and extent of subconjunctival hemorrhage. *Ophthalmologica*. 2010;224(2):90–95.

CODES

ICD10

- H11.30 Conjunctival hemorrhage, unspecified eye
- H11.31 Conjunctival hemorrhage, right eye
- H11.32 Conjunctival hemorrhage, left eye

CLINICAL PEARLS

- SCH is a clinical diagnosis. The condition is typically asymptomatic and will resolve spontaneously in 1–2 weeks.
- Always check BP in a patient with SCH, as HTN is a risk factor.
- Indications for immediate referral to an ophthalmologist are eye pain, change in vision, lack of pupil reactivity, and/or penetrating eye trauma.
- Reassurance and comfort measures are key.
- Contact lens wearers should not wear contacts until the SCH resolves completely.

S

SUBSTANCE USE DISORDERS

S. Lindsey Clarke, MD, FAAFP

 BASICS

DESCRIPTION

A substance use disorder manifests as any pattern of substance use causing significant physical, mental, or social dysfunction:

- Substances of abuse include:
  - Alcohol
  - Tobacco
  - Cannabinoids (marijuana)
  - Synthetic marijuana (Spice, K2)
  - Prescription medications:
    ○ CNS depressants (barbiturates, benzodiazepines, hypnotics)
    ○ Opioids and morphine derivatives (codeine, fentanyl, hydrocodone, hydromorphone, meperidine, methadone, morphine, oxycodone)
    ○ Stimulants (amphetamines, methylphenidate)
    ○ Dextromethorphan
  - Stimulants (cocaine, amphetamines, methamphetamines)
  - Club drugs (MDMA, flunitrazepam, γ-hydroxybutyrate or GHB)
  - Opioids (heroin, opium)
  - Dissociative drugs (ketamine, phencyclidine)
  - Hallucinogens (lysergic acid diethylamide, salvia)
  - Bath salts (synthetic cathinones)
  - Inhalants (glue, paint thinners, nitrous oxide)
  - Anabolic steroids
- For current info see www.drugabuse.gov
- System(s) affected: Cardiovascular; Endocrine/Metabolic; CNS
- Synonym(s): Drug abuse; Drug dependence; Substance abuse

Geriatric Considerations
- Alcohol is the most commonly abused substance, and abuse often goes unrecognized.
- Higher potential for drug interactions

Pregnancy Considerations
Substance abuse may cause fetal abnormalities, morbidity, and fetal or maternal death.

EPIDEMIOLOGY

Incidence
- Predominant age: 16–25 years
- Predominant sex: Male > Female

Prevalence
- 22.5 million (8.7%) Americans reported use of illicit substance in past month in 2011.
- 10.1% for age 12–17 years; 21.4% for age 18–25
- 1:6 males aged 18–25 years use marijuana.

ETIOLOGY AND PATHOPHYSIOLOGY
Multifactorial, including genetic, environmental

Genetics
Substances of abuse affect dopamine, acetylcholine, γ-aminobutyric acid, norepinephrine, opioid, and serotonin receptors. Variant alleles may account for susceptibility to disorders.

RISK FACTORS
- Male gender, young adult
- Depression, anxiety
- Other substance use disorders
- Family history
- Peer or family use or approval
- Low socioeconomic status
- Unemployment
- Accessibility of substances of abuse
- Family dysfunction or trauma
- Antisocial personality disorder
- Academic problems, school dropout
- Criminal involvement

GENERAL PREVENTION
Early identification and aggressive early intervention improve outcomes.

COMMONLY ASSOCIATED CONDITIONS
- Depression
- Personality disorders
- Bipolar affective disorder

ALERT
Prescription narcotic overdose is the leading cause of accidental death between the ages of 25 and 45 in the US; this correlates with increased prescribing of long-acting oxycodone (see www.cdc.gov/Injury/wisqars/pdf/10LCID_All_Deaths_By_Age_Group_2010-a.pdf).

 DIAGNOSIS

- Substance use disorder (DSM-5 criteria): ≥2 of the following in past year, with severity based on number of criteria present:
  - Missed work or school
  - Use in hazardous situations
  - Continued use despite social or personal problems
  - Craving
  - Tolerance (decreased response to effects of drug due to constant exposure)
  - Withdrawal upon discontinuation
  - Using more than intended
  - Failed attempts to quit
  - Increased time spent obtaining, using, or recovering from the substance
  - Interference with important activities
  - Continued use despite health problems

HISTORY
- History of infections (e.g., endocarditis, hepatitis B or C, TB, STI, or recurrent pneumonia)
- Social or behavioral problems, including chaotic relationships and/or employment
- Frequent visits to emergency department
- Criminal incarceration
- History of blackouts, insomnia, mood swings, chronic pain, repetitive trauma
- Anxiety, fatigue, depression, psychosis

PHYSICAL EXAM
- Abnormally dilated or constricted pupils
- Needle marks on skin
- Nasal septum perforation (with cocaine use)
- Cardiac dysrhythmias, pathologic murmurs
- Malnutrition with severe dependence

DIFFERENTIAL DIAGNOSIS
- Depression, anxiety, or other mental states
- Metabolic delirium (hypoxia, hypoglycemia, infection, thiamine deficiency, hypothyroidism, thyrotoxicosis)
- ADHD
- Medication toxicity

DIAGNOSTIC TESTS & INTERPRETATION

ALERT
Screening: A single question: "How many times in the past year have you used an illegal drug or used a prescription medication for nonmedical reasons?": In primary care setting, resulted in sensitivity of 100% and specificity of ~75% (1)[B].

- CRAFFT questionnaire is superior to CAGE for identifying alcohol use disorders in adolescents and young adults; sensitivity is 94% with ≥2 "yes" answers:
  - C: Have you ever ridden in a *car* driven by someone (including yourself) who was "high" or who had been using alcohol or drugs?
  - R: Do you ever use alcohol or drugs to *relax*, feel better about yourself, or fit in?
  - A: Do you ever use alcohol or drugs while you are *alone*?
  - F: Do you ever *forget* things you did while using alcohol or drugs?
  - F: Do your family or *friends* ever tell you that you should cut down on your drinking or drug use?
  - T: Have you gotten into *trouble* while you were using alcohol or drugs?
- Blood alcohol concentration
- Urine drug screen (order qualitative UDS and, if specific drug is in question, a quantitative analysis for specific drug; order confirmatory serum tests if you suspect false-positive)
- Approximate detection limits:
  - Alcohol: 6–10 hours
  - Amphetamines and variants: 2–3 days
  - Barbiturates: 2–10 days
  - Benzodiazepines: 1–6 weeks
  - Cocaine: 2–3 days
  - Heroin: 1–1.5 days
  - LSD, psilocybin: 8 hours
  - Marijuana: 1 day–4 weeks
  - Methadone: 1 day–1 week
  - Opioids: 1–3 days
  - PCP: 7–14 days
  - Anabolic steroids: Oral, 3 weeks; injectable, 3 months; nandrolone, 9 months
- Liver transaminases
- HIV, hepatitis B and C screens
- Echocardiogram for endocarditis
- Head CT scan for seizure, delirium, trauma

TREATMENT

Determine substances abused early (may influence disposition).

GENERAL MEASURES
- Nonjudgmental, medically oriented attitude
- Motivational interviewing and brief interventions can overcome denial and promote change.
- Behavioral and cognitive therapy
- Community reinforcement
- Interventional counseling
- Self-help groups to aid recovery (Alcoholics Anonymous, other 12-step programs)
- Support groups for family (Al-Anon and Alateen)

MEDICATION
- Alcohol withdrawal: See "Alcohol Abuse and Dependence" and "Alcohol Withdrawal."
- Benzodiazepine or barbiturate withdrawal:
  – Gradual taper preferable to abrupt discontinuation
  – Substitution of longer-acting benzodiazepine or phenobarbital
- Nicotine withdrawal: See "Tobacco Use and Smoking Cessation."
- Opioid withdrawal:
  – Buprenorphine: 2–16 mg/d sublingually; use restricted to licensed clinics and certified physicians (2)[A]
  – Methadone: 20–35 mg/d PO; use restricted to inpatient settings and specially licensed clinics (3)[A]
  – Clonidine: 0.1–0.2 mg PO t.i.d. for autonomic hyperactivity (4)[A]
- Stimulant withdrawal:
  – No agent with clear benefit for cocaine
  – Adenovirus-based cocaine vaccine in development
  – Naltrexone: 50 mg PO twice weekly reduces amphetamine use in dependent patients (5)[B].
  – Methylphenidate ER: 54 mg/d PO might enhance abstinence in amphetamine-dependent patients.
- Adjuncts to therapy:
  – Use all medications in conjunction with psychosocial behavioral interventions.
  – Antiemetics, nonaddictive analgesics for opioid withdrawal
  – Nonhabituating antidepressants, mood stabilizers, anxiolytics, and hypnotics for comorbid mood and anxiety disorders and insomnia that persist after detoxification
- Contraindications:
  – Buprenorphine in lactation
  – Naltrexone in pregnancy, liver disease
- Precautions: Clonidine can cause hypotension.
- Significant possible interactions:
  – Buprenorphine and ketoconazole, erythromycin, or HIV protease inhibitors
  – Naltrexone and opioid medications (may precipitate or exacerbate withdrawal)

ISSUES FOR REFERRAL
- Consider addiction specialist, especially for opioid and polysubstance abuse.
- Maintenance therapy for opioid dependence (e.g., methadone) only in licensed clinics
- Psychiatrist for comorbid psychiatric disorders
- Social services

IN-PATIENT CONSIDERATIONS
Admission Criteria/Initial Stabilization
- Indications for inpatient detoxification:
  – History of withdrawal symptoms (e.g., seizures)
  – Disorientation
  – Threat of harm to self or others
  – Obstacles to close monitoring (follow-up)
  – Comorbid medical illness
  – Pregnancy
- For narcotic addiction and withdrawal
- Look for signs of severe infection (e.g., bacterial endocarditis).

IV Fluids
Maintenance until patient is taking fluids well by mouth

Nursing
- Take frequent vital signs during withdrawal.
- Monitor for signs of drug use in the hospital.

Discharge Criteria
Detoxification complete

ONGOING CARE

FOLLOW-UP RECOMMENDATIONS
Restricted if dangerous, psychotic, or disoriented

Patient Monitoring
Verify patient's compliance with the substance abuse treatment program.

DIET
Patients often are malnourished.

PATIENT EDUCATION
- Substance Abuse and Mental Health Services Administration: http://samhsa.gov or 800-662-HELP for information, treatment facility locator
- Alcoholics Anonymous: www.aa.org
- Narcotics Anonymous: www.na.org

PROGNOSIS
- Patients in treatment for longer periods (≥1 year) have higher success rates.
- Behavioral therapy and pharmacotherapy are most successful when used in combination.

COMPLICATIONS
- Serious harm to self and others: Accidents, violence
- Overdoses resulting in seizures, arrhythmias, cardiac and respiratory arrest, coma, death
- Hepatitis, HIV, tuberculosis, syphilis
- Subacute bacterial endocarditis
- Malnutrition
- Social problems, including arrest
- Poor marital adjustment and violence
- Depression, schizophrenia
- Sexual assault (alcohol, flunitrazepam, GHB)

REFERENCES

1. Smith PC, Schmidt SM, Allensworth-Davies D, et al. A single-question screening test for drug use in primary care. *Arch Intern Med.* 2010;170: 1155–1160.
2. Gowing L, Ali R, White JM, et al. Buprenorphine for the management of opioid withdrawal. *Cochrane Database Syst Rev.* 2009;CD002025.
3. Mattick RP, Breen C, Kimber J, et al. Methadone maintenance therapy versus no opioid replacement therapy for opioid dependence. *Cochrane Database Syst Rev.* 2009;CD002209.
4. Gowing L, Farrell M, Ali R, et al. Alpha2-adrenergic agonists for the management of opioid withdrawal. *Cochrane Database Syst Rev.* 2009;CD002024.
5. Jayaram-Lindström N, Hammarberg A, Beck O, et al. Naltrexone for the treatment of amphetamine dependence: A randomized, placebo-controlled trial. *Am J Psychiatry.* 2008;84(11):1442–1448.

ADDITIONAL READING
- Griswold KS, Aronoff H, Kernan JB, et al. Adolescent substance use and abuse: Recognition and management. *Am Fam Physician.* 2008;77: 331–336.
- Standridge JB, Adams SM, Zotos AP, et al. Urine drug screening: A valuable office procedure. *Am Fam Physician.* 2010;81:635–640.
- Substance Abuse and Mental Health Services Administration, *Results from the 2011 National Survey on Drug Use and Health: Summary of National Findings*, NSDUH Series H-44, HHS Publication No. (SMA) 12-4713. Rockville, MD: Substance Abuse and Mental Health Services Administration, 2012. Available at http://www.samhsa.gov/data/NSDUH.aspx.

SEE ALSO

Alcohol Abuse and Dependence; Alcohol Withdrawal; Tobacco Use and Smoking Cessation

CODES

ICD10
- F10.10 Alcohol abuse, uncomplicated
- F12.10 Cannabis abuse, uncomplicated
- F19.10 Other psychoactive substance abuse, uncomplicated

CLINICAL PEARLS
- Substance use disorders are prevalent, serious, and often unrecognized in clinical practice. Comorbid psychiatric disorders are common.
- Substance abuse is distinguished by family, social, occupational, legal, or physical dysfunction that is caused by persistent use of the substance.
- Dependence is characterized by tolerance, withdrawal, compulsive use, and repeated overindulgence.
- Motivational interviewing, brief interventions, and a nonjudgmental attitude can help to promote a willingness to change behavior.

SUDDEN INFANT DEATH SYNDROME (SIDS)

Fern R. Hauck, MD, MS

BASICS

- Leading cause of death in infants 1–12 months of age
- 3rd leading cause of infant mortality overall
- SIDS deaths have been reduced by >50% in the US and other countries that have introduced risk-reduction campaigns, heavily focused on back sleeping for infants (1).
- The condition still remains mysterious, and the exact cause is unknown.

DESCRIPTION

- The sudden death of an infant <1 year of age that remains unexplained after a thorough case investigation, including performance of a complete autopsy, examination of the death scene, and review of the clinical history
- Sudden infant death syndrome (SIDS) was 1st formally defined in 1969. The definition was revised in 1989.
- System(s) affected: Cardiovascular; Endocrine/Metabolic; Nervous; Pulmonary
- Synonym(s): Crib death; Cot death

EPIDEMIOLOGY

- SIDS can affect any infant, but some infants are at higher risk than others, including African Americans and American Indians/Native Americans, males, infants whose mothers smoked/used illegal drugs during pregnancy, and several others described below.
- There is a characteristic age pattern, with deaths peaking at 2–4 months, and more deaths occurring during the colder seasons.

Incidence

- For 2009: All races: 0.54/1,000 live births (2,231 cases/yr):
  - White non-Hispanic: 0.55/1,000 live births (1,213 cases/yr)
  - African American non-Hispanic: 1.01/1,000 live births (614 cases/yr)
  - Hispanic: 0.29/1,000 live births (285 cases/yr)
  - Native American: 1.19/1,000 live births (58 cases/yr)
  - Asian/Pacific Islander: 0.20/1,000 live births (51 cases/yr)
- Predominant age: Uncommon in 1st month of life; peak occurs between 2 and 4 months of age; 90% of deaths occur by 6 months of age.
- Predominant sex: Male > Female (52–60% male)

Pediatric Considerations

Occurs only in infants

ETIOLOGY AND PATHOPHYSIOLOGY

Strong evidence for a respiratory pathway that includes the following stages:

- A life-threatening event causes severe asphyxia and/or brain hypoperfusion. This can include rebreathing exhaled carbon dioxide in a face-down position.
- The vulnerable infant does not wake up or turn his or her head in response to asphyxia, resulting in further rebreathing and inability to recover from apnea.
- Progressive apnea leads to hypoxic coma.

- Bradycardia and hypoxic apnea occur.
- Autoresuscitation fails, resulting in prolonged apnea and death (2).
- There are many theories. There may be subtle developmental abnormalities resulting from pre- and/or perinatal brain injury, which make the infant vulnerable to SIDS.
- Possible causes:
  - Abnormalities in respiratory control and arousal responsiveness
  - Central and peripheral nervous system abnormalities
  - Cardiac arrhythmias
  - Rebreathing in face-down position on soft surface, leading to hypoxia and hypercarbia
  - SIDS may occur when ≥1 environmental risk factors interact with ≥1 genetic risk factors.

Genetics

Emerging evidence for genetic risk factors, especially related to impaired brainstem regulation of breathing or other autonomic control, impaired immune responses, and cardiac ion channelopathies associated with long QT syndrome and fatal arrhythmia

RISK FACTORS

- Although some infants may die from SIDS who have no apparent risk factors, most have ≥1 of the following risk factors associated with SIDS:
  - Race: African Americans and Native Americans have highest incidence.
  - Season: Late fall and winter months
  - Time of day: Between midnight and 6 A.M.
  - Activity: During sleep
  - Low birth weight; intrauterine growth retardation (IUGR)
  - Poverty
- Maternal factors:
  - Younger age
  - Decreased education
  - Maternal use of cigarettes/drugs (e.g., cocaine, opiates) during pregnancy
  - Higher parity
  - Inadequate prenatal care
- Respiratory/GI infection in recent past
- Sleep practices:
  - Prone and side sleep positions
  - Overheating from heavy clothing and bedding and/or elevated room temperature
  - Soft bedding
  - Bed sharing
  - No room sharing
- Passive cigarette smoke exposure after birth
- No pacifier use
- No breastfeeding

GENERAL PREVENTION

Because a SIDS death is sudden and the cause is unknown, SIDS cannot be "treated." However, some measures may be effective in reducing the risk of SIDS (3)[B]:

- Maternal avoidance of cigarette smoking and illicit drug use during pregnancy
- Avoidance of passive cigarette smoke exposure
- Avoidance of the prone (face-down) and side sleep positions, excessive bed clothing, and soft bedding such as pillows, comforters, and bumper pads or a soft mattress

- Avoidance of overheating
- A crib, bassinet, or cradle conforming to federal safety standards is the recommended sleeping location.
- Avoidance of bed sharing with the infant, particularly by adults other than the parent(s) or by other children. Bed sharing should be avoided if the mother/father has used cigarettes, drugs, or alcohol. Bed sharing on couches is very dangerous and should never be done.
- Infants who sleep in the same room as their parents (without bed sharing) have a lower risk of SIDS. It is recommended that infants sleep in a crib/bassinet in their parents' bedroom, which when placed close to their bed will allow for more convenient breastfeeding and contact.
- Breastfeeding is associated with a decreased risk of SIDS and is recommended for all infants (4)[B].
- Pacifier use is associated with a reduced risk of SIDS:
  - Consider offering a pacifier at bedtime and nap time.
  - Delay the introduction of the pacifier among breast-fed infants until 1 month of age (5)[B].
  - Pacifier use has not been found to be detrimental to breastfeeding if it is introduced after the baby is 1 month of age, when breastfeeding is well established (6)[A].
- Avoid commercial devices marketed to reduce the risk of SIDS.
- It is critical that all people caring for infants, including daycare providers, be instructed in these risk-reduction measures.
- Newborn nurseries should implement these recommendations well before discharge so parents see appropriate practices modeled.

COMMONLY ASSOCIATED CONDITIONS

Infants are generally well, or may have had a mild febrile illness (i.e., gastroenteritis or an upper respiratory infection) prior to death.

DIAGNOSIS

The diagnosis of SIDS is made by trained medical examiners/coroners when the death is believed to be from natural causes and after thorough reviews of the medical history, death scene investigation, and postmortem examination do not produce an explanation of the death.

HISTORY

Infant usually found unresponsive by parent/other caregiver without any warning

PHYSICAL EXAM

- These babies generally appear healthy or may have had a minor upper respiratory/GI infection in the last 2 weeks before death.
- Complete postmortem exam to look for signs of possible trauma/child abuse or other cause of death

DIFFERENTIAL DIAGNOSIS
- Suffocation/Accidental asphyxia
- Abnormalities of fatty acid metabolism (e.g., deficiency of medium-chain acyl-coenzyme A dehydrogenase or of carnitine)
- Dehydration/Electrolyte disturbance
- Homicide

DIAGNOSTIC TESTS & INTERPRETATION
Standardized postmortem protocols have been proposed. Although testing varies across sites, common diagnostic tests include electrolytes, toxicology, and microbiology.
- Postmortem laboratory tests are performed to rule out other causes of death (e.g., electrolytes to rule out dehydration and electrolyte imbalance). No consistently abnormal laboratory tests are found.
- Pneumocardiograms have been abandoned in the workup.
- X-rays to rule out possible child abuse

Diagnostic Procedures/Other
Because the diagnosis of SIDS is often one of "exclusion," it is crucial to do a thorough death scene investigation and case review in addition to the autopsy and laboratory tests.

Test Interpretation
Characteristic findings on postmortem examination:
- Frothy discharge, sometimes blood tinged, from nostrils and mouth
- Petechiae on surface of lungs, heart, and thymus gland in 50–85% (but not unique to SIDS)
- Pulmonary congestion and edema often present
- Morphologic markers of hypoxia: Increased gliosis in brain stem, retention of periadrenal brown fat, and hematopoiesis in the liver:
  - Present to varying degrees; not confirmed by all studies

 ## ONGOING CARE

General recommendations for positioning infants:
- Infants frequently should be placed on their bellies when awake and observed by responsible adults to prevent head flattening (plagiocephaly) that can result from infants sleeping supine.
- Avoid placing infants for extended periods in car seat carriers or "bouncers."
- Upright "cuddle time" should be encouraged.
- Alter the side to which the infant places his or her head during sleep.
- Swaddling infants may aid in sleeping more comfortably in the supine position. Infants should never be swaddled if sleeping in the prone position.

FOLLOW-UP RECOMMENDATIONS
- Safe sleep and SIDS risk-reduction messages should be delivered at all well-child checks and by all health professionals in a consistent manner.
- Parents often change from the recommended practices as the baby gets older, often during the peak SIDS incidence period. Thus, it is important to ask about infant care practices at each well-child check.

Patient Monitoring
Although some authorities recommend cardiopulmonary monitoring in siblings of prior SIDS victims, no evidence indicates that the use of monitors prevents SIDS, and they should not be prescribed for that purpose (7)[B].

PATIENT EDUCATION
- Family counseling (see "Prognosis")
- Back to Sleep Information Line (800) 505-CRIB (2742) (sponsored by the Eunice Kennedy Shriver National Institute of Child Health and Human Development, the Maternal and Child Health Bureau, and other organizations to provide information to parents and health providers about their recommendation to place infants on their backs, and general information about SIDS)
- National SUID/SIDS Resource Center, Washington, DC (866) 866-SIDS (7437)
- Association of SIDS and Infant Mortality Programs, East Lansing, MI (800) 930-SIDS (7437)
- First Candle, Bel Air, MD (800) 221-SIDS (7437)
- CJ Foundation for SIDS, Hackensack, NJ (888) 8CJ-SIDS (825-7437)
- Cribs for Kids, Pittsburgh, PA (888) 721-CRIB (2742)

PROGNOSIS
- SIDS deaths have a powerful impact on families and their functioning. Physicians play an important role in providing immediate information about SIDS and sensitive counseling to limit parents' misinformation and feelings of guilt.
- Counseling needs of families vary from the short term to long term:
  - Support groups are helpful to many couples.
  - Physicians need to be familiar with resources available in their communities to help families mourning a SIDS death.
- Follow-up counseling, including review of the autopsy report with the family after some time has passed, is important to help with understanding this condition and to alleviate the tremendous guilt these families experience.
- Parents need to be counseled about subsequent pregnancies:
  - Genetic testing and counseling may be indicated to rule out a metabolic/other genetically acquired disorder.
  - Parents need to be advised of the most current recommendations regarding sleep position and other infant care practices during subsequent pregnancies.

REFERENCES
1. Mitchell EA. SIDS: Past, present and future. *Acta Paediatr*. 2009;98:1712–1719.
2. Kinney HC, Thach BT. The sudden infant death syndrome. *N Engl J Med*. 2009;361:795–805.
3. Task Force on Sudden Infant Death Syndrome, Moon RY. SIDS and other sleep-related infant deaths: Expansion of recommendations for a safe infant sleeping environment. *Pediatrics*. 2011;84(5):1030–1039. Epub 2011 Oct 17.
4. Hauck FR, Thompson JMD, Tanabe KO, et al. Breastfeeding and reduced risk of sudden infant death syndrome: A meta-analysis. *Pediatrics* 2011;128:103–110.
5. Hauck FR, Omojokun OO, Siadaty MS. Do pacifiers reduce the risk of sudden infant death syndrome? A meta-analysis. *Pediatrics*. 2005;84(5): e716–e723. Epub 2005 Oct 10.
6. O'Connor NR, Tanabe KO, Siadaty MS. Pacifiers and breastfeeding: A systematic review. *Arch Pediatr Adolesc Med*. 2009;163:378–382.
7. Committee on Fetus and Newborn. American Academy of Pediatrics. Apnea, sudden infant death syndrome, and home monitoring. *Pediatrics*. 2003; 111:914–917.

 ## CODES

ICD10
R99 Ill-defined and unknown cause of mortality

CLINICAL PEARLS
- Although the exact cause of SIDS is unknown, several risk-reduction measures will significantly reduce an infant's chance of dying from SIDS.
- SIDS incidence has decreased by >50% just by placing infants in a supine position to sleep.
- Breastfeeding is recommended for all infants.
- Safe sleeping arrangements and pacifier use are other ways to reduce the risk of SIDS.

SUICIDE

Irene C. Coletsos, MD • Harold J. Bursztajn, MD

 BASICS

DESCRIPTION
Suicide and attempted suicide are significant causes of morbidity and mortality.

EPIDEMIOLOGY
- Predominant sex:
  - Women *attempt* suicide 1.5× more often than men. Men *complete* suicide 4× more often than women. Men are more likely to choose a means with high lethality.
- Predominant age: Adolescent (3rd leading cause of death in that age group) and geriatric population
- Predominant race: 84% of people who complete suicides are white, non-Hispanic. Native Americans have the next highest rate in the US. Whites have twice the risk of suicide compared with African Americans.
- Marital status: Single > Divorced; widowed > married
- Worldwide, in of all countries, youths (ages 10–24) are the highest risk group.

Incidence
- In 2010, 10th leading cause of death in adults in the US. Military service (not specifically active duty) is associated with increased risk. In 2009, 2010, and 2012, more soldiers died of suicide than in active duty in those years, according to congressional study and National Center for Veterans studies.
- Worldwide, the 3rd leading cause of death.

RISK FACTORS
- "Human understanding is the most effective weapon against suicide. The greatest need is to deepen the awareness and sensitivity of people to their fellow man" (Schneidman, American Association of Suicidology).
- Be alert to a combination of "perturbation" (increased emotional disturbance) and "lethality" (having the potential tools to cause death).
- 80% who complete suicides had a previous attempt.
- 90% who complete suicide meet *Diagnostic and Statistical Manual* criteria for Axis I or II disorders: Major depression; bipolar disorder; schizophrenia; anorexia nervosa; panic disorder; borderline and antisocial personality disorders.
- Substance use (alcohol; "bath salts" and other hallucinogens; opioids)
- Family history of suicide
- Physical illness
- Despair: Feeling unendurable emotional pain *and* has "given up" on self, feels without hope and, consciously or unconsciously, unworthy of help
- Among teenagers: Not feeling "connected" to their peers or family; being bullied; poor grades
- Psychosocial: Recent loss: What may seem to be a small loss (to a medical provider) may be a devastating loss to the patient. *Patient-specific* factors need to be taken into account; social isolation; anniversaries and holidays. Patients who attempt suicide also seem to have impaired decision-making skills and risk awareness, and increased impulsivity, compared with patients who have never attempted suicide (1,2).
- If a patient is incompetent (e.g., too delusional) to inform providers about the potential for suicide, that puts the patient at increased risk; consider hospitalization (3).
- Access to lethal means: Firearms, poisons (including prescription and nonprescription drugs)

GENERAL PREVENTION
- Know how to access resources 24/7 within and outside of the health care institution.
- Screen for risk factors, and consider the overall clinical picture. Screening instruments include the Patient Health Questionnaire-9, the Columbia Suicide Severity Rating Scale, Beck's Scale for Suicidal Ideation, Linehan's Reasons for Living Inventory, and Risk Estimator for Suicide.
- Treat underlying mental illness and substance abuse. Screen for possession of means of harm, including prescription and nonprescription drugs and firearms (encourage these patients to remove guns from their homes and to relinquish gun licenses).
- Women being treated for cancer, chronic obstructive pulmonary disease (COPD), heart disease, osteoporosis, or stroke were found to be at higher risk for suicide (even without a history of depression).
- Create a safety plan for patients at risk for suicide and their families, including education about how to access emergency care 24 hours a day.
- Public education about how to help others access emergency psychiatric care. Suicidal people may 1st confide in those they trust outside health care (e.g., family members, religious leaders, community elders, "healers," hairdressers, and bartenders).
- For the military: Multiple resources available from: www.realwarriors.net. Suggested treatments include cognitive restructuring techniques (that their experience with adversity can be a sources of strength) and help with basic problem-solving skills (so the service member does not feel like a "burden") (4).
- For teens, young adults, and their educators: Multiple programming suggestions and advice for students/families and educators available at: www.cdc.gov/healthyyouth/adolescenthealth; stopbullying.gov
- In developing world countries, pesticide ingestion is a common method of suicide. Limiting free access has led to reduced suicide rates.

 DIAGNOSIS

HISTORY
- Depressed patients should be asked about ideation and about a plan:
  - "Have you ever felt that life isn't worth living? Do you ever wish you could go to sleep and not wake up? Are you having thoughts about killing yourself?"
- Use psychodynamic formulation, which combines mental-state exam (i.e., behavior, mood, mental content, judgment), past history (i.e., what resources has the patient used in the past for support, and are they currently available?), and history of current illness. If the patient is experiencing a loss, is under stress, and does not have access to a previously sustaining resource (e.g., a significant other, a pet, sports ability, a job), that patient is under increased risk for suicide.
- Prior attempts: What precipitated the event, lethality, intent to die, precautions taken to avoid being rescued, reaction to survival (a patient who is upset that the suicide was not completed is at increased risk).
- History of psychiatric symptoms, substance abuse. Also note strengths, such as reasons to live, hopes for future, social supports. A patient without these is at increased risk.
- Collateral history is important (from friends, family, physicians). It may be appropriate to break confidentiality if patient is at imminent risk of suicide.

PHYSICAL EXAM
- Medical conditions: Delirium, intoxication, withdrawal, medication side effects,
- Psychosis: Observe for signs of/ask about command auditory hallucinations to kill oneself, delusional guilt, and persecutory delusions.
- In adults: Observe for signs of hopelessness/despair (see "Risk Factors").
- In teens: Screen for risk factors: Substance abuse, bullying, poor grades, social isolation, because teens may not appear depressed.

DIFFERENTIAL DIAGNOSIS
Differentiate between patients and pseudopatients (i.e., those who are using suicide threats and gestures to manipulate others).

DIAGNOSTIC TESTS & INTERPRETATION
Diagnostic Procedures/Other
Brief tests can help evaluate mood/suicidality as a part of any health assessment, such as the Patient Health Questionnaire-9 (PHQ-9), accessed at www.depression-primarycare.org/clinicians/toolkits/materials/forms/phq9 and www.teenscreen.org; Columbia Suicide Severity Rating Scale, clinical instructions accessed at www.cssrs.columbia.edu/c-ssrs_Triage_guidelines.pdf

TREATMENT

GENERAL MEASURES

- Patients expressing active suicidal thoughts or who made an attempt require an exam for suicide risk factors, mental status exam, and competency test (to determine if they are able/or willing to inform treatment team about ongoing/changing suicidal intentions), as well as a formal psychiatric consultation. Careful primary care screening can be as effective at identifying risk as a psychological assessment (5)[B].
- Cognitive therapy decreased reattempt rate in prior suicide attempters by half (6)[B].
- Psychotherapy with suicidal patients is a challenge even for the most experienced clinicians. The countertransference, a clinician's feelings toward a patient, can evolve into wanting to be rid of the patient. If the patient detects this, the risk of suicide is heightened. The clinician can avoid this by recognizing countertransference and bearing it within so that the patient remains unaware (7)[C].
- Among military personnel: ACE campaign: Ask about suicidal thoughts; care for the person, including removing access to lethal weapons; "escort" the soldier to help: An emergency room, to calling 911 or a support hotline such as (800) 273-TALK (8255)

MEDICATION

- Patients are at increased risk of suicide at the outset of antidepressant treatment and when it is discontinued. Consider tapering/switching medical therapies rather than sudden discontinuation. Monitor carefully at these times.
- Anxiety, agitation, and delusions increasing in intensity are risk factors for suicide and should be treated aggressively.
- In patients with mood disorders, a meta-analysis of randomized, controlled trials found that lithium reduced the risk of death by suicide by 60% (8)[A].
- Agitated or combative patients may require sedation with IV or IM benzodiazepines and/or antipsychotics. Clinical response is typically seen within 20–30 minutes if given IM/IV.

Pediatric Considerations
FDA posted black box warning for antidepressant use in the pediatric population after increased suicidality was noted. If risk of untreated depression is sufficient to warrant treatment with antidepressants, children must be monitored closely for suicidality.

First Line
ECGs before prescribing or continuing antidepressants or antipsychotics to look for QT prolongation

ISSUES FOR REFERRAL
Consider a psychiatric consult. All decisions regarding treatment must be carefully documented and communicated to all involved health care providers

IN-PATIENT CONSIDERATIONS
Admission Criteria/Initial Stabilization
- Inpatient hospitalization if patient is suicidal with a plan to act or is otherwise at high risk; if immediate risk for self-harm, may be hospitalized involuntarily
- Immediately after a suicide attempt, treat the medical problems resulting from the self-harm before attempting to initiate psychiatric care.
- Order lab work (e.g., solvent screen, blood and urine toxicology screen, aspirin and acetaminophen levels). Patients may not disclose ingestions if they wish to succeed in their attempt or if they are undergoing mental status changes.
- Risk for self-harm continues even in hospital setting. Ensure patient safety by least restrictive method (i.e., remove potentially dangerous objects, provide 1-to-1 constant observation, medication). Use mechanical restraints if deemed necessary for patient safety. Trained staff should search patient for dangerous objects as soon as the patient enters the hospital.
- The period after transfer from involuntary to voluntary hospitalization is also a time of high risk.

Discharge Criteria
- No longer considered a danger to self/others
- Clinicians should be aware that a patient may *claim* that he or she is no longer suicidal in order to facilitate discharge—and complete the act. Look for clinical and behavioral signs that the patient truly is no longer in despair and is hopeful, such as improved appetite, sleep, engagement with staff, and group therapy. Clinicians should check with family and ancillary staff to assess patients' conditions because they may share more information with those contacts than with doctors.
- Provide information about 24/7 resources that are available and that patients and those who support them would be willing to access.

 ONGOING CARE

FOLLOW-UP RECOMMENDATIONS
Patient Monitoring
- Increase monitoring at the beginning of treatment, when changing medication regimens, and on discharge. These are times of increased risk.
- Educate family members and other close contacts/confidants to the warning signs of suicidality. For adults: Despair/Hopelessness, isolation, discussing suicide, stating that the world would be a "better place" without them, losses in areas key to the patient's self-worth. For youths: May exhibit the same signs and symptoms, but one should be aware of these additional risks: History of abuse (e.g., sexual, physical), bullying in person or via electronic media (e.g., text messages or social web sites), family stress, changes in eating and sleeping patterns, suicidality of friends, and giving away treasured items.
- Make sure that the patient is willing to accept the type of follow-up offered. Do not assume that just setting it up is sufficient protection.
- Curtail access to firearms.
- Limiting the number of pills may also be appropriate for an impulsive patient. However, clinicians may believe that by simply limiting the number of pills they prescribe, they are preventing further suicide attempts, an example of "magical thinking." Clinicians who find themselves thinking this way can take it as a warning sign that their patients may actually be at increased risk of suicide.

PATIENT EDUCATION
Patients who feel they are in danger of hurting themselves should consider one or several of these options:
- Call 911.
- Go directly to an emergency room.
- If already in counseling, contact that therapist immediately.
- Call the National Suicide Prevention Hotline at (800) 273-TALK (8255).
- Servicemen and servicewomen and their families can call (800) 796-9699; if there is no immediate answer, call (800) 273-TALK (8255).

PROGNOSIS
The key to a favorable course and prognosis is early recognition of risk factors, early diagnosis and treatment of a psychiatric disorder, and appropriate intervention and follow-up.

COMPLICATIONS
- According to the American Association of Suicidality (AAS), the grief process for significant others of suicide victims can be lifelong and can be expressed in emotions ranging from anger to despair. Survivors often attempt to shoulder the burden on their own because of the added guilt and shame of the nature of the attempted death or death.
- The AAS recommends:
  – Counseling: Could include short-term behavioral therapy as well as psychotherapy; some therapy should focus on the survivors' relationships to their current and future significant others. An expert on the lives of adult children of parents/close family members who completed suicides reports that these survivors often seek out life partners as "replacements" for those they lost. This may prevent the survivor from completing his or her mourning (9).

  – Sympathetic listening by friends of the survivors
  – Special support at holiday times, when the loneliness intensifies
  – A web site with links to resources and self-help strategies is www.survivorsofsuicide.com.

REFERENCES

1. Clark L, Dombrovski AY, Siegle GJ, et al. Impairment in risk-sensitive decision-making in older suicide attempters with depression. *Psychol Aging*. 2011;26:321–330.
2. Jollant F, Bellivier F, Leboyer M, et al. Impaired decision making in suicide attempters. *Am J Psychiatry*. 2005;162:304–310.
3. Gutheil TG, Bursztajn H, Brodsky A. The multidimensional assessment of dangerousness: Competence assessment in patient care and liability prevention. *Bull Am Acad Psychiatry Law*. 1986;14(2):123–129.
4. Bryan CJ, Jennings KW, Jobes DA, et al. Understanding and preventing military suicide. *Arch Suicide Res*. 2012;16(2):95–110.
5. O'Connor E, Gaynes BN, Burda BU, et al. Screening for and treatment of suicide risk relevant to primary care. *Ann Intern Med*. 2013;158(10):741–754.
6. Brown GK. Cognitive therapy for the prevention of suicide attempts: A randomized controlled trial. *JAMA*. 2005;295:563–570.
7. Maltsberger JT, Buie DH. Countertransference hate in the treatment of suicidal patients. *Arch Gen Psychiatry*. 1974;30:625–633.
8. Cipriani A, Pretty H, Hawton K, et al. Lithium in the prevention of suicidal behavior and all-cause mortality in patients with mood disorders: A systematic review of randomized trials. *Am J Psychiatry*. 2005;162:1805–1819.
9. Massicotte WJ. Faculty, Canadian Institute of Psychoanalysis; Chair, National Scientific Program Committee. Correspondence, April 24, 2009.

 CODES

ICD10
- R45.851 Suicidal ideations
- T14.91 Suicide attempt
- Z91.5 Personal history of self-harm

CLINICAL PEARLS
- The most important preventative measure is to listen to a patient and take steps to keep him or her safe. This could include immediate hospitalization. Questions to explore include, "Are you thinking of killing yourself?", "Who do you have to live for?", and "What has to change, or what needs to change, for you to live with your suffering?"
- Clozapine, lithium, and cognitive–behavioral therapy are proven to reduce the risk of suicide.
- Family members and contacts of people who have attempted or committed suicide suffer from reactions ranging from rage to despair. Their grief is often longer lasting and less well treated because of the shame and guilt associated with the act. Encourage them to discuss this and consider counseling.
- Resources for clinicians: www.suicidology.com; www.suicideassessment.com

SUPERFICIAL THROMBOPHLEBITIS

Kelly Alberda, MD

BASICS

DESCRIPTION
- Superficial thrombophlebitis is an inflammatory condition of the veins with secondary thrombosis.
- Traumatic thrombophlebitis types:
  - Injury
  - IV catheter related
  - Intentional (i.e., sclerotherapy)
- Septic (suppurative) thrombophlebitis types:
  - Iatrogenic, long-term IV catheter use
  - Infectious, mainly syphilis and psittacosis
- Aseptic thrombophlebitis types:
  - Primary hypercoagulable states: Disorders with measurable defects in the proteins of the coagulation and/or fibrinolytic systems
  - Secondary hypercoagulable states: Clinical conditions with a risk of thrombosis
- Mondor disease:
  - Rare presentation of anterior chest/breast veins of women
- System(s) affected: Cardiovascular
- Synonym(s): Phlebitis; Phlebothrombosis

Geriatric Considerations
Septic thrombophlebitis is more common; prognosis is poorer.

Pediatric Considerations
Subperiosteal abscesses of adjacent long bone may complicate the disorder.

Pregnancy Considerations
- Associated with increased risk of aseptic superficial thrombophlebitis
- NSAIDs are contraindicated.

EPIDEMIOLOGY
- Predominant age:
  - Traumatic/IV related has no predominate age/sex
  - Aseptic primary hypercoagulable state:
    ○ Childhood to young adult
  - Aseptic secondary hypercoagulable state:
    ○ Mondor disease: Women, ages 21–55 years
    ○ Thromboangiitis obliterans onset: Ages 20–50 years
- Predominant sex:
  - Suppurative: Male = Female
  - Aseptic:
    ○ Mondor: Female > Male (2:1)
    ○ Thromboangiitis obliterans: Female > Male (1–19% of clinical cases)

Incidence
- Septic:
  - Incidence of catheter-related thrombophlebitis is 88/100,000 persons.
  - Develops in 4–8% if cutdown is performed
- Aseptic primary hypercoagulable state: Antithrombin III and heparin cofactor II deficiency incidence is 50/100,000 persons.
- Aseptic secondary hypercoagulable state:
  - In pregnancy, 49-fold increased incidence of phlebitis
  - Superficial migratory thrombophlebitis in 27% of patients with thromboangiitis obliterans

Prevalence
- Superficial thrombophlebitis is common.
- 1/3 of patients in a medical ICU develop thrombophlebitis that eventually progresses to the deep veins.

ETIOLOGY AND PATHOPHYSIOLOGY
- Similar to DVT and Virchow triad. A combination of vessel trauma, stasis, and hypercoagulability whether it is genetic, iatrogenic, or idiopathic
- Mondor disease pathophysiology not completely understood
- Septic:
  - *Staphylococcus aureus*, *Pseudomonas*, *Klebsiella*, *Peptostreptococcus* sp.
  - *Candida* sp.
- Aseptic primary hypercoagulable state:
  - Due to inherited disorders of hypercoagulability
- Aseptic secondary hypercoagulable states:
  - Malignancy (Trousseau syndrome: Recurrent migratory thrombophlebitis): Most commonly seen in metastatic mucin or adenocarcinomas of the GI tract (pancreas, stomach, colon, and gallbladder), lung, prostate, and ovary
  - Pregnancy
  - Oral contraceptives
  - Behçet, Buerger, or Mondor disease

Genetics
Not applicable other than hypercoagulable states

RISK FACTORS
- Nonspecific:
  - Immobilization
  - Obesity
  - Advanced age
  - Postoperative states
- Traumatic/Septic:
  - IV catheter (plastic > coated)
  - Lower extremity IV catheter
  - Cutdowns
  - Cancer, debilitating diseases
  - Burn patients
  - AIDS
  - Varicose veins
- Aseptic:
  - Pregnancy
  - Oral contraceptives
  - Surgery, trauma, infection
  - Hypercoagulable state (i.e., factor V, protein C or S deficiency, others)
- Thromboangiitis obliterans: Persistent smoking
- Mondor disease:
  - Breast cancer or breast surgery

GENERAL PREVENTION
- Avoidance of lower extremity cannulations/IV
- Insertion under aseptic conditions, securing cannulas, and replacing q72h
- Avoiding stasis or using usual deep vein thrombosis (DVT) prophylaxis in high-risk patients (i.e., ICU, immobilized)

DIAGNOSIS

HISTORY
Pain along the course of a vein

PHYSICAL EXAM
- Swelling, tenderness, redness along the course of a vein or veins
- May look like localized cellulitis or erythema nodosum
- Fever in 70% of patients in septic phlebitis
- Sign of systemic sepsis in 84% of suppurative cases

DIFFERENTIAL DIAGNOSIS
- Cellulitis
- DVT
- Erythema nodosum
- Cutaneous polyarteritis nodosa

DIAGNOSTIC TESTS & INTERPRETATION
Initial Tests (lab, imaging)
Often none necessary if afebrile, otherwise healthy
- Small or distal veins (i.e., forearms or below the knee): No recommended imaging
- Venous Doppler US to assess extent of thrombosis and rule out DVT

Follow-Up Tests & Special Considerations
- If suspicious for sepsis:
  - Blood cultures (bacteremia in 80–90%)
  - Consider culture of the IV fluids being infused.
  - CBC demonstrates leukocytosis.
- Aseptic: Evaluation for coagulopathy if recurrent or without another identifiable cause (e.g., protein C and S, lupus anticoagulant, anticardiolipin antibody, factor V and VIII, homocysteine)
- In migratory thrombophlebitis, have a high index of suspicion for malignancy.
- Repeat venous ultrasound to assess effectiveness of therapy:
  - If thrombosis is extending, more aggressive therapy required

Test Interpretation
The affected vein is enlarged, tortuous, and thickened with endothelial damage and necrosis.

TREATMENT

GENERAL MEASURES

- Suppurative: Consultation/Evaluation for urgent surgical venous excision
- Local, mild:
  - Nonmedication management crucial, antibiotics not useful
  - For varicosities:
    ○ Compression stockings, maintain activities
  - Catheter/Trauma associated:
    ○ Immediately remove IV and culture tip.
    ○ Elevate with application of warm compresses.
    ○ If slow to resolve, consider LMWH.
- Large, severe, or septic thrombophlebitis:
  - Inpatient care or bedrest with elevation and local warm compress
  - When the patient is ambulating, then start compression stockings or Ace bandages.

MEDICATION

First Line

- Localized, mild (usually self-limited):
  - NSAIDs, ASA for inflammation/pain

- Cochrane Review for superficial thrombophlebitis of lower extremities found benefit in preventing DVT with 6 weeks of LMWH (1)[A].

Second Line

- Septic/Suppurative:
  - May present or be complicated by sepsis
  - Requires IV antibiotics (broad spectrum initially) and anticoagulation
- Large or involving long saphenous vein are at risk for progression into DVT; consider pharmacologic preventive therapies:
  - To prevent venous thromboembolism (VTE), 4 weeks of LMWH; such as enoxaparin (2)[A]
  - 45 days of fondaparinux was found to reduce DVT and VTE by 85% (relative risk reduction) in 1 study (3)[B].
- Superficial thrombophlebitis related to inherited or acquired hypercoagulable states will need to be prevented by treating the related disease.

ISSUES FOR REFERRAL

Varicosities, severely inflamed, or very large phlebitis should be evaluated for excision.

SURGERY/OTHER PROCEDURES

- Septic:
  - Consult/Evaluate for excision of the involved vein segment and all involved tributaries.
  - Drainage of contiguous abscesses
  - Remove all associated cannula and culture tips.
- Aseptic: Management of underlying conditions:
  - Evaluation for saphenous vein ligation to prevent deep vein extension
  - Consider referral for varicosity excision.

IN-PATIENT CONSIDERATIONS

Admission Criteria/Initial Stabilization

- Septic: Inpatient
- Aseptic: Outpatient

 ONGOING CARE

FOLLOW-UP RECOMMENDATIONS

Patient Monitoring

- Septic: Routine WBC count and differential and culture-based treatment
- Severe aseptic:
  - Repeat venous Doppler US in 1–2 weeks to ensure no DVT and assess treatment effectiveness: Do not expect resolution, just nonprogression.
  - Repeat of blood studies for fibrinolytic system, platelets, and factors
- Local, mild: Per clinician judgement, usually PRN if not resolving

DIET

No restrictions

PATIENT EDUCATION

Importance of local care, elevation, and use of compression hose for acute treatment and prevention of recurrence

PROGNOSIS

- Septic/Suppurative:
  - High mortality (50%) if untreated
  - Depends on treatment delay or need for surgery
- Aseptic:
  - Usually benign course; recovery in 2–3 weeks
  - Depends on development of DVT and early detection of complications
  - Aseptic thrombophlebitis can be isolated, recurrent, or migratory.
  - Recurrence likely if related to varicosity or if severely affected vein not removed

COMPLICATIONS

- Septic: Systemic sepsis, bacteremia (84%), septic pulmonary emboli (44%), metastatic abscess formation, pneumonia (44%), subperiosteal abscess of adjacent long bones in children
- Aseptic: DVT, VTE, thromboembolic phenomena

REFERENCES

1. Di Nisio M, Wichers IM, Middeldorp S. Treatment for superficial thrombophlebitis of the leg. *Cochrane Database Syst Rev*. 2013;4:CD004982. Epub 2013 Apr 30.
2. Wichers IM, Di Nisio M, Büller HR, et al. Treatment of superficial vein thrombosis to prevent deep vein thrombosis and pulmonary embolism: A systematic review. *Haematologica*. 2005;90:672–677.
3. Decousus H, Prandoni P, Mismetti P, et al. Fondaparinux for the treatment of superficial-vein thrombosis in the legs. *N Engl J Med*. 2010;363: 1222–1232.

ADDITIONAL READING

- Gillet JL, French P, Hanss M, et al. [Predictive value of D-dimer assay in superficial thrombophlebitis of the lower limbs.] *J Mal Vasc*. 2007;32(2):90–95.
- Samlaska CP, James WD. Superficial thrombophlebitis. I. Primary hypercoagulable states. *J Am Acad Dermatol*. 1990;22:975–989.
- Samlaska CP, James WD. Superficial thrombophlebitis. II. Secondary hypercoagulable states. *J Am Acad Dermatol*. 1990;23(1):1–18.

 SEE ALSO

Deep Vein Thrombosis (DVT)

CODES

ICD10

- I80.00 Phlbts and thombophlb of superfic vessels of unsp low extrm
- I80.8 Phlebitis and thrombophlebitis of other sites
- I80.9 Phlebitis and thrombophlebitis of unspecified site

CLINICAL PEARLS

- Mild disease is self-limiting.
- Severe or lower extreme disease benefits from anticoagulation to prevent DVT.

SURGICAL COMPLICATIONS

Caitlin Bonney, MD • Mitchell A. Cahan, MD, FACS

 BASICS

DESCRIPTION
- Any negative outcome either by surgeon or patient; no consensus on definition
- Multiple classification systems exist based on severity.

EPIDEMIOLOGY
Incidence
Incidence varies with type of operation, operative time, hospital, surgeon, and patient characteristics:
- Mortality rate in general and vascular surgery is 3.5–6.9% (1).
- Overall complication rate in general and vascular surgery is 24.6–26.9% (1).
- Postoperative fever is very common. Incidence ranges (14–91%) (2).
- Rate of venous thromboembolic events: 3/1,000 surgical discharges in the US (3)
- Emergent cases associated with more complications than nonemergent cases (22.8% vs. 14.2%) and have higher mortality rate (6.5% vs. 1.4%) (4)
- Complications after bariatric surgery: Anastamotic leak (0–5.6%), internal hernia (3–4.5%), marginal ulcer (1–16%), GI bleeding (0.6–4%), acute distention of distal stomach
- Surgical infection incidence varies with type of operation:
  - 1–2% clean operative site (e.g., hernia repair)
  - 5–15% clean contaminated site (e.g., cholecystectomy)
  - 10–20% contaminated site (e.g., colectomy)
  - 50% dirty operative site

ETIOLOGY AND PATHOPHYSIOLOGY
- Fever caused by pyrogens (mediated by interleukin-1): Bacteria, viruses, antigen–antibody complexes
- Wound dehiscence: Poor wound healing (malnutrition) or increased intra-abdominal pressure
- Deep vein thrombosis: Blood clot formation incited by Virchow triad:
  - Hypercoagulability
  - Hemodynamic changes (stasis, turbulence)
  - Endothelial injury/dysfunction
- Renal failure:
  - Drug toxicity (commonly antibiotics)
  - Inadequate resuscitation leading to poor perfusion (catecholamine release during surgery and activation of renin-angiotensin-aldosterone system) results in ATN.
- Respiratory:
  - Decreased vital capacity leads to atelectasis, pneumonitis, and acute respiratory distress syndrome (ARDS).
  - Aspiration can occur at any time. Stomach acid/particulate matter causes an inflammatory reaction, leading to respiratory distress or death.
  - Pulmonary edema due to fluid transudation to alveolus from fluid overload or heart failure
  - Pulmonary mechanics are compromised postoperatively. Precipitating factors include pain and altered mental status.

- Cardiac:
  - Postoperative MI occurs within 3 days of surgery; caused by anesthetics and blood loss (loss of as little as 500 mL can cause shock).
  - Arrhythmia is due to destabilization of cardiac membranes or prolongation of conduction.
- Small bowel obstruction: Adhesive bands cause bowel torsion or constriction at any time after intra-abdominal procedures.
- Urinary retention: More frequent in men than women, impaired coordination between α-receptors in the bladder neck and parasympathetic stimulation to the bladder due to anesthetic agents
- Fever in the first 24 hours is usually due to atelectasis. Consider the 5 Ws:
  - Wind—atelectasis, PNA, aspiration
  - Water—UTI
  - Walking—deep venous thrombosis (DVT)
  - Wound—surgical site infection
  - Wonder drugs—drug fever
- Fever >102°F in the first 48 hours is concerning for necrotizing wound infection.
- *Staphylococcus aureus* is the most common cause of wound infection. Others include *Pseudomonas*, *Proteus*, and *Klebsiella*.
- Hematoma: Inadequate hemostasis
- Seroma: Disruption of lymphatics
- UTI: Related to indwelling catheter
- Dehiscence: Increased abdominal pressure, inadequate fascial closure, malnutrition, contamination, and chemotherapy
- Renal failure: Hypovolemia, drug toxicity (commonly due to antibiotics or IV contrast)
- Respiratory: Volume overload, aspiration, and decreased vital capacity lead to decreased diffusion capacity. Pulmonary embolism formation is another possible postoperative etiology.
- Pulmonary embolism: Generally due to thromboembolism from the deep veins of the legs; more rarely from air, fat, or amniotic fluid.
- Cardiac: Arrhythmia occurs due to electrolyte abnormalities, catecholamine release (from pain), hypercapnia, and digitalis.
- Fistula/intestinal leak: Generally occurs at the site of bowel anastomosis due to suture line breakdown
- Stomal complications:
  - More common in obese patients
  - Include fibrosis of bowel at stoma, necrosis, retraction, skin breakdown, and stomal stricture
  - Most complications are due to technical errors at the time of operation.

Genetics
Malignant hyperthermia syndrome (MHS): Skeletal muscle disorder manifested as hypermetabolic crisis following administration of halogenated inhalational anesthetic agents or succinylcholine.
- Incidence: 1/50–100,000; treated with dantrolene
- Autosomal-dominant inheritance with incomplete penetrance
- No practical screening tests for general population available
- Patients with MHS may safely undergo general anesthesia without triggering agents

RISK FACTORS
- People at increased operative risk include those with:
  - Poorly controlled diabetes/obesity
  - Heart disease (especially myocardial infarction [MI] and heart failure)
  - Bleeding disorders
  - Malnutrition
  - Renal failure
  - Liver and pulmonary disease
  - Smoking
  - Immunosuppression
  - Malignancy
- Other risk factors:
  - Prolonged surgery
  - Immobility following surgery
  - Emergency surgery
- Pseudocholinesterase deficiency:
  - Inherited enzyme deficiency resulting in abnormally slow degradation of choline ester drugs
  - Causes prolonged respiratory paralysis following administration of standard doses of succinylcholine
  - Incidence: <0.01% of the general population; may have personal or family history of prolonged postanesthesia wake-up time
- Bleeding disorders, including hemophilia

GENERAL PREVENTION
Preventive measures span entire perioperative period:
- Smoking cessation (5)[A]
- Imaging
- Appropriate fluid/blood resuscitation
- Assessment of underlying risk factors
- Preoperative antibiotics, when appropriate
- Sterile technique
- Warming during surgery
- Clip hair instead of shaving preoperatively (6)[B]

COMMONLY ASSOCIATED CONDITIONS
- Adrenal insufficiency when on chronic steroids preoperatively
- Liver failure in patients with pre-existing disease
- Delirium tremens in alcoholics
- Thyroid storm in patients with undiagnosed hyperthyroidism
- Parotitis in the elderly
- Depression

Pediatric Considerations
Operative procedures can lead to severe anxiety in children aged 1–2 years, with lasting emotional disturbance in 20%.

Geriatric Considerations
90% of patients age >65 years experience depression after surgery, with ADLs impaired in 50%. Increase human contact to prevent withdrawal and reduce symptoms.

 DIAGNOSIS

HISTORY
- Wound infection: History of surgery several days prior to presentation with pain, warmth, redness, or drainage at site of incision
- Expanding mass is consistent with seroma or hematoma. Hematoma more likely if surgery within 2–3 days; seroma more likely if interval is longer.

- Dehiscence/Hernia: Some patients feel sutures "pop." They may complain of a palpable bulge. Attributed to increased abdominal pressure (e.g., coughing, Valsalva maneuver)
- DVT: Pain, swelling, and redness of leg in immobilized patient or with hypercoagulability
- Renal failure: Oliguria or anuria, fatigue
- Pulmonary: Lack of incentive spirometry, narcotics, fluid retention, age >65 years, shortness of breath, chest pain
- Cardiac: Elderly, cardiac dysfunction; chest pain in 27% of perioperative MI (most are pain-free)
- Ileus or small bowel obstruction: Progressive nausea, bilious vomiting, inability to tolerate PO intake, abdominal pain, cessation of flatus
- Fistula or intestinal leak: Severe abdominal pain (leak), fever, nausea/vomiting
- Stomal complications: Pain at stoma site, change in color of stoma
- Urinary retention: Inability to void, suprapubic pain

PHYSICAL EXAM
- Low fevers are not significant until 48 hours postop. Wound infection is most common cause of fever after 72 hours.
- High fever, mental status changes, hypotension, and rigors are associated with severe wound complications or intestinal leak.
- Detection of intra-abdominal complications may be more challenging in obese patients due to body habitus.
- Dolor, tumor, rubor, and calor may indicate a wound infection, as do pus or foul-smelling discharge. The patient may be febrile.
- Hematoma: Expanding, tender mass. Seroma: Slowly expanding, nontender mass
- Dehiscence/Hernia: Salmon-colored drainage on postop days 4–5, evisceration, or later as ventral hernia; may see open incision or palpable fascial edge, rarely tender
- Renal failure: Persistent oliguria; can have pericardial rub, bleeding/hematoma if uremic
- Pulmonary: Dyspnea, cough, fever, basilar crackles, poor inspiratory effort, egophony, dullness to percussion at bases
- Cardiac: Peripheral edema, irregularly irregular heartbeat
- Ileus/Small bowel obstruction: "Tinkling" or absent bowel sounds, tympanitic abdomen, tenderness to palpation, occasionally guarding
- Fistula/Intestinal leak: Feces protruding from skin opening, acute/firm abdomen, fever, guarding, peritoneal signs, hypotension
- Stomal complications are evident when the ostomy appliance is removed: Skin irritation, black/discolored intestinal mucosa, retracted ostomy
- Urinary retention: Suprapubic pain, palpable bladder
- Anastamotic leak: May manifest as isolated tachycardia or patient anxiety in after gastric bypass

DIAGNOSTIC TESTS & INTERPRETATION
Initial Tests (lab, imaging)
- CBC with differential, blood culture and sensitivity (C/S), chemistries, BUN/creatinine, urinalysis (UA), urine C/S, ABG, chest x-ray (CXR)
- Elevated WBC count with wound infections, atelectasis, pneumonia, infected hematoma/seroma, bowel leak, and stomal complications
- Renal failure: BUN, creatinine, urine chemistries, and FE_{NA}
- Pulmonary: Hypoxia, hypercarbia on ABG

- Cardiac: Elevated troponins, creatine kinase (CK), CK-MB
- UTI: UA, urine C/S
- Subcutaneous gas can be seen in necrotizing fasciitis on x-ray or CT.
- CT or ultrasound can be used to diagnose hernia or fascial disruption.
- Small bowel obstruction/ileus: Upright abdominal film shows air–fluid levels, dilated small bowel; transition point may be seen on CT.
- Fistula: Fistulogram aids in diagnosis and is critical for treatment planning.
- Intestinal leak: CXR reveals free air under the diaphragm; CT shows fluid collection in abdomen.
- Bladder scan can help diagnose urinary retention if diagnosis in doubt.
- DVT: Duplex ultrasound
- Pulmonary: CXR, CT pulmonary angiography more sensitive test for suspected pulmonary embolism.

Diagnostic Procedures/Other
- Exploratory laparotomy/laparoscopy if extremely ill/septic and diagnosis is unknown
- Dehiscence is considered a surgical emergency.
- Intra-abdominal abscesses frequently can be drained percutaneously.
- Cardiac: ECG shows signs of ischemia or dysrhythmia.

TREATMENT
MEDICATION
- Opiates for pain control.
- Broad-spectrum antibiotics for sepsis or severe infection (piperacillin/tazobactam and vancomycin).
- Simple wound infections and stomal complications: 1st- or 2nd-generation cephalosporins
- Intestinal leak: Gram-negative and gram-positive coverage (levofloxacin and metronidazole)
- Pneumonia should be treated empirically with antibiotics to cover local flora.
- Cardiac complications can be avoided or treated with β-blockade for rate control.
- Urinary retention: α-blockers (tamsulosin)

SURGERY/OTHER PROCEDURES
- Wound infections often need surgical débridement.
- Hematomas may need re-exploration and hemostasis if progressing.
- Dehiscence/hernia should be repaired. Evisceration is a surgical emergency.
- Small bowel obstruction that fails to resolve with nasogastric decompression should be explored.
- Intestinal leak is a surgical emergency for immediate exploration and repair. Fistulas generally need surgical intervention to resolve.
- Some stomal complications (necrosis, retraction) need surgical revision.

IN-PATIENT CONSIDERATIONS
Admission Criteria/Initial Stabilization
Need for IV fluids/antibiotics and for nasogastric decompression
- Fluid resuscitation, as needed
- Broad-spectrum antibiotics, if the patient is septic
- IV antibiotics for infections

Discharge Criteria
Able to tolerate PO intake, voiding, return of bowel function

ONGOING CARE
DIET
NPO for patients with fistula, intestinal leak, or small bowel obstruction

REFERENCES
1. Ghaferi A. Variation in hospital mortality associated with inpatient surgery. *N Engl J Med*. 2009;361: 1368–1375.
2. Pile JC. Evaluating postoperative fever: A focused approach. *Cleve Clin J Med*. 2006;73(Suppl 1): S62–S66.
3. US Department of Health and Human Services, Agency for Healthcare Research and Quality. National Healthcare Quality Report, 2011. Full Report. Rockville, MD: AHRQ. http://www.ahrq.gov/qual/qrdr11.htm
4. Becher RD, Hoth JJ, Miller PR, et al. A Critical assessment of outcomes in emergency versus nonemergency general surgery using the American College of Surgeons National Surgical Quality Improvement Program Database. *Am Surg*. 2011;77:951–959.
5. Thomsen T, Tønnesen H, Møller AM, et al. Effect of preoperative smoking cessation interventions on postoperative complications and smoking cessation. *Br J Surg*. 2009;96:451–461.
6. Tanner J, Woodings D, Moncaster K. Preoperative hair removal to reduce surgical site infection. *Cochrane Database Syst Rev*. 2006;(3):CD004122. Epub 2006 Jul 19.

CODES
ICD10
- R50.82 Postprocedural fever
- T81.4XXA Infection following a procedure, initial encounter
- T81.31XA Disruption of external operation (surgical) wound, not elsewhere classified, initial encounter

CLINICAL PEARLS
- Smoking cessation at any interval prior to surgery decreases postop complications.
- Surgical site infections are decreased by clipping to remove hair rather than shaving.
- Appropriate antibacterial preparation should be utilized to decrease bacterial counts.
- Amputation sites heal faster with plaster casting than with gauze. No difference found in healing rates with foam vs. gauze dressings, but patients prefer foam.
- 50% of all wound infections are identified after the patient is discharged.
- Treatment of some complications related to hospitalization will no longer be reimbursed by payers, including wrong-site surgery and central venous catheter infections.

SYNCOPE

Santiago O. Valdes, MD, FAAP

BASICS

DESCRIPTION
- Transient loss of consciousness characterized by unresponsiveness, loss of postural tone, and spontaneous recovery; usually caused by cerebral hypoxemia
- System(s) affected: Cardiovascular; Nervous

EPIDEMIOLOGY
Incidence
- Up to 20% of adults will have ≥1 episode by age 75; 15% of children <18 years of age
- Accounts for 1–6% of hospital admissions and ~3% of emergency room visits
- Yearly prevalence of fainting spells resulting in medical evaluation was 9.5/1,000 inhabitants (1).

Prevalence
In institutionalized elderly (>75 years), 6%

ETIOLOGY AND PATHOPHYSIOLOGY
- In some cases, vagal response leads to decreased heart rate.
- Systemic hypotension secondary to decreased cardiac output and/or systemic vasodilation leads to a drop in cerebral perfusion and resulting loss of consciousness.
- Cardiac (obstruction to outflow):
  – Aortic stenosis
  – Hypertrophic cardiomyopathy
  – Pulmonary embolus
- Cardiac arrhythmias:
  – Sustained ventricular tachycardia (VT)
  – Supraventricular tachycardia (atrial fibrillation, atrial flutter, re-entrant SVT)
  – 2nd- and 3rd-degree AV block
  – Sick-sinus syndrome
- Noncardiac:
  – Reflex-mediated vasovagal (neurocardiogenic/neurally mediated), situational (micturition, defecation, cough, hair combing)
  – Orthostatic hypotension
  – Drug-induced
  – Neurologic: Seizures; transient ischemic attack (can in theory cause syncope, but presentation usually markedly clinically different from pure syncope)
  – Carotid sinus hypersensitivity
  – Psychogenic

Genetics
Specific cardiomyopathies and arrhythmias may be familial (i.e., long QT syndrome, catecholaminergic polymorphic ventricular tachycardia, hypertrophic cardiomyopathy).

RISK FACTORS
- Heart disease
- Dehydration
- Drugs:
  – Antihypertensives
  – Vasodilators (including calcium channel blockers, ACE inhibitors, and nitrates)
  – Phenothiazines
  – Antidepressants
  – Antiarrhythmics
  – Diuretics

GENERAL PREVENTION
See "Risk Factors."

COMMONLY ASSOCIATED CONDITIONS
See "Etiology."

DIAGNOSIS

HISTORY
- Careful history, physical exam, and an ECG are more important than other investigations in determining the diagnosis (2)[A]. Syncope associated with physical exertion suggests a potential cardiac etiology.
- Make sure that the patient or witness (if present) is not talking about vertigo (i.e., sense of rotary motion, spinning, and whirling), seizure, or causes of fall without loss of consciousness.
- Even after careful evaluation, including diagnostic procedures and special tests, the cause will be found in only 50–60% of the patients.
- Onset of syncope is usually rapid, and recovery is spontaneous, rapid, and complete. Duration of episodes are typically brief (<60 seconds). The presence of underlying cardiac or neurologic conditions provides the key to diagnosis.
- Ask for family history of long QT syndrome, hypertrophic cardiomyopathy, or unexplained sudden cardiac death in young family members.

PHYSICAL EXAM
- BP and pulse, both lying and standing
- Check for cardiac murmur or focal neurologic abnormality.

DIFFERENTIAL DIAGNOSIS
- Drop attacks
- Coma
- Vertigo
- Seizure disorder

DIAGNOSTIC TESTS & INTERPRETATION
History and physical examination should guide laboratory testing.

Initial Tests (lab, imaging)
Consider (not all indicated in all individuals):
- CBC
- Electrolytes, BUN, creatinine, glucose (rarely helpful: <2% have hyponatremia, hypocalcemia, hypoglycemia, or renal failure causing seizures).
- Cardiac enzymes (only if history suggestive of cardiac ischemia)
- D-dimer (for pulmonary embolism workup)
- hCG
- Lung scan or helical CT scan of thorax if history and physical exam suggest pulmonary embolism (PE)

Follow-Up Tests & Special Considerations
- If history and physical suggest ischemic, valvular, or congenital heart disease:
  – ECG
  – Exercise stress test (if syncope with exertion)
  – Echocardiogram
  – Cardiac catheterization
- If CNS disease suspected:
  – EEG
  – Head CT scan
  – Head MRI/MRA when vascular cause is suspected
  – Do not order these tests without hints of CNS disease on history or physical exam.

- ECG monitoring, either in hospital or ambulatory (Holter) (3)[C]:
  – Useful in 4–15% of patients
  – Should be done in patients with heart disease or recurrent syncope
  – Arrhythmias frequently documented, but not always associated with syncope
- Electrophysiologic studies (3,4)[C]:
  – Have been positive in 18–75% of patients
  – Induction of VT and dysfunction of His-Purkinje system are the 2 most common abnormalities.
  – Should be done in patients with heart disease and recurrent syncope, although they may not show whether arrhythmia noted or induced during study is cause of syncope.
- Carotid hypersensitivity evaluation (3,4)[C]:
  – Carotid hypersensitivity should be considered in patients with syncope during head turning, especially while wearing tight collars, and with neck tumors and neck scars.
  – The technique is not standardized; 1 side at a time is compressed gently at a time for 20 seconds with constant monitoring of pulse and BP/ECG.
  – Atropine should be readily available.
- Tilt-table testing ± isoproterenol infusion (3,4)[C]:
  – Provocative test for vasovagal syncope
  – Perform if cardiac causes have been excluded; role in workup of patients with syncope of unknown origin
  – Protocol is not standardized, but has been reported positive (symptomatic hypotension and bradycardia) in 26–87% of patients; also positive in up to 45% of control subjects
- Psychiatric evaluation: Anxiety, depression, and alcohol and drug abuse can be associated with syncope.

Diagnostic Procedures/Other
Patient-activated implantable loop recorders can record 4–5 minutes of retrograde ECG rhythm. Helpful in selective patients with recurrent syncope, with yield of 32–80% (3,4)[C].

Test Interpretation
Depends on etiology and presence of underlying cardiac or neurologic conditions

TREATMENT

Maintaining good hydration status and normal salt intake are initial therapy. Educate patients of the premonitory signs of syncope (5)[B].

GENERAL MEASURES
- Elderly patients without previously recognized heart disease should be admitted if the physician thinks that the cause of syncope is likely cardiac.
- Patients without heart disease, especially young patients (age <60 years), can be worked up safely as outpatients.
- Prescribe antiarrhythmics for documented arrhythmias occurring simultaneously with syncope or symptoms of presyncope. Asymptomatic arrhythmias do not necessarily require treatment.
- The decision to treat patients on basis of arrhythmias or conduction abnormalities provoked or detected during EPS is even more problematic: Does the arrhythmia or conduction abnormality have anything to do with the patient's symptoms?

- Most would treat patients with provoked sustained VT with an antiarrhythmic drug that suppressed arrhythmia during study.
- Rationale for such treatment: Recurrent syncope is less frequent in patients with positive EPS who are treated than it is in those who have negative EPS.

MEDICATION
First Line
- Geared toward specific underlying cardiac or neurologic abnormalities
- In cases of recurrent vasovagal/neurocardiogenic/neurally mediated syncope (6)[B]:
  – α-Adrenergic agonists (midodrine)
  – Mineralocorticoids (fludrocortisone)
  – β-Adrenergic blockers

Second Line
- SSRIs (paroxetine, sertraline, fluoxetine)
- Vagolytics (disopyramide)

ISSUES FOR REFERRAL
When cardiac or neurologic etiologies are suspected, obtain appropriate consultation, as indicated.

SURGERY/OTHER PROCEDURES
- Implantable cardioverter-defibrillator (ICD) placement for patients with cardiac conditions with high risk of sudden death and/or recurrent syncope on medications (i.e., long QT syndrome, catecholaminergic polymorphic ventricular tachycardia, hypertrophic cardiomyopathy)
- Many recommend pacemaker implantation in patients with:
  – 2nd- (Mobitz type II) and 3rd-degree heart block
  – H-V intervals >100 ms
  – Pacing-induced infranodal block
  – Sinus node recovery time ≥3 seconds

IN-PATIENT CONSIDERATIONS
Admission Criteria/Initial Stabilization
Patients with benign etiologies of syncope with negative ED work ups are associated with benign outcomes, even in the presence of other risk factors (7)[B]. Patients with suspected cardiac or neurologic cause for syncope should be admitted to the hospital for evaluation.

- Support ABCs.
- Stabilize heart rate and BP, typically with IV fluids.

IV Fluids
Use isotonic crystalloid fluids for fluid resuscitation, if needed.

Nursing
Close monitoring of BP and heart rate during initial presentation

Discharge Criteria
- Attainment of hemodynamic stability
- Satisfactory completion of workup for etiology
- Adequate control of specific arrhythmia or seizure, if present

 ## ONGOING CARE

FOLLOW-UP RECOMMENDATIONS
Patient Monitoring
- Frequent follow-up visits for patients with cardiac causes of syncope, especially patients on antiarrhythmics
- Patients with an unknown cause of syncope rarely (5%) are diagnosed during the follow-up.

DIET
- No specific diet unless the patient has heart disease
- Increased fluid and salt intake to maintain intravascular volume in cases of recurrent vasovagal syncope

PATIENT EDUCATION
- Reassure the patient that most cardiac causes of syncope can be treated, and patients with noncardiac causes do well, even if the cause of syncope is never discovered.
- Physical counterpressure maneuvers can prevent recurrences of vasovagal syncope.
- Physician and patient should carefully consider whether the patient should continue to drive while syncope is being evaluated. Physicians should be aware of pertinent laws in their own states.

PROGNOSIS
- Cumulative mortality at 2 years:
  – Low: Young patients (<60 years) with noncardiac or unknown cause of syncope
  – Intermediate: Older patients (>60 years) with noncardiac or unknown cause of syncope
  – High: Patients with cardiac cause of syncope
- Independent predictors of poor short-term outcomes (8,9)[B]:
  – Abnormal ECG
  – Shortness of breath
  – Systolic BP <90 mm Hg
  – Hematocrit <30%
  – Congestive heart failure

COMPLICATIONS
- Trauma from falling
- Death (see "Prognosis")

REFERENCES
1. Malasana G, Brignole M, Daccarett M, et al. The prevalence and cost of the faint and fall problem in the state of Utah. *Pacing Clin Electrophysiol.* 2011;34:278–283.
2. Kessler C, Tristano JM, De Lorenzo R. The emergency department approach to syncope: Evidence-based guidelines and prediction rules. *Emerg Med Clin North Am.* 2010;28:487–500.
3. Task Force for the Diagnosis and Management of Syncope, European Society of Cardiology (ESC), European Heart Rhythm Association (EHRA), et al. Guidelines for the diagnosis and management of syncope (version 2009). *Eur Heart J.* 2009;30: 2631–2671. Epub 2009 Aug 27.
4. Brignole M, Hamdan MH. New concepts in the assessment of syncope. *J Am Coll Cardiol.* 2012;59: 1583–1591.
5. Romme JJ, Reitsma JB, Go-Schön IK, et al. Prospective evaluation of non-pharmacological treatment in vasovagal syncope. *Europace.* 2010; 12:567–573.
6. Kuriachan V, Sheldon RS, Platonov M. Evidence-based treatment for vasovagal syncope. *Heart Rhythm.* 2008;5:1609–1614.
7. Grossman SA, Fischer C, Kancharla A, et al. Can benign etiologies predict benign outcomes in high-risk syncope patients? *J Emerg Med.* 2011; 40: 592–597.
8. Quinn JV, Stiell IG, McDermott DA, et al. Derivation of the San Francisco Syncope Rule to predict patients with short-term serious outcomes. *Ann Emerg Med.* 2004;43:224–232.
9. Saccilotto RT, Nickel CH, Bucher HC, et al. San Francisco Syncope Rule to predict short-term serious outcomes: A systematic review. *CMAJ.* 2011;183:E1116–E1126. Epub 2011 Sep 26.

ADDITIONAL READING
- Parry SW, Tan MP. An approach to the evaluation and management of syncope in adults. *BMJ.* 2010;340:c880.
- Reed MJ, Newby DE, Coull AJ, et al. The ROSE (risk stratification of syncope in the emergency department) study. *J Am Coll Cardiol.* 2010;55: 713–721.
- Strickberger SA, Benson DW, Biaggioni I. AHA/ACCF scientific statement on the evaluation of syncope: From the American Heart Association Councils on Clinical Cardiology, Cardiovascular Nursing, Cardiovascular Disease in the Young, and Stroke, and the Quality of Care and Outcomes Research Interdisciplinary Working Group; and the American College of Cardiology Foundation in Collaboration with the Heart Rhythm Society. *J Am Coll Cardiol.* 2006;47:473–484.

 ## SEE ALSO
- Aortic Valvular Stenosis; Atrial Septal Defect (ASD); Carotid Sinus Hypersensitivity; Idiopathic Hypertrophic Subaortic Stenosis (IHSS); Patent Ductus Arteriosus; Pulmonary Arterial Hypertension; Pulmonary Embolism; Seizure Disorders; Stokes-Adams Attacks
- Algorithms: Syncope; Transient Ischemic Attack, and Transient Neurologic Deficit

 ## CODES

ICD10
R55 Syncope and collapse

CLINICAL PEARLS
- A careful history and physical exam are key to a diagnosis.
- Use the ECG/event-recorder to evaluate for cardiac conditions.
- True neurologic causes of syncope are very rare; by far, cardiac causes are more common.
- <2% of cases are caused by hyponatremia, hypocalcemia, hypoglycemia, or renal failure causing seizures.

SYNCOPE, REFLEX (VASOVAGAL SYNCOPE)

Melinda Y. Kwan, DO, MPH • Norton Winer, MD

BASICS

Syncope is a reversible loss of consciousness and postural tone secondary to systemic hypotension and cerebral hypoperfusion.

The hypotension is due to vasodilation and/or bradycardia (rarely, tachycardia) and results in spontaneous recovery and no neurologic sequelae.

The term *syncope* excludes seizures, coma, shock, or other states of altered consciousness.

DESCRIPTION
- Derived from the Greek term "syncopa," meaning "to cut short"
- Sudden, transient loss of consciousness characterized by unresponsiveness, falling, and spontaneous recovery
- Common cause of syncope in all age groups, especially in patients with no evidence of neurologic or cardiac disease
- 4 types: Vasovagal or neurocardiogenic syncope, situational syncope, orthostatic hypotension, carotid sinus hypersensitivity, and glossopharyngeal/trigeminal neuralgia syncope (uncommon) (1).

EPIDEMIOLOGY
- Mortality: Cardiac-related syncope 20–30% and 5% in idiopathic syncope
- Age: Any age

Incidence
- Ranges from 7.5% in children age <18 years and 15% in adults age >70 years
- 36–62% of all syncopal episodes
- 30% recurrence rate

Prevalence
22% in the general population

ETIOLOGY AND PATHOPHYSIOLOGY
Caused by an abnormal interaction of the normal mechanisms for maintaining BP and upright posture:
- In normal individuals, upright posture results in venous pooling and transient decrease in BP.
- Neurally induced syncope may result from a cardioinhibitory response, a vasodepressor response, or a combination of the 2.
- Cardioinhibitory response results from increase in parasympathetic tone, which may cause bradycardia.
- Vasodepressor response results from decrease in sympathetic tone, which may cause hypotension (2).
- Vasovagal syncope usually has a precipitating event, often related to fright, pain, panic, exercise, noxious stimuli, or heat exposure. Also common in pregnancy when changing from supine to lateral decubitus or upright position (2)
- Carotid sinus syncope is precipitated by position change, turning head, or wearing a tight collar; also possibly from neck tumors or surgical scarring.
- Situational syncope is related to micturition, defecation, postexercise, postprandial, cough, or phobia of needle or blood (3).
- Glossopharyngeal syncope is related to throat or facial pain (4).

Genetics
Vasovagal syncope: Strong heritable component to the etiology of >20% of cases

RISK FACTORS
- Low resting BP
- Age: Older age
- Prolonged supine position with resulting deconditioning of autonomic control

GENERAL PREVENTION
Avoidance of precipitating events or situations. Optimization of diabetes mellitus (DM) control, elastic stockings, adequate hydration. Limited evidence suggests that polydipsia may reduce recurrences.

COMMONLY ASSOCIATED CONDITIONS
- Cardiopulmonary disorders: CHF, MI, arrhythmias, HOCM, HTN, PE
- Neurologic disorders: Autonomic dysfunction, Shy-Drager, PD, MSA, TIA, VBI, PN
- Psychiatric disorders:
  – Generalized anxiety disorder
  – Panic disorder
  – Major depression
  – Alcohol dependence

DIAGNOSIS

History and physical and 12-lead ECG are preliminary tests.

HISTORY
- Evaluation of syncope and presyncope are the same.
- Important 1st to rule out cardiac syncope
- Neurally mediated syncope is preceded by blurred vision, palpitations, nausea, warmth, diaphoresis, or lightheadedness, or there may be history of nausea, warmth, diaphoresis, or fatigue *after* syncope (5)[C].
- Vasovagal syncope:
  – 3 phases: Prodrome, loss of consciousness, and postsyncope
  – Precipitating event or stimulus is usually identified, such as panic, fright, pain, or exercise.
  – Athletes may have syncope after exertion (diagnosis of exclusion)
  – Position: *Can be preceded by prolonged standing, but can occur from any position; generally resolves when the patient becomes supine:*
    ○ Preceding events: As discussed above
    ○ Prodrome: As listed above for neurally mediated syncope
  – Duration: Generally brief (seconds–minutes)
  – Recovery: May be prolonged with persistent nausea, pallor, and diaphoresis, but without neurologic change or confusion
- Carotid sinus syncope is precipitated by position change, after turning head, or wearing a tight collar.
- Situational syncope is related to micturition, defecation, or coughing.
- Glossopharyngeal syncope (less common) is related to throat or facial pain (4)[C]:
  – Precipitating events or situations may include panic, pain, exercise, micturition, defecation, coughing, or swallowing.

PHYSICAL EXAM
- Vital signs, including orthostatics and bilateral BP
- Cardiac exam: Volume status, murmurs, rhythm, carotid bruits
- Neurologic exam: Signs of focal deficit
- Assess for occult blood loss, including guaiac.
- Dix-Hallpike maneuver to rule out benign paroxysmal vertigo

DIFFERENTIAL DIAGNOSIS
- Seizure
- Hypoglycemia
- Cardiac syncope
- Cerebrovascular syncope
- Orthostatic hypotension
- Drop attacks
- Psychiatric illness

DIAGNOSTIC TESTS & INTERPRETATION
As indicated by history and physical
Includes basic tests to rule out the 3 main reasons for syncope: Hypoglycemia, arrhythmia, and anemia

Initial Tests (lab, imaging)
- Blood sugar
- ECG should be ordered for all patients. Abnormal ECG findings are common in patients with cardiac syncope.
- CBC to rule out anemia
- Only obtain Head CT, MRI/MRA, carotid ultrasound in patients whose history or physical exam suggests a neurologic or worrisome cause (i.e., patients with seizures, chest pain, headache, abdominal pain, dyspnea, hemorrhage, hypotension, or a new neurologic deficit):
  – The 2007 American College of Emergency
  – Physicians (ACEP) Guidelines for diagnostic testing (6):
    ○ *Level A recommendations:* Standard 12-lead ECG
    ○ *Level B recommendations:* None specified
    ○ *Level C recommendations:* Laboratory testing and investigations, including echocardiography or head CT, to be performed only if indicated by specific findings in the history or physical exam

Follow-Up Tests & Special Considerations
- 24-hour Holter monitoring only in patients with a high probability of cardiac cause of syncope and/or abnormal ECG findings
- A low hemoglobin without obvious cause of bleed would warrant a guaiac, CT abdomen, CT head to rule out retroperitoneal bleed, subarachnoid hemorrhage (SAH).
- Negative imaging will prompt workup for alternative causes.
- Stroke, bleed, or carotid stenosis will require appropriate disease-oriented management.
- EEG only when history or physical exam is very suggestive of seizure activity

Diagnostic Procedures/Other
- Head-up tilt-table testing:
  – Contraindicated in patients with known cardiac or neurovascular disease or in pregnancy
  – Indicated for recurrent syncope or single episode accompanied by injury or risk to others (e.g., pilots, surgeons)
  – Uses positional changes to reproduce symptoms
  – Positive tests are diagnostic for vasovagal syncope.
- Carotid sinus massage, only in a monitored setting (i.e., BP and HR monitoring, IV access):
  – Contraindicated in patients with carotid disease (careful auscultation prior to massage is essential)
  – Pressure at the angle of the jaw for 5 seconds with simultaneous ECG monitoring
  – Positive tests (causing syncope or cardiac pause >3 seconds) are diagnostic of carotid sinus syncope.
- Psychiatric evaluation: To rule out anxiety, depression, and alcohol abuse

TREATMENT

Therapy is primarily for recurrent syncope. Situational syncope will not warrant any treatment.

GENERAL MEASURES

Recognition and avoidance of precipitating events or situations

MEDICATION

Medical management is based on small, nonrandomized clinical trials.

First Line

- Nonpharmacologic treatment:
  – Includes patient counseling:
  ○ Development of coping skills
  ○ Increased salt and fluid intake
  – Moderate exercise training
  – Tilt-table training:
  ○ Progressively prolonged periods of enforced upright posture
  – Intense gripping of the hands and tensing of the arms for 2 minutes at the onset of tilt-induced symptoms raises systolic BP (7)[C].

Second Line

- α-Agonists are mainly used for orthostatic hypotension:
  – Midodrine is commonly used. It increases peripheral vascular resistance and venous return. Side effects include HTN, paresthesia, urinary retention, "goose bumps," hyperactivity, dizziness, tremor, and nervousness.
- SSRIs: Paroxetine, fluoxetine, and sertraline are SSRIs useful in treating neurocardiogenic/vasovagal syncope:
  – Serotonin induces vagally mediated bradycardia and hypotension.
  – Side effects include weight gain, nausea, anxiety, sexual dysfunction, and insomnia.
- Mineralocorticoids: Fludrocortisone has been found helpful mainly in orthostatic hypotension:
  – Helpful in renal sodium absorption and increasing the vasoconstrictive peripheral vascular response
  – Adverse reactions include fluid retention, HTN, CHF, peripheral edema, and hypokalemia.
- β-Blockers: Metoprolol, atenolol, or pindolol are mainly used for postural tachycardia syndrome (POTS):
  – Block peripheral vasodilators and ventricular mechanoreceptor stimulation
  – Stabilization of HR and BP
  – Side effects: Hypotension and bradycardia (with worsening of syncope), fatigue, depression, and sexual dysfunction
  – Contraindicated in asthma

ISSUES FOR REFERRAL

Neurology or cardiology, as needed

ADDITIONAL THERAPIES

- Increased salt and fluid intake: May include salt tablets or electrolyte/sports drinks
- Moderate exercise training
- Tilt-table training: Involves periods of prolonged, forced upright posture
- Use of support/pressure stockings
- Leg crossing, hand grip, or arm tensing

SURGERY/OTHER PROCEDURES

Pacemaker placement may be of use in patients with frequent neurocardiogenic/vasovagal syncope that is refractory to other therapies (7)[C]:

- Prevents prolonged bradycardia or asystole during syncopal episodes
- Long-term effect
- Invasive placement procedure

COMPLEMENTARY AND ALTERNATIVE MEDICINE

These include treatments for underlying heart disease or precipitating factors like anxiety. None of these is a proven therapy:

- Nutrition and supplements: Omega-3 fatty acids, multivitamin, CoQ10, acetyl-L-carnitine, alpha-lipoic acid, and L-arginine
- Herbs: Green tea (Camellia sinensis), bilberry (Vaccinium myrtillus), ginkgo (Ginkgo biloba)
- Homeopathy: Carbo vegetabilis, opium, sepia
- Acupuncture: An analysis of 102 serious cases showed improvement in most. It may precipitate fainting.

IN-PATIENT CONSIDERATIONS

Admission Criteria/Initial Stabilization

2007 ACEP Guidelines mandate that the patient be admitted if (6):

- Level B recommendations:
  – Admit patients with syncope and evidence of heart failure or structural heart disease.
  – Admit patients with syncope and high-risk factors.
- High-risk stratification is based on following factors:
  – Older age and associated comorbidities
  – Abnormal ECG, hematocrit (Hct) 30 (if obtained)
  – History or presence of heart failure, coronary artery disease, or structural heart disease
- Additional causes to admit:
  – Syncope occurring during exercise
  – Syncope causing severe injury
  – Family history of sudden death

IV Fluids

IV fluids to stabilize HR and BP: Isotonic crystalloids, as needed

Nursing

Vital sign monitoring

Discharge Criteria

Hemodynamically stable and workup satisfactory

 ONGOING CARE

DIET

- Increased salt intake may be helpful if not contraindicated (2)[C].
- Maintain fluid intake.

PATIENT EDUCATION

- To identify and avoid precipitating events or situations
- Avoid dehydration, alcohol consumption, warm environments, tight clothing, and long periods of standing motionless.
- Recognize presyncopal symptoms.
- Use behaviors, such as lying down, to avoid syncope.

PROGNOSIS

May be recurrent, but not life-threatening

COMPLICATIONS

May result in injury from fall

REFERENCES

1. Angaran P, Klein GJ, Yee R, et al. Syncope. Neurol Clin. 2011;29(4):903–925.
2. Nair N. Pathophysiology and management of neurocardiogenic syncope. Am J Managed Care. 2003;9:327–334.
3. Gauer RL. Evaluation of syncope. Am Fam Physician. 2011;84(6):640–650.
4. Chen-Scarabelli C. Neurocardiogenic syncope. Br Med J. 2004;329:336.
5. Chen LY, Benditt DG, Shen WK. Management of syncope in adults: An update. Mayo Clin Proc. 2008;83:1280–1293.
6. Huff S, Decker W. Clinical policy: Critical issues in the evaluation and management of adult patients presenting to the emergency department with syncope. Ann Emerg Med. 2007;49:431–444.
7. Grubb BP. Clinical practice. Neurocardiogenic syncope. N Engl J Med. 2005;352(10):1004–1010.

ADDITIONAL READING

- Lelonek M. [Genetics in neurocardiogenic syncope]. Prz Lek. 2006;63:1310–1312.
- Márquez MF, Urias-Medina K, Gómez-Flores J, et al. [Comparison of metoprolol vs clonazepam as a first treatment choice among patients with neurocardiogenic syncope]. Gac Med Mex. 2008;144:503–507.

 SEE ALSO

Algorithms: Syncope; Transient Ischemic Attack and Transient Neurologic Deficit

 CODES

ICD10

R55 Syncope and collapse

CLINICAL PEARLS

- History should include a careful analysis of the events preceding the attack.
- It is important to rule out cardiologic or neurologic pathology.
- Prodrome is often present.
- Recovery may be prolonged, with persistent symptoms but no neurologic deficit or confusion.
- Test only if worrisome history or PE.
- Counseling patient to avoid precipitating situations or events is first-line treatment.

S

SYPHILIS
Melissa Badowski, PharmD • Mahesh C. Patel, MD

 BASICS

DESCRIPTION
- A chronic, systemic infectious disease caused by *Treponema pallidum*
- Transmitted sexually, maternal–fetal, contact with an active lesion, and via blood transfusions
- Untreated disease includes 4 overlapping stages:
  - Primary: Usually single painless chancre at point of entry; appears in 10–90 days; chancre heals without treatment in 3–6 weeks
  - Secondary: Appears 2–8 weeks after primary chancre. Nonpruritic rash on palms or soles of feet, mucous membrane lesions, headache, fever, lymphadenopathy
  - Latent: Seroreactive without evidence of disease:
    ○ Early latent: Acquired within the last year
    ○ Late latent: Exposure >12 months prior to diagnosis
  - Tertiary (late): Serology may be negative (although fluorescent treponemal antibody absorption [FTA-ABS] test is positive almost 100%):
    ○ Refers to gumma and cardiovascular and late neurosyphilis; may be lethal
  - Neurosyphilis: Represents *any* type of CNS involvement with syphilis and can occur at *any* stage:
    ○ Psychosis, delirium, dementia
- Ability to affect nearly every organ/tissue in the body has led to it being called "the great imitator."

Pediatric Considerations
In noncongenital cases, consider child abuse.

Pregnancy Considerations
- All pregnant patients should have VDRL or rapid plasma reagin (RPR) test at 1st prenatal visit (1). If high exposure risk, repeat the tests at 28 weeks and at delivery (2)[A].
- The same nontreponemal test for initial diagnosis also should be used for follow-up tests.

EPIDEMIOLOGY
Incidence
- Syphilis rate decreased until 2000, increasing primarily in men since then (3).
- In 2010: 14.9/100,000 population (an increase of 2.2% from 2009) (4):
  - Highest in both men and women aged 20–24 years:
    ○ Men: 7.9/100,000
    ○ Women: 1.1/100,000
  - Congenital: 8.7 cases/100,000 live births
- Race/Ethnicity (3):
  - Caucasian, non-Hispanic: 2.1/100,000
  - African American: 16.8/100,000
  - Hispanic: 4.6/100,000
  - Asian/Pacific Islander: 1.3/100,000
  - Native American/Alaska native: 2.5/100,000

Prevalence
- Predominant sex: Male > Female (7:1)
- Increasing male-to-female ratio (was 1.2:1 in 1996) suggests greatest syphilis increase in men having sex with men (MSM).

ETIOLOGY AND PATHOPHYSIOLOGY
T. pallidum subspecies *pallidum*, spirochete

RISK FACTORS
MSM, multiple sexual partners, exposure to infected body fluids, IV drug use, transplacental transmission, adult inmates, high-risk sexual behavior, HIV positive

GENERAL PREVENTION
Education; condoms reduce, but do not eliminate transmission (5)[A].

COMMONLY ASSOCIATED CONDITIONS
HIV infection, hepatitis B, other STIs

 DIAGNOSIS

HISTORY
Previous sexual contact with partner with known infection/partner with high-risk sexual behavior

PHYSICAL EXAM
Signs/Symptoms depend on stage:
- Primary: Single (occasionally multiple), usually painless ulcer (chancre) in groin or at other point of entry
- Secondary:
  - Rash: Skin/Mucous membranes:
    ○ Rough, red–brown macules, usually on palms and soles
    ○ May appear with chancre or after it has healed
  - Nonspecific symptoms: Fever, adenopathy, malaise, headache

DIFFERENTIAL DIAGNOSIS
- Primary: Chancroid, lymphogranuloma venereum, granuloma inguinale, condyloma acuminata, herpes simplex, Behçet syndrome, trauma, carcinoma, mycotic infection, lichen planus, psoriasis, fungal infection
- Secondary: Pityriasis rosea, drug eruption, psoriasis, lichen planus, viral exanthema, Stevens-Johnson syndrome
- Positive serology, asymptomatic: Previously treated syphilis/other spirochetal disease (yaws, pinta)

DIAGNOSTIC TESTS & INTERPRETATION
Initial Tests (lab, imaging)
- Dark-field microscopy demonstrating *T. pallidum* spirochetes in lesion exudate/tissue biopsy: Gold standard, but difficult and not very sensitive
- Nontreponemal tests (VDRL/RPR):
  - Primary screening test: Positive within 7 days of exposure
  - Nonspecific, false-positive results common; must confirm diagnosis with treponemal tests
  - Positive test should be quantified and titers followed at regular intervals after treatment (6):
    ○ Titers usually correlate with disease activity; 4-fold change demonstrates clinically significant difference (6).
    ○ Titer decreases with time/treatment; following adequate treatment for primary/secondary disease, a 4-fold decline is typically seen after 6–12 months.
    ○ Absence of a 4-fold decline may indicate treatment failure.
    ○ >15% of appropriately treated patients do not have a 4-fold decline in titer 12 months after treatment (6). Management is unclear, but consideration should be given to repeat HIV testing and/or examination of the CSF, as well as close follow-up of titers.
    ○ Titers eventually should be negative (see "serofast reaction" below).

- ○ Titers of patients treated in latent stages decline more gradually.
  - Prozone phenomenon: Negative results from high titers of antibody; test diluted serum
  - Serofast reaction: Persistently positive results years after successful treatment; new infection diagnosed by 4-fold rise in titer
  - Disorders that may alter lab results (noting that all stages of syphilis can have a false-negative RPR result, especially in primary syphilis):
    ○ Pregnancy, autoimmune disease, mononucleosis, malaria, leprosy, viral pneumonia, presence of cardiolipin antigens, injection drug use, acute febrile illness, HIV infection; elderly can have false-positive results
- Treponemal tests (*confirmatory test after positive nontreponemal screening test*): FTA-ABS, TP-PA: (*T. pallidum* particle agglutination):
  - FTA-ABS, TP-PA
  - Confirmatory test; not used for screening
  - Usually positive for life after treatment
  - Titers of no benefit
  - 15–25% of patients treated during the primary stage revert to being serologically nonreactive after 2–3 years.
- Lumbar puncture:
  - Indicated if clinical evidence of neurologic involvement or has syphilitic ocular/auditory manifestations
  - Some experts advise in all secondary and early latent cases without neurologic symptoms
  - In some HIV-positive patients with late latent/latent of unknown duration
  - In select patients with late latent/latent of unknown duration/when nonpenicillin therapy is planned
  - In treatment failures
  - If other evidence of active tertiary syphilis is present (e.g., aortitis, gumma, iritis)
  - In children with syphilis, after the newborn period, and to rule out neurosyphilis
  - VDRL, not RPR, used on CSF; may be negative in neurosyphilis; highly specific but insensitive
  - Send fluid for protein, glucose, and cell count.
  - Monitor resolution by cell count at 6 months along with serologies as recommended (see "Patient Monitoring").
  - Negative FTA-ABS or microhemagglutination (MHA)-TP on CSF excludes neurosyphilis (highly sensitive)
  - Positive FTA-ABS or MHA-TP on CSF not diagnostic because of high false-positive rate
  - Bloody tap, tuberculosis (TB), pyogenic/aseptic meningitis can result in false-positive VDRL finding.

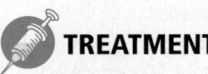 **TREATMENT**

GENERAL MEASURES
- Advise patients to avoid intercourse until treatment is complete and keep track of partners.
- All persons who have syphilis should be tested for HIV.
- Management of sexual contacts:
  - Those exposed within 90 days of diagnosis, treat presumptively.
  - Those exposed >90 days before diagnosis should be treated presumptively if serologic test results are not available immediately and follow-up is uncertain.

– Those exposed to a patient diagnosed with syphilis of unknown duration and who have high treponemal titers (>1:32) should be treated presumptively.
– Long-term sex partners of patients with latent infection should be evaluated clinically and serologically and treated on the basis of findings.

MEDICATION
First Line
Parenteral penicillin G is drug of choice for all stages (6)[A]. Choice of formulation is determined by the disease stage and clinical manifestations.

ALERT
- Bicillin L-A should be used and *not* Bicillin C-R (combination benzathine–procaine penicillin) when penicillin G benzathine is indicated (6)[A].
- Primary, secondary, and early latent <1 year:
  – Benzathine penicillin G 2.4 million units IM for 1 dose (6)[A]
  – Penicillin-allergic patients: Doxycycline 100 mg PO b.i.d. × 2 weeks, or tetracycline 500 mg PO q.i.d. × 2 weeks, or ceftriaxone 1 g IM or IV daily × 10–14 days:
    ○ Azithromycin 2 g PO × 1 dose (early syphilis only; should not be used in MSM or pregnancy).
    ○ Resistance and treatment failures have been noted in several geographical locations in the US.
- Late latent/Latent of unknown duration and tertiary without evidence of neurosyphilis:
  – Benzathine penicillin G 2.4 million units IM weekly × 3 doses (6)[A]
  – Penicillin-allergic patients: Attempt desensitization and treatment with penicillin or doxycycline 100 mg PO 2 b.i.d. × 28 days, *or* tetracycline 500 mg PO q.i.d.× 28 days; compliance may be an issue
- Neurosyphilis:
  – Aqueous crystalline penicillin G 3–4 million units IV q4h or continuous infusion × 10–14 days
  – Procaine penicillin G 2.4 million units IM daily in conjunction with probenecid 500 mg PO q.i.d. × 10–14 days (if compliance can be ensured) (6)[A]
  – Penicillin-allergic patients: Attempt desensitization and treat with penicillin; ceftriaxone 2 g/d IM or IV × 10–14 days
  – If late latent, latent of unknown duration, or tertiary in addition to neurosyphilis, consider also treating as recommended for late latent after completion of neurosyphilis treatment.
- Congenital:
  – Aqueous crystalline penicillin G 50,000 U/kg/dose IV q12h × first 7 days of life and q8h thereafter for a total of 10 days, or procaine penicillin G 50,000 U/kg/dose IM daily × 10 days (6)[A]
  – If negative CSF serologies, normal physical exam, and titer: Maternal titer, then 50,000 U/kg benzathine penicillin G IM in single dose is also alternative (6)[A].
  – If >1 day of drug is missed, restart course.
  – Children (after newborn period): Aqueous crystalline penicillin G 50,000 U/kg/dose IV q4–6h × 10 days; late latent, 50,000 U/kg IM as 3 doses at 1-week intervals (6)[A]

– Epidemiologic treatment for contacts without symptoms: Treat as primary after serologies.
– HIV-infected and pregnant patients may show poor response to recommended IM doses. Use IV therapy for all treatment failures in these patients.
– Do not give benzathine or procaine penicillins IV.
- Children (after newborn period): Aqueous crystalline penicillin G 50,000 U/kg/dose IV q4–6h × 10 days; late latent, 50,000 U/kg IM as 3 doses at 1-week intervals (6)[A]
- Pregnancy:
  – Treatment same as for nonpregnant patients
  – Some specialists recommend 2nd dose of 2.4 million units benzathine penicillin G 1 week after initial dose in 3rd trimester or with primary, secondary, or early latent syphilis
  – Penicillin sensitivity: No proven alternatives to penicillin exist for treatment during pregnancy.
  – Consider desensitization and treatment with penicillin (6)[A].
  – Epidemiologic treatment for contacts without symptoms: Treat as primary after serologies.
  – HIV-infected and pregnant patients may show poor response to recommended IM doses. Use IV therapy for all treatment failures in these patients.
  – Do not give benzathine or procaine penicillins IV.
- Epidemiologic treatment for contacts without symptoms: Treat as primary after serologies.
- Precautions:
  – HIV-infected and pregnant patients may show poor response to recommended IM doses. Use IV therapy for all treatment failures in these patients.
  – Do not give benzathine or procaine penicillins IV.

ONGOING CARE

FOLLOW-UP RECOMMENDATIONS
- Clinical and serologic evaluation at 6 and 12 months after treatment; if >1 year's duration, check at 24 months also.
- In HIV-infected persons, clinical and serologic evaluation at 3, 6, 9, 12, and 24 months after therapy.

Patient Monitoring
- Use VDRL or RPR test to monitor therapy: 4-fold rise in titer indicates new infection, whereas failure to decrease 4-fold in 6–12 months may indicate treatment failure (although definitive criteria for cure not established); titers not consistent between tests; always use same test, preferably same lab, as initially.
- Strongly consider retreatment for persistent clinical signs or recurrence, 4-fold rise in titers, or failure of initially high titer to decrease 4-fold by 6–12 months.
- Labs titer tests to final endpoint (e.g., do not report as ">1:512") to make best use of results in monitoring therapy response.
- Neurosyphilis: Repeat lumbar puncture every 6 months to check for normalization of CSF cell count (± CSF-VDRL and protein evaluation).

PATIENT EDUCATION
No sexual contacts until 4-fold titer drop

PROGNOSIS
- Excellent in all cases except patients with late syphilis complications and with HIV infection
- Syphilis in HIV-infected patient:
  – Treatment same as for HIV-negative patients
  – More often false-negative treponemal and nontreponemal tests or unusually high titers
  – Response to therapy less predictable
  – Early syphilis: Increased risk of neurosyphilis and higher rates of treatment failure
  – Late neurosyphilis: Harder to treat; can occur up to 20+ years after infection

COMPLICATIONS
- Cardiovascular
- Membranous glomerulonephritis
- Paroxysmal cold hemoglobinemia
- Meningitis and tabes dorsalis
- Irreversible organ damage
- Jarisch-Herxheimer reaction:
  – Fever, chills, headache, myalgias, new rash
  – Common when starting treatment (of primary/secondary disease; less common with tertiary) owing to lysis of treponemes
  – Should not be confused with drug reaction
  – Managed with analgesics and antipyretics

REFERENCES
1. U.S. Preventive Services Task Force. Screening for syphilis infection in pregnancy: U.S. Preventive Services Task Force reaffirmation recommendation statement. *Ann Intern Med.* 2009;150:705–709.
2. Gomez GB, Kamb ML, Newman LM, et al. Untreated maternal syphilis and adverse outcomes of pregnancy: A systematic review and meta-analysis. *Bull World Health Org.* 2013;91(3): 217–226.
3. Centers for Disease Control and Prevention. *Sexually Transmitted Disease Surveillance 2007 Supplement, Syphilis Surveillance Report.* Atlanta, GA: U.S. Department of Health and Human Services, Centers for Disease Control and Prevention, March 2009.
4. Centers for Disease Control and Prevention. *2010 Sexually Transmitted Diseases Surveillance.* Atlanta, GA, November 2011.
5. Koss CA, Dunne EF, Warner L, et al. A systematic review of epidemiologic studies assessing condom use and risk of syphilis. *Sex Transm Dis.* 2009;36: 401–405.
6. CDC Sexually Transmitted Diseases Treatment Guidelines, 2010. *MMWR Weekly.* 2010;59(RR-12):26–36.

 SEE ALSO

Chlamydial Sexually Transmitted Diseases; Gonococcal Infections

 CODES

ICD10
- A51.0 Primary genital syphilis
- A53.0 Latent syphilis, unspecified as early or late
- A53.9 Syphilis, unspecified

CLINICAL PEARLS
All patients with high-risk activity or HIV-positive status should be screened for syphilis.

TARSAL TUNNEL SYNDROME

Christie Langenberg, MD • Gregory Murphy, MD • J. Herbert Stevenson, MD

 BASICS

DESCRIPTION
Tarsal tunnel syndrome is a compression neuropathy of the posterior tibial nerve as it passes behind the medial malleolus and under the flexor retinaculum (laciniate ligament) in the medial ankle, a region commonly known as the tarsal tunnel.

Pregnancy Considerations
- Tarsal tunnel syndrome can occur during pregnancy, typically secondary to local compression caused by fluid retention and volume changes.
- Care usually is supportive until after delivery because many cases resolve after pregnancy.

EPIDEMIOLOGY
- Women are slightly more affected than men (56%).
- Individuals in all postpubescent ages can be affected.

ETIOLOGY AND PATHOPHYSIOLOGY
- The posterior tibial nerve passes through the tarsal tunnel, which is formed by the 3 osseus structures—sustentaculum tali, medial calcaneus, and medial malleolus—and covered by the laciniate ligament
- Compression of the posterior tibial nerve within the confined space of the tarsal tunnel results in decreased blood flow and ischemic damage.
- Chronic compression can destroy endoneurial microvasculature, leading to edema and eventually fibrosis and demyelination (1).
- Increased pressure in the tarsal tunnel can be caused by a variety of mechanisms, both mechanical and biochemical. The specific cause for compression is identifiable in only 60–80% of patients (2); causes can be grouped into 3 categories: Trauma, space-occupying lesion, and deformity.
- Most common causes include (2):
  – Trauma including displaced fractures, deltoid ligament sprains, or tenosynovitis
  – Varicosities
  – Hindfoot varus or valgus
  – Fibrosis of the perineurium
- Other causes of compression include:
  – Osseous prominences
  – Ganglia
  – Lipoma
  – Neurolemmoma
  – Inflammatory synovitis
  – Pigmented villonodular synovitis
  – Tarsal coalition
  – Accessory musculature
- In patients with a systemic disease such as diabetes, "double-crush" syndrome should be considered; this refers to the development of a 2nd compression along the same nerve at a site of anatomic narrowing in patients with previous proximal nerve damage (3).
- Tarsal tunnel decompression may improve sensory impairment and restore protective sensation in diabetic peripheral neuropathies where there is nerve entrapment at the tarsal tunnel (4)[C]

RISK FACTORS
- Several have associated tarsal tunnel syndrome with certain occupations and activities, especially those that involve repetitive weight bearing on the foot and ankle, like jogging (5) or dancing (6).
- Other possible risk factors include (3):
  – Diabetes
  – Systemic inflammatory arthritis
  – Connective tissue disorders
  – Obesity
  – Varicosities
  – Heel varus or valgus
  – Bifurcation of the posterior tibial nerve into medial and lateral plantar nerves proximal to the tarsal tunnel

 DIAGNOSIS

Tarsal tunnel syndrome remains largely a clinical diagnosis, with tibial nerve compression indicated by pain and paresthesias along the course of the nerve and a positive Tinel sign (3).

HISTORY
- Often history of trauma to the foot, including trivial trauma that precipitated pain
- Classically, pain and paresthesia on the plantar aspect of the foot and/or posteromedial ankle
- Pain usually worsens during standing or activity.
- Pain can radiate proximally up medial leg (Valleix phenomenon) in 33% of patients with severe compression or distally along the path of involved nerves (2).
- Some patients have substantial night pain, which may be related to venostasis.
- Symptoms improve with rest, wearing loose footwear, and elevation.
- In advanced nerve compression, motor involvement may cause weakness, atrophy, and digital contractures of the intrinsic foot muscles (3).

ALERT
Other neuropathies due to systemic causes, such as diabetes, alcoholism, HIV, or drug reactions, can present with similar symptoms.

PHYSICAL EXAM
- Perform a complete foot and ankle examination
- Foot alignment:
  – Examine for hindfoot varus or valgus abnormalities
  – Exaggerating heel dorsiflexion, inversion, or eversion may reproduce symptoms by stretching or compressing the nerve.
- Palpate the tarsal tunnel and the course of the tibial nerve for:
  – Tenderness
  – Swelling consistent with a space-occupying lesion
- Tinel sign: Percussion over the course of the tibial nerve may produce paresthesia that radiates distally.
- Valleix sign: Percussion over the course of the tibial nerve may produce paresthesia that radiates proximally.

- Cuff test: Using a pneumatic cuff to create a venous tourniquet may cause engorgement of varicosities and reproduce symptoms.
- Compression test: Applying pressure to the tarsal tunnel for 60 seconds may reproduce symptoms.
- Sensory examination:
  – The medial calcaneal nerve usually is spared, but numbness and altered sensation may be present in the distribution of the medial or lateral plantar nerve.
  – Vibratory sensation and 2-point discrimination are decreased early in the disease process.
- Motor examination:
  – Intrinsic weakness is difficult to assess.
  – Rarely, weakness of toe plantarflexion may be present.
  – Atrophy of the abductor hallucis or abductor digiti minimi may be seen late in the disease process.

DIFFERENTIAL DIAGNOSIS
- Peripheral neuropathies (diabetes, alcoholism, HIV, or drug related)
- Inflammatory arthritis (rheumatoid arthritis) (7)
- Morton neuroma
- Metatarsalgia
- Subtalar joint arthritis
- Tibialis posterior tendinitis/dysfunction
- Plantar fasciitis
- Plantar callosities
- Peripheral vascular disease
- Lumbar radiculopathy
- Proximal injury or compression of the tibial branch of the sciatic nerve

DIAGNOSTIC TESTS & INTERPRETATION
Initial Tests (lab, imaging)
Routine lab tests can be used to rule out other conditions that may mimic tarsal tunnel syndrome, including diabetic neuropathy, rheumatoid arthritis, thyroid dysfunction, or other systemic illnesses (8).
- Routine weight-bearing radiographs, followed by CT if necessary to assess for fracture or structural abnormality
- Consider evaluation of lumbar spine x-ray if double-crush (injury to lumbar nerve results in compensatory injury to posterior tibial nerve) is suspected (8).
- MRI: Can be helpful in assessing the tarsal tunnel for soft tissue masses or other sources of nerve compression before surgery (2).
- US: Alternatively, US can be used to check for synovitis or ganglia (8).

Pediatric Considerations
MRI is recommended for evaluating pediatric tarsal tunnel syndrome because compression by a neoplastic mass is not uncommon.

Follow-Up Tests & Special Considerations
Postoperative management includes:
- Non–weight-bearing splint until incision heals (2–3 weeks), followed by progressively increased weight-bearing and range of motion exercises
- RICE protocol (rest, ice, compression, elevation) to limit swelling

Diagnostic Procedures/Other

Electrodiagnostic studies (2):

- According to a systematic review in 2005, electromyography (EMG) of the intrinsic muscles of the foot can be used only to confirm the diagnosis of tarsal tunnel syndrome because there is a large percentage of asymptomatic people with abnormal results (9). However, a normal EMG does not exclude the diagnosis as there is a false-negative rate of around 10% (2).
- A nerve conduction study may reveal slowed conduction of the tibial nerve.
- It is important to evaluate for proximal nerve compression, including a lumbar radiculopathy or a double-crush phenomenon.

Test Interpretation

At the time of surgical exploration, the following may be found:

- Focal swelling, scarring, or nerve abnormalities
- A pathologic source of compression

 TREATMENT

Conservative management is recommended, except for tarsal tunnel syndrome of acute onset or in the setting of a known space-occupying lesion (excluding synovitis).

MEDICATION

First Line

- Analgesics and anti-inflammatories
- Corticosteroid injection
- Medications that alter neurogenic pain (tricyclic antidepressants, antiepileptic drugs, nerve blockers)

ADDITIONAL THERAPIES

- Rest/Immobilization
- Taping and bracing
- Orthotics or shoe modification
- Physical therapy for desensitization (stretching, US, massage, icing)
- Physical therapy to strengthen the intrinsic and extrinsic muscles of the foot and to restore the medial longitudinal arch
- Compression stockings to decrease swelling
- Weight loss in obese patients

SURGERY/OTHER PROCEDURES

- Surgery is indicated (1,2,10):
  - If nonoperative measures fail following a 3–6-month trial
  - In the setting of acute tarsal tunnel syndrome
  - If a space-occupying lesion is identified
- The surgical outcome is dependent on technique and postoperative management. The ability to achieve a good to excellent outcome ranges from 50–95%.

 ONGOING CARE

PATIENT EDUCATION

- An outline of the conservative care modalities available should be presented.
- Use of each of these therapies will depend on patient circumstance.
- A decision about surgical intervention should be made with a clear understanding of limitations of this treatment and the potential adverse outcomes.

PROGNOSIS

The most symptomatic improvement with surgery is expected for (2):

- Young patients
- Short duration of symptoms
- Localized space-occupying lesion identified (10)
- No motor neuron involvement
- Surgical outcomes are dependent on technique and postoperative management.

COMPLICATIONS

- The main adverse outcome is unsuccessful surgical intervention: No improvement, partial/incomplete improvement, or temporary improvement with recurrence of symptoms (2).
- Causes for a failed tarsal tunnel release:
  - Incorrect diagnosis
  - Incomplete release
  - Adhesive neuritis (external scar formation)
  - Intraneural damage (systemic disease, direct nerve injury)
  - Failure to treat all sources of nerve compression in a double-crush phenomenon
- Electrodiagnostic studies are rarely helpful in determining the cause of a failed tarsal tunnel release.
- Revision surgery results are poorer than for the primary surgical release.

REFERENCES

1. Dellon AL. The four medial ankle tunnels: A critical review of perceptions of tarsal tunnel syndrome and neuropathy. *Neurosurg Clin North Am.* 2008;19:629–648.
2. Lau JT, Daniels TR. Tarsal tunnel syndrome: A review of the literature. *Foot Ankle Int.* 1999;20:201–209.
3. Reade BM, Longo DC, Keller MC. Tarsal tunnel syndrome. *Clin Podiatr Med Surg.* 2001;18:395–408.
4. Gondring WH, Tarun PK, Trepman E. Touch pressure and sensory density after tarsal tunnel release in diabetic neuropathy. *Foot Ankle Surg.* 2012;18:241–246.
5. Shapiro BE, Preston DC. Entrapment and compressive neuropathies. *Med Clin North Am.* 2009;93:285–315.
6. Kennedy JG, Baxter DE. Nerve disorders in dancers. *Clin Sports Med.* 2008;27:329–334.
7. Campbell WW, Landau ME. Controversial entrapment neuropathies. *Neurosurg Clin North Am.* 2008;19:597–608.
8. Franson J, Baravarian B. Tarsal tunnel syndrome: A compression neuropathy involving four distinct tunnels. *Clin Podiatr Med Surg.* 2006;23:597–609.
9. Patel AT, Gaines K, Malamut R, et al. Usefulness of electrodiagnostic techniques in the evaluation of suspected tarsal tunnel syndrome: An evidence-based review. *Muscle Nerve.* 2005;32:236–240.
10. Sung KS, Park SJ. Short-term operative outcome of tarsal tunnel syndrome due to benign space-occupying lesions. *Foot Ankle Int.* 2009;30:741–745.

ADDITIONAL READING

- Abouelela AA, Zohiery AK. The triple compression stress test for diagnosis of tarsal tunnel syndrome. *Foot.* 2012;22:146–149.
- Allen JM, Greer BJ, Sorge DG, et al. MR imaging of neuropathies of the leg, ankle, and foot. *Magn Reson Imaging Clin North Am.* 2008;16:117–131.
- Imai K, Ikoma K, Imai R, et al. Tarsal tunnel syndrome in hemodialysis patients: a case series. *Foot Ankle Int.* 2013;34:439–444.

 SEE ALSO

Algorithm: Foot Pain

 CODES

ICD10

- G57.50 Tarsal tunnel syndrome, unspecified lower limb
- G57.51 Tarsal tunnel syndrome, right lower limb
- G57.52 Tarsal tunnel syndrome, left lower limb

CLINICAL PEARLS

- Tinel sign: Percussion over the course of the tibial nerve produces paresthesias and distal symptoms over the plantar aspect of the foot (most sensitive and specific test) (1)
- EMG alone cannot be used to diagnose tarsal tunnel syndrome; it may only be used to confirm clinical diagnosis.
- Conservative management is recommended, except for tarsal tunnel syndrome of acute onset or in the setting of a known space-occupying lesion.

TEETHING
Frank J. Domino, MD

BASICS

DESCRIPTION
- Teething is the eruption of the primary or deciduous teeth, which most children experience without difficulty. It is a natural, gradual, and predictable process, with normal variation among infants.
- Primary (deciduous) teeth:
  - Primary tooth eruption usually begins at 5–7 months of age.
  - The order of primary tooth eruption and average age is:
    - Central mandibular incisors (5–7 months)
    - Central maxillary incisors (6–8 months)
    - Lateral mandibular incisors (7–10 months)
    - Lateral maxillary incisors (8–11 months)
    - Cuspids (16–20 months)
    - 1st molars (10–16 months)
    - 2nd molars (20–30 months)
  - Delayed eruption may be familial or due to systemic syndromes or nutritional deficiencies. Delayed eruption may also be seen with cleft palate (1) and lower birth weight (2,3).
  - Tooth eruption in premature infants occurs according to postconceptual age rather than age since birth (chronological age).
  - Natal/Neonatal teeth:
    - Natal teeth (present at birth) occur in 1/2,000 neonates.
    - Neonatal teeth erupt in the 1st month of life.
    - Natal/Neonatal teeth are most often prematurely erupted primary (deciduous) teeth, but may be supernumerary.
    - 15–20% of cases are familial; also may be secondary to a syndrome or congenital anomalies of the head and neck.
    - Natal/Neonatal teeth may be loose, but most are the normal deciduous lower central incisors and can persist.
    - Natal/Neonatal teeth may be removed if there is an aspiration risk or if they cause trauma to the infant or to the mother (breastfeeding).
- System(s) affected: Gastrointestinal

EPIDEMIOLOGY
Incidence
Predominant age: Birth–3 years of age

ETIOLOGY AND PATHOPHYSIOLOGY
Teething symptoms are more common with eruption of the primary incisors (4)[B].

Genetics
Both premature and delayed tooth eruption may be familial. Primary failure of eruption has been linked to mutations of the *PTHR1* gene (5).

COMMONLY ASSOCIATED CONDITIONS
Teething may be coincident with other conditions, such as common childhood illnesses (e.g., roseola, viral gastroenteritis, upper respiratory infection) and serious bacterial infections, causing local or systemic signs and symptoms (e.g., fever, GI disturbance, fussiness, drooling, rash, and sleep disturbance).

DIAGNOSIS

HISTORY
- Biting
- Drooling
- Rubbing of gingivae
- Sucking
- Irritability
- Wakefulness
- Ear rubbing
- Facial rash
- Decreased appetite for solid foods
- Up to one-third of infants have no symptoms (6)[C]

PHYSICAL EXAM
- Infants may have no signs or symptoms of teething, although symptoms are present in most children (7).
- Excessive drooling and chewing on fingers begins at 3–4 months of age. This is also the time that normal hand–mouth stimulation increases salivation.
- Discomfort may be observed more commonly with the eruption of the 1st tooth, the molars, and/or with the simultaneous eruption of multiple teeth.
- Minor signs and symptoms of biting or chewing, drooling, irritability, facial rash, and low-grade fever (<101.9°F; 38.9°C) have been reported in association with teething, although no evidence identifies specific signs/symptoms caused by teething (8)[B].
- Serious signs and symptoms (e.g., fever >101.9°F; 38.9°C, dehydration) are not caused by teething and warrant evaluation for organic disease (8,9,10,11)[B].
- A small red or white spot may appear over the swollen gingivae just prior to tooth eruption.
- Local inflammation, swelling, or hematoma (bluish swelling) can be found on the involved gingivae overlying the erupting tooth. Gingival irritation was present in 96% of infants in one study (4)[B].

DIFFERENTIAL DIAGNOSIS
Herpetic gingivostomatitis: Infants with fever, irritability, sleeplessness, and difficulty feeding may have underlying infection caused by herpes simplex virus. Some infants with positive culture may not have evidence of inflammation or ulceration expected in gingivostomatitis.

DIAGNOSTIC TESTS & INTERPRETATION
Imaging
Radiographs can distinguish prematurely erupted primary teeth from supernumerary teeth.

TREATMENT

GENERAL MEASURES
- Education of mothers regarding common symptoms of teething and management options resulted in decreased use of pharmacologic treatment and increased use of other methods such as rubbing the gums (12).
- Treatment includes reassurance and symptomatic treatment.
- Provide the infant with a safe, 1-piece teething ring, clean cloth, or pacifier for gumming.
- Apply pressure over involved swollen gingivae with a clean finger or piece of wet gauze.
- May use cool (but not frozen) fluids, cold teething rings, or cold vegetables, such as a peeled cucumber
- Avoid the use of alcohol (historically rubbed on gingivae for an analgesic effect).
- Gingival hematomas that erupt appear as blue cysts. Most do not require medical intervention. Be sure there are no other signs of a bleeding disorder.
- Avoid:
  - Dipping a pacifier or teething ring in sugar or honey
  - Giving an infant a bottle in bed
  - Using fluid-filled teething rings (contents may leak)
  - Using frozen foods or teething rings (these could cause thermal damage to the tissues)
  - Tying a teething ring around infant's neck

MEDICATION
First Line
For an infant with low-grade fever, irritability, and/or inflamed gingivae (where other comforting measures have not been of help), acetaminophen in proper doses (15 mg/kg/dose q4–6h PRN) can be used.

Second Line
Topical analgesics are commonly used by parents (7).

ISSUES FOR REFERRAL
If tooth eruption is significantly delayed, consider referral to pediatric dentist.

Pediatric Considerations
Over-the-counter preparations for teething, such as lidocaine (Xylocaine 2%),or Benzocaine (Baby Ora-Gel, Num-Zit Gel, Num-Zit Liquid, Baby Anbesol), should be AVOIDED. Misuse, overuse, toxicity, and sensitivity have been reported (13):

- These are of questionable benefit because they are washed off quickly by saliva, and the benefit may be due in part to the pressure placed on the gingivae when applied (14).
  - FDA issued a warning about a possible effect of benzocaine, found in OTC teething gels, causing methemoglobinemia (15)

ADDITIONAL THERAPIES
Infants who bite or chew while breastfeeding can be trained not to bite by withdrawing the child from the breast for a moment, and then resume. Resist urge to startle the infant.

COMPLEMENTARY AND ALTERNATIVE MEDICINE
Homeopathy is used to treat teething. Calcarea carbonica (i.e., calcium carbonate) is one recommended treatment (16).

IN-PATIENT CONSIDERATIONS
Admission Criteria/Initial Stabilization
Outpatient

 ONGOING CARE

FOLLOW-UP RECOMMENDATIONS
No restrictions

DIET
Breastfeeding can continue during and after teething. Otherwise, no special diet required.

PATIENT EDUCATION
- Parents should be cautioned not to misinterpret teething as the cause of any systemic manifestation. The health provider should be consulted for any systemic complaints.
- American Dental Association, *For the Dental Patient: Tooth Eruption, the Primary Teeth*, 2005; www.ada.org
- Teething Tots: http://kidshealth.org/parent/pregnancy_newborn/common/teething.html

PROGNOSIS
Normal progression through the teething process without illness

REFERENCES

1. Kobayashi TY, Gomide MR, Carrara CF. Timing and sequence of primary tooth eruption in children with cleft lip and palate. *J Appl Oral Sci.* 2010;18:220–224.
2. Aktoren O, Tuna EB, Guven Y, et al. A study on neonatal factors and eruption time of primary teeth. *Community Dent Health.* 2010;27:52–56.
3. Sajjadian N, Shajari H, Jahadi R, et al. Relationship between birth weight and time of first deciduous tooth eruption in 143 consecutively born infants. *Pediatr Neonatol.* 2010;51:235–237.
4. Kiran K, Swati T, Kamala BK, et al. Prevalence of systemic and local disturbances in infants during primary teeth eruption: A clinical study. *Eur J Paediatr Dent.* 2011;12:249–252.
5. Stellzig-Eisenhauer A, Decker E, Meyer-Marcotty P, et al. Primary failure of eruption (PFE)—clinical and molecular genetics analysis. *J Orofac Orthop.* 2010;71:6–16.
6. Noor-Mohammed R, Basha S. Teething disturbances: Prevalence of objective manifestations in children under age 4 months to 36 months. *Med Oral Patol Oral Cir Bucal.* 2012;17:e491–e494.
7. Feldens CA, Faraco Jr. IM, Ottoni AB, et al. Teething symptoms in the first year of life and associated factors: A cohort study. *J Clin Pediatr Dent.* 2010;34:201–206.
8. Tighe M, Roe MF. Does a teething child need serious illness excluding? *Arch Dis Child.* 2007;92:266–268.
9. Macknin ML, Piedmonte M, Jacobs J, et al. Symptoms associated with infant teething: A prospective study. *Pediatrics.* 2000;105:747–752.
10. Ashley MP. It's only teething: A report on the myths and modern approaches to teething. *Br Dental J.* 2001;191:4–8.
11. Frank J, Drezner J. Is teething in infants associated with fever or other symptoms? *J Fam Pract.* 2001;50:257.
12. Plutzer K, Spencer AJ, Keirse MJ. How first-time mothers perceive and deal with teething symptoms: A randomized controlled trial. *Child Care Health Dev.* 2012;38(2):292–299. Epub 2011 Mar 6.
13. Williams GD, Kirk EP, Wilson CJ, et al. Salicylate intoxication from teething gel in infancy. *Med J Aust.* 2011;194:146–148.
14. McIntyre GT, McIntyre GM. Teething troubles? *Br Dental J.* 2002;192:251–255.
15. FDA Drug Safety Communication: Reports of a rare, but serious and potentially fatal adverse effect with the use of over-the-counter (OTC) benzocaine gels and liquids applied to the gums or mouth. Available at: www.fda.gov/Drugs/DrugSafety/ucm250024.htm.
16. Bergguist P. Therapeutic homeopathy. In: *Integrative Medicine*, 2nd ed. Philadelphia: Saunders; 2007:1181.

 CODES

ICD10
K00.7 Teething syndrome

CLINICAL PEARLS

- Teething is the natural, gradual, and predictable process of eruption of the primary or deciduous teeth, which most children experience without difficulty.
- Teething may cause discomfort, but does not cause significant fevers.
- Teething babies can still breastfeed. Babies can be taught not to bite, and breastfeeding may continue past 12 months of age without difficulty.

TELOGEN EFFLUVIUM
Adarsh K. Gupta, DO, MS, FACOFP

BASICS

Diffuse hair loss or hair thinning; most often an acute self-limited process

DESCRIPTION

Telogen effluvium (TE) is a transient condition in which there is a premature conversion of a significant proportion of anagen (growth phase) hairs into telogen (resting phase) hairs resulting in increased shedding of these resting hair follicles and the clinical appearance of moderate to severe hair thinning:

- 5 proposed types of TE:
  - Immediate anagen release: A highly common form, lasting 3–4 weeks, in which follicles meant to remain in anagen phase enter telogen prematurely due to a signal, including high fever, drug-induced, or stress (1).
  - Delayed anagen release: Occurs most often postpartum, in which a large group of hair follicles that have remained in the anagen phase for an extended period all together enter the telogen phase, resulting in hair loss (1)
  - Short anagen: A somewhat speculative type, in which at least 50% of the hair follicles have an idiopathic shortening of the anagen phase, resulting in a corresponding doubling of the follicles in the telogen phase (1).
  - Immediate telogen release: Normal resting club hairs remain within the hair follicle until an unknown signal causes their release, initiating the anagen stage to begin. In this type, the resting club hairs are prematurely released, ending the telogen phase abruptly and causing diffuse shedding (1).
  - Delayed telogen release: In this type, the presence of increased visible light, whether it be a seasonal or environmental change, is thought to end a prolonged telogen phase and initiate the anagen phase, resulting in diffuse shedding of hair follicles (1).

EPIDEMIOLOGY

Incidence
2nd most common cause of alopecia

Prevalence
Unknown

ETIOLOGY AND PATHOPHYSIOLOGY

The hair cycle consists of 2 predominant phases: The anagen (growth phase) and the telogen (resting phase), lasting ~3 years and 3 months, respectively. On the scalp, ~10–15% of hairs are in the telogen phase normally. Due to the presence of some types of external/internal stress, there may be an increase in the percentage of telogen hairs. As new anagen hairs emerge, these telogen hair follicles are forced out. The preceding event usually occurs 2–3 months prior to the appearance of hair loss.

It is hypothesized that substance P plays a key role in the pathogenesis of TE through various mechanisms. Studies have been conducted on human hair follicles in vitro and mice hair follicles in vivo which support this theory:

- Role of substance P includes:
  - Upregulation of substance P receptor, NK1, at the gene and protein level, leading to premature catagen development and hair growth inhibition (2)
  - Upregulation of nerve growth factor (NGF) and subsequently its hair apoptosis producing receptor, p75NTR (2)
  - Downregulation of hair-growth promoting receptor, TrkA (2)
  - Upregulation of major histocompatibility class (MHC) I and β_2-microglobulin resulting in loss of hair follicle immune-privilege (2)
  - Increase in tumor necrosis factor-α release by mast cells resulting in hair keratinocyte apoptosis (2)
- Decreased cortisol levels in chronic stress states may also enhance the effects of substance P (3).

RISK FACTORS

- Infection
- Trauma
- Major surgery
- Thyroid disorder
- Febrile illness
- Malignancy
- Allergic contact dermatitis (4)
- Iron deficiency anemia (5)
- Excess vitamin A (1)
- Protein-calorie restriction (1)
- End-stage liver or renal disease
- Hormonal changes (including pregnancy, delivery, and estrogen-containing medications) (1)
- Chronic stress
- Drug-induced (β-blockers, anticonvulsants, antidepressants, anticoagulants, retinoids, ACE-inhibitors, etc.) (1)
- Immunizations

DIAGNOSIS

HISTORY

- Commonly, an inciting event 2–6 months previous
- Fear of becoming bald
- Patients often present with bags of hair to emphasize the severity of their hair loss.

PHYSICAL EXAM

- Decreased density of hair on the scalp, most commonly involving the crown
- In rare cases of chronic TE, there is hair loss of eyebrows and pubic region.
- May be able to demonstrate diffuse shedding of hair when running fingers through scalp
- Shed hairs are telogen hairs, which have a small bulb of unpigmented or pigmented keratin on the root end.
- May effect nail growth, resulting in the appearance of Beau lines, which are transverse grooves on the nails of the hands and feet

DIFFERENTIAL DIAGNOSIS

- Hypothyroidism
- Hyperthyroidism
- Alopecia areata (diffuse-pattern)
- Androgenetic alopecia
- Drug-induced alopecia
- Systemic lupus erythematous
- Secondary syphilis
- Trichotillomania

DIAGNOSTIC TESTS & INTERPRETATION

Most often, TE is a clinical diagnosis of exclusion. Blood work may be collected primarily to rule out other possible causes of hair loss and/or to identify a possible cause for TE.

Initial Tests (lab, imaging)
If indicated:

- CBC, ferritin
- TSH
- Creatinine
- Consider hepatic enzymes
- Consider RPR/VDRL

Diagnostic Procedures/Other

- Hair pull test: Unreliable; performed by gently pulling 25–30 hairs from various sites on a patient's scalp. Each pull should elicit <5 normal club hairs; increased quantity may indicate possibility of TE (1).
- Hair clip test: Performed by cutting 25–30 hairs from the patient's scalp and examining them under a microscope. A negative test (not indicative of TE) will demonstrate <10% of hair shafts of small diameter. A positive test will demonstrate >10% of hair shafts of small diameter (1).
- Trichogram: ~50 hairs are plucked from the patient's scalp, and the number of telogen and anagen hairs present are counted. In TE, there will be >10% of hairs in the telogen phase.
- Scalp biopsy: Rarely needed; it is recommended that several 4-mm punch biopsies be obtained, all horizontally embedded to determine an accurate anagen-to-telogen ratio. Histologically, catagen-to-telogen hairs have numerous apoptotic cells in the outer sheath epithelium. >12–15% of hair follicles in telogen phase is consistent with TE (1,6).

TREATMENT

TE is a benign, self-limited process. Patient should be reassured that full hair growth will occur in ~6 months–1 year. No treatment is required.

MEDICATION

- Minoxidil: Stimulates hair regrowth via arteriolar smooth muscle vasodilation; not effective in TE
- Oral zinc therapy: New medication that may have benefits for patients with TE through various mechanisms all essential to hair growth, including (7):
  - Cofactor for enzymes needed in nucleic acid and protein synthesis and cell division
  - Inhibition of the catagen phase by blocking certain enzymes involved in hair apoptosis
  - Involved in hair growth regulation via hedgehog signaling

COMPLEMENTARY AND ALTERNATIVE MEDICINE

A nutritionist may be consulted to help evaluate the deficiencies or excess vitamin and mineral intake in a patient's diet. Rarely, cause of hair loss in well-nourished individuals.

REFERENCES

1. Headington JT. Telogen effluvium. New concepts and review. *Arch Dermatol*. 1993;84(3):356–363.
2. Peters EM, Liotiri S, Bodó E, et al. Probing the effects of stress mediators on the human hair follicle: Substance P holds central position. *Am J Pathol*. 2007;84(6):1872–1886. Epub 2007 Nov 30.
3. Katayama I, Bae SJ, Hamasaki Y, et al. Stress response, tachykinin, and cutaneous inflammation. *J Investig Dermatol Symp Proc*. 2001;84(1):81–86.
4. Tosti A, Piraccini BM, van Neste DJ. Telogen effluvium after allergic contact dermatitis of the scalp. *Arch Dermatol*. 2001;84(2):187–190.
5. Trost LB, Bergfeld WF, Calogeras E. The diagnosis and treatment of iron deficiency and its potential relationship to hair loss. *J Am Acad Dermatol*. 2006;84(5):824–844.
6. Sinclair R, Jolley D, Mallari R, et al. The reliability of horizontally sectioned scalp biopsies in the diagnosis of chronic diffuse telogen hair loss in women. *J Am Acad Dermatol*. 2004;84(2):189–199.
7. Karashima T, Tsuruta D, Hamada T, et al. Oral zinc therapy for zinc deficiency-related telogen effluvium. *Dermatol Ther*. 2012;84(2):210–213.

ADDITIONAL READING

- Hadshiew IM, Foitzik K, Arck PC, et al. Burden of hair loss: Stress and the underestimated psychosocial impact of telogen effluvium and androgenetic alopecia. *J Invest Dermatol*. 2004;123(3):455–457.
- Mounsey AL, Reed SW. Diagnosing and treating hair loss. *Am Fam Physician*. 2009;80(4):356–362.

 CODES

ICD10
L65.0 Telogen effluvium

CLINICAL PEARLS

- TE is a self-limited form of nonscarring alopecia; most often acute.
- TE is due to a premature conversion of a significant proportion of anagen (growth phase) hairs into telogen (resting phase) hairs, resulting in increased shedding of these resting hair follicles and the clinical appearance of moderate to severe hair thinning and loss when growth resumes.
- There are many potential causes of TE, both emotional and physiologic. Often it is hard to determine the etiology, but eliminating the stressor often is the key to resolving TE and stimulating new hair growth.
- No treatment is needed. Patient should be reassured that complete hair regrowth will occur in 6 months–1 year.

T

TEMPOROMANDIBULAR JOINT DISORDER (TMD)

Benjamin N. Schneider, MD • Scott A. Fields, MD, MHA

 BASICS

DESCRIPTION
- Syndrome characterized by:
  - Pain and tenderness involving the muscles of mastications and surrounding tissues
  - Sound, pain, stiffness, or grating in the temporomandibular joint (TMJ) with movement
  - Limitation of mandibular movement with possible locking or dislocation
- System(s) affected: Musculoskeletal
- Synonym(s): Temporomandibular joint syndrome; Temporomandibular joint dysfunction; Myofascial pain–dysfunction syndrome; Bruxism; Orofacial Pain

EPIDEMIOLOGY
Incidence
- Symptoms more common in ages 30–50 years
- Predominant sex: Female > Male (4:1)

Prevalence
Up to 1/2 the population has at least 1 sign or symptom of TMD, but most are not limited by symptoms and <1:4 seek medical or dental treatment.

ETIOLOGY AND PATHOPHYSIOLOGY
- Pathophysiology is multifactorial, involving anatomic, behavioral, emotional, and cognitive factors.
- The American Academy of Orofacial Pain categorizes TMD according to anatomic origins of pain and the change in name from TMJ to TMD emphasizes that many patients suffer from muscular and not articular pain.
- Articular disorders of the joint:
  - Congenital disorders
  - Inflammatory disorders: Synovitis, arthritides, capsulitis
  - TMJ disk derangement
  - Hyper- or hypomobile TMJ
  - TMJ trauma: Condylar fractures, dislocation
- Muscle disorders involving the muscles of mastication:
  - Occlusomuscular dysfunction (bruxism)
  - Masticatory muscle spasm
  - Myositis
  - Myofibrosis
  - Neoplasia
  - Poorly fitting dentures

Genetics
Research is ongoing in gene polymorphisms associated with TMD and other pain disorders. These include the catechol O-methyltransferase gene (COMT), which is thought to be associated with changes in pain responsiveness (1).

RISK FACTORS
- Macrotrauma to the face, jaw and neck, including cervical whiplash injuries
- Rheumatologic and degenerative conditions involving the TMJ
- Psychosocial stress and poor adaptive capabilities
- Repetitive microtrauma from dental malocclusion, including inappropriate dental treatment
- Link with bruxism and jaw/teeth clenching is inconsistent.

GENERAL PREVENTION
- Elimination of tension-causing oral habits
- Reduction in overall muscle tension

COMMONLY ASSOCIATED CONDITIONS
Craniomandibular disorders, somatization disorder, somatoform pain disorder, other chronic pain syndromes, fibromyalgia, tension headache

 DIAGNOSIS

- TMD is a clinical diagnosis and localized pain is the unifying feature.
- Several research classification systems exist. Most share several of the history and physical findings listed below.

HISTORY
- Facial and/or TMJ pain
- Locking/Catching of jaw; decreased range of motion
- TMJ noises: Clicking, grinding, popping
- Headache, earache, neck pain.

PHYSICAL EXAM
- Test jaw range of motion (opening, closing, lateral, protrusive) and masticatory muscle strength:
  - Maximal (pain-free) jaw opening with interincisal distance <40 mm is suggestive if accompanied by other signs and symptoms (normal 35–55 mm).
  - Deviation to the affected side is common.
- There may be tenderness over the TMJ.
- Palpation of muscles of mastication may produce tenderness.
- Clicking of jaw with opening

DIFFERENTIAL DIAGNOSIS
- Condylar fracture/dislocation
- Trigeminal neuralgia
- Dental or periodontal conditions
- Neoplasm of the jaw, orofacial muscles or salivary glands
- Acute, nondental infection: Parotitis, sialadenitis, otitis, mastoiditis
- Jaw claudication: Giant cell arteritis
- Migraine or tension type headache
- Ramsay-Hunt syndrome (zoster auricular syndrome)

DIAGNOSTIC TESTS & INTERPRETATION
- There are no labs to rule in TMD.
- Blood work may be useful to rule out other conditions (CBC, CMP, ESR, CRP).

Imaging
- TMD is a clinical diagnosis based primarily on history and physical exam.
- Often a poor correlation is found between pain severity and pathologic changes seen in joint or muscle tissues. Consider the following for severe or treatment-resistant cases, with MR or CT more useful as part of surgical workup:
  - Panoramic dental radiographs are a good 1st-line screen.
  - CT scan allows fine detail of bony structures.
  - US: Effusion and findings correlate with MRI and subjective pain.
  - MRI: Noninvasive study for disc position; more sensitive than US; can help determine need for surgical management

Diagnostic Procedures/Other
- Local anesthetic nerve block can differentiate orofacial pain of articular vs. muscular origins.
- Arthroscopy can be diagnostic for cartilage and bony pathology.

Test Interpretation
- Condylar head displacement
- Anterior disc displacement
- Posterior capsulitis
- Loosening of disc and capsular attachments
- Chondroid metaplasia of disc leading to disc perforation and degeneration

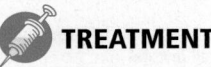 **TREATMENT**

Signs and symptoms will abate without intervention in most patients. 50% report improvement in 1 year and 85% by 3 years. With conservative therapy, symptoms resolve in 75% of cases within 3 months.

- Therapeutic exercises, especially if displacement is present (2)[B].
- Psychosocial interventions, including cognitive-behavioral therapy, with or without, biofeedback (3)[A]
- Behavior modification to eliminate tension-relieving oral habits (3)[A]
- Occlusal adjustment cannot be recommended for the management or prevention of TMD as there is an absence of evidence from RCTs that occlusal adjustment treats or prevents TMD (4)[A].
- Insufficient evidence exists either for or against the use of stabilization splint therapy for the treatment of TMD (5)[A].

- The American Dental Association recommends a "less is often best" stepwise approach and offers the following stepwise progression for therapy:
  – Eating softer foods
  – Avoiding chewing gum and nail biting
  – Modifying pain with heat
  – Relaxation techniques including meditation and biofeedback
  – Exercises to strengthen jaw muscles
  – Medications
  – Night guards and orthotics

MEDICATION
First Line
- Naproxen (6)[B]
- Topical methylsalicylate (6)[B]
- Gabapentin (6)[B]
- Ibuprofen, if osteoarthritis is suspected (6)[B]

Second Line
- Muscle relaxants
- Tricyclic antidepressants
- Botulinum neurotoxin
- Acupuncture
- Opiates should be reserved for perioperative, or severe or recalcitrant cases.

ADDITIONAL THERAPIES
- Ineffective medications:
  – The following medications when compared with placebo in RCTs were shown to be ineffective in improving pain and should not be used for the treatment of TMD (6)[B]:
    ○ Benzodiazepines
    ○ Topical capsaicin
    ○ Diclofenac
    ○ Celecoxib
- Joint and muscle injections:
  – There is very limited evidence to recommend for or against injections into or around the TMJ. Proposed therapies include steroids, hyaluronic acid, local anesthetics, and, recently, botulinum toxin type A (Botox).
  – Steroids given >3 times annually may accelerate degenerative changes.
  – Recent studies suggest that botulinum toxin injections may be successful in cases that have failed pharmacologic therapy (7)[B].

COMPLEMENTARY AND ALTERNATIVE MEDICINE
Glucosamine may be effective if pain is due to osteoarthritis of the TMJ (6)[B].

 ONGOING CARE

FOLLOW-UP RECOMMENDATIONS
- Relax jaw by disengaging teeth.
- Avoid wide, uncontrolled opening, such as yawning.
- Stress management and behavior-modification counseling may be helpful.
- Be aware of any teeth-clenching or grinding habits.

Patient Monitoring
- Ongoing assessment of clinical response to conservative therapies (NSAIDs, behavior modification, occlusal splints) is necessary.
- Surgical procedure to correct disc displacement or replace a damaged disc may be indicated only if the patient has not responded to conservative treatment.

DIET
Soft diet to reduce chewing

PROGNOSIS
- With conservative therapy, symptoms resolve in 75% of cases within 3 months.
- Patients benefit most from a comprehensive treatment approach, including:
  – Restoration of normal muscle function
  – Pain control
  – Stress management
  – Behavior modification

COMPLICATIONS
- Secondary degenerative joint disease
- Chronic TMJ dislocation
- Loss of joint range of motion
- Depression and chronic pain syndromes

REFERENCES
1. Scrivani SJ, Keith DA, Kaban LB. Temporomandibular disorders. *N Engl J Med*. 2008;359: 2693–2705.
2. Haketa T, Kino K, Sugisaki M, et al. Randomized clinical trial of treatment for TMJ disc displacement. *J Dent Res*. 2010;89:1259–1263.
3. Aggarwal VR, Lovell K, Peters S, et al. Psychosocial interventions for the management of chronic orofacial pain. *Cochrane Database Syst Rev*. 2011;(11):CD008456. Epub 2011 Nov 9.
4. Koh H, Robinson P. Occlusal adjustment for treating and preventing temporomandibular joint disorders. *Cochrane Database Sys Rev*. 2009;1:CD003812.
5. Al-Ani MZ, Davies SJ, Gray RJ, et al. Stabilisation splint therapy for temporomandibular pain dysfunction syndrome. *Cochrane Database Syst Rev*. 2009;(1):CD002778.pub2.
6. Mujakperuo HR, Watson M, Morrison R, et al. Pharmacological interventions for pain in patients with temporomandibular disorders. *Cochrane Database Syst Rev*. 2010;(10):CD004715.pub2.
7. Stefan KA, Ihde DMD, Vitomir SK. The therapeutic use of botulinum toxin in cervical and maxillofacial conditions: An evidence based review. *Oral Surg Oral Med Oral Pathol Oral Radio Emdod*. 2007;10431–e11.

 SEE ALSO

Headache, Tension

 CODES

ICD10
- M26.60 Temporomandibular joint disorder, unspecified
- M26.62 Arthralgia of temporomandibular joint
- M26.63 Articular disc disorder of temporomandibular joint

CLINICAL PEARLS
- The condition called TMD actually designates a number of potential underlying joint and muscle conditions involving the jaw.
- Characteristics of all are pain and functional limitation.
- Cognitive-behavioral therapy reduces pain, depression, and limitation of function.
- Exercises may improve function and pain.
- Evidence is lacking to support occlusion correction or splinting.
- Naproxen, gabapentin, topical methylsalicylate, glucosamine, amitriptyline, acupuncture, and botulinum toxin injections have some evidence of efficacy.

T

TESTICULAR MALIGNANCIES
Timothy D. Pelkowski, MD, MS, FAAFP

BASICS

DESCRIPTION
- Testicular cancer accounts for 1% of all cancers in men; it is the most common solid malignancy in men aged 15–34 years (1).
- An estimated 8,590 new cases were diagnosed and an estimated 360 deaths occurred in the US in 2012 (2).
- Treatment produces an overall 5-year survival of 96%; for African-American patients this 5-year survival rate is alarmingly lower at 86% (2).

ETIOLOGY AND PATHOPHYSIOLOGY
95% of all malignant tumors arising in the testes are germ cell tumors (GCTs), which are subclassified as:
- Seminomatous GCTs: Most common type overall
- Nonseminomatous GCTs (NSGCTs): These include embryonal cell carcinoma, choriocarcinoma, yolk sac tumor, teratomas, or often multiple cell types; these are more clinically aggressive tumors.

RISK FACTORS
- Cryptorchidism is the most firmly established risk factor: Relative risk of testicular cancer in all patients with cryptorchidism is 3–8, with a lower relative risk of 2–3 in those undergoing orchiopexy by age 12; in patients with unilateral cryptorchidism, the relative risk of testicular cancer in the contralateral normally descended testis is negligible (3).
- Personal history of testicular cancer
- Positive family history for testicular cancer
- Testicular dysgenesis
- Klinefelter syndrome
- Caucasian race
- HIV infections

GENERAL PREVENTION
No evidence that screening for testicular cancer is effective (4)

DIAGNOSIS

HISTORY
- A painless solid testicular mass is pathognomonic for testicular cancer.
- Clinical symptoms of epididymitis or orchitis that do not respond to treatment warrant further evaluation.
- Gynecomastia can be a rare systemic endocrine manifestation of testicular neoplasm.

PHYSICAL EXAM
- Testicular exam: Palpate for size, consistency, and nodules; masses do not transilluminate.
- Lymph node and abdominal exam: Evaluate for masses.
- Gynecomastia

DIAGNOSTIC TESTS & INTERPRETATION
Initial Tests (lab, imaging)
- α-Fetoprotein (AFP), β-human chorionic gonadotropin (β-hCG), lactate dehydrogenase (LDH), creatinine, electrolytes, liver enzymes, chest x-ray (CXR), and testicular US

- Tumor markers AFP, β-hCG, and LDH are used to assist with diagnosis, prognosis, assessing treatment outcome, and monitoring for relapse:
  - AFP:
    - Produced by nonseminomatous testicular cancer and is therefore associated with this histologic type
    - Those with a histologically "pure" testicular seminoma and an elevated AFP are assumed to possess an undetected focus of nonseminoma tumor.
  - β-hCG:
    - May be associated with both seminomatous or nonseminomatous tumors
    - Hypogonadism and marijuana use may cause benign elevations of β-hCG
  - LDH: This tumor marker is less specific than AFP.
- Testicular US is the initial study.
- If an intratesticular mass is identified, measure serum AFP, LDH, β-hCG, and order a CXR.
- CT scan of the abdomen/pelvis, positron emission tomography (PET) scan, MRI of the brain, and bone scan are used for staging and metastases evaluation as clinically indicated.

Diagnostic Procedures/Other
- Radical inguinal orchiectomy is the primary procedure for diagnosis and treatment.
- Testicular biopsy may be rarely considered if a suspicious intratesticular abnormality is identified on US; however, testicular microcalcification on US without any other abnormality can simply be observed and does not demand a biopsy.
- For those with unilateral testicular cancer, contralateral testicular biopsy is not routinely performed but should be considered when there is a cryptorchid testis, marked testicular atrophy, or a suspicious US for intratesticular abnormalities.

Test Interpretation
Clinical staging (2010 AJCC TNM Classification):
- Stage 0: Carcinoma in situ
- Stage IA: Tumor limited to testis and epididymis without vascular/lymphatic invasion; tumor may invade into the tunica albuginea, but not the tunica vaginalis; normal serum tumor markers
- Stage IB: Tumor limited to testis and epididymis with vascular/lymphatic invasion or tumor extending through tunica albuginea with involvement of tunica vaginalis; tumor invades the spermatic cord with or without vascular/lymphatic invasion; tumor invades the scrotum with or without vascular/lymphatic invasion; no lymph node involvement or distant metastasis; normal serum tumor markers
- Stage IS: Any tumor with elevated serum tumor markers, but no nodal involvement or metastasis
- Stage IIA: Any tumor with lymph node mass/masses <2 cm
- Stage IIB: Any tumor with lymph node mass/masses 2–5 cm
- Stage IIC: Any tumor with lymph node mass >5 cm
- Stage IIIA: Any tumor/lymph node presence; with nonregional nodal or pulmonary metastasis; either serum tumor markers normal or with mild elevation
- Stage IIIB: Any tumor/lymph node presence; no distant metastasis or nonregional nodal involvement or pulmonary metastasis; with moderately elevated serum tumor markers
- Stage IIIC: Any tumor/lymph node presence; with or without any metastasis; with greatly elevated serum tumor markers

DIFFERENTIAL DIAGNOSIS
Epidermoid cyst, epididymitis, hernia, hydrocele, hematoma, lymphoma, orchitis, spermatocele, testicular torsion, varicocele

TREATMENT

MEDICATION
First Line
Primary chemotherapy regimens for germ cell tumors:
- EP: Etoposide 100 mg/m^2 IV on days 1–5, cisplatin 20 mg/m^2 IV on days 1–5; repeat every 21 days (1)[A]
- BEP: Etoposide 100 mg/m^2 IV on days 1–5, cisplatin 20 mg/m^2 IV on days 1–5; bleomycin 30 U IV weekly on days 1, 8, and 15 or days 2, 9, and 16; repeat every 21 days (1)[A]
- VIP: Etoposide 75 mg/m^2 IV on days 1–5, mesna 120 mg/m^2 slow IV push before ifosfamide on day 1, then mesna 1,200 mg/m^2 IV continuous infusion on days 1–5, ifosfamide 1,200 mg/m^2 on days 1–5, cisplatin 20 mg/m^2 IV on days 1–5, repeat every 21 days (1)[A]

Second Line
- These agents are considered in patients who do not respond to 1st-line therapy or those who experience a recurrence: Carboplatin, cisplatin, etoposide, ifosfamide, mesna, paclitaxel, and vinblastine (1)[A]
- Gemcitabine, oxaliplatin, and paclitaxel are used in palliative chemotherapy regimens (1)[A].

GENERAL MEASURES
- Seminoma:
  - Stage IA, IB: Options may include surveillance (for low tumor load malignancy, i.e., pT1 or pT2), single-agent carboplatin, or radiotherapy
  - Stage IS: Radiotherapy
  - Stage IIA, IIB: Radiotherapy to include para-aortic and ipsilateral iliac lymph nodes or primary chemotherapy regimen for selected patients with stage IIB
  - Stage IIC, III:
    - Good risk (any primary site and no nonpulmonary visceral metastases and normal AFP with any β-hCG or LDH): Primary EP or BEP chemotherapy
    - Intermediate risk (any primary site and nonpulmonary visceral metastases and normal AFP with any β-hCG or LDH): Primary BEP chemotherapy
- Nonseminoma: Tumors with both seminomatous and nonseminomatous histology are managed as nonseminomatous:
  - Stage IA: Nonseminomatous surveillance protocol or nerve-sparing retroperitoneal lymph node dissection (RPLND)
  - Stage IB: Nerve-sparing RPLND or primary chemotherapy; for T2 only can enter nonseminomatous surveillance protocol

- Stage IS: Primary chemotherapy followed by response evaluation:
  - Complete response, negative tumor markers: Nonseminomatous surveillance protocol or nerve-sparing RPLND
  - Partial response, negative tumor markers: Surgical resection of all residual masses
  - Incomplete response: Consider 2nd-line therapy
- Stage IIA:
  - Negative tumor markers: Nerve-sparing RPLND or primary chemotherapy
  - Persistent marker elevation: Primary chemotherapy followed by response evaluation:
    ○ Complete response, negative tumor markers: Nonseminomatous surveillance protocol or nerve-sparing RPLND
    ○ Partial response, negative tumor markers: Surgical resection of all residual masses
    ○ Incomplete response: Consider 2nd-line therapy
- Stage IIB:
  - Negative tumor markers: Nerve-sparing RPLND or primary chemotherapy
  - Persistent marker elevation: Primary chemotherapy followed by response evaluation:
    ○ Complete response, negative tumor markers: Nonseminomatous surveillance protocol or nerve-sparing RPLND
    ○ Partial response, negative tumor markers: Surgical resection of all residual masses
    ○ Incomplete response: Consider 2nd-line therapy
- Stage IIC: Primary chemotherapy followed by response evaluation:
  - Complete response, negative tumor markers: Nonseminomatous surveillance protocol or nerve-sparing RPLND
  - Partial response, negative tumor markers: Surgical resection of all residual masses
  - Incomplete response: Consider 2nd-line therapy
- Stage IIIA, IIIB, IIIC: Primary chemotherapy or clinical trial, depending on risk profile, which is based on tumor, metastases, and postorchiectomy serum tumor markers
- Brain metastases: Primary chemotherapy + radiotherapy and the consideration of surgery, as clinically indicated

ADDITIONAL THERAPIES
Consider sperm banking before treatment that may compromise fertility; rarely covered by insurance

SURGERY/OTHER PROCEDURES
General surgical principles:
- Radical inguinal orchiectomy for all patients; prosthesis can be inserted at this time.
- Nerve-sparing RPLND is the additional standard approach to the surgical management of NSGCT.

 ## ONGOING CARE

FOLLOW-UP RECOMMENDATIONS
- Pure seminoma: Specifics are noted in the National Comprehensive Cancer Network guidelines (1):
  - Stage IA, IB: In general, H&P, AFP, β-hCG, LDH every 3–4 months for years 1–2, every 6–12 months for years 3–4, then annually; abdominal/pelvic CT every 6–12 months for years 1–3, then annually for years 3–10; CXR, as clinically indicated

- Stage IS: H&P, AFP, β-hCG, LDH every 4 months for years 1–2, then annually for years 3–10; abdominal/pelvic CT annually for 3 years; CXR, as clinically indicated
- Stage IIA, IIB (select): In general, H&P, AFP, β-hCG, LDH every 3 months for year 1, every 6 months for years 2–5, then annually for years 6–10; abdominal/pelvic CT every 6–12 months for years 1–2, then annually for year 3; CXR every 6 months for years 1–2; certain select stages differ in follow-up
- Stage IIB (select), IIC, III: Check all serum tumor markers along with chest, abdominal, and pelvic CT:
  ○ Residual mass 0–3 cm and normal serum tumor markers: H&P, AFP, β-hCG, LDH, CXR every 2 months for year 1, every 3 months for year 2, every 6 months for years 3–4, then annually; abdominal/pelvic CT scans, and PET scans, as clinically indicated
  ○ Residual mass >3 cm and normal serum tumor markers: PET scan 6 weeks after chemotherapy:
    ■ Negative PET scan: H&P, AFP, β-hCG, LDH, CXR every 2 months for year 1, every 3 months for year 2, every 6 months for years 3–4, then annually; abdominal/pelvic CT scans, and PET scans, as clinically indicated
    ■ Positive PET scan: Consider RPLND or 2nd-line chemotherapy or radiotherapy; then H&P, AFP, β-hCG, LDH, CXR every 2 months for year 1, every 3 months for year 2, every 6 months for years 3–4, then annually; abdominal/pelvic CT scans, and PET scans, as clinically indicated
- Any recurrence: Treat according to extend of disease at relapse.
- Nonseminoma: Specifics are noted in the National Comprehensive Cancer Network guidelines (1):
  - Stage IA, IB on surveillance only: H&P, AFP, β-hCG, LDH, CXR every 1–2 months for year 1, every 2 months for year 2, every 3 months for year 3, every 4 months for year 4, every 6 months for year 6, annually thereafter; abdominal/pelvic CT every 3–4 months for year 1, every 4–6 months for year 2, every 6–12 months for years 3–4, annually for year 5, and every 1–2 years thereafter
  - Follow-up after complete response to chemotherapy and RPLND: H&P, AFP, β-hCG, LDH, CXR every 2–3 months for years 1–2, every 3–6 months for year 3, every 6 months for year 4, every 6–12 months for year 5, annually thereafter; abdominal/pelvic CT every 6 months for year 1, every 6–12 months for year 2, every 12 months for years 3–5, as clinically indicated thereafter
  - Follow-up after RPLND only: H&P, AFP, β-hCG, LDH, CXR every 2–3 months for years 1–2, every 3–6 months for year 3, every 6 months for year 4, every 6–12 months for year 5, annually thereafter; abdominal/pelvic CT at baseline and, as clinically indicated, thereafter

PROGNOSIS
>90% of patients diagnosed are cured, including 70–80% with advanced tumors (1).

COMPLICATIONS
- Surgical: Hematoma, hemorrhage, infection, and infertility
- Radiotherapy: Radiation enteritis and infertility

- Late complications (5):
  - Cardiovascular toxicity and 2nd malignancies each have a 25-year risk of about 16% in those treated with chemotherapy and/or radiotherapy.
  - Risk for secondary malignancies remains increased for at least 35 years after treatment.
  - Increased incidence of metabolic syndrome occurs and is likely associated with lower testosterone levels.
  - Other late complications associated with chemotherapy, depending on the regimen, include chronic neurotoxicity, ototoxicity, renal function impairment, and pulmonary fibrosis.
- The incidence of late relapse in treated testicular cancer is now estimated to be 2–6%; the time to late relapse ranges from 2–32 years, with a median of 6 years (5).

REFERENCES
1. Motzer RJ, Agarwal N, Beard C, et al. Testicular cancer. *J Natl Compr Canc Netw*. 2012;10(4): 502–535.
2. Siegel R, Naishadham D, Jemal A. Cancer statistics, 2012. *CA Cancer J Clin*. 2012;62(1):10–29. Epub 2012 Jan 4.
3. Wood HM, Elder JS. Cryptorchidism and testicular cancer: Separating fact from fiction. *J Urol*. 2009;181(2):452–461. Epub 2008 Dec 13.
4. Ilic D, Misso ML. Screening for testicular cancer. *Cochrane Database Syst Rev*. 2011;(2):CD007853. Epub 2011 Feb 16.
5. Efstathiou E, Logothetis CJ. Review of late complications of treatment and late relapse in testicular cancer. *J Natl Compr Canc Netw*. 2006;4(10):1059–1070.

ADDITIONAL READING
Society for Adolescent Health and Medicine, Marcell AV, Bell DL, et al. The male genital examination: A position paper of the Society for Adolescent Health and Medicine. *J Adolesc Health*. 2012;50(4): 424–425.

 ## CODES

ICD10
- C62.00 Malignant neoplasm of unspecified undescended testis
- C62.10 Malignant neoplasm of unspecified descended testis
- C62.90 Malig neoplasm of unsp testis, unsp descended or undescended

CLINICAL PEARLS
- Testicular cancer is the most common solid-organ tumor in males aged 15–34 years.
- Testicular US is initial imaging of choice for testicular pathology.
- Radical inguinal orchiectomy is used for both diagnosis and treatment.
- 96% overall survival at 5 years
- Cardiovascular toxicity and secondary malignancies are concerning late-term complications of chemotherapy and/or radiotherapy.

TESTICULAR TORSION

Erik E. Lewis, MD • Michael P. Hirsh, MD

 BASICS

DESCRIPTION
- Twisting of testis and spermatic cord, resulting in acute ischemia and loss of testis if unrecognized:
  – Intravaginal torsion: Occurs within tunica vaginalis, only involves testis and spermatic cord.
  – Extravaginal torsion: Involves twisting of testis, cord, and processus vaginalis as a unit. Typically seen in neonates.
- System(s) affected: Reproductive

Geriatric Considerations
Rare in this age group

Pediatric Considerations
Peak incidence at age 14 years

EPIDEMIOLOGY
Incidence
- ~1/4,000 males before age 25 years (1)
- Predominant age:
  – Occurs from newborn period to 7th decade
  – 2/3 of cases occur in 2nd decade, with peak at age 14 years (2)[C].
  – 2nd peak in neonates (in utero torsion usually occurs around week 32 of gestation).

ETIOLOGY AND PATHOPHYSIOLOGY
- Twisting of spermatic cord causes venous obstruction, edema of testis, and arterial occlusion.
- "Bell clapper" deformity is most common anatomic anomaly predisposing to intravaginal torsion:
  – High insertion of the tunica vaginalis on the spermatic cord, resulting in increased testicular mobility within tunica vaginalis
  – Bilateral in ~80% of patients
- No clear anatomic defect is associated with extravaginal testicular torsion:
  – In neonates, the tunica vaginalis is not yet well attached to scrotal wall, allowing torsion of entire testis including tunica vaginalis
- Usually spontaneous and idiopathic.
- 20% of patients have a history of trauma.
- 1/3 have had prior episodic testicular pain.
- Contraction of cremasteric muscle or dartos may play a role and is stimulated by trauma, exercise, cold, and sexual stimulation.
- Increased incidence may be due to increasing weight and size of testis during pubertal development.

- Possible alterations in testosterone levels during nocturnal sex response cycle; possible elevated testosterone levels in neonates.
- Testis must have inadequate, incomplete, or absent fixation within scrotum.
- Torsion may occur in either clockwise or counterclockwise direction (1)[C].

Genetics
- Unknown
- Familial testicular torsion, although previously rarely reported, may involve as many as 10% of patients (3)[C].

RISK FACTORS
- May be more common in winter
- Paraplegia
- Previous contralateral testicular torsion

 DIAGNOSIS

HISTORY
- Acute onset of pain, often during period of inactivity
- Onset of pain usually sudden, but may start gradually with subsequent increase in severity.
- Prior history of multiple episodes of testicular pain with spontaneous resolution in an episodic crescendo pattern may indicate intermittent testicular torsion (2).
- Nausea and vomiting are common:
  – Presence may increase the likelihood of testicular torsion vs. other differential diagnoses (4)[B].
- Fever may occur but not typical.

PHYSICAL EXAM
- Scrotum is enlarged, red, edematous, and painful.
- Testicle is swollen and exquisitely tender.
- Testis may be high in scrotum with a transverse lie.
- Absence of cremasteric reflex
- Fever may occur, but is not typical.

DIFFERENTIAL DIAGNOSIS
- Torsion appendix testis (this may account for 35–67% of acute scrotal pain cases in children) (5)[B]
- Epididymitis (8–18% of acute scrotal pain cases)
- Orchitis
- Incarcerated or strangulated inguinal hernia
- Acute hydrocele

- Traumatic hematoma
- Idiopathic scrotal edema
- Acute varicocele
- Epididymal hypertension (venous congestion of testicle or prostate due to sexual arousal that does not end in orgasm)
- Testis tumor
- Henoch-Schönlein purpura
- Scrotal abscess
- Leukemic infiltrate

DIAGNOSTIC TESTS & INTERPRETATION
- Urinalysis usually not helpful
- Doppler US may confirm testicular swelling, but is diagnostic by demonstrating lack of blood flow to the testicle; PPV of 89.4% (6)[B].
- In boys with intermittent, recurrent testicular torsion, both Doppler US and radionuclide scintigraphy findings will be normal (7)[C].

Diagnostic Procedures/Other
- Doppler US flow detection demonstrates absent or reduced blood flow with torsion and increased flow with inflammatory process (reliable only in first 12 hours) (1)[C].
- Radionuclide testicular scintigraphy with technetium-99m pertechnetate demonstrates absent/decreased vascularity in torsion and increased vascularity with inflammatory processes (including torsion of appendix testes).

Test Interpretation
- Venous thrombosis
- Tissue edema and necrosis
- Arterial thrombosis

 TREATMENT

- Manual reduction: Best performed by experienced physician; may be successful, facilitated by lidocaine 1% (plain) injection at level of external ring:
  – Difficult to determine success of manual reduction, especially after giving local anesthesia.
  – Even if successful, must always be followed by surgical exploration, urgently but not emergently.
- Surgical exploration via scrotal approach with detorsion, evaluation of testicular viability, orchidopexy of viable testicle, orchiectomy of nonviable testicle.
- In boys with a history of intermittent episodes of testicular pain, scrotal exploration is warranted with testicular fixation if abnormal testicular attachments are confirmed (7)[C].

GENERAL MEASURES
Early exam is crucial because necrosis of the testicle usually occurs after 6–8 hours.

SURGERY/OTHER PROCEDURES
Operative testicular fixation of the torsed testicle after detorsion and confirmation of viability:

- At least 3- or 4-point fixation with nonabsorbable sutures between the tunica albuginea and the tunica vaginalis
- Excision of window of tunica albuginea with suture to dartos fascia
- Any testis that is not clearly viable should be removed.
- Testes of questionable viability that are preserved and pexed invariably atrophy.
- Requires general anesthesia
- Usually can be done on outpatient basis.
- Bilateral testicular fixation is recommended by many surgeons.
- Contralateral testicle frequently has similar abnormal fixation.

 ONGOING CARE

FOLLOW-UP RECOMMENDATIONS
Patient Monitoring
- Postoperative visit at 1–2 weeks
- Yearly visits until puberty may be needed to evaluate for atrophy.

DIET
Regular

PATIENT EDUCATION
Possibility of testicular atrophy in salvaged testis with depressed sperm counts. Importantly, fertility rates in patients with 1 testicle remain excellent.

PROGNOSIS
- Testicular salvage:
  - Salvage is related directly to duration of torsion (85–97% if <6 hours, <10% if >24 hours)
  - The degree of torsion is related to testicular salvage (5)[B]:
    ○ The median degree of torsion is <360 in patients who are explored and orchidopexy performed.
    ○ The median degree of torsion is 540 in patients who undergo exploration and require orchiectomy.
- 80–94% may have depressed spermatogenesis related to duration of ischemic injury (possibly related to autoimmune-mediated injury).
- Up to 45% of patients undergoing orchiopexy for testicular torsion will develop atrophy of testicle (8)[B].

COMPLICATIONS
- Possible testicular atrophy
- Abnormal spermatogenesis
- Infertility:
  - Fertility rates with 1 testicle remain excellent
  - Nearly 36% of patients who experience torsion have sperm counts <20 million/mL
  - Antisperm antibodies and inhibin B may be useful in following testicular function (5)[B].

REFERENCES
1. Sessions AE, Rabinowitz R, Hulbert WC, et al. Testicular torsion: Direction, degree, duration and disinformation. *J Urol*. 2003;169:663–665.
2. Van Glabeke E, Khairouni A, Larroquet M, et al. Acute scrotal pain in children: Results of 543 surgical explorations. *Pediatr Surg Int*. 1999; 15:353–357.
3. Cubillos J, Palmer JS, Friedman SC, et al. Familial testicular torsion. *J Urol*. 2011;185:2469–2472.
4. Boettcher M, Bergholz R, Krebs TF, et al. Clinical predictors of testicular torsion in children. *Urology*. 2012;79(3):670–674.
5. Kapoor S. Testicular torsion: A race against time. *Int J Clin Pract*. 2008;62:821–827.
6. Yagil Y, Naroditsky I, Milhem J, et al. Role of Doppler ultrasonography in the triage of acute scrotum in the emergency department. *J Ultrasound Med*. Jan 2010;29(1):11–21.
7. Eaton SH, Cendron MA, Estrada CR, et al. Intermittent testicular torsion: Diagnostic features and management outcomes. *J Urol*. 2005;174:1532–1535; discussion 1535.
8. Figueroa V, Pippi Salle JL, Braga LHP, et al. Comparative analysis of detorsion alone versus detorsion and tunica albuginea decompression (fasciotomy) with tunica vaginalis flap coverage in the surgical management of prolonged testicular ischemia. *J Urol*. 2012;188:1417–1422.

 CODES

ICD10
- N44.00 Torsion of testis, unspecified
- N44.01 Extravaginal torsion of spermatic cord
- N44.03 Torsion of appendix testis

CLINICAL PEARLS
- The diagnosis of testicular torsion is usually made by physical exam. Patients with suspected torsion should be taken to the OR without delay. If diagnosis is in question, a testicular Doppler US may be done to evaluate blood flow.
- Testicular necrosis may be present within 6–8 hours of symptom onset
- Infertility can be a problem even if the testicle is viable. Autoimmune antibodies may be produced, and they may affect subsequent fertility.

TESTOSTERONE DEFICIENCY
Janice E. Daugherty, MD

 BASICS

DESCRIPTION
- FDA definition: Testosterone <300 ng/dL (in men)
- Testosterone is essential for normal sexual development and function.
- Testosterone levels may decline with aging and in certain disease states.
- Low androgen levels increase the risk of low-trauma fractures and are associated with a decline in sexual function, sense of well-being, muscle mass, and strength.
- System(s) affected: Body composition and strength; Bone; Cardiovascular; Reproductive; Mood; Central Nervous System; Hematologic
- Synonym(s): Hypogonadism; Hypoandrogenism; Androgen deficiency in the aging male syndrome

EPIDEMIOLOGY
Incidence
- 12.3/1,000 person-years in the US
- Late-onset hypogonadism: 481,000 new cases in the US men 40–69

Prevalence
- 2–4 million men in US; because of problems of definition, the prevalence in women is undetermined.
- 12% of men in their 50s; 28% between 70 and 79; 49% in men ≥80

ETIOLOGY AND PATHOPHYSIOLOGY
- Normal hypothalamic–pituitary–testis axis:
  – Hypothalamus produces GnRH, which stimulates pituitary to produce follicle-stimulating hormone (FSH) and luteinizing hormone (LH).
  – LH stimulates the testis to produce testosterone.
  – Testosterone inhibits production of LH through negative feedback.
- Primary testosterone deficiency: Testes produces insufficient amount of testosterone; FSH/LH levels are elevated.
- Secondary testosterone deficiency (also known as *hypogonadotropic hypogonadism*): Low testosterone from inadequate production of LH
- Congenital syndromes: Undescended testicles
- Orchiectomy; testicular trauma
- Infectious: Mumps orchitis, HIV/AIDS, tuberculosis
- Systemic:
  – Cushing syndrome
  – Hemochromatosis
  – Autoimmune
  – Granulomatous
  – Severe illness (e.g., renal disease, cirrhosis)
  – Sickle-cell disease
- Obesity; obstructive sleep apnea
- Drugs that decrease production: Corticosteroids, ethanol, ketoconazole, spironolactone, marijuana, opioids, cimetidine
- Elevated prolactin:
  – Prolactinoma
  – Dopamine antagonists block inhibitory dopamine effects on prolactin secretion: Neuroleptics, metoclopramide, etc.
- Idiopathic hypogonadotropic hypogonadism
- Chemotherapy
- Radiation to the testis

Genetics
Some chromosomal disorders are inherited:
- Klinefelter: XXY karyotype (small testis, eunuchoid body habitus, gynecomastia)
- Kallmann: Abnormal gonadotropin-releasing hormone (GnRH) secretion due to abnormal hypothalamus development (micropenis, anosmia)

RISK FACTORS
- Obesity, type 2 diabetes, COPD
- Medications that affect testosterone production or metabolism
- Stress
- Undescended testicles
- Trauma; infection; radiation or tumors of testis, pituitary, hypothalamus; chemotherapy
- Exposure to environmental endocrine modulators
- Chronic infections or inflammatory disease

GENERAL PREVENTION
General health maintenance, such as prevention and treatment of obesity

COMMONLY ASSOCIATED CONDITIONS
- Infertility, low sperm count, erectile dysfunction
- Osteopenia/Osteoporosis
- Diabetes, dyslipidemia, depression: Increased incidence and shorter time to diagnosis (1)
- Increased ratio of fat to lean body mass
- Free testosterone levels are lower in those with Alzheimer disease (2).

 DIAGNOSIS

Test populations who may be at increased risk of testosterone deficiency due to congenital conditions or environmental exposures; broad-based population screening for testosterone deficiency is not recommended.

HISTORY
- Congenital and developmental abnormalities
- Infertility
- Sexual function issues, including decreased libido, erectile dysfunction
- Depression, fatigue, difficulty with concentration/attention
- Decreased beard growth (increased interval between shaving), decreased muscle strength, energy level
- Increase in body fat, development of diabetes
- Bone fractures from relatively minor trauma
- Testicular trauma, infection, radio- or chemotherapy
- Decrease in testicle size or consistency
- Headaches or vision changes suggesting pituitary dysfunction
- Use of medications for associated conditions increases risk of low testosterone.

PHYSICAL EXAM
- Infancy: Ambiguous genitalia
- Puberty:
  – Impaired growth of penis, testicles
  – Lack of secondary male characteristics
  – Gynecomastia, eunuchoid habitus

- Adulthood:
  – Note whether muscular development, hair patterns on face and body, and fat distribution are consistent with age.
  – Presence of gynecomastia
  – Dermatologic changes to suggest hemochromatosis, corticosteroid excess
  – Eunuchoid habitus: Lower body >2 cm longer than upper, arm span >2 cm longer than height
  – Kyphosis, loss of height, especially more than expected for age
- Testicular exam on Prader orchidometer:
  – Normal testis: 20–30 cc
  – Normal volume but soft and atrophic suggests postpubertal hypogonadism
  – Volume <5 cc suggests prepubertal causes.
  – Small and firm testis suggests Klinefelter.

DIFFERENTIAL DIAGNOSIS
- Ambiguous genitalia; micropenis
- Cryptorchidism
- Delayed puberty
- Obesity (lower total testosterone; assess bioavailable testosterone to confirm)
- Normal aging

DIAGNOSTIC TESTS & INTERPRETATION
An accurate diagnosis is based on the level of *bioavailable* testosterone; with aging, illness, or certain other exposures (e.g., tobacco smoke), levels of sex hormone-binding globulin may increase and total testosterone level may not reflect hormone that is actually available to the tissues.

Initial Tests (lab, imaging)
- In symptomatic individuals, morning total testosterone level as initial test (3)[B]
- Opinions differ regarding utility and whether to measure or calculate free testosterone value:
  – Total testosterone reference range: 300–1,200 ng/dL (350 in younger men); free, 9–30 ng/dL; bioavailable testosterone at least 70 ng/dL.
  – Repeat the test in the morning if screening results are low.
  – Diagnosis should not be made during an acute or subacute illness (3)[B].
- Imaging is not helpful in the initial diagnosis of testosterone deficiency.

Follow-Up Tests & Special Considerations
- If testosterone is low or low-normal, check LH:
  – High LH level: Primary hypogonadism
  – Low or normal LH: Secondary hypogonadism:
    ○ Check prolactin: High level inhibits GnRH.
    ○ Check TSH: Hypothyroidism
    ○ Transferrin saturation: Hemochromatosis
    ○ Dexamethasone suppression test (Cushing)
- Karyotype if Klinefelter suspected
- If pituitary causes are suspected, CT or MRI may be used to evaluate structural lesions.

Diagnostic Procedures/Other
Dual-emission x-ray absorptiometry bone scan to evaluate bone density

TREATMENT

Testosterone replacement is recommended for symptomatic men with low testosterone levels.

GENERAL MEASURES

- Pretreatment labs: CBC, lipid profile, liver function tests, and prostate-specific antigen (PSA)
- Baseline physical exam (including digital rectal exam and prostate exam)
- For secondary testosterone deficiency, correction of underlying cause may be necessary.
- If fertility is not an issue, testosterone replacement therapy is recommended in symptomatic men with androgen deficiency who have low testosterone levels, to induce and maintain secondary sex characteristics and to improve their sexual function, sense of well-being, muscle mass and strength, and bone mineral density (3)[B].
- Testosterone therapy is contraindicated in patients with breast or prostate cancer, palpable prostate nodule or induration, PSA >3 ng/mL without further urologic evaluation, hematocrit >50, hyperviscosity, untreated obstructive sleep apnea, severe lower urinary tract symptoms with an International Prostate Symptom Score >19, or class III or IV heart failure (3)[B].
- Testosterone therapy is not recommended for:
  - Mood or strength improvement in otherwise healthy older men (4)[C]
  - Asymptomatic men with low testosterone measurements (3)[B]
- Testosterone-deficient men with HIV infection or receiving high doses of glucocorticoid treatment may benefit from short-term testosterone therapy to promote preservation of lean body mass and bone density (3)[B].

MEDICATION

First Line

- Testosterone gel (AndroGel, Testim, Fortesta, Axiron):
  - 5–10 g containing 50–100 mg of testosterone applied daily

ALERT

- Must avoid transfer of testosterone gel to female partner or children
  - Improvements in sexual function, mood, lean body mass, bone density have been reported (5)[C].
- Oral therapy is not recommended:
  - May cause liver toxicity
  - Physiologic levels are difficult to maintain.
  - Not beneficial in older men

Second Line

- Delatestryl (testosterone enanthate) or Depo-Testosterone (testosterone cypionate) injection:
  - 100 mg/wk or 200 mg every 2 weeks
  - Inexpensive
  - Levels high immediately after injection, fall to very low before next injection is due; may cause mood swings
- Transdermal patch (Androderm, Testoderm):
  - More expensive
  - May cause skin irritation

- Scrotal patch:
  - Applied daily; delivers 6 mg
  - Need to shave scrotum
  - Dihydrotestosterone levels are higher than normal.
  - Nonscrotal patch: 1–2 patches daily
  - Rotate sites to avoid irritation.
- Transbuccal bioadhesive tablets (Striant):
  - 30 mg b.i.d.
  - Gum-related events in 16% of men
- SC pellets (Testopel) or compounded:
  - Last 3–6 months
  - May be difficult to adjust dose; easier to customize with compounded formulation.
  - Requires surgical insertion, which can be done in the office with local anesthesia.

ISSUES FOR REFERRAL

- In prepubertal patients, starting hormonal therapy at the appropriate age is of paramount importance:
  - In hypogonadotropic hypogonadism, testosterone therapy does not confer fertility or stimulate testicular growth.
  - Pulsatile LH–releasing hormone or human chorionic gonadotropin therapy is an option.
- Elevated PSA; abnormal prostate exam

COMPLEMENTARY AND ALTERNATIVE MEDICINE

Dehydroepiandrostenedione supplementation has not been studied adequately in humans to define potential risks vs. benefits (6)[C].

 ONGOING CARE

Monitoring the effectiveness of therapy, as well as surveillance for adverse effects of replacement, is necessary every 6–12 months.

FOLLOW-UP RECOMMENDATIONS

Patient Monitoring

Monitor replacement therapy for 2–4 months initially and then 6–12 months thereafter:

- Digital prostate exam, PSA, lipid profile, CBC, serum glutamic pyruvic transaminase before initiating therapy and at least annually thereafter
- Testosterone levels until stabilized

DIET

- Calcium 1,200 mg/d, vitamin D 800 IU/d
- Hypocaloric diet to reduce weight if obese

PATIENT EDUCATION

- Testosterone deficiency is a chronic condition that is likely to need lifelong replacement therapy.
- Women and children must not be allowed to come in contact with testosterone replacement products.

PROGNOSIS

- Sustained reversal of symptoms is the goal of therapy when adequate serum levels of testosterone are achieved.
- Hypogonadotropic hypogonadism may be reversed successfully in 10% of patients (7).
- Androgen supplementation does not seem to improve any aspects of age-related frailty (6).

COMPLICATIONS

- Decreased sexual desire, muscle mass, bone density, loss of secondary sexual characteristics
- Complications of testosterone replacement:
  - Benign prostate hyperplasia exacerbation
  - Gynecomastia
  - Acne

- Aggressive behavior
- Polycythemia
- Exacerbation of sleep apnea
- Possible increased risk for cardiovascular events (8)[A]
- Hepatotoxicity with prolonged use
- Exacerbation of metastatic prostate cancer

REFERENCES

1. Shores MM, Sloan KL, Matsumoto AM, et al. Increased incidence of diagnosed depressive illness in hypogonadal older men. *Arch Gen Psychiatry*. 2004;61(2):162–167.
2. Moffat SD, Zonderman AB, Metter EJ, et al. Free testosterone and risk for Alzheimer disease in older men. *Neurology*. 2004;62(2):170–171.
3. Bhasin S, Cunningham GR, Hayes FJ, et al. Testosterone therapy in adult men with androgen deficiency syndromes: An Endocrine Society clinical practice guideline. *J Clin Endocrinol Metab*. 2006;91(6):1995.
4. Lawrence D. US panel urges caution on testosterone therapy. Large-scale trials of efficacy and safety are needed before widespread use can be recommended. *Lancet*. 2003;362(9397):1725.
5. Wang C, Cunningham G, Dobs A, et al. Long-term testosterone gel (AndroGel) treatment maintains beneficial effects on sexual function and mood, lean and fat mass, and bone mineral density in hypogonadal men. *J Clin Endocrinol Metab*. 2004;89(5):2085–2098.
6. Muller M, van den Beld AW, van der Schouw YT, et al. Effects of dehydroepiandrosterone and atamestane supplementation on frailty in elderly men. *J Clin Endocrinol Metab*. 2006;91:3988–3991.
7. Raivio T, Falardeau J, Dwyer A, et al. Reversal of idiopathic hypogonadotropic hypogonadism. *N Engl J Med*. 2007;357:863–873.
8. Haddad RM, Kennedy CC, Caples SM, et al. Testosterone and cardiovascular risk in men: A systematic review and meta-analysis of randomized placebo-controlled trials. *Mayo Clin Proc*. 2007;82:29–39.

ADDITIONAL READING

Kumar P, Kumar N, Thakur D, et al. Male hypogonadism: Symptoms and treatment. *J Adv Pharm Technol Res*. 2010;1(3):297–301.

CODES

ICD10

- E29.1 Testicular hypofunction
- E89.5 Postprocedural testicular hypofunction

CLINICAL PEARLS

- Every man presenting with a complaint of erectile dysfunction or with a low-trauma fracture should be assessed for the presence of hypogonadism.
- Initial test of choice is a morning total testosterone; if low, repeat morning total testosterone.

THALASSEMIA

Herbert L. Muncie, Jr., MD

 BASICS

DESCRIPTION

- A group of inherited hematologic disorders that affect the synthesis of adult hemoglobin tetramer (HbA) (1,2)[C]
- α-Thalassemia is due to a deficient synthesis of α-globin chain, whereas β-thalassemia is due to a deficient synthesis of β-globin chain:
  - The synthesis of the unaffected globin chain proceeds normally.
  - The unbalanced globin chain production causes unstable hemoglobin tetramers, which leads to hypochromic, microcytic RBCs, and hemolytic anemia.
- Thalassemia is prevalent in the Mediterranean region, the Middle East, Southeast Asia, and among ethnic groups originating from these areas.
- α-Thalassemia is more common in persons of Mediterranean, African, and Southeast Asian descent, whereas β-thalassemia is more common in patients of African and Southeast Asian descent,.
- Types:
  - Thalassemia (minor) trait (α or β): Absent or mild anemia with microcytosis and hypochromia. No therapy is needed.
  - α-Thalassemia major with hemoglobin Barts usually results in fatal hydrops fetalis (fluid in ≥ 2 fetal compartments secondary to anemia and fetal heart failure).
  - α-Thalassemia intermedia with hemoglobin H (hemoglobin H disease): Hemolytic anemia and splenomegaly
  - β-Thalassemia major: Severe anemia, growth retardation, hepatosplenomegaly, bone marrow expansion, and bone deformities. Transfusion therapy is necessary to sustain life.
  - β-Thalassemia intermedia: Milder form; transfusion therapy may not be needed or may be needed later in life.
- Other variants include hemoglobin E/β-thalassemia in Southeast Asians, which often mimics the severity of α-thalassemia major.
- System(s) affected: Hematologic/Lymphatic/Immunologic; Cardiac; Hepatic
- Synonym(s): Mediterranean anemia; Hereditary leptocytosis; Thalassemia major and minor; Cooley anemia

Pediatric Considerations
- β-Thalassemia major causes symptoms during early childhood, usually starting at 6 months of age, and requires periodic transfusions to sustain life.
- Newborn's cord blood or heel stick should be screened for hemoglobinopathies with hemoglobin electrophoresis or comparably accurate test, although this primarily detects sickle cell disease.

Pregnancy Considerations
- Preconception genetic counseling is advised for couples at risk for having a child with thalassemia and for parents or other relatives of a child with thalassemia (3)[A].
- Once pregnant, a chorionic villus sample at 10–11 weeks' gestation or an amniocentesis at 15 weeks' gestation can be done to detect point mutations or deletions with polymerase chain reaction (PCR) technology.

EPIDEMIOLOGY

Incidence
- Occurs in ~4.4/10,000 live births
- Predominant age: Symptoms start to appear 6 months after birth with β-thalassemia major.
- Predominant sex: Male = Female

Prevalence
- Worldwide ~200,000 people are alive with β-thalassemia major and <1,000 patients are in the US.
- In the worldwide population, an estimated 1.5% are β-thalassemia carriers and 5% α-thalassemia carriers (4).

ETIOLOGY AND PATHOPHYSIOLOGY
Unknown; it is unclear how the imbalance of α-globin in β-thalassemia and β-globulin in α-thalassemia results in ineffective red cell genesis and hemolysis.

Genetics
- Inherited in an autosomal recessive pattern
- α-Thalassemia results from a deletion of ≥ 1 of the 4 genes, 2 on each chromosome 16, responsible for α-globin synthesis. 1-gene deletion is a silent carrier state, 2-gene deletion is the trait, 3-gene deletion results in hemoglobin H, and 4-gene deletion results in hemoglobin Barts causing fatal hydrops fetalis.
- Nondeletional forms do occur rarely. Hemoglobin H Constant Spring is the most common nondeletional hemoglobin H.
- β-thalassemia is caused by any of >200 point mutations and, very rarely, deletions on chromosome 11, although probably 20 alleles account for >80% of the mutations.
- Significantly disparate phenotype with the same genotype occurs because β-globin chain production can range from near normal to absent.

RISK FACTORS
Family history

GENERAL PREVENTION
- Prenatal information: Genetic counseling regarding partner selection and information on the availability of diagnostic tests during the pregnancy
- Complication prevention:
  - For offspring of adult thalassemia patients, an evaluation for thalassemia by 1 year of age
  - Severe forms:
    ○ Avoid exposure to sick contacts.
    ○ Keep immunizations up to date, including pneumococcal vaccine and annual influenza vaccine.
  - Promptly treat bacterial infections (after splenectomy, patients should maintain a supply of an appropriate antibiotic to take at the onset of symptoms of a bacterial infection).
  - Dental checkups every 6 months
  - Avoid activities that could increase the risk of bone fractures.
- Genetic counseling

COMMONLY ASSOCIATED CONDITIONS
See "Complications."

 DIAGNOSIS

Thalassemia trait has no signs or symptoms.

HISTORY
- Poor growth
- Excessive fatigue
- Cholelithiasis
- Pathologic fractures
- Shortness of breath

PHYSICAL EXAM
- Pallor
- Splenomegaly
- Jaundice
- Maxillary hyperplasia/frontal bossing due to massive bone marrow expansion
- Dental malocclusion

DIFFERENTIAL DIAGNOSIS
- Iron deficiency
- Other microcytic anemias: lead toxicity, sideroblastic
- Other hemolytic anemias
- Hemoglobinopathies

DIAGNOSTIC TESTS & INTERPRETATION
Special tests:
- Bone marrow aspiration to evaluate for other causes of microcytic anemia is rarely needed.
- Multiple indices have been evaluated to discriminate β-thalassemia trait from iron deficiency anemia, yet none is sensitive enough to exclude β-thalassemia trait.
- Hemoglobin: Usual range 10–12 g/dL with thalassemia trait and 3–8 g/dL with β-thalassemia major before transfusions
- Hematocrit:
  - 28–40% in thalassemia trait
  - May fall to <10% in β-thalassemia major
- Peripheral blood:
  - Microcytosis (MCV <70 fl)
  - Hypochromia (MCH <20 pg)
  - High percentage of target cells
  - Reticulocyte count elevated
- Red cell distribution width (RDW):
  - A normal RDW with a microcytic hypochromic anemia is almost always thalassemia trait.
  - Although the RDW is usually normal, it can be elevated in ~50% of thalassemia trait patients. This is in contrast to iron-deficiency anemia, where the RDW is almost always elevated (90%).
- Hemoglobin electrophoresis:
  - In α-thalassemia trait, no recognizable electrophoretic pattern occurs in adults.
  - However, in the neonatal period 3–10% of trait patients will have hemoglobin H or hemoglobin Bart at birth, which would confirm α-thalassemia.
  - If HbA$_2$ is below normal (<2.5%) with a normal HbF level, the diagnosis is α-thalassemia intermedia (HbH disease) or, if tested in the neonatal period, 15–30% will have hemoglobin Bart.
  - In the neonatal period with β-thalassemia trait, the electrophoresis is normal. However, in adults, elevated HbA$_2$ levels (>4%) may be present but are usually normal (5).
  - In β-thalassemia major or intermedia, elevated HbA$_2$, elevated HbF, reduced or absent HbA

- DNA analysis:
  - α-Thalassemia can definitively be diagnosed with genetic testing of hemoglobin A1 and A2 (for deletions and point mutations), but this is not routinely done due to the high cost.

Pediatric Considerations
For children, calculate Mentzer index (mean corpuscular volume/RBC count):
- <13: Thalassemia more likely
- >13: Iron deficiency more likely

Test Interpretation
- Bone marrow erythroid hyperplasia
- Iron deposits in heart muscle
- Liver iron concentrations can be assessed with MRI imaging (Ferriscan)
- Hepatic siderosis

 TREATMENT

- Outpatient for mild cases
- Inpatient for transfusion therapy

GENERAL MEASURES
- Mild cases (trait or minor) require no therapy.
- Thalassemia intermedia: Normally, no therapy is necessary unless hemoglobin falls to a level that causes symptoms; then transfusion therapy may be needed. Decision is based primarily on patient's quality of life.
- Iron supplements should not be given unless iron deficiency is confirmed. Supplements can increase the risk of iron overload.
- Thalassemia major:
  - A regular transfusion schedule to increase post transfusion hemoglobin to 13.0–14.0 g/L and maintain a mean hemoglobin level of at least 9.3 g/dL (1.4 mmol/L).
  - Iron overload (6)[C]:
    ○ Patients receiving transfusion therapy increase total-body iron 4× over the normal amount.
    ○ Therapy is iron chelation. (See "Medication.")

MEDICATION
Thalassemia intermedia and major: Folic acid supplements (1 mg/d)

First Line
β-thalassemia major:
- Iron chelation with deferoxamine (Desferal):
  - SC or continuous IV infusion, 20–40 mg/kg over 8–12 hours daily
  - Usually started before 5–8 years of age
  - Treatment lasts 3–5 years to reach serum ferritin <1,000 ng/mL.
- Deferasirox (Exjade): 20–30 mg/kg/d PO acceptable alternative (7); approved for transfusion- and nontransfusion-dependent patients with liver concentrations > 5 mg/g of liver tissue

Second Line
Deferiprone (Ferriprox) 25 mg/kg t.i.d. PO initially is an acceptable alternative for patients who have not responded to deferoxamine; may provide more cardioprotection. A drawback is that ~1% of patients develop agranulocytosis necessitating weekly blood counts.

ISSUES FOR REFERRAL
Thalassemia major usually requires hematology consult.

ADDITIONAL THERAPIES
β-thalassemia intermedia:
- Hydroxyurea may improve hemoglobin 1–2 g/dL.
- Psychological support seems appropriate for this chronic disease. However, no conclusions can be made regarding specific psychological therapies.

SURGERY/OTHER PROCEDURES
- Splenectomy:
  - May be needed if hypersplenism causes a marked increase in the transfusion requirements (>180–200 ml/kg/yr) (8)
  - Defer surgery until patient is at least 4 years of age (due to increased infection risk).
  - Administer pneumococcal polyvalent-23 vaccine 1 month before splenectomy. Children should complete their pneumococcal conjugate vaccine series before surgery.
  - Daily penicillin prophylaxis, 250 mg b.i.d., after splenectomy for 2 years for all patients and for children until age 16.
- Bone marrow transplantation with HLA-identical related donor stem cells in children before developing hepatitis or iron overload has high likelihood of remission but may impair fertility.

 ONGOING CARE

FOLLOW-UP RECOMMENDATIONS
- Thalassemia trait requires no restrictions.
- β-thalassemia major:
  - Avoid strenuous activities (e.g., football, soccer).
  - Acceptable activity levels will be determined on an individual basis depending on the severity of the disorder.

Patient Monitoring
- Thalassemia-trait patients require no special follow-up.
- For β-thalassemia major, lifelong monitoring is necessary because the therapy and disease progression have numerous potential complications.

DIET
- Thalassemia trait requires no restrictions.
- β-thalassemia major:
  - Limit intake of iron-rich foods (e.g., red meats such as liver and some cereals).

PATIENT EDUCATION
Printed patient information available from Cooley Anemia Foundation, 330 7th Ave. Suite 900, New York, NY 10001; www.thalassemia.org or www.cooleysanemia.org

PROGNOSIS
- Outlook varies depending on type.
- Thalassemia-trait patients live a normal lifespan.
- β-Thalassemia major patients live an average of 17 years and usually die by age 30.
- Iron overload causes most of the morbidity and mortality:
  - Cardiac events are the primary cause of death.
  - Effective iron chelation is improving longevity.

COMPLICATIONS
- Chronic hemolysis
- Susceptibility to infections after splenectomy
- Infections from blood transfusion
- Jaundice
- Leg ulcers
- Cholelithiasis
- Osteoporosis and low-trauma fractures
- Impaired growth rate

- Delayed or absent puberty
- Hypogonadism
- Hepatic siderosis
- Splenomegaly
- Cardiac disease from iron overload
- Thromboembolic phenomenon
- Aplastic and megaloblastic crises

REFERENCES

1. Muncie HL, Campbell J. Alpha and beta thalassemia. *Am Fam Physician*. 2009;80: 339–344.
2. Higgs DR, Engel JD, Stamatoyannopoulos G, et al. Thalassaemia. *Lancet*. 2012;379:373–383.
3. Tamhankar PM, Agarwal S, Arya V, et al. Prevention of homozygous beta thalassemia by premarital screening and prenatal diagnosis in India. *Prenat Diagn*. 2009;29:83–88.
4. Peters M, Heijboer H, Smiers F, et al. Diagnosis and management of thalassaemia. *BMJ*. 2012;344: e228. Epub 2012 Jan 25.
5. Mosca A, Paleari R, Ivaldi G, et al. The role of haemoglobin A(2) testing in the diagnosis of thalassaemias and related haemoglobinopathies. *J Clin Pathol*. 2009;62:13–17.
6. Fleming RE, Ponka P. Iron overload in human disease. *N Engl J Med*. 2012;84(4):348–359.
7. Taher A, El-Beshlawy A, Elalfy MS, et al. Efficacy and safety of deferasirox, an oral iron chelator, in heavily iron-overloaded patients with beta-thalassemia: The ESCALATOR study. *Eur J Haematol*. 2009;82:458–465.
8. Galanello R, Origa R. Beta-thalassemia. *Orphanet J Rare Dis*. 2010;5:11.

ADDITIONAL READING

Borgna-Pignatti C. Modern treatment of thalassaemia intermedia. *Br J Haematol*. 2007;84(3):291–304. Epub 2007 Jun 12.

 CODES

ICD10
- D56.0 Alpha thalassemia
- D56.1 Beta thalassemia
- D56.9 Thalassemia, unspecified

CLINICAL PEARLS

- Thalassemia (group of inherited hematologic disorders that affect the synthesis of adult hemoglobin tetramer) is a genetic condition; hemoglobin will not improve over time.
- α-Thalassemia is due to a deficient synthesis of the α-globin chain, whereas β-thalassemia is due to a deficient synthesis of the β-globin chain.
- Hemoglobin electrophoresis is needed for genetic counseling but not to make the diagnosis of thalassemia minor when evaluating a patient with mild hypochromic, microcytic anemia, and normal serum ferritin.
- Anemia from thalassemia minor is not due to inadequate iron availability or iron storage. Therefore, iron supplements will not improve the anemia and could be harmful due to GI distress and iron overload. If coexisting iron deficiency is proven, then iron therapy is appropriate.

THORACIC OUTLET SYNDROME

Muhammad Imran Khan, MD • Najm Hasan Siddiqui, MD

 BASICS

DESCRIPTION

- A constellation of symptoms that affect the head, neck, shoulders, and upper extremities caused by compression of the neurovascular structures (i.e., brachial plexus and subclavian vessels) at the thoracic outlet, specifically in the area superior to the 1st rib and posterior to the clavicle
- 3 forms of thoracic outlet syndrome (TOS) have been described: Neurogenic, vascular (containing venous and arterial symptoms), and nonspecific (includes traumatic and secondary to certain provocative movements).
- Synonym(s): Scalenus anticus syndrome; Cervical rib syndrome; Costoclavicular syndrome

Pregnancy Considerations
Generalized tissue fluid accumulations and postural changes may aggravate symptoms.

EPIDEMIOLOGY

Incidence
- Predominant age:
  – Neurogenic type (95%): 20–60 years
  – Venous type (4%): 20–35 years
  – Arterial type (1%; atherosclerosis): Young adult or >50 years
- Predominant sex:
  – Neurogenic type: Female > Male (3.5:1)
  – Venous type: Male > Female
  – Arterial type: Male = Female
- No objective confirmatory tests available to measure true incidence
- Estimated 3–8/1,000 cases for neurogenic type
- Incidence of other TOS types is unclear.

ETIOLOGY AND PATHOPHYSIOLOGY
The interscalene triangle area is reduced in TOS and may become smaller during certain shoulder and arm movements. Fibrotic bands, cervical ribs, and muscle variations may further narrow the triangle. Trauma or provocative movements affecting the lower brachial plexus have strong implications in TOS pathogenesis.

- 3 known causes of TOS: Anatomic, traumatic/repetitive-movement activities, and neurovascular entrapment
- Anatomic: Variations in the anatomy of the neck scalene muscles may be responsible for presentations of the neurologic type of TOS and may involve the superior border of the 1st rib. Cervical ribs also have been implicated as a cause of neurologic TOS, with subsequent neuronal fibrosing and degeneration associated with arterial hyalinization in the lower trunk of the brachial plexus. Fibrous bands to cervical ribs are often congenital.
- Trauma or repetitive-movement activities: Motor vehicle accidents with hyperextension injury and resulting fibrosis, including fibrous bands to the clavicle; musicians who maintain prolonged positions of shoulder abduction or extension may be at increased risk.
- Neurovascular entrapment: Occurring in the costoclavicular space between the 1st rib and the head of the clavicle

RISK FACTORS
- Trauma, especially to the shoulder girdle
- Presence of a cervical rib
- Posttraumatic, exostosis of clavicle or 1st rib, postural abnormalities (e.g., drooping of shoulders, scoliosis), body building with increased muscular bulk in thoracic outlet area, rapid weight loss with vigorous physical exertion and/or exercise, pendulous breasts
- Occupational exposure: Computer users; musicians; repetitive work involving shoulders, arms, hands
- Young, thin females with long necks and drooping shoulders

GENERAL PREVENTION
Consider observation or further evaluation in patients with cervical ribs.

COMMONLY ASSOCIATED CONDITIONS
- Paget–von Schrötter syndrome: Thrombosis of subclavian vein
- Gilliatt-Sumner hand: Neurogenic atrophy of abductor pollicis brevis

 DIAGNOSIS

HISTORY
- Neurologic type, upper plexus (C4–C7):
  – Pain and paresthesias in head, neck, mandible, face, temporal area, upper back/chest, outer arm, and hand in a radial nerve distribution
  – Occipital and orbital headache
- Neurologic type, lower plexus (C8–T1):
  – Pain and paresthesias in axilla, inner arm, and hand in an ulnar nerve distribution, often nocturnal
  – Hypothenar and interosseous muscle atrophy
- Venous type: Arm claudication, cyanosis, swelling, distended arm veins
- Arterial type: Digital vasospasm, thrombosis/embolism, aneurysm, gangrene

PHYSICAL EXAM
- Positive Adson maneuver (head rotation to the affected side with cervical extension and then deep inhalation); test is positive if paresthesias occur or if radial pulse is not palpable during maneuver.
- Tenderness to percussion or palpation of supraclavicular area
- Worsening of symptoms with elevation of arm, overhead extension of arms, or with arms extended forward (e.g., driving a car, typing, carrying objects); prompt disappearance of symptoms with arm returning to neutral position
- Morley test:
  – Brachial plexus compression test in the supraclavicular area from the scalene triangle
  – Positive with reproduction of an aching sensation and typical localized paresthesia
- Hyperabduction test: Diminishment of radial pulse with elevation of arm above the head

- Military maneuver (i.e., costoclavicular bracing): When patient elevates chin and pushes shoulders posteriorly in an extreme "at-attention" position, symptoms are provoked.
- 1-minute Roos test:
  – A thoracic outlet shoulder girdle stress test
  – Shoulders and arms are braced in a 90-degree abducted and externally rotated position; patient is required to clench and relax fists repetitively for 1 minute.
  – A positive test reproduces the symptom.

DIFFERENTIAL DIAGNOSIS
- Cervical disk or carpal tunnel syndrome
- Orthopedic shoulder problems (shoulder strain, rotator cuff injury, tendonitis)
- Cervical spondylitis
- Ulnar nerve compression at elbow and hand
- Multiple sclerosis
- Spinal cord tumor/disease
- Angina pectoris
- Migraine
- Complex regional pain syndromes
- C3–C5 and C8 radiculopathies

DIAGNOSTIC TESTS & INTERPRETATION
Initial Tests (lab, imaging)
CBC, ESR, and C-reactive protein (CRP) determination may rule out underlying inflammatory conditions.
- Radiograph (chest, C-spine, shoulders) (1)[C] may reveal elongated C7 transverse process or a cervical rib, Pancoast tumor, or healed clavicle fracture.
- Nerve conduction studies and electromyography (EMG)
- CT scan or MRI, although MRI is the method of choice when searching for nerve compression
- Evidence is insufficient to use MR angiography (2)[B].
- Doppler and duplex US if vascular obstruction is suspected
- Arteriogram and venogram have limited roles; useful when symptoms suggestive of arterial insufficiency or ischemia, or in planning surgical intervention (3)[C]

Diagnostic Procedures/Other
No indicated procedures; anesthetic anterior scalene block may relieve pressure by scalene muscles on the brachial plexus, making this type of block diagnostic and potentially therapeutic, but it poses the risk of procedural damage to the brachial plexus.

Test Interpretation
Systematic results of biopsy have not been reported. There is no indication for biopsy unless to investigate another underlying condition.

TREATMENT

GENERAL MEASURES
- Conservative management usually involves approaches to reduce and redistribute pressure and traction through the use of physiotherapy or prosthesis.
- Interscalene injections of botulinum toxin have been shown to decrease symptoms of TOS (4)[C].
- Physical therapy will develop strength in pectoral girdle muscles and achieve normal posture (1)[C].
- Severe cases may use taping, adhesive elastic bandages, moist heat, TENS, or US but should not substitute active exercise and correction of posture and muscle imbalance (5)[B].

MEDICATION
- No firm evidence exists for any approach to the 4 types of TOS.
- Physical therapy is 1st-line treatment (5)[B].
- Anti-inflammatory (ibuprofen):
  – Adult dose: 400–800 mg PO q8h; not to exceed 3,200 mg/d
  – Pediatric dose:
    ○ <12 years: Not recommended
    ○ >12 years: As in adults
  – Contraindications: Documented hypersensitivity, active PUD, renal or hepatic impairment, recent use of anticoagulants, hemorrhagic conditions
- Neuropathic pain: Carbamazepine, gabapentin, phenytoin, pregabalin; muscle relaxants such as baclofen, methocarbamol, or tizanidine may be helpful
- Severe pain: Consider opiates for brachial plexus nerve block, steroid injections

ISSUES FOR REFERRAL
- Neurologic, anesthesiologic, orthopedic, vascular surgery referral(s) may be indicated depending on the type of pathologic condition.
- Physical and rehabilitation physicians

SURGERY/OTHER PROCEDURES
- Operative if vascular involvement is present and/or loss of function or lifestyle occurs secondary to severity of symptoms and if conservative therapy fails after 2–3 months (1)[C]
- Transaxillary 1st rib resection (TFRR) may provide better pain relief than supraclavicular neuroplasty of the brachial plexus (SNBP), although, overall, both treatment options have generally positive outcomes (6)[B].
- Resection of 1st rib or cervical ribs via transaxillary (preferred with good to excellent outcome 80% of patients), supraclavicular (good to excellent outcome 80% of patients), posterior approaches (reserved for complicated TOS due to necessity of large muscle incision)
- Excision of adhesive bands, anterior scalenectomy (7)[B]
- Supra clavicular scalenectomy (8)[C]

IN-PATIENT CONSIDERATIONS
Admission Criteria/Initial Stabilization
Conservative, outpatient, nonpharmacologic treatment is reasonable first-line therapy except in cases of thromboembolic phenomena and acute ischemia, symptoms of chronic vascular occlusion, stenosis, arterial dilatation, or progressive neurologic deficit (5)[B].

ONGOING CARE

FOLLOW-UP RECOMMENDATIONS
Correct improper posture, practice proper posture, exercises to strengthen shoulder elevator and neck extensor muscles, stretching exercises for scalene muscles, support bra for women with pendulous breasts, breast reduction surgery in selected cases; sleep with arms below chest level, avoid/reduce prolonged hyperabduction.

Patient Monitoring
Office follow-up visits every 3–4 weeks

PATIENT EDUCATION
Physical therapy, postural exercises, ergonomic workstation

PROGNOSIS
Follow-up from surgery at mean of 7.5 years showed that functional results were excellent, good, fair, and poor in 87 (49.4%), 61 (34.6%), 14 (8%), and 14 (8%) procedures, respectively (9)[C].

COMPLICATIONS
- Postoperative shoulder, arm, hand pain, and paresthesias in 10%
- Patients who will have symptomatic recurrences at 1 month–7 years postoperatively (usually within 3 months): 1.5–2%
- Patients who will have brachial plexus injury, probably due to intraoperative traction: 0.5–1%
- Reoperation is indicated for symptomatic recurrence with long posterior remnant of 1st rib (posterior approach) or with disrupted fibrous adhesions (transaxillary approach).
- Venous obstruction or arterial emboli; usually responds to thrombolytics

REFERENCES
1. Huang JH, Zager EL. Thoracic outlet syndrome. *Neurosurgery.* 2004;55:897–902; discussion 902–903.
2. Estilaei SK, Byl NN. An evidence-based review of magnetic resonance angiography for diagnosing arterial thoracic outlet syndrome. *J Hand Ther.* 2006;19:410–420.
3. Sanders RJ, Hammond SL, Rao NM. Diagnosis of thoracic outlet syndrome. *J Vasc Surg.* 2007;46: 601–604.
4. Lee GW, Kwon YH, Jeong JH, et al. The efficacy of scalene injection in thoracic outlet syndrome. *J Korean Neurosurg Soc.* 2011;84(1):36–39. Epub 2011 Jul 31.
5. Vanti C, Natalini L, Romeo A. Conservative treatment of thoracic outlet syndrome. A review of the literature. *Eura Medicophys.* 2007;43:55–70.
6. Sheth RN, Campbell JN. Surgical treatment of thoracic outlet syndrome: A randomized trial comparing two operations. *J Neurosurg Spine.* 2005;3:355–363.
7. Urschel HC, Kourlis H. Thoracic outlet syndrome: A 50-year experience at Baylor University Medical Center. *Proc (Bayl Univ Med Cent).* 2007;20: 125–135.
8. Glynn RW, Tawfick W, Elsafty Z, et al. Supraclavicular scalenectomy for thoracic outlet syndrome—functional outcomes assessed using the DASH scoring system. *Vasc Endovascular Surg.* 2012;84(2):157–162. Epub 2012 Feb 5.
9. Degeorges R. Thoracic outlet syndrome surgery: Long-term functional results. *Ann Vas Surg.* 2004;18(5):558–565.

ADDITIONAL READING
- Aralasmak A, Cevikol C, Karaali K, et al. MRI findings in thoracic outlet syndrome. *Skeletal radiology.* 2012 Jul 11. Epub 2012 Jul 11.
- Povlsen B, Belzberg A, Hansson T, et al. Treatment for thoracic outlet syndrome. *Cochrane Database Syst Rev.* 2010;(1):CD007218. Epub 2010 Jan 20.

CODES

ICD10
G54.0 Brachial plexus disorders

CLINICAL PEARLS
- Consider breast reduction for patients with pendulous breasts.
- Avoid opiate dependence.
- Consider pain clinic referral if there are nonsurgical causes.

THROMBOANGIITIS OBLITERANS (BUERGER DISEASE)

Felix B. Chang, MD, DABMA • Alfonso J. Tafur, MD

BASICS

DESCRIPTION
- Nonatherosclerotic vasculitis of small- and medium-sized arteries and veins resulting in segmental occlusion
- Involves arteries, veins, and nerves of extremities
- Characterized clinically by an inflammatory and vaso-occlusive phenomenon, rest pain, unremitting ischemic ulcerations, and gangrene of the digits of hands and feet
- Occurs primarily in men who smoke
- Patients are young smokers who present with distal extremity ischemia, ischemic digit ulcers, or digit gangrene.
- Synonym(s): Buerger disease

EPIDEMIOLOGY
- The prevalence has decreased in North America over the past 30 years.
- Worldwide, but most prevalent in Eastern Europe, Mediterranean, and Asian countries

Incidence
- 11–30/100,000 persons/year
- Predominant age: 20–40 years
- Predominant sex: Male > Female; increasing numbers of women are being diagnosed, possibly due to increased smoking.

Prevalence
- Estimates range from as low as 0.5–5.5% in Western Europe, to 45–63% in India, to 80% in Israel among Jews of Ashkenazi ancestry.
- Accounts for 5% and 16% of patients hospitalized for arterial occlusive disease in Europe and Japan, respectively
- 13/100,000 US population
- Overall occurrence is decreasing worldwide.

Geriatric Considerations
Not common in this age group

Pediatric Considerations
Should be considered in the differential diagnosis of the young patient with claudication.

ETIOLOGY AND PATHOPHYSIOLOGY
- Impaired endothelium-dependent vasorelaxation and decreased peripheral sympathetic outflow
- Segmental infiltration of inflammatory cells in vessel wall leads to thrombotic occlusion of vessel.
- Highly cellular and inflammatory thrombus with relative sparing of the blood vessel wall
- Idiopathic
- Smoking
- Genetic factors
- Autoimmune disorder with cell-mediated sensitivity to types I and III human collagens (both are normal constituents of blood vessels)
- Impaired peripheral endothelium-dependent vasodilation. Nonendothelial mechanisms of vasodilation are intact.
- Arsenic content of tobacco
- Chronic anaerobic periodontal infection

Genetics
- Greater prevalence of HLA-A54, HLA-A9, and HLA-B5
- HLA-B12 antigen may be associated with disease resistance.
- Familial cases reported rarely

RISK FACTORS
- Smoking tobacco, as little as 1–2 cigarettes daily, chewing tobacco, snuff, and nicotine replacement
- Chronic anaerobic periodontal infection also may play a role in the development of Buerger disease.

GENERAL PREVENTION
Never smoke. Tobacco and smoking cessation is the only way to prevent Buerger disease.

DIAGNOSIS

- Point scoring systems may help to clarify clinical diagnosis. Many diagnostic tools are available.
- Criteria proposed by Olin is one most widely accepted:
  – Smoking history
  – Onset <50 years
  – Infrapopliteal arterial occlusions
  – Either upper limb involvement or phlebitis migrans
  – Absence of atherosclerotic risk factors other than smoking
- Disease diagnosis may be made only when all 5 requirements have been fulfilled.
- Symptoms tend to wax and wane in early disease and often are asymmetric. Symptoms may be gradual/have a sudden onset related to impaired vasculature. Usually >1 limb is involved.

HISTORY
- Foot/Arch claudication may be the presenting manifestation (rarely hand, forearm) and is often mistaken for an orthopedic problem.
- Cold sensitivity
- Paresthesias (e.g., numbness, tingling, burning, hypoesthesia) of feet and/or fingers
- Persistent extremity pain (may be worse at rest); pain may be disabling
- Paroxysmal "electric shock" pain of ischemic neuropathy
- Migratory superficial phlebitis

PHYSICAL EXAM
- 76% of patients had ischemic ulcerations at the time of presentation.
- Allen test should be performed.
- Ulceration of digits
- Raynaud phenomenon (~20% of patients)
- Postural color changes: Pallor on elevation; rubor on dependency
- "Buerger color": Cyanosis of hands and feet
- Tender skin nodules on extremities
- Impaired distal pulses
- Proximal pulses normal; Allen test may be abnormal.
- Foot edema
- Gangrene
- Features: Thrombotic, nonatherosclerotic, segmental, chronic, and inflammatory

DIFFERENTIAL DIAGNOSIS
- Peripheral neuropathy, peripheral atherosclerotic disease, arterial embolus and thrombosis, idiopathic peripheral thrombosis
- Takayasu arteritis; CREST syndrome (calcinosis, Raynaud phenomenon, esophageal dysfunction, sclerodactyly, telangiectasia)
- Hypercoagulable states; systemic lupus erythematosus; scleroderma
- Necrotizing arteritis

- Occupational trauma; acrocyanosis; frostbite; neurotrophic ulcers
- Reflex sympathetic dystrophy; metatarsalgia; gout

DIAGNOSTIC TESTS & INTERPRETATION
No specific lab finding is relevant for thromboangiitis obliterans (TAO).

Initial Tests (lab, imaging)
- Noninvasive vascular studies, including transcutaneous oxygen tension ($TcPO_2$), ankle brachial index, and simultaneous brachial pressures
- To rule out diseases in the differential diagnosis, consider CBC, LFTs, creatinine, fasting glucose, erythrocyte sedimentation rate (ESR), antinuclear antibodies (ANA), rheumatoid factor (RF), anticentromere antibody, and Scl70 antibody, as well as a hypercoagulability screen.
- Autoantibodies to collagen and circulating immune complexes may be present, but the significance is still to be determined.
- Increased levels of antiendothelial cell antibodies are seen in patients with active disease.
- Anticardiolipin antibodies may be associated with TAO and may worsen the thrombotic event (1)[A].
- Homocysteine may be elevated, but lacks specificity.
- Toxin screen when appropriate: Cocaine, amphetamines, and cannabis ingestion can mimic TAO.
- A vascular biopsy is usually not necessary unless patients present with unusual characteristics such as large-artery involvement or age >45.
- Doppler US (not specific)
- Arteriogram/Digital subtraction angiography:
  – Multiple areas of segmental occlusion of small- to medium-sized arteries of arms and legs
  – The disease is confined most often to the distal circulation and is almost always infrapopliteal in the lower extremities and distal to the brachial artery in the upper extremities.
  – "Skip" areas may be demonstrated.
  – Numerous collateral vessels around occluded segments may give a characteristic corkscrew appearance (Martorell sign):
    ○ Classification by size and pattern has been proposed:
      ▪ Type I, artery diameter >2 mm, large helical sign
      ▪ Type II, diameter >1.5 mm and ≤2 mm, medium helical sign
      ▪ Type III, diameter ≥1 mm and ≤1.5 mm, small helical sign
      ▪ Type IV, diameter <1 mm, tiny helical sign (2)
  – Larger arteries are spared. More serious disease occurs distally.
  – No apparent source of emboli

Follow-Up Tests & Special Considerations
- The Westergren sedimentation rate and serum C-reactive protein are usually normal.
- Commonly measured autoantibodies (e.g., ANA and RF) are normal/negative.
- Circulating immune complexes, complement levels, and cryoglobulins are normal despite an immune reaction in the arterial intima.
- The prevalence of ischemic ulcers is significantly higher in patients who have small corkscrew patterns (type III and IV) in distal segments of limb collaterals than in patients who have large corkscrew collaterals (2).

Diagnostic Procedures/Other
- Echocardiography (to exclude emboli)
- Biopsy only indicated if there are unusual features:
  – Age >45 at onset
  – Disease in unusual location
  – Proximal disease
  – CNS disease
  – Tobacco history is not consistent with diagnosis.

Test Interpretation
- Segmental inflammatory thrombosis of both arteries and veins
- Histologic findings may vary between acute, intermediate, and chronic stages of the disease.
- Histologic sine qua non: Granulomas with collections of neutrophils in the organizing thrombus:
  – Vessel wall is relatively spared.
  – Wall sparing distinguishes TAO from arteriosclerosis and other systemic vasculitides, which show striking wall disruption.
- Acute lesions show occlusive, highly cellular, inflammatory thrombi with less inflammation in vessel wall. Polymorphonuclear neutrophils, microabscesses, and multinucleated giant cells may be present.
- Intermediate lesions show organizing thrombus.
- Chronic lesions show recanalized thrombus and perivascular fibrosis.

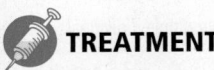
TREATMENT

GENERAL MEASURES
- Stop smoking (mandatory).
- Protect against trauma (poorly fitting shoes) and infections.
- Protect against vasoconstriction from cold/drugs.
- Eliminate exposure to thermal and chemical damage (e.g., iodine, carbolic acid, salicylic acid).
- Thrombolytic therapy of occlusive thrombus and angioplasty are experimental.

MEDICATION
First Line
- Discontinue smoking/tobacco use in any form.
- Wound care
- Amputation for severe disease
- Antibiotics for infected digital ulcers and osteomyelitis
- Urokinase or streptokinase selectively infused into occluded artery
- IM endothelial growth factor gene therapy

Second Line
- If vasospasm is present, trial of dihydropyridine calcium channel blocker such as amlodipine or nifedipine
- Iloprost, a prostacyclin analogue, promotes ulcer healing and decreases analgesic requirement.
- IM gene transfer of vascular growth factors
- Case studies have shown success with phosphodiesterase type 5 inhibitors (3)[C]

ISSUES FOR REFERRAL
Consider referral to nicotine-addiction clinics.

ADDITIONAL THERAPIES
- Initiate a walking program.
- The possibility of distraction osteogenesis as a therapeutic approach is an emergent alternative. This option, however, is an investigational approach (4).

- Intermittent pneumatic compression has been shown to enhance calf circulation and may serve as adjunctive therapy in patients who are not candidates for revascularization.
- Foot care
- Lubricate skin with moisturizer.
- Lamb's wool between toes
- Avoid trauma (e.g., heel protectors, orthotics for shoes, vascular boots).
- Spinal cord stimulation may play a role (5)[C].

SURGERY/OTHER PROCEDURES
- Amputation:
  – For nonhealing ulcers, gangrene, or intractable pain
  – Should preserve as much limb as possible
- Omental autotransplantation has been successful in treating ulcers.
- Infrainguinal bypass
- In severe disease, a lumbar sympathectomy to increase blood supply to the skin (6)[A]
- Surgical revascularization is not usually a viable alternative due to the diffuse segmental involvement and extreme distal nature of the disease.

COMPLEMENTARY AND ALTERNATIVE MEDICINE
Hyperbaric oxygen therapy and autologous bone marrow transplant of mononuclear cells are alternative therapy modalities, with very small studies suggesting potential utility.

IN-PATIENT CONSIDERATIONS
Inpatient nicotine-dependence treatment is an alternative for recidivist smokers.

Admission Criteria/Initial Stabilization
Critical limb ischemia
- Inpatient: gangrene
- Inpatient for dorsal/lumbar sympathectomy

ONGOING CARE

FOLLOW-UP RECOMMENDATIONS
Use a bed cradle (nonheated) to prevent pressure from bed linens.

Patient Monitoring
Frequent history and physical exams

PATIENT EDUCATION
- Remove exposure to others in the environment who smoke.
- Use heel pads/foam rubber boots.

PROGNOSIS
- Average death age 52 ± 8.9 years; significantly lower than matched US population (7)
- In the Cleveland Clinic series, 94% of patients who quit smoking remained free of amputation, whereas 43% of patients who continued smoking required at least 1 amputation.
- Data from Mayo Clinic showed an amputation rate of 25% at 5 years and 38% at 10 years of follow-up (7).
- The risk of amputation is eliminated after 8 years of smoking cessation.

COMPLICATIONS
- Ulcerations, gangrene, need for amputation
- Rare occlusion of cerebral, coronary, renal, splenic, mesenteric, pulmonary, iliac arteries, and aorta

REFERENCES

1. Pereira de Godoy JM, Braile DM. Buerger's disease and anticardiolipin antibodies. *J Cardiovasc Med (Hagerstown)*. 2009;10(10):792–794.
2. Fujii Y, Soga J, Nakamura S, et al. Classification of corkscrew collaterals in thromboangiitis obliterans (Buerger's disease). *Circ J*. 2010;74(8):1684–1688.
3. Abeles AM, Nicolescu M, Pinchover Z, et al. Thromboangiitis obliterans successfully treated with phosphodiesterase type 5 inhibitors. *Vascular*. 2013 Sep 2. Epub ahead of print.
4. Kulkarni S, Kulkarni G, Shyam AK, et al. Management of thromboangiitis obliterans using distraction osteogenesis: A retrospective study. *Indian J Orthop*. 2011;45:459–464.
5. Ryu SW, Jeon HJ, Cho SS, et al. Treatment of digit ulcers in a patient with Buerger's disease by using cervical spinal cord stimulation: A case report-. *Korean J Anesthesiol*. 2013;65(2):167–171.
6. Bozkurt AK, Köksal C, Demirbas MY, et al. A randomized trial of intravenous versus lumbar sympathectomy in the management of Buerger's disease. *Int Angiol*. 2006;25(2):162–168.
7. Cooper LT, Tse TS, Mikhail MA, et al. Long-term survival and amputation risk in thromboangiitis obliterans (Buerger's disease). *J Am Coll Cardiol*. 2004;44:2410–2411.

ADDITIONAL READING

- D'Agargon PT, Landry GJ. Buerger's disease. *Ann Vasc Surg*. 2012;26:871.
- De Haro J, Acin F, Bleda S, et al. Treatment of thromboangiitis obliterans (Buerger's disease) with bosentan. *BMC Cardiovasc Disord*. 2012;12:5.
- Graziani L, Morelli L, Parini F, et al. Clinical outcome after extended endovascular recanalization in Buerger's disease in 20 consecutive cases. *Ann Vasc Surg*. 2012; 26:387.
- Hurelbrink CB, Barnett Y, Buckland ME, et al. Revisiting cerebral thromboangiitis obliterans. *J Neurol Sci*. 2012;317:141–145.

CODES

ICD10
I73.1 Thromboangiitis obliterans [Buerger's disease]

CLINICAL PEARLS
- Stopping the use of tobacco products and smoking cessation is important to decrease the risk for amputation.
- Presence of diabetes mellitus rules out diagnosis of thromboangiitis obliterans.
- Measurement of urinary nicotine and cotinine should be performed if the disease is still active despite patient's claims of tobacco cessation.
- Nicotine replacement may keep the disease active.

THROMBOPHILIA AND HYPERCOAGULABLE STATES

Christopher Hogan, MD

BASICS

DESCRIPTION
- An inherited or acquired disorder of the coagulation system predisposing an individual to thromboembolism (the formation of a venous, or less commonly, an arterial blood clot) (1)
- Venous thrombosis typically manifests as deep venous thrombosis (DVT) of the lower extremity in the legs or pelvis and pulmonary embolism (PE) (1).
- System(s) affected: Cardiovascular; Nervous; Pulmonary; Reproductive; Hematologic
- Synonym(s): Hypercoagulation syndrome, prothrombotic state

EPIDEMIOLOGY
- An inherited thrombophilic defect or risk can be detected in up to 50% of patients with venous thromboembolism (VTE).
- Factor V Leiden is the most common inherited thrombophilia (1/2 of all currently characterizable inherited thrombophilia cases involve the factor V Leiden mutation), and it is present in its heterozygous form in up to ~20% of patients with a 1st VTE.
- Heterozygous prothrombin G20210A mutation, the 2nd most common inherited thrombophilia, is present in up to ~8% of patients with VTE.

Incidence
1st-time thromboembolism:
- ~100/100,000/yr among the general population
- <1/100,000/yr in those age <15 years
- ~1,000/100,000/yr in those age ≥85 years

Prevalence
- 40–80% of lower extremity orthopedic procedures can result in DVT if appropriate prophylaxis is not used.
- VTE accounts for ~1.2–4.7 deaths per 100,000 pregnancies.

ETIOLOGY AND PATHOPHYSIOLOGY
- Virchow's triad as a cause of VTE includes blood stasis, vascular endothelial injury, and abnormalities in circulating blood constituents (i.e., hypercoagulability).
- An imbalance between the hemostatic and fibrinolytic pathways leads to thrombus formation.
- VTE is considered to be the result of genetic tendencies (measurable or not) with other acquired risks.
- Upper extremity DVT: >60% are associated with venous catheters. Malignancy is an additional significant risk (2).

Genetics
- The most common genetic thrombophilias (factor V Leiden, prothrombin G20210A, proteins C and S, and antithrombin III deficiency) are inherited in an autosomal-dominant pattern.
- Homozygous mutations generally have a higher risk of VTE.
- Factor V Leiden/Activated protein C (aPC) resistance is the most common inherited thrombophilia:
  - 2–5% prevalence among Caucasians; rare in African Americans or Asians
  - aPC does not cleave factor Va so thrombin formation continues.
  - Other acquired risks are synergistic (3).
- Prothrombin gene mutation G20210A: Prevalence 6% among Caucasians. Heterozygous carriers have increased risk of thrombosis.

- Hyperhomocysteinemia: 5–6% among the general population. Increases risk of coronary artery disease/myocardial infarction, cerebrovascular accident, deep venous thrombosis or pulmonary embolism (DVT/PE). Acquired in those with folate, vitamin B_{12}, and vitamin B_6 deficiencies.
- Antithrombin deficiency: <0.2% among the general population; produced in the liver; acquired deficiency in disseminated intravascular coagulation (DIC), sepsis, liver disease, nephrotic syndrome.
- Protein C and S deficiencies: 0.5% and 1% incidences, respectively, among the general population. Homozygotes and heterozygotes are hypercoagulable. Vitamin K-dependent, produced in the liver. Protein C inactivates Va and VIIIa. Protein C may become an acquired deficiency in liver disease, sepsis, DIC, acute respiratory distress syndrome, and after surgery. Protein S is a cofactor for protein C, and it may become an acquired deficiency with OCP use, pregnancy, liver disease, sepsis, DIC, HIV, and nephrosis.

RISK FACTORS
- Acquired risk factors:
  - Immobilization
  - Trauma
  - Surgery, especially orthopedic
  - Malignancies (especially pancreatic, ovarian, brain, and lymphoma)
  - Pregnancy
  - Acute medical illness
  - Exogenous female hormones/oral contraceptives (OCP)
  - Obesity
  - Nephrotic syndrome
  - Antiphospholipid syndrome (APS) and lupus anticoagulant
  - Myeloproliferative disorders (polycythemia vera, essential thrombocythemia)
  - Hyperviscosity syndromes (sickle cell, paraproteinemias)
  - Hyperhomocysteinemia secondary to vitamin deficiencies (B_6, B_{12}, folic acid)
  - Tamoxifen, thalidomide, lenalidomide, bevacizumab, L-asparaginase, erythropoietic stimulating agents
  - Previous thromboembolism
  - Prolonged travel
- Established genetic factors:
  - Factor V Leiden
  - Prothrombin G20210A mutation
  - Protein C deficiency
  - Protein S deficiency
  - Antithrombin III deficiency
- Rare genetic factors:
  - Dysfibrinogenemia
  - Hyperhomocysteinemia (methylene tetrahydrofolate reductase mutation)
- Indeterminate factors:
  - Elevated factor VIII
- Age: >60
- Gender: Men
- Race: Incidence is higher among African Americans.

GENERAL PREVENTION
- Consider prophylaxis with medications in any hospitalized patient with VTE risk factors; hospitalized patients should be encouraged to ambulate as soon as possible (4)[A].

- Consider mechanical prophylaxis in patients at low risk for VTE or those in whom anticoagulation may be contraindicated.
- Consider prophylaxis with low-molecular-weight heparin (LMWH) + aspirin in pregnant patients with APS or other thrombophilia.
- Prophylaxis with unfractionated heparin or LMWH should be considered in patients with genetic or acquired risks of thrombosis and an anticipated additional risk, such as the immobilization associated with surgery.
- Use caution with procoagulant medicines (e.g., OCPs) in asymptomatic individuals who have a known hereditary predisposition.

COMMONLY ASSOCIATED CONDITIONS
Advanced age, cancer, pregnancy, obesity, prior history of thrombosis, surgery, immobilization

DIAGNOSIS

HISTORY
Consider prothrombotic assessment for:
- Unprovoked thrombosis at age <45–50 years
- Thrombosis at an unusual anatomic site or recurrent thromboses
- Family history suggesting multiple individuals affected with VTE
- Recurrent pregnancy loss or thrombosis with OCP use

PHYSICAL EXAM
- DVT: Swelling, pain, warmth, and redness, usually of 1 extremity
- PE: Dyspnea, pleurisy, hemoptysis, hypoxia, tachycardia
- Superficial phlebitis: Red, painful cord palpable along the path of thrombosed vein
- Postthrombotic syndrome: Pain, swelling, pigmentation, and/or ulceration

DIAGNOSTIC TESTS & INTERPRETATION
Testing for heritable thrombophilia in all patients with a 1st episode of VTE is not required (2,5)[B].

Initial Tests (lab, imaging)
- CBC
- Activated protein C resistance profile (aPC Profile): ≤2.0 implies factor V Leiden mutation; 95–100% are factor V Leiden positive; false-positive finding in pregnancy or with use of OCPs, confirm with factor V Leiden mutation testing or consider factor V Leiden mutation testing up front:
  - aPC resistance may be unreliable while taking LMWH or unfractionated heparin (UFH).
- Prothrombin G20210A genetic assay
- ATIII functional assay:
  - Will be low with acute thrombosis and on heparin therapy
- Protein C functional assay:
  - May be low with acute thrombosis; will be lower on warfarin
- Protein S antigen and functional assay and free S:
  - May be low with acute thrombosis; will be lower on warfarin
- Antiphospholipid antibodies: Phospholipid-dependent tests and anticardiolipin antibodies, lupus anticoagulant:
  - May be unreliable on heparin

- Consider evaluation for subclinical malignancy in an unprovoked thrombosis in those >50 or at greater risk.
- Consider homocysteine level, although treatment of hyperhomocysteinemia (vitamins B_{12} and B_6, folate) does not alter the thrombophilic risk.

Follow-Up Tests & Special Considerations
Dysfibrinogenemia and plasminogen deficiency are very rare causes of thrombophilia.

TREATMENT

MEDICATION
First Line
- Parenteral anticoagulation: LMWH has largely replaced UFH as first-line therapy for VTE:
  – Enoxaparin (Lovenox): 1 mg/kg SC b.i.d. for at least 5 days (with concomitant warfarin), until international normalized ratio (INR) has reached 2 for at least 24 hours:
    ○ Enoxaparin is preferred in patients with active cancer for a minimum of 3 months (can dose at 1.5 mg/kg SC daily), after which time the patient can be re-evaluated to continue enoxaparin or transition to warfarin.
    ○ Adverse reactions: Bleeding, heparin-induced thrombocytopenia (HIT) <0.5% incidence, bone loss (uncommon)
    ○ Reversal: Stop LMWH
  – UFH: 80 U/kg or 5,000-unit IV bolus, then 18 U/kg/hr or 1,300 U/hr to target the activated partial thromboplastin time (aPTT) to a corresponding anti-Xa level of 0.3–0.7 U/mL. The 1st aPTT should be checked 6 hours after initial therapy and adjusted per standard heparin nomograms, aiming for an adequate level within 24 hours. Transition to warfarin is similar to the recommendations for enoxaparin:
    ○ SC UFH is an alternative and can be given as 5,000 U IV (once) followed by 250 U/kg SC b.i.d., or 250 U/kg bolus followed by 250 U/kg b.i.d. (monitored as for IV UFH), or 333 U/kg once followed by 250 U/kg SC b.i.d. (unmonitored).
    ○ Adverse reactions: Bleeding, HIT 3% incidence, bone loss (long-term use)
    ○ Reversal: Stop heparin, protamine
- Oral anticoagulation:
  – Warfarin (Coumadin): 5 mg/d initially and adjust to INR 2–3 for at least 3 months, potentially indefinitely in those with high risk of recurrence, recurrent or unprovoked VTE:
    ○ Warfarin requires careful and frequent monitoring because of many drug–drug and drug–diet (e.g., vitamin K) interactions.
    ○ Adverse reactions: Bleeding, skin necrosis (rare and early in course)
    ○ Reversal: Fresh frozen plasma and/or vitamin K
- Pregnancy (controversial): Low-dose aspirin and/or LMWH or UFH; warfarin is contraindicated

Second Line
Usually indicated when contraindication to heparin or LMWH, such as heparin-associated thrombosis and thrombocytopenia, if there is an inability to use IV drugs, or renal failure:
- Factor Xa inhibitors (ATIII inhibitor):
  – Fondaparinux: Efficacious for prevention and treatment of acute VTE, postoperative prophylaxis, PE (FDA-approved indications):
    ○ Dose: Acute VTE/PE. Weight <50 kg: 5 mg/d SC; weight 50–100 kg: 7.5 mg/d SC; weight

>100 kg: 10 mg/d SC; use for 5–9 days until oral anticoagulation is therapeutic.
    ○ Prophylaxis: 2.5 mg/d SC
    ○ Dose adjustments: Needed for renal insufficiency; if creatinine clearance is <30 mL/min, use is contraindicated
  – Rivaroxaban: Oral factor Xa inhibitor, FDA approved for postoperative thromboprophylaxis after hip/knee replacement and for thromboembolic prophylaxis in patients with nonvalvular atrial fibrillation. Can be reversed with 4-factor prothrombin complex concentrate (PCC) (6)[C]
- Direct thrombin inhibitors: Most commonly used for anticoagulation in HIT. Representative drugs include:
  – Lepirudin: Excreted by kidneys, crosses the placenta; dosing based on creatinine clearance; therapeutic dose based on aPTT
  – Argatroban: Liver metabolized; may be dose adjusted in liver dysfunction; therapeutic dose based on aPTT
  – Dabigatran: Oral direct thrombin inhibitor, FDA approved for thromboembolic prophylaxis in patients with nonvalvular atrial fibrillation (noninferior to warfarin). Currently no known antidote to anticoagulant effect. May be dialyzable (6)[C]

SURGERY/OTHER PROCEDURES
- Catheter extraction/thrombectomy for extreme emergencies (e.g., massive PE where thrombolysis not feasible)
- Inferior vena cava filter:
  – Reduces short-term risk of PE in those with contraindications to anticoagulation (e.g., GI bleeding, cerebral hemorrhage)
  – May increase long-term risk of recurrent DVT
  – Use for patients with multiple episodes of recurrent thromboembolism despite therapeutic anticoagulation.

ONGOING CARE

FOLLOW-UP RECOMMENDATIONS
Avoid significant risk for trauma (e.g., contact sports, climbing a ladder).

Patient Monitoring
Monitor warfarin as frequently as needed to maintain an INR goal of 2–3 (through an anticoagulation clinic).

DIET
Vitamin K-stable diet if patient is taking warfarin

PATIENT EDUCATION
- Assume that any drug may enhance or attenuate the warfarin effect.
- Increase the frequency of monitoring following any medication change to ensure therapeutic anticoagulation and to avoid over-anticoagulation, especially with antibiotics.
- Many drugs may modulate warfarin effect: Alcohol, antibiotics, aspirin, NSAIDs, acetaminophen

PROGNOSIS
- Patients with a provoked VTE (i.e., surgery, hospitalization) not receiving chronic anticoagulation have a risks of recurrence of 7% (year 1), 16% (year 5), and 23% (year 10).
- Patients with an unprovoked VTE not receiving chronic anticoagulation have risks of recurrence of 15% (year 1), 41% (year 5), and 53% (year 10).

- Currently, there are no data from randomized, controlled trials or controlled clinical trials about the benefits of thrombophilia testing to decrease the risk of recurrent VTE (1).

COMPLICATIONS
Venous or arterial thrombosis; bleeding in anticoagulated patients

REFERENCES
1. Cohn D, Vansenne F, de Borgie C, et al. Thrombophilia testing for prevention of recurrent venous thromboembolism. *Cochrane Database Syst Rev.* 2012;CD007069.
2. Baglin T, Gray E, Greaves M, et al. Clinical guidelines for testing for heritable thrombophilia. *Br J Haematol.* 2010;149:209–220.
3. Anderson JA, Weitz JI. Hypercoagulable states. *Clin Chest Med.* 2010;31:659–673.
4. Hill J, Treasure T, National Clinical Guideline Centre for Acute and Chronic Conditions. Reducing the risk of venous thromboembolism in patients admitted to hospital: Summary of NICE guidance. *BMJ.* 2010;340:c95. Epub 2010 Jan 27.
5. National Clinical Guideline Centre. The management of venous thromboembolic diseases and the role of thrombophilia testing. *NICE Clinical Guidelines.* 2012:144
6. Schulman S, Crowther MA. How I treat with anticoagulants in 2012: New and old anticoagulants, and when and how to switch. *Blood.* 2012;119:3016–3023.

ADDITIONAL READING
- Guyatt GH, Akl EA, Crowther M, et al. Antithrombotic Therapy and Prevention of Thrombosis, 9th edition: American College of Chest Physicians Evidence-Based Clinical Practice Guidelines. *Chest.* 2012;141:1S–70S.
- Hirsh J, Bauer KA, Donati MB, et al. Parenteral anticoagulants: American College of Chest Physicians Evidence-Based Clinical Practice Guidelines (8th ed.). *Chest.* 2008;133(6 Suppl): 141S–159S.

CODES

ICD10
- D68.2 Hereditary deficiency of other clotting factors
- D68.51 Activated protein C resistance
- D68.59 Other primary thrombophilia

CLINICAL PEARLS
- Factor V Leiden (resistance to aPC) is the most common inherited thrombophilia, with a prevalence of 2–7% in the US Caucasian population.
- Test patients <50 years of age with a history of venous thrombosis, and consider testing 1st-degree relatives.
- Rule out malignancy, especially in those >50 years.

THROMBOTIC THROMBOCYTOPENIC PURPURA
Kellie A. Sprague, MD

 BASICS

DESCRIPTION
- An acute syndrome of microangiopathic hemolytic anemia (MAHA) and consumptive thrombocytopenia with deposition of hyaline thrombi in terminal arterioles and capillaries leading to ischemic multiorgan damage
- Thrombotic thrombocytopenic purpura (TTP) is characterized by MAHA and thrombocytopenia, with or without the following signs and symptoms (1):
  – Neurologic symptoms
  – Renal dysfunction
  – Fever
  – Most patients do not show the historic pentad of MAHA, thrombocytopenia, renal dysfunction, neurologic abnormalities, and fever because treatment is initiated before the pentad can develop.

EPIDEMIOLOGY
Incidence
- Predominant age: 30–60 years.
- Predominant sex: Female > Male (2:1)
- Incidence ratio in blacks to whites is 3:1
- The age–sex–race standardized incidence of clinically suspected TTP is 6/million/yr in the US (2).

ETIOLOGY AND PATHOPHYSIOLOGY
- In TTP, the aggregating agent responsible for platelet thrombi is unusually large von Willebrand factor (UL vWF) multimers, which are far larger than those found in normal plasma.
- A metalloproteinase, ADAMTS13, which normally enzymatically cleaves UL vWF multimers to prevent clumping within vessels, is deficient, defective, or absent, allowing UL vWF to react with platelets. This leads to the endothelial cell damage and disseminated thrombi characteristic of TTP.
- Arterioles most often affected are in the brain, kidney, pancreas, heart, and adrenal glands. Lungs and liver are relatively spared.
- In familial TTP, patients have an inherited deficiency of ADAMTS13.
- In acquired idiopathic TTP, autoantibodies are directed against the metalloproteinase ADMATS-3. The trigger is unknown (3).
- Endothelial injury, either directly from a drug/toxin or indirectly via platelet/neutrophil activation, has been proposed as a cause of secondary TTP, especially in those without ADAMTS13 deficiency:
  – Drug-induced (see "Risk Factors")
  – Hematopoietic cell transplantation

Genetics
TTP is most often an acquired disorder. A congenital form of inherited TTP (Schulman-Upshaw syndrome) is due to a mutation at the ADAMTS13 metalloproteinase gene locus on chromosome 9q34. This rare form of TTP has an autosomal-recessive pattern of inheritance.

RISK FACTORS
- Pregnancy and oral contraceptives
- AIDS and early symptomatic HIV infection
- Autoimmune disease:
  – Antiphospholipid antibody syndrome
  – Systemic lupus erythematosus
  – Scleroderma
- Cancer
- Hematopoietic stem cell transplantation
- Drug toxicity:
  – Cancer chemotherapy:
    ○ Mitomycin C and gemcitabine
    ○ Bleomycin and cisplatin
  – Calcineurin inhibitors:
    ○ Tacrolimus and cyclosporine
  – Immune-mediated:
    ○ Quinine and quinidine
    ○ Ticlopidine and clopidogrel

COMMONLY ASSOCIATED CONDITIONS
- TTP/ HUS/atypical HUS (hemolytic uremic syndrome) have similar presentations with MAHA and thrombocytopenia and multiorgan involvement.
- TTP generally presents with minimal renal involvement and may have neurologic abnormalities, whereas the opposite tends to be more characteristic of HUS/atypical HUS.
- However, patients with HUS and TTP may have both prominent renal and neurologic manifestations, often making the distinction unclear, thus leading to the hybrid name "TTP-HUS."
- ADAMTS13 levels are diminished in adults with familial or acquired idiopathic TTP, but are normal in children diagnosed with HUS following infection with *Escherichia coli* (particularly type O157:H7), so-called typical HUS. Atypical HUS is due to complement dysregulation.

 DIAGNOSIS

- Most common symptoms are nonspecific: Nausea, vomiting, weakness, abdominal pain, fatigue, fever
- Related to thrombocytopenia:
  – Easy bruising, purpura, or petechiae
  – Epistaxis, menorrhagia, bleeding gums
  – GI bleeding
  – Intracranial hemorrhage
  – Visual symptoms due to retinal hemorrhage
- Related to hemolytic anemia (MAHA): Jaundice, fatigue
- Related to end-organ ischemia:
  – Neurologic: CNS symptoms occur in 50%:
    ○ Often fluctuating symptoms
    ○ Headache
    ○ Altered mental status: Spectrum runs from behavioral/personality changes to obtundation/stupor/coma.
    ○ Seizures
    ○ Stroke
  – Renal: Hematuria, oliguria, or anuria
  – Cardiac: Arrhythmia, myocardial infarction, heart failure

HISTORY
- Generally acute onset of symptoms, but subacute in about 1/4 of patients
- It is important to assess for potential underlying causes or risk factors (see above).

PHYSICAL EXAM
- Fever
- Mental status/Neurologic: Confusion, coma, stupor, weakness
- HEENT: Retinal hemorrhage, scleral icterus, epistaxis
- Abdomen/GI: Nonspecific tenderness
- Skin: Jaundice, petechiae, purpura, ecchymoses

DIFFERENTIAL DIAGNOSIS
- HUS and atypical HUS: See "Commonly Associated Conditions"
- Antiphospholipid antibody syndrome: Prolonged partial thromboplastin time (PTT) and presence of lupus anticoagulant
- Systemic lupus erythematosus
- Malignant hypertension (HTN): Diastolic > 130 mm Hg, papilledema, retinal hemorrhages
- Pregnancy-associated preeclampsia/eclampsia or HELLP: Low ATIII levels
- Disseminated intravascular coagulation:
  – Prolonged prothrombin time (PT)/PTT, low fibrinogen
  – Low factors V and VIII
  – Secondary to sepsis/shock or widely disseminated malignancy
- Idiopathic thrombocytopenic purpura:
  – No hemolysis, normal LDH and bilirubin
  – Presence of antiplatelet antibodies
- Malignancy-associated microangiopathy
- Evan syndrome (autoimmune hemolytic anemia and thrombocytopenia): Positive direct Coombs' test
- Sclerodermal kidney

DIAGNOSTIC TESTS & INTERPRETATION
Initial Tests (lab, imaging)
- CBC:
  – Hemoglobin (decreased): Average is 8–10 g/dL
  – Platelets decreased: typically in the 10-30,000 range
- Reticulocyte count (increased)
- Haptoglobin decreased (hemolysis)
- Peripheral smear:
  – Schistocytes (prominent)
  – Helmet cells, RBC fragments
  – Nucleated RBCs
  – Polychromasia (reticulocytosis)
- Coagulation studies:
  – Normal in most; mild elevation in 15%
  – Fibrinogen normal
- Coombs' test: Negative direct Coombs' test
- Electrolytes, BUN/creatinine: Mild elevation of BUN and creatinine (creatinine <3 mg/dL)
- Liver function studies: Increased indirect bilirubin (hemolysis)
- Lactate dehydrogenase (LDH): 5–10× normal
- Urinalysis:
  – Proteinuria, microscopic hematuria
  – Positive dipstick for large blood, but minimal RBCs on microscopic exam
- ECG: Sinus tachycardia, heart block
- Troponin: Increased if cardiac involvement
- HIV, Hepatitis A, B, C testing: Exclude underlying viral precipitant

- Pregnancy test
- Pretreatment ADAMTS13 activity level of <5% is useful in distinguishing acquired or familial TTP from other disorders.
- Head CT/MRI scan: Performed if mental status changes are present to rule out possible intracranial hemorrhage or ischemic changes

Test Interpretation
Biopsy of affected organs shows platelet thrombi within or beneath damaged endothelium. However, biopsy is rarely obtained because the diagnosis is made on clinical grounds and laboratory findings.

 TREATMENT

- Prompt treatment of TTP is necessary due to the high mortality (90%).
- In the absence of another apparent cause, the dyad of MAHA and thrombocytopenia is sufficient to begin treatment for TTP while the workup proceeds (3):
  – Plasma exchange transfusion (PEX) is the cornerstone of treatment of classic TTP (3)[A].
  – PEX replaces deficient or defective metalloproteinase (ADAMTS13) and removes UL vWF and antimetalloproteinase antibodies.
  – 1–1.5 plasma volumes/day should be begun immediately and continued daily.
  – Optimal PEX duration is unknown. Convention is to continue for 2 days after platelet count is ≥150,000 (3)[B].
  – Fresh frozen plasma (3)[B]: Temporary measure until PEX can be initiated

MEDICATION
First Line
- Glucocorticoids may be of benefit in some patients. British guidelines recommend its use for all patients (4)[B].
  – Steroids may work by suppressing the autoantibodies inhibiting ADAMTS13 activity.
  – Utility may be in patients with severe ADAMTS13 deficiency, in the setting of exacerbation when PEX is stopped or in relapse after remission.
  – Little benefit of steroids when used as monotherapy
  – Doses: Prednisone 1 mg/kg/d and taper once in remission (4)[B] or methylprednisolone 1 g/d IV × 3 days (4)[B].
- Rituximab, an anti-CD 20 antibody that deletes B cells, may reduce relapse when given in conjunction with PEX and steroids (4)[B]:
  – Dose: 375 mg/m^2 IV weekly × 4 weeks

Second Line
The following medications are used in refractory cases:
- Rituximab (4,5)[B]
- Vincristine, cyclophosphamide (6) cyclosporine (4)
- Intravenous immunoglobulin (IVIG)

ISSUES FOR REFERRAL
- Hematology or blood bank for plasma exchange transfusion
- Nephrology for dialysis
- Cardiology for presence of significant heart block or ischemia
- Neurosurgery for intracranial hemorrhage

SURGERY/OTHER PROCEDURES
Splenectomy is reserved for severe, refractory cases (6).

IN-PATIENT CONSIDERATIONS
Admission Criteria/Initial Stabilization
- ABCs, oxygen, IV access, telemetry
- Volume resuscitation if hypotensive/actively bleeding
- Packed RBCs can be transfused safely.
- Platelet transfusion may be used for the treatment of hemorrhage.

Discharge Criteria
On normalization and stabilization of neurologic symptoms, LDH, platelets, and renal function

 ONGOING CARE

FOLLOW-UP RECOMMENDATIONS
- No maintenance therapy is required. After PEX is discontinued, blood counts should be monitored over a few months. If testing results remain normal, testing interval can be lengthened.
- Promptly evaluate any symptoms of relapse.

PATIENT EDUCATION
- On discharge, advise patients to self-monitor for signs of relapse (e.g., fever, headache, bruising).
- Patients should be advised about prolonged periods of fatigue following the acute phase.
- www.nhlbi.nih.gov/health/dci/Diseases/ttp/ TTP_WhatIs.html

PROGNOSIS
- Most patients recover fully from idiopathic TTP when treated promptly:
  – 30-day mortality is 10% in those who receive PEX.
  – 70% respond within 14 days; 90% respond within 28 days.
  – 80% survival in patients with idiopathic TTP treated with PEX (7)
- Initial LDH and platelet counts are not predictive of the patient's response to treatment.
- Final platelet count and LDH or the length or intensity of treatment does not predict relapse.
- Low levels of ADAMTS13 activity during remission are associated with higher risk of relapse (8,9).
- In patients with severe ADAMTS13 deficiency, the risk of relapse is estimated to be 41% at 7.5 years, with the greatest risk being in the 1st year (7).

COMPLICATIONS
- Patients may experience mild cognitive impairments in attention, concentration, and memory following ≥1 episodes of TTP (10).
- Complications of PEX include:
  – Central line infections and hemorrhage
  – Citrate toxicity
  – Hypersensitivity reactions to frequent plasma

REFERENCES
1. Sadler JE. Von Willebrand factor, ADAMTS13, and thrombotic thrombocytopenic purpura. *Blood*. 2008;112:11–18.
2. Terrell DR, Williams LA, Vesley SK, et al. The incidence for thrombotic thrombocytopenic purpura-hemolytic uremic syndrome: All patients, idiopathic patients, and patients with severe ADAMTS13 deficiency. *J Thromb Heamost*. 2005;3(7):1432–1436.
3. George JN. Clinical practice. Thrombotic thrombocytopenic purpura. *N Engl J Med*. 2006;354:1927–1935.
4. Scully M, Hunt B, Benjamin S et al. Guidelines on the diagnosis and management of thrombotic thrombocytopenic purpura and other thrombotic microangiopathies. *Br J Haematol*. 2012;158:323–355.
5. Scully M, McDonald V, Cavenagh J, et al. A phase 2 study of the safety and efficacy of rituximab with plasma exchange in acute acquired thrombotic thrombocytopenic purpura. *Blood*. 2011;118(7):1746–1753.
6. Beloncle F, Buffet M, Coindre Jean-Phillipe. Splenectomy and/or cyclophosphamide as salvage therapies in thrombotic thrombocytopenic purpura: the French TMA Reference Center experience. *Transfusion*. 2012:52(11):2436–2444.
7. Kremer Hovinga JA, Vesley SK. Survival and relapse in patients with thrombotic thrombocytopenic purpura. *Blood*. 2010;115(8):1500–1511.
8. Jin M, Casper C, Cataland SR, et al. Relationship between ADAMTS13 activity in clinical remission and the risk of TTP relapse. *Br J Haematol*. 2008;141(5):651–658.
9. Peyvandi F, Lavoretano S, Palla R, et al. ADAMTS13 and anti-ADAMTS13 antibodies are markers for recurrence or acquired thrombotic thrombocytopenia purpura during remission. *Haematologica*. 2008;93:69–76.
10. Kennedy AS, Lewis QF, Scott JG et al. Cognitive deficits after recovery from thrombotic thrombocytopenic purpura. *Transfusion*. 2009;49:1092–1001.

ADDITIONAL READING
Diagnostic and therapeutic challenges in the thrombotic thrombocytopenic purpura and hemolytic uremic syndromes. *Hematology Am Soc Hematol Educ Program*. 2012:604–609.

 CODES

ICD10
M31.1 Thrombotic microangiopathy

CLINICAL PEARLS
- The diagnosis of TTP is made clinically; common symptoms are nonspecific: Nausea, vomiting, weakness, abdominal pain, fatigue, fever, and easy bruising, purpura, or petechiae.
- The historical pentad of fever, neurologic symptoms, renal dysfunction, MAHA, and thrombocytopenia is not present in most patients.
- The dyad of MAHA and thrombocytopenia is sufficient to initiate treatment with PEX.
- Do not wait for results of ADAMTS13 determination to initiate therapy.

THYROGLOSSAL DUCT CYST

Felix B. Chang, MD • Nicolas Hernandez, MD

 BASICS

DESCRIPTION
- Cyst composed of epithelial remnants of the thyroglossal tract
- Midline neck mass at the level of the thyrohyoid membrane, closely associated with the hyoid bone, within 2 cm of the midline
- Single, smooth, nontender, and mobile
- 65% infrahyoid, 20% suprahyoid, 15% juxtahyoid, 10% suprasternal
- Intralaryngeal very rare: Suprasternal notch, superior mediastinum
- System(s) affected: Endocrine; Metabolic; Skin; Exocrine

EPIDEMIOLOGY
- Most common form of congenital cyst in the neck
- Accounts for 2–4% of all neck masses

Incidence
- 50% of cases in patients ≤20 years of age
- Peak prevalence in children <10 years
- Predominant sex: Male = Female
- Caucasian race

Prevalence
- Occurs in about 7% of population.
- Thyroglossal duct anomalies are the 2nd most common pediatric neck mass, behind adenopathy.

ETIOLOGY AND PATHOPHYSIOLOGY
- Cystic expansion of a remnant of the thyroglossal duct tract
- Incomplete closure of the thyroglossal duct during gestation
- Persistence of the epithelial tract, the thyroglossal duct, during the descent of the thyroid from the foramen cecum to its final position in the anterior neck
- The thyroglossal duct tract usually atrophies and disappears by the 8th–10th week of gestation.
- Portions of the tract and remnants of thyroid tissue associated with it may persist at any point between the tongue and the thyroid.
- Failure of the thyroglossal duct to atrophy and involute after descent of the thyroid in the 4th–7th week of gestation
- Hypothesis: Lymphoid tissue associated with the tract hypertrophies at the time of a regional infection, thereby occluding the tract with resulting cyst formation.

Genetics
- Usually sporadic; if familial, autosomal-dominant is most common mode of inheritance.
- Familial occurrence is extremely rare.

COMMONLY ASSOCIATED CONDITIONS
- History of a recent upper respiratory tract infection
- Ectopic thyroid tissue in 50% of patients
- Thyroid carcinoma 1%

 DIAGNOSIS

HISTORY
- Most often asymptomatic
- Swelling, dyspnea, dysphagia
- Painful or slightly tender
- Redness
- Neck mass
- 25% present with a draining sinus.
- Foul taste in the mouth if the spontaneous drainage occurred by way of the foramen cecum
- Rare: Severe respiratory distress/sudden infant death syndrome from lesions at the base of the tongue, a lateral cystic neck mass, an anterior tongue fistula, or coexistence with branchial anomalies

PHYSICAL EXAM
- Midline neck mass, usually within 2 cm of the midline
- Nontender/slightly tender, unless infected
- Rises in the neck with tongue protrusion and swallowing
- Infected thyroglossal duct cyst may manifest as tender mass with associated dysphagia, dysphonia, draining sinus, fever, or increasing neck mass.
- Airway obstruction is possible, especially with intralingual cysts.

DIFFERENTIAL DIAGNOSIS
- Ectopic midline thyroid
- Dermoid cyst
- Thyroid adenoma of isthmus/pyramidal lobe
- Lymphadenitis
- Cervical thymic cyst
- Sebaceous (epidermal) cysts
- Medial branchial cleft cyst
- Salivary gland tumor
- Lymphatic malformations
- Lipoma
- Hypertrophic pyramidal lobes of the thyroid

DIAGNOSTIC TESTS & INTERPRETATION
Preoperative US and a screening thyroid-stimulating hormone (TSH) determination
- The wall of a thyroglossal duct is the 2nd most common site for ectopic thyroid tissue.

Initial Tests (lab, imaging)
Assess thyroid function.
- US/CT scan to confirm diagnosis, identify thyroid, and demonstrate relationship to hyoid bone (1)
- Patients with elevated TSH levels suggesting hypothyroidism or a solid mass should undergo scintiscanning to rule out a median ectopic thyroid.
- Thyroid scan if midline ectopic thyroid/thyroid nodule is suspected
- Small roll under shoulders allows exposure of neck in infants.
- Occasionally, if the cyst is infected, hemorrhagic, or has a high protein content, it may appear as hyperdense on CT scan, as an area of high signal intensity on T_1- and T_2-weighted MRI, and have an internal echo on US.
- Malignancy may be suspected if a soft tissue component exists within or around the cyst.

Follow-Up Tests & Special Considerations
- If a solid mass is encountered during excision of a suspected thyroglossal duct cyst, it should be sent for frozen section to rule out a median ectopic thyroid.
- Fine-needle aspiration (FNA) biopsy is the most reliable method for preoperative diagnosis of thyroid carcinoma, especially if done with US guidance.
- FNA can be helpful to decrease cyst size and, in some cases, may lead to identification of thyroglossal duct cyst carcinoma if solid elements of the lesion can be sampled.

Diagnostic Procedures/Other
- FNA for preoperative evaluation of thyroglossal duct cysts may reveal colloid, neutrophils, macrophages, lymphocytes, and ciliated columnar cells.
- If cyst is infected, antibiotic treatment may be required prior to definitive resection.
- Incision and drainage with resulting scarring may complicate resection.

Test Interpretation
- Cyst lined with stratified squamous/pseudostratified ciliated columnar epithelium
- Thyroid tissue is seen in 10–45% of cysts.
- Reports show traces of the thyroglossal duct located near the hyoid bone, superior to the thyroid isthmus, or lingual.
- Less than 1% of thyroglossal duct cysts have malignant tissue, usually well-differentiated thyroid carcinoma.

TREATMENT

Elective surgical excision

GENERAL MEASURES
IV antibiotics for severe infections

MEDICATION
- All thyroglossal duct cysts should be surgically removed.
- Infected cysts/sinuses are first managed by treating the infection.
- The most common organisms are *Haemophilus influenzae*, *Staphylococcus aureus*, and *S. epidermidis*.
- Antibiotics directed toward these organisms should be started.

First Line
For infected cyst: Cephalexin 500 mg PO q6h, amoxicillin-clavulanate 500 mg/125 mg PO q8h, or clindamycin 600 mg PO q8h

Second Line
- Coverage against methicillin-resistant *Staphylococcus aureus* is not recommended, unless identified by culture.
- For severe infections: Cefazolin 1–1.5 g IV q8h in combination with clindamycin (600–900 mg IV) q8h

ADDITIONAL THERAPIES
Sclerotherapy: Percutaneous ethanol injection is an alternative approach in patients who are not surgical candidates if the presence of malignancy can be excluded (2)[B].

IN-PATIENT CONSIDERATIONS
Admission Criteria/Initial Stabilization
- If incision and drainage are necessary, the incision should be placed so that it can be excised completely with an ellipse at the time of definitive resection.
- Formal incision and drainage should be avoided.

ONGOING CARE

If a thyroglossal duct is not removed, as many as half become infected.

FOLLOW-UP RECOMMENDATIONS
- Unrestricted
- Infection before surgery is a well-described cause of recurrence.

Patient Monitoring
1–2 weeks after resection (3)

DIET
Unrestricted

PATIENT EDUCATION
Reassure family about absence of malignancy (if appropriate).

PROGNOSIS
- Recurrence after complete excision using Sistrunk procedure is reported to be 2.6–5% (4)[A].

- Increased risk of recurrence:
  - Failure to excise the cyst completely
  - In children <2 years of age, intraoperative cyst rupture and presence of a cutaneous component
  - Preoperative/concurrent infection of the cyst at the time of the surgery
- After excision, thyroglossal cyst has a high risk for recurrence (20–35%) and requires a wider en bloc resection.
- Most cases of thyroglossal duct cyst carcinoma are treated adequately by Sistrunk procedure, with a reported cure rate of 95%.
- Unless tumor is invasive (which is rare), Sistrunk procedure is usually curative.

COMPLICATIONS
- Infection occurs in up to half of cysts if not excised.
- Malignant degeneration may occur (1–2%) if cyst is not excised.
- Must rule out primary thyroid carcinoma if thyroglossal duct cyst carcinoma is found.
- Reports demonstrate that lingual location of thyroglossal duct cysts can cause not only various respiratory problems, but also infant death.
- Wide local excision is a valuable extension of the Sistrunk operation for the management of recurrent disease.
- Patient may require thyroid medication for life if ectopic midline thyroid is mistakenly removed.
- Thyroglossal duct sinus or a thyroglossal duct fistula
- Sistrunk procedure at an early age may be associated with altered craniofacial growth.

REFERENCES
1. Huoh KC, Durr ML, Meyer AK, et al. Comparison of imaging modalities in pediatric thyroglossal duct cysts. *Laryngoscope*. 2012;122:1405–1408.
2. Chow TL, Choi CY, Yee-Hing Hui J, et al. Thyroglossal duct cysts in adults treated by ethanol sclerotherapy: A pilot study of a nonsurgical technique. *Laryngoscope*. 2012;122:1262–1264.
3. Szybiak B, Golusiski W. Preoperative and postoperative management of patients after neck surgery. *Otolaryngol Pol*. 2012;84(3):201–206.
4. Galuzzi F, Pignataro L. et al. Risk of recurrence in children operated for thyroglossal duct cyst: A systematic review. *J Pediatr Surg*. 2013;48(1):222–227.

ADDITIONAL READING
- LaRiviere C, Waldhausen J. Congenital cervical cysts, sinuses, and fistulae. *Pediatr Surg*. 2012;92(3):583–597.
- Ibrahim, M, Hammoud, K. Congenital cystic lesions of the head and neck. *Med Clin North Am*. 2011; 21(3):621–639.
- Rosenberg TL. Evaluating the adult patient with a neck mass. *Med Clin North Am*. 2010;94(5):1017–1029.

CODES

ICD10
Q89.2 Congenital malformations of other endocrine glands

CLINICAL PEARLS

- Elevation of mass with swallowing or protrusion of tongue.
- FNA biopsy is the most reliable method for preoperative diagnosis of thyroid cancer, especially if done with ultrasound guidance.
- If the cyst is found to contain thyroid carcinoma, the surgeon must be sure that the carcinoma arose from within the cyst and is not a cystic metastasis to a midline lymph node from a primary thyroid carcinoma.
- The carcinoma is considered to have originated in the thyroglossal duct cyst if there is histologic evidence of columnar/squamous epithelial lining in the cyst, normal thyroid follicles in the cyst wall, and complete absence of lymph node tissue, and ultrasonographic evidence of a normal thyroid gland.

THYROID MALIGNANT NEOPLASIA

James P. Miller, MD

 BASICS

DESCRIPTION

Thyroid malignant neoplasia is an autologous growth of thyroid nodules with potential for metastases:

- Papillary carcinoma:
  - Most common variety, 60–70% of thyroid tumors
  - Peak incidence in the 3rd–4th decades
  - 3× more common in women
  - May be associated with radiation exposure
  - Tumor contains psammoma bodies, 50%
  - Metastasizes by lymphatic route (30% at time of diagnosis)
  - Multicentric in ≥20%, especially in children
  - Higher risk in patients with Hashimoto's thyroiditis
- Follicular carcinoma:
  - 10–20% of thyroid tumors
  - Peak incidence in 5th decade of life
  - Incidence has been decreasing since the addition of dietary iodine.
  - Metastasizes by the hematogenous route
- Hürthle cell carcinoma (variant of follicular with poorer prognosis):
  - 2–3% of thyroid malignancies
  - Usually in patients >60 years
  - No gender difference
  - Radioresistant
  - Composed of distinct large eosinophilic cells with abundant cytoplasmic mitochondria
  - Variant of follicular carcinoma with worse prognosis
- Medullary thyroid carcinoma (MCT):
  - Arises from parafollicular cells, C cells
  - Multiple endocrine neoplasia (MEN) syndromes 2A and 2B occur within the first 2 decades of life.
  - 3–4% of all thyroid tumors
  - 25–35% are associated with MEN syndromes (2A more common than 2B), which can be familial or sporadic.
  - Calcitonin is a chemical marker.
  - RET proto-oncogene mutation is screen; family members who carry the RET gene should consider early prophylactic thyroidectomy.
- Anaplastic carcinoma:
  - 3% of thyroid tumors
  - Most aggressive form of thyroid neoplasia
  - More common in females
  - Usually in patients >60 years
- Other: Lymphoma, sarcoma, or metastatic (renal, breast, or lung)
- System(s) affected: Endocrine/Metabolic
- Synonym(s): Follicular carcinoma of the thyroid; Papillary carcinoma of the thyroid; Hürthle cell carcinoma of the thyroid; Anaplastic cell carcinoma of the thyroid

Geriatric Considerations
Risk of malignancy increases at >60 years.

Pediatric Considerations
>60% of thyroid nodules are malignant.

EPIDEMIOLOGY

Incidence
- 10/100,000 per year in the US
- Deaths: 6/1 million per year in the US
- In 2013, estimated 60,220 new cases and 1,850 deaths from thyroid cancer in the US
- Predominant age: Usually >40 years
- Predominant sex: Female > Male (2.6:1).

ETIOLOGY AND PATHOPHYSIOLOGY
Unknown

Genetics
- Familial polyposis of the colon, Turcot syndrome, and Gardner syndrome with the APC gene, 5q21
- Medullary: Autosomal dominant with MEN syndrome
- BRAF mutation
- RET oncogene

RISK FACTORS
- Family history
- Neck irradiation (6–2,000 rads): Papillary carcinoma
- Iodine deficiency: Follicular carcinoma
- Multiple endocrine neoplasia (MEN-2) syndrome: Medullary carcinoma. Autosomal dominant.
- Previous history of subtotal thyroidectomy for malignancy: Anaplastic carcinoma
- Asian race
- Female gender

GENERAL PREVENTION
- Physical exam in high-risk group
- Calcium infusion or pentagastrin stimulation test screening in high-risk MEN patients
- Screen for RET proto-oncogene in groups at risk for MCT.

COMMONLY ASSOCIATED CONDITIONS
Medullary carcinoma: Pheochromocytoma, hyperparathyroidism, ganglioneuroma of the GI tract, neuromata of mucosal membranes

 DIAGNOSIS

HISTORY
- Change in voice (hoarseness)
- Positive family history
- Neck mass
- Dysphagia
- Dyspnea
- Cough
- Difficulty swallowing

PHYSICAL EXAM
- Neck mass: If fixed to surrounding tissue, this finding suggests advanced disease.
- Cervical adenopathy

DIFFERENTIAL DIAGNOSIS
- Multinodular goiter
- Thyroid adenoma
- Thyroglossal duct cyst
- Thyroiditis
- Thyroid cyst
- Ectopic thyroid
- Dermoid cyst

DIAGNOSTIC TESTS & INTERPRETATION
- Medullary carcinoma: Calcitonin level (normal <30 pg/mL [300 ng/L]), pentagastrin stimulation test and RET proto-oncogene
- Thyroglobulin (TG) level: Postoperative tumor marker
- DNA content of tumors from biopsy specimen: Diploid content has a better prognosis.
- Thyroid function tests usually normal
- Thyroid scan: 12–15% of cold nodules are malignant; rate is higher in patients <40 and those with microcalcifications on US.
- US: Solid mass and microcalcifications are more suspicious of malignancy.
- CT scan and MRI can be useful to evaluate large substernal masses and recurrent soft-tissue masses.
- 18F-FDG positron-emission tomographic scan can help if the cytology is inconclusive; helpful with recurrent disease when patient has a negative 131I scan and an elevated TG level (1)[C].

Diagnostic Procedures/Other
- Fine-needle aspiration (FNA).
- Surgical biopsy/excision
- Laryngoscopy if vocal cord paralysis is suspected

Test Interpretation
- Papillary: Psammoma bodies, anaplastic epithelial papillae
- Follicular: Anaplastic epithelial cords with follicles
- Hürthle cell: Large eosinophilic cells with granular cytoplasm
- Medullary: Large amounts of amyloid stroma
- Anaplastic: Small-cell and giant-cell undifferentiated tumors

TREATMENT

MEDICATION

Postoperatively, will require thyroid hormone replacement: Goal is to keep TSH <0.1 mU/L:

- Levothyroxine (T4, Synthroid) 100–200 μg/d, *or*
- Liothyronine (T3, Cytomel) 50–100 μg/d

GENERAL MEASURES

- Papillary/Follicular: [131]I thyroid remnant ablation
- Medullary: Vandetanib has been tried in patients with advanced disease (2)[C].
- Anaplastic: Doxorubicin and cisplatin have achieved partial remission in some patients.
- Recurrent tumor: Sorafenib has been used in patients with recurrent disease.

ADDITIONAL THERAPIES

External-beam radiation for advanced disease

SURGERY/OTHER PROCEDURES

- Papillary carcinoma: Lobectomy with isthmectomy (if lesion <1.5 cm) or total thyroidectomy and removal of suspicious lymph nodes
- Follicular carcinoma and Hürthle cell: Total thyroidectomy and removal of suspicious lymph nodes
- Medullary carcinoma: Total thyroidectomy with central node dissection; unilateral or bilateral modified radical neck dissection if lateral nodes are histologically positive
- Anaplastic carcinoma: Aggressive en bloc thyroidectomy; tracheostomy often required; not responsive to [131]I.

ONGOING CARE

FOLLOW-UP RECOMMENDATIONS
Patient Monitoring

- Thyroid scan at 6 weeks and administration of ^{131}I for any visible uptake; any evidence of residual thyroid tissue (after total thyroidectomy) or lymph node disease noted on scan is treated with radioactive iodine.
- At 6 months and then yearly, the patient should have a thyroid scan and chest x-ray.
- Papillary and follicular: A thyroglobulin (TG) level should be done yearly. Recombinant human thyroid-stimulating hormone (rhTSH)–stimulated TG level may be more sensitive (3,4)[B].
- Medullary: Calcitonin level should be done yearly with pentagastrin stimulation.
- The thyroid scan and TG level should be done with the patient in the hypothyroid state induced by 6-week withdrawal of levothyroxine or 2–3-week withdrawal of liothyronine.
- Decreased incidence of recurrence when TSH is suppressed

DIET

Avoid iodine deficiency.

PATIENT EDUCATION

National Cancer Institute: (301) 496-5583; www.cancer.gov

PROGNOSIS

- Papillary carcinoma: 10-year overall survival is 93%; 30-year cancer related death rate of 6%
- Follicular carcinoma: 10-year overall survival is 85%; histologically, microinvasive tumors parallel papillary tumor results, whereas grossly invasive tumors do far worse. 30-year cancer related death rate of 15%.
- Hürthle cell carcinoma: 93% 5-year survival rate and 83% survival rate overall; grossly invasive tumor survival <25%
- Medullary carcinoma: Negative nodes, 90% 5-year survival rate and 85% 10-year survival rate; with positive nodes, 65% 5-year survival rate and 40% 10-year survival rate. Prognosis worse for MEN 2B compared to MEN 2A. Overall 10-year survival is 75%.
- Anaplastic carcinoma: Survival unexpected. Long-term survivors should have original pathology re-examined.

COMPLICATIONS

- Recurrence of tumor is 10–30%. 80% recur in neck, and 20% recur distally.
- Hoarseness from tumor invasion or operative injury to recurrent laryngeal nerve
- Hypoparathyroidism from operative injury to parathyroid glands

REFERENCES

1. Wang W, Larson SM, Fazzari M, et al. Prognostic value of [18F]fluorodeoxyglucose positron emission tomographic scanning in patients with thyroid cancer. *J Clin Endocrinol Metab*. 2000;85: 1107–1113.
2. Wells SA Jr, Robinson BG, Gagel RF, et al. Vandetanib in patients with locally advanced or metastatic medullary thyroid cancer: A randomized, double-blind phase III trial. *J Clin Oncol*. 2012; 30:134–141.
3. Blamey S, Barraclough B, Delbridge L, et al. Using recombinant human TSH for the diagnosis of recurrent thyroid cancer. *ANZ J Surg*. 2005;75:10–20.
4. Haugen BR, Pacini F, Reiners C, et al. A comparison of recombinant human thyrotropin and thyroid hormone withdrawal for the detection of thyroid remnant or cancer. *J Clin Endocrinol Metab*. 1999;84:3877–3885.

ADDITIONAL READING

- Burns WR, Zeiger MA. Differentiated thyroid cancer. *Semin Oncol*. 2010;37:557–566.
- Cox AE, LeBeau SO. Diagnosis and treatment of differentiated thyroid carcinoma. *Radiol Clin North Am*. 2011;49:453–462, vi.
- Marsh DJ, Gimm O. Multiple endocrine neoplasia: Types 1 and 2. *Adv Otorhinolaryngol*. 2011;70: 84–90.
- Pitt SC, Moley JF. Medullary, anaplastic, and metastatic cancers of the thyroid. *Semin Oncol*. 2010;37:567–579.

SEE ALSO

Multiple Endocrine Neoplasia (MEN)

CODES

ICD10
C73 Malignant neoplasm of thyroid gland

CLINICAL PEARLS

- Standard workup for a patient suspected of having a thyroid cancer is a physical exam, TSH level, neck US, and FNA.
- Thyroglobulin levels can be elevated in several thyroid disorders. Its usefulness comes once the diagnosis of cancer has been made. It serves as a better marker for recurrent disease.
- ~2% of the normal population will have a positive ^{18}F-FDG positron-emission tomographic scan, so it is more useful for postresection follow-up.

THYROIDITIS
Michelle A. Tinitigan, MD

 BASICS

DESCRIPTION
Inflammation of the thyroid gland that may be painful or painless:

- Thyroiditis with thyroid pain:
  - Subacute granulomatous thyroiditis (nonsuppurative thyroiditis, de Quervain thyroiditis, or giant cell thyroiditis): Self-limited; viral URI prodrome, symptoms and signs of thyroid dysfunction (variable) (1)
  - Infectious/Suppurative thyroiditis:
    - Bacterial, fungal, mycobacterial, or parasitic infection of the thyroid
    - Most commonly associated with *Streptococcus pyogenes, Staphylococcus aureus,* and *S. pneumoniae.*
  - Radiation-induced thyroiditis: From radioactive iodine therapy (1%) or external irradiation for lymphoma and head/neck cancers
- Thyroiditis with no thyroid pain:
  - Hashimoto (autoimmune) thyroiditis (chronic lymphocytic thyroiditis): Most common etiology of chronic hypothyroidism; autoimmune disease; 90% of patients with high-serum antithyroid peroxidase (TPO) antibodies
  - Postpartum thyroiditis: Episode of thyrotoxicosis, hypothyroidism, or thyrotoxicosis followed by hypothyroidism in the 1st year postpartum or after spontaneous/induced abortion in women who were without clinically evident thyroid disease before pregnancy.
  - Painless (silent) thyroiditis (subacute lymphocytic thyroiditis): Mild hyperthyroidism, small painless goiter, and no Graves ophthalmopathy/pretibial myxedema (1)
  - Riedel (fibrous) thyroiditis: Rare inflammatory process involving the thyroid and surrounding cervical tissues; associated with various forms of systemic fibrosis (2); presents as a firm mass in the thyroid commonly associated with compressive symptoms (dyspnea, dysphagia, hoarseness, and aphonia) caused by local infiltration of the advancing fibrotic process with hypocalcemia and hypothyroidism (2).
  - Drug-induced thyroiditis: Interferon-α, interleukin-2, amiodarone, or lithium

EPIDEMIOLOGY
- Subacute granulomatous thyroiditis: Most common cause of thyroid pain; peaks during summer; incidence: 3/100,000/year; Female > Male (4:1); peak age: 40–50 years (1)
- Suppurative thyroiditis: Commonly seen with pre-existing thyroid disease/immunocompromise
- Hashimoto thyroiditis: Peak age of onset, 30–50 years; can occur in children; primarily a disease of women; Female > Male (7:1)
- Postpartum thyroiditis: Female only; occurs within 12 months of pregnancy 8–11% of pregnancies; occurs in 25% with type 1 diabetes mellitus; incidence is affected by genetic influences and iodine intake.
- Painless (silent) thyroiditis: Female > Male (4:1) with peak age 30–40; common in areas of iodine sufficiency
- Riedel thyroiditis: Female > Male (4:1); highest prevalence age 30–60 years

ETIOLOGY AND PATHOPHYSIOLOGY
- Hashimoto disease: Antithyroid antibodies may be produced in response to an environmental antigen and cross-react with thyroid proteins (molecular mimicry). Precipitating factors include infection, stress, sex steroids, pregnancy, iodine intake, radiation exposure.
- Subacute granulomatous thyroiditis: Probably viral
- Postpartum thyroiditis: autoimmunity-induced discharge of preformed hormone from the thyroid
- Painless (silent) thyroiditis: Autoimmune

Genetics
Autoimmune thyroiditis is associated with the CT60 polymorphism of cytotoxic T-cell lymphocyte–associated antigen 4. Also associated with HLA-DR4, -DR5, and -DR6 in whites.

RISK FACTORS
- Hashimoto disease: Family history of thyroid/autoimmune disease, personal history of autoimmune disease (type 1 diabetes, celiac disease), high iodine intake, cigarette smoking, selenium deficiency
- Subacute granulomatous thyroiditis: Recent viral respiratory infection
- Suppurative thyroiditis: Congenital abnormalities (persistent thyroglossal duct/piriform sinus fistula), greater age, immunosuppression
- Radiation-induced thyroiditis: High-dose irradiation, younger age, female sex, pre-existing hypothyroidism
- Postpartum thyroiditis: Smoking, history of spontaneous/induced abortion
- Painless (silent) thyroiditis: Iodine-deficient areas

GENERAL PREVENTION
Selenium may decrease inflammatory activity in pregnant women with autoimmune hypothyroidism and may reduce postpartum thyroiditis risk in those positive for TPO antibodies (3)[C].

COMMONLY ASSOCIATED CONDITIONS
Postpartum thyroiditis: Family history of autoimmune thyroid disease; HLA-DRB, -DR4, and -DR5

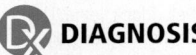 **DIAGNOSIS**

HISTORY
- Hypothyroid symptoms (e.g., constipation, heavy menstrual bleeding, fatigue, weakness, dry skin, hair loss, cold intolerance)
- Hyperthyroid symptoms (e.g., irritability, heat intolerance, increased sweating, palpitations, loose stools, disturbed sleep, and lid retraction)
- Subacute granulomatous thyroiditis: Sudden/gradual onset, with preceding upper respiratory infection/viral illness (fever, fatigue, malaise, anorexia, and myalgia are common); pain may be limited to thyroid region or radiate to upper neck, jaw, throat, or ears.
- Classic triphasic course (thyrotoxic, hypothyroid, recovery), but variable: In subacute, silent, and postpartum thyroiditis (1)[C]

PHYSICAL EXAM
- Examine thyroid size, symmetry, and nodules:
  - Hashimoto disease: 90% have a symmetric, diffusely enlarged, painless gland, with a firm, pebbly texture; 10% have thyroid atrophy.
  - Postpartum thyroiditis: Painless, small, nontender, firm goiter (2–6 months after delivery)

- Reidel thyroiditis: Rock-hard, woodlike, fixed, painless goiter, often accompanied by symptoms of esophageal/tracheal compression (stridor, dyspnea, a suffocating feeling, dysphagia, and hoarseness)
- Signs of hypothyroid: Delayed relaxation phase of deep tendon reflexes, nonpitting edema, dry skin, alopecia, bradycardia
- Signs of hyperthyroid: Moist palms, hyperreflexia, tachycardia/atrial fibrillation

DIFFERENTIAL DIAGNOSIS
Simple goiter; iodine-deficient/lithium-induced goiter; Graves disease; lymphoma; acute infectious thyroiditis; oropharynx and trachea infections; thyroid cancer; amiodarone; contrast dye; amyloid

DIAGNOSTIC TESTS & INTERPRETATION
- Thyroid-stimulating hormone (TSH), anti-TPO antibodies
- Hashimoto disease:
  - High titers of anti-TPO antibodies
  - New subtype: IgG4 thyroiditis, which is histopathologically characterized by lymphoplasmacytic infiltration, fibrosis, increased numbers of IgG4-positive plasma cells, and high serum IgG4 levels; more closely associated with rapid progress, subclinical hypothyroidism, higher levels of circulating antibodies, and more diffuse low echogenicity (4)
- Subacute granulomatous thyroiditis:
  - High T_4, T_3; low TSH during early stages and elevated later; TSH varies with phase (1)
  - High thyroglobulin; normal levels of anti-TPO and antithyroglobulin antibodies (present in 25%, usually low titers)
  - Elevated erythrocyte sedimentation rate (ESR) (usually >50 mm/hr) and C-reactive protein; mild anemia and slight leukocytosis; LFTs frequently abnormal during initial hyperthyroid phase and resolve over 1–2 months
- Suppurative thyroiditis:
  - In the absence of pre-existing thyroid disease, thyroid function normal, but hyper-/hypothyroidism may occur.
  - Elevated ESR and WBC with marked increase in left shift
  - Fine-needle aspiration (FNA) of the lesion with Gram stain and culture is the most useful diagnostic test.
- Postpartum thyroiditis:
  - Anti-TPO antibody positivity is the most useful marker for the prediction of postpartum thyroid dysfunction.
  - Women known to be anti-TPO-Ab+ should have TSH measured at 6–12 weeks' gestation and at 6 months postpartum, or as clinically indicated.
  - Thyrotoxic phase occurs 1 and 6 months postpartum (most commonly at 3 months) and usually lasts only 1–2 months.
  - Hypothyroidism occurs between 3 and 8 months (most commonly at 6 months).
  - Most patients (80%) have normal thyroid function at 1 year (1); 30–50% of patients develop permanent hypothyroidism within 9 years.
  - High thyroglobulin, normal ESR

- Painless (silent) thyroiditis:
  - Hyperthyroid state in 5–20%: Averages 3–4 months, and total duration of illness is <1 year, followed by hypothyroidism and then a return to normal state; some have primary/subclinical hypothyroidism:
    - ~50% have anti-TPO antibodies (1)
- Reidel thyroiditis:
  - Hypothyroidism due to extensive replacement of the gland by scar tissue. Anti-TPO antibodies are present in 2/3 of patients along with low radioactive iodine uptake (RAIU).
- Drug-induced thyroiditis:
  - Hyper-/hypothyroidism, low RAIU, and variable presence of anti-TPO antibodies
- US: Shows variable heterogeneous texture, hypoechogenic in subacute, painless (silent), and postpartum thyroiditis
- Thyroid RAIU scan: Decreased in all forms of thyroiditis, but not helpful in establishing diagnosis of Hashimoto disease. High RAIU in hashitoxicosis, Graves disease
- Random urine iodine measurement may be helpful to distinguish from other causes of low RAIU:
  - Urine iodine <500 µg/L (subacute granulomatous thyroiditis)
  - Urine iodine >1,000 µg/L (in patients with exposure to excess exogenous iodine/radiocontrast material)

Diagnostic Procedures/Other
- Hashimoto with a dominant nodule should have FNA to rule out thyroid carcinoma.
- Open biopsy is necessary for a definitive diagnosis of Reidel thyroiditis.

Test Interpretation
- Hashimoto disease: Lymphocytic infiltration with formation of Askanazy (Hürthle) cells, oxyphilic changes in follicular cells, fibrosis, thyroid atrophy
- Subacute granulomatous thyroiditis: Giant cells, mononuclear cell (granulomatous) infiltrate
- Postpartum thyroiditis: Lymphocytic infiltration, occasional germinal centers, disruption and collapse of thyroid follicles
- Painless (Silent) thyroiditis: Lymphocytic infiltration, but without fibrosis, Askanazy cells, and extensive lymphoid follicle formation (1)

 TREATMENT

GENERAL MEASURES
Analgesics for pain; corticosteroids for severe granulomatous thyroiditis

MEDICATION
- Hashimoto disease:
  - If hypothyroid/goitrous: Levothyroxine (1.7 µg/kg/d for adults <50 years). If no cardiac complications and no adrenal insufficiency, 1/2 replacement dose and increase to full replacement in 10 days:
    - If >50 years of age or heart disease and/or adrenal insufficiency, begin with 25 µg/d and titrate to TSH of lower limit normal range.
  - If thyrotoxic and symptomatic: Propylthiouracil and propranolol
  - An elevated TSH level in a woman who is pregnant or attempting to become pregnant is an indication for thyroid replacement (5)[A].
- Subacute granulomatous thyroiditis:
  - Analgesics for 2–8 weeks (NSAIDs or aspirin)

- Symptomatic hyperthyroidism: β-Blockers while thyrotoxic (propranolol 40–120 mg/d)
- Symptomatic hypothyroid phase: Levothyroxine, as above, target TSH in the normal range
- Pain with no improvement in 2–3 days after NSAID use: Prednisone 40 mg/d; should result in pain relief in 1–2 days; if not, question diagnosis
- Severe pain: Prednisone 40–60 mg/d discontinued over 4–6 weeks. If pain recurs, increase dose for several weeks and then taper.
- Suppurative thyroiditis:
  - Parenteral empiric, broad-spectrum antibiotics and surgical drainage
- Painless (silent) thyroiditis:
  - No treatment needed
  - If symptomatic during hyperthyroid state, treat with β-blocker
  - Prednisone shortens the period of hyperthyroidism. Monitor TSH every 4–8 weeks to confirm resolution.
  - Treat hypothyroid symptoms and asymptomatic patients with TSH >10 mU/L with levothyroxine (50–100 µg/d), to be discontinued after 3–6 months.
- Postpartum thyroiditis:
  - Treat symptomatic hyper-/hypothyroid state. Most do not need treatment.
  - Caution in breastfeeding mothers because β-blockers are secreted into breast milk.
  - For symptomatic hypothyroidism, treat with levothyroxine. Otherwise, remonitor in 4–8 weeks. Taper replacement hormone after 6 months if thyroid function has normalized.
- Reidel thyroiditis:
  - Corticosteroids in early stages, but controversial thereafter. Prednisone 10–20 mg/d for 4–6 months, possibly continued thereafter if effective (6)[C]
  - Long-term anti-inflammatory medications to arrest progression and maintain a symptom-free course (6)[C]
  - Tamoxifen 10–20 mg monotherapy or in conjunction with prednisone reduces mass size and clinical symptoms.
  - Methotrexate is used with some success.
  - Reduction of goiter seen with a combination of mycophenolate mofetil (1 g b.i.d.) and 100 mg/d prednisone.
  - Debulking surgery is limited to isthmusectomy to relieve constrictive pressure when total thyroidectomy is not possible (2)[C].
- Drug-induced thyroiditis:
  - Discontinue offending drug

SURGERY/OTHER PROCEDURES
Enlarged painful thyroid or tracheal compression

 ONGOING CARE

FOLLOW-UP RECOMMENDATIONS
Patient Monitoring
- Hashimoto disease: Repeat thyroid function tests every 3–12 months.
- Subacute granulomatous thyroiditis: Repeat thyroid function tests every 3–6 weeks until euthyroid, then every 6–12 months.
- Postpartum thyroiditis: Check TSH annually
- Reidel thyroiditis: CT of cervical mediastinal region is recommended.
- TSH every 6 months in patients on amiodarone

Pregnancy Considerations
- Avoid radioisotope scanning if possible.

- Keep TSH maximally suppressed.
- If using RAIU scan, discard breast milk for 2 days because RAI is secreted in breast milk.

PROGNOSIS
- Hashimoto disease: Persistent goiter; eventual thyroid failure
- Subacute granulomatous thyroiditis: 5–15% hypothyroid beyond a year: Some with eventual return to normal; remission may be slower in the elderly; recurrence rate: 1–4% after a year (1).
- Painless (silent) thyroiditis: 10–20% hypothyroid beyond a year; recurrence rate 5–10% (much higher in Japan) (1)
- Postpartum thyroiditis: 15–50% hypothyroid beyond a year; women may be euthyroid/continue to be hypothyroid at the end of 1st postpartum year. 70% recurrence rate in subsequent pregnancies (1); substantial risk exists for later development of hypothyroidism/goiter (7).

REFERENCES
1. Samuels MH. Subacute, silent, and postpartum thyroiditis. Med Clin North Am. 2012;84(2):223–233. Epub 2012 Feb 4.
2. Hennessey JV. Clinical review: Riedel's thyroiditis: A clinical review. J Clin Endocrinol Metab. 2011;84(10):3031–3041. Epub 2011 Aug 10.
3. Duntas LH. Selenium and the thyroid: A close-knit connection. J Clin Endocrinol Metab. 2010;95:5180–5188.
4. Li Y. Hashimoto's thyroiditis: Old concepts and new insights. Curr Opin Rheumatol. 2011;23(1):102–107.
5. Reid SM, Middleton P, Cossich MC, et al. Interventions for clinical and subclinical hypothyroidism in pregnancy. Cochrane Database Syst Rev. 2010;7:CD007752.
6. De Groot L, Abalovich M, Alexander EK, et al. Management of thyroid dysfunction during pregnancy and postpartum: An Endocrine Society clinical practice guideline. J Clin Endocrinol Metab. 2012;97(8):2543-65. doi: 10.1210/jc.2011-2803.
7. Stagnaro-Green A, Schwartz A, Gismondi R, et al. High rate of persistent hypothyroidism in a large-scale prospective study of postpartum thyroiditis in southern Italy. J Clin Endocrinol Metab. 2011;96:652–657.

 SEE ALSO

Hyperthyroidism; Hypothyroidism, Adult

 CODES

ICD10
- E06.0 Acute thyroiditis
- E06.1 Subacute thyroiditis
- E06.9 Thyroiditis, unspecified

CLINICAL PEARLS
- TSH elevation above the normal range indicates a hypothyroid state; suppressed TSH indicates hyperthyroid state. Follow up with free T$_3$/T$_4$ determination.
- Follow patients on thyroid replacement with periodic TSH level.

TINEA (CAPITIS, CORPORIS, CRURIS)

Elisabeth Backer, MD

 BASICS

DESCRIPTION

- Superficial fungal infections of the skin/scalp; various forms of dermatophytosis; the names relate to the particular area affected:
  - Tinea cruris: Infection of crural fold and gluteal cleft
  - Tinea corporis: Infection involving the face, trunk, and/or extremities: Often presents with ring-shaped lesions, hence the misnomer *ringworm*.
  - Tinea capitis: Infection of the scalp and hair: Affected areas of the scalp can show characteristic black dots resulting from broken hairs.
- Infections result from contact with infected persons/animals:
  - Zoophilic infections are acquired from animals.
  - Anthropophilic infections are acquired from personal contact (e.g., wrestling) or fomites.
  - Geophile infections are acquired from the soil.
- System(s) affected: Skin; Exocrine
- Synonym(s): Jock itch; ringworm

EPIDEMIOLOGY

Incidence
- Tinea cruris:
  - Predominant age: Any age; rare in children
  - Predominant sex: Male > Female
- Tinea corporis:
  - Predominant age: All ages
  - Predominant sex: Male = Female
- Tinea capitis:
  - Predominant age: 3–9 years; almost always occurs in young children
  - Predominant sex: Male = Female

Prevalence
Common

Pediatric Considerations
- Tinea cruris is rare prior to puberty.
- Tinea capitis is common in young children.

Geriatric Considerations
Tinea cruris is more common in the geriatric population due to an increase in risk factors.

Pregnancy Considerations
Tinea cruris and capitis are rare in pregnancy.

ETIOLOGY AND PATHOPHYSIOLOGY
Superficial fungal infection of skin/scalp

- Tinea cruris: Source of infection is usually the patient's own tinea pedis, with agent being transferred from the foot to the groin via the underwear when dressing; most common causative dermatophyte is *Trichophyton rubrum*; rare cases caused by *Epidermophyton floccosum* and *T. mentagrophytes*.
- Tinea corporis: Most commonly caused by *T. rubrum*; *T. tonsurans* most often found in patients with tinea gladiatorum.
- Tinea capitis: *T. tonsurans* found in 90% and *Microsporum* sp. in 10% of patients.

Genetics
Evidence suggests a genetic susceptibility in certain individuals.

RISK FACTORS
- Warm climates; summer months and/or copious sweating; wearing wet clothing/multiple layers (tinea cruris)
- Daycare centers/Schools/Confined quarters (tinea corporis and capitis)
- Depression of cell-mediated immune response (e.g., individuals with atopy or AIDS)
- Obesity (tinea cruris and corporis)
- Direct contact with an active lesion on a human, an animal, or rarely, from soil; working with animals (tinea corporis)

GENERAL PREVENTION
- Avoidance of risk factors, such as contact with suspicious lesions
- Fluconazole or itraconazole may be useful in wrestlers to prevent outbreaks during competitive season (1).

COMMONLY ASSOCIATED CONDITIONS
Tinea pedis, tinea barbae, tinea manus

 DIAGNOSIS

HISTORY
- Lesions range from asymptomatic to pruritic.
- In tinea cruris, acute inflammation may result from wearing occlusive clothing; chronic scratching may result in an eczematous appearance.
- Previous application of topical steroids, especially in tinea cruris and corporis, may alter the overall appearance, causing a more extensive eruption with irregular borders and erythematous papules. This modified form is called *tinea incognito*.

PHYSICAL EXAM
- Tinea cruris: Well-marginated, erythematous, half-moon–shaped plaques in crural folds that spread to upper thighs; advancing border is well defined, often with fine scaling and sometimes vesicular eruptions. Lesions are usually bilateral and do not include scrotum/penis (unlike with *Candida* infections), but may migrate to perineum, perianal area, and gluteal cleft and onto the buttocks in chronic/progressive cases. The area may be hyperpigmented on resolution.
- Tinea corporis: Scaling, pruritic plaques characterized by a sharply defined annular pattern with peripheral activity and central clearing (ring-shaped lesions); papules and occasionally pustules/vesicles present at border and, less commonly, in center.
- Tinea capitis: Commonly begins with round patches of scale (alopecia less common). In its later stages, the infection frequently takes on patterns of chronic scaling with either little/marked inflammation and alopecia. Less often, patients will present with multiple patches of alopecia and the characteristic black-dot appearance of broken hairs. Extreme inflammation results in kerion formation (exudative, pustular nodulation).

DIFFERENTIAL DIAGNOSIS
- Tinea cruris:
  - Intertrigo: Inflammatory process of moist opposed skin folds, often including infection with bacteria, yeast, and fungi; painful longitudinal fissures may occur in skin folds.
  - Erythrasma: Diffuse brown, scaly, noninflammatory plaque with irregular borders, often involving groin; caused by bacterial infection with *Corynebacterium minutissimum;* fluoresces coral red with Wood's lamp
  - Seborrheic dermatitis of groin
  - Psoriasis of groin ("inverse psoriasis")
  - Candidiasis of groin (typically involves the scrotum)
  - Acanthosis nigricans
- Tinea capitis:
  - Psoriasis
  - Seborrheic dermatitis
  - Pyoderma
  - Alopecia areata and trichotillomania
  - Aplasia cutis congenital
- Tinea corporis:
  - Pityriasis rosea
  - Eczema (nummular)
  - Contact dermatitis
  - Syphilis
  - Psoriasis
  - Seborrheic dermatitis
  - Subacute SLE
  - Erythema annulare centrifugum
  - Erythema multiforme; erythema migrans
  - Impetigo circinatum
  - Granuloma annulare

DIAGNOSTIC TESTS & INTERPRETATION
Wood's lamp exam reveals no fluorescence in most cases (*Trichophyton* sp.); 10% of infections, those caused by *M. rubrum*, will fluoresce with a green light.

Initial Tests (lab, imaging)
- Potassium hydroxide (KOH) preparation of skin scrapings from dermatophyte leading border shows characteristic translucent, branching, rod-shaped hyphae.
- Arthrospores can be visualized within hair shafts. Spores and/or hyphae may be seen on KOH exam.

Follow-Up Tests & Special Considerations
- Re-evaluate to assess response, especially in resistant/extensive cases.
- Fungal culture using Sabouraud dextrose agar/dermatophyte test medium

Test Interpretation
- Skin scrapings show fungal hyphae in epidermis.
- Arthrospores found in hair shafts; spores and/or hyphae seen on KOH exam.

TREATMENT

GENERAL MEASURES

- Careful handwashing and personal hygiene; laundering of towels/clothing of affected individual; no sharing of towels/clothes/headgear
- Evaluate other family members, close contacts, or household pets.
- Avoid predisposing conditions such as hot baths and tight-fitting clothing (boxer shorts are better than briefs) (2)[C].
- Keep area as dry as possible (talcum/powders may be beneficial) (2)[C].
- Itching can be alleviated by OTC preparations such as Sarna or Prax.
- Topical steroid preparations should be avoided (see "Tinea Incognito") (3)[C], unless absolutely needed to control itching and only after definitive diagnosis and initiation of antifungal treatment.
- Nystatin should be avoided in tinea infections, but is indicated for cutaneous candidal infections.
- Avoid contact sports (e.g., wrestling) temporarily while starting treatment.

MEDICATION
First Line

- Tinea cruris/corporis:
  - Topical azole antifungal compounds (3)[B]:
    - Econazole (Spectazole), ketoconazole (Nizoral): Usually applied b.i.d. × 2–3 weeks
    - Terbinafine (Lamisil): Over-the-counter (OTC) compound; can be applied once or b.i.d. × 1–2 weeks
    - Butenafine (Mentax): Applied once daily × 2 weeks; also very effective
  - To prevent relapse, use for 1 week after resolution (4)[C].

- Tinea capitis:
  - PO griseofulvin (2,5)[A] for *Trichophyton* and *Microsporum* sp.; micro-sized preparation available; dosage 125 mg/d in patients weighing 10–20 kg; 250 mg/d if weight is 20–40 kg; 500 mg/d if weight is >40 kg; taken b.i.d. or as a single dose daily × 6–12 weeks
  - PO terbinafine (2,5)[A] can be used for *Trichophyton* sp. at 62.5 mg/d in patients weighing 10–20 kg; 125 mg/d if weight 20–40 kg; 250 mg/d if weight >40 kg; use for 4–6 weeks
  - PO itraconazole (2)[A] can be used for *Microsporum* sp. and matches griseofulvin efficacy while being better tolerated. Dosage of 3–5 mg/kg/d, but most studies have used 100 mg/d × 6 weeks in children >2 years of age.

Second Line
Tinea cruris/corporis:

- Oral antifungal agents are effective, but not indicated in uncomplicated tinea cruris/corporis cases. They can be used for resistant and extensive infections or if the patient is immunocompromised. If topical therapy fails, consider possible oral therapy. Griseofulvin can be given 500 mg/d for 1–2 weeks.

- The following oral regimens have been reported in medical literature as being effective, but currently are not specifically approved by the FDA for tinea cruris:
  - PO terbinafine (Lamisil): 250 mg/d × 1 week
  - PO itraconazole (Sporanox): 100 mg b.i.d. once and repeated 1 week later (6)
  - PO fluconazole (Diflucan): 150 mg once/week × 4 weeks
- Topical terbinafine 1% solution has been studied recently and appears effective as a once-daily application for 1 week.
- Contraindications:
  - PO itraconazole (Sporanox): Contraindicated with astemizole (Hismanal), triazolam (Halcion), lovastatin (Mevacor), simvastatin (Zocor). Pravastatin (Pravachol) can be given with itraconazole.
- Oral antifungals can interact with warfarin, OCPs, alcohol; contraindicated in pregnancy. Monitor for liver toxicity when using oral antifungals.

ISSUES FOR REFERRAL
Refer if disease is nonresponsive/resistant, especially in immunocompromised host.

ADDITIONAL THERAPIES
Treatment of secondary bacterial infections

 ONGOING CARE

FOLLOW-UP RECOMMENDATIONS
Re-evaluate response to treatment.

Patient Monitoring
Liver function testing prior to therapy and at regular intervals during course of therapy for patients requiring oral terbinafine, fluconazole, itraconazole, and griseofulvin

PATIENT EDUCATION
Explain the causative agents, predisposing factors, and prevention measures.

PROGNOSIS
- Excellent prognosis for cure with therapy in tinea cruris and corporis.
- In tinea capitis, lesions will heal spontaneously in 6 months without treatment, but scarring is more likely.

COMPLICATIONS
- Secondary bacterial infection
- Generalized, invasive dermatophyte infection

REFERENCES
1. Kohl TD, Martin DC, Berger MS. Comparison of topical and oral treatments for tinea gladiatorum. *Clin J Sport Med*. 1999;9:161–166.
2. Gonzalez U, Seaton T, Bergus G, et al. Systemic antifungal therapy for tinea capitis in children. *Cochrane Database Sys Rev*. 2007:CD004685.
3. Bonifaz A. Comparative study between terbinafine 1% emulsion-gel versus ketoconazole 2% cream in tinea cruris and corporis. *Eur J Derm*. 2000;10:107.
4. Lesher JL. Butenafine 1% cream in the treatment of tinea cruris: A multicenter, vehicle-controlled, double-blind trial. *J Am Acad Dermatol*. 1997; 36(2 pt 1):S20–S24.
5. Tey HL, Tan AS, Chan YC. Meta-analysis of randomized, controlled trials comparing griseofulvin and terbinafine in the treatment of tinea capitis. *J Am Acad Dermatol* 2011;64:663.
6. Sanmano B, Hiruma M, Mizoguchi M. Abbreviated oral itraconazole therapy for tinea corporis and tinea cruris. *Mycoses*. 2003;46:316–321.

ADDITIONAL READING
- Akinwale SO. Personal hygiene as an alternative to griseofulvin in the treatment of tinea cruris. *Afr J Med Sci*. 2000;29:41.
- Ameen M. Epidemiology of superficial fungal infections. *Clin Dermatol*. 2010;28:197.
- Fuller LC, Smith CH, Cerio R. A randomized comparison of 4 weeks of terbinafine vs. 8 weeks of griseofulvin for the treatment of tinea capitis. *Br J Dermatol*. 2001;144:321–327.
- Gupta AK, Cooper EA. Update in antifungal therapy of dermatophytosis. *Mycopathologia*. 2008;166:353.
- Nozickova M, Koudelkova V, Kulikova Z. A comparison of the efficacy of oral fluconazole, 150 mg/week versus 50 mg/day, in the treatment of tinea corporis, tinea cruris, tinea pedis, and cutaneous candidosis. *Int J Dermatol*. 1998;37:703–705.
- Seebacker C, Bouchara JP, Mignon B. Updates on the epidemiology of dermatophyte infections. *Mycopathologia* 2008;166:335.

CODES

ICD10
- B35.0 Tinea barbae and tinea capitis
- B35.4 Tinea corporis
- B35.6 Tinea cruris

CLINICAL PEARLS
- Tinea corporis is characterized by scaly plaque, with peripheral activity and central clearing.
- Tinea cruris is characterized by erythematous plaque in crural folds, usually sparing the scrotum.
- Tinea capitis is a fungal infection of the scalp, affecting hair growth.

TINEA PEDIS

Elisabeth Backer, MD

 BASICS

DESCRIPTION
- Superficial infection of the feet caused by dermatophytes
- Most common dermatophyte infection encountered in clinical practice
- Often accompanied by tinea manuum, tinea unguium, and tinea cruris
- 2 clinical forms: Acute and chronic; both are contagious
- System(s) affected: Skin/Exocrine
- Synonym(s): Athlete's foot

EPIDEMIOLOGY
- Predominant age: 20–50 years, although can occur at any age
- Predominant gender: Male > Female

Prevalence
4% of population

Pediatric Considerations
Rare in younger children; common in teens

Geriatric Considerations
Elderly are more susceptible to outbreaks because of immunocompromise and impaired perfusion of distal extremities.

ETIOLOGY AND PATHOPHYSIOLOGY
Superficial infection caused by dermatophytes that thrive only in nonviable keratinized tissue
- *Trichophyton mentagrophytes* (acute)
- *T. rubrum* (chronic)
- *T. tonsurans*
- *Epidermophyton floccosum*

Genetics
No known genetic pattern

RISK FACTORS
- Hot, humid weather
- Occlusive/Tight-fitting footwear
- Immunosuppression
- Prolonged application of topical steroids

GENERAL PREVENTION
- Good personal hygiene
- Wearing rubber or wooden sandals in community showers, bathing places, locker rooms
- Careful drying between toes after showering or bathing; blow-drying feet with hair dryer may be more effective than drying with towel
- Changing socks and shoes frequently
- Applying drying or dusting powder
- Applying topical antiperspirants
- Putting on socks before underwear to prevent infection from spreading to groin

COMMONLY ASSOCIATED CONDITIONS
- Hyperhidrosis
- Onychomycosis
- Tinea manuum/unguium/cruris/corporis

 DIAGNOSIS

HISTORY
- Itchy, scaly rash on foot, usually between toes; may progress to fissuring/maceration in toe web spaces
- May be associated with onychomycosis and other tinea infections

PHYSICAL EXAM
- Acute form: Self-limited, intermittent, recurrent; scaling, thickening, and fissuring of sole and heel; scaling or fissuring of toe webs; or pruritic vesicular/bullous lesions between toes or on soles
- Chronic form: Most common; slowly progressive, pruritic erythematous erosion/scales between toes, in digital interspaces; extension onto soles, sides/dorsum of feet (moccasin distribution). If untreated, may persist indefinitely.
- Other features: Strong odor, hyperkeratosis, maceration, ulceration

DIFFERENTIAL DIAGNOSIS
- Interdigital type: Erythrasma, impetigo, pitted keratolysis, candida intertrigo
- Moccasin type: Psoriasis vulgaris, eczematous dermatitis, pitted keratolysis
- Inflammatory/Bullous type: Impetigo, allergic contact dermatitis, dyshidrotic eczema (negative KOH examination of scrapings), bullous disease

DIAGNOSTIC TESTS & INTERPRETATION
Wood's lamp exam will not fluoresce unless complicated by another fungus, which is uncommon; *M. furfur* (yellow to white), *Corynebacterium* (red), or *Microsporum* (blue–green).

Initial Tests (lab, imaging)
Testing is not needed in typical presentation
- Direct microscopic exam (potassium hydroxide)of scrapings of the lesions
- Culture (Sabouraud medium)

Test Interpretation
- Potassium hydroxide preparation: Septate and branched mycelia
- Culture: Dermatophyte

 TREATMENT

Treatment is generally with topical antifungal medications for up to 4 weeks (1) and is more effective than placebo (2)[A]:
- Acute treatment:
  – Aluminum acetate soak (Burow solution; Domeboro, 1 pack to 1 quart warm water) to decrease itching and acute eczematous reaction
  – Antifungal cream of choice b.i.d. after soaks
- Chronic treatment:
  – Antifungal creams b.i.d., continuing for 3 days after the rash is resolved: Terbinafine 1% (possibly most effective topical), clotrimazole 1%, econazole 1%, ketoconazole 2%, tolnaftate 1%, etc. (1)[A]
  – May try systemic antifungal therapy; see below (consider if concomitant onychomycosis or after failed topical treatment)

GENERAL MEASURES
- Soak with aluminum chloride 30% or aluminum subacetate for 20 minutes b.i.d.
- Careful removal of dead/thickened skin after soaking or bathing
- Chronic or extensive disease or nail involvement requires oral antifungal medication and systemic therapy.

MEDICATION
For use when topical therapy has failed

First Line
- Systemic antifungals (3)[A]:
  – Itraconazole (Sporanox): 200 mg PO b.i.d. for 14 days (cure rate >90%)
  – Terbinafine (Lamisil): 250 mg/d PO for 14 days

- If concomitant onychomycosis:
  - Itraconazole: 200 mg PO b.i.d. for 1st week of month for 3 months. Liver function testing is recommended.
  - Terbinafine: 250 mg/d PO for 12 weeks, or pulse dosing: 500 mg/d PO for 1st week of month for 3 months. Not recommended if creatinine clearance <50 mL/min.
- Pediatric dosing options:
  - Griseofulvin: 10–15 mg/kg/d or divided
  - Terbinafine: 10–20 kg: 62.5 mg/d:
    - 20–40 kg: 125 mg/d
    - >40 kg: 250 mg/d
  - Itraconazole: 5 mg/kg/d
  - Fluconazole: 6 mg/kg/week
- Contraindications: Itraconazole, pregnancy Category C
- Precautions: All systemic antifungal drugs may have potential hepatotoxicity.
- Significant possible interactions: Itraconazole requires gastric acid for absorption; effectiveness is reduced with antacids, H$_2$ blockers, proton pump inhibitors, etc. Take with acidic beverage such as soda if on antacids.

Second Line

- Systemic antifungals: Griseofulvin 250–500 mg of microsize b.i.d. daily for 21 days
- Contraindications (griseofulvin):
  - Patients with porphyria, hepatocellular failure
  - Patients with history of hypersensitivity to griseofulvin
- Precautions (griseofulvin):
  - Should be used only in severe cases
  - Periodic monitoring of organ-system functioning, including renal, hepatic, and hematopoietic
  - Possible photosensitivity reactions
  - Lupus erythematosus, lupuslike syndromes, or exacerbation of existing lupus erythematosus has been reported.
- Significant possible interactions (griseofulvin):
  - Decreases activity of warfarin-type anticoagulants
  - Barbiturates usually depress griseofulvin activity.
  - May potentiate effect of alcohol, producing tachycardia and flush

ISSUES FOR REFERRAL

If extensive or resistant disease, especially in immunocompromised host

ADDITIONAL THERAPIES

- Treatment of secondary bacterial infections
- Treatment of eczematoid changes

 ONGOING CARE

FOLLOW-UP RECOMMENDATIONS

Avoid sweating feet.

Patient Monitoring

Evaluate for response, recognizing that infections may be chronic/recurrent.

DIET

No restrictions

PATIENT EDUCATION

See "General Prevention."

PROGNOSIS

- Control, but not complete cure
- Infections tend to be chronic with exacerbations (e.g., in hot weather).
- Personal hygiene and preventive measures such as open-toed sandals, careful drying, and frequent sock changes are essential.

COMPLICATIONS

- Secondary bacterial infections (common portal of entry for streptococcal infections, producing lymphangitis/cellulitis of lower extremity)
- Eczematoid changes

REFERENCES

1. Crawford F, Hollis S. Topical treatments for fungal infections of the skin and nails of the foot. *Cochrane Database Syst Rev.* 2007;CD001434.
2. Rotta I, Sanchez A, Gonçalves PR, et al. Efficacy and safety of topical antifungals in the treatment of dermatomycosis: A systematic review. *Br J Dermatol.* 2012;84(5):927–933.
3. Bell-Syer SE, Hart R, Crawford F, et al. Oral treatments for fungal infections of the skin of the foot. *Cochrane Database Syst Rev.* 2002: CD003584.

ADDITIONAL READING

Ameen M. Epidemiology of superficial fungal infections. *Clin Dermatol.* 2010;28:197.

 SEE ALSO

Dermatitis, Contact; Dyshidrosis

 CODES

ICD10

B35.3 Tinea pedis

CLINICAL PEARLS

- Treatment is generally with topical antifungal medications for up to 4 weeks (1)[A].
- Often is recurrent/chronic in nature
- Careful drying between toes after showering or bathing helps prevent recurrences. (Blow drying feet with hair dryer may be more effective than drying with towel.)
- Socks should be changed frequently. Put on socks before underwear to prevent infection from spreading to groin (tinea cruris).
- Dusting and drying powders (containing antifungal agents) may prevent recurrences.

T

TINEA VERSICOLOR

Elisabeth Backer, MD

 BASICS

DESCRIPTION

- Rash due to a common superficial mycosis with a variety of colors and changing shades of color, predominantly present on trunk and proximal upper extremities; macules usually hypopigmented, light brown, or salmon-colored; fine scale often apparent. It is not a dermatophyte infection.
- System(s) affected: Skin/Exocrine
- Synonym(s): Pityriasis versicolor

EPIDEMIOLOGY

Incidence
- Common, occurs worldwide, especially in tropical climates
- Predominant age: Teenagers and young adults
- Predominant sex: Male = Female

Pediatric Considerations
Usually occurs after puberty (except in tropical areas); facial lesions are more common in children.

Geriatric Considerations
Not common in the geriatric population

ETIOLOGY AND PATHOPHYSIOLOGY
Inhibition of pigment synthesis in epidermal melanocytes, leading to hypomelanosis; in the hyperpigmented type, the melanosomes are large and heavily melanized.

- Saprophytic yeast: *Pityrosporum orbiculare* (also known as *P. ovale*, *Malassezia furfur*, or *M. ovalis*), which is a known colonizer of all humans
- Development of clinical disease associated with transformation of *Malassezia* from yeast cells to pathogenic mycelial form.

Genetics
Genetic predisposition may exist.

RISK FACTORS
- Hot, humid weather
- Use of topical skin oils
- Hyperhidrosis
- HIV infection/Immunosuppression (1)
- High cortisol levels (Cushing, prolonged steroid administration)
- Pregnancy
- Malnutrition
- Oral contraceptives

GENERAL PREVENTION
- Recheck and treat again each spring prior to tanning season.
- Avoid skin oils.

 DIAGNOSIS

HISTORY
- Asymptomatic scaling macules on trunk
- Possible mild pruritus
- More prominent in summer
- Suntanning accentuates lesions because infected areas do not tan.
- Periodic recurrences common

PHYSICAL EXAM
- *Versicolor* refers to the variety and changing shades of colors.
- Sun-exposed areas: Lesions usually white/hypopigmented
- Covered areas: Lesions often brown or salmon-colored
- Distribution (sebum-rich areas): Chest, shoulders, back (also face and intertriginous areas).
  – Face more likely to be involved in children.
- Appearance: Small individual macules that frequently coalesce
- Scale: Fine, more visible with scraping

DIFFERENTIAL DIAGNOSIS
- Other skin diseases with discolored macules and plaques, including:
  – Pityriasis alba/rosea ("Christmas tree-like" distribution visible in *P. rosea*)
  – Vitiligo (presents without scaling)
  – Seborrheic dermatitis (more erythematous; thicker scale)
  – Nummular eczema
  – Secondary syphilis
  – Erythrasma

DIAGNOSTIC TESTS & INTERPRETATION
Wood's lamp: Yellow to yellow–green fluorescence or pigment changes

Initial Tests (lab, imaging)
- Direct microscopy of scales with 10% potassium hydroxide (KOH) preparation to visualize hyphae and spores ("spaghetti and meatballs" pattern)
- Routine lab tests usually not necessary
- Fungal culture not useful

Test Interpretation
- Short, stubby, or Y-shaped hyphae
- Small, round spores in clusters on hyphae

TREATMENT

GENERAL MEASURES
- Apply prescribed topical medications to affected skin with cotton balls.
- Pigmentation may take months to fade or fill in.
- Repeat treatment each spring prior to sun exposure; some may require repeated treatment during the summer as prophylaxis.

MEDICATION
Topical antifungal therapy is the treatment of choice in limited disease. Evidence is generally of poor quality, but data suggest that longer durations of treatment and higher concentrations of active agents produce greater cure rates (2)[A].

First Line
- Ketoconazole 2% shampoo applied to damp skin and left on for 5 minutes × 1–3 days *or*
- Selenium sulfide shampoo 2.5% (Selsun):
  – Allowed to dry for 10 minutes prior to showering: Daily × 1 week *or*
  – Allowed to remain on body for 12–24 hours prior to showering: Once a week × 4 weeks *or*
- Clotrimazole topical (Lotrimin) b.i.d. × 2–4 weeks *or*
- Miconazole (Micatin, Monistat) b.i.d. × 2–4 weeks *or*
- Ketoconazole 2% (Nizoral) cream b.i.d. × 2–4 weeks *or*
- Terbinafine (Lamisil) 1% solution b.i.d. × 1 week *or*
- Terbinafine (Lamisil Derm Gel) once daily × 1 week
- Cure rates of topical antiyeast preparations typically 70–80%; healing continues after active treatment. Resumption of even pigmentation may take months.
- Contraindications: Ketoconazole is contraindicated in pregnancy.
- Newer preparations: 2.25% selenium sulfide foam; ketoconazole gel

Second Line

- Use for extensive disease or nonresponders
- Oral ketoconazole (rarely needed and has significant adverse reactions) 400 mg in single dose or 200 mg/d for 1 week; cure rate >90% (3)[C]
- Oral fluconazole 300 mg once weekly for 2 weeks
- Itraconazole 200 mg/d PO × 1 week; cure rate >90% (3)[C]
- Oral terbinafine or griseofulvin not effective
- Pramiconazole has been studied, but is not yet available for clinical use (4)

ISSUES FOR REFERRAL

- If resistant to treatment
- If extensive disease occurs in immunocompromised host

 ONGOING CARE

- Ketoconazole 2% or selenium sulfide 2.5% shampoo can be used weekly for maintenance or monthly for prophylaxis.
- Itraconazole 400 mg once monthly during the warmer months of the year can also reduce recurrences.

FOLLOW-UP RECOMMENDATIONS

Warn patients that whiteness will remain for several months after treatment.

Patient Monitoring

- Recheck and treat again each spring prior to tanning season.
- Failure to respond should prompt reassessment or dermatology referral.
- Resistance to treatment, frequent recurrences, or widespread disease may point to immunodeficiency.

PATIENT EDUCATION

For patient education materials favorably reviewed on this topic, contact American Academy of Dermatology, 930 N. Meacham Road, P.O. Box 4014, Schaumburg, IL 60168-4014; (708) 330-0230.

PROGNOSIS

- Duration of lesions months/years
- Recurs almost routinely, since this yeast is a known human colonizer

REFERENCES

1. Güleç AT, Demirbilek M, Seçkin D, et al. Superficial fungal infections in 102 renal transplant recipients: A case-control study. *J Am Acad Dermatol*. 2003; 49:187–192.
2. Hu SW, Bigby M. Pityriasis versicolor: A systematic review of interventions. *Arch Dermatol*. 2010; 146:1132.
3. Köse O, Bülent Tatan H, Riza Gür A, et al. Comparison of a single 400 mg dose versus a 7-day 200 mg daily dose of itraconazole in the treatment of tinea versicolor. *J Dermatolog Treat*. 2002;13(2):77–79.
4. Faergemann J, Todd G, Pather S, et al. A double-blind, randomized, placebo-controlled, dose-finding study of oral pramiconazole in the treatment of pityriasis versicolor. *J Am Acad Dermatol*. 2009;61:971.

ADDITIONAL READING

- Bhogal CS, Singal A, Baruah MC. Comparative efficacy of ketoconazole and fluconazole in the treatment of pityriasis versicolor: A one year follow-up study. *J Dermatol*. 2001;28:535–539.
- Gupta AK, Batra R, Bluhm R, Faergemann J. Pityriasis versicolor. *Dermatol Clin* 2003;21:413.
- Morishita N, Sei Y. Microreview of pityriasis versicolor and *Malassezia* species. *Mycopathologia*. 2006;162:373–376.

 CODES

ICD10

B36.0 Pityriasis versicolor

CLINICAL PEARLS

- Noncontagious macules of varying colors, with fine scale
- Recurrence in summer months
- More apparent after tanning. Skin areas with fungal infection do not tan; thus, hypopigmented areas become more visible.
- Warn patients that whiteness will remain for several months after treatment.

TINNITUS
David Holmes, MD

BASICS

DESCRIPTION
- Tinnitus is the perception of sound in the absence of an acoustic stimulus; may be a buzz, ring, roar, chirp, whistle, or hiss. Tinnitus is derived from the Latin word *tinnire* meaning "to ring."
- Subjective tinnitus: Heard only by the patient
- Objective tinnitus: Heard through a stethoscope placed near the patient's ear
- Tinnitus for >6 months is considered chronic.

EPIDEMIOLOGY
Prevalence
- Predominant age: 40–70 years (prevalence increases with age)
- Predominant sex: Males > Females
- 16% of the US population >65 years of age have chronic tinnitus.
- Rare in children with normal hearing; occurs in 33–64% of children who have severe hearing loss.

ETIOLOGY AND PATHOPHYSIOLOGY
- Moderate sounds cause tiny movements of the stereocilia, which are attached to hair cells in the cochlea. This triggers neuronal transmission in CN VIII. Loud sounds (≥85 dB) cause the stereocilia to bend more than they should. Hair cells that respond to higher frequency sounds are located at the base of the cochlea and are the 1st to be damaged. This causes high-pitched ringing. If loud noise exposure is excessive, then stereocilia cannot recover and permanent damage occurs. This results in hearing loss and possibly tinnitus.
- Subjective tinnitus (My AAA NOISE PAIN):
  – Medications and heavy metals that cause or exacerbate tinnitus: Aspirin, aminoglycosides, benzodiazepines, calcium channel blockers, chloroquine, cisplatin, erythromycin, fluoroquinolones, lead, lidocaine, loop diuretics, mercury, methotrexate, NSAIDs, proton pump inhibitors, quinine, sertraline, tetracycline, tricyclic antidepressants, valproate, vancomycin
  – Ménière disease
  – Aging-related hearing loss (presbycusis)
  – Anemia
  – Arterial problems (hypertension [HTN], cerebral aneurysm, cerebrovascular accident)
  – Noise (chronic exposure to loud noise/acoustic trauma due to acute exposure to very loud noise)
  – Otosclerosis and osteogenesis imperfecta
  – Infections (otitis, meningitis, Lyme disease, neurosyphillis, rubella) or impaction (cerumen)
  – Sclerosis (multiple sclerosis)
  – Endocrine (diabetes mellitus [DM], thyroid)
  – Psychogenic (depression, anxiety, psychosis)
  – Autoimmune disease of inner ear
  – Injury (head and neck) and idiopathic
  – Neoplasms (acoustic neuroma/cholesteatoma)
- Objective tinnitus (<1% of all cases of tinnitus; CAGED PETS):
  – Vascular abnormalities:
    ○ Carotid stenosis/CAD
    ○ Arteriovenous shunt/fistula
    ○ Glomus jugulare
    ○ Existing stapedial artery
    ○ Dehiscent jugular bulb/a vascular loop

- Mechanical abnormalities:
  ○ Palatal myoclonus
  ○ Eustachian tube abnormally patent
  ○ TMJ disorder
  ○ Stapedial muscle spasticity

Genetics
Possibly a genetic predisposition, but a tinnitus gene has not yet been discovered. Genes have been identified for temporomandibular joint (TMJ) dysfunction, Ménière disease, and acoustic neuroma.

RISK FACTORS
- Advanced age
- Pregnancy
- Excessive noise exposure
- Hearing loss
- Use of ototoxic medications
- Renal/Hepatic impairment
- White

GENERAL PREVENTION
Avoid prolonged exposure to loud noises, wear hearing protection when loud noises cannot be avoided (e.g., lawn mower, power tools), and avoid overuse of ototoxic medications. Even occasional exposure to loud sounds can cause irreversible damage to the hair cells of the auditory nerve fibers and cochlea resulting in hearing loss and tinnitus (1).

COMMONLY ASSOCIATED CONDITIONS
- Hearing loss (~90% of chronic tinnitus is associated with sensorineural hearing loss):
  – Causes of sensorineural hearing loss: Loud noise, presbycusis, ototoxic medications, Ménière disease, acoustic neuroma
  – Causes of conductive hearing loss: Cerumen, ear infection/effusion, trauma, tumor
- TMJ dysfunction
- Depression, anxiety, insomnia, fibromyalgia (40–60% of patients with tinnitus also have major depressive disorder)
- Psychological disorders can contribute to the distress of tinnitus. Some patients with severe tinnitus contemplate suicide.

DIAGNOSIS

HISTORY
- Onset and duration: Gradual (presbycusis), sudden (recent loud noise exposure)
- Location: Unilateral (cerumen impaction, otitis media), unilateral plus hearing loss (acoustic neuroma, CVA)
- Pattern: Continuous (hearing loss), episodic (Ménière disease), pulsatile (vascular)
- Pitch: Low-pitch, rumbling (Ménière disease); high-pitched (sensorineural hearing loss)
- Severity: Use 1–10 scale (10 = most severe), Visual Analog Scale, Tinnitus Severity Index, or Tinnitus Handicap Inventory.
- Exacerbated by: Fatigue, stress, noise exposure, medications
- Alleviated by: Lying down with head in dependent position, medications, masking sounds
- Sudden hearing loss in 1 ear that progresses to the other ear (autoimmune)

- Hearing loss type: Congenital, sensorineural, conductive, or mixed
- Vertigo (Ménière disease)
- Facial muscle paralysis (cholesteatoma)
- Vestibular disturbances
- Symptoms of depression/anxiety; suicidal thoughts
- Insomnia, difficulty concentrating
- Noise exposure >85 dB (traffic = 85 dB)
- Upper respiratory infection, sinusitis, ear infection, allergic rhinitis
- Otalgia
- Otorrhea
- Head trauma
- Surgery
- Family history of hearing loss/tinnitus
- Medical history/symptoms of: Hypo- or hyperthyroidism, HTN, DM, arteriosclerosis, autoimmune disorders
- Medications (prescription and OTC)
- Exposure to heavy metals (lead/mercury)
- Psychosocial history: Employment, recreational activities, insomnia, anxiety, depression, obsessive–compulsive disorder, psychosis, fibromyalgia

PHYSICAL EXAM
- Otoscopy: Otitis externa/media, cerumen
- Auscultation close to ear for objective tinnitus
- Auscultation of neck (bruits, venous hum)
- Tinnitus of venous origin is suppressed by compression of ipsilateral jugular vein.
- Examine TMJ.
- Air and bone conduction testing with 512- or 1,024-Hz tuning fork (Weber and Rinne tests)
- Neurologic exam: Romberg test, Dix-Hallpike maneuver (if patient has vertigo), gait testing, cranial nerves
- Test hearing (audiology)

DIFFERENTIAL DIAGNOSIS
Auditory hallucinations

DIAGNOSTIC TESTS & INTERPRETATION
- Audiometry
- Tympanometry
- Auditory brain stem response (retrocochlear pathology, such as acoustic neuroma)
- Electrocochleography (endolymphic hydrops)
- Electronystagmography (vestibular disorders)

Initial Tests (lab, imaging)
Lab investigation is not indicated in all patients; use clinical judgment. Consider:
- CBC
- BUN/creatinine
- Fasting glucose
- Fasting lipid profile
- Thyroid-stimulating hormone
- A full clinical evaluation should precede radiologic studies.
- Gadolinium-enhanced MRI (if tinnitus is continuous)
- Contrast-enhanced CT scan/MRI (if tinnitus is pulsatile)
- Sonography, angiography, or MRA (to asses vascular abnormalities in the neck)
- Single-photon emission CT (SPECT) may be more sensitive than CT scan, MRI, or MR angiography (MRA), and it identifies dynamic changes within the brain at the neurotransmitter level.

- Positron emission tomography (PET) scan: Increased activity in the auditory cortex suggests that transcranial magnetic stimulation may effectively treat the tinnitus.

Follow-Up Tests & Special Considerations
Consider HIV, rapid plasma reagin, autoimmune panel

 TREATMENT

GENERAL MEASURES
- Management depends on the severity of tinnitus and may require multiple treatment strategies.
- Traditional management of tinnitus includes education/counseling, stress reduction, and use of therapeutic sound.
- Treat the underlying cause.
- Discontinue ototoxic medications.
- Anxiety, insomnia, and depression may exacerbate tinnitus, which, in turn, may exacerbate the anxiety, insomnia, and/or depression. Treat to stop this vicious cycle.
- Hearing aids/cochlear implants
- Hearing protection during noise exposure
- Compression of myofascial trigger points (2)[B]

MEDICATION
New-onset tinnitus often is associated with hearing loss; steroid pulse/standard-dose therapy is indicated with idiopathic sudden sensorineural hearing loss (ISSHL).

First Line
Antidepressants (SSRIs or tricyclic antidepressant [TCAs], such as amitriptyline): If patients are depressed/anxious or have severe tinnitus; no evidence that 1 antidepressant works best. Caution: Tinnitus can be a side effect of antidepressant medications.

Second Line
- Antihistamines
- Baclofen
- Benzodiazepines
- Hyperbaric oxygen may help to improve hearing of those with early presentation of ISSHL.
- Anticonvulsants, such as gabapentin, are used occasionally, but research has shown that they do not significantly reduce tinnitus (3)[B].

ISSUES FOR REFERRAL
- Refer patients to a comprehensive tinnitus management program (audiologist).
- Neurologist/neurosurgeon, depending on etiology

ADDITIONAL THERAPIES
- Structured tinnitus-specific CBT using standardized tinnitus-specific interventions has been shown to decrease tinnitus, including loudness and annoyance factors (4)[A]. CBT has also been shown to reduce depression and improve quality of life (5)[A].
- Transcranial magnetic stimulation (TMS) and repetitive TMS: A noninvasive method to stimulate neurons in the brain by rapidly changing magnetic fields. This is effective even with patients who have long-term symptoms that are resistant to medications. It also may help treat migraine headaches, strokes, Parkinson disease, dystonia, major depression, and auditory hallucinations (6)[B].

- Acoustic therapy: Listening to relaxing sounds with headphones when the environment is too quiet.
- Biofeedback and stress reduction: Relaxation techniques may help to reduce the severity of the tinnitus.
- Neurofeedback: Many patients with tinnitus have abnormal oscillatory brain activity. Neurofeedback helps to normalize this and treat tinnitus.
- Tinnitus retraining therapy: Uses counseling and sound enrichment to help patients stop their negative reaction to tinnitus and then reduce and eventually end their perception of it (7)[B]. TRT with monaural noise generators significantly improved Tinnitus Handicap Inventory scores in severely distressed patients (8)[B].
- Sound therapy (masking): Patients wear low-level noise generators to mask the tinnitus noise; commonly used, but effectiveness is unknown; may require 1–2 years of therapy.
- Electrical stimulation of the external ear has been shown to reduce severe tinnitus (9)[B].

SURGERY/OTHER PROCEDURES
- Otosclerosis: Stapedectomy surgery with implantation of ossicular prosthesis
- Severe Ménière disease or other forms of endolymphatic hydrops that are not alleviated by medications: Installation of endolymphatic shunt, labyrinthectomy, or vestibular neurectomy
- Auditory neoplasms: Surgical resection/radiation
- Vascular pulsatile tinnitus due to atherosclerotic carotid artery disease: Carotid endarterectomy

COMPLEMENTARY AND ALTERNATIVE MEDICINE
- Zinc: In 1 small study, zinc 50 mg/d for 2 months decreased severity of subjective tinnitus.
- Botulinum toxin
- Acamprosate (a medication used to treat alcohol dependence)
- Hypnosis (10)[B]
- Acupuncture (unknown effectiveness)
- Low-power laser to mastoid bone (unknown effectiveness)
- Gingko biloba, melatonin, lecithin (all are ineffective)

IN-PATIENT CONSIDERATIONS
Admission Criteria/Initial Stabilization
Hospitalization is rarely indicated.

 ONGOING CARE

FOLLOW-UP RECOMMENDATIONS
- Audiologist: For complete evaluation and therapy; specialists as indicated
- Family physician: 1–2 months after therapy initiated and periodically thereafter

PATIENT EDUCATION
- Help patients to understand that tinnitus is not a threat to their physical health.
- American Tinnitus Association: (800) 634-8978; www.ata.org
- National Institute on Deafness and Other Communication Disorders: (800) 241-1044; www.nidcd.nih.gov
- American Academy of Otolaryngology: (703) 836-4444; www.entnet.org

PROGNOSIS
Chronic tinnitus cannot be cured because of association with irreversible sensorineural hearing loss. Focus is on managing the tinnitus and reducing severity, not curing.

REFERENCES
1. Plenkowski M, Egggermont J. Reversible long-term changes in auditory processing in mature and auditory cortex induced by passive, moderate-level sound exposure. *Ear Hear.* 2012;33(3):305–314.
2. Rocha CA, Sanchez TG. Myofascial trigger points: Another way of modulating tinnitus. *Prog Brain Res.* 2007;166:209–214.
3. Hoekstra CE, Rynja SP, van Zanten GA, et al. Anticonvulsants for tinnitus. *Cochrane Database Syst Rev.* 2011:CD007960.
4. Zenne HS, Vonthein R, Zenner B, et al. Standardized tinnitus-specific individual cognitive-behavioral therapy: A controlled outcome study with 286 tinnitus patients. *Hearing Res.* 2013; 298:117–125.
5. Martinez Devesa P, Waddell A, Perera R, et al. Cognitive behavioural therapy for tinnitus. *Cochrane Database Syst Rev.* 2007:CD005233.
6. Anders M, Dvorakova J, Rathova L, et al. Efficacy of repetitive transcranial magnetic stimulation for the treatment of refractory chronic tinnitus: A randomized, placebo controlled study. *Neuroendocrine Letters.* 2010;31(2):238–249.
7. Phillips JS, McFerran D. Tinnitus Retraining Therapy (TRT) for tinnitus. *Cochrane Database Syst Rev.* 2010:CD007330.
8. Oishi N, Shinden S, Kanzaki S, et al. Effects of tinnitus retraining therapy involving monaural noise generators. *Eur Arch Oto-Rhino-Laryngol.* 2013;270(2):443–448.
9. Mielczarek M, Konopka W, Olszewski J. The application of direct current electrical stimulation of the ear and cervical spine kinesitherapy in tinnitus treatment. *Larynx.* 2013;40(1):61–65.
10. Cope TE. Clinical hypnosis for the alleviation of tinnitus. *Int Tinnitus J.* 2008;14:135–138.

ADDITIONAL READING
Hoare DJ, Kowalkowski VL, Kang S, et al. Systematic review and meta-analyses of randomized controlled trials examining tinnitus management. *Laryngoscope.* 2011;121:1555–1564.

 CODES

ICD10
- H93.11 Tinnitus, right ear
- H93.12 Tinnitus, left ear
- H93.19 Tinnitus, unspecified ear

CLINICAL PEARLS
- Tinnitus is rare in children with normal hearing, but common in children with severe hearing loss.
- To keep tinnitus from getting worse, avoid loud noises, reduce stress, control BP, get enough sleep, decrease alcohol and caffeine, and do not smoke.
- People have different levels of tolerance to tinnitus. It may affect sleep, concentration, and emotional state. ~50% of patients with chronic tinnitus also have major depressive disorder.

TOBACCO USE AND SMOKING CESSATION

Cassandra Dorvil, MBS, DO • Felix Chang, MD

 BASICS

DESCRIPTION
- Tobacco use, mostly in the cigarette form, may be defined as any habitual use of the tobacco plant leaf and its products.
- *Smokeless tobacco* refers to tobacco products that are sniffed, sucked, or chewed.
- Nicotine sources: Cigars, pipes, waterpipes, hookahs, and cigarettes

EPIDEMIOLOGY
Incidence
- 2.4 million new smokers annually in the US (2.6% initiation rate)
- 58.8% of new smokers are <18 years of age (5.8% initiation rate for teens).

Prevalence
- 443,000 deaths annually in the US
- Cigarette smoking among adults in the US has decreased from 42.4% to 19.3% (2011 CDC)
- Highest among those aged 18–25 (40.8%)
- Adults aged > 25y/o (28.5%)
- Race: Highest among whites (22.1%) and African Americans (21.3%) and is lower among Hispanics (14.6%) and Asians (12%)
- Gender: Male > Female (21.5 vs. 17.3%)
- Inversely proportional to education level

ETIOLOGY AND PATHOPHYSIOLOGY
- Addiction due to nicotine's rapid stimulation of the brain's dopamine system (teenage brain especially susceptible)
- Atherosclerotic risk due to adrenergic stimulation, endothelial damage, carbon monoxide, and adverse effects on lipids
- Direct airway damage from cigarette tar
- Carcinogens in all tobacco products

RISK FACTORS
- Presence of a smoker in the household
- Easy access to cigarettes
- Perceived parental approval of smoking
- Comorbid stress and psychiatric disorders
- Low self-esteem/self-worth
- Poor academic performance
- Boys: High levels of aggression and rebelliousness
- Girls: Preoccupation with weight and body image

GENERAL PREVENTION
- Most 1st-time tobacco use occurs before high school graduation, so educational interventions should target students in grade and middle schools and must address health consequences and psychosocial aspects of smoking (1)[A].
- The AAFP's Tar Wars program has targeted 4th and 5th graders successfully.
- Other helpful measures include:
  – Smoking bans in public areas and workplaces
  – Restriction of minors' access to tobacco
  – Restrictions on tobacco advertisements
  – Raising prices through taxation
  – Media literacy education
  – Tobacco-free sports initiatives

COMMONLY ASSOCIATED CONDITIONS
- Coronary artery disease
- Cerebrovascular disease
- Peripheral vascular disease
- Abdominal aortic aneurysm (AAA)
- COPD
- Cancer of the lip, oral cavity, pharynx, larynx, lung, esophagus, stomach, pancreas, kidney, bladder, cervix, and blood
- Pneumonia
- Osteoporosis
- Periodontitis
- Alcohol use
- Depression and anxiety
- Reduced fertility

Pregnancy Considerations
- Women who smoke or are exposed to 2nd-hand smoke during pregnancy have increased risks of miscarriage, placenta previa, placental abruption, premature rupture of membranes, preterm delivery, low-birth-weight infants, and stillbirth.

Pediatric Considerations
- 2nd-hand smoke increases the risk of the following in infants and children (2)[A]:
  – Sudden infant death syndrome
  – Acute upper and lower respiratory tract infections
  – More frequent and more severe exacerbations of asthma
  – Otitis media and need for tympanostomies
- Nicotine passes through breast milk, and its effects on the growth and development of nursing infants are unknown.

 DIAGNOSIS

HISTORY
- Ask about tobacco use and 2nd-hand smoke exposure at every physician encounter.
- Type and quantity of tobacco used
- Pack years = packs/day × years
- Awareness of health risks
- Assess interest in quitting.
- Identify triggers for smoking.
- Prior attempts to quit: Method, duration of success, reason for relapse

PHYSICAL EXAM
- General: Tobacco smoke odor
- Skin: Premature face wrinkling
- Mouth: Nicotine-stained teeth; inspect for suspicious mucosal lesions
- Lungs: Crackles, wheezing, increased or decreased volume
- Vessels: Carotid or abdominal bruits, abdominal aortic enlargement, peripheral pulses, stigmata of peripheral vascular disease

DIAGNOSTIC TESTS & INTERPRETATION
- CXR for patients with pulmonary symptoms or signs of cancer but not for screening
- The USPSTF recommends 1-time screening US for AAA in men ≥65 who ever smoked (number needed to screen to prevent 1 AAA = 500)

Diagnostic Procedures/Other
PFTs for smokers with chronic pulmonary symptoms, such as wheezing and dyspnea

 TREATMENT

Both behavioral counseling and pharmacotherapy benefit patients who are trying to quit smoking especially when use in combination (3)[A].

ALERT
Provider recommending smoking cessation at *every clinical visit* improves cessation rates (4)[A].Nonpharmacologic approaches are appropriate for pregnant women and patients who smoke <10 cigarettes/day.

GENERAL MEASURES
- Behavioral Counseling includes the 5 As of promoting smoking cessation:
  – Ask about tobacco use at every office visit.
  – Advise all smokers to quit.
  – Assess the patient's willingness to quit.
  – Assist the patient in his or her attempt to quit.
  – Arrange follow-up.
- Patients ready to quit smoking should set a quit date within the next 2 weeks. No difference in success rates between patients who taper prior to their quit date and those who stop abruptly.
- It might help for patients to have a quitting partner, such as a spouse, friend, or coworker, to provide mutual encouragement.
- Patients desiring to quit should dispose of all smoking paraphernalia (such as lighters) on their quit dates to make relapse more difficult.
- Patients must anticipate and avoid social/environmental triggers for smoking and should have a plan for dealing with the urge to smoke.

MEDICATION
First Line
- Varenicline (Chantix): 0.5 mg/d PO × 3 days, then 0.5 mg b.i.d. × 4 days, then 1 mg b.i.d. for 11 weeks (5,6)[A]:
  – Start 1–4 weeks prior to smoking cessation and continue for 12–24 weeks
  – Superior to placebo and to bupropion; number needed to treat = 7
  – S/E: Nausea, insomnia, headache, depression, suicidal ideation; safety not established in adolescents or patients with psychiatric or cardiovascular disease; pregnancy Category C

- Bupropion SR (Zyban): 150 mg PO × 3 days, then 150 mg b.i.d. (7,8)[A]:
  - Start 1 week prior to smoking cessation, and continue for 7–12 weeks
  - Twice as effective as placebo
  - Drug of choice for patients with depression or schizophrenia
  - S/E: Tachycardia, headache, nausea, insomnia, dry mouth; contraindicated in patients who have seizure disorders or bipolar affective disorder; pregnancy Category C
- Nicotine replacement therapy (e.g., patch, gum, lozenge, inhaler, nasal spray) (4)[A]:
  - Improves quit rates by 50–70% vs. placebo
  - Over-the-counter
  - Patch (NicoDerm CQ 21, 14, and 7 mg):
    - 1 patch q24h
    - Start with 21 mg if smoking ≥10 cigarettes/d; otherwise, start with 14 mg.
    - 6 weeks on initial dose, then taper
    - 2 weeks each on subsequent doses
    - No proven benefit beyond 8 weeks
  - Gum (Nicorette, 2 and 4 mg):
    - Use 4 mg if smoking ≥25 cigarettes/d.
    - Chew 1 piece q1–2h × 6 weeks, then 1 q2–4h × 3 weeks, then 1 q4–8h × 3 weeks.
  - May use in combination with bupropion, monitor for hypertension
  - S/E: Headache, pharyngitis, cough, rhinitis, dyspepsia; all mainly with inhaler and spray forms
  - Pregnancy Category D

Second Line
- Nortriptyline: 25–75 mg/d PO or in divided doses (7)[A]:
  - Start 10–14 days prior to smoking cessation and continue for at least 12 weeks.
  - Efficacy similar to bupropion, but side effects more common; pregnancy Category D
- Clonidine: 0.1 mg PO b.i.d. or 0.1 mg/d transdermal patch weekly (7)[A]:
  - Side effects: Hypotension, bradycardia, depression, fatigue; pregnancy Category C

ADDITIONAL THERAPIES
The following interventions have been shown to be effective in helping patients quit smoking:
- Advice from nurses, especially in hospital
- Individual counseling/group therapy
- Telephone counseling/Web-based cessation programs
- Exercise
- Electronic cigarettes are a type of nicotine delivery system; insufficient data on safety/effectiveness.

COMPLEMENTARY AND ALTERNATIVE MEDICINE
Acupuncture, aversive therapy, and hypnosis have not been proven to enhance long-term smoking cessation (9)[A].

ONGOING CARE

FOLLOW-UP RECOMMENDATIONS
- Follow-up 3–7 days after scheduled quit date and at least monthly for 3 months thereafter.
- Telephone follow-up if office visits not feasible
- Refraining from tobacco products for first 2 weeks is critical to long-term abstinence.
- Encourage patients who relapse to try again. Most smokers experience ≥1 failed attempts before quitting permanently. Reinforce behavioral interventions.

Patient Monitoring
- Short-term withdrawal symptoms include dysphoria, depressed mood, irritability, anxiety, insomnia, increased appetite, and poor concentration.
- Longer-term risks of smoking cessation include weight gain (4–5 kg on average) and depression.
- Quitting also is associated with exacerbations of ulcerative colitis and worsening of cognitive function in patients with schizophrenia.

DIET
Healthy eating for limiting weight gain following smoking cessation.

PATIENT EDUCATION
1-800-QUIT-NOW: Free counseling, resources, and support for quitting

PROGNOSIS
- Measurable cardiovascular benefits of smoking cessation begin as early as 24 hours after quitting and continue to mount until the risk is reduced to that of nonsmokers by 5–15 years.
- People who quit smoking after a heart attack or cardiac surgery reduce their risk of death by 1/3.
- Relapse rates initially >60% but decrease to 2–4% per year after completing 2 years of abstinence.

COMPLICATIONS
- Disability and premature death due to heart attack, stroke, cancer, COPD
- Smoking more than doubles the risk of coronary artery disease and doubles the risk of stroke.
- Smokers are 12–22× more likely than nonsmokers to die from lung cancer.

REFERENCES
1. Substance Abuse and Mental Health Services Administration, *Results from the 2010 National Survey on Drug Use and Health: Summary of National Findings*, NSDUH Series H-41, HHS Publication No. (SMA) 11-4658. Rockville, MD: Substance Abuse and Mental Health Services Administration, 2011. Accessed 7/4/2012 at http://www.samhsa.gov/data/NSDUH.aspx.
2. Jones LL, Hashim A, McKeever T, et al. Parental and household smoking and the increased risk of bronchitis, bronchiolitis and other lower respiratory infections in infancy: Systematic review and meta-analysis. *Respir Res*. 2011;12:5.
3. Stead LF, Lancaster T. Combined pharmacotherapy and behavioural interventions for smoking cessation. *Cochrane Database Syst Rev*. 2012;10:CD008286.
4. Larzelere MM, Williams DE. Promoting smoking cessation. *Am Fam Physician*. 2012;85:591–598.
5. Cahill K, Stead LF, Lancaster T. Nicotine receptor partial agonists for smoking cessation. *Cochrane Database Syst Rev*. 2012;4:CD006103.
6. Hajek P, McRobbie HJ, Myers KE, et al. Use of varenicline for 4 weeks before quitting smoking: Decrease in ad lib smoking and increase in smoking cessation rates. *Arch Intern Med*. 2011;171: 770–777.
7. Cahill K, Stevens S, Perera R, Lancaster T. Pharmacological interventions for smoking cessation: An overview and network meta-analysis. *Cochrane Database Syst Rev*. 2013; doi:10.1002/14651858.CD009329.pub2
8. Giersch JM, Bastian LA, Calhoun PS, et al. Smoking cessation interventions for patients with depression: A systematic review and meta-analysis. *J Gen Intern Med*. 2012;27(3):351.
9. White AR, Rampes H, Liu JP, et al. Acupuncture and related interventions for smoking cessation. *Cochrane Database Syst Rev*. 2011;1:CD000009.

ADDITIONAL READING
- Centers for Disease Control and Prevention. Current Cigarette Smoking Among Adults—United States, 2011. *MMWR*. 2012;61(44):889–994.
- De Flora S, Bartsch H. Genomic and post–genomic effects of cigarette smoke: Mechanisms and implications for risk assessment and prevention strategies. *Int J Cancer*. 2012;131: 2721–2723. doi: 10.1002/ijc.27833
- Quitnet. Available at www.quitnet.com.

SEE ALSO

Nicotine Addiction; Substance Use Disorders

CODES

ICD10
- F17.210 Nicotine dependence, cigarettes, uncomplicated
- F17.211 Nicotine dependence, cigarettes, in remission
- F17.213 Nicotine dependence, cigarettes, with withdrawal

CLINICAL PEARLS
- Quitting smoking has both immediate and long-term health benefits.
- Every patient who uses tobacco should be offered smoking cessation.
- Use the 5 A's: Ask, Advise, Assess, Assist, and Arrange
- Behavioral counseling and medication are most effective for helping patients to quit smoking when they are used in combination.
- Depression with suicidal ideations is a contraindication to use varenicline.

TORCH INFECTIONS

Erin McMaster, MD

 BASICS

DESCRIPTION

- An acronym describing a group of infections that are acquired prenatally or during the birth process and have similar physical findings, including skin and ocular manifestations:
  - *Toxoplasmosis*: Protozoan parasite, *Toxoplasma gondii* (1)
  - *Other (syphilis)*: Spirochete, *Treponema pallidum* (2)
  - *Rubella*: Virus (3)
  - *CMV*: Cytomegalovirus (4)
  - *Herpes*: Herpes simplex virus (HSV) (5,6)
- System(s) affected: Skin/Exocrine; HEENT; Nervous; Gastrointestinal; Lymphatic/Heme; Renal; Cardiac; Pulmonary
- Synonym(s): CMV infection, also known as cytomegalic inclusion disease (CID) or cytoplasmic inclusion body disease

EPIDEMIOLOGY

- Predominant age: Prenatal to infants
- Predominant sex: Male = Female

Incidence

- Toxoplasmosis: 1.1/1,000 live births
- Syphilis: 10.1/100,000 live births
- Rubella: No longer endemic in the US; rare cases seen with immigrant mothers
- CMV: 1/100 live births; defects present in 10% of infected infants
- Herpes: 1/5,000 live births

ETIOLOGY AND PATHOPHYSIOLOGY

- All infections transmitted vertically, either transplacentally or through maternal genital tract
- Toxoplasmosis: *T. gondii* protozoan results in cyst dissemination throughout tissues and host cell death.
- Syphilis: Spirochetes cause inflammatory damage to most organ systems.
- Rubella: Mechanism of damage unclear, possibly secondary to vasculitis
- CMV: Immunosuppressive virus replicates in leukocytes, secretory glands, and kidneys.
- Herpes: Virus replicates in sensory ganglion; inability to control replication results in disseminated infection:
  - Acquired vertically due to maternal infection during pregnancy

RISK FACTORS

- General: Inadequate prenatal care
- Toxoplasmosis: Effects are more severe with 1st- or 2nd-trimester infection; increased risk if mother is of southeast Asian descent or has exposure to raw meat or cat feces
- Rubella: Inadequate maternal vaccination
- CMV: Care for preschool-aged children during pregnancy; initial sexual activity <2 years prior to pregnancy; STD during pregnancy; maternal age <25 years
- Herpes: Positive HSV serology at delivery *and* vaginal delivery; invasive monitoring; initial episode of HSV; premature labor; maternal age <21 years

GENERAL PREVENTION

- Toxoplasmosis: Avoid handling of cat litter; keep cats indoors and feed them canned foods; wear rubber gloves for meat preparation and gardening.
- Syphilis: Screen with VDRL or rapid plasma reagin (RPR) test at 1st prenatal visit, confirm with fluorescent treponemal antibody absorption (FTA-ABS). Give infected, previously untreated pregnant women penicillin G IM, dose 2.4 million units once for primary, secondary, or early latent; 2.4 million units weekly every 3 weeks for late latent (7).
- Rubella: Test IgG titers to determine immunity at initial prenatal visit.
- CMV: Prenatal antibody titers to determine serologic status; avoid prolonged exposure to young children during pregnancy.
- Herpes: Insufficient evidence for antiviral prophylaxis decreasing neonatal herpes incidence, although it does decrease viral shedding, clinical lesions, and number of cesarean sections. Prophylactic treatment with acyclovir 200 mg q.i.d. or 300 mg t.i.d. starting at 36 weeks' gestation

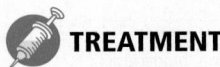 **DIAGNOSIS**

HISTORY

- Toxoplasmosis: No maternal symptoms or history of flulike syndrome
- Syphilis, rubella, and CMV: Maternal history of fever and rash
- Herpes: Infant may present with fever, change in mental status, or seizures.

PHYSICAL EXAM

- Toxoplasmosis: Growth retardation, jaundice, maculopapular rash, microcephaly, chorioretinitis, ascites, hepatosplenomegaly
- Syphilis: Most infants asymptomatic; early signs are snuffles (rhinitis), poor feeding, retinitis, jaundice and hepatosplenomegaly; rash varies from red macular to bullous; chronic infection may present with neurosyphilis (tabes dorsalis, deafness), Hutchinson incisors, mulberry molars, saddle nose deformity, or uveitis.
- Rubella: Classic triad involves sensorineural hearing loss, ocular abnormalities (cataracts, glaucoma, retinopathy), and congenital heart disease (patent ductus arteriosus [PDA]).
- CMV: Most infected infants are asymptomatic; 10% with symptoms including intrauterine growth retardation (IUGR), hepatosplenomegaly, petechiae and purpura (blueberry muffin rash), microcephaly, deafness, chorioretinitis
- Herpes: Vesicular lesions on skin, eyes or mouth, fever, irritability, focal neurologic symptoms

DIFFERENTIAL DIAGNOSIS

- Congenital lymphocytic choriomeningitis virus
- Encephalopathies
- Meningitis
- Parvovirus B19
- Bacterial sepsis
- HIV
- Varicella
- Epstein-Barr virus

DIAGNOSTIC TESTS & INTERPRETATION

Initial Tests (lab, imaging)

- Toxoplasmosis: Newborn serum testing of IgM and IgA antibodies; may also test maternal blood prenatally
- Syphilis: Newborn screen with VDRL or RPR test, confirm with FTA-ABS; CBC with differential and LFTs; CSF for VDRL, cell count, and protein
- Rubella: Viral isolation by polymerase chain reaction (PCR) preferred over serologic testing
- CMV: DNA PCR or viral culture from urine or saliva (8,9)
- Herpes: HSV culture of vesicle, conjunctiva, oropharynx or blood; CSF PCR
- Toxoplasmosis: US at 20–24 weeks' gestation to evaluate for hydrocephalus
- Syphilis: Chest x-ray (CXR) (pneumonia alba); long-bone x-ray (onion-skinning, rat bite tibia)
- CMV: Head CT (periventricular calcifications)
- Herpes: Head CT or MRI if concern for encephalitis (temporal lobe abnormalities)

Follow-Up Tests & Special Considerations

- Toxoplasmosis: Head CT (ring-enhancing lesions)
- Rubella: Echocardiography to diagnose heart defects; head CT may show intracranial calcifications

Diagnostic Procedures/Other

- Rubella and CMV: Ophthalmic and audiology evaluation (10)
- Herpes: Ophthalmic exam

Test Interpretation

- Toxoplasmosis: Tissue with tachyzoites definitive for active infection
- CMV: Presence of inclusion giant cells
- Herpes: Multinucleate giant cells

TREATMENT

GENERAL MEASURES

- Nutritional and respiratory support
- Phototherapy for hyperbilirubinemia

MEDICATION

First Line

- Toxoplasmosis: Pyrimethamine (1 mg/kg/d PO daily for 6 months, then Monday, Wednesday, Friday for 6 months; max 25 mg/d) and sulfadiazine (100 mg/kg/d PO q12h) for 12 months in both symptomatic and asymptomatic infants. Folinic acid (5–10 mg 3×/wk) to reduce hematologic toxicity.
- Syphilis: Aqueous crystalline penicillin G 50,000 U/kg IV q12h for 7 days, then q8h for total treatment of 10 days. Desensitize patient if penicillin allergic.
- Rubella: No specific antiviral agent indicated
- CMV: Ganciclovir may be useful for acutely ill infants.
- Herpes: Insufficient evidence to evaluate antiviral use in neonates; recommended treatment is acyclovir 20 mg/kg IV q8h for 14–21 days.

Second Line
- Toxoplasmosis: Clindamycin if sulfadiazine is not tolerated; corticosteroids for ocular and CNS complications
- Syphilis: Procaine penicillin G 50,000 U/kg IM daily for 10 days

ISSUES FOR REFERRAL
Consider consultation based on organ systems involved (ophthalmology, cardiology, neurology, orthopedics).

SURGERY/OTHER PROCEDURES
- Possibility of gastrostomy placement based on nutritional needs
- Rubella: Repair of congenital heart defects

IN-PATIENT CONSIDERATIONS
Admission Criteria/Initial Stabilization
Infected neonates to remain inpatient from birth; respiratory support

IV Fluids
Indicated if oral feeding is inadequate; determined by weight-based calculations

Discharge Criteria
Once stable and treatment is completed or arranged on outpatient basis; infants infected with rubella must remain hospitalized in isolation until 2 cultures taken 1 month apart are negative.

ONGOING CARE

FOLLOW-UP RECOMMENDATIONS
Patient Monitoring
- Continue to follow neurologic and developmental status.
- Toxoplasmosis: Follow up every 2 weeks until stable, then monthly while being treated; CBC every week for 1 month, then every 2 weeks
- Syphilis: Serologic testing every 2–3 months until nonreactive or 4-fold titer decrease. If CSF is abnormal, repeat LP every 6 months until normal.
- Rubella: Vision and hearing screens

DIET
Normal diet, as tolerated

PATIENT EDUCATION
- An infected mother should be informed of potential harm to the fetus.
- Pregnant women should avoid contact with those infected with rubella.

PROGNOSIS
- Toxoplasmosis: Development and behavior normal with adequate treatment; chorioretinitis in 26% of treated infants (1)
- Syphilis: 6.4% mortality rate
- Rubella: Poor outcome with significant organ damage
- CMV: Normal development if 12-month exam within normal limits; chorioretinitis untreatable
- Herpes: 30% mortality of treated disseminated disease; good outcome with treated mucocutaneous infections

COMPLICATIONS
- Toxoplasmosis: Meningoencephalitis with hydrocephalus, seizure disorder, vision impairment, deafness, mental retardation
- Syphilis: Pneumonia alba, stillbirth, multiple-organ damage
- Rubella: Deafness, vision impairment, skeletal defects, congenital heart defects
- CMV: Hearing loss, chorioretinitis, thrombocytopenia
- Herpes: Seizures, pneumonia, adrenal involvement, respiratory distress, liver dysfunction, eczema herpeticum

REFERENCES

1. McLeod R, Boyer K, Karrison T, et al. Outcome of treatment for congenital toxoplasmosis, 1981–2004: The National Collaborative Chicago-Based, Congenital Toxoplasmosis Study. Clin Infect Dis. 2006;42:1383–1394.
2. French P. Syphilis. BMJ. 2007;334:143–147.
3. Control and prevention of rubella: Evaluation and management of suspected outbreaks, rubella in pregnant women, and surveillance for congenital rubella syndrome. MMWR Recomm Rep. 2001;50:1–23.
4. ACOG practice bulletin. Perinatal viral and parasitic infections. Number 20, September 2000. (Replaces educational bulletin number 177, February 1993). American College of Obstetrics and Gynecologists. Int J Gynaecol Obstet. 2002;76(1):95–107.
5. Anzivino E, Fioriti D, Mischitelli M, et al. Herpes simplex virus infection in pregnancy and in neonate: Status of art of epidemiology, diagnosis, therapy and prevention. Virol J. 2009;6:40.
6. Corey L, Wald A. Maternal and neonatal herpes simplex virus infections. N Engl J Med. 2009; 361:1376–1385.
7. Workowski KA, Berman S, Centers for Disease Control and Prevention (CDC). Sexually transmitted diseases treatment guidelines, 2010. MMWR Recomm Rep. 2010;59(RR-12):1–110.
8. de Vries JJ, van der Eijk AA, Wolthers KC, et al. Real-time PCR versus viral culture on urine as a gold standard in the diagnosis of congenital cytomegalovirus infection. J Clin Virol. 2012;53(2):167–170. Epub 2011 Dec 15.
9. Boppana SB, Ross SA, et al. Saliva polymerase-chain-reaction assay for cytomegalovirus screening in newborns. N Engl J Med. 2011; 364(22):2111–2118.
10. Kadambari S, Williams EJ, Luck S, et al. Evidence based management guidelines for the detection and treatment of congenital CMV. Early Hum Dev. 2011;87(11):723–728. Epub 2011 Sep 29.

CODES

ICD10
- P00.2 Newborn affected by maternal infec/parastc diseases
- P35.1 Congenital cytomegalovirus infection
- P37.1 Congenital toxoplasmosis

CLINICAL PEARLS
- Adequate prenatal care is paramount for prevention of TORCH infections.
- Initial workup includes thorough maternal history and indicated lab tests (CBC, antibodies, viral culture).
- Infants with altered mental status need brain imaging to evaluate for intracranial lesions, hydrocephalus, or other abnormalities.
- After treatment, infants should be regularly monitored for potential sequelae.

TORTICOLLIS

Bryan C. Bordeaux, DO, MPH • Tisamarie B. Sherry, PhD

 BASICS

DESCRIPTION
- Torticollis is a spectrum of disorders characterized by head tilt with rotation or involuntary movement.
- Pediatric disorders include:
  - Congenital muscular torticollis (CMT): 80% of all infants presenting with torticollis are found to have CMT. CMT is seen at birth or early infancy and results from unilateral fibrosis and shortening of the sternocleidomastoid (SCM) muscle.
  - Acquired torticollis
- Adult disorders include:
  - Acquired torticollis (also known as wryneck), which is usually self-limited
  - Spasmodic torticollis, also known as cervical dystonia, is caused by recurrent involuntary muscular contractions.
- Other forms (oculogyric, gastroesophageal reflux, arthritis-related, scoliosis-related, and hysterical torticollis) are not discussed.
- System(s) affected: Musculoskeletal; Nervous.
- Synonym(s): Acute wryneck; Idiopathic generalized torticollis; SCM torticollis; Neonatal torticollis; Idiopathic cervical dystonia; Focal dystonia; Nuchal dystonia.

EPIDEMIOLOGY
- ~90% of cases occur in individuals aged 31–60.
- Predominant age: CMT: Newborn and infants; pediatric acquired torticollis, <10 years; adult acquired torticollis, 30–60 years; spasmodic torticollis, 30–50 years (mean age 40–43) (1)
- Predominant sex: Spasmodic torticollis, Female > Male (1.6:1); CMT, Male > Female (3:2) (2)

Incidence
Congenital: Up to 1/250 births (2); spasmodic, estimated at 1/100,000; overall incidence for torticollis is 24/1 million persons.

Prevalence
All focal dystonias combined: 295/1 million persons; no reliable data for acquired torticollis

ETIOLOGY AND PATHOPHYSIOLOGY
- CMT:
  - Intrauterine malpositioning may lead to trauma of the SCM and fibrosis.
  - Birth trauma, such as a clavicular fracture
- Pediatric acquired torticollis:
  - CNS disorders, increased intracranial pressure
  - Ocular disorders
  - Bony abnormalities, soft tissue pathologies
  - Gastrointestinal disease
  - Drug-induced
  - Conversion disorder
    - Adult acquired torticollis:
  - Emotional stress, postural factors (e.g., work, sleep, lying while reading or watching TV, prolonged unusual positioning of neck), or exposure to cold; many cases are idiopathic
  - Medication reactions (e.g., amphetamines, haloperidol, chlorpromazine, ketamine)
- Spasmodic torticollis:
  - Muscular damage from inflammatory or infectious diseases
  - Cervical spine injuries and spondylosis
  - Ocular disorders
  - Organic CNS disorders

- Psychogenic
- Tumors
- Vestibular dysfunction

Genetics
Some forms may have a genetic basis, such as spasmodic torticollis (1).

RISK FACTORS
- CMT: Intrauterine crowding, breech position, ischemia, birth injury
- Pediatric acquired torticollis: Soft-tissue inflammation or infection, neurologic conditions, visual disturbances, trauma
- Adult acquired torticollis: Stress, unusual positioning (particularly when sleeping), exposure to cold drafts of air, medications, trauma, infection
- Spasmodic: Family history of dystonia, soft-tissue inflammation or infection, neurologic conditions, visual disturbances, trauma

Pediatric Considerations
Congenital: Associated with birth injury that, without treatment, becomes a fibrous cord and may be associated with persistent craniofacial deformities.

COMMONLY ASSOCIATED CONDITIONS
- >80% of infants with CMT also present with craniofacial asymmetry, deformational plagiocephaly of varying degrees, and developmental hip dysplasia.
- Congenital and pediatric acquired torticollis: Consider Klippel-Feil syndrome (congenital fusion of cervical vertebrae).
- Pediatric and adult acquired torticollis: Spinal abnormalities, tumors
- Spasmodic torticollis: Psychiatric disorders

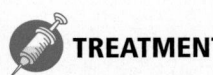 **DIAGNOSIS**

HISTORY
- Abnormal head posture, neck pain, headache, neck muscle stiffness, restricted neck range of motion (ROM), neck mass or swelling
- Birth history in children
- Family history focusing on dystonias
- Medication history
- Recent cervical spine trauma

PHYSICAL EXAM
- Normal ROM: Flexion 60°; extension 75°; rotation 90°; sidebending 45°
- Can present in rotational (twisting), anterocollis (flexion), laterocollis (side bending), and retrocollis (extension) positions with the head tilting to the affected side (80%, to right side) and the chin rotating to the opposite side
- Intermittent painful spasms of trapezius, SCM, and other neck muscles
- There may be tenderness over affected SCM.
- Neck mass, lymphadenopathy in some cases
- Craniofacial asymmetry (plagiocephaly) indicates congenital or chronic torticollis.
- Phasic jerking or tremor of antagonist muscles
- Sensory tricks (*geste antagoniste*), such as touching face, reduce severity in most patients (pathognomonic for spasmodic torticollis) (1,3).
- Ocular irregularities such as diplopia
- Spinal abnormality: Short neck with low posterior hairline may indicate occipitocervical synostosis.
- Structural abnormalities of the hips or feet

- Common presentations:
  - CMT: At birth, there may be firm, nontender, palpable enlargement of the SCM (2). However, the SCM may appear normal at birth, with swelling and tightness developing weeks later.
  - Pediatric and adult acquired torticollis: Unilateral neck stiffness, pain, spasm, or decreased ROM without trauma
  - Spasmodic torticollis may initially present with neck stiffness progressing to pain, head jerking, and neck spasms (1).

DIFFERENTIAL DIAGNOSIS
- Osseous:
  - Atlantoaxial rotatory subluxation
  - Atlantooccipital subluxation
  - Posttraumatic fracture or dislocation
  - Cervical disc disease
  - Congenital scoliosis
  - Klippel-Feil syndrome
  - Occipitocervical synostosis
  - Grisel syndrome (subluxation of C1 on C2, associated with head or neck infection)
  - Syringomyelia
  - Arnold-Chiari malformation
- Nonosseous:
  - Myositis involving cervical muscles
  - Soft-tissue trauma
  - Neoplastic: Spinal cord tumor, acoustic neuroma, osteoblastoma, orbital tumor, fibromatosis, metastasis
  - Infection: Upper respiratory infection, cervical lymph node abscess, epidural abscess, retropharyngeal abscess, vertebral osteomyelitis
  - Vestibular disorders
  - Essential head tremor
  - Basal ganglion diseases
  - Cranial nerve palsy
  - Psychiatric disorders
  - Drugs or toxins
  - Down syndrome
  - Sandifer syndrome (association of gastroesophageal disease with spastic torticollis and dystonic body movements)
  - Myasthenia gravis

DIAGNOSTIC TESTS & INTERPRETATION
Lab studies are generally not helpful and are only needed to evaluate an underlying primary cause.
- Radiographs should be taken to rule out spinal pathology in traumatic and congenital cases.
- Consider MRI or CT scan of cervical spine for patients with neurologic deficits.
- CMT can be confirmed with US of involved SCM.

Follow-Up Tests & Special Considerations
All pediatric patients should have a eye exam.

Diagnostic Procedures/Other
For pediatric-acquired torticollis, response to low-dose levodopa (100–300 mg) with carbidopa suggests that torticollis is secondary to a dopa-responsive dystonia.

TREATMENT

GENERAL MEASURES
- CMT:
  - >90% of children achieve good outcome with conservative treatment when therapy is initiated in first 12 months of life.

- Conservative treatment for CMT includes positioning, environmental adaptations, passive and active stretching of the tight SCM muscle, strengthening of weak neck and trunk muscles, and movement therapy.
- Physical therapy and aggressive stretching should be started before ages 3–6 months (2)[B].
- Place toys on opposite side of bed from rotational deformity to encourage use of affected muscles.
- Surgery is indicated for refractory cases, a tight muscular band or SCM mass.
- Pediatric acquired torticollis:
  - Place a television on opposite side of bed from rotational deformity.
- Adult and pediatric acquired torticollis:
  - Conservative management includes soft cervical collar, intermittent heat or ice, and bed rest.
  - Analgesics are helpful for pain relief.
- Spasmodic:
  - Conservative: Soft cervical collar, intermittent heat or ice, and bed rest.
  - Selective peripheral nerve denervation is a safe procedure with minimal side effects; it is indicated for cervical dystonia.
  - Pallidal deep brain stimulation can achieve lasting improvements in medication-resistant cases of cervical dystonia (4)[B].

MEDICATION

First Line

- Treatment for spasms:
  - Botulinum toxin: Type A and B injections may be more effective than anticholinergic drugs for cervical dystonia (1)[B],(5)[A]. EMG (6)[A] or PET-CT (7)[B] may help guide the injection site Immunoresistance can develop but is rare (8)[A].
    - Congenital muscular: Botulinum toxin type A was found effective in a case series (2,9)[C].
    - Cervical dystonia: Botulinum toxin type A was found effective and safe for treating adults (≥16) with cervical dystonia (1)[B].
  - Botox: Botulinum toxin type A: Adult: Initial 1.25–2.5 units (0.05–0.1 mL) IM into most active neck muscles; repeat every 3–4 months; not to exceed 200 units cumulative dose in 1-month period.
    - Pediatric (<12 years of age): Not established; >12 years, administer as for adults
  - Myobloc: Botulinum toxin type B:
    - Adult: 2,500–5,000 units IM divided among affected muscles in patients treated previously with any type of botulinum toxin; use lower dose in untreated patients.
    - Pediatric: Not established
  - Diazepam:
    - Adult: 2–10 mg PO 2b.i.d./q.i.d.
    - Pediatric: 1–2.5 mg PO t.i.d./q.i.d.; increase gradually as needed or tolerated
  - Diphendydramine or diazepam can be used for torticollis caused by medications (1)[C]:
    - Diphendydramine:
      - Adult: 25–50 mg PO q6–8h PRN, not to exceed 400 mg/d; 10–50 mg IV/IM q6–8h PRN, not to exceed 400 mg/d
      - Pediatric: 12.5–25 mg PO t.i.d./q.i.d. or 5 mg/kg/d or 150 mg/m^2/d divided t.i.d./ q.i.d. PRN, not to exceed 300 mg/d; 5 mg/kg/d IV/IM or 150 mg/m^2/d, divided q.i.d. PRN, not to exceed 300 mg/d
  - Anticholinergics may relieve acute muscle spasms (1)[C]. High doses are usually necessary, and benefit is often delayed by several weeks.

- Carbidopa-levodopa (1)[C] for focal dystonia of unknown cause: Trial might be warranted although some non–dopa-responsive dystonias improve, equal numbers have symptoms worsen.
- Treatment for pain:
  - Analgesics are useful for acquired torticollis and may be helpful in other cases. Consider NSAIDs and acetaminophen for most cases and opiates for only the most severe pain.

ISSUES FOR REFERRAL

- Refer prolonged symptoms of idiopathic spasmodic torticollis to a neurologist.
- Fixed deformities in children may require surgical.
- CMT: Refer if visual dysfunction (ophthalmology), failed hip screen (orthopedics), abnormal neurologic exam (neurology), patient has plagiocephaly (plastic surgery), patient presents with bony prominence (orthopedics) (10,11).

ADDITIONAL THERAPIES

- Osteopathic manipulation may be useful, including the following techniques:
  - Direct myofascial stretching of cervical region with attention to the SCM
  - Occipital-atlantal release
  - V-spread of the occipitomastoid suture on the side of restriction
  - Muscle energy and/or functional positional release at the cervical region
- Physical therapy may be beneficial for acquired childhood and adult torticollis (12)[B].
- If detected early, 90% of CMT responds to stretching exercises.

SURGERY/OTHER PROCEDURES

CMT: Surgical release if physical therapy is unsuccessful by 1 year of age.

COMPLEMENTARY AND ALTERNATIVE MEDICINE

Acupuncture may also provide benefit.

 ONGOING CARE

FOLLOW-UP RECOMMENDATIONS

- Monitor infants with CMT every 2–4 weeks.
- Screen for depression, since this is a common complication in protracted cases.

PROGNOSIS

- CMT: Good for correctable pathologies:
  - 50–70% resolve spontaneously by 1st year
  - >90% of children achieve good to excellent outcome with conservative treatment when therapy is instituted during the first 12 months of life.
- Pediatric acquired torticollis: Good when the underlying pathology is discovered
- Adult acquired torticollis: Excellent; generally resolves in a few days to weeks
- Spasmodic: May wax and wane for years, even with treatment

COMPLICATIONS

- Facial asymmetry in congenital cases; possibly an increased risk of developmental delay/disorders
- Dental malocclusion
- Degenerative osteoarthritis of the cervical spine, hypertrophy of the SCM muscle, and paresthesia due to compressed nerve roots
- Depression

REFERENCES

1. Tarsy D, Simon DK. Dystonia. *N Engl J Med*. 2006;355:818–829.
2. Do TT. Congenital muscular torticollis: Current concepts and review of treatment. *Curr Opin Pediatr*. 2006;18:26–29.
3. Walsh RA, Sidiropoulos C, Lozano AM, et al. Bilateral pallidal stimulation in cervical dystonia: Blinded evidence of benefit beyond 5 years. *Brain*. 2013;136:761–769.
4. Patel S, Martino D. Cervical dystonia: From pathophysiology to pharmacotherapy. *Behav Neurol*. 2012 May 24. Epub 2012 May 24.
5. Nijmeijer SW, Koelman JH, Kamphuis DJ, et al. Muscle selection for treatment of cervical dystonia with botulinum toxin: A systematic review. *Parkinsonism Relat Disord*. 2012;18(6):731–736. Epub 2012 May 8.
6. Lee HB, Young-Sil A, Lee HY et al. Usefulness of ^{18}f-fluorodeoxyglucose positron emission tomography/computed tomography in management of cervical dystonia. *Ann Rehabil Med*. 2012;36:745–755.
7. Coleman C, Hubble J, Schwab J, et al. Immunoresistance in cervical dystonia patients after treatment with botulinum toxin A. *Int J Neurosci*. 2012;122:358–362.
8. Benecke R, Dressler D. Botulinum toxin treatment of axial and cervical dystonia. *Disabil Rehabil*. 2007;29:1769–1777.
9. Lee IJ, Lim SY, Song HS, et al. Complete tight fibrous band release and resection in congenital muscular torticollis. *J Plast Reconstr Aesthet Surg*. 2010;63:947–953.
10. van Vlimmeren LA, Helders PJ, van Adrichem LN, et al. Torticollis and plagiocephaly in infancy: Therapeutic strategies. *Pediatr Rehabil*. 2006;9:40–46.
11. Ribeiro Queiroz MA, Chien HF, Sekeff-Salem FA, et al. Physical therapy program for cervical dystonia: A study of 20 cases. *Funct Neurol*. 2012;27:187–192.
12. Tomczak KK, Rosman NP. Torticollis. *J Child Neurol* 2013;28:365–378.

 CODES

ICD10

- G24.3 Spasmodic torticollis
- M43.6 Torticollis
- Q68.0 Congenital deformity of sternocleidomastoid muscle

CLINICAL PEARLS

- Suspect torticollis in patients with head tilt, chin lift, and restricted movement of the neck.
- Be vigilant for secondary causes in both children and adults.
- Most adult cases of torticollis are self-limiting and resolve within days to weeks.
- In congenital and acquired pediatric cases, rearranging the child's environment by placing items of interest (e.g., TV, toys) on the opposite side of the bed is often beneficial.

TOURETTE SYNDROME
Evan R. Horton, PharmD • Brendan Kelly, MD

BASICS

DESCRIPTION
- A childhood-onset neurobehavioral disorder characterized by the presence of multiple motor and at least 1 phonic tic (see "Physical Exam"):
  - Tics are sudden, brief, repetitive, stereotyped motor movements (motor tics) or sounds (phonic tics) produced by moving air through the nose, mouth, or throat.
  - Tics tend to occur in bouts.
  - Tics can be simple or complex:
    - Motor tics precede vocal tics.
    - Simple tics precede complex tics.
  - Tics often are preceded by sensory symptoms, especially a compulsion to move.
  - Patients are able to suppress their tics, but voluntary suppression is associated with an inner tension that results in more forceful tics when suppression ceases.
- System(s) affected: Nervous

EPIDEMIOLOGY
Incidence
- Predominant age:
  - Average age of onset: 7 years (3–8 years).
  - Tic severity is greatest at ages 7–12 years:
    - 96% present by age 11
  - Of children with Tourette syndrome (TS), 50% will experience complete resolution of symptoms by age 18 (based on self-reporting).
- Predominant sex: Male > Female (3:1)
- Predominant race/ethnicity: Clinically heterogeneous disorder, but non-Hispanic whites 2:1 compared with Hispanics and/or blacks

Prevalence
0.77% overall in children
- 1.66% in boys
- 0.25% in girls

ETIOLOGY AND PATHOPHYSIOLOGY
Abnormalities of dopamine neurotransmission and receptor hypersensitivity, most likely in the ventral striatum, play a primary role in the pathophysiology.
- Abnormality of basal ganglia development
- Mechanism is uncertain; may involve dysfunction of basal ganglia–thalamocortical circuits, likely involving decreased inhibitory output from the basal ganglia, which results in an imbalance of inhibition and excitation in the motor cortex.
- Controversial pediatric autoimmune neuropsychiatric disorder association with *Streptococcus* (PANDAS) (1):
  - TS/OCD cases linked to immunologic response to previous group A β-hemolytic streptococcal infection (GABHS)
  - Thought to be linked to 10% of all TS cases
  - 5 criteria:
    - Presence of tic disorder and/or OCD
    - Prepubertal onset of neuropsychosis
    - History of sudden onset of symptoms and/or episodic course, with abrupt symptom exacerbation, interspersed with periods of partial/complete remission
    - Evidence of a temporal association between onset/exacerbation of symptoms and a prior streptococcal infection
    - Adventitious movements during symptom exacerbation (e.g., motor hyperactivity)

Genetics
- Predisposition: Frequent familial history of tic disorders and obsessive–compulsive disorder (OCD)
- Precise pattern of transmission and genetic origin unknown. Recent studies suggest polygenic inheritance with evidence for a locus on chromosome 17q; sequence variants in *SLITRK1* gene on chromosome 13q also are associated with TS.
- Higher concordance in monozygotic compared with dizygotic twins; wide range of phenotypes

RISK FACTORS
- Risk of TS among relatives: 9.8–15%.
- 1st-degree relatives of individuals with TS have a 10–100-fold increased risk of developing TS.

COMMONLY ASSOCIATED CONDITIONS
- ADHD and OCD are most common.
- Depression and anxiety are also concerns due to disruptive behavior problems that can lead to social difficulties and learning disorders.
- Impairments of visual perception, sleep disorders, restless leg syndrome, and migraine headaches are higher than in the general population.

DIAGNOSIS

HISTORY
Diagnosis of TS is based on history and clinical presentation (i.e., observation of tics with/without presence of coexisting disorders).

PHYSICAL EXAM
- Typically, the physical exam is normal.
- Motor and vocal tics are the clinical hallmarks.
- Tics fluctuate in type, frequency, and anatomic distribution over time.
- Multiple motor tics include facial grimacing, blinking, head/neck jerking, tongue protruding, sniffing, and touching.
- Vocal tics include grunts, snorts, throat clearing, barking, yelling, and hiccupping.
- Tics are exacerbated by anticipation, emotional upset, anxiety, or fatigue.
- Tics subside when patient is concentrating/absorbed in activities.
- Motor and vocal tics may persist during all stages of sleep, especially light sleep.
- Blink-reflex abnormalities may be observed.
- No known clinical measures reliably predict children who will continue to express tics in adulthood; severity of tics in late childhood is associated with future tic severity.
- *Diagnostic and Statistical Manual* (DSM) criteria:
  - Both multiple motor and ≥1 vocal tics have been present at some time during the illness, although not necessarily concurrently.
  - Tics occur many times a day (usually in bouts) nearly every day or intermittently throughout a period of >1 year, with no tic-free period of >3 consecutive months.
  - Onset occurs before age 18 years.
  - Tics are not due to the direct physiologic effects of a substance (e.g., stimulants) or a general medical condition (e.g., Huntington disease or postviral encephalitis).
- The World Health Organization and Tourette Syndrome Classification Group also have classification systems.

DIFFERENTIAL DIAGNOSIS
- Chronic motor/vocal tic disorder
- Transient tic disorder
- Tic disorder not otherwise specified
- Huntington disease
- Stroke
- Lesch-Nyhan syndrome
- Wilson disease
- Sydenham chorea
- Multiple sclerosis
- Postviral encephalitis
- Head injury
- Dystonia
- Myoclonus
- Drug effects (e.g., dopamine agonists)

DIAGNOSTIC TESTS & INTERPRETATION
Initial Tests (lab, imaging)
- No definitive lab tests diagnose TS.
- Thyroid-stimulating hormone (TSH) should be measured because of association of tics with hyperthyroidism.
- No imaging studies diagnose TS.
- EEG shows nonspecific abnormalities; useful only to differentiate tics from epilepsy.

Test Interpretation
- Smaller caudate volumes in patients with TS
- Striatal dopaminergic terminals are increased, as is striatal dopamine transporter (DAT) density.

TREATMENT

GENERAL MEASURES
- Treatment assessment:
  - Yale Global Tic Severity Score
  - Tourette Syndrome Severity Scale
- Educate that tics are neither voluntary nor psychiatric.
- Many patients require no treatment; patient should play an active role in treatment decisions.
- Educate patient, family, teachers, and friends to identify and address psychosocial stressors and environmental triggers.
- No cure for tics: Treatment is purely symptomatic, and multimodal treatment usually is indicated.
- Neurologic and psychiatric evaluation may be useful for other primary disorders and comorbid conditions (especially ADHD, OCD, and depression).
- TS clusters with several comorbid conditions; each disorder must be evaluated for associated functional impairment because patients often are more disabled by their psychiatric conditions than by the tics; choice of initial treatment depends largely on worst symptoms (tics, obsessions, or impulsivity).
- Monotherapy is preferred to polytherapy.

MEDICATION
First Line
- Atypical antipsychotics
  - Risperidone (2)[A]: Now recommended for standard therapy:
    - Initiate 0.25 b.i.d.; titrate to 0.25–6.0 mg/d
    - As effective as haloperidol and pimozide for tics with fewer side effects
    - Effective against comorbidities such as OCD
    - Side effects may limit use: Sedation, weight gain, and fatigue

- α_2-Adrenergic receptor agonists (3)[B]:
  - Historically, first-line agents due to favorable side-effect profile, but suboptimal efficacy in limited clinical trials
  - Side effects: Sedation and hypotension common:
    ○ Initiate therapy gradually and taper when discontinuing to avoid cardiac adverse events.
  - Clonidine 0.1–0.3 mg/d given b.i.d. or t.i.d.:
    ○ 50–75% of subjects report little or no reduction in tics
  - Guanfacine 1–3 mg/d given daily or b.i.d.:
    ○ Less sedating and longer duration of action compared with clonidine
    ○ Improves motor/vocal tics by 30% in some studies, no better than placebo in others

Second Line
- Neuroleptics:
  - Typical antipsychotics (2)[A]:
    ○ Haloperidol 0.5–5.0 mg at bedtime:
      ■ Should be reserved for patients with severe disease due to side effects compared with other neuroleptics: Extrapyramidal symptoms (EPS)
      ■ FDA-approved for treating tics
    ○ Pimozide: Initiate 0.5 mg/d and titrate 0.5 mg/week up to 1–8 mg at bedtime (4)[A]:
      ■ Risk of cardiac toxicity (prolonged Q-T interval and arrhythmias) limits use; must be given under ECG monitoring; long-term use may induce sedation, weight gain, depression, pseudoparkinsonism, and akathisia.
      ■ Found to work better in long-term control of tics vs. acute exacerbations
      ■ FDA-approved for treating tics
    ○ Fluphenazine: 2.5–10 mg/d:
      ■ Effective, but less favored compared with atypicals due to side effects
  - Atypical antipsychotics (2)[C]:
    ○ Olanzapine: Initiate 2.5–5.0 mg/d; titrate up to 20 mg/d:
      ■ Equally effective as haloperidol and pimozide
      ■ 2nd-line due to side effects: Metabolic disturbances and weight gain
    ○ Quetiapine: Initiate 100–150 mg/d; titrate to 100–600 mg/d:
      ■ Well tolerated, but limited data exist
    ○ Ziprasidone: 5–10 mg/d:
      ■ Second-line due to increased side effects: Q-T prolongation
    ○ Aripiprazole: Initiate 2 mg/d; titrate up to 20 or 30 mg/d:
      ■ Few studies, but favorable side-effect profile
- Alternative treatments (3)[C]:
  - Tetrabenazine
  - Topiramate
  - Botulinum toxin
  - Baclofen
  - Clonazepam

- Treatment of ADHD in patients with tics (5)[A]:
  - Stimulants:
    ○ Comorbid tic disorder is not a serious contraindication, as previously held; exacerbation of tics is neither clinically significant nor common.
    ○ Methylphenidate: 2.5–30 mg/d
    ○ Dextroamphetamine: 5–30 mg/d
  - α_2-Adrenergic agonists:
    ○ Guanfacine
    ○ Clonidine
      ■ The combination of methylphenidate and clonidine has shown superior efficacy in treating both ADHD and tic symptoms compared to monotherapy with either agent in 1 trial.
  - Other medications:
    ○ Atomoxetine
    ○ Desipramine
- Treatment of OCD in patients with tics (1)[B]:
  - SSRIs:
    ○ Side effects include nausea, insomnia, sexual dysfunction, headache, and agitation.
    ○ First-line treatment of OCD
    ○ Comorbid tic disorder not a contraindication; exacerbation of tics neither clinically significant nor common
    ○ Some risk of suicidality noted with SSRIs and other antidepressants
    ○ Fluoxetine: 10–80 mg/d
    ○ Fluvoxamine: 50–300 mg/d
    ○ Sertraline: 50–200 mg/d
  - Tricyclic antidepressants:
    ○ Clomipramine: 25–200 mg/d:
      ■ Can be used in patients refractory to SSRIs or to augment SSRIs in partial responders
      ■ Side effects: Weight gain, dry mouth, lowered seizure threshold, and constipation; ECG changes, including Q-T prolongation and tachycardia

ADDITIONAL THERAPIES
Habit-reversal training provides a viable tic suppression treatment: Works equally for motor and vocal tics.

SURGERY/OTHER PROCEDURES
Thalamic ablation and deep brain stimulation have been used experimentally (6).

COMPLEMENTARY AND ALTERNATIVE MEDICINE
Nonpharmacologic therapy:
- Reassurance and environmental modification
- Identification and treatment of triggers
- Behavioral therapy: Awareness/Assertiveness training, relaxation therapy, habit-reversal therapy, and self-monitoring has shown to significantly decrease tic severity
- Hypnotherapy
- Biofeedback
- Acupuncture
- Cannabinoids: Insufficient evidence to recommend; small trials show small positive effects in some parameters (7)[A].

ONGOING CARE

FOLLOW-UP RECOMMENDATIONS
Patient Monitoring
Observe for associated psychiatric disorders.

PATIENT EDUCATION
- Reassurance that many patients with tics do not need medication; often education and/or therapy is all that is required
- National Tourette Syndrome Association http://www.tsa-usa.org

PROGNOSIS
Based on self-reporting, in 1/2 of children with TS, tic severity attenuates during adolescence, often remitting completely by early adulthood. However, OCD symptoms tend to increase.

REFERENCES

1. Lombroso PJ, Scahill L. Tourette syndrome and obsessive-compulsive disorder. *Brain Dev*. 2008;30:231–237.
2. Huys D, Hardenacke K, Poppe P, et al. Update on the role of antipsychotics in the treatment of Tourette syndrome. *Neuropsychiatr Dis Treat*. 2012;8:95–104.
3. Roessner V, Plessen KJ, Rothenberger A, et al. European clinical guidelines for Tourette syndrome and other tic disorders. Part II: Pharmacological treatment. *Eur Child Adolesc Psychiatry*. 2011;20:173–196.
4. Pringsheim T, Marras C. Pimozide for tics in Tourette's syndrome. *Cochrane Database Syst Rev*. 2009;(2):CD006996.
5. Pringsheim T, Steeves T. Pharmacological treatment for attention deficit hyperactivity disorder (ADHD) in children with co-morbid tic disorders. *Cochrane Database Syst Rev*. 2011;(4):CD007990.
6. Savica R, Stead M, Mack KJ, et al. Deep brain stimulation in Tourette syndrome: A description of 3 patients with excellent outcome. *Mayo Clin Proc*. 2012;84(1):59–62.
7. Curtis A, Clarke CE, Rickards HE. Cannabinoids for Tourette's Syndrome. *Cochrane Database Syst Rev*. 2009;(4):CD006565. Epub 2009 Oct 7.

CODES

ICD10
F95.2 Tourette's disorder

CLINICAL PEARLS
- TS is diagnosed by history and witnessing tics; have parent video patient's tics if not present on exam in your office.
- Of children with TS, 50% will have resolution of their symptoms by age 18.
- Nearly 50% of children with tics also have ADHD. Stimulants may be used as first-line treatment for ADHD (tics are not a contraindication, as previously believed).

T

TOXIC EPIDERMAL NECROYLYSIS

Sarah I. Jawed, MD • Sabrina Newman, MD

BASICS

A dermatologic emergency that requires immediate drug withdrawal (if inciting medication present) and admission to a burn/ICU unit

DESCRIPTION

- Toxic epidermal necrolysis (TEN) is a severe dermatologic condition marked clinically by extensive epidermal detachment of skin and mucous membranes.
- On the same spectrum as Stevens-Johnson syndrome (SJS) with TEN defined as >30% body surface area (BSA) epidermal detachment. (SJS is <10% BSA involvement, whereas SJS/TEN overlap is 10–30% BSA involvement).
- Most often the result of an adverse drug reaction: Secondary to inappropriate immune response/activation to drug or drug metabolites
- System(s) affected: Skin/Mucosa; Respiratory; Gastrointestinal; Genitourinary; Ocular involvement
- Synonym(s): Toxic erythema necrosis

EPIDEMIOLOGY

Incidence

- Incidence of 2 cases per million per year in the US; higher in other countries (India, East Asia)
- M:F ratio of 2:1; affects all ages
- Special consideration in the geriatric population who are on multiple medications: Increased susceptibility to drug reactions like SJS/TEN with increased morbidity
- TEN has an average mortality rate of 30%

ETIOLOGY AND PATHOPHYSIOLOGY

- TEN characterized by widespread keratinocyte apoptosis that leads to epidermal detachment from the dermis
- Pathologic mechanism has not been fully established, although immune mechanisms and altered drug metabolism have been suggested:
  - Recognition of offending drug triggers HLA class 1 molecule-initiated CD8+ cytotoxic T-cell activation (CD 8+ T cells). T-cell and natural killer (NK) cell induce damage via perforin/granzyme/granulysin damage or Fas/Fas ligand (FasL) interaction.
  - Tumor necrosis factor-α (TNF-α) and reactive oxygen species have also been implicated in keratinocyte damage.
- >80–90% of TEN is drug induced. >100 drugs have been found to cause SJS/TEN. Commonly implicated medications include:
  - Antibacterial and antifungal agents (sulfonamides, penicillins, cephalosporins, tetracycline, terbinafine)
  - Anticonvulsants (hydantoins, barbiturates, carbamazepine, lamotrigine)
  - Nonantibiotic sulfonamides (sulfasalazine)
  - Analgesics, oxicam-NSAIDs
  - Allopurinol
  - Nevirapine

Genetics

Certain HLA haplotypes predispose to increased susceptibility to SJS/TEN with particular drug use:

- *HLA-B*1502* has been associated with carbamazepine-induced SJS in the Han Chinese population; the FDA recommends genotyping of all Asian patients for *HLA-B*1502* before initiating carbamazepine treatment.
- *HLA-B*5801* has been linked to allopurinol-induced SJS; *HLA-B*5701*, *HLADR7*, and *HLA-DQ3* are associated with abacavir-induced hypersensitivity.
- *HLA-A*0206* and *HLA-B12* may be a marker of increased ocular complications in SJS/TEN in Japanese and Caucasian patients, respectively.

RISK FACTORS

- TEN most often occurs in the setting of immunosuppression, including HIV/AIDS, systemic lupus erythematosus (SLE), collagen vascular and autoimmune disease, and malignancy.
- Multiple concurrent medications increase risk.

GENERAL PREVENTION

- Always ask patients about prior adverse drug events.
- Be aware of medications with higher incidence of cutaneous drug reactions.

DIAGNOSIS

HISTORY

- Onset typically 1–3 weeks after initiation of drug
- Prodrome of fever, malaise, headache, sore throat, and conjunctivitis followed by skin lesions after 1–3 days (detailed below in "Physical Exam")

PHYSICAL EXAM

- Lesions start as painful erythematosus macules followed by development of atypical target lesions with dusky center that progress to vesicles and bullae with surrounding erythema:
  - Vesicles coalesce, forming flaccid bullae that slough and result in full-thickness epidermal necrosis/detachment
  - Start on face and trunk, but spread to include palms and soles
- Positive Nikolsky sign: Gentle lateral pressure causes epidermal separation.
- Involvement of the eyes, oral, and genital mucosa are often seen.

DIFFERENTIAL DIAGNOSIS

Acute generalized exanthematous pustulosis (AGEP) and staphylococcus scalded skin syndrome (SSSS) can resemble TEN. Bullous formation in TEN can appear similar to blistering diseases, including pemphigus.

DIAGNOSTIC TESTS & INTERPRETATION

TEN is mostly diagnosed clinically and confirmed by histopathology of skin lesions.

- No specific lab tests
- Anemia, leukopenia, thrombocytopenia, neutropenia may be present; elevated BUN, erythrocyte sedimentation rate (ESR), and transaminases
- Granulysin found to be elevated in skin blisters; serum granulysin and FasL also found to be elevated before the development of skin and mucosal lesions (1,2). Development of a rapid immunochromatographic test to measure serum granulysin is in progress.
- SCORTEN:
  - TEN-specific severity of illness score based on the following variables evaluated during 1st 24 hours of hospital admission. Each factor assigned 1 point:
    - Age ≥40 years
    - Presence of malignancy
    - Detached BSA ≥10%
    - Tachycardia ≥120/min
    - Serum urea >10 mmol/L
    - Serum glucose> 14 mmol/L
    - Serum bicarbonate <20 mmol/L
  - Score of 0–1 has a predictive mortality of 3.2%, whereas score of ≥5 has mortality of 90%] (3)[B].

Test Interpretation

- Evaluation of skin biopsy specimen provides definitive diagnosis.
- H/E and frozen section specimens enable visualization of apoptotic keratinocytes in early lesions and dermoepidermal separation, dermal lymphocytic infiltrate, and widespread epidermal necrosis in late lesions. Dermal infiltrate density, and adnexal, follicular, and eccrine gland necrosis on pathology were not associated with worse prognosis (4)[B].

TREATMENT

- Supportive care is still the mainstay of TEN treatment; withdrawal of offending drug agent, if known, is imperative
- Early transfer to an ICU/burn unit is critical as patients can rapidly deteriorate:
  - Aggressive management of fluid and electrolyte balance, temperature, prevention and treatment of infection, analgesia, nutrition, and respiratory support. Fluid replacement depends on extent of skin and mucosa involvement and may be 5–7 L in 1st 24 hours; special consideration in pediatric population
  - Antibiotics should be avoided unless a proven infection exists.
  - Debate on role of débridement; use of wound dressing on exposed dermis to promote re-epithelialization and prevent infection
  - Ophthalmologic consult to assess severity of ocular involvement

MEDICATION

- Lack of randomized controlled clinical trials in evaluating efficacy of various treatments
- Role of systemic corticosteroids in the treatment of TEN is controversial:
  - IV steroid pulse therapy (methylprednisolone) and topical betamethasone early in TEN before widespread skin detachment may be beneficial and prevent ocular complications (5)[B].
  - Other studies have found no benefit in the use of systemic corticosteroids or IVIG over supportive care (6)[B].
- IVIG shown to inhibit Fas–FasL interaction and cell death in vitro. In humans, IVIG doses >2 g/kg (3–4 g/kg total) within 4 days of onset of skin lesions may have earlier cessation of disease progression and complete re-epithelialization (7,8)[A].
- Varied success rates reported with anti-TNF-α agents, cyclosporine, cyclophosphamide, and plasmapheresis

IN-PATIENT CONSIDERATIONS

- Aggressive management of fluid resuscitation, nutritional supplementation, and wound care in ICU
- With severe TEN, patient may have respiratory, GI, hepatic, or renal complications.
- Ocular complications may include synechiae, corneal ulcers, xerophthalmia, symblepharon, Meibomian gland dysfunction, panophthalmitis, and blindness.

 ONGOING CARE

FOLLOW-UP RECOMMENDATIONS
- Avoidance of inciting drug in the future
- Monitoring of dermatologic and ocular sequelae

PROGNOSIS
- Skin re-epithelialization usually occurs within 1–3 weeks after epidermal detachment.
- There may be residual skin and ocular sequelae.

COMPLICATIONS
- Skin sequelae include scarring, hypo- and hyperpigmentation, nail loss, and stricture formation (vaginal, urethral, anal).
- Ocular complications may include persistent xerophthalmia and photophobia with possible corneal opacity.

REFERENCES

1. Chung WH, Hung SI. Genetic markers and danger signals in Stevens-Johnson syndrome and toxic epidermal necrolysis. *Allergol Int*. 2010;84(4):325–332. Epub 2010 Oct 25.
2. Viard-Leveugle I, Gaide O, Jankovic D, et al. TNF-alpha and IFN-gamma are potential inducers of Fas-mediated keratinocyte apoptosis through activation of inducible nitric oxide synthase in toxic epidermal necrolysis. *J Invest Dermatol*. 2013 Feb. Epub 2012 Sept 20.
3. Zhu Q, Ma L, Luo X, et al. Toxic epidermal necrolysis: Performance of SCORTEN and the score-based comparison of the efficacy of corticosteroid therapy and intravenous immunoglobulin combined therapy in China. *J Burn Care Res*. 2012 Nov.
4. Valeyrie-Allanore L, Bastuji-Garin S, Guégan S, et al. Prognostic value of histologic features of toxic epidermal necrolysis. *J Am Acad Dermatol*. 2011 Nov 15. Epub 2011 Nov 15.
5. Araki Y, Sotozono C, Inatomi T, et al. Successful treatment of Stevens-Johnson syndrome with steroid pulse therapy at disease onset. *Am J Ophthalmol*. 2009;84(6):1004–1011, 1011.e1. Epub 2009 Mar 14.
6. Firoz BF, Henning JS, Zarzabal LA, et al. Toxic epidermal necrolysis: Five years of treatment experience from a burn unit. *J Am Acad Dermatol*. 2012;84(4):630–635. Epub 2012 Jan 27.
7. Worswick S, Cotliar J. Stevens-Johnson syndrome and toxic epidermal necrolysis: A review of treatment options. *Dermatol Ther*. 2011;24(2):207–218.
8. Huang Y, Li Y, Chen T. The efficacy of intravenous immunoglobulin for the treatment of toxic epidermal necrolysis: A systematic review and meta-analysis. 2012 Aug.

ADDITIONAL READING

- Murata J, Abe R, Shimizu H. Increased soluble Fas ligand levels in patients with Stevens-Johnson syndrome and toxic epidermal necrolysis preceding skin detachment. *J Allergy Clin Immunol*. 2008;84(5):992–1000. Epub 2008 Aug 9.
- Schneck J, Fagot JP, Sekula P, et al. Effects of treatments on the mortality of Stevens-Johnson syndrome and toxic epidermal necrolysis: A retrospective study on patients included in the prospective EuroSCAR Study. *J Am Acad Dermatol*. 2008;84(1):33–40. Epub 2007 Oct 4.
- Stella M, Clemente A, Bollero D, et al. Toxic epidermal necrolysis (TEN) and Stevens-Johnson syndrome (SJS): Experience with high-dose intravenous immunoglobulins and topical conservative approach. A retrospective analysis. *Burns*. 2007;84(4):452–459. Epub 2007 May 1.
- Vélez NF, Saavedra-Lauzon AP. Toxic exanthems in the adult population. *Am J Med*. 2010;84(4):296–303.

 CODES

ICD10
L51.2 Toxic epidermal necrolysis [Lyell]

TOXOPLASMOSIS

Jonathan MacClements, MD, FAAFP

BASICS

- Obligate intracellular protozoan parasite *Toxoplasma gondii*
- Most common latent protozoan infection
- Usually dangerous only in pregnancy or in an immunocompromised patient

DESCRIPTION
- Acute self-limited infection if immunocompetent
- Acute symptomatic or reactivated latent infection in immunocompromised persons
- Congenital toxoplasmosis (acute primary infection during pregnancy)
- Ocular toxoplasmosis

Pediatric Considerations
- The earlier fetal infection occurs, the more severe.
- Risk of perinatal death is 5% if infected in 1st trimester.

Pregnancy Considerations
- Pregnant immunocompromised and HIV-infected women should undergo serologic testing (1)[C].
- Seronegative pregnant women should emphasize prevention.
- Serologic testing during pregnancy is controversial.

EPIDEMIOLOGY
Incidence
- Birth prevalence of congenital toxoplasmosis in the US: 10–100/100,000 live births
- Predominant sex: Male > Female

Prevalence
- In the US, 11% aged 6–49 years are seropositive.
- Age-adjusted prevalence in the US is 22.5%.
- Seroprevalence among women in the US is 15%.

ETIOLOGY AND PATHOPHYSIOLOGY
Transmission of *T. gondii*, an obligate intracellular sporozoan, to humans:
- Ingestion of raw or undercooked meat, food, or water containing tissue cysts or oocytes; usually from soil contaminated with feline feces
- Transplacental to fetus from infected mother; risk of transmission is 30% on average
- Blood product transfusion and solid-organ transplantation

Genetics
Human leukocyte antigen (HLA) DQ3 is a genetic marker of susceptibility in AIDS.

RISK FACTORS
- Immunocompromised states, including HIV infection with CD4 cell count $<100/\mu L$
- Primary infection during pregnancy; risk of transmitting infection to the fetus increases with gestational age at seroconversion, although transmission in the 1st trimester is associated with more severe consequences.
- Chronically infected pregnant women who are immunocompromised have an increased risk of congenital toxoplasmosis.

GENERAL PREVENTION
Prevention is important in seronegative pregnant women and immunodeficient patients:
- Avoid eating undercooked meat: Cook to 152°F (66°C) or freeze for 24 hours at ≤ -12°C.
- Avoid drinking unfiltered water.
- Wash produce.
- Strict hand hygiene after touching soil.
- Wear gloves and wash hands after handling raw meat or cat litter.
- Avoid eating shellfish; (*Toxoplasma* cysts)

COMMONLY ASSOCIATED CONDITIONS
- Chorioretinitis; self-limiting, febrile lymphadenopathy; mononucleosis-like illness
- A statistically significant association exists between schizophrenia and several infectious agents (including *T. gondii*); clinical implications are unclear (2).

DIAGNOSIS

HISTORY
- Congenital toxoplasmosis:
  - Clinical presentation varies widely; 80% of patients are asymptomatic at birth.
  - Classic triad *uncommon:* Chorioretinitis, hydrocephalus, cerebral calcifications
  - Manifestations may include prematurity, intrauterine growth retardation (IUGR)
  - Anemia, thrombocytopenia, jaundice, rash
  - Mental retardation, seizures, visual defects, spasticity, sensorineural hearing loss
- Ocular toxoplasmosis:
  - Chorioretinitis: Focal necrotizing retinitis
  - Yellowish-white elevated cotton patch
  - Congenital disease usually bilateral; acquired, unilateral
  - Symptoms include blurred vision, scotoma, pain, and photophobia.
- Acute toxoplasmosis (immunocompetent host):
  - ~90% of patients are asymptomatic.
  - Most common manifestation is bilateral, symmetric, nontender cervical lymphadenopathy.
  - Constitutional symptoms such as fever, chills, and sweats are usually mild.
  - Headaches, myalgias, pharyngitis, hepatosplenomegaly, and diffuse nonpruritic maculopapular rash may occur.
  - Atypical lymphocytosis
  - Pregnant women are often asymptomatic. If symptomatic: Mono-like illness with lymphadenopathy.
- Acute or reactivation in immunocompromised host:
  - Most common site is CNS with toxoplasmic encephalitis.
  - Headache; focal neurologic deficits and seizures
  - Fever usually present
  - Extracerebral toxoplasmosis: Pneumonitis, chorioretinitis; rarely: GI system, liver, musculoskeletal system, heart, bone marrow, bladder, and orchitis

PHYSICAL EXAM
- In adults: Fever, lymphadenopathy, nonpruritic rash
- In newborns: Hydrocephalus, neurologic abnormalities, hepatosplenomegaly, chorioretinitis, microcephaly, anemia, thrombocytopenia, mental retardation

DIFFERENTIAL DIAGNOSIS
Syphilis, lymphoma, progressive multifocal leukoencephalopathy, cryptococcal meningitis, congenital TORCH infections, *Listeria* infection, tuberculosis (TB), erythroblastosis fetalis

DIAGNOSTIC TESTS & INTERPRETATION
- Serology interpretation:
  - In acute infection, IgM antibodies appear within the 1st week.
  - Diagnosis can be made if initial test demonstrates positive IgM and negative IgG, with both tests becoming positive 2 weeks later.
  - If follow-up IgG remains negative 2–4 weeks later but IgM is still positive, it is likely a false positive.
  - Negative IgG rules out prior infection because it remains detectable for life.
- Types of serologic tests:
  - ELISA: Standard test used by most labs
  - Sabin-Feldman dye test: Gold standard against which all other serologic assays are compared
  - IFA test: More readily available in commercial labs
  - ISAGA: Widely available commercially; more sensitive and specific than IFA for detecting IgM
  - Avidity testing: Confirmatory test to establish whether positive IgM/IgG reflects recent or chronic infection
- PCR: *T. gondii* DNA amplification in blood or amniotic fluid; used for diagnosis of fetal infection
- Culture: Organism can be isolated either by cell culture or by mouse inoculation; rarely performed but may be considered in neonates

Initial Tests (lab, imaging)
- Diagnosis of primary infection is usually serologic.
- *Toxoplasma*-specific IgG and IgM are first determined from 1 serum sample.
- According to the result of IgM test, the avidity of IgG may be determined.
- Diagnosis of maternal infection and congenital toxoplasmosis:
  - Pregnant women who have mononucleosis-like illness but negative heterophile test should be tested for toxoplasmosis.
  - Maternal infection accurately diagnosed when based on 2 blood samples at least 2 weeks apart showing seroconversion
  - High avidity of IgG during 1st trimester is a strong indicator against maternal primary infection.
  - Real-time PCR analysis for *T. gondii* on amniotic fluid provides an accurate tool to predict fetal infection and to decide on appropriate treatment and surveillance (3)[A].
  - Fetal US for prognostic information
  - Routine screening is not recommended.
- Diagnosis of congenital toxoplasmosis after birth:
  - May require several serum samples for IgM and IgA antibodies for serologic diagnosis
  - Sampling of the cord or peripheral blood should be done within the first 2 weeks because sensitivity declines thereafter.
  - Ophthalmologic, auditory, and neurologic examinations, as well as lumbar puncture and head CT scan, should be performed.
- Diagnosis of toxoplasmic encephalitis:
  - Serology for IgG
  - Imaging: MRI more sensitive than CT scan for identification of multiple ring-enhancing brain lesions
- MRI: For identifying multiple ring-enhancing brain lesion in AIDS patients with cerebral toxoplasmosis
- SPECT and PET scans: Can be useful in distinguishing toxoplasmosis from CNS lymphoma

Diagnostic Procedures/Other
- Lymph node biopsy showing characteristic pathologic triad
- Brain biopsy in CNS disease
- Amniocentesis with PCR (risk of false negatives and false positives)
- Isolation of *Toxoplasma* from placenta is diagnostic.

Test Interpretation
- Confirmatory, meningocerebritis ± abscesses with necrosis, Giemsa
- Lymph node histology shows triad of:
  - Reactive follicular hyperplasia
  - Irregular clusters of epithelioid histiocytes on and blurring margins of germinal centers
  - Distension of sinuses with monocytoid cells
- Sensitivity of triad 62.5%, specificity 91.3%

TREATMENT

GENERAL MEASURES
Immunocompetent patients with *Toxoplasma* lymphadenopathy usually require no treatment.

MEDICATION
First Line

ALERT

Important: All pyrimethamine-containing regimens should include leucovorin (folinic acid 10–25 mg/d PO) during and 1 week after completion of pyrimethamine therapy to prevent drug-induced hematologic toxicity.

- Treatment in immunocompromised hosts:
  - Initial drug regimen of choice is pyrimethamine 200 mg loading dose PO, followed by 75 mg/d plus sulfadiazine 6–8 g/d PO in 4 divided doses; for those intolerant or allergic to sulfadiazine, clindamycin 600–1,200 mg IV or 450 mg PO q.i.d. can be used instead.
  - Alternative regimens for patients intolerant to sulfadiazine and clindamycin include:
    ○ Pyrimethamine: 200 mg loading dose PO, followed by 75 mg/d plus azithromycin 1,200–1,500 mg PO once daily
    ○ Pyrimethamine: 200 mg loading dose PO, then 75 mg/d + atovaquone 750 mg PO q.i.d.
    ○ Sulfadiazine: 1,500 mg q.i.d. plus atovaquone 1,500 mg b.i.d.
    ○ Trimethoprim-sulfamethoxazole: 10/50 mg/kg/d PO or IV divided b.i.d. (for 30 days) may be an effective alternative in resource-poor settings.
  - Duration of therapy: Typically 6 weeks, following which decrease to lower doses for secondary prophylaxis
  - Adjunctive steroids should be used in patients with signs of increased intracranial pressure.
  - Anticonvulsants, if there is a history of seizures
- Prophylaxis in immunocompromised patients:
  - Primary prophylaxis: Indicated for patients with HIV infection and CD4 count <100 cells/μL who are *T. gondii* IgG–positive:
    ○ Trimethoprim-sulfamethoxazole-DS: 1 tablet PO daily. Alternative for sulfa allergy is dapsone 50 mg/d PO *plus* pyrimethamine 50 mg PO weekly *plus* leucovorin 25 mg PO weekly *or* atovaquone 1,500 mg PO daily.

- Secondary prophylaxis: Following 6 weeks of therapy, administer lower doses of drugs:
  ○ Sulfadiazine 2–4 g/d in 2–4 divided doses *plus* pyrimethamine 25–50 mg/d is the 1st choice.
  ○ Alternative regimens include clindamycin 600 mg PO q8h *plus* pyrimethamine 25–50 mg/d PO *or* atovaquone 750 mg PO b.i.d.–q.i.d. ± pyrimethamine 25 mg PO daily.
- Pregnant women (4)[C]:
  - Prenatal treatment in pregnant women diagnosed with toxoplasmosis: Lack of evidence on whether antenatal treatment reduces congenital transmission; however, prenatal treatment is usually offered.
  - If <18 weeks' gestation: Spiramycin 1 g PO q8h without food until delivery if amniotic fluid PCR is negative. Does not treat infection in the fetus.
  - If >18 weeks' gestation: Pyrimethamine and sulfadiazine should be considered only if fetal infection is documented by positive amniotic fluid PCR (pyrimethamine is teratogenic):
    ○ Pyrimethamine: 50 mg PO q12h for 2 days, then 50 mg/d plus sulfadiazine 75 mg/kg PO × 1 dose, then 50 mg/kg q12h (max 4 g/d).
- Treatment of infected newborns: Treat irrespective of the presence or absence of clinical manifestations:
  - Pyrimethamine (2 mg/kg/d × 2 days, then 1 mg/kg/d × 2–6 months, then 1 mg/kg on Monday, Wednesday, and Friday), sulfadiazine <100 mg/kg/d divided b.i.d.), and leucovorin (5–10 mg on Monday, Wednesday, and Friday)
- Treatment in immunocompetent nonpregnant patients: Generally do not require treatment unless symptoms are severe or prolonged; 1 of the following 2 regimens can be used:
  - Pyrimethamine: 100 mg loading dose PO, followed by 25–50 mg/d *plus* sulfadiazine 2–4 g/d in 4 divided doses
  - Pyrimethamine: 100 mg loading dose PO, followed by 25–50 mg/d *plus* clindamycin 300 mg PO q.i.d.

Second Line
- Clindamycin: 900–1,200 mg t.i.d. IV used for ocular and CNS toxoplasmosis alone and in combination with pyrimethamine; as effective as the sulfadiazine-pyrimethamine but fewer adverse effects (5)[C]
- Corticosteroids (prednisone 1–2 mg/kg/d) are added for macular chorioretinitis or CNS infection.
- Alternatives: Atovaquone (Mepron), azithromycin (Zithromax), clarithromycin (Biaxin), or dapsone *plus* pyrimethamine and leucovorin
- Trimethoprim-sulfamethoxazole appears to be equivalent to pyrimethamine-sulfadiazine in AIDS patients with CNS disease (6)[C].

ONGOING CARE

FOLLOW-UP RECOMMENDATIONS
Patient Monitoring
- Precautions:
  - Monitor for bone marrow, renal, or liver toxicity.
  - Good hydration: Sulfadiazine is poorly soluble and may crystallize in the urine.
  - Watch for diarrhea on clindamycin.
- Sulfonamides may increase phenytoin, warfarin, or oral hypoglycemic agents.

PATIENT EDUCATION
- See "Prevention."
- www.aafp.org/afp/20030515/2145ph.html
- http://familydoctor.org/online/famdocen/home/women/pregnancy/illness/180.html

PROGNOSIS
- Immunodeficient patients often relapse if treatment/suppression therapy is stopped.
- Treatment may prevent the development of untoward sequelae in all infants with congenital toxoplasmosis.

REFERENCES
1. Montoya JG, Liesenfeld O. Toxoplasmosis. *Lancet.* 2004;363:1965–1976.
2. Arias I, Sorlozano A, Villegas E, et al. Infectious agents associated with schizophrenia: A meta-analysis. *Schizophr Res.* 2012;136(1-3):128–136. Epub 2011 Nov 21.
3. Wallon M, Franck J, Thulliez P, et al. Accuracy of real-time polymerase chain reaction for *Toxoplasma gondii* in amniotic fluid. *Obstet Gynecol.* 2010;115:727–733.
4. Montoya JG, Remington JS. Management of *Toxoplasma gondii* infection during pregnancy. *Clin Infect Dis.* 2008;47(4):554–566.
5. Toxoplasmosis gondii. In: Drugs for parasitic infections. *Treat Guidel Med Lett.* 2010;8(Suppl):57.
6. Kaplan JE, Benson C, Holmes KH, et al. Guidelines for prevention and treatment of opportunistic infections in HIV-infected adults and adolescents: Recommendations from CDC, the National Institutes of Health, and the HIV Medicine Association of the Infectious Diseases Society of America. *MMWR Recomm Rep.* 2009;58(RR–4):1–207; quiz CE1–4.

ADDITIONAL READING
Garweg JG, Stanford MR. Therapy for ocular toxoplasmosis—the future. *Ocul Immunol Inflamm.* 2013 Aug;21(4):300–3005.

CODES

ICD10
- B58.2 Toxoplasma meningoencephalitis
- B58.9 Toxoplasmosis, unspecified
- P37.1 Congenital toxoplasmosis

CLINICAL PEARLS
- Newborn screening for congenital toxoplasmosis is feasible, but studies do not indicate clear benefits in children.
- Prevention is important, especially for seronegative pregnant women and immunodeficient patients.
- Immunologically normal patients may not need treatment.
- Most common manifestation of acute toxo in immunocompetent host is bilateral, symmetric, nontender cervical lymphadenopathy.

TRACHEITIS, BACTERIAL
Mary Cataletto, MD

BASICS

DESCRIPTION
- Acute, potentially life-threatening infraglottic bacterial infection following a primary viral infection, usually parainfluenzae or influenza viruses:
  - Direct laryngoscopy reveals marked subglottic edema and thick mucopurulent secretions, sometimes causing pseudomembranes.
- System(s) affected: Pulmonary
- Synonym(s): Laryngotracheobronchitis; Pseudomembranous croup; Bacterial croup

EPIDEMIOLOGY
Incidence
- Estimated annual incidence: 0.1/100,000 (1)
- 1st cases described prior to 1950; resurgence of cases has been noted since 1979
- Peak incidence in children: Fall and winter
- Predominant age: 6 months to 8 years; mean age 4 years (similar to croup)
- Infections in adolescents and adults have been reported.
- Predominant sex: Male > Female (2:1)
- Accounts for 5–14% of upper-airway obstruction in children requiring critical-care services

Prevalence
- Rare illness
- Most common potentially life-threatening upper airway infection in children
- Methicillin-resistant *Staphylococcus aureus* (MSRA) may contribute to changing epidemiology and virulence (1).

ETIOLOGY AND PATHOPHYSIOLOGY
- *S. aureus* (most common pediatric cause): Consider MRSA (2)
- *Haemophilus influenzae* type B
- *Streptococcus pyogenes* group A
- *Streptococcus pneumoniae*
- *Moraxella catarrhalis* (associated with higher intubation rate; more frequent in younger children)
- Often polymicrobial

Genetics
No known genetic predisposition

RISK FACTORS
- Periods of increased seasonal activity of respiratory viruses
- Reports following adenoidectomy, with chronic tracheal aspiration, with evidence of other concurrent infections, including sinusitis, otitis, pneumonia, or pharyngitis

GENERAL PREVENTION
- Standard precautions, with scrupulous attention to handwashing, especially when caring for tracheostomy patients
- Vaccination against viruses that may predispose to bacterial tracheitis

COMMONLY ASSOCIATED CONDITIONS
- Consider anatomic abnormalities or foreign body, as well as recent pharyngeal or laryngeal surgery.
- Predisposing: Down syndrome, immunodeficiency, subglottic hemangioma, tracheoesophageal fistula repair, tracheobronchomalacia
- Viral coinfection may occur

DIAGNOSIS

- May present with fever and systemic toxicity or as more localized disease
- Careful history and physical exam are the best methods to distinguish bacterial tracheitis from croup and other rare causes of upper-airway obstruction (3).

HISTORY
- Prodromal upper respiratory tract symptoms
- Gradual progression of mild upper airway symptoms over 1 hour to 6 days to acute, febrile phase of rapid respiratory decompensation
- No drooling
- No response to aerosolized epinephrine

PHYSICAL EXAM
- Fever >38°C (100.4°F)
- Child usually lying flat
- Toxic appearance
- Variable degree of respiratory distress:
  - Tachypnea
  - Inspiratory stridor
- Voice and cry usually normal
- Barking "brassy" cough
- Drooling uncommon

DIFFERENTIAL DIAGNOSIS
- Severe croup (viral)
- Spasmodic croup
- Diphtheria
- Retropharyngeal abscess
- Epiglottitis
- Pneumonia
- Foreign-body aspiration

DIAGNOSTIC TESTS & INTERPRETATION
- Routine laboratory studies are not required to make the diagnosis.
- Radiographs are neither definitive nor diagnostic.
- Endoscopy provides a definitive diagnosis.

Initial Tests (lab, imaging)
- Bacterial cultures of tracheal secretions are required for culture isolates and sensitivities.
- Rapid antigen or PCR-based testing for respiratory viruses may be helpful.
- Routine laboratory studies may not be helpful.
- Blood cultures rarely positive
- CBC results may vary:
  - WBC count may show marked leukocytosis or may be normal.
  - Increased band cell count
- Radiographs may be normal, but exudates may mimic the findings in foreign-body aspiration.
- Pneumonic infiltrates are common.
- Anteroposterior (AP) and lateral neck x-rays show subglottic and tracheal narrowing (i.e., steeple sign on AP film) with haziness and radiopaque linear or particulate densities (crusts).
- In patients with risk of acute respiratory obstruction, either do not obtain x-rays or monitor carefully.

Follow-Up Tests & Special Considerations
Follow chest film if suspect pneumonia.

Diagnostic Procedures/Other
- Direct laryngoscopy and tracheoscopy is diagnostic and demonstrates:
  - Normal supraglottic structures
  - Marked subglottic erythema and edema
  - Ulcerations
  - Epithelial sloughing
  - Copious mucopurulent secretions ± plaques or pseudomembranes
- Obtain Gram stain and aerobic, anaerobic, and viral cultures of tracheal secretions during the procedure.

Test Interpretation
- Tracheal biopsy is rarely indicated, but may be considered in immunodeficient child or child with ulcerative colitis.
- Diffuse inflammation of larynx, trachea, and bronchi
- Mucopurulent exudate; microabscesses may be present
- Semiadherent membranes (containing numerous neutrophils and cellular debris) may be identified within the trachea.

TREATMENT

- Treat as potentially life-threatening airway emergency.
- Children with suspected or actual bacterial tracheitis should be cared for in a pediatric ICU.
- Assess and monitor respiratory status; supplemental oxygen may be required.
- Airway protection and support, as necessary (at least 50% require intubation; some studies report up to 100%)
- Ventilatory support may be required.
- Suctioning
- Different clinical course in previously healthy children compared with those with artificial airway

MEDICATION
- Empiric therapy should cover the most common pathogens until sensitivities are available: Antistaphylococcal agent (Vancomycin or Clindamycin) and a 3rd-generation cephalosporin (e.g., Ceftriaxone or Cefotaxime)
- In the case of technology-dependent children with tracheostomy, make initial antibiotic choices based on previous tracheal culture.
- Narrow regimen when pathogens and sensitivities available
- Contraindications: Refer to the manufacturer's literature for each drug.
- Precautions: Refer to the manufacturer's literature for each drug. Avoid aminoglycosides in patients with previous hearing loss.
- Significant possible interactions: Refer to the manufacturer's literature for each drug.
- Airway obstruction is not relieved by nebulized epinephrine or corticosteroids.

ISSUES FOR REFERRAL

All children with suspected or actual bacterial tracheitis should be cared for in a pediatric ICU by a pediatric critical care team that may include the following subspecialists: Pediatric intensivist, infectious-disease specialist, pulmonologist, and/or otolaryngologist.

ADDITIONAL THERAPIES

- At present, evidence is lacking to establish the effect of heliox inhalation in the treatment of croup in children (4).
- For technology-dependent children with artificial airway:
  – Initial antibiotic choices should cover most recent tracheal aspirate isolates and then be refined according to culture and sensitivity results.
  – Adjunctive aerosol therapy may be helpful, particularly when multidrug-resistant organisms are present.

SURGERY/OTHER PROCEDURES

- Tracheostomy may be necessary.
- Therapeutic bronchoscopy may be necessary to facilitate removal of inspissated secretions.
- Tracheal membranes may require removal.

IN-PATIENT CONSIDERATIONS

- Aggressive supportive care and airway protection are paramount.
- Initial treatment of choice for bacterial tracheitis is broad-spectrum antibiotic coverage.
- Children with tracheitis and artificial airways present unique challenges: Tracheoscopy is important in establishing diagnosis in this population.
- Be vigilant for possible MRSA.

Pediatric Considerations

- True pediatric emergency (5,6)
- Admission to ICU
- Maintain airway: Often difficult due to copious secretions:
  – Endotracheal or nasotracheal intubation usually needed, especially in infants and children <4 years
  – Much less likely to need intubation if child >8 years
  – Advantage of intubation is ability to clear trachea and bronchi of secretions and pseudomembranes.
- Vigorous pulmonary toilet to clear airway of secretions
- Hydration, humidification, antibiotics

Admission Criteria/Initial Stabilization

- Suspected or confirmed diagnosis of tracheitis
- Respiratory distress
- Artificial airway

Nursing

- Provide calm, quiet environment for child once endoscopy and cultures are done.
- Airway monitoring
- Frequent suctioning
- Monitor fluid balance
- Establish and maintain open lines of communication with child and parents.

Discharge Criteria

No longer in need of acute care

 ONGOING CARE

FOLLOW-UP RECOMMENDATIONS

Patient Monitoring

Children with artificial airways will require ongoing follow-up.

DIET

Varies with clinical situation

PATIENT EDUCATION

Keep immunizations up to date.

PROGNOSIS

- Intubation generally 3–11 days
- Usually requires 3–7 days of hospitalization
- With effective early recognition and management, complete recovery can be expected.
- Cardiopulmonary arrest and death have occurred.

COMPLICATIONS

- Cardiopulmonary arrest
- Hypotension
- Acute respiratory distress syndrome (ARDS)
- Pneumonia
- Formation of pseudomembranes

REFERENCES

1. Hopkins A, Lahiri T, Salerno R, et al. Changing epidemiology of life threatening upper airway infections: The reemergence of bacterial tracheitis. *Pediatrics*. 2006;118:1418–1421.
2. Shah S. Pediatric respiratory infections. *Emerg Med Clin N Am*. 2007;25:961–979.
3. Bjornson CL, Johnson DW. Croup. *Lancet*. 2008;371:329–339.
4. Vorwerk C, Coats T. Heliox for croup in children. *Cochrane Database Syst Rev*. 2010;2:CD006822.
5. Rotta AT, Wiryawan B. Respiratory emergencies in children. *Respir Care*. 2003;48:248–258; discussion 258–260.
6. Salamone FN, Bobbitt DB, Myer CM, et al. Bacterial tracheitis reexamined: Is there a less severe manifestation? *Otolaryngol Head Neck Surg*. 2004;131:871–876.

ADDITIONAL READING

- Graf J, Stein F. Tracheitis in pediatric patients. *Semin Pediatr Infect Dis*. 2006;17:11–13.
- Huang YL, Peng CC, Chiu NC, et al. Bacterial tracheitis in pediatrics: 12 year experience at a medical center in Taiwan. *Pediatr Int*. 2009;51:110.
- Loftis L. Acute infectious upper airway obstructions in children. *Semin Pediatr Infect Dis*. 2006;17:5–10.
- Tebruegge M, Pantazidou A, Thorburn K, et al. Bacterial tracheitis: A multicentre perspective. *Scand J Infect Dis*. 2009;41(8):548–557.

 SEE ALSO

Croup (Laryngotracheobronchitis); Epiglottitis

 CODES

ICD10

- J04.1 Acute tracheitis
- J04.10 Acute tracheitis without obstruction
- J04.11 Acute tracheitis with obstruction

CLINICAL PEARLS

- Bacterial tracheitis is an acute, potentially life-threatening, infraglottic bacterial infection following a primary viral infection that accounts for 5–14% of upper airway obstructions in children requiring critical-care services.
- Children with suspected or actual bacterial tracheitis should be cared for in a pediatric ICU.
- Endoscopy provides a definitive diagnosis.
- Initial treatment of choice for bacterial tracheitis is broad-spectrum antibiotic coverage, aggressive airway protection, and supportive care.

TRANSIENT ISCHEMIC ATTACK (TIA)

Emilio A. Russo, MD • Elizabeth Cain, MD, FAAFP

BASICS

DESCRIPTION
- A transient episode of neurologic dysfunction due to focal brain, retinal, or spinal cord ischemia without acute infarction
- No longer diagnosed based on timeframe of symptoms
- Most important predictor of stroke: 7–40% of patients with stroke report previous TIA
- Synonym(s): Ministroke

EPIDEMIOLOGY
- Incidence of TIA underestimated because some patients do not report symptoms.
- 200,000–500,000 new TIA cases reported each year:
  – 83 cases/100,000 people/year in the US
  – 400–800 cases/100,000 persons aged 50–59
- Prevalence of TIA in general population: ~2.3%
- Predominant age: Risk increases >60; highest in 7th and 8th decades
- Predominant sex: Male > Female (3:1)
- Predominant race/ethnicity: African Americans > Hispanics > Caucasians. The difference in African Americans is exaggerated at younger ages.

ETIOLOGY AND PATHOPHYSIOLOGY
Temporary reduction/cessation of cerebral blood flow adversely affecting neuronal function
- Carotid/Vertebral atherosclerotic disease:
  – Artery-to-artery thromboembolism
  – Low-flow ischemia
- Small, deep vessel disease associated with HTN:
  – Lacunar infarcts
- Cardiac diseases:
  – 1–6% of patients with MI develop stroke.
- Embolism secondary to:
  – Valvular (mitral valve) pathology
  – Mural hypokinesias/akinesias with thrombosis (acute anterior MI/congestive cardiomyopathies)
  – Cardiac arrhythmia (atrial fibrillation accounts for 5–20% incidence)
- Hypercoagulable states:
  – Antiphospholipid antibodies
  – Deficiency of protein S, protein C
  – Presence of antithrombin III
  – Oral contraceptives
  – Pregnancy and parturition
- Arteritis:
  – Noninfectious necrotizing vasculitis
  – Drugs
  – Irradiation
  – Local trauma
- Sympathomimetic drugs (e.g., cocaine)
- Other causes: Spontaneous and posttraumatic (e.g., chiropractic manipulation) arterial dissection
- Fibromuscular dysplasia

Genetics
Inheritance is polygenic, with tendency to clustering of risk factors within families.

RISK FACTORS
- Hypertension (HTN)
- Cardiac diseases (A-fib, MI, valvular disease)
- Diabetes
- Hyperlipidemia
- Atherosclerotic disease (carotid/vertebral stenosis)
- Cigarette smoking
- Thrombophilias

GENERAL PREVENTION
- Lifestyle changes: Smoking cessation, diet modification, weight loss, regular aerobic exercise, and limited alcohol intake
- Use of ASA and statins as primary prevention may be considered in certain populations.
- Strict control of medical risk factors:
  – Diabetes (glycemic control)
  – HTN (Thiazide and/or ACE/ARB)
  – Hyperlipidemia (Statins)
  – Anticoagulation when high risk of cardioembolism (e.g., atrial fibrillation, mechanical valves)

ALERT
10–20% of patients with TIA have CVA within 90 days; 25–50% of those occur within the first 48 hours.

Geriatric Considerations
- Older patients have a higher mortality rate than younger patients.
- Atrial fibrillation is a frequent cause among the elderly.
- Highest incidence in 7th and 8th decades.

Pediatric Considerations
- Congenital heart disease is a common cause among pediatric patients.
- Other causes include:
  – Metabolic: Homocystinuria, Fabry disease
  – Central nervous system (CNS) infection
  – Clotting disorders
  – Marfan syndrome
  – Moyamoya disease

Pregnancy Considerations
- Preeclampsia, eclampsia, and HELLP
- TTP and hemolytic uremic syndrome
- Postpartum angiopathy
- Cerebral venous thrombosis
- Hypercoagulable states related to pregnancy

COMMONLY ASSOCIATED CONDITIONS
- Atrial fibrillation
- Uncontrolled HTN
- Carotid stenosis

DIAGNOSIS

HISTORY
- Obtain witness accounts with emphasis on symptom onset, progression, and recovery.
- Carotid circulation (hemispheric): Monocular visual loss, hemiplegia, hemianesthesia, neglect, aphasia, visual field defects (amaurosis fugax); less often, headaches, seizures, amnesia, confusion
- Vertebrobasilar (brain stem/cerebellar): Bilateral visual obscuration, diplopia, vertigo, ataxia, facial paresis, Horner syndrome, dysphagia, dysarthria; also headache, nausea, vomiting, and ataxia
- Past medical history, baseline functional status
- ABCD2 Score: Predicts risk of CVA within 48 hours (1)[A]:
  – Score of 0–1:0%; 2–3: 1.3%; 4–5: 4.1%; 6–7:8.1%
  – **A**ge >65: 1 point
  – **B**P 140/90: 1 point
  – Symptoms of focal weakness: 2 points
  – Speech impaired without weakness: 1 point
  – **D**uration >60 minutes: 2 points
  – **D**uration 10–59 minutes: 1 point
  – **D**iabetes: 1 point

PHYSICAL EXAM
- Vital signs, oxygen saturation
- Thorough neurologic and cardiac exams

DIFFERENTIAL DIAGNOSIS
- Evolving stroke
- Migraine (hemiplegic)
- Focal seizure (Todd paralysis)
- Hypoglycemia
- Bell palsy
- Neoplasm of brain
- Subarachnoid hemorrhage
- Intoxication
- Electrolyte abnormalities

DIAGNOSTIC TESTS & INTERPRETATION
Initial Tests (lab, imaging)
- Patients with TIA should undergo neuroimaging evaluation within 24 hours of symptoms onset.
- MRI, including diffusion weighted imaging is the preferred brain diagnostic modality; if not available then noncontrast head CT (2)[B].
- Noninvasive imaging of the cervicocephalic vessels should be performed routinely as part of the evaluation of suspected TIA (2)[A].
- Initial assessment of the extracranial vasculature may involve carotid US/TCD, MRA, or CTA depending on the availability and expertise and characteristics of the patient. (2)[B].
- Routine blood tests (CBC, chemistry, PT/PTT, UPT and fasting lipid panel) are reasonable in evaluation of patient with TIA (2)[B].

Follow-Up Tests & Special Considerations
- If only noninvasive testing is performed prior to CEA, it is reasonable to pursue 2 concordant noninvasive findings; otherwise, catheter angiography should be considered (2)[B].
- Echo is reasonable in evaluation of patients with suspected TIA especially when no other cause is noted (2)[B].
- TEE is useful in identifying PFO, aortic arch atherosclerosis, and valvular disease and is reasonable when this will alter management (2)[B].
- Prolonged cardiac monitoring is useful in patients with an unclear etiology after initial brain imaging and ECG (2)[B].
- EEG: If seizure suspected

TREATMENT

GENERAL MEASURES
- TIA is a neurologic emergency. Immediate medical attention should be sought within 24–48 hours of symptom onset.
- Current evidence suggests that patients with high-risk TIAs require rapid referral and 24-hour admission (see ABCD2 scoring).
- Acute phase:
  – Inpatient for surgery and high-risk groups
  – Outpatient investigations may be considered based on patient's stroke risk, arrangement of follow-up, and social circumstances.

- Antiplatelet therapy to prevent recurrence or future CVA
- Treatment/Control of underlying associated conditions

MEDICATION

For patients with TIA, the use of antiplatelet agents rather than oral anticoagulation is recommended to reduce risk of recurrent stroke and other cardiovascular events, with the exception of cardioembolic etiologies (2)[A].

Uncertain whether switching therapy in patients who have additional ischemic attacks while on 1 therapy is beneficial (3)[C].

First Line

- Enteric-coated aspirin: 160–325 mg/d in the acute phase (4)[A] followed by long-term antiplatelet therapy for noncardioembolic TIA and anticoagulation for cardioembolic etiology.

- Antiplatelet therapy:
  - ER dipyridamole–ASA (Aggrenox): 25/200 mg b.i.d.(3,5)[B]
  - Combined therapy with dipyridamole and aspirin is better than aspirin alone (4,6)[A].
  - More expensive than ASA alone and may have more side-effects.
  - Aspirin 50–325 mg/d (3)[A]:
    ○ Contraindications: Active PUD and hypersensitivity to ASA or NSAIDs
    ○ Precautions: May aggravate preexisting peptic ulcer disease; may worsen symptoms of asthma
    ○ Significant possible interactions: May potentiate effects of anticoagulants and sulfonylurea analogues
  - Clopidogrel 75 mg/d (3)[B]:
    ○ Can be used in patients who are allergic to ASA (3)[B]
    ○ Precautions: Thrombotic thrombocytopenic purpura (TTP) can occur and increases risk of bleeding when combined with aspirin.
    ○ May be very slightly more effective than aspirin alone (4)[B]; more expensive and more side effects than aspirin.

- Anticoagulation therapy:
  - Factor Xa Inhibitors (rivaroxaban, apixaban, dabigatran) (7)[B]:
    ○ Noninferior to warfarin in nonvalvular AF
    ○ Precautions: Avoid in CKD
    ○ Expensive
  - Warfarin (INR-adjusted dose) (3,8)[A]:
    ○ Contraindications: Intolerance/Allergy, active liver disease, active bleeding, pregnancy
    ○ Significant possible interactions: Antibiotics, antiepileptics, antifungals, and many others
    ASA 325 mg/d or ASA 81/clopidrigel 75 mg/d (3)[A]:
    ○ Patients who cannot take anticoagulation for reasons other than bleeding risk

nd Line
pidine (Ticlid): 250 mg PO b.i.d.:
 patients who cannot tolerate other agents
 ntraindications: Hypersensitivity, presence of
 atopoietic/hemostatic disorders, conditions
 ciated with bleeding, severe liver dysfunction
 utions: Neutropenia (0.8% severe), which is
 ible with cessation of the drug. Monitor
 counts every 2 weeks for first 3 months. TTP
 cur.
 nt possible interactions: Digoxin plasma
 creased 15%; theophylline half-life
 d from 8.6–12.2 hours

ISSUES FOR REFERRAL
- Neurology for ongoing workup and treatment
- Cardiology if cardiac cause suspected
- Vascular surgery if carotid endarterectomy appropriate

ADDITIONAL THERAPIES
- Secondary prevention of TIA should be initiated as noted above.
- Venous thromboembolism (VTE) prophylaxis
- Patients with TIA or ischemic stroke should be started on a statin (9,10)[A].
- BP should be reduced when appropriate after 24 hours. ACE inhibitors/thiazide have shown to be of benefit (9)[A].

SURGERY/OTHER PROCEDURES
- Consider carotid endarterectomy in patients with a high degree of carotid artery stenosis (9)[A].
- When CEA is indicated for patients with TIA, surgery within 2 weeks is reasonable if there are no contraindications to early revascularization (9)[B].

IN-PATIENT CONSIDERATIONS
Admission Criteria/Initial Stabilization
- Hospitalize if symptoms <72 hours and the following (11)[C]:
  - ABCD2 score of ≥3
  - ABCD2 score of 0–2 and uncertainty that diagnostic workup can be completed within 2 days as outpatient
  - ABCD2 score of 0–2 and evidence that indicates the patient's event was caused by focal ischemia
- Correct fluid and electrolyte imbalances.

Discharge Criteria
Consider safety at home if another incident occurs.

 ONGOING CARE

FOLLOW-UP RECOMMENDATIONS

PATIENT MONITORING
- Follow-up every 3 months for 1st year; then yearly.
- Close attention to recurrence or subsequent CVA

DIET
- As appropriate for underlying medical problems; see section on prevention.

PROGNOSIS
- The risk of stroke on the ipsilateral side within 90 days and cumulative thereafter is 10–20%.
- Frequency increases with the addition of multiple risk factors and severity of carotid stenosis.
- Patients with larger artery occlusion or cardioembolic etiology are at increased risk of recurrence.
- The major cause of death in the first 5 years is cardiac disease.

COMPLICATIONS
- Stroke
- Functional impairment

REFERENCES

1. Tsivgoulis G, Stamboulis E, Sharma VK. Multicenter external validation of the ABCD2 score in triaging TIA patients. *Neurology.* 2010;74:1351–1357.
2. Adams RJ, Albers G, Alberts MJ, e the AHA/ASA recommendations for Update to of stroke in patients with stroke and prevention ischemic attack. *Stroke.* 2008; 39(5):16 1652.
3. Lansberg MG, O'Donnell MJ, Khatri P, et al. Antithrombotic and thrombolytic therapy for ischemic stroke: Antithrombotic therapy and prevention of thrombosis, 9th ed.: American College of Chest Physicians Evidence-Based Clinical Practice Guidelines. *Chest.* 2012;141; e601S–e636S.
4. Albers GW, Amarenco P, Easton JD, et al. Antithrombotic and thrombolytic therapy for ischemic stroke: American College of Chest Physicians Evidence-Based Clinical Practice Guidelines (8th ed.). *Chest.* 2008;133: 630S–669S.
5. De Schryver EL, Algra A, van Gijn J. Dipyridamole for preventing stroke and other vascular events in patients with vascular disease. *Cochrane Database Syst Rev.* 2007;CD001820.
6. Yip S, Benavente O. Antiplatelet agents for stroke prevention. *Neurotherapeutics.* 2011;8(3): 475–487.
7. Nagarakanti R, Ellis CR. Dabigatran in clinical practice. *Clin Ther.* 2012;34(10):2051–2060.
8. Aguilar MI, Hart R, Pearce LA. Oral anticoagulants versus antiplatelet therapy for preventing stroke in patients with non-valvular atrial fibrillation and no history of stroke or transient ischemic attacks. *Cochrane Database Syst Rev.* 2007;CD006186.
9. Furie KL, Kasner SE, Adams RJ, et al. Guidelines for the prevention of stroke in patients with stroke or transient ischemic attack. A guideline for healthcare professionals from the American Heart Association/American Stroke Association. *Stroke.* 2011;42:227–276.
10. Manktelow BN, Potter JF. Interventions in the management of serum lipids for preventing stroke recurrence. *Cochrane Database Syst Rev.* 2009;CD002091.
11. Adams H, del Zoppo G, Alberts M, Bhatt D, et al. Guidelines for the early management of adults with ischemic stroke. *Circulation.* 2007;115 e478–e534.

 SEE ALSO

Algorithms: Stroke; TIA and Transient Neurologic Deficit

 CODES

ICD10
- G45.0 Vertebro-basilar artery syndrome
- G45.1 Carotid artery syndrome (hemispheric)
- G45.9 Transient cerebral ischemic attack, unspecified

CLINICAL PEARLS

- Primary/Secondary prevention is important, stressing smoking cessation, exercise, weight loss, limited ETOH intake, and control of HTN, hyperlipidemia, and diabetes.
- Antiplatelet therapy (e.g., aspirin or clopidogrel or aspirin-dipyridamole) should be initiated.
- Warfarin should be initiated in patients with atrial fibrillation or cardioembolic risk factors.
- A 30% risk of stroke exists within 5 years of a TIA.

T

TRANSIENT STRESS CARDIOMYOPATHY

Timothy Fitzgibbons, MD, PhD • Gerard P. Aurigemma, MD

BASICS

DESCRIPTION
- Transient stress cardiomyopathy (TSC) is a unique cause of reversible left ventricle (LV) dysfunction with a clinical presentation indistinguishable from the acute coronary syndromes (ACS), particularly ST-segment elevation myocardial infarction (MI).
- Typically, the patient is a postmenopausal woman who presents with acute chest pain or dyspnea after an identifiable "trigger" (i.e., an acute emotional or physiologic stressor).
- 1st reported by authors from Japan (1,2), TSC was known initially as the *takotsubo syndrome* because the typical LV morphology (i.e., apical ballooning) resembled that of a Japanese octopus trap or *takotsubo*.
- Presenting clinical features include:
  - Chest symptoms and/or dyspnea
  - ECG changes, including ST-segment elevations or diffuse T-wave inversions
  - Mild elevation in cardiac biomarkers (creatine kinase [CK], troponin)
  - Transient wall motion abnormalities that may involve the base, midportion, and/or lateral walls of the LV
  - The apex of the right ventricle (RV) may be affected in up to 25% of cases (3).
- Clinical features may vary on a case-by-case basis, and formal diagnostic criteria have not been established.
- Authors from the Mayo Clinic have proposed that 3 of the 4 following criteria establish the diagnosis (4):
  - Transient akinesis or dyskinesis of the LV apical and midventricular segments with regional wall motion abnormalities extending beyond a single epicardial vascular distribution
  - Absence of obstructive coronary artery disease (CAD) or angiographic evidence of acute plaque rupture
  - New ECG abnormalities, either ST-segment elevation or T-wave inversion
  - Absence of:
    - Recent significant head trauma
    - Intracranial bleeding
    - Pheochromocytoma
    - Obstructive epicardial CAD
    - Myocarditis
    - Hypertrophic cardiomyopathy
- Synonym(s) (5): Takotsubo cardiomyopathy; Apical ballooning syndrome; Stress cardiomyopathy; Broken heart syndrome; Ampulla cardiomyopathy

EPIDEMIOLOGY
Incidence
- TSC accounts for a small percentage (1–3%) of ACS (5).
- In a recent prospective evaluation of patients admitted to the ICU, as many as 28% had apical ballooning, often in association with sepsis (5).
- Predominant sex: 82–100% of cases occur in women (4).
- Predominant age: Mean age of patients is 62–75 years.

Prevalence
2.2% of patients presenting to a referral hospital with ST-segment MIs were found to have TSC (4).

ETIOLOGY AND PATHOPHYSIOLOGY
- The exact pathophysiology is not known.
- It has been speculated that overwhelming activation of the sympathetic nervous system incites a cascade of events, including:
  - Catecholamine-induced LV dysfunction: "Biased agonism" of epinephrine for β2AR receptors, located predominantly at the cardiac apex (6).
  - Endothelial dysfunction and vasospasm: Prolonged TIMI frame counts and diffuse multivessel spasm have been observed in the acute phase, but more recent studies do not support this mechanism.
  - Cellular metabolic injury:
    - Myocardial norepinephrine release
    - Calcium overload
    - Contraction band necrosis

Genetics
No genetic associations have been described to date.

RISK FACTORS
- Female sex
- Postmenopausal state
- Emotional stress (i.e., argument, death of family member)
- Physiologic stress (i.e., acute medical illness)

COMMONLY ASSOCIATED CONDITIONS
Death from TSC is rare, and most cases resolve rapidly, within 2–3 days. Reported complications include:
- Left-sided heart failure
- Pulmonary edema
- Cardiogenic shock and hemodynamic compromise
- Dynamic LV outflow tract gradient complicated by hypotension
- Mitral regurgitation
- Ventricular arrhythmias
- LV thrombus formation
- LV free wall rupture
- Death (rare, 0–8%)

DIAGNOSIS

Because TSC often is indistinguishable from an ACS, it should be treated initially as such:
- Activate emergency medical services or report to emergency department.
- Oxygen, IV access, and ECG monitoring
- Urgent cardiology consultation

HISTORY
- Exposure to a "trigger event":
  - Emotional stress: Argument, death of family member, divorce, public speaking, etc.
  - Physiologic stress: Acute medical condition such as head trauma, asthma attack, seizure, etc.
- Acute onset of dyspnea or chest pain
- Palpitations
- Syncope

PHYSICAL EXAM
Exam may be unremarkable or may include any of the following:
- Tachypnea
- Tachycardia
- Hypotension
- Jugular venous distension
- Bibasilar rales
- S_3 gallop
- Systolic ejection murmur due to dynamic LV outflow tract gradient
- Holosystolic murmur of mitral regurgitation

DIFFERENTIAL DIAGNOSIS
- Acute ST-segment elevation MI
- Pulmonary embolism
- Myopericarditis
- Pheochromocytoma
- Hypertrophic cardiomyopathy
- Subarachnoid hemorrhage or stroke

DIAGNOSTIC TESTS & INTERPRETATION
- ECG should be done urgently and may show:
  - Diffuse ST-segment elevations
  - Diffuse and often dramatic T-wave inversions
  - QTc interval prolongation
  - Q waves
- Laboratory tests typically reveal a mild elevation in cardiac biomarkers, such as:
  - CK (rarely >500 U/mL)
  - Troponin I
  - B-type natriuretic peptide
- Chest radiograph:
  - Cardiomegaly
  - Pulmonary edema
- Echocardiogram:
  - Reduced LV systolic function
  - Abnormal diastolic function, including evidence of increased filling pressures
  - Regional wall motion abnormalities in 1 of the following patterns:
    - Classic or "takotsubo-type" ballooning of the apex with a hypercontractile base
    - "Reverse takotsubo": Apical hypercontractility with basal akinesis
    - "Midventricular" akinesis with apical and basal hypercontractility
    - Focal or localized akinesis of an isolated segment
  - Dynamic intracavitary LV gradient
  - Mitral regurgitation
  - Variable involvement of the right ventricle
- Cardiac MRI:
  - Reduced LV function
  - Wall motion abnormalities as described transthoracic echocardiography
  - Absence of delayed hyperenhancement gadolinium

Sec
- Tick
  - Fo
  - Co
  her
  ass
  - Prec
  rever
  blood
  can oc
  - Signific
  levels c
  increase

Diagnostic Procedures/Other

- Because ST-segment elevation MI is the diagnosis of exclusion, patients typically are referred for urgent cardiac catheterization.
- Coronary angiography:
  – Nonocclusive CAD
  – Rarely, epicardial coronary spasm
  – Endothelial dysfunction, as measured by fractional flow reserve or TIMI frame counts
- Left-sided heart catheterization: Increased LV end-diastolic pressure
- Ventriculography: Wall motion abnormalities as described for transthoracic echocardiography
- Right-sided heart catheterization:
  – Increased pulmonary capillary wedge pressure
  – Secondary pulmonary hypertension
  – Increased right ventricular filling pressures
  – Reduced cardiac output or cardiogenic shock (cardiac index <2 and mean arterial pressure [MAP] <60 mm Hg)

Test Interpretation

Characteristic pathologic findings of involved myocardium have not been described.

TREATMENT

- Activation of emergency medical services
- Advanced cardiac life support therapies as needed
- Oxygen
- IV access
- ECG monitoring

MEDICATION

After diagnostic cardiac catheterization, empirical treatment goals are:

- Management of hypotension: Differentiation between cardiogenic shock or dynamic LV cavity gradient
- Management of increased filling pressures and congestive states
- Attenuation of sympathetic drive

First Line

- Consideration should be given to β-blockers in all patients (e.g., metoprolol 12.5–75 mg PO b.i.d. or carvedilol 6.25–25 mg PO b.i.d.) if tissue perfusion is adequate.
- If there is evidence of congestive heart failure (CHF) or pulmonary edema, consider:
  – Furosemide: 20–40 mg IV b.i.d. as needed to reduce LV filling pressures and dyspnea
  – ACE inhibitors: Lisinopril 10–40 mg/d PO or equivalent

Second Line

Short-term anticoagulation should be considered in patients with severely reduced LV function to prevent LV thrombus formation. Unfractionated heparin 80 U/kg IV bolus followed by 18 U/kg/hr IV or Lovenox 1 mg/kg SC b.i.d.

ISSUES FOR REFERRAL

All patients with TSC generally should be co-managed with cardiology while inpatient and referred to cardiology as an outpatient.

ADDITIONAL THERAPIES

- Urgent cardiology consultation and consideration of cardiac catheterization
- Hypotension may require:
  – Vasopressors (e.g., dopamine or Levophed) if there is no LV outflow tract gradient
  – Phenylephrine and IV fluids to increase afterload in the presence of an LV outflow tract gradient
  – Cardiogenic shock that is not due to an LV outflow tract gradient may require placement of an intraaortic balloon pump.

IN-PATIENT CONSIDERATIONS

Admission Criteria/Initial Stabilization

- 12-lead ECG
- Chest radiograph
- Laboratory testing
- Echocardiography
- Patients with TSC usually are admitted for observation because the differential diagnosis includes ACS.

IV Fluids

Normal saline infusion to support BP, if necessary, and no evidence of heart failure

Discharge Criteria

Generally considered after exclusion of ACS and resolution of:

- Congestive state
- Hypotension
- Profound impairments of systolic function

ONGOING CARE

FOLLOW-UP RECOMMENDATIONS

- Impairments in systolic function typically resolve in 2–3 days, but may last as long as 1 month.
- Patients should follow-up with cardiology and serial echocardiography to document improved LV function.

PROGNOSIS

- Prognosis is excellent. Inpatient mortality is rare and ranges from 0–8%.
- Recurrence is rare; it also has been reported in 0–8% of patients.

REFERENCES

1. Dote K, Sato H, Tateishi H, et al. [Myocardial stunning due to simultaneous multivessel coronary spasms: A review of 5 cases]. *J Cardiol*. 1991;21:203–214.
2. Tsuchihashi K, Ueshima K, Uchida T, et al. Transient left ventricular apical ballooning without coronary artery stenosis: A novel heart syndrome mimicking acute myocardial infarction. Angina pectoris—Myocardial Infarction Investigations in Japan. *J Am Coll Cardiol*. 2001;38:11–18.
3. Fitzgibbons TP, Madias C, Seth A, et al. Prevalence and clinical characteristics of right ventricular dysfunction in transient stress cardiomyopathy. *Am J Cardiol*. 2009;104:133–136.
4. Bybee KA, Kara T, Prasad A, et al. Systematic review: Transient left ventricular apical ballooning: A syndrome that mimics ST-segment elevation myocardial infarction. *Ann Intern Med*. 2004;141:858–865.
5. Aurigemma GP. Acute stress cardiomyopathy and reversible left ventricular dysfunction. *Cardiol Rounds*. 2006;10(10). http://www.cardiologyrounds.org/crus/cardus1206.pdf
6. Paur H, Wright PT, Sikkel MB, et al. High levels of circulating epinephrine trigger apical cardiodepression in a β2-adrenergic receptor/Gi dependent manner: A new model of takotsubo cardiomyopathy. *Circulation*. 2012; 126: 697–706.

ADDITIONAL READING

- Bybee KA, Prasad A. Stress-related cardiomyopathy syndromes. *Circulation*. 2008;118:397–409.
- Madias C, Fitzgibbons TP, Alsheikh-Ali AA, et al. Acquired long QT syndrome from stress cardiomyopathy is associated with ventricular arrhythmias and torsades de pointes. *Heart Rhythm*. 2011;8:555–561.
- Wittstein IS, Thiemann DR, Lima JA, et al. Neurohumoral features of myocardial stunning due to sudden emotional stress. *N Engl J Med*. 2005;352:539–548.

 SEE ALSO

Algorithm: Chest Pain/Acute Coronary Syndrome

 CODES

ICD10

I51.81 Takotsubo syndrome

CLINICAL PEARLS

- TSC is a cause of reversible LV dysfunction with a clinical presentation indistinguishable from the ACSs, particularly ST-segment elevation MI.
- Echocardiography may strongly suggest the diagnosis.
- Treatment is supportive and should include β-blockers in most patients, and diuretics and ACE inhibitors in patients with CHF.

TRICHOMONIASIS

Adriana C. Linares, MD, MPH, DrPH

BASICS

DESCRIPTION
- Sexually transmitted urogenital infection caused by a pear-shaped, parasitic protozoan
- A cause of nongonococcal urethritis (NGU) in men
- System(s) affected: Genitourinary
- Synonym(s): Trich; Trichomonal urethritis

EPIDEMIOLOGY
Incidence
- Affects >120 million women worldwide
- Estimated 7.4 million new cases annually in the US among men and women
- 10–25% of vaginal infections
- 1–17% of cases of NGU; reported prevalence rates among men without urethritis have ranged from 0–8%.
- Predominant age: Young and middle-aged adults:
  – Rare until onset of sexual activity
  – Not uncommon in postmenopausal women; age is not protective, and long-term carriage is possible.
- Predominant sex: Male = Female, but women are more commonly symptomatic.

Pediatric Considerations
Rare in prepubertal children; confirmed diagnosis should raise concern of sexual abuse

Prevalence
- 2.3% of young adults:
  – 2.8% of women
  – 1.7% of men
- 3.1% of all US women
- Racial disparity exists (1):
  – 1.3% of white, non-Hispanic women
  – 1.8% of Mexican American women
  – 13.3% of black, non-Hispanic women

ETIOLOGY AND PATHOPHYSIOLOGY
- *Trichomonas vaginalis*: A pear-shaped, flagellated, parasitic protozoan
- Grows best at 35–37°C in anaerobic conditions at pH of 5.5–6
- STI
- Transmission via a nonvenereal route is possible because the organism survives for several hours in a moist environment.

Genetics
No known genetic considerations

RISK FACTORS
- Multiple sexual partners
- Unprotected intercourse
- Lower socioeconomic status
- Other STIs
- Untreated partner with previous infection

GENERAL PREVENTION
- Use of male or female condoms
- Reducing exposure by limiting numbers of partners
- Male circumcision may be protective (2).

COMMONLY ASSOCIATED CONDITIONS
- Other STIs, including HIV
- Bacterial vaginosis

DIAGNOSIS

HISTORY
- Women:
  – Yellow–green, malodorous vaginal discharge
  – Vulvovaginal pruritus
  – Dysuria
  – 50–75% are asymptomatic.
- Men:
  – Dysuria
  – Urethral discharge
  – 80% are asymptomatic.

PHYSICAL EXAM
- Women:
  – Vaginal erythema
  – Yellow–green, frothy, malodorous vaginal discharge
  – Petechiae on cervix (strawberry cervix; seen in ~10% of patients)
  – Basic medium: usually pH >4.5; however, it is not very specific since pH is also elevated in BV
- Men: Penile discharge, spontaneous and with expression

DIFFERENTIAL DIAGNOSIS
- Women (other vaginitides):
  – Bacterial vaginosis
  – Vaginal candidiasis
  – Chlamydial infection
  – Gonorrheal infection
  – Mixed vaginitis
- Men (other urethritides):
  – Chlamydial infection
  – Gonorrheal infection

DIAGNOSTIC TESTS & INTERPRETATION
Initial Tests (lab, imaging)
- Wet mount of vaginal or urethral discharge (3)[A]: Direct visualization of motile trichomonads:
  – Sensitivity: 60–70%
  – Specificity: 99.8%
- Gram stain
- Culture: Sensitivity: >95%; can take 4–7 days:
  – ELISA and direct fluorescent antibody tests: Sensitivity of 80–90%
  – Rapid diagnostic kits using polymerase chain reaction DNA probes: Sensitivity, 97%; specificity, 98%

Follow-Up Tests & Special Considerations
Detection on Papanicolaou smear (3)[A]:
- Sensitivity: 57–98%
- Specificity: 97%

Diagnostic Procedures/Other
Detection on self-obtained sample

TREATMENT

- Symptomatic individuals require treatment.
- Asymptomatic partners should be treated presumptively.
- Complete screening for other STIs, including HIV, gonorrhea, chlamydia, syphilis, hepatitis B, and hepatitis C, should be considered part of required treatment.
- Patients should abstain from sexual intercourse during treatment and until they are asymptomatic.

GENERAL MEASURES
If metronidazole resistance is suspected, use tinidazole.

MEDICATION
First Line
- Metronidazole: 2 g PO, 1 dose (4)[A]
- Metronidazole: 1.5 g PO, 1 dose:
  – FDA pregnancy risk Category B
  – American Association of Pediatrics recommends abstaining from breastfeeding during treatment and for 12–24 hours after last dose, but this is an old recommendation not supported by current evidence (5).
- Tinidazole: 2 g PO, 1 dose:
  – FDA pregnancy risk Category C
  – Abstain from breastfeeding during treatment and for 3 days after the dose.

Second Line
- Only if still symptomatic after initial treatment
- Metronidazole: 500 mg PO b.i.d. for 7 days (4)[A]

Pregnancy Considerations
Metronidazole is effective against a trichomoniasis infection during pregnancy, but may increase the risk of preterm and low-birth-weight babies (6)[A].

ISSUES FOR REFERRAL
- Multidrug-resistant organism
- Patient allergy to metronidazole: Desensitization to metronidazole is possible.

ADDITIONAL THERAPIES
- Men:
  – None currently available in the US
- Women (4)[A]:
  – Clotrimazole: 100 mg PO b.i.d. for 7 days
  – Sulfanilamide-aminacrine-allantoin vaginal suppositories b.i.d. for 7 days
  – Nonoxynol 9
  – Povidone-iodine douche

COMPLEMENTARY AND ALTERNATIVE MEDICINE

Not sufficiently investigated to be recommended

IN-PATIENT CONSIDERATIONS

Admission Criteria/Initial Stabilization

Admission may be necessary for resistant organisms because IV therapy provides higher tissue concentrations.

Discharge Criteria

Clearance of infection

 ONGOING CARE

FOLLOW-UP RECOMMENDATIONS

- If symptoms persist after initial treatment, reculture and/or repeat wet mount.
- No need for test of cure in asymptomatic individuals (4)[A].

DIET

Abstain from alcohol while being treated with 5-nitroimidazole derivatives, such as metronidazole, due to disulfiramlike reaction.

PATIENT EDUCATION

Educate about the sexually transmitted aspect of the infection:

- Inform partner so that partner can be treated.
- Discuss safe sex during health maintenance visits.
- Abstain from intercourse while undergoing treatment; use condoms if abstention is not feasible/possible.
- Avoid alcohol during treatment with metronidazole or tinidazole.
- Condom use can prevent recurrence.

PROGNOSIS

- Excellent
- Usually treated after 1 course, but increasing number of metronidazole-resistant cases

COMPLICATIONS

Pregnancy Considerations

Linked to low birth weight, preterm/premature rupture of membranes, and preterm birth (6)

REFERENCES

1. Sutton M, Sternberg M, Koumans EH, et al. The prevalence of *Trichomonas vaginalis* infection among reproductive-age women in the United States, 2001–2004. *Clin Infect Dis*. 2007;45: 1319–1326.
2. Sobngwi-Tambekou J, Taljaard D, Nieuwoudt M, et al. Male circumcision and *Neisseria gonorrhoeae, Chlamydia trachomatis* and *Trichomonas vaginalis*: Observations after a randomised controlled trial for HIV prevention. *Sex Transm Infect*. 2009;85: 116–120.
3. Wiese W, Patel SR, Patel SC, et al. A meta-analysis of the Papanicolaou smear and wet mount for the diagnosis of vaginal trichomoniasis. *Am J Med*. 2000;108:301–308.
4. Forna F, Gülmezoglu AM. Interventions for treating trichomoniasis in women. *Cochrane Database Syst Rev*. 2003:CD000218.
5. Hale T. *Medications and mothers milk: A manual of lactational pharmacology (medications and mother's milk)*, 14th ed. Amarillo, TX: Pharmasoft Medical Pub, 2009.
6. Gülmezoglu AM, Azhar M. Interventions for trichomoniasis in pregnancy. *Cochrane Database Syst Rev*. 2011:CD000220. Epub 2011 May 11.

ADDITIONAL READING

- Allsworth JE, Ratner JA, Peipert JF, et al. Trichomoniasis and other sexually transmitted infections: Results from the 2001–2004 National Health and Nutrition Examination Surveys. *Sex Transm Dis*. 2009;36:738–744.
- Centers for Disease Control and Prevention, Workowski KA, Berman SM. Sexually transmitted diseases treatment guidelines, 2006. *MMWR Recomm Rep*. 2006;55:1–94.
- Centers for Disease Control and Prevention. Trichomoniasis. Available at: www.cdc.gov/std/trichomonas.

- Helms DJ, Mosure DJ, Secor WE, et al. Management of *Trichomonas vaginalis* in women with suspected metronidazole hypersensitivity. *Am J Obstet Gynecol*. 2008;198:370e1–370e7.
- Klebanoff MA, Carey JC, Hauth JC, et al. Failure of metronidazole to prevent preterm delivery among pregnant women with asymptomatic *Trichomonas vaginalis* infection. *N Engl J Med*. 2001;345: 487–493.
- McClelland RS, Sangare L, Hassan WM, et al. Infection with *Trichomonas vaginalis* increases the risk of HIV-1 acquisition. *J Infect Dis*. 2007;195: 698–702.
- Miller M, Liao Y, Gomez AM, et al. Factors associated with the prevalence and incidence of *Trichomonas vaginalis* infection among African American women in New York City who use drugs. *J Infect Dis*. 2008;197:503–509.
- Saperstein AK, Firnhaber GC. Clinical inquiries. Should you test or treat partners of patients with gonorrhea, chlamydia, or trichomoniasis? *J Fam Pract*. 2010;59:46–48.
- Wendel KA, Workowski KA. Trichomoniasis: Challenges to appropriate management. *Clin Infect Dis*. 2007;44(Suppl 3):S123–129.

 CODES

ICD10

- A59.01 Trichomonal vulvovaginitis
- A59.03 Trichomonal cystitis and urethritis
- A59.9 Trichomoniasis, unspecified

CLINICAL PEARLS

- Both partners need to be treated for trichomoniasis.
- Test of cure is unnecessary.
- Avoid alcohol during treatment with standard agents.
- Treatment does not reduce risk of adverse pregnancy outcomes.
- Male circumcision may be protective.

TRICHOTILLOMANIA

Carol Hustedde, PhD • William G. Elder, Jr., PhD

BASICS

- Trichotillomania (TTM) is a hair-pulling disorder characterized by self-induced, repeated, and often noticeable hair loss. It can become severe and difficult to control.
- TTM has been conceptualized as an anxiety disorder and as a disorder of habits. It is now classified as an impulse control disorder because many individuals experience a sense of relief or gratification once the hair is pulled.

DESCRIPTION

- TTM causes uncontrollable hair pulling from anywhere on the body, although the scalp is the most common area followed by the eyelashes, eyebrows, pubic/perirectal area, axilla, and face. It usually results in variable degrees of alopecia.
- TTM usually presents in childhood or early adolescence.
- Denial and hiding of hair pulling is common.
- Recurrence or worsened hair pulling is associated with increased stress/anxiety, but trichotillomania can also occur at times of relaxation and distraction, such as when reading.
- The 3 subtypes of trichotillomania: Early onset, automatic, and focused (1).
- When TTM is associated with trichophagia, it may also result in GI complaints secondary to bezoars.
- TTM has frequent comorbidity with other psychiatric diagnoses.

EPIDEMIOLOGY

- It is difficult to assess the exact number of individuals affected by trichotillomania because of the social stigma associated with it. Small studies have estimated a range of 1–3.5% for late adolescents and young adults (2).
- It is possible that up to 1 of 50 individuals are affected by TTM at least once in their lifetime.
- The mean age of onset is at 13 years.
- During childhood, males and females are equally affected by TTM. During adulthood, females are far more affected than males.

ETIOLOGY AND PATHOPHYSIOLOGY

- Serotonin deficiency
- Tension relief
- Habitual behavior
- There is currently a significant flux in the conceptualizations of the mechanisms and causes of impulse control, behavior, anxiety, and OCDs. Brain imaging, and biochemical and neuropsychological studies should help to resolve this issue. It can be expected that there will be increased differentiation as well as redefinitions of disorders that are based on neurophysiology and brain circuitry.

Genetics

Genetics appears to contribute to the development of TTM, as demonstrated by a higher rate of concordance in monozygotic twins (38.1%) vs. dizygotic twins (0%) (3). Genetic involvement is multifaceted and not clearly understood at this time (4).

RISK FACTORS

- Positive family history
- Other psychiatric disorders: Depression, obsessive–compulsive disorder (OCD), anxiety, posttraumatic stress disorder (PTSD), eating disorders, nail biting, skin picking

COMMONLY ASSOCIATED CONDITIONS

- Depression
- Anxiety
- Impulse control disorder
- OCD
- Eating disorders

DIAGNOSIS

- Trichotillomania may be difficult to diagnose because individuals may deny it because of the social stigma and embarrassment (5)[C].
- Several TTM-specific assessment tools have been developed that further understanding about psychopathology of TTM (6).
- Assessment should include multiple sources of information to provide understanding of TTM in context (7)[C].

HISTORY

- TTM most commonly manifests as hair pulling from any part of the body, resulting in alopecia of variable severity.
- The scalp is the most common area from which hair is pulled, but can also involve other parts of the body, such as eyebrows and eyelashes.
- Individuals may deny the hair pulling because of embarrassment, making it hard to diagnose because the hair pulling may be done in private and is unwitnessed by others (7)[C].
- TTM may also cause social isolation because individuals may withdraw from friends and family to engage in hair-pulling behavior.
- If TTM is associated with trichophagia (compulsive eating of hair), it may present with various GI symptoms with variable severity, from acute generalized abdominal pain to a bowel obstruction secondary to a trichobezoar.
- TTM is not always associated with anxiety and stress, but it is commonly precipitated by highly stressful situations. The action of hair pulling may be associated with tension relief.

PHYSICAL EXAM

- The most common manifestation of TTM is alopecia.
- The severity of the alopecia is variable, from isolated areas of hair loss to complete baldness.
- Hair loss can be from any part of the body.
- The Friar Tuck sign may be seen, which consists of hair loss seen in a circular pattern with varying lengths of broken hairs (8)[C].
- There is also a lack of dermatologic abnormalities associated with the hair loss.
- In addition to the hair loss, hair abnormalities consisting of damaged hair follicles, broken hairs of varying lengths
- When TTM is associated with trichophagia and, consequently, trichobezoars, there may be symptoms of abdominal pain, nausea, vomiting, obstructive jaundice, bowel obstruction symptoms, and anemia (7)[C].
- Patients with TTM may also pull hairs from other people and pets, sometimes surreptitiously. They may also pull fibers from carpets and fabrics.

DIFFERENTIAL DIAGNOSIS

- Alopecia areata
- Tinea capitis
- Traction alopecia
- Loose anagen syndrome
- OCD
- Schizophrenia or other psychotic disorders
- Stereotypic movement disorders
- Factitious behaviors

DIAGNOSTIC TESTS & INTERPRETATION

US or CT scan for trichobezoar detection

Diagnostic Procedures/Other

- Trichotillomania Scale for Children
- Trichotillomania Diagnostic Interview
- National Institute of Mental Health Trichotillomania Questionnaire
- Premonitory Urge for Tics Scale

Test Interpretation

- Punch biopsy: High frequency of telogen hairs; deformed, noninflamed catagen hairs; melanin pigment casts
- Trichogram
- Referrals:
  - Some diagnostic procedures may require a dermatology referral. In the presence of missing hair follicles or other hair disorder, a dermatology consult will allow for visual and/or microscopic (trichogram) analysis to determine structure and cycle of the hair disorder.
  - A referral to a psychiatrist, psychologist, or psychopharmacologist who specializes in impulse control and OCD may be helpful. He or she will have access to the specialized symptoms scales described above and also is likely to have professional relationships with psychotherapists who can provide specific therapies, such as habit–reversal training. Such referral may also allow for stepped treatment including aggressive use of SSRIs and other antidepressants with combinations of 2nd-line pharmacologic options sometimes tried for impulse control and OCD disorders.

TREATMENT

Treatment of TTM involves both pharmacologic treatment and psychological methods that include specific psychotherapies, support groups, and combined approaches.

MEDICATION
First Line
- SSRIs remain the first-line pharmacologic option, with a dosing strategy similar to that for OCD.
- SSRIs:
  – Fluoxetine (Prozac): 20–80 mg/d
  – Sertraline (Zoloft): 50–200 mg/d
  – Paroxetine (Paxil): 10–50 mg/d
  – Citalopram (Celexa): 20–60 mg/d
  – Escitalopram (Lexapro): 10–20 mg/d

Second Line
- Tricyclic antidepressants
- Atypical antipsychotics
- Opioid blockers
- Glutamate modulators

ADDITIONAL THERAPIES
Psychological treatment of TTM may be the primary treatment and is almost always needed in addition to medications.
- Habit-reversal training:
  – Habit-reversal training is a behavioral therapy that is effective in reducing troublesome behaviors associated with impulse control disorders. It consists of 4 main components: Awareness training, development of a competing response, building motivation, and generalization of skills
- Relaxation training (when stress is high)
- Support groups to deal with stigma and denial
- Treatment of comorbid psychiatric condition
- Unlikely to be helpful:
  – Undifferentiated, nonspecific psychotherapy
  – Hypnosis
  – Acupuncture
- A nutritional supplement, N-Acetylcysteine (1,200–2,400 mg/d), shows some benefit (9)[C].

SURGERY/OTHER PROCEDURES
Surgery is only warranted for removal of trichobezoars.

IN-PATIENT CONSIDERATIONS
Inpatient admission is usually not due to TTM itself, but either treatment of comorbid psychiatric conditions or a bowel obstruction secondary to trichobezoar.

 ONGOING CARE

DIET
No special diet required for trichotillomania

PATIENT EDUCATION
- Trichotillomania is a multifactorial condition. Not only do medications aid in the treatment of TTM, but psychological therapies have a benefit as well.
- Online resource: www.trich.org

PROGNOSIS
TTM tends to be a chronic disorder; however, it can be transient in childhood.

COMPLICATIONS
- Trichobezoars
- Alopecia

REFERENCES
1. Duke DC, Keeley ML, Geffken GR, et al. Trichotillomania: A current review. *Clin Psychol Rev*. 2010;30:181–193.
2. Christenson GA, Pyle RL, Mitchell JE. Estimated lifetime prevalence of trichotillomania in college students. *J Clin Psychiatry*. 1991;52(10):415–417.
3. Novak CE, Keuthen NJ, Stewart SE, et al. A twin concordance study of trichotillomania. *Am J Med Genet B Neuropsychiatr Genet*. 2009;150B(7):944–949.
4. Chatterjee K. The genetic factors influencing the development of trichotillomania. *J Genet*. 2011;90:259–262.
5. Tolin DF, Franklin ME, Diefenbach GJ, et al. Pediatric trichotillomania: Descriptive psychopathology and an open trial of cognitive behavioral therapy. *Cogn Behav Ther*. 2007;36(3):129–144.
6. Harrison JP, Franklin ME. Pediatric trichotillomania. *Curr Psychiatry Rep*. 2012;14(3):188–196.
7. Franklin ME, Zagrabbe K, Benavides KL, et al. Trichotillomania and its treatment: A review and recommendations. *Expert Rev Neurother*. 2011;11:1165–1174.
8. Springer K, Brown M, Stulberg DL, et al. Common hair loss disorders. *Am Fam Physician*. 2003;68:93–102.
9. Grant J, Odlaug B, Kim S. N-Acetylcysteine, a glutamate modulator in the treatment of trichotillomania. *Arch Gen Psychiatry*. 2009;66(7):756–763.

ADDITIONAL READING
Trichotillomania Learning Center: www.trich.org. Expert Consensus Guidelines on Treatment of TTM and Skin Picking at http://www.trich.org/dnld/ExpertGuidelines_000.pdf.

 CODES

ICD10
F63.3 Trichotillomania

CLINICAL PEARLS
- Etiology of TTM is multifactorial and differs among individuals. It is important to distinguish between different etiologies.
- Patients may benefit from both medications and psychotherapy.
- It is important to realize that TTM is underreported and underdiagnosed because of the social stigma.
- TTM can have a significant impact on psychological, social, academic, and occupational functions.

TRIGEMINAL NEURALGIA
Noah M. Rosenberg, MD • Stacy Potts, MD, MEd

 BASICS

DESCRIPTION
- Disorder of the sensory nucleus of the trigeminal nerve (cranial nerve [CN] V) that produces episodic, paroxysmal, severe, lancinating facial pain lasting seconds to minutes in the distribution of ≥1 divisions of the nerve
- Often precipitated by stimulation of well-defined, ipsilateral trigger zones: Usually perioral, perinasal, and, occasionally, intraoral (e.g., by washing, shaving)
- System(s) affected: Nervous
- Synonym(s): Tic douloureux; Fothergill neuralgia; Trifacial neuralgia; Prosopalgia

EPIDEMIOLOGY
Incidence
- Women: 5.9/100,000/yr
- Men: 3.4/100,000/yr
- >70 years of age: ~25.6/100,000/yr
- Predominant age:
  - >50 years; incidence increases with age
  - Rare <35 years of age (consider another primary disease; see "Etiology").
- Predominant sex: Female > Male (~2:1)

Prevalence
16/100,000

Pediatric Considerations
Unusual during childhood

Pregnancy Considerations
Teratogenicity limits therapy for 1st and 2nd trimesters.

ETIOLOGY AND PATHOPHYSIOLOGY
- Demyelination around the compression site seems to be the mechanism by which compression of nerves leads to symptoms.
- Demyelinated lesions may set up an ectopic impulse generation causing erratic responses: Hyperexcitability of damaged nerves and transmission of action potentials along adjacent, undamaged, unstimulated sensory fibers.
- Compression of trigeminal nerve by anomalous arteries or veins of posterior fossa, compressing trigeminal root
- Etiologic classification:
  - Idiopathic (classic)
  - Secondary: Cerebellopontine angle tumors (e.g., meningioma); tumors of CN V (e.g., neuroma, vascular malformations), trauma, demyelinating disease (e.g., multiple sclerosis [MS])

RISK FACTORS
Unknown

COMMONLY ASSOCIATED CONDITIONS
- Sjögren syndrome; Rheumatoid arthritis
- Chronic meningitis
- Acute polyneuropathy
- MS
- Hemifacial spasm
- Charcot-Marie-Tooth neuropathy
- Glossopharyngeal neuralgia

 DIAGNOSIS

HISTORY
Paroxysms of pain in the distribution of the trigeminal nerve

PHYSICAL EXAM
All exam findings typically are negative due to the paroxysmal nature of the disorder.

DIFFERENTIAL DIAGNOSIS
- Other forms of neuralgia usually have sensory loss. Presence of sensory loss nearly excludes the diagnosis of TN (if younger patient, frequently MS).
- Neoplasia in cerebellopontine angle
- Vascular malformation of brain stem
- Demyelinating lesion (MS is diagnosed in 2–4% of patients with trigeminal neuralgia.)
- Vascular insult
- Migraine, cluster headache
- Giant cell arteritis
- Postherpetic neuralgia
- Chronic meningitis
- Acute polyneuropathy
- Atypical odontalgia
- SUNCT syndrome (short-lasting, unilateral, neuralgiform pain with conjunctival injection, and tearing)

DIAGNOSTIC TESTS & INTERPRETATION
- The International Headache Society diagnostic criteria for classic trigeminal neuralgia (TN):
  - Paroxysmal attacks of pain lasting from a fraction of 1 second to 2 minutes, affecting ≥1 divisions of the trigeminal nerve
  - Pain has at least an intense, sharp, superficial, or stabbing characteristic or is precipitated from trigger areas or by trigger factors.
  - Attacks are stereotyped in the individual patient.
  - No clinically evident neurologic deficit found.
  - Not attributed to another disorder
- Secondary trigeminal neuralgia is characterized by pain that is indistinguishable from classic TN but is caused by a demonstrable structural lesion other than vascular compression.
  - Indicated in all 1st-time presenting patients to rule out secondary causes
- MRI vs. CT scan: MRI, with and without contrast, offers more detailed imaging and is preferred, if not contraindicated.
- Routine head imaging identifies structural causes in up to 15% of patients.
- No positive findings are significantly correlated with diagnosis.

Test Interpretation
- Trigeminal nerve: Inflammatory changes, demyelination, and degenerative changes
- Trigeminal ganglion: Hypermyelination and microneuromata

 TREATMENT

GENERAL MEASURES
- Outpatient
- Drug treatment is 1st approach.
- Invasive procedures are reserved for patients who cannot tolerate, fail to respond to, or relapse after chronic drug treatment.
- Avoid stimulation (e.g., air, heat, cold) of trigger zones, including lips, cheeks, and gums.

MEDICATION
First Line
- Carbamazepine (Tegretol) (1,2)[A]: Start at 100–200 mg b.i.d.; effective dose usually 200 mg q.i.d.; max dose 1,200 mg/d:
  - 70–90% of patients respond initially.
  - By 3 years, 30% are no longer helped (number needed to treat [NNT] = 1.7) (1)[A]
  - Most common side effect: Sedation
- Contraindications: Concurrent use of monoamine oxidase inhibitors (MAOIs)
- Precautions: Caution in the presence of liver disease
- Significant possible medication interactions: Macrolide antibiotics, oral anticoagulants, anticonvulsants, tricyclics, oral contraceptives, steroids, digitalis, isoniazid, MAOIs, methyprylon, nabilone, nizatidine, other H_2 blockers, phenytoin, propoxyphene, benzodiazepines, and calcium channel blockers
- Oxcarbazepine (Trileptal): Start at 150–300 mg b.i.d.; effective dose usually 375 mg b.i.d.; max dose 1,200 mg/d:
  - Efficacy similar to carbamazepine (2)[B],(3)[A]
  - Faster, with less drowsiness and fewer drug interactions than carbamazepine
  - Decreases serum sodium
  - Most common side effect: Sedation

Second Line
- Antiepileptic drugs: Insufficient evidence from randomized, controlled trials to show significant benefit from antiepileptic drugs in trigeminal neuralgia (4)[A]
- Phenytoin (Dilantin): 300–400 mg/d (synergistic with carbamazepine):
  - Potent P450 inducer (enhanced metabolism of many drugs)
  - Various CNS side effects (sedation, ataxia)
- Baclofen (Lioresal): 10–80 mg/d; start at 5–10 mg t.i.d. with food (as an adjunct to phenytoin or carbamazepine); side effects: Drowsiness, weakness, nausea, vomiting
- Gabapentin (Neurontin): Start at 100 mg t.i.d. or 300 mg at bedtime; can increase dose up to 300–600 mg t.i.d.–q.i.d. Can be used as monotherapy or in combination with other medications and reduces the cost of illness.
- Lamotrigine: Titrate up to 200 mg b.i.d. over weeks; side effect: 10% experience rash

- Chlorphenesin carbamate (Maolate): 800–2,400 mg/d (as an adjunct to phenytoin and/or carbamazepine); drowsiness is side effect
- Antidepressants, including amitriptyline, fluoxetine, trazodone:
  – Used especially with anticonvulsants
  – Particularly effective for atypical forms of trigeminal neuralgia
- Clonazepam (Klonopin) frequently causes drowsiness and ataxia.
- Sumatriptan (Imitrex) 3 mg SC reduces acute symptoms and may be helpful after failure of conventional medical therapy.
- Capsaicin cream topically
- Botulinum toxin injection into zygomatic arch
- Valproic acid (Depakene, Depakote)

ISSUES FOR REFERRAL
Initial treatment failure or positive findings on imaging studies

ADDITIONAL THERAPIES
- Radiotherapy
- Stereotactic radiosurgery, such as gamma knife radiosurgery, has been shown to be effective after drug failure:
  – Produces lesions with focused gamma knife radiation
  – Therapy aimed at the proximal trigeminal root
  – Minimal clinically effective dose: 70 Gy
  – ~60–80% of patients achieve complete relief within 1 year; by 3 years, ~40% maintain complete relief (NNT = 2.9) (5)[B].
  – Most common side effect: Sensory disturbance (corneal numbness)
  – Failure rates are higher in patients with past TN-related invasive procedures

SURGERY/OTHER PROCEDURES
- Microvascular decompression of CN V at its entrance to (or exit from) brain stem:
  – 98% of patients achieve initial pain relief; by 20 months, 86% maintain complete relief (NNT = 2) (6)[B].
  – Surgical mortality across studies was 0.3–0.4%.
  – Most common side effect: Transient facial numbness and diplopia, headache, nausea, vomiting
  – Pain relief after procedure strongly correlates with the type of TN pain: Type 1 (shocklike pain) results in better outcomes than type 2 (constant pain) (7).
- Peripheral nerve ablation (multiple methods):
  – Higher rates of failure and facial numbness than decompression surgery
  – Radiofrequency thermocoagulation
  – Neurectomy
  – Cryotherapy: High relapse rate
  – Partial sensory rhizotomy
- 4% tetracaine dissolved in 0.5% bupivacaine nerve block (only a few case reports to date; ropivacaine)
- Alcohol block or glycerol injection into trigeminal cistern: Unpredictable side effects (dysesthesia and anesthesia dolorosa); temporary relief
- Peripheral block or section of 5th nerve proximal to Gasserian ganglion
- Balloon compression of Gasserian ganglion
- Evidence supporting destructive procedures for benign pain conditions remains limited (8)[A].

COMPLEMENTARY AND ALTERNATIVE MEDICINE
Acupuncture, moxibustion (herb): Weak evidence for efficacy (9)[B]

 ONGOING CARE

FOLLOW-UP RECOMMENDATIONS
Regular outpatient follow-up to monitor symptoms and therapeutic failure

Patient Monitoring
- Carbamazepine and/or phenytoin serum levels
- If carbamazepine is prescribed: CBC and platelets at baseline, then weekly for a month, then monthly for 4 months, then every 6–12 months if dose is stable (regimens for monitoring vary)
- Reduce drugs after 4–6 weeks to determine whether condition is in remission; resume at previous dose if pain recurs. Withdraw drugs slowly after several months, again to check for remission or if lower dose of drugs can be tolerated.

DIET
No special diet

PATIENT EDUCATION
- Instruct patient regarding medication dosage and side effects, risk-to-benefit ratios of surgery or radiation therapy.
- Support organizations:
  – The Facial Pain Association (formerly the Trigeminal Neuralgia Association): www.fpa-support.org
  – Living with Trigeminal Neuralgia: www.livingwithtn.org

PROGNOSIS
- 50–60% eventually fail pharmacologic treatment (2)[B].
- After having microvascular decompression surgery, most patients wish they had undergone the procedure sooner (73%; NNT = 1.4) (10)[A].
- Of those, relapse is seen in ~50% of stereotactic radiosurgeries and ~27% of surgical microvascular decompressions (2)[B].

COMPLICATIONS
- Mental and physical sluggishness; dizziness with carbamazepine (2)
- Paresthesias and corneal reflex loss with stereotactic radiosurgery
- Surgical mortality and morbidity associated with microvascular decompression

REFERENCES
1. Wiffen PJ, Derry S, Moore RA, et al. Carbamazepine for acute and chronic pain in adults. *Cochrane Database Syst Rev.* 2011;(1):CD005451. Epub 2011 Jan 19.
2. Beniczky S, Tajti J, Tímea Varga E, et al. Evidence-based pharmacological treatment of neuropathic pain syndromes. *J Neural Transm.* 2005;112:735–749.
3. Attal N, Cruccu G, Baron R, et al. EFNS guidelines on the pharmacological treatment of neuropathic pain: 2010 revision. *Eur J Neurol.* 2010;17: 1113–e1188.
4. Yang M, Zhou M, He L, et al. Non-antiepileptic drugs for trigeminal neuralgia. *Cochrane Database Syst Rev.* 2011;1:CD004029.
5. Elaimy AL, Hanson PW, Lamoreaux WT, et al. Clinical outcomes of gamma knife radiosurgery in the treatment of patients with trigeminal neuralgia. *Int J Otolaryngol.* 2012;2012:919186. Epub 2011 Oct 25.
6. Sekula RF, Frederickson AM, Jannetta PJ, et al. Microvascular decompression for elderly patients with trigeminal neuralgia: A prospective study and systematic review with meta-analysis. *J Neurosurg.* 2011;114:172–179.
7. Miller JP, Acar F, Burchiel KJ, et al. Classification of trigeminal neuralgia: Clinical, therapeutic, and prognostic implications in a series of 144 patients undergoing microvascular decompression. *J Neurosurg.* 2009;111:1231–1234.
8. Zakrzewska JM, Akram H. Neurosurgical interventions for the treatment of classical trigeminal neuralgia. *Cochrane Database Syst Rev.* 2011;(9):CD007312. Epub 2011 Sep 7.
9. Liu H, Li H, Xu M, et al. A systematic review on acupuncture for trigeminal neuralgia. *Altern Ther Health Med.* 2010;16:30–35.
10. Cetas JS, Saedi T, Burchiel KJ. Destructive procedures for the treatment of nonmalignant pain: A structured literature review. *J Neurosurg.* 2008;109:389–404.

ADDITIONAL READING
Gronseth G, Cruccu G, Alksne J, et al. Practice parameter: The diagnostic evaluation and treatment of trigeminal neuralgia (an evidence-based review): Report of the Quality Standards Subcommittee of the American Academy of Neurology and the European Federation of Neurological Societies. *Neurology.* 2008;71:1183–1190.

 CODES

ICD10
G50.0 Trigeminal neuralgia

CLINICAL PEARLS
- Patients with TN typically have a normal physical exam.
- The long-term efficacy of pharmacotherapy for TN is 40–50%.
- If pharmacotherapy fails, stereotactic radiosurgery or surgical microvascular decompression often is successful.

TRIGGER FINGER (DIGITAL STENOSING TENOSYNOVITIS)

Alan M. Ehrlich, MD • Robert A. Yood, MD

 BASICS

DESCRIPTION
Trigger finger manifests in a clicking, snapping, or locking of a finger/thumb after full flexion ± associated pain.

EPIDEMIOLOGY
Incidence
- Adult population: 28/100,000/year:
  – Rare in children
- Diabetics have up to 4× the risk of the general population (1)[B].
- Predominant age:
  – Childhood form presents typically with thumb involvement in the 1st decade of life.
  – Adult form typically presents in the 5th and 6th decades of life.
- Predominant sex:
  – Children: Female = Male
  – Adults: Female > Male (6:1)

Prevalence
Lifetime prevalence in the general population is 2.6%.

Pediatric Considerations
- The thumb is more commonly involved in children (2)[C].
- When children have a trigger finger instead of a trigger thumb, surgery is often more complicated.
- Release of the A1 pulley alone is often insufficient, and other procedures may be necessary at the time of surgery.

ETIOLOGY AND PATHOPHYSIOLOGY
- Narrowing around the A1 pulley usually is due to either thickening from inflammation or protein deposits or thickening of the tendon per se; with prolonged inflammation, fibrocartilaginous metaplasia of the tendon sheath occurs.
- The flexor tendon may become distorted with nodule formation, which can give rise to the triggering because the nodule has difficulty passing through the tunnel under the A1 pulley.
- Because flexors are stronger than extensors, the finger can get stuck in the flexed position.
- Most cases are idiopathic, and no known prevention exists.
- No clear association with repetitive movements

RISK FACTORS
- Diabetes mellitus (DM)
- Rheumatoid arthritis (RA)
- Hypothyroidism
- Mucopolysaccharide disorders
- Amyloidosis

GENERAL PREVENTION
Most cases are idiopathic, and no known prevention exists. No clear association with repetitive movements

COMMONLY ASSOCIATED CONDITIONS
- De Quervain tenosynovitis
- Carpal tunnel syndrome
- Dupuytren contracture (usually occurs in 4th/5th digit; thickening of palmar connective tissue results in a flexion contracture of the distal digit)
- DM
- RA
- Hypothyroidism
- Amyloidosis

 DIAGNOSIS

Diagnosis is based on clinical presentation.

HISTORY
History of clicking, snapping, or locking of a finger/thumb after full flexion ± associated pain

PHYSICAL EXAM
- A palpable nodule may be present.
- Snapping/Locking may be present, but neither is necessary for the diagnosis.
- Tenderness to palpation is variable.

DIAGNOSTIC TESTS & INTERPRETATION
Test Interpretation
- Thickening of the A1 pulley with fibrocartilaginous metaplasia
- Thickening/Nodule formation of flexor tendon

 ONGOING CARE

FOLLOW-UP RECOMMENDATIONS
- Follow-up is needed only if symptoms persist or if complications of surgery develop.
- Splinting of the affected digit to minimize flexion/extension of the MCP joint can lead to resolution of symptoms (1)[B],(3)[C].

PROGNOSIS
Prognosis for resolution of symptoms is excellent with either conservative or surgical intervention. Recurrence following corticosteroid injection is more likely for patients with type 1 DM, younger age, involvement of multiple digits, and history of other upper-extremity tendinopathies (4)[C].

COMPLICATIONS
- Complications from surgery include infection, bleeding, digital nerve injury, and persistent pain and loss of range of motion of the affected finger. The rate of major complications is low (3%), but the rate of minor complications (including loss of range of motion) can be significantly higher (up to 28%) (5).
- Injury to the A2 pulley may result in bowstringing, which is a bulging of the flexor tendon in the palm with flexion. This can be associated with pain.
- Diabetic patients may have significantly increased blood sugar levels for up to 5 days following steroid injection.

 TREATMENT

- Splinting the metacarpophalangeal (MCP) joint at 10–15 degrees of flexion for 6 weeks with the distal joints free to move has been reported to be effective:
  – Splinting is more effective for treating fingers than thumbs (70% vs. 50%).
  – Less effective with severe symptoms, symptoms >6 months, and multiple digits involved (1)[B]
- Long-acting corticosteroids may be injected several times to achieve relief of symptoms, although subsequent injections often are less likely to work than the initial injection.
- Surgery has high success rate for patients unresponsive to splinting/corticosteroid injections.

GENERAL MEASURES

Splinting/Steroid injection should be tried before surgery. Splinting may be more effective for preventing recurrence than as initial treatment (6)[B].

MEDICATION

First Line

- Steroid injection of the tendon sheath/surrounding SC tissue has 57–90% success rate (4)[B],(7)[C].
- Injection in surrounding tissues is as efficacious as injecting into the tendon sheath (1,8)[B]. Injection into the palmar surface at the midproximal phalanx is associated with less pain than injection of tendon sheath at MCP joint (9)[B].
- Corticosteroid injection has higher success rate than splinting (6)[B]. Higher success rates are associated with a shorter duration of symptoms.

Second Line

- Oral NSAIDs may reduce pain and discomfort, but they have not been shown to reduce the underlying cause. They do not reduce symptoms of snapping/locking.
- Injection with diclofenac may be an alternative to corticosteroid for patients with diabetes mellitus where increase in blood sugar may be a concern.
- Corticosteroids appear more effective during the first 3 weeks postinjection but efficacy appears similar by 3 months post injection (10)[B].

ISSUES FOR REFERRAL

Refer to a hand surgeon if the patient is not responding to splinting and/or steroid injections.

ADDITIONAL THERAPIES

Physiotherapy has been used in the treatment of trigger digits in children.

SURGERY/OTHER PROCEDURES

- Surgical release can be done as an open procedure or percutaneously (11).
- Success rates with either procedure are very high; no apparent significant differences in terms of treatment success or rates of complications (11)[A].
- Most hand surgeons still prefer the open release because of concern about avoiding nerve injury with the blind procedure.

IN-PATIENT CONSIDERATIONS

Admission Criteria/Initial Stabilization

Day surgery for trigger finger release

Discharge Criteria

Absence of complications

REFERENCES

1. Akhtar S, Bradley MJ, Quinton DN. Management and referral for trigger finger/thumb. *BMJ.* 2005; 331:30–33.
2. Cardon LJ, Ezaki M, Carter PR. Trigger finger in children. *J Hand Surg Am.* 1999;84(6): 1156–1161.
3. Ryzewicz M, Wolf JM. Trigger digits: Principles, management, and complications. *J Hand Surg Am.* 2006;84(1):135–146.
4. Rozental TD, Zurakowski D, Blazar PE. Trigger finger: Prognostic indicators of recurrence following corticosteroid injection. *J Bone Joint Surg Am.* 2008;84(8):1665–1672.
5. Will R, Lubahn J. Complications of open trigger finger release. *J Hand Surg Am.* 2010;84(4):594–596. Epub 2010 Feb 26.
6. Salim N, Abdullah S, Sapuan J, et al. Outcome of corticosteroid injection versus physiotherapy in the treatment of mild trigger fingers. *J Hand Surg Eur* 2012;84(1):27–34.
7. Fleisch SB, Spindler KP, Lee DH. Corticosteroid injections in the treatment of trigger finger: A level I and II systematic review. *J Am Acad Orthop Surg.* 2007;84(3):166–171.
8. Kazuki K, Egi T, Okada M, et al. Clinical outcome of extrasynovial steroid injection for trigger finger. *Hand Surg.* 2006;84(1–2):1–4.
9. Pataradool K, Buranapuntaruk T. Proximal phalanx injection for trigger finger: Randomized controlled trial. *Hand Surg.* 2011;84(3):313–317.
10. Shakeel H, Ahmad TS. Steroid injection versus NSAID injection for trigger finger: A comparative study of early outcomes. *J Hand Surg Am.* 2012;37(7):1319–1323.
11. Wang J, Zhao JG, Liang CC. Percutaneous release, open surgery, or corticosteroid injection, which is the best treatment method for trigger digits? *Clin Orthop Relat Res.* 2013 Jun;471(6):1879–1886.

ADDITIONAL READING

- Moore JS. Flexor tendon entrapment of the digits (trigger finger and trigger thumb). *J Occup Environ Med.* 2000;42:5.
- Moore JS. Flexor tendon entrapment of the digits (trigger finger and trigger thumb). *J Occup Environ Med.* 2000;84(5):526–545.

CODES

ICD10

- M65.30 Trigger finger, unspecified finger
- M65.319 Trigger thumb, unspecified thumb
- M65.329 Trigger finger, unspecified index finger

CLINICAL PEARLS

- This condition is caused by narrowing of the A1 pulley, usually due to either thickening from inflammation or protein deposits or thickening of the tendon per se; with prolonged inflammation, fibrocartilaginous metaplasia of the tendon sheath occurs.
- Splinting the MCP joint at 10–15 degrees flexion for 6 weeks with the distal joints free to move has been reported effective. Splinting is more effective for treating fingers than thumbs (70% vs. 50%). This is less effective with severe symptoms, symptoms >6 months, and multiple digits involved (1)[B].
- Long-acting corticosteroids may be injected several times to achieve the relief of symptoms, although subsequent injections often are less likely to work than the initial injection.
- Both open and percutaneous surgery have high success rates with a low risk of complications (10).
- Most hand surgeons still prefer the open release because of concern about avoiding nerve injury with the blind procedure.

TROCHANTERIC BURSITIS (GREATER TROCHANTERIC PAIN SYNDROME)

David W. Kruse, MD • Joann Chang, MD

 BASICS

The name *trochanteric bursitis* has been used in the historical literature to refer to pain at the lateral hip with tenderness over the greater trochanter. As more continues to be learned about potential sources of pain at the lateral hip and the discovery that many patients lack an inflammatory process, this condition has been referred to as *greater trochanteric pain syndrome* (GTPS) in the more recent literature (1).

DESCRIPTION
- Bursae are fluid-filled sacs found at bony protuberances, typically at tendon attachment sites:
  - Multiple bursae are described in the area of the greater trochanter of the femur.
  - These bursae correspond to the tendons of the gluteus muscles, iliotibial band (ITB), and tensor fasciae latae.
  - The subgluteus maximus bursa is implicated most commonly in lateral hip pain (1).
- Other structures that surround the lateral hip include:
  - ITB
  - Tensor fasciae latae
  - Gluteus maximus tendon
  - Gluteus medius tendon
  - Gluteus minimus tendon
  - Quadratus femoris muscle
  - Vastus lateralis tendon
  - Piriformis tendon.
- *Bursitis* refers to inflammation of the bursa.
- *Tendinopathy* refers to any abnormality of a tendon, inflammatory or degenerative.

EPIDEMIOLOGY
Incidence
- In primary-care setting: 1.8 patients/1,000 persons/yr
- Predominant age: All ages:
  - Peak incidence in 4th–6th decades

Prevalence
- Predominant sex: Female > Male
- Sports:
  - Running
  - Contact sports: Football, rugby, soccer

ETIOLOGY AND PATHOPHYSIOLOGY
- Acute: Abnormal gait or poor muscle flexibility and strength lead to:
  - Friction on bursa, causing inflammatory response
  - Tendon overuse and inflammation
  - Direct trauma from contact or frequently lying with body weight on hip can cause an inflammatory response.
- Chronic:
  - Fibrosis and thickening of bursal sac due to chronic inflammatory process
  - Tendinopathy due to chronic overuse and degeneration: Gluteus medius and minimus (1)
- See "Risk Factors" and "Pathophysiology" sections.

Genetics
No known genetic factors

RISK FACTORS
Multiple factors have been implicated (1,2):
- Female
- Obesity
- Tight hip musculature or ITB
- Direct trauma
- Total hip arthroplasty
- Abnormal biomechanics or gait:
  - Leg-length discrepancy
  - Sacroiliac (SI) joint dysfunction
  - Knee or hip osteoarthritis
  - Abnormal foot mechanics (e.g., pes planus, overpronation)
  - Neuromuscular disorder

GENERAL PREVENTION
- Maintain ITB, hip, and lower-back flexibility and strength.
- Avoid direct trauma (use of appropriate padding in contact sports).
- Avoid banked running.
- Wear appropriate shoes.
- Weight loss, if appropriate

COMMONLY ASSOCIATED CONDITIONS
- Many biomechanical factors can be associated with this condition (1):
  - Tight ITBs
  - Leg-length discrepancy
  - SI joint dysfunction
  - Pes planus
  - Width of greater trochanters greater than width of iliac wings (3)[B]
- Other associated pathology (1):
  - Low-back pain
  - Knee and hip osteoarthritis
  - Obesity

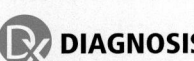 **DIAGNOSIS**

HISTORY
General historical points on presentation (1):
- Pain localized to the lateral aspect of the hip or buttock
- May radiate to groin or lateral thigh (pseudoradiculopathy)
- Exacerbated by:
  - Prolonged walking or standing
  - Rising after prolonged sitting
  - Sitting with legs crossed
  - Lying on affected side
- Other possible points:
  - Direct trauma to affected hip
  - Chronic low-back pain
  - Chronic leg/knee/ankle/hip pain
  - Recent increase in running distance or intensity
  - Change in running surfaces

PHYSICAL EXAM
- Point tenderness with direct palpation over the lateral hip is the most characteristic sign for GTPS (1)[B].
- Other tests have been described but lack sensitivity (1)[B]:
  - May have pain with extremes of passive rotation, abduction, or adduction
  - Pain with resisted hip abduction and external or internal rotation
  - Trendelenburg sign
- Other testing to evaluate for associated conditions:
  - Positive Patrick-FABERE (flexion, abduction, external rotation, extension) testing for SI joint dysfunction
  - Ober test for ITB pathology
  - Flexion and extension of hip for osteoarthritis
  - Leg-length measurement
  - Foot inspection for pes planus or overpronation
  - Lower extremity neurologic assessment for lumbar radiculopathy or neuromuscular disorders

DIFFERENTIAL DIAGNOSIS
Multiple conditions should be considered (1)[C]:
- ITB syndrome
- Gluteus medius or minimus tendinopathy
- Osteoarthritis or avascular necrosis of the hip
- Lumbosacral osteoarthritis/disc disease causing nerve root compression
- If associated trauma: Fracture or contusion of the hip or pelvis
- Stress reaction/fracture of femoral neck, especially in female runners
- Septic bursitis/arthritis

DIAGNOSTIC TESTS & INTERPRETATION
No routine lab testing is recommended.

Imaging
Diagnosis can be made by history and exam, but radiologic imaging can be helpful to evaluate for other associated conditions.

Initial approach
If imaging is ordered:
- Anteroposterior and frog-leg views of affected hip
- Consider lumbar spine radiographs if back pain is thought to be a contributing factor.
- Musculoskeletal US also can provide accurate imaging of potential pathology.
- For recalcitrant pain, MRI can be utilized to view direct and indirect signs of GTPS and to rule out other causes of refractory pain (4).

Follow-Up Tests & Special Considerations
- If there is a concern for a septic bursitis, then aspiration or incision and drainage may be necessary.
- Advanced imaging rarely necessary; detection of abnormalities on MRI is a poor predictor of GTPS (5)[B].

TREATMENT

- Weight loss (if applicable)
- Minimize aggravating activities such as prolonged walking or standing.
- Avoid lying on affected side.
- Runners:
  – May need to decrease distance and/or intensity of runs during treatment period of 2–4 weeks
  – May need a period of cessation of running; amount of time is case specific but may range from 2–4 weeks
  – Should avoid banked tracks or roads with excessive tilt

MEDICATION
First Line
- NSAIDs (1)[B]: Treat for 2–4 weeks:
  – Naprosyn: 500 mg PO b.i.d.
  – Ibuprofen: 800 mg PO t.i.d.
- Corticosteroid injection is effective for pain relief (6)[C]. In certain cases, injection can be considered first-line therapy:
  – Dexamethasone: 4 mg/mL or
  – Kenalog: 40 mg/mL 1–2 mL
  – Consider adding a local anesthetic (short- and/or long-acting) for more immediate pain relief.
  – Can be repeated for recurrence with similar effect if original treatment showed a strong response
  – Goal is acute or subacute pain relief (7)[A].

ISSUES FOR REFERRAL
- Septic bursitis
- Recalcitrant bursitis

ADDITIONAL THERAPIES
- Ice
- Physical therapy to address underlying dysfunction and rebuild atrophic muscle mass
- Low-energy shock-wave therapy has been shown to be superior to other nonoperative modalities (8)[A].
- Focus on achieving flexibility of hip musculature, particularly the ITB.
- Correct pelvic/hip instability.
- Correct lower limb biomechanics.
- Address contributing factors:
  – Low-back flexibility
  – If leg-length discrepancy, may need heel lift
  – If pes planus or overpronation, may need arch supports or custom orthotics

SURGERY/OTHER PROCEDURES
- Rarely requires surgery, but effective in refractory cases (8)[A]
- If surgery is indicated, potential options include:
  – Arthroscopic bursectomy (9,10)[B]
  – Release of the ITB
  – Gluteus medius tendon repair

COMPLEMENTARY AND ALTERNATIVE MEDICINE
Other techniques have been described for the treatment of chronic fibrosis and tendinopathy and may play a role in the treatment of GTPS:
- Acupuncture
- Prolotherapy
- Growth factor injection techniques

 ONGOING CARE

FOLLOW-UP RECOMMENDATIONS
4 weeks posttreatment, sooner if significant worsening

PATIENT EDUCATION
- Avoid lying on affected side.
- Minimize prolonged standing or walking.
- Maintain hip musculature flexibility, including ITB.
- Correct issues that may cause abnormal gait:
  – Low back pain
  – Knee pain
  – Leg-length discrepancy
  – Foot mechanics
- Gradual return to physical activity

PROGNOSIS
Depends on chronicity and recurrence, with more acute cases having an excellent prognosis

COMPLICATIONS
Bursal thickening and fibrosis

REFERENCES
1. Williams BS, Cohen SP. Greater trochanteric pain syndrome: A review of anatomy, diagnosis and treatment. *Anesth Analg.* 2009;108:1662–1670.
2. Farmer KW, Jones LC, Brownson KE, et al. Trochanteric bursitis after total hip arthroplasty: Incidence and evaluation of response to treatment. *J Arthroplasty.* 2010;25:208–212.
3. Viradia NK, Berger AA, Dahners LE, et al. Relationship between width of greater trochanters and width of iliac wings in trochanteric bursitis. *Am J Orthop.* 2011;40:E159–E162.
4. McMahon SE, Smith TO, Hing CB. A systematic review of imaging modalities in the diagnosis of greater trochanteric pain syndrome. *Musculoskelet Care.* 2012;10:232–239.
5. Blankenbaker DG, Ullrick SR, Davis KW, et al. Correlation of MRI findings with clinical findings of trochanteric pain syndrome. *Skeletal Radiol.* 2008;37(10):903–909.
6. Stephens MB, Beutler AI, O'Connor FG. Musculoskeletal injections: A review of the evidence. *Am Fam Physician.* 2008;78:971–976.
7. Brinks A, van Rijn RM, Willemsen SP, et al. Corticosteroid injections for greater trochanteric pain syndrome: A randomized controlled trial in primary care. *Ann Fam Med.* 2011;9:226–234.
8. Lustenberger DP, Ng VY, Best TM, et al. Efficacy of treatment of trochanteric bursitis: A systematic review. *Clin J Sport Med.* 2011;21:447–453.
9. Baker CL, Massie RV, Hurt WG, et al. Arthroscopic bursectomy for recalcitrant trochanteric bursitis. *Arthroscopy.* 2007;23:827–832.
10. Pretell J, Ortega J, García-Rayo R, et al. Distal fascia lata lengthening: An alternative surgical technique for recalcitrant trochanteric bursitis. *Int Orthop.* 2009;33:1223–1227.

ADDITIONAL READING
- Barnthouse NC, Wente TM, Voos JE. Greater trochanteric pain syndrome: Endoscopic treatment options. *Oper Tech Sports Med.* 2012;20:320–324.
- Hugo D, de Jongh HR. Greater trochanteric pain syndrome. *SA Orthopaedic Journal.* 2012;11(1):28–33.

 CODES

ICD10
- M70.60 Trochanteric bursitis, unspecified hip
- M70.61 Trochanteric bursitis, right hip
- M70.62 Trochanteric bursitis, left hip

CLINICAL PEARLS
- One of the most common complaints from a patient with GTPS is inability to lie on the affected side.
- Thorough knowledge of associated conditions ensures accurate diagnosis and effective treatment.
- Corticosteroid injection can be considered first-line therapy for some patients.
- Aggressively use physical therapy in treatment to address underlying dysfunction and rebuild weakened muscle mass.

TUBERCULOSIS

Brandon M. Weeks DO, MPH • Swati B. Avashia, MD

BASICS

DESCRIPTION
- Usually acquired by inhalation of airborne bacilli from a person with active tuberculosis (TB). Bacilli multiply in alveoli and spread via macrophages, lymphatics, and blood. 3 possible outcomes:
  - Eradication: Tissue hypersensitivity halts infection within 10 weeks.
  - Primary infection
  - Latent infection: Asymptomatic with positive purified protein derivative (PPD), negative chest radiograph, noninfectious
- Active tuberculosis:
  - Occurs from primary infection or reactivation of latent infection
  - Affects 10% of infected individuals without preventive therapy
  - Risk increases with immunosuppression: Highest the first 2 years after infection
  - Well-described forms: Pulmonary (85% of cases), miliary (disseminated), meningeal, abdominal
  - Abdominal TB more common in the 3rd or 4th decade in women.

Pediatric Considerations
Children <4 years have higher risk for disseminated TB (lower-lobe infections more common); also more likely to have immediate clinical or radiographic signs. Treat with 4 drugs. Older children and adolescents develop upper-lobe infiltrates; can re-occur in adulthood.

EPIDEMIOLOGY
Incidence
- Worldwide (2011): 8.7 million (13% HIV co-infected)
- US (2012): 9,951 (3.2/100,000), 127 were multidrug resistant (MDR), and 107 of those were foreign born (1)

Prevalence
Worldwide (2011): 170 cases/100,000 population (36% decrease since 1990); highest burden in Asia and Africa

ETIOLOGY AND PATHOPHYSIOLOGY
- Cell-mediated response by the body causes activated T lymphocytes and macrophages to form a "granuloma" that limits organism replication. Destruction of the macrophages produces early "solid necrosis." In 2–3 weeks, "caseous necrosis" develops, establishing latency. In immunocompetent, granuloma undergoes "fibrosis" and calcification; in immunocompromised, primary progressive tuberculosis develops.
- *Mycobacterium tuberculosis, M. bovis,* or *M. africanum*

RISK FACTORS
- For infection: Homeless, minority, institutionalized settings; close contact with infected individual; persons from areas with high incidence of active tuberculosis (Asia, Africa, Latin America, former Soviet Union states); health care workers; frequent or prolonged visits to high-prevalence areas; and populations with locally increased incidence (e.g., medically underserved, low income, substance abusers)

- For development of disease once infected: HIV; lymphoma; silicosis; diabetes mellitus; chronic renal failure; cancer of head, neck, or lung; children <5 years of age; malnutrition; systemic corticosteroids, immunosuppressive drugs; IV drug abuse, alcohol abuse, cigarette smokers; <2 years since infection with *M. tuberculosis*; history of gastrectomy or jejunal bypass; <90% of ideal body weight; tuberculin skin test (PPD) or interferon-γ release assay (IGRA) conversion within previous 2 years

GENERAL PREVENTION
- Treat latent infection and report to health department for identification; test and treat all close contacts.
- Bacille Calmette Guérin (BCG) vaccine: Live attenuated *M. bovis,* prevents 50% of pulmonary disease and 80% of meningitis and miliary disease in children. Used more in countries with endemic TB. In the US, consider BCG for high-risk children with negative PPD and HIV tests for health care workers at high risk for drug-resistant infection.

COMMONLY ASSOCIATED CONDITIONS
HIV infection: Emphasize direct observed therapy (DOT) and early initiation of ART.

DIAGNOSIS

HISTORY
- Known exposure
- HIV status/risk factors
- Signs and symptoms:
  - General: Fever, night sweats, weight loss, malaise, painless adenopathy
  - Pulmonary TB: Cough, hemoptysis, pleuritic chest pain
  - Abdominal TB: Acute presentation often as surgical emergencies such as peritonitis or acute abdomen, obstruction, or perforation; chronic presentation may be doughy abdomen, vague abdominal symptoms, abdominal mass.
  - Meningitis: See "Tuberculosis, CNS."
  - Miliary: See "Tuberculosis, Miliary."

PHYSICAL EXAM
- Often entirely normal. Specific findings depend on organs involved: adenopathy, rales, or hepatosplenomegaly.
- Late findings: Renal, bone, or CNS disease

DIFFERENTIAL DIAGNOSIS
Other pneumonias, malignancies, fungal infections, other atypical *Mycobacteria* or *Nocardia*

DIAGNOSTIC TESTS & INTERPRETATION
Initial Tests (lab, imaging)
- Chest radiograph:
  - Primary TB: Infiltrate with or without effusion, atelectasis, or adenopathy
  - Recrudescent TB: Cavitary lesions and upper-lobe disease with hilar adenopathy
  - HIV: Atypical findings with primary infection, right upper-lobe atelectasis
- CT chest: Good sensitivity
- 3 consecutive sputum samples (8–24-hour intervals with at least 1 in early AM) for acid-fast bacilli (AFB) stain and culture by aerosol induction, gastric aspirate (children), or bronchoalveolar lavage:
  - Positive AFB: Treat immediately. Culture and sensitivity guide treatment.

- Tuberculin skin test (TST) (e.g., PPD): 5 U (0.1 mL) intermediate-strength intradermal injection into volar forearm. Measure induration at 48–72 hours:
  - PPD positive if induration:
    - >5 mm and HIV infection, recent TB contact, immunosuppressed, disease on x-ray
    - >10 mm and age <4 years or other risk factors
    - >15 mm and age >4 years and no risk factors
    - 2-step test if no recent PPD, age >55, nursing home resident, prison inmate, or health care worker. 2nd test 1–3 weeks after initial test; interpret as usual.
  - Context of PPD results:
    - False positive: BCG (unreliable, should not affect decision to treat)
    - False negative: HIV, steroids, gastrectomy, alcoholism, renal failure, sarcoidosis, malnutrition, hematologic or lymphoreticular disorder, very recent exposure
    - If positive once, not necessary to repeat
    - No need for control with candida/other

- Interferon-γ release assays (IGRAs) measure interferon release after stimulation in vitro by *M. tuberculosis* antigens (2)[A]:
  - Lack of cross-reaction with BCG and most nontuberculous mycobacteria:
    - Preferred (better specificity) for testing persons who have had BCG (vaccine or for cancer therapy)
  - Can be used in settings in which skin testing is recommended, except tuberculin skin test (TST) is preferred in children age <5 years
  - May substitute for TST in shortage (3)[A]

Follow-Up Tests & Special Considerations
- Baseline CBC, creatinine, AST, ALT, bilirubin, alkaline phosphatase, visual acuity, and red–green color discrimination
- HIV: If positive, get baseline CD4 count.
- High risk: Check hepatitis B and C (injection drug users, Africa or Asia born, HIV infected).
- Extrapulmonary: Urine, CSF, bone marrow, and liver biopsy for culture as indicated
- Nonspecific laboratory findings: Anemia, monocytosis, thrombocytosis, hypergammaglobulinemia, syndrome of inappropriate secretion of antidiuretic hormone (SIADH), sterile pyuria

Diagnostic Procedures/Other
Biopsy: Granulomas with central caseating necrosis

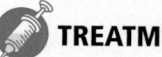

TREATMENT

GENERAL MEASURES
- If clinical suspicion, treat immediately. Prescribing physician is responsible for treatment completion.
- Ambulatory patients: Use mask and tissues.
- Not infectious if favorable clinical response after 2–3 weeks of therapy and 3 negative AFB smears

MEDICATION
Ideal body weight used for dosing. DOT required for children, institutionalized patients, risk for nonadherence, and nondaily regimens. DOT is strongly recommended for all regimens (4)[C].

First Line

- Latent TB infection:
  - Isoniazid (INH) for 9 months at 5 mg/kg/d *or* 15 mg/kg 2×/wk (5)[A] *or*
  - INH 15 mg/kg + rifapentine 300–900 mg weekly for 12 weeks given by DOT for patients age ≥12 years (5),(6)[A]
- Active TB infection:
  - Regimen 1 (preferred) (7)[A]:
    - Initial phase:
      - INH 5 mg/kg, rifampin (RIF) 10 mg/kg, pyrazinamide (PZA) 15–30 mg/kg, and ethambutol (EMB) 15–20 mg/kg daily for 8 weeks, *or*
      - INH/RIF/PZA/EMB 5 d/wk for 8 weeks
    - Continuation phase:
      - INH/RIF daily for 18 weeks; or, if DOT, INH/RIF 5 days/week for 18 weeks (recommended for HIV + with CD4 <100 cells/mm^3 due to increased risk of resistance), *or*
      - INH/RIF 2–3×/wk for 18 weeks (not used if HIV+ with CD4 <100; may have increased risk of relapse), *or*
      - INH/rifapentine once weekly for 18 weeks (acceptable only for HIV–patients without cavitary disease, may have increase risk of relapse) (7)[A]
  - Regimen 2:
    - Initial phase:
      - INH/RIF/PZA/EMB daily for 2 weeks, then twice weekly for 6 weeks, *or*
      - INH/RIF/PZA/EMB 5 d/wk for 2 weeks, then twice weekly for 6 weeks
    - Continuation phase:
      - INH/RIF 2–3×/wk for 18 weeks (not recommended if HIV+ with CD4 <100; may have increased risk of relapse), *or*
      - INH/RIF once weekly for 18 weeks (acceptable only for HIV–patients without cavitary disease; may have increase risk of relapse) (7)[A]
      - Treat TB in pregnancy with INH, RIF, and EMB; supplement with pyridoxine 25 mg/d.

Pregnancy Considerations

- Streptomycin: Ototoxic and nephrotoxic; do not use in pregnancy. Pyrazinamide not used in pregnant women in the US.
- Congenital infection: From maternal miliary or endometrial TB. If suspected, get PPD, chest x-ray (CXR), lumbar puncture, and culture placenta. Start treatment promptly.
- Breastfeeding: OK while taking TB drugs; supplement with pyridoxine 25 mg/d

Pediatric Considerations

- Children: Ethambutol is not used.
- Children on medication may attend school.

ALERT

- Maximum drug doses: INH 300 mg/d or 900 mg 2–3×/wk, RIF 600 mg all regimens, PZA 2,000 mg/d or 4,000 mg 2×/wk, EMB, 600 mg/d or 4,000 mg 2×/wk
- If patient does not receive PZA during entire first 2 months, extend treatment to 9 months.
- *M. bovis* is resistant to PZA; must be treated 9 months.
- Continue EMB until organism susceptibility to INH+RIF is determined (7)[A].

Second Line

Include fluoroquinolones and injectable aminoglycosides. Use when MDR is suspected or patient intolerance (see "Tuberculosis, MDR").

ISSUES FOR REFERRAL

ALERT

Refer drug-resistant TB and HIV-positive patients on antiretroviral therapy to an infectious disease specialist.

ADDITIONAL THERAPIES

- Pyridoxine: 50 mg prophylaxis with each dose may prevent INH-associated peripheral neuropathy, especially for those who are malnourished or have comorbidities that increase risk of neuropathy (6)[A].
- Steroids: Recommended for TB meningitis or pericarditis, use only with concomitant anti-TB therapy (4)[B].

SURGERY/OTHER PROCEDURES

For extrapulmonary complications (e.g., spinal cord compression, intestinal obstruction, constrictive pericarditis)

COMPLEMENTARY AND ALTERNATIVE MEDICINE

Vitamin D deficiency may increase susceptibility to TB and development of active TB. Supplementation may be beneficial (8)[C].

IN-PATIENT CONSIDERATIONS

- Place on airborne infection isolation.
- Use personal sealed respirators.
- 3 consecutive negative sputum AFB smears for release from isolation

Discharge Criteria

Once a diagnosis of TB is excluded or the patient has (1) effective therapy and is clinically improving; (2) outpatient follow-up with a provider who will manage TB; (3) case management from the local public health department and they agree with plan, and (4) enough anti-TB medication in hand until outpatient appointment

 ONGOING CARE

FOLLOW-UP RECOMMENDATIONS

Patient Monitoring

- Assess monthly for treatment adherence and adverse effects.
- HIV+: CD4 count, CBC, and liver enzymes every 1–3 months
- Liver enzymes monthly if chronic liver disease, alcohol use, pregnant, or postpartum. Temporarily discontinue medications if asymptomatic and enzymes ≥5× normal or if symptomatic and enzymes ≥3× normal.
- Visual acuity and red–green color discrimination monthly if on ethambutol >2 months or doses >20 mg/kg/d
- If culture positive after 2 months of therapy, reassess drug sensitivity and initiate DOT.
- Chest radiograph at 3 months

PATIENT EDUCATION

- Emphasize adherence to drug therapy.
- Identify exposed contacts.
- Notify patient that treating physician must inform the local health department.
- Tuberculosis General Information, 2011: http://www.cdc.gov/tb/publications/factsheets/general/tb.htm

PROGNOSIS

Few complications and full resolution of infection if drugs taken for full course as prescribed. Untreated, leads to multiple complications, including death.

COMPLICATIONS

- Cavitary lesions can become secondarily infected.
- Risk for drug resistance: HIV positive, treatment nonadherence, or from area with high incidence of resistance
- MDR-TB: resistance to INH and rifampicin
- XDR-TB: resistant to fluoroquinolones (9% of MDR)

REFERENCES

1. World Health Organization. *WHO global tuberculosis report 2012: Global tuberculosis control*. Available at: http://apps.who.int/iris/bitstream/10665/75938/1/9789241564502_eng.pdf.
2. Mazurek GH, Jereb J, Vernon A, et al. Updated Guidelines for using interferon gama release assays to detect *Mycobacterium tuberculosis* infection–United States. *MMWR Recomm Rep*. 2010; 59(RR05):1–25.
3. Centers for Disease Control and Prevention (CDC). National shortage of purified-protein derivative tuberculin products. *MMWR*. April 26, 2013; 62(16):312.
4. Golden MP, Vikram HR. Extrapulmonary tuberculosis: An overview. *Am Fam Physician*. 2005;72:1761–1768.
5. Drugs for tuberculosis. *Treat Guidel Med Lett*. 2012;10(116):29–36; quiz 37–38.
6. Centers for Disease Control and Prevention (CDC). Recommendations for use of an isoniazid-rifapentine regimen with direct observation to treat latent Mycobacterium tuberculosis infection. *MMWR Morb Mortal Wkly Rep*. 2011;60(48): 1650–1653.
7. Hall RG, Leff RD, Gumbo T. Treatment of active pulmonary tuberculosis in adults: Current standards and recent advances. *Pharmacotherapy*. 2009;29(12):1468–1481.
8. Luong KVQ, Nguyen LTH. Impact of vitamin D in the treatment of tuberculosis. *Am J Med Sci*. 2011; 341(6):493–498.

ADDITIONAL READING

Centers for Disease Control and Prevention (CDC). Trends in tuberculosis: United States 2012. *MMWR*. March 22, 2013;62(11):201–205.

 SEE ALSO

- Tuberculosis, CNS; Tuberculosis, Latent; Tuberculosis, Miliary
- Algorithm: Weight Loss

CODES

ICD10

- A15.9 Respiratory tuberculosis unspecified
- A17.9 Tuberculosis of nervous system, unspecified
- A19.9 Miliary tuberculosis, unspecified

CLINICAL PEARLS

- Have high suspicion for TB in patients with chronic cough and 1 additional risk factor.
- Patients ≥65 years have few classic features of TB.

TUBERCULOSIS, LATENT
Kay A. Bauman, MD, MPH

 BASICS

DESCRIPTION
- Tuberculosis (TB) is a common infection transmitted by inhaling airborne bacilli from a person with active TB. The bacilli multiply in the alveoli and are carried by macrophages, lymphatics, and blood to distant sites (e.g., lung, pleura, brain, kidney, bone). Tissue hypersensitivity halts infection within 10 weeks.
- Latent TB infection (LTBI) is asymptomatic, noninfectious, and usually detected by a positive skin test (i.e., purified protein derivative [PPD]) or chest x-ray (CXR), which is evidence of prior TB infection; acid-fast bacilli smear and culture are negative, and CXR does not suggest active TB.
- TB: Active disease occurs in 5–10% of infected individuals without preventive therapy. Chance of disease increases with immunosuppression and is highest for all individuals within 2 years of infection; 85% of the cases are pulmonary, which is infectious.
- LTBI treatment is a key component of the TB elimination strategy of the US. For example, an estimated 4,000–11,000 active TB cases were prevented by LTBI treatment in 2002 (1).

ALERT
A key alert to health care providers is to test for LTBI (PPD) and treat latent infection, with special attention to persons born in countries with high incidence. In the US, foreign-born persons have 11.5× the rate of active TB as the rate of US-born persons, comprising 63% of the total US cases. US TB rates from the highest 5 countries of immigration are Mexico (20.9%), Philippines (12.3%), India (8.5%), Vietnam (7.2%), and China (5.6%) (2,3)
- System(s) affected: Asymptomatic

EPIDEMIOLOGY
- High-risk groups include immigrants from Asia, Latin America, Africa, and the Pacific Basin; homeless persons; persons with a history of drug use or history of incarceration; HIV-infected individuals.
- Also at high risk are those newly exposed, including the pediatric population.
- In 2012, Asians had the highest active TB case rate of all groups, 25.0× the rate in whites. Hispanic rate is 6.6× that in whites; and for non-Hispanic blacks, the rate is 7.3× that in whites.
- Of active TB cases in 2012 in ethnic minorities, 95.7% of Asian cases, 75% of Hispanic cases, 39.7% of black cases, and 19.1% of white cases were foreign born. This emphasizes the need to screen foreign-born persons for latent TB and treat those who are positive.
- In 2012, 7.7% of active TB cases in the US were HIV positive, 5.6% were homeless, and 12.1% reported excessive alcohol use.

Prevalence
- In the US, 4% of the population has latent TB infection.
- Worldwide, it is estimated that 1/3 of the population harbors latent TB.
- Predominant gender: Male > Female

ETIOLOGY AND PATHOPHYSIOLOGY
Mycobacterium tuberculosis, *M. bovis*, and *M. africanum*

RISK FACTORS
- HIV infection, immunosuppression
- Immigrants (from Asia, Africa, Latin America, Pacific Islands, or area with high rate of TB), including migrant workers
- Close contact with infected individual
- Institutional environment (e.g., prison, nursing home)
- Use of illicit drugs
- Lower socioeconomic status or homeless
- Health care workers
- Chronic disease, such as diabetes mellitus (DM), end-stage renal disease, cancer, or silicosis; organ transplant
- Persons with fibrotic changes on CXR consistent with previous TB infection (4)
- Recent TB skin test (TST) converters (4)
- Personnel from mycobacteriology laboratories
- Patients with organ transplants

GENERAL PREVENTION
Treatment of LTBI is preventive: The goal is to decrease the incidence of active TB in the individuals treated and decrease the risk to close contacts should active TB occur.

COMMONLY ASSOCIATED CONDITIONS
- HIV infection (see "Initial Tests")
- Immune suppression

 DIAGNOSIS

HISTORY
History of immigration from a high-risk area, history of IV drug use and/or drug treatment, HIV, homelessness, recent incarceration

PHYSICAL EXAM
No signs of infection

DIFFERENTIAL DIAGNOSIS
Fungal infections; atypical mycobacteria or *Nocardia*

DIAGNOSTIC TESTS & INTERPRETATION
Initial Tests (lab, imaging)
- None routinely recommended
- In higher risk patients: Liver profile, hepatitis C virus (HCV), and hepatitis B virus (HBV) screening
- HIV test recommended to assess risk for active TB in men who have sex with men or persons with a history of IV drug use
- CXR required to rule out TB in asymptomatic infected persons
- CT scan of the chest has good sensitivity.

Diagnostic Procedures/Other
- PPD: 5 U (0.1 mL) intermediate-strength intradermal volar forearm. Measure induration at 48–72 hours:
  - Positive if induration is:
    - >5 mm and patient has HIV infection (or suspected) (4), is immunosuppressed, had recent close TB contact, or has clinical evidence of active or old disease on CXR
    - >10 mm and patient age <4 years or has other risk factors noted above
    - >15 mm and patient age >4 years and has no risk factors (4)
  - Negative if induration <5 mm on initial test and, if indicated, on 2nd test
  - Use the 2-step test (administer a 2nd intradermal test 1–3 weeks after initial test; measure and interpret as usual) if patient has had no recent PPD and is age >55 years or is a nursing home resident, prison inmate, or health care worker.
- The interferon blood test or QuantiFERON-TB and QuantiFERON-TB GOLD measure the release of interferon by sensitized lymphocytes when exposed to antigens of *M. tuberculosis*. It is unaffected by prior BCG vaccination, requires only 1 patient visit, and has improved sensitivity and specificity, but is costly (1).
- Special considerations:
  - Steroids: False-negative skin test
  - Measles vaccine: May suppress tuberculin activity; simultaneous PPD and measles vaccine recommended; if not simultaneous, defer PPD 4–6 weeks after measles vaccine.
  - The multiple-puncture tine test is not recommended.
  - Do not use history of BCG vaccination as a reason to ignore a positive PPD in adults and forego recommendation for treatment.
  - Disorders that may alter results and give a false-negative skin test:
    - Recent viral infection
    - New (<10 weeks) infection
    - Severe malnutrition
    - HIV
    - Anergy
    - Age <6 months
    - Overwhelming TB

 TREATMENT

GENERAL MEASURES
- Must exclude active TB
- Treatment for LTBI is crucial to control and eliminate TB disease in the US because it both decreases the risk of active TB in those treated and decreases risks to those potentially infected by those same people (4).
- Treat LTBI at any age if patient has HIV, has had close TB contact, is a recent converter (<2 years), is an IV drug user, has an abnormal CXR, has a high-risk medical condition, or is in another high-risk group:
  - Use isoniazid (INH) for 9 months.
  - Preferred: INH 300 mg/d or 900 mg twice weekly × 9 months (4)
  - Acceptable alternative: INH 300 mg/d or 900 mg twice weekly × 6 months (4)
  - Directly observed therapy (DOT) is recommended if patient adherence is not assured.

- Treat LTBI during pregnancy if patient has recent infection or is HIV positive (use INH with pyridoxine and monitor liver enzymes); otherwise, treatment may be postponed until postpartum (4).
- Special considerations for HIV infection and suspected INH resistance (4)
- *Note:* Because of severe liver injury and death associated with rifampin and pyrazinamide, these medications are no longer recommended for LTBI (4).
- Exclusions: Cirrhosis, active hepatitis, history of excessive alcohol consumption (4)

MEDICATION
First Line
- INH scored tablets: 100 mg, 300 mg, or syrup 10 mg/mL:
  - Daily: Adult 300 mg; pediatric 10–15 mg/kg (maximum 300 mg) (5)
  - Twice weekly: Adult 15 mg/kg; pediatric 20–30 mg/kg (maximum 900 mg) (5)
  - Treatment for 9 months; typical completion rates of ≤60%.
- Precautions:
  - Follow liver function if the patient has history of alcoholism, HBV, HCV or other liver dysfunction, or new signs of liver injury.
  - INH: Peripheral neuritis and hypersensitivity are possible. Consider pyridoxine.
  - INH: An idiosyncratic drug reaction that results in INH-associated severe liver injury has been reported by the CDC in 17 patients in years 2004–2008. These included 15 adults and 2 children; 5 underwent liver transplantation and 5 subsequently died (1 of the liver transplant recipients). Thus, monitoring of patients while on treatment is recommended, looking for symptoms of liver injury (all were symptomatic!), and not be limited to laboratory monitoring. The rate of this reaction is difficult to calculate, as unknown numbers of patients are treated for LTBI, but 1 estimate is 291,000–433,000/year in the US (6).

Second Line
- Patients >12 years: Rifapentine, a rifampinlike drug used to treat active TB, 900 mg weekly and INH, 15–25 mg/kg weekly for 12 weeks. This new and shorter treatment has increased rates of completion compared with 9 months of INH (82% compared with 69% in 1 trial), slightly more adverse effects (4.9% vs. 3.7%), and is more costly (approximately $160 vs. $6 for course of treatment):
  - Contraindications to rifapentine: Alcoholism, renal failure, HIV infection, pregnancy. Can cause hyperuricemia and hematuria (2).
- Rifampin alone: Adults 600 mg/d for 4 months; children 10–20 mg/kg/d for 6 months. Fewer data exist for efficacy of this regimen, but can be considered for contacts of INH-resistant TB or patients with INH contraindications. In 1 study, the 4-month course increased compliance from 62.6% with INH to 71.6% with rifampin (7).

ADDITIONAL THERAPIES
Pediatric Considerations
Protocol for newborn with mother/household contact with infection or disease
- If mother or household contact has LTBI, skin test all household contacts and treat any with positive PPD.
- If contact has abnormal CXR, separate infant until infectious status known; if not contagious, monitor infant PPD (5).
- If mother has disease and is possibly contagious, evaluate infant for congenital TB and test for HIV; separate newborn until mother is noninfectious (5).
- If congenital TB is suspected, treat.
- If no congenital disease, start INH and repeat PPD after 3–4 months. If positive, reassess infant and finish 9 months of INH. If PPD is negative and source is noninfectious, stop INH and monitor infant (5).
- BCG vaccine, live-attenuated *M. bovis:* Used more commonly in developing countries in children to prevent complications of TB

IN-PATIENT CONSIDERATIONS
Geriatric Considerations
- Before entering a chronic-care facility, patients should have a PPD using 2-step protocols.
- INH side effects are more pronounced.

Discharge Criteria
- Activity, as tolerated
- No isolation required

ONGOING CARE
FOLLOW-UP RECOMMENDATIONS
Patient Monitoring
- During preventive therapy for LTBI: Initial monthly visits to assess adherence to regimen and to monitor for hepatitis and neuropathy; if stable, can monitor less frequently.
- If patient remains asymptomatic, repeat CXR is not needed.
- Check liver enzymes if patient is symptomatic, is HIV positive, has chronic liver disease, uses alcohol, or is pregnant or postpartum, and modify drugs, if needed.

DIET
Regular; consider pyridoxine supplement, 10–50 mg/d.

PROGNOSIS
- Generally, there are few complications, and treatment is effective if drugs are taken for full course as prescribed.
- Retreatment is not necessary.

COMPLICATIONS
Recrudescent TB

REFERENCES

1. Campos-Outcalt D. When, and when not, to use the interferon-gamma TB test. *J Fam Pract.* 2005;54:873–875.
2. Centers for Disease Control and Prevention (CDC). Recommendations for use of an isoniazid-rifapentine regimen with direct observation to treat latent *Mycobacterium* tuberculosis infection. *MMWR Morb Mortal Wkly Rep.* 2011;60(48): 1650–1653.
3. Centers for Disease Control and Prevention (CDC). Trends in tuberculosis–United States, 2012. *MMWR Morb Mortal Wkly Rep.* 2013;62(11):201–205.
4. Centers for Disease Control and Prevention. Guidelines for preventing the transmission of *Mycobacterium* TB in health-care settings, 2005. *MMWR Recomm Rep.* 2005;54(RR-17):53–55.
5. American Academy of Pediatrics. *Report of the Committee on Infectious Diseases (Red Book).* Elk Grove Village, IL: American Academy of Pediatrics; 2003.
6. Centers for Disease Control and Prevention (CDC). Severe isoniazid-associated liver injuries among persons being treated for latent tuberculosis infection—United States, 2004–2008. *MMWR Morb Mortal Wkly Rep.* 2010;59(8):224–229.
7. Page KR, Sifakis F, Montes de Oca R, et al. Improved adherence and less toxicity with rifampin vs isoniazid for treatment of latent tuberculosis: A retrospective study. *Arch Intern Med.* 2006;166: 1863–1870.

ADDITIONAL READING

- Centers for Disease Control and Prevention (CDC), American Thoracic Society. Update: Adverse event data and revised American Thoracic Society/CDC recommendations against the use of rifampin and pyrazinamide for treatment of latent tuberculosis infection—United States, 2003. *Morb Mortal Wkly Rep.* 2003;52:735–739.
- Young DB, Gideon HP, Wilkinson RJ. Eliminating latent tuberculosis. *Trends Microbiol.* 2009;17(5): 183–188.

SEE ALSO

Tuberculosis; Tuberculosis, Miliary

CODES

ICD10
- R76.1 Nonspecific reaction to test for tuberculosis
- R76.11 Nonspecific reaction to skin test w/o active tuberculosis
- R76.12 Nonspecific reaction to cell mediated immunity measurement of gamma interferon antigen response without active tuberculosis

CLINICAL PEARLS
- Treatment for latent TB is crucial to control and eliminate TB disease in the US; an estimated 4% of the US population has LTBI.
- Test household contacts of PPD-positive patients.
- History of BCG vaccination, especially >10 years before PPD testing, should not be considered the cause of a positive PPD. The interferon-γ blood test is unaffected by prior BCG vaccination.
- Treat all HIV-positive patients with latent TB with a prophylactic regimen.
- Screen foreign-born persons for latent TB and treat those who are positive.

TURNER SYNDROME
Rayna Goldstein, MD • Michele Roberts, MD, PhD

BASICS

DESCRIPTION
- Turner syndrome (TS) is a condition characterized by ovarian dysgenesis and short stature in phenotypic females who have only 1 sex chromosome, an X; although a partial 2nd sex chromosome, X or Y, may be present
- The most common sex chromosome abnormality syndrome in females
- System(s) affected: Cardiovascular; Reproductive; Endocrine/Metabolic; Musculoskeletal; Nervous; Renal/Urologic
- Synonym(s): Ullrich-Turner syndrome; Bonnevie-Ullrich syndrome; Monosomy X; Sexual infantilism; Gonadal dysgenesis

EPIDEMIOLOGY
Incidence
- Occurs in 1/2,500 live female births
- ~1–3% of all conceptuses affected, of whom <1% will survive to term
- Accounts for 15% of all spontaneously aborted fetuses
- Predominant sex: Female only

Prevalence
Estimated 50,000–75,000 females in the US

ETIOLOGY AND PATHOPHYSIOLOGY
Haploinsufficiency of *SHOX* (short stature homeobox-containing gene), located in the pseudoautosomal region of the X chromosome, is thought to be responsible for short stature and skeletal abnormalities in TS.

Monosomy for all or part of the X chromosome can result in features of TS. Genes located mainly in Xp11.2–p22.1.

Genetics
- 50% of patients have 45,X karyotype (sporadic nondisjunction). Translocations involving the X chromosome may result in TS.
- 80% of girls with 45,X have maternal X, although phenotype is identical if X is paternal.
- TS occurs with a deletion of the *SRY* segment of the Y chromosome in 46,XY karyotype, with resulting female phenotype (5–6%).
- FISH or PCR may be necessary to identify Y material because of increased risk of gonadoblastoma (7–10%) if Y material is present; indicated if signs of virilization or marker chromosome present.
- Also may be mosaic for 45,X/46,XY, 45,X/46,XX, or 45,X/47,XXX

COMMONLY ASSOCIATED CONDITIONS
- Gonadal dysgenesis (infertility 98%)
- Short stature (100%), usually not GH deficient. Height is generally 20 cm below that expected for family.
- Hearing loss (50%), otitis media (70–100%)
- Frequent (>5–10% but <50% of individuals):
  - Cardiovascular abnormalities, including coarctation of the aorta (15–30%), aortic valvular disease (1/3 have bicuspid aortic valve), mitral valve prolapse (25%), aortic root dilatation (8–29%), aortic dissection, ECG abnormalities
  - Renal abnormalities
  - Hypertension (HTN; >30%)
  - Glucose intolerance
  - Hyperlipidemia
  - Ocular abnormalities
  - Hypothyroidism, autoimmune thyroiditis
  - GI vascular malformations
  - Glucose intolerance
  - Gonadoblastoma in 8% of individuals with Y chromosomal material
- Occasional: Inflammatory bowel disease, celiac disease, colon cancer, neuroblastoma, juvenile rheumatoid arthritis, liver disease (especially cirrhosis)

DIAGNOSIS

HISTORY
- Increasingly diagnosed prenatally. When karyotype is obtained in response to suggestive US findings, result is highly specific. When karyotype obtained for other reasons, false-positive results or mosaicism may be found.
- Noninvasive prenatal testing for aneuploidy may increase prenatal diagnosis.
- Edema of hands and feet and redundant skin of the neck (webbing) are presenting features during infancy. Lymphedema is the most common reason to test for TS during infancy.
- 50% of girls are <5th percentile in height by 1.5 years; 75% by 3.5 years. Short stature is the most common reason to test for TS during childhood and adolescence. Diagnosis of TS should be considered in any girl with an unexplained short stature.
- During adolescence, primary amenorrhea, short stature, and infantile secondary sex characteristics are presenting features.

PHYSICAL EXAM
Frequencies are for classic 45,X and vary with other chromosomal abnormalities associated with TS:
- Intelligence is usually normal.
- Very frequent (>50% of individuals):
  - Short stature: Use the Turner growth chart.
  - Lymphedema of hands and feet present at birth, and may recur
  - Deep-set hyperconvex nails
  - Unusual shape and rotation of ears
  - Narrow maxilla and dental crowding, micrognathia
  - Low posterior hairline
  - Broad chest with widely spaced, inverted, or hypoplastic nipples
  - Cubitus valgus
  - Short 4th metacarpals and/or metatarsals
  - Tibial exostosis
  - Tendency to obesity
  - Recurrent otitis media
  - Frequent (<50% of individuals): Pigmented nevi, webbed neck, keloid formation, scoliosis (10–12%), hip dysplasia
  - Occasional (<5% of individuals): Kyphosis, lordosis

DIFFERENTIAL DIAGNOSIS
- Short stature: Noonan syndrome (a genetic condition that shares some facial and other physical characteristics with TS); hypothyroidism, familial short stature, dyschondrosteosis (Léri-Weill syndrome), brachydactyly, growth hormone deficiency, glucocorticoid excess, Klippel-Feil anomaly, short stature due to chronic disease
- Amenorrhea or delayed puberty: Pure gonadal dysgenesis, polycystic ovary syndrome (Stein-Leventhal syndrome), primary/secondary amenorrhea
- Lymphedema: Hereditary congenital lymphedema, Milroy disease, lymphedema with recurrent cholestasis, lymphedema with intestinal lymphangiectasia
- Other: Multiple pterygium syndrome, pseudo-hypoparathyroid syndrome

DIAGNOSTIC TESTS & INTERPRETATION
Initial Tests (lab, imaging)
- Chromosome analysis: A buccal smear is not adequate to rule out TS. An analysis of at least 20–30 cells is required. Analysis of 2 cell types (e.g., blood and skin) may be necessary if peripheral blood karyotype is normal in those in whom there is clinical suspicion of Turner syndrome.
- Thyroid function tests, celiac screening
- MR aortography and echocardiography to evaluate cardiovascular system (1)[C]
- Renal US to evaluate structural renal abnormalities

Follow-Up Tests & Special Considerations
- With prenatal diagnosis, counseling is important due to high rate of spontaneous fetal loss.
- Postnatal karyotype required for confirmation of prenatal diagnosis.
- At puberty, follicle-stimulating hormone (FSH) and luteinizing hormone levels may approach levels consistent with the absence of ovaries. FSH may be transiently high in infancy.
- Annual evaluation of thyroid function
- Continued follow-up in adulthood for cardiac pathology including bicuspid aortic valve, conduction defects, and aortic dissection (2)

Diagnostic Procedures/Other
Upper and lower extremity BP; ENT/audiology for hearing test; assess for congenital hip dislocation

Test Interpretation
- Ovarian dysgenesis (>90%): Streak gonads, atretic follicles, or no follicles present
- Renal: Horseshoe kidney, double collecting system (60%)
- Cardiac (20–40% of patients): Coarctation of the aorta, bicuspid aortic valve, valvular aortic stenosis (70% of TS patients with heart defects also have coarctation), HTN
- Bone dysplasia (>50%), osteoporosis
- Gonadoblastomas in patients with X/XY mosaicism
- Ocular abnormalities: Amblyopia, ptosis, strabismus, red/green color blindness
- GI: Increased incidence of celiac disease
- CNS abnormalities: ADHD, decreased visuospatial organization, impaired social cognition

TREATMENT

MEDICATION
- Recombinant human growth hormone (rhGH) (3)[C]
- Treat in evidence of growth failure (4)[C], if height falls below 5th percentile by 18 months of age. Adult height is maximized if GH is initiated at a young age: 0.375–0.400 mg/kg/wk. rhGH improves body proportions, may help to lower diastolic BP, and improve lipid panel and insulin resistance.

- Anabolic steroids in conjunction with GH. Consider oxandrolone in girls ≥9 years or those with extreme short stature.
- Estrogen: Promotes sexual development and bone maturation, optimizes peak bone mass, and may benefit cognitive development in young girls (5)[C]:
  – Due to accelerated follicular atresia, most girls with TS undergo ovarian failure prior to or around the time of puberty. Treat gonadal failure in girls who do not enter puberty spontaneously.
  – Replacement therapy: Starting at age 12 years, continuing to age 50. Begin with 1–2 years of low-dose estrogen, followed by larger dose estrogens cycled with progesterone. Do not delay puberty to promote statural growth (1)[C].
- β-Blockers for blood pressure control if aortic dilatation is present.

ADDITIONAL THERAPIES
Pregnancy Considerations
- Although pregnancy is rare, sexually active girls and women should receive contraception counseling.
- Infertility is the general rule; <2% of pregnancies are achieved without medical assistance:
  – In vitro fertilization and embryo transfer
  – Successful ovarian transplants have been reported in teenage girls with TS.
  – In mosaic TS: Ovarian hyperstimulation and oocyte cryopreservation to preserve fertility
- High risk of maternal mortality due to cardiac complications, especially aortic dissection. Aortic root dimensions must be monitored throughout pregnancy by echo. Pregnancy contraindications: Previous aortic coarctation or dissection and aortic size >25 mm/m² (2)
- Increased risk of fetal malformations, chromosome anomalies, cephalopelvic disproportion

ISSUES FOR REFERRAL
- Genetics
- Congenital heart disease, bicuspid aortic valve, coarctation of the aorta, aortic dissection (especially with valvular abnormalities or coarctation, or systemic HTN); close cardiology follow-up in pregnancy
- Pediatric endocrinologist for GH and estrogen
- Response to growth hormone is variable.
- Orthodontic evaluation
- Psychiatric/Educational: May have problems in nonverbal areas such as evaluating objects in relationship to one another. Evaluate school performance. Patients may be at risk for ADHD or impaired social cognition (5).

SURGERY/OTHER PROCEDURES
- Removal of gonads is recommended in patients with X/XY mosaicism due to risk of gonadoblastoma.
- Angioplasty or surgical correction of coarctation of the aorta
- Reconstructive surgery is possible, if desired to enhance physical appearance.

 ## ONGOING CARE

FOLLOW-UP RECOMMENDATIONS
Patient Monitoring
- For complete health supervision guidelines, see Frias et al. (6)[C].
- Multidisciplinary evaluation, supplementing screening tests as informed by expert opinion guidelines, can aid in the interpretation of test results, optimize medical care, and thus may reduce morbidity and mortality in TS (7)[C].
- Regular cardiac exams; US/MRI at pubertal induction
- Height, weight, BP, pubertal staging (after age 10)
- Every 12–18 months: Thyroid function and IGF-1, bone age, hearing and vision assessment
- Every 3–5 years: Dual-energy x-ray absorptiometry scan for bone density
- FSH, liver function tests (LFTs), and pelvic US prior to pubertal induction
- Regular visits to primary care physicians are recommended. Be aware of the social and emotional problems associated with issues such as short stature and infertility.
- Adults with TS should be monitored for cardiovascular disease, including HTN, conduction abnormalities, and valve disease.
- Cardiac imaging (preferably MRI) every 5–10 years for aortic root dilatation/aortic dissection; frequent imaging during pregnancy
- Adults also should be monitored for thyroid disease, liver disease, diabetes, obesity, and dyslipidemia (8).

PATIENT EDUCATION
- Provide a thorough explanation of the condition and its management, especially about sexual development and growth. Support groups may be helpful.
- Genetics Home Reference http://ghr.nlm.nih.gov/condition/turner-syndrome
- Turner Syndrome Society of the United States: (800) 365-9944; www.turnersyndrome.org. "Turner Syndrome: A Guide for Families" (2002) is downloadable from this site.
- Magic Foundation: www.magicfoundation.org
- Human Growth Foundation: www.hgfound.org

PROGNOSIS
- Most girls lead reasonably normal lives with appropriate medical management; however, mortality was found to be 3-fold higher in women with TS than in the general population. Medical follow-up is important in adulthood; some deaths are preventable.
- Infertility: Most women with TS are infertile; however, pregnancy without medical assistance has been documented. Successful pregnancy following oocyte donation is well described. A thorough cardiovascular evaluation should be performed because the risk of aortic dissection is greatly increased during pregnancy.
- The overall risk of cancer is not increased in TS; however, risk may be increased for meningioma, childhood brain tumors, and possibly bladder cancer, melanoma, and uterine cancer. Risk of breast cancer is decreased in TS.
- 45,X/46,XY mosaicism confers increased risk for gonadoblastoma.

REFERENCES
1. Bondy CA, Turner Syndrome Study Group. Care of girls and women with Turner syndrome: A guideline of the Turner Syndrome Study Group. J Clin Endocrinol Metab. 2007;92:10–25.
2. Turtle EJ, Sule AA, Bath LE, et al. Assessing and addressing cardiovascular risk in adults with Turner syndrome. Clin Endocrinol. 2013;78:639–645.
3. Collett-Solberg PF. Update in growth hormone therapy of children. J Clin Endocrinol Metab. 2011;96:573–579.
4. Davenport ML. Approach to the patient with Turner syndrome. J Clin Endocrinol Metab. 2010;95: 1487–1495.
5. Hong DS, Dunkin B, Reiss AL, et al. Psychosocial functioning and social cognitive processing in girls with Turner syndrome. J Dev Behav Pediatr. 2011;32:512–520.
6. Frías JL, Davenport ML. Committee on Genetics and Section on Endocrinology. Health supervision for children with Turner syndrome. Pediatrics. 2003;111:692–702.
7. Pinsker E. Turner Syndrome: Updating the paradigm of clinical care. J Clin Endocrin Metab. 2012;97: 1–10.
8. Trolle C, Mortensen KH, Hjerrildl BE, et al. Clinical care of adult Turner syndrome-new aspects. Pediatr Endocrinol Rev. 2012;9 Suppl 2: 736–745.

 ## SEE ALSO

Amenorrhea; Coarctation of the Aorta; Hypothyroidism

 ## CODES

ICD10
- Q96.0 Karyotype 45, X
- Q96.3 Mosaicism, 45, X/46, XX or XY
- Q96.9 Turner's syndrome, unspecified

CLINICAL PEARLS
- TS is the most common sex chromosome abnormality syndrome in females.
- Edema of the hands and feet and redundant skin of the neck (webbing) are presenting features during infancy. In school-aged girls, the triad of short stature, social issues, and frequent ear infections should be investigated. During adolescence, primary amenorrhea, short stature, and infantile secondary sex characteristics are presenting features.
- Much of the treatment for TS is not evidence-based, and there is much controversy, especially in hormone replacement therapy, although this is the subject of current investigation.

TYPHOID FEVER

Douglas W. MacPherson, MD, MSc(CTM), FRCPC

 BASICS

- Typhoid fever is a rare enteric infectious syndrome in the US.
- Most cases reported in the US are imported from endemic areas of the world, particularly from South and Southeast Asia, or Latin America.

DESCRIPTION

- Typhoid fever is an acute systemic illness in humans caused by *Salmonella typhi*:
  – Classic example of enteric fever caused by the *Salmonella* bacterium
- Enteric fevers due to *S. paratyphi* can present in a similar manner as classic typhoid fever.
- Typhoid is endemic in some developing nations where sanitation is poor. Most cases in North America and other developed nations are acquired after travel to disease-endemic areas.
- "Visiting family or friends" travelers may be at greater risk of typhoid than other travelers.
- Mode of transmission is fecal–oral through ingestion of contaminated food (commonly poultry or milk) or water.
- Incubation period varies from 7–21 days.
- System(s) affected: Gastrointestinal; Pulmonary; Skin/Exocrine
- Synonym(s): Typhoid; Typhus abdominalis; Enteric fever

Geriatric Considerations
Disease is more serious in the elderly.

Pediatric Considerations
Disease is more serious in infants, but may be milder in children.

EPIDEMIOLOGY
Although typhoid outbreaks have been described in the US, most cases are reported in international travelers who have been exposed in endemic transmission zones (in particular, South and Southeast Asia, parts of Latin America) (1):
- Predominant age: All ages
- Predominant sex: Male = Female

Incidence
In the US, 300–500 new cases per year

ETIOLOGY AND PATHOPHYSIOLOGY
- Acute typhoid and other enteric fevers are seen most commonly in international travelers to endemic *S. typhi* regions of the world.
- The initial infection is transmitted via the fecal–oral route, with a GI source of the bacterium resulting in bacteremia and sepsis. Involvement of the bowel wall (Peyer patch) rarely may be associated with bleeding from the bowel or bowel perforation.
- *S. typhi* chronic carrier state may occur with shedding of the bacterium in the stools. Potential for person-to-person transmission may occur. In a chronic carrier state, *S. typhi* appears to locate in the biliary tract and, in particular, the gallbladder. Chronic suppressive antimicrobials may clear a carrier state. In extreme cases, cholecystectomies have been performed to attempt to clear carriage of *S. typhi*.

RISK FACTORS
Must be considered in any patient presenting with fever after tropical travel or exposure to a chronic carrier

GENERAL PREVENTION
- Food and water consumption precautions are paramount in the prevention of all enteric infections, including typhoid fever.
- Avoid tap water, salad/raw vegetables, unpeeled fruits, and dairy products in tropical travel.
- Avoid undercooked poultry or poultry products left unrefrigerated for prolonged periods.
- Wash hands before and after food preparation.
- For high-risk travel to an endemic area, consider vaccination against typhoid:
  – Parenteral ViCPS or capsular polysaccharide typhoid vaccine (Typhim Vi) *or*
  – Ty21a or live oral typhoid vaccine (Vivotif Berna), particularly if traveler will be at prolonged risk (>4 weeks)
- Consider vaccination for workers exposed to *S. typhi* or those with household or intimate exposure to a carrier of *S. typhi* (2).
- Occupational health and safety precautions, including screening of domestic and commercial food handlers, may be considered in some situations.

 DIAGNOSIS

Assessment of the clinical presentation and exposure history, including endemic zone travel and known chronic *S. typhi* carrier exposure

HISTORY
Patient presentation: Fever, headache, constipation with:
- Travel history to an endemic region and exposure to contaminated food or water
- Exposure to a chronic *S. typhi* carrier

PHYSICAL EXAM
- Fever
- Headache
- Malaise
- Abdominal discomfort/bloating/constipation
- Diarrhea (less common)
- Dry cough
- Confusion/Lethargy
- Rose spot (transient erythematous maculopapular rash in anterior thorax or upper abdomen)
- Splenomegaly
- Hepatomegaly
- Cervical adenopathy
- Relative bradycardia
- Conjunctivitis
- Constitutionally unwell, fever, relative bradycardia, rose spots, abdominal pain, hepatosplenomegaly

DIFFERENTIAL DIAGNOSIS
- Malaria
- "Enteric fever-like" syndrome caused by *Yersinia enterocolitica*, pseudotuberculosis, and *Campylobacter* spp.
- Enteric fever caused by nontyphoid *Salmonella* spp.
- Infectious hepatitis

- Dengue
- Atypical pneumonia
- Infectious mononucleosis
- Subacute bacterial endocarditis
- Tuberculosis
- Brucellosis
- Q fever
- Toxoplasmosis
- Typhus
- Viral infections: Epstein-Barr virus (EBV), cytomegalovirus (CMV), viral hemorrhagic agents

DIAGNOSTIC TESTS & INTERPRETATION
Due to the rarity of enteric fevers/typhoid syndromes in the US, a high level of clinical suspicion must be present. A travel history to a known typhoid-endemic zone or exposure to a known chronic carrier of *S. typhi* will contribute to the clinical and laboratory diagnosis of typhoid fever.
- Definitive diagnosis is by culture of *S. typhi* from blood or other sterile body fluid.
- Isolation of *S. typhi* in sputum, urine, or stool is a presumptive diagnosis in typical clinical presentation.
- Serology is nonspecific and usually not useful.
- If there are multiple negative blood cultures, or in patients with prior antibiotic therapy, diagnostic yield is better with bone marrow culture.
- Anemia, leukopenia (neutropenia), thrombocytopenia, or evidence of disseminated intravascular coagulopathy are supportive. Elevated liver enzymes are common.
- Drugs that may alter lab results:
  – Prior antibiotic therapy
  – Vaccination
- Have a high clinical suspicion for intestinal perforation or consider serial plain abdominal films for evidence of perforation.

Diagnostic Procedures/Other
- Bone marrow aspirate for culture of *S. typhi* has been reported to be more sensitive than blood cultures, but is rarely indicated as a primary investigation.
- A bone marrow aspiration may be done for evaluation of a persistent fever in a clinically suspect situation with negative cultures or for investigation of a "pyrexia/fever of unknown origin."

Test Interpretation
Classically, pathology of the bowel shows mononuclear proliferation involving lymphoid tissue of intestinal tract, especially Peyer patch in terminal ileum.

 TREATMENT

Awareness of emerging drug-resistant *S. typhi* strains globally and the epidemiology of the patient's exposure may direct primary therapy. Knowledge of local resistance patterns for presumptive treatment or laboratory sensitivity should guide therapy. Fluoroquinolone-resistant *S. typhi* is becoming very common in Asia.

GENERAL MEASURES
- Fluid and electrolyte support
- Strict isolation of patient's linen, stool, and urine
- Monitor clinically and consider serial plain abdominal films for evidence of perforation, usually in the 3rd–4th week of illness.
- Indications and contraindications for specific treatment of typhoid disease and chronic carrier states must be determined on an individual basis. Factors to be considered are age, public health and occupational health risk (e.g., food handler, chronic care facilities, medical personnel), intolerance to antibiotics, and evidence of biliary tract disease.
- For hemorrhage: Blood transfusion and management of shock

MEDICATION
See below for treatment recommendations for acute typhoid fever and chronic carrier states.

First Line
- Chloramphenicol: Pediatric 50 mg/kg/d PO q.i.d. × 2 weeks; adult dose 50 mg/kg/d divided q6h for 2 weeks *or*
- Ampicillin: Pediatric 100 mg/kg/d q.i.d. PO × 2 weeks; adults 500 mg q6h for 2 weeks *or*
- Ciprofloxacin: 500 mg PO b.i.d. × 2 weeks, *indicated in multiple-drug-resistant typhoid:*
  – Has been used successfully and safely in children; WHO recommends as first-line in areas with drug resistance to older first-line antibiotics (3)[A]
  – Fluoroquinolones may prevent clinical relapse better than chloramphenicol (4)[A].
- Ceftriaxone: 1–2 g IV once daily × 2 weeks *or*
- Furazolidone: 7.5 mg/kg/d PO × 10 days; in uncomplicated multidrug-resistant typhoid; safe in children; efficacy >85% cure
- Chronic carrier state:
  – Ampicillin: 4–5 g/d plus probenecid 2 g/d q.i.d. × 6 weeks (for patients with normally functioning gallbladder without evidence of cholelithiasis)
  – Ciprofloxacin: 500 mg PO b.i.d. for 4–6 weeks is also efficacious. Chloramphenicol resistance has been reported in Mexico, South America, Central America, Southeast Asia, India, Pakistan, Middle East, and Africa.
- Contraindications: Refer to manufacturer's profile for each drug.
- Precautions: Rarely, Jarisch-Herxheimer reaction appears after antimicrobial therapy.
- Significant possible interactions: Refer to manufacturer's profile for each drug.

Second Line
Trimethoprim–sulfamethoxazole

Pregnancy Considerations
Ciprofloxacin therapy is relatively contraindicated in pregnant patients.

ISSUES FOR REFERRAL
Complications of sepsis, bowel perforation

SURGERY/OTHER PROCEDURES
- Complications: Bowel perforation
- Cholecystectomy may be warranted in carriers with cholelithiasis, relapse after therapy, or intolerance to antimicrobial therapy.

IN-PATIENT CONSIDERATIONS
Admission Criteria/Initial Stabilization
- Inpatient if acutely ill
- Outpatient for less ill patient or for carrier
- Clinical severity

Nursing
Observe enteric precautions.

 ## ONGOING CARE

FOLLOW-UP RECOMMENDATIONS
Bed rest initially, then activity as tolerated

Patient Monitoring
See "General Measures."

DIET
NPO if abdominal symptoms are severe. With improvement, begin normal low-residue diet, possibly high-calorie.

PATIENT EDUCATION
- Discuss chronic carrier state and its complications.
- For family members, travelers, or workers at risk, provide hygiene education and possibly vaccination.
- Educate patients that the typhoid vaccines do not protect against *S. paratyphi* infection (5).
- Typhoid vaccines protect 50–80% of recipients (not 100%) with diminishing effectiveness over 2–4 years.
- CDC Patient Handout: www.cdc.gov/vaccines/pubs/vis/downloads/vis-typhoid.pdf (6)

PROGNOSIS
Overall prognosis is good with therapy; <2% mortality rate; 15% relapse rate with some antibiotic treatments; 3% bowel perforation

COMPLICATIONS
- Intestinal hemorrhage and perforation in distal ileum
- Patients may become chronic carriers (up to 3%), defined as persistent stool excretor of *S. typhi* for >1 year.
- Predilection for seeding in the biliary tract exists and may become a focus for relapse of typhoid fever: Most common in females and older patients (>50)
- Osteomyelitis is found especially in patients with sickle cell anemia, systemic lupus erythematosus, and hematologic neoplasms, as well as in immunosuppressed hosts.
- Endovascular infection in the elderly and in patients with a history of bypass operation or aneurysm
- Rarely, endocarditis or meningitis

REFERENCES
1. Sánchez-Vargas FM, Abu-El-Haija MA, Gómez-Duarte OG. Salmonella infections: An update on epidemiology, management, and prevention. *Travel Med Infect Dis*. 2011;9(6): 263–277. Epub 2011 Nov 25.
2. Kroger AT, Atkinson WL, Marcuse EK, et al. General recommendations on immunization. Recommendations of the Advisory Committee on Immunization Practices (ACIP). *MMWR*. 2006; 55(RR15):1–48.
3. Effa EE, Lassi ZS, Critchley JA, et al. Fluoroquinolones for treating typhoid and paratyphoid fever (enteric fever). *Cochrane Database Syst Rev*. 2011;(10):CD004530. Epub 2011 Oct 5.
4. Thaver D, Zaidi AK, Critchley J, et al. A comparison of fluoroquinolones versus other antibiotics for treating enteric fever: Meta-analysis. *BMJ*. 2009; 338:b1865. Epub 2009 Jun 3.
5. Centers for Disease Control and Prevention. Typhoid fever. Available at: www.cdc.gov/ncidod/dbmd/diseaseinfo/typhoidfever_g.htm.
6. Centers for Disease Control and Prevention. Vaccines and preventable diseases: Typhoid. Available at: www.cdc.gov/vaccines/vpd-vac/typhoid/default.htm.

ADDITIONAL READING
- Basnyat B. Typhoid fever in the United States and antibiotic choice. *JAMA*. 2010;303:34; author reply 34–35.
- Butler T. Treatment of typhoid fever in the 21st century: Promises and shortcomings. *Clin Microbiol Infect*. 2011;17(7):959–963.
- Centers for Disease Control and Prevention. *The pre-travel consultation. Travel-related vaccine preventable diseases*. Chapter 2. Typhoid and Paratyphoid Fever. Available at: wwwnc.cdc.gov/travel/yellowbook/2010/chapter-2/typhoid-paratyphoid-fever.htm.
- Chalya PL, Mabula JB, Koy M, et al. Typhoid intestinal perforations at a University teaching hospital in Northwestern Tanzania: A surgical experience of 104 cases in a resource-limited setting. *World J Emerg Surg*. 2012;7:4. Epub 2012 Mar 8.
- Clark TW, Daneshvar C, Pareek M, et al. Enteric fever in a UK regional infectious diseases unit: A 10 year retrospective review. *J Infect*. 2010;60(2): 91–98. Epub 2009 Dec 3.
- Crump JA, Mintz ED. Global trends in typhoid and paratyphoid Fever. *Clin Infect Dis*. 2010;50(2): 241–246.
- Kaurthe J. Increasing antimicrobial resistance and narrowing therapeutics in typhoidal salmonellae. *J Clin Diagn Res*. 2013;7:576–579.

 ## CODES

ICD10
- A01.00 Typhoid fever, unspecified
- A01.09 Typhoid fever with other complications
- Z22.0 Carrier of typhoid

CLINICAL PEARLS
- Along with malaria and other regionally defined exotic infections, including dengue, enteric fevers, and others, typhoid should be considered as a possible diagnosis for any febrile traveler from endemic areas such as Latin America, sub-Saharan Africa, or South Asia.
- Routine blood cultures will detect *S. typhi*, but may be negative if antibiotics have been taken prior to testing.
- A history or documentation of vaccination against *S. typhi* does not exclude the diagnosis of typhoid fever.

TYPHUS FEVERS

Douglas W. MacPherson, MD, MSc(CTM), FRCPC

BASICS

Typhus is an infectious disease syndrome caused by several bacterial organisms resulting in acute, chronic, and recrudescing disease.

DESCRIPTION
- Acute infectious diseases caused by 3 species of *Rickettsiae*:
  – Epidemic typhus: Human-to-human transmission by body louse vector. Primarily in circumstances such as refugee camps, war, famine, and disaster. Recrudescent disease, occurring years after initial infection, can be a source of human outbreak. Flying squirrels are also a reservoir.
  – Endemic (murine) typhus: Infection by rodents to humans by rat flea bite
  – Scrub typhus: Infection and infestation of chiggers and of rodents to humans by the chigger; primarily in Asia and western Pacific areas
- System(s) affected: Endocrine/Metabolic; Hematologic/Lymphatic/Immunologic; Pulmonary; Skin/Exocrine
- Synonym(s): Louse-borne typhus; Brill-Zinsser disease; Murine typhus

EPIDEMIOLOGY
- Epidemic and endemic typhus: Rare in the US (outside of south Texas)
- Scrub typhus: Travelers returning from endemic areas only (rare)

Incidence
Endemic typhus: <100 cases annually, primarily in states around the Gulf of Mexico, especially south Texas; underreporting suspected

ETIOLOGY AND PATHOPHYSIOLOGY
- Epidemic typhus by *R. prowazekii*
- Endemic typhus by *R. typhi*
- Scrub typhus by *R. tsutsugamushi*

RISK FACTORS
Exposure to vectors (e.g., during travel to countries where endemic)

Geriatric Considerations
Elderly may have more severe disease.

GENERAL PREVENTION
Avoid vectors for each disease:
- Scrub typhus: Wear protective clothing and use insect repellents.
- Endemic typhus: Practice ectoparasite and rodent control.
- Epidemic typhus: Delousing and cleaning of clothing; vaccine may be considered for those at high risk of exposure (typhus vaccine production has been discontinued in the US).

DIAGNOSIS

Given the rarity of typhus syndromes in the US, a high level of clinical suspicion is necessary to make the diagnosis.

HISTORY
Travel or other risk exposure

PHYSICAL EXAM
- General:
  – Acute onset
  – Fever
  – Chills
  – Headache
  – Myalgia
  – Malaise
  – Diffuse organ involvement (e.g., intestine, liver, heart, kidneys, brain)
- Epidemic typhus:
  – Incubation period ~1 week
  – Macular or maculopapular rash beginning on trunk ~5th day of illness
  – Nonproductive cough
  – Pulmonary infiltrates
- Endemic typhus:
  – Incubation period 1–2 weeks
  – Macular or maculopapular rash beginning on trunk 3rd–5th day of illness
- Scrub typhus:
  – Incubation period 1–3 weeks
  – Eschar at bite site
  – Regional lymphadenopathy
  – Generalized lymphadenopathy
  – Splenomegaly
  – Macular or maculopapular rash beginning on trunk approximately 5th day of illness
  – Relative bradycardia early in disease
  – Ocular pain
  – Conjunctival injection

DIFFERENTIAL DIAGNOSIS
- Any acute febrile disease
- Rocky Mountain spotted fever
- Meningococcemia
- Bacterial meningitis
- Mediterranean spotted fever (boutonneuse fever) (*R. conorii*)
- Measles
- Rubella
- Toxoplasmosis
- Leptospirosis
- Typhoid fever
- Dengue
- Malaria
- Relapsing fever
- Secondary syphilis
- Viral syndromes: Mononucleosis, acute retroviral syndrome

DIAGNOSTIC TESTS & INTERPRETATION
- Specific serologic test showing a rising antibody titer
- Isolation of *Rickettsia* should be undertaken only in special laboratories to minimize the risk of laboratory-acquired infection.

Initial Tests (lab, imaging)
- Leukocyte findings usually normal
- Abnormalities reflecting the particular organs affected
- Weil-Felix serologic reaction may be positive; test value hampered to mid-illness or after and by low sensitivity and nonspecificity; epidemic and endemic typhus, 4-fold titer rise or titer >1/320 to OX-19; scrub typhus, 4-fold rise in titer to OX-K
- Hyponatremia in severe cases
- Hypoalbuminemia in severe cases
- Drugs that may alter lab results: Prior antibiotic use

Test Interpretation
Diffuse vasculitis on skin biopsy

TREATMENT

Treatment should be started based on strong epidemiologic risk assessment and clinical presentation:
- One study has suggested that treatment of Mediterranean spotted fever with a fluoroquinolone may result in a more severe clinical course (1).

GENERAL MEASURES
- Protect agitated patient from injury.
- Skin and mouth care
- Supportive care for the severely ill, directed at complications

MEDICATION
First Line
- Treatment should begin when diagnosis is reasonably likely and continue until the patient's state is improved and the patient is afebrile for a minimum of 48 hours; usual treatment course is 5–7 days.
- Children ≥8 years of age and adults:
  – Tetracycline: 25 mg/kg PO initially, then 25 mg/kg/d in equally divided doses q6h
  – If severely ill, may use doxycycline IV: Adults 100 mg q12h, children ≥8 years of age 5 mg/kg in 24 hours (maximum of 200 mg/24 hours)
- Children ≤8 years of age, pregnant women, or if typhoid fever is possible cause of illness:
  – Chloramphenicol: 50 mg/kg PO initially, then 50 mg/kg/d in equally divided doses q6h
  – If severely ill, chloramphenicol sodium succinate: 20 mg/kg IV initially, infused over 30–45 minutes, then 50 mg/kg/d infused in equally divided doses q6h until orally tolerable
- Precautions: Refer to the manufacturer's profile for each drug.
- Significant possible interactions: Refer to the manufacturer's profile for each drug.

Second Line

- Doxycycline: Single oral dose of 100 or 200 mg for those in refugee camps, victims of disasters, or in the presence of limited medical services
- Isolated reports indicate that erythromycin and ciprofloxacin are effective.
- Azithromycin 3-day course is effective for scrub typhus; better tolerated than doxycycline but more expensive (2)[B].
- Rifampin may be effective in areas where scrub typhus responds poorly to standard antirickettsial drugs (3)[A].

ISSUES FOR REFERRAL

Due to the rarity of typhus syndromes in the US, consider a tropical medicine or infectious disease physician consultation for diagnosis and/or management.

IN-PATIENT CONSIDERATIONS

Admission Criteria/Initial Stabilization

- Outpatient care unless severely ill
- Severely ill or constitutionally unstable (e.g., shock)

ONGOING CARE

FOLLOW-UP RECOMMENDATIONS

Bed rest during acute stages; otherwise, as tolerated

Patient Monitoring

- Severely ill patients should be admitted and observed regularly in the hospital.
- Outpatients should be checked as clinically indicated until improving.

DIET

As tolerated

PATIENT EDUCATION

Provide prevention information to travelers (geographic distribution, exposure risks, vector avoidance).

PROGNOSIS

- Recovery is expected if treatment is instituted before the onset of complications.
- Relapses may follow treatment, especially if initiated within 48 hours of onset (this is *not* an indication to delay treatment). Relapses are treated the same as primary disease.
- Without treatment, the mortality rate of typhus is 40–60% for epidemic, 1–2% for endemic, and up to 30% for scrub disease.
- Mortality is higher among the elderly.

COMPLICATIONS

- Consequences of specific organ-system involvement in the 2nd week (e.g., azotemia, meningoencephalitis, seizures, delirium, coma, myocardial failure, hyponatremia, hypoalbuminemia, hypovolemia, and shock)
- Death

REFERENCES

1. Botelho-Nevers E, Rovery C, Richet H, et al. Analysis of risk factors for malignant Mediterranean spotted fever indicates that fluoroquinolone treatment has a deleterious effect. *J Antimicrob Chemother*. 2011;66(8):1821–1830. Epub 2011 Jun 4.
2. Phimda K, Hoontrakul S, Suttinont C, et al. Doxycycline versus azithromycin for treatment of leptospirosis and scrub typhus. *Antimicrob Agents Chemother*. 2007;51:3259–3263.
3. Panpanich R, Garner P. Antibiotics for treating scrub typhus. *Cochrane Database Syst Rev*. 2002;CD002150.

ADDITIONAL READING

- Adjemian J, Eremeeva ME, Dasch GA. Rickettsial (spotted and typhus fevers) and related infections (anaplasmosis and ehrlichiosis). Chapter 5. Other infectious disease related to travel. Available at: wwwnc.cdc.gov/travel/yellowbook/2010/chapter-5/rickettsial-and-related-infections.htm.
- Botelho-Nevers E, Raoult D. Host, pathogen and treatment-related prognostic factors in rickettsioses. *Eur J Clin Microbiol Infect Dis*. 2011;30:1139–1150.
- Botelho-Nevers E, Socolovschi C, Raoult D, Parola P. Treatment of Rickettsia spp. infections: A review. *Expert Rev Anti Infect Ther*. 2012;10:1425–1437.
- Graham J, Stockley K, Goldman RD. Tick-borne illnesses: A CME update. *Pediatr Emerg Care*. 2011;27(2):141–147; quiz 148–150.
- Green JS, Singh J, Cheung M, et al. A cluster of pediatric endemic typhus cases in Orange County, California. *Pediatr Infect Dis J*. 2011;30:163–165.
- Hendershot EF, Sexton DJ. Scrub typhus and rickettsial diseases in international travelers: A review. *Curr Infect Dis Rep*. 2009;11:66–72.

- Jensenius M, Fournier PE, Raoult D. Rickettsioses and the international traveler. *Clin Infect Dis*. 2004;39:1493–1499.
- Molina N. Borders, laborers, and racialized medicalization Mexican immigration and US public health practices in the 20th century. *Am J Public Health*. 2011;101:1024–1031.
- Walker DH, Paddock CD, Dumler JS, et al. Emerging and re-emerging tick-transmitted rickettsial and ehrlichial infections. *Med Clin North Am*. 2008;92:1345–1361, x.

CODES

ICD10

- A75.0 Epidemic louse-borne typhus fever d/t Rickettsia prowazekii
- A75.2 Typhus fever due to Rickettsia typhi
- A75.9 Typhus fever, unspecified

CLINICAL PEARLS

- Along with malaria or dengue, consider a typhus diagnosis with any febrile traveler from endemic areas, including sub-Saharan Africa and Asia.
- Rickettsial infections typically present within 2–14 days, so febrile illnesses onset >18 days after travel are unlikely to be rickettsial.
- Routine blood cultures will not detect *Rickettsia* bacteria.
- Vaccination against travel diseases does not exclude the diagnosis of typhus.
- Severe headache is often intractable and not eased by the standard drugs.
- Report case to appropriate public health department or other agency.

ULCER, APHTHOUS

Elenee M.P. Raudenbush, DO • Louis D. Leone, DO

 BASICS

DESCRIPTION

- Self-limited, painful ulcerations of the nonkeratinized oral mucosa that are often recurrent
- Synonyms: Canker sores; aphthae; aphthous stomatitis:
  – Comes from *aphth* meaning "ulcer" in Greek; 1st used by Hippocrates between 460 and 370 BC to categorize oral disease (1,2)
- Referred to as recurrent aphthous stomatitis (RAS) if a patient has at least 3 episodes within 3 years in varying locations of the mouth (1)
- Categorization:
  – Minor aphthous ulcers:
    ○ Usually <10 mm in diameter
    ○ Self-limited, healing within 1–2 weeks
    ○ Rarely effect the dorsum of the mouth.
    ○ Nonscarring
  – Major aphthous ulcers (Sutton disease):
    ○ Usually >10 mm in diameter
    ○ Can effect the dorsum of the mouth.
    ○ May take weeks–months to heal.
    ○ Generally more painful than minor aphthous ulcers
    ○ May cause scarring.
  – Herpetiform ulcers (HU):
    ○ Unrelated to viral-caused herpetic stomatitis
    ○ Occur in small clusters in 10s–100s, lasting 1–4 weeks
    ○ Generally more painful than minor aphthous ulcers
    ○ May cause scarring.

EPIDEMIOLOGY

- Usually, the initial episode occurs in childhood, then begins to taper after the 3rd decade (3).
- More common in women, Caucasians, and nonsmoking patients
- More common in patients of higher socioeconomic status
- Most frequent inflammatory disorder of the oral mucosa:
  – Minor aphthous ulcers:
    ○ Most common: 70–90% of all aphthae
  – Major aphthous ulcers:
    ○ 10–15% of all aphthae
  – Herpetiform:
    ○ Least common: 7–10% of all aphthae

Prevalence

Lifetime prevalence of 25–40%

ETIOLOGY AND PATHOPHYSIOLOGY

Likely multifactorial; exact etiology unknown

RISK FACTORS

- Genetics:
  – 40% of patients have family history of RAS.
  – If familial, attacks are usually more severe and begin earlier in life.
  – Possible HLA antigen associations
- Trauma: Sharp teeth, dental treatments, mucosa toothbrush injury, and so forth
- Increased stress
- Nutritional deficiencies: Iron, vitamin B, and folate
- Immunodeficiency
- Recent cessation of tobacco use
- Food sensitivity: To benzoic acid/cinnamaldehyde

 DIAGNOSIS

Diagnosis is made by history and clinical presentation.

HISTORY

- Prodrome of burning/pricking sensation of oral mucosa 1–2 days prior to appearance of ulcers
- Patients typically complain of oral ulcerations, which are painful and exacerbated by movement of the mouth. Exacerbation may also be reported with certain foods (hot, spicy, acidic, or carbonated foods or drinks).
- Ask about other ulcerative lesions of other anatomic areas.
- Ask about family history of RAS.
- Ask about patient medical history of prior aphthous stomatitis.

PHYSICAL EXAM

- Round/Ovoid ulcerations generally <10 mm in size. Usually have a white, gray, or yellow base with inflammatory/erythematous halo.
- Ulcers are typically found in the buccal and lip mucosa, ventral tongue, soft palate, or oral vestibule; rarely, on the dorsum of the mouth/lips.
- Evaluate for signs of secondary infection, including elevated temperature, increased surrounding edema, or pus drainage.

DIFFERENTIAL DIAGNOSIS

- Important to rule out possibility of underlying systemic disease, causing aphthous-like ulcerations:
  – Highest suspicion in adult patients with their initial episode, or in individuals with additional lesions elsewhere in the body
- Trauma:
  – Biting
  – Dentures
- Infection:
  – Herpes virus (herpetic stomatitis):
    ○ Vesicular lesions
  – HIV:
    ○ Ulcerations have lengthened healing time.
    ○ History of oral candidiasis/hairy leukoplakia

- Mucocutaneous disease; especially if chronic or nonhealing:
  – Lichens planus
  – Pemphigus
- Malignancy: Further investigate and closely monitor nonhealing lesions, especially those with ipsilateral cervical lymphadenopathy (3)[C].
- Underlying secondary conditions (causing aphthous-like ulceration):
  – Behcet syndrome: Autoimmune systemic vasculitis usually involving mucous membranes:
    ○ Genital and oral ulceration
    ○ Uveitis
  – Reiter syndrome: Reactive arthritis, preceded by infection, usually of the genital tract:
    ○ Uveitis
    ○ Urethritis
    ○ HLA-B27–associated arthritis
  – Sweet syndrome: Acute neutrophilic dermatitis:
    ○ Fever, sudden onset
    ○ Erythematous skin plaques/papules, well-demarcated
    ○ Leukocytosis
    ○ 50% of patients have an associated malignancy.
    ○ Most often in middle-aged females
  – Inflammatory bowel disease (IBD): Crohn disease, ulcerative colitis:
    ○ 10% of patients with Crohn disease experience recurrent oral ulcers.
    ○ Bloody/Persistent diarrhea
    ○ Weight loss
  – Cyclic neutropenia:
    ○ Recurrent fevers associated with infections, occasionally intraoral
    ○ Begins in childhood.
  – Systemic lupus erythematosus (SLE): Autoimmune vascular collagen disease
    ○ Oral lesions have great variability, including recurrent ulceration.
  – Gluten-sensitive enteropathy (celiac disease):
    ○ Weight loss and signs of malabsorption
    ○ Bloating and diarrhea
  – Medication effects:
    ○ NSAIDs: Patients may also have an associated dermatitis.
    ○ β-Blocker medications
    ○ Alendronate (Fosamax)

DIAGNOSTIC TESTS & INTERPRETATION

Lab workup is rarely helpful to diagnose aphthous ulceration.

Follow-Up Tests & Special Considerations

- If lesions are solitary and have persisted >3 weeks, consider (3)[C]:
  – CBC
  – Vitamin B$_{12}$
  – Iron studies
  – Folate
- HIV
- Biopsy and viral cultures
- Rheumatologic serology

TREATMENT

GENERAL MEASURES

- Avoid potential irritating food or drink:
  - Spicy
  - Acidic
  - Hot food or drink
  - Carbonated beverages.
  - Abrasive/hard foods (i.e. chips, nuts, etc.)
- Recommend avoiding dental trauma with toothbrush/biting.

MEDICATION

In general, the goals of treatment rely on the extent of ulceration and the level of recurrence.

First Line

- Immunomodulators:
  - Amlexanox (Aphthasol) (improves healing time, reduces symptoms, and prevents recurrence) (4)[A]:
    ○ 5% topical oral paste, apply to ulcers q.i.d. for up to 2 weeks or until ulcer resolution.
    ○ Adverse effect: May cause stinging sensation.
- Topical corticosteroid (to improve healing time and symptoms) (5)[A]:
  - Adverse effect: May increase risk of oral candidiasis (more likely with higher potency formulations)
  - Preparations:
    ○ Triamcinolone 0.1% dental paste (Adcortyl or Kenalog in Orabase):
      ■ Apply sparingly to ulcers q.i.d. for up to 2 weeks or until ulcer resolution.
    ○ Hydrocortisone (Corlan):
      ■ 2.5-mg pellets applied to ulcer q.i.d. for up to 2 weeks or until ulcer resolution
    ○ Fluocinonide (Lidex):
      ■ 0.05% gel/ointment, apply sparingly to ulcer q.i.d. daily for up to 2 weeks or until ulcer resolution.
    ○ Dexamethasone (Decadron) (6)[B]:
      ■ 5 mg/5 mL elixer: Rinse for 3 minutes and spit q.i.d. until ulcer resolution.
- Topical anesthetics (to reduce symptoms only) (7)[A]:
  - Apply q.i.d. as needed for pain, for up to 2 weeks or until ulcer resolution.
  - Adverse effects: May cause numbness/stinging.
  - Preparations available as 2% lidocaine gel (viscous Xylocaine), benzydamine oral rinse (Difflam, Tantum).
  - Antimicrobial mouth rinses (improve healing time and prevent recurrence) (8)[A]:
    ○ Use q.i.d. for up to months at a time.
    ○ Adverse effects: May cause superficial tooth staining.
    ○ Preparations available as Chlorhexidine gluconate aqueous mouth wash in 0.12% or 0.2% (Peridex).
  - Penicillin G (improves healing time and reduces symptoms) (9)[A]

Second Line

- Systemic corticosteroids (10)[B]
- Colchicine (11)[B]
- Dapsone (12)[B]
- Thalidomide (Thalomid) (12)[A]:
  - 50–200 mg daily for 4–8 weeks
  - Adverse effects:
    ○ Neuropathy (monitor every 3 months)
    ○ Drowsiness
    ○ Known teratogen, Category X

ISSUES FOR REFERRAL

Otolaryngology referral if lesions have not resolved as expected

ADDITIONAL THERAPIES

Vitamin B$_{12}$ supplementation has been shown to decrease burden of outbreaks and recurrence, independent of preexisting deficiency (13)[A].

SURGERY/OTHER PROCEDURES

Chemical cautery with silver nitrate (reduces ulcer pain) (14)[A]

COMPLEMENTARY AND ALTERNATIVE MEDICINE

Recent randomized controlled trials have shown promise for several herbal and alternative treatments (15,16)[B]:

- *Glycyrrhiza* (licorice); *Myrtus communis* (myrtle); *Eupatorium laevigatum* paste; bee propolis

REFERENCES

1. Preeti L, Magesh K, Rajkumar K, et al. Recurrent aphthous stomatitis. *J Oral Maxillofac Pathol*. 2011;84(3):252–256.
2. Chavan M, Jain H, Diwan N, et al. Recurrent aphthous stomatitis: A review. *J Oral Pathol Med*. 2012;84(8):577–583. Epub 2012 Mar 13.
3. Scully C. Clinical practice. Aphthous ulceration. *N Engl J Med*. 2006;84(2):165–172.
4. Binnie WH, Curro FA, Khandwala A, et al. Amlexanox oral paste: A novel treatment that accelerates the healing of aphthous ulcers. *Compend Contin Educ Dent*. 1997;84(11):1116–1118, 1120–1122, 1124.
5. Quijano D, Rodríguez M. [Topical corticosteroids in recurrent aphthous stomatitis. Systematic review]. *Acta Otorrinolaringol Esp*. 2008;84(6):298–307.
6. Liu C, Zhou Z, Liu G, et al. Efficacy and safety of dexamethasone ointment on recurrent aphthous ulceration. *Am J Med*. 2012;84(3):292–301.
7. Hopper SM, Babl FE, McCarthy M, et al. A double blind, randomised placebo controlled trial of topical 2% viscous lidocaine in improving oral intake in children with painful infectious mouth conditions. *BMC Pediatr*. 2011;11:106. Epub 2011 Nov 21.
8. Gorsky M, Epstein J, Rabenstein S, et al. Topical minocycline and tetracycline rinses in treatment of recurrent aphthous stomatitis: A randomized cross-over study. *Dermatol Online J*. 2007;84(2):1. Epub 2007 May 1.
9. Zhou Y, Chen Q, Meng W, et al. Evaluation of penicillin G potassium troches in the treatment of minor recurrent aphthous ulceration in a Chinese cohort: A randomized, double-blinded, placebo and no-treatment-controlled, multicenter clinical trial. *Oral Surg Oral Med Oral Pathol Oral Radiol Endod*. 2010;84(4):561–566. Epub 2010 Feb 26.
10. Pakfetrat A, Mansourian A, Momen-Heravi F, et al. Comparison of colchicine versus prednisolone in recurrent aphthous stomatitis: A double-blind randomized clinical trial. *Clin Invest Med*. 2010;84(3):E189–E195. Epub 2010 Jun 1.
11. Fontes V, Machet L, Huttenberger B, et al. [Recurrent aphthous stomatitis: Treatment with colchicine. An open trial of 54 cases]. *Ann Dermatol Venereol*. 2002;84(12):1365–1369.
12. Mimura MA, Hirota SK, Sugaya NN, et al. Systemic treatment in severe cases of recurrent aphthous stomatitis: An open trial. *Clinics (Sao Paulo)*. 2009;84(3):193–198.
13. Carrozzo M. Vitamin B12 for the treatment of recurrent aphthous stomatitis. *Evid Based Dent*. 2009;84(4):114–115.
14. Alidaee MR, Taheri A, Mansoori P, et al. Silver nitrate cautery in aphthous stomatitis: A randomized controlled trial. *Br J Dermatol*. 2005;84(3):521–525.
15. Martin MD, Sherman J, van der Ven P, et al. A controlled trial of a dissolving oral patch concerning glycyrrhiza (licorice) herbal extract for the treatment of aphthous ulcers. *Gen Dent*. 84(2):206–210; quiz 211–212, 224.
16. Babaee N, Mansourian A, Momen-Heravi F, et al. The efficacy of a paste containing *Myrtus communis* (myrtle) in the management of recurrent aphthous stomatitis: A randomized controlled trial. *Clin Oral Investig*. 2010;84(1):65–70. Epub 2009 Mar 21.

CODES

ICD10

K12.0 Recurrent oral aphthae

CLINICAL PEARLS

- Aphthous ulcers are the most common inflammatory disorder of the oral mucosa.
- Most cases are mild, self-limited episodes. Appropriate treatment should be aimed at symptom control and promotion of healing.
- If lesions are nonhealing, simultaneously occur elsewhere in the body, or when patients present with their initial episode in adulthood, it is imperative to rule out secondary causes of oral aphthouslike ulcers.

ULCERATIVE COLITIS
Jill A. Grimes, MD, FAAFP

 BASICS

DESCRIPTION
- Idiopathic inflammatory disease of the colonic mucosa that can affect any section of the colon from the rectum to the cecum
  - >95% of patients have rectal involvement, with 50% of cases limited to rectum and sigmoid.
  - 20% have pancolitis.

EPIDEMIOLOGY
Incidence
- US: 9–12 new cases/100,000 persons/year
- Predominant age: 15–35 years; 2nd and smaller peak in the 7th decade
- Predominant sex: Female > Male (slight)

Prevalence
205–240/100,000 persons

Pregnancy Considerations
- Similar to general population; 1 study showed 30% with inactive disease at onset of pregnancy relapsed.
- Treatment with sulfasalazine does not seem to affect pregnancy outcome.
- Patients should delay pregnancy until disease is inactive.

ETIOLOGY AND PATHOPHYSIOLOGY
Unknown; hypotheses include allergy to dietary components and abnormal immune responses to bacterial or "self" antigens; final outcome is mucosal inflammation secondary to immune cell infiltration.

Genetics
- Family history in 5–10% in population surveys and 20–30% in referral-based studies
- More common in the Jewish population

RISK FACTORS
- Better sanitation, indoor work environments, and fatty foods increase risk.
- NSAIDs can activate disease.
- Appendectomy is protective against later development of disease.
- Negative association with smoking: Relative risk of smokers is 40% of nonsmokers.

GENERAL PREVENTION
- Patients with long-term disease who do not have colectomy are at increased risk for colon cancer.
- Aspirin (≥300 mg/d) and ursodeoxycholic acid (10 mg/kg) have been shown to be preventive.

Pediatric Considerations
Breastfeeding may be protective for pediatric inflammatory bowel disease (IBD).

COMMONLY ASSOCIATED CONDITIONS
- Extracolonic manifestations in 10–15%
- Arthritic conditions, including large joint arthritis, sacroiliitis, and ankylosing spondylitis
- Pyoderma gangrenosum
- Episcleritis and uveitis
- Sclerosing cholangitis
- Asymptomatic fatty liver (common); occasional hepatomegaly
- Primary sclerosing cholangitis: 1–4%
- Cirrhosis of liver: 1–5%
- Bile duct carcinoma
- Thromboembolic disease: 1–6%

 DIAGNOSIS

HISTORY
Bloody diarrhea (watery stool accompanied by blood, pus, and mucus); tenesmus; abdominal pain (tenderness in severe disease); rectal urgency, occasional fecal incontinence; weight loss; arthralgias

PHYSICAL EXAM
- Arthralgias and arthritis: 15–40%
- Spondylitis: 3–6%
- Ocular: 4–10%; includes uveitis, cataracts, keratopathy, and central serous retinopathy
- Erythema nodosum
- Pyoderma gangrenosum
- Aphthous ulcers of mouth: 5–10%

DIFFERENTIAL DIAGNOSIS
- Other sources of rectal bleeding: Hemorrhoids, neoplasms, colonic diverticula, arteriovenous malformation, Crohn disease
- Infectious diarrhea, including bacterial (enterotoxigenic *Escherichia coli*), *Clostridium difficile* colitis, and parasitic (*Entamoeba histolytica*)
- Herpes simplex, *Chlamydia trachomatis*, *Cryptosporidium, Isospora belli*, cytomegalovirus
- Radiation proctitis; ischemic colitis

DIAGNOSTIC TESTS & INTERPRETATION
- Anemia (chronic disease ± iron deficiency from blood loss)
- Leukocytosis during exacerbation
- Elevated ESR and CRP
- Electrolyte abnormalities, especially hypokalemia
- Hypoalbuminemia, elevated LFTs
- Perinuclear antineutrophil cytoplasmic antibody (pANCA) is elevated in 85% of cases.
- Anti-*Saccharomyces cerevisiae* antibodies (ASCA—more common in Crohn disease) or pANCA can diagnose, but not rule out IBD.
- Antiglycan antibody is elevated in 75% of Crohn disease and 5% of ulcerative colitis cases.

Initial Tests (lab, imaging)
- Plain abdominal films:
  - Obtain immediately in patients with significant abdominal tenderness, fever, and leukocytosis for early diagnosis of toxic megacolon and perforation
- Upper GI series with small bowel follow-through to rule out Crohn disease
- Ultrasound, MRI, scintigraphy, and CT may have similar accuracy in diagnosis of IBD (1)[A].

Diagnostic Procedures/Other
- Sigmoidoscopy (2) (may include biopsy): Should be sufficient to make initial diagnosis
- Colonoscopy (2) (may include biopsy):
  - For evaluation of premalignant features; to differentiate from Crohn disease; to investigate suspected stricture/mass; to define the extent and location of involvement
- Full colonoscopy contraindicated in severely active disease/colonic dilatation (risk of perforation)

Test Interpretation
Inflammation of the colonic mucosa with ulcerations:
- Ulcerations are hyperemic and hemorrhagic.
- Rectum is involved 95% of the time.
- Extends proximally, without skips
- May affect terminal ileum, so-called backwash ileitis
- Colonic strictures are rare with ulcerative colitis.

TREATMENT
Management involves acute treatment of inflammatory symptoms, followed by maintenance of remission; therapeutic approach determined by symptom severity and the degree of colonic involvement:

- 5-aminosalicylic acid (5-ASA) therapies are effective in inducing remission in mild to moderately active disease (number needed to treat [NNT] = 6) and are very effective at preventing relapse in quiescent disease (NNT = 4) (2)[A]:
  - Topical mesalamine agents may be superior to oral aminosalicylates or topical steroids for proctitis but often have systemic side effects due to mucosal absorption (2)[A].
  - Combination of oral and topical aminosalicylates is more effective than either alone (2)[A].
- Corticosteroid therapies are effective at inducing remission in active disease (NNT = 3) (2)[A].
- Azathioprine or 6-mercaptopurine (6-MP) are not recommended for inducing remission in active disease, but are effective as steroid-sparing agents or to "hold" the response from steroids as the steroids are tapered (2)[C].
- Methotrexate is not recommended for inducing remission in active disease or for preventing relapse in quiescent disease (2)[C]. (It is only indicated in Crohn disease.)

- Maintenance of remission in mild to moderate distal disease with the use of the following: Mesalamine suppositories for proctitis or enemas for distal colitis, sulfasalazine, balsalazide, or combination oral and topical mesalamine (2)[A]
- Maintenance of remission in mild to moderate extensive disease with the use of the following: Sulfasalazine, olsalazine, mesalamine, and balsalazide (2)[A]
- Infliximab is effective at inducing remission in ambulatory patients with moderate to severely active disease (2)[A] and for symptomatic improvement of hospitalized patients with severely active disease (2)[C].

GENERAL MEASURES
Control inflammation, prevent complications, and replace nutritional losses and blood volume.

MEDICATION
First Line
- Sulfasalazine:
  - Uncoated tablets. Adults: Initial: 1 g PO q6–8h; maintenance: 500 mg PO q6h. Children ≥6 years: Initial: 40–60 mg/kg/d PO in 3–6 divided doses; maintenance: 30 mg/kg/d PO divided q6h (max 2 g/d)
  - Enteric-coated tablets. Adults: Initial: 3–4 g/d PO in divided doses; maintenance: 2 g/d PO in divided doses. Children ≥6 years: Initial: 40–60 mg/kg/d PO in 3–6 divided doses; maintenance: 30 mg/kg/d PO in 4 divided doses (max 2 g/d)
- Mesalamine:
  - Oral delayed-release tablets (Asacol) for induction of remission. Adults: 800 mg PO t.i.d. × 6 weeks
  - Oral controlled-release tablets (Pentasa) for maintenance of remission. Adults: 1 g PO q.i.d.

- Single daily dose available for mesalamine under brand Lialda (acute therapy 4.8 g once daily or 2.4 g once daily for maintenance) and brand name Apriso (1.5 g once daily; approved in the US ONLY for maintenance).
- Once daily dosing is as effective as conventional t.i.d. dosing for mild to moderately active ulcerative colitis treatment and for maintenance of remission (3)[A].
- 5-ASA (e.g., mesalamine) enemas and suppositories can be used to treat proctitis/proctosigmoiditis:
  - Suppositories: (Canasa) Adults: 1,000 mg per rectum at bedtime
  - Enemas: Adults: 4 g per rectum, retained for 8 hours each night; use for 3–6 weeks or until remission is achieved.
- Balsalazide: Adults: 2,250 mg PO t.i.d. for total daily dose of 6.75 g for 8–12 weeks. Children/Adolescents: 2,250 mg PO t.i.d. for total daily dose of 6.75 g or 750 mg PO t.i.d. for total daily dose of 2.25 g for 8 weeks
- Olsalazine: Adults: 500 mg PO b.i.d. (up to 3 g/d). Children/Adolescents: 30 mg/kg/d in 2 divided doses (up to 2 g/d), primarily used for maintenance

Second Line
- Prednisone for severe exacerbations: Adult dosage: Initial: 40–60 mg/d PO (max 1 mg/kg/d) × 7–10 days; taper over 2–3 months; can be given IV in hospitalized patients
- Infliximab is effective in patients whose disease is refractory to conventional treatment (2,4)[A]:
  - Adult dose: 5 mg/kg IV at weeks 0, 2, and 6 for induction, then maintenance of 5 mg/kg IV is given every 8 weeks
- Adalimumab: For moderate to severe ulcerative colitis refractory to steroids and azathioprine/6-MP. Initial dose: 160 mg; 2nd dose 2 weeks later: 80 mg, and maintenance: 40 mg every other week thereafter. Should only be continued if evidence of remission by 8 weeks (4).

Pediatric Considerations
- Infliximab can increase the risk of cancer in children and adolescents; weigh risks vs. benefits.
- Immunomodulators can be used in patients unresponsive to steroids and aminosalicylates or who cannot be weaned from high-dose steroids:
  - Daily plain films of the abdomen are obtained until improvement occurs.
  - If dilatation of colon increases/treatment has failed to attain reversal in 72 hours, emergency colectomy is indicated.

SURGERY/OTHER PROCEDURES
- Indicated for medically refractory disease/when treatment side effects are unacceptable (high-dose steroids)
- May be emergent for massive hemorrhage, perforation, and toxic dilatation of the colon
- Surgery also indicated for cancer/multisite mucosal dysplasia
- Total colectomy with ileostomy is *curative*. An alternative is total colectomy with ileoproctostomy.
- Regular proctoscopic surveillance is required if a colonic mucosal cuff is retained, thereby leaving a risk of future cancer development.

COMPLEMENTARY AND ALTERNATIVE MEDICINE
- Insufficient evidence exists to support the efficacy of probiotics for maintenance of remission (5)[A].

- Encouraging results but limited studies for aloe vera gel, wheat grass juice, *Andrographis paniculata* extract (HMPL-004), topical Xilei-san, Curcumin, *Boswellia serrata* gum resin, *Plantago ovata* seeds, evening primrose oil, wormwood, and *Tripterygium wilfordii* (6)[A]

IN-PATIENT CONSIDERATIONS
Admission Criteria/Initial Stabilization
- Obtain imaging studies to assess disease activity
- Initiate IV corticosteroids and rule out infectious etiologies (clostridium difficile infection, cytomegalovirus) as well as bacterial infections (e.g., shigella)/ameba with acute presentations.

 ONGOING CARE

FOLLOW-UP RECOMMENDATIONS
Patient Monitoring
- Surveillance colonoscopy. Recommendations vary with different GI societies. Most recommend beginning a surveillance program after 7–8 years of disease with involvement beyond the splenic flexure and that total colonoscopy should be performed every 1–2 years.
- Controversial if low-grade dysplasia is found on surveillance biopsy, although most recommend total colectomy if low-grade dysplasia is found in a surgical candidate.
- Magnification chromoendoscopy may detect significantly more intraepithelial neoplasias than conventional colonoscopy.
- Annual LFTs
- Patients on long-term mesalamine need annual BUN/creatinine.
- Cholangiography for cholestasis

Pediatric Considerations
Cancer surveillance is important because occurrence of cancer relates to the duration and extent of disease, whether or not frequently symptomatic.

DIET
- NPO during acute exacerbations
- Lactose-free diet is often recommended; evidence-based support is lacking without an associated lactase deficiency.
- Omega-3 fatty acids, seal and cod liver oil, dietary lactulose, wheat grass juice, vitamin D, and diets with decreased meat and alcohol have been recommended to reduce relapses and improve systemic symptoms (evidence conflicting) (7)[A].

PATIENT EDUCATION
- Discuss the importance of adherence to drug therapy to induce and maintain remission.
- Self-help organizations such as Crohn and Colitis Foundation of America (CCFA) www.ccfa.org

PROGNOSIS
- Variable; mortality for initial attack is ~5%; 75–85% experience relapse; and up to 20% eventually require colectomy.
- Colon cancer risk is the single most important risk factor affecting long-term prognosis.
- Primary sclerosing cholangitis increases the risk of colon cancer in patients with ulcerative colitis (8).
- Left-sided colitis and ulcerative proctitis have favorable prognoses with probable normal lifespan.

Geriatric Considerations
Increased mortality if 1st presentation occurs after 60 years of age

COMPLICATIONS
Perforation; toxic megacolon; liver disease; stricture formation (<Crohn disease); colon cancer

REFERENCES
1. Horsthuis K, Bipat S, Bennink RJ, et al. Inflammatory bowel disease diagnosed with US, MR, scintigraphy, and CT: Meta-analysis of prospective studies. *Radiology*. 2008;247:64–79.
2. Talley NJ, Abreu MT, Achkar JP, et al. An evidence-based systematic review on medical therapies for inflammatory bowel disease. *Am J Gastroenterol*. 2011;106:S2–S2.
3. Feagan BG, MacDonald JK. Once daily oral mesalamine compared to conventional dosing for induction and maintenance of remission in ulcerative colitis: A systematic review and meta-analysis. *Inflamm Bowel Dis*. 2012;84: 1785–1794.
4. Sandborn WJ, van Assche G, Reinisch W, et al. Adalimumab induces and maintains clinical remission in patients with moderate-to-severe ulcerative colitis. *Gastroenterology*. 2012;84: 257–265.e1–e3.
5. Jonkers D, Penders J, Masclee A, et al. Probiotics in the management of inflammatory bowel disease: A systematic review of intervention studies in adult patients. *Drugs*. 2012;72:803–823.
6. Ng SC, Lam YT, Tsoi KK, et al. Systematic review: the efficacy of herbal therapy in inflammatory bowel disease. *Aliment Pharmacol Ther*. 2013;38: 854–863.
7. Nicholson I, Dalzell AM, El-Matary W, et al. Vitamin D as a therapy for colitis: A systematic review. *J Crohns Colitis*. 2012;6:405–411.
8. Soetikno RM, Lin OS, Heidenreich PA, et al. Increased risk of colorectal neoplasia in patients with primary sclerosing cholangitis and ulcerative colitis: A meta-analysis. *Gastrointest Endosc*. 2002;84:48–54.

ADDITIONAL READING
Huang X, Lv B, Jin HF, et al. A meta-analysis of the therapeutic effects of tumor necrosis factor-α blockers on ulcerative colitis. *Eur J Clin Pharmacol*. 2011;84: 759–766.

 SEE ALSO

Algorithm: Hematemesis (Bleeding, Upper GI)

 CODES

ICD10
- K51.80 Other ulcerative colitis without complications
- K51.90 Ulcerative colitis, unspecified, without complications
- K51.919 Ulcerative colitis, unspecified with unspecified complications

CLINICAL PEARLS
- Treat proctitis with 5-ASA suppositories (not oral).
- Normal screening lab tests (ESR, hemoglobin, platelets, and albumin) do NOT rule out IBD regardless of disease severity.
- Colectomy is curative.

UPPER RESPIRATORY INFECTION

Lisa M. Schroeder, MD

 BASICS

Upper respiratory infections (URIs) are the 2nd most common medical diagnosis, contributing to ~20 million/year office visits.

DESCRIPTION
- Inflammation of nasal passages resulting from infection with various respiratory viruses
- Most cases are self-treated.
- Usually mild–moderate severity, self-limited
- System(s) affected: ENT; Pulmonary

EPIDEMIOLOGY
- Each virus has different seasonal peaks (e.g., rhinovirus: Late spring, fall)
- Cold climates do not increase susceptibility.
- Transmission:
  - Hand contact with contaminated skin/surface followed by contact with mucous membranes
  - Aerosolized particles from sneezing and coughing
- Viral shedding peaks after 48–72 hours of illness and can last up to 2 weeks.
- Virus may last up to 2 hours on skin or longer on environmental surfaces.

Incidence
- Predominant age: Children > Adults:
  - Preschool children: 6–10 colds/year
  - Kindergarten: 12/year
  - Schoolchildren: 7/year
  - Adolescents/Adults: 2–4/year
- Predominant sex: Male = Female

ETIOLOGY AND PATHOPHYSIOLOGY
Rhinoviruses infect the ciliated epithelium lining the nose, resulting in edema and hyperemia of nasal mucous membranes.
- 1/200 virus strains from different virus families; many strains present within the same geographic region or patient family:
  - Rhinovirus, with >100 serotypes: 30–50%
  - Influenzavirus types A, B, C: 15%
  - Coronaviruses: 15%
  - Parainfluenza, respiratory syncytial virus (RSV): 10%; more common in children
  - Enteroviruses, adenoviruses: <10%
- In 30% of cases, no pathogen is identified.

RISK FACTORS
- Exposure to infected people
- Allergic disorders
- Smoking
- Immunosuppression
- Malnutrition

GENERAL PREVENTION
- Frequent handwashing, especially in children (1)[A]
- Limiting exposure to infected persons/children

COMMONLY ASSOCIATED CONDITIONS
- Pharyngitis
- Sinusitis
- Otitis media
- Bronchitis
- Bronchiolitis
- Pneumonia
- Croup
- Asthma

 DIAGNOSIS

HISTORY
- Onset of symptoms is 1–3 days after exposure.
- Nasal stuffiness and/or obstruction: 80–100%
- Sneezing: 50–70%
- Scratchy throat: 50%
- Cough: 40%
- Hoarseness: 30%
- Malaise: 20–25%
- Headache: 25%
- Fever >100°F (37.7°C): 0–1%

PHYSICAL EXAM
- Low-grade temperature/afebrile
- Stable vital signs
- Rhinorrhea (clear, yellow, or green)
- Inflamed mucosa
- Postnasal drainage
- Erythema of the throat
- Dull tympanic membranes

DIFFERENTIAL DIAGNOSIS
- Allergic rhinitis
- Acute sinusitis
- Strep pharyngitis
- Infectious mononucleosis
- Influenza
- Pertussis

DIAGNOSTIC TESTS & INTERPRETATION
Initial Tests (lab, imaging)
- No routine lab testing is needed.
- For pharyngitis, use a lab test (rapid strep antigen/culture) to rule out group A streptococcal infection.
- Rapid flu test if influenza suspected
- Imaging is not necessary to distinguish URI from acute bacterial sinusitis in children (2)[C].

Follow-Up Tests & Special Considerations
Patients should contact the primary care physician's office for fever >101°F associated with systemic symptoms, difficulty breathing, or purulent drainage >2 days.

Test Interpretation
- Exudation of serous and mucinous fluid containing immunoglobulins
- Histology: Edema of subepithelial connective tissue and a scanty cellular infiltrate containing neutrophils, plasma cells, lymphocytes, and eosinophils
- Rhinovirus causes a "nondestructive" inflammation of the mucous membranes.
- Influenza and parainfluenza denude epithelium to the basement membrane.

TREATMENT

GENERAL MEASURES
- Smoking cessation
- Vaporizer/Humidifier: No consistent benefit proven (3)[A]

MEDICATION
Primarily for supportive therapy

First Line
- Avoid Antibiotics – more harm than good (4)[A]
- Analgesics: Acetaminophen, ASA, and NSAIDs for relieving discomfort or pain caused by the common cold (5)[A]
- Topical decongestants (sympathomimetics) reduce nasal mucosa swelling and airflow resistance, promote drainage. Topicals have minimal systemic effects. Sprays preferred over drops in patients >6 years of age:
  - Rebound congestion may occur after 72 hours of use:
    - Oxymetazoline:
      - Adults and children aged 6–12 years: 0.05% solution, 2–3 sprays in each nostril b.i.d.
      - Children aged 2–6 years: 0.025% solution, 2–3 drops in each nostril b.i.d.
- Inhaled anticholinergics:
  - Ipratropium inhaler: A bronchodilator; recommended by the American College of Chest Physicians for use as a cough suppressant in URIs (ACCP Grade A):
    - Adults and children age >14 years: 2 sprays (17 µg/spray) 4×/d.
- Topical anticholinergics may improve rhinorrhea and sneezing, but do not relieve nasal congestion:
  - Ipratropium: Adults and children >11 years of age: 0.06% solution, 2 sprays to each nostril t.i.d. × 4 days (6)[A]
- Oral decongestants (sympathomimetic) advantages over topical decongestants: Longer duration of action, lack of local irritation, and no risk of rebound congestion:
  - Pseudoephedrine: Potential for abuse/misuse for methamphetamine production:
    - Adults: 60 mg q4–6h (120 mg sustained-release q12h) superior to placebo in short-term use (7)[A]
    - Children aged 6–12 years: 30 mg q4–6h; 2–5 years: 15 mg q4–6h
  - Acute cough, postnasal drip, and throat clearing associated with the common cold can be treated with a 1st-generation antihistamine/decongestant preparation (brompheniramine and sustained-release pseudoephedrine) (ACCP Grade A) (8)[A].
  - A single oral dose of phenylephrine 10 mg is an effective decongestant in adults with acute nasal congestion associated with the common cold (9)[A].
- Antihistamines: Safe and mildly effective for sneezing and rhinorrhea. Only 1st-generation (sedating) antihistamines show any symptomatic relief, but sedation may be worse than relief:
  - Chlorpheniramine:
    - Adults: 4 mg q.i.d., 8 mg t.i.d., 12 mg b.i.d.
    - Children age 6–12: 2 mg q4–6h
    - Children age 2–6: 1 mg q4–6h
  - Brompheniramine
- Cough suppressants: Not recommended for use by the ACCP (ACCP Grade D) due to limited efficacy:
  - Codeine: Side effects of sedation and GI upset:
    - Adults: 10–20 mg q4–6h PRN
  - Dextromethorphan:
    - Adults: 10–30 mg q4–6h
    - Children age 6–12: 15 mg q4–6h

- Children age 2–6: 2.5–7.5 mg q4–6h
  - Nasal steroids: Current evidence does not support the use of intranasal corticosteroids for symptomatic relief from the common cold (10)[A].
- Expectorants:
  - Guaifenesin (no evidence in children, some evidence in adults):
    - Adults: 100–400 mg q4h
    - Children age 6–12: 100–200 mg q4h
    - Children age 2–6: 50–100 mg q4h
- Common combinations: Most cold medicines come in combinations: Not recommended for use by ACCP (Grade D):
  - Dextromethorphan/Phenylephrine/Guaifenesin: 10/5/100 mg, pediatric: 5/2.5/50
  - Dextromethorphan/Guaifenesin: 10/100 mg
  - Acetaminophen/Chlorpheniramine/Dextromethorphan/Phenylephrine: 160/1/5/2.5 mg
  - Chlorpheniramine/Dextromethorphan/Phenylephrine: 4/15/12.5 mg
  - Chlorpheniramine/Dextromethorphan: 1/7.5 mg

Pediatric Considerations
In 2007, the FDA issued a warning on all cough and cold preparations for children age ≤2 due to risk of overdose.

Second Line
- Many mouthwashes, gargles, and lozenges are promoted to relieve the pain of sore throat. The demulcent effects of hard candy, gargling with warm saline, and products with anesthetics (benzocaine/phenol) may provide pain relief.
- Aromatic oils (menthol, camphor, eucalyptus), in topical/lozenge form, produce a sensation of increased airflow in the absence of a significant change in airflow resistance.
- Saline nasal irrigation is safe for adults and children.
- *Antibiotics are not recommended. They produce minimal to no reduction in symptoms or duration, with greater risk of side effects from usage.*

COMPLEMENTARY AND ALTERNATIVE MEDICINE
- Zinc prevents viral replication in vitro:
  - Avoid intranasal preparations of zinc: Risk of potential permanent loss of smell
  - Has shown moderate benefit in reducing symptoms and duration, but proper dosing has not been determined (11)[A]
- Echinacea has not proven effective for treatment of common cold symptoms (12)[A].
- Probiotics may decrease severity and duration of URIs and possibly reduce episodes (13)[A].
- Vitamin C (ascorbic acid):
  - Regular supplementation trials have shown that vitamin C may reduce the duration of colds (14)[A].
  - Vitamin C prophylaxis *not* recommended for general use, but may be beneficial in those exposed to severe physical exertion and cold environments (14)[A].
  - Precipitation of urate, oxalate, or cystine stones has been seen. Urine glucose monitoring may be inaccurate in people taking large doses of vitamin C.

Geriatric Considerations
Cold medications, especially decongestants and antihistamines, commonly produce adverse effects in older people.

Pregnancy Considerations
- Ipratropium is category B.
- Decongestants: No clear association has been determined between use of this drug group and congenital defects.
- Antihistamines: No clear association has been confirmed between use of this drug group and congenital defects.
- Codeine: Indiscriminate use during pregnancy may pose a risk to the fetus.

ONGOING CARE

FOLLOW-UP RECOMMENDATIONS
Contact the primary care physician's office for fever, difficulty breathing, or symptoms persisting beyond expected course.

DIET
Encourage fluids and adequate hydration (15)[C].

PATIENT EDUCATION
- Discuss with patients the difference between viral and bacterial infections; instruct about appropriate and inappropriate antibiotic use.
- Frequent hand washing (1)[A]
- Symptomatic treatment; no cure
- Reinfection is possible with reexposure.
- Patient information: www.niaid.nih.gov/factsheets/cold.htm

PROGNOSIS
- Excellent; expect full recovery. Usual duration 5–7 days, but may last up to 2 weeks. For smokers, 3–4 additional days.
- Cough may persist after other symptoms have resolved.

COMPLICATIONS
Small percentage may develop worsening symptoms leading to otitis media, sinusitis, bronchitis, or pneumonia.

REFERENCES

1. Jefferson T, Del Mar CB, Dooley L, et al. Physical interventions to interrupt or reduce the spread of respiratory viruses. *Cochrane Database Syst Rev.* 2011;CD006207.
2. Walder ER, Applegate KE, Bordley C, et al. Clinical practice guideline for diagnosis and management of acute bacterial sinusitis in children aged 1–18 years. *Pediatrics.* 2013;132(1):e262–e280.
3. Singh M, Singh M. Heated, humidified air for the common cold. *Cochrane Database Syst Rev.* 2013; 6:CD001728.
4. Kenealy T, Arroll B. Antibiotics for the common cold and acute purulent sinusitis. *Cochrane Database Syst Rev.* 2013;6 CD000247.
5. Kim SY, Chang YJ, Cho HM, et al. Non-steroidal anti-inflammatory drugs for the common cold. *Cochrane Database Syst Rev.* 20134;6: CD006362.
6. Al Balawi ZH, Othman SS, Alfaleh K. Intranasal ipratropium bromide for the common cold. *Cochrane Database Syst Rev.* 2013;6:CD008231.
7. Eccles R, Jawad MS, Jawad SS. Efficacy and safety of single and multiple doses of pseudoephedrine in the treatment of nasal congestion associated with common cold. *Am J Rhinol.* 2005;19:25–31.
8. De Sutter AI, van Driel ML, Kumar AA, et al. Oral antihistamine-decongestant-analgesic combinations for the common cold. *Cochrane Database Syst Rev.* 2012;2:CD004976.
9. Kollar C, Schneider H, Waksman J. Meta-analysis of the efficacy of a single dose of phenylephrine 10 mg compared with placebo in adults with acute nasal congestion due to the common cold. *Cl Therapeutics.* 2007;29(6):1057–1070.
10. Hayward G, Thompson MJ, Perera R, et al. Corticosteroids for the common cold. *Cochrane Database Syst Rev.* 2012;8:CD008116.
11. Singh M, Das RR. Zinc for the common cold. *Cochrane Database Syst Rev.* 2013;6:CD001364.
12. Linde K, Barrett B, Wolkart K, et al. Echinacea for preventing and treating the common cold. Cochrane Acute Respiratory Infections Group. *Cochrane Database Syst Rev.* 2006;4.
13. Hao Q, Lu Z, Dong BR, et al. Probiotics for preventing acute upper respiratory tract infections. *Cochrane Database Syst Rev.* 2011;(9):CD006895.
14. Hemilä H, Chalker E. Vitamin C for preventing and treating the common cold. *Cochrane Database Syst Rev.* 2013;1:CD000980.
15. Guppy MP, Mickan SM, Del Mar CB, et al. Advising patients to increase fluid intake for treating acute respiratory infections. *Cochrane Database Syst Rev.* 2011;(2):CD004419.

ADDITIONAL READING

- CDC. Treatment Guidelines for Upper Respiratory Tract Infections. Available at: www.cdc.gov.
- Li S, Yue J, Dong BR, et al. Acetaminophen (paracetamol) for the common cold in adults. *Cochrane Database Syst Rev.* 20131;7:CD008800.
- National Guideline Clearinghouse. 2008 diagnosis and treatment of respiratory illness in children and adults. Available at: www.guideline.gov.
- National Guideline Clearinghouse. Cough suppressant and pharmacologic protussive therapy: ACCP evidence-based clinical practice guidelines and cough and the common cold. Available at: www.guideline.gov.

SEE ALSO

Bronchitis, Acute; Pharyngitis; Rhinitis, Allergic

CODES

ICD10
- B34.8 Other viral infections of unspecified site
- J06.9 Acute upper respiratory infection, unspecified
- J11.1 Influenza due to unidentified influenza virus with other respiratory manifestations

CLINICAL PEARLS
- Supportive therapy is mainstay; many commonly recommended treatments lack medical evidence.
- If pharyngitis is the primary complaint, diagnose group A streptococcus with lab testing.
- Limit unnecessary use of antibiotics.
- Patient education is key.
- Smokers have symptoms that last 3–4 more days than nonsmokers.

URETHRITIS

Karen Cherian, MD • David O Parrish, MD

 BASICS

DESCRIPTION
- Urethral inflammation marked by dysuria, pruritus, mucopurulent discharge, and/or hematuria
- Usually a result of an STI or, less commonly, autoimmune disorders (Reiter syndrome), trauma, or chemical irritation
- Complications include epididymitis, endocarditis, meningitis, or disseminated gonococcal infection.
- Risk factors:
  - Women and men <25
  - Patients with history of prior STIs
  - Patients with new and/or multiple sexual partners
  - Sex workers
  - Drug users
  - African Americans
  - Men who have sex with men
  - Patients with inconsistent condom use

EPIDEMIOLOGY
Incidence
- In 2011, 1.4 million new cases of chlamydia and 321,000 cases of gonorrhea were reported by the CDC. Prevalence varies by region, with highest incident in southern US; racial discrepancies include an 8× higher rate for African Americans and a 2.7× higher rate for Hispanic patients compared with whites (1,2).
- Predominant age: 15–24 years, sexually active, following trends for STI
- Predominant sex: Men report symptoms more frequently, but similar incidence is likely.

ETIOLOGY AND PATHOPHYSIOLOGY
- Predominantly *Neisseria gonorrhoeae* and *Chlamydia trachomatis* infection, increased transmission among HIV-positive persons
- Less common infectious agents include:
  - *Ureaplasma urealyticum*
  - *Trichomonas vaginalis*
  - Herpesvirus
  - *Mycoplasma genitalium*
  - Viral: Conflicting data on HPV, herpes simplex
- Noninfectious causes (generally rare): Foreign bodies, soaps, shampoos, douches, spermicides, urethral instrumentation

RISK FACTORS
- Multiple sexual partners and unprotected intercourse
- African American, Native American, or Hispanic ethnicity
- History of STIs, bacterial vaginosis, recurrent candidiasis
- Excessive use of chemical lubricants or powders

GENERAL PREVENTION
- Safer sex techniques and treatment of all partners
- Abstinence
- Avoidance of excessive lubricants, powders, or chemical irritants

COMMONLY ASSOCIATED CONDITIONS

ALERT
Patients with any suspected STI should undergo testing for syphilis, hepatitis B and C, *Trichomonas*, and HIV.
Gonorrhea and *Chlamydia* are reportable to the Health Department.

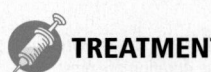 DIAGNOSIS

- Important to take detailed sexual and travel history; increased incidence seen with travel to some regions with resistance to cephalosporins in Asian countries (1,3)
- In men:
  - Abrupt onset of dysuria symptoms 3–14 days after exposure to an infected sexual partner
  - Urethral discharge: May be profuse and purulent in acute gonorrhea
  - Urethral itching or tenderness
  - Proctitis, pharyngitis, and conjunctivitis also may be present (sexual history is important).
- In women: Classic urethral syndrome often is not present:
  - Tenderness, edema, and inflammation of the urethral meatus, especially in women
  - Dyspareunia
  - Vaginitis, cystitis, cervicitis
- Fever is not part of the syndrome and usually suggests another diagnosis.
- Bloody discharge: Rarely seen and suggests another diagnosis
- Suprapubic or abdominal pain suggests another diagnosis or the emergence of complications (e.g., PID, prostatitis, or cystitis).
- Key physical exam points:
  - Expression of purulent urethral discharge
  - Palpate scrotum to check for epididymitis or orchitis.
  - Check for ulcers.
  - Check for inguinal lymphadenopathy.

Pediatric Considerations
In pediatric patients, proven cases of gonorrhea, chlamydia, and trichomoniasis require evaluation for sexual abuse.

DIFFERENTIAL DIAGNOSIS
- Other genitourinary tract diseases:
  - Cystitis/urinary tract infection
  - Epididymitis
  - Prostatitis
  - PID
  - Pyelonephritis
- Vaginal atrophy, especially in postmenopausal women
- Stevens-Johnson syndrome
- Reiter syndrome: Uveitis, urethritis, arthritis (can't see, can't pee, can't climb a tree)
- Wegener granulomatosis

DIAGNOSTIC TESTS & INTERPRETATION
- For patients who present without symptoms and state that a sexual partner was treated for this problem, obtain specimens for lab tests, but also provide immediate treatment.
- Check culture and antibiotic susceptibilities in patients suspected of having resistant infections.
- Evidence is insufficient to recommend for or against screening in asymptomatic men at increased risk.

ALERT
The US Preventative Services Task Force recommends screening all sexually active women until age 25 years and all women at increased risk of infection.
- Gram stain of discharge: ≥5 WBCs per high-power field (HPF) indicates urethritis. Intracellular gram-negative diplococci strongly indicate gonorrhea.
- Cultures of the intraurethral/endocervical swabs:
  - Gonorrhea and chlamydia cultures should be obtained in all symptomatic patients.
  - Culture may be performed on urethral exudates if they are present.
- Nucleic acid amplification test (NAAT) using polymerase chain reaction assay on urine is very sensitive and specific but costly. Also test for other, less common pathogens if negative.
- Urinalysis:
  - Usually normal in cases of simple urethritis
  - 1st-void urine often is positive for leukocyte esterase and should have ≥10 WBCs per HPF in urethritis.
  - Men should not have urinated for at least 4 hours prior.
- Urine culture: Performed only if Gram stain of discharge is unremarkable or unobtainable
- Wet prep: May reveal *Trichomonas*; trichomoniasis, bacterial vaginosis, and *Candida* infection; need to be evaluated for persistent symptoms after antibiotic course
- Syphilis, HIV, and hepatitis B serology as indicated to rule out concomitant STIs

Initial Tests (lab, imaging)

ALERT
When an STI is suspected, provide informed consent and recommend HIV testing at initial presentation.

Follow-Up Tests & Special Considerations
Test of cure for chlamydia and gonorrhea is recommended in pregnant women or when treatment noncompliance is suspected.

Diagnostic Procedures/Other
Urethrocystoscopy for cases with suspected foreign body, intraurethral warts, urethral stricture

Test Interpretation
Urethral strictures (untreated gonorrhea), intraurethral lesions (venereal warts, congenital anomalies), PID, or tubo-ovarian abscesses possible

TREATMENT

GENERAL MEASURES
All sexual partners who came in contact with the patient within 60 days should be evaluated, tested, and treated for both gonorrhea and chlamydia.

MEDICATION
First Line
- Most cases can be treated in the outpatient setting.
- Single-dose regimens, directly observed in office for noncompliant or high-risk patients
- Antibiotics should not be withheld from symptomatic patients until culture results are known if there is a convincing clinical presentation.

- Treatment should cover both gonorrhea and chlamydia and any other suspected pathogens.
- Gonorrhea (3,4):
  - Ceftriaxone 250 mg IM *and* either doxycycline 100 mg PO b.i.d. for 7 days *or* azithromycin 1 g PO
  - For children ≤45 kg: Ceftriaxone 125 mg IM single dose
  - If ceftriaxone is not an option: Cefixime 400 mg PO single dose *and* either doxycycline 100 mg PO b.i.d. × 7 days *or* azithromycin 1 g PO followed by a test-of-cure in 1 week
  - If patient has high-risk allergy to cephalosporins, azithromycin 2 g PO can be given, followed by a test-of-cure in 1 week. This should be limited due to increasing resistance.
- Chlamydia:
  - Doxycycline: 100 mg PO b.i.d. for 7 days *or*
  - Azithromycin: 1 g PO single dose
- Trichomoniasis:
  - Metronidazole: 2 g PO single dose *or* metronidazole 250 mg t.i.d. for 7 days
- Recurrent and resistant urethritis:
  - Metronidazole: 2 mg PO single dose *or* tinidazole 2 g PO single dose *and* azithromycin 1 g PO single dose, if not already used for initial episode
  - Erythromycin 500 mg PO q.i.d. for 7 days *and* valacyclovir 400 mg PO t.i.d. for 5 days if suspicious for herpes simplex virus (HSV)
- Contraindications: Sensitivity to any of the indicated medications
- Precautions: Patients taking tetracyclines may have increased photosensitivity.
- Significant possible interactions:
  - Tetracyclines should not be taken with milk products or antacids.
  - Oral contraceptives may be rendered less effective by oral antibiotics. Patients and partners should use a backup method of birth control for the remainder of the cycle.

Pregnancy Considerations
- Tetracyclines and quinolones are contraindicated.
- Avoid erythromycin estolate because of an increased risk of cholestatic jaundice; otherwise, use the standard treatment recommendations.
- Single-dose therapy is recommended.

Second Line
- Gonorrhea (3):
  - Fluoroquinolones were previously considered second-line treatment options; however, due to reported worldwide resistance, they are no longer recommended by the CDC.
  - Resistance to penicillin and tetracycline has been reported in up to 1/3 of isolates of *N. gonorrhoeae*.
  - Gonococcal treatment resistance noted to be more common among men who have sex with men, when compared to men who have sex with women (5).
- Chlamydia:
  - Erythromycin base 500 mg PO q.i.d. for 7 days *or* erythromycin ethylsuccinate 800 mg PO q.i.d. for 7 days: If intolerant of high-dose erythromycin, then erythromycin base 250 mg PO q.i.d. for 14 days *or* erythromycin ethylsuccinate 400 mg PO q.i.d. for 14 days *or*
  - Ofloxacin 300 mg PO b.i.d. for 7 days *or*
  - Levofloxacin 500 mg/d PO for 7 days

- Patients with persistent symptoms and signs after adequate treatment should be evaluated for other causes of urethritis:
  - Resistant strains of *Ureaplasma urealyticum* or *Mycoplasma genitalium*
  - *Trichomonas vaginalis*
  - Herpes simplex virus
  - Adenovirus
  - Enteric bacteria
  - Chronic nonbacterial prostatitis
  - Chronic pelvic pain syndrome

 ## ONGOING CARE

FOLLOW-UP RECOMMENDATIONS
- Full activity
- Sexual activity should be avoided until both partners complete treatment and are symptom-free or 7 days after single-dose therapy.
- Patients should refer their sexual partners for evaluation if they had sexual contact within 60 days of symptom onset. If the last sexual encounter was >60 days prior to symptom onset, the last sex partner should still be referred for diagnosis.
- If sexual partner is unlikely to follow-up, consider giving the patient antibiotic therapy to give to the partner.

Patient Monitoring
Instruct patients to return if symptoms persist or recur after completing treatment. Test-of-cure cultures usually are not required unless the patient is pregnant.

DIET
Avoid alcohol when taking metronidazole.

PATIENT EDUCATION
Most important to emphasize the need for compliance with therapy, treatment of sexual partners, and use of safer sex practices; patients should be urged to undergo screening for other STIs.

PROGNOSIS
If the diagnosis is firmly established, appropriate medications are prescribed, and the patient is compliant with treatment, relief of symptoms occurs within days and the problem will resolve without sequelae.

COMPLICATIONS
- Stricture formation
- Epididymitis
- Prostatitis
- Proctitis
- PID in women
- Disseminated gonococcal infection
- Gonococcal meningitis
- Gonococcal endocarditis
- Perinatal transmission (chlamydial conjunctivitis, chlamydial pneumonia, ophthalmia neonatorum)
- Reiter syndrome

REFERENCES
1. Ansart S, Hochedez P, Perez L, et al. Sexually transmitted diseases diagnosed among travelers returning from the tropics. *J Travel Med*. 2009;16:79–83.
2. Centers for Disease Control and Prevention. Sexually transmitted diseases treatment guidelines. *MMWR*. 2006;55(No. RR-11).
3. Workowski KA, Berman S. Sexually transmitted diseases treatment guidelines. *MMWR Recomm Rep*. 2010:59(No. RR-12).
4. Berg AO. Screening for chlamydia infections: Recommendations and rationale. *Am J Prev Med*. 2001;20:90–94.
5. Kirkcaldy RD, Zaidi A, Hook EW 3rd, et al. Neisseria gonorrhoeae antimicrobial resistance among men who have sex with men and men who have sex exclusively with women: The Gonococcal Isolate Surveillance Project, 2005–2010. *Ann Intern Med*, 2013;158:321–328.

ADDITIONAL READING
- Centers for Disease Control and Prevention. *Sexually transmitted disease surveillance, 2007*. Atlanta, GA: U.S. Department of Health and Human Services; December 2008.
- Centers for Disease Control and Prevention. Sexually transmitted diseases treatment guidelines, 2010. Gonococcal infections. Atlanta, GA: U.S. Department of Health and Human Services.
- Wetmore CM, Manhart LE, Lowens MS, et al. *Ureaplasma urealyticum* is associated with nongonococcal urethritis among men with fewer lifetime sexual partners: A case-control study. *J Infect Dis*. 2011;204:1274–1282.

 ## SEE ALSO
- Chlamydial Sexually Transmitted Diseases; Epididymitis; Gonococcal Infections; Pelvic Inflammatory Disease (PID); Prostatitis; Urinary Tract Infection in Females; Urinary Tract Infection in Males; Vulvovaginitis, Estrogen Deficient; Vulvovaginitis, Prepubescent
- Algorithms: Dysuria; Genital Ulcers; Urethral Discharge

 ## CODES

ICD10
- A54.01 Gonococcal cystitis and urethritis, unspecified
- A56.01 Chlamydial cystitis and urethritis
- N34.2 Other urethritis

CLINICAL PEARLS
- Urethral inflammation marked by painful urination, pruritus, hematuria, and/or discharge
- Usually a result of an STI or, less commonly, autoimmune disorders (Reiter syndrome), trauma, or chemical irritation
- Complications such as urethral stricture in men or PID in women may occur if untreated.

U

URINARY TRACT INFECTION (UTI) IN FEMALES
Akhil Das, MD, FACS

BASICS

DESCRIPTION
- Urinary tract infection (UTI) is the presence of pathogenic microorganisms within the urinary tract with concomitant symptoms.
- This topic refers primarily to infectious cystitis; other complicated UTIs, such as pyelonephritis, are discussed elsewhere.
- Uncomplicated UTI: Occurs in patients who have a normal, unobstructed urinary tract, who have no history of recent instrumentation, and whose symptoms are confined to the lower urinary tract. Uncomplicated UTIs are most common in young, sexually active women.
- Complicated UTI: An infection of the lower or upper urinary tract in the presence of an anatomic abnormality, a functional abnormality, or a urinary catheter
- Recurrent UTI: Symptomatic UTIs that follow resolution of an earlier episode, usually after appropriate treatment:
  - No single definition of the frequency of recurrent UTI exists, but a pragmatic definition is ≥3 infections per year.
  - Most recurrences are thought to represent reinfection rather than relapse.
  - No evidence indicates that recurrent UTIs lead to health problems such as hypertension or renal disease, in the absence of anatomic or functional abnormalities of the urinary tract (1).
- System(s) affected: Renal/Urologic
- Synonym(s): Cystitis; Infectious cystitis

EPIDEMIOLOGY
Incidence
- Accounts for 8 million doctor visits and 1 million emergency room visits, and contributes to >100,000 hospital admissions each year
- 11% of women have UTIs in any given year.
- Predominant age: Young adults and older
- Predominant sex: Female > Male

Prevalence
- >50% of females have at least 1 UTI in their lifetime.
- 1 in 4 women have recurrent UTIs.

ETIOLOGY AND PATHOPHYSIOLOGY
- Bacteria and subsequent infection in the urinary tract arise chiefly via ascending bacterial movement and propagation.
- Pathogenic organisms (*Escherichia coli*) possess adherence factors and toxins that allow initiation and propagation of genitourinary infections:
  - Type 1 and *P. pili (pyelonephritis-associated pili)*
  - Lipopolysaccharide
- Most UTIs are caused by bacteria originating from bowel flora:
  - *E. coli* is the causative organism in 80% of cases of uncomplicated cystitis.
  - *Staphylococcus saprophyticus* accounts for 15% of infections.
  - Enterobacteriaceae (i.e., *Klebsiella, Proteus, Enterobacter, Pseudomonas)* also contribute.
- *Candida* is associated with nosocomial UTI.

Genetics
Women with HLA-3 and nonsecretor Lewis antigen have an increased bacterial adherence, which may lead to an increased risk in UTI.

RISK FACTORS
- Previous UTI
- Diabetes mellitus (DM)
- Pregnancy
- Sexual activity
- Use of spermicides or diaphragm
- Underlying abnormalities of the urinary tract, such as tumors, calculi, strictures, incomplete bladder emptying, urinary incontinence, neurogenic bladder
- Catheterization
- Recent antibiotic use
- Poor hygiene
- Estrogen deficiency
- Inadequate fluid intake

GENERAL PREVENTION
- Maintain good hydration.
- Women with frequent or intercourse-related UTI should empty bladder immediately before and following intercourse; consider postcoital antibiotic.
- Avoid feminine hygiene sprays and douches.
- Wipe urethra from front to back.
- Cranberry juice (not cranberry juice cocktail) consumption may prevent recurrent infections.

COMMONLY ASSOCIATED CONDITIONS
See "Risk Factors."

Geriatric Considerations
- Elderly patients are more likely to have underlying urinary tract abnormality.
- Acute UTI may be associated with incontinence or mental status changes in the elderly.

DIAGNOSIS

HISTORY
Note: Any or all may be present:
- Burning during urination
- Pain during urination (dysuria)
- Urgency (sensation of need to urinate often)
- Frequency
- Sensation of incomplete bladder emptying
- Blood in urine
- Lower abdominal pain or cramping
- Offensive odor of urine
- Nocturia
- Sudden onset of urinary incontinence
- Dyspareunia

PHYSICAL EXAM
- Suprapubic tenderness
- Urethral and/or vaginal tenderness
- Fever or costovertebral angle tenderness indicates upper UTI.

DIFFERENTIAL DIAGNOSIS
- Vaginitis
- Asymptomatic bacteriuria
- STDs causing urethritis or pyuria
- Hematuria from causes other than infection (e.g., neoplasia, calculi)
- Interstitial cystitis
- Psychological dysfunction

DIAGNOSTIC TESTS & INTERPRETATION
Initial Tests (lab, imaging)
- No lab testing is necessary in women with high likelihood of lower UTI based on classic symptoms.
- Urinalysis:
  - Pyuria (>10 neutrophils/high-power field [HPF])
  - Bacteriuria (any amount on unspun urine, or 10 bacteria/HPF on centrifuged urine)
  - Hematuria (>5 RBCs/HPF)
- Dipstick urinalysis:
  - Leukocyte esterase (75–96% sensitivity, 94–98% specificity, when >100,000 colony-forming units [CFU])
  - Nitrite tests useful with nitrite-reducing organisms (e.g., Enterococci, *S. saprophyticus, Acinetobacter)*
- Urine culture: *Only* indicated if diagnosis is unclear or patient has recurrent infections and resistance is suspected:
  - Presence of 100,000 CFU/mL of organism indicates infection.
  - Identification of a single organism at lower CFU/mL likely also represents infection in the presence of appropriate symptoms.
  - Suspect a contaminated specimen when culture shows multiple types of bacteria.
- Imaging studies are often not required in most cases of UTI.

Follow-Up Tests & Special Considerations
- In nonpregnant, premenopausal women with symptoms of UTI, positive urinalysis, and no risks for complicated infection, empirical treatment may be given without obtaining a urine culture.
- Dipstick urinalysis may be helpful, but not necessary in patients with characteristic symptoms (i.e., high pretest probability).
- Imaging may be indicated for UTIs in men, infants, immunocompromised patients, febrile infection, signs or symptoms of obstruction, failure to respond to appropriate therapy, and in patients with recurrent infections.
- CT scan and MRI provide the most complete anatomic data in adults.

Pediatric Considerations
For infants and children, obtain US; if ureteral dilatation is detected, obtain either voiding cystourethrogram or isotope cystogram to evaluate for reflux.

Diagnostic Procedures/Other
- Urethral catheterization maybe necessary to obtain a urine specimen from children and adults if the voided urine is suspected of being contaminated.
- Suprapubic bladder aspiration or urethral catheterization can be used to obtain specimens from infants.
- Cystourethroscopy may be indicated for patients with recurrent UTIs and previous anti-incontinence surgery or hematuria.

TREATMENT

GENERAL MEASURES
- Maintain good hydration.
- Maintain good hygiene.
- 1/4 of women with uncomplicated UTI experience a 2nd UTI within 6 months and 1/2 at some time during their lifetime.

MEDICATION

First Line

- The urinary tract topical analgesic phenazopyridine 100–200 mg t.i.d. produces rapid relief of symptoms and should be offered to patients with more than minor discomfort; it is available over-the-counter. This medication is not a substitute for definitive treatment.
- Uncomplicated UTI (adolescents and adults who are nonpregnant, nondiabetic, afebrile, immunocompetent, and without genitourinary anatomic abnormalities) (2):
  - TMP-SMZ (Bactrim): 160/800 mg PO b.i.d. × 3 days (3,4)[A], best where resistance of *E. coli* strains <20%
  - 5-day course of nitrofurantoin or 3-day fluoroquinolone course should be used in patients with allergy to TMP-SMZ and in areas where *E. coli* resistance to TMP-SMZ >20% (3, 4)[A]
- Lower UTI in pregnancy:
  - Nitrofurantoin (Macrobid): 100 mg PO b.i.d. × 7 days (5)[C]
  - Cephalexin (Keflex): 500 mg PO b.i.d. × 7 days (5)[C]
- Postcoital UTI: Single-dose TMP-SMX or cephalexin may reduce frequency of UTI in sexually active women.
- Complicated UTI (pregnancy, diabetes, febrile, immunocompromised patient, recurrent UTIs): Extend course to 7–10 days of treatment with antibiotic chosen based on culture results; may begin with fluoroquinolone, TMP-SMX, or cephalosporin while awaiting results:
  - Fluoroquinolones are not safe during pregnancy and are usually avoided in treatment of children.
  - TMP-SMX use in pregnancy is not desirable (especially in 3rd trimester), but is appropriate in some circumstances.

Second Line

- Uncomplicated UTI:
  - Ciprofloxacin: 250 mg PO b.i.d. × 3 days; should be reserved for complicated UTIs
  - Fosfomycin (Monurol): 3 g PO single dose (expensive)
- Chronic UTIs:
  - Women with recurrent symptomatic UTIs can be treated with continuous or postcoital prophylactic antibiotics. Treatment duration guided by the severity of patient symptoms and by physician and patient preference: Consider 6 months of therapy, followed by observation for reinfection after discontinuing prophylaxis (1):
    - Continuous antimicrobial prophylaxis involves daily administration of low-dose TMP-SMX 40/200 mg or nitrofurantoin 50–100 mg, among others (1,6).
  - Another treatment option is self-started antibiotics.

Pediatric Considerations

Long-term antibiotics appear to reduce the risk of recurrent symptomatic UTI in susceptible children, but the benefit is small and must be considered together with the increased risk of microbial resistance (7).

ISSUES FOR REFERRAL

Men with uncomplicated UTI and most other patients with complicated UTI should be referred to a urologist for evaluation.

Pediatric Considerations

UTI in children, especially <1 year of age, should prompt workup for urinary tract anomalies.

SURGERY/OTHER PROCEDURES

- Urinary tract obstruction with urosepsis requires urgent drainage of obstructed system.
- Patients with emphysematous pyelonephritis or pyonephrosis may need immediate surgical intervention.

COMPLEMENTARY AND ALTERNATIVE MEDICINE

- Preliminary studies indicate that *Vaccinium macrocarpon* (cranberry) juice may help to prevent and treat UTIs by inhibiting bacterial adherence to the bladder epithelium.
- Cranberry juice may decrease the number of symptomatic UTIs over a 1-year period, particularly for women with recurrent UTIs. The optimal dosage or method of administration (e.g., juice, tablets, or capsules) is still unclear (8).

IN-PATIENT CONSIDERATIONS

Outpatient treatment, except for complicated or upper UTIs

 ## ONGOING CARE

FOLLOW-UP RECOMMENDATIONS

- 1st or rare UTI: Young or middle-aged, nonpregnant adult females require no follow-up if UTI is clinically cured after 3-day therapy.
- If symptoms persist after 2–3 days of therapy, obtain culture/sensitivity and change antibiotic accordingly.

Pregnancy Considerations

- UTI during pregnancy always requires culture/sensitivity and usually requires a 7–14-day treatment.
- Following the treatment of acute infection, pregnant women warrant surveillance urine cultures every trimester. They may receive prophylactic antibiotics for the remainder of pregnancy for recurrent or upper tract disease.

PATIENT EDUCATION

- Although no controlled studies support this intervention, postcoital voiding is commonly advised.
- FamilyDoctor.org: http://familydoctor.org/online/famdocen/home/women/gen-health/190.html

PROGNOSIS

Symptoms resolve within 2–3 days of antibiotic treatment in almost all patients.

COMPLICATIONS

- Pyelonephritis or sepsis
- Renal abscess
- Acute urinary outlet obstruction

Pregnancy Considerations

Pregnant females, infants, and young children with cystitis are at higher risk of pyelonephritis.

REFERENCES

1. Kodner CM, Thomas Gupton EK. Recurrent urinary tract infections in women: Diagnosis and management. *Am Fam Physician*. 2010;82: 638–643.
2. Litza JA, Brill JR. Urinary tract infections. *Prim Care*. 2010;37:491–507, viii.
3. Gupta K, Hooton TM, Naber KG, et al. International clinical practice guidelines for the treatment of acute uncomplicated cystitis and pyelonephritis in women: a 2010 update by the Infectious Diseases Society of America and the European Society for Microbiology and Infectious Diseases. *Clin Infect Dis*. 2011;52:e103–e120.
4. Zalmanovici Trestioreanu A, et al. Antimicrobial agents for treating uncomplicated urinary tract infection in women. *Cochrane Database Syst Rev*. 2010;10:CD007182.
5. Mehnert-Kay SA. Diagnosis and management of uncomplicated urinary tract infections. *Am Fam Physician*. 2005;72:451–456.
6. Stapleton A, Stamm WE. Prevention of urinary tract infection. *Infect Dis Clin N Am*. 1997;11:719–733.
7. Williams G, Craig JC. Long-term antibiotics for preventing recurrent urinary tract infection in children. *Cochrane Database Syst Rev*. 2011: CD001534.
8. Jepson RG, Craig JC. Cranberries for preventing urinary tract infections. *Cochrane Database Syst Rev*. 2008:CD001321.

ADDITIONAL READING

Hooten TM. Uncomplicated urinary tract infection. *N Engl J Med*. 2012; 366:1028–1037.

 ### SEE ALSO

Algorithm: Dysuria

 ### CODES

ICD10

- N30.90 Cystitis, unspecified without hematuria
- N30.91 Cystitis, unspecified with hematuria
- N39.0 Urinary tract infection, site not specified

CLINICAL PEARLS

- Uncomplicated UTIs cause significant morbidity but generally do not cause renal damage.
- Treatment of uncomplicated UTIs reduces morbidity, but the risk of recurrence stays the same.
- Bacteria originating from intestinal tract cause most UTIs, especially *E. coli*.
- Imaging studies are not required for most women with UTIs.
- Uncomplicated UTIs should be treated for 3 days (TMP-SMX) or 5 days (nitrofurantoin).
- All pregnant women with bacteriuria should be treated.

URINARY TRACT INFECTION (UTI) IN MALES

Holly Milne Hofkamp, MD • Scott A. Fields, MD

BASICS

DESCRIPTION
- Cystitis is an infection of the lower urinary tract, usually resulting from a single gram-negative enteric bacteria. (See also "Prostatitis," "Pyelonephritis," and "Urethritis.")
- System(s) affected: Renal/Urologic
- Synonym(s): Urinary tract infection (UTI); cystitis

EPIDEMIOLOGY
Incidence
- Predominant age: Increases with age
- Uncommon in men <50 years of age.
- 6–8 infections/10,000 men aged 21–50 years (1)

Prevalence
Not common

ETIOLOGY AND PATHOPHYSIOLOGY
- *Escherichia coli* (70–95% of infections) (1)
- *Klebsiella*
- *Enterobacter*
- *Enterococcus*
- Proteus
- Pseudomonas
- Serratia
- *Streptococcus faecalis* and *Staphylococcus* sp.
- *Pseudomonas* and *Morganella* (more common in elderly and catheterized patients) (2)

Genetics
Not applicable

RISK FACTORS
(3,4)
- Age
- Obesity (3)
- History of prior UTI
- Outlet obstruction
  - Benign prostatic hypertrophy (BPH)
  - Urethral stricture
  - Calculi
- Cognitive impairment
- Fecal incontinence
- Urinary incontinence
- Anal intercourse
- Recent urologic surgery
- Infection of the prostate/kidney
- Urinary tract instrumentation, catheterization
- Immunocompromised host
- Diabetes
- Bladder diverticula
- Neurogenic bladder
- Institutionalization
- Uncircumcised

GENERAL PREVENTION
- Prompt treatment of predisposing factors
- Use a catheter only when necessary; if needed, use aseptic technique and closed system, and remove as soon as possible.
- Currently cranberry products are not recommended for preventing UTIs in men (5)[A]

COMMONLY ASSOCIATED CONDITIONS
- Acute bacterial pyelonephritis
- Chronic bacterial pyelonephritis
- Urethritis
- Prostatitis
- Prostatic hypertrophy
- Prostate cancer

Geriatric Considerations
Bacteriuria is common among the elderly; may be related to functional status and usually is transient. Of men over 65, 10% have asymptomatic bacteriuria (ASB). If ASB is noted, no treatment is needed (2)[A]

Pediatric Considerations
Can be associated with obstruction to normal flow of urine, such as vesicoureteral reflux. Unique diagnostic criteria and evaluation recommendations exist (see below).

DIAGNOSIS

HISTORY
- Urinary frequency
- Urinary urgency
- Dysuria
- Hesitancy
- Slow urinary stream
- Dribbling of urine
- Nocturia
- Suprapubic discomfort
- Low back pain
- Hematuria
- Systemic symptoms (chills, fever) present with concomitant pyelonephritis or prostatitis

PHYSICAL EXAM
- Suprapubic tenderness
- Costovertebral angle (CVA) tenderness and/or fever may be present with concomitant pyelonephritis/prostatitis.

DIFFERENTIAL DIAGNOSIS
- Anatomic/Functional pathology of the urinary tract
- Urethritis/STIs
- Infections in other sites of the genitourinary tract (e.g., epididymis, prostatitis)

DIAGNOSTIC TESTS & INTERPRETATION
Initial Tests (lab, imaging)
- Urine dipstick/manual microscopy showing:
  - Pyuria (>10 WBCs)
  - Bacteriuria
  - Positive leukocyte esterase (in males: sensitivity, 54%; specificity, 55%; PPV, 65%; NPV, 44%) (6)[C]
  - Positive nitrite (in males: sensitivity, 38%; specificity, 84%; PPV, 78%; NPV, 46%) (6)[C]
  - In general, leukocyte esterase is more sensitive and nitrite is more specific in detecting UTI.
- Automated microscopy/flow cytometry that measures cell counts and bacterial counts can be used to improve screening characteristics (sensitivity, 92%; specificity, 55%; PPV, 47%; NPV, 97%). The high NPV of these screening tests allows for more judicious use of urine culture (7)[C].
- Urine culture: >100,000 colony-forming units (CFU; >10^5 CFU) of bacteria/mL of urine confirm diagnosis. Lower counts also may be indicative of infection, especially in the presence of pyuria (1,8,9)[C]. Diagnosis in infants and children <24 months made on the basis of both pyuria and 50,000 CFU on culture (10)[C].
- Renal and bladder ultrasound recommended in infants and young children after first confirmed UTI (10)[C].

Follow-Up Tests & Special Considerations
- Consider assessing for risk factors for STIs as chlamydial/gonococcal urethritis can mimic a UTI. If risk factors are present, use urine nucleic acid amplification tests to identify gonococcal and chlamydia infections and treat as necessary.
- Further urologic evaluation is warranted to rule out other disorders in men with recurrent UTI, febrile UTI, or pyelonephritis (1)[C]. This may include:
  - Ultrasound
  - Cystoscopy
  - Urodynamics
  - IV pyelography
- Antibiotics prior to culture or phenazopyridine prior to urine dipstick can alter results.

Test Interpretation
Depends on site of infection

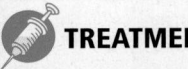 **TREATMENT**

GENERAL MEASURES
- Hydration
- Analgesia, if required
- Patient with indwelling catheters:
  - If asymptomatic bacterial colonization, no need to treat (sterilization of urine is not possible, and resistant organisms may take up residence).
  - If symptomatic of acute infection, institute treatment.

MEDICATION
First Line
- Acute, uncomplicated cystitis:
  - Treat empirically or based on culture and sensitivity results for 7 days (1)[B,C]. For empirical therapy, a fluoroquinolone or trimethoprim-sulfamethoxazole DS usually used to treat the most likely pathogens (1)[C].
- Complicated, febrile, or recurrent infection:
  - Prescribe a minimum of 2 weeks antibiotics based on antimicrobial sensitivities with repeat urine check after the treatment (1)[C]. In men with febrile UTI or pyelonephritis, prostatic involvement also has to be considered. Treatment of concomitant prostatitis requires antimicrobials with good prostatic tissue and fluid penetration (fluoroquinolones) (1)[C].

Second Line
According to culture and sensitivity results and patient's history

ISSUES FOR REFERRAL
Further urologic evaluation and referral are warranted to rule out other disorders in men with recurrent UTI, febrile UTI, or pyelonephritis (1)[C].

IN-PATIENT CONSIDERATIONS
Admission Criteria/Initial Stabilization
- Inability to tolerate oral medications
- Acute renal failure
- Suspected sepsis

 ONGOING CARE

FOLLOW-UP RECOMMENDATIONS
Patient Monitoring
Close follow-up until clinically well

DIET
Encourage adequate fluid intake

PATIENT EDUCATION
For patient education materials about this topic that have been reviewed favorably, contact the National Kidney Foundation, 30 E. 33rd Street, Suite 1100, New York, NY 10016; 212-889-2210.

PROGNOSIS
Clearing of infections with appropriate antibiotic treatment

COMPLICATIONS
- Pyelonephritis
- Ascending infection
- Recurrent infection

REFERENCES
1. Uncomplicated urinary tract infections in adult. In: Grabe M, Bishop MC, Bjerklund-Johansen TE, et al. *Guidelines on urological infections*. Arnhem, The Netherlands: European Association of Urology (EAU); 2013:15–25.
2. Matthews SJ, Lancaster JW. Urinary tract infections in the elderly population. *Am J Geriatr Pharmacother*. 2011;9:286–309.
3. Semins MJ, Shore AD, Makary MA, et al. The impact of obesity on urinary tract infection risk. *Urology*. 2012;79:266–269.
4. Drekonja DM, Rector TS, Cutting A, et al. Urinary tract infection in male veterans: Treatment patterns and outcomes. *JAMA Intern Med*. 2013;173:62–68.
5. Jepson R, Williams G, Craig J. Cranberries for preventing urinary tract infections. *Cochrane Database Syst Rev*. 2012;10:CD001321.
6. Hummers-Pradier E, Ohse AM, Koch M, et al. Urinary tract infection in men. *Int J Clin Pharmacol Ther*. 2004;42:360–366.
7. Evans R, Davison M, Sim L, et al. Testing by Sysmex UF-100 flow cytometer and with bacterial culture in a diagnostic laboratory: A comparison. *J Clin Pathol*. 2006;59:661–662.
8. Koeijers JJ, Verbon A, Kessels AG, et al. Urinary tract infection in male general practice patients: Uropathogens and antibiotic susceptibility. *Urology*. 2010;76:336–340.
9. van Pinxteren B, van Vliet SM, Wiersma TJ, et al. [Summary of the practice guideline 'Urinary-tract infections' (second revision) from the Dutch College of General Practitioners]. *Ned Tijdschr Geneeskd*. 2006;150:718–722.
10. Clinical Practice Guideline: Urinary tract infection: Clinical practice guideline for the diagnosis and management of the initial UTI in febrile infants and children 2 to 24 Months. Subcommittee on Urinary Tract Infection, Steering Committee on Quality Improvement and Management. *Pediatrics*. 2011;128:3 595–610.

ADDITIONAL READING
- Gerber GS, Brendler CB. Evaluation of the urologic patient: History, physical examination, and urinalysis. In: Campbell MF, Walsh PC, Retik AB, eds., *Campbell's urology*. 8th ed. Philadelphia: Saunders; 2002:107.

 SEE ALSO

- Prostate Cancer; Prostatic Hyperplasia, Benign (BPH); Prostatitis; Pyelonephritis; Urethritis
- Algorithms: Dysuria; Urethral Discharge

 CODES

ICD10
- N30.90 Cystitis, unspecified without hematuria
- N30.91 Cystitis, unspecified with hematuria
- N39.0 Urinary tract infection, site not specified

CLINICAL PEARLS
- Cystitis is an infection of the lower urinary tract, usually resulting from a single gram-negative enteric bacteria.
- Risk factors/causes: Age, history of UTI, obesity, BPH, cognitive impairment, fecal incontinence, urinary incontinence, anal intercourse, recent urologic surgery, catheterization, infection of the prostate/kidney, urinary tract instrumentation, immunocompromised host, diabetes, neurogenic bladder, outlet obstruction
- Evaluation: Urinalysis, urine culture, STI testing (e.g., gonorrhea, chlamydia by culture/DNA probe)
- Treat empirically with fluoroquinolones or trimethoprim-sulfamethoxazole DS for 7 days.

U

UROLITHIASIS

Phillip Fournier, MD

 BASICS

DESCRIPTION
- Stone formation within the urinary tract: Urinary crystals bind to form a nidus, which grows to form a calculus (stone).
- Range of symptoms: Asymptomatic to obstructive; febrile morbidity if result of infection

EPIDEMIOLOGY
- The worldwide epidemiology differs according to both geographic area (higher prevalence in hot, arid, or dry climates) and socioeconomic conditions (dietary intake and lifestyle). Radiolucent stones and stones secondary to infection are less influenced by environmental conditions.
- Vesical calculosis (bladder stones) due to malnutrition during early life is frequent in Middle Eastern and Asian countries.
- Incidence in industrialized countries seems to be increasing, probably due to improved diagnostics, as well as to increasingly rich diets.
- Increased incidence in patients with surgically induced absorption issues, such as Crohn disease and gastric bypass surgery (1)[B]

Incidence
- In industrialized countries: 100–200/100,000/year (2)
- Predominant age: Mean age is 40–60 years.
- Predominant sex: Male > Female (~2:1)

ETIOLOGY AND PATHOPHYSIOLOGY
- Supersaturation and dehydration lead to high salt content in urine, which congregates.
- Stasis of urine:
  - Renal malformation (e.g., horseshoe kidney, ureteropelvic junction obstruction)
  - Incomplete bladder emptying (e.g., neurogenic bladder, prostate enlargement, multiple sclerosis)
- Crystals may form in pure solutions (homogeneous) or on existing surfaces, such as other crystals or cellular debris (heterogeneous).
- Balance of promoters and inhibitors: Organic (Tamm-Horsfall protein, glycosaminoglycan, uropontin, nephrocalcin) and inorganic (citrate, pyrophosphate)
- Calcium oxalate and/or phosphate stones (80%):
  - Hypercalciuria:
    - Absorptive hypercalciuria: Increased jejunal calcium absorption
    - Renal leak: Increased calcium excretion from renal proximal tubule
    - Resorptive hypercalciuria: Mild hyperparathyroidism
  - Hypercalcemia:
    - Hyperparathyroidism
    - Sarcoidosis
    - Malignancy
    - Immobilization
    - Paget disease
- Hyperoxaluria:
  - Enteric hyperoxaluria:
    - Intestinal malabsorptive state associated with irritable bowel disease, celiac sprue, or intestinal resection
    - Bile salt malabsorption leads to formation of calcium soaps.
  - Primary hyperoxaluria: Autosomal-recessive, types I and II

  - Dietary hyperoxaluria: Overindulgence in oxalate-rich food
- Hyperuricosuria:
  - Seen in 10% of calcium stone formers
  - Caused by increased dietary purine intake, systemic acidosis, myeloproliferative diseases, gout, chemotherapy, Lesch-Nyhan syndrome
  - Thiazides, probenecid
- Hypocitraturia:
  - Caused by acidosis: Renal tubular acidosis, malabsorption, thiazides, enalapril, excessive dietary protein
- Uric acid stones (10–15%): Hyperuricemia causes as above
- Struvite stones (5–10%): Infected urine with urease-producing organisms (most commonly *Proteus* sp.)
- Cystine stones (<1%): Autosomal-recessive disorder of renal tubular reabsorption of cystine
- Bladder stones: Seen with chronic bladder catheterization and some medications (indinavir)
- In children: Usually due to malnutrition

Genetics
- Up to 20% of patients have a family history. However, spouses of those who form stones have higher calcium excretion rates than controls, suggesting strong dietary–environmental factors.
- Autosomal-dominant: Idiopathic hypercalciuria
- Autosomal-recessive:
  - Cystinuria, Lesch-Nyhan syndrome, hyperoxaluria types I and II
  - Ehlers-Danlos syndrome, Marfan syndrome, Wilson disease, familial renal tubular acidosis

RISK FACTORS
- White > African American in regions with both populations
- Family history
- Previous history of nephrolithiasis
- Diet rich in protein, refined carbohydrates, and sodium
- Occupations associated with a sedentary lifestyle or with a hot, dry workplace
- Incidence rates peak during summer secondary to dehydration
- Obesity
- Surgically/Medically induced malabsorption (Crohn disease, gastric bypass, celiac)

GENERAL PREVENTION
- Hydration (3)[A]
- Decrease salt and meat intake.
- Avoid oxalate-rich foods.

Pediatric Considerations
Rare: More common in men; in those with low socioeconomic status

Pregnancy Considerations
- Pregnant women have the same incidence of renal colic as do nonpregnant women.
- Most symptomatic stones occur during the 2nd and 3rd trimesters, heralded by symptoms of flank pain/hematuria.
- Most common differential diagnosis is physiologic hydronephrosis of pregnancy. Use US to avoid irradiation. Noncontrast-enhanced CT scan also is diagnostic.

- Treatment goals:
  - Control pain, avoid infection, and preserve renal function until birth or stone passage.
  - 30% require intervention, such as stent placement.

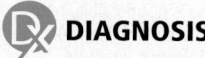 **DIAGNOSIS**

HISTORY
- Pain:
  - Renal colic: Acute onset of severe groin and/or flank pain
  - Distal stones may present with referred pain in labia, penile meatus, or testis.
- Microscopic/Gross hematuria occurs in 95% of patients.
- Nonspecific symptoms of nausea, vomiting, tachycardia, diaphoresis
- Low-grade fever without signs of infection
- Infectious origin: Associated with high-grade fevers require more urgent treatment (see below)
- Frequency and dysuria especially occur with stones at the vesicoureteric junction (VUJ).
- Asymptomatic: Nonobstructing stones within the renal calyces

PHYSICAL EXAM
Tender costovertebral angle with palpation/percussion and/or iliac fossa

DIFFERENTIAL DIAGNOSIS
- Appendicitis
- Ruptured aortic aneurysm
- Musculoskeletal strain
- Pyelonephritis (upper UTI)
- Pyonephrosis (obstructed upper UTI; emergency)
- Perinephric abscess
- Ectopic pregnancy
- Salpingitis

DIAGNOSTIC TESTS & INTERPRETATION
- Urinalysis for RBCs, leukocytes, nitrates, pH (acidic urine <5.5 is associated with uric acid stones; alkaline >7 with struvite stones)
- Midstream urine for microscopy, culture, and sensitivity
- Blood: Urea, creatinine, electrolytes, calcium, and urate; consider CBC.
- Parathyroid hormone only if calcium elevated
- Stone analysis if/when stone passed

Initial Tests (lab, imaging)
- Noncontrast-enhanced helical CT scan of the abdomen and pelvis has replaced IV pyelogram as the investigation of choice (4)[A]:
  - Stone is found most commonly at levels of ureteric luminal narrowing: Pelviureteric junction, pelvic brim, and VUJ.
  - Acute obstruction: Proximal ureter and renal pelvis are dilated to the level of obstruction, and perinephric stranding is possible on imaging.
- X-ray of kidneys, ureter, and bladder to determine if stone is radiopaque or lucent:
  - Calcium oxalate/phosphate stones are radiopaque.
  - Uric acid stones are radiolucent.
  - Staghorn calculi (that fill the shape of the renal calyces) are usually struvite and opaque.
  - Cystine stones are faintly opaque (ground-glass appearance).

- US has low sensitivity and specificity, but is often the 1st choice for pregnant women.

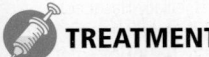 ## TREATMENT

GENERAL MEASURES
- 75% of patients are successfully treated conservatively and pass the stone spontaneously.
- Stones that do not pass usually require surgical intervention.
- 30–50% of patients will have recurrent stones.

MEDICATION
- Medical expulsive therapy: α_1-Antagonists (e.g., terazosin) and calcium channel blockers (e.g., nifedipine) improve likelihood of spontaneous stone passage with a number needed to treat (NNT) of ~5.
- Class C in pregnancy

ISSUES FOR REFERRAL
- Urgent referral of patients with UTI/sepsis or acute renal failure/solitary kidney
- Early referral of pregnant patients, large stones (>8 mm), chronic renal failure, children
- Refer patients if no passage at 2–4 weeks or poorly controlled pain.

ADDITIONAL THERAPIES
- Uric acid stone dissolution therapy:
  - Alkalinize urine with potassium citrate; keep pH >6.5.
  - Allopurinol: 100–300 mg/d PO
- Cystine stone dissolution/prevention:
  - Alkalinize urine with potassium citrate; keep pH >6.5
  - Chelating agents: Captopril, α-mercapto propionylglycine, D-penicillamine
- Consider altering medications that increase risk of stone formation: Probenecid, loop diuretics, salicylic acid, salbutamol, indinavir, triamterene, acetazolamide.
- Vitamin D supplementation has not been proven to induce stone formation.
- Treat hypercalciuria with thiazides on an acute basis only.
- Treat hypocitraturia with potassium citrate and high-citrate juices (e.g., orange, lemon).
- Treat enteric hyperoxaluria with oral calcium/magnesium, cholestyramine, and potassium citrate.

SURGERY/OTHER PROCEDURES
- Immediate relief of obstruction is required for patients with the following conditions:
  - Sepsis
  - Renal failure (obstructed solitary kidney, bilateral obstruction)
  - Uncontrolled pain, despite adequate analgesia
- Emergency surgery for obstruction:
  - Placement of a retrograde stent (i.e., endoscopic surgery, usually requires an anesthetic)
  - Radiologic placement of a percutaneous nephrostomy tube
- Elective surgery for stone treatment:
  - Extracorporeal shock-wave lithotripsy
  - Ureteroscopy with basket extraction/lithotripsy (laser/pneumatic)
  - Percutaneous nephrolithotomy
- Open surgery is uncommon.

IN-PATIENT CONSIDERATIONS
Admission Criteria/Initial Stabilization
- Analgesia:
  - Combination of NSAIDs (ketorolac 30–60 mg) and oral opiate
  - Parenteral narcotic if vomiting or if preceding fails to control pain (morphine 5–10 mg IV or IM q4h)
  - Antiemetic if required or prophylactically with parenteral narcotics
- Septic patients with urosepsis or pyonephrosis may require IV antibiotics (once blood and urine cultures are taken), IV fluids and, in severe cases, cardiorespiratory support in intensive care during recovery.

 ## ONGOING CARE

FOLLOW-UP RECOMMENDATIONS
- Patients with ureteric stones who are being treated conservatively should be followed until imaging is clear or stone is visibly passed:
  - Strain urine and send stone for composition.
  - Tamsulosin and nifedipine in selected patients to speed passage
  - Present to the hospital if pain worsens/signs of infection.
  - If pain management is suboptimal or stone does not progress or pass within 2–4 weeks, patient should be referred to a urologist and imaging should be repeated.
- Patients with recurrent stone formation should have metabolic workup: 24-hour urine for volume, pH, creatinine, calcium, cystine, phosphate, oxalate, uric acid, magnesium.
- Recurrent calcium stones: Consider using thiazide diuretics, citrates, or allopurinol (5)[A].

DIET
- Increased fluid intake for life cannot be overemphasized for decreasing recurrence. Encourage intake of 2–3 L/d; advise patient to have clear urine rather than yellow.
- Limit or eliminate carbonated soft drinks.
- Patients who form calcium stones should minimize high-oxalate foods such as green leafy vegetables, rhubarb, peanuts, chocolates, and beer.
- Decrease protein and salt intake.
- Lowering calcium intake is inadvisable and even may increase urine calcium excretion.

PROGNOSIS
- Spontaneous stone passage depends on stone location (proximal vs. distal) and stone size (<5 mm, 90% pass; >8 mm, 10% pass).
- Stone recurrence: 50% of patients at 10 years

REFERENCES
1. Matlaga BR, Shore AD, Magnuson T, et al. Effect of gastric bypass surgery on kidney stone disease. *J Urol.* 2009;181:2573–2577.
2. Tiselius HG. Epidemiology and medical management of stone disease. *BJU Int.* 2003;91:758–767.
3. Qiang W, Ke Z. Water for preventing urinary calculi. *Cochrane Database Sys Rev.* 2004;3:CD004292.
4. Worster A, Preyra I, Weaver B, et al. The accuracy of noncontrast helical computed tomography versus intravenous pyelography in the diagnosis of suspected acute urolithiasis: A meta-analysis. *Ann Emerg Med.* 2002;40:280–286.
5. Fink, HA. Medical management to prevent recurrent nephrolithiasis: a systematic review. *Ann Intern Med* 2013;158(7):535–43.

ADDITIONAL READING
- Hollingsworth JM, Rogers MA, Kaufman SR, et al. Medical therapy to facilitate urinary stone passage: A meta-analysis. *Lancet.* 2006; 368;1171–1179.
- Penniston KL, Jones AN, Nakada SY, et al. Vitamin D repletion does not alter urinary calcium excretion in healthy postmenopausal women. *BJU Int.* 2009;104:1512–1516.

 ## SEE ALSO

Algorithms: Dysuria; Renal Calculi; Urethral Discharge

 ## CODES

ICD10
- N20.9 Urinary calculus, unspecified
- N21.0 Calculus in bladder
- N21.8 Other lower urinary tract calculus

CLINICAL PEARLS
- Incidence in industrialized countries seems to be increasing, probably due to improved diagnostics, as well as to increasingly rich diets.
- Vesical calculosis (bladder stones) due to malnutrition during early life is frequent in Middle Eastern and Asian countries.
- Medical expulsive therapy: α_1-Antagonists (e.g., terazosin) and calcium channel blockers (e.g., nifedipine) improve likelihood of spontaneous stone passage with NNT of ~5.
- Increased fluid intake for life cannot be overemphasized for decreasing recurrence. Encourage 2–3 L/d intake; advise patient to have clear urine rather than yellow.
- Patients who form calcium stones should minimize high-oxalate foods such as green leafy vegetables, rhubarb, peanuts, chocolates, and beer.
- Decrease protein and salt intake.
- Lowering calcium intake is inadvisable and even may increase urine calcium excretion.

U

URTICARIA

M. Tye Haeberle, MD • William B. Adams, MD

BASICS

DESCRIPTION

- A cutaneous lesion involving transient edema of the epidermis and/or dermis characterized by the acute onset of a polymorphic lesion with central pallor and edema with an erythematous flare ranging in size from millimeters to centimeters.
- Pathophysiology is primarily mast cell degranulation and subsequent histamine release.
- Lesions subside within 24 hours, whereas angioedema, a dermal lesion of similar pathophysiology, may take up to 72 hours to remit.
- Pruritus and burning are more commonly associated with urticaria; pain more often with angioedema.
- Spontaneous urticaria:
  - Acute: Persists <6 weeks:
    - Specific extrinsic triggers commonly are the cause, although a vast number of possible causes exist (e.g., drugs, foods, infections [esp. *Streptococci*], envenomation, allergens)
    - Underlying etiology may be difficult to pinpoint
  - Chronic: Persists >6 weeks with >2 episodes/week off treatment:
    - Unlike acute urticaria, 80% of cases have no obvious external stimulus.
    - If symptoms occur less than twice a week, this is more likely recurrent acute urticaria and should be approached as such.
    - For those with chronic urticaria, 40% have concurrent angioedema.
    - Chronic infection, pseudoallergy, malignancy including mastocytosis, autoimmunity (esp. thyroid), and medications may underlie the remaining 20%.
    - 1/2 of those with chronic idiopathic urticaria have sera positive for IgG that releases histamine through binding of IgE or its receptor.
    - The other 50% are truly idiopathic.
  - Physical urticaria: Urticaria due to mechanical stimuli:
    - Dermatographism: "Skin writing" or the appearance of linear wheals at the site of friction, scratching, or any type of irritation. This is the most common physical urticaria.
    - Cold urticaria: Wheals occur within minutes of rewarming after cold exposure; 95% idiopathic, but can be due to infections (mononucleosis, HIV), neoplasia, or autoimmune diseases.
    - Delayed pressure urticaria: Urticaria occurs 0.5–12 hours after pressure to skin (e.g., from elastic or shoes), may be pruritic and/or painful, and may not subside for several days.
    - Solar urticaria: From sunlight exposure, usually UV; onset in minutes; subsides within 2 hours
    - Heat urticaria: From direct contact with warm objects or air; rare
    - Vibratory urticaria/angioedema: Very rare; secondary to vibrations (e.g., motorcycle)
  - Special forms of urticaria:
    - Cholinergic urticaria: Due to brief increase of core body temperature from exercise, baths, or emotional stress; small pin-sized (5–10-mm) wheals surrounded by an erythema, but also can have larger wheals. This is the 2nd most common form.
    - Adrenergic urticaria: Also caused by stress; extremely rare; vasoconstricted, blanched skin around pink wheals as opposed to cholinergic's erythematous surrounding

  - Contact urticaria: Wheals at sites where chemical substances contact the skin, may be either IgE dependent (e.g., latex) or IgE independent (e.g., stinging nettle)
  - Aquagenic and solar urticaria: Small wheals after contact with water of any temperature or UV light, respectively; rare
  - Urticarial vasculitis: Urticaria >24 hours and more painful than pruritic. A leukocytoclastic vasculitis; may be palpable and purpuric; arthralgias
- System(s) affected: Integumentary
- Synonym(s): Hives, Wheals

EPIDEMIOLOGY

Incidence

- Equally distributed across all ages: Children more likely to have acute, whereas adults and elderly predisposed to chronic urticaria.
- Predominant gender: Female > Male (2:1 in chronic urticaria)
- In 20% of patients, chronic urticaria lasts >10 years.

Prevalence

- Affects anywhere from 5–25% of the population
- Of people with urticaria, 40% have no angioedema, 40% have urticaria and angioedema, and 20% have angioedema with no urticaria (1).
- Up to 3% of the population at some point has chronic idiopathic urticaria.
- Chronic urticaria affects only 0.1–3% of children.

ETIOLOGY AND PATHOPHYSIOLOGY

- Mast cell degranulation with release of inflammatory reactants, which leads to vascular leakage, inflammatory cell extravasation, and dermal (angioedema) and/or epidermal (wheals/hives) edema
- Histamine, cytokines, leukotrienes, and proteases are main active substances released.
- Mast cell degranulation may be caused by allergen cross-linkage of IgE, autoimmune activation of FcεRI (IgE receptor), substance P, C5a, opiates, or physical stimuli.
- Spontaneous acute urticaria:
  - Bacterial infections: Strep throat, sinusitis, otitis, urinary tract
  - Viral infections: Rhinovirus, rotavirus, hepatitis B, mononucleosis, herpes
  - Foods: Peanuts, tree nuts, seafood, milk, soy, fish, wheat, and eggs; tend to be IgE-mediated; pseudoallergenic foods, such as strawberries, tomatoes, preservatives, and coloring agents contain histamine.
  - Drugs: IgE-mediated (e.g., penicillin and other antibiotics), direct mast cell stimulation (e.g., aspirin, NSAIDs, opiates)
  - Inhalant, contact, ingestion, or occupational exposure (e.g., latex, cosmetics)
  - Parasitic infection; insect bite/sting
  - Transfusion reaction
- Spontaneous chronic urticaria:
  - Chronic subclinical allergic rhinitis, eczema, and other atopic disorders
  - Chronic indolent infections: *Helicobacter pylori*, fungal, parasitic (*Anisakis simplex*, strongyloidiasis), and chronic viral infections (hepatitis)
  - Collagen-vascular disease (cutaneous vasculitis, serum sickness, lupus)

  - Thyroid autoimmunity, especially Hashimoto
  - Hormonal: Pregnancy and progesterone
  - Autoimmune antibodies to the IgE receptor α chain on mast cells and to the IgE antibody
  - Chronic medications (e.g., NSAIDs, hormones, ACE inhibitors)
  - Malignancy
  - Physical stimuli (cold, heat, vibration, pressure) in physical urticaria

Genetics

No consistent pattern known: Chronic urticaria has increased frequency of HLA-DR4 and HLA-D8Q MHC II alleles.

RISK FACTORS

- Atopic diseases, asthma, allergic rhinitis, other allergies
- Of patients, >50% possess an atopic disease, >40% with allergic rhinitis, and >15% have atopic dermatitis or allergic asthma in chronic urticaria (1).

GENERAL PREVENTION

Treatment of any underlying atopic or other disease; avoidance of known triggers

COMMONLY ASSOCIATED CONDITIONS

- Angioedema
- Anaphylaxis

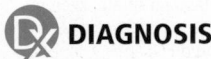 DIAGNOSIS

HISTORY

- Duration, timing (onset/offset), and distribution of lesions; exacerbating and alleviating factors, and history of atopy and/or autoimmune diseases
- Potential trigger exposure
- Concomitance of angioedema: Pruritus in urticarial wheals vs. pain in angioedema
- Urticaria may be an initial symptom of a generalized anaphylactic reaction.
- Fast onset; resolves in <24–48 hours

PHYSICAL EXAM

- Single/Multiple raised, polymorphic indurated plaques with central pallor and edema with an erythematous flare
- Variably sized: ≥1–20 cm
- Evaluate for underlying conditions including thyroid abnormalities (nodules), bacterial, viral, or fungal infection (e.g., fever).
- Often, lesions have cleared and patient's photographs may be useful.

DIFFERENTIAL DIAGNOSIS

- Anaphylaxis (may present with urticaria)
- Morbilliform or fixed drug eruptions
- Erythema multiforme
- Systemic lupus erythematous (SLE), vasculitis, and polyarteritis
- Angioedema without urticaria
- Urticaria pigmentosa/systemic mastocytosis
- Bullous pemphigoid (urticarial stage)
- Arthropod bite
- Atopic/contact dermatitis
- Viral exanthem

DIAGNOSTIC TESTS & INTERPRETATION

- Acute urticaria: Testing should be directed by clinical suspicion of underlying cause:
  - Full lab workups provide little except in cases of a failed trial of antihistamines, lesions that last >24 hours, lesions that do not blanch on pressure or leave pigmentary changes
  - Allergy skin tests and radioallergosorbent test (RAST) for inhaled allergens, insects, drugs, or foods
  - Infection: Consider pharyngeal culture, LFTs, mononucleosis test, urinalysis in appropriate setting.
- Chronic urticaria: "In the overwhelming majority of patients with chronic urticaria, a definite etiology is not identified. Limited laboratory testing may be warranted to exclude underlying causes. Targeted laboratory testing based on clinical suspicion is appropriate. Routine extensive testing is neither cost effective nor associated with improved clinical outcomes. Skin or serum-specific IgE testing for inhalants or foods is not indicated, unless there is a clear history implicating an allergen as a provoking or perpetuating factor for urticaria" (2).
  - CBC with differential, ESR, and/or CRP are recommended by most guidelines.
  - Thyroid function tests, LFTs, and urinalysis are recommended by several guidelines.
  - Consider allergy skin tests and RAST for inhaled allergens, insects, drugs, or foods; total IgE level
  - Autoimmune: ESR, ANA, RF, complement (e.g., CH50, C3, C4), cryoglobulins in urticarial vasculitis
  - Tests for *H. pylori* (e.g., antibodies) in dyspeptic patients. Consider stool for ova and parasites in at-risk individuals.
  - Autologous serum skin testing: Injection of serum under skin to test for presence of IgE receptor-activating antibodies
  - Consider malignancy workup, including serum protein electrophoresis and immunofixation in the proper setting.

  Indicated only if clinical suspicion for underlying indolent infections/malignancy

Diagnostic Procedures/Other

- Food and drug reactions: Elimination of (or challenges with) suspected agents
- Physical and special forms of urticaria: Challenge tests:
  - Dermatographism: Stroke skin lightly with rounded object and observe for surrounding urticaria.
  - Cold urticaria: Ice cube test: Place ice cube on skin for 5 minutes; observe for 10–15 minutes.
  - Cholinergic: Exercise to the point of sweating/partial immersion in 42°C bath for 10 minutes
  - Solar: Exposure to different wavelengths of light
  - Delayed pressure: Apply 5 lb. sandbag to back for 20 minutes, observe 6 hours later.
  - Aquagenic: Apply water at various temperatures.
  - Vibratory: Apply vibration 4–5 minutes with a lab mixing device; observe.
- Skin biopsy to rule out urticarial vasculitis in cases of lesions lasting >24 hours

Test Interpretation

- Early lesions: Dermal edema with intravascular margination of neutrophils
- Late lesions: Scant polymorphous perivascular and interstitial infiltrate, with no expansion of cell walls/fibrin deposition

 TREATMENT

GENERAL MEASURES

- Calamine or 1% topical menthol may be useful.
- Avoid the eliciting stimulus (e.g., diet modification, pressure, temperature changes/extremes).
- NSAIDs and alcohol may exacerbate symptoms.

ISSUES FOR REFERRAL

Referral to an allergist, immunologist, or dermatologist for recalcitrant cases, complex management, testing for potential triggers, and anaphylaxis

MEDICATION

First Line

- 2nd-generation antihistamine (H_1) blockers are the first-line treatment of any urticaria in which avoidance of stimulus is impossible or not feasible (3,4)[A]. Higher than typical ($4\times$) 2nd-generation H_1 blocker dosages should be attempted before adding 1st-generation H_1 or H_2 blockers (5)[C]:
  - Fexofenadine (Allegra): 180 mg/d
  - Loratadine (Claritin): 10 mg/d, increasing as above; only medication studied for safe use in pregnancy
  - Desloratadine (Clarinex): 5 mg/d
  - Cetirizine (Zyrtec): 10 mg/d, increasing as above
  - Levocetirizine (Xyzal): 5 mg/d; requires weight-based dosing in children
  - Rupatadine: Novel H_1 antagonist with antiplatelet-activating factor activity
- 1st-generation antihistamines (H_1; for patients with sleep disturbed by itching) (3,4)[A]:
  - Older children and adults: Hydroxyzine or diphenhydramine 25–50 mg q6h
  - Children <6 years of age: Diphenhydramine 12.5 mg q6–8h (5 mg/kg/d) or hydroxyzine (10 mg/5 mL) 2 mg/kg/d divided q6–8h
- H_2-specific antihistamines (beneficial as adjuvants) (3,4)[C]: Cimetidine, ranitidine, nizatidine, famotidine
- Precautions and notes: Drowsiness and dry mouth and eyes in 1st-generation H_1 blockers (elderly)

Second Line

- Omalizumab: Anti-IgE; effective, although expensive. 150–375 mg SQ q2–4wk. Restricted to allergists only (4,6)[A]
- Leukotriene antagonists (montelukast, zileuton, and zafirlukast): Safe and worth trying in chronic, unresponsive cases; useful alone, but best used in addition to antihistamines (3,4,5)[C]
- Corticosteroids: Prednisolone 2×20 mg/d $\times$ 4 days; best used only for exacerbations; avoid chronic use (4)[C]
- Cyclosporine: Well-studied, effective (2.5–5 mg/kg/d); best used in combination with antihistamines in cases recalcitrant to $4\times$ dosing; significant renal side effects (3,5)[C]
- Doxepin: Tricyclic antidepressant with strong H_1- and H_2-blocking properties; 10–30 mg at bedtime; sedation limits usefulness; useful in treating concomitant depression (3,4)[C]
- Methotrexate: Antifolate; proven useful in recalcitrant cases; GI upset most common complaint; long-term requires LFT monitoring
- UV therapy decreases number of mast cells; has shown promise in the treatment of mastocytosis-induced urticaria (3)[C]

IN-PATIENT CONSIDERATIONS
Admission Criteria/Initial Stabilization
Educating patient on use of EpiPen as pathophysiology similar. If the airway is threatened, immediate consult to evaluate for laryngeal edema and need for airway access

 ONGOING CARE

FOLLOW-UP RECOMMENDATIONS
Patient Monitoring
A diary of potential triggers (e.g., foods, activities) may help in recalcitrant/persistent cases.

PROGNOSIS
Resolution of acute symptoms: 70% <72 hours. Of patients with chronic urticaria, 35% will be symptom-free in a year; another 30% will see symptom reduction. Not life threatening, but 18% will have decreased quality of life (1).

REFERENCES

1. Zuberbier T, Balke M, Worm M, et al. Epidemiology of urticaria: A representative cross-sectional survey. *Clin Exp Dermatol*. 2010;35:869–873.
2. Choosing Wisely initiative of ABIM: American Academy of Allergy, Asthma and Immunology Recommendation http://choosingwisely.org/wp-content/uploads/2012/04/5things_12_factsheet_AAAAI.pdf
3. Poonawalla T, Kelly B. Urticaria: A review. *Am J Clin Dermatol*. 2009;10(1):9–21.
4. Zuberbier T, Asero R, Bindslev-Jensen C, et al. EAACI/GA(2)LEN/EDF/WAO guideline: Management of urticaria. *Allergy*. 2009;84(10):1427–1443.
5. Maurer M, Weller K, et al. Unmet clinical needs in chronic spontaneous urticaria. A GA²LEN task force report. *Allergy*. 2011;66:317–330.
6. Maurer M, Rosen K, Hsieh HJ et al. Omalizumab for the treatment of chronic idiopathic or spontaneous urticaria. *N Engl J Med*. 2013;368(10):924-35

 CODES

ICD10
- L50.1 Idiopathic urticaria
- L50.8 Other urticaria
- L50.9 Urticaria, unspecified

CLINICAL PEARLS

- "Chronic urticaria" with <2 episodes/week should be approached as acute.
- Antihistamines are the best studied and most efficacious therapy, but may require higher-than-normal doses for efficacy.
- Lesions lasting >24 hours should be evaluated for urticarial vasculitis.

UTERINE MYOMAS

Laura K. Randolph, DO, MS • Michael P. Hopkins, MD, MEd

 BASICS

DESCRIPTION
- Uterine leiomyomas are well-circumscribed, pseudoencapsulated, benign monoclonal tumors composed mainly of smooth muscle with varying amounts of fibrous connective tissue (1,2).
- 3 major subtypes:
  – Subserous: Common; external; may become pedunculated
  – Intramural: Common; within myometrium; may cause marked uterine enlargement
  – Submucous: ~5% of all cases; internal, evoking abnormal uterine bleeding and infection; occasionally protruding from cervix
- Rare locations: Broad, round, and uterosacral ligaments
- System affected: Reproductive
- Synonym(s): Fibroids; Myoma; Fibromyoma; Myofibroma; Fibroleiomyoma

EPIDEMIOLOGY
Incidence
- Cumulative incidence up to 80%
  – 60% in African American women by age 35, 80% by age 50
  – 40% in Caucasian women by age 35, 70% by age 50 (1,3)
- Incidence increases with each decade during reproductive years
- Rarely seen in premenarchal females
- Predominant sex: Females only

ETIOLOGY AND PATHOPHYSIOLOGY
Enlargement of benign smooth muscle tumors that may lead to symptoms affecting the reproductive, GI, or genitourinary system

Complex multifactorial process involving transition from normal myocyte to abnormal cells and then to visibly evident tumor (monoclonal expansion):
- Hormones (1): Increases in estrogen and progesterone are correlated with myoma formation (i.e., rarely seen before menarche). Estrogen receptors in myomas bind more estradiol than normal myometrium (2).
- Growth factors (1):
  – Increased smooth muscle proliferation (transforming growth factor β [TGF-β], basic fibroblast growth factor [bFGF])
  – Increase DNA synthesis (epidermal growth factor [EGF], platelet-derived growth factor [PDGF], activin, myostatin)
  – Stimulate synthesis of extracellular matrix (TGF-β)
  – Promote mitogenesis (TGF-β, EGF, insulin-like growth factor [IGF], prolactin)
  – Promote angiogenesis (bFGF, vascular endothelial growth factor [VEGF])
- Vasoconstrictive hypoxia (1): Proposed, but not confirmed, mechanism of myometrial injury during menstruation

Genetics
- A variety of somatic chromosomal rearrangements have been described in 40% of uterine myomas.
  – Mutations in the gene encoding mediator complex subunit 12 (MED12) on the X chromosome were found in 70% of myomas in one study (3).

- Higher levels of aromatase and therefore estrogen have been found in myomas in African American women (3).

RISK FACTORS
- African American heritage
  – 2.9× greater risk than Caucasian women; occur at a younger age, are more numerous, larger, and more symptomatic (1)
- Early menarche (<10 years)
- Nulliparous
- Hypertension
- Familial predisposition
  – 2.5× more likely in women with a 1st degree relative with myomas (1)
- Obesity
  – Risk increases by 21% with each 10 kg of weight gain (1).
- Alcohol

COMMONLY ASSOCIATED CONDITIONS
Endometrial and breast cancer also associated with high unopposed estrogen stimulation.

 DIAGNOSIS

HISTORY
- Usually asymptomatic, 30% present with abnormal symptoms (2)
- Symptoms include:
  – Abnormal uterine bleeding, usually heavy/prolonged menses
  – Pain: Infrequent, usually associated with torsion of pedunculated myoma, degeneration, or cervical dilation by submucous myoma near cervical os
  – Pressure on bladder: Suprapubic discomfort, urinary frequency/obstruction
  – Pressure on rectosigmoid: May cause low back pain, constipation
  – Infertility: Rare, estimated 1–2.5% (2). Usually from submucous myoma distorting the uterine cavity or interference with implantation.

ALERT
Rapid growth, particularly in perimenopausal/postmenopausal patients, may indicate sarcoma. Extremely rare, 0.1–0.3% of cases (2)

PHYSICAL EXAM
- Usually incidental finding on abdominal and pelvic exam
- Firm, smooth nodules/masses arising from uterus
- Masses are mobile without tenderness.

DIFFERENTIAL DIAGNOSIS
- Intrauterine pregnancy
- Cancer, including ovarian, uterine, or leiomyosarcoma
- Cecal/Sigmoid tumor
- Appendiceal abscess
- Diverticulitis
- Pelvic kidney
- Urachal cyst

DIAGNOSTIC TESTS & INTERPRETATION
Initial Tests (lab, imaging)
- Pregnancy test
- Hemoglobin

- Pelvic ultrasound: Shows characteristic hypoechoic appearance (4).
- Saline-infusion hysterosonography: Helps to distinguish submucosal myomas (4).
- Hysterosalpingogram: Evaluates the contour of the endometrial cavity (4).
- CT scan or MRI: May help to differentiate complex cases or used when uterine artery embolization is planned (4)[B].

Follow-Up Tests & Special Considerations
Consider CA-125: May be slightly elevated in some cases of uterine myoma, but generally more useful in differentiating myomas from various gynecologic adenocarcinomas
- IV pyelogram: If suspect ureteral distortion (4)
- Barium enema

Diagnostic Procedures/Other
- Fractional dilation and curettage: Aids in ruling out cervical/uterine carcinomas when clinically suspicious.
- Hysteroscopy: Helps to diagnose submucosal/intracavitary myomas.
- Laparoscopy: Useful in complex cases and to rule out other pelvic diseases/disorders.

Test Interpretation
- Myomas are usually multiple and vary in size and location; have been reported up to 100 lb.
- Gross pathology: Firm tumors with characteristic whorl-like trabeculated appearance; a thin pseudocapsular layer is present.
- Microscopic: Bundles of smooth muscle mixed with varying amounts of connective tissue elements running in different directions
- Cellular variant has a preponderance of muscle cells. Mitoses are rare.
- May undergo various types of degeneration:
  – Hyaline degeneration: Very common
  – Calcification: Late result of circulatory impairment to myomas
  – Infection and suppuration: Most common with submucosal myomas
  – Necrosis: Most common with pedunculated myomas secondary to torsion

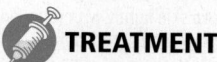 TREATMENT

- Treatment must be individualized.
- Medical therapy may be of benefit.
- Patients with minimal symptoms may be treated with iron preparations and analgesics.
- Conservative management of asymptomatic myomas:
  – Pelvic exams and ultrasounds at ≥3-month intervals if size remains stable
  – Substantial regression usually occurs after menopause.
- Surgical options should be considered if symptomatic or worrisome myomas are unresponsive to conservative/medical management.

GENERAL MEASURES
Patients not desiring pharmacologic therapy or surgery may consider:

- Uterine artery embolization: Averages 50% shrinkage of myomas (4)[A]; painful and may cause ovarian failure (1–2%), amenorrhea, or other complications; shorter hospital stay and quicker recovery, but no difference in satisfaction compared with hysterectomy (2,5)[B]
- MRI-guided focused ultrasound (MRgFUS): Noninvasive, ultrasound transducer passes through abdominal wall and causes coagulative necrosis of fibroid. Up to 98% reduction in myoma volume and symptoms. Not appropriate for some types of myomas (2)[B]. Efficacy may be comparable with other hysterectomy-sparing procedures (6)[B]. Fertility has been shown to be preserved (7)[A].

MEDICATION
- Progestins may reduce overall uterine size (4)[B]:
  - Norethindrone 10 mg/d
  - Medroxyprogesterone 200 mg IM monthly
  - Levonorgestrel intrauterine device (2)[B]
- Combination oral contraceptives: May help prevent development of new fibroids:
  - Contraindications: History of thromboembolic events
- Luteinizing hormone-releasing hormone:
  - Nafarelin (nasal spray), goserelin acetate, and leuprolide
  - Induces abrupt artificial menopause; may reduce myoma symptoms dramatically; induces atrophy of myomas by up to 40% in 2–3 months (4)[B].
  - May be valuable as preoperative adjunct to myomectomy/hysterectomy by allowing recovery of anemia, donation of autologous blood, and possibly converting abdominal to vaginal hysterectomy (4)[B].
  - Not recommended for use >6 months because of osteoporosis risk.
  - Following discontinuation, myomas return within 60 days to pretherapy size.
- Antiprogesterones:
  - Mifepristone:
    ○ Shown to have similar reduction in myoma size as gonadotropin-releasing hormone agonists (6)[B]
  - Selective progesterone receptor modulator (SPRM):
    ○ Ulipristal acetate: May be as effective as gonadotropin-releasing hormones with fewer side effects (8)[B]

ISSUES FOR REFERRAL
- Medical therapy may be initiated by a primary care physician/gynecologist after adequate pelvic examination.
- Surgical considerations may be pursued with gynecologic consultation.
- Uterine embolization may be discussed with an interventional radiologist.

SURGERY/OTHER PROCEDURES
- Surgical management is indicated in the following situations (4)[B]:
  - Excessive uterine size or excessive rate of growth (except during pregnancy)
  - Submucosal myomas when associated with hypermenorrhea
  - Pedunculated myomas that are painful or undergo torsion, necrosis, and hemorrhage
  - If a myoma causes symptoms from pressure on bladder/rectum
  - If differentiation from ovarian mass is not possible
  - If associated pelvic disease is present (endometriosis, pelvic inflammatory disease)
  - If infertility/habitual abortion is likely due to the anatomic location of the myoma
- Surgical procedures:
  - Preliminary pelvic examination, Pap smear, and endometrial biopsy should be performed to rule out malignant/premalignant conditions.
  - Hysterectomy: May be performed vaginally, laparoscopically, robotically, or by laparotomy:
    ○ Effective in relieving symptoms and improving quality of life (6)[B]
    ○ Similar fertility and live-birth rates between laparoscopic and abdominal myomectomy (2)[B]
  - Abdominal, laparoscopic, or robotic myomectomy may be performed in younger women who want to maintain fertility (4)[B].
  - Hysteroscopic/laparoscopic cautery/laser myoma resection can be performed in selected patients.
  - Endometrial ablation: For small submucosal myomas

IN-PATIENT CONSIDERATIONS
Admission Criteria/Initial Stabilization
- Usually outpatient
- Inpatient for some surgical procedures

 ONGOING CARE

FOLLOW-UP RECOMMENDATIONS
Patient Monitoring
- Pelvic examination and ultrasound: Every 2–3 months for newly diagnosed symptomatic/excessively large myomas
- Hemoglobin and hematocrit: If uterine bleeding is excessive
- Once uterine size and symptoms stabilize, monitor every 6–12 months.

DIET
No restrictions

PATIENT EDUCATION
- Society of Interventional Radiology: http://sirweb.org/patients/uterine-fibroids/
- US Department of Health and Human Services: http://womenshealth.gov/faq/uterine-fibroids.cfm
- American Congress of Obstetricians and Gynecologists (ACOG): www.acog.org

PROGNOSIS
- Resection of submucosal fibroids has been associated with increased fertility (6)[B].
- At least 10% of myomas recur after myomectomy; however, most women will not require further treatment (6)[B].

COMPLICATIONS
- May mask other gynecologic malignancies (e.g., uterine sarcoma, ovarian cancer)
- Degenerating fibroids may cause pain and bleeding.
- May rarely prolapse through the cervix

Pregnancy Considerations
- Rapid growth of fibroids is common.
- Pregnant women may need additional fetal testing if placenta is located over or near fibroid.
- Complications during pregnancy: Abortion, premature labor, 2nd-trimester rapid growth leading to degeneration and pain, and 3rd-trimester fetal malpresentation and dystocia during labor and delivery
- Cesarean section is recommended if the endometrial cavity was entered during myomectomy due to increased risk of uterine rupture.

Geriatric Considerations
In postmenopausal patients with newly diagnosed uterine myoma/enlarging uterine myomas, have a high suspicion of uterine sarcoma/other gynecologic malignancy.

REFERENCES
1. Parker WH. Etiology symptomatology, and diagnosis of uterine myomas. *Fertil Steril*. 2007;87:725–736.
2. Duhan N, Sirohiwal D. Uterine myomas revisited. *Eur J Obstet Gynecol Reprod Biol*. 2010;152: 119–125.
3. Bulun, SE. Uterine fibroids. *N Engl J Med* 2013:369; 1344–1355.
4. Wallace EE, Vlahos NF. Uterine myomas: An overview of development, clinical features and management. *Obstetrics Gynecol*. 2004;104(2):393–406.
5. Freed MM, Spies JB. Uterine artery embolization for fibroids: A review of current outcomes. *Semin Reprod Med*. 2010;28:235–241.
6. Parker WH. Uterine myomas: Management. *Fertil Steril*. 2007;88:255–271.
7. Hesley GK, Gorny KR, Woodrum DA. MR-guided focused ultrasound for the treatment of uterine fibroids. *Cardiovasc Intervent Radiol*. 2012;Mar 28. Epub 2012 Mar 28.
8. Donnez J, Tomaszewski J, Vázquez F, et al. Ulipristal acetate versus leuprolide acetate for uterine fibroids. *N Engl J Med*. 2012;84(5): 421–432.

ADDITIONAL READING
Laughlin SK, Schroeder JC, Baird DD, et al. New directions in the epidemiology of uterine fibroids. *Semin Reprod Med*. 2010;28:204–217.

 CODES

ICD10
- D25.1 Intramural leiomyoma of uterus
- D25.2 Subserosal leiomyoma of uterus
- D25.9 Leiomyoma of uterus, unspecified

CLINICAL PEARLS
- Uterine myomas are benign smooth muscle tumors composed mainly of fibrous connective tissue.
- Usually incidental finding on pelvic exam or ultrasound, but may cause pelvic pain and pressure, abnormal uterine bleeding, and/or infertility.
- Management ranges from conservative to medical to surgical.

UTERINE PROLAPSE

Jowhara Al-Qahtani, MD • Kristeina Sole. MD

 BASICS

DESCRIPTION

- Uterine prolapse occurs when the integrity of pelvic supporting structures is lost. This allows the uterus to descend into the vagina. In advanced cases, complete protrusion with inversion of the vagina occurs, known as procidentia.
- Before menopause, the degree and severity of prolapse are usually related to the number of pregnancies and the difficulty of childbirth. After menopause, atrophy and loss of tissue integrity can lead to further prolapse.
- System(s) affected: Gastrointestinal; Renal/Urologic; Reproductive
- Synonym(s): Uterine prolapse; Genital prolapse; Genital relaxation; Uterine descensus; Total or partial procidentia; Dropped uterus

Geriatric Considerations
This is largely a disease of aging, and incidence will be much higher as the median age of the population increases.

Pediatric Considerations
Prolapse in newborns has been reported, but it is rare and usually associated with congenital disorders and neuropathies.

EPIDEMIOLOGY

Incidence
- Annual incidence ~2%
- Predominant age: Perimenopausal and postmenopausal women
- Predominant sex: Female only

Prevalence
- ~30–50% of women experience some degree of prolapse (24% in stage 0, 38% in stage I, 35% in stage II, while 2–6% in stage III).
- The relative prevalence of pelvic organ prolapse (POP) in the general population increases by about 40% with every additional decade of life.

ETIOLOGY AND PATHOPHYSIOLOGY
- Advancing age and vaginal childbirth are the most important factors.
- Incidence of prolapse increases with frequency and difficulty of vaginal deliveries (e.g., operative vaginal delivery); <2% of prolapse occurs in nulliparous women.
- Although this disorder in large part results from the distension and distortion of supporting tissues with vaginal childbirth, pregnancy, regardless of mode of delivery, may contribute to prolapse.
- Other less common causes of prolapse include connective tissue disorders with lax tissue (e.g., Marfan syndrome), neurogenic disorders (e.g., multiple sclerosis), cloacal agenesis, chronic constipation, pelvic tumors or ascites, and chronic coughing resulting from chronic lung disease.
- Patients who have undergone radical vulvectomy with loss of the external supporting structures have a higher rate of prolapse.

Genetics
- More common among Caucasians
- Less common among Asians and African Americans, and particularly uncommon in South African Bantus and West Africans

- Some genetic predisposition, which is proven in twin studies and other families who share certain single nucleotide polymorphisms.
- Suggested genes were found on chromosome 9q21 (i.e., type VI college protein encoding gene).

RISK FACTORS
- Childbirth, particularly multiple parity, accounts for 20–40% as a risk factor.
- Vaginal delivery, especially operative vaginal delivery
- Advancing age
- Caucasian or Hispanic (4–5-fold increased risk compared with African Americans)
- Tobacco use
- Occupations requiring heavy lifting
- Various connective tissue and neurogenic disorders
- Conditions resulting in increased intra-abdominal pressure (e.g., obesity, abdominal or pelvic tumors, pulmonary disease with chronic coughing, chronic constipation)
- Estrogen-deficient state

GENERAL PREVENTION
- Kegel exercises increase the strength of the pelvic diaphragm muscles and may provide some pelvic support.
- Weight loss and proper management of conditions that increase abdominal pressure help to prevent prolapse.
- Tobacco cessation
- Postmenopausal estrogen replacement therapy

COMMONLY ASSOCIATED CONDITIONS
Cystocele, rectocele, enterocele, and vaginal vault prolapse are often associated with uterine prolapse.

 DIAGNOSIS

HISTORY
- Patients are often asymptomatic. They may experience the following:
  - Pelvic pressure and low back pain
  - Bulging sensation in vagina or at introitus
  - Vaginal bleeding (mucosal irritation)
- They may also experience symptoms related to bowel, bladder and sexual dysfunction:
  - Dyspareunia
  - Difficulty with urination or defecation
  - Symptoms often worsen following long periods of standing
  - Constipation:
- Inquiry should be made as to:
  - The number of pregnancies, mode of deliveries, episiotomies, extent and repair of vaginal/perineal lacerations
  - Previous pelvic surgery
  - Congenital abnormalities
  - Medical conditions that chronically increase intra-abdominal pressure (e.g., chronic obstructive pulmonary disease [COPD])

PHYSICAL EXAM
- Diagnosis is confirmed by a pelvic exam. With coughing and straining, the cervix will prolapse toward introitus or beyond.
- Use only 1 blade of speculum during pelvic exam to better appreciate prolapse.

ALERT
- The patient needs to be examined while standing as well as lying down to confirm diagnosis.
- Severity of symptoms and degree of prolapse are not strongly correlated.
- Can use 1 of many evaluation systems to describe extent of prolapse:
  - Baden-Walker classification system has been widely replaced by the Pelvic Organ Prolapse Quantification (POP-Q)
  - The POP-Q (1) system is more accurate and more complex:
    - Stage 0: No prolapse
    - Stage 1: >1 cm above the hymen
    - Stage 2: ≤1 cm proximal or distal to the plane of the hymen
    - Stage 3: >1 cm below the plane of the hymen, but protrudes no further than 2 cm less than the total vaginal length
    - Stage 4: Eversion of the lower genital tract is complete.

DIFFERENTIAL DIAGNOSIS
- Other pelvic organ prolapse (e.g., cystocele, rectocele, enterocele)
- Pelvic mass, benign or malignant

DIAGNOSTIC TESTS & INTERPRETATION
- Evaluation of renal function (BUN and creatinine) to rule out ureteral obstruction
- Urinalysis to rule out UTI
- IV pyelogram to rule out ureteral obstruction in complete uterine prolapse (optional)
- Pelvic US or CT to rule out other pelvic pathology, if suspected (optional)

Diagnostic Procedures/Other
- If surgical correction is planned, urodynamic studies should be performed to evaluate for potential urinary incontinence masked by the prolapse (2)[B].
- If ulceration or bleeding is present, Pap smears and appropriate cervical and endometrial biopsies should be done to rule out concomitant malignancies.

Test Interpretation
Hyperkeratosis of the cervical and vaginal tissues occurs with prolapse beyond the introitus due to chronic irritation and drying. As the irritation becomes more pronounced, bleeding and ulceration occur.

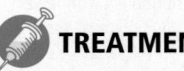 **TREATMENT**

GENERAL MEASURES
- Treatment depends on multiple variables, including the severity of prolapse, age, sexual activity, associated pelvic pathology, and desire for future fertility.
- Treatment of stage I or II prolapse is expectant unless patient is symptomatic.
- Conservative therapies include vaginal estrogen replacement, mechanical support using pessary, and physical therapy (3)[C].
- Pessaries are indicated for women who are unfit for, or decline, surgery. Proper fitting and maintenance are required (4)[C].
- Pessaries also may be used in the preoperative evaluation of prolapse (4)[C].

- Surgery is indicated for women who fail conservative therapies and/or desire definitive treatment (2)[B].

MEDICATION

- Vaginal estrogen therapy can increase blood supply to the vagina and supporting tissue, which may improve tissue strength; may also be beneficial for mild urinary incontinence. This is especially important in postmenopausal women using pessaries or undergoing reconstructive pelvic surgery (2)[B].
- Progestin therapy or monitoring of endometrial status in a woman with an intact uterus is not generally necessary with vaginal estrogen therapy.
- Estrogen therapy should be used in the lowest possible dose for the shortest time. However, women may need long-term therapy due to the chronic nature of uterine prolapse.
- 3 forms of vaginal estrogen therapy:
  - Vaginal cream (conjugated equine estrogen or estradiol cream): Insert via applicator each night × 14 days and then 2–3 times/wk.
  - Vaginal estradiol tablet: Insert via preloaded applicator each night × 14 days and then 2–3 times/wk.
  - Estradiol-containing vaginal ring: Insert into vagina and replace every 3 months.
- Contraindications:
  - Breast- or estrogen-dependent carcinoma
  - Undiagnosed vaginal bleeding
  - Thromboembolic disorders
  - Thrombophlebitis
  - Pregnancy
- Precautions: Any abnormal vaginal bleeding must be evaluated.

ISSUES FOR REFERRAL
Urogynecology evaluation for patients who may be surgical candidates

ADDITIONAL THERAPIES
Physical therapy, including biofeedback, electrical stimulation, and pelvic muscle training (Kegels), may be an option for women with mild prolapse and/or those wishing conservative therapy (4)[C].

SURGERY/OTHER PROCEDURES

- Surgical candidates without additional pelvic pathology: Vaginal or abdominal hysterectomy ± enterocele, cystocele, rectocele, paravaginal repair, urethral suspension, and culdoplasty depending on coexisting pelvic organ prolapse (2)[B]
- Incontinence procedure is often done at same time as prolapse repair, although almost 1/3 of women are relieved of stress urinary incontinence by prolapse surgery alone (5)[B].
- Vault suspension is typically necessary with hysterectomy:
  - Vaginal procedures include sacrospinous ligament fixation, uterosacral ligament fixation, and endopelvic fascial suspension.
- Sacral colpopexy can be performed via laparoscopic or open abdominal approach.
- The abdominal approach (sacral colpopexy) has a decreased risk of recurrent apical prolapse and less postoperative dyspareunia and stress incontinence compared with the vaginal approach (sacrospinous ligament fixation). However, the abdominal approach is associated with longer operative and recovery times (6)[A].

- Uterine suspension is an option for patients who desire to maintain reproductive function (2)[B].
- In elderly women, uterine conservation with sacrospinous fixation is comparable with vaginal hysterectomy but with fewer postoperative complications (6)[B].
- Older women who are not sexually active can be treated with colpocleisis or vaginal obliteration procedure.
- Current recommendations from the American Urogynecologic Society about the use of transvaginal mesh include that it may improve an anterior compartment repair, but the risk–benefit ratio must balance improved support with cost of the devices and complications.

IN-PATIENT CONSIDERATIONS
Admission Criteria/Initial Stabilization
- Outpatient
- Inpatient when surgery is necessary

 ONGOING CARE

FOLLOW-UP RECOMMENDATIONS
- Heavy lifting, sexual intercourse, and other activities that increase intra-abdominal pressure should be avoided for 6–12 weeks after surgical correction.
- Maintain ideal body weight

Patient Monitoring
- Expectant management is appropriate, with periodic follow-up exams.
- If a pessary is placed, it should be removed, cleaned, and replaced every 3–6 months (4)[C].

DIET
Avoid constipation by increasing dietary fiber and fluid intake.

PATIENT EDUCATION
- Kegel exercises when applicable
- American College of Obstetricians and Gynecologists (ACOG), 409 12th St., SW, Washington, DC 20024-2188; 800-762-ACOG; www.acog.org

PROGNOSIS
- It is expected that the incidence and severity of prolapse will increase as patients age.
- Although surgical correction is usually successful initially, reoperation rate is ~29% (2)[B].

COMPLICATIONS
- Ureteral obstruction and renal failure
- Incarceration of bowel herniations
- Pessary use may not always be effective and may cause discomfort, ulcers, and infection
- Mesh erosion

Pregnancy Considerations
- Management:
  - Bed rest in a moderately Trendelenburg position
  - Good genital hygiene with local antiseptics
  - Continuous usage of a pessary is recommended until labor
- If conservative solutions have failed, minimally invasive surgery in the gravid patient may be considered such as Gilliam suspension.
- Labor induction with misoprostol and oxytocin should be avoided as well as manual uterine fundal pressure.

REFERENCES

1. Kow, N. Goldman H, Rideway B. Management options for women with uterine prolapse interested in uterine preservation. *Curr Urol Rep*. 2013;14: 395–402.
2. Tsikouras P, Dafopoulos A, Varchnis N, et al. Uterine prolapse in pregnancy: Risk factors, complications and management. *J Matern Fetal Neonatal Med*. 2013, in press.
3. Trowbridge ER, Fenner DE. Conservative management of pelvic organ prolapse. *Clin Obstet Gynecol*. 2005;48:668–681.
4. Borstad E, Abdelnoor M, Staff AC. Surgical strategies for women with pelvic organ prolapse and urinary stress incontinence. *Int Urogynecol J Pelvic Floor Dysfunct*. 2010;21:179–186.
5. Maher C, Feiner B, Baessler K. Surgical management of pelvic organ prolapse in women. *Cochrane Database Syst Rev*. 2010;4:CD004014.
6. Hefni M, El-Toukhy T. Sacrospinous cervicocolpopexy with uterine conservation for uterovaginal prolapse in elderly women: An evolving concept. *Am J Obstet Gynecol*. 2003;188: 645–650.

ADDITIONAL READING

- Baden WF. Fundamentals, symptoms and classification. In: Baden WF, et al., eds. *Surgical repair of vaginal defects*. Philadelphia: Lippincott; 1992:1.
- Committee on Gynecologic Practice. Vaginal placement of synthetic mesh for pelvic organ prolapse. *Female Pelvic Med Reconstr Surg*. 2012;18:5–9.
- Doshani A, Teo RE, Mayne CJ, et al. Uterine prolapse. *BMJ*. 2007;335:819–823.
- Onwude JL. Genital prolapse in women. *Clin Evid (Online)*. 2012;2012:pii 0817.
- Society of Obstetricians and Gynaecologists of Canada. SOGC clinical practice guidelines. The detection and management of vaginal atrophy. *Number 145*, May 2004. *Int J Gynaecol Obstet*. 2005;88:222–228.

 CODES

ICD10
- N81.2 Incomplete uterovaginal prolapse
- N81.3 Complete uterovaginal prolapse
- N81.4 Uterovaginal prolapse, unspecified

CLINICAL PEARLS

- Uterine prolapse occurs when the integrity of pelvic supporting structures is lost.
- Advancing age and vaginal childbirth (including the number of pregnancies and the difficulty of childbirth) are the most important factors that contribute to uterine prolapse.
- Conservative therapies include vaginal estrogen replacement, pessary use, and physical therapy.
- Surgery is indicated for women who fail conservative therapies and/or desire definitive treatment.

U

UTERINE SYNECHIAE

Virginia Van Duyne, MD

 BASICS

DESCRIPTION
- Uterine synechiae are intrauterine adhesions (IUAs).
- Symptoms may include secondary amenorrhea, pelvic pain, recurrent spontaneous abortions (SABs), and/or infertility in a female of child-bearing age.
- When specific symptoms are present it is called Asherman syndrome: IUAs associated with menstrual disturbances (amenorrhea, hypomenorrhea, or dysmenorrhea), infertility, and/or recurrent SABs (1,2).
- Severity of disease ranges from mild to moderate to severe, depending on the degree of adhesions (e.g., number, density, thickness, quality).
- 7 different classification systems to categorize disease severity:
  - Each system includes consideration of adhesion characteristics on hysteroscopy (1).
  - Important to classify severity because it has prognostic value for fertility (1); however, currently no single uniform system is endorsed.
  - Difficult to compare studies due to variety of classification systems (1).

EPIDEMIOLOGY
Incidence
1.5% of all hysterosalpingographies (3).
Prevalence
- Varies with geography, population profile, availability of diagnostic devices
- Asymptomatic population: 0.3% incidental finding of uterine adhesions
- After postpartum curettage: 22% (2)
- After postabortion curettage: 37% (3)

ETIOLOGY AND PATHOPHYSIOLOGY
- Endometrial injury stimulates fibrosis. See "Risk Factors" for specific types of injury.
- Fibrous tissue replaces endometrial stroma and glands, replacing normal, vascular tissue with denser, less vascular tissue.
- Eventually endometrial lining becomes atrophic and inert (2,4).

RISK FACTORS
Any damage to endometrium:
- Cesarean section
- Postpartum curettage especially after initial 48 hours postpartum
- Postabortion curettage
- Pelvic radiation
- Polypectomy
- Intrauterine device (IUD) insertion
- Diagnostic curettage
- Myomectomy (2,3,4)
- Postpartum hemorrhage
- Recurrent SABs
- Pelvic infection (e.g., endometrial tuberculosis or pelvic inflammatory disease)—controversial (2,3,4)

GENERAL PREVENTION
- Minimize intrauterine operative interventions while women are fertile and desire pregnancy.
- Expectant or medical management rather than surgical management of SABs.

 DIAGNOSIS

HISTORY
- Infertility
- Menstrual abnormalities:
  - Amenorrhea or hypomenorrhea
  - Menstrual pattern does not correlate with severity of adhesions
  - Endometriosis
- Hematometra and/or hematosalpinx
- Recurrent SABs
- Cyclic pelvic pain (2,4)

PHYSICAL EXAM
- Usually no abnormalities.
- Occasionally, cervical obstruction may be present on blind transcervical uterine sounding (1,2).

DIFFERENTIAL DIAGNOSIS
Differential diagnosis is same as for amenorrhea, infertility, recurrent SABs, and cyclic pelvic pain.

DIAGNOSTIC TESTS & INTERPRETATION
Initial Tests (lab, imaging)
- Hysteroscopy is gold standard for diagnosis. Allows direct visualization of adhesions to diagnose, stratify severity, and treat the adhesions (1,2)[B].
- If hysteroscopy unavailable locally, hysterosalpingogram and hysterosonography are reasonable alternatives for interim evaluation to decide if referral to distant hysteroscopy is indicated (1)[B].

- Hysteroscopy compared with other diagnostic sources (1,2):
  - Hysterosalpingography: Sensitivity 75–81%; specificity 80%; positive predictive value (PPV) 50%; high false–positive rate (up to 38%)
  - Sonohysterography/Saline infusion sonography: Sensitivity 75%; specificity 43%
  - Transvaginal ultrasound: Sensitivity 52%; specificity 11%
  - 3D ultrasound: Compared to 3D sonohysterography only: Sensitivity 87%; specificity 45%
- Consider also evaluating for other causes of infertility, menstrual abnormalities, recurrent SABs.

Follow-Up Tests & Special Considerations
Assess patient's goals for fertility and/or pelvic pain control in order to properly counsel on benefits and risks of hysteroscopy for diagnosis and/or treatment.

Test Interpretation
Diagnosis confirmed on hysteroscopy by:
- Visualization of IUAs
- Volume and quality of adhesions
- Areas of occlusion (e.g., fundus, ostia, portion of uterine cavity)
- Quality of endometrial lining

 TREATMENT

GENERAL MEASURES
Counsel on option of expectant management (i.e., observation) which confers:
- Spontaneous return of menses in 78% within 7 years
- Spontaneous pregnancy in 46%
- Limited data and no randomized controlled trials (RCTs) for expectant vs. hysteroscopic lysis (1)[C]

MEDICATION
First Line
No role for medical treatments in absence of primary surgical intervention (1).

Second Line
There are a few postoperative ancillary treatments to help prevent recurrence of disease; many are still under investigation. No RCTs exist to compare (1):
- Estrogen ± progestin (1,2)[C].
- Nonhormonal medications: Increase vascular flow to endometrial tissue; aspirin, nitroglycerin, sildenafil. Only used in research with rigorous protocols (1)[C].
- IUDs: Goal is to provide physical barrier between uterine walls to prevent adhesion formation:
  - Pediatric Foley catheter
  - Amnion graft
  - Adhesion barrier films with hyaluronic acid (currently under research)
  - Lippes loop (trapezoidal-shaped IUD, not commercially available) (1)[C]

ALERT

Modern contraceptive IUDs, such as Mirena IUD or Paragard copper IUD, are *not* appropriate for IUA postoperative management. They are pro-inflammatory and the surface area is too small to be effective physical barrier.

ISSUES FOR REFERRAL

Offer referral to gynecologist with expertise in hysteroscopy (1)[C].

SURGERY/OTHER PROCEDURES

Hysteroscopy with lysis of adhesions is gold standard. Various techniques exist, however, no RCTs to compare them (1,2)[B]:

- Hysteroscopy with myometrial scoring: For severe IUAs when hysteroscopic adhesiolysis cannot be safely performed.
- Open laparotomy followed by hysterotomy and subsequent blunt dissection of adhesions with finger or curette (used rarely in severe cases).
- Alternative visualizing methods, such as fluoroscopy, transabdominal ultrasound, and laparoscopy: Higher rates of uterine perforation and expense (1)[C].

IN-PATIENT CONSIDERATIONS

Typically managed as outpatient same-day surgical procedure in absence of complications.

ONGOING CARE

FOLLOW-UP RECOMMENDATIONS

- Routine visits at 2 and 6 weeks after surgery
- Repeat hysteroscopy or 2nd-line hysterosalpingography at 2–3 menstrual cycles postsurgery to assess for adhesion recurrence (1)[B].

DIET

Routine same-day surgery care: Advance diet as tolerated to preoperative baseline.

PATIENT EDUCATION

- Resources for patients may include: American Academy of Family Physicians (www.familydoctor.org)
- American Congress of Obstetricians and Gynecologists (www.acog.org/For_Patients)
- American Society for Reproductive Medicine (www.asrm.org)

PROGNOSIS

- Mild-to-moderate disease: Adhesion recurrence rate after lysis of adhesions is 1 of 3 women.
- Severe disease: Adhesion recurrence rate is 2 of 3 women.

COMPLICATIONS

For hysteroscopy:
- Uterine perforation
- Recurrence of adhesions
- Visceral organ injury
- Bleeding
- Infection

REFERENCES

1. AAGL practice report: Practice guidelines for management of intrauterine synechiae. *J Minim Invasive Gynecol*. 2010;17:1–7.
2. Deans R, Abbott J. Review of intrauterine adhesions. *J Minim Invasive Gyencol*. 2010;17:555–556.
3. Dawood A, Al-Talib A, Tulandi T. Predisposing factors and treatment outcome of different stages of intrauterine adhesions. *J Obstet Gynaecol Can*. 2010;32:767–777.
4. March CM. Asherman's syndrome. *Semin Reprod Med*. 2011;29:83–94.

ADDITIONAL READING

- Myers EM, Hurst BS. Comprehensive management of severe Asherman syndrome and amenorrhea. *Fertil Steril*. 2012;97:160–164.
- Socolov R, Anton E, Butureanu S, et al. The endoscopic management of uterine synechiae. A clinical study of 78 cases. *Chirurgia (Bucur)*. 2010;105:515–518.
- Thomson AJ, Abbott JA, Deans R, et al. The management of intrauterine synechiae. *Curr Opin Obstet Gynecol*. 2009;21:335–341.

 SEE ALSO

Algorithm: Amenorrhea, Secondary; Infertility; Pelvic Pain

 CODES

ICD10

N85.6 Intrauterine synechiae

CLINICAL PEARLS

- Typical symptoms: Secondary amenorrhea, infertility, recurrent SABs, and/or cyclic pelvic pain.
- Prevention of adhesions is key by minimizing intrauterine operative interventions while women are fertile and desire pregnancy.
- Hysteroscopy is the gold standard for both diagnosis (adhesion visualization) and therapy (adhesion lysis).

U

UVEITIS

Shailendra K. Saxena, MD, PhD • Mikayla Spangler, PharmD, BCPS • Laura K. Klug, PharmD

 BASICS

DESCRIPTION
- A nonspecific term used to describe any intraocular inflammatory disorder.
- Symptoms vary, depending on depth of involvement and associated conditions.
- The uvea is the middle layer of the eye between the sclera and retina. The anterior part of the uvea includes the iris and ciliary body. The posterior part of the uvea is the choroid:
  - Anterior uveitis: Refers to ocular inflammation limited to the iris (iritis) alone or iris and ciliary body (iridocyclitis)
  - Intermediate uveitis: Refers to inflammation of the structures just posterior to the lens (pars planitis or peripheral uveitis)
  - Posterior uveitis: Refers to inflammation of the choroid (choroiditis), retina (retinitis), or vitreous near the optic nerve and macula
- System(s) affected: Nervous
- Synonym(s): Iritis; Iridocyclitis; Choroiditis; Retinochoroiditis; Chorioretinitis; Anterior uveitis; Posterior uveitis; Pars planitis; Panuveitis. Synonyms are anatomic descriptions of the focus of the uveal inflammation.

Geriatric Considerations
The inflammatory response to systemic disease may be suppressed.

Pediatric Considerations
- Infection should be the primary consideration.
- Allergies and psychologic factors (depression, stress) may serve as a trigger.
- Trauma is also a common cause in this population.

Pregnancy Considerations
May be of importance in the selection of medications

EPIDEMIOLOGY
- Predominant age: All ages
- Predominant sex: Male = Female, except for HLA-B27 anterior uveitis: Male > Female (2.5:1)

Incidence
Anterior uveitis most common (8.2 cases/100,000 annual incidence)

Prevalence
Iritis is 4× more prevalent than posterior uveitis.

ETIOLOGY AND PATHOPHYSIOLOGY
- Infectious: May result from viral, bacterial, parasitic, or fungal etiologies
- Suspected immune-mediated: Possible autoimmune or immune-complex–mediated mechanism postulated in association with systemic (especially rheumatologic) disorders
- Isolated eye disease
- Idiopathic (~25%)
- Autoimmune uveitis (AIU) patients should be referred to an ophthalmologist for local treatment.
- Some medications may cause uveitis. The most causative medications include rifabutin, bisphosphonates, sulfonamides, metipranolol, topical corticosteroids, brimonidine, prostaglandin analogs, anti-VEGF agents, bacillus Calmette-Guerin (BCG) vaccination, and systemic and intraocular cidofovir.
- Masquerade syndromes: Diseases such as malignancies that may be mistaken for primary inflammation of the eye

Genetics
- No specific pattern for uveitis in general
- Iritis: Of patients, 50–70% are HLA-B27–positive.

RISK FACTORS
- No specific risk factors
- Higher incidence seen with specific associated conditions

COMMONLY ASSOCIATED CONDITIONS
- Viral infections: Herpes simplex, herpes zoster, HIV, cytomegalovirus
- Bacterial infections: Brucellosis, leprosy, leptospirosis, Lyme disease, propionibacterium infection, syphilis, tuberculosis (TB), Whipple disease
- Parasitic infections: Acanthamebiasis, cysticercosis, onchocerciasis, toxocariasis, toxoplasmosis
- Fungal infections: Aspergillosis, blastomycosis, candidiasis, coccidioidomycosis, cryptococcosis, histoplasmosis, sporotrichosis
- Suspected immune-mediated: Ankylosing spondylitis, Behçet disease, Crohn disease, drug or hypersensitivity reaction, interstitial nephritis, juvenile rheumatoid arthritis, Kawasaki disease, multiple sclerosis, psoriatic arthritis, Reiter syndrome, relapsing polychondritis, sarcoidosis, Sjögren syndrome, systemic lupus erythematosus, ulcerative colitis, vasculitis, vitiligo, Vogt-Koyanagi (Harada) syndrome
- Isolated eye disease: Acute multifocal placoid pigmentary epitheliopathy, acute retinal necrosis, bird-shot choroidopathy, Fuchs heterochromatic cyclitis, glaucomatocyclitic crisis, lens-induced uveitis, multifocal choroiditis, pars planitis, serpiginous choroiditis, sympathetic ophthalmia, trauma
- Masquerade syndromes: Leukemia, lymphoma, retinitis pigmentosa, retinoblastoma

℞ DIAGNOSIS

HISTORY
- Decreased visual acuity
- Pain, photophobia, blurring of vision:
  - Usually acute
- Anterior uveitis (~80% of patients with uveitis):
  - Generally acute in onset
  - Deep eye pain
  - Photophobia (consensual)
- Intermediate and posterior uveitis:
  - Unresolving floaters
  - Generally insidious in onset
  - More commonly bilateral

PHYSICAL EXAM
Slit-lamp exam and indirect ophthalmoscopy are necessary for precise diagnosis:
- Anterior uveitis (~80% of patients with uveitis):
  - Conjunctival vessel dilation
  - Perilimbal (circumcorneal) dilation of episcleral and scleral vessels (ciliary flush)
  - Small pupillary size of affected eye
  - Hypopyon or hyphema (WBCs or RBCs pooled in the anterior chamber)
  - Frequently unilateral (95% of HLA-B27–associated cases)
  - Bilateral involvement and systemic symptoms (fever, fatigue, abdominal pain) may be associated with interstitial nephritis.
  - Systemic disease is most likely to be associated with anterior uveitis (in 1 study, 53% of patients were found to have systemic disease).
- Intermediate and posterior uveitis:
  - More commonly bilateral
  - Posterior inflammation will generally cause minimal pain or redness unless associated with an iritis.

DIFFERENTIAL DIAGNOSIS
- Acute angle-closure glaucoma
- Conjunctivitis
- Episcleritis
- Keratitis
- Scleritis

DIAGNOSTIC TESTS & INTERPRETATION
No specific test for the diagnosis of uveitis. Tests for etiologic factors or associated conditions should be based on history and physical exam.

Initial Tests (lab, imaging)
- CBC, BUN, creatinine (interstitial nephritis)
- HLA-B27 typing (ankylosing spondylitis, Reiter syndrome)
- Antinuclear antibody, ESR (systemic lupus erythematosus, Sjögren syndrome)
- Venereal disease research laboratory (VDRL) test, fluorescent titer antibody (syphilis)
- Purified protein derivative (PPD) tuberculin skin test (TB)
- Lyme serology (Lyme disease)
- Disorders that may alter lab results: Immunodeficiency
- Chest x-ray (sarcoidosis, histoplasmosis, TB, lymphoma)
- Sacroiliac radiograph (ankylosing spondylitis)

Diagnostic Procedures/Other
Slit-lamp exam

Test Interpretation
- Keratic precipitates
- Inflammatory cells in anterior chamber or vitreous
- Synechiae (fibrous tissue scarring between iris and lens)
- Macular edema
- Perivasculitis of retinal vessels

TREATMENT

GENERAL MEASURES
- Outpatient care with urgent ophthalmologic consultation
- Medical therapy best initiated following full ophthalmologic evaluation
- Treatment of underlying cause, if identified
- Anti-inflammatory therapy

MEDICATION
First Line
- The treatment depends on the etiology, location, and severity of the inflammation.
- Homatropine hydrobromide (Isopto) 2% or 5% ophthalmic solution: 1–2 drops to the affected eye b.i.d., or as often as q3h if necessary; PLUS
- Prednisolone acetate 1% ophthalmic suspension: 2 drops to the affected eye q1h initially, tapering to once a day with improvement (1,2)[C]:
  - Contraindications:
    o Hypersensitivity to the medication or component of the preparation
    o Cycloplegia is contraindicated in patients known to have, or be predisposed to, glaucoma.
    o Topical corticosteroid therapy is contraindicated in uveitis secondary to infectious etiologies, unless used in conjunction with appropriate anti-infectious agents (3)[C].
  - Precautions:
    o Homatropine hydrobromide may produce adverse systemic antimuscarinic effects. Use extreme caution in infants and young children because of increased susceptibility to systemic effects.
    o Topical corticosteroids may increase intraocular pressure. Prolonged use may cause cataract formation and exacerbate existing herpetic keratitis, which may masquerade as iritis.
  - Significant possible interactions
  - Refer to manufacturer's profile for each drug.
- Systemic corticosteroids are useful for maintenance therapy for patients with noninfectiouos uveitis. These should always be used with other immunosuppressive medications for steroid sparing effects. Prednisone 5–10 mg daily. (4)[C].
- Intravitreous corticosteroid deposits may also be used for long-term maintenance. Fluocinolone acetonide (Retisert) 590 mcg released over 30 months, dexamethasone (Ozurdex) 0.7 mg released slowly over 3–6 months (4)[C].
- Retisert has caused all patients to develop cataracts and significant increased in intraocular pressure in about 2/3 of patients, whereas Ozurdex had only 1/4 of patients require medication for increased intraocular pressure and 15% develop cataracts (4)[C].

Second Line
- Cycloplegia: Scopolamine hydrobromide 0.25% (Isopto Hyoscine) up to q.i.d. or cyclopentolate hydrochloride 1% (Cyclogyl) or atropine 1% (2)[C]
- Anti-inflammatory: Prednisolone sodium phosphate 1%, dexamethasone sodium phosphate 0.1%, dexamethasone suspension, rimexolone 1% (Vexol), and loteprednol etabonate 0.5% (Lotemax) (2)[C]

- Rimexolone 1% (Vexol) may be equally effective as prednisolone acetate 1% for short-term treatment of anterior uveitis (5)[B].
- Loteprednol etabonate (Lotemax) may not be as effective as prednisolone acetate 1%, but may be less likely to increase intraocular pressure in cases of acute anterior uveitis (5)[B].
- Periocular corticosteroids may be injected with triamcinolone acetonide being most commonly used. 40 mg/1 mL (4).
- Intravitreal corticosteroid injections are used only in severe cases of recurrence. Triamcinolone acetonide 4–20 mg/0.1 mL, dexamethasone phosphate 0.4 mg/0.1 mL, dexamethasone implant (Ozurdex) (4)
- Ozurdex has a longer effect than triamcinolone acetonide (4)
- Cyclosporine 3–5 mg/kg/day or methotrexate 7.5–15 mg/wk have also been used second line (4).
- Systemic NSAIDs may provide some benefit (2)[C].

ISSUES FOR REFERRAL
Caution should be used when using empiric treatment; referral to an ophthalmologist is recommended in most cases.

ONGOING CARE

FOLLOW-UP RECOMMENDATIONS
Patient Monitoring
- Complete history and physical to evaluate for associated systemic disease
- Ophthalmologic follow-up as recommended by consultant

PATIENT EDUCATION
- Instruct on proper method for instilling eye drops.
- Wear dark glasses if photophobia is a problem.

PROGNOSIS
- Depends on the presence of causal diseases or associated conditions
- Uveitis resulting from infections (systemic or local) tends to resolve with eradication of the underlying infection.
- Uveitis associated with seronegative arthropathies tends to be acute (lasting <3 months) and frequently recurrent.

COMPLICATIONS
- Cycloplegia: Paralysis of the ciliary muscle of the eye, resulting in a loss of accommodation
- Loss of vision as a result of the following:
  - Keratic precipitate deposition on the corneal or lens surfaces
  - Increased intraocular pressure, acute angle-closure glaucoma
  - Formation of synechiae
  - Cataract formation
  - Vasculitis with vascular occlusion, retinal infarction
  - Macular edema
  - Optic nerve damage

REFERENCES
1. Audio PA. A review of evidence guiding the use of corticosteroids in the treatment of intraocular inflammation. Oculi Immunol Inflame. 2004;12(3):169–192.
2. American Optometric Association. Optomeric clinical practice guideline: Care of the patient with anterior uveitis. Available at: http://www.aoa.org/documents/CPG-7.pdf.
3. McCluskey PJ, Towler HM, Lightman S. Management of chronic uveitis. BMJ. 2000;320(7234):555–558.
4. Gallego-Pinazo R, Dolz-Marco R, Martinez-Castillo S, et al. Update on the principles and novel local and systemic therapies for the treatment of non-infectious uveitis. Inflamm Allergy Drug Targets. 2013;12:38–45.
5. Jabs DA. Treatment of ocular inflammation. Ocular Immunol Inflame. 2004;12(3):163–168.

ADDITIONAL READING
- de Smet MD, Taylor SR, Bodaghi B, et al. Understanding uveitis: The impact of research on visual outcomes. Prog Retin Eye Res. 2011;30:452–470.
- Levy RA, de Andrade FA, Foeldvari I, et al. Cutting-edge issues in autoimmune uveitis. Clin Rev Allergy Immunol. 2011;41:214–223.
- Patel H, Goldstein D. Pediatric uveitis. Pediatr Clin North Am. 2003;50(1):125–136.
- Smith JR, Rosenbaum JT. Management of uveitis: A rheumatologic perspective. Arthritis Rheum. 2002;84(2):309–318.

SEE ALSO
Conjunctivitis, Acute; Glaucoma, Primary Closed-Angle; Scleritis

CODES
ICD10
- H20.9 Unspecified iridocyclitis
- H20.019 Primary iridocyclitis, unspecified eye
- H30.90 Unspecified chorioretinal inflammation, unspecified eye

CLINICAL PEARLS
- Symptoms vary, depending on depth of involvement and associated conditions, but should be suspected when eye pain is associated with visual changes.
- Severe or unresponsive uveitis may require therapy, including periocular injection of corticosteroids, sustained-release corticosteroid implants, systemic corticosteroids, cytotoxic agents, immunosuppressive agents, immunomodulatory agents, or tumor necrosis factor inhibitors.

U

VAGINAL ADENOSIS

Laura K. Randolph, DO, MS • Michael P. Hopkins, MD, MEd

 BASICS

DESCRIPTION
- The normal vagina is lined with squamous epithelium. Adenosis is characterized by the presence of columnar epithelium or glandular tissue in the wall of the vagina.
- At about the 15th week of embryologic development, the Müllerian system, which forms the upper 2/3 of the vagina, fuses with the invaginating cloaca or urogenital sinus to form the lower 1/3 of the vagina. Squamous metaplasia from the cloacal region then produces a squamous epithelium through the vagina.
- Adenosis occurs when this squamous epithelium fails to epithelialize the vagina completely.
- 3 main types of adenosis epithelium described:
  - Endocervical
  - Endometrial
  - Tubal
- System(s) affected: Reproductive

Geriatric Considerations
- Adenosis is a disorder of the young female. By menopause, the vagina and cervix should be completely epithelialized.
- The presence of glandular epithelium in the postmenopausal patient is an indication for excision and close evaluation for the possibility of a well-differentiated adenocarcinoma.

Pregnancy Considerations
Pregnancy produces a wide eversion of the transformation zone of the cervix. This occasionally will become so widely everted that it will extend onto the vaginal fornices, leading to the impression of adenosis. This will resolve after the pregnancy is completed.

EPIDEMIOLOGY
Incidence
- Although the cumulative incidence of vaginal adenosis is unknown, the incidence of cloacal malformations is 1/20,000–1/25,000 live births.
- Although spontaneous vaginal adenosis appears to be fairly common (10% of adult women), it is mostly an insignificant coincidental finding. Widespread symptomatic involvement is rare (1).

Prevalence
- In the US: Adenosis is relatively common, affecting 10–20% of young females studied. As maturation progresses with puberty, epithelialization occurs (2).
- Predominant age:
  - Age <1 month: 15%
  - Prepubertal: typically absent
  - Age 13–25 years: 13%
  - Age >25 years: decreasing prevalence, uncommon beyond age 30 years (1)

ETIOLOGY AND PATHOPHYSIOLOGY
- In most young females, the etiology is incomplete squamous metaplasia or epithelialization. This occurs as a natural phenomenon and resolves with age.
- Described as congenital or acquired (3):
  - Congenital: Proliferation of the remnant Müllerian epithelium in the vagina due to exposure to diethylstilbestrol (DES) in utero (DES daughters)
  - Transformation related protein 63 (TRP63/p63) marks the cell fate decision of Müllerian duct epithelium to become squamous epithelium in the cervix and vagina. DES disrupts the TRP63 expression and induces adenosis lesions (4).
  - Acquired: Trauma and inflammation causing spontaneous de novo changes or changes in an acquired lesion in the vaginal epithelium:
    - Trauma: Carbon dioxide laser, 5-fluorouracil, vaginal packs, chronic pessary use
    - Proliferation of the glandular cells in the remnant Müllerian epithelium of the vagina due to sex hormones
    - Idiopathic spontaneous change in epithelium; no cause has been identified.

RISK FACTORS
Adenosis of the vagina/cervix may arise in up to 90% of DES daughters and there is a 40-fold increased risk of the subsequent development of clear cell adenocarcinoma (5).

GENERAL PREVENTION
None: Last DES exposure in the 1970s

COMMONLY ASSOCIATED CONDITIONS
DES exposure:
- Adenosis from DES exposure should lead to an evaluation of other DES-related abnormalities.
- Müllerian tract anomalies associated with DES exposure include cervical hood, cervical ridge, shortened cervix, incompetent cervix, and T-shaped uterine cavity.
- Patients with known DES exposure should have their reproductive tract evaluated prior to conception.
- Most patients with adenosis have not been DES exposed and do not require evaluation of the reproductive system.
- DES is a synthetic, nonsteroidal estrogen that was used to prevent spontaneous abortions or premature deliveries from 1938 to 1971 (5). An estimated 5 million women were prescribed DES during this period (4).
- The FDA issued a drug bulletin in 1971 advising physicians to stop prescribing DES to pregnant women because of its link to vaginal clear cell adenocarcinoma in DES daughters (5).

 DIAGNOSIS

HISTORY
- Maternal DES exposure
- Complaints of:
  - Profuse mucoid vaginal discharge from the glandular epithelium
  - Pruritus
  - Pain/soreness of the vaginal introitus
  - Postcoital bleeding
  - Dyspareunia

PHYSICAL EXAM
On pelvic exam, adenosis appearance is varied: Patchy or diffuse red stippling, granularity or nodularity, single or multiple cysts, erosions, ulcers, or warty protuberances that may even extend to the vulva (1)

DIFFERENTIAL DIAGNOSIS
- Erosive lichen planus
- Fixed drug eruption
- Erythema multiforme
- Bullous skin disease
- Adenocarcinoma:
  - A thorough evaluation for adenocarcinoma of the vagina arising in adenosis should be done.
  - A biopsy may be necessary to ensure that the process represents only benign adenosis.

DIAGNOSTIC TESTS & INTERPRETATION
Initial Tests (lab, imaging)
4-quadrant Pap smear should be used liberally to isolate quadrants of the vagina that may contain abnormalities. None, unless diagnosed with underlying malignancy

Follow-Up Tests & Special Considerations
Pap smear can be followed by colposcopy and biopsy.

Diagnostic Procedures/Other
Colposcopy should be used to outline areas of adenosis to ensure that no malignancy is present.

Test Interpretation
- Biopsy will show benign glandular epithelium.
- Biopsies in the areas of ongoing squamous metaplasia will be typical for this process (3).

TREATMENT

GENERAL MEASURES
- Unless malignancy is present, conservative treatment is indicated.
- In most young females with this condition, it will resolve with expectant management (1)[C].
- Treatment is warranted in women with severe subjective symptoms that impair the quality of life (6).

ISSUES FOR REFERRAL
Malignancy found on biopsy warrants referral to gynecologic oncology specialist.

SURGERY/OTHER PROCEDURES
- Aggressive therapy, such as laser or surgical excision, is necessary if premalignant or malignant changes arise (3)[C].
- Symptomatic treatment with carbon dioxide laser coagulation, unipolar coagulation, or, lastly, vaginal resection (1)

IN-PATIENT CONSIDERATIONS
Admission Criteria/Initial Stabilization
Outpatient management

ONGOING CARE

FOLLOW-UP RECOMMENDATIONS
Patient Monitoring
If the initial colposcopy is normal, a yearly 4-quadrant Pap smear of the vagina and of the cervix is all that is necessary.

DIET
No special diet

PATIENT EDUCATION
- No limitations
- It is not necessary to avoid intercourse or placing objects in the vagina.
- The patient should be educated to keep annual pelvic and Pap smear appointments. In most situations, this is benign, and expectant management is all that is necessary.
- www.acog.org

PROGNOSIS
- It is expected that most patients will have squamous metaplasia and epithelialization with complete resolution of the adenosis.
- The rare patient, 1/1,000–1/10,000, may develop adenocarcinoma in the adenosis and will require definitive therapy as for vaginal cancer.
  - Cumulative incidence of progression of adenosis to adenocarcinoma is 1.5/1,000 for DES daughters (5)

COMPLICATIONS
- Infertility with DES association
- Adverse pregnancy outcome with DES association
- Adenocarcinoma of vagina

REFERENCES

1. Kranl C, Zelger B, Kofler H, et al. Vulval and vaginal adenosis. *Br J Dermatol*. 1998;139:128–131.
2. Sandberg EC. The incidence and distribution of occult vaginal adenosis. *Am J Obstet Gynecol*. 1968;101:322–334.
3. Chattopadhyay I, Cruickshan DJ, Packer M. Non diethylstilbestrol induced vaginal adenosis—A case series and review of literature. *Eur J Gynaecol Oncol*. 2001;22(4):260–262.
4. Laronda MM, Unno K, Butler LM, et al. The development of cervical and vaginal adenosis as a result of diethylstilbestrol exposure in utero. *Differentiation* 2012;84(3):252–260.
5. National Toxicology Program, Department of Health and Human Services. Diethylstilbestrol. *Report on Carcinogens, 12th Ed.* 2011:159–161.
6. Cebesoy FB, Kutlar I, Aydin A. Vaginal adenosis successfully treated with simple unipolar cauterization. *J Natl Med Assoc.* 2007;99(2):166–167.

ADDITIONAL READING

Bamigboye AA, Morris J. Oestrogen supplementation, mainly diethylstilbestrol, for preventing miscarriages and other adverse pregnancy outcomes. *Cochrane Database Syst Rev*. 2003:CD004271.

 SEE ALSO

Vaginal Malignancy; DES Exposure

 CODES

ICD10
Q52.4 Other congenital malformations of vagina

CLINICAL PEARLS

- Adenosis is characterized by the presence of columnar epithelium or glandular tissue in the wall of the vagina.
- Adenosis is more common among women exposed to DES in utero.
- Adenosis is rarely associated with an underlying vaginal malignancy.

VAGINAL BLEEDING DURING PREGNANCY

Virginia Van Duyne, MD

 BASICS

DESCRIPTION
- Vaginal bleeding during pregnancy has many causes and ranges in severity from benign with normal pregnancy outcome to life-threatening for both infant and mother.
- Etiology can be from the vagina, cervix, uterus, fetus, or placenta. The differential diagnosis is guided by the gestational age of the fetus.

EPIDEMIOLOGY
Prevalence
- In early pregnancy: 7–25% of patients
- In late pregnancy: 0.3–2% of patients

ETIOLOGY AND PATHOPHYSIOLOGY
- Many times the cause is unknown.
- Anytime in pregnancy:
  - Cervicitis (infectious or noninfectious)
  - Vaginal or cervical trauma (including postcoital)
  - Cervical lesion or neoplasia
  - Hyperemia of cervix (increased blood flow from pregnancy)
- Early pregnancy:
  - For up to 50% of early-pregnancy bleeding, no cause is ever found.
  - Ectopic pregnancy: Leading cause of 1st-trimester maternal death in the US. Risk factors: Previous ectopic, trauma to fallopian tubes (tubal surgery, infection, tumor), congenital anomaly of tubes, in utero diethylstilbestrol (DES) exposure, current use of IUD, history of infertility, tobacco use
  - Spontaneous abortion: Risk factors: Advanced maternal age (AMA), alcohol use, tobacco use, anesthetic gas, heavy caffeine use, cocaine use, chronic maternal diseases (poorly controlled diabetes mellitus (DM), celiac disease, autoimmune diseases such as antiphospholipid syndrome), short interconceptional time (3–6 months), current use of IUD, maternal infection (e.g., herpes simplex virus [HSV], gonorrhea, chlamydia, toxoplasmosis, listeriosis, HIV, syphilis, malaria), medications (e.g., retinoids, methotrexate, NSAIDs), multiple previous therapeutic abortions, previous spontaneous abortion, toxins (arsenic, lead, polyurethane), uterine abnormalities (congenital, adhesions, fibroids)
  - Implantation bleeding: Benign, about 6 days after fertilization
  - Uterine fibroids
  - Subchorionic bleed: In late 1st trimester
  - Low-lying placenta
  - Gestational trophoblastic disease: Hydatidiform mole (most common), choriocarcinoma, or placental-site trophoblastic tumors

- Late pregnancy:
  - Bloody show of labor
  - Placenta previa: Painless bleeding; occurs in 0.4% deliveries in the US. Risk factors: Previous history of placenta previa, previous uterine surgery (cesarean section, D&C), chronic hypertension, multiparity, multiple gestation, tobacco use, AMA
  - Placental abruption: Painful bleeding; occurs in 1–2% deliveries in the US. Risk factors: Previous placental abruption, 1st-trimester bleeding, hypertension, preeclampsia, multiple gestation, tobacco, cocaine or methamphetamine use, unexplained elevated maternal α-fetoprotein, poly- or oligohydramnios, AMA, trauma to abdomen, premature rupture of membranes, thrombophilia, short umbilical cord, male fetus, chorioamnionitis, nutritional deficiency
  - Vasa previa: Minimal bleeding with fetal distress; rare (1:2,500 deliveries). Risk factors: In vitro fertilization, multiple gestation, placental abnormalities (low-lying position, bilobate, succenturiate lobe, velamentous insertion of umbilical cord)
  - Placenta accreta, increta, percreta: Risk factors: Uterine scar (e.g., from cesarean section, endometrial ablation or D&C), current placenta previa, AMA, tobacco use, multiparity, uterine anomalies, uterine fibroids, hypertension
  - Uterine rupture: Vaginal bleeding, abnormal fetal heart rate, and disordered or hypertonic uterine contractions with or without pain. Risk factors: Previous cesarean section (most common), trauma, use of oxytocin or prostaglandins, multiparity, external cephalic version, placental abruption, shoulder dystocia, placenta percreta, Müllerian duct anomalies, history of pelvic radiation

RISK FACTORS
See specific etiologies above

GENERAL PREVENTION
- Address modifiable risk factors, such as domestic violence, tobacco and drug use
- If placenta or vasa previa, nothing per vagina

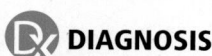 **DIAGNOSIS**

HISTORY
- Anytime in pregnancy: Quality of pregnancy dating, context (e.g., following bowel movement, during voiding, after intercourse, drug use, or trauma including domestic violence), amount of bleeding, obstetrical history, personal or family history of inherited bleeding disorders.
- Early pregnancy: Severe nausea/vomiting (can be associated with molar pregnancy); amount of bleeding, pelvic pain, or suprapubic cramping (e.g., spontaneous abortion, ectopic) complications in previous pregnancies (e.g., spontaneous abortion, abruption, 1st-trimester vaginal bleeding).
- Late pregnancy: Contractions (labor), abdominal pain especially between contractions (abruption, uterine rupture), presence or absence of fetal movement, rupture of membranes.
- See "Etiology and Pathophysiology" for additional pertinent history.

PHYSICAL EXAM
- Vital signs: When present, signs of hemodynamic instability are 1st tachycardia and tachypnea, then hypotension and thready pulse.
- Abdomen: Uterine tenderness, fundal height (increasing fundal height may be associated with placental abruption).
- Speculum: Visualize cervix, identify source of bleeding (from cervical os or from within vagina).
- Cervix: Assess for dilation; required to assess for labor, but should not be performed until placenta previa ruled out via ultrasound.
- Fetal monitoring: Doppler heart tones in early pregnancy; external fetal monitoring for gestational age >26 weeks.

DIFFERENTIAL DIAGNOSIS
- Hematuria (UTI, kidney stones)
- Rectal bleeding

DIAGNOSTIC TESTS & INTERPRETATION
Initial Tests (lab, imaging)
- CBC
- Blood type and screen; if significant hemorrhage, type and cross-match
- Quantitative β-human chorionic gonadotropin (β-hCG):
  - Prior to 12 weeks, levels can be followed serially every 2 days with following trends:
    - Doubles or at least 66% rise in 48 hours in normal pregnancy
    - Falls in spontaneous abortion
    - Extremely high in molar pregnancy
    - Rises gradually (<50% in 48 hours) or plateaus in ectopic pregnancy

- Transvaginal US should be used to confirm an intrauterine pregnancy (IUP) when the quantitative β-hCG >2,000 (1)[A].

- Other lab tests based on clinical scenario:
  - Wet mount, gonorrhea/chlamydia, Pap smear
  - Progesterone level occasionally used to determine viability in threatened abortion (<5 indicates not viable, >25 indicates viability, 5–25 is equivocal)
  - Bleeding time, fibrinogen, and fibrin split products: If suspect coagulopathy or abruption
  - Kleihauer-Betke: Low sensitivity and specificity for abruption; helpful for dosing Rho(d) immunoglobulin (RhoGAM)
- US is the preferred imaging modality:
  - Early pregnancy:
    - Gestational sac seen at 5–6 weeks; fetal heartbeat observed by 8–9 weeks
  - Diagnostic of ectopic with nearly 100% sensitivity when β-hCG level 1,500–2,000 mIU/mL. If no IUP is present and US does not confirm ectopic pregnancy, serial quantitative β-hCG values should be followed (2)[C]
  - Late pregnancy:

ALERT
Confirm fetal presentation and placental position prior to cervical exam.
- Proceed to rule out:
- Placenta previa with US
  - Labor with serial cervical exams
  - Abruption with external fetal monitoring
- Ultrasound is *not* used to diagnose or exclude placental abruption

TREATMENT

MEDICATION

First Line
- Treat underlying cause of bleeding, if identified.
- If mother is Rh negative, give RhoGAM to prevent autoimmunization. In late pregnancy, dose according to the amount of estimated fetomaternal hemorrhage.
- If cause of bleeding is preterm labor, consider betamethasone for fetal lung maturity if <34 weeks' gestation. Tocolytics may be used to prolong pregnancy to allow for course of steroids.
- If threatened abortion: Consider progesterone (relative risk 0.53) (3)[A].
- If mother has an inherited bleeding disorder or if bleeding is severe, consider recombinant or donor blood products.

SURGERY/OTHER PROCEDURES
- Cesarean section may be indicated for recurrent or uncontrolled bleeding with placenta or vasa previa.
- If ectopic is diagnosed, immediate surgical treatment may be needed. Some early ectopic pregnancies can be treated medically if certain criteria are met (2)[C].
- Surgical uterine evacuation is necessary for molar pregnancy due to malignant potential (4)[C].
- Incomplete or inevitable spontaneous abortion: Management is patient centered. In the absence of infection, patient may elect expectant, medical, or surgical management. If expectant management, typically wait 2 weeks for patient to complete abortion; most complete by 9 days. If at 2 weeks abortion is not completed or medical management has failed, surgical intervention (D&C or aspiration) is generally indicated. May send tissue to pathology to confirm (5)[A].

IN-PATIENT CONSIDERATIONS

Admission Criteria/Initial Stabilization
- In early pregnancy: Based on quantity of bleeding, need for surgical treatment for ectopic pregnancy, or presence of infection in case of spontaneous abortion.
- In late pregnancy, if significant bleeding and/or presence of maternal or fetal compromise.
- In late pregnancy with trauma, if ≥2 contractions/10 minutes.

Discharge Criteria
- In case of trauma in late pregnancy, may discharge home if normal fetal heart tracing for ≥4 hours with <2 contractions/10 minutes.
- In late pregnancy, may discharge when bleeding has stopped; labor, previa, and abruption have been ruled out; and fetal heart tracing is normal.

ONGOING CARE

PATIENT MONITORING
- Patient should be instructed to report any increase in the amount or frequency of bleeding and to seek immediate care if experiencing fever, abdominal pain, or sudden increased bleeding. Patient should save any tissue passed vaginally for examination.
- Frequency of outpatient follow-up as indicated based on etiology of bleeding.

PATIENT EDUCATION
- American Academy of Family Physicians (AAFP): www.familydoctor.org
- American College of Obstetricians & Gynecologists (ACOG): www.acog.org

PROGNOSIS
- Prognosis depends on the etiology of vaginal bleeding, severity of bleeding, and rapidity of diagnosis.
- Maternal mortality is 31.9 deaths/100,000 ectopic pregnancies.
- 1/2 of patients with early pregnancy bleeding miscarry. If fetal heart tones are present in 1st-trimester bleed, there is <10% chance of pregnancy loss.
- Heavy bleeding in early pregnancy, particularly when accompanied by pain, is associated with higher risk of spontaneous abortion. Spotting and light episodes are not, especially if lasting only 1–2 days.
- Subchorionic hemorrhage has about 2–3-fold increased risk of spontaneous abortion. Smaller hemorrhage and presence of viable fetal heart rate confer lower risk of loss. Most resolve spontaneously.
- Women with early pregnancy bleeding have an increased risk of preterm delivery, premature rupture of membranes, manual removal of placenta, placental abruption, elective cesarean delivery, and term labor induction later in the same pregnancy. These women also have an increased risk of adverse pregnancy outcomes, including hyperbilirubinemia, congenital anomalies, NICU admission, and reduced neonatal birth weight. Finally, there is an increased risk in subsequent pregnancies of recurrence of early pregnancy bleeding.
- Bed rest has not been shown to affect the outcome of bleeding in early pregnancy, but may be indicated for bleeding in late pregnancy with placenta or vasa previa or with maternal hypertension.

REFERENCES

1. Crochet JR, Bastien LA, Chireau MV. Does this woman have an ectopic pregnancy?: The rational clinical examination systematic review. *JAMA.* 2013;209:1722–1729.
2. Deutchman M, Tubay AT, Turok D, et al. First trimester bleeding. *Am Fam Physician.* 2009;79: 985–994.
3. Wahabi HA, Fayed AA, Esmaeil SA, et al. Progestogen for treating threatened miscarriage. *Cochrane Database Syst Rev.* 2011;12:CD005943.
4. Snell BJ. Assessment and management of bleeding in the first trimester of pregnancy. *J Midwifery Womens Health.* 2009;54:483–491.
5. Nanda K, Lopez LM, Grimes DA, et al. Expectant care versus surgical treatment for miscarriage. *Cochrane Database Syst Rev.* 2012;3:CD003518.

ADDITIONAL READING

- Chi C, Kadir RA et al. Inherited bleeding disorders in pregnancy. *Best Pract Res Clin Obstet Gynaecol.* 2012;26:103–117.
- Dadkhah F, Kashanian M, Eliasi G. A comparison between the pregnancy outcome in women both with or without threatened abortion. *Early Hum Dev.* 2010;86:193–196.
- Griebel CP, Halvorsen J, Golemon TB, et al. Management of spontaneous abortion. *Am Fam Physician.* 2005;72:1243–1250.
- Grimes DA. Estimation of pregnancy-related mortality risk by pregnancy outcome United States, 1991 to 1999. *Am J Obstet Gynecol.* 2006;194: 92–94.
- Hasan R, Baird DD, Herring AH, et al. Association between first-trimester vaginal bleeding and miscarriage. *Obstet Gynecol.* 2009;114:860–867.
- Lykke JA, Dideriksen KL, Lidegaard O, et al. First-trimester vaginal bleeding and complications later in pregnancy. *Obstet Gynecol.* 2010;115: 935–944.
- Magann EF, Cummings JE, Niederhauser A, et al. Antepartum bleeding of unknown origin in the second half of pregnancy: A review. *Obstet Gynecol Surv.* 2005;60:741–745.
- Mercier FJ, Van De Velde M. Major obstetric hemorrhage. *Anesthesiol Clin.* 2008;26:53–66.
- Mukul LV, Teal SB. Current management of ectopic pregnancy. *Obstet Gynecol Clin North Am.* 2007; 34:403–419.
- Oyelese Y, Ananth CV. Placental abruption. *Obstet Gynecol.* 2006;108:1005–1016.
- Publications Committee, Society for Maternal-Fetal Medicine, Belfort MA, et al. Placenta accrete. *Am J Obstet Gynecol.* 2010;203:430-439.
- Sakornbut E, Leeman L, Fontaine P. Late pregnancy bleeding. *Am Fam Physician.* 2007;75:1199–1206.
- Walfish M, Neuman A, Wlody D, et al. Maternal haemorrhage. *Br J Anaesth.* 2009;84(Suppl 1): i47–i56.
- Wijesiriwardana A, Bhattacharya S, Shetty A, et al. Obstetric outcome in women with threatened miscarriage in the first trimester. *Obstet Gynecol* 2006;107:557–562.

SEE ALSO

Abnormal Pap and Cervical Dysplasia; Abortion, Spontaneous (Miscarriage); Abruptio Placentae; Cervical Malignancy; Cervical Polyps; Cervicitis, Ectropion, and True Erosion; Chlamydial Sexually Transmitted Diseases; Ectopic Pregnancy; Placenta Previa; Preterm Labor; Trichomoniasis; Vaginal Malignancy

CODES

ICD10
- O20.0 Threatened abortion
- O20.9 Hemorrhage in early pregnancy, unspecified
- O46.91 Antepartum hemorrhage, unspecified, first trimester

CLINICAL PEARLS
- Obtain blood type and screen on all women presenting with vaginal bleeding in pregnancy and administer RhoGAM to all Rh-negative patients.
- For up to 50% of early pregnancy bleeding, no cause is ever found.
- Always consider ectopic pregnancy in 1st-trimester bleeding.
- Do not perform digital exam in late pregnancy bleeding until placenta has been located on US.

VAGINAL MALIGNANCY

Laura K. Randolph, DO, MS • Michael P. Hopkins, MD, MEd

 BASICS

DESCRIPTION
- Carcinomas of the vagina are uncommon: 3% of gynecologic malignancies (1)
- Vaginal intraepithelial neoplasia (VAIN), defined by squamous cell atypia, is classified by the depth of epithelial involvement:
  – VAIN 1: 1/3 thickness
  – VAIN 2: 2/3 thickness
  – VAIN 3 and carcinoma in situ (CIS): More than 2/3 with CIS, designating full thickness neoplastic changes without invasion through the basement membrane
- Invasive malignancies: Vaginal malignancies include squamous cell carcinoma (85–90%), adenocarcinoma (5–10%), sarcoma (2–3%), and melanoma (2–3%). Clear cell carcinoma is a subtype of adenocarcinoma. Invasive squamous cell carcinoma has the potential for metastasis to the lungs and liver.
- To be classified as a vaginal malignancy, only the vagina can be involved. If the cervix or vulva is involved, then the tumor is classified as a primary cancer arising from the cervix or the vulva.
- Most vaginal malignancies are metastatic (e.g., cervix, vulva, endometrium, breast, ovary).

Pregnancy Considerations
This malignancy is not associated with pregnancy.

EPIDEMIOLOGY
Incidence
- An estimated 2,890 new cases will be diagnosed in 2013 with 840 resulting deaths (1)
- Predominant age:
  – Carcinoma in situ: Mid-40s–60s
  – Invasive squamous cell malignancy: Mid-60s–70s
  – Adenocarcinoma: Any age; 50s is mean age. Peak incidence is between 17–21 years of age.
  – Clear cell adenocarcinoma occurs most often in females <30 with a history of exposure to diethylstilbestrol (DES) in utero.
  – Mixed müllerian sarcomas and leiomyosarcomas in the adult population: Mean age 60 years

Pediatric Considerations
Vaginal tumors are extremely rare. Rhabdomyosarcoma (botryoid and embryonal subtype) is the most common malignant neoplasm of the vagina. Less common entities are germ cell tumor and clear cell adenocarcinoma.

Prevalence
In the US, it is 1 of the rarest of all gynecologic malignancies (3%).

ETIOLOGY AND PATHOPHYSIOLOGY
- Women with a history of cervical malignancy have a higher probability of developing squamous cell malignancy in the vagina even after hysterectomy.
- Human papillomavirus (HPV) is found in 80–93% of patients with vaginal CIS and 50–65% of the patients with invasive vaginal carcinoma (2,3).
- HPV-16 is the most common, found in 66% of CIS and 55% of invasive vaginal cancers (3)
- Smokers have a higher incidence.
- Clear cell adenocarcinoma of the vagina in young women has been associated with DES exposure. The incidence, however, is exceedingly rare, estimated at 1/1,000–1/10,000 exposed females.

- Metastatic lesions can involve the vagina, spreading from the other gynecologic organs.
- Although rare, renal cell carcinoma, lung adenocarcinoma, GI cancer, pancreatic adenocarcinoma, ovarian germ cell cancer, trophoblastic neoplasm, and breast cancer can all metastasize to the vagina.

Genetics
No known genetic pattern

RISK FACTORS
- Similar risk factors as cervical cancer
- Age
- African American
- Smoking
- Multiple sex partners, early age of 1st sexual intercourse
- History of squamous cell cancer of the cervix or vulva
- HPV infection
- Vaginal adenosis
- Vaginal irritation
- DES exposure in utero

COMMONLY ASSOCIATED CONDITIONS
Due to the field effect, patients with vaginal cancer are more likely to develop malignancy in the cervix or vulva and should be followed closely.

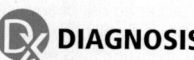 **DIAGNOSIS**

HISTORY
- Abnormal bleeding is the most common symptom.
- Postcoital bleeding can result from direct trauma to the tumor.
- Vaginal discharge
- Dyspareunia
- Urinary symptoms, including hematuria and increased frequency
- Constipation
- Pain along with symptoms and signs of hydroureter are late findings when the tumor has spread into the paravaginal tissues and extends to the pelvic sidewall.

Pediatric Considerations
In children, sarcomas can present either as a mass protruding from the vagina or as abnormal genital bleeding.

PHYSICAL EXAM
Pelvic examination:
- The vagina, uterus, adnexa (fallopian tubes and ovaries), bladder, and rectum should be evaluated for unusual changes.
- Vaginal malignancies are found most commonly on the posterior wall in the upper 1/3 of the vagina.

DIFFERENTIAL DIAGNOSIS
- Premalignant changes: VAIN 1, 2, 3, and CIS
- Adequate biopsies ensure that invasive lesions are not overlooked. Invasive lesions penetrate the basement membrane and cannot be treated conservatively.
- Other malignancies, such as endometrial, cervix, bladder, or colon cancer, can invade directly into the vagina or metastasize to the vagina.

- In the child-bearing years, trophoblastic disease should be considered:
  – The vagina is a common site of metastases, however, biopsy should typically be avoided because the implants are very vascular and may hemorrhage if sampled.
  – The clinical presentation is typically obvious so histopathologic confirmation before treatment is not required.

DIAGNOSTIC TESTS & INTERPRETATION
Initial Tests (lab, imaging)
- Pap smear may incidentally detect asymptomatic lesions.
- Biopsy suspicious lesions.
- Chest x-ray (CXR): To evaluate for metastatic disease
- IV pyelogram (IVP) to evaluate for ureteral obstruction
- CT scan and MRI to evaluate the liver and retroperitoneum, especially the lymph nodes in the pelvic and periaortic area
- Barium enema to rule out rectal invasion
- PET scan detects primary and secondary metastatic lesions more often than CT scan.

ALERT
PET scan correlation with CT scan lesions strongly suggests malignancy.

Follow-Up Tests & Special Considerations
- Lymphoscintigraphy as part of the pretreatment evaluation: Can result in a change in the radiation fields and improve comprehensive treatment planning in women with vaginal cancer.
- HPV vaccination: Implementation of prophylactic HPV vaccination could prevent ~2/3 of the intraepithelial lesions in the lower genital tract, but as yet unproven.

Diagnostic Procedures/Other
- Colposcopy with directed biopsies for small lesions
- Wide excision under anesthesia of superficial disease may be necessary to ensure that invasive cancer is not present.
- Cystoscopy to rule out bladder invasion
- Sigmoidoscopy to rule out rectal invasion

Test Interpretation
Tumors are staged clinically:
- Stage 0: VAIN and CIS
- Stage I: Carcinoma limited to the vaginal wall (26%)
- Stage II: Involves the subvaginal tissues but has not extended to the pelvic wall (37%)
- Stage III: Extends to the pelvic wall (24%)
- Stage IV: Extends beyond the true pelvis (13%)
  – IVa: Tumor invades bladder and/or rectal mucosa and/or direct extension beyond the true pelvis
  – IVb: Spread to distant organs

 TREATMENT

GENERAL MEASURES
Treatment methods for VAIN and CIS include:
- Wide local excision
- Partial or total vaginectomy
- Intravaginal chemotherapy with 5% fluorouracil cream
- Laser therapy
- Intracavitary radiation therapy

MEDICATION

- Imiquimod:
  - In a review of the effectiveness of 5% imiquimod cream in the treatment of vaginal intraepithelial neoplasia, the following results were reported (4)[C]:
    - 26–100% of patients had complete regression
    - 0–60% of patients had partial regression
    - 0–37% experienced recurrence
- Contraindications:
  - The diagnosis must be established with certainty prior to treatment.
  - If there is any doubt that a process beyond in situ disease exists, vaginectomy must be performed. These patients are often elderly, and aggressive therapy is limited by the patient's performance status and ability to tolerate radical surgery, chemotherapy, or radiation.

ISSUES FOR REFERRAL

Patients should be treated by a gynecologic oncologist and/or a radiation oncologist.

ADDITIONAL THERAPIES

- Treatment with radiotherapy depends on the stage of disease. This treatment option should be discussed with physicians experienced with this malignancy.
- It is common to use radiotherapy and chemotherapy (chemoradiation) for better cancer control.
- Early-stage primary squamous cell carcinoma treated with radiation alone has shown good results (5)[A].
- Stage III vaginal cancer may benefit from combined radiation and hyperthermia (6)[C].
- Patients with advanced squamous cell carcinoma or adenocarcinoma receive concurrent irradiation and cisplatin-based chemotherapy (7)[B].
- Neoadjuvant chemotherapy followed by radical surgery may benefit select patients (8)[C].
- In most tumor types, metastatic disease from the vagina to other sites is only minimally responsive to chemotherapy.
- With 1 exception, no chemotherapeutic agents have shown a survival advantage. The exception is childhood sarcomas, which have been treated with combinations of:
  - Vincristine
  - Dactinomycin (actinomycin-D)
  - Cyclophosphamide (Cytoxan)
  - Cisplatin
  - Etoposide (VP-16)

SURGERY/OTHER PROCEDURES

- Whenever there is a doubt as to the presence or absence of invasive disease, vaginectomy must be performed.
- Invasive lesions usually are treated by radiation therapy, but stage I lesions can be treated with radical hysterectomy or radical vaginectomy with pelvic lymph node dissection (9)[A].
- If the lesion involves the lower vagina, inguinal node dissection also must be done because cancer involving the lower vagina can metastasize to the groin region.
- Premenopausal women who desire to retain ovarian function are better candidates for radical surgery for early-stage disease, with vaginal reconstruction possible afterward.

- Patients who have not completed their family occasionally can be treated with limited resection and localized radiation to the area.
- Sarcomas are treated by radiation therapy followed by pelvic exenteration if persistent disease is present.

Pediatric Considerations

The treatment of vaginal tumors today mainly consists of neoadjuvant chemotherapy followed by local control with surgery or radiotherapy.

Geriatric Considerations

Older patients, many with a long history of smoking, are at a higher risk for malignancies requiring surgical treatments.

ONGOING CARE

FOLLOW-UP RECOMMENDATIONS

- Patients are usually ambulatory and able to resume full activity by 6 weeks after surgery.
- Most patients are fully active while receiving chemotherapy and radiation therapy.

Patient Monitoring

- Pelvic examination and Pap smear every 3 months for 2 years, then every 6 months for the next 3 years, and then yearly thereafter
- Annual CXR

PATIENT EDUCATION

- Printed patient information available from American College of Obstetricians and Gynecologists, 409 12th St., SW, Washington, DC 20024-2188; 800-762-ACOG; www.acog.org
- American Cancer Society: www.cancer.gov
- Medline Plus: www.nlm.nih.gov/medlineplus/vaginalcancer.html

PROGNOSIS

Stage and 5-year survival (10):
- I: 77.6%
- II: 52.2%
- III: 42.5%
- IVA: 20.5%
- IVB: 12.9%

COMPLICATIONS

- Those typically associated with major abdominal surgery or radiation therapy
- Common complications of treatment include rectovaginal or vesicovaginal fistulas, rectal/vaginal strictures, radiation cystitis, and/or proctitis.

REFERENCES

1. Siegel R, Naishadham D, Jemal A. Cancer statistics. *CA Cancer J Clin.* 2013;63:11.
2. Daling J, Madeleine MM, Schwartz SM, et al. A population-based study of squamous cell vaginal cancer: HPV and cofactors. *Gynecol Oncol.* 2002;97:1816.
3. Smith J, Backes D, Hoots B, et al. Human papillomavirus type-distribution in vulvar and vaginal cancers and their associated precursors. *Obstet Gynecol.* 2009;113:917–924.
4. Iavazzo C, Pitsouni E, Athanasiou S, et al. Imiquimod for treatment of vulvar and vaginal intraepithelial neoplasia. *Int J Gynaecol Obstet.* 2008;101:3–10.
5. Tran PT, Su Z, Lee P, et al. Prognostic factors for outcomes and complications for primary squamous cell carcinoma of the vagina treated with radiation. *Gynecol Oncol.* 2007;105:641–649.
6. Franckena M, van der Zee J. Use of combined radiation and hyperthermia for gynecological cancer. *Curr Opin Obstet Gynecol.* 2010;22:9–14.
7. Dalrymple JL, Russell AH, Lee SW, et al. Chemoradiation for primary invasive squamous carcinoma of the vagina. *Int J Gynecol Cancer.* 2004;14:110–117.
8. Benedetti Panici P, Bellati F, Plotti F, et al. Neoadjuvant chemotherapy followed by radical surgery in patients affected by vaginal carcinoma. *Gynecol Oncol.* 2008;111:307–311.
9. Tjalma WA, Monaghan JM, de Barros Lopes A, et al. The role of surgery in invasive squamous carcinoma of the vagina. *Gynecol Oncol.* 2001;81:360–365.
10. Beller U, Benedet J, Creasman W, et al. Carcinoma of the vagina. FIGO 26th annual report on the results of treatment in gynecological cancer. *Int J Gynaecol Obstet.* 2006;95:S29–S42.

ADDITIONAL READING

- Creasman WT. Vaginal cancers. *Curr Opin Obstet Gynecol.* 2005;17:71–76.
- Fernandez-Pineda I, Spunt SL, Parida L, et al. Vaginal tumors in childhood: The experience of St. Jude Children's Research Hospital. *J Pediatr Surg.* 2011;46:2071–2075.
- Frumovitz M, Gayed IW, Jhingran A, et al. Lymphatic mapping and sentinel lymph node detection in women with vaginal cancer. *Gynecol Oncol.* 2008;108:478–481.
- Gray HJ. Advances in vulvar and vaginal cancer treatment. *Gynecol Oncol.* 2010;118:3–5.
- Hampl M, Sarajuuri H, Wentzensen N, et al. Effect of human papillomavirus vaccines on vulvar, vaginal, and anal intraepithelial lesions and vulvar cancer. *Obstet Gynecol.* 2006;108:1361–1368.

SEE ALSO

Algorithm: Metrorrhagia (Intermenstrual Bleeding)

CODES

ICD10

- C52 Malignant neoplasm of vagina
- D07.2 Carcinoma in situ of vagina
- N89.3 Dysplasia of vagina, unspecified

CLINICAL PEARLS

- Vaginal cancer is rare; 85–90% of vaginal cancers are squamous cell.
- Vaginal malignancies are found most commonly on the posterior wall in the upper 1/3 of the vagina.
- Most vaginal malignancies are metastatic (from cervix, vulva, endometrium, breast, or ovary).

VAGINITIS AND VAGINOSIS

Rachel Sneed, MD • Bita Haji Zadeh, MD

BASICS

DESCRIPTION
- Vulvovaginal candidiasis (VVC): Inflammation of the vagina and vulva caused by infection with *Candida* species.
- Bacterial vaginosis (BV): A polymicrobial syndrome in which the hydrogen peroxide–producing lactobacilli normally found in the vagina are replaced by other bacteria. VVC and BV are not generally considered STIs.
- Desquamative vaginitis (DV): A rare inflammatory vaginitis of unknown etiology.
- Other causes of vaginitis include allergic and contact dermatitis from feminine hygiene products (fragrances, creams, douches, lubricants, and their preservatives). Atrophic vaginitis is caused by estrogen deficiency.
- A number of dermatoses, such as lichen planus, lichen sclerosus, and psoriasis, may mimic vaginitis symptoms.
- System(s) affected: Reproductive; Skin/Exocrine
- Synonym(s): VVC: Monilial vulvovaginitis; Vaginal yeast infection; BV: *Gardnerella* vaginosis; Nonspecific vaginitis; *Haemophilus* vaginitis; *Corynebacterium* vaginitis

EPIDEMIOLOGY
- Both VVC and BV are common among reproductive-age females, whereas DV is more common in postmenopausal women
- Most cases of VVC are related to *Candia albicans*, but may be caused by other *Candida* sp. (e.g., *C. glabrata* and *C. krusei*)

Prevalence
- VVC: 2nd most common cause of vaginitis after BV:
  - 75% of women diagnosed at least once with VVC; up to 45% diagnosed more than once
  - <5% of females are diagnosed with recurrent VVC (defined as ≥4 episodes of VVC in 1 year).
  - Studies have shown that up to 72% of females may be colonized with *Candida* but do not exhibit symptoms of vaginitis.
- BV: Prevalence varies based on age, race/ethnicity, and socioeconomic status:
  - Most common vaginal infection among reproductive-aged women
  - The National Health and Nutrition Examination Survey (NHANES) data reported an overall prevalence of 29%, with the highest rates (50%) among black women.

Pediatric Considerations
VVC and BV are less common before the onset of puberty and after menopause.

ETIOLOGY AND PATHOPHYSIOLOGY
- VVC: Overgrowth of yeast in the vagina
- BV: Shift from a healthy lactobacilli-based endogenous flora to an anaerobically based endogenous flora, including *Gardnerella vaginalis*, *Mobiluncus* sp., *Mycoplasma hominis*, *Peptostreptococcus*, *Prevotella*, *Bacteroides*, and *Atopobium vaginae*; the rectum may be a reservoir of organisms leading to autoinfection.
- Aerobic vaginitis has been described in which lactobacilli are decreased in number and aerobic organisms including *Escherichia coli*, group B streptococci, and *Staphylococcus aureus* predominate (1).

- Newer data suggest that BV in not a single entity; at least 4 different microbiologic profiles have been identified (2).

RISK FACTORS
- VVC: Diabetes mellitus (DM) with poor glycemic control, antibiotic therapy, immunosuppression (e.g., corticosteroid therapy, HIV infection), high-estrogen states (e.g., pregnancy, oral contraceptive use, hormone-replacement therapy); *C. albicans* accounts for 85–90% of vaginitis cases in pregnancy.
- BV: Black race, lower socioeconomic status, smoking, new or multiple sex partner(s), female sex partners, spermicide use, vaginal douching

GENERAL PREVENTION
- Vulvar hygiene (see "General Measures"); avoid implicated feminine hygiene products
- Maintenance therapy for recurrent cases
- Treatment of sexual partners generally is not recommended, but may be considered in recurrent cases.

COMMONLY ASSOCIATED CONDITIONS
- STIs
- Balanitis may rarely occur among male partners of females with VVC.
- Research is limited in same-sex partners. Symptomatic partners should be evaluated.

DIAGNOSIS

HISTORY
- VVC: Vaginal and vulvar pruritus, vulvar pain, external dysuria, and dyspareunia; thick, curd-like vaginal discharge
- BV: 50% of women are asymptomatic. Unpleasant musty or fishy vaginal odor, exacerbated by intercourse. 10–30% may have vaginal/vulvar irritation; thin gray–white or frothy vaginal discharge
- DV: vaginal pain or burning with yellow to gray discharge, and pruritus

PHYSICAL EXAM
- VVC: Thick, curd-like vaginal discharge; vulvar erythema and edema; vulvar fissures and excoriations; normal vaginal pH (<4.5)
- BV: 10–30% may have vaginal/vulvar irritation. Thin gray–white vaginal discharge is mildly adherent to vaginal walls; 10% have frothy discharge; pH >4.5
- DV: Diffuse exudative vaginitis with epithelial exfoliation without vulvar or perineal disease; pH >4.5

DIFFERENTIAL DIAGNOSIS
- Physiologic discharge and cervical ectropion
- Trichomoniasis
- Contact dermatitis
- Mechanical/Chemical irritation
- Cervicitis (chlamydial or gonococcal)
- Urinary tract infection (UTI)
- Atrophic vaginitis
- Dermatoses: Lichen sclerosus, lichen planus, seborrheic dermatitis, psoriasis

DIAGNOSTIC TESTS & INTERPRETATION
- Wet mount: Prepare 2 slides, both with fresh vaginal discharge: 1 with sodium chloride (NaCl) and 1 with 10% potassium hydroxide (KOH):
  - The presence of budding yeasts and hyphae consistent with VVC (may be more easily seen on KOH prep)
  - Clue cells: At least 20% of total epithelial cells considered clinically significant for diagnosis of BV (saline)
  - WBCs are not numerous in BV but may be present in large numbers in candidiasis.
  - Increased parabasal and inflammatory cells indicative of DV
- Amsel's diagnostic criteria for BV (need 3 out of 4): Clue cells, characteristic vaginal discharge, vaginal pH >4.5, and positive "whiff test" (transient but potent amine or fishy odor with the addition of 10% KOH); vaginal pH also may suggest need for testing for *Trichomonas*. In cases of aerobic vaginitis, clue cells may be <20%.
- Diagnosis of DV requires all of the following: symptoms (discharge, dyspareunia, pruritus, burning, or irritation), vaginal inflammation, pH >4.5, and appropriate wet prep findings.
- Consider vaginal culture for VVC when characteristic symptoms are present, vaginal pH is normal, and no yeast are present on wet mount or to identify species if no improvement with treatment or relapse occurs within 2 months.
- Positive culture for *Candida* sp. or other yeast species may only indicate colonization; clinical correlation is required.
- VVC or BV: May be noted on cytology but must be correlated with clinical symptoms; asymptomatic women generally do not need treatment.
- DNA probe–based tests are available (Affirm VP III, Becton Dickinson, Sparks, MD), but it is unclear whether identification of the presence of yeast (or low numbers of *G. vaginalis*) indicates that the organism is the cause of symptoms. Use may not be cost-effective.
- Over-the-counter tests are available that may suggest the diagnosis of BV or VVC (3).

TREATMENT

GENERAL MEASURES
- Avoid douching, use of panty liners, pantyhose, occlusive pants, and undergarments.
- Regular use of condoms may help to prevent BV, as exposure to semen may trigger symptoms for some women.

MEDICATION
First Line
- VVC (4):
  - Fluconazole 150 mg PO once; use with caution in patients with liver disease and with coadministration of other drugs (2)[C]
    - Short-course therapy with topical azoles is effective in 80–90% of patients.
  - Many topical therapies are available over the counter:
    - Butoconazole 2% cream 5 g intravaginally × 3 days
    - Clotrimazole 1% cream 5 g intravaginally × 7–14 days *or* 2% cream 5 g intravaginally × 3 days (2)[C]

○ Miconazole 2% cream 5 g intravaginally ×
7 days; *or* 4% cream 5 g intravaginally × 3 days;
or 100 mg vaginal suppository, 1 suppository ×
7 days; *or* 200 mg vaginal suppository,
1 suppository × 3 days; *or* 1,200 mg vaginal
suppository, 1 suppository × 1 day (2)[C]

○ Tioconazole 6.5% ointment 5 g intravaginally in
a single application

– Prescription therapies include:

○ Butoconazole 2% cream (single-dose
bioadhesive) 5 g intravaginally × single
application

○ Nystatin 100,000-unit vaginal tablet, 1 tablet ×
14 days

○ Terconazole 0.4% cream 5 g intravaginally ×
7 days; *or* 0.8% cream 5 g intravaginally ×
3 days; *or* 80 mg vaginal suppository,
1 suppository × 3 days

• BV (4):

– Metronidazole (Flagyl) 500 mg PO b.i.d. ×
7 days (1)[A] *or*

– Metronidazole 0.075% vaginal gel 5 g
intravaginally daily × 5 days.

○ 85–90% of women respond to initial treatment;
however, recurrence rates may be as high as
80%.

– Clindamycin 300 mg PO b.i.d. × 7 days (1)[A]

○ Antibiotic resistance against clindamycin and
metronidazole has been reported and may be
responsible for some cases of recurrent BV (1).

• DV (5):

– Clindamycin 2% vaginal gel 4–5 gm daily ×
4–6 weeks (2)[C]

– Hydrocortisone 10% 3–5 gm daily × 4–6 weeks
(2)[C]

ALERT
Oil-based preparations may weaken latex condoms.

Second Line

• VVC:

– Recurrent VVC: Obtain cultures. Infections
associated with *C. glabrata* (5–15%) are less
responsive to first-line therapies (6).

– Consider longer duration therapy (7–14 days of
topical or oral fluconazole every 3rd day for a total
of 3 doses) (2)[C]

– Suppressive maintenance therapy (oral
fluconazole weekly × 6 months or topical
treatments weekly) (7)[B]

– Women with recurrent candidiasis may benefit
from fluconazole 150 mg/wk plus cetirizine
10 mg/d for allergy or itching.

– Boric acid: 600 mg gelatin capsule inserted
vaginally daily × 2 weeks (indicated for
non-*Albicans* disease; 70% clinical and mycologic
cure rate) (6)[C]

• BV:

– Metronidazole 2 g PO single dose (less effective
than alternative regimens)

– Clindamycin 300 mg PO daily × 7 days

– Clindamycin ovules 100 g intravaginally at
bedtime × 3 days

– Tinidazole 2 g PO daily for 2 days or 1 g PO once
daily for 5 days are options for patients who do
not tolerate metronidazole or have difficulty with
compliance.

– Regimens for treating recurrent BV involve use of
metronidazole PO × 7 days and vaginal boric
acid 600 mg × 21 days. (2)[B]

ALERT
Avoid any alcohol-containing product while taking
metronidazole.

Pregnancy Considerations
• VVC: Topical therapy preferred over oral therapy
• BV: Associated with preterm delivery; however, it is
unclear whether the treatment of BV prevents
preterm delivery. All symptomatic women should be
treated; screening is reserved for women at high risk
for preterm delivery. Avoid creams; metronidazole
500 mg PO b.i.d. × 7 days or clindamycin 300 mg
PO b.i.d. × 7 days. Package labeling of
metronidazole indicates that it is contraindicated in
the 1st trimester of pregnancy, but this is not
supported by recent meta-analyses of available data.

ISSUES FOR REFERRAL
Treating male sexual partners does not reduce
symptoms or prevent recurrence, but this may be
considered in patients who have recurrent infection.

COMPLEMENTARY AND ALTERNATIVE
MEDICINE
• A Cochrane analysis reviewed the use of probiotics
for BV and found inconclusive evidence to
recommend probiotics as primary treatment or as a
preventive strategy. Further study was
recommended (8)[A]

• Acidification of the vagina has not been proven
beneficial.

 ## ONGOING CARE

FOLLOW-UP RECOMMENDATIONS
• Delay sexual relations until symptoms
clear/discomfort resolves
• Use of condoms may reduce recurrence of BV

Patient Monitoring
• Generally, no specific follow-up needed; if symptoms
persist or recur within 2 months, repeat pelvic exam
and culture.
• Consider suppressive therapy for women with
recurrent infection.

DIET
Reduction of sugar intake has been recommended but
is not supported by evidence.

PATIENT EDUCATION
• American College of Obstetricians and Gynecologists
(ACOG), 409 12th St., SW, Washington, DC
20024-2188; 800-762-ACOG; www.acog.org
• American Academy of Family Physicians:
www.familydoctor.org

PROGNOSIS
VVC: 80–90% of uncomplicated cases cured with
appropriate treatment; 30–50% of recurrent
infections return after discontinuation of maintenance
therapy; there is a relatively high spontaneous
remission rate of untreated symptoms as well.

COMPLICATIONS
• VVC may occur following treatment of BV.
• BV has been associated with an increased risk of
acquisition and transmission of STIs, including HIV.
• BV has been associated with increased risk of
pregnancy complications, including preterm birth,
chorioamnionitis, postpartum and postabortal
endometritis, and pelvic inflammatory disease.

REFERENCES

1. Donders G. Diagnosis and management of bacterial
vaginosis and other types of abnormal vaginal
bacterial flora: A review. *Obstet Gynecol Surv.*
2010;65:462–473.
2. Li J, McCormick J, Bocking A, et al. Importance of
vaginal microbes in reproductive health. *Reprod
Sci.* 2012;19:235–242.
3. Hainer BL, Gibson MV. *Vaginitis. Am Fam
Physician.* 2011;83:807–815.
4. Workowski KA, Berman S, Centers for Disease
Control and Prevention (CDC), et al. Sexually
transmitted diseases treatment guidelines, 2010.
MMWR Recomm Rep. 2010;59:1–110.
5. Sobel JD, Reichman O, Misra D, et al. Prognosis
and treatment of desquamative inflammatory
vaginitis. *Obstet Gynecol.* 2011;117:850–855.
6. Ray D, Goswami R, Banerjee U, et al. Prevalence of
Candida glabrata and its response to boric acid
vaginal suppositories in comparison with oral
fluconazole in patients with diabetes and
vulvovaginal candidiasis. *Diabetes Care.* 2007;30:
312–317.
7. Pappas PG, Kauffman CA, Andes D, et al. Clinical
practice guidelines for the management of
candidiasis: 2009 update by the Infectious Disease
Society of America. *Clin Infect Dis.* 2009;48:
503–535.
8. Senok AC, Verstraelen H, Temmerman M, et al.
Probiotics for the treatment of bacterial vaginosis.
Cochrane Database Syst Rev. 2009;4:CD006289.

ADDITIONAL READING
American Congress of Obstetricians and Gynecologists
(ACOG) FAQ028, Aug. 2011. Available at:
www.acog.org/~/media/For%20Patients/
faq028.pdf?dmc=1&ts=20131111T1039456914

 ## SEE ALSO

Algorithm: Discharge, Vaginal

 ## CODES

ICD10
• B37.3 Candidiasis of vulva and vagina
• N76.0 Acute vaginitis
• N95.2 Postmenopausal atrophic vaginitis

CLINICAL PEARLS
• Clinical symptoms, signs, and microscopy have
relatively poor performance compared with so-called
gold standards such as culture and DNA probe
assays, but these more sensitive assays can detect
organisms that may not be causing symptoms.
• Most women experience relief of symptoms with
therapy chosen without such gold standard tests,
even when the treatment does not correspond with
the underlying infection.
• Vaginal pH is underused as a diagnostic tool for
evaluation of vaginitis.
• Treatment of sexual partners is not currently the
standard of care for either BV or VVC.

VARICOSE VEINS

Joseph A. Florence, MD • Thomas R. Avonda, MD

 BASICS

DESCRIPTION
- Superficial venous disease causing a permanent dilatation and tortuosity of superficial veins, usually occurring in the legs and feet; caused by systemic weakness in the vein wall, and may result from congenitally incomplete valves or valves that have become incompetent
- Affects legs where reverse flow occurs when dependent
- Truncal varices involve the great and small saphenous veins; branch varicosities involve the saphenous vein tributaries.
- Categorized as (1):
  - Uncomplicated (cosmetic)
  - With local symptoms (pain confined to the varices, not diffuse)
  - With local complications (superficial thrombophlebitis, may rupture causing bleeding)
  - Complex varicose disease (diffuse limb pain, swelling, skin changes/ulcer)
- System(s) affected: Cardiovascular; Skin

ALERT
Ulceration of varicose veins has a high rate of infection, which can lead to sepsis.

Geriatric Considerations
- Common; usually valvular degeneration, but may be secondary to chronic venous deficiency
- Elastic support hose and frequent rests with legs elevated rather than ligation and stripping

Pregnancy Considerations
- Frequent problem
- Elastic stockings are recommended for those with a history of varicosities or if a great deal of standing is involved.

EPIDEMIOLOGY
Incidence
- Predominant age: Middle age
- Predominant gender: Female > Male (2:1) (2)
- National Women's Health Information Center estimates that 50% of women have varicose veins.

ETIOLOGY AND PATHOPHYSIOLOGY
- Varicose veins are caused by venous insufficiency from faulty valves in ≥1 perforator veins in the lower leg, causing secondary incompetence at the saphenofemoral junction (valvular reflux).
- Valvular dysfunction causing venous reflux and subsequently venous hypertension (HTN)
- Failed valves allow blood to flow in the reverse direction (away from the heart), from deep to superficial and from proximal to distal veins.
- Deep thrombophlebitis
- Increased venous pressure from any cause
- Congenital valvular incompetence
- Trauma (consider arteriovenous fistula; listen for bruit)
- Presumed to be due to a loss in vein wall elasticity with failure of the valve leaflets

Genetics
Autosomal-dominant with incomplete penetrance (3)

RISK FACTORS
- Increasing age (4)
- Pregnancy, especially multiple pregnancies
- Occupations that require prolonged standing, restrictive clothing (e.g., very tight girdles)
- Obesity
- History of phlebitis (postthrombotic syndrome)
- Family history
- Female sex
- Increased height
- Congenital valvular dysfunction

COMMONLY ASSOCIATED CONDITIONS
- Stasis dermatitis
- Large varicose veins may lead to skin changes and eventual stasis ulceration.

 DIAGNOSIS

HISTORY
- Symptoms range from minor annoyance/cosmetic problem to a lifestyle-limiting problem.
- Localized symptoms: Pain, burning, itching
- Generalized symptoms:
  - Leg muscular cramp, aching
  - Leg fatigue/swelling
- Pain if varicose ulcer develops
- Symptoms often worse at the end of the day, especially after prolonged standing
- Women are more prone to symptoms due to hormonal influences: Worse during menses
- No direct correlation with the severity of varicose veins and the severity of symptoms

PHYSICAL EXAM
- Inspect lower extremities while the patient is standing. Varicose veins in the proximal femoral ring and distal portion of the legs may not be visible when the patient is supine.
- Varicose veins are:
  - Dilated, tortuous, superficial veins, chiefly in the lower extremities
  - Dark purple/blue in color, raised above the surface of the skin
  - Often twisted, bulging, and can look like cords
  - Most commonly found on the posterior/medial lower extremity
- Edema of the affected limb may be present
- Skin changes may include:
  - Eczema
  - Hyperpigmentation
  - Lipodermatosclerosis
- Spider veins (idiopathic telangiectases):
  - Fine intracutaneous angiectasis
  - May be extensive/unsightly
- Neurologic sensory and motor exam:
- Peripheral arterial vasculature; pulses
- Musculoskeletal exam for associated rheumatologic/orthopedic issues

DIFFERENTIAL DIAGNOSIS
- Nerve root compression
- Arthritis
- Peripheral neuritis
- Telangiectasia: Smaller, visible blood vessels that are permanently dilated
- Deep vein thrombosis
- Inflammatory liposclerosis

DIAGNOSTIC TESTS & INTERPRETATION
Duplex ultrasound: Formal noninvasive imaging of the venous system with duplex ultrasound will confirm the etiology, anatomy, and pathophysiology of segmental venous reflux.

Diagnostic Procedures/Other
- Tourniquet tests (Trendelenburg test for varicose veins, Perthes test for assessing the patency of the deep femoral veins) have been replaced by ultrasound techniques for assessing varicose veins before treatment.
- Duplex scanning, venous Doppler study, photoplethysmography, light-reflection rheography, air plethysmography, and other vascular testing should be reserved for patients who have venous symptoms and/or large (>4 mm in diameter) vessels or large numbers of spider telangiectasia indicating venous HTN.

Test Interpretation
- Varicose veins are classified using the CEAP system (Class, Etiology, Anatomy, and Pathophysiology): Not often used in general clinical practice but valuable in comparative clinical trials (5)
- A clinical classification illustrating the current physical state is useful in clinical practice (4)[C]:
  - 0: No visible or palpable signs of venous disease
  - 1: Spider veins or telangiectasias
  - 2: Varicose veins
  - 3: Edema
  - 4: Skin changes (pigmentation, eczema, lipodermatosclerosis, atrophie blanche)
  - 5: Healed ulcer
  - 6: Active ulcer

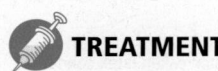 **TREATMENT**

- Ambulatory, conservative, hemodynamic management of varicose veins is more effective than stripping with clinical marking or stripping with duplex marking to treat varicose veins (6)[B].
- Conservative therapy (e.g., elevation, external compression, weight loss) may be helpful (7)[A]
- When comparing quality of life, pain relief, and long-term relief, surgery is favored (5)[A]
- Endovenous laser ablation, radiofrequency ablation, foam sclerotherapy, and surgical stripping for great saphenous varicose veins are all efficacious (8)[A].
- Long-term safety and efficacy of surgery for varicose veins is supported by low-quality evidence; short-term studies support the efficacy of less-invasive treatments that are associated with less periprocedural disability and pain (6)[A].
- Endovenous ablation (radiofrequency and laser) is at least as effective as surgery in the treatment of great saphenous varicose veins; however, ultrasound-guided foam sclerotherapy has insufficient support from available data (8)[A].
- Technical failure rate is highest after foam sclerotherapy; both radiofrequency ablation and foam are associated with faster recovery and less postoperative pain than endovenous laser ablation and stripping.

GENERAL MEASURES
Patients with unsightly varicose veins often seek treatment for cosmetic reasons.

MEDICATION
Superficial thrombophlebitis is not an infective condition and does not require antibiotic treatment.

ISSUES FOR REFERRAL
- Emergency: Bleeding from a varicosity that has eroded the skin
- Urgent: Varicosity that has bled and is at risk for bleeding again
- Soon: Ulcer that is progressive/painful despite treatment
- Routine:
  - Active/healed ulcer/progressive skin changes that may benefit from surgery
  - Recurrent superficial thrombophlebitis
  - Troublesome symptoms attributable to varicose veins, or patient and provider feel that the extent, site, and size of the varicosities are having a severe impact on quality of life

ADDITIONAL THERAPIES
- Apply elastic stockings before lowering legs from the bed
- Activity:
  - Frequent rest periods with legs elevated
  - If standing is necessary, frequently shift weight from side to side.
  - Appropriate exercise routine as part of conservative treatment
  - Walking regimen after sclerotherapy is important to help promote healing.
  - Never sit with legs hanging down.
- Physical therapy

SURGERY/OTHER PROCEDURES
- Surgery:
  - Improved quality-adjusted life-years and symptoms compared to conservative management at 2 years (4)[A]
  - Surgery is indicated if there is pain, recurrent phlebitis, or skin changes/ulceration, or for cosmetic improvement for severe cases.
  - Minimally invasive techniques include:
    - Radiofrequency ablation (RFA): Compared with surgery provides a faster return to work; less pain, better short-term quality of life; less bruising and tenderness compared with endovenous laser therapy (4)[A]
    - Endovenous laser ablation (EVLA) therapy: Produced the same clinical benefits as conventional surgery but was more effective in addressing the underlying pathophysiology and was associated with less periprocedural morbidity and faster recovery (9)[A]
    - Transilluminated power phlebectomy
  - Traditional surgical methods include:
    - Ligation and stripping of the varicose vein
    - Stab avulsion phlebectomy
  - Surgical treatment of clinically symptomatic varicose veins involves treatment of the saphenous vein reflux as well as the varicosities.
- Sclerotherapy:
  - Randomized, controlled trials suggest that the choice of sclerosant, dose, formulation (foam vs. liquid), local pressure dressing, and degree and length of compression has no significant effect on the efficacy of sclerotherapy (8)[A].
  - Sclerosing solution is injected into varicosities, causing vein walls to swell, adhere, and scar; 50–90% improvement can be expected.

- Radiotherapy:
  - RFA takes longer to perform, but a has better early outcome than conventional surgery in patients with great saphenous varicose veins.
  - Radiofrequency and laser treatments replace "stripping"; however, most varicosities still require phlebectomy/sclerotherapy.

 ## ONGOING CARE

DIET
- No special diet
- Weight-loss diet is recommended if obesity is a problem.

PATIENT EDUCATION
- Avoid long periods of standing and crossing legs when sitting
- Exercise (walking, running) regularly to improve leg strength and circulation
- Maintain an appropriate weight
- Wear elastic support stockings
- Avoid clothing that constricts legs
- Surgery/Sclerotherapy may not prevent development of varicosities and the procedure may need to be repeated in later years.
- National Heart, Lung and Blood Institute, Communications and Public Information Branch, National Institutes of Health, Building 31, Room 41–21, 9000 Rockville Pike, Bethesda, MD 20892; 301-496-4236. www.nhlbi.nih.gov

PROGNOSIS
- Usual course: Chronic
- Favorable with appropriate treatment
- Quality of surgical treatment is less satisfactory if significant deep venous reflux, history of ulceration, or congenital arteriovenous malformation exists.
- Surgery has a nonsignificant reduction in the risk of varicose vein recurrence compared with liquid sclerotherapy and endoluminal interventions (6)[A].

COMPLICATIONS
- Complications with sclerotherapy include: Hyperpigmentation, matting, local urticaria, cutaneous necrosis, microthrombi, accidental intra-arterial injection, phlebitis, deep vein thrombosis, thromboembolism, scintillating scotomas, nerve damage, and allergic reactions.
- Petechial hemorrhages
- Chronic edema
- Superimposed infection
- Varicose ulcers
- Pigmentation
- Eczema
- Recurrence after surgical treatment
- Scarring/Nerve damage from stripping technique
- Neurologic complications after sclerotherapy are rare (10)[B].

REFERENCES
1. Raju S, Neglén P. Clinical practice. Chronic venous insufficiency and varicose veins. N Engl J Med. 2009;360:2319–2327.
2. Ruckley CV, Evans CJ, Allan PL, et al. Telangiectasia in the Edinburgh vein study. Eur J Vasc Endovasc Surg. 2008;36:719–724.
3. Cornu-Thenard A, Boivin P, Baud JM, et al. Importance of the familial factor in varicose disease. J Dermatol Surg Oncol. 1994;20:318–326.
4. Hamdan A. Management of varicose veins and venous insufficiency. JAMA. 2012;308:2612–2621.
5. Kistner RL, Eklof B, Masuda EM. Diagnosis of chronic venous disease of the lower extremities: The "CEAP" classification. Mayo Clin Proc. 1996;71:338–345.
6. Murad MH, Coto-Yglesias F, Zumaeta-Garcia M, et al. A systematic review and meta-analysis of the treatments of varicose veins. J Vasc Surg. 2011;53:49S–65S.
7. Palfreyman SJ, Michaels JA. A systematic review of compression hosiery for uncomplicated varicose veins. Phlebology. 2009;24(Suppl 1):13–33.
8. Nesbitt C, Eifell RK, Coyne P, et al. Endovenous ablation (radiofrequency and laser) and foam sclerotherapy versus conventional surgery for great saphenous vein varices. Cochrane Database Syst Rev. 2011;10:CD005624.
9. Carradice S, Mekako W, Hatfield J. Randomized clinical trial of endovenous laser ablation versus conventional surgery for small saphenous varicose veins. Ann Surg. 2013;257:419–426.
10. Kalodiki E, Lattimer CR, Azzam M, et al. Long-term results of a randomized controlled trial on ultrasound-guided foam sclerotherapy combined with saphenofemoral ligation vs standard surgery for varicose veins. J Vasc Surg. 2012;84:451–457.
11. Brar R, Nordon IM, Hinchliffe RJ, et al. Surgical management of varicose veins: Meta-analysis. Vascular. 2010;18:205–220.

ADDITIONAL READING
O'Hare JL, Stephens J, Parkin D, et al. Randomized clinical trial of different bandage regimens after foam sclerotherapy for varicose veins. Br J Surg. 2010;97:650–656.

 ## CODES

ICD10
- I83.009 Varicose veins of unsp lower extremity w ulcer of unsp site
- I83.10 Varicose veins of unsp lower extremity with inflammation
- I83.90 Asymptomatic varicose veins of unspecified lower extremity

CLINICAL PEARLS
- Long-term safety and efficacy of surgery for the treatment of varicose veins is supported by low-quality evidence. Less-invasive treatments, which are associated with less periprocedural disability and pain, are supported by short-term studies (6)[A].
- Endovascular treatment of varicose veins is safe and effective and has a rapid recovery (11)[A].
- Insufficient evidence exists to prefer sclerotherapy over surgery (8)[A].
- The efficacy of sclerotherapy is not significantly affected by the choice of sclerosant, dose, formulation (foam vs. liquid), local pressure dressing, or degree and length of compression (8)[A].

VASCULITIS

Irene J. Tan, MD, FACR

BASICS

DESCRIPTION
Vasculitis is an inflammatory disease of the blood vessels:
- Clinical features result from the destruction of blood vessel walls, with subsequent thrombosis, ischemia, bleeding, and/or aneurysm formation.
- Consists of a large, heterogeneous group of diseases classified by the predominant size, type, and the location of the blood vessels involved (1):
  - Small-vessel vasculitis:
    - Microscopic polyangiitis (MPA)
    - Granulomatosis with polyangiitis (GPA, formerly Wegener's granulomatosis)
    - Eosinophilic granulomatosis with polyangiitis (EGPA, formerly Churg-Strauss syndrome)
    - Anti-glomerular basement membrane disease (anti-GBM)
    - Cryoglobulinemic vasculitis
    - IgA vasculitis (Henoch-Schönlein purpura)
    - Hypocomplementemic urticarial vasculitis
  - Medium-vessel vasculitis:
    - Polyarteritis nodosa (PAN)
    - Kawasaki disease (KD)
  - Large-vessel vasculitis:
    - Takayasu arteritis (TAK)
    - Giant cell arteritis (GCA)
- Occurs as primary disorders or secondary to infection, a drug reaction, malignancy, or connective tissue disorder:
  - Variable vessel vasculitis:
    - Behçet disease
    - Cogan syndrome
  - Single-organ vasculitis:
    - Cutaneous leukocytoclastic angiitis
    - Cutaneous arteritis
    - Primary CNS vasculitis
  - Vasculitis associated with systemic disease
    - Lupus vasculitis
    - Rheumatoid vasculitis
    - Sarcoid vasculitis
  - Vasculitis associated with probable etiology:
    - Hepatitis C-associated cryoglobulinemic vasculitis
    - Hepatitis B-associated vasculitis
    - Syphilis-associated aortitis
    - Drug-induced immune complex vasculitis
    - Drug-associated antineutrophil cytoplasmic antibodies (ANCA)-associated vasculitis
    - Cancer-associated vasculitis
- Protean features often delay the diagnosis.

EPIDEMIOLOGY
Highly variable, depending on the vasculitic syndrome:
- *Hypersensitivity vasculitis is the most commonly encountered vasculitis in clinical practice.*
- Kawasaki disease, Henoch-Schönlein purpura, and dermatomyositis are more common in children.
- Takayasu arteritis is most prevalent in young Asian women.
- Wegener granulomatosis, microscopic polyangiitis, and Churg-Strauss syndrome are more common in middle-aged males.
- Giant cell arteritis occurs exclusively in those >50 years of age and is rare in the African American population.

Incidence
The annual incidence in adults unless otherwise specified:
- Hypersensitivity vasculitis: Depends on drug exposure patterns
- Connective tissue disorder–associated vasculitis: Variable
- Henoch-Schönlein purpura: 200–700/1 million in children <17 years of age
- Giant cell arteritis: 170/1 million
- Kawasaki disease: Depends on race/age; ~170/1 million
- Polyarteritis nodosa: 2–33/1 million
- Wegener granulomatosis: 4–15/1 million
- Microscopic polyangiitis: 1–24/1 million
- Churg-Strauss arteritis: 1–3/1 million
- Viral-/retroviral-associated vasculitis: Unknown; >90% of cases of cryoglobulinemic vasculitis are associated with hepatitis C.
- Polyarteritis nodosa: 2–33/1 million
- Takayasu arteritis: 2/1 million

ETIOLOGY AND PATHOPHYSIOLOGY
- 3 major immunopathogenic mechanisms have been proposed:
  - Immune-complex formation: Systemic lupus erythematosus (SLE), IgA vasculitis (HSP), and cryoglobulinemic vasculitis.
  - ANCAs: GPA (formerly Wegener granulomatosis), MPA, and EGPA (formerly Churg-Strauss syndrome)
  - Pathogenic T-lymphocyte response: Giant cell arteritis and Takayasu arteritis
- Not well understood in most forms of vasculitis, except where known drug triggers have been identified (e.g., antibiotics, sulfonamides, and hydralazine)

Genetics
- A number of the vasculitic syndromes have been linked to candidate genes.
- No single gene has been found to cause vasculitis.
- Angiotensin-converting enzyme insertion/deletion polymorphism is associated with susceptibility to vasculitis, especially in Behçet disease and Henoch-Schönlein purpura (2)[A]

RISK FACTORS
A combination of genetic susceptibility and environmental exposure is presumed to play a role in disease onset.

GENERAL PREVENTION
- None
- Early identification is the key to prevent irreversible organ damage in severe forms of systemic vasculitis.

COMMONLY ASSOCIATED CONDITIONS
Hepatitis C (cryoglobulinemic vasculitis), hepatitis B (PAN), SLE, rheumatoid arthritis (RA), Sjögren syndrome, mixed connective tissue disease (MCTD), dermatomyositis, ankylosing spondylitis, Behçet disease, relapsing polychondritis (CTD-associated vasculitis), HIV, cytomegalovirus (CMV), Epstein-Barr virus (EBV), hepatitis B and C (viral-/retroviral-associated vasculitis), respiratory tract methicillin-resistant *Staphylococcus aureus* (MRSA) (Wegener granulomatosis [WG]).

DIAGNOSIS

HISTORY
- Consider patient's age, sex, and ethnicity
- Note the organs affected and estimate the size of blood vessels involved
- Use the pattern of demographics, clinical features, and the predominant vessel size/organ involvement to narrow down the specific type of vasculitis.

PHYSICAL EXAM
- Constitutional symptoms: Fever, weight loss, malaise, fatigue, diminished appetite, sweats
- Skin findings: Palpable purpura, livedo reticularis, nodules, ulcers, gangrene, nail bed capillary changes
- CNS findings: Mononeuritis multiplex, polyneuropathy, headaches, visual loss, tinnitus, stroke, seizure, encephalopathy
- Heart/Lung findings: Myocardial infarction, cardiomyopathy, pericarditis, arrhythmia, cough, chest pain, hemoptysis, dyspnea
- Renal manifestations: Hypertension, proteinuria, hematuria, renal insufficiency
- GI manifestations: Abdominal pain, hematochezia, perforation
- Musculoskeletal manifestations: Arthralgia, myalgia
- Miscellaneous: Unexplained ischemic or hemorrhagic events, chronic sinusitis, scleritis, episcleritis, and recurrent epistaxis

DIFFERENTIAL DIAGNOSIS
- Fibromuscular dysplasia
- Embolic disease (atheroma, cholesterol emboli, atrial myxoma, mycotic aneurysm with embolization)
- Vasospasm, drug-induced (cocaine, amphetamines, ergots)
- Thrombotic thrombocytopenic disorders (disseminated intravascular coagulation [DIC], thrombotic thrombocytopenic purpura [TTP], antiphospholipid syndrome, heparin- or warfarin-induced thrombosis)
- Systemic infection (infective endocarditis, fungal infections, disseminated gonococcal infection, Lyme disease, syphilis, Rocky Mountain spotted fever [RMSF], bacteremia)
- Malignancy (lymphomatoid granulomatosis, angioimmunoblastic T-cell lymphoma, intravascular lymphoma)
- Miscellaneous (Goodpasture syndrome, sarcoidosis, amyloidosis, Whipple disease, congenital coarctation of aorta)

DIAGNOSTIC TESTS & INTERPRETATION

ALERT
- Clinically silent kidney involvement warrants both a routine serum creatinine and urinalysis with microscopy for underlying glomerulonephritis.
- *Labs are required to exclude alternate diagnosis, which has major treatment implications.*

Initial Tests (lab, imaging)
- Routine tests:
  - CBC
  - Liver enzymes
  - Serum creatinine
  - Urinalysis with microscopy

- Serology:
  – Antinuclear antibodies (ANA)
  – Rheumatoid factor (RF)
  – Rapid plasma reagin/venereal disease reaction level (RPR/VDRL)
  – RMSF titer
  – Lyme test
  – Complements C3,C4
  – ANCA
  – Anti-Proteinase-3 antibodies (anti-P3)
  – Anti-Myeloperoxidase antibodies (anti-MPO)
  – Hepatitis screen for B and C
  – Cryoglobulin
  – Antiglomerular basement membrane titer
  – HIV
  – Serum protein electrophoresis
- Miscellaneous:
  – Drug screen
  – ESR
  – C-reactive protein
  – Creatine kinase (CK)
  – Blood culture
  – ECG

Chest x-ray (CXR), CT scan, MRI, and arteriography may be required to delineate extent of organs involved.

Diagnostic Procedures/Other
- Electromyography with nerve conduction studies may be useful for documenting neuropathy and to target affected nerve for biopsy.
- Biopsy of the affected tissue/organ is essential to substantiate diagnosis (e.g., temporal artery, sural nerve, renal biopsy).
- If biopsy is not practical, angiography may be diagnostic for large- and medium-vessel vasculitides.
- Bronchoscopy may be required to differentiate pulmonary infection from potentially life-threatening hemorrhagic vasculitis in patients with hemoptysis.

Test Interpretation
Immune cell infiltration into the blood vessel wall layers with varying degrees of necrosis and granuloma formation, depending on the type of vasculitis

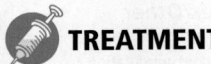 **TREATMENT**

GENERAL MEASURES
- Discontinue the offending drug for hypersensitivity vasculitis.
- Simple observation for mild cases of Henoch-Schönlein purpura.

MEDICATION
First Line
Corticosteroids are the initial systemic anti-inflammatory agent (3)[A],(4)[C] with rapid onset of action.

Second Line
Cytotoxic medications (e.g., cyclophosphamide (5,6)[A], methotrexate, azathioprine (6)[A], mycophenolate mofetil (6)[A], and rituximab (6)[A]) are often required in combination with corticosteroids for rapidly progressive vasculitis with significant organ involvement or inadequate response to corticosteroids.

ISSUES FOR REFERRAL
- Rheumatology referral for complicated cases where newer or more toxic treatments are required.
- Nephrology referral for persistent hematuria or proteinuria, rising creatinine, or a positive ANCA titer

- Pulmonary referral for persistent pulmonary infiltrate unresponsive to antibiotic therapy or gross hemoptysis

ADDITIONAL THERAPIES
- IVIG and aspirin for Kawasaki disease, but corticosteroids are contraindicated
- Plasma exchange appears to improve recovery of patients with severe acute renal failure secondary to vasculitis (7)[A] and pulmonary hemorrhage.

SURGERY/OTHER PROCEDURES
Rarely, corrective surgery is required to repair tissue damage as a result of aggressive vasculitis.

IN-PATIENT CONSIDERATIONS
Admission Criteria/Initial Stabilization
- Hemoptysis, acute renal failure, intestinal ischemia, any organ-threatening symptoms or signs, and/or need for biopsy
- Initial therapy is guided by the organ system involved:
  – If pulmonary hemorrhage is present, life-saving measures may include mechanical ventilation, plasmapheresis, and immunosuppression.
  – If acute renal failure is present, electrolyte and fluid balance as well as plasma exchange and immunosuppression should be considered.
  – If signs of intestinal ischemia, patient should be NPO and be considered for plasmapheresis, immunosuppression, and parenteral nutrition.

Discharge Criteria
Stabilization or resolution of potential life-threatening symptoms

 ONGOING CARE

FOLLOW-UP RECOMMENDATIONS
If significant coronary artery disease is involved in Kawasaki disease, moderate activity restriction may be of benefit.

Patient Monitoring
Frequent clinical follow-up supported by patient self-monitoring is the key to the timely identification of disease relapse.

DIET
Special diet for patients with renal involvement or those with hyperglycemia/dyslipidemia as a result of therapeutic corticosteroids

PROGNOSIS
Prognosis is good, particularly vasculitis with limited organ involvement. Relapsing courses, renal, intestinal, or extensive lung involvement portend the worst prognosis.

COMPLICATIONS
- Varying degrees of persistent organ dysfunction may be the result of the disease, medications, or scarring in the more serious forms of vasculitis.
- Early death is due to active vasculitic disease, and late death may be a result of complications of therapy (corticosteroids and cytotoxic medications).

REFERENCES
1. Jennette JC, Falk RJ, Bacon PA, et al. 2012 revised International Chapel Hill Consensus Conference Nomenclature of Vasculitides. *Arthritis Rheum.* 2013;65:1–11.
2. Lee YH, Choi SJ, Ji JD, et al. Associations between the angiotensin-converting enzyme insertion/deletion polymorphism and susceptibility to vasculitis: A meta-analysis. *J Renin Angiotensin Aldosterone Syst.* 2012;13:196–201.
3. Weiss PF, Feinstein JA, Luan X, et al. Effects of corticosteroid on Henoch-Schönlein purpura: A systematic review. *Pediatrics.* 2007;120: 1079–1087.
4. Wood L, Tulloh R. Kawasaki disease: Diagnosis, management and cardiac sequelae. *Expert Rev Cardiovasc Ther.* 2007;5:553–561.
5. Bertsias G, Ioannidis JP, Boletis J, et al. EULAR recommendations for the management of systemic lupus erythematosus. Report of a Task Force of the EULAR Standing Committee for International Clinical Studies Including Therapeutics. *Ann Rheum Dis.* 2008;67:195–205.
6. Smith RM, Jones RB, Jayne DR. Progress in treatment of ANCA-associated vasculitis. *Arthritis Res Ther.* 2012;14:210.
7. Walters GD, Willis NS, Craig JC. Interventions for renal vasculitis in adults. A systematic review. *BMC Nephrol.* 2010;11:12.

ADDITIONAL READING
- Appel GB, Contreras G, Dooley MA, et al. Mycophenolate mofetil versus cyclophosphamide for induction treatment of lupus nephritis. *J Am Soc Nephrol.* 2009;20:1103–1112.
- Bosch X, Guilabert A, Espinosa G, et al. Treatment of antineutrophil cytoplasmic antibody associated vasculitis: A systematic review. *JAMA.* 2007;298:655–669
- Gatto M, Iaccarino L, Canova M, et al. Pregnancy and vasculitis: A systematic review of the literature. *Autoimmun Rev.* 2012;11:A447–459.
- National Heart Lung and Blood Institute Diseases and Conditions Index: Vasculitis: www.nhlbi.nih. gov/health/dci/Diseases/vas/vas_whatis.html
- Stone JH, Merkel PA, Spiera R, et al. Rituximab versus cyclophosphamide for ANCA-associated vasculitis. *N Engl J Med.* 2010;363:221–232.
- The Vasculitis Foundation: www. vasculitisfoundation.org/

 CODES

ICD10
- D69.0 Allergic purpura
- I77.6 Arteritis, unspecified
- M31.30 Wegener's granulomatosis without renal involvement

CLINICAL PEARLS
- Suspect a vasculitic process in patients with unexplained ischemia or multiorgan involvement, particularly presence of petechial rash or palpable purpura, glomerulonephritis, pulmonary-renal syndrome, intestinal ischemia, or mononeuritis multiplex.
- Look for clinically silent kidney involvement with serum creatinine and urinalysis with microscopy.
- Vasculitis tends to have "skip" lesions, so a generous specimen may be needed for diagnostic biopsy.
- A pitfall in vasculitis is the failure to exclude a primary process, such as infection, thrombosis, or malignancy.

V

VENOUS INSUFFICIENCY ULCERS

Barbara Provo, MSN, RN, FNP, CWON • SreyRam Kuy, MD, MHS

 BASICS

- Venous insufficiency disorders include simple spider veins, varicose veins, and leg edema.
- In the US, 23% of adults have varicose veins, an estimated 22 million women, 11 million men.
- Venous leg ulcers are the most serious consequence of venous insufficiency.
- 500,000 people in the US have chronic venous ulcers, with an estimated treatment cost of >$3 billion per year.

DESCRIPTION

- Full-thickness skin defect with surrounding pigmentation and dermatitis
- Most frequently located in ankle region of lower leg ("gaiter region")
- Present for >30 days and fails to heal spontaneously
- May only have mild pain unless infected
- Other signs of chronic venous insufficiency include edema/brawny edema and chronic skin changes (i.e., hyperpigmentation and/or fibrosis).

EPIDEMIOLOGY
Up to 80% of leg ulcers are caused by venous disease; arterial disease accounts for 10–25%, which may coexist with venous disease.

Incidence
- Overall incidence of venous ulcers is 18/100,000 persons.
- Prevalent sex: Women > Men (20.4 vs. 14.6 per 100,000 for venous ulcer); increased with age for both sexes

Prevalence
- Seen in ~1% of adult population in industrialized countries, increased to 5% in patients ≥80 years old
- Prevalence studies only available for Western countries
- Point prevalence underestimates the extent of the disease because ulcers often recur.
- 70% of ulcers recur within 5 years of closure

ETIOLOGY AND PATHOPHYSIOLOGY
- In a diseased venous system, venous pressure in the deep system fails to fall with ambulation, causing venous hypertension.
- Venous hypertension comes from:
  – Venous obstruction
  – Incompetent venous valves in the deep or superficial system
  – Inadequate muscle contraction (e.g., arthritis, myopathies, neuropathies) so that the calf pump is ineffective
- Venous pressure transmitted to capillaries leading to venous hypertensive microangiopathy and extravasation of RBCs and proteins (especially fibrinogen)
- Increased RBC aggregation leads to reduced oxygen transport, slowed arteriolar circulation, and ischemia at the skin level, contributing to ulcers.
- Leukocytes aggregate to hypoxic areas and increase local inflammation.
- Factors promoting persistence of venous ulcers:
  – Prolonged chronic inflammation
  – Bacterial infection, critical colonization

RISK FACTORS
- History of leg injury
- Obesity
- Congestive heart failure (CHF)
- History of deep venous thrombosis (DVT)
- Failure of calf muscle pump (e.g., ankle fusion, inactivity) is a strong independent predictor of poorly healing wounds.
- Previous varicose vein surgery
- Family history

GENERAL PREVENTION
- Primary prevention after symptomatic DVT: Prescribe compression hose to be used as soon as feasible for at least 2 years (≥20–30 mm Hg compression).
- Secondary prevention of recurrent ulceration includes compression, correction of the underlying problem, and surveillance. Circumstantial evidence from 2 RCTs showed those who stopped wearing compression hose were more likely to recur (1)[A].
- Compression hose reduce rates of recurrence compared with no compression (2).
- Because most ulcers develop following some type of trauma, avoiding lower leg trauma may help to prevent ulceration.

COMMONLY ASSOCIATED CONDITIONS
Up to 50% of patients have allergic reactions to topical agents commonly used for treatment:
- Contact sensitivity was more common in patients with stasis dermatitis (62% vs. 38%).
- Avoid neomycin sulfate in particular (including triple antibiotic ointment).

 DIAGNOSIS

A diagnosis of venous reflux or obstruction must be established by an objective test beyond the routine clinical examination of the extremity.

HISTORY
- Family history of venous insufficiency and ulcers
- Recent trauma
- Nature of pain: Achy (better with leg elevation)
- Wound drainage
- Duration of wound and over-the-counter (OTC) treatments already attempted
- History of DVTs (especially factor V Leiden mutation; strongly associated with ulceration)
- History of leg edema that improves over night.
- Edema that does not improve over night is more likely lymphedema.

PHYSICAL EXAM
- Look for evidence of venous insufficiency:
  – Pitting edema
  – Hemosiderin staining (red and brown spotty or diffuse pigment changes)
  – Stasis dermatitis
  – White skin lesions (atrophie blanche)
  – Lipodermatosclerosis ("bottle neck" narrowing in the lower leg from fibrosis and scarring)
- Look for evidence of significant lymphedema (i.e., dorsal foot or toe edema, edema that does not resolve overnight or with elevation). This may require referral for special comprehensive lymph therapy.
- Examine for palpable pulses.

ALERT
- Examine wound for:
  – Length, width, depth, to monitor wound healing rate
  – Presence of necrotic tissue
  – Presence of infection: Purulent material in the wound, spreading cellulitis, fever and chills
  – Extent and type of drainage
- Get initial and interim girth measurements (at ankle and midcalf) to monitor edema.
- Important to rule out poor arterial circulation:
  – Compression dressings cannot be used in patients with ankle brachial index (ABI) <0.8.

DIFFERENTIAL DIAGNOSIS
- Arterial insufficiency ulcer
- Neuropathic ulcer
- Malignancy
- Sickle cell ulcer
- Vasculitic ulcer
- Calciphylaxis
- Cryoglobulinemia
- Pyoderma gangrenosum
- Collagen vascular disease
- Leishmaniasis
- Cutaneous tuberculosis

DIAGNOSTIC TESTS & INTERPRETATION
- Consider prothrombin time (PT)/international normalization ratio (INR) and partial thromboplastin time (PTT) if patient is anticoagulated
- Consider biopsy of leg ulcers that fail to heal or have atypical features
- Consider factor V Leiden mutation; strongly associated with venous ulcers
- Test for diabetes as necessary with fasting glucose
- Use duplex imaging to diagnose anatomic and hemodynamic abnormalities with venous insufficiency. It will also identify any DVT present.

Diagnostic Procedures/Other
- Check ABI for evidence of arterial disease
- An ABI <0.8 is a relative contraindication to compression therapy.
- Duplex imaging for evaluation of superficial and deep venous reflux and incompetent perforator veins.
- With concomitant severe arterial insufficiency, refer to a vascular surgeon for revascularization.

Test Interpretation
Strongly consider biopsy on wounds with atypical locations, failure to heal, or any suspicion of malignancy.

 TREATMENT

GENERAL MEASURES
Dressings: All wounds need some kind of a dressing underneath the compression system:
- Wound dressings: No single type of dressing proved superior (3)[B]
- Maintain moist wound environment: Not excessively wet or dry

- Wounds are often exudative until edema is decreased: Use absorptive dressings (calcium alginate or absorptive pads). Both superabsorbent diapers and female protection pads are cost-effective alternatives.
- Consider using barrier ointment/cream to prevent maceration of surrounding skin.
- If wound tends to be dry, use a hydrogel.
- A hydrocolloid dressing may be used with minimal exudate, if skin adhesive is tolerated.

MEDICATION

- Effective compression management is the cornerstone of therapy (1)[A].
- Diuretics may help to reduce edema, but compression is the mainstay.
- Pentoxifylline 400 mg PO t.i.d., in addition to local care and compression, improves cure rates. There is some response even without compression. GI side effects are common (4)[B].

ISSUES FOR REFERRAL

- With prominent toe or foot edema, consider lymphedema. Refer to certified lymphedema therapist (CLT).
- Refer to a wound clinic for complex or poorly healing ulcers
- Refer to a vein clinic or vascular specialist for recurrent ulcers
- Use home health nurses to help with immobile patients needing frequent wrapping/dressing changes

ADDITIONAL THERAPIES

- Edema management: Reduce venous hypertension and improve venous return to reduce inflammation, pain, and improve healing:
  - Compression therapy for edema management is the cornerstone of treatment for venous insufficiency with or without ulcers (1)[A].
  - Short-stretch multilayer bandages are ideal for acute phase, until edema is stable, and the patient can be fitted for compression hose.
  - Long-term compression hose (fit once edema is reduced). Aim for a minimum pressure 20–30 mm Hg, preferably 30–40 mm Hg.
  - Elevation of legs to heart level for 30 minutes 3–4 times per day.
  - Exercise to strengthen calf muscle pump is also effective.
- Infection control:
  - Debride necrotic tissue
  - Treat cellulitis (usually gram-positive bacteria) with bactericidal systemic antibiotics. Suspect local infection when there is pain or no improvement in the wound after 2 weeks of compression. Consider deep quantitative swab, after thorough cleansing, or tissue biopsy for culture.
  - Treat critical colonization with topical antimicrobials, especially cadexomer iodine (5)[A]. (Silver dressings are widely used, but definitive data are lacking.)
  - For venous ulcers resistant to healing with wound care and compression, consider adding an intermittent compression pump 1–4 hr/d (6)[B].
- Encourage exercise (e.g., activation of calf muscle pump with ankle flexion and extension) in conjunction with leg compression and elevation.
- Vacuum-assisted closure (VAC) dressings may be beneficial, but a Cochrane review indicates no clear benefit over optimal traditional wound care (7)[A].

SURGERY/OTHER PROCEDURES

- Necrotic tissue impedes healing:
  - Consider sharp debridement.
  - Other methods include enzymatic ointments (collagenase), low-frequency ultrasound, and wet-to-dry dressings.
  - Avoid using collagenase with silver dressings because silver inactivates the enzyme.
- Allografts made of synthetic skin bilayered with living keratinocytes and fibroblasts improve healing at 6 months; insufficient evidence to support use of autografts.
- In patients with incompetent perforator veins and ulcers refractory to conservative therapy, surgical options for venous reflux include open and minimally invasive ligation of incompetent perforator veins.

COMPLEMENTARY AND ALTERNATIVE MEDICINE

- Chestnut seed extract (50 mg b.i.d.) is effective for venous insufficiency but not ulceration.
- Topical medicinal honey used on wounds shows no evidence of improved healing.

IN-PATIENT CONSIDERATIONS

For those with acute significant cellulitis

Admission Criteria/Initial Stabilization

Infected wounds requiring IV antibiotics, especially in diabetics

 ONGOING CARE

- Venous insufficiency is a lifelong issue.
- After resolution of an ulcer, edema management must be maintained lifelong.

FOLLOW-UP RECOMMENDATIONS

When ulcers are nearly healed and edema is controlled, switch from compression bandages to compression hose:

- Insurance may not reimburse for compression hose unless an ulcer is present.
- Referral for hose fitting must be done just prior to the ulcer being healed.

Patient Monitoring

Monitor the ulcer for healing by measuring its area. Expect at least 10% reduction every 2 weeks.

DIET

- Obese patients may benefit from weight loss
- Low-salt diets help fluid retention

PATIENT EDUCATION

- Patient education for understanding of underlying mechanism is important for long-term management:
  - Develop long-term plan for edema management and instruction on compression therapy.
  - Instruct the patient on topical wound therapy.
  - Teach early recognition and treatment of new ulcers or cellulitis.

PROGNOSIS

- Ulcers recur frequently. Early identification and immediate treatment are essential.
- Ongoing diligence, with edema control, avoiding infections, and avoiding trauma, are important.

REFERENCES

1. O'Meara S, Cullen NA, Nelson EA, et al. Compression for venous leg ulcers. *Cochrane Database Syst Rev.* 2012;11:CD000265.
2. Nelson EA, Bell-Syer SE. Compression for preventing recurrence of venous ulcers. *Cochrane Database Syst Rev.* 2012;8:CD002303.
3. Palfreyman SJ, Nelson EA, Lochiel R, et al. Dressings for healing venous leg ulcers. *Cochrane Database Syst Rev.* 2006;3:CD001103.
4. Jull A, Arroll B, Parag V, et al. Pentoxifylline for treating venous leg ulcers. *Cochrane Database Syst Rev.* 2007;3:CD001733.
5. O'Meara S, Al-Kurdi D, Ovington LG. Antibiotics and antiseptics for venous leg ulcers. *Cochrane Database Syst Rev.* 2008;1:CD003557.
6. Kearon C, Kahn SR, Agnelli G, et al. Antithrombotic therapy for venous thromboembolic disease: American College of Chest Physicians Evidence-Based Clinical Practice Guidelines (8th Edition). *Chest.* 2008;133:454S–545S.
7. Ubbink DT, Westerbos SJ, Evans D, et al. Topical negative pressure for treating chronic wounds. *Cochrane Database Syst Rev.* 2008;3:CD001898.

ADDITIONAL READING

- Hamden A. Management of Varicose Veins and Venous Insufficiency. *JAMA.* 2012;208:2612–2621.
- O'Brien JF, Grace PA, Perry IJ, et al. Randomized clinical trial and economic analysis of four-layer compression bandaging for venous ulcers. *Br J Surg.* 2003;90:794–798.
- Rueda C, Bittenbinder E, Buckley C, et al. The management of chronic venous insufficiency with ulceration: the role of minimally invasive perforator interruption. *Ann Vasc Surg.* 2013;27:89–95.

 SEE ALSO

Algorithm: Leg Ulcer

 CODES

ICD10

- I83.008 Varicos vn unsp low extrm w ulcer oth part of lower leg
- I83.009 Varicose veins of unsp lower extremity w ulcer of unsp site
- I87.2 Venous insufficiency (chronic) (peripheral)

CLINICAL PEARLS

- Initial diagnostic workup should include venous duplex scan and arterial evaluation.
- Refer patients with ABI <0.8 to vascular surgery specialist.
- Refer patients with recurrent or poor healing venous ulcers to venous specialist or wound specialist.
- Compression is essential for edema management with or without wounds.
- Treat critical colonization with topical antimicrobials (avoid neomycin).
- Make sure that the diagnosis is correct, and biopsy when in doubt.

VENTRICULAR SEPTAL DEFECT

Jamie Nicole Colombo, DO • Brent Barber, MD

BASICS

DESCRIPTION
- Congenital or acquired defect of the interventricular septum that allows communication of blood between the left and the right ventricles
- Other than bicuspid aortic valve, this is the most common congenital heart malformation reported in infants and children. It also occurs as a complication of acute myocardial infarction (MI).
- Blood flow across the defect typically is left to right and depends on the size of the defect and the pulmonary vascular resistance (PVR).
- Prolonged shunting of blood can lead to pulmonary hypertension (HTN) and eventual reversal of flow across the defect, as well as to cyanosis (Eisenmenger complex).
- System(s) affected: Cardiovascular

Geriatric Considerations
In this population, almost entirely associated with MI

Pediatric Considerations
Congenital

ALERT
- Pregnancy may exacerbate symptoms and signs of a ventricular septal defect (VSD).
- Tolerated during pregnancy if the septal defect is small
- May be associated with an increased risk of preeclampsia in women with an unrepaired VSD (1)

EPIDEMIOLOGY
Incidence
- Predominant sex: No gender predilection
- Males are affected more than females if associated with MI
- Occurs in ~2/1,000 live births (2)

Prevalence
In the US:
- Acute MI: Estimated to complicate 1–3%
- Lowered prevalence in adults due to spontaneous closure of defects

ETIOLOGY AND PATHOPHYSIOLOGY
- Congenital
- In adults, secondary to MI

Genetics
Multifactorial etiology; autosomal-dominant and recessive transmissions have been reported

RISK FACTORS
- Congenital:
  - Risk of sibling being affected: 4.2%
  - Risk of offspring being affected: 4%
  - Prematurity
- Postacute MI:
  - First MI
  - HTN
  - Most frequent within 1st week after MI
  - Occurs in 1–3% of MIs, most commonly after anterior MI

GENERAL PREVENTION
For adults, avoid risk factors for MI and obtain evaluation before pregnancy.

COMMONLY ASSOCIATED CONDITIONS
- Congenital:
  - Tetralogy of Fallot
  - Aortic valvular deformities, especially aortic insufficiency and bicuspid aortic valve
  - Down syndrome (trisomy 21), endocardial cushion defect
  - Transposition of great arteries
  - Coarctation of aorta
  - Tricuspid atresia
  - Truncus arteriosus
  - Patent ductus arteriosus
  - Atrial septal defect
  - Pulmonic stenosis
  - Subaortic stenosis
- Adult: Coronary artery disease

DIAGNOSIS

HISTORY
- Depends on the degree of shunting across the defect; may be completely asymptomatic with small defects
- Respiratory distress, tachypnea, tachycardia
- Diaphoresis with feeds, poor weight gain in infants

PHYSICAL EXAM
- Small defect:
  - Harsh holosystolic murmur loudest at left lower sternal border
  - Detected after pulmonary vascular resistance drops at 4–8 weeks of life
- Moderate defect:
  - Harsh holosystolic murmur at left lower sternal border associated with a thrill
  - Forceful apical impulse with lateral displacement
  - Increased intensity of P_2
  - Diastolic rumble at apex due to increased flow across the mitral valve
- Large defect:
  - Holosystolic murmur heard throughout the precordium with diastolic rumble at apex with precordial bulge and hyperactivity, although large defects may have little or no murmur initially
  - If congestive heart failure (CHF) exists: Tachycardia, tachypnea, and hepatomegaly
  - If pulmonary HTN exists: Cyanosis with exertion
  - If Eisenmenger complex is present: Cyanosis and clubbing

DIFFERENTIAL DIAGNOSIS
- Any defect with left-to-right shunt, such as patent ductus arteriosus, atrial septal defect
- Children: Tetralogy of Fallot
- Adults: Mitral regurgitation

DIAGNOSTIC TESTS & INTERPRETATION
Initial Tests (lab, imaging)
- A 12-lead ECG may suggest severity of VSD. Initially, left ventricular hypertrophy and left atrial enlargement may be evident. With pulmonary HTN, right ventricular hypertrophy and right atrial enlargement may be seen.
- After surgical repair, right bundle-branch block is common.
- A chest x-ray (CXR) may demonstrate increased pulmonary vascularity and/or cardiomegaly.
- A 2D echocardiogram for visualization of location and size of defect.

- Color-flow Doppler for direction and velocity of VSD jet; may be used to estimate right ventricular pressure.

Follow-Up Tests & Special Considerations
- Weight and hematocrit check
- Cardiac catheterization performed occasionally for perioperative planning or to assess need for closure of defect

Diagnostic Procedures/Other
- Cardiac catheterization (left and right sides of heart) can confirm the diagnosis, document number of defects, quantify ratio of pulmonary blood flow to systemic blood flow (Qp/Qs), and determine pulmonary vascular resistance.
- Demonstration of an oxygen saturation step up from the right atrium to the distal pulmonary artery

Test Interpretation
- Congenital VSD (4 major anatomic types):
  - Membranous (70%)
  - Muscular (20%)
  - Atrioventricular canal type (5%)
  - Supracristal (5%; higher in Asians)
- Post-MI VSD predominantly involves muscular septum

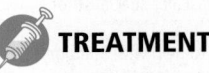

TREATMENT

- Start diuretic therapy if overload signs present
- Minimize IV fluids
- Consider ACE inhibitor and/or digoxin
- Nasogastric feeds
- Correct anemia via iron supplementation or a possible RBC transfusion

GENERAL MEASURES
- Appropriate health care
- Outpatient, until surgical repair is indicated
- Inpatient in setting of acute MI
- Inpatient for treatment of severe CHF

MEDICATION
First Line
- Endocarditis antibiotic prophylaxis is no longer recommended for most VSDs. Antibiotic prophylaxis is recommended for VSDs associated with complex cyanotic heart disease, during the 1st 6 months after surgical repair, or for residual VSDs located near the patch following surgery (3).
- Pediatric: Medications aim to control pulmonary edema, decrease work of breathing, and allow for growth:
  - Furosemide 1–2 mg/kg PO/IV once to twice a day (4)[A]
  - Digoxin: Infants <2 years of age, 10 mcg/kg/d PO divided b.i.d.; children, 2–10 years of age, 5–10 mcg/kg/d PO divided b.i.d.; children >10 years of age, 2–5 mcg/kg/d PO divided b.i.d.
  - Spironolactone 1–2 mg/kg/d divided b.i.d.
  - Captopril 0.1–0.4 mg/kg PO given q6–24h (maximum 6 mg/kg/24 hr)
- Adults: Digoxin and diuretics may be beneficial in some circumstances
- Side effects:
  - Drugs that increase systemic vascular resistance may increase left-to-right shunting and cause signs and symptoms of pulmonary overcirculation
  - HTN

Second Line

- Surgical closure is generally indicated if the pulmonic-to-systemic flow is >2:1 or with poorly controlled pulmonary overcirculation despite maximal medical and dietary interventions.
- If an infant with a VSD has persistent pulmonary HTN or failure to grow, surgical repair generally is recommended prior to 6 months of age even if patient is asymptomatic.
- In the post-MI setting, afterload reduction, inotropic support, intra-aortic balloon pump, and left ventricular assist device may be used to stabilize the patient prior to surgery. Surgical repair includes debridement and patch placement.

ISSUES FOR REFERRAL

Close follow-up of a congenital VSD is necessary until primary intracardiac repair is performed to ensure that significant pulmonary HTN does not develop.

ADDITIONAL THERAPIES

- Caloric requirements up to 150 kcal/kg/d for adequate weight gain
- Treatment of iron-deficiency anemia to increase oxygen-carrying capacity

SURGERY/OTHER PROCEDURES

- Surgical correction with either a VSD patch or repair is commonly utilized. Postsurgical outcomes for isolated VSD are excellent. Complications are rare and include reoperation for residual VSD, extended hospital stay, arrhythmias, valve injury, depressed ventricular function, and heart block (5).
- Percutaneous transcatheter device closure of muscular defects is an option (6). The closure of membranous defects with septal occluders is currently under research protocols. Complications include embolization of the device, residual defects, and complete heart block.
- Periventricular device closure of isolated VSDs without cardiopulmonary bypass is feasible and safe under transesophageal echocardiographic (TEE) guidance. However, further evaluation of intermediate and long-term results is necessary.

IN-PATIENT CONSIDERATIONS

Admission Criteria/Initial Stabilization

- Failure to thrive
- Pulmonary overcirculation/CHF
- Stabilize airway
- Reduce temperature stress

Nursing

Frequent vital sign monitoring; daily weight and calorie counts

Discharge Criteria

CHF stabilization, weight gain, or successful repair

 ONGOING CARE

FOLLOW-UP RECOMMENDATIONS

- Small VSDs without evidence of CHF or pulmonary HTN generally can be followed every 1–5 years after the neonatal period
- Moderate to large VSDs require more frequent follow-up
- Potential complications of VSDs include right ventricular outflow obstruction and aortic valve prolapse

Patient Monitoring

- Physical growth and development monitoring
- Influenza vaccine for children >6 months of age
- Palivizumab to children <2 years of age with hemodynamically significant lesions

DIET

- Low-sodium in heart failure
- High-calorie in failure to thrive

PATIENT EDUCATION

- No activity restriction in absence of pulmonary HTN
- Parents need support and instructions for prevention of complications until the child is ready for surgery

PROGNOSIS

- Congenital:
  - Course is variable depending on the size of the VSD.
  - Small VSD: 25–45% will close spontaneously by age 3 years. Muscular defects are more likely to close spontaneously.
  - Large VSD: CHF or failure to thrive in infancy necessitating surgical repair.
  - 20-year survival rate for isolated VSD: 98.3% (7).
  - Progressive pulmonary vascular disease and pulmonary HTN are the most feared complications of VSD caused by left-to-right shunting and may eventually lead to reversal of the shunt (Eisenmenger complex). Death usually occurs in the 4th decade of life if untreated.
- Post-MI:
  - With medical management alone, 80–90% mortality in the first 2 weeks
  - Prognosis worse with inferior MI compared with anterior MI

COMPLICATIONS

- CHF
- Aortic insufficiency
- Sudden death
- Hemoptysis
- Cerebral abscess
- Paradoxical emboli
- Cardiogenic shock
- Heart block rarely may accompany surgical closure.
- Pulmonary HTN

REFERENCES

1. Yap S-C, Drenthen W, Pieper P. Pregnancy outcome in women with repaired versus unrepaired isolated ventricular septal defect. *BJOG*. 2010;117: 683–689.
2. Mitchell SC, Korones SB, Berendes HW. Congenital heart disease in 56,109 births: Incidence and natural history. *Circulation*. 1971;43:323–332.
3. Wilson W. Prevention of infective endocarditis. Guidelines From the American Heart Association. A guideline From the American Heart Association Rheumatic Fever, Endocarditis, and Kawasaki Disease Committee, Council on Cardiovascular Disease in the Young, and the Council on Clinical Cardiology, Council on Cardiovascular Surgery and Anesthesia, and the Quality of Care and Outcomes Research Interdisciplinary Working Group. *Circulation*. 2007;116:1736–1754.
4. Faris R, Flather MD, Purcell H. Diuretics for heart failure. *Cochrane Database Sys Rev*. 2006;2: CD003838.
5. Scully BB, Morales DL, Zafar F, et al. Current expectations for surgical repair of isolated ventricular septal defects. *Ann Thorac Surg*. 2010;89:544.
6. Knauth AL, Lock JE, Perry SB. Transcatheter device closure of congenital and postoperative residual ventricular septal defects. *Circulation*. 2004; s110:501–507.
7. Tennant PW, Pearce MS, Bythell M, et al. 20-year survival of children born with congenital anomalies: A population-based study. *Lancet*. 2010;375:649.

ADDITIONAL READING

- Patanè F, Centofanti P, Zingarelli E. Potential role of the Impella Recover left ventricular assist device in the management of postinfarct ventricular septal defect. *J Thorac Cardiovasc Surg*. 2009;137: 1288–1289.
- Quansheng X, Silin P, Zhongyun Z. Minimally invasive perventricular device closure of an isolated perimembranous ventricular septal defect with a newly designed delivery system: Preliminary experience. *J Thorac Cardiovasc Surg*. 2009; 137:556–559.

 SEE ALSO

Down Syndrome; Myocardial Infarction, Myocardial Infarction, ST-Segment Elevation (STEMI); Non–ST-Segment Elevation (NSTEMI); Tetralogy of Fallot

 CODES

ICD10

- I51.0 Cardiac septal defect, acquired
- Q21.0 Ventricular septal defect

CLINICAL PEARLS

- A loud 2–3/6 low-pitched harsh holosystolic murmur at the left lower sternal border is typical.
- A diastolic rumble at the apex indicates moderate-to-large VSD or Qp:Qs >2:1.
- Disappearance of the murmur could be secondary to spontaneous closure of the defect or the development of pulmonary HTN.
- Development of a new murmur of semilunar valve insufficiency should be further evaluated. Pulmonary regurgitation may occur as PVR increases, and the development of aortic regurgitation usually will require early surgery.

VERTIGO
Robert A. Baldor, MD, FAAFP

BASICS

DESCRIPTION
- Sensation of movement ("room spinning") when no movement is actually occurring; results from peripheral/central causes, or may be induced by medications/anxiety disorders
- Important to distinguish between vertigo and presyncope (patient feels lightheaded; vision and hearing may become obscured)
- System(s) affected: Nervous
- Synonym(s): Dizziness; Acute vestibular neuronitis; Labyrinthitis; Benign paroxysmal positional vertigo (BPPV)

EPIDEMIOLOGY
Incidence
- Vertigo accounts for 54% of cases of dizziness reported in primary care; >90% of these patients are diagnosed with peripheral causes, such as BPPV.
- Predominant sex: Female = Male; women are more likely to experience central causes, particularly vertiginous migraine.

Geriatric Considerations
Patients who are elderly and have risk factors for cerebrovascular disease (CVD) are more likely to experience central causes.

Prevalence
- Ranges from 5–10% within the general population
- Lifetime prevalence for BPPV is 2.4%.

ETIOLOGY AND PATHOPHYSIOLOGY
Dysfunction of the rotational velocity sensors of the inner ear results in asymmetric central processing.
    This is related to the combination of sensory disturbance of motion and malfunction of the central vestibular apparatus.
- Peripheral causes: Acute labyrinthitis, acute vestibular neuronitis, BPPV, herpes-zoster oticus, cholesteatoma, Ménière disease, otosclerosis
- Central causes: Cerebellar tumor, CVD, migraine, multiple sclerosis
- Drug causes: Psychotropic agents (antipsychotics, antidepressants, anxiolytics, anticonvulsants, mood stabilizers), aspirin, aminoglycosides, furosemide, amiodarone
- Other causes: Cervical, psychological

Genetics
Family history of CVD/migraines may indicate higher risk of central causes.

RISK FACTORS
- History of migraines
- History of CVD/risk factors for CVD
- Use of ototoxic medications
- Trauma/Barotrauma
- Perilymphatic fistula
- Heavy weight bearing
- Psychosocial stress/depression
- Exposure to toxins

GENERAL PREVENTION
- Precautions to avoid injuries from falls that may occur secondary to imbalance
- If due to motion sickness, consider pretreatment with anticholinergics, such as scopolamine.

DIAGNOSIS

HISTORY
- Determine whether true vertigo exists vs. other causes of dizziness by asking the patient if he/she feels lightheaded OR sees the world spinning around during a dizzy spell. Spinning is indicative of true vertigo (1)[C].
- Ask about the presence of the following symptoms: Dizziness, rotary illusions, nystagmus, nausea and vomiting, hearing loss, diaphoresis, pain, neurologic symptoms (e.g., ataxia).
- Factors that may help to distinguish between peripheral and central causes:
  - Timing and duration:
    ○ Seconds–minutes: Peripheral
    ○ Minutes–hours: Peripheral/Central
    ○ Days: Peripheral/Central
    ○ Weeks: Central/Psychological
  - Provoking factors:
    ○ Changes in head position: Peripheral/Central
    ○ Spontaneous episodes: Peripheral/Central
    ○ Recent upper viral respiratory infection: Peripheral
    ○ Stress: Central/Psychological
    ○ Immunosuppression: Peripheral
    ○ Changes in ear pressure: Peripheral
  - Associated symptoms:
    ○ Rotary illusions with nausea and vomiting: Peripheral
    ○ Horizontal and rotational nystagmus: Peripheral
    ○ Horizontal, vertical, or rotational nystagmus: Central
    ○ Hearing loss: Peripheral
    ○ Neurologic symptoms: Central
- Obtain medical and medication history:
  - Recent use of ototoxic medications (e.g., aminoglycosides)
  - History of alcohol, nicotine, and caffeine use
  - Sexual history
  - History of CVD/risk factors for CVD

PHYSICAL EXAM
- Neurologic: Cranial nerves for signs of palsies, nystagmus
- Balance:
  - Peripheral: Mild to moderate, able to walk
  - Central: Severe, unable to walk
- Dix-Hallpike maneuver (PPV 83%, NPV 52%), performed by rapidly moving the patient from a sitting position to the supine position with the head turned 45° to the right. After waiting 20–30 seconds, observe for nystagmus, the patient is returned to the sitting position. If no nystagmus was observed, the procedure then is repeated on the left side:
  - The presence of nystagmus indicates a positive test, implying that peripheral causes should be investigated.
  - If induced nystagmus does not subside, consider central causes.

- Head and neck: Tympanic membranes:
  - Vesicles: Herpes-zoster oticus
  - Cholesteatoma
- Cardiovascular: Orthostatic changes in BP, dehydration/autonomic dysfunction

DIFFERENTIAL DIAGNOSIS
- Acoustic neuroma
- Anxiety disorder
- BPPV
- Cerebellar degeneration, hemorrhage, or tumor
- Labyrinthitis/Labyrinthine concussion
- Ménière disease
- Multiple sclerosis
- Perilymphatic fistula
- Syphilis
- Vascular ischemia
- Vertiginous migraine
- Vestibular neuronitis/ototoxicity

DIAGNOSTIC TESTS & INTERPRETATION
Initial Tests (lab, imaging)
- Consider CBC/chemistry panel in the absence of clinical findings pointing to a specific cause. Not routinely necessary.
- Consider MRI in the presence of other neurologic symptoms, risk factors for CVD, or progressive unilateral hearing loss.

Diagnostic Procedures/Other
Audiometry if acoustic neuroma or Ménière disease is suspected

TREATMENT

- Epley maneuver for BPPV (2)[A] (Video of technique available at www.youtube.com.)
- Modified Epley maneuver for BPPV (3)[B]
- Vestibular exercises for acute vestibular neuronitis (3)[B]
- Low-salt diet and diuretics for Ménière disease (3)[B]
- Migraine prophylaxis, migraine abortive medications, and vestibular exercises for vertiginous migraines (3)[B]
- SSRIs when associated with anxiety disorders (3)[B]
- Vestibular-suppressant medications for symptom relief in acute vestibular neuronitis (3,4)[C]

GENERAL MEASURES
- Provide an explanation and offer assurance to avoid anxiety that may exacerbate symptoms.
- Treatments depend on cause:
  - BPPV: Epley maneuver/modified Epley maneuver (2)[A]
  - Vestibular neuronitis and labyrinthitis:
    ○ Vestibular-suppressant medications (3,4)[C]
    ○ Vestibular rehabilitation exercises (3)[B]
  - Ménière disease (see separate topic):
    ○ Low-salt diet (<1–2 g/d) (3)[B]
    ○ Diuretics, such as hydrochlorothiazide (3)[B]
  - Vascular ischemia: Prevention of future events through BP reduction, lipid lowering, smoking cessation, antiplatelet therapy, and anticoagulation, if necessary
  - Vertiginous migraines: Dietary and lifestyle modifications, vestibular rehabilitation exercises, prophylactic and migraine abortive medications (3)[B]
  - Drug-induced vertigo: Discontinue causative agent.
  - Psychological: SSRIs (3)[B]

MEDICATION
Avoid use of medication in mild cases. Use for acute phase only (few days at most) as longer-term use may impair adaptation/compensation by the brain. Medications not recommended for BPPV:
- Meclizine: 12.5–50 mg PO q4–8h (3,4)[C]
- Dimenhydrinate: 25–100 mg PO, IM, or IV q4–8h (3,4)[C]:
  - Precautions: Concomitant use of CNS depressants, prostatic hyperplasia, glaucoma
  - Adverse effects: Sedation, xerostomia
  - Interactions: CNS depressants
  - Prochlorperazine: 5–10 mg PO or IM q6–8h; 25 mg rectally q12h; 5–10 mg by slow IV over 2 minutes (3,4)[C]:
    ○ Contraindications: Blood dyscrasias, age <2 years, severe hypotension
    ○ Precautions: Children with acute illness, glaucoma, history of breast cancer, impaired cardiovascular function, pregnancy, prostatic hyperplasia
    ○ Adverse effects: Sedation, xerostomia, hypotension, extrapyramidal effects
    ○ Interactions: Phenothiazines, tricyclic antidepressants
  - Metoclopramide: 5–10 mg PO q6h, 5–10 mg slow IV q6h:
    ○ Contraindications: Concomitant use of drugs with extrapyramidal effects, seizure disorders
    ○ Precautions: History of depression, Parkinson disease, hypertension
    ○ Adverse effects: Sedation, fluid retention, constipation
    ○ Interactions: Linezolid, cyclosporine, digoxin, levodopa

  - Benzodiazepines (3,4)[C]:
    ○ Diazepam: 2–10 mg PO or IV q4–8h
    ○ Lorazepam: 0.5–2 mg PO, IM, or IV q4–8h:
      ■ Contraindications: Acute angle-closure glaucoma, age <6 months
      ■ Precautions: Concomitant use of CNS depressants, hepatic insufficiency, pregnancy
      ■ Adverse effects: Sedation, respiratory depression, hypotension
      ■ Interactions: CNS depressants

Geriatric Considerations
Use vestibular-suppressant medications with caution due to increased risk of falls and urinary retention.

Pregnancy Considerations
Meclizine and dimenhydrinate are pregnancy Category B.

ISSUES FOR REFERRAL
Consider referral to otolaryngologist, ENT specialist, vestibular rehabilitation therapist, or neurologist if patient requires further care.

ADDITIONAL THERAPIES
- Epley maneuver/modified Epley maneuver for BPPV to displace calcium deposits in the semicircular canals (2)[A]:
  - Effective for short-term symptomatic improvement and for converting patient from positive to negative Dix-Hallpike maneuver
  - Contraindications: Carotid stenosis, unstable cardiac disease, severe neck disease
- Vestibular rehabilitation exercises (3)[B]: Ball toss, lying-to-standing, target-change, thumb-tracking, tightrope, walking turns

 ## ONGOING CARE

FOLLOW-UP RECOMMENDATIONS
Balance exercises should be adhered to for symptom reduction and return to normal activities of daily living (ADLs).

Patient Monitoring
After 1–2 weeks, assess for the following:
- Recurrence of symptoms
- New-onset symptoms
- Medication-related adverse effects
- Relief from vestibular rehabilitation exercises

DIET
- Restricted salt intake for Ménière disease
- Dietary modifications for vertiginous migraine

PATIENT EDUCATION
- Reduce sodium intake (Ménière disease).
- Avoid triggers, such as caffeine/alcohol (vertiginous migraine).

PROGNOSIS
Depends on diagnosis and response to treatment

COMPLICATIONS
- Anxiety
- Depression
- Disability
- Injuries from falls

REFERENCES
1. Labuguen RH. Initial evaluation of vertigo. *Am Fam Physician*. 2006;73:244–251.
2. Hilton M, Pinder D. The Epley (canalith repositioning) maneuver for benign paroxysmal positional vertigo. *Cochrane Database Syst Rev*. 2007;(3):CD003162.
3. Swartz R, Longwell P. Treatment of vertigo. *Am Fam Physician*. 2005;71:1115–1122.
4. Hain TC, Uddin M. Pharmacological treatment of vertigo. *CNS Drugs*. 2003;17:85–100.

ADDITIONAL READING
- Bhattacharyya N, Baugh RF, Orvidas L. Clinical practice guideline: Benign paroxysmal positional vertigo. *Otolaryngol Head Neck Surg*. 2008;139: S47–S81.
- Fife TD, Iverson DJ, Lempert T. Practice parameter: Therapies for benign paroxysmal positional vertigo (an evidence-based review): Report of the Quality Standards Subcommittee of the American Academy of Neurology. *Neurology*. 2008;70:2067–2074.

 ## SEE ALSO
- Ménière Disease, Motion Sickness
- Algorithm: Vertigo

 ## CODES

ICD10
- H81.10 Benign paroxysmal vertigo, unspecified ear
- H81.10 Benign paroxysmal vertigo, unspecified ear
- R42 Dizziness and giddiness

CLINICAL PEARLS
- Risk factors include history of migraines, history of CVD/CVD risk factors, use of ototoxic medications, trauma/barotrauma, perilymphatic fistula, heavy weight bearing, psychosocial stress, and exposure to toxins.
- The presence of nystagmus indicates a positive Dix-Hallpike test, implies a peripheral causes. If nystagmus persists, investigate a central cause.
- The Epley maneuver is recommended for the treatment of BPPV; this maneuver repositions calcium debris within the semicircular canals to provide relief from vertigo; a modified version of the maneuver can be performed at home.
- Medications are not recommended for BPPV.

V

VERTIGO, BENIGN PAROXYSMAL POSITIONAL

Janet Odry Helminski, PT, PhD • Mark A. Sanders, DO, JD, MPH, LLM, FACOFP • Tinh Le, DO, MBA

 BASICS

DESCRIPTION
- Benign paroxysmal positional vertigo (BPPV) is a mechanical disorder of the inner ear characterized by a brief period of vertigo experienced when the position of the patient's head is changed relative to gravity.
- The brief period of vertigo is caused by abnormal stimulation of ≥1 of the 3 semicircular canals of the inner ear, with the posterior canal most commonly affected.
- BPPV is the single most common cause of vertigo.

EPIDEMIOLOGY
- The lifetime prevalence of BPPV is 2.4% and the 1-year incidence is 0.6% (1). The age of onset is most commonly between the 5th and 7th decades of life, and the incidence of BPPV increases with each decade of life, peaking in the 6th and 7th decades (1).
- Prevalent sex: Female > Male (1).
- BPPV affects the quality of life of elderly patients and is associated with reduced activities of daily living scores, falls, and depression (2).

Prevalence
Common

ETIOLOGY AND PATHOPHYSIOLOGY
- In BPPV, calcite particles (otoconia) that normally weight the sensory membrane of the maculae become dislodged and settle into the canals, changing the dynamics of the canals. Reorientation of the canal relative to gravity causes the otoconia to move to the lowest part of the canal, creating a drag on the endolymph and activating the primary afferent sensory apparatus. This results in the generation of nystagmus and the associated sensation of vertigo.
- BPPV may be idiopathic, posttraumatic, or associated with viral neurolabyrinthitis.

 DIAGNOSIS

The diagnosis is established based on history and findings on positional testing (3,4)[B]. Positional tests place the plane of the canal being tested into the plane parallel with gravity.

HISTORY
- Brief episodes of vertigo (sensation that the room is spinning) associated with:
  – Rolling over in bed
  – Getting out of bed
  – Looking up (referred to as "top-shelf syndrome")
  – Bending forward
  – Quick head movements
- Patients may also complain of lightheadedness or feeling "off balance."
- Frequently patients complain of nausea and, if severe enough, vomiting.

PHYSICAL EXAM
- The Dix-Hallpike Test (DHT) is used to diagnosis BPPV (3,4)[A]. The test provokes the characteristic nystagmus associated with the symptoms of vertigo.
- To perform the DHT, the patient is positioned in long-sitting on the exam table with the knees extended. If testing the right posterior canal, the head is rotated 45° to the right. The patient is then lowered to supine with the head 20° below the horizontal, over the edge of the exam table. The position is maintained for a minimum of 45 seconds. The patient is then returned to the seated position. The procedure is repeated toward the left.
- For each position, the clinician notes the direction of the fast phase of the nystagmus and the latency and duration of the nystagmus. For posterior canal BPPV, in the head hanging position, the superior poles of the eyes beat up and rotate toward the lower-most ear, the involved ear. On return to the seated position, the nystagmus reverses direction. The latency of onset of nystagmus is 1–45 seconds, and the duration is usually <1 minute. The nystagmus fatigues (reduction in the severity of symptoms) with repeated positioning. For anterior canal BPPV, in the head hanging position, the eyes will beat down and rotate toward the involved ear. For lateral canal BPPV, a directional changing positional nystagmus is observed. The eyes will beat horizontally toward the lower-most ear or will beat away from the floor in the head left and right position.
- Alternative positional tests are available if the patient is unable to assume the test positions (side-lying test) or if the lateral canal is involved (supine roll test).
- No further testing is indicated unless the diagnosis is uncertain or there are additional symptoms and signs unrelated to BPPV that warrant testing (3)[C].

DIFFERENTIAL DIAGNOSIS
- Orthostatic hypotension and other disorders that cause low BP; symptoms usually occur when the patient stands up
- Damage to the brainstem or cerebellum can cause positional vertigo, but is accompanied by other neurologic signs and usually has a different pattern of nystagmus.
- Low spinal fluid pressure may cause positional symptoms that are worse when lying down.
- Migraine-associated vertigo

 TREATMENT

- The Canalith Repositioning Procedure (CRP) or Epley maneuver is effective in the treatment of posterior canal BPPV (3,4)[A]. The clinician moves the patient through a series of positions. With each position, the otoconia settles to the lowest part of the canal. The debris is moved around the arc of the canal into the vestibule. In randomized controlled trials, the average short-term success rate of the CRP following 1 treatment session is 80 ± 9% (4)[A]. Contraindications are carotid stenosis, unstable cardiac disease, and severe neck disease. If the CRP is ineffective, self-administered CRP is performed at home (3,4)[A]. The patient performs the CRP on the bed over the edge of the pillow. Better outcomes are achieved with a combination of CRP with self-administered CPR (4,5)[A].
- CRP illustrated for right posterior canal BPPV. The clinician moves the patient through a series of 4 provoking positions, starting with the placement of the right posterior canal (involved canal) in the right head-hanging position of the DHT. The head is then rotated a total of 90° toward the left (uninvolved side) into 45° of left head rotation. Maintaining 45° of left head rotation, the patient is rolled onto the left side (uninvolved side) with the head slightly elevated from the supporting surface. The patient then sits up. Each position is maintained for a minimum of 45 seconds or as long as the nystagmus lasts. The procedure is repeated 3 times.
- Postmaneuver activity restrictions are often advocated (4)[C]. For 1 week following the maneuver, patients should avoid lying on the involved side, use 2 pillows to sleep slightly elevated, and avoid up-and-down movements of the head.

MEDICATION

- Vestibular suppressant medications are not recommended for treatment of BPPV, other than for the short-term management of vegetative symptoms (3)[C].
- Antiemetics such as ondansetron (Zofran) may be considered for prophylaxis for patients who have had severe nausea or vomiting with the DHT.
- Vestibular suppressants such as benzodiazepines and antihistamines should be avoided because they may suppress nystagmus during the DHT and treatment.

ISSUES FOR REFERRAL

Consider a referral to a specialist if BPPV is unresponsive to treatment or if the patient is diagnosed with atypical BPPV involving the anterior or lateral canal. Other maneuvers are available for treatment of typical and atypical BPPV. Consider referring to a physical therapist, ENT specialist, or neurologist.

ADDITIONAL THERAPIES

- Brandt-Daroff exercises are not as effective as self-administered CRP. At 1 week, the average success rate for the Brandt-Daroff exercise is 23–24% compared with 90% for self-administered CRP (4)[A].
- Surgical intervention is rarely indicated, except for refractory BPPV, and includes posterior canal occlusion and singular neurectomy.

 ONGOING CARE

FOLLOW-UP RECOMMENDATIONS
The patient should follow-up within a week after treatment to ensure resolution.

PATIENT EDUCATION
A number of illustrative videos are available on www.youtube.com

PROGNOSIS
- 30% of patients diagnosed with BPPV will spontaneously resolve within 1 week.
- BPPV often recurs. Of patients treated successfully, 25% redevelop BPPV within 1 year and 44% redevelop BPPV within 2 years.

COMPLICATIONS
During the maneuvers, a canal conversion may occur. The debris from the canal being treated may reflux into another canal.

REFERENCES

1. von Brevern M, Radtke A, Lezius F, et al. Epidemiology of benign paroxysmal positional vertigo: A population based study. *J Neurol Neurosurg Psychiatry*. 2007;78:710–715.
2. Oghalai JS, Manolidis S, Barth JL, et al. Unrecognized benign paroxysmal positional vertigo in elderly patients. *Otolaryngol Head Neck Surg*. 2000;122:630–634.
3. Bhattacharyya N, Baugh RF, Orvidas L, et al. Clinical practice guideline: Benign paroxysmal positional vertigo. *Otolaryngol Head Neck Surg*. 2008;139(Suppl 4):S47–S81.
4. Helminski JO, Zee DS, Janssen I, et al. Effectiveness of particle repositioning manuevers in the treatment of benign paroxysmal positional vertigo: A systematic review. *Phys Ther*. 2010;90:663–678.
5. Radtke A, von Brevern M, Tiel-Wilck K, et al. Self-treatment of benign paroxysmal positional vertigo: Semont maneuver vs Epley procedure. *Neurology*. 2004;63:150–152.

ADDITIONAL READING

Fife TD, Iverson DJ, Lempert T, et al. Practice parameter: Therapies for benign paroxysmal positional vertigo (an evidence-based review): Report of the Quality Standards Subcommittee of the American Academy of Neurology. *Neurology*. 2008;70: 2067–2074.

 CODES

ICD10
- H81.10 Benign paroxysmal vertigo, unspecified ear
- H81.11 Benign paroxysmal vertigo, right ear
- H81.12 Benign paroxysmal vertigo, left ear

CLINICAL PEARLS

- The diagnosis of BPPV is based on history and findings on positional testing (Dix-Hallpike test).
- The typical presentation is reports of brief episodes of vertigo (sensation that the room is spinning) associated with head movements.
- BPPV may be treated effectively with particle-repositioning maneuvers.
- Vestibular suppressant medications are not recommended for treatment of BPPV, other than for the short-term management of symptoms.

V

VINCENT STOMATITIS

Robert A. Baldor, MD

BASICS

DESCRIPTION
- Inflammatory oral infection of the gingiva
- Disease caused by *Fusobacterium,* spirochetes, and heavy growth of oral flora (1)
- Concomitant infection with Epstein-Barr virus, herpes simplex virus, and type 1 human cytomegalovirus is common (2).
- Organisms invade gingiva and oral papillae with the formation of a pseudomembranous exudate.
- Clinical presentation includes ulceration, halitosis, pain, bleeding, and necrosis.
- Synonym(s): Vincent angina; Trench mouth; Acute necrotizing ulcerative gingivitis

EPIDEMIOLOGY
Incidence
- Predominant age: 18–21 years in developed countries (3)
- 3–14 years of age among malnourished children

Prevalence
- A Chilean study of 9,203 students aged 12–21 years revealed a prevalence of 6.7% (3).
- Overall prevalence decreases with age

ETIOLOGY AND PATHOPHYSIOLOGY
- Impaired host immunologic response due to immunocompromise or malnutrition
- Loss of integrity of the oral mucosa
- Increased bacterial attachment with herpesvirus active infection

RISK FACTORS
- Poor oral hygiene
- Infrequent or absent dental care
- Malnutrition
- Tobacco use
- Herpesvirus infection
- Immunosuppression
- Psychological stress
- Diabetes
- Down syndrome

GENERAL PREVENTION
- Regular dental care
- Proper oral hygiene
- Appropriate nutrition
- Prompt recognition and institution of therapy
- Stress management

COMMONLY ASSOCIATED CONDITIONS
- Bacteremia
- Osteomyelitis
- Tooth loss
- Noma/Cancrum oris, which can be life-threatening
- Aspiration pneumonia (4)

DIAGNOSIS

HISTORY
- Acute onset of gingival ulcer
- Halitosis (5)[C]
- Painful, bleeding, and inflamed gingiva
- Fever
- Malaise
- History of immunosuppression chemotherapy, HIV infection
- History of herpesvirus infection

PHYSICAL EXAM
- Ulceration of the oral papillae
- Inflamed, erythematous gingiva
- Formation of gray, pseudomembranous exudate
- Necrotic tissue on gingiva and surrounding structures
- Cervical lymphadenopathy

DIFFERENTIAL DIAGNOSIS
- Herpes simplex virus
- Periodontitis
- Pericoronitis
- Medication side effects
- Oral malignancy
- Xerostomia
- Diphtheria (6)
- Lymphoma (6)
- Primary syphilis (6)

DIAGNOSTIC TESTS & INTERPRETATION
Initial Tests (lab, imaging)
- Aerobic and anaerobic cultures of inflamed or débrided tissue
- Group A strep rapid antigen detection assay (7)[C]
- Group A strep throat culture (7)[C]
- Blood cultures if systemic involvement
- Dental radiographs
- Facial radiographs or CT of the neck and sinuses if infection has progressed

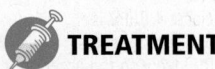

TREATMENT

MEDICATION
- Decision regarding locus of treatment (outpatient or inpatient) and route (PO or IV) depends on the degree of systemic illness present and on the involvement of structures in the neck.
- Medication regimens provided below are for outpatient treatment.
- The same antibiotics may be used IV.

First Line
- Penicillin V K 500 mg q6h for 7–10 days (8)[C]
- Amoxicillin-clavulanate 875 mg q12h for 7–10 days

Second Line
- Metronidazole 500 mg q12h for 7–10 days
- Clindamycin 450 mg q8h for 7–10 days

ISSUES FOR REFERRAL
Patients can be evaluated and treated by oral surgeon, dentist/periodontist, or ear, nose, and throat specialist depending on patient preference and severity of infection.

ADDITIONAL THERAPIES
- Chlorhexidine gluconate or salt water rinses
- Pain management with NSAIDs

SURGERY/OTHER PROCEDURES
- Debridement of inflamed and necrotic tissue
- Dental extraction

IN-PATIENT CONSIDERATIONS
Admission Criteria/Initial Stabilization
- Failure of oral antibiotics and disease progression
- Need for parenteral antibiotics and analgesia
- Inability to meet nutritional needs

IV Fluids
May be required if patient is unable to tolerate oral fluids

Discharge Criteria
- Arrest of disease progression and improvement at site
- Ability to tolerate oral antibiotics and fluids
- Oral analgesia is effective.

ONGOING CARE

FOLLOW-UP RECOMMENDATIONS
Frequent dental cleanings and examinations

DIET
- Proper nutrition
- Multivitamin supplementation

PATIENT EDUCATION
- Proper nutrition
- Appropriate oral hygiene
- Tobacco cessation
- Stress management

COMPLICATIONS
- Malnutrition
- Pain
- Poor dentition, tooth loss
- Systemic infection
- Involvement of soft tissues and structures of the neck

REFERENCES

1. Miyairi I, Franklin JA, Andreansky M, et al. Acute necrotizing ulcerative gingivitis and bacteremia caused by *Stenotrophomonas maltophilia* in an immunocompromised host. *Pediatr Infect Dis J*. 2005;24:181–183.
2. Slots J. Herpesviral-bacterial synergy in the pathogenesis of human periodontitis. *Curr Opin Infect Dis*. 2007;20:278–283.
3. Lopez R, Fernandez O, Jara G, et al. Epidemiology of necrotizing ulcerative gingival lesions in adolescents. *J Periodont Res*. 2002;37:439–444.
4. Marik PE. Pulmonary aspiration syndromes. *Curr Opin Pulm Med*. 2011;84:148–154.
5. Porter SR. Diet and halitosis. *Curr Opin Clin Nutr Metab Care*. 2011;14:463–468.
6. Carlson JA, Dabiri G, Cribier B, et al. The immunopathobiology of syphilis: The manifestations and course of syphilis are determined by the level of delayed-type hypersensitivity. *Am J Dermatopathol*. 2011;84: 433–460.
7. Bisno AL, Gerber MA, Gwaltney JM, et al. Practice guidelines for the diagnosis and management of group A streptococcal pharyngitis. Infectious Diseases Society of America. *Clin Infect Dis*. 2002;84:113–125.
8. Edwards PC, Kanjirath P. Recognition and management of common acute conditions of the oral cavity resulting from tooth decay, periodontal disease, and trauma: An update for the family physician. *J Am Board Fam Med*. 2010;23: 285–294.

CODES

ICD10
A69.1 Other Vincent's infections

CLINICAL PEARLS
- Poor oral hygiene and immunosuppression are key factors in infection.
- Early recognition and institution of therapy decrease complications.
- Penicillin is the drug of choice for patients not systemically ill.

VITAMIN B$_{12}$ DEFICIENCY
Catherine Chamberlain, MD • Edward Feller, MD

BASICS

- Vitamin deficiency related to inadequate intake or inability to absorb cobalamin (vitamin B$_{12}$).
- Cobalamin is critical for CNS functioning.
- Deficiency can cause megaloblastic anemia and diverse neurologic disorders
  - Neurologic disorders are due to demyelination of cervical, thoracic dorsal and lateral spinal cords, demyelination of white matter, and demyelination of cranial and peripherial nerves

DESCRIPTION
Normal B$_{12}$ absorption:

- B$_{12}$ present in animal-source foods (meat, fish, eggs, milk) and foods fortified with B$_{12}$
- Dietary vitamin B$_{12}$ (cobalamin) bound to food is cleaved by acids in stomach and bound to haptocorrin (commonly known as R-factor)
- Duodenal proteases cleave B$_{12}$ from haptocorrin.
- In duodenum, B$_{12}$ uptake depends on binding to intrinsic factor (IF) secreted by gastric parietal cells.
- B$_{12}$-IF complex is absorbed by terminal ileum into portal circulation.
- Body's B$_{12}$ stored in liver = 50%:
  - B$_{12}$ secreted into bile from liver recycled via enterohepatic circulation
  - Delay 5–10 years from onset of B$_{12}$ deficiency to clinical symptoms due to hepatic stores and enterohepatic circulation
- Typical Western diet: 3–30 mcg/d (1):
  - Recommend 2.4 mcg/d for adults and 2.6–2.8 mcg/d during pregnancy (most prenatal vitamins contain B$_{12}$).

EPIDEMIOLOGY
Prevalence
- Endemic area: Northern Europe, including Scandinavia; more common in those of African ancestry.
- Prevalence 5–20% in developed countries (2):
  - 12% in elderly living in community
  - 30–40% in elderly in institutions, sick, or malnourished
  - 5% patients in tertiary reference hospitals
- Prevalence by age group (2):
  - 20–39 years old: Prevalence 3%
  - 40–59 years old: Prevalence 4%
  - >70 years old: Prevalence 6%

ETIOLOGY AND PATHOPHYSIOLOGY
- Decreased oral intake:
  - Vegetarians and vegans: B$_{12}$ is found in animal-source foods; however, strict vegetarians uncommonly develop deficiency because only 1 mg/d is needed, with adequate amounts present in legumes.

- Decreased intrinsic factor:
  - Pernicious anemia (PA): Autoantibodies directed toward gastric intrinsic factors
  - Chronic atrophic gastritis: Autoimmune attack on gastric parietal cells causing autoimmune gastritis and leading to decreased IF production
  - Gastrectomy: Removal of entire or part of stomach decreases amount of parietal cells
- Decreased ileal absorption:
  - Crohn disease: Terminal ileal inflammation decreases body's ability to absorb B$_{12}$
  - Chronic alcoholism: Decreases body's ability to absorb B$_{12}$
  - Ileal resection
  - Pancreatic insufficiency: Pancreatic proteases are required to cleave the vitamin B$_{12}$-haptocorrin bond to allow vitamin B$_{12}$ to bind to intrinsic factor.
  - *Helicobacter pylori* infection: Impairs release of B$_{12}$ from bound proteins
- Medications: Proton pump inhibitors (PPIs), H$_2$ antagonists, antacids decrease gastric acidity, inhibiting B$_{12}$ release from dietary protein; metformin
- Hereditary (rare):
  - Imerslund-Grasbeck disease (juvenile megaloblastic anemia)
  - Congenital deficiency of transcobalamin
  - Severe methylene tetrahydrofolate reductase deficiency
  - Abnormalities of methionine synthesis

  Causes:
- Food-cobalamin malabsorption syndrome (1,2):
  - As many as 50% of cases
  - Primary cause in elderly
  - Pathophysiology: Inability to release cobalamin from food or binding protein, especially if in the setting of hypochlorhydria
  - Causes: Atrophic gastritis, long-term ingestion of antacids and biguanides, possible relationship to *H. pylori* infection
- PA (1,3):
  - 1/3 of all cases; most frequent cause of severe disease. Neurologic disorders are common presenting complaints.
  - Common in elderly, as high as 20%, with mild atrophic gastritis, hypochlorhydria, and impaired release of dietary vitamin B$_{12}$
  - Autoimmune disease with destruction of gastric fundal mucosa cells via a cell-mediated process
  - Antigastric parietal cell antibodies: Sensitivity >90%, specificity 50%; use for screening test
  - Anti-intrinsic factor antibodies: Sensitivity 50%
  - Associated with other autoimmune diseases
- Insufficient dietary intake: 2% of cases; vegans or long-standing vegetarians (1)
- Infants born to vitamin B$_{12}$ deficient mothers may have deficiency or develop it if breastfed exclusively (4).

- Intestinal causes (1,3):
  - 1% of cases; prevalence depends on risk factors, such as surgical conditions noted below.
  - Gastrectomy: Due to decreased production of intrinsic factor
  - Gastric bypass: Appears 1–9 years after surgery, prevalence 12–33%
  - Ileal resection or disease
  - Fish tapeworm
  - Severe pancreatic insufficiency
- Undetermined etiology (1):
  - 1/10 of cases

Genetics
Imerslund-Grasbeck disease (juvenile megaloblastic anemia): Inadequate uptake of B$_{12}$-IF complex

GENERAL PREVENTION
Risk factors: Vegan diet, age >65, female, chronic atrophic gastritis, Crohn disease or other ileal disorders, chronic PPI, or metformin use

DIAGNOSIS

Symptoms and physical exam findings:

- Asymptomatic patients may be diagnosed by the incidental finding of anemia or an elevated mean corpuscular volume (MCV) during routine testing or evaluation of unassociated disorders.
- Hematological (1):
  - Frequent: Macrocytosis, hypersegmentation of neutrophils, spinal cord medullar megaloblastosis (blue spinal cord)
  - Rare: Isolated thrombocytopenia and neutropenia, pancytopenia
  - Very rare: Hemolytic anemia, thrombotic microangiopathy with schistocytes
- Neuropsychiatric (2,5):
  - Frequent: Sensory polyneuritis, paresthesias, positive Babinski sign, weakness, gait unsteadiness, loss of proprioception (impaired vibratory sensation, positive Romberg, ataxia, hyperreflexia)
  - Classic, but uncommon: Subacute combined degeneration of spinal cord associated with PA; myelin in the lateral and posterior columns degenerates; ataxia, proprioception and vibration loss, bowel and bladder incontinence, orthostatic hypotension, decreased memory (4)
  - Under investigation: Dementia, stroke, atherosclerosis, mania
- Digestive (1):
  - Classic: Hunter glossitis, jaundice, and high lactate dehydrogenase and bilirubin
  - Possible: Abdominal pain, dyspepsia, nausea, vomiting, diarrhea
  - Rare: Mucocutaneous ulcers
- Other (1):
  - Frequent: pallor, edema, jaundice
  - Under investigation: Chronic vaginal and urinary infections, atrophy of vaginal mucosa, hypofertility, venous thromboembolism, angina, miscarriages
  - Commonly insidious and nonspecific; thus, delay in diagnosis is common.

HISTORY
- Underlying disease associated with vitamin B_{12} deficiency
- Fatigue, anorexia
- Depression
- Falls (due to diminished proprioception)
- Loss of sensation in "stocking-glove" distribution
- Glossitis/loss of sense of taste, and other subtle, nonspecific neurologic symptoms

DIAGNOSTIC TESTS & INTERPRETATION
- Measurement of vitamin B_{12}, methylmalonic acid (MMA), and homocysteine, CBC (MCV)(2,6).
- Measurement of B_{12} may be low or low normal depending on institution's cutoff value (2,6)
  - 65–95% sensitivity levels <200 pg/mL
  - May need additional tests such as MMA and homocysteine depending on clinical suspicion
- MCV often increased
- Measurement of MMA
  - 98% sensitive
  - Levels increased in renal failure
- Measurement of homocysteine
  - 96% sensitive
  - Levels increased in folate deficiency and renal failure
- Other tests: Folate and other markers of anemia (iron studies)
- Other tests: Complete blood count. Low hemoglobin and hematocrit, MCV >95–100 fL
- MCV may be normal, decreased, or increased if vitamin B_{12} deficiency coexists with other forms of anemia, such as iron deficiency or hemolysis. Thus, RBCs may be normochromic, normocytic, or hypochromic microcytic.

ALERT
- Low levels of vitamin B_{12} are seen in folate deficiency, HIV, and multiple myeloma (6)
- Elevated levels of vitamin B_{12} are seen in renal disease, occult malignancy, alcoholic liver disease, and a result of technical error (2)
- Macrocytosis may be due to folate deficiency, reticulocytosis, medications, bone marrow dysplasia, hypothyroidism, or be masked by concomitant microcytic anemia (2,6)
- Serum homocysteine and MMA:
  - Elevated in B_{12} deficiency secondary to decreased metabolism
  - If both are normal, B_{12} deficiency is effectively ruled out.
  - If MMA is normal and homocysteine is increased, think folate deficiency.
- PA:
  - Check antibody to intrinsic factor; positive test is confirmatory for PA, but sensitivity is only 50–70%.
  - Anti-parietal cell antibody positivity indicated pernicious anemia
  - For patients who are antibody positive, consider screening for autoimmune thyroid disease

Pregnancy Considerations
Because B_{12} crosses the placenta, pregnant women with low levels of B_{12} are at higher risk of having children with neural tube defects or developmental delays and failure to thrive (5).

Diagnostic Procedures/Other
- Bone marrow exam, in selected cases, may help confirm the diagnosis of megaloblastic anemia.
- Spinal cord imaging is not standard; MRI in selected cases, especially with severe myelopathy

TREATMENT

MEDICATION
- Consider giving folate and vitamin B_{12} repletion together.
- IM cyanocobalamin (2):
  - 1,000 mcg/d for 7 days, *then*
  - 1,000 mcg weekly for 4 weeks, *then*
  - 1,000 mcg monthly for life
- Sublingual tablets, transdermal patches, oral or nasal sprays are investigational.
- High-dose, daily oral vitamin B_{12} at doses of 1,000–2,000 mcg may be as effective as monthly intramuscular injection. Long-term trials are in progress.

ALERT
Folic acid without vitamin B_{12} in patients with PA is contraindicated; will not correct neurologic abnormalities.

IN-PATIENT CONSIDERATIONS
Admission Criteria/Initial Stabilization
- Consider blood transfusion for severe anemia
- Draw blood for hematologic parameters before transfusing

ONGOING CARE

FOLLOW-UP RECOMMENDATIONS
Patient Monitoring
- Hematologic:
  - Reticulocytosis in 3–4 days
  - Rise in hemoglobin beginning at 10 days; usually will return to normal in ~8 weeks
  - Monitor potassium in profoundly anemic patients (hypokalemia due to potassium utilization)
  - Serum methylmalonic acid decreases with replacement therapy.
- Neurologic: Symptoms may be irreversible.

DIET
Meat, animal protein, and legumes unless contraindicated

REFERENCES
1. Allen LH. How common is vitamin B_{12} deficiency? *Am J Clin Nutr*. 2009;84: 693S–696S.
2. Stabler SP. Vitamin B_{12} deficiency. *N Engl J Med*. 2013;368:149–160.
3. Fernández- Bañares F, Monzón H, Forné M. A short review of malabsorption and anemia. *World J Gastroenterol*. 2009;84:4644–4652.
4. Hinton CF, Ojodu JA, Fernhoff PM, et al. Maternal and neonatal vitamin B_{12} deficiency detected through expanded newborn screening—United States, 2003–2007. *J Pediatr*. 2010;157:162–163.
5. Lachner C, Steinle NI, Regenold WT. The neuropsychiatry of vitamin B_{12} deficiency in elderly patients. *J Neuropsychiatry Clin Neurosci*. 2012; 24:5–15.
6. Oberley MJ, Yang DT. Laboratory testing for cobalamin deficiency in megaloblastic anemia. *Am J Hematol*. 2013;88:522–526.

ADDITIONAL READING
Langan RC, Zawistoski KJ. Update on vitamin B_{12} deficiency. *Am Fam Phys*. 2011;83:1425–1430.

CODES

ICD10
- D51.0 Vitamin B12 defic anemia due to intrinsic factor deficiency
- D51.3 Other dietary vitamin B12 deficiency anemia
- E53.8 Deficiency of other specified B group vitamins

CLINICAL PEARLS
- Schilling test, the classic procedure to diagnose PA, is no longer available in many parts of the country.
- Consider monitoring B_{12} levels annually if on metformin.
- Correcting folate deficiency without treating with vitamin B_{12} in megaloblastic anemia may correct hematologic, but not neurologic, disorders.
- Vitamin B_{12} deficiency can coexist with other causes of anemia, including iron deficiency or hemolysis; thus, MCV can be normal, decreased, or increased.
- For patients with pernicious anemia, vitamin B_{12} replacement must be lifelong.

V

VITAMIN D DEFICIENCY

Frank J. Domino, MD • Samir Malkani, MD, MRCP (UK)

 BASICS

This topic covers the commonly acquired vitamin D deficiency and not type II vitamin D–resistant rickets/type I pseudovitamin D–resistant rickets (both rare autosomal–recessive disorders).

DESCRIPTION
- Vitamin D is both a hormone and a vitamin.
- Cholecalciferol (D3) is synthesized in the skin by exposure to ultraviolet B (UV-B) radiation. Ergocalciferol (D2) and D3 are present in foods.
- D2 and D3 are hydroxylated in the liver to 25 vitamin D (calcidiol), its major circulating form.
- Calcidiol is further hydroxylated in the kidney to the active metabolite 1,25 vitamin D (calcitriol).
- Hypocalcemia stimulates parathyroid hormone (PTH) to be secreted, which prompts the increased conversion of 25 vitamin D to 1,25 vitamin D.
  - 1,25 vitamin D decreases renal calcium and phosphorus excretion, increases intestinal calcium and phosphorus absorption, and increases osteoclast activity. These effects increase serum calcium.

EPIDEMIOLOGY
- Unclear in general population
- In the community, a cohort study of asymptomatic adolescents in Boston found 24.1% were deficient, with 4.6% severely deficient (1).
- A study of hospitalized patients in Massachusetts found 57% vitamin D deficient (VDD).
- Women with history of osteoporosis/osteoporotic fracture have high prevalence of vitamin D deficiency.
- A cross-sectional study of patients with persistent, nonspecific pain in an urban Minneapolis primary care clinic found 93% deficient and 28% severely deficient (2).
- A cohort study in Arizona found >25% of adults were VDD; highest rates among African Americans and Hispanics (3).
- Prevalence of vitamin D Deficiency is increased in obese individuals (4).

Pediatric Considerations
NHANES data found 70% of children did not have sufficient 25 OH vitamin D serum levels (9% deficient and 61% insufficient), which was associated with an increase in BP and decrease in high-density lipoprotein (HDL) cholesterol (5)[B].

ETIOLOGY AND PATHOPHYSIOLOGY
- Insufficient dietary intake of vitamin D and/or lack of UV-B exposure results in low levels of vitamin D.
  - This limits calcium absorption, causing excess PTH to be released.
- PTH stimulates osteoclast activity, which helps to normalize calcium and phosphorous, but results in osteomalacia.
- Dietary deficiency:
  - Inadequate vitamin D intake
- Inadequate sunlight exposure:
  - Institutionalized/Hospitalized patients
  - Chronic illness: Liver/Kidney disease
- Malabsorptive states

Genetics
Vitamin D–dependant rickets type 1 occurs due to inactivating mutation of the 1 alpha hydroxylase gene; as a result calcidiol is not hydroxyated to calcitriol.

RISK FACTORS
- Inadequate sun exposure
- Female
- Dark skin
- Immigrant populations
- Low socioeconomic status
- Latitudes higher than 38°
- Elderly
- Institutionalized
- Depression
- Medications (phenobarbital, phenytoin)
- Gastric bypass surgery
- Obesity

GENERAL PREVENTION
- Adequate exposure to sunlight and dietary sources of vitamin D (plants, fish); many foods are fortified with vitamin D2 and D3.
- Recommended daily allowance from the 2010 Institute of Medicine Report is minimally 600 IU/d for those 1–70 years of age and 800 IU/d for those >70 years. Up to 4,000 IU/d is safe in healthy adults without risk of toxicity (6)[C].
- Higher intake of vitamin D recommended for age >50 years

- 2005 and 2009: Meta-analysis demonstrated for ages 51–70, minimally recommended supplementation is 800 IU/d to prevent nonvertebral fractures (7,8)[A].

Pediatric Considerations
The American Academy of Pediatrics recommends all breast-fed babies receive 400 IU/d of vitamin D beginning "within the 1st few days of life."

Pregnancy Considerations
ACOG recommends data insufficient to screen all pregnancies; only those "at risk" and states it is safe to take 1,000–2,000 IU/d during pregnancy (9)[B].

Geriatric Considerations
US Preventive Services Task Force recommends seniors take at least 800 IU/d vitamin D to reduce risk of falls in community-dwelling older adults (10)[A].

COMMONLY ASSOCIATED CONDITIONS
- Osteomalacia, osteoporosis
- Premenstrual syndrome
- Rickets
- Celiac disease
- Gastric bypass
- Chronic renal disease
- Bacterial vaginosis in pregnant women
- Hypertension

ALERT
VDD is associated with risk of myocardial infarction (MI): (11)[B] and all-cause mortality (12)[B].

 DIAGNOSIS

- Nonspecific musculoskeletal complaints
- Weak antigravity muscles
- Fracture with minimal trauma

HISTORY
- Senior citizens at risk of falling
- Renal disease
- GI (malabsorption) disorders
- Liver dysfunction
- Immigration from tropical to colder climates
- Dark-skinned/veiled individuals
- Housebound patients
- Women at perimenopause

PHYSICAL EXAM
- Vague neurologic signs: Numbness, proximal myopathy, paresthesias, muscle cramps, laryngospasm
- Chvostek sign: Contraction of the facial muscles by tapping along the facial nerve
- Trousseau phenomenon: Carpal spasms and paraesthesia produced by pressure on nerves and vessels of the upper arm, by inflation of a BP cuff
- Tetany, seizures

DIAGNOSTIC TESTS & INTERPRETATION
Initial Tests (lab, imaging)
- 25 OH vitamin D (most sensitive measure of vitamin D status)
- Vitamin D deficiency:
  - <20 ng/mL (13)
- PTH elevation: Not routinely obtained unless severe deficiency
- Low-normal/low calcium and phosphorous
- Elevated alkaline phosphatase (in later disease)
- Plain radiographs: If atypical fracture, radiographs may show osteomalacia (pseudofractures/looser zones) in pelvis, femur, and fibula.
- Osteoporosis screen (14)[C]:
  - Women ≥65 years with no risk factors
  - Women ≥60 years at risk: Body weight <70 kg (best predictor)
  - Less evidence: Smoking, low body mass index, family history, decreased activity, alcohol or caffeine use
  - African American women have higher bone density than Caucasians.

TREATMENT

- Treatment goals remain unclear, but current "normal" 25 OH vitamin D levels are based on suppression of PTH.
- Obesity: Treatment of VDD in obesity, especially those who are obese and depressed, improves outcomes.
- Hypertension: Vitamin D supplementation, especially those with dark skin, lowers BP in those with hypertension.

ALERT
All-cause mortality: Cochrane Systematic Review found vitamin D supplementation lowers all-cause mortality (15)[A].

Geriatric Considerations
In senior citizens, serum 25 OH vitamin D of 50 nmol/L resulted in optimal hip and greater trochanter BMD, and in best physical performance scores.

MEDICATION
- Vitamin D sufficient (25 OH Vitamin D ≥20 ng/mL):
  – Vitamin D 800–4,000 IU/d D2/D3
  – D3 (animal derived) may be slightly more effective than D2 (plant derived), but clinical significance is uncertain.
  – Calcium supplementation: Unclear benefit and may increase some CHD risk in patients. No supplementation currently required (see below).
- Vitamin D deficiency (25 OH vitamin D <20 ng/mL):
  – Ergocalciferol 50,000 IU/wk for 8–12 weeks, followed by 2,000–4,000 IU/d of vitamin D3
- Calcium: Meta-analysis data support:
  – Dietary intake of ~700 mg/d leads to best outcomes; higher doses did NOT decrease risk of osteoporotic fractures.
  – Only dietary, not supplementary, found to be beneficial
  – Supplementary calcium associated with an increased risk of MI, especially in women(16)[A].

ISSUES FOR REFERRAL
Endocrinology if no response to treatment

ADDITIONAL THERAPIES
Aggressive calcium in ICU patients with ionized calcium <3.2 mg/dL or if symptomatic (tetany, seizures, QT prolongation, bradycardia, or hypotension, or ventilated patient with decreased diaphragmatic function)

IN-PATIENT CONSIDERATIONS
Admission Criteria/Initial Stabilization
- Symptoms of severe hypocalcemia *or*
- Malabsorption syndromes

ONGOING CARE

FOLLOW-UP RECOMMENDATIONS
Follow-up of abnormal 25 OH vitamin D not currently required.

DIET
- Cod liver oil is most potent source of vitamin D and has ~1,300 IU vitamin D/tablet
- Fatty fish (tuna, salmon)
- Fortified milk (100 IU/8 oz), cereal, and foods

PROGNOSIS
- Systematic review of 63 observational studies found adequate 25 vitamin D levels correlated with lower rates of colon, breast, and prostate cancer.
- Cohort study found that vitamin D deficiency is correlated with increased risk of all-cause mortality (12)[B].

ALERT
Meta-analysis of 57,000 patients found supplementation of >500 IU/d lowered the risk of all-cause mortality (17)[A].

REFERENCES

1. Gordon CM, DePeter KC, Feldman HA, et al. Prevalence of vitamin D deficiency among healthy adolescents. *Arch Pediatr Adolesc Med.* 2004; 158:531–537.
2. Plotnikoff GA, Quigley JM. Prevalence of severe hypovitaminosis D in patients with persistent, nonspecific musculoskeletal pain. *Mayo Clin Proc.* 2003;78:1463–1470.
3. Jacobs ET, Alberts DS, Foote JA, et al. Vitamin D insufficiency in southern Arizona. *Am J Clin Nutr.* 2008;87:608–613.
4. Vimaleswaran KS, Berry DJ, Lu C et al. Causal relationship between obesity and vitamin D status: Bi-directional mendelian randomization analysis of multiple cohorts. *PLOS Medicine.* 2013;10:e1001383.
5. Kumar J, Muntner P, Kaskel FJ, et al. Prevalence and associations of 25-hydroxyvitamin D deficiency in US children: NHANES 2001–2004. *Pediatrics.* 2009;124(3):e362–e370.
6. Ross AC, Manson JE, Abrams SA, et al. The 2011 report on dietary reference intakes for calcium and vitamin D from the Institute of Medicine: What clinicians need to know. *J Clin Endocrinol Metab.* 2011;96:53–58.
7. Bischoff-Ferrari HA, Willett WC, Wong JB, et al. Fracture prevention with vitamin D supplementation: A meta-analysis of randomized controlled trials. *JAMA.* 2005;293:2257–2264.
8. Bischoff-Ferrari HA, Willett WC, Wong JB, et al. Prevention of nonvertebral fractures with oral vitamin D and dose dependency: A meta-analysis of randomized controlled trials. *Arch Intern Med.* 2009;169:551–561.
9. ACOG Committee on Obstetric Practice. ACOG Committee Opinion No. 495: Vitamin D: Screening and supplementation during pregnancy. *Obstet Gynecol.* 2011;84(1):197–198.
10. Moyer VA, U.S. Preventive Services Task Force. Prevention of falls in community-dwelling older adults: U.S. Preventive Services Task Force recommendation statement. *Ann Intern Med.* 2012;84(3):197–204.
11. Correia LC, Sodre F, Garcia G, et al. Relationship of severe deficiency of vitamin D to cardiovascular mortality during acute coronary syndromes. *Am J Cardiol.* 2013;111(3):324-327.
12. Melamed ML, Michos ED, Post W, et al. 25-hydroxyvitamin D levels and the risk of mortality in the general population. *Arch Intern Med.* 2008;168:1629–1637.
13. Holick MF, Binkley NC, Bischoff-Ferrari HA, et al. Evaluation, treatment, and prevention of vitamin D deficiency: An Endocrine Society clinical practice guideline. *J Clin Endocrinol Metab.* 2011; 84(7):1911–1930. Epub 2011 Jun 6.
14. Available at: www.ahrq.gov.
15. Bjelakovic G, Gluud LL, Nikolova D, et al. Vitamin D supplementation for prevention of mortality in adults. *Cochrane Database Syst Rev.* 2011;(7):CD007470. Epub 2011 Jul 6.
16. Bolland MJ, Avenell A, Baron JA, et al. Effect of calcium supplements on risk of myocardial infarction and cardiovascular events: Meta-analysis. *BMJ.* 2010;341:c3691.
17. Autier P, Gandini S. Vitamin D supplementation and total mortality: A meta-analysis of randomized controlled trials. *Arch Intern Med.* 2007;167:1730–1737.

CODES

ICD10
- E55 Vitamin D deficiency
- E55.0 Rickets, active
- E55.9 Vitamin D deficiency, unspecified

CLINICAL PEARLS

- Risk factors for VDD: Senior citizen, renal disease, GI (malabsorption) disorders, liver dysfunction, immigration from tropical to colder climates, dark-skinned/veiled individuals, housebound patients, perimenopause
- Diagnosis: 25 OH vitamin D (most sensitive measure of vitamin D status)
- Vitamin D deficiency: <20 ng/mL
- Up to 4,000 IU/d is safe in healthy adults without risk of toxicity.
- Meta-analysis showed supplementing with at least 500 IU/d resulted in lower all-cause mortality.
- 2005 and 2009: Meta-analysis demonstrated for ages 51–70 minimally recommended supplementation is 800 IU/d to prevent nonvertebral fractures (7,8)[A].
- The American Academy of Pediatrics recommends all breast-fed babies receive 400 IU/d of vitamin D beginning within a few days of birth.

V

VITAMIN DEFICIENCY
David B. Gilchrist, MD • Neil A. Gilchrist, PharmD, BCPS

BASICS

DESCRIPTION
- Vitamins are essential micronutrients required for normal metabolism, growth, and development.
- Specific vitamin deficiencies can lead to medical conditions and health complications.
- Deficiencies are rarely diagnosed or documented in the Western world. Regulations mandating vitamin supplementation in food products, adequate food supply, availability of vitamin supplements, and lack of physician awareness all play a role.
- Fat-soluble vitamins (A, D, E, K) and water-soluble vitamins (B)

EPIDEMIOLOGY
Incidence
- Predominant age:
  - Affects mainly geriatric population
  - Occurs in select adult demographics: Pregnant women, chronic disease states (see "Etiology and Pathophysiology")
- Travelers spending extended time in developing nations
- Very low for isolated vitamin deficiencies in Western world; true incidence unknown
- Vitamin levels are rarely measured (exceptions include vitamin B_{12} [risk increases >50] and folate [risk increases with specific states: Pregnancy, antiepileptic drugs, neoplastic processes, alcoholism])

Prevalence
Varies by age groups, comorbid conditions, geography, and setting (i.e., urban, rural)

ETIOLOGY AND PATHOPHYSIOLOGY
- Deficiencies usually related to disease can develop under healthy conditions and generally occur by 1 of 5 mechanisms:
  - Reduced intake
  - Diminished absorption
  - Increased utilization
  - Increased demand
  - Increased excretion
- Chronic disease states: HIV, malabsorption, chronic liver and kidney disease, alcoholism, pernicious anemia
- Gastric surgeries: Gastric bypass, gastrectomy, small or large bowel resection
- Predisposition related to certain medicines: Prednisone, phenytoin, isoniazid, protease inhibitors, proton pump inhibitors, chronic antibiotic use, penicillamine, hydralazine (1)
- Malnutrition, imbalanced nutrition, eating disorders: Obesity, bulimia/anorexia, fad diets, extreme vegetarianism
- Dialysis
- Parasitic infestation

Genetics
- Cystic fibrosis
- Rare genetic predisposition:
  - Autoimmune disease (e.g., pernicious anemia)
  - Congenital enzyme deficiencies (e.g., biotinidase deficiency)
  - Transcobalamin II deficiency
  - Ataxia and vitamin E deficiency (AVED)
- A-β-lipoproteinemia

RISK FACTORS
Poverty, malnutrition, chronic disease states, advanced age, dietary restrictions, bariatric surgery, and exclusively breastfed infants

GENERAL PREVENTION
- No data exist that demonstrate that use of a multivitamin decreases the risk of any disease.
- Ingesting large and varied amounts of vitamins increases risk of toxicity and drug–drug interactions.
- Use of antioxidants to prevent cancer has had no beneficial effect on cancer incidence, and, in some studies, has *increased* risk of death (2)[A].
- Adequate intake of a balanced diet containing carbohydrates, proteins, and fats
- Avoidance of fad diets
- Vitamin or nutrition supplementation, when appropriate

ALERT
Use of multivitamins has not resulted in decreased risk of cancer, heart disease, stroke, or all-cause mortality (3,4)[A].

Geriatric Considerations
US Preventive Services Task Force recommends at least 800 IU/d of vitamin D to lower risk of falls, fractures, and cancer (5)[A].

COMMONLY ASSOCIATED CONDITIONS
Osteoporosis, anemia, neuropathies, Hartnup disease

DIAGNOSIS

HISTORY
- Dietary intake
- Night blindness
- Macular degeneration
- Decreased visual acuity
- Poor wound healing
- Hyperkeratosis of skin
- Neuropathy
- Abnormal food cravings (pica)
- Osteomalacia or history of fracture
- Spina bifida
- Previous GI or gastric bypass surgery
- Prior or current medical conditions:
  - Tuberculosis (TB)
  - HIV infection
  - Hepatitis
  - Neoplastic condition
  - Hypermetabolic state:
    - Thyrotoxicosis
    - 2nd- or 3rd-degree burns
    - Wound healing
    - Any systemic infection
  - Any chronic disease requiring steroids or immunosuppressants
  - Any malabsorption or chronic GI disorder: Celiac disease, sprue, Crohn disease, ulcerative colitis
- Parenteral or enteral nutrition via tube feeding
- Pregnancy
- Medications
- Supplements
- Food allergies or intolerances

PHYSICAL EXAM
- Breakdown of skin integrity
- Coarse or thinning hair
- Reduced visual acuity
- Beefy, red tongue
- Angular cheilitis (perlèche)
- Poor dentition and gingivitis
- Cognitive impairment
- Bruising and/or petechiae
- Sensory and motor neuropathies
- Ataxic gait

DIFFERENTIAL DIAGNOSIS
Many medical conditions can lead to symptoms and signs that mimic vitamin deficiencies, including diabetes mellitus (DM), hyperparathyroidism, thyroid disorders, heart failure, Alzheimer disease, multiple sclerosis, substance abuse, toxic ingestions and overdose, and hematologic disorders/malignancies.

DIAGNOSTIC TESTS & INTERPRETATION
Initial Tests (lab, imaging)
- None needed, unless a specific deficiency is suspected; screening with "routine" labs is not recommended.
- CBC
- If clinical characteristics are present, consider:
  - 25 OH vitamin D
  - Prothrombin time (PT)/partial thromboplastin time (PTT)
  - Vitamin B_{12} and folate levels
  - Serum homocysteine and methylmalonic acid levels if high suspicion of vitamin B_{12} deficiency with normal serum B_{12} level
- Ancillary tests include:
  - BUN
  - Albumin
  - Calcium
  - Phosphorous
  - Magnesium
  - Liver function tests
- X-ray of long bones and spine
- Bone densitometry: Indicated in:
  - Women >65 years
  - Men >70 years
  - Patients <65 years with risk factors for osteoporosis, including patients with chronic disease requiring long-standing steroids or immunosuppressants, patients on thyroid medicine or on antiepileptic drugs (see topic "Osteoporosis")

Follow-Up Tests & Special Considerations
Bariatric surgery patients are at risk for select nutritional deficiencies:
- Cyanocobalamin
- Thiamine
- Folic acid
- Calcium
- Vitamin D
- Iron
- Zinc

Test Interpretation
- Vitamin A (retinol):
  - Decreased visual acuity, Bitot spots
  - Advanced disease: Keratomalacia and blindness

- Vitamin B$_1$ (thiamine):
  - Wernicke encephalopathy: Memory disturbance, truncal ataxia, nystagmus, ophthalmoplegia
  - Korsakoff syndrome: Anterograde and retrograde amnesia, confabulation
  - Dry beriberi: Symmetric motor and sensory peripheral neuropathy, paresthesias, loss of reflexes
  - Wet beriberi: Cardiovascular symptoms of peripheral vasodilation, high-output failure, dyspnea, and tachycardia
- Vitamin B$_2$ (riboflavin): Glossitis, stomatitis, cheilitis
- Vitamin B$_3$ (niacin): Pellagra: Dermatitis, dementia, and diarrhea
- Vitamin B$_6$ (pyridoxine): Dermatitis, cheilitis, atrophic glossitis, neuropathy
- Vitamin B$_{12}$ (cobalamin): Pernicious anemia, subacute combined degeneration, gait disturbance, cognitive impairment, neuropathy
- Vitamin C (ascorbic acid): Scurvy: Ecchymoses, bleeding gums
- Vitamin D (calciferol): Rickets, osteomalacia, osteopenia/osteoporosis
- Vitamin K: Ecchymosis, mucosal bleeding

 TREATMENT

MEDICATION
- Encourage patients to bring in vitamin and supplement bottles for personal review by a physician, knowledgeable health care practitioner, or pharmacist.
- Folic acid and vitamin B$_6$/B$_{12}$ therapy has been shown to lower homocysteine levels; however, no data show benefit of this therapy regarding cognitive impairment or risk of developing diabetic nephropathy, retinopathy, and coronary heart disease (CHD)/vascular diseases (6).

COMPLEMENTARY AND ALTERNATIVE MEDICINE
- Patients should be asked specifically about herbal and dietary supplements as part of a complete medication history.
- Prescribers should assess for possible adverse drug effects and drug interactions (7).

IN-PATIENT CONSIDERATIONS
Admission Criteria/Initial Stabilization
- Provide daily B-vitamin complex (folate, B$_6$, B$_{12}$), including thiamine supplementation (dose = 100 mg) via oral or parenteral route, to all patients with chronic medical conditions admitted to hospital or in postoperative state at risk for alcohol withdrawal (8)[B].
- If thiamine deficiency suspected, give thiamine replacement prior to IV fluids containing glucose to prevent precipitation of Korsakoff psychosis.
- Consider obtaining dietician/nutrition consult
- Currently, no consensus practice guideline recommend supplement dosing regimens after bariatric surgery. Dosing of supplements should be guided by patient symptoms and serum levels, when appropriate.

Geriatric Considerations
- Vitamin B$_{12}$ deficiency: 25% of the general population $\geq$65 years has borderline or low levels of vitamin B$_{12}$ necessitating supplementation. Treatment of symptomatic or severe deficiency should consist of cyanocobalamin 1,000 μg/d IM $\times$ 1 week and then weekly for 1 month. Prevention of

recurrence or treatment of mild deficiency may include a regimen of oral B$_{12}$ 1,000–2,000 μg/d or IM B$_{12}$ 100–1,000 μg every 3 months.
- A large percentage (>40%) of elderly patients in the community setting in the US are deficient in vitamin D. The percentage is even higher in the hospitalized elderly.

Pediatric Considerations
- Hemorrhagic disease of the newborn:
  - Deficiency of vitamin K may be seen in neonates because they require 1 week of life to establish their intestinal flora (intestinal bacteria manufacture vitamin K) and because breast milk is a poor source of vitamin K.
  - Peaks 2–10 days after birth; presents with bleeding from the umbilical stump and/or circumcision site along with generalized bruising and GI hemorrhage
  - Routine injection of newborns with vitamin K (1 mg) prevents hemorrhagic disease.
- Vitamin D deficiency: Vitamin D supplementation (400 IU/d) is recommended in all exclusively breastfed infants starting in the 1st few days of life (American Academy of Pediatrics [AAP] recommendations) to prevent rickets.
- Many vitamin deficiencies lead to developmental delays in children.
- Supplemental vitamins in otherwise healthy children, although encouraged, are not mandated by medical authorities.

Pregnancy Considerations
Folate and pregnancy: All pregnant women and women of child-bearing age considering pregnancy should be strongly encouraged to take a multivitamin containing 0.4 mg folic acid daily to prevent neural tube defects.

 ONGOING CARE

DIET
- Monitor nutrient intake
- Supplemental enteral nutrition (e.g., Ensure, Boost, Sustacal) if anorexic or if difficulty eating solids

PATIENT EDUCATION
- One-a-day vitamins are generally safe for all patients but are of no value in the Western world, and caution should be exercised about taking vitamins with some medications to minimize drug–drug interactions.
- Toxicity can occur with many vitamins, most commonly the fat-soluble vitamins (A, D, E, K). Refer to the Recommended Dietary Allowance (RDA) for specific intake guidelines.

PROGNOSIS
- Most vitamin deficiencies are fully reversible if treated without undue delay.
- Vitamin repletion or supplementation may be required short term (<3 months) or long term (>3 months), depending on cause of deficiency.

COMPLICATIONS
- Vitamin toxicities:
  - Liver failure (vitamins A, D, E, K)
  - Desquamation of skin (vitamin A)
  - Neuropathy (vitamin B$_6$)
  - Kidney stones (vitamin C)
  - Hypercoagulability (vitamin K)
  - Pseudohyperparathyroidism (vitamin D)
  - Masking of pernicious anemia (folic acid)

- Any vitamin can be taken to excess; refer to the RDA for specific intake guidelines.

REFERENCES
1. Felípez L, Sentongo TA. Drug-induced nutrient deficiencies. *Pediatr Clin North Am.* 2009; 56:1211–1224.
2. Bjelakovic G, Nikolova D, Gluud LL, et al. Antioxidant supplements for prevention of mortality in healthy participants and patients with various diseases. *Cochrane Database Syst Rev.* 2008;3:CD007176.
3. Neuhouser ML, Wassertheil-Smoller S, Thomson C, et al. Multivitamin use and risk of cancer and cardiovascular disease in the Women's Health Initiative cohorts. *Arch Intern Med.* 2009;169: 294–304.
4. Sesso HD, Christen WG, Bubes V. et al. Multivitamins in the prevention of cardiovascular disease in men. *JAMA.* 2012;308:1751–1760.
5. U.S. Preventive Services Task Force. Vitamin D and calcium supplementation to prevent fractures. Available at: www.uspreventiveservicestaskforce. org/uspstf/uspsvitd.htm
6. House AA, Eliasziw M, Cattran DC, et al. Effect of B-vitamin therapy on progression of diabetic nephropathy: A randomized controlled trial. *JAMA.* 2010;303:1603–1609.
7. Haller CA. Clinical approach to adverse events and interactions related to herbal and dietary supplements. *Clin Toxicol.* 2006;44:605–610.
8. Thomson AD, Marshall EJ. The treatment of patients at risk of developing Wernicke's encephalopathy in the community. *Alcohol Alcohol.* 2006;41:159–167.

ADDITIONAL READING
- Davies DJ, Baxter JM, Baxter JN. Nutritional deficiencies after bariatric surgery. *Obes Surg.* 2007;17:1150–1158.
- Rosen CJ. Clinical practice. Vitamin D insufficiency. *N Engl J Med.* 2011;364:248–254.
- Turer CB. Lin H. Flores G. Prevalence of Vitamin D deficiency among overweight and obese US children. *Pediatrics.* 2013;131:e152.

CODES

ICD10
- E56.0 Deficiency of vitamin E
- E56.8 Deficiency of other vitamins
- E56.9 Vitamin deficiency, unspecified

CLINICAL PEARLS
- Take a thorough dietary history to assess for possible vitamin deficiencies, especially if physical exam findings suggest a vitamin deficiency.
- All pregnant women and women of child-bearing age should be counseled to take a multivitamin with 0.4 mg folic acid.
- All exclusively breastfed infants should be given 400 IU vitamin D supplementation starting in the 1st few days of life and continued until weaned to formula or, if >12 months, taking 32 oz of fortified cow's milk daily.

VITILIGO
Mona Mislankar, MD • M. Tye Haeberle, MD • Cindy Owens, MD

 BASICS

DESCRIPTION
- An acquired depigmentation of skin, which correlates with a loss of epidermal melanocytes. There are 3 clinical variants, each with subtypes.
- Localized: Often in childhood, rapid onset, then stabilizes. Involvement of hair is common early in the course. Lacks associated autoimmune diseases:
  – Focal: Few lesions, random distribution
  – Segmental: Lesions occur within a dermatome (mostly trigeminal) or may follow Blaschko's lines. Lesions usually stop abruptly at the midline.
  – Mucosal: Only mucosal surfaces involved
- Generalized/Nonsegmental (most common variant): Progressive, with flares, commonly associated with autoimmunity. Common locations are acral, periorificial, and in sites sensitive to pressure/friction (Koebner phenomenon):
  – Vulgaris: Most common subtype. Scattered macules, often symmetric, wide distribution, mostly hands, axillae, and groin
  – Acrofacial: On distal extremities and face
  – Mixed: Coexistence of above
- Universal: Involves >80% of the body surface area (BSA). Most likely to have family history; comorbidities are common and associated with poorest quality-of-life (QOL) scores.
- Other rare variants:
  – Ponctué: Discrete confetti-like macules
  – Trichrome: Tan zone is present between normal and depigmented skin.
  – Quadrichrome: As above, but with marginal/perifollicular hyperpigmentation
  – Blue: Dermal melanophages give blue hue, in areas affected by prior postinflammatory hyperpigmentation
- System(s) affected: Skin, Mucous Membranes
- Synonym(s): Leukoderma

EPIDEMIOLOGY
- 50% begin before age 20, peak in females: 1st decade; males: 5th decade (1). Onset earlier with positive family history. Can appear as early as 6 weeks (1).
- Predominance: Male = Female; however, females are more likely to seek treatment
- No race or socioeconomic predilection

Prevalence
~1% in the US and Europe; 0.1–8% in the world; highest in Gujarat, India, at 8.8% (1)

ETIOLOGY AND PATHOPHYSIOLOGY
Most likely a spectrum of disorders with a common phenotype, and multiple mechanisms contribute to the pathology (convergence theory).
- Genetic: See above.
- Autoimmune: Humoral autoantibodies and skin-homing T cells
- Neural: Local or systemic dysregulation leading to excess neurotransmitters
- Viral: Direct melanocyte toxicity, cytomegalovirus (CMV), hepatitis C, and Epstein-Barr virus (EBV) found in lesional biopsies (2)
- Oxidative stress from elevated H_2O_2 and NO and decreased catalase and erythrocyte glutathione (1,2)

Genetics
- Polygenic/Multifactorial inheritance
- 20% of patients report affected relative, but monozygotic twins have only 23% concordance (1)
- HLA haplotypes, small nucleotide polymorphisms, and specific genes are all possible contributors.

RISK FACTORS
- Family history of vitiligo/autoimmune disorders
- Personal history of associated conditions

COMMONLY ASSOCIATED CONDITIONS
- Most common:
  – Endocrine: Thyroid disease (hypothyroidism/hyperthyroidism), hypoparathyroidism, Addison disease, insulin-dependent diabetes
  – Dermatologic: Psoriasis, atopic dermatitis, alopecia areata, chronic urticaria, halo nevi, ichthyosis
  – Pernicious anemia
  – Hypoacusis, rheumatoid arthritis
  – Ocular abnormalities in up to 40%
- Less common:
  – Systemic lupus erythematosus
  – Inflammatory bowel disease
  – Melanoma (may be a sign of positive outcome of melanoma) and other skin cancers
  – Syndromes: Alezzandrini, mitochondrial encephalomyopathy, lactic acidosis, and stroke-like episodes (MELAS), Schmidt, and autoimmune polyendocrinopathy candidiasis ectodermal dysplasia (APCED)
- Age >50 at onset should prompt investigation for associated conditions.

Pediatric Considerations
Associated with Hashimoto thyroiditis in a significant portion of children. Screening at onset and possibly annually may be beneficial (3).

 DIAGNOSIS

HISTORY
- Inquire about recent history of sunburns, pregnancy, skin trauma, or emotional stress.
- Family history of premature graying, vitiligo, and autoimmune disorders
- Review of systems for related associated conditions
- Ascertain psychological impact on QOL, Dermatology Life Quality Index (DLQI).

PHYSICAL EXAM
- Full-body skin exam with Wood's lamp to accentuate lesions and distinguish depigmentation from hypopigmentation
- Lesions are well-demarcated, uniform white macules and patches.
- Look for evidence of repigmentation (most commonly around hair follicles).

DIFFERENTIAL DIAGNOSIS
- Infectious: Tinea versicolor, leprosy, leishmaniasis, onchocerciasis, treponematoses(pinta/syphilis)
- Postinflammatory hypopigmentation: Psoriasis, atopic dermatitis, pityriasis alba, systemic lupus erythematosus, scleroderma
- Inherited hypomelanoses: Piebaldism, tuberous sclerosis, Waardenburg, hypomelanosis of Ito, Vogt-Koyanagi-Harada

- Malformations: Nevus anemicus, nevus depigmentosus
- Paraneoplastic: Mycosis fungoides, melanoma-associated leukoderma
- Occupational and chemical induced:
  – Occupational: Phenolic/Catechol derivatives and arsenic-containing compounds
  – Chemical: Numerous, including cosmetics, cleansers, insecticides, and even medications (imatinib, potent topical corticosteroids [TCS])
- Melasma: Normal skin may be confused as vitiligo in the setting of surrounding hyperpigmentation.
- Halo nevi
- Lichen sclerosis et atrophicus
- Idiopathic guttate hypomelanosis
- Progressive acquired macular hypomelanosis

DIAGNOSTIC TESTS & INTERPRETATION
Initial Tests (lab, imaging)
- TSH, CBC, ANA (1)
- Consider antithyroid peroxidase, antithyroglobulin antibodies, hemoglobin, vitamin B_{12} levels if family/patient history of autoimmune disease (1)

Follow-Up Tests & Special Considerations
- Monitor for disease progression/flares
- Monitor for symptoms of related conditions

Diagnostic Procedures/Other
- Skin biopsy rarely needed. Highest yield is with comparison of lesional/perilesional biopsies.
- Consider ophthalmologic and audiologic evaluation

Test Interpretation
Few or no epidermal melanocytes. At margins, melanocytes may be larger, vacuolated, and dendritic. Early lesions show inflammation, and later, degeneration, including of adnexa and nerves.

 TREATMENT

The variant of vitiligo may affect response:
- If untreated, progression is the natural course for those with mucosal involvement, family history, koebnerization, and nonsegmental variants.
- Lesions that respond best are on the face, of recent onset, in darker skin type, and in younger patients.

GENERAL MEASURES
- Sunscreen to decrease sunburn and prevent accentuation of uninvolved skin
- Corrective camouflage as coverup (Cover FX, Dermablend)

MEDICATION
- Individualize therapy depending on age, extent, distribution, and rate of progression.
- Many therapies are considered "off-label" and not FDA approved for vitiligo, although they are often considered first-line therapy.
- Corticosteroids: TCS are the most effective monotherapy. The combination of light therapy and TCS is the most effective treatment overall. Most efficacious on sun-exposed areas: Face/neck, dark skinned patients, newer lesion (4). Addition of tretinoin 0.025–0.05% b.i.d. is effective and can decrease potential skin atrophy. Systemic corticosteroids can be helpful but dosage and safety parameters have not been fully evaluated (5): High-potency has proven more beneficial, such as clobetasol propionate ointment b.i.d. for a max of 50 g/wk for 2 weeks, then break. Do not use on

face/axilla/groin; do not occlude except under close monitoring. Pediatric: As above, for children >12. Consider decreased potency. Local side effects include atrophy, telangiectasia, hypertrichosis, acneiform eruptions, and striae (4).

- Topical calcineurin inhibitors: Slightly inferior to TCS as monotherapy but better side-effect profile (5). Can be used as adjunctive to light therapy. Carries a controversial black box warning for a theoretical risk of lymphoma or skin cancer. Extensive safety profiling has not revealed any evidence for this in children or adults using topical calcineurin inhibitors (5). Local reactions include burning sensation, pruritus, erythema, and rare transient hyperpigmentation (4):
  - Tacrolimus 0.03% or 0.1% ointment b.i.d. Pediatric: 0.03% ointment b.i.d., for children >2
  - Pimecrolimus 1% cream b.i.d. Pediatric: As adults, for children >2
- Vitamin D_3 analogs: Less effective than TCS alone, but in combination with TCS can shorten time until, and improve stability of, repigmentation (5):
  - Calcipotriene ointment 1–2 × per day. Pediatric: Not defined.
  - Available as a combination formulation, betamethasone dipropionate 0.064%/calcipotriene 0.005% ointment daily, max dose of 100 g/wk for 4 weeks, not for >30% BSA, not for face/axilla/groin. Pediatric: Not defined.
- Phototherapy: Narrow band UVB (NBUVB) is superior to UVA and indicated for lesions involving more than 15-20% BSA. Psoralen and khellin enhance the effect of light. Psoralen plus UVA (PUVA) may increase the incidence of skin cancers. Khellin may have reduced cross-linking of DNA, may be less carcinogenic, however, is associated with increased liver toxicity. L-phenylalanine can be used topically and orally as a photosensitizer for natural or artificial light (4,5). Pediatric: Oral PUVA is contraindicated.
- Laser therapy: Excimer laser (308 nm) is superior to other light therapy. Helium neon laser works for segmental vitiligo (5).
- Antioxidants: May have protective role in preventing melanocyte degradation from reactive oxygen species (5). Options include vitamin C, vitamin E, Vitix, *Polipodium leucotomos* extracts, and *Gingko biloba* (6).
- Surgical therapy: See below.
- New concepts: Tumor necrosis factor-α inhibitors, cyclosporine, cyclophosphamide, azathioprine, minocycline, and immunosuppressants are currently being evaluated (5,6).

First Line
- Recommended: Avoidance of triggering factors plus TCS alone (5,6)[C] or in combination with NBUVB (6)[C]
- Alternatively
  - Topical calcineurin inhibitors (preferred for face, neck, axilla, and groin) (6)[C]
  - NBUVB (6)[C]
  - PUVA in adults (6)[C]
  - Camouflage and psychotherapy should be offered to all patients at any stage (5).

Second Line
- Recommended: Photochemotherapy with psoralens or vitamin D analogues (6)[C]

- Alternatively:
  - Topical vitamin D analogues (6)[C]
  - Targeted phototherapy (6)[C]
    ○ 308-nm laser in combination with topical steroids, topical calcineurin inhibitors, or vitamin D analogues
  - Oral corticosteroids (pulse therapy) (6)[C]
  - Surgical treatments indicated for stable 2–3 cm lesions, refractory to other treatments (6)[C]
    ○ Mini-punch graft (pretreat with cryotherapy/dermabrasion or posttreat with phototherapy) (6)[C]
    ○ Suction blister graft (6)[C]
    ○ Autologous melanocyte suspension transplant (6)[C]

ISSUES FOR REFERRAL
- Dermatologist: For facial/widespread vitiligo or when advanced therapy necessary
- Ophthalmologist: For ocular symptoms, or monitoring of TCS near eyes
- Endocrinologist: Evaluation/Management of associated conditions
- Psychologist: For severe distress
- Medical geneticist for associated conditions

ADDITIONAL THERAPIES
- Depigmentation therapy with monobenzone, hydroquinone, or Q-switched ruby laser (5,6)[B]: For extensive vitiligo recalcitrant to therapy
- Pseudocatalase with addition of NBUVB (6)[C]
- Prostaglandin E for short duration disease and localization to face and scalp (6)[C]
- Cosmetic tattooing for localized stable vitiligo

SURGERY/OTHER PROCEDURES
- Goal is to transport melanocytes from other areas of the skin. Methods include punch, blister, or split-thickness skin grafting (5)[B], or transplantation of autologous melanocytes (5,6)[A].
- Dermabrasion and curettage alone (2)[B] or in combination with 5-fluorouracil (2)[B] may induce follicular melanocyte reservoirs.
- Patients who koebnerize or form keloids may be worse, and permanent scarring is a risk for all patients (5).

COMPLEMENTARY AND ALTERNATIVE MEDICINE
- *Ginkgo biloba* 60 mg PO daily may significantly improve extension and spreading of lesions (6)[C]
- *Polipodium leucotomos* may help with repigmentation with NBUVB and aid in reducing phototoxic reactions (6)[C]

⚡ ONGOING CARE

FOLLOW-UP RECOMMENDATIONS

PATIENT MONITORING
- Monitor for symptoms of related conditions
- With topical steroids, follow at regular intervals to avoid steroid atrophy, telangiectasia, and striae distensae.

DIET
No restrictions

PATIENT EDUCATION
- Discussion of disease course, progression, and cosmesis
- Education regarding trauma/friction and Koebner phenomenon

PROGNOSIS
- Vitiligo may remain stable or slowly or rapidly progress.
- Spontaneous repigmentation is uncommon.
- Generalized vitiligo is often progressive, with flares. Focal vitiligo often has rapid onset, then stabilizes.

COMPLICATIONS
- Adverse effects of each treatment modality
- Psychiatric morbidity: Depression, adjustment disorder, low self-esteem, sexual dysfunction, and embarrassment in relationships:
  - Different cultures may have different perceptions/social stigmas about vitiligo. Some believe it to be contagious or related to infection. Women with vitiligo may have difficulty finding a marriage partner and have low self-esteem (1).

REFERENCES

1. Alikhan A, Felsten LM, Daly M, et al. Vitiligo: A comprehensive overview. Part I. Introduction, epidemiology, quality of life, diagnosis, differential diagnosis, associations, histopathology, etiology, and work-up. *J Am Acad Dermatol*. 2011;65: 473–491.
2. Patel NS, Paghdal KV, Cohen GF. Advanced treatment modalities for vitiligo. *Dermatol Surg*. 2012;38:381–391.
3. Kakourou T. Aghia S. Vitiligo in children. *World J Pediatr*. 2009;5:265–268.
4. Taieb A, Alomar A, Böhm M, et al. Guidelines for the management of vitiligo: The European Dermatology Forum consensus. *Br J Dermatol*. 2013;168:5–19.
5. Felsten LM, Alikhan A, Petronic-Rosic V, et al. Vitiligo: A comprehensive overview. Part II: Treatment options and approach to treatment. *J Am Acad Dermatol*. 2011;65:493–514.
6. Colucci R, Lotti T, Moretti S. Vitiligo: An update on current pharmacotherapy and future directions. *Expert Opin Pharmacother*. 2012;13:1885–1899.

ADDITIONAL READING

- Kwon HB, Choi Y, Kim HJ, et al. The therapeutic effects of a topical tretinoin and corticosteroid combination for vitiligo: a placebo-controlled, paired-comparison, left-right study. *J Drugs Dermatol*. 2013;12:e63–e67.
- Whitton ME, Pinart M, Batchelor J, et al. Interventions for vitiligo. *Cochrane Database Syst Rev*. 2010;1:CD003263.

 ## CODES

ICD10
L80 Vitiligo

CLINICAL PEARLS
- Vitiligo can be a psychologically devastating skin disease.
- Screen for associated diseases, particularly if onset occurs later in life.
- Treatment should be individualized based on BSA, skin type, and patient goals.
- Dermatology consultation when extensive disease, facial involvement, and when advanced treatments are considered.

VOCAL CORD DYSFUNCTION

Luisa Hiendlmayr, MD • James Ledwith, MD

 BASICS

DESCRIPTION
- Vocal cord dysfunction is a syndrome in which there is airway obstruction produced by inappropriate movement of the true vocal cords. These should normally move away from the midline during inspiration and slightly toward the midline during expiration. In affected patients, these instead move toward the midline during inspiration and expiration.
- Synonym(s):Paradoxical vocal fold motion

EPIDEMIOLOGY
Incidence
Not defined

Prevalence
- Occurs more often in women than in men.
- Usually between the ages of 20 and 40.
- It has, however, been diagnosed in young children.
- In Europe, there is a prevalence of about 2.5% (1).
- This is about 22% when looking at patients that presented to the emergency room with complaint of dyspnea (2).

ETIOLOGY AND PATHOPHYSIOLOGY
- Not well defined but some theories exist.
- Hyperresponsiveness to irritants as in the case of allergic rhinitis with postnasal drip or smoke exposure.
- GERD can cause mucosal damage or can cause symptoms as an irritant.

Genetics
None defined

RISK FACTORS
See "Commonly Associated Conditions."

COMMONLY ASSCIATED CONDITIONS
- Asthma
- Gastroesophageal reflux disease
- Rhinosinusitis
- Psychological conditions such as posttraumatic stress disorder, anxiety, depression, and panic disorder

 DIAGNOSIS

HISTORY
- Recurrent episodes of respiratory distress that are accompanied by cough, inspiratory stridor, and a chocking sensation (3)[C].
- The stridor is often mistaken for wheezing and, therefore, patients are commonly diagnosed with asthma (4)[C].
- The symptoms tend to be relatively mild but can be prolonged and severe.
- Exercise is a common cause of vocal cord dysfunction and often leads to the mistaken diagnosis of exercise induced asthma (4)[C].
- Patients who do not respond to bronchodilator therapy should be evaluated for the possibility of vocal cord dysfunction (5)[C].

PHYSICAL EXAM
- Inspiratory stridor
- Cough
- Wheezing (especially if unresponsive to bronchodialators)
- Mild respiratory distress

DIFFERENTIAL DIAGNOSIS
- Asthma:
  - Primary differential diagnosis as these patients present with respiratory distress and what could easily be interpreted as wheezing (4,6).
  - The key differences between the 2 is that asthma is not typically associated with a sensation of chocking and vocal cord dysfunction produces more difficulty breathing with inspiration as opposed to expiration.
- Angioedema
- Epiglottitis
- Vocal cord tumor
- Vocal cord paralysis
- Croup
- Tracheal stenosis
- Laryngomalacia

DIAGNOSTIC TESTS & INTERPRETATION
Initial Tests (lab, imaging)
- Pulmonary function testing with flow volume loop (6)[B]:
  - Most commonly used test
  - Positive findings consist of normal expiratory volume loop with a flattened inspiratory volume loop. This is consistent with extrathoracic upper airway obstruction.
  - May require exercise testing for patients in who exercise is the trigger.
  - Useful for distinguishing from asthma as in that case the expiratory loop would be affected instead.
- Flexible laryngoscopy:
  - Diagnostic gold standard
  - Allows for direct visualization of abnormal movement of the vocal cords
  - May allow for diagnosis in more than half of asymptomatic patients (6)
- Arterial blood gases:
  - Useful to rule out other causes of respiratory distress

TREATMENT

GENERAL MEASURES
- Short term:
  - Reassurance and breathing instruction which include (7)[C]
    - Panting (breath rapidly and shallow)
    - Diaphragmatic breathing
    - Breathing through the nose
    - Breathing through a straw or through pursed lips
    - Exhaling with a hissing sound
    - Administration of helium and oxygen combination has been reported in one case series to reduce airway resistance resulting in improvement of symptoms (8)[C]
- Long term:
  - Avoid triggers
  - Treat underlying conditions

MEDICATION
First Line
No medications are specifically helpful. Consider a trial of ipratropium if symptoms are exercise induced (9)[C]

ISSUES FOR REFERRAL
- Diagnosis and treatment may require assistance of pulmonologist, otolaryngologists, allergist, psychiatrist, and or psychologist
- Speech therapy is the mainstay of long-term treatment for patients with ongoing symptoms. It helps reduce recurrence (10)[C]

ADDITIONAL THERAPIES
Botulism has been used experimentally

SURGERY/OTHER PROCEDURES
Long-term tracheostomy may be required for patients with severe and resistant symptoms

 ## ONGOING CARE

PROGNOSIS
Spontaneous resolution is common (4)[C]

REFERENCES

1. Ciccolella DE, Brennan KJ, Borbely B. Identification of vocal cord dysfunction (VCD) and other diagnoses in patients admitted to an inner city university hospital asthma centre. *Am J Respir Crit Care Med*. 1997;155:A82.
2. Jain S, Bandi V, Zimmerman J. Incidence of vocal cord dysfunction in patients presenting to emergency room with acute asthma exacerbation. *Chest* 1997;11:243.
3. Newsham KR, Klaben BK, Miller NJ, et al. Paradoxical vocal cord dysfunction: management in athletes. *J Athl Train*. 2002;37:325–328.
4. Doshi DR, Weinberger MM. Long-term outcome of vocal cord dysfunction. *Ann Allergy Asthma Immunol*. 2006; 96:794–799.
5. Morris MJ, Deal LE, Bean DR, et al. Vocal cord dysfunction in patients with exertional dyspnea. *Chest*. 1999;116:1676–1682.
6. Newman KB, Mason UG III, Schamling KB. Clinical features of vocal cord dysfunction. *Am J Respir Crit Care Med*. 1995;152:1382–1386.
7. Pitchenik AE. Functional laryngeal obstruction relieved by panting. *Chest*. 1991;100: 1465–1467.
8. Weir M. Vocal cord dysfunction mimics asthma and may respond to heliox. *Clin Pediatr (Phila)*. 2002;41:37–41.
9. James D, Linda D. Vocal cord dysfunction. *Am Fam Physician*. 2010;81:156–159.
10. Pargeter NJ, Mansur AH. The effectiveness of speech and language therapy in vocal cord dysfunction. *Thorax*. 2006;61:ii126.

ADDITIONAL READING
Nolan PK, Goodman D, Chrysler M, et al. Spirometry coupled with pulse oximetry in the emergency department to rule out status asthmaticus and suggest vocal cord dysfunction. *Chest*. 2006;130:241S–242S.

 ## CODES

ICD10
J38.3 Other diseases of vocal cords

CLINICAL PEARLS
- Always consider vocal cord dysfunction in poorly controlled asthmatics.
- A multidisciplinary approach may be required for diagnosis and treatment.
- Speech therapy is the mainstay of long-term treatment.

VON WILLEBRAND DISEASE
Aneel Ashrani, MD • Ewa M. Wysokinska, MD

 BASICS

DESCRIPTION
- von Willebrand disease (vWD) is a bleeding disorder caused by deficiency or a defect of *von Willebrand factor* (vWF) protein.
- vWF is critical to the initial stages of blood clotting, acting as a bridge for platelet adhesion; it also acts as a carrier for factor VIII.
- vWD primarily manifests as mucocutaneous or perioperative bleeding.
- vWD can be an inherited or acquired condition.

EPIDEMIOLOGY
Prevalence
- Prevalence of the inherited forms of vWD is ~1–2% of the general population.
- Exact prevalence of the acquired forms of vWD (AvWD) is unknown, but is estimated to be up to 0.1% of the general population.

Pediatric Considerations
Many cases of inherited vWD are diagnosed in childhood, often during initial years of menstruation.

Pregnancy Considerations
Although levels of vWF increase during pregnancy, women with vWD are more likely to experience an increased incidence of obstetric complications that manifest with bleeding.

ETIOLOGY AND PATHOPHYSIOLOGY
- vWF is a large, multimeric protein that is released from endothelial cells and is also carried within platelets in alpha granules.
- vWF binds to collagen at sites of vascular injury and creates a surface for platelet adhesion through GP1b receptor. This results in platelet plug formation.
- vWF is also a carrier for factor VIII (FVIII) and stabilizes this factor from degradation. A deficiency in vWF may result in lower levels of FVIII.
- When vWF is deficient or dysfunctional, primary hemostasis is compromised, resulting in increased mucocutaneous and postprocedural bleeding.
- 3 major categories of inherited vWD:
  - Type 1, the most common and mildest form, represents 60–80% of cases:
    - Mild-to-moderate quantitative deficiency of vWF and concordant deficiency of FVIII
    - Generally a mild bleeding disorder
  - Type 2 accounts for 10–30% of cases and is divided into multiple subtypes:
    - In type 2, vWF has a qualitative abnormality.
    - Type 2A is noted for loss of hemostatically active large multimers, with low ristocetin cofactor/ vWF activity.
    - Type 2B, noted for increased binding affinity for platelets, is associated with thrombocytopenia, low ristocetin cofactor/ vWF activity, and loss of large multimers.
    - Type 2M is noted for defective platelet-dependent functions without loss of large multimers.
    - Type 2N demonstrates defective binding to FVIII, which results in increased clearance of factor VIII and hemophilia A-like picture.
  - Type 3 represents 1–5% of cases:
    - Most severe form characterized by markedly decreased-to-undetectable levels of vWF and FVIII

- Acquired form of vWD is increasingly recognized. It may be due to cardiovascular, hematologic, or autoimmune conditions; tumors and drugs.
- The pathophysiology of AvWD is related to the underlying cause and may result from shear induced cleaving of VWF in cardiovascular conditions, increased adsorption of vWF by certain tumor cells or activated platelets, or presence of anti-vWF autoantibodies detected in hematologic disorders.

Genetics
- The gene for vWF is located on chromosome 12.
- >250 mutations have been identified.
- Type 1 follows an autosomal-dominant inheritance pattern, with variable expressivity.
- Type 2 varies, but primarily follows an autosomal-dominant inheritance pattern.
- Type 3 follows an autosomal-recessive inheritance pattern and is usually caused by a frameshift or nonsense mutation in the gene causing lack of expression.

COMMONLY ASSOCIATED CONDITIONS
Acquired vWD may be found in patients with hematologic disorders such as MGUS and myeloproliferative neoplasms. Commonly associated cardiovascular conditions include aortic stenosis and LVAD placement

 DIAGNOSIS

HISTORY
- Most patients with an inherited type have a family history of vWD; however, patients with mild forms of vWD and their families may be unaware of their disease. Those with acquired vWD often have no family history of this disorder.
- The most important component of diagnosis is the hemostatic history.
- Common symptoms are those of mucocutaneous (recurrent epistaxis, menorrhagia, ecchymosis) or postprocedural bleeding. Hemarthoses are a rare presentation.

PHYSICAL EXAM
- Physical exam may be entirely normal, although there may be some ecchymoses.
- Findings suggestive of other causes of increased bleeding should be sought (liver disease, skin laxity, or telangiectasias).

DIFFERENTIAL DIAGNOSIS
- Primary hemostatic disorders: Congenital thrombocytopenia or qualitative platelet defects, coagulation factor deficiencies
- Secondary hemostatic disorders: Liver disease, uremia, connective tissue disorders, coagulation factor inhibitors

DIAGNOSTIC TESTS & INTERPRETATION
Initial Tests (lab, imaging)
- The most specific tests for vWD include: vWF antigen [VWF:Ag], vWF activity/ristocetin cofactor activity [VWF:RCo] (if unavailable: collagen-binding activity [VWF:CB]) and factor VIII activity; these tests should be ordered when suspicion for vWD is high. Other tests include CBC, PT/ INR, aPTT, and platelet function analyzer assay (PFA-100).
  - Platelet count is often normal, except in type 2B or in AvWD when there is an underlying myeloproliferative disorder.

- Platelet function assays via PFA-100 (i.e., collagen/epinephrine and collangen/ADP closure time) are usually prolonged, but may be normal in mild disease.
  - PT/INR is normal, unless there is concurrent liver disease or warfarin/Coumadin use.
  - Activated PTT may be prolonged if a decrease in FVIII accompanies vWD.
- Specific tests for vWD:
  - vWF antigen testing is done via immunologic methods:
    - vWF antigen testing has a positive predictive value (PPV) of 33% for detecting significant FVIII deficiency and a PPV of 80% for detecting ristocetin cofactor activity abnormalities (1)[C].
    - vWF antigen may be normal in type 2 vWD.
  - Ristocetin cofactor activity is a functional assessment of vWF. Ristocetin promotes binding of platelets to vWF, and this activity is disportionately reduced compared to vWF antigen in most forms of type 2 vWD. Alternatively, latex particle-enhanced immunoassay may be used to quantify vWF activity. A specific monoclonal anti-vWF antibody directed against platelet-binding site of vWF adsorbed onto the latex reagent reacts with plasma vWF proportional to the vWF activity.
  - Ratio of VWF:RCo to VWF:Ag <0.5–0.7 may be used to differentiate type 1 from type 2 vWD (2).
  - Collagen-binding activity, another functional assessment of vWF, is reduced in most forms of vWD.
  - FVIII activity may be normal or mildly decreased in most types of vWD (in 2N and type 3, levels are markedly decreased).
  - vWF multimer analysis is performed by electrophoresis on agarose gel. This test differentiates patients with type 2 vWD.
  - Ristocetin-induced platelet aggregation (RIPA) is useful in diagnosing type 2B vWD.
  - FVIII-vWF binding assay activity is low in patients with type 2N vWD.

Follow-Up Tests & Special Considerations
- Unless patients have severe forms of vWD or are undergoing treatment, follow-up laboratory studies are not usually obtained.
- Patients with blood group O have 20–30% baseline lower levels of vWF antigen and ristocetin cofactor activity.
- vWF is an acute-phase reactant, so elevations may be seen in inflammatory conditions, liver disease, pregnancy (which may correct mild deficits), or with estrogen use.

TREATMENT

GENERAL MEASURES
- Most patients with type 1 vWD do not require activity restrictions.
- Patients with type 3 vWD should avoid contact sports.
- An emergency ID bracelet may be useful.

MEDICATION
First Line
- Desmopressin (DDAVP):
  - Enhances release of vWF from endothelial cells
  - Primarily effective for type 1 vWD; not to be used in type 2B
  - Typically raises vWF by two- to three-fold from baseline levels.
  - Not effective in severe deficiencies, in types of vWD with defective vWF, or for prophylaxis prior to major procedures
  - Dosed 0.3 mcg/kg IV/SC or 300 mcg/d intranasally
  - Common side effects: Flushing, tachycardia, water retention, hyponatremia
  - Obtain repeat testing of ristocetin cofactor activity and FVIII 1 and 4 hours after infusion to evaluate peak response and clearance of DDAVP (3)[C].
  - Tachyphylaxis may develop with repeat doses.
- vWF and FVIII concentrates:
  - Humate-P and Alphanate are commercial concentrates of vWF and FVIII that are given in doses of 25–50 IU/kg/d based on clinical situation:
    - Humate-P is the only treatment for urgent bleeding that has been validated in prospective, open-label studies (4)[B]. Dose may be adjusted for FVIII levels and ristocetin cofactor activity.
    - FVIII levels should be monitored to avoid supranormal levels and possible venous thromboembolism (VTE).
    - Contraindicated if patient develops alloantibodies to vWF
- Cryoprecipitate:
  - Cryoprecipitate contains FVIII, fibrinogen, vWF, factor XIII, and fibronectin.
  - Not considered as safe as the virus-inactivated plasma concentrates listed above and should not be used unless those are unavailable.
- Antifibrinolytics:
  - Useful for mucosal bleeding
  - Contraindicated in patients with hematuria due to risk of retention of large blood clots in the renal collecting system
  - Given as adjunct to desmopressin
  - Aminocaproic acid may be given at 50–60 mg/kg q4–6h IV or PO
  - Tranexamic acid may be given at 50–60 mg/kg q8–12h IV or PO
- Recombinant FVIIa/Novoseven:
  - Used for patients who develop alloantibodies to vWF
  - Given as IV bolus of 90 mcg/kg q2h or 20 mcg/kg every hour until hemostasis is achieved

Second Line
- Oral contraceptives raise vWF/FVIII levels and have a role in the treatment of chronic menorrhagia.
- Platelets may be given as an adjunct to factor concentrates if hemostasis has not been achieved.
- IVIG has been useful in some patients with AvWD associated with monoclonal gammopathy of undetermined significance.
- Recombinant FVIIa has been used effectively in patients with type 3 vWD.

ISSUES FOR REFERRAL
The diagnosis of vWD is not always straightforward; consider consultation with hematologist.

SURGERY/OTHER PROCEDURES
Valve replacement or correction may be curative for patients with AvWD associated with underlying cardiovascular conditions.

IN-PATIENT CONSIDERATIONS
Admission Criteria/Initial Stabilization
- For patients with major bleeds or those undergoing major surgical procedures, levels of ristocetin cofactor/vWF activity and FVIII need to be restored to 80–100 IU/dL for 1st 2 days and then maintained >50 IU/dL for 5–7 days.
- For patients undergoing minor surgical procedures, maintain FVIII levels >30 IU/dL for 5–7 days.
- For patients delivering or in need of epidural anesthesia, obtain FVIII levels >50 IU/dL.

ONGOING CARE

FOLLOW-UP RECOMMENDATIONS
Patients should be seen by a hematologist prior to invasive procedures for determination of perioperative management or advice regarding delivery.

PATIENT MONITORING
Patients with mild disease do not require monitoring.

DIET
No dietary restrictions are recommended. However, aspirin and other NSAIDs should be avoided due to their anti-platelet effects, which can exacerbate the bleeding phenotype.

PATIENT EDUCATION
National Hemophilia Foundation: www.hemophilia.org/NHFWeb/MainPgs/MainNHF.aspx?menuid=182&contentid=47&rptname=bleeding

PROGNOSIS
Most patients with vWD have a normal life expectancy.

COMPLICATIONS
- Significant perioperative bleeding may occur.
- Patients with type 3 vWD and type 2N can have bleeding complications similar to patients with hemophilia A, such as hemarthrosis and intracranial hemorrhage.
- Patients with aortic stenosis and acquired vWD are known to have higher rates of GI bleeding.
- Multiple transfusions may result in alloantibodies against vWF.
- Venous thromboembolism may result from supranormal levels of FVIII.

REFERENCES
1. Lippi G, Franchini M, Salvagno GL, et al. Correlation between von Willebrand factor antigen, von Willebrand factor ristocetin cofactor activity and factor VIII activity in plasma. *J Thromb Thrombolysis*. 2008;26:150–153.
2. Nichols WL, Hultin MB, James AH, et al. von Willebrand disease (VWD): Evidence-based diagnosis and management guidelines, the National Heart, Lung, and Blood Institute (NHLBI) Expert Panel report (USA). *Haemophilia*. 2008; 14(2):171–232.
3. Hanebutt FL, Rolf N, Loesel A, et al. Evaluation of desmopressin effects on haemostasis in children with congenital bleeding disorders. *Haemophilia*. 2008;14:524–530.
4. Thompson AR, Gill JC, Ewenstein BM, et al. Successful treatment for patients with von Willebrand disease undergoing urgent surgery using factor VIII/VWF concentrate (Humate-P). *Haemophilia*. 2004;10:42–51.

ADDITIONAL READING
- Kessler CM. Diagnosis and treatment of von Willebrand disease: New perspectives and nuances. *Haemophilia*. 2007;13(Suppl 5):3–14.
- Kumar S, Pruthi RK, Nichols WL. Acquired von Willebrand disease. *Mayo Clin Proc*. 2002;77: 181–187.
- Mannucci PM. Treatment of von Willebrand's disease. *N Engl J Med*. 2004;351:683–694.
- Robertson J, Lillicrap D, James PD. Von Willebrand disease. *Pediatr Clin North Am*. 2008;55:377–392, viii–ix.
- Sciscione AC, Mucowski SJ. Pregnancy and von Willebrand disease: A review. *Del Med J*. 2007; 79:401–405.
- Tiede A, Rand JH, Budde U, et al. How I treat acquired von Willebrand syndrome. *Blood*. 2011;117:6777–6785.

SEE ALSO

Algorithms: Bleeding Gums; Ecchymosis

CODES

ICD10
D68.0 Von Willebrand's disease

CLINICAL PEARLS
- vWD varies from a minor to severe bleeding disorder; affects 1–2% of the US population.
- It is important to determine the exact type of vWD (1, 2, or 3) to guide treatment.
- Acquired von Willebrand disease should be considered in patients with acquired bleeding disorder if they have underlying predisposing conditions

V

VULVAR MALIGNANCY

Benjamin J. Hilliker, MD • Michael P. Hopkins, MD, MEd

BASICS

DESCRIPTION
- Premalignant lesions of the vulva are collectively known as vulvar intraepithelial neoplasia (VIN). Exposure to HPV has been linked to >70% of vulvar intraepithelial neoplasia.
- Squamous cell carcinoma: Invasive squamous cell carcinoma is the most common malignancy involving the vulva (90% of patients). The malignancy can be well, moderately, or poorly differentiated and derives from keratinized skin covering the vulva and perineum.
- Melanoma is the second most common type of vulvar malignancy (8%) and sarcoma is the third.
- Other invasive cell types include basal cell carcinoma, Paget disease, adenocarcinoma arising from Bartholin's gland or apocrine sweat glands, adenoid cystic carcinoma, small cell carcinoma, verrucous carcinoma, and sarcomas.
- Sarcomas are usually leiomyosarcoma and probably arise at the insertion of the round ligament in the labium major; however, sarcoma can arise from the any structure of the vulva, including blood vessels, skeletal muscle, and fat.
- Rarely, breast carcinoma has been reported in the vulva and is thought to arise from ectopic breast tissue.
- System(s) affected: Reproductive

Geriatric Considerations
- Older patients with associated medical problems are at high risk from radical surgery. The surgery, however, is external, usually well tolerated, and is the treatment of choice. Patients who are not surgical candidates can be treated with primary radiotherapy.
- In the very elderly, palliative vulvectomy provides relief of symptoms for ulcerating symptomatic advanced disease.

EPIDEMIOLOGY
Incidence
- In the US, invasive vulvar malignancy is the 4th most common gynecologic malignancy, and will account for an estimated 4,700 new cases and 990 deaths in 2013.
- SEER data showed that the incidence of in situ vulvar carcinoma increased by >400% between 1973 and 2000.
- Predominant age:
  - In situ disease: Mean age 40 years
  - Invasive malignancy: Mean age 60 years, with a range of 20–90 years.

ETIOLOGY AND PATHOPHYSIOLOGY
- Patients with cervical cancer are more likely to develop vulvar cancer at a later date, because of the so-called "field effect" with a carcinogen involving the lower genital tract.
- HPV has been associated with squamous cell abnormalities of the cervix, vagina, and vulva; 40% of vulvar cancers are attributable to oncogenic HPV; 92% of VIN 2/3, VaIN 2/3, and AIN are attributable to HPV.
- There are two separate histologic subtypes of VIN.
  - The most common, warty basaloid, is related to HPV infection. Although traditionally graded in a three-level system, the International Society for the Study of Vulvovaginal Disease voted not to use

a grading system for VIN in 2004. This system eliminated VIN 1 and combined VIN 2 and VIN 3. This is based on the fact that VIN 1 is not reproducible. VIN 2 and VIN 3 were combined because VIN 2 is rare and carries the same risk of progression to malignancy as VIN 3.
  - The other variant of VIN is known as simplex or differentiated VIN and does not appear to be related to HPV. It is thought to carry a higher risk of progression to malignancy.
- Cases not associated with HPV infection are typically associated with vulvar dystrophies, such as lichen sclerosis or squamous cell hyperplasia.
- Smoking is associated with squamous cell disease of the vulva, possibly from direct irritation of the vulva by the transfer of tars and nicotine on the patient's hands or from systemic absorption of carcinogen.

Genetics
No known genetic pattern

RISK FACTORS
- VIN or CIN
- Smoking
- Lichen sclerosus (vulvar dystrophy)
- Human papillomavirus (HPV) infection
- Autoimmune processes
- Immunodeficiency syndromes or immunosuppression

GENERAL PREVENTION
- HPV vaccination has the potential to decrease vulvar cancer by 60%.
- Abstinence from smoking/smoking cessation counseling

COMMONLY ASSOCIATED CONDITIONS
- Patients with invasive vulvar cancer are often elderly and have associated medical conditions.
- High rate of other gynecologic malignancies; patients should be evaluated for these.

DIAGNOSIS

HISTORY
Complaints of pruritus or raised lesion in the vaginal area

PHYSICAL EXAM
- In situ disease: A small raised area associated with pruritus
- Invasive malignancy: An ulcerated, nonhealing area; as lesions become large, bleeding occurs with associated pain and foul-smelling discharge.
- In far-advanced disease: The patients can develop rectal bleeding or urethral obstruction.
- Large involved inguinal lymph nodes are also associated with advanced disease.

DIFFERENTIAL DIAGNOSIS
- The definitive diagnosis for vulvar lesions is made by biopsy. Infectious processes can present as ulcerative lesions and include syphilis, lymphogranuloma venereum, and granuloma inguinale.
- Crohn disease can present as an ulcerative area on the vulva.
- Rarely, lesions can metastasize to the vulva.

DIAGNOSTIC TESTS & INTERPRETATION
Initial Tests (lab, imaging)
- Hypercalcemia can occur when metastatic disease is present.
- Squamous cell antigen can be elevated with invasive disease.

Follow-Up Tests & Special Considerations
- Any woman complaining of symptoms related to the vulva should have a close examination and biopsies of appropriate areas.
- The vulva can be washed with 3% acetic acid to highlight areas. Areas of white, raised epithelium should be biopsied.
- For patients with new onset of pruritus, the area of pruritus should be biopsied.
- Liberal biopsies must be used to diagnose in situ disease prior to invasion and to diagnose early invasive disease.
- The patient should not be treated for presumed benign conditions of the vulva without full exam and biopsy, including Pap smear and colposcopy of cervix, vagina, and vulva.
- When symptoms persist, re-examine and rebiopsy.
- Treatment of benign condyloma of the vulva has not been shown to decrease the eventual incidence of in situ or invasive disease of the vulva.
- CXR to evaluate for metastatic disease
- CT scan to evaluate pelvic and periaortic lymph node status if tumor >2 cm or if suspicion of metastatic disease.

Diagnostic Procedures/Other
Office vulvar biopsy is done to establish the diagnosis.

Test Interpretation
A surgical staging system is used for vulvar cancer (International Federation of Obstetrics and Gynecology Classification):
- Stage I: Tumor confined to the vulva:
  - Stage IA: Lesions ≤2 cm in size, confined to the vulva or perineum, and with stromal invasion ≤1 mm, no node metastasis
  - Stage IB: Lesions >2 cm in size or with stromal invasion >1 mm, confined to the vulva or perineum, with negative nodes
- Stage II: Tumor of any size with extension to adjacent perineal structures (1/3 lower urethra, 1/3 lower vagina, anus) with negative nodes
- Stage III: Tumor of any size with or without extension to adjacent perineal structures (1/3 lower urethra, 1/3 lower vagina, anus) with positive inguinofemoral lymph nodes:
  - Stage IIIA:
    ○ With 1 lymph node metastasis (≥5 mm), or
    ○ 1–2 lymph node metastasis(es) (<5 mm)
  - Stage IIIB:
    ○ With ≥2 lymph node metastases (≥5 mm), or
    ○ ≥3 lymph node metastases (<5 mm)
  - Stage IIIC: With positive nodes with extracapsular spread
- Stage IV: Tumor invades other regional (2/3 upper urethra, 2/3 upper vagina) or distant structures
  - Stage IVA: Tumor invades any of the following:
    ○ Upper urethral and/or vaginal mucosa, bladder mucosa, rectal mucosa, or fixed to pelvic bone, or
    ○ Fixed or ulcerated inguinofemoral lymph nodes
  - Stage IVB: Any distant metastasis, including pelvic lymph nodes

TREATMENT

There are no curative drugs.

GENERAL MEASURES

- Wide excision can be performed for carcinoma in situ, and any lesion about which there is doubt should be further excised for definitive diagnosis to ensure that invasive disease is not coexistent with the carcinoma in situ.
- Cystoscopy and sigmoidoscopy should be performed if there is a question of invasion into the urethra, bladder, or rectum.

MEDICATION

- As an adjuvant therapy, fluorouracil (Efudex) cream for in situ disease can produce occasional results, but is not well tolerated because of irritation of the vulva.
- Chemoradiotherapy with cisplatin and 5-fluorouracil (5-FU) has been successful in advanced or recurrent disease, although local morbidity is increased (1)[B].
- Adjuvant chemotherapy has not proved to be effective in this disease (2)[A].
- Contraindications: Elderly patients: If chemotherapeutic agents are used, pay close attention to the patient's performance status and ability to tolerate aggressive chemotherapy.
- Precautions: The usual precautions for chemotherapy agents.

ISSUES FOR REFERRAL

Patients may need care from a gynecologic oncologist and/or a radiation oncologist.

ADDITIONAL THERAPIES

- Radiation therapy is used as adjuvant therapy for patients with positive inguinal lymph nodes.
- Preoperative radiation/chemotherapy may allow for a less radical surgical procedure in patients with advanced disease (3,4)[B].
- Postoperative radiation as an adjuvant treatment decreases recurrence frequency and may improve survival (3)[B].
- Radiation is contraindicated with verrucous carcinoma because it induces anaplastic transformation and increases metastases.

SURGERY/OTHER PROCEDURES

- In situ disease can be treated with wide excision or laser vaporization of the affected area. Laser vaporization is preferable in the younger patient, whereas wide excision is preferable in the elderly patient, in whom the risk of invasive disease is also higher.
- 0.5 mm of negative margin is adequate for in situ disease (1)[C].
- Stage IA: Radical local excision without lymph node dissection because lymph node metastases are <1%. (1)[C]
- Stage IB: Radical local excision with inguinofemoral lymph node dissection because the risk of metastases increases to 8% (1)[C]
- Stage II: Modified radical vulvectomy and groin node dissection are recommended (1)[C].
- Stage III and IVA: Radical vulvectomy and bilateral inguinal lymph node dissection are recommended (1)[C].
- Bulky advanced-stage lesions are often treated initially with chemoradiation followed by less radical surgery (4)[B].

- Adjuvant radiation therapy is recommended with microscopically positive lymph nodes (1)[C].
- Pelvic exenteration after radiation provides effective therapy for advanced or recurrent malignancies involving the bladder or rectum.
- More limited surgery:
  - Has been undertaken for early invasive lesions, especially in young patients, to preserve the clitoris and sexual function
  - Sentinel lymph node (SLN) biopsy also has been advocated for early invasive lesion; however, data show lower accuracy compared with complete dissection (5)[C].
  - Radical vulvectomy with bilateral groin node dissection through separate incisions provides better cosmetic results than the en bloc technique.
  - Radical hemivulvectomy and unilateral groin node dissection also can be used for smaller unilateral lesions.

IN-PATIENT CONSIDERATIONS

Typically inpatient for treatment

Admission Criteria/Initial Stabilization

In advanced malignancy involving the urethra and rectum, concomitant cisplatin/5-FU chemotherapy with radiation produces a significant decrease in size of the primary tumor, usually obviating the need for pelvic exenteration.

ONGOING CARE

FOLLOW-UP RECOMMENDATIONS

Patient Monitoring

- Early stage, treated with surgery alone: Clinical exam of the groin nodes and vulvar area every 6 months for 2 years; then annually
- Advance stage, treated with surgery + chemo/radiation: Clinical exam of the groin nodes and vulvar area every 3 months for 2 years; then every 6 months for 3 years, then annually
- Annual CXR
- Majority of relapses occur within first year.

DIET

As tolerated and according to comorbid conditions

PATIENT EDUCATION

- American College of Obstetricians and Gynecologists (ACOG), 409 12th St., SW, Washington, DC 20024-2188; (800) 762-ACOG; www.acog.org
- American Cancer Society: www.cancer.org
- Medline Plus: www.nlm.nih.gov/medlineplus/vulvarcancer.html

PROGNOSIS

The 5-year survival is based on stage:
- Stage I: 78.5%
- Stage II: 58.8%
- Stage III: 43.2%
- Stage IV: 13%

COMPLICATIONS

- The major complications from radical vulvectomy and groin node dissection are:
  - Wound breakdown
  - Lymphocysts
  - Lymphedema
  - Urinary stress incontinence
  - Psychosexual consequences

- 2 common complications with radical vulvectomy and bilateral groin node dissection:
  - In the immediate postoperative period, ~50% of patients experience breakdown of the wound. This requires aggressive wound care by visiting nurses as often as twice a day. The wounds usually granulate and heal over a period of 6–10 weeks.
  - ~15–20% of patients experience some form of mild-to-moderate lymphedema after the groin node dissection. These patients should be instructed in the use of leg elevation and support hose. <1% of patients experience severe, debilitating lymphedema.

REFERENCES

1. de Hullu JA, van der Zee AG. Surgery and radiotherapy in vulvar cancer. *Crit Rev Oncol Hematol*. 2006;60:38–58.
2. Shylasree TS, Bryant A, Howells RE. Chemoradiation for advanced primary vulval cancer. *Cochrane Database Syst Rev*. 2011;(4):CD003752.
3. Montana GS. Carcinoma of the vulva: Combined modality treatment. *Curr Treat Options Oncol*. 2004;5:85–95.
4. de Hullu JA, van der Avoort IA, Oonk MH, et al. Management of vulvar cancers. *Eur J Surg Oncol*. 2006;32(8):825–831.
5. Radziszewski J, Kowalewska M, Jedrzejczak T, et al. The accuracy of the sentinel lymph node concept in early stage squamous cell vulvar carcinoma. *Gynecol Oncol*. 2010;116:473–477.

ADDITIONAL READING

- Crosbie EJ, Slade RJ, Ahmed AS, et al. The management of vulval cancer. *Cancer Treat Rev*. 2009;35:533–539.
- Hampl M, Sarajuuri H, Wentzensen N, et al. Effect of human papillomavirus vaccines on vulvar, vaginal, and anal intraepithelial lesions and vulvar cancer. *Obstet Gynecol*. 2006;108(6):1361–1368.
- Markowitz LE, Dunne EF, Saraiya M, et al. Quadrivalent human papillomavirus vaccine: Recommendations of the Advisory Committee on Immunization Practices (ACIP). *MMWR Recomm Rep*. 2007;56(RR-2):1–24.

CODES

ICD10
- C51.0 Malignant neoplasm of labium majus
- C51.9 Malignant neoplasm of vulva, unspecified
- D07.1 Carcinoma in situ of vulva

CLINICAL PEARLS

- 60% of vulvar cancers are attributable to oncogenic HPV, and 92% of all VIN 2/3, VaIN 2/3, and AIN are attributable to HPV. Therefore, HPV vaccination has the potential to decrease vulvar cancer by 1/3.
- Biopsy all suspicious or nonhealing vulvar lesions.

VULVODYNIA

Tara J. Neil, MD

 BASICS

DESCRIPTION

- Vulvar discomfort, often described as burning. Occurs in the absence of relevant visible findings, relevant lab abnormalities, or a clinically identifiable neurologic disorder
- Classification is based on whether pain is generalized or localized and whether it is provoked (by physical contact), spontaneous, or mixed:
  - Generalized: Involvement of majority of the vulva; usually persistent or spontaneous pain
  - Localized: Severe pain of certain vulvar areas, such as the vestibule (formerly known as *vestibulodynia*), usually provoked with touch or attempted vaginal entry; thought to be the leading cause of painful intercourse among premenopausal women:
    - Primary: Introital dyspareunia from 1st episode of intercourse or 1st insertion of tampon or vaginal speculum
    - Secondary: Introital dyspareunia developing after a period of painless intercourse, tampon use, or speculum exams

EPIDEMIOLOGY

- Most women diagnosed between the ages of 20 and 80.
- Patients are psychologically comparable with asymptomatic controls and have similar marital satisfaction.

Incidence

- Recent retrospective study estimates annual rate of new onset vulvodynia to be 1.8% (1).
- Evidence indicates lifetime cumulative incidence approaches 15%, suggesting nearly 14 million US women will experience persistent vulvar discomfort at some point in their lives (2).

Prevalence

- Reports between 3.1% and 15%; nonclinical-based studies approximate a prevalence of 7% with validation by exam.
- Studies show Hispanics 80% are more likely to present with vulvar pain compared with Caucasians and African Americans (3).

ETIOLOGY AND PATHOPHYSIOLOGY

- Vulvodynia is likely to be neuropathically mediated:
  - Allodynia and hyperalgesia are thought to result from neurogenic inflammation, leading to sensitization of primary afferents by inflammatory peptides, prostaglandins, and cytokines. Impulses transmitted to the CNS, where reinforcing signals sustain pain loop.
  - In recent investigations of vulvar biopsy specimens, increased neuronal proliferation and branching in vulvar tissue are evident when compared with tissue of asymptomatic women (4).
- Pelvic floor pathology also should be considered: In one study, the vulvodynia group showed an increase in pelvic floor hypertonicity at the superficial muscle layer, less vaginal muscle strength with contraction, and decreased relaxation of pelvic floor muscles after contraction (2).
- No cause of vulvodynia has been established. It is most likely a neuropathic pain caused by:
  - Recurrent vulvovaginal candidiasis or other infections

- Chemical exposure (trichloroacetic acid) or physical trauma
- Reduced estrogen receptor expression/changes in estrogen concentration
- CNS etiology, similar to other regional pain syndromes

RISK FACTORS

- Vulvovaginal infections, specifically candidiasis. Unclear if infection, treatment, or underlying hypersensitivity is the cause (5)
- Hormonal factors: Controversial evidence proposes increased risk with use of oral contraception pills (OCPs); early age at 1st use of OCPs and longer duration of use have been associated with increased risk.
- Pelvic floor dysfunction: Increased instability of pelvic floor muscles may perpetuate vulvar tissue inflammation, leading to vascular changes and histamine release.
- Comorbid interstitial cystitis and painful bladder syndrome; potentially related to common embryological origin of structures
- Abuse: Increased risk of vulvodynia if childhood physical or sexual abuse by a primary family member; causal relationship remains unclear (2)
- Depression and anxiety (5)
- Other neuropathic disorders, including regional pain syndrome

Genetics

Proposed genetic deficiency impairing one's ability to stop the inflammatory response triggered by infection or chemicals; homozygosity of the 2 alleles of the interleukin-1 receptor antagonist occurs in 25–50% of vestibulodynia patients, compared with <10% in controls (4).

GENERAL PREVENTION

- Wear 100% cotton underwear in the daytime and no underwear to sleep.
- Avoid douching and other vulvar irritants such as perfumes, dyes, detergents.
- Avoid abrasive activities and tight, synthetic clothing.
- Avoid panty liners.
- Clean the vulva with water only and pat area dry after bathing.
- Avoid use of hairdryers in the vulvar area.

COMMONLY ASSOCIATED CONDITIONS

Higher incidence of chronic pain syndromes associated with vulvodynia, including chronic cystitis, irritable bowel syndrome (IBS), fibromyalgia, migraines, depression, endometriosis, low back pain

℞ DIAGNOSIS

- Vulvodynia is a clinical diagnosis and should be suspected in any women with chronic pain at the introitus and vulva (4)[B].

- Pain should be characterized using a standard measure, such as the McGill Pain Questionnaire; duration and nature of the pain should be established. Use physical exam to rule out other causes of vulvovaginal pain. Negative fungal culture, along with relevant history and positive cotton swab test (see below), confirm diagnosis.

HISTORY

Adequate sexual, social, and pain history should be taken to assess degree of symptoms. Visual pain scales and pain diaries may be helpful (6)[C]:

- Specifically ask about bowel and bladder habits, history of trauma or abuse, history of infections, including herpes, and personal hygiene.
- Onset of vulvodynia often sudden and without precedents
- Pain often described as generalized, unprovoked
- Specific skin complaints may suggest alternate diagnosis; a history of allergies may suggest vulvar dermatitis.
- Assess for precipitants of vulvar pain: Tight garments, bicycle riding, tampon use, prolonged sitting, perfumed or deodorant soaps, douching
- Assess for complaints of dyspareunia:
  - Presence of vaginismus (involuntary vaginal muscle spasm), adequate lubrication, anorgasmia, partner problems, abuse
  - Psychosexual morbidity significantly higher in patients with vulvodynia; counseling may complement medical interventions.

PHYSICAL EXAM

- Ask patient to show where pain is localized or most painful.
- Mouth and skin exams to assess for lesions suggestive of lichen planus or lichen sclerosis
- Vaginal exam should be done to exclude other causes of vulvovaginal pain, including external inspection, palpation, and single digit, speculum, and bimanual exams:
  - The vulva may be erythematous, especially at the vestibule. Discomfort with separation of the labia minora is common.
  - Spontaneous or elicited pain at the lower 1/2 of anterior vaginal wall suggests bladder etiology.
- Bulbocavernosus and anal wink reflexes should be checked to assess for peripheral neuropathy.

DIFFERENTIAL DIAGNOSIS

- Infections: Candidiasis, herpes, human papillomavirus (HPV), bacterial vaginosis, trichomoniasis, dermatophytes
- Inflammation: Lichen planus, immunobullous disorder, allergic vulvitis, lichen sclerosis, atrophic vaginitis
- Neoplasia: Paget disease, vulvar or vaginal intraepithelial neoplasia, squamous cell carcinoma
- Neurologic/Muscular: Herpes neuralgia, spinal nerve compression, vaginismus

DIAGNOSTIC TESTS & INTERPRETATION

Cotton swab or Q-tip test: Vulva tested for localized areas of pain beginning at thighs and continuing medially toward vestibule using the soft end and broken sharp end of the cotton swab. 5 distinct positions (2, 4, 6, 8, and 10 o'clock) surveyed using light palpation. Pain rated on a scale from 0 (none) to 10 (most severe). Posterior introitus and posterior hymenal remnants most common sites of increased sensitivity

Initial Tests (lab, imaging)

- Vaginal pH, wet mount, and yeast culture are recommended to rule out vaginitis.
- Gonorrhea and chlamydia testing done at physician's discretion
- HPV screening is unnecessary; no association has been identified between HPV and vulvodynia.

Follow-Up Tests & Special Considerations
- Varicella-zoster and herpes simplex virus should be considered if ulcers or vesicular eruptions are present.
- Biopsy should be considered if concerned about neoplasm or dermatophyte infection or if the patient is resistant to treatment.

Diagnostic Procedures/Other
Colposcopy can be helpful if epidermal abnormalities are present. This should be done with caution because acetic acid worsens vulvar pain.

Test Interpretation
No specific histologic features are associated with vulvodynia, although reactive squamous atypia has been observed. Biopsies are unnecessary for diagnosis. Presence of rash/altered mucosa is not consistent with vulvodynia; this requires further evaluation (6)[C].

TREATMENT

A trial of several medications for at least 3 months is usually needed.

GENERAL MEASURES
Combining treatments should be encouraged when treating women with vulvodynia (6)[C]: Various reports on use of a combination of medical treatments, psychotherapy, and dietary intervention reveal women on these combinations do significantly better compared with those who receive medication only.

MEDICATION
- Oral therapies:
  - Tricyclic antidepressants (TCAs): First-line treatment for unprovoked vulvodynia (6)[B]; do not stop use abruptly; contraindicated in patients with cardiac abnormalities and those taking MAOIs; fatigue, constipation, sweating, palpitations, and weight gain are most common side effects:
    - Amitriptyline, Nortriptyline: Most widely studied; start at 10 mg daily; dose should be titrated to pain control. Average effective dose is 60 mg daily. In one study, a 47% complete response rate was recorded (7)[B].
  - SSRIs/SSNRIs: Not commonly used; however, have been helpful in those who cannot tolerate TCAs:
    - Venlafaxine is currently being prescribed more frequently with good results.
  - Gabapentin: Started at 300 mg daily and increased by 300 mg every 3 days. Maximum recommended dose is 3,600 mg daily divided into 3 doses. Dosing regimen limits popularity.
  - Narcotics/NSAIDs: Consistently have not been helpful in relieving vulvar pain
- Topical therapies:
  - Lidocaine 5% ointment: For provoked vestibulodynia; application advised 15–20 minutes prior to intercourse. Penile numbness and possible toxicity with ingestion can occur:
    - A trial of local anesthetics may be recommended for all patients who present with vulvodynia. Use judiciously to avoid increased irritation (6)[C].
    - In one study, lidocaine 5% ointment was left in vestibule overnight (average of 8 hours) for a period of 6–8 weeks; at follow-up, up to 76% of women reported no discomfort with intercourse (2)[C].

  - Cromolyn 4% cream: Decreases mast cell degranulation in vulvar tissue; recommended application t.i.d. (5)[C]
  - Capsaicin 0.025%: Decreases in discomfort and increases in frequency of intercourse with 20-minute daily application (2)[B]
  - Topical amitriptyline 2% combined with baclofen 2% is helpful in patients with comorbid vaginismus.
  - Topical corticosteroids and testosterone creams have not been shown to alleviate symptoms of vulvodynia.
  - Gabapentin 3% ointment or gabapentin 6% (must be compounded)
  - Topical nitroglycerin may be helpful, but may cause headaches
  - Topical estrogen
- Injectable therapies:
  - Triamcinolone acetonide 0.1%: No more than 40 mg should be injected monthly; is best when combined with 0.25–0.5% bupivacaine.
  - Submucosal methylprednisone and lidocaine: Reports of up to 68% response rate with weekly injections (6)[B]
  - Interferon-α: Useful in treatment of vestibulodynia. Side effects (myalgias, fever, malaise) limit use.
  - Botulinum toxin A injectable

ISSUES FOR REFERRAL
A team approach is recommended for most effective management. Triage to psychosexual medicine, psychology, and pain management teams should be strongly considered (6)[B].

ADDITIONAL THERAPIES
- Biofeedback/Physical therapy: Useful with concomitant vaginismus. Treats both generalized and localized vulvar pain; treatment value for unprovoked pain remains unclear. Most studies report an average of 12–16-week treatment time.
- Surface electromyography (sEMG): Efficacious for pelvic floor rehabilitation. Patients are more likely to endure pain-free sexual intercourse after sEMG. Significant reductions seen on pain measures at long-term follow-up.
- Cognitive-behavioral therapy (CBT): One randomized trial revealed that CBT is associated with a 30% decrease in vulvar discomfort with sexual intercourse. CBT is the recommended treatment for patients who present with dyspareunia as a main complaint (4)[B].

COMPLEMENTARY AND ALTERNATIVE MEDICINE
Acupuncture: Small studies of women with unprovoked vulvodynia who did not respond to conventional treatment reported significant decreases in pain severity with acupuncture; treatment value with provoked pain is unknown (6)[C].

SURGERY/OTHER PROCEDURES
- Surgery may be considered for patients who have failed to respond to other measures. Use of surgical treatment is not recommended for generalized vulvodynia (6)[B].
- 60–80% of women who undergo surgery report a significant reduction in pain symptoms; however, when surveyed, patients prefer behavioral therapies to surgical intervention.

- A 3-armed randomized trial in 2001 found that women who underwent surgical intervention were more satisfied than those treated with biofeedback or CBT (4)[B].
- All patients who are considering surgical intervention should be tested for vaginismus. Vestibulectomy is less successful in this subgroup.
- Surgical approaches:
  - Local excision: Precise localization of painful areas; tissue closed in elliptical fashion
  - Total vestibulectomy: Incision is made and tissue is removed from Skene ducts to perineum. The vagina is then brought down to cover defect.
  - Perineoplasty: Vestibulectomy plus removal of perineal tissue; incision usually terminated above the anal orifice; reserved for severe cases (4)[B]

ONGOING CARE

PATIENT EDUCATION
Patients should be reassured that this condition is not infectious, nor does it predispose to cancer (6)[C]. Emphasize self-hygiene. Encourage treatment with home remedies, including ice packs, sitz baths, and barrier cream to preserve moisture after bathing.

PROGNOSIS
Traditionally viewed as a chronic pain disorder, new evidence of remission has been documented; recent 2-year follow-up study revealed 1 in 10 vulvodynia patients reported remission.

REFERENCES

1. Reed B, Haefner H, Sen A, et al. Vulvodynia incidence and remission rates among adult women: A 2-year follow-up study. *Obstet Gynecol.* 2008; 112:231–237.
2. Boardman L, Stockdale C. Sexual pain. *Clin Obstet Gynecol.* 2009;52:682–690.
3. Harlow BL, Stewart EG. A population-based assessment of chronic unexplained vulvar pain: Have we underestimated the prevalence of vulvodynia? *J Am Med Womens Assoc.* 2003; 58:82–88.
4. Reed B. Vulvodynia: Diagnosis and management. *Am Fam Physician.* 2006;73:1231–1239.
5. Groysman V. Vulvodynia: New concepts and review of the literature. *Dermatol Clin.* 2010;28:681–696.
6. Mandal D, Nunns M, Byrne J, et al. Guidelines for the management of vulvodynia. *BJD.* 2010; 162:1180–1185.
7. Haefner H, Collins M, Davis G, et al. The vulvodynia guideline. *J Low Genit Tract Dis.* 2005;9:40–51.

 # CODES

ICD10
- N94.810 Vulvar vestibulitis
- N94.818 Other vulvodynia
- N94.819 Vulvodynia, unspecified

CLINICAL PEARLS

Vulvodynia is a clinical diagnosis; it should be suspected in any woman with chronic pain at the introitus and vulva.

V

VULVOVAGINITIS, ESTROGEN DEFICIENT
Maria de La Luz Nieto, MD

 BASICS

DESCRIPTION
- Vaginal atrophy is due to decreased blood flow to vaginal epithelium, resulting in thinning of the female genital tissues.
- Estrogen deficiency affects all tissues in the female body; however, the genital tissues are especially hormone responsive and are most affected, leading to atrophy.
- Patients with estrogen-deficient vulvovaginitis may present with urinary incontinence, vaginal burning and itching, dyspareunia, increased urinary frequency, or recurrent UTIs.
- System(s) affected: Reproductive

EPIDEMIOLOGY
Incidence
- Predominant age: Postmenopausal females. The average age of menopause in the US is 51.3 years.
- May affect lactating women
- Predominant sex: Female only
- May occur in younger women with premature ovarian failure

Prevalence
- Most postmenopausal women are affected to some degree.
- Up to 40% of postmenopausal women experience symptoms severe enough to seek treatment.

ETIOLOGY AND PATHOPHYSIOLOGY
- Decreased estrogen levels in the vagina and vulva result in decreased blood flow and decreased lubrication of vaginal and vulvar tissue.
- Vaginal and vulvar tissues become thin secondary to decreased vaginal cell maturation.
- Decreased cellular maturation results in decreased glycogen stores, which affects the normal vaginal flora and pH.
- Estrogen deficiency due to:
  – Menopause (surgical or natural)
  – Premature ovarian failure (chemotherapy, irradiation, autoimmune, anorexia, genetic)
  – Postpartum, lactation
  – Medications that alter hormonal concentration, such as gonadotropin-releasing hormone agonists, and antiestrogens, such as tamoxifen and danazol
  – Elevated prolactin from hypothalamic-pituitary disorders

Genetics
No known pattern

RISK FACTORS
Estrogen-deficient states

COMMONLY ASSOCIATED CONDITIONS
- Urge and stress urinary incontinence
- Pelvic organ prolapse
- Frequent UTIs
- Bacterial vaginosis or yeast infections

 DIAGNOSIS

HISTORY
- All female patients should be asked about symptoms because many women are embarrassed to discuss these issues with their health care providers:
  – Vaginal dryness
  – Dyspareunia
  – Pruritus
  – Burning
  – Pressure
  – Tenderness
  – Malodorous discharge
  – Urinary symptoms: Dysuria, hematuria, frequency, infections, stress and urge urinary incontinence
- Ask about self-treatment and products used
- Determine exposure to irritants (e.g., soaps, feminine sprays, lotions, lubricants, constant pad use).

PHYSICAL EXAM
Evidence for the diagnosis includes the following (1):
- Loss of pubic hair
- Decreased vulvar and vaginal fullness
- Decreased vulvar subcuticular fat and moisture
- Pale-appearing, shiny, smooth vaginal and urethral epithelium
- Vaginal shortening, intolerance to speculum exams
- Loss of vaginal rugation
- Pelvic organ prolapse

DIFFERENTIAL DIAGNOSIS
- Malignancy
- Dermatologic conditions of vulva and vagina:
  – Dermatitis
  – Lichen sclerosis
  – Lichen planus
- Bacterial or yeast vulvovaginitis

DIAGNOSTIC TESTS & INTERPRETATION
Because vulvovaginitis is a clinical diagnosis, labs are not always necessary.

Initial Tests (lab, imaging)
However, the following labs may be obtained as corroborative of clinical impression:
- Check follicle-stimulating hormone (FSH) and estrogen levels. FSH rises and estrogen drops with menopause.
- Evaluate for infections via wet preparation and vaginal pH (usually >5).
- Urine dip and urinalysis if suspected concomitant UTI
- Perform cytology for maturation index: Higher proportion of parabasal cells and lower proportion of intermediate and superficial cells indicate decreased maturation index.

Follow-Up Tests & Special Considerations
Drugs that may alter lab results:
- Estrogen therapy will alter the maturation index.
- Digoxin has estrogen-like properties.
- Tamoxifen may produce menopausal-type symptoms, but also may act on genital tissues as a weak estrogen agonist.
- Progestins, danazol, and gonadotropin-releasing hormone agonists may produce a reversible pseudomenopause state.

Test Interpretation
- Thinning of the cornified squamous layer of both the vulva and the vagina
- Increased parabasal cells
- Compact underlying collagenous tissue

TREATMENT

GENERAL MEASURES
- Wear loose-fitting, undyed cotton underwear
- Avoid prolonged pad use, especially scented pads
- Avoid feminine deodorant sprays and douching
- Use over-the-counter water-based lubricants, as needed
- Symptomatic relief, if needed (e.g., cool baths or compresses)

MEDICATION
- Vaginal estrogen can reverse atrophic changes and help to alleviate symptoms (2,3)[A]:
  - Vaginal cream 1 g (conjugated equine estrogens or estradiol cream): Insert via applicator each night × 14 days and then 2–3 × per week.
  - Vaginal estradiol 10-μg tablet: Insert via preloaded applicator each night × 14 days and then 2–3 × per week.
  - Estradiol-containing vaginal ring 2 mg: Insert into vagina, and replace every 3 months.
- Estrogen therapy should be used in the lowest possible dose for the shortest duration of time.
- Long-term therapy may be necessary owing to the chronic nature of estrogen-deficient vulvovaginitis.
- Systemic therapy typically is used as hormonal treatment of vasomotor symptoms and not for the primary treatment of estrogen-deficient vulvovaginitis.
- Contraindications:
  - Breast or estrogen-dependent carcinoma
  - Undiagnosed vaginal bleeding
  - Thromboembolic disorders
  - Thrombophlebitis
  - Pregnancy
- Precautions: Any abnormal vaginal bleeding must be evaluated.

ISSUES FOR REFERRAL
- Refer to urogynecologist for evaluation if symptomatic due to pelvic organ prolapse and/or stress and urge urinary incontinence.
- Recurrent UTIs should be referred to urogynecology and/or urology for evaluation.

IN-PATIENT CONSIDERATIONS
Admission Criteria/Initial Stabilization
Outpatient treatment

ONGOING CARE

FOLLOW-UP RECOMMENDATIONS
No restrictions

Patient Monitoring
Instruct the patient that symptoms should improve within 30–60 days. If they do not, re-evaluate and re-examine for other causes.

DIET
No special diet

PATIENT EDUCATION
- American College of Obstetricians and Gynecologists (ACOG), 409 12th St., SW, Washington, DC 20024-2188; 800-762-ACOG; www.acog.org
- Lactating postpartum women with high levels of prolactin are in a hypoestrogenic state. These women should be instructed to use lubrication for symptoms of dyspareunia and reassured that the symptoms will resolve when they are no longer breastfeeding.

PROGNOSIS
The prognosis is excellent. Most symptoms will be alleviated with vaginal estrogen replacement therapy.

COMPLICATIONS
- Recurrent UTIs may occur in women with vaginal atrophy.
- Vaginal atrophy predisposes patients to vaginal infections.

REFERENCES

1. Johnston SL, Farrell SA, Bouchard C, et al. The detection and management of vaginal atrophy. *J Obstet Gynaecol Can*. 2004;26:503–515.
2. Suckling J, Lethaby A, Kennedy R. Local oestrogen for vaginal atrophy in postmenopausal women. *Cochrane Database Syst Rev*. 2006;4:CD001500.
3. Farquhar CM, Marjoribanks J, Lethaby A, et al. Long-term hormone therapy for perimenopausal and postmenopausal women. *Cochrane Database Syst Rev*. 2005;3:CD004143.

ADDITIONAL READING
- Ibe C, Simon JA. Vulvovaginal atrophy: Current and future therapies (CME). *J Sex Med*. 2010;7: 1042–1050; quiz 1051.
- Mehta A, Bachmann G. Vulvovaginal complaints. *Clin Obstet Gynecol*. 2008;51:549–555.

CODES

ICD10
- N95.2 Postmenopausal atrophic vaginitis
- N76.0 Acute vaginitis

CLINICAL PEARLS
- Estrogen-deficient vulvovaginitis affects virtually all postmenopausal women to some degree.
- This disorder is often associated with urinary incontinence, increased urinary frequency, and recurrent UTIs.
- Lab tests are generally unnecessary to make the diagnosis.
- Vaginal estrogen preparations, rather than systemic preparations, should be 1st-line therapy in a woman whose primary complaint is associated with vaginal atrophy.

V

VULVOVAGINITIS, PREPUBESCENT
Katherine M. Callaghan, MD • Dawn S. Tasillo, MD

 BASICS

DESCRIPTION
- Vulvitis is inflammation of the external genitals.
- Vaginitis, often associated with vaginal discharge, is inflammation involving the vaginal mucosa.
- In premenarchal girls, vulvitis is usually primary with secondary extension into the vagina.
- System(s) affected: Reproductive; Skin/Exocrine
- Synonym(s): Vaginitis; Vulvitis

EPIDEMIOLOGY
Incidence
Unknown
Prevalence
Most common gynecologic problem in prepubertal girls

ETIOLOGY AND PATHOPHYSIOLOGY
- In the prepubertal child, the levels of estrogen are low.
- Due to the low levels of estrogen, the vaginal epithelium is thin, immature, and fragile.
- Absence of pubic hair and a well-developed labia, as well as close proximity of the anus and vagina, make contamination more likely.
- The prepubertal child also has an absence of lactobacilli, creating a neutral to alkaline vaginal pH.
- Neutral pH, atrophic mucosa, and moist environment of the vagina increases the risk of infection.
- Most cases of pediatric vulvovaginitis are nonspecific inflammation.
- Specific infections that occur are typically respiratory, enteric, or sexually transmitted.
- Nonspecific vulvovaginitis:
  - Poor perineal hygiene
  - Nonspecific chemical irritants (bubble baths, scented soaps, shampoos)
  - Tight-fitting clothing

Genetics
Understudied

RISK FACTORS
- Prepubertal girls are particularly susceptible due to behavioral and anatomic reasons:
  - Inadequate hand washing or perineal cleansing after urination and defecation
  - Tight-fitting clothing
  - Proximity of the vagina to the anus, lack of protective hair, and labial fat pads
  - Trauma
- Obese girls are also susceptible to nonspecific vulvovaginitis (1).

GENERAL PREVENTION
- Good perineal hygiene (including wiping from front to back)
- Urination with legs spread apart and labia separated
- Avoidance of tight-fitting clothing and nonabsorbent underwear
- Avoidance of irritants such as harsh soaps and bubble baths
- The most common respiratory pathogen is *Streptococcus pyogenes*. Vulvitis may occur in the absence of respiratory symptoms.
- *Shigella* vaginitis is associated with mucopurulent bloody discharge and likewise is not always accompanied by a history of diarrhea.

Respiratory	Enteral	Sexually transmitted
Streptococcus pyogenes	*Shigella*	*Neisseria gonorrhoeae*
Staphylococcus aureus	*Yersinia enterocolitica*	*Chlamydia trachomatis*
Haemophilus influenzae		*Trichomonas vaginalis*
Moraxella catarrhalis		*Papilloma* virus
Streptococcus pneumoniae		*Herpes* virus
Neisseria meningitidis		

- *Enterobius vermicularis* (pinworms):
  - Very common in young children and certain populations
  - Should be considered in children with vaginal itching and irritation
  - Most common symptom is nocturnal perineal itching
- Foreign body:
  - Presents with foul-smelling, bloody, or brown discharge from the vagina
  - Should be considered with recurrent vulvovaginitis where other causes have been eliminated
- Other:
  - With chronic vulvovaginitis, anatomic abnormalities or systemic disease should be considered:
    - Anatomic abnormalities include double vagina with fistula, ectopic ureter, and urethral prolapse.
  - Systemic disease (inflammatory diseases)
  - Other conditions, such as lichen sclerosus, vitiligo, psoriasis, and atopic dermatitis, should be considered.

ALERT
Cultures of sexually transmitted organisms in prepubertal children warrant investigations of sexual abuse.

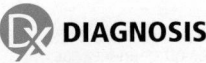 **DIAGNOSIS**

HISTORY
- Irritation and erythema of vulva
- Itching
- Bleeding
- Vaginal discharge
- Unpleasant odor
- Dysuria
- Soreness

PHYSICAL EXAM
- Look for evidence of chronic illness or dermatologic disease
- Look for trauma or other signs that may correlate with abuse
- Inspect the genital area in the supine position:
  - Excoriation of the genital area
  - Inflammation (erythema, swelling) of the introitus
  - Inspect the vagina and cervix in the knee–chest position
  - Perform rectal exam if vaginal bleeding or abdominal pain

DIFFERENTIAL DIAGNOSIS
- Contact dermatitis
- Eczema
- Psoriasis
- Lichen sclerosus

DIAGNOSTIC TESTS & INTERPRETATION
Initial Tests (lab, imaging)
- Culture for bacteria, fungi (yeast), or viruses (herpes).
- Urinalysis, urine culture, and urine for STI; via nucleic acid amplification test)
- Tape exam for pinworms
- Potassium hydroxide and saline smears of vaginal discharge, if present
- If an anatomic abnormality is suspected, imaging may be necessary to confirm.
- Consider consultation with a pediatric or adult gynecologist to determine the most appropriate imaging study.

Follow-Up Tests & Special Considerations
Exploration of the vagina for a foreign body may be necessary in cases of persistent, recurrent vulvitis.

Diagnostic Procedures/Other
If blood or foul-smelling discharge is present, visualization is mandatory:
- Place the child in the knee–chest position for best results. Hold the buttocks apart and slightly upward.
- Visualization of the vagina may be necessary by using a nasal speculum or infant laryngoscope.
- If available, consider referral to a provider with specific training/experience in this specialized exam.

TREATMENT

- The definitive diagnosis of bacterial vulvitis requires a culture of vulva and vaginal secretions.
- The typical colony count and bacterial mix are unknown in prepubescent girls. Antibiotic use should be directed against the species with the highest colony count.
- General hygiene always should be recommended, particularly in cases of a retained foreign body (e.g., toilet paper).
- When no cause is identified, treatment should focus on hygiene as well as minimizing soap exposure and tight-fitting clothes (2).

GENERAL MEASURES
- Appropriate health care: Outpatient (except where systemic illness requires hospital care)
- Soak the vulva/perineum in a small amount of clear, warm water for 15 minutes b.i.d.
- If smegma is present in the labial folds, clean the area gently with a mild soap (1).

MEDICATION
First Line
- To break the itching–scratching–infection cycle, use a low-dose topical hydrocortisone cream for a limited time (3).
- Estrogen deficiency with labial adhesion/agglutination: Estrogen cream 0.625 mg to fused area nightly for 2 weeks (4).
- Antibiotic use should be restricted to cases of bacterial infection only (3).
- For empirical treatment of suspected bacterial infection, use amoxicillin 20 mg/kg/d for 7 days (4).
- Specific organisms on culture:
  – Group A *Streptococcus*, *S. pneumoniae*: Penicillin V (Pen Vee K) 250 mg PO b.i.d.–t.i.d. for 10 days (5)
  – *H. influenzae*: Amoxicillin, 20–40 mg/kg/d PO for 7 days (5)
  – *S. aureus*: Cephalexin, 25–50 mg/kg/d PO q.i.d. for 7–10 days *or* dicloxacillin, 25 mg/kg/d for 7–10 days *or*, amoxicillin-clavulanate, 20–40 mg/kg/d for 7–10 days (5)
  – *S. pyogens*: Amoxicillin, 50 mg/kg/d PO divided into 3 doses/d for 10 days (3)
  – *Candida* sp.: Topical nystatin (Mycostatin), miconazole, clotrimazole, or terconazole
  – *Shigella*: Trimethoprim/sulfamethoxazole or ampicillin for 5 days
  – Pinworms: Mebendazole, 100 mg PO, repeated in 2 weeks
  – *Chlamydia trachomatis*: ≤45 kg: Erythromycin, 50 mg/kg/d t.i.d. for 14 days; ≥45 kg: Azithromycin, 1 g PO or doxycycline 100 mg b.i.d. for 7 days (5)

  – *Neisseria gonorrhoeae*: ≤45 kg: Ceftriaxone, 125 mg IM plus medication for chlamydia if not ruled out (5); >45 kg: Ceftriaxone, 250 mg IM × 1
  – *Trichomonas*: Metronidazole, 15 mg/kg/d t.i.d. (max 250 mg t.i.d.) for 7 days (5)
- Contraindications: Allergy to proposed treatment
- Precautions: Avoid potential allergens and topical sensitizers if possible.

ISSUES FOR REFERRAL
- Suspected sexual abuse
- Suspected anatomic abnormality (except minor labial agglutination)
- Persistent, severe, or recurrent infections

 ONGOING CARE

FOLLOW-UP RECOMMENDATIONS
Patient Monitoring
Monitor for fever, pruritus, and vaginal discharge.

DIET
- Healthy balanced diet, high in fiber to prevent constipation
- Adequate fluid intake

PATIENT EDUCATION
Hygiene:
- Wipe front to back after elimination
- Avoid bubble baths and other irritating products
- Clean daily with mild soap and water and dry gently with soft towel or cool hair dryer
- Apply bland ointments for skin protection, if necessary

PROGNOSIS
Excellent

COMPLICATIONS
- If an STI is identified and not treated effectively, the patient is at risk for pelvic inflammatory disease (PID).
- Vaginismus

REFERENCES

1. Van Eyk N, Allen L, Giesbrecht E, et al. Pediatric vulvovaginal disorders: A diagnostic approach and review of the literature. *J Obstet Gynaecol Can*. 2009;31:850–862.
2. Delago C, Finkel MA, Deblinger E. Urogenital symptoms in premenarchal girls: Parents' and girls' perceptions and associations with irritants. *J Pediatr Adolesc Gynecol*. 2012;25:67–73.
3. Dei M, DiMaggio F, DiPaolo G. Vulvovaginitis in childhood. *Best Pract Res Clin Obstet Gynaecol*. 2010;24:129–137.
4. Velander MH, Mikkelsen DB, Bygum A. Labial agglutination in a prepubertal girl: effect of topical oestrogen. *Acta Derm Venereol*. 2009;89:198–199.
5. Emans JS. Vulvovaginal problems in the prepubertal child. In: *Pediatric & adolescent gynecology*, 5th ed. Philadelphia: Lippincott Williams & Wilkins; 2005:83–99.

ADDITIONAL READING

- Joishy M. Do we need to treat vulvovaginitis in prepubertal girls? *Br Med J*. 2005;22:330:186–188.
- Merkley K. Vulvovaginitis and vaginal discharge in the pediatric patient. *J Emerg Nurs*. 2005;31:400–402.
- Rome ES. Vulvovaginitis and other common vulvar disorders in children. *Endocr Dev*. 2012;22:72–83.
- Sticker T. Vulvovaginitis. *Ped Child Health*. 2009;20:143–145.

 CODES

ICD10
N76.0 Acute vaginitis

CLINICAL PEARLS
- Vulvovaginitis is the most common gynecologic problem in prepubescent girls.
- The hypoestrogenic state and prepubescent anatomy may increase susceptibility to vulvar and vaginal infection.
- Treatment is typically supportive (avoid scratching, warm soaks), but may require antibiotics if a bacterial infection is suspected.
- Isolating an infection with known sexual transmission should prompt further investigation.
- Recurrent or persistent vulvitis, especially with foul-smelling discharge, should prompt a skilled exam of the vagina for a retained foreign body.
- Good perineal hygiene will limit this condition.

WARTS

Herbert P. Goodheart, MD

BASICS

- Warts (verrucae) are benign growths that are confined to the epidermis. All warts are caused by the human papillomavirus (HPV). Warts can appear on any area of the skin or mucous membranes. Common warts are predominantly seen in children and young adults.
- Clinically, warts are rather arbitrarily described as:
  – Common warts (verrucae vulgaris)
  – Plantar warts (verrucae plantaris)
  – Flat warts (verrucae plana)
  – Venereal warts (condyloma acuminatum)
  – Epidermodysplasia verruciformis is a rare, lifelong hereditary disorder characterized by chronic infection with HPV.
- System(s) affected: Skin/Exocrine

DESCRIPTION
- Common warts are most often found at sites subject to frequent trauma, such as the hands and feet. Since warts often vary widely in shape, size, and appearance, the various descriptive names for them generally reflect their clinical appearance, location, or both.
- For example, filiform (fingerlike) warts are threadlike, planar warts are flat, and plantar warts are located on the plantar surfaces (soles) of the feet.
- Genital warts, or condyloma acuminata, may be large and cauliflower-like, or they may consist of small papules.
- Warts on mucous membranes (mucosal papillomas), such as those in the mouth or vagina, tend to be white in color due to moisture retention.

EPIDEMIOLOGY
Incidence
- Predominant age: Young adults and children
- Predominant sex: Female = Male

Prevalence
- ~7–10% of the US population
- Common warts appear ~2 times as frequently in whites as in blacks or Asians.

ETIOLOGY AND PATHOPHYSIOLOGY
- HPV is a double-stranded, circular, supercoiled DNA virus.
- The virus infects epidermal keratinocytes, stimulating cell proliferation.
- Various strains of DNA HPV: To date, >150 different subtypes have been identified.
- Common warts: HPV types 2 and 4 (most common), followed by types 1, 3, 27, 29, and 57
- Palmoplantar warts: HPV type 1 (most common), followed by types 2, 3, 4, 27, 29, and 57
- Flat warts: HPV types 3, 10, and 28
- Butcher warts: HPV type 7
- The virus is passed primarily through skin-to-skin contact or from the recently shed virus kept intact in a moist, warm environment.

RISK FACTORS
- HIV/AIDS and other immunosuppressive diseases (e.g., lymphomas)
- Immunosuppressive drugs that decrease cell-mediated immunity (e.g., prednisone, cyclosporine, and chemotherapeutic agents)
- Pregnancy
- Handling raw meat, fish, or other types of animal matter in one's occupation (e.g., butchers)
- Previous wart infection

GENERAL PREVENTION
There is no known way to prevent warts.

DIAGNOSIS

- Most often made on clinical appearance
- Skin biopsy, if necessary

PHYSICAL EXAM
- Distribution of warts is generally asymmetric, and lesions are often clustered or may appear in a linear configuration due to scratching (autoinoculation).
- Common wart: Rough-surfaced, hyperkeratotic, papillomatous, raised, skin-colored to tan papules, 5–10 mm in diameter; several may coalesce into a cluster (mosaic wart) 1–3 cm in diameter; most frequently seen on hands, knees, and elbows; usually asymptomatic but may cause cosmetic disfigurement or tenderness
- Filiform warts: These are long, slender, delicate, fingerlike growths, usually seen on the face around the lips, eyelids, or nares.
- Plantar warts often have a rough surface and appear on the plantar surface of the feet in children and young adults:
  – Can be tender and painful, and extensive involvement on the sole of the foot may impair ambulation, particularly when present on a weight-bearing surface.
  – Most often seen on the metatarsal area, heels, and toes in an asymmetric distribution (pressure points)
  – Pathognomonic "black dots" (thrombosed dermal capillaries); punctate bleeding becomes more evident after paring with a no. 15 blade
  – Both common and plantar warts generally demonstrate the following clinical findings:
    ○ A loss of normal skin markings (dermatoglyphics) such as finger, foot, and hand prints
    ○ Lesions may be solitary or multiple, or they may appear in clusters (mosaic warts).
- Flat warts: Slightly elevated, flat-topped, skin-colored or tan papules, small (1–3 mm) in diameter:
  – Commonly found on the face, arms, dorsa of hands, shins (women)
  – Sometimes exhibit a linear configuration caused by autoinoculation
  – In men, shaving spreads flat warts.
  – In women, they often occur on the shins, where leg shaving spreads lesions.
- Epidermodysplasia verruciformis (rare): Widespread flat, reddish brown pigmented papules and plaques that present in childhood with lifelong persistence on the trunk, hands, upper and lower extremities, and face are characteristic.

DIFFERENTIAL DIAGNOSIS
- Molluscum contagiosum
- Seborrheic keratosis
- Epidermal nevus
- Acrochordon (skin tag)
- Solar keratosis and cutaneous horn
- Acquired digital fibrokeratoma
- Squamous cell carcinoma (SCC)
- Keratoacanthoma
- Subungual SCC can easily be misdiagnosed as a subungual wart or onychomycosis.
- Corns/Calluses:
  – Corns (clavi) are sometimes difficult to distinguish from plantar warts. Like calluses, corns are thickened areas of the skin and most commonly develop at sites subjected to repeated friction and pressure, such as the tops and the tips of toes and along the sides of the feet:
    ○ They are usually hard and circular, with a polished or central translucent core, like the kernel of corn from which they take their name.
    ○ Corns do not have "black dots," and skin markings are retained except for the area of the central core.

ALERT
- A melanoma on the plantar surface of the foot can mimic a plantar wart.
- Verrucous carcinoma, a slow-growing, locally invasive, well-differentiated SCC, also may be easily mistaken for a common or plantar wart.

DIAGNOSTIC TESTS & INTERPRETATION
Diagnosis:
- HPV cannot be cultured, and lab testing is rarely necessary.
- Definitive HPV diagnosis can be achieved by:
  – Electron microscopy
  – Viral DNA identification employing Southern blot hybridization is used to identify the specific HPV type present in tissue.
  – Polymerase chain reaction may be used to amplify viral DNA for testing.

Follow-Up Tests & Special Considerations
Skin biopsy if unusual presentation or if diagnosis is unclear

Test Interpretation
- Histopathologic features of common warts include digitated epidermal hyperplasia, acanthosis, papillomatosis, compact orthokeratosis, hypergranulosis, dilated tortuous capillaries within the dermal papillae, and vertical tiers of parakeratotic cells with entrapped red blood cells above the tips of the digitations.
- In the granular layer, HPV-infected cells may have coarse keratohyaline granules and vacuoles surrounding wrinkled-appearing nuclei. These koilocytic (vacuolated) cells are pathognomonic for warts.

TREATMENT

The abundance of therapeutic modalities described below is a reflection of the fact that none of them is uniformly or even clearly effective in trials. Placebo treatment response rate is significant and quality of evidence in general is poor. Beyond topical salicylates, there is no clear evidence-based rationale for choosing 1 method over another (1)[A]. The choice of method of treatment depends on:

- Age of the patient
- Cosmetic and psychological considerations
- Relief of symptoms
- Patient's pain threshold
- Type of wart
- Location of the wart
- Experience of the physician

GENERAL MEASURES
- There is no ideal treatment.
- In children, most warts tend to regress spontaneously.
- In many adults and immunocompromised patients, warts are often difficult to eradicate.
- Painful, aggressive therapy should be avoided unless there is a need to eliminate the wart(s).
- For surgical procedures, especially in anxious children, pretreat with anesthetic cream such as EMLA (emulsion of lidocaine and prilocaine).

MEDICATION
First Line
- Self-administered topical therapy: Keratolytic (peeling) agents: The affected area(s) should be hydrated first by soaking in warm water for 5 minutes before application. Most over-the-counter agents contain salicylic acid and/or lactic acid; agents such as Duofilm, Occlusal-HP, Trans-Ver-Sal, and Mediplast (1)[A].
- Office-based:
  – Cantharidin 0.7%, an extract of the blister beetle that causes epidermal necrosis and blistering
  – Combination cantharidin 1%, salicylic acid 30%, podophyllin resin 5% in flexible collodion; applied in a thin coat, occluded 4–6 hours, then washed off

Second Line
- Home-based:
  – Imiquimod 5% (Aldara) cream, a local inducer of interferon, is applied at home by the patient. It is approved for external genital and perianal warts and is used off-label and may be applied to warts under duct-tape occlusion. It is applied at bedtime and washed off after 6–10 hours. Applied to flat warts without occlusion.
  – Topical retinoids (e.g., tretinoin 0.25–0.1% cream or gel) for flat warts
- Immunotherapy: Induction of delayed-type hypersensitivity with:
  – Diphenylcyclopropenone (DCP)
  – Dinitrochlorobenzene (DNCP)
  – Squaric acid dibutylester (SADBE): There is possible mutagenicity and side effects with this agent.
- Intralesional injections:
  – Mumps or Candida antigen
  – Bleomycin: Intradermal injection is expensive and usually causes severe pain.
  – Interferon-α-2b

- Oral therapy:
  – Oral high-dose cimetidine: Possibly works better in children (2)
  – Acitretin (an oral retinoid)
- Other treatments (all have all been used with varying results):
  – Dichloroacetic acid, trichloroacetic acid, podophyllin, formic acid, aminolevulinic acid in combination with blue light (3), 5-fluorouracil, silver nitrate, formaldehyde, levamisole, topical or IV cidofovir for recalcitrant warts in the setting of HIV, and glutaraldehyde

COMPLEMENTARY AND ALTERNATIVE MEDICINE
- Duct tape: Cover wart with waterproof tape (e.g., duct tape). Leave the tape on for 6 days, and then soak, pare with emery board, and leave uncovered overnight; then reapply tape cyclically for 8 cycles; 85% resolved compared with 60% efficacy with cryotherapy (4,5).
- Hyperthermia: Safe and inexpensive approach; immerse affected area into 45°C water bath for 30 minutes 3 × per week
- Hypnotherapy (6)
- Raw garlic cloves have demonstrated some antiviral activity.
- Vaccines are currently in development.

Pregnancy Considerations
The use of some topical chemical approaches may be contraindicated during pregnancy or in women who are likely to become pregnant during the treatment period.

SURGERY/OTHER PROCEDURES
- Cryotherapy with liquid nitrogen (LN_2) may be applied with a cotton swab or with a cryotherapy gun (Cryogun). Aggressive cryotherapy may be more effective than salicylic acid, but it is associated with increased adverse effects (blistering and scarring) (7):
  – Best for warts on hands; also during pregnancy and breastfeeding
  – Fast; can treat many lesions per visit
  – Painful; not tolerated well by young children
  – Freezing periungual warts may result in nail deformation.
  – In darkly pigmented skin, treatment can result in hypo- or hyperpigmentation.
- Light electrocautery with or without curettage:
  – Best for warts on the knees, elbows, and dorsa of hands
  – Also good for filiform warts
  – Tolerable in most adults
  – Requires local anesthesia
  – May cause scarring
- Photodynamic therapy: Topical 5-aminolevulinic acid is applied to warts followed by photoactivation.
- CO_2 or pulse-dye laser ablation: Expensive and requires local anesthesia
- For filiform warts: Dip hemostat into LN_2 for 10 seconds, then gently grasp the wart for 10 seconds and repeat. Wart sheds in 7–10 days.

ONGOING CARE

FOLLOW-UP RECOMMENDATIONS
Patient Monitoring
1/3 of the warts of epidermodysplasia may become malignant.

PROGNOSIS
- More often than not (especially in children), warts tend to "cure" themselves over time.
- In many adults and immunocompromised patients, warts often prove difficult to eradicate.
- Rarely, certain types of lesions may transform into carcinomas.

COMPLICATIONS
- Autoinoculation (pseudo-Koebner reaction)
- Scar formation
- Chronic pain after plantar wart removal or scar formation
- Nail deformity after injury to nail matrix

REFERENCES

1. Gibbs S, Harvey I. Topical treatments for cutaneous warts. Cochrane Database Syst Rev. 2006;3:CD001781.
2. Rogers CJ, Gibney MD, Siegfried EC, et al. Cimetidine therapy for recalcitrant warts in adults: Is it any better than placebo? J Am Acad Dermatol. 1999;41:123–127.
3. Ohtsuki A, Hasegawa T, Hirasawa Y, et al. Photodynamic therapy using light-emitting diodes for the treatment of viral warts. J Dermatol. 2009;36:525–528.
4. de Haen M, Spigt MG, van Uden CJ, et al. Efficacy of duct tape vs placebo in the treatment of verruca vulgaris (warts) in primary school children. Arch Pediatr Adolesc Med. 2006;160:1121–1125.
5. Wenner R, Askari SK, Cham PM, et al. Duct tape for the treatment of common warts in adults: A double-blind randomized controlled trial. Arch Dermatol. 2007;143:309–313.
6. Ewin DM. Hypnotherapy for warts (verruca vulgaris): 41 consecutive cases with 33 cures. Am J Clin Hypn. 1992;35:1–10.
7. Kwok CS, Holland R, Gibbs S. Efficacy of topical treatments for cutaneous warts: A meta-analysis and pooled analysis of randomized controlled trials. Br J Dermatol. 2011;84:233–246.

CODES

ICD10
- A63.0 Anogenital (venereal) warts
- B07.0 Plantar wart
- B07.9 Viral wart, unspecified

CLINICAL PEARLS

- No single therapy for warts is uniformly effective or superior; thus, treatment involves a certain amount of trial and error.
- Since most warts in children tend to regress spontaneously within 2 years, benign neglect is often a prudent option.
- Conservative, nonscarring, least painful, least expensive treatments are preferred.
- Freezing and other destructive treatment modalities do not kill the virus, but merely destroy the cells that harbor HPV.

WILMS TUMOR

John K Uffman, MD, MPH

 BASICS

DESCRIPTION
- An embryonal renal neoplasm containing blastema, stromal, or epithelial cell types, usually affecting children <5 years of age
- Most common renal tumor in children; 5th most common pediatric malignancy
- Staging: In the US, National Wilms Tumor Study Group (NWTSG) staging is done pretreatment based on radiographic imaging and surgery, whereas in Europe/Asia, Société Internationale d'Oncologie Pédiatrique (SIOP) staging is done *after* neoadjuvant chemotherapy is administered (1):
  - I: Tumor limited to kidney; completely excised
  - II: Tumor extends beyond kidney; completely excised
  - III: Residual nonhematogenous tumor confined to abdomen (lymph nodes positive, spillage of tumor, peritoneal implants, extension beyond resection region)
  - IV: Hematogenous metastases
  - V: Bilateral renal involvement
- System(s) affected: Renal/Urologic
- Synonym(s): Nephroblastoma

Pediatric Considerations
- Occurs only in children
- Most common renal malignancy in childhood

EPIDEMIOLOGY
Incidence
- Frequency rarer in East Asian populations than whites
- Frequency higher in black children than in whites
- Predominant age: Median age of 36.5 months
- Predominant sex: Female > Male (1.1:1)
- Represents 6–7% of all childhood cancers:
  - >80% are diagnosed before 5 years of age (median age is 3.5 years at diagnosis).
  - Wilms tumor makes up 95% of all renal cancers in children <15 years (2)

Prevalence
US: 0.69/100,000; 7.6 cases/1 million children <15 years

ETIOLOGY AND PATHOPHYSIOLOGY
- Hereditary or sporadic forms of genetic mutation
- Familial form: Autosomal-dominant trait with incomplete penetrance (1%)
- Potential of parental occupational exposure (machinists, welders, motor vehicle mechanics, auto body repairmen)

Genetics
- Several congenital anomalies are known to be associated with Wilms tumor. A 2-stage mutational model has been proposed: Occurrence in either hereditary form or sporadic form. Patients with aniridia have a deletion of the short arm of chromosome 11 (11p13).
- Abnormalities of chromosome 11 at the 11p15 locus are associated with Beckwith-Wiedemann syndrome. Wilms tumor-suppressor gene (*WT1*) has been identified, as well as additional candidates for another suppressor gene (*WT2*). Chromosome band 17q12–21 has been linked to 2 kindreds with Wilms tumor, and other kindred are associated with a Wilms tumor predisposition gene at 19q13.3–q13.4. Loss of heterozygosity at chromosomes 16q and 1p is associated with adverse outcome (1)[C].
- p53 is associated with anaplastic Wilms tumors (2)

RISK FACTORS
- Familial occurrence (5%) (1):
  - These patients tend to have earlier age of onset.
  - Familial patients have greater risk of bilateral disease.
- Parental occupation (machinists, welders, motor vehicle mechanics, auto body repairmen)
- Maternal exposure to pesticides prior to child's birth (3)
- High birth weight or preterm birth (3)
- Compared with firstborn, being a 2nd or later birth may be associated with significantly decreased risk of Wilms tumor (3).

GENERAL PREVENTION
- Routine surveillance in patients with syndromes associated with Wilms tumor
- Routine screening with serial renal US at 3–4-month intervals has been recommended in children who have syndromes associated with Wilms tumor >5% (4)[C].
- Routine screening with serial renal US also recommended for infants born to kindreds with familial Wilms (every 3–4 months until age 7) (4)[C].

COMMONLY ASSOCIATED CONDITIONS
- Aniridia (partial or complete absence of iris) 600 × normal risk
- Hemihypertrophy (100 × normal risk)
- Cryptorchidism
- Hypospadias
- Duplicated renal collecting systems
- Denys-Drash syndrome (nephropathy, renal failure, male pseudohermaphroditism, Wilms tumor)
- Klippel-Trenaunay syndrome
- WAGR complex (Wilms tumor, aniridia, genitourinary malformations, and mental retardation)
- Beckwith-Wiedemann syndrome (visceromegaly, macroglossia, omphalocele, hyperinsulinemic hypoglycemia)

DIAGNOSIS
- Symptoms of pain, anorexia, vomiting, malaise in 30% (1)
- >90% present with asymptomatic abdominal mass (5).

HISTORY
- History of increasing abdominal size
- Usually asymptomatic; may have fever, abdominal pain

PHYSICAL EXAM
- Palpable upper abdominal mass
- Fever, hepatosplenomegaly
- Rarely, signs of acute abdomen with free intraperitoneal rupture
- Cardiac murmur
- Ascites, prominent abdominal wall veins, varicocele
- Gonadal metastases
- Aniridia (present in 1.1% of Wilms tumor patients)
- Hypertension (20–65%) (1)

DIFFERENTIAL DIAGNOSIS
- Neuroblastoma
- Hepatic tumor
- Sarcoma
- Rhabdoid tumor
- Cystic nephroma
- Renal cell carcinoma (generally occurs in older children)
- Mesoblastic nephroma: Distinguished only by histology. Age usually <6 months, essentially benign, although metastases have been reported; tend to be locally invasive
- Nephroblastomatosis: Considered premalignant; may present as nodularity of 1 or both kidneys.

DIAGNOSTIC TESTS & INTERPRETATION
- Urinalysis (occasional hematuria, proteinuria)
- CBC (anemia)
- Lactate dehydrogenase
- Plasma renin (rarely helpful)
- Urine catecholamines
- Serum creatinine and calcium
- Coagulation factors
- Chest radiograph
- Abdominal US (with Doppler imaging): Best initial test. Gives best information about tumor and extension into inferior vena cava
- CT scan (with IV and oral contrast material) of chest and abdomen. Allows anatomical visualization and excludes synchronous bilateral disease with a high degree of sensitivity (2).
- CT may have high sensitivity and specificity for atriocaval thrombus and obviate the needs for US (2).
- Chest lesions only identified on CT have improved event-free survival with 3 drug treatment regimens (6)[B].

Diagnostic Procedures/Other
Occasionally, bone marrow aspiration is necessary to distinguish from neuroblastoma.

Test Interpretation
- Favorable findings (mortality of 7%):
  - Bulky lesion, well encapsulated
  - Focal areas of hemorrhage and necrosis
  - Absence of anaplasia and sarcomatous cell types
  - Presence of blastema, stomal, and epithelial elements (5):
    ○ Predominance of epithelial elements usually are less aggressive when diagnosed early, but tend to be resistant to treatment when diagnosed late.
    ○ Predominance of blastemal elements indicate more aggressive tumors.
- Unfavorable histology (mortality rate of 57%):
  - Anaplasia: Markedly enlarged and multipolar mitotic figures, 3-fold enlargement of nuclei in comparison with adjacent similar nuclei, hyperchromasia of enlarged nuclei; anaplasia may be diffuse or focal
  - Sarcomatous changes: Now considered to be separate from Wilms, not subtypes (mortality 64%)
  - Rhabdoid tumor of the kidney: Now considered to be separate tumor from Wilms
- Nephroblastomatosis: Considered premalignant
- Nephrogenic rests (5): These are precursor lesions found in 25–40% of Wilms. Found in 1% of infants at autopsy, but most do not develop into malignancy

TREATMENT

GENERAL MEASURES

- Appropriate health care: Inpatient workup and treatment until stable postoperatively and induction chemotherapy completed
- Chemotherapy; some recommend pretreatment with neoadjuvant chemotherapy (1):
  - May decrease incidence of intraoperative tumor rupture (debatable)
  - May result in inappropriate treatment with chemotherapeutic agents of non-Wilms tumors (5%) or benign lesions (1.6%)
  - Results in the inability to directly compare treatment results worldwide
- Radiation therapy in stage II (unfavorable histology), stage III, and stage IV

MEDICATION

First Line

- Dactinomycin (Actinomycin-D)
- Vincristine
- Doxorubicin
- Cyclophosphamide (Cytoxan)
- Iphosphamide
- Etoposide
- Topotecan
- Irinotecan

Second Line

- Doxorubicin (Adriamycin)
- Cyclophosphamide

SURGERY/OTHER PROCEDURES

- Exploration of contralateral kidney no longer required if adequate CT done preoperatively
- Radical nephroureterectomy and lymph node sampling are needed to provide precise staging information.
- Renal sparing resection:
  - Tumors usually too large, but 10–15% may be amenable to partial nephrectomy if given preoperative chemotherapy (4)[C]
  - May be recommended for patients with high risk of bilateral disease or renal failure (4)[C]
- Sampling of any enlarged lymph nodes (absence of any lymph nodes in the surgical specimen mandates treatment as stage III disease) (5)[B]
- Identification of any retained tumor with titanium clips
- Tumor should be given to pathologist fresh, not in formalin.
- Vertical midline incision if tumor extension to right atrium; increased morbidity (2)
- Bilateral Wilms tumors (represent 4–6% of Wilms) (5)[B]:
  - Preoperative chemotherapy with re-evaluation by CT or MRI after 6 weeks (some are biopsied prior to chemotherapy)
  - Renal-sparing operation at 6 weeks if good response to chemotherapy:
    - Partial nephrectomy or wedge excision of tumor preferred, but only if it does not compromise tumor resection
    - Kidney with lowest tumor burden is addressed 1st. If successful resection accomplished, radical nephrectomy can be done on the contralateral kidney. Bilateral partial nephrectomy may be possible in some cases.

- Preoperative treatment also generally is accepted in a solitary kidney, horseshoe kidneys, intravascular extension of tumor above the intrahepatic vena cava, and in the case of respiratory distress from extensive metastatic tumor.
- Treatment of patients with relapsed Wilms (7)[B]: Current treatment is either with chemotherapy with or without radiation therapy alone or high-dose chemotherapy followed by autologous stem cell rescue.

ONGOING CARE

FOLLOW-UP RECOMMENDATIONS

Patient Monitoring

- Multidrug chemotherapy every 3–4 weeks for 16 weeks–15 months depending on stage
- Every 4 months for 1 year, every 6 months for 2nd to 3rd year; yearly after that
- CBC, CT of chest and abdomen with each visit
- Patients at high risk for developing Wilms tumor should be monitored with renal US every 3–4 months until 5 years of age. Patients with Beckwith-Wiedemann syndrome or Simpson-Golabi-Behmel syndrome should have yearly US until 7 years of age (8)[C].

PATIENT EDUCATION

- Possibility of 2nd malignancy (up to 12% by age 50)
- Side effects of chemotherapy, radiation therapy

PROGNOSIS

- With favorable histology (1):
  - Children <2 years of age and stage I, favorable histology: 98% survival in NWTSG 1–3 studies
  - Children with stage III, favorable histology tumor: Overall survival of 89% in NWTSG 3–4 studies
- With diffuse anaplasia (1):
  - Children with stage I, diffuse or focal anaplasia: Overall survival 82.6%
  - Stage II tumors with anaplasia: Overall survival 81.5%
  - Stage III tumors with anaplasia: Overall survival 66.7%
  - Stage IV tumors with anaplasia: Overall survival 33.3%
- With bilateral involvement (stage V): 4-year survival 81.7% (1)
- With rhabdoid features: 19% 3-year survival
- Survival of patients with relapsed Wilms tumor is 40–70% (8)[B]:
  - Patients with pulmonary relapse only had higher 4-year survival rate (77.7%) compared with other sites (41.6%).

COMPLICATIONS

- Complication rate of 6–10%
- 1–2% will develop 2nd malignant neoplasms (leukemia, lymphoma, hepatocellular carcinoma, soft tissue sarcoma): 12.2% by 50 years of age
- High risk of delivering low-birth-weight infants, perinatal mortality in offspring of female survivors of Wilms tumor
- Chest is usual site of recurrence.
- Occurrence of 2nd malignant neoplasms in 2% of patients 7–34 years after treatment:
  - Bone and soft tissue sarcomas, breast cancer, hepatocellular carcinoma, lymphoma, gastrointestinal tract tumors, melanoma, leukemias

- Surgical complications:
  - Postoperative small bowel obstruction (5–7%)
  - Tumor rupture with spillage in 15.3% according to NWTSG-5; this may be spontaneous or surgical and results in upstaging the tumor. Only 2.7% of spills are considered avoidable. Incidence of tumor spillage is reported at 2.2% by SIOP following preoperative neoadjuvant chemotherapy (5)[B].
- Local tumor recurrence:
  - Abdominal tumor recurrence after tumor spillage is reduced by radiation therapy (10 or 20 Gy)
- Renal failure
- Cardiomyopathy (usually related to doxorubicin and radiation therapy)
- Impaired pulmonary function (radiation therapy)

REFERENCES

1. Sonn G, Shortliffe LM. Management of Wilms tumor: Current standard of care. *Nat Clin Pract Urol.* 2008;5:551–560.
2. Davidoff, AM. Wilms tumor. *Adv Pediatr.* 2012;59:247–267.
3. Chu A, Heck JE, Ribeiro KB, et al. Wilms tumour: A systematic review of risk factors and meta-analysis. *Paediatr Perinat Epidemiol.* 2010;24:449–469.
4. Nakamura L, Ritchey M. Current management of Wilms' tumor. *Curr Urol Rep.* 2010;11:58–65.
5. Ko EY, Ritchey ML. Current management of Wilms tumor in children. *J Pediatr Urol.* 2009;5:56–65.
6. Grundy PE, Green DM, Dirks AC, et. al. Clinical significance of pulmonary nodules detected by CT and not CXR in patients treated for favorable histology wilms tumor on national Wilms tumor studies-4 and -5: A report from the Children's Oncology Group. *Pediatr Blood Cancer.* 2012;59:631–635.
7. Presson A, Moore TB, Kempert P. Efficacy of high-dose chemotherapy and autologous stem cell transplant for recurrent Wilms tumor: A meta-analysis. *J Pediatr Hematol Oncol.* 2010;32:454–461.
8. Scott RH. Surveillance for Wilms tumor in at-risk children: Pragmatic recommendations for best practice. *Arch Dis Child.* 2006;91:995–999.

CODES

ICD10

- C64.1 Malignant neoplasm of right kidney, except renal pelvis
- C64.2 Malignant neoplasm of left kidney, except renal pelvis
- C64.9 Malignant neoplasm of unsp kidney, except renal pelvis

CLINICAL PEARLS

- Wilms is the most common renal tumor in children; it is an embryonal renal neoplasm containing blastema, stromal, or epithelial cell types, usually affecting children <5 years of age.
- Risks include parental occupation (machinists, welders, motor vehicle mechanics, auto body repairmen) and maternal exposure to pesticides prior to child's birth.
- Nephrectomy performed as soon as possible after completing radiographic evaluation is the major component in tumor staging.

W

ZINC DEFICIENCY

Adarsh K. Gupta, DO, MS, FACOFP

 BASICS

DESCRIPTION

- Nutritional condition whose manifestations may involve growth retardation; hypogonadism; cell-mediated immune dysfunction; poor wound healing; poor appetite; hair loss; depression; and increased incidence of infection, anorexia, diarrhea, and eye and skin lesions related to decreased zinc levels.
- System(s) affected: Endocrine/Metabolic; Nervous; Skin/Exocrine; Hematologic/Oncologic; Gastroenterologic

Geriatric Considerations

- Zinc deficiency may cause poor night vision, leading to falls; poor wound healing or chronic ulcer; or loss of smell and taste, which may worsening nutrition.
- Elderly persons living in institutions may have low zinc intake.

Pediatric Considerations

Zinc deficiency may cause failure to thrive and diarrhea and may impair growth and development of secondary sexual characteristics.

Pregnancy Considerations

Requirements increase; deficiency may cause spontaneous abortion, inadequate weight gain

EPIDEMIOLOGY

Prevalence

- In the US: Rare in general population
- High prevalence in developing countries
- Predominate age: All ages
- Predominant sex: Male = Female

ETIOLOGY AND PATHOPHYSIOLOGY

- Increased requirements:
  - Pregnancy
  - Lactation
  - Rapid growth phase in childhood
  - Burns
  - Major trauma
- Increased losses:
  - Diabetes
  - Cirrhosis
  - Renal disease
  - Malabsorption states (e.g., inflammatory bowel diseases)
  - Sickle cell anemia
  - Diuretics: Thiazides, chlorthalidone

- Decreased absorption:
  - Acrodermatitis enteropathica, an autosomal-recessive deficiency in the enzyme required for intestinal absorption
  - Geophagia
  - Chelating agents
  - Parasitism
  - Diet high in phytates (plant fiber)
  - Drugs: Penicillamines, tetracyclines, quinolones, bisphosphonates
- Insufficient dietary intake:
  - Vegetarianism
  - Parenteral hyperalimentation without zinc supplementation
  - Breastfeeding
  - Suboptimal zinc conditions in diet (rare)
  - Alcoholism

Genetics

- Usually acquired
- Rarely caused by acrodermatitis enteropathica (autosomal recessive inheritance)
- Associated with sickle cell anemia (autosomal recessive)

RISK FACTORS

- Drugs: Diuretics, penicillamine, sodium valproate, and ethambutol
- Low socioeconomic status
- Malabsorption syndromes
- Living in developing nations
- Hyperalimentation with zinc supplementation
- Thermal burns
- Strict vegetarian diet
- Alcoholism
- Chronic renal failure patients on hemodialysis

GENERAL PREVENTION

- Adequate diet
- Supplementation when indicated (see "Medication")

COMMONLY ASSOCIATED CONDITIONS

- Sickle cell anemia
- Malabsorption
- Parenteral hyperalimentation
- In the older patient: Those taking diuretics, those with diabetes mellitus, cirrhosis
- In hemodialysis patients, zinc deficiency is associated with depression.

 DIAGNOSIS

HISTORY

- Mild deficiency:
  - Hypogeusia (lack of taste)
  - Decreased dark adaptation
  - Decreased lean body mass
- Moderate deficiency:
  - All of the above
  - Diarrhea
  - Growth retardation
  - Hypogonadism (especially male)
  - Mental lethargy
  - Anergy
  - Rough skin
  - Delayed wound healing
  - Glucose intolerance
  - Impaired cell-mediated immunity
- Severe deficiency:
  - All of the above
  - Bullous pustular dermatitis
  - Weight loss
  - Dwarfism
  - Emotional instability
  - Tremors
  - Ataxia
  - Alopecia
  - Death

PHYSICAL EXAM

- Depends on level of deficiency
- Acrodermatitis enterohepatica: Erythema, scales, erosions, and/or vesiculobullous eruptions often quite dramatic in diaper area

DIFFERENTIAL DIAGNOSIS
- Congenital dwarfism
- Failure to thrive in infants
- Multiple micronutrient deficiencies
- Primary hypogonadism
- Mental retardation

DIAGNOSTIC TESTS & INTERPRETATION
- Plasma zinc levels decreased (in moderate-to-severe zinc deficiency). Levels <60 g/L are strongly suggestive, but correction may be needed for low albumin because most serum zinc is bound to albumin.
- Erythrocyte or leukocyte zinc levels more adequately reflect tissue stores, but are not widely available.
- Hair and fingernail levels are not useful.

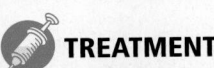 TREATMENT

MEDICATION
- Zinc supplements (take at least 1 hour before or 2 hours after meals high in calcium, fiber, and phytates)
- Oral form: Zinc gluconate (lozenges, tablets), zinc sulfate (capsules, tablets, extended-release tablets)
- Injectable form: Zinc chloride, zinc sulfate
- Use the recommended dietary allowance (RDA) as a guideline for dosing (see "Diet").
- In adult patient, 4–6 mg/d of elemental zinc added to hyperalimentation; may increase to 12 mg q.i.d. if suspect ongoing heavy zinc losses (e.g., burns or major trauma)
- Precautions: Avoid large (>20 mg elemental zinc) parenteral doses.

 ONGOING CARE

FOLLOW-UP RECOMMENDATIONS
Full activity

Patient Monitoring
Clinical status such as improved energy, weight gain, resolution of symptoms

DIET
- Balanced omnivorous diet or vegetarian diet with supplementation
- Avoid excessive intake of foods with high phytate content (e.g., raw cereals, but ready-to-eat cereal may be the richest source of zinc from a plant product).
- Lean beef and pork, oysters, poultry, soybeans, pumpkin, sunflower seeds, seafood, milk, eggs, grains, legumes, nuts, and wheat bran are rich in zinc.
- RDA for zinc:
  – Men: 15 mg/d
  – Women: 12 mg/d
  – Pregnant women: 15 mg/d
  – Breastfeeding women: 19 mg/d

PROGNOSIS
Immediate improvement in clinical status with treatment; full resolution in signs and symptoms

ADDITIONAL READING
- Hambidge KM, Krebs NF. Zinc deficiency: A special challenge. *J. Nutr.* 2007;137:1101–1105.
- Lukacik M, Thomas RL, Aranda JV. A meta-analysis of the effects of oral zinc in the treatment of acute and persistent diarrhea. *Pediatrics.* 2008;121: 326–336.
- Office of Dietary Supplements. National Institutes of Health. Zinc. Available at: http://ods.od.nih.gov/factsheets/zinc.asp#en2

 SEE ALSO

Alcohol Abuse and Dependence; Anemia, Sickle Cell; Failure to Thrive (FTT)

 CODES

ICD10
- E60 Dietary zinc deficiency

CLINICAL PEARLS
- Zinc deficiency is uncommon in the US.
- Elderly persons living in long-term facilities may have diets deficient in zinc.
- Zinc deficiency may cause poor wound healing; consider supplementation when treating chronic skin ulcers.

Z

ZOLLINGER-ELLISON SYNDROME

Douglas S. Parks, MD

 BASICS

DESCRIPTION
- Zollinger-Ellison Syndrome triad:
  - Markedly elevated gastric acid secretion
  - Peptic ulcer disease
  - A gastrinoma or non-β islet cell tumor of the pancreas or duodenal wall that produces gastrin
- Gastrinomas (at the time of diagnosis) may be single or multiple (1/2–2/3), large or small, benign or malignant (2/3), sporadic (70–75%) or associated with MEN1 *(multiple endocrine neoplasia type 1)* (25–30%).
- System(s) affected: Endocrine/Metabolic; Gastrointestinal
- Synonym(s): Z-E syndrome; Pancreatic ulcerogenic tumor syndrome; Multiple endocrine neoplasia, partial; Ulcerogenic islet cell tumor

EPIDEMIOLOGY
Incidence
- 1–3 per million per year
- Predominant age: Middle age (30–65 years)
- Predominant sex: Male > Female (1.3:1)

Pediatric Considerations
Very aggressive cases have been reported in teenagers.

Pregnancy Considerations
Cases reported; influences medication choices and surgical timing

ETIOLOGY AND PATHOPHYSIOLOGY
- Gastrinoma is equally distributed between the head of the pancreas and the 1st or 2nd portion of the duodenum; if in the pancreas, the lesion is more likely to metastasize to the liver.
- Also may be found rarely in the mesentery, peritoneum, spleen, skin, or mediastinum (possibly metastasis with primary not identified)

Genetics
~25–30% of cases occur in association with the MEN1 syndrome.

RISK FACTORS
- MEN1
- Family history of ulcer disease

GENERAL PREVENTION
Screen 1st-degree relatives of patients with MEN1.

COMMONLY ASSOCIATED CONDITIONS
- MEN1: Hyperparathyroidism, prolactinomas, other pituitary tumors
- Insulinoma
- Carcinoid tumors

 DIAGNOSIS

HISTORY
Average of 5 years of symptoms, including recurrent ulcers, before diagnosis is made:
- Abdominal pain (80%)
- Diarrhea, including while fasting (70%)
- Heartburn (60%)
- Nausea (30%)
- Reflux esophagitis
- Vomiting that is unresponsive to standard therapy
- Weight loss
- Steatorrhea

PHYSICAL EXAM
- Peptic ulcer disease
- Hepatomegaly with metastasis
- Endoscopic findings, including esophagitis, duodenal ulceration with multiple ulcers, and prominent gastric and duodenal folds
- Complications of severe peptic ulcer disease, including hemorrhage, perforation, and obstruction
- Signs of MEN1 are hypercalcemia, hyperparathyroidism, and Cushing syndrome.

Geriatric Considerations
Consider the diagnosis in a patient with persistent or recurring peptic ulcer disease; it is a less aggressive disease if it appears after 65 years.

DIFFERENTIAL DIAGNOSIS
- Elevated serum gastrin with hypochlorhydria/achlorhydria:
  - Atrophic gastritis
  - Drug-induced (associated with PPIs)
  - Gastric cancer
  - Pernicious anemia
  - Postvagotomy
- Elevated serum gastrin with normal or increased gastric acid:
  - Antral G-cell hyperfunction
  - Chronic renal failure
  - *Helicobacter pylori* infection
  - Gastric outlet obstruction
  - Retained gastric antrum
- Consider gastrinoma in all patients with the following symptoms:
  - Recurrent or refractory ulcer disease
  - Gastric hypertrophy and ulcers
  - Duodenal and jejunal ulcers
  - Ulcers and diarrhea
  - Ulcers and kidney stones
  - Hypercalcemia and ulcers
  - Pituitary disease
  - Family history of ulcer disease or endocrine tumors suggestive of MEN1

DIAGNOSTIC TESTS & INTERPRETATION
- Preferred test is secretion stimulation test: Gastrin level >100 pg/mL (>100 ng/L) (1)[A],(2)[B]
- Some gastrin assays undermeasure serum gastrin. If have strong index of suspicion but gastrin levels low, may need to repeat with a different lab (3)[B]
- Gastric secretory studies: Basal acid output
- Alternative test is calcium infusion test: Gastrin level >400 pg/mL (test is less specific and more dangerous because of IV calcium infusion)
- Elevated serum gastrin fasting level: >1,000 pg/mL with ulcers diagnostic; >200 pg/mL with ulcers is suggestive
- Elevated basal gastric acid output: >15 mEq/hr (>15 mmol/hr)
- Gastric pH <2 with elevated gastrin
- Check serum calcium, phosphorus, cortisol, and prolactin to rule out MEN1.

- Drugs may alter lab results:
  - Histamine (H_2) blockers and proton-pump inhibitors (PPIs) may increase gastric pH and serum gastrin.
  - Hold PPIs 7 days and H_2 blockers 2 days prior to drawing gastrin level.
- Used to localize tumor for possible resection
- Much more likely to find tumors >3 cm (95%) than <1 cm (<15%) (4)[B]
- Abdominal CT scan: Most useful for pancreatic tumors and metastasis >3 cm
- Abdominal US: Not useful except in large tumors
- Abdominal angiography: Not useful except in large tumors
- Endoscopic US: Finds 24–38% of primary tumors
- Abdominal MRI: Not very useful except in large tumors
- Somatostatin receptor scintigraphy (SRS): More sensitive than radiologic studies but still only finds 30% of small tumors
- Portal venous sampling and selective venous sampling for gastrin can localize the area of tumor and metastasis (80–90% sensitivity)
- Sella turcica imaging may help if MEN1 is suspected, to look for pituitary tumors.
- Because pancreatic tumors are most likely to be large and to metastasize to the liver, which worsens prognosis, SRS and an abdominal CT scan are suggested to look for resectable tumors. Both studies are much more sensitive for pancreatic tumors, and surgical resection may improve prognosis considerably (5)[B].

Diagnostic Procedures/Other
Endoscopy may reveal tumors in the duodenal wall; multiple ulcers, including jejunal ulcers; and prominent gastric and duodenal folds.

Test Interpretation
- 90% of gastrinomas are found in the gastric triangle (the borders are the bile duct, the junction of 2nd and 3rd portions of the duodenum, and the junction of the head and body of pancreas).
- ~50% of gastrinomas are in the head of the pancreas (more likely >3 cm, metastasis to liver).
- ~50% of gastrinomas are in the wall of the 1st or 2nd portion of duodenum (more likely to be small, solitary).
- 2/3 of gastrinomas are malignant in both sites (defined by tendency for metastasis).
- 50% of gastrinomas stain positive for adrenocorticotropic hormone (ACTH), vasoactive intestinal polypeptide, insulin, or neurotensin (in decreasing order of incidence).
- 1/3 of patients have metastasis on presentation with regional nodes > liver > bone, rarely to peritoneum, spleen, skin, and mediastinum.
- Duodenal, jejunal, and gastric ulcers; often multiple
- Gastric and duodenal mucosal fold thickening
- Hyperplasia of antral gastrin-producing cells
- Histology similar in appearance to carcinoid

TREATMENT

GENERAL MEASURES
- Advanced imaging initially to assess for possible resection
- Surgical removal when primary tumor can be identified and as an adjunct to symptom control
- Medical treatment for symptom control when primary tumor is not found or metastasis is present on diagnosis

MEDICATION
- PPIs are the first-line treatment; H_2 blockers may need to be added.
- Medications heal 80–85% of ulcers, however,
- the ulcers nearly always recur. Although doses may be adjusted, the patient should plan on lifelong use of medication.
- Dosages frequently exceed usual doses for treatment of ulcers by 4–8-fold:
  – Start at a lower recommended dose given below, and titrate up to resolution of symptoms or the maximum listed subsequently.
- If hyperparathyroidism is present because of MEN1, hypercalcemia must be corrected.

First Line
- PPIs:
  – Omeprazole 60–120 mg/d
  – Lansoprazole 60–180 mg/d (doses >120 mg need to be divided b.i.d.)
  – Rabeprazole 60–100 mg/d up to 60 mg b.i.d.
  – Pantoprazole 40–240 mg/d PO; 80–120 mg q12h IV
- H_2 blockers:
  – Cimetidine 300 mg q6h up to 1.25–5 g/d
  – Ranitidine 150 mg q12h up to 6 g/d
  – Famotidine 20–800 mg at bedtime
- Contraindications:
  – Known hypersensitivity to the drug
  – H_2 blockers: Androgen effects, drug interactions due to cytochrome P450 stimulation
  – PPIs: None
- Precautions:
  – Adjust the doses for renal and geriatric patients depending on the drug.
  – Gynecomastia has been reported with high-dose cimetidine (>2.4 g/d).
  – PPIs may induce a profound and long-lasting effect on gastric acid secretion, thereby affecting the bioavailability of drugs depending on low gastric pH (e.g., ketoconazole, ampicillin, iron).
- Significant possible interactions: Refer to the drug manufacturers' literature.

Second Line
- Octreotide appears helpful in slowing the growth of a liver metastasis, and it may produce regression in some cases. Octreotide LAR can be given every 28 days (4)[B].
- Chemotherapy regimens using streptozocin, 5-fluorouracil, and doxorubicin show only limited response.
- Interferon shows a limited response but may be useful in combination with octreotide.

SURGERY/OTHER PROCEDURES
- Laparotomy to search for resectable tumors (especially in the pancreas and duodenal wall), unless patient has liver metastasis on presentation or MEN1; improves outcome (6)[B]

- Definitive therapy: Removal of gastrinomas when found (surgery finds 95% of tumors; 5-year cure is 40% when all can be removed)
- Total gastrectomy was formerly used to stop acid production before pharmacologic therapy became available; now it is seldom done.
- In MEN1, parathyroidectomy, by lowering calcium, may decrease acid production and decrease antisecretory drug use. Gastrinomas are generally small, benign, and multiple and not usually cured by surgery.

IN-PATIENT CONSIDERATIONS
Admission Criteria/Initial Stabilization
- Advise daily care based on symptoms.
- Appropriate surveillance of basal gastric acid output to monitor antacid secretory therapy
- Appropriate surveillance postoperatively to look for metastasis

 ONGOING CARE

FOLLOW-UP RECOMMENDATIONS
Patient Monitoring
- The patient must be monitored over time for evidence of metastasis.
- Careful dose titration of medical therapy is necessary to control symptoms.
- Advise patients of potential danger of stopping antisecretory treatment (7).
- Gastric acid analysis to maintain basal gastric acid output at <10 mEq/hr (<2 mEq/hr if patient has complications such as perforation or esophagitis)

DIET
Restrict foods that aggravate symptoms.

PATIENT EDUCATION
Inform patients as to the nature of disease and prognosis.

PROGNOSIS
- Overall survival rate: 5–10 years: 69–94%
- The prognosis improves if complete surgical removal of the tumor is possible.
- If liver metastasis is present on initial surgery, 5-year survival is 30–40%; 10-year survival is 25%.
- Mortality is directly related to liver metastasis associated with larger tumors and pancreatic tumors (4,5)[B].

COMPLICATIONS
- Complications of peptic ulcer disease (bleeding, perforation, obstruction)
- 2/3 of gastrinomas are malignant with metastasis.
- A tumor may produce other substances, such as ACTH (5–8% of patients), with resulting Cushing syndrome.
- Decrease in vitamin B12 levels are possible with long-term PPI use (8)[A].

REFERENCES
1. Berna MJ, Hoffmann KM, Long SH, et al. Serum gastrin in Zollinger-Ellison syndrome: II. Prospective study of gastrin provocative testing in 293 patients from the National Institutes of Health and comparison with 537 cases from the literature. evaluation of diagnostic criteria, proposal of new criteria, and correlations with clinical and tumoral features. *Medicine (Baltimore)*. 2006;85:331–364.

2. Kuiper P, Biemond I, Masclee AA, et al. Diagnostic efficacy of the secretin stimulation test for the Zollinger-Ellison syndrome: An intra-individual comparison using different dosages in patients and controls. *Pancreatology*. 2010;10:14–18.

3. Rehfeld JF, Bardram L, Hilsted L, et al. Pitfalls in diagnositic gastrin measurements. *Clin Chem*. 2012;58(5):831–836.

4. Hoffmann KM, Furukawa M, Jensen RT. Duodenal neuroendocrine tumors: Classification, functional syndromes, diagnosis and medical treatment. *Best Pract Res Clin Gastroenterol*. 2005;19:675–697.

5. Jensen RT. Gastrinomas: Advances in diagnosis and management. *Neuroendocrinology*. 2004; 80(Suppl 1):23–27.

6. Morrow EH, Norton JA. Surgical management of Zollinger-Ellison syndrome; state of the art. *Surg Clin North Am*. 2009;89:1091–1103.

7. Poitras P, Gingras MH, Rehfeld JF. The Zollinger-Ellison syndrome: dangers and consequences of interrupting antisecretory treatment. *Clin Gastroenterol Hepatol*. 2012;10(2): 199–202. Epub 2011 Aug 24.

8. Thomson AB, Sauve MD, Kassam N, et al. Safety of the long-term use of proton pump inhibitors. *World J Gastroenterol*. 2010;16(19):2323–2330.

ADDITIONAL READING
- Hirschowitz BI, Fineberg N, Wilcox CM, et al. Costs and risks in the management of patients with gastric acid hypersecretion. *J Clin Gastroenterol*. 2010;44: 28–33.
- Mortellaro VE, Hochwald SN, McGuigan JE, et al. Long-term results of a selective surgical approach to management of Zollinger-Ellison syndrome in patients with MEN-1. *Am Surg*. 2009;75:730–733.
- Smallfield GB, Allison J, Wilcox CM, et al. Prospective evaluation of quality of life in patients with Zollinger-Ellison syndrome. *Dig Dis Sci*. 2010; 55:3108–3112.

 CODES

ICD10
- E16.4 Increased secretion of gastrin

CLINICAL PEARLS
- ~25–30% of cases of Z-E syndrome occur in association with MEN1.
- Once diagnosed, look for the gastrinoma; gastrinoma location is equally distributed between the head of the pancreas and the 1st or 2nd portion of the duodenum.
- PPIs heal ulcers, but think of Z-E syndrome if peptic ulcers recur or if high doses are needed to control symptoms/ulcers.

Z

INDEX